Neurobiology of Mental Illness

NEUROBIOLOGY OF MENTAL ILLNESS

Third Edition

Edited by

DENNIS S. CHARNEY, M.D.
Dean, Mount Sinai School of Medicine
Executive Vice President for Academic Affairs
The Mount Sinai Medical Center
Anne and Joel Ehrenkranz Professor
Departments of Psychiatry, Neuroscience,
and Pharmacology & Systems Therapeutics
Mount Sinai School of Medicine
New York, New York

ERIC J. NESTLER, M.D., PH.D.
Chair of Neuroscience
Director of the Mount Sinai Brain Institute
Nash Family Professor of Neuroscience
Mount Sinai School of Medicine
New York, New York

SECTION EDITORS

Eric J. Nestler, M.D., Ph.D.
Carol A. Tamminga, M.D.
Jeffrey A. Lieberman, M.D.
Charles B. Nemeroff, M.D., Ph.D.
Antonia S. New, M.D.
Steven E. Hyman, M.D.
Mary Sano, Ph.D.
Daniel S. Pine, M.D.

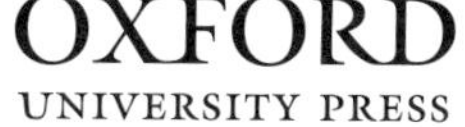
OXFORD
UNIVERSITY PRESS

OXFORD
UNIVERSITY PRESS

Oxford University Press, Inc., publishes works that further
Oxford University's objective of excellence
in research, scholarship, and education.

Oxford New York
Auckland Cape Town Dar es Salaam Hong Kong Karachi
Kuala Lumpur Madrid Melbourne Mexico City Nairobi
New Delhi Shanghai Taipei Toronto

With offices in
Argentina Austria Brazil Chile Czech Republic France Greece
Guatemala Hungary Italy Japan Poland Portugal Singapore
South Korea Switzerland Thailand Turkey Ukraine Vietnam

Published by Oxford University Press, Inc.
198 Madison Avenue, New York, New York 10016
www.oup.com

First issued as an Oxford University Press paperback, 2011

Library of Congress Cataloging-in-Publication Data
Neurobiology of mental illness /
edited by Dennis S. Charney, Eric J. Nestler. — 3rd ed.
p. ; cm. Includes bibliographical references and index.
ISBN 978-0-19-979826-1
1. Neuropsychiatry. 2. Mental illness—Physiological aspects.
I. Charney, Dennis S. II. Nestler, Eric J. (Eric Jonathan), 1954-
[DNLM: 1. Mental Disorders—etiology. 2. Mental Disorders—physiopathology.
3. Mental Disorders—therapy. 4. Neurobiology. WM 140 N9495 2009]
RC341.N393 2009
616.8—dc22
2008025739

9 8 7 6 5 4 3 2 1

Printed in the United States of America
on acid-free paper

Preface

Psychiatry stands poised to make dramatic advances in defining disease pathogenesis, developing diagnostic methods capable of identifying specific and valid disease entities, discovering novel and more effective treatments, and ultimately preventing psychiatric disorders. Publishing the third edition of *Neurobiology of Mental Illness* within 5 years of publication of the second edition is a testament to the progress that has been made in our field.

For this third edition, all the chapters have been thoroughly updated and new chapters have been added in areas where significant advances have been made. As before, Part I provides an overview of basic neuroscience that is relevant to clinical psychiatry or to expanding its foundations. Molecular neurobiology and molecular genetics are emphasized in the context of brain development, neuronal function, and neural networks and their contribution to complex behaviors. A chapter has been added on epigenetic mechanisms in psychiatry based on recent advances in understanding the influence of chromatin regulation on normal behavior as well as abnormalities in behavior seen in major psychiatric disorders.

Part II reviews and evaluates the methods used to examine the neurobiological basis of mental illness in humans. This part has been expanded to reflect critically important advances in the techniques of cognitive neuroscience, procedures for the postmortem investigation of the human brain, and current approaches to drug discovery. The chapters in this part provide a context for recent findings from neuroimaging studies that have related specific genes to the regulation of emotion. Further, an understanding of the methods underlying drug discovery will facilitate the translation of preclinical and clinical neuroscience research into badly needed breakthroughs in our therapeutic toolkit.

The remaining parts of the book cover the neurobiology of psychiatric disorders: psychoses, mood disorders, anxiety disorders, substance abuse disorders, dementias, disorders of childhood onset, and special topic areas. These parts have been augmented in several different areas as a reflection of research progress. New chapters have been added on epidemiology, animal models, different forms of dementia, mental retardation, neuropsychiatry, and developmental therapeutics. Current diagnostic classification systems are limited because they are based primarily on phenomenology rather than etiology and pathophysiology. We predict that the research advances reviewed in the parts on psychiatric disorders will ultimately lead to diagnostic systems in which genetic and neurobiological abnormalities have a primary role.

This edition of *Neurobiology of Mental Illness* reflects the continuing reintegration of psychiatry into the mainstream of biomedical science. The research tools that are transforming other branches of medicine—epidemiology, genetics, molecular biology, imaging, and medicinal chemistry—are also transforming psychiatry. It is our hope that, like us, the reader is optimistic that the progress in molecular, cellular, and behavioral neuroscience described in this textbook will eventually break new ground in the diagnosis, treatment, and prevention of disabling psychiatric disorders.

D.S.C.
New York, New York

E.J.N.
New York, New York

Contents

PART VI SUBSTANCE ABUSE DISORDERS

Section Editor: Steven E. Hyman
Introduction: Steven E. Hyman

PART VII DEMENTIA

Section Editor: Mary Sano
Introduction: Mary Sano

PART VIII PSYCHIATRIC DISORDERS OF CHILDHOOD ONSET

Section Editor: Daniel S. Pine
Introduction: Daniel S. Pine

Contributors*

Anissa Abi-Dargham, M.D.
Departments of Psychiatry and Radiology
Columbia University College of Physicians and Surgeons
New York, NY

George K. Aghajanian, M.D.
Departments of Psychiatry and Pharmacology
Yale School of Medicine
New Haven, CT

Stewart A. Anderson, M.D.
Departments of Psychiatry and Neuroscience
Weill Cornell Medical College
Cornell University
Ithaca, NY

Victoria Arango, Ph.D.
Department of Psychiatry
Columbia University College of Physicians and Surgeons
New York, NY

Neil Archibald, M.A., B.M.B.Ch., MRCP
Institute for Ageing and Health
Newcastle University
Newcastle upon Tyne, UK

Clive G. Ballard, M.D.
Institute for Ageing and Health
Newcastle University
Newcastle upon Tyne, UK

Deanna M. Barch, Ph.D.
Departments of Psychiatry and Psychology
Washington University in St. Louis
St. Louis, MO

Aysenil Belger, Ph.D.
Department of Psychiatry
University of North Carolina at Chapel Hill
Chapel Hill, NC

Monica Beneyto, Ph.D.
Department of Psychiatry
University of Pittsburgh School of Medicine
Pittsburgh, PA

Tami D. Benton, M.D.
Department of Psychiatry
University of Pennsylvania
Philadelphia, PA

Joanne Berger-Sweeney, Ph.D.
Department of Neuroscience
Wellesley College
Wellesley, MA

Christine Bergmann, M.D., Ph.D.
Department of Psychiatry
Mount Sinai School of Medicine
New York, NY

Robert M. Berman, M.D.
Department of Psychiatry
Columbia University
New York, NY

Wade H. Berrettini, M.D., Ph.D.
Department of Psychiatry
University of Pennsylvania School of Medicine
Philadelphia, PA

Olivier Berton, Ph.D.
Department of Psychiatry
University of Texas Southwestern Medical Center at Dallas
Dallas, TX

O. Joseph Bienvenu, M.D., Ph.D.
Department of Psychiatry and Behavioral Science
Johns Hopkins University School of Medicine
Baltimore, MD

R.J.R. Blair, Ph.D.
National Institute of Mental Health
National Institutes of Health
Bethesda, MD

Randy D. Blakely, Ph.D.
Departments of Pharmacology and Psychiatry
Vanderbilt University
Nashville, TN

* Visit www.NMI3_disclosures.com for details of contributors' disclosures.

MICHAEL H. BLOCH, M.D.
Department of Psychiatry
Yale School of Medicine
New Haven, CT

HILARY BLUMBERG, M.D.
Departments of Psychiatry and Diagnostic Radiology
Yale School of Medicine
New Haven, CT

MATTHEW BOBINSKI, M.D., PH.D.
Department of Radiology
University of California Davis Health System
Sacramento, CA

J. DOUGLAS BREMNER, M.D.
Departments of Psychiatry and Radiology
Emory University School of Medicine
Atlanta, GA

ADAM BRICKMAN, PH.D.
Department of Neurology
Columbia University College of Physicians and Surgeons
New York, NY

MIROSLAW BRYS, M.D., PH.D.
Department of Research
New York University School of Medicine
New York, NY

MONTE S. BUCHSBAUM, M.D.
Department of Psychiatry
Mount Sinai School of Medicine
New York, NY

DAVID J. BURN, M.D.
Institute for Ageing and Health
Newcastle University
Newcastle upon Tyne, UK

DAVID E. A. BUSH
Center for Neural Science
New York University
New York, NY

TIZIANO COLIBAZZI, M.D.
Department of Psychiatry
Columbia University
New York, NY

WILLIAM A. CARLEZON, JR., PH.D.
Departments of Psychiatry and Neuroscience
Harvard Medical School
Belmont, MA

CAMERON S. CARTER, M.D.
Department of Psychiatry and Behavioral Sciences
University of California, Davis
Sacramento, CA

B.J. CASEY, PH.D.
Department of Psychiatry
Weill Cornell Medical College
New York, NY

LISA A. CATAPANO, PH.D.
National Institute of Mental Health
National Institutes of Health
Bethesda, MD

MARK CELANO
National Institute of Mental Health
National Institutes of Health
Bethesda, MD

JOAQUIM CEREJEIRA
President
Associação Portuguesa de Internos de Psiquiatria
Coimbra, Portugal

STEVEN Z. CHAO, M.D., PH.D.
Department of Neurology
University of California, San Francisco
San Francisco, CA

DENNIS S. CHARNEY, M.D.
Department of Psychiatry, Neuroscience, and
Pharmacology & Systems Therapeutics
Mount Sinai School of Medicine
New York, NY

GUANG CHEN, M.D., PH.D.
National Institute of Mental Health
National Institutes of Health
Bethesda, MD

XIANGNING CHEN, PH.D.
Department of Psychiatry
Virginia Commonwealth University
Richmond, VA

PEARL H. CHIU, PH.D.
Department of Neuroscience
Baylor College of Medicine
Houston, TX

HELENA C. CHUI, M.D.
Department of Neurology
School of Medicine of University of Southern California
Los Angeles, CA

Chiara Cirelli, M.D., Ph.D.
Department of Psychiatry
University of Wisconsin, Madison
Madison, WI

Jonathan D. Cohen, M.D., Ph.D.
Princeton Neuroscience Institute
Princeton University
Princeton, NJ

Tiziano Colibazzi, M.D.
Department of Psychiatry
Columbia University College of Physicians and Surgeons
New York, NY

Daniel Collerton, M.Sc.
Newcastle Biomedicine
Newcastle University
Newcastle upon Tyne, UK

Kevin P. Conway, Ph.D.
National Institute of Drug Abuse
National Institute of Mental Health
Bethesda, MD

Edwin H. Cook, Jr., M.D.
Department of Psychiatry
University of Illinois at Chicago
Chicago, IL

Nicole S. Cooper, Ph.D.
Department of Psychiatry
Mount Sinai School of Medicine
New York, NY

Paul Crits-Christoph, Ph.D.
Department of Psychiatry
University of Pennsylvania Medical School
Philadelphia, PA

Dean G. Cruess, Ph.D.
Department of Psychology
University of Connecticut
Storrs, CT

Charles Dackis, M.D.
Department of Psychiatry
University of Pennsylvania
Philadelphia, PA

Jacek Debiec, M.D., Ph.D.
Center for Neural Science
New York University
New York, NY

Steven T. DeKosky, M.D.
Department of Neurology
University of Pittsburgh School of Medicine
Pittsburgh, PA

Mony J. de Leon, Ed.D
Department of Psychiatry
New York University School of Medicine
New York, NY

Susan DeSanti, Ph.D.
Department of Psychiatry
New York University School of Medicine
New York, NY

Ariel Y. Deutch, Ph.D.
Departments of Psychiatry and Pharmacology
Vanderbilt University Medical Center
Nashville, TN

Ralph J. DiLeone, Ph.D.
Department of Psychiatry
Yale School of Medicine
New Haven, CT

Wayne C. Drevets, M.D.
National Institute of Mental Health
National Institutes of Health
Bethesda, MD

Jing Du, M.D., Ph.D.
National Institute of Mental Health
National Institutes of Health
Bethesda, MD

Benoit Dube, M.D.
Department of Psychiatry
University of Pennsylvania
Philadelphia, PA

Ronald S. Duman, Ph.D.
Departments of Psychiatry and Pharmacology
Yale School of Medicine
New Haven, CT

Boadie W. Dunlop, M.D.
Department of Psychiatry & Behavioral Sciences
Emory University School of Medicine
Atlanta, GA

Sarah Durston, Ph.D.
Department of Child and Adolescent Psychiatry
University Medical Center Utrecht
Utrecht, The Netherlands

Andrew J. Dwork, M.D.
Departments of Pathology and Psychiatry
Columbia University
New York, NY

Gregory A. Elder, M.D.
Department of Psychiatry
Mount Sinai School of Medicine
New York, NY

Dwight L. Evans, M.D.
Departments of Psychiatry, Medicine, and Neuroscience
University of Pennsylvania
Philadelphia, PA

Michael B. First, M.D.
Department of Psychiatry
Columbia University College of Physicians and Surgeons
New York, NY

Joanna S. Fowler, Ph.D.
Chemistry Department
Brookhaven National Laboratory
Upton, NY

Karyn M. Frick, Ph.D.
Department of Psychology
Yale University
New Haven, CT

Abby J. Fyer, M.D.
Department of Psychiatry
Columbia University College of Physicians and Surgeons
New York, NY

Kishore M. Gadde, M.D.
Department of Psychiatry
Duke University Medical Center
Durham, NC

Amir Garakani, M.D.
Department of Psychiatry
Mount Sinai School of Medicine
New York, NY

Eliot L. Gardner, M.D.
National Institute on Drug Abuse
National Institutes of Health
Bethesda, MD

Steven J. Garlow, M.D., Ph.D.
Department of Psychiatry & Behavioral Sciences
Emory University School of Medicine
Atlanta, GA

Joel Gelernter, M.D.
Department of Psychiatry
Yale School of Medicine
New Haven, CT

David R. Gettes
Department of Psychiatry
University of Pennsylvania
Philadelphia, PA

S. Nassir Ghaemi, M.D.
Department of Psychiatry
Emory University
Atlanta, GA

Jay N. Giedd, M.D.
National Institute of Mental Health
National Institutes of Health
Bethesda, MD

Jean-Antoine Girault, M.D., Ph.D.
Inserm and Pierre & Marie Curie University
Institut du Fer a Moulin
Paris, France

Lidia Glodzik-Sobanska, M.D., Ph.D.
Department of Psychiatry
NYU Center for Brain Health
New York, NY

Nitin Gogtay, M.D.
National Institute of Mental Health
National Institutes of Health
Bethesda, MD

Martin Goldstein, M.D.
Department of Neurology
Mount Sinai School of Medicine
New York, NY

Marianne Goodman, M.D.
Department of Psychiatry
Mount Sinai School of Medicine
New York, NY

Frederick K. Goodwin, M.D.
Department of Psychiatry
George Washington University
Washington, DC

Paul Grant, M.D.
National Institute of Mental Health
National Institutes of Health
Bethesda, MD

Michael F. Green, Ph.D.
Department of Psychiatry and Biobehavioral Sciences
University of California, Los Angeles
Los Angeles, CA

Paul Greengard, Ph.D.
Laboratory of Molecular and Cellular Neuroscience
The Rockefeller University
New York, NY

Margaret Haglund, M.D.
Department of Psychiatry
Mount Sinai School of Medicine
New York, NY

Steven P. Hamilton, M.D., Ph.D.
Department of Psychiatry
University of California, San Francisco
San Francisco, CA

Antonio Y. Hardan, M.D.
Department of Psychiatry and Behavioral Science
Stanford University School of Medicine
Stanford, CA

John A. Hardy, Ph.D.
National Institute on Aging
National Institutes of Health
Bethesda, MD

Veronica Harsh, M.D.
National Institute of Mental Health
National Institutes of Health
Bethesda, MD

Erin A. Hazlett, Ph.D.
Department of Psychiatry
Mount Sinai School of Medicine
New York, NY

Ellen J. Hoffman, M.D.
Department of Psychiatry
Mount Sinai School of Medicine
New York, NY

Florian Holsboer, M.D., Ph.D.
Max Planck Institute of Psychiatry
Munich, Germany

Matthew J. Hoptman, Ph.D.
Department of Psychiatry
New York University
New York, NY

Thomas M. Hyde, M.D., Ph.D.
National Institute of Mental Health
National Institutes of Health
Bethesda, MD

Steven E. Hyman, M.D.
Office of the Provost
Harvard University
Cambridge, MA

Thomas R. Insel, M.D.
National Institute of Mental Health
National Institutes of Health
Bethesda, MD

Evelyn Jaros, Ph.D.
Institute for Ageing and Health
Newcastle University
Newcastle upon Tyne, UK

David Jimerson, M.D.
Department of Psychiatry
Harvard Medical School
Boston, MA

Amanda Kalaydjian, Ph.D.
Department of Mental Health at the Bloomberg School of Public Health
Johns Hopkins University
Baltimore, MD

Daniel I. Kaufer, M.D.
Department of Neurology
University of North Carolina, Chapel Hill
Chapel Hill, NC

Joan Kaufman, Ph.D.
Department of Psychiatry
Yale University School of Medicine
New Haven, CT

Walter Kaye, M.D.
Department of Psychiatry
University of Pittsburgh Medical School
Pittsburgh, PA

Brendan J. Kelley, M.D.
Department of Neurology
May Medical School
Rochester, MN

Kenneth S. Kendler, M.D.
Departments of Psychiatry and Human and Molecular Genetics
Virginia Commonwealth University
Richmond, VA

Justine M. Kent, M.D.
Department of Psychiatry
Columbia University College of Physicians and Surgeons
New York, NY

Robert S. Kern, Ph.D.
Department of Psychiatry and Biobehavioral Sciences
University of California, Los Angeles
Los Angeles, CA

John G. Kerns, Ph.D.
Department of Psychological Sciences
University of Missouri-Columbia
Columbia, MO

Byeong-Chae Kim, M.D., Ph.D.
Department of Neurology
Chonnam National University Medical School
Korea

Jong-Hoon Kim, M.D.
Department of Psychiatry
Columbia University College of Physicians and Surgeons
New York, NY

Barry E. Kosofsky, M.D., Ph.D.
Department of Pediatrics
Weill Cornell Medical College
New York, NY

K. Ranga R. Krishnan, M.D.
Department of Psychiatry and Behavioral Sciences
Duke University School of Medicine
Durham, NC

Evelyn K. Lambe, Ph.D.
Departments of Physiology and Obstetrics and Gynaecology
University of Toronto
Toronto, Canada

Jaakko Lappalainen, M.D., Ph.D.
Pharmacogenetics and Clinical Research, Discovery Medicine
AstraZeneca Pharmaceuticals
Wilmington, DE

James F. Leckman, M.D.
Department of Psychiatry
Yale School of Medicine
New Haven, CT

Joseph E. LeDoux, Ph.D.
Center for Neural Science
New York University
New York, NY

Junghee Lee, Ph.D.
Department of Psychology
Vanderbilt University
Nashville, TN

Ellen Leibenluft, M.D.
National Institute of Mental Health
National Institutes of Health
Bethesda, MD

Yi Li, M.D.
Department of Psychiatry
New York University School of Medicine
New York, NY
Department of Radiology
Qi Lu Hospital Shandog University
China

Jeffrey A. Lieberman, M.D.
Department of Psychiatry
Columbia University College of Physicians
and Surgeons
New York, NY

Barry M. Lester, Ph.D.
Department of Psychiatry
Brown University
Providence, RI

David A. Lewis, M.D.
Departments of Psychiatry and Neuroscience
University of Pittsburgh School of Medicine
Pittsburgh, PA

Falk W. Lohoff, M.D.
Department of Psychiatry
University of Pennsylvania
Philadelphia, PA

Paul J. Lombroso, M.D.
Departments of Psychiatry and Neurobiology
Yale School of Medicine
New Haven, CT

Hanzhang Lu, Ph.D.
Advance Imaging Research Center
University of Texas Southwestern
Medical Center
Dallas, TX

David M. Lyons, Ph.D.
Department of Psychiatry and Behavioral Sciences
Stanford University School of Medicine
Stanford, CA

Husseini K. Manji, M.D.
National Institute of Mental Health
National Institutes of Health
Bethesda, MD

J. John Mann, M.D.
Department of Psychiatry
Columbia University College of Physicians and Surgeons
New York, NY

Andrés Martin, M.D., M.P.H.
Department of Psychiatry
Yale School of Medicine
New Haven, CT

Diana Martinez, M.D.
Department of Psychiatry
Columbia University Medical Center
New York, NY

Sanjay J. Mathew, M.D.
Department of Psychiatry
Mount Sinai School of Medicine
New York, NY

William M. McDonald, M.D.
Department of Psychiatry and Behavioral Sciences
Emory University
Atlanta, GA

Bruce S. McEwen, Ph.D.
Harold and Margaret Milliken Hatch Laboratory of Neuroendocrinology
The Rockefeller University
New York, NY

Bryan E. McGill, M.D., Ph.D.
Department of Pediatrics
Washington University
St. Louis School of Medicine
St. Louis, MO

Ian G. McKeith, M.D.
Institute for Ageing and Health
Newcastle University
Newcastle upon Tyne, UK

Andrew McLaren, MRCP
Institute for Ageing and Health
Newcastle University
Newcastle upon Tyne, UK

Samantha Meltzer-Brody, M.D.
Department of Psychiatry
University of North Carolina at Chapel Hill School of Medicine
Chapel Hill, NC

Kathleen R. Merikangas, Ph.D.
National Institute of Mental Health
National Institutes of Health
Bethesda, MD

Bruce L. Miller, M.D.
Departments of Neurology and Psychiatry
University of California, San Francisco
San Francisco, CA

Effie M. Mitsis
Department of Psychiatry
Mount Sinai School of Medicine
New York, NY

Christopher S. Monk, Ph.D.
Department of Psychology
University of Michigan
Ann Arbor, MI

P. Read Montague, Ph.D.
Departments of Neuroscience and Psychiatry
Baylor College of Medicine
Houston, TX

Lisa M. Monteggia, Ph.D.
Department of Psychiatry
The University of Texas Southwestern Medical Center
Dallas, TX

Chris M. Morris, Ph.D.
Institute for Ageing and Health
Newcastle University
Newcastle upon Tyne, UK

Lisa Mosconi, Ph.D.
Department of Psychiatry
New York School of Medicine
New York, NY

Elizabeta B. Mukaetova-Ladinska, M.D., Ph.D.
Institute for Ageing and Health
Newcastle University
Newcastle upon Tyne, UK

James W. Murrough, M.D.
Department of Psychiatry
Mount Sinai School of Medicine
New York, NY

Charles B. Nemeroff, M.D., Ph.D.
Department of Psychiatry and Behavioral Sciences
Emory University School of Medicine
Atlanta, GA

Paul Nestadt, B.S.
School of Medicine
New York Medical College
New York, NY

Eric J. Nestler, M.D., Ph.D.
Department of Neuroscience
Mount Sinai School of Medicine
New York, NY

Antonia S. New, M.D.
Department of Psychiatry
Mount Sinai School of Medicine
New York, NY

Nancy Nielsen-Brown, M.S., PA-C
College of Allied Health Professions
Western University of Health Sciences
Pomona, CA

Charles P. O'Brien, M.D., Ph.D.
Department of Psychiatry
University of Pennsylvania
Philadelphia, PA

John T. O'Brien, M.D.
Institute for Ageing and Health
Newcastle University
Newcastle upon Tyne, UK

Michael S. Okun, M.D.
Departments of Neurology and Neurosurgery
University of Florida
Gainesville, FL

C. Warren Olanow, M.D.
Department of Neurology
Mount Sinai School of Medicine
New York, NY

Daniel P. Perl, M.D.
Department of Neuropathology
Mount Sinai School of Medicine
New York, NY

Elaine K. Perry, BSc, Ph.D., DSc
Institute for Ageing and Health
Newcastle University
Newcastle upon Tyne, UK

Robert Perry, PRCP, FRCPath
Institute for Ageing and Health
Newcastle University
Newcastle upon Tyne, UK

Ronald C. Petersen, M.D., Ph.D.
Department of Neurology
Mayo Medical School
Rochester, MN

Bradley S. Peterson, M.D.
Department of Psychiatry
Columbia College of Physicians and Surgeons
New York, NY

John M. Petitto, M.D.
Departments of Psychiatry, Nueroscience and Pharmacology
University of Florida College of Medicine
Gainesville, FL

Margaret A. Piggott, Ph.D.
Institute for Ageing and Health
Newcastle University
Newcastle upon Tyne, UK

Daniel S. Pine, M.D.
National Institute of Mental Health
National Institutes of Health
Bethesda, MD

Kerstin J. Plessen, M.D., Ph.D.
Center for Child and Adolescent Mental Health
University of Bergen
Bergen, Norway

Judith Rapoport, M.D.
National Institute of Mental Health
National Institutes of Health
Bethesda, MD

Scott L. Rauch, M.D.
Department of Psychiatry
Harvard Medical School
Boston, MA

Allan L. Reiss, M.D.
Department of Psychiatry and Behavioral Sciences
Stanford University School of Medicine
Stanford, CA

Martin J. Repetto, M.D., Ph.D.
Department of Psychiatry
University of Florida College of Medicine
Gainesville, FL

Brien Riley, Ph.D.
Department of Psychiatry
Virginia Commonwealth University
Richmond, VA

Steven P. Roose, M.D.
Department of Psychiatry
Columbia University College of Physicians and Surgeons
New York, NY

Raymond C. Rosen, Ph.D.
Department of Psychiatry
University of Medicine and Dentistry of New Jersey
Piscataway, NJ

Robert H. Roth, Ph.D.
Departments of Psychiatry and Pharmacology
Yale School of Medicine
New Haven, CT

John L.R. Rubenstein, M.D., Ph.D.
Langley Porter Psychiatric Institute
University of California, San Francisco
San Francisco, CA

David R. Rubinow, M.D.
Department of Psychiatry
University of North Carolina at Chapel Hill School of Medicine
Chapel Hill, NC

Michael Rutter, M.D.
Institute of Psychiatry
King's College, London
London, UK

Mary Sano, Ph.D.
Department of Psychiatry
Mount Sinai School of Medicine
New York, NY

Laura R. Schaevitz, Ph.D.
Department of Biological Sciences
Wellesley College
Wellesley, MA

Peter J. Schmidt, M.D.
National Institute of Mental Health
National Institutes of Health
Bethesda, MD

Stuart N. Seidman, M.D.
Department of Psychiatry
Columbia University College of Physicians and Surgeons
New York, NY

Etienne Sibille, Ph.D.
Department of Psychiatry
University of Pittsburgh
Pittsburgh, PA

Inge Sillaber, Ph.D.
Behavioural Pharmacology
Affectis Pharmaceuticals
Munich, Germany

Mark Slifstein, Ph.D.
Department of Psychiatry
Columbia University College of Physicians and Surgeons
New York, NY

John F. Smiley, Ph.D.
Nathan S. Kline Institute for Psychiatric Research
Orangeburg, NY

Steven Southwick, M.D.
Department of Psychiatry
Yale School of Medicine
New Haven, CT

Sarah Spence, M.D.
National Institute of Mental Health
National Institutes of Health
Bethesda, MD

Jonathan Sporn, M.D.
Department of Psychiatry
Massachusetts General Hospital
Boston, MA

Murray B. Stein, M.D., M.P.H.
Department of Psychiatry
University of California, San Diego
La Jolla, CA

Michael Strober, Ph.D.
Department of Psychiatry
David Geffen School of Medicine at UCLA
Los Angeles, CA

Gregory M. Sullivan, M.D.
Department of Psychiatry
Columbia University College of Physicians
and Surgeons
New York, NY

Susan E. Swedo, M.D.
National Institute of Mental Health
National Institutes of Health
Bethesda, MD

Carol A. Tamminga, M.D.
Department of Psychiatry
The University of Texas Southwestern Medical Center
Dallas, TX

Audrey Thurm, Ph.D.
National Institute of Mental Health
National Institutes of Health
Bethesda, MD

GARY D. TOLLEFSON, M.D., PH.D.
Department of Psychiatry
Indiana School of Medicine
Indianapolis, IN

GIULIO TONONI, M.D., PH.D.
Department of Psychiatry
University of Wisconsin, Madison
Madison, WI

JOSEPH TRIEBWASSER, M.D.
Bronx Veterans Administration Medical Center
Bronx, NY

JEREMY M. VEENSTRA-VANDERWEELE, M.D.
Department of Psychiatry
Vanderbilt University
Nashville, TN

INDRE VISKONTAS, PH.D.
Department of Neurology
University of California, San Francisco
San Francisco, CA

DAVID W. VOLK, M.D., PH.D.
Department of Psychiatry
University of Pittsburgh School of Medicine
Pittsburgh, PA

NORA D. VOLKOW, M.D.
National Institute on Drug Abuse
National Institutes of Health
Bethesda, MD

GARY L. WENK, PH.D.
Department of Psychology and Neuroscience
The Ohio State University
Columbus, OH

SAMANTHA L. WHITE, M.D.
National Institute of Mental Health
National Institutes of Health
Bethesda, MD

DANIEL R. WILSON, M.D., PH.D.
Department of Psychiatry
Creighton University
Omaha, NE

JAMES T. WINSLOW, M.D.
National Institute of Mental Health
National Institutes of Health
Bethesda, MD

ROY A. WISE, M.D.
National Institute on Drug Abuse
National Institutes of Health
Bethesda, MD

CARSTEN T. WOTJAK, PH.D.
Neuronal Plasticity
Max Planck Institute of Psychiatry
Munich, Germany

YIHONG YANG, PH.D.
National Institute on Drug Abuse
National Institutes of Health
Bethesda, MD

CARLOS A. ZARATE, JR., M.D.
National Institute of Mental Health
National Institutes of Health
Bethesda, MD

JING ZHANG, M.D.
National Institute on Aging
National Institutes of Health
Bethesda, MD

HUDA Y. ZOGHBI, M.D.
Department of Neuroscience
Baylor College of Medicine
Houston, TX

I INTRODUCTION TO BASIC NEUROSCIENCE

ERIC J. NESTLER

THE first part of this book provides an overview of basic neuroscience and molecular biology. Each chapter represents an enormous body of material that could itself be the subject of an entire textbook. Accordingly, these chapters are not intended to be comprehensive reviews, but rather concise summaries of the fields that lay the foundation of basic biological principles required for the clinical material that is the main focus of the book.

Chapter 1 provides an overview of brain development. There is increasing evidence that certain neuropsychiatric disorders may involve abnormalities in the formation of the nervous system. Although the details of such abnormalities remain obscure, the chapter provides insights into the cellular and molecular processes that may be involved and the ways in which such processes can be influenced by genetic and external factors.

Chapter 2 describes the neurochemical organization of the brain. It summarizes the diverse types of molecules that neurons in the brain use as neurotransmitters and neurotrophic factors, and how these molecules are synthesized and metabolized. The chapter also presents the array of receptor proteins through which these molecules regulate target neuron functioning and the reuptake proteins that generally terminate the neurotransmitter signal. Today a large majority of all drugs used to treat psychiatric disorders, as well as most drugs of abuse, still have as their initial targets proteins involved directly in neurotransmitter function.

Chapter 3 summarizes the electrophysiological basis of neuronal function. Ultimately, brain function is mediated by interactions between nerve cells, and the readout of such interactions is an alteration in the electrical properties of the cells. The chapter reviews the several types of recording techniques that are commonly used to measure neuronal activity, followed by a presentation of the many types of ion channels and receptors that control a neuron's electrophysiological responses.

Chapter 4 covers postreceptor intracellular messenger cascades through which neurotransmitters and neurotrophic factors, and their receptors, produce their diverse physiological effects. A major advance over the past generation of research has been an appreciation of the complex webs of intracellular signaling pathways that control every aspect of a neuron's functioning, from neurotransmitter signaling to cell shape and motility to gene expression. Although only a small number of medications used in psychiatry today have as their initial target intracellular signaling proteins, it is likely that drug development efforts will look increasingly to such proteins for the discovery of novel medications with fundamentally new mechanisms of action.

Chapter 5 describes prominent mechanisms of neural plasticity, that is, ways in which neurons adapt over time in response to environmental perturbations. It is this capacity for adaptation (or maladaptation) that makes it possible for the brain to not only learn and think but also for the brain to get sick. The chapter focuses on protein phosphorylation as a prominent molecular basis of neural plasticity. The ways in which protein phosphorylation mechanisms contribute to adaptive and maladaptive changes in the brain are discussed.

Chapter 6 provides an overview of the genetic basis of the nervous system. The chapter covers the structure of DNA and chromatin in the nucleus, how genes encode messenger RNAs and proteins, and the mechanisms (for example, alternative splicing and posttranslational processing) by which numerous proteins can be generated from individual genes. The chapter also describes how this process of gene expression is under dynamic regulation throughout the adult life of an organism via the regulation of transcription factors and other nuclear proteins, and how such mechanisms contribute in important ways to long-lived neural plasticity.

Chapter 7 offers a progress report on new tools developed by molecular biologists to manipulate the expression of genes in the nervous system. Through the use of tools such as viral-mediated gene transfer and inducible mutations in mice, scientists are able to manipulate genes in the brain with increasing spatial and temporal precision. Such tools are essential as we strive to better understand the contribution of individual genes to complex behavior.

Chapter 8, new to this third edition, covers epigenetic mechanisms in psychiatry. Epigenetic regulation in neurons describes a process in which the activity of a particular gene is controlled by the structure of chromatin in that gene's proximity. Recent work has demonstrated the dynamic nature of chromatin remodeling in the nervous system and its importance for the normal development of the nervous system as well as the brain's capacity to adapt over time to environmental challenges. Abnormalities in chromatin remodeling have also been implicated in several neurological and psychiatric disorders.

A great deal has been written recently about the need for translational research in psychiatry. Yet we all know how uniquely difficult translational research is in our field. This is due to several factors, including the unique complexity of the brain, the lack of ready access to the brains of our patients, and the apparent complexity of at least some psychiatric disorders with respect to etiology and pathophysiology. As a result, it is currently difficult, if not impossible, to relate most of the material covered in this first part of the book to studies of the clinical disorders. How does one study, for example, the transcription factor *cyclic adenosine monophosphate response element binding protein* (CREB) or changes in dendritic spine density implicated in animal models of several psychiatric conditions, in living patients? We view this difficulty, though very real today, as a time-limited obstacle. As advances in human genetics and brain imaging progress, it will become possible to analyze diverse neurotransmitter and neurotrophic factor systems, intracellular signaling proteins, and even gene expression profiles in our patients and ultimately within discrete brain regions implicated in disease pathophysiology. Such methodologies will complete psychiatry's transformation into a field of modern molecular medicine.

1 Overview of Brain Development

JOHN L.R. RUBENSTEIN AND STEWART A. ANDERSON

There is increasing evidence that abnormalities in the development of the brain either predispose or directly cause certain psychiatric disorders. Although it is not surprising that childhood disorders, such as autism, are caused by neurodevelopmental abnormalities, disorders that display their most characteristic symptoms during or after adolescence also may be influenced by developmental abnormalities that occurred in utero. For instance, numerous lines of evidence suggest that some cases of schizophrenia are the result of abnormal neurodevelopment. Thus, there is a compelling rationale for behavioral scientists and clinicians to understand the basic mechanisms that regulate assembly of the brain, as this information may be key to understanding the etiology and perhaps even the prevention and treatment of major psychiatric disorders.

This chapter highlights the major processes involved in development of the brain to provide the reader with a foundation for understanding developmental neuroscience. The chapter briefly surveys neurodevelopment, from induction of the central nervous system (CNS) to patterning of the primordia of major brain regions, proliferation of neuroepithelial cells, differentiation and migration of immature neurons and glia, formation of axon tracts and synapses, and concludes with the establishment and plasticity of neuronal networks. Although most of the information described in this chapter is based upon studies in nonprimate mammals, it is likely that these findings are also true in the developing human brain.

INDUCTION AND PATTERNING OF THE EMBRYONIC CNS

Early CNS development involves an ordered sequence of inductive processes that begin with the formation of the neural plate followed by a hierarchical series of inductions that lead to regionally distinct developmental programs (for a more extensive review on this subject, see Rubenstein and Puelles, 2003). Inductive processes generally involve two tissues. One tissue is the target of the induction; the other, called the *organizer*, produces the molecular signals that carry out the induction. These molecular signals, which generally are proteins, induce in the target tissues a new pattern of gene expression that dictates their subsequent developmental program.

Development of the CNS begins during gastrulation by a process called *neural induction*. Proteins produced by organizer tissues cause the embryonic ectoderm to differentiate into a neural fate. This process involves activation of receptor tyrosine kinases, perhaps through fibroblast growth factors (FGFs) and/or insulin-like growth factors (IGFs) (Streit et al., 2000; Wilson and Rubenstein, 2000; Pera et al., 2001) and inhibition of transforming growth factor-b (TGF-b) signaling through the noggin and chordin proteins that bind to bone morphogenetic proteins (BMPs) (de Robertis et al., 2000; Wilson and Edlund, 2001). In addition, wingless (WNT) signaling is implicated in inhibiting neural induction in some species (Wilson and Edlund, 2001). Induction of the neural ectoderm leads to the formation of the neural plate, which will give rise to the entire CNS (Fig. 1.1); its lateral edges will give rise to the neural crest, which gives rise to most of the peripheral nervous system (PNS) and contributes to the head skeleton.

Beginning during neural induction, inductive processes subdivide the neural plate into molecularly distinct domains that are the primordia of the major subdivisions of the CNS. One can distinguish three types of inductive processes during CNS regionalization: (*1*) anterior-posterior or A-P, (*2*) mediolateral or M-L, and (*3*) local. The A-P regionalization subdivides the neural plate into transverse domains. The principal transverse subdivisions of the brain are the prosencephalon (forebrain), mesencephalon (midbrain), and rhombencephalon (hindbrain) (Fig. 1.2). Further refinements of A-P regionalization subdivide the rhombencephalon into segment-like domains called *neuromeres* (*rhombomeres*). The forebrain may also have neuromeric subdivisions called *prosomeres*. The inductive mechanisms underlying A-P regionalization are poorly understood but probably include vertical inductions (from underlying tissues) from mesoderm and endoderm (via substances such as the protein cereberus) and planar inductions (from substances that transmit their effects in the plane of the neural plate), perhaps from the node (via substances such as retinoids).

The M-L regionalization produces distinct tissues that are longitudinally aligned along the long axis of the CNS (Fig. 1.1). Medial inductions are regulated by

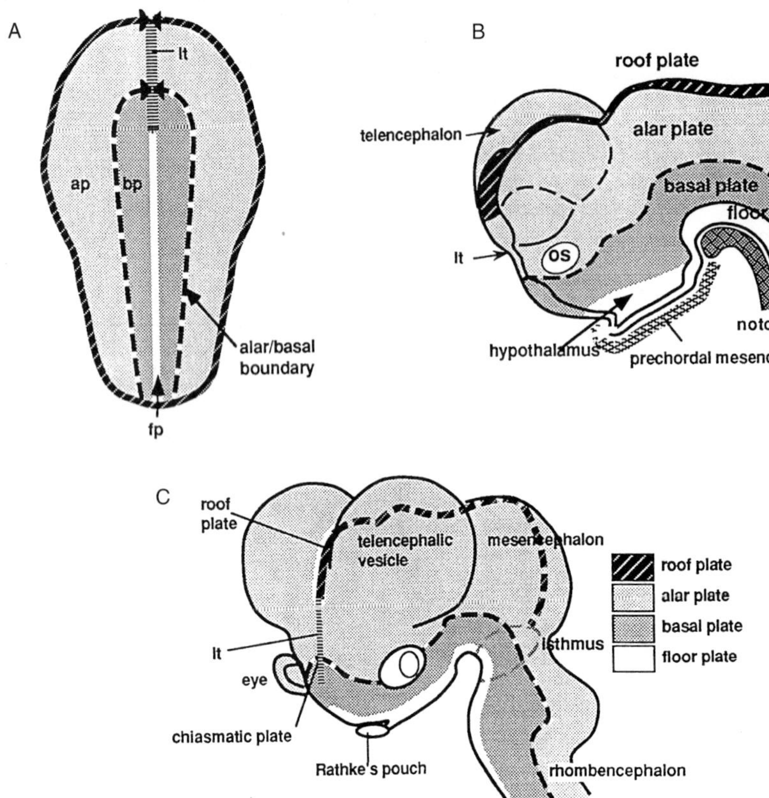

FIGURE 1.1 Schemes of the longitudinal organization of the forebrain proposed in Shimamura et al. (1995; see Rubenstein and Shimamura, 1997). (*A*) Model of the longitudinal domains in the neural plate, including the primordia of the floor, basal, alar, and roof plates (fp, bp, ap). Beneath the medial neural plate are the notochord and the prechordal plate. (*B*) Medial view of the neural tube. (*C*) Rostrolateral view of the neural tube. lt, lamina terminalis; os, optic stalk.

substances produced by axial mesodermal organizers: the notochord and prechordal plate. These organizers are midline structures that lie underneath the middle of the neural plate and produce substances, such as sonic hedgehog, that induce the medial neural plate to form the primordia of the floor plate and basal plate (Fig. 1.1). Lateral inductions are believed to be mediated by substances such as TGF-bs that include the BMPs that are produced along the rim of the neural plate by the non-neural ectoderm. Lateral inductions are likely to be essential for development of the neural crest, roof plate, and alar plate (Fig. 1.1).

The combination of A-P and M-L patterning generates a checkerboard organization of brain subdivisions (Fig. 1.2), each of which expresses a distinct combination of regulatory genes. Superimposed on this pattern are the local inductive signals that are essential for the formation of the vesicles that evaginate from the brain such as the telencephalon, eyes, and posterior pituitary. Evidence suggests that signals originating from ectodermal tissues (lens placode, anterior neural ridge, and anterior pituitary, respectively) adjacent to these structures produce signals that induce their formation.

Although the process of regionalization subdivides the neural plate into the primordia of the major brain regions, the process of morphogenesis transforms the shape of the neural plate into a tube that additionally has flexures and evaginations. Note that the folding of the neural plate into the neural tube converts the lateromedial dimension of the neural plate into the dorsoventral (D-V) dimension of the neural tube (Fig. 1.1).

A cross section through the D-V axis of the neural tube transects its four primary longitudinal subdivisions (Fig. 1.3). From ventral to dorsal, these longitudinal

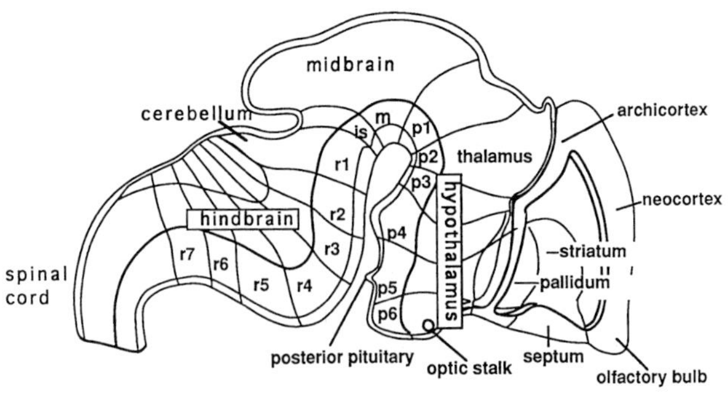

FIGURE 1.2 Schemes of the embryonic 12.5-day mouse brain, in which the primordia of some forebrain structures are labeled. In addition, longitudinal and transverse subdivisions are indicated. The paired telencephalic vesicles make up the majority of the forebrain and can be subdivided into the cortical and subcortical areas. The cortical region includes the neocortex, archicortex (hippocampus), and paleocortex (olfactory bulb and olfactory cortex). The subcortical areas include the striatum, globus pallidus, septum, and parts of the amygdala (not shown). Ventral to the telencephalon are the eyes and hypothalamic areas. Neuromeric (transverse) components are labeled in their basal plate: r1–r7: rhombomeres; p1–p6 are the theoretical prosomeres. This drawing is a modified version of the prosomeric model (e.g., see Rubenstein and Shimamura, 1997). is, isthmus; m, midbrain.

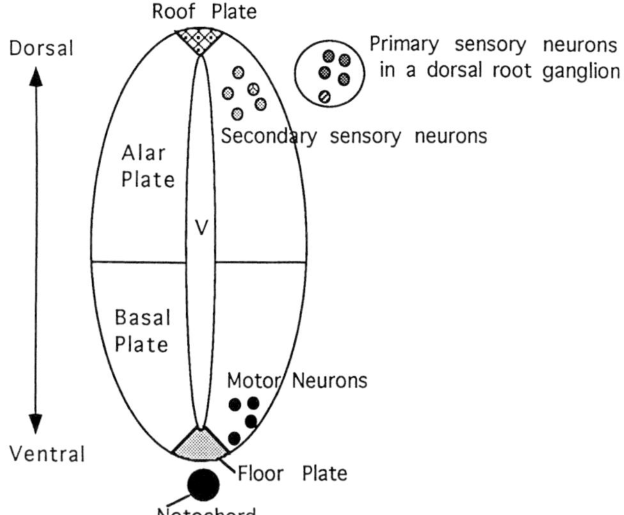

FIGURE 1.3 Cross section of the D-V organization of the neural tube at the level of the spinal cord. The floor plate is induced by the notochord; together they produce sonic hedgehog protein, which induces motor neurons in the basal plate. Neural crest cells from the most dorsal alar plate form the spinal ganglia, including the dorsal root ganglia, which contain the primary sensory neurons. Secondary sensory neurons are in the alar plate. v, ventricle.

columns are the floor, basal, alar, and roof plates. Each of these longitudinal columns may extend along the entire A-P axis of the CNS and contribute to distinct functional elements of the nervous system. The basal plate is the primordia for the motor neurons. The alar plate is the primordia for the secondary sensory neurons. The floor plate, which does not produce any neurons, has several functions that are required during development. Like the notochord, the floor plate produces sonic hedgehog and is believed to serve as a secondary ventral (medial) organizer where it also, in combination with chemotropic molecules such as netrins, guides the growth of axon tracts (Okada et al., 2006). Most of the roof plate forms the nonneuronal dorsal midline, which in some regions gives rise to specialized structures such as the choroid plexus and the pineal gland. The roof plate is marked by its high expression of BMPs and WNTs.

The regionalization process continues after neurulation (neural tube formation) to further subdivide large primordial regions into their constituent domains. These aspects of regionalization are probably carried out by planar inductive mechanisms via organizers that are within the neural tube. For example, secondary D-V patterning can be regulated by the floor plate (see the next section), whereas secondary A-P patterning can be regulated by the isthmus. The isthmus is a region between the mid- and hindbrain that produces inductive substances such as FGFs and WNT that regulate development of the midbrain and cerebellum.

HISTOGENESIS OF BRAIN REGIONS: PROLIFERATION, CELL FATE DETERMINATION, MIGRATION, AND DIFFERENTIATION

The process of regionalization subdivides the CNS into the primordia of its major structures (for example, cerebral cortex, striatum, thalamus, cerebellum) and initiates within these primordia their genetic programs of histogenesis. Histogenesis is a complex process that can be subdivided into two general parts: proliferation and differentiation (for more extensive reviews of this subject, see Rakic, 1995; Alvarez-Buylla et al., 2001; Marin and Rubenstein, 2001; Kriegstein et al., 2006). In general, each of these processes takes place in distinct zones within the wall of the neural tube. Proliferation takes place in the ventricular zone (VZ), which lines the inner surface of the neural tube and is adjacent to the ventricular cavity, whereas differentiation takes place largely in the mantle, which surrounds the VZ (see Fig. 1.4).

The VZ cells are undifferentiated and mitotically active. Each brain region has a distinct proliferation program that regulates the rate of cell division, the number of times VZ cells divide, and the character of the cell division. Cell division can be symmetrical, producing daughter cells that are identical, or asymmetrical, producing daughter cells that are nonidentical. Symmetrical divisions produce daughter cells that, like their mother, continue to proliferate or, unlike their mother, differentiate or die. Asymmetric division can produce one daughter cell that differentiates and one daughter cell that continues to proliferate. The regulation of these processes is integral to controlling how many cells are produced in each region

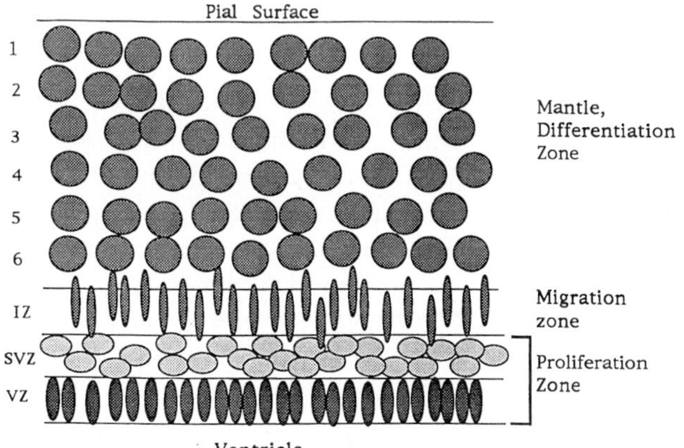

FIGURE 1.4 Organization of proliferative and differentiation zones within the wall of the neural tube. This scheme shows developing cerebral neocortex. The proliferative zones (ventricular zone [VZ] and subventricular zone [SVZ]) are adjacent to the ventricle. Postmitotic cells migrate from the proliferation zones, through the intermediate zone (IZ), and stop migrating in the mantle, where differentiation is completed. The cerebral cortex is a laminar structure (six major layers); cells in the deeper layers (for example, layer 6) are generally born before cells in the superficial layers.

and when these cells are made. For example, the expansion of the cerebral cortex in primates may relate to increased numbers of symmetrical divisions of neuron-producing progenitors in the cortical subventricular zone (Kriegstein et al., 2006).

There are many types of cells that make up the CNS. The two major classes are neurons and glia (Lemke, 2001). There are two major types of neurons: projection neurons, whose axons migrate to distant territories, and local circuit neurons (interneurons), whose processes ramify nearby. Within these general categories, there are many distinct types of projection and local circuit neurons that differ by neurochemistry, firing characteristics, and connectivity (Wonders and Anderson, 2006). There are two types of CNS-derived glia, astrocytes and oligodendrocytes, whereas the other major glial type, the microglia, is mesodermally derived (Colognato and French-Constant, 2004). Astrocytes regulate the local chemical milieu and appear to play a role in synaptogenesis (Allen and Barres, 2005). Oligodendrocytes produce the myelin sheaths that surround many axons; these sheaths function as insulators that increase the velocity of action potentials. Microglia are related to macrophages and subserve a phagocytic role in removing dead cells from the CNS.

Early in development, the VZ contains proliferative cells that have the potential to produce neurons and glia. In general, neurogenesis precedes gliogenesis. Whereas most regions of the CNS can produce neurons and astrocytic glia, some regions are specialized for producing oligodendroglia. For instance, a small region of the ventral spinal cord that initially generates motor neurons later converts to producing oligodendrocytes (Richardson et al., 2006).

Different types of neurons are generated at distinct D-V positions in the CNS. For instance, within the spinal cord, motor neurons are generated by ventral progenitors, whereas sensory neurons are generated by dorsal progenitors (Shirasaki and Pfaff, 2002). Likewise, in the telencephalon, ventral progenitors produce neurons of the basal ganglia, whereas dorsal progenitors produce cortical neurons. This arrangement is the result of the D-V patterning mechanisms described earlier in this chapter. Although patterning of the nervous system produces separate primordia of major brain regions (for example, cerebral cortex and basal ganglia), cell migration processes "mix" certain cell types between these primordia.

The mechanisms underlying cell fate decisions in the nervous system involve molecules within the cells (intrinsic signals controlled by proteins such as transcription factors; see Chapter 6) as well as molecules outside of the cells (extrinsic signals controlled by proteins such as growth/differentiation factors and their receptors). These proteins have integral roles in regulating whether a cell continues to divide, whether it undergoes symmetrical or asymmetrical division, whether the daughter cells go on to differentiate, and what lineage they will differentiate along.

Notch signaling is an example of extrinsic control of differentiation and is mediated by *Notch* receptors and their ligands (for example, Delta) (Justice and Jan, 2002). Activation of *Notch* by its ligand biases a cell not to differentiate; thus neurogenesis requires inhibition of *Notch* signaling (Gaiano and Fishell, 2002). Thus, *Notch* signaling can control the rate and timing of neuron production. Furthermore, high levels of *Notch* signaling bias progenitors toward an astrocytic fate. *Notch* signaling activates a cascade of molecular switches that culminates in the induction of transcription factors that change gene expression in the differentiating cell (Bertrand et al., 2002).

Although *Notch* signaling largely operates through basic helix-loop-helix transcription factors, many other types of transcription factors have central roles in brain development. These include *Homeobox*, *Sox*, *T-box*, *Winged-Helix*, and *HMG*-box families. Each family consists of subfamilies; for instance, key homeobox genes include *Dlx*, *Emx*, *Nkx*, *Otx*, *Pax*, and *POU*, which control such processes as regional fate, cell type identity, neuronal maturation, and cell migration (Briscoe et al., 2000; Wilson and Rubenstein, 2000).

Once neurons are generated, the next step in their differentiation is migration to the appropriate destination (Ayala et al., 2007). Each brain region has a specific migration program. In cortical structures (for example, cerebral cortex and superior colliculus), migrations are orchestrated to form layered or laminar structures. In most subcortical regions, migrations form nuclear structures that generally are not laminar. There are two general types of migration: radial and tangential. Radial migration is movement perpendicular to the plane of the ventricle toward the pial surface; tangential migration is movement parallel to the plane of the ventricle.

Radial migration involves the interaction between the elongated processes of radial glial cells and the migrating immature neurons. The immature neurons migrate to a specified location within the wall of the neural tube where they disengage from the radial glial cell and continue to differentiate. One of the key molecules regulating this process was identified through analysis of the *reeler* mutant mouse (Rice and Curran, 2001). In the cerebral cortex of *reeler* mice, later-born neurons fail to migrate past their earlier-born siblings, leading to partial inversion of the usual inside-out lamination. The *reeler* gene encodes a large, secreted molecule named *reelin* that appears to promote dissociation of neuroblasts from radial glia. Further mouse genetic studies have implicated two low-density lipoprotein receptors (VLDLR and ApoER2) as the receptors for the reelin molecule.

In addition to radial migration of neurons, it is now clear that nervous system development also depends on tangential migration. Tangential migration of neurons has long been known to occur in the cerebellum and in the rostral migratory stream (RMS) of the olfactory bulb, where adult neurogenesis is best characterized. Now it appears that many GABAergic local circuit neurons of the telencephalon are generated in the basal ganglia primordia and then tangentially migrate to the cerebral cortex and hippocampus (Marin and Rubenstein, 2001). This process results in mixing of gamma-aminobutyric acid (GABA)ergic neurons from the basal ganglia anlage with glutamatergic projection neurons of the cerebral cortex, thus allowing inhibitory regulation of excitatory transmission. Neuregulin1, a candidate gene for contributing risk of schizophrenia, has been identified as providing critical guidance cues for tangenially migrating interneurons (Flames et al., 2004).

Progress has also been made in identifying genes that control cytoskeletal processes that are essential for migration. Several of these genes were first identified as causing neuronal migration defects in humans, including *Lisencephaly-1*, *Doublecortin*, and *Filamin* (Mochida and Walsh, 2004).

The time when a neuron is born (the cell is no longer mitotically active and migrates away from the VZ) has an important influence on its fate (the type of neuron it becomes and its location within the brain). For instance, in the cerebral cortex, there are seven layers: layers 1, 2, 3, 4, 5, 6, and the subplate. Layer 1 is the most superficial, and the subplate is closest to the VZ. In the cerebral cortex, cells that are born first populate the deepest layers; this produces the so-called inside-out pattern of histogenesis. Each layer has distinct functions. For instance, the subplate is believed to provide signals that direct the incoming thalamic axons to their appropriate cortical target zone; layers 5 and 6 contain neurons that project out of the cortex; neurons in layer 4 receive input from the thalamus; neurons in layers 2 and 3 have intracortical projections; reelin-secreting layer 1 neurons participate in regulating cortical histogenesis by modulating the radial migration process (Tissir and Goffinet, 2003).

WIRING OF THE BRAIN: FORMATION OF AXON PATHWAYS AND SYNAPSES

As the immature neurons and glia migrate from the proliferative zone to the differentiation zone (the mantle), they elaborate more complex cellular structures. Neurons extend several thin processes away from their cell body; these include multiple dendrites and a single axon. Perhaps the most distinctive feature of the nervous system is how axon processes navigate long distances to find their targets (for a more extensive review of this subject see Tessier-Lavigne and Goodman, 1996; Grunwald and Klein, 2002; Charron and Tessier-Lavigne, 2005). The growing tip of the axon is called the *growth cone.* This dynamic web-like structure extends filopodia that appear to explore their environment, searching for cues that either attract or repel them.

Molecules and their receptors have been identified that serve as chemoattractants or repellents for growing axons. Some of these molecules are long-range signals that instruct growing axons from a distance where to project. Other signals have local effects and provide more specific information to the axon concerning the path it should take. Some of these signals are found on the surface of glial cells that serve as guideposts for the axons. The first axon pathways that develop create a scaffold for later-arriving axons. Through a process called *fasciculation*, later-arriving axons can adhere to axons that are already in an axon pathway. Molecules on the surface of the axons, some of which are related to immunoglobulins, can regulate selective fasciculation to generate axon bundles with common properties. When an axon has reached its target, a process called *defasciculation* enables the axon to separate from the axon bundle.

As axons grow and navigate, they express receptors for guidance molecules expressed by neighboring cells (Tessier-Lavigne and Goodman, 1996; Brose and Tessier-Lavigne, 2000; Yu and Bargmann, 2001). These processes operate as growth cones grow along specific pathways that in many cases involve crossing midline structures (commissures), such as the optic chiasm and corpus callosum. Activation of these receptors determines whether an axon grows toward or away from a target cell. At least four conserved families of guidance molecules have been identified. The semaphorins comprise a large 20-member family of soluble and membrane-bound molecules that elicit repulsive signals through two receptor families, neuropilins and plexins. The slit family of proteins consists of three members in mammals and acts through Robo receptors in commissural axons to prevent these axons from recrossing the midline. Whereas the slits and semaphorins are repulsive, members of the netrin family can be repulsive or attractive for a growth cone, depending upon the types of receptors expressed by the axon (receptor complexes containing either the colorectal cancer [DCC] or the neogenin protein lead to attraction; UNC-5-related protein leads to repulsion). Members of the ephrin family of ligands are membrane-bound and interact with two families of receptors, EphA and EphB (Kullander and Klein, 2002). EphrinB ligands, when bound to EphB receptors, are capable of bidirectional signaling whereby the cytoplasmic domain of the ephrin ligand transmits a phosphorylation signal. In addition to regulating axon pathfinding, semaphorins, slits, netrins, and ephrins control neuronal migrations.

Upon reaching its target, the growth cone is further modified as it forms a part of the synapse (Sanes and Lichtman, 2001). Reciprocal signals between the growth cone and the postsynaptic target cell induce the production of molecules and membranous specializations found in synapses (Benson et al., 2001). For instance, the presynaptic cells produce synaptic vesicles filled with neurotransmitters, and the postsynaptic cells form dendrites with specialized domains containing neurotransmitter receptors (Jan and Jan, 2001). Both cells express the channels and other components required for the initiation and propagation of action potentials. In the 1950s, Levi Montalcini discovered nerve growth factor (NGF), the first of four so-called neurotrophins that provide signals that control such processes as neuronal survival and synapse strength (Huang and Reichardt, 2001). By the end of the 1980s the neurotrophic hypothesis was firmly entrenched, and it suggested that postsynaptic cells are responsible for releasing neurotrophins that the presynaptic neuronal process was attracted to via its expression of a so-called Trk receptor. The amount of neurotrophin released by a given cell determined whether a cell reached a given target and formed a synapse or otherwise was destined for "programmed death." The mechanisms underlying programmed cell death, or apoptosis, have recently been elucidated (Kuan et al., 2000).

The biochemical nature of apoptosis was first discovered by studying the nematode *Caenorhabditis elegans*. A genetic analysis identified a cascade of proteases, known as *caspases*, that control programmed cell death in all animals. Subsequently, mitochondrial-associated proteins have also emerged as important regulators of apoptosis including the Bcl-2 family, APAF, and cytochrome C. Apoptosis is recognized as a fundamental process that, together with progenitor cell proliferation, controls neuronal numbers during development. Presently, researchers are investigating whether some neurodegenerative disorders may be the result of aberrant apoptosis or neurotrophin signaling and whether neurotrophins or apoptosis inhibitors can be used clinically to treat neurodegenerative abnormalities.

The wiring of complex CNS systems requires the connection of multiple cell types that are located in different positions. The wiring diagram of the visual system is an instructive example of this process. The neural retina contains primary sensory receptor neurons (rods and cones), interneurons (for example, amacrine, bipolar, and horizontal cells), glia (Müller cells), and projection neurons called *retinal ganglion cells*. The retinal ganglion cells extend axons that must make several choices on the path to their targets. First, they exit the eye through the optic nerve and confront the optic chiasmatic plate, a structure at the front of the hypothalamus. Axons from the temporal retina do not cross at the chiasm, whereas axons from the nasal retina do cross. Intrinsic signals that distinguish nasal and temporal cells (for example, the brain factor-1 and -2 transcription factors) permit the growing axons to sort themselves out to follow the correct pathway. There appear to be signals that the axons detect in the chiasmatic plate that direct the axon traffic. Upon exiting the chiasm, the optic axons grow posteriorly toward their two main targets: the thalamus and the superior colliculus. The optic tracts grow along the surface of the hypothalamic mantle zone, passing many nuclei, until they reach the thalamus. Branches perpendicular to the trajectory of the optic tracts grow out from the axons. These branches then specifically enter the visual centers of the thalamus, principally the lateral geniculate nucleus (LGN), where they form synapses with the LGN neurons. Before describing the LGN in greater detail, it is important to point out that some optic axons continue to grow more posteriorly into the midbrain, where they form branches into the superior colliculus (or optic tectum). Here, the optic axons synapse in specific locations; axons from the temporal retina synapse in the anterior tectum, whereas axons from the nasal retina synapse in the posterior tectum. Molecules that may regulate this retinotopic map on the optic tectum are membrane-bound *Eph*-type receptors (found on the axons) and their membrane-bound protein ligands (found on the target cells). The *Eph* proteins probably make up part of the molecular system that orchestrates the precise mapping of axonal projections onto the target tissues in all CNS regions.

In the LGN, the optic axons also form a retinotopic map. In higher mammals, the LGN is a laminar structure; each layer in the adult is connected with only one eye. However, during development, axons from both eyes have processes that extend into many LGN layers. Experimental evidence suggests that neuronal activity is required for the sorting-out process that eliminates branches in some layers and strengthens the synapses in others. Neuronal activity–dependent processes appear to have an essential role in many steps that refine the patterns of connections in the CNS; this is addressed further below.

The projection neurons in the LGN send axons anteriorly into the telencephalon, where they traverse the striatum in the internal capsule and enter their target: the cerebral neocortex. The thalamocortical fibers enter the cortex while neurogenesis is still actively occurring and grow into a layer called the *intermediate zone* that is interposed between the proliferative (VZ and subventricular zone [SVZ]) and mantle (cortical plate) zones. The thalamocortical fibers' next task is to innervate the correct region of the neocortex. The neocortex is subdivided into functionally distinct areas, each with a distinctive set of inputs. The LGN axons must innervate the primary visual cortex. Evidence suggests that some of the positional information that regulates this process is found in a transient layer of cortical neurons called the *subplate cells*. These are among the first cortical neurons to differentiate, and they are located in the deepest layer of the cortical plate, adjacent to the intermediate zone. The axons from different thalamic nuclei form transient synapses with the subplate cells in distinct cortical domains. The LGN fibers grow to a caudal position in the cortex, which will become the primary visual cortex. There the LGN axons form synapses with the subplate cells and wait in this location until the cerebral cortex has further matured. Then the LGN fibers leave the subplate, grow into the cortex, and form synapses with neurons in layer 4. After the axons leave the subplate, most of these cells die, leaving no trace of this important step in neurodevelopment.

Initially, inputs from both eyes converge within the same areas in layer 4 of the primary visual cortex. Then the axons from each eye segregate into distinct alternating domains called the *ocular dominance columns*. Evidence suggests that formation of these columns requires neuronal activity and that correlated activity from subregions of each eye plays a role in this process (see Katz and Shatz, 1996, for a review of this subject). Because ocular dominance formation occurs in utero, the neuronal activity is not induced by visual experience but is probably regulated by intrinsic neuronal discharges within the retina.

As the thalamocortical circuit is maturing, local connections between cortical layers 1–6 form a columnar intracortical circuit that is the basic unit of cortical function. Each region of visual space is represented in these cortical columns, and the ensemble of these columns becomes the primary visual cortex. Through processes that are beyond the scope of this chapter, the primary visual cortex regulates the development of secondary visual centers that are concerned with more complex aspects of processing and integrating visual information. These areas project to cortical association areas that integrate visual and other information, which then influences motor output areas of the cortex. Forming and refining of these more complex intracortical circuits continues into postnatal life. These postnatal aspects of CNS development are greatly influenced by visual experience.

POSTNATAL DEVELOPMENTAL PROCESSES

Many aspects of neuronal development continue during postnatal life. As noted above, there is the continued elaboration and refinement of neuronal connections. Indeed, neocortical connectivity remains plastic into adulthood. For instance, in adult animals, when peripheral sensory inputs are eliminated, such as through amputation of a finger, the cortical regions that previously received input from the now-removed finger now receive sensory inputs from the adjacent fingers. There is evidence that this alteration in the neocortical sensory map results from changes in the sizes and shapes of axonal processes and the distribution of synapses. Thus, the synaptic connectivity of the adult neocortex is capable of a significant level of reorganization.

In addition to the ability of neuronal processes to continue to grow and change in shape in postnatal animals, there are several brain regions that postnatally continue to produce new cells, probably neurons and glia. For instance, the SVZ of the lateral ventricles produces interneurons of the olfactory bulb, and the subgranular zone of the dentate gyrus in the hippocampus continues to make new granular neurons postnatally. Recent studies suggest that adult neurogenesis in the hippocampal dentate gyrus mediates aspects of spatial memory as well as aspects of antidepressant response and is negatively affected by certain forms of stress (Dranovsky and Hen, 2006; Perera et al., 2007).

Gliogenesis is also active in many brain regions, including the cerebral cortex, where the cells differentiate into oligodendrocytes that actively continue to myelinate axons postnatally. In primates, some central circuits are not fully myelinated (and hence are not fully functional) until late adolescence or young adulthood. Thus, brain development does not end following birth, and several aspects of development are perhaps maintained throughout life.

As newborns become exposed to sensory information, experience-driven influences gain increasing importance in molding the structure and function of the CNS. Although experience-based learning involves alterations in the structure of the brain (through physical changes that affect the number and distribution of synapses), it is likely that other mechanisms also have important roles. For instance, there are models that suggest that learning may include changes in the strength of synaptic signaling (via processes called *long-term potentiation* and *long-term depression*) accomplished at the molecular level (Chapter 5). It will not be surprising if such a complex process as learning turns out to involve multiple mechanisms.

In sum, CNS development is probably a lifelong process requiring a precise order of events to occur at particular times. When a genetic or other influence eliminates, alters, or postpones (during a critical period) a specific developmental step, it is likely that optimal function of the CNS may be forever impaired. This may lead either to overt psychopathology or to a predisposition for later psychopathological problems.

Postnatal development involves the melding of genetically driven events with those influenced by experience. How abnormalities in the developmental program lead to psychiatric disorders remains a mystery, probably due to the staggering complexity of the problem. Progress will, however, result eventually from further investigation, and the potential benefits of further study are many. Establishing the mechanisms underlying psychiatric disorders offers the potential of more rational diagnoses through genetic, molecular, histological, neuroimaging, and other methods. If we can identify individuals who are carriers of genes, or gene combinations, that predispose to neuropsychiatric disorders, we can offer genetic counseling and intervene early in the cases of their children who may be at risk for psychopathology. Finally, through an understanding of disease mechanisms, there is hope for the development of better therapies. Although most developmental abnormalities probably cannot be precisely repaired, one can be optimistic that rational molecular, cellular, and psychotherapeutic interventions will ameliorate CNS dysfunction—in part due to the plasticity of the mature brain.

REFERENCES

Allen, N.J., and Barres, B.A. (2005) Signaling between glia and neurons: focus on synaptic plasticity. *Curr. Opin. Neurobiol.* 15:542–548

Alvarez-Buylla, A., Garcia-Verdugo, J.M., and Tramontin, A.D. (2001) A unified hypothesis on the lineage of neural stem cells. *Nat. Rev. Neurosci.* 2:287–293.

Ayala, R., Shu, T., and Tsai, L.H. (2007) Trekking across the brain: the journey of neuronal migration. *Cell* 128:29–43.

Benson, D.L., Colman, D.R., and Huntley, G.W. (2001) Molecules, maps and synapse specificity. *Nat. Rev. Neurosci.* 2:899–909.

Bertrand, N., Castro, D.S., and Guillemot, F. (2002) Proneural genes and the specification of neural cell types. *Nat. Rev. Neurosci.* 7:517–530.

Briscoe, J., Pierani, A., Jessell, T.M., and Ericson, J. (2000) A homeodomain protein code specifies progenitor cell identity and neuronal fate in the ventral neural tube. *Cell* 101:435–445.

Brose, K., and Tessier-Lavigne, M. (2000) Slit proteins: key regulators of axon guidance, axonal branching, and cell migration. *Curr. Opin. Neurobiol.* 10:95–102.

Charron, F., and Tessier-Lavigne, M. (2005) Novel brain wiring functions for classical morphogens: a role as graded positional cues in axon guidance. *Development* 132:2251–2262.

Colognato, H., and French-Constant, C. (2004) Mechanisms of glial development. *Curr. Opin. Neurobiol.* 14:37–44.

De Robertis, E.M., Larrin, J., Oelgeschläger, M., and Wessely, O. (2000) The establishment of Spemann's organizer and patterning of the vertebrate embryo. *Nat. Genet.* 3:171–181.

Dranovsky, A., and Hen, R. (2006) Hippocampal neurogenesis: regulation by stress and antidepressants. *Biol. Psychiatry* 59(12): 1136–1143.

Flames, N., Long, J.E., Garratt, A.N., Fischer, T.M., Gassmann, M., Birchmeier, C., Lai, C., Rubenstein, J.L., and Marin, O. (2004) Short- and long-range attraction of cortical GABAergic interneurons by neuregulin-1. *Neuron* 44(2):251–261.

Gaiano, N., and Fishell, G. (2002) The role of notch in promoting glial and neural stem cell fates. *Annu. Rev. Neurosci.* 25:471–490.

Gleeson, J.G., and Walsh, C.A. (2000) Neuronal migration disorders: from genetic diseases to developmental mechanisms. *Trends Neurosci.* 23:352–359.

Greer, J.M., and Capecchi, M.R. (2002) Hoxb8 is required for normal grooming behavior in mice. *Neuron* 33:23–34.

Grunwald, I.C., and Klein, R. (2002) Axon guidance: receptor complexes and signaling mechanisms. *Curr. Opin. Neurobiol.* 12:250–259.

Harrison, P.J., and Law, A.J. (2006) Neuregulin 1 and schizophrenia: genetics, gene expression, and neurobiology. *Biol. Psychiatry* 60(2):131–140.

Hoogenraad, C.C., Koekkoek, B., Akhmanova, A., Krugers, H., Dortland, B., Miedema, M., van Alphen, A., Kistler, W.M., Jaegle, M., Koutsourakis, M., Van Camp, N., Verhoye, M., van der Linden, A., Kaverina, I., Grosveld, F., De Zeeuw, C.I., and Galjart, N. (2002) Targeted mutation of Cyln2 in the Williams syndrome critical region links CLIP-115 haploinsufficiency to neurodevelopmental abnormalities in mice. *Nat. Genet.* 32:116–127.

Huang, E.J., and Reichardt, L.F. (2001) Neurotrophins: roles in neuronal development and function. *Annu. Rev. Neurosci.* 24: 677–736.

Jan, Y.N., and Jan, L.Y. (2001) Dendrites. *Genes Dev.* 15:2627–2641.

Jessell, T.M. (2000) Neuronal specification in the spinal cord: inductive signals and transcriptional codes. *Nat. Rev. Genet.* 1:20–29.

Jessell, T.M., and Sanes, J.R. (2000) Development. The decade of the developing brain. *Curr. Opin. Neurobiol.* 10:599–611.

Justice, N.J., and Jan, Y.N. (2002) Variations on the Notch pathway in neural development. *Curr. Opin. Neurobiol.* 2:64–70.

Katz, L.C., and Shatz, C.J. (1996) Synaptic activity and the construction of cortical circuits. *Science* 274:1133–1138.

Kriegstein, A., Noctor, S., and Martinez-Cerdeno, V. (2006) Patterns of neural stem and progenitor cell division may underlie evolutionary cortical expansion. *Nat. Rev. Neurosci.* 7:883–890.

Kuan, C.Y., Roth, K.A., Flavell, R.A., and Rakic, P. (2000) Mechanisms of programmed cell death in the developing brain. *Trends Neurosci.* 23:291–297.

Kullander, K., and Klein, R. (2002) Mechanisms and functions of Eph and ephrin signalling. *Nat. Rev. Mol. Cell Biol.* 7:475–486.

Lemke, G. (2001) Glial control of neuronal development. *Annu. Rev. Neurosci.* 24:87–105.

Lumsden, A., and Krumlauf, R. (1996) Patterning the vertebrate neur-axis. *Science* 274:1109–1114.

Marin, O., and Rubenstein, J.L.R. (2001) A long remarkable journey: tangential migration in the telencephalon. *Nat. Rev. Neurosci.* 2:780–790.

Meng, Y., Zhang, Y., Tregoubov, V., Janus, C., Cruz, L., Jackson, M., Lu, W.Y., MacDonald, J.F., Wang, J.Y., Falls, D.L., and Jia, Z. (2002) Abnormal spine morphology and enhanced LTP in LIMK-1 knockout mice. *Neuron* 35:121–133.

Mochida, G.H., and Walsh, C.A (2004) Genetic basis of developmental malformations of the cerebral cortex. *Arch. Neurol.* 61:637–640.

Okada, A., Charron, F., Morin, S., Shin, D.S., Wong, K., Fabre, P.J, Tessier-Lavigne, M., and McConnell, S.K. (2006) Boc is a receptor for sonic hedgehog in the guidance of commissural axons. *Nature* 444:369–373.

Pera, E.M., Wessely, O., Li, S.Y., and De Robertis, E.M. (2001) Neural and head induction by insulin-like growth factor signals. *Cell* 5:655–665.

Perera, T.D., Coplan, J.D., Lisanby, S.H., Lipira, C.M., Arif, M., Carpio, C., Spitzer, G., Santarelli, L., Scharf, B., Hen, R., Rosoklija, G., Sackeim, H.A., and Dwork, A.J. (2007) Antidepressant-induced neurogenesis in the hippocampus of adult nonhuman primates. *J. Neurosci.* 27:4894–4901.

Rakic, P. (1995) A small step for the cell, a giant leap for mankind: a hypothesis of neocortical expansion during evolution. *Trends Neurosci.* 18:383–388.

Rice, D.S., and Curran, T. (2001) Role of the reelin signaling pathway in central nervous system development. *Annu. Rev. Neurosci.* 24: 1005–1039.

Richardson, W.D., Kessaris, N., and Pringle, N. (2006) Oligodendrocyte wars. *Nat. Rev. Neurosci.* 7(1):11–18.

Rubenstein, J.L.R., and Puelles, L. (2003) Development of the nervous system. In: Epstein, C.J., Erikson, R.P., and Wynshaw-Boris, A., eds. *Inborn Errors of Development.* New York: Oxford University Press, pp. 75–88.

Rubenstein, J.L.R., and Shimamura, K. (1997) Regulation of patterning and differentiation in the embryonic vertebrate forebrain. In: Cowan, W.M., Jessel, T.M., and Zipursky, S.L., eds. *Molecular and Cellular Approaches to Neural Development.* Oxford, UK: Oxford University Press, pp. 356–390.

Sanes, J.R., and Lichtman, J.W. (2001) Development, induction, assembly, maturation and maintenance of a postsynaptic apparatus. *Nat. Rev. Neurosci.* 2:791–805.

Shahbazian, M., Young, J., Yuva-Paylor, L., Spencer, C., Antalffy, B., Noebels, J., Armstrong, D., Paylor, R., and Zoghbi, H. (2002) Mice with truncated MeCP2 recapitulate many Rett syndrome features and display hyperacetylation of histone H3. *Neuron* 35:243–254.

Shimamura, K., Hartigan, D.J., Martinez, S., Puelles, L., and Rubenstein, J.L.R. (1995) Longitudinal organization of the anterior neural plate and neural tube. *Development* 121:3923–3933.

Shirasaki, R., and Pfaff, S.L. (2002) Transcriptional codes and the control of neuronal identity. *Annu. Rev. Neurosci.* 25:251–281.

Streit, A., Berliner, A.J., Papanayotou, C., Sirulnik, A., and Stern, C.D. (2000) Initiation of neural induction by FGF signalling. *Nature* 406(6791):74–78.

Tessier-Lavigne, M., and Goodman, C. (1996) The molecular biology of axon guidance. *Science* 274:1123–1131.

Tissir, F., and Goffinet, A.M. (2003) Reelin and brain development. *Nat. Rev. Neurosci.* 4:496–505.

Wilson, S.I., and Edlund, T. (2001) Neural induction: toward a unifying mechanism. *Nat. Neurosci.* 4(Suppl):1161–1168.

Wilson, S.W., and Rubenstein, J.L.R. (2000) Induction and dorsoventral patterning of the telencephalon. *Neuron* 28:641–651.

Wonders, C.P., and Anderson, S.A. (2006) The origin and specification of cortical interneurons. *Nat. Rev. Neurosci.* 7:687–696.

Yu, T.W., and Bargmann, C.I. (2001) Dynamic regulation of axon guidance. *Nat. Neurosci.* 4(Suppl):1169–1176.

2 Neurochemical Systems in the Central Nervous System

ARIEL Y. DEUTCH AND ROBERT H. ROTH

More than a century ago the introduction of the neuron doctrine by Santiago Ramon y Cajal marked the beginning of modern neuroscience and positioned the neuron as the individual unit of the brain. The modes of communication between neurons have occupied the subsequent century. Although battles on the nature of the primary mode of communication, electrical or chemical, raged on for more than 50 years, by the mid-20th century there was widespread acceptance that chemical signals were the primary means of interaction between two neurons (see Valenstein, 2005). The "classic" view of transmission of signals between neurons was that transmitter molecules that are synthesized by the presynaptic neurons are released into the synaptic cleft when the neuronal membrane is depolarized, with the transmitter subsequently binding to specific postsynaptic receptors that are coupled to intracellular second messengers.

Although many thought the defining principles of neural transmission had been worked out by the beginning of the 21st century, the past decade has been as scientifically tumultuous as any of the last 100 years, with several findings challenging certain long-held and cherished beliefs about neurotransmitters. We examine the basic underpinnings of classical neurotransmitters and then explore new notions of chemical transmission brought about by the discovery of several decidedly unclassical chemical messengers.

WHAT DEFINES A NEUROTRANSMITTER?

Several criteria have been established that define a *neurotransmitter* (Cooper et al., 2002). These include the following: (*1*) a neurotransmitter should be synthesized in the neuron from which it is released; (*2*) the substance released from neurons should be present in a chemically or pharmacologically identifiable form, that is, should be capable of being measured and identified; (*3*) exogenous application of the neurotransmitter in physiologically relevant concentrations should cause changes in the postsynaptic neuron that mimic the effects of stimulation of the presynaptic neuron; (*4*) the effects of the neurotransmitter should act on specific receptor sites on neurons and should therefore be blocked by administration of specific antagonists; and (*5*) there should be appropriate active mechanisms to terminate the actions of the neurotransmitter; these can include high-affinity reuptake processes or enzymatic degradation.

These criteria are based largely on studies of acetylcholine (ACh), the first neurotransmitter identified. The experimental steps required to advance a transmitter role for ACh were relatively simple because ACh was initially studied at the neuromuscular junction rather than in the brain. The ability to expose and maintain preparations of the neuromuscular junction, a peripheral site, permitted electrophysiological and biochemical studies of synaptic transmission. Physiological studies revealed fast excitatory responses of muscle fibers in response to stimulation of the nerve innervating the muscle, similar to the effects of ACh. Moreover, miniature end-plate potentials were observed, which Fatt and Katz (1952) demonstrated to be due to the slow "leakage" of individual vesicles' contents of ACh from the presynaptic terminal. In contrast, overt depolarization is due to an increased number of quanta released over a set period of time. Finally, studies of the neuromuscular junction and another peripheral site, the superior cervical ganglion, allowed detailed analyses of the enzymatic inactivation of ACh. These studies of ACh established the standard to which subsequent studies of neurotransmitters would be held.

Many of the rules that were uncovered in studies of ACh apply to other transmitters. For example, the concept of the quantal nature of neurotransmission is central to current ideas of transmitter release. However, in the past generation, our ideas about the defining characteristics and functions of neurotransmitters have been eroded by the discovery of a number of chemical messengers that do not meet the criteria established for classical transmitters but have been clearly demonstrated to convey information from one neuron to another.

FUNCTIONAL ASPECTS OF MULTIPLE NEUROTRANSMITTER

Why are there so many neurotransmitters? In early years it seemed as if simple excitatory or inhibitory transmission would suffice, thus requiring two, or at least few, transmitters. More careful consideration reveals that several factors may contribute to the need for multiple chemical messengers (Deutch and Roth, 2008).

The simplest explanation is that many afferents terminate on a single postsynaptic neuron, which must be able to distinguish between these multiple inputs. Although multiple inputs terminate on different parts of the postsynaptic neuron (such as different dendritic spines), many inputs to a neuron arrive in such close apposition that spatial segregation of inputs using the same transmitter will not allow accurate discrimination between incoming signals. Multiple transmitters allow the postsynaptic cell to distinguish differences in inputs by chemically coding the information, with the receptive neurons having distinct receptors and intracellular signaling pathways.

A second reason for multiple transmitters may be related to the number of chemical messengers found in a single neuron. Thirty years ago, it was commonly thought that each neuron had but a single neurotransmitter; it is now clear that most if not all neurons have two or more chemical messengers (Deutch and Bean, 1995). Multiple transmitters in a single neuron permit the information transmitted by a neuron to a postsynaptic target to be encoded by different chemical messengers for different functional states. For example, the firing rates of neurons differ widely, and thus it may be useful for a neuron to encode a high-frequency discharge by one transmitter and a lower-frequency discharge by another transmitter. Similarly, differences in firing pattern convey different information; for example, classical and peptide transmitters are differentially released by different patterns of discharge.

A third reason for multiple transmitters is that different types of transmitters are depleted at different rates. Classical transmitters are synthesized in the nerve terminal by enzymatic processing of a precursor; this process allows these transmitters to be released over extended periods of time while simultaneously being replenished at the terminal. In contrast, peptide transmitters are synthesized in the cell body and transported long distances to the axon terminal. Peptides can therefore be depleted by repetitive firing of neurons before new stores of the peptide are synthesized and transported to the nerve terminal for use.

Still another reason for multiple transmitters is that transmitters are released from different parts of a neuron. The prototypic site of release is the axon terminal. However, transmitters are also released from dendrites, or at least escape from dendrites to function as chemical messengers, and can also be released from varicosities present on the axon. It has been suggested that these different sites of release may be occupied by different transmitters.

The types of spatial arrangements between neurons may dictate yet another reason for multiple transmitters. We generally consider synapses to be the structural specializations for intercellular communication. However, transmitters may also be released from nonjunctional appositions between two neurons. Multiple transmitters may allow the postsynaptic cell to distinguish between transmitters released from nonjunctional appositions and areas of synaptic specializations.

Another factor that may contribute to the need for multiple transmitters is that postsynaptic responses to transmitters occur over different time frames. Such temporal differences allow the postsynaptic cell to respond in a manner that takes into account antecedent activity in the presynaptic neuron. Thus, one transmitter can set the stage for the response of a particular cell to subsequent stimuli, which can occur on the order of seconds, or even minutes, independent of changes in gene expression.

So many substances are now commonly accepted as neurotransmitters that one cannot discuss them all, much less new transmitter candidates. We therefore review in some detail the principles of neurotransmission for one group of classical neurotransmitters. A representative peptide transmitter is then discussed, emphasizing similarities and differences between neuropeptide and classical transmitters. Finally, we briefly touch on unconventional transmitters, a growing group that includes such unexpected members as soluble gases (for example, nitric oxide and carbon monoxide).

CLASSICAL TRANSMITTERS

Classical is a relative term in science, and particularly in neuroscience, where it can refer to a year, a decade, or a century. Despite the use of the term *classical* to define certain neurotransmitters, some of these were unknown 50 years ago. Nonetheless, there is a wealth of information concerning virtually every step in the biosynthetic and catabolic processes of the classical transmitters. One characteristic of classical transmitters, shared only by some of the more recently defined transmitters, is that the final synthesis of classical transmitters occurs in the axon terminal. Another defining characteristic of classical transmitters is that they (or their metabolic products) are accumulated by the presynaptic cell via an active process; there is no energy-dependent, high-affinity reuptake process for nonclassical transmitters.

The catecholamines are a group of three related classical transmitters that are synthesized in certain central neurons, as well as the peripheral nervous system, where they can have hormonal functions. Because of the involvement of the catecholamines in several neuropsychiatric disorders, ranging from schizophrenia and depression to Parkinson's disease and dystonias, these transmitters have been the focus of extensive investigation. A detailed description of the life cycle of catecholamine transmitters offers an excellent appreciation of the basic characteristics of classical transmitters.

Catecholamines

Catecholamines are organic compounds with a catechol nucleus (a benzene ring with two adjacent hydroxyl substitutions) and an amine group (Fig. 2.1). The term *catecholamine* is used more loosely to describe dopamine (DA; dihydroxyphenylethylamine) and its metabolic products norepinephrine and epinephrine. These three transmitters are generated by successive enzymatic modification of the amino acid *tyrosine*, each step requiring a different enzyme. The three catecholamines are found as transmitters in distinct dopamine-, norepinephrine-, and epinephrine-containing neurons because the biosynthetic enzymes that sequentially form these transmitters are localized to different cells.

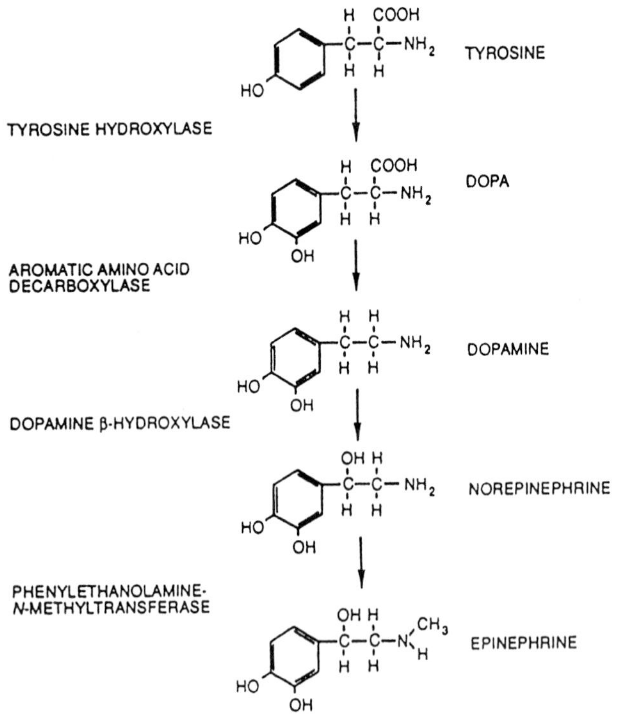

FIGURE 2.1 Synthetic pathway for catecholamines. From Hyman and Nestler (1993).

Catecholamine synthesis

The amino acids *phenylalanine* and *tyrosine* are present in high concentration in plasma and brain and are precursors for catecholamine synthesis. Under most conditions the starting point of catecholamine synthesis is tyrosine, which is derived from dietary phenylalanine by the hepatic enzyme *phenylalanine hydroxylase*. Decreased levels of this enzyme cause phenylketonuria, a disorder that results in severe intellectual deficits if not treated.

The amino acid *tyrosine* is accumulated by catecholamine neurons and then hydroxylated by the enzyme *tyrosine hydroxylase* (TH) to 3,4-dihydroxyphenylalanine (L-DOPA); this intermediary is immediately metabolized to DA by L-aromatic amino acid decarboxylase (AADC). In DA-containing neurons, this is the final synthetic step. However, neurons that use norepinephrine (NE) or epinephrine as transmitters contain the enzymes *dopamine-β-hydroxylase* (DBH) as well as *TH*, and DBH acts on DA to yield NE. Finally, brain stem neurons that use epinephrine as a transmitter, and adrenal medullary chromaffin cells that release epinephrine, contain phenylethanolamine-*N*-methyltransferase (PNMT), which is responsible for the formation of epinephrine from norepinephrine (Fig. 2.1).

The entry of tyrosine into the brain depends on an energy-dependent uptake process for large neutral amino acids; tyrosine competes with other large neutral amino acids at this transporter. Under normal conditions, brain levels of tyrosine are high enough to saturate TH, and thus changes in precursor availability do not affect catecholamine synthesis. As a result, TH is considered the rate-limiting step in catecholamine synthesis. There are, however, certain exceptions to this rule, including in poorly controlled diabetes, in which the size of the large neutral amino acid pool is altered.

Tyrosine hydroxylase. A single TH gene in humans gives rise to four TH messenger ribonucleic acids (mRNAs) through alternative splicing. In most non-human primates, two mRNA species are present, whereas in the rat there is but a single transcript. The functional significance of multiple transcripts is unknown, although it has been speculated that there may be subtle differences in enzyme activity in the different protein species.

The amount of TH protein and the activity of the enzyme determine TH function. Enzyme activity is dependent upon phosphorylation of the enzyme at four distinct serine residues by different protein kinases. This provides remarkably specific control over TH activity. In addition to regulation of the enzyme by phosphorylation, TH activity can be regulated by end product (DA in the case of dopaminergic neurons) inhibition. Catecholamines inhibit the activity of TH through competition for tetrahydrobiopterin, a required cofactor for TH. Levels of reduced tetrahydrobiopterin are not saturated under basal conditions and thus play an important role in regulating TH activity. This is best illustrated by DOPA-responsive dystonia, which is due to mutations in the gene encoding GTP-cyclohydrolase I, which is the rate-limiting enzyme in the synthesis of tetrahydrobiopterin (Ichinose et al., 1994).

The two means by which catecholamine neurons can cope with an increased demand for synthesis are by inducing TH protein or by activating (phosphorylating) existing enzyme (Kumer and Vrana, 1996). The degree to which catecholamine synthesis depends on de novo synthesis of enzyme protein or changes in enzymatic activity differ in various catecholamine neurons. Noradrenergic neurons of the brainstem nucleus locus coeruleus respond to increased demands for synthesis primarily by increasing TH gene expression, ultimately leading to an increase in TH protein levels. However, in midbrain DA neurons changes in TH mRNA levels are rarely seen; synthesis in these DA cells is thought to occur primarily by altering the activity of TH, that is, by posttranslational events such as phosphorylation.

L-Aromatic amino acid decarboxylase. The product of tyrosine hydroxylation is the formation of L-DOPA, which in turn is immediately decarboxylated to form DA. This latter step requires the enzyme AADC (also referred to as *DOPA decarboxylase*). AADC has low substrate specificity: because the enzyme decarboxylates tryptophan as well as tyrosine, it is a key step in the synthesis of serotonin and catecholamines. The activity of AADC is so high that L-DOPA is almost instantaneously converted to DA.

A single AADC gene encodes multiple transcripts that are differentially expressed in the central nervous system (CNS) and peripheral tissues. L-Aromatic amino acid decarboxylase mRNA is enriched in catecholamine- and indoleamine-containing neurons in the CNS but is also found at low levels in other cell types.

Dopamine has very poor blood-brain barrier penetrability. In contrast, the DA precursor L-DOPA readily enters the brain and has therefore become the mainstay in the treatment of Parkinson's disease, the proximate cause of which is striatal DA insufficiency. Administration of L-DOPA to parkinsonian patients quickly increases brain DA levels and improves symptomatology.

Dopamine-β-hydroxylase. Noradrenergic and adrenergic neurons, but not dopaminergic neurons, contain DBH, the enzyme that converts DA to norepinephrine. In noradrenergic neurons this is the final step of catecholamine synthesis. Two different human DBH mRNAs are generated from a single gene.

Dopamine-β-hydroxylase has relatively poor substrate specificity and can oxidize *in vitro* almost any phenylethylamine to its corresponding phenylethanolamine. Thus, in addition to the oxidation of DA to form NE, DBH promotes the conversion of tyramine to octopamine and α-methyldopamine to α-methylnorepinephrine. This lack of substrate specificity has been exploited in the laboratory: several structurally analogous compounds can replace NE function as "false transmitters," providing useful experimental tools. Specific receptors have now been identified for the trace amines, including octopamine (Zucchi et al., 2006). These receptors are expressed in brain and gut and may in part be responsible for the "cheese" effect seen in patients treated with monoamine oxidase inhibitors (see below).

Contrary to the usual situation in which TH is the rate-limiting step in catecholamine synthesis, when the activity of locus coeruleus noradrenergic neurons is increased, DBH is saturated and becomes the rate-limiting step. Because DBH is localized to the vesicle, if DBH is saturated then DA can accumulate, and thus when the vesicles dock with the plasma membrane NE *and* DA and DA metabolites are released, that is, the noradrenergic cell becomes a source of DA. Under sustained periods of activation, there is a compensatory increase in DBH expression in these cells.

Phenylethanolamine-N-methyltransferase. The enzyme *phenylethanolamine-N-methyltransferase* methylates NE to epinephrine. Epinephrine neurons are clustered into two groups of brainstem cells. In addition, high levels of PNMT are present in the adrenal medulla. The enzyme has relatively poor substrate specificity and will transfer methyl groups to the nitrogen atom on a variety of β-hydroxylated amines. Nonspecific *N*-methyltransferases are also found in the lung and will methylate many indoleamines. The high levels of PNMT in the adrenal gland, coupled with relatively easy access to the adrenal, have led to an extensive characterization of the enzyme in this gland, where enzyme activity and expression are tightly regulated by glucocorticoids and nerve growth factor.

Storage of catecholamines: Synaptic vesicles and vesicular transporters

Catecholamine transmitters are stored in small vesicles located near the synapse and poised for fusion with the neuronal membrane and subsequent exocytosis. In addition to serving as a storage depot for catecholamines, vesicles sequester catecholamines from cytosolic enzymes and from some toxins that enter the neuron.

Dopamine-β-hydroxylase differs from other catecholamine-synthesizing enzymes by being localized to the vesicle, rather than neuronal cytosol. Thus, DA must be accumulated by noradrenergic vesicles through an active uptake process prior to being converted to norepinephrine. The vesicular storage of DBH also means that the enzyme is released from neurons when norepinephrine is released. Moreover, because DBH is the rate-limiting enzyme for activated noradrenergic neurons, DA accumulates in the vesicles when catecholamine neurons are activated, culminating in release of DA along with norepinephrine.

The accumulation of DA by vesicles depends on a vesicular monoamine transporter protein (VMAT). Two VMAT genes have been cloned: one is in the adrenal medulla, and the other (called *VMAT2*) is found in catecholamine and serotonin neurons of the CNS. VMAT2 broadly accumulates monoamines, including catecholamines and indoleamines.

The VMATs are targets of some psychotropic drugs. Reserpine, a blocker of VMAT, has been used for decades to treat hypertension and psychosis. Studies of reserpine shed light on how this drug can reduce psychotic symptoms (by decreasing DA accumulation into vesicles and thereby decreasing DA availability) and hypertension (by disrupting catecholamine synthesis in the adrenal medulla and thereby decreasing circulating catecholamine levels).

Regulation of catecholamine synthesis and release by autoreceptors

We have shown how catecholamines are synthesized, and some of the regulatory features that govern synthesis of these transmitters. Another way in which the synthesis of catecholamines can be regulated is by the catecholamine transmitter that is released from the neuron. Once released, the transmitter (for example, DA) interacts with a receptor located on the catecholamine axon that binds the transmitter (for example, a DA D_2 receptor). This nerve terminal "autoreceptor" provides a feedback loop that controls release of the transmitter. This feedback can be a negative feedback, in which released transmitter shuts down further transmitter release; drugs that are antagonists of the autoreceptor can promote transmitter release. There are several types of autoreceptors. In addition to autoreceptors that regulate transmitter release, there are autoreceptors that regulate transmitter synthesis, and still another type that regulates the firing rate of the neuron. Thus, the transmitter regulates its own synthesis and release and determines the firing rate of the neuron from which it is released.

Dopamine autoreceptors, which are among the best-characterized autoreceptors, are found on the cell bodies, dendrites, and nerve terminals of dopaminergic neurons. The different sites correspond to the different end points of autoreceptor tone. Release- and synthesis-modulating autoreceptors are present on axon terminals and somatodendritic regions of DA neurons. In addition, impulse-modulating autoreceptors that govern the firing rate of the neuron are present on somatodendritic regions of the neuron. All three types of DA autoreceptors are D_2-like receptors. Although once suspected that different types of DA receptors subserve the different autoreceptor functions, it appears that there may be, to some degree, distinct transduction mechanisms, all operating through a D_2 receptor.

Release-modulating autoreceptors are present on all DA neurons. However, synthesis-modulating autoreceptors are not. For example, DA neurons that innervate the prefrontal cortex and hypothalamic tuberoinfundibular DA neurons do not have functional synthesis-modulating autoreceptors. Impulse-modulating autoreceptors are also present on most but not all DA neurons. Such differences in the localization of autoreceptors to different types of neurons are thought to confer regional specificity on the function of DA neurons.

Autoreceptors for norepinephrine are also well characterized. Although noradrenergic autoreceptors that regulate release of NE are well known, and are important targets for drugs used to treat cardiovascular and neuropsychiatric disorders, the presence of synthesis-modulating autoreceptors on NE neurons is not well established. Norepinephrine autoreceptors in brain are α_2-adrenergic receptors, the activation of which serves to inhibit norepinephrine release. In contrast, autoreceptors on peripheral nerves are β-adrenergic receptors and facilitate norepinephrine release. There is almost no information concerning autoreceptor-mediated release function of central epinephrine neurons.

Inactivation of released catecholamine neurotransmitters

Continuous (as opposed to discrete pulsatile) release of a transmitter does not provide target neurons with appropriate information about the dynamic state of the presynaptic neuron. Accordingly, there is a need for mechanisms to inactivate the released transmitter. The importance of this process can be easily appreciated by considering the consequences of unrestrained stimulation of ion channel-forming receptors that allow calcium entry into the neuron: if intracellular Ca^{2+} levels increase too much, excitotoxic cell death results.

There are several specific mechanisms for terminating transmitter actions. Diffusion contributes to inactivation of a transmitter. However, functional receptors are often present on the axon as well as in the immediate synaptic region, making diffusion a poor means for terminating transmitter action. The primary mode of inactivation appears to be uptake by neurons of the released transmitter by a plasma membrane-associated transporter protein. Inactivation by means of transporter-mediated reuptake is efficient, and often allows for recycling of the transmitter or metabolites to lower energy demands on the neuron. A second way for transmitter actions to be terminated is by catabolic enzymes located either extra- or intracellularly.

Enzymatic inactivation of catecholamines. Two enzymes sequentially metabolize catecholamines. Monoamine oxidases (MAO) deaminate catecholamines to yield aldehyde derivatives; these are further catabolized by dehydrogenases and reductases. Catechol-O-methyltransferase (COMT) methylates the meta-hydroxy group on catechols, and these methylated intermediaries are further oxidized by MAO. Enzymatic inactivation, particularly by COMT, is the primary mode of terminating the actions of catecholamines circulating in the blood. In the brain, termination of catecholamine actions by reuptake mechanisms appears to be more important. Nevertheless, drugs that target the enzymatic inactivation of catecholamines have been very useful therapeutic strategies for several disorders, including depression.

Two MAO genes have been cloned, and two isoforms of the enzyme can be distinguished by substrate specificities. Both isoforms are present in the CNS and peripheral tissues. MAO_A displays high affinities for NE and serotonin, whereas MAO_B has a higher affinity for β-phenylethylamines. Drugs that inhibit MAO_A (*clorgyline, tranylcypromine*) are among the most effective antidepressant drugs. However, these agents have serious side effects, including development of hypertensive crisis. Thus, patients treated with MAO_A inhibitors who eat foods high in tyramine content (for example, aged cheeses and Chianti, a particularly appetizing combination) do not effectively metabolize tyramine, which releases catecholamines from nerve endings and thereby sharply and dangerously increases blood pressure. Recently, novel receptors for which tyramine and other trace amines have high affinity have been identified and may be targets for drugs that prevent or treat the side effects of MAO_A inhibitors (Zucchi et al., 2006). Interestingly, amphetamine and lysergic acid diethylamide (LSD) are also agonists at one of these receptors.

Deprenyl is a specific inhibitor of MAO_B and is sometimes used in the treatment of early-stage Parkinson's disease (PD). The use of deprenyl in PD derived from studies of the neurotoxin 1-methyl-4-phenyl-1,2,3,6-tetrahydropyridine (MPTP), which causes a parkinsonian syndrome. 1-Methyl-4-phenyl-1,2,3,6-tetrahydropyridine itself is not toxic, but the active metabolite MPP^+ that is generated by the actions of MAO_B is highly toxic. Because the MAO_B inhibitor deprenyl blocks the formation of MPP^+ from MPTP, pretreatment with deprenyl prevents MPTP-induced parkinsonism. Genetic defects that cause PD account for a small percentage of the total cases of PD, leading to the suggestion that an environmental toxin similar to MPTP might cause parkinsonism. Studies of the ability of deprenyl to slow progression of PD in newly diagnosed patients ensued. Early analysis of these studies suggested that the drug did slow disease progression, but longer term analyses failed to sustain the early enthusiasm, although it does appear that deprenyl may offer some symptomatic relief. This probably occurs by increasing DA levels secondary to the inhibition of MAO_B-mediated catabolism of DA. In addition, small amounts of amphetamine and methamphetamine, potent DA releasers, are generated by the metabolism of deprenyl and may contribute to symptomatic improvement in parkinsonian symptoms.

Catecholamine reuptake: Membrane transporter. The reuptake of transmitters released into the extracellular space via specific cell membrane proteins is thought to be the major mode of inactivation of classical transmitters. The accumulation of transmitters in the presynaptic neuron may also permit intracellular degradative enzymes to act and further contribute to transmitter inactivation, particularly if the transmitter is not rapidly accumulated by vesicles.

Neuronal reuptake of catecholamines and other classical transmitters has several characteristics: the process is energy dependent, saturable, involves Na^+ cotransport, and requires extracellular Cl^- (Zahniser and Doolen, 2001). It is worthwhile to note that transporters can operate bidirectionally and under certain conditions may paradoxically transport in the "wrong" direction, thereby "releasing" a transmitter.

Catecholamine transporters are found in catecholamine but not other neurons. There appears to be some catecholamine uptake by glial cells, but this is not a high-affinity reuptake process and the functional significance of this process remains obscure. However, extracellular levels of amino acid transmitters such as γ-aminobutyric acid (GABA) and glutamate are strongly regulated by glial (astrocytic) uptake.

In mammals, two different catecholamine transporters, the DA (DAT) and NE (NET) transporters, have been identified. An amphibian epinephrine transporter has been cloned, but a mammalian homologue of this gene has not been identified. Both DAT and NET transporters have significant sequence homology. They also share relatively poor substrate specificity; in fact, NET has a higher affinity for DA than for NE.

Anatomical studies have revealed that DAT and NET are restricted to DA- and norepinephrine-containing cells, respectively. However, DAT is not present in measurable levels in all DA neurons. For example, the hypothalamic neurons that release DA into the pituitary portal blood supply do not express detectable levels of DAT mRNA or protein. Because DA released from these neurons is rapidly carried away in the portal vasculature, there is probably no need for inactivation of DA by reuptake into tuberoinfundibular neurons.

Immunohistochemical studies have revealed that under basal conditions, DAT, as well as other transmitter transporters, is localized to the extrasynaptic region of the axon terminal (Hoffman et al., 1998), suggesting that the transporter may be important in clearing DA that has diffused from the synaptic region. When one considers that DA receptors are also found adjacent to the synapse rather than at the synaptic junction, extrasynaptic (so-called paracrine) transmission may be of greater importance than was previously realized for catecholaminergic transmission (Wickens and Arbuthnott, 2005).

Just as there is a tight process of regulation over enzyme activity, there are regulatory controls for neurotransmitter transporters. Chronic administration of catecholamine reuptake inhibitors decreases the number of transporter sites, consistent with a decrease in gene expression. In addition, the activity of catecholamine transporters appears to be regulated acutely by several mechanisms (Zahniser and Doolen, 2001). The recognition that transporter expression is dynamically regulated has broad implications for *in vivo* imaging studies of transporters (such as studies of DAT in PD) because drug treatments that patients receive may alter the apparent density of the transporter.

The generation of mice lacking DAT has revealed that a remarkably broad array of DA neuron functions is disrupted by loss of the transporter (Sotnikova et al., 2006). It is therefore not surprising that transporters are key targets of psychoactive drugs. Cocaine increases extracellular monoamine levels by blocking the transporters for DA, NE, and serotonin. The tricyclic antidepressants potently inhibit NE and serotonin reuptake, with significantly weaker effects on DAT, and are one of the major means of treating certain types of depression. The newer serotonin-selective reuptake blockers, such as fluoxetine, are now the most widely prescribed antidepressant medications.

Anatomy of catecholamine neurons

Neurons expressing DA, NE, and epinephrine are found in a wide variety of species, although there are some major differences in the anatomical organization of these neurons between species. For example, midbrain DA neurons are present in all vertebrates except bony fish (*teleosts*), and dopaminergic cells (although few in number) are present in flies and worms. There are some differences in the anatomy of the catecholaminergic neurons between primate and lower mammalian species, but these differences are mainly quantitative rather than qualitative, and the general organization of the catecholamine systems of primates and lower mammalian species is quite similar.

Dopamine neurons in the ventral midbrain cells project to several forebrain sites, including the caudate nucleus and putamen (striatum), limbic sites such as the amygdala, septum, and hippocampus, and certain cortical sites (Fig. 2.2). The cortical DA innervation in primates is much broader than that seen in rodents. In addition to the midbrain DA neurons, several clusters of DA neurons are found in the diencephalon, including hypothalamic cells with long axons that innervate the spinal cord as well as intrahypothalamic projections. Still another set of DA neurons is found in the olfactory bulb. The reader is referred to the review by Moore and Bloom (1978) for a more comprehensive discussion of the anatomy of DA neurons.

Norepinephrine-containing cells are located in the medulla and pons (Fig. 2.3). In the rostral pons, a small but important group of cells is found in the nucleus locus coeruleus. These neurons give rise to most of the noradrenergic innervation of the forebrain, as well as of the brain stem and spinal cord. Pontine and lower brain stem NE-containing cells project to ventral forebrain and diencephalic sites, including certain nuclei in the hypothalamus and thalamus, and limbic areas such as the amygdala, hippocampus, and septum.

Epinephrine-containing cells are found in two nuclei in the medulla and provide descending projections as well as an important projection to the pons that regulates the activity of the locus coeruleus NE-containing cells.

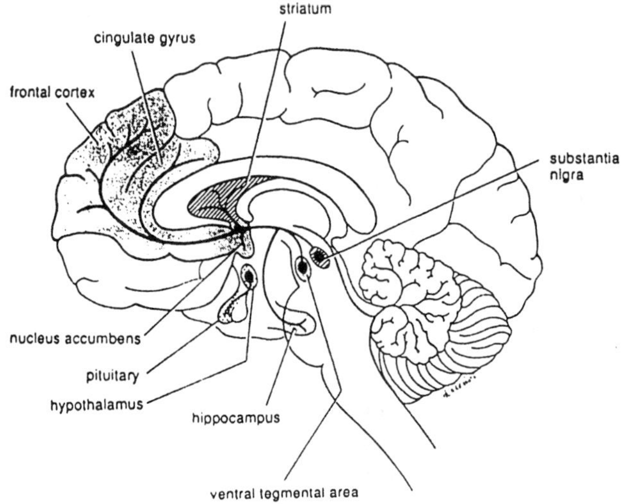

FIGURE 2.2 Dopaminergic projection systems in the brain. The major dopaminergic nuclei in the brain are the substantia nigra pars compacta (*hatched*), shown projecting to the striatum (also *hatched*); the ventral tegmental area (*fine stipple*), shown projecting to the frontal and cingulate cortex, nucleus accumbens, and other limbic structures (*fine stipple*); and the arcuate nucleus of the hypothalamus (*coarse stipple*), which provides dopaminergic regulation to the pituitary. From Hyman and Nestler (1993).

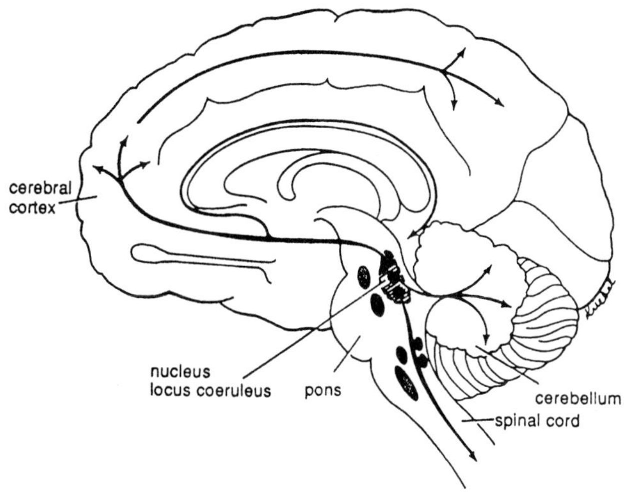

FIGURE 2.3 Noradrenergic projection systems in the brain. Shown are the major noradrenergic nuclei of the brain, the locus coeruleus (*hatched*), and the lateral tegmental nuclei (*fine stipple*). Epinephrine-containing nuclei are shown in black. The projections from the locus coeruleus (as described in the text) are markedly simplified. Projections from the other noradrenergic nuclei are not shown. From Hyman and Nestler (1993).

Serotonin

The major processes that regulate catecholamine synthesis and degradation are common to all classical transmitters, including serotonin. Nonetheless, there are some relatively minor differences among the classical transmitters. The following discussion focuses on the differences between serotonin and catecholamine neurotransmitters.

Synthesis of serotonin

The synthesis of serotonin (5-hydroxytryptamine) follows the basic scheme laid out for catecholamine transmitters: the uptake of a precursor amino acid (tryptophan) into the neuron, the sequential enzymatic formation of serotonin from tryptophan, the accumulation of serotonin by VMAT2 and its storage by vesicles, and active reuptake of extracellular serotonin as the primary mode of inactivation of the transmitter.

The precursor amino acid *tryptophan* enters the CNS on a large neutral amino acid transporter, where it competes with other amino acids (including phenylalanine and tyrosine). In serotonergic neurons, tryptophan is a substrate for tryptophan hydroxylase, which results in the formation of 5-hydroxytryptophan (5-HTP), the immediate serotonin precursor (Fig. 2.4). Tryptophan hydroxylase is not saturated; therefore, peripheral, including dietary, sources of tryptophan have a major influence on central serotonin synthesis.

Tryptophan hydroxylase is found in the CNS and the periphery. There are some biochemical differences between the central and peripheral forms, which appear to be due to posttranslational modifications. Situations requiring increased synthesis of serotonin are dealt with mainly by increasing the activity of the enzyme through phosphorylation; some long-term changes in demand may lead to increases in tryptophan hydroxylase gene expression.

5-Hydroxytryptophan is metabolized to serotonin by L-aromatic amino acid decarboxylase, the same enzyme that converts L-DOPA to DA. With one prominent exception, serotonin is the end point of indoleamine synthesis in the brain. That exception is in the pineal gland, where serotonin is metabolized to form the hormone *melatonin*. There is also a kynurenic acid shunt from tryptophan metabolism that results in the formation of several compounds, including quinolinic acid and kynurenic acid. Quinolinic acid is a potent *N*-methyl-D-aspartate (NMDA) receptor agonist and can cause convulsions and neurotoxicity. In contrast, kynurenine is an NMDA antagonist (Schwarcz, 2004). It has been suggested that the ratio of the two substances may be of significance in clinical conditions such as stroke, where cell death is mediated in part by NMDA receptors.

Storage and release of serotonin

Serotonin is stored intraneuronally in vesicles. The accumulation of serotonin by vesicles is accomplished by VMAT2. There is one major difference between serotonin and catecholamine neurons: serotonin synthesis is not regulated by end product inhibition *in vivo*. Otherwise, the regulatory features are quite similar, including serotonin autoreceptors that regulate serotonin release and synthesis, acting through functionally distinct somatodendritic and terminal autoreceptors. The release and impulse-modulating autoreceptor in

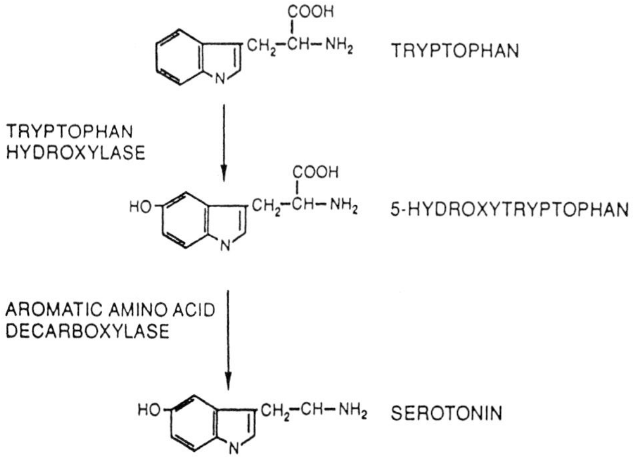

COOH
CH_2–CH–NH_2 TRYPTOPHAN

TRYPTOPHAN HYDROXYLASE

COOH
HO– CH_2–CH–NH_2 5-HYDROXYTRYPTOPHAN

AROMATIC AMINO ACID DECARBOXYLASE

HO– CH_2–CH–NH_2 SEROTONIN

FIGURE 2.4 Synthetic pathway for serotonin. From Hyman and Nestler (1993).

serotonin neurons is a 5-HT_1 receptor. The 5-HT_{1A} receptor is an autoreceptor present on the somatodendritic region of the serotonin neurons, whereas the 5-HT_{1B} receptor is an autoreceptor found on serotonin nerve terminals. In addition, the 5-HT_{1A} receptor is also found on some nonserotonergic neurons.

Inactivation of released serotonin

Reuptake of released serotonin by a specific serotonin transporter (SERT) is the major means of terminating serotonin's actions. The SERT is a member of the same molecular family as the catecholamine transporters and has the same requirements for action (Zahniser and Doolen, 2001). The SERT, like DAT and NET, is a major target for psychotropic drugs, including the most commonly used antidepressants, which are serotonin-selective reuptake inhibitors (Blakely, 2001). Like the catecholamines, serotonin can be inactivated enzymatically by MAO.

Anatomy of serotonin-containing neurons

Serotonergic cells are present in distinct groups of brain stem neurons, which are found from the caudal medulla to the caudal midbrain level (Fig. 2.5). Pontine serotonin cells in the dorsal and median raphe nuclei are the source of diencephalic and telencephalic sites; cells in the medulla provide important descending serotonin projections to the spinal cord.

Amino Acid Transmitters

The excitatory and inhibitor amino acid transmitters glutamate and GABA, respectively, are the most abundant transmitters in the brain. Monoamine-containing neurons are discretely localized in the brain, but glutamatergic and GABAergic neurons are found in virtually all areas of the brain. Although there are some significant differences between amino acid and monoamine transmitters, most of the major principles discussed in the section on catecholamine transmitters are applicable to amino acid transmitters.

The amino acid transmitters are derived from intermediary glucose metabolism. This dual role for GABA and glutamate as transmitters and metabolic intermediaries requires some mechanisms for segregating the transmitter and metabolic pools (Hassel and Dingledine, 2006; Olsen and Betz, 2006). The other major difference between amino acid and monoamine transmitters is that the former are subject to uptake by high-affinity transporters expressed by glial cells as well as by transporters localized to neurons. This discussion focuses on those aspects of amino acid transmitters that differ from monoamine transmitters, as enumerated above. Although glycine is also an inhibitory transmitter, particularly in the spinal cord, GABA is discussed as the major inhibitory transmitter. Glutamate is discussed as the major excitatory transmitter, although other excitatory amino acids, including aspartate, *N*-acetylaspartylglutamate, and sulfur-containing amino acids such as homocysteic acid, also have key roles.

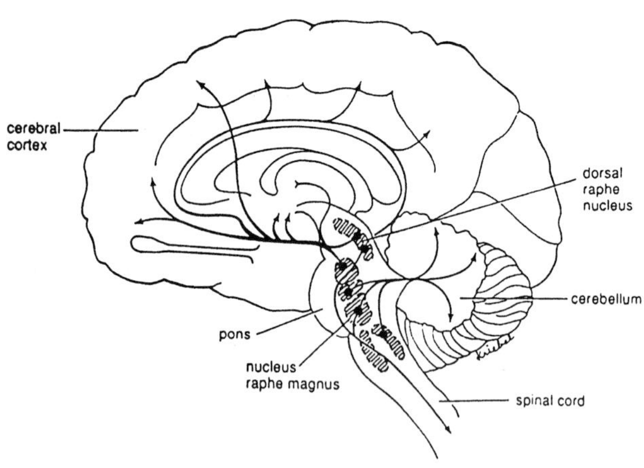

FIGURE 2.5 Serotonergic projection systems in the brain. The major serotonergic nuclei in the brain are the brain stem raphe nuclei (*hatched*). The nuclei are shown slightly enlarged, and their diffuse projections (as described in the text) are markedly simplified. From Hyman and Nestler (1993).

Amino acid transmitter synthesis

γ-Aminobutyric acid is derived from glucose metabolism, with α-ketoglutarate from the Krebs (tricarboxylic acid) cycle being transaminated to glutamate by GABA α-oxoglutarate transaminase (GABA-T). The key step for the generation of the transmitter pool of GABA is the action of the enzyme *glutamic acid decarboxylase* (GAD), which converts glutamate to GABA. Glutamic acid decarboxylase is found almost exclusively in neurons that use GABA as a transmitter and thus serves as a marker for GABAergic neurons.

Two isoforms of GAD are encoded by two different genes. The two GAD species (designated *GAD65 and GAD67* on the basis of their mass) have somewhat different intracellular distributions and are differently regulated; thus, the processes that govern GABA synthesis may be specialized to some degree in different parts of the neuron. Glutamic acid decarboxylase requires a pyridoxal phosphate cofactor for activity. The lower-mass enzyme, GAD65, has a high affinity for the cofactor, but GAD67 does not. The high affinity of GAD65 for cofactor provides a way in which enzyme activity can be quickly and efficiently regulated. However, GAD67 activity is not as readily regulated, although the amount of enzyme can be regulated at the transcriptional level.

As noted above, GAD is an excellent marker for cells in which GABA is a transmitter. Glutamic acid decarboxylase is a cytosolic protein. However, GABA-T, which synthesizes the GABA precursor glutamate from α-ketoglutarate, is a mitochondrial enzyme. Thus, there is a metabolic pool of GABA that is mitochondrial. The process by which glutamate destined for the transmitter pool is exported from the mitochondria is not well understood.

Glutamate is the immediate precursor to the inhibitory transmitter GABA, but it has a major independent role as an excitatory transmitter in different neurons. Neurons must therefore have some mechanisms to prevent GABA neurons from using glutamate as a transmitter. Glutamic acid decarboxylase is not found in neurons that use glutamate as a transmitter, thus ensuring that GABAergic neurons use GABA but not glutamate as a transmitter. The process that sequesters glutamate from the transmitter pathway in GABA neurons is less clear. It has been proposed that synthesis of glutamate destined for the transmitter pool may require a special form of glutaminase. Although GABA and glutamate are not cotransmitters, it is interesting to note that a recent report suggested that some reports indicate that single neurons may contain an excitatory and an inhibitory transmitter (Salter and De Koninck, 1999).

Glutamate can also be formed directly from glutamine, which is synthesized in glial cells. The glutamine that is formed in glia can be transported into nerve terminals and then locally converted by glutaminase into glutamate. Thus, glial cells may in part regulate glutamate synthesis. This underscores the complex functions of glia, which are now recognized to play several critical roles in brain fuction in addition to the support role previously envisioned (Volterra and Meldolesi, 2005).

Storage of amino acid transmitters: Vesicular transporters

Although vesicular storage of amino acid transmitters has been known for some time, only very recently were the vesicular transporters cloned. A vesicular transporter that accumulates GABA and glycine has been cloned and characterized (McIntire et al., 1997). This vesicular transporter is expressed in GABA and glycine neurons, where it is enriched in axon terminals. In contrast to the monoamine vesicular transporters, which use a pH gradient to transport monoamines into the cell, the vesicular GABA transporter uses electrochemical and pH gradients to drive transport.

Three vesicular glutamate transporters have recently been identified and cloned (Fremeau et al., 2004). These proteins also transport inorganic phosphate, on which basis they were first identified, and accumulate glutamate by an electrochemical gradient. The expression of these transporters is the definitive marker for a neuron that uses glutamate as a transmitter.

Regulation of amino acid transmitter release by autoreceptors

Autoreceptor-mediated regulation of GABA neurons occurs through $GABA_B$ receptors, which in contrast to the postsynaptic ionotropic $GABA_A$ receptors are G protein–coupled. $GABA_B$ receptors are also found on non-GABA cells, where they may regulate the release of glutamate and other transmitters. The release of glutamate from nerve terminals is also subject to autoreceptor regulation, a function subserved by G protein–coupled metabotropic glutamate receptors (mGluR). There are three groups of mGluR receptors that include eight different receptors; one group of mGluRs are autoreceptors. In addition to the well-characterized release-modulating mGluRs, electrophysiological studies have suggested the presence of a glutamate impulse–modulating autoreceptor. Drugs that target metabotropic glutamate receptors are a target for the development of new drugs to treat a variety of neuropsychiatric disorders, including schizophrenia and Parkinson's disease

Inactivation of released GABA and glutamate

The uptake of released GABA and glutamate is the primary means of terminating the actions of these transmitters. High-affinity GABA and glutamate uptake by neurons and glia has long been known and distinguishes these transmitters from the monoamines, which are not accumulated by high-affinity glial transporters (Zahniser and Doolen, 2001).

In contrast to monoamine transporters, which include a single transporter for each of the monoamines, at least three transporters accumulate GABA (Kanner, 2006); other transporters present in the brain, such as a betaine transporter, can also accumulate GABA. The three types of GABA transporters (GATs) do not readily correspond to different subtypes in glia and neurons. Early pharmacological studies defined two GATs that could be distinguished in part on the basis of glial and neuronal uptake. However, the cloning of GAT genes and subsequent generation of specific probes to mark these transporters revealed that a cloned GAT, which on pharmacological grounds corresponded to the classical glial transporter, was present mainly on neurons. Other GATs are expressed in neurons and glia. Although it is possible to distinguish glial from neuronal uptake of GABA pharmacologically, the inability to ascribe glial and neuronal transporters to specific cell types suggests that still other GATs may be present.

Glial and neuronal expression of glutamate transporters also occurs. Two glutamate transporters are primarily expressed in glia, with a third glutamate transporter being predominantly neuronal. The glutamate transporters accumulate L-glutamate and D- and L-aspartate; all three of these transporters have similar affinities for glutamate, but there are substantial differences in affinities for other amino acids.

Anatomy of amino acid transmitters

GABA- and glutamate-containing neuronal elements can be found in almost every area of the brain. Nonetheless, certain discrete projections for excitatory and inhibitory neurons have been identified. For example, inhibitory GABAergic cells are often found as local circuit neurons. However, some GABA neurons are projection neurons; among these are cells that project from the basal forebrain to the cortex and striatal GABAergic neurons that innervate the globus pallidus and substantia nigra. Among the many glutamatergic neurons are the pyramidal cells of the cortex, as well as a variety of long-axoned projection neurons in subcortical sites.

Diversity of amino acid transmitters

More so than other classical transmitters, GABA and glutamate as transmitters are marked by a complexity and diversity of function. There are multiple membrane transporters for GABA and glutamate, and multiple vesicular glutamate transporters. GABA and glutamate play transmitter and metabolic roles in neurons. There are a diverse group of receptors for GABA and glutamate, including ionotropic and metabotropic receptors. GABA and glutamate involve more than just neurons but critically bring into play glial cells.

We focused this brief discussion of the amino acid transmitters on GABA and glutamate, but there are other amino acids that are transmitters or have been proposed to be neurotransmitters; these include *N*-acetylaspartylglutamate, glycine, and sulfur-containing amino acids. Among the most surprising of the amino acids transmitter candidates are D-amino acids (Snyder and Ferris, 2000; Martineau et al., 2006). Conventional wisdom has held that L- but not D-enantiomers of amino acids are active; D-amino acids were relegated to their functions in bacteria and invertebrates. However, D-serine and D-aspartate are present in relatively high concentrations in the human brain. D-Serine is heterogeneously distributed, with the highest concentrations in regions with a high density of NMDA glutamate receptors. An enzyme, *serine racemase*, which converts L-serine to D-serine, has been found in glia but not neurons, suggesting that glia may synthesize and release D-serine. However, classical considerations of transmitters hold that neurons but not glia communicate via release of transmitters. This conundrum has been resolved by noting that certain types of glia express α-amino-3-hydroxy-5-methyl-4-isoxasolepropionic acid (AMPA)-type glutamate receptors and respond to glutamate stimulation by releasing D-serine onto NMDA-receptor-bearing neurons. Thus, in this case, glia serve as intermediate functional links between two neurons, and D-amino acids may be neurotransmitters, albeit uncoventional ones (see below).

PEPTIDE TRANSMITTERS

Peptides have become firmly established as neurotransmitters only over the past 30 years. The notion that there are peptide transmitters initially met with resistance because peptides did not appear to meet some of the criteria developed for classical transmitters. Some of these missing steps were subsequently shown to be due to methodological issues, including sensitivity of assay techniques.

There are two major differences between classical and peptide transmitters. The first is the intraneuronal site(s) of synthesis of the transmitter. Synthetic enzymes for classical transmitters are present in axon terminals as well as cell body regions, allowing a rapid response to increased demand for transmitter release from axon terminals. In contrast, peptide transmitters are typically synthesized in the cell body but not in axons. As such, increased demand for the peptide transmitter requires *de novo* protein synthesis and transport of the peptide to the terminal. The second major difference is that peptides are inactivated almost exclusively by enzymatic means; there are no high-affinity transporters that accumulate neuropeptides. Despite the failure of peptide transmitters to meet all of the classical criteria for transmitters, neuropeptides clearly convey information between neurons. Such information is not simply generalized information about the milieu, but temporally and spatially coded information transfer. Table 2.1 lists some of the peptide transmitters in the brain.

The general principles of the peptide transmitters are discussed below. The discussion focuses on specific examples drawn from one widely distributed peptide, *neurotensin*.

Synthesis and Storage of Peptide Transmitters

Classical transmitters are typically synthesized by enzymatic processing of precursor(s) in the vicinity of the release site, often the axon terminal. In contrast, peptide transmitters are formed from a prohormone precursor that is transcribed and translated in the cell body of the neuron, where it is then incorporated into vesicles. Thus, most peptide transmitters are formed from a single precursor from which active peptides are cleaved, in contrast to the successive enzymatic modifications of a precursor amino acid that give rise to most classical transmitters.

The general process can be easily understood by examining the case of the peptide transmitter *neurotensin* (NT). A large (170 amino acid) prohormone precursor of NT and a related peptide, *neuromedin N* (NMN), are encoded by a single gene that is transcribed

TABLE 2.1. *Examples of Peptide Transmitters*

Opioid and related peptides
Dynorphin
Endorphin
Enkephalin
Nociceptin (orphanin FQ)
Gut-brain peptides[a]
Cholecystokinin (CCK)
Gastrin
Secretin
Somatostatin
Vasoactive intestinal polypeptide (VIP)
Tachykinin peptides
Substance K
Substance P
Neuromedin N
Pituitary peptides[b]
Adrenal corticotropic hormone (ACTH)
Melanocyte stimulating hormone (MSH)
Oxytocin
Vasopressin
Hypothalamic releasing factors[c]
Corticotropin releasing hormone (CRH)
Growth hormone releasing factor (GHRF)
Luteinizing hormone releasing hormone (LHRH)
Thyrotropin releasing hormone (TRH)
Others
Angiotensin
Calcitonin gene-related peptide (CGRP)
Cocaine- and amphetamine-related transcript (CART)
Melanocyte concentration hormone (MCH)
Neurotensin
Hypocretin/Orexin

[a] Peptides first found in the gut and later shown to serve as neurotransmitters in the brain.

[b] Peptides first discovered as pituitary hormones and later shown to serve as neurotransmitters in the brain.

[c] Peptides first discovered for their role as hypothalamic release hormones and later shown to serve as neurotransmitters in the brain.

to yield two mRNAs. The two transcripts are present in equal abundance in most brain areas. Different molar ratios of NT and NMN are found in some tissues because of differential processing of the prohormone (Kitabgi et al., 1992).

Classical neurotransmitters are usually packaged in small (<50 nm) synaptic vesicles, while neuropeptide transmitters are localized to large (<100 nm) dense-core vesicles. Because peptides are often released at higher neuronal firing rates than classical transmitters, it has been assumed that there are differences between the processes that subserve vesicular release of peptides and classical transmitters (Bean et al., 1995); recent data have begun to untangle the mechanisms responsible (Sieburth et al., 2007).

Release of Peptides

The depolarization-elicited release of peptides from dense-core vesicular stores is calcium dependent. The amount of peptide transmitter that is released from neurons varies as a function of the firing rate and firing pattern of the neuron. For example, studies of neurons that use both DA and NT as transmitters have found that higher firing frequencies are required to elicit release of the peptide. The temporal pattern of impulses arriving at the nerve terminal also determines release characteristics: The release of many peptides is most prominent under conditions of burst firing, where neurons fire in very rapid succession (Bean and Roth, 1992).

Inactivation of Peptide Transmitters

Peptides are inactivated enzymatically; there do not appear to be conventional transporters that accumulate released peptides. The enzymes that metabolize peptides are specific for certain dipeptide sites along the peptide chain. Thus, the same enzymes can catabolize any peptide with the requisite dipeptide linkages. An example is a metallo-endopeptidase that inactivates the small opioid transmitters called *enkephalins*. Although this enzyme is often called *enkephalinase*, it also participates in the enzymatic processing of other peptides, including NT. Three endopeptidases enzymatically inactivate NT. Enkephalinase cleaves NT at two sites, Pro10-Tyr11 and Tyr11-Ile12, to yield a decapeptide. Another peptidase acts at the Arg8-Arg9 site, and the third at the same Pro10-Tyr11 site as enkephalinase. Such processing can give rise to multiple metabolic products of the parent peptide.

The enzymatic inactivation of classical transmitters results in products that are not active at the transmitter's receptors. However, this is not necessarily the case for peptide transmitters, in which the products of enzymatic breakdown may retain activity at the receptor site. Indeed, some peptide fragments that are generated by the actions of peptidases may even have a higher affinity for the receptor than the parent peptide.

Newer Peptide Transmitters

There have been no additions to the list of classical transmitters for some time, although new receptors for these transmitters have been uncovered at a rapid rate. In contrast to the stable number of classical or conventional transmitters, the number of peptide transmitters continues to grow. The increased number of peptide transmitters is due in part to molecular biological strategies aimed at identifying novel genes. Many peptides have been identified in this manner, and of these, a considerable number have subsequently been shown to be neuroactive and meet criteria for a transmitter. One recent example stands out. Two groups simultaneously and independently identified a novel gene encoding a prohormone that gave rise to two isoforms of a peptide, designated *hypocretin* (de Lecea et al., 1998) or *orexin* (Sakurai et al., 1998). These peptides are expressed only in a small number of lateral hypothalamic neurons. Despite the small number of hypocretin/orexin neurons, these cells send axons to cover almost the entire brain. Two G protein–coupled hypocretin/orexin receptors are widely but differentially distributed in the brain. One of the most interesting aspects of these cells is that among the functions ascribed to them is arousal (Sutcliffe and de Lecea, 2002). Degeneration of hypocretin/orexin neurons in humans is the cause of narcolepsy, a disorder marked by excessive daytime sleepiness, while in narcoleptic dogs there is a mutation in one of the hypocretin/orexin receptors. Since the discovery of the hypocretins/orexins, it has become apparent that they are critically involved in attention and cognition, reward and motivated behavior, and feeding behavior and metabolism.

UNCONVENTIONAL TRANSMITTERS

Technical approaches limit advances in any scientific endeavor, including neuroscience. For example, prior to the development of radioimmunoassays, it was difficult to detect peptides in the brain, and hence peptides were not considered serious transmitter candidates. The development of contemporary analytical methods, which are capable of reliably measuring substances at attomole levels, has opened the door to the identification of many new neurotransmitters.

The criteria necessary for establishment of a neuroactive substance as a neurotransmitter may need to be reconsidered. We previously discussed the idea that a very simple definition of *neurotransmitter* would be a neuroactive substance that allows information to flow from one neuron to another (Deutch and Roth, 2008). This definition avoids the issues of glial contribution to the milieu of the neuron, despite the fact that glia may convey important information and play an active role in the CNS (Haydon and Carmignoto, 2006). One problem with this definition is that it does not specify either the temporal or spatial characteristics of a transmitter and thus could define as a neurotransmitter a hormone, which typically acts over an extended time course across relatively large distances. Nor does this definition cover roles for transmitters that are only now starting to be uncovered, such as soluble gases and neurotrophic factors. And D-serine, which we already discussed, can hardly be considered conventional, being synthesized in glia and posing as an intermediate between pre- and postneurons, with even the synapse almost seeming to be an outdated concept.

In view of our inability to arrive at a satisfactory definition for transmitters, we suggest the term "unconventional transmitters." Because the unconventional may soon become conventional, it is likely that our choice of terms will bring only temporary relief.

Nitric Oxide and the Gas Neurotransmitters

Nitric oxide (NO) is perhaps best known as an air pollutant and thus would not immediately come to mind as a neurotransmitter. Indeed, it is difficult to envision gases as neurotransmitters because a gas cannot be conventionally stored or released in an impulse-dependent manner. Nitric oxide is not stored and thus does not meet one of the key criteria for a neurotransmitter. Other gases, including carbon monoxide and hydrogen sulfide, also appear to have a transmitter function (Boehning and Snyder, 2003). Because NO is not stored in cells, it cannot be released by exocytosis. Nitric oxide also lacks an active process to terminate its action, and its "receptors" are intracellular signaling proteins such as guanylyl cyclase. Finally, NO appears to regulate the function of presynaptic terminals. As one reviews these characteristics, it becomes apparent that "unconventional" is a very conservative designation. Despite some hesitancy to embrace fully NO as a neurotransmitter, there are now ample data on the processes that control the synthesis, "release," and termination of action of NO to consider gases as transmitters (Boehning and Snyder, 2003).

There is only one step in the synthesis of NO: the conversion of L-arginine by the enzyme nitric oxide synthase (NOS) to yield NO and citrulline. Three forms of NOS have been identified. *Macrophage-inducible NOS* (iNOS) is present in microglia, *endothelial NOS* (eNOS) is found in cells that line blood vessels, and *neuronal NOS* (nNOS) is indeed neuronal. All three NOS isoforms can be regulated, despite the use of the adjective *inducible* only for iNOS. Among the regulatory processes are phosphorylation (which decreases NOS activity) and hormonal control. In addition, levels of NOS can be modified by direct inhalation of NO as a feedback mechanism.

Nitric oxide is an uncharged molecule that diffuses freely across cell membranes. This ability allows NO to play a role in interneuronal communication. For example, NO may pass from one cell through an adjacent cell to influence a third neuron, which is not even a next-door neighbor of—much less synaptically coupled with—the original neuron. Indeed, recent data suggest that NO may act primarily as a retrograde messenger, modifying transmitter release and metabolism from presynaptic terminals. This situation has been most thoroughly explored in the hippocampus, where NMDA-evoked NO release from pyramidal neurons increases glutamate release from presynaptic elements and may thereby influence long-term potentiation (and, by extension, learning and memory). Although one would suspect that a transmitter that acts by diffusion could not regulate other cells phasically, neuronal stimulation elicits NO release and therefore suggests phasic signaling capacity.

There is no active mechanism to terminate the effects of NO. However, the half-life of NO is only about 30 seconds, and thus this spontaneous decay to nitrite limits the duration of action of NO. In addition, NO can react with iron-containing compounds, such as hemoglobin, which effectively terminate the actions of NO.

Neurotrophic Factors

Neurotrophic or growth factors are a diverse group of proteins that are critical for the survival and differentiation of neurons (Huang and Reichardt, 2001). There are many different classes of neurotrophic factors, and within each class several members can be identified (Table 2.2). Although there are differences in the effects of members of a given class of growth factors, and differences in the receptors through which these growth factors may exert their effects, there are broad similarities in the basic principles concerning synthesis, release, and termination of action of these growth factors (Huang and Reichardt, 2001).

Neurotrophic factors are unconventional in several ways, including their synthesis and release characteristics. In addition, the target neurons of the neurotrophic factors are often presynaptic to the cell in which the factor is found consistent with neurotrophic factors providing trophic support for developing axons.

Current appreciation of the synthesis and regulation of neurotrophic factors has been gained almost entirely through molecular biological studies. Neurotrophic factors are often translated from multiple mRNAs. An example is brain-derived neurotrophic factor (BDNF), which contains five different exons that encode BDNF protein. Four of the five exons are controlled by separate promotors, the alternative use of which generates eight different BDNF mRNAs. Yet there appears to be only one mature BDNF protein! Because the different promotors are regulated through different means, an intricate cascade of events may lead to mature BDNF production, and different transcripts may differ in stability or translatability and thereby yield different amounts of protein (Aid et al., 2007).

Our knowledge of the posttranslational processing of neurotrophic factors is relatively poor compared to that of peptide transmitters. Perhaps the best-known situation is that of nerve growth factor (NGF), where the mature protein is cleaved from a prohormone, somewhat analogous to the situation seen in peptides. However, the NGF prohormone is quite different from neuropeptide prohormones: three subunits of the prohormone are present, one of which is catalytic and cleaves the prohormone to generate NGF. An interesting twist in the synthesis of neurotrophins is the necessity for dimerization of neurotrophins to form active species. It was originally thought that neurotrophins were exclusively present as homodimers *in vivo*, in contrast to studies in vitro, which indicated heterodimer assembly.

TABLE 2.2. *Examples of Neurotrophic Factors in Brain*

Neurotrophins
Brain-derived neurotrophic factor (BDNF)
Nerve growth factor (NGF)
Neurotrophin-3 (NT-3)
Neurotrophin-4 (NT-4)
Glial-derived neurotrophic factor (GDNF) family[a]
GDNF
Neurturin
Persephin
Tumor growth factor-β (TGFβ) family
TGFβ1-3
Bone morphogenic proteins (BMPs)
Myostatin
Sonic hedgehog
Insulin family
Insulin
Insulin-like growth factor-I (IGF-I)
Insulin-like growth factor-II (IGF-II)
Fibroblast growth factor (FGF) family
FGF (acidic)
FGF (basic)
Epidermal growth factor (EGF) family
ACh-receptor-inducing activity (ARIA)
Amphiregulin
EGF
Heregulin
TGF[a]
Cytokines[b]
Ciliary neurotrophic factor (CIF), leukemia inhibitory factor (LIF), cardiotrophin, interleukin-6 (IL-6) (gp 130-linked receptor)
Granulocyte colony stimulating factor (G-CSF) (G-CSF receptor)
IL-2, IL-4 others (CD132 receptor)
IL-3, IL-5, others (CDw131 receptor)
Leptin (OB-receptor)

[a] This family of neurotrophic factors interacts with the Ret signaling pathway (see Chapter 4).

[b] Cytokines are categorized according to the receptor with which they interact; all couple ultimately to the JAK-STAT signaling pathway (see Chapter 4).

However, recent data suggest that heterodimers of BDNF and NGF can be formed in mammalian cells in vivo.

There are two different pathways through which proteins, including neurotrophins, may be secreted or released. The constitutive pathway for secretion is not driven by extracellular stimulation and is used to secrete membrane components, viral proteins, and extracellular matrix molecules; in other words, the constitutive pathway is not the pathway generally associated with neurotransmitters. Yet neurotrophic factors have typically been considered to be secreted by the constitutive pathway, in contrast to the release of more conventional peptide transmitters (e.g., those shown in Table 2.1) through the regulated pathway. Prohormones have an N-terminal signal sequence, which targets the protein to the endoplasmic reticulum and then to the Golgi network, from where it is ultimately packaged into vesicles. Because many neurotrophic factors lack a signal sequence, the idea that growth factors are secreted by the constitutive pathway occurred by default. However, specific antibodies used for immunohistochemical studies have revealed that BDNF is present in chromogranin-containing secretory granules and thus can secrete through the regulated pathway as well as the constitutive pathway.

The pathway through which neurotrophic factors are secreted has immediate relevance to the issue of whether the release can be evoked by neuronal depolarization. It now appears that under basal conditions BDNF and NGF are constitutively released from somatodendritic regions of the neuron, but that depolarization leads to regulated release, although it is unclear if this release is calcium dependent.

Among the functions subserved by neurotrophic factors are those commonly ascribed to growth factors, including involvement in development, differentiation, and survival of neurons. However, there are other more "transmitter"-like functions. Neurotrophic factor expression and release from neurons, like transmitter expression and release, are regulated by afferent signals. For example, NGF and BDNF expression are increased by the excitatory transmitter glutamate and decreased by the inhibitory transmitter GABA. In addition, the regulation of BDNF by events such as seizures is regionally, spatially, and temporally distinct, with seizures leading to BDNF induction in different types of hippocampal neurons and with specific patterns of promotor activation (Kokaia et al., 1994).

Finally, a transmitter role for neurotrophic factors is suggested by their ability to regulate other neurons. Neurotrophic factors activate receptor proteins on target cells, which then initiate complex cascades of intracellular signaling pathways leading to their diverse biological effects. These effects include not only the more traditional growth factor responses but also the same types of changes that are seen in response to classical transmitters, such as regulation of ion channels (albeit on a different time scale). This underscores the notion that neurotrophic factors can serve as transmitters, just as more conventional transmitters (for example, monoamines) can exert some trophic effects on target cells.

Endocannabinoids

Marijuana has been used as a recreational drug and a therapeutic agent for thousands of years and remains a popular but illicit drug in the United States. The name *marijuana* is derived from the Mexican word *maraguanquo*, meaning "intoxicating plant." The behavioral effects of marijuana vary widely across individuals, with some becoming giddy and euphoric, while others become sedated and depressed. Use of the drug may lead to distortion of sensory perceptions and time. Potential adverse effects following acute administration include impairment of short-term memory and impaired motor coordination and tracking during the performance of certain tasks such as driving. The psychoactive properties of marijuana suggest that there is a specific brain receptor for the drug.

Δ-9-Tetrahydrocannabinol (THC) is the major psychoactive constituent in marijuana. It binds to two G-protein–coupled receptors that are found in the brain and periphery, both of which couple to $G_{i/o}$ and inhibit adenylyl cyclase. Initially it was thought that the CB_1 receptor is neuronal and the CB_2 receptors are localized to peripheral sites. It is now clear that although CB_1 is the major cannabinoid receptor in brain, it is also found in the periphery, and there are CB_2 sites in brain.

The term *cannabinoid receptor* is based on the active ingredient of marijuana, THC. However, this is a misnomer: Cannabinoids are not the natural ligand for these receptors. The presence of receptors for the active constituent of marijuana sparked interest in endogenous ligands for these receptors. The search for the endogenous ligands resulted in the discovery of not one but two lipid transmitters, the "endocannabinoids" *anandamide* (*N*-arachidonylethanolamine) and *2-arachidonylglycerol.*

These lipids are derived from cleavage from a membrane-bound phospholipid precursor, which occurs in a calcium-dependent manner upon neuronal activation, generating the release of anandamide. Anandamide is produced by hydrolysis of *N*-arachidonyl-phosphotidylethanolamine (PE), with phospholipase D catalyzing the process. The synthesis of anandamide is in essence the same step as release, as we have seen previously in the case of NO. Once released, anandamide is rapidly inactivated by carrier-mediated uptake and enzymatic hydrolysis. Inhibitors of this carrier have been identified that potentiate the actions of anandamide. The endocannabinoids are also inactivated intracellularly by a membrane-bound hydrolase, anandamide amidohydrolase (FAAH). Several high-potency compounds have been identified that irreversibly inhibit FAAH and have proven useful research tools.

The endocannabinoids differ in several critical aspects from classical and peptide neurotransmitters and modulators. Endocannabinoids are lipid products and highly hydrophobic; they cannot be stored in vesicles because they easily diffuse through membranes. Instead of being released conventionally, endocannabinoids are produced upon demand via receptor-stimulated enzymatic breakdown of specific membrane lipids and thus "released" from the cell. It is also clear that anandamide influences the function of presynaptic as well as postsynaptic neurons (Chevaleyre et al., 2006).

Because of the psychoactive effects of marijuana, there has been considerable interest in determining the functions of the endogenous cannabinoids. It has often been speculated that cannabinoid receptors or cannabinoid ligands may be dysregulated in certain psychiatric disorders, particularly schizophrenia. Several indirect lines of evidence are consistent with a possible role of endogenous cannabinoids in the pathophysiology of schizophrenia. Chronic marijuana use has been associated with cognitive deficits that progressively worsen with continued drug use and resemble to some degree the cognitive deficits of schizophrenia, and elevated cerebrospinal fluid levels of anandamide have been reported in patients with schizophrenia. A study of a small group of participants has reported an increase in the density of CB_1 receptors in the dorsolateral prefrontal cortex of patients with schizophrenia. Although many of these clinical data await independent verification, studies in laboratory animals are consistent with THC-induced cognitive deficits and transmitter changes. In particular, chronic administration of THC causes a decrease in DA turnover and ACh release in the prefrontal cortex that persists upon discontinuation of the drug treatment; during this drug-free period, attention and short-term memory deficits are present.

NEUROTRANSMITTERS AND THEIR EVOLVING ROLES

Our views of what constitutes a neurotransmitter are in a state of flux. We have moved from being limited to classical transmitters such as acetylcholine to accepting peptides as transmitters, and have grown comfortable with gases and lipids, which are neither stored nor actively released. Having considered these changes in our views of neurotransmitters, it is not surprising to learn that interneuronal communication may be only one of multiple roles played by transmitters. For example, mRNAs that encode enzymes involved in transmitter synthesis, such as the ACh-synthesizing enzyme *choline acetyltransferase*, are found in lymphocytes. The ACh-inactivating enzyme *acetylcholinesterase* is also expressed in lymphocytes, as are certain acetylcholine receptors. The expression of these markers of transmitter systems is not restricted to lymphocytes but is seen across different tissues: choline acetyltransferase is even found in spermatazoa! When one considers that so many different aspects of acetylcholine synthesis and action are found in blood cells, it is reasonable to speculate that changes in these factors in peripheral cells may reflect central changes that are present in neuropsychiatric disorders such as Alzheimer's disease. This tantalizing notion has been repeatedly explored, but no such simple peripheral marker has yet emerged from these studies.

There is inevitably strong resistance to change in scientific thinking, as Kuhn so compelling discussed. Just as inevitably, our conventional wisdom changes and gives rise to new dogma. The consideration of interneuronal messengers such as NO and the endocannabinoids as neurotransmitters is indicative that we have entered an era of new dogma. Just as surely, however, our most cherished beliefs will be challenged soon by new data, which will cause us to revise (and ultimately overthrow) our current views. This should not be a cause for alarm. As we have advanced in our understanding of the nature of neurotransmitters, so have we discovered new potential targets for the treatment of psychiatric disorders. An understanding of transmitters and their receptor partners, as well as other near and distant relations such as transporters and transduction mechanisms, is essential to our approaches to defining and treating psychiatric disorders.

REFERENCES

Aid, T., Kazantseva, A., Piirsoo, M., Palm, K., and Timmusk, T. (2007) Mouse and rat BDNF gene structure and expression revisited. *J. Neurosci. Res.* 85:525–535.

Bean, A.J., and Roth, R.H. (1992) Dopamine-neurotensin interactions in mesocortical neurons: evidence from microdialysis studies. *Ann. N.Y. Acad. Sci.* 668:43–53.

Bean, A.J., Zhang, X., and Hökfelt, T. (1995) Peptide secretion: what do we know? *FASEB J.* 8:630–638.

Blakely, R.D. (2001) Physiological genomics of antidepressant targets: keeping the periphery in mind. *J. Neurosci.* 21:8319–8323.

Boehning, D., and Snyder, S.H. (2003) Novel neural modulators. *Ann. Rev. Neurosci.* 26:105–131.

Chevaleyre, V., Takahashi, K.A., and Castillo, P.E. (2006) Endocannabinoid-mediated synaptic plasticity in the CNS. *Ann. Rev. Neurosci.* 29:37–76.

Cooper, J.R., Bloom, F.E., and Roth, R.H. (2002) *The Biochemical Basis of Neuropharmacology, 8th ed.* New York: Oxford University Press.

de Lecea, L., Kilduff, T.S., Peyron, C., Gao, X., Foye, P.E., Danielson, P.E., Fukuhara, C., Battenberg, E.L., Gautvik, V.T., Bartlett, F.S. II, Frankel, W.N., van den Pol, A.N., Bloom, F.E., Gautvik, K.M., and Sutcliffe, J.G. (1998) The hypocretins: hypothalamus-specific peptides with neuroexcitatory activity. *Proc. Natl. Acad. Sci. USA* 95:322–327.

Deutch, A.Y., and Bean, A.J. (1995) Colocalization in dopamine neurons. In: Bloom, F.E., and Kupfer, D.J., eds. *Psychopharmacology: The Fourth Generation of Progress*. New York: Raven Press, pp. 197–206.

Deutch, A.Y., and Roth, R.H. (2008) Neurotransmitters. In: Squire, L.R., Bloom, F.E., Berg, D.K., Du Lac, S., Ghosh, A., and Spitzer, N. C., eds. *Fundamental Neuroscience, 3rd ed.* San Diego, CA: Academic Press, pp. 133–156.

Fatt, P., and Katz, B. (1952) Spontaneous subthreshold activity at motor nerve endings. *J. Physiol. (Lond.)* 117:109–128.

Fremeau, R.T., Voglmaier, S., Seal, R.P., and Edwards, R.H. (2004) VGLUTs define subsets of excitatory neurons and suggest novel roles for glutamate. *TINS* 27:98–102.

Hassel, B., and Dingledine, R. (2006) Glutamate. In: Siegel, G. J., Albers, R. W., Brady, S., and Price, D. L., eds. *Basic Neurochemistry, 7th ed.* San Diego, CA: Elsevier–Academic Press, pp. 267–290.

Haydon, P.G., and Carmignoto, G. (2006) Astrocyte control of synaptic transmission and neurovascular coupling. *Physiol. Rev.* 86:1009–1031.

Hoffman, B.J., Hansson, S.R., Mezey, E., and Palkovits, M. (1998) Localization and dynamic regulation of biogenic amine transporters in the mammalian central nervous system. *Front. Neuroendocrinol.* 19:187–231.

Huang, E.J., and Reichardt, L.F. (2001) Neurotrophins: roles in neuronal development and function. *Annu. Rev. Neurosci.* 24: 677–736.

Hyman, S.E., and Nestler, E.J. (1993) *The Molecular Foundations of Psychiatry*. Washington, DC: American Psychiatric Press.

Ichinose, H., Ohye, T., Takahashi, E., Seki, N., Hori, T., Segawa, M., Nomura, Y., Endo, K., Tanaka, K., Tanaka, H., and Tsuji, S. (1994) Hereditary progressive dystonia with marked diurnal fluctuation caused by mutations in the GTP cyclohydrolase I gene. *Nat. Genet.* 8:236–242.

Kanner, B.I. (2006) Structure and function of sodium-coupled GABA and glutamate transporters. *J. Membr. Biol.* 213:89–100.

Kitabgi, P., De Nadal, F., Rovere, C., and Bidard, J.N. (1992) Biosynthesis, maturation, release, and degradation of neurotensin and neuromedin N. *Ann. N.Y. Acad. Sci.* 668:30–42.

Kokaia, Z., Metsis, M., Kokaia, M., Bengzon, J., Elmer, E., Smith, M.L., Timmusk, T., Siesjo, B.K., Persson, H., and Lindvall, O. (1994) Brain insults in rats induce increased expression of the BDNF gene through differential use of multiple promoters. *Eur. J. Neurosci.* 6:587–596.

Kumer, S.C., and Vrana, K.E. (1996) Intricate regulation of tyrosine hydroxylase activity and gene expression. *J. Neurochem.* 67: 443–462.

Martineau, M., Baux, G., and Mothet, J.P. (2006) D-serine signalling in the brain: friend and foe. *Trends Neurosci.* 29:481–491.

McIntire, S.L., Reimer, R.J., Schuske, K., Edwards, R.H., and Jorgensen, E.M. (1997) Identification and characterization of the vesicular GABA transporter. *Nature* 389:870–876.

Moore, R.Y., and Bloom, F.E. (1978) Central catecholamine neuron systems: anatomy and physiology of the dopamine systems. *Annu. Rev. Neurosci.* 1:129–169.

Olsen, R.W., and Betz, H. (2006) GABA and glycine. In: Siegel, G.J., Albers, R.W., Brady, S., and Price, D.L., eds. *Basic Neurochemistry (7th ed.)*. San Diego, CA: Elsevier–Academic Press, pp. 291–302.

Sakurai, T., Amemiya, A., Ishii, M., Matsuzaki, I., Chemelli, R.M., Tanaka, H., Williams, S.C., Richardson, J.A., Koslowski, G.P., Wilson, S., Arch, J.R., Buckingham, R.E., Haynes, A.C., Carr, S.A., Annan, R.S., McNulty, D.E., Liu, W.S., Terrett, J.A., Elshourbagy, N.A., Bergsma, D.J., and Yanagisawa, M. (1998) Orexins and orexin receptors: a family of hypothalamic neuropeptides and G protein–coupled receptors that regulate feeding behavior. *Cell* 92:573–585.

Salter, M.W., and De Koninck, Y. (1999) An ambiguous fast synapse: a new twist in the tale of two transmitters. *Nat. Neurosci.* 2: 199–200.

Schwarcz, R. (2004) The kynurenine pathway of tryptophan degradation as a drug target. *Curr. Opin. Pharmacol.* 4:12–17.

Sieburth, D., Madison, J.M., and Kaplan, J. M. (2007) PKC-1 regulates secretion of neuropeptides. *Nat. Neurosci.* 10:49–57.

Snyder, S.H., and Ferris, C.D. (2000) Novel neurotransmitters and their neuropsychiatric relevance. *Am. J. Psychiat.* 157:1738–1751.

Sotnikova, T.D., Beaulieu, J.M., Gainetdinov, R.R., and Caron, M.G. (2006) Molecular biology, pharmacology and functional role of the plasma membrane dopamine transporter. *CNS Neurol. Disord. Drug. Targets* 5:45–56.

Sutcliffe, J.G., and de Lecea, L. (2002) The hypocretins: setting the arousal threshold. *Nat. Rev. Neurosci.* 3:339–349.

Valenstein, E.S. (2005) *The War of the Soups and the Sparks*. New York: Columbia University Press.

Volterra, A., and Meldolesi, J. (2005) Astrocytes, from brain glue to communication elements: the revolution continues. *Nat. Rev. Neurosci.* 6:626–640.

Wickens, J.R., and Arbuthnott, G.W. (2005) Structural and functional interactions in the striatum at the receptor level. In: Dunnett, S.B., Bentivoglio, M., Bjorklund, A., and Hokfelt, T., eds. *Handbook of Chemical Neuroanatomy: Vol. 21. Dopamine*. Amsterdam: Elsevier, pp. 199–239.

Zahniser, N.R., and Doolen, S. (2001) Chronic and acute regulation of Na1/Cl-dependent neurotransmitter transporters: drugs, substrates, presynaptic receptors, and signaling systems. *Pharmacol. Ther.* 92:21–55.

Zucchi, R., Chiellini, G., Scanlan, T.S., and Grandy, D.K. (2006) Trace amine-associated receptors and their ligands. *Br. J. Pharmacol.* 149:967–978.

3 Using Basic Electrophysiology to Understand the Neurobiology of Mental Illness

EVELYN K. LAMBE AND GEORGE K. AGHAJANIAN

Neurons communicate with each other through electrochemical signaling. Their electrical state is vital to their ability to respond to stimuli and to release neurotransmitter, the chemical signal that is the main form of communication between neurons. Although we have understood for a long time how neurons send signals, we are only beginning to understand how this signaling in different brain regions is affected by prior activity and by the presence of neuromodulators. Mental illness is a compelling example of a subtle dysfunction of neuronal communication that has dramatic consequences for how a person perceives and responds to the world. In the treatment of psychiatric illnesses such as depression and schizophrenia, certain drugs have been shown to be able to ameliorate some of the symptoms, although often with serious side effects. Despite understanding certain properties of these drugs (for example, their acute ability to block a certain type of receptor), we do not fully appreciate how these properties change activity of brain systems over time in terms of bringing about improved function and in terms of causing side effects.

Electrophysiologists examine how neurons communicate with each other and how different drugs affect this signaling. *Electrophysiology* as a subject covers a broad range of techniques, but all give access to a higher level of resolution than most brain-imaging methods. To understand the meaning of electrophysiological data, it is critical to understand how neurons work and to know about the typical electrophysiological methods. This chapter begins with a review of neuronal physiology, discusses the typical tools electrophysiologists use, and then gives examples of how electrophysiological approaches are relevant to understanding neurobiology of mental illness.

HOW NEURONS WORK

Neurons are encased in phospholipid membranes in which proteins are embedded. The proteins of greatest relevance to electrophysiology are ion channels and receptors. The latter group falls into two types that are discussed in detail later in this chapter: receptors that are ligand-gated ion channels and receptors that couple to G proteins. The membrane is impermeable to charged particles unless they travel passively through ion channels or are actively moved by another group of proteins called *ion pumps*. Together, ion pumps and ion channels lead to the creation of concentration and electrical gradients across the membrane. We now discuss mechanisms by which these gradients are created and how they serve the neuron's ability to communicate.

Resting Potential

To understand the baseline or resting condition of a neuron, one must appreciate how ions are distributed. The solution surrounding neurons, called *extracellular fluid*, is essentially like seawater. There is a high level of sodium and a low level of potassium. Neurons spend a lot of energy pumping sodium out of and potassium into their intracellular space. As depicted in Figure 3.1, neurons thus have low internal sodium and high internal potassium levels. In addition to sodium and potassium ions that are positively charged, neurons also contain negatively charged ions, most of which are membrane-impermeable anions (abbreviated as A^- on figures) such as sulfate. At rest, the membrane is permeable to potassium because of "leak" potassium channels; by contrast, there is very low permeability to sodium.

The array of channels that are open at a given time determines the membrane potential. Since the sodium-potassium pump has increased the internal potassium above the extracellular concentration, potassium ions flow out of the cell through leak potassium channels. As illustrated in Figure 3.2, this potassium ion movement leads to a local buildup of positive charge on the outside of the cell membrane near the potassium channels, and a local buildup of negative charge on the inside of

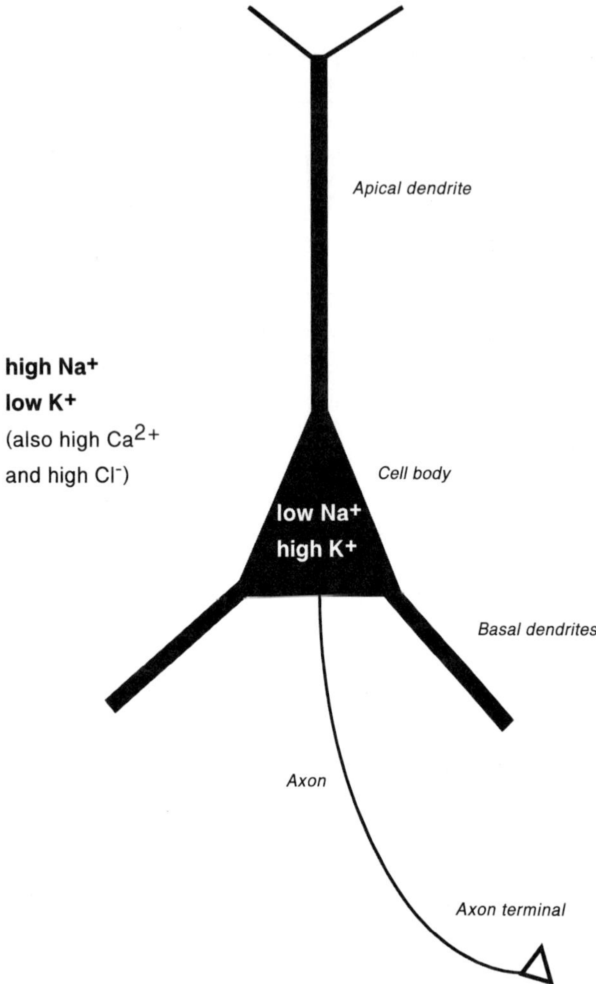

FIGURE 3.1 Schematic of a neuron showing concentration differences for various ions across the cellular membrane. The cytoplasm of the neuron is high in potassium ions (K^+) and low in sodium ions (Na^+), whereas the extracellular solution is high in sodium ions and low in potassium ions. Chloride and calcium ions also occur at high concentrations in the extracellular space compared to the intracellular space. Neurons receive inputs to their dendrites and send out information in the form of action potentials through their axons.

the membrane. This electrical gradient opposes the concentration gradient (also known as the driving force). Rather than flowing through their ion channel from a place of high concentration to one of low concentration, the intracellular potassium ions are attracted to the buildup of negatively charged ions on the inside of the membrane and repelled by the local buildup of positively charged ions on the outside. So, the net flow of potassium ions stops. This steady state is called the *resting potential*. The word *potential* refers to the difference in charge. At rest, the neuron is hyperpolarized; the inside of the membrane is more negative than the outside of the membrane. While the leak potassium channels are integral to setting a hyperpolarized resting potential, the exact resting potential is a function of the permeability of that neuron to potassium, sodium, and chloride. A typical membrane potential for a cortical pyramidal neuron at rest is –70 mV.

It is important to remember that this resting state is a dynamic process. Ion channels that are open have ions flowing through all the time; at rest, there is no net flow. Under most conditions, the flow of ions through ion channels has negligible effects (less than 0.01%) on the total concentrations of ions inside and outside the cell. The energy-driven pumps are the main players at setting the intracellular concentration of ions and the volume of extracellular fluid can be presumed to be infinite

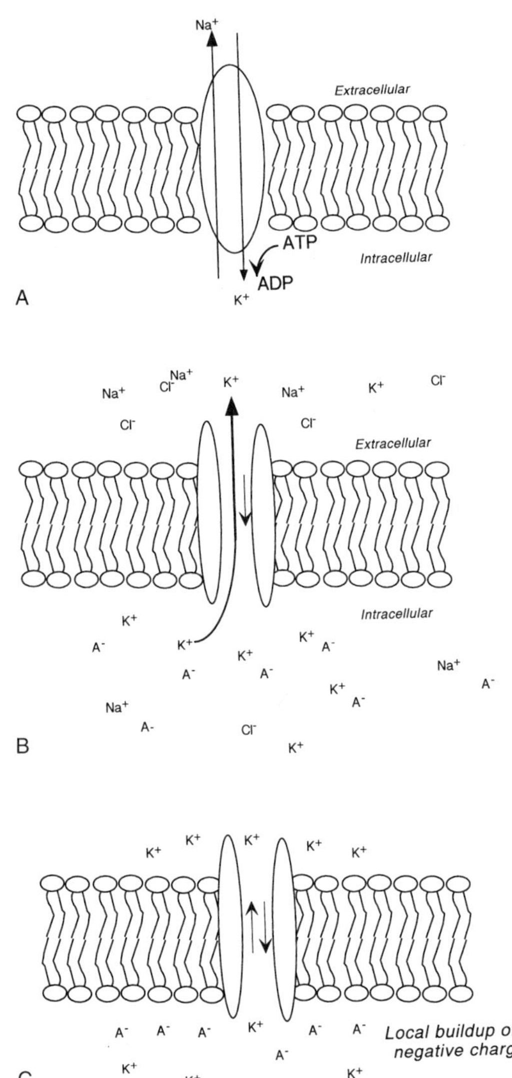

FIGURE 3.2 Schematic of a portion of the phospholipid membrane. (*A*) Depiction of the sodium-potassium pump. This protein uses energy to create concentration gradients by pumping sodium out of the neuron and potassium into the neuron. (*B*) The leak potassium channels are open at rest. Through these channels, potassium diffuses out of the neuron along its concentration gradient. This diffusion creates a local electrical gradient that opposes the concentration gradient. (*C*) A schematic of the separation of charge across the membrane created by diffusion through leak potassium channels. This separation of charge contributes to the resting potential, in which the inside of the cell membrane is more negative than the outside.

compared to that of the neuron. The ion channels lead to charge separations across the membrane, as illustrated in part C of Figure 3.2.

Calcium is another positively charged ion that is at a higher concentration in the extracellular fluid than in the cytoplasm (mostly because the neuron spends energy sequestering calcium in intracellular storage compartments). At rest, the cell membrane has very low permeability to calcium ions. Calcium can enter the neuron through a variety of channels, some opened by neurotransmitters (usually also permeable to other cations such as sodium and potassium) and some opened by changes in membrane potential. Calcium is very important for many aspects of neuronal signaling. It is discussed in detail later.

How Neurons Communicate: Spikes

The negative resting potential, together with the concentration gradient of sodium across the cell membrane, allows the neuron the ability to communicate rapidly. At the resting potential, sodium ions don't have open ion channels to travel through because channels that are permeable to sodium are either ligand gated (for example, by glutamate) or are voltage gated (that is, the neuron has to become less negative before these channels will open). Activation of glutamate receptors opens channels that allow sodium and calcium to flow along their concentration gradients into the cell, which makes the neuron less negative transiently—known as an *excitatory postsynaptic potential* or EPSP. If a given cell is sufficiently depolarized by the summation of several EPSPs arriving close together in time, the voltage-gated sodium channels will open. This level of depolarization is called *threshold* because once a few voltage-gated sodium channels open, sodium rushes in down its concentration gradient, leading to more depolarization, which opens more voltage-gated sodium channels, and so on. Threshold is thus the start of a positive-feedback "all-or-nothing process" that is the action potential, as illustrated in Figure 3.3.

In an action potential, sodium rushes in through voltage-gated sodium channels, and this makes the membrane go from being negative relative to the local extracellular environment to being positive (remember: this is

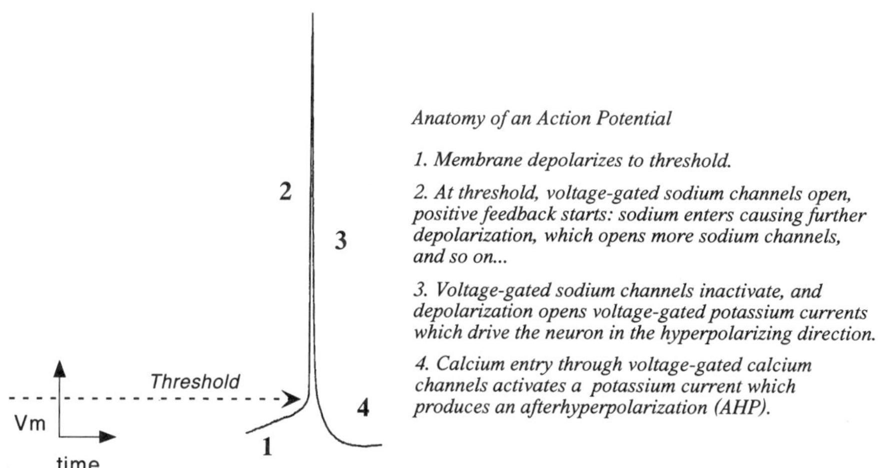

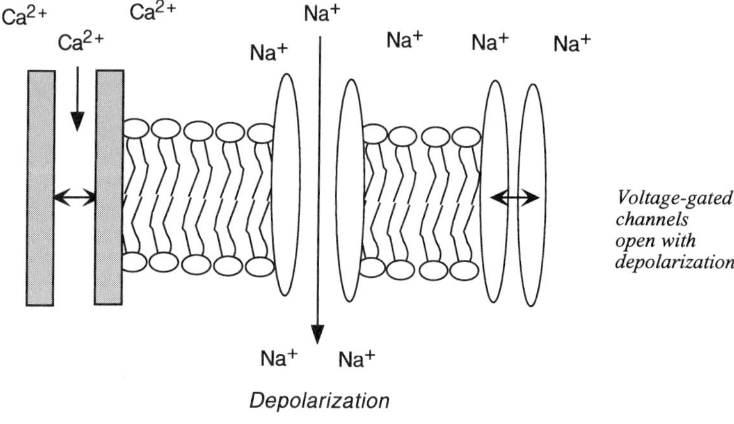

FIGURE 3.3 Action potentials are all-or-nothing events. When the membrane is depolarized to the threshold point, either by inputs from other neurons or through intrinsic mechanisms, voltage-gated sodium channels open, letting sodium flow down its concentration gradient into the cell, further depolarizing the cell and opening more voltage-gated sodium channels. This depolarization also opens voltage-gated calcium channels.

about local changes in electrical charge, not major changes in total intracellular or extracellular ion concentrations). As the cell membrane becomes more positive, however, two changes happen that tend to restore the neuron to its resting potential. First, voltage-gated potassium channels begin to open. The outward flow of potassium ions down their concentration gradient tends to bring the membrane potential to a more negative level. Second, voltage-gated sodium channels begin to inactivate. When they are inactivated, they are open but blocked. For this block to be relieved and the channels to close, the membrane potential must again become hyperpolarized. So with a hyperpolarizing force and the loss of the depolarizing force, the cell membrane becomes even more negative than the resting potential (calcium-activated potassium channels play an important role in this phenomenon called after *hyperpolarization* that is discussed further later) and then returns to the resting potential as the voltage-gated potassium channels slowly close.

Voltage-gated sodium channel opening and inactivation explain much about how action potentials are generated and travel. Summation of several EPSPs arriving close together in time is usually required to trigger a spike. A spike then depolarizes the entire neuron as the wave of depolarization opens more and more voltage-gated sodium channels. The axon, the output branch of the neuron, has evolved to enable particularly fast conduction. This thin branch is coated in myelin, which is similar in principle to the insulation that is used to increase the efficiency of electrical wires. Because the wave of depolarization is not substantially decreased between the gaps in myelin, it essentially "jumps" between the gaps or nodes (which have clusters of voltage-gated sodium channels). The action potential keeps traveling along neuronal structures toward their ends because sodium channel inactivation prevents sodium influx in a portion of the cell where the spike has already passed through. This phenomenon also limits how closely together spikes can be fired; this is known as the *refractory period*.

Release of Neurotransmitter

When the action potential reaches the end of the axon, it reaches a structure specialized for chemical transmission. Axon terminals have vesicles of neurotransmitter that are docked and ready to be released. Most axon terminals are the presynaptic structure of a synapse. Figure 3.4 shows a glutamatergic synapse. *Synapses* are an anatomical specialization for chemical

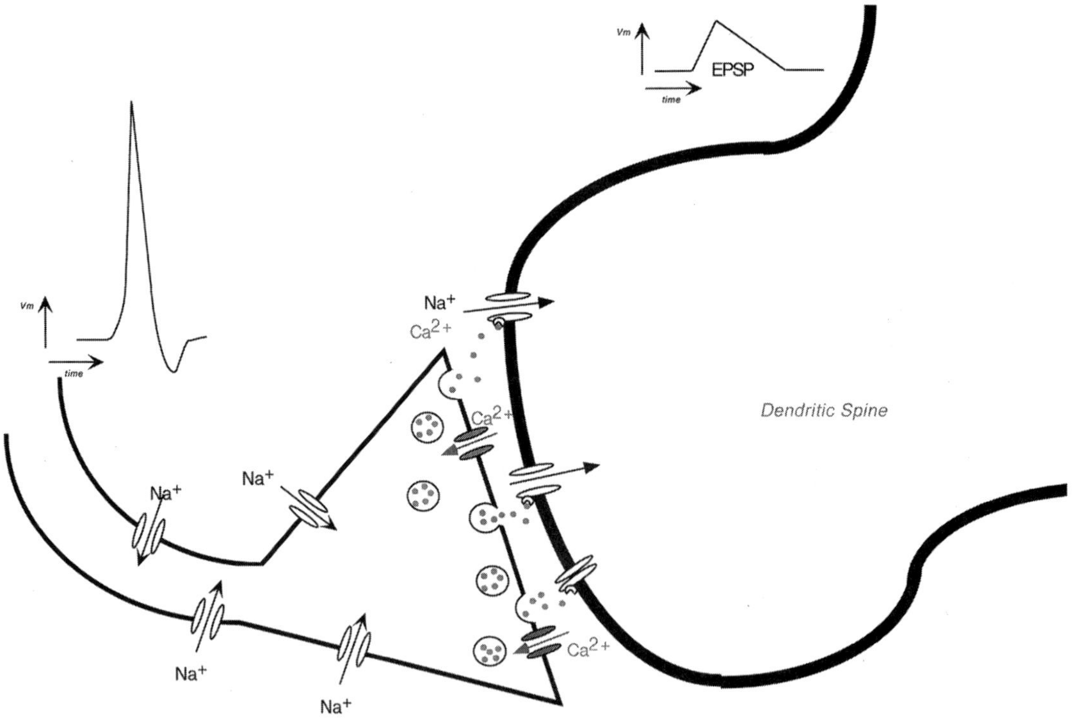

FIGURE 3.4 When an action potential reaches the end of an axon, the flood of calcium into the terminal through voltage-gated calcium channels results in the fusion of vesicles with the cell membrane and the release of neurotransmitter. Molecules of neurotransmitter diffuse across the synaptic cleft and bind to receptors on the postsynaptic membrane. The binding of the neurotransmitter glutamate to AMPA receptors opens these ligand-gated ion channels to allow sodium and potassium to pass through. This mixed cation current (mainly sodium diffusing into the neuron) is depolarizing and results in an excitatory postsynaptic potential (EPSP). If this EPSP depolarizes the postsynaptic neuron to threshold, perhaps through summation with another EPSP close together in time and space, it could cause a spike in this postsynaptic neuron.

neurotransmission, involving a presynaptic portion that releases the neurotransmitter and a postsynaptic portion that has a high density of relevant receptors and ion channels. The trigger for release of neurotransmitter is the influx of calcium through voltage-gated calcium channels in the axon terminal. Although there are such channels in many parts of the neuron, only in the axon terminal does calcium influx trigger neurotransmitter release. Once released, the neurotransmitter diffuses across the synapse to receptors on the postsynaptic cell. For example, if the transmitter is glutamate, it brings about an EPSP in the postsynaptic cell, as previously described.

Effect of Neurotransmitters on Postsynaptic Neurons: Fast, Ionotropic Receptors

The major way neurons communicate with each other is through chemical transmission, by releasing neurotransmitters from their axon terminal onto the dendrites of the target neuron where it binds to specialized receptors. It is important to appreciate how the resting potential of a given cell is affected by the neurons that communicate with it. When an excitatory neuron sends a signal down its axon to the postsynaptic neuron, it can excite the cell (make it less negative). When an inhibitory cell sends a signal to this neuron, it can inhibit the cell (make it more negative). In both cases, this is accomplished by neurotransmitters binding to a receptor that is directly coupled to an ion channel (referred to as fast neurotransmission). The two major fast neurotransmitters are *glutamate* and *γ-aminobutyric acid* (GABA). Neurons are excited by glutamate binding and inhibited by GABA binding. As mentioned previously and shown in Figure 3.5, activation of glutamate receptors creates an EPSP by opening channels that allow sodium and calcium to flow along their concentration gradients into the cell, which makes the neuron less negative transiently. By contrast, GABA binding opens a channel that allows negatively charged chloride ions to flow along their concentration gradient into the neuron, which makes it more negative transiently—known as an *inhibitory postsynaptic potential* (IPSP). Waves of potential spread passively along the dendrite. If many inputs to a neuron are active within a narrow time window, these waves summate (or cancel in the case of concurrent excitatory and inhibitory potentials). In the special case when several excitatory neurons release glutamate onto a neuron nearly simultaneously, the EPSPs or waves of positive potential raise the potential difference of the membrane to the level that can trigger an action potential.

The ligand-gated channels represent the most direct form of coupling between a receptor and effector where both components are part of the same protein complex. This group of channels is described further in Table 3.1. Binding of the agonist results in a conformational change of the channel protein complex, resulting in a rapid and marked increase in the permeability of the channel to the ion or ions for which it is selective. For example, when glutamate binds to an α-amino-3-hydroxy-5-methyl-4-isoxasolepropionic acid (AMPA) receptor as shown in Figure 3.5, it opens a channel that is permeable to sodium and calcium. Some ligand-gated channels also have a component of voltage gating. For example, glutamate is an agonist for the *N*-methyl-D-aspartate (NMDA) receptor as well; however, glutamate binding alone will not open the NMDA channel at hyperpolarized voltages. When the membrane is hyperpolarized, a magnesium ion blocks the channel from the extracellular side. The membrane must be depolarized to free the magnesium ion and allow sodium and calcium ions to pass through the NMDA channel into the neuron. In essence, this means that presynaptic axons must release

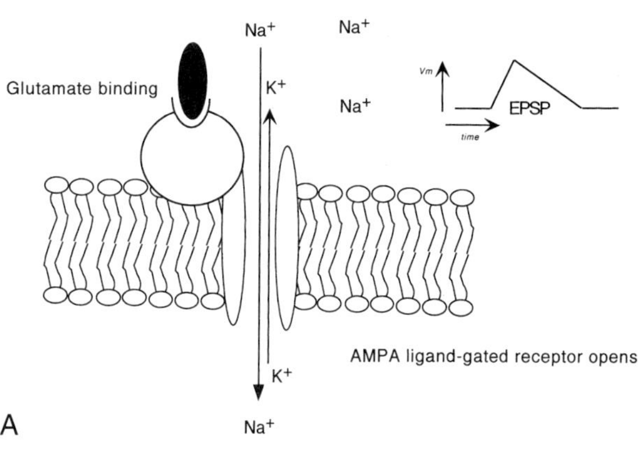

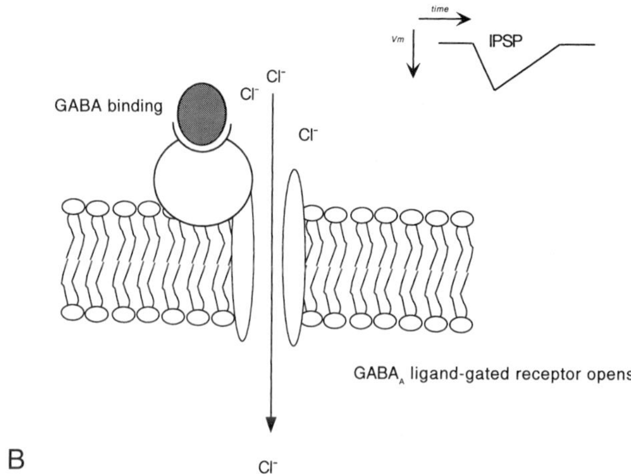

FIGURE 3.5 Schematic of postsynaptic effects. (*A*) If glutamate is released and binds to postsynaptic α-amino-3-hydroxy-5-methyl-4-isoxasolepropionic acid (AMPA) receptors, it will open and allow a mixed cation current to depolarize the neuron, producing a subthreshold wave of depolarization called an *excitatory postsynaptic potential* (EPSP). (*B*) By contrast, if γ-aminobutyric acid (GABA) binds to a postsynaptic $GABA_A$ receptor, it will open to allow chloride to flow down its concentration gradient into the cell. This current hyperpolarizes the neuron in a wave of negative potential called an *inhibitory postsynaptic potential* (IPSP).

TABLE 3.1. *Ligand-Gated Ion Channels*

Neurotransmitter	*Receptor Subtype*	*Ion Channel Permeability*	*Physiological Response*
Acetylcholine	nicotinic	Na^+, K^+, Ca^{2+}	Fast excitation
Glutamate	AMPA	Na^+, K^+ (Ca^{2+})	Fast excitation
	kainate	Na^+, K^+ (Ca^{2+})	Fast excitation
	NMDA	Na^+, K^+, Ca^{2+}	Slow excitation
Glycine	GlyRα/β	Cl^-	Fast inhibition
GABA	$GABA_A$	Cl^-	Fast inhibition
Serotonin	5-HT_3	Na^+, K^+, Ca^{2+}	Fast excitation

AMPA: α-amino-3-hydroxy-5-methyl-4-isoxasoleproptonic acid; GABA: γ-aminobutyric acid; NMDA: *N*-methyl-D-aspartate.

sufficient glutamate onto the neuron not only to bind to NMDA receptors but also to depolarize that region of the cell (through activation of AMPA receptors and influx of sodium). So the NMDA receptor is thought to act as a coincidence detector, and its permeability to calcium allows for long-term changes in the cell through mobilization of second messenger systems.

Effect of Neurotransmitters on Postsynaptic Neurons: G Protein-Coupled Receptors

In addition to glutamate and GABA, there are many other transmitters. So far, we have only discussed ligand-gated channels also known as *ionotropic receptors* (those where the receptor directly opens an ion channel). However, there are also metabotropic receptors. The latter are coupled to G proteins and can affect cellular processes quickly or over a longer time period through activation of second messenger systems. Glutamate, GABA, serotonin, and acetylcholine have both ionotropic and metabotropic receptors. Other neurotransmitters, such as dopamine and norepinephrine, appear to only have metabotropic receptors. All of these are further described in Table 3.2.

Most neurotransmitter receptors found in the brain are not an intrinsic component of ion channels but are coupled to ion channels through a class of proteins whose functional properties are intimately related to their ability to bind guanosine-5′ triphosphate (GTP) and who are known as *G proteins*. These metabotropic receptors can up- or down-regulate the excitability of neurons in the short term and over a longer time period.

G protein activation can also have a relatively rapid direct effect, where the $\beta\gamma$ subunit of the activated G protein dissociates and interacts directly with an ion channel. A group of inwardly rectifying potassium channels (Kir3 or GIRKs) are directly activated by $\beta\gamma$ subunits from G_i/G_o proteins. Their activation tends to hyperpolarize the neuron. The alpha subunit of G_q is thought also to interact with ion channels.

G protein activation is often coupled to ion channels through one or more second messenger molecules. The specific type of second messenger activated depends on the type of G protein. Three major types of G proteins include G_s (which stimulates the production of cyclic adenosine monophosphate [cAMP]), G_i/G_o (which inhibits the production of cAMP), and G_q (which stimulates the phosphoinositol pathway).

Through these mechanisms, G proteins can modulate the fast, ionotropic transmission described in Table 3.1 and the previous section. However, through activation of second messenger systems, they can also have long-term effects on neuronal physiology through covalent modification of ion channels and intermediate and long-term changes in gene expression of receptors.

THE BASIC TOOLS OF THE ELECTROPHYSIOLOGIST

Electrophysiology is the study of the electrical properties of neurons and how these properties change under different conditions. Such recording can be performed in vivo, in brain slice, or in isolated cells (possibly from dissociated brain slice or primary culture of neurons or another cell type). Each of these types of recordings has benefits and limitations in terms of the types of questions that can be addressed.

In vivo electrophysiologists record neuronal activity in certain regions of the brain to answer the question of how small groups of neurons respond during the performance of a task or when another brain area is stimulated. Data about individual neurons are extracted mathematically from the recordings of electrical activity at the place where the electrode was positioned. These experiments are extremely difficult logistically and are limited in terms of controlling different variables.

Questions about local circuitry can be better explored with slice physiology. This technique relies on the fact that it is possible under special conditions to keep a slice of brain alive and healthy for many hours. The investigator

TABLE 3.2. *G Protein–Coupled Receptors*

Neurotransmitter	*Receptor Subtype*	*G Protein*	*Second Messenger*	*Ion Channel*	*Physiological Response*
Acetylcholine	M_1, M_5	G_q/G_{11}	⇑ IP_3 & DAG	⇓ K^+ currents	excitation
	M_2, M_3, M_4	G_i/G_o	⇓ cAMP	⇑ Kir3[a], ⇓ Ca^{2+}	inhibition
Serotonin	5-HT_1 family	G_i/G_o	⇓ cAMP	⇑ Kir3, ⇓ Ca^{2+}	inhibition
	5-HT_2 family	G_q/G_{11}	⇑ IP_3 & DAG	⇓ K^+ currents	excitation
	5-$HT_{4,6,7}$	G_s	⇑ cAMP		variable
Norepinephrine	α_1	G_q/G_{11}	⇑ IP_3 & DAG	⇓ K^+ currents	excitation
	α_2	G_i/G_o	⇓ cAMP	⇑ Kir3, ⇓ Ca^{2+}	inhibition
	β_1, β_2	G_s	⇑ cAMP		variable
Dopamine	D_1, D_5	G_s/G_{olf}	⇑ cAMP		variable
	D_2, D_3, D_4	G_i/G_o	⇓ cAMP	⇑ Kir3, ⇓ Ca^{2+}	inhibition
GABA	$GABA_B$	G_i/G_o	⇓ cAMP	⇑ Kir3, ⇓ Ca^{2+}	inhibition
Somatostatin	—	G_i/G_o	⇓ cAMP	⇑ Kir3, ⇓ Ca^{2+}	inhibition
Tachykinins	NK_1, NK_2, NK_3	G_q/G_{11}	⇑ IP_3 & DAG	⇓ K^+ currents ⇑ cationic	excitation
Neuropeptide Y	Neuropeptide Y	G_i/G_o	⇓ cAMP	⇑ Kir3, ⇓ Ca^{2+}	inhibition
VIP	VIP_1, VIP_2	G_s	⇑ cAMP	⇑ cationic	excitation
Opiate	μ, δ, κ	G_i/G_o	⇓ cAMP	⇑ Kir3, ⇓ Ca^{2+}	inhibition
Hypocretin/Orexin	Hcrt1, Hcrt2	G_q/G_{11}	⇑ IP_3 & DAG	⇓ K^+ currents ⇑ cationic	excitation
Glutamate	mGlu group1	G_q/G_{11}	⇑ IP_3 & DAG	⇓ K^+ currents	excitation
	mGlu groups 2&3	G_i/G_o	⇓ cAMP	⇑ Kir3, ⇓ Ca^{2+}	inhibition

[a] Kir3 is also known as GIRK (G protein–activated inwardly rectifying potassium current).

cAMP: cyclic adenosine monophosphate; DAG: diacylglycerol; GABA: γ-aminobutyric acid; 5HT: 5-hydroxytryptamine; IP_3: intestinal peptide-3; VIP: vasoactive intestinal peptide.

records from individual neurons and can examine how this neuron's electrical activity is affected by different conditions. Yet here too, there can be logistical difficulties accounting for so many variables.

Some investigators want to understand how one type of ion channel behaves under different conditions. To answer this sort of question, there are electrophysiologists who record from a small section of membrane from either a neuron or a cell from a line that has been molecularly altered such that it contains one channel or receptor of interest.

The brain is so complicated that any one level of electrophysiology will not answer all our questions. But the interplay of answers from labs using different techniques gives us unparalleled information about how neurons communicate with each other.

In Vivo Recording

The spiking activity of individual neurons can be studied in vivo with extracellular recording via a microelectrode in the brain. This form of recording is referred to as *extracellular* because the electrode picks up signals from outside a cell. Recording in awake animals, termed *chronic unit recording*, allows for correlations between neuronal activity and behavioral state. If the animal is doing a task, patterns of neuronal activity correlated with correct performance can be contrasted with activity correlated with making a mistake. Patterns of activity can be correlated with broader behavioral states such as the different stages of sleep. Chronic unit recording is also performed sometimes in people with intractable epilepsy to better localize seizure foci before surgery. Extracellular recording is generally used to measure changes in firing activity. Some investigators will apply small quantities of a drug that affects a certain type of receptor, to see how either stimulating or blocking this receptor will change the firing pattern of a neuron or group of neurons. This is known as *microiontophoresis*.

Neurons can be further studied in vivo with multiphoton imaging. The longer wavelengths of light used for this imaging can penetrate deeply into thick, scattering brain tissue. As a result, multiphoton microscopy can be used to visualize fluorescent molecules hundreds of microns deep in the cortex. Usually the fluorescent dyes or calcium indicators have been infused with a pipette or were genetically expressed. Transgenic animals expressing green fluorescent protein (GFP) in a Golgi-like pattern in a population of neurons can be used to assess developmental or environmental changes in dendritic branches and spines.

Slice Recording

Recording from individual neurons in brain slice is used to measure changes in membrane potential affected by the behavior of different ion channels. The slice is kept alive in a chamber under conditions that mimic those in vivo as closely as possible. The state of the art is to use an infrared camera that allows the visualization of the neurons in the slice so the experimenter can select a healthy neuron and guide the pipette up to the selected neuron under carefully controlled conditions, as illustrated in Figure 3.6. When the pipette is brought into contact with the neuron, a small amount of suction is applied. This induces the formation of a strong seal between the glass of the pipette and the cell membrane. At this point, further suction is applied and the small patch of membrane is opened. The pipette then has complete physical and electrical access to the neuron; this is known as *whole-cell patch recording*.

Slice physiologists can then look at changes in membrane potential or firing in response to certain treatments, such as application of a drug in the bath or more locally through another pipette. When reading about slice physiology experiments, it is interesting to note whether the recordings were made in current clamp or voltage clamp. In the former, either depolarizing or hyperpolarizing current is injected and the effect on the membrane potential is assessed. This is similar to mimicking the effects of synaptic input. In voltage clamp, by contrast, the experimenter controls the membrane potential and measures the amount of current needed to maintain this "holding" potential. This is particularly useful for assessing the effects of some treatment on different voltage-gated ion channels because membrane potential is the key variable for this type of channel gating. Synaptic potentials are best measured in voltage clamp (they are measured as opposing currents needed to hold the membrane at the set potential) because they are relatively small and brief events that would be obscured by capacitive transients.

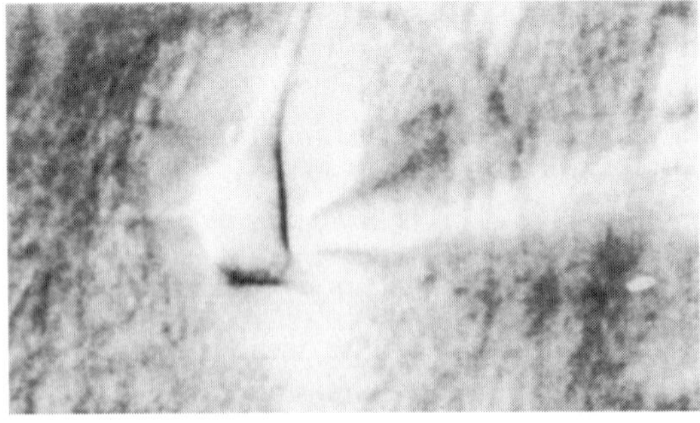

FIGURE 3.6 Visualization of a pyramidal neuron in a slice of cerebral cortex using infrared-differential interference contrast optics. The pipette, shown to the right, will be brought into contact with the neuron. After formation of a gigaohm seal, a small amount of suction will be applied to allow recording in the whole-cell configuration.

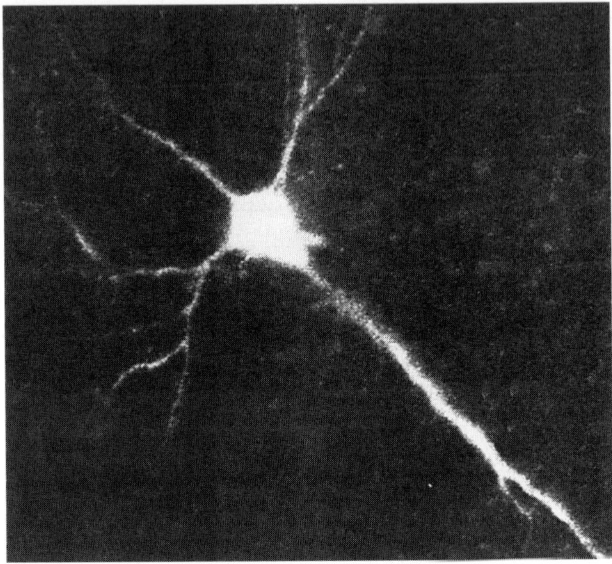

FIGURE 3.7 A cortical pyramidal neuron previously filled with a fluorescent indicator through whole cell patch clamp. The membrane reseals after the patch pipette is pulled away.

The complete physical access permitted in whole-cell recording allows the neuron to be filled with a fluorescent dye so that it can be visualized as shown in Figure 3.7. There are indicators available that change their level of fluorescence depending on the concentration of calcium. These calcium indicators allow us to "watch" the effects of calcium channels being opened by an action potential as it back-propagates through the dendritic arbor. The wave of depolarization opens voltage-gated calcium channels, increasing the concentration of calcium in spines and dendrites as shown in Figure 3.8.

Beyond Slice

There are many reasons why experimenters would like to reduce the complexity of the preparation they record in. For example, they might want to minimize inputs to the neuron they record from, to record from a small piece of membrane, or to record from a cell that has been genetically altered. Various possibilities for simplifying the system exist. These include mechanically dissociating a slice, creating a primary culture of the slice (though it is not possible to have neurons replicate themselves the way other cell types will under cell culture conditions, it is feasible to create conditions where neurons from a brain slice will live for weeks rather

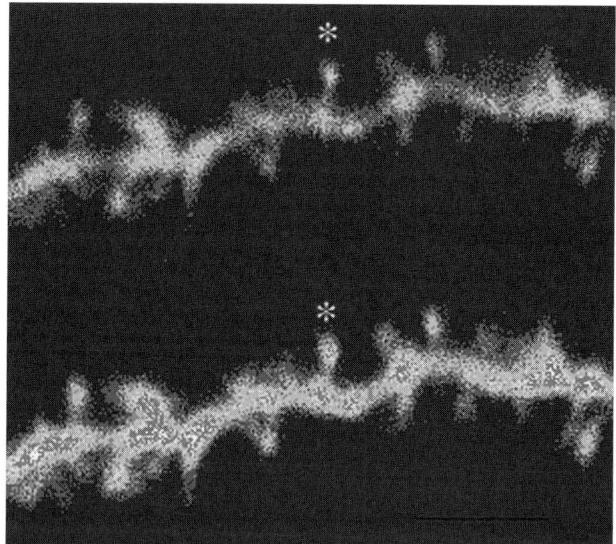

FIGURE 3.8 Two photon images of spines on a dendritic branch. The fluophore is Oregon Green BAPTA-1, a calcium indicator that becomes more intensely fluorescent when the level of calcium in the neuron increases. The upper image is this portion of the branch under baseline conditions of slice physiology. The lower image shows when the neuron is induced to fire repeated action potentials with injection of positive current. Action potentials open voltage-gated calcium channels along the dendrites and in the spines. One spine is marked by an asterisk to facilitate comparisons between low and high conditions of calcium influx. The influx of calcium raises the intensity of the indicator.

than the hours they usually survive under typical slice conditions), or working with "neuronal-like" cell lines (cells originally from a tumor that will replicate themselves). The last are frequently transformed genetically so that they express certain receptors or ion channels that an electrophysiologist wishes to further characterize. For example, transfecting a cell line with different subunits of a particular channel in varying proportions permits one to investigate the kinetic properties of channels with different combinations of subunits. One way one could approach this question would be with single-channel recording. Generally, one patches onto a cell, much the same way one would patch onto a neuron in slice. Then the electrode is pulled away. Depending on the technique, this can enable one to record from a small piece of membrane in several possible configurations. The single-channel approach allows the detailed examination of the kinetics of channel gating by different modulators and, in combination with genetically altered amino acids in channel subunits, the ability to understand which amino acids are critical for ion permeability through the pore or which endow vulnerability to various ion channel toxins.

ELECTROPHYSIOLOGY OF PSYCHOTROPIC DRUG ACTION

Mental illness is an example of a subtle dysfunction of normal neuronal communication. Our understanding of what triggers and perpetuates these illnesses is still in its infancy. Most medicines for psychiatric illness have been found serendipitously and not by design. Although these drugs effectively resolve many psychiatric symptoms, we are unclear how they work for the most part. Although the initial receptor targets of drugs are known, the mechanisms through which they have their chronic therapeutic effects are not clear. In this section, several classes of psychoactive drugs are explored from the perspective of basic electrophysiology. In each case, a brief example is given of how we have come to better understand the initial or chronic action of such drugs using electrophysiological techniques. Because it is not feasible to study the neurophysiology of mental illness directly, where relevant, we also briefly describe possible animal models that may be helpful in the study of neuronal physiology relevant to mental illness.

Anxiolytics

Several drugs to relieve anxiety—such as benzodiazepines, barbiturates, and even alcohol—work by enhancing inhibitory neurotransmission through the GABA system. They are the rare psychoactive drugs in which the acute action is also the therapeutic one; their therapeutic effects are directly correlated to the current blood level of the drug in the person taking it. Anxiolytics work by potentiating the $GABA_A$ receptor. As described in a previous section, the $GABA_A$ receptor is an ionotropic receptor that opens a chloride channel, tending to make the neuron less excitable, partly through hyperpolarization, and therefore less likely to be brought to spike threshold by an excitatory stimulus.

Benzodiazepines bind to a site on the $GABA_A$ receptor that increases the probability that GABA binding will open the chloride channel. They increase the chance that chloride can flow down its concentration gradient and hyperpolarize the neuron. In short, benzodiazepines potentiate the effect of synaptically released GABA. Barbiturates take this action one step further by increasing the duration of individual channel openings. Because GABA is the major inhibitory neurotransmitter in the brain, the anticonvulsant and sleep-inducing properties of these drugs are not surprising. Side effects such as withdrawal insomnia and withdrawal convulsions can be serious. Currently, dose level and metabolic clearance of the drug are the variables that are manipulated to try to maximize the therapeutic effect while minimizing side effects.

It is not well understood which regions of the brain are particularly involved in the antianxiety action of these drugs. Yet it appears that $GABA_A$ receptors are actually a heterogeneous population made up of different combinations of subunits. Certain combinations appear to be limited to regions of the brain, such as the amygdala and the limbic circuit, that are particularly involved in generating anxiety disorders. This may allow for the modification of the drugs to create compounds affecting the GABA system that are able to discriminate between anxiolytic, anticonvulsant, and sleep-inducing effects.

Another approach to anxiety disorders is through manipulating neuromodulatory systems such as serotonin or norepinephrine. One reason to focus on these systems is not necessarily because they are thought to be involved in the etiology of the illness, but because they are more limited in their actions. They modulate glutamate and GABA transmission, which means through neuromodulators one can manipulate glutamate and GABA transmission indirectly. Such indirect manipulation has less potential for extreme side effects (precipitating seizures or unconsciousness) than drugs that affect the glutamate or GABA systems directly.

Psychotomimetics

Psychotomimetics or hallucinogens are not used to treat mental illness; in fact, they can exacerbate schizophrenia and other types of psychosis. However, they give us an interesting window into the neurobiology of hallucinations and sensory perturbations. The effects of hallucinogens on an array of complex integrative processes such as cognition, perception, and mood suggest the involvement of the cerebral cortex. There are two major classes of psychotomimetics: psychedelics and NMDA antagonists. Both have been considered relevant animal models of psychosis.

The psychotomimetic effect of psychedelic hallucinogens depends on their stimulation of serotonin 5-HT_{2A} receptors. Slice physiology experiments in cerebral cortex have shown that selective stimulation of 5-HT_{2A} receptors decreases the threshold for recurrent network activity and enhances its duration far beyond that normally seen (Lambe and Aghajanian, 2007). This effect of selective 5-HT_{2A} stimulation in cortex might be responsible for the sensory perturbations that people experience after taking psychedelic hallucinogens. Network activity has been suggested to provide a "context" in which information is interpreted and decisions are made. It has been hypothesized that aberrations in the modulation of network activity may account for the perceptual and cognitive abnormalities in schizophrenia. Normal modulation of network activity may work to enhance cortical efficiency by changing the signal-to-noise ratio.

The results of brain imaging studies by Vollenweider and colleagues tend to support this hypothesis (Vollenweider and Geyer, 2001; Vollenweider et al., 1997). They show that psilocybin, another 5-HT_{2A} receptor agonist, tends to activate the frontal cortex, and this activation correlates with the onset of sensory perturbations. Serotonin, the endogenous agonist of this receptor, does not cause this phenomenon. Most likely, this is due to its opposing actions through other receptors, such as the 5-HT_{1A} receptor. Whereas the 5-HT_{2A} receptor tends to inactivate potassium conductances and make neurons more excitable, 5-HT_{1A} receptor tends to activate potassium currents and make neurons less excitable. These opposing actions appear to have ramifications for psychoactive drugs such as the selective serotonin reuptake inhibitors (SSRIs) that tend to increase serotonin at synapses in the brain.

NMDA antagonists such as phencyclidine (PCP) and ketamine are dissociative anesthetics. In short, at high concentrations they are anesthetic and at lower concentrations they produce psychosis in adults (these psychiatric side effects do not occur in children, and ketamine is routinely used in pediatric anesthesia). Phencyclidine intoxication causes effects in otherwise healthy people that mimic positive and negative symptoms of schizophrenia, and it exacerbates psychotic symptoms in people with schizophrenia. Phencyclidine and ketamine are known to act as noncompetitive antagonists of the NMDA receptor, a subtype of glutamate receptor discussed previously. These antagonists bind to the open pore NMDA receptors and block the flow of cations through the channels. However, they do not block the AMPA subtype of glutamate receptors. It appears that blocking glutamate transmission through NMDA receptors increases glutamate release and excessively stimulates AMPA receptors in certain regions of the brain, including the prefrontal cortex. Although this increased stimulation of glutamate receptors in prefrontal cortex appears to differ from that induced by psychedelic hallucinogens, suppressing excessive glutamate release ameliorates many of the adverse behavioral effects in both cases.

Antidepressants

The most commonly prescribed antidepressants, the SSRIs, increase serotonin in the brain by blocking the mechanism that actively removes serotonin from synapse. Over a period of chronic administration, this tends to desensitize the autoreceptors on serotonergic neurons, such that the feedback mechanism that normally limits the release of serotonin requires much higher levels of serotonin to be activated. It has been suggested that one possible explanation why some people may be vulnerable to developing depression is that their 5-HT_{1A} autoreceptors might be hypersensitive, which would tend to clamp down on the release of serotonin into the cortex. The time lag required for desensitization of the autoreceptors might explain why a therapeutic improvement is not observed until 2–3 weeks after onset of drug treatment. Single-cell recordings suggest that repeated daily administration of antidepressants enhances the effects of 5-HT in the forebrain with a time course that parallels the therapeutic effects of antidepressants (Mongeau et al., 1997).

Stress can be used to produce animal models of depression. Preclinical and clinical studies have demonstrated that stress and depression result in cell atrophy and loss in limbic and cortical brain regions (Duman and Monteggia, 2006). These effects can be reversed with such diverse antidepressant treatments as SSRIs, electroconvulsive shock, and exercise. Interestingly, a number of gene products that mediate neurotrophin and growth factor signaling are reduced in depressed patients and in stressed animals. Antidepressant treatments, by contrast, elevate the expression of multiple genes involved in neurotrophin signaling pathways. Together, these findings implicate neurotrophic factors in the etiology and treatment of depression. Some electrophysiology studies of the neurotrophic hypothesis of depression have examined the properties of new neurons generated in the dentate through adult neurogenesis (van Praag et al., 2002) and their contributions to synaptic plasticity in the hippocampus (Ge et al., 2007). Other electrophysiology studies have used transgenic mice with alterations of neurotrophic factors or receptors to assess the effects of long-term changes in these systems on brain physiology (Rios et al., 2006).

Antipsychotics

Like most psychoactive drugs, antipsychotic drugs were discovered serendipitously. Although chlorpromazine, the original antipsychotic, had actions at many receptors, its ability to act as an antagonist at the dopamine D_2 receptor turned out to be critical. Although there are many antipsychotic drugs today, almost every single one has some ability to downregulate the activation of D_2 receptors by endogenous dopamine, either by direct antagonism or by partial agonism (Kapur and Remington, 2001). Positron emission tomography (PET) imaging studies have used radiolabeled versions of these drugs to assess the degree and length of binding. For the typical antipsychotic, reduction of "positive" symptoms (for example, *pychosis, hallucinations, delusions*) requires the antipsychotic drug to have bound to ~65% of D_2 receptors. However, there is a very narrow window of binding before motor side effects, called *extrapyramidal symptoms*, set in at binding higher than 70%. A major development in psychiatry has been the emergence of an antipsychotic drug, *clozapine*, that does not cause these motor side effects. It is often referred to as an atypical antipsychotic in contrast to previous "typical" antipsychotics such as chlorpromazine and haloperidol. Of perhaps even greater significance is the fact that clozapine, unlike typical antipsychotics, treats negative symptoms of schizophrenia (for example, *flat affect, anhedonia, withdrawal*).

The emergence of clozapine has focused more recent research on differences between typical antipsychotics and clozapine. The latter has a very complicated profile of action that includes effects at dopamine, norepinephrine, serotonin, acetylcholine, and histamine receptors. Clozapine is a significantly more potent 5-HT_{2A} antagonist and a significantly less potent D_2 antagonist compared to the typical antipsychotics. This pattern, together with the large body of work on the psychotomimetic effects of 5-HT_{2A} agonists, awakened interested in the therapeutic effects of a pure 5-HT_{2A} antagonist. However, this drug did not succeed in clinical trials. It may be clozapine's more moderate action at D_2 receptors, rather than its ability to block pure 5-HT_{2A} receptors, which is responsible for its ability to improve negative symptoms as well as its reduced propensity to induce motor side effects.

One hypothesis that has been proposed to explain the clinical efficacy of antipsychotic drugs relates to the "depolarization block" of midbrain dopamine neurons projecting to the prefrontal cortex (Bunney, 1992). The blockade of autoreceptors on dopaminergic neurons leads to chronic depolarization of these neurons, which prevents the relief from sodium channel inactivation. Electrophysiological experiments revealed that one difference between clozapine and typical antipsychotics is that chronic administration of clozapine results in depolarization block only of the midbrain dopaminergic cells that project to the medial prefrontal cortex, whereas chronic administration of typical antipsychotics results in depolarization block of the neostriatum as well as the medial prefrontal cortex. This former is thought to account for the extrapyramidal symptoms associated with typical antipsychotics.

There have been several animal models postulated for schizophrenia. The psychotomimetic drug model of the disease has proved informative about what types of neurotransmission are involved in acute psychosis. The amphetamine model has proved useful for understanding the paranoid state. However, given the evidence for neurodevelopmental abnormalities in schizophrenia, several groups of researchers have tried to model this illness in rodents through lesions early in development (Lipska and Weinberger, 2000). One such model, involving lesions to the ventral-hippocampus, has been shown to result in the postpubertal onset of dopaminergic abnormalities (Goto and O'Donnell, 2002) similar to what is hypothesized to occur in schizophrenia. These animal models will allow the in vivo electrophysiological examination of how an early brain lesion alters interactions between the dopaminergic and glutamatergic systems in adulthood.

OVERVIEW AND FUTURE DIRECTIONS

This chapter explored how basic electrophysiology can be used to clarify how neurons communicate with each other and how different drugs affect this signaling. Appreciating how a neuron maintains its electrical state and ability to release neurotransmitter onto other cells is critical to appreciating the many subtle ways that thought can be influenced by psychoactive drugs. However, an understanding of neurophysiological mechanisms mediating the action of psychotropic drugs can provide only limited insight into the underlying factors involved in the development and expression of psychiatric disorders. Recent progress in the molecular genetics of schizophrenia and mood disorders promises to provide new opportunities for targeting electrophysiological studies toward uncovering the role of susceptibility genes in these illnesses. Notable examples include studies on neuregulin 1 (NRG1) and its receptor erbB4, which have been associated robustly with schizophrenia through linkage analysis. Several recent electrophysiological studies in brain slice or primary culture preparations have shown that NRG1 and erbB4 regulate transmission at glutamate and GABA synapses (Fischbach, 2007). These findings raise the possibility of investigating, directly or indirectly, synaptic defects underlying the clinical phenotype of schizophrenia as well as other psychiatric disorders.

REFERENCES

Aghajanian, G.K., and Marek, G.J. (1999) Serotonin and hallucinogens. *Neuropsychopharm.* 21:16S–23S.

Bunney, B.S. (1992) Clozapine: a hypothesized mechanism for its unique clinical profile. *Br. J. Psychiatry* 160 (Suppl. 17):17–21.

Duman, R.S., and Monteggia, L.M. (2006) A neurotrophic model for stress-related mood disorders. *Biol. Psychiatry* 59:1116–1127

Fischbach, G.D. (2007) NRG1 and synaptic function in the CNS. *Neuron* 54:495–497.

Ge, S., Yang, C.H., Hsu, K.S., Ming, G.L., and Song, H. (2007) A critical period for enhanced synaptic plasticity in newly generated neurons of the adult brain. *Neuron* 54:559–566.

Goto, Y., and O'Donnell, P. (2002) Delayed mesolimbic system alteration in a developmental animal model of schizophrenia. *J. Neurosci.* 22:9070–9077.

Kapur, S., and Remington, G. (2001) Dopamine D(2) receptors and their role in atypical antipsychotic action: still necessary and may even be sufficient. *Biol. Psychiatry* 50:873–883.

Lambe, E.K., and Aghajanian, G.K. (2007) Prefrontal cortical network activity: opposite effects of psychedelic hallucinogens and D1/D5 dopamine receptor activation. *Neuroscience* 145: 900–910.

Lipska, B.K., and Weinberger, D.R. (2000) To model a psychiatric disorder in animals: schizophrenia as a reality test. *Neuropsychopharm.* 23:223–239.

Mongeau, R., Blier, P., and de Montigny, C. (1997) The serotonergic and noradrenergic systems of the hippocampus: their interactions and the effects of antidepressant treatments. *Brain Res. Reviews* 23:145–195.

Rios, M., Lambe, E.K., Liu, R., Teillon, S., Liu, J., Akbarian, S., Roffler-Tarlov, S., Jaenisch, R., and Aghajanian, G.K. (2006) Severe deficits in 5-HT2A-mediated neurotransmission in BDNF conditional mutant mice. *J. Neurobiol.* 66:408–420.

van Praag, H., Schinder, A.F., Christie, B.R., Toni, N., Palmer, T.D., and Gage, F.H. (2002) Functional neurogenesis in the adult hippocampus. *Nature* 415:1030–1034.

Vollenweider, F.X., and Geyer, M.A. (2001) A systems model of altered consciousness: integrating natural and drug-induced psychoses. *Brain Res. Bull.* 56:495–507.

Vollenweider, F.X., Leenders, K.L., Scharfetter, C., Maguire P., Stadelmann, O., and Angst, J. (1997) Positron emission tomography and fluorodeoxyglucose studies of metabolic hyperfrontality and psychopathology in the psilocybin model of psychosis. *Neuropsychopharm.* 16:357–372.

4 Principles of Signal Transduction

JEAN-ANTOINE GIRAULT AND PAUL GREENGARD

SIGNAL TRANSDUCTION

All cells react to changes in their environment and to clues that may be important for their survival and/or function. This is true for unicellular as well as multicellular organisms. Unicellular organisms react to light, to chemical gradients of nutrients, and to specific molecules released by other cells from the same species. In multicellular organisms, the harmonious functioning of billions of cells, assembled in tissues as sophisticated as the human brain, requires a highly complex network of intercellular signaling involving molecules known as *hormones, neurotransmitters, cytokines, growth factors*, etc. Yet the molecular mechanisms by which these signals are perceived and interpreted by individual cells are quite similar to those used by much simpler unicellular beings. Indeed, work over the past few years has demonstrated an amazing degree of conservation of many of these molecular mechanisms among brewer's yeast (*Saccharomyces*), nematode worms (*Caenorhabditis elegans*), fruit flies (*Drosophila*), and mammals, including humans. In addition, specialized cells, such as the cones or the rods in the retina, or the olfactory epithelial cells, have retained the ability to perceive changes in the physical or chemical environment. These specialized cells translate information from the external world into changes in neuronal activity that can be communicated to the rest of the organism.

The term *signal transduction* is used to describe the cascades of biochemical reactions by which cells translate various extracellular signals into appropriate responses, whether the primary extracellular signal comes from other cells or from the external world. Signal transduction involves a number of key players and reactions that we examine successively. The initial reaction involves a "receptor," the protein that interacts with the extracellular signal and triggers its effects. Subsequently, a series of reactions of varying degrees of complexity ensues, resulting in a vast array of physiological responses. In many instances, the coupling between receptors and effector pathways requires an intermediate agent, a guanosine 5′-triphosphate (GTP)-binding protein or *G protein*, which acts as a molecular switch, and the generation of a second messenger. Second messengers are small molecules that are generated within cells in response to extracellular signals (the latter correspond to "first messengers"). One particular class of signaling molecules comprises small molecules that can readily cross biological membranes and act as intercellular messengers and second messengers. Such molecules include fatty acids such as arachidonic acid, and the gas nitric oxide. The major covalent modification of proteins involved in signal transduction is phosphorylation. This modification has been shown to result in changes of innumerable biological properties of nerve cells, such as activation of biosynthetic enzymes, activation of transcription factors, regulation of the permeability of ion channels, regulation of neurotransmitter release, and alteration of the sensitivity to neurotransmitters.

GENERAL PROPERTIES OF SIGNAL TRANSDUCTION PATHWAYS

Signal transduction pathways have a number of important properties in common that are interesting to consider before describing these pathways in details.

First, many signaling cascades have a tremendous capability of signal amplification. This explains why, in some instances, cells are able to detect only a single photon—in the case of retina photoreceptor cells—or a few molecules in their environment. A second property is specificity. Cells are able to discriminate between a virtually unlimited number of extracellular molecules and to react to very few of them. Moreover, different signals acting on the same cells will have different effects. This is true in spite of the fact that receptor proteins belong to a limited number of classes and that many of the components of the signaling cascades are rather ubiquitous. Thus, during development, a characteristic set of genes, the products of which are involved in signal transduction, is selected in each cell type, providing it with the capability to react in an appropriate way to specific signals. A third important characteristic of signal transduction pathways is their pleiotropy. Thus, a single extracellular signal can generate multiple responses in the cell. For instance, a single neurotransmitter can trigger the opening of some ion channels and the closing of others, the activation of multiple enzymes, the modification of cytoskeletal organization, and the stimulation of the expression of specific genes.

Another property of signal transduction pathways is that they allow the integration of several simultaneous or successive signals. The cascades of reactions triggered by each signal interact with the others at many levels, sometimes reinforcing each other, sometimes canceling each other. As a result, the final output in terms of cellular response is a subtle combination of what would have been induced by each extracellular signal separately and may indeed be quite different from responses to individual signals. Some signals may, for instance, have little effect by themselves yet inhibit or potentiate considerably the response to other signals. In the nervous system this property is called *neuromodulation*. These properties of integration and transformation of multiple signaling pathways are often quite complex, and computer modeling is necessary to help predict their output.

Finally, the response to extracellular signals can have long-lasting effects on cells and modify their subsequent response to the same or other signals. One obvious example involves gene expression: One hormone, for instance, will induce the expression of a gene necessary for the response to a neurotransmitter. In fact, there are many different ways by which such long-lasting changes in cellular responses can be implemented. They represent the molecular basis for "cellular" learning and memory, a capacity that all cells possess to some extent. Thus at any given time the response of a cell to external signals depends on its previous history. Such mechanisms have a special importance in neurons in which they represent the cellular basis for synaptic plasticity, which is thought to underlie "psychological" learning and memory (Chapter 5).

THE IMPORTANCE OF ELUCIDATING SIGNAL TRANSDUCTION PATHWAYS

Deciphering the complex networks of reactions that constitute signal transduction pathways is important for understanding the physiology of cells and multicellular organisms, including the human brain. Moreover, such understanding is certainly critical for elucidating the mechanisms of diseases that are still elusive, and eventually treating them. It is easy to understand that dysfunctions of signal transduction pathways will have profound and deleterious consequences on the properties of cells. This point is well illustrated by the fact that cancers result from the dysfunction of signaling pathways that regulate cell growth and division. Similarly, many naturally occurring toxins exert their effects by interrupting or diverting normal intracellular signaling pathways. The causes of several types of mental retardation of genetic origin have been identified as mutations in genes' coding for signaling proteins. It seems likely that, as our knowledge of signal transduction in neurons progresses, we will discover that alterations of signal transduction pathways play an important role in a number of neurological or psychiatric diseases. In addition, the multiple enzymes involved in these pathways represent potential targets for therapeutic drugs. Lithium is one example of a drug that is already used in psychiatry and is thought to exert its effect by acting on signal transduction mechanisms (see below). The study of complete genomes sequences, including those of brewers yeast (*Saccharomyces cerevisiae*), a plant (*Arabidopsis thaliana*), a round worm (*Caenorhabditis elegans*), fruit fly (*Drosophila melanogaster*), and human (*Homo sapiens*), allows an estimation of the number of genes devoted to signal transduction in various eukaryotic organisms (Table 4.1). Comparison of signaling networks in organisms of various complexities provides useful information about their organizing and functioning principles. Exhaustive identification of the components of such networks in humans pinpoints potential candidates for genetic alterations that may underlie neurological or psychiatric disease, or more likely enhance the susceptibility to such diseases. It also provides novel targets for designing new pharmacological tools aimed at modifying specific signaling pathways either to correct natural deficits or to counteract the consequences of their alterations, regardless of the cause of these alterations.

RECEPTORS: HOW CELLS DETECT EXTRACELLULAR SIGNALS

Cells can detect chemical as well as physical signals from their environment. We concentrate on chemical signals that are the more relevant for understanding brain physiology. The first step in signal transduction is the interaction of the extracellular signaling molecule with a receptor. A receptor is a protein that is able to bind the signaling molecule with high affinity and specificity and to trigger a biological response in reaction to this binding. Extracellular signaling molecules include neurotransmitters, hormones, growth factors, and related substances and can be divided into two broad categories: those that do not penetrate the cells and act at the level of the plasma membrane and those that readily penetrate the cells and act on intracellular targets. It should be emphasized that these two mechanisms of action are not always exclusive and that compounds such as steroid hormones appear to have membrane receptors in addition to their well-characterized intracellular receptors.

Signals That Act at the Level of the Plasma Membrane

Receptors that have been characterized at the level of the plasma membrane can be divided into several classes depending on their organization and properties. Representatives of each of these classes of receptors are present in neurons, where they play diverse roles.

TABLE 4.1. *Estimated Number of Genes Coding for Proteins Involved in Signal Transduction*

Protein family	*Human*	*Fly*	*Worm*	*Yeast*	*Mustard Weed*
Eukaryotic protein kinases[a]	575	319	437	121	1049
Ser/Thr and dual specificity protein kinases[b]	395	198	315	114	1102
Tyr protein kinases[b]	106	47	100	5	16
Ser/Thr protein phosphatases[b]	15	19	51	13	29
Tyr and dual specificity protein phosphatases[a]	112	35	108	12	21
Cyclic nucleotide phosphodiesterases[b]	25	8	6	1	0
G protein–coupled receptors[a]	569	97	358	0	16
G protein alpha[b]	27	10	22	2	5
G protein beta[b]	5	3	2	1	1
G protein gamma[b]	13	2	2	0	0
Ras superfamily[b]	141	64	62	26	86
SH2 domains	119[a]	39[b]	48[b]	1	3[b]
SH3 domains	215[a]	75[b]	62[a]	27[b]	4[b]
Voltage–gated Ca^{2+} channels alpha subunits[b]	32	7	10	2	2
Caspases[b]	13	7	3	0	0
Nuclear hormone receptors[b]	59	25	183	1	4

Note: The numbers are given for human (*Homo sapiens*), fly (*Drosophila melanogaster*), round worm (*Caenorhabditis elegans*), yeast (*Saccharomyces cerevisiae*), and mustard weed (*Arabidopsis thaliana*). Because the sequencing and analysis of the genomes of these organisms is not fully complete, these numbers represent only lower limits. Data in human are based on the publications by the International Human Genome Sequencing Consortium (*Nature*, 2001 409:860–921) indicated by [a] and by Celera genomics and associates (*Science*, 2001 291:1304–1351) indicated by [b].

Neurotransmitter-gated ion channels

Biological membranes are impermeable to small ions including Na^+, K^+, Ca^{2+}, and Cl^- (Chapter 3). The concentrations of these ions are very different in the intracellular and extracellular compartments, due to the existence of active transport mechanisms. Ion channels are proteins that form pores within the membranes and allow the selective flow of specific ions to which they are permeable. The magnitude and direction of ion flow depend on two forces: the concentration gradient and the electrical potential difference between the two sides of the membrane. Opening or closing of one class of channels allows or blocks flow of ions to which this class of channels is permeable. This, in turn, regulates the electrical potential across the membrane. At rest, the intracellular side of the membrane is electronegative as compared to the extracellular side (usually −60 to −80 mV).

The opening of several ion channels is directly regulated by neurotransmitters. Such channels are called *neurotransmitter-gated channels* or *ionotropic receptors* (Box 4.1). The neurotransmitter binds to the ion channel and triggers its opening by inducing a change in its conformation. Since no intermediate biochemical reaction is involved, the effects of neurotransmitters on ligand-gated channels are very fast. This type of receptor underlies most of the fast synaptic excitatory or inhibitory transmission in brain. In addition, the response of ionotropic receptors to neurotransmitters can be regulated by several extracellular or intracellular signals, providing a fine tuning of their properties (see the examples of glutamate *N*-methyl-D-aspartate [NMDA] receptor and γ-aminobutyric acid [GABA-A] receptor, Box 4.1). Such modulatory sites are targets for molecules of great pharmacological importance, including benzodiazepines and barbiturates which increase the response to GABA (Box 4.1).

G protein-coupled receptors

A large number of receptors work in close association with heterotrimeric GTP-binding proteins or G proteins that are composed of three subunits (α, β, and γ; Box 4.2). Although these receptors belong to several different gene families, they have a major structural feature in common, which has been conserved throughout evolution: *the polypeptide chain of these receptors crosses the plasma membrane seven times*. Therefore, these receptors are called *7-transmembrane domain receptors* or *serpentine receptors*. When these receptors bind their specific ligand, they undergo a conformational change that has consequences for the associated G protein (Box 4.2), leading to the dissociation of a GTP-bound α subunit and β/γ complex, each of which is able to interact with various targets including ion channels and enzymes (Box 4.7). Interestingly, these G protein–coupled receptors are also involved in the detection of clues from the environment: receptors for odors, pheromones, and light belong to this category.

BOX 4.1 *Neurotransmitter-Gated Ion Channels*

The neurotransmitter receptors responsible for fast synaptic transmission are ligand-gated ion channels. They comprise several subunits arranged in such a way as to form a central pore through which ions can cross the plasma membrane. Binding of the neurotransmitter triggers the opening of this pore. Neurotransmitter-gated ion channels are specific for one or several ions, the nature of which is responsible for their excitatory or inhibitory effects.

Receptors for excitatory neurotransmitters such as acetylcholine (nicotinic subtype), or glutamate (subtypes named after chemicals not present in the brain but which are specific agonists: [RS]-alpha-amino-3-hydroxy-5-methyl-4-isoxazolepropionic acid [AMPA] and kainate), let Na^+ ions flow into the neuron, and K^+ ions flow out (Fig. 4.1A). At resting potential, the Na^+ influx predominates and is responsible for the depolarizing, excitatory effects of these neurotransmitters. The open state of neurotransmitter-gated ion channels is usually unstable. They switch spontaneously to a desensitized state, in which the ion channel is closed, although the neurotransmitter is still bound with high affinity. Desensitization is thought to be a protective mechanism against overstimulation.

NMDA receptors are a subtype of glutamate receptors, named after their specific synthetic agonist (N-*methyl-D-aspartate*), that have a number of unique properties (Fig. 4.1B). First, glycine must also be bound to these receptors for them to open in response to glutamate. Second, at resting membrane potential, when NMDA receptors open, they are obstructed by Mg^{2+} ions. This block is relieved only when the membrane is depolarized simultaneously by another mechanism (for example, stimulation of nearby glutamate receptors of the AMPA subtype). Finally, in addition to Na^+ and K^+, NMDA receptors are highly permeable to Ca^{2+}. The resulting Ca^{2+} influx is responsible for the role of NMDA receptors in synaptic plasticity and also for its deleterious, excitotoxic effects in pathological conditions.

Receptors for GABA (GABA-A subtype, Fig. 4.1C) and glycine (not shown) are selectively permeable to Cl^- ions. In most instances, the resulting Cl^- influx is responsible for the inhibitory effects of these neurotransmitters. GABA-A receptors account for most of the inhibitory receptors in the central nervous system, whereas glycine receptors are restricted to the brain stem and spinal cord. GABA-A receptors are modulated by two drugs that have important clinical applications. Benzodiazepines (for example, diazepam) or barbiturates (for example, phenobarbital), although they cannot open the GABA-A ion channel by themselves, increase the response to GABA. The existence and the nature of endogenous ligands for the benzodiazepine and barbiturate modulatory sites on GABA-A receptors are still a matter of dispute.

Other abbreviations: GABA: γ-aminobutyric acid.

Further reading: Cull-Candy et al., 2001; Nutt and Malizia, 2001; Mohler et al., 2002; Johnston, 2005; Mayer, 2005; Benarroch, 2007; Dani and Bertrand, 2007; Derkach et al., 2007.

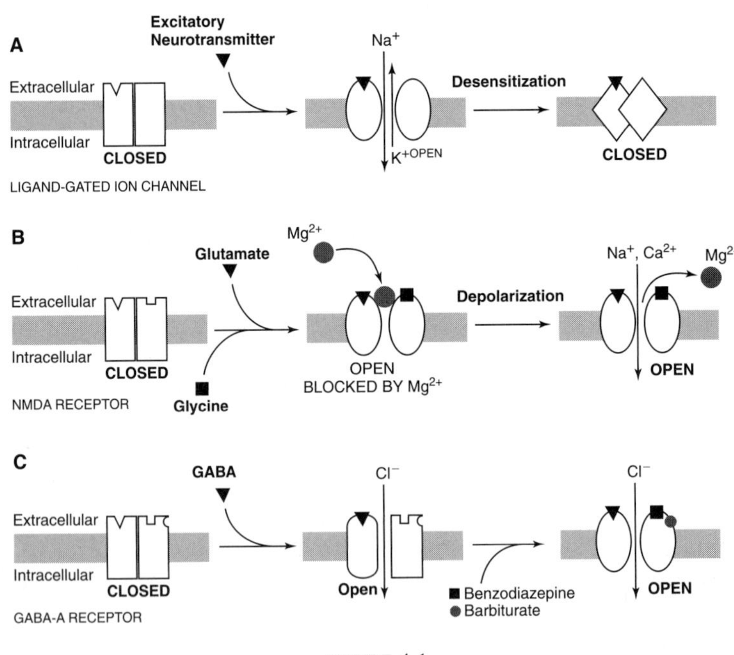

FIGURE 4.1

BOX 4.2 *G Protein–Coupled Receptors*

A large number of neurotransmitter receptors belong to the category of seven transmembrane domain *G protein–coupled receptors*, which also includes receptors for hormones, light, odorants, pheromones, and Ca^{2+}. These receptors are associated with heterotrimeric G proteins (see Box 4.7). Heterotrimeric G proteins comprise three subunits: α, β, and γ. They are not transmembrane proteins but are associated with the membrane by covalently bound fatty acid molecules. In the resting state, GDP is bound to the α subunit, which is closely attached to the β/γ complex. When the neurotransmitter binds to the receptor, the conformation of the receptor changes, inducing a change in the conformation of the α subunit, which expels GDP and replaces it by GTP. GTP-bound α subunit is no longer capable of interacting with the receptor or β/γ. Instead, GTP-bound α and β/γ diffuse away from each other and from the receptor, while still attached to the membrane, and interact with specific targets. After a short time GTP is hydrolyzed to GDP, and GDP-bound α reassociates with β/γ. At about the same time, the neurotransmitter leaves its receptor, which returns to its resting state and reassociates with α-GDP and β/γ.

There are several different types of α, β, and γ subunits, encoded by different genes. The nature of the α subunit that associates with a given receptor determines the actions that can be triggered by this receptor. β/γ subunits have their own effects on similar targets that can be in the same direction as that of their cognate α subunit, or, sometimes, in the opposite direction. β/γ subunits have additional specific properties, such as recruiting to the membrane a protein kinase (*G protein–coupled receptor kinase* or GRK) which phosphorylates the receptor and prevents its further interaction with G proteins. This represents an important mechanism of desensitization of G protein–coupled receptors.

Other abbreviations: G protein: guanine nucleotide binding protein; GDP: guanosine 5′-diphosphate; GTP: guanosine 5′-triphosphate; Pi: inorganic phosphate.

Further reading: Bockaert and Pin, 1999; Gainetdinov et al., 2004; DeWire et al., 2007; May et al., 2007; Moore et al., 2007.

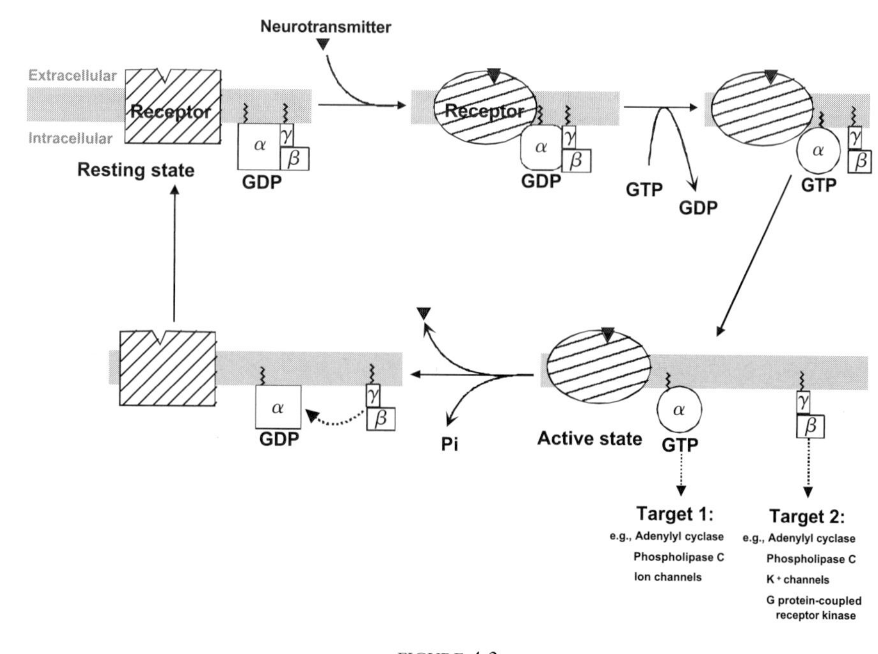

FIGURE 4.2

Receptors that are themselves enzymes

Some receptors are transmembrane proteins that are composed of an extracellular domain that binds the extracellular signaling molecule, a single transmembrane domain, and an intracellular domain that possesses an enzymatic activity. Binding of the ligand to the extracellular domain dramatically alters the activity of the intracellular enzymatic domain. This activation often results from the dimerization of the receptor.

The best known receptors in this category are tyrosine kinase receptors for polypeptide growth factors, including nerve growth factor (NGF) and related neurotrophins (Box 4.3). Their ligands are polypeptides that are often soluble but can also be attached to the membrane of other cells. The intracellular domain of this type of receptor is a protein kinase, which is able to phosphorylate itself and other proteins on tyrosines (see Box 4.14). Phosphorylation on tyrosine triggers cascades of reactions that are detailed in Boxes 4.3, 4.4, and 4.8.

A variation on the same theme is represented by receptors that do not possess an enzymatic activity by

BOX 4.3 *Protein Tyrosine Kinase Receptors*

Receptors for many polypeptide growth factors, including nerve growth factor and related neurotrophins, are transmembrane tyrosine kinases. These receptors are composed of a single peptide chain whose extracellular domain can bind the growth factor, whereas the intracytoplasmic domain is a protein tyrosine kinase (see Box 4.14). In the absence of growth factor, the tyrosine kinase is inactive. In the presence of growth factor, two identical receptors interact with each other (*homodimerization*), and this results in the activation of the tyrosine kinase domains. They phosphorylate several tyrosine residues located in each other's sequence (*autophosphorylation*). Autophosphorylation on tyrosine provides docking sites for a number of proteins that possess SH2 domains (see Box 4.4), resulting in the phosphorylation-dependent clustering of several important proteins around the growth factor receptor. These proteins, many of which become phosphorylated on tyrosine, include phospholipase C γ(PLCγ) that hydrolyzes phosphatidylinositol 4,5 bisphosphate into diacylglycerol and inositol 1,4,5 trisphosphate (IP_3, see Boxes 4.10 and 4.12), phosphatidylinositol 3 kinase (PI3 kinase) that phosphorylates phosphatidylinositol at position 3 and activates its own signal transduction pathway, phosphotyrosine phosphatases (PTP), adaptor molecules, and others. Adaptor molecules are proteins that possess, in addition to an SH2 domain, SH3 domains (see Box 4.4). By these SH3 domains the adaptors are bound to proline-rich regions of guanine nucleotide exchange factors (GEF; see Box 4.7). GEF are enzymes that catalyze the exchange of GDP for GTP on small G proteins of the Ras family. Their recruitment to the membrane, mediated by the adaptor, brings them in contact with Ras, which they put in its GTP-bound, active form (see Boxes 4.7 and 4.8). The precise nature of the SH2-containing enzymes or adaptor molecules that are recruited varies from one growth factor receptor to another; however, the principles of signaling are the same in all cases.

Other abbreviations: G protein: guanine nucleotide binding protein; GDP: guanosine 5′-diphosphate; GTP: guanosine 5′-triphosphate; P: phosphate group; SH2: Src-homology domain 2; SH3: Src-homology domain 3.

Further reading: Schlessinger, 2002; Schlessinger and Lemmon, 2003; Kalb, 2005; Papin et al., 2005.

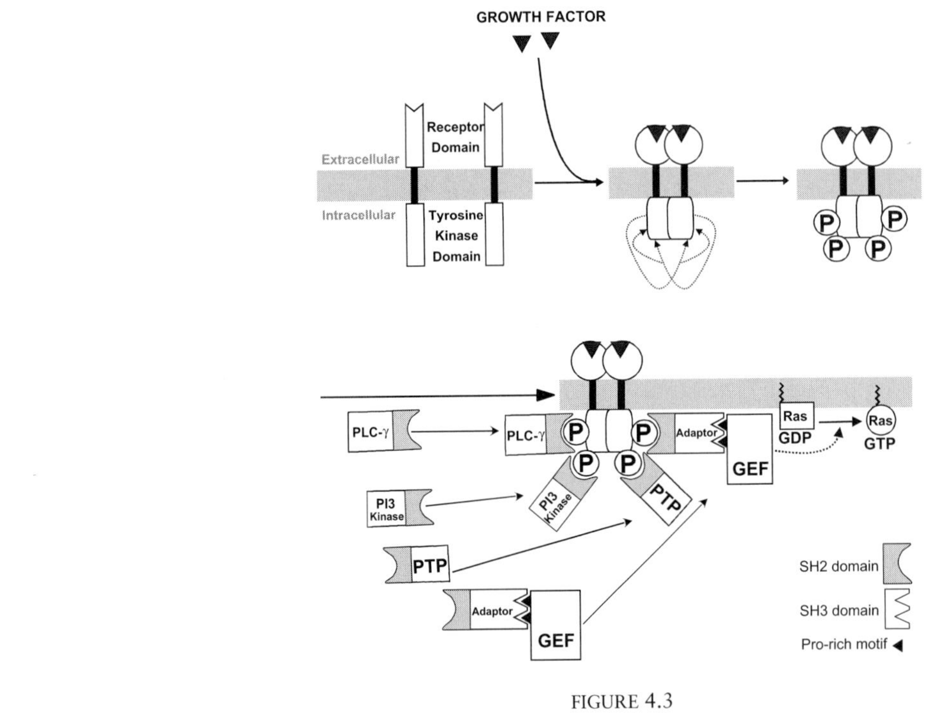

FIGURE 4.3

themselves but that associate with tyrosine kinases. For example, receptors for some neurotrophic factors, such as glial derived neurotrophic factor (GDNF), are extracellular proteins attached to the membrane by a lipid anchor (*glycosyl-phosphatidyl inositol*). Due to their localization, they cannot transduce the signal directly to the interior of the cell. They do it by virtue of their association to a transmembrane protein whose intracellular domain is a tyrosine kinase (c-Ret in the case of GDNF receptor). An important class of receptor comprises transmembrane proteins that have the capability to associate with intracytoplasmic tyrosine kinase. This class includes receptors for key messengers in the immune response (for example, cytokines, interferon),

BOX 4.4 *SH2 and SH3 Domains*

SH2 (Src-homology domain 2) and SH3 (Src-homology domain 3) were first identified in the cytoplasmic tyrosine kinase Src. They have now been recognized in a large number of proteins, many of which are involved in signal transduction.

SH2 domains bind to peptide sequences within proteins that contain a phosphorylated tyrosine. In the absence of phosphorylation, there is no binding. In addition, SH2 domains recognize a few amino acids located on the carboxy-terminal side of the phosphorylated tyrosine, thus providing specificity to this type of interaction: each SH2 domain binds preferentially to specific protein regions phosphorylated on tyrosine.

SH3 domains bind to proline-rich regions that adopt a characteristic conformation. Each SH3 domain reacts preferentially with particular proline-rich sequences, providing specificity to this type of interaction. SH3-mediated interactions are constitutive and do not depend on phosphorylation. In fact, SH3 and proline-rich regions are one example of a large number of pairs of protein domains that are able to interact with each other with high affinity and specificity. These protein–protein interactions are important in signal transduction and in other neuronal functions, such as the clustering of receptors at the postsynaptic sites.

Other abbreviations: P: phosphate group; Tyr: tyrosine.

Further reading: Kuriyan and Cowburn, 1997; Pawson and Scott, 1997; Pawson, 2004.

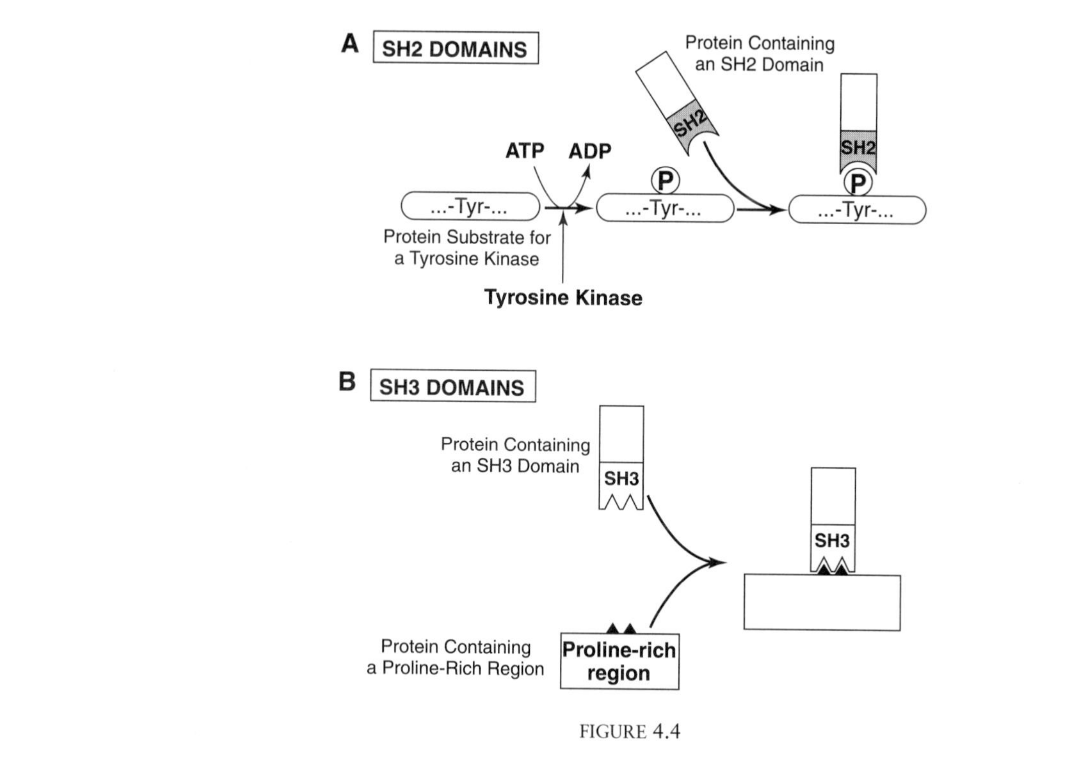

FIGURE 4.4

hormones (for example, growth hormone, prolactin, leptin), and polypeptides that have growth factor activity (for example, erythropoietin, ciliary-derived neurotrophic factor). The intracellular segment of these receptors binds a tyrosine kinase of the JAK family (*Janus kinase*; see Box 4.5). Other types of receptors, including the receptors for the antigen of lymphocytes, have a similar, although more complicated, organization. In this case the enzyme is a member of the Src family of tyrosine kinases. Similarly, integrins, which are receptors for extracellular matrix proteins, associate on their intracellular side with a tyrosine kinase called *FAK* (focal adhesion kinase).

Several other families of receptors are transmembrane proteins that possess other types of enzymatic activities. One group corresponds to receptors for transforming growth factor beta (TGFβ), activin, and inhibin, the intracellular domain of which possesses a protein serine/threonine kinase activity. Another group of receptors, including the receptor for atrial natriuretic factor (ANF), have an intracellular domain that is a guanylyl cyclase, an enzyme that generates the second messenger cyclic guanosine 3′,5′-monophosphate (cGMP). Other receptors, such as those for Fas and tumor necrosis factor α (TNFα), which are able to trigger programmed cell death (apoptosis), associate with various intracellular

BOX 4.5 *JAK-STAT-Coupled Receptors*

A large number of receptors for polypeptide messengers (for example, *cytokines, interferon, growth hormone, prolactin, leptin, erythropoietin, ciliary derived neurotrophic factor*) utilize a tyrosine phosphorylation signaling mechanism. In contrast to the growth factor receptors depicted in Box 4.3, the cytoplasmic domain of these receptors does not possess tyrosine kinase activity. However, this domain is associated with a cytoplasmic tyrosine kinase belonging to the JAK subfamily (these kinases have two tyrosine kinase domains, only one of which is catalytically active, and are called *Janus tyrosine kinase* after the two-faced Roman god). When the receptor binds its ligand, it dimerizes and becomes phosphorylated by the associated JAK tyrosine kinases. Remarkably, activation of this class of receptor can regulate gene expression via a single family of intermediary proteins called *STAT* (signal transducer and activator of transcription). One important consequence of the phosphorylation of the receptor is the recruitment of STAT, which possesses an SH2 domain (Box 4.4). When STAT molecules are bound to the phosphorylated receptor by their SH2 domain, they become phosphorylated by the JAK kinases. This allows a switch in the interaction of the SH2 domain of the two molecules of STAT that, instead of binding to the receptor, bind to each other. The resulting dimer detaches from the receptor and enters the nucleus, where it binds to the promoter region of specific genes and, in combination with several other proteins, induces their transcription (Chapter 6).

Other abbreviations: P: phosphate group; SH2: Src-homology domain 2.

Further reading: Imada and Leonard, 2000; Seidel et al., 2000; Yamaoka et al., 2004; O'Shea et al., 2005.

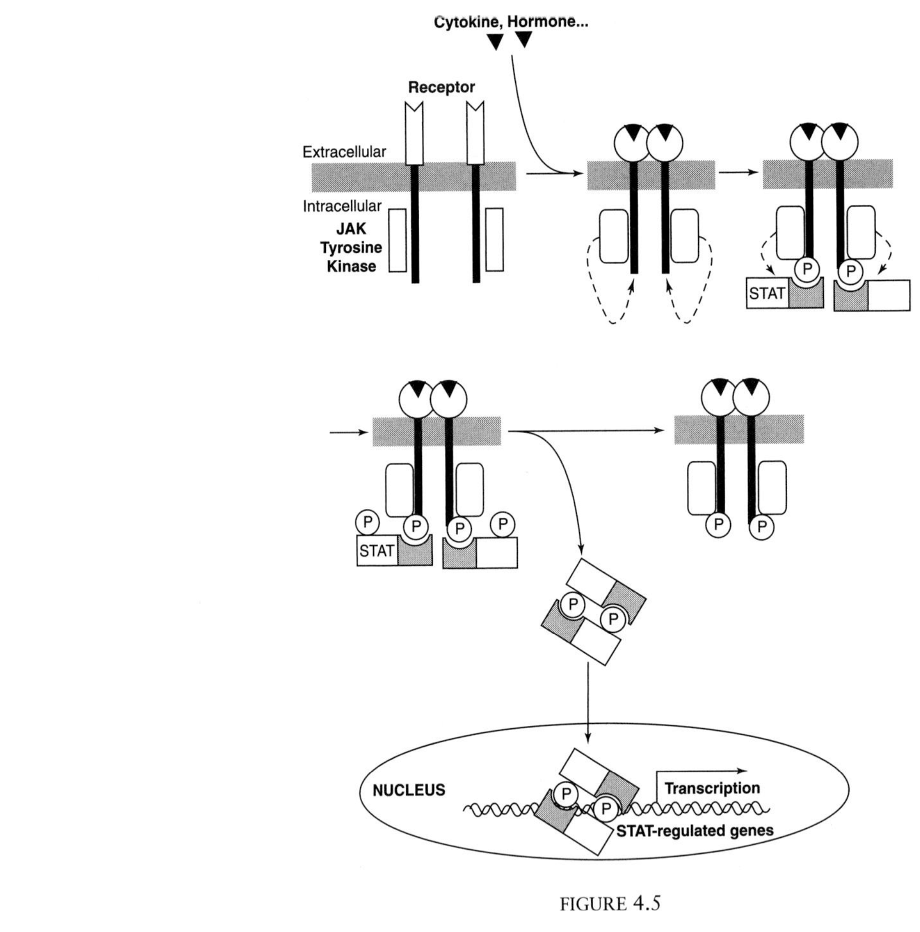

FIGURE 4.5

proteins that, among other things, activate proteolytic enzymes.

Extracellular Signals That Penetrate Cells

Most of the molecules that act on membrane receptors cannot cross the plasma membrane because of their charge, which makes them highly hydrophilic, or their size. On the other hand, some signaling molecules are readily able to cross the lipid bilayer of the plasma membrane because of their hydrophobic nature and/or their small size. These molecules include steroid hormones and the related vitamin D derivatives, thyroid hormones, and retinoic acid. Steroid hormones bind to

BOX 4.6 *Receptors for Steroid Hormones*

In contrast to other intercellular messengers such as neurotransmitters, peptide hormones, or growth factors, steroid hormones are capable of readily penetrating the target cells. This is due to their lipophilic nature that allows them to cross the plasma membrane. The glucocorticoid receptor (GR) is a protein located in the cytoplasm, where it is sequestered by association with several proteins, including one called *heat shock protein 90* (HSP90). When the GR has bound cortisol, it undergoes a conformational change that releases it from the associated proteins. The hormone-bound receptor then diffuses into the nucleus where, as a dimer, it binds to specific DNA sequences in the promoter region of glucocorticoid-responsive genes. The hormone-bound receptor stimulates the transcription of these genes. Other steroid hormones have similar mechanisms of action, except that in some instances their receptor is always located within the nucleus but becomes capable of activating transcription only in the presence of the hormone. Thyroid hormones, vitamin D metabolites, and retinoic acid (a compound important for the regulation of development) have similar mechanisms of action.

Further reading: Weatherman et al., 1999; Dilworth and Chambon, 2001; Mark et al., 2006.

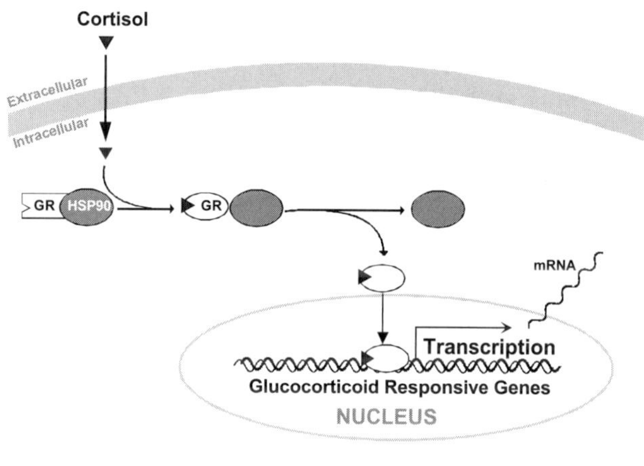

FIGURE 4.6

intracellular receptors that, in addition to the hormone binding domain, contain a deoxyribonucleic acid (DNA) binding domain, and a domain capable of stimulating messenger ribonucleic acids (mRNA) transcription of specific genes (Box 4.6 and Chapter 6). In the absence of hormone, the receptor is in an inactive conformation, unable to enhance transcription, and, usually, sequestered in the cytoplasm. In the presence of steroid hormone, the receptor switches to an active form, which translocates to the nucleus where it binds to the promoter region of specific genes and activates their transcription. Retinoic acid and thyroid hormones have similar modes of action.

G PROTEINS: MOLECULAR SWITCHES IN SIGNAL TRANSDUCTION

G proteins are proteins that possess a specific domain capable of binding GTP or guanosine 5′-diphosphate (GDP). In general, the GDP-bound form is inactive and the GTP-bound form is active (Box 4.7). G proteins act as molecular switches that can be turned on by replacement of GDP by GTP, or turned off by hydrolysis of GTP to GDP. They belong to two classes: small G proteins that contain little more than the GDP/GTP binding domain, and large heterotrimeric G proteins in which the GDP/GTP interacting subunit α is associated with two other subunits, β and γ. Small G proteins are involved in many cellular functions (Box 4.7). The role of the small G protein *Ras* in the action of growth factors is depicted in Box 4.8. Heterotrimeric G proteins are important in the action of seven transmembrane domain receptors (Box 4.2) and are also coupled to multiple effectors (Box 4.7).

SECOND MESSENGERS

Cyclic Nucleotides

Cyclic adenosine 3′-5′-monophosphate (cAMP) was the initial second messenger to be identified. It is generated by a class of enzymes called *adenylyl cyclases* that form cAMP

BOX 4.7 *G Proteins*

G proteins can bind GDP or GTP. They act as molecular switches that are active in the GTP bound form and inactive in the GDP-bound form. Although G proteins are not transmembrane proteins, they are attached to the membrane by various lipid molecules covalently bound to the protein and inserted into the membrane.

Small G proteins are simple molecular switches. In the resting state they are bound to GDP and are inactive. The exchange of GDP for GTP is catalyzed by a guanine nucleotide exchange factor (GEF). In the case of Ras, the GEF is brought into play by its adaptor-mediated attachment to phosphorylated growth factor receptors (Box 4.3). In its GTP-bound form, Ras is active and triggers a cascade of phosphorylation reactions (Box 4.8). The inactivation of Ras requires a specific type of protein, called *GAP* (GTPase activating protein). GAP allows Ras to hydrolyze GTP and to return to the inactive, GDP-bound state.

Although the principle of their function is similar to that of small G proteins, large G proteins are more complicated.

These heterotrimeric G proteins are composed of 3 subunits (α, β, and γ). The α subunit is the one that binds GDP and GTP. The exchange of GDP for GTP is triggered by seven transmembrane domain receptors, when they are bound to their ligand, a neurotransmitter or hormone (Box 4.2). Then, α-GTP and β/γ can diffuse freely at the level of the membrane and act on various targets (Box 4.2). The α subunit has the ability to hydrolyze GTP and to return spontaneously to the inactive GDP-bound form, behaving as a time device. α subunits are the targets of bacterial toxins: α_s is irreversibly activated by cholera toxin, whereas α_i and α_o are irreversibly inhibited by the toxin of *Bordetella pertussis*, the agent of whooping cough.

A

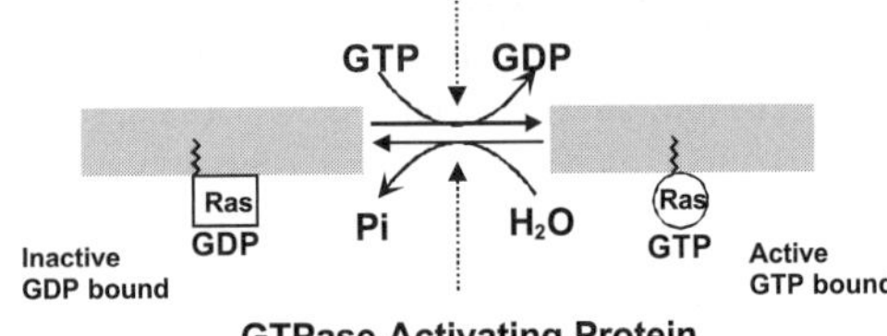

B

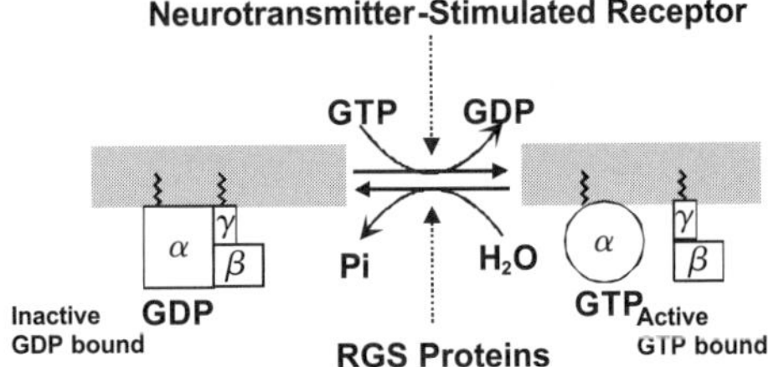

FIGURE 4.7

Recently, GAPs for some α subunits have been identified. They are called *RGS* (regulator of G protein signaling) and facilitate the return to the inactive GDP-bound form of the G protein.

Other abbreviations: G protein: guanine nucleotide binding protein; GDP: guanosine 5′-diphosphate; GTP: guanosine 5′-triphosphate; Pi: inorganic phosphate.

Further reading: Bourne, 1995, 1997; Jaffe and Hall, 2005; Koelle, 2006; Luttrell, 2006.

TABLE 4.2. *Examples of GTP-Biding Proteins*

GTP-Binding Protein Class	*Name*	*Function*
Small G protein	Ras	Responds to growth factors, activates Raf/MAP-kinase pathway
	Rho	Regulates actin filaments
	Rab	Regulates vesicle trafficking, including synaptic vesicles
Heterotrimeric G proteins:		
α subunit (binds GTP)	α_s and α_{Olf}	Activate adenylyl cyclase
	α_i	Inhibits adenylyl cyclase, activates K^+ channels
	α_t	Stimulates cGMP phosphodiesterase (retina)
	α_q and $\alpha_{11, 14\text{–}16}$	Stimulate phospholipase C
	α_O	Inhibits Ca^{2+} channels
	$\alpha_{12, 13}$	Activate Na^+/H^+ exchanger
β/γ (does not bind GTP directly, but associates to α subunits)	$\beta_{1\text{–}5}$, $\gamma_{1\text{–}8}$	Activate or inhibit adenylyl cyclase and phospholipase C, activate K^+ channels, MAP-kinase pathway, recruit β-adrenoceptor kinase

cGMP: cyclic guanosine 3′-5′-monophosphate; GTP: guanosine 5′-triphosphate; MAP-kinase: mitogen-activated protein kinase.

BOX 4.8 *The Ras/MAP-Kinase Pathway*

Stimulation of growth factor receptors results in the conversion of Ras to its active GTP-bound form (Boxes 4.3 and 4.7). Ras exerts its effects by triggering a protein kinase cascade that results, among other things, in the increased transcription of specific genes. The first step is the recruitment to the membrane, by Ras-GTP, of a protein kinase called *Raf*, which, thus, becomes activated. Raf phosphorylates a second protein kinase called *MEK* (MAP-kinase/ERK kinase). Phosphorylation of MEK activates it, making it capable of phosphorylating ERK (extracellular signal-regulated kinase) also called *MAP-kinase* (mitogen-activated protein kinase). MEK is an unusual protein kinase that is able to phosphorylate ERK on threonine and tyrosine residues. This double phosphorylation activates ERK that can phosphorylate cytoplasmic substrates such as phospholipase A2 (Box 4.10) or enter the nucleus. In the nucleus, ERK phosphorylates transcription factors, including Elk-1, a component of the ternary complex factor, thus increasing the transcription of specific genes. This cascade of biochemical reactions is important in the regulation of cell growth and differentiation. In fact, it represents one example of a highly conserved set of kinase cascades that are involved in signal transduction in all eukaryotic cells. For example, two other pathways leading to the activation of MAPKs termed *JNK* and *p38-MAPK* are organized in a very similar manner.

Other abbreviations: ERK: extracellular signal regulated kinase; GTP: guanosine 5′-triphosphate; JNK: *c-Jun* N-terminal kinase; P: phosphate group.

Further reading: Lu et al., 2006; Shalin et al., 2006; Girault et al., 2007; Zebisch et al., 2007.

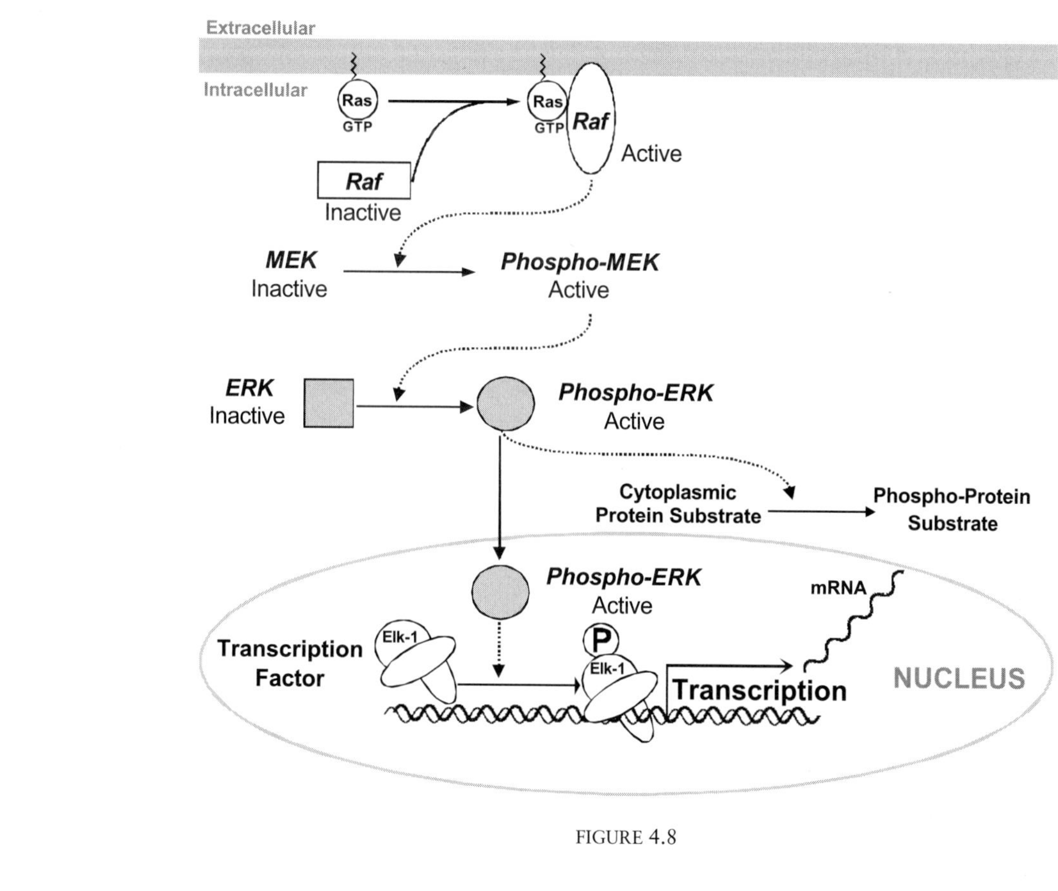

FIGURE 4.8

using adenosine 5′-triphosphate (ATP) as a precursor. The major action of cAMP is to activate a protein kinase called *cAMP-dependent protein kinase*. The metabolism and actions of cAMP are detailed in Box 4.9. cGMP is also a second messenger. It is formed by guanylyl cyclases that belong to two groups: as mentioned above, some are transmembrane receptors for polypeptides such as atrial natriuretic factor (ANF); others are soluble enzymes activated by nitric oxide (Box 4.13). cGMP has several targets in mammalian cells, one of which is cGMP-dependent protein kinase.

BOX 4.9 *cAMP*

Cyclic adenosine 3′-5′-monophosphate (cAMP) is formed from ATP by a class of transmembrane enzymes, *adenylyl cyclases.* Adenylyl cyclases are activated by two related subtypes of α subunits of G protein: α_s (stimulatory) and α_{olf} (olfactory, which is found in olfactory epithelium and some brain neurons such as striatal neurons). Adenylyl cyclases are inhibited by α_i (inhibitory). In addition, some adenylyl cyclases can be stimulated or inhibited by β/γ, or Ca^{2+} combined with calmodulin. cAMP is inactivated by hydrolysis into AMP by phosphodiesterases, a family of enzymes that are inhibited by theophylline and related methylxanthines. cAMP has very few targets in vertebrates, including a cAMP-gated ion channel that is most prominently found in olfactory neurons, cAMP-regulated guanine nucleotide exchange factors (GEF; see Box 4.7), and the cAMP-dependent protein kinase that is present in all cells. cAMP-dependent protein kinase is a tetramer composed of two catalytic subunits and two regulatory subunits (only one of each is shown on the figure). When cAMP binds to the regulatory subunits (two molecules of cAMP bind to each regulatory subunit), they dissociate from the catalytic subunits that, once free, are active as protein kinases. The catalytic subunit phosphorylates numerous specific substrates including ion channels, receptors, and enzymes synthesizing neurotransmitters. In addition, the catalytic subunit can enter the nucleus, where it phosphorylates transcription factors. One well-characterized transcription factor phosphorylated in response to cAMP is CREB (cAMP-responsive element binding protein). CREB forms a dimer that binds to a specific DNA sequence in the promoter region of cAMP-responsive genes, called *CRE* (cyclic AMP-responsive element). However CREB is unable to promote transcription when it is not phosphorylated, whereas phospho-CREB strongly stimulates transcription. Genes regulated by CREB include immediate early genes *c-Fos* and *c-Jun* (Box 4.16). It should be noted that CREB is also activated by Ca^{2+}/calmodulin dependent protein kinases and by protein kinases downstream from MAP-kinases (see Table 4.3, Box 4.11).

Other abbreviations: ATP: adenosine 5′-triphosphate.

Further reading: Smith et al., 1999; Michel and Scott, 2002; Arnsten et al., 2005.

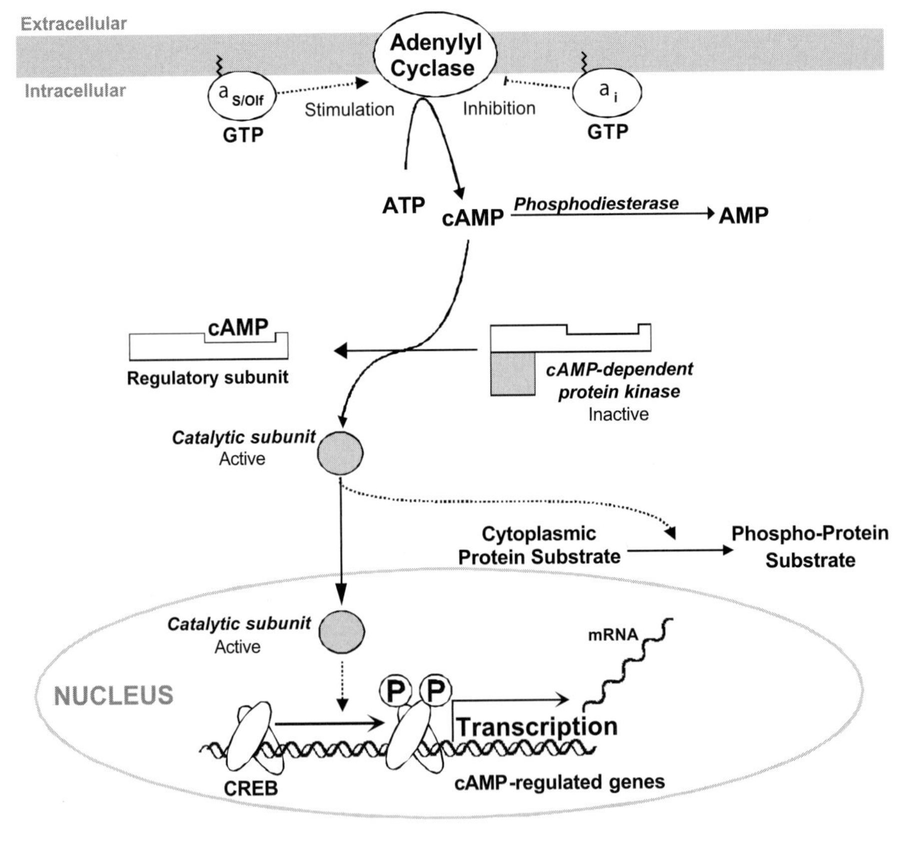

FIGURE 4.9

BOX 4.10 *Phospholipid Metabolites*

The basic backbone of phospholipids is made up of glycerol that is esterified on positions 1 and 2 by fatty acids and on position 3 by a phosphate group, forming phosphatidic acid. The two fatty acids are inserted into the membrane to which they attach the phospholipid. A water-soluble molecule is linked to the phosphate, giving rise to various types of phospholipids such as phosphatidylcholine, phosphatidylethanolamine, or phosphatidylinositol. Enzymes called *phospholipases* are capable of hydrolyzing specific chemical bonds within these phospholipids, as indicated by solid arrows in the figure.

Phospholipase A2 (PLA2) releases the fatty acid located in position 2 of the glycerol backbone. PLA2 acts preferentially on phosphatidylcholine or phosphatidylethanolamine, in which the fatty acid in position 2 is arachidonic acid, releasing a lysophospholipid and free arachidonic acid. Arachidonic acid is moderately hydrophobic and can diffuse within the cell in which it has been formed, or to neighboring cells. It has several intrinsic biological activities by itself and is also a precursor for many active molecules called *eicosanoids*, including prostaglandins, thromboxanes, and hydroperoxy-metabolites. PLA2 is activated by many extracellular signals including neurotransmitters, although the mechanism of its regulation is still incompletely understood.

Phospholipase C (PLC) hydrolyzes the bond between the phosphate group and the glycerol backbone. PLC acts preferentially on phosphatidylinositol 4,5 bisphosphate and generates diacylglycerol and inositol 1,4,5 trisphosphate (IP_3; see Box 4.11). Diacylglycerol stays in the membrane and participates in the activation of protein kinase C. IP_3 is very water-soluble and diffuses in the cytosol. It binds to a receptor located on the endoplasmic reticulum and triggers the release of Ca^{2+} from internal stores (Box 4.11). Among many other actions, Ca^{2+} participates in the activation of protein kinase C. PLC is activated by many neurotransmitters that act on G protein–coupled, 7 transmembrane domain receptors. PLC is stimulated by α_q-GTP and α_{11}-GTP as well as by some β/γ complexes (Box 4.2 and 4.7).

Phospholipase D (PLD) acts preferentially on phosphatidylcholine and hydrolyzes the bond between the phosphate group and the water-soluble molecule that esterifies it. Thus, it releases phosphatidic acid and choline. It is not known if choline has a role in signal transduction. On the other hand, phosphatidic acid stimulates protein kinase C subtypes. Although PLD is activated by several extracellular signals, including neurotransmitters, the mechanism of its activation is still incompletely understood.

Other abbreviations: G protein: guanine nucleotide binding protein.

Further reading: Cockcroft, 2006; Farooqui et al., 2006.

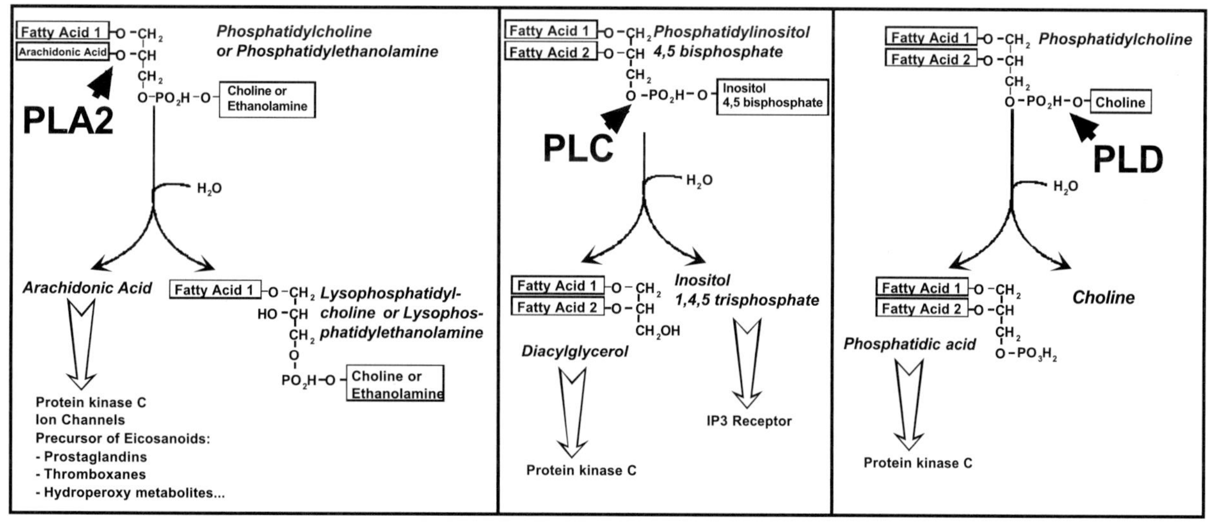

FIGURE 4.10

Phospholipid Metabolites

In addition to their importance in the structure of membranes, phospholipids are precursors for many signaling molecules. The structures of some glycerophospholipids are depicted in Box 4.10. These phospholipids generate signaling molecules under the control of different classes of phospholipases, each of which cleaves the precursor at a specific position (Box 4.10). In addition to glycerophospholipids, other membrane lipids such as sphingomyelin have been found to be involved in signal transduction. A breakdown product of sphingomyelin, ceramide, may play a role of second messenger.

Ca^{2+}

Normal concentrations of Ca^{2+} in the cytosol are very low, due to the impermeability of membranes to this ion and the efficiency of the mechanisms of extrusion (Box 4.11). Ca^{2+} can flow into the cytosol either from the outside through neurotransmitter- or voltage-operated Ca^{2+} channels, or from internal stores through Ca^{2+} channels called *inositol-trisphosphate* (IP_3) receptors and *ryanodine receptors* (see Box 4.11). Ca^{2+} has many biological effects that are brought about by its binding to a number of enzymes and their subsequent activation (see Table 4.3 in Box 4.11). Ca^{2+} binds directly to some of these enzymes that contain specific Ca^{2+}-binding domains. In many cases, however, Ca^{2+} interacts first with a small protein, *calmodulin*. The Ca^{2+}/calmodulin complex binds to many proteins, including signaling enzymes, and alters their properties. An important class of such enzymes is the Ca^{2+}/calmodulin-dependent protein kinases.

Depolarization of neurons triggers the opening of voltage-gated Ca^{2+} channels, leading to an increase in intracellular Ca^{2+}. In nerve terminals, this is the signal responsible for neurotransmitter release. Ca^{2+} influx also provides a mechanism by which nerve cell stimuli, such as the action potential, can be transduced into biochemical signals important for the regulation of neurotransmitter synthesis, gene expression, and many other responses in neurons. Ca^{2+} is an essential trigger of the biochemical reactions that result in long-term depression and long-term potentiation of synaptic efficacy. These forms of synaptic plasticity are thought to be important cellular bases of learning and memory. In addition to its paramount role in neuronal physiology, Ca^{2+} is a key player in the induction of neuronal death in pathological circumstances. For instance, during hypoxia extracellular glutamate levels increase, leading to an abnormal stimulation of glutamate NMDA receptors. This, in combination with the partial depolarization of neuronal membranes and impairment of Ca^{2+} extrusion mechanisms (due to an energy deficiency), leads to a prolonged increase in cytosolic Ca^{2+} concentrations. Ca^{2+} triggers several cascades of reactions that can lead to neuronal death. Such reactions are the subject of intense investigations, with the hope that their pharmacological inhibition will improve survival and recovery in stroke and other neurological diseases.

DIFFUSIBLE MOLECULES ACTING AS INTERCELLULAR AND INTRACELLULAR MESSENGERS

Arachidonic Acid and its Metabolites

Arachidonic acid is a 20-carbon fatty acid with four double bonds. It is released from precursor phospholipids by phospholipase A2 (Box 4.10). It can act in the cells in which it has been produced, for instance, by stimulating protein kinase C. Arachidonic acid can also diffuse to neighboring cells or nerve terminals and act as a local intercellular messenger. In addition, it is a precursor for a large family of signaling molecules called *eicosanoids* (*eicosi* is the Greek radical for 20, referring to the length of the carbon chain). Such molecules include prostaglandins, thromboxanes, and hydroperoxymetabolites. A particular class of interesting derivatives of arachidonic acid is composed of endogenous ligands for brain cannabinoid receptors, referred to as *endocannabinoids*. Cannabinoid receptors are the targets of $\Delta 9$-tetrahydrocannabinol, the active substance in hashish and marijuana. Endocannabinoids include arachidonoylethanolamine, also called *anandamide* (from *ananda*, the Sanskrit word for "bliss"), and 2-arachidonoylglycerol, which are released from specific phospholipid precursors in a Ca^{2+}-dependent manner. Endocannabinoids seem to be intercellular messengers, rather than second messengers, and are implicated in important aspects of neuromodulation, as retrograde signaling from postsynaptic to presynaptic sites.

Nitric oxide

Nitric oxide (NO) is a gas molecule that has important biological functions. On the one hand, it is a highly reactive chemical species that is used by macrophages to destroy exogenous substances. On the other hand, it is a chemical messenger, which can diffuse freely, over a short range, through cellular membranes. Nitric oxide was originally discovered as a vasodilator substance generated by endothelial cells that acts on smooth muscle cells of blood vessels. In neurons, *NO synthase*, the enzyme that generates NO, is activated by Ca^{2+} (Box 4.13). A well-characterized effect of NO is to increase cGMP by activation of soluble guanylyl cyclase. Because of its diffusible nature, NO is a retrograde messenger in the nervous system, diffusing from the postsynaptic to the presynaptic side of synapses, and thus plays a role in synaptic plasticity (Chapter 5).

PROTEIN PHOSPHORYLATION

Protein phosphorylation is a reversible covalent chemical modification of proteins that plays a central role in signal transduction (Box 4.14). The vast majority of known signal transduction pathways involve the activation of one or several protein kinases. In most instances, it is by altering the state of phosphorylation of key intracellular proteins that intercellular messengers including neurotransmitters, hormones, growth factors, and others ultimately exert their effects. The amino acids whose side chains are phosphorylated in the context of signal transduction in metazoans are predominantly *serine, threonine*, and *tyrosine*. The presence of a bulky and negatively charged phosphate group on the side chain of these amino acids can change dramatically

BOX 4.11 *Ca^{2+}*

Ca^{2+} is a divalent cation whose concentrations are relatively high in the extracellular space (around 1.2 mM) and more than 10,000 times lower within the cytosol (around 100 nM) (Berridge, 1998; Berridge et al., 2000). Some intracellular organelles, however, namely *mitochondria* and *endoplasmic reticulum*, contain high concentrations of Ca^{2+}. In resting conditions the plasma membrane is impermeable to Ca^{2+}. Ca^{2+} can penetrate neurons through specific channels, which include voltage-gated Ca^{2+} channels (VGCC) and glutamate receptors of the NMDA subtype. When these channels are open, in response to depolarization in the case of VGCC or in the presence of glutamate in the case of *N*-methyl-D-aspartate (NMDA) receptor (see Box 4.1), Ca^{2+} flows readily into the cytosol following its concentration gradient and the electrical potential. Ca^{2+} can also be released into the cytosol from internal stores that are mostly located in the endoplasmic reticulum. Two types of Ca^{2+} channels are responsible for the release of Ca^{2+} from internal stores. One is the inositol 1,4,5 trisphosphate (IP_3) receptor whose opening is triggered by IP_3, a second messenger generated by phospholipase C (Boxes 4.10 and 4.12). The other is the ryanodine receptor, named after *ryanodine*, a drug that triggers its opening, although it is not a physiological ligand. In fact, opening of ryanodine receptors is triggered by Ca^{2+} itself by a mechanism called *Ca^{2+}-induced Ca^{2+} release*, which can give rise to propagation of waves of Ca^{2+} release along the endoplasmic reticulum. In the cytosol, Ca^{2+} is mostly bound to specific binding proteins. Some of them appear to play a role primarily as buffering proteins, preventing excessive rises in cytosolic free Ca^{2+}. Other proteins are the actual targets of Ca^{2+}, which account for its potent biological effects. Among the best characterized targets are calmodulin and calmodulin-related proteins. When they are bound to Ca^{2+}, calmodulin and the related proteins undergo a conformational change that enables them to interact with, and activate, a number of enzymes (Table 4.3). Ca^{2+} can also bind to another type of protein domain called C2 that is found in several different proteins (Table 4.3). Free Ca^{2+} in the cytosol is maintained at very low levels by several highly active processes, which include Ca^{2+} pumps and Ca^{2+} exchangers. Ca^{2+} pumps have a high affinity but a low capacity for Ca^{2+} and are used for fine tuning Ca^{2+} levels. They are located on the plasma membrane and the membrane of the endoplasmic reticulum, and their energy is provided by ATP hydrolysis. Na^+/Ca^{2+} exchangers, whose driving force is provided by the Na^+ gradient, have a large capacity, but a low affinity for Ca^{2+}.

Other abbreviations: C2: second constant domain within protein kinase C sequence; cAMP: cyclic adenosine 3′-5′-monophosphate; ER: endoplasmic reticulum; NMDA-R: *N*-methyl-D-aspartate subtype of glutamate receptor.

Further reading: Berridge, 2005; Collin et al., 2005; Pietrobon, 2005; Iino, 2007.

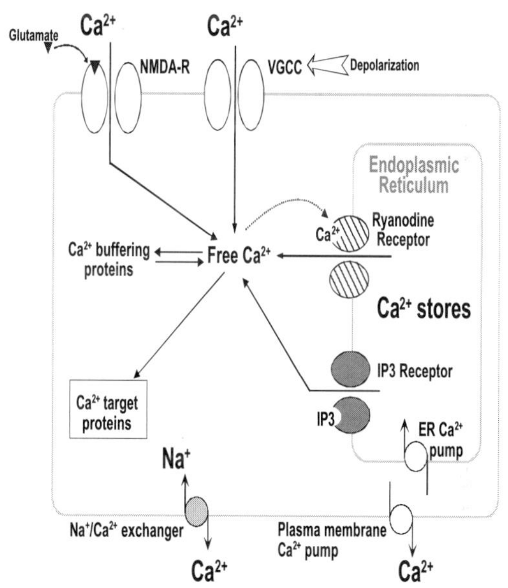

FIGURE 4.11

TABLE 4.3. *Examples of Target Proteins for Cytosolic Free Ca^{2+}*

Ca^{2+}-Binding Domain	*Target Protein*	*Function*
Calmodulin	Ca^{2+}/calmodulin kinases I, II, IV	Protein kinases that increase phosphorylation of multiple proteins
	Elongation factor 2 (EF2) kinase	Protein kinase that phosphorylates EF2 and inhibits protein synthesis
	Calcineurin (Phosphatase 2B)	Protein phosphatase that decreases phosphorylation of specific proteins
	Adenylyl cyclase	Increases cAMP
	Phosphodiesterase	Decreases cAMP
	NO synthase	Triggers NO production
Calmodulin-like	Calpains	Proteases that cut specific proteins
C2 domains	Protein kinase C	Increases phosphorylation of multiple proteins
	Phospholipase A2	Releases arachidonic acid
	Synaptotagmin	Regulates neurotransmitter release

cAMP: cyclic adenosine 3′-5′-monophosphate; NO: nitric oxide.

BOX 4.12 *Inositol-Trisphosphate*

Inositol 1,4,5 trisphosphate (IP_3) is an important second messenger. It is generated by the enzyme phospholipase C (PLC) that hydrolyzes a membrane phospholipid, *phosphatidylinositol 4,5 bisphosphate* (see Box 4.10). PLC is activated by neurotransmitters that act on G protein–coupled, 7-transmembrane domain receptors (Box 4.2). PLC generates diacylglycerol and IP_3. IP_3 is very water soluble and diffuses in the cytosol. It binds to a receptor located on the endoplasmic reticulum and thereby triggers the release of Ca^{2+} from internal stores (Box 4.11). Inositol 1,4,5 trisphosphate is inactivated by several phosphoinositol phosphatases that remove successively the phosphate molecules from the inositol backbone. These phosphatases can act in various sequences, not necessarily that depicted in the figure. The phosphatase that removes the phosphate in position 1 of the inositol backbone is inhibited by lithium (Li^+). Inositol can be reincorporated into membrane phospholipids by its coupling to an activated form of diacylglycerol (CDP-diacylglycerol) and phosphorylated on positions 4 and 5 by specific kinases to regenerate phosphatidylinositol 4,5 bisphosphate (broken arrow in the figure). Chronic treatment with lithium may decrease the amount of inositol that can be incorporated into neuronal phospholipids and thus dampen the effects of neurotransmitters that activate PLC. This property of lithium may participate in its mood stabilizing effects.

Other abbreviations: CDP: cytosine 5′-diphosphate; G protein: guanine nucleotide binding protein; Pi: inorganic phosphate.

Further reading: Mikoshiba and Hattori, 2000; Berridge, 2005.

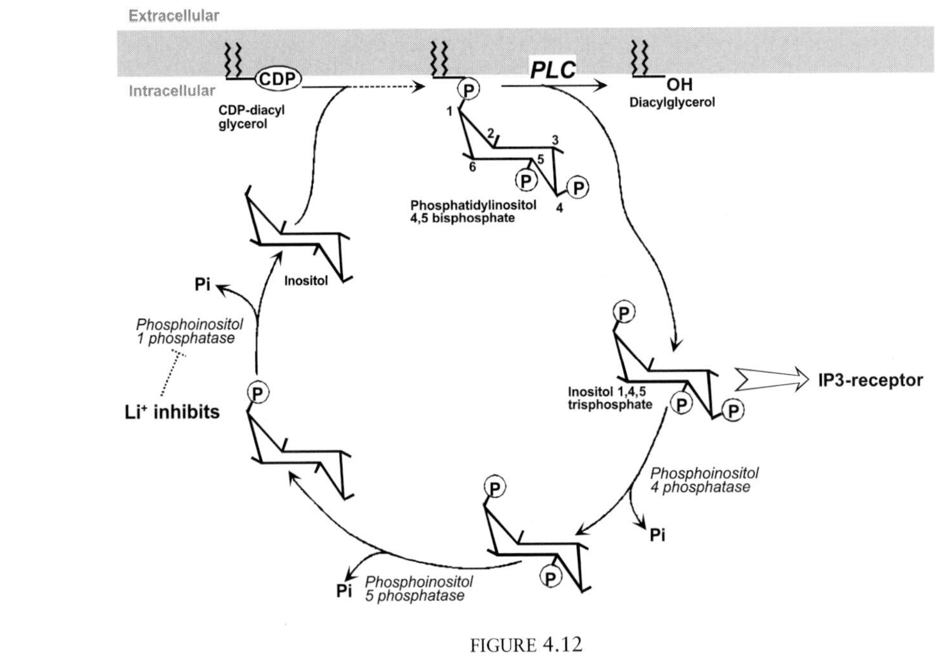

FIGURE 4.12

the properties of the protein, leading to the activation or inhibition of enzymes, opening or closing of ion channels, modulation of neurotransmitter receptors, activation of transcription factors, etc. Thus, phosphorylation reactions play an effector role when the substrate proteins are critical components for the behavior of cells (see Box 4.14). In addition, protein phosphorylation is involved in cascades of signal transduction in two ways. First, phosphorylation of amino acid residues can promote the recruitment of proteins important for signal transduction, as exemplified by interaction of protein regions phosphorylated on tyrosine with Src-homology-2 (SH2) domains (Boxes 4.3, 4.4, 4.5). Second, many signaling pathways involve protein kinase cascades in which a first kinase activates a second kinase, which activates a third one, and so on. Functions of such kinase cascades (see Box 4.8 for an example) are to provide amplification and, in some cases, to turn graded inputs into switch-like all-or-none responses (bistable systems).

The state of phosphorylation of a protein is determined by its relative rates of phosphorylation and dephosphorylation. The enzymes that remove phosphate groups from proteins are called *phosphoprotein*

BOX 4.13 *Nitric Oxide*

Nitric oxide (NO) is a gas that is highly diffusible and chemically reactive. In the nervous system it is used as a locally active intra- or intercellular messenger. The enzyme responsible for the formation of NO is NO synthase (NOS). It is activated by Ca^{2+} associated to calmodulin. In neurons, opening of glutamate receptors of the *N*-methyl-D-aspartate (NMDA) subtype is a major source of Ca^{2+} influx (Box 4.1) that can lead to the activation of NOS. NOS is a complex enzyme that uses molecular oxygen, O_2, to generate NO by transforming arginine into citrulline. NO can cross membranes readily and diffuse to neighboring cells or nerve endings. Thus, the rest of the cascade depicted in the figure can take place in a cell different from that in which NO was generated, as symbolized by the dotted pair of lines in the figure. A major target of NO is soluble guanylyl cyclase. This enzyme is activated by NO and uses guanosine 5′-triphosphate (GTP) to form cyclic guanosine 3′,5′-monophosphate (cGMP), a second messenger which remains within the cell in which it is produced. cGMP exerts its effects by activating several enzymes, one of which is cGMP-dependent protein kinase. Phosphorylation of specific proteins by cGMP-dependent protein kinase accounts for some of the physiological effects of NO.

Other abbreviations: GC: guanylyl cyclase; NMDA-R: *N*-methyl-D-aspartate subtype of glutamate receptor; PKG: cGMP-dependent protein kinase.

Further reading: Snyder et al., 1998; Iino, 2006.

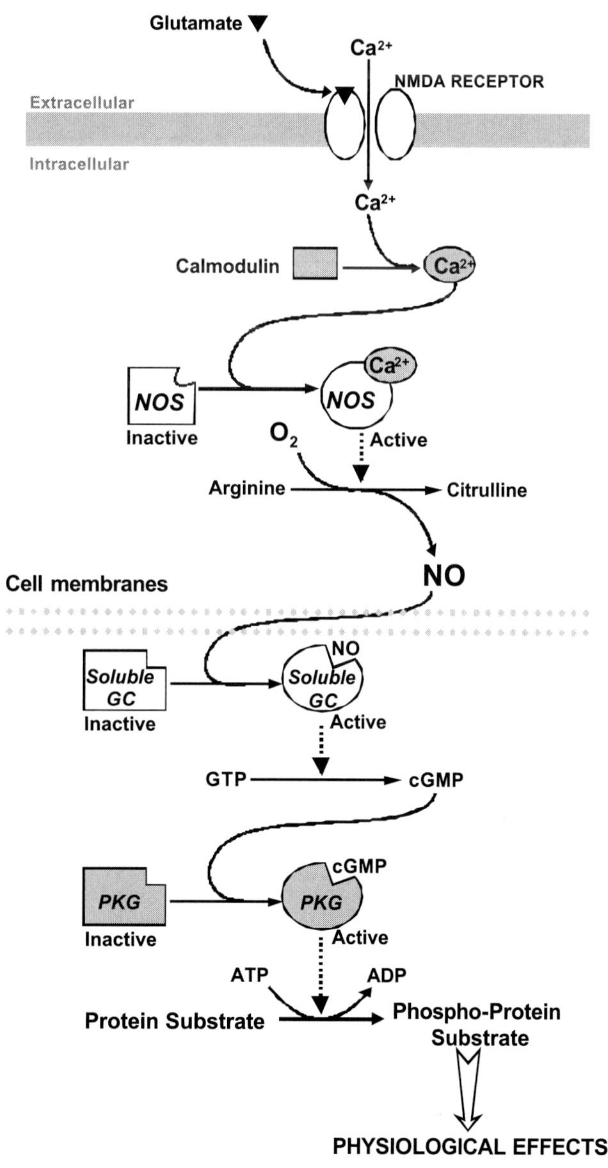

FIGURE 4.13

BOX 4.14 *Protein Phosphorylation*

Phosphorylation is carried out by protein kinases, which, in the presence of Mg^{2+}, transfer a phosphoryl group from ATP to serine, threonine, or tyrosine residues. Because these kinases often recognize the amino acid sequence surrounding the serine, threonine, or tyrosine to be phosphorylated, protein kinases have a high degree of substrate specificity. Protein kinases form a very large group of related enzymes, each of which has its own localization, regulation, and substrate specificity (Table 4.4). Some protein kinases are either receptors for extracellular signals (Box 4.3) or are associated with such receptors (Box 4.5). Several protein kinases are activated directly by second messengers and account for most of the effects of these second messengers. These include cAMP- and cGMP-dependent protein kinases (Boxes 4.9 and 4.13), protein kinases activated by Ca^{2+} associated to calmodulin (Box 4.11), and protein kinase C which is activated by Ca^{2+}, diacylglycerol, and/or several other lipid derivatives (Box 4.10). Some protein kinases are themselves regulated by phosphorylation and participate in kinase cascades (see Box 4.8).

The reverse reaction, the removal of the phosphate group, is catalyzed by phosphoprotein phosphatases. This class of enzymes, if not quite as large as that of protein kinases, includes many members belonging to several gene families (Table 4.5). Different types of phosphatases are responsible for the removal of phosphate groups from serine and threonine side chains and from tyrosine side chains. A very large number of important neuronal proteins are regulated by phosphorylation/dephosphorylation (Table 4.6).

Other abbreviations: ATP: adenosine 5′-triphosphate; cAMP: cyclic adenosine 3′-5′-monophosphate; cGMP: cyclic guanosine 3′-5′-monophosphate.

Further reading: Johnson and Hunter, 2005; Papin et al., 2005; Mansuy and Shenolikar, 2006.

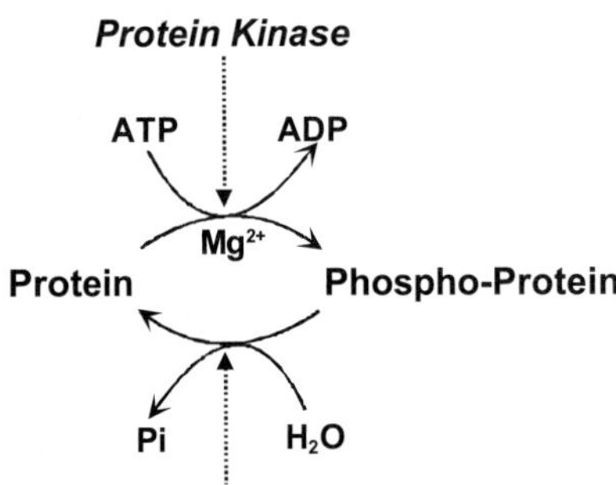

FIGURE 4.14

TABLE 4.4. *Examples of Protein Kinases*

Amino Acid Phosphorylated	*Activation Mechanism*	*Protein Kinase*
Serine and/or threonine	cAMP	cAMP-dependent protein kinase
	cGMP	cGMP-dependent protein kinase
	Ca^{2+}-calmodulin	Ca^{2+}/calmodulin kinases I, II, IV
		Elongation Factor 2 kinase
	Ca^{2+}, DAG, arachidonic acid	Protein kinase C
	Interaction with Ras-GTP	Raf
	Recruitment to the membrane by phosphoinositides	AKT (or PKB)
	Phosphorylation	MAP-kinases (ERK, JNK, p38-MAP-kinase)
	Phosphorylation, dephosphorylation, cyclin binding	Cyclin-dependent kinases
	Extracellular ligand binding	Receptors for TGFβ, activin, inhibin, etc.
Tyrosine	Extracellular ligand binding	Receptors for insulin or growth factors
	Interaction with a receptor	JAK, Src family kinases
Threonine and tyrosine	Phosphorylation	MAP-kinase kinase (or MEK)

cAMP: cyclic adenosine 3′-5′-monophosphate; cGMP: cyclic guanosine 3′-5′-monophosphate; DAG: diacylglycerol; ERK: extracellular signal-related kinase; GTP: guanosine 5′-triphosphate; JAK: Janus kinase; JNK: *c-Jun* N-terminal kinase; MAP-Kinase: mitogen-activated protein kinase; MEK: MAP-kinase/ERK kinase; PKB: protein kinase B; TGFβ: transforming growth factor-beta.

TABLE 4.5. *Classification of Phosphoprotein Phosphatases*

Target Phospho-Amino Acid	*Properties*	*Protein Phosphatase*
Phosphoserine and/or phosphothreonine	Sensitive to specific protein inhibitors (phospho-inhibitor 1, phospho-DARPP-32, inhibitor 2):	Phosphatase 1
	Insensitive to these inhibitors:	
	Insensitive to divalent cations	Phosphatase 2A
	Activated by Ca^{2+}	Calcineurin (phosphatase 2B)
	Requires Mg^{2+}	Phosphatase 2C
Phosphotyrosine	Transmembrane “receptor-like” proteins	
	Cytoplasmic proteins (usually possess targeting domains)	
Phosphoserine and/or phosphothreonine and/or phosphotyrosine	Phosphatases acting on MAP-kinase or cyclin-dependent kinases	Dual specificity phosphatases

DARPP: dopamine- and cAMP-regulated phosphoprotein of 32 kDa; MAP-Kinase: mitogen-activated protein kinase.

TABLE 4.6. *Examples of Neuronal Proteins Regulated by Phosphorylation/Dephosphorylation*

Regulated Protein	*Protein Kinase*	*Effect*
Ion channels:		
Ca^{2+} (L type)	cAMP-dependent	Increases Ca^{2+} permeability
K^+ (Kv1.2, 1.3)	Tyrosine kinase	Closes the channel
Na^+	PKC, cAMP-dependent	Decreases Na^+ permeability
Neurotransmitter-gated ion channels:		
Glutamate (AMPA-subtype)	cAMP-dependent	Increases response
Glutamate (NMDA-subtype)	PKC, tyrosine kinase	Increases response
GABA-A	Tyrosine kinase	Increases response
G protein-coupled receptors:		
β-Adrenoceptor	β-Adrenoceptor kinase	Desensitization, recruitment of partners
Neurotransmitter synthesizing enzymes:		
Tyrosine hydroxylase	cAMP-, Ca^{2+}/calmodulin-dependent, MAP-kinase	Increases catecholamine synthesis
Tryptophan hydroxylase	Ca^{2+}/calmodulin dependent	Increases serotonin synthesis
Synaptic vesicle proteins:		
Synapsins	Ca^{2+}/calmodulin dependent	Facilitates neurotransmitter release
Transcription factors:		
CREB	cAMP-dependent, kinases activated by MAP-kinases	Increases transcription

AMPA: α-amino-3-hydroxy-5-methyl-4-isoxasolepropionic acid; cAMP: cyclic adenosine 3′-5′-monophosphate; CREB: cAMP-response element binding protein; GABA: γ-amino butyric acid; MAP-kinase: mitogen-activated protein kinase; NMDA: *N*-methyl-D-aspartate; PKC: protein kinase C.

phosphatases (Box 4.14) and may be as important in signal transduction as protein kinases. The regulation of protein phosphatases is, in general, not as well understood as that of protein kinases. There are nevertheless well-documented examples of protein phosphatases whose activity is regulated by neurotransmitters, as illustrated in Box 4.15.

SIGNALING BY PROTEOLYSIS

In contrast to noncovalent protein–protein interactions and to protein phosphorylation that are reversible, proteolysis is irreversible. In addition to its obvious role in the degradation of proteins, proteolysis is involved in intracellular signaling cascades. For example, signals that lead to programmed cell death, or *apoptosis*, activate a set of proteases, *the caspases*. Caspases activate each other in an ordered manner by limited proteolysis and also contribute directly to cell death by cleaving a number of cellular proteins (Box 4.16). Other types of intracellular proteases can play a role in signaling, outside of the context of cell death. For example, calpains are proteases activated by increased levels of cytosolic free Ca^{2+} (Table 4.3). One important system for the degradation of cellular proteins is a large multiprotein complex called *proteasome*. Proteins are targeted to the proteasome by conjugation to a small polypeptide termed *ubiquitin*, under the action of specific enzymes and cofactors. The ubiquitin "tag" triggers the degradation of improperly folded proteins but also has a role in signaling (Box 4.16). Thus, recently several pathways of regulated proteolysis of specific proteins have been identified as important components of signal transduction not only for programmed cell death, but also during development as well as in the mature nervous system. Moreover, abnormal regulation of proteolysis is likely to be a key aspect in pathological conditions such as Alzheimer's disease.

REGULATION OF GENE EXPRESSION

Regulation of gene expression is an important target of signal transduction in neurons, as in other cells. Because of its long-lasting effects, it is important in mediating the actions of neurotrophins, as well as in learning and memory (Chapter 5). Signaling pathways involving growth factor receptors and the mitogen-activated protein (MAP) kinase cascade (Boxes 4.3, 4.8), JAK-STAT-associated receptors (Box 4.5), steroid hormones (Box 4.6), cAMP (Box 4.9), and proteolysis (Box 4.16) lead to changes in gene expression. Other pathways involving Ca^{2+}/calmodulin-activated protein kinases or protein kinase C also exert profound effects on gene expression, via similar mechanisms. In fact, the promoter region of regulated genes often contains several consensus DNA sequences capable of interacting with specific transcription factors (see Chapter 6). The overall rate of transcription of such genes depends on the interaction between various transcription factors and the housekeeping proteins involved in mRNA synthesis. The nuclear localization, DNA-binding, and activity of transcription factors can be modulated by phosphorylation. In addition, signaling pathways regulate histones, which are basic proteins associated to DNA to form the chromatin, thereby facilitating or preventing the accessibility and transcription of specific genes. These regulations include different types of modification of histones such as phosphorylation, methylation, and acetylation. Thus, several signal transduction pathways can converge to modulate precisely the levels of gene expression. Some transcription factors are present at low levels in basal conditions but can be rapidly induced in response to extracellular signals. These transcription factors belong to the class of immediate early genes, which include *c-Fos* and *c-Jun* and are useful markers of neuronal activity (Box 4.17).

TERMINATION OF SIGNALS

Intuitively, for cells to adapt swiftly to changes in their environment or incoming signals, it seems critical that they are able to stop rapidly the responses they started. This may be appropriate either when the external signal itself is off, or when the signal is too intense or too prolonged, so that excessive responding could become deleterious. In fact, most reactions of signal transduction are reversible and cells have developed highly sophisticated ways to control the duration and intensity of their responses. Most receptors go through several types of inactivation that prevent excessive stimulation. Many ligand-gated ion channels undergo desensitization. This means that in the presence of the neurotransmitter the receptor switches spontaneously into a closed (that is, inactive) conformation, which is usually rather stable and corresponds to a state of high affinity for the neurotransmitter (see Box 4.1). G protein–coupled receptors also undergo desensitization, a process that involves phosphorylation of the receptor. Many serpentine receptors are regulated by phosphorylation by a specific class of protein kinases (*G protein–coupled receptor kinases*, GRKs) that act specifically on the active, neurotransmitter-bound form of the receptor. Phosphorylation of the receptor by GRKs decreases or blocks its ability to interact with G proteins and facilitates its endocytosis. Indeed, most receptors, including G protein–coupled receptors, as well as tyrosine kinase receptors and many others, are subjected to endocytosis when they are activated by their cognate ligand. Internalization of the receptor may lead to its degradation

BOX 4.15 *Regulation of Neuronal Phosphoprotein Phosphatases*

The regulation of protein phosphatase activity by neurotransmitters is best understood in striatonigral neurons. These neurons receive a glutamatergic input from the cerebral cortex, as well as a rich dopaminergic innervation from the substantia nigra. Dopamine regulates the efficacy and plasticity of corticostriatal transmission. Dopamine, acting on D1 dopamine receptors, stimulates adenylyl cyclase via a G protein (not shown in the figure; see Box 4.9). Increased cAMP levels activate cAMP-dependent protein kinase. A major substrate for cAMP kinase in these neurons is DARPP-32 (*dopamine- and cAMP-regulated phosphoprotein with an apparent molecular weight of 32,000*). When it is phosphorylated, DARPP-32 becomes a potent inhibitor of protein phosphatase 1 (Box 4.14). On the other hand, glutamate acting on NMDA receptors (Box 4.1) gives rise to a large influx of Ca^{2+}. This results in the stimulation of a protein phosphatase activated by Ca^{2+} and calmodulin, called *calcineurin or phosphatase 2B* (Box 4.14). One of the actions of calcineurin is to dephosphorylate DARPP-32, and thus to relieve the inhibition of phosphatase 1. In this system, the activities of two phosphatases, *calcineurin and phosphatase 1*, are regulated by the neurotransmitters *dopamine* and *glutamate*. In turn, phosphatase 1 is important for the regulation of several targets including Na^+ and Ca^{2+} channels, and glutamate receptors. The scheme presented here is a simplification since DARPP-32 is, in reality, regulated by several phosphorylation sites and many neurotransmitters and neuromodulators.

Other abbreviations: cAMP: cyclic adenosine 3′-5′-monophosphate; G protein: guanine nucleotide binding protein; NMDA: *N*-methyl-D-aspartate.

Further reading: Girault and Greengard, 2004; Nairn et al., 2004; Svenningsson et al., 2004.

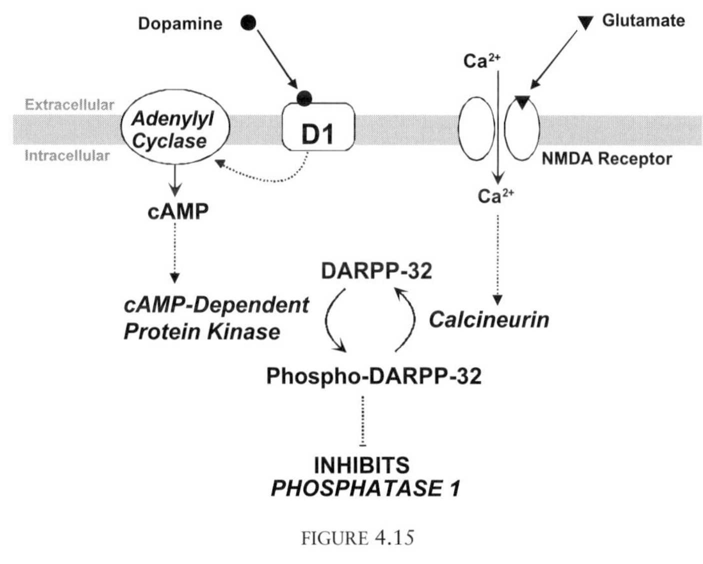

FIGURE 4.15

or to its recycling to the membrane. In fact, regulation of the number of receptors present at the membrane, by adjustment of their endocytosis and exocytosis rates, appears to be an important mechanism by which cells alter their sensitivity to external signals. For example, regulation of the number of glutamate receptors in the postsynaptic membrane is an important aspect of synaptic plasticity.

G proteins have built-in inactivating mechanisms: spontaneous or induced GTP hydrolysis leads to the inactivation of the G protein (see Box 4.7). The importance of this mechanism is underlined by the dramatic consequences of its blockade. Cholera toxin–induced blockade of GTP hydrolysis by $G\alpha_s$ in the intestinal epithelium is responsible for a potentially lethal water loss, while mutations that hamper the GTPase activity of Ras are potently oncogenic. Second messengers themselves are rapidly degraded by specific enzymes. Phosphodiesterases transform cAMP and cGMP into inactive AMP and GMP, respectively (see Box 4.9). Inositol phosphates are dephosphorylated by specific phosphatases (see Box 4.12). Free cytosolic Ca^{2+} is buffered by binding proteins and rapidly eliminated by various pumps and exchangers either to the outside of the cell or into intracellular stores (see Box 4.11). These various mechanisms can be important pharmacological targets. For example, lithium inhibits phospho-inositol-phosphatases, while inhibitors of cGMP phosphodiesterase have attracted a lot of public attention for their effects on sexual performance.

Protein phosphorylation reactions are also reversible, due to the presence of protein phosphatases (see Box 4.14), and the tightly regulated activity of these enzymes is an integral part of signaling mechanisms (see Box 4.15).

BOX 4.16 *Signaling by Proteolysis*

In contrast to phosphorylation, which is reversible, proteolysis is irreversible. Nevertheless it is an important component of several signaling pathways. All cells can undergo a programmed cell death or apoptosis, which is a way to control precisely cell numbers during development and to eliminate abnormal cells. Excessive apoptosis is also a mechanism underlying many neurological diseases. A specific group of evolutionarily conserved proteases are termed *caspases* because they contain a cysteine residue in their active site and cleave their substrates in the vicinity of aspartate residues. Caspases are the final common pathway of apoptosis (Fig. 4.16A). Caspases exist as inactive precursors, the pro-caspases that become active following limited proteolysis. Upstream caspases are activated by autocleavage following interaction with specific factors in response to various signals. For example, pro-caspase-8 is activated by ligation of "death receptors" such as Fas and the p75 neurotrophin receptor, while pro-caspase-9 is activated by the release of proapoptotic factors from mitochondria. Once in their active form, these caspases cleave and activate effector caspases, such as caspase-3, which contribute to cell death by cutting multiple cellular proteins.

Degradation of proteins by the proteasome is important for the elimination of abnormal or improperly folded proteins. It is also involved in some signaling pathways. Proteins are targeted for degradation in the proteasome by the attachment to their lysine side chains of one or several polypeptides called *ubiquitin*. This mechanism is important for the activation of the transcription factor NFκB (*nuclear factor κB*, named because of its role in the regulation of κ immunoglobulin light chains in B lymphocytes) (Fig. 4.16B). NFκB plays a role in many biological responses ranging from early development to inflammation. NFκB is a dimer of two subunits maintained in an inactive state in the cytoplasm by interaction with an inhibitor protein termed *IκB*. Activation of NFκB in response to stimulation of various receptors involves its dissociation from IκB, triggered by phosphorylation. IκB is then ubiquitinated and degraded by the proteasome, allowing NFκB to translocate to the nucleus and activate transcription of multiple genes, some of which may have antiapoptotic effects.

Other abbreviation: TNFα: tumor necrosis factor alpha.

Further reading: Baud and Karin, 2001; Jiang and Wang, 2004; Yan and Shi, 2005; Patrick, 2006.

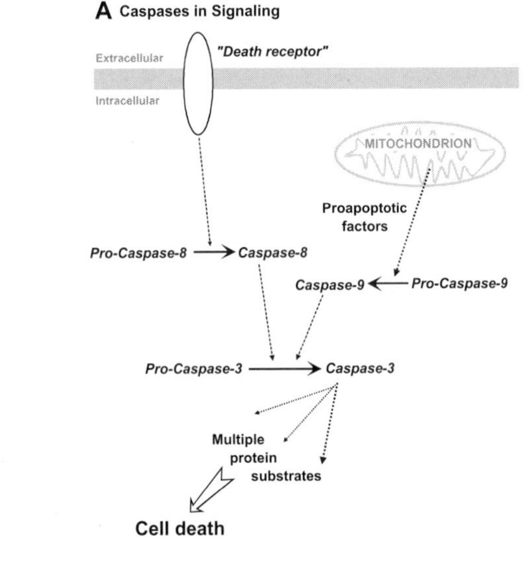

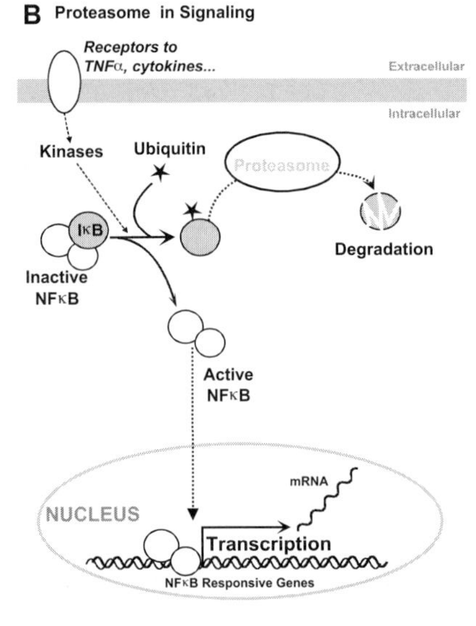

FIGURE 4.16

It is worth mentioning that in many cases signaling pathways appear to be active to some degree even in the absence of extracellular signals, but that inactivation mechanisms (for example, GTPases, phosphodiesterases, or phosphatases) counteract this spontaneous activity. What the extracellular signal does is to tilt the balance by enhancing the rate of activation and/or decreasing the rate of inactivation of the signaling. Although this permanent bustle of signaling pathways may, at first sight, appear costly for the cell, it may be advantageous by providing the capability to react very rapidly to extracellular signals.

PSYCHOTHERAPEUTIC AGENTS AND SIGNAL TRANSDUCTION

Most of the therapeutic agents used at present in psychiatry act at the level of synaptic transmission by altering either the reuptake of neurotransmitters into

BOX 4.17 *Immediate Early Genes*

The transcription of genes encoding certain transcription factors, such as c-Fos and c-Jun depicted here, is readily regulated by extracellular signals that act by various signal transduction pathways involving cAMP, Ca^{2+}, or phosphorylation cascades (see Boxes 4.9, 4.12, and 4.8, respectively). The levels of c-Fos and c-Jun are very low in basal conditions, but their transcription increases dramatically and transiently in many neurons within minutes following various extracellular signals or depolarization. The increased transcription of these genes is the consequence of the phosphorylation of transcription factors that are already present in the cell under an inactive form, and which are activated by phosphorylation (examples of such factors are Elk-1, see Box 4.8, and cAMP-responsive element binding protein [CREB], see Box 4.9). Such genes are called *immediate early genes*, and stimulation of their transcription does not require protein synthesis to occur. When c-Fos and c-Jun messenger ribonucleic acids (mRNAs) are translated into proteins, they dimerize and form an active transcription factor that binds to specific DNA sequences in the promoter region of other genes and stimulates their transcription. Transcription of these latter genes occurs several hours after the initial stimuli and is prevented by protein synthesis inhibitors that block the synthesis of c-Fos and c-Jun proteins (Chapter 6).

Other abbreviations: cAMP: cyclic adenosine 3′-5′-monophosphate.

Further reading: Guzowski et al., 2005; Hyman et al., 2006; Girault et al., 2007.

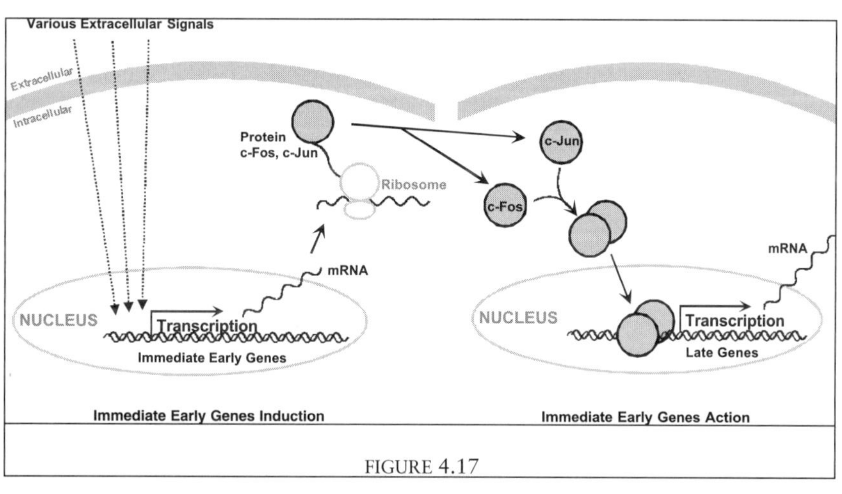

FIGURE 4.17

presynaptic terminals, their degradation, or their action on target nerve cells. Benzodiazepines are potent modulators of GABA-A receptors. Most neuroleptics are antagonists at dopamine receptors. Most antidepressants are inhibitors of the plasma membrane transporters for norepinephrine and/or serotonin. Other drugs have intracellular targets such as the monoamine oxidase inhibitor class of antidepressants, which inhibit an enzyme that degrades catecholamines and serotonin. In contrast to agents that act at the level of neurotransmitters, lithium is thought to exert its mood-stabilizing effects in part by dampening phosphatidylinositol turnover. It provides an example of a psychotherapeutic agent that appears to act directly at the level of a signal transduction pathway. Recent work has identified other signaling pathways as potential additional targets for lithium, including the protein kinase *glycogen-synthase kinase-3*. Although few psychotherapeutic drugs used at present act directly on signaling mechanisms, several compounds have already proven their usefulness in other fields of medicine, including cancer treatment and immunosuppression. It is safe to predict that due to the intense research in this field, new classes of drugs with interesting applications in psychiatry will be developed.

The antipsychotic effects of neuroleptics, as well as the therapeutic effects of antidepressants, take several days to appear, whereas their actions on receptors, transporters, or enzymes are immediate. This discrepancy indicates that many biochemical steps are probably involved between the primary targets of these drugs and the biological changes responsible for their clinically useful effects. These steps may include signal transduction pathways, which have started to be studied only very recently. It is likely that elucidation of such signaling pathways will be required to explain the therapeutic effects of neuroleptics and antidepressants and will be helpful in the design of new and more rapid active treatments. Likewise the signaling pathways underlying learning and memory at the cellular level are being deciphered at a rapid pace. Recent work has shown that abnormal incentive learning plays an important role in drug addiction (see Chapters 45 and 46), and possibly in other psychiatric diseases. The understanding of intracellular signaling pathways involved in the action of drugs of abuse is progressing rapidly and sheds light on the molecular basis of this frequent condition.

CONCLUSIONS

Signal transduction pathways form a complex network of biochemical reactions that allow cells to translate changes in their environment into appropriate responses. In spite of their complexity, these pathways have been highly conserved during evolution, and neurons use the same types of signaling cascades as other cells. In neurons, they are important for the modulation of the fast reactions involved in neuronal activity. They also provide the basis for the reactions that lead to neuronal and synaptic plasticity, and thus for the development of the nervous system, as well as for learning and memory. It is likely that, in the near future, environmental or genetic alterations of signal transduction pathway components will be found to be important in some psychiatric diseases. The understanding of these pathways is just at its beginning. To date, a few compounds acting on signal transduction mechanisms have already found clinical application. Moreover, this is an area of intense research, and it is likely that an increasing number of psychotherapeutic agents will be discovered that act by altering signal transduction mechanisms.

REFERENCES

Arnsten, A.F., Ramos, B.P., Birnbaum, S.G., and Taylor, J.R. (2005) Protein kinase A as a therapeutic target for memory disorders: rationale and challenges. *Trends Mol. Med.* 11:121–128.

Baud, V., and Karin, M. (2001) Signal transduction by tumor necrosis factor and its relatives. *Trends Cell Biol.* 11:372–377.

Benarroch, E.E. (2007) GABAA receptor heterogeneity, function, and implications for epilepsy. *Neurology* 68:612–614.

Berridge, M.J. (1998) Neuronal calcium signaling. *Neuron* 21:13–26.

Berridge, M.J. (2005) Unlocking the secrets of cell signaling. *Annu. Rev. Physiol.* 67:1–21.

Berridge, M.J., Lipp, P., and Bootman, M.D. (2000) The versatility and universality of calcium signalling. *Nat. Rev. Mol. Cell Biol.* 1:11–21.

Bockaert, J., and Pin, J.P. (1999) Molecular tinkering of G protein-coupled receptors: an evolutionary success. *Embo. J.* 18:1723–1729.

Bourne, H.R. (1995) GTPases: a family of molecular switches and clocks. *Philos. Trans. R. Soc. Lond. B Biol. Sci.* 349:283–289.

Bourne, H.R. (1997) How receptors talk to trimeric G proteins. *Curr. Opin. Cell Biol.* 9:134–142.

Cockcroft, S. (2006) The latest phospholipase C, PLCeta, is implicated in neuronal function. *Trends Biochem. Sci.* 31:4–7.

Collin, T., Marty, A., and Llano, I. (2005) Presynaptic calcium stores and synaptic transmission. *Curr. Opin. Neurobiol.* 15:275–281.

Cull-Candy, S., Brickley, S., and Farrant, M. (2001) NMDA receptor subunits: diversity, development and disease. *Curr. Opin. Neurobiol.* 11:327–335.

Dani, J.A., and Bertrand, D. (2007) Nicotinic acetylcholine receptors and nicotinic cholinergic mechanisms of the central nervous system. *Annu. Rev. Pharmacol. Toxicol.* 47:699–729.

Derkach, V.A., Oh, M.C., Guire, E.S., and Soderling, T.R. (2007) Regulatory mechanisms of AMPA receptors in synaptic plasticity. *Nat. Rev. Neurosci.* 8:101–113.

DeWire, S.M., Ahn, S., Lefkowitz, R.J., and Shenoy, S.K. (2007) Beta-arrestins and cell signaling. *Annu. Rev. Physiol.* 69:483–510.

Dilworth, F.J., and Chambon, P. (2001) Nuclear receptors coordinate the activities of chromatin remodeling complexes and coactivators to facilitate initiation of transcription. *Oncogene.* 20:3047–3054.

Farooqui, A.A., Ong, W.Y., and Horrocks, L.A. (2006) Inhibitors of brain phospholipase A2 activity: their neuropharmacological effects and therapeutic importance for the treatment of neurologic disorders. *Pharmacol. Rev.* 58:591–620.

Gainetdinov, R.R., Premont, R.T., Bohn, L.M., Lefkowitz, R.J., and Caron, M.G. (2004) Desensitization of G protein-coupled receptors and neuronal functions. *Annu. Rev. Neurosci.* 27:107–144.

Girault, J.A., and Greengard, P. (2004) The neurobiology of dopamine signaling. *Arch. Neurol.* 61:641–644.

Girault, J.A., Valjent, E., Caboche, J., and Herve, D. (2007) ERK2: a logical and gate critical for drug-induced plasticity? *Curr. Opin. Pharmacol.* 7:77–85.

Guzowski, J.F., Timlin, J.A., Roysam, B., McNaughton, B.L., Worley, P.F., and Barnes, C.A. (2005) Mapping behaviorally relevant neural circuits with immediate-early gene expression. *Curr. Opin. Neurobiol.* 15:599–606.

Hyman, S.E., Malenka, R.C., and Nestler, E.J. (2006) Neural mechanisms of addiction: the role of reward-related learning and memory. *Annu. Rev. Neurosci.* 29:565–598.

Iino, M. (2006) Ca2+-dependent inositol 1,4,5-trisphosphate and nitric oxide signaling in cerebellar neurons. *J. Pharmacol. Sci.* 100:538–544.

Iino, M. (2007) Regulation of cell functions by Ca2+ oscillation. *Adv. Exp. Med. Biol.* 592:305–312.

Imada, K., and Leonard, W.J. (2000) The Jak-STAT pathway. *Mol. Immunol.* 37:1–11.

Jaffe, A.B., and Hall, A. (2005) Rho GTPases: biochemistry and biology. *Annu. Rev. Cell Dev. Biol.* 21:247–269.

Jiang, X., and Wang, X. (2004) Cytochrome C-mediated apoptosis. *Annu. Rev. Biochem.* 73:87–106.

Johnson, S.A., and Hunter, T. (2005) Kinomics: methods for deciphering the kinome. *Nat. Methods* 2:17–25.

Johnston, G.A. (2005) GABA(A) receptor channel pharmacology. *Curr. Pharm. Des.* 11:1867–1885.

Kalb, R. (2005) The protean actions of neurotrophins and their receptors on the life and death of neurons. *Trends Neurosci.* 28: 5–11.

Koelle, M.R. (2006) Heterotrimeric G protein signaling: Getting inside the cell. *Cell* 126:25–27.

Kuriyan, J., and Cowburn, D. (1997) Modular peptide recognition domains in eukaryotic signaling. *Annu. Rev. Biophys. Biomol. Struct.* 26:259–288.

Lu, L., Koya, E., Zhai, H., Hope, B.T., and Shaham, Y. (2006) Role of ERK in cocaine addiction. *Trends Neurosci.* 29:695–703.

Luttrell, L.M. (2006) Transmembrane signaling by G protein-coupled receptors. *Methods Mol. Biol.* 332:3–49.

Mansuy, I.M., and Shenolikar, S. (2006) Protein serine/threonine phosphatases in neuronal plasticity and disorders of learning and memory. *Trends Neurosci.* 29:679–686.

Mark, M., Ghyselinck, N.B., and Chambon, P. (2006) Function of retinoid nuclear receptors: lessons from genetic and pharmacological dissections of the retinoic acid signaling pathway during mouse embryogenesis. *Annu. Rev. Pharmacol. Toxicol.* 46:451–480.

May, L.T., Leach, K., Sexton, P.M., and Christopoulos, A. (2007) Allosteric modulation of G protein-coupled receptors. *Annu. Rev. Pharmacol. Toxicol.* 47:1–51.

Mayer, M.L. (2005) Glutamate receptor ion channels. *Curr. Opin. Neurobiol.* 15:282–288.

Michel, J.J., and Scott, J.D. (2002) Akap mediated signal transduction. *Annu. Rev. Pharmacol. Toxicol.* 42:235–257.

Mikoshiba, K., and Hattori, M. (2000) IP_3 receptor-operated calcium entry. *Sci. STKE* 2000:E1.

Mohler, H., Fritschy, J.M., and Rudolph, U. (2002) A new benzodiazepine pharmacology. *J. Pharmacol. Exp. Ther.* 300:2–8.

Moore, C.A., Milano, S.K., and Benovic, J.L. (2007) Regulation of receptor trafficking by GRKs and arrestins. *Annu. Rev. Physiol.* 69:451–482.

Nairn, A.C., Svenningsson, P., Nishi, A., Fisone, G., Girault, J.A., and Greengard, P. (2004) The role of DARPP-32 in the actions of drugs of abuse. *Neuropharmacology* 47 (Suppl 1):14–23.

Nutt, D.J., and Malizia, A.L. (2001) New insights into the role of the GABA(A)-benzodiazepine receptor in psychiatric disorder. *Br. J. Psychiatry* 179:390–396.

O'Shea, J.J., Park, H., Pesu, M., Borie, D., and Changelian, P. (2005) New strategies for immunosuppression: interfering with cytokines by targeting the Jak/Stat pathway. *Curr. Opin. Rheumatol.* 17: 305–311.

Papin, J.A., Hunter, T., Palsson, B.O., and Subramaniam, S. (2005) Reconstruction of cellular signalling networks and analysis of their properties. *Nat. Rev. Mol. Cell Biol.* 6:99–111.

Patrick, G.N. (2006) Synapse formation and plasticity: recent insights from the perspective of the ubiquitin proteasome system. *Curr. Opin. Neurobiol.* 16:90–94.

Pawson, T. (2004) Specificity in signal transduction: from phosphotyrosine-SH2 domain interactions to complex cellular systems. *Cell* 116:191–203.

Pawson, T., and Scott, J.D. (1997) Signaling through scaffold, anchoring, and adaptor proteins. *Science* 278:2075–2080.

Pietrobon, D. (2005) Function and dysfunction of synaptic calcium channels: insights from mouse models. *Curr. Opin. Neurobiol.* 15:257–265.

Schlessinger, J. (2002) Ligand-induced, receptor-mediated dimerization and activation of EGF receptor. *Cell* 110:669–672.

Schlessinger, J., and Lemmon, M.A. (2003) SH2 and PTB domains in tyrosine kinase signaling. *Sci. STKE* 2003:RE12.

Seidel, H.M., Lamb, P., and Rosen, J. (2000) Pharmaceutical intervention in the JAK/STAT signaling pathway. *Oncogene.* 19: 2645–2656.

Shalin, S.C., Egli, R., Birnbaum, S.G., Roth, T.L., Levenson, J.M., and Sweatt, J.D. (2006) Signal transduction mechanisms in memory disorders. *Prog. Brain Res.* 157:25–41.

Smith, C.M., Radzio-Andzelm, E., Madhusudan, Akamine, P., and Taylor, S.S. (1999) The catalytic subunit of cAMP-dependent protein kinase: prototype for an extended network of communication. *Prog. Biophys. Mol. Biol.* 71:313–341.

Snyder, S.H., Jaffrey, S.R., and Zakhary, R. (1998) Nitric oxide and carbon monoxide: parallel roles as neural messengers. *Brain Res. Brain Res. Rev.* 26:167–175.

Svenningsson, P., Nishi, A., Fisone, G., Girault, J.A., Nairn, A.C., and Greengard, P. (2004) DARPP-32: an integrator of neurotransmission. *Annu. Rev. Pharmacol. Toxicol.* 44:269–296.

Weatherman, R.V., Fletterick, R.J., and Scanlan, T.S. (1999) Nuclear-receptor ligands and ligand-binding domains. *Annu. Rev. Biochem.* 68:559–581.

Yamaoka, K., Saharinen, P., Pesu, M., Holt, V.E. III, Silvennoinen, O., and O'Shea, J.J. (2004) The Janus kinases (Jaks). *Genome Biol.* 5:253.

Yan, N., and Shi, Y. (2005) Mechanisms of apoptosis through structural biology. *Annu. Rev. Cell Dev. Biol.* 21:35–56.

Zebisch, A., Czernilofsky, A.P., Keri, G., Smigelskaite, J., Sill, H., and Troppmair, J. (2007) Signaling through RAS-RAF-MEK-ERK: from basics to bedside. *Curr. Med. Chem.* 14:601–623.

5 Mechanisms of Neural Plasticity

ERIC J. NESTLER AND STEVEN E. HYMAN

The human brain is remarkably plastic. It adapts to a wide variety of circumstances, forms memories of experiences, and learns motor programs and complex behavioral strategies; it can become dependent on drugs or produce disabling psychopathology; and it can recover. The plasticity of our brains and, therefore, our ability to learn and adapt is at the heart of our evolutionary success in nature and of our cultural evolution as well.

The plasticity of the brain is based on the ability of a host of external or environmental factors, and an array of internal factors (including hormones, neurotransmitters, and neurotrophic factors), to produce relatively stable changes in neural and glial cells throughout the nervous system and thus to alter neural circuits. Such changes underlie alterations in the ways in which neurons process information.

Many types of plasticity have been documented in the nervous system. In several model systems, memory formation has been shown to be dependent on altering the strength of synaptic connections between neurons. Other forms of plasticity can be viewed as compensatory homeostatic responses to return the system to baseline function in the continued presence of the initiating stimulus. Such adaptations, referred to as *negative feedback*, could easily explain, for example, tolerance to a drug or desensitization to some behavioral challenge. Yet other neural plastic events represent positive feedback in that they serve to increase the sensitivity of the system to continued presence of the initiating stimulus. Such changes could explain various forms of sensitization, such as the production of psychotic symptoms by even small doses of cocaine in individuals with heavy abuse histories. In addition to these quantitative neural plastic events, which involve conceptually simple up- or down-regulation of signaling through a given pathway in response to a certain stimulus, the brain exhibits the ability to change qualitatively. That is, some stimuli, after repeated application, alter the brain's response to the same stimulus as well as to other stimuli, resulting in a new functional state. It may be that such qualitative, and more complex, forms of neural plasticity are particularly relevant to the pathogenesis and treatment of psychiatric disorders (Hyman and Nestler, 1996).

Because virtually all functions in a nerve cell are subserved by proteins, plasticity must ultimately be mediated by alterations in the functioning of individual proteins. There are three general ways in which this can occur: allosteric regulation, covalent modification, and changes in the total amount of a protein at its site of action in the cell.

ALLOSTERIC REGULATION

Allosteric regulation of proteins is one of the fundamental processes of cell regulation. It involves alterations in a protein's function upon binding another molecule, which in some cases is another protein. A classical example of allosteric regulation is an alteration in an enzyme's activity by a small molecule. As just one example, tyrosine hydroxylase (the rate-limiting enzyme in catecholamine biosynthesis) exhibits end-product inhibition, wherein enzyme activity is inhibited upon binding specific products of its biosynthetic pathway (for example, dihydroxyphenylalanine [DOPA], dopamine). However, allosteric regulation is far more pervasive than enzyme regulation. Thus, activation of all receptors by their specific neurotransmitter, hormone, or other ligand represents allosteric regulation. Similarly, protein–protein interactions between subunits of a multimeric protein complex or between successive steps in signal transduction pathways (Chapter 4) represent allosteric regulation as well. Nevertheless, though allosteric regulation is widespread, it is almost always relatively transient and therefore mediates particularly short-lived forms of plasticity in the nervous system. More long-lived changes occur via other mechanisms.

COVALENT MODIFICATION

Covalent modification is a process wherein proteins are modified by the formation of new chemical bonds. Of the numerous forms of covalent modification, protein phosphorylation is by far the most significant (Chapter 4). Virtually every type of neural protein, and therefore every type of neural process, is regulated by phosphorylation; moveover, such phosphorylation reactions are regulated by virtually every type of external and internal stimulus. As a result, protein phosphorylation can be viewed as the major molecular currency of intracellular regulation and one of the central mechanisms underlying diverse types of neural plasticity (Greengard, 2001). Some examples of phosphorylation-mediated neural plasticity include phosphorylation of ion channels (which alters the electrical excitability of target neurons), phosphorylation of neurotransmitter receptors and postreceptor signaling proteins (which alters the responsiveness of target neurons to synaptic inputs), and phosphorylation of neurotransmitter synthetic enzymes and of proteins that control neurotransmitter storage and release (which alters a neuron's capacity for neurotransmission, that is, its ability to influence target neurons).

There are many other types of covalent modification of proteins (for example, acylation, glycosylation, adenosine diphosphate [ADP]-ribosylation, carboxymethylation), which in a relatively small number of cases provide additional mechanisms of plasticity. As one example, the addition of various fatty acid groups (*myristoylation, palmitoylation*, etc.) can alter the ability of a protein to associate with a cell membrane. Another example is the acetylation and methylation of histone proteins (nuclear proteins that bind DNA), which regulates the transcription of nearby genes (Chapter 8).

REGULATION OF THE TOTAL AMOUNT OF A PROTEIN

The other general mechanism underlying neural plasticity is alteration in the amount of a specific protein in a cell. This can result in quantitative and even qualitative changes in the innumerable protein components of neurons. Some examples include alterations in the numbers and types of ion channels and receptors present on the cell membrane, levels of proteins involved in postreceptor signal transduction in neurons, and even the morphology of neurons and the number of synaptic connections they form. Regulation of the types and amounts of proteins expressed by a neuron occurs on a continual basis to fine-tune the functional state of the neuron in response to complex synaptic inputs.

There are many ways in which the total amount of a protein in a neuron can be altered. Most work to date has focused on the regulation of gene expression, that is, the rate at which a particular gene is transcribed. Indeed, the mechanisms by which neurotransmitters and other extracellular stimuli result in alterations at the transcriptional level are becoming increasingly well understood. Changes at the level of transcription can exhibit a prolonged time course, which makes them attractive candidates as mediators of long-lasting plasticity in the brain.

However, it is important to emphasize from the outset that the total amount of a protein can be altered at a number of other levels. The level of a protein will change, despite a constant rate of transcription, if its mRNA is degraded or translated at a different rate. Similarly, the level of a protein will change, despite a constant rate of messenger ribonucleic acid (mRNA) translation, if it is degraded at a different rate. In recent years, it has become apparent that changes in mRNA and protein stability probably do contribute in important ways to neurotransmitter-induced changes in protein levels. For example, the stability and translatability of specific mRNAs have been shown to be regulated via the phosphorylation of several types of ribosome-associated proteins by various protein kinases. mRNA stability is also regulated by microRNAs (miRNAs), which bind to specific mRNAs and induce their degradation (Cao et al., 2006). As another example, a family of proteases (enzymes that degrade proteins) have been shown to be specifically activated by increases in cellular Ca^{2+} levels. In addition, the proteolysis of certain proteins via their ubiquitinylation and subsequent degradation in proteasomes is subject to dynamic regulation. The importance of posttranscriptional mechanisms is highlighted by the growing number of cases where changes in the level of a protein in response to some perturbation are not associated with changes in that protein's mRNA. These posttranscriptional mechanisms now warrant much greater attention as mechanisms of neural plasticity.

Another way the function of a protein can be altered is by controlling its distribution within the cell, that is, controlling what fraction of the protein present in a cell is localized to its site of action. There are highly regulated processes governing the translocation of a newly translated protein to its site of action. Moreover, once positioned at its site of action, a protein can be reversibly moved to and from this position. This is best illustrated by G protein–coupled receptors, many of which, upon persistent activation by ligand, become sequestered into intracellular membrane vesicles. The receptor proteins can remain sequestered for a period of time, during which they can be reinserted into the plasma membrane as a functional receptor upon removal of the ligand. After prolonged periods of agonist exposure, however, this process becomes irreversible as the receptors are digested via the lysosomal pathway. Another illustration of this general mechanism is anchoring proteins, which serve to scaffold specific signaling proteins (*receptors, protein kinases, protein phosphatases*) to specific subcellular domains. Efforts to understand the contribution of these anchoring proteins to neural plasticity represent an exciting area of current research (Scannevin and Huganir, 2000).

The multitude of mechanisms by which total amounts of proteins can be regulated in a neuron (*transcriptionally, pretranslationally,* and *posttranslationally*) underscores the complex mechanisms used by neurons to maintain their homeostatic balance.

BEHAVIORAL PLASTICITY

Ultimately, the long-term effects of environmental stimuli on the brain, ranging from long-term memory to altered patterns of behavior, are mediated by these complex processes involving regulation of the covalent modification and total amounts of numerous proteins in specific types of neurons in the brain. These biochemical changes lead successively to changes in the function or efficacy of synapses, changes in the way individual neurons process information, and, ultimately, changes in communication among neural networks that underlie complex behaviors. The purpose of this chapter is to illustrate some of the basic mechanisms by which protein phosphorylation, the predominant form of covalent modification of proteins, contributes to the extraordinary plasticity evident in the adult brain. The role played by the regulation of gene expression is covered in Chapter 6.

NEURAL PLASTICITY MEDIATED BY PROTEIN PHOSPHORYLATION

As stated above, virtually every type of neuronal protein undergoes phosphorylation, and the vast majority of neuronal process can be regulated by this process. Evidence accumulated over the past 20 years has indicated ways in which phosphorylation alters the functional activity of specific proteins and has established the precise mechanisms by which their phosphorylation, in response to neurotransmitters and other extracellular stimuli, mediates short- and long-term effects of those extracellular stimuli on neuronal function (Fig. 5.1). Illustrative examples are provided below. A more complete description of the pathways that control individual phosphorylation reactions can be found in Chapter 4.

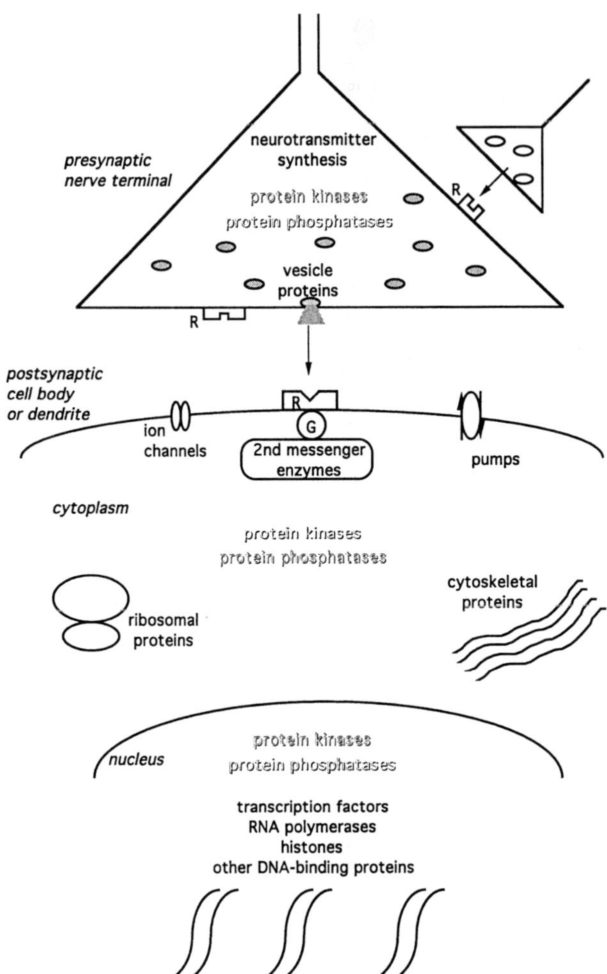

FIGURE 5.1 Schematic illustration of the types of neuronal proteins regulated by phosphorylation. The figure shows that virtually every class of protein, and therefore every type of neural process, is influenced by protein phosphorylation mechanisms. From Hyman and Nestler (1993).

Regulation of Receptors by Phosphorylation

Most neurotransmitter receptors are regulated by phosphorylation. Such phosphorylation alters the functional activity of G protein–coupled receptors, for example, by altering their ability to be activated by their endogenous ligand or to activate their G protein effectors. Phosphorylation of ionotropic receptors can, in addition, alter the properties of their intrinsic ion channels (e.g., Swope et al., 1999; Malenka and Bear, 2004).

Stimulation of most G protein–coupled receptors by their ligands leads to decreased sensitivity of the receptor to subsequent stimulation, a process called *homologous desensitization* (Fig. 5.2). In all cases of homologous desensitization studied to date, this is due to receptor-mediated activation of protein kinases leading to phosphorylation of the receptor. A receptor can also be phosphorylated by a protein kinase activated by stimulation of another receptor type on the same cell. This is described as heterologous desensitization (Fig. 5.2).

The best-studied example of receptor phosphorylation involves the β-adrenergic receptor (Fig. 5.3) (Kohout and Lefkowitz, 2003). Activation of this receptor leads, via coupling with stimulatory G proteins (Gs), to activation of adenylyl cyclase, as well as increased levels of cyclic adenosine monophosphate (cAMP) and of activated cAMP-dependent protein kinase (PKA), which then phosphorylates the receptor on several serine residues in its cytoplasmic domains. This appears to reduce the ability of the receptor to bind ligand or

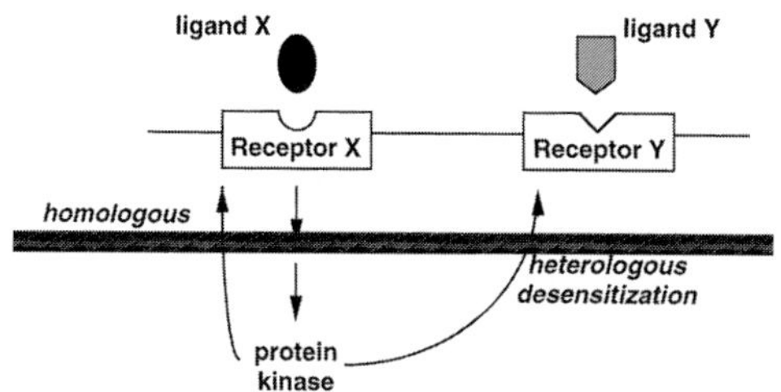

FIGURE 5.2 Schematic illustration of homologous and heterologous desensitization of G protein–coupled receptors. Homologous desensitization occurs when a protein kinase activated by a particular ligand–receptor interaction feeds back and phosphorylates (and inhibits the further activation of) that receptor. Heterologous desensitization occurs when a protein kinase activated by a particular ligand–receptor interaction phosphorylates (and inhibits the further activation of) a receptor for a different ligand.

activate its associated G protein. Phosphorylation of the β-adrenergic receptor by PKA could also mediate heterologous desensitization of the receptor: any neurotransmitter–receptor system that works through cAMP would be expected to stimulate β-adrenergic receptor phosphorylation via PKA and lead to receptor desensitization.

In addition, the β-adrenergic receptor is phosphorylated on several distinct serine residues by another protein kinase physically associated with the receptor (Fig. 5.3). This kinase was originally termed β-adrenergic receptor kinase (βARK) but is now referred to as a G protein receptor kinase (GRK), which along with numerous other GRK subtypes phosphorylates many types of Gs (Kohout and Lefkowitz, 2003; von Zastrow et al., 2003). GRKs can phosphorylate the β-adrenergic receptor and other receptors only when they are bound to ligand; that is, the binding of ligand to the receptors alters the receptors' conformation such that they are rendered good substrates for the kinases. Upon phosphorylation by a GRK, the receptors can bind an additional protein, from a family called the *arrestins*, which renders the receptors unable to interact further with ligand or G protein. This process involves the sequestration of the receptor via an active endocytic process mediated via the protein dynamin.

Regulation of Ion Channels and Pumps by Phosphorylation

Like receptors, most ion channels and pumps can be phosphorylated by one or more protein kinases (Cantrell and Catterall, 2001). In most cases, phosphorylation of the channels modifies their probability of opening or closing in response to their primary gating mechanism. This is illustrated by the L-type voltage-dependent Ca^{2+} channel, the type of channel inhibited by the dihydropyridine Ca^{2+} channel blocker drugs such as verapamil. When the L-type channel is phosphorylated by PKA, it is rendered more likely to open in response to membrane depolarization (Fig. 5.4). This mechanism plays an important role in the regulation of cardiac function: stimulation of β-adrenergic receptors by norepinephrine or epinephrine causes phosphorylation of the channel by increasing levels of cAMP and of activated PKA. Because the phosphorylated L-type channel opens more readily, a greater amount of Ca^{2+} enters the cell. In the heart, this mechanism is responsible for catecholamine-induced increases in cardiac rate and contractility. In a smaller number of cases, phosphorylation of ion

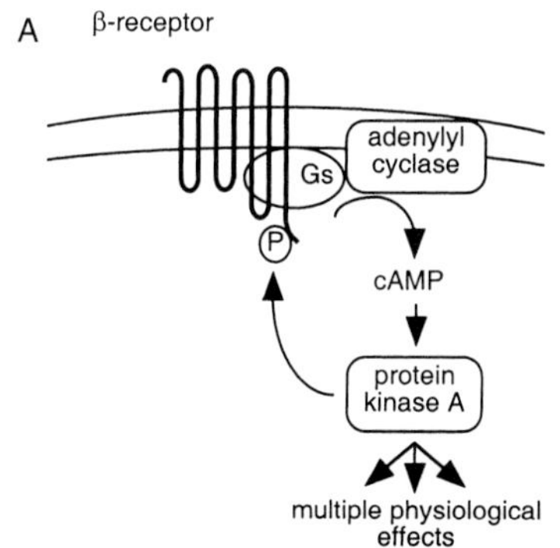

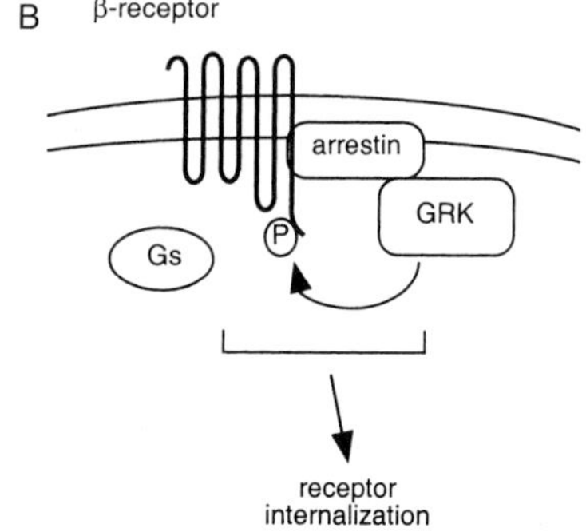

FIGURE 5.3 Scheme illustrating desensitization of the β-adrenergic receptor mediated by receptor phosphorylation. (*A*) Activation of the β-adrenergic receptor by its ligand results, via coupling with stimulatory G proteins (Gs), in stimulation of adenylyl cyclase, increased levels of cyclic adenosine monophosphate (cAMP), and stimulation of cAMP-dependent protein kinase, which mediates the physiological effects of β-receptor activation through the phosphorylation of numerous cellular proteins. The protein kinase also phosphorylates several serine residues in cytoplasmic domains of the receptor, which results in receptor desensitization. (*B*) Activation of the β-adrenergic receptor also results in a conformational change in the receptor, which renders it an effective substrate for a G protein receptor kinase (GRK). This GRK phosphorylates the receptor at distinct serine residues, which leads to the functional "uncoupling" of the receptor from Gs, thereby resulting in receptor desensitization. This uncoupling requires the action of an additional protein, termed *arrestin*, which interacts preferentially with the phosphorylated receptor to prevent its activation of Gs.

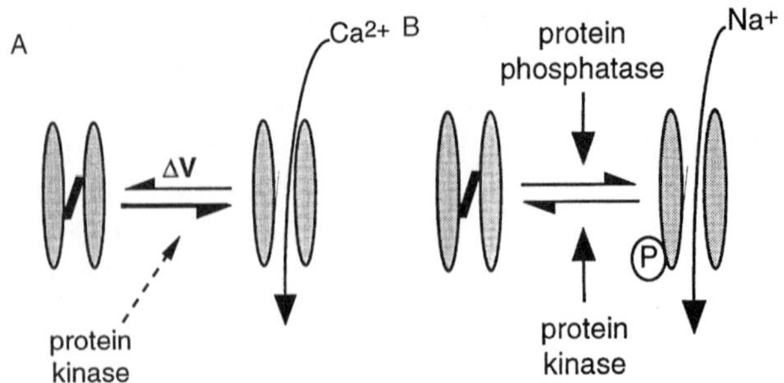

FIGURE 5.4 Schematic diagram of the regulation of ion channels by phosphorylation. For most channels, phosphorylation modulates channel function by altering the probability of opening in response to the primary gating mechanism. For example, (*A*) shows a voltage-gated l-type Ca21 channel that opens or closes in response to a change in membrane potential (DV). Phosphorylation increases the likelihood of channel opening upon membrane depolarization. In other cases, as shown in (*B*), phosphorylation can gate (open or close) a channel.

channels may represent the primary gating mechanism that determines their opening or closing, although this has yet to be demonstrated with certainty.

Most types of electrogenic pumps, which maintain stable levels of ions inside and outside of the neuronal membrane, also undergo phosphorylation by second messenger–dependent protein kinases (Lopina, 2000). For example, phosphorylation and regulation of the activity of the Na^+,$K^{\+}$- pump alters the rate at which the normal distribution of ions can be restored after a train of action potentials. This would be expected to alter the excitability of the neurons.

Regulation of Intracellular Messenger Pathways by Phosphorylation

Many of the protein components of intracellular messenger systems are themselves phosphoproteins (that is, substrates for protein kinases) (Nestler and Greengard, 1984). This permits extraordinarily complex cross-talk between signaling pathways, which enables cells to coordinate their responses to multiple environmental stimuli. Numerous G protein subunits undergo phosphorylation by a variety of protein kinases. Proteins that control the synthesis of the cyclic nucleotide second messengers (*adenylyl cyclase* and *guanylyl cyclase*), as well as the degradation of cyclic nucleotides (*phosphodiesterases*), are regulated by phosphorylation. Similarly, proteins that lead to increases in intracellular Ca^{2+} or phosphatidylinositol turnover (for example, phospholipase C, Ca^{2+} channels, the inositol 1,4,5 triphosphate [IP_3] receptor), as well as proteins that decrease Ca^{2+} levels (for example, the Ca^{2+},Mg^{2+}-ATPase pump), are regulated by phosphorylation. Many protein kinases are themselves phosphorylated and regulated by other protein kinases. For example, as described in Chapter 4, MAP-kinases (mitogen-activated protein kinases; also called extracellular signal regulated kinases or ERKs) are activated by MAP-kinase kinases, which in turn are activated by MAP-kinase kinase kinases. These successive phosphorylation events enable a high degree of amplification of a signal in response to an extracellular stimulus. Likewise, protein phosphatases are regulated by phosphorylation: protein phosphatase type 1 (one of a family of enzymes that removes phosphate groups from other proteins; Chapter 4) is regulated by protein phosphatase inhibitor proteins, which themselves are regulated by phosphorylation. An example is provided by dopamine- and cAMP-regulated phosphoprotein of 32 kDa (DARPP32), which is highly enriched in striatal neurons. Phosphorylation of DARPP32 by PKA, and by several other protein kinases, modulates protein phosphatase 1 activity and thereby potently influences the ability of several neurotransmitters and psychotropic drugs to regulate striatal function (Greengard, 2001).

In addition, most, and possibly all, protein kinases undergo autophosphorylation, whereby they phosphorylate and regulate themselves. In most cases, such autophosphorylation appears to facilitate activation of the enzyme. For example, autophosphorylation of Ca^{2+}/calmodulin-dependent protein kinase II (Cam-kinase II) renders the protein kinase independent of Ca^{2+}. This means that the enzyme, activated originally in response to elevated levels of cellular Ca^{2+}, remains active after Ca^{2+} levels have returned to normal. By this mechanism, neurotransmitters that activate Cam-kinase II can produce relatively long-lived alterations in neuronal function.

It is clear from the above discussion that each second messenger system in the brain influences many others. This means that these systems operate as a complex web of interacting pathways. Thus, any time a neurotransmitter produces its primary effect on one second messenger system, many other systems will also be influenced eventually, with such interactions mediated for the most part through protein phosphorylation.

Regulation of Neurotransmitter Metabolism by Phosphorylation

Many neurotransmitter synthetic enzymes are regulated by phosphorylation. The best-studied example is tyrosine hydroxylase, which is phosphorylated and activated by PKA, Cam-kinase II, protein kinase C, and MAP-kinases, among others, with distinct serine residues phosphorylated by each of these kinases (Kumer and Vrana, 1996). In general, phosphorylation increases the V_{max} of tyrosine hydroxylase (that is, increases the maximal catalytic activity of a single enzyme molecule), as well as the affinity of the enzyme for its pterin cofactor (which would make the enzyme more active at subsaturating concentrations of cofactor). Such phosphorylation of the enzyme has been shown to mediate the ability of many types of neurotransmitters (acting through the cAMP and/or Ca^{2+} systems) and neurotrophic factors (acting ultimately through MAP-kinases) to rapidly increase tyrosine hydroxylase activity and, as a result, the capacity of catecholaminergic neurons to synthesize their neurotransmitter. This provides a critical homeostatic control mechanism that enables catecholaminergic neurons to alter their functional activity in response to a variety of synaptic inputs.

Regulation of Neurotransmitter Release by Phosphorylation

As discussed earlier, many ion channels are regulated by phosphorylation, and such phosphorylation at nerve terminals would be expected to alter neurotransmitter release by influencing the amount of Ca^{2+} that enters the terminals during an action potential. There are also recent reports that transporters, proteins that mediate the reuptake of neurotransmitter from the synapse back into nerve terminals, can also be regulated by phosphorylation (e.g., Prasad et al., 2005). Such reactions regulate the duration and extent of a neurotransmitter signal. Additional mechanisms by which neurotransmitter release is regulated in the brain involve the phosphorylation of a variety of synaptic vesicle–associated proteins (Lin and Scheller, 2000; Jahn et al., 2003). Examples include SNAP25 (synaptosomal associated protein 25), syntaxin 1, and synaptobrevin, which are key mediators of neurotransmitter release. These proteins are phosphorylated by several Ca^{2+}-dependent and -independent protein kinases, which influences the proteins' interactions with two other phosphoproteins, NSF (N-ethylmaleimide-sensitive fusion protein) and SNAP (soluble NSF attachment protein). These interactions in turn influence docking of synaptic vesicles with the nerve terminal plasma membrane and for subsequent membrane fusion, which underlies neurotransmitter release. These various mechanisms of regulating neurotransmitter release are important steps by which behavioral stimuli and psychotropic drugs modulate the strength of specific synaptic connections in specific neural circuits.

Regulation of Neuronal Growth and Differentiation by Phosphorylation

Alterations in neural shape and structure occur not only during development, but continually throughout the adult life of an organism. The retraction (or elimination) of synapses in specific brain regions, or the formation of new synapses, is a major form of neural plasticity in the adult brain. This has been highlighted in recent years by the finding that dendritic spines, which receive incoming synaptic contacts, can be extended or retracted to a remarkable extent over a relatively short time period—for example, in response to stress, learning, or drug treatments (Robinson and Kolb, 2004; Yuste and Bonhoeffer, 2004; Korte et al., 2005). This seems to involve the formation or dissolution of large multiprotein complexes that mediate neurotransmission at the synapse. Understanding the molecular basis of this form of plasticity, which has been implicated in many neuropsychiatric disorders, is a major challenge of the next decade of psychiatric neuroscience. Although details of the molecular mechanisms involved remain incompletely understood, protein phosphorylation appears to play a central role.

As described in Chapter 4, all neurotrophic factors activate, either directly or indirectly, protein tyrosine kinases, which, in turn, trigger complex cascades that lead to the activation of many types of protein serine-threonine kinases, such as the MAP-kinases and Akt (also called *protein kinase B*). Akt is particularly interesting because regulation of its levels has been shown in several systems to control the size of neuronal cell bodies. Increased Akt function, for example, increases neuronal size and has been implicated in rare forms of mental retardation and autism. Progress has been made in recent years in identifying the proteins whose phosphorylation mediates the myriad trophic actions of these factors, as well as the trophic actions of more traditional neurotransmitters. Virtually all cytoskeletal and contractile proteins are heavily phosphorylated by numerous protein kinases, and, in many cases, their functional activity is known to be altered upon phosphorylation. Specific types of protein kinases are induced in cells, including neurons, at precise points during the cell cycle. An example is the cyclin-dependent kinases (Cdks). Similarly, specific types of protein kinases and substrate proteins are expressed in brain at particular stages during development and differentiation. Neural cell adhesion molecules and proteins (for example, growth-associated protein of 43 kD [GAP-43]) expressed specifically in axonal growth cones (the leading tips of growing axons), which are important for cell-cell interactions in the brain and the formation of synaptic connections, are also regulated by phosphorylation. Finally, as is seen in Chapter 6, many proteins that control gene expression are regulated by phosphorylation. As complex neural functions are described increasingly in terms of the molecular events that underlie them, it will be possible to understand the basis on which growth and motility are regulated in the nervous system and result in important forms of neural plasticity.

Regulation of Gene Expression by Phosphorylation

In recent years, it has become clear that protein phosphorylation also plays a fundamental role in the regulation of neuronal gene expression, in a sense the ultimate end point of signal transduction in the brain (e.g., Hyman and Nestler, 1996; Mayr and Montminy, 2001). Such regulation appears to be achieved through the phosphorylation of subsets of proteins that regulate every step involved in transcribing the genetic code from DNA to protein (Chapter 6).

NEURAL PLASTICITY MEDIATED BY ALTERED PROTEIN EXPRESSION

As mentioned above, changes in the levels of specific proteins in response to extracellular signals, which occur continually to adapt brain function to complex environmental cues, can potentially produce long-lasting alterations in virtually all aspects of a neuron's functioning. Altered levels of channels alter the electrical properties and excitability of a neuron; altered levels of receptors alter the neuron's responsiveness to the relevant neurotransmitter inputs; altered levels of peptide neurotransmitters (or of enzymes that synthesize small-molecule neurotransmitters) alter the neuron's capacity for neurotransmission; altered levels of presynaptic reuptake transporters alter the duration of the relevant neurotransmitter signals; and altered levels of enzymes in the glutathione pathway (a neuron's major protective mechanism against oxidative injury) alter the neuron's vulnerability to excitotoxicity. Indeed, almost all proteins in brain are probably subject to dynamic regulation under particular circumstances.

There are now many well described examples of altered levels of a particular protein after chronic perturbations, such as drug treatments, electrical stimulation, stress, and so on, as seen throughout this textbook. In most cases, however, the mechanisms underlying such in vivo changes (whether transcriptional, posttranscriptional, or posttranslational) remain poorly understood. It also has been difficult to relate changes in a specific protein to changes in the functional activity of a neuron and in the behavioral output in which that neuron plays a role.

Building such causal bridges between molecular, cellular, and behavioral levels represents one of the foremost challenges in the neurosciences today. Genetic mutant mice and viral-mediated gene transfer are promising new tools with which to establish such information. For example, it is now possible to construct mice in which a particular gene of interest can be turned on or off selectively in specific subpopulations of neurons at any time in the life of the animal (e.g., Kelz et al., 1999; Mayford and Kandel, 1999). As another example, neurotropic viruses (*adeno-associated virus, herpes simplex virus*) can be injected into specific brain regions, where they infect neurons in the vicinity of the injection site and express an exogenous protein of interest (Neve et al., 2005). By combining these new approaches of molecular neurobiology (which are described in greater detail in Chapter 7) with the more traditional disciplines of neuropharmacology and behavioral neuroscience, it will be possible over the next several decades to build a progressively more sophisticated and complete understanding of the ways in which molecular and cellular plasticity summates to behavioral plasticity.

MOLECULAR BASIS OF LEARNING AND MEMORY

Understanding how the brain learns and stores memories is one of the ultimate goals of neuroscience. Each of the neurotransmitter, neurotrophic factor, and drug-induced changes in protein phosphorylation and expression discussed in this chapter and elsewhere (Chapters 4 and 6) represents a form of molecular "memory" within individual neurons. In all likelihood, learning and memory at the behavioral level are mediated by complex accumulations of these basic types of changes to produce alterations in the number, structure, and efficacy of synapses within particular neural circuits. Changes in synaptic efficacy may be due to altered patterns of neurotransmitter release by the presynaptic neuron or changes in the effect of a neurotransmitter on the postsynaptic cell. Because alterations in protein phosphorylation tend to be more readily reversible than alterations in protein expression, it is often hypothesized that regulation of the phosphorylation state of particular proteins may underlie short-term memory, whereas changes in protein expression may be required for longer term memory. As mentioned above, a major objective of current research is to relate specific alterations in the phosphorylation or expression of proteins to specific behavioral phenomena.

Long-term potentiation and long-term depression are particularly well-studied forms of synaptic plasticity. Although they have not been related beyond doubt to specific forms of behaviorally relevant memory, these processes provide important model systems in which long-term changes in the efficacy of synaptic transmission can be elicited and maintained in the nervous system.

Long-Term Potentiation and Depression

Long-term potentiation (LTP) and long-term depression (LTD) are the most widely studied forms of activity-dependent synaptic plasticity in the mammalian nervous system (Malenka and Bear, 2004). Both have been best characterized in area CA1 of the hippocampus but demonstrated at numerous other locations as well. Hippocampal neurons have been intensively studied for several reasons. First, the hippocampus has a relatively simple and orderly architecture that permits physiological experimentation on intact synapses within brain slices. Second, clinical-pathological correlations in humans, following stroke, anoxic injury, or viral infections, have demonstrated that the hippocampus is required for the formation of new declarative memory (Squire and Zola, 1996).

Long-term potentiation can be induced experimentally in vivo, as well as in vitro in brain slices, in area CA1 of the hippocampus by stimulating presynaptic fibers (the Schaeffer collateral pathway) with a brief (1 second) train of high-frequency electrical impulses (referred to as a tetanus) resembling impulse trains that can occur physiologically. The result of the tetanus is a marked and long-lasting enhancement in the functional responsiveness of postsynaptic cells to subsequent low-frequency stimulation (that is, presynaptic stimuli produce a much larger synaptic current after induction of LTP than before). Long-term potentiation induced in vivo in the CA1 region of hippocampus can last for weeks.

Hippocampal synapses that express LTP utilize glutamate as their neurotransmitter. As described in Chapter 2, glutamate receptor types (named for their selective agonists) include *N*-methyl-D-aspartate (NMDA) receptors and two types of non-NMDA receptors (α-amino-3-hydroxy-5-methyl-4-isoxasolepropionic acid [AMPA] and kainate). To a first approximation, activation of AMPA and kainate receptors causes increased permeability predominantly to Na^+ and, hence, depolarization of the postsynaptic neuron. The NMDA receptors permit entry of Na^+ and Ca^{2+} but are activated only by glutamate if the postsynaptic cell has already been depolarized. This is because depolarization is required to relieve a block of the NMDA receptor channel by Mg^{2+}. Thus, the NMDA receptor channel is ligand- and voltage-gated.

In hippocampal CA1 neurons, LTP can be generated only if Ca^{2+} enters the postsynaptic neuron via NMDA channels (Luscher et al., 2000). Compounds that selectively block the glutamate binding site on NMDA receptors (for example, 2-amino-5-phosphonovalerate [APV]) or that block the NMDA receptor channel (for example, MK801 or dizocilpine) block the initiation of LTP. The NMDA receptors detect coincident activity among presynaptic inputs: depolarization of the postsynaptic cell (for example, by AMPA or kainate receptors) followed closely by activation of the NMDA receptor itself. As a result, Ca^{2+} entry into the postsynaptic cell depends on a close association between two events. A neural mechanism that detects coincident events (associations) is an attractive model of memory because association is the essence of classical conditioning in animals and of the inference of causal relations in humans.

Experimentally, initiation of LTP can be separated from its long-term maintenance. For example, compounds that inhibit protein synthesis have no effect on the initiation of LTP in CA1 neurons but appear to block its maintenance. Increasing evidence indicates that entry of Ca^{2+} through NMDA receptor channels initiates LTP in CA1 neurons by activating protein kinases, in particular, Cam-kinase II (Fig. 5.5). The phosphoprotein targets of these kinases that mediate LTP have not yet been identified with certainty. One possibility is that the AMPA glutamate receptors themselves are phosphorylated by the protein kinases, and that this results in an enhancement of receptor function. There is also evidence that phosphorylation of "silent" AMPA receptors, which are sequestered intracellularly, causes their redistribution to the plasma membrane, where they become functional (Malinow and Malenka, 2002).

Distinct but related processes may underlie the maintenance of LTP so that it can last for days, weeks, or even longer. It is currently believed that this long-term maintenance of LTP requires new protein synthesis and regulation of gene transcription, perhaps via a protein kinase cascade. A role for certain transcription factors has been proposed but remains hypothetical. Transcription factors are proteins that bind to specific sequences of DNA in the promoters of certain genes and control the rate at which those genes are transcribed (Chapter 6). Attention has focused mainly on the transcription factor *CREB* (cAMP-response element binding protein) (Marie et al., 2005), although numerous other transcription factors also may be involved. It is not yet clear whether the very-long-lasting change in synaptic efficacy requires synaptic modifications in addition to, or in place of, those caused by the early activation of protein kinases. Possible functional changes implicated in this long-lasting enhancement of synaptic efficacy include (*1*) enhancement of glutamate receptor function achieved via receptor phosphorylation or (*2*) an increased number of glutamate receptor subunits achieved via altered gene expression (Fig. 5.5).

Long-term potentiation has been described at many other synapses in the brain. Importantly, different mechanisms may be involved in mediating the initiation and expression of LTP compared to those established for the CA1 neurons of the hippocampus. For example, activation of NMDA receptors is not required for the production of LTP in CA3 pyramidal neurons. In addition, in many brain regions, LTP appears to involve primarily presynaptic alterations, such as an enhancement in the amount of glutamate released from glutamatergic nerve terminals in response to a nerve impulse. One mechanism underlying such presynaptic LTP is the

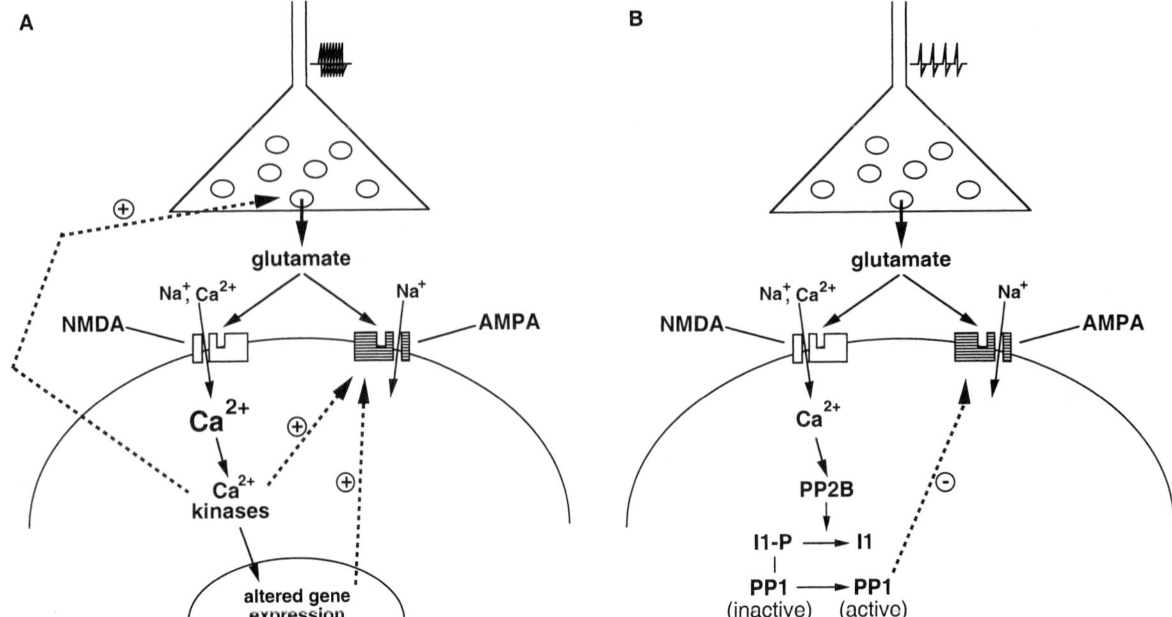

FIGURE 5.5 Schematic illustration of possible mechanisms underlying long-term potentiation (LTP) and long-term depression (LTD) in CA1 of hippocampus. (*A*) *Long-term potentiation* refers to a long-lasting enhancement of synaptic efficacy in response to a brief period of intense stimulation. Stimulation of the presynaptic nerve results in release of glutamate, which acts on α-amino-3-hydroxy-5-methyl-4-isoxasolepropionic acid (AMPA) glutamate receptors to depolarize the postsynaptic dendritic element. Upon high-frequency stimulation, this depolarization becomes sufficient to relieve Mg21 blockade (not shown) of the *N*-methyl-D-aspartate (NMDA) glutamate receptor to enable glutamate to also activate this receptor, which leads to the influx of Ca21 into the neuron. Ca21 serves as the critical signal to then initiate LTP, probably via the activation of Ca21-dependent protein kinases, such as Ca21/calmodulin-dependent protein kinase II (Cam-kinase II). Once activated, the protein kinases may phosphorylate AMPA glutamate receptors and thereby increase the physiological responsiveness of the receptors to subsequent signals. Receptor phosphorylation also appears to stimulate the insertion of "silent" AMPA receptors (sequestered intracellularly) into the plasma membrane, where they become functional (not shown). The protein kinases also may phosphorylate transcription factors (for example, cAMP-responsive element binding protein [CREB]) and thereby increase the expression of AMPA glutamate receptor subunits, which also increase their physiological responsiveness to subsequent signals. (*B*) *Long-term depression* refers to a long-lasting decrease in synaptic efficacy caused by sustained low-frequency stimulation. In CA1 pyramidal neurons, LTD is mediated via smaller NMDA receptor-dependent increases in intracellular Ca21 levels, which activate the Ca21/calmodulin-dependent protein phosphatase, calcineurin (or PP2B). Calcineurin then dephosphorylates inhibitor 1 (I1), which in its phosphorylated form is an inhibitor of protein phosphatase 1 (PP1). This leads to the activation of PP1, which reduces postsynaptic excitability in part via dephosphorylation of AMPA receptors. It should be emphasized that the mechanisms shown here for LTP and LTD refer to the CA1 region of hippocampus only, as LTP- and LTD-like processes are mediated by very different mechanisms at other synapses. Based on information reviewed by Nicoll and Malenka (1995).

phosphorylation of the synaptic vesicle protein, RIM1 (rab3A interacting molecule) (Kaeser and Sudhof, 2005). Knockout of RIM1 causes loss of presynaptic LTP at CA3 synapses and also results in severe deficits in learning and memory.

The mechanisms of LTD are also best established in the hippocampal CA1 region. Interestingly, LTD, like LTP, is mediated via NMDA-dependent increases in intracellular Ca^{2+} levels. The main distinction between LTD and LTP is the frequency of the incoming synaptic stimulation and, therefore, the extent of rises in intracellular Ca^{2+} (Fig. 5.5). Long-term potentiation involves high-frequency stimulation and large increases in intracellular Ca^{2+} levels, sufficient to activate Cam-kinase II. In contrast, LTD involves lower frequency stimulation and smaller increases in intracellular Ca^{2+} levels, which are capable of activating calcineurin (also called *protein phosphatase 2B*), a Ca^{2+}- and calmodulin-activated protein phosphatase. Activated calcineurin seems to depress postsynaptic function by catalyzing the dephosphorylation of glutamate receptors.

The discovery of LTP and LTD makes it clear that at many if not all excitatory synapses in the brain, synaptic strength (*efficacy*) can be modified bidirectionally by electrical activity. This ability to modulate synaptic strength up and down likely contributes to the enormous information storage capacity of the brain and its adaptability to the continual multitude of environmental stimuli that each of us experiences during a lifetime. A major challenge for current research is to understand how processes like LTP, LTD, and other forms of cellular plasticity summate in the brain to mediate complex behavioral memory critical for normal brain function and how abnormalities in these processes contribute to the pathophysiology of many neuropsychiatric disorders.

REFERENCES

Cantrell, A.R., and Catterall, W.A. (2001) Neuromodulation of Na^+ channels: an unexpected form of cellular plasticity. *Nature Rev. Neurosci.* 2:397–407.

Cao, X., Yeo, G., Muotri, A.R., Kuwabara, T., and Gage, F.H. (2006) Noncoding RNAs in the mammalian central nervous system. *Annu. Rev. Neurosci.* 29:77–103.

Greengard, P. (2001) The neurobiology of slow synaptic transmission. *Science* 294:1024–1030.

Hyman, S.E., and Nestler, E.J. (1993) *The Molecular Foundations of Psychiatry*. Washington, DC: American Psychiatric Press.

Hyman, S.E., and Nestler, E.J. (1996) Initiation and adaptation: a paradigm for understanding psychotropic drug action. *Am. J. Psychiatry* 153:151–162.

Jahn, R., Lang, T., and Sudhof, T.C. (2003) Membrane fusion. *Cell* 112:519–533.

Kaeser, P.S., and Sudhof, T.C. (2005) RIM function in short- and long-term synaptic plasticity. *Biochem. Soc. Trans.* 33(Pt 6): 1345–1349.

Kelz, M.B., Chen, J.S., Carlezon, W.A., Whisler, K., Gilden, L., Beckmann, A.M., Steffen, C., Zhang, Y.-J., Marotti, L., Self, D.W., Tkatch, R., Baranauskas, G., Surmeier, D.J., Neve, R.L., Duman, R.S., Picciotto, M.R., and Nestler, E.J. (1999) Expression of the transcription factor DFosB in the brain controls sensitivity to cocaine. *Nature* 401:272–276.

Kohout, T.A., and Lefkowitz, R.J. (2003) Regulation of G protein-coupled receptor kinases and arrestins during receptor desensitization. *Mol. Pharmacol.* 63:9–18.

Korte, S.M., Koolhaas, J.M., Wingfield, J.C., and McEwen, B.S. (2005) The Darwinian concept of stress: benefits of allostasis and costs of allostatic load and the trade-offs in health and disease. *Neurosci. Biobehav. Rev.* 29:3–38.

Kumer, S.C., and Vrana, K.E. (1996) Intricate regulation of tyrosine hydroxylase activity and gene expression. *J. Neurochem.* 67: 443–462.

Lin, R.C., and Scheller, R.H. (2000) Mechanisms of synaptic vesicle exocytosis. *Annu. Rev. Cell Dev. Biol.* 16:19–49.

Lopina, O.D. (2000) Na^+,K^+-ATPase: structure, mechanism, and regulation. *Membr. Cell Biol.* 13:721–744.

Luscher, C., Nicoll, R.A., Malenka, R.C., and Muller, D. (2000) Synaptic plasticity and dynamic modulation of the postsynaptic membrane. *Nature Neurosci.* 3:545–550.

Malenka, R.C., and Bear, M.F. (2004) LTP and LTD: an embarrassment of riches. *Neuron* 44:5–21.

Malinow, R., and Malenka, R.C. (2002) AMPA receptor trafficking and synaptic plasticity. *Annu. Rev. Neurosci.* 25:103–126.

Marie, H., Morishita, W., Yu, X., Calakos, N., and Malenka, R.C. (2005) Generation of silent synapses by acute in vivo expression of CaMKIV and CREB. *Neuron* 45:741–752.

Mayford, M., and Kandel, E.R. (1999) Genetic approaches to memory storage. *Trends Genet.* 15:463–470.

Mayr, B., and Montminy, M. (2001) Transcriptional regulation by the phosphorylation-dependent factor CREB. *Nature Rev. Mol. Cell Biol.* 2:599–609.

Nestler, E.J., and Greengard, P. (1984) *Protein Phosphorylation in the Nervous System*. New York: Wiley.

Nestler, E.J., Hyman, S.E., and Malenka, R.C. (2001) *Molecular Basis of Neuropharmacology*. New York: McGraw-Hill.

Neve, R.L., Neve, K.A., Nestler, E.J., and Carlezon, W.A., Jr. (2005) Use of herpes virus amplicon vectors to study brain disorders. *BioTechniques* 39:381–391.

Nicoll, R.A., and Malenka, R.C. (1995) Contrasting properties of two forms of long-term potentiation in the hippocampus. *Nature* 377:115–118.

Prasad, H.C., Zhu, C.B., McCauley, J.L., Samuvel, D.J., Ramamoorthy, S., Shelton, R.C., Hewlett, W.A., Sutcliffe, J.S., and Blakely, R.D. (2005) Human serotonin transporter variants display altered sensitivity to protein kinase G and p38 mitogen-activated protein kinase. *Proc. Natl. Acad. Sci. USA* 102:11545–11550.

Robinson, T.E., and Kolb, B. (2004) Structural plasticity associated with exposure to drugs of abuse. *Neuropharmacology* 47: S33–S46.

Scannevin, R.H., and Huganir, R.L. (2000) Postsynaptic organization and regulation of excitatory synapses. *Nature Rev. Neurosci.* 1: 133–141.

Squire, L.R., and Zola, S.M. (1996) Structure and function of declarative and nondeclarative memory systems. *Proc. Natl. Acad. Sci. USA* 93:13515–13522.

Swope, S.L., Moss, S.I., Raymond, L.A., and Huganir, R.L. (1999) Regulation of ligand-gated ion channels by protein phosphorylation. *Adv. Second Messenger Phosphoprotein Res.* 33:49–78.

von Zastrow, M., Svingos, A., Haberstock-Debic, H., and Evans, C. (2003) Regulated endocytosis of opioid receptors: cellular mechanisms and proposed roles in physiological adaptation to opiate drugs. *Curr. Opin. Neurobiol.* 13:348–353.

Yuste, R., and Bonhoeffer, T. (2004) Genesis of dendritic spines: insights from ultrastructural and imaging studies. *Nature Rev. Neurosci.* 5:24–34.

6 Principles of Molecular Biology

STEVEN E. HYMAN AND ERIC J. NESTLER

Recent advances in molecular biology and in understanding the genetics of complex human phenotypes have opened a new world of possibilities for research on mental disorders and their treatment. Scientific and technological developments in genetics and molecular biology have been rapid and profound during the past 15 years; as a result, the use of molecular tools should drive a great deal of progress in research on mental disorders and their treatments in the foreseeable future. Because, however, the diseases with which psychiatry is ultimately charged are expressed at the level of behavior, molecular work must be complemented by ongoing research in the more integrative aspects of neuroscience and behavioral science described elsewhere in this textbook. Thus, for example, the pathophysiology of mental disorders depends on the complex interaction of genetic (bottom-up) factors and environmental (top-down) factors affecting the development and subsequent function of the brain. Many scientific disciplines must contribute to that understanding.

Despite substantial evidence that genes and environment are inseparable partners in brain development and plasticity—and therefore in the formation of personalities, talents, and all other aspects of behavior, including vulnerability to mental illness and very likely responsiveness to treatments for mental illness—simplistic versions of the nature–nurture debate never seem to disappear. It is true that from the time a one-cell embryo is formed from the fusion of sperm and egg, the genetic endowment of that individual is fixed. An important focus of current research, however, is to find out precisely what that means with respect to behavioral traits. It is now becoming increasingly clear that behavioral phenotypes, including vulnerability to serious mental disorders such as schizophrenia, manic–depressive illness, and autism, result from the interaction of multiple genes, very likely acting at different times during brain development in interaction with the environment. Thus, an important goal of psychiatric research is to understand how genetic information is read out during development and how the brain changes as a result of stochastic or random processes during development, as well as in response to experience of the sensory world and other environmental inputs, such as drugs, infections, and injuries.

The goal of this chapter is to describe the fundamental molecular processes by which information is encoded in the genome and how this information is expressed within an environmental context. We describe what genes are, how they function, and how their expression is regulated by signals from outside the cell. This chapter shows that the control of gene expression by extracellular signals is a critical arena for gene–environment interactions relevant to psychiatry (Hyman and Nestler, 1993). Chapter 8 builds on this foundation by describing epigenetic regulation in psychiatry, namely, how stable changes in genes—and hence in the behaviors they regulate—can be produced without changes in the genetic code itself.

NUCLEIC ACIDS

Deoxyribonucleic acid (DNA) contains the genetic blueprints of cells, that is, the information to produce ribonucleic acid (RNA) and proteins, that in turn create the fundamental structural and functional properties of our cells. The latest estimate is that the human genome contains approximately 30,000 genes, which use about 1.5% of ~3,000,000,000 base pairs of DNA. Deoxyribonucleic acid exists as a double helix, each strand of which is an unbranched chain built out of small building blocks called *nucleotide bases*. DNA and RNA are synthesized out of only four types of nucleotide bases. The four nucleotides that make up DNA are the *purines*, *adenine* (A) and *guanine* (G), and the *pyrimidines*, *cytosine* (C) and *thymine* (T), each containing a deoxyribose sugar group. In RNA the pyrimidine uracil (U) takes the place of thymine, and the sugar group is ribose instead of deoxyribose. Individual nucleotides are joined into strands of DNA or RNA via the phosphate groups that form a phosphodiester linkage.

The alternating deoxyribose sugar and phosphate groups that connect the bases of each DNA strand form a "sugar-phosphate backbone" on the outside of the double helix with the bases arrayed on the inside of the double helix (Fig. 6.1). In DNA, the nucleotide base A is always paired with (or is complementary to) T on the opposite strand, and G is paired with C. In RNA, U is structurally quite similar to T and is also complementary to A. The rules of base pairing observed in DNA result from the fact that only complementary pairs of nucleotides form a maximum number of stabilizing hydrogen bonds. Any other arrangement of bases destabilizes the structure of the DNA. A critical property of a linear polymer such as DNA (or RNA) is that it can serve as a template for the synthesis of other macromolecules. The principle of complementary base pairing provides the mechanism by which information can be transferred. An enzyme, a DNA polymerase in the case of DNA replication, or RNA polymerase in the case of transcription of DNA into RNA, can proceed down a template strand of DNA, adding a nucleotide base complementary to the base on the template strand as it forms a new strand of nucleic acid (Fig. 6.1).

Although the actual enzymatic steps involved in the replication of DNA are quite complex, the overall principles are simple. Replication begins with separation of the two complementary DNA strands in a local region.

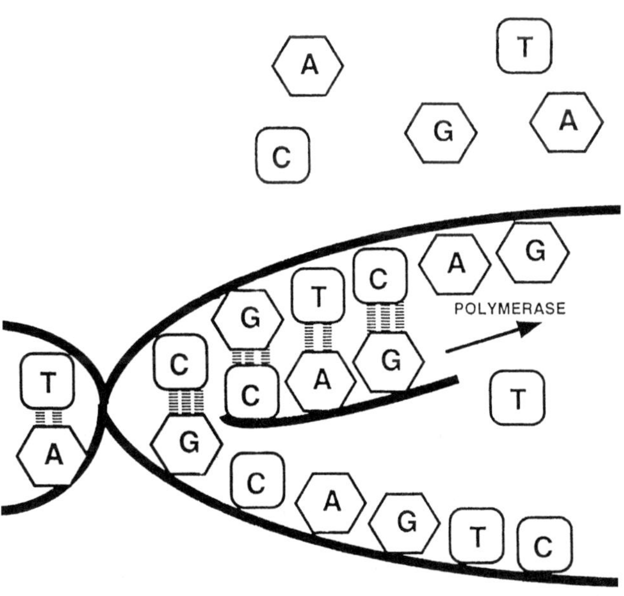

FIGURE 6.1 Schematic of complementary base pairing of deoxyribonucleic acid (DNA). Two complementary strands of DNA hybridize with one another to form a double helix. The sugar-phosphate backbones of the two strands are found on the outside of the double helix; the bases are found on the inside. Formation of a DNA double helix is stabilized when hydrogen bonds form between complementary bases of the two strands. Two hydrogen bonds form when A is across from T; three hydrogen bonds form when G is across from C. Other appositions of bases are destabilizing and do not occur. A strand of DNA can serve as a template for a second strand of nucleic acid (DNA or ribonucleic acid [RNA]). A polymerase enzyme assembles individual nucleotides into a new strand using the first strand as a template. The sequence of the new strand is therefore determined by the template, permitting the transfer of information across generations. Complementary base pairing is also the fundamental principle in the synthesis of RNA from DNA and in many experimental situations in which it is desirable to detect the presence of a specific DNA or RNA strand.

Each strand then serves as a template for a new DNA molecule by the sequential polymerization of nucleotides. Eventually the replication process generates two complete DNA double helices, each identical in sequence to the original. Replication of DNA is said to be semiconservative because each daughter DNA molecule contains one of the original parental strands plus one newly synthesized strand. Transcription of DNA into RNA is conceptually similar except that only one DNA strand serves as a template, and when synthesis of the RNA is complete, it is released and the DNA strands can reanneal into their stable double-helical structure.

INFORMATION FLOWS FROM DNA TO RNA TO PROTEIN

As was described, DNA carries information in its linear sequence of nucleotides. Although the linear polynucleotide structure of DNA is well suited for the stable storage of information and for self-replication, its chemical simplicity and its relatively rigid helical structure limit its biological functions. Thus, the information contained within DNA must be read out to yield RNA and proteins. Like DNA, RNA is chemically quite simple (that is, composed of four nucleotides), but because it is a flexible single strand, free to fold into a variety of conformations, it is functionally more versatile than DNA.

Messenger RNA (mRNA) functions as an intermediate between the sequence of DNA that comprises the transcribed regions of genes and the sequence of proteins. Not all RNA serves as mRNA, however. Other RNAs function in varied roles in cells. Ribosomes, the organelles on which proteins are synthesized, are constructed out of complexes of several types of ribosomal RNA (rRNAs) with proteins. Transfer RNA (tRNAs) transport specific amino acids to the ribosomes for incorporation into proteins during the process in which mRNA is translated into protein. In recent years, scientists have discovered several types of small RNAs, such as microRNAs (miRNAs) or small interfering RNAs (siRNAs), which bind to specific mRNAs and inhibit their translation (Cao et al., 2006). This discovery has been translated into a new powerful tool, which uses small RNAs, called *RNA interference* or *RNAi*, to experimentally suppress expression of a targeted mRNA and protein.

Like DNA, mRNA carries information encoded in its linear sequence of nucleotides. DNA and mRNA specify amino acid building blocks for proteins in linear stretches of three nucleotides. Proteins consist of unbranched chains of amino acid building blocks. An amino acid is a small molecule that contains an amino group (NH_2) and a carboxylic acid or carboxy group (COOH) plus a variable side chain. The side chains used by the 20 common amino acids differ markedly in size, shape, hydrophobicity, and charge. Amino acids are linked to each other by peptide bonds that join the amino group of one amino acid to the carboxy group of another amino acid.

Within the portion of an mRNA that is translatable into a protein, each successive group of three nucleotide bases (called a *codon*) specifies either one amino acid or termination of the protein chain. The rules specifying the correspondence between a codon and an amino acid are called the *genetic code*. Because RNA is a linear polymer of 4 nucleotides, there are 4^3 or 64 possible codons but only 20 amino acids. As a result, although each codon specifies only a single amino acid, most amino acids are specified by more than one codon. The genetic code is therefore said to be degenerate. With only a few minor exceptions, the code has been conserved across evolution. The codons in an mRNA molecule do not interact directly with the amino acids they specify; the translation of mRNA into protein depends on the presence of tRNAs that serve as adapter molecules that recognize a specific codon and the corresponding amino acid (Fig. 6.2).

The ribosome is a structure composed of proteins and structural RNAs; these organelles provide a structure on which tRNAs can interact (via their anticodons) with the codons of an mRNA in sequential order. The ribosome finds a specific start site on the mRNA that sets the reading frame and then moves along the mRNA molecule progressively, translating the nucleotide sequence one codon at a time, using tRNAs to add amino acids to the growing end of the polypeptide chain (Fig. 6.3).

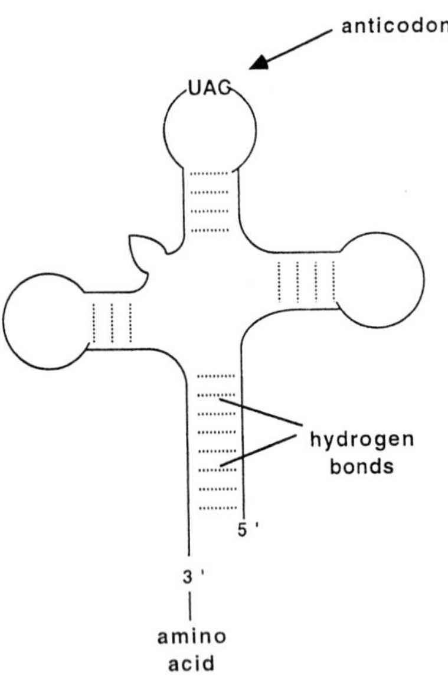

FIGURE 6.2 Transfer RNA (tRNA). Transfer RNA (tRNA) is a single strand of RNA that folds on itself through the apposition of complementary base pairs and the subsequent formation of hydrogen bonds, indicated by the dashed lines in the figure. One of the loops formed contains the anticodon, the sequence of three nucleotides on the tRNA that binds to the complementary codon on a messenger RNA molecule. For the anticodon AGA shown in the figure, the corresponding codon on the mRNA would be UCU. The free end of the tRNA binds to a specific amino acid. Each tRNA, with a given anticodon, binds only one type of amino acid determined by the genetic code. In the case shown in the figure, the amino acid bound would be serine. From Hyman and Nestler (1993).

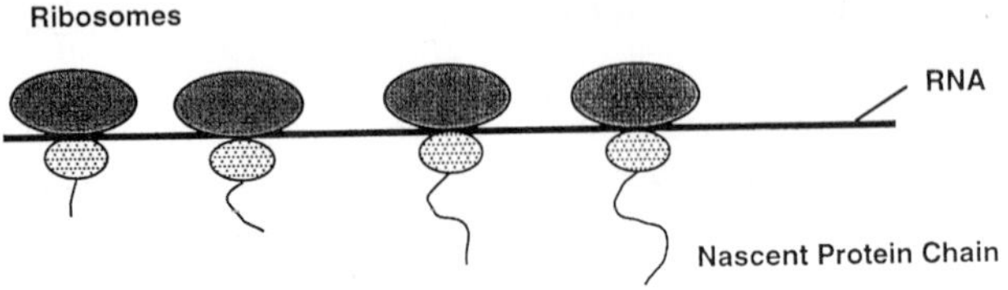

FIGURE 6.3 Protein translation. Ribosomal subunits bind together on mature messenger ribonucleic acids (mRNAs) to form actively translating ribosomes. The ribosome begins adding amino acids when it reaches a start codon on the mRNA and processes down the mRNA, one codon at a time, adding the appropriate amino acid as it is delivered by a transfer RNA (tRNA). When a stop codon is reached, the ribosome releases the polypeptide chain and dissociates from the mRNA. Each mRNA that is being actively translated has multiple ribosomes moving sequentially down its length, forming a polyribosome complex. From Hyman and Nestler (1993).

In contrast with nucleic acids, which are constructed of four bases that are chemically similar, proteins are constructed out of 20 quite different amino acids. By incorporating so many different types of amino acids, each with its chemically diverse side chains, proteins have extraordinary functional versatility, unlike DNA or RNA. The specific properties of proteins depend not only on the linear sequence of their amino acid building blocks (primary structure), but also on the tendency of certain combinations of amino acids to form intrinsic structural motifs (secondary structures, for example, α helices or β sheets) and by their folded three-dimensional characteristics (*tertiary structure*). In addition, proteins form stable interactions (*complexes*) with other proteins (*quaternary structure*). In such cases, the individual polypeptide chains are called *subunits*. The folding of proteins, and the interactions of proteins with each other and with other molecules such as nucleic acids, may also be regulated by chemical modification of the protein, most often of particular side chains. For example, one ubiquitous mechanism of regulation of protein function is by the covalent addition of a phosphate group (by specific enzymes called *protein kinases*) to the hydroxyl groups found in serine, threonine, or tyrosine side chains (Chapters 4 and 5). Cells may contain tens of thousands of distinct proteins, each with unique structural and functional properties, including neurotransmitter receptors, neuropeptides, ion channels, enzymes, and a very large number of other types of proteins.

GENES AND CHROMOSOMES

As a first approximation, genes were initially defined as stretches of DNA that encode a single protein or a single functional RNA, such as an rRNA or a tRNA. This rule breaks down quickly, however, because there are mechanisms, such as alternative splicing of the primary RNA transcript into different mRNAs, that may intervene between a given gene and a finished protein. Moreover, individual protein precursors may be cleaved into numerous functionally active peptides. As a result of these and other processes, many individual genes actually encode multiple proteins, although we still do not know what fraction of all genes function in this manner.

Genes are arrayed on extremely long chains of DNA called *chromosomes*. Eukaryotic chromosomes contain not only genes, but also large amounts of intergenic DNA. Indeed, within the human genome, the 30,000 genes take up perhaps only 3% of chromosomal DNA. Moreover, genes are not distributed equally along the chromosomes but are often found in clusters. Some chromosomes are "gene rich" and others are relatively "gene poor." Within intergenic regions there is a great deal of DNA with unique sequences of unknown function, as well as long stretches of tandemly repeated sequences known as *satellite DNA*. These tandem repeats, which show a great deal of variability in length from person to person, are the basis of commonly used genetic markers for research on the pattern of heritability of traits, such as in linkage analysis, and for the identification of individuals in forensic investigations (see Chapter 10).

The chromosomes of eukaryotic cells are so long that they would not fit in the nucleus in their extended form. Thus stretches of the DNA that are not being actively transcribed are tightly packed into a conformation described as a coiled coil, which permits the chromosomes to fit within the nucleus. To create packed conformations, lengths of DNA are coiled around structural and regulatory proteins, of which the most important are the histones. These structures are termed *nucleosomes*. Regions of DNA that are being actively transcribed into RNA may be greater than 1000-fold more extended than regions that are transcriptionally quiescent. The unwinding of tightly packed nucleosomes, which enables their expression, appears to be mediated in part via histone acetylation and other modifications, which are discussed in detail in Chapter 8 (Lachner et al., 2003; Hake et al., 2004).

GENE EXPRESSION

As described above, proteins are not synthesized directly from the DNA that encodes them, but in two sequential processes, *transcription of DNA into mRNA*, which occurs in the nucleus, and *translation of the mRNA into protein* according to the rules of the genetic code, which occurs in the cytoplasm. Transcription of protein-coding genes can be divided into three major steps. First, the enzyme primarily involved in RNA synthesis, *RNA polymerase*, must interact with the gene at an appropriate transcription start site and begin transcribing (*initiation*). Second, the RNA polymerase must successfully transcribe an appropriate length of RNA (*elongation*). Third, transcription of the RNA must terminate appropriately. The resulting RNA is then posttranscriptionally processed. It receives a stretch of adenines, a poly-(A) tail, which makes it more stable in the cell. It is also spliced to remove internal sequences (*introns*) that are not appropriate for translation into protein in that particular cell. The spliced "exportable" sequences (*exons*) exit the nucleus to be translated into protein in the cytoplasm (Fig. 6.4).

TRANSCRIPTIONAL CONTROL

We have now reviewed the flow of information from gene to protein. Every step along the way can be regulated, but the major control point in reading out the information contained within the genome is transcription initiation. Indeed, this is the step at which environmental signals often exert powerful regulatory control on gene expression, during development and in mature cells. How does this come about?

In addition to encoding information that ultimately directs the synthesis of proteins, genes contain regulatory information. Every cell in our bodies contains all of our genes in its nucleus, but not every gene is active in every cell. Our cells differ—indeed, their identity is defined—by the fact that each type of cell in the body expresses only a subset of the entire complement of genes. In any given cell, some genes are "on," being read out to make mRNA and hence proteins, and the rest are silent. Thus, for example, in the red blood cell precursors of the bone marrow, the genes that encode globins, proteins that are the critical building blocks of hemoglobin, are actively making globin-encoding mRNA. In our midbrains, a subset of cells are making a protein called *tyrosine hydroxylase*, the rate-limiting enzyme for the synthesis of dopamine. It would not be adaptive for these cells to synthesize large amounts of hemoglobin, just as red blood cell precursors need not use energy to synthesize tyrosine hydroxylase. The processes by which certain genes are "silenced" in a tissue-specific manner during development are now increasingly understood and involve epigenetic mechanisms (Chapter 8).

Regulatory sequences within genes work by virtue of their ability to bind specific proteins. Certain regulatory

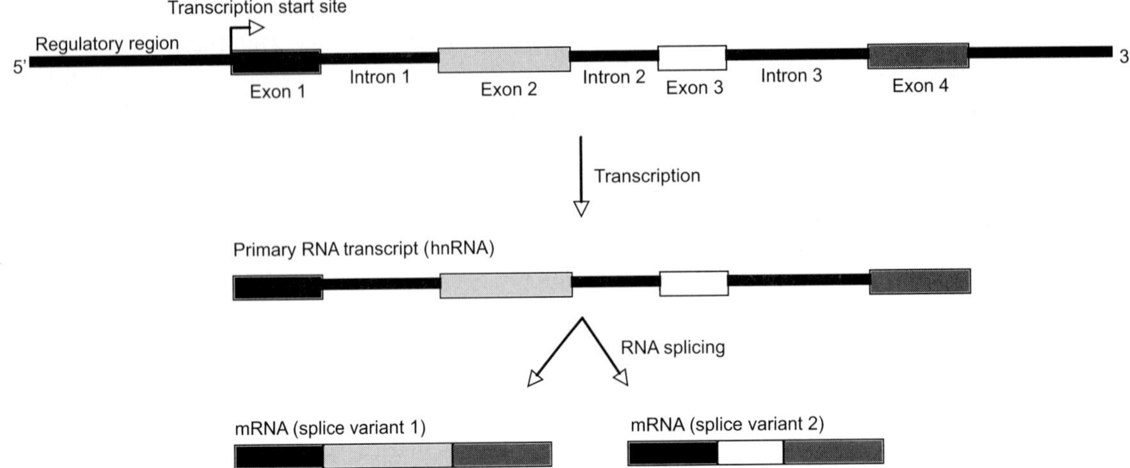

FIGURE 6.4 NA splicing. Horizontal black lines represent deoxyribonucleic acid (DNA) regulatory regions and introns. Black, gray, and white rectangles represent exons. The region to the left of the first exon is the 5′ regulatory region of the gene, but cis-regulatory elements are also found in introns and sometimes even downstream of the last exon. The primary transcript, also known as *heterogeneous ribonucleic acid* (hnRNA), contains exons and introns and gives rise, in the case shown, to two alternatively spliced messenger ribonucleic acids (mRNAs): one containing exons 1, 2, and 4, and one containing exons 1, 3, and 4. These splice variants, after export from the nucleus and translation in the cytoplasm, give rise to distinct proteins.

sequences specify the beginnings and ends of segments of DNA that can be transcribed into RNA. Other regulatory sequences determine in what cell types and under what circumstances their gene can be read out. DNA sequences that subserve such control functions are often called *cis-regulatory elements* (Fig. 6.5). The term *cis* refers to the fact that the relevant regulatory sequences are physically linked, on the DNA, to the region being controlled, which is usually a segment of DNA that can be transcribed into RNA. The proteins that bind to cis elements have been described as *trans-acting* factors because they may be encoded anywhere in the genome

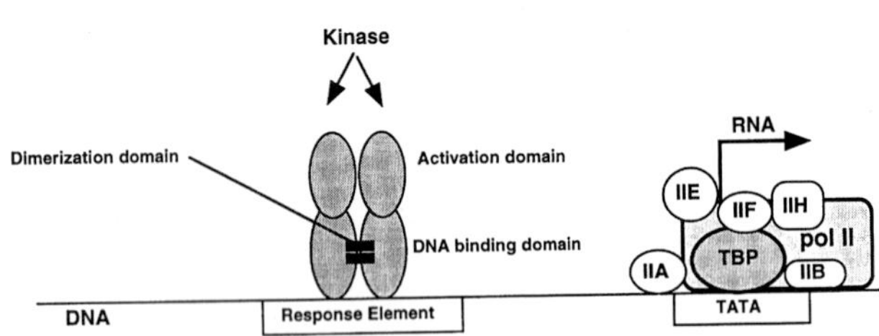

FIGURE 6.5 Cis and transregulation. The figure shows two cis-regulatory elements (open rectangles) along the stretch of deoxyribonucleic acid (DNA) (thin line). The element to the left represents a response element that serves as a binding site for a hypothetical transcription factor that binds as a homodimer. The other is the thymine adenine thymine adenine (TATA) element, shown binding the TATA binding protein (TBP). Multiple general transcription factors and ribonucleic acid (RNA) polymerase II (pol II) associate with TBP. This basal transcription apparatus recruits RNA polymerase II into the complex and also forms the substrate for interactions with activator proteins, such as those binding to the activator elements shown. The transcription factor shown binding to the response element is a substrate for a protein kinase that phosphorylates its activation domain (see text).

rather than on the same stretch of DNA that they regulate. Those proteins that are involved in specifying whether, and under what circumstances, a gene will be transcribed are more generally known as *transcription factors*. Many transcription factors bind DNA directly; others interact only indirectly via protein–protein interactions with factors that bind DNA.

Those cis-regulatory elements that specify the site within a gene at which transcription starts, and upon which the complex of proteins that forms the basal transcription apparatus is assembled, are called the *basal or core promoter*. The core promoters for many protein-encoding genes consist of a sequence motif rich in the nucleotides A and T, called the *TATA box*. The TATA box is generally located between 25 and 30 nucleotides upstream of the actual site at which transcription of DNA into RNA is initiated. In the nervous system, however, numerous genes do not contain identifiable TATA boxes, which means that their transcription start sites are defined differently. In eukaryotes, transcription of protein-coding genes is carried out by the enzyme RNA polymerase II, which does not directly contact DNA but interacts with the complex of proteins that assembles at the TATA box or distinct transcription start site (Fig. 6.5).

Sequence-Specific Transcription Factors Interact with the Basal Transcription Apparatus to Produce Significant Levels of Transcription

The basal transcription complex assembled at the TATA box or other transcription start site is only sufficient to initiate low levels of transcription of DNA into RNA.

To achieve significant levels of gene expression, the basal transcription complex requires help from additional transcription factors that recognize and bind to cis-regulatory elements found elsewhere within the gene. Cis-elements that exert control near the core promoter itself have been called *promoter elements*, and those that act at a distance—often several hundred to more than 1000 nucleotide base pairs away—have been called *enhancer elements*, but the commonly made distinction between promoter and enhancer elements is artificial. Both are composed of small "modular" sequences of DNA (generally 7–12 base pairs in length), each of which is a specific binding site for one or more transcription factors. Multiple cis-regulatory elements arrayed throughout the control regions of a gene, and the proteins they bind, act in combinatorial fashion to give each gene its distinct patterns of expression and regulation.

Transcription factors that are tethered to DNA by binding cis-elements are often described as sequence-specific transcription factors (Herdegen and Leah, 1998). Most such proteins have a modular structure composed of physically separate domains: a domain that recognizes and binds a specific DNA sequence, an activation domain that interacts with the basal transcription complex to activate or inhibit it, and a multimerization domain that permits the formation of homo- and heteromultimers with other transcription factors (Fig. 6.5). Many transcription factors are active only as dimers or higher order complexes. Within transcription factor dimers, whether homodimers or heterodimers, it is common for both partners to contribute jointly to the DNA binding domain and the activation domain. Sequence-specific transcription factors may contact the basal transcription complex directly; in many cases, they interact through the mediation of adapter proteins. In either case, transcription factors that bind cis-regulatory elements at a distance from the core promoter can interact with the basal transcription apparatus because the DNA forms loops that bring distant regions in contact with each other (Fig. 6.6A,B).

Regulation of Gene Expression by Extracellular Signals

All regulation of gene expression by extracellular signals requires a mechanism that carries a signal from the cell membrane to the nucleus. In many cases, intracellular signaling molecules, such as protein kinases, serve this function. This is illustrated by CREB (cAMP-response element binding protein), which mediates many of the effects of the cyclic adenosine monophosphate (cAMP) system, and other intracellular pathways, on gene expression (Shaywitz and Greenberg, 1999; Mayr and Montminy, 2001). CREB is bound under basal cellular conditions to its cognate cis-regulatory element (the cyclic AMP-response element, or CRE). Stimuli that increase levels of cAMP activate cAMP-dependent protein kinase (PKA), which results in liberation of the kinase's catalytic subunits. A portion of the free catalytic subunit then enters the nucleus, where it phosphorylates CREB, permitting it to activate transcription. Similarly, stimuli that activate other intracellular signaling cascades (for example, Ca^{2+} or mitogen-activated protein [MAP]-kinase pathways)

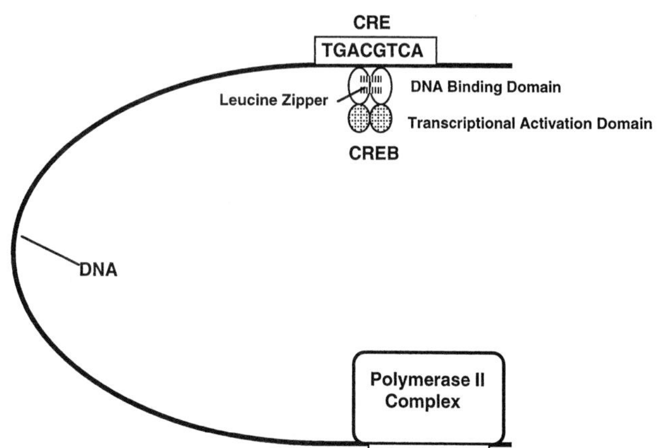

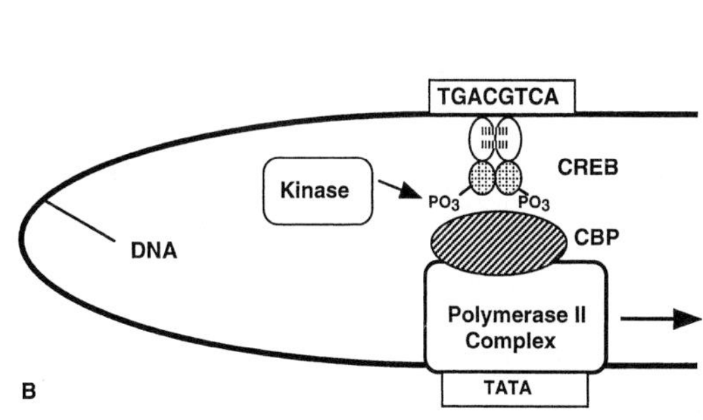

FIGURE 6.6 Looping of deoxyribonucleic acid (DNA) permits activator (or repressor) proteins binding at a distance to interact with the basal transcription apparatus. In the figure, the basal transcription apparatus is shown as a single box bound at the thymine adenine thymine adenine (TATA) element. The activator protein, cyclic adenosine monophosphate (cAMP)-response element binding protein (CREB), is shown bound as a homodimer to its cognate cis-regulatory element, the cAMP-response element (CRE), at a distance from the TATA element (panels *A* and *B*). Upon phosphorylation, many activators such as CREB are able to recruit adapter proteins that mediate between the activator and the basal transcription apparatus. An adapter protein that binds phosphorylated CREB is called *CREB binding protein* (CBP). With the recruitment of the adapter, a mature transcription complex forms that permits the synthesis of ribonucleic acid (RNA) by RNA polymerase II (panel *B*).

lead to the activation of other protein kinases, which also phosphorylate and activate CREB.

In other cases, a transcription factor, itself activated at the cell membrane or in the cytoplasm, then translocates to the nucleus. This is illustrated by the transcription factor NF-κB (nuclear factor κB), which is involved, among other things, in the activation of genes involved in inflammatory responses (Ghosh and Karin, 2002). Under basal conditions, NF-κB is retained in the cytoplasm by its inhibitory binding protein (IκB); this interaction masks a protein sequence within the NF-κB molecule that serves as a nuclear localization signal. Phosphorylation of IκB by IκB-kinase (IκK) leads to dissociation of NF-κB, which permits it to enter the nucleus, where it binds to its response elements; IκB is then digested within the cytoplasm.

The above discussion highlights that the critical nuclear translocation step can involve the transcription factor itself or another signaling molecule. Either mechanism can activate a third scenario: Some transcription factors are expressed only at very low levels when cells are in their unstimulated state. Their genes contain response elements that lead to their synthesis when cells are activated. Thus, gene expression may occur in cascades, with the stimulation of preexisting transcription factors leading to the expression of genes encoding (among many other genes) additional transcription factors, which can then stimulate yet other genes. Activation of genes by preexisting transcription factors occurs more rapidly than activation of genes by factors that must be synthesized de novo. Thus, not surprisingly, different neurotransmitters, drugs, and other stimuli may activate gene expression with widely varying time courses ranging from minutes to many hours.

Many transcription factors are members of families, presumably related by evolution, with related structures and functions. Below we illustrate the function of representative families of transcription factors, which serve as instructive examples of the diverse mechanisms governing the regulation of transcription in the nervous system.

The CREB Family of Transcription Factors

CREB was the first-discovered and best-characterized member of a family of related proteins that bind to a particular DNA sequence termed the *CRE*, as mentioned above (Shaywitz and Greenberg, 1999; Mayr and Montminy, 2001). The family is composed of CREB, the ATFs (activating transcription factors), and the CREMs (cAMP-response element modulators). CREB itself plays a major role in mediating the effects of cAMP and Ca^{2+} and of those neurotransmitters that act through cAMP or Ca^{2+}, on gene expression. A large number of genes contain CREs, including the gene encoding the transcription factor c-Fos and the genes encoding proenkephalin, somatostatin, tyrosine hydroxylase, and VIP (vasoactive intestinal polypeptide). Members of the CREB/ATF family bind to CREs as dimers. The dimerization domain used by the CREB/ATF proteins and several other families of transcription factors is called a *leucine zipper*, an alpha helical motif in which every seventh residue is a leucine. The proteins form a coil in which electrostatic interactions stabilize dimer formation.

The methods used to characterize CREs, and indeed all cis-regulatory elements, involve deleting them, or mutating them more subtly, and then reintroducing them into eukaryotic cells in culture by transfection. When a critical base in a DNA regulatory element is mutated, it weakens or destroys the binding site for the relevant transcription factor. If the protein can no longer bind, the gene can no longer be activated by the physiological stimulus under investigation, such as cAMP. By comparing response element sequences that have been investigated by mutagenesis within many genes, an idealized consensus sequence can be derived. The consensus nucleotide sequence of the CRE is TGACGTCA, with the nucleotides CGTCA absolutely required.

The consensus CRE sequence illustrates an important principle, the palindromic nature of many transcription factor binding sites. In the sequence TGACGTCA, it can be readily observed that the sequence on the two complementary strands, which run in opposite directions, is identical. Many cis-regulatory elements are perfect or approximate palindromes permitting binding of transcription factors in the form of dimers, where each member of the dimer recognizes one of the half-sites.

The primary mechanism by which CREB is regulated is through its phosphorylation on a single serine residue (ser133) by any of several protein kinases, including PKA, Ca^{2+}/calmodulin-dependent protein kinase IV (Cam-kinase IV), and several kinases in the MAP-kinase cascade. CREB is constitutively synthesized so that it exists in neurons under basal conditions, although its expression can be regulated under certain circumstances, such as in response to psychotropic drug treatments. Nonphosphorylated CREB is localized to the nucleus, where it is bound to its response elements without considerable transcriptional activity (Fig. 6.6A). Phosphorylation of CREB activates its transcriptional activity by permitting CREB to interact with another protein, *CBP* (CREB binding protein) (Fig. 6.6B) (Vo and Goodman, 2001). CBP is called an *adapter protein* because it intervenes between a sequence-specific transcription factor CREB and the basal transcription apparatus, thus activating transcription. Despite its name, CBP provides this adapter function for several regulated transcription factors in addition to CREB family proteins. Moreover, it functions in part by acetylating nearby histones, as discussed in Chapter 8.

The mechanism by which neurotransmitters that increase cAMP levels regulate gene expression via CREB is straightforward. Neurotransmitter-receptor stimulation increases levels of cAMP and of activated PKA. Activated PKA (that is, free catalytic subunits of the enzyme) is then translocated into the nucleus, where it phosphorylates and activates CREB. Phosphorylation of CREB, in turn, serves to activate the expression of genes that contain CREB bound to their promoter regions. Similar mechanisms operate for neurotransmitters (or nerve impulses) that activate CREB via stimulation of cellular Ca^{2+} signals and for neurotrophic factors that activate CREB via stimulation of MAP-kinase signals.

The convergence of multiple signaling pathways on CREB may be very significant for the function of the nervous system. For example, associative memory appears to result from the integration of multiple signals that converge on target neurons, integration that could be achieved in part via CREB phosphorylation. Indeed, experiments performed by numerous laboratories in *Drosophila* and in mice, in which CREB was inactivated by different experimental methods, yield organisms with deficits in long-term memory, while increases in CREB function produce animals with enhanced memory (e.g., Tully et al., 2003; Josselyn et al., 2004; Marie et al., 2005; Pittenger et al., 2006). CREB has also been implicated in many additional psychiatric phenomena including drug addiction and depression (Carlezon et al., 2005; Blendy, 2006).

CREB illustrates yet another important principle of transcriptional regulation. As described above, CREB is a member of a larger family of related proteins. The ATFs and CREMs (distinct CREM products are generated from a single CREM gene via alternative splicing) bind CREs as dimers; many can dimerize with CREB itself. Activating transcription factor-1 (ATF-1) appears to be very similar to CREB; it can be activated by the cAMP and Ca^{2+} pathways. Many of the other ATF proteins and CREM isoforms appear to activate transcription; however, certain CREMs, such as one called *ICER* (inducible cAMP repressor), may act to repress it. Inhibitory CREM isoforms lack a glutamine-rich transcriptional activation domain found in CREB. Thus, certain CREB–CREM heterodimers might bind CREs but fail to activate transcription. Some inhibitory CREMs (for example, ICER) are induced by CREB itself but with a delayed time course. In this way, these proteins may help terminate genes that had been activated by a CREB signal. Work in recent years has begun to demonstrate the involvement of ATFs and CREMs in an individual's adaptations to environmental stimuli, such as stress and drugs of abuse (Conti et al., 2004; Green et al., 2006).

The AP-1 Family of Transcription Factors

Another group of transcription factors that plays a central role in the regulation of neural gene expression by extracellular signals is the AP-1 proteins (Morgan and Curran, 1995; Herdegen and Leah, 1998). The name *AP-1* was originally applied to a transcriptional activity, then called *Activator Protein-1*, that was subsequently found to be composed of multiple proteins that bind as heterodimers (and a few as homodimers) to the DNA sequence TGACTCA, the AP-1 sequence. The AP-1 proteins are actually divided into two groups, the *Fos* and *Jun* families. Like the CREB/ATF family, the AP-1 proteins dimerize via a leucine zipper. The consensus AP-1 sequence is a heptamer, which forms a palindrome flanking a central C or G. The AP-1 sequence differs from the CRE sequence by only a single base. Yet this one base difference strongly biases protein binding away from CREB (which requires an intact CGTCA motif) to the AP-1 family of proteins and means that, under most circumstances, this sequence will not confer cAMP responsiveness on a gene. Instead, AP-1 sequences tend to confer responsiveness to growth factor–stimulated signaling pathways such as the Ras/MAP-kinase pathways and to the protein kinase C pathway. Indeed, the AP-1 sequence is sometimes described as a TPA-response element (TRE) because the phorbol ester *12-O-tetradecanoyl-phorbol-13-acetate* (TPA), which activates protein kinase C, strongly induces gene expression via AP-1 proteins. It is a staggering illustration of the specificity of cellular regulation that a single base change (from a CRE to an AP-1 site) in a gene thousands of bases long can result in such a profound change in gene regulation.

The AP-1 proteins generally bind DNA as heterodimers composed of one member each of the Fos and Jun families. The Fos family includes c-Fos, Fra-1 (Fos-related antigen-1), Fra-2, and FosB (which gives rise to full-length FosB plus a truncated splice variant termed *ΔFosB*). The Jun family includes c-Jun, JunB, and JunD. Heterodimers form between members of the Fos and Jun families via the leucine zipper. The potential complexity of transcriptional regulation is greater still because some AP-1 proteins can heterodimerize via the leucine zipper with members of the CREB–ATF family (for example, ATF2 with c-Jun).

Among the known Fos and Jun proteins, only JunD is expressed constitutively at high levels in many cell types. The other AP-1 proteins tend to be expressed at low or even undetectable levels under basal conditions, but with stimulation, they may be induced to high levels of expression. Thus, unlike genes that are regulated by constitutively expressed transcription factors such as CREB, genes that are regulated by c-Fos/c-Jun heterodimers require new transcription and translation of these AP-1 proteins.

Genes encoding Fos and Jun family proteins are often termed immediate early genes

Genes, such as the c-Fos gene itself, that are activated rapidly (within minutes), transiently, and without requiring new protein synthesis are frequently referred to as *cellular immediate early genes* (IEGs) (Morgan and Curran, 1995; Herdegen and Leah, 1998). Genes that are induced or repressed more slowly (over hours), and are dependent on new protein synthesis, may be described as *late response genes*. The term *IEG* was initially applied to describe viral genes that are activated immediately upon infection of eukaryotic cells by commandeering host cell transcription factors for their expression. Viral IEGs generally encode transcription factors needed to activate viral late gene expression. This terminology has been extended to cellular (that is, nonviral) genes with varying success. The terminology is problematic because there are many cellular genes induced independently of protein synthesis, but with a time course intermediately between those of classical IEGs and late response genes. In fact, some genes may be regulated with different time courses or requirements for protein synthesis in response to different extracellular signals. Moreover, it must be recalled that many cellular genes regulated as IEGs encode proteins that are not transcription factors. Despite these caveats, the concept of IEG-encoded transcription factors in the nervous system has been useful heuristically. Because of their rapid induction from low basal levels in response to neuronal depolarization (the critical signal being Ca^{2+} entry) and to second messenger and growth factor pathways, several IEGs have been used as cellular markers of neural activation, permitting novel approaches to functional neuroanatomy. This includes not only the Fos and Jun families of transcription factors, but also Zif268 (also called *Egr1*), which belongs to a distinct family of transcription factors that binds to its own response elements. Examples of the use of c-Fos as a marker of neuronal activation include induction of c-Fos in dorsal horn of the spinal cord by nociceptive stimuli, in motor and sensory thalamus by stimulation of sensory cortex, in supraoptic/paraventricular nuclei by water deprivation, and in numerous brain regions by acute and chronic opiate and cocaine administration, as well as in response to a number of other psychotropic drug treatments.

The composition of AP-1 complexes changes over time

Following acute stimulation of cells, different members of the Fos family are induced with varying time courses of expression, which leads to a progression of distinct AP-1 protein complexes over time (Sonnenberg et al., 1989). Under resting conditions, c-Fos mRNA and protein are barely detectable in most neurons; however, c-Fos gene expression can be induced dramatically in response to a variety of stimuli. As just one example, experimental induction of a grand mal seizure causes marked increases in levels of c-Fos mRNA in rat brain within 30 minutes and induces substantial levels of c-Fos protein within 2 hours. c-Fos is highly unstable and is degraded back to low, basal levels within 4–6 hours. Administration of cocaine or amphetamine causes a similar pattern of c-Fos expression in the rat striatum. In either of these stimulus paradigms, other Fos-like proteins are also induced, but with a longer temporal latency than c-Fos; their peak levels of expression lag behind c-Fos by approximately 1 hour. Moreover, expression of these proteins persists a bit longer than that of c-Fos but still returns to basal levels within 8–12 hours.

With repeated stimulation, however, the c-Fos gene, and to a lesser extent the genes for other Fos-like proteins, become refractory to further activation (that is, their expression becomes desensitized). However, in most systems, isoforms of ΔFosB continue to be expressed (McClung et al., 2004). These isoforms exhibit very long half-lives in brain (1–2 weeks). As a result, ΔFosB accumulates in specific neurons in response to repeated perturbations and persists long after cessation of these perturbations (Fig. 6.7). As discussed in Chapter 46, it has been proposed that ΔFosB thereby plays an important role in mediating some of the long-term effects of drugs of abuse and other treatments on the nervous system.

Although the biological significance of these changes in the composition of AP-1 complexes over time is not yet fully appreciated, it is believed that these changes can produce precisely varying patterns of expression of AP-1-regulated genes, thereby permitting neurons to adapt to the pattern of stimulation to which they are being subjected.

The c-Fos gene is activated by multiple signaling pathways

The precise intracellular mechanisms by which extracellular stimuli induce c-Fos expression are becoming increasingly well understood. Stimuli that depolarize neurons (for example, seizure activity, glutamate) induce c-Fos through a Ca^{2+}-dependent mechanism that involves the phosphorylation, by a Cam-kinase, of a CREB protein that is already present in the cell and bound to CREs in the c-Fos gene. Neurotransmitters that activate the cAMP pathway in target neurons phosphorylate CREB on the same amino acid residue via PKA. Phosphorylation of CREB, as outlined above, activates its transcriptional activity and leads to increased c-Fos expression.

The c-Fos gene can also be induced by the Ras/MAP-kinase pathway, which is activated by many types of

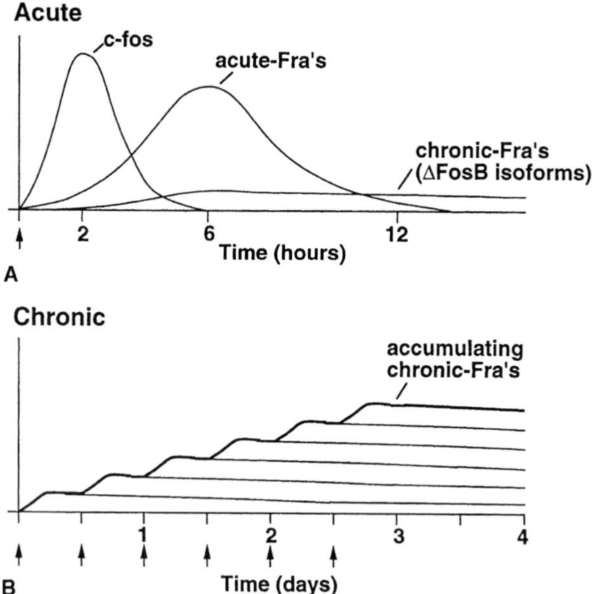

FIGURE 6.7 Scheme for the gradual accumulation of ΔFosB versus the rapid and transient induction of c-Fos and several other Fos family proteins in the brain. (*A*) Several waves of Fos family proteins are induced by many acute stimuli in neurons. c-Fos is induced rapidly and degraded within several hours of the acute stimulus, whereas others (FosB, ΔFosB, FRA-1 [Fos-related antigen-1], FRA-2) are induced somewhat later and persist somewhat longer than c-Fos. In contrast, ΔFosB is induced (although at low levels) following a single acute simulus but persists in brain with a half-life of 1–2 weeks due to its unique stability. In a complex with Jun family proteins, these waves of Fos family proteins form AP-1 binding complexes with shifting composition over time. (*B*) With repeated (twice daily) stimulation, each acute stimulus induces a low level of ΔFosB. This is indicated by the lower set of overlapping lines, which indicate ΔFosB induced by each acute stimulus. The result is a gradual increase in the total levels of ΔFosB with repeated stimuli during a course of chronic treatment. This is indicated by the increasing stepped line in the graph. The increasing levels of ΔFosB with repeated stimulation result in the gradual induction of a long-lasting AP-1 complex, which underlies persisting forms of neural plasticity in the brain. From Hope et al. (1994).

growth factors, via at least two distinct mechanisms, which may operate to different extents in different cell types. One mechanism, discussed above in the description of CREB, involves the phosphorylation of CREB by a MAP-kinase-activated CREB-kinase called *Rsk2*. A second mechanism involves the phosphorylation and activation, also by MAP-kinase, of a different transcription factor termed *Elk-1*. Elk-1 binds, along with still another transcription factor, serum response factor (SRF), to the serum response element (SRE) within the c-Fos gene. Similar mechanisms hold for the regulation of many other genes by growth factors. In comparison with cAMP- and Ca^{2+}-dependent phosphorylation of CREB, regulation of transcription by the Ras/MAP-kinase pathway depends on a complex cascade of multiple phosphorylation events, which can nonetheless occur very rapidly to induce gene expression.

The activation of IEG products such as c-Fos in response to a large number of stimuli raises the question of how specificity of response is achieved. First, specificity is partly achieved by the particular neural circuitry involved; that is, c-Fos and the other proteins are induced only along those particular neural pathways activated in response to some stimulus. Second, specificity is achieved by specialization within neuronal cell types. For example, in particular cell types not every gene that contains an appropriate binding site (for example, an AP-1 site) to which c-Fos can bind is in a chromatin configuration that permits access to c-Fos-containing complexes (Chapter 8). Third, individual transcription factors generally cannot act alone to induce or repress the expression of a given gene. Multiple types of transcription factors, binding to distinct regulatory elements within a gene's promoter region, must often act in concert to produce significant effects on gene expression.

Fourth, as alluded to above, protein products of many IEGs including c-Fos can bind DNA with high affinity only after binding to other transcription factors to form heterodimers. Such interactions are well exemplified by c-Fos and c-Jun. By itself, c-Fos is unable to bind DNA with high affinity. c-Jun homodimers can bind DNA but do so with relatively low affinity. However, c-Fos/c-Jun heterodimers bind to the AP-1 site with high affinity to regulate transcription. In contrast, heterodimers of c-Fos and JunB appear to be relatively inactive. Because there appear to be many members of the Fos and Jun families, complex regulatory schemes can readily be imagined by which a great deal of specificity in regulating cellular genes can be attained (Herdegen and Leah, 1998).

Although the primary mechanism by which Fos family members are regulated appears to be at the level of their transcription, the proteins are probably also regulated by phosphorylation. This is best illustrated by c-Fos itself, which is heavily phosphorylated on several closely spaced serine residues in the C-terminal region of the protein by PKA and Cam-kinases and by protein kinase C. c-Fos phosphorylation appears to be a critical regulatory mechanism for the protein: The difference between normal c-Fos (cellular Fos) and its viral counterpart v-Fos (which is oncogenic) is a frame-shift mutation that deletes the serine residues from the viral protein. It has been suggested that phosphorylation of c-Fos triggers the protein's ability to suppress its own transcription, thereby providing key regulatory feedback control of the expression of this transcription factor. Another example is the phosphorylation of Jun proteins by Jun-kinases (JNKs). Jun-kinases are activated by cellular forms of stress via MAP-kinase cascades. The resulting phosphorylation of Jun transcription factors is thought to be an important part of a cell's adaptation to stress.

Regulation of Gene Expression by Cytokines and Nonreceptor Protein Tyrosine Kinases

A series of cytokines subserve a wide array of functions within and outside of the nervous system (Chapters 1 and 2). Such cytokines include leukemia inhibitory factor (LIF), ciliary neurotrophic factor (CNTF), and interleukin-6 (IL-6). Recall from Chapter 4 that each of these cytokines produces its biological effects through activation of the gp130 class of plasma membrane receptor and the subsequent activation of the JAK (Janus kinase)-STAT (signal transducers and activators of transcription) pathway (Horvath, 2000; Ihle, 2001). The crucial feeding peptide, *leptin*, also acts via a JAK-STAT linked receptor.

The gp130-linked receptors for these cytokines and related signals do not contain protein kinase domains. Rather, the cytoplasmic portions of the receptors interact with nonreceptor protein tyrosine kinases of the JAK family, which include JAK1, JAK2, and Tyk2. Cytokine receptors show some specificity for the types of JAKs activated in a given cell type. Signal transduction to the nucleus involves the tyrosine phosphorylation, by the JAKs, of one or more of a family of proteins called *STATs*. Upon phosphorylation, STAT proteins translocate to the nucleus, where they bind appropriate cytokine response elements present in target genes.

The transcriptional activity of STAT proteins can be illustrated by regulation of c-Fos. Cytokines are known to induce c-Fos expression in target cells via activation of the JAK-STAT pathway. The c-Fos gene contains a response element called the SIE (sis-inducible element), which binds STAT proteins and mediates STAT induction of gene expression. Cytokine response elements have now been identified within many neural genes, including those for VIP and several other neuropeptides.

Steroid Hormone Receptors Are Ligand-Activated Transcription Factors

The differentiation of many cell types in the brain is established by exposure to steroids. For example, exposure to estrogen or testosterone during critical developmental periods results in sexually dimorphic development of certain nuclei. The steroid hormone receptor superfamily (also called the *nuclear receptor superfamily*), which includes the receptors for glucocorticoids, gonadal steroids, mineralocorticoids, retinoids, thyroid hormone, vitamin D, and cholesterol-related steroids, consists of lipid-soluble molecules that diffuse readily across cell membranes. They act on their receptors within the cell cytoplasm, in marked distinction to the other types of intercellular signals described above that act on plasma membrane receptors. Another unique feature of the nuclear receptor superfamily is that their receptors are actually transcription factors (Lin et al., 1998). Like other transcription factors described above, the steroid hormone receptors are modular in nature. Each has a transcriptional activation domain at its amino terminus, a DNA binding domain, and a hormone binding domain at its carboxy terminus. The DNA binding domains recognize different types of steroid hormone response elements within the regulatory regions of genes. The DNA binding domains of the steroid hormone receptors are described as zinc finger domains, a cysteine-rich motif that contains a zinc ion. This motif is used by many other transcription factors, but by few factors that are regulated by extracellular signals.

Once bound by hormone, activated steroid hormone receptors translocate into the nucleus where they bind to their cognate response elements. Such binding then increases or decreases the rate at which these target genes are transcribed, depending on the precise nature and DNA sequence context of the element. Steroid hormone receptors can therefore be considered ligand-activated transcription factors. In recent years, steroid hormone receptors have been shown to regulate the transcription of genes that do not contain steroid response elements by forming protein-protein interactions with other transcription factors, for example, AP-1 and CREB proteins. This discovery reveals highly complex regulatory mechanisms by which steroid hormones control gene expression (Karin and Chang, 2001).

Although the primary mechanism by which the transcriptional activity of steroid hormone receptors is regulated is through their ligand binding and consequent nuclear translocation, the receptors are also regulated in vivo at transcriptional and posttranslational levels. The total amount of the receptors expressed in specific target tissues can be altered by various hormonal and drug treatments, including in vivo treatment of animals with antidepressant medications (Chapter 29). Steroid hormone receptors are also known to be phosphorylated by PKA and Ca^{2+}-dependent protein kinases and by protein tyrosine kinases. The physiological role of receptor phosphorylation remains unknown but could alter the affinity of the receptors for their ligands, their translocation into the nucleus, or their binding to their DNA response elements.

REFERENCES

Blendy, J.A. (2006) The role of CREB in depression and antidepressant treatment. *Biol. Psychiatry* 59:1144–1150.

Cao, X., Yeo, G., Muotri, A.R., Kuwabara, T., and Gage, F.H. (2006) Noncoding RNAs in the mammalian central nervous system. *Annu. Rev. Neurosci.* 29:77–103.

Carlezon, W.A., Jr., Duman, R.S., and Nestler, E.J. (2005) The many faces of CREB. *Trends Neurosci.* 28:436–445.

Chawla, A., Repa, J.J., Evans, R.M., and Mangelsdorf, D.J. (2001) Nuclear receptors and lipid physiology: opening the X-files. *Science* 294:1866–1870.

Conti, A.C., Juo, Y.C., Valentino, R.J., and Blendy, J.A. (2004) Inducible cAMP early repressor regulates corticosterone suppression after tricyclic antidepressant treatment. *J. Neurosci.* 24: 1967–1975.

Ghosh, S., and Karin, M. (2002) Missing pieces in the NF-kappaB puzzle. *Cell* 109:S81–S96.

Green, T.A., Alibhai, I.N., Hommel, J.D., DiLeone, R.J., Kumar, A., Theobald, D.E., Neve, R.L., and Nestler, E.J. (2006) Induction of ICER expression in nucleus accumbens by stress or amphetamine increases behavioral responses to emotional stimuli. *J. Neurosci.* 26:8235–8242.

Hake, S.B., Xiao, A., and Allis, C.D. (2004) Linking the epigenetic "language" of covalent histone modifications to cancer. *Br. J. Cancer* 90:761–769.

Herdegen, T., and Leah, J.D. (1998) Inducible and constitutive transcription factors in the mammalian nervous system: control of gene expression by Jun, Fos and Krox, and CREB/ATF proteins. *Brain Res. Rev.* 28:370–490.

Hope, B.T., Nye, H.E., Kelz, M.B., Self, D.W., Iadarola, M.J., Nakabeppu, Y., Duman, R.S., and Nestler, E.J. (1994) Induction of a long-lasting AP-1 complex composed of altered Fos-like proteins in brain by chronic cocaine and other chronic treatments. *Neuron* 13:1235–1244.

Horvath, C.M. (2000) STAT proteins and transcriptional responses to extracellular signals. *Trends Biochem. Sci.* 25:496–502.

Hyman, S.E., and Nestler, E. (1993) *The Molecular Foundations of Psychiatry*. Washington, DC: American Psychiatric Association.

Ihle, J.N. (2001) The Stat family in cytokine signaling. *Curr. Opin. Cell Biol.* 13:211–217.

Impey, S., McCorkle, S.R., Cha-Molstad, H., Dwyer, J.M., Yochum, G.S., Boss, J.M., McWeeney, S., Dunn, J.J., Mandel, G., and Goodman, R.H. (2004) Defining the CREB regulon: a genome-wide analysis of transcription factor regulator regions. *Cell* 119:1041–1054.

Josselyn, S.A., Kida, S., and Silva, A.J. (2004) Inducible repression of CREB function disrupts amygdala dependent memory. *Neurobiol. Learn. Mem.* 82:159–163.

Karin, M., and Chang, L. (2001) AP-1–glucocorticoid receptor cross-talk taken to a higher level. *J. Endocrinol.* 169:447–451.

Lachner, M., O'Sullivan, R.J., and Jenuwein, T. (2003) An epigenetic road map for histone lysine methylation. *J. Cell Sci.* 116: 2117–2124.

Lin, R.J., Kao, H.Y., Ordentlich, P., and Evans, R.M. (1998) The transcriptional basis of steroid physiology. *Cold Spring Harbor Symp. Quant. Biol.* 63:577–585.

Marie, H., Morishita, W., Yu, X., Calakos, N., and Malenka, R.C. (2005) Generation of silent synapses by acute in vivo expression of CaMKIV and CREB. *Neuron* 45:741–752.

Mayr, B., and Montminy, M. (2001) Transcriptional regulation by the phosphorylation-dependent factor CREB. *Nature Rev. Mol. Cell Biol.* 2:599–609.

McClung, C.A., Ulery, P.G., Perrotti, L.I., Zachariou, V., Berton, O., and Nestler, E.J. (2004) ΔFosB: A molecular switch for long-term adaptation in the brain. *Mol. Brain Res.* 132:146–154.

Morgan, J.I., and Curran, T. (1995) Immediate-early genes: ten years on. *Trends Neurosci.* 18:66–77.

Nestler, E.J., Hyman, S.E., and Malenka, R.C. (2001) *Molecular Basis of Neuropharmacology*. New York: McGraw-Hill.

Pittenger, C., Fasano, S., Mazzocchi-Jones, D., Dunnett, S.B., Kandel, E.R., and Brambilla, R. (2006) Impaired bidirectional synaptic plasticity and procedural memory formation in striatum-specific cAMP response element-binding protein-deficient mice. *J. Neurosci.* 26:2808–2813.

Shaywitz, A.J., and Greenberg, M.E. (1999) CREB: a stimulus-induced transcription factor activated by a diverse array of extracellular signals. *Annu. Rev. Biochem.* 68:821–861.

Sonnenberg, J.L., Macgregor-Leon, P.F., Curran, T., and Morgan, J.I. (1989) Dynamic alterations occur in the levels and composition of transcription factor AP-1 complexes after seizure. *Neuron* 3: 359–365.

Tully, T., Bourtchouladze, R., Scott, R., and Tallman, J. (2003) Targeting the CREB pathway for memory enhancers. *Nature Rev. Drug Discov.* 2:267–277.

Vo, N., and Goodman, R.H. (2001) CREB-binding protein and p300 in transcriptional regulation. *J. Biol. Chem.* 276:13505–13508.

7 Functional Genomics and Models of Mental Illness

LISA M. MONTEGGIA, WILLIAM A. CARLEZON, JR., AND RALPH J. DILEONE

Genetics relies upon the study of mutants to better understand the function of genes. For many decades, the field used mutation analysis to identify important genes. However, the completion of the genome project and the development of high-throughput genomic techniques have made it possible to rapidly evaluate expression of hundreds of genes. These approaches can be used on populations of ribonucleic acid (RNA) or protein from specific tissue sources, such as the brain, and have resulted in a massive influx of gene regulatory data. Although expression changes under different conditions may suggest a function, it is necessary to conduct more traditional genetic analysis in model organisms to define gene function. This conversion of extensive genomic data to *functional* genomic understanding is multidisciplinary and has implications for many fields, including psychiatry.

Mutant analysis in model systems has helped to define and elucidate signal transduction pathways and transcriptional hierarchies. While yeast, flies, and worms have helped define basic genetic pathways, mice have become a powerful genetic organism that is representative of complex mammalian systems. The mouse is particularly relevant in neuroscience and psychiatry, where the development of effective models is dependent on complex mammalian brain circuitry and behavior. Although the current technology is emphasized here, the infrastructure established over decades of work made the modern techniques possible and more powerful.

The extensive history of mouse studies has enabled large-scale efforts to understand gene function. A consortium of mutagenesis centers has recently been organized and will likely result in the generation of useful mouse models for neurobiological and psychiatric research. However, modern mouse research also takes advantage of transgenics and targeted gene knockouts, where specific genes are added or removed from the mouse genome. This "reverse genetic" strategy (from a cloned gene to mutant animal) has redefined experimental possibilities and has dominated the landscape of mouse genetics for the last 20 years. As new genes are implicated in a biological process, it is possible to directly assess their relevance in a complete animal system. The reverse genetic approach is increasingly needed because the completion of the genome project has shown that a large number of genes cannot be placed into a functional category from their primary sequence information.

This chapter focuses on how genetic animal models are relevant for advancing our understanding of psychiatric disorders. The creation of genetically modified animal models has led to our ability to study the contribution of individual genes and their products in the brain. These genetic models have also complemented and extended our understanding of heuristic and pharmacological models of psychiatric diseases. We discuss conventional approaches to generate transgenic mice, in which a gene of interest is added to the animal, and knockout mice, in which a gene of interest is disrupted or inactivated. We also address more recent technologies such as viral-mediated gene transfer that allow for spatial and temporal control over gene function. The use of these technical advances has elevated the use of the rat, another well-studied model in neurobiology and behavioral studies, as a genetic model.

TRANSGENIC MICE

Transgenic mice are created by adding deoxyribonucleic acid (DNA) directly to the genome (Box 7.1). As the first efficient approach for taking previously isolated genes and evaluating possible functions in vivo, this technique revolutionized mouse genetics by allowing for direct tests of gene function in an entire animal system. Transgenic experiments are often used to (*1*) overexpress a gene at high levels, (*2*) misexpress a gene in the wrong place or at the wrong time, (*3*) express a mutant or modified form or a gene, or

BOX 7.1 *Transgenic Mice Production: Transgenic Disease Models*

Transgenic mice are commonly used to model human disease states and to test hypotheses concerning the genetic causes of the disease. The isolation of genes that cause neurological disease has allowed transgenic mice to be used to model the disease by directly mimicking the genetic cause found in patients. For example, mice overexpressing mutant forms of superoxide dismutase (SOD1) developed muscle atrophy, neurodegeneration, and death as seen in human amyotrophic lateral sclerosis (ALS) cases (Gurney et al., 1994). Similarly, the cellular and molecular mechanisms of polyglutamine disorders, such as spinocerebellar ataxia, have been modeled and better understood by studying mouse models generated via transgenic expression of mutant proteins (N. Heintz and Zoghbi, 2000). In the case of Alzheimer's disease, overexpression of mutant forms of amyloid precursor protein (APP) has been used to test hypotheses and generate powerful disease models (Box 7.2).

Adapted from Richardson et al. (1997).

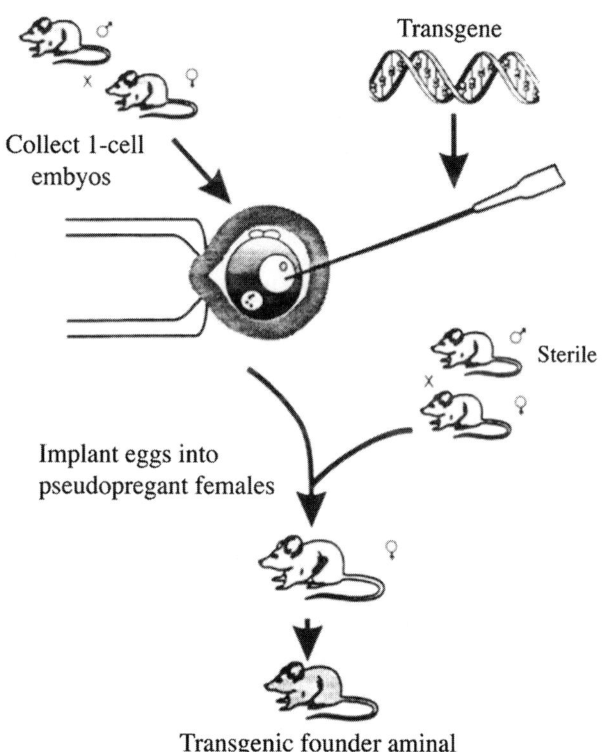

(*4*) study gene regulation via reporter gene constructs. Gene overexpressing can yield important information of the dosage sensitivity of the gene product while misexpression experiments can indicate whether or not a gene will cause defects when abnormally expressed. Overexpression of certain mutant forms can also be used to reduce the function of the endogenous gene ("dominant negative").

Transgenic mouse lines can be made and established rapidly. Transgenic mice are generated via nuclear microinjection of cloned DNA into fertilized mouse eggs. The DNA construct usually inserts into a single random site of the genome as multiple copies (usually between 5–50). Because this transgene integration often occurs at the one- or two-cell stage, the transgenic founder mouse contains the transgenes in most cell types and can pass the transgene directly to progeny. Expression is then mediated by regulatory elements contained within the original construct (Box 7.1). However, transgene expression is usually influenced by DNA sequences surrounding the insertion site, which necessitates the creation and characterization of multiple founder mice to find lines with the desired expression patterns. This concern is mitigated by use of larger pieces of DNA as described below.

Large-Clone Transgenics and Disease Models

Traditional transgenics are made with relatively small DNA constructs (3–25 kilobases) that can be generated

BOX 7.2 *Transgenics and Alzheimer's Disease*

Alzheimer's disease (AD) is a neurodegenerative disease characterized by a gradual decline in cognition and memory over a period of years. The neuropathology of AD is marked by the presence of extracellular senile plaques and intracellular neurofibrillary tangles. Although the debate over the causative factor for AD remains controversial, growing evidence suggests plaques are required for the development of AD. Plaques are generated by accumulation of a 42 amino acid amyloid ß protein (Aß), which is derived from the amyloid precursor protein (APP). Genetic studies have identified mutations in the APP gene and in the presenilin genes (*PS1* and *PS2*) in familial forms of AD. Disorders that lead to the oversecretion of APP result in Alzheimer's disease-like syndromes.

Transgenic mice overexpressing APP and presenilin mutations have been used to model AD. The first successful attempt, using a platelet-derived growth factor promoter to drive expression of a familial APP mutation, resulted in mice with elevated levels of APP as well as increased amyloid deposits (Games et al., 1995; Masliah et al., 1996). More recently, transgenics have been generated that link the elevated APP to learning and memory deficits (Moran et al., 1995; Hsiao et al., 1996). Transgenic mice coexpressing the wild-type human APP gene and various *PS1* mutations exhibited high levels of Aß in the brain, suggesting the *PS1* mutations may influence Aß production and contribute to the pathology of the disease (Citron et al., 1997). This model has recently been used to test the effectiveness of immunomodulatory therapy (Janus et al., 2000; Morgan et al., 2000). The ability of transgenic mice to model aspects of AD represents a major advancement toward understanding the pathophysiology of this disease.

through standard cloning techniques. Although sufficient for many experiments, the complexity of gene regulation, and the large size of mammalian genes, often demands the use of larger fragments of DNA to effectively model gene regulation and disease states. Large-clone transgenics are made using bacterial artificial chromosomes (BACs) and yeast artificial chromosomes (YACs) (N. Heintz, 2001). Bacterial artificial chromosomes can be used to successfully propagate up to 300 kilobases (300,000 base pairs) of mammalian DNA in bacteria while YACs can propagate over 1000 kilobases (1,000,000 base pairs) of mammalian DNA in yeast, allowing for transgenics to be made with entire genes and surrounding genomic regulatory sequences. Large-clone transgenics have been used to effectively model diseases that are caused by mutations in large genes. The accurate expression of the mutant form is likely to yield models that most closely mimic the human pathology. For example, YACs containing the entire human Huntingtin protein have been used to model Huntington's disease (Hodgson et al., 1999). The YACs were modified to express the glutamine repeats that are found in individuals with the disease. Mice transgenic for these constructs developed the cellular, physiological, and behavioral characteristics similar to human patients with Huntington's disease, including selective striatal neurodegeneration. Transgenic approaches have also been useful in delineating the role of the amyloid precursor protein (APP) in Alzheimer's disease (Box 7.2).

Large clone transgenics have also been used to determine the significance of gene dosage effects on behavior and disease states. For example, DNA around the Down's syndrome candidate region was introduced via large-clone transgenics and mice were screened for learning abnormalities. This led to identification of the minibrain-related gene, *Dyrk-1*, as a candidate gene for Down's syndrome (Smith et al., 1997). The large size of most mammalian genes necessitates the large-clone approach for these studies.

BAC Transgenics as Reporter Genes

Another powerful application of large-scale clones has been the generation of reporter lines that express readily detectable marker proteins, such as green fluorescent protein (GFP). By using BACs surrounding specific genes, a series of mouse lines has been generated that allow researchers to detect, study, and isolate specific neuron populations that are otherwise difficult to detect (H. Heintz, 2004). These BAC reporter mice have been used to distinguish direct and indirect output neurons within the striatum, allowing for definitive characterization of different electrophysiological properties in these important neurons (Kreitzer and Malenka, 2007).

Rat Transgenic Models

Although less common, transgenic rats have been made and are powerful tools for assessing physiology or behavior that is better characterized in rat models. For example, a transgenic model of Huntington's disease was generated in rats to allow for longitudinal imaging studies in a larger brain (von Hörsten et al., 2003). Working memory deficits have been characterized in transgenic rats overexpressing the adenosine receptor (A_{2A}) in rat brain (Giménez-Llort et al., 2007). In addition, transgenic reporter rats have been generated for the study of circadian rhythms (Yamazaki et al., 2000). As the generation of transgenic rats becomes more efficient, including application of large-clone techniques, rat reporter and disease models will become more common and more powerful for behavioral and psychiatric research.

CONVENTIONAL KNOCKOUT MICE

Transgenic mice created via microinjection allow for efficient gain-of-function analysis or expression of exogenous molecules. Although this approach is powerful and can be used to model a subset of diseases, there was still a need to test the necessity of gene products via loss-of-function analysis. The goal of removing genes in a directed fashion motivated a number of approaches to modify the endogenous genes within the mouse genome. Ultimately, the knockout strategy depended upon modifying the genome of embryonic stem (ES) cell lines and subsequently generating a mouse from the modified cell lines.

Early research on cell lines derived from early embryos and embryonic carcinomas indicated that these lines could retain totipotency, or the ability to give rise to all differentiated cell types of the mouse. Cells derived from the inner cell mass of a mouse blastula were used to establish the first ES cell lines. Importantly, ES cell lines could be cultured and frozen, and they allowed recombination to occur between introduced DNA and homologous sequences in the cellular genome (Fig. 7.1). However, the rates of recombination that occur in ES cells are very low compared to random insertion events. To select for the rare recombination event, a "positive-negative" strategy was developed to select for inserts into the desired (homologous) position, while selecting against random insertions (Mansour et al., 1988). After a single copy (maternal or paternal) of the gene is modified, the cells are expanded and introduced into a developing mouse embryo. The cells become incorporated into the developing embryo, and the resulting founder mouse is a mosaic of wild-type cells and mutant cells. This founder must be bred to confirm the presence of the transgene in the progeny. Finally, progeny are mated to generate mice that are missing both copies of the gene (homozygous mutants).

Knockouts originally used a replacement strategy to exchange an endogenous gene with a neomycin-resistance gene cassette (PGK-neo^r). Later generation knockouts took advantage of the recombination event to replace the original gene with a reporter gene or a mutated version of an original gene. These "knock-in" studies yielded powerful data on gene expression and gene redundancy and are now standard practice in current gene analysis. This strategy could be used to misexpress a gene as with transgenic microinjections. Although more time-consuming than traditional transgenic approaches, no knowledge of regulatory elements is required because placing the new gene into the same position of the genome should ensure correct expression.

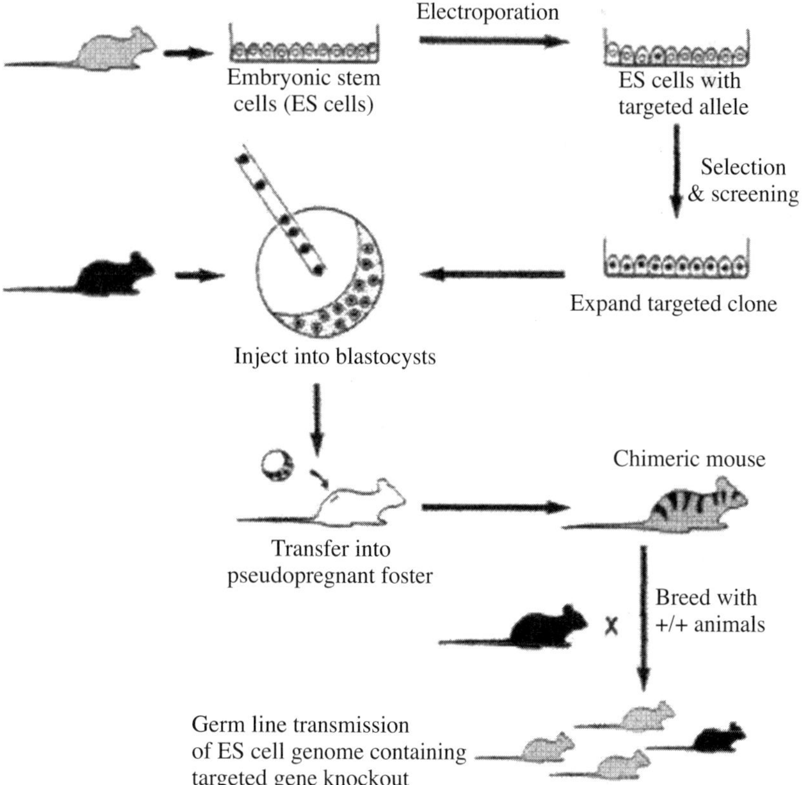

FIGURE 7.1 Knockout mouse production. Adapted from Joyner (2000).

BOX 7.3 *Knockouts and the Dopaminergic System*

Dopamine (DA) plays an important role in Parkinson's disease, drug addiction, and schizophrenia among other neuropsychiatric diseases. However, the role of individual components of the dopaminergic system in these disorders remains unknown. The ability to knockout specific genes involved in DA synthesis, release, signaling, and reuptake allows for a comparison of specific genetic alterations with pharmacological models of these disorders

Dopamine is synthesized from tyrosine by tyrosine hydroxylase (TH) in the nerve cell cytoplasm and then loaded onto vesicles by vesicular monoamine transporters (VMATs). Once DA is released from the synapse it can (*1*) activate either presynaptic (D2) or postsynaptic (D1-D5) DA receptors, (*2*) be degraded by catechol-O-methyltransferase (COMT) or monoamine oxidase (MAO), or (*3*) be taken up by a dopamine transporter (DAT).

Mice that lack TH die at birth, implicating catecholamines in fetal development (Zhou & Palmiter, 1995). The loss of VMAT disrupts the ability of DA to be loaded in the synaptic vesicles and results in mice that die shortly after birth (Takahashi et al., 1997; Wang et al., 1997). In contrast, knockouts of all of the DA receptor genes (D1–D5) are viable with mild alterations in locomotor activity (Xu et al., 1994; Baik et al., 1995; Accili et al., 1996; Rubinstein et al., 1997; Xu et al., 1997; Clifford et al., 1998; Kelly et al., 1998; Dulawa et al., 1999; Holmes et al., 2001). The loss of the DA degradative enzymes does not produce alterations in locomotor activity but does result in increased aggression and reactivity to stress (Gogos et al., 1998; Shih et al., 1999). The DAT knockouts have high extracellular DA concentration and display alterations in various behavioral abnormalities including deficits in spatial cognitive function and sensorimotor gating (Giros et al., 1996; Jones et al., 1998). These knockouts of the dopaminergic system allow for a comparison of specific genetic alterations with pharmacological models of psychiatric and neurological disorders and may contribute to new therapeutic approaches in drug discovery.

Knockout Disease Models

Many human neurological and psychiatric diseases are likely to be due to loss of gene function that cannot be readily modeled with transgenics. For example, a subset of dominant human mutations is caused by loss of function of only one gene copy. This is known as *haplo-insufficiency* and is best modeled by evaluating heterozygote mice that are missing only one copy of a gene. This is particularly relevant and best studied in cancer models, where heterozygote mutant mice are more prone to tumor formation due to somatic loss of the normal copy. However, it is also possible that a loss of a single copy of a gene is sufficient to recapitulate aspects of psychiatric diseases in animal models. Recently, it was found that animals missing only one copy of the Reeler gene displayed gene expression changes as well as dendritic defects similar to those found in postmortem tissue from patients with schizophrenia (Liu et al., 2001). It may be useful to conduct more widespread and thorough behavioral testing on heterozygous mice to evaluate the effects of reduced gene expression on behavior.

Like transgenic mice, knockout mice can be used to target specific genes to test a hypothesis or model a disease state. Box 7.3 and Table 7.1 highlight results obtained from knockout studies on molecules related to the dopamine system, which have clearly helped to elucidate the specific role of receptors, enzymes, and proteins.

TABLE 7.1. *Knockouts and the Dopaminergic System*

Knockout Mice	*Phenotypes*
Tyrosine hydroxylase (TH)	Lethal (Zhou and Palmiter, 1995)
VMAT2	Lethal (Takahashi et al., 1997; Wang et al., 1997)
D1 DA receptor	Hyperactivity, spatial learning deficit (Xu et al., 1994; Clifford et al., 1998)
D2 DA receptor	Hypoactive, some dysfunction of prepulse inhibition (PPI) sensorimotor gating (Baik et al., 1995; Kelly et al., 1998)
D3 DA receptor	Hyperactive (Accili et al., 1996; Xu et al., 1997)
D4 DA receptor	Hypoactive (Rubinstein et al., 1997; Dulawa et al., 1999)
D5 DA receptor	Normal (Holmes et al., 2001)
COMT	Normal activity; increased aggression, impairment of emotional reactivity (Gogos et al., 1998)
MAO-A	Normal activity; increased aggression, more reactive to stress (for review, see Shih et al., 1999)
MAO-B	Normal activity; more reactive to stress (for review, see Shih et al., 1999)
DAT	Hyperactive, deficits in PPI sensorimotor gating and spatial cognitive impairments (Giros et al., 1996; Jones et al., 1998)

VMAT2: Vesicular monoamine transporter type 2; COMT: catechol-O-methyltransferase; MAO-A: monoamine oxidase A; MAO-B: monoamine oxidase B; DAT: dopamine transporter; PPI: prepulse inhabition.

Knockouts have also been useful in testing the specificity and effects of pharmacological agents. By completely removing a receptor, for example, knockout mice can be screened for the effects of various drugs. For example, mice missing the 5-HT_{2C} receptor have a paradoxical locomotor increase in response to the nonselective serotonin agonist, *m-chlorophenlypiparazine*, which normally induces a locomotor decrease (Heisler and Tecott, 2000). It was subsequently discovered that the agonist was acting on 5-HT_{1B} receptors in the absence of 5-HT_{2C}, revealing the dependence of drug response on the genetic constitution of the individual.

Although genetic knockout studies have traditionally focused on the use of mice, the completion of the rat genome project (Gibbs et al., 2004) and the extensive history and use of rats in studying behavior and modeling psychiatric disease have motivated efforts for generating rat knockouts. There are mutagenesis strategies being used to systematically generate a large set of rat knockouts (Smits et al., 2006). This will undoubtedly lead to more use of rat knockouts for modeling behavior and psychiatric disease.

Limitations of Knockout Mice

Early studies with knockout mice produced many surprises while also exposing a number of limitations. One major limitation was the occurrence of lethal mutations. Because developmental biologists did most of the early work, the early terminal phenotypes were of interest. However, early lethality precludes studies of gene function in adult animals demanding use of conditional mutagenesis strategies that are outlined in the next section.

Combining knockouts and transgenics can be used to overcome this limitation. By generating a tyrosine hydroxylase (TH) knockout mouse that has been genetically engineered to express the TH gene only in noradrenergic cells, it's possible to generate a mouse that is missing DA and yet creates normal norepinephrine (Zhou and Palmiter, 1995). These DA-deficient mice survive until birth, indicating that the fetal lethality of TH mutant mice was caused by the lack of norepinephrine. These mice can be kept alive via daily injections of 3,4-dihydroxyphenylalanine (L-DOPA) and have been used extensively to better evaluate the function of DA in locomotion, nest building, and feeding.

Although this strategy was used successfully, it is not always possible to develop effective rescue experiments. More recent work has established strategies for better control of transgenic and knockout effects.

CONDITIONAL CONTROL OF GENE EXPRESSION

The ideal system to control gene expression would be a "genetic switch" that can be operated at will to turn genes on or off. Newer transgenic models are taking advantage of these inducible systems to clearly define the relationship between the transgene expression and the phenotype. In these models, the transgenic expression is regulated temporally by administration of an exogenous agent. Most approaches involve the use of a binary system, or two-gene system, in which one transgene controls the expression of a second. Binary systems that control gene expression can be classified into two groups: (*1*) transcriptional transactivator systems, to overexpress a gene of interest, and (*2*) site-specific recombination systems, to knockout a gene of interest (Fig. 7.2).

Transcriptional Transactivator Systems

There are many different types of transcriptional transactivator systems; here we focus on the most commonly used system, the *tetracycline gene regulation system* (Gossen and Bujard, 1992). In this system, the first transgene encodes the tetracycline transactivator (tTA) under the control of enhancer sequences that dictate expression patterns. The second transgene encodes the gene of interest to be overexpressed under the control of a tetracycline responsive promoter (TetOp) (Fig 7.2A). In this system, tTA binds to TetOp and results in

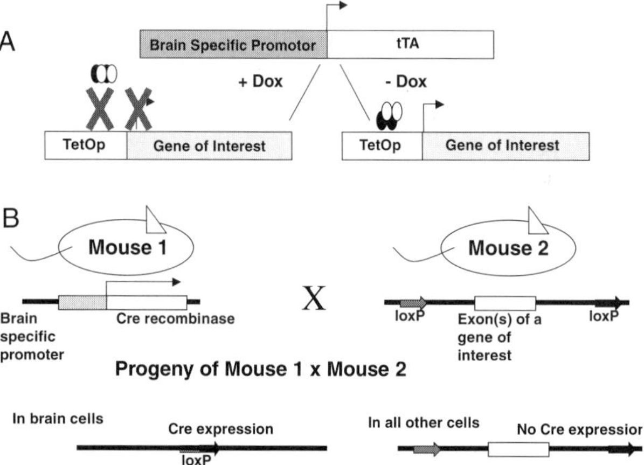

FIGURE 7.2 Binary systems for gene induction and removal. (*A*) Schematic of the tetracycline transactivator system for the generation of double transgenic animals. In this system, a brain-specific promotor drives expression of the tetracycline transactivator (tTA) gene selectively to the brain. In the presence of doxycycline (dox), a tetracycline analog, tTA can not bind to its promotor (TetOp) and the gene of interest is not expressed. In the absence of dox, tTA binds to TetOp and results in transcription of the gene of interest selectively to the brain. (*B*) Schematic of the CRE-loxP system for conditional knockouts: Genetic techniques are used to express CRE recombinase under the control of a brain-specific promotor. A second construct contains loxP sites flanking a critical region of the gene to be knocked out. The two lines of mice are crossed, and resulting bigenic mice show a loss of the gene of interest, which occurs at the time of development and selectively in those cells in the brain in which the brain-specific promotor is active. The gene of interest is expressed at wild-type levels in cells not expressing CRE recombinase.

BOX 7.4 *Overexpression of ΔFosB and the Link to Drug Abuse*

Chronic exposure to many drugs of abuse (for example, *cocaine, amphetamine, morphine*, and *nicotine*) results in the accumulation of the transcription factor ΔFosB in the striatum. ΔFosB is a protein that, once induced, persists for a very long time in the brain. The striatum regions are important for mediating many behavioral aspects of addiction. The molecular mechanisms that are responsible for the long-term induction of ΔFosB in the striatum may represent one biological basis underlying the transition from a nonaddicted to an addicted state.

The tetracycline gene–regulated system has been used to successfully overexpress the transcription factor ΔFosB to the striatum region of the brain (J. Chen et al., 1998). The resulting mice were more responsive to the rewarding effects of cocaine (Kelz et al., 1999). The use of additional genomic technologies (that is, *viral-mediated gene transfer*) has provided evidence that ΔFosB-associated upregulation of GluR2 (an α-amino-3-hydroxy-5-methyl-4-isoxasolepropionic acid [AMPA] glutamate receptor) causes, at least in part, the increases in sensitivity to cocaine (Kelz et al., 1999) and other types of rewards (Todtenkopf et al., 2006) (see Fig. 7.3). Interestingly, in a parallel set of experiments with the tetracycline gene–regulated system, mice were generated that overexpressed a dominant negative inhibitor of ΔFosB in the striatum, and these mice were less responsive to cocaine (Peakman et al., 2000). These findings demonstrate a direct role for ΔFosB in the rewarding properties of cocaine and may suggest a role for this molecule in promoting a switch from casual drug use to addiction. By limiting overexpression of ΔFosB in adult mice, this molecular phenotype is mimicked without the potential developmental effects that might have been caused by more traditional transgenic analysis.

transcription on the gene of interest unless tetracycline (or doxycycline, a tetracycline analog that can cross the blood-brain barrier) is present. Tetracycline interferes with the ability of tTA to bind to TetOp and drive expression of the gene of interest and is referred to as the "tet-off" system. Thus, mice remain treated with doxycycline until the time the researcher wants to study the overexpression of the gene. This is an inducible system because the gene of interest is controlled by the presence or absence of doxycycline. It is also a cell-targeted system because the transgene of interest will only be expressed in those cells that express tTA, which is controlled by the choice of promoter in the first transgene construct.

Inducible Transgenics and Disease Models

The tetracycline gene regulation system has been used to successfully overexpress genes in the central nervous system. The first published report overexpressed the calcium-calmodulin-dependent protein kinase II (CaMKII) selectively within the hippocampus of adult mice (Mayford et al., 1996). The resulting mice had cellular phenotypes including impaired functioning of place cells as well as decrements in long-term potentiation within the hippocampus. These mice also had a decrement in spatial learning, which is thought to be a hippocampal-dependent task. These findings suggest that CaMKII in an important step in cellular and behavioral forms of plasticity and highlight the functional importance of the gene in the hippocampus.

Other studies have direct implications for better understanding of brain disease. For example, Yamamoto et al. (2000) found that the neuropathology and motor dysfunction caused by overexpression of Huntingtin was reversible by simply turning off the transgene. This has important mechanistic implications that are relevant to the development of effective therapeutics. In contrast, the inducible transgenic strategy has been used to show that 5-HT_{1A} serotonin receptor function is required during development, and not in the adult, to produce normal anxiety responses in mice (Gross et al., 2002). Another use of inducible transgenic technology is to mimic molecular changes that may be seen in psychiatric disease states as exemplified in Box 7.4.

There are many advantages of the tetracycline gene-regulated system including the reversibility of the system and the ability to target it to a specific cell type with the use of a cell type–specific enhancer/promoter. There are, however, also limitations to the system. First, the dynamics of gene induction are relatively slow because this system requires the mice to be removed from doxycycline to induce expression of the target gene of interest. Second, transgene expression can be influenced by the position that it has inserted into the genome and not just by the promoter that is driving its expression (Box 7.5). Although these concerns are of importance, the tetracycline gene-regulated system is still being used with remarkable success to study the function of genes in the adult nervous system. These inducible transgenic systems are of particular use in psychiatry where minor developmental disturbances could have subtle but persistent repercussions.

Site-Specific Recombination Systems

One way to target a genetic deletion in a regionally and temporally dependent manner is with site-specific recombination. Site-specific recombinases are enzymes that catalyze recombination between specific DNA sites. The CRE recombinase from P1 bacteriophage is the most widely used enzyme. CRE recognizes a 34 bp site (*loxP*, or *locus of recombination*) to catalyze recombination.

BOX 7.5 *cAMP-Response Element (CRE)-Driven Lines Can Influence the Phenotype of the Conditional Knockout*

Recently, conditional knockouts of neurotrophin 3 (NT-3) were generated to study the role of this growth factor in adult brain. Traditional knockouts of NT-3 die shortly after birth. Two independent groups have generated conditional NT-3 knockouts in which the loss of NT-3 is restricted to the brain and the conditional NT-3 knockouts survive into adulthood. The first group generated conditional NT-3 knockouts by crossing floxed NT-3 mice with animals expressing CRE recombinase under the control of the neural specific promoter, *synapsin 1* (Ma et al., 1999). The conditional knockouts had an ablation of NT-3 in many regions of the brain including the hippocampus. These conditional knockouts were examined in several parameters of synaptic transmission and displayed no difference between wild-type controls, suggesting that NT-3 does not play a role in synaptic transmission and some forms of hippocampus dependent learning. The second group used the neural specific nestin promoter to drive CRE expression in floxed NT-3 mice (Akbarian et al., 2001). These nestin-CRE expressing mice caused a more widespread pattern of NT-3 loss in the brain than the synapsin I-CRE expressing mice. In contrast to the synapsin-CRE results, the nestin-CRE NT-3 conditional knockouts established a role for this growth factor in modulating noradrenergic function and opiate withdrawal in the brain.

The conditional knockouts generated by the two different groups resulted in progeny with different patterns of NT-3 loss in the brain and different reported phenotypes. This example illustrates the importance of using different CRE-driven expression lines to elucidate "gene-function" relationships in conditional knockouts. However, there are many important limitations with the currently available CRE driven expression lines. First, there are not many enhancer and promoter sequences that are successful in expressing CRE recombinase specifically to the brain, let alone to particular regions or cell types. Second, many of these promoters do not express the CRE recombinase in the predicted locations. One approach is to identify better regulatory sequences to drive recombinase expression. Alternatively, knocking the recombinase directly into a known genetic locus by homologous recombination may allow for better control of its expression.

If two loxP sites are placed in the same orientation on a piece of DNA, the region between the two sites will be excised by the recombinase (Nagy, 2000).

Recombinase sites are not normally found in the mammalian genome. The recombinase sites are inserted into the genome of ES cells by homologous recombination such that the sites flank an exon (or exons) of a gene of interest. The gene with flanking recombinase sites is referred to as a "floxed" gene. The recombinase sites should be placed in the genome so as not to interfere with the expression or function of the gene of interest before the recombination event. A selection strategy is employed to identify those ES cells containing the floxed gene in a similar manner as that used to generate a conventional knockout (see Fig. 7.1). The resulting floxed mice still have the functional endogenous gene because the CRE recombinase has not yet been introduced into the system. To obtain a knockout of the targeted gene, the floxed mouse is bred to a second mouse in which a regional or cell type–specific transcriptional promoter controls CRE recombinase expression (Fig. 7.2B). These mice are referred to as "conditional" knockouts because the knockout occurs only in certain regions and is dependent on CRE recombinase expression. This approach has proved quite useful in the development of adult knockout mice where the traditional knockout of the gene is fatal and has moved us closer to understanding the function of specific genes (in the brain) and modeling human genetic diseases.

The first successful attempt of a conditional brain-specific gene knockout was the ionotropic glutamate receptor *N*-methyl-D-aspartate (*NMDAR1*) gene. The *NMDAR1* gene is an obligatory subunit of NMDA receptors. A floxed *NMDAR1* mouse was crossed with a transgenic line expressing CRE under the control of the *CaMKII* promoter. The *CaMKII* promoter turns on CRE recombinase in specific regions of the brain without any peripheral expression. The resulting mice displayed a relatively selective knockout of *NMDAR1* in the hippocampus that resulted in an impairment in hippocampal long-term potentiation and spatial memory. These cellular and behavioral phenotypes provided support for the view that endogenous *NMDAR1* is important in hippocampal dependent tasks (McHugh et al., 1996; Tsien, Chen, et al., 1996; Tsien, Huerta, et al., 1996; Shimizu et al., 2000).

Conditional Knockouts and Disease Models

Conditional knockouts have also been used to model aspects of Rett syndrome (RTT), a childhood neurological disorder that occurs almost exclusively in females. An exciting recent discovery has been the identification of the gene responsible for RTT (Amir et al., 1999). The majority of RTT is caused by mutations in the methyl-CpG-binding protein (*MeCP2*) gene located on the X-chromosome (Wan et al., 1999). The *MeCP2* gene encodes a protein that binds to methylated DNA.

Original attempts to knockout the *MeCP2* gene by traditional knockout approaches resulted in early lethality of the mice. Conditional knockout techniques resulted in the generation of viable mice that have a neurological phenotype similar to human RTT (R. Z. Chen et al., 2001; Guy et al., 2001). Behavioral characterization of the conditional *MeCP2* knockout mice showed that the loss of this gene in broad forebrain regions was sufficient to mediate behavioral aspects of the disorder and starts to provide a framework of the brain regions that may be important in mediating some of these behavioral components of the disease (Gemelli et al., 2006). A mouse model that recapitulates aspects of a human disorder is a major advancement in studying this disease and may provide a model in which pharmacological agents can be tested for prevention or possible reversal of the behavioral phenotypes.

Conditional knockouts are showing great promise in elucidating the genetics of synaptic vesicle function. Synaptic vesicles influence neurotransmitter release and thus play important roles in mediating synaptic transmission. There are a vast number of synaptic vesicle proteins, of which the majority have been knocked out by traditional genetic approaches. Traditional knockouts have provided support for the role of many of these proteins in neurotransmitter release, but their functional redundancy and lack of regional specificity make it difficult to assess their role to individual neurotransmitter systems. This limitation is particularly important in diseases that are thought to be due to imbalances of particular neurotransmitter systems such as schizophrenia that may be due to an elevated dopaminergic and reduced glutaminergic transmission. The ability to target a knockout to a particular brain region in delineating the role of these particular proteins to specific neurotransmitter systems may contribute to our understanding particular molecular mechanisms of psychiatric illnesses (Fernandez-Chacon and Sudhof, 1999).

VIRAL-MEDIATED GENE TRANSFER

Another strategy for genetic intervention in the brain is to engineer viral vectors that carry a specific gene (or coding sequence) of interest. These constructs can then be microinjected directly into discrete brain regions. This technique exploits the natural ability of viruses to deliver genetic material to cells. When delivered to the brain, these vectors cause infected cells to express (or, in the case of endogenous genes, overexpress) transferred genes (*transgenes*) or sequences. Vectors can be used to increase the expression of endogenous genes, mutated genes (for example, encoding dominant-negative proteins), or small interfering RNA (siRNA). As such, viral-mediated gene transfer complements the use of mutant (knockout or transgenic) mice in neuropsychiatric research and is particularly useful when the goal is to manipulate expression of a single gene (*1*) in a specific brain region (*2*) at a specific time (*3*) in animals that developed normally.

There are several types of viruses that can be adapted for use as viral vectors, including those based on herpes simplex virus (HSV-1), adenovirus (AV), adeno-associated virus (AAV), and lentivirus (LV). Considering that each type of vector has unique advantages and disadvantages (see Carlezon, Nestler, et al., 2000; Neve et al., 2005), the selection of the most appropriate viral backbone depends upon the goals of the experiment. For example, HSV (Fig. 7.3) is an excellent vector when targeting neurons because it is naturally neurotropic and accommodates relatively large foreign complementary deoxyribonucleic acid (cDNA) sequences, but it is associated with a short duration (~5 days) of transgene expression. Adenovirus, on the other hand, is associated with a longer duration of transgene expression (months), but it is not selective for neurons and can elicit immune responses in the host. Adeno-associated virus elicits less of an immune response, but it can accommodate only small foreign cDNA sequences, thereby restricting the genes that can be transferred. Lentivirus vectors—which belong to the same class of viruses as human immunodeficiency virus (HIV)—integrate into the host DNA and cause permanent increases in transgene expression but are often associated with biosafety concerns.

Generally, viral vectors are replication deficient: they transfer the gene (or sequence) of interest into cells, but they lack the genes that enable the wild-type virus to

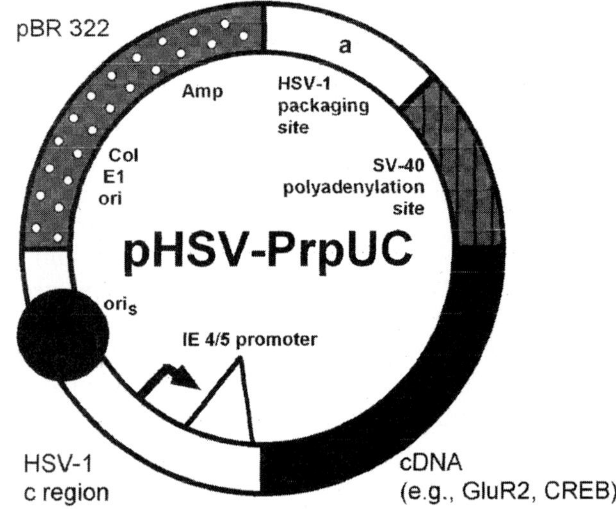

FIGURE 7.3 The amplicon (plasmid-based) vector HSV-PrpUC, into which foreign complementary deoxyribonucleic acid (cDNA) (for example, that encoding GluR2, cAMP-responsive element binding protein [CREB]) is subcloned. The viral backbone contains minimal with-type viral genes and relies upon specially engineered cell lines for propagation and helper virus to produce the proteins needed for packaging.

replicate or cause a destructive (lytic) infection. Currently, there are two types of replication-deficient vectors. *Genomic* vectors can be conceptualized as "gutted" viruses; the starting point is a competent virus from which harmful (lytic) genes have been removed, and to which the foreign cDNA has been added (for review, see Fink et al., 1996). Conversely, *amplicon* vectors (see Fig. 7.3) can be conceptualized as "modular" viruses; the starting point is a plasmid (*amplicon*) carrying the exogenous gene, to which minimal viral sequences are added that allow it to be packaged into virus particles with the aid of a helper virus and specialized cell lines (for review, see Carlezon, Nestler, et al., 2000; Neve et al., 2005).

Typically in neuropsychiatric research, small quantities of viral vectors (for a rat or mouse, 1-2 μl) are microinjected directly into discrete brain regions during stereotaxic surgery. Following a period of time that allows transgene expression to increase (or to increase and then wane), the consequences of increased transgene expression are evaluated in biochemical or behavioral assays. For a viral vector to have utility for this type of research (or ultimately, for gene therapy), the consequences of increased transgene expression must be detectable against the damage caused by the delivery procedure and any cytopathic effects of the viral vector (Fig. 7.4). Theoretically, it is possible to engineer viral vectors that express any biological entity with a known sequence. For example, vectors have been used that encode enzymes (for example, TH, CRE recombinase), transcription factors (for example, cAMP-response element binding protein [CREB], nucleus accumbens 1 [NAC-1]), receptors (for example, dopamine [DA] D1), receptor subunits (for example, GluRs), growth-associated proteins (for example, GAP43), and reporter proteins (β-galactosidase, GFP). Moreover, vectors encoding antisense sequences, dominant negative mutations (assuming that they exist), or siRNA for any of these entities can be engineered. There are some practical limitations, including the size of the foreign cDNA and the ease with which it can be subcloned into the viral backbone. The larger the cDNA construct, the less efficient the amplification will be during replication, which leads to less favorable amplicon-to-helper virus ratios and lower titers of the vector (see Carlezon, Nestler, et al., 2000). Assuming that the sequence of the construct is known, the cDNA itself is available, and that no untoward complications are encountered during subcloning, new HSV vectors can be engineered and generated usually within a period of several weeks, and sometimes within days.

Early Applications of Viral-Mediated Gene Transfer

During et al. (1994) performed one of the first in vivo applications of viral-mediated gene transfer. The goal in this study was to use the vectors as gene therapy to elicit behavioral recovery in an animal model of Parkinson's disease. In this model, rats were given unilateral, intrastriatal microinjections of the neurotoxin 6-hydroxydopamine (6-OHDA) to deplete local concentrations of DA. Viral-mediated gene transfer (by stereotaxic microinjections of vector) was then used to convert the endogenous cells of the striatum (primarily γ-aminobutyric acid [GABA]ergic medium spiny neurons) into L-DOPA-producing cells by delivering the gene for TH, the rate-limiting enzyme in the synthesis of DA. Hypothetically, increased expression of TH would lead to restored striatal DA levels and recovery of function. During et al. (1994) reported significant increases in the expression of TH within the striatum accompanied by partial behavioral recovery after viral-mediated gene transfer and concluded that TH gene therapy was

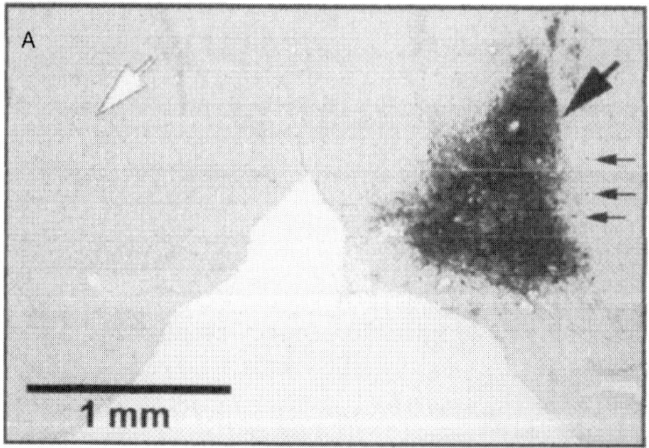

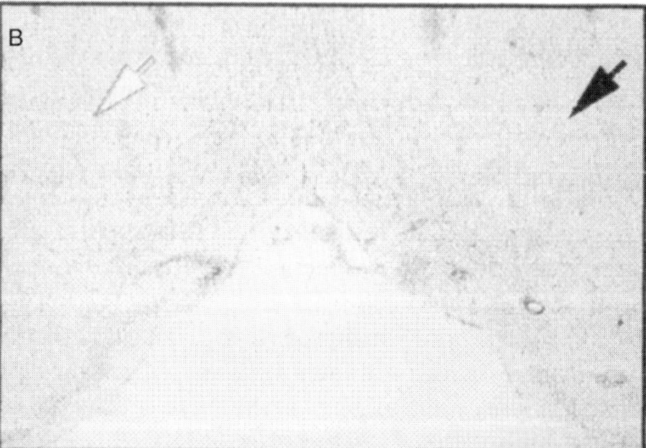

FIGURE 7.4 Histological examination of nucleus accumbens (NAc) tissue 3 days after gene transfer. (*A*) Large solid arrow: brain site at which the viral vector herpes simplex virus (HSV)-LacZ was microinjected. This vector encodes the reporter protein *Escherichia coli* β-galactosidase, which causes a dark blue reaction product in the presence of substrate. Small solid arrows: individual cells expressing β-galactosidase. Open arrow: noninjected NAc. (*B*) An adjacent, Nissl-stained slice from the same brain, showing minimal evidence of toxicity or damage despite strong transgene expression. Damage produces gliosis and darker Nissl staining.

effective in this model. Although other investigators (Isacson, 1995) who used the same viral vector preparations in their studies proposed alternative explanations for the behavioral data of During et al. (1994), this early work highlighted the theoretical potential of viral-mediated gene transfer to facilitate recovery from neurodegenerative processes and, more generally, the use of viral vectors to study how gene expression in discrete brain regions can influence behavior.

More recently, viral-mediated gene transfer has been used to study complex motivational states associated with neuropsychiatric disorders such as addiction and depression. The use of viral vectors is particularly well-suited to the study of addiction because exposure to drugs of abuse causes many changes in gene expression within the brain (Nestler, 2005). Because viral vectors offer the capability to study individual changes in gene expression in discrete brain regions, it is possible to mimic certain aspects of the drug-exposed state without ever administering the drugs themselves. For example, repeated exposure to drugs of abuse can cause increases in sensitivity ("sensitization") to the rewarding effects of drugs (Lett, 1989; Piazza et al., 1990), a phenomenon that may contribute to the addiction process (Robinson and Berridge, 2001). Because the DA projection from the ventral tegmental area (VTA) of the midbrain to the nucleus accumbens (NAc) of the basal forebrain has been implicated in the habit-forming (rewarding) effects of virtually all abused drugs, many studies on the molecular basis of addiction have focused on this circuitry. Repeated intermittent exposure to morphine or cocaine can increase expression of the α-amino-3-hydroxy-5-methyl-4-isoxasolepropionic acid (AMPA) (glutamate) receptor subunit GluR1 within the VTA and NAc (Fitzgerald et al., 1996; Churchill et al., 1999). To directly test the hypothesis that these drug-induced molecular adaptations cause drug-induced behavioral adaptations (including sensitization), viral vectors were used to elevate GluR1 levels within the VTA of rats not exposed previously to drugs. Rats with viral-mediated elevations in GluR1 expression within anterior portions of the VTA showed dramatic increases in sensitivity to the rewarding effects of morphine (Carlezon et al., 1997; Carlezon, Haile, et al., 2000). These data suggest that the behavioral consequences of repeated exposure to morphine are mimicked by gene transfer of GluR1 into the VTA and support a causal relation between previously disparate drug-induced molecular and behavioral adaptations. Remarkably, elevated expression of GluR1 in the NAc appears to have the opposite effect—reduced sensitivity to reward (Todtenkopf et al., 2006)—highlighting the fact that altered expression of any given gene cannot be assumed to have uniform functional consequences from brain region to brain region (Carlezon et al., 2005).

Hints about the genes and intracellular mechanisms involved in depressive disorders have also evolved from this type of addiction research. Exposure to drugs of abuse increases the function of the transcription factor cAMP response element binding protein (CREB) in striatal regions, including the NAc (Cole et al., 1995; Turgeon et al., 1997). cAMP response element binding protein regulates the expression of many genes (Shaywitz and Greenberg, 1999), including that for dynorphin (Hurd et al., 1992), an opioid peptide implicated in dysphoric (aversive) states (Pfeiffer et al., 1986). Viral vector-mediated elevations of CREB in the NAc of rats make low doses of cocaine aversive, and higher doses of cocaine less rewarding (Carlezon et al., 1998). In addition to producing these signs of anhedonia—a hallmark symptom of depression characterized by a diminished ability to experience rewarding stimuli as rewarding—elevations of CREB in the NAc also produce other symptoms of depression in animal models (Pliakas et al., 2001). Antagonists of brain receptors for dynorphin (κ-opioid receptors) eliminate the signs of aversion and depression (Carlezon et al., 1998; Pliakas et al., 2001; Mague et al., 2003), suggesting that CREB-mediated induction of dynorphin contributes directly to these complex behavioral states.

Together, these types of "biobehavioral" studies demonstrate how viral-mediated gene transfer offers a unique methodology with which to examine how alterations in a single, localized gene product can lead to changes in behaviors that reflect complex motivational states. Moreover, they may help to identify intracellular pathways and alterations in gene expression that are potential targets for new generations of pharmacotherapies for addiction, depression, and possibly other neuropsychiatric disorders (see Box 7.6).

RECENT DEVELOPMENTS IN VIRAL-MEDIATED GENE TRANSFER

Transgene Tagging

A general improvement to gene transfer methods has been the incorporation of "tags" onto the transgene product to facilitate its detection in brain, and to differentiate between endogenous gene expression and viral-mediated transgene expression. One increasingly popular and powerful strategy is to incorporate the gene for the GFP into the vectors. Coexpression of GFP enables researchers to visually detect cells infected by the vector against a background of endogenous gene expression. There are numerous engineering strategies that can be used to tag vector-infected cells (see Neve et al., 2005). The advantages of tagging proteins are obvious: for example, in cases where viral-mediated elevations in

BOX 7.6 *Complementary Genomic Strategies to Study ΔFosB and GluR2*

As described in Box 7.4, mice engineered to overexpress ΔFosB in the ventral striatum (NAc) are more sensitive to the stimulant and rewarding effects of cocaine (Kelz et al., 1999). Presumably, the proximal cause of heightened drug sensitivity is not increased expression of ΔFosB per se, but rather increased expression of a target gene (or genes) regulated by this long-lasting transcription factor. Protein immunoblotting studies revealed that the ΔFosB-overexpressing mice also had large increases in GluR2 expression in the NAc, raising the possibility that local alterations in the expression of this AMPA receptor subunit contribute to increased drug sensitivity. To test the hypothesis that elevated GluR2 expression in the NAc is sufficient to cause increased sensitivity to the rewarding effects of cocaine, rats were given stereotaxic microinjections of an herpes simplex virus (HSV) vector encoding GluR2 (HSV-GluR2) into this brain region. Rats that received this manipulation showed dramatic increases in sensitivity to the rewarding effects of cocaine in place conditioning studies, mimicking the effects of increased expression of ΔFosB in mice (Kelz et al., 1999). They also showed heightened sensitivity to the rewarding effects of electrical stimulation of the medial forebrain bundle (Todtenkopf et al., 2006). These findings provide strong evidence that the increases in cocaine reward seen in ΔFosB transgenic mice are attributable, at least in part, to elevated expression of GluR2 in the NAc.

The use of additional viral vector constructs provided strong evidence that elevated expression of GluR2 in the NAc increases cocaine reward because of effects on calcium (Ca^{2+}) permeability of neurons within this region. There are numerous possible explanations for how local alterations in Ca^{2+} flux might influence drug reward, considering the role of Ca^{2+} in cellular functions including membrane depolarization, neurotransmitter release, signal transduction, and plasticity (Zucker, 1999; Malinow and Malenka, 2002). Regardless, the combined use of complementary genomic techniques allowed the testing of complex working hypotheses and led not only to the elucidation of drug reward mechanisms, but also to the identification of potential targets for new generations of medications for addiction.

transgene expression have been found to have biobehavioral significance (for example, GluR2 in the NAc), electrophysiologists can visually identify infected neurons for study. An added advantage of the GFP tag is the ability to track the subcellular location of the transgene product, which may increase interest in the use of viral vectors for anatomical studies. Additionally, any of several nonfluorescent tags can be fused to the transgene product because they are not expressed in the brain endogenously, including -HA (hemaglutinen), -FLAG (Asp-Tyr-Lys-Asp-Asp-Asp-Asp-Lys), and -myc (an epitope of the avian myelocytomatosis oncogene). This type of work comes with an important caveat, however: it is imperative to demonstrate that the addition of the tag directly to the transgene product does not affect the native function of the protein.

Neuronal Specificity and Duration of Expression

Current limitations of many viral vectors include their lack of selectivity for neuronal subtypes (for example, neurotransmitter-specific) and the transient nature of their effects. Reportedly, substitution of a viral transgene promoter with a neuronal promoter can solve both of these limitations. For example, HSV vectors that contain a fragment of the TH promoter cause increased transgene expression selectively in TH-positive (for example, dopaminergic) neurons, and the expression has been observed for months after infection (Jin et al., 1996). However, the size of neuronal promoters can make packaging less efficient, thereby causing significant reductions in viral titers. Application of neuronal promoters to AV vectors—which do not have issues associated with short duration of expression—might also make them more specific for certain types of neurons (Hwang et al., 2001). Similar techniques have been utilized to restrict LV-mediated transgene expression to neurons (Jakobsson et al., 2006). Regardless, this is one avenue of viral vector design and construction that requires significant improvement, such that the ability to control transgene expression becomes routine. Ultimately, the ability to target specific cell types within discrete brain regions (for example, dynorphin-containing GABAergic medium spiny neurons within the NAc) will likely dramatically extend the utility (and acceptance) of viral vectors in neuropsychiatric research.

Deactivation and Activation of Genes

One intriguing possibility is to use viral vectors in conjunction with other genomic technologies, such as mutant (knockout) mice. A current limitation of knockout mice (inducible knockouts notwithstanding) is that they lack the gene under study for their entire lives, raising the possibility of developmental adaptations that may complicate interpretation of results (Gingrich and Hen, 2000). However, the use of viral vectors that express CRE recombinase can eliminate this limitation. The general strategy is to engineer mutant mice such that the gene (or genes) to be knocked out is flanked by loxP sites ("floxed"), molecular targets for CRE recombinase (Nagy, 2000). Microinjection of a vector expressing CRE recombinase can then cut and fuse the DNA at the loxP sites, permanently knocking out the gene flanked by the sites. This approach enables regional and temporal selectivity to the genetic manipulation—two current limitations of mutant mouse technology, and two current advantages of viral-mediated gene transfer. Viral vector–induced excision of floxed genes has been used to demonstrate that expression of brain-derived neurotrophic factor (BDNF) in the mesolimbic system plays an essential role in stress-induced development of depressive-like behaviors (Berton et al., 2006) and self-administration and relapse to drugs of abuse (Graham et al., 2007). Viral vectors have also been utilized together with siRNA to achieve gene knockdown with spatial and temporal specificity (Hommel et al., 2003). This approach has also applied to generate conditional knockdown rats with gene loss restricted to the midbrain region (Hommel et al., 2006). The use of viral vectors to deliver siRNA is not trivial, however, and often requires additional engineering of the viral backbone and siRNA oligonucleotide (Sandy et al., 2005; Saydam et al., 2005).

It may also be possible to design viral vectors that cause transgene expression that is subject to pharmacological regulation. For example, a vector has been created that expresses an RU486 (*mifepristone*)-inducible transactivator (Oligino et al., 1998). Transgenes under control of this transactivator are expressed only in the presence of RU486. Similarly, inducible LV vectors have been created that contain promoter elements that render transgene expression sensitive to doxycycline (Markusic et al., 2005). This strategy is analogous to the use of inducible promoters to regulate gene expression in mutant mice, which dramatically improves the temporal resolution of altered gene expression and facilitates the identification of causal relations between altered gene expression and altered behavior.

Limitations of Viral-Mediated Gene Transfer

As an in vivo technique for neuropsychiatry research, viral-mediated gene transfer has two main limitations. First, the vectors must be injected directly into the brain region of interest. This involves anesthesia, stereotaxic microinjections, damage to brain regions dorsal to the injection sites from the injection track, damage to the injection sites themselves from the hydraulic pressure of the microinjection, and several days recovery time for the animal. The size and shape of the targeted brain region can make the microinjection procedure difficult, or prevent certain regions from being targeted with specificity. Many of these limitations are similar to those encountered with other brain manipulations (for example, lesions), and their severity is often associated with the skill and experience of the researchers performing the in vivo procedures. Historically, cytotoxic effects of the viral vectors themselves or from an immune response from the host are also concerns, although improvements in vector engineering and purification (see Carlezon, Nestler, et al., 2000) have greatly diminished their severity. The second limitation is that, in general, the vectors do not target specific types of cells. Whereas vectors such as HSV target neurons, others such as AV, AAV, and LV are not naturally selective for neurons or glia. More importantly, none of the current vectors can selectively target specific types of neurons (for example, dynorphin-containing GABAergic medium spiny neurons). Manipulations to the vector promoters may eventually offer the ability to target virtually any cell phenotype (see below and Hwang et al., 2001), although in most cases this theoretical feasibility is not yet routine. As such, viral-mediated gene transfer into regions with significant cell heterogeneity can cause ectopic transgene expression (expression of the exogenous gene within cell population that do not normally express the endogenous gene). This limitation is like that often encountered with mutant mice. As with any technique, these limitations of viral-mediated gene transfer must be weighed against its advantages and potential.

THE FUTURE OF VIRAL-MEDIATED GENE TRANSFER

Gene therapy is an obvious medical application for viral vectors. The use of viral vectors to transfer therapeutic genes or siRNA to treat neurological conditions (for example, brain tumors) shows great promise (Saydam et al., 2005). However, gene therapy for neuropsychiatric disorders must overcome several technological challenges before it can become a reality (Neve et al., 2005). As emphasized above, the ability to control the efficacy of the vectors will continue to be a critical consideration. In the past, most vectors have utilized strong or "promiscuous" promoters that tend to drive gene expression beyond physiological levels, raising the possibility of unwanted—and possibly detrimental—effects on cell function. An improved ability to target specific cell types while tightly regulating the timing and strength of gene expression will open up a wealth of opportunities for clinical applications. There are also conceptual hurdles. Aside from the fact that it seems unlikely that any neuropsychiatric disorder is due to alterations in a single gene, the brain is not particularly accessible or hospitable to genetic intervention. In addition, neuropsychiatric disorders such as schizophrenia may have their origins in molecular processes that occur transiently in small subsets of cells at very specific times during development. Once established, these molecular misadaptations may be difficult or impossible to correct with delayed interventions. Thus though viral-mediated gene transfer is presently well-suited for brain research in animals, a substantial amount of work is needed before it can be determined whether it has practical applications in evolving fields of molecular medicine.

REFERENCES

Accili, D., Fishburn, C.S., Drago, J., Steiner, H., Lachowicz, J.E., Park, B.H., Gauda, E.B., Lee, E.J., Cool, M.H., Sibley, D.R., Gerfen, C.R., Westphal, H., and Fuchs, S. (1996) A targeted mutation of the D3 dopamine receptor gene is associated with hyperactivity in mice. *Proc. Natl. Acad. Sci. USA* 93:1945–1949.

Akbarian, S., Bates, B., Liu, R.J., Skirboll, S.L., Pejchal, T., Coppola, V., Sun, L.D., Fan, G., Kucera, J., Wilson, M.A., Tessarollo, L., Kosofsky, B.E., Taylor, J.R., Bothwell, M., Nestler, E.J., Aghajanian, G.K., and Jaenisch, R. (2001) Neurotrophin-3 modulates noradrenergic neuron function and opiate withdrawal. *Mol. Psychiatry* 6:593–604.

Amir, R.E., Van den Veyver, I.B., Wan, M., Tran, C.Q., Francke, U., and Zoghbi, H.Y. (1999) Rett syndrome is caused by mutations in X-linked MECP2, encoding methyl-CpG-binding protein 2. *Nat. Genet.* 23:185–188.

Baik, J.H., Picetti, R., Saiardi, A., Thiriet, G., Dierich, A., Depaulis, A., Le Meur, M., and Borrelli, E. (1995) Parkinsonian-like locomotor impairment in mice lacking dopamine D2 receptors. *Nature* 377:424–428.

Berton, O., McClung, C.A., Dileone, R.J., Krishnan, V., Renthal, W., Russo, S.J., Graham, D., Tsankova, N.M., Bolanos, C.A., Rios, M., Monteggia, L.M., Self, D.W., and Nestler, E.J. (2006) Essential role of BDNF in the mesolimbic dopamine pathway in social defeat stress. *Science* 311:864–868.

Carlezon, W.A., Jr., Boundy, V.A., Haile, C.N., Lane, S.B., Kalb, R.G., Neve, R.L., and Nestler, E.J. (1997) Sensitization to morphine induced by viral-mediated gene transfer. *Science* 277:812–814.

Carlezon, W.A., Jr., Duman, R.S., and Nestler, E.J. (2005) The many faces of CREB. *Trends Neurosci.* 28:436–445.

Carlezon, W.A., Jr., Haile, C.N., Coopersmith, R., Hayashi, Y., Malinow, R., Neve, R.L., and Nestler, E.J. (2000) Distinct sites of opiate reward and aversion within the midbrain identified by a herpes simplex virus vector expressing GluR1. *J. Neurosci.* 20: RC62, 1–5.

Carlezon, W.A., Jr., Nestler, E.J., and Neve, R.L. (2000) Herpes simplex virus-mediated gene transfer as a tool for neuropsychiatric research. *Crit. Rev. Neurobiol.* 14:47–67.

Carlezon, W.A., Jr., Thome, J., Olson, V.G., Lane-Ladd, S.B., Brodkin, E.S., Hiroi, N., Duman, R.S., Neve, R.L., and Nestler, E.J. (1998) Regulation of cocaine reward by CREB. *Science* 282: 2272–2275.

Chen, J., Kelz, M.B., Zeng, G., Sakai, N., Steffen, C., Shockett, P.E., Picciotto, M.R., Duman, R.S., and Nestler, E.J. (1998) Transgenic animals with inducible, targeted gene expression in brain. *Mol. Pharmacol.* 54:495–503.

Chen, R.Z., Akbarian, S., Tudor, M., and Jaenisch, R. (2001) Deficiency of methyl-CpG binding protein-2 in CNS neurons results in a Rett-like phenotype in mice. *Nat. Genet.* 27: 327–331.

Churchill, L., Swanson, C.J., Urbina, M., and Kalivas, P.W. (1999) Repeated cocaine alters glutamate receptor subunit levels in the nucleus accumbens and ventral tegmental area of rats that develop behavioral sensitization. *J. Neurochem.* 72:2397–2403.

Citron, M., Westaway, D., Xia, W., Carlson, G., Diehl, T., Levesque, G., Johnson-Wood, K., Lee, M., Seubert, P., Davis, A., Kholodenko, D., Motter, R., Sherrington, R., Perry, B., Yao, H., Strome, R., Lieberburg, I., Rommens, J., Kim, S., Schenk, D., Fraser, P., St. George-Hyslop, P., and Selkoe, D.J. (1997) Mutant presenilins of Alzheimer's disease increase production of 42- residue amyloid beta-protein in both transfected cells and transgenic mice. *Nat. Med.* 3:67–72.

Clifford, J.J., Tighe, O., Croke, D.T., Sibley, D.R., Drago, J., and Waddington, J.L. (1998) Topographical evaluation of the phenotype of spontaneous behaviour in mice with targeted gene deletion of the D1A dopamine receptor: paradoxical elevation of grooming syntax. *Neuropharmacology* 37:1595–1602.

Cole, R.L., Konradi, C., Douglass, J., and Hyman, S.E. (1995) Neuronal adaptation to amphetamine and dopamine: molecular mechanisms of prodynorphin gene regulation in rat striatum. *Neuron* 14:813–823.

Dulawa, S.C., Grandy, D.K., Low, M.J., Paulus, M.P., and Geyer, M.A. (1999) Dopamine D4 receptor-knock-out mice exhibit reduced exploration of novel stimuli. *J. Neurosci.* 19:9550–9556.

During, M.J., Naegele, J.R., O'Malley, K.L., and Geller, A.I. (1994) Long-term behavioral recovery in Parkinsonian rats by an HSV vector expressing tyrosine hydroxylase. *Science* 266:1399–1403.

Fernandez-Chacon, R., and Sudhof, T.C. (1999) Genetics of synaptic vesicle function: toward the complete functional anatomy of an organelle. *Annu. Rev. Physiol.* 61:753–776.

Fink, D.J., DeLuca, N.A., Goins, W.F., and Glorioso, J.C. (1996) Gene transfer to neurons using herpes simplex virus-based vectors. *Annu. Rev. Neurosci.* 19:265–287.

Fitzgerald, L.W., Ortiz, J., Hamedani, A.G., and Nestler, E.J. (1996) Drugs of abuse and stress increase the expression of GluR1 and NMDAR1 glutamate receptor subunits in the rat ventral tegmental area: common adaptations among cross-sensitizing agents. *J. Neurosci.* 16:274–282.

Games, D., Adams, D., Alessandrini, R., Barbour, R., Berthelette, P., Blackwell, C., Carr, T., Clemens, J., Donaldson, T., Gillespie, F., et al. (1995) Alzheimer-type neuropathology in transgenic mice overexpressing V717F beta-amyloid precursor protein. *Nature* 373:523–527.

Gemelli, T., Berton, O., Nelson, E., Perroti, L.I., Jaenisch, R., and Monteggia, L.M. (2006) Postnatal loss of MeCP2 in the forebrain is sufficient to mediate behavioral aspects of Rett syndrome in mice. *Biol. Psychiatry* 59(5):468–476.

Gibbs, R.A., et al., Rat Genome Sequence Project Consortium. (2004) Genome sequence of the brown Norway rat yields insights into mammalian evolution. *Nature* 428:493–521.

Giménez-Llort, L., Schiffmann, S.N., Shmidt, T., Canela, L., Camón, L., Wassholm, M., Canals, M., Terasmaa, A., Fernández-Teruel, A., Tobeña, A., Popova, E., Ferré, S., Agnati, L., Ciruela, F., Martínez, E., Scheel-Kruger, J., Lluis, C., Franco, R., Fuxe, K., and Bader, M. (2007) Working memory deficits in transgenic rats overexpressing human adenosine A2A receptors in the brain. *Neurobiol. Learn. Mem.* 87:42–56.

Gingrich, J.A., and Hen, R. (2000) The broken mouse: the role of development, plasticity and environment in the interpretation of phenotypic changes in knockout mice. *Curr. Opin. Neurobiol.* 10:146–152.

Giros, B., Jaber, M., Jones, S.R., Wightman, R.M., and Caron, M.G. (1996) Hyperlocomotion and indifference to cocaine and amphetamine in mice lacking the dopamine transporter. *Nature* 379: 606–612.

Gogos, J.A., Morgan, M., Luine, V., Santha, M., Ogawa, S., Pfaff, D., and Karayiorgou, M. (1998) Catechol-O-methyltransferase-deficient mice exhibit sexually dimorphic changes in catecholamine levels and behavior. *Proc. Natl. Acad. Sci. USA* 95: 9991–9996.

Gossen, M., and Bujard, H. (1992) Tight control of gene expression in mammalian cells by tetracycline- responsive promoters. *Proc. Natl. Acad. Sci. USA* 89:5547–5551.

Graham, D.L., Edwards, S., Bachtell, R.K., Dileone, R.J., Rios, M., and Self, D.W. (2007) Dynamic BDNF activity in nucleus accumbens with cocaine use increases self-administration and relapse. *Nat. Neurosci.* 10:1029–1037.

Gross, C., Zhuang, X., Stark, K., Ramboz, S., Oosting, R., Kirby, L., Santarelli, L., Beck, S., and Hen, R. (2002) Serotonin1A receptor acts during development to establish normal anxiety-like behaviour in the adult. *Nature* 416(6879):396–400.

Gurney, M.E., Pu, H., Chiu, A.Y., Dal Canto, M.C., Polchow, C.Y., Alexander, D.D., Caliendo, J., Hentati, A., Kwon, Y.W., Deng, H.X., et al. (1994) Motor neuron degeneration in mice that express a human Cu,Zn superoxide dismutase mutation. *Science* 264(5166):1772–1775.

Guy, J., Hendrich, B., Holmes, M., Martin, J.E., and Bird, A. (2001) A mouse Mecp2-null mutation causes neurological symptoms that mimic Rett syndrome. *Nat. Genet.* 27:322–326.

Heintz, H. (2004) Gene expression nervous system atlas (GENSAT). *Nat. Neurosci.* 7:483.

Heintz, N. (2001) BAC to the future: the use of bac transgenic mice for neuroscience research. *Nat. Rev. Neurosci.* 2(12): 861–870.

Heintz, N., and Zoghbi, H.Y. (2000) Insights from mouse models into the molecular basis of neurodegeneration. *Annu. Rev. Physiol.* 62:779–802.

Heisler, L.K., and Tecott, L.H. (2000) A paradoxical locomotor response in serotonin 5-HT(2C) receptor mutant mice. *J. Neurosci.* 20(8):RC71.

Hodgson, J.G., Agopyan, N., Gutekunst, C.A., Leavitt, B.R., LePiane, F., Singaraja, R., Smith, D.J., Bissada, N., McCutcheon, K., Nasir, J., Jamot, L., Li, X.J., Stevens, M.E., Rosemond, E., Roder, J.C., Phillips, A.G., Rubin, E.M., Hersch, S.M., and Hayden, M.R. (1999) A YAC mouse model for Huntington's disease with full-length mutant huntingtin, cytoplasmic toxicity, and selective striatal neurodegeneration. *Neuron* 23(1):181–192.

Holmes, A., Hollon, T.R., Gleason, T.C., Liu, Z., Dreiling, J., Sibley, D.R., and Crawley, J.N. (2001) Behavioral characterization of dopamine D5 receptor null mutant mice. *Behav. Neurosci.* 115:1129–1144.

Hommel, J.D., Sears, R.M., Georgescu, D., Simmons, D.L., and DiLeone, R.J. (2003) Local gene knockdown in the brain using viral-mediated RNA interference. *Nat. Med.* 9:1539–1544.

Hommel, J.D., Trinko, R., Sears, R.M., Georgescu, D., Liu, Z.W., Gao, X.B., Thurmon, J.J., Marinelli, M., and DiLeone, R.J. (2006) Leptin receptor signaling in midbrain dopamine neurons regulates feeding. *Neuron* 51:801–810.

Hsiao, K., Chapman, P., Nilsen, S., Eckman, C., Harigaya, Y., Younkin, S., Yang, F., and Cole, G. (1996) Correlative memory deficits, Abeta elevation, and amyloid plaques in transgenic mice. *Science* 274:99–102.

Hurd, Y.L., Brown, E.E., Finlay, J.M., Fibiger, H.C., and Gerfen, C.R. (1992) Cocaine self-administration differentially alters mRNA expression of striatal peptides. *Brain Res. Mol. Brain Res.* 13: 165–170.

Hwang, D.Y., Carlezon, W.A., Jr., Isacson, O., and Kim, K.S. (2001) A high-efficiency synthetic promoter that drives transgene expression selectively in noradrenergic neurons. *Human Gene Ther.* 12:1731–1740.

Isacson, O. (1995) Behavioral effects and gene delivery in a rat model of Parkinson's disease. *Science* 269:856–857.

Jakobsson, J., Nielsen, T.T., Staflin, K., Georgievska, B., and Lundberg, C. (2006) Efficient transduction of neurons using Ross River glycoprotein-pseudotyped lentiviral vectors. *Gene Therapy* 13:966–973.

Janus, C., Pearson, J., McLaurin, J., Mathews, P.M., Jiang, Y., Schmidt, S.D., Chishti, M.A., Horne, P., Heslin, D., French, J., Mount, H.T., Nixon, R.A., Mercken, M., Bergeron, C., Fraser, P.E., St. George-Hyslop, P., and Westaway, D. (2000) A beta peptide immunization reduces behavioural impairment and plaques in a model of Alzheimer's disease. *Nature* 408(6815):979–982.

Jin, B.K., Belloni, M., Conti, B., Federoff, H.J., Starr, R., Son, J.H., Baker, H., and Joh, T.H. (1996) Prolonged in vivo gene expression by a tyrosine hydroxylase promoter in a defective herpes simplex virus amplicon vector. *Hum. Gene Ther.* 7:2015–2024.

Jones, S.R., Gainetdinov, R.R., Jaber, M., Giros, B., Wightman, R.M., and Caron, M.G. (1998) Profound neuronal plasticity in response to inactivation of the dopamine transporter. *Proc. Natl. Acad. Sci. USA* 95:4029–4034.

Joyner, A. (2000). *Gene Targeting: A Practical Approach*. New York: Oxford University Press.

Kelly, M.A., Rubinstein, M., Phillips, T.J., Lessov, C.N., Burkhart-Kasch, S., Zhang, G., Bunzow, J.R., Fang, Y., Gerhardt, G.A., Grandy, D.K., and Low, M.J. (1998) Locomotor activity in D2 dopamine receptor-deficient mice is determined by gene dosage, genetic background, and developmental adaptations. *J. Neurosci.* 18:3470–3479.

Kelz, M.B., Chen, J., Carlezon, W.A., Jr., Whisler, K., Gilden, L., Beckmann, A.M., Steffen, C., Zhang, Y.J., Marotti, L., Self, D.W., Tkatch, T., Baranauskas, G., Surmeier, D.J., Neve, R.L., Duman, R.S., Picciotto, M.R., and Nestler, E.J. (1999) Expression of the transcription factor deltaFosB in the brain controls sensitivity to cocaine. *Nature* 401:272–276.

Kreitzer, A.C., and Malenka, R.C. (2007) Endocannabinoid-mediated rescue of striatal LTD and motor defects in Parkinson's disease models. *Nature* 445:643–647.

Lett, B.T. (1989) Repeated exposures intensify rather than diminish the rewarding effects of amphetamine, morphine, and cocaine. *Psychopharmacol.* 98:357–362.

Liu, W.S., Pesold, C., Rodriguez, M.A., Carboni, G., Auta, J., Lacor, P., Larson, J., Condie, B.G., Guidotti, A., and Costa, E. (2001) Down-regulation of dendritic spine and glutamic acid decarboxylase 67 expressions in the reelin haploinsufficient heterozygous reeler mouse. *Proc. Natl. Acad. Sci. USA* 98(6):3477–3482.

Ma, L., Reis, G., Parada, L.F., and Schuman, E.M. (1999) Neuronal NT-3 is not required for synaptic transmission or long-term potentiation in area CA1 of the adult rat hippocampus. *Learn. Mem.* 6:267–275.

Mague, S.D., Pliakas, A.M., Todtenkopf, M.S., Tomasiewicz, H.C., Zhang, Y., Stevens, W.C., Jr., Jones, R.M., Portoghese, P.S., Carlezon,W.A., Jr. (2003) Antidepressant-like effects of k-opioid receptor antagonists in the forced swim test in rats. *Journal of Pharmacology and Experimental Therapeutics* 305:323–330.

Malinow, R., and Malenka, R.C. (2002) AMPA receptor trafficking and synaptic plasticity. *Annu. Rev. Neurosci.* 25:103–125.

Mansour, S.L., Thomas, K.R., and Capecchi, M.R. (1988) Disruption of the proto-oncogene int-2 in mouse embryo-derived stem cells: a general strategy for targeting mutations to non-selectable genes. *Nature* 336(6197):348–352.

Markusic, D., Oude-Elferink, R., Das, A.T., Berkhout, B., and Seppen, J. (2005) Comparison of single regulated lentiviral vectors with rtTA expression driven by a autoregulatory loop or a constitutive promoter. *Nucleic Acid Research* 33:e63.

Masliah, E., Sisk, A., Mallory, M., Mucke, L., Schenk, D., and Games, D. (1996) Comparison of neurodegenerative pathology in transgenic mice overexpressing V717F beta-amyloid precursor protein and Alzheimer's disease. *J. Neurosci.* 16:5795–5811.

Mayford, M., Bach, M.E., Huang, Y.Y., Wang, L., Hawkins, R.D., and Kandel, E.R. (1996) Control of memory formation through regulated expression of a CaMKII transgene. *Science* 274:1678–1683.

McHugh, T.J., Blum, K.I., Tsien, J.Z., Tonegawa, S., and Wilson, M.A. (1996) Impaired hippocampal representation of space in CA1-specific NMDAR1 knockout mice. *Cell* 87:1339–1349.

Moran, P.M., Higgins, L.S., Cordell, B., and Moser, P.C. (1995) Age-related learning deficits in transgenic mice expressing the 751-amino acid isoform of human beta-amyloid precursor protein. *Proc. Natl. Acad. Sci. USA* 92:5341–5345.

Morgan, D., Diamond, D.M., Gottschall, P.E., Ugen, K.E., Dickey, C., Hardy, J., Duff, K., Jantzen, P., DiCarlo, G., Wilcock, D.,

Connor, K., Hatcher, J., Hope, C., Gordon, M., and Arendash, G.W. (2000) A beta peptide vaccination prevents memory loss in an animal model of Alzheimer's disease. *Nature* 408(6815): 982–985.

Nagy, A. (2000) Cre recombinase: the universal reagent for genome tailoring. *Genesis* 26: 99–109.

Nestler, E.J. (2005) Is there a common molecular pathway for addiction? *Nat. Neurosci.* 8:1445–1449.

Neve, R.L., Neve, K.A., Nestler, E.J., and Carlezon, W.A., Jr. (2005) Use of herpesvirus vectors to study brain function. *BioTechniques* 31:381–391.

Oligino, T., Poliani, P.L., Wang, Y., Tsai, S.Y., O'Malley, B.W., Fink, D.J., and Glorioso, J.C. (1998) Drug inducible transgene expression in brain using a herpes simplex virus vector. *Gene Ther.* 5: 491–496.

Peakman, M.-C., Colby, C., Duman, C., Allen, M.R., Stock, J.L., McNeish, J.D., Kelz, M., Chen, J.S., Nestler, E.J., and Schaeffer, E. (2000) Inducible, brain-region specific expression of Δc-Jun in transgenic mice decreases sensitivity to cocaine. *Soc. Neurosci. Abs.* 26:49.10

Pfeiffer, A., Brantl, V., Herz, A., and Emrich, H.M. (1986) Psychotomimesis mediated by kappa opiate receptors. *Science* 233:774–776.

Piazza, P.V., Deminiere, J.M., le Moal, M., and Simon, H. (1990) Stress- and pharmacologically-induced behavioral sensitization increases vulnerability to acquisition of amphetamine self-administration. *Brain Res.* 514:22–26.

Pliakas, A.M., Carlson, R., Neve, R.L., Konradi, C., Nestler, E.J., Carlezon, W.A., Jr. (2001) Altered responsiveness to cocaine and increased immobility in the forced swim test associated with elevated cAMP response element binding protein expression in nucleus accumbens. *J. Neurosci.* 21:7397–7403.

Richardson, A., Heydari, A.R., Morgan, W.W., Nelson, J.F., Sharp, Z.D., and Walter, C.A. (1997). The use of transgenic mice in aging research. *Inst. Lab. Anim. Res. J.* 38:124–127.

Robinson, T.E., and Berridge, K.C. (2001) Incentive-sensitization and addiction. *Addiction* 96:103–114.

Rubinstein, M., Phillips, T.J., Bunzow, J.R., Falzone, T.L., Dziewczapolski, G., Zhang, G., Fang, Y., Larson, J.L., McDougall, J.A., Chester, J.A., Saez, C., Pugsley, T.A., Gershanik, O., Low, M.J., and Grandy, D.K. (1997) Mice lacking dopamine D4 receptors are supersensitive to ethanol, cocaine, and methamphetamine. *Cell* 90:991–1001.

Sandy, P., Ventura, A., and Jacks, T. (2005) Mammalian RNAi: a practical guide. *BioTechniques* 39:1–10.

Saydam, O., Glauser, D.L., Heid, I., Turkeri, G., Hilbe, M., Jacobs, A.H., Ackermann, M., and Fraefel, C. (2005) Herpes simplex virus 1 amplicon vector-mediated siRNA targeting epidermal growth factor receptor inhibits growth of human glioma cells in vivo. *Mol. Ther.* 12:803–812.

Shaywitz, A.J., and Greenberg, M.E. (1999) CREB: a stimulus-induced transcription factor activated by a diverse array of extracellular signals. *Annu. Rev. Biochem.* 68:821–861.

Shih, J.C., Chen, K., and Ridd, M.J. (1999) Monoamine oxidase: from genes to behavior. *Annu. Rev. Neurosci.* 22:197–217.

Shimizu, E., Tang, Y.P., Rampon, C., and Tsien, J.Z. (2000) NMDA receptor-dependent synaptic reinforcement as a crucial process for memory consolidation. *Science* 290:1170–1174.

Smith, D.J., Stevens, M.E., Sudanagunta, S.P., Bronson, R.T., Makhinson, M., Watabe, A.M., O'Dell, T.J., Fung, J., Weier, H.U., Cheng, J.F., and Rubin, E.M. (1997) Functional screening of 2 Mb of human chromosome 21q22.2 in transgenic mice implicates minibrain in learning defects associated with Down syndrome. *Nat. Genet.* 16(1):28–36.

Smits, B.M., Mudde, J.B., van de Belt, J., Verheul, M., Olivier, J., Homberg, J., Guryev, V., Cools, A.R., Ellenbroek, B.A., Plasterk, R.H., and Cuppen, E. (2006). Generation of gene knockouts and mutant models in the laboratory rat by ENU-driven target-selected mutagenesis. *Pharmacogenet. Genomics* 16:159–169.

Takahashi, N., Miner, L.L., Sora, I., Ujike, H., Revay, R.S., Kostic, V., Jackson-Lewis, V., Przedborski, S., and Uhl, G.R. (1997) VMAT2 knockout mice: heterozygotes display reduced amphetamine-conditioned reward, enhanced amphetamine locomotion, and enhanced MPTP toxicity. *Proc. Natl. Acad. Sci. USA* 94: 9938–9943.

Todtenkopf, M.S., Parsegian, A., Neve, R.L., Carlezon, W.A., Jr. (2006) Brain reward regulated by glutamate receptor subunits in the nucleus accumbens shell. *J. Neurosci.* 26:11665–11669.

Tsien, J.Z., Chen, D.F., Gerber, D., Tom, C., Mercer, E.H., Anderson, D.J., Mayford, M., Kandel, E.R., and Tonegawa, S. (1996) Subregion- and cell type-restricted gene knockout in mouse brain. *Cell* 87:1317–1326.

Tsien, J.Z., Huerta, P.T., and Tonegawa, S. (1996) The essential role of hippocampal CA1 NMDA receptor-dependent synaptic plasticity in spatial memory. *Cell* 87:1327–1338.

Turgeon, S.M., Pollack, A.E., and Fink, J.S. (1997) Enhanced CREB phosphorylation and changes in c-Fos and FRA expression in striatum accompany amphetamine sensitization. *Brain Res.* 749:120–126.

von Hörsten, S., Schmitt, I., Nguyen, H.P., Holzmann, C., Schmidt, T., Walther, T., Bader, M., Pabst, R., Kobbe, P., Krotova, J., Stiller, D., Kask, A., Vaarmann, A., Rathke-Hartlieb, S., Schulz, J.B., Grasshoff, U., Bauer, I., Vieira-Saecker, A.M., Paul, M., Jones, L., Lindenberg, K.S., Landwehrmeyer, B., Bauer, A., Li, X.J., and Riess, O. (2003) Transgenic rat model of Huntington's disease. *Hum. Mol. Gen.* 12:617–624.

Wan, M., Lee, S.S., Zhang, X., Houwink-Manville, I., Song, H.R., Amir, R.E., Budden, S., Naidu, S., Pereira, J.L., Lo, I.F., Zoghbi, H.Y., Schanen, N.C., and Francke, U. (1999) Rett syndrome and beyond: recurrent spontaneous and familial MECP2 mutations at CpG hotspots. *Am. J. Hum. Genet.* 65: 152–1529.

Wang, Y.M., Gainetdinov, R.R., Fumagalli, F., Xu, F., Jones, S.R., Bock, C.B., Miller, G.W., Wightman, R.M., and Caron, M.G. (1997) Knockout of the vesicular monoamine transporter 2 gene results in neonatal death and supersensitivity to cocaine and amphetamine. *Neuron* 19:1285–1296.

Xu, M., Koeltzow, T.E., Santiago, G.T., Moratalla, R., Cooper, D.C., Hu, X.T., White, N.M., Graybiel, A.M., White, F.J., and Tonegawa, S. (1997) Dopamine D3 receptor mutant mice exhibit increased behavioral sensitivity to concurrent stimulation of D1 and D2 receptors. *Neuron* 19:837–848.

Xu, M., Moratalla, R., Gold, L.H., Hiroi, N., Koob, G.F., Graybiel, A.M., Tonegawa, S. (1994) Dopamine D1 receptor mutant, Moratal mice are deficient in striatal expression of dynorphin and in dopamine-mediated behavioral responses. *Cell* 79:729–742.

Yamamoto, A., Lucas, J.J., and Hen, R. (2000) Reversal of neuropathology and motor dysfunction in a conditional model of Huntington's disease. *Cell* 101(1):57–66.

Yamazaki, S., Numano, R., Abe, M., Hida, A., Takahashi, R., Ueda, M., Block, G.D., Sakaki, Y., Menaker, M., and Tei, H. (2000) Resetting central and peripheral circadian oscillators in transgenic mice. *Science* 288:682–685.

Zhou, Q.Y., and Palmiter, R.D. (1995) Dopamine-deficient mice are severely hypoactive, adipsic, and aphagic. *Cell* 83:1197–1209.

Zucker, R.S. (1999) Calcium- and activity-dependent synaptic plasticity. *Curr. Opin. Neurobiol.* 9: 305–313.

8 Epigenetics of Psychiatric Diseases

BRYAN E. MCGILL AND HUDA Y. ZOGHBI

Coined by Conrad Waddington in 1946, the term *epigenetic* was originally used to describe the effect of gene-environment interactions on the expression of particular phenotypes. Today, the same word commonly refers to stable changes in gene expression that occur without altering the underlying deoxyribonucleic acid (DNA) sequence (Haig, 2004). Epigenetic changes are characterized by being mitotically stable, meaning that they can be faithfully inherited through generations of somatic cell division. Furthermore, epigenetic changes result in stable phenotypic alterations for the organism.

In recent years, a number of molecular pathways have been identified that mediate the establishment, maintenance, and interpretation of the epigenetic code (Allis et al., 2007). Although the underlying mechanisms regulating the epigenome might differ, they all share a common final pathway that converges on regulating gene expression by manipulating chromatin structure. *Chromatin* is a word used to describe the form that DNA takes in eukaryotic cells. Chromatin is composed of repeating units called *nucleosomes*, each of which consist of 147 base pairs of DNA wrapped around a complex of 8 histone proteins, including 2 copies each of histone 2A, histone 2B, histone 3, and histone 4 (Kornberg, 1974; Kornberg and Thomas, 1974; Luger et al., 1997). Broadly, nuclear chromatin is divided into two categories: euchromatin and heterochromatin. *Euchromatin* refers to chromatin in its more open state, wherein the DNA double helix is accessible to the transcriptional machinery. Because of its association with active transcription, euchromatin is often referred to as "active" chromatin. In contrast, *heterochromatin* describes chromatin in a highly condensed state that is largely resistant to transcription. Thus, heterochromatin is described as being "silent." Thus, altering the chromatin structure at a particular allele of a gene is an effective way of regulating its transcription.

In this chapter, we provide a brief primer on some of the epigenetic mechanisms that are currently known to exist in humans: DNA methylation, covalent histone modification, chromatin remodeling by Polycomb-Group (PcG) and trithorax-Group (trxG) proteins, ribonucleic acid (RNA) interference, and imprinting. Next, we discuss examples whereby errors in these processes either correlate with or contribute to the pathogenesis of psychiatric diseases. We also discuss emerging studies from research in animals and in vitro systems. We conclude the chapter by discussing mechanisms of epigenetic inheritance and the plasticity of epigenetic marks and their relevance to psychiatric disorders.

MECHANISMS OF EPIGENETICS

DNA Methylation and Methyl-Binding Proteins

In humans (and other mammals), the cytosine base in DNA can be covalently modified at the carbon-5 position of its ring structure by the addition of a methyl group. The modified bases, designated 5-methylcytosines, are found exclusively in symmetric CpG dinucleotide pairs (Bird, 2002). In most cases, CpG methylation represses gene expression. Thus, the vast majority of methyl-CpGs are found near retrotransposons, endogenous retroviruses, and repetitive elements, where they are involved in setting up a transcriptionally repressive environment (Li and Bird, 2007). The remaining CpGs are found in clusters called *CpG islands*, which are primarily located in the promoters of genes and are largely unmethylated (Caiafa and Zampieri, 2005). When cytosine methylation occurs in these regions it can have a profound negative impact on downstream gene expression (for examples, see discussion of the role of methylation in schizophrenia and Fragile X syndrome below).

DNA methylation is mediated by a class of proteins known as DNA methyltransferases (DNMTs). In mammals, this family of proteins includes five polypeptides that function to establish and maintain DNA methylation: DNMT1, DNMT2, DNMT3a, DNMT3b, and DNMT3L (Bestor, 2000; Siedlecki and Zielenkiewicz, 2006). DNMT3a and DNMT3b are de novo methyltransferases that function to establish the initial pattern of DNA methylation during embryogenesis (Okano et al., 1998; Okano et al., 1999). DNMT3L is a related protein that was identified by its similarity to DNMT3a and DNMT3b (Aapola et al., 2000). Although it is unable to methylate DNA on its own, it is required for proper DNA methylation to occur in developing embryos (Bourc'his et al., 2001; Hata et al., 2002). DNMT3L appears to function by forming protein complexes with DNMT3a and DNMT3b and enhancing their DNA methylation activity (Suetake et al., 2004). DNMT2 preferentially methylates transfer RNA (tRNA) (Goll et al., 2006) and only weakly methylates DNA (Hermann et al., 2003). Thus, its contribution to DNA methylation as an epigenetic phenomenon appears to be negligible. The final member of this protein family, DNMT1, maintains DNA methylation patterns during cell division. DNA methylation patterns are replicated in a semiconservative manner. That is, the two parental DNA strands are separated, and each provides a template that DNMT1 uses to duplicate the methylation pattern on the newly synthesized DNA strand (Bestor and Ingram, 1983; Bird, 2002). Loss of DNMT1 function results in a nearly 10-fold increase in the overall transcriptional activity of cells (Jackson-Grusby et al., 2001), thereby illustrating the critical role for DNA methylation in maintaining gene silencing under normal circumstances.

DNA methyltransferases obtain the methyl group used to methylate DNA from the methyl donor S-adenosyl-methionine (SAM) (Fig. 8.1). SAM is produced from methionine by the enzyme *methionine adenosyl transferase*. Deoxyribonucleic acid methylation depletes the available pool of SAM and generates the metabolite S-adenosyl-homocysteine, which is converted to homocysteine. The ultimate source of methionine, the precursor of SAM, is the diet. However, methionine can also be regenerated from homocysteine by the enzyme *methionine synthase*. This reaction requires the methyl donor *5-methyl tetrahydrofolate* (5MTHF), the major circulating form of the nutrient folic acid (folate). As with methionine, dietary intake is the ultimate source of folate. In this way, levels of DNA methylation are closely linked to the nutritional status of the organism (Muskiet and Kemperman, 2006).

DNA methylation inhibits gene expression via at least two mechanisms (Fig. 8.2). First, methyl-CpGs can directly interfere with the binding of some transcription factors (Watt and Molloy, 1988). Second, DNA methylation can block gene expression via the methyl-CpG-directed recruitment of one of a family of proteins that contains a conserved methyl-binding domain (MBD), including MBD1, MBD2, MBD3, MBD4, and MeCP2. Another methyl-CpG binding protein, Kaiso, lacks an MBD and instead uses a series of zinc finger protein motifs to interact with methylated cytosines.

The MBD proteins differ from one another with respect to their binding preferences and their preferred corepressors. For example, MBD1 can bind either methylated or unmethylated CpG dinucleotides. MBD2 binds single methylated CpGs, while Kaiso requires a sequence containing a pair of adjacent methylated CpGs. MBD3 is unable to bind methylated CpGs at all and instead works as a cofactor in a complex of proteins that represses transcription (Jorgensen and Bird, 2002; Klose and Bird, 2006). MBD4 binds methyl-CpG in the context of G:T mismatches that occur as a result of cytosine deamination. It contains a DNA glycosylase domain and is involved in the repair of these mismatches (Walsh and Xu, 2006). The final MBD protein, MeCP2, binds methylated CpG dinucleotides located in proximity to a run of at least four adenine or thymine nucleotides (Klose et al., 2005). Once bound to methylated DNA, MBD proteins recruit corepressor proteins that promote the transcriptional repression of nearby DNA sequences. For example, MeCP2 interacts with a wide variety of corepressor complexes, including one containing Sin3a and the histone deacetylases HDAC1 and HDAC2 (Jones et al., 1998; Nan et al., 1998), as well as histone methyltransferases (Lunyak et al., 2002; Fuks et al., 2003), DNA methyltransferases (Kimura and Shiota, 2003), ATP-dependent chromatin remodeling

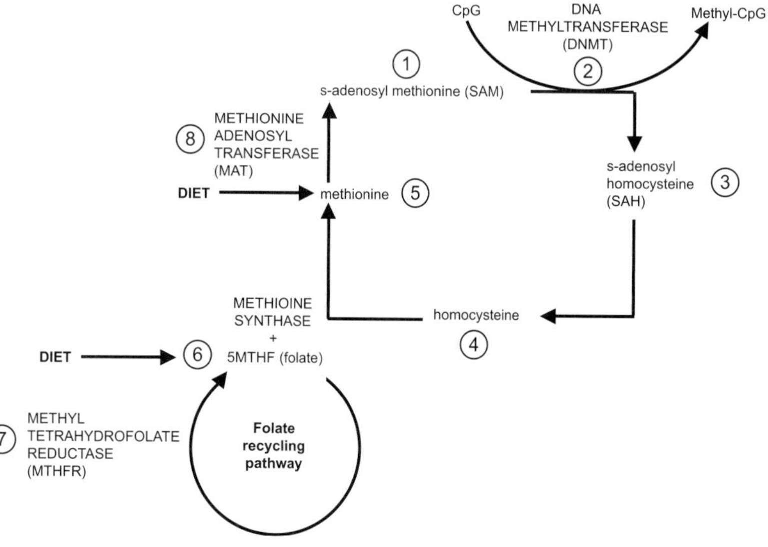

FIGURE 8.1 Biochemical pathways link dietary folic acid and methionine to DNA methylation. (*1*) S-adenosyl methionine (SAM) provides the methyl group that (2) DNA methyltransferase (DNMT) uses to methylate CpG dinucleotides in DNA. When SAM donates its methyl group to DNMT, it is converted to S-adenosyl homocysteine (SAH) (*3*). Then, SAH is converted to homocysteine (*4*). Homocysteine is converted to methionine (*5*) by methionine synthase in a reaction that consumes 5-methyltetrahydrofolate (5MTHF), the major circulating form of the nutrient folic acid (*6*). Folate itself can be regenerated in a series of enzymatic reactions, the last of which is carried out by methylene tetrahydrofolate reductase (MTHFR) (*7*). Then, SAM is generated from the methionine by the enzyme methionine adenosyl transferase (MAT) (*8*). The diet is the ultimate source of methionine and folic acid.

A

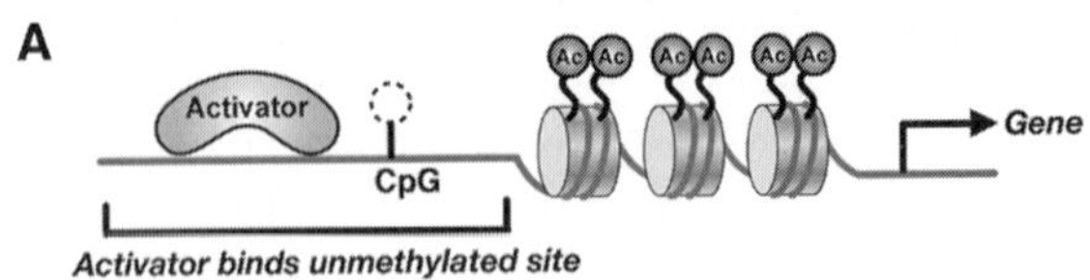

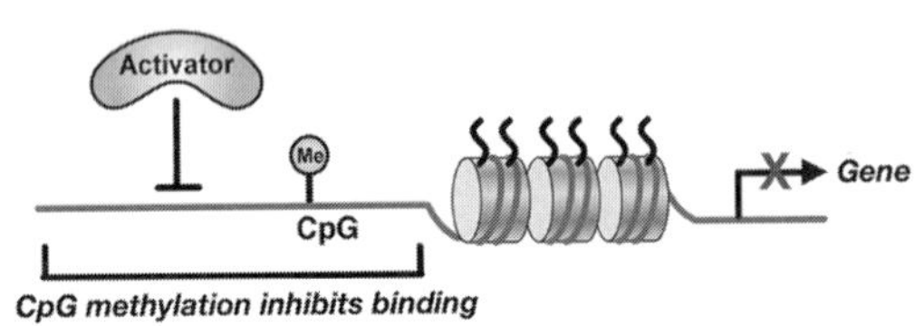

B

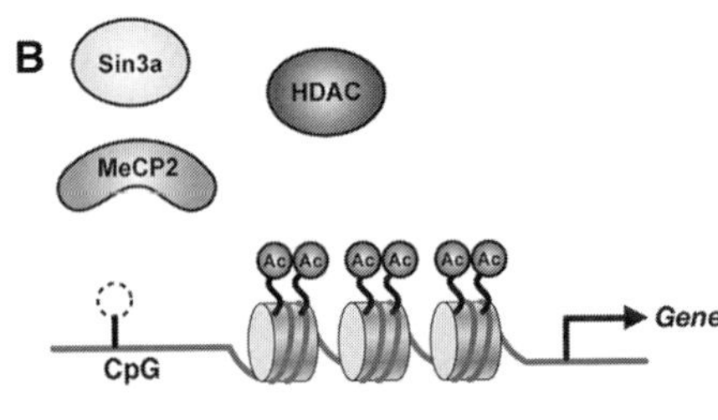

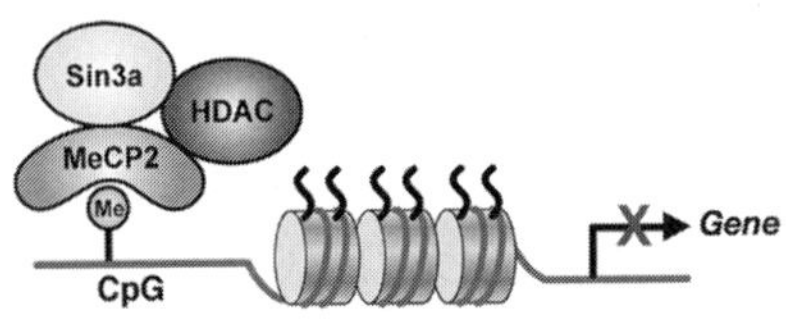

FIGURE 8.2 Mechanisms of epigenetic gene regulation by DNA methylation. (*A*) Deoxyribonucleic acid (DNA) methylation may lead to gene repression by interfering with transcription factor binding. (*B*) Alternatively, DNA methylation may recruit methyl-CpG binding proteins and their attendant corepressors. For example, MeCP2 binds a single methyl-CpG and recruits Sin3a and histone deacetylases (HDACs). In this figure, the DNA strand is represented by a dark gray line, nucleosomes are represented by gray cylinders, histone tails are represented by squiggly lines, and histone modifications (here, acetylation) are represented by circles atop the squiggly lines. DNA methylation of CpG sites is represented by shaded lollipops. The absence of DNA methylation is represented by dotted lollipops.

proteins (Harikrishnan et al., 2005), and the protein CoREST (Lunyak et al., 2002).

Although much is known about the proteins that methylate DNA and interpret DNA methylation, far less is understood about DNA demethylation. DNA demethylation occurs during early embryonic development and resets the offspring's genome to a totipotent state. Two methods of DNA demethylation exist: active and passive demethylation. Passive DNA demethylation is accomplished by preventing DNMT1 from interacting with replicating DNA. Because the duplication of DNA methylation patterns occurs in a semiconservative manner, each successive round of DNA replication further dilutes the original complement of methylated cytosines, resulting in demethylation (Morgan et al., 2005).

The exact mechanism by which active DNA demethylation occurs is still an area of active investigation (Morgan et al., 2005). However, a few studies have identified biochemical pathways that may function in humans. One study examined the proteins Activation-induced cytidine deaminase (Aid) and Apolipoprotein B mRNA editing enzyme, catalytic polypeptide 1 (Apobec1), both of which are expressed in mammalian oocytes. These proteins were found to deaminate 5-methylcytosine to produce thymine. Base excision repair of the resulting thymine:guanine mismatch by either thymine DNA glycosylase (TDG) or MBD4, both of which can replace thymine with an unmethylated cytosine, may be one mechanism by which active DNA demethylation occurs (Morgan et al., 2004). More recently, Barreto et al. (2007) found that the protein Gadd45a promotes DNA demethylation in oocytes from the aquatic frog, *Xenopus laevis*, by interacting with elements of the base excision repair pathway. Gadd45a recruits XPB, a DNA helicase, and XPG, a 3' endonuclease. These proteins work together to excise individual methylated cytosines (Barreto et al., 2007). Whether either of these mechanisms actually operates in mammals during embryogenesis is still a subject of active research, as is the search for more DNA demethylases.

The processes of DNA methylation and demethylation have long been thought to be limited to periods of embryogenesis and cell differentiation, when DNA methylation patterns are initially established, as well as periods of cell division, when DNA methylation patterns are replicated. However, recent evidence suggests that DNA methylation may be more dynamic than previously appreciated. For example, Levenson et al. (2006) demonstrated that rapid changes in DNA methylation and DNMT protein expression—on a time scale of hours—occur in vitro. Similarly, changes in DNA methylation levels (*hypermethylation* and *demethylation*) occur over a similar time scale in vivo in rodents exposed to a simple conditioned learning paradigm (Miller and Sweatt, 2007). Thus, the stage seems to be set to uncover a broader role for DNA methylation in the regulation of gene expression.

Covalent Histone Modification

Covalent posttranslational modification of histone proteins is another major mechanism by which epigenetic information is encoded. Each of the histone proteins is composed of a compact globular core, around which the DNA is wrapped, and a flexible N-terminal "tail" domain. Primarily, it is this histone tail that is recognized by a variety of proteins that add either small chemical groups or large peptides to individual amino acid residues. Covalent modifications that can be posttranslationally added to histone tails include acetylation, methylation, phosphorylation, ubiquitination, sumoylation, and ADP-ribosylation of discrete amino acids (Nightingale et al., 2006).

These modifications have the potential to exert multiple effects on chromatin structure. Indeed, three general models have been proposed to explain the effects of these modifications (Fig. 8.3). First, by altering the charge of the histone tails, the addition and subtraction of these chemical groups changes the binding affinity of histones for DNA, thereby changing local chromatin structure and making it more or less transcriptionally permissive. Second, histone tail modifications may block binding of certain proteins to chromatin. The third model proposes the reverse effect, that histone tail modifications may recruit proteins to a particular site on the chromatin (Kouzarides and Berger, 2007). Based on the multitude of potentially modifiable sites on the histone tails and the various effects that these modifications can have, covalent histone modifications have been proposed to form the basis of a combinatorial "histone code," an epigenetic system that stores and transmits information about the activity state of genes in individual cells (Strahl and Allis, 2000; Jenuwein and Allis, 2001).

Of the known covalent histone modifications, acetylation, methylation, and phosphorylation are three with suspected roles in psychiatric disease (see below). Lysine (K) residues on histone tails are acetylated by histone acetyltransferases (HATs). Histone deacetylases (HDACs) remove these acetyl groups. Histone acetylation marks regions of chromatin that are actively transcribed. Thus, it follows that deacetylated histones are a sign of transcriptional repression (Kouzarides and Berger, 2007).

Methylation of histone tails occurs at lysine (K) and arginine (R) residues and is catalyzed by histone methyltransferases (HMTs) (Martin and Zhang, 2005; Wysocka et al., 2006). Histone methylation was long thought to be a permanent mark, but the recent identification of lysine demethylases has demonstrated that this is not the case (Shi et al., 2004). Arginine demethylases have not been identified yet. However, the methylation of arginine residues can be eliminated by deiminase enzymes that convert methylated arginine to the amino acid citrulline (Klose and Zhang, 2007). In contrast to acetylation, histone methylation can identify chromatin as either transcriptionally active or inactive, depending on the residue involved. For example, methylated histone H3 lysine 9 marks silenced genes, while methylated histone H3 lysine 4 marks actively transcribed genes (Martin and Zhang, 2005).

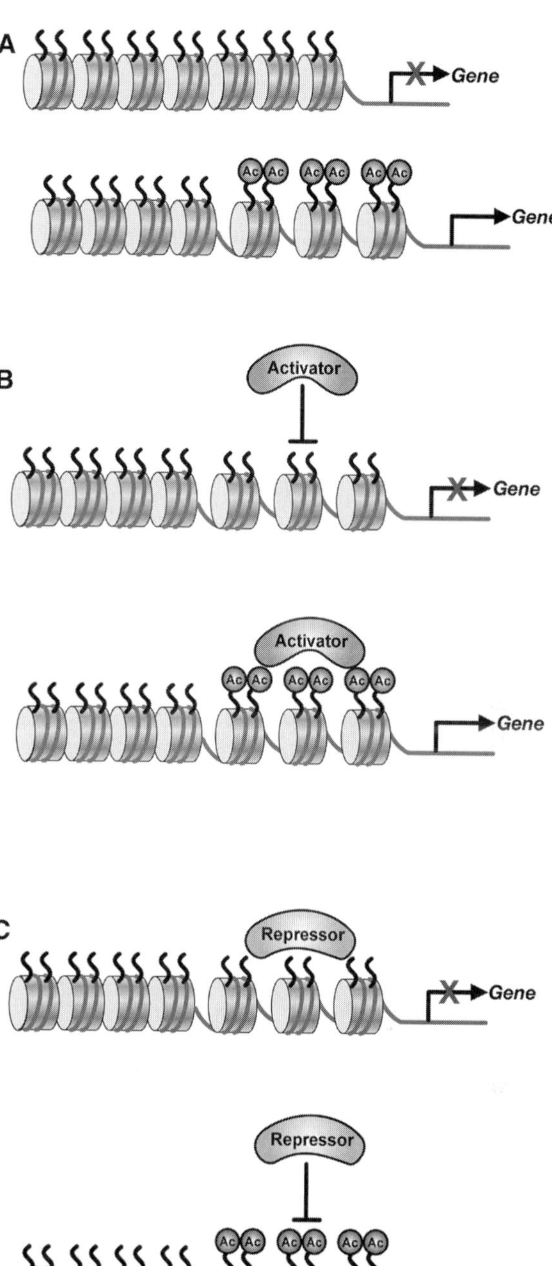

FIGURE 8.3 Mechanisms of epigenetic gene regulation by covalent histone modification. (*A*) Covalent histone modification may directly alter chromatin compaction by altering the affinity of histone proteins for one another or for DNA. (*B*) Alternatively, modifications may attract transcriptional activators that recognize particular chemical moieties (*C*) or repel transcriptional repressors that ordinarily bind histones in the absence of a particular modification. In this figure, the deoxyribonucleic acid (DNA) strand is represented by a dark gray line, nucleosomes are represented by gray cylinders, histone tails are represented by squiggly lines, and histone modifications (here, acetylation) are represented by circles atop the squiggly lines.

Phosphorylation of histone tails occurs at serine residues. As with other cellular proteins, kinases phosphorylate histones while phosphatases remove these marks from histones. Similar to histone methylation, phosphorylation of some histone tail residues promotes transcriptional activation, while the phosphorylation of other residues promotes transcriptional repression (Bode and Dong, 2005).

Chromatin Remodeling by Polycomb- and Trithorax-Group Proteins

A third mechanism of epigenetic gene regulation involves the manipulation of chromatin structure by Polycomb-Group (PcG) and trithorax-Group (trxG) proteins (Grimaud et al., 2006). Both groups of proteins were initially discovered in the fruit fly, *Drosophila melanogaster*, where they organize development along the anterior-posterior axis by regulating the expression of a cluster of genes known as homeotic genes. PcG and trxG proteins are involved in gene regulation in mammals as well, making them relevant to epigenetic processes occurring in humans.

Like covalent posttranslational modification of histone proteins, PcG and trxG proteins target chromatin structure at the level of the nucleosome. PcG proteins form two protein complexes, Polycomb Repressive Complex 1 (PRC1) and Polycomb Repressive Complex 2 (PRC2). A component of PRC2, Ezh1/2, trimethylates the lysine 27 residue of histone H3, which leads to the recruitment of PRC1 to DNA. PRC1 is involved in repressing gene activity, but the exact mechanism by which this occurs is currently unknown (Schwartz and Pirrotta, 2007). trxG proteins have a variety of functions. Of particular importance are those that mediate adenosine tri-phosphate (ATP)-dependent chromatin remodeling, in which the chemical energy stored in ATP is used to alter chromatin structure. These alterations include sliding nucleosomes along the DNA double helix, disrupting DNA–histone interactions, and ejecting entire nucleosomes, all of which serve to expose regions of DNA to proteins that activate gene expression. ATP-dependent chromatin remodeling complexes are organized in three categories, based on the protein family to which the ATPase subunit belongs. These include SWI/SNF (Switch2/Sucrose Non-Fermentable 2), ISWI (Imitation Switch), and CHD (Chromodomain Helicase DNA-binding) complexes (Johnson et al., 2005; de la Serna et al., 2006).

RNA Interference

Ribonucleic acid interference (RNAi) is an epigenetic mechanism that relies on the production of small, single-stranded RNA molecules 21–22 nucleotides (nt) in length (Fig. 8.4). These are generated from two types of RNA precursors, microRNAs (miRNAs) and small interfering RNAs (siRNAs). MicroRNAs and siRNAs are members of a larger class of noncoding RNAs, or RNAs that are not translated into proteins. miRNAs are encoded by discrete genes (Lagos-Quintana et al., 2001; Lau et al., 2001; R. C. Lee and Ambros, 2001) that are transcribed by RNA polymerases II (Y. Lee et al., 2004) and III (Borchert et al., 2006). The initial double-stranded transcript is known as a pri-miRNA, and it is processed within the nucleus by the microprocessor protein complex (Denli et al., 2004; Gregory et al., 2004; Han et al., 2004), which includes Drosha (Y. Lee et al., 2003) and DGCR8 (Landthaler et al., 2004). The product of this initial processing step is a pre-miRNA, which is exported from the cell nucleus into the cytoplasm by the RAN (ras-related nuclear protein)-guanosine-5′ triphosphate (GTP)ase exportin 5 (Lund et al., 2004). Once there, the pre-miRNA is further processed by a protein complex containing Dicer, transactivation-responsive binding protein (TRBP) and Argonaute 2 (Ago2) to produce the 21–22nt miRNA (Hutvagner et al., 2001; Y. Lee et al., 2002; Chendrimada et al., 2005; Gregory et al., 2005). The double-stranded miRNA is separated into its component strands, and one of these strands, *the guide strand*, is loaded onto Ago2 (Gregory et al., 2005). The guide strand–bound Ago2, together with Dicer, TRBP, and the protein PACT (Y. Lee et al., 2006), make up the RNA-induced silencing complex (RISC). RNA-induced silencing complex uses the guide strand to find mRNA targets that will be silenced. These targets are identified by complementary base pairing between the guide strand and the target. Targets that are completely complementary to the guide strand are rapidly cleaved by the endonuclease, or “slicer” activity of the argonaute protein in RISC (Hutvagner and Zamore, 2002; Zeng et al., 2003; Liu et al., 2004; Meister et al., 2004; Song et al., 2004). However, most targets are not fully complementary with the guide strand. Instead of being cleaved outright, the translation of these mRNAs is suppressed (Doench et al., 2003; Zeng et al., 2003), which requires interaction between RISC and the protein RCK/p54 (Chu and Rana, 2006). Translationally suppressed mRNAs may be degraded by the mRNA decay pathway or held in stasis for later translation into protein (Chu and Rana, 2006).

In contrast with miRNAs, siRNAs are not produced from discrete genes but are instead created by transcription of repetitive DNA sequences, such as transposons or centromeric repeats (Billy et al., 2001; Provost et al., 2002; H. Zhang et al., 2002). siRNAs undergo a single processing step by Dicer to generate a double-stranded siRNA. Similar to miRNA, RISC forms by the addition of TRBP, Ago2, and Dicer to the siRNA, and a guide strand is selected (Chendrimada et al., 2005).

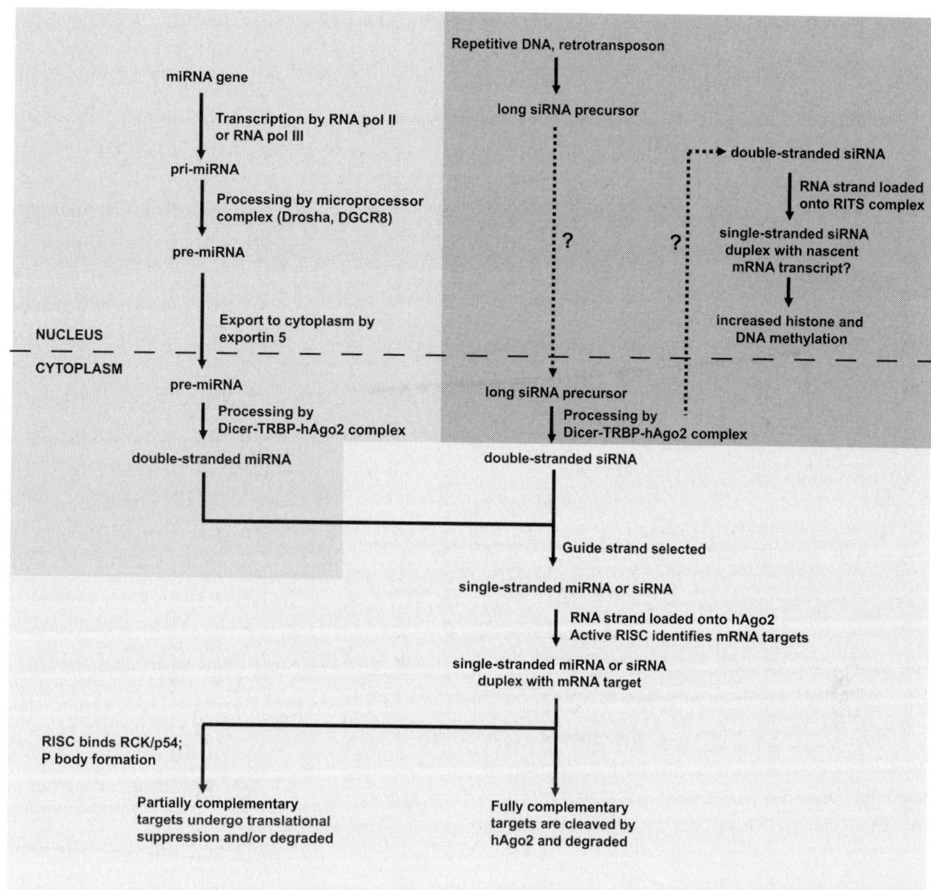

FIGURE 8.4 The ribonucleic acid (RNA) interference pathways. Major steps in the biochemical processing of microRNA (miRNA) are shaded in medium gray, major steps in the biochemical processing of small interfering RNA (siRNA) are shaded in dark gray, and steps that are common to the biochemical processing of miRNA and siRNA are shaded in light gray. Dotted lines marked with question marks represent pathways that remain hypothetical or are supported by limited evidence (see text for details).

In addition to interfering with mRNA translation, siRNAs are also play a role in blocking transcription. After cleavage by Dicer, siRNAs may associate with a different group of proteins collectively known as the RNA-induced transcriptional suppressor (RITS) complex (Verdel et al., 2004). Similar to RISC, RITS uses the siRNA guide strand to identify its targets, which are thought to be newly transcribed RNA sequences (Buhler et al., 2006). These targets localize RITS to the correct location of the chromatin strand, which in mammals includes centromeric regions (Kanellopoulou et al., 2005). The mechanism by which RITS blocks transcription in mammals at these locations is still being worked out, but the preponderance of evidence indicates that it involves histone H3 K9 and K27 methylation (Castanotto et al., 2005; Kanellopoulou et al., 2005; Weinberg et al., 2006), although there is still some dispute (Murchison et al., 2005). In addition, RITS may or may not suppress transcription by promoting DNA methylation (Morris et al., 2004; Park et al., 2004; Svoboda et al., 2004; Kanellopoulou et al., 2005).

Imprinting

The term *imprinting* describes an epigenetic phenomenon in which a gene is expressed differentially (often monoallelically) in a parent-of-origin-specific manner (Reik and Walter, 2001; Delaval and Feil, 2004; Wood and Oakey, 2006). DNA methylation, covalent histone modification, and RNA interference are used to regulate the expression of imprinted genes. Approximately 80 imprinted genes have been identified (Morison et al., 2005), and the existence of many more has been predicted (Luedi et al., 2005; Wood and Oakey, 2006). The majority of imprinted genes are localized in close physical proximity to one another in a handful of clusters that are scattered throughout the chromosomes. The remaining imprinted genes exist in isolation within the introns of larger genes.

In general, imprinted gene expression is regulated by the differential methylation of DNA regions known as imprinting control elements (singular: imprinting control element, or ICE). ICE methylation modulates imprinted gene expression via three known mechanisms (Fig. 8.5). The simplest mechanism is utilized by a handful of genes including *Nnat*, *Nap1l5*, *Peg13*, *Inpp5f_v2*, and *U2af1-rs1*. Expression of the maternal alleles of these genes is blocked by methylation of the promoter region, whereas the paternal allele is unmethylated and expressed (Nabetani et al., 1997; Evans et al., 2001; Smith et al., 2003; Choi et al., 2005).

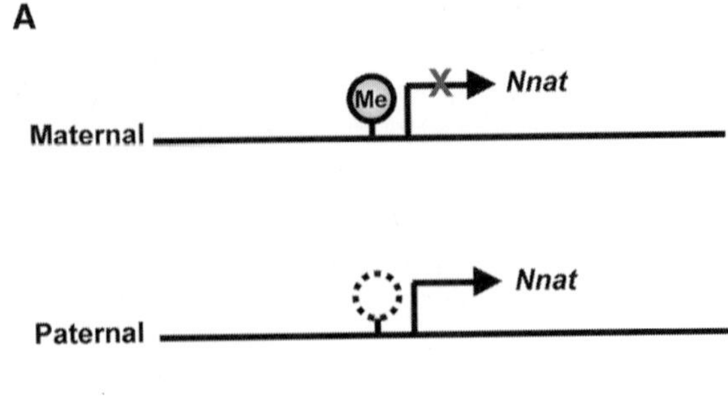

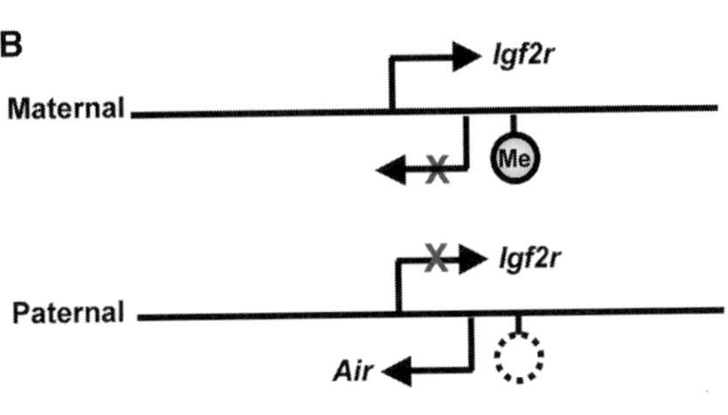

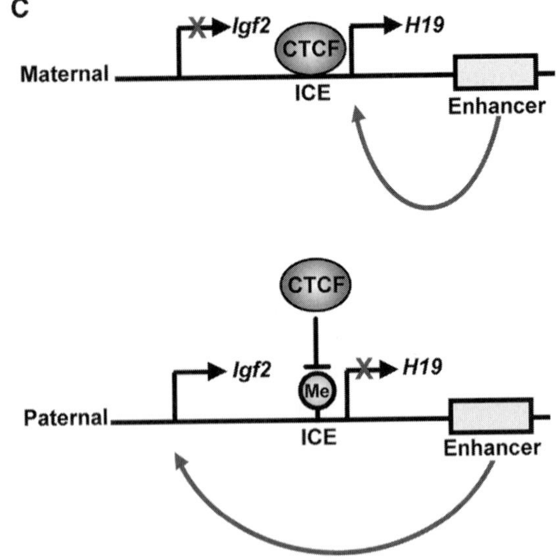

FIGURE 8.5 Mechanisms of imprinting. There are three general mechanisms by which genes are imprinted. (*A*) In the simplest model, deoxyribonucleic acid (DNA) methylation alone is sufficient to achieve allele-specific repression of a gene. For example, methylation suppresses *Nnat* expression. (*B*) In some cases, DNA methylation regulates the expression of a noncoding ribonucleic acid (RNA) that is antisense to another gene. In the absence of DNA methylation, the noncoding RNA is transcribed and interferes with the expression of the gene on the opposite strand. For example, expression of the noncoding RNA *Air* is regulated by methylation. Unmethylated *Air* is expressed and interferes with *Igf2r* expression. (*C*) Yet other imprinted gene clusters rely on a DNA binding protein that binds unmethylated, but not methylated alleles. The presence of this protein allows the expression of a noncoding RNA, which regulates the expression of other genes in the cluster. For example, methylation of the imprinting control element (ICE) upstream of *H19* interferes with the binding of the protein, CCCTC-binding factor (CTCF). This allows the enhancer element to interact with the *Igf2* gene. In this figure, DNA methylation of CpG sites is represented by shaded lollipops (see text for details).

Another imprinting mechanism utilizes DNA methylation to achieve allele-specific suppression of a noncoding RNA, which in turn controls the expression of its target gene. Typically, the target gene is transcribed from the opposite strand as the noncoding RNA. In the absence of the noncoding RNA, the target gene is expressed. However, production of the noncoding RNA disrupts expression of the target gene via RNAi. Imprinting at the *Igf2r* locus is illustrative of this mechanism. On the maternal chromosome, methylation of an ICE on the *Igf2r* antisense strand suppresses transcription of the noncoding RNA, *Air*. On the paternal chromosome, however, the ICE is unmethylated, and *Air* is transcribed. *Air* then blocks expression of *Igf2r* by RNAi (Sleutels et al., 2002).

The third mechanism operates similarly, but in addition to DNA methylation and RNAi requires a DNA binding protein. Imprinting at the *H19/Igf2* gene cluster is illustrative of this mechanism. There, differential methylation of the ICE regulates interaction with a protein, CCCTC-binding factor (CTCF). CTCF readily binds an unmethylated ICE on the maternal allele that is located upstream of *H19*, between *Igf2* and its transcriptional enhancer. This blocks interaction between *Igf2* and the enhancer and instead promotes the expression of the *H19* noncoding RNA. However, ICE methylation on the paternal allele blocks CTCF binding, preventing *H19* expression and permitting expression of *Igf2* (Hark et al., 2000). Recently, covalent histone modification also was shown to have a role in the imprinting process at this locus. Specifically, dimethyl histone H4 arginine 3 (H4R3me2) was shown to be necessary for the proper methylation of the paternal ICE, which is carried out by the de novo methyltransferases DNMT3a, DNMT3b, and DNMT3L (Jelinic et al., 2006).

NEUROPSYCHIATRIC DISORDERS ASSOCIATED WITH EPIGENETIC DEFECTS

Schizophrenia

Emerging evidence suggests a possible role for altered DNA methylation in the development of schizophrenia.

As described above, the production of SAM, which donates the methyl group used to methylate DNA, requires 5MTHF, the circulating form of folic acid. Today, poor nutrition during gestation is recognized as a risk factor for the development of schizophrenia. The most dramatic examples of this association come from observational studies of the offspring of victims of 20th century famines in China and the Netherlands. Children born to women who became pregnant during these disasters had a significantly higher risk of developing schizophrenia later in life (Susser et al., 1996; St. Clair et al., 2005). These children were also at higher risk for the development of neural tube defects, which other studies have linked to folic acid deficiency. Thus, it has been hypothesized that low serum folate levels during pregnancy contribute to an increased risk for developing schizophrenia (Susser et al., 1996).

One reason why gestational folate status may be an important risk factor for the development of schizophrenia could be that DNA methylation patterns are initially established during pregnancy in humans (Morgan et al., 2005). Malnutrition, due to famine or other causes, may lead to a folic acid deficiency that interferes with the establishment of a normal pattern of DNA methylation during prenatal development. Indeed, studies in rodents demonstrate that altering the amount of folic acid available to pregnant dams affects the degree of DNA methylation that is observed in their pups (Cooney et al., 2002; Waterland et al., 2006).

Although the ultimate source of 5MTHF is dietary folic acid, 5MTHF can also be recycled in the cell through a series of enzymatic reactions, the last of which is catalyzed by the enzyme methylenetetrahydrofolate reductase (MTHFR), which is encoded by the *MTHFR* gene (Fig. 8.1). A common polymorphism in *MTHFR*, C677T, causes an alanine to valine missense mutation at amino acid 222 of the MTHFR protein. This mutation impairs the enzymatic activity of MTHFR, particularly in the context of low serum folate levels (Frosst et al., 1995). Higher concentrations of folate stabilize MTHFR and normalize its activity levels (Guenther et al., 1999). Thus, TT homozygotes must ingest more folic acid to meet their needs for this nutrient. Not surprisingly, TT homozygotes with low-serum folic acid levels have significantly decreased amounts of DNA methylation in their peripheral leukocytes (Friso et al., 2002). Interestingly, a higher incidence of psychiatric illness, including schizophrenia, is also observed in TT homozygotes (Lewis et al., 2005; Muntjewerff et al., 2006; Gilbody et al., 2007). This may be related to the fact that people with schizophrenia consume significantly less folic acid (Henderson et al., 2006) and tend to have lower levels of serum folate than members of matched control populations (Regland et al., 1995; Levine et al., 2002; Applebaum et al., 2004; Goff et al., 2004). It is unknown whether levels of DNA methylation in leukocytes and neurons are closely correlated in MTHFR TT homozygotes. However, these results suggest that this population may have reduced levels of DNA methylation in neurons, which could contribute to an increased risk for developing schizophrenia.

Given the importance of folic acid to DNA methylation, one might expect malnutrition to lead to altered levels of DNA methylation. In fact, folate depletion leads to hypomethylation of some genes and hypermethylation of others, at least in vitro (Jhaveri et al., 2001). Consistent with this, there is evidence that DNA hypomethylation and DNA hypermethylation may contribute to schizophrenia. *COMT* is an example of a gene for which there is a correlation between DNA hypomethylation and schizophrenia. *COMT* encodes a soluble (*S-COMT*) and a membrane-bound (*MB-COMT*) isoform of catechol-O-methyltransferase, an enzyme that degrades the synaptic catecholamines *dopamine, epinephrine,* and *norepinepherine.* Some studies have found evidence of a genetic linkage between chromosome 22q11, the region containing *COMT*, and schizophrenia (Ross et al., 2006). In addition, there is a high rate of schizophrenia in 22q11 deletion syndrome, a genetic disorder caused by deletions of this same chromosomal region (Arinami, 2006). Two recent studies examined *COMT* promoter methylation in schizophrenia. The first found a correlation between promoter hypomethylation and increased *MB-COMT* expression in a set of postmortem tissue samples collected from the prefrontal cortex of patients with schizophrenia (Abdolmaleky et al., 2006). The second examined *S-COMT* promoter methylation in tissue samples collected from twins discordant for schizophrenia. Although differences in *S-COMT* promoter methylation were not observed between discordant twins, one patient was identified with a particularly severe case of schizophrenia in which the *S-COMT* promoter was completely methylated (Murphy et al., 2005). These results suggest the possibility of a link between methylation of the *COMT* promoter and schizophrenia.

RELN provides an example of a gene for which there is a correlation between DNA hypermethylation and schizophrenia. *RELN* encodes a glycoprotein, reelin, that is secreted by cortical γ-aminobutyric acid (GABA)-ergic interneurons and binds to the very low density lipoprotein receptor (VLDLR) and apolipoprotein E receptor 2 (APOER2). Reelin is instrumental in positioning cortical neurons during brain development. Later in life, reelin functions to enhance synaptic plasticity, a process important to learning and memory formation (Herz and Chen, 2006). Multiple investigations have identified decreased *RELN* expression in postmortem brain tissue collected from patients with schizophrenia (Fatemi et al., 2000; Guidotti et al., 2000; Eastwood and Harrison, 2003; Veldic et al., 2007). In addition, two independent studies found evidence of *RELN* promoter hypermethylation in other postmortem tissue samples collected from the prefrontal cortex of schizophrenic patients (Abdolmaleky et al., 2005; Grayson et al., 2005).

Promoter hypermethylation typically suppresses gene expression. Indeed, this seems to be the case for *RELN*, at least in vitro, as cell lines expressing low levels of *RELN* have increased promoter methylation compared with cell lines expressing higher levels of *RELN* (Chen et al., 2002). This has led to speculation that reduced levels of *RELN* expression in schizophrenia are due to *RELN* promoter hypermethylation (Grayson et al., 2006). However, currently there is little direct evidence to support this claim. *RELN* expression and methylation have been examined together in only a few ($n = 3$) prefrontal cortical tissue samples from schizophrenic patients. An inverse relationship between the degree of *RELN* hypermethylation and the level of *RELN* expression was observed in these samples (Abdolmaleky et al., 2005). Otherwise, analyses of *RELN* methylation have been limited to mouse and in vitro cell culture systems, making it difficult to estimate the actual coincidence of *RELN* hypermethylation with reduced *RELN* expression in humans brain tissue.

In addition to DNA methylation, a few studies have examined covalent histone modifications in schizophrenia. Aston et al. (2004) identified decreased expression of the histone modifying enzyme, histone deacetylase 3 (HDAC3), in the temporal gyrus of schizophrenics compared to controls. In another study, Akbarian et al. (2005) examined covalent histone modifications in postmortem prefrontal cortex tissue from schizophrenics. They found evidence of increased levels of histone H3 arginine 17 methylation in a subgroup of patients with schizophrenia with reduced metabolic gene expression. Another subgroup, this one with increased expression of the ornithine aminotransferase (*OAT*) gene, was found to have increased levels of histone H3 serine 10 phosphorylation and histone H3 lysine 17 acetylation (Akbarian et al., 2005). Clearly, further study will be required to determine whether these results are reproducible. In addition, the significance of abnormal histone modification to the pathogenesis schizophrenia remains to be determined.

Addiction

Studies in animals suggest that covalent histone modifications may play a role in regulating the brain's response to drugs of abuse and thus may prove relevant to understanding and treating addiction. Kumar et al. (2005) found that acute and chronic cocaine use by rats altered histone acetylation at genes that undergo characteristic expression changes in response to drug use. Acetylated histones were detected after acute cocaine treatment at the promoter of *cfos*, an immediate early gene activated by acute but not chronic cocaine. *Bdnf* and *Cdk5*, two genes induced by chronic but not acute exposure to cocaine, were found to have acetylated histones only after chronic cocaine treatment. Finally, acetylated histones were present following acute and chronic cocaine delivery at *fosB*, a gene that is activated by acute and chronic cocaine. Thus, the presence of acetylated histones at genes regulated by cocaine use correlates with the time frame at which they are known to be activated (Kumar et al., 2005). In addition to changes in histone acetylation, another recent study identified decreased levels of histone H3 methylation at lysine 4 and lysine 27 in the brains of rats following binge cocaine use (Black et al., 2006). Together, these studies suggest that the addictive effects of cocaine, and perhaps other drugs of abuse, are the result of changes in gene expression mediated by covalent histone modification.

Rett Syndrome

Evidence of the role of epigenetic processes in psychiatric disease comes from genetic disorders with prominent psychiatric phenotypes. Some of these disorders are caused by mutations in genes encoding components of epigenetic systems (Table 8.1). For example, mutations in *MeCP2*, the X-linked gene that encodes MeCP2, cause Rett syndrome (RTT) (Amir et al., 1999). To summarize the typical features of the disease, children with RTT suffer from cognitive impairment and motor dysfunction. Ataxia is common, and locomotion may be severely impaired. Purposeful hand movements are characteristically replaced by stereotypies, which are frequently described as hand-washing or wringing movements. Abnormal breathing patterns and vasomotor disturbances are also commonly observed. Other aspects of RTT include seizures, sleep disturbances, and reduced pain sensitivity, and a variety of behavioral abnormalities (Trevethan and Moser, 1988; Hagberg et al., 2002). Importantly, RTT also has a significant behavioral phenotype. Autistic features, including absence of speech, indifference to others, avoidance of eye contact, and social withdrawal, are commonly reported in patients with RTT (Mount et al., 2001; Mount et al., 2003). Anxiety and fearfulness are also major components of the RTT behavioral phenotype, occurring in up to 75% of children with RTT (Coleman et al., 1988; Sansom et al., 1993; Mount et al., 2002).

Besides classic RTT, mutations in *MeCP2* cause a wide spectrum of neuropsychiatric phenotypes in females. Because *MeCP2* is located on the X chromosome and is subject to X chromosome inactivation (XCI), females, who carry two X chromosomes, will manifest partial features depending on XCI patterns. Favorable XCI, which occurs when a majority of cells express the wild type (WT) *MeCP2* allele instead of the mutated *MeCP2* allele, accounts for the partial neuropsychiatric

TABLE 8.1. *Syndromes with Prominent Neuropsychiatric Phenotypes that are Linked to Mutations in Genes Regulating Epigenetic Processes*

Disease	*Gene(s)*	*Neuropsychiatric phenotype(s)*
Rett syndrome	*MeCP2*	Anxiety, autism, childhood-onset schizophrenia
Rubinstein–Taybi syndrome	*CREBBP, EP300*	Hyperactivity, mood lability, obsessive behaviors, autistic features
α-thalassemia/mental retardation syndrome, X-linked	*ATRX*	Autistic features, mood lability, emotional outbursts, self-injurious and obsessive behaviors
Angelman syndrome	*UBE3A*	Autistic features
Prader–Willi syndrome	Unknown. Linked to paternally expressed genes at 15q11-q13.	Autistic features
Fragile X syndrome	*FMR1*	Autistic features, attention deficit/hyperactivity

phenotypes in females (Archer et al., 2006). Males with severe *MeCP2* mutations suffer from early lethality because they have only one X chromosome (Wan et al., 1999; Villard et al., 2000; Hoffbuhr et al., 2001; Kankirawatana et al., 2006). However, males with mild *MeCP2* mutations may develop less severe disease manifesting as a neuropsychiatric disorder compatible with life.

A phenotype commonly linked to *MeCP2* mutations is autism. In a screen of 69 females diagnosed with autism, Carney et al. (2003) identified two girls with *MeCP2* mutations (a 2.8% hit rate). A similar screen found a slightly higher rate of *MeCP2* mutations in series of females with autism (4.8%, or 1 out of 21) (Lam et al., 2000). *MeCP2* mutations have also been found in males clinically diagnosed with autism (Shibayama et al., 2004).

Other neuropsychiatric phenotypes have been associated with *MeCP2* mutations, particularly in males. These include childhood-onset schizophrenia, alcoholism, phobia, and attention-deficit/hyperactivity disorder (ADHD) (Shibayama et al., 2004). The A140V *MeCP2* mutation in particular seems closely linked to psychotic behavior. Klauck et al. (2002) linked this mutation to the PPM-X syndrome, which is characterized by manic-depressive psychosis, pyramidal signs, and macroorchidism. In addition, Couvert et al. (2001) describe a frankly psychotic male with the same mutation.

Although there is no doubt that *MeCP2* mutations cause a variety of neuropsychiatric disorders, the molecular basis of these phenotypes is only now being uncovered. In general, it is thought that in the absence of functional MeCP2 the normal pattern of DNA methylation is not interpreted correctly. As a result, genes that would normally be repressed by DNA methylation via MeCP2 are instead expressed (Willard and Hendrich, 1999). *UBE3A*, a gene linked to autism and Angelman syndrome, a genetic disorder with prominent autistic features (discussed below), is one such proposed MeCP2 target (Makedonski et al., 2005; Samaco et al., 2005), although not all laboratories have found evidence of this (Jordan and Francke, 2006). *Crh*, the gene encoding corticotropin-releasing hormone, a neuropeptide with anxiogenic properties (Bale and Vale, 2004), is another MeCP2 target that is relevant to the anxiety phenotype observed in RTT (McGill et al., 2006). These findings suggest that further study of RTT may provide insight into the epigenetic and molecular basis of several psychiatric diseases.

Rubinstein–Taybi Syndrome (RTS)

Errors in covalent histone modification have been linked to the pathogenesis of Rubinstein–Taybi syndrome (RTS), a genetic disorder characterized by mental retardation, microcephaly, facial abnormalities, broad thumbs, and broad great toes (Hennekam, 2006). RTS also has a significant psychiatric component characterized in part by hyperactivity and short attention span. Mood lability and repetitive and obsessive behaviors also occur frequently in RTS. In addition, autistic behaviors, such as a preference for being alone, are described in RTS (Rubinstein and Taybi, 1963; Gotts and Liemohn, 1977; Stevens et al., 1990; Hennekam et al., 1992; Levitas and Reid, 1998; Hellings et al., 2002).

Mutations in the genes encoding cAMP-response element binding (CREB) binding protein (CBP) and E1A binding protein p300, as well as microdeletions of chromosome 16p13.3 (the location of the gene encoding CBP), account for approximately 55% of RTS cases (Hennekam, 2006). The cause of the remaining 45% of cases is unknown but could be due to further genetic heterogeneity. CBP and its homolog, p300, are histone acetyltransferases that interact with the phosphorylated form of CREB, a transcriptional activator. Thus, the HAT activity of CBP and p300 helps promote the transcription of CREB-responsive genes. A subset of these genes is critical for long-term memory formation, as is evident from the study of genetically engineered mice containing mutations in CBP. Mice lacking normal CBP levels have significant learning deficits, as one might predict given the mental retardation phenotype of humans with RTS (Oike et al., 1999; Bourtchouladze et al., 2003; Alarcon et al., 2004). Similarly, the disruption of transcription of a subset of CBP/p300-regulated genes in RTS may account for the behavioral features of this disease. Further research will be required to identify the genes in question.

α-Thalassemia/Mental Retardation Syndrome, X-linked (ATRX)

As its name implies, α-thalassemia and mental retardation are features of ATRX. In addition, other common features of ATRX include facial dysmorphism, abnormal genitalia, skeletal abnormalities, and microcephaly. Anecdotal evidence suggests that ATRX has a behavioral phenotype, also. The majority of patients with ATRX have a happy disposition, but a subset is socially withdrawn and exhibit behaviors reminiscent of autism. Emotional outbursts, sudden mood changes, and self-injurious and obsessive behaviors are observed in this disorder (Gibbons, 2006).

α-Thalassemia/Mental Retardation syndrome, X-linked is caused by mutations in the *ATRX* gene (formerly *XNP*). *ATRX* encodes a protein that is a member of the SWI/SNF family of chromatin remodeling enzymes (Gibbons et al., 1995), and it interacts with other chromatin structural proteins including HP1 (Gibbons et al., 1997) and EZH2 (Cardoso et al., 1998). Moreover, the ATRX protein was recently found to interact with MeCP2, thereby linking the chromatin modifying activity of ATRX to the protein machinery that interprets DNA methylation (Nan et al., 2007). The exact molecular mechanisms linking *ATRX* mutation with the behavioral phenotype of the disease remain obscure but are likely due to alterations in downstream gene expression that occur as a result of *ATRX* loss of function.

Neuropsychiatric Phenotypes Caused by Imprinting Defects on Chromosome 15q11-q13

Imprinting errors at chromosome 15q11-q13 cause two neurobehavioral disorders, Angelman syndrome (AS) and Prader–Willi syndrome (PWS), both of which are associated with a significant psychiatric phenotype, *autism* (Schanen, 2006). Moreover, cytogenetic abnormalities involving this chromosomal region, the most common of which is the isodicentric chromosome 15 (idic[15]), are also linked to autism (Schanen, 2006).

Angelman syndrome is identified by a constellation of features including mental retardation, impaired speech, movement disorders including ataxia and/or tremor, and seizures. Excessive or inappropriate laughter and a happy disposition are also common features, as are hyperactivity and hand-flapping or waving movements (Williams et al., 2006). Features of autism are prevalent in AS. For example, Steffenburg et al. (1996), evaluated four patients with AS for the presence of autism and found that all of them met the *DSM-IV* (American Psychiatric Association, 1994) criteria for the disease. Similarly, Trillingsgaard diagnosed 13 of 16 patients with AS and autism according to the ADOS-G (Autism Diagnostic Observation Schedule, Generic) criteria for the disease (Trillingsgaard and Ostergaard, 2004). A third population-based study of patients with AS found that 42% (8 out of 19 AS patients) met criteria for autism by the ADOS-G and the ADI-R (Autism Diagnostic Interview, Revised) (Peters et al., 2004). In contrast, a recent systematic review of the literature estimated that only about 2% of people with AS exhibit autism (Veltman et al., 2005). However, the authors did not include the studies by Trillingsgaard and by Peters in their analysis. Regardless of the exact coincidence of AS and autism, it is clear that in at least some instances the AS phenotype includes features of autism.

PWS is characterized by a different set of clinical findings than AS. Initially, children with PWS present with hypotonia and failure to thrive. As they develop, other features become prominent, including mental retardation, hypogonadism, and hyperphagia that results in severe obesity if left unchecked (Goldstone, 2004). Autistic features are also associated with PWS. A recent extensive literature review estimated the prevalence of autism in PWS at 25% (Veltman et al., 2005), whereas a direct examination of a PWS patient population indicated a slightly higher figure of 36% (Descheemaeker et al., 2006).

In addition to PWS and AS, cytogenetic abnormalities involving chromosome 15q11-q13, including duplications, triplications, and deletions, are also linked to autism spectrum disorders (ASDs). The most common cytogenetic abnormality involving this region is an inverted duplication that creates a supernumerary dicentric chromosome 15 (Battaglia, 2005). As a group, these abnormalities cause as many as 4% of cases of ASDs in various case series (Schroer et al., 1998). Cytogenetic abnormalities of 15q11-q13 that are associated with ASDs are primarily maternally inherited, suggesting that maternally expressed genes are involved in the development of the autistic features that are observed (Browne et al., 1997; Cook et al., 1997; Schroer et al., 1998; Bolton et al., 2001).

AS is caused by loss of function of the maternal copy of the ubiquitin E3 ligase gene (*UBE3A*), which encodes the E6-associated protein (E6-AP), an enzyme that participates in the ubiquitin–proteasome protein degradation pathway (Kishino et al., 1997; Matsuura et al., 1997). *UBE3A* is only imprinted in the brain (Vu and Hoffman, 1997) and is biallelically expressed elsewhere (Nakao et al., 1994). In mice, paternal uniparental disomy results in a marked reduction of *UBE3A* expression in hippocampal neurons and cerebellar Purkinje cells (Albrecht et al., 1997), suggesting an important role for E6-AP in the function of these cells. Indeed, mice with maternal *Ube3a* deficiency have memory deficits and motor dysfunction, as would be expected from derangements of these neurons (Jiang et al., 1998).

There are four known mechanisms by which maternal *UBE3A* loss of function occurs (Fig. 8.6). First, deletion of the maternal copy of *UBE3A* eliminates E6-AP from cells that express predominantly the maternal allele. Second, mutations in the maternal copy of *UBE3A* that eliminate the protein's catalytic activity result in a functional null for maternal *UBE3A*. Third, paternal disomy for chromosome 15 leads to the inheritance of 2 silenced copies of *UBE3A*. Finally, imprinting center defects on the maternal chromosome can repress maternal *UBE3A* expression (Williams et al., 2006).

PWS is caused by loss of function of imprinted genes on the paternal copy of 15q11-q13 (Fig. 8.6). Unlike AS, no single gene deletions have been shown to cause PWS. However, the critical region has been narrowed to a 1.5Mb area that includes 10 paternally expressed loci (Stefan et al., 2005), and growing evidence suggests that the disruption of the *Pwcr1/MBII-85* snoRNA cluster is responsible for the disease (Gallagher et al., 2002; Ding et al., 2005; Schule et al., 2005). Similar to AS, multiple mechanisms lead to paternal loss of function of 15q11-q13. These include the following: paternal deletion of 15q11-q13, maternal uniparental disomy of chromosome 15, and imprinting errors that silence expression of the paternal allele. Rarely, balanced translocations may cause PWS, but the molecular mechanism responsible for disease in these cases has not been conclusively identified. Interestingly, autistic features are significantly more common in PWS caused by maternal uniparental disomy as compared to PWS caused by deletion events, suggesting that increased dosage of an imprinted gene on maternal 15q11-q13 may contribute to autism (Veltman et al., 2004; Milner et al., 2005; Veltman et al., 2005; Descheemaeker et al., 2006).

Careful study of the imprinting process at chromosome 15q11-q13 has provided insight into the molecular mechanisms that underlie AS and PWS. Gene expression at chromosome 15q11-q13 is under the control of a bipartite imprinting control region (ICR) that includes the AS-ICR, the loss of which causes Angelman syndrome, and the PWS-ICR, deletion of which results in Prader–Willi syndrome (Buiting et al., 1995). The AS-ICR has been mapped to an 880bp stretch of DNA located 35kb upstream of the *SNURF-SNRPN* gene (Buiting et al., 1999), while the PWS-ICR has been localized to a 4kb region that includes the promoter and the first exon of *SNURF-SNRPN* (Ohta et al., 1999). The two ICRs are differentially methylated according to parent of origin early in development. The PWS-ICR is unmethylated on the paternal allele and methylated on the maternal allele (Kantor, Kaufman, et al., 2004; Kantor, Makedonski, et al., 2004). Methylation of the maternal PWS-ICR is permanent and functions to silence expression of the *SNRPN* transcript (Shemer et al., 1997). In contrast, differential methylation of the AS-ICR occurs only transiently during early embryogenesis. Experiments in mice suggest that the AS-ICR primarily functions to regulate the imprinting of the PWS-ICR (Kantor, Kaufman, et al., 2004). The AS-ICR is methylated in sperm and male embryos, but it remains unmethylated in oocytes and female embryos. However, in adult mice the AS-ICR is not differentially methylated on the maternal and paternal chromosomes (Kantor, Kaufman, et al., 2004).

Covalent histone modification also plays a role in establishing imprinting at chromosome 15q11-q13. Saitoh and Wada (2000) found evidence that the transcriptionally active paternal *SNRPN* promoter, the site of the PWS-ICR, in addition to being unmethylated, is also enriched for acetylated histone H3 and acetylated histone H4. On the other hand, the inactive maternal *SNRPN* promoter, which is completely methylated in vivo, is hypoacetylated and enriched for methylated histone H3 lysine 9. Similarly, differences in histone methylation are also observed at the *SNRPN* promoter, with methylated histone H3 lysine 4 present at the active paternal allele and methyl-histone H3 lysine 9 present at the inactive maternal allele (Xin et al., 2001). Histones at the AS-ICR are similarly covalently modified according to the activity state of the parental allele. That is, the active maternal AS-ICR contains acetyl-histone H3 and H4 as well as methyl-histone H3 lysine 4. None of these modifications are found at the inactive paternal AS-ICR (Perk et al., 2002). Considered together, these covalent histone modifications are consistent with what is known about the activity state of each ICR. Thus, covalent histone modifications contribute to the imprinting of 15q11-q13 by maintaining and reinforcing the activity states of the AS-ICR and the PWS-ICR.

In addition to DNA methylation and covalent histone modification, antisense RNA also contributes to imprinting at 15q11-q13. The extreme 3' end of the paternally expressed *SNRPN* transcript extends into the *UBE3A* locus to generate an *UBE3A* antisense transcript (*UBE3A-AS*) (Runte et al., 2001). *UBE3A-AS* is produced only in neurons in the brain (Yamasaki et al., 2003; Landers et al., 2004), suggesting that it functions to silence the paternal *UBE3A* allele. In support of this model, mutations in the PWS-IC relieve *UBE3A* repression and lead to decreased production of the *UBE3A-AS* transcript (Chamberlain and Brannan, 2001). Although the exact role of antisense RNA in the control of *UBE3A* expression remains controversial (Landers et al., 2005), the involvement of DNA methylation and covalent histone modification in the regulation of imprinted gene expression at 15q11-q13 nevertheless provides an important example of the role of epigenetic processes in the pathogenesis of genetic disorders with major psychiatric components.

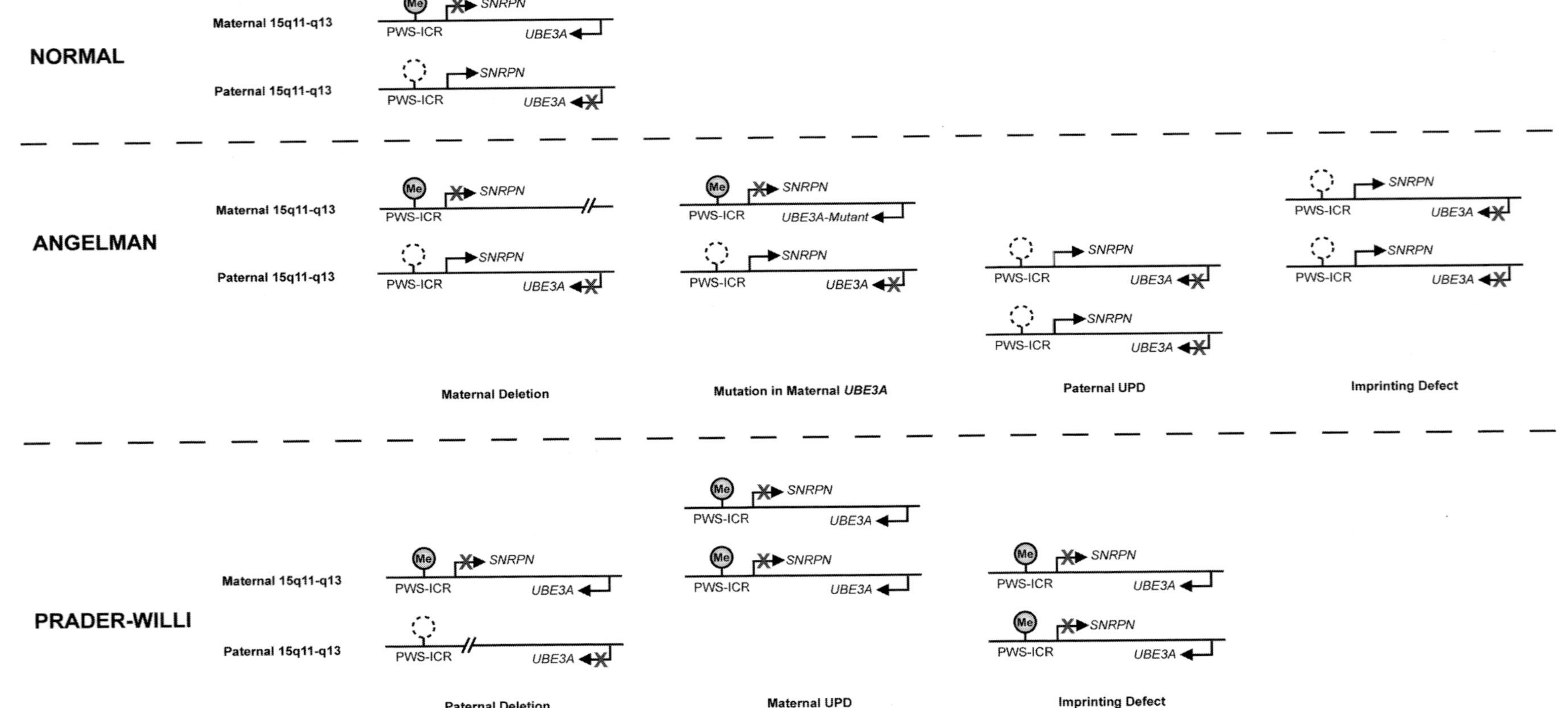

FIGURE 8.6 Causes of Angelman syndrome and Prader-Willi syndrome. Angelman syndrome (AS) and Prader–Willi syndrome (PWS) are caused by mutations and imprinting errors at chromosome 15q11-q13. Normally, *UBE3A* is expressed from the maternal chromosome, while a group of 10 genes, including *SNRPN*, are expressed from the paternal chromosome. Expression of *UBE3A*, *SNRPN*, and the other nine paternally expressed genes is regulated by the differential methylation of the Angelman syndrome imprinting control region (AS-ICR) and the PWS imprinting control region (PWS-ICR). Differential methylation of the AS-ICR occurs transiently during embryonic development and is not shown here. DNA methylation at the PWS-ICR is represented by shaded lollipops, whereas unmethylated DNA at this site is indicated by dotted lollipops. Angelman syndrome is caused by mutations and epimutations that result in decreased expression of the maternal copy of *UBE3A* or the function of its protein product, *UBE3A*. Prader–Willi syndrome is caused by mutations and epimutations, including balanced translocations (not shown), that disrupt the expression of paternally imprinted genes at chromosome 15q11-q13 (see text for more details).

Fragile X Syndrome

The most common cause of intellectual disability, Fragile X syndrome (FXS) occurs in approximately 1 in 4000 males and 1 in 8000 females (Crawford et al., 2001). In addition to mental retardation, the FXS phenotype includes macroorchidism in males, hypotonia, joint hyperextensibility, and dysmorphic facial features (Terracciano et al., 2005). Behavioral abnormalities, including repetitive speech and stereotyped behaviors, occur frequently in FXS (Baumgardner et al., 1995). Features of ADHD have also been repeatedly observed (Fryns et al., 1984; Bregman et al., 1988; Baumgardner et al., 1995; Backes et al., 2000; Hatton et al., 2002; Sullivan et al., 2006). Moreover, autism is a significant component of the FXS behavioral phenotype. Two studies of patients with FXS using the current gold standard metrics for diagnosing autism, the Autism Diagnostic Observation Scale-Generic (ADOS-G) and the Autism Diagnostic Interview (ADI-R), one by Rogers et al. (2001), and another by Clifford et al. (2007), found that 33%–67% of males with FXS met criteria for autism by at least one of these tools. The study by Clifford et al. also examined females with FXS and found that fewer (23%) demonstrated evidence of autism. This observation is consistent with the generally milder course of FXS in females, which is the result of FXS being an X-linked disorder.

Fragile X syndrome is caused by expansion of a cytosine-guanine-guanine (CGG) repeat in the first exon of the *FMR1* gene (Verkerk et al., 1991). Normal alleles of *FMR1* contain between 5 and 50 CGG repeats, unstable premutation alleles contain 50 to 200 CGG repeats, and mutant alleles of *FMR1* contain more than 200 repeats (Terracciano et al., 2005). Through a mechanism that remains unclear, CGG repeat expansion leads to abnormal methylation of an upstream CpG island in the *FMR1* promoter (Verkerk et al., 1991). In response, the *FMR1* gene is repressed, its protein product, the Fragile X mental retardation protein (FMRP) is not produced, and FXS is the result (Sutcliffe et al., 1992).

In addition to abnormal DNA methylation, altered covalent histone modifications and chromatin remodeling figure prominently in FXS. Consistent with decreased *FMR1* expression in FXS, reduced levels of covalent histone modifications linked to transcriptional activity have been observed at the *FMR1* promoter in FXS patient-derived cell lines, including acetyl-histone H3, acetyl-histone H4, and dimethyl-histone H3 lysine 4 (Coffee et al., 1999; Coffee et al., 2002). Furthermore, increased levels of dimethyl-histone H3 lysine 9, a histone modification associated with transcriptional inhibition, have also been observed at the *FMR1* locus in FXS (Coffee et al., 2002).

Chromatin structural changes are also relevant to the pathogenesis of FXS. Harikrishnan et al. (2005) showed that a protein complex containing MeCP2 and the SWI/SNF family ATP-dependent chromatin remodeling enzyme, Brm, localize to the hypermethylated *FMR1* promoter in FXS. Importantly, *FMR1* expression was enhanced when the expression of the Brm parent gene, *SMARCA2*, was blocked (Harikrishnan et al.), suggesting a possible therapeutic approach to this disorder.

In addition to the epigenetic errors described above, abnormal RNA interference also contributes to FXS. *FMR1* encodes the FMRP, an RNA binding protein (Ashley et al., 1993; Siomi et al., 1993; Feng et al., 1997). FMRP interacts with translating polyribosomes at the base of dendritic spines, the primary sites of synaptic plasticity in neurons (Khandjian et al., 2004; Stefani et al., 2004). Furthermore, FMRP suppresses RNA translation in vitro (Laggerbauer et al., 2001; Z. Li et al., 2001). Among the known targets of FMRP is MAP1B, a microtubule-associated protein that helps form the scaffolding of dendritic spines (Zhang et al., 2001). Thus, FMRP is thought to control synaptic structure and function by regulating mRNA translation at dendritic spines.

Recent evidence indicates that FMRP controls mRNA translation via post-transcriptional gene silencing (PTGS). Fragile X mental retardation protein interacts with eIF2C2, the mammalian homolog of AGO1, and it associates with Dicer activity in vivo as well (Jin, Zarnescu, et al., 2004). FMRP protein preferentially binds Dicer-generated miRNAs via its KH domain but can also bind single-stranded siRNAs. Indeed, deletion of FMR1 disrupts RNAi mediated by miRNA and siRNA (Plante et al., 2006). Still, the exact targets of FMRP translational suppression and the exact mechanisms by which their aberrant translation in FXS contributes to the disease phenotype remain unknown.

In addition to the involvement of RNAi-mediated PTGS in FXS, Jin et al. recently hypothesized that RNAi-induced transcriptional gene silencing (TGS) may also contribute to the pathogenesis of this disease (Jin, Alisch, and Warren, 2004). This hypothesis was based on the finding that RNA transcribed from the mutated FMR1 allele forms a hairpin structure capable of being cleaved by Dicer to produce small RNAs (Handa et al., 2003). Jin, Alisch, and Warren (2004) proposed that these small RNAs target the RITS complex to the *FMR1* promoter, which in turn recruits DNMTs that methylate the CpG island there. Although this hypothesis has yet to be tested, the fact that RNAi-directed DNA methylation was recently identified in mammalian cells (Morris et al., 2004) makes this theory plausible. If it turns out to be true, it would be yet another example of the involvement of epigenetic mechanisms in FXS.

EPIGENETIC INHERITANCE, METASTABLE EPIALLELES, AND ENVIRONMENTALLY INDUCED EPIGENETIC PLASTICITY: POTENTIAL RELEVANCE TO PSYCHIATRIC DISEASE

So far in our discussion of epigenetic mechanisms in psychiatric disease, we have confined our examples to those involving epigenetic marks that are established early in development and then propagated by somatic cell division as the body grows. These modifications, which include the majority of epigenetic marks, affect only the individual possessing them. This is due to the fact that epigenetic marks made by DNA methylation are erased from all but a few sequences shortly after fertilization, preventing the transfer of this epigenetic information to the offspring (Morgan et al., 2005). However, new research indicates that at least for some genes, epigenetic inheritance exists, in which epigenetic states can be inherited across multiple generations (Fig. 8.7).

Although the phenomenon of epigenetic inheritance has been known to exist in plants and lower animals for some time, the first definitive evidence of epigenetic inheritance in humans came to light only recently. Chan et al. (2006) described a three-generation family in which individuals who inherited a specific epimutation were predisposed to develop colon and endometrial cancers. In this case, the epimutation consisted of a hypermethylated region in the promoter of the mutS homolog 2 colon cancer nonpolyposis type 1 (*MSH2*) gene, a tumor suppressor gene that encodes a DNA mismatch repair enzyme. The authors hypothesized that *MSH2* expression was effectively repressed from the methylated allele, predisposing carriers to cancer as a result of a second environmentally acquired mutation in the remaining allele (Chan et al., 2006). Epigenetic inheritance was also recently described for another tumor suppressor gene, the mutL homolog 1 colon cancer nonpolyposis type 2 (*MLH1*) gene (Hitchins et al., 2007). In both of these cases, the epimutation was transmitted maternally, but the identification of sperm carrying epimutations in the *MLH1* gene suggests that paternal transmission is also possible (Suter et al., 2004).

A further wrinkle to the concept of epigenetic inheritance comes from the fact that some genes have multiple alleles that differ only in their epigenetic features, which are heritable. These alleles are termed *metastable epialleles*. The word *epiallele* refers to the different epigenetic states that these alleles can acquire, while the term *metastable* refers to the fact that these alleles can undergo epigenetic modification during early embryonic development that is faithfully propagated through mitotic cell division. In this way, the phenotype of the offspring may differ from that of the parent as a result of epigenetic changes, even though the inherited genetic information is identical (Fig. 8.8) (Rakyan and Beck, 2006).

A classic example of epigenetic metastability concerns *agouti*, a gene with multiple alleles that determines coat color in mice. Mice homozygous for the dominant *A* allele of this gene have a yellow coat, whereas mice homozygous for the *a* allele have a black coat. Heterozygous mice have an agouti coat, which is brown. The expression of another allele, A^{vy}, is controlled by a nearby methylatable retrotransposon. Decreased methylation leads to enhanced expression of A^{vy}, to the point that A^{vy}/a mice with low levels of A^{vy} methylation have a yellow coat whereas A^{vy}/a mice with higher levels of A^{vy} methylation have an agouti coat; this latter group is described as pseudoagouti (Morgan et al., 1999). Evidence for metastability of the *agouti* gene comes from examining the offspring of A^{vy}/a males crossed to *a/a* females. Normally, a significant number of these offspring are yellow. However, *a/a* dams fed diets rich in methyl donors bear fewer yellow offspring and more

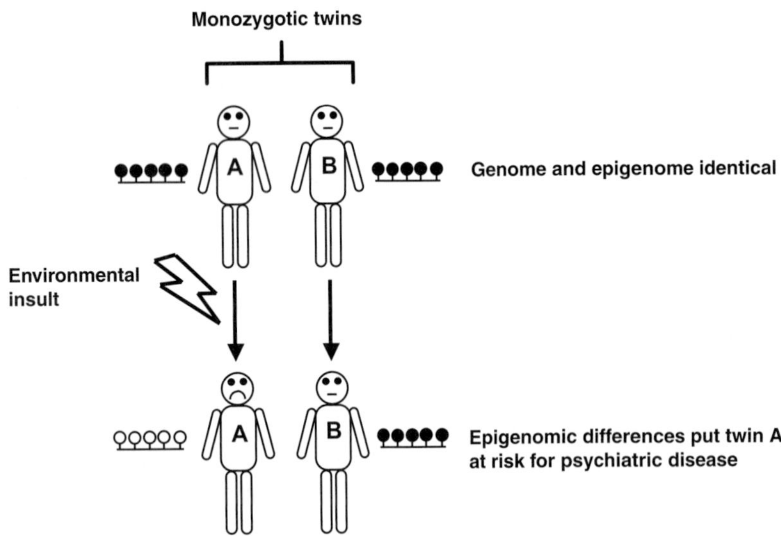

FIGURE 8.7 Epigenetic plasticity. Epigenetic plasticity may explain twin discordance for schizophrenia and other psychiatric diseases. In this figure, a pair of monozygotic twins begins life with identical genomes and epigenomes (signified by filled-in lollipops, representing deoxyribonucleic acid (DNA) methylation, on a black line, representing the DNA strand). However, twin A is exposed to an environmental insult (represented by the lightening bolt) that alters his epigenome (signified by empty lollipops, representing absent DNA methylation), putting him at increased risk for the development of schizophrenia later in life.

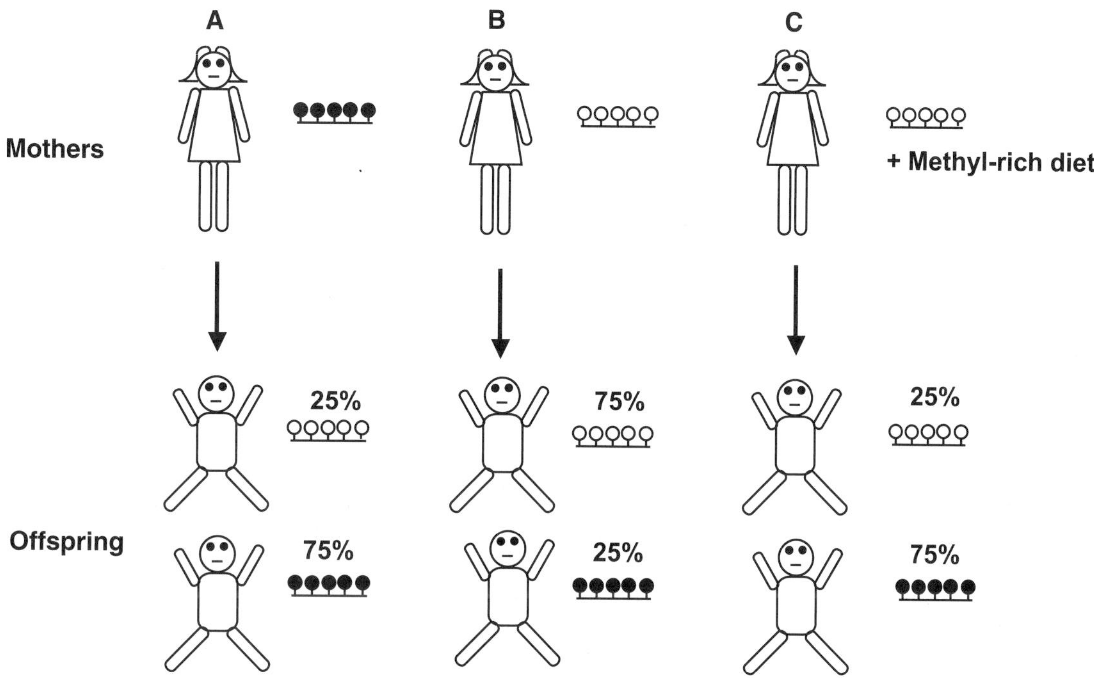

FIGURE 8.8 Epigenetic metastability. In epigenetic metastability, the maternal epigenome influences the epigenetic characteristics of the offspring. In this hypothetical example, mothers with a methylated epigenome (signified by filled-in lollipops, representing deoxyribonucleic acid [DNA] methylation, on a black line, representing the DNA strand) primarily have offspring with a methylated epigenome (*A*), whereas mothers with an unmethylated epigenome primarily have offspring with an unmethylated epigenome (*B*) (signified by empty lollipops, representing absent DNA methylation, on a black line, representing the DNA strand). However, mothers with an unmethylated epigenome that consume a diet rich in methyl donors primarily give birth to offspring with a methylated epigenome (*C*).

pseudoagouti offspring due to increased methylation of the A^{vy} retrotransposon upstream of the allele (Waterland and Jirtle, 2003).

Not all epigenetic marks are set early in development. At least in some cases, epigenetic modifications may be altered even after terminal cell differentiation has already occurred. For example, the maternal behavior of rat dams alters DNA methylation patterns in their offspring. Pups raised by dams that frequently lick, groom, and nurse them, so-called high licking and grooming (hereafter, HLG) mothers, have decreased CpG methylation in the exon 1_7 promoter of the glucocorticoid receptor (*Nr3c1*) gene compared to offspring of low licking and grooming (hereafter, LLG) dams that only rarely lick, groom, and nurse their offspring. In particular, demethylation of a cytosine residue within an NGFI-A transcription factor binding site in the *Nr3c1* exon 1_7 promoter enhances transcription of *Nr3c1*, resulting in increased levels of the glucocorticoid receptor protein in the hippocampus. This enables the adult offspring of HLG dams to more efficiently suppress stress-induced activation of the hypothalamic-pituitary-adrenal axis. As a result, rats raised by HLG dams have lower serum glucocorticoid levels and decreased anxiety-like behavior compared with rats raised by LLG dams (Weaver et al., 2004).

Interestingly, some evidence suggests that similar processes might also exist in humans. For example, in a prospective study of 170 mother–infant pairs, Huizink et al. (2002) found that various forms of maternal anxiety, including perceived maternal stress and pregnancy anxiety, predicted the temperament of infants at 3 and 8 months of age. Likewise, Austin et al. (2005) observed that maternal trait anxiety, as measured by psychological self-questionnaire during the third trimester of pregnancy, accurately predicted the temperament of infants at 4–6 months of age. Maternal anxiety in humans also affects stress hormone levels in offspring. Yehuda et al. (2005) identified a relationship between cortisol levels during pregnancy in women with post-traumatic stress disorder and cortisol levels in their infant offspring. These effects appear to be long lasting, similar to the effects observed in rats. Gutteling et al. (2005), analyzing the same cohort as Huizink et al. (2002), found that children of women with higher levels of pregnancy anxiety had higher cortisol responses on their first day of school for the year. Moreover, maternal cortisol levels during pregnancy were directly correlated with cortisol levels in their children (Gutteling et al., 2005). Although definitive evidence is still lacking, results like these suggest the possibility that epigenetic mechanisms might regulate human susceptibility to anxiety disorders.

Still, there is evidence that epigenetic differences exist between individuals and that these differences are acquired over the course of a lifetime. For example, a study that examined the DNA methylation status of over 250 unique amplicons in the human major histocompatibility complex (MHC) found that 46% of the regions analyzed demonstrated evidence of interindividual variation (Rakyan et al., 2004). Another study examined DNA methylation and histone H3 and H4 acetylation patterns in lymphocytes from monozygotic twin pairs. Although most twins had similar epigenetic profiles, 35% of the pairs were discordant for all three epigenetic modifications. Furthermore, the authors found a significant association between age and epigenetic discordance, with older twin pairs more discordant than younger twin pairs. As well, they found a significant association between life history and epigenetic discordance, with twins that lived in different environments or had different medical histories also presenting with higher levels of epigenetic discordance (Fraga et al., 2005).

Currently there is no evidence that epigenetic inheritance, epigenetic metastability, or epigenetic plasticity contributes to the development of psychiatric disease. However, Petronis (2004) speculated that such mechanisms might play a significant role in the development of schizophrenia, which could explain some aspects of its epidemiology, including the incidence of monozygotic twin discordance for the disease, its variable age of onset, and the waxing and waning of its clinical course. Similarly, Jiang et al. (2004) proposed that a mixed epigenetic and genetic and mixed de novo and inherited (MEGDI) model might explain a fraction of cases of autism. The MEGDI model predicts that epigenetic mutations, or epimutations, in addition to genetic mutations, cause autism, and it suggests that epigenetic inheritance and metastable epialleles contribute to the development and complex epidemiology of autism. Intriguingly, it has been further suggested that a MEGDI model could help explain other neuropsychiatric disorders (Jiang et al.). For the moment though, the involvement of epigenetic inheritance, epigenetic metastability, and epigenetic plasticity in psychiatric disease remains an interesting hypothesis, the merits of which must be put to the test through more research.

INTERVENTIONAL EPIGENETIC MODIFICATION

Epigenetic plasticity of the type described in the examples above is important because it provides the potential for a link between environmental insults and phenotypes, including behavioral phenotypes. One important implication of epigenetic plasticity is that, at least in some cases, there may be an opportunity to perform interventions directed at preventing or reversing deleterious epigenetic modifications. Alternatively, it may be possible to promote or even augment protective or advantageous epigenetic modifications. The most obvious intervention is pharmacologic therapy or prophylaxis using drugs tailored to affect a particular epigenetic modification. Indeed, much research is currently being devoted toward the development of drugs that target DNA methylation and histone modification.

One potentially useful class of drugs is DNMT inhibitors, which interfere with DNA methylation, thereby promoting the activation of epigenetically repressed genes. Representative DNMT inhibitors include the chemotherapeutic agents *doxorubicin, azacytidine,* and *zebularine.* Mice treated with these agents show increased expression of *RELN* and *GAD67*, two genes downregulated in schizophrenics, suggesting that DNMT inhibitors might be useful for treating this devastating psychiatric disease if toxic effects can be avoided (Kundakovic et al., 2007).

Another important class of drugs under development is HDAC inhibitors, which promote the activation of epigenetically repressed genes by interfering with histone deacetylation. Preclinical studies using this class of drugs suggest that they may prove to be useful in treating a variety of psychiatric conditions. For example, the anxiety phenotype of LLG rat offspring is reversed by treatment with the HDAC inhibitor *trichostatin A* (Weaver et al., 2006), as is the hyperactive stress response in these animals (Weaver et al., 2004). Similarly, sodium butyrate, another HDAC inhibitor, is an effective anxiolytic in mice and has a synergistic effect when combined with fluoxetine (Schroeder et al., 2006). Of particular interest are newer HDAC inhibitors that concentrate in specific brain regions, such as MS-275, a frontal cortex-selective agent that may prove useful for the treatment of schizophrenia (Simonini et al., 2006).

It is interesting that new evidence indicates that the mechanism of action of some current psychiatric medications involves altering covalent histone modifications. For example, valproic acid, a commonly used mood stabilizer, is an HDAC antagonist (Phiel et al., 2001). In addition to its use in treating bipolar disease, valproate has also been shown to be effective in treating schizophrenia (Casey et al., 2003). This may be due to its effects on the expression of *RELN* and *GAD67*. In mice, valproate promotes the expression of both genes, the expression of which is reduced in a putative mouse model of schizophrenia, *the heterozygous reeler mouse* (Tremolizzo et al., 2002).

Antidepressants are also proving to have unexpected effects on epigenetic processes. Chronic treatment with the tricyclic antidepressant imipramine promoted increased acetylation of histone H3 at lysine 9 and lysine 14 at the *Bdnf* locus of chronically stressed mice.

This was accompanied by increased *Bdnf* expression and an antidepressant effect (Tsankova et al., 2006). In another study, Cassel et al. (2006) found that the antidepressant effect of chronic fluoxetine treatment was associated with increased HDAC expression and reduced overall levels of histone acetylation in GABAergic interneurons in the rat striatum, dentate gyrus, and frontal cortex. This was also accompanied by increased expression of the genes *MeCP2* and *MBD1* in the same neurons, suggesting that fluoxetine may also have an indirect effect on DNA methylation. Curiously, the data from these studies indicate that HDAC inhibition (by butyrate and imipramine) and HDAC enhancement (by fluoxetine) produce an identical therapeutic result (antidepressant effect). A variety of hypotheses have been proposed to explain these inconsistencies (Newton and Duman, 2006), but they have yet to be explored.

Besides pharmacotherapy, dietary modification may be a cheap and effective method whereby the epigenetic code can be modified, especially with respect to DNA methylation. Supplementation with either folic acid or methionine has been hypothesized to alter DNA methylation, and it has been suggested that such alterations might affect psychiatric symptoms (Tremolizzo et al., 2002; Peedicayil and Subbanna, 2007). In support of this concept, folate administration relieves some psychiatric symptoms in schizophrenia (Godfrey et al., 1990) and depression (Young and Ghadirian, 1989; Bottiglieri et al., 2000). On the other hand, methionine supplementation exacerbates symptoms of psychosis (Cohen et al., 1974) and mania (Mischoulon and Fava, 2002; Pancheri et al., 2002). Although these studies demonstrate a correlation between specific dietary modifications and symptomatic outcomes in psychiatric disease, it is important to keep in mind that neither these nor any other study has yet provided clear-cut evidence of changes in DNA methylation patterns in a population of psychiatric patients after treating them with dietary modification.

CONCLUSION

Although epigenetics as a field of study is young, the discipline of psychiatric epigenetics can genuinely be described as in its infancy. Fundamental questions regarding the exact role of epigenetic processes in the development and pathogenesis of psychiatric disease remain unanswered. How are global and local patterns of epigenetic modification different in patients with psychiatric diseases as compared to the general population? Are epigenomic changes the cause or the consequence of psychiatric disease? Are any psychiatric diseases epigenetically inherited? Do environmental effects on the epigenome contribute to the development of psychiatric disease? Can treatments that modify epigenetic marks be used to successfully treat psychiatric conditions? Although there are many unknowns one thing is certain: As our understanding of the basic mechanisms controlling the establishment, maintenance, interpretation, and modification of the epigenetic code increases, so too will our ability to apply this knowledge to answer these and other questions.

REFERENCES

Aapola, U., Kawasaki, K., Scott, H. S., Ollila, J., Vihinen, M., Heino, M., Shintani, A., Minoshima, S., Krohn, K., Antonarakis, S.E., Shimizu, N., Kudoh, J. and Peterson, P. (2000) Isolation and initial characterization of a novel zinc finger gene, DNMT3L, on 21q22.3, related to the cytosine-5-methyltransferase 3 gene family. *Genomics* 65(3):293–298.

Abdolmaleky, H.M., Cheng, K.H., Faraone, S.V., Wilcox, M., Glatt, S.J., Gao, F., Smith, C.L., Shafa, R., Aeali, B., Carnevale, J., Pan, H., Papageorgis, P., Ponte, J.F., Sivaraman, V., Tsuang, M. T., and Thiagalingam, S. (2006) Hypomethylation of MB-COMT promoter is a major risk factor for schizophrenia and bipolar disorder. *Hum. Mol. Genet.* 15(21):3132–3145.

Abdolmaleky, H.M., Cheng, K.H., Russo, A., Smith, C.L., Faraone, S.V., Wilcox, M., Shafa, R., Glatt, S.J., Nguyen, G., Ponte, J.F., Thiagalingam, S., and Tsuang, M.T. (2005) Hypermethylation of the reelin (RELN) promoter in the brain of schizophrenic patients: a preliminary report. *Am. J. Med. Genet. B Neuropsychiatr. Genet.* 134(1):60–66.

Akbarian, S., Ruehl, M.G., Bliven, E., Luiz, L.A., Peranelli, A.C., Baker, S.P., Roberts, R.C., Bunney, W.E., Jr., Conley, R.C., Jones, E.G., Tamminga, C.A., and Guo, Y. (2005) Chromatin alterations associated with down-regulated metabolic gene expression in the prefrontal cortex of subjects with schizophrenia. *Arch. Gen. Psychiatry* 62(8):829–840.

Alarcon, J. M., Malleret, G., Touzani, K., Vronskaya, S., Ishii, S., Kandel, E.R., and Barco, A. (2004) Chromatin acetylation, memory, and LTP are impaired in CBP+/– mice: a model for the cognitive deficit in Rubinstein-Taybi syndrome and its amelioration. *Neuron* 42(6):947–959.

Albrecht, U., Sutcliffe, J.S., Cattanach, B.M., Beechey, C.V., Armstrong, D., Eichele, G., and Beaudet, A.L. (1997) Imprinted expression of the murine Angelman syndrome gene, UBE3A, in hippocampal and Purkinje neurons. *Nat. Genet.* 17(1):75–78.

Allis, C. D., Jenuwein, T., and Reinberg, D. (2007) Overview and concepts. In: Allis, C. D., Jenuwein, T., Reinberg, D., and Caparros, M.L., eds. *Epigenetics*. Cold Spring Harbor, NY: Cold Spring Harbor Laboratory Press, pp. 23–62.

American Psychiatric Association. (1994) *Diagnostic and Statistical Manual of Mental Disorders* (4th ed.). Washington, DC: Author.

Amir, R.E., Van den Veyver, I.B., Wan, M., Tran, C.Q., Francke, U. and Zoghbi, H.Y. (1999) Rett syndrome is caused by mutations in X-linked MECP2, encoding methyl-CpG-binding protein 2. *Nat. Genet.* 23(2):185–188.

Applebaum, J., Shimon, H., Sela, B.A., Belmaker, R.H., and Levine, J. (2004) Homocysteine levels in newly admitted schizophrenic patients. *J. Psychiatr. Res.* 38(4):413–416.

Archer, H.L., Whatley, S.D., Evans, J.C., Ravine, D., Huppke, P., Kerr, A., Bunyan, D., Kerr, B., Sweeney, E., Davies, S.J., Reardon, W., Horn, J., MacDermot, K.D., Smith, R.A., Magee, A., Donaldson, A., Crow, Y., Hermon, G., Miedzybrodzka, Z., Cooper, D.N., Lazarou, L., Butler, R., Sampson, J., Pilz, D.T., Laccone, F., and Clarke, A.J. (2006) Gross rearrangements of the MECP2 gene are found in both classical and atypical Rett syndrome patients. *J. Med. Genet.* 43(5):451–456.

Arinami, T. (2006) Analyses of the associations between the genes of 22q11 deletion syndrome and schizophrenia. *J. Hum. Genet.* 51(12):1037–1045.

Ashley, C.T., Jr., Wilkinson, K.D., Reines, D., and Warren, S.T. (1993) FMR1 protein: conserved RNP family domains and selective RNA binding. *Science* 262(5133):563–566.

Aston, C., Jiang, L., and Sokolov, B.P. (2004) Microarray analysis of postmortem temporal cortex from patients with schizophrenia. *J. Neurosci. Res.* 77(6):858–866.

Austin, M.P., Hadzi-Pavlovic, D., Leader, L., Saint, K., and Parker, G. (2005) Maternal trait anxiety, depression and life event stress in pregnancy: relationships with infant temperament. *Early Hum. Dev.* 81(2):183–190.

Backes, M., Genc, B., Schreck, J., Doerfler, W., Lehmkuhl, G., and von Gontard, A. (2000) Cognitive and behavioral profile of fragile X boys: correlations to molecular data. *Am. J. Med. Genet.* 95(2):150–156.

Bale, T.L., and Vale, W.W. (2004) CRF and CRF receptors: role in stress responsivity and other behaviors. *Annu. Rev. Pharmacol. Toxicol.* 44:525–557.

Barreto, G., Schafer, A., Marhold, J., Stach, D., Swaminathan, S. K., Handa, V., Doderlein, G., Maltry, N., Wu, W., Lyko, F., and Niehrs, C. (2007) Gadd45a promotes epigenetic gene activation by repair-mediated DNA demethylation. *Nature* 445(7128):671–675.

Battaglia, A. (2005) The inv dup(15) or idic(15) syndrome: a clinically recognisable neurogenetic disorder. *Brain Dev.* 27(5):365–369.

Baumgardner, T.L., Reiss, A.L., Freund, L.S., and Abrams, M.T. (1995) Specification of the neurobehavioral phenotype in males with fragile X syndrome. *Pediatrics* 95(5):744–752.

Bestor, T. H. (2000) The DNA methyltransferases of mammals. *Hum. Mol. Genet.* 9(16):2395–2402.

Bestor, T.H., and Ingram, V.M. (1983) Two DNA methyltransferases from murine erythroleukemia cells: purification, sequence specificity, and mode of interaction with DNA. *Proc. Natl. Acad. Sci. USA* 80(18):5559–5563.

Billy, E., Brondani, V., Zhang, H., Muller, U., and Filipowicz, W. (2001) Specific interference with gene expression induced by long, double-stranded RNA in mouse embryonal teratocarcinoma cell lines. *Proc. Natl. Acad. Sci. USA* 98(25):14428–14433.

Bird, A. (2002) DNA methylation patterns and epigenetic memory. *Genes Dev.* 16(1):6–21.

Black, Y.D., Maclaren, F. R., Naydenov, A.V., Carlezon, W.A., Jr., Baxter, M.G., and Konradi, C. (2006) Altered attention and prefrontal cortex gene expression in rats after binge-like exposure to cocaine during adolescence. *J. Neurosci.* 26(38):9656–9665.

Bode, A.M., and Dong, Z. (2005) Inducible covalent posttranslational modification of histone H3. *Sci. STKE* 2005(281):RE4.

Bolton, P.F., Dennis, N.R., Browne, C.E., Thomas, N.S., Veltman, M.W., Thompson, R.J., and Jacobs, P. (2001) The phenotypic manifestations of interstitial duplications of proximal 15q with special reference to the autistic spectrum disorders. *Am. J. Med. Genet.* 105(8):675–685.

Borchert, G.M., Lanier, W., and Davidson, B.L. (2006) RNA polymerase III transcribes human microRNAs. *Nat. Struct. Mol. Biol.* 13(12):1097–1101.

Bottiglieri, T., Laundy, M., Crellin, R., Toone, B.K., Carney, M.W., and Reynolds, E.H. (2000) Homocysteine, folate, methylation, and monoamine metabolism in depression. *J. Neurol. Neurosurg. Psychiatry* 69(2):228–232.

Bourc'his, D., Xu, G.L., Lin, C.S., Bollman, B., and Bestor, T.H. (2001) Dnmt3L and the establishment of maternal genomic imprints. *Science* 294(5551):2536–2539.

Bourtchouladze, R., Lidge, R., Catapano, R., Stanley, J., Gossweiler, S., Romashko, D., Scott, R., and Tully, T. (2003) A mouse model of Rubinstein-Taybi syndrome: defective long-term memory is ameliorated by inhibitors of phosphodiesterase 4. *Proc. Natl. Acad. Sci. USA* 100(18):10518–10522.

Bregman, J.D., Leckman, J.F., and Ort, S.I. (1988) Fragile X syndrome: genetic predisposition to psychopathology. *J. Autism Dev. Disord.* 18(3):343–354.

Browne, C.E., Dennis, N.R., Maher, E., Long, F.L., Nicholson, J.C., Sillibourne, J., and Barber, J.C. (1997) Inherited interstitial duplications of proximal 15q: genotype-phenotype correlations. *Am. J. Hum. Genet.* 61(6):1342–1352.

Buhler, M., Verdel, A., and Moazed, D. (2006) Tethering RITS to a nascent transcript initiates RNAi- and heterochromatin-dependent gene silencing. *Cell* 125(5):873–886.

Buiting, K., Lich, C., Cottrell, S., Barnicoat, A., and Horsthemke, B. (1999) A 5-kb imprinting center deletion in a family with Angelman syndrome reduces the shortest region of deletion overlap to 880 bp. *Hum. Genet.* 105(6):665–666.

Buiting, K., Saitoh, S., Gross, S., Dittrich, B., Schwartz, S., Nicholls, R.D., and Horsthemke, B. (1995) Inherited microdeletions in the Angelman and Prader-Willi syndromes define an imprinting centre on human chromosome 15. *Nat. Genet.* 9(4):395–400.

Caiafa, P., and Zampieri, M. (2005) DNA methylation and chromatin structure: the puzzling CpG islands. *J. Cell Biochem.* 94(2): 257–265.

Cardoso, C., Timsit, S., Villard, L., Khrestchatisky, M., Fontes, M., and Colleaux, L. (1998) Specific interaction between the XNP/ATR-X gene product and the SET domain of the human EZH2 protein. *Hum. Mol. Genet.* 7(4):679–684.

Carney, R.M., Wolpert, C.M., Ravan, S.A., Shahbazian, M., Ashley-Koch, A., Cuccaro, M.L., Vance, J.M., and Pericak-Vance, M.A. (2003) Identification of MeCP2 mutations in a series of females with autistic disorder. *Pediatr. Neurol.* 28(3):205–211.

Casey, D.E., Daniel, D.G., Wassef, A.A., Tracy, K.A., Wozniak, P., and Sommerville, K.W. (2003) Effect of divalproex combined with olanzapine or risperidone in patients with an acute exacerbation of schizophrenia. *Neuropsychopharmacology* 28(1):182–192.

Cassel, S., Carouge, D., Gensburger, C., Anglard, P., Burgun, C., Dietrich, J. B., Aunis, D., and Zwiller, J. (2006) Fluoxetine and cocaine induce the epigenetic factors MeCP2 and MBD1 in adult rat brain. *Mol. Pharmacol.* 70(2):487–492.

Castanotto, D., Tommasi, S., Li, M., Li, H., Yanow, S., Pfeifer, G. P., and Rossi, J. J. (2005) Short hairpin RNA-directed cytosine (CpG) methylation of the RASSF1A gene promoter in HeLa cells. *Mol. Ther.* 12(1):179–183.

Chamberlain, S.J., and Brannan, C.I. (2001) The Prader-Willi syndrome imprinting center activates the paternally expressed murine Ube3a antisense transcript but represses paternal Ube3a. *Genomics* 73(3):316–322.

Chan, T.L., Yuen, S.T., Kong, C.K., Chan, Y.W., Chan, A.S., Ng, W.F., Tsui, W.Y., Lo, M.W., Tam, W.Y., Li, V.S., and Leung, S.Y. (2006) Heritable germline epimutation of MSH2 in a family with hereditary nonpolyposis colorectal cancer. *Nat. Genet.* 38(10): 1178–1183.

Chen, Y., Sharma, R.P., Costa, R.H., Costa, E., and Grayson, D.R. (2002) On the epigenetic regulation of the human reelin promoter. *Nucleic Acids Res.* 30(13):2930–2939.

Chendrimada, T.P., Gregory, R.I., Kumaraswamy, E., Norman, J., Cooch, N., Nishikura, K., and Shiekhattar, R. (2005) TRBP recruits the Dicer complex to Ago2 for microRNA processing and gene silencing. *Nature* 436(7051):740–744.

Choi, J.D., Underkoffler, L.A., Wood, A.J., Collins, J.N., Williams, P.T., Golden, J.A., Schuster, E.F., Jr., Loomes, K.M., and Oakey, R.J. (2005) A novel variant of Inpp5f is imprinted in brain, and its expression is correlated with differential methylation of an internal CpG island. *Mol. Cell Biol.* 25(13):5514–5522.

Chu, C.Y., and Rana, T.M. (2006) Translation repression in human cells by microRNA-induced gene silencing requires RCK/p54. *PLoS Biol.* 4(7):E210.

Clifford, S., Dissanayake, C., Bui, Q.M., Huggins, R., Taylor, A.K., and Loesch, D.Z. (2007) Autism spectrum phenotype in males and females with fragile x full mutation and premutation. *J. Autism Dev. Disord.* 37(4):738–747.

Coffee, B., Zhang, F., Ceman, S., Warren, S.T., and Reines, D. (2002) Histone modifications depict an aberrantly heterochromatinized FMR1 gene in fragile x syndrome. *Am. J. Hum. Genet.* 71(4): 923–932.

Coffee, B., Zhang, F., Warren, S.T., and Reines, D. (1999) Acetylated histones are associated with FMR1 in normal but not fragile X-syndrome cells. *Nat. Genet.* 22(1):98–101.

Cohen, S.M., Nichols, A., Wyatt, R., and Pollin, W. (1974) The administration of methionine to chronic schizophrenic patients: a review of ten studies. *Biol. Psychiatry* 8(2):209–225.

Coleman, M., Brubaker, J., Hunter, K., and Smith, G. (1988) Rett syndrome: a survey of North American patients. *J. Ment. Defic. Res.* 32(Pt 2):117–124.

Cook, E.H., Jr., Lindgren, V., Leventhal, B. L., Courchesne, R., Lincoln, A., Shulman, C., Lord, C., and Courchesne, E. (1997) Autism or atypical autism in maternally but not paternally derived proximal 15q duplication. *Am. J. Hum. Genet.* 60(4):928–934.

Cooney, C.A., Dave, A.A., and Wolff, G.L. (2002) Maternal methyl supplements in mice affect epigenetic variation and DNA methylation of offspring. *J. Nutr.* 132(8 Suppl):2393S–2400S.

Couvert, P., Bienvenu, T., Aquaviva, C., Poirier, K., Moraine, C., Gendrot, C., Verloes, A., Andres, C., Le Fevre, A.C., Souville, I., Steffann, J., des Portes, V., Ropers, H.H., Yntema, H.G., Fryns, J. P., Briault, S., Chelly, J., and Cherif, B. (2001) MECP2 is highly mutated in X-linked mental retardation. *Hum. Mol. Genet.* 10(9):941–946.

Crawford, D.C., Acuna, J.M., and Sherman, S.L. (2001) FMR1 and the fragile X syndrome: human genome epidemiology review. *Genet. Med.* 3(5):359–371.

de la Serna, I.L., Ohkawa, Y., and Imbalzano, A.N. (2006) Chromatin remodelling in mammalian differentiation: lessons from ATP-dependent remodellers. *Nat. Rev. Genet.* 7(6):461–473.

Delaval, K., and Feil, R. (2004) Epigenetic regulation of mammalian genomic imprinting. *Curr. Opin. Genet. Dev.* 14(2):188–195.

Denli, A.M., Tops, B.B., Plasterk, R.H., Ketting, R.F., and Hannon, G.J. (2004) Processing of primary microRNAs by the microprocessor complex. *Nature* 432(7014):231–235.

Descheemaeker, M.J., Govers, V., Vermeulen, P., and Fryns, J.P. (2006) Pervasive developmental disorders in Prader-Willi syndrome: the Leuven experience in 59 subjects and controls. *Am. J. Med. Genet. A* 140(11):1136–1142.

Ding, F., Prints, Y., Dhar, M.S., Johnson, D.K., Garnacho-Montero, C., Nicholls, R.D., and Francke, U. (2005) Lack of Pwcr1/MBII-85 snoRNA is critical for neonatal lethality in Prader-Willi syndrome mouse models. *Mamm. Genome* 16(6):424–431.

Doench, J.G., Petersen, C.P., and Sharp, P.A. (2003) siRNAs can function as miRNAs. *Genes Dev.* 17(4):438–442.

Eastwood, S.L., and Harrison, P.J. (2003) Interstitial white matter neurons express less reelin and are abnormally distributed in schizophrenia: towards an integration of molecular and morphologic aspects of the neurodevelopmental hypothesis. *Mol. Psychiatry* 8(9):769, 821–831.

Evans, H.K., Wylie, A.A., Murphy, S.K., and Jirtle, R.L. (2001) The neuronatin gene resides in a "micro-imprinted" domain on human chromosome 20q11.2. *Genomics* 77(1-2):99–104.

Fatemi, S.H., Earle, J.A., and McMenomy, T. (2000) Reduction in Reelin immunoreactivity in hippocampus of subjects with schizophrenia, bipolar disorder and major depression. *Mol. Psychiatry* 5(6):654–663.

Feng, Y., Absher, D., Eberhart, D.E., Brown, V., Malter, H.E., and Warren, S.T. (1997) FMRP associates with polyribosomes as an mRNP, and the I304N mutation of severe fragile X syndrome abolishes this association. *Mol. Cell* 1(1):109–118.

Fraga, M.F., Ballestar, E., Paz, M.F., Ropero, S., Setien, F., Ballestar, M.L., Heine-Suner, D., Cigudosa, J.C., Urioste, M., Benitez, M., Boix-Chornet, M., Sanchez-Aguilera, A., Ling, C., Carlsson, E., Poulsen, P., Vaag, A., Stephan, Z., Spector, T.D., Wu, Y. Z., Plass, C., and Esteller, M. (2005) Epigenetic differences arise during the lifetime of monozygotic twins. *Proc. Natl. Acad. Sci. USA* 102(30):10604–10609.

Friso, S., Choi, S.W., Girelli, D., Mason, J.B., Dolnikowski, G.G., Bagley, P.J., Olivieri, O., Jacques, P.F., Rosenberg, I.H., Corrocher, R., and Selhub, J. (2002) A common mutation in the 5,10-methylenetetrahydrofolate reductase gene affects genomic DNA methylation through an interaction with folate status. *Proc. Natl. Acad. Sci. USA* 99(8):5606–5611.

Frosst, P., Blom, H.J., Milos, R., Goyette, P., Sheppard, C.A., Matthews, R.G., Boers, G.J., den Heijer, M., Kluijtmans, L.A., van den Heuvel, L.P., et al. (1995) A candidate genetic risk factor for vascular disease: a common mutation in methylenetetrahydrofolate reductase. *Nat. Genet.* 10(1):111–113.

Fryns, J.P., Jacobs, J., Kleczkowska, A., and van den Berghe, H. (1984) The psychological profile of the fragile X syndrome. *Clin. Genet.* 25(2):131–134.

Fuks, F., Hurd, P.J., Wolf, D., Nan, X., Bird, A.P., and Kouzarides, T. (2003) The methyl-CpG-binding protein MeCP2 links DNA methylation to histone methylation. *J. Biol. Chem.* 278(6):4035–4040.

Gallagher, R.C., Pils, B., Albalwi, M., and Francke, U. (2002). Evidence for the role of PWCR1/HBII-85 C/D box small nucleolar RNAs in Prader-Willi syndrome. *Am. J. Hum. Genet.* 71(3): 669–678.

Gibbons, R. (2006) Alpha thalassaemia-mental retardation, X linked. *Orphanet. J. Rare Dis.* 1:15.

Gibbons, R.J., Bachoo, S., Picketts, D.J., Aftimos, S., Asenbauer, B., Bergoffen, J., Berry, S.A., Dahl, N., Fryer, A., Keppler, K., Kurosawa, K., Levin, M.L., Masuno, M., Neri, G., Pierpont, M.E., Slaney, S.F., and Higgs, D.R. (1997) Mutations in transcriptional regulator ATRX establish the functional significance of a PHD-like domain. *Nat. Genet.* 17(2):146–148.

Gibbons, R.J., Picketts, D.J., Villard, L., and Higgs, D.R. (1995) Mutations in a putative global transcriptional regulator cause X-linked mental retardation with a-thalassemia (ATR-X syndrome). *Cell* 80:837–845.

Gilbody, S., Lewis, S., and Lightfoot, T. (2007) Methylenetetrahydro folate reductase (MTHFR) genetic polymorphisms and psychiatric disorders: a HuGE review. *Am. J. Epidemiol.* 165(1):1–13.

Godfrey, P.S., Toone, B.K., Carney, M.W., Flynn, T.G., Bottiglieri, T., Laundy, M., Chanarin, I., and Reynolds, E.H. (1990) Enhancement of recovery from psychiatric illness by methylfolate. *Lancet* 336(8712):392–395.

Goff, D.C., Bottiglieri, T., Arning, E., Shih, V., Freudenreich, O., Evins, A.E., Henderson, D.C., Baer, L., and Coyle, J. (2004) Folate, homocysteine, and negative symptoms in schizophrenia. *Am. J. Psychiatry* 161(9):1705–1708.

Goldstone, A.P. (2004) Prader-Willi syndrome: advances in genetics, pathophysiology and treatment. *Trends Endocrinol. Metab.* 15(1):12–20.

Goll, M.G., Kirpekar, F., Maggert, K.A., Yoder, J.A., Hsieh, C.L., Zhang, X., Golic, K.G., Jacobsen, S.E., and Bestor, T.H. (2006) Methylation of tRNAAsp by the DNA methyltransferase homolog Dnmt2. *Science* 311(5759):395–398.

Gotts, E.E., and Liemohn, W.P. (1977) Behavioral characteristics of three children with the broad thumb-hallux (Rubinstein-Taybi) syndrome. *Biol. Psychiatry* 12(3):413–423.

Grayson, D.R., Chen, Y., Costa, E., Dong, E., Guidotti, A., Kundakovic, M., and Sharma, R.P. (2006) The human reelin gene: transcription factors (+), repressors (-) and the methylation switch (+/–) in schizophrenia. *Pharmacol. Ther.* 111(1):272–286.

Grayson, D.R., Jia, X., Chen, Y., Sharma, R.P., Mitchell, C.P., Guidotti, A., and Costa, E. (2005) Reelin promoter hypermethylation in schizophrenia. *Proc. Natl. Acad. Sci. USA* 102(26): 9341–9346.

Gregory, R.I., Chendrimada, T.P., Cooch, N., and Shiekhattar, R. (2005) Human RISC couples microRNA biogenesis and posttranscriptional gene silencing. *Cell* 123(4):631–640.

Gregory, R.I., Yan, K.P., Amuthan, G., Chendrimada, T., Doratotaj, B., Cooch, N., and Shiekhattar, R. (2004) The microprocessor complex mediates the genesis of microRNAs. *Nature* 432(7014): 235–240.

Grimaud, C., Negre, N., and Cavalli, G. (2006) From genetics to epigenetics: the tale of polycomb group and trithorax group genes. *Chromosome Res.* 14(4):363–375.

Guenther, B.D., Sheppard, C.A., Tran, P., Rozen, R., Matthews, R.G., and Ludwig, M.L. (1999) The structure and properties of methylenetetrahydrofolate reductase from Escherichia coli suggest how folate ameliorates human hyperhomocysteinemia. *Nat. Struct. Biol.* 6(4):359–365.

Guidotti, A., Auta, J., Davis, J.M., Di-Giorgi-Gerevini, V., Dwivedi, Y., Grayson, D.R., Impagnatiello, F., Pandey, G., Pesold, C., Sharma, R., Uzunov, D., and Costa, E. (2000) Decrease in reelin and glutamic acid decarboxylase67 (GAD67) expression in schizophrenia and bipolar disorder: a postmortem brain study. *Arch. Gen. Psychiatry* 57(11):1061–1069.

Gutteling, B.M., de Weerth, C., and Buitelaar, J.K. (2005) Prenatal stress and children's cortisol reaction to the first day of school. *Psychoneuroendocrinology* 30(6):541–549.

Hagberg, B., Hanefeld, F., Percy, A., and Skjeldal, O. (2002) An update on clinically applicable diagnostic criteria in Rett syndrome. Comments to Rett Syndrome Clinical Criteria Consensus Panel Satellite to European Paediatric Neurology Society Meeting, Baden Baden, Germany, 11 September 2001. *Eur. J. Paediatr. Neurol.* 6(5):293–297.

Haig, D. (2004) The (dual) origin of epigenetics. *Cold Spring Harb. Symp. Quant. Biol.* 69:67–70.

Han, J., Lee, Y., Yeom, K.H., Kim, Y.K., Jin, H., and Kim, V.N. (2004) The Drosha-DGCR8 complex in primary microRNA processing. *Genes Dev.* 18(24):3016–3027.

Handa, V., Saha, T., and Usdin, K. (2003) The fragile X syndrome repeats form RNA hairpins that do not activate the interferon-inducible protein kinase, PKR, but are cut by Dicer. *Nucleic Acids Res.* 31(21):6243–6248.

Harikrishnan, K.N., Chow, M.Z., Baker, E.K., Pal, S., Bassal, S., Brasacchio, D., Wang, L., Craig, J.M., Jones, P.L., Sif, S., and El-Osta, A. (2005) Brahma links the SWI/SNF chromatin-remodeling complex with MeCP2-dependent transcriptional silencing. *Nat. Genet.* 37(3):254–264.

Hark, A.T., Schoenherr, C.J., Katz, D.J., Ingram, R.S., Levorse, J.M., and Tilghman, S.M. (2000) CTCF mediates methylation-sensitive enhancer-blocking activity at the H19/Igf2 locus. *Nature* 405(6785):486–489.

Hata, K., Okano, M., Lei, H., and Li, E. (2002) Dnmt3L cooperates with the Dnmt3 family of de novo DNA methyltransferases to establish maternal imprints in mice. *Development* 129(8): 1983–1993.

Hatton, D.D., Hooper, S.R., Bailey, D.B., Skinner, M.L., Sullivan, K.M., and Wheeler, A. (2002) Problem behavior in boys with fragile X syndrome. *Am. J. Med. Genet.* 108(2):105–116.

Hellings, J.A., Hossain, S., Martin, J.K., and Baratang, R.R. (2002) Psychopathology, GABA, and the Rubinstein-Taybi syndrome: a review and case study. *Am. J. Med. Genet.* 114(2):190–195.

Henderson, D.C., Borba, C.P., Daley, T.B., Boxill, R., Nguyen, D.D., Culhane, M.A., Louie, P., Cather, C., Eden Evins, A., Freudenreich, O., Taber, S.M., and Goff, D.C. (2006) Dietary intake profile of patients with schizophrenia. *Ann. Clin. Psychiatry* 18(2):99–105.

Hennekam, R.C. (2006) Rubinstein-Taybi syndrome. *Eur. J. Hum. Genet.* 14(9):981–985.

Hennekam, R.C., Baselier, A.C., Beyaert, E., Bos, A., Blok, J.B., Jansma, H.B., Thorbecke-Nilsen, V.V., and Veerman, H. (1992) Psychological and speech studies in Rubinstein-Taybi syndrome. *Am. J. Ment. Retard.* 96(6):645–660.

Hermann, A., Schmitt, S., and Jeltsch, A. (2003) The human Dnmt2 has residual DNA-(cytosine-C5) methyltransferase activity. *J. Biol. Chem.* 278(34):31717–31721.

Herz, J., and Chen, Y. (2006) Reelin, lipoprotein receptors and synaptic plasticity. *Nat. Rev. Neurosci.* 7(11):850–859.

Hitchins, M.P., Wong, J.J., Suthers, G., Suter, C.M., Martin, D.I., Hawkins, N.J., and Ward, R.L. (2007) Inheritance of a cancer-associated MLH1 germ-line epimutation. *N. Engl. J. Med.* 356(7):697–705.

Hoffbuhr, K., Devaney, J.M., LaFleur, B., Sirianni, N., Scacheri, C., Giron, J., Schuette, J., Innis, J., Marino, M., Philippart, M., Narayanan, V., Umansky, R., Kronn, D., Hoffman, E.P., and Naidu, S. (2001) MeCP2 mutations in children with and without the phenotype of Rett syndrome. *Neurology* 56(11):1486–1495.

Huizink, A.C., de Medina, P.G., Mulder, E.J., Visser, G.H., and Buitelaar, J.K. (2002) Psychological measures of prenatal stress as predictors of infant temperament. *J. Am. Acad. Child Adolesc. Psychiatry* 41(9):1078–1085.

Hutvagner, G., McLachlan, J., Pasquinelli, A.E., Balint, E., Tuschl, T., and Zamore, P.D. (2001) A cellular function for the RNA-interference enzyme Dicer in the maturation of the let-7 small temporal RNA. *Science* 293(5531):834–838.

Hutvagner, G., and Zamore, P.D. (2002) A microRNA in a multiple-turnover RNAi enzyme complex. *Science* 297(5589):2056–2060.

Jackson-Grusby, L., Beard, C., Possemato, R., Tudor, M., Fambrough, D., Csankovszki, G., Dausman, J., Lee, P., Wilson, C., Lander, E., and Jaenisch, R. (2001) Loss of genomic methylation causes p53-dependent apoptosis and epigenetic deregulation. *Nat. Genet.* 27(1):31–39.

Jelinic, P., Stehle, J.C., and Shaw, P. (2006) The testis-specific factor CTCFL cooperates with the protein methyltransferase PRMT7 in H19 imprinting control region methylation. *PLoS Biol.* 4(11): E355.

Jenuwein, T., and Allis, C.D. (2001) Translating the histone code. *Science* 293(5532):1074–1080.

Jhaveri, M.S., Wagner, C., and Trepel, J.B. (2001) Impact of extracellular folate levels on global gene expression. *Mol. Pharmacol.* 60(6):1288–1295.

Jiang, Y.H., Armstrong, D., Albrecht, U., Atkins, C.M., Noebels, J.L., Eichele, G., Sweatt, J.D., and Beaudet, A.L. (1998) Mutation of the Angelman ubiquitin ligase in mice causes increased cytoplasmic p53 and deficits of contextual learning and long-term potentiation. *Neuron* 21(4):799–811.

Jiang, Y.H., Sahoo, T., Michaelis, R.C., Bercovich, D., Bressler, J., Kashork, C.D., Liu, Q., Shaffer, L.G., Schroer, R.J., Stockton, D.W., Spielman, R.S., Stevenson, R.E., and Beaudet, A. L. (2004) A mixed epigenetic/genetic model for oligogenic inheritance of autism with a limited role for UBE3A. *Am. J. Med. Genet. A* 131(1):1–10.

Jin, P., Alisch, R.S., and Warren, S.T. (2004) RNA and microRNAs in fragile X mental retardation. *Nat. Cell Biol.* 6(11):1048–1053.

Jin, P., Zarnescu, D.C., Ceman, S., Nakamoto, M., Mowrey, J., Jongens, T.A., Nelson, D.L., Moses, K., and Warren, S.T. (2004) Biochemical and genetic interaction between the fragile X mental retardation protein and the microRNA pathway. *Nat. Neurosci.* 7(2):113–117.

Johnson, C.N., Adkins, N.L., and Georgel, P. (2005) Chromatin remodeling complexes: ATP-dependent machines in action. *Biochem. Cell Biol.* 83(4):405–417.

Jones, P.L., Veenstra, G.J., Wade, P.A., Vermaak, D., Kass, S.U., Landsberger, N., Strouboulis, J., and Wolffe, A.P. (1998) Methylated DNA and MeCP2 recruit histone deacetylase to repress transcription. *Nat. Genet.* 19(2):187–191.

Jordan, C., and Francke, U. (2006) Ube3a expression is not altered in Mecp2 mutant mice. *Hum. Mol. Genet.* 15(14):2210–2215.

Jorgensen, H.F., and Bird, A. (2002) MeCP2 and other methyl-CpG binding proteins. *Ment. Retard. Dev. Disabil. Res. Rev.* 8(2): 87–93.

Kanellopoulou, C., Muljo, S.A., Kung, A.L., Ganesan, S., Drapkin, R., Jenuwein, T., Livingston, D.M., and Rajewsky, K. (2005) Dicer-deficient mouse embryonic stem cells are defective in differentiation and centromeric silencing. *Genes Dev.* 19(4): 489–501.

Kankirawatana, P., Leonard, H., Ellaway, C., Scurlock, J., Mansour, A., Makris, C.M., Dure, L.S. 4th, Friez, M., Lane, J., Kiraly-Borri, C., Fabian, V., Davis, M., Jackson, J., Christodoulou, J., Kaufmann, W.E., Ravine, D., and Percy, A.K. (2006) Early progressive encephalopathy in boys and MECP2 mutations. *Neurology* 67(1):164–166.

Kantor, B., Kaufman, Y., Makedonski, K., Razin, A., and Shemer, R. (2004) Establishing the epigenetic status of the Prader-Willi/Angelman imprinting center in the gametes and embryo. *Hum. Mol. Genet.* 13(22):2767–2779.

Kantor, B., Makedonski, K., Green-Finberg, Y., Shemer, R., and Razin, A. (2004) Control elements within the PWS/AS imprinting box and their function in the imprinting process. *Hum. Mol. Genet.* 13(7):751–762.

Khandjian, E.W., Huot, M.E., Tremblay, S., Davidovic, L., Mazroui, R., and Bardoni, B. (2004) Biochemical evidence for the association of fragile X mental retardation protein with brain polyribosomal ribonucleoparticles. *Proc. Natl. Acad. Sci. USA* 101(36): 13357–13362.

Kimura, H., and Shiota, K. (2003) Methyl-CpG-binding protein, MeCP2, is a target molecule for maintenance DNA methyltransferase, Dnmt1. *J. Biol. Chem.* 278(7):4806–4812.

Kishino, T., Lalande, M., and Wagstaff, J. (1997) UBE3A/E6-AP mutations cause Angelman syndrome. *Nat. Genet.* 15(1): 70–73.

Klauck, S.M., Lindsay, S., Beyer, K.S., Splitt, M., Burn, J., and Poustka, A. (2002) A mutation hot spot for nonspecific X-linked mental retardation in the MECP2 gene causes the PPM-X syndrome. *Am. J. Hum. Genet.* 70(4):1034–1037.

Klose, R.J., and Bird, A.P. (2006) Genomic DNA methylation: the mark and its mediators. *Trends Biochem. Sci.* 31(2):89–97.

Klose, R.J., Sarraf, S.A., Schmiedeberg, L., McDermott, S.M., Stancheva, I., and Bird, A.P. (2005) DNA binding selectivity of MeCP2 due to a requirement for A/T sequences adjacent to methyl-CpG. *Mol. Cell* 19(5):667–678.

Klose, R.J., and Zhang, Y. (2007) Regulation of histone methylation by demethylimination and demethylation. *Nat. Rev. Mol. Cell Biol.* 8(4):307–318.

Kornberg, R.D. (1974) Chromatin structure: a repeating unit of histones and DNA. *Science* 184(139):868–871.

Kornberg, R.D., and Thomas, J.O. (1974) Chromatin structure: oligomers of the histones. *Science* 184(139):865–868.

Kouzarides, T., and Berger, S.L. (2007) Chromatin modifications and their mechanism of action. In: Allis, C.D., Jenuwein, T., Reinberg, D., and Caparros, M.L., eds. *Epigenetics*. Cold Spring Harbor, NY: Cold Spring Harbor Laboratory Press, pp. 191–210.

Kumar, A., Choi, K.H., Renthal, W., Tsankova, N.M., Theobald, D.E., Truong, H.T., Russo, S.J., Laplant, Q., Sasaki, T.S., Whistler, K.N., Neve, R.L., Self, D.W., and Nestler, E.J. (2005) Chromatin remodeling is a key mechanism underlying cocaine-induced plasticity in striatum. *Neuron* 48(2):303–314.

Kundakovic, M., Chen, Y., Costa, E., and Grayson, D.R. (2007) DNA methyltransferase inhibitors coordinately induce expression of the human reelin and glutamic acid decarboxylase 67 genes. *Mol. Pharmacol.* 71(3):644–653.

Laggerbauer, B., Ostareck, D., Keidel, E.M., Ostareck-Lederer, A., and Fischer, U. (2001) Evidence that fragile X mental retardation protein is a negative regulator of translation. *Hum. Mol. Genet.* 10(4):329–338.

Lagos-Quintana, M., Rauhut, R., Lendeckel, W., and Tuschl, T. (2001) Identification of novel genes coding for small expressed RNAs. *Science* 294(5543):853–858.

Lam, C.W., Yeung, W.L., Ko, C.H., Poon, P.M., Tong, S.F., Chan, K.Y., Lo, I.F., Chan, L.Y., Hui, J., Wong, V., Pang, C.P., Lo, K.M., and Fok, T.F. (2000) Spectrum of mutations in the MECP2 gene in patients with infantile autism and Rett syndrome. *J. Med. Genet.* 37(12):E41.

Landers, M., Bancescu, D.L., Le Meur, E., Rougeulle, C., Glatt-Deeley, H., Brannan, C., Muscatelli, F., and Lalande, M. (2004) Regulation of the large (approximately 1000 kb) imprinted murine Ube3a antisense transcript by alternative exons upstream of Snurf/Snrpn. *Nucleic Acids Res.* 32(11):3480–3492.

Landers, M., Calciano, M.A., Colosi, D., Glatt-Deeley, H., Wagstaff, J., and Lalande, M. (2005) Maternal disruption of Ube3a leads to increased expression of Ube3a-ATS in trans. *Nucleic Acids Res.* 33(13):3976–3984.

Landthaler, M., Yalcin, A., and Tuschl, T. (2004) The human DiGeorge syndrome critical region gene 8 and Its D. melanogaster homolog are required for miRNA biogenesis. *Curr. Biol.* 14(23):2162–2167.

Lau, N.C., Lim, L.P., Weinstein, E.G., and Bartel, D.P. (2001) An abundant class of tiny RNAs with probable regulatory roles in Caenorhabditis elegans. *Science* 294(5543):858–862.

Lee, R.C., and Ambros, V. (2001) An extensive class of small RNAs in Caenorhabditis elegans. *Science* 294(5543):862–864.

Lee, Y., Ahn, C., Han, J., Choi, H., Kim, J., Yim, J., Lee, J., Provost, P., Radmark, O., Kim, S., and Kim, V.N. (2003) The nuclear RNase III Drosha initiates microRNA processing. *Nature* 425(6956):415–419.

Lee, Y., Hur, I., Park, S.Y., Kim, Y.K., Suh, M.R., and Kim, V.N. (2006) The role of PACT in the RNA silencing pathway. *Embo. J.* 25(3):522–532.

Lee, Y., Jeon, K., Lee, J.T., Kim, S., and Kim, V.N. (2002) MicroRNA maturation: stepwise processing and subcellular localization. *Embo. J.* 21(17):4663–4670.

Lee, Y., Kim, M., Han, J., Yeom, K.H., Lee, S., Baek, S.H., and Kim, V.N. (2004) MicroRNA genes are transcribed by RNA polymerase II. *Embo. J.* 23(20):4051–4060.

Levenson, J.M., Roth, T.L., Lubin, F.D., Miller, C.A., Huang, I.C., Desai, P., Malone, L. M., and Sweatt, J.D. (2006) Evidence that DNA (cytosine-5) methyltransferase regulates synaptic plasticity in the hippocampus. *J. Biol. Chem.* 281(23):15763–15773.

Levine, J., Stahl, Z., Sela, B.A., Gavendo, S., Ruderman, V., and Belmaker, R.H. (2002) Elevated homocysteine levels in young male patients with schizophrenia. *Am. J. Psychiatry* 159(10): 1790–1792.

Levitas, A.S., and Reid, C.S. (1998) Rubinstein-Taybi syndrome and psychiatric disorders. *J. Intellect. Disabil. Res.* 42(Pt 4):284–292.

Lewis, S.J., Zammit, S., Gunnell, D., and Smith, G.D. (2005) A meta-analysis of the MTHFR C677T polymorphism and schizophrenia risk. *Am. J. Med. Genet. B Neuropsychiatr. Genet.* 135(1):2–4.

Li, E., and Bird, A. (2007) DNA methylation in mammals. In: Allis, C.D., Jenuwein, T., Reinberg, D., and Caparros, M.L., eds. *Epigenetics*. Cold Spring Harbor, NY: Cold Spring Harbor Laboratory Press, pp. 341–356.

Li, Z., Zhang, Y., Ku, L., Wilkinson, K.D., Warren, S.T., and Feng, Y. (2001) The fragile X mental retardation protein inhibits translation via interacting with mRNA. *Nucleic Acids Res.* 29(11): 2276–2283.

Liu, J., Carmell, M.A., Rivas, F.V., Marsden, C.G., Thomson, J.M., Song, J.J., Hammond, S.M., Joshua-Tor, L., and Hannon, G.J. (2004) Argonaute2 is the catalytic engine of mammalian RNAi. *Science* 305(5689):1437–1441.

Luedi, P.P., Hartemink, A.J., and Jirtle, R.L. (2005) Genome-wide prediction of imprinted murine genes. *Genome Res.* 15(6): 875–884.

Luger, K., Mader, A.W., Richmond, R.K., Sargent, D.F., and Richmond, T.J. (1997) Crystal structure of the nucleosome core particle at 2.8 A resolution. *Nature* 389(6648):251–260.

Lund, E., Guttinger, S., Calado, A., Dahlberg, J.E., and Kutay, U. (2004) Nuclear export of microRNA precursors. *Science* 303 (5654):95–98.

Lunyak, V.V., Burgess, R., Prefontaine, G.G., Nelson, C., Sze, S.H., Chenoweth, J., Schwartz, P., Pevzner, P.A., Glass, C., Mandel, G., and Rosenfeld, M.G. (2002) Corepressor-dependent silencing of chromosomal regions encoding neuronal genes. *Science* 298 (5599):1747–1752.

Makedonski, K., Abuhatzira, L., Kaufman, Y., Razin, A., and Shemer, R. (2005) MeCP2 deficiency in Rett syndrome causes epigenetic aberrations at the PWS/AS imprinting center that affects UBE3A expression. *Hum. Mol. Genet.* 14(8):1049–1058.

Martin, C., and Zhang, Y. (2005) The diverse functions of histone lysine methylation. *Nat. Rev. Mol. Cell Biol.* 6(11):838–849.

Matsuura, T., Sutcliffe, J.S., Fang, P., Galjaard, R.J., Jiang, Y.H., Benton, C.S., Rommens, J.M., and Beaudet, A.L. (1997) De novo truncating mutations in E6-AP ubiquitin-protein ligase gene (UBE3A) in Angelman syndrome. *Nat. Genet.* 15(1): 74–77.

McGill, B.E., Bundle, S.F., Yaylaoglu, M.B., Carson, J.P., Thaller, C., and Zoghbi, H.Y. (2006) Enhanced anxiety and stress-induced corticosterone release are associated with increased Crh expression in a mouse model of Rett syndrome. *Proc. Natl. Acad. Sci. USA* 103(48):18267–18272.

Meister, G., Landthaler, M., Patkaniowska, A., Dorsett, Y., Teng, G., and Tuschl, T. (2004) Human Argonaute2 mediates RNA cleavage targeted by miRNAs and siRNAs. *Mol. Cell.* 15(2): 185–197.

Miller, C.A., and Sweatt, J.D. (2007) Covalent modification of DNA regulates memory formation. *Neuron* 53(6):857–869.

Milner, K.M., Craig, E.E., Thompson, R.J., Veltman, M.W., Thomas, N.S., Roberts, S., Bellamy, M., Curran, S.R., Sporikou, C.M., and Bolton, P.F. (2005) Prader-Willi syndrome: intellectual abilities and behavioural features by genetic subtype. *J. Child Psychol. Psychiatry* 46(10):1089–1096.

Mischoulon, D., and Fava, M. (2002) Role of S-adenosyl-L-methionine in the treatment of depression: a review of the evidence. *Am. J. Clin. Nutr.* 76(5):1158S–1161S.

Morgan, H.D., Dean, W., Coker, H.A., Reik, W., and Petersen-Mahrt, S.K. (2004) Activation-induced cytidine deaminase deaminates 5-methylcytosine in DNA and is expressed in pluripotent tissues: implications for epigenetic reprogramming. *J. Biol. Chem.* 279(50):52353–52360.

Morgan, H.D., Santos, F., Green, K., Dean, W., and Reik, W. (2005) Epigenetic reprogramming in mammals. *Hum. Mol. Genet.* 14(Spec No 1):R47–58.

Morgan, H.D., Sutherland, H.G., Martin, D.I., and Whitelaw, E. (1999) Epigenetic inheritance at the agouti locus in the mouse. *Nat. Genet.* 23(3):314–318.

Morison, I.M., Ramsay, J.P., and Spencer, H.G. (2005) A census of mammalian imprinting. *Trends Genet.* 21(8):457–465.

Morris, K.V., Chan, S.W., Jacobsen, S.E., and Looney, D.J. (2004) Small interfering RNA-induced transcriptional gene silencing in human cells. *Science* 305(5688):1289–1292.

Mount, R.H., Charman, T., Hastings, R.P., Reilly, S., and Cass, H. (2002) The Rett Syndrome Behaviour Questionnaire (RSBQ): refining the behavioural phenotype of Rett syndrome. *J. Child Psychol. Psychiatry* 43(8):1099–1110.

Mount, R.H., Charman, T., Hastings, R.P., Reilly, S., and Cass, H. (2003) Features of autism in Rett syndrome and severe mental retardation. *J. Autism Dev. Disord.* 33(4):435–442.

Mount, R.H., Hastings, R.P., Reilly, S., Cass, H., and Charman, T. (2001) Behavioural and emotional features in Rett syndrome. *Disabil. Rehabil.* 23(3/4):129–138.

Muntjewerff, J.W., Kahn, R.S., Blom, H.J., and den Heijer, M. (2006) Homocysteine, methylenetetrahydrofolate reductase and risk of schizophrenia: a meta-analysis. *Mol. Psychiatry* 11(2):143–149.

Murchison, E.P., Partridge, J.F., Tam, O.H., Cheloufi, S., and Hannon, G.J. (2005) Characterization of Dicer-deficient murine embryonic stem cells. *Proc. Natl. Acad. Sci. USA* 102(34):12135–12140.

Murphy, B.C., O'Reilly, R.L., and Singh, S.M. (2005) Site-specific cytosine methylation in S-COMT promoter in 31 brain regions with implications for studies involving schizophrenia. *Am. J. Med. Genet. B Neuropsychiatr. Genet.* 133(1):37–42.

Muskiet, F.A., and Kemperman, R.F. (2006) Folate and long-chain polyunsaturated fatty acids in psychiatric disease. *J. Nutr. Biochem.* 17(11):717–727.

Nabetani, A., Hatada, I., Morisaki, H., Oshimura, M., and Mukai, T. (1997) Mouse U2af1-rs1 is a neomorphic imprinted gene. *Mol. Cell Biol.* 17(2):789–798.

Nakao, M., Sutcliffe, J.S., Durtschi, B., Mutirangura, A., Ledbetter, D.H., and Beaudet, A.L. (1994) Imprinting analysis of three genes in the Prader-Willi/Angelman region: SNRPN, E6-associated protein, and PAR-2 (D15S225E). *Hum. Mol. Genet.* 3(2):309–315.

Nan, X., Hou, J., Maclean, A., Nasir, J., Lafuente, M.J., Shu, X., Kriaucionis, S., and Bird, A. (2007) Interaction between chromatin proteins MECP2 and ATRX is disrupted by mutations that cause inherited mental retardation. *Proc. Natl. Acad. Sci. USA* 104(8):2709–2714.

Nan, X., Ng, H.H., Johnson, C.A., Laherty, C.D., Turner, B.M., Eisenman, R.N., and Bird, A. (1998) Transcriptional repression by the methyl-CpG-binding protein MeCP2 involves a histone deacetylase complex. *Nature* 393(6683):386–389.

Newton, S.S., and Duman, R.S. (2006) Chromatin remodeling: a novel mechanism of psychotropic drug action. *Mol. Pharmacol.* 70(2):440–443.

Nightingale, K.P., O'Neill, L.P., and Turner, B.M. (2006) Histone modifications: signalling receptors and potential elements of a heritable epigenetic code. *Curr. Opin. Genet. Dev.* 16(2): 125–136.

Ohta, T., Gray, T.A., Rogan, P.K., Buiting, K., Gabriel, J.M., Saitoh, S., Muralidhar, B., Bilienska, B., Krajewska-Walasek, M., Driscoll, D.J., Horsthemke, B., Butler, M.G., and Nicholls, R.D. (1999) Imprinting-mutation mechanisms in Prader-Willi syndrome. *Am. J. Hum. Genet.* 64(2):397–413.

Oike, Y., Hata, A., Mamiya, T., Kaname, T., Noda, Y., Suzuki, M., Yasue, H., Nabeshima, T., Araki, K., and Yamamura, K. (1999) Truncated CBP protein leads to classical Rubinstein-Taybi syndrome phenotypes in mice: implications for a dominant-negative mechanism. *Hum. Mol. Genet.* 8(3):387–396.

Okano, M., Bell, D.W., Haber, D.A., and Li, E. (1999) DNA methyltransferases Dnmt3a and Dnmt3b are essential for de novo methylation and mammalian development. *Cell* 99(3): 247–257.

Okano, M., Xie, S., and Li, E. (1998) Cloning and characterization of a family of novel mammalian DNA (cytosine-5) methyltransferases. *Nat. Genet.* 19(3):219–220.

Pancheri, P., Scapicchio, P., and Chiaie, R.D. (2002) A double-blind, randomized parallel-group, efficacy and safety study of intramuscular S-adenosyl-L-methionine 1,4-butanedisulphonate (SAMe) versus imipramine in patients with major depressive disorder. *Int. J. Neuropsychopharmacol.* 5(4):287–294.

Park, C.W., Chen, Z., Kren, B.T., and Steer, C.J. (2004) Double-stranded siRNA targeted to the huntingtin gene does not induce DNA methylation. *Biochem. Biophys. Res. Commun.* 323(1): 275–280.

Peedicayil, J., and Subbanna, P.K. (2007) Revisiting the methylation hypothesis for the psychoses. *Med. Hypotheses* 68(3):721.

Perk, J., Makedonski, K., Lande, L., Cedar, H., Razin, A., and Shemer, R. (2002) The imprinting mechanism of the Prader-Willi/Angelman regional control center. *Embo. J.* 21(21):5807–5814.

Peters, S.U., Beaudet, A.L., Madduri, N., and Bacino, C.A. (2004) Autism in Angelman syndrome: implications for autism research. *Clin. Genet.* 66(6):530–536.

Petronis, A. (2004) The origin of schizophrenia: genetic thesis, epigenetic antithesis, and resolving synthesis. *Biol. Psychiatry* 55(10):965–970.

Phiel, C.J., Zhang, F., Huang, E.Y., Guenther, M.G., Lazar, M.A., and Klein, P.S. (2001) Histone deacetylase is a direct target of valproic acid, a potent anticonvulsant, mood stabilizer, and teratogen. *J. Biol. Chem.* 276(39):36734–36741.

Plante, I., Davidovic, L., Ouellet, D.L., Gobeil, L.A., Tremblay, S., Khandjian, E.W., and Provost, P. (2006) Dicer-derived micrornas Are utilized by the fragile x mental retardation protein for assembly on target RNAs. *J. Biomed. Biotechnol.* 2006(4):64347.

Provost, P., Dishart, D., Doucet, J., Frendewey, D., Samuelsson, B., and Radmark, O. (2002) Ribonuclease activity and RNA binding of recombinant human Dicer. *Embo. J.* 21(21):5864–5874.

Rakyan, V.K., and Beck, S. (2006) Epigenetic variation and inheritance in mammals. *Curr. Opin. Genet. Dev.* 16(6):573–577.

Rakyan, V.K., Hildmann, T., Novik, K.L., Lewin, J., Tost, J., Cox, A.V., Andrews, T.D., Howe, K.L., Otto, T., Olek, A., Fischer, J., Gut, I.G., Berlin, K., and Beck, S. (2004) DNA methylation profiling of the human major histocompatibility complex: a pilot study for the human epigenome project. *PLoS Biol.* 2(12):E405.

Regland, B., Johansson, B.V., Grenfeldt, B., Hjelmgren, L.T., and Medhus, M. (1995) Homocysteinemia is a common feature of schizophrenia. *J. Neural Transm. Gen. Sect.* 100(2):165–169.

Reik, W., and Walter, J. (2001) Genomic imprinting: parental influence on the genome. *Nat. Rev. Genet.* 2(1):21–32.

Rogers, S.J., Wehner, D.E., and Hagerman, R. (2001) The behavioral phenotype in fragile X: symptoms of autism in very young children with fragile X syndrome, idiopathic autism, and other developmental disorders. *J. Dev. Behav. Pediatr.* 22(6):409–417.

Ross, C.A., Margolis, R.L., Reading, S.A., Pletnikov, M., and Coyle, J.T. (2006) Neurobiology of schizophrenia. *Neuron* 52(1): 139–153.

Rubinstein, J.H., and Taybi, H. (1963) Broad thumbs and toes and facial abnormalities. A possible mental retardation syndrome. *Am. J. Dis. Child.* 105:588–608.

Runte, M., Huttenhofer, A., Gross, S., Kiefmann, M., Horsthemke, B., and Buiting, K. (2001) The IC-SNURF-SNRPN transcript serves as a host for multiple small nucleolar RNA species and as an antisense RNA for UBE3A. *Hum. Mol. Genet.* 10(23): 2687–2700.

Saitoh, S., and Wada, T. (2000) Parent-of-origin specific histone acetylation and reactivation of a key imprinted gene locus in Prader-Willi syndrome. *Am. J. Hum. Genet.* 66(6):1958–1962.

Samaco, R.C., Hogart, A., and LaSalle, J.M. (2005) Epigenetic overlap in autism-spectrum neurodevelopmental disorders: MECP2 deficiency causes reduced expression of UBE3A and GABRB3. *Hum. Mol. Genet.* 14(4):483–492.

Sansom, D., Krishnan, V.H., Corbett, J., and Kerr, A. (1993) Emotional and behavioural aspects of Rett syndrome. *Dev. Med. Child Neurol.* 35(4):340–345.

Schanen, N.C. (2006) Epigenetics of autism spectrum disorders. *Hum. Mol. Genet.* 15(Spec No 2):R138–150.

Schroeder, F.A., Lin, C.L., Crusio, W.E., and Akbarian, S. (2006) Antidepressant-like effects of the histone deacetylase inhibitor, sodium butyrate, in the mouse. *Biol. Psychiatry* 62:55–64.

Schroer, R.J., Phelan, M.C., Michaelis, R.C., Crawford, E.C., Skinner, S.A., Cuccaro, M., Simensen, R.J., Bishop, J., Skinner, C., Fender, D., and Stevenson, R. E. (1998) Autism and maternally derived aberrations of chromosome 15q. *Am. J. Med. Genet.* 76(4):327–336.

Schule, B., Albalwi, M., Northrop, E., Francis, D.I., Rowell, M., Slater, H.R., Gardner, R.J., and Francke, U. (2005) Molecular breakpoint cloning and gene expression studies of a novel translocation t(4;15)(q27;q11.2) associated with Prader-Willi syndrome. *BMC Med. Genet.* 6:18.

Schwartz, Y.B., and Pirrotta, V. (2007) Polycomb silencing mechanisms and the management of genomic programmes. *Nat. Rev. Genet.* 8(1):9–22.

Shemer, R., Birger, Y., Riggs, A.D., and Razin, A. (1997) Structure of the imprinted mouse Snrpn gene and establishment of its parental-specific methylation pattern. *Proc. Natl. Acad. Sci. USA* 94(19): 10267–10272.

Shi, Y., Lan, F., Matson, C., Mulligan, P., Whetstine, J.R., Cole, P.A., and Casero, R.A. (2004) Histone demethylation mediated by the nuclear amine oxidase homolog LSD1. *Cell* 119(7):941–953.

Shibayama, A., Cook, E.H., Jr., Feng, J., Glanzmann, C., Yan, J., Craddock, N., Jones, I.R., Goldman, D., Heston, L.L., and Sommer, S.S. (2004) MECP2 structural and 3'-UTR variants in schizophrenia, autism and other psychiatric diseases: a possible association with autism. *Am. J. Med. Genet. B Neuropsychiatr. Genet.* 128(1):50–53.

Siedlecki, P., and Zielenkiewicz, P. (2006) Mammalian DNA methyltransferases. *Acta Biochim. Pol.* 53(2):245–256.

Simonini, M.V., Camargo, L.M., Dong, E., Maloku, E., Veldic, M., Costa, E., and Guidotti, A. (2006) The benzamide MS-275 is a potent, long-lasting brain region-selective inhibitor of histone deacetylases. *Proc. Natl. Acad. Sci. USA* 103(5):1587–1592.

Siomi, H., Siomi, M.C., Nussbaum, R.L., and Dreyfuss, G. (1993) The protein product of the fragile X gene, FMR1, has characteristics of an RNA-binding protein. *Cell* 74(2):291–298.

Sleutels, F., Zwart, R., and Barlow, D.P. (2002) The non-coding Air RNA is required for silencing autosomal imprinted genes. *Nature* 415(6873):810–813.

Smith, R.J., Dean, W., Konfortova, G., and Kelsey, G. (2003) Identification of novel imprinted genes in a genome-wide screen for maternal methylation. *Genome Res.* 13(4):558–569.

Song, J.J., Smith, S.K., Hannon, G.J., and Joshua-Tor, L. (2004) Crystal structure of Argonaute and its implications for RISC slicer activity. *Science* 305(5689):1434–1437.

St. Clair, D., Xu, M., Wang, P., Yu, Y., Fang, Y., Zhang, F., Zheng, X., Gu, N., Feng, G., Sham, P., and He, L. (2005) Rates of adult schizophrenia following prenatal exposure to the Chinese famine of 1959–1961. *JAMA* 294(5):557–562.

Stefan, M., Portis, T., Longnecker, R., and Nicholls, R.D. (2005) A nonimprinted Prader-Willi Syndrome (PWS)-region gene regulates a different chromosomal domain in trans but the imprinted pws loci do not alter genome-wide mRNA levels. *Genomics* 85(5): 630–640.

Stefani, G., Fraser, C.E., Darnell, J.C., and Darnell, R.B. (2004) Fragile X mental retardation protein is associated with translating polyribosomes in neuronal cells. *J. Neurosci.* 24(33):7272–7276.

Steffenburg, S., Gillberg, C.L., Steffenburg, U., and Kyllerman, M. (1996) Autism in Angelman syndrome: a population-based study. *Pediatr. Neurol.* 14(2):131–136.

Stevens, C.A., Carey, J.C., and Blackburn, B.L. (1990) Rubinstein-Taybi syndrome: a natural history study. *Am. J. Med. Genet. Suppl.* 6:30–37.

Strahl, B.D., and Allis, C.D. (2000) The language of covalent histone modifications. *Nature* 403(6765):41–45.

Suetake, I., Shinozaki, F., Miyagawa, J., Takeshima, H., and Tajima, S. (2004) DNMT3L stimulates the DNA methylation activity of Dnmt3a and Dnmt3b through a direct interaction. *J. Biol. Chem.* 279(26):27816–27823.

Sullivan, K., Hatton, D., Hammer, J., Sideris, J., Hooper, S., Ornstein, P., and Bailey, D., Jr. (2006) ADHD symptoms in children with FXS. *Am. J. Med. Genet. A* 140(21):2275–2288.

Susser, E., Neugebauer, R., Hoek, H.W., Brown, A.S., Lin, S., Labovitz, D., and Gorman, J.M. (1996) Schizophrenia after prenatal famine. Further evidence. *Arch. Gen. Psychiatry* 53(1):25–31.

Sutcliffe, J.S., Nelson, D.L., Zhang, F., Pieretti, M., Caskey, C.T., Saxe, D., and Warren, S.T. (1992) DNA methylation represses FMR-1 transcription in fragile X syndrome. *Hum. Mol. Genet.* 1(6):397–400.

Suter, C.M., Martin, D.I., and Ward, R.L. (2004) Germline epimutation of MLH1 in individuals with multiple cancers. *Nat. Genet.* 36(5):497–501.

Svoboda, P., Stein, P., Filipowicz, W., and Schultz, R.M. (2004) Lack of homologous sequence-specific DNA methylation in response to stable dsRNA expression in mouse oocytes. *Nucleic Acids Res.* 32(12):3601–3606.

Terracciano, A., Chiurazzi, P., and Neri, G. (2005) Fragile X syndrome. *Am. J. Med. Genet. C Semin. Med. Genet.* 137(1):32–37.

Tremolizzo, L., Carboni, G., Ruzicka, W.B., Mitchell, C.P., Sugaya, I., Tueting, P., Sharma, R., Grayson, D.R., Costa, E., and Guidotti, A. (2002) An epigenetic mouse model for molecular and behavioral neuropathologies related to schizophrenia vulnerability. *Proc. Natl. Acad. Sci. USA* 99(26):17095–17100.

Trevethan, E., and Moser, H. (1988) Diagnostic criteria for Rett syndrome. *Ann. Neurol.* 23:425–428.

Trillingsgaard, A., and Ostergaard, J.R. (2004) Autism in Angelman syndrome: an exploration of comorbidity. *Autism* 8(2):163–174.

Tsankova, N.M., Berton, O., Renthal, W., Kumar, A., Neve, R.L., and Nestler, E.J. (2006) Sustained hippocampal chromatin regulation in a mouse model of depression and antidepressant action. *Nat. Neurosci.* 9(4):519–525.

Veldic, M., Kadriu, B., Maloku, E., Agis-Balboa, R.C., Guidotti, A., Davis, J.M., and Costa, E. (2007) Epigenetic mechanisms expressed in basal ganglia GABAergic neurons differentiate schizophrenia from bipolar disorder. *Schizophr. Res.* 91(1/3): 51–61.

Veltman, M.W., Craig, E.E., and Bolton, P.F. (2005) Autism spectrum disorders in Prader-Willi and Angelman syndromes: a systematic review. *Psychiatr. Genet.* 15(4):243–254.

Veltman, M.W., Thompson, R.J., Roberts, S.E., Thomas, N.S., Whittington, J., and Bolton, P.F. (2004) Prader-Willi syndrome—a study comparing deletion and uniparental disomy cases with reference to autism spectrum disorders. *Eur. Child Adolesc. Psychiatry* 13(1):42–50.

Verdel, A., Jia, S., Gerber, S., Sugiyama, T., Gygi, S., Grewal, S.I., and Moazed, D. (2004) RNAi-mediated targeting of heterochromatin by the RITS complex. *Science* 303(5658):672–676.

Verkerk, A.J., Pieretti, M., Sutcliffe, J.S., Fu, Y.H., Kuhl, D.P., Pizzuti, A., Reiner, O., Richards, S., Victoria, M.F., Zhang, F.P., et al. (1991) Identification of a gene (FMR-1) containing a CGG repeat coincident with a breakpoint cluster region exhibiting length variation in fragile X syndrome. *Cell* 65(5):905–914.

Villard, L., Kpebe, A., Cardoso, C., Chelly, P.J., Tardieu, P.M., and Fontes, M. (2000) Two affected boys in a Rett syndrome family: clinical and molecular findings. *Neurology* 55(8):1188–1193.

Vu, T.H., and Hoffman, A.R. (1997) Imprinting of the Angelman syndrome gene, UBE3A, is restricted to brain. *Nat. Genet.* 17(1):12–13.

Walsh, C.P., and Xu, G.L. (2006) Cytosine methylation and DNA repair. *Curr. Top. Microbiol. Immunol.* 301:283–315.

Wan, M., Lee, S.S., Zhang, X., Houwink-Manville, I., Song, H.R., Amir, R.E., Budden, S., Naidu, S., Pereira, J.L., Lo, I.F., Zoghbi, H.Y., Schanen, N.C., and Francke, U. (1999) Rett syndrome and beyond: recurrent spontaneous and familial MECP2 mutations at CpG hotspots. *Am. J. Hum. Genet.* 65(6):1520–1529.

Waterland, R.A., Dolinoy, D.C., Lin, J.R., Smith, C.A., Shi, X., and Tahiliani, K.G. (2006) Maternal methyl supplements increase offspring DNA methylation at Axin Fused. *Genesis* 44(9): 401–406.

Waterland, R.A., and Jirtle, R.L. (2003) Transposable elements: targets for early nutritional effects on epigenetic gene regulation. *Mol. Cell Biol.* 23(15):5293–5300.

Watt, F., and Molloy, P.L. (1988) Cytosine methylation prevents binding to DNA of a HeLa cell transcription factor required for optimal expression of the adenovirus major late promoter. *Genes Dev.* 2(9):1136–1143.

Weaver, I.C., Cervoni, N., Champagne, F.A., D'Alessio, A.C., Sharma, S., Seckl, J.R., Dymov, S., Szyf, M., and Meaney, M.J. (2004) Epigenetic programming by maternal behavior. *Nat. Neurosci.* 7(8):847–854.

Weaver, I.C., Meaney, M.J., and Szyf, M. (2006) Maternal care effects on the hippocampal transcriptome and anxiety-mediated behaviors in the offspring that are reversible in adulthood. *Proc. Natl. Acad. Sci. USA* 103(9):3480–3485.

Weinberg, M.S., Villeneuve, L.M., Ehsani, A., Amarzguioui, M., Aagaard, L., Chen, Z.X., Riggs, A.D., Rossi, J.J., and Morris, K.V. (2006) The antisense strand of small interfering RNAs directs histone methylation and transcriptional gene silencing in human cells. *Rna* 12(2):256–262.

Willard, H.F., and Hendrich, B.D. (1999) Breaking the silence in Rett syndrome. *Nat. Genet.* 23(2):127–128.

Williams, C.A., Beaudet, A.L., Clayton-Smith, J., Knoll, J.H., Kyllerman, M., Laan, L.A., Magenis, R.E., Moncla, A., Schinzel, A.A., Summers, J.A., and Wagstaff, J. (2006) Angelman syndrome 2005: updated consensus for diagnostic criteria. *Am. J. Med. Genet. A* 140(5):413–418.

Wood, A.J., and Oakey, R.J. (2006) Genomic imprinting in mammals: emerging themes and established theories. *PLoS Genetics* 2(11):E147.

Wysocka, J., Allis, C.D., and Coonrod, S. (2006) Histone arginine methylation and its dynamic regulation. *Front. Biosci.* 11:344–355.

Xin, Z., Allis, C.D., and Wagstaff, J. (2001) Parent-specific complementary patterns of histone H3 lysine 9 and H3 lysine 4 methylation at the Prader-Willi syndrome imprinting center. *Am. J. Hum. Genet.* 69(6):1389–1394.

Yamasaki, K., Joh, K., Ohta, T., Masuzaki, H., Ishimaru, T., Mukai, T., Niikawa, N., N. Ogawa, N., Wagstaff, J., and Kishino, T. (2003) Neurons but not glial cells show reciprocal imprinting of sense and antisense transcripts of Ube3a. *Hum. Mol. Genet.* 12(8): 837–847.

Yehuda, R., Engel, S.M., Brand, S.R., Seckl, J., Marcus, S.M., and Berkowitz, G.S. (2005) Transgenerational effects of posttraumatic stress disorder in babies of mothers exposed to the World Trade Center attacks during pregnancy. *J. Clin. Endocrinol. Metab.* 90(7):4115–4118.

Young, S.N., and Ghadirian, A.M. (1989) Folic acid and psychopathology. *Prog. Neuropsychopharmacol. Biol. Psychiatry* 13(6):841–863.

Zeng, Y., Yi, R., and Cullen, B.R. (2003) MicroRNAs and small interfering RNAs can inhibit mRNA expression by similar mechanisms. *Proc. Natl. Acad. Sci. USA* 100(17):9779–9784.

Zhang, H., Kolb, F.A., Brondani, V., Billy, E., and Filipowicz, W. (2002) Human Dicer preferentially cleaves dsRNAs at their termini without a requirement for ATP. *Embo. J.* 21(21):5875–5885.

Zhang, Y.Q., Bailey, A.M., Matthies, H.J., Renden, R.B., Smith, M.A., Speese, S.D., Rubin, G. M., and Broadie, K. (2001) Drosophila fragile X-related gene regulates the MAP1B homolog Futsch to control synaptic structure and function. *Cell* 107(5): 591–603.

II METHODS OF CLINICAL NEUROBIOLOGICAL RESEARCH

CAROL A. TAMMINGA

NEUROSCIENCE discoveries of the future are built on the novel technologies and methodologies we advance today. This is especially true for the study of human brain diseases, where novel technologies are critical in exposing unanticipated functions, and creative methodologies demonstrate subtle but pivotal disease differences. Dr. Julie Axelrod, the first modern psychiatric neuroscientist to win the Nobel Prize, is credited with expressing the opinion that the biggest advances in science always come from new methodologies that permit measuring things simply and rapidly.

For many years there were almost no informative technical approaches that were sensitive enough or sufficiently selective to provide critical new knowledge of normal brain function, let alone data to inform disease pathophysiology. The situation has changed. Now, basic neuroscience has developed at such a pace that knowledge of fundamental brain function and the methodologies to examine complex neural phenomena are available to human research. This situation has revolutionized human brain research and provided considerable hope for future discovery. The examples are already legendary. The first papers identifying neurotransmitter receptors and their quantification in laboratory animals have led to routine applications of receptor pharmacology in drug discovery. The discovery of deoxyribonucleic acid (DNA) structure and methods for its analysis along with clever mathematical approaches for sequence reconstruction allowed the sequencing of the human genome, knowledge that is fundamental in disease research today. Even the most routine techniques used in molecular discovery today, like the polymerase chain reaction (PCR) and ribonucleic acid (RNA) interference (RNAi), have revolutionized not only the process of translational research but also the kind of questions that can be posed and the nature of the data collected. This critical flow of new methodologies is the fundamental machine for current discovery.

This section is designed to present and examine some of the best and most forward-looking methodologies for brain research, especially translational methodologies for human discovery. Merikangas and Kalaydjian define, describe, and illustrate what is arguably one of the most basic of clinical methodologies, *epidemiology*. They describe the orientation and goal of epidemiology as the study of illness distribution and determinants in humans; the identification of disease etiology and ultimately prevention are its major goals. Epidemiological methods are the basic tools for estimating prevalence of mental illness in community populations, as well as genetic and environmental risk factors for mental illnesses. It is the foundation methodology for all clinical genetics, as well as for almost all assessment methodologies. Following that presentation, Gelernter and Lappalainen present the basic methodological considerations of *clinical molecular genetics* in mental illnesses. The most extraordinary advance in our knowledge of human genetics has been provided by the Human Genome Project. To capitalize on that advance for the advantage of mental illness, neuroscientists will have to understand the basic steps in localizing unknown genes and determining which genes influence a phenotype. Genetic linkage, linkage disequilibrium, genetic association, and now whole-genome association are methodologies that this chapter defines, describes, and illustrates, with considerable clarity and vision.

In developing the concept of phenotype for mental illness further, Green, Lee, and Kern, discuss the basic human behavioral methodologies used in virtually all human discovery research: behavioral evaluation using neuropsychological assessments. Assessing cognition with standardized tests provides information on brain-mediated behaviors; cognitive dysfunctions differ across mental illnesses hence can be used to define and characterize an illness or a subdomain of function. Cognition has been used to dissect mental diagnoses into component symptom complexes and to examine these symptom complexes as phenotypes, predictors, and treatment targets. Thus, tools to reliably and quantitatively measure aspects of cognition in humans are critical to discovery in mental illness. This same line of inquiry is continued in the next chapter by Carter, Kerns, and Cohen, who present the basic methodologies and conceptual approaches of cognitive neuroscience. They describe *cognitive neuroscience* as an integrative and new field, directed toward understanding how mental processes emerge from brain mechanisms. They emphasize three critical and intersecting elements: cognition models, functional brain imaging, and animal cognition models, used together to meet the overall goal of understanding brain behavior mechanistically. The chapter presents concepts and liberally uses illustrations to enable readers to understand the direction and limits of the field.

The next chapter, by Lu and Yang, provides a clear and detailed description of human brain imaging methodologies based on magnetic resonance (MR). The diversity of MR measures is vast, and their application provides an array of sensitive and selective outcomes of clear relevance for human brain research: regional perfusion measures, functional magnetic resonance imaging (MRI) blood oxygen level–dependent (BOLD) assessment, resting connectivity, diffusion-based imaging, and neurochemical examination with spectroscopy. This chapter presents the conceptual basis and technical process as well as illustrations of data from these methods to introduce and encourage any translational neuroscientist around these MR imaging approaches. Molecular brain imaging using positron emission tomography (PET) is almost another field of brain imaging with its own hardware, methods, and study designs. Kim, Martinez, Slifstein, and Abi-Dargham describe the use of radio-labeled chemical compounds with PET or single photon emission computed tomography (SPECT) to measure protein molecules recognized by the radiolabeled tracer to examine the functions of these proteins and examine differences across types of mental illness. The logical development, detailed explanations, and illustrations from the field enable a reader to understand relevance as well as the methodological approaches afforded by molecular imaging; receptor occupancy has become a near requirement in the area of drug development, described in this chapter.

Beneyto, Sibille, and Lewis provide an excellent update on the methods of human postmortem brain tissue analysis in mental illness, arguing that an understanding of the molecular and cellular pathways of mental illness can be most directly approached by using postmortem brain tissue from normal and illness cases. The chapter provides the kind of experimental detail necessary for users to become informed about the proper use of human postmortem resource and the vast range of techniques for study. The translational nature of these tissue approaches, making animal model discoveries directly translatable into human experiments, is obvious. The chapter proposes, explains and illustrates postmortem tissue method. Petitto, Cruess, Repetto, Gettes, Benton, and Evans review methodologies involved in neuroimmunological approaches to neural discovery, how various behavioral states influence the immune system, and how the immune system affects brain function. It is the common signals and receptors of the immune, endocrine, and brain systems that have suggested an association and the role of cytokines as mediators. In the last chapter, Tollefson presents a rare practical and conceptual view of the process of drug discovery, one of the main practical goals of all of these methodologies for mental illness research. Although it is easy to conceptualize the goal of pharmaceutical development as seeking novel pharmacological approaches to unmet clinical needs, the challenge is daunting. This chapter reviews both theoretical aspects, including the importance of a focused strategy, as well as very practical components of the drug development process, including work with regulatory agencies, as only an "insider" can do.

The scientific approaches and methodologies presented in this section are used to provide incremental knowledge to advance disease constructs as well as to transform patho-etiological concepts and test creative novel hypotheses. Whether readers are gaining general familiarity with methods outside of their own expertise, updating their own techniques, evaluating novel approaches to test a hypothesis, or seeking a detailed methodology to apply in their research, this section will satisfy; it represents a range of methodologies available for human neurobiology research in mental illness, with each chapter providing the concepts and many of the details for application. Basic scientists, clinical scholars, and students of translational clinical neuroscience have a source book in this section, authored by the best scientists in these fields, to index and expand their own methodological approaches.

9 Contributions of Epidemiology to the Neurobiology of Mental Illness

KATHLEEN R. MERIKANGAS AND AMANDA KALAYDJIAN

OVERVIEW OF THE DISCIPLINE OF EPIDEMIOLOGY

Definition and Study Designs

The field of epidemiology is defined as the study of the distribution and determinants of diseases in human populations. Epidemiologic studies are concerned with the extent and types of illnesses in groups of people and with the factors that influence their distribution (Gordis, 2000). Epidemiologists investigate the interactions that may occur among the host, agent, and environment (the classic epidemiologic triangle) to produce a disease state. The chief goal of epidemiologic studies is to identify the etiology of a disease to prevent or intervene in the progression of the disorder. To achieve this goal, epidemiologic studies generally proceed from studies that specify the amount and distribution of a disease within a population by person, place, and time (that is, descriptive epidemiology), to more focused studies of the determinants of disease in specific groups (that is, analytic epidemiology) (Gordis, 2000).

Descriptive epidemiologic studies are important in specifying the rates and distribution of disorders in the general population. These data can be applied to identify biases that may exist in treated populations and to construct case registries from which persons may serve as probands for analytic epidemiologic studies. Such attention to sampling issues is a major contribution of the epidemiologic approach, as individuals identified in clinical settings often constitute the biased tip of the iceberg of the disease and may not be representative of the general population of similarly affected individuals with respect to demographic, social, or clinical characteristics. Associations that are identified at the descriptive level may then be tested systematically with case-control designs that compare the relationship between a particular risk factor or disease correlate and the presence or absence of a given disease, after controlling for relevant confounding variables. Case-control studies involve a retrospective design to investigate these particular associations. Researchers then proceed to prospective cohort studies, which can formally test the temporal direction of such associations.

The identification of risk factors for a disease includes an intermediate step in the process of identifying a discrete and valid disorder in the general population and culminates in analytic studies that attempt to identify etiologic factors. There are several criteria for assessing the extent to which a risk factor is causally involved in a trait or disease.

These include the strength of the association, a dose-response effect, and a lack of temporal ambiguity. Broader criteria that can be applied to a set of studies on a putative etiologic risk factor include consistency of the findings, biologic plausibility of the hypothesis, and a specificity of association (Hill, 1953; Kleinbaum et al., 1982). Each of these analytic approaches is germane to epidemiologic research and can be applied to the field of psychiatry to identify risk factors for mental disorders and potential mechanisms of etiology.

Goals of Epidemiology

Whether descriptive or analytic, the ultimate goal of epidemiologic investigations is prevention. The traditional epidemiologic concept of prevention is comprised of three levels: (*1*) primary prevention to reduce the incidence of a disease, (*2*) secondary prevention to reduce the risk of disease among susceptible individuals, and (*3*) tertiary prevention to reduce the impact or consequences of a disease.

Despite its clear implications for prevention, there is nonetheless growing controversy regarding the role of epidemiology in contemporary society (Susser and Susser, 1996). As advances in biomedicine unlock the secrets of the development and function of the human organism, epidemiology has followed these advances, parting from the traditional emphasis on infectious disease models to focus on identifying environmental risk factors such as diet or exposure to environmental toxins for chronic human diseases such as cancer and heart disease. The increasing focus on chronic human diseases (which are characterized by etiologic complexity) has diminished the potential contributions of the epidemiologic method because these diseases are likely to be etiologically heterogeneous and attributable to combinations of environmental and genetic factors, each with small effects. This complexity reduces the chance that any one study will have a major impact in identifying disease etiology. The increasing focus on risk factor research and molecular epidemiology has led to criticism by some public health leaders that the narrow disease-focused route has led to neglect of a public health perspective (Susser and Susser, 1996). Similar criticism has been leveled against psychiatry with its increasing focus on neurobiology rather than on community mental health.

APPLICATION OF EPIDEMIOLOGY TO PSYCHIATRY

The first formal use of the term *epidemiology* with respect to psychiatric disorders can be traced to a conference of the Milbank Memorial Fund in 1949, in which there was a consensus regarding the value of the application of the epidemiologic approach to causal research and its implications for administrative policy (Milbank Memorial Fund, 1950; Shepherd, 1984). Prior to 1949, however, there were many classic descriptive epidemiologic studies of psychiatric disorders throughout the world, and epidemiology as applied to this domain rapidly had become synonymous with large-scale studies deriving population base rates and demographic correlates of mental disorders. It should be emphasized, however, that this is only one application of the epidemiologic method. Table 9.1 presents a more complete description of the major goals of epidemiologic investigations in psychiatry.

DEFINITIONS AND ASSESSMENT OF PSYCHIATRIC DISORDERS

The traditional contributions of the application of the tools of epidemiology to psychiatry comprised methodologic developments including the introduction of structured and semistructured diagnostic interviews, statistical methods for estimating prevalence and correlates of mental disorders, and the focus on population-based samples to obtain estimates of the magnitude and correlates of mental disorders unbiased by treatment seeking.

TABLE 9.1. *Goals of Psychiatric Epidemiologic Studies*

Develop standardized assessments of psychiatric disorders
Establish validity of diagnostic nomenclature
Estimate magnitude of psychiatric disorders in the general population
Identify risk and protective factors for psychopathology
Collect information on patterns of use and adequacy of psychiatric services
Provide empirical basis for timing and targets for prevention

The results of recent epidemiologic studies have illustrated the need for further development of the psychiatric diagnostic system (Regier et al., 1990; Kessler et al., 1994; First et al., 2004). The dimensional classification of disorders, inclusion of subthreshold diagnostic categories and diagnostic spectra, and pervasive comorbidity between purportedly distinct diagnostic entities, has generated widespread concern about the lack of validity of the current categorical classification system in psychiatry (Angst and Merikangas, 1997; Angst et al., 1997; Judd et al., 1998).

In his discussion of the validity of psychiatric disorders, Kendell (1989) noted that it is unlikely that the etiologic secrets of the major psychiatric disorders will be unlocked without accurate and valid identification of the syndromes themselves. Such validation has particular relevance for the search for biological markers, which depends in large part on the identification of discrete and homogeneous forms of disorders (Freedman, 1984). However, as noted by Jablensky (2005), if the variation in psychiatric symptomatology is continuous and does not coalesce into well-defined clusters, it may be difficult for genetic and neuroscience research using these categorical definitions to generate meaningful information.

Recent studies have begun to expand the diagnostic criteria for mental disorders to collect information on the spectra of expression of particular conditions. Several studies have begun to deconstruct psychiatric phenotypes by their component features or subtypes, including bipolar disorder (Angst, 1997), general anxiety disorder (Angst et al., 2006), obsessive compulsive disorder (Eapen et al., 2006), schizophrenia (Braff et al., 2007), and panic disorder (Smoller and Tsuang, 1998). For example, recent findings from the National Comorbidity Survey-Replication demonstrated the validity of the spectrum concept of bipolar disorder (Merikangas et al., 2007) that had been proposed by clinicians for more than a decade (Benazzi and Akiskal, 2005).

RATES OF PSYCHIATRIC DISORDERS IN THE GENERAL POPULATION

During the last decade, the results of several surveys of mental disorders in the U.S. population using contemporary diagnostic criteria have become available. Table 9.2 presents findings from four large-scale epidemiologic surveys of the lifetime prevalence of adult psychiatric disorders that have used structured diagnostic interviews. The first of the studies, the Epidemiologic Catchment Area (ECA) program, sampled community and institutionalized residents from numerous cities across the United States (representing a nearly fivefold increase in sample size over previous North American studies; see Freedman, 1984). The results of the National Comorbidity Survey (NCS) and

TABLE 9.2. *Lifetime Prevalence Rates (% [SE]) by Investigation*

Disorders	*ECA (Robins et al., 1984)*	*NCS (Kessler et al., 1994)*	*NCS-R (Kessler et al., 2005)*	*NESARC (Conway et al., 2006)*
Anxiety disorders	15.5 (0.7)[a]	24.9 (0.8)	28.8 (0.9)	16.16 (0.42)
Affective disorders	7.9 (0.6)	19.3 (0.7)	20.8 (0.6)	19.54 (0.38)
Psychosis (nonaffective)	1.7 (0.3)	0.7 (0.1)	1.5 (—)	—
Substance use disorders	16.7 (0.8)	26.6 (1.0)	14.6 (0.6)	10.33 (0.32)[b]
Any disorder	32.6 (1.0)	48.0 (1.1)	46.4 (1.1)	—

ECA: Epidemiologic Catchment Area; NCS: National Comorbidity Survey; NCS-R: National Comorbidity Survey-Replication; NESARC: National Epidemiologic Survey on Alcohol and Related Conditions.

[a] Includes somatoform disorders.

[b] Includes drug use disorders only.

the National Comorbidity Survey-Replication (NCS-R) conducted a decade later have provided the first estimates of mental disorders in a probability sample of the general population of the United States. Another large study focused on the epidemiology of alcoholism has also provided information on base rates of mental disorders and their association with substance use disorders (NESARC).

Perhaps the most basic finding from these diverse investigations is the high prevalence of psychiatric disorders in community residents. As demonstrated by Table 9.2, the recent lifetime prevalence rates range from approximately 33% to 48% of the general population. The generally higher NCS and NCS-R rates are likely to be due to the application of increasingly sophisticated interview methods that minimize biases in retrospective recall. Nonetheless, the high prevalence rates across sites underscore the magnitude of psychopathology in nonclinically derived samples. These investigations have added to psychiatry not only by portraying the natural history of these disorders in a descriptive sense, but also by raising important issues about the comparability of clinical and community samples concerning treatment utilization and the universal nature of psychiatric conditions.

INTERNATIONAL RESEARCH

The results of numerous studies of the magnitude of mental disorders in other continents have also recently been published. The Netherlands Mental Health Survey and Incidence Study (NEMESIS) began in 1996 to measure the prevalence and incidence of psychiatric disorders in adults who were noninstitutionalized in the Netherlands (Bijl et al., 1998). This was followed by the German National Health Interview and Examination Survey (GHS), the first government-mandated nationwide study to investigate jointly the prevalence of somatic and mental disorders within one study in the general adult population in Germany (Jacobi et al., 2004). Another study to follow was the Health 2000 project, in which a representative sample of Finland's general adult population was interviewed with the Composite International Diagnostic Interview (CIDI; World Health Organization, 1990; Wittchen, 1994) for presence of *Diagnostic and Statistical Manual of Mental Disorders* (*DSM-IV*; American Psychiatric Association, 1994) mental disorders during the last 12 months (Pirkola et al., 2005). These efforts continue to expand across the globe; the Australian National Survey of Mental Health and Well-Being survey was implemented to estimate the 1-month and 1-year prevalence, disability, and health utilization attributable to mental disorders in the general adult population (Henderson et al., 2000), and the New Zealand Mental Health Survey was carried out in 2003–2004 to estimate the lifetime prevalence of *DSM-IV* Disorders and projected lifetime risk at age 75 years (Oakley Browne et al., 2006). Assessments of mental disorders in the general population have also been completed in Nigeria (Gureje et al., 2006), Mexico (Medina-Mora et al., 2005), Chile (Vicente et al., 2006), Japan (Kawakami et al., 2004), China (Shen et al., 2006), and the United Arab Emirates (Abou-Saleh et al., 2001) among others.

With the development of standardized assessment instruments and common diagnostic criteria, there has been increasing collaboration among investigators in epidemiology across international settings. The International Consortium in Psychiatric Epidemiology (ICPE) was established to facilitate global research using the WHO CIDI. This effort has taken the critical step of taking psychiatric epidemiology beyond the United States and Europe to the global population and to minority populations within the United States. During the first phase, 33,638 participants in seven nations were surveyed and data prepared for analysis (Merikangas, Mehta, et al., 1998; Kessler, 1999; Kessler et al., 2001). The work group continues to coordinate the WHO World Mental Health 2000 Initiative (WMH2000). Results are now available from the WMH studies in Belgium (Bonnewyn et al., 2007), Ukraine (Bromet et al., 2005), and Lebanon (Karam et al., 2006). A recent publication also compiled results from 15 surveys carried out in 14 countries in the Americas (Colombia, Mexico, United States), Europe (Belgium, France, Germany, Italy, Netherlands, Spain, Ukraine), the Middle East and Africa (Lebanon, Nigeria), and Asia (Japan, separate surveys in Beijing and Shanghai in the People's Republic of China) (Demyttenaere et al., 2004). These international and cross-cultural samples continue to expand our understanding of the validity and correlates of psychiatric disorders as well as the differential expression of disorders across the globe.

EPIDEMIOLOGY OF MENTAL DISORDERS IN CHILDREN AND ADOLESCENTS

Several years ago, the landmark U.S. surgeon general's report on mental health (U.S. Department of Health and Human Services, 2001) cited the urgent need for information tracking knowledge on the prevalence and distribution of mental disorders and patterns of service utilization in the United States, yet there is still a striking lack of information on the prevalence and distribution of mental disorders in children in the U.S. population. However, aggregation of the findings of several population-based studies of children and adolescents in specific regions of the United States, including Connecticut (Schwab-Stone et al., 1995), Illinois (Buka, Tsuang, Torrey, Klebanoff, Beinstein, and Yolken 2001), Massachusetts (Reinherz and Griffin, 1977), Missouri (Kashani et al., 1987), New York State (Cohen et al., 1993), North Carolina (Costello et al., 1996), and Oregon (Lewinsohn et al., 1993), has provided a range of estimates of the magnitude and socioeconomic correlates of mental disorders in youth. A recent summary by Costello et al. (2005) yielded the following estimates of the median and range of the prevalence of disorders in youth: any disorder–26% (8%–45%); any anxiety–8% (2%–33%); attention deficit disorder–3.5% (1%–14%); disruptive behavior disorders–6% (4%–20%); drug abuse/dependence–4% (2%–24%); and mood disorders–4% (1%–17%). The most important finding was that in any given year, approximately 12% of children in the United States suffer from a serious emotional disturbance that led to functional impairment. This implies that one out of every eight children in the United States is in need of mental health treatment.

Unfortunately, the results of these epidemiologic surveys also reveal that the vast majority of children with serious emotional disturbances do not receive treatment for their condition. Of particular concern is the finding that service use is particularly low among ethnic minority youth (Costello et al., 1993).

IMPACT OF MENTAL DISORDERS

One of the major advances in epidemiology during the past decade has been the increasing focus on the impact and burden of mental disorders. The importance of role disability has become increasingly recognized as a major source of indirect costs of illness because of its high economic impact on ill workers, their employers, and society (Verbrugge and Patrick, 1995; Goetzel et al., 2004; Lerner et al., 2005).

The introduction of the concept of *disability adjusted life years*, which estimate the disease-specific reduction in life expectancy attributable to disability and increased mortality, has highlighted the dramatic public health impact of mental disorders (Murray and Lopez, 1996). By the year 2020, it is estimated that psychiatric and neurologic disorders will account for 15% of the total burden of all diseases. According to WHO estimates from 2001, unipolar depressive disorders are the leading causes of years lived with disability in the world (YLDs) and the third leading source of disability adjusted life year (DALY) disease burden in high-income countries, surpassing dementia, lung cancer, and diabetes (Colin et al., 2007). By the year 2030, unipolar depressive disorders are projected to become the second leading cause of worldwide DALY burden, surpassed only by HIV/AIDS (Lopez and Mathers, 2006). The dramatic impact of mood disorders, schizophrenia, substance abuse, and anxiety disorders on lifetime disability highlights the importance of epidemiology in surveillance, understanding, and control of the major mental disorders. Comparative studies of role disability reveal that the effects of mental conditions are as large as those of most chronic physical conditions (Wells et al., 1988; Stewart-Brown and Layte, 1997; Kessler et al., 2003; Buist-Bouwman et al., 2005).

The global burden of mental disorders in children and adolescents up to 24 years of age has also been examined. Similar to studies within the United States, there is a broad range to estimates of the rates of mental disorders. A recent review reported estimates that ranged from 8% (in the Netherlands) to 57% (for young people receiving services in five sectors of care in San Diego, California) (Patel et al., 2007). Results from the Australian National Survey of Mental Health and Well-Being showed that at least 14% of adolescents younger than age 18 years had a diagnosable mental or substance use disorder within the previous 12 months, and this figure rose to 27% in the age 18–24 year group (Sawyer et al., 2000). A review of the childhood and adolescent data by Patel and colleagues (Patel et al., 2007) showed that at least one out of every four to five young people in the general population will suffer from at least one mental disorder in any given year. However, there is much less information on the burden of mental disorders in developing countries, and substantial cross-cultural variations are likely.

RISK FACTORS AND CORRELATES OF MENTAL DISORDERS

Although epidemiologic investigations may appear distant from the immediate goals of biological and laboratory-based studies of psychopathology, differential distribution of disorders may provide clues regarding etiologic factors underlying diseases. For example, there are large sex differences in the rates of several psychiatric disorders, with women having greater rates of anxiety, affective, and eating disorders, whereas men report more substance-related and other behavioral disorders. Although the sex ratio for the major psychoses is approximately equal, research has revealed gender differences in the age of onset of schizophrenia (Hafner et al., 1993; Thorup et al., 2007). Furthermore, investigations across the life span reveal that sex differences in the affective and emotional disorders tend to emerge during adolescence, whereas males tend to have increased rates of behavior and attention problems throughout life (Costello, 1989; Loeber, 1991). In addition, studies of the longitudinal evolution of psychopathology have revealed that anxiety states and depression may result from common underlying biological and cultural factors with age-dependent expression (Merikangas and Angst, 1996).

IDENTIFICATION OF ENVIRONMENTAL RISK FACTORS

The bulk of the work on environmental risk factors has been based on retrospective and ecological data; prospective confirmation of putative associations is still lacking. Longitudinal studies are critical to evaluate the order of onset of putative risk factors and diseases, as well as to characterize the evolution, course, and sequelae of psychiatric disorders. However, the lack of specific environmental factors that play an etiologic rather than provocative role in mental disorders is a major gap. A recent review of prospective evidence for environmental risk factors for mental disorders concluded that evidence for causal environmental risk factors is still forthcoming (Eaton, 2004).

Some of the prospective studies of mental disorders in community samples that may identify environmental risk factors include the Zurich Study of Young Adults that surveyed a probability sample of adults from age 20, with six follow-up interviews over 15 years (Angst et al., 1984; Merikangas, Avenevoli, et al., 2002). Its detailed attention to symptoms permits investigators to address the longitudinal stability of disorders, changing levels of subthreshold disease, and sequences of risk factor expression (Angst and Merikangas, 1997; Merikangas, Avenevoli, et al., 2002). The Baltimore site of the ECA recently completed a fourth wave of follow-up, results of which promise to produce a more comprehensive longitudinal picture of psychopathology (W. Eaton, principal investigator). Likewise, results from the 10-year follow-up of the NCS-R were recently released (R. Kessler, principal investigator). The National Institute on Alcohol Abuse and Alcoholism's (NIAAA) National Longitudinal Alcohol Epidemiologic Survey (NLAES), completed in 1991–1992, and the subsequent NESARC study, completed in 2001–2002, have also provided a wealth of data on the epidemiology of mental disorders in large nationally representative data sets of the U.S. population (B. F. Grant, 1997; B. F. Grant et al., 2004). Such studies will provide data to validate and correct current nosology.

One additional source of identification of environmental risk factors is cross-cultural studies that elucidate cultural differences in rates and patterns of disorders. These studies can provide clues regarding the context, assessment, and risk factors for the major categories of psychopathology. Studies of migration have been particularly informative in identifying environmental contributions to the etiology of cancer and cardiovascular disease. Recent studies of migrants have also demonstrated the importance of environmental exposure to schizophrenia. Numerous studies have reported an increased risk for the development of schizophrenia among immigrants in several different countries including East African immigrants to Sweden (Selten et al., 2002), Surinamese immigrants to the Netherlands (Hanoeman et al., 2002), Afro Caribbean immigrants to the United Kingdom (Cooper, 2005), Finnish immigrants to Sweden (Leao et al., 2006), and European immigrants to Canada (Smith et al., 2006). Although selective migration may be one explanation, there is converging evidence that socially disrupted environments may trigger the onset of schizophrenia in susceptible individuals.

In contrast to most other mental disorders, there is a growing body of evidence on specific environmental risk factors for schizophrenia. An increased incidence of numerous neurodevelopmental abnormalities among high-risk compared to low-risk offspring of patients with schizophrenia (Brewer et al., 2006; Owens and Johnstone, 2006) has led to a focus on early developmental factors in the etiology of schizophrenia. Some of the specific environmental risk factors currently under investigation include obstetric complications (Clarke et al., 2006), childhood trauma (Morgan and Fisher, 2007), prenatal factors such as nutritional deficiencies (Ludvigsson et al., 2007), increased paternal age (Malaspina et al., 2002), family interactions (McGuffin,

2004), maternal infections (Buka, Tsuang, Torrey, Klebanoff, Bernstein, and Yolken, 2001), maternal cytokines (Buka, Tsuang, Torrey, Klebanoff, Wagner, and Yolken, 2001), gluten sensitivity (Kalaydjian et al., 2006), and cannabis use (Arseneault et al., 2002; Dean and Murray, 2005). In summary, schizophrenia is now widely viewed as a neurodevelopmental disorder comprising a confluence of vulnerability genes and environmental exposures (Dealberto, 2007).

GENETIC RISK FACTORS: GENETIC EPIDEMIOLOGY

The wealth of data from family, twin, and adoption studies of the major mental disorders exceeds that of all other chronic human diseases. The increased recognition of the role of biologic and genetic vulnerability factors for mental disorders has led to research with increasing methodologic sophistication that has spanned the second half of the 20th century (Rosenthal, 1959; Kety et al., 1968; Reich et al., 1969; Tsuang et al., 1977; Gershon et al., 1982; Weissman et al., 1982; Winokur et al., 1982; Andreasen et al., 1987; Kendler, 2001). There are numerous comprehensive reviews of genetic research on specific disorders of interest as well as on psychiatric genetics in general (Kendler et al., 1993; McGuffin et al., 1994; Merikangas and Swendsen, 1996; Plomin et al., 1997; "A Full Genome Screen," 1998; Kendler and Prescott, 1998a, 1998b; Sullivan and Kendler, 1998; Szatmari et al., 1998; Moldin, 1999; Risch et al., 1999; Rutter et al., 1999; Thapar et al., 1999; Nestadt et al., 2000; Smoller et al., 2000; Sullivan et al., 2000; van den Heuvel et al., 2000; Craddock and Jones, 2001; McGuffin et al., 2002; Merikangas, 2002; Rice et al., 2002; Thapar and Scourfield, 2002; Uhl et al., 2002).

There is a wide range of estimates of magnitude of familial aggregation of the most common mental disorders from controlled studies. The risk ratios comparing the proportion of affected relatives of cases versus controls are greatest for autism (50–100), bipolar disorder (7–10), and schizophrenia (8–10); intermediate for substance dependence (4–8) and subtypes of anxiety (4–6), particularly panic (3–8); and lowest for major depression (2–3). The estimates of heritability (that is, the proportion of variance attributable to genetic factors) derived from twin studies, which compare rates of disorders in monozygotic and dizygotic twins, demonstrate that a substantial proportion of the familial aggregation of mental disorders can be attributed to genetic factors. Heritability estimates are greatest for autism (.90) and schizophrenia (.80), followed by bipolar disorder (.65) and panic disorder (.60), followed by substance dependence (.40), anxiety disorders (.35), and major depression (.30). Furthermore, adoption and half-sibling studies also support a genetic basis for the observed familial aggregation.

SOURCES OF COMPLEXITY IN GENETICS OF MENTAL DISORDERS

The major impediments to gene identification for psychiatric disorders are the *lack of validity of the classification* of psychiatric disorders (for example, phenotypes, or observable aspects of diseases) and the *complexity of the pathways from genotypes to psychiatric phenotypes* (that is, heterogeneity).

Lack of Validity of the Classification System

Psychiatric disorder phenotypes, based solely on clinical manifestations without pathognomonic markers, still lack conclusive evidence for the validity of classification (Kendell, 1989). Recent studies have attempted to identify more valid phenotypic constructs for genetic studies. Phenotypic traits or markers that may represent intermediate forms of expression between the output of underlying genes and the broader disease phenotype have been termed *endophenotypes* (Gottesman and Gould, 2003). Studies of the role of genetic factors involved in these systems may be more informative than studies of the aggregate psychiatric phenotypes because they may more closely represent expression of underlying biologic systems. To the extent that particular endophenotypes more clearly represent expression of genotypes, they may help to unravel the complexity of transmission of mental disorders. For example, some of the endophenotypes that may underlie mood disorders include circadian rhythm, stress reactivity, and mood, sleep, and appetite regulation (Lenox et al., 2002). However, before applying endophenotypes in gene identification studies, there should be evidence that the endophenotype has a stronger genetic signal than the broader phenotype. A recent meta-analysis of psychiatric endophenotypes (Flint and Munafo, 2007) and a review of the genetic architecture of traits in model organisms do not provide evidence that endophenotypes are superior to current phenotypic disease definitions (Valdar et al., 2006).

Complex Patterns of Transmission

The application of advances in genomics to mental disorders is still limited by the complexity of the process through which genes exert their influence on mental disorders. There is substantial evidence that a lack of one-to-one correspondence between the genotype and phenotype exists for most of the major mental disorders. Phenomena such as *penetrance* (that is, probability of phenotypic expression among individuals with susceptibility gene), *variable expressivity* (that is, variation in clinical expression associated with a particular gene), *gene-environment interaction* (that is, expression of genotype only in the presence of particular environmental exposures), *pleiotropy* (that is, capacity of genes to manifest several different phenotypes simultaneously), *genetic heterogeneity* (that is, different genes leading to indistinguishable phenotypes), *gene-environment correlation* (Dick et al., 2006), and *polygenic and oligogenic modes of inheritance* (that is, simultaneous contributions of multiple genes rather than Mendelian single gene models) are characteristic of the mental disorders, as they are of numerous other complex disorders for which susceptibility genes have been identified (Gottesman and Shields, 1972; Risch, 1990). Other complex genetic processes include mitochondrial inheritance, imprinting, and epigenetic phenomena (Guttmacher and Collins, 2002).

The high magnitude of comorbidity and coaggregation of index disorders with other major psychiatric disorders (that is, bipolar disorder and alcoholism, major depression and anxiety disorders, schizophrenia and drug dependence), in part induced by the classification system, has been demonstrated in clinical and community studies (Merikangas, 1990; Maier et al., 1993; Merikangas, Stevens, et al., 1998; Maier et al., 2002). For example, alcoholism, a well-established complication of bipolar illness, may mask the underlying features of bipolarity, leading to phenotypic misclassification in genetic studies (Merikangas and Gelernter, 1990). Nonrandom mating is also a common phenomenon in mental disorders that impedes evaluation of patterns of familial transmission (Merikangas, 1982). Assortative mating is particularly pronounced for substance use disorders for which substance dependence among spouses of substance-dependent probands may be as high as 90% (Galbaud du Fort et al., 1998). These phenomena serve to decrease the signal-to-noise ratio in defining the mental disorders for genetic studies. Studies that attempt to identify the impact of these phenomena on phenotypic and endophenotypic expression in individuals and families will bring us closer to understanding the role of the underlying genes on the components of mental disorders.

Identification of Genes for Mental Disorders

Although the mapping of the human genome has led to the discovery of genes for most of the Mendelian diseases, identification of genes for complex disorders has been far more difficult, and few of the genes that have been identified through the candidate gene approach have withstood the ultimate test of replication (Altmuller et al., 2001; Ioannidis et al., 2001; Hirschhorn et al., 2002; Ott, 2004a; Hirschhorn and Daly, 2005). There is widespread agreement regarding the chief obstacles to identifying genes for complex diseases with the candidate gene approach. These include the lack of validity of phenotype characterization, biased sampling, inadequate controls, failure to correct for multiple tests, high false-positive rates due to low a priori probability, use of an overly liberal alpha value, and the lack of adequate power of gene-searching approaches (Risch, 2000; Wacholder et al., 2002; Wacholder et al., 2004; Todd, 2006). To offset the high false-positive rate that has plagued the literature on complex disease genetics, journals in nearly all fields of medicine have published editorials detailing these issues or adopted policies to restrict publication to only the most well designed studies (Ott, 2004b; Begg, 2005).

As the lack of replication of association studies using the candidate gene approach has become increasingly apparent, the genome-wide association method (Risch and Merikangas, 1996) has been proposed as the most promising approach to gene identification in future studies of complex diseases (Botstein and Risch, 2003; Hirschhorn and Daly, 2005). The identification and replication of genes for complex disorders with the genome-wide association approach has proceeded far more rapidly than was anticipated. Since the initial successful identification of genes for macular degeneration (Edwards et al., 2005; Haines et al., 2005; Klein et al., 2005), genes for several other disorders including inflammatory bowel diseases (Crohn's disease and ulcerative colitis) (Duerr et al., 2006), prostate cancer (Amundadottir et al., 2006; M.L. Freedman et al., 2006), and genes underlying diabetes Type I and Type II (S.F. Grant et al., 2006; Groves et al., 2006; Field et al., 2007; Scott et al., 2007; Sladek et al., 2007; Zeggini et al., 2007) have been located. The most exciting finding of this work is the nearly universally accepted independent replications of these findings that have confirmed the potential yield of this approach (Couzin and Kaiser, 2007). Although the results of genome-wide association studies of mental disorders such as bipolar disorder are beginning to emerge, replications of these findings are still forthcoming.

FUTURE APPROACHES

The importance of epidemiology to the future of genetics has been described by numerous geneticists and epidemiologists who conclude that the best strategy for gene identification for complex disorders will ultimately involve large epidemiologic studies from diverse populations (Risch and Merikangas, 1996; Khoury and Yang, 1998; Risch, 2000; Thomas, 2000; Yang et al., 2000; Merikangas, 2002; Merikangas, Chakravarti, et al., 2002; Khoury et al., 2003). It is likely that population-based studies will assume increasing importance in translating the products of genomics to public health. Because current knowledge of genes as risk factors is based nearly exclusively on clinical and nonsystematic samples, it will be essential to assess the generalizability of genetic and environmental risk factors in the general population. To obtain accurate risk estimates, it will be necessary to move beyond samples identified through individuals who are affected to the population to obtain estimates of the risk of specific polymorphisms for the population as a whole. Similar to the role of epidemiology in quantifying risk associated with traditional disease risk factors, applications of human genome epidemiology can provide information on the specificity, sensitivity, and impact of genetic tests to inform science and the individual (Yang et al., 2000). Some of the areas where epidemiology can contribute to future genetic studies are described below.

Samples

The shift from systematic large-scale family studies to linkage studies in psychiatry has led to the collection of families according to very specific sampling strategies (for example, many affected relatives, affected sibling pairs, affected relatives on one side of the family only, availability of parents for study) to maximize the power of detecting genes according to the assumed model of familial transmission. Despite the increase in power for detecting genes, these sampling approaches have diminished the generalizability of the study findings and will contribute little else to the knowledge base if genes are not discovered. Future studies will attempt to collect families and controls from representative samples of the population to enable estimation of population risk parameters, enhance generalizability, and examine the specificity of endophenotypic transmission.

Selection of Controls

The most serious problem in the design of association studies is the failure to select controls who are comparable to the cases on all factors except the disease of interest (Wacholder et al., 2000; Ott, 2004). Controls should be drawn from same population as cases, and must have the same probability of exposure (that is, genes) as cases. Controls should be selected to ensure the validity rather than representativeness of a study. Failure to equate cases and controls may lead to confounding (that is, a spurious association due to an unmeasured factor that is associated with the candidate gene and the disease). In genetic case-control studies, the most likely source of confounding is ethnicity because of differential gene and disease frequencies in different ethnic subgroups.

Risk Estimation

Because genetic polymorphisms involved in complex diseases are likely to be nondeterministic (that is, the marker neither predicts disease nor nondisease with certainty), traditional epidemiologic risk factor designs can be used to estimate their impact. As epidemiologists add genes to their risk equations, it is likely that the contradictory findings from studies that have generally employed solely environmental risk factors, such as diet, smoking, alcohol use, and so on, will be resolved. Likewise, the studies that seek solely to identify genes will also continue to be inconsistent without considering the effects of nongenetic biologic parameters as well as environmental factors that contribute to the diseases of interest.

Identification of Environmental Risk Factors

Over the next decades, it will be important to identify and evaluate the effects of specific environmental factors on disease outcomes and to refine measurement of environmental exposures to evaluate specificity of effects. Once susceptibility genes have been identified, it will be important to identify environmental factors that operate either specifically or nonspecifically on those with susceptibility to mental disorders to develop effective prevention and intervention efforts. Study designs and statistical methods should focus increasingly on gene-environment interaction (Ottman, 1990; Beaty, 1997; Yang and Khoury, 1997).

Although numerous recent studies have reported gene-environment interaction between several genes that interact with nonspecific environmental exposures such as life stress, childhood adversity, and a range of outcomes including depression, cannabis dependence, and conduct disorder (Caspi et al., 2003), replication of these findings is still forthcoming (Zammit and Owen, 2006). Increased knowledge of the developmental pathways of *emotion, cognition,* and *behavior* will expand our ability to identify specific environmental factors such as infection, poor diet, prenatal environment, and early life experiences that interact with the genetic architecture of mood regulation and cognition (Meaney, 2001).

SUMMARY: RELEVANCE OF EPIDEMIOLOGY TO NEUROSCIENCE

A summary of the major contributions of epidemiologic research to neuroscience is presented in Table 9.3. As indicated in this chapter, there has been substantial progress made within the last decade in the development of large-scale nationally representative data sets. Information obtained from these studies will be used to refine estimates of mental disorders within countries as well as to facilitate cross-cultural comparisons of the rates, onset, progression, and course of mental disorders. Results will also be used to generate more valid diagnostic criteria, which will aid in the identification of environmental, social, and genetic risk factors.

TABLE 9.3. *Relevance of Epidemiology to Neurosciences*

Establishment of generalizability of clinical samples
Identification of clues to etiology of psychiatric disorders:
Sex differences in psychiatric disorders
Age-specific patterns of onset and offset
Cohort effects
Derivation of attributable risk of neurobiologic and genetic risk factors
Identification of environmental agents (for example, viral exposure, toxins, diet)
Geographic patterns (for example, cultural patterns of expression, risk factors, migration)

Sociodemographic factors such as gender and age provide important clues regarding underlying biologic mechanisms for emotional, cognitive, and behavioral regulation, which could be far more intensively studied in the future. Additionally, epidemiologists need to expand their tools to include environmental and biologic measures as reliable and valid correlates of psychiatric disorders.

This chapter suggests that epidemiology can contribute to our understanding of the etiology and prevention of mental disorders through the following steps: (*1*) incorporate the results of international prospective population-based studies along with other study designs to refine the current nosological conceptions of mental disorders; (*2*) conduct prospective population-based studies of children and adolescents to fill the tremendous gaps in our knowledge about the prevalence, course, and service patterns of mental disorders in youth; (*3*) apply within-family study designs to identify the core components of mental disorders that are attributable to genetic and environmental risk factors; and (*4*) incorporate genetic risk factors from the rapidly growing genetics knowledge base along with sociodemographic and environmental vulnerability factors in the construction of comprehensive risk profiles for the development of mental disorders.

There is an increasing awareness of the importance of population, samples both efforts in terms of understanding the etiology of disorders but also as the context for intervention (Susser and Susser, 1996). As the neurosciences continue to advance knowledge regarding human brain structure and function, the relevance of neurobiologic factors to psychiatric disorders at the population level is likely to increase as we attempt to identify the extent to which basic sciences explain chronic human disease.

REFERENCES

A full genome screen for autism with evidence for linkage to a region on chromosome 7q. International Molecular Genetic Study of Autism Consortium. (1998) *Hum. Mol. Genet.* 7:571–578.

Abou-Saleh, M.T., Ghubash, R., and Daradkeh, T.K. (2001) A1 Ain Community Psychiatric Survey. I. Prevalence and sociodemographic correlates. *Soc. Psychiatry Psychiatr. Epidemiol.* 36:20–28.

Altmuller, J., Palmer, L.J., Fischer, G., Scherb, H., and Wjst, M. (2001) Genomewide scans of complex human diseases: true linkage is hard to find. *Am. J. Hum. Genet.* 69:936–950.

American Psychiatric Association. (1994). *Diagnostic and Statistical Manual of Mental Disorders* (4th ed.). Washington, DC: Author.

Amundadottir, L.T., Sulem, P., and Gudmundsson, J., et al. (2006) A common variant associated with prostate cancer in European and African populations. *Nat. Genet.* 38:652–658.

Andreasen, N.C., Rice, J., Endicott, J., Coryell, W., Grove, W.M., and Reich, T. (1987) Familial rates of affective disorder. A report from the National Institute of Mental Health Collaborative Study. *Arch. Gen. Psychiatry* 44:461–469.

Angst, J. (1997) The bipolar spectrum. *Br. J. Psychiatry* 190:189.

Angst, J., Dobler-Mikola, A., and Binder, J. (1984) The Zurich study—a prospective epidemiological study of depressive, neurotic and psychosomatic syndromes. I. Problem, methodology. *Eur. Arch. Psychiatry Neurol. Sci.* 234:13–20.

Angst, J., Gamma, A., Joseph Bienvenu, O., et al. (2006) Varying temporal criteria for generalized anxiety disorder: prevalence and clinical characteristics in a young age cohort. *Psychol. Med.* 36:1283–1292.

Angst, J., and Merikangas, K. (1997) The depressive spectrum: diagnostic classification and course. *J. Affect. Disord.* 45:31–39; discussion 39–40.

Angst, J., Merikangas, K.R., and Preisig, M. (1997) Subthreshold syndromes of depression and anxiety in the community. *J. Clin. Psychiatry* 58:6–10.

Arseneault, L., Cannon, M., Poulton, R., Murray, R., Caspi, A., and Moffitt, T.E. (2002) Cannabis use in adolescence and risk for adult psychosis: longitudinal prospective study. *BMJ* 325:1212–1213.

Beaty, T.H. (1997) Evolving methods in genetic epidemiology. I. Analysis of genetic and environmental factors in family studies. *Epidemiol. Rev.* 19:14–23.

Begg, C.B. (2005) Reflections on publication criteria for genetic association studies. *Cancer Epidemiol. Biomarkers Prev.* 14:1364–1365.

Benazzi, F., and Akiskal, H.S. (2005) A downscaled practical measure of mood lability as a screening tool for bipolar II. *J. Affect. Disord.* 84:225–232.

Bijl, R.V., Ravelli, A., and van Zessen, G. (1998) Prevalence of psychiatric disorder in the general population: results of The Netherlands Mental Health Survey and Incidence Study (NEMESIS). *Soc. Psychiatry Psychiatr. Epidemiol.* 33:587–595.

Bonnewyn, A., Bruffaerts, R., Vilagut, G., Almansa, J., and Demyttenaere, K. (2007) Lifetime risk and age-of-onset of mental disorders in the Belgian general population. *Soc. Psychiatry Psychiatr. Epidemiol.* 42:522–529.

Botstein, D., and Risch, N. (2003) Discovering genotypes underlying human phenotypes: past successes for Mendelian disease, future approaches for complex disease. *Nat. Genet.* 33:S228–S237.

Braff, D.L., Freedman, R., Schork, N.J., and Gottesman, I.I. (2007) Deconstructing schizophrenia: an overview of the use of endophenotypes in order to understand a complex disorder. *Schizophr. Bull.* 33:21–32.

Brewer, W.J., Wood, S.J., Phillips, L.J., et al. (2006) Generalized and specific cognitive performance in clinical high-risk cohorts: a review highlighting potential vulnerability markers for psychosis. *Schizophr. Bull.* 32:538–555.

Bromet, E.J., Gluzman, S.F., Paniotto, V.I., et al. (2005) Epidemiology of psychiatric and alcohol disorders in Ukraine: findings from the Ukraine World Mental Health survey. *Soc. Psychiatry Psychiatr. Epidemiol.* 40:681–690.

Buist-Bouwman, M.A., de Graaf, R., Vollebergh, W.A., and Ormel, J. (2005) Comorbidity of physical and mental disorders and the effect on work-loss days. *Acta Psychiatr. Scand.* 111:436–443.

Buka, S.L., Tsuang, M.T., Torrey, E.F., Klebanoff, M.A., Bernstein, D., and Yolken, R.H. (2001) Maternal infections and subsequent psychosis among offspring. *Arch. Gen. Psychiatry* 58:1032–1037.

Buka, S.L., Tsuang, M.T., Torrey, E.F., Klebanoff, M.A., Wagner, R. L., and Yolken, R.H. (2001) Maternal cytokine levels during pregnancy and adult psychosis. *Brain Behav. Immun.* 15:411–420.

Caspi, A., Sugden, K., Moffitt, T.E., et al. (2003) Influence of life stress on depression: moderation by a polymorphism in the 5-HTT gene. *Science* 301:386–389.

Clarke, M.C., Harley, M., and Cannon, M. (2006) The role of obstetric events in schizophrenia. *Schizophr. Bull.* 32:3–8.

Cohen, P., Cohen, J., Kasen, S., et al. (1993) An epidemiological study of disorders in late childhood and adolescence—I. Age- and gender-specific prevalence. *J. Child Psychol. Psychiatry* 34:851–867.

Colin, X., Lafuma, A., and Gueron, B. (2007) Costs of cardiovascular events of diabetic patients in the French hospitals. *Diabetes Metab.* 33(4):310–313.

Cooper, B. (2005) Schizophrenia, social class and immigrant status: the epidemiological evidence. *Epidemiol. Psichiatr. Soc.* 14:137–144.

Costello, E.J. (1989) Developments in child psychiatric epidemiology. *J. Am. Acad. Child Adoles. Psychiatry* 28:836–841.

Costello, E.J., Angold, A., Burns, B.J., Erkanli, A., Stangl, D.K., and Tweed, D.L. (1996) The Great Smoky Mountains Study of Youth. Functional impairment and serious emotional disturbance. *Arch. Gen. Psychiatry* 53:1137–1143.

Costello, E.J., Burns, B.J., Angold, A., and Leaf, P.J. (1993) How can epidemiology improve mental health services for children and adolescents? *J. Am. Acad. Child Adoles. Psychiatry* 32:1106–1114.

Costello, E.J., Egger, H., and Angold, A. (2005) 10-year research update review: the epidemiology of child and adolescent psychiatric disorders: I. Methods and public health burden. *J Am Acad Child Adolesc Psychiatry.* 44:972–986.

Couzin, J., and Kaiser, J. (2007) Genome-wide association. Closing the net on common disease genes. *Science* 316:820–822.

Craddock, N., and Jones, I. (2001) Molecular genetics of bipolar disorder. *B. J. Psychiatry* 41:S128–S133.

Dealberto, M.J. (2007) Why are immigrants at increased risk for psychosis? Vitamin D insufficiency, epigenetic mechanisms, or both? *Med. Hypotheses* 68:259–267.

Dean, K., and Murray, R.M. (2005) Environmental risk factors for psychosis. *Dialogues Clin. Neurosci.* 7:69–80.

Demyttenaere, K., Bruffaerts, R., Posada-Villa, J., et al. (2004) Prevalence, severity, and unmet need for treatment of mental disorders in the World Health Organization World Mental Health Surveys. *JAMA* 291:2581–2590.

Dick, D.M., Rose, R.J., and Kaprio, J. (2006) The next challenge for psychiatric genetics: characterizing the risk associated with identified genes. *Ann. Clin. Psychiatry* 18:223–231.

Duerr, R.H., Taylor, K.D., Brant, S.R., et al. (2006) A genome-wide association study identifies IL23R as an inflammatory bowel disease gene. *Science* 314:1461–1463.

Eapen, V., Pauls, D.L., and Robertson, M.M. (2006) The role of clinical phenotypes in understanding the genetics of obsessive-compulsive disorder. *J. Psychosom. Res.* 61:359–364.

Eaton, W.W. (2004). *Risk Factors for Mental Health Disorders.* National Institute of Mental Health unpublished report.

Edwards, A., Ritter, R., and Abel, K. (2005) Complement factor H polymorphism and age-related macular degeneration. *Science* 308:421.

Field, S.F., Howson, J.M., Smyth, D.J., Walker, N.M., Dunger, D.B., and Todd, J.A. (2007) Analysis of the type 2 diabetes gene, TCF7L2, in 13,795 type 1 diabetes cases and control subjects. *Diabetologia* 50:212–213.

First, M.B., Pincus, H.A., Levine, J.B., Williams, J.B., Ustun, B., and Peele, R. (2004) Clinical utility as a criterion for revising psychiatric diagnoses. *Am. J. Psychiatry* 161:946–954.

Flint, J., and Munafo, M.R. (2007) The endophenotype concept in psychiatric genetics. *Psychol. Med.* 37:163–180.

Freedman, D.X. (1984) Psychiatric epidemiology counts. *Arch. Gen. Psychiatry* 41:931–933.

Freedman, M.L., Haiman, C.A., Patterson, N., et al. (2006) Admixture mapping identifies 8q24 as a prostate cancer risk locus in African-American men. *Proc. Natl. Acad. Sci. USA* 103:14068–14073.

Galbaud du Fort, G., Bland, R.C., Newman, S.C., and Boothroyd, L.J. (1998) Spouse similarity for lifetime psychiatric history in the general population. *Psychol. Med.* 28:789–802.

Gershon, E.S., Hamovit, J., and Guroff, J.J. (1982) A family study of schizoaffective, bipolar I, bipolar II, unipolar, and normal control probands. *Arch. Gen. Psychiatry* 39:1157–1167.

Goetzel, R.Z., Long, S.R., Ozminkowski, R.J., Hawkins, K., Wang, S., and Lynch, W. (2004) Health, absence, disability, and presenteeism cost estimates of certain physical and mental health conditions affecting U.S. employers. *J. Occup. Environ. Med.* 46:398–412.

Gordis, L. (2000) *Epidemiology*. Philadelphia: W.B. Saunders.

Gottesman, I.I., and Gould, T.D. (2003) The endophenotype concept in psychiatry: etymology and strategic intentions. *Am. J. Psychiatry* 160:636–645.

Gottesman, I., and Shields, J. (1972) *Schizophrenia and Genetics: A Twin Study Vantage Point*. New York: Academic Press.

Grant, B.F. (1997) Prevalence and correlates of alcohol use and DSM-IV alcohol dependence in the United States: results of the National Longitudinal Alcohol Epidemiologic Survey. *J. Stud. Alcohol* 58:464–473.

Grant, B.F., Dawson, D.A., Stinson, F.S., Chou, S.P., Dufour, M.C., and Pickering, R.P. (2004) The 12-month prevalence and trends in DSM-IV alcohol abuse and dependence: United States, 1991-1992 and 2001-2002. *Drug Alcohol. Depend.* 74:223–234.

Grant, S.F., Thorleifsson, G., Reynisdottir, I., et al. (2006) Variant of transcription factor 7-like 2 (TCF7L2) gene confers risk of type 2 diabetes. *Nat. Genet.* 38:320–323.

Groves, C.J., Zeggini, E., Minton, J., et al. (2006) Association analysis of 6,736 U.K. subjects provides replication and confirms TCF7L2 as a type 2 diabetes susceptibility gene with a substantial effect on individual risk. *Diabetes* 55:2640–2644.

Gureje, O., Lasebikan, V.O., Kola, L., and Makanjuola, V.A. (2006) Lifetime and 12-month prevalence of mental disorders in the Nigerian Survey of Mental Health and Well-Being. *Br. J. Psychiatry* 188:465–471.

Guttmacher, A.E., and Collins, F.S. (2002) Genomic medicine—a primer. *N. Engl. J. Med.* 347:1512–1520.

Hafner, H., Riecher-Rossler, A., An Der Heiden, W., Maurer, K., Fatkenheuer, B., and Loffler, W. (1993) Generating and testing a causal explanation of the gender difference in age at first onset of schizophrenia. *Psychol. Med.* 23:925–940.

Haines, J.L., Hauser, M.A., Schmidt, S., et al. (2005) Complement factor H variant increases the risk of age-related macular degeneration. *Science* 308:419–421.

Hanoeman, M., Selten, J.P., and Kahn, R.S. (2002) Incidence of schizophrenia in Surinam. *Schizophr. Res.* 54:219–221.

Henderson, S., Andrews, G., and Hall, W. (2000) Australia's mental health: an overview of the general population survey. *Aust. N. Z. J. Psychiatry* 34:197–205.

Hill, A.B. (1953) Observation and experiment. *N. Engl. J. Med.* 248:995–1001.

Hirschhorn, J.N., and Daly, M.J. (2005) Genome-wide association studies for common diseases and complex traits. *Nat. Rev. Genet.* 6:95–108.

Hirschhorn, J.N., Lohmueller, K., Byrne, E., and Hirschhorn, K. (2002) A comprehensive review of genetic association studies. *Genet. Med.* 4:45–61.

Ioannidis, J.P., Ntzani, E.E., Trikalinos, T.A., and Contopoulos-Ioannidis, D.G. (2001) Replication validity of genetic association studies. *Nat. Genet.* 29:306–309.

Jablensky, A. (2005) Categories, dimensions and prototypes: critical issues for psychiatric classification. *Psychopathology* 38:201–205.

Jacobi, F., Wittchen, H.U., Holting, C., et al. (2004) Prevalence, co-morbidity and correlates of mental disorders in the general population: results from the German Health Interview and Examination Survey (GHS). *Psychol. Med.* 34:597–611.

Judd, L.L., Akiskal, H.S., Maser, J.D., et al. (1998) A prospective 12-year study of subsyndromal and syndromal depressive symptoms in unipolar major depressive disorders. *Arch. Gen. Psychiatry* 55:694–700.

Kalaydjian, A.E., Eaton, W., Cascella, N., and Fasano, A. (2006) The gluten connection: the association between schizophrenia and celiac disease. *Acta Psychiatr. Scand.* 113:82–90.

Karam, E.G., Mneimneh, Z.N., Karam, A.N., et al. (2006) Prevalence and treatment of mental disorders in Lebanon: a national epidemiological survey. *Lancet* 367:1000–1006.

Kashani, J.H., Beck, N.C., Hoeper, E.W., et al. (1987) Psychiatric disorders in a community sample of adolescents. *Am. J. Psychiatry* 144:584–589.

Kawakami, N., Shimizu, H., Haratani, T., Iwata, N., and Kitamura, T. (2004) Lifetime and 6-month prevalence of DSM-III-R psychiatric disorders in an urban community in Japan. *Psychiatry Res.* 121:293–301.

Kendell, R.E. (1989) Clinical validity. *Psychol. Med.* 19:45–55.

Kendler, K., and Prescott, C. (1998a) Cannabis use, abuse and dependence in a population-based sample of female twins. *Am. J. Psychiatry* 155:1016–1022.

Kendler, K., and Prescott, C. (1998b) Cocaine use, abuse and dependence in a population-based sample of female twins. *B. J. Psychiatry* 173:345–350.

Kendler, K.S. (2001) Twin studies of psychiatric illness: an update. *Arch. Gen. Psychiatry* 58:1005–1014.

Kendler, K.S., Neale, M.C., and Kessler, R.C. (1993) Panic disorder in women: a population-based twin study. *Psychol. Med.* 23:397–406.

Kessler, R.C. (1999) The World Health Organization International Consortium in Psychiatric Epidemiology (ICPE): initial work and future directions—the NAPE Lecture 1998. Nordic Association for Psychiatric Epidemiology. *Acta Psychiatr. Scand.* 99:2–9.

Kessler, R.C., Aguilar-Gaxiola, S., Andrade, L., Bijl, R., Borges, G., Caraveo-Anduaga, J.J., DeWit, D.J., Kology, B., Merikangas, K. R., Molnar, B.E., Vega, W.A., Walters, E.E., Wittchen, H.-U., and Ustun, T.B. (2001) Mental-substance comorbities in the ICPE surveys (English). *Psychiatria Fennica* 32(Suppl 2):62–79.

Kessler, R.C., McGonagle, K.A., Zhao, S., et al. (1994) Lifetime and 12-month prevalence of DSM-III-R psychiatric disorders in the United States. Results from the National Comorbidity Survey. *Arch. Gen. Psychiatry* 51:8–19.

Kessler, R.C., Ormel, J., Demler, O., and Stang, P.E. (2003) Comorbid mental disorders account for the role impairment of commonly occurring chronic physical disorders: results from the National Comorbidity Survey. *J. Occup. Environ. Med.* 45:1257–1266.

Kety, S.S., Rosenthal, D., Wender, P.H., and Schulsinger, F. (1968) The types of prevalence of mental illness in the biological and adoptive families of adopted schizophrenics. In: Rosenthal, D. and Kety, S.S., eds. *The Transmission of Schizophrenia*. Oxford, UK: Pergamon Press.

Khoury, M.J., McCabe, L.L., and McCabe, E.R. (2003) Population screening in the age of genomic medicine. *N. Engl. J. Med.* 348:50–58.

Khoury, M.J., and Yang, Q. (1998) The future of genetic studies of complex human disease. An epidemiologic perspective. *Epidemiol.* 9:350–354.

Klein, R.J., Zeiss, C., Chew, E.Y., et al. (2005) Complement factor H polymorphism in age-related macular degeneration. *Science* 308:385–389.

Kleinbaum, D.G., Kupper, L.L., and Morgenstern, H. (1982) *Epidemiologic Research: Principles and Quantitive Methods*. Belmont, CA: Wadsworth.

Leao, T.S., Sundquist, J., Frank, G., Johansson, L.M., Johansson, S.E., and Sundquist, K. (2006) Incidence of schizophrenia or other psychoses in first- and second-generation immigrants: a national cohort study. *J. Nerv. Ment. Dis.* 194:27–33.

Lenox, R.H., Gould, T.D., and Manji, H.K. (2002) Endophenotypes in bipolar disorder. *Am. J. Med. Genet.* 114:391–406.

Lerner, D., Allaire, S.H., Reisine, S.T. (2005) Work disability resulting from chronic health conditions. *J. Occup. Environ. Med.* 47:253–264.

Lewinsohn, P.M., Hops, H., Roberts, R.E., Seeley, J.R., Andrews, J.A. (1993) Adolescent psychopathology: I. Prevalence and incidence of depression and other DSM-III-R disorders in high school students. *J. Abnorm. Psychol.* 102:133–144.

Loeber, R. (1991) Antisocial behavior: more enduring than changeable? *J. Am. Acad. Child Adoles. Psychiatry* 30:393–397.

Lopez, A.D., and Mathers, C.D. (2006) Measuring the global burden of disease and epidemiological transitions: 2002-2030. *Ann. Trop. Med. Parasitol.* 100:481–499.

Ludvigsson, J.F., Osby, U., Ekbom, A., and Montgomery, S.M. (2007) Coeliac disease and risk of schizophrenia and other psychosis: A general population cohort study. *Scand. J. Gastroenterol.* 49:179.

Maier, W., Lichtermann, D., Franke, P., Heun, R., Falkai, P., and Rietschel, M. (2002) The dichotomy of schizophrenia and affective disorders in extended pedigrees. *Schizophr. Res.* 57:259–266.

Maier, W., Minges, J., and Lichtermann, D. (1993) Alcoholism and panic disorder: co-occurrence and co-transmission in families. *Eur. Arch. Psychiatry Clin. Neurosci.* 243:205–211.

Malaspina, D., Brown, A., Goetz, D., et al. (2002) Schizophrenia risk and paternal age: a potential role for de novo mutations in schizophrenia vulnerability genes. *CNS Spectr.* 7:26–29.

McGuffin, P. (2004) Nature and nurture interplay: schizophrenia. *Psychiatr. Prax.* 31(Suppl 2):S189–S193.

McGuffin, P., Asherson, P., Owen, M., and Farmer, A. (1994) The strength of the genetic effect. Is there room for an environmental influence in the aetiology of schizophrenia? *B. J. Psychiatry* 164: 593–599.

McGuffin, P., Owen, M.J., and Gottesman, I.I. (2002) *Psychiatric Genetics and Genomics*. Oxford, UK: Oxford University Press.

Meaney, M.J. (2001) Maternal care, gene expression, and the transmission of individual differences in stress reactivity across generations. *Annu. Rev. Neurosci.* 24:1161–1192.

Medina-Mora, M.E., Borges, G., Lara, C., et al. (2005) Prevalence, service use, and demographic correlates of 12-month DSM-IV psychiatric disorders in Mexico: results from the Mexican National Comorbidity Survey. *Psychol. Med.* 35:1773–1783.

Merikangas, K.R. (1982) Assortative mating for psychiatric disorders and psychological traits. *Arch. Gen. Psychiatry* 39:1173–1180.

Merikangas, K.R. (1990). *Comorbity for Anxiety and Depression: Review of Family and Genetic Studies*. Washington, DC: American Psychiatric Press.

Merikangas, K.R. (2002a) Genetic epidemiology: Bringing genetics to the population-the NAPE Lecture 2001. *Acta Psychiatr. Scand.* 105:3–13.

Merikangas, K.R. (2002b) Genetic epidemiology of substance-use disorders. In: D'haenen, D. Boer, J., Willner, P., eds. *Textbook of Biological Psychiatry*. New York: John Wiley & Sons, pp. 537–546.

Merikangas, K.R., Akiskal, H.S., Angst, J., et al. (2007) Lifetime and 12-month prevalence of bipolar spectrum disorder in the national comorbidity survey replication. *Arch. Gen. Psychiatry* 64: 543–552.

Merikangas, K.R., and Angst, J. (1996) The challenge of depressive disorders in adolescence. In Rutter, M., ed. *Psychosocial Disturbances in Young People: Challenges for Prevention*. New York: Cambridge University Press, pp. 131–165.

Merikangas, K.R., Avenevoli, S., Acharyya, S., Zhang, H., and Angst, J. (2002) The spectrum of social phobia in the Zurich cohort study of young adults. *Biol. Psychiatry* 51:81–91.

Merikangas, K.R., Chakravarti, A., Moldin, S.O., et al. (2002) Future of genetics of mood disorders research: Workgroup on genetics for NIMH strategic plan for mood disorders. *Biol. Psychiatry* 52:457–477.

Merikangas, K.R., and Gelernter, C.S. (1990) Comorbidity for alcoholism and depression. *Psychiatr. Clin. North Am.* 13:613–632.

Merikangas, K.R., Mehta, R.L., Molnar, B.E., et al. (1998) Comorbidity of substance use disorders with mood and anxiety disorders: results of the International Consortium in Psychiatric Epidemiology. *Addict. Behav.* 23:893–907.

Merikangas, K.R., Stevens, D.E., Fenton, B., et al. (1998) Comorbidity and familial aggregation of alcoholism and anxiety disorders. *Psychol. Med.* 28:773–788.

Merikangas, K.R., and Swendsen, J.D. (1996) Genetic epidemiology of psychiatric disorders. *Epidemiol. Rev.* 19:1–12.

Milbank Memorial Fund. (1950) *Epidemiology of Mental Disorder*. New York: Author.

Moldin, S.O. (1999) Summary of research—appendix to the report of the NIMH's Genetics Workgroup. *Biol. Psychiatry* 45:573–602.

Morgan, C., and Fisher, H. (2007) Environment and schizophrenia: environmental factors in schizophrenia: childhood trauma—a critical review. *Schizophr. Bull.* 33:3–10.

Murray, C.J., and Lopez, A.D. (1996) The incremental effect of age-weighting on YLLs, YLDs, and DALYs: a response. *Bull. World Health Organ.* 74:445–446.

Nestadt, G., Samuels, J., Riddle, M., et al. (2000) A family study of obsessive-compulsive disorder. *Arch. Gen. Psychiatry* 57:358–363.

Oakley Browne, M.A., Wells, J.E., Scott, K.M., and McGee, M.A. (2006) Lifetime prevalence and projected lifetime risk of DSM-IV disorders in Te Rau Hinengaro: the New Zealand Mental Health Survey. *Aust. N. Z. J. Psychiatry* 40:865–874.

Ott, J. (2004a) Association of genetic loci: Replication or not, that is the question. *Neurology* 63:955–958.

Ott, J. (2004b) Issues in association analysis: error control in case-control association studies for disease gene discovery. *Hum. Hered.* 58:171–174.

Ottman, R. (1990) An epidemiologic approach to gene-environment interaction. *Genet. Epidemiol.* 7:177–185.

Owens, D.G., and Johnstone, E.C. (2006) Precursors and prodromata of schizophrenia: findings from the Edinburgh High Risk Study and their literature context. *Psychol. Med.* 36:1501–1514.

Patel, V., Flisher, A.J., Hetrick, S., and McGorry, P. (2007) Mental health of young people: a global public-health challenge. *Lancet* 369:1302–1313.

Pirkola, S.P., Isometsa, E., Suvisaari, J., et al. (2005) DSM-IV mood-, anxiety- and alcohol use disorders and their comorbidity in the Finnish general population—results from the Health 2000 Study. *Soc. Psychiatry Psychiatr. Epidemiol.* 40:1–10.

Plomin, R., Fries, J.C., and McClearn, G.E. (1997) *Behaviorial Genetics*. London: St. Martin's Press.

Regier, D.A., Burke, J.D., and Bruke, K.C. (1990) *Comorbity of Affective and Anxiety Disorders in the NIMH Epidemiologic Catchment Area (ECA) Program*. Washington, DC: American Psychiatric Press.

Reich, T., Clayton, P. J., and Winokur, G. (1969) Family history studies: V. The genetics of mania. *Am. J. Psychiatry* 125:1358–1369.

Reinherz, H., and Griffin, C.L. (1977) Identifying children at risk: a first step to prevention. *Health Education* 8:14–16.

Rice, F., Harold, G., and Thapar, A. (2002) The genetic aetiology of childhood depression: a review. *J. Child Psychol. Psychiatry* 43:65–79.

Risch, N. (1990) Linkage strategies for genetically complex traits. I. Multilocus models. *Am. J. Hum. Genet.* 46:222–228.

Risch, N.J. (2000) Searching for genetic determinants in the new millennium. *Nature* 405:847–856.

Risch, N., and Merikangas, K. (1996) The future of genetic studies of complex human diseases. *Science* 273:1516–1517.

Risch, N., Spiker, D., Lotspeich, L., et al. (1999) A genomic screen of autism: evidence for a multilocus etiology. *Am. J. Hum. Genet.* 65:493–507.

Robins, L.N., Helzer, J., Weissman, M., et al. (1984) Lifetime prevalence of specific psychiatric disorders in three sites. *Arch. Gen. Psychiatry* 41:949–958.

Rosenthal, D. (1959) Some factors associated with concordance and discordance with respect to schizophrenia in monozygotic twins. *J. Nerv. Ment. Dis.* 129:1–10.

Rutter, M., Silberg, J., O'Connor, T., and Simonoff, E. (1999) Genetics and child psychiatry: II Empirical research findings. *J. Child Psychol. Psychiatry* 40:19–55.

Sawyer, M.B., Baghurst, P.A., and Clark, J.J. (2000) *The Mental Health of Young People in Australia*. Canberra, Australia: Canberra Mental Health and Special Programs Branch, Commonwealth Department of Health and Aged and Care.

Schwab-Stone, M.E., Ayers, T.S., Kasprow, W., et al. (1995) No safe haven: a study of violence exposure in an urban community. *J. Am. Acad. Child Adoles. Psychiatry* 34:1343–1352.

Scott, L.J., Mohlke, K.L., Bonnycastle, L.L., et al. (2007) A genome-wide association study of type 2 diabetes in Finns detects multiple susceptibility variants. *Science* 316:1341–1345.

Selten, J.P., Cantor-Graae, E., Slaets, J., and Kahn, R.S. (2002) Odegaard's selection hypothesis revisited: schizophrenia in Surinamese immigrants to The Netherlands. *Am. J. Psychiatry* 159:669–671.

Shen, Y.C., Zhang, M.Y., Huang, Y.Q., et al. (2006) Twelve-month prevalence, severity, and unmet need for treatment of mental disorders in metropolitan China. *Psychol. Med.* 36:257–267.

Shepherd, M. (1984) The contribution of epidemiology to clinical psychiatry. *Am. J. Psychiatry* 141:1574–1576.

Sladek, R., Rocheleau, G., Rung, J., et al. (2007) A genome-wide association study identifies novel risk loci for type 2 diabetes. *Nature* 445:881–885.

Smith, G.N., Boydell, J., Murray, R.M., et al. (2006) The incidence of schizophrenia in European immigrants to Canada. *Schizophr. Res.* 87:205–211.

Smoller, J.W., Finn, C., and White, C. (2000) The genetics of anxiety disorders: An overview. *Psychiatric Annals* 30:745–753.

Smoller, J.W., and Tsuang, M.T. (1998) Panic and phobic anxiety: defining phenotypes for genetic studies. *Am. J. Psychiatry* 155: 1152–1162.

Stewart-Brown, S., and Layte, R. (1997) Emotional health problems are the most important cause of disability in adults of working age: a study in the four counties of the old Oxford region. *J. Epidemiol. Community Health* 51:672–675.

Sullivan, P.F., and Kendler, K.S. (1998) Typology of common psychiatric syndromes: An empirical study. *B. J. Psychiatry* 173:312–319.

Sullivan, P.F., Neale, M.C., and Kendler, K.S. (2000) Genetic epidemiology of major depression: Review and meta-analysis. *Am. J. Psychiatry* 157:1552–1562.

Susser, M., and Susser, E. (1996) Choosing a future for epidemiology: I. Eras and paradigms. *Am. J. Public Health* 86:668–673.

Szatmari, P., Jones, M.B., Zwaigenbaum, L., and MacLean, J.E. (1998) Genetics of autism: overview and new directions. *J. Autism Dev. Disord.* 28:351–368.

Thapar, A., Holmes, J., Poulton, K., and Harrington, R. (1999) Genetic basis of attention deficit and hyperactivity. *Br. J. Psychiatry* 174:105–111.

Thapar, A., and Scourfield, J. (2002) Childhood disorders. In: McGuffin, P., Owen, M.J., Gottesman, I.I., eds. *Psychiatric Genetics and Genomics.* Oxford, UK: Oxford University Press, pp. 147–180.

Thomas, D.C. (2000) Genetic epidemiology with a capital "E." *Genet. Epidemiol.* 19:289–300.

Thorup, A., Waltoft, B.L., Pedersen, C.B., Mortensen, P.B., and Nordentoft, M. (2007) Young males have a higher risk of developing schizophrenia: a Danish register study. *Psychol. Med.* 37:479–484.

Todd, J.A. (2006) Statistical false positive or true disease pathway? *Nat. Genet.* 38:731–733.

Tsuang, M., Dempsey, G., Dvoredsky, A., and Strauss, A. (1977) A family history study of schizoaffective disorder. *Biol. Psychiatry* 12:331–338.

Uhl, G.R., Liu, Q.R., and Naiman, D. (2002) Substance abuse vulnerability loci: converging genome scanning data. *Trends Genet.* 18:420–425.

U.S. Department of Health and Human Services. (2001) *Mental Health: A Report of the Surgeon General.* http://www.surgeongeneral.gov/library/mentalhealth/home.html.

Valdar, W., Solberg, L.C., Gauguier, D., et al. (2006) Genome-wide genetic association of complex traits in heterogeneous stock mice. *Nat. Genet.* 38:879–887.

van den Heuvel, O.A., van de Wetering, B.J., Veltman, D.J., and Pauls, D.L. (2000) Genetic studies of panic disorder: a review. *J. Clin. Psychiatry* 61:756–766.

Verbrugge, L.M., and Patrick, D.L. (1995) Seven chronic conditions: their impact on US adults' activity levels and use of medical services. *Am. J. Public Health* 85:173–182.

Vicente, B., Kohn, R., Rioseco, P., Saldivia, S., Levav, I., and Torres, S. (2006) Lifetime and 12-month prevalence of DSM-III-R disorders in the Chile psychiatric prevalence study. *Am. J. Psychiatry* 163: 1362–1370.

Wacholder, S., Chanock, S., Garcia-Closas, M., El Ghormli, L., and Rothman, N. (2004) Assessing the probability that a positive report is false: an approach for molecular epidemiology studies. *J. Natl. Cancer Inst.* 96:434–442.

Wacholder, S., Garcia-Closas, M., and Rothman, N. (2002) Study of genes and environmental factors in complex diseases. *Lancet* 359:1155; author reply 1157.

Wacholder, S., Rothman, N., and Caporaso, N. (2000) Population stratification in epidemiologic studies of common genetic variants and cancer: quantification of bias. *J. Natl. Cancer Inst.* 92: 1151–1158.

Weissman, M.M., Gershon, E.S., Kidd, K.K., et al. (1984) Psychiatric disorder in relatives of probands with affective disorders: The Yale-NIMH collaborative family study. *Arch. Gen. Psychiatry* 41:13–21.

Weissman, M.M., Kidd, K.K., and Prusoff, B.A. (1982) Variability in rates of affective disorders in relatives of depressed and normal probands. *Arch. Gen. Psychiatry* 39:1397–1403.

Wells, K.B., Golding, J.M., and Burnam, M.A. (1988) Psychiatric disorder in a sample of the general population with and without chronic medical conditions. *Am. J. Psychiatry* 145:976–981.

Winokur, G., Tsuang, M.T., and Crowe, R.R. (1982) The Iowa 500: Affective disorder in relatives of manic and depressed patients. *Am. J. Psychiatry* 139:209–212.

Wittchen, H.-U. (1994) Reliability and validity studies of the WHO Composite International Diagnostic Interview (CIDI): a critical review. *J Psychiatr Res.* 28:57–84

World Health Organization. (1990) *Composite International Diagnostic Interview (CIDI, Version 1.0).* Geneva: World Health Organization.

Yang, Q., and Khoury, M.J. (1997) Evolving methods in genetic epidemiology. III. Gene-environment interaction in epidemiologic research. *Epidemiol. Rev.* 19:33–43.

Yang, Q., Khoury, M.J., Coughlin, S.C., Sun, F., and Flanders, W.D. (2000) On the use of population-based registries in the clinical validation of genetic tests for disease susceptibility. *Genet. Med.* 2:186–192.

Zammit, S., and Owen, M.J. (2006) Stressful life events, 5-HTT genotype and risk of depression. *Br. J. Psychiatry* 188:199–201.

Zeggini, E., Weedon, M.N., Lindgren, C.M., et al. (2007) Replication of genome-wide association signals in UK samples reveals risk loci for type 2 diabetes. *Science* 316:1336–1341.

10 Basic Methods for Clinical Molecular Genetics of Psychiatric Illness

JOEL GELERNTER AND JAAKKO LAPPALAINEN

The fact of a genetic contribution to the development of certain psychiatric disorders has been appreciated for over a century, and a genetic contribution can be supported for a broad range of behavioral phenotypes, from level of neuroticism (Lesch et al., 1996) to self-esteem (Roy et al., 1995). Our understanding of the genetics of major mental illness over the past three decades has paralleled enormous progress in molecular and statistical methods. The field experienced the extraordinary leap in our knowledge of human genetics created by the Human Genome Project (Lander et al., 2001; Venter et al., 2001), and now the International HapMap project (The International HapMap Consortium, 2005; http://www.hapmap.org) is having enormous impact. Very broadly, the arc can be traced as follows: in the 1950s and 1960s, the introduction of effective pharmacological treatments for the symptoms of psychiatric illness altered perceptions of these disorders, with a revision in focus away from psychoanalysis and toward biology. This represented a progression from studying the final behavioral output of the organism toward trying to understand the biological events underlying behavior. A second shift in viewpoint occurred when the tools became available to study the genetic events underlying these biological events—that is, the action of genes influencing behavior, including psychopathology. The molecular tools necessary to operationalize this next step (principally, molecular deoxyribonucleic acid [DNA] markers) started to become available in 1980s, but with many quantum steps since then in ease of data generation. In the early 1990s a state-of-the-art genetic study might have employed 10 different polymorphic genetic markers; at the time of this writing, it could easily employ a million, in the form of the newly practical *genomewide association study* design.

The first major successes for gene mapping (that is, assigning a gene to a particular location on a particular chromosome) using molecular markers were all for Mendelian disorders, for example, the localization of a gene predisposing to Huntington's disease in 1983 by genetic linkage (Gusella et al., 1983) (see below). Methods widely applicable to gene mapping for "complex" genetic disorders—in this context, *complex* means a genetic disorder not following simple (Mendelian) rules of inheritance such as dominant, recessive, or X-linked—did not become available until much more recently. With such methods, we have evidence of genes mapped, or located, by linkage for schizophrenia (e.g., Straub et al., 1995; S. Wang et al., 1995), bipolar affective disorder (e.g., Freimer et al., 1996), and alcohol dependence (Long et al., 1998; Reich et al., 1998). Association studies, and related methods, have produced evidence for relationships of specific genes with psychiatric phenotype; examples of these findings include linkage disequilibrium (LD) of an allele at the γ-aminobutyric acid (GABA) A receptor, alpha 2 locus (*GABRA2*) with alcohol dependence (Edenberg et al., 2004), and association of variation at the catechol-O-methyltransferase (*COMT*) locus with cognitive function and schizophrenia (Egan et al., 2001). (*LD* refers to nonrandom association of genetic traits, which can be markers or phenotypes; two traits in LD are expected to be molecularly close to each other. A gene in LD with a phenotype, such as alcohol dependence, is either close to a gene influencing the trait or is influencing the trait itself.) Such findings should lead to a richer understanding of disease pathophysiology and may eventually apply to a broader range of psychiatric pathology.

BASIC ISSUES

Variation in DNA sequences between individuals is called *polymorphism* if the most common allele (or version of a gene or sequence) is observed no more than 99% of the time. The process of identifying genes related to illness (once the illness has been established to be genetically influenced) usually relies initially on statistical analysis of frequencies of polymorphic variants in certain specialized samples including affected individuals (Table 10.1). A basic division in approach to this problem opposes candidate gene studies (testing a single gene or sets of specific genes, which might be selected for study based on the function of the proteins they encode or based on their position) and genomewide scanning studies (querying the entire genome, using either linkage or association methods). Both have advantages and disadvantages; genome scanning is a more general solution but is not always applicable and is usually resource intensive; candidate gene studies have the potential to be more efficient. Although the two approaches diverge in philosophy initially, eventually they converge on the study of specific genes, where some variant in a specific gene must be shown to be consistent with an effect on the phenotype through function or to be strongly associated with the phenotype statistically.

This chapter reviews some of the basic methods used, first, in localizing unknown genes (by genetic linkage or genomewide association) and in determining if specified "candidate" genes influence a certain phenotype. The genetic raw data for these kinds of studies are made up of genetic marker data, or "genotype" data: information about what alleles of genes or markers occur in families or individuals. The behavioral, or phenotypic, data comprises information about a set of participants regarding diagnosis, behavior, or some "intermediate phenotype" such as a neuroimaging measure. This chapter also discusses molecular methods used to identify and characterize genetic variation and, finally, examples of studies that applied some of these techniques.

IDENTIFYING GENES RELATED TO PHENOTYPES: LINKAGE, ASSOCIATION, AND RELATED ISSUES

Genetic Linkage

Genetic linkage refers to cotransmission of genetic markers or traits, one of which might be a phenotype such as a disease state, in families. If a genetic marker of known chromosomal location is linked to a certain trait, and a certain form of the marker is therefore usually inherited with the trait in a family, then the location of a gene influencing the trait may be inferred, and it is said to be mapped, or localized (Fig. 10.1). (A genetic marker could be, for example, a polymorphic short tandem repeat—that is, a series of repeated units of the DNA sequence "CA" repeated different numbers of times in different individuals. A single nucleotide polymorphism, or SNP, is a kind of variation that affects only a single base in the DNA sequence. Issues relating to types of genetic markers are discussed in greater detail below.) Linkage, when applicable, provides a general solution to the problem of localization of genetic susceptibility loci, the only necessary prior knowledge being that the phenotype studied has at least a partially genetic basis (for nonparametric analyses) and sometimes an idea of how the disorder is transmitted (for parametric analyses) (discussed below). Prior to the recent advent of practical genomewide association study methodology, linkage was the only truly genomewide method available. Moreover, a genomewide linkage scan can be completed with a limited marker set, that is, about 400 marker genotypes per individual studied; standard marker sets are available, and this is a straightforward process for many laboratories.

This approach is not universally applicable. The linkage approach poses difficult challenges when applied to complex traits. The clinical material required extends from the specialized (affected sibling pairs, preferably with their biological parents) to the highly specialized (large extended pedigrees). If linkage is used to map a disease susceptibility locus for a complex disorder, and

TABLE 10.1. *Strategies Used in Locating and Identifying Genes*

Strategy	*Application*	*Comments*	*Examples of Uses in Psychiatry (See text for specifics)*
Linkage analysis	Gene mapping	May use extended pedigrees or relative pairs Many statistical variants Usually provides a gene location without specifically identifying the gene	Bipolar affective disorder Schizophrenia Alcohol dependence
Family association	Identification of phenotypic effects of specific genes	Uses affected probands plus relatives (usually parents) Several statistical variants Identifies linkage disequilibrium of a gene with a phenotype, which does not necessarily identify the specific polymorphism responsible for the effect	Schizophrenia Nicotine dependence
Candidate gene association	Identification of phenotypic effects of specific genes	Uses sets of unrelated affected individuals and sets of unrelated controls Subject to population stratification artifact and other biases	*ADH2*, *ALDH2*, and alcohol dependence
Genomewide association	Gene mapping (with greater power than via linkage analysis)	Uses sets of unrelated affected individuals and sets of unrelated controls Subject to population stratification artifact and other biases	Nicotine dependence

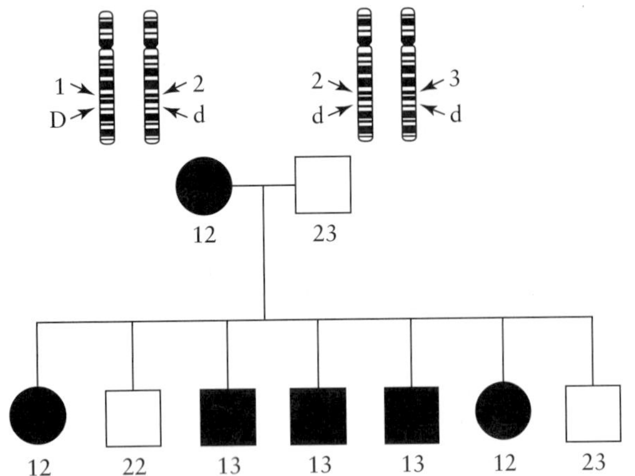

FIGURE 10.1 Linkage. Dark symbols mean "ill," white symbols mean "well." In this example, *D* is the "disease" allele, and *d* is the "normal" allele, at the "disease" locus. We cannot observe this (disease) locus directly, but we can observe genotypes at the "marker" locus, which in this case are designated 1, 2, and 3. Every person with marker allele 1 has the disease. If this family were considerably larger and the same pattern held, we would be able to conclude that the marker locus was linked to the disease locus, and we could then infer that the disease locus was somewhere near the marker locus (which is how it is drawn).

if the gene mapped accounts for a small proportion of illness, it may be very difficult to obtain sufficient family material to permit the eventual identification of the gene. Positional cloning (that is, identifying and isolating a disease-influencing gene given its approximate location) is difficult even for a homogeneous disorder with a known mode of inheritance (and was famously difficult for Huntington's disease, where it took 10 years from identification of linkage to identification of the gene; Huntingtons Disease Collaborative Research Group, 1993). It is an even greater problem for genes localized through affected sibling pair strategies, and this imprecise localization sometimes has made it difficult even to establish if a result has actually been replicated (Risch and Botstein, 1996). A positive linkage genome scan result leaves one with a gene location (that is, a position for a gene on a particular chromosome) rather than a gene.

Lod score (parametric) methods

Lod (or log of odds ratio) score linkage analysis is most clearly suitable for Mendelian diseases occurring in extended pedigrees (Ott, 1991). The standard measure of statistical significance for linkage analysis is the lod score, where the odds ratio in question compares the likelihood of a particular set of marker data arising under the condition of linkage to that of the same set of data arising in the absence of linkage. Higher lod scores mean stronger evidence for linkage, and because the scale is logarithmic, each increase in lod score of 1 corresponds to 10 times better evidence. Analyses are conducted under certain assumptions of mode of inheritance (for example, dominant or recessive), differences in liability for illness based on age and sex, and so on. The lod score necessary to establish linkage of genomewide significance (that is, significant when corrected for the multiple comparisons engendered by the examination of hundreds of markers in a genomewide linkage scan) is generally taken as 3.3 (Lander and Kruglyak, 1995).

Nonparametric methods

Replicable parametric linkage results for purely psychiatric illnesses were sparse initially. Several features of psychiatric illness and of the initial published studies contributed to this difficulty, including the genetic complexity of these disorders (Risch, 1990a), difficulties with establishing diagnosis (Tsuang et al., 1993), and small sample size resulting in insufficient power in the context of genetic complexity. Additionally, linkage analysis was sometimes applied in nonconservative ways—that is, under numerous models of diagnostic spectrum—that increased the risk of a chance false-positive finding. The resulting disappointments were among the factors that eventually led to innovation in linkage analysis, spawning a more recent series of positive results that found a higher degree of consistency across studies.

A key step in modifying the linkage approach so that it could be applied more robustly was to address two key questions of classical linkage analysis: who has the disorder? and how exactly is it transmitted? The importance of the former question was demonstrated because in trying to make the best use possible of the linkage information that could be extracted from extended pedigrees, analyses were often performed under several sets of disease definition, some of which would require inclusion of less severe forms of the illness than the core phenotype—or at least that was the intention. This approach was particularly common when the disorder under study had a low recurrence risk, such as schizophrenia; even high-density pedigrees where schizophrenia appears to be transmitted tend not to contain a large number of individuals with the full syndrome. Those analyses including more "affected" individuals tended to be the most "powerful" (as they would include the largest number of highly informative individuals) and therefore could generate the most impressive lod scores, but they would also be most likely to include in the "affected" class individuals who did not really have an illness genetically related to the core phenotype under study. The latter question was important because conventional lod score linkage analyses require specification of a "disease model," that is how the disorder is inherited. Although this is straightforward for classical (Mendelian) disorders such as Huntington's disease (single major locus [SML] dominant) and cystic fibrosis (SML recessive), it is not straightforward for common, genetically complex disorders such as schizophrenia and bipolar affective disorder. The realization that these disorders are genetically complex and must be treated as such began to take over after publication of a series of articles by Risch, one of which (Risch, 1990b) demonstrated, through consideration of risk ratios in different classes of relatives (λ_R), that schizophrenia is likely to be caused by several genetic loci, and that single locus models are therefore unlikely to succeed in identifying genes related to illness.

For the common psychiatric illnesses, it is difficult to specify which individuals in a pedigree have an illness genetically related to, but not identical to, the one under study. Furthermore, it is impossible in most cases to state an accurate genetic model for the common psychiatric illnesses. Methods of analysis were needed that eliminated the need to broaden disease definition (that is, that studied unambiguously affected individuals only) and that did not require specification of genetic models (that is, were nonparametric). Such methods had been under development for some time; when applied to psychiatric illness, they provided a powerful tool to add to lod score linkage methods.

Sibling pair (Suarez et al., 1978; Kruglyak and Lander, 1995; Risch and Zhang, 1995) and affected pedigree member (APM) (Weeks and Lange, 1988, 1992) methods are frequently used nonparametric strategies for linkage analysis. The sibling pair strategy, as employed by Suarez et al. (1978), makes use of marker data from affected siblings and biological parents to identify *identical-by-descent* genetic markers in the siblings. Allele sharing is increased when the marker studied is linked to illness. Various nonparametric, or model-free, linkage analysis methods are incorporated in popular linkage analysis programs such as SOLAR (which implements variance components analysis methods; Almasy and Blangero, 1998; http://www.sfbr.org/solar/) and MERLIN (Abecasis et al., 2002; http://www.sph.umich.edu/csg/abecasis/Merlin/).

Linkage Disequilibrium and Genetic Association

Genetic linkage identifies a chromosomal region (in geographic terms, a part of a specific interstate highway, so to speak) and not a gene (a particular exit on the highway), and it is therefore necessary to have additional methods available for identifying actual susceptibility loci and particular alleles once a linkage has been found. Association methods, which usually rely upon LD, have the potential to locate genes influencing traits much more finely than linkage methods. As discussed briefly above, *LD* refers to nonindependence of alleles that are located on the same chromosome and usually in close proximity to each other. LD reflects "historical" recombination events between two alleles on the same chromosomal segments. Recombination is the only major factor attempting to shuffle the co-occurrence of the alleles that are located on the same chromosome (another phenomenon, *gene conversion*, appears to be quite rare). However, this "shuffling" is not complete, and alleles, especially if they are located close to each other, still tend to co-occur in unrelated individuals more often than just by random chance. In other words, these alleles have been "fellow travelers" throughout the generations.

The following paragraph contains details about LD and may be skipped by casual readers. Suppose that allele A at locus 1 and allele B at locus 2 occur at frequencies pA and pB in the population. If the two alleles are independent, then we would expect to see the AB haplotype at frequency of pApB. If the population frequency is either higher or lower than pApB, implying that particular alleles tend to be observed together, then the loci are said to be in LD (assumptions for this example are randomly mating population and population homogeneity). The length of a chromosomal segment where LD can be detected is related to the population age and historical events, such as population bottlenecks (periods of contraction of the population size followed by expansion) and genetic drift. In general, younger populations have longer LD segments. The population LD length, however, is always shorter than the length of an average segment shared between affected siblings at a complex trait locus.

LD methods therefore provide an approach complementary to linkage for gene identification. Samples for case-control association studies comprise unrelated individuals. Allele frequencies at candidate or marker loci are compared between affected and unaffected participants. If a particular allele occurs more frequently in one of the groups, it is said to be associated with the trait. Difference in allele frequency between cases and controls might be attributable to a relationship between the allelic variant studied (or another variant in LD with it) and the phenotype. It might also be attributable to population subdivision (or stratification).

Population stratification is thought to be a cause of some false-positive results in association studies. This can happen when both (*1*) allele frequencies for markers under study and (*2*) the phenotypes under study differ by population group; in this case, differences in allele frequency seen in different groups (which might also be classified as "ill" or "well") may arise from broadly observable population differences rather than phenotypic differences. Although population stratification is clearly a possible confounder for genetic association studies of conventional design (Gelernter et al., 1993), it can be overcome or minimized by certain study designs. The first widely used such design was the haplotype relative risk (HRR) method (Falk and Rubinstein, 1987; Terwilliger and Ott, 1992), a family-based genetic association method using participants and their parents, that compares allele frequency in a set of ill participants with the set of nontransmitted parental alleles.

The closely related transmission/disequilibrium test (TDT) also uses parent offspring trios; TDT uses parents heterozygous for the disease-associated marker and considers observed transmission versus nontransmission of the alleles at a locus to affected offspring. The family-based association test (FBAT) approach implements a more general strategy to test for genetic association, or LD, with family controls, including use of affected–unaffected sibling pairs, and this software is now used widely (Laird et al., 2000; http://www.biostat.harvard.edu/~fbat/default.html).

Families are much more difficult to collect than case-control samples; the ideal method would allow valid use of easily collected series of unrelated affecteds and unaffecteds by correcting for, or accounting for, population stratification. Several methods have been described; the first to be implemented widely were the structured association (SA) method (Pritchard and Rosenberg, 1999; Pritchard, Stephens, and Donnelly, 2000; Pritchard, Stephens, et al., 2000) and genomic control (GC) (Devlin and Roeder, 1999) method. Both SA and GC methods involve genotyping unlinked markers in case and control samples. Genomic control uses data from a set of unlinked SNP-type markers to, in effect, adjust required significance levels to account for stratification. Structured association uses data from a set of unlinked markers (not necessarily SNPs) to, in effect, adjust for population structure inferred on the basis of the marker genotypes. These methods generated tremendous interest and enthusiasm; available statistical methodology to deal with stratification is currently evolving rapidly, and newer approaches, including, for example, EIGENSTRAT (Price et al., 2006), which implements a principal components analysis method, have been demonstrated to gain power or computation efficiency.

Association approaches are well-suited for testing of candidate genes. Candidate gene studies may be physiologically motivated (based on hypotheses about relationships between specific known loci and particular phenotypes) or positionally motivated (based on prior evidence that a gene affecting the phenotype of interest maps to a certain genomic region). Although candidate gene studies in psychiatry based on purely physiologic hypotheses have sometimes been criticized because of our limited knowledge of the underlying pathophysiology of illness (and this is a real and significant impediment), there is also much we do know; this is borne out by the existence of several well replicated candidate gene findings in psychiatry (see below). Moreover, it is not necessary to identify the cause of a disease to advance knowledge of genetic influences on phenotype. With recent enormous advances in mutational analysis techniques and in the availability of sequence information from multiple individuals, it has become clear that genetic variation affecting protein function is not at all rare and in some cases (for example, serotonin transporter protein, genetic locus *SLC6A4*; Lesch et al., 1996), functional variation in important genes is common. This means that, within a population expressing genetic polymorphism in a brain protein that corresponds to functional polymorphism, individuals who are genetically different could process any brain events relating to the functional polymorphism differently. As such they might carry out neurotransmission, process information, or in some way—perhaps important, perhaps barely perceptible—experience reality differently. It would therefore be very surprising if genetic variation in some of these genes known to play a major role in neurotransmission, and (for example) in the action or metabolism of psychotropic drugs, did not affect psychiatric phenotype in some way.

One early validation for the candidate gene idea in psychiatry was found in a linkage study that landed on a candidate gene. Genetic linkage was used to identify the location of a gene causing an unusual syndrome involving violence and impulsivity; molecular and biochemical methods (Brunner, Nelen, Breakefield, et al., 1993) identified the mutated gene as *MAOA*, which encodes monoamine oxidase A. This enzyme constitutes a major catabolic pathway for catecholamines and serotonin, and it has been intensively studied by biological psychiatrists for decades. In this case, the data led back to a well-known metabolic mechanism and a well-known gene.

Some of the earliest consistent findings of association between candidate genes and a psychiatric diagnosis describe a relationship between alcohol dependence (AD) and genes encoding alcohol metabolizing enzymes, alcohol dehydrogenases (*ADH* genes) and acetaldehyde dehydrogenases (*ALDH* genes). The *ADH* genes metabolize ethanol to acetaldehyde, and *ALDH* genes (of which *ALDH2* is thought to be the most important in this context) metabolize acetaldehyde to acetate. Acetaldehyde has dysphoric and toxic effects. Numerous genotype/phenotype relationships in this system have been described. For example, an inactive *ALDH2* variant, common in some Asian populations, causes a significant reduction in risk for alcoholism because of buildup of acetaldehyde and a consequent aversive "Antabuse-like" reaction to alcohol drinking. Heterozygotes for this allele are about one third as likely to be alcohol dependent as those without this allele, and homozygotes are nearly immune to developing alcoholism (Thomasson et al., 1991, Chen et al., 1999). Recent years have seen a major resurgence in interest in variants at alcohol-metabolizing enzyme loci, with, for example, demonstration that *ADH4* is an important AD risk locus (Luo et al., 2005; Edenberg et al., 2006; Luo, Kranzler, Zuo, Lappalainen, et al., 2006), and that in fact many genes that map to an *ADH* gene cluster influence AD risk independently (Edenberg et al., 2006; Luo, Kranzler, Zuo, Wang, et al., 2006).

Whole-genome association methods

As discussed above, association (LD) methods can locate genes influencing traits much more finely than linkage methods. But what if the LD approach could be used for a genomewide scan, in the manner of a linkage study? Whole-genome association studies (WGASs) may be more useful for mapping genes influencing complex traits than conventional extended-pedigree linkage studies. The major problem with the application of such approaches was initially a practical one, of the requirement for a very large number of genotypes for such a study to be completed. This is the case because markers studied must be close enough together such that every spot in the genome is in LD with at least one marker. There has been spirited discussion in the field regarding how many markers are actually required for such an analysis to be truly comprehensive.

Recent developments have provided the technology to support true WGAS. Two companies, Illumina and Affymetrix, now provide genotyping microarrays that can provide genotypes at large numbers of marker loci—presently, up to about 1,000,000 or so—using array-based technology, and at relatively low pergenotype cost. Such a study is a large undertaking in populations of European ancestry; it is an even larger undertaking in populations of African ancestry, due to lower LD (in general) and consequent need to use a denser marker set to achieve the same power. Nevertheless, WGAS designs are unique in their potential to identify risk loci of relatively small effect, much smaller than may be detected through linkage strategies. Further, linkage requires family sampling schemes, which bias toward detection of loci of relatively high attributable familial relative risk; other loci may, however, be more important on a population level. WGAS designs are starting to fulfill their potential.

Molecular Methods

The most fundamental method: The polymerase chain reaction (PCR)

Polymerase chain reaction is the key molecular method used for most of the kinds of studies discussed above and below. Introduction of PCR (Saiki et al., 1988) revolutionized research in molecular biology; PCR is required to genotype most of the currently used polymorphisms and is used in sequencing reactions also. By means of this reaction, specific segments of DNA can be amplified in vitro 10 million-fold (Saiki et al., 1988) (Fig. 10.2). This makes it easy to study those very specific parts of the genome in greater detail. The genomic regions studied may include polymorphic markers (as part of a process of mapping disease genes), or segments of genes as part of a process of identifying specific DNA variants that give rise to variation in phenotype.

Deoxyribonucleic acid segments are amplified using unique oligonucleotides called *PCR primers*, which are short synthetic pieces of DNA (usually about 20 nucleotides long) flanking the desired sequence. DNA containing the

A Template DNA (e.g., genomic DNA)

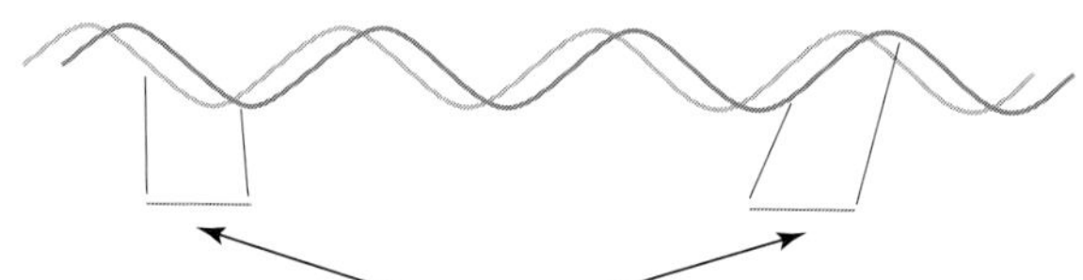

Synthetic oligonucleotides (about 20 bases of single stranded DNA) flanking the region to be amplified, complementary to known sequence

B

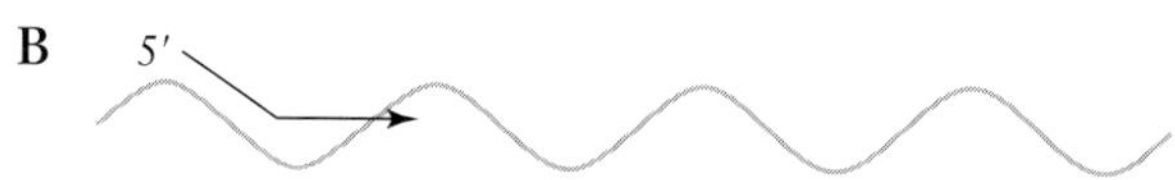

Direction of new DNA synthesis

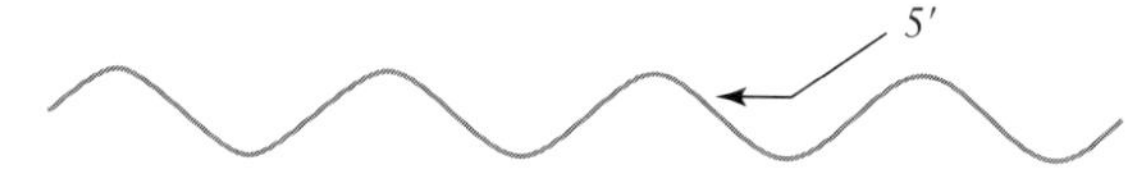

C

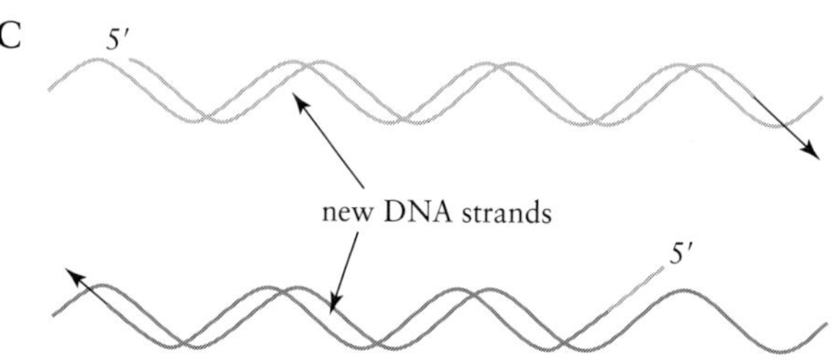

D

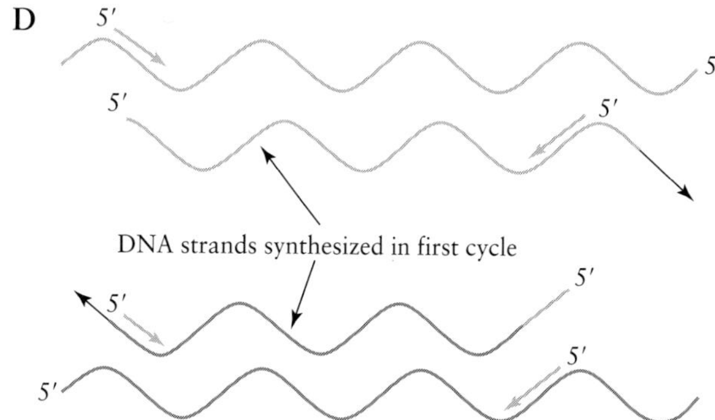

FIGURE 10.2 The polymerase chain reaction (PCR). (*A*) Synthetic oligonucleotides complementary to sequence of template DNA are designed. (*B*) Template DNA is denatured and oligonucleotides anneal (the first cycle thus starts with two strands) (*C*) New DNA strands are synthesized by polymerase's action of placing deoxynucleotides (dATP, dCTP, dGTP and dTTP) complementary to the template sequentially into the elongating DNA strand. (*D*) The DNA is denatured again, and the starting point for the next cycle is four strands.

sequence to be amplified ("template") is denatured—that is, the two strands are made to separate; the oligonucleotides anneal to the target DNA, and synthesis of new DNA begins at the oligonucleotides, catalyzed by a thermostable DNA polymerase (a DNA-synthesizing enzyme that retains its function even after it is exposed to the high temperatures needed to denature DNA). This cycle is repeated about 30 times; for the first cycles, the quantity of PCR product doubles with each cycle, but later the amplification process is exponential. Figure 10.2 illustrates the first few steps of this process. Following PCR and electrophoresis, the position and quality of the amplified DNA can be determined by direct staining, for example, with ethidium bromide or through use of a radioactive or fluorescent label.

Sequencing technology

Genetic studies on identifying genes that contribute to a risk for an illness have as their ultimate goal the discovery of what it is about the gene—specifically—that leads to the relationship between the gene and illness. Finding out what it is about the gene that is different among those at risk may serve as a critical point to begin understanding the biology and pathways behind the disease process. In the past decade, several methods, such as single-strand conformation polymorphism (SSCP) analysis and denaturing high-pressure liquid chromatography (dHPLC), were developed for rapid scanning of genes for mutations. However, owing to the decreasing cost and higher level of automation, direct gene sequencing, the method of breaking down the genetic code base-by-base at a molecular level, has almost entirely replaced other methods of detecting mutations in the genetic code.

The most common method for gene sequencing at this moment is cycle sequencing (but the technologies that will replace it are already starting to be adopted at some centers). This technology combines the use of fluorescent technologies and dideoxynucleotides (ddNTPs), which have the unique capacity to interrupt DNA elongation if placed on the DNA strand by polymerase. In principle, with the exception of the presence of ddNTPs, cycle sequencing is very similar to PCR. The reaction mixture contains the template to be sequenced, a polymerase, an oligonucleotide primer, and deoxynucleotides (dA, dC, dG, and dT). The reaction is controlled by repeated cycles of heating and cooling. For the purpose of detection, each ddNTP base (ddA, ddC, ddG, and ddT) is labeled with a different fluorescent dye (for example, green, blue, yellow, and red). Because billions of DNA molecules are present in the reaction, ddNTPs can interrupt the elongation of a PCR strand at any position of the template resulting in a collection of DNA fragments of differing lengths each labeled with a specific ddNTP at their ultimate base position. The fragment mixture is electrophoresed through a polyacrylamide gel or a capillary, which separates the fragments by length; the shortest fragment will reach the end of the capillary first, where laser detection of the fluorescence takes place. The second shortest will reach the end of the capillary second, and so forth. For example, if the first and second base of a template were A and G, the first two sequencer electropherogram peaks would be distinct colors corresponding to the colors labeling the complementary ddT and ddC (Fig. 10.3).

Molecular methods used for detection of known genetic variants

Polymorphisms used in genetic mapping fall into two main categories: single nucleotide polymorphisms (SNPs) and short tandem repeats (STRs). Other kinds of variants, such as variable number of tandem repeats (VNTR) and insertion/deletion polymorphisms, are sometimes of great importance for disease association but are less commonly used as genetic markers than SNPs and STRs.

Single nucleotide polymorphisms (SNPs). Single nucleotide polymorphisms are substitutions or deletions of a single base pair in the genetic code. Most SNPs do not reside in coding regions of genes but are located in introns, promoters, and regions intervening genes. The most common SNPs that are found in the coding sequence of genes are nucleotide substitutions that do not change amino acid sequence of the genes they encode. Many SNPs, however, do change the function of the gene and the protein they encode (either by changing amino acid sequence or by altering regulatory elements). Good examples of such SNPs are the Val$^{108/158}$Met in the catechol-O-methyltransferase gene (*COMT*) and Val^{66}Met in the brain-derived neurotrophic factor gene (*BDNF*), which influence the function of the protein and cause subtle differences in brain function. Single nucleotide polymorphisms are rapidly becoming the most valuable asset for

T G G A T G T C A A C T A C G C G T T T C T C C A T G C A A

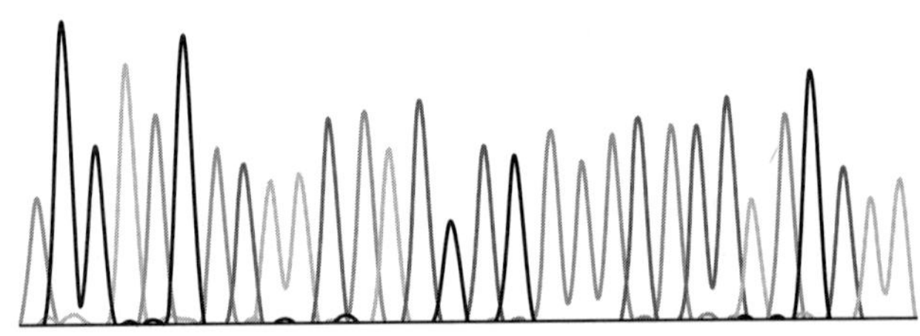

FIGURE 10.3 Sequencing results. The end result of cycle sequencing is an electropherogram showing the order of nucleotides (bases) in the genetic code. The sequence in this illustration is part of the gene encoding glutamate decarboxylase-65 (GAD65).

genetic mapping of complex traits. Although SNPs are not as polymorphic as the STRs, the lack of variation is compensated by their more frequent occurrence in the human genome (roughly every 100–500 base pairs). More importantly, it is thought that SNPs, but not STRs, are the primary source of common functional variation in the human genome, and thus, they may be directly relevant to understanding disease risk mechanisms.

A wide array of techniques have been developed to detect SNPs. Restriction fragment-length polymorphism (RFLP) analysis, the oldest molecular SNP genotyping method, is still in use in many laboratories because of its relative ease of use and robustness. The technique is based on bacterial restriction enzyme's capacity to digest DNA only at specific DNA sequence. Single nucleotide polymorphisms can be detected as RFLPs if they change the sequence recognized by the restriction enzyme; altered restriction pattern can be easily observed by electrophoresing the enzyme-digested PCR product on a size-fractionating gel. The problem with the PCR-RFLP method is that it does not allow high-throughput genotyping. In recent years, many high-throughput SNP genotyping methods have been described, which are based on different biochemical platforms; perhaps the most popular technique presently is the 5′ nuclease method (Shi et al., 1999) (implemented commercially in the "TaqMan" system). The essence of this technique is in the use of DNA probes that are specifically complementary to the alleles of the SNP. When hybridized to the template, an exact match between the probe and SNP allele results in a higher affinity pairing as compared to the opposite situation where there is a mismatch. During PCR amplification, as the flanking PCR primers are elongated across the template, the probe, if it is specific to the allele and thus bound with a high affinity, will be degraded by the 5′ nuclease activity of the polymerase. Degradation of the probe results in a release of light, which is detected by the instrument. If the probe is not specific to the template, the probe is displaced from the site rather than degraded, and no signal is emitted.

In terms of sheer numbers of genotypes acquired, we have now reached the point where array-based (or "chip") genotyping is responsible for the greatest data production. There are two major competing systems for array-based genotyping, marketed by Affymetrix and Illumina. Both systems are capable of creating hundreds of thousands of genotypes (at least) per sample at costs in the range of <$0.001 per genotype, if fixed arrays of predetermined SNPs are used. These arrays are very suitable for applications like whole-genome association studies, and less applicable for studies where the investigator selects a small set of specific SNPs. However, other array-based methods are gaining adherents for medium-sized genotyping projects, at per-SNP costs that are more favorable than the older, individual-genotype methods. It is beyond the scope of this chapter to discuss the methods involved in detail.

Short tandem repeats (STRs). The human genome contains many types of repeat sequences; the repeat polymorphisms that are most commonly used in genetic mapping are short, typically only 2–4 nucleotides long (for example, CA CA CA CA CA CA is a STR). These kinds of repeats are highly polymorphic in humans, making them very useful for genetic mapping and for identification of population structure (a key step in correcting for population stratification) (Yang et al., 2005). For example, some STRs are so polymorphic that up to 80%–90% of humans are heterozygotes for the alleles of the STR. Short tandem repeats have been invaluable tools for linkage mapping because linkage information can be derived only from families in which a parent is a heterozygote at the genetic marker locus, and these markers ensure that many parents will be heterozygous. The vast majority of the repeat sequences do not affect predisposition for any disease directly, and they are therefore useful only as genetic markers in linkage and population studies. However, some neuropsychiatric diseases, the best example being Huntington's disease, are due to aberrant elongation of trinucleotide repeat elements. Although repeat polymorphisms continue to be used in genetic linkage mapping of monogenic diseases, they are rapidly becoming pedestrian as a tool for linkage disequilibrium mapping (that is, association), largely due to the development of high-throughput SNP detection methods, which are more suitable for these kinds of studies.

Short tandem repeat polymorphism detection is based on differences in the number of repeats between individuals. Therefore, available methods to genotype STRs are based on detecting differences in the length of a PCR product generated using PCR amplification and primers flanking the STR sequence. The detection of length differences is achieved by electrophoresing the PCR product through denaturing polyacrylamide gel or a capillary. This is now generally accomplished by means of semiautomated high-throughput genotyping, including robot-assisted setting up of the PCR reactions and use of fluorescently labeled primers, and detection of the electrophoresis results using laser detection.

APPLICATIONS OF METHODS USED TO LOCATE AND CHARACTERIZE GENES RELATED TO PSYCHIATRIC ILLNESS

Linkage Studies

The parametric linkage approach is applicable for Mendelian traits but has also been successful for certain complex traits. Genetic linkage was used to identify the location of a gene causing an unusual X-linked syndrome involving violence, mild mental retardation, and impulsivity (Brunner, Nelen, van Zandvoort, 1993). First, the locus for the disorder was mapped to the X chromosome, with a maximum lod score of 3.7 at the *MAOA* gene locus (Brunner, Nelen, Breakefield, et al., 1993). Biochemical data also implicated a defect in *MAOA*. Subsequent sequencing identified the mutation in exon 8 of the *MAOA* structural gene (Brunner, Nelen, van Zandvoort, et al., 1993) that abolished the function of the protein. Although to date no other families with members with this syndrome have been identified, this was a very important finding, in that it established a clear genotype-phenotype relationship for violence and impulsivity-related behaviors. Parametric linkage analysis is often deployed as a tool in the context of linkage analysis of complex traits, as well, but usually not as the only analysis method (cf. Gelernter et al., 2005).

Genome scan linkage mapping projects have identified promising map positions for genes for most major psychiatric traits. We will consider AD as an example where linkage results led to gene identification, but reasonably similar examples can also be cited for, for example, schizophrenia and nicotine dependence. Linkage studies of AD published by the Collaborative Study of the Genetics of Alcoholism (COGA) group (Reich et al., 1998) and the National Institute on Alcohol Abuse and Alcoholism (NIAAA) group (Long et al., 1998) provided several chromosomal locations with promising lod scores. Both studies relied primarily on nonparametric analysis methods. Encouragingly, there were regions of possible linkage in common between the studies, despite the use of vastly different populations, including regions of chromosome 4. It is the nature of complex trait-linkage analysis that identical results cannot be expected of all studies of a certain trait (owing to sampling random and systematic differences, genetic heterogeneity, and methodological differences, among other explanations), but certain genomic regions have tended to be endorsed in multiple studies. For example, Ehlers et al. (2004) published an AD linkage study that endorsed loci on chromosomes 4 and 12, and Prescott et al. (2006) published a study where the strongest linkage results observed were, again, on chromosome 4. There is now very good evidence for specific risk genes in several of these regions.

Fine Mapping by Linkage Disequilibrium

As noted previously, linkage analysis does not provide sufficient chromosomal resolution to identify genes influencing risk for a phenotype; it only provides a general location. Linkage disequilibrium mapping may often be used to locate a specific gene, sometimes even a specific polymorphism, that acts to influence risk. Linkage disequilibrium mapping may be used to locate genes within a previously linked region or within the context of a whole-genome or whole-chromosome LD scan. The case of *GABRA2*, a chromosome 4 AD risk gene, is discussed below. Another report provided moderately strong support for muscarinic acetylcholine receptor M2 (genetic locus *CHRM2*) as an AD susceptibility locus (J.C. Wang et al., 2004). Like the ADH cluster loci and *GABRA2*, *CHRM2* maps into a chromosomal region that had been identified as being "of interest" based on an AD linkage study (Reich et al., 1998). Luo et al. (2005) have replicated this finding.

Other than the alcohol-metabolizing enzymes, the locus probably most studied with respect to AD is the D2 dopamine receptor locus, *DRD2*. Whether variation in this particular gene actually contributes to risk of alcoholism remains controversial. Interestingly, a variant previously claimed to be associated to AD and thought to map to *DRD2* was recently shown to map within the gene *ANKK1* (Neville et al., 2004). *DRD2* in fact maps close to three other genes, in the order: *NCAM1/TTC12/ANKK1/DRD2*. Based on the premise that observed weak and inconsistent *DRD2* association signals might be better explained through LD with another gene in this cluster (the initial hypothesis was that this might be the *NCAM1* gene), we recently studied a set of SNPs that span this region. We found very strong evidence of association of nicotine dependence with SNPs that map to a haplotype block that includes parts of *ANKK1* and *TTC12* (Gelernter et al., 2006). This region coincides with a linkage peak we observed for nicotine dependence (Gelernter et al., 2007).

Study of "Endophenotypes"

To understand better the multifactorial nature of psychiatric illnesses, many researchers have turned to identifying genes contributing to heritable personality, biochemical, cognitive, and physiological traits associated with a disorder of interest in lieu of the clinical diagnosis itself. These kinds of traits are often called *endophenotypes*. Endophenotypes have the potential to be closer to the gene action compared to the clinical (i.e., *Diagnostic and Statistical Manual of Mental Disorders*) diagnosis, and in the event of such a proximal relationship, the association or linkage signal detected should be robust. We discuss below two successful examples of identification of an association between a polymorphism and an endophenotype trait. In both cases, the initial genetic discoveries spurred research into completely new directions, and a myriad of critically important findings about neurobiological underpinnings of affective illness and schizophrenia have resulted from these studies.

The discovery of a functional 5′ promoter region VNTR polymorphism in the serotonin transporter gene (*SLC6A4*) in 1996 led to a series of genetic studies seeking to associate this polymorphism with endophenotypes related to disorders with postulated serotonergic dysfunction, such as anxiety and depression. The shorter of the two common alleles of this repeat polymorphism was reported to have lower transcriptional activity, leading to decreases in messenger ribonucleic acid (mRNA) levels, serotonin binding, and serotonin uptake (Lesch et al., 1996). Initial studies attempting to establish an association between broad clinical diagnoses and this variant did not lead to a consistent picture of the effect this gene. More recently, the field has moved into examining the effect of this gene variant on emotional reactivity and gene × environment interaction, with very interesting results. Studies using functional magnetic resonance imaging (fMRI) techniques have provided replicated evidence that the short allele is associated with heightened activation of amygdala in response to emotionally provocative stimuli, a response thought to be central to vulnerability to affective illness (Hariri and Holmes, 2006). A repeated environmental stress could thereby invoke an emotional response sufficient to precipitate affective illness among individuals with the short allele; the long allele, on the contrary, may correspond to greater resilience against the disorder. An interesting new line of research has recently emerged suggesting that this may in fact be the case. Caspi et al. (2003) reported that the short allele increases susceptibility to depression. However, the effect of the genotype is seen only if the participant has been exposed to stressful events and maltreatment as a child implicating an interaction between the transporter genotype and environment (Caspi et al., 2003; Kaufman et al., 2004).

Another interesting line of research concerns the gene encoding catechol-*O*-methyltransferase (COMT), a common Val$^{108/158}$Met polymorphism in the *COMT* gene, and dopamine function in prefrontal cortex. COMT is very important in metabolism of various neuropsychiatrically important biochemicals, including dopamine. In 1995, Lotta et al. (1995) showed that the Val and Met alleles are functionally different—the enzyme containing Met is unstable at 37° C and has only about one fourth of the dopamine-catabolizing activity of the enzyme containing Val. Egan et al. (2001) studied this polymorphism in relation to performance on prefrontally mediated cognition-related tasks and prefrontal neurophysiology in healthy controls and in individuals with schizophrenia. They discovered that the Met allele was associated with fewer perseverative errors on the Wisconsin Card Sorting task and what was judged to be more effective physiological response in prefrontal cortex, as assessed by fMRI. These findings were consistent with other evidence showing that increased dopamine activity enhances prefrontal function. Then, using a family-based association analysis, they showed that the Val allele was preferentially transmitted from parents to offspring with schizophrenia, suggesting that the Val allele increases risk for schizophrenia. A robust genotype effect was seen when the polymorphism was correlated to the endophenotype, whereas the genotype effect on the risk for a broad diagnosis of schizophrenia was less evident, using these particular markers. Consistent with this finding, the effect of the Val$^{108/158}$Met genotype on prefrontally mediated tasks has been replicated many times, whereas the association between Val$^{108/158}$Met and schizophrenia has not been demonstrated consistently. (This may be because variants besides Val$^{108/158}$Met are important in modulating schizophrenia risk; cf. Shifman et al., 2002.) Further, two studies reported that participants with schizophrenia with the Met allele have superior improvement in prefrontally mediated cognitive tasks after treatment with antipsychotic medications, extending the importance of these findings to understanding factors that influence response to pharmacotherapy in schizophrenia (Bertolino et al., 2004; Weickert et al., 2004). This is one locus for which the plot seems to thicken continuously; Nackley et al. (2006) demonstrated a new source of functional variation caused by *COMT* polymorphism, through effects on mRNA secondary structure.

Association Studies: GABRA2/GABRG1 and Alcohol Dependence

Compelling recent work has supported associations between specific loci and risk for AD. Porjesz et al. (2002) demonstrated genetic linkage of EEG β frequencies (a quantitative trait) to chromosome 4p, then LD to a GABA-A receptor cluster, in a sample ascertained through pedigrees with multiple individuals with AD. Fine mapping of this region with a dense SNP map showed allelic and haplotypic association to *GABRA2* (Edenberg et al., 2004). Several research groups have replicated this finding using case-control association approaches, in three different populations (Covault et al., 2004; Lappalainen et al., 2005; Fehr et al., 2006). Although this can now be regarded as a replicated finding, no specific causative variant has been reported. And notwithstanding the replication with *GABRA2* markers, the most recent evidence (Covault et al., 2008) suggests that there is either an additional association signal that derives from the adjacent *GABRG1* locus or that that gene could be the source of the association signal detected through *GABRA2* markers.

Whole-Genome Association Studies (WGAS)

Whole-genome association studies have now been completed for numerous complex traits, and results from some of them have been extremely striking. For example, in one of the first such studies, Klein et al. (2005) reported that the gene-encoding complement factor H influences risk for age-related macular degeneration. This study was based on a 100k SNP set, which would nowadays be considered very small. Duerr et al. (2006) used a 300k array in a WGAS of inflammatory bowel disease, a study that had the dramatic result of identifying *IL23R* as a novel risk locus. Results for neuropsychiatric illness have been more mixed. Bierut et al. (2007) reported a WGAS for the trait of tobacco dependence; interesting results were reported for numerous loci, many of which would have been considered strong candidates a priori. However, very strong association signals were lacking. Presumably the lessons of the first such studies will allow improvements in designs, as has happened for, for example, the linkage approach. By the time this volume is published, many more such results will be available from several large initiatives, including the Genetic Association Information Network project, sponsored by the National Institutes of Health and several private companies. Genetic Association Information Network has funded large genomewide association studies of schizophrenia, attention deficit/hyperactivity disorder, bipolar affective disorder, and depression. These studies, and studies like them, have the potential to revolutionize our understanding of the genetics and the physiology of these disorders.

CONCLUSION

Studies in molecular psychiatric genetics have advanced greatly in the past decades. Genetic findings will provide the means for much more nuanced understanding of the pathophysiological processes in the relevant behaviors than was possible previously. It is apparently the case that genetic contributions to behavioral phenotype are not only widespread, but (in a sense) disturbingly so. There are now numerous findings that force us to come to terms with the existence of single-gene switches with small but measurable effects on a person's normal experience of life.

Many genes have been proven (or at least replicated in different labs) to influence behavior, usually with small effect size. Identifying genes of even small effect can, however, be extremely helpful, for beginning to understand basic disease pathophysiology, and for advancing future work. When studying a genetically heterogeneous disorder, it is of great heuristic value to be able to identify a genetically homogeneous subset that, when removed from all known cases, decreases the heterogeneity of what remains. The next steps are to learn more about the specific genotype-phenotype relationships for genes of known effect, to find many more of them, and to design interventions based on these findings for treatment or prevention.

ACKNOWLEDGMENTS

This work was supported in part by National Institute on Drug Abuse grants DA12849, DA12690, and DA15105; the U.S. Department of Veterans Affairs (the VA Medical Research Program, the VA Connecticut-Massachusetts Mental Illness Research, Education and Clinical Center [MIRECC], and the Research Enhancement Award Program [REAP]).

REFERENCES

Abecasis, G.R., Cherny, S.S., Cookson, W.O., and Cardon, L.R. (2002) Merlin-rapid analysis of dense genetic maps using sparse gene flow trees. *Nat. Genet.* 30:97–101.

Almasy, L., and Blangero, J. (1998) Multipoint quantitative trait linkage analysis in general pedigrees. *Am. J. Hum. Genet.* 62: 1198–1211.

Bertolino, A., Caforio, G., Blasi, G., De Candia, M., Latorre, V., Petruzzella, V., Altamura, A., Nappi, G., Papa, S., Callicott, J.H., Mattay, V.S., Bellomo, A., Scarabino, T., Weinberger, D.R., and Nardini, M. (2004) Interaction of COMT $Val^{108/158}$ Met genotype and olanzapine treatment on prefrontal cortical function in patients with schizophrenia. *Am. J. Psychiatry* 161:1798–1805.

Bierut, L.J., Madden, A.F., Breslau, N., Johnson, E.O., Hatsukami, D., Pomerleau, O.F., Swan, G.E., Rutter, J., Bertelsen, S., Fox, L., Fugman, D., Goate, A.M., Hinrichs, A.L., Konvicka, K., Martin, N.G., Montgomery, G.W., Saccone, N.L., Saccone, S.F., Wang, J.C., Chase, G.A., Rice, J.P., and Ballinger, D.G. (2007) Novel genes identified in a high-density genome wide association study for nicotine dependence. *Hum. Mol. Genet.* 16(1):24–35.

Brunner, H.G., Nelen, M., Breakefield, X.O., Ropers, H.H., and van Oost, B.A. (1993) Abnormal behavior associated with a point mutation in the structural gene for monoamine oxidase A. *Science* 262:578–580.

Brunner, H.G., Nelen, M., van Zandvoort, P., Abeling, N.G.G.M., van Gennip, A.H., Wolters, E.C., Kuiper, M.A., Ropers, H.H., and van Oost, B.A (1993) X-linked borderline mental retardation with prominent behavioral: phenotype, genetic localization, and evidence for disturbed monoamine metabolism. *Am. J. Hum. Genet.* 52:1032–1039.

Caspi, A., Sugden, K., Moffitt, T. E., Taylor, A., Craig, I.W., Harrington, H., McClay, J., Mill, J., Martin, J., Braithwaite, A., and Poulton, R. (2003) Influence of life stress on depression: moderation by a polymorphism in the 5-HTT gene. *Science* 301: 386–389.

Chapman, N.H., and Wijsman, E.M. (1998) Genome screens using linkage disequilibrium tests: optimal marker characteristics and feasibility. *Am. J. Hum. Genet.* 63:1872–1885.

Chen, C.C., Lu, R.B., Chen, Y.C., Wang, M.F., Chang, Y.C., Li, T. K., and Yin, S.J. (1999) Interaction between the functional polymorphisms of the alcohol-metabolism genes in protection against alcoholism. *Am. J. Hum. Genet.* 65:795–807.

Covault, C., Gelernter, J., Hesselbrock, V., Nellissery, M., and Kranzler, H.R. (2004) Allelic and haplotypic association of GABRA2 with alcohol dependence. *Am. J. Med. Genet.* 129B:104–109.

Covault, J., Gelernter, J., Jensen, K., Anton, R., and Kranzler, H.R. (2008) Markers in the 5′ Region of GABRG1 associate to alcohol dependence and are in linkage disequilibrium with markers in the adjacent GABRA2 gene. *Neuropsychopharmacology* 33: 837–848. [Epub ahead of print] doi: 10.1038/sj.npp.1301456.

Devlin, B., and Roeder, K. (1999) Genomic control for association studies. *Biometrics* 55:997–1004.

Duerr, R.H., Taylor, K.D., Brant, S.R., Rioux, J.D., Silverberg, M.S., Daly, M.J., Steinhart, A.H., Abraham, C., Regueiro, M., Griffiths, A., Dassopoulos, T., Bitton, A., Yang, H., Targan, S., Datta, L. W., Kistner, E.O., Schumm, L.P., Lee, A., Gregersen, P.K., Barmada, M.M., Rotter, J.I., Nicolae, D.L., and Cho, J.H. (2006)

A genome-wide association study identifies IL23R as an inflammatory bowel disease gene. *Science* 314(5804):1461–1463.

Edenberg, H.J., Dick, D.M., Xuei, X., Tian, H., Almasy, L., Bauer, L.O., Crowe, R.R., Goate, A., Hesselbrock, V., Jones, K., Kwon, J., Li, T.K., Nurnberger, J.I., Jr., O'Connor, S.J., Reich, T., Rice, M., Schuckit, M.A., Porjesz, B., Foroud, T., and Begleiter, H. (2004) Variations in GABRA2, encoding the 2 subunit of the GABAA receptor, are associated with alcohol dependence and with brain oscillations. *Am. J. Hum. Genet.* 74:705–714.

Edenberg, H.J., Xuei, X., Chen, H.J., Tian, H., Wetherill, L.F., Dick, D.M., Almasy, L., Bierut, L., Bucholz, K.K., Goate, A., Hesselbrock, V., Kuperman, S., Nurnberger, J., Porjesz, B., Rice, J., Schuckit, M., Tischfield, J., Begleiter, H., and Foroud, T. (2006) Association of alcohol dehydrogenase genes with alcohol dependence: a comprehensive analysis. *Hum. Mol. Genet.* 15:1539–1549.

Egan, M.F., Goldberg, T.E., Kolachana, B.S., Callicott, J.H., Mazzanti, C.M., Straub, R.E., Goldman, D., and Weinberger, D.R. (2001) Effect of COMT Val108/158 Met genotype on frontal lobe function and risk for schizophrenia. *Proc. Natl. Acad. Sci. USA* 98:6917–6922.

Ehlers, C.L., Gilder, D.A., Wall, T.L., Phillips, E., Feiler, H., and Wilhelmsen, K.C. (2004) Genomic screen for loci associated with alcohol dependence in Mission Indians. *Am. J. Med. Genet. (Neuropsychiatr. Genet.)* 129:110–115.

Falk, C.T., and Rubinstein, P. (1987) Haplotype relative risks: an easy reliable way to construct a proper control sample for risk calculations. *Ann. Hum. Genet.* 51:227–233.

Fehr, C., Sander, T., Tadic, A., Lenzen, K.P., Anghelescu, I., Klawe, C., Dahmen, N., Schmidt, L.G., and Szegedi, A. (2006) Confirmation of association of the GABRA2 gene with alcohol dependence by subtype-specific analysis. *Psychiatr. Genet.* 16:9–17.

Freimer, N.B., Reus, V.I., Escamilla, M.A., McInnes, L.A., Spesny, M., Leon, P., Service, S.K., Smith, L.B., Silva, S., Rojas, E., Gallegos, A., Meza, L., Fournier, E., Baharloo, S., Blankenship, K., Tyler, D.J., Batki, S., Vinogradov, S., Weissenbach, J., Barondes, S.H., and Sandkuijl, L.A. (1996) Genetic mapping using haplotype, association and linkage methods suggests a locus for severe bipolar disorder (BPI) at 18q22-q23. *Nat. Genet.* 12:436–441.

Gelernter, J., Goldman, D., and Risch, N. (1993) The A1 allele at the D_2 dopamine receptor gene and alcoholism: a reappraisal. *JAMA* 269:1673–1677.

Gelernter, J., Panhuysen, C., Weiss, R., Brady, K., Hesselbrock, V., Rounsaville, B., Poling, J., Wilcox, M., Farrer, L., and Kranzler, H.R. (2005) Genomewide linkage scan for cocaine dependence and related traits: Linkages for a cocaine-related trait and cocaine-induced paranoia. *Am. J. Med. Genet. (Neuropsych. Genet.)* 136B:45–52.

Gelernter, J., Panhuysen, C., Weiss, R., Brady, K., Poling, J., Krauthammer, M., Farrer, L., and Kranzler, H.R. (2007) Genomewide linkage scan for nicotine dependence: identification of a chromosome 5 risk locus. *Biol. Psych.* 61:119–126.

Gelernter, J., Yu, Y., Weiss, R., Brady, K., Panhuysen, C., Yang, B. Z., Kranzler, H.R., and Farrer, L. (2006) Haplotype spanning TTC12 and ANKK1, flanked by the DRD2 and NCAM1 loci, is strongly associated to nicotine dependence in two distinct American populations. *Hum. Mol. Genet.* 15:3498–3507.

Gusella, J.F., Wexler, N.S., Conneally, P.M., Naylor, S.L., Anderson, M.A., Tanzi, R.E., Watkins, P.C., Ottina, K., Wallace, M.R., Sakaguchi, A.Y., et al. (1983) A polymorphic DNA marker genetically linked to Huntington's disease. *Nature* 306:234–238.

Hariri, A.R., and Holmes, A. (2006) Genetics of emotional regulation: the role of the serotonin transporter in neural function. *Trends Cogn. Sci.* 10:182–191.

Huntington's Disease Collaborative Research Group (1993) A novel gene containing a trinucleotide repeat that is expanded and unstable on Huntington's disease chromosomes. *Cell* 72:971–983.

The International HapMap Consortium (2005) A haplotype map of the human genome. *Nature* 437:1299–1320.

Kaufman, J., Yang, B.Z., Douglas-Palumberi, H., Houshyar, S., Lipschitz, D., Krystal, J.H., and Gelernter, J. (2004) Social supports and serotonin transporter gene moderate depression in maltreated children. *Proc. Natl. Acad. Sci. USA* 101:17316–17321.

Klein, R.J., Zeiss, C., Chew, E.Y., Tsai, J.-Yn., Sackler, R.S., Haynes, R.S., Henning, A.K., SanGiovanni, J.P., Mane, S.M., Mayne, S.T., Bracken, M.B., Ferris, F.L., Ott, J., Barnstable, C., and Hoh, J. (2005) Complement factor H polymorphism in age-related macular degeneration. *Science* 308:385–389.

Kruglyak, L., and Lander, E.S. (1995) Complete multipoint sib-pair analysis of qualitative and quantitative traits. *Am. J. Hum. Genet.* 57:439–454.

Laird, N., Horvath, S., and Xu, X. (2000) Implementing a unified approach to family based tests of association. *Genet. Epidemiol.* 19(Suppl 1):S36–S42.

Lander, E., and Kruglyak, L. (1995) Genetic dissection of complex traits: guidelines for interpreting and reporting linkage results. *Nat. Genet.* 11:241–247.

Lander, E.S., Linton, L.M., Birren, B., Nussbaum, C., Zody, M.C., Baldwin, J., Devon, K., Dewar, K., Doyle, M., FitzHugh, W., Funke, R., Gage, D., Harris, K., Heaford, A., Howland, J., Kann, L., Lehoczky, J., LeVine, R., McEwan, P., McKernan, K., Meldrim, J., Mesirov, J.P., Miranda, C., Morris, W., Naylor, J., Raymond, C., Rosetti, M., Santos, R., Sheridan, A., Sougnez, C., Stange-Thomann, N., Stojanovic, N., Subramanian, A., Wyman, D., Rogers, J., Sulston, J., Ainscough, R., Beck, S., Bentley, D., Burton, J., Clee, C., Carter, N., Coulson, A., Deadman, R., Deloukas, P., Dunham, A., Dunham, I., Durbin, R., French, L., Grafham, D., Gregory, S., Hubbard, T., Humphray, S., Hunt, A., Jones, M., Lloyd, C., McMurray, A., Matthews, L., Mercer, S., Milne, S., Mullikin, J.C., Mungall, A., Plumb, R., Ross, M., Shownkeen, R., Sims, S., Waterston, R.H., Wilson, R.K., Hillier, L.W., McPherson, J.D., Marra, M.A., Mardis, E.R., Fulton, L. A., Chinwalla, A.T., Pepin, K.H., Gish, W.R., Chissoe, S.L., Wendl, M.C., Delehaunty, K.D., Miner, T.L., Delehaunty, A., Kramer, J.B., Cook, L.L., Fulton, R.S., Johnson, D.L., Minx, P.J., Clifton, S.W., Hawkins, T., Branscomb, E., Predki, P., Richardson, P., Wenning, S., Slezak, T., Doggett, N., Cheng, J.F., Olsen, A., Lucas, S., Elkin, C., Uberbacher, E., Frazier, M., Gibbs, R.A., Muzny, D.M., Scherer, S.E., Bouck, J.B., Sodergren, E.J., Worley, K.C., Rives, C.M., Gorrell, J.H., Metzker, M.L., Naylor, S.L., Kucherlapati, R.S., Nelson, D.L., Weinstock, G.M., Sakaki, Y., Fujiyama, A., Hattori, M., Yada, T., Toyoda, A., Itoh, T., Kawagoe, C., Watanabe, H., Totoki, Y., Taylor, T., Weissenbach, J., Heilig, R., Saurin, W., Artiguenave, F., Brottier, P., Bruls, T., Pelletier, E., Robert, C., Wincker, P., Smith, D.R., Doucette-Stamm, L., Rubenfield, M., Weinstock, K., Lee, H.M., Dubois, J., Rosenthal, A., Platzer, M., Nyakatura, G., Taudien, S., Rump, A., Yang, H., Yu, J., Wang, J., Huang, G., Gu, J., Hood, L., Rowen, L., Madan, A., Qin, S., Davis, R.W., Federspiel, N.A., Abola, A.P., Proctor, M.J., Myers, R.M., Schmutz, J., Dickson, M., Grimwood, J., Cox, D.R., Olson, M.V., Kaul, R., Raymond, C., Shimizu, N., Kawasaki, K., Minoshima, S., Evans, G.A., Athanasiou, M., Schultz, R., Roe, B.A., Chen, F., Pan, H., Ramser, J., Lehrach, H., Reinhardt, R., McCombie, W.R., de la Bastide, M., Dedhia, N., Blocker, H., Hornischer, K., Nordsiek, G., Agarwala, R., Aravind, L., Bailey, J.A., Bateman, A., Batzoglou, S., Birney, E., Bork, P., Brown, D.G., Burge, C.B., Cerutti, L., Chen, H.C., Church, D., Clamp, M., Copley, R.R., Doerks, T., Eddy, S.R., Eichler, E.E., Furey, T.S., Galagan, J., Gilbert, J.G., Harmon, C., Hayashizaki, Y., Haussler, D., Hermjakob, H., Hokamp, K., Jang, W., Johnson, L.S., Jones, T.A., Kasif, S., Kaspryzk, A., Kennedy, S., Kent, W.J., Kitts, P., Koonin, E.V., Korf, I., Kulp, D., Lancet, D., Lowe, T.M., McLysaght, A., Mikkelsen, T., Moran,

J.V., Mulder, N., Pollara, V.J., Ponting, C.P., Schuler, G., Schultz, J., Slater, G., Smit, A.F., Stupka, E., Szustakowski, J., Thierry-Mieg, D., Thierry-Mieg, J, Wagner, L., Wallis, J., Wheeler, R., Williams, A., Wolf, Y.I., Wolfe, K.H., Yang, S.P., Yeh, R.F., Collins, F., Guyer, M.S., Peterson, J., Felsenfeld, A., Wetterstrand, K.A., Patrinos, A., Morgan, M.J., de Jong, P., Catanese, J.J., Osoegawa, K., Shizuya, H., Choi, S., Chen, Y.J., and International Human Genome Sequencing Consortium (2001) Initial sequencing and analysis of the human genome. *Nature* 409:860–921.

Lappalainen, J., Krupitsky, E., Remizov, M., Pchelina, S., Taraskina, A., Zvartau, E., Somberg, L.K., Covault, J., Kranzler, H.R., Krystal, J., and Gelernter, J. (2005) Association between alcoholism and GABRA2 in a Russian population. *Alcohol Clin. Exp. Res.* 29:493–498.

Lautenberger, J.A., Stephens, J.C., O'Brien, S.J., and Smith, M.W. (2000) Significant disequilibrium across 30 cM around the FY locus in African-Americans. *Am. J. Hum. Genet.* 66:969–978.

Lesch, K.-P., Bengel, D., Heils, A., Sabol, S.Z., Greenberg, B., Petri, S., Benjamin, J., Müller, C.R., Hamer, D.H., and Murphy, D.L. (1996) Association of anxiety-related traits with a polymorphism in the serotonin transporter gene regulatory region. *Science* 274:1527–1531.

Long, J.C., Knowler, W.C., Hanson, R.L., Robin, R.W., Urbanek, M., Moore, E., Bennett, P.H., and Goldman, D. (1998) Evidence for genetic linkage to alcohol dependence on chromosomes 4 and 11 from an autosome-wide scan in an American Indian population. *Am. J. Med. Genet.* 81:216–221.

Lotta, T., Vidgren, J., Tilgmann, C., Ulmanen, I., Melen, K., Julkunen, I., and Taskinen, J. (1995) Kinetics of human soluble and membrane-bound catechol-O-methyltransferase: a revised mechanism and description of the thermolabile variant of the enzyme. *Biochemistry* 34:4202–4210.

Luo, X., Kranzler, H.R., Zuo, L., Lappalainen, J., Yang, B.Z., and Gelernter, J. (2006) ADH4 gene variation is associated with alcohol and drug dependence in European Americans: results from HWD tests and case-control association studies. *Neuropsychopharmacology* 31:1085–1095.

Luo, X., Kranzler, H.R., Zuo, L., Wang, S., Schorck, N.J., and Gelernter, J. (2006) Diplotype trend regression (DTR) analysis of the ADH gene cluster and ALDH2 gene: multiple significant associations for alcohol dependence. *Am. J. Hum. Genet.* 78:973–987.

Luo, X., Kranzler, H.R., Zuo, L., Yang, B.Z., Lappalainen, J., and Gelernter, J. (2005) ADH4 gene variation is associated with alcohol and drug dependence in European Americans: results from family-controlled and population-structured association studies. *Pharmacogenet. Genomics* 15:755–768.

Nackley, A.G., Shabalina, S.A., Tchivileva, I.E., Satterfield, K., Korchynskyi, O., Makarov, S.S., Maixner, W., and Diatchenko, L. (2006) Human catechol-O-methyltransferase haplotypes modulate protein expression by altering mRNA secondary structure. *Science* 314(5807):1930–1933.

Neville, M.J., Johnstone, E.C., and Walton, R.T. (2004) Identification and characterization of ANKK1: a novel kinase gene closely linked to DRD2 on chromosome band 11q23.1. *Hum. Mutat.* 23:540–545.

Ott, J. (1991) *Analysis of Human Genetic Linkage* (rev. ed.). Baltimore: Johns Hopkins University Press.

Porjesz, B., Almasy, L., Edenberg, H.J., Wang, K., Chorlian, D.B., Foroud, T., Goate, A., Rice, J.P., O'Connor, S.J., Rohrbaugh, J., Kuperman, S., Bauer, L.O., Crowe, R.R., Schuckit, M.A., Hesselbrock, V., Conneally, P.M., Tischfield, J.A., Li, T.K., Reich, T., and Begleiter, H. (2002) Linkage disequilibrium between the beta frequency of the human EEG and a $GABA_A$ receptor gene locus. *Proc. Natl. Acad. Sci. USA* 99:3729–3733.

Prescott, C.A., Sullivan, P.F., Kuo, P.H., Webb, B.T., Vittum, J., Patterson, D.G., Thiselton, D.L., Myers, J.M., Devitt, M., Halberstadt, L.J., Robinson, V.P., Neale, M.C., van den Oord, E.J., Walsh, D., Riley, B.P., and Kendler, K.S. (2006) Genomewide linkage study in the Irish affected sib pair study of alcohol dependence: evidence for a susceptibility region for symptoms of alcohol dependence on chromosome 4. *Mol. Psych.* 11:603–611.

Price, A.L., Patterson, N.J., Plenge, R.M., Weinblatt, M.E., Shadick, N.A., and Reich, D. (2006) Principal components analysis corrects for stratification in genome-wide association studies. *Nat. Genet.* 38:904–909.

Pritchard, J.K., and Rosenberg, N.A. (1999) Use of unlinked genetic markers to detect population stratification in association studies. *Am. J. Hum. Genet.* 65:220–228.

Pritchard, J.K., Stephens, M., and Donnelly, P. (2000) Inference of population structure using multilocus genotype data. *Genetics* 155:945–959.

Pritchard, J.K., Stephens, M., Rosenberg, N.A., and Donnelly, P. (2000) Association mapping in structured populations. *Am. J. Hum. Genet.* 67:170–181.

Reich, T., Edenberg, H.J., Goate, A., Williams, J.T., Rice, J.P., Van Eerdewegh, P., Foroud, T., Hesselbrock, V., Schuckit, M.A., Bucholz, K., Porjesz, B., Li, T.K., Conneally, P.M., Nurnberger, J.I., Jr., Tischfield, J.A., Crowe, R.R., Cloninger, C.R., Wu, W., Shears, S., Carr, K., Crose, C., Willig, C., and Begleiter, H. (1998) Genome-wide search for genes affecting the risk for alcohol dependence. *Am. J. Med. Genet. (Neuropsychiat. Genet.)* 81:207–215.

Risch, N. (1990a) Genetic linkage and complex diseases, with special reference to psychiatric disorders. *Genet. Epidemiol.* 7:3–16.

Risch, N. (1990b) Linkage strategies for genetically complex traits. I. Multilocus models. *Am. J. Hum. Genet.* 46:222–228.

Risch, N., and Botstein, D.L. (1996) A manic depressive history. *Nat. Genet.* 12:351–353.

Risch, N., and Zhang, H. (1995) Extreme discordant sib pairs for mapping quantitative trait loci in humans. *Science* 268:1584–1589.

Roy, M.A., Neale, M.C., and Kendler, K.S. (1995) The genetic epidemiology of self-esteem. *Br. J. Psychiatry* 166:813–820.

Saiki, R.K., Gelfand, D.H., Stoffel, S., Scharf, S.J., Higuchi, R., Horn, G.T., Mullis, K.B., and Erlich, H.A. (1988) Primer-directed enzymatic amplification of DNA with a thermostable DNA polymerase. *Science* 239:487–491.

Shi, M.M., Myrand, S.P., Bleavins, M.R., and de la Iglesia, F.A. (1999) High throughput genotyping for the detection of a single nucleotide polymorphism in NADPH quinone oxidoreductase DT diaphorase using TaqMan probes. *Mol. Pathol.* 52:295–299.

Shifman, S., Bronstein, M., Sternfeld, M., Pisante-Shalom, A., Lev-Lehman, E., Weizman, A., Reznik, I., Spivak, B., Grisaru, N., Karp, L., Schiffer, R., Kotler, M., Strous, R.D., Swartz-Vanetik, M., Knobler, H.Y., Shinar, E., Beckmann, J.S., Yakir, B., Risch, N., Zak, N.B., and Darvasi, A. (2002) A highly significant association between a COMT haplotype and schizophrenia. *Am. J. Hum. Genet.* 71(6):1296–1302.

Spielman, R.S., McGinnis, R.E., and Ewens, W.J. (1993) Transmission test for linkage disequilibrium: the insulin gene region and insulin-dependent diabetes mellitus (IDDM). *Am. J. Hum. Genet.* 52:506–516.

Straub, R.E., MacLean, C.J., O'Neill, F.A., Burke, J., Murphy, B., Duke, F., Shinkwin, R., Webb, B.T., Zhang, J., Walsh, D., et al. (1995) A potential vulnerability locus for schizophrenia on chromosome 6p24-22: evidence for genetic heterogeneity. *Nat. Genet.* 3:287–293.

Suarez, B.K., Rice, J., and Reich, T. (1978) The generalized sib-pair IBD distribution: its use in the detection of linkage. *Ann. Hum. Genet.* 42:87–94.

Terwilliger, J.D., and Ott, J. (1992) A haplotype-based "haplotype relative risk" approach to detecting allelic associations. *Hum. Hered.* 42:337–346.

Thomasson, H.R., Edenberg, H.J., Crabb, D.W., Mai, X.L., Jerome, R.E., Li, T.K., Wang, S.P., Lin, Y.T., Lu, R.B., and Yin, S.J. (1991) Alcohol and aldehyde dehydrogenase genotypes and alcoholism in Chinese men. *Am. J. Hum. Genet.* 48:677–681.

Tsuang, M.T., Faraone, S.V., and Lyons, M.J. (1993) Identification of the phenotype in psychiatric genetics. *Eur. Arch. Psychiatry Clin. Neurosci.* 243:131–142.

Venter, J.C., Adams, M.D., Myers, E.W., Li, P.W., Mural, R.J., Sutton, G.G., Smith, H.O., Yandell, M., Evans, C.A., Holt, R.A., Gocayne, J.D., Amanatides, P., Ballew, R.M., Huson, D.H., Wortman, J.R., Zhang, Q., Kodira, C.D., Zheng, X.H., Chen, L., Skupski, M., Subramanian, G., Thomas, P.D., Zhang, J., Gabor Miklos, G.L., Nelson, C., Broder, S., Clark, A.G., Nadeau, J., McKusick, V.A., Zinder, N., Levine, A.J., Roberts, R.J., Simon, M., Slayman, C., Hunkapiller, M., Bolanos, R., Delcher, A., Dew, I., Fasulo, D., Flanigan, M., Florea, L., Halpern, A., Hannenhalli, S., Kravitz, S., Levy, S., Mobarry, C., Reinert, K., Remington, K., Abu-Threideh, J., Beasley, E., Biddick, K., Bonazzi, V., Brandon, R., Cargill, M., Chandramouliswaran, I., Charlab, R., Chaturvedi, K., Deng, Z., Di Francesco, V., Dunn, P., Eilbeck, K., Evangelista, C., Gabrielian, A.E., Gan, W., Ge, W., Gong, F., Gu, Z., Guan, P., Heiman, T.J., Higgins, M.E., Ji, R.R., Ke, Z., Ketchum, K.A., Lai, Z., Lei, Y., Li, Z., Li, J., Liang, Y., Lin, X., Lu, F., Merkulov, G.V., Milshina, N., Moore, H.M., Naik, A.K., Narayan, V.A, Neelam, B., Nusskern, D., Rusch, D.B., Salzberg, S., Shao, W., Shue, B., Sun, J., Wang, Z., Wang, A., Wang, X., Wang, J., Wei, M., Wides, R., Xiao, C., Yan, C., Yao, A., Ye, J., Zhan, M., Zhang, W., Zhang, H., Zhao, Q., Zheng, L., Zhong, F., Zhong, W., Zhu, S., Zhao, S., Gilbert, D., Baumhueter, S., Spier, G., Carter, C., Cravchik, A., Woodage, T., Ali, F., An, H., Awe, A., Baldwin, D., Baden, H., Barnstead, M., Barrow, I., Beeson, K., Busam, D., Carver, A., Center, A., Cheng, M.L., Curry, L., Danaher, S., Davenport, L., Desilets, R., Dietz, S., Dodson, K., Doup, L., Ferriera, S., Garg, N., Gluecksmann, A., Hart, B., Haynes, J., Haynes, C., Heiner, C., Hladun, S., Hostin, D., Houck, J., Howland, T., Ibegwam, C., Johnson, J., Kalush, F., Kline, L., Koduru, S., Love, A., Mann, F., May, D., McCawley, S., McIntosh, T., McMullen, I., Moy, M., Moy, L., Murphy, B., Nelson, K., Pfannkoch, C., Pratts, E., Puri, V., Qureshi, H., Reardon, M., Rodriguez, R., Rogers, Y.H., Romblad, D., Ruhfel, B., Scott, R., Sitter, C., Smallwood, M., Stewart, E., Strong, R., Suh, E., Thomas, R., Tint, N.N., Tse, S., Vech, C., Wang, G., Wetter, J., Williams, S., Williams, M., Windsor, S., Winn-Deen, E., Wolfe, K., Zaveri, J., Zaveri, K., Abril, J.F., Guigo, R., Campbell, M.J., Sjolander, K.V., Karlak, B., Kejariwal, A., Mi, H., Lazareva, B., Hatton, T., Narechania, A., Diemer, K., Muruganujan, A., Guo, N., Sato, S., Bafna, V., Istrail, S., Lippert, R., Schwartz, R., Walenz, B., Yooseph, S., Allen, D., Basu, A., Baxendale, J., Blick, L., Caminha, M., Carnes-Stine, J., Caulk, P., Chiang, Y.H., Coyne, M., Dahlke, C., Mays, A., Dombroski, M., Donnelly, M., Ely, D., Esparham, S., Fosler, C., Gire, H., Glanowski, S., Glasser, K., Glodek, A., Gorokhov, M., Graham, K., Gropman, B., Harris, M., Heil, J., Henderson, S., Hoover, J., Jennings, D., Jordan, C., Jordan, J., Kasha, J., Kagan, L., Kraft, C., Levitsky, A., Lewis, M., Liu, X., Lopez, J., Ma, D., Majoros, W., McDaniel, J., Murphy, S., Newman, M., Nguyen, T., Nguyen, N., Nodell, M., Pan, S., Peck, J., Peterson, M., Rowe, W., Sanders, R., Scott, J., Simpson, M., Smith, T., Sprague, A., Stockwell, T., Turner, R., Venter, E., Wang, M., Wen, M., Wu, D., Wu, M., Xia, A., Zandieh, A., and Zhu, X. (2001) The sequence of the human genome. *Science* 291: 1304–1351.

Wang, J.C., Hinrichs, A.L., Stock, H., Budde, J., Allen, R., Bertelsen, S., Kwon, J.M., Wu, W., Dick, D.M., Rice, J., Jones, K., Nurnberger, J.I., Jr., Tischfield, J., Porjesz, B., Edenberg, H.J., Hesselbrock, V., Crowe, R., Schuckit, M., Begleiter, H., Reich, T., Goate, A.M., and Bierut, L.J. (2004) Evidence of common and specific genetic effects: association of the muscarinic acetylcholine receptor M2 (CHRM2) gene with alcohol dependence and major depressive syndrome. *Hum. Mol. Genet.* 13:1903–1911.

Wang, S., Sun, S.E., Walczak, C.A., Ziegle, J.S., Kipps, B.R., Goldin, L.R., and Diehl, S.R. (1995) Evidence for a susceptibility locus for schizophrenia on chromosome 6pter-p22. *Nat. Genet.* 10: 41–46.

Weeks, D.E., and Lange, K. (1988) The affected-pedigree-member method of linkage analysis. *Am. J. Hum. Genet.* 42:315–326.

Weeks, D.E., and Lange, K. (1992) A multilocus extension of the affected-pedigree-member method of linkage analysis. *Am. J. Hum. Genet.* 50:859–868.

Weickert, T., Goldberg, T., Mishara, A., Apud, J., Kolachana, B., Egan, M., and Weinberger, D. (2004) Catechol-O-methyltransferase val108/158met genotype predicts working memory response to antipsychotic medications. *Biol. Psychiatry* 56:677–682.

Yang, B.Z., Zhao, H., Kranzler, H.R., and Gelernter, J. (2005) Practical population group assignment with selected informative markers: characteristics and properties of Bayesian clustering via STRUCTURE. *Genet. Epidemiol.* 28:302–312.

11 Neurocognitive Assessment for Psychiatric Disorders

MICHAEL F. GREEN, JUNGHEE LEE, AND ROBERT S. KERN

NEUROCOGNITIVE ASSESSMENT: BACKGROUND AND ORIGINS

Although current clinical neurocognitive assessment is a highly quantitative and technical endeavor, its roots go back very far. The earliest written record for the study of brain-behavior relationships appears to extend back to the 17th century B.C., and perhaps as early as 2500 to 3000 B.C. (Walsh, 1978). The Edwin Smith Surgical Papyrus has been described as the earliest known scientific document (Breasted, 1930). It contains reports of 48 patients treated by an Egyptian physician, several of which include descriptions of head trauma suffered by victims of wars during the period. The graphic reports provide details of the injury, treatment procedures, and the consequences of the injury on behavior. An excerpt from one of the cases translated in 1862 is provided below:

> If thou examinest a man with a gaping wound in his head, penetrating to the bone, (and) splitting his skull, thou shouldst palpate his wound. Shouldst thou find something disturbing therein under thy fingers, (and) he shudders exceedingly. (cited in Walsh, 1978, p. 2)

In the fourth and fifth centuries B.C., Hippocrates and his contemporaries recognized the importance of the brain's functioning on human behavior. The brain was believed to be the seat of the soul and housed one's mental functions. Knowledge about brain-behavior relationships grew from the study of patients with differing brain pathologies, with an emphasis on head injury and epilepsy. This early version of the case study approach gave rise to a number of key discoveries. For example, it was learned that damage to one hemisphere of the brain produced spasms or convulsions to the contralateral side of the body. Through the centuries, many key figures contributed to the evolution of neurocognitive assessment, including Aristotle, Galen, Vesalius, Descartes, Gall, Broca, and Wernicke.

Perhaps the person most often associated with modern neuropsychological assessment is Alexander Luria. His examination of thousands of Russian patients who suffered head injuries in World War II provided the foundation for modern methods of neurocognitive assessment. Luria's early work ranged from studies of cultural development of undereducated minorities (under Lev Vygotsky) to twin studies of the cultural and genetic factors involved in human cognitive development. During World War II, Luria led a team at an army hospital looking for ways to compensate for behavioral dysfunction in patients who were suffering from various war-related brain injuries. The resulting hundreds of case studies contributed significantly to knowledge of assessment and treatment (that is, cognitive remediation) of brain-injured patients. Luria believed that neuropsychology as a field of study could provide early diagnosis and localization of brain injuries, as well as a better understanding of complex psychological functions for which specific brain regions are responsible (Luria, 1970).

These accounts of head injury from the case study method led to a nomenclature for specific regions of the brain affected by insult so that these areas could be identified across cases, and they also led to the discovery that damage to specific regions was tied to specific behavioral dysfunctions. These accomplishments laid the foundation for modern methods of neurocognitive assessment.

Previous Applications of Neurocognitive Assessment in Clinical Settings

Throughout the early to mid-20th century, brain damage was generally viewed as a unitary phenomenon (that is, "organicity"). Organic conditions were thought to reflect a central behavioral defect that was common across patients with different types of brain damage (K. Goldstein, 1939). When applied to patients with psychiatric disorders, a primary use of neurocognitive assessment was to assist in differential diagnosis, particularly in distinguishing between "organic (neurological)" versus "functional (psychiatric)" conditions (G. Goldstein, 1978). A number of tests were developed in an effort to distinguish brain-damaged patients from psychiatric patients and healthy adults. This particular goal for neurocognitive assessment has gradually decreased and largely disappeared as the field's knowledge of neurological and psychiatric conditions has increased. An understanding of psychiatric conditions from a brain-based neurodevelopmental perspective replaced assumptions that had their roots in psychoanalytic traditions.

Standardized and Nonstandardized Neurocognitive Approaches

The methods of neurocognitive assessment have progressed in terms of their ability to quantify and provide clinically meaningful information on differing brain functions. In the 1970s and 1980s, standardized batteries, such as the Luria–Nebraska Neuropsychological Battery (Golden et al., 1985) or the Halstead–Reitan Battery (Reitan and Wolfson, 1978), were a preferred approach. These batteries can assess a wide range of cognitive functions using a standardized set of tests with accompanying norms. Despite their initial appeal, a number of limitations were cited for specific batteries in particular, and for a highly standardized approach in general (Lezak, 1995). Subsequently, preference has grown for process approach methods that included flexible batteries which varied according to the clinical questions posed by a particular patient.

Measurement of Key Cognitive Domains

In evaluating patients with psychiatric disorders, neurocognitive assessment is now rarely used for diagnostic purposes. Instead, the primary purpose is to quantify the severity of impairment in clinically relevant domains of cognitive functioning. The cognitive domains of interest for psychopathology, for the most part, are the same domains that are of interest for other conditions such as neurological disorders or learning disabilities. Because terminology varies considerably, Table 11.1 includes a listing and definition of commonly measured domains.

Traditionally, neurocognitive assessment has been conducted using paper-and-pencil tests, but computerized tests and batteries are growing in popularity and offer advantages and disadvantages (Kern et al., 2004). Computerized tests can be particularly advantageous in measuring cognitive domains such as attention and speed of processing that require sophisticated methods of stimuli presentation and precise measurement of reaction time. They also offer advantages in reliability of test administration and can provide automated data scoring and saving. On the other hand, because of technical malfunction or operation error, computerized assessment measures are frequently the single largest source of missing data in research studies.

Normative data from large demographically representative samples are now available for a number of neurocognitive tests. Normative data bases allow the examiner to quantify the level of neurocognitive impairment compared to persons of similar demographic characteristics (for example, age, gender, education), as well as identify areas of relative strength across separate cognitive domains. The increasing emphasis in neurological and psychiatric disorders in understanding the consequences of cognitive impairment for community functioning (see below) has led to an emphasis in measuring areas of cognitive functioning linked to functional outcome. The results from such neurocognitive assessments can be used to inform patients, families, and clinicians on the likely impact on daily functioning, and they help to identify treatment targets for pharmacological or nonpharmacological intervention that may improve the patient's level of functioning.

VALUE OF NEUROCOGNITIVE ASSESSMENTS FOR PSYCHIATRIC DISORDERS

Neurocognitive assessments can provide valuable information with respect to the nature, genetics, disability, and prognosis of psychiatric disorders. For example, neurocognitive information can reveal core aspects on an illness, provide endophenotypes for use in genetic studies, and help to determine obstacles to community reentry. The empirical literature for these areas is particularly well-established for schizophrenia, and we use that illness as an example. Similar applications of neurocognitive measures are likely to be found for other major psychiatric disorders.

Cognition as a Core Feature of Schizophrenia

Cognition is generally considered to be a core feature of schizophrenia. The meaning of a core deficit in this context is that the impairment does not derive from other clinical features of schizophrenia (for example, psychotic symptoms of hallucinations and delusions), and it is not strictly a result of the psychiatric medications. There are several lines of evidence that lead to this conclusion (Braff, 1993; Nuechterlein et al., 1994; Gold, 2004; Gold and Green, 2004), including the following:

- A different time course of cognitive impairment from that of clinical symptoms. Patients can demonstrate cognitive or intellectual impairments long before the onset of psychotic symptoms and other clinical features (Nuechterlein, 1983; Cornblatt et al., 1992; Cornblatt et al., 1999; Davidson et al., 1999; Reichenberg et al., 2002; Niendam et al., 2003).
- Detection of attenuated cognitive impairment in unaffected first-degree relatives of patients with schizophrenia. Measurable, but comparatively mild, impairments in first-degree relatives suggest that some aspects of neurocognition indicate genetic vulnerability to schizophrenia (Cannon et al., 1994; Kremen et al., 1994; Green et al.,

TABLE 11.1 *Common Neurocognitive Constructs*

Attention

Vigilance/Sustained attention

The ability to maintain readiness to respond and focused mental effort over time.

Selective attention

The ability to maintain focused mental effort in the presence of distraction.

Perception

The transformation of sensory input into meaningful knowledge about one's immediate environment.

Memory

Declarative/Explicit

Involves the ability to retain and revive impressions, or to recall or recognize previous experiences; always with conscious awareness.

Working/Short-term Memory: The transient storage of information in the service of other mental operations (for example, planning); serves as a stepping stone to long-term memory.

Long-term/Secondary/Episodic Memory: The ability to acquire and store information over extended periods of time (at least several minutes).

Both of these forms of memory can be separated into verbal and visual/spatial components.

Non-declarative/Implicit

Learning that does not require the conscious recollection of past events or even an awareness that learning is taking place; typically evidenced through improved task performance (for example, when learning to play sports like tennis or golf). Examples of non-declarative learning include procedural learning, priming, classical conditioning, and non-associative learning.

Motor functioning

Measures within this domain typically assess one of three types of responses:

(*a*) reaction time: the ability to execute a fast response to an environmental stimulus;

(*b*) fine motor speed: the ability to execute rapid fine motor movements;

(*c*) manual dexterity: the ability to carry out rapid coordinated fine motor movements.

Reasoning and Problem Solving

The ability to engage in strategic planning and carry out decision-making activities for the purpose of meeting a desired goal. This domain overlaps with executive functioning.

1997; Cannon et al., 2000; Asarnow et al., 2002; Snitz et al., 2006).

• Relative stability of the cognitive impairment across clinical state. On some cognitive measures, level of impairment during a psychotic episode is similar to that seen when their symptoms are under control or when they are in full remission (Finkelstein et al., 1997; Nuechterlein et al., 1998). Hence, cognitive impairment can occur with reduced, or absent, clinical symptoms of schizophrenia.

• Low cross-sectional correlations between cognitive performance and ratings of psychotic symptom severity. These correlations are typically very small (Goldberg et al., 1993; Mohamed et al., 1999; Bilder et al., 2000; Nieuwenstein et al., 2001; Heydebrand et al., 2004) for psychotic symptoms (that is, hallucinations and delusions). Findings are inconsistent regarding disorganized symptoms (for example, formal thought disorder) with some studies showing relationships and others not (Perry and Braff, 1994; Spitzer, 1997; Mohamed et al., 1999). Cognitive performance tends to have modest relationships to negative symptoms, with typically about 15% of variance overlap.

• Discrepancy between effects of antipsychotic medications on psychotic symptoms versus cognition. This pattern is true for first- and second-generation antipsychotic medications, and the discrepancy suggests that antipsychotic medications act on different neural systems from those that underlie the cognitive impairments. Even if differences in neurocognitive effects exist between first- and second-generation medications, which is a matter of some debate, the impact is rather small compared with the clinical impact of medications on psychotic symptoms (Harvey and Keefe, 2001; Woodward et al., 2005).

Cognition and Functional Outcome

Functional outcome in schizophrenia has been consistently disappointing, even after the introduction of efficacious antipsychotic medications (Helgason, 1990; Hegarty et al., 1994; Wiersma et al., 2000). Antipsychotic medications control psychotic symptoms for the majority of patients, yet only a minority of individuals with schizophrenia can achieve adequate community functioning, including finding a job, forming a network of friends, or living independently. Schizophrenia remains one of the largest causes of disability among all factors (including illnesses, accidents, and wars) for young adults (Murray and Lopez, 1996). Psychotic symptoms in optimally treated people with schizophrenia are not strong or consistent determinants of community functioning for these patients, but cognitive impairments are.

The empirical literature on cognition–function relationships is quite large and well-established. Several reviews of this literature have shown that cognitive deficits have highly consistent relationships to functional outcomes, including social functioning, vocational outcome, degree of independent living, and the ability to acquire skills in psychosocial rehabilitation (Green, 1996; Green et al., 2000; Green, Kern, and Heaton, 2004). The strengths of the associations tend to be medium for individual cognitive domains but can be large when multiple cognitive domains are combined into a global score (Green et al., 2000). Although many of the studies have been cross-sectional, a review of prospective studies also showed that cognitive impairment at a baseline point is a reasonable predictor of later community functioning (Green, Kern, and Heaton, 2004). Several studies reported good associations with outcome 2 to 4 years after baseline assessment (Dickerson et al., 1999; Friedman et al., 2002; Gold et al., 2002; Stirling et al., 2003; Robinson et al., 2004).

There are several remaining questions in this area that are actively under investigation. For example, we do not know yet whether specific neurocognitive domains relate to certain types of functional outcome. In addition, the intervening variables that act between the neurocognitive measures and functional outcome are only now starting to be identified. Two potential intervening variables, *social cognition* and *functional capacity*, appear to act as mediators in models of outcome (Brekke et al., 2005; Bowie et al., 2006; Sergi et al., 2006), meaning that they are related to basic neurocognition, related to functional outcome, and help to account for the direct relationships between the two. Hence, they are considered to be important factors for understanding the pathways to successful outcome, and they may become treatment targets in their own right.

Neurocognitive Endophenotypes

Schizophrenia and other psychotic illness are believed to be complex heritable disorders. The conventional approach of genetic linkage studies is to use clinical features (for example, the diagnosis of schizophrenia) as the primary phenotype. With a clinical diagnosis, members of a pedigree are identified who are, or are not, affected with the illness. An alternative approach for genetic studies is to examine endophenotypes that are thought to be more stable than clinical features and closer to neurobiological processes (Braff and Freedman, 2002; Gottesman and Gould, 2003). Endophenotypes (also called *intermediate phenotypes*) are reliably measured quantitative features that are associated with the illness but are also found in first-degree relatives who do not have the illness.

Cognitive impairments have several characteristics that make them promising endophenotypes for studies of the genetics of schizophrenia. Specifically, they are generally heritable, they can be measured reliably over time and across sites, they are not dependent on a specific clinical state, and they are found (in attenuated form) in first-degree relatives of patients with schizophrenia. For these reasons, there is now considerable interest in examining the genetic basis of cognitive endophenotypes of schizophrenia and other psychiatric disorders. The National Institute of Mental Health (NIMH) Consortium on the Genetics of Schizophrenia is currently examining such endophenotypes in families who include a member with schizophrenia (Calkins et al., 2007). Three of the primary endophenotypes from this study are neurocognitive measures: assessments of verbal learning, working memory, and attention/vigilance (Gur et al., 2007).

The genetic architecture for these endophenotypes is presumed to be simpler than for the clinical disorder of schizophrenia, but that has not been determined yet. The hope is that this approach will provide genetic endophenotypes that are more amenable to genetic dissection. Hence, the idea is to work with an intermediate phenotype that can be more easily mapped on the genome. This genetic approach will likely suggest candidate genes and pathophysiological processes that currently are not being considered for schizophrenia. Importantly for data analysis, endophenotypes can be treated as either continuous or discrete variables (for example, performance below or above a certain cut-off score). Because many more family members are expected to have reduced performance on the endophenotype than have clinical schizophrenia, this approach yields better statistical power for linkage studies. Essentially, this approach is one that seeks the genetics of risk factors for schizophrenia and other psychotic disorders, as opposed to the presence of illness.

Neurocognitive Applications to Other Psychiatric Disorders

Although the lion's share of published research on these topics comes from schizophrenia, much of the same conclusions appear to be applicable to schizoaffective disorder and bipolar disorder. The pattern and magnitude of neurocognitive impairment in schizoaffective disorder are not distinguishable from that of schizophrenia (Miller et al., 1996; Evans et al., 1999; Buchanan et al., 2005; Fiszdon et al., 2007). Also the level of community adaptation is comparable between schizophrenia and schizoaffective disorder (Lysaker and Davis, 2004; Hofer et al., 2006). Patients with schizoaffective disorder are frequently included with patients with schizophrenia in studies of neurocognition and functional outcome, as well as in studies of genetics. Hence, the conclusions from studies of schizophrenia probably apply equally well to schizoaffective disorder.

Cognitive impairment is present in depression and bipolar disorder, but the magnitude and pattern tend to be different from that seen in schizophrenia. Similar to schizophrenia, cognitive impairment might be considered a core feature of bipolar disorder, at least for a subgroup of patients. The impairment is present even when patients with bipolar disorder are out of a mood episode (van Gorp et al., 1998; Fleck et al., 2001; Altshuler et al., 2004; Buchanan et al., 2005), and cognitive impairment is found in some first-degree relatives (Glahn et al., 2004). Some studies, but not others, have reported cognitive impairment in national samples of army recruits before the onset of bipolar disorder (Reichenberg et al., 2002; Tiihonen et al., 2005).

Although relatively few published studies have examined the associations between neurocognition and functional outcome for other psychiatric disorders, some recent findings suggest that similar relationships exist for bipolar disorder (Dickerson et al., 2004; Martínez-Arán et al., 2004; Green, 2006). It is possible that distinct patterns of relationships will characterize different disorders depending on the typical demands for each group of patients. For example, one study found that verbal memory was particularly important for social functioning in schizophrenia, and executive functions were relatively more important for bipolar disorder (Laes and Sponheim, 2006).

There is limited, but increasing, evidence that cognitive impairment is a potential endophenotype for bipolar disorder (Gourovitch et al., 1999; Glahn et al., 2004). A review suggested some criteria for establishing valid endophenotypes for bipolar disorder and concluded that there is already sufficient evidence for the domains of executive function, working memory, and verbal learning (Glahn et al., 2004). Hence, the available evidence suggests that cognitive impairment generally can serve as a reasonable endophenotype for bipolar disorder and schizophrenia, though the specific cognitive domains may turn out to be different for each illness.

Neurocognitive impairment is also clearly present in major depression. Patients with depression complain of cognitive impairments in everyday life (for example, trouble concentrating, reduced ability to make a decision, psychomotor retardation). Studies also have shown deficits of patients with depression in the domains of speed of processing, attention, verbal/visual memory, and executive function using neuropsychological tests (Elliott et al., 1996; Tavares et al., 2003; Chamberlain and Sahakian, 2005), though neurocognitive impairments tend to be less severe than subjective complaints would indicate (O'Connor et al., 1990). The level of these impairments, based on meta-analytic studies, is smaller than those found in other major mental illness (that is, $<$ 1.0 standard deviation below healthy participants) (Christensen et al., 1997; Veiel, 1997). At this point, it is not clear whether neurocognitive impairments are a core feature of depression. For example, it is not known if impaired performance lasts beyond the depressive episode (Christensen et al., 1997; Paradiso et al., 1997). Psychomotor slowing or amotivation may contribute to poor performance. Considering the importance of cognitive impairments in everyday life, it will be critical to understand better whether the cognitive impairment in depression is limited to the clinical episode, or if it has trait-like features in a subgroup of patients.

APPLICATIONS OF NEUROCOGNITIVE ASSESSMENT TO NEW DRUG DEVELOPMENT

Because neurocognitive impairment is considered to be a core feature of illness and is related to community functioning, cognition is now seen as an important treatment target in schizophrenia. In fact, cognitive impairment is frequently identified as a critical unmet need in schizophrenia. However, no drug so far has been approved for cognition enhancement in schizophrenia.

Given this gap between an identified unmet need and the lack of approved treatments, the NIMH launched the Measurement and Treatment Research to Improve Cognition in Schizophrenia (MATRICS) Initiative. The goal of MATRICS was to address and overcome the obstacles to drug approval in this area in an effort to stimulate the development of new drugs to improve cognitive impairment in schizophrenia (Hyman and Fenton, 2003; Marder and Fenton, 2004).

MATRICS used a consensus-building process that included representatives from the pharmaceutical industry, the academic community, the NIMH, and the U.S. Food and Drug Administration (Green, Neuchterlein, et al., 2004; Buchanan et al., 2005). One of the key obstacles to address was the absence of an accepted, consensus-based assessment of cognition that can serve as an endpoint for clinical trials. Prior to selection of a battery, it was first necessary to identify the key cognitive domains that should be represented in a consensus battery. Based on a review of the empirical (mainly factor analytic) literature and discussion at a consensus meeting, seven cognitive domains were selected: *speed of processing, attention/vigilance, working memory, verbal learning, visual learning, reasoning and problem solving,* and *social cognition* (Nuechterlein et al., 2004). Next, tests were selected to represent each of these domains through a lengthy consensus and data collection process (Green, Neuchterlein, et al., 2004; Nuechterlein et al., 2008). The resulting tests that constitute the MATRICS Consensus Cognitive Battery (MCCB) are shown in Table 11.2. The MCCB has been recommended as the standard outcome measure for clinical trials of cognition enhancement in schizophrenia.

As the field starts to focus on cognition enhancement as a treatment target, it creates new challenges at

TABLE 11.2. *MATRICS Domains, Performance Tests, and Animal Models*

Cognitive Domain	*Human Performance Measures*	*Animal Models*
Speed of processing	Category Fluency Trail Making A BACS—Symbol Coding	5-Choice Serial Reaction Time Task Simple reaction time tasks
Attention/vigilance	Identical Pairs Continuous Performance Test	5-Choice Serial Reaction Time Task Latent inhibition Prepulse inhibition and auditory gating
Working memory	Wechsler Memory Scale–III Spatial Span Letter–Number Span	Operant or T-maze Delayed Nonmatch to Position/Delayed Match to Position Radial Arm Maze
Verbal learning	Hopkins Verbal Learning Test–Revised	
Visual learning	Brief Visuospatial Memory Test–Revised	Novel object recognition Social recognition
Reasoning and problem solving	NAB—Mazes	Attentional set shifting Maze tasks
Social cognition	Mayer-Salovey-Caruso Emotional Intelligence Test (MSCEIT)—Managing Emotions	Social interaction/social recognition?

Source: Adapted from Hagan and Jones (2005).
NAB: Neuropsychological assessment battery.

two levels. As described above, one level is how to assess neurocognition in humans who are part of clinical trials. Another level involves animal models of neurocognition at the preclinical level. Clearly animal models that are used to screen compounds for psychosis will not be ideal to screen compounds for procognitive effects. A discussion of animal models is beyond the scope of this chapter (see special issue of *Psychopharmacology,* vol. 174[1], 2004). However, in the context of drug discovery, discussions about human neurocognitive assessment will need to interface with discussions about animal models that map onto the key constructs. The MATRICS discussions about human neurocognition generated considerable interest in the selection of animal models for preclinical screening. Table 11.2 shows a notable attempt to link animal models to the MATRICS cognitive domains (Hagan and Jones, 2005). A systematic approach to identify and organize animal models along these lines will be one of the products of a clinical trial network that was recently funded by NIMH: Treatment Units for Neurocognition and Schizophrenia (TURNS: www.turns.ucla.edu).

INFLUENCES ON FUTURE ASSESSMENT: SOCIAL/EMOTION PROCESSES AND COGNITIVE NEUROSCIENCE

Neurocognitive assessment for psychiatric disorders is being influenced by an infusion of methods and concepts from other areas, including social cognition and cognitive neuroscience. We briefly describe both developments.

Social Cognition

Assessments of neurocognition are typically considered to be measures of "cold cognition," meaning that they do not include measures of social or emotional factors but instead intentionally use neutral numbers, letters, or shapes. However, social and emotional factors are increasingly important considerations for research in nonclinical samples and have generated impressive literatures. The area of social cognition has emerged in recent years as an important component to better understand the nature of major psychiatric illnesses and the associated social dysfunction.

Social cognition refers to an ability to recognize, understand, manipulate, regulate, and behave with respect to socially relevant information (Fiske and Taylor, 1991; Kunda, 1999; Adolphs, 2001), and it is critical for adaptive social interaction. As a result, social cognition may provide a way to more fully explain impaired community function in patients with psychiatric disorder. Problems that seem to be attributable to social cognition are frequently described as part of the clinical phenomenology of major psychiatric disorders, such as inappropriate affect, misinterpretation, and lack of relatedness. When applied to major mental illness, research on social cognition has typically included assessment of one or more of the following areas: emotional processing, mental state attribution (that is, theory of mind), social perception, and attribution bias (Green et al., 2005).

Using objective measures, impaired social cognition has been well-documented in schizophrenia. Assessments of social cognition are designed to measure how we process social information in "real" social situations, and they tend to use more real-life stimuli such as facial photographs and video clips, as well as vignettes describing diverse social situations. These characteristics can yield tests that are more engaging for patients, perhaps minimizing other confounding factors such as motivation. Nonetheless, patients with schizophrenia have deficits in a range of social cognitive abilities, including recognizing facial emotion expressions, understanding others' mental state, social perception, and self-perception (Penn et al., 1997; Penn et al., 2006). There is increasing evidence that social cognition is important for functional outcome in schizophrenia (Mueser et al., 1996; Penn et al., 1996; Kee et al., 2003; Sergi et al., 2006). Social cognition may act as a mediator between basic neurocognition and functional outcome in schizophrenia and can explain independent variance in outcome, above and beyond neurocognitive deficits (Vauth et al., 2004; Brekke et al., 2005; Addington et al., 2006; Sergi et al., 2006). These studies suggest that social cognition may be a valuable target for intervention strategies as a way to improve functional outcome in schizophrenia. The importance of social cognition is further supported by its inclusion by MATRICS as one of the cognitive domains assessed in the MCCB (Nuechterlein et al., 2004).

One limitation of the social cognitive measures is that their psychometric properties are typically not as well established as those for neurocognitive tests. For example, several measures of mental state attribution were adopted from developmental psychology or studies for autism. Scaling problems (for example, ceiling effects) make it difficult to find patient–control differences and also to see and interpret patterns of performance impairments. Hence, the development of social cognitive measures with good psychometric properties is a priority. New tests with stronger normative bases (Mayer et al., 2002) or with wider ranges for levels of performance (McDonald et al., 2002) are starting to be used with psychiatric samples.

Cognitive Neuroscience

In addition to influences from developments in social cognition, neurocognitive assessment in psychiatric disorders can be influenced by developments in cognitive neuroscience. There is typically a trade-off between tests that come from a clinical neuropsychology approach and those that come from a cognitive neuroscience approach. Clinical neuropsychology tends to emphasize psychometrics and norming, whereas cognitive neuroscience tends to emphasize construct validity. We can use the MCCB as an example.

The selection criteria for the MCCB included features such as good test–retest reliability, demonstrated utility as a repeated measure (for example, manageable practice effects), practicality for use in clinical trials (for example, ease of setup, administration, and scoring), and tolerability for the participant (for example, acceptable duration and difficulty). All of these criteria are essential for clinical trials. Candidate tests from the clinical neuropsychology approach tend to be more established and to have clear standardized administration guidelines, demonstrated reliability, and existence of normative databases that made them somewhat easier to evaluate. In contrast, candidate tests from the cognitive neuroscience approach tend to have less (or less compelling) psychometric data, or to be more complicated to administer in the context of a clinical trial. However, these tests often had an advantage over clinical neuropsychological tests in terms of their ability to assess a particular cognitive process (that is, construct validity). Based on recommendations from MATRICS, the NIMH has launched a follow-up series of consensus meetings, Cognitive Neuroscience Treatment Research to Improve Cognition in Schizophrenia (CNTRICS), to evaluate and develop new or modified measures from cognitive neuroscience that can be psychometrically honed so they can be used in clinical trials of cognition enhancing drugs. The goal is to have assessments that combine the best of both worlds.

Overall, neurocognitive assessment in psychiatric disorders represents a methodology with very deep roots, but one that is also moving in new directions as it borrows from neighboring fields. Information gained from neurocognitive methods will provide a better understanding of the nature of psychiatric illnesses, a clearer delineation of the determinants of community outcome, and eventually, ways to advance drug development.

REFERENCES

Addington, J., Saeedi, H., and Addington, D. (2006) Facial affect recognition: a mediator between cognitive and social functioning in schizophrenia? *Schizophr. Res.* 85:142–150.

Adolphs, R. (2001) The neurobiology of social cognition. *Curr. Opin. Neurobiol.* 11:231–239.

Altshuler, L.L., Ventura, J., van Gorp, W.G., Green, M.F., Theberge, D.C., and Mintz, J. (2004) Neurocognitive function in clinically stable men with bipolar I disorder or schizophrenia and normal control subjects. *Biol. Psychiatry* 56:560–569.

Asarnow, R.F., Nuechterlein, K.H., Subotnik, K.L., Fogelson, D., Torquato, R., Payne, D., Asamen, J., Mintz, J., and Guthrie, D. (2002) Neurocognitive impairments in non-psychotic parents of children with schizophrenia and attention deficit hyperactivity disorder: The UCLA Family Study. *Arch. Gen. Psychiatry* 59:1053–1060.

Bilder, R.M., Goldman, R.S., Robinson, D., Reiter, G., Bell, L., Bates, J.A., Pappadopulos, E., Wilson, D.F., Alvir, J.M., Woerner, M.G.,

Geisler, S., Kane, J.M., and Lieberman, J.A. (2000) Neuropsychology of first-episode schizophrenia: initial characterization and clinical correlates. *Am. J. Psychiatry* 157:549–559.

Bowie, C.R., Reichenberg, A., Patterson, T.L., Heaton, R.K., and Harvey, P.D. (2006) Determinants of real-world functional performance in schizophrenia subjects: Correlations with cognition, functional capacity, and symptoms. *Am. J. Psychiatry* 163:418–425.

Braff, D. (1993) Information processing and attention dysfunctions in schizophrenia. *Schizophr. Bull.* 19:233–259.

Braff, D.L., and Freedman, R. (2002). The importance of endophenotypes in studies of the genetics of schizophrenia. In: Davis, K.L., Charney, D., Coyle, J.T., and Nemeroff, C., eds. *5th Generation of Progress.* Philadelphia: Lippincott, Williams & Wilkins, pp. 703–716.

Breasted, J.H. (1930) *The Edwin Smith Surgical Papyrus.* Chicago: University of Chicago Press.

Brekke, J.S., Kay, D.D., Kee, K.S., and Green, M.F. (2005) Biosocial pathways to functional outcome in schizophrenia. *Schizophr. Res.* 80:213–225.

Buchanan, R.W., Davis, M., Goff, D., Green, M.F., Keefe, R.S.E., Leon, A.C., Nuechterlein, K.H., Laughren, T., Levin, R., Stover, E., Fenton, W., and Marder, S.R. (2005) A summary of the FDA-NIMH-MATRICS workshop on clinical trial design for neurocognitive drugs for schizophrenia. *Schizophr. Bull.* 31:5–19.

Calkins, M.E., Dobie, D.J., Cadenhead, K.S., Olincy, A., Freedman, R., Green, M.F., Greenwood, T.A., Gur, R.E., Gur, R.C., Light, G.A., Mintz, J., Nuechterlein, K.H., Radant, A.D., Schork, N.J., Seidman, L.J., Siever, L.J., Silverman, J.M., Stone, W.S., Swerdlow, N.R., Tsuang, D.W., Tsuang, M.T., Turetsky, B.I., and Braff, D.L. (2007) The Consortium on the Genetics of Endophenotypes in Schizophrenia: model recruitment, assessment, and endophenotyping methods for a multisite collaboration. *Schizophr. Bull.* 33:33–48.

Cannon, T.D., Eyler-Zorrilla, L., Shtasel, D., Gur, R.C., Marco, E.J., Moberg, P., and Price, R.A. (1994) Neuropsychological functioning in siblings discordant for schizophrenia and healthy volunteers. *Arch. Gen. Psychiatry* 51:651–661.

Cannon, T.D., Huttunen, M.O., Lonnqvist, J., Tuulio-Henriksson, A., Pirkola, T., Glahn, D., Finkelstein, J., Hietanen, M., Kaprio, J., and Kosenvuo, M. (2000) The inheritance of neuropsychological dysfunction in twins discordant for schizophrenia. *Am. J.Hum. Genet.* 67:369–382.

Chamberlain, S.R., and Sahakian, B.J. (2005) Neuropsychological assessment of mood disorder. *Clinical Neuropsychiatry* 2:137–148.

Christensen, H., Griffiths, K., Mackinnon, A., and Jacomb, P. (1997) A quantitative review of cognitive deficits in depression and Alzheimer-type dementia. *J. Int. Neuropsychol. Soc.* 3:631–651.

Cornblatt, B., Lenzenweger, M.F., Dworkin, R., and Erlenmeyer-Kimling, L. (1992) Childhood attentional dysfunction predicts social deficits in unaffected adults at risk for schizophrenia. *Br. J. Psychiatry* 161:59–64.

Cornblatt, B., Obuchowski, M., Roberts, S., Pollack, S., and Erlenmeyer-Kimling, L. (1999) Cognitive and behavioral precursors of schizophrenia. *Dev. Psychopathol.* 11:487–508.

Davidson, M., Reichenberg, A., Rabinowitz, J., Weiser, M., Kaplan, Z., and Mark, M. (1999) Behavioral and intellectual markers for schizophrenia in apparently healthy male adolescents. *Am. J. Psychiatry* 156:1328–1335.

Dickerson, F., Boronow, J.J., Ringel, N., and Parente, F. (1999) Social functioning and neurocognitive deficits in outpatients with schizophrenia: A 2-year follow-up. *Schizophr. Res.* 37:13–20.

Dickerson, F.B., Boronow, J.J., Stallings, C.R., Origoni, A.E., Cole, S., and Yolken, R.H. (2004) Association between cognitive functioning and employment status of persons with bipolar disorder. *Psychiatr. Serv.* 55:54–58.

Elliott, R., Sahakian, B.J., McKay, A.P., Herrod, J.J., Robbins, T.W., and Paykel, E.S. (1996) Neuropsychological impairments in unipolar depression: the influence of perceived failure on subsequent performance. *Psychol. Med.* 26:975–989.

Evans, J.D., Heaton, R.K., Paulsen, J.S., McAdams, L.A., Heaton, S.C., and Jeste, D.V. (1999) Schizoaffective disorder: a form of schizophrenia or affective disorder? *J. Clin. Psychiatry* 60:874–882.

Finkelstein, J.R.J., Cannon, T.D., Gur, R.E., Gur, R.C., and Moberg, P. (1997) Attentional dysfunctions in neuroleptic-naive and neuroleptic-withdrawn schizophrenic patients and their siblings. *J. Abnorm. Psychol.* 106:203–212.

Fiske, S.T., and Taylor, S.E. (1991) *Social Cognition*, 2nd ed. New York: McGraw-Hill.

Fiszdon, J.M., Richardson, R., Greig, T., and Bell, M.D. (2007) A comparison of basic and social cognition between schizophrenia and schizoaffective disorder. *Schizophr. Res.* 91:117–121.

Fleck, D.E., Sax, K.W., and Strakowski, S.M. (2001) Reaction time measures of sustained attention differentiate bipolar disorder from schizophrenia. *Schizophr. Res.* 52:251–259.

Friedman, J.I., Harvey, P.D., McGurk, S.R., White, L., Parrella, M., Raykov, T., Coleman, T., Adler, D.N., and Davis, K.L. (2002) Correlates of change in functional status of institutionalized geriatric schizophrenic patients: focus on medical comorbidity. *Am. J. Psychiatry* 159:1388–1394.

Glahn, D.C., Bearden, C.E., Niendam, T.A., and Escamilla, M.A. (2004) The feasibility of neuropsychological endophenotypes in the search for genes associated with bipolar affective disorder. *Bipolar Disord.* 6:171–182.

Gold, J.M. (2004) Cognitive deficits as treatment targets in schizophrenia. *Schizophr. Res.* 72:21–28.

Gold, J.M., Goldberg, R.W., McNary, S.W., Dixon, L., and Lehman, A.F. (2002) Cognitive correlates of job tenure among patients with severe mental illness. *Am. J. Psychiatry* 159:1395–1401.

Gold, J.M., and Green, M.F. (2004). Neurocognition in schizophrenia. In: Sadock, B.J., and Sadock, V.A., eds. *Comprehensive Textbook of Psychiatry*, 8th ed. Baltimore: Lippincott, Williams & Wilkins, pp. 1436–1448.

Goldberg, T.E., Gold, J.M., Greenberg, R., and Griffin, S. (1993) Contrasts between patients with affective disorders and patients with schizophrenia on a neuropsychological test battery. *Am. J. Psychiatry* 150:1355–1362.

Golden, C.J., Purisch, A.D., and Hammeke, T.A. (1985) *Luria-Nebraska Neuropsychological Battery: Forms I and II.* Los Angeles: Western Psychological Services.

Goldstein, G. (1978) Cognitive and perceptual differences between schizophrenics and organics. *Schizophr. Bull.* 4:160–185.

Goldstein, K. (1939) *The Organism.* New York: American Book Co.

Gottesman, I.I., and Gould, T.D. (2003) The endophenotype concept in psychiatry: etymology and strategic intentions. *Am. J. Psychiatry* 160:636–645.

Gourovitch, M.L., Torrey, E.F., Gold, J.M., Randolph, C., Weinberger, D.R., and Goldberg, T.E. (1999) Neuropsychological performance of monozygotic twins discordant for bipolar disorder. *Biol. Psychiatry* 45:639–646.

Green, M.F. (1996) What are the functional consequences of neurocognitive deficits in schizophrenia? *Am. J. Psychiatry* 153:321–330.

Green, M.F. (2006) Cognitive impairment and functional outcome in schizophrenia and bipolar disorder. *J. Clin. Psychiatry* 67 (Suppl 9):3–8; discussion 36–42.

Green, M.F., Kern, R.S., Braff, D.L., and Mintz, J. (2000) Neurocognitive deficits and functional outcome in schizophrenia: Are we measuring the "right stuff"? *Schizophr. Bull.* 26:119–136.

Green, M.F., Kern, R.S., and Heaton, R.K. (2004) Longitudinal studies of cognition and functional outcome in schizophrenia: implications for MATRICS. *Schizophr. Res.* 72:41–51.

Green, M.F., Nuechterlein, K.H., and Breitmeyer, B. (1997) Backward masking performance in unaffected siblings of schizophrenia patients: Evidence for a vulnerability indicator. *Arch. Gen. Psychiatry* 54:465–472.

Green, M.F., Nuechterlein, K.H., Gold, J.M., Barch, D.M., Cohen, J., Essock, S., Fenton, W.S., Frese, F., Goldberg, T.E., Heaton, R.K., Keefe, R.S.E., Kern, R.S., Kraemer, H., Stover, E., Weinberger, D.R., Zalcman, S., and Marder, S.R. (2004) Approaching a consensus cognitive battery for clinical trials in schizophrenia: the NIMH-MATRICS conference to select cognitive domains and test criteria. *Biol. Psychiatry* 56:301–307.

Green, M.F., Olivier, B., Crawley, J.N., Penn, D.L., and Silverstein, S. (2005) Social cognition in schizophrenia: recommendations from the MATRICS New Approaches Conference. *Schizophr. Bull.* 31:882–887.

Gur, R.E., Calkins, M.E., Gur, R.C., Horan, W.P., Nuechterlein, K.H., Seidman, L.J., and Stone, W.S. (2007) The Consortium on the Genetics of Schizophrenia: neurocognitive endophenotypes. *Schizophr. Bull.* 33:49–68.

Hagan, J.J., and Jones, D.N. (2005) Predicting drug efficacy for cognitive deficits in schizophrenia. *Schizophr. Bull.* 31:830–853.

Harvey, P.D., and Keefe, R.S.E. (2001) Studies of the cognitive change in patients with schizophrenia following novel antipsychotic treatment. *Am. J. Psychiatry* 158:176–184.

Hegarty, J.D., Baldessarini, R.J., Tohen, M., Waternaux, C., and Oepen, G. (1994) One hundred years of schizophrenia: a meta-analysis of the outcome literature. *Am. J. Psychiatry* 151: 1409–1416.

Helgason, L. (1990) Twenty years' follow-up of first psychiatric presentation for schizophrenia: what could have been prevented? *Acta Psychiatr. Scand.* 81:231–235.

Heydebrand, G., Weiser, M., Rabinowitz, J., Hoff, A.L., DeLisi, L.E., and Csernansky, J.G. (2004) Correlates of cognitive deficits in first episode schizophrenia. *Schizophr. Res.* 68:1–9.

Hofer, A., Rettenbacher, M.A., Widschwendter, C.G., Kemmler, G., Hummer, M., and Fleischhacker, W.W. (2006) Correlates of subjective and functional outcomes in outpatient clinic attendees with schizophrenia and schizoaffective disorder. *Eur. Arch. Psychiatry Clin. Neurosci.* 256:246–255.

Hyman, S.E., and Fenton, W.S. (2003) What are the right targets for psychopharmacology? *Science* 299:350–351.

Kee, K.S., Green, M.F., Mintz, J., and Brekke, J.S. (2003) Is emotion processing a predictor of functional outcome in schizophrenia? *Schizophr. Bull.* 29:487–497.

Kern, R.S., Green, M.F., Nuechterlein, K.H., and Deng, B.H. (2004) NIMH-MATRICS survey on assessment of neurocognition in schizophrenia. *Schizophr. Res.* 72:11–19.

Kremen, W.S., Seidman, J., Pepple, J.R., Lyons, M.J., Tsuang, M.T., and Faraone, S.V. (1994) Neuropsychological risk indicators for schizophrenia: a review of family studies. *Schizophr. Bull.* 20:103–119.

Kunda, Z. (1999) *Social Cognition: Making Sense of People.* Cambridge, MA: MIT Press.

Laes, J.R., and Sponheim, S.R. (2006) Does cognition predict community function only in schizophrenia?: a study of schizophrenia patients, bipolar affective disorder patients, and community control subjects. *Schizophr. Res.* 84:121–131.

Lezak, M.D. (1995) *Neuropsychological Assessment,* 3rd ed. New York: Oxford University Press.

Luria, A.R. (1970) The functional organization of the brain. *Sci. Am.* 222:66–72.

Lysaker, P.H., and Davis, L.W. (2004) Social function in schizophrenia and schizoaffective disorder: associations with personality, symptoms and neurocognition. *Health Qual. Life Outcomes* 2:15.

Marder, S.R., and Fenton, W.S. (2004) Measurement and treatment research to improve cognition in schizophrenia: NIMH MATRICS Initiative to support the development of agents for improving cognition in schizophrenia. *Schizophr. Res.* 72:5–10.

Martínez-Arán, A., Vieta, E., Colom, F., Torrent, C., Sánchez-Moreno, J., Reinares, M., Benabarre, A., Goikolea, J.M., Brugué, E., Daban, C., and Salamero, M. (2004) Cognitive impairment in euthymic bipolar patients: implications for clinical and functional outcome. *Bipolar Disord.* 6:224–232.

Mayer, J.D., Salovey, P., and Caruso, D.R. (2002) *Mayer-Salovey-Caruso Emotional Intelligence Test (MSCEIT) User's Manual.* Toronto, Canada: MHS Publishers.

McDonald, S., Flanagan, S., and Rollins, J. (2002) *The Awareness of Social Inference Test.* Suffolk, UK: Thames Valley Test Company, Ltd.

Miller, L.S., Swanson-Green, T., Moses, J.A., and Faustman, W.O. (1996) Comparison of cognitive performance in RDC-diagnosed schizoaffective and schizophrenic patients with the Luria-Nebraska Neuropsychological Battery. *J. Psychiatr. Res.* 30:277–282.

Mohamed, S., Paulsen, J.S., O'Leary, D.S., Arndt, S., and Andreasen, N.C. (1999) Generalized cognitive deficits in schizophrenia. *Am. J. Psychiatry* 156:749–754.

Mueser, K.T., Doonan, R., Penn, D.L., Blanchard, J.J., Bellack, A.S., Nishith, P., and DeLeon, J. (1996) Emotion recognition and social competence in chronic schizophrenia. *J. Abnorm. Psychol.* 105:271–275.

Murray, C.J.L., and Lopez, A.D., eds. (1996) *The Global Burden of Disease.* Boston: Harvard School of Public Health.

Niendam, T.A., Bearden, C.E., Rosso, I.M., Sanchez, L.E., Hadley, T., Nuechterlein, K.H., and Cannon, T.D. (2003) A prospective study of childhood neurocognitive functioning in schizophrenic patients and their siblings. *Am. J. Psychiatry* 160:2060–2062.

Nieuwenstein, M.R., Aleman, A., and de Haan, E.H.F. (2001) Relationship between symptom dimensions and neurocognitive functioning in schizophrenia: a meta-analysis of WCST and CPT studies. *J. Psychiatr. Res.* 35:119–125.

Nuechterlein, K.H. (1983) Signal detection in vigilance tasks and behavioral attributes among offspring of schizophrenic mothers and among hyperactive children. *J. Abnorm. Psychol.* 92:4–28.

Nuechterlein, K.H., Asarnow, R.F., Subotnik, K.L., Fogelson, D.L., Ventura, J., Torquato, R., and Dawson, M.E. (1998). Neurocognitive vulnerability factors for schizophrenia: convergence across genetic risk studies and longitudinal trait/state studies. In: Lenzenweger, M.F., and Dworkin, R.H., eds. *Origins and Development of Schizophrenia: Advances in Experimental Psychopathology.* Washington, DC: American Psychological Association, pp. 299–327.

Nuechterlein, K.H., Barch, D.M., Gold, J.M., Goldberg, T.E., Green, M.F., and Heaton, R.K. (2004) Identification of separable cognitive factors in schizophrenia. *Schizophr. Res.* 72:29–39.

Nuechterlein, K.H., Dawson, M.E., and Green, M.F. (1994) Information-processing abnormalities as neuropsychological vulnerability indicators for schizophrenia. *Acta Psychiatr. Scand.* 90:71–79.

Nuechterlein, K.H., Green, M.F., Kern, R.S., Baade, L.E., Barch, D., Cohen, J., Essock, S., Fenton, W.S., Frese, F.J., Gold, J.M., Goldberg, T., Heaton, R., Keefe, R.S.E., Kraemer, H., Mesholam-Gately, R., Seidman, L.J., Stover, E., Weinberger, D., Young, A.S., Zalcman, S., and Marder, S.R. (2008) The MATRICS Consensus Cognitive Battery: part 1. test selection, reliability, and validity. *Am. J. Psychiatry* 165:203–213.

O'Connor, D.W., Pollitt, P.A., Roth, M., Brook, P.B., and Reiss, B.B. (1990) Memory complaints and impairment in normal, depressed, and demented elderly persons identified in a community survey. *Arch. Gen. Psychiatry* 47:224–227.

Paradiso, S., Lamberty, G.J., Garvey, M.J., and Robinson, R.G. (1997) Cognitive impairment in the euthymic phase of chronic unipolar depression. *J. Nerv. Ment. Dis.* 185:748–754.

Penn, D.L., Addington, J., and Pinkham, A. (2006). Social cognitive impairments. In: Lieberman, J.A., Stroup, T.S., and Perkins, D.O., eds. *American Psychiatric Association Textbook of Schizophrenia.* Arlington, VA: American Psychiatric Publishing Press, Inc., pp. 261–274.

Penn, D.L., Corrigan, P.W., Bentall, R.P., Racenstein, J.M., and Newman, L. (1997) Social cognition in schizophrenia. *Psychol. Bull.* 121:114–132.

Penn, D.L., Spaulding, W., Reed, D., and Sullivan, M. (1996) The relationship of social cognition to ward behavior in chronic schizophrenia. *Schizophr. Res.* 20:327–335.

Perry, W., and Braff, D.L. (1994) Information-processing deficits and thought disorder in schizophrenia. *Am. J. Psychiatry* 151: 363–367.

Reichenberg, A., Weiser, M., Rabinowitz, J., Caspi, A., Schmeidler, J., Mark, M., Kaplan, Z., and Davidson, M. (2002) A population-based cohort study of premorbid intellectual, language, and behavioral functioning in patients with schizophrenia, schizoaffective disorder, and nonpsychotic bipolar disorder. *Am. J. Psychiatry* 159:2027–2035.

Reitan, R.M., and Wolfson, D. (1978) *The Halstead-Reitan Neuropsychological Test Battery: Theory and Clinical Interpretation.* Tucson, AZ: Neuropsychology Press.

Robinson, D.G., Woerner, M.G., McMeniman, M., Mendelowitz, A., and Bilder, R.M. (2004) Symptomatic and functional recovery from a first episode of schizophrenia or schizoaffective disorder. *Am. J. Psychiatry* 161:473–479.

Sergi, M.J., Rassovsky, Y., Nuechterlein, K.H., and Green, M.F. (2006) Social perception as a mediator of the influence of early visual processing on functional status in schizophrenia. *Am. J. Psychiatry* 163:448–454.

Snitz, B.E., MacDonald, A.W., and Carter, C.S. (2006) Cognitive deficits in unaffected first-degree relatives of schizophrenia patients: a meta-analytic review of putative endophenotypes. *Schizophr. Bull.* 32:179–194.

Spitzer, M. (1997) A cognitive neuroscience view of schizophrenic thought disorder. *Schizophr. Bull.* 23:29–50.

Stirling, J., White, C., Lewis, S., Hopkins, R., Tantam, D., Huddy, A., and Montague, L. (2003) Neurocognitive function and outcome in first-episode schizophrenia: a 10-year follow-up of an epidemiological cohort. *Schizophr. Res.* 65:75–86.

Tavares, J.V., Drevets, W.C., and Sahakian, B.J. (2003) Cognition in mania and depression. *Psychol. Med.* 33:959–967.

Tiihonen, J., Haukka, J., Henriksson, M., Cannon, M., Kieseppa, T., Laaksonen, I., Sinivuo, J., and Lonnqvist, J. (2005) Premorbid intellectual functioning in bipolar disorder and schizophrenia: results from a cohort study of male conscripts. *Am. J. Psychiatry* 162:1904–1910.

van Gorp, W.G., Altshuler, L., Theberge, D.C., Wilkins, J., and Dixon, W. (1998) Cognitive impairment in euthymic bipolar patients with and without prior alcohol dependence: a preliminary study. *Arch. Gen. Psychiatry* 55:41–46.

Vauth, R., Rusch, N., Wirtz, M., and Corrigan, P.W. (2004) Does social cognition influence the relation between neurocognitive deficits and vocational functioning in schizophrenia? *Psychiatry Res.* 128:155–165.

Veiel, H.O. (1997) A preliminary profile of neuropsychological deficits associated with major depression. *J. Clin. Exp. Neuropsychol.* 19:587–603.

Walsh, K.W. (1978). *Neuropsychology—A Clinical Approach.* Edinburgh, UK: Churchill Livingstone.

Wiersma, D., Wanderling, J., Dragomirecka, E., Ganev, K., Harrison, G., An der Heiden, W., Nienhuis, F.J., and Walsh, D. (2000) Social disability in schizophrenia: its development and prediction over 15 years in incidence cohorts in six European centres. *Psychol. Med.* 30:1155–1167.

Woodward, N.D., Purdon, S.E., Meltzer, H.Y., and Zald, D.H. (2005) A meta-analysis of neuropsychological change to clozapine, olanzapine, quetiapine, and risperidone in schizophrenia *Int. J. Neuropsychopharmacol.* 8:457–472.

12 Cognitive Neuroscience: Bridging Thinking and Feeling to the Brain, and its Implications for Psychiatry

CAMERON S. CARTER, JOHN G. KERNS, AND
JONATHAN D. COHEN

Over the past 20 years a new integrative discipline, *cognitive neuroscience*, has emerged and begun to have a major impact on the way we think about the neural basis of human cognition and behavior. Considered historically, cognitive neuroscience developed as a convergence of psychology and neuroscience (Gazzaniga, 1995; Cowan et al., 2000; Kandel and Squire, 2000). The field of *cognitive neuroscience* is defined as the effort to understand how mental processes emerge from the function of the brain (Albright et al., 2000). The scope of cognitive neuroscience extends from efforts to understand the neural basis of the simplest perceptual events to efforts to understand the neural regulation of complex human behaviors.

Cognitive neuroscience is an integrative scientific discipline. Models of the neural basis of mental events are developed from data collected across multiple levels of analysis, from cellular and molecular to overt behavior. Most critically for psychiatry and psychology, human experimentation, using rigorous cognitive experimental methods and noninvasive neuroscientific tools such as functional brain imaging, is a critical element of the cognitive neuroscience approach. These noninvasive methods and the normative data that they have provided present a vast array of opportunities for developing a new level of understanding of the neural basis of disordered thinking and behavior. In this chapter we review several of the exciting developments in cognitive neuroscience, in particular as they relate to the study of psychopathology. Collectively, these indicate that the time is ripe for a fuller incorporation of the tools and constructs of cognitive neuroscience—specifically those involving noninvasive human experimentation—into clinical neuroscience research and practice. We believe that this will not only bring a new clarity and rigor to our understanding of psychopathology and its neural underpinnings, but will also facilitate the integration of knowledge about potential disease mechanisms derived from animal models. Figure 12.1 shows how the three critical elements (rigorous cognitive models and methods, noninvasive functional brain imaging, and experimentation with animal models) that form the basis of the cognitive neuroscience approach can also serve as the basis for a truly translational approach (that is, from the bench to the bedside and back again) to understanding the mechanisms and genetics, and for the development of targeted treatments in mental disorders. This approach will take us closer to a cellular and molecular level of understanding of the neural basis of mental disorders, and this is an essential step if we are to begin to develop treatments based on pathophysiology and understand their genetic underpinnings.

THREE MAJOR RESEARCH METHODS IN COGNITIVE NEUROSCIENCE

In general, successful scientific research involves two interactive activities: (*1*) building theories that capture important facets of the real world and (*2*) testing those theories with data that are powerful enough to rule out alternative, competing theories. For cognitive neuroscience research there are significant challenges to building theories and to acquiring powerful data. Psychological activity can be highly complex (for example, consider the myriad processes that are involved in being able to read and understand the words you see on this page). Furthermore, this complex mental activity is somehow instantiated in the brain by billions of individual neurons interacting with one another on the time scale of tens of milliseconds. Thus, successful cognitive neuroscience research must have a theoretical framework that is sophisticated enough to be able to address this complexity and have empirical tools that can collect

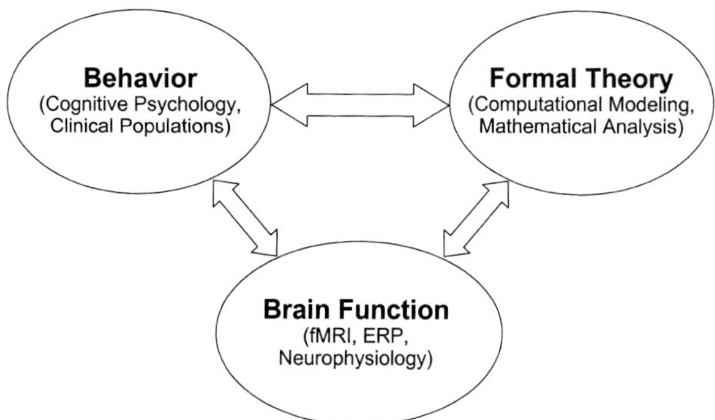

FIGURE 12.1 The application of cognitive neuroscience methods to clinical research involves a close interaction between behavioral methods, measurements of brain function, and the use of such data to constrain the development of formally explicit theories about the relationship between psychological processes and underlying neural mechanisms.

data precise enough to support or disconfirm its theories. To address these challenges, cognitive neuroscience has developed as an integrative discipline that combines cognitive testing, neuroscientific measurements, and computer simulation modeling. We discuss examples of each of these three key methods below, chosen to be relevant to clinical neuroscience research. Each is discussed from a historical and theoretical perspective and illustrated by a set of related examples from the literature.

Experimental Cognitive Methods: Identification and Measurement of the Behavioral Building Blocks of Normal and Disordered Cognition

To conceptualize and measure cognitive mechanisms, cognitive neuroscience draws on the theories of *perception, attention, memory,* and *higher cognitive functions* such as language and problem solving that were developed during the "cognitive revolution" of experimental psychology in the second half of the 20th century. The theoretical approach of cognitive psychology is supported by a rich scientific technology, with experimental and statistical approaches approximating the sophistication of those used in the physical sciences. Cognitive neuroscience emerged as a discipline when cognitive scientists began using these methods to test their theories in individuals with focal brain injuries or using noninvasive neuroscience methods such as scalp electrical recording (or event-related potentials, ERPs) and positron emission tomography (PET) and, convergently, neuroscientists recording from the brains of behaving animals began to relate their results to theories about mental function developed within cognitive psychology. For example, it became clear relatively early on in neuroimaging research that the meaning of a pattern of brain activity observed (or its disturbance in a patient) could not be properly interpreted without a clear conception of the cognitive or emotional processes engaged by the task(s) used to produce that pattern of brain activity.

It is important to note that to apply a cognitive experimental approach to understanding psychopathology we may need to undergo a change in how we think about mental disorders. In current practice, there is a strong effort to segregate different mental disorders into distinct categories. However, in actuality, these disorders may reflect a complex combination of disturbances in more fundamental processes, or dimensions of function, that do not necessarily align with currently identified categories of disorder. For example, schizophrenia and depression may ultimately be better understood as particular changes in the functioning of underlying cognitive and emotional systems (such as executive control and reinforcement learning), with different combinations of deficits in these underlying systems producing the different behavior deficits that are categorized clinically as two distinct illnesses. If this is so, then it suggests that a more powerful way of characterizing and understanding these illnesses is to draw on the conceptual and experimental framework provided by cognitive psychology by developing behavioral paradigms that can sensitively and specifically measure the critical functions of interest. This also promises a more direct path toward relating clinical disturbance to underlying neurobiological pathology, insofar as fundamental cognitive processes are more likely to map onto specific, identifiable neurobiological mechanisms. Such an approach can be informed by a variety of cognitive neuroscientific methods, such as noninvasive neuroimaging for studying brain activity and its response to psychopharmacological intervention, as well as by parallel, invasive animal studies.

Two central assumptions of the cognitive psychological approach are that mental function is composed of distinguishable fundamental processes and that these processes can be selectively engaged by properly designed experimental task manipulations. A critical corollary to this approach is that a theoretically guided task analysis is a precursor to the design of any experiment. A *task analysis* is simply a clear specification of the processes thought to be engaged by the experimental task and how these processes will be influenced by the variables to be manipulated in the experiment. For example, an experimental task might require participants to observe letters presented visually one at a time and to respond to any repeats by pressing a button. The task analysis for this design might identify the following processes: attention to the visual display, encoding of each stimulus into a short-term memory store, identification of the stimulus as a letter, comparison of this letter to ones seen previously and maintained in memory, generation of an appropriate motor response based on the outcome of the comparison process, encoding and/or maintenance of the current stimulus in memory, and preparation for the next stimulus. With this task analysis in mind and a theory about the functioning of the processes involved, the experimenter can now identify experimental variables that are predicted to selectively influence different processes. For example, by manipulating the number of previous stimuli over which a repeat might occur, the experimenter can selectively probe memory processes without affecting sensory or motor processes.

It should be evident why this approach is valuable to the cognitive neuroscientist with an interest in basic and disordered function: It provides a way of interpreting the influence of experimental variables on specific cognitive processes and thereby differentially engaging these cognitive processes so that they can be related to measurements of brain activity. It is important, however, to note several things about this approach. First, as noted above, it requires and is driven by a prior theory about the processes needed to perform a task. In the example given above, the theory assumed that sensory encoding and encoding into short-term memory are separate processes. However, in principle, these might actually be closely related processes or even part of a single process. This highlights an important value of the cognitive psychological approach. By emphasizing a theoretically motivated experimental design, it provides a way of testing specific hypotheses about the architecture of cognitive processes. Thus, for example, a failure to confirm behavioral predictions generated by a task analysis that assumes that sensory and memory encoding are distinct processes may lead to a revision of the theory in which they are construed as related processes.

A similar issue concerns the grain of the task analysis. For example, the identification of the visual stimulus as a particular letter could be decomposed into a more detailed set of processes involving feature identification, object recognition, and so on. Again, the iterative cycle of theory construction, task analysis, experimental design, behavioral testing coupled with neurobiological measurements, and then theory revision provides a way of refining our understanding of the processes that make up mental function and how these relate to underlying neural mechanisms.

Finally, it is important to recognize that psychological processes, neural mechanisms, and, in particular, the dynamics of their operation may be quite complex. This, and the added complexity of the interaction among different processes and mechanisms, may exceed our ability to reason intuitively about them or describe them in strictly verbal terms. To address this complexity, some investigators have turned to computer simulation modeling. This is a tool that was first advocated as part of the cognitive science revolution (Newell and Simon, 1972; Anderson, 1983) as a way of helping to make theories about cognitive processes explicitly mechanistic. This approach, using neural network models, has also been extremely useful for exploring the connection between cognitive processes and underlying brain mechanisms (Rumelhart and McClelland, 1986). We consider an example of this below.

The cognitive neuroscience approach, as described above, contrasts with and complements more traditional neuropsychological approaches to relating behavior—normal and disordered—to the brain. Neuropsychology, growing out of the Luria tradition, has sought to identify correlations between well-characterized patterns of neurological damage and performance on standard behavioral instruments. This approach has the advantage of a large body of normative data that has been collected over several decades and has generated important insights into the relationship between cognitive function and the brain—for example, the importance of the frontal lobes to executive functions (Stuss and Benson, 1986). As noted, however, the use of standardized instruments is at the core of this approach. These instruments contrast with the approach to behavioral research taken by cognitive neuroscientists in two respects.

First, by their very nature, standardized instruments are not subject to modification because the goal of such research is to compare the performance of a large group of participants on the same tasks. In contrast, as described above, cognitive neuroscientists specifically seek to design new tasks and then modify these from experiment to experiment, as a way of testing and refining theories about underlying cognitive processes. Second, from the cognitive psychological perspective, the behavioral tasks used in standard neuropsychological batteries are often overly complex, engaging a variety of cognitive processes that are difficult to dissociate from one another within the context of those tasks. For example, though neuropsychological studies have clearly demonstrated that the Wisconsin Card Sorting Task is highly sensitive to frontal lobe damage, this task has been less useful in determining which specific components of executive function may be impaired. This is because the task engages a variety of processes, including categorization, decision making, hypothesis testing, and reinforcement learning, among others, in ways that are difficult to separate from one another in the context of this task.

Because of their complexity, neuropsychological tasks also often confound specific cognitive processes with nonspecific factors such as motivation, generalized disturbances of attention, and so on (Chapman and Chapman, 1978; Knight and Silverstein, 2001). In contrast, drawing on an appropriate task analysis and corresponding experimental design, cognitive psychological instruments can be designed that provide sensitive and specific measures of cognitive processes while controlling for generalized deficits. Not all studies using cognitive experimental methods demonstrate such a high level of specificity; however, the potential for specificity, as well as for sensitivity, invites more widespread use of this approach in psychiatry (A.W. MacDonald and Carter, 2002).

Finally, it is important to note that, as its name implies, the cognitive neuroscience approach has focused largely on identifying and analyzing cognitive processes and their relationship to brain function. However, the same theoretical and empirical methods can be and have begun to be applied to the analysis of emotional and social processes (Ochsner and Lieberman, 2001). Indeed, such an approach is increasingly revealing that the distinction between cognitive and emotional processes is not as fundamental as is commonly thought. However, even if such a distinction is meaningful, there is growing recognition of the intimate relationship between cognitive, emotional, and social processes, which, of course, has profound relevance to psychiatric research. We believe that the next several years will see an explosion of research using cognitive neuroscience methods to explore the nature of the interaction between these various processes.

Example: Experimental cognitive studies of context processing in schizophrenia

The notion that executive functions may be disrupted in schizophrenia has formed the basis of many general theories of impaired cognition in this illness (Calloway and Naghdi, 1982; Braff, 1993; Posner and Abdullaev, 1996; Barch and Carter, 1998). Indeed, this is an informative and parsimonious way of understanding the range of cognitive deficits seen in this illness. However, the term *executive functions* needs clarification because it refers to a broad set of complex processes across a number of domains of cognition (Tranel et al., 1994). A disturbance in the ability to initiate and maintain controlled information processing can account for the pattern of deficits of selective attention, working memory, and declarative memory performance seen in patients with this illness. Building on ideas articulated by Shakov in the 1960s and Calloway in the 1970s and 1980s, Cohen and Servan-Schreiber (1992a, 1992b) hypothesized that a deficit in a specific cognitive function, referred to as *context processing*, could account for impaired executive functions in schizophrenia.

Context processing refers to the maintenance of task-relevant information in working memory and its influence on other processes required to perform a task. Context information may include a representation of stimuli, rules specifying how to respond to these stimuli, or the set of possible responses. Cohen and Servan-Schreiber hypothesized that patients with schizophrenia are impaired in their ability to represent and maintain context, and that this can account for a wide range of cognitive deficits in schizophrenia. To test this hypothesis, they used a variant of the continuous performance test (CPT) referred to as the *modified AX-CPT task* (Fig. 12.2). In this test, single letters appear one at a time on a computer screen, and participants are required to give a target response to any appearance of an *X* that follows an *A* and a nontarget response to any other stimulus. This task engages context processing insofar as participants must actively maintain a representation of context provided by the prior stimulus (*A* or non-*A*) to know how to respond to the subsequent appearance of an *X* (target if preceded by an *A*, nontarget otherwise). A critical experimental manipulation involves the frequency of the AX trials. These occur 70% of the time. This leads to the development of two habitual response tendencies as subjects perform this task. The first is that participants develop a strong tendency to make a target response to an *X* whenever it occurs (that is, irrespective of the preceding stimulus) because it is almost always a target. On trials in which an *X* follows some other letter (referred to as *BX trials*), participants must use the context provided by the preceding letter to overcome this otherwise very strong tendency to give a target response to the *X*. The second habitual response tendency is a target response to any stimulus that follows an *A* because on a majority of trials this is an *X*. When *A* is followed by a non-*X* stimulus (referred to as AY trials), participants must overcome this tendency to produce a target response. Thus, for AY trials, context processing produces a bias toward incorrect responding. As a result of this experimental design, a degradation in context processing should result in two disordinal effects: worse performance on BX trials (that is, the production of a larger number of nontarget responses) but better performance on AY trials (fewer incorrect target responses). This pattern of performance has in fact been observed in a number of different populations of patients with schizophrenia, medicated and unmedicated and at different stages of the illness (Cohen et al., 1999; Servan-Schreiber et al., 1996; Barch et al., 2003). Importantly, this pattern of performance can be interpreted as reflecting a specific deficit in context processing and not a generalized performance deficit, as a generalized deficit would predict poor performance on both difficult trial types, BX and AY, in the patient group. Recently, a variant of this task was used to show that a specific context-processing deficit was observed in the unaffected first-degree relatives of patients with schizophrenia, suggesting that this cognitive deficit is likely to reflect genetic liability to the illness (A. MacDonald et al., 2003). When the relationship between symptoms and impaired context processing (worse performance on BX relative to AY trials) was examined, consistent (and specific) correlations were seen with ratings of behavioral disorganization obtained at the time of testing (Cohen

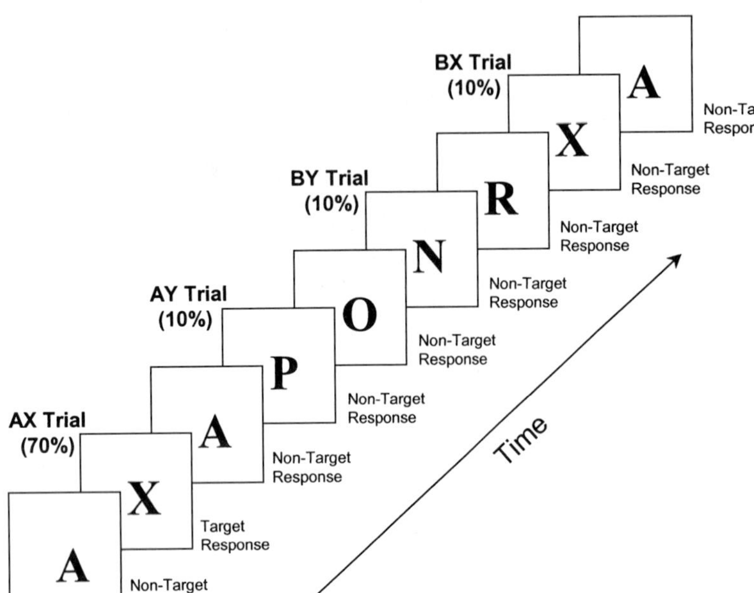

FIGURE 12.2 Variant of the AX-CPT, designed to elicit selective performance deficits associated with a disturbance in the processing of context (continuous performance test [CPT]). The stimulus sequence shown was chosen to illustrate each trial type (AX, AY, BX, and BY) but does not reflect their actual proportions (which are indicated in the labels). See Servan-Schreiber et al. (1996) for more details.

et al., 1999; Barch et al., 2003; Berenbaum et al., 2007). This work is presented as an example of how a theoretically based approach to understanding impaired cognition in schizophrenia can guide the design of cognitive experimental studies that, in turn, may lead to an increased understanding of the mechanisms underlying behavioral disturbances in schizophrenia. The incorporation of this approach into hypothesis-driven functional imaging studies is discussed later in this chapter.

Noninvasive Functional Brain Imaging: New and Powerful Tools for the In Vivo Study of the Disordered Human Brain

A second, core cognitive neuroscience research methodology is functional brain imaging techniques. Typically in functional brain imaging studies, participants perform a behavioral task that engages the psychological activity of interest. As noted above, cognitive neuroscience emphasizes the importance of a theoretically motivated task analysis in experimental design. This is particularly important in the context of a functional neuroimaging study as a way of ensuring that patterns of brain activity observed under different experimental conditions can be related to the cognitive processes of interest. Cognitive tasks can be combined with a variety of measures of brain function. For example, functional magnetic resonance imaging (fMRI) involves measuring changes in the MR signal that reflect the amount of deoxygenated blood in brain tissue, indirectly indexing neural activity–dependent blood flow in the brain. Another example of a functional brain imaging technique is ERP recording. This involves measuring electrical activity at the scalp that is time locked to events of interest within the behavioral paradigm.

Each of these functional imaging techniques has strengths and weaknesses. Relative to earlier neuroimaging methods, fMRI has the advantage of providing excellent spatial localization of brain activity (on the order of millimeters) and temporal resolution (on the order of seconds). This has permitted the development of event-related designs (e.g., Rosen et al., 1998; D'Esposito et al., 1999) that can measure changes in brain activity associated with psychological events of interest on a trial-to-trial basis. However, relative to the time scale of psychological processes that transpire within a trial (occurring over tens to hundreds of milliseconds), the temporal resolution of fMRI is limited. Similarly, fMRI cannot tell us about spatial organization at the level of local neural circuits (10–100 mm). Finally, present MRI-based methods cannot tell us about neurotransmitter function. However, other methods are available that overcome each of these limitations. The recording of scalp electrical potentials, or ERPs, provides temporal resolution on the order of milliseconds and can thus easily track brain activity on the time scale over which psychological processes occur. Event-related potentials studies have limited spatial resolution. However, a newly developed method, magnetoencephaloscopy (MEG) offers promise at providing good spatial resolution along with the temporal resolution of ERP. Invasive single-unit recordings can be used in nonhuman species to provide precise temporal and spatial information about brain activity but are generally not suitable for human studies. Finally, PET can be used, in humans and in nonhuman species, to measure the functioning of specific neurotransmitter systems while participants perform cognitive tasks, but it lacks the temporal or spatial resolution of fMRI.

Given that individual imaging techniques have complementary strengths and weaknesses, one promising approach to functional neuroimaging research is to use more than one imaging technique in the same study (Dale and Sereno, 1993; Luck, 1999). For example, fMRI and ERP have been used in conjunction with one another, capitalizing on the strengths of each approach, the spatial resolution of fMRI, and the temporal resolution of ERP to obtain a spatiotemporal map of brain activity associated with cognitive processes of interest.

Example: Functional imaging studies of impaired context processing in schizophrenia

The first functional imaging study in schizophrenia, conducted by Ingvar and Franzen (1974), reported that patients with schizophrenia showed a loss of the normal hyperfrontal pattern of blood flow while performing a neuropsychological task. Since that time, many, but certainly not all, studies of schizophrenia have reported reduced blood flow or metabolism in the dorsolateral prefrontal cortex (DLPFC) in schizophrenia (Weinberger, Berman, and colleagues completed several such studies; see Buchsbaum, 1990; Andreasen et al., 1992; Taylor et al., 1996, for reviews). This finding is not as reliable when patients are studied at rest (Gur and Gur, 1995). Indeed, many have noted that it is most reliably present when patients are performing tasks that engage cognitive systems known to reflect neural activity in this region of the brain (Goldman-Rakic, 1987, 1991; Carter et al., 1998; Perlstein et al., 2001).

An important prediction of the context-processing theory of cognitive dysfunction in schizophrenia is that the representation and maintenance of context depend on the integrity of the PFC, and that a disturbance in this process is related to impaired executive functions (Cohen and Servan-Schreiber, 1992a). During the past several years, basic cognitive neuroscience studies have confirmed a role for the DLPFC in context processing. This was shown initially with relatively nonspecific tasks, such as the N-Back task (Braver et al., 1997; Cohen et al., 1997), and then with more specific context-processing tasks, such as the AX-CPT (Barch et al., 1997) and an instructed version of the Stroop task (A. M. MacDonald et al., 2000). Using the N-Back task during fMRI, Perlstein et al. (2001) showed that DLPFC activation was impaired in schizophrenia. In that study, failure to increase activity in DLPFC was correlated with poor task performance and increased clinical ratings of behavioral disorganization. Using the AX-CPT task, Barch et al. (2001) showed impairment of DLPFC activity when never-medicated, first-episode patients with schizophrenia had to maintain context representations. This finding was specific to DLPFC, with Broca's area showing normal activation in patients. Finally, a recent fully event-related analysis of a large group of never-medicated, first-episode patients confirmed that hypofrontality was specific to schizophrenia (compared to nonschizophrenia-related first-episode psychosis) and was correlated with poor performance and ratings of disorganization (A. MacDonald et al., 2005). The important point to note is that as the cognitive experimental approach has become more rigorous and focused on specific cognitive deficits, the specificity of the results to schizophrenia and the ability to relate impaired cognition, hypofrontality, and behavioral disorganization have become more reliable. Over time, this approach offers the promise of developing more sensitive clinical instruments that can be used in other forms of research (for example, the identification of genetic markers) and clinical practice (for example, diagnosis, treatment evaluation).

Functional magnetic resonance imaging is a powerful method for noninvasively imaging the activity across the human brain associated with specific cognitive mechanisms such as the examples related to context processing described above. In recent years investigators have been able to acquire fMRI data in behaving nonhuman primates undergoing simultaneous intracranial recording that has provided new insights in the neurophysiology of cognition and suggested new hypotheses regarding the underlying pathophysiology of disordered cognition in schizophrenia. The hemodynamically based blood oxygen level–dependent (BOLD) response measured during fMRI has been shown to be most strongly related to population neuronal activity, particularly synchronous activity in the high (40 Hz) or gamma band (Logothetis et al., 2001, Niessing et al., 2005). This is relevant for understanding hypofrontality in schizophrenia because postmortem studies in schizophrenia have consistently suggested abnormalities in two key neural substrates of gamma oscillations in the PFC, alterations in thalamocortical connectivity (suggested by reduced volumes and cell counts in the dorsomedial thalamus and reductions in dendritic spines in the thalamic recipient zones of BA area 9) and altered synchronization of the local circuit in the PFC due to reductions in key elements of γ-aminobutyric acid (GABA)-ergic neurotransmission (Jones, 1997, Lewis et al., 2004). Alterations in stimulus-driven gamma (40 Hz activity in the electroencephalogram [EEG] evoked by 40 Hz sensory stimulation; e.g., Kwon et al., 1999) have been reported for a number of years. Cho et al. (2006) reported that gamma band activity induced in the PFC as context-processing demands increased was reduced over the PFC in schizophrenia. As previously reported using fMRI and the AX-CPT task in patients; PFC gamma synchrony was associated with measures of behavioral disorganization in the schizophrenia group. This result, using spectral temporal analysis of cognition-related EEG recordings, suggests an understanding of impaired cognition in schizophrenia that bridges postmortem findings involving local cortical networks in the PFC, local circuit function (high-frequency thalamocortical oscillatory activity involving populations of PFC neurons), hypofrontality measured using fMRI, impaired context processing, and disorganized thinking and behavior in schizophrenia.

Computational Modeling: Building and Testing Precise Theories that Link Disordered Brain and Behavior

A third and equally important research method is computational modeling. Computer simulations of connectionist or neural network models involve the formal specification of the psychological processes involved in cognition and behavior in terms of explicit, biologically plausible computational mechanisms (Rumelhart and McClelland, 1986). Such models are designed to simulate human cognitive-task performance. These models are useful in part because simulations are another way of testing the validity of the model, as well as generating novel theoretical predictions. Moreover, neural network models involve properties that are thought likely to be true about information processing in the brain. For example, neural network models represent information as distributed graded patterns of activity over a collection of simple processing units, processing as the continuous flow of activity over the connections from one set of units to another, and learning as changes in the strength of these connections. Thus, neural network models implement psychological processes in terms of computational mechanisms that capture fundamental features of information processing as it occurs in the brain. In this way, these models have the potential to provide an important bridge between the neural and behavioral levels of analysis (Cohen et al., 1992b; McClelland, 1993; Braver and Cohen, 1999). Critically, they help make explicit the hypotheses about the relationship of psychological function to brain mechanisms. Sometimes such models have been criticized as requiring too many unwarranted assumptions. However, a virtue of computational modeling in general is that it helps bring such assumptions into view. Every theory makes assumptions. The danger is not that these assumptions are wrong but that they go undetected. Indeed, one useful way to view the assumptions made by a computational model is as a set of hypotheses that can be tested in subsequent experiments.

Example: Computational modeling of impaired context processing in schizophrenia

Neural network models of schizophrenia have attempted to capture important aspects of disordered cognition (for example, impaired context processing) as well as disordered biology (for example, impaired DLPFC and dopamine function) (Cohen and Servan-Schreiber, 1992b; Cohen and Servan-Schreiber, 1993; Braver and Cohen, 1999; for related examples, see Hoffman, 1987; Dehaene and Changeux, 1992). Figure 12.3 presents one example of such a model. Important elements of the model are that it includes units that represent and maintain context information, thus instantiating the proposed function of the DLPFC, and that changes in the model can be used to simulate the effects of dopamine. In the model, context information biases the processing in other parts of the model to select task-appropriate responses. Changes in the responsivity (or gain) of processing units in the model are used to simulate the effects of dopamine (Cohen and Servan-Schreiber, 1992a, 1993). To simulate the behavior of persons with schizophrenia, the gain was decreased in the model, thus simulating a hypodopaminergic state in the DLPFC (Davis et al., 1991). This model of impaired cognition was able to simulate the specific pattern of behavioral deficits observed in persons with schizophrenia in three cognitive tasks: the Stroop task, the CPT, and a lexical disambiguation task (Cohen and Servan-Schreiber, 1992a). Thus, the model provided not only a well-specified theory of impaired cognition in schizophrenia, but also its relationship to underlying biological disturbances.

After initial work with this model, it was refined by elaborating the role of dopamine in accordance with more recent research on the role of dopamine in the brain (Braver & Cohen, 1999, 2000). In the modified version of the model, phasic dopamine signals provide a gating mechanism, which allows for the selective and task-appropriate updating of context representations in PFC, whereas tonic dopamine levels support maintenance of these representations. The revised model has been used to simulate more detailed features of the behavioral performance of persons with schizophrenia in the AX-CPT, including increased BX trial response time and errors as well as decreased AY trial reaction time and errors. This more detailed model also makes a number of novel predictions regarding the dynamics of PFC activity, and its relationship to task performance, that are currently being tested.

Important Methodological Considerations in Clinical Cognitive Neuroscience Research

Although cognitive neuroscience has a great deal to offer the study of psychopathology, there are important methodological challenges in research on clinical populations that need to be considered to conduct successful clinical research. These methodological issues have plagued clinical research using cognitive assessments and functional imaging since their beginning. An important strength of the cognitive neuroscience approach is that it provides solutions to each of these problems. In this last section, we discuss some important methodological issues and confounds and their potential solutions through the application of cognitive neuroscience methods to clinical research.

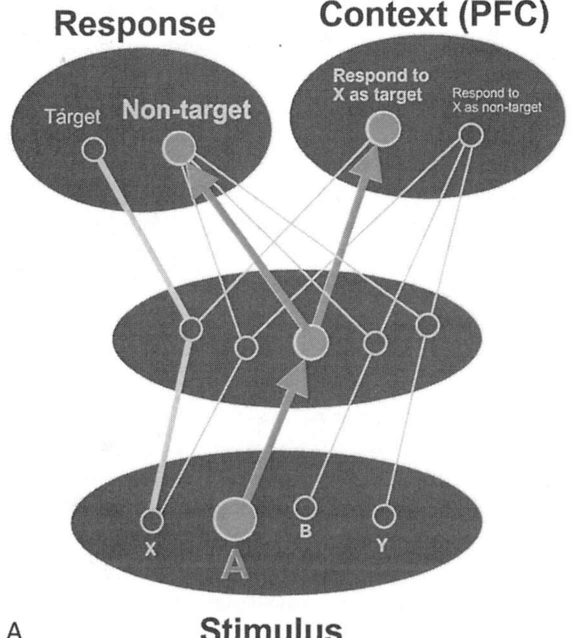

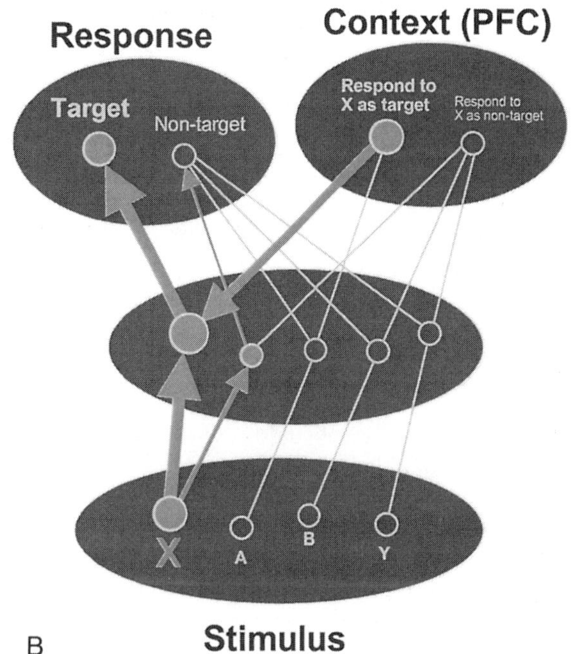

FIGURE 12.3 A model of the AX-CPT (continuous performance test [CPT]). Panel A depicts the state of the network while processing the letter *A* as the stimulus. Panel B depicts the state of the network while processing the letter *X* after processing the letter *A*. Currently activated nodes are shown as medium gray and a larger size. Medium gray arrows designate cascade of activity. Stronger connections are shown with heavier line weights. Note that the connections are strongest from the node representing the letter *X* in the input to the intermediate and response nodes representing a target response. This captures the increased strength of these associations as a result of the high frequency of target trials (70% of trials). Note also that, in Panel B, prior presentation of the letter A has activated the "Respond to X as target" node in the context layer. This, coupled with input from the stimulus node for the letter *X*, activates the target node in the response layer. If the previous letter had been other than *A* (for example, *B*), the "Respond to X as nontarget" context node would have been activated. This, in turn, would have activated the associative node connecting the stimulus node for *X* to the nontarget response. See Braver and Cohen (2001) for more details.

A crucial issue in clinical research is the effects of generalized performance deficits. For example, on average, a group of persons with schizophrenia will perform worse than controls on a majority of cognitive tasks. Thus, although one might like to infer that if people with schizophrenia show deficits on a particular task, these deficits are due to a unique association between this task and schizophrenia, an alternative interpretation is that persons with schizophrenia perform poorly on most difficult tasks. This is especially true for task conditions that are the most difficult for control groups—which are often just those conditions that are thought to be specifically sensitive to schizophrenia. Hence, poor performance by persons with schizophrenia on a particular task may not provide compelling evidence for a unique association between that task and schizophrenia because the a priori expectation would be that persons with schizophrenia would perform worse on most challenging tasks anyway. Although this issue is most frequently discussed in connection with schizophrenia, it is relevant to research on nearly all clinical populations in which poor performance could be attributed to general performance deficits (for example, persons with depressive disorders). Overcoming this problem, and demonstrating the specificity of a deficit to a particular patient population, can be achieved by using psychometrically matched tasks (Chapman and Chapman, 1973, 1978). Thus, if persons with schizophrenia perform more poorly on one task than controls, but do not perform more poorly than controls on a second task that is psychometrically matched to the first task (in terms of difficulty, reliability, and variance, or, in other words, true score variance), then it can be inferred that persons with schizophrenia have a specific deficit on that task (e.g., Oltmanns and Neale, 1975). Demonstrating a specific deficit can also be achieved by devising hypotheses and empirical patterns of behavioral performance (for example, better performance of a clinical population on a predicted task condition, such as fewer AY trial errors in persons with schizophrenia on the AX-CPT) that cannot be accounted for by generalized poor performance.

Another issue in clinical cognitive research is interpreting brain activity changes in the context of impaired behavioral performance. For example, persons with schizophrenia exhibit decreased DLPFC activity compared to controls on the N-Back task (Perlstein et al., 2001). This is consistent with DLPFC dysfunction in persons with schizophrenia. However, persons with schizophrenia also perform worse on the task than controls. Thus, it might be argued that decreased DLPFC activity may not be a function of impaired DLPFC but instead is a by-product of poor behavioral performance. That is, reduced DLPFC may be a result of impaired behavioral performance rather than its cause. At one level, this merely reflects the correlational nature of this research. Further evidence is needed to establish that DLPFC is a causal factor in behavioral impairments. Such evidence can be sought from a variety of converging sources. For example, one additional piece of convergent evidence is impaired DLPFC structural integrity in persons with schizophrenia (Glantz and Lewis, 2000). Another is the ability of computational models that simulate impairments of DLPFC to accurately predict the particular pattern of behavioral deficits in persons with schizophrenia (Braver and Cohen, 2001). It is also possible to conduct analogue studies with participants who are nonpsychiatric that simulate DLPFC dysfunction, for example, by manipulating cognitive demands (Barch and Berenbaum, 1994; Sher and Trull, 1996; Kerns and Berenbaum, 2003; Kerns, 2007) or through pharmacological challenge (Servan-Schreiber et al., 1998). If these simulated deficits in participants who are nonpsychiatric result in behavior and brain activity similar to that of persons with schizophrenia, this lends support to the hypothesis that a disruption of DLPFC is a cause of behavioral deficits in the illness. A new method, *transcranial magnetic stimulation* (TMS), which can activate or inactivate specific brain areas and thereby explore the causal role they have in behavior, may help resolve these issues in the future. In summary, given a finding of changes in brain activity associated with impaired behavioral performance, there are a variety of ways to obtain compelling convergence evidence that establishes a causal role of identified aspects of brain dysfunction in producing impaired behavior among psychiatric populations.

Another important issue in functional brain imaging studies is that psychiatric populations might exhibit increased movement or other sources of variability compared to control participants. This can cause problems for a number of brain imaging methods. For example, in fMRI research, increased movement in patients might reduce the ability to detect focused, localizable brain activity from a particular brain region. Thus, a finding of decreased brain activity in patients might be attributable simply to increased movement in patients. One potential way of dealing with increased movement in patients is to exclude participants with a high level of movement to examine whether this would change the results. For example, Barch et al. (2001) found that decreased DLPFC activity in persons with schizophrenia remained unchanged even after participants with excessive movement were eliminated. For ERP studies, increased blink rates in patients could differentially decrease the number of valid trials for patients. Given the importance of averaging signal intensity across a number of trials in ERP research, a finding of decreased intensity of an ERP component might be attributable simply to fewer valid trials in patients. One way to deal with increased blink rates is to use sophisticated regression-based correction algorithms. A complementary approach is to include a sufficiently large number of trials for each condition (for example, $N = 200$) so that increased blink rates in patients would not result in too few trials.

CONCLUSIONS

The emergence of cognitive neuroscience as an important mainstream scientific discipline provides an unprecedented opportunity for clinical neuroscientists interested in understanding the mechanisms and etiology of major psychiatric diseases. In this chapter we presented a related set of examples to illustrate this point. These are intended to be representative of the growing number of studies that use cognitive neuroscience methods in clinical research. This approach can provide new insights into the cognitive and emotional mechanisms that produce psychopathological symptoms. It can also provide detailed information regarding the neural circuitry that is disturbed in mental disorders. This analysis can be elaborated to the cellular and molecular levels by developing animal models and studying them using methods that parallel those used in the human studies. Formally specified and parametrically measured cognitive and emotional traits and deficits can also be used as phenotypes in the search for liability genes contributing to mental disorders. Finally, cognitive neuroscience research can serve as a valuable new source of data for understanding mechanisms of treatment effects and can suggest new directions for therapeutic research. Leading neuroscientists now recognize that "cognitive neuroscience, with its concern about perception, action, memory, language and selective attention, will increasingly come to represent the central focus of all neurosciences in the 21st century" (Kandel and Squire, 2000). We believe that this appraisal applies equally well to clinical neuroscience, for which our understanding of the neural underpinnings of the disturbances in perception, action, memory, language, and selective attention that characterize the severe mental disorders is still rudimentary. Cognitive neuroscience provides us with a powerful new set of empirical tools and theoretical constructs, together with a growing knowledge of the neural basis of normal cognition, that provide an ideal point of departure for developing a truly detailed understanding of the mechanisms and etiology of disturbed cognition and behavior in mental disorders.

REFERENCES

Albright, T., Kandel, E., and Posner, M. (2000) Cognitive neuroscience. *Curr. Opin. Neurobiol.* 10:612–624.

Anderson, J. (1983) *The Architecture of Cognition*. Cambridge, MA: Harvard University Press.

Andreasen, N.C., Rezai, K., Alliger, R., et al. (1992) Hypofrontality in neuroleptic naive patients and in patients with chronic schizophrenia: assessment with xenon 133 single photon emission computed tomography and the Tower of London. *Arch. Gen. Psychiatry* 49:943–958.

Barch, D.M., and Berenbaum, H. (1994) The relationship between information processing and language production. *J. Abnorm. Psychol.* 103:241–251.

Barch, D.M., Braver, T.S., Nystrom, L.E., et al. (1997) Dissociating working memory from task difficulty in human prefrontal cortex. *Neuropsychologia* 35(10):1373–1380.

Barch, D.M., and Carter, C.S. (1998) Selective attention in schizophrenia: relationship to verbal working memory. *Schizophr. Res.* 33:53–61.

Barch, D.M., Carter, C.S., Braver, T.S., et al. (2001) Selective deficits in prefrontal cortex function in medication naive patients and schizophrenia. *Arch. Gen. Psychiatry* 58:280–288.

Barch, D.M., Carter, C., MacDonald, A., et al. (2003) Context processing deficits in schizophrenia: diagnostic specificity, four-week course, and relationships to clinical symptoms. *J. Abnorm. Psychol.* 112:132–143.

Berenbaum, H., Kerns, J.G., Vernon, L.L., and Gomez, J.J. (2007) *Cognitive correlates of schizophrenia signs and symptoms: I. Verbal communication disturbances*. Manuscript submitted for publication.

Braff, D. (1993) Information processing and attention dysfunction in schizophrenia. *Schizophr. Bull.* 19:233–259.

Braver, T.S., and Cohen, J.D. (1999) Dopamine, cognitive control, and schizophrenia: the gating model. *Prog. Brain Res.* 121:327–349.

Braver, T.S., and Cohen, J.D. (2000) On the control of control: the role of dopamine in regulating prefrontal function and working memory. In: Monsell, S., and Driver, J., eds. *Attention and Performance XVIII*. Cambridge, MA: MIT Press, pp. 713–737.

Braver, T.S., and Cohen, J.D. (2001) Working memory, cognitive control, and the prefrontal cortex: computational and empirical studies. *Cogn. Proc.* 2:25–55.

Braver, T.S., Cohen, J.D., Nystrom, L.E., et al. (1997) A parametric study of prefrontal cortex involvement in human working memory. *NeuroImage* 5:49–62.

Buchsbaum, M. (1990) The frontal lobes, basal ganglia and temporal lobes as sites for schizophrenia. *Schizophr. Bull.* 16:379–389.

Calloway, E., and Naghdi, S. (1982) An information processing model for schizophrenia. *Arch. Gen. Psychiatry* 39:339–347.

Carter, C.S., Braver, T.S., Barch, D.M., et al. (1998) Anterior cingulate cortex, error detection, and the on line monitoring of performance. *Science* 280(5364):747–749.

Chapman, L.J., and Chapman, J.P. (1973) Problems in the measurement of cognitive deficit. *Psychol. Bull.* 79:380–385.

Chapman, L.J., and Chapman, J.P. (1978) The measurement of differential deficit. *J. Psychiatr. Res.* 14:303–311.

Cho, R.Y., Konecky, R.O., and Carter, C.S. (2006) Impairments in frontal cortical gamm synchrony and cognitive control in schizophrenia. *Proc. Natl. Acad. Sci. USA* 103(52):19878–19883.

Cohen, J.D., Barch, D.M., Carter, C.S., et al. (1999) Schizophrenic deficits in the processing of context: converging evidence from three theoretically motivated cognitive tasks. *J. Abnorm. Psychol.* 108:120–133.

Cohen, J.D., Perlstein, W.M., Braver, T.S., et al. (1997) Temporal dynamics of brain activation during a working memory task. *Nature* 386: 604–608.

Cohen, J.D., and Servan-Schreiber, D. (1992a) Context, cortex and dopamine: a connectionist approach to behavior and biology in schizophrenia. *Psychol. Rev.* 99(1):45–77.

Cohen, J.D., and Servan-Schreiber, D. (1992b) Introduction to neural network models in psychiatry. *Psychiatr. Ann.* 22(3):113–118.

Cohen, J.D., and Servan-Schreiber, D. (1993) A theory of dopamine function and its role in cognitive deficits in schizophrenia. *Schizophr. Bull.* 19(1):85–104.

Cowan, W.M., Harter, D.H., and Kandel, E.R. (2000) The emergence of modern neuroscience: some implications for neurology and psychiatry. *Annu. Rev. Neurosci.* 23:343–391.

Dale, A.M., and Sereno, M.I. (1993) Improved localization of cortical activity by combining EEG and MEG with MRI cortical surface reconstruction: a linear approach. *J. Cogn. Neurosci.* 5(2): 162–176.

Davis, K., Kahn, R., Ko, G., et al. (1991) Dopamine in schizophrenia: a review and reconceptualization. *Am. J. Psychiatry* 148:1474–1486.

Dehaene, S., and Changeux, J.P. (1992) The Wisconsin Card Sorting Test: theoretical analysis and modeling in a neuronal network. *Cerebral Cortex* 1:62–79.

D'Esposito, M., Zarahn, E., and Aguirre, G.K. (1999) Event-related functional MRI: implications for cognitive psychology. *Psychol. Bull.* 125(1):155–164.

Gazzaniga, M. (1995). *The Cognitive Neurosciences*. Cambridge, MA: MIT Press.

Glantz, L.A., and Lewis, D.A. (2000) Decreased dendritic spine density on prefrontal cortical pyramidal neurons in schizophrenia [see comments]. *Arch. Gen. Psychiatry* 57(1):65–73.

Goldman-Rakic, P.S. (1987) Circuitry of primate prefrontal cortex and regulation of behavior by representational memory. In: Plum, F., ed. *Handbook of Physiology: The Nervous System*. Bethesda, MD: American Physiological Society, pp. 373–417.

Goldman-Rakic, P.S. (1991) Prefrontal cortical dysfunction in schizophrenia: the relevance of working memory. In: Carroll, B.J., and Barrett, J.E., eds. and trans. *Psychopathology and the Brain*. New York: Raven Press, pp. 1–23.

Gur, R.C., and Gur, R.E. (1995) Hypofrontality in schizophrenia: RIP. *Lancet* 345:1383–1384.

Hoffman, R.E. (1987) Computer simulations of neural information processing and the schizophrenia-mania dichotomy. *Arch. Gen. Psychiatry* 44:178–188.

Ingvar, D.H., and Franzen, G. (1974) Abnormalities of cerebral blood flow distribution in patients with chronic schizophrenia. *Acta Psychiatr. Scand.* 50:425–462.

Jones, E.G. (1997) Cortical development and thalamic pathology in schizophrenia. *Schizophr. Bull.* 23(3):483–501.

Kandel, E., and Squire, L. (2000) Neuroscience: breaking down scientific barriers to the study of brain and mind. *Science* 290:1113–1120.

Kerns, J.G. (2007) Experimental manipulation of cognitive control processes causes an increase in communication disturbances in healthy volunteers. *Psychol. Med.* 37:995–1004.

Kerns, J.G., and Berenbaum, H. (2003) The relationship between formal thought disorder and executive functioning component processes. *J. Abnorm. Psychol.* 112:339–352.

Knight, R.A., and Silverstein, S.M. (2001) A process-oriented approach for averting confounds resulting from general performance deficiencies in schizophrenia. *J. Abnorm. Psychol.* 110:15–30.

Kwon, J.S., et al. (1999) Gamma frequency-range abnormalities to auditory stimulation in schizophrenia. *Arch. Gen. Psychiatry* 56 (11):1001–1005.

LeDoux, T.S. (2000) Emotion circuits in the brain. *Annu. Rev. Neurosci.* 23:155–184.

Lewis, D.A., Volk, D.W., and Hashimoto, T. (2004) Selective alterations in prefrontal cortical GABA neurotransmission in schizophrenia: a novel target for the treatment of working memory dysfunction. *Psychopharmacology* 174:143–150.

Logothetis, N.K., et al. (2001) Neurophysiological investigation of the basis of the fMRI signal. *Nature* 412(6843):150–157.

Luck, S.J. (1999) Direct and indirect integration of event-related potentials, functional magnetic resonance images, and single-unit recordings [review]. *Hum. Brain Mapp.* 8(2–3):115–201.

MacDonald, A., Carter, C., Kerns, J., et al. (2005) Specificity of prefrontal dysfunction and context processing deficits to schizophrenia in never-medicated patients with first-episode psychosis. *Am. J. Psychiatry* 162:475–484.

MacDonald, A., Pogue-Geile, M.F., Johnson, M., et al. (2003) A specific deficit in context processing in the unaffected siblings of patients with schizophrenia. *Arch. Gen. Psychiatry* 60:57–65.

MacDonald, A.W., and Carter, C.S. (2002) Cognitive experimental approaches to investigating impaired cognition in schizophrenia: a paradigm shift. *J. Clin. Exp. Neuropsychol.* 24:7, 873–882.

MacDonald, A.W., Cohen, J.D., Stenger, V.A., et al. (2000) Dissociating control processes of dorsolateral prefrontal cortex and anterior cingulate cortex with fMRI and the stroop task. *Science* 288:1835–1838.

McClelland, J.L. (1993) Toward a theory of information processing in graded, random, and interactive networks. In: Meyer, D.E., and Kornblum, S., eds. *Attention and Performance XIV: Synergies in Experimental Psychology, Artificial Intelligence, and Cognitive Neuroscience.* Cambridge, MA: MIT Press, pp. 655–688.

Niessing, J., et al. (2005) Hemodynamic signals correlate tightly with synchronized gamma oscillations. *Science* 309(5736):948–951.

Newell, A., and Simon, H. (1972) *Human Problem Solving.* Englewood Cliffs, NJ: Prentice Hall.

Ochsner, K., and Lieberman, M. (2001) The emergence of social cognitive neuroscience. *Am. Psychol.* 56:717–734.

Oltmanns, T.F., and Neale, J.M. (1975) Schizophrenic performance when distractors are present: attentional deficit or differential task difficulty? *J. Abnorm. Psychol.* 84:205–209.

Perlstein, W.M., Carter, C.S., Noll, D.C., et al. (2001) fMRI evidence of prefrontal cortex dysfunction in schizophrenia during parametric manipulation of working memory load. *Am. J. Psychiatry* 158(7):1105–1113.

Posner, M.I., and Abdullaev, Y.G. (1996) What to image? Anatomy, circuitry and plasticity of human brain function. In: Toga, A.W., and Mazziota, J.C., eds. *Brain Mapping: The Methods.* New York: Academic Press, pp. 408–419.

Rosen, B.R., Buckner, R.L., and Dale, A.M. (1998) Event-related functional MRI: past, present, and future. *Proc. Natl. Acad. Sci. USA* 95:773–780.

Rumelhart, D.E., and McClelland, J.L. (1986) *Parallel Distributed Processing: Explorations in the Microstructure of Cognition, Vol. I and II.* Cambridge, MA: MIT Press.

Servan-Schreiber, D., Carter, C., Bruno, R., et al. (1998) Dopamine and the mechanisms of cognition. Part II: D-amphetamine effects in human subjects performing a selective attention task. *Biol. Psychiatry* 43:723–729.

Servan-Schreiber, D., Cohen, J., and Steingard, S. (1996) Schizophrenic deficits in the processing of context: a test of a theoretical model. *Arch. Gen. Psychiatry* 53:1105–1112.

Sher, K., and Trull, T. (1996) Methodological issues in psychopathology research. *Annu. Rev. Psychol.* 47:371–400.

Stuss, D.T., and Benson, D. (1986) *The Frontal Lobes.* New York: Raven Press.

Taylor, S., Kornblum, S., and Tandon, R. (1996) Facilitation and interference of selective attention in schizophrenia. *J. Psychiatr. Res.* 30:251–259.

Tranel, D., Anderson, S., and Benton, A. (1994) Development of the concept of "executive functions" and its relationship to the frontal lobes. In: Boller, F., and Spinnler, H., eds. and trans. *Handbook of Neuropsychology: Vol. 9, Sec. 12: The Frontal Lobes.* New York: Academic Press, pp. 123–149.

13 Neuroimaging Methods using Nuclear Magnetic Resonance

HANZHANG LU AND YIHONG YANG

Neuroimaging allows the study of psychiatric disorders on a systems level and is typically conducted under in vivo conditions. This chapter focuses on methodologies using magnetic resonance (MR) spectroscopy and imaging techniques. The most important advantage of MR methods is that they are minimally invasive and do not use radioactive materials. Many magnetic resonance imaging (MRI) studies can be performed noninvasively, as the source of the signal is the nuclei of biological molecules. For many years, MRI has been a useful diagnostic tool for focal brain diseases such as tumor and stroke, but its utility for psychiatric disorders has been limited. Recently, with the advances in MR technology and quantitative measures of brain physiology, MRI is becoming a key component in psychiatric studies, in particular for human studies. Six topics assessing different aspects of the brain are described in this chapter.

MEASUREMENT OF CEREBRAL PERFUSION USING MRI

Estimation of cerebral perfusion parameters provides a useful means to evaluate tissue integrity and viability (Harris et al., 1996; de Crespigny et al., 1998; Loeber et al., 1999; Alsop et al., 2000). Various MRI techniques can be used to quantitatively study perfusion parameters, including cerebral blood flow (CBF), cerebral blood volume (CBV), and mean transit time (MTT).

Dynamic susceptibility contrast (DSC) MRI uses a Food and Drug Administration (FDA)-approved MR contrast reagent (namely, the *gadolinium complex of diethylenetriamine pentaacetic acid, Gd-DTPA*) administered intravenously and employs rapid image acquisitions (for example, 1 image/second) to monitor the first passage of the reagent in the brain (Rosen et al., 1990; Ostergaard, Weisskoff, et al., 1996). Unlike perfusion tracers used in positron emission tomography (PET), the Gd-DTPA reagent is a nondiffusable tracer and does not penetrate the blood-brain-barrier (BBB). However, using a model that accounts for the input–output functions of the vasculature, it is still possible to estimate the perfusion parameters, including CBV, CBF, and MTT (Ostergaard, Sorensen, et al., 1996; Ostergaard, Weisskoff, et al., 1996). One important requirement to accurately determine perfusion using DSC MRI is the estimation of arterial input function (AIF), which describes the time course of the reagent concentration in the incoming arterial blood (Rausch et al., 2000; van Osch et al., 2003; Calamante et al., 2004). This is typically done by selecting pixels containing large arteries and using the averaged time course as the AIF (Law et al., 2004; Cha et al., 2005). If absolute quantification is not necessary, one can calculate the relative perfusion parameters by normalizing the values against the value in a region-of-interest (ROI), often the white matter.

A steady-state (SS) contrast MRI approach can also be used to evaluate cerebral perfusion, in this case only the CBV. This method acquires two MRI images before and after the contrast reagent injection and utilizes the fact that Gd-DTPA is an intravascular reagent and only occupies the vascular space (Moseley et al., 1992; Schwarzbauer et al., 1993; Kuppusamy et al., 1996; Lu et al., 2005). As a result, the difference signal is proportional to the CBV. Several variants of the technique are available, and their main differences reside in the use of different methods to normalize the signal, thereby converting the dimensionless MRI signal to physiologic values. Figure 13.1 shows a CBV map using the vascular-space-occupancy (VASO) approach, in which the normalization factor was obtained from a cerebrospinal fluid (CSF) region (Lu et al., 2005). In comparison with DSC MRI, the SS contrast MRI has the advantages that the model is relatively simple and does not require the knowledge of the AIF. In addition, the SS approach does not require rapid acquisitions; therefore higher spatial resolution can be achieved, and the image distortion is minimal. A pitfall is that this technique only estimates CBV (Lu et al., 2005) but not other parameters such as CBF, which is believed to be more useful in predicting tissue viability.

Cerebral blood flow can also be evaluated noninvasively using a technique called *arterial spin labeling*

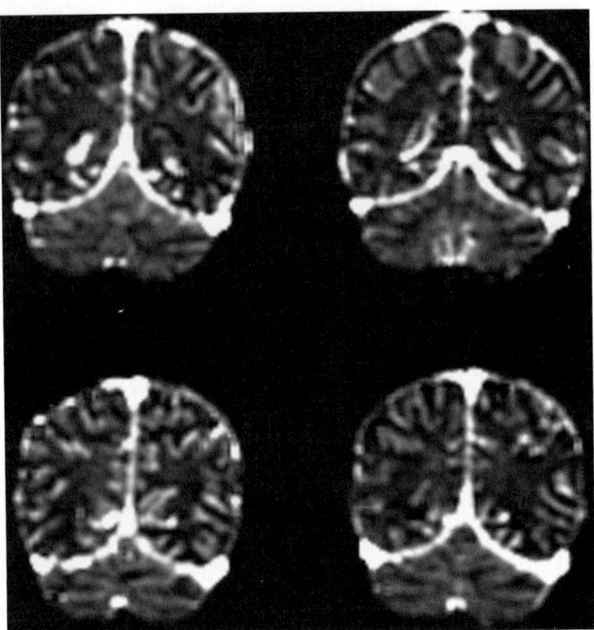

FIGURE 13.1 Absolute cerebral blood volume maps using vascular-space-occupancy (VASO) magnetic resonance imaging (MRI). Imaging parameters: coronal slices, resolution 1.5 × 1.5 mm², acquisition time 5 minutes.

(ASL) MRI (Detre et al., 1992; S.G. Kim, 1995; Kwong et al., 1995; Golay et al., 1999). The ASL pulse sequence starts with a radiofrequency (RF) pulse to magnetically label the incoming blood in the arterial vessels. Then, after a certain waiting period (1–2 seconds) to allow the blood to flow into the perfused tissue, an image is taken that contains signal from labeled blood and static tissue. In a second scan, the blood is not labeled, and similar waiting and acquisition schemes are undertaken. By subtracting one image from the other, the static tissue signal is canceled out, and the remaining difference image reflects the amount of labeled blood water that has flowed into the tissue, which can be used to calculate CBF. The main advantage of the ASL technique is that the experimental procedure is noninvasive and straightforward. A pitfall is that the quantification is not trivial, and it involves several confounding factors, including arterial transit time and vessel signal contributions (Calamante et al., 1996; Buxton, Frank, et al., 1998; Yang et al., 2000; Hendrikse et al., 2003).

ASSESSING BRAIN FUNCTIONS USING MRI

Neuronal activity in the brain is accompanied by an increased consumption of glucose and oxygen. In addition, there are pronounced changes in blood supply to the activated regions, characterized by increased CBF and CBV (Roy and Sherrington, 1890). The precise mechanism of this neurovascular coupling is not clear. But it is thought to be mediated by one or more factors related to metabolism and/or neurotransmitters (Iadecola, 2004). Regardless of the mechanism, it is important to note that the increase in blood supply overcompensates for the increase in oxygen metabolism. As a result, the blood oxygenation in the draining veins and the capillaries is actually more oxygenated during the stimulation period compared to the resting state. This forms the basis of blood oxygenation level dependent (BOLD) functional magnetic resonance imaging (fMRI) signal (Kwong et al., 1992; Ogawa et al., 1992). The hemoglobin in erythrocytes has different MR properties during the oxygenated and deoxygenated states. Deoxygenated blood is paramagnetic, which reduces the transverse relaxation times (T2 and T2*) of the water signal (inside the blood compartment and outside the blood compartment), whereas oxygenated blood is not paramagnetic. As a result, the MR signal is directly correlated with the amount of deoxyhemoglobin in the voxel (Ogawa et al., 1993). The BOLD effect on T2* is more pronounced than that on T2. As a result, the T2* weighted gradient-echo echo-planar-imaging (EPI) sequence is the most widely used pulse sequence.

It is important to note that the BOLD signal is an indirect assessment of underlying neuronal activity, and its spatial and temporal characteristics will not completely match those of the neuronal activity (Logothetis et al., 2001; Logothetis, 2002). To gain further understanding of the mechanism of the BOLD fMRI signal, it is helpful to discuss the different stages of the signal time-course. Figure 13.2 illustrates a typical BOLD response to a 10-second stimulus (Boynton et al., 1996; X. Hu et al., 1997; Yacoub and Hu, 1999; Janz et al., 2000; Lu et al., 2006).

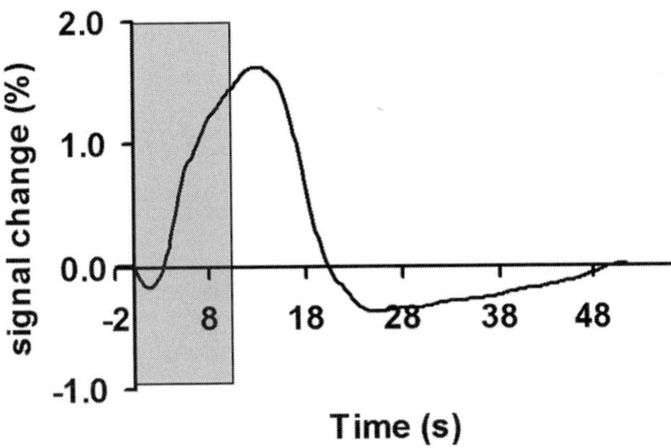

FIGURE 13.2 Illustration of a blood oxygenation level dependent (BOLD) functional magnetic resonance imaging (fMRI) response to a 10-second visual stimulation. The percentage signal change is plotted as a function of time. The stimulation period is shown by the shadowed rectangle. Phase 1 corresponds to 0–3 seconds. Phase 2 corresponds to 3–20 seconds. Phase 3 corresponds to 20–50 seconds.

Phase 1: Initial Dip

Within the first 3 seconds of stimulation, the BOLD signal does not show any increase. Instead, several groups have reported a signal decrease, often termed *initial dip* (Ernst and Hennig, 1994; Menon et al., 1995; X. Hu et al., 1997; Yacoub and Hu, 1999). This early response is thought to be caused by rapid rise in oxygen consumption before the CBF starts to increase. Because the oxygen consumption change should be localized to the activated tissue, the initial dip is believed to have better spatial specificity and has been used to study fine cortical organizations (Duong et al., 2000; D.S. Kim et al., 2000). However, such a signal reduction is only observed in a limited number of studies and, therefore, has caused some controversies (Buxton, 2001; Ances, 2004). Recently, several studies have measured changes of different physiological parameters during this initial period, and the majority of the results suggest that there indeed exists such a period in which the hemodynamic response undercompensates the oxygen metabolism. Thompson et al. (2003) performed simultaneous recording of neuronal activity and tissue oxygen pressure in cat visual cortex; they found that the tissue oxygen pressure clearly showed a initial drop, which is only localized in the stimulated orientation column. Similar findings were noted by Ances et al. (2001) who showed a mismatch between CBF and oxygen pressure in rats using forepaw stimulation. Using optical intrinsic signals, several groups have shown a transient decrease in blood oxygenation in microvasculatures (Malonek and Grinvald, 1996; Vanzetta and Grinvald, 1999; Devor et al., 2003; Sheth et al., 2004). In addition, using multimodality fMRI, Lu et al. (2004) showed that the cerebral metabolic rate of oxygen ($CMRO_2$) increases more rapidly than CBF or CBV during the initial period, again supporting the hypothesis that increased oxygen consumption preceding the vascular response may be responsible for the BOLD initial dip. Therefore, current evidence supports the existence of the initial dip during functional activation. However, whether such a small and transient signal can be routinely detected in fMRI experiments is still questionable. Most studies that report the detection of the initial dip were carried out at high field (4 Tesla [T] and up) (Menon et al., 1995; X. Hu et al., 1997; Duong et al., 2000; D.S. Kim et al., 2000; Yacoub et al., 2001). In the majority of fMRI experiments performed at low or intermediate field strength (1.5T–3.0T), the initial dip is often not observed.

Phase 2: Positive BOLD Response

The signal increase following the initial dip is the most robust part of the BOLD time course and is the basic signal for the vast majority of the fMRI studies. It is caused by a mismatch between a mildly elevated oxygen metabolism and an overcompensating CBF (P.T. Fox and Raichle, 1986; P.T. Fox et al., 1988). As shown in Figure 13.2, the positive BOLD signal lasts many seconds after the stimulation was stopped, suggesting a temporal smoothing effect of the brain vasculature. Interestingly, the time between the end of stimulus and the end of positive BOLD signal appears to be relatively independent of the stimulus duration. For a stimulus duration of 2 to 30 seconds, the BOLD signal always continues for 8–10 seconds after the cessation of the stimulation (Boynton et al., 1996; Janz et al., 2000; Lu et al., 2002; Lu et al., 2004; Lu et al., 2006). This probably reflects the time constant for the vessels to recover.

Phase 3: Poststimulus Undershoot

The positive BOLD response is often followed by an undershoot, which is larger in amplitude and longer in duration than the initial dip. Because the BOLD signal is determined by the amount of deoxyhemoglobin in the voxel, which is the product of the deoxyhemoglobin concentration in the blood and the venous blood volume, different hypotheses have proposed explanations for the poststimulus undershoot. One hypothesis is that a delayed return of venous blood volume (Buxton, Wong, and Frank, 1998; Mandeville et al., 1999) may be the reason for the BOLD poststimulus undershoot, often known as the *balloon model*. The balloon model hypothesizes that, after the stimulation is stopped, the oxygen consumption and blood supply return and stay at baseline. On the other hand, venous blood vessels are compliant, and it would take longer for these balloon-like vessels to "deflate" back to the resting level. As a result, there is a period during poststimulation that the blood oxygenation is at baseline but the venous blood volume is elevated, thereby causing the BOLD signal to appear as an undershoot. Another hypothesis is that the poststimulus undershoot is caused by a transient decrease in venous oxygenation (Frahm et al., 1996; Janz et al., 2001; Lu et al., 2004). In this model, it is hypothesized that, after the stimulation is stopped, the blood flow and volume return to baseline level while the oxygen consumption is still elevated to restore the ion gradients that are dissipated during the neural activation. Because the blood oxygenation is determined by the balance between blood flow and oxygen consumption, such a condition will cause the venous oxygenation to decrease below baseline, similar to the mechanism of the initial dip. Both hypotheses are supported by respective data in literature, and there is also the suggestion that the two mechanisms may be responsible for the observed BOLD undershoot in a spatial specific manner (Yacoub et al., 2006).

In addition to BOLD fMRI, alternative techniques are available that are sensitive to other activation-evoked changes. Examples are CBF-based fMRI (S.G. Kim, 1995),

CBV-based fMRI (Lu et al., 2003), and diffusion-based fMRI (Darquie et al., 2001). However, these techniques tend to have lower sensitivity and poorer spatial coverage, and they have only been used for special brain-mapping applications (Duong et al., 2001).

RESTING-STATE FUNCTIONAL CONNECTIVITY

Intrinsic brain activity can be investigated using spontaneous fluctuations in resting-state fMRI signal (Biswal et al., 1995). As illustrated in Figure 13.3 (see also COLOR FIGURE 13.3 in separate insert), fMRI signals from the left and right primary sensorimotor cortices show highly synchronized fluctuations at rest, and "functional connectivity" maps based on the synchrony can be obtained by cross-correlation analysis using signal from a selected brain area as a "seed point" or reference. Brain connectivity maps in the absence of task performance have been reported to follow specific brain circuits, including sensorimotor, visual, auditory, and language processing networks (Biswal et al., 1995; Lowe et al., 1998; Xiong et al., 1999; Cordes et al., 2000; Greicius et al., 2003; Beckmann et al., 2005; M.D. Fox et al., 2005). Among these observations, the existence of a brain network including posterior cingulate cortex (PCC) and medial prefrontal cortex (MPF) has been reported (Greicius et al., 2003; M.D. Fox et al., 2005). This finding supports previous suggestions that there is a functionally significant "default brain mode" in the awake resting state (Gusnard et al., 2001; Raichle et al., 2001). Because the brain expends a considerable amount of energy for neuronal-signaling processes in the absence of a particular task (Sibson et al., 1998; Shulman et al., 2004),

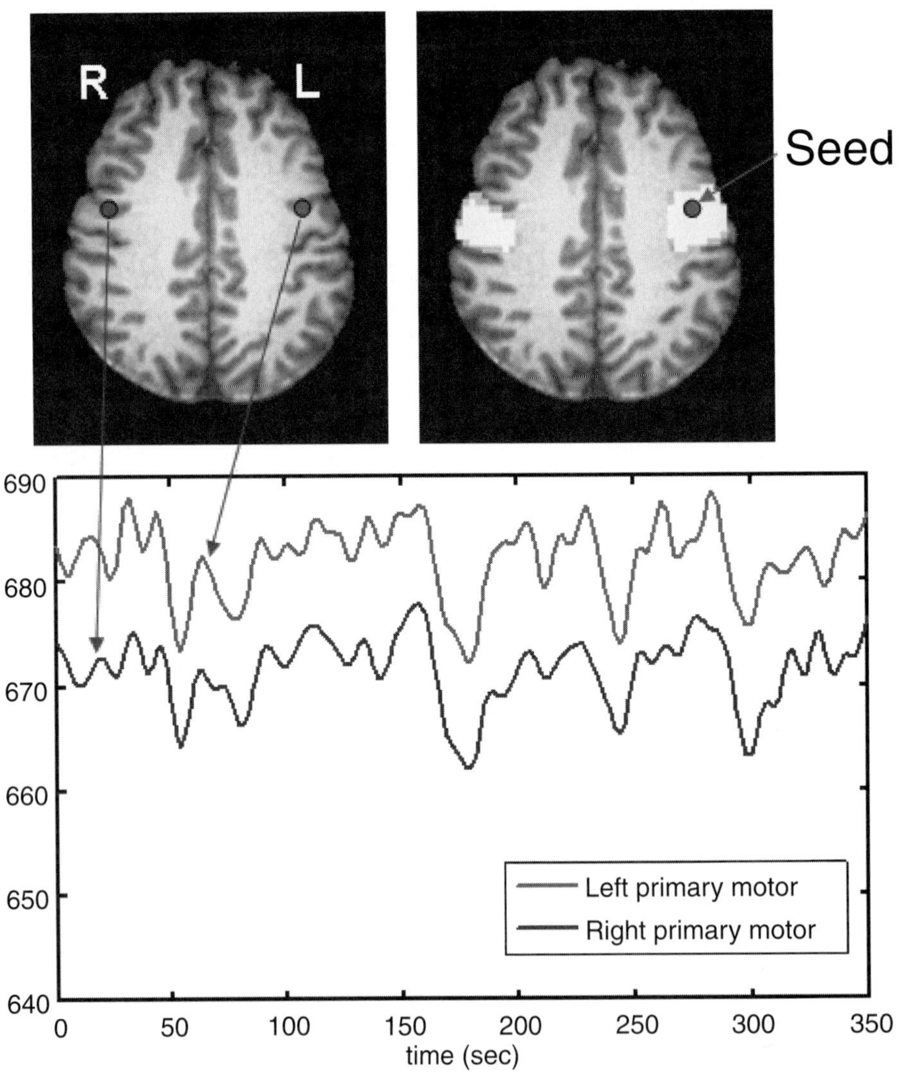

FIGURE 13.3 Functional magnetic resonance imaging (fMRI) signals at rest (bottom) from the left and right primary sensorimotor cortices (upper left), and functional connectivity map (upper right) obtained from cross-correlation analysis using the left sensorimotor cortex as a reference.

it is further argued that, in pursuit of better understanding of brain functions, observation of intrinsic brain activity may be at least as important as that of evoked activity (Gusnard et al., 2001; Raichle et al., 2001).

Recently, various applications of resting-state fMRI to brain diseases have been demonstrated, including studies of Alzheimer's disease (Li et al., 2002; Greicius et al., 2003), schizophrenia (Liang et al., 2006), epilepsy (Waites et al., 2006), cocaine dependence (Li et al., 2000), and antidepressant effects (Anand et al., 2005). Using a cross-correlation–based analysis method, Li et al. (2002) quantified functional synchrony in the hippocampus of patients with Alzheimer's disease and demonstrated lower correlation of signals in patients with Alzheimer's disease compared to age-matched mild cognitive impairment (MCI) participants and healthy controls. Their study suggested that resting-state synchrony may be used as a quantitative marker for diagnosis and stage of Alzheimer's disease. Greicius et al. (2003) investigated the default brain mode activity in patients with Alzheimer's disease using independent component analysis (ICA). They found that patients with Alzheimer's disease showed decreased resting-state activity in the posterior cingulate and hippocampus, suggesting disrupted connectivity between these two brain regions, consistent with the posterior cingulated hypometabolism commonly found in previous PET studies of early Alzheimer's disease. These studies demonstrated the utility of resting-state functional connectivity in the study of neurological and neuropsychiatric disorders.

DIFFUSION-BASED MRI TECHNIQUES

Diffusion occurs as a result of random thermal motion of small particles such as water molecules in a given medium. The effects of molecular diffusion on MR signals have been studied since the 1950s (Hahn, 1950; Carr and Purcell, 1954). A significant improvement of diffusion measurement using MR techniques was made in the 1960s (Stejskal and Tanner, 1965) by utilizing magnetic gradient pulses to encode the phase dispersion caused by diffusion. Diffusion-weighted imaging (DWI) was developed in the 1980s (Le Bihan et al., 1986) as an integration of MRI and diffusion-sensitive magnetic gradients. In ideal free diffusion, the diffusivity is uniform along all directions or *isotropic*. However, a diffusion process in biological tissue, such as brain white matter, could be *anisotropic* because the diffusive molecules may experience direction-dependent restrictions due to specific arrangements of tissue structures. Diffusion tensor imaging (DTI) was developed in the 1990s (Basser et al., 1994) as a tool to quantify the anisotropy of diffusion in biological tissue. An important advantage of DTI is that it provides rotation-invariant measurements, which means that the measurements are independent from participant positions, thus making longitudinal and group comparisons possible (Basser and Pierpaoli, 1996). In recent years, "beyond tensor" imaging techniques (Tuch et al., 2003) have been proposed to overcome challenges encompassed in DTI, such as the handling of complex white matter structures. Tractography, a promising technique to delineate neuronal pathways based on DTI or beyond tensor techniques, has also been developed (Xue et al., 1999).

Principles of Diffusion MRI

For unrestricted diffusion in a three-dimensional space, the displacements of an ensemble of molecules can be described by the Einstein equation (Einstein, 1926),

$$\langle r^2 \rangle = 6D\tau_D$$

where $<r^2>$ is the mean-squared displacement, τ_D is the diffusion time, and D is the diffusion coefficient. Fundamental principles of diffusion MRI can be illustrated by the traditional pulsed gradient experiment (Stejskal and Tanner, 1965) designed to measure the spin-echo signal attenuation caused by phase dispersion of diffusive nuclear spins in the presence of diffusion-sensitive gradients. As illustrated in Figure 13.4, in a spin-echo pulse sequence, a pair of identical gradients is placed on both sides of the 180-degree refocus RF pulse. For a static spin, the two gradients would result in phase shifts with the same magnitude but opposite signs, respectively, leading to cancellation of the phase change at the echo time. However, for a diffusive spin, the gradients would produce a net phase shift, and phase dispersion in an ensemble of spins would cause signal attenuation at the echo time. The spin-echo signal in the presence of diffusion gradients, $S(b)$, with respect to that in the absence of the gradients, $S(0)$, can be expressed as

$$S(b) = S(0)\exp(-bD)$$

where b is called "b factor," a measure of the strength of the diffusion-weighting gradients, and is determined by the duration of the gradients δ, separation of the gradients Δ, and the amplitude of the gradient G. For the setting in Figure 13.4, $b = \gamma^2G^2\Delta^2(\Delta - \delta/3)$, where γ is the gyromagnetic ratio. Diffusion MRI can be implemented by a combination of an imaging sequence with the diffusion-sensitive gradients to map diffusion coefficient in an object. Diffusion coefficient measured in biological tissue is often influenced by restricted diffusion due to complex microscopic structures as well as macroscopic motion such as blood perfusion, and therefore diffusion strength measured in biological systems

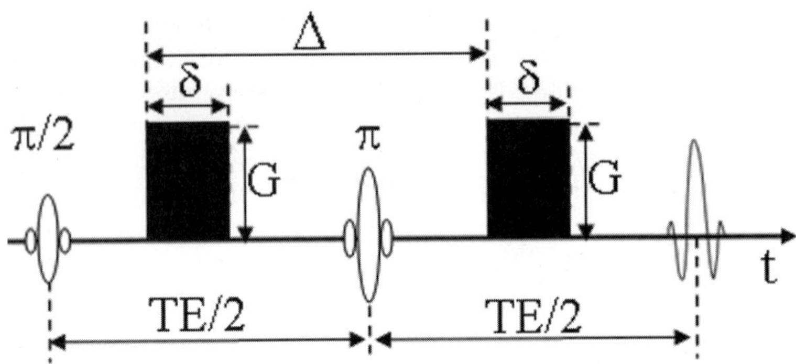

FIGURE 13.4 Schematic diagram of the Stejskal–Tanner pulsed gradient diffusion experiment.

is generally termed "*apparent diffusion coefficient*" or ADC.

Diffusion Tensor Imaging

Diffusion tensor imaging (DTI) is a diffusion-imaging technique to characterize diffusion anisotropy (Basser et al., 1994). Molecular diffusion in biological tissue is often anisotropic due to varied restriction along different directions. For instance, water molecules in a white matter fiber fascicle typically diffuse faster along the fibers compared to that cross the fibers. Diffusion in such an anisotropic medium needs to be described by multiple diffusion coefficients accounting for the direction dependence. In the formulation of DTI (Basser et al., 1994), the diffusion coefficient is no longer characterized by a scalar parameter D, but rather by a 3 × 3 tensor D:

$$D = \begin{pmatrix} D_{xx} & D_{xy} & D_{xz} \\ D_{yx} & D_{yy} & D_{yz} \\ D_{zx} & D_{zy} & D_{zz} \end{pmatrix}$$

where D_{ij} $(i,j = x,y,z)$ denotes the cross-correlation of the diffusion coefficient between the i and j axis, and thus D is always symmetric, that is, $D_{ij} = D_{ji}$. Similarly, a 3 × 3 matrix b is employed in DTI with elements b_{ij} representing the b-factor corresponding to the element D_{ij} in D. Thus, the diffusion-weighted signal attenuation can be expressed in the DTI formulation

$$S(b) = S(0)\exp\left(-\sum_{i=x,y,z}\sum_{j=x,y,z} b_{ij}D_{ij}\right)$$

To determine the six independent elements in D, one needs to perform at least six diffusion-weighted measurements with the b matrices independent from each other. An additional experiment is also needed to provide a nondiffusion-weighted reference image. Therefore, a minimum of seven measurements are required to determine the diffusion tensor D. Recent studies have indicated that using more directions for diffusion encoding generally helps to improve the accuracy and/or the efficiency of the DTI technique, if these directions are appropriately optimized (Le Bihan et al., 2001).

Diffusion tensor can be analyzed based on the eigenanalysis theorem (Golub and Van Loan, 1996). Several rotation-invariant indices have been widely used to visualize and quantify diffusion tensor maps in biological applications. These include (Basser et al., 1994) the mean diffusivity (MD), the average diffusion strength in all directions,

$$MD = \langle D \rangle = \frac{\lambda_1 + \lambda_2 + \lambda_3}{3}$$

and the fractional anisotropy (FA), a *normalized* ($0 \le FA < 1$) degree of the diffusion anisotropy:

$$FA = \sqrt{\frac{3\left((\lambda_1 - \langle D \rangle)^2 + (\lambda_2 - \langle D \rangle)^2 + (\lambda_3 - \langle D \rangle)^2\right)}{2\left(\lambda_1^2 + \lambda_2^2 + \lambda_3^2\right)}}$$

where λ_1, λ_2, and λ_3 are eigenvalues of the diffusion tensor. Figure 13.5 illustrates maps of MD and FA calculated from the diffusion tensor map acquired from a human brain. In general, the MD map shows high intensities in ventricles and gray matter, where the diffusion is relatively isotropic with higher strength. The FA map highlights the white matter tracts in the brain, where the diffusion is highly anisotropic. The primary eigenvector of the diffusion tensor is useful to indicate the orientation of the well-organized tissue, such as fiber boundless in white matter, and can be used to track neural pathways.

"Beyond-Tensor" Diffusion Techniques

Despite the success of DTI in a variety of applications, challenges exist in handling complex brain structures, in which diffusion patterns are far more complicated than a tensor model can deal with. For instance, DTI often fails to correctly describe diffusion patterns in brain areas with fiber crossings. In the case of multiple

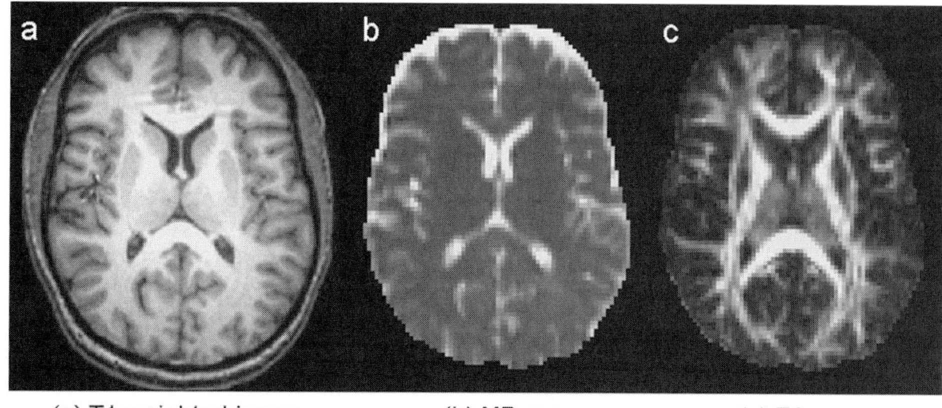

FIGURE 13.5 T1-weighted image (*A*) and corresponding mean diffusivity (*B*) and fractional anisotropic (*C*) images of a brain section.

fiber components sharing a single voxel, the major eigenvector of the diffusion tensor could be substantially biased from the actual fiber orientation, resulting in misleading fiber tracing. This is fundamentally limited by the tensor model because the diffusion tensor is only a second-order approximation (in terms of mean square fitting) to the real three-dimensional diffusion process (Basser et al., 2000). "Beyond tensor" diffusion techniques based on higher-order mathematical models, such as high angular resolution diffusion (HARD) and q-space imaging (QSI), have been proposed recently to overcome these difficulties (Frank, 2001; Tuch et al., 2003; Zhan et al., 2004; Jensen et al., 2005).

MAGNETIC RESONANCE SPECTROSCOPY

Magnetic resonance spectroscopy (MRS) is a noninvasive technique that can be used to investigate biochemistry of living systems. The first in vivo ^{31}P MRS experiment was conducted on a mouse head using a conventional spectrometer with a RF coil surrounding the entire head (Chance et al., 1978). Spectra of brain without contamination from other tissues were first obtained using a localization technique with a surface coil (Ackerman et al., 1980). In the past decades, MRS has evolved into a powerful tool for biological research and clinical diagnosis. Unlike MRI that measures the signal from protons in water molecules, MRS usually detects the signal from compounds in much lower concentrations. Besides the most sensitive nuclear ^{1}H, MRS can also detect a range of nuclei including ^{31}P, ^{13}C, ^{19}F, ^{15}N, ^{23}Na, and ^{7}Li.

Spatial Localization

The simplest way to obtain a localized spectrum is to use a surface coil, which produces a limited excitation volume close to the coil (Ackerman et al., 1980). The sensitivity distribution of the volume depends on the shape and orientation of the coil. For a single-loop coil, the selective volume is roughly a cylindrical region with a radius and length about the same as the coil radius. A disadvantage of using surface coils for localization is that the sensitivity is extremely inhomogeneous in the volume, which makes quantification of spectroscopic data difficult.

Single-volume spectroscopy techniques use shaped RF pulses along with field gradients to selectively excite the spins in a defined volume. The most commonly used approaches in this category are point resolved spectroscopy (PRESS) (Bottomley, 1987), and stimulated echo acquisition mode (STEAM) (Frahm et al., 1987). Similar to slice selection in imaging, these techniques select a volume using three slab-selective RF pulses in the presence of field gradients in three orthogonal directions. A spin echo or stimulated echo is formed by the signal from the intersection of the three selected slabs.

Spectroscopic imaging (SI) or chemical shift imaging (CSI) uses phase encoding and/or frequency encoding to obtain spatial and spectroscopic information (Lauterbur et al., 1975; Brown et al., 1982). Like imaging, this technique acquires spectroscopic data in a matrix of spatially resolved voxels, allowing for observation of spectra in multiple regions simultaneously.

^{1}H MRS

Proton MRS can reliably detect *N*-acetylaspartate (NAA), creatine (Cr)/phosphocreatine (PCr), choline (Cho)-containing compounds including phosphocholine (PC) and glycerophosphocholine (GPC), and *myo*-inositol (Ins) in the brain. At high field strengths (> 7 T), glutamate (Glu), glutamine (Gln), and other metabolites can be resolved. A spectrum acquired from the cingulate of a rat brain at 9.4 T is illustrated in Figure 13.6.

Brain metabolites measured by ^{1}H MRS are involved in cellular metabolism, neurotransmission, cell membrane synthesis, or serve as a marker specific to neurons or glia (de Graaf, 1998; Govindaraju et al., 2000). NAA is commonly believed to be a marker of mature neurons, and a reduction of NAA level in the brain is indicative

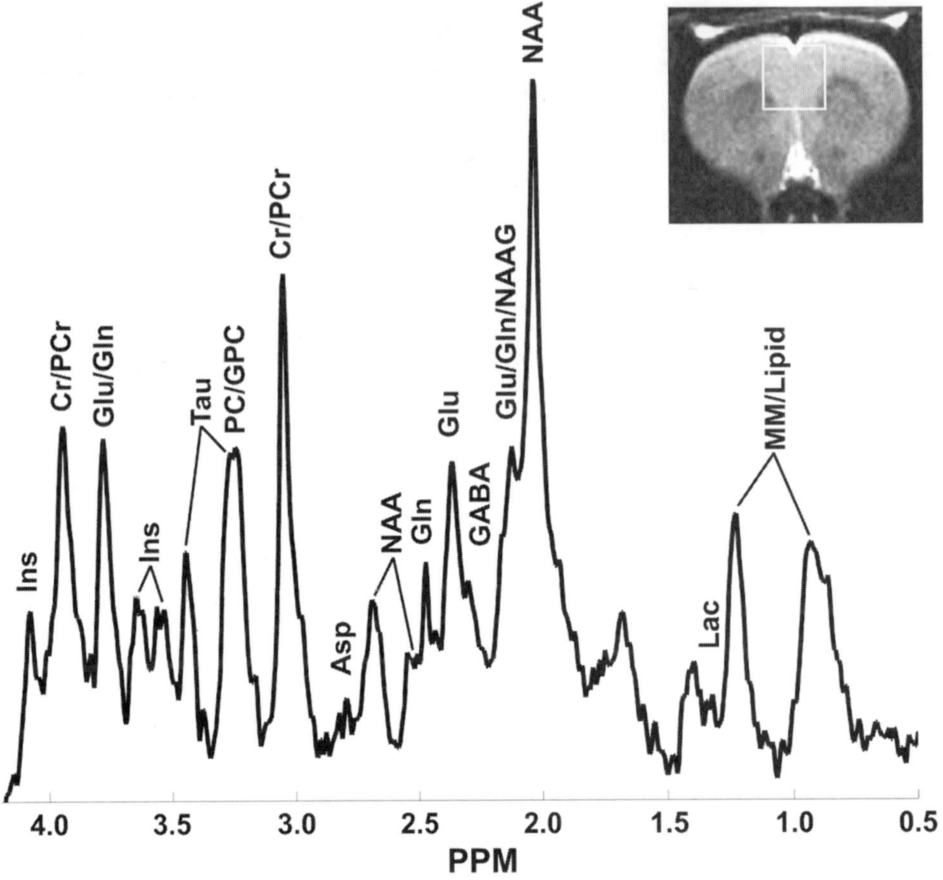

FIGURE 13.6 A stimulated echo acquisition mode (STEAM) spectrum from the rat cingulate, volume size = 3 × 3 × 3 mm^3, repetition time/echo time/mixing time (TR/TE/TM) = 3000/9.1/10 ms, number of average = 300. Asp = aspartate, Cr = creatine, GABA = γ-aminobutyric acid, Gln = glutamine, GPC = glycerophosphocholine, Glu = glutamate, Gln = glutamine, Lac = lactate, Ins = *myo*-inositol, NAA = *N*-acetylaspartate, NAAG = *N*-acetylaspartyglutamate, PC = phosphocholine, PCr = phosphocreatine, Tau = taurine, MM = macromolecules.

of neuronal loss and/or dysfunction. The protons of an *N*-acetyl CH_3 group provide the most prominent singlet resonance at 2.02 ppm, which can be measured robustly. Cr and PCr are observed as a strong singlet resonance at 3.03 pm. The Cr/PCr level is relatively stable across the brain and is therefore often used as an internal concentration reference. This measure should be used with caution because reduced levels of Cr are observed in some pathological conditions, such as tumors and stroke. Cho is an important precursor of cell membrane synthesis, and increases of Cho indicate membrane damage to myelin or neuron. Cho, PC, and GPC give rise to a prominent singlet resonance at 3.20 ppm. Ins is believed to be a glial marker, and an increase of Ins reflects gliosis. This compound has a prominent doublet-of-doublet centered at 3.52 ppm and a triplet at 3.61 ppm.

Glu is the major excitatory neurotransmitter in the central nervous system (CNS). Closely coupled to Glu, Gln is mostly located in glial cells as the end product of Glu catabolism and is a reservoir for Glu production in the neuron. γ-aminobutyric acid (GABA) is the major inhibitory neurotransmitter in CNS. These neurotransmitters play important roles in many neurological and psychiatric disorders, such as epilepsy, depression, and drug addiction. However, reliable detection and accurate quantification of Glu, Gln, or GABA in vivo remains challenging using proton ^{1}H MRS at low and middle magnetic field strengths (1.5–4.7 T), primarily due to spectral overlap of these compounds. Recently, new techniques such as echo time (TE)-averaged PRESS (Hurd et al., 2004) and STEAM with optimized timing parameters (J. Hu et al., 2007) have been developed to deal with this problem. An example of resolved Glu and Gln STEAM spectrum on the human brain with optimized TE and mixing time (TM) at 3 T is illustrated in Figure 13.7. Glu and Gln peaks at 2.35–2.45 ppm are well resolved and can be accurately quantified.

Spectral Quantification

The goal of spectral quantification is to estimate metabolite concentrations from spectroscopic data. Although the area underneath a spectrum is directly proportional to the number of nuclei within the sensitive volume of

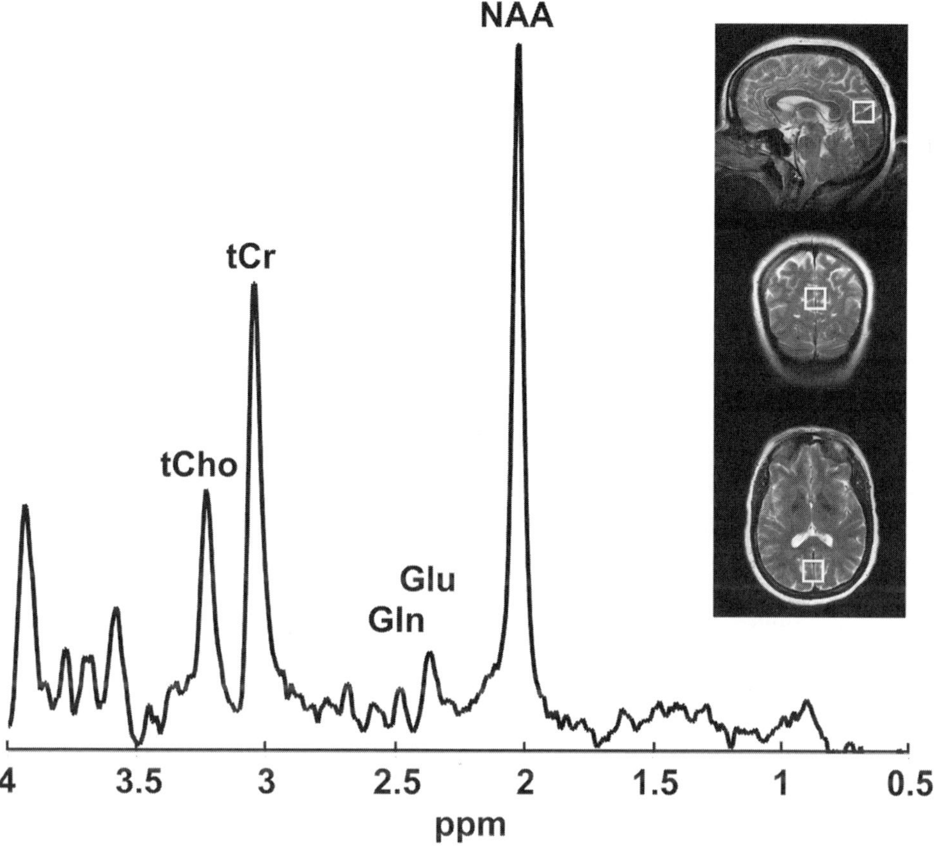

FIGURE 13.7 A stimulated echo acquisition mode (STEAM) spectrum with optimized echo time/mixing time (TE/TM) (72/6 ms) in the medial occipitoparietal junction of the human brain (voxel size = 20 × 20 × 20 mm3). Glu and Gln peaks are well resolved at 2.35–2.45 ppm. Glu = glutamate, Gln = glutamine.

the coil, it is not straightforward to achieve this goal. A number of factors have to be taken into account in quantifying spectroscopic data (Kauppinen and Williams, 1994).

Spectroscopic signal intensity is related to relaxation times and equilibrium magnetization. Magnetization recovers during a repetition time (TR) with longitudinal relaxation time (T1) and decays during a TE with transverse relaxation time (T2). Effects of T1 and T2 can be minimized using long TR and short TE. In many circumstances, however, knowledge of the relaxation times is needed to correct for these effects.

Spectral peak intensities can be affected by data acquisition and processing strategies as well as the existence of macromolecules in the sensitive volume. For instance, in chemical shift imaging using phase encoding for spatial localization (Brown et al., 1982), the early data points in the free induction decay (FID) are not collected, resulting in baseline and line-shape distortions in the spectrum. Appropriate processing techniques are needed to estimate the missing data points and thus to correct for spectral distortions. Macromolecules contribute to a broad baseline in a spectrum, which has to be removed in data acquisition or processing. Techniques to extract signal intensities, such as LCModel (Provencher, 1993) and jMRUI (Naressi et al., 2001), have been developed and widely used for spectral quantification.

Metabolite concentrations can be presented as ratios, for example, relative to Cr that is thought to be relatively stable in normal brains. Recent studies demonstrated that absolute quantification of metabolites has added value for unambiguous data interpretation (Jansen et al., 2006). However, extra calibration steps are required to achieve absolute quantification. Several strategies have been developed for this purpose, including internal endogenous marker, external reference, replace-and-match method, water signal reference, and principle of reciprocity (Jansen et al., 2006). Although absolute quantification requires more time and expertise, it can improve the diagnosis utility of MR spectroscopy.

STRUCTURAL IMAGING USING MRI

With recent advances in high field MR imaging technology and the development of parallel imaging acquisitions, structural MR images can be obtained with higher spatial resolutions and signal-to-noise ratio (SNR). Whole brain images with a resolution of $1 \times 1 \times 1$ mm^3 are now routinely acquired with scan durations of 4 to 8 minutes. This renders to MRI the capability of evaluating regional volumetric changes for various tissue types, such as gray matter, white matter, and CSF; this is especially useful for studies of psychiatric disorders because the involved brain regions may be relatively diffused and changes can be subtle. The typical MR pulse sequence used is called magnetization-prepared rapid acquisitions of gradient-echo (MPRAGE) (Mugler and Brookeman, 1991) and the resulting images are T1-weighted, with clear contrast between gray and white matters. This technique is increasingly used to assess brain atrophy in longitudinal and cross-sectional studies. The MRI data can be analyzed using one of three different methods.

One method is to manually draw ROI on a slice-by-slice basis and to calculate the volume for each tissue type (Convit et al., 1997). The intersubject variability in head size can be corrected by dividing the ROI volume by the total intracranial volume. The advantage of such a method is that the procedure is relatively straightforward, and the results are less sensitive to SNR and image inhomogeneity. However, this approach is very time-consuming, and the operators need to be well-trained to produce consistent results. A less labor-intensive ROI approach is to use a semi-automatic procedure, in which a large ROI is selected based on simple landmarks and an algorithm is applied to segment the ROI into gray matter, white matter, and CSF, and the normalized tissue volume is used for atrophy comparison (Rusinek et al., 2003).

A second method is voxel-based morphometry (VBM). This processing strategy first uses spatial coregistration to normalize individual brains into the coordinates of a brain template (Wright et al., 1995; Ashburner and Friston, 2000; Rombouts et al., 2000), so that equivalent structures in different brains are roughly in the same location. Image segmentation is then performed to partition the normalized brain image into gray matter, white matter, and CSF. It is important to note that, after the segmentation, the signal intensity in the original image is replaced by a value between 0 and 1, indicating the probability that the voxel belongs to gray matter, white matter, or CSF. These values are not influenced by the actual signal intensity in the raw MPRAGE image. This conversion from MRI signal to brain mask value is crucial in VBM as the scaling factor of the raw MRI signal is arbitrary and may be different for different participants. Therefore, a comparison of the signals in the MPRAGE image across participants is not meaningful. The next key step in VBM processing is the smoothing of the mask images. It is this step that creates the contrast between a normal brain and an atrophic brain, which can be used for statistical comparison. The spatial smoothing in effect allows the signal in a single voxel to reflect the concentration of the tissue in its surrounding areas. Therefore, a voxel in a thick gray matter layer will have a larger value than a voxel in a thin layer after smoothing, even though their values before smoothing were identical (for example, both 1). In addition, the smoothing also reduces the effect of regional brain-shape differences, which cannot be compensated for in the normalization step. Following smoothing, statistical comparison is performed on a voxel-by-voxel basis to detect the regions that show significant changes in tissue concentration. The advantage of the VBM method is that the processing steps are highly automated, and one can assess the atrophy for the entire brain easily. One disadvantage is that this processing requires the anatomical data to be of high quality, in terms of resolution and SNR, and data acquired using different MRI scanners or different imaging parameters may yield drastically different results.

A third method for analyzing structural images is deformation-based morphometry (Freeborough and Fox, 1998; Shen and Davatzikos, 2002). In this method, the brain image is transformed into the coordinates of a template brain or a baseline brain image. Then the information in the transformation matrix is used to determine whether the position of a particular brain structure is shifted or the shape has changed. Certain indices are often obtained from the transformation matrix (for example, the Jacobian determinant), and they can be used for statistical analysis. The advantage of the deformation-based approach is that it does not use spatial smoothing to generate the volumetric information. On the other hand, the performance of this method would require the algorithm to be able to detect deformations at a very small scale.

SUMMARY

It is clear that neuroimaging using MR methods will continue to contribute to our understanding of mental disorders and may emerge as a diagnostic tool and eventually be used for monitoring treatments. Many MRI biomarkers have already been proposed for the evaluation of diseases and to guide therapeutic procedures. MRI is a versatile technique in that it provides a variety of tools for in vivo assessment of human brain, ranging from anatomical structure, neuronal functions to cerebral perfusion. Meanwhile, it is necessary to be cautious in interpreting and understanding MR data. Although MR images are often shown in high resolution and sometimes labeled in colors, investigators should always try to gain a full understanding of the results and be informed about potential uncertainties in the measurements and confounding factors in the quantification.

REFERENCES

Ackerman, J.J., Grove, T.H., Wong, G.G., Gadian, D.G., and Radda, G.K. (1980) Mapping of metabolites in whole animals by 31P NMR using surface coils. *Nature* 283:167–170.

Alsop, D.C., Detre, J.A., and Grossman, M. (2000) Assessment of cerebral blood flow in Alzheimer's disease by spin-labeled magnetic resonance imaging. *Ann. Neurol.* 47:93–100.

Anand, A., Li, Y., Wang, Y., Wu, J., Gao, S., Bukhari, L., Mathews, V.P., Kalnin, A., and Lowe, M.J. (2005) Antidepressant effect on connectivity of the mood-regulating circuit: an fMRI study. *Neuropsychopharmacology* 30:1334–1344.

Ances, B.M. (2004) Coupling of changes in cerebral blood flow with neural activity: what must initially dip must come back up. *J. Cereb. Blood Flow Metab.* 24:1–6.

Ances, B.M., Buerk, D.G., Greenberg, J.H., and Detre, J.A. (2001) Temporal dynamics of the partial pressure of brain tissue oxygen during functional forepaw stimulation in rats. *Neurosci. Lett.* 306:106–110.

Ashburner, J., and Friston, K.J. (2000) Voxel-based morphometry—the methods. *Neuroimage* 11:805–821.

Basser, P.J., Mattiello, J., and LeBihan, D. (1994) MR diffusion tensor spectroscopy and imaging. *Biophys. J.* 66:259–267.

Basser, P.J., Pajevic, S., Pierpaoli, C., Duda, J., and Aldroubi, A. (2000) In vivo fiber tractography using DT-MRI data. *Magn. Reson. Med.* 44:625–632.

Basser, P.J., and Pierpaoli, C. (1996) Microstructural and physiological features of tissues elucidated by quantitative-diffusion-tensor MRI. *J. Magn. Reson. B* 111:209–219.

Beckmann, C.F., DeLuca, M., Devlin, J.T., and Smith, S.M. (2005) Investigations into resting-state connectivity using independent component analysis. *Philos. Trans. R. Soc. Lond. B Biol. Sci.* 360:1001–1013.

Biswal, B., Yetkin, F.Z., Haughton, V.M., and Hyde, J.S. (1995) Functional connectivity in the motor cortex of resting human brain using echo-planar MRI. *Magn. Reson. Med.* 34:537–541.

Bottomley, P.A. (1987) Spatial localization in NMR spectroscopy in vivo. *Ann. N Y Acad. Sci.* 508:333–348.

Boynton, G.M., Engel, S.A., Glover, G.H., and Heeger, D.J. (1996) Linear systems analysis of functional magnetic resonance imaging in human V1. *J. Neurosci.* 16:4207–4221.

Brown, T.R., Kincaid, B.M., and Ugurbil, K. (1982) NMR chemical shift imaging in three dimensions. *Proc. Natl. Acad. Sci. USA* 79:3523–3526.

Buxton, R.B. (2001) The elusive initial dip. *Neuroimage* 13:953– 958.

Buxton, R.B., Frank, L.R., Wong, E.C., Siewert, B., Warach, S., and Edelman, R.R. (1998) A general kinetic model for quantitative perfusion imaging with arterial spin labeling. *Magn. Reson. Med.* 40:383–396.

Buxton, R.B., Wong, E.C., and Frank, L.R. (1998) Dynamics of blood flow and oxygenation changes during brain activation: the balloon model. *Magn. Reson. Med.* 39:855–864.

Calamante, F., Morup, M., and Hansen, L.K. (2004) Defining a local arterial input function for perfusion MRI using independent component analysis. *Magn. Reson. Med.* 52:789–797.

Calamante, F., Williams, S.R., van Bruggen, N., Kwong, K.K., and Turner, R. (1996) A model for quantification of perfusion in pulsed labelling techniques. *NMR Biomed.* 9:79–83.

Carr, H.Y., and Purcell, E.M. (1954) Effects of diffusion on free precession in nuclear magnetic resonance experiments. *Physics Review* 94:630–638.

Cha, S., Tihan, T., Crawford, F., Fischbein, N.J., Chang, S., Bollen, A., Nelson, S.J., Prados, M., Berger, M.S., and Dillon, W.P. (2005) Differentiation of low-grade oligodendrogliomas from low-grade astrocytomas by using quantitative blood-volume measurements derived from dynamic susceptibility contrast-enhanced MR imaging. *AJNR Am. J. Neuroradiol.* 26:266–273.

Chance, B., Nakase, Y., Bond, M., Leigh, J.S., Jr., and McDonald, G. (1978) Detection of 31P nuclear magnetic resonance signals in brain by in vivo and freeze-trapped assays. *Proc. Natl. Acad. Sci. USA* 75:4925–4929.

Convit, A., De Leon, M.J., Tarshish, C., De Santi, S., Tsui, W., Rusinek, H., and George, A. (1997) Specific hippocampal volume reductions in individuals at risk for Alzheimer's disease. *Neurobiol. Aging* 18:131–138.

Cordes, D., Haughton, V.M., Arfanakis, K., Wendt, G.J., Turski, P.A., Moritz, C.H., Quigley, M.A., and Meyerand, M.E. (2000) Mapping functionally related regions of brain with functional connectivity MR imaging. *AJNR Am. J. Neuroradiol.* 21:1636–1644.

Darquie, A., Poline, J.B., Poupon, C., Saint-Jalmes, H., and Le Bihan, D. (2001) Transient decrease in water diffusion observed in human occipital cortex during visual stimulation. *Proc. Natl. Acad. Sci. USA* 98:9391–9395.

de Crespigny, A., Rother, J., van Bruggen, N., Beaulieu, C., and Moseley, M.E. (1998) Magnetic resonance imaging assessment of cerebral hemodynamics during spreading depression in rats. *J. Cereb. Blood Flow Metab.* 18:1008–1017.

de Graaf, R.A. (1998) *In Vivo NMR Spectroscopy*. New York: John Wiley.

Detre, J.A., Leigh, J.S., Williams, D.S., and Koretsky, A.P. (1992) Perfusion imaging. *Magn. Reson. Med.* 23:37–45.

Devor, A., Dunn, A.K., Andermann, M.L., Ulbert, I., Boas, D.A., and Dale, A.M. (2003) Coupling of total hemoglobin concentration, oxygenation, and neural activity in rat somatosensory cortex. *Neuron* 39:353–359.

Duong, T.Q., Kim, D.S., Ugurbil, K., and Kim, S.G. (2000) Spatiotemporal dynamics of the BOLD fMRI signals: toward mapping submillimeter cortical columns using the early negative response. *Magn. Reson. Med.* 44:231–242.

Duong, T.Q., Kim, D.S., Ugurbil, K., and Kim, S.G. (2001) Localized cerebral blood flow response at submillimeter columnar resolution. *Proc. Natl. Acad. Sci. USA* 98:10904–10909.

Einstein, A. (1926) *Investigations on the Theory of Brownian Motion*. New York: Dover.

Ernst, T., and Hennig, J. (1994) Observation of a fast response in functional MR. *Magn. Reson. Med.* 32:146–149.

Fox, M.D., Snyder, A.Z., Vincent, J.L., Corbetta, M., Van Essen, D. C., and Raichle, M.E. (2005) The human brain is intrinsically organized into dynamic, anticorrelated functional networks. *Proc. Natl. Acad. Sci. USA* 102:9673–9678.

Fox, P.T., and Raichle, M.E. (1986) Focal physiological uncoupling of cerebral blood flow and oxidative metabolism during somatosensory stimulation in human subjects. *Proc. Natl. Acad. Sci. USA* 83:1140–1144.

Fox, P.T., Raichle, M.E., Mintun, M.A., and Dence, C. (1988) Nonoxidative glucose consumption during focal physiologic neural activity. *Science* 241:462–464.

Frahm, J., Kruger, G., Merboldt, K.D., and Kleinschmidt, A. (1996) Dynamic uncoupling and recoupling of perfusion and oxidative metabolism during focal brain activation in man. *Magn. Reson. Med.* 35:143–148.

Frahm, J., Merboldt, K.D., and Hanicke, W. (1987) Localized proton spectroscopy using stimulated echoes. *J. Magn. Reson.* 72: 502–508.

Frank, L.R. (2001) Anisotropy in high angular resolution diffusion-weighted MRI. *Magn. Reson. Med.* 45:935–939.

Freeborough, P.A., and Fox, N.C. (1998) Modeling brain deformations in Alzheimer disease by fluid registration of serial 3D MR images. *J. Comput. Assist. Tomogr.* 22:838–843.

Golay, X., Stuber, M., Pruessmann, K.P., Meier, D., and Boesiger, P. (1999) Transfer insensitive labeling technique (TILT): application to multislice functional perfusion imaging. *J. Magn. Reson. Imaging* 9:454–461.

Golub, G.H., and Van Loan, C.F. (1996). *Matrix Computations.* Baltimore: Johns Hopkins University Press.

Govindaraju, V., Young, K., and Maudsley, A.A. (2000) Proton NMR chemical shifts and coupling constants for brain metabolites. *NMR Biomed.* 13:129–153.

Greicius, M.D., Krasnow, B., Reiss, A.L., and Menon, V. (2003) Functional connectivity in the resting brain: a network analysis of the default mode hypothesis. *Proc. Natl. Acad. Sci. USA* 100: 253–258.

Gusnard, D.A., Raichle, M.E., and Raichle, M.E. (2001) Searching for a baseline: functional imaging and the resting human brain. *Nat. Rev. Neurosci.* 2:685–694.

Hahn, E.L. (1950) Spin echo. *Physics Review* 80:580–594.

Harris, G.J., Lewis, R.F., Satlin, A., English, C.D., Scott, T.M., Yurgelun-Todd, D.A., and Renshaw, P.F. (1996) Dynamic susceptibility contrast MRI of regional cerebral blood volume in Alzheimer's disease. *Am. J. Psychiatry* 153:721–724.

Hendrikse, J., Lu, H., van der Grond, J., Van Zijl, P.C., and Golay, X. (2003) Measurements of cerebral perfusion and arterial hemodynamics during visual stimulation using TURBO-TILT. *Magn. Reson. Med.* 50:429–433.

Hu, J., Yang, S., Xuan, Y., Jiang, Q., Yang, Y., and Haacke, E.M. (2007) Simultaneous detection of resolved glutamate, glutamine, and gamma-aminobutyric acid at 4 Tesla. *J. Magn. Reson.* 185: 204–213.

Hu, X., Le, T.H., and Ugurbil, K. (1997) Evaluation of the early response in fMRI in individual subjects using short stimulus duration. *Magn. Reson. Med.* 37:877–884.

Hurd, R., Sailasuta, N., Srinivasan, R., Vigneron, D.B., Pelletier, D., and Nelson, S.J. (2004) Measurement of brain glutamate using TE-averaged PRESS at 3T. *Magn. Reson. Med.* 51:435–440.

Iadecola, C. (2004) Neurovascular regulation in the normal brain and in Alzheimer's disease. *Nat. Rev. Neurosci.* 5:347–360.

Jansen, J.F., Backes, W.H., Nicolay, K., and Kooi, M.E. (2006) 1H MR spectroscopy of the brain: absolute quantification of metabolites. *Radiology* 240:318–332.

Janz, C., Schmitt, C., Kornmayer, J., Speck, O., and Hennig, J. (2001) Decoupling of the short-term hemodynamic response and the blood oxygen concentration. *NMR Biomed.* 14:402–407.

Janz, C., Schmitt, C., Speck, O., and Hennig, J. (2000) Comparison of the hemodynamic response to different visual stimuli in single-event and block stimulation fMRI experiments. *J. Magn. Reson. Imaging* 12:708–714.

Jensen, J.H., Helpern, J.A., Ramani, A., Lu, H., and Kaczynski, K. (2005) Diffusional kurtosis imaging: the quantification of non-gaussian water diffusion by means of magnetic resonance imaging. *Magn. Reson. Med.* 53:1432–1440.

Kauppinen, R.A., and Williams, S.R. (1994) Nuclear magnetic resonance spectroscopy studies of the brain. *Prog. Neurobiol.* 44:87–118.

Kim, D.S., Duong, T.Q., and Kim, S.G. (2000) High-resolution mapping of iso-orientation columns by fMRI. *Nat. Neurosci.* 3:164–169.

Kim, S.G. (1995) Quantification of relative cerebral blood flow change by flow-sensitive alternating inversion recovery (FAIR) technique: application to functional mapping. *Magn. Reson. Med.* 34:293–301.

Kuppusamy, K., Lin, W., Cizek, G.R., and Haacke, E.M. (1996) In vivo regional cerebral blood volume: quantitative assessment with 3D T1-weighted pre- and postcontrast MR imaging. *Radiology* 201:106–112.

Kwong, K.K., Belliveau, J.W., Chesler, D.A., Goldberg, I.E., Weisskoff, R.M., Poncelet, B.P., Kennedy, D.N., Hoppel, B.E., Cohen, M.S., Turner, R., et al. (1992) Dynamic magnetic resonance imaging of human brain activity during primary sensory stimulation. *Proc. Natl. Acad. Sci. USA* 89:5675–5679.

Kwong, K.K., Chesler, D.A., Weisskoff, R.M., Donahue, K.M., Davis, T.L., Ostergaard, L., Campbell, T.A., and Rosen, B.R. (1995) MR perfusion studies with T1-weighted echo planar imaging. *Magn. Reson. Med.* 34:878–887.

Lauterbur, P.C., Kramer, C.D., House, W.V., and Chen, C.N. (1975) Zeugmatographic high-resolution nuclear magnetic resonance spectroscopy - imaging of chemical inhomogeneity within macroscopic object. *J. Am. Chem. Soc.* 97:6866–6868.

Law, M., Yang, S., Babb, J.S., Knopp, E.A., Golfinos, J.G., Zagzag, D., and Johnson, G. (2004) Comparison of cerebral blood volume and vascular permeability from dynamic susceptibility contrast-enhanced perfusion MR imaging with glioma grade. *AJNR Am. J. Neuroradiol.* 25:746–755.

Le Bihan, D., Breton, E., Lallemand, D., Grenier, P., Cabanis, E., and Laval-Jeantet, M. (1986) MR imaging of intravoxel incoherent motions: application to diffusion and perfusion in neurologic disorders. *Radiology* 161:401–407.

Le Bihan, D., Mangin, J.F., Poupon, C., Clark, C.A., Pappata, S., Molko, N., and Chabriat, H. (2001) Diffusion tensor imaging: concepts and applications. *J. Magn. Reson. Imaging* 13:534–546.

Li, S.J., Biswal, B., Li, Z., Risinger, R., Rainey, C., Cho, J.K., Salmeron, B.J., and Stein, E.A. (2000) Cocaine administration decreases functional connectivity in human primary visual and motor cortex as detected by functional MRI. *Magn. Reson. Med.* 43:45–51.

Li, S.J., Li, Z., Wu, G., Zhang, M.J., Franczak, M., and Antuono, P.G. (2002) Alzheimer disease: evaluation of a functional MR imaging index as a marker. *Radiology* 225:253–259.

Liang, M., Zhou, Y., Jiang, T., Liu, Z., Tian, L., Liu, H., Hao, Y. (2006) Widespread functional disconnectivity in schizophrenia with resting-state functional magnetic resonance imaging. *Neuroreport* 17:209–213.

Loeber, R.T., Sherwood, A.R., Renshaw, P.F., Cohen, B.M., and Yurgelun-Todd, D.A. (1999) Differences in cerebellar blood volume in schizophrenia and bipolar disorder. *Schizophr. Res.* 37: 81–89.

Logothetis, N.K. (2002) The neural basis of the blood-oxygen-level-dependent functional magnetic resonance imaging signal. *Philos. Trans. R. Soc. Lond. B Biol. Sci.* 357:1003–1037.

Logothetis, N.K., Pauls, J., Augath, M., Trinath, T., and Oeltermann, A. (2001) Neurophysiological investigation of the basis of the fMRI signal. *Nature* 412:150–157.

Lowe, M.J., Mock, B.J., and Sorenson, J.A. (1998) Functional connectivity in single and multislice echoplanar imaging using resting-state fluctuations. *Neuroimage* 7:119–132.

Lu, H., Donahue, M.J., and van Zijl, P.C. (2006) Detrimental effects of BOLD signal in arterial spin labeling fMRI at high field strength. *Magn. Reson. Med.* 56:546–552.

Lu, H., Golay, X., Pekar, J.J., and van Zijl, P.C.M. (2003) Functional magnetic resonance imaging based on changes in vascular space occupancy. *Magn. Reson. Med.* 50:263–274.

Lu, H., Golay, X., Pekar, J.J., and van Zijl, P.C. (2004) Sustained post-stimulus elevation in cerebral oxygen utilization following vascular recovery. *J. Cereb. Blood Flow Metab.* 24:764–770.

Lu, H., Golay, X., and van Zijl, P.C. (2002) Inter-voxel heterogeneity of event-related fMRI responses as a function of T1-weighting. *Neuroimage* 17:943–955.

Lu, H., Law, M., Johnson, G., Ge, Y., van Zijl, P.C., and Helpern, J.A. (2005) Novel approach to the measurement of absolute cerebral blood volume using vascular-space-occupancy magnetic resonance imaging. *Magn. Reson. Med.* 54:1403–1411.

Malonek, D., and Grinvald, A. (1996) Interactions between electrical activity and cortical microcirculation revealed by imaging spectroscopy: implications for functional brain mapping. *Science* 272:551–554.

Mandeville, J.B., Marota, J.J., Ayata, C., Zaharchuk, G., Moskowitz, M.A., Rosen, B.R., and Weisskoff, R.M. (1999) Evidence of a cerebrovascular postarteriole windkessel with delayed compliance. *J. Cereb. Blood Flow Metab.* 19:679–689.

Menon, R.S., Ogawa, S., Hu, X., Strupp, J.P., Anderson, P., and Ugurbil, K. (1995) BOLD based functional MRI at 4 Tesla includes a capillary bed contribution: echo-planar imaging correlates with previous optical imaging using intrinsic signals. *Magn. Reson. Med.* 33:453–459.

Moseley, M.E., Chew, W.M., White, D.L., Kucharczyk, J., Litt, L., Derugin, N., Dupon, J., Brasch, R.C., and Norman, D. (1992) Hypercarbia-induced changes in cerebral blood volume in the cat: a 1H MRI and intravascular contrast agent study. *Magn. Reson. Med.* 23:21–30.

Mugler, J.P., 3rd, and Brookeman, J.R. (1991) Rapid three-dimensional T1-weighted MR imaging with the MP-RAGE sequence. *J. Magn. Reson. Imaging* 1:561–567.

Naressi, A., Couturier, C., Devos, J.M., Janssen, M., Mangeat, C., de Beer, R., and Graveron-and Demilly, D. (2001) Java-based graphical user interface for the MRUI quantitation package. *MAGMA* 12:141–152.

Ogawa, S., Menon, R.S., Tank, D.W., Kim, S.G., Merkle, H., Ellermann, J.M., and Ugurbil, K. (1993) Functional brain mapping by blood oxygenation level-dependent contrast magnetic resonance imaging. A comparison of signal characteristics with a biophysical model. *Biophys. J.* 64:803–812.

Ogawa, S., Tank, D.W., Menon, R., Ellermann, J.M., Kim, S.G., Merkle, H., and Ugurbil, K. (1992) Intrinsic signal changes accompanying sensory stimulation: functional brain mapping with magnetic resonance imaging. *Proc. Natl. Acad. Sci. USA* 89: 5951–5955.

Ostergaard, L., Sorensen, A.G., Kwong, K.K., Weisskoff, R.M., Gyldensted, C., and Rosen, B.R. (1996) High resolution measurement of cerebral blood flow using intravascular tracer bolus passages. Part II: Experimental comparison and preliminary results. *Magn. Reson. Med.* 36:726–736.

Ostergaard, L., Weisskoff, R.M., Chesler, D.A., Gyldensted, C., and Rosen, B.R. (1996) High resolution measurement of cerebral blood flow using intravascular tracer bolus passages. Part I: Mathematical approach and statistical analysis. *Magn. Reson. Med.* 36:715–725.

Provencher, S.W. (1993) Estimation of metabolite concentrations from localized in vivo proton NMR spectra. *Magn. Reson. Med.* 30:672–679.

Raichle, M.E., MacLeod, A.M., Snyder, A.Z., Powers, W.J., Gusnard, D.A., and Shulman, G.L. (2001) A default mode of brain function. *Proc. Natl. Acad. Sci. USA* 98:676–682.

Rausch, M., Scheffler, K., Rudin, M., and Radu, E.W. (2000) Analysis of input functions from different arterial branches with gamma variate functions and cluster analysis for quantitative blood volume measurements. *Magn. Reson. Imaging* 18:1235–1243.

Rombouts, S.A., Barkhof, F., Witter, M.P., and Scheltens, P. (2000) Unbiased whole-brain analysis of gray matter loss in Alzheimer's disease. *Neurosci. Lett.* 285:231–233.

Rosen, B.R., Belliveau, J.W., Vevea, J.M., and Brady, T.J. (1990) Perfusion imaging with NMR contrast agents. *Magn. Reson. Med.* 14:249–265.

Roy, C.S., and Sherrington, C.S. (1890) On the regulation of the blood-supply of the brain. *J. Physiol.* 11:85–108.

Rusinek, H., De Santi, S., Frid, D., Tsui, W.H., Tarshish, C.Y., Convit, A., and de Leon, M.J. (2003) Regional brain atrophy rate predicts future cognitive decline: 6-year longitudinal MR imaging study of normal aging. *Radiology* 229:691–696.

Schwarzbauer, C., Syha, J., and Haase, A. (1993) Quantification of regional blood volumes by rapid T1 mapping. *Magn. Reson. Med.* 29:709–712.

Shen, D., and Davatzikos, C. (2002) HAMMER: hierarchical attribute matching mechanism for elastic registration. *IEEE Trans. Med. Imaging* 21:1421–1439.

Sheth, S.A., Nemoto, M., Guiou, M., Walker, M., Pouratian, N., Hageman, N., and Toga, A.W. (2004) Columnar specificity of microvascular oxygenation and volume responses: implications for functional brain mapping. *J. Neurosci.* 24:634–641.

Shulman, R.G., Rothman, D.L., Behar, K.L., and Hyder, F. (2004) Energetic basis of brain activity: implications for neuroimaging. *Trends Neurosci.* 27:489–495.

Sibson, N.R., Dhankhar, A., Mason, G.F., Rothman, D.L., Behar, K. L., and Shulman, R.G. (1998) Stoichiometric coupling of brain glucose metabolism and glutamatergic neuronal activity. *Proc. Natl. Acad. Sci. USA* 95:316–321.

Stejskal, E.O., and Tanner, J.E. (1965) Spin diffusion measurement: spin echoes in the presence of a time-dependent field gradient. *J. Chem. Phys.* 42:288–292.

Thompson, J.K., Peterson, M.R., and Freeman, R.D. (2003) Single-neuron activity and tissue oxygenation in the cerebral cortex. *Science* 299:1070–1072.

Tuch, D.S., Reese, T.G., Wiegell, M.R., and Wedeen, V.J. (2003) Diffusion MRI of complex neural architecture. *Neuron* 40: 885–895.

van Osch, M.J., Vonken, E.J., Viergever, M.A., van der Grond, J., and Bakker, C.J. (2003) Measuring the arterial input function with gradient echo sequences. *Magn. Reson. Med.* 49:1067–1076.

Vanzetta, I., and Grinvald, A. (1999) Increased cortical oxidative metabolism due to sensory stimulation: implications for functional brain imaging. *Science* 286:1555–1558.

Waites, A.B., Briellmann, R.S., Saling, M.M., Abbott, D.F., and Jackson, G.D. (2006) Functional connectivity networks are disrupted in left temporal lobe epilepsy. *Ann. Neurol.* 59:335–343.

Wright, I.C., McGuire, P.K., Poline, J.B., Travere, J.M., Murray, R. M., Frith, C.D., Frackowiak, R.S., and Friston, K.J. (1995) A voxel-based method for the statistical analysis of gray and white matter density applied to schizophrenia. *Neuroimage* 2:244–252.

Xiong, J., Parsons, L.M., Gao, J.H., and Fox, P.T. (1999) Interregional connectivity to primary motor cortex revealed using MRI resting state images. *Hum. Brain Mapp.* 8:151–156.

Xue, R., van Zijl, P.C., Crain, B.J., Solaiyappan, M., and Mori, S. (1999) In vivo three-dimensional reconstruction of rat brain axonal projections by diffusion tensor imaging. *Magn. Reson. Med.* 42:1123–1127.

Yacoub, E., and Hu, X. (1999) Detection of the early negative response in fMRI at 1.5 Tesla. *Magn. Reson. Med.* 41:1088–1092.

Yacoub, E., Shmuel, A., Pfeuffer, J., Van De Moortele, P.F., Adriany, G., Ugurbil, K., and Hu, X. (2001) Investigation of the initial dip in fMRI at 7 Tesla. *NMR Biomed.* 14:408–412.

Yacoub, E., Ugurbil, K., and Harel, N. (2006) The spatial dependence of the poststimulus undershoot as revealed by high-resolution BOLD- and CBV-weighted fMRI. *J. Cereb. Blood Flow Metab.* 26:634–644.

Yang, Y., Engelien, W., Xu, S., Gu, H., Silbersweig, D.A., and Stern, E. (2000) Transit time, trailing time, and cerebral blood flow during brain activation: measurement using multislice, pulsed spin-labeling perfusion imaging. *Magn. Reson. Med.* 44:680–685.

Zhan, W., Stein, E.A., and Yang, Y. (2004) Mapping the orientation of intravoxel crossing fibers based on the phase information of diffusion circular spectrum. *Neuroimage* 23:1358–1369.

14 Molecular Brain Imaging Research in Mental Illness

JONG-HOON KIM, DIANA MARTINEZ, MARK SLIFSTEIN, AND ANISSA ABI-DARGHAM

Molecular imaging is a rapidly emerging field aiming to evaluate biological processes at a molecular level. In the realm of psychiatry, the term *in vivo molecular imaging* generally refers to the use of radiolabeled chemical compounds (radiotracers) with positron emission tomography (PET) and single photon emission computed tomography (SPECT) to measure protein molecules such as receptors, transporters, and enzymes, as well as cellular processes such as transmitter synthesis and release. At a more fundamental level, molecular imaging has the potential to measure the most basic processes of intracellular signaling including gene expression either by measuring the translation into a protein product of an endogenous gene or the de novo effects of a transplanted gene (Phelps, 2000; Jacobs et al., 2003). As the contribution of genetically determined molecular alterations to the pathogenesis of psychiatric diseases is unraveled with their corresponding intracellular signaling–associated changes, molecular imaging of these genes and their by-products will play a crucial role in the future.

The main contributions of PET and SPECT so far have been in two broad areas: unraveling molecular biomarkers for psychiatric disease, and aiding in drug discovery for treatment of these diseases. Biomarkers are biological alterations that are reliably and selectively associated with a disease process. Although no biomarkers as such have been established and validated in psychiatric research, some have emerged as promising leads. Nevertheless, and for simplicity of expression, we refer to those as *biomarkers* in this review, with the understanding that studies of specificity and selectivity are still needed. These putative biomarkers consist in replicated observations using molecular imaging of alterations in receptor expression or measures of endogenous transmitter via pharmacological or nonpharmacological challenges. Studies of dopaminergic parameters in schizophrenia and addiction have been the most yielding in this regard and are described.

Positron emission tomography and SPECT molecular imaging can also aid drug development by demonstrating that drugs reach their receptor and enzyme targets and by defining dose occupancy curves for phase 1 and phase 2 studies and thereby rationalizing choice of dosing in clinical trials (Brooks, 2005).

An important property of PET and SPECT is that they can measure molecules present in the brain in the nanomolar to picomolar range of concentrations (Talbot and Laruelle, 2002), allowing a level of sensitivity unmatched by any other method currently available to investigators. The major disadvantages of PET and SPECT are the radiation exposure involved, limiting the number of scans that a participant may have, and the dependence of the technique on the availability of appropriate radioligands to label molecules of interest. To date, the neurochemical systems most widely studied in humans are the dopamine (DA) and serotonin systems, although entire neurochemical systems are implicated in the pathophysiology of psychiatric disorders. Nevertheless, ligand development is proceeding at a rapid pace, and as new radiotracers are available for use in human studies, more information will be revealed about the pathophysiology of psychiatric disorders and the targets for successful therapeutic interventions.

In this chapter we describe the important methodological concepts relevant to the design of PET and SPECT studies, and some existent applications in the two areas outlined above of biomarker development and drug discovery; then we describe the potentials of these techniques for future developments and applications as more probes for novel targets become available. The purpose of this chapter is to provide a general overview of the important issues in designing a molecular imaging study and the main applications, but it is not intended to be an in-depth review of all these aspects, and the reader is encouraged to go to more specialized sources for each topic.

METHODOLOGICAL CONSIDERATIONS

Measurement of Receptor Parameters

Positron emission tomography and SPECT are most typically used to assess neuroreceptors. Although PET is more expensive than SPECT, it allows more versatility, meaning a larger number of candidate targets in the brain can be visualized. Positron emission tomography produces higher quality images due to higher resolution and sensitivity of the scanner. Positron emission tomography is also more quantitatively informative because tissue attenuation can be more accurately measured with PET technology and the associated radioisotopes than with SPECT. Fewer academic centers have PET compared to SPECT because it necessitates an on-site cyclotron to produce the radioactive isotopes used in the synthesis of the radiochemicals to be injected to visualize the sites in the brain that are under investigation. SPECT, due to the longer half-lives of radioisotopes used for the scanner, does not necessitate an on-site cyclotron. Isotopes can be shipped because they decay more slowly.

A crucial step in this technology is the synthesis of radiotracers. To be successfully used for in vivo molecular imaging, the chemical properties of a radiotracer must fall within a fairly narrow range of appropriate combinations of lipophilicity, affinity/selectivity, specificity, reversibility, and toxicity (Halldin et al., 2001). In addition, slow metabolism during the time frame of the experiment is desirable to avoid radiolabeled metabolites crossing into the brain. In case of metabolism, the absence of radiolabeled metabolites crossing the blood-brain-barrier (BBB) is necessary for accurate quantification; otherwise the modeling will have to account for an additional and changing source of radioactive input to the brain. Radiotracer production is the most challenging step of imaging and has been the rate-limiting step in terms of exploring new targets in the brain. As an example we have tracers for dopaminergic and serotonergic sites, but very few for sites outside of these systems that are available for use in humans.

Once produced successfully, the radiotracer is injected into a vein, travels throughout the body, crosses the BBB, and binds to the receptor (referred to as *specific binding*). The radiotracer also binds to other nonreceptor proteins in the brain (termed *nonspecific binding*). The radioactivity that accumulates in a receptor-rich region contains specific and nonspecific binding, while the activity that is measured in a region devoid of receptors is used to measure nonspecific binding, more accurately designated as nondisplaceable binding, as these regions contain not only nonspecific signal but also the signal originating from the free unbound radiotracer. The scanner takes serial images of the radioactive signal emitted by the tracer. Typically arterial samples are also obtained serially as brain data acquisition is occurring. The purpose is to obtain the concentration of radioactive tracer that the brain is exposed to after injection, called the "input" to the brain, while the scanner measures the "response" of the brain. The input function and response function are used to calculate the receptor parameters of interest.

The outcome measure in PET studies is termed *receptor availability* or "binding potential" (BP), which is equivalent in pharmacological terms to the product of receptor density and affinity of the radiotracer for the receptor. Different iterations of BP correspond to the presence of correction for nonspecific binding in the brain and/or in the plasma (Table 14.1 and Fig. 14.1). These are termed differently by different groups; however, a consensus emerged on using similar terminology (Innis, 2007). In this terminology the terms BP_F, BP_P, and BP_{ND} are used to refer to BP relative to the free tracer concentration in the plasma (BP_F, which is B_{max}, and K_D), BP relative to the total tracer concentration in the plasma (BP_P, which is $f_P B_{max}/K_D$, f_P being the free fraction in the plasma or fraction of ligand that is not bound to plasma proteins), and BP relative to the concentration of radiotracer in a region with nondisplaceable activity (that is, a reference region) (BP_{ND}, which is $f_{ND}B_{max}/K_D$, with f_{ND}) the free fraction of the free plus nonspecifically bound ligand in the nondisplaceable compartment). The latter two incorporate measures of nonspecific binding in the plasma and the brain, respectively. If these are used to compare population samples to each other and if they show differences among these samples, one cannot be certain if the differences are related to specific versus nonspecific factors. However, the reason the latter two are used is the fact that correction for nonspecific binding can be either

TABLE 14.1. *On the Meaning of Binding Potential ($\approx B_{max}/K_D$)*

= BP in Literature (%)	*Kinetic Derivation*	*Relation to Receptor Parameters*	*Arterial Sampling*	*f_p measurement*	*Assumption*
90	k_3/k_4	$f_{ND}\ B_{max}/K_D$	No	No	f_{ND}=constant
9	$(K_1k_3)/(k_2k_4)$	$f_p\ B_{max}/K_D$	Yes	No	f_p=constant
1	$(K_1k_3)/(f_pk_2k_4)$	B_{max}/K_D	Yes	Yes	*

f_{ND} = free fraction in C_{ND} (nondisplaceable compartment); f_p = free fraction in C_P (arterial plasma); * = no assumption.

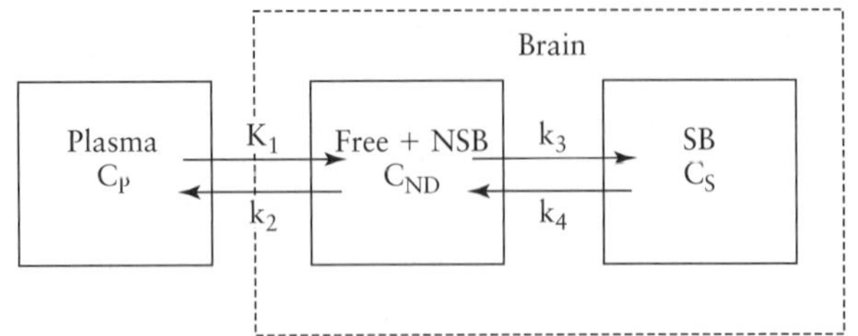

f_{ND} = free fraction in C_{ND} (nondisplaceable compartment)
f_P = free fraction in C_P (arterial plasma)
$BP_{ND} = k_3/k_4 = f_{ND}B_{max}/K_D$

FIGURE 14.1 Representation of a classic three-compartment model used in analysis of positron emission tomography (PET) or single photon emission computed tomography (SPECT) data to derive receptor parameters. See text for details.

difficult or can introduce excess noise in the outcome measure. A reference region devoid of receptors will provide a measure of the nondisplaceable binding of the tracer denoted as the distribution volume of the nonspecific compartment V_{ND}. For a region containing specific and nonspecific binding, one can also refer to the sum of BP_P and V_{ND} as the total distribution volume or V_T. V_T is defined as the ratio of radioligand concentration in a brain region to that in the arterial plasma at equilibrium. The name is a historical holdover from more conventional pharmacology, and in fact the quantity does not have units of volume—its units are mL/cm^3, due to the fact that concentrations are measured per unit of fluid volume in plasma and per unit of spatial volume in images.

These quantitative estimates of receptor parameters are independent of effects such as clearance and regional cerebral blood flow because they are obtained by fitting brain and blood data collected during the scan to a mathematical model (a "compartment model") that takes these factors into account. The standard compartment model incorporates transport of ligand into brain tissue and subsequent binding of ligand to receptors into a coupled set of differential equations. The model is based on certain assumptions about the experimental conditions that are necessary for the outcome to be valid. These include tracer dose injection of the compound (very low mass, or high specific activity of the tracer, leading to an occupancy of the receptor well below 5%), constant regional cerebral blood flow and an available receptor population that is unchanged during the course of the scan. Under these conditions, outcome measures that are proportional to available receptor density can be estimated. Good understanding of the approximations and assumptions that are incorporated in the models and the relationships between the various components of the measured signal will lead to more insightful interpretation of data obtained using PET and SPECT.

It should be emphasized that the quantity of interest, *receptor density or B_{max}*, is proportional to the various forms of BP, but the quantity that can be reliably measured directly is V_T that contains information about nonspecific binding as well. If an independent estimation of V_{ND} is available, then one would think that BP_P and BP_{ND} can be reliably inferred for any brain region with receptors, regardless of receptor density. For idealized, noise-free data, this would be true. But given the inherently stochastic nature of the signal being measured, the relative sizes of V_{ND} and BP_P ($V_T = V_{ND} + BP_P$) will play a role in determining the utility of a radioligand. The overall variance in PET and SPECT image data increases when mean activity increases. The decay process that generates signal is independent of ligand binding; nonspecific binding generates the same rate of decay as specific binding. If a ligand has a large V_{ND} relative to BP_P in a given brain region, then the nonspecific binding will make a large contribution to the overall variance without any contribution to the ability to detect specific binding. The effect is to reduce ability to detect specific binding. As an example, consider the two serotonin transporter (SERT) ligands [^{11}C]McNeil 5625 (MCN) (Suehiro et al., 1993; Szabo et al., 1995; Buck et al., 2000; Parsey et al., 2000; Ikoma et al., 2002) and [^{11}C]DASB (DSB) (Houle et al., 2000; Wilson et al., 2000; Ginovart et al., 2001; Meyer et al., 2001; Huang et al., 2002; Szabo et al., 2002). Both are specific for serotonin reuptake sites, but nonspecific binding comprises a greater fraction of the signal from MCN than DSB. Cerebellum is often used as a reference region for SERT ligands. Human cerebellar V_{ND} is approximately 20 for MCN and 10 for DSB. In high receptor-density regions such as midbrain, V_T is approximately 50 for MCN and 30 for DSB, so that BP_{ND} is approximately 1.5 for MCN and 2 for DSB. Both ligands are suitable for SERT quantification in midbrain. But in regions that have relatively low SERT density, such as hippocampus or anterior cingulate, BP_{ND} values are approximately 0.2 for MCN and 0.3 for DSB. This increase in BP_{ND} will allow for more reliable quantification in these regions with DSB compared to MCN. Better signal-to-noise characteristics, as embodied in the relative sizes of V_{ND} and BP_P, will determine whether a ligand is suitable for interrogation of regions that are small or that have low receptor density but are still of clinical relevance.

It should be noted that the majority of PET studies conducted in humans do not differentiate between receptor density and affinity because the outcome measure is the product of both parameters. In other words, a difference in BP seen between two study groups could reflect either a difference in receptor density or receptor affinity. It is possible to obtain estimates of B_{max} and K_D separately, but this requires scans with pharmacological doses (high receptor occupancy) of the radioligand. For this reason, such studies are rarely performed with human participants.

Positron emission tomography studies performed with receptor antagonists are not affected by differences in the affinity state of the receptor because an antagonist binds similarly to both states of the receptor. On the other hand, PET studies performed with an agonist can provide information regarding receptor affinity states. In terms of agonist tracers, the first available for human use are agonists at the $D_{2/3}$ system. D_2 receptors, like all G-protein–linked receptors, exist in states of high or low affinity for agonists (denoted D_{2high} and D_{2low}, respectively). Antagonists, such as [^{11}C]raclopride and [^{123}I]IBZM, bind to both configurations with similar affinity. Thus, the in vivo binding of these antagonists does not provide information about the affinity of D_2 receptors for agonists. In contrast, PET studies performed with a radiolabeled D_2 agonist tracer would allow the direct in vivo measurement of the affinity of D_2 receptors for agonists, allowing researchers to control for this important variable in clinical studies. As the high-affinity state of DA D_2 receptors, D_{2high} is the functional state of D_2 and relates to DA behavioral supersensitivity and intracellular signaling, it is important to assess the proportion of D_2 receptors in the high-affinity state in diseases involving alterations in DA transmission, such as schizophrenia and addiction. [^{11}C]PHNO is a new tracer developed by Wilson (Wilson et al., 2005) and already used in humans (Willeit et al., 2005) to quantify D_{2high}. [^{11}C]NPA is another one that has been extensively characterized in nonhuman primates (Hwang et al., 2004; Narendran et al., 2004) and is currently being examined in humans.

Measurement of Endogenous Transmitters

Over the last decade, strong evidence has emerged demonstrating that in vivo neuroreceptor imaging with PET and SPECT can be used to measure acute fluctuations in synaptic concentration of neurotransmitters. This application of neuroreceptor imaging enables direct measurement of synaptic transmission in the living brain and correlations of these dynamic measurements with behaviors and symptoms. It has been most successfully applied to the measurements of changes in dopamine synaptic concentration. Some work has been done to image changes in acetylcholine and endorphins levels by imaging the muscarinic (Dewey et al., 1990; Tsukada et al., 2000; Skaddan et al., 2001), nicotinic (Ding et al., 1998; Ding et al., 2000), and opiate systems (Frost, 1992; Zubieta et al., 2001; Zubieta et al., 2003). This line of research has emerged under a theorical framework referred to as the *occupancy model*. The occupancy model predicts that challenges that increase the synaptic concentration of a transmitter will result in increased occupancy of receptors by the transmitter, and reduced availability of these receptors for binding to the radiotracer. Conversely, manipulations that decrease synaptic concentration of the transmitter will reduce receptor occupancy by the transmitter and increase receptor availability to radiotracer binding.

The best illustration and the most validated example of such a use is measuring DA transmission using the radiotracers [^{123}I]IBZM and [^{11}C]raclopride, which are benzamides. The binding of these tracers is sensitive to acute changes in endogenous DA in the brain: increases in extraneuronal DA using a psychostimulant (such as methylphenidate or amphetamine) decrease their binding. Therefore, in the same individual, a comparison of baseline (that is, prestimulant administration) binding potential and BP following the stimulant provides an indirect measure of DA transmission. Studies in nonhuman primates combining this imaging technique with microdialysis have shown a linear correlation between the stimulant-induced change in BP and extracellular DA increase (Breier et al., 1997; Laruelle, Iyer, et al., 1997). However, there is a significant loss of sensitivity: as an example, each percent decrease in [^{11}C]raclopride BP corresponds to a 54% increase in extracellular DA measured with microdialysis (Breier et al., 1997). The exact mechanism behind the decrease in these tracers' binding is not known. Although competition between extracellular DA and the radiotracer for the receptor has been used as a model to explain the decrease in radiotracer binding, it is not sufficient to explain all aspects observed with the imaging paradigm, such as the prolonged effect of a transient change in transmitter level on the radiotracer binding, paradoxical effects of these manipulations on certain tracers, and the lack of observable effects with many others. For these reasons, other phenomena, such as receptor affinity state, internalization, or polymerization, have also been implicated (Laruelle, 2000; Logan et al., 2001), and it is accepted that changes in DA occupancy may not be the only factors playing a role in the modulation of receptor availability following changes in DA synaptic concentration. Regardless of the exact mechanisms that underlie the change in radiotracer binding related to acute changes in DA, the phenomenon measured remains tightly related to the change in DA. Thus it would not invalidate the conclusions drawn from clinical studies using these challenges because binding of DA to D_2 receptors is the first step in the cascade of events leading to D_2 receptor internalization and changes in BP. To this extent, these challenges provide a noninvasive measure of D_2 receptor stimulation by DA, even if receptor internalization or trafficking contribute to some extent to the observed effect.

Cocaine was also reported to affect [^{11}C]raclopride uptake in chronic cocaine abusers (Schlaepfer et al., 1997). The hallucinogen *psilocybin*, a potent $5HT_{2A}$ agonist, decreased [^{11}C]raclopride BP by 20% (Vollenweider et al., 1999) as well as alcohol (Boileau et al., 2003). Fingers or feet movements were shown to decrease [^{11}C]raclopride

(Ouchi et al., 2002; Goerendt et al., 2003). Dopamine depletion studies in humans showed that acute alpha-methyl-para-tyrosine AMPT challenge resulted in significant increase in [^{123}I]IBZM and [^{11}C]raclopride BP (Laruelle, D'Souza, et al., 1997; Verhoeff et al., 2001). The only major inconsistency in the [^{11}C]raclopride literature is related to the effect of ketamine: three studies showed that ketamine decreased [^{11}C]raclopride BP (Breier et al., 1998; Smith et al., 1998; Vollenweider et al., 2000), whereas two studies, using similar doses, failed to observe this effect (Aalto et al., 2002; Kegeles et al., 2002). In addition, the elucidation of the exact mechanism(s) underlying the "benzamide effect" is important to the development of this field of brain imaging. So far, imaging studies of dynamic neurotransmission have been essentially restricted to the study of DA transmission at the D_2 receptors with substituted benzamides. Clinical results obtained with this "benzamide effect" highlight the promises of this technique for the field and motivate the extension of this technique to other receptor systems. As mentioned earlier, encouraging observations have been reported for the muscarinic (Dewey et al., 1990; Tsukada et al., 2000; Skaddan et al., 2001), nicotinic (Ding et al., 1998; Ding et al., 2000), and opiate systems (Frost, 1992; Zubieta et al., 2001; Zubieta et al., 2003), but these observations require considerable validation before maturing into clinical research tools. On the other hand, results obtained so far with D_1, dopamine transporter (DAT) and serotonin $5HT_{1A}$ and 5HT transporter ligands are disappointing (Gatley, Ding, et al., 1995; Gatley, Volkow, et al., 1995; Parsey et al., 1998; Abi-Dargham et al., 1999). We propose that a better understanding of the multiple factors that determine radiotracer binding vulnerability to changes in endogenous transmitter levels will be essential to realize the unique potential of these techniques for measurement of synaptic transmission in the living human brain. Furthermore, conducting these studies using tracers that are agonists will potentiate the signal. As an example, it is predicted that DA would be more potent at inhibiting binding of an agonist compared to that of [^{11}C]raclopride. Thus, conducting these studies with a radiolabeled agonist like [^{11}C]NPA or [^{11}C]PHNO would increase the signal-to-noise ratio of the amphetamine effect. Finally an important methodological point is that a challenge may induce changes in blood flow that could represent a violation of the assumptions inherent to the modeling approaches used to the quantification of binding. For these reasons, imaging under conditions of true equilibrium where the tracer is administered as a bolus followed by a constant infusion to achieve steady state has been a preferred method for these challenges.

Use of Molecular Imaging in Nonpharmacological Challenges

Molecular imaging can also be used to assess the effects of stress or a challenging task on radiotracer binding. Transmagnetic stimulation (Strafella et al., 2003), anticipation of a challenge (Boileau et al., 2007), monetary rewards (Zald et al., 2004), as well as stress (Pruessner et al., 2004) have also been shown to affect binding. However, replications under better controlled conditions (for example, controlling for effects of challenge on blood flow) and assessment of reliability of the measurements are needed. Nevertheless these applications are very exciting as they allow measuring transmitter release during cognitive tasks or nonpharmacological manipulations.

Use of Molecular Imaging to Probe Transmitter Interactions

Molecular imaging has been used to image interactions at the system level between different transmitters. One of the most studied has been the effect of *N*-methyl-D-aspartate (NMDA) blockade on DA release in the striatum, and on amphetamine-induced DA release. Three PET studies found a significant reduction in striatal D_2 receptor availability following ketamine in healthy human participants (Breier et al., 1998; Smith et al., 1998; Vollenweider et al., 2000), but others did not (Aalto et al., 2002; Kegeles et al., 2002). However, a more reliable probe may be the effect of ketamine on amphetamine-induced DA release (Kegeles et al., 2002). This study showed that NMDA deficit produced by ketamine in healthy controls results in a dysregulation of striatal DA transmission similar to that seen in schizophrenia, thus validating the relevance of an NMDA dysfunction model to the study of schizophrenia. Furthermore, LY354740, a highly selective agonist at $mGlu_{2/3}$ receptors (Schoepp et al., 1997) enhanced amphetamine-induced DA release measured with PET and the [^{11}C]raclopride displacement paradigm in baboons (van Berckel et al., 2006). Because the effects of LY354740 on glutamic acid (GLU) transmission are inhibitory, this study provided the clearest evidence that inhibition of GLU transmission increases amphetamine-induced DA release and provided additional support to the hypothesis that the dysregulation of DA function revealed by the amphetamine challenge in schizophrenia might stem from a deficit in GLU transmission.

Similarly one can design challenges to assess 5HT-DA interactions or if tracers for glutamatergic and cannabinoid system become available; these may be relevant to many disease processes.

APPLICATIONS

Biomarkers

Studies of dopaminergic parameters in schizophrenia and addiction have yielded the most replicated set of findings. These observations have now been replicated enough that they can be considered established phenotypes found commonly in most patients and produce potential biomarkers for the disease.

In schizophrenia, evidence of increased striatal DA transmission derives from studies of [^{18}F]DOPA or [^{11}C]DOPA (dihydroxyphenylalanine), which examine the activity of DOPA decarboxylase (AADC) by measuring the accumulation of radiotracer in the brains of patients with schizophrenia compared to controls, studies of striatal DA release, as well as measurements of expression of striatal D_2. All these are increased in schizophrenia (Guillin et al., 2007). This set of convergent findings suggest that increased striatal DA transmission could be used as a biomarker for psychosis risk in vulnerable prodromal populations and guide the choice of treatment. [^{18}F]DOPA imaging could be acquired in large sets of patients and in centers that do not have on-site cyclotrons due to the long half-life of [^{18}F], thus representing the most feasible approach.

In addiction, low striatal D_2 as well as low DA release have been observed in cocaine (Volkow et al., 2003) and alcohol addiction (Martinez et al., 2005). Low D_2 seems to be associated with risk for addictive disorders, while high D_2 may have a protective effect (Volkow et al., 2006).

Measurement of Occupancy by Drugs

Methods

Molecular PET and SPECT can be used to measure occupancy by drugs. The term *occupancy* refers to the fraction of a receptor population that is bound by a ligand (drug or endogenous transmitter) under equilibrium conditions. Occupancy can be completely characterized by a single parameter: under equilibrium conditions, the relationship between bound and free ligand is given by

$$Bound = B_{max}\frac{Free / K_D}{1 + Free / K_D} = B_{max} \times occupancy$$

Here, B_{max} is the concentration of receptors and K_D, the equilibrium dissociation constant, is the ratio of the "off rate" to the "on rate" for the reversible bimolecular reaction between the ligand and receptor. Occupancy ranges from 0 (when *Free* = 0) to 100% (when *Free* >> K_D). The equation shows that, given knowledge of K_D, occupancy will be known if the free drug concentration is known, and conversely, any desired level of occupancy can be attained by adjusting the free level appropriately. Thus the goal of an occupancy study is to estimate the K_D or some surrogate for K_D, so that in clinical applications, receptor occupancy can be maintained within an appropriate therapeutic window. In the in vitro setting, it is possible to directly measure free concentrations and therefore estimate the K_D. In the in vivo setting, either in humans or nonterminal animal experiments, it is not possible to directly measure drug concentration in brain tissue, so that some surrogate marker for the K_D must be estimated. If blood plasma levels of the drug can be measured, the estimated quantity is referred to as the *EC50* (expected concentration for 50% occupancy); if only the administered doses are known, the parameter is called the *ED50* (*D* for dose). The equations for EC50 or ED50 are of the same form as the one for K_D. This follows from the assumed linear relationship between dose, plasma concentration, and concentration of free ligand in brain tissue. That is, given a particular dose and the resultant plasma and brain concentrations, changing the dose by some proportionality will cause the plasma and brain concentrations to change by the same proportionality.

To estimate K_D, occupancy must be measured over a range of free concentrations; the plot of bound versus free is then fitted by a statistical procedure to obtain estimates of K_D and B_{max}. Positron emission tomography–based estimates of occupancy, however, are rarely obtained by directly radiolabeling the drug because labeling a compound is not always practical and because the kinetic properties that are desirable for a therapeutic agent are not usually conducive to quantitative imaging. Rather, a reporter ligand that binds specifically to the same target receptor as the drug and has kinetic properties appropriate for imaging is utilized. It can be shown that if the drug and radioligand compete for the same receptor site and the radioligand is administered at tracer dose, the occupancy can be inferred from the relative difference in binding potential (BP_P or BP_{ND}) of the radioligand between a baseline scan and one with drug on board. That is,

$$\frac{BP(baseline) - BP(with\ drug)}{BP(baseline)} = \frac{(Free\ Drug / E50)}{1 + (Free\ Drug / E50)} = occupancy$$

where the free concentration and the E50 are in the same units (*dose* for ED50 or *plasma* concentration for EC50). The E50 is estimated by repeating the experiment with multiple drug levels and fitting the data to Equation 2. For statistical reasons, it is more common to plot the left-hand side of Equation 2 against the logarithm of the free drug concentration, leading to a sigmoidal curve (Fig. 14.2). Log(E50) is then estimated as the log of the drug concentration associated with the occupancy halfway between the minimum and maximum values.

Occupancy Studies in Drug Development

Positron emission tomography occupancy studies can inform and streamline the drug development process in the early phase and, following proof of concept, in the late development phase. In the early phase, a pharmaceutical manufacturer may have developed several candidate compounds with demonstrated specificity for a target receptor, as demonstrated in vitro or in small animal assays. Specificity, however, is only one component of a successful therapeutic agent. Frequently, there is a "therapeutic window," a range of occupancies given by the combination of the minimal occupancy necessary to be effective, and the maximal occupancy that, if exceeded, will lead to undesirable side effects. There will also be a maximally allowable mass dose associated with the onset of toxicity. It would be prohibitively expensive for the manufacturer to proceed with each of the candidates all the way through human trials to determine which, if any, meet all these criteria. Rather, the compound with the most potential for success must be selected early on in the process. Positron emission tomography–based occupancy studies in nonhuman primates provide valuable information for making this kind of assessment. The pharmacokinetic, anatomic, and neurochemical conditions are far more similar to humans than are small animal models such as rodents. On the other hand, it is relatively inexpensive, fast, and more feasible to do occupancy studies in primates compared to humans. For these reasons, PET image–based occupancy studies in nonhuman primates are increasingly becoming a routine part of the early drug-development process. Positron emission tomography occupancy studies can also provide important information in the late, premarket phase of drug development. When drugs have progressed to the level of human trials, PET occupancy studies can be used to determine the dose associated with a desired level of occupancy. Or, by correlating efficacy or side effects to dose and occupancy, PET studies can be used to help define windows for therapeutic effects or side effects. An important example is the definition of 80% threshold occupancy by D_2 antagonists as the threshold needed for emergence of extrapyramidal symptoms (EPS). This observation first reported by Farde et al. (1989) has remained true for all antipsychotics. $5HT_{2A}$ binding of atypical antipsychotics did not affect this threshold, allowing some insights into the mechanisms of atypicality (Abi-Dargham and Laruelle, 2005). This threshold also provided in vivo evidence for partial agonism at the D_2 receptor for aripiprazole as no EPS are observed despite higher than 80% occupancy with this drug (Yokoi et al., 2002).

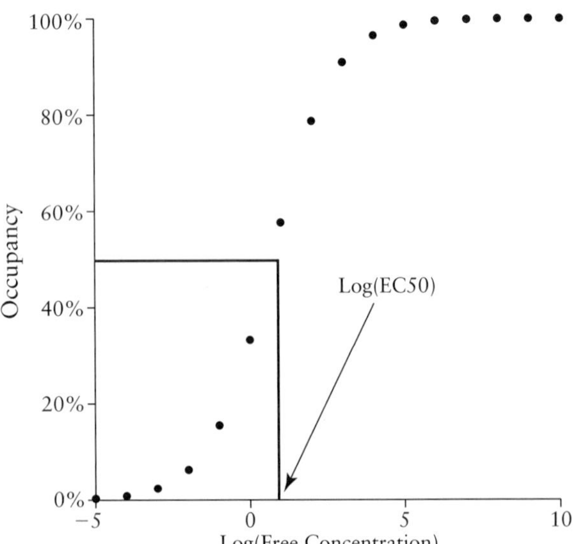

FIGURE 14.2 Idealized occupancy graph. EC50 is estimated as the concentration associated with 50% occupancy.

IMAGING INTRACELLULAR PROCESSES

Imaging intracellular signaling pathways, among which is gene expression, is ultimately the goal needed for an in-depth understanding of cellular processes underlying diseases and their therapies. Imaging gene expression has become possible because of the explosion of knowledge of genome structure and the genetic basis for cellular processes in normal and pathological conditions, as well as in relation to therapies. This area is a new emerging field with most applications in oncology (Phelps, 2000; Jacobs et al., 2003), and few in neurology and other fields. Genetically engineered mice are the primary focus so far. The main available methods can visualize gene expression by introducing radioprobes, typically a radiolabeled oligonucleotide that contain a sequence complementary to the messenger ribonucleic acid (mRNA) of interest and that measures the translation of this mRNA by the accumulation of the radioactive protein. It is equivalent to imaging in vivo hybridization. An indirect approach involves introducing an exogenous gene via a vector or virus to measure the effects of this gene onto the expression of a protein that can be labeled with a PET radiotracer. This has been applied to the study of addiction, where researchers showed that transient overexpression of D_2 receptor gene in the nucleus accumbens of ethanol-preferring rats using an adenoviral vector decreased alcohol intake (Thanos et al., 2004).

The future of gene expression studies in psychiatry will depend on the development of the correct probes and their correct validation and quantification. In this process, the availability of molecular imaging in mice is a crucial development as it allows testing the numerous animal models of psychiatric disorders that are emerging. By going back and forth between the animal models and the actual patients to test the genetic underpinnings of biological findings, imaging will play a crucial role in translational research and will ultimately lead to new discoveries.

FUTURE DIRECTIONS

Single photon emission computed tomography and PET imaging studies have revealed a consistent pattern of alterations in a set of mental illnesses: schizophrenia and addiction. However, the contributions to other areas have been more modest and limited by inconsistencies and lack of replication of findings. The reasons may relate to differences in techniques among imaging groups or to the nature of the illness itself and how strongly it is associated with some static alterations in the brain that could be measured and thought of as biomarkers. One way to address some of these issues is to move toward multisite well-coordinated imaging protocols using similar methods and outcome measures, where the data can be merged to provide bigger samples and comparable results. Another issue that needs to be addressed to have a more effective impact on the field is the rapid development and sharing of new tracers to assess the vast amount of unexplored but crucial systems such as the glutamatergic, cannabinoid, and noradrenergic systems, to cite only a few. Tracers for some of these sites are becoming available. Tracers that bind preferentially to the high-affinity states of receptors are needed to probe the functional state of the receptor in addition to the expression level that can be assessed with antagonists. Furthermore, tracers that allow exploration of intracellular processes and gene expression would allow greater knowledge regarding physiological and pathological brain processes in various mental disorders. Imaging of gene expression has been applied to cancer research (Blasberg, 2002) and is a relatively new tool for neuroscience research. Ultimately molecular imaging holds great promise for the understanding of cellular processes and systems interactions in mental illness, its prevention through biomarkers development, and in guiding treatment development.

REFERENCES

Aalto, S., Hirvonen, J., Kajander, J., Scheinin, H., Nagren, K., Vilkman, H., Gustafsson, L., Syvalahti, E., and Hietala, J. (2002) Ketamine does not decrease striatal dopamine D2 receptor binding in man. *Psychopharmacology (Berl)* 164:401–406.

Abi-Dargham, A., and Laruelle, M. (2005) Mechanisms of action of second generation antipsychotic drugs in schizophrenia: insights from brain imaging studies. *Eur. Psychiatry* 20:15–27.

Abi-Dargham, A., Simpson, N., Kegeles, L., Parsey, R., Hwang, D.R., Anjilvel, S., Zea-Ponce, Y., Lombardo, I., Van Heertum, R., Mann, J.J., Foged, C., Halldin, C., and Laruelle, M. (1999) PET studies of binding competition between endogenous dopamine and the D1 radiotracer [11C]NNC 756. *Synapse* 32:93–109.

Blasberg, R. (2002) Imaging gene expression and endogenous molecular processes: molecular imaging. *J. Cereb. Blood Flow Metab.* 22:1157–1164.

Boileau, I., Assaad, J.M., Pihl, R.O., Benkelfat, C., Leyton, M., Diksic, M., Tremblay, R.E., and Dagher, A. (2003) Alcohol promotes dopamine release in the human nucleus accumbens. *Synapse* 49:226–231.

Boileau, I., Dagher, A., Leyton, M., Welfeld, K., Booij, L., Diksic, M., and Benkelfat, C. (2007) Conditioned dopamine release in humans: a positron emission tomography [11C]raclopride study with amphetamine. *J. Neurosci.* 27:3998–4003.

Breier, A., Adler, C.M., Weisenfeld, N., Su, T.P., Elman, I., Picken, L., Malhotra, A.K., and Pickar, D. (1998) Effects of NMDA antagonism on striatal dopamine release in healthy subjects: application of a novel PET approach. *Synapse* 29:142–147.

Breier, A., Su, T.P., Saunders, R., Carson, R.E., Kolachana, B.S., deBartolomeis, A., Weinberger, D.R., Weisenfeld, N., Malhotra, A.K., Eckelman, W.C., and Pickar, D. (1997) Schizophrenia is associated with elevated amphetamine-induced synaptic dopamine concentrations: Evidence from a novel positron emission tomography method. *Proc. Natl. Acad. Sci. USA* 94:2569–2574.

Brooks, D.J. (2005) Positron emission tomography and single-photon emission computed tomography in central nervous system drug development. *NeuroRx* 2:226–236.

Buck, A., Gucker, P.M., Schonbachler, R.D., Arigoni, M., Kneifel, S., Vollenweider, F.X., Ametamey, S.M., and Burger, C. (2000) Evaluation of serotonergic transporters using PET and [C-11](+)McN-5652: Assessment of methods. *J. Cereb. Blood Flow Metab.* 20: 253–262.

Dewey, S.L., Brodie, J.D., Fowler, J.S., MacGregor, R.R., Schyler, D.J., King, P.T., Alexoff, D.L., Volkow, N.D., Shiue, C.Y., Wolf, A.P., and Bendriem, B. (1990) Positron emission tomography (PET) studies of dopamine/cholinergic interaction in the baboon brain. *Synapse* 6:321–327.

Ding, Y.S., Fowler, N.D., Volkow, N.D., Logan, J., Dewey, S.L., Carroll, F.I., and Kuhar, M.J. (1998) Dopamine D2 receptor mediated regulation of central cholinergic activity: PET studies with [18F]fluoroepibatidine. *J. Nucl. Med.* 39:12P.

Ding, Y.S., Logan, J., Bermel, R., Garza, V., Rice, O., Fowler, J.S., and Volkow, N.D. (2000) Dopamine receptor-mediated regulation of striatal cholinergic activity: positron emission tomography studies with norchloro[18F]fluoroepibatidine. *J. Neurochem.* 74:1514–1521.

Farde, L., Wiesel, F.A., Nordström, A.L., and Sedvall, G. (1989) D1- and D2-dopamine receptor occupancy during treatment with conventional and atypical neuroleptic. *Psychopharmacology* 99:S28–S31.

Frost, J.J. (1992) Receptor imaging by positron emission tomography and single-photon emission computed tomography. *Invest. Radiol.* 27(Suppl. 2):S54–S58.

Gatley, S.J., Ding, Y.S., Volkow, N.D., Chen, R., Sugano, Y., and Fowler, J.S. (1995) Binding of d-threo-[^{11}C]methylphenidate to the dopamine transporter in vivo: insensitivity to synaptic dopamine. *Eur. J. Pharmacol.* 281:141–149.

Gatley, S.J., Volkow, N.D., Fowler, J.S., Dewey, S.L., and Logan, J. (1995) Sensitivity of striatal [11C]cocaine binding to decreases in synaptic dopamine. *Synapse* 20:137–144.

Ginovart, N., Wilson, A.A., Meyer, J.H., Hussey, D., and Houle, S. (2001) PET quantification of C-11-DASB binding to the serotonin transporter in human. *J. Nucl. Med.* 42:105p–105p.

Goerendt, I.K., Messa, C., Lawrence, A.D., Grasby, P.M., Piccini, P., and Brooks, D.J. (2003) Dopamine release during sequential finger movements in health and Parkinson's disease: a PET study. *Brain* 126:312–325.

Guillin, O., Abi-Dargham, A., and Laruelle, M. (2007) Neurobiology of dopamine in schizophrenia. *Int. Rev. Neurobiol.* 78:1–39.

Halldin, C., Gulyas, B., Langer, O., and Farde, L. (2001) Brain radioligands—state of the art and new trends. *Q. J. Nucl. Med.* 45: 139–152.

Houle, S., Ginovart, N., Hussey, D., Meyer, J.H., and Wilson, A.A. (2000) Imaging the serotonin transporter with positron emission tomography: initial human studies with [C-11]DAPP and [C-11] DASB. *Eur. J. Nucl. Med.* 27:1719–1722.

Huang, T.Y., Hwang, D.R., Narendran, R., Sudo, Y., Chatterjee, R., Bae, S.A., Mawlawi, T., Kegeles, T.S., Wilson, A.A., Kung, H.F., and Laruelle, M. (2002) Comparative evaluation in nonhuman primates of five PET radiotracers for imaging the serotonin transporters: [C-11]McN 5652, [C-11]ADAM, [C-11]DASB, [C-11]DAPA, and [C-11]AFM. *J. Cereb. Blood Flow Metab.* 22:1377–1398.

Hwang, D.R., Narendran, R., Huang, Y., Slifstein, M., Talbot, P.S., Sudo, Y., Van Berckel, B.N., Kegeles, L.S., Martinez, D., and Laruelle, M. (2004) Quantitative analysis of (-)-N-(11)C-propyl-norapomorphine in vivo binding in nonhuman primates. *J. Nucl. Med.* 45:338–346.

Ikoma, T., Suhara, T., Toyama, H., Ichimiya, T., Takano, A., Sudo, T., Inoue, M., Yasuno, T., and Suzuki, K. (2002) Quantitative analysis for estimating binding potential of the brain serotonin transporter with [C-11]McN5652. *J. Cereb. Blood Flow Metab.* 22:490–501.

Innis, R. (2007) Consensus nomenclature for in vivo imaging of reversibly binding radioligands. *J. Cereb. Blood Flow Metab.* 9:1533–1539

Jacobs, A.H., Li, H., Winkeler, A., Hilker, R., Knoess, C., Ruger, A., Galldiks, N., Schaller, B., Sobesky, J., Kracht, L., Monfared, P., Klein, M., Vollmar, S., Bauer, B., Wagner, R., Graf, R., Wienhard, K., Herholz, K., and Heiss, W.D. (2003) PET-based molecular imaging in neuroscience. *Eur. J. Nucl. Med. Mol. Imaging* 30:1051–1065.

Kegeles, L.S., Martinez, D., Kochan, L.D., Hwang, D.R., Huang, Y., Mawlawi, O., Suckow, R.F., Van Heertum, R.L., and Laruelle, M. (2002) NMDA antagonist effects on striatal dopamine release: positron emission tomography studies in humans. *Synapse* 43:19–29.

Laruelle, M. (2000) Imaging synaptic neurotransmission with in vivo binding competition techniques: a critical review. *J. Cereb. Blood Flow Metab.* 20:423–451.

Laruelle, M., D'Souza, C.D., Baldwin, R.M., Abi-Dargham, A., Kanes, S.J., Fingado, C.L., Seibyl, J.P., Zoghbi, S.S., Bowers, M.B., Jatlow, P., Charney, D.S., and Innis, R.B. (1997) Imaging D-2 receptor occupancy by endogenous dopamine in humans. *Neuropsychopharmacology* 17:162–174.

Laruelle, M., Iyer, R.N., Al-Tikriti, M.S., Zea-Ponce, Y., Malison, R., Zoghbi, S.S., Baldwin, R.M., Kung, H.F., Charney, D.S., Hoffer, P.B., Innis, R.B., and Bradberry, C.W. (1997) Microdialysis and SPECT measurements of amphetamine-induced dopamine release in nonhuman primates. *Synapse* 25:1–14.

Logan, J., Fowler, J.S., Dewey, S.L., Volkow, N.D., and Gatley, S.J. (2001) A consideration of the dopamine D2 receptor monomer-dimer equilibrium and the anomalous binding properties of the dopamine D2 receptor ligand, N-methyl spiperone. *J. Neural Transm.* 108:279–286.

Martinez, D., Gil, R., Slifstein, M., Hwang, D.R., Huang, Y., Perez, A., Kegeles, L., Talbot, P., Evans, S., Krystal, J., Laruelle, M., and Abi-Dargham, A. (2005) Alcohol dependence is associated with blunted dopamine transmission in the ventral striatum. *Biol. Psychiatry* 58:779–786.

Meyer, J.H., Wilson, A.A., Ginovart, N., Goulding, V., Hussey, D., Hood, K., and Houle, S. (2001) Occupancy of serotonin transporters by paroxetine and citalopram during treatment of depression: A [C-11]DASB PET imaging study. *Am. J. Psychiatry* 158: 1843–1849.

Narendran, R., Hwang, D.R., Slifstein, M., Talbot, P.S., Erritzoe, D., Huang, Y., Cooper, T.B., Martinez, D., Kegeles, L.S., Abi-Dargham, A., and Laruelle, M. (2004) In vivo vulnerability to competition by endogenous dopamine: comparison of the D2 receptor agonist radiotracer (-)-N-[11C]propyl-norapomorphine ([11C]NPA) with the D2 receptor antagonist radiotracer [11C]-raclopride. *Synapse* 52:188–208.

Ouchi, Y., Yoshikawa, E., Futatsubashi, M., Okada, H., Torizuka, T., and Sakamoto, M. (2002) Effect of simple motor performance on regional dopamine release in the striatum in Parkinson disease patients and healthy subjects: a positron emission tomography study. *J. Cereb. Blood Flow Metab.* 22:746–752.

Parsey, R.V., Hwang, D., Simpson, N., Kegeles, L., Anjilvel, S., Zea-Ponce, Y., Lombardo, I., Popilskis, S., van Heerthum, R., Mann, J.J., and Laruelle, M. (1998) Kinetic derivation of serotonin 5HT-1A receptor binding potential with [11C]carbonylway 100635 and competition studies with endogenous serotonin. *Neuroimage* 7:A10.

Parsey, R.V., Kegeles, L., Hwang, D.R., Simpson, N., Abi-Dargham, A., Mawlawi, O., Sfistein, M., Van Heertum, R., Mann, J.J., and Laruelle, M. (2000) Quantification of brain serotonin transporters in humans with (+) and (-)McNeil 5652. *J. Nucl. Med.* 41:1465–1477.

Phelps, M.E. (2000) PET: the merging of biology and imaging into molecular imaging. *J. Nucl. Med.* 41:661–681.

Pruessner, J.C., Champagne, F., Meaney, M.J., and Dagher, A. (2004) Dopamine release in response to a psychological stress in humans and its relationship to early life maternal care: a positron emission tomography study using [11C]raclopride. *J. Neurosci.* 24:2825–2831.

Schlaepfer, T.E., Pearlson, G.D., Wong, D.F., Marenco, S., and Dannals, R.F. (1997) PET study of competition between intravenous cocaine and [C-11]raclopride at dopamine receptors in human subjects. *Am. J. Psychiatry* 154:1209–1213.

Schoepp, D.D., Johnson, B.G., Wright, R.A., Salhoff, C.R., Mayne, N.G., Wu, S., Cockerman, S.L., Burnett, J.P., Belegaje, R., Bleakman, D., and Monn, J.A. (1997) LY354740 is a potent and highly selective group II metabotropic glutamate receptor agonist in cells expressing human glutamate receptors. *Neuropharmacology* 36:1–11.

Skaddan, M.B., Kilbourn, M.R., Snyder, S.E., and Sherman, P.S. (2001) Acetylcholinesterase inhibition increases in vivo N-(2-[18F]fluoroethyl)-4-piperidyl benzilate binding to muscarinic acetylcholine receptors. *J. Cereb. Blood Flow Metab.* 21:144–148.

Smith, G.S., Schloesser, R., Brodie, J.D., Dewey, S.L., Logan, J., Vitkun, S.A., Simkowitz, P., Hurley, A., Cooper, T., Volkow, N.D., and Cancro, R. (1998) Glutamate modulation of dopamine measured in vivo with positron emission tomography (PET) and 11C-raclopride in normal human subjects. *Neuropsychopharmacology* 18:18–25.

Strafella, A.P., Paus, T., Fraraccio, M., and Dagher, A. (2003) Striatal dopamine release induced by repetitive transcranial magnetic stimulation of the human motor cortex. *Brain* 126:2609–2615.

Suehiro, M., Scheffel, U., Dannals, R.F., Ravert, H.T., Ricaurte, G.A., and Wagner, H., Jr. (1993) A PET radiotracer for studying serotonin uptake sites: carbon-11-McN-5652Z. *J. Nucl. Med.* 34: 120–127.

Szabo, Z., McCann, U.D., Wilson, A.A., Scheffel, U., Owonikoko, T., Mathews, W.B., Ravert, H.T., Hilton, J., Dannals, R.F., and Ricaurte, G.A. (2002) Comparison of (+)-C-11-McN5652 and C-11-DASB as serotonin transporter radioligands under various experimental conditions. *J. Nucl. Med.* 43:678–692.

Szabo, Z., Scheffel, U., Suehiro, M., Dannals, R.F., Kim, S.E., Ravert, H.T., Ricaurte, G.A., and Wagner, H., Jr. (1995) Positron emission tomography of 5-HT transporter sites in the baboon brain with [11C]McN5652. *J. Cereb. Blood Flow Metab.* 15:798–805.

Talbot, P.S., and Laruelle, M. (2002) The role of in vivo molecular imaging with PET and SPECT in the elucidation of psychiatric drug action and new drug development. *Eur. Neuropsycho-pharmacol.* 12:503–511.

Thanos, P.K., Taintor, N.B., Rivera, S.N., Umegaki, H., Ikari, H., Roth, G., Ingram, D.K., Hitzemann, R., Fowler, J.S., Gatley, S.J., Wang, G.J., and Volkow, N.D. (2004) DRD2 gene transfer into the nucleus accumbens core of the alcohol preferring and nonpreferring rats attenuates alcohol drinking. *Alcohol. Clin. Exp. Res.* 28:720–728.

Tsukada, H., Sato, K., Nishiyama, S., and Harada, N. (2000) Development of muscarinic cholinergic receptor ligands with various affinities for receptors. *Neuroimage* 11:S51.

van Berckel, B.N., Kegeles, L.S., Waterhouse, R., Guo, N., Hwang, D.R., Huang, Y., Narendran, R., Van Heertum, R., and Laruelle, M. (2006) Modulation of amphetamine-induced dopamine release by group II metabotropic glutamate receptor agonist LY354740 in non-human primates studied with positron emission tomography. *Neuropsychopharmacology* 31:967–977.

Verhoeff, N.P., Kapur, S., Hussey, D., Lee, M., Christensen, B., Papatheodorou, G., and Zipursky, R.B. (2001) A simple method to measure baseline occupancy of neostriatal dopamine D2 receptors by dopamine in vivo in healthy subjects. *Neuropsychopharmacology* 25:213–223.

Volkow, N.D., Fowler, J.S., and Wang, G.J. (2003) The addicted human brain: insights from imaging studies. *J. Clin. Invest.* 111: 1444–1451.

Volkow, N.D., Wang, G.J., Begleiter, H., Porjesz, B., Fowler, J.S., Telang, F., Wong, C., Ma, Y., Logan, J., Goldstein, R., Alexoff, D., and Thanos, P.K. (2006) High levels of dopamine D2 receptors in unaffected members of alcoholic families: possible protective factors. *Arch. Gen. Psychiatry* 63:999–1008.

Vollenweider, F.X., Vontobel, P., Hell, D., and Leenders, K. (1999) 5-HT modulation of dopamine release in basal ganglia in psilocybin-induced psychosis in man—a PET study with [11C]raclopride. *Neuropsychopharmacology* 20:424–433.

Vollenweider, F.X., Vontobel, P., Oye, I., Hell, D., and Leenders, K.L. (2000) Effects of (S)-ketamine on striatal dopamine: a [11C]raclopride PET study of a model psychosis in humans. *J. Psychiatr. Res.* 34:35–43.

Willeit, M., Ginovart, N., Kapur, S., Houle, S., Hussey, D., Seeman, P., and Wilson, A.A. (2005) High-affinity states of human brain dopamine D2/3 receptors imaged by the agonist [(11)C]-(+)-PHNO. *Biol. Psychiatry* 59(5):389–394.

Wilson, A.A., Ginovart, N., Schmidt, M., Meyer, J.H., Threlkeld, P.G., and Houle, S. (2000) Novel radiotracers for imaging the serotonin transporter by positron emission tomography: synthesis, radiosynthesis, and in vitro and ex vivo evaluation of C-11-labeled 2-(phenylthio)araalkylamines. *J. Med. Chem.* 43:3103–3110.

Wilson, A.A., McCormick, P., Kapur, S., Willeit, M., Garcia, A., Hussey, D., Houle, S., Seeman, P., and Ginovart, N. (2005) Radiosynthesis and evaluation of [11C]-(+)-4-propyl-3,4,4a,5,6,10b-hexahydro-2H-naphtho[1,2-b][1,4]oxazin-9-ol as a potential radiotracer for in vivo imaging of the dopamine D2 high-affinity state with positron emission tomography. *J. Med. Chem.* 48:4153–4160.

Yokoi, F., Grunder, G., Biziere, K., Stephane, M., Dogan, A.S., Dannals, R.F., Ravert, H., Suri, A., Bramer, S., and Wong, D.F. (2002) Dopamine D2 and D3 receptor occupancy in normal humans treated with the antipsychotic drug aripiprazole (OPC 14597): a study using positron emission tomography and [11C]raclopride. *Neuropsychopharmacology* 27:248–259.

Zald, D.H., Boileau, I., El-Dearedy, W., Gunn, R., McGlone, F., Dichter, G.S., and Dagher, A. (2004) Dopamine transmission in the human striatum during monetary reward tasks. *J. Neurosci.* 24:4105–4112.

Zubieta, J.K., Heitzeg, M.M., Smith, Y.R., Bueller, J.A., Xu, K., Xu, Y., Koeppe, R.A., Stohler, C.S., and Goldman, D. (2003) COMT val158met genotype affects mu-opioid neurotransmitter responses to a pain stressor. *Science* 299:1240–1243.

Zubieta, J.K., Smith, Y.R., Bueller, J.A., Xu, Y., Kilbourn, M.R., Jewett, D.M., Meyer, C.R., Koeppe, R.A., and Stohler, C.S. (2001) Regional mu opioid receptor regulation of sensory and affective dimensions of pain. *Science* 293:311–315.

15 Human Postmortem Brain Research in Mental Illness Syndromes

MONICA BENEYTO, ETIENNE SIBILLE, AND DAVID A. LEWIS

Substantial advances in basic neuroscience, including understanding the molecular and cellular pathways of neural transmission and plasticity, offer new insights into the mechanisms that underlie brain dysfunction in psychiatric illnesses. However, testing of these ideas requires the examination of the human brain at the molecular, cellular, and circuitry levels, a resolution that can currently be obtained only by direct examination of brain tissue. Unlike other organ systems, brain tissue cannot be assessed via biopsy in the living patient with a psychiatric disorder; therefore, the availability of brain samples obtained at autopsy is critical for advancing the field. As a result, interest in postmortem studies has been renewed over the last two decades, despite previous criticisms that the problems and confounds were too numerous or challenging to control (Plum, 1972). Pioneering work by the leaders of the renaissance in postmortem studies of psychiatric illness (Bracha and Kleinman, 1984; Kleinman et al., 1985; Bracha and Kleinman, 1986; Kovelman and Scheibel, 1986; Benes and Bird, 1987; Benes, Majocha, et al., 1987; Benes, Matthysse, et al., 1987; Mann, Arango, et al., 1989; Mann, Marzuk, et al., 1989; Arango et al., 1990; Benes, 1998) and the application of new investigational techniques and more rigorous methods of quantification have led to the continuing improvement in the design and conduct of postmortem studies.

The critical levels of resolution provided by postmortem studies are complementary to genetic and brain imaging approaches to the study of mental illnesses. For example, for many types of genetic findings, the potential biological significance of a putative susceptibility genetic variant is strengthened by evidence that the expression level of the encoded transcription product is altered in the brain. Similarly, findings from neuroimaging studies of regional patterns of functional activation, ligand receptor binding, or volumetric differences depend upon postmortem studies to identify or confirm the neurobiological basis for the observations.

Advances in understanding the molecular, cellular, and circuitry alterations in psychiatric illnesses depend directly upon the number and quality of available brain specimens and the appropriate implementation of experimental designs that maximize the yield of interpretable data and minimize the influence of confounding factors. For example, a recent study of the methodological considerations for gene expression profiling in postmortem human brain found that clinical data, tissue, RNA, and technique quality must all be considered as potential confounding factors (Atz et al., 2007). Consequently, advances in postmortem human brain studies require (*1*) well-characterized brain specimens, (*2*) well-conceptualized or designed studies, and (*3*) well-controlled confounds (Lewis, 2002). In the following sections, we discuss the approaches that can facilitate the achievement of these goals.

CHARACTERIZATION OF THE SUBJECTS

Clinical Diagnosis

As with any area of investigation of psychiatric disorders, postmortem studies depend upon syndromal diagnoses based on clinical features. Thus, as in genetic neuroimaging or other studies, the information value of a postmortem study is only as good as the amount and accuracy of the knowledge that supports the presence of the disorder under investigation. Consequently, the same emphasis on the systematic acquisition of clinical data and of reliability in the diagnostic process that characterizes state-of-the-art clinical studies must be applied in postmortem investigations. In addition, it is also essential to know, with a similar level of certainty, that the normal comparison subjects do not have a history of a psychiatric disorder. For example, in our experience with subjects identified through a medical examiner's office, subjects for whom the initially available clinical records indicated no history of psychiatric illness are commonly found to have a diagnosable psychiatric disorder, especially substance abuse or dependence.

Just as structured interviews, with documented reliability, are state-of-the-art for clinical studies, the same diagnostic rigor is an essential element in the characterization of subjects for postmortem studies. Structured, antemortem diagnostic assessments have been used quite effectively in postmortem studies of subjects who are elderly, chronically hospitalized, and with schizophrenia (Arnold et al., 1998; Sokolov et al., 2000). The course of illness and substantial cognitive impairment of many of these subjects suggest that they represent a unique and important subgroup of subjects with schizophrenia, but their distinctive clinical features limit the extent to which findings from these studies can be generalized to other forms or earlier stages of the illness.

Such prospective, antemortem assessments are not possible for studies of individuals in the early to mid-stages of a psychiatric disorder who are most likely to die by suicide, or by accidental or natural causes apparently unrelated to the primary disease process. Using chart review to obtain clinical information on these subjects has several limitations. First, the amount and detail of the available information depend upon the approach used by the clinicians recording the data and the extent to which the full chart history is actually available for review. Second, chart review is limited to subjects who have been seen by the medical profession. However, medical records can be a valuable source of information in concert with "psychological autopsies" that involve structured interviews of surviving relatives and friends and directed questioning of health care providers. Consequently, the use of psychological autopsies represents the most effective approach at present for the study of subjects who are nonelderly, noninstitutionalized, and with psychiatric disorders and comparison subjects. The value of this approach has been demonstrated by Kelly and Mann (1996), who found that comparison of research diagnoses made solely by psychological autopsy with diagnoses made antemortem by a clinician generated a kappa coefficient of 0.85 for Axis I diagnoses, a degree of agreement similar to that found in reliability studies involving direct interviews with patients. However, it may be that for certain disorders, chart review can provide a reliable research diagnosis. For example, Deep-Soboslay et al. (2005) found that for subjects with schizophrenia, the agreement was high between chart review alone and interview with a surviving relative (kappa coefficient = 0.94), whereas the agreement was much lower for bipolar disorder (0.58) and major depressive disorder (0.68).

The information obtained from antemortem assessments or psychological autopsies requires formulation into consensus *Diagnostic and Statistical Manual of Mental Disorders* (*DSM-IV*; American Psychiatric Association, 1994) diagnoses. Using an independent panel of experienced research clinicians to make these diagnoses avoids the potential biases of investigators who will be studying the postmortem tissue and provides additional parallels to the approaches that produce high diagnostic reliability in clinical studies.

Neuropathological Assessment

Although psychiatric disorders do not have stigmata that can be detected by standard neuropathological examination, these assessments are clearly important to exclude other diseases that may mimic the clinical features of psychiatric disorders and to characterize the presence of brain abnormalities that might affect study design or interpretation. Clearly, the types and incidence of neuropathological abnormalities are likely to differ across psychiatric subjects as a function of a variety of factors (for example, age, cause and manner of death). However, not every abnormality detected on neuropathological exam necessarily represents an exclusion condition, an important consideration given the importance of maximizing the sample sizes utilized in postmortem studies. Thus, the goal of neuropathological inquiry is to ascertain the presence of all abnormalities so that the potential impact of each can be considered in the design of each study. At the same time, it is important to minimize the impact that neuropathological assessment has on the availability of brain tissue for subsequent studies. The involvement of an interested neuropathologist in the brain collection process makes it possible to approach the assessment on an individualized basis, guided by the clinical record and gross tissue inspection to obtain standard tissue samples and additional ones as appropriate, with minimal disruption of the preferred tissue blocking approach.

Design of postmortem studies

The design of postmortem studies requires attention to a number of important issues that may affect outcome and interpretation, some of which are unique to these types of studies. One of the most difficult issues is whether the available postmortem tissue specimens will actually support the type of investigation under consideration. That is, the investigator must decide, independent of the interest or importance of the question to be addressed, if the characteristics of the available tissue specimens can actually provide interpretable data. If the available tissue specimens are poorly characterized or suboptimal in some respect (for example, poor ribonucleic acid [RNA] integrity), then the investigator must decide if potentially flawed or misleading data are better than no data at all.

Statistical methods can be used to correct for certain differences in demographic (for example, age, sex) or other (for example, brain pH, postmortem interval [PMI], tissue storage time) variables across subject groups. However, the matching of individual pairs (or triads) of subjects from each diagnostic group as closely as possible on these variables has several advantages. First, matching helps ensure that the mean and variance for a given independent measure will be comparable across subject groups. Second, for assays in which tissue samples from all subjects cannot be processed together, matching of subjects across diagnostic groups, and always processing tissue from matched subjects together, helps reduce the potentially confounding influence of interassay variation. Third, matching subjects makes it possible to compare the results of different statistical models, in which subject pair and/or one or more of the matching variables are entered as blocking variables or covariates (e.g., see Pierri et al., 2001). Comparable results across models provide additional support for the finding of interest. However, this strategy requires the availability of a large number of subjects in the comparison groups of interest to adequately match subjects on the relevant variables.

The development of stereological methods has clearly demonstrated the importance of using systematic uniform random sampling to obtain valid estimates of the density or absolute number of objects in a region (Dorph-Petersen et al., 2004; Dorph-Petersen et al., 2007). That is, ideally the entire region of interest is sampled in a fashion such that every object of interest has an equal probability of being counted or measured. By extrapolation, estimates of the tissue concentration of a given molecule would also benefit from a similar approach to selecting the bits of tissue to be sampled. However, limitations in tissue specimens can present problems in this area so that the best possible sampling (for example, systematic and random, even if the lack of availability of the entire structure of interest prevents uniform sampling) procedure should be used, with explicit acknowledgment of the resulting limitations in interpretation. Because using a larger sample of subjects may help mitigate the problems associated with less precise measurements, the clear solution for advancing the field is to increase the availability of resources so that an appropriate number of brains is adequately sampled in all studies.

MEASURES OF INTEREST

Numerous techniques are currently used to study disease-related abnormalities in the levels of gene products in postmortem human brain samples. The first step in protein synthesis is the expression of a unique gene; this is achieved by the production of a primary RNA transcript by gene transcription that is complementary to the entire gene sequence. This primary transcript is intermediate and contains sequences encoding introns and exons. Additional processing removes the intronic sequences, and the exon-complementary regions are spliced together to generate the final messenger RNA (mRNA). Following transcription, mature mRNA is translated into a protein molecule on ribosomes at the endoplasmic reticulum. Proteins then may undergo extensive post-translational modifications (glycosylation, phosphorylation, etc.), proteolysis, or assembly into protein complexes. Each of these processes has an intermediate product that can be directly measured in postmortem brain tissue; however, it is important to consider the factors that can affect those measurements in ways not related to the disease process of interest. Each technique has its strengths and limitations in the analysis of gene products that must be kept in mind in designing studies and interpreting results.

Messenger Ribonucleic Acid (mRNA)

Isolation of intact mRNA is essential for many techniques used in gene expression analysis. Northern analysis, in situ hybridization, and microarray analysis (especially when priming with oligo [dT] sequences) require RNA of extremely high integrity. Reverse transcriptase-polymerase chain reaction (RT-PCR), however, involves analysis of smaller regions of RNA (generally from fewer than 100 to 1000 nucleotides) and may be more tolerant of partially degraded RNA. A recent study, in which critical factors in gene expression in postmortem human studies were analyzed, showed that the strongest predictor of gene expression was total RNA quality (Lipska et al., 2006). Other significant factors included pH, PMI, age, and the duration of the agonal state, but their importance depended on the transcript measured, brain region analyzed, and diagnosis. Thus, it is essential to check RNA integrity before gene expression analysis in all postmortem studies (see RNA integrity estimates below) and include the other potential confounding factors as regressors in the statistical analysis of the data. Although used as a matching factor in postmortem studies of transcript expression, previous reports have shown that PMI is not predictive of RNA stability (Trotter et al., 2002; Stan et al., 2006).

Protein

Evaluating the protein product(s) of a given gene provides an important and complementary approach to assessments of the expression level of the cognate mRNA. The level of transcription of a gene gives only a rough estimate of its level of expression into a protein. An mRNA produced in abundance may be degraded rapidly or translated inefficiently, resulting in a small amount of protein. In addition, many transcripts give rise to more than one protein through alternative splicing or post-translational modifications. Immunocytochemistry, Western blot analysis, radioimmunoassay, and immunoprecipitation are some of the methods used in proteomics to study the translation of mRNAs into the final gene product. These techniques use specific antibodies to assess qualitatively the cellular and regional expression patterns of proteins (for example, immunocytochemistry) or to determine quantitatively the amount of protein in a given sample (for example, Western blots). Other protocols, such as autoradiography, use specific ligands which by binding to proteins (for example, receptors) can provide quantitative data on the expression and functional integrity of the targeted molecules.

A special consideration for immunocytochemistry in postmortem brain studies is the method of tissue fixation, which prevents the diffusion and degradation of the protein to be detected. Immunoreactivity can be affected by the type of fixative and by the duration of fixation. Antigen-retrieval techniques, such as exposure of tissue specimens to elevated temperature or microwave irradiation, have produced remarkable recovery of immunoreactivity (Rangell and Keller, 2000). However, limited data exist about whether this recovery is consistent across samples with different fixation exposure times. It is also important to note that fixation and other processing and storage conditions of tissue can produce substantial tissue shrinkage (Dorph-Petersen et al., 2005) that may be difficult to assess or account for, depending upon the type of study to be conducted, and that can substantially bias measures of regional brain volumes or density of neural structures. Interestingly, no studies to date have examined whether the amount of tissue shrinkage differs as a function of diagnosis.

Many proteins undergo post-translational modifications that profoundly affect their activities; for example, some proteins are not active until they become phosphorylated. Phosphoproteomics and glycoproteomics, which assess these post-translational modifications, are currently being evaluated in postmortem human brain research. However, the phosphorylation state of proteins can change very rapidly after death (Li et al., 2003), raising concerns about the potential yield of such studies. Most proteins function in collaboration with other proteins, and one goal of proteomics is to identify which proteins interact. Methods to probe protein–protein interactions include protein microarrays, immunoaffinity chromatography followed by mass spectrometry, and combinations of experimental methods such as phage display and computational methods. For example, two recent papers assessed the functional integrity of proteins and the activation of their signaling cascades in postmortem tissue (Hahn et al., 2006; Dwivedi et al., 2007). In these kinds of studies, the protein extracts from the postmortem tissues need to be prepared under conditions in which protein–protein interactions are maintained, which requires, among other things, the availability of tissue samples in which protein degradation is limited. Furthermore, the degree to which the results of these protocols correspond to *in vivo* measurements is unclear.

POTENTIAL CONFOUNDS

Premortem, perimortem, and postmortem factors can affect the quality of the results in mRNA and protein detection studies in human brain research. Thus, it is essential to determine as fully as possible the presence of such factors and to systematically assess their potential impact on the biological measures of interest.

Premortem Factors

Comorbid conditions, such as alcohol, nicotine, or other substance abuse, are common in many psychiatric disorders. Prevalence of current abuse/dependence in psychiatric inpatients ranges from 12% to 60% (Brady et al., 1991; Havassy and Arns, 1998; Cantwell et al., 1999), and from 48% to 64% for lifetime abuse/dependence (Brady et al., 1991; Dixon et al., 1991). Among outpatients, rates of lifetime and current abuse/dependence vary from 6% to 60% (Gogek, 1991; el Guebaly and Hodgins, 1992; Fowler et al., 1998). In particular, the lifetime prevalence rate of substance abuse among people with schizophrenia is close to 50% (Dixon et al., 1991; Mueser et al., 1995), with prevalence rates for current substance abuse as high as 65% in some samples (Mueser, Bellack, and Blanchard, 1992; Mueser, Yarnold, and Bellack, et al., 1992). Similarly, individuals with schizophrenia and bipolar disorder have extremely high rates of nicotine use, 2 to 3 times higher than seen in the general population and considerably higher than among subjects with other psychiatric illnesses. In the United States, about one fourth of the population are smokers (Hymowitz et al., 1997), whereas more than 70% of patients with schizophrenia are nicotine dependent (Ziedonis and George, 1997; Van Dongen, 1999). Among other drugs, cannabis and cocaine are the most commonly used in the dual-diagnosis population (Soyka et al., 1993; Dixon et al., 1991; Hambrecht and Hafner, 2000; Duke et al., 2001).

Each of these comorbid conditions can affect measures of interest in postmortem studies. For example, drugs of abuse such as cocaine and amphetamine produce an experience-dependent structural plasticity that alters dendritic length and complexity in certain brain areas (Robinson et al., 2001; Robinson et al., 2002; Crombag et al., 2005). Alcohol abuse and smoking have documented effects on the expression of specific gene products (Liu et al., 2004; Flatscher-Bader et al., 2005; Flatscher-Bader and Wilce, 2006; Flatscher-Bader et al., 2006). Chronic alcoholism affects a number of signaling cascades and transcription factors, which in turn result in distinct gene expression patterns, such as pronounced differences in expression of myelin-related genes and genes involved in protein trafficking in the cerebral cortex (Liu et al., 2004). Significant changes in the expression of known alcohol-responsive genes, and genes involved in calcium, cyclic adenosine monophosphate (cAMP), and thyroid signaling pathways, have also been identified (Mayfield et al., 2002). Nicotine administration also modulates the expression level of a variety of genes, including those involved in transcriptional activation and in catecholamine and neuropeptide synthesis. In animal models, chronic exposure to nicotine induces long-term increases in the mRNA expression levels of genes involved in the regulation of food intake and energy expenditure, such as neuropeptide Y (NPY), orexins, and their receptors (Kane et al., 2000; Li et al., 2000).

The exclusion of all subjects with any history of a substance abuse disorder, though seemingly ideal from the perspective of eliminating the impact of confounding factors, is problematic from other perspectives. For example, the high incidence of these confounds in the subject populations of interest, and the limited availability of postmortem tissue, means that the resulting studies would likely have very small sample sizes. In addition, the resulting sample would be highly biased to only a certain subpopulation of individuals with the diagnosis of interest. Thus, a better alternative is the comparison within and across diagnostic groups of subjects with and without comorbid substance use histories. Within the diagnostic group of interest, if the subgroups with and without substance use do not differ on the measure of interest, and both show similar divergence from a normal comparison group, then one can provisionally conclude that the comorbid factor does not influence the measure of interest, and thus that the observed alteration reflects the underlying disease process.

Clearly, assessment of the potential impact of psychotropic agents in postmortem studies requires knowledge of the presence of such agents. At present, this assessment is usually limited to assays of blood or other bodily fluids. The extension of such evaluations to brain tissue and hair would, respectively, provide data that may be more biologically relevant and that would reflect exposure over the several months preceding death.

Similarly, the interpretation of findings from a postmortem study requires determining whether the measure of interest is influenced by the pharmacological treatment of the illness under investigation. This determination depends upon knowledge of which medications the subject received, for how long, and at what dosage. However, such detailed information is difficult to obtain, frequently incomplete, confounded by adherence issues, and usually not available to the same degree across subjects (with the possible exception of individuals who have been chronically hospitalized). Even when such information is available, it is difficult to know how to make comparisons across subjects: for example, is the relevant measure dose at time of death, total life time dose, and so on? Finally, a substantial percentage of subjects have received more than one psychotropic medication, and the extent to which drug interactions confound the picture is difficult to assess.

Because adequate samples of postmortem brain specimens from subjects who were never medicated with a given psychiatric disorder are not available, several less direct approaches must be used to address the influence of psychotropic medications. These approaches include (*1*) the comparison of data from subjects who were on or off the medications of interest at the time of death, (*2*) the examination of subjects with other disorders who were treated with the same medications, and (*3*) the use of animal models that mimic the clinical treatment of the disorder under investigation.

Certainly, the first two approaches have obvious, and difficult to control, potential confounds. Long-term exposure to psychotropic medications, as is typical in the treatment of most psychiatric disorders, may have effects on brain morphology, neurochemistry, or gene expression that persist for a substantial period of time after the drug is discontinued. In addition, even though the same agents are utilized, the pharmacological treatment of other disorders may be different than that of the disease of interest. For example, compared with schizophrenia, the treatment of other psychotic disorders with antipsychotic medications tends to be more intermittent or for a shorter duration of time.

In the case of animal models of drug effects, studies in rodents frequently involve dosage and/or length of treatment parameters that do not reflect the human treatment condition. These limitations can be overcome through studies in nonhuman primates that involve extended periods of treatment with medication-dosing regimens that produce serum drug levels demonstrated to be therapeutic in humans. For example, chronic exposure to antipsychotic medications, in particular haloperidol and olanzapine, in macaque monkeys was associated with an 8%–11% reduction in mean fresh brain weights, with the differences between treatment conditions most robust in the frontal and parietal lobes (Dorph-Petersen et al., 2005). However, the potential problem of species differences, and the possibility that the medications of interest may have different effects on the brain of an individual with a psychiatric illness than on the normal brain, must be kept in mind. Despite the limitations of each of these three approaches individually, convergent findings across them should lead to reasonable conclusions about the extent to which psychotropic medications account for any observed brain differences between subjects who are psychiatrically ill and normal comparisons.

Perimortem Factors

The manner and cause of death also have potential influences on the measures of interest. For example, in cases of prolonged agonal state and terminal stress, conditions such as hypoxia or ischemia activate anaerobic metabolic pathways, predominantly the lactic acid cycle, resulting in an increased production of acid equivalents, responsible for inter- and intracellular acidosis (Rehncrona et al., 1985; Yates et al., 1990). Evidence from analyses of postmortem human brain has shown that brain tissue pH is decreased by prolonged agonal states accompanied by hypoxia (Hardy et al., 1985; Kingsbury et al., 1995). Furthermore, a recent study suggests that increased levels of lactate, possibly due to antipsychotic medications, are associated with decreased pH in postmortem human brains of patients with schizophrenia (Halim et al., 2007). On the other hand, brain tissue pH appears to remain constant across postmortem delays (Kingsbury et al., 1995) and has also been reported to be unaffected by freezer storage time (Stan et al., 2006). Brain tissue pH also seems to be similar across different regions within a given brain (Harrison et al., 1995; Mexal et al., 2005; Mexal et al., 2006). Although protein immunoreactivity and ligand binding to receptors show no change related to brain pH (Harrison et al., 1995), brain pH does predict enzymatic activity (Perry et al., 1982; Stan et al., 2006), RNA yield (Taylor et al., 1986; Yates et al., 1990), and mRNA integrity (Harrison et al., 1995; Kingsbury et al., 1995; Johnston et al., 1997; Bahn et al., 2001; Tomita et al., 2004).

Interestingly, a recent microarray study revealed a functional specificity of changed genes related to pH. With lower pH values, the expression of transcripts encoding stress-response proteins and transcription factors was altered, suggesting that the change in their tissue levels is not simply due to an overall RNA degradation in response to low pH but reflected a biological response in living cells in response to stress (Li et al., 2004; Vawter et al., 2006).

Reliable RNA expression and protein data can be obtained from postmortem brains with relatively long PMIs (see below) if the agonal factors and acidosis are not severe. Although pH values are correlated with RNA integrity, a higher pH does not guarantee intact RNA. For example, an analysis of a large brain collection revealed that several diagnostic groups had significantly lower pH values than other groups, but they did not have significantly lower RNA integrity (Webster, 2006). Consequently, RNA integrity must be assessed for every case before it is included in a postmortem study.

Measurement of mRNA levels in postmortem tissue is based on the assumption that these levels reflect the amount of transcripts in vivo. The kinetics of degradation of newly synthesized cytoplasmic poly(A)-bearing RNA have been examined in resting human lymphocytes (Berger and Cooper, 1975). Two classes were identified, a labile component with a short half-life and a very stable component that remains undiminished across long time periods. These findings raise the possibility that partial degradation could cause a variable bias in the quantification of different transcripts (Auer et al., 2003). Furthermore, in the case of postmortem samples, the integrity of RNA molecules results from a combination of circumstances that can include in vivo, in situ, and in vitro events. Indeed, active exo- and endonuclease activity may occur in live tissue during early postmortem periods, and autocatalytic degradation generates random fragmentation at later times in dead tissue or during extraction/storage of RNA material.

18S/28S ratio

Because mRNA comprises only 1%–3% of total RNA, it is difficult to detect. Ribosomal RNA (rRNA), on the other hand, makes up more than 80% of the total RNA sample, with the majority of that comprising the 28S and 18S rRNA species. Messenger ribonucleic acid quality traditionally has been assessed by electrophoresis of total RNA followed by staining with ethidium bromide. This method relies on the assumption that rRNA quality and quantity reflect that of the underlying mRNA population. According to this, intact total RNA run on a denaturing gel will have sharp, clear 28S and 18S rRNA bands (Fig. 15.1, Panel A). The 28S rRNA band should be approximately twice as intense as the 18S rRNA band.

With increasing degradation, heights of 18S and 28S peaks gradually decrease and additional "degradation peak signals" appear in a molecular weight range between small RNAs and the 18S peak (Fig. 15.1, Panel B). The ratio of the average degradation peak signal to the 18S peak signal multiplied by 100 is referred to as the *degradation factor*. This analysis has been tested on 19 tissues of seven organisms, and it is a reproducible parameter for degradation of mammalian RNA (Auer et al., 2003).

A 2:1 ratio (28S:18S) is a good indication that the RNA is completely intact. Because mammalian 28S and 18S rRNAs are approximately 5 kb and 2 kb in size, the theoretical 28S:18S ratio is approximately 2.7:1; but a 2:1 ratio has long been considered the benchmark for intact RNA. Partially degraded RNA will have a smeared appearance, will lack the sharp rRNA bands, or will not exhibit the 2:1 ratio of high-quality RNA. Completely degraded RNA will appear as a very low molecular weight smear (Fig. 15.1, Panel A).

Isolating RNA from human tissue presents challenges that are not always present in experimental animal work. Confounding factors almost guarantee that human total RNA will rarely have a 28S:18S rRNA ratio of 2:1.

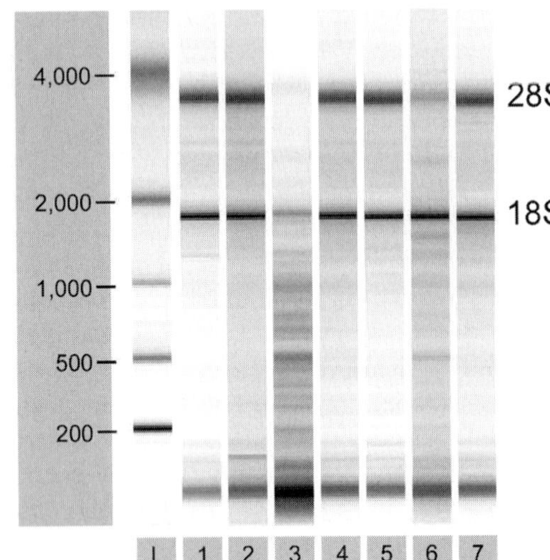

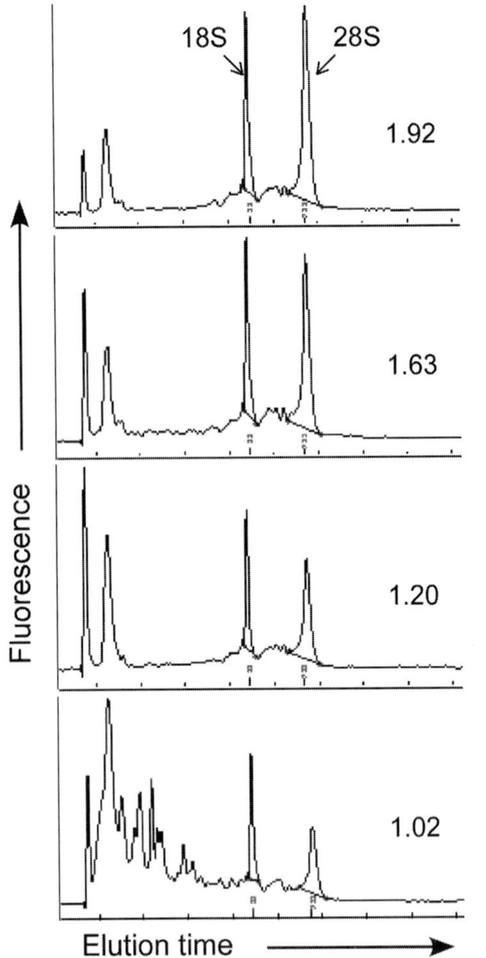

FIGURE 15.1 Ribonucleic acid (RNA) integrity profile. (*A*) Virtual gel from human brain RNA samples run on an Agilent 2100 Bioanalyzer. 28S and 18S ribosomal RNAs are clearly visible in high quality samples (lanes 1, 2, 4, 5, 7, and 8; 28S/18S ratios in 1.30 to 1.54 range; RNA integrity number [RIN] in 7.3 to 8.5 range). Lanes 3 and 6 show degradation with shifts toward lower molecular weight and laddering appearance (Lane 3, 28S/18S n/a; RIN = 3; Lane 6, 28S/18S = 0.51; RIN = 5.7). Lane L, molecular weight markers. Low molecular weight RNA species are present in the lower part of the gel lanes. (*B*) Bioanalyzer chromatograms of RNA samples with decreasing 28S/18S ratio (values indicated in graphs). Note the progressive shift to the left in peak heights from 18S and 28S to lower molecular weight with decreasing RNA quality.

Although crisp 28S and 18S rRNA bands are indicative of intact RNA, it is less clear how these long-lived and abundant molecules actually reflect the quality of the underlying mRNA population, which turns over much more rapidly.

A drawback to using denaturing agarose gels to assess integrity RNA is the amount of RNA required for visualization. Generally, at least 200 ng to 1 μg of RNA must be loaded onto a denaturing agarose gel to be visualized with ethidium bromide. Some small RNA preparations, such as those from laser capture microdissected samples, produce very low yields. In these cases, it may be impossible to spare 200 ng of RNA to assess integrity before proceeding with the expression profiling application. Alternative nucleic acid stains, such as SYBR Gold and SYBRï Green II RNA gel stain from Molecular Probes (Eugene, OR), offer a significant increase in sensitivity compared to the traditional ethidium bromide stain in agarose gels.

RNA integrity number (RIN)

An alternative to traditional gel-based analysis that integrates the quantification of RNA samples with quality assessment in a quick and simple assay uses a combination of microfluidics, capillary electrophoresis, and fluorescent dyes that bind to nucleic acid to simultaneously evaluate RNA concentration and integrity. Automated determination of RIN has provided a direct measure of RNA quality requiring as little as 10 ng of RNA per analysis. In addition to assessing RNA integrity, this automated system also provides a good estimate of RNA concentration and purity (that is, rRNA contamination in mRNA preparations) in a sample. In this system, an integrity number is automatically assigned to a eukaryote total RNA sample. The 28S:18S rRNA ratio is calculated by integrating the areas of 18S and 28S rRNA peaks and then dividing the area of the 18S rRNA peak into the area of the 28S rRNA peak. Using this tool, sample integrity is no longer determined by the ratio of the ribosomal bands, but by the entire electrophoretic trace of the RNA sample. This includes the presence or absence of degradation products. In this way, interpretation of an electropherogram is facilitated, comparison of samples is enabled, and replication of experiments is ensured. The assigned RIN is independent of sample concentration, instrument, and analyst, and therefore represents a legitimate standard for RNA integrity. It correlates with tissue pH and incorporates the extent of RNA degradation with the presence of 28S/18S peaks (Ross et al., 1992; Colangelo et al., 2002; Jones et al., 2006) (Fig. 15.1, Panel B). However, there is a limitation in the use of RIN as an indicator of mRNA quality. Under certain circumstances, some specific transcripts show special degradation rates (Buesa et al., 2004; Barrachina et al., 2006); this suggests the necessity of verifying individual mRNA quality within an experiment.

3′/5′ ratio

3′/5′ ratios are measurements of RNA quality that relate to specific technical aspects of oligonucleotide microarrays. Deoxyribonucleic acid microarray technology relies on the monitoring of relative changes in RNA abundance between samples. Microarrays investigate changes in transcriptomes (the set of mRNA expressed in a tissue sample), and results are therefore particularly dependent on RNA quality. Here we briefly describe how 3′/5′ ratios are generated, how they are influenced by RNA quality, and how 28S/18S ratios and RIN numbers correlate with 3′/5′ ratios and can predict the quality of array results.

The array technology is essentially an extension of Southern hybridization, in which the labeled probe is free in solution and the target mRNA sequence is fixed on a solid phase. To generate probes corresponding to expressed mRNAs, total RNA is reverse-transcribed and converted into double-stranded complementary

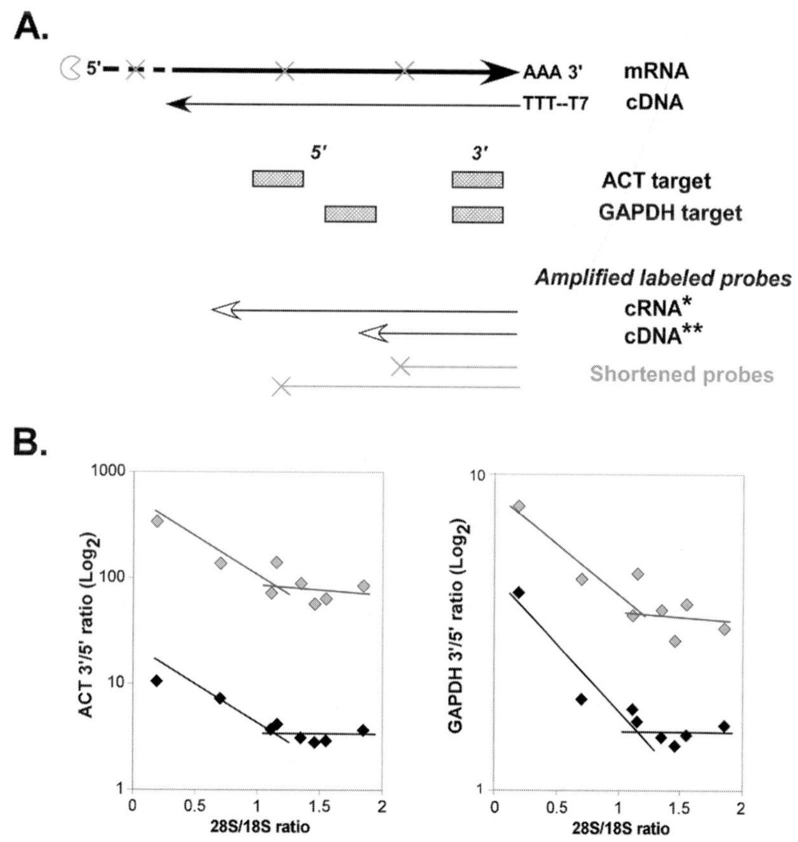

FIGURE 15.2 3′/5′ ratio and ribonucleic acid (RNA) integrity correspondence. (*A*) Messenger ribonucleic acid (mRNA) are reverse-transcribed using poly-A primers that also incorporate promoter sequences (for example, T7) used for "copying" or amplifying labeled probes (double-stranded complementary deoxyribonucleic acid [cDNA] step is omitted for clarity). Labeled probes "recognize" or hybridize to targets for control genes (*ACT* and *GAPDH*) that correspond to sequences on the mRNA located at increasing distances from the 3′ tail of transcripts. Relevant degradation mechanisms are illustrated on the mRNA strand (5′ exonuclease and endonuclease/fragmentation; Red). Labeled probes generated with the standard Affymetrix protocol (cRNA*) average ~2KB in size. Alternate protocols commonly used with low amount of starting RNA (for example, laser-capture RNA material) generate shorter probes (cDNA*) that average ~1kb in size (Nugen Ovations amplification system). Depending on the site of fragmentation on the RNA template, shortened or truncated cRNA*/cDNA* labeled probes are produced. (*B*) 3′/5′ ratios obtained from cRNA* (black squares) and cDNA* (grey squares) generated from eight different human brain RNA samples with variable levels of RNA integrity (X-axis). Low 28S/18S ratios (< ~1.2) correspond to higher fragmentation levels, which resulted in lower hybridization at 5′ targets, higher 3′/5′ ratios, and arrays with poor quality control parameters. Typically, cDNA* generate higher 3′/5′ ratios due to shorter probes that only rarely cover the 5′ target regions of control genes. Importantly, cRNA* and cDNA** displayed similar biphasic curves with adequate overall array quality only in the 1.2 to 2 28S/18S ratio range.

deoxyribonucleic acid (cDNA), using primers that are complementary to the poly(A) tails located at the 3′ end of mRNAs (Fig. 15.2, Panel A). The length of the labeled probes will depend on the integrity of the RNA template and on the reverse transcription and amplification steps (Fig. 15.2, Panel A). Thus, this labeling protocol is sensitive to 5′-end degradation and internal fragmentation. For instance, fragmented mRNA will limit the extent of reverse-transcription and yield short labeled probes, while intact mRNA will allow for longer probes to be generated. Oligonucleotide microarrays from Affymetrix, Inc (Santa Clara, CA) have incorporated in their array designs different sets of targets for several control genes. These different targets are located at different distances from the 3′-end of the respective control mRNAs. Differences in intensity of hybridization at proximal (3′) versus distal (5′) probes can therefore be used to estimate the proportion of intact to truncated or shortened RNA templates, as the probability of an internal break being present in the template increases with the distance of the target from the 3′-end poly(A) tail. Targets have been designed for the actin and glyceraldehyde-3-phosphate dehydrogenase (GAPDH) genes so that values for 3′/5′ ratios that are close to 1 correspond to optimal RNA integrity for array experiments, while ratios higher than 3 are indicative of levels of RNA degradation that will compromise the reliability of the array results (Figure 15.2, Panel B).

Postmortem Factors

Factors that occur after death can also affect the measures of interest in postmortem human studies. For example, the PMI, the elapsed time between death and the freezing or immersion of brain tissue in fixative, is a frequently employed measure of the quality of postmortem brain specimens. The effect of PMI on a given dependent variable may be complex, and it is not always the case that a short PMI ensures a valid assessment of the measure of interest. The nonlinear nature of PMI effects has been demonstrated in several studies. For example, a study of the impact of PMI on the somal size of a specific subtype of interneurons in adjacent blocks of monkey neocortex revealed that PMI predicted somal size between 30 minutes to 12 hours, but not between 12 and 48 hours (Hayes et al., 1991). The tissue concentrations of certain members of a family of proteins may also change in different ways as a function of PMI. Figure 15.3 compares the tissue concentrations of three pro-somatostatin-derived peptides in biopsy samples of monkey prefrontal cortex frozen at different time intervals after removal, creating a range of PMIs (Hayes et al., 1991). The concentration of one peptide, somatostatin-28, declined to 10%–20% of baseline levels at the 10-minute PMI, whereas the concentrations of two other peptides, somatostatin-14 and somatostatin-28 (1-12), actually increased during the same time interval, presumably as a consequence of the cleaving of somatostatin-28. However, by 12-hour PMI, each of these peptides showed a different relative tissue concentration compared with its baseline level. That is, somatostatin-28 levels remained stable at about 20% of baseline, somatostatin-14 levels were approximately 60% of baseline, and somatostatin-28 (1-12) levels had returned to baseline levels. Similarly complex PMI-related effects have also been observed for different isoforms of the same protein (Lewis et al., 1993, 1994).

Postmortem interval may also have a differential effect on immunoreactivity for the same protein in different brain structures, and even across layers within the same region of the cerebral cortex. For example, an antibody directed against nonphosphorylated epitopes of neurofilament proteins (NFP) identifies a subpopulation of neurons in the human entorhinal cortex with characteristic regional and laminar patterns of distribution (Beall and Lewis, 1992). In the intermediate subdivision of the human entorhinal cortex, intensely immunoreactive NFP-positive neurons are present in layers 2 and 5 (Fig. 15.4, panel A). Interestingly, in a pilot study of schizophrenia, NFP-immunoreactive neurons were absent in layer 2 but were clearly detectable in layer 5 (Fig. 15.4, panel B), suggesting the possibility of laminar- and neuron-specific disturbance in this illness (Lewis and Akil, 1997). However, in adjacent thin tissue blocks of monkey entorhinal cortex fixed at varying PMIs, NFP-immunoreactive neurons were clearly present in layers 2 and 5 following a 30-minute PMI (Fig. 15.4, panel C), but in layer 2 the overall

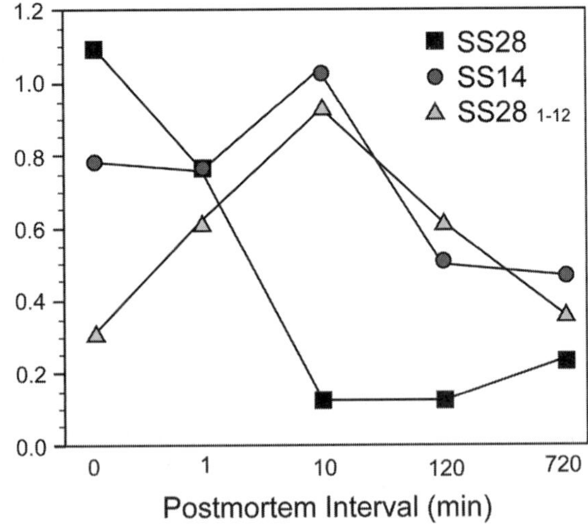

FIGURE 15.3 Tissue concentrations (ng/mg protein) of three pro-somatostatin-derived peptides in biopsied tissue from area 9 of monkey prefrontal cortex following different "postmortem intervals." Note the complex and distinctive patterns of change in the concentrations of somatostatin-28 (SS28), somatostatin-14 (SS14), and somatostatin-28(1-12). Data adapted from Hayes et al. (1991).

intensity of immunoreactivity was substantially reduced at 12-hour PMI and was undetectable following a 24-hour PMI (Fig. 15.4, panel D). In contrast, layer 5 neurons remained clearly immunoreactive up to a 48-hour PMI. These findings demonstrate that PMI effects on the same protein can differ across cortical layers within the same brain region, and they illustrate how such complex effects could be misinterpreted as the result of a disease-specific process.

Freezer storage time for fresh-frozen tissue has been reported to be negatively correlated with tissue levels of some, but not all, mRNA transcripts (Burke et al., 1991; Harrison et al., 1995). However, immunoreactivity does not appear to be altered in tissue fixed for a standard period of time and then stored in cryoprotectant at -30°C (Erickson et al., 1998).

CONCLUSIONS

Postmortem human brain research is a fundamental component in the study of the neurobiology of mental disorders and is essential in characterizing potential drug targets for treatment of these conditions. Two of the most critical variables in selecting the subjects for inclusion in a postmortem study are diagnostic verification and exclusion of brains with coexisting pathology or confounding factors that will severely limit the investigation of the primary disease pathology. The next step is to evaluate the integrity of the biological material. New RNA integrity measures have become available, like RIN and 3′/5′ ratio, and offer a more reliable and accurate evaluation of postmortem tissue quality. Together, the multiple confounds in postmortem research require

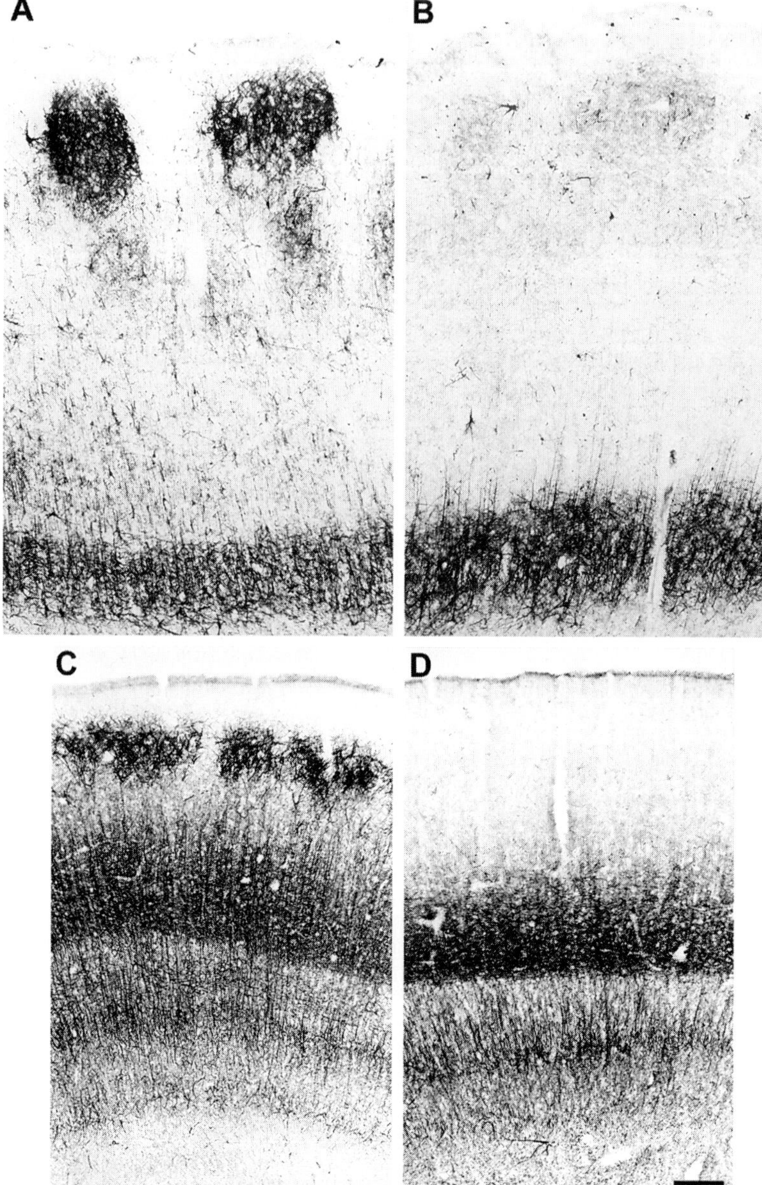

FIGURE 15.4 Brightfield photomicrographs comparing nonphosphorylated neurofilament protein (NFP) immunoreactivity in the intermediate subdivision (EI) of human entorhinal cortex from a normal control subject (*A*) and a subject with schizophrenia (*B*). Note the absence of NFP immunoreactivity in layer II clusters of neurons in the subject with schizophrenia, despite the presence of these neurons on an adjacent Nissl-stained section (not shown) and the presence of intensely immunoreactive neurons and dendrites in the deep cortical layers, similar to that of the normal control subject. However, the decreased NFP immunoreactivity in layer II of panel *A* appears to represent a postmortem effect rather than a schizophrenia-related change as indicated by the result of experiments summarized in panels C and *D*. These panels show NFP immunoreactivity in sections from adjacent tissue blocks, containing the same subdivision of monkey entorhinal cortex, that were processed following postmortem intervals of 0.5 (*C*) and 24 (*D*) hours. Note that the longer postmortem interval (PMI) (*D*) results in a loss of NFP immunoreactivity that is restricted to layer II. Scale bar = 150 μm and applies to all panels. Figure reprinted from Lewis and Akil (1997).

the use of convergent approaches to explicate and minimize the potential influence of these confounds. The use of animal models in parallel studies provides one means to assess potential confounds in a systematic fashion.

In summary, reliable postmortem studies are based on an appropriate understanding of potential confounds prior to the experimental procedure and the inclusion of well-designed controls to assess the potential impact of confounds on the measures of interest. Appropriate tissue preparation allows the maintenance of the structural and molecular integrity of postmortem tissue permitting detailed morphological and molecular investigations. Continued advances in the estimation of tissue quality and the impact of confounds will help increase the potential clinical value of the observations made through the direct investigation of the postmortem human brain.

ACKNOWLEDGMENTS

Cited work conducted by the authors was supported by National Institutes of Health Grants MH045156, MH043784 and MH067721, and by a National Alliance for Research on Schizophrenia and Depression (NARSAD) Young Investigator Award.

REFERENCES

American Psychiatric Association. (1994) *Diagnostic and Statistical Manual of Mental Disorders*, 4th ed. Washington, DC: Author.

Arango, V., Ernsberger, P., Marzuk, P.M., Chen, J.S., Tierney, H., Stanley, M., Reis, D.J., and Mann, J.J. (1990) Autoradiographic demonstration of increased serotonin 5-HT2 and beta-adrenergic receptor binding sites in the brain of suicide victims. *Arch. Gen. Psychiatry* 47:1038–1047.

Arnold, S.E., Trojanowski, J.Q., Gur, R.E., Blackwell, P., Han, L.Y., and Choi, C. (1998) Absence of neurodegeneration and neural injury in the cerebral cortex in a sample of elderly patients with schizophrenia. *Arch. Gen. Psychiatry* 55:225–232.

Atz, M., Walsh, D., Cartagena, P, Li, J., Evans, S., Choudary, P., Overman, K., Stein, R., Tomita, H., Potkin, S., Myers, R., Watson, S.J., Jones, E.G., Akil, H., Bunney, W.E., Jr., and Vawter, M.P. (2007) Methodological considerations for gene expression profiling of human brain. *J Neurosci Methods* 163:295–309.

Auer, H., Lyianarachchi, S., Newsom, D., Klisovic, M.I., Marcucci, G., and Kornacker, K. (2003) Chipping away at the chip bias: RNA degradation in microarray analysis. *Nat. Genet.* 35:292–293.

Bahn, S., Augood, S.J., Ryan, M., Standaert, D.G., Starkey, M., and Emson, P.C. (2001) Gene expression profiling in the post-mortem human brain—no cause for dismay. *J. Chem. Neuroanat.* 22:79–94.

Barrachina, M., Castano, E., and Ferrer, I. (2006) TaqMan PCR assay in the control of RNA normalization in human post-mortem brain tissue. *Neurochem. Int.* 49:276–284.

Beall, M.J., and Lewis, D.A. (1992) Heterogeneity of layer II neurons in human entorhinal cortex. *J. Comp. Neurol.* 321:241–266.

Benes, F.M. (1998) Model generation and testing to probe neural circuitry in the cingulate cortex of postmortem schizophrenic brain. *Schizophr. Bull.* 24:219–230.

Benes, F.M., and Bird, E.D. (1987) An analysis of the arrangement of neurons in the cingulate cortex of schizophrenic patients. *Arch. Gen. Psychiatry* 44:608–16.

Benes, F.M., Majocha, R., Bird, E.D., and Marotta, C.A. (1987) Increased vertical axon numbers in cingulate cortex of schizophrenics. *Arch. Gen. Psychiatry* 44:1017–1021.

Benes, F.M., Matthysse, S.W., Davidson, J., and Bird, E.D. (1987) The spatial distribution of neurons and glia in human cortex based on the Poisson distribution. *Anal. Quant. Cytol. Histol.* 9:531–534.

Berger, S.L., and Cooper, H.L, (1975) Very short-lived and stable mRNAs from resting human lymphocytes. *Proc. Natl. Acad. Sci. USA* 72:3873–3877.

Bracha, H.S., and Kleinman, J.E. (1984) Postmortem studies in psychiatry. *Psychiatr. Clin. North Am.* 7:473–485.

Bracha, H.S., and Kleinman, J.E. (1986) Postmortem neurochemistry in schizophrenia. *Psychiatr. Clin. North Am.* 9:133–141.

Brady, K., Casto, S., Lydiard, R.B., Malcolm, R., and Arana, G. (1991) Substance abuse in an inpatient psychiatric sample. *Am. J. Drug Alcohol Abuse* 17:389–397.

Buesa, C., Maes, T., Subirada, F., Barrachina, M., and Ferrer, I. (2004) DNA chip technology in brain banks: confronting a degrading world. *J. Neuropathol. Exp. Neurol.* 63:1003–1014.

Burke, W.J., O'Malley, K.L., Chung, H.D., Harmon, S.K., Miller, J.P., and Berg, L. (1991) Effect of pre- and postmortem variables on specific mRNA levels in human brain. *Brain Res. Mol. Brain Res.* 11:37–41.

Cantwell, R., Brewin, J., Glazebrook, C., Dalkin, T., Fox, R., Medley, I., and Harrison, G. (1999) Prevalence of substance misuse in first episode psychosis. *Br. J. Psychiatry* 174:150–153.

Colangelo, V., Schurr, J., Ball, M.J., Pelaez, R.P., Bazan, N.G., and Lukiw, W.J. (2002) Gene expression profiling of 12633 genes in Alzheimer hippocampal CA1: transcription and neurotrophic factor down-regulation and up-regulation of apoptotic and proinflammatory signaling. *J. Neurosci. Res.* 70:462–473.

Crombag, H.S., Gorny, G., Li, Y., Kolb, B., and Robinson, T.E. (2005) Opposite effects of amphetamine self-administration experience on dendritic spines in the medial and orbital prefrontal cortex. *Cereb. Cortex* 15:341–348.

Deep-Soboslay, A., Akil, M., Martin, C.E., Bigelow, L.B., Herman, M.M., Hyde, T.M., and Kleinman, J.E. (2005) Reliability of psychiatric diagnosis in postmortem research. *Biol. Psychiatry* 57:96–101.

Dixon, L., Haas, G., Weiden, P.J., Sweeney, J., and Frances, A.J. (1991) Drug abuse in schizophrenic patients: clinical correlates and reasons for use. *Am. J. Psychiatry* 148:224–230.

Dorph-Petersen, K.A., Pierri, J.N., Sun, Z., Sampson, A.R., and Lewis, D.A. (2004) Stereological analysis of the mediodorsal thalamic nucleus in schizophrenia: volume, neuron number, and cell types. *J. Comp. Neurol.* 472:449–462.

Dorph-Petersen, K.A., Pierri, J.N., Perel, J.M., Sun, Z., Sampson, A.R., and Lewis, D.A. (2005) The influence of chronic exposure to antipsychotic medications on brain size before and after tissue fixation: a comparison of haloperidol and olanzapine in macaque monkeys. *Neuropsychopharm.* 30:1649–1661.

Dorph-Petersen, K.A., Pierri, J.N., Wu, Q., Sampson, A.R., and Lewis, D.A. (2007) Primary visual cortex volume and total neuron number are reduced in schizophrenia. *J. Comp. Neurol.* 501:290–301.

Drake, R.E., Alterman, A.I., and Rosenberg, S.R. (1993) Detection of substance use disorders in severely mentally ill patients. *Community Ment. Health J.* 29:175–192.

Drake, R.E., Osher, F.C., and Wallach, M.A. (1989) Alcohol use and abuse in schizophrenia. A prospective community study. *J. Nerv. Ment. Dis.* 177:408–414.

Drake, R.E., and Wallach, M.A. (1989) Substance abuse among the chronic mentally ill. *Hosp. Community Psychiatry* 40: 1041–1046.

Duke, P.J., Pantelis, C., McPhillips, M.A., and Barnes, T.R. (2001) Comorbid non-alcohol substance misuse among people with schizophrenia: epidemiological study in central London. *Br. J. Psychiatry* 179:509–513.

Dwivedi, Y., Rizavi, H.S., Teppen, T., Zhang, H., Mondal, A., Roberts, R.C., Conley, R.R., Pandey, G.N. (2007) Lower phosphoinositide 3-kinase (PI 3-kinase) activity and differential expression levels of selective catalytic and regulatory PI 3-kinase subunit isoforms in prefrontal cortex and hippocampus of suicide subjects. *Neuropsychopharmacology*. [Epub ahead of print]

el Guebaly, N., and Hodgins, D.C. (1992) Schizophrenia and substance abuse: prevalence issues. *Can. J. Psychiatry* 37:704–710.

Erickson, S.L., Akil, M., Levey, A.I., and Lewis, D.A. (1998) Postnatal development of tyrosine hydroxylase- and dopamine transporter-immunoreactive axons in monkey rostral entorhinal cortex. *Cereb. Cortex* 8:415–427.

Flatscher-Bader, T., van der Brug, M., Hwang, J.W., Gochee, P.A., Matsumoto, I., Niwa, S., and Wilce, P.A. (2005) Alcohol-responsive genes in the frontal cortex and nucleus accumbens of human alcoholics. *J. Neurochem.* 93:359–370.

Flatscher-Bader, T., van der Brug, M.P., Landis, N., Hwang, J.W., Harrison, E., and Wilce, P.A. (2006) Comparative gene expression in brain regions of human alcoholics. *Genes Brain Behav.* 5(Suppl 1):78–84.

Flatscher-Bader, T., and Wilce, P.A. (2006) Chronic smoking and alcoholism change expression of selective genes in the human prefrontal cortex. *Alcohol. Clin. Exp. Res.* 30:908–915.

Fowler, I.L., Carr, V.J., Carter, N.T., and Lewin, T.J. (1998) Patterns of current and lifetime substance use in schizophrenia. *Schizophr. Bull.* 24:443–455.

Gogek, E.B. (1991) Prevalence of substance abuse in psychiatric patients. *Am. J. Psychiatry* 148:1086.

Hahn, C.G., Wang, H.Y., Cho, D.S., Talbot, K., Gur, R.E., Berrettini, W.H., Bakshi, K., Kamins, J., Borgmann-Winter, K.E., Siegel, S.J., Gallop, R.J., and Arnold, S.E. (2006) Altered neuregulin 1-erbB4 signaling contributes to NMDA receptor hypofunction in schizophrenia. *Nat. Med.* 12(7):734–735.

Halim, N.D., Lipska, B.K., Hyde, T.M, Deep-Soboslay, A., Saylor, E. M., Herman, M.M., Thakar, J., Verma, A., and Kleinman, J.E. (2007) Increased lactate levels and reduced pH in postmortem brains of schizophrenics: Medication confounds. *J. Neurosci. Methods* [Epub ahead of print].

Hambrecht, M., and Hafner, H. (1996) Substance abuse and the onset of schizophrenia. *Biol. Psychiatry* 40:1155–1163.

Hambrecht, M., and Hafner, H. (2000) Cannabis, vulnerability, and the onset of schizophrenia: an epidemiological perspective. *Aust. N. Z. J. Psychiatry* 34:468–475.

Hardy, J.A., Wester, P., Winblad, B., Gezelius, C., Bring, G., and Eriksson, A. (1985) The patients dying after long terminal phase have acidotic brains: implications for biochemical measurements on autopsy tissue. *J. Neural Transm.* 61:253–264.

Harlan, R.E., and Garcia, M.M. (1998) Drugs of abuse and immediate-early genes in the forebrain. *Mol. Neurobiol.* 16:221–267.

Harrison, P.J., Heath, P.R., Eastwood, S.L., Burnet, P.W., McDonald, B., and Pearson, R.C. (1995) The relative importance of premortem acidosis and postmortem interval for human brain gene expression studies: selective mRNA vulnerability and comparison with their encoded proteins. *Neurosci. Lett.* 200:151–154.

Havassy, B.E., and Arns, P.G. (1998) Relationship of cocaine and other substance dependence to well-being of high-risk psychiatric patients. *Psychiatr. Serv.* 49:935–940.

Hayes, T.L., Cameron, J.L., Fernstrom, J.D., and Lewis, D.A. (1991) A comparative analysis of the distribution of prosomatostatin-derived peptides in human and monkey neocortex. *J. Comp. Neurol.* 303:584–599.

Horowitz, J.M., Goyal, A., Ramdeen, N., Hallas, B.H., Horowitz, A.T., and Torres, G. (2003) Characterization of fluoxetine plus olanzapine treatment in rats: a behavior, endocrine, and immediate-early gene expression analysis. *Synapse* 50:353–364.

Hymowitz, N., Jaffe, F.E., Gupta, A., and Feuerman, M. (1997) Cigarette smoking among patients with mental retardation and mental illness. *Psychiatr. Serv.* 48:100–102.

Johnston, N.L., Cervenak, J., Shore, A.D., Torrey, E.F., and Yolken, R.H. (1997) Multivariate analysis of RNA levels from postmortem human brains as measured by three different methods of RT-PCR. Stanley Neuropathology Consortium. *J. Neurosci. Methods* 77: 83–92.

Jones, C., Simpson, P., Mackay, A., and Lakhani, S.R. (2006) Expression profiling using cDNA microarrays. *Methods Mol. Med.* 120:403–414.

Kane, J.K., Parker, S.L., Matta, S.G., Fu, Y., Sharp, B.M., and Li, M.D. (2000) Nicotine up-regulates expression of orexin and its receptors in rat brain. *Endocrinology* 141:3623–3629.

Kelly, T.M., and Mann, J.J. (1996) Validity of DSM-III-R diagnosis by psychological autopsy: a comparison with clinician antemortem diagnosis. *Acta Psychiatr. Scand.* 94:337–343.

Kingsbury, A.E., Foster, O.J., Nisbet, A.P., Cairns, N., Bray, L., Eve, D. J., Lees, A.J., and Marsden, C.D. (1995) Tissue pH as an indicator of mRNA preservation in human post-mortem brain. *Brain Res. Mol. Brain Res.* 28:311–318.

Kleinman, J.E., Hong, J., Iadarola, M., Govoni, S., and Gillin, C.J. (1985) Neuropeptides in human brain--postmortem studies. *Prog. Neuropsychopharmacol. Biol. Psychiatry* 9:91–95.

Kovelman, J.A., and Scheibel, A.B. (1986) Biological substrates of schizophrenia. *Acta Neurol. Scand.* 73:1–32.

Lewis, D.A. (2002) The human brain revisited: opportunities and challenges in postmortem studies of psychiatric disorders. *Neuropsychopharmacology* 26:143–154.

Lewis, D.A., and Akil, M. (1997) Cortical dopamine in schizophrenia: strategies for postmortem studies. *J. Psychiatry Res.* 31:175–195.

Lewis, D.A., Melchitzky, D.S., and Haycock, J.W. (1993) Four isoforms of tyrosine hydroxylase are expressed in human brain. *Neuroscience* 54:477–492.

Lewis, D.A., Melchitzky, D.S., and Haycock, J.W. (1994) Expression and distribution of two isoforms of tyrosine hydroxylase in macaque monkey brain. *Brain Res.* 656:1–13.

Li, J., Gould, T.D., Yuan, P., Manji, H.K., and Chen, G. (2003) Post-mortem interval effects on the phosphorylation of signaling proteins. *Neuropsychopharmacology* 28:1017–1025.

Li, J.Z., Vawter, M.P., Walsh, D.M., Tomita, H., Evans, S.J., Choudary, P.V., Lopez, J.F., Avelar, A., Shokoohi, V., Chung, T., Mesarwi, O., Jones, E.G., Watson, S.J., Akil, H., Bunney, W.E., Jr., and Myers, R.M. (2004) Systematic changes in gene expression in postmortem human brains associated with tissue pH and terminal medical conditions. *Hum. Mol. Genet.* 13: 609–616.

Li, M.D., Kane, J.K., Parker, S.L., McAllen, K., Matta, S.G., and Sharp, B.M. (2000) Nicotine administration enhances NPY expression in the rat hypothalamus. *Brain Res.* 867:157–164.

Lipska, B.K., Deep-Soboslay, A., Weickert, C.S., Hyde, T.M., Martin, C. E., Herman, M.M., and Kleinman, J.E. (2006) Critical factors in gene expression in postmortem human brain: focus on studies in schizophrenia. *Biol. Psychiatry* 60:650–658.

Liu, J., Lewohl, J.M., Dodd, P.R., Randall, P.K., Harris, R.A., and Mayfield, R.D. (2004) Gene expression profiling of individual cases reveals consistent transcriptional changes in alcoholic human brain. *J. Neurochem.* 90:1050–1058.

Mann, J.J., Arango, V., Marzuk, P.M., Theccanat, S., and Reis, D.J. (1989) Evidence for the 5-HT hypothesis of suicide. A review of post–mortem studies. *Br. J. Psychiatry* 8(Suppl):7–14.

Mann, J.J., Marzuk, P.M., Arango, V., McBride, P.A., Leon, A.C., and Tierney, H. (1989) Neurochemical studies of violent and nonviolent suicide. *Psychopharmacol. Bull.* 25:407–413.

Mayfield, R.D., Lewohl, J.M., Dodd, P.R., Herlihy, A., Liu, J., and Harris, R.A. (2002) Patterns of gene expression are altered in the frontal and motor cortices of human alcoholics. *J. Neurochem.* 81:802–813.

Mexal, S., Berger, R., Adams, C.E., Ross, R.G., Freedman, R., and Leonard, S. (2006) Brain pH has a significant impact on human postmortem hippocampal gene expression profiles. *Brain Res.* 1106:1–11.

Mexal, S., Frank, M., Berger, R., Adams, C.E., Ross, R.G., Freedman, R., and Leonard, S. (2005) Differential modulation of gene expression in the NMDA postsynaptic density of schizophrenic and control smokers. *Brain Res. Mol. Brain Res.* 139:317–32.

Mueser, K.T., Bellack, A.S., and Blanchard, J.J. (1992) Comorbidity of schizophrenia and substance abuse: implications for treatment. *J. Consult. Clin. Psychol.* 60:845–856.

Mueser, K.T., Nishith, P., Tracy, J.I., DeGirolamo, J., and Molinaro, M. (1995) Expectations and motives for substance use in schizophrenia. *Schizophr. Bull.* 21:367–378.

Mueser, K.T., Yarnold, P.R., and Bellack, A.S. (1992) Diagnostic and demographic correlates of substance abuse in schizophrenia and major affective disorder. *Acta Psychiatr. Scand.* 85:48–55.

Nisell, M., Nomikos, G.G., Chergui, K., Grillner, P., and Svensson, T.H. (1997) Chronic nicotine enhances basal and nicotine-induced Fos immunoreactivity preferentially in the medial prefrontal cortex of the rat. *Neuropsychopharmacology* 17:151–161.

Perry, E.K., Perry, R.H., and Tomlinson, B.E. (1982) The influence of agonal status on some neurochemical activities of post-mortem human brain tissue. *Neurosci. Lett.* 29:303–307.

Pich, E.M., Pagliusi, S.R., Tessari, M., Talabot-Ayer, D., van Huijsduijnen Hooft, R., and Chiamulera, C. (1997) Common neural substrates for the addictive properties of nicotine and cocaine. *Science* 275:83–86.

Pierri, J.N., Volk, C.L., Auh, S., Sampson, A., and Lewis, D.A. (2001) Decreased somal size of deep layer 3 pyramidal neurons in the prefrontal cortex of subjects with schizophrenia. *Arch. Gen. Psychiatry* 58:466–473.

Plum, F. (1972) Prospects for research on schizophrenia. 3. Neurophysiology. Neuropathological findings. *Neurosci. Res. Program Bull.* 10:384–388.

Rangell, L.K., and Keller, G.A. (2000) Application of microwave technology to the processing and immunolabeling of plastic-embedded and cryosections. *J. Histochem. Cytochem.* 48: 1153–1159.

Ravid, R., Van Zwieten, E.J., and Swaab, D.F. (1992) Brain banking and the human hypothalamus—factors to match for, pitfalls and potentials. *Prog. Brain Res.* 93:83–95.

Rehncrona, S., Rosen, I., and Smith, M.L. (1985) Effect of different degrees of brain ischemia and tissue lactic acidosis on the short-term recovery of neurophysiologic and metabolic variables. *Exp. Neurol.* 87:458–473.

Robinson, T.E., Gorny, G., Mitton, E., and Kolb, B. (2001) Cocaine self-administration alters the morphology of dendrites and dendritic spines in the nucleus accumbens and neocortex. *Synapse* 39:257–266.

Robinson, T.E., Gorny, G., Savage, V.R., and Kolb, B. (2002) Widespread but regionally specific effects of experimenter- versus self-administered morphine on dendritic spines in the nucleus accumbens, hippocampus, and neocortex of adult rats. *Synapse* 46:271–279.

Ross, B.M., Knowler, J.T., and McCulloch, J. (1992) On the stability of messenger RNA and ribosomal RNA in the brains of control human subjects and patients with Alzheimer's disease. *J. Neurochem.* 58:1810–1819.

Sokolov, B.P., Tcherepanov, A.A., Haroutunian, V., and Davis, K.L. (2000) Levels of mRNAs encoding synaptic vesicle and synaptic plasma membrane proteins in the temporal cortex of elderly schizophrenic patients. *Biol. Psychiatry* 48:184–96.

Soyka, M., Albus, M., Kathmann, N., Finelli, A., Hofstetter, S., Holzbach, R., Immler, B., and Sand, P. (1993) Prevalence of alcohol and drug abuse in schizophrenic inpatients. *Eur. Arch. Psychiatry Clin. Neurosci.* 242:362–372.

Stan, A.D., Ghose, S., Gao, X.M., Roberts, R.C., Lewis-Amezcua, K., Hatanpaa, K.J., and Tamminga, C.A. (2006) Human postmortem tissue: what quality markers matter? *Brain Res.* 1123:1–11.

Swaab, D.F., and Boer, K. (1972) The presence of biologically labile compounds during ischemia and their relationship to the EEG in rat cerebral cortex and hypothalamus. *J. Neurochem.* 19: 2843–2853.

Taylor, G.R., Carter, G.I., Crow, T.J., Johnson, J.A., Fairbairn, A.F., Perry, E.K., and Perry, R.H. (1986) Recovery and measurement of specific RNA species from postmortem brain tissue: a general reduction in Alzheimer's disease detected by molecular hybridization. *Exp. Mol. Pathol.* 44:111–116.

Tomita, H., Vawter, M.P., Walsh, D.M., Evans, S.J., Choudary, P.V., Li, J., Overman, K.M., Atz, M.E., Myers, R.M., Jones, E.G., Watson, S.J., Akil, H., and Bunney, W.E., Jr. (2004) Effect of agonal and postmortem factors on gene expression profile: quality control in microarray analyses of postmortem human brain. *Biol. Psychiatry* 55:346–352.

Trotter, S.A., Brill, L.B., and Bennett, J.P., Jr. (2002) Stability of gene expression in postmortem brain revealed by cDNA gene array analysis. *Brain Res.* 942:120–123.

Van Dongen, C.J. (1999) Smoking and persistent mental illness: an exploratory study. *J. Psychosoc. Nurs. Ment. Health Serv.* 37:26–34.

Vawter, M.P., Tomita, H., Meng, F., Bolstad, B., Li, J., Evans, S., Choudary, P., Atz, M., Shao, L., Neal, C., Walsh, D.M., Burmeister, M., Speed, T., Myers, R., Jones, E.G., Watson, S.J., Akil, H., and Bunney, W.E. (2006) Mitochondrial-related gene expression changes are sensitive to agonal-pH state: implications for brain disorders. *Mol. Psychiatry* 11:663–679.

Webster, M.J. (2006) Tissue preparation and banking. *Prog. Brain Res.* 158:3–14.

Yates, C.M., Butterworth, J., Tennant, M.C., and Gordon, A. (1990) Enzyme activities in relation to pH and lactate in postmortem brain in Alzheimer-type and other dementias. *J. Neurochem.* 55:1624–1630.

Ziedonis, D.M., and George, T.P. (1997) Schizophrenia and nicotine use: report of a pilot smoking cessation program and review of neurobiological and clinical issues. *Schizophr. Bull.* 23:247–254.

16 Neuroimmunology

JOHN M. PETITTO, DEAN G. CRUESS, MARTIN J. REPETTO, DAVID R. GETTES, TAMI D. BENTON, AND DWIGHT L. EVANS

The scope of neuroimmunology is growing, and many of the methods and approaches used in this field are now being used in other areas of neuroscience as well. Understanding of how various behavioral states and the underlying central nervous system (CNS) pathways influence the immune systems, and how peripheral immune processes affect brain function and behavior, was the initial focus of mental health–related studies (and is frequently referred to as *psychoneuroimmunology*). The traditional approach in medical research was to study individual organ systems in isolation. As noted in the sections that follow, there is now considerable evidence that immune, endocrine, and central nervous systems share some common signals and receptors. Thus, neuroimmunology research also encompasses the study of endogenous "immunological" gene products in the brain, and of "neural" or "endocrine" gene products in organs outside of the CNS (for example, the gastrointestinal [GI] tract). In Alzheimer's disease research, for example, the role of proinflammatory immune cytokines that are produced in the brain are proteins that appear to be involved in the neuropathophysiology of the disease. In many instances, endogenous brain cytokines are produced at very low levels but have significantly higher affinities for their respective receptors than neurotransmitters and neuromodulators. Knowledge of fundamental neuroimmunology and research approaches used in neuroimmunology has important implications for neuroscience and mental health research. In this chapter, we seek to convey some of the issues and ideas guiding ongoing and future research relevant to mental illness. We cite some selected studies to illustrate particular examples and principles, and where possible, reviews of larger bodies of literature for selected topics. We wish to acknowledge that the limited scope of this chapter does not seek to review the entire literature.

PERTINENT HISTORY

Nearly 40 years ago, two psychiatrists performed groundbreaking research demonstrating that the brain could modulate parameters of the immune response. Research psychiatrists and experimental psychologists were among the first scientists to appreciate that changes in immune function may be associated with changes in brain function and behavior. The late George Solomon and his colleagues (1968) published a landmark study showing that early experience could produce long-term changes in immune physiology in animals. In a series of mechanistic studies, Marvin Stein et al. (1969) demonstrated that hypothalamic lesions could modify immune processes and anaphylactic responses across animal species. Their studies led to the hypothesis (now supported by a large body of research) that the hypothalamus transmits signals to the immune system via its control of neuroendocrine and autonomic activity that could modulate immune physiology. Robert Ader and Nicholas Cohen provided the most compelling illustration of the ability of the brain to modify immune responses. In a pioneering collaborative study, Ader (an experimental psychologist) and Cohen (a comparative immunologist) behaviorally conditioned mice by pairing saccharin (a conditioned stimulus that has no intrinsic immunomodulatory actions) with an immunosuppressant, cyclophosphamide (an unconditioned stimulus). They showed that when behaviorally conditioned mice were exposed to only saccharin at a later point in time, saccharin itself led to inhibition of antibody production following immunization with sheep red blood cells (Ader and Cohen, 1975). Because of the long-held view by immunologists that the immune system was an autonomous system, these scientists initially faced considerable skepticism. In subsequent experiments they set out to demonstrate further that the changes in immune physiology elicited by behavioral conditioning were clinically meaningful and could alter the health status of the organism. In their classic *Science* article that propelled research efforts in the field of pyschoneuroimmunology, they subsequently showed that exposure to saccharin alone could modify the course of murine systemic lupus erythematosus (Ader and Cohen, 1982).

NEURAL AND ENDOCRINE MODULATION OF IMMUNE FUNCTION

Prompted by the compelling studies noted above, researchers sought to uncover the outflow pathways from the CNS involved in the neuromodulation of immune physiology. Figure 16.1 is a simple schematic diagram showing the various levels of neuroimmunological communication between and within systems. The brain's modulation of other systemic homeostatic processes such as blood pressure regulation were recognized for a number of years prior and set a precedent for research to elucidate the basic mechanisms underlying brain–immune system interactions. It is now appreciated that lymphoid organs such as the spleen and thymus are innervated by sympathetic efferent fibers, where noradrenergic nerve terminals are found in close proximity to lymphocytes forming functional neuroeffector contacts (Felten and Felten, 1987). Various hormonal signals of the hypothalamic-pituitary-adrenal (HPA) axis have also been shown to possess modulatory properties on some immune cell subsets (Dunn, 1995).

Much attention has been given to the role of the HPA axis on immune parameters. Although preclinical studies have documented select immunomodulatory effects of various HPA neuropeptides (for example, adrenocorticotrophic hormone [ACTH], corticotrophin releasing factor [CRF], endorphins), most emphasis has been given to the role of adrenal steroids. The known immunosuppressive effects of high doses of synthetic steroids (Cupps and Fauci, 1982) led to the commonly held view that behavioral state–induced (for example, stress, bereavement, depression) elevations in adrenal corticosteroids would suppress immune activity. Under physiological conditions, however, endogenous adrenal steroids have bidirectional immunomodulatory actions on immune cell trafficking and function (Ottoway and Husband, 1992; Miller et al., 1993). Although HPA axis dysregulation has been studied extensively in the field of biological psychiatry (for example, major depression), the neuroimmunomodulatory actions of adrenal cortisol in association with psychiatric disorders including depression and stressful events has yielded mixed results. The need for multidisciplinary research strategies to disentangle the complex interactive mechanisms between systems (for example, central nervous, endocrine, and immune systems) has become increasingly apparent.

The neural modulation of immune activity was shown to involve limbic, forebrain, and cortical regions, areas involved in expression of emotional, cognitive, and motor processes, respectively. Researchers therefore tested hypotheses that neurobiological changes in these brain areas associated with various behavioral states such as stress and mental illness may result in alterations in the activity of the HPA axis and/or descending sympathetic autonomic pathways that innervate immune organs (for example, spleen). These alterations in turn can modify immune status and susceptibility to disease in individuals who are vulnerable. There are many excellent studies that have used animal models to elucidate the neural pathways involved in modulating components of the immune system. Extending the behavioral conditioning research of Ader and Cohen described earlier, for example, Lysle and Coussons-Read (1995) showed that conditioned environmental stimuli (inherently nonaversive stimuli) previously paired with an aversive event (footshock stress) can themselves induce pronounced changes in immune status and modify disease course in animals. Tracing the step(s) involved in a series of studies using this model, they showed that central opioid systems activate descending sympathetic pathways that transduce the effects to cells of the immune system (for example, subsets of splenic lymphocytes).

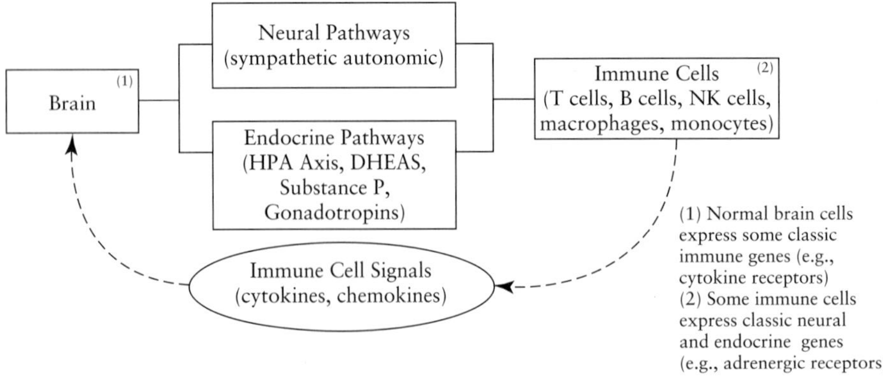

FIGURE 16.1 Neurological communication between and within central nervous and immune systems. Neural and endocrine pathways may modulate parameters of immune physiology. The peripheral immune system can signal the brain (for example, cytokines can cross the blood-brain-barrier and, in some cases, may activate vagal nerve afferents). The central nervous (CNS) and immune systems are known to share particular endogenous signaling molecules that were once thought to be exclusive to either the CNS or peripheral immune cells. HPA: hypothalmic-pituitary-adrenal; DHEA-S: dehydroepiandrosterone sulfate; NK: natural killer.

SHARED SIGNALS AND RECEPTORS, AND BIDIRECTIONAL COMMUNICATION

Considerable evidence has established that immune, endocrine, and central nervous systems share some common signals and receptors. Seminal studies by Besedovsky et al. (1991) indicating that peripheral immunization led to activation of hypothalamic neurons and Blalock (1994) showing that lymphocytes had the capacity to produce neuropeptides sparked research efforts that have established that some immune cell–derived signals (for example, cytokines) communicate with endocrine and brain cells. Just as scientists were surprised decades ago to discover digestive peptides such as CCK and VIP in the brain, cytokines and chemokines and their receptors have been identified in the brain. Many cytokines and their receptors once thought to be derived solely from lymphoid cells have been shown to be regulated by genes in the brain, and they function as neuromodulators, growth factors, as well as mediators of immune-like responses in the CNS in various neuropathological states. How these factors affect neurodevelopmental, neuronal regeneration, and infection-induced CNS processes is the focus of ongoing investigation. Conversely, the role of immunomodulators (interleukin, for example, IL-1, IL-2, IL-6) on brain cells and neuromodulators (for example, norepinepherine) on immune cells are questions being explored to understand their physiological significance and relation to pathological events seen in clinical diseases. Cytokines derived from peripheral immune cells (and in some cases perhaps other tissues) can cross the blood-brain-barrier (BBB), although the mechanisms by which this occurs differs for different cytokines (for example, active vs. passive transport) and influences the degree to which they pass into the CNS. In general, most peripheral cytokines do not readily cross the BBB. Work from the laboratories of Maier and Watkins (1998) shows that the afferent sensory fibers of the vagus can carry signals initiated by interleukin-1 to brain stem areas (for example, nucleus tractus solitarius).

In a review, Dantzer and Kelley (2007) described the considerable advances that have been made in understanding the mechanisms by which increased levels of certain peripheral cytokines (for example, IL-1, IL-2) elicit sickness behavior in animals. The sickness syndrome includes mild leukocytosis, fever, increased levels of slow-wave sleep, increased production of acute phase proteins by the liver, decreased activity and exploration, reduced social interaction, increased sensitivity to pain, and depressive-like symptoms. It has been theorized that this immune system signal provides an adaptive message to the brain. This message is thought to aid in the initiation of a recuperative process by modifying the organism's physiology (for example, fever can act to reduce severity of infection by a subset of microorganisms) and behavior (for example, decreased exploration of the environment to preserve energy). Psychological and physical stressors activate much of the same neurobiological circuitry that is activated by infectious agents or immune cell–derived products that elicit the sickness syndrome. This intriguing avenue of investigation may provide new insights into some of the enigmatic immune and acute phase-like changes described in some individuals experiencing major depression or other neuropsychiatric conditions (discussed briefly in a subsequent section). Dantzer and Kelley (2007) proposed how available pharmacological agents may advance this avenue of research from the bench to the bedside.

NEUROIMMUNOLOGY AND GENETICS

The genetic mechanisms underlying brain–immune system interactions are not well understood because studies in this area have been more limited. We very briefly describe a few of the highlights and refer the interested reader to a more comprehensive evaluation of this area of inquiry (Petitto, 2001). The available literature suggests that subsets of genes involved in the expression of complex behavioral and immunological traits may be physically linked, interactive at the level of the genome, or shared by the brain and immune system. Only a few clinical studies on the topic have been published. Narcolepsy, for example, has been found to be associated with specific human leukocyte antigen (HLA) alleles (Kadotani et al., 1998). Functional genetic relationships between behavior and immunity are precedented. Several lines of investigation address the potential evolutionary significance of genetic mechanisms linking adaptive behavioral and immunological processes in vertebrate species. Diverse major histocompatibility complex (MHC) allelic polymorphisms controlling individual odor profiles function as chemosensory signals. These chemosensory signals appear to play a role in mating preference (acting against inbreeding depression and promoting diversity of the gene pool) and communal behaviors (to ensure that related individuals share in the survival of their offspring) in animals (Apanius et al., 1997). We sought to assess whether known candidate immunological genes and/or immune-related disease susceptibility loci (an interval on a chromosome where the gene[s] involved have not been identified or definitively determined) might be physically linked to behavioral quantitative trait loci. Quantitative trait loci (QTL) are individual loci involved in controlling complex traits where none of the individual genes involved is sufficient for the expression of the complex trait. To determine if specific candidate immunological genes and/or immune disease susceptibility loci might be physically linked to QTL for emotional or cognitive behavioral traits in animals, we recently examined the Mouse Genome Database for possible linkages. This assessment provided intriguing evidence that a handful of behavioral QTLs involved in emotionality, learning, and memory may be linked to a subset of immune genes or susceptibility loci (Petitto, 2001). The functional significance of these potential linkages remains to be determined. A gene (or set of genes) may be involved in encoding a process common to the expression of a behavioral and immunological trait (pleitropic gene effects that influence both traits). The simplest example of this is where a particular gene is experimentally deleted or "knocked out" in mice, and the loss of this gene product is found to result in alterations in the central nervous and immune systems. In our studies, for example, we have demonstrated that in addition to producing marked effects on the immune system, IL-2 gene deletion produces impairments in endogenous hippocampal cytokines (Beck et al., 2005) and neurodevelopmental changes in hippocampal cytoarchitecture that correlates with spatial learning and memory abnormalities in these animals (Beck et al., 2002). Abnormalities in "immunological" genes involved in neurodevelopemental processes could have particular relevance for neuropsychiatric disorders such as autism, where neuroimmunological and neurodevelopmental alterations could be associated with one another.

PSYCHOSOCIAL FACTORS AND DEPRESSION TO IMMUNITY AND DISEASE

There is evidence that psychosocial factors such as life stress and clinical depression may be predictive cofactors of human morbidity and mortality (Evans and Charney, 2003). An excellent review by Irwin and Irwin (2007) describes the history of research that has examined the association between depressive disorders and immunity. There is evidence on the one hand that clinical depression may influence immune-related diseases (as noted below), and that altered immune function could play a role in the pathogenesis of clinical depression. Emotional factors may influence the onset and course of immune-based diseases under certain circumstances. Extensive investigation has been devoted to the effects of stress on immunity in humans, and excellent summaries and assessments of this body of research exist (Ader et al., 2001; Glaser and Kiecolt-Glaser, 2005). Several notable studies pertaining to psychosocial factors and disease are highlighted in this section.

Considerable evidence indicates that psychosocial factors can influence the course of general medical illnesses (Evans et al., 2005). Thus, it is not surprising that psychosocial factors might also influence the course of immune-based diseases (Evans et al., 2002). There has been much interest in cancer research. In one longitudinal study, for example, it was found that severe life stress increased the likelihood of relapse in women with breast cancer by nearly sixfold (Ramirez et al., 1989). Psychosocial interventions have also been reported, for example, to increase survival in men with malignant melanoma (Fawzy et al., 1993). Some of the best evidence relating psychosocial events to susceptibility and clinically meaningful end points comes from experimental laboratory studies in humans. Cohen et al. (1991) inoculated participant volunteers with cold virus (for example, rhinovirus) and found that psychosocial stress preceding inoculation was associated with an increased rate of acute respiratory infection. Moreover, their data suggested that this relationship was dose-dependent. Whereas Cohen et al. (1991) showed that psychosocial factors were associated with an increase in infection rates among experimentally inoculated participants, Stone et al. (1992) showed that psychosocial factors were correlated with increased cold symptoms in participants with confirmed rhinovirus infection following experimental inoculation.

ILLUSTRATION OF A PSYCHONEUROIMMUNOLOGY (PNI) RESEARCH MODEL USING HIV INFECTION

Human immunodeficiency virus (HIV) infection is now commonly seen as a chronic disease, often consisting of a wide array of recurrent and sometimes severe psychosocial stressors (Schneiderman et al., 1997). Some of the most studied variables include stressful life events, distress states, and anxious and depressive symptoms (Leserman et al., 2006). How patients respond to and cope with these many challenges may ultimately affect disease processes and overall health status. A number of researchers have studied HIV infection within a PNI framework as a way to help understand the potential mechanisms underlying the effects that psychosocial factors and psychological states might have on the physiological functioning and disease status of individuals who are HIV-positive (Evans et al., 2002). This is illustrated in the model seen in Figure 16.2. Using such a model, our HIV research group has followed longitudinally a cohort of homosexual men who are HIV-positive. In this research, we have found that severe life stress was associated with lower natural killer (NK) and $CD8^+$ T-cell counts at the time of entry into the study (Evans et al., 1995), and similar associations were found after 2 years (Leserman et al., 1997). Men reporting more stress also had faster HIV disease progression over a 7½ year period (Leserman et al., 2000). Progression to Acquired Immune Deficiency Syndrome (AIDS) was related to more stressful life events, greater use of denial coping, higher cortisol level, and less

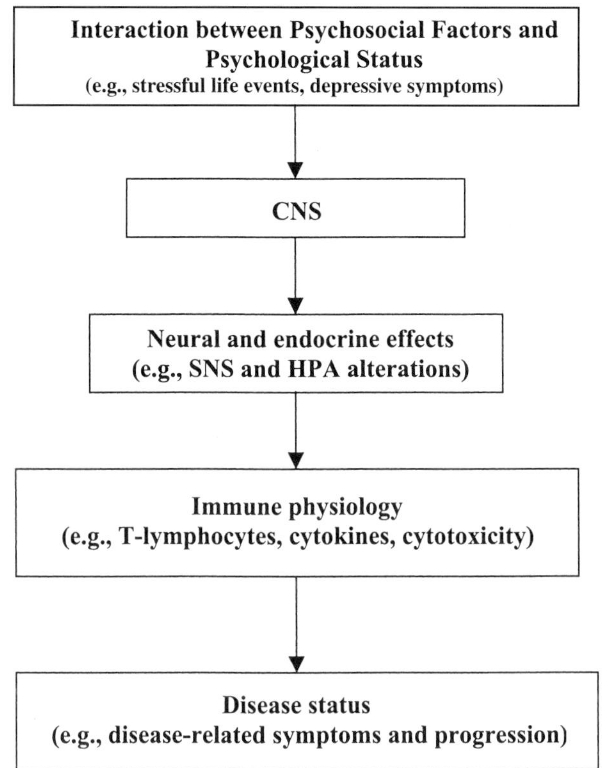

FIGURE 16.2 Psychoneuroimmunology schema depicting how psychological and psychosocial factors may influence immune-based disease processes such as in cancer and HIV. SNS: sympathetic nervous system; HPA: hypothalmic-pituitary-adrenal axis.

social support. The effects that certain psychosocial factors have on immune functioning and disease progression might operate, at least partially, through underlying alterations in neural and endocrine processes.

Chronic distress states can often lead to persistent elevations in sympathetic nervous system (SNS) activity that are involved in the human stress response. There is some evidence that elevations in norepinephrine might alter cytokine production relevant for cytotoxic functioning during HIV disease, which may impair an infected person's ability to control HIV replication. One study recently found that homosexual men who were HIV-positive randomly assigned to a 10-week, group-based stress management intervention had significantly lower 24-hour urinary norepinephrine levels and anxious mood than men assigned to a waitlist control group (Antoni, Cruess, Cruess, et al., 2000). Norepinephrine reductions were associated with decreases in anxious mood across the intervention period, and men with the largest reductions in distress and norepinephrine levels had greater numbers of $CD8^+$ T cells at 1-year follow-up following the behavioral intervention. This study was among the first to show that a brief stress reduction intervention can help reduce distress, decrease stress hormone levels, and enhance the immune status of individuals who are HIV-positive over time.

Alterations in HPA axis functioning are observed among individuals who are HIV-positive. In a recent study, men participating in a stress management intervention showed significant reductions in 24-hour urinary cortisol levels and depressed mood compared to men assigned to a control group (Antoni, Cruess, and Cruess, 2000). Cortisol reductions were associated with decreases in depressed mood across the intervention period. Further analysis revealed that mood improvement across the 10-week intervention was related to reductions in salivary cortisol achieved during relaxation training within the individual sessions (Cruess, Antoni, Kumar, and Schneiderman, 2000). Men at 1-year follow-up assigned to stress management had higher levels of transitional naive T-cells ($CD45^+CD29^+$) thought to reflect evidence of immune system reconstitution (Antoni et al., 2002), benefits attributable in part to the reductions in depressed mood and cortisol levels achieved during the 10-week intervention (Cruess, Antoni, Klimas, et al., 2000). These intervention studies point to the efficacy of stress management strategies to reduce distress and cortisol levels and to enhance immune status of individuals who are HIV-positive.

In conclusion, in studies of homosexual men who are HIV-positive, there is some evidence that psychosocial factors seem to operate, at least partially, through underlying stress-related alterations in endocrine regulation that subsequently affect immune functioning and potentially affect physical health and survival. There is a need for more scientific research focused on the physiological mechanisms that may help explain the detrimental effects of psychosocial factors during HIV disease, especially among women. Longitudinal studies that repeatedly and systematically assess relevant psychosocial factors, endocrine and immune parameters, and disease status, either through a naturalistic design or through a stress management intervention study, are key to elucidating these types of PNI mechanisms during HIV disease.

BRAIN DEVELOPMENT AND CYTOKINES: A ROLE IN NEUROPATHOLOGY AND MENTAL ILLNESS?

Understanding the neurobiological function of certain cytokines and brain cytokine receptors could provide important new clues to unravel the etiology and pathogenesis of major neuropsychiatric diseases such as schizophrenia and Alzheimer's disease. The prototypical immunoregulatory cytokine, *IL-2*, an interest of our lab, provides a good example that may be relevant to disorders such as schizophrenia where neurodevelopmental abnormalities are believed to play an important role in the pathogenesis. IL-2 has been detected in cerebrospinal fluid (CSF) of patients with schizophrenia manifesting symptoms of psychosis (Licinio et al., 1993; McAllister et al., 1995), and in treatment trials in cancer patients, where administration of this cytokine induces side effects including psychotic symptoms (Denicoff et al., 1987). Receptors for IL-2 have been cloned and sequenced in the brain and are expressed in limbic areas where this cytokine can modulate the release of the neurotransmitter *dopamine* and related behaviors (Petitto et al., 1997; Petitto and Huang, 2001; Zalcman et al., 1994; Zalcman et al., 1998). IL-2 has also been shown to have trophic effects on fetal glial cells and neurons as well as to possess a variety of other actions (for example, effects on myelin basic protein expression), and it is plausible, for example, that during early development an event such as viral infection in a genetically susceptible individual could disrupt the normal timing at which IL-2 may stimulate neuronal growth and migration. As noted earlier, loss of the IL-2 gene in mice during development results in cytoarchitectural abnormalities in the hippocampus (Beck et al., 2002). If such events occurred in a region like the hippocampus where IL-2 receptors are enriched, this could contribute to the alterations in this region (for example, abnormal orientation of subsets of hippocampal neurons) that are seen in postmortem brains of individuals with schizophrenia.

AUTOIMMUNITY OR EPIPHENOMENA?

It is noteworthy that findings such as elevations in acute phase reactants, increased levels of inflammatory cytokines, and certain behavioral characteristics (for example, reduced activity and social interaction) fit within the theoretical framework of the sickness syndrome described earlier (Maier and Watkins, 1998; Dantzer et al., 1998). There has been much interest in the theory that autoimmune processes may underlie some neuropathological processes associated with certain neuropsychiatric disorders.

In major depression, for example, the research of Maes (1995) and others suggests that, at least in subgroups of patients who are depressed, the reduced NK activity and altered T-cell proliferation described earlier are accompanied by measures of immune activation and inflammatory or autoimmune-like laboratory correlates. Reduced NK activity and altered T-cell activity together with estimates of immune activation (for example, nonspecific antinuclear and antiphospholipid antibodies, acute phase reactants, and increased production of some proinflammatory cytokines) are sometimes exhibited by individuals diagnosed with systemic autoimmune diseases. There is a lack of compelling evidence, however, that activation markers on peripheral blood lymphocytes or serum soluble immune activation markers (for example, IL-2 receptor-α chain) are a valid reflection of prior or ongoing autoimmune-like processes affecting the brain in individuals with neuropsychiatric disorders. Nonetheless, it is noteworthy that lymphocytes expressing activation markers and certain adhesion molecules (molecules on the surface of lymphocytes that allow them to pass across endothelial cells into organ tissues including brain) are the cells that have the capacity to cross the BBB and enter the nondiseased brain (Hickey et al., 1991). In those subsets of individuals with neuropsychiatric conditions that exhibit increased levels of activated lymphocytes and expression of certain adhesion molecules, it is therefore plausible that these lymphocytes have a greater opportunity to enter the brain.

The potential role of autoantibodies in this area of research is also a topic of interest. Because there is not evidence that the BBB is disrupted in individuals with neuropsychiatric conditions such as in patients with schizophrenia or depression (vs. multiple sclerosis, for example), the question arises as to whether putative autoantibodies postulated to be involved in CNS pathogenesis could access the brain. Recent evidence has shown that under certain conditions, B lymphocytes may traffic into the normal, nondiseased brain and engage in intrathecal antibody synthesis (Knopf et al., 1998). It remains to be determined whether such processes may be operative in neuropsychiatric syndromes suspected of having immunopathogenic involvement. Conversely, it should be noted that there is emerging new evidence that peripheral immune cells may aid in processes such as neuronal regeneration under some conditions (Schwartz et al., 1999), further confounding our ability to interpret how changes in immune measures in the peripheral blood observed in various neuropsychiatric syndromes might influence the brain.

Support for the theory that autoimmune-like processes may be involved in the pathogenesis of various neuropsychiatric diseases (for example, schizophrenia) comes largely from nonspecific correlative data. Frequently, the mean values of patient groups for various laboratory measures of immune status (for example, proinflammatory cytokines, subsets of activated lymphocytes) differ significantly from the group means of normal control participants, but the actual values themselves fall within the range of normal limits. By the same token, many questions that we as neuroscientists are asking are actually the same questions being asked by our colleagues studying systemic autoimmune disorders. Using studies of schizophrenia as an example again, subsets of individuals with schizophrenia (including never-medicated participants) have been found to have a significantly higher frequency of antinuclear antibodies than control participants (Spivak et al., 1995). Non-specific antinuclear antibodies are also found in certain systemic autoimmune disorders, and it is often unclear if they are involved in the pathogenesis of auto-immunity (such as inflammation and destruction of the pancreas in autoimmune diabetes, renal pathology in lupus). Thus, it is unclear if these nonspecific, autoimmune-like laboratory estimates observed in schizophrenia or other neuropsychiatric disorders represent evidence of pathophysiological steps involved in autoimmunity or are epiphenomena.

Data that are unfolding from molecular genetic research of complex autoimmune traits provide an interesting basis for speculation in this regard. Intriguing hypotheses relating autoimmune-like processes and neuropsychiatric conditions may be posed from our current knowledge of the genetics of complex autoimmune diseases. Experimental models in animals (that nicely reflect related work in humans) are being used to identify the relative contribution of the multiple genes required for the expression of complex, polygenic autoimmune diseases like insulin dependent diabetes mellitis (IDDM). Different genomic intervals have been found to contribute component phenotypes (for example, autoantibodies, amplification of T helper cells). Drawing parallels to neuropsychiatric disorders, it is plausible that subgroups of individuals exhibiting schizophrenia, for example, could possess several of the autoimmune susceptibility intervals common to systemic autoimmune diseases. Thus, they may exhibit a laboratory correlate (for example, a nonspecific autoantibody) but lack the necessary complement of other autoimmune genes necessary to express systemic autoimmune disease (for example, diabetes, systemic lupus erythematosus [SLE]). Moreover, it is also possible that susceptibility genes unique to schizophrenia in concert with one or more autoimmune susceptibility intervals may result in immune-associated abnormalities of brain development.

NEUROIMMUNOLOGICAL METHODS: USE IN NEUROPSYCHIATRIC RESEARCH

Clinical research studies of immune function in individuals with neuropsychiatric disorders most commonly have sought to determine how the disease state (for example, active depression) correlates with peripheral immune function. The measurements typically quantify numbers of certain cell types in the peripheral blood (for example, T-cell subsets), the activity of particular immune cell subtypes (for example, NK cells against a tumor cell, how T cells respond to a specific antigen), or concentrations of cytokines or other immune mediators or antibodies in blood. Various immune challenges can be performed, such as immunizing participants of interest with a specific vaccine and determining how a certain manipulation (for example, a laboratory stress paradigm) or a psychological state (for example, active clinical depression) may influence the immune system's response to immunization.

A few of the more common research laboratory techniques employed by psychoneuroimmunologists include radio immune assays (RIAs, for example, for endocrine hormones, cortisol, ACTH, dehydroepiandrosterone sulfate [DHEA-S]); Enzyme Linked ImmunoSorbent Assay (ELISAs, for example, for various cytokines); polymerase chain reaction (PCR, for example, for mRNA, gene work); Natural Killer Cell Assay (NKA, for example, for number and functional strength of NK cells). In many laboratories, investigators separate specific cells from whole blood (for example, ficoll separation of monocytes), grow them (for example, monocyte-derived macrophages), and then use various challenges (for example, virus, oxidative stress) and measure the output of multiple compounds or functions (for example, chemokine and cytokine concentrations, viral entry, viral replication). Flow cytometric methods and analyses may be performed to phenotype and quantify populations of T lymphocytes, B cells, monocytes, and subpopulations of NK cells. A relatively new instrument called a Luminex (Luminex Corp., Austin, Texas) is able to measure up to 100 different analytes from a few microliters of serum, plasma, or supernatant sample and is therefore generating much interest in the field of neuroimmunology, where understanding the relationship between multiple compounds is helpful. In sum, there are a plethora of assays and methods used in clinical and basic neuroimmunology research (an excellent, comprehensive, detailed guide is *Current Protocols in Immunology* [2007] John Wiley and Sons Inc.). We wish to emphasize that there are unique methodological issues that are essential to consider and standardize to draw sound conclusions from interpretation of the data obtained.

For example, discrepancies in the literature may, in part, stem from differences across studies including duration and severity of symptoms, temporal parameters (for example, when samples are drawn for assays), and subject variables such as gender, age, and trait (for example, heritable personality characteristics) among others. Certain methodological factors that have differed among existing studies may account, in part, for some of these conflicting findings in the literature. Alterations in sleep could be a salient variable that may induce changes in measures of cellular immune physiology in depression. Studies show that altered sleep patterns can have profound effects on measures of cellular immune status (Irwin et al., 1996). Moreover, in normal control participants, subsets of circulating lymphocytes exhibit different circadian rhythms that coincide with the rhythms of HPA hormones such as cortisol (Kronfol et al., 1997). This is one reason why it is critical to standardize the time of the day when samples are drawn for immune assays comparing participant groups (for example, depressed vs. normal comparison groups). Preclinical studies indicate that immunological rhythms may be entrained to CNS rhythms (Ottoway and Husband, 1992). It is well established that circadian (or ultradian) rhythms are often disrupted in major depression, and that these depression-related rhythm abnormalities include parameters of the neural and endocrine functions implicated as immunomodulators (for example, cortisol, melatonin, and estimates of noradrenergic activity). We compared circulating NK cell phenotypes and NK activity in participants with major depression and normal control participants at 8 a.m. and 4 p.m. during the same 24-hour period. These times approximate the diurnal peak and nadir respectively of NK cell functional activity in healthy, normal individuals on a schedule of nocturnal rest and diurnal activity. Compared to normal control participants, participants with major depression exhibited significantly reduced diurnal variation in levels of Leu-11 NK cells and NK cytotoxic activity between 8 a.m. and 4 p.m. (Petitto et al., 1992). Findings such as this may represent a phase shift in a circadian rhythm, rather than a reduction or increase in the measure of immune status. Other factors that are important to control for include immunosuppressive drugs such as steroids and nonsteroid anti-inflammatory medications. In general, clinical researchers view reductions in in vitro laboratory immune measures cautiously because substantive data supporting the idea that these reductions correlate with immunocompetence in vivo are lacking.

CONCLUSIONS

The rapidly expanding evidence base and the new technologies in neuroimmunology research continue to inform our understanding of the common signals and receptors shared by the immune, endocrine, and central nervous systems. Recent research suggests that alterations in the HPA axis and the SNS serve as mediators for immune cell functions, and that their products may serve as neuromodulators and immunomodulators for pathological events seen in psychiatric illness. Genetic research suggests that subsets of genes involved in the expression of complex behavioral and immunological traits may be linked at the genome level or shared by the brain and immune systems.

Recent studies utilizing multidisciplinary research strategies continue to further our understanding of the complex interactions between the central nervous, endocrine, and immune systems. New technologies in neuroimmunology and genetics may allow us to better examine the complex relationships between endocrine–immune mediators and their genetic determinants, and also improve the efficiency of data collection and analysis, that is, luminex technology. Answers are still needed to explain how these neuroimmune findings in altered behavioral states affect the etiologies, prognosis, or treatments of physical illness. Prospective longitudinal studies examing these neuromodulators and immunomodulators in individuals with neuropsychiatric disorders over time might allow us to understand their roles in the development of disease states. Future studies should focus on the translation of these findings into novel treatments for neuropsychiatric conditions, for example, targeting specific neuroimmune mediators such as the proinflammatory cytokines in the "sickness syndrome," or the use of antidepressants targeting corticotrophin-releasing hormone (CRH) and the use of CRH antagonists (CRH secretion is increased by cytokines that mediate innate immunity, and the hypersecretion of CRH is increased in patients with depression). Furthermore, preventive or interventional studies aimed at cognitive and behavioral interventions for individuals with medical diseases might favorably modify the relationships between neuroimmune mediators and disease expression. Research in neuroimmunology provides a valuable framework for understanding the effects of neuropsychiatric disorders and psychosocial factors on the pathophysiology of medical illness.

REFERENCES

Ader, R., and Cohen, N. (1975) Behaviorally conditioned immunosuppression. *Psychosom. Med.* 37:333–340.

Ader, R., and Cohen, N. (1982) Behaviorally conditioned immunosuppression and murine systemic lupus erythematosus. *Science* 215:1534.

Ader, R., Felten, D., and Cohen, N. (Eds.). (2001). *Psychoneuroimmunology*, 3rd ed. New York: Academic Press.

Antoni, M.H., Cruess, D.G., Cruess, S., Lutgendorf, S., Kumar, M., Ironson, G., Klimas, N., Fletcher, M.A., and Schneiderman, N. (2000) Cognitive behavioral stress management intervention effects on anxiety, 24-hour urinary norepinephrine output, and T-cytotoxic/suppressor cells over time among symptomatic HIV-infected gay men. *J. Consult. Clin. Psychol.* 68:31–45.

Antoni, M.H., Cruess, D.G., Klimas, N., Maher, K., Cruess, S., Kumar, M., Lutgendorf, S., Ironson, G., Schneiderman, N., and Fletcher, M.A. (2002) Stress management and immune system reconstitution in symptomatic HIV-infected gay men over time: effects on transitional naive T cells (CD4(+)CD45RA(+)CD29(+). *Am. J. Psychiatry* 159(1):143–145.

Antoni, M.H., Cruess, S.E., and Cruess, D.G. (2000) Cognitive behavioral stress management reduces distress and 24-hour urinary free cortisol output among symptomatic HIV-infected gay men. *Ann. Behav. Med.* 22:29–37.

Apanius, V., Penn, D., Slev, P.R., Ruff, L.R., and Potts, W.K. (1997) The nature of selection on the major histocombatibility complex. *Crit. Rev. Immunol.* 17:179–224.

Beck, R.D., King, M.A., Huang, Z., and Petitto, J.M. (2002) Alterations in septohippocampal cholinergic neurons resulting from interleukin-2 gene knockout. *Brain Res.* 955:16–23.

Beck, R.D., Waserfall, C., Ha, G.K., Cushman, J.D., Huang, Z., and Petitto, J.M. (2005) Changes in hippocampal IL-15, related cytokines and neurogenesis in IL-2 deficient mice. *Brain Res.* 1041:223–230.

Besedovsky, H.O., del Rey, A., Klusman, I., Furukawa, H., Monge Arditi, G., and Kabiersch, A. (1991) Cytokines as modulators of the hypothalamus-pituitary-adrenal axis. *J. Steroid Biochem. Mol. Biol.* 40:613–618.

Blalock, J.E. (1994) The syntax of immune-neuroendocrine communications. *Immunol. Today* 15:504–511.

Cohen, S., Tyrrell, D.A.J., and Smith, A.P. (1991) Psychological stress and susceptibility to the common cold. *N. Eng. J. Med.* 325:606–612.

Cruess, D.G., Antoni, M.H., Klimas, N., Maher, K., Cruess, S.E., Kumar, M., Lutgendorf, S.K., Ironson, G., Schneiderman, N., and Fletcher, M.A. (2000) Stress management and immune system reconstitution in symptomatic HIV-positive men: effects on transitional naïve T-cells. *Psychosom. Med.* 62:102.

Cruess, D.G., Antoni, M.H., Kumar, M., and Schneiderman, N. (2000) Reductions in salivary cortisol are associated with mood improvement during relaxation training among HIV-seropositive men. *J. Behav. Med.* 23:107–122.

Cupps, T.R., and Fauci, A.S. (1982) Corticosteroid-mediated immunoregulation in man. *Immunol. Rev.* 65:133–155.

Dantzer, R., Bluthe, R.M., Gheusi, G., Cremona, S., Laye, S., Parnet, P., and Kelley, K.W. (1998) Molecular basis of sickness behavior. *Ann. N. Y. Acad. Sci.* 856:132–138.

Dantzer, R., and Kelley, K.W. (2007) Twenty years of research on cytokine-induced sickness behavior. *Brain Behav. Immun.* 21(2): 153–160.

Denicoff, K.D., Rubinow, D.R., Papa, M.Z., Simpson, C., Seipp, C., Lotze, M.T., Chang, A.E., Rosenstein, D., and Rosenberg, S.A. (1987) The neuropsychiatric effects of treatment with interleukin-2 and lymphokine-activated killer cells. *Ann. Intern. Med.* 107: 293–300.

Dunn, A.J. (1995) Interactions between the nervous system and the immune system: implications for psychopharmacology. In: Bloom, F.E., and Kupfer, D.J., eds. *Psychopharmacology: The Fourth Generation of Progress*. New York: Raven Press, p. 719.

Evans, D.L., and Charney, D.S. (2003) Mood disorders and medical Illness: a major public health problem. *Biol. Psychiatry* 54(3):177–180.

Evans, D.L., Charney, D.S., Lewis, L., Golden, R.N., Gorman, J.M., Krishnan, K.R., Nemeroff, C.B., Bremner, J.D., Carney, R.M., Coyne, J.C., Delong, M.R., Frasure-Smith, N., Glassman, A.H., Gold, P.W., Grant, I., Gwyther, L., Ironson, G., Johnson, R.L., Kanner, A.M., Katon, W.J., Kaufmann, P.G., Keefe, F.J., Ketter, T., Laughren, T.P., Leserman, J., Lyketsos, C.G., McDonald, W.M., McEwen, B.S., Miller, A.H., Musselman, D., O'Connor, C., Petitto, J.M., Pollock, B.G., Robinson, R.G., Roose, S.P., Rowland, J., Sheline, Y., Sheps, D.S., Simon, G., Spiegel, D., Stunkard, A., Sunderland, T., Tibbits, P., Jr., and Valvo, W.J. (2005) Mood disorders in the medically ill: scientific review and recommendations. *Biol. Psychiatry* 58(3): 175–189.

Evans, D.L., Leserman, J., Perkins, D.O., Stern, R.A., Murphy, C., Tamul, K., Lioa, D., Van der Horst, C.M., Hall, C.D., Folds, J.D., Golden, R.N., and Petitto, J.M. (1995) Stress associated reductions of cytotoxic T lymphocytes and natural killer cells in asymptomatic human immunodeficiency virus infection. *Am. J. Psychiatry* 152:543–550.

Evans, D.L., Mason, K.R., Leserman J., and Petitto, J.M. (2002) Neuropsychiatric manifestations of HIV-1 infection and AIDS. In: Charney, D., Coyle, J., Davis, K., and Nemeroff, C. eds. *Neuropsycho-pharmacology: The Fifth Generation of Progress*. New York: Raven Press, pp. 1281–1299.

Fawzy, F.I., Fawzy, N.W., Hyun, C.S., Eashoff, R., Guthrie, D., Fahey, J.L., and Morton, D.L. (1993) Malignant melanoma effects of an early structured psychiatric intervention, coping, and affective state on recurrence and survival 6 years later. *Arch. Gen. Psychiatry* 50:681–689.

Felten, D.L., and Felten, S.Y. (1987) Immune interactions with specific neural structures. *Brain Behav. Immunity* 1:287–289.

Glaser, R., and Kiecolt-Glaser, J.K. (2005) Stress-induced immune dysfunction: implications for health. *Nat. Rev. Immunol.* 5: 243–251.

Herbert, T.B., and Cohen, S. (1993) Depression and immunity: a meta-analytic review. *Psychol. Bull.* 1133:472–486.

Hickey, W.F., Hsu, B.L., and Kimura, H. (1991) T-lymphocyte entry into the central nervous system. *J. Neurosci. Res.* 28:254–260.

Irwin, M., McClintick, J., Costlow, C., Fortner, M., White, J., and Gillin, J.C. (1996) Partial night sleep deprivation reduces natural killer and cellular immune responses in humans. *FASEB J.* 10:643–653.

Irwin, M.R., and Irwin, A.H. (2007) Depressive disorders and immunity: 20 years of progress and discovery. *Brain Behav. Immun.* 21(4):374–383.

Kadotani, H., Faraco, J., and Mignot, E. (1998) Genetic studies in the sleep disorder narcolepsy. *Research* 8:427–434.

Knopf, P.M., Harling-Berg, C.J., Cserr, H.F., Basu, D., Sirulnick, E. J., Nolan, S.C., Park, J.T., Keir, G., Thompson, E.J., and Hickey, W.F. (1998) Antigen-dependent intrathecal antibody synthesis in the normal rat brain: tissue entry and local retention of antigen-specific B cells. *J. Immunology* 161(2):692–701.

Kronfol, Z., Nair, M., Zhang, Q., Hill, E.E., and Brown, M.B. (1997) Circadian immune measures in healthy volunteers: relationship to hypothalamic-pituitary axis hormones and sympathetic neurotransmitters. *Psychosom. Med.* 59(1):42–50.

Leserman, J., Cruess, D.G., and Petitto, J.M., (2006) HIV/AIDS and mood disorders. In: Evans, D.L., Charney, D.S., and Lewis, L., eds. *Physician's Guide to Depression and Bipolar Disease*. New York: McGraw Hill.

Leserman, J., Petitto, J.M., Golden, R.N., Gaynes, B.N., Gu, H., Perkins, D.O., Silva, S.G., Folds, J.D., and Evans, D.L. (2000) Impact of stressful life events, depression, social support, coping, and cortisol on progression to AIDS. *Am. J. Psychiatry* 157: 1221–1228.

Leserman, J. Petitto, J.M., Perkins, D.O., Folds, J.D., Golden, R.N., and Evans, D.L. (1997) Severe stress, depressive symptoms, and changes in lymphocyte subsets in human immunodeficiency virus-infected men. A 2-year follow-up study. *Arch. Gen. Psychiatry* 54(3):279–285.

Licinio, J., Seibyl, J.P., Altemus, M., Charney, D.S., and Krystal, J.H. (1993) Elevated CSF levels of interleukin-2 in neuroleptic-free schizophrenic patients. *Am. J. Psychiatry* 150:1408–1410.

Lysle, D.T., and Coussons-Read, M.E. (1995) Mechanisms of conditioned immunomodulation. *Int. J. Immunopharmacol.* 17:641–647.

Maes, M. (1995) Evidence for an immune response in major depression: a review and hypothesis. *Prog. Neuropsychopharmacol. Biol. Psychiatry* 19:11–38.

Maier, S.F., and Watkins, L.R. (1998) Cytokines for psychologists: implications of bidirectional immune-to-brain communication for understanding behavior, mood and cognition. *Psychological Rev.* 105:83.

McAllister, C.G., van-Kammen, D.P., Rehn, T.J., Miller, A.L., Gurklis, J., Kelley, M.E., Yao, J., and Peters, J.L. (1995) Increases in CSF levels of interleukin-2 in schizophrenia: effects of recurrence of psychosis and medication status. *Am. J. Psychiatry* 152: 1291–1297.

Miller, A.H., Spencer, R.L., McEwen, B.S., and Stein, M. (1993) Depression, adrenal steroids, and the immune system. *Ann. Med.* 25:481–487.

Ottaway, C.A., and Husband, H.A. (1992) Central nervous system influence of lymphoid migration. *Brain Behav. Immun.* 6:97–116.

Petitto, J.M. (2001) Behavioral genetics and immunity. In: Ader, R., Felten, D., and Cohen, N., eds. *Psychoneuroimmunology*, 3rd ed. New York: Academic Press, pp. 173–186.

Petitto, J.M., Folds, J.D., Ozer, H., Quade, D., and Evans, D.L. (1992) Abnormal diurnal variation in circulating natural killer cell phenotypes and cytotoxic activity in major depression. *Am. J. Psychiatry* 149:694–696.

Petitto, J.M., and Huang, Z. (2001) Cloning of the full-length IL-2/ IL-15 receptor-beta cDNA sequence from mouse brain: evidence of enrichment in hippocampal formation neurons. *Regul. Pepti.* 98:77–97.

Petitto, J.M., McCarthy, D.B., Rinker, C.M., Huang, Z., and Getty, T. (1997) Modulation of behavioral and neurochemical measures of forebrain dopamine function in mice by species-specific interleukin-2. *J. Neuroimmunol.* 73:183–190.

Ramirez, A.J., Craig, K.J.T., Watson, J.P., Fentiman, I.S., North, W.R.S., and Rubens, R.D. (1989) Stress and relapse of breast cancer. *BMJ* 298:291–293.

Schneiderman, N., Antoni, M.H., and Ironson, G. (1997) Cognitive behavioral stress management and secondary prevention in HIV/ AIDS. *Psychology & AIDS Exchange* 22:1–8.

Schwartz, M., Cohen, I., Lazarov-Spiegler, O., Moalem, G., and Yoles, E. (1999) The remedy may lie in ourselves: prospects for immune cell therapy in central nervous system protection and repair. *J. Mol. Med.* 77:713–717.

Solomon, G.F., Levine, S., and Kraft, J.K. (1968) Early experience and immunity. *Nature* 220:821–822.

Spivak, B., Radwan, M., Bartur, P., Mester, R., and Weizman, A. (1995) Antinuclear autoantibodies in chronic schizophrenia. *Acta Psychiatr. Scand.* 92:266–269.

Stein, M., Schiavi, R.C., and Luparello, T.J. (1969) The hypothalamus and immune process. *Ann. N.Y. Acad. Sci.* 164(2): 464–472.

Stone, A.A., Bovbjerg, D.H., Neale, J.M., Napoli, A., Valdimarsdottir, H., Cox, D., Hayden, F.G., and Gwaltney, J.M. (1992) Development of common cold symptoms following experimental rhinovirus infection is related to prior stressful life events. *Behav. Med.* 18(3):115–120.

Zalcman, S.S., Green-Johnson, J.M., Murray, L., Nance, D.M., and Greenberg, A.H. (1994) Cytokine-specific central monoamine alterations induced by interleukin-1, -2, and -6. *Brain Res.* 643: 40–49.

Zalcman, S.S., Murray, L., Dyck, D.G., Greenberg, A.H., and Nance, D.M. (1998) Interleukin-2 and -6 induce behavioral-activating effects in mice. *Brain Res.* 811:111–121.

17 Drug Discovery and Development Methods for Mental Illness

GARY D. TOLLEFSON

The pharmaceutical industry and its life blood of drug discovery, development, and commercialization are sustained by a continuous process of innovation and opportunism. A key "value driver" in this pursuit is the identification of novel approaches to unmet medical needs: what is the clinician and/or the patient asking for that will improve clinical and functional treatment outcomes? Given the inherent complexity and breadth of such a task, success mandates that those interested in drug development start with a focused strategy. Stated another way, this means achieving the critical mass, within a few strategically defined therapeutic areas, necessary to deliver the number of targets and compound screens required to find an eventual commercial candidate.

To discover and develop a drug, why is it necessary to have a strategy? The discovery strategy benefits by having (*1*) an innovative platform, (*2*) relevant information on the external or competitive environment, (*3*) the right people (addressing the capacity and capabilities necessary for the task), (*4*) effective processes in place that enable the right work to get done within an acceptable time frame and financial outlay, and (*5*) the best enabling technologies or informatics systems. Winning drug discovery strategies most often succeed when they are coordinated, leverage more than one approach, retain planning flexibility, and welcome challenge to the status quo of how things get done (Goldsbrough et al., 1999).

To deliver the broad portfolio of drug development candidates necessary to sustain a large drug discovery operation, one needs to have multiple biological platforms, robust chemistry support for synthesis, and sophisticated technological means for lead candidate screening/optimization. It is becoming increasingly difficult for a single company or institution to sustain such an effort. Thus, the field is headed toward much greater "outside-in" reliance. Stated another way, drug discovery will be increasingly reliant on networking to leverage external technical expertise, the outsourcing of certain development activities, and the creation of virtual global discovery networks connected by state-of-the-art information technology.

The current challenges confronting research-based pharmaceutical companies are many; however, none is greater than the skyrocketing costs associated with drug discovery/development. In any drug discovery setting, resources are finite. Thus, a premium is placed on those individuals who can focus discovery/development efforts, effectively prioritize among myriad targets, allocate resources in a cost-effective manner, and make unequivocal decisions early in the process, that is, fail fast. Yet another challenge in drug discovery is the ability to translate the plethora of revolutionary findings in neurobiology into pragmatic clinical opportunities: for example, what is the relevant clinical target for the newly cloned serotonin "9xyz" receptor? Especially vexing to drug discovery in the neurosciences is the identification of animal models that accurately portray human disorders of the brain. Moreover, we find ourselves still in a primitive stage of biomarker development (disease state surrogates, evidence of central drug penetration, genomic-based drug response predictors, etc.).

HISTORICAL BASIS

One relative constant in the discovery/development enterprise has been the sequence of (*1*) identifying a target (for example, a receptor), (*2*) screening novel compounds against that target, and (*3*) choosing the best candidate to move into testing. However, the means to accomplish this have been, and still are, labor intensive, resulting a time frame that has been just too long. Unfortunately, scant progress has been made in this area recently. Historically, stellar pharmaceutical development careers were based on years of effort yielding identification of only one or two realized discovery targets. Such successes were in large part the by-product of serendipity or phenomenology. Subsequently, drug discovery has moved through several eras (Fig. 17.1).

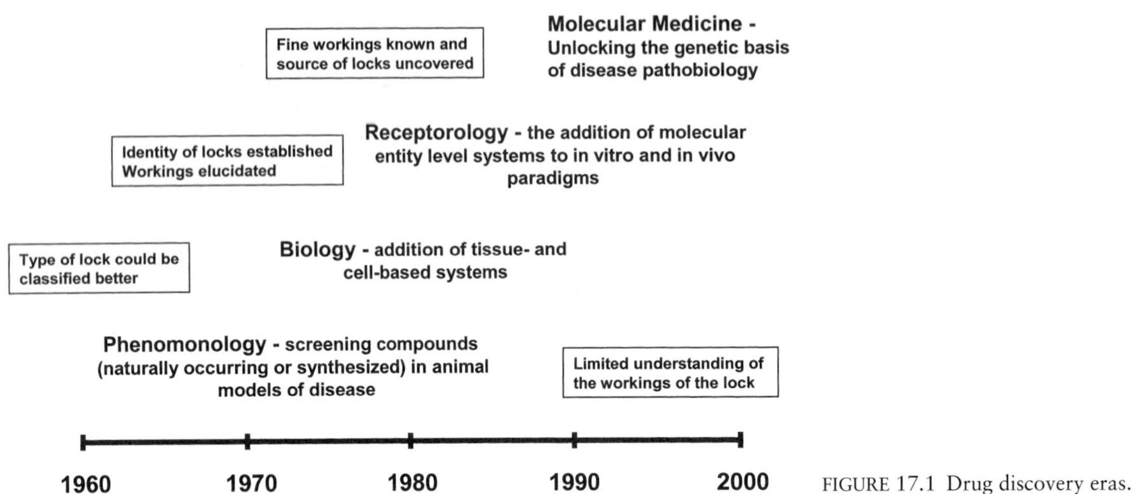

FIGURE 17.1 Drug discovery eras.

Regardless of the era, success has been defined by the discovery of a "blockbuster"—a drug that has the potential to address a highly prevalent unmet medical need and that can be successfully commercialized for those treating and/or manifesting a well-defined condition. Large sales generated by a small number of such products sustain many large pharmaceutical companies. Such blockbuster products are required to offset the enormous costs of pharmaceutical research and development, which are further magnified by the hit-or-miss nature of clinical drug development. Burrill & Co., a life science investment bank based in California, has identified several disadvantages of the blockbuster business model:

- enormous, fully capitalized development costs of approximately US $802 million per drug
- long development times: 8–12 years from the laboratory to the pharmacy
- large clinical studies to demonstrate statistically relevant effectiveness
- high attrition rates: only 5–9 of 100 preclinical substances reach the status of "new drug application" (NDA)
- the drugs are only effective in 40%–60% of patients
- the risk of severe side effects that are only recognized when large patient numbers are involved in the trials
- the development of "me-too" preparations and generic drugs reduce the period in which the original drugs generate high profit (within the next 6 years, all 20 of today's best-selling drugs will have lost patent protection.)
- higher expenditures do not necessarily lead to better drugs or to better investment returns

As stated above, winning in the past with a blockbuster drug was often the by-product of serendipity and translational clinical powers of observation. However, such a formula has been slow and unpredictable. Today it is quite simply inadequate. For example, a single chemist might take a year to synthesize 50 candidate compounds. Moreover, the screening of those candidates was a manual exercise consuming weeks to identify a lead molecule. Today many of the functions required to identify disease targets and screen drug candidates are systematized and automated. These automated modeling techniques test many different scenarios that would have required untold person-hours in the past to reach similar conclusions. Thus, in today's drug discovery world, we see far greater efforts to introduce a more rational approach to drug discovery, leveraging the profound advances made in the fields of molecular biology, informatics, and genomics (Fig. 17.2). However, though the promise is great, the tangible output of this tremendous investment in technology has yet to reach the level of sustained productivity necessary for pharmaceutical companies to stay competitive.

The Role of Biotechnology and Specialty Pharma in Pipeline Enrichment

Given the overall lack of productivity from large pharmaceutical company pipelines, one might assume some rather ominous consequences. However, in-house challenges with innovation and productivity do not mean that fewer products are on the way to the market. Rather, large companies have started to include more diverse and economical approaches to developing new products. Perhaps the best example, where we see today an expansion on an already existing trend, is to buy or license intellectual property rather than develop it entirely in-house. The source of that innovation is principally from the biotechnology/specialty pharmaceuticals arena. It is standard practice for large companies to have specialized "drug hunting" teams to go find opportunity wherever it resides. Such "find-it" teams routinely set out to acquire the intellectual property needed to develop new tools, processes, or products. Although a principal driver for such initiatives relates back to a basic lack of productivity and inefficiency, financial considerations aren't alone

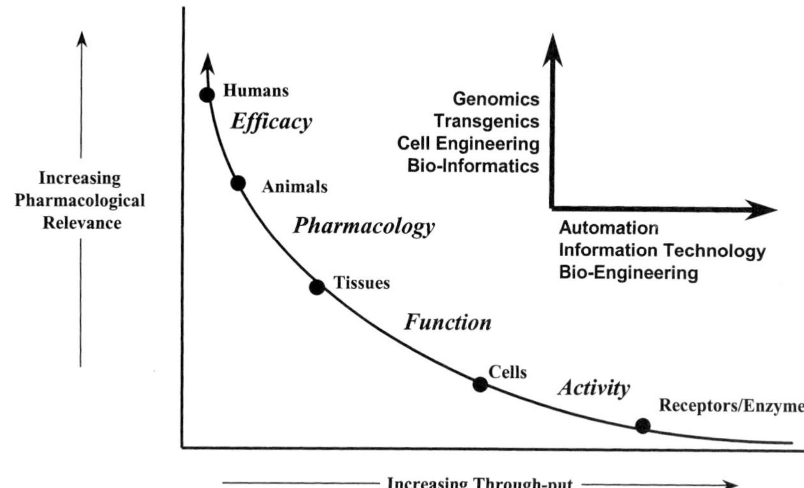

FIGURE 17.2 The path of drug discovery in the future: How is the curve shifting up and to the right?

in forcing firms to consider licensing or acquiring intellectual property. With the rapid explosion of knowledge in the life sciences arena, companies that develop new products and tools increasingly find themselves working in novel fields in which they have scant experience. In those circumstances, collaboration with biotech or academic groups is an essential business practice. So increasingly we are seeing partnerships between large pharma and biotech, academic departments, or research institutions that foster cooperative projects designed to take novel research findings from the laboratory and convert them to viable drug candidates. More and more, these partnerships cross national boundaries. As biotechnology clusters spring up in new locations, pharmaceutical firms are moving rapidly to take advantage of local expertise resident in their research institutions or early stage "start-ups."

This approach may represent a win-win strategy. The benefit to the large pharma is access to candidate compounds. The benefit to the academic or biotech partner is experience and strength of a multinational development organization. But are such partnerships more likely to be successful? A recent review titled "Biotech-Pharma Alliances as a Signal of Asset and Firm Quality" (Nicholson et al., 2005) that was based in part on a study of 539 licensing deals made between 1988 and 2000 reported that drugs produced by a codevelopment partnership were more likely to succeed in winning approval from the Food and Drug Administration (FDA) than those developed by a sole company. Of 691 new chemical entities approved by the FDA from 1963 to 1999, 38% evolved out of alliances. So, not surprisingly with success, the average number of biotech alliances per pharmaceutical firm has grown consistently over the past 15 years.

THE DISCOVERY OF DRUGS

The drug development continuum consists of a series of steps or development stages (Fig. 17.3). The exercise begins with the discovery. There are three key steps in the drug discovery process: (*1*) discovery of relevant biological targets, (*2*) generation of lead candidates, and (*3*) optimization of those leads to deliver potent, safe, and effective therapeutics.

Targets

One way to accelerate the effort to generate a sufficient candidate list to satisfy the ever-growing demand

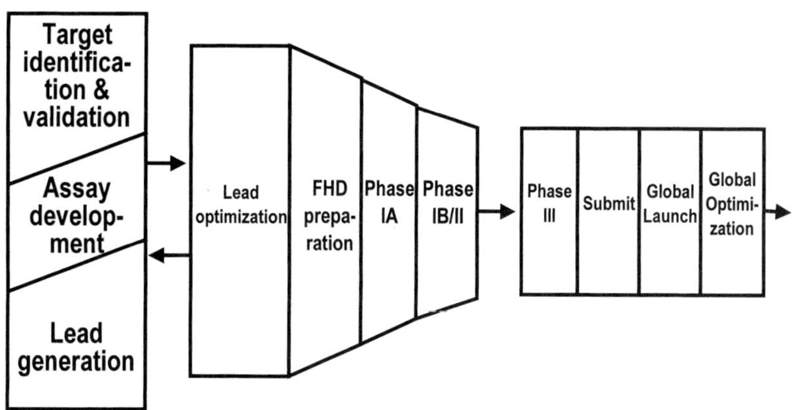

FIGURE 17.3 The research and development process: discovery and commercialization.

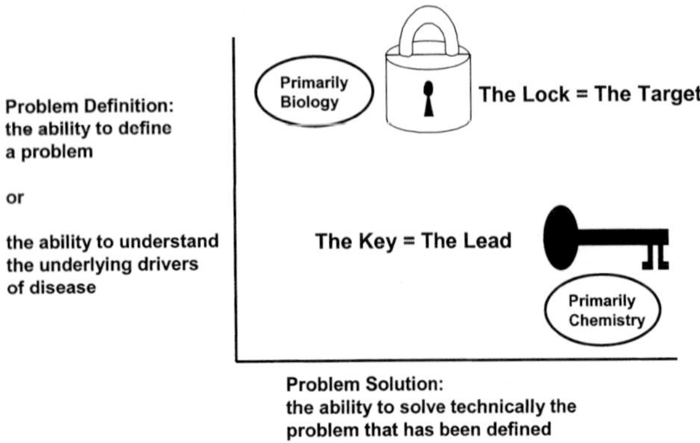

FIGURE 17.4 The drug discovery process: a framework.

for new drugs is to find and leverage the best of the new technologies (M.J. Ashton et al., 1996). These technologies represent the means to discover new targets. A drug target is a potential site of action with presumed etiopathologic relevance. One can think of the target as a lock (Fig. 17.4). The discovery of new targets (*target identification*) is primarily in the domain of the biologist. The present revolution in neurobiology is expanding the universe of potential new targets by unraveling cellular mechanisms associated with clinical disorders (Fig. 17.5). Tests are conducted to confirm the relevance to the disease state. Target prioritization looks across the universe of available targets and, based on the strength of their relative associations with one or more specific disease states or conditions, selects those that will be the basis for delivering a series of drug candidates (Schreiber, 2000). Once targets are identified and prioritized, an iterative process of finding molecular drug candidates or potential leads commences (*lead identification*).

Screens

Modern drug discovery involves screening small molecular weight molecules for their ability to bind (interface) to a preselected target (often a protein). The chemist's role is to identify the key to the lock (see Fig. 17.4).

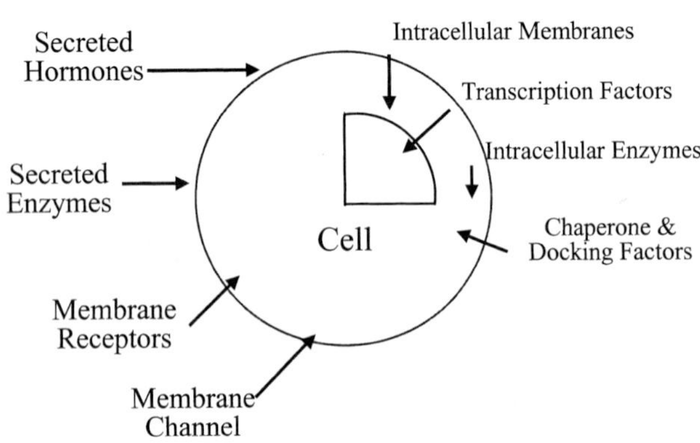

FIGURE 17.5 The discovery of new drug targets.

That task is often akin to finding the proverbial needle in the haystack. The lock, or novel chemical entity or biological product (for example, novel protein), is thus a search exercise. Given the large number of potential locks, this was a time-consuming process in the past. Initial selection, once a painstaking manual exercise, has been replaced with automated processes such as high-throughput screening (HTS) of extensive molecular libraries. These require days instead of weeks or months to perform. These automated experiments often model systems designed to resemble the human disease state of interest. Such advances in the drug discovery effort have included the marriage of combinatorial chemistry with HTS. Combinatorial chemistry literally "throws" thousands of small molecules at the target. It can be employed in an iterative series of steps in the service of lead optimization. The HTS procedure employs robotics, coupled with miniaturization, to run much larger series of screens in shorter periods of time. Today, laboratories are realizing a 10-fold increase in the number of compounds (keys) generated for assay and a near 100-fold increase in the overall number of compounds screened. This can mean a 50% reduction in costs and time to market. It is hoped that through the use of novel technologies, the ultimate hit rate, that is, identification of viable drug candidates, will become less a game of chance and, in turn, a more cost-effective process (PriceWaterhouseCoopers, 1998).

The objective of the screening process is to identify those leads with the best binding (activity) characteristics to the target. However, many of the properties desired for an ultimate candidate may not be achieved through HTS. Within existing drug leads, one may have to "engineer" additional chemical changes to a molecule to enhance its profile (for example, absorption or metabolism). Computer-based design is one tool that has accelerated this process and has led to the term *in silico* research to capture modeled experimentation within the computer. This is becoming an increasingly important tool that complements more traditional in vitro and in vivo methods. The advantage of a sophisticated drug discovery engine is the speed with which one can iterate around the initial chemical structure to refine the drug candidate's characteristics. This can be referred to as *lead optimization*, a process that compares and contrasts the properties of various compounds in terms of key success factors to select those molecules with the greatest potential to become drugs for humans. During this stage, studies may be conducted for the first time in living organisms as well as in vitro.

Beyond the scope of a detailed discussion in this chapter, but critical during this phase of development, are the functions of toxicology and chemical manufacturing. The former includes a number of essential steps to determine the safety and product characteristics of a lead compound using well-harmonized animal models. Key exclusions include carcinogenicity, organ toxicity, and fetal (offspring) genetic anomaly. Chemical manufacturing can also provide critical go or no-go observations determining the fate of a new drug candidate. The complexity and/or number of synthetic steps, the costs associated with the bulk drug (precursor), the yield in the synthetic route, the exposure safety profile to manufacturing staff, and so on are essential steps in determining the viability of a drug to move forward in the development continuum.

Although we often visualize the process of drug discovery as a rational, sophisticated effort, as outlined above, attractive therapeutic indications may become evident only later in the life cycle of a molecule, that is, well after its discovery. For example, it may only be after a Phase 2 trial in indication A that a certain profile emerges in the safety assessment—for example, a reduction in headache frequency from baseline. Such an observation by an astute clinician/researcher may lead to a proof-of-concept trial for the compound for pain relief. A recent real-world example of such a phenomenon is Viagra. This molecule began its development as a cardiovascular disease candidate and ended up as a commercial blockbuster in the treatment of male erectile dysfunction. The point is that despite the profound research breakthroughs in basic neurobiology and chemistry, a number of seminal drug discoveries continue to be the product of clinical observation and creative hypothesis generation. Diligent observation during early clinical trials for "signals" on how a particular drug performs may still create the highest probability of ultimate commercial success. Stated another way, there is no substitute for the well-thought-out collection, analysis, and interpretation of clinical data in making the right choices in drug development.

THE TRANSITION FROM ANIMAL TO HUMAN STUDIES

Investigational New Drug Application

During a new drug's preclinical development, the primary goals are to determine (*1*) if the product is acceptably safe for initial studies in humans and (*2*) whether the compound exhibits the pharmacological activity necessary to justify its commercial development (FDA, 2003). When a product is identified as a viable candidate to move into Phase 1 development (limited, early-stage clinical studies), the focus shifts to the collection of sufficient data to establish that the product will not expose humans to unreasonable risks. Generally, this includes data and information in three broad areas:

- Animal pharmacology and toxicology studies: preclinical data to permit an assessment of whether the product is reasonably safe for initial testing in humans.
- Manufacturing information: information pertaining to the composition, manufacture, stability, and controls used for manufacturing the drug substance and the drug product. This information is assessed to ensure that the company can adequately produce and supply consistent batches of the drug.
- Clinical protocols and investigator information: detailed protocols for proposed clinical studies to assess whether the initial-phase trials will expose participants to unnecessary risks. Also included is information on the qualifications of clinical investigators—professionals (generally physicians) who oversee the administration of the experimental compound—to assess whether they are qualified to fulfill their clinical trial duties.

The investigational new drug (IND) application can be thought of as the culmination of a successful preclinical development program. The IND is a required vehicle for the sponsor to advance to the next stage of drug development: human clinical trials. The IND is not an application to commercialize a new drug. Rather, it is a request for an exemption from the federal statute that prohibits an unapproved drug from being shipped via interstate commerce (FDA, 2003). Current federal law requires that a drug have an approved marketing application before it is transported or distributed across state lines. The sponsor technically obtains this exemption from the FDA for this purpose; however, its real purpose is to provide summary documentation necessary to determine the safety of the drug candidate to move into human studies.

Clinical Drug Development in Humans

Phase 1 includes the initial introduction of an IND into human beings. These studies entail comprehensive evaluations of study participants and may be conducted in patients or (more typically) in healthy volunteers. Trials at this stage of drug development are designed to determine the absorption, distribution, metabolic, and excretory (ADME) profile of the test compound. More and more in neuroscience, pharmacodynamic studies are also being conducted in this early phase of development to ensure central activity and characterize the central structural-activity actions (for example, regional activity). Phase 1 also includes careful observation and recording of the side effects associated with increasing doses and, if possible, early evidence of possible effectiveness signals. These data are crucial to assess whether the molecule has those attributes desired for commercialization. They also serve as a cornerstone for the design of Phase 2 proof-of-efficacy studies. The total number of participants included in Phase 1 studies varies with the drug but is generally in the range of 20 to 80. During Phase 1 studies, the FDA's reviewing division can impose a "clinical hold" if there are potential new and serious risks to humans.

Phase 2 includes early placebo-controlled clinical studies, which are designed to obtain preliminary data on the effectiveness of the drug within a particular indication or indications and are conducted in patients with the disease or condition. This phase of testing also helps determine the more common short-term side effects and risks associated with the drug. Phase 2 studies are typically well controlled, closely monitored, and conducted in a relatively small number of patients, usually several hundred people. Placebo controls are often used to provide for assay sensitivity (is the population being studied actually more responsive to the active intervention?) and to provide a base rate of treatment-associated adverse events that may be part of the disease state in question.

Phase 3 studies are expanded in scope relative to Phase 2 and consist of controlled and uncontrolled trials. They are performed after preliminary evidence suggesting effectiveness of the drug has been obtained in Phase 2 and are intended to gather the additional information about effectiveness and safety that is needed to evaluate the overall benefit–risk relationship of the drug. Phase 3 studies also provide an adequate basis for extrapolating the results to the general population and transmitting that information to the physician via product labeling. Phase 3 studies usually include several hundred to several thousand people. Safety exposures, as an offshoot of recent international regulatory harmonization efforts, usually require at least 1500 exposures (one dose or more) and 6 ($N = 500$) and 12 ($N = 100$) months of continuation treatment. Special population analyses are typically derived from this data set as well.

In Phase 2 and Phase 3, the FDA reviews proposed clinical protocols before they are sent to Institutional Review Boards for ethical approval. If the protocol is clearly deficient in design or in the proposed analytic methods, thus limiting its ability to achieve its stated objectives, revision will be requested.

New Drug Application

The regulation and control of new drugs in the United States have been based on the NDA process since 1938. When the Food, Drug, and Cosmetic Act (FD&C Act) was passed in 1938, NDAs were only required to contain information pertaining to the product's safety profile. However, in 1962, the Kefauver–Harris Amendments to the FD&C Act introduced the requirement that an NDA must also contain evidence that the drug candidate is effective for its intended use. Thus, it established the concept of benefit:risk assessment. Today's NDA is a summary encompassing the entire continuum of data gathered during preclinical animal studies as well as that from the conduct of Phase 1–3 human clinical trials. These data are supplemented by toxicological studies, chemical manufacturing reports, and so on to form the foundation of the NDA (see below). More recently, in 1985, the FDA revised the NDA regulations in what was called the *NDA Rewrite*. This was primarily intended to restructure data organization within the NDA to facilitate the review process.

Although the quantity of information and data submitted in NDAs can vary significantly, the components of NDAs are more uniform. These are well detailed on the FDA's relevant Website. As outlined in Form FDA-356h, the Application to Market a New Drug for Human Use or as an Antibiotic Drug for Human Use, NDAs can consist of as many as 15 different sections:

- Index
- Summary
- Chemistry, Manufacturing, and Control
- Samples, Methods Validation Package, and Labeling
- Nonclinical Pharmacology and Toxicology
- Human Pharmacokinetics and Bioavailability
- Microbiology (for antimicrobial drugs only)
- Clinical Data
- Safety Update Report (typically submitted 120 days after the NDA's submission)
- Statistical
- Case Report Tabulations
- Case Report Forms
- Patent Information
- Patent Certification
- Other Information

SPECIAL TOPICS

In recent years a huge variety of powerful new tools and technologies has become available for life scientists, enabling them to make key advances and discoveries in biotechnology, drug discovery, and other industrial and academic fields. Tools such as deoxyribonucleic acid (DNA) and protein arrays, small interfering ribonucleic acid (RNA) (siRNA), stem cells, and methods of transferring genes from one species to another, combined with high throughput instruments and other systems for laboratory automation, have increased productivity in many laboratories. The field is moving incredibly quickly.

Genomics

Genomics, simply understood, is the effort to establish the relationships between genes and diseases. Recent advances in the sequencing of the genome point to a universe of some 500–1000 genes believed to be associated with one or more disease states. Previously, our screening technology in drug discovery was limited by our marginal understanding of these disease pathways. Genomic research has opened a new front in the search for novel drugs by better enabling us to understand variations in the course of a disease across patients, patterns of symptomatic expression, and interindividual differences in pharmacological response (G.H.S. Ashton et al., 2002).

The relevance of genomics to the drug discovery/development process extends across the entire product life cycle (Fig. 17.6). For example, genomics may (1) facilitate identification of a predisposition among normals (for example, the gene for Huntington's disease), (2) be used to screen and identify those with an early preclinical disease process (for example, glucose-processing irregularities), (3) establish prognostic guidelines for those already diagnosed (for example, tumor grading), (4) serve as a biomarker of disease progression (for example, prostate-specific antigen), or (5) identify those at risk for a nonresponse or patient intolerance (a serious adverse event) related to a drug's chemical structure/mechanism of action (for example, the CD4 count).

During the past decade, pharmaceutical companies have searched for new drug candidates from a universe of some 500 targets. The seductive promise of functional genomics, and perhaps even more exciting proteonomics, is the potential identification of many more new disease-associated targets, perhaps representing as much as a 500-fold increase. For discovery research, techniques such as transcription profiling integrate polymerase chain reaction array elements, array production, hybridization, and image analysis under one roof and increase the probability of technical success. Critical success factors when applying such genomically based technologies to drug discovery include

- integration of DNA, RNA, and protein technology platforms
- knowledge of biology and drug response mechanisms for a target disease
- highly annotated clinical samples
- bioinfomatics
- clinical study methods expertise; biogenetic statistical experience.

With the introduction of gene chip technologies, many drug discovery efforts today are based on characterizing the range of disease expression among populations and understanding patterns of transmission. Microarrays have emerged as key tools for research in all sectors of life science, including large and small pharmas, biotechnology firms, and academic departments. One of the major advances we've seen in the last couple of years is the move from microarrays being a very specialized research tool applied only in top academic labs and a few large corporate centers to being a very robust, high-quality tool available to a wide number of researchers around the globe. As preclinical surrogates are discovered, we will increasingly see their use to validate animal models, accelerate candidate selection, and better inform first human-dose studies. Genomically derived targets are currently evident across such disease states as Alzheimer's disease (for example, beta amyloid), obesity, and breast cancer.

Although most of the benefits have yet to be realized (or perhaps even conceived), the recent investment in the genomic revolution is already paying dividends. Examples include an improved understanding of the molecular basis of some diseases, as well as a glimpse into why and how certain individuals respond to or tolerate a particular pharmaceutical treatment, whereas others do not. Thus, one can envision a growing movement in drug discovery/development to identify more individualized or customized pharmacological solutions. Such "patient-segmented" solutions create internal debate on the market-size ramifications: Will pharmacogenomics fragment a disease state into commercially less attractive (that is, smaller) segments? The real sales impact of a pharmacogenomic marker associated with a high-response/remission rate to a specific drug is a function of the size of that targeted population, the market share the drug can command within that segment, the price premium associated with the delivery of a superior outcome, and the degree to which improved treatment adherence can be anticipated relative to the better response/tolerability of the product within that segment.

Pharmacogenomics also has the potential to revolutionize clinical trials necessary to register a drug (that

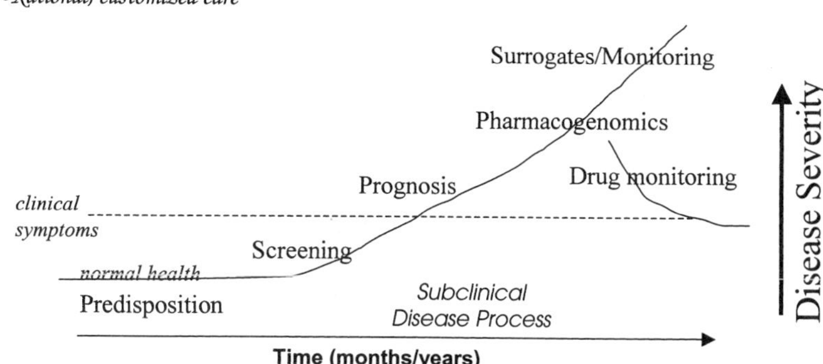

FIGURE 17.6 Molecular medicine: benefits and process.

is, Phase 2/3 studies). Valid clinical surrogates for a disease may accelerate early dose finding and the Phase 2 (proof of concept) to Phase 3 (demonstration of the benefit:risk ratio) transition. This plays into the need to reduce cycle times and drive down unnecessary development expenses/delays.

In summary, genomics has application to drug discovery/ development through

- an increased probability of finding a disease-relevant drug candidate
- more efficient drug development through focused, smaller clinical trials
- enhanced efficacy (effect sizes) based on a better patient-selection process
- improved patient safety by screening out patients with at-risk genotypes
- the identification of additional indications to expand a drug's marketplace utility.

Examples of applying such techniques to drug development include candidate safety and efficacy. An example of the former is "toxicogenomics." This is a new enabling technology that allows for early assessment of a candidate compound's potential toxicity. One example of a company working in this arena is Gene Logic, which is developing a primary rat hepatocyte system as a new assay platform for the prediction of human liver toxicity. In their system, they employ a robust 96-well high-throughput cell culture and microarray assay platform to screen panels of compounds with a high throughput mind-set. The promise of a discipline such as toxicogenomics is to analyze predictive biomarkers early on in the drug development process. On the efficacy side of the equation, gene-based applications have seen their greatest utility in the development of novel oncolytics. The key to understanding the genome is understanding how cells work using the gene products: in other words, a means to manipulate certain elements within the cell and then make systems cell biology measurements. For example, the role of *p53* in as many as one-half of all cancers has been suggested. Cancer drug discovery researchers can now manipulate the levels of *p53* and actually profile drug candidates for their ability to induce apoptosis, metabolic changes, multiple organelle functions, or other desired specific biochemical changes. An example of the increased sophistication in leveraging genomics in a next generation of targeted oncolytics is a molecule like SJG-136. Whereas conventional chemotherapy drugs interact with many areas of DNA to prevent cancer cells from reproducing, SJG-136 has the ability to recognize and bind fewer DNA sequences in a way that may be able to prevent cancer cells from reproducing. This drug candidate has been "engineered" to cross-link the two strands of the DNA double helix at specific sites, effectively "handcuffing" certain parts of the DNA vital to the cancer cells' reproduction. This project is also a nice illustration of the concept of *partnering* mentioned earlier as it brings together Cancer Research UK, the UK biotech company Spirogen, the National Cancer Institute (NCI), and now licensee Ipsen.

Even in neuroscience the concept of *genetic susceptibility factors* has generated interest. At Psychiatric Genomics, researchers start by evaluating postmortem samples of the human brain to discover the changes in gene expression in target individuals compared with normal controls (the disease signature). There is also the opportunity to work backward, that is, to identify the genetic signature within cultured human neurons when exposed to known effective therapeutics. By combining these approaches, drug discoverers hope to identify genes whose changes in expression overlap between disease and drug treatments and, in turn, are interesting targets for novel chemical entities.

RNA Interference

Yet another hot topic in life science laboratories is RNA interference (RNAi), the process that introduces double-stranded RNA into a cell to inhibit gene expression in a sequence-dependent fashion. Much of the excitement here is RNAi participation in antiviral defense and regulation of gene expression. Small interfering RNA (siRNA) or silencing RNA represents a class of 20–25 nucleotide-long double-stranded RNA molecules that play a variety of roles in biology. Most notably, siRNA is involved in the RNAi pathway where the siRNA interferes with the expression of a specific gene. In addition to its role in the RNAi pathway, siRNA can induce gene silencing in mammalian cells. Thus exogenous siRNA holds great promise as a new tool in functional genomics. One of the inherent challenges will be to develop functional assays and employ siRNAs to identify genes in relevant pathways. A leader in this area is Sirna, whose lead clinical development candidate, Sirna-027, is a chemically optimized siRNA currently moving into Phase 2 development for the treatment of the wet-form of age related macular degeneration (AMD). In addition to the collaboration with Allergan, Sirna has established a strategic alliance with GlaxoSmithKline for the development of siRNA compounds for the treatment of respiratory diseases. Yet another example of large pharmas' appetite for biotech innovation was the recent acquisition of Sirna, by Merck, for over $1 billion.

Transgenics and Stem Cells

There is an increasing trend in the pharmaceutical industry to supplement traditional small-molecule research with an increased focus on larger "natural" products, for example, antibodies. Another example of work in this area is under way at Scotland's Roslin Institute, where one transgenic program aims to develop the idea of transgenic chickens that produce human antibodies in quantity and at a reasonable price. Of interest, drug discovery in this area already encompasses some 250 treatments for disease that are actively under development throughout the world and that use human antibodies as their targets. One interesting example is a novel osteoporosis treatment now in final testing among some 9000 patients by Amgen. This new drug, *AMG 162*, isn't a pill but rather a monoclonal antibody created in the laboratory that mimics a beneficial bone protein called *OPG*. OPG neutralizes a second protein that causes bone decay. Amgen researchers reportedly discovered a version of the OPG gene a decade ago, oddly enough, in the intestines of rat fetuses. The new drug may one day transform the osteoporosis market.

In Silico Tools

Efforts to revolutionize cycle times includes efforts that are referred to as *in silico*. In the search for new drug candidates, in silico tries to optimize leads with a team approach that combines computational as well as medicinal chemists. Whereas lead optimization typically requires the synthesis of hundreds of compounds over several years until the desired pharmacological profile is obtained, in silico three-dimensional models and the virtual ADME profiles are especially important because they help disclose what to synthesize and, just as important, what not to synthesize. As an example, Predix Pharmaceuticals reported a recent success in developing a lead candidate for treatment of anxiety and depression where the candidate that was discovered and optimized, from beginning to end, used an in silico model-based approach. This candidate reached clinical trials fewer than 2 years from project initiation including fewer than 6 months in lead optimization. Predix started by modeling the three-dimensional structure of the 5-HT (serotonin) receptor and identified a binding pocket in the extracellular domain. In silico screening identified 78 virtual hits and eventually a lead compound.

High-content Cellular Imaging

High-content imaging permits researchers to validate whether they have "hit" their intended biological target in the cell. It provides an important link between molecular screening and functional cellular assays. Researchers at Boehringer-Ingelheim are employing high-content cellular imaging to support compound prioritization and timely decision making during the hit-to-lead and lead-optimization phases of their drug discovery projects. Among other things, high-content cellular imaging also provides tools to quantitatively analyze cellular events to evaluate compound potency and verify structure-activity relationships. Think of this new tool as a means to preview a look at a complex cellular response to a drug candidate, for example, cytoxicity, apoptosis, and cell cycle.

Have these and other techniques really made a difference? The jury is out, and arguments pro and con exist. Regardless, it has been an expensive bet placed on ensuring survival of pharmaceutical companies going forward, large and small. Stay tuned.

Cycle-Time Reduction

Within drug discovery and development, significant attention has been directed at shortening cycle times, that is, reducing the amount of unnecessary time spent getting from one stage to the next (see Fig. 17.3). Through the mid-1990s, the average cycle time from filing an IND to completion of Phase 3 and submission of the NDA to regulators was approximately 55 months. The best in class experiences were, however, as short as 39 months. Although the length of this process certainly varies by therapeutic area, diagnosis, indication sought, and novelty of the associated mechanism of action, opportunities to eliminate non-value-adding activities are increasingly being sought. Case studies have revealed that drug discovery/development efforts associated with proper allocation of resources, quality leadership and decision making, strong information support, and improved trial design are more likely to deliver new products to the market sooner.

So, not surprisingly, the drug development engine is being asked to increase its productivity. What trends are emerging among drug discovery scientists and clinician researchers? Efforts designed to reduce cycle times include (*1*) acceleration of molecules in the discovery pipeline through efforts to streamline the process, (*2*) increasing or jump starting the number of "shots on goal" within a portfolio through aggressive alliance formation to license novel discovery platforms or new chemical entities, (*3*) more effective implementation of clinical trials with core objectives defined a priori and analysis/reports of trial results, (*4*) reducing regulatory approval times by more effective data presentation and faster response times, and (*5*) being more thoroughly prepared for a product launch.

Of note, every month earlier a new drug is approved is one additional month of sales before the end of the product's patent life cycle.

Intellectual Property

No discussion of drug discovery and development is complete without a few words on intellectual property. No discovery generates revenue for the inventor unless it is protected under a patent. In discovery, though there are many types of patent filings, the more relevant ones for this discussion include the molecular patent (structure), the method of use (for example, the indication treated by drug), and the process for the drug's synthesis. Method of use has to be thought of early in the context of drug development as part of the molecule's life cycle (for example, additional indications after its first commercialization). Otherwise, the developer may have the experience encountered with fluoxetine (Prozac), where its registration and commercialization for premenstrual dysphoric disorder required that the use patent be licensed from an independent group who originally had filed and were issued a patent for that indication.

However, protecting intellectual property is more than just a simple matter of whether the discoverer has a patent. Past drug discovery efforts include numerous situations where a serendipitous observation, in an environment of cost containment and timeline acceleration, led to the generation of a narrow scope of data to support a patent application. Such patents often failed to restrict competitors, who 18 months after the U.S. patent filing had access to critical information about the innovation. Once competitors understood the basic approach and chemical structure of the discoverer's patent, they could identify a related drug candidate from their own chemical library. In turn, they become "fast followers" with the introduction of a related compound. Only some 5 years ago, 42 of the best-selling 100 pharmaceuticals were such follow-up compounds.

Thus, in today's discovery environment, we are seeing a trend in the opposite direction toward the filing of "larger" patent spaces around candidate molecules. For example, companies or academic centers claim that their proprietary technologies and/or databases identify entire classes of drugs or broad gene-based therapeutic strategies. Although the defense of such patents as valid remains a question, it is an important consideration in protecting the company's research investment and challenging future competitors. Thus, intellectual property planning is a cornerstone of the early drug discovery strategy.

The Role of the Patient

Increasingly, drug development and commercialization are being conducted with the customer in mind. The unmet medical needs of patients in a particular disease state serve as the basis for determining the opportunities and technical probabilities for success and, in turn, strategic prioritizations within a therapeutic area.

Examples of patient-centered questions relevant in drug development and commercialization might include the following sequence: (*1*) How prevalent is the problem? (*2*) How aware are individuals of having the problem? (*3*) If they are aware, how likely are they to seek treatment? (*4*) Once engaged in the health care system, how likely are clinicians to identify the problem accurately? (*5*) Once the problem is identified, what is the threshold for deciding to initiate a treatment? (*6*) Finally, what is the patient–physician dynamic in selecting one option over another? This series is sometimes referred to as the *health care transaction model* (Fig. 17.7).

If the patient is the driver in defining drug development targets of interest, we can expect that shifting demographics (for example, aging) and personal expectations (for example, lifestyle optimization) will take on more prominent roles. We have already seen, with respect to the former, increased interest in diseases such as osteoporosis, Alzheimer's dementia, and arthritis. Male erectile dysfunction (the "Viagra phenomenon") perhaps best illustrates the increased attention to lifestyle-enhancing products. However, in that same spectrum are other contemporary indication targets such as urinary incontinence, age-associated memory impairment, physical frailty, and so on.

Proof of efficacy in registering a drug for a new indication requires evidence of superiority on one or more patient-focused disease severity measures. The pharmaceutical industry is familiar with the use of rating instruments such as the Hamilton Depression Rating Scale and the Brief Psychiatric Rating Scale. Although these reflect a historic focus in drug development on treatment efficacy (for example, baseline to end point rating scale score changes achieved during a predefined treatment interval) obtained from a controlled clinical trial, increasing attention is currently evident in the disciplines of health economics and functional well-being. In addition to conventional controlled studies, large-scale naturalistic trials are being used to address these topics. Health economic assessment of a drug development candidate includes efforts to support a product's cost-effectiveness. For example, is there evidence that use of the novel treatment candidate is associated with a reduction in disease-associated direct and/or indirect health costs that exceeds its cost of acquisition relative to the existing standard of care? This assessment focuses on patients in the real world and expands the health care transactional model to include concepts of treatment effectiveness. For example, once written, is a prescription

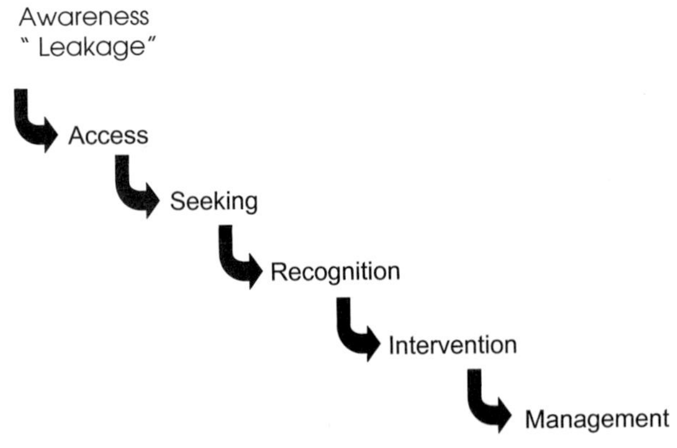

FIGURE 17.7 The health care transaction model.

filled? Once it is filled, is the course of therapy initiated? If it is initiated, how adherent to the recommended schedule and length of treatment is the individual? Each of these questions is becoming increasingly critical when designing clinical trials or commercialization programs to evaluate a new drug's relative impact.

Another aspect of drug therapy is the patient's and the family's increased desire to participate in the selection of the treatment. In the process of rendering an informed consent decision, clinical trials that generate patient-relevant answers will favorably position the new product to be selected. In other words, studies that deliver answers that matter will benefit consumers and better inform their drug choices. The commercialization phase of drug development is currently being challenged to find targeted and impactful communication vehicles to distribute such product-related information. One example, direct-to-consumer advertising in the United States, is on the rise. Thus, a clear trend emerging in the pharmaceutical business is the increased availability/distribution of customer information pertaining to disease, diagnostics, or targeted solutions.

Maximizing the Value Associated with a Drug Discovery

Given the extraordinary challenges in finding and developing a successful drug, it is surprising how often the return on that investment is not optimized. Optimizing a drug discovery can occur through several different pathways: (*1*) an effective launch strategy, (*2*) the reduction of between-country share-of-market variance, and (*3*) superior product life-cycle management.

Preparing for the launch of a product is critical. In the past, the launch may even have been somewhat of an afterthought. Today, months or even years before the receipt of a regulatory authorization to commercialize a drug, detailed launch strategies are begun. These can include preparation of the medical community for a novel mechanism of action, enhanced consumer awareness of a disease, establishment of sales force relationships with key customers/opinion leaders, and so on. All of this effort is designed to accelerate the slope of the product's sales curve during the first 5 years on the market. This parameter has been shown to correlate robustly with the peak sales achieved by the product. Figure 17.8 illustrates some successful recent launch slopes.

Historically, drug candidates were launched in a sequential manner around the world—starting in a test market, learning from that experience, refining a marketing/sales strategy, and then moving to the next country. However, this approach may limit the resources behind the product at any one time, waste precious and finite patent protection, and give competitors more time to prepare a counterpromotional strategy. In some cases, it has taken over a decade for a drug to be commercialized in each of its 10 largest pharmaceutical markets. In reaction, we now see a greater effort to speed the pace of new product globalization via global branding, simultaneous launches, and the use of centralized regulatory reviews such as those of the European Medicines Agency for member-states of the European Union. Such approaches can also accelerate the time to peak global sales for a drug. Even a 2-year acceleration can generate an additional 10% in annual sales for each of the first 5 years postlaunch.

It is amazing to see the wide variance in a drug's share of market by country, despite a fairly consistent set of patient needs and opportunities. Some of the variables identified are the sales and marketing infrastructure investment made by the country, the degree of shared learning by local organizations, the ability to retain experienced persons in key roles, the investment in local drug experience programs, and support of opinion leader investigator-initiated trials. When key opinion leaders are not engaged in a therapeutic area (for example, via an opportunity to work with the new drug), it has been demonstrated that initial product uptake and excitement will be not be optimized. Strategies to reduce variance in

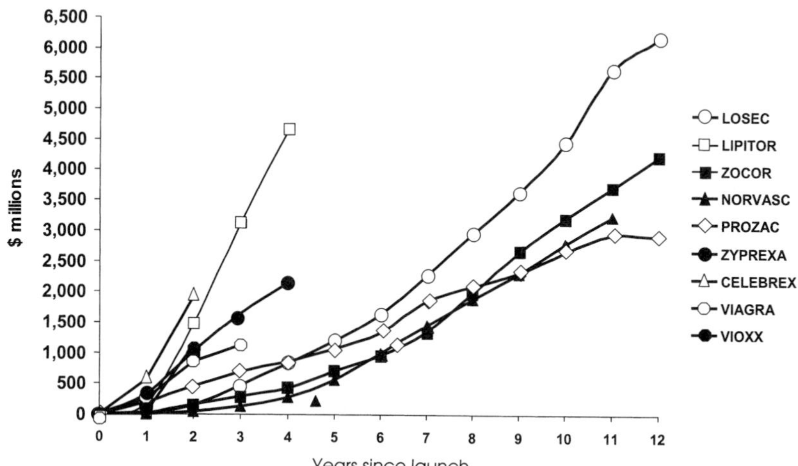

FIGURE 17.8 Sales development of top brands.

market penetration across launch countries provide a significant opportunity to improve the investment return.

Enhanced product life-cycle management is the third means to optimize commercial success. This is achieved by new (additional) indications and/or alternative product formulations. In addition to expanding the scope of the drug's target market, such strategies are tailored to address unique patient needs. A collateral benefit of post-launch development activities is the continued flow of new drug information/studies that increase promotional access time and, in turn, product excitement (noise). As a benchmark, the best in class at life-cycle management average three to five subsequent indications during the patent life of the molecule.

The Role of Strategy

Often there is no one strategy that can be singled out as clearly superior to another. What differentiates a winning approach is often based on how well the enterprise has defined its own capabilities and networking and then how effectively the strategic plan is implemented. A.T. Kearney (1999) commented that companies with winning strategies tend to share four characteristics:

- ensuring that all internal and external activities complement each other and are well coordinated
- building many technology platforms rather than betting on only one approach
- encouraging change within the organization
- challenging the way routine business is conducted (continuous process improvement)

The key strategic questions when formulating a development strategy can be captured in four steps (Table 17.1). The first three enable the company to develop a hypothesis or propose strategic options for the development program, and the fourth focuses on implementation. The first step, "analyses and givens," includes a definition of the market (for example, the disease state or indication sought) and its relevant subsegments. What are the greatest treatment needs for a given disease? What are the significant trends characterizing that disease state? How might the program seize a competitive advantage? This step also surveys the competitors, analyzing their strengths and weaknesses relative to the company's strategic position. It leads to the identification of methods to ensure a sustained competitive advantage. The second step is the "strategic ends" of the development effort: what will the seminal areas of investigation be and why? It considers the disease state, customer or patient groups, and geographic differences in the identification of the project's critical success factors. These project-specific factors can be translated into a set of metrics that permit measurement along the project's development timeline; they are a series of milestones deemed essential to achieve the ultimate strategic product intent. Last, this step considers any asset gaps in the program and proposes solutions. The third step consists of "strategic means." It includes consideration of a value proposition describing what the development opportunity will provide to make a difference for key customers or stakeholders. Last, it considers current resource gaps. Here one must decide which of those gaps will be addressed and which will not. For the latter, this implies the opportunity to determine the consequences of not addressing them. The final or fourth strategic planning step consists of the "operational plan." For example, what are the key decisions/milestones that will define the project's success? What are the key supporting activities necessary to enable decision making? At this stage, the strategy is translated into a business plan, ideally one that can be implemented. In summary, having a strategy is important; implementing it in an efficient manner is essential.

TABLE 17.1. *Strategic Planning Framework*

(1) *Analyses and Givens*	*(2)* *Strategic Ends*	*(3)* *Strategic Means*	*(3)* *Operational Plan*
Markets	Mission	Image of value Cycle	Targets Tasks
Key players	Vision	Key value proposition	Resources
Business fundamentals	Strategic intent		Schedules
		Relationship to key players	
Key externalities	Core		Processes
Critical trends	Competencies		
Key uncertainities		Product programs	Sites
Competitor positioning	Key metrics	Capabilities and key relationships	Budgets
Strengths and weaknesses	Business lines	Organizational architecture	Other resources

SUMMARY

In conclusion, the top-performing groups involved in drug discovery and clinical product development will be those that successfully focus on information, people, and processes. Information is the cornerstone of any business steeped in intellectual property. In drug development, this includes integration of critical players, top-tier bioinformatics support, competent technology assessment (licensing necessary supplemental tools and talent), and competitive analysis (external environmental awareness). Of note, pharmaceutical product development will not be able to realize the advantages provided by the technological revolution without the requisite processes in place that foster use and exchange of that information, that is, unleash the potential of the talent base within the enterprise. In the discovery of drugs, necessary processes that facilitate successful implementation of work efforts include portfolio management, program assessment, project management, resource management, and adherence to predesignated critical success factors (the ability to fail fast). In drug development, many of the same processes are leveraged; however, an even greater premium is placed on having milestone-driven timelines and external benchmarking comparisons. On approaching the launch of a new drug, premarket preparation including an understanding of the customer, disease-relevant patient segments, health economic rationale, and an effective communication process with key customers (for example, regulators, payors, advocates) is essential.

Last, a company or academic center will not achieve success in the highly complicated world of drug discovery/development without the brightest and best people. Necessary skills include innovation, technology development, project management (implementation), networking, and portfolio management (prioritization). Critical issues are not limited to their recruitment but also include retention. The latter is facilitated by reward and recognition programs and a work environment that offers flexible career development opportunities.

REFERENCES

Ashton, G.H.S., McGrath, J.A., and South, A.P. (2002) Strategies to identify disease genes. *Drugs of Today* 38(4):235–244.

Ashton, M.J., Jaye, M., and Mason, J.S. (1996) New perspectives in lead generation I: discovery of biologic targets. *Drug Discov. Today* 1:11–15.

Food and Drug Administration, Center for Drug Evaluation and Research Regulatory (2003) http://www.fda.gov/cder/regulatory/default.htm.

Goldsbrough, P., Lawyer, P., and Sondhi, G. (1999) *The Pharmaceutical Industry into its Second Century: From Serendipity to Strategy*. Boston: Boston Consulting Group.

Kearney, A.T. (1999) *Sharpening Discovery and Development Skills–Quickly Adjusting to a New Paradigm*. A.T. Kearney.

Nicholson, S., Danzon, P.M., and McCullogh, J. (2005, July) Biotech-pharma alliances as a signal of asset and firm quality. *Journal of Business*.

PriceWaterhouseCoopers. (1998) *Pharma 2005 An Industrial Revolution in R & D*. http://www.pwc.com/gx/eng/about/ind/pharma/industrial_revolution.pdf.

Schreiber, S.L. (2000) Target-oriented and diversity oriented organic synthesis in drug discovery. *Science* 287:1964–1969.

III PSYCHOSES

JEFFREY A. LIEBERMAN

THIS section describes what is known and has been learned about schizophrenia and related psychotic disorders since the publication of the second edition of the *Neurobiology of Mental Illness*. It includes three revised chapters (Genetics of Schizophrenia, Neurobiological Theories of Schizophrenia, and Pharmacotherapy of Schizophrenia) and four new chapters (Diagnosis of Schizophrenia, Postmortem and In Vivo Structural Pathology in Schizophrenia, Cognitive Neuroscience and Neuroimaging in Schizophrenia, and The Neurochemistry of Schizophrenia: A Focus on Dopamine and Glutamate) all authored by leading researchers in these respective disciplines. The expansion of this section in some ways reflects the growing knowledge base and increased traction that we have developed in the field of schizophrenia research.

Schizophrenia is the most dramatic and disabling of mental diseases, almost always chronic and devastating in its social and psychological impact. It represents what might be considered the prototype for brain disorders that are manifest through disturbances in mental functions (of perception, cognition, and emotion) and behavior. We have chosen to consider this illness and discuss its associated phenomenology and underlying neurobiology in the context of the broader rubric of schizophrenia and related psychotic disorders, as the nosologic boundaries are not sharply defined or definitively validated. Ultimately, it will be from the data which emerges from studies of these investigative approaches that the precise definition and even the etiology of schizophrenia will be determined.

No chapter can be completely comprehensive in covering all of the relevant information and theories. However, this section is representative of our knowledge about schizophrenia and includes the most current and important lines of investigation, and illuminating and influential theoretical formulations on this topic. We hope that readers will find this section of interest and beneficial in their effort to understand and combat this mysterious and ancient illness.

18 Diagnosis of Schizophrenia

MICHAEL B. FIRST

Although there have been impressive discoveries in schizophrenia research over the past three decades, there is still a glaring lack of progress in answering some of the most basic questions about the etiology and pathophysiology of this illness. For example, it is not known if neurodevelopmental versus neurodegenerative processes (or both) underlie the illness, what gene (or family of genes) is (are) causative, how environmental factors affect disease progression, or what are the key neurochemical processes responsible for symptom manifestation. For this reason, schizophrenia is still best understood as a clinical syndrome, that is, a collection of mental and behavioral phenomena that co-occur in individuals and that have a characteristic course, treatment response, and family history.

Attempts to find valid criteria to classify the psychoses are centuries old. In the past 40 years, great progress has been made in the diagnostic classification of schizophrenia and the other psychotic disorders. Worldwide, the *Diagnostic and Statistical Manual of Mental Disorders*'s (*DSM-IV*; American Psychiatric Association [APA], 1994) definition of *schizophrenia* is the most influential in clinical practice and research (Mezzich, 2002). Its operationalized criteria facilitate communication among clinicians and researchers and promote reliable assessment methods (Bertelsen, 2002). It has high clinical utility, providing nontrivial information about course, outcome, and likely treatment response (e.g., Bromet, Naz, et al., 2005). However useful the *DSM-IV* construct of *schizophrenia* is, it does not provide information about the fundamental etiology or pathophysiology of the illness. On the contrary, some have argued that the hegemony and reification of the *DSM-IV* diagnostic definitions may be hindering, rather than advancing, research into our understanding of mental disorders (Charney, Barlow, et al., 2002). Hyman (2003) cautioned that

> scientists attempting to discover genetic or neural underpinnings of disease have all too often reified the disorders listed in DSM-IV-TR as "natural kinds." . . In reifying DSM-IV-TR diagnoses, one increases the risk that science will get stuck, and the very studies that are needed to define phenotypes are held back. (p. xix)

This chapter begins with a review of the historical roots of the concept and definition of *schizophrenia*. Next, the current "official" diagnostic criteria for schizophrenia (that is, *DSM-IV* and International Classification of Diseases [ICD]-10) will be examined. Then the potential advantages of alternative psychopathological approaches including broad inclusion criteria (that is, the schizophrenia spectrum) and more discrete subtyping approaches based on symptom clusters will be examined. Last, the issue of whether schizophrenia is best conceptualized as a categorical versus dimensional construct, an issue that will be addressed during the next revision of the *DSM* and ICD classifications, is discussed.

HISTORICAL OVERVIEW

In ancient Greece, Hippocrates (460–377 B.C.) (Hippocrates, 1950) in his medical writings identified six conditions based on the observed phenomenology of mental disorders: (*1*) phrenitis (acute mental disturbance with fever); (*2*) mania (acute mental disturbance without fever); (*3*) melancholia (all kinds of chronic mental disturbances); (*4*) epilepsy (same as current meaning); (*5*) hysteria (paroxysmic dyspnea, pain, convulsions); and (*6*) Scythian disease (comparable to transvestitism). In addition, Hippocrates provided what amounted to a second diagnostic axis for noting the four temperaments by relating them to internal imbalances of the four bodily humors: (*1*) choleric (angry, hostile traits related to an excess of yellow bile); (*2*) sanguine (optimistic cheerful traits related to an excess of blood); (*3*) melancholic (pessimistic, depressed traits related to excess of black bile); and (*4*) phlegmatic (apathetic, indifferent traits related to an excess of lymph). He speculated that our emotions, joyous and sorrowful, come from the brain and posited that madness arises from the diseased brain.

Galen (129–216), a prominent physician in the first century A.D., also attributed mental illness to the disturbances of the humors. He expanded upon the Aristotelian notion of mania and melancholia and described abnormalities in emotion and thought as a result of spirits and temperature alterations in the brain. He extended the notion that mental illnesses can be divided into subtypes, including aspects of paranoia and despair.

Sydenham (1624–1663), the father of modern medical thinking, rejected the notion that there was a single dysfunction at the root of all ailments (for example, distorted humeral balance) and postulated that each disease has an independent existence with a uniform presentation in different individuals so that the same phenomena that you would observe in the sickness of a Socrates you would observe in the sickness of a simpleton (Latham, 1848). He proposed that diseases should be carefully observed and reduced to species in the same way as the emerging science of botany was beginning to classify plants.

Philippe Pinel (1745–1820), a prominent French physician, was one of a growing list of clinical scientists who proposed that mental illness is a disease of the central nervous system and can be caused by hereditary and environmental factors. He classified mental illness into four fundamental clinical types: (*1*) mania (all conditions with acute excitement or fury); (*2*) melancholia (depressive conditions, delusions with limited topics); (*3*) dementia (lack of cohesion in the ideas); and (*4*) idiotism (including idiocy and organic dementia). He also grouped patients into those who had continuous symptoms and those who had signs of intermittent madness.

In 1857, the British neurologist Sir John Russell first differentiated positive and negative symptoms in patients with epilepsy (Berrios, 1985). This early symptom dichotomy became an important subtyping approach that is reflected in the current nosology of schizophrenia. In the psychiatric literature, positive symptoms have come to mean those that are actively expressed, such as hallucinations, thought disorder, delusions, and bizarre behavior, whereas the negative symptoms reflect deficit states such as avolition, flattened affect, and alogia.

Benedict-Augustin Morel (1809–1873) was the first to describe a mental illness primarily on the basis of course. This illness, which he referred to as *demence precoce,* was characterized by mental deterioration with an early onset that evolved rapidly (that is, over a few months to a few years). Emil Kraepelin (1856–1926) made a distinction between what he called *dementia praecox* and manic depression (Kraepelin, 1919). *Dementia* referred to the progressive deteriorating course of emotional and cognitive processes, whereas *praecox* indicated the early age of onset in previously healthy individuals. Kraepelin differentiated the generally deteriorating course of dementia praecox from the more episodic and customarily better outcome seen in manic depressive disorder, although he later came to believe that not all patients with dementia praecox ended in a demented state and that a few even recovered. Kraepelin observed, however, that a common pattern among these patients was that they experienced a withdrawn state with concomitant hallucinations or bizarre delusions with no impairment of consciousness, sensorium, or memory. He divided patients into three subtypes—hebephrenic, catatonic, and paranoid—and later described paraphrenia, a separate clinical entity resembling paranoia with either systematized or nonsystematized beliefs and not characterized by the deterioration of personality that occurred in dementia praecox.

Eugen Bleuler (1857–1937) introduced the term *schizophrenia,* which means "split brain," because he was impressed with the dissociation between the cognitive and affective features of patients with this illness (Bleuler, 1950). He differed from Kraepelin in believing that schizophrenia is not typically characterized by an early onset and a terminal dementia, and that delusions and hallucinations were accessory symptoms because they also occurred in other illnesses. Bleuler developed the notion that patients with schizophrenia had at least one primary symptom (one of the "four A's") and other secondary symptoms. Bleuler's diagnostic "four A's" consisted of: profound ambivalence, looseness of associations, disturbance of affect (either excitation or withdrawal), and autism, which he described as living in an internal, unrealistic world, separated from normal social interaction. Secondary symptoms included delusions and hallucinations. His description of *schizophrenia* described a much broader and more heterogeneous group of patients as compared to Kraepelins, many of whom were less ill. Bleuler's career overlapped with Sigmund Freud's, and he, like Freud, believed that factors at work underneath the explicit manifestation of behavior were important determinants of illness.

American psychiatrists in the middle of the 20th century were using a relatively broad definition of *schizophrenia* based largely on the Bleulerian four A's. At its broadest, the boundaries of the concept of *schizophrenia* included Kasanin's (1993) schizoaffective disorder, Hoch and Polatin's (1949) pseudoneurotic schizophrenia, and "good prognosis" schizophrenia (Vaillant, 1964), as well as nonpsychotic variants such as simple and latent schizophrenia.

Kurt Schneider (1887–1967), partly in response to diagnostic uncertainties inherent in Bleuler's broadly defined concepts, formulated a list of first- and second-rank symptoms that he thought captured the essence of schizophrenia and would help differentiate it from other forms of psychosis (Schneider, 1959). According to Schneider, the diagnosis of *schizophrenia* is appropriate if the patient experiences just one first-rank symptom, while the second-rank symptoms, although common in schizophrenia, are not as specific to this illness. These so-called pathognomonic first-rank symptoms included delusions of thoughts being broadcast, feelings of an external force inserting thoughts or withdrawing them from the mind, thought interference, and the sensation of forces influencing behavior, will, or bodily functions. The first-rank symptoms also included specific hallucinatory experiences, such as hearing voices, often two or more, commenting on the patient's behavior, or criticizing the patient. The second-rank symptoms included paranoia, affective extremes, apathy or absence of emotions, and any hallucinatory experience other than those described above. Schneider's description of schizophrenia emphasized the presence of one or more of these psychotic symptoms and was cross-sectional in its definition of the illness. He defined an acutely ill group of patients significantly different from either those described by Kraepelin (who were more chronic) or Bleuler (who were less psychotic). The validity of using first-rank symptoms to diagnose schizophrenia, however, has been questioned (Bertelsen, 2002).

An important research development that had a significant impact on the diagnostic conceptualization of schizophrenia came from the United States-United Kingdom Diagnostic Project (Zubin and Gurland, 1977). It had been observed that although the total admission rates for functional psychoses were nearly identical in the two countries, the relative admission rates for schizophrenia and affective disorders were strikingly different; namely, that schizophrenia was diagnosed 4 times more often in the United States as compared to the United Kingdom, with the opposite being true for a diagnosis of affective disorder. To determine whether these diagnostic discrepancies were due to differences intrinsic to the patient populations or to differences in the diagnostic concepts, the same structured interview that combined items from the Present State Examination (Wing, Cooper, et al., 1974) and the Psychiatric Status Schedule (Spitzer, Endicott, et al., 1970) was administered to patients in both countries. The study found that the differences were not in the patients themselves or even in the symptoms observed by the clinicians but rather in the way that the symptoms were interpreted and classified; specifically, it was the very broad concept of *schizophrenia* used by the American psychiatrists compared to the much narrower concept used by their British counterparts that was responsible for the apparent diagnostic differences.

At the time of the U.S.-U.K. study, psychiatrists' definitions of *schizophrenia* and *affective disorder* were based on relatively broad glossary definitions that lent themselves to potentially idiosyncratic interpretations. For example, *DSM-II* (APA, 1968) defined *schizophrenia* as follows:

> This large category includes a group of disorders manifested by characteristic disturbances of thinking, mood and behavior. Disturbances in thinking are marked by alternations of concept formation which may lead to misinterpretation of reality and sometimes to delusions and hallucinations, which frequently appear to be psychologically self-protective. Corollary mood changes include ambivalent, constructed, and inappropriate emotional responsiveness and loss of empathy with others. Behavior may be withdrawn, regressive and bizarre. (p. 33)

The U.S.-U.K. study underscored the importance of adopting well-operationalized definitions for *schizophrenia* and *affective disorder* to ensure that diagnoses are made in a standardized manner. Furthermore, another consequence of these findings was that a narrower definition of schizophrenia and a broader construct for *psychotic mood disorder* were subsequently adopted in the United States.

The first widely adopted operationalized definition of *schizophrenia* was put forth by a group of researchers at the Washington University School of Medicine, led by Robins and Guze, as part of the so-called Feighner criteria, which were named after the senior author of the paper that presented the criteria (Feighner, Robins, et al., 1972). Research criteria were provided for 16 diagnostic categories and listed those features required for each (known as *inclusion criteria*) and those features whose presence would rule out each diagnosis (known as *exclusion criteria*). The Feighner criteria for schizophrenia are shown in Table 18.1. Central to the definition was the requirement that it be a chronic illness with a minimum 6-month duration with a deteriorating level of functioning (that is, without a return to the premorbid level of psychosocial adjustment). Unlike later definitions of *schizophrenia*, few specifics regarding the nature of the required positive symptoms were indicated; essentially any type of delusions, hallucinations, or thought disorder was sufficient to meet criteria. The Feighner criteria proved to be enormously popular with the re-

TABLE 18.1 *Feighner Criteria for Schizophrenia*

For a diagnosis of schizophrenia, A through C are required:

A. Both of the following are necessary:
   (*1*) a chronic illness with at least 6 months of symptoms prior to the index evaluation without return to the premorbid level of psychosocial adjustment
   (*2*) absence of a period of depressive or manic symptoms sufficient to quality for affective disorder or probable affective disorder
B. The patient must have at least one of the following:
   (*1*) delusions or hallucinations without significant perplexity or disorientation associated with them
   (*2*) verbal production that makes communication difficulty because of a lack of logical or understandable organization
C. At least three of the following must be present for a diagnosis of "definite" schizophrenia and two for a diagnosis of "probable" schizophrenia
   (*1*) single
   (*2*) poor premorbid social adjustment or work history
   (*3*) family history of schizophrenia
   (*4*) absence of alcoholism or drug abuse within 1 year of onset of psychosis
   (*5*) onset of illness prior to age 40

From Feighner et al. (1972), p. 59.

search community as indicated by the fact that they were cited 1157 times from 1972 through 1980, which was more than 70 times the citation rate of an average article published in the *Archives of General Psychiatry* during that same time (Blashfield, 1982).

A "successor" to the Feighner criteria, in the sense that they were similarly widely adopted by psychiatric researchers, were the Research Diagnostic Criteria (RDC) (Spitzer, Endicott, et al., 1978) that were developed in 1975 to meet the needs of a National Institute of Mental Health–sponsored collaborative project on the psychobiology of depression. The RDC criteria for schizophrenia (see Table 18.2) differed from the Feighner criteria in several important ways. First of all, the 6-month duration requirement was dropped, greatly broadening the definition to include nonchronic cases. Secondly, the criteria relied "heavily on the presence of Schneiderian first-rank symptoms in order to exclude borderline and paranoid states" (p. 776). Finally, in contrast to *DSM-II* and ICD-9, which included schizoaffective disorder as a subtype of schizophrenia, the RDC included a separate category for schizoaffective disorder, reflected in the "C" criterion exclusion.

With the publication of *DSM-III* in 1980 (APA, 1980), operationalized diagnostic criteria (mostly based on the RDC definitions) were provided for each disorder in the classification. Although the cross-sectional symptom criteria for schizophrenia in *DSM-III* were largely the same as the RDC definition (that is, relying heavily on Schneiderian symptoms), *DSM-III* returned to the Feighner requirement that the duration of the disturbance be at least 6 months to "define a group that is more homogeneous with regard to familial pattern and course" (Williams and Spitzer, 1982, p. 1284) (see Table 18.3) Changes to the definition of schizophrenia in the next revision, *DSM-III-R* (APA, 1987), were relatively modest: the list of active phase symptoms was reorganized in order to give the Schneiderian symptoms less prominence, the word "deterioration" was removed from the definition because of the incorrect implication that recovery never occurs, and the requirement that the onset be before age 45 was eliminated since studies demonstrated the existence of late onset cases (see Table 18.4).

THE DIAGNOSIS OF SCHIZOPHRENIA IN *DSM-IV*

The most recent major revision of the *DSM*, *DSM-IV*, was published in 1994 (a text revision, *DSM-IV-TR*, was published in 2000, but, with few exceptions, no changes were made to the diagnostic criteria sets) (First and Pincus, 2002). Table 18.5 presents the *DSM-IV* diagnostic criteria for schizophrenia. Going back to the RDC definition, schizophrenia has been divided into one or more active phases (generally lasting at least 1 month) that may be interspersed with one or more residual phases consisting of attenuated forms of the active phase symptoms. Furthermore, prior to the onset of the first active phase, there may be a period of similarly attenuated symptoms, known as the *prodromal phase*.

TABLE 18.2 *The Research Diagnostic Criteria (RDC) for Diagnosis of Schizophrenia*

A through C are required for the period of illness being considered.

A. During an active phase of the illness (may or may not now be present), at least two of the following are required for definite and one for probable:
   (*1*) thought broadcasting, insertion or withdrawal
   (*2*) delusions of being controlled (or influenced), other bizarre delusions, or multiple delusions
   (*3*) somatic, grandiose, religious, nihilistic, or other delusions without persecutory or jealous content lasting at least 1 week
   (*4*) delusions of any type if accompanied by hallucinations of any type for at least 1 week
   (*5*) auditory hallucinations in which either a voice keeps up a running commentary on the patient's behavior or thoughts as they occur, or two or more voices conversing with each other
   (*6*) nonaffective verbal hallucinations spoken to the patient
   (*7*) hallucinations of any type throughout the day for several days or intermittently for at least 1 month
   (*8*) definite instances of marked formal thought disorder accompanied by either blunted or inappropriate affect, delusions or hallucinations of any type, or grossly disorganized behavior

B. Signs of the illness lasted at least 2 weeks from the onset of a noticeable change in the patient's usual condition (current signs of the illness may not now meet criterion A and may be residual symptoms only, such as extreme social withdrawal, blunted or inappropriate affect, mild formal thought disorder, or unusual thoughts or perceptual experiences).

C. At no time during the active period of illness being considered (delusions, hallucinations, marked formal thought disorder, bizarre behavior, etc.) did the patient meet full criteria for either probable or definite manic or depressive syndrome to such a degree that it was a prominent part of the illness.

From Spitzer, Endicott, and Robins (1978).

TABLE 18.3 DSM-III *Criteria for Schizophrenia*

A. At least one of the following during a phase of the illness:

(*1*) bizarre delusions (content is patently absurd and has no possible basis in fact, such as delusions of being controlled, thought broadcasting, thought insertion, or thought withdrawal)

(*2*) somatic, grandiose, religious, nihilistic, or other delusions without persecutory or jealous content

(*3*) delusions with persecutory or jealous content if accompanied by hallucinations of any type

(*4*) auditory hallucinations in which either a voice keeps up a running commentary on the individual's behavior or thoughts, or two or more voices conversing with each other

(*5*) auditory hallucinations on several occasions with content of more than one or two words, having no apparent relation to depression or elation

(*6*) incoherence, marked loosening of associations, markedly illogical thinking or marked poverty of content of speech if associated with at least one of the following:

(*a*) blunted, flat, or inappropriate affect

(*b*) delusions or hallucinations

(*c*) catatonic or other grossly disorganized behavior

B. Deterioration from a previous level of functioning such as work, social relations, and self-care

C. Duration. Continuous signs of the illness for at least 6 months at some time during the patient's life with some signs of the illness at present. The 6-month period must include an active phase during which there were symptoms from A with or without a prodrome or residual phase.

D. The full depressive or manic syndrome if present developed after any psychotic symptoms or was brief in duration relative to the duration of the psychotic symptoms in A.

E. Onset of the prodrome or active phase of the illness before age 45

F. Not due to any organic mental disorder or mental retardation

TABLE 18.4 DSM-III-R *Criteria for Schizophrenia*

A. Presence of characteristic psychotic symptoms in the active phase: either (*1*), (*2*), or (*3*) for at least 1 week (unless the symptoms are successfully treated):

(*1*) two of the following:

(*a*) delusions

(*b*) prominent hallucinations (throughout the day for several days or several times a week for several weeks, each hallucinatory experience not being limited to a few brief moments)

(*c*) incoherence or marked loosening of associations

(*d*) catatonic behavior

(*e*) flat or grossly inappropriate affect

(*2*) bizarre delusions (that is, involving a phenomenon that the person's culture would regard as totally implausible, for example, thought broadcasting, being controlled by a dead person)

(*3*) prominent hallucinations of a voice with content having no apparent relation to depression or elation or a voice keeping up a running commentary on the person's behavior or thoughts or two or more voices conversing with each other

B. During the course of the disturbance, functioning in such areas as work, social relations, and self-care is markedly below the highest level achieved before the onset of the disturbance.

C. Schizoaffective and mood disorder with psychotic features has been ruled out, that is, if a major depressive or manic syndrome has ever been present during an active phase of the disturbance, the total duration of all episodes of a mood syndrome has been brief relative to the total duration of the active and residual phases of the disturbance.

D. Continuous signs of the disturbance for at least 6 months. The 6-month period must include an active phase (of at least 1 week or less if symptoms have been successfully treated) during which there were psychotic symptoms characteristic of schizophrenia (symptoms in A), with or without a prodromal or residual phase.

E. It cannot be established that an organic factor initiated and maintained the disturbance.

F. If there is a history of autistic disorder, the additional diagnosis of schizophrenia is made only if prominent delusions or hallucinations are also present.

TABLE 18.5 DSM-IV *Criteria for Schizophrenia*

A. *Characteristic symptoms*: Two (or more) of the following, each present for a significant portion of time during a 1-month period (or less if successfully treated):
   (*1*) delusions
   (*2*) hallucinations
   (*3*) disorganized speech (for example, frequent derailment or incoherence)
   (*4*) grossly disorganized or catatonic behavior
   (*5*) negative symptoms, that is, affective flattening, alogia or avolition

Note: Only one A symptom is required if delusions are bizarre or hallucinations consist of a voice keeping up a running commentary on the person's behavior or thoughts, or two or more voices conversing with each other.

B. *Social/occupational dysfunction:* For a significant portion of the time since the onset of the disturbance, one or more major areas of functioning such as work, interpersonal relations, or self-care are markedly below the level achieved prior to the onset (or when the onset is in childhood or adolescence, failure to achieve expected level of interpersonal, academic, or occupational achievement).

C. *Duration:* Continuous signs of the disturbance persist for at least 6 months. This 6-month period must include at least 1 month of symptoms (or less if successfully treated) that meet criterion A (that is, active phase symptoms), and may include periods of prodromal or residual symptoms. During these prodromal or residual periods, the signs of the disturbance may be manifested by only negative symptoms (that is, affective flattening, alogia, avolition) or two or more symptoms listed in criterion A present in an attenuated form (for example, odd beliefs, unusual perceptual experiences).

D. *Schizoaffective and mood disorder exclusion:* Schizoaffective disorder and mood disorder with psychotic features have been ruled out because either: (*1*) no major depressive, manic or mixed episodes have occurred concurrently with the active phase symptoms (that is, the "A" symptoms listed above) or (*2*) the total duration of mood episodes (occurring during the disturbance) has been brief relative to the total duration of the active and residual phases.

E. *Substance/general medical condition exclusion:* The disturbance is not due to the direct physiological effects of a substance (for example, a drug of abuse, a medication) or to a general medical condition.

F. *Relationship to a pervasive developmental disorder:* If there is a history of autistic disorder or another pervasive developmental disorder, the additional diagnosis of schizophrenia is made only if prominent delusions or hallucinations are also present for at least a month (or less if successfully treated).

Criterion A, which specifies the symptoms characteristic of the active phase of the illness, defines a remarkably heterogeneous group of schizophrenic symptom presentations, consistent with the wide range of presentations that have been observed historically. Those patients who qualify by virtue of having delusions and hallucinations (criteria A[1] and A[2]) manifest the most typically Kraepelinin form of the disorder; those with disorganized speech, disorganized behavior, and negative symptoms (criteria A[3], A[4], and A[5]) have a more typically Bleulerian form of schizophrenia, whereas those patients who qualify under the "note" (indicating that the criterion is satisfied by virtue of either bizarre delusions or hallucinations of a voice keeping up a running commentary or two or more voices conversing) correspond to Schneider's definition of the disorder. Among the changes introduced to the criteria in *DSM-IV* was the increase in the minimum duration of symptoms from 1 week to 1 month and the addition of negative symptoms to the roster of active phase symptoms in recognition of their correlation with cognitive impairment, imaging findings, differential treatment response, and poor outcome (Carpenter, Bartko, et al., 1978; Angrist, Rotrosen, et al., 1980; Breier, Wolkowitz, et al., 1987; Andreasen, Flaum, et al., 1990).

Criterion B establishes a definition of *schizophrenia* that requires major impairment in functioning during a significant portion of the current episode. This impairment can arise from either the impact of the delusions or hallucinations on the person's functioning (for example, refusal to leave the house because of persecutory delusions), from the disorganized speech or behavior, or most commonly from the negative symptoms. This requirement helps to differentiate schizophrenia from delusional disorder, in which the individual's functioning is largely preserved apart from the impact of the delusions. Criterion C requires that the duration of the disturbance (adding up the prodromal, active, and residual phases) must have lasted for 6 months or longer to qualify for a diagnosis of *schizophrenia.* Illness durations of between 1 month and 6 months are diagnosed as *schizophreniform disorder,* and durations of less than 1 month are diagnosed as *brief psychotic disorder*.

Although pure forms of schizophrenia and episodic mood disorders are certainly quite common, there are a large number of individuals who have a mixture of mood and psychotic symptoms. The categorical nature of the *DSM* and ICD forces the clinician to choose among three mutually exclusive categories for classifying such individuals: schizophrenia, schizoaffective disorder, or mood disorder with psychotic features (see below for a critique of this categorical requirement). Criterion D delineates between schizophrenia and the other two disorders by establishing rules concerning the temporal overlap of the mood and psychotic symptoms and the relative proportion of time during the disturbance that the individual is experiencing mood symptoms versus psychotic symptoms. Schizoaffective disorder and mood disorder with psychotic features require the concurrent occurrence of psychotic symptoms and mood symptoms; in the absence of such overlap (that is, mood symptoms occurring only during nonpsychotic phases of the disturbance), schizophrenia is diagnosed regardless of how long the mood symptoms have lasted. In those cases in which there is an overlap between active phase and mood symptoms, the decision as to whether to diagnose schizophrenia versus schizoaffective disorder/mood disorder with psychotic features depends on a consideration of the duration of mood symptoms versus the total duration of the disturbance. If the relative duration of mood symptoms is brief (that is, the mood symptoms are only a minor part of the overall picture), then the diagnosis is schizophrenia; otherwise, the disorder is schizoaffective disorder or mood disorder with psychotic features (the choice depending essentially on whether the psychotic symptoms have occurred exclusively in the context of a mood episode, in which case the diagnosis is mood disorder with psychotic features).

Criterion E is meant to exclude cases in which the symptoms are due to the direct physiological effects of a substance or a general medical condition on the central nervous system. In *DSM-IV*, the term *substance-induced* is used broadly to include the effects of intoxication or withdrawal from drugs of abuse (for example, phencyclidine intoxication, alcohol withdrawal) as well as from prescribed medications (for example, corticosteroid-induced psychosis). Although it is usually a relatively straightforward matter to rule out an etiological substance or general medical condition in a patient with chronic psychotic symptoms, this task can be considerably more challenging with individuals who may be experiencing their first psychotic episode, especially when the psychotic symptoms emerge during a period of chronic, heavy drug use. To differentiate between a substance-induced and primary psychotic disorder, it is important to identify a period of time during which the individual was experiencing psychotic symptoms while not using drugs. If no such period of abstinence exists, the individual may have to be observed for a period of time off drugs to see if the psychotic symptoms resolve (First and Gladis, 1993).

Finally, criterion F helps to clarify the relationship between autism and schizophrenia. *DSM-I* and *DSM-II* did not include autism but instead included a category for "childhood type" of schizophrenia that was characterized by "autistic, atypical, and withdrawn behavior, failure to develop identity separate from mother's and general unevenness, gross immaturity and inadequacy in development" (APA, 1968, p. 35). The fact that autism was a category distinct from schizophrenia came from large studies of "psychotic" children demonstrating that such children fell into two groups, an early-onset group (that is, before age 6) that resemble what is now recognized as *autistic disorder*, and a later-onset group who presented with delusions and hallucinations. Thus, individuals with autism can also qualify for a later diagnosis of *schizophrenia* if they develop delusions or hallucinations.

To deal with the vast heterogeneity in the diagnosis, since the time of Kraepelin and Bleular *schizophrenia* has been categorized into a number of subtypes, including latent, simple, catatonic, paranoid, hebephrenic, undifferentiated, and residual (Morrison, 1974). *DSM-III* dropped simple schizophrenia and reformulated latent schizophrenia into schizotypal personality disorder. The other classical subtypes have been retained, however, despite questions about their validity (Carpenter, Bartko, et al., 1976; Carpenter and Stephens, 1979). *DSM-IV* introduced an alternative to this subtyping scheme in its appendix for "Criteria Sets and Axes Provided for Further Study" based on evidence suggesting that they may have different implications for treatment and pathophysiology (Buchanan and Carpenter, 1994; Johnstone and Frith, 1996). This alternative dimensional description of *schizophrenia* suggests that clinicians and researchers describe the extent to which psychotic (hallucinations and delusions), disorganized, and negative (deficit) symptoms have been prominent within the past 6 months or over the course of the disorder. They were purposely conceptualized as dimensions (as opposed to categories) because various combinations along each dimension may occur, and it is rare for one dimension to be elevated without an elevation on another.

ICD-10 DEFINITION OF SCHIZOPHRENIA

The ICD-10 (see Table 18.6) and *DSM-IV* criteria sets have many basic similarities but differ in a number of ways. Symptomatically, the ICD-10 and *DSM-IV* are quite comparable. The ICD-10 and *DSM-IV* offer two ways to satisfy the symptom requirement for schizophrenia: either having one symptom from a list of especially characteristic symptoms (i.e., Schneiderian first-rank symptoms and others) or alternatively having two from a second list of psychotic symptoms. However, the specific symptoms constituting the lists differ among the two systems. ICD-10 offers a list of very specific types of symptoms, including thought echo, thought insertion or withdrawal, or thought broadcasting; delusions of

TABLE 18.6 *ICD-10 Diagnostic Criteria for Research for Schizophrenia*

G1. Either at least one of the syndromes, symptoms, and signs listed under (*1*) below or at least two of the symptoms and signs listed under (2) should be present for most of the time during an episode of psychotic illness lasting for at least 1 month (or at some time during most of the days):

(*1*) at least one of the following must be present:

(*a*) thought echo, thought insertion or withdrawal, or thought broadcasting

(*b*) delusions of control, influence, or passivity, clearly referred to body or limb movements or specific thoughts, actions or sensations; delusional perceptions

(*c*) hallucinatory voices giving a running commentary on the patient's behavior or discussing the patient among themselves or other types of hallucinatory voices coming from some part of the body

(*d*) persistent delusions of other kinds that are culturally inappropriate and completely impossible (for example, being able to control the weather, or being in communication with aliens from another world)

(2) or at least two of the following:

(*a*) persistent hallucinations in any modality, when occurring every day for at least 1 month, when accompanied by delusions (which may be fleeting or half-formed) without clear affective content, or when accompanied by persistent overvalued ideas

(*b*) neologisms, breaks, or interpolations in the train of thought, resulting in incoherence or irrelevant speech

(*c*) catatonic behavior, such as excitement, posturing, or waxy flexibility, negativism, mutism, and stupor

(*d*) "negative" symptoms such as marked apathy, paucity of speech, and blunting or incongruity of emotional responses

G2. Most commonly used exclusion clauses:

(*1*) if the patient also meets criteria for a manic episode or depressive episode, the criteria in G1(*1*) and G1(2) must have been met before the disturbance in mood developed

(2) the disorder is not attributable to organic brain disease or to alcohol or drug-related intoxication or withdrawal

From World Health Organization (1993).

control, influence, or passivity; hallucinatory voices giving a running commentary or discussing the patient among themselves, or persistent delusions of other kinds that are "completely impossible." The corresponding list in *DSM-IV* offers only two items: bizarre delusions (which would cover the three delusional symptoms in the ICD-10 list) and auditory hallucinations also of the type described in ICD-10. The second list in ICD-10 includes four items: hallucinations accompanied by delusions or overvalued ideas; incoherence or irrelevant speech; catatonic behavior; and "negative" symptoms. In contrast, *DSM-IV* offers a choice of five symptoms: delusions of any type; hallucinations of any type; disorganized speech; catatonic or grossly disorganized behavior; and negative symptoms. Both systems require these symptoms to be present for most of the time for at least 1 month.

Perhaps the most significant difference between the ICD-10 and *DSM-IV* definitions is duration. Although both definitions require at least 1 month of psychotic symptoms, *DSM-IV* requires that the total duration of the illness be at least 6 months (which can include prodromal and residual symptoms). Even though the *DSM-IV* and ICD-10 symptom definitions differ in form and content, the *DSM-IV* field trial showed that based on symptoms, the ICD-10 and *DSM-IV* definitions identified mostly the same patients (Flaum, Amador, et al., 1998). The main reason for discordance in diagnoses is based on the duration requirement. Both systems generally concur on the diagnosis of individuals whose symptoms persist for 6 months or longer. The difference occurs in those patients with a typically first onset of psychotic symptoms lasting for at least 1 month but fewer than 6 months. In ICD-10, such individuals would be diagnosed as schizophrenia, whereas in *DSM-IV* the diagnosis would be schizophreniform disorder.

DIAGNOSTIC ALTERNATIVES FOR SCHIZOPHRENIA

There is much debate regarding whether the standard diagnostic criteria for schizophrenia are appropriate for neurobiological studies. Some researchers argue that they are too broad, and others that they are too narrow. Genetic studies suggest that this definition is too narrow and should be expanded to encompass additional psychotic disorders.

Lumping Disorders into a Schizophrenia Spectrum

Evidence from family studies suggests that current diagnostic criteria for schizophrenia may be too narrow and that genetic vulnerability encompasses a broad spectrum of schizophrenic-like psychopathology including schizophrenia, schizoaffective disorder, delusional disorder, and schizotypal personality disorder. Thus, from the perspective of trying to detect an underlying genetic diathesis to psychosis, a broad definition that would lump together those disorders that have been shown to be part of this schizophrenia spectrum would be optimal for research in this area.

A large body of family, twin, and adoption studies has confirmed a genetic basis for schizophrenia (Kendler and Diehl, 1993). In addition to observing increased rates of schizophrenia among biological relatives of patients with schizophrenia, other disorders have been found to coaggregate in these families. This observation has supported the notion of a schizophrenia spectrum, or a family of disorders that share clinical and perhaps etiological (that is, genetic) characteristics with schizophrenia. In particular, studies have demonstrated that other nonaffective psychotic disorders (that is, schizophreniform disorder, delusional disorder, schizoaffective disorder, atypical psychosis) occur in biological relatives of patients with schizophrenia at rates greater than those in control families and the general population, suggesting that they may share a similar familial liability and perhaps etiology with schizophrenia. For example, Gershon and colleagues (Gershon, DeLisi, et al., 1988) reported that the first-degree family risk for schizoaffective disorder and atypical psychosis was 7.1% in families with schizophrenic members and 0.9% in control families, a highly significant difference. In contrast, the majority of family studies have failed to find increased rates of primary affective disorder among biological relatives of schizophrenia probands. Furthermore, in a review of family and adoption studies of paranoid and schizotypal disorders, Kendler and colleagues (Kendler, McGuire, et al., 1993) in the Roscommon Family Study also found compelling support for including paranoid and schizotypal personality disorders in the schizophrenia spectrum. They found a paranoid/schizotypal prevalence of 8.2% in families of schizophrenia probands and 1.7% in families of controls, a difference that was strongly significant. This association was specific to schizophrenia, that is, they found a significantly higher prevalence in relatives of schizophrenia probands as compared to relatives of probands with primary affective disorder.

Symptom-Based Subtypes/Dimensions

Given the premise that schizophrenia may have a heterogeneous etiology and pathophysiology (that is, be made up of multiple discrete disease entities) and that this heterogeneity may account for the varied clinical manifestations of this illness, it has been argued that schizophrenia should be split into more etiologically homogeneous subtypes. One proposal has been to split the disorder into positive versus negative symptoms. Crow (1980) first proposed that schizophrenia could be divided into two syndromes based on positive and negative symptoms. Type I schizophrenia presents with a predominantly positive symptom profile and is characterized by acute onset, a good prognosis, a favorable response to neuroleptics, and possibly dopaminergic dysfunction as its core pathophysiological feature. In contrast, type II schizophrenia has a predominance of negative symptoms. It is characterized by a chronic course, a poor prognosis, an inadequate response to antipsychotic drugs, and evidence of intellectual impairment, enlarged ventricular size, and cortical atrophy.

Andreasen and colleagues (Andreasen, Olsen, et al., 1982) proposed that positive and negative symptoms may be overlapping end points along a single continuum of biological and clinical manifestations. In their study of 52 patients with schizophrenia, they found that negative symptoms correlated with the presence of ventricular enlargement, while patients with small ventricles were more likely to manifest positive symptoms.

A categorical scheme for differentiation of primary and secondary negative symptoms was developed by Carpenter and colleagues (Carpenter, Bartko, et al., 1976). Negative symptoms that are a core element of schizophrenia are deemed primary or deficit symptoms. Deficit-type schizophrenia has been related to specific attentional (Buchanan, Strauss, et al., 1997) and other neurocognitive abnormalities (Buchanan, Strauss, et al., 1994), a poorer outcome (Fenton and McGlashan, 1991), and brain metabolic (Tamminga, Thaker, et al., 1992) and structural abnormalities (Buchanan, Breier, et al., 1993). Secondary negative symptoms are seen in depression and medical illness, as a result of positive symptoms, or of medication side effects.

Although the dichotomous positive/negative distinction has gained wide clinical and research recognition, factor analytic studies suggest that schizophrenia is subdivided into three dimensions: a psychotic symptom dimension (including hallucinations and delusions), a disorganization symptom dimension (including thought disorder, bizarre behavior, and inappropriate affect), and a negative symptom dimension (essentially splitting the positive dimension into two finer grained dimensions) (Grube, Bilder, et al., 1998).

Categorical versus Dimensional Conceptualizations

The *DSM* and the ICD conceptualize schizophrenia as a categorical diagnosis, that is, according to these systems, a particular individual either has or does not have schizophrenia. This categorical approach has been roundly criticized, however, especially by those in the research community; for example, Cloninger (1998) noted that the assumption that psychiatric disorders are discrete entities that can be categorically defined is "inconsistent with available knowledge of the psychobiology, genetics, development, and evolution of thoughts, emotions, and behavior" (p. 174).

Studies that assume schizophrenia represents a "real" construct in nature will not delineate the true underlying pathology and causal mechanisms (Allardycce, Gaebel, et al., 2007). The categorical definition of *schizophrenia* sets artificial boundaries on two fronts: between schizophrenia and "normality" and between schizophrenia and other disorders that are characterized by psychotic symptoms, like schizoaffective disorder and bipolar disorder with psychotic features. Mounting evidence suggests that rather than there being a discrete demarcation in the distribution of psychotic phenomena in the general population (as would be suggested by a categorical conceptualization of schizophrenia), delusions and hallucinations have a continuous distribution in the general population (Kendler, Gallagher, et al., 1996; Van Os, Hanssen, et al., 2000; Johns, Cannon, et al., 2004). Furthermore, the Kraepelinian separation of schizophrenia and bipolar disorder into discrete categories has also been challenged (Dutta, Greene, et al., 2007). Notably, Kraepelin himself came to doubt the validity of his own approach and in his later writings suggested replacing this dichotomy with a dimensional model more appropriate to the heterogeneity of clinical presentations (Kraepelin, 1992). Evidence that schizophrenia and bipolar disorder may share important underlying elements comes from treatment studies and genetic studies. For example, a study by Casey and colleagues (Casey, Daniel, et al., 2003) showed that treatment with a mood stabilizer (that is, divalproex) in combination with an atypical antipsychotic agent resulted in earlier improvements in a range of psychotic symptoms among acutely hospitalized patients with schizophrenia. The fact that schizophrenia, schizoaffective disorder, and bipolar disorder share genetic risk is illustrated by a twin study (Cardno, Rijsdijk, et al., 2002) showing that if one member of a twin pair has schizophrenia, there is an 8% chance of the other twin being diagnosed with bipolar disorder and an 8% chance of being diagnosed with schizoaffective disorder.

In recognition of the limitations of the categorical approach, the next revision of *DSM* and ICD will likely seriously consider incorporating dimensionality into the definition of *schizophrenia* and other psychotic disorders to facilitate research into the etiology and pathophysiology of these disorders (Regier, 2007). Whether such approaches can be successfully integrated into the classification in such a way as to be clinically useful or else presented as an alternative for research use only (First, 2006) remains to be seen.

CONCLUSION

DSM-IV, the current classification system used for schizophrenia in the United States, has many advantages, including being founded on strong historical roots and containing clear symptom definitions, useful clinical information pertaining to age, duration of symptoms, and social and occupational dysfunction. The limitation of the *DSM-IV* definition is that it does not provide vitally important information to patients, clinicians, and researchers related to distinct pathophysiological subtypes, long-term prognosis, and/or predictability of response to treatment. This is contrasted with classification systems used in other medical areas such as oncology, where tumors are typed and graded (for example, from benign to very aggressive).

It is clear that the diagnosis, classification, and phenotypic description of schizophrenia and the related psychoses is an evolving process that is far from complete. The explosion of new information from genetics, brain imaging, postmortem, and other neurobiological studies is dramatically shaping the way we conceive of the psychotic disorders. The challenge for descriptive and nosological research is to integrate new research findings and use them to establish the most valid and clinically meaningful classification schemas for these complicated illnesses.

ACKNOWLEDGMENTS

Portions of this chapter were adapted from the corresponding chapter written by Alan Breier that was included in the prior edition of the *Neurobiology of Mental Illness*.

REFERENCES

Allardycce, J., Gaebel, W., et al. (2007) Deconstructing Psychosis Conference February 2006: the validity of schizophrenia and alternative approaches to the classification of psychosis. *Schizophr. Bull.* 33(4):863–867.

American Psychiatric Association. (1968) *Diagnostic and Statistical Manual of Mental Disorders*, 2nd ed. Washington, DC: Author.

American Psychiatric Association. (1980) *Diagnostic and Statistical Manual of Mental Disorders*, 3rd ed. Washington, DC: Author.

American Psychiatric Association. (1987) *Diagnostic and Statistical Manual of Mental Disorders*, 3rd ed., rev. Washington, DC: Author.

American Psychiatric Association. (1994) *Diagnostic and Statistical Manual of Mental Disorders*, 4th ed. Washington, DC: Author.

Andreasen, N., Flaum, M., et al. (1990) Positive and negative symptoms in schizophrenia. A critical reappraisal. *Arch. Gen. Psychiatry* 47:615–621.

Andreasen, N., Olsen, S., et al. (1982) Ventricular enlargement in schizophrenia: relationship to positive and negative symptoms. *Am. J. Psychiatry* 139:297–302.

Angrist, B., Rotrosen, J., et al. (1980) Differential effects of amphetamine and neuroleptics on negative vs. positive symptoms in schizophrenia. *Psychopharmacology* 72:17–19.

Berrios, G.E. (1985) Positive and negative symptoms and Jackson: a conceptual history. *Arch. Gen. Psychiatry* 42:95–97.

Bertelsen, A. (2002) Schizophrenia and related disorders: experience with current diagnostic systems. *Psychopathology* 35(2/3):89–93.

Blashfield, R. (1982) Feighner et al., invisible colleges, and the Matthew effect. *Schizophr. Bull.* 8(1):1–12.

Bleuler, E. (1950) *Dementia Praecox or the Group of Schizophrenics* (J. Zinkin, Trans.) New York: International Universities Press.

Breier, A., Wolkowitz, O., et al. (1987) Neuroleptic responsivity of negative and positive symptoms in schizophrenia. *Am. J. Psychiatry* 144:1549–1555.

Bromet, E., Naz, B., et al. (2005) Long-term diagnostic stability and outcome in recent first-episode cohort studies of schizophrenia. *Schizophr. Bull.* 31:639–649.

Buchanan, R., Breier, A., et al. (1993) Structural abnormalities in deficit and nondeficit schizophrenia. *Am. J. Psychiatry* 150:59–65.

Buchanan, R., and Carpenter, W. (1994) Domains of psychopathology: an approach to the reduction of heterogeneity in schizophrenia. *J. Nerv. Ment. Dis.* 182:193–204.

Buchanan, R., Strauss, M., et al. (1994) Neuropsychological impairments in deficit vs. nondeficit forms of schizophrenia. *Arch. Gen. Psychiatry* 51:804–812.

Buchanan, R., Strauss, M., et al. (1997) Attentional impairments in deficit and nondeficit forms of schizophrenia. *Am. J. Psychiatry* 154:363–370.

Cardno, A., Rijsdijk, F., et al. (2002) A twin study of genetic relationships between psychotic symptoms. *Am. J. Psychiatry* 159:539–545.

Carpenter, W., Bartko, J., et al. (1976) Another view of schizophrenia subtypes. A report from the International Pilot Study of Schizophrenia. *Arch. Gen. Psychiatry* 33:508–516.

Carpenter, W., Bartko, J., et al. (1978) Signs and symptoms as predictors of outcome: a report from the International Pilot Study of Schizophrenia. *Am. J. Psychiatry* 135:940–944.

Carpenter, W., and Stephens, J. (1979) An attempted integration of information relevant to schizophrenia subtypes. *Schizophr. Bull.* 5:490–506.

Casey, D., Daniel, D., et al. (2003) Effect of divalproex combined with olanzapine or risperidol in patients with an acute exacerbation of schizophrenia. *Neuropsychopharmacology* 28:182–192.

Charney, D., Barlow, D., et al. (2002) Neuroscience research agenda to guide development of a pathophysiologically based classification system. In: Kupfer, D., First, M., and Regier, D, eds. *A Research Agenda for DSM-V*. Washington, DC: American Psychiatric Association, pp. 31–84.

Cloninger, C. (1998) A new conceptual paradigm from genetics and psychobiology for the science of mental health. *Aust. N. Z. J. Psychiatry* 33:174–186.

Crow, T. (1980) Molecular pathology of schizophrenia: more than one disease process? *BMJ* 280:66–68.

Dutta, R., Greene, T., et al. (2007) Biological, life course, and cross-cultural studies all point toward the value of dimensional and developmental ratings in the classification of psychosis. *Schizophr. Bull.* 33:868–876.

Feighner, J., Robins, E., et al. (1972) Diagnostic criteria for use in psychiatric research. *Arch. Gen. Psychiatry* 26:57–63.

Fenton, W., and McGlashan, T. (1991) Natural history of schizophrenia subtypes. II. Positive and negative symptoms and long-term course. *Arch. Gen. Psychiatry* 48:978–986.

First, M. (2006) Beyond clinical utility: broadening the DSM-V research appendix to include alternative diagnostic constructs. *Am. J. Psychiatry* 163:1679–1681.

First, M., and Gladis, M. (1993) Diagnosis and differential diagnosis of psychiatric and substance use disorders. In: Solomon, J., Zimberg, S., and Shollar, E., eds. *Dual Diagnosis: Evaluation, Treatment, Training, and Program Development*. New York: Plenum, pp. 23–38.

First, M., and Pincus, H. (2002) The DSM-IV text revision: rationale and potential impact on clinical practice. *Psychiatr. Serv.* 53(3):288–292.

Flaum, M., Amador, X., et al. (1998) DSM-IV field trial for schizophrenia and other psychotic disorders. In: Widiger, T., Frances, A., Pincus, H., et al., eds. *DSM-IV Sourcebook Volume 4*. Washington, DC: American Psychiatric Association, pp. 687–713.

Gershon, E., DeLisi, L., et al. (1988) A controlled family study of chronic psychoses. *Arch. Gen. Psychiatry* 45:328–333.

Grube, B., Bilder, R., et al. (1998) Meta-analysis of symptom factors in schizophrenia. *Schizophr. Res.* 31(2/3):113–120.

Hippocrates. (1950) *The Medical Works of Hippocrates*. Oxford, UK: Blackwell.

Hoch, P., and Polatin, P. (1949) Pseudoneurotic forms of schizophrenia. *Psychiatr. Q.* 23:248–276.

Hyman, S. (2003) Foreword. In: Phillips, K., First, M., and Pincus, H., eds. *Advancing DSM: Dilemmas in Psychiatric Diagnosis*. Washington, DC: American Psychiatric Association, pp. xi–xix.

Johns, L., Cannon, M., et al. (2004) Prevalence and correlates of self-reported psychotic symptoms in the British population. *Br. J. Psychiatry* 185:298–305.

Johnstone, B., and Frith, C. (1996) Validation of three dimensions of schizophrenic symptoms in a large unselected sample of patients. *Psychol. Med.* 26:669–679.

Kasanin, J. (1933) The acute schizoaffective psychosis. *Arch. Gen. Psychiatry* 90:97–126.

Kendler, K., and Diehl, S. (1993) The genetics of schizophrenia; a current, genetic-epidemiologic perspective. *Schizophr. Bull.* 19:261–285.

Kendler, K., Gallagher, T., et al. (1996) Lifetime prevalence, demographic risk factors, and diagnostic validity of nonaffective psychosis as assessed in a US community sample. The National Comorbidity Study. *Arch. Gen. Psychiatry* 53:1022–1031.

Kendler, K., McGuire, M., et al. (1993) The Roscommon Family Study, I: Methods, diagnosis of probands and risk of schizophrenia in relatives. *Arch. Gen. Psychiatry* 50:527–540.

Kraepelin, E. (1919) *Dementia Praecox and Paraphrenia*. Huntington, NY: Robert E. Krieger Publishing.

Kraepelin, E. (1992) Die Erscheinungsformen des Irreseins [The manifestations of insanity]. *Hist. Psychiatry* 3:509–529.

Latham, R.G. (1848) Medical observations, 3rd edition, Preface. *The Works of Thomas Sydenham, M.D.* London: Sydenham Society, pp. 11–22.

Mezzich, J.E. (2002) International surveys on the use of ICD-10 and related diagnostic systems. *Psychopathology* 35(2/3):72–75.

Morrison, J. (1974) Changes in subtype diagnosis of schizophrenia: 1920-1966. *Am. J. Psychiatry* 136:674–677.

Regier, D. (2007) Time for a fresh start? Rethinking psychosis in DSM-V. *Schizophr. Bull.* 33:843–845.

Schneider, K. (1959) *Clinical Psychopathology*. New York: Grune and Stratton.

Spitzer, R., Endicott, J., et al. (1970) The Psychiatric Status Schedule. A technique for evaluating psychopathology and impairment in role functioning. *Arch. Gen. Psychiatry* 23:41–55.

Spitzer, R. L., Endicott, J., and Robins, E. (1978) Research diagnostic criteria: rationale and reliability. *Arch. Gen. Psychiatry* 35: 773–782.

Tamminga, C., Thaker, G., et al. (1992) Limbic system abnormalities identified in schizophrenia using PET/FDG and neocortical alterations with deficit syndrome. *Arch. Gen. Psychiatry* 49:522–530.

Vaillant, G. (1964) Prospective prediction of schizophrenia remission. *Arch. Gen. Psychiatry* 11:509–518.

Van Os, J., Hanssen, M., et al. (2000) Strauss (1969) revisited: a psychosis continuum in the general population? *Schizophr. Res.* 45: 11–20.

Williams, J., and Spitzer, R. (1982, November) Research diagnostic criteria and DSM-III. *Arch. Gen. Psychiatry* 39:1283–1289.

Wing, J., Cooper, J., et al. (1974) *The Measurement and Classification of Psychiatric Symptoms*. New York: Cambridge University Press.

World Health Organization. (1993) *The ICD-10 Classification of Mental and Behavioral Disorders: Diagnostic Criteria for Research*. Geneva, Switzerland: Author, pp. 64-65.

Zubin, J., and Gurland, B. (1977) The United States-United Kingdom Project on diagnosis of the mental disorders. *Ann. N. Y. Acad. Sci.* 285(1):676–686.

19 | Genetics of Schizophrenia

XIANGNING CHEN, BRIEN RILEY, AND KENNETH S. KENDLER

This chapter provides an overview of the rapidly evolving field of the genetics of schizophrenia. It covers the genetic epidemiology of schizophrenia but focuses more on recent work in the molecular genetics—specifically linkage and association studies. Due to the large volume of literature, the review is selective.

GENETIC EPIDEMIOLOGY OF SCHIZOPHRENIA

Schizophrenia is a strongly familial disorder. Modern studies suggest that the risk of schizophrenia is increased 10-fold in first-degree relatives of schizophrenic probands. Family, twin, and adoption studies have consistently suggested that most of this increased risk is genetic.

Family Studies

The combined results of many European studies (Gottesman, 1991) yield a lifetime morbid risk (MR) in the general population of about 1%. The risk to siblings or offspring of people with schizophrenia has been reported in the older literature to be ~10-fold greater or 10%. The risk in parents is lower because having schizophrenia reduces the chances that an individual will successfully find a mate and reproduce. Smaller but consistent increases in MR are seen in second-degree and third-degree relatives, and the risk increases as more relatives are affected. Methodological criticisms of early family studies included lack of proper controls, nonsystematic methods of sampling, lack of standardized diagnostic criteria, and failure to diagnose family members blind to the status of the index case (or proband). However, data from seven studies designed to answer these criticisms, when pooled and reanalyzed, yielded estimates for a lifetime MR of narrowly defined schizophrenia of 0.5% for relatives of controls and 4.8% for relatives of people with schizophrenia (Kendler and Diehl, 1993).

Twin Studies

Historically, twin studies are used to assess whether a phenotype, such as schizophrenia, has a genetic component. The basic rationale is that monozygotic and dizygotic twins share 100% and 50% genetic material, respectively; therefore, if the phenotype is 100% genetic, we would expect 100% and 50% concordance, respectively, for the monozygotic and dizygotic twins. The deviation of observed concordance from the expectation would be attributed to environmental factors. Many twin studies (D.C. Rao et al., 1981; Kendler, 1983; McGuffin et al., 1995) have been reported in the literature, and the consensus of these studies is that schizophrenia is highly heritable (heritability estimated ~80%). In a meta-analysis of twin studies (Sullivan et al., 2003), shared environmental factors were shown to have a small but significant influence on disease risk.

Although we do not review them here, a range of high-quality adoption studies performed in the United States, Denmark, and Finland are congruent with twin studies in suggesting that genetic factors play a major role in the etiology of schizophrenia.

Sex Differences in Schizophrenia

Whether there are sex differences in schizophrenia remains controversial. For a long time, many researchers believed that schizophrenia affected males and females equally. However, in recent publications, consistent reports have begun to emerge showing significant differences in the two sexes. These differences can be summarized as follows: (*1*) males have a higher prevalence rate (Aleman et al., 2003; McGrath et al., 2004); (*2*) males have a younger age of onset than females (Leung and Chue, 2000; Seeman, 2000; M.L. Rao and Kolsch, 2003); (*3*) females have a better course and treatment response; and (*4*) sex-specific associations are reported for several candidate genes (Shifman et al., 2002; Sazci et al., 2005; Tan et al., 2005; Thomson et al., 2005).

The mechanisms whereby sex contributes to these differences in schizophrenia are not clear. There is no evidence that direct, X-linked genes contribute to a risk for schizophrenia. One of the mechanisms for sex influence could be mediated through sex hormones. There are extensive reviews that sex hormones affect the development of the brain (Marchetti et al., 2000; Gooren and Toorians, 2003; R. Li and Shen, 2005) and that these influences relate to the differences observed in male and female patients with schizophrenia (Leung and Chue, 2000; Halbreich and Kahn, 2003; M.L. Rao and Kolsch, 2003). Estrogen, the most powerful female hormone, exerts its influence on many organs, including the brain. This influence is achieved through regulation of gene expression via binding to its receptors (Kushner et al., 2000; O'Lone et al., 2004; Bjornstrom and Sjoberg, 2005). The diverse signaling pathways and mechanisms of estrogen-mediated gene regulation may explain the variations in phenotype differences observed in patients with schizophrenia. At the physiological level, there is evidence that estrogen affects the development and function of the brain dopamine and γ-aminobutyric acid systems, which play a role in cognition, memory, stress response, and reward and motivational behaviors (Malyala et al., 2005; Kipp et al., 2006). Of particular interest, estrogen has a protective effect against Parkinson's and other neuro-degenerative disorders (Morale et al., 2006; Dhandapani and Brann, 2007), and some researchers have suggested that it may have the same protective effect on schizophrenia (Kolsch and Rao, 2002; Halbreich and Kahn, 2003; M.L. Rao and Kolsch, 2003).

Spectrum Disorders and Risk in Relatives

Debate continues about the boundaries of the schizophrenia spectrum. Because accurate definition of the affected phenotype is crucial in genetic investigations, a major area of interest has been to use genetically informative designs to determine which psychiatric syndromes reflect the transmitted liability to schizophrenia. Substantial evidence suggests that the phenotype transmitted in families includes other psychotic and schizophrenia-like personality disorders (Kendler et al., 1993). Considerable controversy (and variability between studies) remains about the diagnosis of persons considered "affected."

LINKAGE STUDIES OF SCHIZOPHRENIA

Linkage is a phenomenon in which genetic traits travel together on the same chromosomal region in a family. The chance that two traits on the same chromosome are separated is a function of distance between the two genetic loci responsible for the two traits. This separation is a consequence of recombination occurred during meiosis. If we place genetic markers roughly evenly across the human genome and obtain the genotypes for families with affected and unaffected individuals, we can correlate the affection status with recombination sites in the families. Linkage analysis is a statistical method to estimate the likelihood where a genetic locus responsible for the affection status is located by summing up information obtained from multiple families. Linkage results are commonly reported as a statistic called *lod score*—for log of the odds. A lod score is the logarithm, to the base 10, of the likelihood of the observed data given linkage divided by the likelihood of those same data given no linkage. So, lod scores of 3 and –2 mean that the likelihood that the observed families are linked is 10^3 or 1000:1 and 10^{-2} or 0.01:1, respectively. The lod scores require the specification of a genetic model and are thus termed parametric. Variations of the lod score that allow for heterogeneity, or that assess only the individuals who are affected in a sample, have been applied to address some of the problems outlined above, but we do not distinguish between these in the discussion that follows. An alternative approach, widely used in complex traits, is *nonparametric linkage analysis*. All classes of relatives have predefined probabilities of sharing zero, one, or two marker alleles identical by descent at any random locus. These nonparametric methods are based on testing for deviations from expected allele-sharing distributions and avoid the problem of specifying a genetic model, which, as we saw above, is very difficult for complex traits, including schizophrenia.

Of the many linkage studies performed, a few studies show linkage with genome-wide significance. Many chromosomal regions showed suggestive linkages to schizophrenia. We summarize these studies in Table 19.1. The main conclusions we can draw from these studies are:

1. Of all reported linkage studies, no Mendelian-like major effect genes have been found. A majority of these studies reported multiple linkages. These results suggest that the genetic structure of schizophrenia is most likely oligogenic or polygenic, and the effects of individual genes on risk of illness are likely small.
2. Only a few regions were found to reach genome-wide significance. In the Lewis et al. (2003) meta-analysis, 2q was the only region reaching genome-wide significance. In some more recent linkage studies, 6q23, 10q22-25, and 22q11 also reached genome-wide significance.
3. Many more regions showed suggestive linkage; some of them were implicated in two or more independent studies. These regions are 1p34-11, 1q33-42, 2p14-12, 2q14-37, 3q13-28, 4q21-35, 5q21-33, 6p22-21, 6q23-25, 7p22-14, 7q11-31, 8p23-21, 9q21-31, 10p24-11, 10q22-25, 13q12-28, 14q11-13, 15q11-26, 17p22-11, and 22q11-13. In Lewis et al.'s (2003) meta-analysis, 2q (D2S2254), 5q (D5S422), 3p (D3S3521), 11q (D11S1316), 6p (D6S274), 1q (D1S2705), 22q (D22S424), 8q (D8S1809), 20q (D20S190), and 14p (D14S70) showed most consistent results. The variations in these linkage studies may be due to the differences in sample sizes, ascertainments, and methodologies. Despite these differences, it may be reasonable to conclude that linkage regions reaching global significance and those implicated in more than one study are likely to harbor susceptibility genes for schizophrenia.

TABLE 19.1 *A Summary of Linkage Studies of Schizophrenia*

Author	*Ethnicity*	*Sample Size*	*Linkage Region*	*Statistics*	*Reference*
Coon, H.	Caucasian	9 families	22q13 (D22S276)	lod = 2.09	*Am. J. Med. Genet.* 1994. 54(1):72–79
Moises, H.W.	Caucasian	stage 1: 5 families	6p (D6S274)	$p = 0.005$	*Nat. Genet.* 1995. 11(3):321–324
		stage 2: 65 families	9q (D9S175)	$p = 0.009$	
			20p11 (D20S40)	$p = 0.0008$	
Pulver, A.E.	Caucasian	57 families	8p22	$p = 0.0001$	*Am. J. Med. Genet.* 1995. 60(3):252–260
Blouin, J.L.	Caucasian	stage 1: 54 families	13q32	NPL = 4.18	*Nat. Genet.* 1998. 20(1):70–73
		stage 2: 51 families	8p21-22	NPL = 3.64	
			14q13	NPL = 2.57	
			7q11	NPL = 2.50	
			22q11	NPL = 2.42	
Faraone, S.V.	Caucasian	43 families	10p12 (D10S1423)	NPL = 3.40	*Am. J. Med. Genet.* 1998. 81(4):290–295
Kaufmann, C.A.	African American	30 families	8p23 (D8S439)	NPL = 2.27	*Am. J. Med. Genet.* 1998. 81(4):282–289
			9q34 (D9S1830)	NPL = 2.17	
Levinson, D.F.	Caucasian	43 families	10q23(D10S1239)	NPL = 2.01	*Am. J. Psychiatry.* 1998. 155(6):741–750
Shaw, S.H.	Caucasian	70 families	11p11 (D11S1393)	NPL = 2.30	*Am. J. Med. Genet.* 1998. 81(5):364–376
			13q12-13 (D13S1293)	NPL = 2.85	
Hovatta, I.	Caucasian	69 families	1q32-41	NPL = 3.82	*Am. J. Hum. Genet.* 1999. 65(4): 1114–1124
			4q31	NPL = 2.74	
			9q21	NPL = 1.95	
			Xp11	NPL = 2.01	
Williams, N.M.	Caucasian	196 sibpairs	4p15 (D4S403)	MLS = 1.73	*Hum. Mol. Genet.* 1999. 8(9):1729–1739
			10p24 (D10S542)	MLS = 1.92	
			Xp11 (DXS993)	MLS = 1.45	
Brzustowicz, L.M.	Caucasian	22 families	1q22 (D1S1679)	$Z_{max} = 5.77$	*Am. J. Hum. Genet.* 1999. 65(4): 1096–1103
			12q22 (PAH)	$Z_{max} = 2.31$	
			3q13 (D3S3045)	$Z_{max} = 2.11$	
			8p21 (D8S136)	$Z_{max} = 2.09$	
Ekelund, J.	Caucasian	134 sibpairs	7q31 (D7S486)	lod = 3.18	*Hum. Mol. Genet.* 2000. 9(7):1049–1057
			1q41 (D1S439)	lod = 2.62	
Schwab, S.G.	Caucasian	71 families	6p22 (D6S274)	lod = 2.20	*Mol. Psychiatry.* 2000. 5(6):638–649
			10p13 (D10S1714)	lod = 2.1	
Gurling, H.M.	Caucasian	13 families	1q33	lod = 3.2	*Am. J. Hum. Genet.* 2001. 68(3): 661–673
			5q33	lod = 3.6	
			8p22	lod = 3.6	
			11q21	lod = 3.18	
Straub, R.E.	Caucasian	270 families	2p14-13	NPL = 2.08	*Mol. Psychiatry.* 2002. 7(6):542–559
			5q21-31	NPL = 2.65	
			6p23-22	NPL = 3.59	
			8p22-21	NPL = 2.56	
			10p1-11	NPL = 2.04	
Lindholm, E.	Caucasian	1 family	6q25.2 (D6S264)	lod = 3.45	*Am. J. Hum. Genet.* 2001. 69(1):96–105
DeLisi, L.E.	Caucasian	382 sibpairs	10p15-13(D10S189)	lod = 3.60	*Am. J. Psychiatry.* 2002. 159(5):803–812
			2p12 (D2S139)	lod = 2.99	
			22q12 (D22S283)	lod = 2.00	

TABLE 19.1 *A Summary of Linkage Studies of Schizophrenia (Continued)*

Author	*Ethnicity*	*Sample Size*	*Linkage Region*	*Statistics*	*Reference*
Jang, Y.L.	Asian / Korean	46 families	1q41 (D1S2891)	NPL = 2.67	*Am. J. Med. Genet.* 2007. 144(3):279–284
Bulayeva, K.B.	Caucasian	4 families	17p11-12	lod = 3.73	*Genomics.* 2007. 89(2):167–177
			22q11	lod = 4.4	
Escamilla, M.A.	Mexican	99 families	1pter-p36	NPL = 3.42, $p = 0.00003$	*Am. J. Med. Genet.* 2007. 144(2):193–199
			18p11	NPL = 3.14, $p = 0.00015$	
			5q35	NPL = 3.09, $p = 0.00020$	
Faraone, S.V.	Asian / Chinese	606 families	1p31 (D1S551)	NPL = 2.08	*Am. J. Psychiatry.* 2006. 163(10):1760–1766
			2q14 (D2S410)	NPL = 2.31	
			4q21 (D4S2361)	NPL = 2.00	
			15q14 (D15S1012)	NPL = 2.07	
			10q22 (D10S2327)	NPL = 2.88	
Fallin, M.D.	Caucasian	29 families	10q22 (D10S1774)	NPL = 4.27	*Am. J. Hum. Genet.* 2003. 73(3):601–611
			1p34 (D1S2729)	NPL = 2.45	
			4q35 (D4S1535)	NPL = 2.30	
			6p21 (D6S1610)	NPL = 2.37	
			7p14 (D7S510)	NPL = 2.09	
			15q11 (D15S128)	NPL = 2.15	
			21q21 (D21S1914)	NPL = 2.04	
Vazza, G.	Caucasian	16 families	15q26 (D15S1014)	NPL = 3.05	*Mol. Psychiatry.* 2007. 12:87–93
Zheng, Y.	Asian / Chinese	25 families	5q35 (D5S408)	NPL = 1.88	*Biochem. Biophys. Res. Commun.* 2006. 342(4):1049–1057
			1p21 (D1S206)	NPL = 2.27	
			6p21 (D6S1610)	NPL = 2.08	
			22q13 (D22S274)	NPL = 2.56	
Suarez, B.K.	Caucasian / African American	263 Caucasian families, 146 African American families	8p23 (D8S1771)	lod = 2.30	*Am. J. Hum. Genet.* 2006. 78(2):315–333
			11p11 (D11S2371)	lod = 1.63	
Arinami, T.	Asian / Japanese	286 sibpairs	1p21 (rs2048839)	lod = 3.39	*Am. J. Hum. Genet.* 2005. 77(6):937–944
			14q11 (rs1319956)	lod = 2.87	
			20p12 (rs7988)	lod = 2.33	
Hamshere, M.L.	Caucasian	24 families	1q42 (D1S2800)	lod = 3.54	*Arch. Gen. Psychiatry.* 2005. 62(10):1081–1088
			22q11 (D22S420)	lod = 1.96	
			19p13 (19S221)	lod = 1.85	
Faraone, S.V.	Caucasian / African American	166 families	18pter (D18S59)	lod = 2.96	*Am. J. Med. Genet.* 2005. 139(1):91–100
			6p	lod = 2.11	
			14p	lod = 2.13	
Klei, L.	Oceanic / Palau	13 families	3q28 (D3S2418)	lod = 3.03	*Hum. Genet.* 2005. 117(4):349–356
			17q32 (D17S1290)	lod = 2.80	

TABLE 19.1 *A Summary of Linkage Studies of Schizophrenia (Continued)*

Author	*Ethnicity*	*Sample Size*	*Linkage Region*	*Statistics*	*Reference*
			Xq27 (CXS318)	lod = 2.13	
Liu, C.M.	Asian / Chinese	52 families	8p22 (D8S1222)	lod = 2.45	*Am. J. Med. Genet.* 2005. 134(1):79–83
Cooper-Casey, K.	Hispanic	1 family	5p13 (D5S426)	lod = 2.70	*Mol. Psychiatry.* 2005. 10(7):651–656
Macgregor, S.	Caucasian	35 families	1q42 (D1S103)	lod = 2.77	*Mol. Psychiatry.* 2004. 9(12):1083–1090
Abecasis, G.R.	African	143 families	1p (D1S1612)	NPL = 3.30	*Am. J. Hum. Genet.* 2004. 74(3):403–417
Sklar, P.	Caucasian	29 families	5q31-35 (D5S820)	NPL = 3.28	*Mol. Psychiatry.* 2004. 9(2):213–218
Williams, N.M.	Caucasian	353 sibpairs	10q25	lod = 3.87	*Am. J. Hum. Genet.* 73(6):1355–1367
			17p11	lod = 3.35	
			22q11	lod = 2.29	
Wijsman, E.M.	Caucasian	1 family	2q37 (D2S2176)	Z_{max} = 2.07	*Mol. Psychiatry.* 2003. 8(7):695–705, 643
Lerer, B.	Caucasian	21 families	6q23 (D6S292)	lod = 4.60	*Mol. Psychiatry.* 2003. 8(5):488–498
			10q24 (D10S187)	lod = 3.24	
			7p22 (D7S531)	lod = 2.21	
			2q37 (D2S345)	lod = 2.42	

lod: log of the odds; NPL: Non-parametric linkage; MLS: Multipoint linkage score; Z_{max}: Maximal Z score

ASSOCIATION STUDIES

The other major technique that has been widely used to identify susceptibility genes for schizophrenia is association studies, or, as it is sometimes called, *linkage disequilibrium* (LD) studies. *Linkage disequilibrium* refers to the nonrandom association of alleles of different loci, that is, some alleles associate with each other more or less than expected by chance given their frequencies. Association studies take advantage of LD phenomenon and use genetic markers in LD with the causative mutations to identify genes responsible for the traits of interest. This is a quite different method from linkage analysis, with different strengths and weaknesses. Linkage is a within-pedigree phenomenon and is relatively immune to population structure and stratification. Association studies are based on the principle of LD, which is a population-level phenomenon and relies on the population history of the markers and disease mutations. Linkage is immune to allelic heterogeneity (disease risk resulting from different variants in the same gene) whereas association studies are very sensitive to its effects.

Compared to linkage scans, association studies have much higher resolution. This is because genetic markers separated by large distances tend to have higher probability to be separated by recombination during meiosis sometime during evolution. As pointed out by Risch and Merikangas (1996), another potentially important advantage of association studies is their substantially greater power to detect susceptibility genes of modest effect. However, for the same reason, association studies are very sensitive to population stratification and evolutionary history. To evaluate results obtained from association studies, therefore, appropriate measurements, such as evaluation of ethnicities and population substructure of the cases and controls, and utilization of admixture models in association analysis should be applied.

In the last several years, the Human Genome Project produced millions of single nucleotide polymorphisms (SNPs). More recently, the international HapMap project genotyped millions of SNPs for several populations. Data from the HapMap are deposited at dbSNP (http://www.ncbi.nlm.nih.gov/SNP/index.html), and these data are valuable resources for association studies.

Traditionally, association studies for schizophrenia are conducted for candidate genes selected from linkage regions and from pharmacological studies of drugs used to treat schizophrenia and other psychotic disorders. In the last several years, many candidate genes have been studied, and some promising candidates have been identified. However, it is very difficult to interpret the results, as many studies of the same candidate genes produce inconsistent and even conflicting results. How to evaluate association studies is beyond the scope of this chapter, but we touch on some of the issues in the next section. Typically, association studies begin with selection of candidate and genetic markers (SNPs). To cover a gene sufficiently, many SNPs are needed to include all major haplotypes—a combination of alleles from multiple loci transmitting together to the offspring—in the gene. Because the size and LD vary from gene to gene, a common approach is to include all known variants with pairwise LD greater than a selected threshold. In our laboratory, the threshold is r^2 (a measurement of LD) ≥ 0.8–0.85.

Another factor that affects association studies is the development of genotyping technologies. In recent years, high throughput SNP typing techniques have been developed. As a result of these developments, it is now practical to scan the whole genome with hundreds of thousands of SNP markers. In fact, as this chapter is written, two such studies for schizophrenia are being conducted.

Whole-genome association studies for other complex phenotypes have been reported (Smyth et al., 2006; Saxena et al., 2007; Scott et al., 2007; Sladek et al., 2007; The Wellcome Trust Consortium, 2007; Zeggini et al., 2007). Based on these studies of diabetes and other complex diseases, highly significant associations were found for all phenotypes studied. Several independent studies validated each other (Saxena et al., 2007; Scott et al., 2007; Sladek et al., 2007; Steinthorsdottir et al., 2007; Zeggini et al., 2007). This is encouraging news. However, for bipolar disorder—a disease often discussed and studied with schizophrenia side-by-side—a very large study did not identify any apparent candidates. As this chapter is written, one whole-genome association study of schizophrenia has been reported. In this study, only one SNP reached genome-wide significance (Lencz et al., 2007). Because the association studies literature in schizophrenia is quite large and growing rapidly, our review of candidate genes is necessarily selective.

Promising Candidates

In recent years, a large number of candidates for schizophrenia have been identified and studied, including those from major linkage regions. However, the results have generally been quite mixed. In the recent literature, there are several discussions regarding the criteria of replication in association studies. It was argued that a replication could be made at the levels of markers, haplotypes, or the gene (Neale and Sham, 2004; Sullivan, 2007). Depending on the criteria used, the same study can be viewed as either replicated or not replicated. Using the stringent criteria, that is, replication at same markers, same allele (haplotype), and same sex (Sullivan, 2007), without exception, all candidate genes identified so far have inconsistent or conflict results. For these reasons, the validity of most candidates is subject to debate, and our selection here is somewhat subjective.

The neuregulin 1 (NRG1) *gene*

The association of *NRG1* with schizophrenia was first identified in Icelandic families (Stefansson et al., 2003). *NRG1* is located at 8p12, a linkage region implicated in linkage studies (Lewis et al., 2003). *NRG1* is a very large gene, spanning over 1 million base pairs of genomic DNA, with multiple transcripts and splicing variants. Since the first report of association, many replication studies have been published, some positive and others negative. Recently, two meta-analyses have been conducted for *NRG1* (D. Li et al., 2006; Munafo et al., 2006). One study found that there is no association in the most studied polymorphism (SNP8NRG221533). But in haplotype analyses, significant association was found (Munafo et al., 2006). The other analysis found significant associations at single markers and haplotypes (D. Li et al., 2006). Based on this evidence, it is reasonable to conclude that *NRG1* is associated with schizophrenia and is one of the best candidates reported so far. The effect size is, however, modest. The odds ratio for the risk haplotype in this gene with schizophrenia has been estimated at 1.22, 95% confidence interval 1.15–1.30 (D. Li et al., 2006).

The dystrobrevin binding protein 1 (DTNBP1) *gene*

The *DTNBP1* gene was identified in the Irish Study of High Density Schizophrenia Families (ISHDSF) in 2002 (Straub et al., 2002). *DTNBP1* is located at 6p22, another region showing evidence of linkage to schizophrenia. The biological functions of this gene are largely unknown. In a subsequent haplotype analysis, a minor haplotype with a frequency of ~8% was found to increase the risk to schizophrenia (van den Oord et al., 2003). Since the first publication, a total of 14 studies have been published attempting to replicate this finding. Of these studies, some provided supporting evidence, while in others the results were negative. When the patterns of association are examined, the markers and haplotypes showing associations vary across studies and ethnic groups. Due to these inconsistencies, a meta-analysis is needed to clarify whether *DTNBP1* is associated with schizophrenia.

Disrupted in schizophrenia 1 (DISC1) *gene*

The *DISC1* gene was first identified in a large pedigree with multiple individuals diagnosed with schizophrenia and other psychiatric disorders (Millar et al., 2000). In this pedigree, a balanced translocation between chromosome 1 and 11 disrupts this gene. The function of this gene is not well understood, but it has been shown to interact with phosphodiesterase-4 and modulate cyclic adenosine monophosphate (cAMP) in the cell (Millar et al., 2005). It has a broad distribution in the cell (James et al., 2004). Since the first report, multiple association studies have been conducted, and as with other candidate genes, positive and negative evidence has been found (Owen et al., 2005). In addition, *DISC1* is one of the best studied candidate genes in neurobiology and animal models (Clapcote et al., 2007; Mackie et al., 2007; Roberts, 2007).

The regulator of G-protein signaling 4 (RGS4) *gene*

RGS4 is located at 1q23, encoding a protein belonging to the guanine triphosphatase activating protein family. Its function involves the regulation of G protein–coupled receptors upon binding of neurotransmitters. It was first identified in a postmortem expression study that showed differential expression between patients with schizophrenia and healthy controls. The association with schizophrenia was reported in 2003 with three different family samples (Chowdari et al., 2002). Replication studies report positive and negative results. Meta-analysis with 13 samples did not show significant association at individual markers. Similar to the *NRG1* gene, significant haplotype association was found in this meta-analysis (Talkowski et al., 2006).

The catechol-O-methyl transferase (COMT) gene

The *COMT* gene is one of the most widely studied candidate genes for schizophrenia. The function of *COMT* is to degrade dopamine, a neurotransmitter and precursor of noradrenaline and adrenaline. The gene is widely expressed in the central nervous system and has a soluble form and a membrane form. *COMT* is located at 22q11, a region that has been implicated in linkage studies of schizophrenia. There is a functional polymorphism, $Val^{158/108}Met$ (rs4680), showing direct impact on the activities of the enzyme (Lachman et al., 1996). The enzyme carrying the Val allele has significantly lower enzyme activities than that carrying the Met allele.

The association studies of $Val^{158/108}Met$ with schizophrenia have been conducted with case-control samples and family samples. These studies also include several ethnic groups. However, the results are not always consistent. Several meta-analyses have also been reported, and these meta-analyses did not arrive at similar conclusions. In one meta-analysis, it was concluded that the Val allele carries a small but consistent risk for schizophrenia in studies with subjects of European ancestry (Glatt et al., 2003). However, more recent analyses including one meta-analysis concluded that there was no association between the $Val^{158/108}Met$ polymorphism and schizophrenia (Fan et al., 2005; Munafo et al., 2005; Williams et al., 2005).

There are other polymorphisms studied for their association with schizophrenia in the *COMT* gene. But the number of studies including other markers is relatively small, and there is no meta-analysis reported on other markers. Is it possible that the $Val^{158/108}Met$ polymorphism is not associated with schizophrenia, but *COMT* is? The answer is not clear. In addition to the affection status, *COMT* is also studied for other endophenotypes (Bramon et al., 2006; Lu et al., 2007) and executive functions (Barnett et al., 2007).

Other Candidates

In addition to those genes mentioned above, there are other candidate genes identified from linkage regions; these include the *G72/G30* genes (Chumakov et al., 2002), *Epsin 4* (Pimm et al., 2005), *CAPON* (Brzustowicz et al., 2004), *TRAR4* (Duan et al., 2004), *synapsin II* (Q. Chen et al., 2004), *GABAA* (Petryshen et al., 2005), *CHI3L1* (Zhao et al., 2007), *PIP5K2A* (Schwab et al., 2006), *SPEC2/PDZ-GEF2/ACSL6* (X. Chen et al., 2006), *GRM3* (Egan et al., 2004), *PPP3CC* (Gerber et

TABLE 19.2 *A Summary of Candidate Genes and Their Functions*

Gene	*Location (hg 18 positions)*	*Function*	*Reference*
NRG1	chr8:31,616,810-32,720312	Growth factor essential for neuronal development and synaptic plasticity	Stefansson, H. *Am. J. Hum. Genet.* 2002. 71:877–892.
DTNBP1	chr6:15,631,018-15,771,250	Structural protein with no clearly defined functions.	Straub et al., 2002
DISC1	chr1:229,829,184-230,243,614	Structural protein modulating cytoskeleton and cAMP, and influencing the development of cerebral cortex.	St. Clair, D. *Lancet*. 1990. 336: 13–16
RGS4	chr1:161,305,285-161,313,216	Regulator of G protein–coupled signal transduction	Chowdari et al., 2002
COMT	chr22:18,309,309-18,336,530	Enzyme catalyzing the transfer of a methyl group from S-adenosylmethionine to catecholamines, including dopamine, epinephrine, and norepinephrine	Li, T. *Psychiatr. Genet.* 1996. 6:131–133.
DAOA (G72/G30)	chr13:104,916,217-104,941,384	D-amino acid oxidase	Cloninger, C.R. *Proc. Natl. Acad. Sci. USA*. 2002. 99:13365–13367.
CLINT1 (Epsin 4)	chr5:157,145,875-157,218,746	Clathrin interactor binding to membranes enriched in phosphatidylinositol-4,5-biphosphate	Pimm, J. *Am. J. Hum. Genet.* 2005, 76:902–907.

TABLE 19.2 *A Summary of Candidate Genes and Their Functions (Continued)*

Gene	*Location (hg 18 positions)*	*Function*	*Reference*
NOS1AP (CAPON)	chr1:160,306,205-160,604,854	Adaptor protein involved in neuronal nitric oxidase synthesis	Brzustowicz et al., 2004
TAAR6 (TRAR4)	chr6:132,933,154-132,934,191	Trace amine receptor	Duan et al., 2004
SYN2	chr3:12,020,862-12,208,532	Phosphoprotein involved in synaptogenesis and modulation of neurotransmitter release	Q. Chen et al., 2004
CHI3L1	chr1:201,414,553-201, 422,500	Unknown, possibly in the immune system	X. Zhao et al., 2007
PIP5K2A	chr10:22,865,828-23,043,490	Catalyzing the phosphorylation of phosphatidylinositol-4-phosphate on the fifth hydroxyl of the myo-inositol ring, to form phosphatidylinositol-4, 5-biphosphate	Stopkova, P. *Am. J. Med. Genet. B. Neuropsychiatr. Genet.* 2003. 123:50–58.
SPEC2/PDZ-GEF2/ACSL6	SPEC2, chr5:130,672, 601-130,758,260	Small effector protein of CDC42 Rac GTPase	X. Chen et al., 2006
	PDZ-GEF2, chr5:130,789, 503-131,160,655	Guanine nucleotide exchange factor for Rap1A, Rap2A and M-Ras GTPase.	
	ACSL6, chr5:131,317, 051-131,375,248	Acyl-CoA synthetase involved in long chain fatty acid metabolism	
IL3	chr5:131,424,246-131,426,795	Multi-potent growth factor	X. Chen et al., 2007
CSF2RA/IL3RA	CSF2RA, chrX:1,347, 701-1,388,827	Cytokine specific receptor for CSF2	Lencz et al., 2007
	IL3RA, chrX:1,415, 509-1,461,582	Cytokine specific receptor for IL3	
CSF2RB	chr22:35,639,621-35,664,764	Common receptor for interleukin 3, 5 and CSF2	Q. Chen et al., in press
GRM3	chr7:86,111,166-86,332,128	Metabotropic glutamate receptor	Egan et al., 2004
PPP3CC	chr8:22,354541-22,454582	Calcium-dependent protein phosphatase	Gerber et al., 2003
ZDHHC8	chr22:18,499,365-18,515,529	Palmitoyltransferase involved in protein palmitoylation	Mukai et al., 2003
FXYD6	chr11:117,212,903-117,252,577	Regulator of tissue specific Na, K-ATPase	Choudhury et al., 2007

ATP: adenosine tri-phosphate; cAmp: cyclic adenosine monophosphate; GTP: guanosine 5'-diphosphate; IL: interleukin.

al., 2003), *ZDHHC8* (Mukai et al., 2004), and *FXYD6* (Choudhury et al., 2007). The associations of these genes with schizophrenia are difficult to evaluate at this time due largely to the lack of replication studies. Table 19.2 lists the genomic location and function of these and other candidate genes.

Many more candidates selected from a variety of criteria have been tested for their roles in schizophrenia. The literature on these genes is large (see http://www.schizophreniaforum.org/res/sczgene/default.asp), and we do not intend to cover these genes extensively. However, a few themes recurring in the testing hypotheses are worth mentioning:

1. Genes involved in the metabolic pathways of neurotransmitters such as dopamine, γ-aminobutyric acid, and their respective receptors and transporters.

2. Genes involved in immune responses, such as interleukins and their receptors. An example is the interleukin 3 pathway, where all three essential components of the pathway are now reported to be associated with schizophrenia (Lencz et al., 2007; X. Chen et al., 2007; Q. Chen et al., in press).

3. Genes involved in the signal transduction networks. Genes in these groups are selected largely by their plausible biological functions. However, with exception of a few genes, many do not show consistent associations with schizophrenia.

CONCLUSIONS AND FUTURE DIRECTIONS

In the last several years, we have witnessed substantial progress in the genetics of schizophrenia. Thanks to the

Human Genome and the HapMap Projects, millions of SNPs are publicly available. These resources significantly speed up the identification of many candidate genes that potentially contribute to the risk of schizophrenia. The progress in high-throughput genotyping technologies now makes it practical to conduct whole genome associations with 500,000–1,000,000 genetic markers. It is likely (but by no means certain) that many candidate genes with modest effects will be identified in the near future by the ongoing whole-genome associations. A critical question remains as to how well genes found in one whole-genome association will be replicated in other studies. The fields of genetics studies of complex diseases, including the genetics studies of schizophrenia, are now facing a transition from identification of candidate genes to functional studies to understand the pathophysiology of these complex diseases. Specific to the genetics studies of schizophrenia, we anticipate that these areas will attract more attention and research activities:

To Identify and Understand the Genetic Mechanisms of Causative Variants

As mentioned above, several promising candidate genes have been identified. In the coming years, we have good reasons to believe that more candidate genes will be identified and verified. Once these candidate genes are identified, the next logical step is to find out what variants in the genes cause the dysfunction. In several promising candidates, such as *NRG1* and *DTNBP1*, such efforts have already begun. However, the results to date are not very clear. Several factors may be contributing to these results. In the next phase of causative variant studies, these areas should be considered carefully.

1. Deoxyribonucleic acid (DNA) sequencing alone may not be sufficient to discover the causative mutations. From the experience learned from Mendelian disorders, where a single or a few genes cause the diseases, sequencing the entire gene is the routine procedure to identify causative mutations once the candidate gene is identified. Although DNA sequencing may be a necessary step, it alone may not be sufficient to discover the causative variants in complex diseases. There is accumulating evidence that the causes of complex diseases may be much more complex than those that have been found for single gene diseases. This may require us to adapt new techniques and explore new approaches. In the last few years, many studies have been conducted for the human genome, and many surprising discoveries have been made (Redon et al., 2006; Birney et al., 2007). These new studies indicate that the human genome is much more dynamic than we thought. For example, it was not too long ago that we believed that the structure of human genome was more or less the same across individuals and ethnic groups. We now know there are many structural variants in the human genome; these include segmental duplication, copy number variation, large translocation, inversion, and so on, and their frequencies are much higher than previously acknowledged (Sebat et al., 2004; Freeman et al., 2006; Redon et al., 2006). These variants involve thousands to millions of base pairs, much larger than the polymerase chain reaction (PCR) fragment routinely used in direct DNA sequencing. If the sequencing efforts are within a duplication, for example, we would not be able to find the duplication unless we come across the duplication boundaries. Due to the fact that there are substantial structure differences between people, structural studies of candidate genes should be included in the plan to discover causative variants. Relying on the reference genome solely may be naive and could hinder these efforts.

2. Regulatory elements may not be in the immediate vicinity of the candidate gene. More and more evidence indicates that many genes are regulated by elements far away from the gene. The distance may be several hundreds of kilo-bases (Kleinjan and van Heyningen, 2005). These regulatory elements include DNA binding proteins and micro ribonucleic acids (RNAs). DNA binding proteins can bring genes far apart together, and put them under similar regulatory controls. Micro RNA can modulate the accessibility of transcribed messenger ribonucleic acid (mRNA), alternative splicing, and expression (Mendell, 2005; Krutzfeldt et al., 2006; Ying and Lin, 2006; Zhang and Coukos, 2006). The obvious implication of these discoveries is that if we only focus on the candidate gene itself, we may miss these regulatory elements and, therefore, may not find the causes of disease. How to identify these remote controlling elements remains a challenge. In those studies that identify long-distance regulators, the approaches used are diverse, and no generalized methods yet exist.

3. The causes of complex diseases, including schizophrenia, can be epigenetic. If that is the case, the likelihood that they can be discovered by direct DNA sequencing is very low. There is evidence that epigenetic factors, such as methylation and acetylation, can significantly alter the accessibility and expression of targeted genes (Feinberg, 2007; Reik, 2007). In many psychiatric illnesses, including schizophrenia, there is evidence that for at least some cases environmental factors can trigger the onset of the disease. Although there may be other mechanisms to respond to environmental factors, DNA methylation, histone protein acetylation, and immune responses can all be triggered by environmental factors and can lead to the activation and repression of gene transcription that may be related to disease onset. Of particular interest is that DNA methylation, histone acetylation/deacetylation, and the immune systems are interlinked. Of the many hypotheses of the etiology of

schizophrenia, the dysregulation of the immune system is one of them. Therefore, it is plausible that epigenetics may be involved in schizophrenia, and so our search for causative variants should include epigenetic systems.

To Understand the Biology and Physiology of Candidate Genes

With a few exceptions, most candidate genes identified do not have well-characterized functions. To understand the functions of candidate genes, in vitro cell culture and in vivo animal models are necessary tools. Using these tools, we can discover where the proteins—the products of the candidate genes—are located in a cell and what other proteins they interact with. This information will provide some insight into the biological pathways in which the candidates are likely involved. It is of particular interest to determine whether several distinct candidate genes are involved in the same biological pathways, as for example have been found for Alzheimer's and Crohn's disease.

To use animal models to study schizophrenia is not without controversy. Although it is nearly certain that we cannot usefully model the key symptoms of schizophrenia in animal models, given the conservation in evolution, we have good reasons to believe that the fundamental biological processes in which the candidate genes are involved (such as cognition) might be sufficiently similar between humans and animal models. The reelin gene mouse model (Fatemi, 2001; Pappas et al., 2003; D'Arcangelo, 2006) and behavioral studies of *DISC1* (Clapcote et al., 2007) are good examples. The key advantage of animal models is that we can introduce and test genetic variants directly in living animals and follow the development of the pathophysiology. There is also a potential that animal model studies could validate endophenotypes and biomarkers that can be used for genetics studies in humans.

In conclusion, genetic epidemiological studies clearly show that genetic risk factors play a key role in the etiology of schizophrenia. The field is now very actively trying to move from the latent level of aggregate "genes" to specific molecular variants. The task has not been easy. It is now increasingly clear that the illness of schizophrenia typically requires the effects of multiple genes with environmental risks, the nature of which we still poorly understand. The field is now poised for a tidal wave of new data from whole-genome associations. Will this new method allow us to find and replicate susceptibility genes for schizophrenia? However, gene identification is only the beginning of the process. To understand the relationship among the candidates, their biological function, and their roles in the pathophysiology of schizophrenia will require the cooperation and integration of multiple disciplines. Geneticists will need to work closely with statisticians, neurobiologists, biochemists, and experts in bioinformatics, animal models, and systems biology, and use techniques in these fields to understand the biology of candidate genes. Only these functional studies can demonstrate beyond reasonable doubt that variants in a candidate gene lead to the development of schizophrenia.

REFERENCES

Aleman, A., Kahn, R.S., and Selten, J.P. (2003) Sex differences in the risk of schizophrenia: evidence from meta-analysis. *Arch. Gen. Psychiatry* 60:565–571.

Barnett, J.H., Jones, P.B., Robbins, T.W., and Muller, U. (2007) Effects of the catechol-O-methyltransferase Val158Met polymorphism on executive function: a meta-analysis of the Wisconsin Card Sort Test in schizophrenia and healthy controls. *Mol. Psychiatry* 12:502–509.

Birney, E., Stamatoyannopoulos, J.A., Dutta, A., Guigo, R., Gingeras, T.R., Margulies, E.H., Weng, Z., Snyder, M., Dermitzakis, E.T., Thurman, R.E., Kuehn, M.S., Taylor, C.M., Neph, S., Koch, C.M., Asthana, S., Malhotra, A., Adzhubei, I., Greenbaum, J.A., Andrews, R.M., Flicek, P., Boyle, P.J., Cao, H., Carter, N.P., Clelland, G. K., Davis, S., Day, N., Dhami, P., Dillon, S.C., Dorschner, M.O., Fiegler, H., Giresi, P.G., Goldy, J., Hawrylycz, M., Haydock, A., Humbert, R., James, K.D., Johnson, B.E., Johnson, E.M., Frum, T.T., Rosenzweig, E.R., Karnani, N., Lee, K., Lefebvre, G.C., Navas, P.A., Neri, F., Parker, S.C., Sabo, P.J., Sandstrom, R., Shafer, A., Vetrie, D., Weaver, M., Wilcox, S., Yu, M., Collins, F.S., Dekker, J., Lieb, J.D., Tullius, T.D., Crawford, G.E., Sunyaev, S., Noble, W.S., Dunham, I., Denoeud, F., Reymond, A., Kapranov, P., Rozowsky, J., Zheng, D., Castelo, R., Frankish, A., Harrow, J., Ghosh, S., Sandelin, A., Hofacker, I.L., Baertsch, R., Keefe, D., Dike, S., Cheng, J., Hirsch, H.A., Sekinger, E.A., Lagarde, J., Abril, J.F., Shahab, A., Flamm, C., Fried, C., Hackermuller, J., Hertel, J., Lindemeyer, M., Missal, K., Tanzer, A., Washietl, S., Korbel, J., Emanuelsson, O., Pedersen, J.S., Holroyd, N., Taylor, R., Swarbreck, D., Matthews, N., Dickson, M.C., Thomas, D.J., Weirauch, M.T., Gilbert, J., Drenkow, J., Bell, I., Zhao, X., Srinivasan, K.G., Sung, W.K., Ooi, H.S., Chiu, K.P., Foissac, S., Alioto, T., Brent, M., Pachter, L., Tress, M.L., Valencia, A., Choo, S.W., Choo, C.Y., Ucla, C., Manzano, C., Wyss, C., Cheung, E., Clark, T.G., Brown, J.B., Ganesh, M., Patel, S., Tammana, H., Chrast, J., Henrichsen, C.N., Kai, C., Kawai, J., Nagalakshmi, U., Wu, J., Lian, Z., Lian, J., Newburger, P., Zhang, X., Bickel, P., Mattick, J.S., Carninci, P., Hayashizaki, Y., Weissman, S., Hubbard, T., Myers, R.M., Rogers, J., Stadler, P.F., Lowe, T.M., Wei, C.L., Ruan, Y., Struhl, K., Gerstein, M., Antonarakis, S.E., Fu, Y., Green, E.D., Karaoz, U., Siepel, A., Taylor, J., Liefer, L. A., Wetterstrand, K.A., Good, P.J., Feingold, E.A., Guyer, M.S., Cooper, G.M., Asimenos, G., Dewey, C.N., Hou, M., Nikolaev, S., Montoya-Burgos, J.I., Loytynoja, A., Whelan, S., Pardi, F., Massingham, T., Huang, H., Zhang, N.R., Holmes, I., Mullikin, J.C., Ureta-Vidal, A., Paten, B., Seringhaus, M., Church, D., Rosenbloom, K., Kent, W.J., Stone, E.A., Batzoglou, S., Goldman, N., Hardison, R.C., Haussler, D., Miller, W., Sidow, A., Trinklein, N.D., Zhang, Z.D., Barrera, L., Stuart, R., King, D.C., Ameur, A., Enroth, S., Bieda, M.C., Kim, J., Bhinge, A.A., Jiang, N., Liu, J., Yao, F., Vega, V.B., Lee, C.W., Ng, P., Shahab, A., Yang, A., Moqtaderi, Z., Zhu, Z., Xu, X., Squazzo, S., Oberley, M.J., Inman, D., Singer, M.A., Richmond, T.A., Munn, K.J., Rada-Iglesias, A., Wallerman, O., Komorowski, J., Fowler, J.C., Couttet, P., Bruce, A.W., Dovey, O.M., Ellis, P.D., Langford, C. F., Nix, D.A., Euskirchen, G., Hartman, S., Urban, A.E., Kraus, P., Van Calcar, S., Heintzman, N., Kim, T.H., Wang, K., Qu, C., Hon, G., Luna, R., Glass, C.K., Rosenfeld, M.G., Aldred, S.F., Cooper, S.J., Halees, A., Lin, J.M., Shulha, H.P., Zhang, X., Xu, M., Haidar,

J.N., Yu, Y., Ruan, Y., Iyer, V.R., Green, R.D., Wadelius, C., Farnham, P.J., Ren, B., Harte, R.A., Hinrichs, A.S., Trumbower, H., and Clawson, H. (2007) Identification and analysis of functional elements in 1% of the human genome by the ENCODE pilot project. *Nature* 447:799–816.

Bjornstrom, L., and Sjoberg, M. (2005) Mechanisms of estrogen receptor signaling: convergence of genomic and nongenomic actions on target genes. *Mol. Endocrinol.* 19:833–842.

Bramon, E., Dempster, E., Frangou, S., McDonald, C., Schoenberg, P., MacCabe, J.H., Walshe, M., Sham, P., Collier, D., and Murray, R.M. (2006) Is there an association between the COMT gene and P300 endophenotypes? *Eur. Psychiatry* 21:70–73.

Brzustowicz, L.M., Simone, J., Mohseni, P., Hayter, J.E., Hodgkinson, K.A., Chow, E.W., and Bassett, A.S. (2004) Linkage disequilibrium mapping of schizophrenia susceptibility to the CAPON region of chromosome 1q22. *Am. J. Hum. Genet.* 74:1057–1063.

Chen, Q., He, G., Qin, W., Chen, Q.Y., Zhao, X.Z., Duan, S.W., Liu, X.M., Feng, G.Y., Xu, Y.F., St. Clair, D., Li, M., Wang, J.H., Xing, Y.L., Shi, J.G., and He, L. (2004) Family-based association study of synapsin II and schizophrenia. *Am. J. Hum. Genet.* 75:873–877.

Chen, Q., Wang, X., O'Neill, F.A., Walsh, D., Fanous, A., Kendler, K.S., and Chen, X. (in press) Association study of CSF2RB with schizophrenia in Irish family and case - control samples. *Mol. Psychiatry.*

Chen, X., Wang, X., Hossain, S., O'Neill, F.A., Walsh, D., van den Oord, E.J., Fanous, A., and Kendler, K.S. (2007) Interleukin 3 and schizophrenia: the impact of sex and family history. *Mol. Psychiatry* 12:273–282.

Chen, X., Wang, X., Hossain, S., O'Neill, F.A., Walsh, D., Pless, L., Chowdari, K.V., Nimgaonkar, V.L., Schwab, S.G., Wildenauer, D.B., Sullivan, P.F., van den, O.E., and Kendler, K.S. (2006) Haplotypes spanning SPEC2, PDZ-G EF2 and ACSL6 genes are associated with schizophrenia. *Hum. Mol. Genet.* 15:3329–3342.

Choudhury, K., McQuillin, A., Puri, V., Pimm, J., Datta, S., Thirumalai, S., Krasucki, R., Lawrence, J., Bass, N.J., Quested, D., Crombie, C., Fraser, G., Walker, N., Nadeem, H., Johnson, S., Curtis, D., St. Clair, D., and Gurling, H.M. (2007) A genetic association study of chromosome 11q22-24 in two different samples implicates the FXYD6 gene, encoding phosphohippolin, in susceptibility to schizophrenia. *Am. J. Hum. Genet.* 80:664–672.

Chowdari, K.V., Mirnics, K., Semwal, P., Wood, J., Lawrence, E., Bhatia, T., Deshpande, S.N., Thelma, B.K., Ferrell, R.E., Middleton, F.A., Devlin,B., Levitt, P., Lewis, D.A., and Nimgaonkar, V. L. (2002) Association and linkage analyses of RGS4 polymorphisms in schizophrenia. *Hum. Mol. Genet.* 11:1373–1380.

Chumakov, I., Blumenfeld, M., Guerassimenko, O., Cavarec, L., Palicio, M., Abderrahim, H., Bougueleret, L., Barry, C., Tanaka, H., La Rosa, P., Puech, A., Tahri, N., Cohen-Akenine, A., Delabrosse, S., Lissarrague, S., Picard, F.P., Maurice, K., Essioux, L., Millasseau, P., Grel, P., Debailleul, V., Simon, A.M., Caterina, D., Dufaure, I., Malekzadeh, K., Belova, M., Luan, J.J., Bouillot, M., Sambucy, J.L., Primas, G., Saumier, M., Boubkiri, N., Martin-Saumier, S., Nasroune, M., Peixoto, H., Delaye, A., Pinchot, V., Bastucci, M., Guillou, S., Chevillon, M., Sainz-Fuertes, R., Meguenni, S., Aurich-Costa, J., Cherif, D., Gimalac, A., Van Duijn, C., Gauvreau, D., Ouellette, G., Fortier, I., Raelson, J., Sherbatich, T., Riazanskaia, N., Rogaev, E., Raeymaekers, P., Aerssens, J., Konings, F., Luyten, W., Macciardi, F., Sham, P.C., Straub, R.E., Weinberger, D.R., Cohen, N., Cohen, D., Ouelette, G., and Realson, J. (2002) Genetic and physiological data implicating the new human gene G72 and the gene for D-amino acid oxidase in schizophrenia. *Proc. Natl. Acad. Sci USA* 99:13675–13680.

Clapcote, S.J., Lipina, T.V., Millar, J.K., Mackie, S., Christie, S., Ogawa, F., Lerch, J.P., Trimble, K., Uchiyama, M., Sakuraba, Y., Kaneda, H., Shiroishi, T., Houslay, M.D., Henkelman, R.M., Sled, J.G., Gondo, Y., Porteous, D.J., and Roder, J.C. (2007) Behavioral phenotypes of Disc1 missense mutations in mice. *Neuron* 54:387–402.

D'Arcangelo, G. (2006) Reelin mouse mutants as models of cortical development disorders. *Epilepsy Behav.* 8:81–90.

Dhandapani, K. M., and Brann, D. W. (2007) Role of astrocytes in estrogen-mediated neuroprotection. *Exp. Gerontol.* 42:70–75.

Duan, J., Martinez, M., Sanders, A.R., Hou, C., Saitou, N., Kitano, T., Mowry, B.J., Crowe, R.R., Silverman, J.M., Levinson, D.F., and Gejman, P.V. (2004) Polymorphisms in the trace amine receptor 4 (TRAR4) gene on chromosome 6q23.2 are associated with susceptibility to schizophrenia. *Am. J. Hum. Genet* 75:624–638.

Egan, M.F., Straub, R.E., Goldberg, T.E., Yakub, I., Callicott, J.H., Hariri, A.R., Mattay, V.S., Bertolino, A., Hyde, T.M., Shannon-Weickert, C., Akil, M., Crook, J., Vakkalanka, R.K., Balkissoon, R., Gibbs, R.A., Kleinman, J.E., and Weinberger, D.R. (2004) Variation in GRM3 affects cognition, prefrontal glutamate, and risk for schizophrenia. *Proc. Natl. Acad. Sci. USA* 101:12604–12609.

Fan, J.B., Zhang, C.S., Gu, N.F., Li, X.W., Sun, W.W., Wang, H.Y., Feng, G.Y., St Clair, D., and He, L. (2005) Catechol-O-methyltransferase gene Val/Met functional polymorphism and risk of schizophrenia: a large-scale association study plus meta-analysis. *Biol. Psychiatry* 57:139–144.

Fatemi, S.H. (2001) Reelin mutations in mouse and man: from reeler mouse to schizophrenia, mood disorders, autism and lissencephaly. *Mol. Psychiatry* 6:129–133.

Feinberg, A.P. (2007) Phenotypic plasticity and the epigenetics of human disease. *Nature* 447:433–440.

Freeman, J.L., Perry, G.H., Feuk, L., Redon, R., McCarroll, S.A., Altshuler, D.M., Aburatani, H., Jones, K.W., Tyler-Smith, C., Hurles, M.E., Carter, N.P., Scherer, S.W., and Lee, C. (2006) Copy number variation: new insights in genome diversity. *Genome Res.* 16: 949–961.

Gerber, D.J., Hall, D., Miyakawa, T., Demars, S., Gogos, J.A., Karayiorgou, M., and Tonegawa, S. (2003) Evidence for association of schizophrenia with genetic variation in the 8p21.3 gene, PPP3CC, encoding the calcineurin gamma subunit. *Proc. Natl. Acad. Sci. USA* 100:8993–8998.

Glatt, S.J., Faraone, S.V., and Tsuang, M.T. (2003) Association between a functional catechol-O-methyltransferase gene polymorphism and schizophrenia: meta-analysis of case-control and family-based studies. *Am. J. Psychiatry* 160:469–476.

Gooren, L. J., and Toorians, A. W. (2003) Significance of oestrogens in male (patho)physiology. *Ann. Endocrinol. (Paris)* 64:126–135.

Gottesman, I.I. (1991) *Schizophrenia Genesis.* New York: W.H. Freeman.

Halbreich, U., and Kahn, L.S. (2003) Hormonal aspects of schizophrenias: an overview. *Psychoneuroendocrinology* 28(Suppl 2): 1–16.

James, R., Adams, R.R., Christie, S., Buchanan, S.R., Porteous, D.J., and Millar, J.K. (2004) Disrupted in schizophrenia 1 (DISC1) is a multicompartmentalized protein that predominantly localizes to mitochondria. *Mol. Cell Neurosci.* 26:112–122.

Kendler, K.S. (1983) Overview: a current perspective on twin studies of schizophrenia. *Am. J. Psychiatry* 140:1413–1425.

Kendler, K.S., and Diehl, S.R. (1993) The genetics of schizophrenia: a current, genetic-epidemiologic perspective. *Schizophr. Bull.* 19:261–285.

Kendler, K.S., McGuire, M., Gruenberg, A.M., O'Hare, A., Spellman, M., and Walsh, D. (1993) The Roscommon Family Study. III. Schizophrenia-related personality disorders in relatives. *Arch. Gen. Psychiatry* 50:781–788.

Kipp, M., Karakaya, S., Pawlak, J., Araujo-Wright, G., Arnold, S., and Beyer, C. (2006) Estrogen and the development and protection of nigrostriatal dopaminergic neurons: concerted action of a multitude of signals, protective molecules, and growth factors. *Front. Neuroendocrinol.* 27:376–390.

Kleinjan, D.A., and van Heyningen, V. (2005) Long-range control of gene expression: emerging mechanisms and disruption in disease. *Am. J. Hum. Genet.* 76:8–32.

Kolsch, H., and Rao, M.L. (2002) Neuroprotective effects of estradiol-17beta: implications for psychiatric disorders. *Arch. Womens Ment. Health* 5:105–110.

Krutzfeldt, J., Poy, M.N., and Stoffel, M. (2006) Strategies to determine the biological function of microRNAs. *Nat. Genet.* 38:S14–S19.

Kushner, P.J., Agard, D.A., Greene, G.L., Scanlan, T.S., Shiau, A.K., Uht, R.M., and Webb, P. (2000) Estrogen receptor pathways to AP-1. *J. Steroid. Biochem. Mol. Biol.* 74:311–317.

Lachman, H.M., Papolos, D.F., Saito, T., Yu, Y.M., Szumlanski, C. L., and Weinshilboum, R.M. (1996) Human catechol-O-methyltransferase pharmacogenetics: description of a functional polymorphism and its potential application to neuropsychiatric disorders. *Pharmacogenetics* 6:243–250.

Lencz, T., Morgan, T.V., Athanasiou, M., Dain, B., Reed, C.R., Kane, C.R., Kucherlapati, R., and Malhotra, A.K. (2007) Converging evidence for a pseudoautosomal cytokine receptor gene locus in schizophrenia. *Mol. Psychiatry* 12:572–580.

Leung, A., and Chue, P. (2000) Sex differences in schizophrenia, a review of the literature. *Acta Psychiatr. Scand. Suppl.* 401:3–38.

Lewis, C.M., Levinson, D.F., Wise, L.H., DeLisi, L.E., Straub, R.E., Hovatta, I., Williams, N.M., Schwab, S.G., Pulver, A.E., Faraone, S.V., Brzustowicz, L.M., Kaufmann, C.A., Garver, D.L., Gurling, H.M., Lindholm, E., Coon, H., Moises, H.W., Byerley, W., Shaw, S.H., Mesen, A., Sherrington, R., O'Neill, F.A., Walsh, D., Kendler, K.S., Ekelund, J., Paunio, T., Lonnqvist, J., Peltonen, L., O'Donovan, M.C., Owen, M.J., Wildenauer, D.B., Maier, W., Nestadt, G., Blouin, J.L., Antonarakis, S.E., Mowry, B.J., Silverman, J.M., Crowe, R.R., Cloninger, C.R., Tsuang, M.T., Malaspina, D., Harkavy-Friedman, J.M., Svrakic, D.M., Bassett, A.S., Holcomb, J., Kalsi, G., McQuillin, A., Brynjolfson, J., Sigmundsson, T., Petursson, H., Jazin, E., Zoega, T., and Helgason, T. (2003) Genome scan meta-analysis of schizophrenia and bipolar disorder, part II: Schizophrenia. *Am. J. Hum. Genet.* 73:34–48.

Li, D., Collier, D.A., and He, L. (2006) Meta-analysis shows strong positive association of the neuregulin 1 (NRG1) gene with schizophrenia. *Hum. Mol. Genet.* 15:1995–2002.

Li, R., and Shen, Y. (2005) Estrogen and brain: synthesis, function and diseases. *Front. Biosci.* 10:257–267.

Lu, B.Y., Martin, K.E., Edgar, J.C., Smith, A.K., Lewis, S.F., Escamilla, M.A., Miller, G.A., and Canive, J.M. (2007) Effect of catechol o-methyltransferase Val(158)Met polymorphism on the P50 gating endophenotype in schizophrenia. *Biol. Psychiatry* 62(7):822–825.

Mackie, S., Millar, J.K., and Porteous, D.J. (2007) Role of DISC1 in neural development and schizophrenia. *Curr. Opin. Neurobiol.* 17:95–102.

Malyala, A., Kelly, M.J., and Ronnekleiv, O.K. (2005) Estrogen modulation of hypothalamic neurons: activation of multiple signaling pathways and gene expression changes. *Steroids* 70:397–406.

Marchetti, B., Gallo, F., Farinella, Z., Tirolo, C., Testa, N., Caniglia, S., and Morale, M.C. (2000) Gender, neuroendocrine-immune interactions and neuron-glial plasticity. Role of luteinizing hormone-releasing hormone (LHRH). *Ann. N. Y. Acad. Sci.* 917: 678–709.

McGrath, J., Saha, S., Welham, J., El Saadi, O., MacCauley, C., and Chant, D. (2004) A systematic review of the incidence of schizophrenia: the distribution of rates and the influence of sex, urbanicity, migrant status and methodology. *BMC. Med.* 2:13.

McGuffin, P., Owen, M.J., and Farmer, A.E. (1995) Genetic basis of schizophrenia. *Lancet* 346:678–682.

Mendell, J.T. (2005) MicroRNAs: critical regulators of development, cellular physiology and malignancy. *Cell Cycle* 4:1179–1184.

Millar, J.K., Pickard, B.S., Mackie, S., James, R., Christie, S., Buchanan, S.R., Malloy, M.P., Chubb, J.E., Huston, E., Baillie, G. S., Thomson, P.A., Hill, E.V., Brandon, N.J., Rain, J.C., Camargo, L.M., Whiting, P.J., Houslay, M.D., Blackwood, D.H., Muir, W. J., and Porteous, D.J. (2005) DISC1 and PDE4B are interacting genetic factors in schizophrenia that regulate cAMP signaling. *Science* 310:1187–1191.

Millar, J.K., Wilson-Annan, J.C., Anderson, S., Christie, S., Taylor, M.S., Semple, C.A., Devon, R.S., Clair, D.M., Muir, W.J., Blackwood, D.H., and Porteous, D.J. (2000) Disruption of two novel genes by a translocation co-segregating with schizophrenia. *Hum. Mol. Genet.* 9:1415–1423.

Morale, M.C., Serra, P.A., L'Episcopo, F., Tirolo, C., Caniglia, S., Testa, N., Gennuso, F., Giaquinta, G., Rocchitta, G., Desole, M. S., Miele, E., and Marchetti, B. (2006) Estrogen, neuroinflammation and neuroprotection in Parkinson's disease: glia dictates resistance versus vulnerability to neurodegeneration. *Neuroscience* 138:869–878.

Mukai, J., Liu, H., Burt, R.A., Swor, D.E., Lai, W.S., Karayiorgou, M., and Gogos, J.A. (2004) Evidence that the gene encoding ZDHHC8 contributes to the risk of schizophrenia. *Nat. Genet.* 36:725–731.

Munafo, M.R., Bowes, L., Clark, T.G., and Flint, J. (2005) Lack of association of the COMT (Val158/108 Met) gene and schizophrenia: a meta-analysis of case-control studies. *Mol. Psychiatry* 10:765–770.

Munafo, M.R., Thiselton, D.L., Clark, T.G., and Flint, J. (2006) Association of the NRG1 gene and schizophrenia: a meta-analysis. *Mol. Psychiatry* 11:539–546.

Neale, B.M., and Sham, P.C. (2004) The future of association studies: gene-based analysis and replication. *Am. J. Hum. Genet.* 75: 353–362.

O'Lone, R., Frith, M.C., Karlsson, E.K., and Hansen, U. (2004) Genomic targets of nuclear estrogen receptors. *Mol. Endocrinol.* 18:1859–1875.

Owen, M.J., Craddock, N., and O'Donovan, M.C. (2005) Schizophrenia: genes at last? *Trends Genet.* 21:518–525.

Pappas, G.D., Kriho, V., Liu, W.S., Tremolizzo, L., Lugli, G., and Larson, J. (2003) Immunocytochemical localization of reelin in the olfactory bulb of the heterozygous reeler mouse: an animal model for schizophrenia. *Neurol. Res.* 25:819–830.

Petryshen, T.L., Middleton, F.A., Tahl, A.R., Rockwell, G.N., Purcell, S., Aldinger, K.A., Kirby, A., Morley, C.P., McGann, L., Gentile, K.L., Waggoner, S.G., Medeiros, H.M., Carvalho, C., Macedo, A., Albus, M., Maier, W., Trixler, M., Eichhammer, P., Schwab, S. G., Wildenauer, D.B., Azevedo, M.H., Pato, M.T., Pato, C.N., Daly, M.J., and Sklar, P. (2005) Genetic investigation of chromosome 5q GABAA receptor subunit genes in schizophrenia. *Mol. Psychiatry* 10:1074–1088, 1057.

Pimm, J., McQuillin, A., Thirumalai, S., Lawrence, J., Quested, D., Bass, N., Lamb, G., Moorey, H., Datta, S.R., Kalsi, G., Badacsonyi, A., Kelly, K., Morgan, J., Punukollu, B., Curtis, D., and Gurling, H. (2005) The epsin 4 gene on chromosome 5q, which encodes the clathrin-associated protein enthoprotin, is involved in the genetic susceptibility to schizophrenia. *Am. J. Hum. Genet.* 76: 902–907.

Rao, D.C., Morton, N.E., Gottesman, I.I., and Lew, R. (1981) Path analysis of qualitative data on pairs of relatives: application to schizophrenia. *Hum. Hered.* 31:325–333.

Rao, M.L., and Kolsch, H. (2003) Effects of estrogen on brain development and neuroprotection—implications for negative symptoms in schizophrenia. *Psychoneuroendocrinology* 28(Suppl 2): 83–96.

Redon, R., Ishikawa, S., Fitch, K.R., Feuk, L., Perry, G.H., Andrews, T.D., Fiegler, H., Shapero, M.H., Carson, A.R., Chen, W., Cho, E.K., Dallaire, S., Freeman, J.L., Gonzalez, J.R., Gratacos, M., Huang, J., Kalaitzopoulos, D., Komura, D., MacDonald, J.R., Marshall, C.R., Mei, R., Montgomery, L., Nishimura, K., Okamura, K., Shen, F., Somerville, M.J., Tchinda, J., Valsesia, A., Woodwark, C., Yang, F., Zhang, J., Zerjal, T., Zhang, J., Armengol, L., Conrad, D.F., Estivill, X., Tyler-Smith, C., Carter,

N.P., Aburatani, H., Lee, C., Jones, K.W., Scherer, S.W., and Hurles, M.E. (2006) Global variation in copy number in the human genome. *Nature* 444:444–454.

Reik, W. (2007) Stability and flexibility of epigenetic gene regulation in mammalian development. *Nature* 447:425–432.

Risch, N., and Merikangas, K. (1996) The future of genetic studies of complex human diseases. *Science* 273:1516–1517.

Roberts, R.C. (2007) Schizophrenia in translation: disrupted in schizophrenia (DISC1): integrating clinical and basic findings. *Schizophr. Bull.* 33:11–15.

Saxena, R., Voight, B.F., Lyssenko, V., Burtt, N.P., de Bakker, P.I., Chen, H., Roix, J.J., Kathiresan, S., Hirschhorn, J.N., Daly, M. J., Hughes, T.E., Groop, L., Altshuler, D., Almgren, P., Florez, J. C., Meyer, J., Ardlie, K., Bengtsson, B.K., Isomaa, B., Lettre, G., Lindblad, U., Lyon, H.N., Melander, O., Newton-Cheh, C., Nilsson, P., Orho-Melander, M., Rastam, L., Speliotes, E.K., Taskinen, M. R., Tuomi, T., Guiducci, C., Berglund, A., Carlson, J., Gianniny, L., Hackett, R., Hall, L., Holmkvist, J., Laurila, E., Sjogren, M., Sterner, M., Surti, A., Svensson, M., Svensson, M., Tewhey, R., Blumenstiel, B., Parkin, M., DeFelice, M., Barry, R., Brodeur, W., Camarata, J., Chia, N., Fava, M., Gibbons, J., Handsaker, B., Healy, C., Nguyen, K., Gates, C., Sougnez, C., Gage, D., Nizzari, M., Gabriel, S.B., Chirn, G.W., Ma, Q., Parikh, H., Richardson, D., Ricke, D., and Purcell, S. (2007) Genome-wide association analysis identifies loci for type 2 diabetes and triglyceride levels. *Science* 316:1331–1336.

Sazci, A., Ergul, E., Kucukali, I., Kara, I., and Kaya, G. (2005) Association of the C677T and A1298C polymorphisms of methylenetetrahydrofolate reductase gene with schizophrenia: association is significant in men but not in women. *Prog. Neuropsychopharmacol. Biol. Psychiatry.* 29:1113–1123.

Schwab, S.G., Knapp, M., Sklar, P., Eckstein, G.N., Sewekow, C., Borrmann-Hassenbach, M., Albus, M., Becker, T., Hallmayer, J.F., Lerer, B., Maier, W., and Wildenauer, D.B. (2006) Evidence for association of DNA sequence variants in the phosphatidylinositol-4-phosphate 5-kinase IIalpha gene (PIP5K2A) with schizophrenia. *Mol. Psychiatry* 11:837–846.

Scott, L.J., Mohlke, K.L., Bonnycastle, L.L., Willer, C.J., Li, Y., Duren, W.L., Erdos, M.R., Stringham, H.M., Chines, P.S., Jackson, A. U., Prokunina-Olsson, L., Ding, C.J., Swift, A.J., Narisu, N., Hu, T., Pruim, R., Xiao, R., Li, X.Y., Conneely, K.N., Riebow, N.L., Sprau, A.G., Tong, M., White, P.P., Hetrick, K.N., Barnhart, M. W., Bark, C.W., Goldstein, J.L., Watkins, L., Xiang, F., Saramies, J., Buchanan, T.A., Watanabe, R.M., Valle, T.T., Kinnunen, L., Abecasis, G.R., Pugh, E.W., Doheny, K.F., Bergman, R.N., Tuomilehto, J., Collins, F.S., and Boehnke, M. (2007) A genome-wide association study of type 2 diabetes in Finns detects multiple susceptibility variants. *Science* 316:1341–1345.

Sebat, J., Lakshmi, B., Troge, J., Alexander, J., Young, J., Lundin, P., Maner, S., Massa, H., Walker, M., Chi, M., Navin, N., Lucito, R., Healy, J., Hicks, J., Ye, K., Reiner, A., Gilliam, T.C., Trask, B., Patterson, N., Zetterberg, A., and Wigler, M. (2004) Large-scale copy number polymorphism in the human genome. *Science* 305:525–528.

Seeman, M.V. (2000) Women and schizophrenia. *Medscape. Womens Health* 5:2.

Shifman, S., Bronstein, M., Sternfeld, M., Pisante-Shalom, A., Lev-Lehman, E., Weizman, A., Reznik, I., Spivak, B., Grisaru, N., Karp, L., Schiffer, R., Kotler, M., Strous, R.D., Swartz-Vanetik, M., Knobler, H.Y., Shinar, E., Beckmann, J.S., Yakir, B., Risch, N., Zak, N.B., and Darvasi, A. (2002) A highly significant association between a COMT haplotype and schizophrenia. *Am. J. Hum. Genet.* 71:1296–1302.

Sladek, R., Rocheleau, G., Rung, J., Dina, C., Shen, L., Serre, D., Boutin, P., Vincent, D., Belisle, A., Hadjadj, S., Balkau, B., Heude, B., Charpentier, G., Hudson, T.J., Montpetit, A., Pshezhetsky, A.V., Prentki, M., Posner, B.I., Balding, D.J., Meyre, D., Polychronakos, C., and Froguel, P. (2007) A genome-wide association study identifies novel risk loci for type 2 diabetes. *Nature* 445:881–885.

Smyth, D.J., Cooper, J.D., Bailey, R., Field, S., Burren, O., Smink, L.J., Guja, C., Ionescu-Tirgoviste, C., Widmer, B., Dunger, D.B., Savage, D.A., Walker, N. M., Clayton, D.G., and Todd, J.A. (2006) A genome-wide association study of nonsynonymous SNPs identifies a type 1 diabetes locus in the interferon-induced helicase (IFIH1) region. *Nat. Genet.* 38:617–619.

Stefansson, H., Sarginson, J., Kong, A., Yates, P., Steinthorsdottir, V., Gudfinnsson, E., Gunnarsdottir, S., Walker, N., Petursson, H., Crombie, C., Ingason, A., Gulcher, J.R., Stefansson, K., and St. Clair, D. (2003) Association of neuregulin 1 with schizophrenia confirmed in a Scottish population. *Am. J. Hum. Genet.* 72:83–87.

Steinthorsdottir, V., Thorleifsson, G., Reynisdottir, I., Benediktsson, R., Jonsdottir, T., Walters, G.B., Styrkarsdottir, U., Gretarsdottir, S., Emilsson, V., Ghosh, S., Baker, A., Snorradottir, S., Bjarnason, H., Ng, M.C., Hansen, T., Bagger, Y., Wilensky, R.L., Reilly, M.P., Adeyemo, A., Chen, Y., Zhou, J., Gudnason, V., Chen, G., Huang, H., Lashley, K., Doumatey, A., So, W.Y., Ma, R.C., Andersen, G., Borch-Johnsen, K., Jorgensen, T., Vliet-Ostaptchouk, J.V., Hofker, M.H., Wijmenga, C., Christiansen, C., Rader, D.J., Rotimi, C., Gurney, M., Chan, J.C., Pedersen, O., Sigurdsson, G., Gulcher, J.R., Thorsteinsdottir, U., Kong, A., and Stefansson, K. (2007) A variant in CDKAL1 influences insulin response and risk of type 2 diabetes. *Nat. Genet.* 39:770–775.

Straub, R.E., Jiang, Y., MacLean, C.J., Ma, Y., Webb, B.T., Myakishev, M.V., Harris-Kerr, C., Wormley, B., Sadek, H., Kadambi, B., Cesare, A.J., Gibberman, A., Wang, X., O'Neill, F.A., Walsh, D., and Kendler, K.S. (2002) Genetic variation in the 6p22.3 gene DTNBP1, the human ortholog of the mouse dysbindin gene, is associated with schizophrenia. *Am. J. Hum. Genet.* 71:337–348.

Sullivan, P.F. (2007) Spurious genetic associations. *Biol. Psychiatry* 61:1121–1126.

Sullivan, P.F., Kendler, K.S., and Neale, M.C. (2003) Schizophrenia as a complex trait: evidence from a meta-analysis of twin studies. *Arch. Gen. Psychiatry* 60:1187–1192.

Talkowski, M.E., Seltman, H., Bassett, A.S., Brzustowicz, L.M., Chen, X., Chowdari, K.V., Collier, D.A., Cordeiro, Q., Corvin, A.P., Deshpande, S.N., Egan, M.F., Gill, M., Kendler, K.S., Kirov, G., Heston, L.L., Levitt, P., Lewis, D.A., Li, T., Mirnics, K., Morris, D.W., Norton, N., O'Donovan, M.C., Owen, M.J., Richard, C., Semwal, P., Sobell, J.L., St. Clair, D., Straub, R.E., Thelma, B.K., Vallada, H., Weinberger, D.R., Williams, N.M., Wood, J., Zhang, F., Devlin, B., and Nimgaonkar, V.L. (2006) Evaluation of a susceptibility gene for schizophrenia: genotype based meta-analysis of RGS4 polymorphisms from thirteen independent samples. *Biol. Psychiatry* 60:152–162.

Tan, E.C., Chong, S.A., Wang, H., Chew-Ping, L.E., and Teo, Y.Y. (2005) Gender-specific association of insertion/deletion polymorphisms in the nogo gene and chronic schizophrenia. *Brain Res. Mol. Brain Res.* 139:212–216.

The Wellcome Trust Consortium. (2007) Genome-wide association study of 14,000 cases of seven common diseases and 3,000 shared controls. *Nature* 447:661–678.

Thomson, P.A., Wray, N.R., Thomson, A.M., Dunbar, D.R., Grassie, M.A., Condie, A., Walker, M.T., Smith, D.J., Pulford, D.J., Muir, W., Blackwood, D.H., and Porteous, D.J. (2005) Sex-specific association between bipolar affective disorder in women and GPR50, an X-linked orphan G protein-coupled receptor. *Mol. Psychiatry* 10:470–478.

van den Oord, E.J., Sullivan, P.F., Jiang, Y., Walsh, D., Neill, F.A., Kendler, K.S., and Riley, B.P. (2003) Identification of a high-risk haplotype for the dystrobrevin binding protein 1 (DTNBP1) gene in the Irish study of high-density schizophrenia families. *Mol. Psychiatry* 8:499–510.

Williams, H.J., Glaser, B., Williams, N.M., Norton, N., Zammit, S., Macgregor, S., Kirov, G.K., Owen, M.J., and O'Donovan, M.C.

(2005) No association between schizophrenia and polymorphisms in COMT in two large samples. *Am. J. Psychiatry* 162:1736–1738.

Ying, S.Y., and Lin, S.L. (2006) Current perspectives in intronic micro RNAs (miRNAs). *J. Biomed. Sci.* 13:5–15.

Zeggini, E., Weedon, M.N., Lindgren, C.M., Frayling, T.M., Elliott, K.S., Lango, H., Timpson, N.J., Perry, J.R., Rayner, N.W., Freathy, R.M., Barrett, J.C., Shields, B., Morris, A.P., Ellard, S., Groves, C.J., Harries, L.W., Marchini, J.L., Owen, K.R., Knight, B., Cardon, L.R., Walker, M., Hitman, G.A., Morris, A.D., Doney, A.S., Burton, P.R., Clayton, D.G., Craddock, N., Deloukas, P., Duncanson, A., Kwiatkowski, D.P., Ouwehand, W.H., Samani, N.J., Todd, J.A., Donnelly, P., Davison, D., Easton, D., Evans, D., Leung, H.T., Spencer, C.C., Tobin, M.D., Attwood, A.P., Boorman, J.P., Cant, B., Everson, U., Hussey, J.M., Jolley, J.D., Knight, A.S., Koch, K., Meech, E., Nutland, S., Prowse, C.V., Stevens, H.E., Taylor, N.C., Walters, G.R., Walker, N.M., Watkins, N.A., Winzer, T., Jones, R.W., McArdle, W.L., Ring, S.M., Strachan, D.P., Pembrey, M., Breen, G., St Clair, D., Caesar, S., Gordon-Smith, K., Jones, L., Fraser, C., Green, E.K., Grozeva, D., Hamshere, M.L., Holmans, P.A., Jones, I.R., Kirov, G., Moskvina, V., Nikolov, I., O'Donovan, M.C., Owen, M.J., Collier, D.A., Elkin, A., Farmer, A., Williamson, R., McGuffin, P., Young, A.H., Ferrier, I.N., Ball, S.G., Balmforth, A.J., Barrett, J.H., Bishop, D.T., Iles, M.M., Maqbool, A., Yuldasheva, N., Hall, A.S., Braund, P.S., Dixon, R. J., Mangino, M., Stevens, S., Thompson, J.R., Bredin, F., Tremelling, M., Parkes, M., Drummond, H., Lees, C.W., Nimmo, E.R., Satsangi, J., Fisher, S.A., Forbes, A., Lewis, C.M., Onnie, C.M., Prescott, N.J., Sanderson, J., Mathew, C.G., Barbour, J., Mohiuddin, M.K., Todhunter, C.E., Mansfield, J.C., Ahmad, T., Cummings, F.R., Jewell, D.P., Webster, J., Brown, M.J., Lathrop, G.M., Connell, J., Dominiczak, A., Braga Marcano, C.A., Burke, B., Dobson, R., Gungadoo, J., Lee, K.L., Munroe, P.B., Newhouse, S.J., Onipinla, A., Wallace, C., Xue, M., Caulfield, M., Farrall, M., Barton, A., Bruce, I.N., Donovan, H., Eyre, S., Gilbert, P.D., Hider, S.L., Hinks, A.M., John, S.L., Potter, C., Silman, A.J., Symmons, D.P., Thomson, W., Worthington, J., Dunger, D.B., Widmer, B., Newport, M., Sirugo, G., Lyons, E., Vannberg, F., Hill, A.V., Bradbury, L.A., Farrar, C., Pointon, J.J., Wordsworth, P., Brown, M. A., Franklyn, J.A., Heward, J.M., Simmonds, M.J., Gough, S.C., Seal, S., Stratton, M.R., Rahman, N., Ban, M., Goris, A., Sawcer, S.J., Compston, A., Conway, D., Jallow, M., Rockett, K.A., Bumpstead, S.J., Chaney, A., Downes, K., Ghori, M.J., Gwilliam, R., Hunt, S.E., Inouye, M., Keniry, A., King, E., McGinnis, R., Potter, S., Ravindrarajah, R., Whittaker, P., Widden, C., Withers, D., Cardin, N.J., Ferreira, T., Pereira-Gale, J., Hallgrimsdottir, I.B., Howie, B.N., Su, Z., Teo, Y.Y., Vukcevic, D., Bentley, D., Compston, A., Ouwehand, N.J., Samani, M.R., Isaacs, J.D., Morgan, A.W., Wilson, G.D., Ardern-Jones, A., Berg, J., Brady, A., Bradshaw, N., Brewer, C., Brice, G., Bullman, B., Campbell, J., Castle, B., Cetnarsryj, R., Chapman, C., Chu, C., Coates, N., Cole, T., Davidson, R., Donaldson, A., Dorkins, H., Douglas, F., Eccles, D., Eeles, R., Elmslie, F., Evans, D.G., Goff, S., Goodman, S., Goudie, D., Gray, J., Greenhalgh, L., Gregory, H., Hodgson, S.V., Homfray, T., Houlston, R.S., Izatt, L., Jackson, L., Jeffers, L., Johnson-Roffey, V., Kavalier, F., Kirk, C., Lalloo, F., Langman, C., Locke, I., Longmuir, M., Mackay, J., Magee, A., Mansour, S., Miedzybrodzka, Z., Miller, J., Morrison, P., Murday, V., Paterson, J., and Pichert, G. (2007) Replication of genome-wide association signals in UK samples reveals risk loci for type 2 diabetes. *Science* 316:1336–1341.

Zhang, L., and Coukos, G. (2006) MicroRNAs: a new insight into cancer genome. *Cell Cycle* 5:2216–2219.

Zhao, X., Tang, R., Gao, B., Shi, Y., Zhou, J., Guo, S., Zhang, J., Wang, Y., Tang, W., Meng, J., Li, S., Wang, H., Ma, G., Lin, C., Xiao, Y., Feng, G., Lin, Z., Zhu, S., Xing, Y., Sang, H., St. Clair, D., and He, L. (2007) Functional variants in the promoter region of Chitinase 3-like 1 (CHI3L1) and susceptibility to schizophrenia. *Am. J. Hum. Genet.* 80:12–18.

20 Neurobiological Theories of Schizophrenia

DAVID A. LEWIS AND DAVID W. VOLK

The clinical picture recognized as *schizophrenia* includes symptoms that reflect disturbances in a range of brain functions and signs indicative of alterations in cognitive, emotional, perceptual, and motor processes (D.A. Lewis and Lieberman, 2000). The initial formal descriptions of this disorder highlighted the substantial interindividual variability in the specific constellation of clinical features, and the severity and course of the illness, manifested by persons with schizophrenia. This clinical heterogeneity, in concert with the identification of differences across individuals in the presence and magnitude of various brain abnormalities, supports the idea that what we diagnose clinically as schizophrenia is likely to encompass a set of disorders that differ with respect to their underlying etiologies, pathogenetic mechanisms, and pathological features. However, the extent to which the heterogeneity of the illness reflects diversity (different disease processes) versus variability (variance within a given disease process) remains unclear.

This complexity has made the exploration of the underlying neurobiology of schizophrenia very challenging. Available data indicate that genetic, environmental, and developmental influences all contribute to the risk of developing schizophrenia (D.A. Lewis and Levitt, 2002). However, the precise details of how these factors combine to give rise to the illness continue to be elusive, and how they become instantiated in specific abnormalities of brain structure and function remains an unanswered question. The apparent discrepancies in the literature, in terms of failures to replicate particular positive findings regarding the neurobiology of schizophrenia, likely reflects, at least to some degree, the complex and diverse nature of the disorder. Thus, as is the case for many human disease states, the clinical syndrome termed *schizophrenia* may represent the end point of many different pathogenetic paths and types of neurobiological disturbances.

Although clearly not mutually exclusive perspectives, hypotheses regarding the nature of this illness have tended to emphasize alterations in brain structure, in particular populations of cells, in neurotransmitter systems, or in molecular and genetic factors. Consequently, in this chapter, we consider examples of each of these views of the neurobiology of schizophrenia.

NEUROANATOMICAL HYPOTHESES

Since Johnstone and colleagues (1976) reported the first computed tomography (CT) brain-imaging evidence of ventricular enlargement, this finding has continued to be one of the most robust findings of structural brain abnormalities in schizophrenia. Fully 80% of 55 magnetic resonance imaging (MRI) studies examining ventricular size found increased volumes in subjects with schizophrenia (Shenton et al., 2001). Notably, only 11 of 50 studies assessing whole-brain volumes found decrements, suggesting that the magnitude of any such differences may be closely approximated by the present limits of MRI sensitivity. Indeed, a meta-analysis (Ward et al., 1996) that estimated the effect size for brain volume reductions found it to be relatively small (–0.26). Assuming that these subtle differences at the whole-brain scale do not reflect generalized pathology uniformly affecting all neuroanatomic regions, it is reasonable to expect that examination of more circumscribed areas might reveal more substantial relative decreases in volume (Dorph-Petersen et al., 2007).

One of the brain regions that has received the greatest attention in this regard is the prefrontal cortex (PFC), the association areas of the frontal lobe located rostral to the premotor and motor regions. Interest in the PFC has been driven by the convergence of observations that (*1*) the activation of this region is impaired when individuals with schizophrenia perform certain cognitive tasks, such as those that require working memory or cognitive control (Weinberger et al., 1986), and (2) PFC circuit integrity is required for working-memory performance in nonhuman primates (Goldman-Rakic, 1994). Despite this evidence implicating PFC dysfunction in schizophrenia, structural imaging studies of the PFC have been equivocal, with only 60% of 50 studies showing gray matter deficits (Shenton et al., 2001). The negative findings have been attributed to various reasons

(McCarley et al., 1999) including the possibility that MRI sensitivity may be inadequate to detect relatively subtle decrements in PFC volume, estimated at 3%–12% by postmortem studies (Pakkenberg, 1993; Daviss and Lewis, 1995; Selemon et al., 1995; Woo et al., 1997). Importantly, volumetric reductions in PFC gray matter have been reported in first-episode, neuroleptic-naïve patients, suggesting that these changes were extant prior to the potential confounds of illness chronicity and treatment (Lim et al., 1996).

Of the potential neurobiological sources for these subtle volume differences, dendritic spines, the principal targets of excitatory synapses to pyramidal neurons, have received substantial attention. Approximately 75% of the dendritic spines present in the mouse cortex are stable over adulthood (Zuo et al., 2005), but their number and morphology can be altered by a number of neuroplastic changes, such as a loss of their presynaptic excitatory input (DeFelipe and Farinas, 1992). In schizophrenia, dendritic spine density in pyramidal neurons has been reported to be decreased in the PFC and other cortical regions by a number of research groups (Garey et al., 1998; Glantz and Lewis, 2000; Kalus et al., 2000; Broadbelt et al., 2002; Black et al., 2004; Broadbelt et al., 2006). In addition, studies of basilar dendritic spine density on Golgi-impregnated pyramidal neurons in each cortical layer of the PFC in the same subjects found a significant ~20% lower spine density for pyramidal neurons in deep layer 3. In contrast, spine density on pyramidal neurons in superficial layer 3 was reduced to a lesser degree, whereas the density of those on the basilar dendrites of pyramidal neurons in layer 5 or 6 did not differ across subject groups (Glantz and Lewis, 2000; Kolluri et al., 2005).

The functional integrity of the pyramidal neurons with lower dendritic spine densities may be reflected by changes in their somal volume. For example, shifts in somal size may indicate disturbances in neuronal connectivity, given that somal size has been shown to be correlated with measures of a neuron's dendritic tree (Hayes and Lewis, 1996; Jacobs et al., 1997) and axonal arbor (C.D. Gilbert and Kelly, 1975; Lund et al., 1975). Indeed, the mean cross-sectional somal area of the Golgi-impregnated, deep layer 3 pyramidal neurons was 9.1% smaller in subjects with schizophrenia relative to normal control subjects, although this difference did not achieve statistical significance (Glantz and Lewis, 2000). Consistent with this observation, the mean somal volume of Nissl-stained pyramidal neurons in PFC deep layer 3 was 9.2% smaller in a different cohort of subjects with schizophrenia, relative to matched normal comparison subjects, a decrease that was not explained by either antipsychotic medication history or duration of illness (Pierri et al., 2001). Similarly, in another study, the mean somal size of all layer 3 neurons in PFC area 9 was smaller in subjects with schizophrenia and was accompanied by a decrease in the density of the largest neurons in deep layer 3, without a change in somal volume in layer 5 (Rajkowska et al., 1998). Furthermore, in primary and association auditory cortices, somal volumes of deep layer 3, but not of layer 5, pyramidal neurons were smaller in schizophrenia (Sweet et al., 2003; Sweet et al., 2004). Together, these findings suggest that in schizophrenia, basilar dendritic spine density is lower and somal volume is smaller in pyramidal neurons, that these alterations are specific to or at least most prominent in deep layer 3, that this pattern of alterations is not restricted to the PFC, and that these findings reflect the underlying disease process and not confounding factors. However, understanding the significance of these findings requires knowledge of the role of the affected pyramidal neurons in cortical circuitry.

Pyramidal neurons can be divided into subgroups based on the brain region targeted by their principal axonal projection and the sources of their excitatory inputs; both of these characteristics are associated with the laminar location of pyramidal cell bodies. For example, many pyramidal cells in layers 2–3 send axonal projections to other cortical regions, pyramidal neurons in layer 5 tend to project to the striatum and other subcortical structures, and pyramidal neurons in layer 6 furnish projections primarily to the thalamus (Jones, 1984). Furthermore, even within the same cortical layer, different subpopulations of pyramidal neurons exhibit quantitative differences in dendritic morphology and qualitative differences in the gene products that they express, and these subpopulations of pyramidal neurons tend to differ in the targets of their principal axon projections. For example, pyramidal neurons in layer 3 of the primate PFC that send axons to the other cerebral hemisphere have larger dendritic arbors and exhibit a greater density of dendritic spines than do neighboring pyramidal cells that furnish axons to the adjacent regions of the same hemisphere (Soloway et al., 2002). Pyramidal neurons that furnish axonal projections to distant cortical regions also tend to have larger cell bodies and to express high levels of nonphosphorylated epitopes of neurofilament proteins (NNFP) compared to pyramidal cells in the same location that provide shorter corticocortical projections (Hof et al., 1996). Attempts to identify the affected pyramidal neurons based on such markers have not yet yielded fruit. For example, the somal volumes of NNFP-containing layer 3 neurons were reported to be unaltered in schizophrenia (Law and Harrison, 2003; Pierri et al., 2003), but these studies appear to have been subject to a methodological confound that resulted in an overestimation of somal volumes in schizophrenia (Maldonado-Aviles et al., 2006). Furthermore, the ability to distinguish other subpopulations of pyramidal neurons based on their molecular phenotype still awaits the types of gene expression profiling studies that have been successfully utilized for characterizing subclasses of cortical interneurons (Sugino et al., 2006).

Excitatory projections from the mediodorsal thalamus, the principal source of thalamic inputs to the PFC (Giguere and Goldman-Rakic, 1988), synapse primarily on dendritic spines (Melchitzky et al., 1999). These axons densely arborize in PFC layers deep 3 and 4 but do not innervate the deep cortical layers (Erickson and Lewis, 2004). Because the basilar dendrites of PFC deep layer 3 pyramidal neurons are present in the same location, a reduction in the number or activity of mediodorsal thalamic afferents could contribute to the observed decrement in spine density in schizophrenia. Initial reports indicated that the total number of neurons with this nucleus was lower in schizophrenia (Pakkenberg, 1990; Popken et al., 2000; Young et al., 2000; Byne et al., 2002), suggesting that a reduced number of these afferents might contribute to lower spine density in the PFC in schizophrenia. However, more recent studies, including some from the same research groups that reported the initial positive findings, have failed to find a decrement in thalamic neuron number (Cullen et al., 2003; Dorph-Petersen et al., 2004; Young et al., 2004). Some neuroimaging studies have reported smaller thalamic volumes, altered shape, and decreased activity (Manoach et al., 1999) in subjects with schizophrenia, including studies in first-episode subjects in whom the potential confounds of medication effects and illness chronicity are mitigated (Ettinger et al., 2001; A.R. Gilbert et al., 2001). Furthermore, reduced volume of the total thalamus has been suggested to mark the genetic contribution to the illness in studies of twin pairs concordant or discordant for schizophrenia (Ettinger et al., 2007). Thus, even in the face of a normal number of thalamic neurons, these observations might suggest that the nature, if not the number, of thalamic projections is altered in schizophrenia.

Two other major sources provide excitatory inputs to deep layer 3 PFC pyramidal neurons, although these inputs are less laminarly restricted than those from the mediodorsal thalamus. First, the axons of pyramidal neurons in layers 2 and 3, which project to other cortical regions, also give rise to neighboring and long-range axon collaterals that travel through the gray matter for up to several millimeters before arborizing in discrete stripe-like clusters in the same cortical region (Levitt et al., 1993; Pucak et al., 1996). The extrinsic and long-range intrinsic collaterals of these neurons target almost exclusively the dendritic spines of other pyramidal cells, whereas the synaptic targets of the local axon collaterals are equally divided between dendritic spines and the dendritic shafts of the parvalbumin-containing class of γ-aminobutyric acid (GABA) neurons (Melchitzky et al., 1998; Melchitzky et al., 2001; Melchitzky and Lewis, 2003). Second, associational or callosal projections from other cortical regions also terminate in these layers (Barbas, 1992; Pucak et al., 1996). Thus, the smaller decrease in spine density on superficial layer 3 pyramidal cells raises the possibility that abnormalities in thalamocortical afferents to deep layer 3 have an additive effect to a disturbance in cortical axon terminals that are distributed across layer 3. However, even if these interpretations are correct, they do not reveal the direction of the pathogenetic mechanisms. For example, the inputs to dorsolateral prefrontal cortex (DLPFC) layer 3 pyramidal cells might not be reduced due to a more primary disturbance in the source of the inputs, but because an abnormality intrinsic to these pyramidal cells renders them unable to support a normal complement of excitatory inputs.

CELLULAR HYPOTHESES

As indicated in the preceding section, alterations in pyramidal neurons appear to contribute to the pathology of schizophrenia. Other studies suggest that glial cells, the most numerous type of brain cells, may also be altered in the illness. Although proliferation of glia to form a glial scar (termed *gliosis*) was initially reported in postmortem studies of schizophrenia, cortical gliosis is no longer considered a characteristic feature of the illness (Harrison, 1999; Cotter, Pariante, and Everall, 2001). However, convergent lines of evidence from postmortem, genetic association, and imaging studies suggest that oligodendrocytes, determinants of white matter myelination and regulators of grey matter neuronal development and support, may be dysfunctional in schizophrenia. For example, a decreased density of Nissl-stained oligodendrocytes has been reported in PFC area 9 in layers 3 and 6 and in the subjacent white matter (Orlovskaya et al., 2000; Hof et al., 2003; Uranova et al., 2004). Other studies have reported lower glial cell number in the orbitofrontal, anterior cingulate, and primary motor cortices (Benes et al., 1986; Benes et al., 1991; Rajkowska et al., 1999; Cotter, Mackay, et al., 2001) of subjects with schizophrenia. However, some studies have not detected significant changes in glial cell number or density changes in prefrontal, anterior cingulate, and occipital cortices in individuals with schizophrenia (Selemon et al., 1995, 1998; Cotter, Pariante, and Everall, 2001). Furthermore, studies in monkeys found that chronic exposure to haloperidol or olanzapine in a manner that mimics the clinical treatment of schizophrenia was associated with lower total glia cell number, without a change in neuron number, raising the question of the extent to which the treatment of the illness contributes to the postmortem human findings (Konopaske et al., 2007).

However, other studies have found alterations in the tissue levels of some, but not all, transcripts expressed by oligodendrocytes, suggesting that the cells are still present but dysfunctional. For example, decreased messenger ribonucleic acids (mRNA) levels for genes encoding myelin-related products in the PFC in schizophrenia including 2', 3'-cyclic nucleotide 3'-phosphodiesterase (CNP), which maintains microtubular function of oligodendrocytes, and myelin-associated glycoprotein (MAG), which supports the myelin-axonal interface and structure of myelin sheaths, have been reported in microarray and quantitative polymerase chain reaction (PCR) studies (Hakak et al., 2001; Tkachev et al., 2003). Decreased expression of CNP and MAG have been observed at the protein level as well in the PFC (Flynn et al., 2003; Hof et al., 2003; Dracheva et al., 2006). Furthermore, allelic association studies have found some evidence of an association between individual single nucleotide polymorphisms (SNP) and schizophrenia for CNP and MAG (Wan et al., 2005; Peirce et al., 2006), although these findings have not been independently replicated yet.

Alterations in oligodendrocytes in schizophrenia are supported by reports of smaller frontal and temporal lobe white matter volume in imaging studies of schizophrenia (for review, see Walterfang et al., 2006). Furthermore, proton magnetic resonance spectroscopy studies have reported reduced levels of *N*-acetylaspartate (NAA), a marker of neuronal and axonal integrity, in frontal white matter (for review, see Steen et al., 2005). In addition, diffusion tensor imaging studies have revealed disruption of white matter fiber organization in frontal cortex, and these abnormalities do not appear to be the result of antipsychotic medication because they are present in first-episode subjects with schizophrenia (Szeszko et al., 2005; Hao et al., 2006).

NEUROTRANSMITTER HYPOTHESES

Abnormalities in Dopamine (DA) Neurotransmission

The initial dopamine (DA) hypothesis of schizophrenia posited that the psychotic features of the illness resulted from a functional excess of DA neurotransmission. This hypothesis was principally based on two pharmacological observations. First, DA agonists, such as amphetamine, can induce psychotic symptoms in control subjects and exacerbate psychosis in individuals with schizophrenia. Second, the potency of antipsychotic medications is proportional to the ability to block DA D_2 receptors (for review, see Seeman, 2006). Subsequent imaging studies demonstrated that amphetamine induces a greater amount of DA release in the striatum in subjects who are drug-free and have schizophrenia than in control subjects (Laruelle et al., 1997). However, in the PFC, DA neurotransmission appears to be diminished in schizophrenia and appears to contribute to working-memory dysfunction in schizophrenia (Davis et al., 1991). For example, lesions of the PFC DA system (Brozoski et al., 1979) and antagonists of the DA D_1 receptor (Sawaguchi and Goldman-Rakic, 1991), the predominant DA receptor expressed in the PFC (Goldman-Rakic et al., 1990), are associated with impaired working-memory performance in monkeys. Consistent with these observations, the density of axons with detectable levels of the rate-limiting enzyme in DA synthesis and of the transporter responsible for its reuptake is decreased in the PFC of subjects with schizophrenia (Akil et al., 1999). In addition, positron emission tomography (PET) studies of subjects who are drug-free with schizophrenia found elevated levels of D_1 receptor in the PFC, suggesting that it was upregulated in response to a deficit in DA. In addition, D_1 receptor levels were inversely correlated with cognitive performance (Abi-Dargham et al., 2002). Taken together, these data suggest that reduced DA neurotransmission in the PFC may contribute to impaired cognitive performance in schizophrenia.

This interpretation has been further supported by studies of catechol-O-methyltransferase (COMT), which regulates the metabolic degradation of DA in the PFC (Tunbridge et al., 2004). A single guanine to adenosine transition in the COMT gene produces a change in amino acids from valine (val) to methionine (met) at codon 108 or 158 (for the soluble and membrane-bound forms of COMT, respectively). The met-containing COMT enzyme has 25% of the activity of val-containing COMT, resulting in substantially lower DA metabolism by the met-containing COMT enzyme. Thus, the presence of the high-activity val-containing COMT allele, which results in lower DA levels, may contribute to impaired cognitive function in schizophrenia (Chen et al., 2004). Because COMT appears to be substantially more important for DA metabolism in the PFC than in other brain regions such as the striatum (Gogos et al., 1998), the presence of the val allele would be predicted to produce lower extrasynaptic DA levels predominantly in cortical regions. Consistent with this prediction, DA levels are elevated by over 200% in frontal cortex, but not in striatum or hypothalamus, of COMT knock-out mice (Gogos et al., 1998). Furthermore, some studies, though not all (Ho et al., 2005), have found that subjects with schizophrenia and control subjects homozygous for the val allele perform more poorly on measures of working-memory and other cognitive functions than either individuals heterozygoues or homozygous for the met genotype (Egan et al., 2001). Thus, even though changes in levels of COMT protein (Tunbridge et al., 2006) or mRNA expression (Tunbridge et al., 2004) have not been found in postmortem studies of schizophrenia, the presence of the val allele could adversely affect DA neurotransmission in the PFC. However, a recent meta-analysis found a small effect of COMT genotype on executive function (as measured by the Wisconsin Card Sorting Test) in healthy individuals, but not in subjects with schizophrenia (Barnett et al., 2007).

Abnormalities in Glutamate Neurotransmission

Pyramidal neurons, the principal class of cortical excitatory neurons, use glutamate as a neurotransmitter. Pharmacological data suggest that glutamatergic neurotransmission through the *N*-methyl-D-aspartate (NMDA) receptor is altered in schizophrenia. For example, phenylcyclidine and ketamine, noncompetitive antagonists of the NMDA receptor, induce or exacerbate positive symptoms, negative symptoms, and cognitive deficits in control and schizophrenia subjects, respectively (Krystal et al., 1994; Coyle, 2007). Conversely, initial clinical trials found that treatment with NMDA receptor-enhancing agents such as (*1*) glycine, which facilitates NMDA receptor function by binding to a modulatory site; (*2*) D-cycloserine, a selective partial agonist at the glycine modulatory site; or (*3*) *N*-methyl-glycine (sarcosine), a glycine transporter I inhibitor, might each improve positive and negative symptoms and cognitive dysfunction in subjects with schizophrenia (Goff et al., 1995; Leiderman et al., 1996; Lane et al., 2005). However, these results have not been consistently replicated (Goff et al., 2005; Coyle, 2007).

Similarly, in animal models, systemic administration of NMDA receptor antagonists to rodents impairs performance on working-memory tasks (Verma and Moghaddam, 1996). Deficits in working memory can also be induced in monkeys by selective injections of NMDA receptor antagonists into the PFC (Dudkin et al., 2001), which contains a relatively high density of NMDA receptors compared to other neocortical regions in humans (Scherzer et al., 1998). These data are at least consistent with the hypothesis that NMDA receptor hypofunction in the PFC might contribute to working-memory impairments in schizophrenia.

Despite the strength of these findings for the theory of NMDA receptor hypofunction in schizophrenia, direct evidence of a substantial decrease in NMDA receptor expression has not been consistently found in subjects with schizophrenia (Akbarian et al., 1996; Kristiansen et al., 2006). Furthermore, though some genetic studies have found statistically significant associations between individual NMDA receptor subunit allelic variants and schizophrenia (Tang et al., 2006; Zhao et al., 2006), it is unclear if these genetic variations have any detrimental effects on NMDA receptor function.

However, NMDA receptor hypofunction in schizophrenia may still occur even without direct alterations in either NMDA receptor levels or in the genetic sequence of the NMDA receptor itself. For example, neuregulin 1 (*NRG1*), which acts through the receptor ErbB4, has been implicated as a susceptibility gene in schizophrenia (see following section). Interestingly, *NRG1*-ErbB4 signaling has been shown to reduce NMDA receptor-mediated currents in PFC pyramidal neurons (Gu et al., 2005) and to regulate the maturation and plasticity of glutamatergic synapses (Li et al., 2007). Application of *NRG1* to postmortem human brain tissue resulted in increased tyrosine phosphorylation of ErbB4 and decreased tyrosine phosphorylation of the NMDAR2A receptor subunit, which is a measure of NMDA receptor activation (Hahn et al., 2006). Thus, even in the absence of changes of overall NMDA receptor levels, changes in *NRG1* signaling might still affect NMDA receptor activation.

Abnormalities in GABA Neurotransmission

Recent studies suggest that disturbances in inhibitory (GABA) neurons play a prominent role in the dysfunction of cortical circuitry in schizophrenia. For example, one of the most consistently reported alterations in postmortem studies of schizophrenia is lower levels of the mRNA for glutamate decarboxylase (GAD_{67}), the principal enzyme responsible for GABA synthesis (Akbarian and Huang, 2006). Expression of the mRNA for the GABA membrane transporter (GAT-1), which is responsible for the reuptake of GABA into the nerve terminal, is similarly reduced in subjects with schizophrenia (Volk et al., 2001). Indeed, earlier studies reported that presynaptic markers of the synthesis, release, and reuptake of GABA were decreased in postmortem samples from schizophrenia subjects (Simpson et al., 1989; Sherman et al., 1991; Impagnatiello et al., 1998). Furthermore, allelic variants in the gene (*GAD1*) for GAD_{67} have been reported to be associated with increased risk for schizophrenia (Addington et al., 2005; Straub et al., 2007; Zhao et al., 2007) (although other studies have failed to find such an association; De Luca et al., 2004; Lundorf et al., 2005; Ikeda et al., 2007), and an SNP in the 5′ untranslated region, which is predicted to be in the promoter, was associated with reduced GAD_{67} mRNA in the DLPFC of individuals with schizophrenia (Straub et al., 2007). Interestingly, injection of GABA antagonists into the PFC disrupts working-memory performance in monkeys (Sawaguchi et al., 1989). Given the role that GABA neurons play in the PFC circuitry that subserves working-memory function (for review, see D.A. Lewis et al., 2005), these data suggest that deficient GABA signaling in PFC may contribute to cognitive impairment in schizophrenia.

Cortical GABA neurons are composed of heterogenous subpopulations of neurons that exhibit unique anatomical, biochemical, and electrophysiological properties (Markram et al., 2004) reflecting specialized functional roles in the regulation of neuronal activity (D.A. Lewis et al., 2005). For example, chandelier neurons provide a linear array of axon terminals (cartridges) that exclusively synapse along the axon initial segment of pyramidal neurons, the site of action potential generation. Chandelier neurons are also among the minority of GABA neurons that express the calcium-binding protein *parvalbumin* and that exhibit a fast-spiking, nonadapting firing pattern. These characteristics suggest that chandelier neurons are specially adapted to powerfully regulate the output of pyramidal neurons. In contrast, double bouquet neurons, which express the calcium-binding protein calretinin and exhibit a regular-spiking, adaptive firing pattern, provide axon terminals that target more distal dendritic sites on pyramidal cells or other GABA neurons.

Interestingly, recent studies have indeed found that alterations in inhibitory neurotransmission in schizophrenia appear to be most prominent in a subset of PFC GABA neurons that includes chandelier cells. For example, the protein level of GAT-1 appears to be selectively reduced in the axon terminals of chandelier cells (Woo et al., 1998; Pierri et al., 1999). In addition, in PFC area 9, the relative cellular levels of expression of GAD_{67} and GAT-1 mRNAs are actually normal in the majority of inhibitory neurons but are undetectable in a subset of neurons in the same cortical layers where chandelier cells are located (Volk et al., 2000, 2001). Furthermore, parvalbumin, but not calretinin, mRNA expression levels are reduced in the PFC in schizophrenia (T. Hashimoto et al., 2003). In subjects with schizophrenia, ~50% of parvalbumin mRNA-expressing neurons do not express detectable levels of GAD_{67} mRNA, suggesting that parvalbumin neurons, which include chandelier neurons, are part of the subset of functionally impaired GABA neurons in schizophrenia (T. Hashimoto et al., 2003).

The nature of the disturbances in GABA neurotransmission in chandelier neurons in schizophrenia is evident from the status of $GABA_A$ receptors specifically located at the principal postsynaptic targets of chandelier cells, the axon initial segments (AIS) of pyramidal cells. The density of pyramidal neuron axon initial segments immunoreactive for the $GABA_A$ receptor α_2 subunit was markedly increased in the PFC of subjects with schizophrenia, but not in subjects with major depression, and the density of α-labeled axon initial segments was inversely correlated to the density of GAT-1-labeled cartridges in subjects with schizophrenia (Volk et al., 2002). Thus, $GABA_A$ receptors appear to be up-regulated at pyramidal neuron axon initial segment in response to deficient GABA neurotransmission at chandelier axon terminals in schizophrenia.

These schizophrenia-related disturbances in PFC chandelier neurons may be a contributing factor to working-memory deficits in schizophrenia. For example, gamma band oscillations, which reflect synchronized firing of neuronal networks at 30–80 Hz, are induced and sustained during the delay period of working-memory tasks (Tallon-Baudry et al., 1998), and the amplitude of gamma band oscillations in the PFC also increases in proportion to working-memory load in control subjects (Howard et al., 2003). However, gamma synchrony is reduced in the PFC of individuals with schizophrenia during cognitive tasks (Cho et al., 2006). Furthermore, parvalbumin neurons, in particular chandelier neurons, are critically involved in initiating and maintaining the oscillatory, synchronous discharges of pyramidal neurons at gamma frequency. Indeed, a single chandelier neuron, whose axon terminals synapse on the axon initial segment of hundreds of pyramidal neurons (Somogyi, 1977), can synchronize the firing of multiple pyramidal neurons in rat hippocampus (Cobb et al., 1995). Thus, impaired perisomatic inhibition from parvalbumin neurons in the PFC may result in deficient pyramidal neuron synchronization, abnormalities in electroencephalogram (EEG)-measured gamma band oscillations, and consequently working-memory dysfunction in subjects with schizophrenia.

Interestingly, some evidence suggests that NMDA receptor hypofunction (see above) may be an upstream contributor to the molecular alterations in parvalbumin neurons. For example, application of NMDA receptor antagonists to cell cultures reduces parvalbumin and GAD_{67} immunoreactivity in a subset of GABA neurons (Kinney et al., 2006). In addition, systemic administration of phencyclidine (PCP) to rodents does not affect the density of parvalbumin mRNA-containing neurons but reduces parvalbumin mRNA expression level per neuron by approximately 25% (Cochran et al., 2003), a pattern very similar to that reported in schizophrenia (T. Hashimoto et al., 2003). Thus, selective alterations in the PFC GABA system in schizophrenia may represent a downstream consequence of deficient NMDA receptor signaling in schizophrenia.

Abnormalities in Cholinergic Neurotransmission

Sensory gating abnormalities are well-documented in individuals with schizophrenia (see Braff and Geyer, 1989, for review). That is, individuals with schizophrenia appear to have deficits in the ability to gate, or internally screen, sensory stimuli. In humans, the gating of auditory stimuli is reflected in a smaller evoked electroencephalographic response to the second of two consecutive auditory stimuli. That is, when two paired tones are delivered 500 msec apart, the amplitude of the P50 auditory evoked potential (a positive response that occurs 50 msec after a tone) to the second tone normally decreases to less than 40% of the P50 following the first tone. In contrast, in over 75% of individuals with schizophrenia, and in about 50% of their unaffected family members, the response to the second tone fails to show this normal decrease in amplitude and may actually increase (Adler et al., 1982).

This deficit in the P50 is transmitted as an autosomal dominant in families with schizophrenia, and a study found that this trait was linked to a dinucleotide repeat polymorphism (D15S1360) located at chromosome 15q14

(Freedman et al., 1997). Evidence for linkage of the locus to schizophrenia was also positive, but not as strong; as expected, attempts to replicate the linkage to schizophrenia have produced positive and negative findings (Leonard et al., 1998; Neves-Pereira et al., 1998; Curtis et al., 1999; Riley et al., 2000; Freedman et al., 2001).

The relevance of this locus for the pathophysiological mechanism of auditory gating deficits and possibly for the pathogenesis of schizophrenia is supported by the fact that the gene (*CHRNA7*) for the α_7 subunit of the nicotinic acetylcholine receptor (nAChR) is located <120kb from the dinucleotide marker (Freedman et al., 1997; Leonard et al., 1998). Several lines of evidence support a role for the nAChR α_7 subunit in the pathophysiology of sensory-gating deficits in schizophrenia. In humans, the binding of bungarotoxin, which probably corresponds to nAChRs containing the α_7 subunit (Leonard et al., 2000), is reduced in postmortem studies of individuals with schizophrenia (Freedman et al., 1995). In addition, the P50 deficit is improved by nicotine in subjects with schizophrenia and their unaffected family members (Adler et al., 1998). However, in contrast to control subjects, who show an upregulation of nicotinic receptors in association with smoking, individuals with schizophrenia exhibit lower binding at every level of smoking history (Breese et al., 2000). Furthermore, in sensory-gating paradigms in rats, the N40 wave is thought to be the analogue of the human P50. Interestingly, the administration of specific antagonists of the α_7 nAChR, and the use of antisense oligonucleotides complementary to the α_7 translation start site, blocked the gating of the N40 wave in rats (Leonard et al., 1996).

These observations are of particular clinical interest because smoking and other uses of nicotine-containing tobacco products are much more common in schizophrenia than in the general population, and individuals with schizophrenia appear to extract more nicotine from each cigarette than unaffected smokers (Olincy et al., 1997). These observations suggest that individuals with schizophrenia use tobacco excessively as a means of self-medication. That is, by stimulating deficient α_7-containing nAChRs, they are able to transiently reduce the subjective distress associated with sensory-gating disturbances (Adler et al., 1998). Consistent with this hypothesis, a recent proof-of-principle study demonstrated that acute, systemic administration of a partial α_7 agonist to subjects with schizophrenia resulted in a normalization of auditory-evoked P50 measures (Olincy et al., 2006).

GENETIC HYPOTHESES

The genetic liability to schizophrenia appears to be transmitted in a polygenic, non-Mendelian fashion (Risch and Baron, 1984; Risch, 2000), and a number of chromosomal loci have been reported to be associated with schizophrenia (Badner and Gershon, 2002; C.M. Lewis et al., 2003). Although individual SNPs and haplotypes have been associated with an increased risk for developing schizophrenia, in many cases these findings have proven to be difficult to replicate in subsequent cohorts of subjects. This phenomenon may highlight the genetic complexity of schizophrenia, with different subtypes or etiologies of schizophrenia produced by different fundamental molecular defects. Consequently, it is not possible at present to point to single genes that have been unequivocally implicated as susceptibility factors for schizophrenia (Harrison and Weinberger, 2005), although emerging evidence continues to support an etiologic role for the following well-studied genes (Ross et al., 2006).

Neuregulin

Neuregulin 1 (*NRG1*), a large 1.4 megabase gene at chromosome 8p13, encodes at least 15 distinct peptides derived from six different isoforms (I-VI). *NRG1* was initially identified as a potential susceptibility gene in an Icelandic population (Stefansson et al., 2002), with a core risk haplotype involving five SNPs. Subsequent case-control and family-based genetic studies in other population samples have also reported associations between schizophrenia and various SNPs located within the same Icelandic haplotype as well as with additional *NRG1* haplotypes (for review, see Harrison and Law, 2006). However, it is important to note that no single SNP or haplotype of *NRG1* has been consistently reported across sample populations to be associated with an increased risk of schizophrenia, and a few studies have failed to find any *NRG1* allelic variants associated with the disease.

A recent study identified a particular allelic variation in the *NRG1* promoter (SNP8NRG243177), part of the original Icelandic risk haplotype (Stefansson et al., 2002), that was associated with a higher rate of conversion to psychosis and with impaired PFC activation during a cognitive task in individuals at high risk for schizophrenia (Hall et al., 2006). Furthermore, this same allelic variant was associated with elevated mRNA levels of the type IV isoform of *NRG1* in the hippocampus (Law et al., 2006), but type IV *NRG1* mRNA levels were actually not different between subjects with schizophrenia and control subjects (R. Hashimoto et al., 2004; Law et al., 2006). In addition, although type I *NRG1* mRNA expression levels were reported to be increased in schizophrenia subjects in hippocampus and PFC, SNP8NRG243177 was not associated with the level of type I *NRG1* mRNA expression in schizophrenia (Law et al., 2006). Thus, the consistent identification of specific SNPs or risk haplotypes of *NRG1* that clearly associate with the pathology and the clinical phenotype of schizophrenia remains elusive.

NRG1 and its receptor tyrosine kinase, ErbB4, are involved in multiple aspects of neural development and functioning including neuronal migration, synaptogenesis, myelination, and GABA and NMDA receptor function (for review, see Corfas et al., 2004). Many of these same processes have been implicated in schizophrenia as described above. Thus, the identification of *NRG1* as a susceptibility gene in schizophrenia is at least consistent with the concept that reported deficiencies in *NRG1* signaling (Hahn et al., 2006) may be a contributory factor to a broad range of pathological abnormalities reported in schizophrenia.

Dysbindin

Dysbindin (dystrobrevin binding protein or *DTNBP1*), a 140-kilobase gene located in chromosomal region 6p22.3, was identified as a susceptibility gene for schizophrenia in a family-based genetic association analysis of 270 Irish families (Straub et al., 2002). Multiple risk haplotypes were initially identified in this cohort, and one particular haplotype was found to confer the highest risk for schizophrenia, although this haplotype contained only intronic SNPs and was present in a small number (6%) of subjects (van den Oord et al., 2003). Subsequent studies identified additional risk haplotypes for schizophrenia (Numakawa et al., 2004; Williams et al., 2004). However, no single risk haplotype for schizophrenia has been consistently reported across studies (Mutsuddi et al., 2006), and both alleles at the same SNP site have been associated with increased risk for schizophrenia (Schwab et al., 2003).

As with *NRG1*, the functional consequences of these genetic variants have not yet been determined. However, some of the risk variants have been linked to certain clinical features of schizophrenia. For example, schizophrenia-associated SNPs have been reported to correlate with altered PFC activation during a cognitive task in normal control subjects (Fallgatter et al., 2006). In subjects with schizophrenia, one particular risk haplotype has been associated with greater severity of lifetime negative symptoms (DeRosse et al., 2006), lower performance on tasks measuring general cognitive ability (Burdick et al., 2006), and possibly a greater degree of cognitive decline through the course of the illness (Burdick et al., 2007).

DTNBP1 may play a role in glutamatergic neurotransmission as suggested by findings that *DTNBP1* (*1*) is largely localized to presynaptic axon terminals forming asymmetric synapses onto spines and (*2*) associates with synaptic vesicles in human hippocampus (Talbot et al., 2006). In human PFC, *DTNBP1* mRNA expression has been reported in pyramidal neurons as well (Weickert et al., 2004). In addition, overexpression of *DTNBP1* results in increased evoked glutamate release, and RNA silencing of *DTNBP1* results in decreased evoked glutamate release in rodent cortical neuron cultures (Numakawa et al., 2004). In subjects with schizophrenia, decreased *DTNBP1* mRNA expression levels have been reported in the PFC (Weickert et al., 2004), and decreased *DTNBP1* protein levels have been reported in glutamatergic terminal fields in the hippocampus (though no difference was found in the anterior cingulate cortex) (Talbot et al., 2004). Taken together, these data at least suggest that altered *DTNBP1* levels, and perhaps inherited sequence variations in the *DTNBP1* gene, may contribute to alterations in glutamate neurotransmission in schizophrenia.

DISC1

DISC1, or disrupted in schizophrenia 1, was initially identified as a susceptibility gene by its localization to the breakpoint of a balanced chromosomal translocation t(1;11)(q42;q14.3) that significantly cosegregated with several major mental illnesses, including schizophrenia (St. Clair et al., 1990). Although the breakpoint at chromosome 11 did not involve any genes, the breakpoint at chromosome 1 was found to directly "disrupt" two genes later identified as *DISC1* and *DISC2* (Millar et al., 2000). In addition, some SNPs and haplotypes of *DISC1* have been linked to an increased risk for developing schizophrenia, and these same risk variants are associated with greater severity of some of the clinical, endophenotypic, and pathological features of schizophrenia. For example, in the same Scottish family described above, carriers of the chromosome 1:11 translocation were reported to have a reduced magnitude of the event-related potential P300, a physiologically relevant EEG measure associated with information processing that is decreased in subjects with schizophrenia (Blackwood et al., 2001). Furthermore, in Finnish populations, *DISC1* risk variants (Hennah et al., 2003) were also associated with poorer cognitive performance and reduced grey matter volume (Cannon et al., 2005). In addition, a nonconservative *DISC1* SNP encoding a serine-cysteine substitution was reported to be associated with an increased risk for schizophrenia, and carriers of the Ser allele were found to have smaller hippocampal volume, lower hippocampal NAA content, and altered activation of the hippocampus during cognitive tasks (Callicott et al., 2005), all features previously reported in schizophrenia.

However, not all genetic association studies have found positive relationships between various *DISC1* SNPs and schizophrenia (Devon et al., 2001), and the same allelic variants have not been consistently reported across study populations to be associated with schizophrenia (e.g., see Liu et al., 2006). Furthermore, it remains unclear whether the schizophrenia risk alleles actually represent functional variants or perhaps might be in linkage disequilibrium with another functional variant. Indeed, postmortem studies of schizophrenia subjects generally have not reported changes in the expression levels of *DISC1* mRNA or protein in hippocampus, PFC, or orbitofrontal cortex (Lipska et al., 2006; Sawamura et al., 2005).

Interestingly, mRNA expression levels for some of the proteins that interact with *DISC1* such as fasciculation and elongation protein zeta-1 (FEZ1), nuclear-distribution element-like (NUDEL), and lissencephaly 1 protein (LIS1) have been reported to be decreased in the hippocampus and PFC in subjects with schizophrenia, and these decreased mRNA expression levels were associated with some of the schizophrenia-linked SNPs located near the binding sites for these proteins (Lipska et al., 2006), suggesting a possibly defective interaction between *DISC1* and its binding partners. These *DISC1* binding partners are involved in neurite outgrowth, neuronal migration, and a wide variety of other functions. Thus, even without evidence of a direct change in *DISC1* mRNA or protein levels in schizophrenia, alterations in the level of *DISC1* binding partners, and, possibly, their impaired interactions with *DISC1*, may affect *DISC1* function in schizophrenia.

CONCLUSION

As summarized above, recent findings have generated and supported a number of neurobiologically plausible hypotheses that might account for alterations in aspects of brain dysfunction in schizophrenia, and potential avenues of convergence across these hypotheses is also beginning to emerge. It should be noted, though, that the hypotheses reviewed here are by no means exhaustive, and a number of other possibilities have been suggested (see, e.g., Costa et al., 2001; Mirnics et al., 2001). Future studies are certain to lead to refinements in these hypotheses that will increase their falsifiability and enhance their utility in guiding the pursuit of novel therapeutic interventions for the illness.

REFERENCES

Abi-Dargham, A., Mawlawi, O., Lombardo, I., Gill, R., Martinez, D., Huang, Y., Hwang, D.R., Keilp, J., Kochan, L., van Heertum, R., Gorman, J.M., and Laruelle, M. (2002) Prefrontal dopamine D1 receptors and working memory in schizophrenia. *J. Neurosci.* 22:3708–3719.

Addington, A.M., Gornick, M., Duckworth, J., Sporn, A., Gogtay, N., Bobb, A., Greenstein, D., Lenane, M., Gochman, P., Baker, N., Balkissoon, R., Vakkalanka, R.K., Weinberger, D.R., Rapoport, J.L., and Straub, R.E. (2005) GAD1 (2q31.1), which encodes glutamic acid decarboxylase (GAD(67)), is associated with childhood-onset schizophrenia and cortical gray matter volume loss. *Mol. Psychiatry* 10:581–588.

Adler, L.E., Olincy, A., Waldo, M.C., Harris, J.G., Griffith, J., Stevens, K., Flach, K., Nagamoto, H., Bickford, P., Leonard, S., and Freedman, R. (1998) Schizophrenia, sensory gating, and nicotinic receptors. *Schizophr. Bull.* 24:189–202.

Adler, L.E., Pachtman, E., Franks, R., Pecevich, M., Waldo, M.C., and Freedman, R. (1982) Neurophysiological evidence for a defect in neuronal mechanisms involved in sensory gating in schizophrenia. *Biol. Psychiatry* 17:639–654.

Akbarian, S., and Huang, H.S. (2006) Molecular and cellular mechanisms of altered GAD1/GAD67 expression in schizophrenia and related disorders. *Brain Res. Rev.* 52:293–304.

Akbarian, S., Sucher, N.J., Bradley, D., Tafazzoli, A., Trinh, D., Hetrick, W.P., Potkin, S.G., Sandman, C.A., Bunney, W.E., Jr., and Jones, E.G. (1996) Selective alterations in gene expression of NMDA receptor subunits in prefrontal cortex of schizophrenics. *J. Neurosci.* 16:19–30.

Akil, M., Pierri, J.N., Whitehead, R.E., Edgar, C.L., Mohila, C., Sampson, A.R., and Lewis, D.A. (1999) Lamina-specific alterations in the dopamine innervation of the prefrontal cortex in schizophrenic subjects. *Am. J. Psychiatry* 156:1580–1589.

Badner, J.A., and Gershon, E.S. (2002) Meta-analysis of whole-genome linkage scans of bipolar disorder and schizophrenia. *Mol. Psychiatry* 7:405–411.

Barbas, H. (1992) Architecture and cortical connections of the prefrontal cortex in the Rhesus monkey. *Adv. Neur.* 57:91–115.

Barnett, J.H., Jones, P.B., Robbins, T.W., and Muller, U. (2007) Effects of the catechol-O-methyltransferase Val(158)Met polymorphism on executive function: a meta-analysis of the Wisconsin Card Sort Test in schizophrenia and healthy controls. *Mol. Psychiatry* 12:502–509.

Benes, F.M., Davidson, J., and Bird, E.D. (1986) Quantitative cytoarchitectural studies of the cerebral cortex of schizophrenics. *Arch. Gen. Psychiatry* 43:31–35.

Benes, F.M., McSparren, J., Bird, E.D., SanGiovanni, J.P., and Vincent, S.L. (1991) Deficits in small interneurons in prefrontal and cingulate cortices of schizophrenic and schizoaffective patients. *Arch. Gen. Psychiatry* 48:996–1001.

Black, J.E., Kodish, I.M., Grossman, A.W., Klintsova, A.Y., Orlovskaya, D., Vostrikov, V., Uranova, N., and Greenough, W.T. (2004) Pathology of layer V pyramidal neurons in the prefrontal cortex of patients with schizophrenia. *Am. J. Psychiatry* 161:742–744.

Blackwood, D.H., Fordyce, A., Walker, M.T., St. Clair, D.M., Porteous, D.J., and Muir, W.J. (2001) Schizophrenia and affective disorders—cosegregation with a translocation at chromosome 1q42 that directly disrupts brain-expressed genes: clinical and P300 findings in a family. *Am. J. Hum. Genet.* 69:428–433.

Braff, D.L., and Geyer, M.A. (1989) Sensorimotor gating and the neurobiology of schizophrenia: human and animal model studies. In: Schulz, S.C., and Tamminga, C.A., eds. *Schizophrenia: Scientific Progress*. New York: Oxford University Press, pp. 124–136.

Breese, C.R., Lee, M.J., Adams, C.E., Sullivan, B., Logel, J., Gillen, K.M., Marks, M.J., Collins, A.C., and Leonard, S. (2000) Abnormal regulation of high affinity nicotinic receptors in subjects with schizophrenia. *Neuropsychopharmacology* 23:351–364.

Broadbelt, K., Byne, W., and Jones, L.B. (2002) Evidence for a decrease in basilar dendrites of pyramidal cells in schizophrenic medial prefrontal cortex. *Schizophr. Res.* 58:75–81.

Broadbelt, K., Ramprasaud, A., and Jones, L.B. (2006) Evidence of altered neurogranin immunoreactivity in areas 9 and 32 of schizophrenic prefrontal cortex. *Schizophr. Res.* 87:6–14.

Brozoski, T.J., Brown, R.M., Rosvold, H.E., and Goldman, P.S. (1979) Cognitive deficit caused by regional depletion of dopamine in prefrontal cortex of rhesus monkeys. *Science* 205:929–932.

Burdick, K.E., Goldberg, T.E., Funke, B., Bates, J.A., Lencz, T., Kucherlapati, R., and Malhotra, A.K. (2007) DTNBP1 genotype influences cognitive decline in schizophrenia. *Schizophr. Res.* 89:169–172.

Burdick, K.E., Lencz, T., Funke, B., Finn, C.T., Szeszko, P.R., Kane, J.M., Kucherlapati, R., and Malhotra, A.K. (2006) Genetic variation in DTNBP1 influences general cognitive ability. *Hum. Mol. Genet.* 15:1563–1568.

Byne, W., Buchsbaum, M.S., Mattiace, L.A., Hazlett, E.A., Kemether, E., Elhakem, S.L., Purohit, D.P., Haroutunian, V., and Jones, L. (2002) Postmortem assessment of thalamic nuclear volumes in subjects with schizophrenia. *Am. J. Psychiatry* 159:59–65.

Callicott, J.H., Straub, R.E., Pezawas, L., Egan, M.F., Mattay, V.S., Hariri, A.R., Verchinski, B.A., Meyer-Lindenberg, A., Balkissoon, R., Kolachana, B., Goldberg, T.E., and Weinberger, D.R. (2005) Variation in DISC1 affects hippocampal structure and function and increases risk for schizophrenia. *Proc. Natl. Acad. Sci. USA* 102:8627–8632.

Cannon, T.D., Hennah, W., Van Erp, T.G., Thompson, P.M., Lonnqvist, J., Huttunen, M., Gasperoni, T., Tuulio-Henriksson, A., Pirkola, T., Toga, A.W., Kaprio, J., Mazziotta, J., and Peltonen, L. (2005) Association of DISC1/TRAX haplotypes with schizophrenia, reduced prefrontal gray matter, and impaired short- and long-term memory. *Arch. Gen. Psychiatry* 62:1205–1213.

Chen, J., Lipska, B.K., Halim, N., Ma, Q.D., Matsumoto, M., Melhem, S., Kolachana, B.S., Hyde, T.M., Herman, M.M., Apud, J., Egan, M.F., Kleinman, J.E., and Weinberger, D.R. (2004) Functional analysis of genetic variation in catechol-O-methyltransferase (COMT): effects on mRNA, protein, and enzyme activity in postmortem human brain. *Am. J. Hum. Genet.* 75:807–821.

Cho, R.Y., Konecky, R.O., and Carter, C.S. (2006) Impairments in frontal cortical gamma synchrony and cognitive control in schizophrenia. *Proc. Natl. Acad. Sci. USA* 103:19878–19883.

Cobb, S.R., Buhl, E.H., Halasy, K., Paulsen, O., and Somogyi, P. (1995) Synchronization of neuronal activity in hippocampus by individual GABAergic interneurons. *Nature* 378:75–78.

Cochran, S.M., Kennedy, M., McKerchar, C.E., Steward, L.J., Pratt, J.A., and Morris, B.J. (2003) Induction of metabolic hypofunction and neurochemical deficits after chronic intermittent exposure to phencyclidine: differential modulation by antipsychotic drugs. *Neuropsychopharmacology* 28:265–275.

Corfas, G., Roy, K., and Buxbaum, J.D. (2004) Neuregulin 1-erbB signaling and the molecular/cellular basis of schizophrenia. *Nat. Neurosci.* 7:575–580.

Costa, E., Davis, J., Grayson, D.R., Guidotti, A., Pappas, G.D., and Pesold, C. (2001) Dendritic spine hypoplasticity and downregulation of reelin and GABAergic tone in schizophrenia vulnerability. *Neurobiol. Dis.* 8:723–742.

Cotter, D., Mackay, D., Landau, S., Kerwin, R., and Everall, I. (2001) Reduced glial cell density and neuronal size in anterior cingulate cortex in major depressive disorder. *Arch. Gen. Psychiatry* 58:545–553.

Cotter, D.R., Pariante, C.M., and Everall, I.P. (2001) Glial cell abnormalities in major psychiatric disorders: the evidence and implications. *Brain Res. Bull.* 55:585–595.

Coyle, J.T. (2007) Glutamate and schizophrenia: beyond the dopamine hypothesis. *Cell. Mol. Neurobiol.* 26:365–384.

Cullen, T.J., Walker, M.A., Parkinson, N., Craven, R., Crow, T.J., Esiri, M.M., and Harrison, P.J. (2003) A postmortem study of the mediodorsal nucleus of the thalamus in schizophrenia. *Schizophr. Res.* 60:157–166.

Curtis, L., Blouin, J.-L., Radhakrishna, U., Gehrig, C., Lasseter, V.K., Wolyniec, P., Nestadt, G., Dombroski, B., Kazazian, H.H., Pulver, A.E., Housman, D., Bertrand, D., and Antonarakis, S.E. (1999) No evidence for linkage between schizophrenia and markers at chromosome 15q13-14. *Am. J. Med. Genet. (Neuropsych. Genet.)* 88:109–112.

Davis, K.L., Kahn, R.S., Ko, G., and Davidson, M. (1991) Dopamine in schizophrenia: a review and reconceptualization. *Am. J. Psychiatry* 148:1474–1486.

Daviss, S.R., and Lewis, D.A. (1995) Local circuit neurons of the prefrontal cortex in schizophrenia: selective increase in the density of calbindin-immunoreactive neurons. *Psychiatry Res.* 59:81–96.

DeFelipe, J., and Farinas, I. (1992) The pyramidal neuron of the cerebral cortex: morphological and chemical characteristics of the synaptic inputs. *Prog. Neurobiol.* 39:563–607.

De Luca, V., Muglia, P., Masellis, M., Jane, D.E., Wong, G.W., and Kennedy, J.L. (2004) Polymorphisms in glutamate decarboxylase genes: analysis in schizophrenia. *Psychiatr. Genet.* 14:39–42.

DeRosse, P., Funke, B., Burdick, K.E., Lencz, T., Ekholm, J.M., Kane, J.M., Kucherlapati, R., and Malhotra, A.K. (2006) Dysbindin genotype and negative symptoms in schizophrenia. *Am. J. Psychiatry* 163:532–534.

Devon, R.S., Anderson, S., Teague, P.W., Burgess, P., Kipari, T.M., Semple, C.A., Millar, J.K., Muir, W.J., Murray, V., Pelosi, A.J., Blackwood, D.H., and Porteous, D.J. (2001) Identification of polymorphisms within disrupted in schizophrenia 1 and disrupted in schizophrenia 2, and an investigation of their association with schizophrenia and bipolar affective disorder. *Psychiatr. Genet.* 11:71–78.

Dorph-Petersen, K.A., Pierri, J.N., Sun, Z., Sampson, A.R., and Lewis, D.A. (2004) Stereological analysis of the mediodorsal thalamic nucleus in schizophrenia: volume, neuron number, and cell types. *J. Comp. Neurol.* 472:449–462.

Dorph-Petersen, K.A., Pierri, J.N., Wu, Q., Sampson, A.R., and Lewis, D.A. (2007) Primary visual cortex volume and total neuron number are reduced in schizophrenia. *J. Comp. Neurol.* 501:290–301.

Dracheva, S., Davis, K.L., Chin, B., Woo, D.A., Schmeidler, J., and Haroutunian, V. (2006) Myelin-associated mRNA and protein expression deficits in the anterior cingulate cortex and hippocampus in elderly schizophrenia patients. *Neurobiol. Dis.* 21:531–540.

Dudkin, K.N., Kruchinin, V.K., and Chueva, I.V. (2001) Neurophysiological correlates of delayed visual differentiation tasks in monkeys: the effects of the site of intracortical blockade of NMDA receptors. *Neurosci. Behav. Physiol.* 31:207–218.

Egan, M.F., Goldberg, T.E., Kolachana, B.S., Callicott, J.H., Mazzanti, C.M., Straub, R.E., Goldman, D., and Weinberger, D.R. (2001) Effect of COMT Val 108/158 Met genotype on frontal lobe function and risk for schizophrenia. *Proc. Natl. Acad. Sci. USA* 98: 6917–6922.

Erickson, S.L., and Lewis, D.A. (2004) Cortical connections of the lateral mediodorsal thalamus in cynomolgus monkeys. *J. Comp. Neurol.* 473:107–127.

Ettinger, U., Chitnis, X.A., Kumari, V., Fannon, D.G., Sumich, A.L., O'Ceallaigh, S., Doku, V.C., and Sharma, T. (2001) Magnetic resonance imaging of the thalamus in first-episode psychosis. *Am. J. Psychiatry* 158:116–118.

Ettinger, U., Picchioni, M., Landau, S., Matsumoto, K., van Haren, N.E., Marshall, N., Hall, M.H., Schulze, K., Toulopoulou, T., Davies, N., Ribchester, T., McGuire, P.K., and Murray, R.M. (2007) Magnetic resonance imaging of the thalamus and adhesio interthalamica in twins with schizophrenia. *Arch. Gen. Psychiatry* 64:401–409.

Fallgatter, A.J., Herrmann, M.J., Hohoff, C., Ehlis, A.C., Jarczok, T.A., Freitag, C.M., and Deckert, J. (2006) DTNBP1 (dysbindin) gene variants modulate prefrontal brain function in healthy individuals. *Neuropsychopharmacology* 31:2002–2010.

Flynn, S.W., Lang, D.J., Mackay, A.L., Goghari, V., Vavasour, I.M., Whittall, K.P., Smith, G.N., Arango, V., Mann, J.J., Dwork, A.J., Falkai, P., and Honer, W.G. (2003) Abnormalities of myelination in schizophrenia detected in vivo with MRI, and post-mortem with analysis of oligodendrocyte proteins. *Mol. Psychiatry* 8:811–820.

Freedman, R., Coon, H., Myles-Worsley, M., Orr-Urtreger, A., Olincy, A., Davis, A., Polymeropoulos, M., Holik, J., Hopkins, J., Hoff, M., Rosenthal, J., Waldo, M.C., Reimherr, R., Wender, P., Yaw, J., Young, D.A., Breese, C.R., Adams, C., Patterson, D., Adler, L.E., Kruglyak, L., Leonard, S., and Byerly, W. (1997) Linkage of a neurophysiological deficit in schizophrenia to a chromosome 15 locus. *Proc. Natl. Acad. Sci. USA* 94:587–592.

Freedman, R., Hall, M., Adler, L.E., and Leonard, S. (1995) Evidence in postmortem brain tissue for decreased numbers of hippocampal nicotinic receptors in schizophrenia. *Biol. Psychiatry* 38:22–33.

Freedman, R., Leonard, S., Gault, J.M., Hopkins, J., Cloninger, C.R., Kaufmann, C.A., Tsuang, M.T., Faraone, S.V., Malaspina, D., Svrakic, D.M., Sanders, A., and Gejman, P. (2001) Linkage disequillibrium for schizophrenia at the chromosome 15q13-14 locus of the a7-nicotinic acetylcholine receptor subunit gene (CHRNA7). *Am. J. Med. Genet.* 105:20–22.

Garey, L.J., Ong, W.Y., Patel, T.S., Kanani, M., Davis, A., Mortimer, A.M., Barnes, T.R.E., and Hirsch, S.R. (1998) Reduced dendritic spine density on cerebral cortical pyramidal neurons in schizophrenia. *J. Neurol. Neurosurg. Psychiatry* 65:446–453.

Giguere, M., and Goldman-Rakic, P.S. (1988) Mediodorsal nucleus: areal, laminar, and tangential distribution of afferents and efferents in the frontal lobe of rhesus monkeys. *J. Comp. Neurol.* 277:195–213.

Gilbert, A.R., Rosenberg, D.R., Harenski, K., Spencer, S., Sweeney, J.A., and Keshavan, M.S. (2001) Thalamic volumes in patients with first-episode schizophrenia. *Am. J. Psychiatry* 158:618–624.

Gilbert, C.D., and Kelly, J.P. (1975) The projections of cells in different layers of the cat's visual cortex. *J. Comp. Neurol.* 63:81–106.

Glantz, L.A., and Lewis, D.A. (2000) Decreased dendritic spine density on prefrontal cortical pyramidal neurons in schizophrenia. *Arch. Gen. Psychiatry* 57:65–73.

Goff, D.C., Herz, L., Posever, T., Shih, V., Tsai, G., Henderson, D.C., Freudenreich, O., Evins, A.E., Yovel, I., Zhang, H., and Schoenfeld, D. (2005) A six-month, placebo-controlled trial of D-cycloserine co-administered with conventional antipsychotics in schizophrenia patients. *Psychopharmacology (Berl)* 179:144–150.

Goff, D.C., Tsai, G., Manoach, D.S., and Coyle, J.T. (1995) Dose-finding trial of D-cycloserine added to neuroleptics for negative symptoms in schizophrenia. *Am. J. Psychiatry* 152:1213–1215.

Gogos, J.A., Morgan, M., Luine, V., Santha, M., Ogawa, S., Pfaff, D., and Karayiorgou, M. (1998) Catechol-O-methyltransferase-deficient mice exhibit sexually dimorphic changes in catecholamine levels and behavior. *Proc. Natl. Acad. Sci. USA* 95:9991–9996.

Goldman-Rakic, P.S. (1994) Working memory dysfunction in schizophrenia. *Journal of Neuropsychiatry and Clinical Neuroscience* 6:348–357.

Goldman-Rakic, P.S., Lidow, M.S., and Gallagher, D.W. (1990) Overlap of dopaminergic, adrenergic, and serotoninergic receptors and complementarity of their subtypes in primate prefrontal cortex. *J. Neurosci.* 10:2125–2138.

Gu, Z., Jiang, Q., Fu, A.K., Ip, N.Y., and Yan, Z. (2005) Regulation of NMDA receptors by neuregulin signaling in prefrontal cortex. *J. Neurosci.* 25:4974–4984.

Hahn, C.G., Wang, H.Y., Cho, D.S., Talbot, K., Gur, R.E., Berrettini, W.H., Bakshi, K., Kamins, J., Borgmann-Winter, K.E., Siegel, S. J., Gallop, R.J., and Arnold, S.E. (2006) Altered neuregulin 1-erbB4 signaling contributes to NMDA receptor hypofunction in schizophrenia. *Nat. Med.* 12:734–735.

Hakak, Y., Walker, J.R., Li, C., Wong, W.H., Davis, K.L., Buxbaum, J.D., Haroutunian, V., and Fienberg, A.A. (2001) Genome-wide expression analysis reveals dysregulation of myelination-related genes in chronic schizophrenia. *Proc. Natl. Acad. Sci. USA* 98:4746–4751.

Hall, J., Whalley, H.C., Job, D.E., Baig, B.J., McIntosh, A.M., Evans, K.L., Thomson, P.A., Porteous, D.J., Cunningham-Owens, D.G., Johnstone, E.C., and Lawrie, S.M. (2006) A neuregulin 1 variant associated with abnormal cortical function and psychotic symptoms. *Nat. Neurosci.* 9:1477–1478.

Hao, Y., Liu, Z., Jiang, T., Gong, G., Liu, H., Tan, L., Kuang, F., Xu, L., Yi, Y., and Zhang, Z. (2006) White matter integrity of the whole brain is disrupted in first-episode schizophrenia. *NeuroReport* 17:23–26.

Harrison, P.J. (1999) The neuropathology of schizophrenia: a critical review of the data and their interpretation. *Brain* 122:593–624.

Harrison, P.J., and Law, A.J. (2006) Neuregulin 1 and schizophrenia: genetics, gene expression, and neurobiology. *Biol. Psychiatry* 60:132–140.

Harrison, P.J., and Weinberger, D.R. (2005) Schizophrenia genes, gene expression, and neuropathology: on the matter of their convergence. *Mol. Psychiatry* 10:40–68.

Hashimoto, R., Straub, R.E., Weickert, C.S., Hyde, T.M., Kleinman, J.E., and Weinberger, D.R. (2004) Expression analysis of neuregulin-1 in the dorsolateral prefrontal cortex in schizophrenia. *Mol. Psychiatry* 9:299–307.

Hashimoto, T., Volk, D.W., Eggan, S.M., Mirnics, K., Pierri, J.N., Sun, Z., Sampson, A.R., and Lewis, D.A. (2003) Gene expression deficits in a subclass of GABA neurons in the prefrontal cortex of subjects with schizophrenia. *J. Neurosci.* 23:6315–6326.

Hayes, T.L., and Lewis, D.A. (1996) Magnopyramidal neurons in the anterior motor speech region: dendritic features and inter hemispheric comparisons. *Arch. Neurol.* 53:1277–1283.

Hennah, W., Varilo, T., Kestila, M., Paunio, T., Arajarvi, R., Haukka, J., Parker, A., Martin, R., Levitzky, S., Partonen, T., Meyer, J., Lonnqvist, J., Peltonen, L., and Ekelund, J. (2003) Haplotype transmission analysis provides evidence of association for DISC1 to schizophrenia and suggests sex-dependent effects. *Hum. Mol. Genet.* 12:3151–3159.

Ho, B.C., Wassink, T.H., O'Leary, D.S., Sheffield, V.C., and Andreasen, N.C. (2005) Catechol-O-methyl transferase Val158Met gene polymorphism in schizophrenia: working memory, frontal lobe MRI morphology and frontal cerebral blood flow. *Mol. Psychiatry* 10: 287–298.

Hof, P.R., Haroutunian, V., Friedrich, V.L., Jr., Byne, W., Buitron, C., Perl, D.P., and Davis, K.L. (2003) Loss and altered spatial distribution of oligodendrocytes in the superior frontal gyrus in schizophrenia. *Biol. Psychiatry* 53:1075–1085.

Hof, P.R., Ungerleider, L.G., Webster, M.J., Gattass, R., Adams, M.M., Sailstad, C.A., and Morrison, J.H. (1996) Neurofilament protein is differentially distributed in subpopulations of corticocortical projection neurons in the macaque monkey visual pathways. *J. Comp. Neurol.* 376:112–127.

Howard, M.W., Rizzuto, D.S., Caplan, J.B., Madsen, J.R., Lisman, J., Aschenbrenner-Scheibe, R., Schulze-Bonhage, A., and Kahana, M.J. (2003) Gamma oscillations correlate with working memory load in humans. *Cereb. Cortex* 13:1369–1374.

Ikeda, M., Ozaki, N., Yamanouchi, Y., Suzuki, T., Kitajima, T., Kinoshita, Y., Inada, T., and Iwata, N. (2007) No association between the glutamate decarboxylase 67 gene (GAD1) and schizophrenia in the Japanese population. *Schizophr. Res.* 91:22–26.

Impagnatiello, F., Guidotti, A.R., Pesold, C., Dwivedi, Y., Caruncho, H., Pisu, M.G., Uzunov, D.P., Smalheiser, N.R., Davis, J.M., Pandey, G.N., Pappas, G.D., Teuting, P., Sharma, R.P., and Costa, E. (1998) A decrease of reelin expression as a putative vulnerability factor in schizophrenia. *Proc. Natl. Acad. Sci. USA* 95:15718–15723.

Jacobs, B., Driscoll, L., and Schall, M. (1997) Life-span dendritic and spine changes in areas 10 and 18 of human cortex: a quantitative Golgi study. *J. Comp. Neurol.* 386:661–680.

Johnstone, E.C., Crow, T.J., Frith, C.D., Husband, J., and Kreel, L. (1976) Cerebral ventricular size and cognitive impairment in chronic schizophrenia. *Lancet* 2:924–926.

Jones, E.G. (1984) Laminar distribution of cortical efferent cells. In: Jones, E.G., and Peters, A., eds. *Cerebral Cortex* Vol. 1. New York: Plenum, pp. 521–553.

Kalus, P., Müller, T.J., Zuschratter, W., and Senitz, D. (2000) The dendritic architecture of prefrontal pyramidal neurons in schizophrenic patients. *NeuroReport* 11:3621–3625.

Kinney, J.W., Davis, C.N., Tabarean, I., Conti, B., Bartfai, T., and Behrens, M.M. (2006) A specific role for NR2A-containing NMDA receptors in the maintenance of parvalbumin and GAD67 immunoreactivity in cultured interneurons. *J. Neurosci.* 26:1604–1615.

Kolluri, N., Sun, Z., Sampson, A.R., and Lewis, D.A. (2005) Lamina-specific reductions in dendritic spine density in the prefrontal cortex of subjects with schizophrenia. *Am. J. Psychiatry* 162:1200–1202.

Konopaske, G.T., Dorph-Petersen, K.A., Pierri, J.N., Wu, Q., Sampson, A.R., and Lewis, D.A. (2007) Effect of chronic exposure to antipsychotic medication on cell numbers in the parietal cortex of macaque monkeys. *Neuropsychopharmacology* 32:1216–1223.

Kristiansen, L.V., Beneyto, M., Haroutunian, V., and Meador-Woodruff, J.H. (2006) Changes in NMDA receptor subunits and interacting PSD proteins in dorsolateral prefrontal and anterior cingulate cortex indicate abnormal regional expression in schizophrenia. *Mol. Psychiatry* 11:737–747.

Krystal, J.H., Karper, L.P., Seibyl, J.P., Freeman, G.K., Delaney, R., Bremner, J.D., Heninger, G.R., Bowers, M.B., Jr., and Charney, D.S. (1994) Subanesthetic effects of the noncompetitive NMDA antagonist, ketamine, in humans. Psychotomimetic, perceptual, cognitive, and neuroendocrine responses. *Arch. Gen. Psychiatry* 51:199–214.

Lane, H.Y., Chang, Y.C., Liu, Y.C., Chiu, C.C., and Tsai, G.E. (2005) Sarcosine or D-serine add-on treatment for acute exacerbation of schizophrenia: a randomized, double-blind, placebo-controlled study. *Arch. Gen. Psychiatry* 62:1196–1204.

Laruelle, M., Abi-Dargham, A., van Dyck, C.H., Gil, R., D'Souza, C.D., Erdos, J., McCance, E., Rosenblatt, W., Fingado, C., Zoghbi, S.S., Baldwin, R.M., Seibyl, J.P., Krystal, J.H., Charney, D.S., and Innis, R.B. (1997) Single photon emission computerized tomography imaging of amphetamine-induced release in drug-free schizophrenic subjects. *Proc. Natl. Acad. Sci. USA* 93:9235–9240.

Law, A.J., and Harrison, P.J. (2003) The distribution and morphology of prefrontal cortex pyramidal neurons identified using anti-neurofilament antibodies SMI32, N200 and FNP7. Normative data and a comparison in subjects with schizophrenia, bipolar disorder or major depression. *J. Psychiatr. Res.* 37:487–499.

Law, A.J., Lipska, B.K., Weickert, C.S., Hyde, T.M., Straub, R.E., Hashimoto, R., Harrison, P.J., Kleinman, J.E., and Weinberger, D.R. (2006) Neuregulin 1 transcripts are differentially expressed in schizophrenia and regulated by 5' SNPs associated with the disease. *Proc. Natl. Acad. Sci USA* 103:6747–6752.

Leiderman, E., Zylberman, I., Zukin, S.R., Cooper, T.B., and Javitt, D.C. (1996) Preliminary investigation of high-dose oral glycine on serum levels and negative symptoms in schizophrenia: an open-label trial. *Biol. Psychiatry* 39:213–215.

Leonard, S., Adams, C., Breese, C.R., Adler, L.E., Bickford, P., Byerley, W., Coon, H., Griffith, J.M., Miller, C., Myles-Worley, M., Nagamoto, H.T., Rollins, Y., Stevens, K.E., Waldo, M., and Freedman, R. (1996) Nicotinic receptor function in schizophrenia. *Schizophr. Bull.* 22:431–445.

Leonard, S., Breese, C., Adams, C., Benhammou, K., Gault, J., Stevens, K., Lee, M., Adler, L., Onlincy, A., Ross, R., and Freedman, R. (2000) Smoking and schizophrenia: abnormal nicotinic receptor expression. *Eur. J. Pharm.* 393:237–242.

Leonard, S., Gault, J., Moore, T., Hopkins, J., Robinson, M., Olincy, A., Adler, L.E., Cloninger, C.R., Kaufmann, C.A., Tsuang, M.T., Faraone, S.V., Malaspina, D., Svrakic, D.M., and Freedman, R. (1998) Further investigation of a chromosome 15 locus in schizophrenia: analysis of affected sibpairs from the NIMH Genetics Initiative. *Am. J. Med. Genet.* 81:308–312.

Levitt, J.B., Lewis, D.A., Yoshioka, T., and Lund, J.S. (1993) Topography of pyramidal neuron intrinsic connections in macaque monkey prefrontal cortex (areas 9 & 46). *J. Comp. Neurol.* 338:360–376.

Lewis, C.M., Levinson, D.F., Wise, L.H., DeLisi, L.E., Straub, R.E., Hovatta, I., Williams, N.M., Schwab, S.G., Pulver, A.E., Faraone, S.V., Brzustowicz, L.M., Kaufmann, C.A., Garver, D.L., Gurling, H.M., Lindholm, E., Coon, H., Moises, H.W., Byerley, W., Shaw, S.H., Mesen, A., Sherrington, R., O'Neill, F.A., Walsh, D., Kendler, K.S., Ekelund, J., Paunio, T., Lonnqvist, J., Peltonen, L., O'Donovan, M.C., Owen, M.J., Wildenauer, D.B., Maier, W., Nestadt, G., Blouin, J.L., Antonarakis, S.E., Mowry, B.J., Silverman, J.M., Crowe, R.R., Cloninger, C.R., Tsuang, M.T., Malaspina, D., Harkavy-Friedman, J.M., Svrakic, D.M., Bassett, A.S., Holcomb, J., Kalsi, G., McQuillin, A., Brynjolfson, J., Sigmundsson, T., Petursson, H., Jazin, E., Zoega, T., and Helgason, T. (2003) Genome scan meta-analysis of schizophrenia and bipolar disorder, part II: Schizophrenia. *Am. J. Hum. Genet.* 73:34–48.

Lewis, D.A., Hashimoto, T., and Volk, D.W. (2005) Cortical inhibitory neurons and schizophrenia. *Nat. Rev. Neurosci.* 6:312–324.

Lewis, D.A., and Levitt, P. (2002) Schizophrenia as a disorder of neurodevelopment. *Ann. Rev. Neurosci.* 25:409–432.

Lewis, D.A., and Lieberman, J.A. (2000) Catching up on schizophrenia: natural history and neurobiology. *Neuron* 28:325–334.

Li, B., Woo, R.S., Mei, L., and Malinow, R. (2007) The neuregulin-1 receptor erbB4 controls glutamatergic synapse maturation and plasticity. *Neuron* 54:583–597.

Lim, K.O., Tew, W., Kushner, M., Chow, K., Matsumoto, B., and DeLisi, L.E. (1996) Cortical gray matter volume deficit in patients with first-episode schizophrenia. *Am. J. Psychiatry* 153:1548–1553.

Lipska, B.K., Peters, T., Hyde, T.M., Halim, N., Horowitz, C., Mitkus, S., Weickert, C.S., Matsumoto, M., Sawa, A., Straub, R.E., Vakkalanka, R., Herman, M.M., Weinberger, D.R., and Kleinman, J.E. (2006) Expression of DISC1 binding partners is reduced in schizophrenia and associated with DISC1 SNPs. *Hum. Mol. Genet.* 15:1245–1258.

Liu, Y.L., Fann, C.S., Liu, C.M., Chen, W.J., Wu, J.Y., Hung, S.I., Chen, C.H., Jou, Y.S., Liu, S.K., Hwang, T.J., Hsieh, M.H., Ouyang, W.C., Chan, H.Y., Chen, J.J., Yang, W.C., Lin, C.Y., Lee, S. F., and Hwu, H.G. (2006) A single nucleotide polymorphism fine mapping study of chromosome 1q42.1 reveals the vulnerability genes for schizophrenia, GNPAT and DISC1: association with impairment of sustained attention. *Biol. Psychiatry* 60:554–562.

Lund, J.S., Lund, R.D., Hendrickson, A.E., Bunt, A.H., and Fuchs, A.F. (1975) The origin of efferent pathways from the primary visual cortex, area 17, of the macaque monkey as shown by retrograde transport of horseradish peroxidase. *J. Comp. Neurol.* 164:287–304.

Lundorf, M.D., Buttenschon, H.N., Foldager, L., Blackwood, D.H., Muir, W.J., Murray, V., Pelosi, A.J., Kruse, T.A., Ewald, H., and Mors, O. (2005) Mutational screening and association study of glutamate decarboxylase 1 as a candidate susceptibility gene for bipolar affective disorder and schizophrenia. *Am. J. Med. Genet. B Neuropsychiatr. Genet.* 135:94–101.

Maldonado-Aviles, J.G., Wu, Q., Sampson, A.R., and Lewis, D.A. (2006) Somal size of immunolabeled pyramidal cells in the prefrontal cortex of subjects with schizophrenia. *Biol. Psychiatry* 60:226–234.

Manoach, D.S., Press, D.Z., Thangaraj, V., Searl, M.M., Goff, D.C., Halpern, E., Saper, C.B., and Warach, S. (1999) Schizophrenic subjects activate dorsolateral prefrontal cortex during a working memory task, as measured by fMRI. *Biol. Psychiatry* 45:1128–1137.

Markram, H., Toledo-Rodriguez, M., Wang, Y., Gupta, A., Silberberg, G., and Wu, C. (2004) Interneurons of the neocortical inhibitory system. *Nat. Rev. Neurosci.* 5:793–807.

McCarley, R.W., Wible, C.G., Frumin, M., Hirayasu, Y., Levitt, J.J., Fischer, I.A., and Shenton, M.E. (1999) MRI anatomy of schizophrenia. *Biol. Psychiatry* 45:1099–1119.

Melchitzky, D.S., González-Burgos, G., Barrionuevo, G., and Lewis, D.A. (2001) Synaptic targets of the intrinsic axon collaterals of supragranular pyramidal neurons in monkey prefrontal cortex. *J. Comp. Neurol.* 430:209–221.

Melchitzky, D.S., and Lewis, D.A. (2003) Pyramidal neuron local axon terminals in monkey prefrontal cortex: differential targeting of subclasses of GABA neurons. *Cereb. Cortex* 13:452–460.

Melchitzky, D.S., Sesack, S.R., and Lewis, D.A. (1999) Parvalbumin-immunoreactive axon terminals in macaque monkey and human prefrontal cortex: laminar, regional and target specificity of Type I and Type II synapses. *J. Comp. Neurol.* 408:11–22.

Melchitzky, D.S., Sesack, S.R., Pucak, M.L., and Lewis, D.A. (1998) Synaptic targets of pyramidal neurons providing intrinsic horizontal connections in monkey prefrontal cortex. *J. Comp. Neurol.* 390:211–224.

Millar, J.K., Wilson-Annan, J.C., Anderson, S., Christie, S., Taylor, M.S., Semple, C.A., Devon, R.S., Clair, D.M., Muir, W.J., Blackwood, D.H., and Porteous, D.J. (2000) Disruption of two novel genes by a translocation co-segregating with schizophrenia. *Hum. Mol. Genet.* 9:1415–1423.

Mirnics, K., Middleton, F.A., Lewis, D.A., and Levitt, P. (2001) Analysis of complex brain disorders with gene expression microarrays: schizophrenia as a disease of the synapse. *Trends Neurosci.* 24:479–486.

Mutsuddi, M., Morris, D.W., Waggoner, S.G., Daly, M.J., Scolnick, E.M., and Sklar, P. (2006) Analysis of high-resolution HapMap of DTNBP1 (Dysbindin) suggests no consistency between reported common variant associations and schizophrenia. *Am. J. Hum. Genet.* 79:903–909.

Neves-Pereira, M., Bassett, A.S., Honer, W.G., Lang, D., King, N.A., and Kennedy, J.L. (1998) No evidence for linkage of the CHRNA7 gene region in Canadian schizophrenia families. *Am. J. Med. Genet. (Neuropsych. Genet.)* 81:361–363.

Numakawa, T., Yagasaki, Y., Ishimoto, T., Okada, T., Suzuki, T., Iwata, N., Ozaki, N., Taguchi, T., Tatsumi, M., Kamijima, K., Straub, R.E., Weinberger, D.R., Kunugi, H., and Hashimoto, R. (2004) Evidence of novel neuronal functions of dysbindin, a susceptibility gene for schizophrenia. *Hum. Mol. Genet.* 13:2699–2708.

Olincy, A., Harris, J.G., Johnson, L.L., Pender, V., Kongs, S., Allensworth, D., Ellis, J., Zerbe, G.O., Leonard, S., Stevens, K.E., Stevens, J.O., Martin, L., Adler, L.E., Soti, F., Kem, W.R., and Freedman, R. (2006) Proof-of-concept trial of an alpha7 nicotinic agonist in schizophrenia. *Arch. Gen. Psychiatry* 63:630–638.

Olincy, A., Young, D.A., and Freedman, R. (1997) Increased levels of the nicotine metabolite cotinine in schizophrenic smokers compared to other smokers. *Biol. Psychiatry* 42:1–5.

Orlovskaya, D.D., Vikhreva, O.V., Zimina, I.S., Denisov, D.V., and Uranova, N.A. (2000) Ultrastructural dystrophic changes of oligodendroglial density cells in the prefrontal cortex area 9 in schizophrenic and mood disorders: a study of brain collection from the Stanley Foundation Neuropathology Consortium. *Schizophr. Res.* 41:105–106.

Pakkenberg, B. (1990) Pronounced reduction of total neuron number in mediodorsal thalamic nucleus and nucleus accumbens in schizophrenics. *Arch. Gen. Psychiatry* 47:1023–1028.

Pakkenberg, B. (1993) Total nerve cell number in neocortex in chronic schizophrenics and controls estimated using optical disectors. *Biol. Psychiatry* 34:768–772.

Peirce, T.R., Bray, N.J., Williams, N.M., Norton, N., Moskvina, V., Preece, A., Haroutunian, V., Buxbaum, J.D., Owen, M.J., and O'Donovan, M.C. (2006) Convergent evidence for 2',3'-cyclic nucleotide 3'-phosphodiesterase as a possible susceptibility gene for schizophrenia. *Arch. Gen. Psychiatry* 63:18–24.

Pierri, J.N., Chaudry, A.S., Woo, T.-U., and Lewis, D.A. (1999) Alterations in chandelier neuron axon terminals in the prefrontal cortex of schizophrenic subjects. *Am. J. Psychiatry* 156:1709–1719.

Pierri, J.N., Volk, C.L.E., Auh, S., Sampson, A., and Lewis, D.A. (2001) Decreased somal size of deep layer 3 pyramidal neurons in the prefrontal cortex of subjects with schizophrenia. *Arch. Gen. Psychiatry* 58:466–473.

Pierri, J.N., Volk, C.L., Auh, S., Sampson, A., and Lewis, D.A. (2003) Somal size of prefrontal cortical pyramidal neurons in schizophrenia: differential effects across neuronal subpopulations. *Biol. Psychiatry* 54:111–120.

Popken, G.J., Bunney, W.E., Jr., Potkin, S.G., and Jones, E.G. (2000) Subnucleus-specific loss of neurons in medial thalamus of schizophrenics. *Proc. Natl. Acad. Sci. USA* 97:9276–9280.

Pucak, M.L., Levitt, J.B., Lund, J.S., and Lewis, D.A. (1996) Patterns of intrinsic and associational circuitry in monkey prefrontal cortex. *J. Comp. Neurol.* 376:614–630.

Rajkowska, G., Miguel-Hidalgo, J.J., Wei, J., Dilley, G., Pittman, S.D., Meltzer, H.Y., et al. (1999) Morphometric evidence for neuronal and glial prefrontal cell pathology in major depression. *Biol. Psychiatry* 45:1085–1098.

Rajkowska, G., Selemon, L.D., and Goldman-Rakic, P.S. (1998) Neuronal and glial somal size in the prefrontal cortex: a postmortem morphometric study of schizophrenia and Huntington disease. *Arch. Gen. Psychiatry* 55:215–224.

Riley, B.P., Makoff, A., Mogudi-Carter, M., Jenkins, T., Williamson, R., Collier, D., and Murray, R. (2000) Haplotype transmission disequillibrium and evidence for linkage of the CHRNA7 gene region to schizophrenia in Southern African Bantu families. *Am. J. Med. Genet. (Neuropsych. Genet.)* 96:196–201.

Risch, N., and Baron, M. (1984) Segregation analysis of schizophrenia and related disorders. *Am. J. Hum. Genet.* 36:1039–1059.

Risch, N.J. (2000) Searching for genetics determinants in the new millenium. *Nature* 405:847–856.

Ross, C.A., Margolis, R.L., Reading, S.A., Pletnikov, M., and Coyle, J.T. (2006) Neurobiology of schizophrenia. *Neuron* 52:139–153.

Sawaguchi, T., and Goldman-Rakic, P.S. (1991) D1 dopamine receptors in prefrontal cortex: involvement in working memory. *Science* 251:947–950.

Sawaguchi, T., Matsumura, M., and Kubota, K. (1989) Delayed response deficits produced by local injection of bicuculline into the dorsolateral prefrontal cortex in Japanese macaque monkeys. *Exp. Brain Res.* 75:457–469.

Sawamura, N., Sawamura-Yamamoto, T., Ozeki, Y., Ross, C.A., and Sawa, A. (2005) A form of DISC1 enriched in nucleus: altered subcellular distribution in orbitofrontal cortex in psychosis and substance/alcohol abuse. *Proc. Natl. Acad. Sci. USA* 102:1187–1192.

Scherzer, C.R., Landwehrmeyer, G.B., Kerner, J.A., Counihan, T.J., Kosinski, C.M., Standaert, D.G., Daggett, L.P., Velicelebi, G., Penney, J.B., and Young, A.B. (1998) Expression of *N*-methyl-D-aspartate receptor subunit mRNAs in the human brain: hippocampus and cortex. *J. Comp. Neurol.* 390:75–90.

Schwab, S.G., Knapp, M., Mondabon, S., Hallmayer, J., Borrmann-Hassenbach, M., Albus, M., Lerer, B., Rietschel, M., Trixler, M., Maier, W., and Wildenauer, D.B. (2003) Support for association of schizophrenia with genetic variation in the 6p22.3 gene, dysbindin, in sib-pair families with linkage and in an additional sample of triad families. *Am. J. Hum. Genet.* 72:185–190.

Seeman, P. (2006) Targeting the dopamine D2 receptor in schizophrenia. *Expert. Opin. Ther. Targets* 10:515–531.

Selemon, L.D., Rajkowska, G., and Goldman-Rakic, P.S. (1995) Abnormally high neuronal density in the schizophrenic cortex: a morphometric analysis of prefrontal area 9 and occipital area 17. *Arch. Gen. Psychiatry* 52:805–818.

Selemon, L.D., Rajkowska, G., and Goldman-Rakic, P.S. (1998) Elevated neuronal density in prefrontal area 46 in brains from schizophrenic patients: application of a three-dimensional, stereologic counting method. *J. Comp. Neurol.* 392:402–412.

Shenton, M.E., Dickey, C.C., Frumin, M., and McCarley, R.W. (2001) A review of MRI findings in schizophrenia. *Schizophr. Res.* 49:1–52.

Sherman, A.D., Davidson, A.T., Baruah, S., Hegwood, T.S., and Waziri, R. (1991) Evidence of glutamatergic deficiency in schizophrenia. *Neurosci. Lett.* 121:77–80.

Simpson, M.D.C., Slater, P., Deakin, J.F.W., Royston, M.C., and Skan, W.J. (1989) Reduced GABA uptake sites in the temporal lobe in schizophrenia. *Neurosci. Lett.* 107:211–215.

Soloway, A.S., Pucak, M.L., Melchitzky, D.S., and Lewis, D.A. (2002) Dendritic morphology of callosal and ipsilateral projection neurons in monkey prefrontal cortex. *Neuroscience* 109:461–471.

Somogyi, P. (1977) A specific axo-axonal interneuron in the visual cortex of the rat. *Brain Res.* 136:345–350.

St. Clair, D., Blackwood, D., Muir, W., Carothers, A., Walker, M., Spowart, G., Gosden, C., and Evans, H.J. (1990) Association within a family of a balanced autosomal translocation with major mental illness. *Lancet* 336:13–16.

Steen, R.G., Hamer, R.M., and Lieberman, J.A. (2005) Measurement of brain metabolites by 1H magnetic resonance spectroscopy in patients with schizophrenia: a systematic review and meta-analysis. *Neuropsychopharmacology* 30:1949–1962.

Stefansson, H., Sigurdsson, E., Steinthorsdottir, V., Bjornsdottir, S., Sigmundsson, T., Ghosh, S., Brynjolfsson, J., Gunnarsdottir, S., Ivarsson, O., Chou, T.T., Hjaltason, O., Birgisdottir, B., Jonsson, H., Gudnadottir, V.G., Gudmundsdottir, E., Bjornsson, A., Ingvarsson, B., Ingason, A., Sigfusson, S., Hardardottir, H., Harvey, R. P., Lai, D., Zhou, M., Brunner, D., Mutel, V., Gonzalo, A., Lemke, G., Sainz, J., Johannesson, G., Andresson, T., Gudbjartsson, D., Manolescu, A., Frigge, M.L., Gurney, M.E., Kong, A., Gulcher, J.R., Petursson, H., and Stefansson, K. (2002) *Neuregulin 1* and susceptibility to schizophrenia. *Am. J. Hum. Genet.* 71:877–892.

Straub, R.E., Jiang, Y., MacLean, C.J., Ma, Y., Webb, B.T., Myakishev, M.V., Harris-Kerr, C., Wormley, B., Sadek, H., Kadambi, B., Cesare, A.J., Gibberman, A., Wang, X., O'Neill, F.A., Walsh, D., and Kendler, K.S. (2002) Genetic variation in the 6p22.3 gene DTNBP1, the human ortholog of the mouse dysbindin gene, is associated with schizophrenia. *Am. J. Hum. Genet.* 71:337–348.

Straub, R.E., Lipska, B.K., Egan, M.F., Goldberg, T.E., Callicot, J.H., Mayhew, M.B., Vakkalanka, R.K., Kolachana, B.S., Kleinman, J.E., and Weinberger, D.R. (2007) Allelic variation in GAD1 (GAD67) is associated with schizophrenia and influences cortical function and gene expression. *Mol. Psychiatry* 12:854–869.

Sugino, K., Hempel, C.M., Miller, M.N., Hattox, A.M., Shapiro, P., Wu, C., Huang, Z.J., and Nelson, S.B. (2006) Molecular taxonomy of major neuronal classes in the adult mouse forebrain. *Nat. Neurosci.* 9:99–107.

Sweet, R.A., Bergen, S.E., Sun, Z., Sampson, A.R., Pierri, J.N., and Lewis, D.A. (2004) Pyramidal cell size reduction in schizophrenia: evidence for involvement of auditory feedforward circuits. *Biol. Psychiatry* 55:1128–1137.

Sweet, R.A., Pierri, J.N., Auh, S., Sampson, A.R., and Lewis, D.A. (2003) Reduced pyramidal cell somal volume in auditory association cortex of subjects with schizophrenia. *Neuropsychopharmacology* 28:599–609.

Szeszko, P.R., Ardekani, B.A., Ashtari, M., Kumra, S., Robinson, D.G., Sevy, S., Gunduz-Bruce, H., Malhotra, A.K., Kane, J.M., Bilder, R.M., and Lim, K.O. (2005) White matter abnormalities in first-episode schizophrenia or schizoaffective disorder: a diffusion tensor imaging study. *Am. J. Psychiatry* 162:602–605.

Talbot, K., Cho, D.S., Ong, W.Y., Benson, M.A., Han, L.Y., Kazi, H.A., Kamins, J., Hahn, C.G., Blake, D.J., and Arnold, S.E. (2006) Dysbindin-1 is a synaptic and microtubular protein that binds brain snapin. *Hum. Mol. Genet.* 15:3041–3054.

Talbot, K., Eidem, W.L., Tinsley, C.L., Benson, M.A., Thompson, E. W., Smith, R.J., Hahn, C.G., Siegel, S.J., Trojanowski, J.Q., Gur, R.E., Blake, D.J., and Arnold, S.E. (2004) Dysbindin-1 is reduced in intrinsic, glutamatergic terminals of the hippocampal formation in schizophrenia. *J. Clin. Invest.* 113:1353–1363.

Tallon-Baudry, C., Bertrand, O., Peronnet, F., and Pernier, J. (1998) Induced gamma-band activity during the delay of a visual short-term memory task in humans. *J. Neurosci.* 18:4244–4254.

Tang, J., Chen, X., Xu, X., Wu, R., Zhao, J., Hu, Z., and Xia, K. (2006) Significant linkage and association between a functional (GT)n polymorphism in promoter of the *N*-methyl-D-aspartate receptor subunit gene (GRIN2A) and schizophrenia. *Neurosci. Lett.* 409:80–82.

Tkachev, D., Mimmack, M.L., Ryan, M.M., Wayland, M., Freeman, T., Jones, P.B., Starkey, M., Webster, M.J., Yolken, R.H., and Bahn, S. (2003) Oligodendrocyte dysfunction in schizophrenia and bipolar disorder. *Lancet* 362:798–805.

Tunbridge, E.M., Bannerman, D.M., Sharp, T., and Harrison, P.J. (2004) Catechol-*O*-methyltransferase inhibition improves set-shifting performance and elevates stimulated dopamine release in the rat prefrontal cortex. *J. Neurosci.* 24:5331–5335.

Tunbridge, E.M., Weinberger, D.R., and Harrison, P.J. (2006) A novel protein isoform of catechol-O-methyltransferase (COMT): brain expression analysis in schizophrenia and bipolar disorder and effect of Val158Met genotype. *Mol. Psychiatry* 11:116–117.

Uranova, N.A., Vostrikov, V.M., Orlovskaya, D.D., and Rachmanova, V.I. (2004) Oligodendroglial density in the prefrontal cortex in schizophrenia and mood disorders: a study from the Stanley Neuropathology Consortium. *Schizophr. Res.* 67:269–275.

van den Oord, E.J., Sullivan, P.F., Jiang, Y., Walsh, D., O'Neill, F.A., Kendler, K.S., and Riley, B.P. (2003) Identification of a high-risk haplotype for the dystrobrevin binding protein 1 (DTNBP1) gene in the Irish study of high-density schizophrenia families. *Mol. Psychiatry* 8:499–510.

Verma, A., and Moghaddam, B. (1996) NMDA receptor antagonists impair prefrontal cortex function as assessed via spatial delayed alternation performance in rats: modulation by dopamine. *J. Neurosci.* 16:373–379.

Volk, D.W., Austin, M.C., Pierri, J.N., Sampson, A.R., and Lewis, D.A. (2000) Decreased glutamic acid decarboxylase67 messenger RNA expression in a subset of prefrontal cortical gamma-aminobutyric acid neurons in subjects with schizophrenia. *Arch. Gen. Psychiatry* 57:237–245.

Volk, D.W., Austin, M.C., Pierri, J.N., Sampson, A.R., and Lewis, D.A. (2001) GABA transporter-1 mRNA in the prefrontal cortex in schizophrenia: decreased expression in a subset of neurons. *Am. J. Psychiatry* 158:256–265.

Volk, D.W., Pierri, J.N., Fritschy, J.-M., Auh, S., Sampson, A.R., and Lewis, D.A. (2002) Reciprocal alterations in pre- and post-synaptic inhibitory markers at chandelier cell inputs to pyramidal neurons in schizophrenia. *Cereb. Cortex* 12:1063–1070.

Walterfang, M., Wood, S.J., Velakoulis, D., and Pantelis, C. (2006) Neuropathological, neurogenetic and neuroimaging evidence for white matter pathology in schizophrenia. *Neurosci. Biobehav. Rev.* 30:918–948.

Wan, C., Yang, Y., Feng, G., Gu, N., Liu, H., Zhu, S., He, L., and Wang, L. (2005) Polymorphisms of myelin-associated glycoprotein gene are associated with schizophrenia in the Chinese Han population. *Neurosci. Lett.* 388:126–131.

Ward, K.E., Friedman, L., Wise, A., and Schulz, S.C. (1996) Meta-analysis of brain and cranial size in schizophrenia. *Schizophr. Res.* 22:197–213.

Weickert, C.S., Straub, R.E., McClintock, B.W., Matsumoto, M., Hashimoto, R., Hyde, T.M., Herman, M.M., Weinberger, D.R., and Kleinman, J.E. (2004) Human dysbindin (DTNBP1) gene expression in normal brain and in schizophrenic prefrontal cortex and midbrain. *Arch. Gen. Psychiatry* 61:544–555.

Weinberger, D.R., Berman, K.F., and Zec, R.F. (1986) Physiologic dysfunction of dorsolateral prefrontal cortex in schizophrenia. I. Regional cerebral blood flow evidence. *Arch. Gen. Psychiatry* 43:114–124.

Williams, N.M., Preece, A., Morris, D.W., Spurlock, G., Bray, N.J., Stephens, M., Norton, N., Williams, H., Clement, M., Dwyer, S., Curran, C., Wilkinson, J., Moskvina, V., Waddington, J.L., Gill, M., Corvin, A.P., Zammit, S., Kirov, G., Owen, M.J., and O'Donovan, M.C. (2004) Identification in 2 independent samples of a novel schizophrenia risk haplotype of the dystrobrevin binding protein gene (DTNBP1). *Arch. Gen. Psychiatry* 61:336–344.

Woo, T.-U., Miller, J.L., and Lewis, D.A. (1997) Schizophrenia and the parvalbumin-containing class of cortical local circuit neurons. *Am. J. Psychiatry* 154:1013–1015.

Woo, T.-U., Whitehead, R.E., Melchitzky, D.S., and Lewis, D.A. (1998) A subclass of prefrontal gamma-aminobutyric acid axon terminals are selectively altered in schizophrenia. *Proc. Natl. Acad. Sci. USA* 95:5341–5346.

Young, K.A., Holcomb, L.A., Yazdani, U., Hicks, P.B., and German, D.C. (2004) Elevated neuron number in the limbic thalamus in major depression. *Am. J. Psychiatry* 161:1270–1277.

Young, K.A., Manaye, K.F., Liang, C.-L., Hicks, P.B., and German, D.C. (2000) Reduced number of mediodorsal and anterior thalamic neurons in schizophrenia. *Biol. Psychiatry* 47:944–953.

Zhao, X., Li, H., Shi, Y., Tang, R., Chen, W., Liu, J., Feng, G., Shi, J., Yan, L., Liu, H., and He, L. (2006) Significant association between the genetic variations in the 5' end of the *N*-methyl-D-aspartate receptor subunit gene GRIN1 and schizophrenia. *Biol. Psychiatry* 59:747–753.

Zhao, X., Qin, S., Shi, Y., Zhang, A., Zhang, J., Bian, L., Wan, C., Feng, G., Gu, N., Zhang, G., He, G., and He, L. (2007) Systematic study of association of four GABAergic genes: glutamic acid decarboxylase 1 gene, glutamic acid decarboxylase 2 gene, GABA(B) receptor 1 gene and GABA(A) receptor subunit beta2 gene, with schizophrenia using a universal DNA microarray. *Schizophr. Res.* 93:374–384.

Zuo, Y., Lin, A., Chang, P., and Gan, W.B. (2005) Development of long-term dendritic spine stability in diverse regions of cerebral cortex. *Neuron* 46:181–189.

21 Postmortem and In Vivo Structural Pathology in Schizophrenia

ANDREW J. DWORK, JOHN F. SMILEY, TIZIANO COLIBAZZI, AND MATTHEW J. HOPTMAN

The usual purpose of a neuropathological or radiological examination is to make a diagnosis. We begin by acknowledging that our current knowledge of schizophrenia does not allow this, although anatomical examinations may be useful to exclude rare conditions that can bear a clinical resemblance to schizophrenia. The studies described in this chapter, and hundreds of others that could not be included for want of space, were conducted to obtain measurements that might provide some insight into the cause or pathophysiology of schizophrenia. Even when differences were found between schizophrenia and nonpsychiatric groups, the range of values in the groups usually overlapped. Furthermore, when studies include other psychiatric diagnoses, these often yield similar group differences (for a summary of many such studies, see Torrey et al., 2005), so in the absence of a psychiatric comparison group, one cannot assume that an effect is specific for schizophrenia. Psychiatric comparison groups also allow some degree of control for the effects of antipsychotic and other medications. Additionally, one can control for antipsychotic effects by covarying for lifetime or current dosage or including subjects who never received these medications. Experimental animals are also useful for identifying medication effects. None of these methods is definitive. Most of the authors cited herein have considered and discussed this confound.

We attempted to organize this chapter into sections that separately consider imaging and autopsy studies of related phenomena, but a one-to-one correspondence is not always feasible. We focus on topics that are influencing current thought about biology and schizophrenia. More detailed and inclusive discussions are available in review articles (Heckers et al., 1991; Dwork, 1997; Harrison, 1999; Heckers, 2001; Shenton et al., 2001; Harrison and Weinberger, 2005; Walterfang et al., 2006; Dwork et al., 2007).

METHODOLOGICAL CONSIDERATIONS

Postmortem

Histological measurements commonly include estimates of tissue volume, cell density, and total cell number. *Cell density* is the number of cells (usually neurons) per unit volume. *Total cell number*, equal to cell density multiplied by volume, is the number of such cells in an entire anatomic structure. Volume of a neuroanatomic structure is usually estimated by measuring its cross-sectional area in several parallel planes and multiplying the sum of areas by the distance between the planes. For meaningful measurements of volume, it is essential that the cross sections include the entire length of the structure of interest. As long as measurements are made through the entire structure, orientation will not affect the volume measurement.

Estimates of neuronal density depend upon counting all neurons with equal probability, regardless of size or shape. This is best achieved with three-dimensional counting methods, such as the optical disector (Gundersen, 1986). Two-dimensional density measurements can be adjusted for cell size with the Abercrombie correction factor, but there are inherent uncertainties in the precision of this method (Williams and Rakic, 1988). Estimates of tissue volume and cell density are affected by artefactual shrinkage or swelling of tissue during fixation or processing. However, because these effects are inversely proportional, total cell number is not affected. Unbiased estimates of cell size require that the tissue be sectioned in a suitably random plane, which appears not to have been done in any of the studies that we have reviewed; hence, comparisons of neuronal size may be influenced by neuronal orientation.

In Vivo

The most common method to examine differences in brain morphometry in vivo is the use of T1-weighted magnetic resonance images. Most morphometric studies have depended on manual measurements of regions of interest (ROI). These studies provide measures of the volume of specific brain areas and have the advantage that the boundaries used are typically guided by relevant neuroanatomical parameters. The reliability of such measures tends to be high.

Voxel-based morphometry (VBM) (Ashburner and Friston, 2000) is a newer analytic method in which anatomical scan data are coregistered into a standard space, so that comparisons can be made at homologous locations across images. Prior to analysis, the images typically are segmented into grey matter, white matter, and cerebrospinal fluid components and spatially transformed to fit a standard brain template. The findings from these studies are generally interpreted as differences in tissue density, which is roughly analogous to the number of voxels of grey or white matter in the transformed image that correspond to a voxel of grey or white matter, respectively, in the template. The advantage of VBM is the ease with which it can be carried out, as well as its ability to interrogate the entire brain at once, meaning that novel findings can be more easily detected. However, the quality of intersubject image registration can significantly influence results (Bookstein, 2001), and VBM is more sensitive to localized changes than to diffuse differences (Davatzikos, 2004). Another shortcoming is that the large number of statistical tests inherent in the comparisons have necessitated the development of novel techniques to avoid type I error.

NEURONAL DENSITY AND CORTICAL THICKNESS

Postmortem

Two articles by Selemon et al. (1995, 1998) reported significantly greater numerical density of neurons in prefrontal (BA9 and BA46) and primary visual (BA17) cortex, by 17%, 21%, and 10%, respectively, and nonsignificantly thinner cortical ribbons in these regions (by ~10%), in subjects with schizophrenia compared with nonpsychiatric subjects. These studies are currently among the most influential postmortem studies of schizophrenia, giving rise to the hypothesis that a reduction in cortical neuropil, without loss of neurons, is a critical anatomical substrate of schizophrenia. The magnitude of these changes was similar to that observed by Pakkenberg (1993), who found that total neuron number was not changed, but neuronal density was increased by 13% in the frontal lobe, 38% in temporal lobe, 6% in parietal lobe, and 14% in occipital lobe, although only the temporal difference was statistically significant. Selemon et al. (2003) subsequently replicated their results for BA9, finding a 12% greater neuronal density, and found no difference in neuronal density in Broca's area (BA44). Diagnostic specificity was supported by similar studies showing lowered neuronal cell densities in major depression (Rajkowska et al., 1999) and bipolar disorder (BPD) (Rajkowska et al., 2001). Other investigators, however, have found prefrontal neuronal density to be lower (Benes et al., 1986) or unchanged (Akbarian et al., 1995; Cotter, Mackay, et al., 2002; Cullen et al., 2006) in schizophrenia. The negative study of Cullen et al. (2006) is of particular interest because it employed virtually identical three-dimensional counting methodology to the Selemon studies. Thune et al. (2001), using three-dimensional methods, found no significant differences between subjects with schizophrenia and nonpsychiatric subjects in volume, neuronal density, or total neuronal number in prefrontal cortex (PFC), although neuronal density was nominally 5% lower in schizophrenia. Immunohistochemical studies of BA9 found no change in density of neurons (mainly pyramidal) expressing various neurofilament epitopes (Law and Harrison, 2003; Miguel-Hidalgo et al., 2005). In primary visual cortex (BA17), a careful study using three-dimensional counting found, in contrast to Selemon et al. (1995), no difference in cell density, but lower volume and total neuronal number in schizophrenia (Dorph-Petersen et al., 2007).

In anterior cingulate (BA24b) and orbitofrontal cortex (OFC), Cotter et al. (2001) applied stereological methods and found no difference in neuron density in schizophrenia, BPD, or major depression. However, using two-dimensional counting methods in the same brains, they found evidence for increased neuron density in cingulate (BA24c) layers 5 and 6 (Chana et al., 2003). Other studies of cingulate cortex found no change or a slight reduction in neuron density (Benes et al., 1986; Benes, McSparren et al., 1991; Kalus et al., 1997). In the hippocampus, Zaidel, Esiri, Harrison, Zaidel, et al. (1997) found significantly greater densities of pyramidal neurons in hippocampal subfields CA1 and CA3 on the right side, by ~25%, but not on the left side. Benes, Sorensen, and Bird (1991) found a 36% decrease in density of CA1 pyramidal neurons in subjects with schizophrenia without superimposed mood disorders. Auditory cortex is discussed below.

Woo et al. (1997) reported cortical thickness (nonsignificantly) decreased by only 3.2% in BA9, 4.7% in BA46, and 5.9% in BA17, and Beasley, Zhang, et al. (2002) found a nonsignificant decrease of 6.5% in cortical thickness of BA9. Significant decreases of 5%–10% were found in cortical width of BA9 and anterior cingulate cortex in one study (Kreczmanski et al., 2005), whereas Radewicz et al. (2000) reported no difference in cortical thickness in BA9, anterior cingulate, or superior temporal gyrus.

In summary, results on neuronal density are inconsistent in every area studied. Most studies of cortical thickness show small, statistically insignificant differences, on the order of 5% (100–200 microns) thinner in schizophrenia, comparable to results obtained in vivo (see below).

In Vivo

Smaller frontal lobe volumes have been reported in chronic schizophrenia and in first-episode psychosis, but there have also been negative studies. In a comprehensive review of magnetic resonance imaging (MRI) reports published between 1988 and 2000, Shenton et al. (2001) concluded that findings in the frontal lobe were equivocal, possibly because of small effect sizes, and possibly because measurements of the whole frontal lobe obscured localized effects. Comparison of subjects with schizophrenia with their unaffected monozygotic twins found grey matter deficits specifically localized within dorsolateral prefrontal cortex (DLPFC) (Cannon et al., 2002).

Several studies have shown decreased cortical thickness and grey matter concentration, most evident in lateral prefrontal and in the right medial prefrontal cortices (Sanfilipo et al., 2002; Kuperberg et al., 2003; Farrow et al., 2005; Narr, Bilder, et al., 2005). An important question is whether these grey matter differences are progressive or stable over time. Hirayasu et al. (2001) reported smaller prefrontal grey matter volumes in first-episode schizophrenia relative to affective psychoses and normal controls. Rescanning the same subjects approximately 18 months later confirmed this finding, and there was no evidence of progression (Dickey et al., 2004). A longitudinal study in first-episode patients did not reveal any changes over time (typically 2–3 years) in hippocampal volume or total volume of neocortex plus white matter (Lieberman et al., 2001). Others have reported smaller grey matter volumes in the DLPFC of patients with chronic schizophrenia compared with first-episode patients (Premkumar et al., 2006) and progressive neocortical volume reduction in patients with first-episode schizophrenia followed over 1.5 years (Nakamura, Salisbury, et al., 2007). A longitudinal study of childhood-onset schizophrenia showed severe and progressive grey matter loss occurring early in adolescence within medial frontal regions (Vidal et al., 2006).

Smaller prefrontal cortical volumes in patients with stable schizophrenia have been associated with poorer insight (Sapara et al., 2007), impaired social cognition (Yamada et al., 2007), apathy (Roth et al., 2004), overall impaired cognitive performance (Antonova et al., 2004), and worse functional outcome (Prasad et al., 2005).

In the cingulate gyrus, initial reports on grey matter volume were divided, possibly because morphological variability of the cingulate gyrus rendered regional definitions inconsistent. By simultaneously assessing cingulate volume, surface area, and cortical thickness, Wang et al. (2007) showed cortical thinning along the entire contour of the cingulate gyrus. Morphological alterations and thinning of the anterior portion have also been reported in the absence of volumetric reductions (Fornito et al., 2007). These studies generally support prior findings of prominent bilateral reduction of anterior cingulate volumes (Yamasue et al., 2004), as well as of cortical thinning within the supragenual anterior and posterior cingulate cortices in first-episode patients (Narr, Toga, et al., 2005) and in childhood-onset schizophrenia (Vidal et al., 2006), where the difference from controls appeared later in cingulate cortex than in frontal cortex. Decreased grey matter density in the cingulate gyrus has been noted in high-risk populations (Job et al., 2003).

Cingulate morphological measurements have been correlated with poor performance on emotion attribution tasks in subjects with schizophrenia (Fujiwara et al., 2007; Yamada et al., 2007).

The few structural neuroimaging studies of the orbitofrontal region in schizophrenia have yielded inconsistent results. Szeszko et al. (1999) found that male first-episode patients who were treated with typical neuroleptic drugs had larger right orbitofrontal volumes than did healthy controls. On the other hand, Convit et al. (2001) found smaller orbitofrontal volumes in chronically ill male patients than in healthy controls. Lower orbitofrontal grey matter volumes or densities have been found in high-risk individuals who went on to develop schizophrenia (Pantelis et al., 2002), in subjects with schizophrenia but not in subjects with schizotypal disorder (Kawasaki et al., 2004), and in female but not male subjects with schizophrenia (Gur et al., 2000), but other studies are negative (Baare et al., 1999; Rupp et al., 2005). Nakamura, Nestor, et al. (2007) found that certain sulcal patterns were more or less common in schizophrenia, suggesting a developmental effect.

In a study of subjects who were poorly responsive to treatment, Hoptman et al. (2005) found that smaller OFC volumes were associated with better neuropsychological performance and lower levels of aggression. Similar associations were also found for the caudate nucleus (Hoptman, Volavka, et al., 2006). The authors suggested that their results might be due to ineffective long-term treatment with typical neuroleptics. On the other hand, smaller orbitofrontal volume has been associated with better response to olanzapine (Molina et al., 2004).

In summary, imaging studies generally report thinner dorsal prefrontal and anterior cingulate cortices in schizophrenia. These deficits correlate with function and may be progressive. Specificity for schizophrenia is not established.

HIPPOCAMPAL VOLUMES AND NEURONAL COUNTS

Postmortem

In 1997, we reviewed the autopsy studies of the hippocampal formation in schizophrenia and concluded that although many studies reported positive findings, the studies were mutually inconsistent, with a larger temporal horn of the lateral ventricle being the only consistent finding in this region (Dwork, 1997). Since then, only a handful of structural studies have appeared, all of them negative: Most significantly, a thorough, bilateral stereologic study of 30 subjects with schizophrenia and 29 nonpsychiatric subjects revealed no difference in volume, neuronal density, or total neuronal number in any hippocampal subfield (Walker et al., 2002). Amygdala volume bilaterally (Chance et al., 2002), fiber content of the fornix bilaterally (Chance et al., 1999), and densities and total numbers of parvalbumin neurons in the entorhinal cortex (Pantazopoulos et al., 2007) were also unaffected.

In Vivo

The original finding of smaller medial temporal volumes in schizophrenia (Bogerts et al., 1990) has been replicated, even in first-episode patients (Ohnuma et al., 1997). Negative findings have been reported in studies of first-episode (Laakso et al., 2001) and chronic patients (Kalus et al., 2004). In a meta-analysis of MRI studies on first-episode patients, Steen et al. (2006) found reduced hippocampal and whole brain volumes.

Earlier studies, which employed slice thicknesses of at least 3.1 mm, combined hippocampal and amygdala regions, despite the highly differentiated function of these structures. More recent studies, with greater resolution, generally indicate that it is the anterior hippocampal volumes that are reduced in subjects with schizophrenia (O'Driscoll et al., 2001; Szeszko et al., 2003), although this has not always been found (Weiss et al., 2005).

In first-episode subjects, lower anterior hippocampal volumes were more strongly associated with poor executive and motor function (Bilder et al., 1995) than with impairments of memory or language function (Szeszko et al., 2002).

In summary, the majority of imaging studies suggest lower hippocampal volumes in schizophrenia, probably present at first episode, more pronounced in the anterior hippocampus, and correlated with poorer performance on neuropsychological tasks sensitive to frontal lobe damage. The contrast between the imaging and autopsy studies is striking and without obvious explanation. Perhaps the process that causes in vivo volume loss is sensitive to changes that occur during death or tissue processing. Alternatively, some abnormal property of the tissue in schizophrenia, or the larger adjacent temporal horns, may be artefactually affecting the MRI signal to create the appearance of decreased hippocampal volume.

AUDITORY CORTEX IN SCHIZOPHRENIA

Although studies of schizophrenia historically focused on the frontal and temporolimbic areas, accumulating evidence has demonstrated changes across the entire cerebral cortex. Even in early stages of cortical sensory-information processing, evoked potential studies have demonstrated irregularities in visual and auditory modalities (Javitt et al., 2000; Butler et al., 2007).

Auditory cortex offers distinct advantages as a site for investigating neuropathology. Functionally distinct areas can be confidently identified, and pathology can be evaluated across cortical types including primary sensory and association areas. Additionally, auditory cortex has pronounced hemispheric asymmetry, and schizophrenia is characterized by altered functional and anatomical asymmetries. For example, in vivo imaging has repeatedly shown altered asymmetry of glucose metabolism and functional magnetic resonance imaging (fMRI) activation in the middle and superior temporal gyri (Gur and Chin, 1999). Crow (1997) argued that failure of language lateralization may be a key causative factor of schizophrenia.

Postmortem

Cytoarchitectonic studies of auditory areas in schizophrenia are still few in number compared to other areas of cortex. Sweet et al. (2004) reported a 10%–13% decrease in the volume of neurons, selected by their pyramidal shape, from layer 3 of primary auditory and association areas of auditory cortex. This change was comparable to reduced pyramidal cell size in prefrontal area 9 in the same brains (Pierri et al., 2001), suggesting that the pathological processes that affect pyramidal cell size are similar across areas of cortex. Two studies did not find altered size, sampling primary and secondary auditory cortex, but these sampled all neurons, without selecting by shape (Beasley et al., 2005; Smiley et al., 2005).

Konapaske et al. (2006) measured the density of synaptic cartridges immunoreactive for the γ-aminobutyric acid (GABA) transporter and found evidence that these were modestly reduced in auditory association cortex, similar to their reduction in prefrontal area 46. Cotter and coworkers (Cotter et al., 2004; Beasley et al., 2005) found neuron density unchanged in Heschl's gyrus (HG) and the adjacent planum temporale (PT), as it was in their studies of BA9 and BA24 in the same brains. Smiley et al. (2005), using stereological methods, also found neuron density in primary and secondary auditory areas to be unchanged from control levels in primary and secondary auditory areas.

Smiley et al. (2007), measuring auditory cortical thickness bilaterally, found evidence for reduced thickness in schizophrenia, especially in the supragranular layers. The reduction was approximately 3%–7% of the upper layers and reached statistical significance only in the left PT. Similar width measurements by Cotter and collaborators from mixed left and right hemispheres showed a nonsignificant 5% decrease in the supragranular layers (Beasley et al., 2005). Chance et al. (2004) measured cortical width in the walls and depths of Heschl's sulcus and did not find a significant difference in schizophrenia. Postmortem findings of reduced cortical thickness are consistent with MRI findings of thinner cortex, usually by about 9%, in several cortical areas including the superior temporal plane.

In summary, initial investigations of auditory areas have provided evidence that some changes found in other areas, such as decreased size of large neurons, cortical thinning, and changes in GABA-receptor synapses are also likely to be present even in early stages of auditory information processing. At present, most findings need to be considered with caution until they are further replicated.

In Vivo

Heschl's gyrus is the most prominent transverse gyrus on the ventral surface of the lateral sulcus and contains the primary auditory cortex on its caudal-medial part (Fig. 21.1). There is some variability in the morphology of HG, and the different methods used to identify its borders probably have contributed some inconsistency to the findings. Left>right asymmetry in the size of HG is a common but not universal finding (see below).

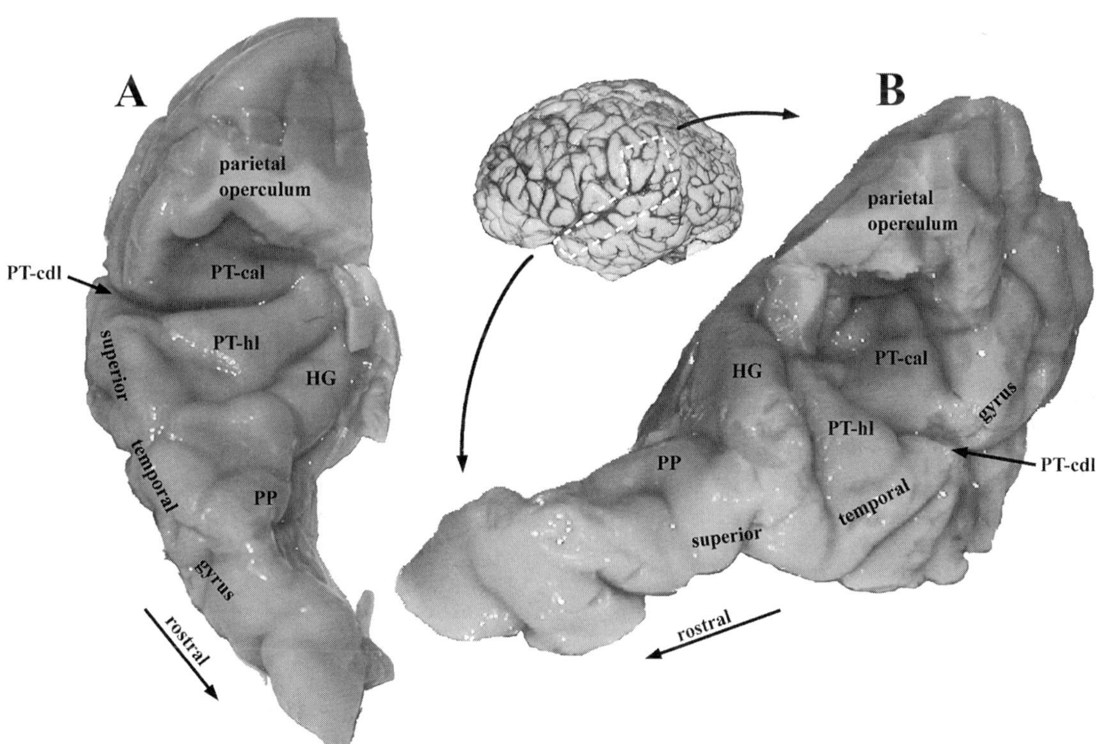

FIGURE 21.1 Dissections of the superior temporal planes from the right (*A*) and left (*B*) hemisphere of one subject illustrate the structure of this region. The viewer's perspective in *A* is from anterior and dorsal, and in *B* is from lateral. The inset shows the approximate source of the dissected tissue from the whole brain. Numerous structural studies have measured the superior temporal gyrus or its component parts. The dorsal surface of this gyrus is composed of Heschl's gyrus (HG), the planum temporale (PT) caudal to HG, and the planum polare (PP) rostral to HG. The PT is frequently parcellated into a horizontal limb (PT-hl), a caudal ascending limb (PT-cal), and, in cases where it is present, a caudal descending limb (PT-cdl). In practice, the precise borders of these structures can be ambiguous, due to the highly variable gyrification of this region, and different investigators have used different criteria to define them. In this example, the left HG (in *B*) is clearly separated from the PT by a sulcus that extends to the lateral surface of the superior temporal gyrus, but the right HG (in *A*) ends before reaching the lateral surface. The PT on the right (*A*) clearly splits into caudal ascending and descending limbs. In the left (*B*), the caudal descending limb is poorly developed, and the caudal ascending limb does not angle up sharply from the horizontal limb. On average, the caudal limb angles up more steeply on the right, but it is common to see a steep upward angle on the left.

A number of recent in vivo MRI studies of HG have reported reductions of grey matter volume in schizophrenia, although some earlier studies did not find this change. Among the studies that reported significant decrease, the difference was in the range of 6%–30%, with a mean difference of about 15% (Takahashi et al., 2006; Salisbury et al., 2007, and citations therein). It is striking that most of these studies also reported a left>right asymmetry of HG (nearly 20%). The extent of hemispheric asymmetry was similar or only modestly reduced in the subjects with schizophrenia compared with controls, although one study of subjects with schizotypal disorder found decreases only in the left hemisphere (Dickey et al., 2002). In contrast, those studies that did not find volume reductions in schizophrenia did not report hemispheric asymmetry even in the controls (Barta et al., 1997; Frangou et al., 1997; Kwon et al., 1999).

Most studies of HG volume in schizophrenia used mainly or exclusively male subjects. Takahashi et al. (2006) found similar volume reductions in male and female subjects with schizophrenia. In contrast, a study of subjects with paranoid schizophrenia found reduced volume of HG in males but not females (Rojas et al., 1997).

Correlations with behavioral changes and symptoms provide insights into the significance of HG volume changes. Sumich et al. (2002) reported a striking correlation of decreased volume with hallucinations and delusions in first-episode patients, and Kasai et al. (2003) found a correlation with suspicious thinking, but other studies did not find similar correlations (Kwon et al., 1999; Hirayasu et al., 2000; Crespo-Facorro et al., 2004). A link between HG and positive symptoms is also suggested by fMRI studies that found increased activation in the region of HG during auditory hallucinations (Dierks et al., 1999). Decreased HG volume also has been found to correlate with P300 and mismatch negativity electrophysiological deficits (Salisbury et al., 2007).

The planum temporale (PT) is the superior temporal plane lateral and caudal to HG (Fig. 21.1) and includes auditory association areas as well as multimodal association cortex. Findings of altered PT structure in schizophrenia have included reduced or reversed hemispheric asymmetry, or bilateral reductions in volume. These findings are not replicated by all laboratories, and the literature is complicated by the variety of definitions used to define the borders of the PT. A few studies found altered hemispheric asymmetry of the length of the lateral sulcus at its lateral surface, but this was not replicated in later studies (Shapleske et al., 2001). Most of the earlier structural MRI studies measured cortical surface area, typically measuring only the horizontal limb of the PT, before the dorsal upturn of the more caudal ascending limb. Although some groups found striking loss of asymmetry mainly due to a reduction of left PT, a number of subsequent studies did not find significant changes (reviewed in Shapleske et al., 1999).

More recent studies have measured cortical volume, and these can be divided into those that measured only the horizontal limb and those that measured the whole planum (horizontal plus vertical limbs). Falkai et al. (1995) used postmortem brains to measure the horizontal limb and found a loss of asymmetry due to a 20% reduction in volume in the left hemisphere. More recently, a structural MRI study of first-episode patients found bilateral reduction of the PT that reached significance only in the left hemisphere (Sumich et al., 2002). Several other studies that measured the horizontal limb did not find significant differences (Sallet et al., 2003; Crespo-Facorro et al., 2004, and included citations). Fewer studies have measured the volume of the combined horizontal and vertical limbs of the PT. A series of studies from McCarley's group (see Kasai et al., 2003) have consistently found a significant loss of asymmetry due to 20%–30% volume decreases only in the left hemisphere. Similar findings were obtained in both chronic and first-episode patients, and a follow-up study on the same subjects showed evidence that this volume reduction is progressive over the first 1.5 years after disease onset (Kasai et al., 2003). Recently, another research group measured the whole PT and also found about a 20% reduction in the left hemisphere, but the right hemisphere reduction was nearly as large (Takahashi et al., 2006). In contrast to these positive findings, Meisenzahl et al. (2002) did not find altered volumes or asymmetry in the whole PT. The reason for the discrepancy is not obvious, but it is notable that in the studies with positive findings the control groups have a striking asymmetry, and this was not found by Meisenzhal et al. (2002).

The superior temporal gyrus includes HG and the PT plus cortex extending laterally to the superior temporal sulcus. Shenton et al. (2001) reviewed MRI findings across brain regions and concluded that this region had the most consistently reported decreases in cortical volume, followed closely by the medial temporal lobe. Nearly all MRI studies found decreased volumes, usually in the range of about 10% compared with controls. The specificity of this finding to schizophrenia is supported by negative findings in subjects with BPD, and by similar reductions in unmedicated subjects with schizotypal disorder (Hirayasu et al., 1998; Dickey et al., 1999). Several studies (e.g., Onitsuka et al., 2004) found that the volume decrease was mainly or exclusively localized to the left hemisphere, but others (e.g., Gur et al., 2000; Sanfilipo et al., 2000) found comparable decrease in the left and right hemispheres. Several studies found that left hemisphere reductions were correlated with positive but not negative symptoms (Shenton et al., 2001; Onitsuka et al., 2004), but not all studies found this correlation (Gur et al., 2000; Sanfilipo et al., 2000).

In summary, MRI findings have rather consistently found reduced cortical volume in the auditory regions. Reductions of HG are consistent with deficits in early sensory processing. There are some findings that the changes are especially pronounced in the left hemisphere, and that left hemisphere changes are associated with positive symptoms.

SIZE OF PYRAMIDAL NEURONS

There are several reports of smaller neuronal cell bodies in schizophrenia, a finding that has been interpreted as supportive of the reduced neuropil hypothesis (Selemon et al., 1998). An important confound in such studies, recently elucidated, is that immunoperoxidase stains give apparently larger cell measurements than do Nissl stains because the diaminobenzidine reaction product is deposited beyond the confines of the cell membrane (Maldonado-Aviles et al., 2006). Furthermore, for reasons that are unclear, this effect was greater for schizophrenia cases than for nonpsychiatric cases. In light of this uncertainty with respect to immunoperoxidase results, the following considers only studies using Nissl stained cells.

Prefrontal studies are divided, with reports of 5%–6% reduction of neuron size in BA9 (Rajkowska et al., 1998), 14% smaller volumes of deep layer 3 pyramidal-shaped neurons in BA9 (Pierri et al., 2003), no change in BA9 in schizophrenia, but decreased neuronal size in major depression and BPD (Cotter, Mackay, et al., 2002), and absence of differences in the PFC (Benes et al., 1996; Benes et al., 2000).

In the anterior cingulate cortex, there are several negative studies (Benes et al., 1992, Benes et al., 2000; Cotter et al., 2001). In auditory association cortex (BA42), mean volume of pyramidal neurons in deep layer 3 was 13% lower in schizophrenia, and there was a significant correlation of somal volumes with those previously measured (Pierri et al., 2003) in BA9 (Sweet et al., 2003).

Positive findings in the hippocampal formation include smaller pyramidal neurons (typically 10%–15% smaller cross-sectional area) in all hippocampal sectors (Benes, Sorensen, and Bird, 1991), significantly in CA1, subiculum, and entorhinal cortex, but nonsignificantly elsewhere (Arnold et al., 1995), and only in left CA1, left CA2, and right CA3 (Zaidel, Esiri, and Harrison, 1997). Negative studies include two comprehensive surveys (Benes et al., 1998; Highley et al., 2003) and a study restricted to CA1 (Christison et al., 1989).

In summary, one can conclude that pyramidal neurons in the areas studied are probably not larger in schizophrenia, but it is not clear that they are smaller. In view of the inconsistencies of the results, it would be important to perform studies without the bias of a predetermined plane of section.

VOLUME AND NEURONAL NUMBER IN MEDIAL DORSAL THALAMUS

Postmortem

Several stereological studies have found smaller volume and fewer neurons in the medial dorsal nucleus of the thalamus in schizophrenia (Pakkenberg, 1992; Popken et al., 2000; Young et al., 2000; Byne et al., 2002). Until recently, this was one of the most consistently replicated histological findings in schizophrenia, leading to the postulate of reduced thalamic input to prefrontal and anterior cingulate cortices (e.g., Lewis et al., 2001). Recently, however, several stereological studies failed to replicate these results (Cullen et al., 2003; Dorph-Petersen et al., 2004; Kreczmanski et al., 2007).

In Vivo

Andreasen et al. (1990, 1994) first reported magnetic resonance abnormalities and lower signal intensity in the thalami of subjects with schizophrenia. Buchsbaum et al. (1996) confirmed this, although subsequent studies suggested only localized changes (Hazlett et al., 1999; Brickman et al., 2004) or none (Deicken et al., 2002). Smaller thalamic volumes have also been reported in high-risk individuals (Lawrie et al., 2001) and in relatives of individuals with schizophrenia (Seidman et al., 1997; Staal et al., 1998).

Byne and colleagues (2001; Kemether et al., 2003) examined the mediodorsal (MDN), pulvinar (PUL), and centromedian (CMN) nuclei in subjects with schizophrenia by using image filtering to enhance contrast (Fig. 21.2). In schizophrenia, all three nuclei were

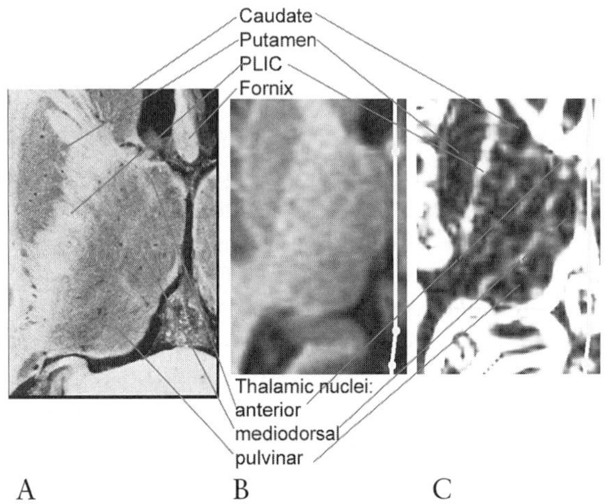

FIGURE 21.2 Horizontal sections through thalamus. (*A*) Autopsy specimen, unstained fixed tissue. (*B*) T1 MRI scan of live subject. (*C*) Application of Sobel intensity gradient filter to scan shown in *B* allows demarcation of thalamic nuclei. PLIC, posterior limb of internal capsule. White lines (in *B* and *C*) mark anatomical midline. (Courtesy Drs. William Byne and Monte Buchsbaum.)

smaller than in controls, in absolute terms and relative to total brain volume. There were no differences in effects across the three nuclei, and the reduction in their volumes appeared to account for an overall reduction in thalamic volume. Moreover, the effects were similar for subjects who were exposed or naïve to neuroleptics. Reduced thalamic volume in subjects who were naïve to neuroleptics was also observed by Gur et al. (1998), who found that typical neuroleptics were associated with larger thalamic volumes.

A meta-analysis of MRI studies of thalamic volume computed an effect size of 0.35 (Konick and Friedman, 2001); subsequent studies are consistent with this (for example, for medial dorsal nucleus, Kemether et al., 2003, obtained an effect size of 0.3 on the right and 0.5 on the left). Thus, the inconsistencies among the postmortem studies could be attributed to lack of statistical power. For instance, if 0.35 is the true effect size, the 11 controls and 9 subjects with schizophrenia studied by Dorph-Petersen et al. (2004) would give a power of 0.1 for a two-tailed test with $\alpha = 0.05$. There may be other reasons for inconsistencies in postmortem results, but larger studies are clearly indicated.

PATHOLOGY OF DENDRITES

Decreased density of dendritic spines (that is, decreased numbers of spines per unit length of dendrite) is one of the most robust neuropathological abnormalities in schizophrenia. Golgi techniques (Fig. 21.3; see also COLOR FIGURE 21.3 in separate insert) are the primary methods for observing the anatomy of neuronal processes in brain tissue, and they are essentially the only methods that have been used for this purpose in human tissue.

Garey et al. (1998) found spine densities 59% lower in temporal cortex and 31% lower in frontal cortex in formaldehyde-fixed tissue from subjects with schizophrenia. Glantz and Lewis (2000) used similar Golgi methods to study BA46 and BA17. There was a significant effect of diagnosis on basilar dendritic spine density only for neurons of deep layer 3 of BA46, with subjects with schizophrenia 23% lower than nonpsychiatric subjects. Values for the other psychiatric subjects fell between those of the nonpsychiatric and control subjects and did not differ significantly from either. Although the schizophrenia means were nominally lower than the nonpsychiatric means in superficial layer 3 of BA46 and in layer 3 of BA17, regional specificity is further supported by a significant difference in spine density between superficial and deep layer 3 in BA46 for subjects with schizophrenia, while the spine densities at both depths were virtually the same for nonpsychiatric subjects. Furthermore, these slides were revisited in a subsequent study (Kolluri et al., 2005), which found no differences between groups in layers 5/6 of BA46. In a subsequent study of a partially overlapping sample, Hill et al. (2006) measured messenger ribonucleic acid (mRNA) in BA9 for several proteins involved in assembly, stabilization, and disassembly of the actin skeleton of spines. Subjects with schizophrenia had lower levels than nonpsychiatric subjects, and mRNA for two of these proteins, Cdc42 and Duo, correlated with deep layer 3 spine density previously measured in BA46. However, unlike the difference for spine density, the difference in mRNA was present in deep layer 3 and layer 6. The authors suggest that the localized deficit in spines could result from an interaction between decreased synthesis of these proteins and decreased excitatory input from the medial dorsal nucleus of the thalamus, which projects primarily to cortical layers 3 and 4. They point out that this hypothesis would predict a decrease in spine density on apical dendrites of layer 6 neurons as they pass through layers 3 and 4, a testable hypothesis.

Rosoklija et al. (2000) used a similar Golgi protocol to study neurons in the deep pyramidal layer of the subiculum. The density of spines on apical dendrites was markedly (73%) lower in subjects with schizophrenia than in nonpsychiatric subjects, with no overlap between the two groups. A similar study (Rosoklija et al., 2004), employed the same region of interest and similar counting methods on Golgi–Kopsch stained hippocampal blocks in a younger sample. Spine density was ~80% lower in schizophrenia and mood disorders, with no overlap between psychiatric and nonpsychiatric subjects.

It is notable that none of these studies found any effect of neuroleptic exposure. However, most or all of the psychiatric subjects died in institutions or by suicide, and it is possible that medications could affect spine density when treatment is more successful.

Five Golgi studies, including two of the above, have addressed other aspects of dendritic morphology in schizophrenia. Kolluri et al. (2005) found no differences in lengths or branching parameters in individual basilar dendrites in BA46, layers 5 and 6. Rosoklija et al. (2000) found less extensive subicular apical dendritic arbors in the schizophrenia cases than in the nonpsychiatric cases. There was no effect of diagnosis on subicular basilar dendrites or on apical or basilar dendrites in layer 5 of the adjacent fusiform gyrus.

Kalus et al. (2000) used the Golgi modification of Bubenaite to stain fresh tissue from BA11 of five age- and sex-matched pairs of subjects with schizophrenia and nonpsychiatric subjects, aged 37 to 84. They found ~30% smaller basilar dendritic arbors of layer 3 pyramidal neurons in schizophrenia, with no differences in apical dendrites. Decreased basilar dendritic arbors were also reported in BA32 (Broadbelt et al., 2002) and BA10 (Black et al., 2004).

A potential limitation of most of these studies is the notorious unreliability of Golgi impregnations, particularly

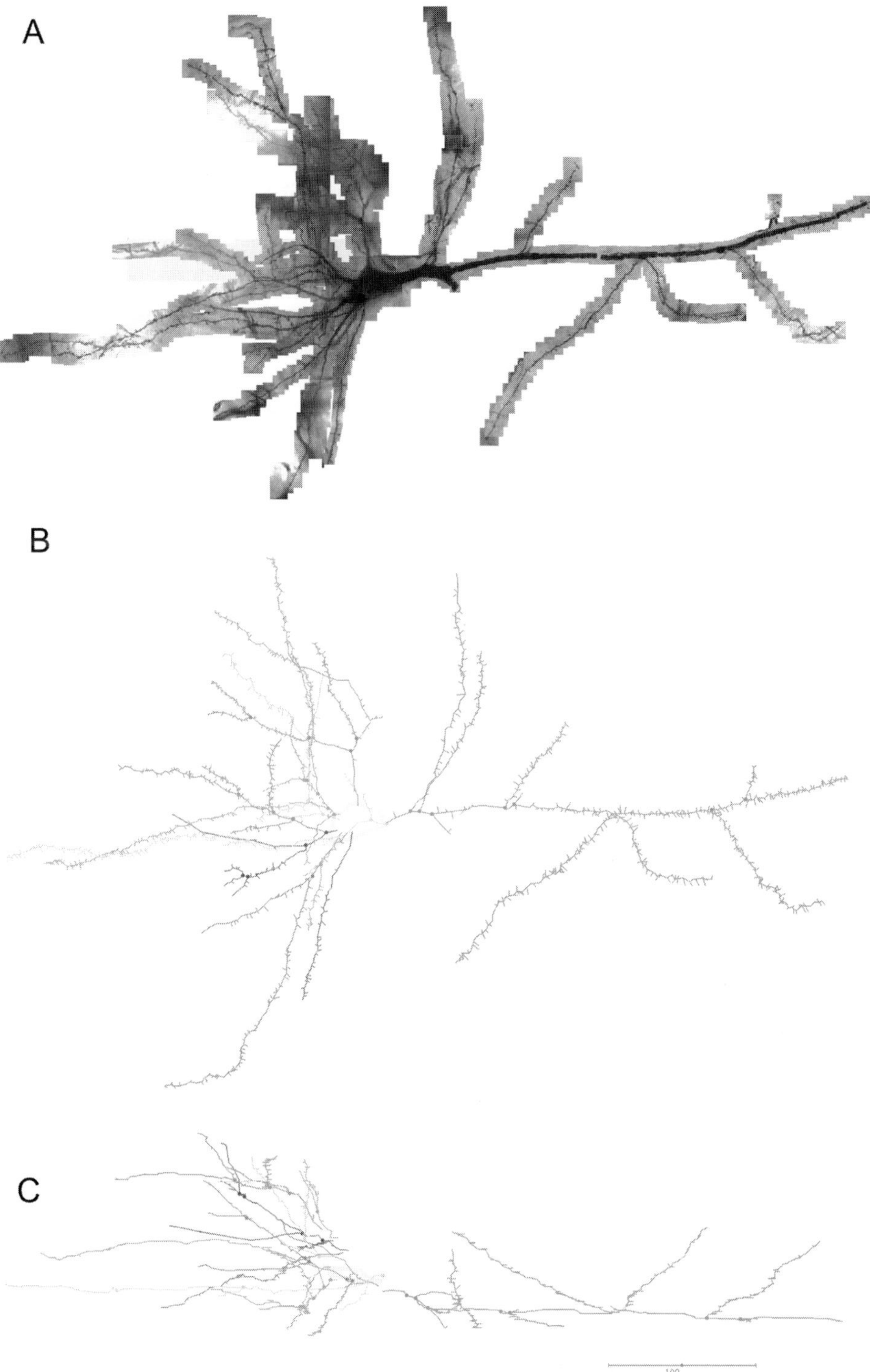

FIGURE 21.3 (*A*) Photomontage and (*B*) computer-recorded tracing of Golgi stain (on unfixed autopsy specimen) of a subicular pyramidal neuron. (C) Rotation of tracing perpendicular to the plane of section demonstrates that several dendrites, including the main shaft of the apical dendrite, were truncated at the cut surface of the 200 micron-thick section. Scale bar = 100 microns. (Thanks to Tatiana Schnieder.)

when applied to previously fixed tissue (Fig. 21.3) (Rosoklija et al., 2003). This excludes inclusion of all available cases, analysis of multiple regions from all included cases, and application of systematic uniform random sampling of neurons within a region of interest. Most seriously, it can sometimes be difficult to distinguish pathological changes from poor impregnation. In our own experience, despite considerable effort to optimize these procedures and to match the procedure to the condition of the tissue (Rosoklija et al., 2003), the familiar difficulties could not be entirely eliminated in fixed human tissue. Considerably more reliable staining can be obtained if impregnation is performed on freshly collected tissue, which will no doubt become the standard for future studies.

Spines and synapses in schizophrenia have also been studied by electron microscopy. Roberts et al. (1996) reported that striatal spines were 30% smaller in schizophrenia. In hippocampal area CA3, Kolomeets et al. (2005) found that the ratio of volumes of spines to their synaptic partner mossy fiber terminals was 40% lower, and the number of spines with synaptic contacts with each mossy fiber terminal was reduced by 32%, only in subjects with schizophrenia with predominantly positive symptoms. The number of synapses per mossy fiber terminal was 22% lower than in nonpsychiatric subjects, independent of symptom pattern. In layer 2 of anterior cingulate cortex, area densities of axodendritic synapses are reportedly decreased, and axospinous increased, in schizophrenia (Aganova and Uranova, 1992).

In summary, lower dendritic spine density appears to be a robust finding in schizophrenia, although confirmation awaits examination of equivalent dendrites by different laboratories. Fewer or smaller dendritic spines are consistent with other evidence for decreased glutamatergic neurotransmission. There are myriad mechanisms by which glutamatergic activity sustains spines or promotes their growth (Park et al., 2006); conversely, spines are important for efficient excitatory transmission. Hence, lowered spine density in schizophrenia could be a primary cause of impaired transmission, a secondary effect, or a self-perpetuating process.

PATHOLOGY OF INHIBITORY INTERNEURONS

GABAergic transmission in schizophrenia has been studied extensively (reviewed in Blum and Mann, 2002). A series of studies (Benes, McSparren, et al., 1991; Benes et al., 1992; Benes et al., 1996; Benes et al., 2000) of prefrontal and anterior cingulate cortex in schizophrenia found the density of small neurons (presumed GABAergic interneurons) lower selectively in layer 2, with more GABA-A receptor binding sites on pyramidal neurons in layers 2 and 3. In PFC only, the density of pyramidal neurons was increased in layer 6, and GABA-A binding sites on pyramidal neurons were increased in layers 5 and 6. The GABA-A receptor findings were interpreted as a compensatory response to a locally decreased ratio of interneurons to pyramidal cells. However, there was no effect of schizophrenia on the numerical density of 65 kD form of glutamic acid decarboxylase (GAD65)-immunoreactive terminals on neurons in any layer. Because GAD65 is the predominant isoform in axons, this was inconsistent with the hypothesized GABAergic deficit, leading to the speculation that a deficit might be selective for the 67 kD isoform (GAD67; predominant form in neuronal cell bodies).

Other studies failed to replicate the differences in small neuron density (Akbarian et al., 1995; Benes et al., 2001), and one (Rajkowska et al., 1998) found substantially higher densities of small prefrontal neurons.

In PFC, several laboratories have shown markedly lower levels of mRNA for GAD67 (Akbarian et al., 1995; Guidotti et al., 2000; Volk et al., 2000) and GAD67 protein (Guidotti et al., 2000). Volk et al. (2000, 2001) found fewer neurons expressing mRNA for GAD67 or the GABA transporter, GAT1, with unchanged expression per positive neuron. The numerical density of GAT1-immunoreactive cartridges (specialized axonal terminals of GABAergic chandelier neurons on initial axon segments from pyramidal neurons) was decreased by 40%–45% (Woo et al., 1998). This decrease was correlated with an increase (~100%) in the density of initial segments immunoreactive for the GABA-A-α2 (high-affinity) receptor subunit (Volk et al., 2002).

Cortical GABA neurons can be divided into three separate populations with antibodies to the calcium-binding proteins *parvalbumin, calbindin,* and *calretinin*, which together label about 90% of the cortical interneurons (Conde et al., 1994). Hashimoto et al. (2003) found that mRNA for parvalbumin was approximately 30% lower in neurons of layers 3 and 4 in schizophrenia PFC, even though the numerical density of parvalbumin-expressing neurons (by in situ hybridization and immunohistochemistry) was unaffected. Unchanged parvalbumin cell density was also reported in previous studies (Woo et al., 1997; Tooney and Chahl, 2004), although there are reports of decreased density (Beasley and Reynolds, 1997; Reynolds and Beasley, 2001). Hashimoto et al. (2003) also reported that the parvalbumin mRNA expression per neuron was strongly correlated with the density of GAD67-expressing neurons. In schizophrenia, 45% of neurons expressing parvalbumin mRNA lacked GAD67 mRNA, compared with 10% in controls, although it was not determined whether parvalbumin and GAD67 mRNA expression were correlated at the level of individual neurons.

Calbindin-containing interneurons are especially concentrated in layer 2 of cortex. The density of these cells was found to be reduced about 34% in cingulate cortex (Cotter, Landau, et al., 2002), 26% in PFC (Beasley,

Zhang, et al., 2002), and about 15% in auditory association cortex (Chance et al., 2005). In prefrontal and cingulate cortex, there was some evidence for selectivity of this reduction, as the densities of calretinin and parvalbumin cells were not significantly reduced.

In the hippocampal formation, there may be even greater abnormalities of GABAergic neurons, although the results of different types of studies vary widely. Benes et al. (1998), using cresyl violet stains, reported a 50% decrease of nonpyramidal neurons, only in CA2, in schizophrenia and BPD. Zhang and Reynolds (2002) showed numerical densities of parvalbumin-immunoreactive neurons lower by at least 50% in each subfield, with larger effects in males than in females. Heckers et al. (2002), using in situ hybridization, found no significant effect of schizophrenia in any region of the hippocampal formation, but significantly lower densities of GAD67- and GAD65-expressing cells in BPD. Preliminary data from microarrays demonstrate lower levels of GAD67 mRNA in the stratum oriens (where most hippocampal interneurons are located) of CA2/3 by ~60% in schizophrenia and ~90% in BPD (Benes et al., 2007). These studies suggest an association of psychosis with interneuron pathology in CA2/3.

In summary, though there are some discrepancies regarding counts of small neurons, which can be difficult to distinguish from glia in Nissl stains, these and other measures are generally consistent with lower densities or activities of prefrontal and possibly hippocampal and anterior cingulate GABAergic neurons in schizophrenia and BPD. There is a clear indication for stereological studies that will determine total numbers of different classes of interneurons, defined by morphology and calcium-binding protein expression, in specific anatomical structures.

"INTERSTITIAL" NEURONS IN WHITE MATTER

The distribution of neurons in the white matter in schizophrenia is controversial with respect to the findings and their interpretation. Isolated, so-called interstitial neurons in subcortical white matter are readily observed in humans and other mammals; they are most numerous immediately deep to the cortex but are also present at greater depths. Several studies have examined the distribution of these neurons, as visualized with different markers and in different brain regions. Although all of the studies report abnormalities in schizophrenia, there are important inconsistencies in the results: studies by Akbarian et al. (Akbarian, Bunney, et al. 1993; Akbarian, Vinuela, et al. 1993; Akbarian et al., 1996) consistently found schizophrenia to be associated with a lower density of neurons in superficial (immediately subcortical) white matter and a higher density in deeper white matter; this applied to nicotinamide-adenine dinucleotide phosphate-diaphorase (NADPH-d)-expressing cells in the white matter of hippocampal formation and adjacent temporal neocortex, NADPH-d cells in prefrontal white matter, and prefrontal white matter neurons immunoreactive for microtubule-associated protein 2 (MAP2) and nonphosphorylated neurofilament heavy chain. Other investigators have found a greater density of interstitial neurons in superficial layers of subcortical white matter in schizophrenia, and little or no difference in deeper compartments. These studies include MAP2-immunoreactive neurons in prefrontal (Anderson et al., 1996; Kirkpatrick et al., 2003) and inferior parietal (Kirkpatrick et al., 1999) white matter, and NeuN (a presumably pan-neuronal marker)-immunoreactive neurons in superior temporal gyrus (Eastwood and Harrison, 2003). One study found no effect of schizophrenia or other psychiatric disorders on the distribution of MAP2-immunoreactive neurons in prefrontal white matter (Beasley, Cotter, et al., 2002). These inconsistencies cannot be readily explained by methodological differences, as the superficial compartment was defined relatively consistently across studies.

Further controversy surrounds the embryological origin of the interstitial neurons or their significance as indicators of impaired migration during corticogenesis. Although traditionally considered remnants of the embryological subplate (Kostovic and Rakic, 1980; Chun and Shatz, 1989; Kostovic and Rakic, 1990), Meyer et al. (1992) contended that the pyramidal morphology of most of these neurons, particularly those immunoreactive for MAP2 and located superficially, is more consistent with an extension of cortical layer 6. To the extent that aberrantly located white matter neurons may represent subplate remnants, it seems unlikely that they represent a major disruption of the subplate, which should create an obvious cortical abnormality (Kostovic and Rakic, 1990). They could represent aberrant dissolution of the subplate, a process that is poorly understood. Kostovic and Rakic (1990) proposed a role for the subplate in preserving cortical integrity in the face of developmental insult; one could speculate that such a process would lead to aberrant subplate remnants.

WHITE MATTER IN SCHIZOPHRENIA

Postmortem

Imaging and genetic association studies have suggested that myelination of white matter may be abnormal in schizophrenia (reviewed in Dwork et al., 2007). If this is so, the abnormalities are sufficiently subtle to have escaped histological detection so far and may in fact be discernable only by morphometry of myelin sheaths in electron micrographs or semithin sections. In a large sample of subjects who were elderly, we found no histological evidence for loss of integrity of myelin as evaluated by conventional (Verhoeff) myelin stains, in the dorsal prefrontal white matter in schizophrenia (Mancevski et al., 2007). Falkai et al. (1999) found no evidence for astrocytosis in the white matter of the premotor cortex or the subventricular zone of the third ventricle, which suggests that at least in these structures, a demyelinating process is unlikely.

Hof et al. (2002, 2003), with small groups (N = 4–7) of subjects who were elderly and chronically institutionalized, found 15%–28% lower density of oligodendrocytes in layer 3 of BA9 and in the underlying white matter. Uranova et al. (2004), in a younger sample, reported a similar loss of oligodendroglial density in layer 6 of BA9, in mood disorders as well as schizophrenia, but not in the underlying white matter. Because the lower oligodendrocyte densities found by Hof et al. (2003) tended to be in the older subjects with schizophrenia, it could be that the loss of white matter oligodendrocytes, or of their immunoreactivity for cyclic nucleotide 3'-phosphodiesterase (CNP)ase, or both occur in schizophrenia only at advanced ages, or that these few cases had undetected cerebrovascular disease that was not present in the few nonpsychiatric subjects of similar age. Marner and Pakkenberg (2003) compared eight schizophrenia and nine nonpsychiatric subjects with a mean age of 60 and found no difference in the total length of myelinated axons in the prefrontal white matter, nor in the diameters of these axons. Differences might have been found in an older sample, and they did not measure the thickness of the myelin sheaths, which could have revealed hypomyelination.

The other structural postmortem studies of white matter in schizophrenia focused on fiber tracts. Two studies of the corpus callosum found no schizophrenia-associated differences in fiber density or glial density (Nasrallah et al., 1983; Casanova et al., 1989), whereas one found lower fiber densities in females with schizophrenia (Highley, Esiri, McDonald, Cortina-Borja, et al., 1999). Fiber densities were decreased in the anterior commissure among females with schizophrenia (Highley, Esiri, McDonald, Roberts, et al., 1999), increased in the fornix among males with schizophrenia (Chance et al., 1999), and unaffected in the uncinate fasciculus (Highley et al., 2002). One study used in situ hybridization to quantify mRNA levels for myelin-associated proteins and found lower levels (by 14%–22%) of message for several myelin-related proteins in anterior cingulate white matter of 41 elderly subjects with schizophrenia, both medicated and unmedicated, compared with 34 elderly subjects without psychiatric illness (McCullumsmith et al., 2007). No changes were found in mRNA for a variety of other myelin-related proteins, and no message was significantly altered in cingulate grey matter. Diminished expression of myelin-associated genes in schizophrenia has been reported in other studies of grey matter, as have associations between gene expression and schizophrenia-associated polymorphisms of some of these genes (reviewed in Dwork et al., 2007).

Electron microscopic studies of cortical oligodendrocytes may be revealing. A study of BA10 biopsies found lipofuscin deposits in oligodendroglial cytoplasm and increased numbers of electron-dense granules in neuronal cytoplasm, axon-oligodendrocyte interfaces, and myelin sheaths (Miyakawa et al., 1972). A study of autopsy material (Uranova et al., 2001) showed subtle abnormalities in oligodendroglia and myelin sheaths of cortical layer 6 of BA10 and the caudate nucleus in schizophrenia. These included decreased cross-sectional areas of nuclei and decreased fraction of cytoplasmic volume occupied by mitochondria. In the caudate nucleus, there were apoptotic oligodendroglia, splitting of myelin lamellae, and concentric lamellar bodies consistent with myelin breakdown. Neither study included white matter or measured the diameters of myelin sheaths. Furthermore, there appears to have been no effort in either study to mask the observers to the source of the specimens. Nonetheless, these abnormalities bear intriguing similarities to "dying back oligodendrogliopathies" in certain animal models in which interactions of axons and myelin are impaired (in processes involving genes that may be linked to schizophrenia), such as mutant mice lacking myelin-associated glycoprotein (Montag et al., 1994; Lassmann et al., 1997) or in which a dominant negative mutation of ErbB4 in oligodendrocytes and Schwann cells prevents neuregulin signaling (Roy et al., 2007).

In Vivo

Diffusion tensor imaging (DTI) offers a promising new technique for the identification of cerebral networks critical to schizophrenia (Basser et al., 1994). This method measures the diffusion of water and gives a measure of the directionality and organization of diffusion barriers in the brain. The main cause of anisotropic diffusion in fascicles of parallel axons appears to be the organization and integrity of cell membranes, with myelin playing a modulatory role (Beaulieu and Allen, 1994; Beaulieu, 2002). Several metrics of diffusion anisotropy are used, including fractional anisotropy (FA), which ranges from 0 (*perfectly isotropic diffusion*) to 1 (*perfectly unidirectional diffusion*). Additionally, it has been suggested that diffusivity perpendicular to (radial diffusivity [D_{RA}]) and parallel to (axial diffusivity [D_{AX}]) the direction of principal diffusion may be sensitive to different aspects of white matter pathology (see Dwork et al., 2007, for discussion). These measures might prove helpful in clarifying the relative roles of myelin and axonal integrity in white matter changes in schizophrenia. As an example, Kitamura et al. (2005) found increased radial diffusivity in frontal regions in subjects with schizophrenia without a concomitant decrease in axial diffusivity.

Recent literature reviews concluded that, although most studies have found significant reductions in FA (Fig. 21.4; see also COLOR FIGURE 21.4 in separate insert), the location of these reductions has been variable between studies (Kanaan et al., 2005; Dwork et al., 2007; Kubicki et al., 2007). Whole brain surveys found widespread FA reductions in white matter, using either voxel-wise (Ardekani et al., 2003) or ROI-based analyses (Minami et al., 2003). Lim et al. (1999) found widespread reductions in FA despite apparently normal white matter volumes. Several findings have examined FA by placing ROIs in specific tracts. Among the positive findings, reduced FA in the cingulate white matter appears to be a rather consistent finding (e.g., Kubicki et al., 2003; Sun et al., 2003). Two studies found differences in the splenium, but not the genu of the corpus callosum (Foong et al., 2000; Agartz et al., 2001). Other studies found reduced FA in the optic radiations (Butler et al., 2006), in the cerebellar peduncles (Okugawa et al., 2005), in the fornix (Kuroki et al., 2006), and in the uncinate and arcuate fasciculi (Burns et al., 2003).

The changes in FA appear to be present early in the disease and cannot be entirely attributed to medication effects. Two studies reported that first-episode patients had widespread decreases in FA (Hao et al., 2006; Szeszko et al., 2007), with similar findings in early-onset subjects (Kumra et al., 2005; Ashtari et al., 2007).

Relationships between FA and function have been shown in a number of domains including impulsivity (Hoptman et al., 2002; Hoptman et al., 2004), cognitive function (Kubicki et al., 2003; Nestor et al., 2004; Kuroki et al., 2006; Lim et al., 2006; Szeszko et al., 2007), and negative symptomatology (Wolkin et al., 2003; Szeszko et al., 2007). Fractional anisotropy in optic radiations has been correlated with increased amplitude of steady-state evoked potentials that are sensitive to the function of the magnocellular visual pathway, which appears to be perturbed in schizophrenia (Butler et al., 2005). Auditory hallucinations may be associated with increased FA in left superior temporal gyrus (Hubl et al., 2004) and inferior fronto-occipital fasciculus (Szeszko et al., 2007).

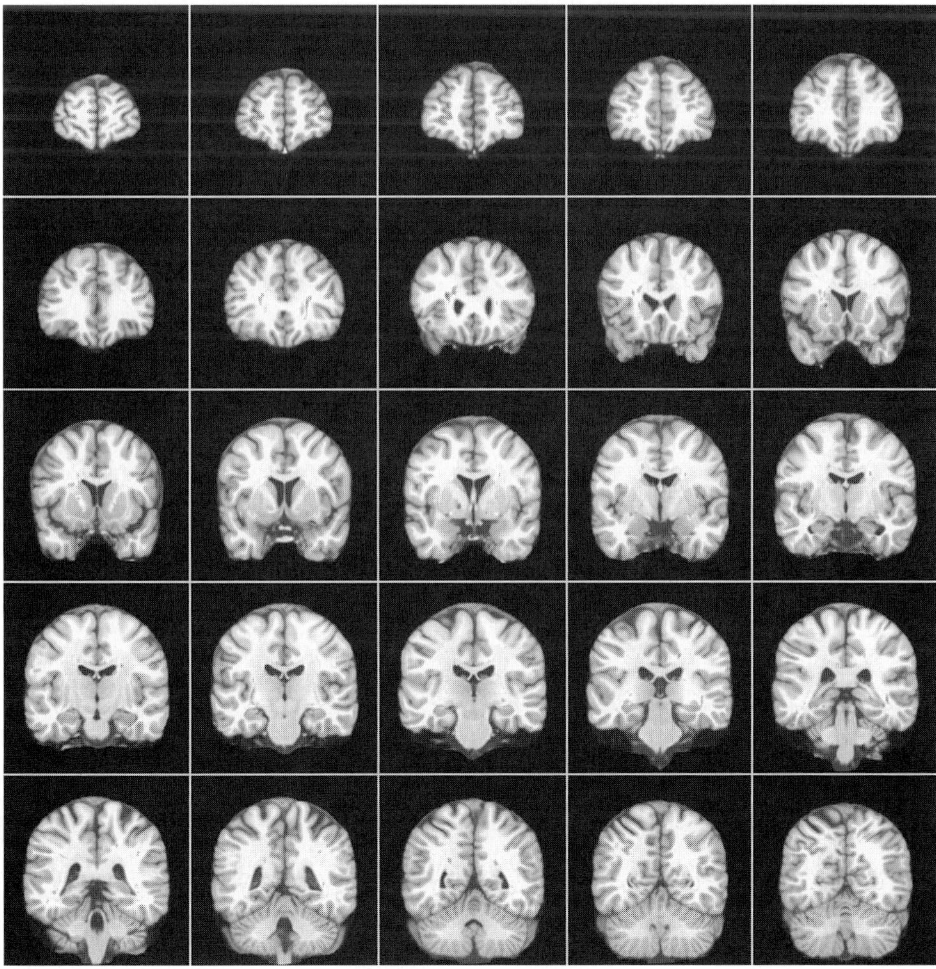

FIGURE 21.4 Widespread differences in white matter fractional anisotropy (FA) between 43 subjects with schizophrenia or schizoaffective disorder and 47 healthy comparison subjects. Yellow = areas in which FA is higher in controls, Blue = areas in which FA is higher in subjects. Images are thresholded at $p = .0065$ (false discovery rate $q = .05$), with a 50mm^3 extent threshold. Every fifth coronal millimeter is shown, from anterior to posterior (see Figure 21.4 in color insert).

A potentially promising application of DTI is fiber tractography (Mori et al., 1999; Wieshmann et al., 1999), wherein directional information from the diffusion tensor can be used to map out putative fiber tracts. Tractography also provides another way to examine group differences between patients and healthy controls. For instance, Kanaan et al. (2006) used tractography to define the genu of the corpus callosum and found reduced FA within that tract. A second study by the same group (Shergill et al., 2007) found reduced FA in the superior longitudinal fasciculus and genu of the corpus callosum. In addition, within the patient group, the propensity for auditory hallucinations was correlated with increased FA in the superior longitudinal fasciculus and anterior cingulum.

Magnetization transfer imaging (MTI; Henkelman et al., 2001) offers another method to assess the role of white matter in schizophrenia. Magnetization transfer imaging provides contrast based on the suppression of the normally observed tissue water signal by excitation of protons contained in large macromolecules (including components of myelin) in tissue. In this imaging modality, two sequences are used, one of which is essentially proton density–weighted. In the other sequence, a special radiofrequency pulse is placed before the original sequence to excite hydrogen protons bound to macromolecules, which then exchange with the free water protons and consequently suppress the MR signal. The contrast difference between the two image sets is given by the magnetization transfer ratio (MTR). Greater MTR values presumably represent greater interactions of free water with macromolecules and possibly indicate a greater abundance of macromolecules. Studies conducted in early development, aging, and multiple sclerosis suggest that DTI and MTR may provide complementary information about white matter integrity, with DTI primarily reflecting organization of fibers tracts and MTR being particularly sensitive to myelin and axonal integrity (Hoptman, Gunning-Dixon, et al., 2006; Wozniak and Lim, 2006).

In schizophrenia, lower MTR has been found in many of the same regions as lower FA (Foong et al., 2001; Bagary et al., 2003; Kubicki et al., 2005) although discrepancies were found in a study employing both measures (Price et al., 2006). In a voxelwise study of chronic schizophrenia, Antosik-Biernacka et al. (2006), after correcting for multiple comparisons, found no significant reductions in MTR compared to healthy controls.

In summary, DTI and MTI appear to indicate white matter abnormalities in young subjects with schizophrenia. The most consistent sites of localization are the cingulum bundle and uncinate fasciculus. In general, the histological bases of DTI and MTI abnormalities are poorly understood, and this is particularly true in schizophrenia because very few pathological studies of white matter have been conducted.

ACKNOWLEDGMENTS

We thank Jan Hrabe, PhD for helpful comments about the physics of MTI. Research support was provided by MH60877, MH64168, the National Alliance for Research on Schizophrenia and Depression, and the Lieber Center for Schizophrenia Research at Columbia University (all to AJD), grants from the Stanley Medical Research Institute (to AJD and JFS), MH67138 (to JFS), MH64783 (to MJH), and MH15144 (supporting TC).

REFERENCES

Aganova, E.A., and Uranova, N.A. (1992) Morphometric analysis of synaptic contacts in the anterior limbic cortex in the endogenous psychoses. *Neurosci. Behav. Physiol.* 22:59–65.

Agartz, I., Andersson, J.L., and Skare, S. (2001) Abnormal brain white matter in schizophrenia: a diffusion tensor imaging study. *Neuroreport* 12:2251–2254.

Akbarian, S., Bunney, W.E., Jr., Potkin, S.G., Wigal, S.B., Hagman, J.O., Sandman, C.A., and Jones, E.G. (1993) Altered distribution of nicotinamide-adenine dinucleotide phosphate-diaphorase cells in frontal lobe of schizophrenics implies disturbances of cortical development. *Arch. Gen. Psychiatry* 50:169–177.

Akbarian, S., Kim, J.J., Potkin, S.G., Hagman, J.O., Tafazzoli, A., Bunney, W.E., Jr., and Jones, E.G. (1995) Gene expression for glutamic acid decarboxylase is reduced without loss of neurons in prefrontal cortex of schizophrenics. *Arch. Gen. Psychiatry* 52:258–266.

Akbarian, S., Kim, J.J., Potkin, S.G., Hetrick, W.P., Bunney, W.E., Jr., and Jones, E.G. (1996) Maldistribution of interstitial neurons in prefrontal white matter of the brains of schizophrenic patients. *Arch. Gen. Psychiatry* 53:425–436.

Akbarian, S., Vinuela, A., Kim, J.J., Potkin, S.G., Bunney, W.E., Jr., and Jones, E.G. (1993) Distorted distribution of nicotinamide-adenine dinucleotide phosphate-diaphorase neurons in temporal lobe of schizophrenics implies anomalous cortical development. *Arch. Gen. Psychiatry* 50:178–187.

Anderson, S.A., Volk, D.W., and Lewis, D.A. (1996) Increased density of microtubule associated protein 2-immunoreactive neurons in the prefrontal white matter of schizophrenic subjects. *Schizophr. Res.* 19:111–119.

Andreasen, N.C., Arndt, S., Swayze, V., 2nd, Cizadlo, T., Flaum, M., O'Leary, D., Ehrhardt, J.C., and Yuh, W.T. (1994) Thalamic abnormalities in schizophrenia visualized through magnetic resonance image averaging [see comment]. *Science* 266:294–298.

Andreasen, N.C., Ehrhardt, J.C., Swayze, V.W., Alliger, R.J., Yuh, W.T., Cohen, G., and Ziebell, S. (1990) Magnetic resonance imaging of the brain in schizophrenia. The pathophysiologic significance of structural abnormalities. *Arch. Gen. Psychiatry* 47:35–44.

Antonova, E., Sharma, T., Morris, R., and Kumari, V. (2004) The relationship between brain structure and neurocognition in schizophrenia: a selective review. *Schizophr. Res.* 70:117–145.

Antosik-Biernacka, A., Peuskens, H., De Hurt, M., Peuskens, J., Sunaert, S., Van, H.P., and Goraj. B. (2006) Magnetization transfer imaging in chronic schizophrenia. *Med. Sci. Mon.* 12:17–21.

Ardekani, B.A., Nierenberg, J., Hoptman, M.J., Javitt, D.C., and Lim, K.O. (2003) MRI study of white matter diffusion anisotropy in schizophrenia. *Neuroreport* 14:2025–2029.

Arnold, S.E., Franz, B.R., Gur, R.C., Gur, R.E., Shapiro, R.M., Moberg, P.J., and Trojanowski, J.Q. (1995) Smaller neuron size in schizophrenia in hippocampal subfields that mediate cortical-hippocampal interactions. *Am. J. Psychiatry* 152:738–748.

Ashburner, J., and Friston, K.J. (2000) Voxel based morphometry—the methods. *Human Brain Mapp.* 7:254–266.

Ashtari, M., Cottone, J., Ardekani, B.A., Cervellione, K., Szeszko, P.R., Wu, J., Chen, S., and Kumra, S. (2007) Disruption of white matter integrity in the inferior longitudinal fasciculus in adolescents with schizophrenia as revealed by fiber tractography. *Arch. Gen. Psychiatry* 64:1270–1280.

Baare, W.F., Hulshoff Pol, H.E., Hijman, R., Mali, W.P., Viergever, M.A., and Kahn, R.S. (1999) Volumetric analysis of frontal lobe regions in schizophrenia: relation to cognitive function and symptomatology. *Biol. Psychiatry* 45:1597–1605.

Bagary, M.S., Symms, M.R., Barker, G.J., Mutsatsa, S.H., Joyce, E. M., and Ron, M.A. (2003) Gray and white matter brain abnormalities in first-episode schizophrenia inferred from magnetization transfer imaging. *Arch. Gen. Psychiatry* 60:779–788.

Barta, P.E., Pearlson, G.D., Brill, L.B., Royall, R., McGilchrist, I.K., Pulver, A.E., Powers, R.E., Casanova, M.F., Tien, A.Y., Frangou, S., and Petty, R.G. (1997) Planum temporale asymmetry reversal in schizophrenia: replication and relationship to gray matter abnormalities. *Am. J. Psych.* 154:661–667.

Basser, P., Mattiello, J., and LeBihan, D. (1994) MR diffusion tensor spectroscopy and imaging. *Biophys. J.* 66:259–267.

Beasley, C.L., Chana, G., Honavar, M., Landau, S., Everall, I.P., and Cotter, D. (2005) Evidence for altered neuronal organisation within the planum temporale in major psychiatric disorders. *Schizophr. Res.* 73:69–78.

Beasley, C.L., Cotter, D.R., and Everall, I.P. (2002) Density and distribution of white matter neurons in schizophrenia, bipolar disorder and major depressive disorder: no evidence for abnormalities of neuronal migration. *Mol. Psychiatry* 7:564–570.

Beasley, C.L., and Reynolds, G.P. (1997) Parvalbumin-immunoreactive neurons are reduced in the prefrontal cortex of schizophrenics. *Schizophr. Res.* 24:349–355.

Beasley, C.L., Zhang, Z.J., Patten, I., and Reynolds, G.P. (2002) Selective deficits in prefrontal cortical GABAergic neurons in schizophrenia defined by the presence of calcium-binding proteins. *Biol. Psychiatry* 52:708–715.

Beaulieu, C. (2002) The basis of anisotropic water diffusion in the nervous system—a technical review. *NMR in Biomedicine* 15:435–455.

Beaulieu, C., and Allen, P.S. (1994) Water diffusion in the giant axon of the squid: implications for diffusion-weighted MR imaging of the human brain. *Magn. Reson. Med.* 32:579–583.

Benes, F., Lim, B., Matzilevich, D., and Walsh, J. (2007) Abnormal maintenance of the gabaergic phenotype in hippocampal neurons of schizophrenics and bipolars through different molecular mechanisms. *Schizophr. Bull.* 33:256–257.

Benes, F.M., Davidson, J., Bird, E.D., Benes, F.M., Davidson, J., and Bird, E.D. (1986) Quantitative cytoarchitectural studies of the cerebral cortex of schizophrenics. *Arch. Gen. Psychiatry* 43: 31–35.

Benes, F.M., Kwok, E.W., Vincent, S.L., and Todtenkopf, M.S. (1998) A reduction of nonpyramidal cells in sector CA2 of schizophrenics and manic depressives. *Biol. Psychiatry* 44:88–97.

Benes, F.M., McSparren, J., Bird, E.D., SanGiovanni, J.P., and Vincent, S.L. (1991) Deficits in small interneurons in prefrontal and cingulate cortices of schizophrenic and shizoaffective patients. *Arch. Gen. Psych.* 48:996–1001.

Benes, F.M., Sorensen, I., and Bird, E.D. (1991) Reduced neuronal size in posterior hippocampus of schizophrenic patients. *Schizophr. Bull.* 17:597–608.

Benes, F.M., Todtenkopf, M.S., Logiotatos, P., and Williams, M. (2000) Glutamate decarboxylase(65)-immunoreactive terminals in cingulate and prefrontal cortices of schizophrenic and bipolar brain. *J. Chem. Neuroanatomy* 20:259–269.

Benes, F.M., Vincent, S.L., Alsterberg, G., Bird, E.D., and SanGiovanni, J.P. (1992) Increased GABAA receptor binding in superficial layers of cingulate cortex in schizophrenics. *J. Neuroscience* 12:924–929.

Benes, F.M., Vincent, S.L., Marie, A., and Khan, Y. (1996) Up-regulation of GABAA receptor binding on neurons of the prefrontal cortex in schizophrenic subjects. *Neuroscience* 75:1021–1031.

Benes, F.M., Vincent, S.L., and Todtenkopf, M. (2001) The density of pyramidal and nonpyramidal neurons in anterior cingulate cortex of schizophrenic and bipolar subjects. *Biol. Psychiatry* 50:395–406.

Bilder, R.M., Bogerts, B., Ashtari, M., Wu, H., Alvir, J.M., Jody, D., Reiter, G., Bell, L., and Lieberman, J.A. (1995) Anterior hippocampal volume reductions predict "frontal lobe" dysfunction in first episode schizophrenia. *Schizophrenia Research* 17(1): 47–58.

Black, J.E., Kodish, I.M., Grossman, A.W., Klintsova, A.Y., Orlovskaya, D., Vostrikov, V., Uranova, N., and Greenough, W.T. (2004) Pathology of layer V pyramidal neurons in the prefrontal cortex of patients with schizophrenia. *Am. J. Psychiatry* 161:742–744.

Blum, B.P., and Mann, J.J. (2002) The GABAergic system in schizophrenia. *Int. J. Neuropsychopharmacol.* 5:159–179.

Bogerts, B., Falkai, P., Haupts, M., Greve, B., Ernst, S., Tapernon-Franz, U., and Heinzmann, U. (1990) Post-mortem volume measurements of limbic system and basal ganglia structures in chronic schizophrenics: initial results from a new brain collection. *Schizophr. Res.* 3:295–301.

Bookstein, F.L. (2001) "Voxel-based morphometry" should not be used with imperfectly registered images. *Neuroimage* 14:1452–1462.

Brickman, A.M., Buchsbaum, M.S., Shihabuddin, L., Byne, W., Newmark, R.E., Brand, J., Ahmed, S., Mitelman, S.A., and Hazlett, E.A. (2004) Thalamus size and outcome in schizophrenia. *Schizophr. Res.* 71:473–484.

Broadbelt, K., Byne, W., and Jones, L.B. (2002) Evidence for a decrease in basilar dendrites of pyramidal cells in schizophrenic medial prefrontal cortex. *Schizophr. Res.* 58:75–81.

Buchsbaum, M.S., Someya, T., Teng, C.Y., Abel, L., Chin, S., Najafi, A., Haier, R.J., Wu, J., and Bunney, W.E., Jr. (1996) PET and MRI of the thalamus in never-medicated patients with schizophrenia. *Am. J. Psychiatry* 153:191–199.

Burns, J., Job, D., Bastin, M.E., Whalley, H., Macgillivray, T., Johnstone, E.C., and Lawrie, S.M. (2003) Structural disconnectivity in schizophrenia: a diffusion tensor magnetic resonance imaging study. *Br. J. Psychiatry* 182:439–443.

Butler, P.D., Hoptman, M.J., Nierenberg, J., Foxe, J.J., Javitt, D.C., and Lim, K.O. (2006) Visual white matter integrity in schizophrenia. *Am. J. Psychiatry* 163:2011–2013.

Butler, P.D., Martinez, A., Foxe, J.J., Kim, D., Zemon, V., Silipo, G., Mahoney, J., Shpaner, M., Jalbrzikowski, M., and Javitt, D.C. (2007) Subcortical visual dysfunction in schizophrenia drives secondary cortical impairments. *Brain* 130:417–430.

Butler, P.D., Zemon, V., Schechter, I., Saperstein, A.M., Hoptman, M.J., Lim, K.O., Revheim, N., Silipo, G., and Javitt, D.C. (2005) Early-stage visual processing and cortical amplification deficits in schizophrenia. *Arch. Gen. Psychiatry* 62:495–504.

Byne, W., Buchsbaum, M.S., Kemether, E., Hazlett, E.A., Shinwari, A., Mitropoulou, V., and Siever, L.J. (2001) Magnetic resonance imaging of the thalamic mediodorsal nucleus and pulvinar in schizophrenia and schizotypal personality disorder. *Arch. Gen. Psychiatry* 58:133–140.

Byne, W., Buchsbaum, M.S., Mattiace, L.A., Hazlett, E.A., Kemether, E., Elhakem, S.L., Purohit, D.P., Haroutunian, V., and Jones, L. (2002) Postmortem assessment of thalamic nuclear volumes in subjects with schizophrenia. *Am. J. Psychiatry* 159:59–65.

Cannon, T.D., Thompson, P.M., van Erp, T.G., Toga, A.W., Poutanen, V.P., Huttunen, M., Lonnqvist, J., Standerskjold-Nordenstam, C.G., Narr, K.L., Khaledy, M., Zoumalan, C.I., Dail, R., and Kaprio, J. (2002) Cortex mapping reveals regionally specific patterns of genetic and disease-specific gray-matter deficits in twins discordant for schizophrenia. *Proc. Natl. Acad. Sci. USA* 99:3228–3233.

Casanova, M.F., Zito, M., Bigelow, L.B., Berthot, B., Sanders, R.D., and Kleinman, J.E. (1989) Axonal counts of the corpus callosum of schizophrenic patients. *J. Neuropsychiatry Clin. Neurosci.* 1: 391–393.

Chana, G., Landau, S., Beasley, C., Everall, I.P., Cotter, D., Chana, G., Landau, S., Beasley, C., Everall, I.P., and Cotter, D. (2003) Two-dimensional assessment of cytoarchitecture in the anterior cingulate cortex in major depressive disorder, bipolar disorder, and schizophrenia: evidence for decreased neuronal somal size and increased neuronal density. *Biol. Psychiatry* 53:1086–1098.

Chance, S.A., Esiri. M.M., Crow, T.J., Chance, S.A., Esiri, M.M., and Crow, T.J. (2002) Amygdala volume in schizophrenia: post-mortem study and review of magnetic resonance imaging findings [see comment]. *Br. J. Psychiatry* 180:331–338.

Chance, S.A., Highley, J.R., Esiri, M.M., and Crow, T.J. (1999) Fiber content of the fornix in schizophrenia: lack of evidence for a primary limbic encephalopathy. *Am. J. Psychiatry* 156:1720–1724.

Chance, S.A., Tzotzoli, P.M., Vitelli, A., Esiri, M.M., and Crow, T.J. (2004) The cytoarchitecture of sulcal folding in Heschl's sulcus and the temporal cortex in the normal brain and schizophrenia: lamina thickness and cell density. *Neurosci. Lett.* 367:384–388.

Chance, S.A., Walker, M., and Crow, T.J. (2005) Reduced density of calbindin-immunoreactive interneurons in the planum temporale in schizophrenia. *Brain Res.* 1046:32–37.

Christison, G.W., Casanova, M.F., Weinberger, D.R., Rawlings, R., and Kleinman, J.E. (1989) A quantitative investigation of hippocampal pyramidal cell size, shape, and variability of orientation in schizophrenia. *Arch. Gen. Psychiatry* 46:1027–1032.

Chun, J.J., and Shatz, C.J. (1989) Interstitial cells of the adult neocortical white matter are the remnant of the early generated subplate neuron population. *J. Comp. Neurol.* 282:555–569.

Conde, F., Lund, J.S., Jacobowitz, D.M., Baimbridge, K.G., and Lewis, D.A. (1994) Local circuit neurons immunoreactive for calretinin, calbindin D-28k or parvalbumin in monkey prefrontal cortex: distribution and morphology. *J. Comp. Neurol.* 341:95–116.

Convit, A., Wolf, O.T., de Leon, M.J., Patalinjug, M., Kandil, E., Caraos, C., Scherer, A., Saint Louis, L.A., and Cancro, R. (2001) Volumetric analysis of pre-frontal regions: findings in aging and schizophrenia. *Psychiatry Research: Neuroimaging* 107:61–73.

Cotter, D., Landau, S., Beasley, C., Stevenson, R., Chana, G., MacMillan, L., and Everall, I. (2002) The density and spatial distribution of GABAergic neurons, labelled using calcium binding proteins, in the anterior cingulate cortex in major depressive disorder, bipolar disorder, and schizophrenia. *Biol. Psychiatry* 51:377–386.

Cotter, D., Mackay, D., Chana, G., Beasley, C., Landau, S., and Everall, I.P. (2002) Reduced neuronal size and glial cell density in area 9 of the dorsolateral prefrontal cortex in subjects with major depressive disorder. *Cereb. Cortex* 12:386–394.

Cotter, D., Mackay, D., Frangou, S., Hudson, L., and Landau, S. (2004) Cell density and cortical thickness in Heschl's gyrus in schizophrenia, major depression and bipolar disorder. *Br. J. Psychiatry* 185:258–259.

Cotter, D., Mackay, D., Landau, S., Kerwin, R., and Everall, I. (2001) Reduced glial cell density and neuronal size in the anterior cingulate cortex in major depressive disorder. *Arch. Gen. Psychiatry* 58:545–553.

Crespo-Facorro, B., Kim, J.J., Chemerinski, E., Magnotta, V., Andreasen, N.C., and Nopoulos, P. (2004) Morphometry of the superior temporal plane in schizophrenia: relationship to clinical correlates. *J. Neuropsychiatry Clin. Neurosci.* 16:284–294.

Crow, T.J. (1997) Schizophrenia as failure of hemispheric dominance for language. *TINS* 20:339–343.

Cullen, T.J., Walker, M.A., Eastwood, S.L., Esiri, M.M., Harrison, P.J., and Crow, T.J. (2006) Anomalies of asymmetry of pyramidal cell density and structure in dorsolateral prefrontal cortex in schizophrenia. *Br. J. Psychiatry* 188:26–31.

Cullen, T.J., Walker, M.A., Parkinson, N., Craven, R., Crow, T.J., Esiri, M.M., and Harrison, P.J. (2003) A postmortem study of the mediodorsal nucleus of the thalamus in schizophrenia. *Schizophr. Res.* 60:157–166.

Davatzikos, C. (2004) Why voxel-based morphometric analysis should be used with great caution when characterizing group differences. *Neuroimage* 23:17–20.

Deicken, R.F., Eliaz, Y., Chosiad, L., Feiwell, R., and Rogers, L. (2002) Magnetic resonance imaging of the thalamus in male patients with schizophrenia. *Schizophr. Res.* 58(2/3):135–144.

Dickey, C.C., McCarley, R.W., Voglmaier, M.M., Frumin, M., Niznikiewicz, M.A., Hirayasu, Y., Fraone, S., Seidman, L.J., and Shenton, M.E. (2002) Smaller left Heschl's gyrus volume in patients with schizotypal personality disorder. *Am. J. Psychiatry* 159:1521–1527.

Dickey, C.C., McCarley, R.W., Voglemaier, M.M., Niznikiewicz, M. A., Seidman, L.J., Hirayasu, Y., Fischer, I., Teh, E.K., van Rhoads, R., Jakab, M., Kikinis, R., Jolesz, F.A., and Shenton, M.E. (1999) Schizotypal personality disorder and MRI abnormalities of temporal lobe gray matter. *Biol. Psch.* 45:1393–1402.

Dickey, C.C., Salisbury, D.F., Nagy, A.I., Hirayasu, Y., Lee, C.U., McCarley, R.W., and Shenton, M.E. (2004) Follow-up MRI study of prefrontal volumes in first-episode psychotic patients. *Schizophr. Res.* 71:349–351.

Dierks, T., Linden, D.E., Jandl, M., Formisano, E., Goebel, R., Lanfermann, H., and Singer, W. (1999) Activation of Heschl's gyrus during auditory hallucinations. *Neuron* 22:615–621.

Dorph-Petersen, K.A., Pierri, J.N., Sun, Z., Sampson, A.R., and Lewis, D.A. (2004) Stereological analysis of the mediodorsal thalamic nucleus in schizophrenia: volume, neuron number, and cell types. *J. Comp. Neurol.* 472:449–462.

Dorph-Petersen, K.A., Pierri, J.N., Wu, Q., Sampson, A.R., Lewis, D.A., Dorph-Petersen, K.-A., Pierri, J.N., Wu, Q., Sampson, A.R., and Lewis, D.A. (2007) Primary visual cortex volume and total neuron number are reduced in schizophrenia. *J. Comp. Neurol.* 501:290–301.

Dwork, A.J. (1997) Postmortem studies of the hippocampal formation in schizophrenia. *Schizophr. Bull.* 23:385–402.

Dwork, A.J., Mancevski, B., and Rosoklija, G. (2007) White matter and cognitive function in schizophrenia. *Int. J. Neuropsychopharmacol.* 10(4):516–536.

Eastwood, S.L., and Harrison, P.J. (2003) Interstitial white matter neurons express less reelin and are abnormally distributed in schizophrenia: towards an integration of molecular and morphologic aspects of the neurodevelopmental hypothesis. *Mol. Psychiatry* 8:821–831.

Falkai, P., Bogerts, B., Schneider, T., Greve, B., Pfeiffer, U., Pilz, K., Gonsiorzcyk, C., Majtenyi, C., and Ovary, I. (1995) Disturbed planum temporale asymmetry in schizophrenia. A quantitative post-mortem study. *Schiz. Res.* 14:161–176.

Falkai, P., Honer, W.G., David, S., Bogerts, B., Majtenyi, C., and Bayer, T.A. (1999) No evidence for astrogliosis in brains of schizophrenic patients. A post-mortem study. *Neuropath. Appl. Neurobio.* 25:48–53.

Farrow, T.F., Whitford, T.J., Williams, L.M., Gomes, L., and Harris, A.W. (2005) Diagnosis-related regional gray matter loss over two years in first episode schizophrenia and bipolar disorder. *Biol. Psychiatry* 58:713–723.

Foong, J., Maier, M., Clark, C.A., Barker, G.J., Miller, D.H., and Ron, M.A. (2000) Neuropathological abnormalities of the corpus callosum in schizophrenia: a diffusion tensor imaging study. *J. Neuro., Neurosurg. Psychiatry* 68:242–244.

Foong, J., Symms, M.R., Barker, G.J., Maier, M., Woermann, F.G., Miller, D.H., and Ron, M.A. (2001) Neuropathological abnormalities in schizophrenia: evidence from magnetization transfer imaging. *Brain* 124:882–892.

Fornito, A., Yucel, M., Wood, S.J., Adamson, C., Velakoulis, D., Saling, M.M., McGorry, P.D., and Pantelis, C. (2007) Surface-based morphometry of the anterior cingulate cortex in first episode schizophrenia. *Hum. Brain Mapp* 29(4):478–489.

Frangou, S., Sharma, T., Sigmudsson, T., Barta, P., Pearlson, G., and Murray, R.M. (1997) The Maudsley family study 4. Normal planum temporale asymmetry in familial schizophrenia. *Br. J. Psych.* 170:328–333.

Fujiwara, H., Hirao, K., Namiki, C., Yamada, M., Shimizu, M., Fukuyama, H., Hayashi, T., and Murai, T. (2007) Anterior cingulate pathology and social cognition in schizophrenia: a study of gray matter, white matter and sulcal morphometry. *Neuroimage* 36:1236–1245.

Garey, L.J., Ong, W.Y., Patel, T.S., Kanani, M., Davis, A., Mortimer, A.M., Barnes, T.R., and Hirsch, S.R. (1998) Reduced dendritic spine density on cerebral cortical pyramidal neurons in schizophrenia. *J. Neurol. Neurosur. Psychiatry* 65:446–453.

Glantz, L.A., and Lewis, D.A. (2000) Decreased dendritic spine density on prefrontal cortical pyramidal neurons in schizophrenia. *Arch. Gen. Psychiatry* 57:65–73.

Guidotti, A., Auta, J., Davis, J.M., DiGiorgi, G.V., Dwivedi, Y., Grayson, D.R., Impagnatiello, F., Pandey, G., Pesold, C., Sharma, R., Uzunov, D., and Costa, E. (2000) Decrease in reelin and glutamic acid decarboxylase67 (GAD67) expression in schizophrenia and bipolar disorder: a postmortem brain study. *Arch. Gen. Psychiatry* 57:1061–1069.

Gundersen, H.J. (1986) Stereology of arbitrary particles. A review of unbiased number and size estimators and the presentation of some new ones, in memory of William R. Thompson. *J. Microsc.* 143:3–45.

Gur, R.E., and Chin, S. (1999) Laterality in functional brain imaging studies of schizophrenia. *Schizophren. Bull.* 25:141–156.

Gur, R.E., Maany, V., Mozley, P.D., Swanson, C., Bilker, W., and Gur, R.C. (1998) Subcortical MRI volumes in neuroleptic-naive and treated patients with schizophrenia [see comment]. *Am. J. Psychiatry* 155:1711–1717.

Gur, R.E., Turetsky, B.I., Cowell, P.E., Finkelman, C., Maany, B., Grossman, R.I., Arnold, S.E., Bilker, W.B., and Gur, R.C. (2000) Temporolimbic volume reductions in schizophrenia. *Arch. Gen. Psych.* 57:769–775.

Hao, Y., Liu, Z., Jiang, T., Gong, G., Liu, H., Tan, L., Kuang, F., Xu, L., Yi, Y., and Zhang, Z. (2006) White matter integrity of the whole brain is disrupted in first-episode schizophrenia. *Neuroreport* 17:23–26.

Harrison, P.J. (1999) The neuropathology of schizophrenia. A critical review of the data and their interpretation. *Brain* 122:593–624.

Harrison, P.J., and Weinberger, D.R. (2005) Schizophrenia genes, gene expression, and neuropathology: on the matter of their convergence [erratum appears in *Mol. Psychiatry*. 2005 10(4):420]. *Mol. Psychiatry* 10:40–68.

Hashimoto, T., Volk, D.W., Eggan, S.M., Mirnics, K., Pierri, J.N., Sun, Z., Sampson, A.R., and Lewis, D.A. (2003) Gene expression deficits in a subclass of GABA neurons in the prefrontal cortex of subjects with schizophrenia. *J. Neurosci.* 23:6315–6326.

Hazlett, E., Buchsbaum, M.S., Byne, W., Wei, T.C., Spiegel-Cohen, J., Geneve, C., Kinderlehrer, R., Haznedar, M.M., Shihabuddin, L., and Siever, L.J. (1999) Three-dimensional analysis with MRI and PET of the size, shape, and function of the thalamus in the schizophrenia spectrum. *Am. J. Psychiatry* 156:1190–1199.

Heckers, S. (2001) Neuroimaging studies of the hippocampus in schizophrenia. *Hippocampus* 11:520–528.

Heckers, S., Heinsen, H., Heinsen, Y., and Beckmann, H. (1991) Cortex, white matter, and basal ganglia in schizophrenia: a volumetric postmortem study. *Biol. Psychiatry* 29:556–566.

Heckers, S., Stone, D., Walsh, J., Shick, J., Koul, P., and Benes, F.M. (2002) Differential hippocampal expression of glutamic acid decarboxylase 65 and 67 messenger RNA in bipolar disorder and schizophrenia. *Arch. Gen. Psychiatry* 59:521–529.

Henkelman, R.M., Stanisz, G.J., and Graham, S.J. (2001) Magnetization transfer in MRI: a review. *NMR in Biomedicine* 14:57–64.

Highley, J.R., Esiri, M.M., McDonald, B., Cortina-Borja, M., Herron, B.M., and Crow, T.J. (1999) The size and fibre composition of the corpus callosum with respect to gender and schizophrenia: a post-mortem study. *Brain* 122(Pt 1):99–110.

Highley, J.R., Esiri, M.M., McDonald, B., Roberts, H.C., Walker, M.A., and Crow, T.J. (1999) The size and fiber composition of the anterior commissure with respect to gender and schizophrenia. *Biol. Psychiatry* 45:1120–1127.

Highley, J.R., Walker, M.A., Esiri, M.M., Crow, T.J., and Harrison, P.J. (2002) Asymmetry of the uncinate fasciculus: a post-mortem study of normal subjects and patients with schizophrenia. *Cereb. Cortex* 12:1218–1224.

Highley, J.R., Walker, M.A., McDonald, B., Crow, T.J., and Esiri, M.M. (2003) Size of hippocampal pyramidal neurons in schizophrenia. *Br. J. Psychiatry* 183:414–417.

Hill, J.J., Hashimoto, T., and Lewis, D.A. (2006) Molecular mechanisms contributing to dendritic spine alterations in the prefrontal cortex of subjects with schizophrenia. *Mol. Psychiatry* 11:557–566.

Hirayasu, Y., McCarley, R.W., Salizbury, D.F., Tanaka, S., Kwon, J. S., Frumin, M., Snyderman, D., Yurgelun-Todd, D., Kikinis, R., Jolesz, F.A., and Shenton, M.E. (2000) Planum temporale and Heschl gyrus volume reduction in schziophrenia. *Arch. Gen. Psych.* 57:692–699.

Hirayasu, Y., Shenton, M.E., Salisbury, D.F., Dickey, C.C., Fischer, I.A., Mazzoni, P., Kisler, T., Arakaki, H., Kwon, J.S., Anderson, J.E., Yurgelun-Todd, D., Tohen, M., and McCarley, R.W. (1998) Lower left temporal lobe MRI volumes in patients with first-episode schizophrenia compared with psychotic patients with first-episode affective disorder and normal subjects. *Am. J. Psychiatry* 155:1384–1391.

Hirayasu, Y., Tanaka, S., Shenton, M.E., Salisbury, D.F., DeSantis, M.A., Levitt, J.J., Wible, C., Yurgelun-Todd, D., Kikinis, R., Jolesz, F.A., and McCarley, R.W. (2001) Prefrontal gray matter volume reduction in first episode schizophrenia. *Cereb. Cortex* 11:374–381.

Hof, P.R., Haroutunian, V., Copland, C., Davis, K.L., and Buxbaum, J.D. (2002) Molecular and cellular evidence for an oligodendrocyte abnormality in schizophrenia. *Neurochem. Res.* 27:1193–1200.

Hof, P.R., Haroutunian, V., Friedrich, V.L., Jr., Byne, W., Buitron, C., Perl, D.P., and Davis, K.L. (2003) Loss and altered spatial distribution of oligodendrocytes in the superior frontal gyrus in schizophrenia. *Biol. Psychiatry* 53:1075–1085.

Hoptman, M.J., Ardekani, B.A., Butler, P.D., Nierenberg, J., Javitt, D.C., and Lim, K.O. (2004) DTI and impulsivity in schizophrenia: a first voxelwise correlational analysis. *Neuroreport* 15:2467–2470.

Hoptman, M.J., Gunning-Dixon, F.M., Murphy, C.F., Lim, K.O., and Alexopoulos, G.S. (2006) Structural neuroimaging research methods in geriatric depression. *Am. J. Geriatr. Psychiatry* 14:812–822.

Hoptman, M.J., Volavka, J., Czobor, P., Gerig, G., Chakos, M., Blocher, J., Citrome, L.L., Sheitman, B., Lindenmayer, J.P., Lieberman, J. A., and Bilder, R.M. (2006) Aggression and quantitative MRI measures of caudate in chronic schizophrenia and schizoaffective disorder. *J. Neuropsychiatry and Clin. Neurosci.* 18:509–515.

Hoptman, M.J., Volavka, J., Johnson, G., Weiss, E., Bilder, R.M., and Lim, K.O. (2002) Frontal white matter microstructure, aggression, and impulsivity in men with schizophrenia: a preliminary study. *Biol. Psychiatry* 52:9–14.

Hoptman, M.J., Volavka, J., Weiss, E.M., Czobor, P., Szeszko, P.R., Gerig, G., Chakos, M., Blocher, J., Citrome, L.L., Lindenmayer, J.P., Sheitman, B., Lieberman, J.A., and Bilder, R.M. (2005) Quantitative MRI measures of orbitofrontal cortex in patients with chronic schizophrenia or schizoaffective disorder. *Psychiatry Research: Neuroimaging* 140:133–145.

Hubl, D., Koenig, T., Strik, W., Federspiel, A., Kreis, R., Boesch, C., Maier, S.E., Schroth, G., Lovblad, K., and Dierks, T. (2004) Pathways that make voices: white matter changes in auditory hallucinations. *Arch. Gen. Psychiatry* 61:658–668.

Javitt, D.C., Shelley, A.-M., and Ritter, W. (2000) Associated deficits in mismatch negativity generation and tone matching in schizophrenia. *Clin. Neuropsych.* 111:1733–1737.

Job, D.E., Whalley, H.C., McConnell, S., Glabus, M., Johnstone, E.C., and Lawrie, S.M. (2003) Voxel-based morphometry of grey matter densities in subjects at high risk of schizophrenia. *Schizophr. Res.* 64:1–13.

Kalus, P., Buri, C., Slotboom, J., Gralla, J., Remonda, L., Dierks, T., Strik, W.K., Schroth, G., and Kiefer, C. (2004) Volumetry and diffusion tensor imaging of hippocampal subregions in schizophrenia. *Neuroreport* 15:867–871.

Kalus, P., Muller, T.J., Zuschratter, W., and Senitz, D. (2000) The dendritic architecture of prefrontal pyramidal neurons in schizophrenic patients. *Neuroreport* 11:3621–3625.

Kalus, P., Senitz, D., and Beckmann, H. (1997) Altered distribution of parvalbumin-immunoreactive local circuit neurons in the anterior cingulate cortex of schizophrenic patients. *Psychiatry Res.* 75:49–59.

Kanaan, R.A., Shergill, S.S., Barker, G.J., Catani, M., Ng, V.W., Howard, R., McGuire, P.K., and Jones, D.K. (2006) Tract-specific anisotropy measurements in diffusion tensor imaging. *Psychiatry Res.* 146:73–82.

Kanaan, R.A.A., Kim, J.S., Kaufmann, W.E., Pearlson, G.D., Barker, G.J., and McGuire, P.K. (2005) Diffusion tensor imaging in schizophrenia. *Biol. Psychiatry* 58:921–929.

Kasai, K., Shenton, M.E., Salisbury, D.F., Hirayasu, Y., Onitsuka, T., Spencer, M.H., Yurgelun-Todd, D.A., Kikinis, R., Jolesz, F.A., and McCarley, R.W. (2003) Progressive decrease of left Heschl gyrus and planum temporale gray matter volume in first-episode schizophrenia: a longitudinal magnetic resonance imaging study. *Arch. Gen. Psychiatry* 60:766–775.

Kawasaki, Y., Suzuki, M., Nohara, S., Hagino, H., Takahashi, T., Matsui, M., Yamashita, I., Chitnis, X.A., McGuire, P.K., Seto, H., and Kurachi, M. (2004) Structural brain differences in patients with schizophrenia and schizotypal disorder demonstrated by voxel-based morphometry. *Eur. Arch. Psychiatry Clin. Neurosci.* 254:406–414.

Kemether, E.M., Buchsbaum, M.S., Byne, W., Hazlett, E.A., Haznedar, M., Brickman, A.M., Platholi, J., and Bloom, R. (2003) Magnetic resonance imaging of mediodorsal, pulvinar, and centromedian nuclei of the thalamus in patients with schizophrenia. *Arch. Gen. Psychiatry* 60:983–991.

Kirkpatrick, B., Conley, R.C., Kakoyannis, A., Reep, R.L., and Roberts, R.C. (1999) Interstitial cells of the white matter in the inferior parietal cortex in schizophrenia: an unbiased cell-counting study. *Synapse* 34:95–102.

Kirkpatrick, B., Messias, N.C., Conley, R.R., and Roberts, R.C. (2003) Interstitial cells of the white matter in the dorsolateral prefrontal cortex in deficit and nondeficit schizophrenia. *J. Nerv. Ment. Dis.* 191:563–567.

Kitamura, H., Matsuzawa, H., Shioiri, T., Someya, T., Kwee, I.L., and Nakada, T. (2005) Diffusion tensor analysis in chronic schizophrenia. A preliminary study on a high-field (3.0T) system. *Eur. Arch. Psychiatry Clin. Neurosci.* 255:313–318.

Kolluri, N., Sun, Z., Sampson, A.R., and Lewis, D.A. (2005) Lamina-specific reductions in dendritic spine density in the prefrontal cortex of subjects with schizophrenia. *Am. J. Psychiatry* 162:1200–1202.

Kolomeets, N.S., Orlovskaya, D.D., Rachmanova, V.I., and Uranova, N.A. (2005) Ultrastructural alterations in hippocampal mossy fiber synapses in schizophrenia: a postmortem morphometric study. *Synapse* 57:47–55.

Konick, L.C., and Friedman, L. (2001) Meta-analysis of thalamic size in schizophrenia. *Biol. Psychiatry* 49:28–38.

Konopaske, G.T., Sweet, R.A., Wu, Q., Sampson, A., and Lewis, D.A. (2006) Regional specificity of chandelier neuron axon terminal alterations in schizophrenia. *Neuroscience* 138:189–196.

Kostovic, I., and Rakic, P. (1980) Cytology and time of origin of interstitial neurons in the white matter in infant and adult human and monkey telencephalon. *J. Neurocytol.* 9:219–242.

Kostovic, I., and Rakic, P. (1990) Developmental history of the transient subplate zone in the visual and somatosensory cortex of the macaque monkey and human brain. *J. Comp. Neurol.* 297:441–470.

Kreczmanski, P., Heinsen, H., Mantua, V., Woltersdorf, F., Masson, T., Ulfig, N., Schmidt-Kastner, R., Korr, H., Steinbusch, H.W., Hof, P.R., and Schmitz, C. (2007) Volume, neuron density and total neuron number in five subcortical regions in schizophrenia. *Brain* 130:678–692.

Kreczmanski, P., Schmidt-Kastner, R., Heinsen, H., Steinbusch, H.W., Hof, P.R., and Schmitz, C. (2005) Stereological studies of capillary length density in the frontal cortex of schizophrenics. *Acta Neuropathologica* 109:510–518.

Kubicki, M., McCarley, R., Westin, C.F., Park, H.J., Maier, S., Kikinis, R., Jolesz, F.A., and Shenton, M.E. (2007) A review of diffusion tensor imaging studies in schizophrenia. *J. Psychiatr. Res.* 41:15–30.

Kubicki, M., Park, H., Westin, C.F., Nestor, P.G., Mulkern, R.V., Maier, S.E., Niznikiewicz, M., Connor, E.E., Levitt, J.J., Frumin, M., Kikinis, R., Jolesz, F.A., McCarley, R.W., and Shenton, M.E. (2005) DTI and MTR abnormalities in schizophrenia: analysis of white matter integrity. *Neuroimage* 26:1109–1118.

Kubicki, M., Westin, C.F., Nestor, P.G., Wible, C.G., Frumin, M., Maier, S.E., Kikinis, R., Jolesz, F.A., McCarley, R.W., and Shenton, M.E. (2003) Cingulate fasciculus integrity disruption in schizophrenia: a magnetic resonance diffusion tensor imaging study. *Biol. Psychiatry* 54:1171–1180.

Kumra, S., Ashtari, M., Cervellione, K.L., Henderson, I., Kester, H., Roofeh, D., Wu, J., Clarke, T., Thaden, E., Kane, J.M., Rhinewine, J., Lencz, T., Diamond, A., Ardekani, B.A., and Szeszko, P.R. (2005) White matter abnormalities in early-onset schizophrenia: a voxel-based diffusion tensor imaging study. *J. Am. Acad. Child Adolesc. Psychiatry* 44:934–941.

Kuperberg, G.R., Broome, M.R., McGuire, P.K., David, A.S., Eddy, M., Ozawa, F., Goff, D., West, W.C., Williams, S.C., van der Kouwe, A.J., Salat, D.H., Dale, A.M., and Fischl, B. (2003) Regionally localized thinning of the cerebral cortex in schizophrenia. *Arch. Gen. Psychiatry* 60:878–888.

Kuroki, N., Kubicki, M., Nestor, P.G., Salisbury, D.F., Park, H.J., Levitt, J.J., Woolston, S., Frumin, M., Niznikiewicz, M., Westin, C.F., Maier, S.E., McCarley, R.W., and Shenton, M.E. (2006) Fornix integrity and hippocampal volume in male schizophrenic patients. *Biol. Psychiatry* 60:22–31.

Kwon, J.S., McCarley, R.W., Hirayasu, Y., Anderson, J.E., Fischer, I.A., Kikinis, R., Jolesz, F.A., and Shenton, M.E. (1999) Left planum temporale volume reduction in schizophrenia. *Arch. Gen. Psychiatry* 56:142–148.

Laakso, M.P., Tiihonen, J., Syvalahti, E., Vilkman, H., Laakso, A., Alakare, B., Rakkolainen, V., Salokangas, R.K., Koivisto, E., and Hietala, J. (2001) A morphometric MRI study of the hippocampus in first-episode, neuroleptic-naive schizophrenia. *Schizophr. Res.* 50:3–7.

Lassmann, H., Bartsch, U., Montag, D., and Schachner, M. (1997) Dying-back oligodendrogliopathy: a late sequel of myelin-associated glycoprotein deficiency. *Glia* 19:104–110.

Law, A.J., and Harrison, P.J. (2003) The distribution and morphology of prefrontal cortex pyramidal neurons identified using anti-neurofilament antibodies SMI32, N200 and FNP7. Normative data and a comparison in subjects with schizophrenia, bipolar disorder or major depression. *J. Psychiatr. Res.* 37:487–499.

Lawrie, S.M., Whalley, H.C., Abukmeil, S.S., Kestelman, J.N., Donnelly, L., Miller, P., Best, J.J., Owens, D.G., and Johnstone, E.C.

(2001) Brain structure, genetic liability, and psychotic symptoms in subjects at high risk of developing schizophrenia. *Biol. Psychiatry* 49:811–823.

Lewis, D.A., Cruz, D.A., Melchitzky, D.S., and Pierri, J.N. (2001) Lamina-specific deficits in parvalbumin-immunoreactive varicosities in the prefrontal cortex of subjects with schizophrenia: evidence for fewer projections from the thalamus. *Am. J. Psychiatry* 158:1411–1422.

Lieberman, J., Chakos, M., Wu, H., Alvir, J., Hoffman, E., Robinson, D., and Bilder, R. (2001) Longitudinal study of brain morphology in first episode schizophrenia. *Biol. Psychiatry* 48:487–499.

Lim, K.O., Ardekani, B.A., Nierenberg, J., Butler, P.D., Javitt, D.C., and Hoptman, M.J. (2006) Voxelwise correlational analyses of white matter integrity in multiple cognitive domains in schizophrenia. *Am. J. Psychiatry* 163:2008–2010.

Lim, K.O., Hedehus, M., Moseley, M., de Crespigny, A., Sullivan, E.V., and Pfefferbaum, A. (1999) Compromised white matter tract integrity in schizophrenia inferred from diffusion tensor imaging. *Arch. Gen. Psychiatry* 56:367–374.

Maldonado-Aviles, J.G., Wu, Q., Sampson, A.R., and Lewis, D.A. (2006) Somal size of immunolabeled pyramidal cells in the prefrontal cortex of subjects with schizophrenia. *Biol. Psychiatry* 60:226–234.

Mancevski, B., Ilievski, B., Trencevska, I., Ortakov, V., Serafimova, T., Rosoklija, G., Keilp, J., and Dwork, A.J. (2007) Frontal myelin histology and cognitive function in schizophrenia. *Schizophr. Bull.* 33:270.

Marner, L., and Pakkenberg, B. (2003) Total length of nerve fibers in prefrontal and global white matter of chronic schizophrenics. *J. Psychiatr. Res.* 37:539–547.

McCullumsmith, R.E., Gupta, D., Beneyto, M., Kreger, E., Haroutunian, V., Davis, K.L., and Meador-Woodruff, J.H. (2007) Expression of transcripts for myelination-related genes in the anterior cingulate cortex in schizophrenia. *Schizophr. Res.* 90:15–27.

Meisenzahl, E.M., et al. (2002) Does the definition of borders of the planum temporale influence the results in schizophrenia? *Am. J. Psych.* 159:1198–1200.

Meyer, G., Wahle, P., Castaneyra-Perdomo, A., and Ferres-Torres, R. (1992) Morphology of neurons in the white matter of the adult human neocortex. *Exp. Brain Res.* 88:204–212.

Miguel-Hidalgo, J.J., Dubey, P., Shao, Q., Stockmeier, C., and Rajkowska, G. (2005) Unchanged packing density but altered size of neurofilament immunoreactive neurons in the prefrontal cortex in schizophrenia and major depression. *Schizophr. Res.* 76:159–171.

Minami, T., Nobuhara, K., Okugawa, G., Takase, K., Yoshida, T., Sawada, S., Ha-Kawa, S., Ikeda, K., and Kinoshita, T. (2003) Diffusion tensor magnetic resonance imaging of disruption of regional white matter in schizophrenia. *Neuropsychobiology* 47:141–145.

Miyakawa, T., Sumiyoshi, S., Deshimaru, M., Suzuki, T., and Tomonari, H. (1972) Electron microscopic study on schizophrenia. Mechanism of pathological changes. *Acta Neuropathologica* 20:67–77.

Molina, V., Sanz, J., Benito, C., and Palomo, T. (2004) Direct association between orbitofrontal atrophy and the response of psychotic symptoms to olanzapine in schizophrenia. *Intl. Clin. Psychopharmacol.* 19:221–228.

Montag, D., Giese, K.P., Bartsch, U., Martini, R., Lang, Y., Bluthmann, H., Karthigasan, J., Kirschner, D.A., Wintergerst, E.S., Nave, K.A., et al. (1994) Mice deficient for the myelin-associated glycoprotein show subtle abnormalities in myelin. *Neuron* 13:229–246.

Mori, S., Crain, B.J., Chacko, V.P., and van Zijl, P.C.M. (1999) Three-dimensional tracking of axonal projections in the brain by magnetic resonance imaging. *Ann. Neurol.* 45:265–269.

Nakamura, M., Nestor, P.G., McCarley, R.W., Levitt, J.J., Hsu, L., Kawashima, T., Niznikiewicz, M., and Shenton, M.E. (2007) Altered orbitofrontal sulcogyral pattern in schizophrenia. *Brain* 130:693–707.

Nakamura, M., Salisbury, D.F., Hirayasu, Y., Bouix, S., Pohl, K.M., Yoshida, T., Koo, M.S., Shenton, M.E., and McCarley, R.W. (2007) Neocortical gray matter volume in first-episode schizophrenia and first-episode affective psychosis: a cross-sectional and longitudinal MRI study. *Biol. Psychiatry* 62(7):773–783.

Narr, K.L., Bilder, R.M., Toga, A.W., Woods, R.P., Rex, D.E., Szeszko, P.R., Robinson, D., Sevy, S., Gunduz-Bruce, H., Wang, Y.P., DeLuca, H., and Thompson, P.M. (2005) Mapping cortical thickness and gray matter concentration in first episode schizophrenia. *Cereb. Cortex* 15:708–719.

Narr, K.L., Toga, A.W., Szeszko, P., Thompson, P.M., Woods, R.P., Robinson, D., Sevy, S., Wang, Y., Schrock, K., and Bilder, R.M. (2005) Cortical thinning in cingulate and occipital cortices in first episode schizophrenia. *Biol. Psychiatry* 58:32–40.

Nasrallah, H.A., McCalley-Whitters, M., Bigelow, L.B., and Rauscher, F.P. (1983) A histological study of the corpus callosum in chronic schizophrenia. *Psychiatry Res.* 8:251–260.

Nestor, P.G., Kubicki, M., Gurrera, R.J., Niznikiewicz, M., Frumin, M., McCarley, R.W., and Shenton, M.E. (2004) Neuropsychological correlates of diffusion tensor imaging in schizophrenia. *Neuropsychology* 18:629–637.

O'Driscoll, G.A., Florencio, P.S., Gagnon, D., Wolff, A.V., Benkelfat, C., Mikula, L., Lal, S., and Evans, A.C. (2001) Amygdala-hippocampal volume and verbal memory in first-degree relatives of schizophrenic patients. *Psychiatry Res.* 107:75–85.

Ohnuma, T., Kimura, M., Takahashi, T., Iwamoto, N., and Arai, H. (1997) A magnetic resonance imaging study in first-episode disorganized-type patients with schizophrenia. *Psychiatry Clin. Neurosci.* 51:9–15.

Okugawa, G., Nobuhara, K., Sugimoto, T., and Kinoshita, T. (2005) Diffusion tensor imaging study of the middle cerebellar peduncles in patients with schizophrenia. *Cerebellum* 4:123–127.

Onitsuka, T., Shenton, M.E., Salisbury, D.F., Dickey, C.C., Kasai, K., Toner, S.K., Frumin, M., Kikinis, R., Jolesz, F.A., and McCarley, R.W. (2004) Middle and inferior temporal gyrus gray matter volume abnormalities in chronic schizophrenia: an MRI study. *Am. J. Psychiatry* 161:1603–1611.

Pakkenberg, B. (1992) Stereological quantitation of human brains from normal and schizophrenic individuals. *Acta Neurol. Scand. Supplementum* 137:20–33.

Pakkenberg, B. (1993) Total nerve cell number in neocortex in chronic schizophrenics and controls estimated using optical disectors. *Biol. Psychiatry* 34:768–772.

Pantazopoulos, H., Lange, N., Baldessarini, R.J., and Berretta, S. (2007) Parvalbumin neurons in the entorhinal cortex of subjects diagnosed with bipolar disorder or schizophrenia. *Biol. Psychiatry* 61:640–652.

Pantelis, C., Velakoulis, D., McGorry, P.D., Wood, S.J., Suckling, J., Phillips, L.J., Yung, A.R., Bullmore, E.T., Brewer, W., Soulsby, B., Desmond, P., and McGuire, P.K. (2002) Neuroanatomical abnormalities before and after onset of psychosis: a cross-sectional and longitudinal MRI comparison. *Lancet* 361:281–288.

Park, M., Salgado, J.M., Ostroff, L., Helton, T.D., Robinson, C.G., Harris, K.M., and Ehlers, M.D. (2006) Plasticity-induced growth of dendritic spines by exocytic trafficking from recycling endosomes. *Neuron* 52:817–830.

Pierri, J.N., Volk, C.L., Auh, S., Sampson, A., and Lewis, D.A. (2001) Decreased somal size of deep layer 3 pyramidal neurons in the prefrontal cortex of subjects with schizophrenia. *Arch. Gen. Psychiatry* 58:466–473.

Pierri, J.N., Volk, C.L., Auh, S., Sampson, A., and Lewis, D.A. (2003) Somal size of prefrontal cortical pyramidal neurons in schizophrenia: differential effects across neuronal subpopulations. *Biol. Psychiatry* 54:111–120.

Popken, G.J., Bunney, W.E., Jr., Potkin, S.G., and Jones, E.G. (2000) Subnucleus-specific loss of neurons in medial thalamus of schizophrenics. *Proc. Natl. Acad. Sci. USA* 97:9276–9280.

Prasad, K.M., Sahni, S.D., Rohm, B.R., and Keshavan, M.S. (2005) Dorsolateral prefrontal cortex morphology and short-term outcome in first-episode schizophrenia. *Psychiatry Res.* 140:147–155.

Premkumar, P., Kumari, V., Corr, P.J., and Sharma, T. (2006) Frontal lobe volumes in schizophrenia: effects of stage and duration of illness. *J. Psychiatr. Res.* 40:627–637.

Price, G., Cercignani, M., Bagary, M.S., Barnes, T.R., Barker, G.J., Joyce, E.M., and Ron, M.A. (2006) A volumetric MRI and magnetization transfer imaging follow-up study of patients with first-episode schizophrenia. *Schizophr. Res.* 87:100–108.

Radewicz, K., Garey, L.J., Gentleman, S.M., and Reynolds, R. (2000) Increase in HLA-DR immunoreactive microglia in frontal and temporal cortex of chronic schizophrenics. *J. Neuropathol. Experim. Neurol.* 59:137–150.

Rajkowska, G., Halaris, A., and Selemon, L.D. (2001) Reductions in neuronal and glial density characterize the dorsolateral prefrontal cortex in bipolar disorder. *Biol. Psychiatry* 49:741–752.

Rajkowska, G., Miguel-Hidalgo, J.J., Wei, J., Dilley, G., Pittman, S.D., Meltzer, H.Y., Overholser, J.C., Roth, B.L., and Stockmeier, C.A. (1999) Morphometric evidence for neuronal and glial prefrontal cell pathology in major depression. *Biol. Psychiatry* 45:1085–1098.

Rajkowska, G., Selemon, L.D., and Goldman-Rakic, P.S. (1998) Neuronal and glial somal size in the prefrontal cortex: a postmortem morphometric study of schizophrenia and Huntington disease. *Arch. Gen. Psychiatry* 55:215–224.

Reynolds, G.P., and Beasley, C.L. (2001) GABAergic neuronal subtypes in the human frontal cortex--development and deficits in schizophrenia. *J. Chem. Neuroanat.* 22:95–100.

Roberts, R.C., Conley, R., Kung, L., Peretti, F.J., and Chute, D.J. (1996) Reduced striatal spine size in schizophrenia: a postmortem ultrastructural study. *Neuroreport* 7:1214–1218.

Rojas, D.C., Teale, P., Sheeder, J., Simon, J., and Reite, M. (1997) Sex-specific expression of Heschl's gyrus functional and structural abnormalities in paranoid schizophrenia. *Am. J. Psychiatry* 154:1655–1662.

Rosoklija, G., Mancevski, B., Ilievski, B., Perera, T., Lisanby, S.H., Coplan, J.D., Duma, A., Serafimova, T., and Dwork, A.J. (2003) Optimization of Golgi methods for impregnation of brain tissue from humans and monkeys. *J. Neurosci. Methods* 131:1–7.

Rosoklija, G., Rauski, S., Mancevski, B., Berman, R., Duma, A., Serafimova, T., Filipovska, A., Kurzon, M., Mann, J.J., and Dwork, A.J. (2004) Spine loss on subicular apical dendrites in schizophrenia and mood disorders is not the result of medications or age. *Soc. Neurosci. Abstracts* #1022.8.

Rosoklija, G., Toomayan, G., Ellis, S.P., Keilp, J., Mann, J.J., Latov, N., Hays, A.P., and Dwork, A.J. (2000) Structural abnormalities of subicular dendrites in subjects with schizophrenia and mood disorders: preliminary findings. *Arch. Gen. Psychiatry* 57:349–356.

Roth, R.M., Flashman, L.A., Saykin, A.J., McAllister, T.W., and Vidaver, R. (2004) Apathy in schizophrenia: reduced frontal lobe volume and neuropsychological deficits. *Am. J. Psychiatry* 161:157–159.

Roy, K., Murtie, J.C., El-Khodor, B.F., Edgar, N., Sardi, S.P., Hooks, B.M., Benoit-Marand, M., Chen, C., Moore, H., O'Donnell, P., Brunner, D., and Corfas, G. (2007) Loss of erbB signaling in oligodendrocytes alters myelin and dopaminergic function, a potential mechanism for neuropsychiatric disorders. *Proc. Natl. Acad. Sci. USA* 104(9):8131–8136.

Rupp, C.I., Fleischhacker, W.W., Kemmler, G., Kremser, C., Bilder, R.M., Mechtcheriakov, S., Szeszko, P.R., Walch, T., Scholtz, A. W., Klimbacher, M., Maier, C., Albrecht, G., Lechner-Schoner, T., Felber, S., and Hinterhuber, H. (2005) Olfactory functions and volumetric measures of orbitofrontal and limbic regions in schizophrenia. *Schizophr. Res.* 74:149–161.

Salisbury, D.F., Kuroki, N., Kasai, K., Shenton, M.E., and McCarley, R.W. (2007) Progressive and interrelated functional and structural evidence of post-onset brain reduction in schizophrenia. *Arch. Gen. Psychiatry* 64:521–529.

Sallet, P.C., Elkis, H., Alves, T.M., Oliveira, J.R., Sassi, E., de Castro, C.C., Busatto, G.F., and Gattaz, W.F. (2003) Rightward cerebral asymmetry in subtypes of schizophrenia according to Leonhard's classification and to DSM-IV: a structural MRI study. *Psychiatry Res.* 123:65–79.

Sanfilipo, M., Lafargue, T., Rusinek, H., Arena, L., Loneragan, C., Lautin, A., Feiner, D., Rotrosen, J., and Wolkin, A. (2000) Volumetric measure of the frontal and temporal lobe regions of schizophrenia. *Arch. Gen. Psych.* 57:471–480.

Sanfilipo, M., Lafargue, T., Rusinek, H., Arena, L., Loneragan, C., Lautin, A., Rotrosen, J., and Wolkin, A. (2002) Cognitive performance in schizophrenia: relationship to regional brain volumes and psychiatric symptoms. *Psychiatry Res.* 116:1–23.

Sapara, A., Cooke, M., Fannon, D., Francis, A., Buchanan, R.W., Anilkumar, A.P., Barkataki, I., Aasen, I., Kuipers, E., and Kumari, V. (2007) Prefrontal cortex and insight in schizophrenia: a volumetric MRI study. *Schizophr. Res.* 89:22–34.

Seidman, L.J., Goldstein, J.M., Goodman, J.M., Koren, D., Turner, W.M., Faraone, S.V., and Tsuang, M.T. (1997) Sex differences in olfactory identification and Wisconsin Card Sorting performance in schizophrenia: relationship to attention and verbal ability. *Biol. Psychiatry* 42:104–115.

Selemon, L.D., Mrzljak, J., Kleinman, J.E., Herman, M.M., Goldman-Rakic, P.S., Selemon, L.D., Mrzljak, J., Kleinman, J.E., Herman, M.M., and Goldman-Rakic, P.S. (2003) Regional specificity in the neuropathologic substrates of schizophrenia: a morphometric analysis of Broca's area 44 and area 9. *Arch. Gen. Psychiatry* 60:69–77.

Selemon, L.D., Rajkowska, G., and Goldman-Rakic, P.S. (1995) Abnormally high neuronal density in the schizophrenic cortex. A morphometric analysis of prefrontal area 9 and occipital area 17. *Arch. Gen. Psychiatry* 52:805–818; discussion 819–820.

Selemon, L.D., Rajkowska, G., and Goldman-Rakic, P.S. (1998) Elevated neuronal density in prefrontal area 46 in brains from schizophrenic patients: application of a three-dimensional, stereologic counting method. *J. Comp. Neurol.* 392:402–412.

Shapleske, J., Rossell, S.L., Simmons, A., David, A.S., and Woodruff, P.W. (2001) Are auditory hallucinations the consequence of abnormal cerebral lateralization? A morphometric MRI study of the sylvian fissure and planum temporale. *Biol. Psychiatry* 49: 685–693.

Shapleske, J., Rossell, S.L., Woodruff, P.W.R., David, A.S. (1999) The planum temporale: a systematic quantitative review of its structural, functional and clinical significance. *Brain Res. Rev.* 29: 26–49.

Shenton, M.E., Dickey, C.C., Frumin, M., and McCarley, R.W. (2001) A review of MRI findings in schizophrenia. *Schizophr. Res.* 49: 1–52.

Shergill, S.S., Kanaan, R.A., Chitnis, X.A., O'Daly, O., Jones. D.K., Frangou, S., Williams, S.C., Howard, R.J., Barker, G.J., Murray, R.M., and McGuire, P. (2007) A diffusion tensor imaging study of fasciculi in schizophrenia. *Am. J. Psychiatry* 164:467–473.

Smiley, J.F., Dwork, A.J., Mancevski, B., Rosoklija, G., Duma, A., and Javitt, D.C. (2005) Neuron number, density and size in the primary auditory cortex in schizophrenia. *Schizophr. Bull.* 31: 183.

Smiley, J.F., Dwork, A.J., Mancevski, B., Rosoklija, G., Duma, A., and Javitt, D.C. (2007) Auditory cortex width, hemispheric asymmetry and schizophrenia. *Schizophrenia Bull.* 33:272.

Staal, W.G., Pol, H.E.H., Schnack, H., van der Schot, A.C., and Kahn, R.S. (1998) Partial volume decrease of the thalamus in relatives of patients with schizophrenia. *Am. J. Psychiatry* 155: 1784–1786.

Steen, R.G., Mull, C., McClure, R., Hamer, R.M., and Lieberman, J.A. (2006) Brain volume in first-episode schizophrenia: systematic review and meta-analysis of magnetic resonance imaging studies. *Br. J. Psychiatry* 188:510–518.

Sumich, A., Chitnis, X.A., Fannon, D.G., O'Ceallaigh, S., Doku, V. C., Falrowicz, A., Marshall, N., Matthew, V.M., Potter, M., and Sharma, T. (2002) Temporal lobe abnormalities in first-episode psychosis. *Am. J. Psychiatry* 159:1232–1235.

Sun, Z., Wang, F., Cui, L., Breeze, J., Du, X., Wang, X., Cong, Z., Zhang, H., Li, B., Hong, N., and Zhang, D. (2003) Abnormal anterior cingulum in patients with schizophrenia: a diffusion tensor imaging study. *Neuroreport* 14:1833–1836.

Sweet, R.A., Bergen, S.E., Sun, Z., Sampson, A.R., Pierri, J.N., and Lewis, D.A. (2004) Pyramidal cell size reduction in schizophrenia: evidence for involvement of auditory feedforward circuits. *Biol. Psychiatry* 55:1128–1137.

Sweet, R.A., Pierri, J.N., Auh, S., Sampson, A.R., and Lewis, D.A. (2003) Reduced pyramidal cell somal volume in auditory association cortex of subjects with schizophrenia. *Neuropsychopharmacology* 28:599–609.

Szeszko, P.R., Bilder, R.M., Dunlop, J.A., Walder, D.J., and Lieberman, J.A. (1999) Longitudinal assessment of methylhenidate effects on oral word production and symptoms in first-episode schizophrenia at acute and stabilized phases. *Biol. Psychiatry* 45: 680–686.

Szeszko, P.R., Goldberg, E., Gunduz-Bruce, H., Ashtari, M., Robinson, D., Malhotra, A.K., Lencz, T., Bates, J., Crandall, D.T., Kane, J.M., and Bilder, R.M. (2003) Smaller anterior hippocampal formation volume in antipsychotic-naive patients with first-episode schizophrenia. *Am. J. Psychiatry* 160:2190–2197.

Szeszko, P.R., Robinson, D.G., Ashtari, M., Vogel, J., Betensky, J., Sevy, S., Ardekani, B.A., Lencz, T., Malhotra, A.K., McCormack, J., Miller, R., Lim, K.O., Gunduz-Bruce, H., Kane, J.M., and Bilder, R.M. (2007) Clinical and neuropsychological correlates of white matter abnormalities in recent onset schizophrenia. *Neuropsychopharmacology* 33(5):976–984.

Szeszko, P.R., Strous, R.D., Goldman, R.S., Ashtari, M., Knuth, K. H., Lieberman, J.A., and Bilder, R.M. (2002) Neuropsychological correlates of hippocampal volumes in patients experiencing a first episode of schizophrenia. *Am. J. Psychiatry* 159:217–226.

Takahashi, T., Suzuki, M., Zhou, S.Y., Tanino, R., Hagino, H., Kawasaki, Y., Matsui, M., Seto, H., and Kurachi, M. (2006) Morphologic alterations of the parcellated superior temporal gyrus in schizophrenia spectrum. *Schizophr. Res.* 83:131–143.

Thune, J.J., Uylings, H.B., Pakkenberg, B., Thune, J.J., Uylings, H.B., and Pakkenberg, B. (2001) No deficit in total number of neurons in the prefrontal cortex in schizophrenics. *J. Psychiatr. Res.* 35: 15–21.

Tooney, P.A., and Chahl, L.A. (2004) Neurons expressing calcium-binding proteins in the prefrontal cortex in schizophrenia. *Progr. Neuro-Psychopharmacol. Biol. Psychiatry* 28:273–278.

Torrey, E.F., Barci, B.M., Webster, M.J., Bartko, J.J., Meador-Woodruff, J.H., and Knable, M.B. (2005) Neurochemical markers for schizophrenia, bipolar disorder, and major depression in postmortem brains. *Biol. Psychiatry* 57:252–260.

Uranova, N., Orlovskaya, D., Vikhreva, O., Zimina, I., Kolomeets, N., Vostrikov, V., and Rachmanova, V. (2001) Electron microscopy of oligodendroglia in severe mental illness. *Brain Res. Bull.* 55:597–610.

Uranova, N.A., Vostrikov, V.M., Orlovskaya, D.D., and Rachmanova, V.I. (2004) Oligodendroglial density in the prefrontal cortex in schizophrenia and mood disorders: a study from the Stanley Neuropathology Consortium. *Schizophr. Res.* 67:269–275.

Vidal, C.N., Rapoport, J.L., Hayashi, K.M., Geaga, J.A., Sui, Y., McLemore, L.E., Alaghband, Y., Giedd, J.N., Gochman, P., Blumenthal, J., Gogtay, N., Nicolson, R., Toga, A.W., and Thompson, P.M. (2006) Dynamically spreading frontal and cingulate deficits mapped in adolescents with schizophrenia. *Arch. Gen. Psychiatry* 63:25–34.

Volk, D., Austin, M., Pierri, J., Sampson, A., and Lewis, D. (2001) GABA transporter-1 mRNA in the prefrontal cortex in schizophrenia: decreased expression in a subset of neurons. *Am. J. Psychiatry* 158:256–265.

Volk, D.W., Austin, M.C., Pierri, J.N., Sampson, A.R., and Lewis, D.A. (2000) Decreased glutamic acid decarboxylase67 messenger RNA expression in a subset of prefrontal cortical gamma-aminobutyric acid neurons in subjects with schizophrenia. *Arch. Gen. Psychiatry* 57:237–245.

Volk, D.W., Pierri, J.N., Fritschy, J.M., Auh, S., Sampson, A.R., and Lewis, D.A. (2002) Reciprocal alterations in pre- and postsynaptic inhibitory markers at chandelier cell inputs to pyramidal neurons in schizophrenia. *Cereb. Cortex* 12:1063–1070.

Walker, M.A., Highley, J.R., Esiri, M.M., McDonald, B., Roberts, H.C., Evans, S.P., Crow, T.J., Walker, M.A., Highley, J.R., Esiri, M.M., McDonald, B., Roberts, H.C., Evans, S.P., and Crow, T.J. (2002) Estimated neuronal populations and volumes of the hippocampus and its subfields in schizophrenia [see comment]. *Am. J. Psychiatry* 159:821–828.

Walterfang, M., Wood, S.J., Velakoulis, D., and Pantelis, C. (2006) Neuropathological, neurogenetic and neuroimaging evidence for white matter pathology in schizophrenia. *Neuroscience and Biobehavioral Reviews* 30(7):918–948.

Wang, L., Hosakere, M., Trein, J.C., Miller, A., Ratnanather, J.T., Barch, D.M., Thompson, P.A., Qiu, A., Gado, M.H., Miller, M. I., and Csernansky, J.G. (2007) Abnormalities of cingulate gyrus neuroanatomy in schizophrenia. *Schizophr. Res.* 93:66–78.

Weiss, A.P., DeWitt, I., Goff, D., Ditman, T., and Heckers, S. (2005) Anterior and posterior hippocampal volumes in schizophrenia. *Schizophr. Res.* 73(1):103–112.

Wieshmann, U.C., Symms, M.R., Clark, C.A., Lemieux, L., Franconi, F., Parker, G.J., Barker, G.J., and Shorvon, S.D. (1999) Wallerian degeneration in the optic radiation after temporal lobectomy demonstrated in vivo with diffusion tensor imaging. *Epilepsia* 1155–1158.

Williams, R.W., and Rakic, P. (1988) Three-dimensional counting: An accurate and direct method to estimate numbers of cells in sectioned material. *J. Comp. Neurol.* 278:344–352.

Wolkin, A., Choi, S.J., Szilagyi, S., Sanfilipo, M., Rotrosen, J.P., and Lim, K.O. (2003) Inferior frontal white matter anisotropy and negative symptoms of schizophrenia: a diffusion tensor imaging study. *Am. J. Psychiatry* 160:572–574.

Woo, T.U., Miller, J.L., and Lewis, D.A. (1997) Schizophrenia and the parvalbumin–containing class of cortical local circuit neurons. *Am. J.Psychiatry* 154:1013–1015.

Woo, T.U., Whitehead, R.E., Melchitzky, D.S., and Lewis, D.A. (1998) A subclass of prefrontal gamma-aminobutyric acid axon terminals are selectively altered in schizophrenia. *Proc. Natl. Acad. Sci. USA* 95:5341–5346.

Wozniak, J.R., and Lim, K.O. (2006) Advances in white matter imaging: a review of in vivo magnetic resonance methodologies and their applicability to the study of development and aging. *Neurosci. Biobehav. Rev.* 30:762–774.

Yamada, M., Hirao, K., Namiki, C., Hanakawa, T., Fukuyama, H., Hayashi, T., and Murai, T. (2007) Social cognition and frontal lobe pathology in schizophrenia: a voxel-based morphometric study. *Neuroimage* 35:292–298.

Yamasue, H., Iwanami, A., Hirayasu, Y., Yamada, H., Abe, O., Kuroki, N., Fukuda, R., Tsujii, K., Aoki, S., Ohtomo, K., Kato, N., and Kasai, K. (2004) Localized volume reduction in prefrontal, temporolimbic, and paralimbic regions in schizophrenia: an MRI parcellation study. *Psychiatry Res.* 131:195–207.

Young, K.A., Manaye, K.F., Liang, C., Hicks, P.B., German, D.C. (2000) Reduced number of mediodorsal and anterior thalamic neurons in schizophrenia. *Biol. Psychiatry* 47:944–953.

Zaidel, D.W., Esiri, M.M., and Harrison, P.J. (1997) Size, shape, and orientation of neurons in the left and right hippocampus: investigation of normal asymmetries and alterations in schizophrenia. *Am. J. Psychiatry* 154:812–818.

Zaidel, D.W., Esiri, M.M., Harrison, P.J., Zaidel, D.W., Esiri, M.M., and Harrison, P.J. (1997) The hippocampus in schizophrenia: lateralized increase in neuronal density and altered cytoarchitectural asymmetry. *Psychol. Med.* 27:703–713.

Zhang, Z.J., and Reynolds, G.P. (2002) A selective decrease in the relative density of parvalbumin-immunoreactive neurons in the hippocampus in schizophrenia. *Schizophr. Res.* 55:1–10.

22 Cognitive Neuroscience and Neuroimaging in Schizophrenia

AYSENIL BELGER AND DEANNA M. BARCH

Cognitive impairments represent a core feature of schizophrenia. They are not a consequence of clinical positive and negative symptoms, and their course follows a characteristic pattern independent of changes in the severity of these clinical symptoms. Cognitive deficits have been demonstrated at multiple levels in schizophrenia and range from early sensory-processing deficits, reported in the auditory and more recently in the visual processing domains, to higher order information-processing deficits, reported in the domains of attention, executive function, working and episodic memory, and affective processing. It is now widely accepted that in addition to treatment of the positive and negative symptoms of schizophrenia, it is equally important to treat cognitive deficits in these patients. These cognitive deficits are recognized as major obstacles to the social and professional reentry of patients with schizophrenia (Green, 2006). Although the literature suggests that neurocognitive impairments may not strongly correlate with the clinical symptoms of schizophrenia, there is ample evidence that they relate to social functioning, unemployment, quality of life, relapse prevention, medical comorbidity, and economic cost. Hence, understanding the neurobiological underpinning of these cognitive deficits and their responses to treatment holds a unique promise for the field and for the welfare of individuals with schizophrenia.

DOMAINS OF COGNITIVE DYSFUNCTION IN SCHIZOPHRENIA

Cognitive neuroscience provides a unique framework within which we can study the neural basis of cognitive deficits in schizophrenia. This interdisciplinary field, reviewed in Chapter 68 by Casey and Durston, relies on the converging evidence obtained through a multitude of methodologies to understand how mental and behavioral functions are related to brain processes (Fig. 22.1; see also COLOR FIGURE 22.1 in separate insert). Each of these methodologies provides a unique insight and approach to the study of the neural mechanisms that underlie simple as well as complex thoughts and behaviors, such as perception, attention, emotions, and memory. Information processing deficits span multiple levels in schizophrenia, from early sensory gating deficits to higher order cognitive deficits in domains including attention, working memory, affective perception and expression, and episodic memory. This section presents an overview of the major deficits, with the aim of linking these deficits to selected cortical and subcortical neural circuits. Figure 22.2 (see also COLOR FIGURE 22.2 in separate insert) outlines the three clusters of regions that have been frequently implicated in the three levels of processing deficits that we review.

Early sensory processing deficits have been associated with aberrant neural activity in auditory and visual cortical regions, and their associative cortices. Executive processing and attention deficits typically have been associated with a dorsal brain circuitry consisting of frontal-striate and frontal-parietal regions, in particular the dorsolateral prefrontal cortex (DLPFC), posterior parietal cortex, and basal ganglia. Deficits in episodic memory and affective regulation and social cognition have implicated pathology in ventral prefrontal and limbic cortical regions, in particular the amygdala/hippocampal (AMY/HIP) complex and its ventral prefrontal connections. The observation of abnormal function and structure across such distributed cortical and subcortical circuits reflects the complex neurobiological underpinnings of schizophrenia and the heterogeneity and diversity of the symptoms observed across patients.

Early Sensory Processing and Feature Encoding Deficits

Much of the evidence for early sensory processing and integration deficits has been through electrophysiological studies of surface event-related potentials (ERPs) and electrophysiological studies (electroencephalogram; EEG) of brain activity in response to stimuli and cognitive tasks. Many of the early reported deficits have been with respect to auditory evoked potentials (AEPs). Abnormal auditory sensory information filtering and processing has been proposed as one of the characteristic deficits in schizophrenia (Siegel et al., 1984; Adler et al., 1985;

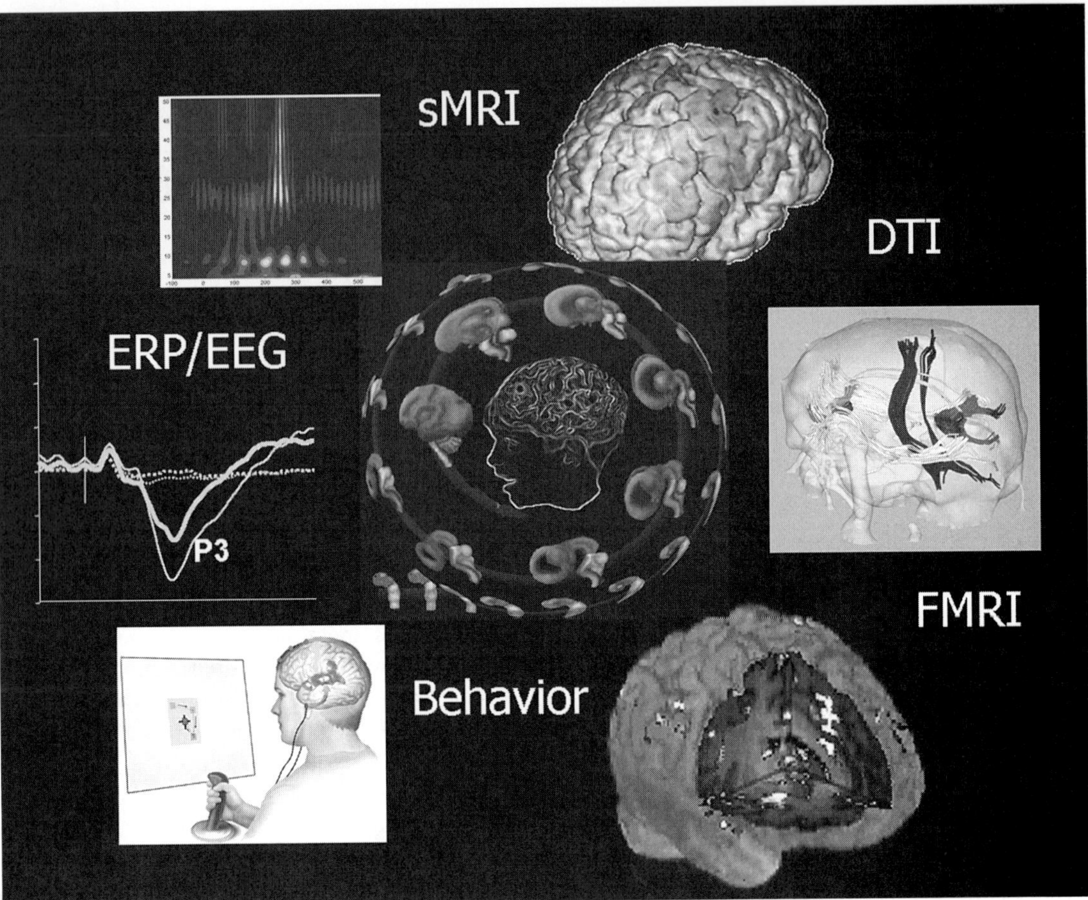

FIGURE 22.1 Representation of converging methods and techniques typically used by cognitive neuroscientists to study behaviors, associated brain functions, and their underlying neuroanatomy. Many of these methods are non invasive, and can be implemented repeated times to enable longitudinal assessments to track disease progression and treatment effects.

Muller et al., 1986; Freedman et al., 1987). These deficits have been described as impairments in inhibitory gating of auditory evoked responses demonstrated using a conditioning-testing paradigm with the P50 wave of the auditory evoked response. In electrophysiological paradigms using paired stimuli, the P50 wave evoked by the second stimulus is reduced to less than 20% because of inhibitory mechanisms activated during the response to the first stimulus in healthy participants. In individuals with schizophrenia, the mean amplitude

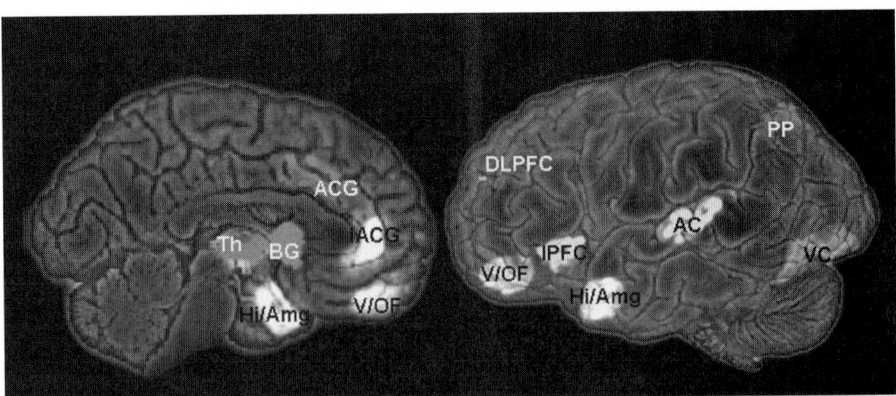

FIGURE 22.2 Neural circuits associated with the three primary domains of information processing deficits in schizophrenia: green: sensory cortices; red: fronto-striate and fronto-parietal executive and attention control regions; yellow: fronto-limbic affective processing and episodic memory regions (see Figure 22.2 in color insert).

of the second response has been reported to be more than 85% of the first, implicating a deficit in inhibition. Furthermore, studies have revealed that approximately one half of the first-degree relatives, generally including at least one parent, had a similar deficit (Siegel et al., 1984; Freedman et al., 1987; Waldo et al., 1991). Presence of this deficit in the parents has further been associated with a family history of schizophrenia (Siegel et al., 1984; Freedman et al., 1991). More recent studies have shed some doubt on the validity and reproducibility of the P50 abnormality in schizophrenia, reporting increased variability and lower reliability of the P50 in individuals with schizophrenia (Guterman and Josiassen, 1994; Jin et al., 1997; Patterson et al., 2000) suggesting that background noise levels are indeed higher in the patient groups. Several studies, however, have reported that the P50 evoked by S1 is smaller in patients with schizophrenia (Clementz et al., 1997; Jin et al., 1997; Patterson et al., 2000), which suggests that overall response amplitudes may be lower and/or response latencies more variable in these patients. In addition, it has been reported that patients with schizophrenia showing the most severe perceptual anomalies did not differ from healthy controls in their P50 refractory effects (Jin et al., 1998). Thus, there seems to be significant controversy surrounding the reduced P50 refractoriness in schizophrenia, including whether it is related to the selective gating or filtering of irrelevant sensory information in the auditory cortical pathways.

The possibility has recently been raised that the mismatch negativity (MMN) component of the ERP could offer a biological marker of postonset progressive cognitive and cortical deterioration in schizophrenia (Javitt et al., 1995; Salisbury et al., 2002). If empirically validated, the MMN could have profound theoretical and clinical implications for understanding and treating schizophrenia. The MMN refers to a scalp-negative ERP component that is usually recorded in a "passive" auditory oddball paradigm (Naatanen, 1992; Umbricht et al., 1997) in response to "deviant" stimuli embedded in a background of homogeneous stimuli. In this paradigm, participants passively listen to a series of frequent standard and infrequent deviant auditory stimuli while they are resting or are involved in the attentive processing of visual information, such as reading a book or performing a visual discrimination task. The MMN typically occurs between about 100 ms and 250 ms following the infrequent, physically deviant auditory stimuli and reaches maximal voltages over frontal and central scalp locations. Although this ERP component may be affected by participant's attention in certain situations (Yucel et al., 2005a, 2005b) the MMN is essentially an automatic, preattentive brain response because its generation is not dependent on the participant's attention toward the eliciting deviant auditory stimuli. As such, the MMN provides a window on auditory sensory or "echoic memory" because it is initiated by a mismatch with the memory traces of the preceding sounds. Deficits in the MMN and other neural indices of "passive" change and novelty detection (Javitt et al., 1993; Javitt et al., 1995; Salisbury et al., 2002) associated with involuntary attention deployment and stimulus deviance detection have been documented in schizophrenia. Recent studies have proposed that these deficits may be related to illness chronicity or severity (Salisbury et al., 2002). These findings provide clear evidence for a deficit in preattentive auditory processing in schizophrenia, although there is some debate about whether the impairment is primarily in temporal processing (Michie et al., 2000) or auditory encoding and trace formation (Javitt, 2000).

The findings support the presence of early auditory sensory-processing deficits in schizophrenia. However evidence is accumulating that patients with schizophrenia also exhibit relatively severe deficits in early visual sensory processing in visual evoked potentials (VEPs) (Foxe et al., 2005). These deficits have been demonstrated primarily within the dorsal stream, in particular in visual pathways preferentially carrying information from the magnocellular pathway, while processing within the ventral stream appears to be relatively more intact. These deficits have been demonstrated in studies using illusory contour (IC) processing to evaluate early processing within regions of the ventral visual stream. The findings revealed a robust decrement in the amplitude of the P1 sensory component in patients and a large topographic difference between groups for this component (54–104 ms), indicating that early dorsal stream processing was severely impaired in this population, while early ventral stream processing is essentially normal. Source analysis further confirmed that the flow of activity into the dorsal stream was substantially decreased in patients. Similar deficits in early visual processing potentially implicating selective dysfunction of the magnocellular visual pathway have been replicated using transient visual evoked potential (tVEP) responses to stimuli biased toward the magnocellular (M) versus parvocellular (P) systems in patients with schizophrenia. Further, this research indicated that P1 amplitude reductions in response to stimuli biased toward the M condition correlated with a proxy measure of global outcome and level of community functioning (Schechter et al., 2005).

Pervasive and subtle alterations of perception in schizophrenia have been further supported by electrophysiological studies of neural synchrony. Event-related neuronal oscillations, in particular in the gamma-band frequency range, have been hypothesized to be fundamental to normal brain function and cognition (Basar and Bullock, 1992; Basar et al., 2001; Basar-Eroglu and Demiralp, 2001; Tallon-Baudry, 2003), and to cognitive dysfunctions in schizophrenia (Green and Nuechterlein, 1999; D. Lee, 2003; van der Stelt et al., 2004). Gamma band responses (GBRs) have been observed during various types of information processing across sensory modalities, across species, and at multiple levels of spatial analysis, from microscopic (for example, single unit) to macroscopic (for example, scalp EEG) measurements. According to Galambos et al. (1981), three types of GBRs may be distinguished: first, the steady-state–evoked GBR to repetitive stimulation at different frequencies; second, the transient-evoked GBR that is phase locked to the onset of a transient stimulus; and last, the induced GBR that is not phase locked to stimulus onset. It is generally assumed that evoked GBRs primarily index sensory processing and reflect cortical responses due to changes in afferent activity, whereas induced GBRs are cognitive in nature and generated by changes in functional connectivity within neuronal networks (Karakas and Basar, 1998; Pfurtscheller and Lopes da Silva, 1999; Tallon-Baudry, 2003).

Several studies have shown that patients with schizophrenia display reduced power and phase synchronization of steady-state auditory-evoked GBRs to clicks, tone pips, or amplitude-modulated tones presented at 40 Hz but not at lower rates of stimulation (Kwon et al., 1999; Brenner et al., 2003). A slower buildup of steady-state visual-evoked potential amplitudes following stimulus onset has also been reported in schizophrenia (Clementz et al., 2004) as well as a significant relationship between the latency of the steady-state VEP and auditory hallucinations in patients with schizophrenia (Line et al., 1998). Deficits in steady-state auditory-evoked GBRs have also been reported to be markedly enhanced in patients with schizophrenia taking new-generation or atypical antipsychotic medications as compared with patients on conventional or typical antipsychotics (Hong et al., 2004). Results have been mixed as to whether the deficits observed in patients with schizophrenia are also present in persons with schizotypal personality traits (Brenner et al., 2003).

Several studies have found that the integrity of stimulus-evoked GBRs in patients with schizophrenia varies according to the nature and severity of their current clinical symptoms. Reduced auditory-evoked GBRs have been noted in nonparanoid, but not in paranoid, schizophrenia subtypes (Johannesen et al., 2005). Similarly, increased levels of negative symptoms in patients with schizophrenia seem to be associated with diminished auditory-evoked GBRs, whereas increased positive symptoms are associated with enlarged auditory-evoked GBRs (K.H. Lee et al., 2003; Herrmann and Demiralp, 2005). Moreover, exceptionally large gamma-band rhythms have been measured simultaneously during the occurrence of somatic hallucinations in a patient with schizophrenia (Baldeweg et al., 1998). Furthermore, it has been demonstrated that patients with schizophrenia exhibit impaired phase locking and phase coherence of early visual transient-evoked GBRs over the occipital scalp during the perception of visual Gestalt patterns (Spencer et al., 2003), suggesting that the temporal synchronization of stimulus-evoked gamma oscillations within the visual cortex is disrupted in schizophrenia. A subsequent study confirmed these findings and also demonstrated that the degree of phase locking of the occipital GBR phase locked to reaction time is positively related to the severity of clinical symptoms, in particular visual hallucinations, thought disorder, and disorganization (Spencer et al., 2004). A recent study observed that visual-induced GBRs, but not evoked GBRs, are disrupted in patients with schizophrenia (Cho et al., 2006). Another study, however, found that visual-induced GBRs during a Gestalt perception task are not abnormal in patients with schizophrenia (Uhlhaas et al., 2006). Instead, this study found that the synchronization of oscillations in the lower, beta frequency range is reduced and accompanies performance deficits in patients with schizophrenia. Although the basis for the discrepancy between results remains to be elucidated, these findings underline the importance of assessing evoked and induced variants of oscillatory neuronal responses in multiple frequency bands in schizophrenia. Finally, abnormalities of evoked and induced GBRs do not appear to be diagnostically specific to schizophrenia but can be found in several other psychiatric and neurological disorders, including attention-deficit/hyperactivity disorder, autism, epilepsy, and Alzheimer's disease (van der Stelt et al., 2004; Herrmann and Demiralp, 2005).

In sum, several studies have reported abnormalities in the enhancement and phase synchronization of GBRs during various types of sensory and cognitive information-processing in patients with schizophrenia. These results provide supporting evidence for the view that neural synchrony is disrupted in schizophrenia. An intriguing finding is the observed relationship in patients with schizophrenia between sensory-evoked GBRs and the severity of clinical positive symptoms, particularly hallucinations (D. Lee, 2003; Spencer et al., 2004; Herrmann and Demiralp, 2005; Johannesen et al., 2005). These data suggest that GBRs could provide important theoretical insights into the generative brain mechanisms that give rise to perceptual disturbances and hallucinations in schizophrenia. Correspondingly, it has been hypothesized that the correlations between enlarged GBRs and hallucinations in schizophrenia reflect cortical hyperexcitability and abnormally increased neural synchrony of thalamocortical networks, leading to incoherent or "underconstrained" perception and disturbed conscious experience (Behrendt and Young, 2004). Gamma-band frequency range alterations in schizophrenia, however, are not invariant across studies but seem to vary as a function of stimulus and task-specific factors and patient sample characteristics (van der Stelt et al., 2004) including the type of antipsychotic medication being used by patients (Hong et al., 2004) and the nature and severity of their current clinical symptoms (D. Lee, 2003; Spencer et al., 2004; Herrmann and Demiralp, 2005; Johannesen et al., 2005). Accordingly, although the study of GBRs in schizophrenia is relatively recent, the currently available data seem to suggest that GBR abnormalities represent a clinical state marker, rather than a trait marker, of schizophrenia.

Executive Function, Attention and Working Memory in Schizophrenia: The Role of Dorsal Frontal, Parietal, and Striatal Circuit Deficits

There is considerable evidence that individuals with schizophrenia experience disturbances in the dorsal frontal-parietal circuit (including projections to and from the caudate) that is thought to subserve a number of different components of cognitive function. In particular, this circuit is thought to support the central executive functions of the working memory system (Baddeley and Logie, 1999), as well as a range of other executive functions that may not be specific to working memory, including task preparation, set-shifting, updating, and temporal ordering. At the behavioral level, there is very consistent evidence that individuals with schizophrenia have difficulty with executive function. For example, individuals with schizophrenia show deficits on (*1*) working memory tasks with all different material types (e.g., Gooding and Tallent, 2004; Kim et al., 2004) with little evidence for differential deficits across material types; (*2*) measures of a range of central executive functions, including manipulation (Gold et al., 1997; Kim et al., 2004; Cannon et al., 2005), interference control and/or dual-task coordination (e.g., Fleming et al., 1995), and information updating and temporal indexing (e.g., Goldberg et al., 2003; Perlstein et al., 2003). In addition, the first-degree relatives of individuals with schizophrenia also show evidence of consistent impairments in central executive components of working memory and other executive functions (Snitz et al., 2006).

At the neurobiological level, numerous studies have identified deficits in the functional activation of DLPFC, one of the key structures in the dorsal frontal-parietal circuit, during performance of a range of tasks thought to assess various components of executive function (for reviews, see Davidson and Heinrichs, 2003; Barch, 2005; Glahn et al., 2005). Importantly, however, the nature of the impaired DLPFC activation has varied across studies, with some studies finding decreased activation, and some studies finding increased activation in patients versus controls. One interesting hypothesis put forth to explain these differential findings of hypo- versus hyper-DLPFC activity is the idea that the memory load–DLPFC response curve may be different for individuals with schizophrenia as compared to healthy controls. Specifically, it may be that at low load levels, individuals with schizophrenia need to devote more resources to working memory, leading to hyperactivation, but that higher load levels exceed their capacity, leading to reduced DLPFC activity (Callicott et al., 1999; Callicott et al., 2000; Callicott et al., 2003). Consistent with this hypothesis, there is evidence that the level of performance impairment among individuals with schizophrenia is related to the likelihood of finding hypo- versus hyper-DLPFC activation. A recent meta-analysis (Van Snellenberg et al., 2006) found that greater performance impairments among individuals with schizophrenia were associated with the presence of hypofrontality. However, the definition of *DLPFC* used in this meta-analysis was a very broad one that includes functionally diverse areas. Thus, it is not yet clear whether the same regions of DLPFC show hypo- and hyperactivation in patients as load level and behavioral performance vary (though see Johnson et al., 2006).

In addition to evidence for impaired DLPFC activation during performance of working memory and executive function tasks, there is growing evidence of impaired posterior parietal cortex (PPC) activation in patients during performance of this same domain of tasks (e.g., Menon et al., 2001; Meyer-Lindenberg et al., 2001; Barch et al., 2002; Kim et al., 2003; Quintana et al., 2003). Importantly, the region of PPC that seems to be impaired in schizophrenia is a more dorsal region that has been specifically associated with load effects in working memory, and which may help to subserve either (or both) temporal ordering and updating executive functions (Ravizza et al., 2004; Barch and Csernanksy, 2007). As with the DLPFC literature, there is some evidence for hypo- and hyper-PPC activity in schizophrenia (e.g., Barch and Csernanksy, 2007; Quintana et al., 2003), though more work is needed to understand the relationship of these patterns to behavioral demand (for example, load and difficulty) and performance level. In addition to impaired DLPFC and dorsal PPC activation, a growing number of studies point to impaired basal ganglia function in schizophrenia during working memory and executive control tasks (e.g., Manoach et al., 2000; Morey et al., 2005; Camchong et al., 2006). This is an important finding, as the caudate is a critical node in the circuit connecting DLPFC and dorsal PPC functions. Consistent with the description of DLPFC, dorsal PPC, and basal ganglia regions as a circuit, there are also findings of altered functional connectivity among these regions in schizophrenia (Meyer-Lindenberg et al., 2001; Kim et al., 2003; Schlosser et al., 2003; Ahveninen et al., 2006), further evidence pointing to a circuit-level abnormality underlying deficits in executive control and working memory in this debilitating illness.

There are a number of other sources besides functional imaging studies that provide evidence for impairments in DLPFC, PPC, and striatal regions in schizophrenia. For example, a number of structural studies have found alterations in gray matter volume in DLPFC (Condray et al., 1996; Shenton et al., 2001; Selemon and Rajkowska, 2003), in some cases specifically associated with altered executive function (Rusch et al., 2007). Studies have also found a variety of cellular and molecular abnormalities in regions of DLPFC, although the precise nature of these abnormalities has varied across studies (Selemon et al., 1995; Rajkowska et al., 1998; Pierri et al., 2001; Selemon and Rajkowska, 2003; Cullen et al., 2006). In addition, magnetic resonance spectroscopy studies have found reductions in *N*-acetylaspartate (NAA) concentrations (a measure of the metabolic integrity of neurons) in PFC among individuals with schizophrenia (Bertolino et al., 1996; Bertolino, Callicott, Elman, et al., 1998; Bertolino, Callicott, Nawroz, et al., 1998; Velligan et al., 1998; Cecil et al., 1999; Sigmundsson et al., 2003), particularly in dorsal as compared to ventral regions (Bertolino et al., 1996; Bertolino, Callicott, Elman, et al., 1998; Bertolino, Callicott, Nawroz, et al., 1998). However, there have been a few nonreplications of these NAA findings as well (Delamillieure et al., 2002; Wood et al., 2003), and some suggestions that reduced NAA may result from antipsychotic treatment (Bustillo et al., 2002). There is also evidence for altered volumes and shapes of basal ganglia structures, including caudate and putamen (Laywer et al., 2006; Mamah et al., 2007), though some of these changes may be related to medication effects (Scherk and Falkai, 2006), and there are also a number of negative findings (Gunduz et al., 2002; Crespo-Facorro et al., 2007). Not surprisingly, there is also evidence for altered volumes in PPC regions in schizophrenia (Zhou et al., 2007), though there is also evidence for less structural change in parietal than prefrontal regions (Kuperberg et al., 2003).

Importantly, there is growing evidence that impairments in the dorsal frontal, parietal, and striatal circuits supporting executive function and working memory may be endophenotypic markers of risk for schizophrenia. There is ample evidence for behavioral impairments in working memory and executive function among individuals at risk for schizophrenia, but who do not yet have the illness, such as first-degree relatives (Glahn et al., 2003; Seidman, Giuliano, et al., 2006; Snitz et al., 2006) and individuals with schizotypal personality disorder (Park et al., 1995; Park and McTigue, 1997; Farmer et al., 2000; Roitman et al., 2000; Mitropoulou et al., 2002; Barch et al., 2004). Further, some evidence suggests that the stronger the genetic risk, the greater the impairment in working memory function in first-degree relatives. For example, siblings from families with more than one affected member do worse on visual working memory tasks than siblings from families with a single affected member (Tuulio-Henriksson et al., 2003). In addition, the performance of unaffected monozygotic twins on a spatial delayed-response tasks was as poor as their affected cotwins, while the performance of unaffected dyzygotic twins was intermediate between their affected cotwins and controls (Glahn et al., 2003).

Although there have been fewer functional and structural imaging studies in at-risk populations, as compared to behavioral studies, there is evidence for neurobiological impairments that are intermediate between the level of deficit shown by ill probands controls. For example, a number of functional imaging studies of working memory and executive function demonstrate abnormalities in activation of DLPFC, dorsal PPC, and basal ganglia (Raemaekers et al., 2002; Thermenos et al., 2004; Brahmbhatt et al., 2006; Seidman, Thermenos, et al., 2006; Snitz et al., 2006; Vink et al., 2006; Delawalla et al., 2008) in at-risk populations. There is also some evidence for structural abnormalities in these regions in at-risk populations, though results are more variable than in patients who are ill (Boos et al., 2007). Further, there is recent evidence that deficits in posterior parietal activation may predict later conversion to psychosis (Whalley et al., 2006).

Episodic Memory: The Role of Frontal-Posterior Limbic Circuitry

Another domain in which individuals with schizophrenia show robust deficits is episodic memory, or the ability to learn and retrieve new information. For many years we have known that the HIP plays a critical role in the formation of long-term memories, based on studies with amnesic patients such as H.M., who have had lesions to the HIP and/or surrounding medial temporal areas (Scoville and Milner, 1957) and nonhuman primate models demonstrating that lesions within HIP and adjacent medial temporal cortex lead to impairments in the ability to retrieve newly learned information (Murray, 1996). More specifically, it has been suggested that the HIP formation is critical for the rapid binding of novel configurations of information (Honer et al., 1995; McClelland et al., 1995; N.J. Cohen and Eichenbaum, 2001). Although the HIP clearly plays an important role in episodic memory function, prefrontal structures also make important contributions to episodic memory. Studies with individuals who have damage to PFC have shown that although individuals do not exhibit classic amnesia, they do experience deficits in episodic memory, including differentially impaired recall as compared to recognition (Janowsky and Shimamura, 1989; Janowsky et al., 1989). Many of these studies have focused on individuals with DLPFC damage, but individuals with damage to ventrolateral PFC also show episodic memory impairments (Alexander et al., 2003). Importantly, a number of researchers have suggested that one of the reasons that PFC damage impairs episodic memory is that it alters the ability to either generate or apply effective encoding strategies (e.g., Stuss et al., 1994; Alexander et al., 2003). In addition, functional imaging studies of episodic memory in healthy participants have elucidated a role for PFC in episodic memory. These studies have demonstrated that PFC regions (anterior BA 44, BA 45/47) are sensitive to semantic processing and preferentially activate during deep semantic elaboration (e.g., Otten et al., 2001; McDermott et al., 2003). Further, areas of left inferior PFC (BA 44, 45, 47), left fusiform gyrus, and left HIP consistently show greater activity during encoding of stimuli that are subsequently remembered, as compared to those forgotten (Brewer et al., 1998; Wagner, Desmond, et al., 1998; Wagner, Poldrack, et al., 1998; Kirchhoff et al., 2000; Braver et al., 2001; Otten et al., 2001). Importantly, activity in these regions (at least the PFC and HIP regions) predicts successful subsequent memory for single items and relational information (Prince et al., 2005). Many of the same brain regions associated with semantic processing at encoding and which predict subsequent memory are also active during retrieval of learned information, including BA 44/45/47 and regions of the HIP and parahippocampal gyrus. However, several additional PFC regions are active during retrieval, including more dorsal and anterior regions such as BA 46/9 and 10.

A large body of literature suggests that deficits in episodic memory are present even at the first episode of illness in individuals with schizophrenia (Saykin et al., 1991; Hoff et al., 1992; Saykin et al., 1994) and that the course of such deficits is relatively stable across time (Censits et al., 1997; Hoff et al., 1999). Further, there is some evidence that individuals with schizophrenia may have particular difficulties with the binding together of novel configurations of information, as they show evidence of greater impairment in associative as compared to item memory (Muller et al., 1986), suggesting that HIP deficits are a source of episodic memory impairment in schizophrenia. However, many tests of associative memory are also tests of source memory, which has been associated with prefrontal function. More recently, researchers have begun to use tasks derived from the animal literature on HIP function in schizophrenia. One such measure is the transitive interference test, which measures the ability to learn the relationships among hierarchically arranged pairs of stimuli (Eichenbaum and Cohen, 2001). Titone et al. (2004) showed that individuals with schizophrenia are impaired on the critical conditions of this task that require relational processing, but not on conditions that require the learning of simpler associative reinforcement mappings. Results such as these begin to provide stronger evidence for disturbances in the type of relational processing or binding of novel pairings thought to be specifically supported by the HIP formation.

At the same time, there are many lines of research suggesting that individuals with schizophrenia also have deficits in the ability to use beneficial strategies during episodic memory. For example, individuals with schizophrenia are impaired in their ability to generate effective mnemonic strategies (Koh, 1978; Iddon et al., 1998; Hill et al., 2004), and they encode information less elaborately than controls (Larsen and Fromholt, 1976; Traupmann et al., 1976; Brebion et al., 1998; Elvevag et al., 2004). Importantly, however, when provided with strategies that promote successful episodic encoding (such as semantic elaboration or categorization), individuals with schizophrenia are typically able to benefit as much as controls from these strategies (Koh and Peterson, 1978; Heckers et al., 1998; Salisbury et al., 2002; Hofer, Weiss, Golaszewski, Siedentopf, Kremser, et al., 2003; Ragland et al., 2003; Weiss et al., 2003; Ragland et al., 2005). Such findings are consistent with the hypothesis that deficits in prefrontal functional also contribute to episodic memory deficits in schizophrenia.

At the neurobiological level, a number of functional imaging studies have provided evidence for abnormal HIP activation in individuals with schizophrenia, at encoding (Barch et al., 2002; Leube et al., 2002; Jessen et al., 2003) and retrieval (Heckers et al., 1998; Barch et al., 2002; Jessen et al., 2003; Weiss et al., 2003; Heckers et al., 2004). These failures to show task-related HIP activity at retrieval have been interpreted as reflecting a failure in explicit recollection among individuals with schizophrenia (Heckers et al., 1998; Weiss et al., 2003). In addition to data from functional imaging studies of episodic memory processing, there are a number of other sources of evidence that individuals with schizophrenia have deficits in HIP volume and shape (Csernansky et al., 1998; Shenton et al., 2001; Wang et al., 2001), particularly for those individuals with schizophrenia who have experienced obstetric or birth complications (van Erp et al., 2002; van Erp et al., 2004). Further, there is some evidence for a relationship between the severity of HIP volume reductions in schizophrenia and the severity of episodic memory deficits (Nestor et al., 1993; Goldberg et al., 1994; Boyer et al., 2007; Nestor et al., 2007), though there are a number of negative findings in this area as well (Torres et al., 1997; Szeszko et al., 2002). The evidence for HIP abnormalities in schizophrenia extends to the cellular level as well, including a variety of cellular and molecular abnormalities (Knable et al., 2004) as well as reductions in NAA (Yurgelun-Todd et al., 1996; Callicott et al., 1998; Deicken et al., 1999), though there is some evidence for greater HIP NAA reductions in chronic as opposed to first-episode patients (Molina et al., 2002).

Although the results across studies have been variable, a recent meta-analysis (Muller et al., 1986) identified consistent impairments in several regions of PFC during encoding in schizophrenia. Specifically, individuals with schizophrenia show deficits in the activation of dorsal and anterior regions of PFC (BA 10 and 9). Given the hypothesized role of DLPFC in executive control and strategy generation/application, such deficits in PFC may be related to the strategic impairment often seen in schizophrenia and may contribute to deficits in the ability to generate or apply effective strategies. In addition, individuals with schizophrenia show deficits in the activation of left inferior frontal cortex (BA 45), a region associated with semantic processing and which predicts successfully memory retrieval. However, studies that have constrained individuals to use "deep" processing during encoding have tended to find relatively intact activity in left BA 45 and 9 (Salisbury et al., 2002; Ragland et al., 2005), coupled with some evidence for enhanced activity in right BA 45 and more anterior regions of BA 10 (Salisbury et al., 2002). However, at least one study of deep processing still found reduced BA 45 activity in males with schizophrenia (Kubicki et al., 2003), and other studies using an encoding task that is somewhat semantic (for example, liking judgments) still sometimes identify abnormal activity in BA 10 and 9 during encoding, even when BA 45 activity is intact (Hofer, Weiss, Golaszewski, Siedentopf, Brinkhoff, et al., 2003; Hofer, Weiss, Golaszewski, Siedentopf, Kremser, et al., 2003), Thus, studies of encoding related activity in schizophrenia using paradigms in which individuals are not constrained to use any particular encoding strategy find reduced BA 45, 9, and 10 activity, as well as reduced HIP activity. However, there is some evidence for "normalization" of activity in PFC regions (BA 45, 9, 10) and some evidence for enhanced HIP activation (Ragland et al., 2005) when individuals with schizophrenia are oriented to use more effective encoding strategies.

At retrieval, individuals with schizophrenia show impairments in brain activation in many of the same regions identified during encoding, including left BA 46/9, left BA 45, and HIP (Muller et al., 1986; Lepage et al., 2006), even when they have been constrained to use effective strategies at encoding (Heckers et al., 1998; Weiss et al., 2003). As noted above, activity in left DLPFC has been associated with retrieval success (Prince et al., 2005), and reduced activity in this region among individuals with schizophrenia may be associated with their less accurate performance and perhaps less reliance on explicit recollection for retrieval. The pattern of activity in BA 10 in schizophrenia during retrieval is less clear. Reduced activation in a very medial region of BA 10 was identified in the Achim and Lepage (2005) meta-analysis. However, several other studies have identified enhanced activity in BA 10 (bilateral or left), either in the region typically associated with retrieval related activity or a somewhat more medial region (Heckers et al., 1998; Hofer, Weiss, Golaszewski, Siedentopf, Brinkhoff, et al., 2003; Weiss et al., 2003; Ragland et al., 2005). Interestingly, these were studies that provided some support for encoding in the form of either orientation toward semantic elaboration or repeated-item presentation, and this enhanced activity has been interpreted as reflecting either greater retrieval effort or monitoring of retrieval output (Weiss et al., 2003). Even with encoding support, individuals with schizophrenia can still show reduced BA 46 activity at retrieval, which may be associated with reduced retrieval success (Hofer, Weiss, Golaszewski, Siedentopf, Brinkhoff, et al., 2003; Hofer, Weiss, Golaszewski, Siedentopf, Kremser, et al., 2003), and still show reduced HIP activity (e.g., Heckers et al., 1998; Jessen et al., 2003; Weiss et al., 2003).

A large number of studies have shown that the unaffected first-degree relatives of individuals with schizophrenia show deficits on episodic memory tasks (Goldberg et al., 1993; Gur et al., 1994; Kremen et al., 1994; Faraone et al., 1995; Toomey et al., 1998; Lawrie et al., 1999; Laurent et al., 2000; Toulopoulou et al., 2003; Delawalla et al., 2006), that are stable over time (Faraone et al., 1999), and seem to be worse in relatives from multiplex as compared to singleplex families (Faraone et al., 2000). Further, several studies have shown abnormal PFC activation in first-degree relatives of individuals with schizophrenia during performance of episodic encoding tasks, particularly in inferior frontal gyrus regions (BA 44/45/57) (Salisbury et al., 2002; Whyte et al., 2004). There is also evidence for HIP NAA reductions in relatives of individuals with schizophrenia (Callicott et al., 1998), as well as HIP volume reductions (Seidman et al., 1999; Keshavan et al., 2002; Seidman et al., 2002) and shape abnormalities (Nelson, 1979), that are sometimes correlated with the severity of episodic memory deficits (O'Driscoll et al., 2001; Seidman et al., 2002). Individuals with schizotypal personality disorder also demonstrate reliable episodic memory deficits (Bergman et al., 1998; Voglmaier et al., 2000; Mitropoulou et al., 2002), though the evidence for altered HIP volume is mixed (Siever et al., 2002). As a whole, the results of studies in high-risk individuals suggest that episodic deficits may be linked to HIP and prefrontal abnormalities, and thus may be vulnerability factors for schizophrenia. However, there are also a number of studies clearly suggesting that factors other than genetics influence the severity of episodic memory and/or HIP abnormalities in schizophrenia (Casanova et al., 1990; Goldberg et al., 1993; van Erp et al., 2004), though the finding that unaffected high-risk relatives show disturbances intermediate between their relatives who are ill and controls is not novel by any means.

Affective Processing Deficits: The Role of Frontal-Anterior Limbic Circuitry

Much of the functional neuroimaging literature in schizophrenia has focused on elucidating the neural basis of a range of cognitive deficits, as described above. However, deficits in emotional processing are also a core feature of schizophrenia. For example, blunted affect is a core feature of schizophrenia, and many individuals with schizophrenia report reductions in the ability to experience pleasure, a symptom referred to as anhedonia. Individuals with schizophrenia also commonly experience deficits in motivation, which may also reflect abnormalities in the processing of internal experiences of emotional information. Interestingly, however, many individuals with schizophrenia report intact experience of pleasure and emotion when provided with emotionally evocative stimuli, suggesting a dissociation between anticipatory pleasure and consummatory pleasure (Kring et al., 1993; Kring and Neale, 1996; Kring, 1999; Burbridge and Barch, 2002; Heerey and Gold, 2007). A growing number of neuroimaging studies have also begun to examine functional brain responses to affect-eliciting stimuli in schizophrenia, positive and negative. These studies have sometimes provided results different from the behavioral studies. For example, Crespo-Facarro et al. (2001) found abnormal affective responses to pleasant, but not unpleasant odors, coupled with abnormal frontal and limbic (including nucleus accumbens) responses to unpleasant odors. Similarly, Paradiso et al. (2003) found abnormal subjective responses to pleasant, but not unpleasant pictures, coupled with reduced frontal activations to pleasant pictures. In addition, Juckle et al. (2006) found reduced ventral striatal responses to cues predicting reward in patients with schizophrenia, though there was some evidence that this reflected typical antipsychotic medication influences (Juckel et al., 2006). The results of such studies suggest that individuals with schizophrenia may experience deficits in the neural circuits supporting the processing of pleasant stimuli, or cues that predict rewards, though they sometimes report intact subjective experiences of pleasant and unpleasant stimuli. Clearly, however, more work is needed to understand the relationships between subjective responses to pleasant stimuli, the anticipation of reward or pleasure, and motivation and hedonic capacity in schizophrenia.

Many individuals with schizophrenia demonstrate deficits in social cognition. *Social cognition* can be broadly described as the mental operations underlying social interactions and strongly relies upon the ability to perceive, interpret, and generate responses to the intentions, dispositions, and behaviors of others (Brothers, 1990; Fiske and Taylor, 1991; Kunda, 1999). In other words, social-cognitive processes enable us to draw inferences about other people's beliefs and intentions. Impaired social cognition has been demonstrated repeatedly in schizophrenia and has emerged as one of the most significant contributors to poor clinical and functional outcome (Penn et al., 1997). Deficits in social cognition may reflect disturbances in the accurate perception of emotion and motivations in others (Brunet-Gouet and Decety, 2006; Couture et al., 2006). Consistent with this hypothesis, individuals with schizophrenia demonstrate reliable deficits in the detection and labeling of facial affect, though it is not clear that this deficit is specific to emotional versus other aspects of facial emotion processing (Maric et al., 2003). Individuals with schizophrenia also show robust deficits in a range of other social-cognitive processes that have been linked to functional outcome in this disorder (Couture et al., 2006). One hypothesis in the literature is that deficits in the processing of facial emotion and social interactions, particularly negatively valenced ones, reflect an abnormality in AMY function in schizophrenia. Ventral limbic structures involved in emotional processing, such as the AMY (Packard et al., 1994; Packard and Teather, 1998; Packard and Cahill, 2001; Kilpatrick and Cahill, 2003; Habel et al., 2004; Packard and Wingard, 2004) and the HIP, provide important modulatory or gating inputs to the PFC and as such play an important role in the regulation of prefrontal executive functions. Suppressed AMY-PFC circuits have been associated with reductions in incentive motivational signals and decreased prefrontal activity (Grossberg, 2000; Shenton et al., 2001; Grady and Keightley, 2002; Paradiso et al., 2003). Research has shown that AMY activity is consistently modulated by the degree of arousal or motivation, such that highly arousing stimuli (either positive or negative) elicited greater AMY activity than low arousal stimuli (Snitz et al., 1999). These findings suggest that the AMY plays a role in assessing the intensity of emotional arousal or the salience of stimuli. However, the literature on AMY function in schizophrenia is extremely mixed. Some studies have found that the AMY demonstrates increased activation to emotional stimuli (faces and pictures) in individuals with schizophrenia compared to healthy controls (e.g., Kosaka et al., 2002; Taylor et al., 2005; Holt et al., 2006). In contrast, other studies have shown either decreased AMY activation to emotional stimuli (e.g., Gur et al., 2002; Hempel et al., 2003; Habel et al., 2004; Takahashi et al., 2004; Williams et al., 2004; Das et al., 2007), or no differences in AMY activation compared to healthy controls when viewing emotional stimuli (faces and pictures) (e.g., Surguladze et al., 2001; Plailly et al., 2006). Some of these differences across studies may reflect differences in the severity of different types of symptoms among the individuals with schizophrenia, as the severity of paranoia symptoms may be particularly associated with abnormal AMY function. In addition, there is evidence that individuals with schizophrenia may also show abnormal medial PFC function, which interacts with AMY during socioemotional processing (Brunet-Gouet and Decety, 2006). For example, Taylor et al. (2005) found that individuals with schizophrenia who rated high on reality distortion symptoms (hallucinations and delusions) showed hyperactivity of medial PFC. More recently, Williams et al. (2004) demonstrated abnormal connectivity between AMY and medial prefrontal regions (Das et al., 2007), suggesting a circuit-level abnormality associated with social-cognitive deficits in schizophrenia. In sum, there is growing evidence that abnormalities in the neural systems underlying the evaluation of aversive stimuli and social-emotional stimuli may contribute to deficits in social cognition and perhaps delusion formation in schizophrenia.

CLINICAL RELEVANCE OF COGNITIVE AND AFFECTIVE DEFICITS IN SCHIZOPHRENIA

If cognitive deficits are a core component of schizophrenia, it is important to ask whether these cognitive deficits contribute to the behavioral and symptomatic manifestations of this illness. Importantly, research over the last 10 years has revealed that the severity of cognitive deficits in schizophrenia may be one of the most important factors limiting functional outcome in this debilitating disorder (Green, 1996; Green, Kern, et al., 2004). This has led to an increased emphasis on treatment approaches, behavioral and pharmacological, specifically targeted at enhancing cognitive function (Green, Nuechterlein, et al., 2004; Marder, 2006). It is also clear that studies of cognitive function in schizophrenia also need to examine and understand individual differences in symptom severity. For example, there is evidence that cognitive deficits in schizophrenia may be more related to the severity of certain types of symptoms and not others. As described above, deficits in early sensory processing and neural synchrony may be particularly important for understanding positive symptoms such as hallucinations. In addition, a number of studies have suggested that deficits in working memory, executive control, and prefrontal dysfunction are strongly related to the severity of disorganization symptoms, but not to the severity of hallucinations and delusions (Barch, Carter, Hachten, et al., 1999; J.D. Cohen et al., 1999; Barch, Carter, Perlstein, et al., 1999; Stratta et al., 2000; Perlstein et al., 2001; Kerns and Berenbaum, 2002; Barch et al., 2003; Kerns and Berenbaum, 2003; Kuperberg et al., 2003; Kostova et al., 2005). The evidence for a relationship between cognitive deficits and negative symptoms is more mixed, with some studies finding relationships and others not. This variability may in part reflect the difficulty of assessing negative symptoms unconfounded by medication effects.

Although there has been less research on the neural circuits underlying emotion and motivational processing in schizophrenia, there are growing suggestions that the severity of hallucinations and/or delusions may be particularly relevant for understanding AMY and medial PFC function, as described earlier in this chapter. Further, individual differences in the severity of negative symptoms such as amotivation and anhedonia will likely be important for understanding the function of reward and pleasure processing systems in schizophrenia, such as dopaminergic systems involving reward prediction (Schultz et al., 1997; Crawford et al., 1998). To more fully understand such individual differences, the nature of functional imaging studies in schizophrenia and at-risk populations may need to change. Specifically, larger sample sizes are needed to powerfully assess individual differences, and greater emphasis is needed on functional imaging measures that demonstrate sufficient reliability and validity for use in individual differences studies.

COGNITIVE DEFICITS AS ENDOPHENOTYPES OF SCHIZOPHRENIA: EXPLORING COGNITIVE DEFICITS IN CLINICAL AND GENETIC HIGH-RISK POPULATIONS

Research strategies focusing on high-risk populations hold a special promise for the exploration of neurobiological changes that may constitute "risk markers" in vulnerable populations. Although schizophrenia is not a monogenetic disorder, genetic epidemiological findings point to a significant heritable component that accounts for about 70% of the risk (Tsuang, 2000). Although early efforts to characterize patients at risk for schizophrenia focused mainly on the biological offspring of patients (Erlenmeyer-Kimling, 2000), the advent of the *prodromal strategy* and its emphasis on early detection as a basis for interventions has provided a new approach for identifying an "enriched" population of patients at imminent risk for psychosis. Indeed, the prodromal stage is a critical juncture in the course of schizophrenia heralding the onset of psychosis and signaling clinical deterioration (Carpenter et al., 1991; McGlashan, 1998). Because of ethical concerns about the preclinical diagnosis of patients and their potential exposure to treatments with side effects, there is a critical need for more specific and reliable diagnostic markers of pending disease onset (Lieberman and Fenton, 2000).

Neurocognitive deficits in attention functions have been identified as one of the most replicated premorbid factors indicating increased risk for schizophrenia. Studies have demonstrated that offspring and siblings with genetically heightened risk for schizophrenia showed significantly impaired attention, working memory, and episodic memory functions compared with normal-risk relatives (Schubert and McNeil, 2005; Snitz et al., 2006). Some measures of early attentional suppression have also been reported to show significant reduction mainly in at-risk individuals with a first-degree relative with schizophrenia (Cadenhead et al., 2005). Neurocognitive and affective impairment also has clinical importance, as it has been consistently related to social and occupational outcome (McGurk and Meltzer, 2000; Rosenheck et al., 2006), functional impairment (Green, 2006; Keefe et al., 2006), quality of life, relapse prevention

(Fenton et al., 1997), medication compliance (Jarboe and Schwartz, 1999) and clinical outcome (Gur et al., 2006) in individuals with schizophrenia as well as genetic high-risk individuals (Cannon et al., 1999; Glatt et al., 2006). Numerous studies have also demonstrated a strong association between executive functioning with community functioning (Lysaker et al., 1995; Bellack et al., 1999; Bilder et al., 2000) and have further demonstrated that neurocognition does in fact have long-term predictive validity for quality of life (Fujii and Wylie, 2003). The contributions of cognitive deficits to poor functional outcomes have made them reasonable treatment targets in individuals with schizophrenia. Much fewer data are available however about the potential role of neural biomarkers, such as functional neuroimaging and electrophysiological measures as treatment targets. The P300 deficits have been shown to be stable longitudinally in schizophrenia, with hallucinations being associated with the frontal P3 (Turetsky et al., 1998), and MMN deficits have been associated with poor functioning in schizophrenia (Light and Braff, 2005). A better understanding of these measures and their characteristics in genetic and clinical high-risk individuals will help bridge the gaps between preclinical and clinical assessments.

Recent studies of individuals with prodromal symptoms and genetic high risk (Morey et al., 2005; Seidman, Thermenos, et al., 2006) have demonstrated abnormal engagement of fronto-striate and fronto-parietal regions during attention and executive function tasks. In fact, a recent meta-analysis of unaffected relatives of individuals with schizophrenia reported that deficits in voluntary (controlled) attention functions represent one of the most valuable endophenotypes in search for genetic factors related to schizophrenia (Snitz et al., 2006). Thus, much evidence suggests that neural circuits engaged during attention tasks may be already deregulated prior to illness onset and such brain/behavior measures may represent useful "risk markers" for schizophrenia. More specifically, the presence of cognitive deficits in the domains of executive processing, attention, working memory, and social cognitions in genetic and clinical high-risk populations indicate that these deficits may serve as an endophenotype for the illness in studies of genetics. Endophenotypes are characteristics that reflect the actions of genes predisposing an individual to a disorder, even in the absence of diagnosable pathology. Individual endophenotypes are presumably determined by fewer genes than the more complex phenotype of schizophrenia and would, therefore, reduce the complexity of genetic analyses. Many of the biological measures of information processing reviewed above, including electrophysiological measures of sensory processing, inhibition, and integration (for example, P50, MMN, and P300) and functional imaging measures of dorsolateral prefrontal cortical activation during working memory and attention tasks have been suggested as endophenotypes for schizophrenia.

SUMMARY

Converging evidence from numerous studies using cognitive neuroscience methodologies have revealed that information-processing deficits are core to schizophrenia and point to a distributed network of pathology involving fronto-parietal, fronto-striate, and fronto-limbic regions. Clearly, imaging and genetic techniques will continue to inform us about the neurobiological underpinning of schizophrenia. Biological and child psychiatry is in a new era, moving from solely behavioral and psychopharmacological investigations of biological substrates of disorders toward a more unified understanding of neural mechanisms involved in neurodevelopmental psychiatric disorders with the use of imaging and genetic methods from a cognitive neuroscience approach. Advances in the development of new methods in cognitive neurosciences and neuroimaging, and the utilization of combined multimodal techniques to achieve converging evidence, have enabled the identification of meaningful intermediate phenotypes in schizophrenia, such as the ones reviewed in this chapter. Combining methodologies such as electrophysiological recordings and functional brain imaging during the same task paradigm will serve to enhance the spatial resolution of the latter with the high temporal resolution of the former. As such, the approach of cognitive neuroscience promises to open up new avenues for therapeutic intervention for clinical populations at the pharmacological, genetic, and behavioral levels and identify windows of development that may be most optimal to treatment.

REFERENCES

Achim, A.M., and Lepage, M. (2005) Episodic memory-related activation in schizophrenia: meta-analysis. *Br. J. Psychiatry* 187:500–509.

Adler, L.E., Waldo, M.C., and Freedman, R. (1985) Neurophysiologic studies of sensory gating in schizophrenia: comparison of auditory and visual responses. *Biol. Psychiatry* 20:1284–1296.

Ahveninen, J., Jaaskelainen, I.P., Osipova, D., Huttunen, M.O., Ilmoniemi, R.J., Kaprio, J., et al. (2006) Inherited auditory-cortical dysfunction in twin pairs discordant for schizophrenia. *Biol. Psychiatry* 60:612–620.

Alexander, M.P., Stuss, D.T., and Fansabedian, N. (2003) California Verbal Learning Test: Performance by patients with focal frontal and non-frontal lesions. *Brain* 126:1493–1503.

Baddeley, A.D., and Logie, R.H. (1999) Working memory: The multiple-component model. In: Miyake, A., and Shah, P., eds. *Models of Working Memory: Mechanisms of Active Maintenance and Executive Control.* Cambridge, UK: Cambridge University Press, pp. 28–61.

Baldeweg, T., Spence, S., Hirsch, S.R., and Gruzelier, J. (1998) Gamma-band electroencephalographic oscillations in a patient with somatic hallucinations. *Lancet* 352:620–621.

Barch, D.M. (2005) The cognitive neuroscience of schizophrenia. In: Cannon, T., and Mineka, S., eds. *Annual Review of Clinical Psychology*, Vol 1. Washington, DC: American Psychological Association, pp. 321–353.

Barch, D.M., Carter, C.S., and Cohen, J.D. (2003) Context processing deficit in schizophrenia: Diagnostic specificity, 4-week course, and relationships to clinical symptoms. *J. Abnorm. Psychol.* 112: 132–143.

Barch, D.M., Carter, C.S., Hachten, P.C., and Cohen, J.D. (1999) The "benefits" of distractibility: The mechanisms underlying increased Stroop effects in schizophrenia. *Schizophr. Bull.* 24:749–762.

Barch, D.M., Carter, C., Perlstein, W., Baird, J., Cohen, J., and Schooler, N. (1999) Increased Stroop facilitation effects in schizophrenia are not due to increased automatic spreading activation. *Schizophr. Res.* 39:51–64.

Barch, D.M., and Csernanksy, J.G. (2007) Abnormal parietal cortex activation during working memory in schizophrenia: verbal phonological coding disturbances versus domain-general executive dysfunction. *Am. J. Psychiatry* 164(7):1090–1098.

Barch, D.M., Csernansky, J., Conturo, T., Snyder, A.Z., and Ollinger, J. (2002) Working and long-term memory deficits in schizophrenia. Is there a common underlying prefrontal mechanism? *J. Abnorm. Psychol.* 111:478–494.

Barch, D.M., Mitropoulou, V., Harvey, P.D., New, A.S., Silverman, J.M., and Siever, L.J. (2004) Context-processing deficits in schizotypal personality disorder. *J. Abnorm. Psychol.* 113:556–568.

Basar, E., Basar-Eroglu, C., Karakas, S., and Schurmann, M. (2001) Gamma, alpha, delta, and theta oscillations govern cognitive processes. *Int. J. Psychophysiol.* 39:241–248.

Basar, E., and Bullock, T.H., eds. (1992) *Induced Rhythms in the Brain.* Boston: Birkhauser.

Basar-Eroglu, C., and Demiralp, T. (2001) Event-related theta oscillations: an integrative and comparative approach in the human and animal brain. *Int. J. Psychophysiol.* 39:167–195.

Behrendt, R.P., and Young, C. (2004) Hallucinations in schizophrenia, sensory impairment, and brain disease: a unifying model. *Behav. Brain Sci.* 27:771–787; discussion 787–830.

Bellack, A.S., Gold, J.M., and Buchanan, R.W. (1999) Cognitive rehabilitation for schizophrenia: problems, prospects, and strategies. *Schizophr. Bull.* 25:257–274.

Bergman, A.J., Harvey, P.D., Roitman, S.L., Mohs, R.C., Marder, D., Silverman, J.M., and Siever, L.J. (1998) Verbal learning and memory in schizotypal personality disorder. *Schizophr. Bull.* 24: 635–641.

Bertolino, A., Callicott, J.H., Elman, I., Mattay, V.S., Tedeschi, G., Frank, J.A., et al. (1998) Regionally specific neuronal pathology in untreated patients with schizophrenia: a proton magnetic resonance spectroscopic imaging study. *Biol. Psychiatry* 43:641–648.

Bertolino, A., Callicott, J.H., Nawroz, S., Mattay, V.S., Duyn, J.H., Tedeschi, G., et al. (1998) Reproducibility of proton magnetic resonance spectroscopic imaging in patients with schizophrenia. *Neuropsychopharmacology* 18:1–9.

Bertolino, A., Nawroz, S., Mattay, V.S., Barnett, A.S., Duyn, J.H., Moonen, C.T., et al. (1996) Regionally specific pattern of neurochemical pathology in schizophrenia as assessed by multislice proton magnetic resonance spectroscopic imaging. *Am. J. Psychiatry* 153:1554–1563.

Bilder, R.M., Goldman, R.S., Robinson, D., Reiter, G., Bell, L., Bates, J.A., et al. (2000) Neuropsychology of first-episode schizophrenia: initial characterization and clinical correlates. *Am. J. Psychiatry* 157:549–559.

Boos, H.B., Aleman, A., Cahn, W., Pol, H.H., and Kahn, R.S. (2007) Brain volumes in relatives of patients with schizophrenia: a meta-analysis. *Arch. Gen. Psychiatry* 64:297–304.

Boyer, P., Phillips, J.L., Rousseau, F.L., and Ilivitsky, S. (2007) Hippocampal abnormalities and memory deficits: New evidence of a strong pathophysiological link in schizophrenia. *Brain Res. Rev.* 54:92–112.

Brahmbhatt, S.B., Haut, K., Csernansky, J.G., and Barch, D.M. (2006) Neural correlates of verbal and nonverbal working memory deficits in individuals with schizophrenia and their high-risk siblings. *Schizophr. Res.* 87:191–204.

Braver, T.S., Barch, D.M., Kelley, W.M., Buckner, R.L., Cohen, N.J., Miezin, F.M., et al. (2001) Direct comparison of prefrontal cortex regions engaged by working and long-term memory tasks. *Neuroimage* 14:48–59.

Brebion, G., Amador, X., Smith, M.J., and Gorman, J.M. (1998) Memory impairment and schizophrenia: the role of processing speed. *Schizophr. Res.* 30:31–39.

Brenner, C.A., Sporns, O., Lysaker, P.H., and O'Donnell, B.F. (2003) EEG synchronization to modulated auditory tones in schizophrenia, schizoaffective disorder, and schizotypal personality disorder. *Am. J. Psychiatry* 160:2238–2240.

Brewer, J.B., Zhao, Z., Desmond, J.E., Glover, G.H., and Gabrieli, J.D. (1998) Making memories: brain activity that predicts how well visual experience will be remembered [see comments]. *Science* 281:1185–1187.

Brothers, L. (1990) The social brain: a project for integrating primate behavior and neurophysiology in a new domain. *Concepts in Neuroscience* 1:27–61.

Brunet-Gouet, E., and Decety, J. (2006) Social brain dysfunctions in schizophrenia: a review of neuroimaging studies. *Psychiatry Res.* 148:75–92.

Burbridge, J.A., and Barch, D.M. (2002) Emotional valence and reference disturbance in schizophrenia. *J. Abnorm. Psychol.* 111:186–191.

Bustillo, J.R., Lauriello, J., Rowland, L.M., Thomson, L.M., Petropoulos, H., Hammond, R., et al. (2002) Longitudinal follow-up of neurochemical changes during the first year of antipsychotic treatment in schizophrenia patients with minimal previous medication exposure. *Schizophr. Res.* 58:313–321.

Cadenhead, K.S., Light, G.A., Shafer, K.M., and Braff, D.L. (2005) P50 suppression in individuals at risk for schizophrenia: the convergence of clinical, familial, and vulnerability marker risk assessment. *Biol. Psychiatry* 57:1504–1509.

Callicott, J.H., Bertolino, A., Mattay, V.S., Langheim, F.J., Duyn, J., Coppola, R., et al. (2000) Physiological dysfunction of the dorsolateral prefrontal cortex in schizophrenia revisited. *Cereb. Cortex* 10:1078–1092.

Callicott, J.H., Eagan, M.F., Bertolino, A., Mattay, V.S., Langhein, F.J.P., Frank, J.A., and Weinberger, D.R. (1998) Hippocampal N-acetyl apartate in unaffected siblings of patients with schizophrenia: a possible intermediate neurobiological phenotype. *Biol. Psychiatry* 44:941–950.

Callicott, J.H., Mattay, V.S., Bertolino, K.F., Coppola, R., Frank, J.A., Goldberg, T.E., and Weinberger, D.R. (1999) Physiological characteristics of capacity constraints in working memory as revealed by functional MRI. *Cereb. Cortex* 9:20–26.

Callicott, J.H., Mattay, V.S., Verchinski, B.A., Marenco, S., Egan, M.F., and Weinberger, D.R. (2003) Complexity of prefrontal cortical dysfunction in schizophrenia: more than up or down. *Am. J. Psychiatry* 160:2209–2215.

Camchong, J., Dyckman, K.A., Chapman, C.E., Yanasak, N.E., and McDowell, J.E. (2006) Basal ganglia-thalamocortical circuitry disruptions in schizophrenia during delayed response tasks. *Biol. Psychiatry* 60(3):235–241.

Cannon, T.D., Glahn, D.C., Kim, J., van Erp, T.G., Karlsgodt, K., Cohen, M.S., et al. (2005) Dorsolateral prefrontal cortex activity during maintenance and manipulation of information in working memory in patients with schizophrenia. *Arch. Gen. Psychiatry* 62:1071–1080.

Cannon, T.D., Rosso, I.M., Bearden, C.E., Sanchez, L.E., and Hadley, T. (1999) A prospective cohort study of neurodevelopmental processes in the genesis and epigenesis of schizophrenia. *Dev. Psychopathol.* 11:467–485.

Carpenter, W.T., Jr., Buchanan, R.W., Breier, A., Kirkpatrick, B., Thaker, G., and Tamminga, C. (1991) Psychopathology and the question of neurodevelopmental or neurodegenerative disorder. *Schizophr. Res.* 5:192–194.

Casanova, M.F., Goldberg, T.E., Suddath, R.L., Daniel, D.G., Rawlings, R., Lloyd, D.G., et al. (1990) Quantitative shape analysis of the temporal and prefrontal lobes of schizophrenic patients: a magnetic resonance image study. *J. Neuropsychiatry Clin. Neurosci.* 2:363–372.

Cecil, K.M., Lenkinski, R.E., Gur, R.E., and Gur, R.C. (1999) Proton magnetic resonance spectroscopy in the frontal and temporal lobes of neuroleptic naive patients with schizophrenia. *Neuropsychopharmacology* 20:131–140.

Censits, D.M., Ragland, J.D., Gur, R.C., and Gur, R.E. (1997) Neuropsychological evidence supporting a neurodevelopmental model of schizophrenia: a longitudinal study. *Schizophr. Res.* 24:289–298.

Cho, R.Y., Konecky, R.O., and Carter, C.S. (2006) Impairments in frontal cortical gamma synchrony and cognitive control in schizophrenia. *Proc. Natl. Acad. Sci. USA* 103:19878–19883.

Clementz, B.A., Geyer, M.A., and Braff, D.L. (1997) P50 suppression among schizophrenia and normal comparison subjects: a methodological analysis. *Biol. Psychiatry* 41:1035–1044.

Clementz, B.A., Keil, A., and Kissler, J. (2004) Aberrant brain dynamics in schizophrenia: delayed buildup and prolonged decay of the visual steady-state response. *Brain Res. Cogn. Brain Res.* 18: 121–129.

Cohen, J.D., Barch, D.M., Carter, C., and Servan-Schreiber, D. (1999) Context-processing deficits in schizophrenia: converging evidence from three theoretically motivated cognitive tasks. *J. Abnorm. Psychol.* 108:120–133.

Cohen, N.J., and Eichenbaum, H. (2001) *From Conditioning to Conscious Recollection.* New York: Oxford University Press.

Condray, R., Steinhauer, S.R., van Kammen, D.P., and Kasparek, A. (1996) Working memory capacity predicts language comprehension in schizophrenic patients. *Schizophr. Res.* 20:1–13.

Couture, S.M., Roberts, D.L., Penn, D.L., Cather, C., Otto, M., and Goff, D.A. (2006) Do baseline client characteristics predict the therapeutic alliance in the treatment of schizophrenia? *J. Nerv. Ment. Dis.* 194(1):10–14

Crawford, T.J., Sharma, T., Puri, B.K., Murray, R.M., Berridge, D. M., and Lewis, S.W. (1998) Saccadic eye movements in families multiply affected with schizophrenia: the Maudsley Family Study. *Am. J. Psychiatry* 155:1703–1710.

Crespo-Facorro, B., Paradiso, S., Andreasen, N.C., O'Leary, D.S., Watkins, G.L., Ponto, L.L.B., and Hichwa, R.D. (2001) Neural mechanisms of anhedonia in schizophrenia. *JAMA* 286:427–435.

Crespo-Facorro, B., Roiz-Santianez, R., Pelayo-Teran, J.M., Gonzalez-Blanch, C., Perez-Iglesias, R., Gutierrez, A., et al. (2007) Caudate nucleus volume and its clinical and cognitive correlations in first episode schizophrenia. *Schizophr. Res.* 91:87–96.

Csernansky, J.G., Joshi, S., Wang, L., Haller, J.W., Gado, M., Miller, J.P., et al. (1998) Hippocampal morphometry in schizophrenia by high dimensional brain mapping. *Proc. Natl. Acad. Sci. USA* 95:11406–11411.

Cullen, T.J., Walker, M.A., Eastwood, S.L., Esiri, M.M., Harrison, P.J., and Crow, T.J. (2006) Anomalies of asymmetry of pyramidal cell density and structure in dorsolateral prefrontal cortex in schizophrenia. *Br. J. Psychiatry* 188:26–31.

Das, P., Kemp, A.H., Flynn, G., Harris, A.W.F., Liddell, B.J., Whitford, T.J., et al. (2007) Functional disconnections in the direct and indirect amygdala pathways for fear processing in schizophrenia. *Schizophr. Res.* 90:284–294.

Davidson, L.L., and Heinrichs, R.W. (2003) Quantification of frontal and temporal lobe brain-imaging findings in schizophrenia: a meta-analysis. *Psychiatry Res.* 122:69–87.

Deicken, R.F., Pegues, M., and Amend, D. (1999) Reduced hippocampal N-acetylaspartate without volume loss in schizophrenia. *Schizophr. Res.* 37:217–223.

Delamillieure, P., Constans, J.M., Fernandez, J., Brazo, P., Benali, K., Courtheoux, P., et al. (2002) Proton magnetic resonance spectroscopy (1H MRS) in schizophrenia: investigation of the right and left hippocampus, thalamus, and prefrontal cortex. *Schizophr. Bull.* 28:329–339.

Delawalla, Z., Barch, D.M., Fisher Eastep, J.L., Thomason, E.S., Hanewinkel, M.J., Thompson, P.A., and Csernansky, J.G. (2006) Factors mediating cognitive deficits and psychopathology among siblings of individuals with schizophrenia. *Schizophr. Bull.* 32(3):525–537.

Delawalla, Z., Csernanksy, J.G., and Barch, D.M. (2008) Prefrontal cortex function in nonpsychotic siblings of individuals with schizophrenia. *Biol. Psychiatry* 63(5):490–497.

Eichenbaum, H., and Cohen, N.J. (2001) *From Conditioning to Conscious Recollection: Memory Systems of the Brain.* New York: Oxford University Press.

Elvevag, B., Fisher, J.E., Weickert, T.W., Weinberger, D.R., and Goldberg, T.E. (2004) Lack of false recognition in schizophrenia: a consequence of poor memory? *Neuropsychologia* 42:546–554.

Erlenmeyer-Kimling, L. (2000) Neurobehavioral deficits in offspring of schizophrenic parents: liability indicators and predictors of illness. *Am. J. Med. Genet.* 97:65–71.

Faraone, S.V., Kremen, W.S., Lyons, M.J., Pepple, J.R., et al. (1995) Diagnostic accuracy and linkage analysis: how useful are schizophrenia spectrum phenotypes? *Am. J. Psychiatry* 152:1286–1290.

Faraone, S.V., Seidman, L.J., Kremen, W.S., Toomey, R., Pepple, J.R., and Tsuang, M.T. (1999) Neuropsychological functioning among the nonpsychotic relatives of schizophrenic patients: a 4-year follow-up study. *J. Abnorm. Psychol.* 108:176–181.

Faraone, S.V., Seidman, L.J., Kremen, W.S., Toomey, R., Pepple, J.R., and Tsuang, M.T. (2000) Neuropsychologic functioning among the nonpsychotic relatives of schizophrenic patients: the effect of genetic loading. *Biol. Psychiatry* 48:120–126.

Farmer, C.M., O'Donnell, B.F., Niznikiewicz, M.A., Voglmaier, M.M., McCarley, R.W., and Shenton, M.E. (2000) Visual perception and working memory in schizotypal personality disorder. *Am. J. Psychiatry* 157:781–788.

Fenton, W.S., Blyler, C.R., and Heinssen, R.K. (1997) Determinants of medication compliance in schizophrenia: empirical and clinical findings. *Schizophr. Bull.* 23:637–651.

Fiske, S.T., and Taylor, S. (1991) *Social Cognition.* New York: McGraw-Hill.

Fleming, K., Goldberg, T.E., Gold, J.M., and Weinberger, D.R. (1995) Verbal working memory dysfunction in schizophrenia: use of a Brown-Peterson paradigm. *Psychiatry Res.* 56:155–161.

Foxe, J.J., Murray, M.M., and Javitt, D.C. (2005) Filling-in in schizophrenia: a high-density electrical mapping and source-analysis investigation of illusory contour processing. *Cereb. Cortex* 15:1914–1927.

Freedman, R., Adler, L.E., Gerhardt, G.A., Waldo, M., Baker, N., Rose, G.M., et al. (1987) Neurobiological studies of sensory gating in schizophrenia. *Schizophr. Bull.* 13:669–678.

Freedman, R., Waldo, M., Bickford-Wimer, P., and Nagamoto, H. (1991) Elementary neuronal dysfunctions in schizophrenia. *Schizophr. Res.* 4:233–243.

Fujii, D.E., and Wylie, A.M. (2003) Neurocognition and community outcome in schizophrenia: long-term predictive validity. *Schizophr. Res.* 59:219–223.

Galambos, R., Makeig, S., and Talmachoff, P.J. (1981) A 40-Hz auditory potential recorded from the human scalp. *Proc. Natl. Acad. Sci. USA* 78:2643–2647.

Glahn, D.C., Ragland, J.D., Abramoff, A., Barrett, J., Laird, A.R., Bearden, C.E., and Velligan, D.I. (2005) Beyond hypofrontality: A quantitative meta-analysis of functional neuroimaging studies of working memory in schizophrenia. *Hum. Brain Mapp.* 25:60–69.

Glahn, D.C., Therman, S., Manninen, M., Huttunen, M., Kaprio, J., Lonnqvist, J., and Cannon, T.D. (2003) Spatial working memory as an endophenotype for schizophrenia. *Biol. Psychiatry* 53:624–626.

Glatt, S.J., Stone, W.S., Faraone, S.V., Seidman, L.J., and Tsuang, M.T. (2006) Psychopathology, personality traits and social development of young first-degree relatives of patients with schizophrenia. *Br. J. Psychiatry* 189:337–345.

Gold, J.M., Carpenter, C., Randolph, C., Goldberg, T.E., and Weinberger, D.R. (1997) Auditory working memory and Wisconsin Card Sorting Test performance in schizophrenia. *Arch. Gen. Psychiatry* 54:159–165.

Goldberg, T.E., Egan, M.F., Gscheidle, T., Coppola, R., Weickert, T., Kolachana, B.S., et al. (2003) Executive subprocesses in working memory: relationship to catechol-O-methyltransferase Val158Met genotype and schizophrenia. *Arch. Gen. Psychiatry* 60:889–896.

Goldberg, T.E., Hyde, T.M., Kleinman, J.E., and Weinberger, D.R. (1993) Course of schizophrenia: neuropsychological evidence for a static encephalopathy. *Schizophr. Bull.* 19:797–804.

Goldberg, T.E., Torrey, E.F., Berman, K.F., and Weinberger, D.R. (1994) Relations between neuropsychological performance and brain morphological and physiological measures in monozygotic twins discordant for schizophrenia. *Psychiatry Res.* 55:51–61.

Gooding, D.C., and Tallent, K.A. (2004) Nonverbal working memory deficits in schizophrenia patients: evidence of a supramodal executive processing deficit. *Schizophr. Res.* 68:189–201.

Grady, C.L., and Keightley, M.L. (2002) Studies of altered social cognition in neuropsychiatric disorders using functional neuroimaging. *Can. J. Psychiatry* 47:327–336.

Green, M.F. (1996) What are the functional consequences of neurocognitive deficits in schizophrenia? *Am. J. Psychiatry* 153:321–330.

Green, M.F. (2006) Cognitive impairment and functional outcome in schizophrenia and bipolar disorder. *J. Clin. Psychiatry* 67(Suppl 9):3–8; discussion 36–42.

Green, M.F., Kern, R.S., and Heaton, R.K. (2004) Longitudinal studies of cognition and functional outcome in schizophrenia: implications for MATRICS. *Schizophr. Res.* 72:41–51.

Green, M.F., and Nuechterlein, K.H. (1999) Cortical oscillations and schizophrenia: timing is of the essence. *Arch. Gen. Psychiatry* 56:1007–1008.

Green, M.F., Nuechterlein, K.H., Gold, J.M., Barch, D.M., Cohen, J., Essock, S., et al. (2004) Approaching a consensus cognitive battery for clinical trials in schizophrenia: the NIMH-MATRICS conference to select cognitive domains and test criteria. *Biol. Psychiatry* 56:301–307.

Grossberg, S. (2000) The imbalanced brain: from normal behavior to schizophrenia. *Biol. Psychiatry* 48:81–98.

Gunduz, H., Wu, H., Ashtari, M., Bogerts, B., Crandall, D., Robinson, D.G., et al. (2002) Basal ganglia volumes in first-episode schizophrenia and healthy comparison subjects. *Biol. Psychiatry* 51: 801–808.

Gur, R.E., Kohler, C.G., Ragland, J.D., Siegel, S.J., Lesko, K., Bilker, W.B., and Gur, R.C. (2006) Flat affect in schizophrenia: relation to emotion processing and neurocognitive measures. *Schizophr. Bull.* 32:279–287.

Gur, R.E., McGrath, C., Chan, R.M., Schroeder, L., Turner, T., Turetsky, B.I., et al. (2002) An fMRI study of facial emotion processing in patients with schizophrenia. *Am. J. Psychiatry* 159:1992–1999.

Gur, R.E., Mozley, P.D., Shtasel, D.L., Cannon, T.D., Gallacher, F., Turetsky, B., et al. (1994) Clinical subtypes of schizophrenia: differences in brain and CSF volume. *Am. J. Psychiatry* 151:343–350.

Guterman, Y., and Josiassen, R.C. (1994) Sensory gating deviance in schizophrenia in the context of task related effects. *Int. J. Psychophysiol.* 18(1):1–12.

Habel, U., Klein, M., Shah, N.J., Toni, I., Zilles, K., Falkai, P., and Schneider, F. (2004) Genetic load on amygdala hypofunction during sadness in nonaffected brothers of schizophrenia patients. *Am. J. Psychiatry* 161:1806–1813.

Heckers, S., Rauch, S.L., Goff, D., Savage, C.R., Schacter, D.L., Fischman, A.J., and Alpert, N.M. (1998) Impaired recruitment of the hippocampus during conscious recollection in schizophrenia. *Nat. Neurosci.* 1:318–323.

Heckers, S., Weiss, A.P., Deckersbach, T., Goff, D.C., Morecraft, R.J., and Bush, G. (2004) Anterior cingulate cortex activation during cognitive interference in schizophrenia. *Am. J. Psychiatry* 161: 707–715.

Heerey, A., and Gold, J.M. (2007) Patients with schizophrenia demonstrate dissociation between affective experience and motivated behavior. *J. Abnorm. Psychol.* 116(2):268–278.

Hempel, A., Hempel, E., Schonknecht, P., Stippich, C., and Schroder, J. (2003) Impairment in basal limbic function in schizophrenia during affect recognition. *Psychiatry Res.* 122:115–124.

Herrmann, C.S., and Demiralp, T. (2005) Human EEG gamma oscillations in neuropsychiatric disorders. *Clin. Neurophysiol.* 116: 2719–2733.

Hill, S.K., Beers, S.R., Kmiec, J.A., Keshavan, M.S., and Sweeney, J.A. (2004) Impairment of verbal memory and learning in antipsychotic-naive patients with first-episode schizophrenia. *Schizophr. Res.* 68:127–136.

Hofer, A., Weiss, E.M., Golaszewski, S.M., Siedentopf, C.M., Brinkhoff, C., Kremser, C., et al. (2003) Neural correlates of episodic encoding and recognition of words in unmedicated patients during an acute episode of schizophrenia: a functional fMRI study. *Am. J. Psychiatry* 160:1802–1808.

Hofer, A., Weiss, E.M., Golaszewski, S.M., Siedentopf, C.M., Kremser, C., Felber, S., and Fleischhacker, W.W. (2003) An fMRI study of episodic encoding and recognition of words in patients with schizoprenia in remission. *Am. J. Psychiatry* 160:911–918.

Hoff, A.L., Riordan, H., O'Donnell, D.W., Morris, L., and DeLisi, L.E. (1992) Neuropsychological functioning of first-episode schizophreniform patients. *Am. J. Psychiatry* 149:898–903.

Hoff, A.L., Sakuma, M., Wieneke, M., Horon, R., Kushner, M., and DeLisa, L.E. (1999) Longitudinal neuropsychological follow-up study of patients with first-episode schizophrenia. *Am. J. Psychiatry* 156:1336–1341.

Holt, D.J., Kunkel, L., Weiss, A.P., Goff, D.C., Wright, C.I., Shin, L.M., et al. (2006) Increased medial temporal lobe activation during the passive viewing of emotional and neutral facial expressions in schizophrenia. *Schizophr. Res.* 82:153–162.

Honer, W.G., Bassett, A.S., Squires-Wheeler, E., Falkai, P., Smith, G.N., Lapointe, J.S., et al. (1995) The temporal lobes, reversed asymmetry and the genetics of schizophrenia. *Neuroreport* 7:221–224.

Hong, L.E., Summerfelt, A., McMahon, R., Adami, H., Francis, G., Elliott, A., et al. (2004) Evoked gamma band synchronization and the liability for schizophrenia. *Schizophr. Res.* 70:293–302.

Iddon, J.L., McKenna, P.J., Sahakian, B.J., and Robbins, T.W. (1998) Impaired generation and use of strategy in schizophrenia: evidence from visuospatial and verbal tasks. *Psychol. Med.* 28:1049–1062.

Janowsky, J., and Shimamura, A.P. (1989) Cognitive impairment following frontal lobe damage and its relevance to human amnesia. *Behav. Neurosci.* 103:548–560.

Janowsky, J.S., Shimamura, A.P., and Squire, L.R. (1989) Source memory impairment in patients with frontal lobe lesions. *Neuropsychologia* 27:1043–1056.

Jarboe, K., and Schwartz, W. (1999) The relationship between medication noncompliance and cognitive function in patients with schizophrenia. *J. Am. Psychiatr. Nurses Assoc.* 5:S2–S8.

Javitt, D.C. (2000) Intracortical mechanisms of mismatch negativity dysfunction in schizophrenia. *Audiol. Neuro-Otol.* 5:207–215.

Javitt, D.C., Doneshka, P., Grochowski, S., and Ritter, W. (1995) Impaired mismatch negativity generation reflects widespread dysfunction of working memory in schizophrenia. *Arch. Gen. Psychiatry* 52:550–558.

Javitt, D.C., Doneshka, P., Zylberman, I., Ritter, W., and Vaughan, H.G., Jr. (1993) Impairment of early cortical processing in schizophrenia: an event-related potential confirmation study. *Biol. Psychiatry* 33:513–519.

Jessen, F., Scheef, L., Germeshausen, L., Tawo, Y., Kockler, M., Kuhn, K.U., et al. (2003) Reduced hippocampal activation during encoding and recognition of words in schizophrenia patients. *Am. J. Psychiatry* 160:1305–1312.

Jin, Y., Potkin, S.G., Patterson, J.V., Sandman, C.A., Hetrick, W.P., and Bunney, W.E., Jr. (1997) Effects of P50 temporal variability on sensory gating in schizophrenia. *Psychiatry Res.* 70:71–81.

Jin, Y., Bunney, W.E., Jr., Sandman, C.A., Patterson, J.V., Fleming, K., Moenter, J.R., Kalali A.H., Hetrick, W.P., and Potkin, S.G. (1998) Is P50 suppression a measure of sensory gating in schizophrenia? *Biol. Psychiatry* 43(12):873–878.

Johannesen, J.K., Kieffaber, P.D., O'Donnell, B.F., Shekhar, A., Evans, J.D., and Hetrick, W.P. (2005) Contributions of subtype and spectral frequency analyses to the study of P50 ERP amplitude and suppression in schizophrenia. *Schizophr. Res.* 78:269–284.

Johnson, M.R., Morris, N.A., Astur, R.S., Calhoun, V.D., Mathalon, D.H., Kiehl, K.A., and Pearlson, G.D. (2006) A functional magnetic resonance imaging study of working memory abnormalities in schizophrenia. *Biol. Psychiatry* 60:11–21.

Juckel, G., Schlagenhauf, F., Koslowski, M., Filonov, D., Wustenberg, T., Villringer, A., et al. (2006) Dysfunction of ventral striatal reward prediction in schizophrenic patients treated with typical, not atypical, neuroleptics. *Psychopharmacology (Berl)* 187: 222–228.

Karakas, S., and Basar, E. (1998) Early gamma response is sensory in origin: a conclusion based on cross-comparison of results from multiple experimental paradigms. *Int. J. Psychophysiol.* 31:13–31.

Keefe, R.S., Poe, M., Walker, T.M., Kang, J.W., and Harvey, P.D. (2006) The Schizophrenia Cognition Rating Scale: an interview-based assessment and its relationship to cognition, real-world functioning, and functional capacity. *Am. J. Psychiatry* 163:426–432.

Kerns, J.B., and Berenbaum, H. (2002) Cognitive impairments associated with formal thought disorder in people with schizophrenia. *J. Abnorm. Psychol.* 111:211–224.

Kerns, J.G., and Berenbaum, H. (2003) The relationship between formal thought disorder and executive functioning component processes. *J. Abnorm. Psychol.* 112:339–352.

Keshavan, M.S., Dick, E., Mankowski, I., Harenski, K., Montrose, D.M., Diwadkar, V., and DeBellis, M. (2002) Decreased left amygdala and hippocampal volumes in young offspring at risk for schizophrenia. *Schizophr. Res.* 58:173–183.

Kilpatrick, L., and Cahill, L. (2003) Amygdala modulation of parahippocampal and frontal regions during emotionally influenced memory storage. *Neuroimage* 20:2091–2099.

Kim, J., Glahn, D.C., Nuechterlein, K.H., and Cannon, T.D. (2004) Maintenance and manipulation of information in schizophrenia: further evidence for impairment in the central executive component of working memory. *Schizophr. Res.* 68:173–187.

Kim, J., Kwon, J.S., Park, H.J., Youn, T., Kang, D.H., Kim, M.S., et al. (2003) Functional disconnection between the prefrontal and parietal cortices during working memory processing in schizophrenia. *Am. J. Psychiatry* 160:919–923.

Kirchhoff, B.A., Wagner, A.D., Maril, A., and Stern, C.E. (2000) Prefrontal-temporal circuitry for episodic encoding and subsequent memory. *J. Neurosci.* 20:6173–6180.

Knable, M.B., Barci, B.M., Webster, M.J., Meador-Woodruff, J., and Torrey, E.F. (2004) Molecular abnormalities of the hippocampus in severe psychiatric illness: postmortem findings from the Stanley Neuropathology Consortium. *Mol. Psychiatry* 9:609–620, 544.

Koh, S.D. (1978) Remembering of verbal material by schizophrenic young adults. In: Schwartz, S., ed. *Language and Cognitive in Schizophrenia.* Hillsdale, NJ: Lawrence Erlbaum, pp. 55–99.

Koh, S.D., and Peterson, R.A. (1978) Encoding orientation and the remembering of schizophrenic young adults. *J. Abnorm. Psychol.* 87:303–313.

Kosaka, H., Omori, M., Murata, T., Iidaka, T., Yamada, H., Okada, T., et al. (2002) Differential amygdala response during facial recognition in patients with schizophrenia: an fMRI study. *Schizophr. Res.* 57:87–95.

Kostova, M., Passerieux, C., Laurent, J.P., and Hardy-Bayle, M.C. (2005) N400 anomalies in schizophrenia are correlated with the severity of formal thought disorder. *Schizophr. Res.* 78:285–291.

Kremen, W.S., Seidman, L.J., Pepple, J.R., Lyons, M.J., Tsuang, M. T., and Faraone, S.V. (1994) Neuropsychological risk indicators for schizophrenia: a review of family studies. *Schizophr. Bull.* 20:103–119.

Kring, A.M. (1999) Emotion in schizophrenia: old mystery, new understanding. *Current Directions in Psychological Science* 8:160–163.

Kring, A.M., Kerr, S.L., Smith, D.A., and Neale, J.M. (1993) Flat affect in schizophrenia does not reflect diminished subjective experience of emotion. *J. Abnorm. Psychol.* 102:507–517.

Kring, A.M., and Neale, J.M. (1996) Do schizophrenic patients show a disjunctive relationship among expression, experiential, and psychophysiological components of emotion? *J. Abnorm. Psychol.* 105:249–257.

Kubicki, M., McCarley, R.W., Nestor, P.G., Huh, T., Kikinis, R., Shenton, M.E., and Wible, C.G. (2003) An fMRI study of semantic processing in men with schizophrenia. *Neuroimage* 20:1923–1933.

Kunda, Z. (1999) *Social cognition: Making sense of people.* Cambridge, MA: MIT Press.

Kuperberg, G.R., Broome, M.R., McGuire, P.K., David, A.S., Eddy, M., Ozawa, F., et al. (2003) Regionally localized thinning of the cerebral cortex in schizophrenia. *Arch. Gen. Psychiatry* 60:878–888.

Kwon, J.S., O'Donnell, B.F., Wallenstein, G.V., Greene, R.W., Hirayasu, Y., Nestor, P.G., et al. (1999) Gamma frequency-range abnormalities to auditory stimulation in schizophrenia. *Arch. Gen. Psychiatry* 56:1001–1005.

Larsen, S.F., and Fromholt, P. (1976) Mnemonic organization and free recall in schizophrenia. *J. Abnorm. Psychol.* 85:61–65.

Laurent, A., Biloa-Tang, M., Bougerol, T., Duly, D., Anchisi, A.M., Bosson, J.L., et al. (2000) Executive/attentional performance and measures of schizotypy in patients with schizophrenia and in their nonpsychotic first-degree relatives. *Schizophr. Res.* 46:269–283.

Lawrie, S.M., Whalley, H., Kestelman, J.N., Abukmeil, S.S., Byrne, M., Hodges, A., et al. (1999) Magnetic resonance imaging of brain in people at high risk of developing schizophrenia. *Lancet* 353:30–33.

Laywer, G., Nyman, H., Agartz, I., Arnborg, S., Jonsson, E.G., Sedvall, G.C., and Hall, H. (2006) Morphological correlates to cognitive dysfunction in schizophrenia as studied with Bayesian regression. *BMC Psychiatry* 6:31.

Lee, D. (2003) Coherent oscillations in neuronal activity of the supplementary motor area during a visuomotor task. *J. Neurosci.* 23:6798–6809.

Lee, K.H., Williams, L.M., Breakspear, M., and Gordon, E. (2003) Synchronous gamma activity: a review and contribution to an integrative neuroscience model of schizophrenia. *Brain Res. Rev.* 41:57–78.

Lepage, M., Montoya, A., Pelletier, M., Achim, A.M., Menear, M., and Lal, S. (2006) Associative memory encoding and recognition in schizophrenia: an event-related fMRI study. *Biol. Psychiatry* 60: 1215–1223.

Leube, D.T., Rapp, A., Buchkremer, G., Bartels, M., and Kircher, T. T.J. (2002) Hippocampal dysfunction during episodic memory encoding in patients with schizophrenia—an fMRI study. *Schizophr. Res.* 64:83–85.

Lieberman, J.A., and Fenton, W.S. (2000) Delayed detection of psychosis: causes, consequences, and effect on public health. *Am. J. Psychiatry* 157:1727–1730.

Light, G.A., and Braff, D.L. (2005) Mismatch negativity deficits are associated with poor functioning in schizophrenia patients. *Arch. Gen. Psychiatry* 62:127–136.

Line, P., Silberstein, R.B., Wright, J.J., and Copolov, D.L. (1998) Steady state visually evoked potential correlates of auditory hallucinations in schizophrenia. *Neuroimage* 8:370–376.

Lysaker, P.H., Bell, M.D., and Bioty, S.M. (1995) Cognitive deficits in schizophrenia. Prediction of symptom change for participators in work rehabilitation. *J. Nerv. Ment. Dis.* 183:332–336.

Mamah, D., Wang, L., Barch, D., de Erausquin, G.A., Gado, M., and Csernansky, J.G. (2007) Structural analysis of the basal ganglia in schizophrenia. *Schizophr. Res.* 89:59–71.

Manoach, D.S., Gollub, R.L., Benson, E.S., Searl, M.M., Goff, D.C., Halpern, E., et al. (2000) Schizophrenic subjects show aberrant fMRI activation of dorsolateral prefrontal cortex and basal ganglia during working memory performance. *Biol. Psychiatry* 48:99–109.

Marder, S.R. (2006) Initiatives to promote the discovery of drugs to improve cognitive function in severe mental illness. *J. Clin. Psychiatry* 67:e03.

Maric, N., Kamer, T., Schneider Axmann, T., Dani, I., Jasovic Gasic, M., Paunovic, V.R., and Falkai, P. (2003) Volumetric analysis of gray matter, white matter and cerebrospinal fluid space in schizophrenia. *Srp. Arh. Celok. Lek.* 131:26–30.

McClelland, J.L., McNaughton, B.L., and O'Reilly, R.C. (1995) Why there are complementary learnings systems in the hippocampus and neocortex: insights from the successes and failures of connectionist models of learning and memory. *Psychol. Rev.* 102: 419–457.

McDermott, K.B., Petersen, S.E., Watson, J.M., and Ojemann, J.G. (2003) A procedure for identifying regions preferentially activated by attention to semantic and phonological relations using functional magnetic resonance imaging. *Neuropsychologia* 41:293–303.

McGlashan, T.H. (1998) Early detection and intervention of schizophrenia: rationale and research. *Br. J. Psychiatry Suppl.* 172:3–6.

McGurk, S.R., and Meltzer, H.Y. (2000) The role of cognition in vocational functioning in schizophrenia. *Schizophr. Res.* 45:175–184.

Menon, V., Anagnoson, R.T., Mathalon, D.H., Glover, G.H., and Pfefferbaum, A. (2001) Functional neuroanatomy of auditory working memory in schizophrenia: relation to positive and negative symptoms. *Neuroimage* 13:433–446.

Meyer-Lindenberg, A., Poline, J.B., Kohn, P.D., Holt, J.L., Egan, M.F., Weinberger, D.R., and Berman, K.F. (2001) Evidence for abnormal cortical functional connectivity during working memory in schizophrenia. *Am. J. Psychiatry* 158:1809–1817.

Michie, P.T., Budd, T.W., Todd, J., Rock, D., Wichmann, H., Box, J., and Jablensky, A.V. (2000) Duration and frequency mismatch negativity in schizophrenia. *Clin. Neurophysiol.* 111(6):1054–1065.

Mitropoulou, V., Harvey, P.D., Maldari, L.A., Moriarty, P.J., New, A.S., Silverman, J.M., and Siever, L.J. (2002) Neuropsychological performance in schizotypal personality disorder: evidence regarding diagnostic specificity. *Biol. Psychiatry* 52:1175–1182.

Molina, V., Reig, S., Desco, M., Gispert, J.D., Sanz, J., Sarramea, F., et al. (2002) Multimodal neuroimaging studies and neurodevelopment and neurodegeneration hypotheses of schizophrenia. *Neurotox. Res.* 4:437–451.

Morey, R.A., Inan, S., Mitchell, T.V., Perkins, D.O., Lieberman, J. A., and Belger, A. (2005) Imaging frontostriatal function in ultra-high-risk, early, and chronic schizophrenia during executive processing. *Arch. Gen. Psychiatry* 62:254–262.

Muller, H.F., Achim, A., Laur, A., and Buchbinder, A. (1986) Topography and possible physiological significance of EEG amplitude variability in psychosis. *Acta Psychiatr. Scand.* 73:665–675.

Murray, E.A. (1996) What have ablation studies told us about neural substrates of stimulus memory? *Seminars in the Neurosciences* 8:13–22.

Naatanen, R. (1992) *Attention and Brain Function.* Hillsdale, NJ: Lawrence Erlbaum.

Nelson, D.L. (1979) Remembering pictures and words: Appearance, significance, and name. In: Cermak, L.S., and Craik, F.I.M., eds. *Levels of Processing in Human Memory.* Hillsdale, NJ: Lawrence Erlbaum, pp. 45–76.

Nestor, P.G., Kubicki, M., Kuroki, N., Gurrera, R.J., Niznikiewicz, M., Shenton, M.E., and McCarley, R.W. (2007) Episodic memory and neuroimaging of hippocampus and fornix in chronic schizophrenia. *Psychiatry Res.* 155:21–28.

Nestor, P.G., Shenton, M.E., McCarley, R.W., Haimson, J., Smith, R.S., O'Donnell, B., et al. (1993) Neuropsychological correlates of MRI temporal lobe abnormalities in schizophrenia. *Am. J. Psychiatry* 150:1849–1855.

O'Driscoll, G.A., Florencio, P.S., Gagnon, D., Wolff, A.V., Benkelfat, C., Mikula, L., et al. (2001) Amygdala-hippocampal volume and verbal memory in first-degree relatives of schizophrenic patients. *Psychiatry Res.* 107:75–85.

Otten, L.J., Henson, R.N.A., and Rugg, M.D. (2001) Depth of processing effects on neural correlates of memory encoding. *Brain* 124:399–412.

Packard, M.G., and Cahill, L. (2001) Affective modulation of multiple memory systems. *Curr. Opin. Neurobiol.* 11:752–756.

Packard, M.G., Cahill, L., and McGaugh, J.L. (1994) Amygdala modulation of hippocampal-dependent and caudate nucleus-dependent memory processes. *Proc. Natl. Acad. Sci. USA* 91:8477–8481.

Packard, M.G., and Teather, L.A. (1998) Amygdala modulation of multiple memory systems: hippocampus and caudate-putamen. *Neurobiol. Learn. Mem.* 69:163–203.

Packard, M.G., and Wingard, J.C. (2004) Amygdala and "emotional" modulation of the relative use of multiple memory systems. *Neurobiol. Learn. Mem.* 82:243–252.

Paradiso, S., Andreasen, N.C., Crespo-Facorro, B., O'Leary, D.S., Watkins, G.L., Boles Ponto, L.L., and Hichwa, R.D. (2003) Emotions in unmedicated patients with schizophrenia during evaluation with positron emission tomography. *Am. J. Psychiatry* 160: 1775–1783.

Park, S., Holzman, P.S., and Lenzenweger, M.F. (1995) Individual differences in spatial working memory in relation to schizotypy. *J. Abnorm. Psychol.* 104:355–363.

Park, S., and McTigue, K. (1997) Working memory and the syndromes of schizotypal personality. *Schizophr. Res.* 26:213–220.

Patterson, J.V., Jin, Y., Gierczak, M., Hetrick, W.P., Potkin, S., Bunney, W.E., Jr., and Sandman, C.A. (2000) Effects of temporal variability on p50 and the gating ratio in schizophrenia: a frequency domain adaptive filter single-trial analysis. *Arch. Gen. Psychiatry* 57:57–64.

Penn, D.L., Spaulding, W., Reed, D., Sullivan, M., Mueser, K.T., and Hope, D.A. (1997) Cognition and social functioning in schizophrenia. *Psychiatry* 60(4):281–291.

Perlstein, W.M., Carter, C.S., Noll, D.C., and Cohen, J.D. (2001) Relation of prefrontal cortex dysfunction to working memory and symptoms in schizophrenia. *Am. J. Psychiatry* 158:1105–1113.

Perlstein, W.M., Dixit, N.K., Carter, C.S., Noll, D.C., and Cohen, J.D. (2003) Prefrontal cortex dysfunction mediates deficits in working memory and prepotent responding in schizophrenia. *Biol. Psychiatry* 53:25–38.

Pfurtscheller, G., and Lopes da Silva, F.H. (1999) Event-related EEG/MEG synchronization and desynchronization: basic principles. *Clin. Neurophysiol.* 110:1842–1857.

Pierri, J.N., Volk, C.L., Auh, S., Sampson, A., and Lewis, D.A. (2001) Decreased somal size of deep layer 3 pyramidal neurons in the prefrontal cortex of subjects with schizophrenia. *Arch. Gen. Psychiatry* 58:466–473.

Plailly, J., d'Amato, T., Saoud, M., and Royet, J.P. (2006) Left temporo-limbic and orbital dysfunction in schizophrenia during odor familiarity and hedonicity judgments. *Neuroimage* 29:302–313.

Prince, S.E., Daselaar, S.M., and Cabeza, R. (2005) Neural correlates of relational memory: successful encoding and retrieval of semantic and perceptual associations. *J. Neurosci.* 25:1203–1210.

Quintana, J., Wong, T., Ortiz-Portillo, E., Kovalik, E., Davidson, T., Marder, S.R., and Mazziotta, J.C. (2003) Prefrontal-posterior parietal networks in schizophrenia: primary dysfunctions and secondary compensations. *Biol. Psychiatry* 53:12–24.

Raemaekers, M., Jansma, J.M., Cahn, W., Van der Geest, J.N., van der Linden, J.A., Kahn, R.S., and Ramsey, N.F. (2002) Neuronal substrate of the saccadic inhibition deficit in schizophrenia investigated with 3-dimensional event-related functional magnetic resonance imaging. *Arch. Gen. Psychiatry* 59:313–320.

Ragland, J.D., Gur, R.C., Valdez, J.N., Loughead, J., Elliott, M., Kohler, C., et al. (2005) Levels-of-processing effect on frontotemporal function in schizophrenia during word encoding and recognition. *Am. J. Psychiatry* 162:1840–1848.

Ragland, J.D., Moelter, S.T., McGrath, C., Hill, S.K., Gur, R.E., Bilker, W.B., et al. (2003) Levels-of-processing effect on word recognition in schizophrenia. *Biol. Psychiatry* 54:1154–1161.

Rajkowska, G., Selemon, L.D., and Goldman-Rakic, P.S. (1998) Neuronal and glial somal size in the prefrontal cortex: a postmortem morphometric study of schizophrenia and Huntington's disease. *Arch. Gen. Psychiatry* 55:215–224.

Ravizza, S.M., Delgado, M.R., Chein, J.M., Becker, J.T., and Fiez, J.A. (2004) Functional dissociations within the inferior parietal cortex in verbal working memory. *Neuroimage* 22:562–573.

Roitman, S.E., Mitropoulou, V., Keefe, R.S., Silverman, J.M., Serby, M., Harvey, P.D., et al. (2000) Visuospatial working memory in schizotypal personality disorder patients. *Schizophr. Res.* 41:447–455.

Rosenheck, R., Leslie, D., Keefe, R., McEvoy, J., Swartz, M., Perkins, D., et al. (2006) Barriers to employment for people with schizophrenia. *Am. J. Psychiatry* 163:411–417.

Rusch, N., Spoletini, I., Wilke, M., Bria, P., Di Paola, M., Di Iulio, F., et al. (2007) Prefrontal-thalamic-cerebellar gray matter networks and executive functioning in schizophrenia. *Schizophr. Res.* 93: 79–89.

Salisbury, D.F., Shenton, M.E., Griggs, C.B., Bonner-Jackson, A., McCarley, R.W. (2002) Mismatch negativity in chronic schizophrenia and first-episode schizophrenia. *Arch. Gen. Psychiatry* 59:686–694.

Saykin, A.J., Gur, R.C., Gur, R.E., Mozley, P.D., Mozley, L.H., Resnick, S.M., et al. (1991) Neuropsychological function in schizophrenia. Selective impairment in memory and learning. *Arch. Gen. Psychiatry* 48:618–624.

Saykin, A.J., Shtasel, D.L., Gur, R.E., Kester, D.B., Mozley, L.H., Stafiniak, P., and Gur, R.C. (1994) Neuropsychological deficits in neuroleptic naive patients with first-episode schizophrenia. *Arch. Gen. Psychiatry* 51:124–131.

Schechter, I., Butler, P.D., Zemon, V.M., Revheim, N., Saperstein, A.M., Jalbrzikowski, M., et al. (2005) Impairments in generation of early-stage transient visual evoked potentials to magno- and parvocellular-selective stimuli in schizophrenia. *Clin. Neurophysiol.* 116:2204–2215.

Scherk, H., and Falkai, P. (2006) Effects of antipsychotics on brain structure. *Curr. Opin. Psychiatry* 19:145–150.

Schlosser, R., Gesierich, T., Kaufmann, B., Vucurevic, G., and Stoeter, P. (2003) Altered effective connectivity in drug free schizophrenic patients. *Neuroreport* 14:2233–2237.

Schubert, E.W., and McNeil, T.F. (2005) Neuropsychological impairment and its neurological correlates in adult offspring with heightened risk for schizophrenia and affective psychosis. *Am. J. Psychiatry* 162:758–766.

Schultz, W., Dayan, P., and Montague, P.R. (1997) A neural substrate of prediction and reward. *Science* 275:1593–1599.

Scoville, W.B., and Milner, B. (1957) Loss of recent memory after bilateral hippocampal lesions. *J. Neurol. Neurosurg. Psychiatry* 20:11–21.

Seidman, L.J., Faraone, S.V., Goldstein, J.M., Goodman, J.M., Kremen, W.S., Toomey, R., et al. (1999) Thalamic and amygdala-hippocampal volume reductions in first-degree relatives of patients with schizophrenia: an MRI-based morphometric analysis. *Biol. Psychiatry* 46:941–954.

Seidman, L.J., Faraone, S.V., Goldstein, J.M., Kremen, W.S., Horton, N.J., Makris, N., et al. (2002) Left hippocampal volume as a vulnerability indicator for schizophrenia: a magnetic resonance imaging morphometric study of nonpsychotic first-degree relatives. *Arch. Gen. Psychiatry* 59:839–849.

Seidman, L.J., Giuliano, A.J., Smith, C.W., Stone, W.S., Glatt, S.J., Meyer, E., et al. (2006) Neuropsychological functioning in adolescents and young adults at genetic risk for schizophrenia and affective psychoses: results from the Harvard and Hillside Adolescent High Risk Studies. *Schizophr. Bull.* 32:507–524.

Seidman, L.J., Thermenos, H.W., Poldrack, R.A., Peace, N.K., Koch, J.K., Faraone, S.V., and Tsuang, M.T. (2006) Altered brain activation in dorsolateral prefrontal cortex in adolescents and young adults at genetic risk for schizophrenia: an fMRI study of working memory. *Schizophr. Res.* 85:58–72.

Selemon, L.D., and Rajkowska, G. (2003) Cellular pathology in the dorsolateral prefrontal cortex distinguishes schizophrenia from bipolar disorder. *Curr. Mol. Med.* 3:427–436.

Selemon, L.D., Rajkowska, G., and Goldman-Rakic, P.S. (1995) Abnormally high neuronal density in the schizophrenic cortex. A morphometric analysis of prefrontal area 9 and occipital area 17. *Arch. Gen. Psychiatry* 52:805–818; discussion 819–820.

Shenton, M.E., Dickey, C.C., Frumin, M., and McCarley, R.W. (2001) A review of MRI findings in schizophrenia. *Schizophr. Res.* 49:1–52.

Siegel, C., Waldo, M., Mizner, G., Adler, L.E., and Freedman, R. (1984) Deficits in sensory gating in schizophrenic patients and their relatives. Evidence obtained with auditory evoked responses. *Arch. Gen. Psychiatry* 41:607–612.

Siever, L.J., Koenigsberg, H.W., Harvey, P.D., Mitropoulou, V., Laruelle, M., Abi-Dargham, A., et al. (2002) Cognitive and brain function in schizotypal personality disorder. *Schizophr. Res.* 54:157–167.

Sigmundsson, T., Maier, M., Toone, B.K., Williams, S.C., Simmons, A., Greenwood, K., and Ron, M.A. (2003) Frontal lobe N-acetylaspartate correlates with psychopathology in schizophrenia: a proton magnetic resonance spectroscopy study. *Schizophr. Res.* 64: 63–71.

Snitz, B.E., Curtis, C.E., Zald, D.H., Katsanis, J., and Iacono, W.G. (1999) Neuropsychological and oculomotor correlates of spatial working memory performance in schizophrenia patients and controls. *Schizophr. Res.* 38:37–50.

Snitz, B.E., Macdonald, A.W., 3rd, and Carter, C.S. (2006) Cognitive deficits in unaffected first-degree relatives of schizophrenia patients: a meta-analytic review of putative endophenotypes. *Schizophr. Bull.* 32:179–194.

Spencer, K.M., Nestor, P.G., Niznikiewicz, M.A., Salisbury, D.F., Shenton, M.E., and McCarley, R.W. (2003) Abnormal neural synchrony in schizophrenia. *J. Neurosci.* 23:7407–7411.

Spencer, K.M., Nestor, P.G., Perlmutter, R., Niznikiewicz, M.A., Klump, M.C., Frumin, M., et al. (2004) Neural synchrony indexes disordered perception and cognition in schizophrenia. *Proc. Natl. Acad. Sci. USA* 101:17288–17293.

Stratta, P., Daneluzzo, E., Bustini, M., Prosperini, P., and Rossi, A. (2000) Processing of context information in schizophrenia: relation to clinical symptoms and WCST performance. *Schizophr. Res.* 44:57–67.

Stuss, D.T., Alexander, M.P., Palumbo, C.L., Buckle, L., Sayer, L., and Pogue, J. (1994) Organizational strategies of patients with unilateral or bilateral frontal lobe injury in word list learning tasks. *Neuropsychology* 8:355–373.

Surguladze, S.A., Calvert, G.A., Brammer, M.J., Campbell, R., Bullmore, E.T., Giampietro, V., and David, A.S. (2001) Audio-visual speech perception in schizophrenia: an fMRI study. *Psychiatry Res.* 106: 1–14.

Szeszko, P.R., Strous, R.D., Goldman, R.S., Ashtari, M., Knuth, K. H., Lieberman, J.A., and Bilder, R.M. (2002) Neuropsychological correlates of hippocampal volumes in patients experiencing a first episode of schizophrenia. *Am. J. Psychiatry* 159:217–226.

Takahashi, H., Koeda, M., Oda, K., Matsuda, T., Matsushima, E., Matsuura, M., et al. (2004) An fMRI study of differential neural response to affective pictures in schizophrenia. *Neuroimage* 22: 1247–1254.

Tallon-Baudry, C. (2003) Oscillatory synchrony and human visual cognition. *J. Physiol. Paris* 97:355–363.

Taylor, S.F., Phan, K.L., Britton, J.C., and Liberzon, I. (2005) Neural response to emotional salience in schizophrenia. *Neuropsychopharmacology* 30:984–995.

Thermenos, H.W., Seidman, L.J., Breiter, H., Goldstein, J.M., Goodman, J.M., Poldrack, R., et al. (2004) Functional magnetic resonance imaging during auditory verbal working memory in nonpsychotic relatives of persons with schizophrenia: a pilot study. *Biol. Psychiatry* 55:490–500.

Titone, D., Ditman, T., Holzman, P.S., Eichenbaum, H., and Levy, D.L. (2004) Transitive inference in schizophrenia: impairments in relational memory organization. *Schizophr. Res.* 68:235–247.

Toomey, R., Faraone, S.V., Seidman, L.J., Kremen, W.S., Pepple, J.R., and Tsuang, M.T. (1998) Association of neuropsychological vulnerability markers in relatives of schizophrenic patients. *Schizophr. Res.* 31:89–98.

Torres, I.J., Flashman, L.A., O'Leary, D.S., Swayze, V., 2nd, and Andreasen, N.C. (1997) Lack of an association between delayed memory and hippocampal and temporal lobe size in patients with schizophrenia and healthy controls. *Biol. Psychiatry* 42:1087–1096.

Toulopoulou, T., Morris, R.G., Rabe-Hesketh, S., and Murray, R. M. (2003) Selectivity of verbal memory deficit in schizophrenic patients and their relatives. *Am. J. Med. Genet.* 116B:1–7.

Traupmann, K.L., Berzofsky, M., and Kesselman, M. (1976) Encoding of taxonomic word categories by schizophrenics. *J. Abnorm. Psychol.* 85:350–355.

Tsuang, M. (2000) Schizophrenia: genes and environment. *Biol. Psychiatry* 47:210–220.

Turetsky, B., Colbath, E.A., and Gur, R.E. (1998) P300 subcomponent abnormalities in schizophrenia: II. Longitudinal stability and relationship to symptom change. *Biol. Psychiatry* 43:31–39.

Tuulio-Henriksson, A., Arajarvi, R., Partonen, T., Haukka, J., Varilo, T., Schreck, M., et al. (2003) Familial loading associates with impairment in visual span among healthy siblings of schizophrenia patients. *Biol. Psychiatry* 54:623–628.

Uhlhaas, P.J., Linden, D.E., Singer, W., Haenschel, C., Lindner, M., Maurer, K., and Rodriguez, E. (2006) Dysfunctional long-range coordination of neural activity during Gestalt perception in schizophrenia. *J. Neurosci.* 26:8168–8175.

Umbricht, D., Javitt, D.C., Bates, J., Pollak, S.D., Lieberman, J., and Kane, J.M. (1997) Auditory event related potentials (ERP) in first episode and chronic schizophrenia. *Biol. Psychiatry* 41:46S.

van der Stelt, O., Belger, A., and Lieberman, J.A. (2004) Macroscopic fast neuronal oscillations and synchrony in schizophrenia. *Proc. Natl. Acad. Sci. USA* 101:17567–17568.

van Erp, T.G., Saleh, P.A., Huttunen, M., Lonnqvist, J., Kaprio, J., Salonen, O., et al. (2004) Hippocampal volumes in schizophrenic twins. *Arch. Gen. Psychiatry* 61:346–353.

van Erp, T.G., Saleh, P.A., Rosso, I.M., Huttunen, M., Lonnqvist, J., Pirkola, T., et al. (2002) Contributions of genetic risk and fetal hypoxia to hippocampal volume in patients with schizophrenia or schizoaffective disorder, their unaffected siblings, and healthy unrelated volunteers. *Am. J. Psychiatry* 159:1514–1520.

Van Snellenberg, J.X., Torres, I.J., and Thornton, A.E. (2006) Functional neuroimaging of working memory in schizophrenia: task performance as a moderating variable. *Neuropsychology* 20:497–510.

Velligan, D.I., Bow-Thomas, C.C., Mahurin, R., Miller, A., Dassori, A., and Erdely, F. (1998) Concurrent and predictive validity of the Allen Cognitive Levels Assessment. *Psychiatry Res.* 80:287–298.

Vink, M., Ramsey, N.F., Raemaekers, M., and Kahn, R.S. (2006) Striatal dysfunction in schizophrenia and unaffected relatives. *Biol. Psychiatry* 60:32–39.

Voglmaier, M.M., Seidman, L.J., Niznikiewicz, M.A., Dickey, C.C., Shenton, M.E., and McCarley, R.W. (2000) Verbal and nonverbal neuropsychological test performance in subjects with schizotypal personality disorder. *Am. J. Psychiatry* 157:787–793.

Wagner, A.D., Desmond, J.E., Glover, G.H., and Gabrieli, J.D. (1998) Prefrontal cortex and recognition memory. Functional-MRI evidence for context-dependent retrieval processes. *Brain* 121:1985–2002.

Wagner, A.D., Poldrack, R.A., Eldridge, L.L., Desmond, J.E., Glover, G.H., and Gabrieli, J.D. (1998) Material-specific lateralization of prefrontal activation during episodic encoding and retrieval. *Neuroreport* 9:3711–3717.

Waldo, M.C., Carey, G., Myles-Worsley, M., Cawthra, E., Adler, L. E., Nagamoto, H.T., et al. (1991) Codistribution of a sensory gating deficit and schizophrenia in multi-affected families. *Psychiatry Res.* 39:257–268.

Wang, L., Joshi, S.C., Miller, M.I., and Csernansky, J.G. (2001) Statistical analysis of hippocampal asymmetry in schizophrenia. *Neuroimage* 14:531–545.

Weiss, A.P., Schacter, D.L., Goff, D.C., Rauch, S.L., Alpert, N.M., Fischman, A.J., and Heckers, S. (2003) Impaired hippocampal recruitment during normal modulation of memory performance in schizophrenia. *Biol. Psychiatry* 53:48–55.

Whalley, H., Simonotto, E., Moorhead, W., McIntosh, A.M., Marshall, I., Ebmeier, K.P., et al. (2006) Functional imaging as a predictor of schizophrenia. *Biol. Psychiatry* 60:454–462.

Whyte, E.M., Dew, M.A., Gildengers, A., Lenze, E.J., Bharucha, A., Mulsant, B.H., and Reynolds, C.F. (2004) Time course of response to antidepressants in late-life major depression: therapeutic implications. *Drugs Aging* 21:531–554.

Williams, L.M., Das, P., Harris, A.W., Liddell, B.B., Brammer, M.J., Olivieri, G., et al. (2004) Dysregulation of arousal and amygdala-prefrontal systems in paranoid schizophrenia. *Am. J. Psychiatry* 161:480–489.

Wood, S.J., Berger, G., Velakoulis, D., Phillips, L.J., McGorry, P.D., Yung, A.R., et al. (2003) Proton magnetic resonance spectroscopy in first episode psychosis and ultra high-risk individuals. *Schizophr. Bull.* 29:831–843.

Yucel, G., Petty, C., McCarthy, G., and Belger, A. (2005a) Graded visual attention modulates brain responses evoked by task-irrelevant auditory pitch changes. *J. Cogn. Neurosci.* 17:1819–1828.

Yucel, G., Petty, C., McCarthy, G., and Belger, A. (2005b) Visual task complexity modulates the brain's response to unattended auditory novelty. *Neuroreport* 16:1031–1036.

Yurgelun-Todd, D.A., Renshaw, P.F., Gruber, S.A., Ed, M., Waternaux, C., and Cohen, B.M. (1996) Proton magnetic resonance spectroscopy of the temporal lobes in schizophrenics and normal controls. *Schizophr. Res.* 19:55–59.

Zhou, S.Y., Suzuki, M., Takahashi, T., Hagino, H., Kawasaki, Y., Matsui, M., et al. (2007) Parietal lobe volume deficits in schizophrenia spectrum disorders. *Schizophr. Res.* 89:35–48.

23 The Neurochemistry of Schizophrenia: A Focus on Dopamine and Glutamate

ANISSA ABI-DARGHAM

THE NEUROBIOLOGY OF SCHIZOPHRENIA

Schizophrenia presents with multiple clinical features, ranging from positive symptoms (hallucinations, delusions, and thought disorder) to negative symptoms (social withdrawal, poverty of speech and thought, flattening of affect, and lack of motivation) and disturbances in cognitive processes (attention, some types of memory, and executive function). The neurobiology of schizophrenia can be similarly conceptualized in different components: the neurobiology of psychosis or positive symptoms on one hand and that of cognitive disturbances and negative symptoms on the other. The neurobiology of psychosis has been clarified to some extent and involves essentially but not exclusively excess stimulation of striatal D_2 receptors, however, the neurobiology of cognitive and negative symptoms is much more complex, involving multiple neurotransmitter systems, and is less well understood (Fig. 23.1). We review here the current state of knowledge from neuropathology and imaging studies relevant to the understanding of the neurobiology and neurocircuitry underlying these different symptom domains.

Circuits

Evidence derived from neuropathological and functional studies shows that certain brain regions are central to the pathophysiology of schizophrenia (Fig. 23.2). These are the dorsolateral prefrontal cortex (DLPFC), hippocampus, striatum, and thalamus. These regions are also intimately interconnected within the cortico-striato-pallido-thalamo-cortical loops, and via projections from the hippocampus to the frontal cortex and to the ventral striatum, suggesting that alterations in one region are likely to affect another and lead to alterations in the functions subserved by the circuit.

In neuropathological studies of the DLPFC of participants with schizophrenia, pyramidal neurons exhibit decreased soma size, dendritic length, and spine density (Pierri et al., 2001). These alterations contribute to increased neuronal density (Selemon et al., 1995) and suggest a "misconnectivity" that could underlie the cortical dysfunction observed with imaging studies and with the clinical symptoms. Multiple alterations related to γ-aminobutyric acid (GABA)ergic transmission within the DLPFC have been reported, including decreases in GABA-synthesizing enzyme GAD67 messenger ribonucleic acid (mRNA) and protein levels, decreases in the GABA transporter, GAT, and increases in the $\alpha 2$ subunit of the GABA-A receptor (Lewis et al., 2005). The thalamus has decreased cell numbers and fewer projections to the DLPFC (Pakkenberg, 1990). Likewise, dopaminergic projections from the ventral tegmental area (VTA) to the DLPFC are also decreased (Akil et al., 2000). The hippocampus shows decreased volume and exhibits cytoarchitectural, neurochemical, and synaptic alterations (Harrison, 1999). These various observations can all result in alterations in connectivity and circuitry affecting the processing and flow of information within and between regions. For example, alterations in connectivity within the DLPFC result in cognitive deficits such as working memory impairment, and in alterations in output of pyramidal cells to other regions of the brain, such as the striatum, with dysregulation of striatal dopamine (DA) function. In turn, increased DA activity induces perturbation in the information flow within this circuit, in the modulation of this information by hippocampus and amygdala, and in the gating of sensory information by the thalamus carried forward to the cortex.

Along this dysfunctional circuit multiple neurochemical alterations in DA have been now documented. These dopaminergic alterations are most likely downstream events to alterations involving other transmitter systems (Lewis and Gonzalez-Burgos, 2006). We review here DA and glutamate (Glu) alterations as well as their interrelatedness.

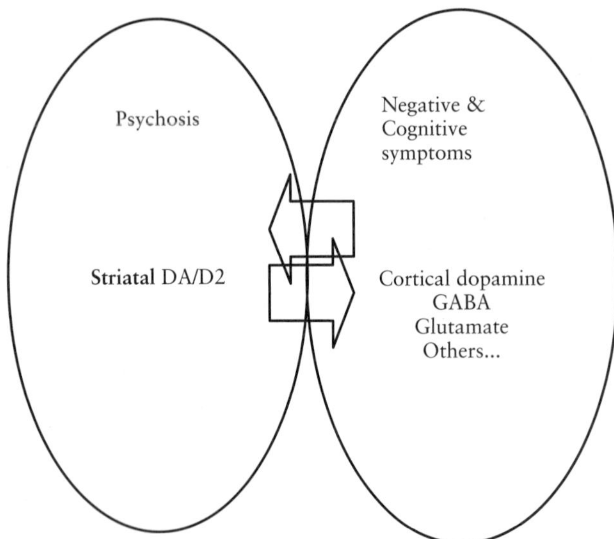

FIGURE 23.1 In schizophrenia, positive symptoms are mostly related to hyperstimulation of striatal D_2 receptors, while cognitive deficits and negative symptoms are multifactorial and mostly related to cortical dysfunction in multiple systems. Furthermore, these areas are linked, as hyperstimulation of D_2 receptors can lead to cortical dysfunction, and cortical dysfunction can itself dysregulate subcortical dopamine; see text for details.

Transmitter Systems

Dopamine

The work of Arvid Carlsson characterizing the presence of DA in the brain and the effects of neuroleptics on monoaminergic indices (Carlsson and Lindqvist, 1963) led to the first formulation of the DA hypothesis of schizophrenia proposing that hyperactivity of DA transmission was responsible for the disorder (Rossum, 1966).

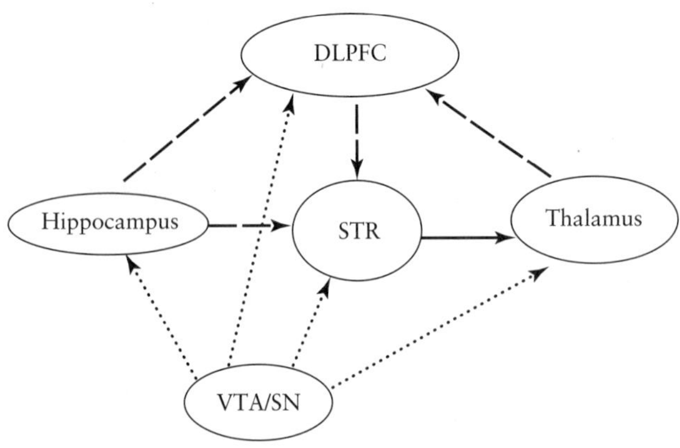

FIGURE 23.2 Schematic representation of the main brain regions involved in the pathophysiology of schizophrenia from postmortem and brain imaging studies and their relationship. Solid lines are GABAergic projections, dashed lines are glutamatergic projections, and dotted lines are dopaminergic. These regions form cortico-striato-thalamo-cortical loops, and all receive dopaminergic projections.

This received further support from the correlation between clinical doses of antipsychotic drugs and their potency to block DA D_2 receptors (Seeman et al., 1975; Creese et al., 1976) and from studies confirming the psychotogenic effects of DA-enhancing drugs (for review, see Angrist and van Kammen, 1984; Lieberman, Kane, and Alvir, 1987). Given the predominant localization of DA terminals and D_2 receptors in subcortical regions such as the striatum and the nucleus accumbens, the classical DA hypothesis of schizophrenia focused on subcortical regions.

Over the years, the increasing awareness of the importance of enduring negative and cognitive symptoms in this illness and of their resistance to D_2 receptor antagonism led to a reformulation of the classical DA hypothesis. Functional brain imaging studies suggested that these symptoms might arise from altered prefrontal cortex (PFC) functions (for reviews, see Knable and Weinberger, 1997). A wealth of preclinical studies emerged documenting the importance of prefrontal DA transmission at D_1 receptors (the main DA receptor in the neocortex) for optimal PFC performance (for review, see Goldman-Rakic et al., 2000). As a result, an imbalance in DA with hyperactive subcortical mesolimbic projections (resulting in hyperstimulation of D_2 receptors and positive symptoms) and hypoactive mesocortical DA projections to the PFC (resulting in hypostimulation of D_1 receptors, negative symptoms, and cognitive impairment) became the predominant hypothesis (Weinberger, 1987; Davis et al., 1991). In addition, a relationship between these two was suggested by the initial observation of Pycock et al. (1980) and subsequent literature (for review, see Tzschentke, 2001) showing that prefrontal DA activity exerts an inhibitory influence on subcortical DA such that a deficiency in mesocortical DA function might translate into disinhibition of mesolimbic DA activity (Weinberger, 1987).

Pharmacological studies, reviewed by Lieberman, Kane, Sarantakos, et al. (1987) showed that patients with schizophrenia, as a group, display increased sensitivity to the psychotogenic effects of acute psychostimulant administration. Postmortem measurements of indices of DA transmission generated a number of consistent observations in the striatum, such as an increase in D_2-like receptors in the striatum of patients with schizophrenia in the absence of change in dopamine transporter (DAT) and D_1 receptors. An increase in D_3 receptors in the ventral striatum (Gurevich et al., 1997) and alteration in tyrosine hydroxylase (TH) immunolabeling in several cortical regions were also observed (Akil et al., 1999) and did not appear to be a consequence of premortem neuroleptic exposure.

The most compelling evidence in support of dopaminergic alterations derived from positron emission tomography (PET) and single photon emission computed tomography (SPECT) imaging in patients with schizophrenia. Four converging lines of evidence have demonstrated the presence of excessive D_2 stimulation by DA:

Striatal D_2 receptors. A meta-analysis of 17 imaging studies comparing D_2 receptor parameters in patients with schizophrenia and controls (Weinberger and Laruelle, 2001) revealed a small (12%) but significant elevation of striatal D_2 receptors in untreated patients with schizophrenia. No alterations in striatal D_1 receptors were reported (Okubo et al., 1997; Abi-Dargham et al., 2002; Karlsson et al., 2002).

Striatal amphetamine-induced DA release is increased. Three studies (Laruelle et al., 1996; Breier et al., 1997; Abi-Dargham et al., 1998) have shown that amphetamine-induced decrease in [^{11}C]raclopride or [^{123}I]IBZM binding, a validated measure of DA release, is elevated in untreated patients with schizophrenia compared to well-matched controls. These studies showed that the increase in DA response is observed in never-treated patients, is related to the transient induction or worsening of positive symptoms by amphetamine, is larger in patients experiencing an episode of illness exacerbation, and is unrelated to stress (Laruelle et al., 1999). Furthermore, it is present in patients with schizotypal personality disorders, albeit to a smaller extent, suggesting that at least, in part, it is mediated by genetic factors, and it is absent in nonpsychotic participants with

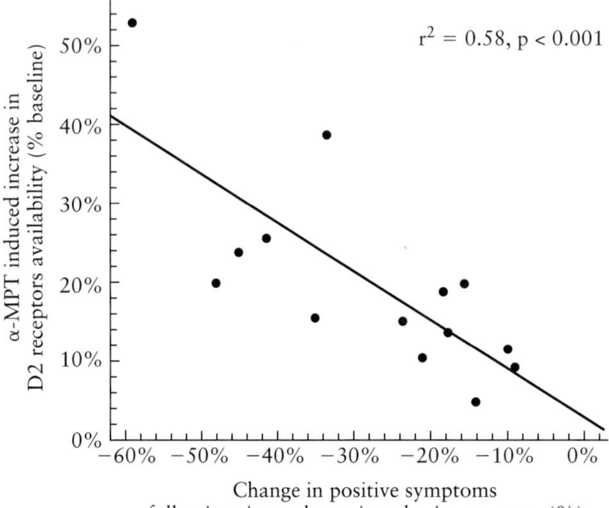

FIGURE 23.3 Excess stimulation of striatal D_2 and positive symptoms. Relationship between dopamine synaptic levels at baseline, as estimated by the α-MPT effect on [^{123}I]IBZM BP, and the decrease in positive symptoms measured after 6 weeks of antipsychotic treatment, which provides D_2 blockade. Patients with high DA synaptic levels, or excess D_2 stimulation, showed larger decrease in positive symptoms following treatment than patients with DA levels similar to controls (effect of α-MPT on [^{123}I]IBZM BP in control subjects was 9% ± 7%).

unipolar depression (Parsey et al., 2001), showing specificity to psychosis and schizophrenia spectrum disorders.

Baseline occupancy of striatal D_2 receptors by DA. Two studies reported higher occupancy of D_2 receptors by DA in patients with schizophrenia (Abi-Dargham et al., 2000; Kegeles et al., 2006). Assuming normal affinity of D_2 receptors for DA, the data are consistent with higher DA synaptic levels in patients with schizophrenia. Furthermore, higher synaptic DA levels were predictive of good therapeutic response of positive symptoms following 6 weeks of treatment with antipsychotics (Fig 23.3). In the most recent study, we observed that the increase in DA transmission within the striatum affects mostly the area that receives projections from the DLPFC, confirming and further localizing the dysfunction along the cortico-striato-pallido-thalamic loops that project back to the cortex discussed earlier.

Striatal DOPA decarboxylase activity. Studies of striatal DA synthesis estimated via the activity of the enzymatic step involving dihydroxyphenylalanine (DOPA) decarboxylase (AADC) in patients with schizophrenia compared to controls using [^{18}F]DOPA or [^{11}C]DOPA were very contributive to the understanding of the DA alteration in the illness. Six reported increased accumulation of DOPA in the striatum of patients with schizophrenia (Reith et al., 1994; Hietala et al., 1995; Dao-Castellana et al., 1997; Hietala et al., 1999; Lindstrom et al., 1999; Elkashef et al., 2000; Meyer-Lindenberg et al., 2002; McGowan et al., 2004), one reported no change (Dao-Castellana et al., 1997), and one study reported reduced uptake (Elkashef et al., 2000). Interestingly, poor prefrontal activation was related to elevated [^{18}F]DOPA accumulation in the striatum, adding evidence to the link between cortical and subcortical dysfunction in schizophrenia (Meyer-Lindenberg et al., 2002). Grunder et al. (2003) reported a decrease in [^{18}F]DOPA uptake following subchronic treatment with haloperidol, suggesting that chronic neuroleptic administration will tend to decrease AADC activity and hence DA synthesis.

In summary, these studies all converge to demonstrate an increase in presynaptic DA synthesis and transmission in the striatum, and in particular most predominantly the head of the caudate within the striatum, in patients with schizophrenia. This is potentiated by an additional increase in D_2 density, leading to excess D_2 stimulation (Fig 23.4). The presence of this excess confers good therapeutic response of positive symptoms to antipsychotics.

Prefrontal DA function and schizophrenia

Evidence for prefrontal DA dysfunction is somewhat indirect. Preclinical studies have documented the importance of prefrontal DA function for cognition (for

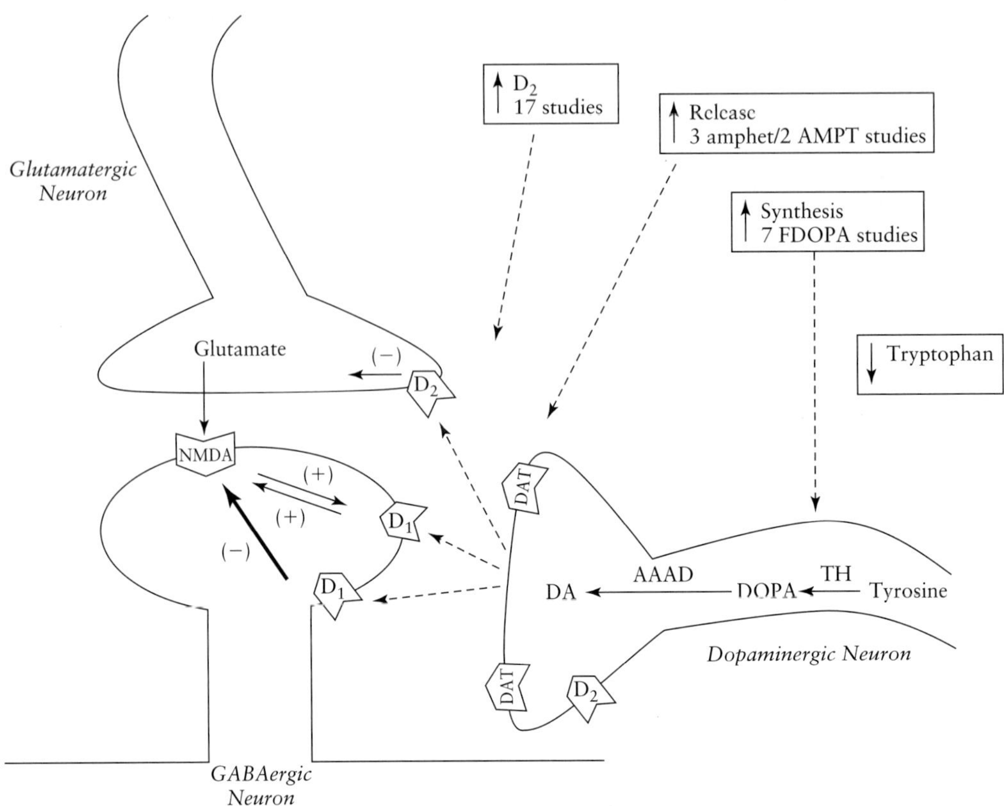

FIGURE 23.4 Illustration of all studies showing excess presynaptic and postsynaptic indices of dopamine transmission in the striatum and their putative effect on cortical glutamatergic flow of information. Dashed arrows represent dopamine release. Dotted arrows show sites of action. (AAAD = Aromatic L-Amino Acid Decarboxolase, TH = Tyrosine Hydroxolase)

review, see Goldman-Rakic, 1994; Goldman-Rakic et al., 2000). This important role has been recently confirmed in humans by the repeated observation that carriers of the high-activity allele of cathecol-O-methyltransferase (COMT), an enzyme involved in DA metabolism, display lower performance in various cognitive tasks compared to carriers of the lower activity allele associated with higher concentration of DA in PFC (for review, see Goldberg and Weinberger, 2004). Clinical studies have suggested a relationship between low cerebro-spinal fluid (CSF) *homovanillic acid*, a measure reflecting low DA activity in the prefrontal cortex, and poor performance at tasks involving working memory in schizophrenia (Weinberger et al., 1988; Kahn et al., 1994). Administration of DA agonists showed beneficial effects on the pattern of prefrontal activation measured with PET during these tasks (Daniel et al., 1991; Dolan et al., 1995). Tyrosine hydroxylase immunolabeling, as an index of DA innervation, is decreased. These observations are all consistent with a hypodopaminergic state in the PFC of patients with schizophrenia but do not represent evidence for it.

Cortical D_1 receptors

The main parameter of extrastriatal DA transmission that is currently quantifiable using noninvasive in vivo studies is D_1 receptor availability. Three PET studies of prefrontal D_1 receptor availability in patients with schizophrenia have recently been published, using [^{11}C]SCH 23390 (Okubo et al., 1997; Karlsson et al., 2002) or [^{11}C]NNC 112 (Abi-Dargham et al., 2002), and yielded discrepant findings. Studies with both radiotracers in the same patients are required to clarify the reasons for the discrepancies. Nevertheless, despite the unsolved issues, and using the same tracer [^{11}C]NNC 112, a convincing pattern has emerged that indirectly supports the findings of alterations in D_1 receptors in the DLPFC of patients with schizophrenia. This consists of the observation of small but significant increases in D_1 receptors in conditions of low DA transmission (Guo et al., 2003; Narendran et al., 2005) consistent with the concept of compensatory upregulation in D_1 receptors in schizophrenia as a response to a deficit of endogenous stimulation.

Extrastriatal D_2 receptors

The recent availability of high-affinity D_2 radiotracers allowed the study of D_2 receptors in low-density regions such as the substantia nigra, thalamus, and temporal cortex in patients with schizophrenia compared to controls. Lower D_2 receptor density has been described in untreated schizophrenia in the thalamus (Suhara et al.,

2002; Talvik et al., 2003; Tuppurainen et al., 2003; Yasuno et al., 2004; Talvik et al., 2006), as well as in the midbrain (Tuppurainen et al., 2006), in temporal cortex (Tuppurainen et al., 2003), and cingulated cortex (Suhara et al., 2002; Glenthoj et al., 2006). Additional studies are needed to replicate and extend these findings and explore their pathophysiological basis and significance.

In summary, imaging studies of dopaminergic indices in schizophrenia have conclusively shown that schizophrenia is associated with hyperactivity of subcortical transmission at D_2 receptors. The findings represent robust evidence for a presynaptic dysregulation (as evidenced by the [^{18}F]DOPA studies). In addition, stimulated (amphetamine challenge studies) and baseline intrasynaptic release (AMPT [alpha-methyl-p-tyrosine] depletion studies) is increased. A potential alternative interpretation for the two latter sets of findings is a higher affinity of D_2 receptors for DA in schizophrenia in the face of normal release. This potential interpretation is testable in future studies using a D_2 agonist radiotracer that allows measurement of the D_2 receptors in the high-affinity state, as opposed to antagonists that measure all available D_2 receptors regardless of their affinity state.

Future investigations should also explore the D_3 receptor, postulated to play an important role in the pathophysiology and treatment of schizophrenia (Sokoloff et al., 2006). Until recently, imaging D_3 receptor was not feasible: positron emission tomography radiotracers commonly used to study D_2 and D_3 receptors exhibit similar affinities for both receptors, and the concentration of D_3 receptors in the human striatum is lower than that of D_2 receptors. The recent discovery that [^{11}C]PHNO is a D_3-preferring imaging agent that might allow the in vivo study of this important target (Narendran et al., 2006). The D_4 has been largely unexplored, but D_4 antagonists have failed as therapeutic agents (Kramer et al., 1997). Finally, more selective tracers and more direct ways of measuring cortical dopaminergic transmission are needed.

Glutamate

A role for a Glu dysfunction at the *N*-methyl-D-aspartate (NMDA) receptor in the pathophysiology of schizophrenia has been suggested by the behavioral effects of NMDA receptor antagonists such as phencyclidine (PCP) or ketamine. These have been shown to produce positive, negative, and cognitive symptoms in healthy individuals and exacerbate preexisting symptoms in patients with schizophrenia even after one single use (Javitt and Zukin, 1991; Krystal et al., 1994). Neurophysiological measures, including alterations in N1 and mismatch negativity (MMN) generation, P50 gating and prepulse inhibition (PPI) deficits, which are among the most consistent and robust indices of brain dysfunction in schizophrenia, can be observed in humans after single administration of NMDA antagonists (Umbricht et al., 2000). The NMDA hypofunction hypothesis of schizophrenia received further support from postmortem studies showing a multitude of alterations that could provide a neuroanatomical and neurochemical substrate for it. These alterations have been described in the main brain regions along the circuit of pathology described earlier, including frontal cortex, hippocampus, and thalamus, and affect directly or indirectly multiple aspects associated with NMDA transmission, from the morphology of the cell to the plasma surface receptor expression, to the intracellular processes of transmission or degradation of signaling. Some of these findings include the following: *(1)* changes in cytoarchitecture of pyramidal neurons in DLPFC of brains of patients with schizophrenia (Pierri et al., 2001); *(2)* changes in Glu receptor binding, transcription, and subunit protein expression in the prefrontal cortex, thalamus, and hippocampus of participants with schizophrenia (Meador-Woodruff and Healy, 2000); *(3)* decreases in NR1 subunits of the NMDA receptor in hippocampus (Gao et al., 2000), and frontal cortical areas (Meador-Woodruff and Healy, 2000); *(4)* high expression of excitatory amino acid transporters (EAAT), which remove Glu from the synapse, in the thalamus (Meador-Woodruff et al., 2003); *(5)* changes in the NMDA receptor-affiliated intracellular proteins such as PSD95 and SAP102 in the prefrontal cortex and thalamus (Meador-Woodruff et al., 2003)—these proteins modulate Glu-associated intracellular signaling events, by anchoring the receptor, modulating its sensitivity, and assembling the intracellular complex needed for signaling; *(6)* alterations in levels of amino acids *N-acethylaspartate* (NAA) and *N-acethylaspartylglutamate* (NAAG), an endogenous ligand for the mGlu3 subtype of Glu receptor, and in the activity of the enzyme that cleaves NAA to NAAG and Glu in the CSF and postmortem tissue from individuals with schizophrenia have all been reported (Tsai, 2005). These observations affect different aspects of glutamatergic transmission but could all be associated with deficits in NMDA function.

Furthermore, the imbalance in DA transmission described with imaging studies and NMDA dysfunction can be conceptually linked, inasmuch as altered prefrontal connectivity involving Glu transmission at (NMDA) receptors could translate into a failure of the PFC to appropriately modulate DA function. In turn, the DA imbalance exacerbates PFC deficits, forming positive feedback loops that underlie the symptomatology and suggest a vicious circle of three main dysfunctions: excess striatal D_2, deficit in cortical D_1 and NMDA function (Fig 23.5). In support of this interrelatedness, in vivo imaging studies have shown that an acute challenge with ketamine can produce increased subcortical DA release (Kegeles et al., 2002) and chronic recreational use of ketamine leads to alterations in DLPFC D_1 simi-

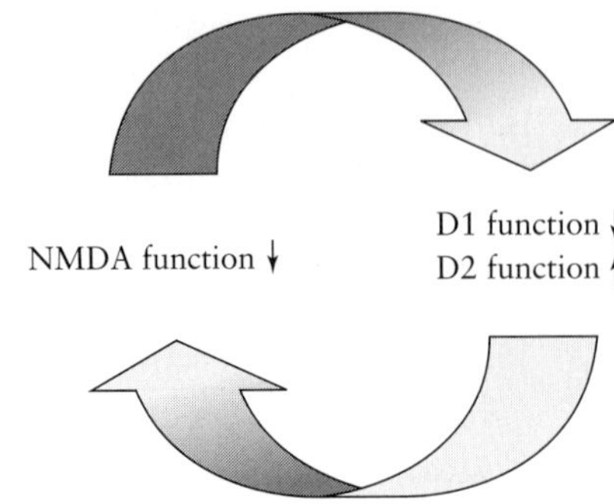

FIGURE 23.5 Dopamine and glutamate alterations in schizophrenia form an interactive and vicious circle.

lar to those observed in schizophrenia (Narendran et al., 2005). Similar findings were reported in a preclinical model of schizophrenia involving chronic administration of MK801, an NMDA antagonist, to nonhuman primates (Tsukada et al., 2005). Furthermore, D_2 overexpression in the striatum in genetically altered mice (Kellendonk et al., 2006) induces long-lasting prefrontal cognitive deficits, presumably via an opposing effect of D_2 stimulation on cortical glutamatergic projections onto the striatal GABAergic or medium spiny neurons, resulting in altered flow of information along cortico-striatal loops.

The final line of evidence implicating glutamatergic transmission in schizophrenia consists in the number of genes recently linked to an increased risk for schizophrenia and that can influence the function of modulatory sites on the NMDA receptor or the intrasynaptic Glu transmission processes such as neuregulin 1, GRM3, and DISC1 (Moghaddam, 2003; Hahn et al., 2006).

These studies overall lend strong support to the concept of broad alterations in NMDA transmission in schizophrenia and suggest these may lead to additional downstream effects on DA. In vivo evidence for alterations in Glu and NMDA transmission is still missing at this point as radiotracers for these systems are not available.

SUMMARY

The neurobiology of schizophrenia can be broadly divided in two components, excess striatal D_2 stimulation underlying psychosis and multiple cortical interactive neurochemical alterations underlying negative symptoms and cognitive disturbances. These remain to be clarified, but at least two factors have emerged and have been reviewed here: a dysfunction of DA and of the Glu NMDA system. Imaging and preclinical studies have shown convergence between these alterations and have highlighted one major dysfunctional axis of pathology in schizophrenia, made up of the hippocampus, cortex, striatum, and thalamus, contributing to disruption of information flow along the cortico-striato-thalamo-cortical loops. Better knowledge of the circuit and cellular alterations will ultimately pave the way to better and more targeted treatment strategies.

REFERENCES

Abi-Dargham, A., Gil, R., Krystal, J., Baldwin, R.M., Seibyl, J.P., Bowers, M., van Dyck, C.H., Charney, D.S., Innis, R.B., and Laruelle, M. (1998) Increased striatal dopamine transmission in schizophrenia: confirmation in a second cohort. *Am. J. Psychiatry* 155:761–767.

Abi-Dargham, A., Mawlawi, O., Lombardo, I., Gil, R., Martinez, D., Huang, Y., Hwang, D.R., Keilp, J., Kochan, L., Van Heertum, R., Gorman, J.M., and Laruelle, M. (2002) Prefrontal dopamine D1 receptors and working memory in schizophrenia. *J. Neurosci.* 22:3708–3719.

Abi-Dargham, A., Rodenhiser, J., Printz, D., Zea-Ponce, Y., Gil, R., Kegeles, L.S., Weiss, R., Cooper, T.B., Mann, J.J., Van Heertum, R.L., Gorman, J.M., and Laruelle, M. (2000) Increased baseline occupancy of D2 receptors by dopamine in schizophrenia. *Proc. Natl. Acad. Sci. USA* 97:8104–8109.

Akil, M., Edgar, C.L., Pierri, J.N., Casali, S., and Lewis, D.A. (2000) Decreased density of tyrosine hydroxylase-immunoreactive axons in the entorhinal cortex of schizophrenic subjects. *Biol. Psychiatry* 47:361–370.

Akil, M., Pierri, J.N., Whitehead, R.E., Edgar, C.L., Mohila, C., Sampson, A.R., and Lewis, D.A. (1999) Lamina-specific alterations in the dopamine innervation of the prefrontal cortex in schizophrenic subjects. *Am. J. Psychiatry* 156:1580–1589.

Angrist, B., and van Kammen, D.P. (1984) CNS stimulants as a tool in the study of schizophrenia. *Trends Neurosci.* 7:388–390.

Breier, A., Su, T.P., Saunders, R., Carson, R.E., Kolachana, B.S., de Bartolomeis, A., Weinberger, D.R., Weisenfeld, N., Malhotra, A.K., Eckelman, W.C., and Pickar, D. (1997) Schizophrenia is associated with elevated amphetamine-induced synaptic dopamine concentrations: evidence from a novel positron emission tomography method. *Proc. Natl. Acad. Sci. USA* 94:2569–2574.

Carlsson, A., and Lindqvist, M. (1963) Effect of chlorpromazine or haloperidol on formation of 3-methoxytyramine and normetanephrine in mouse brain. *Acta Pharmacol. Toxicol.* 20:140–144.

Creese, I., Burt, D.R., and Snyder, S.H. (1976) Dopamine receptor binding predicts clinical and pharmacological potencies of antischizophrenic drugs. *Science* 19:481–483.

Daniel, D.G., Weinberger, D.R., Jones, D.W., Zigun, J.R., Coppola, R., Handel, S., Bigelow, L.B., Goldberg, T.E., Berman, K.F., and Kleinman, J.E. (1991) The effect of amphetamine on regional cerebral blood flow during cognitive activation in schizophrenia. *J. Neurosci.* 11:1907–1917.

Dao-Castellana, M.H., Paillere-Martinot, M.L., Hantraye, P., Attar-Levy, D., Remy, P., Crouzel, C., Artiges, E., Feline, A., Syrota, A., and Martinot, J.L. (1997) Presynaptic dopaminergic function in the striatum of schizophrenic patients. *Schizophr. Res.* 23:167–174.

Davis, K.L., Kahn, R.S., Ko, G., and Davidson, M. (1991) Dopamine in schizophrenia: a review and reconceptualization. *Am. J. Psychiatry* 148:1474–1486.

Dolan, R.J., Fletcher, P., Frith, C.D., Friston, K.J., Frackowiak, R.S., and Grasby, P.M. (1995) Dopaminergic modulation of impaired cognitive activation in the anterior cingulate cortex in schizophrenia. *Nature* 378:180–182.

Elkashef, A.M., Doudet, D., Bryant, T., Cohen, R.M., Li, S.H., and Wyatt, R.J. (2000) 6-(18)F-DOPA PET study in patients with schizophrenia. Positron emission tomography. *Psychiatry Res.* 100: 1–11.

Gao, X.M., Sakai, K., Roberts, R.C., Conley, R.R., Dean, B., and Tamminga, C.A. (2000) Ionotropic glutamate receptors and expression of *N*-methyl-D-aspartate receptor subunits in subregions of human hippocampus: effects of schizophrenia. *Am. J. Psychiatry* 157:1141–1149.

Glenthoj, B.Y., Mackeprang, T., Svarer, C., Rasmussen, H., Pinborg, L.H., Friberg, L., Baare, W., Hemmingsen, R., and Videbaek, C. (2006) Frontal dopamine D(2/3) receptor binding in drug-naive first-episode schizophrenic patients correlates with positive psychotic symptoms and gender. *Biol. Psychiatry* 60:621–629.

Goldberg, T.E., and Weinberger, D.R. (2004) Genes and the parsing of cognitive processes. *Trends Cogn. Sci.* 8:325–335.

Goldman-Rakic, P. (1994) Working memory dysfunction in schizophrenia. *J. Neuropsychiatry Clin. Neurosci.* 6:348–357.

Goldman-Rakic, P.S., Muly, E.C., 3rd, and Williams, G.V. (2000) D(1) receptors in prefrontal cells and circuits. *Brain Res. Rev.* 31:295–301.

Grunder, G., Vernaleken, I., Muller, M.J., Davids, E., Heydari, N., Buchholz, H.G., Bartenstein, P., Munk, O.L., Stoeter, P., Wong, D. F., Gjedde, A., and Cumming, P. (2003) Subchronic haloperidol downregulates dopamine synthesis capacity in the brain of schizophrenic patients in vivo. *Neuropsychopharmacology* 28:787–794.

Guo, N., Hwang, D.R., Lo, E.S., Huang, Y.Y., Laruelle, M., and Abi-Dargham, A. (2003) Dopamine depletion and in vivo binding of PET D1 receptor radioligands: implications for imaging studies in schizophrenia. *Neuropsychopharmacology* 28:1703–1711.

Gurevich, E.V., Bordelon, Y., Shapiro, R.M., Arnold, S.E., Gur, R. E., and Joyce, J.N. (1997) Mesolimbic dopamine D3 receptors and use of antipsychotics in patients with schizophrenia. A postmortem study. *Arch. Gen. Psychiatry* 54:225–232.

Hahn, C.G., Wang, H.Y., Cho, D.S., Talbot, K., Gur, R.E., Berrettini, W.H., Bakshi, K., Kamins, J., Borgmann-Winter, K.E., Siegel, S. J., Gallop, R.J., and Arnold, S.E. (2006) Altered neuregulin 1-erbB4 signaling contributes to NMDA receptor hypofunction in schizophrenia. *Nat. Med.* 12:824–828.

Harrison, P.J. (1999) The neuropathology of schizophrenia. A critical review of the data and their interpretation. *Brain* 122:593–624.

Hietala, J., Syvalahti, E., Vilkman, H., Vuorio, K., Rakkolainen, V., Bergman, J., Haaparanta, M., Solin, O., Kuoppamaki, M., Eronen, E., Ruotsalainen, U., and Salokangas, R.K. (1999) Depressive symptoms and presynaptic dopamine function in neuroleptic-naive schizophrenia. *Schizophr. Res.* 35:41–50.

Hietala, J., Syvalahti, E., Vuorio, K., Rakkolainen, V., Bergman, J., Haaparanta, M., Solin, O., Kuoppamaki, M., Kirvela, O., Ruotsalainen, U., et al. (1995) Presynaptic dopamine function in striatum of neuroleptic-naive schizophrenic patients. *Lancet* 346:1130–1131.

Javitt, D.C., and Zukin, S.R. (1991) Recent advances in the phencyclidine model of schizophrenia. *Am. J. Psychiatry* 148:1301–1308.

Kahn, R.S., Harvey, P.D., Davidson, M., Keefe, R.S., Apter, S., Neale, J.M., Mohs, R.C., and Davis, K.L. (1994) Neuropsychological correlates of central monoamine function in chronic schizophrenia: relationship between CSF metabolites and cognitive function. *Schizophr. Res.* 11:217–224.

Karlsson, P., Farde, L., Halldin, C., and Sedvall, G. (2002) PET study of D(1) dopamine receptor binding in neuroleptic-naive patients with schizophrenia. *Am. J. Psychiatry* 159:761–767.

Kegeles, L., Frankle, W., Gil, R., Narendran, R., Slifstein, M., Hwang, D.-R., Cangiano, C., Haber, S., Abi-Dargham, A., and Laruelle, M. (2006) Schizophrenia is associated with increased synaptic dopamine in associative rather than limbic regions of the striatum: implications for mechanisms of action of antipsychotic drugs. *J. Nucl. Med.* 47(Suppl. 1):139P.

Kegeles, L.S., Martinez, D., Kochan, L.D., Hwang, D.R., Huang, Y., Mawlawi, O., Suckow, R.F., Van Heertum, R.L., and Laruelle, M. (2002) NMDA antagonist effects on striatal dopamine release: Positron emission tomography studies in humans. *Synapse* 43:19–29.

Kellendonk, C., Simpson, E.H., Polan, H.J., Malleret, G., Vronskaya, S., Winiger, V., Moore, H., and Kandel, E.R. (2006) Transient and selective overexpression of dopamine D2 receptors in the striatum causes persistent abnormalities in prefrontal cortex functioning. *Neuron* 49:603–615.

Knable, M.B., and Weinberger, D.R. (1997) Dopamine, the prefrontal cortex and schizophrenia. *J. Psychopharmacol.* 11:123–131.

Kramer, M.S., Last, B., Getson, A., Reines, S.A., Silva, J.A., Wirshing, W., Conley, R., Allan, E., Cheng, H.Y., and ChavezEng C. (1997) The effects of a selective D-4 dopamine receptor antagonist (L-745,870) in acutely psychotic inpatients with schizophrenia. *Arch. Gen. Psychiatry* 54:567–572.

Krystal, J.H., Karper, L.P., Seibyl, J.P., Freeman, G.K., Delaney, R., Bremner, J.D., Heninger, G.R., Bowers, M.B., Jr., and Charney, D. S. (1994) Subanesthetic effects of the noncompetitive NMDA antagonist, ketamine, in humans. Psychotomimetic, perceptual, cognitive, and neuroendocrine responses. *Arch. Gen. Psychiatry* 51: 199–214.

Laruelle, M., Abi-Dargham, A., Gil, R., Kegeles, L., and Innis, R. (1999) Increased dopamine transmission in schizophrenia: relationship to illness phases. *Biol. Psychiatry* 46:56–72.

Laruelle, M., Abi-Dargham, A., van Dyck, C.H., Gil, R., D'Souza, C.D., Erdos, J., McCance, E., Rosenblatt, W., Fingado, C., Zoghbi, S.S., Baldwin, R.M., Seibyl, J.P., Krystal, J.H., Charney, D.S., and Innis, R.B. (1996) Single photon emission computerized tomography imaging of amphetamine-induced dopamine release in drug-free schizophrenic subjects. *Proc. Natl. Acad. Sci. USA* 93: 9235–9240.

Lewis, D.A., and Gonzalez-Burgos, G. (2006) Pathophysiologically based treatment interventions in schizophrenia. *Nat. Med.* 12:1016–1022.

Lewis, D.A., Hashimoto, T., and Volk, D.W. (2005) Cortical inhibitory neurons and schizophrenia. *Nat. Rev. Neurosci.* 6:312–324.

Lieberman, J.A., Kane, J.M., and Alvir, J. (1987) Provocative tests with psychostimulant drugs in schizophrenia. *Psychopharmacology* 91:415–433.

Lieberman, J.A., Kane, J.M., Sarantakos, S., Gadaleta, D., Woerner, M., Alvir, J., and Ramos-Lorenzi, J. (1987) Prediction of relapse in schizophrenia. *Arch. Gen. Psychiatry* 44:597–603.

Lindstrom, L.H., Gefvert, O., Hagberg, G., Lundberg, T., Bergstrom, M., Hartvig, P., and Langstrom, B. (1999) Increased dopamine synthesis rate in medial prefrontal cortex and striatum in schizophrenia indicated by L-(beta-11C) DOPA and PET. *Biol. Psychiatry* 46:681–688.

McGowan, S., Lawrence, A.D., Sales, T., Quested, D., and Grasby, P. (2004) Presynaptic dopaminergic dysfunction in schizophrenia: a positron emission tomographic [18F]fluorodopa study. *Arch. Gen. Psychiatry* 61:134–142.

Meador-Woodruff, J.H., Clinton, S.M., Beneyto, M., and McCullumsmith, R.E. (2003) Molecular abnormalities of the glutamate synapse in the thalamus in schizophrenia. *Ann. NY Acad. Sci.* 1003: 75–93.

Meador-Woodruff, J.H., and Healy, D.J. (2000) Glutamate receptor expression in schizophrenic brain. *Brain Res. Rev.* 31:288–294.

Meyer-Lindenberg, A., Miletich, R.S., Kohn, P.D., Esposito, G., Carson, R.E., Quarantelli, M., Weinberger, D.R., and Berman, K.F. (2002) Reduced prefrontal activity predicts exaggerated striatal dopaminergic function in schizophrenia. *Nat. Neurosci.* 5:267–271.

Moghaddam, B. (2003) Bringing order to the glutamate chaos in schizophrenia. *Neuron* 40:881–884.

Narendran, R., Frankle, W.G., Keefe, R., Gil, R., Martinez, D., Slifstein, M., Kegeles, L.S., Talbot, P.S., Huang, Y., Hwang, D. R., Khenissi, L., Cooper, T.B., Laruelle, M., and Abi-Dargham, A. (2005) Altered prefrontal dopaminergic function in chronic recreational ketamine users. *Am. J. Psychiatry* 162:2352–2359.

Narendran, R., Slifstein, M., Guillin, O., Hwang, Y., Hwang, D.R., Scher, E., Reeder, S., Rabiner, E., and Laruelle, M. (2006) Dopamine (D2/3) receptor agonist positron emission tomography radiotracer [11C]-(+)-PHNO is a D3 receptor preferring agonist in vivo. *Synapse* 60:485–495.

Okubo, Y., Suhara, T., Suzuki, K., Kobayashi, K., Inoue, O., Terasaki, O., Someya, Y., Sassa, T., Sudo, Y., Matsushima, E., Iyo, M., Tateno, Y., and Toru, M. (1997) Decreased prefrontal dopamine D1 receptors in schizophrenia revealed by PET. *Nature* 385:634–636.

Pakkenberg, B. (1990) Pronounced reduction of total neuron number in mediodorsal thalamic nucleus and nucleus accumbens in schizophrenics. *Arch. Gen. Psychiatry* 47:1023–1028.

Parsey, R.V., Oquendo, M.A., Zea-Ponce, Y., Rodenhiser, J., Kegeles, L.S., Pratap, M., Cooper, T.B., Van Heertum, R., Mann, J.J., and Laruelle, M. (2001) Dopamine D(2) receptor availability and amphetamine-induced dopamine release in unipolar depression. *Biol. Psychiatry* 50:313–322.

Pierri, J.N., Volk, C.L., Auh, S., Sampson, A., and Lewis, D.A. (2001) Decreased somal size of deep layer 3 pyramidal neurons in the prefrontal cortex of subjects with schizophrenia. *Arch. Gen. Psychiatry* 58:466–473.

Pycock, C.J., Kerwin, R.W., and Carter, C.J. (1980) Effect of lesion of cortical dopamine terminals on subcortical dopamine receptors in rats. *Nature* 286:74–77.

Reith, J., Benkelfat, C., Sherwin, A., Yasuhara, Y., Kuwabara, H., Andermann, F., Bachneff, S., Cumming, P., Diksic, M., Dyve, S.E., et al. (1994) Elevated dopa decarboxylase activity in living brain of patients with psychosis. *Proc. Natl. Acad. Sci. USA* 91:11651–11654.

Rossum, V. (1966) The significance of dopamine receptor blockade for the mechanism of action of neuroleptic drugs. *Arch. Int. Pharmacodyn. Therapy* 160:492–494.

Seeman, P., Chau-Wong, M., Tedesco, J., and Wong, K. (1975) Brain receptors for antipsychotic drugs and dopamine: direct binding assays. *Proc. Natl. Acad. Sci. USA* 72:4376–4380.

Selemon, L.D., Rajkowska, G., and Goldman-Rakic, P.S. (1995) Abnormally high neuronal density in the schizophrenic cortex. A morphometric analysis of prefrontal area 9 and occipital area 17. *Arch. Gen. Psychiatry* 52:805–818.

Sokoloff, P., Diaz, J., Le Foll, B., Guillin, O., Leriche, L., Bezard, E., and Gross, C. (2006) The dopamine D3 receptor: a therapeutic target for the treatment of neuropsychiatric disorders. *CNS Neurol. Disord. Drug Targets* 5:25–43.

Suhara, T., Okubo, Y., Yasuno, F., Sudo, Y., Inoue, M., Ichimiya, T., Nakashima, Y., Nakayama, K., Tanada, S., Suzuki, K., Halldin, C., and Farde, L. (2002) Decreased dopamine D2 receptor binding in the anterior cingulate cortex in schizophrenia. *Arch. Gen. Psychiatry* 59:25–30.

Talvik, M., Nordstrom, A.L., Okubo, Y., Olsson, H., Borg, J., Halldin, C., and Farde, L. (2006) Dopamine D2 receptor binding in drug-naive patients with schizophrenia examined with raclopride-C11 and positron emission tomography. *Psychiatry Res.* 148:165–173.

Talvik, M., Nordstrom, A.L., Olsson, H., Halldin, C., and Farde, L. (2003) Decreased thalamic D2/D3 receptor binding in drug-naive patients with schizophrenia: a PET study with [11C]FLB 457. *Int. J. Neuropsychopharmacol.* 6:361–370.

Tsai, S.J. (2005) Central N-acetyl aspartylglutamate deficit: a possible pathogenesis of schizophrenia. *Med. Sci. Monit.* 11:HY39–45.

Tsukada, H., Nishiyama, S., Fukumoto, D., Sato, K., Kakiuchi, T., and Domino, E.F. (2005) Chronic NMDA antagonism impairs working memory, decreases extracellular dopamine, and increases D1 receptor binding in prefrontal cortex of conscious monkeys. *Neuropsychopharmacology* 30:1861–1869.

Tuppurainen, H., Kuikka, J., Viinamaki, H., Husso-Saastamoinen, M., Bergstrom, K., and Tiihonen, J. (2003) Extrastriatal dopamine D 2/3 receptor density and distribution in drug-naive schizophrenic patients. *Mol. Psychiatry* 8:453–455.

Tuppurainen, H., Kuikka, J.T., Laakso, M.P., Viinamaki, H., Husso, M., and Tiihonen, J. (2006) Midbrain dopamine D2/3 receptor binding in schizophrenia. *Eur. Arch. Psychiatry Clin. Neurosci.* 256:382–387.

Tzschentke, T.M. (2001) Pharmacology and behavioral pharmacology of the mesocortical dopamine system. *Prog. Neurobiol.* 63:241–320.

Umbricht, D., Schmid, L., Koller, R., Vollenweider, F.X., Hell, D., and Javitt, D.C. (2000) Ketamine-induced deficits in auditory and visual context-dependent processing in healthy volunteers: implications for models of cognitive deficits in schizophrenia. *Arch. Gen. Psychiatry* 57:1139–1147.

Weinberger, D., and Laruelle, M. (2001) Neurochemical and neuropharmachological imaging in schizophrenia. In: Davis, K.L., Charney, D.S., Coyle, J., et al., eds. *Neuropsychopharmacology-The Fifth Generation of Progress*. Philadelphia, PA: Lippincott Williams & Wilkins.

Weinberger, D.R. (1987) Implications of the normal brain development for the pathogenesis of schizophrenia. *Arch. Gen. Psychiatry* 44:660–669.

Weinberger, D.R., Berman, K.F., and Chase, T.N. (1988) Mesocortical dopaminergic function and human cognition. *Ann. NY Acad. Sci.* 537:330–338.

Yasuno, F., Suhara, T., Okubo, Y., Sudo, Y., Inoue, M., Ichimiya, T., Takano, A., Nakayama, K., Halldin, C., and Farde, L. (2004) Low dopamine d(2) receptor binding in subregions of the thalamus in schizophrenia. *Am. J. Psychiatry* 161:1016–1022.

24 Principles of the Pharmacotherapy of Schizophrenia

CAROL A. TAMMINGA

Schizophrenia is an illness that has been recognized for millennia; despite this, the discovery of antipsychotic medications for its treatment has occurred only in the past half-century (Davis, 1969). Although no etiology, pathophysiology, or illness definition for *schizophrenia* has been clarified, empirically derived treatments provide considerable symptomatic benefit for psychosis (Davis, 1969; Tamminga, 1997) and have been naturalistically evaluated (Lieberman et al., 2005; Jones et al., 2006). Effective antipsychotic drugs (APDs) have vastly improved some symptom manifestations and outcomes in schizophrenia, but not others. Further promise exists for the development of new therapies, targeting new symptom domains for drug development, such as cognition enhancement; efforts to identify new molecular targets in cognition are active (Hyman and Fenton, 2003; Geyer and Tamminga, 2007). This chapter focuses first on a review of the symptomatic dysfunctions that are the target for schizophrenia treatment, then on the pharmacology of representative traditional and second-generation drugs and their optimal "real-world" use in patients, and finally on directions being pursued for treating cognition in schizophrenia.

TARGET SYMPTOMS FOR PHARMACOTHERAPY

Symptoms of schizophrenia include positive psychotic symptoms that are prominent during acute periods, and also cognitive dysfunction and enduring negative symptoms that are more persistent. The World Health Organization (WHO), in its 1971 pilot study, looked at schizophrenia symptom type and frequency in several countries (Sartorius et al., 1974). The WHO ranking of the most frequent acute psychotic symptoms (Table 24.1) identifies characteristics of the illness in all of the above domains. The symptom identified as "lack of insight" is nearly ubiquitous among people with the illness and is one of the most crippling. This descriptor means that persons with schizophrenia experience their psychotic perceptions as real sensory information. Not only are people troubled by involuntary thoughts and sensory experiences, but also they identify the psychotic experiences as true events in their lives. Treatments that could merely convert these "real-life experiences" into symptoms, and dissociate their meaning from relevance to the person with schizophrenia, could vastly improve the patient's outcome. Traditional antipsychotics can do this to some extent; clozapine may be superior in this regard.

Several large-factor analytic studies of symptoms in representative treated and stable schizophrenic populations have consistently reported three clusters of symptoms in the illness: (*1*) positive psychotic symptoms (for example, hallucinations, delusions, and paranoia, including thought disorder and bizarre behavior), (*2*) cognitive dysfunction (for example, reductions in attention and executive function), and (*3*) negative symptoms (for example, anhedonia, asociality, and alogia) (Carpenter and Buchanan, 1994; Freedman, 2003). Evidence of cognitive dysfunction and negative symptoms in schizophrenia are ubiquitous and often precede illness onset, as defined by the psychotic symptoms. Any one of these symptom clusters can predominate in individuals with schizophrenia. Whether these clusters represent distinct but symptomatically similar illnesses (for example, like symptoms of chronic heart failure) or a single illness

TABLE 24.1 *Frequency of Psychotic Symptoms in Schizophrenia (WHO International Pilot Study)*

Symptom	Frequency
Lack of insight	97%
Auditory hallucinations	74%
Verbal hallucinations	70%
Ideas of reference	70%
Suspiciousness	65%
Flatness of affect	65%
Voices speaking	65%
Paranoid state	64%
Thought alienation	52%
Thoughts spoken aloud	50%

Source: Sartorius et al. (1974).

with multiple manifestations (for example, like symptoms of diabetes) is frequently debated.

Psychosis is the defining feature of schizophrenia. Its hallmark feature is reality distortion, including hallucinations and delusions; thought disorder is a further deterioration in the structure of language and communication manifest in psychosis. These are the most prominent and the defining characteristics of schizophrenia, whether or not they are the most important pathophysiologically. Psychotic symptoms are particularly impairing because they are accompanied by "lack of insight" (Sartorius et al., 1974), meaning that patients do not have a way of regarding them as nonreality. Observers rarely see the psychotic symptoms in their full manifestation because antipsychotic treatments are so ubiquitous. However, the historical reports of psychotic illness provide a reminder of the impact of this symptom domain on function (Tamminga, 1994). Based on course severity and pharmacology, psychosis is considered to be an independent symptom domain from cognition.

Cognitive disabilities in schizophrenia have a different disease course, often beginning before psychosis onset and persisting across disease years (Cornblatt and Erlenmeyer-Kimling, 1985). Cognitive dysfunction is similar in new persons and chronic persons with schizophrenia (Bilder et al., 1991; Saykin et al., 1994; Gur et al., 1998; Gur et al., 1999; Hill et al., 2004), between adult-onset and adolescent-onset schizophrenia (Kravariti et al., 2003; Brickman et al., 2004), and to some degree, similar in family members (Myles-Worsley and Park, 2002; Niendam et al., 2003; Hoff et al., 2005) and in persons who are high risk but not yet ill (Brewer et al., 2005). But the profile of cognitive disabilities may be largely distinct in schizophrenic compared with nonschizophrenic psychosis (Barch et al., 2003; Fitzgerald et al., 2004). Moreover, cognitive deficits show only small to moderate correlations with clinical state (Censits et al., 1997), no change with APD treatment (Goldberg and Weinberger, 1996), and small gender effects (Carpenter and Buchanan, 1994; Kurtz et al., 2001; Tamminga and Holcomb, 2004). The nature of this dysfunction, thought to be basic to the illness (Elvevag et al., 2004), has been extensively examined in schizophrenia (Braff, 1993; D'Esposito, 1998; Heinrichs and Zakzanis, 1998; Gur et al., 2001; Dickinson et al., 2004; Flashman and Green, 2004; Nuechterlein et al., 2004). It is in the areas of memory and attention that deficits are most pronounced (Flashman and Green, 2004). Although a generalized compromise in cognition in the illness is widely acknowledged, certain domains of function stand out as particularly affected, including visual and verbal declarative memory, working memory, and processing speed (Saykin et al., 1991; Saykin et al., 1994; Heinrichs and Zakzanis, 1998; Cannon et al., 2000; Green et al., 2000; Egan et al., 2001; Dickinson et al., 2004). The degree to which these distinct cognitive profiles result from a general or from distinct etiologies has been argued (Goldman-Rakic, 1994; Andreasen et al., 1998; Cohen et al., 1999) and is an issue important for therapeutics (Nuechterlein et al., 2004). Because the nonpsychotic symptoms of schizophrenia are powerful determinants of poor psychosocial function, specific treatments are being sought. Cognitive dysfunction, particularly poor verbal memory and/or reduced vigilance, predicts broad overall failure in long-term psychosocial rehabilitation. Negative symptoms predict poor social problem solving, but not necessarily poor community functioning or low skill acquisition (Green, 1996).

With respect to treatment, different symptom tracts in schizophrenia respond differently to pharmacotherapy. Hallucinations, delusions, paranoia, and thought disorder show an overall good response to first- (FGA) and second-generation antipsychotics (SGA). Cognitive dysfunction and negative symptoms are poorly responsive, if at all, to these treatments. Because enduring negative symptoms and cognitive dysfunction critically affect overall recovery and rehabilitation, these symptom domains have become targets for treatment development. Depressive symptoms in schizophrenia are variably responsive to antipsychotic treatments. Depression that accompanies an acute psychotic relapse resolves with the acute episode; depression occurring outside of an acute psychosis can be enduring and can critically affect relapse in schizophrenia (Geddes et al., 1994). New neuroleptics may impart benefit in any of these areas.

Treatment of schizophrenia with APDs rarely, if ever, produces a cure or entirely reverses symptoms of the illness. Only 5%–10% of persons with schizophrenia go on to achieve a full recovery with or without these medications. Some 30% show a good but partial response, and another 30% show an inadequate but partial response. The remaining 20%–25% of persons with schizophrenia are resistant to treatment with any APDs. These treatment-resistant individuals suffer continuously without relief and use a disproportionate amount of health care services. Thus their treatment is a priority.

Antipsychotic drugs, as their name implies, treat psychosis in multiple diagnostic categories. Positive psychotic symptoms in bipolar mania, psychotic depression, and dementia with psychosis all respond positively to the antipsychotic treatments described here and are the indicated drugs in these disorders. Schizophrenia characteristically requires continuous treatment for decades, whereas these other psychotic illnesses may require only targeted treatment during active psychotic phases (Tamminga and Davis, 2007). Moreover, certain patient groups are more susceptible to the motor side effects of APDs, such as the elderly and those with mood disorder diagnoses (Kane and Smith, 1982). Dosing considerations are comparable, with accommodation for age and size, especially in the elderly and in children.

TRADITIONAL ANTIPSYCHOTIC DRUGS

The antipsychotic action of the first neuroleptic, *chlorpromazine*, was discovered serendipitously by Delay and Deniker (1952). Its selective antipsychotic properties were quickly noted. In the decade following this discovery, not only was the probable mechanism of APD action articulated as monoamine (especially dopamine [DA]) receptor blockade (Carlsson and Lindquist, 1963), but many additional antipsychotic compounds were generated. These drugs have formed the traditional APD armamentarium for psychiatrists throughout the past half-century. Each of the traditional antipsychotics is associated with a different side-effect profile but with the same primary antipsychotic actions (Davis, 1969).

Chlorpromazine (Thorazine)

Chlorpromazine was first tested in the United States in the early 1950s in several large multicenter trials (Davis, 1969). These trials inevitably included drug-naïve individuals because this was the first effective drug treatment for psychosis. The response was brisk and extensive; full improvement gradually occurred over several weeks. Reductions of 80% or more in symptom profiles occurred commonly, including hallucinations, delusions, and thought disorder. The residual symptoms in the negative and cognitive domains were not immediately noted because of the dramatic overall improvement.

Side effects of chlorpromazine included not only parkinsonism and akathisia, but also hypotension, sedation, constipation, weight gain, and amenorrhea. Hepatotoxicity, electrocardiographic changes, and seizures were less frequent but more serious side effects. Changes in skin color with sun exposure and retinal changes were described. Tardive dyskinesia occurred as well. Today the use of chlorpromazine has gradually diminished, based mostly on its sedation, cardiovascular side effects, and still significant parkinsonism, but it has not disappeared entirely.

Haloperidol (Haldol)

Haloperidol was developed in the 1950s. Until very recently, it was the most widely used antipsychotic for the treatment of schizophrenia. Its potent antipsychotic action with little sedation, despite considerable motor side effects, has sustained its widespread use. Today, these same characteristics, coupled with its relative economic advantage, keep it a viable antipsychotic treatment. It remains to be seen if the new neuroleptics will offer such side-effect advantages over haloperidol to increase compliance and reduce relapse sufficiently to balance their increased cost.

Pharmacology

Haloperidol has a high affinity for the D_2 family of DA receptors (D_2, D_3, and D_4) and for the sigma binding site; it possesses measurable affinity for the 5-hydroxytryptamine2_A (5-HT2_A) serotonin and a1-noradrenergic receptors, but these affinities may not be relevant at doses used clinically (Table 24.2). Haloperidol possesses all the classic pharmacological properties of an antipsychotic agent: it inhibits conditioned-avoidance responding, blocks apomorphine- and amphetamine-induced behaviors, and induces catalepsy in animal preparations. It elevates DA metabolites in the rat dorsal striatum and nucleus accumbens with acute administration (Fink-Jensen and Kristensen, 1994). It causes depolarization blockade in the the nigrostriatal (A9) and mesolimbic (A10) DA neurons with subchronic treatment (Grace et al., 1997); moreover, it stimulates Fos protein expression in striatal DA terminal areas as well as in limbic target regions with acute administration (Robertson et al., 1994). Subchronic treatment in laboratory animals up-regulates D_2 DA receptors in striatum, increases γ-aminobutyric $acid_A$ ($GABA_A$) receptor sites in the substantia nigra pars reticulata, and modifies $GABA_A$ receptor binding in thalamus (Shirakawa and Tamminga, 1994). Several of these pharmacological actions of haloperidol in animals have been linked with its ability to induce parkinsonism and akathisia in humans, such as catalepsy, nonselective (that is, A9 and A10 DA neurons) depolarization blockade, and striatal Fos stimulation.

Metabolism and pharmacokinetics

Reduced-haloperidol is the major single metabolite of haloperidol, and its affinity at the DA receptors is low. Haloperidol's half-life ($T_{B1/2}$) is 12–22 hours in a mixed schizophrenic population; in "good" metabolizers, haloperidol has a half-life of 12–22 hours in a mixed population; in "good" metabolizers, haloperidol's half life is 12.2 +/– 2.6 hours. In a typical population ($N = 10$), the time to maximum concentration (T_{max}) of haloperidol was found to be 5 +/– 2 hours, and its distribution half-life ($T_{a1/2}$) was 1.3 +/–.03 hours; the peak plasma level (C_{max}) after a 10 mg oral concentrate was 12.3 +/– 6.7 ng/ml; the elimination half-life ($T_{B1/2}$) was 21.7 +/– 20 hours. None of these acute or chronic kinetic parameters correlates with the clinical response to the drug. Multiple treatment studies suggest that effective steady-state drug plasma levels are 4–16 ng/ml (VanPutten et al., 1991).

In vivo imaging

Haloperidol at clinically effective doses fully occupies the striatal D_2 receptors, 80%–95%. This level of occupancy

TABLE 24.2 *In Vitro Receptor Binding (Affinity Values Ki in nM)*

	Haloperidol	*Clozapine*	*Olanzapine*	*Seroquel*	*Risperidone*	*Ziprasidone*
D_1	210	85	31	460	430	525
D_2	1	160	44	580	2	4
D_3	2	170	50	940	10	7
D_4	3	50	50	1,900	10	32
5-HT_{2A}	45	16	5	300	0.5	0.4
5-HT_{1A}	1,100	200	>10,000	720	210	3
5-HT_{2C}	>10,000	10	11	5,100	25	1
5-HT_{1D}	>10,000	1,900	800	6,200	170	2
5-HT reuptake	1,700	5,000	ND	ND	1,300	50
NE reuptake	4,700	500	ND	ND	>10,000	50
a_1	6	7	19	7	1	10
a_2	360	8	230	90	1	200
H_1	440	1	3	11	20	50
5-HT_6	9,600	14	10	33	2,200	130
5-HT_7	1,200	100	150	130	2	23
Muscarinic	5,500	2	2	>1,000	>1,000	>1,000

Source: The data in this table were taken from the following references and compiled by Dr. Robert A. Lahti (Leysen et al., 1994; Bymaster et al., 1996; Lahti et al., 1996).

5-HT: 5-hydroxytryptamine; NE: norepinephrine.

has been documented in all patient groups evaluated, even in treatment-resistant persons with schizophrenia. The high D_2 occupancy of haloperidol has suggested this as a mechanism not only for its antipsychotic action but also for its parkinsonism and akathisia side effects. Haloperidol occupancy of the striatal D_2 receptor in schizophrenic patients is dose-dependent; measurable occupancy of the D_2 receptor with chronic treatment remains extends approximately 1 week after drug withdrawal and is not detectable in vivo at 2 weeks (Tamminga et al., 1993). Haloperidol lacks measurable occupancy at the cortical 5-HT_2 receptor using PET with ^{11}C-N-methylspiperone (^{11}C-NMSP).

Functional imaging studies have addressed the question of where in the central nervous system (CNS) haloperidol exerts its therapeutic actions (Holcomb et al., 1996). Our own work in this area has shown that haloperidol increases neuronal activity as measured by regional cerebral blood flow (rCBF) in the human striatum, in dorsal and ventral regions. In addition, haloperidol increases neuronal activity in the thalamus and decreases glucose metabolism in the frontal cortex and anterior cingulate with minimal regional alterations in other CNS areas (Holcomb et al., 1996). We have speculated that haloperidol reduces psychosis by exerting its initial action in the striatum at the D_2 DA receptors and than by transmitting this action to thalamus and frontal and limbic cortex using the well-described neuronal circuits connecting the basal ganglia, thalamus, and cortex (Alexander and Crutcher, 1990). Although actions of other antipsychotics at other receptor sites (for example, serotonin receptors) may be exerted primarily in neocortex, we speculate that the antidopaminergic actions of antipsychotics are initiated in the striatum and then transmitted in a secondary and tertiary manner to cortex through the brain's own neural pathways (Alexander and Crutcher, 1990). In addition, haloperidol could have primary actions in multiple different brain regions to deliver its clinical effect.

Efficacy

The antipsychotic efficacy of haloperidol was initially established in controlled trials in the early 1960s (Davis, 1969); it is a highly effective antipsychotic, useful at low doses. But it was not until recently that a dose-response study was conducted across the apparent dose-sensitive range for haloperidol. Three doses of haloperidol (4, 8, and 16 mg/day) were tested against placebo in a multicenter controlled trial (Zimbroff et al., 1997). The study results showed haloperidol to be highly effective in schizophrenia. There was no linear dose-response relationship with any symptom or symptom cluster across this dose range, as has been previously suggested for APDs.

Side effects and safety

In the above dose study, haloperidol produced significant parkinsonism on the Simpson–Angus Scale (SAS) and akathisia on the Barnes Akathisia Scale (BAS) across all the doses used, even at the lowest dose of 4 mg/day. There were no relationships between drug dose and motor side effects in the 4–16 mg/day range. Other side effects of haloperidol were low, including cardiovascular, anticholinergic, and hematological. No QTc prolongation occurs with haloperidol. Hepatotoxicity is a rare side effect. These safety results are consistent with years of clinical experience using haloperidol.

SECOND-GENERATION ANTIPSYCHOTICS: BROAD PROFILE RECEPTOR ANTAGONISTS

Some second-generation APDs block many monoamine and other G protein–coupled receptors in brain and have a broad receptor affinity profile (Table 24.2). Their spectrum of receptor antagonist activity is extensive, and their overall clinical action is neurochemically complex. The APDs described here are available for prescription in the United States; additional compounds may be available in other countries (for example, amisulpride), even though not described in detail here.

Clozapine (Clozaril)

Clozapine is an APD that, although it has led the "second-generation drug" era, is not itself new. Its demonstration of superior efficacy over chlorpromazine in treatment-resistant patients with schizophrenia spurred subsequent research in this area (Kane et al., 1988). It is the only antipsychotic shown so far to have superior antipsychotic action in schizophrenia compared with the traditional and the new compounds. Its mechanism in this regard remains unknown.

Pharmacology

Clozapine has a broad affinity for many receptors in brain. Not only the DA receptors (D_1, D_5, D_2, D_3, D_4) but also serotonin (5-HT_{2A}, 5-HT_{2C}, 5-HT_6, 5-HT_7), noradrenergic (a_1 and a_2), cholinergic (nicotine and muscarinic), and histamine (H_1) receptors are blocked by clozapine. Clozapine affinities are generally low at all sites (Table 24.2). Consistent with this profile, clozapine blocks not only DA agonist–stimulated behaviors but also cholinergic-, serotonergic-, and noradrenergic-stimulated neurochemical and behavioral actions in animals. Clozapine inhibits conditioned-avoidance behavior but does not produce catalepsy. Clozapine does not measurably alter DA metabolite concentrations in striatum but does increase metabolites (DOPAC) in the rat nucleus accumbens (Coward, 1992).

Clozapine was the first antipsychotic shown to have anatomically restricted electrophysiological actions on DA neurons; clozapine induces depolarization blockade in the mesolimbic (A10) DA neurons but not in the nigrostriatal (A9) cells (Grace et al., 1997). The association of this distinctive preclinical characteristic with the drug's low motor side-effect profile in humans is broadly consistent with the idea that antipsychotic actions are generally mediated through the A10 dopaminergic neurons and motor side effects through the A9 group. Consistent with clozapine's action in the depolarization inactivation model has been its selective functional anatomy using cFos in situ hybridization autoradiography and Fos protein immunohistochemistry (Robertson et al., 1994). These studies show that clozapine stimulates immediate early gene (IEG) expression in rats in mesolimbic projection fields of the DA cell bodies (nucleus accumbens, ventral striatum, anterior cingulate, and medial prefrontal cortex) but not in the nigrostriatal projections to the dorsal striatum (A9). The mechanism subserving this anatomical selectivity of clozapine's action remains unknown. Nonetheless, the principle that limited regional drug action in CNS is important to schizophrenia pharmacology has been repeatedly demonstrated. Moreover, the failure of clozapine to induce dyskinesias in the neuroleptic-sensitized monkey (Casey, 1996) or to cause oral dyskinesias in chronically treated rats (Gunne et al., 1982) is consistent with these observations.

Metabolism and pharmacokinetics

Clozapine has several metabolites, the two most abundant of which are norclozapine and *N*-desmethylclozapine. Too little data are available concerning clozapine catabolism and the activity of its metabolites. *N*-desmethylclozapine has been identified as an active clozapine metabolite with a clozapine-like affinity profile, except for showing muscarinic cholinergic agonist activity instead of anticholinergic activity (Weiner et al., 2004). This compound, known as *ACP104*, is being developed for psychosis and for cognitive dysfunction in schizophrenia. For clozapine, single-dose kinetic analysis with a 200 mg oral dose found the T_{max} to be 3 +/– 1.5 hours and the C_{max} to be 386 +/– 249 ng/ml. The distribution half-life ($T_{a1/2}$) is 0.1 +/–.12 hours, and the elimination half-life ($T_{B1/2}$) is 10.3 +/– 2.9 hours. Plasma concentrations show a linear relationship to dose with multiple dose kinetics. Interindividual variability in metabolism is high. Terminal elimination is linear.

In vivo imaging

Clozapine occupies measurably fewer striatal DA receptors at clinically effective doses than do traditional neuroleptics (Farde et al., 1992). Using ^{11}C-Rac and positron emission tomography (PET), occupancy is 40%–60%; with ^{11}C-NMSP, occupancy is 15%–30%. At the same doses, clozapine occupies 80%–90% of serotonin receptors in cortex, consistent with its in vitro affinity profile. The profile of reduced DA receptor occupancy in striatum and increased serotonin receptor occupancy in cortex is characteristic of second-generation antipsychotics (Kapur et al., 1999).

Functional imaging data show that clozapine, like haloperidol, increases rCBF in striatum, but clozapine does this only in the ventral striatum and to a lesser degree. Moreover, clozapine differs from haloperidol in that it increases (not decreases) neuronal activation in the anterior cingulate cortex and in the middle frontal gyrus, areas that are important to core cognitive functions such as attention and working memory. During task performance, clozapine "normalizes" rCBF in several areas of frontal cortex, especially in the anterior cingulate cortex (Lahti et al., 2003). These broad differences in cerebral activation patterns between clozapine and haloperidol likely represent in some way the unique clinical action of clozapine in schizophrenia and could, with further study, be developed as a surrogate marker of that action.

Efficacy

The general antipsychotic efficacy of clozapine was established more than 20 years ago. However, because of clozapine's higher side-effect burden, including agranulocytosis, the Food and Drug Administration (FDA) required Sandoz to demonstrate its superiority to traditional antipsychotics. Kane and colleagues (1988) demonstrated clozapine to be superior to chlorpromazine in treating treatment-refractory inpatients with schizophrenia. Subsequently, several additional studies confirmed this unique action (Conley, Carpenter, and Tamminga, 1997). Moreover, its superior efficacy in treating partial nonresponding populations was also demonstrated (Kane et al., 2001). Arguably the most convincing demonstration recently of clozapine superiority was in Phase 2 of the Clinical Antipsychotic Trials of Intervention Effectiveness (CATIE) trial where the time to treatment discontinuation and the decrease in Positive and Negative Syndrome Scale (PANSS) scores was greatest by a substantial margin for clozapine compared with three other second-generation antipsychotics (SGAs) (McEvoy et al., 2006). Whether clozapine has superior efficacy in treating primary negative symptoms has been widely debated; the answer is suggested but is still not clear (Davis et al., 2003). Optimal studies where drug action on negative symptoms can be clearly differentiated from secondary effects or lack of drug side effects have not yet been reported. Some cognitive dysfunctions are improved by clozapine, and others are worsened. In clinical populations with drug abuse comorbidity, clozapine is also more effective. Although the final composite outcomes remain to be demonstrated, the long-term psychosocial improvement with clozapine suggests cognitive improvement. There is no doubt that clozapine increases discharge rates from hospital care and improves community function after discharge (Rosenheck et al., 1997; Love et al., 1999).

Side effects and safety

Acute motor side effects with clozapine are very low, if detectable at all, including parkinsonism and akathisia. In addition, clozapine appears by all estimates to have an extremely low (if any) incidence of tardive dyskinesia. Moreover, clozapine treatment of tardive dyskinesia allows dyskinetic symptoms to fade gradually over 6–12 months (Tamminga et al., 1994).

With respect to other side effects, clozapine is at the top of any list. It causes agranulocytosis with an incidence of 0.5%–1%, a condition that has 3%–15% mortality. The risk of agranulocytosis is highest in the 2nd and 3rd months after beginning treatment; the risk is reduced after the first 6 months and remains flat and relatively low (comparable to other APDs) after the first 12 months of treatment. In addition, the drug can induce seizures, increase heart rate, and stimulate cardiac arrhythmias. It causes weight gain, substantial in some instances, and alters carbohydrate metabolism and plasma lipid levels producing the metabolic syndrome (Allison et al., 1999; Wirshing et al., 1999; Henderson et al., 2000; McEvoy et al., 2006). It also causes other, less medically significant but bothersome side effects like sedation and drooling. It is surprising that, with this serious side-effect profile, clozapine is used at all. Its superior efficacy is the reason, in those situations where efficacy is needed, that the drug's substantial side-effect profile is tolerated. Moreover, many clinicians contend that the drug is underused.

Olanzapine (Zyprexa)

Olanzapine is a structural congener of clozapine. It is the third of the new antipsychotics available in the United States, preceded to market by clozapine and risperidone. As would be predicted from its pharmacology, olanzapine has many of the same pharmacological characteristics as clozapine (for example, its affinity at multiple receptors) with several significant exceptions in terms of pharmacology (for example, high not low receptor affinities), side effects (for example, no agranulocytosis) and efficacy (equal, but not superior).

Pharmacology

Olanzapine has a high affinity for a broad range of CNS receptors at clinically relevant concentrations, including DA (D_1–D_5), serotonin (5-HT_{2A}, 5-HT_{2C}, 5-HT_6), noradrenalin (a_1), acetylcholine (muscarinic, particularly M_1), and histamine (H_1) receptors. It is a potent ligand at all of these receptors, with a high affinity at each site (Table 24.2). Different from clozapine, it lacks high affinity for the 5-HT_7, a_2, and other cholinergic receptors (Bymaster et al., 1996). Olanzapine blocks conditioned avoidance responding in rats but causes catalepsy only at high doses.

Olanzapine increases DA and norepinephrine metabolite levels in nucleus accumbens and reduces acetylcholine levels in striatum. Moreover, unlike haloperidol, olanzapine also increases DA and norepinephrine release in frontal cortex (Bymaster et al., 1996). Olanzapine blocks DA and serotonin-stimulated biochemical changes and animal behaviors; its antiserotonin actions are more potent than its antidopaminergic actions. With chronic treatment, olanzapine significantly but minimally upregulates D_2 receptors in striatum (Sakai, Gao, Hashimoto, and Tamminga, 2001); in addition, olanzapine, like clozapine, exerts a regional action on DA-containing neurons. With chronic treatment, olanzapine produces depolarization blockade in A10 DA neurons but not in the A9 cells (Skarsfeldt, 1995). Olanzapine also shows selective activation of the c-Fos IEG gene in ventral striatum and in medial prefrontal cortex without inducing c-Fos messenger ribonucleic acid (mRNA) in the dorsal striatum (Robertson and Fibiger, 1996). Consistent with this regional action, olanzapine produces dystonias in neuroleptic-sensitized monkeys only at high doses, above its clinically effective dose ranges (Casey, 1996) and fails to produce a high rate of oral dyskinesias (purposeless chewing) in chronically treated rats (Sakai Gao, and Tamminga 2001).

Metabolism and pharmacokinetics

Olanzapine has two primary metabolites, 4-N-desmethyl olanzapine and 10-N-glucuronide olanzapine, both of which are inactive as antipsychotics. The parent drug has weak affinity for several different hepatic isoenzyme systems, including CYP-2D6, –1A2, –34A, and –2C19; thus, significant drug–drug interactions on this basis are minimal. T_{max} for olanzapine is 5 hours, and the drug has a mean plasma elimination half-life ($T_{B1/2}$) of 31 hours (range: 21–54 hours). Plasma kinetic studies suggest linear dose proportionality. Female participants show slower metabolism and consequently higher plasma levels than male participants. Concurrent cigarette smoking and carbamezapine use accelerate metabolism and lower olanzapine levels modestly.

In vivo imaging

In preliminary human PET studies, olanzapine shows approximately 60% occupancy at the striatal D_2 receptors when evaluated with ^{11}C-Rac/PET after an acute 10 mg dose (Farde et al., 1997), a lower striatal DA receptor occupancy than that of the traditional antipsychotics. The low motor side effects seen with olanzapine are consistent with the Farde et al. (1992) proposition that it takes a D_2 occupancy greater than 70% to induce acute motor side effects. More recent occupancy studies with olanzapine are consistent with these early data (Kapur et al., 1998).

In preliminary studies comparing the functional activation properties of olanzapine to those of haloperidol, it is easy to see that olanzapine is associated with reduced rCBF activation in basal ganglia and thalamus, like clozapine, and increased rCBF activation in anterior cingulate and temporal cortex, also like clozapine.

Efficacy

Olanzapine's efficacy is based on four large placebo- and haloperidol-controlled multicenter registration trials (Beasley et al., 1997; Tamminga and Kane, 1997). Consistently in all of these trials, olanzapine showed a substantial antipsychotic response in patients with actively psychotic schizophrenia, significantly greater than that of placebo on positive and negative symptoms, and equivalent to that of haloperidol on positive symptoms. There was an indication that olanzapine is more effective than haloperidol in treating negative symptoms. Whether the antinegative symptom response to olanzapine involves primary or secondary negative symptoms has been debated, although the results of a path analysis are consistent with a drug action on primary negative symptoms (Tollefson et al., 1997). Further work in this area is needed to distinguish the primary from the secondary nature of its negative symptom action. In treatment-resistant inpatients with schizophrenia, olanzapine has been compared to chlorpromazine in a trial design mimicking the clozapine-chlorpromazine trial (Kane et al., 1988). At a fixed dose of 25 mg/day, the action of olanzapine on psychotic symptoms was found to be similar to the action of chlorpromazine; no significant differences in efficacy on psychosis emerged between the two drugs in this population, except that olanzapine imparted a significant antianxiety effect (Conley, Tamminga and Beasley, 1997). In addition to schizophrenia, olanzapine currently has an indication in the treatment of mania (Tohen and Zarate, 1998).

Several non-industry-sponsored, naturalistic studies have been conducted to answer the question of comparative efficacy across the SGA compared with FGA. CATIE found that olanzapine, in modal daily doses of 20.1 mg, showed the greatest improvement in effectiveness, including a low rate of discontinuation, a greater initial reduction in psychopathology, a longer duration of successful treatment, and a lower rate of hospitalization for relapse among SGAs (Lieberman et al., 2005). The Cost Utility of the Latest Antipsychotic Drugs in Schizophrenia Study (CUtLASS) study contrasted a group of FGAs with SGAs (including olanzapine) and showed no difference between the two groups of drugs on Quality of Life or on any of their secondary outcome measures;

individual analyses were not done for each drug (Jones et al., 2006). A meta-analysis of FGA and SGA efficacy studies reports that olanzapine shows a modest but significant overall advantage over FGAs with an effect size of 0.21 but is not significantly different from the other SGAs (Davis et al., 2003). Leucht found that, as a group, the SGAs were modestly but significantly better on rate of relapse and failure to respond than the FGAs (Leucht et al., 2003). Rosenheck has found no advantage of olanzapine on overall cost effectiveness in treating chronic schziophrenia (Rosenheck et al., 2003; Rosenheck et al., 2006).

Side effects and safety

Motor side effects with olanzapine are remarkably and significantly diminished from those seen with haloperidol (Beasley et al., 1996; Tamminga and Kane, 1997). This finding is consistent across studies, thus providing confidence from replication. On average in the controlled trials, parkinsonism (SAS) and akathisia (BAS) were equivalent to placebo and lower than with haloperidol use. At the highest olanzapine dose, mild akathisia was evident, along with a low rate of anticholinergic drug use to treat motor side effects. Some evidence exists that this will translate into lower rates of tardive dyskinesia (Tollefson et al., 1997)

Weight gain and other metabolic side effects occur with olanzapine treatment; these changes pose a substantial risk factor for diabetes and heart disease. The metabolic side effects (weight gain, increases in cholesterol, triglycerides, and glycosylated hemoglobin) have been widely documented (Osser et al., 1999; Bettinger et al., 2000; Lieberman et al., 2005; McEvoy et al., 2006). Relative to other SGAs, olanzapine shows the greatest metabolic syndrome burden along with clozapine, followed by quetiapine and then risperidone. In addition, mild anticholinergic actions are evident with olanzapine treatment, including dry mouth and constipation. Few cardiac side effects have been noted with olanzapine, including no blood pressure elevations, tachycardia, electrocardiographic changes, or significant QTc prolongation (Glassman and Bigger, 2001). In addition, no blood dyscrasias have been associated with olanzapine use, a side effect closely evaluated because of the structural similarity between olanzapine and clozapine. Transient dose-sensitive increases in hepatic transaminanses have been noted, but these occur infrequently and attenuate with continued treatment. Initial prolactin elevations occur but are lower than those seen with haloperidol and showed almost complete tolerance over time.

Quetiapine (Seroquel)

Although from a different chemical class, quetiapine displays many biochemical and behavioral similarities to clozapine. Quetiapine has broad and low receptor affinity characteristics and many of the behavioral actions of clozapine. Quetiapine is the fourth antipsychotic marketed in the United States and has become widely prescribed. Its sleep-enhancing properties probably deriving from its potent 5-HT_{2A} activity determine some portion of its prescription base.

Pharmacology

Quetiapine comes from the chemical class of dibenzothiazapine drugs. The drug binds to the D_1, D_5, D_2, D_3, D_4, 5-HT_2, 5-HT_{1A}, a_1, and a_2 receptors, as does clozapine, but lacks clozapine-like affinity for the muscarinic cholinergic receptors. Its affinity to all of these receptors is low, similar to clozapine (Table 24.2). Quetiapine fails to potently upregulate D_2 DA receptors in striatum with chronic treatment, suggesting its low affinity as a DA antagonist. But it increases DA metabolites in striatum as well as in nucleus accumbens with acute administration; it shows an acute but short-lived action on increasing plasma prolactin in rats. The anatomical selectivity of quetiapine in the depolarization block model is not yet clear (conflicting study findings have been reported). However, it shows selective action on regional c-Fos activation, similar to that of clozapine, in that it fails to activate Fos proteins in the dorsal striatum. Quetiapine inhibits conditional avoidance responding at high concentrations; it blocks DA agonist–induced behaviors in rats such as eye blink, climbing, and locomotor activity. Quetiapine induces catalepsy only at very high doses that are no longer clinically relevant (Saller and Salama, 1993). In neuroleptic sensitized Cebus monkeys, quetiapine induces mild dystonias only in a high dose range, which is probably not clinically significant (Casey, 1996).

Metabolism and pharmacokinetics

Acute kinetics are linear; the drug shows good oral bioavailability. The elimination half-life ($T_{B1/2}$) is approximately 6 hours. Plasma concentrations at steady state are linear up to a dose of 600 mg/day; for example, daily doses of 75, 300, and 600 mg produce steady-state (trough) plasma levels of 13.9, 43.9, and 91.1 ng/ml, respectively. Drug clearance is reduced in elderly persons with schizophrenia, perhaps by 50%; therefore, in elderly patients, the dose should be reduced.

In vivo imaging

Preliminary imaging studies of quetiapine using ^{11}C-Rac/PET show occupancy in striatum at 2 hours of 44% and at 12 hours of 27% at the DA receptor. With ^{11}C-NMSP/PET, quetiapine shows occupancy in cortex at the serotonin receptor of 72% (2 hours), and 50% (at 24 hours). More recent imaging studies are consistent but show short-lived occupancy (Kapur et al., 2000).

Efficacy

Quetiapine demonstrates antipsychotic action significantly greater than that of placebo in several placebo-controlled trials at doses of 150–750 mg/day and action equivalent to that of haloperidol. Although this drug was initially recommended for use in schizophrenia at 300 mg/day, many clinicians suspect that a much higher dose is optimal, closer to or above 750 mg/day. Therapeutic action on positive and negative symptoms of psychosis has been demonstrated, with the magnitude of its antipsychotic effect significantly greater than that of placebo in each domain and equivalent to that of haloperidol (Arvanitis and Miller, 1997). The CATIE-1 study showed that quetiapine, in a modal dose of 543.4 mg/day, showed effectiveness outcomes similar to the other SGAs (except clozapine and olanzapine) but had the largest percentage of volunteers who dropped the study before its 18-month end (82%) (Lieberman et al., 2005). In CATIE-2, quetiapine was modestly but significantly less effective than olanzapine or risperidone (Stroup et al., 2006). Studies show that quetiapine has actions on promoting sleep quality and efficacy in Bipolar-2 Disorder depression.

Side effects and safety

Routine safety parameters show a relatively benign safety profile for quetiapine in many respects. Almost no motor side effects accompany its use; no episodes of extrapyramidal adverse events beyond placebo levels have been reported. No anticholinergic medication use beyond that of placebo has been necessary in any dose group. No akathisia is apparent. The most frequently observed side effects are sedation, somnolence, and headache. Significant weight gains occur accompanied by hyper-cholesterolemia and -triglyceridemia, although to a lesser degree than with olanzapine or clozapine (Lieberman et al., 2005). Alterations in cholesterol metabolism are being studied. Transient and reversible increases in hepatic transaminase levels can be seen. No prolactin elevations are apparent in the 6–8-week parallel group studies comparing any dose group to placebo use. Although cataracts have been observed in some animal studies, no evidence to support the onset of cataracats has been found in humans. No significant QTc prolongtion occurs with quetiapine (Glassman and Bigger, 2001).

NEW ANTIPSYCHOTICS: SELECTIVE DOPAMINE AND SEROTONIN RECEPTOR ANTAGONISTS

Selective DA and serotonin receptor blockers show effective antipsychotic action and preserve advantageous motor side-effect profiles. These second-generation drugs show greater serotonin than DA blockade, pharmacologically and in occupancy studies.

Risperidone (Risperdol)

Risperidone was the first second-generation drug presented to the FDA and reviewed by them in approximately 15 years. This long hiatus without new drug products for treating psychosis made clinicians and consumers eager to use this first new drug. Risperidone has been well received and widely prescribed for schizophrenia. It is approved for bipolar disorder with psychosis as well.

Pharmacology

Risperidone is a benzisoxazol derivative with high affinity for the 5-HT_{2A} and D_2 receptors. Its in vitro affinity for 5-HT_{2A} is 20 times higher than for D_2 receptors; its affinity for other serotonin receptor subtypes is lower by two or more orders of magnitude (Table 24.2). Risperidone has moderate affinity for a_1 noradrenergic and H_1 histamine receptors and even lower affinity for a_2 sites. It lacks significant affinity for cholinergic receptors, for the sigma site, and for the D_1 receptor family. The major metabolite of risperidone, *9-hydroxy-risperidone*, is active and has a receptor affinity profile similar to that of its parent compound (Leysen et al., 1994). The pharmacology of 9-OH risperidone accounts for many of the actions of risperidone itself given its extensive metabolism and the long half-life of the metabolite.

Risperidone blocks serotonin and DA agonist–induced behaviors in animal paradigms, with greater serotonergic than dopaminergic potency. It has no anticholinergic activity in behavioral or neurochemical tests. Risperidone increases DA turnover in frontal cortex and in the olfactory area but is less active in striatum (Fink-Jensen and Kristensen, 1994). It induces catalepsy in rats only at relatively high doses, but it induces dystonias in sensitized Cebus monkeys at clinically relevant concentrations (Casey, 1996). Risperidone has a similar effect on A9 and A10 DA neurons in the depolarization inactivation model, but its actions on both cell groups are atypical. At low dose levels, risperidone fails to stimulate c-Fos expression in the dorsal striatum, whereas it activates the IEG briskly in the nucleus accumbens. Preclinically, the profile for anatomical selectivity is mixed and leaves questions about predictions for human motor side effects.

Metabolism and pharmacokinetics

Risperidone is metabolized by the liver isoenzyme CYP2D6. Its major metabolite is 9-hydroxyrisperidone (9-OH-R) and is pharmacologically active. Because the metabolite is renally excreted, hepatic and renal metabolism is important to overall risperidone clearance. Individual genetic variation of the CYP2D6 isoenzyme and other concomitant 2D6-metabolized medications (for example, fluoxetine) significantly alter drug clearance and plasma concentrations.

After a single 1 mg dose of risperidone, T_{max} is 1 hour for risperidone and 3 hours for 9-OH-R; $T_{B1/2}$ for risperidone is 3.6 hours, and for 9-OH-R it is 22 hours. Kinetics are dose proportional up to 10 mg. In extensive metabolizers, $T_{B1/2}$ is 2.8 hours, whereas for poor metabolizers it is 21.0 hours. The $T_{B1/2}$ of 9-OH-R remains 20–22 hours in both groups of metabolizers because its excretion is renally dependent. Also, in individuals who are renally impaired and in the elderly, overall risperidone metabolism and excretion are reduced (Ereshefsky and Lacombe, 1993).

In vivo imaging

With a 1 mg oral dose of risperidone, D_2 occupancy measured in striatum with ^{11}C-Rac/PET was 50% (range: 40%–64%). The 5-HT_{2A} occupancy measured in cortex using ^{11}C-NMSP/PET was 60% (range: 45%–68%). Occupancy is dose proportional; thus, risperidone shows high occupancy with high doses (Kapur et al., 1999). Chronic risperidone treatment at low but clinically effective doses results in D_2 occupancy in striatum of less than 70% (Nyberg et al., 1993).

Efficacy

Risperidone has been studied worldwide in patients who are actively psychotic with schizophrenia. Its actions have been evaluated on positive and negative psychotic symptoms across a broad dose range (2–16 mg/day) in several large multicenter trials, with largely consistent findings. Risperidone treatment results in a significant reduction in positive and negative symptoms compared to placebo; positive symptoms respond to risperidone to a similar extent as haloperidol; the negative symptom response may be greater (Marder and Meibach, 1994). A risperidone dose of 3–6 mg/day produces the best overall outcome of the doses tested, including its effects on positive and negative symptoms. These results are consistent across several risperidone efficacy studies, suggesting a *U*-shaped dose-response curve, with the greatest psychosis response occurring at a daily dose of 3–6 mg/day. Moreover, population survey data confirm physician use of lower doses of risperidone preferentially, with a good outcome (Love et al., 1999).

In the CATIE-1 study, risperidone showed a modest but significantly lower effectiveness than olanzapine (Lieberman et al., 2005), whereas in CATIE-2, it showed equivalent effectiveness (Stroup et al., 2006); in treatment nonresponders, risperidone was less effective than clozapine (McEvoy et al., 2006). In the Davis (Davis et al., 2003) meta-analysis, comparing SGAs to efficacy of FGAs, risperidone showed a modest but significant positive difference from FGAs with an effect size of 0.25.

The 9-OH metabolite of risperidone (developed as *paliperidone*; marketed as *Invega*) has pharmacological effects that largely match those of risperidone, as expected (Kane et al., 2007; Kramer et al., 2007; Marder et al., 2007).

Side effects and safety

Motor side effects with risperidone are at placebo levels at doses below 6 mg/day. At doses above 10 mg/day, parkinsonism and akathisia are significant and probably similar to those with haloperidol. Anticholinergic drug use is also at placebo levels below 6 mg/day but progressively approaches the haloperidol use rate above 10 mg/day. Thus, below 6 mg/day of risperidone, parkinsonian motor side effects are minimal but rise thereafter. Agitation, anxiety, sedation, and insomnia have been reported with risperidone, but at rates similar to those of haloperidol. Hypotension was noted in normal volunteer studies but was not selectively noted in volunteers with schizophrenia. The QTc is not affected by risperidone. Hyperprolactinemia is common, and frank galactorrhea can occur with risperidone. Mild weight gain occurs; alterations in carbohydrate or lipid metabolism should be monitored.

Ziprasidone (Geodon)

Ziprasidone was the fifth new antipsychotic to come to market. It was developed on the basis not only of its aminergic receptor binding profile (5-HT_2.DA_2) but also its unique reuptake blockade property with the serotonin and noradrenergic reuptake proteins. This has encouraged the speculation that ziprasidone will treat schizophrenia with depression and/or anxiety, a question still not fully answered. The side-effect profile of ziprasidone has received considerable attention: on the negative side, due to the QTc prolongation, and on the positive side, due to the lack of any significant weight gain or alterations of cholesterol or lipid metabolism.

Pharmacology

The receptor binding profile of ziprasidone is distinctive in several respects. Its affinity for the D_2 family of receptors is high; 10-fold higher is its affinity for the 5-HT_{2A} receptor. Thus, the 5-HT_{2A}/DA ratio is the highest among the second-generation drugs. Moreover, it has significant affinity for several additional serotonin receptors, including 5-HT_{1A}, 5-HT_{2C}, and 5-HT_{1D} (Table 24.2). Ziprasidone is a partial agonist at the 5-HT_{1A} receptor and thereby increases extracellular DA levels in medial frontal cortex (Sharma and Shapiro, 1996; Daniel et al., 1999). It also acts as an antagonist at its other receptors. It is unique among the new antipsychotics in showing moderate affinity for and inhibition of the 5-HT and norepinephrine receptor proteins, comparable to the action of amitriptyline (Seeger et al., 1995). Moreover, it lacks significant affinity for the muscarinic M_1 receptor (Seeger et al., 1995).

Behaviorally, ziprasidone is a potent inhibitor of DA- and serotonin-mediated behaviors; it is sixfold more potent in inhibiting serotonergic than dopaminergic behaviors. It inhibits conditioned avoidance responding in rats. It decreases spontaneous locomotor activity and causes catalepsy, but the latter only at relatively high doses, thought to be no longer clinically relevant. Ziprasidone appears to affect equally DA cell firing in A9 and A10 neurons with chronic administration; therefore, it lacks the clozapine-like anatomical selectivity on dopaminergic function.

Metabolism and pharmacokinetics

Ziprasidone is metabolized by several hepatic and extrahepatic enzyme systems; hence, its plasma levels are relatively unaffected by other concomitant medications. In metabolic inhibition studies with ketoconasole, the P450 enzyme inhibitor of CYP3A4, ziprasidone plasma levels were unaffected. Additional safety is imparted by ziprasidone's multiple degratory drug routes. There appear to be no active metabolites of ziprasidone. The kinetics of ziprasidone are dose proportional at steady-state kinetics. At therapeutic doses, the T_{max} is 4.7 +/– 1.5 hours and the elimination half-life ($T_{B1/2}$) is 10 hours.

In vivo imaging

Full assessment of ziprasidone occupancy at the D_2 receptor using PET (with ^{11}C-Rac in striatum) and at the 5-HT_2 receptor (with ^{18}F-septoperone in cortex) was carried out in normal human volunteers prior to patient studies to allow rational dose selection. Participants received 40 mg of oral ziprasidone, and neurochemical scans were obtained at regular intervals over the next 36 hours, beginning at T_{max}. At 4 hours, D_2 occupancy in striatum was 79.4% and 5-HT occupancy in cortex was 98.5%. At 12 hours, D_2 occupancy was 52.8% and 5-HT_2 occupancy was 73.1%. Calculations from the model based on all the data predicted that at steady state with 40 mg ziprasidone administered bid, 5-HT_2 occupancy would remain at 90% and D_2 occupancy would average 75% (Bench et al., 1993; Bench et al., 1996).

Efficacy

Results from Phase II and III efficacy studies have been published. In these studies, ziprasidone was compared across a dose range of 40–160 mg/day to placebo and haloperidol at 15 mg/day. Ziprasidone demonstrated significant antipsychotic actions over the dose range of 80–160 mg/day (40–80 mg bid). Therapeutic action on positive symptoms was equivalent to that of haloperidol and comparable to that of other second-generation antipsychotics; significant antinegative effects occurred compared to those of placebo (O'Connor et al., personal communication, 1997; Daniel et al., 2001). In patients with clinically significant depressive symptomatology at baseline, ziprasidone produced an antidepressant effect (Daniel et al., 2001). In the CATIE-1 study, ziprasidone at a modal dose of 112.8 mg/day showed modestly but significantly lower effectiveness than olanzapine (Lieberman et al., 2005), and in CATIE-2, when contrasted with olanzapine, risperidone, and quetiapine in a similar dose range, showed a similar level of low effectiveness (Stroup et al., 2006).

Side effects and safety

Ziprasidone has been associated with a low rate of motor side effects at all of the doses tested, indistinguishable from placebo on SAS and BAS rating scales. The drug produced significantly lower levels of parkinsonism and akathisia than haloperidol. Moreover, anticholinergic drug prescriptions for motor side effects were at placebo levels (10%–15%) across the range of ziprasidone doses and were lower than with haloperidol at any dose (Daniel et al., 2001). Moreover, in contrast to several other new antipsychotics, ziprasidone causes no significant weight gain, either in the short term (Daniel et al., 2001) or in extended (12-month) trials. This advantage in avoiding weight gain is substantial relative to the other new antipsychotics in terms of cardiovascular health (Allison et al., 1999; Bettinger et al., 2000) and compliance (Silverstone et al., 1988). The advantage of ziprasidone on metabolic side effects and weight gain was also documented in the CATIE trials (Lieberman et al., 2005; Stroup et al., 2006).

The most significant ziprasidone side effect is its mild but unequivocal effect on the QTc interval (Glassman and Bigger, 2001). In a rigorously conducted study to evaluate the extent of this drug side effect, the average QTc prolongation time with ziprasidone at peak plasma levels, at its highest recommended dose, was 20.3 ms (95% Confidence Interval [CI]: 14.2–26.4), and this was not increased with a specific metabolic inhibitor (with ketoconazole: QTc520.0 ms; 95% CI: 13.7–26.2). However, in its registration safety database of 7876 electrocardiograms from 3095 patients, only 2 individuals had a QTc interval of over 500 ms (a lower rate than with placebo). Last, the all-cause mortality for ziprasidone in its registration safety database was 1.6 deaths per 100 patient treatment years, well within the range of 1.0–2.0 for all antipsychotics. Of additional and critical relevance is that ziprasidone has multiple routes of metabolic degradation, providing patients with a protection against a drug–drug interactions increasing ziprasidone plasma levels. Ziprasidone is currently marketed with the warning that it not be used in individuals with preexisting heart disease. Ziprasidone use should not be restricted further than the FDA guidelines recommend, especially because its other effects and side-effect advantages are substantial.

Aripiprazole (Abilify)

Aripiprazole was developed as a partial DA agonist with a high affinity for the D_2 DA receptor (>90%) and low intrinsic activity (<20%) (Jordan et al., 2006). As such, the drug should have the capacity to block D_2 receptors at synapses where DA concentrations are characteristically high and to stimulate D_2 receptors in the face of low synaptic transmitter concentrations. The theoretical advantages of this action should be to improve cognition and to decrease long-term motor side effects like tardive dyskinesia.

Pharmacology

Aripiprazole has affinities for several monoaminergic receptors with a novel intrinsic activity (as a partial agonist) at the D_2 DA and the 5-HT_{1A} receptors. It displays high affinity for DA and serotonin receptors, moderate affinity at the alpha-1 adrenergic and H_1 histamine receptors and no appreciable affinity for the cholinergic receptors at therapeutic doses. Its intrinsic activity as an agonist at the D_2 and 5-HT_{1A} receptors is low but measurable. It inhibits prolactin secretion at isolated pituitary slices, like a DA agonist, and blocks DA agonist–induced motor behaviors (for example, stereology), like an antagonist (Inoue et al., 1997). In DA-depleted animals, aripiprazole inhibits the presynaptic DA receptor, like an agonist. Aripiprazole is a high-affinity, low intrinsic activity, DA partial agonist (Kikuchi et al., 1995).

Metabolism and pharmacokinetics

Aripiprazole is extensively metabolized in liver by way of two metabolic pathways: one involving the CYP 3A4 and, the other, CYP 2D6 enzymes. Aripiprazole is the predominant active drug form in systemic circulation. At steady state, the active metabolite, dehydro-aripiprazole (OPC-14857), makes up about 39% of aripiprazole concentrations in plasma. At therapeutic concentrations, aripiprazole and its major metabolite are greater than 99% bound to serum proteins, primarily to albumin (Bristol-Myers Squibb Company, 2004). After a 30 mg dose, the T_{max} is 2 hours and the C_{max} is approximately 400 ng/ml (Citrome et al., 2005). Plasma levels of aripiprazole are decreased significantly by carbamazepine but not altered by lithium or valproate (Citrome et al., 2007).

Efficacy

Aripiprazole has an antipsychotic effect significantly better than placebo and equivalent to either risperidone or haloperidol as demonstrated in several short-term trials in individuals with acute schizophrenic psychosis at doses of 15–30 mg/day (Kane et al., 2002; Marder et al., 2003). In long-term maintenance trials tested in people with chronic schizophrenia, aripiprazole showed similar efficacy to haloperidol, but with greater improvement in depression and in negative symptoms; time-to-drug discontinuation was significantly better for aripiprazole (Kasper et al., 2003). Aripiprazole effects on cognition, as evaluated using measures of general function, executive function, and verbal learning were similar to those of olanzapine and not significantly better (Kern et al., 2006). Overall, consensus recommendations in the United Kingdom find that, despite initial symptoms of nausea, insomnia, and agitation in 10%–20% of patients (these tolerate within 3–7 days), treatment with aripiprazole is recommended and may have an overall long-term side-effect advantage over other SGAs (Sullivan et al., 2007).

Side effects and safety

In registration trials, aripiprazole produced significantly lower motor side effects and prolactin elevation than haloperidol (Kane et al., 2002; Kasper et al., 2003). No QTc increases were associated with aripiprazole administration, nor any weight gain significantly different from the placebo (Kane et al., 2002; Marder et al., 2003). Possibly because of the intrinsic agonist properties of aripiprazole, several of the usual adverse side effects of APDs do not obtain: there is no prolactin elevation, QTc prolongation, weight gain, or changes in cholesterol and triglyceride levels. This side-effect profile is advantageous for the drug.

NONDOPAMINE ANTIPSYCHOTIC TREATMENTS

The first report of potent antipsychotic activity of a drug not acting directly on the DA system came in 2006. The $mGluR_{2/3}$ agonist LY 2140023 showed significant and substantial antipsychotic activity in a controlled trial, although presenting a challenging side-effect profile (Kinon, 2007). Although its mechanisms still need to be fully defined, the compound has been shown to increase the release of glutamate presynaptically, putatively increasing transmission at the *N*-methyl-D-aspartate (NMDA) receptor.

FUTURE PHARMACOTHERAPIES: FOCUS ON COGNITION

The importance of cognitive dysfunction in poor psychosocial outcome in schizophrenia has been documented (Green, 1996) This observation motivated the National Institute of Mental Health (NIMH) to address the unanswered questions of cognition treatment in schizophrenia, in part by forming the Measurement and Treatment Research to Improve Cognition in Schizophrenia (MATRICS) committees. Among the varied tasks of the MATRICS committees was a review of the published scientific literature to detail the major dimensions of cognitive pathology in schizophrenia. Seven separable cognitive dimensions were identified as abnormal in schizophrenia: speed of processing, attention and vigilance, working memory, verbal learning and memory, visual learning and memory, reasoning and problem solving, and social cognition.

Molecular Targets for Cognition in Schizophrenia

No treatments exist for cognitive dysfunction in schizophrenia. Moreover, there are no direct clues from human paradigms regarding rational molecular targets for drug development. Without a molecular target, drug development can only advance serendipitously. The search for molecular targets for cognition in schizophrenia currently relies extensively on animal studies where pharmacology can generate clues to relevant molecular systems.

The role of the hippocampal alpha-7 nicotinic receptor in sensory gating and attention and its alteration in schizophrenia provide the basis for strategies augmenting alpha-7 nicotinic signaling in schizophrenia (Martin et al., 2004). And the delineation of selective deficits in GABA receptor subunits within subpopulations of GABA-containing neurons in the prefrontal cortex has led to the strategy of augmenting GABA signaling in prefrontal cortex pharmacologically (Lewis et al., 2004). These strategies are currently being tested with pharmacologic probes.

Using nonhuman primate models of working memory, Goldman-Rakic elegantly established the importance of D_1 DA signaling in working memory, a key area of dysfunction in schizophrenia (Goldman-Rakic et al., 2004). Dopamine signaling at the D_1 receptor may be deficient in persons with schizophrenia, as supported by diverse sources of data and specific hypotheses (Selemon et al., 1995; Okubo et al., 1997; Karlsson et al., 2002; Akil et al., 2003; Potkin et al., 2003). Moreover, animal studies show that D_1 but not D2 antagonists disrupt working memory and D_1 agonists promote cognition (Goldman-Rakic et al., 2004). Therefore, the augmentation of D_1 signaling in schizophrenia is one of the most viable approaches for improving cognition, especially for augmenting working memory.

The pharmacology of the NMDA-sensitive glutamate receptor suggests that a reduction in glutamate signaling at this site mimics not only some of the psychotic symptoms of schizophrenia (Tamminga, 1999), but also its cognitive symptoms in normal human volunteers (Krystal et al., 1994). Postmortem and genetic studies have detected molecular alterations in postmortem tissue that could impair signaling at this receptor (Gao et al., 2000; Tsai et al., 1995). And there exist some data, even though not entirely consistent, suggesting that agonists at the NMDA receptor can ameliorate symptoms of the illness, including negative and cognitive symptoms (Tamminga, 1999). Therefore, molecular targets making up the NMDA receptor complex have become interesting targets for drug development for cognition.

Serotonin uses many different CNS receptors in for its signaling pathways. Evidence supports a role for the 5-HT_{1A}, 5-HT_{2A}, 5-HT_4, and 5-HT_6 receptor systems as potential targets for schizophrenia cognition (Roth et al., 2004). 5-HT_{1A} receptors are located in regions of brain that subserve learning and memory, including hippocampus and neocortex. Considerable preclinical evidence suggests that 5-HT_{1A} active drugs could be cognitively enhancing; clinical evidence also supports this idea, but without being clear if it is a 5-HT_{1A} partial agonist or a 5-HT_{1A} full antagonist that would have the best action (Roth et al., 2004). Modest but indirect evidence supports the role of the 5-HT_2, 5-HT_4 and 5-HT_6 receptors in cognition enhancement as well. Studies are being carried out in humans with cognitive disorders testing candidates from each of these families.

Additional data (mostly preclinical) exist to support several other molecular targets for cognitive enhancements in schizophrenia, including the muscarinic cholinergic receptors (Friedman, 2004), the metabotopic glutamate receptor (Moghaddam, 2004), and adrenergic receptors (Arnsten, 2004).

It is an era of discovery for schizophrenia therapeutics. The possibility that multiple, dimension-specific cotreatments could be necessary for full response in the illness will be tested.

Complementary Therapies: Cognitive Remediation and Training

An accumulating literature suggests the possibility that cognitive training strategies could improve performance on information processing, including verbal learning and memory, working memory, motor dexterity, and attention and serve to augment APD action in the illness. For example, Wexler et al. (2000) demonstrated that extensive practice resulted in substantial improvement on a motor dexterity task, a visual reading task, and a dot spatial memory task. Kern et al. (1995) employed instructions and monetary reinforcement to produce significant improvements on a measure of span of apprehension, a putative trait marker of schizophrenia that is known to be highly stable. Other studies have shown modest improvements on a variety of attention tasks using practice, shaping, and errorless learning, a behavioral strategy designed to minimize failure experiences (Silverstein et al., 2001). In a comparison of different teaching strategies, O'Carroll et al. (1999) demonstrated that errorless learning was differentially effective in improving verbal memory.

Much of the work to date has involved analogue studies in which brief interventions (one or a few sessions of training and/or practice) have been shown to produce short-term improvements on neuropsychological tests. Their primary significance is in demonstrating that change is possible. However, there is an accumulating literature on clinically relevant interventions suggesting that meaningful change is possible (Wykes and van der Gaag, 2001; Twamley et al., 2003; Bellack, 2004). Moreover, support for the timeliness and significance of a current focus on remediation is provided by several recent uncontrolled reports in the literature that suggest that even brief interventions of this type may be associated with changes in cerebral blood flow (Penades et al., 2000; Wexler et al., 2000; Wykes et al., 2002). Notably, Wexler et al. (2000) demonstrated that 10 weeks of verbal memory exercises normalized activation patterns in some patients. These findings need to be replicated and examined in greater detail in a controlled trial with a more focused rehabilitation program that teaches patients to use normative cognitive strategies. Moreover, the possibility that these cognitive treatments will potentate APDs in improving psychosocial outcome is being tested. It is the ultimate contribution of cognitive training to practical psychosocial outcomes that is impressive (McGurk et al., 2007)

TREATING THE PERSON WITH SCHIZOPHRENIA

Given these new groups of treatments and rehabilitation approaches, the implications for schizophrenia therapeutics are broad. Treating physicians are likely to see their armamentarium of traditional antipsychotic compounds shift even more in the next few years from the FGA to the SGA. More drugs will be available to treat not only patients with schizophrenia but also patients with other psychotic conditions, including persons who are psychotic with a poor drug response, children and adolescents, the elderly, and people with episodic or affective psychoses. Moreover, drugs selective for treating symptom domains within the diagnosis of schizophrenia (for example, cognitive dysfunction) are likely to be developed. Motor side effects at present levels will hopefully become a complication of the past. This will happen none too quickly for the millions of persons with schizophrenia who have had to trade a reduction in the symptoms of psychosis for the difficult motor side effects of traditional antipsychotics.

Optimal application of the new pharmaceuticals will require expanded knowledge not only of their clinical efficacy and safety, but also of their pharmacology, metabolism, pharmacokinetics, and in vivo behavior in brain. Much of these data were unavailable when traditional antipsychotics were characterized. This current expanded database for the new antipsychotics allows their administration and dosing with more precision and discrimination than was previously possible.

The practical considerations of deciding between new and traditional neuroleptics and among new neuroleptics in the clinical situation still need to be articulated. Recommended treatment algorithms already exist (American Psychiatric Association Workgroup on Schizophrenia, 1997). Economic advantage will always rest with the traditional drugs. Where efficacy is equivalent and motor side effects are minimal, traditional antipsychotics are adequate treatment choices. However, given the significant advantage of the new neuroleptics in reducing motor side effects, this characteristic may be paramount with respect to patient comfort, better medication compliance, and subsequent reduced psychosis relapse. Articulating principles to decide rationally among the new neuroleptics will require more clinical experience and data. The new drugs will probably differ in their motor side-effect profile, cardiovascular actions, metabolism effects and weight gain, cognitive actions and side effects, negative symptom actions, and actions on depressive symptoms. All drugs have known kinetic profiles that may be decisive in a particular situation. However, direct comparative studies are necessary to provide a discriminatory clinical pharmacology for each compound.

Clozapine is still being underutilized in the United States. Larger numbers of neuroleptic-resistant patients who are psychotic exist than are being treated with clozapine. Factors including high cost and medical risk have no doubt diminished enthusiasm for this drug. Practical management techniques, such as increasing the clozapine dose slowly, transferring between drugs slowly, and treating benign side effects symptomatically, will maximize clozapine's effectiveness in individual persons. In responding patients, clozapine acts at a given dose within 12 weeks and at an average dose of 450 mg/day. Only 20% of treatment-refractory patients who are ultimately responsive to clozapine require doses higher than 600 mg/day to respond (Conley, Carpenter, et al., 1997). This information suggests fixed time and dose limits for broader clozapine testing in persons with schizophrenia who are full and partial treatment resistant. In an acute psychotic episode, the treating physician can chose between low-dose traditional or new drug treatment. The response to treatment in schizophrenia should be evaluated over many weeks. However, nonresponse to a regimen of traditional antipsychotic treatment even in early-break persons with schizophrenia predicts subsequent nonresponse to other traditional antipsychotics in over 70% of persons. Thus, drug nonresponse can be characterized early in the illness.

This is a time of opportunity in schizophrenia treatment and research. We can anticipate that patient response and outcome will improve. New cotreatments for cognition and negative symptoms are being developed. However, current treatments, even with the new antipsychotics, do not cure psychosis or schizophrenia. Full psychosis treatment will probably have to await a correct articulation of schizophrenia's pathophysiology. This is an area where discovery could translate broadly into patient advantage.

REFERENCES

Akil, M., Kolachana, B.S., Rothmond, D.A., Hyde, T.M., Weinberger, D.R., and Kleinman, J.E. (2003) Catechol-O-methyltransferase genotype and dopamine regulation in the human brain. *J. Neurosci.* 23:2008–2013.

Alexander, G.E., and Crutcher, M.D. (1990) Functional architecture of basal ganglia circuits: neural substrates of parallel processing (review]. *Trends Neurosci.* 13:266–271.

Allison, D.B., Mentore, J.L., Heo, M., Chandler, L.P., Cappelleri, J.C., Infante, M.C., and Weiden, P.J. (1999) Antipsychotic-induced weight gain: a comprehensive research synthesis. *Am. J. Psychiatry* 156:1686–1696.

American Psychiatric Association Workgroup on Schizophrenia. (1997) Practice guidelines for the treatment of patients with schizophrenia. *Am. J. Psychiatry* 54:S1–S33.

Andreasen, N.C., Paradiso, S., and O'Leary, D.S. (1998) "Cognitive dysmetria" as an integrative theory of schizophrenia: a dysfunction in cortical-subcortical-cerebellar circuitry? *Schizophr. Bull.* 24(2):203–218.

Arnsten, A. F. T. (2004) Adrenergic targets for the treatment of cognitive deficits in schizophrenia. *Psychopharmacology* 174(1):25–31.

Arvanitis, L.A., and Miller, B.G. (1997) Multiple fixed doses of "Seroquel" (quetiapine) in patients with acute exacerbation of schizophrenia: a comparison with haloperidol and placebo. *Biol. Psychiatry* 42:233–246.

Barch, D.M., Sheline, Y.I., Csernansky, J.G., and Snyder, A. Z. (2003) Working memory and prefrontal cortex dysfunction: specificity to schizophrenia compared with major depression. *Biol. Psychiatry* 53(5):376–384.

Beasley, C.M., Jr., Tollefson, G., Satterlee, W., Sanger, G., and Hamilton, S. (1997) Olanzapine versus placebo and haloperidol: acute phase results of the North American double-blind olanzapine trial. *Neuropsychopharmacology* 14:111–123.

Beasley, C.M., Tollefson, G.D., Tran, P., Satterlee, W., Sanger, T., and Hamilton, S. (1996) Olanzapine versus placebo and haloperidol. Acute phase results of the North American double-blind olanzapine trial. *Neuropsychopharmacology* 14:111–123.

Bellack, A.S. (2004) Skills training for people with severe mental illness. *Psychiatr. Rehabil. J.* 27(4):375–391.

Bench, C.J., Lammertsma, A.A., Dolan, R.J., Grasby, P.M., Warrington, S.J., Gunn, K., Cuddigan, M., Turton, D.J., Osman, S., and Frackowiak, R.S. (1993) Dose dependent occupancy of central dopamine D2 receptors by the novel neuroleptic CP-88,059-01: a study using positron emission tomography and 11C-raclopride. *Psychopharmacology (Berl.)* 112:308–314.

Bench, C.J., Lammertsma, A.A., Grasby, P.M., Dolan, R.J., Warrington, S.J., Boyce, M., Gunn, K.P., Brannick, L.Y., and Frackowiak, R.S. (1996) The time course of binding to striatal dopamine D2 receptors by the neuroleptic ziprasidone (CP-88,059-01) determined by positron emission tomography. *Psychopharmacology (Berl.)* 124:141–147.

Bettinger, T.L., Mendelson, S.C., Dorson, P.G., and Crismon, M.L. (2000) Olanzapine-induced glucose dysregulation. *Ann. Pharmacother.* 34:865–867.

Bilder, R.M., Lipschutz-Broch, L., Reiter, G., Geisler, S., Mayerhoff, D., and Lieberman, J.A. (1991) Neuropsychological deficits in the early course of first episode schizophrenia. *Schizophr. Res.* 5(3):198–199.

Braff, D.L. (1993) Information processing and attention dysfunctions in schizophrenia. *Schizophr. Bull.* 19(2):233–259.

Brewer, W.J., Francey, S.M., Wood, S.J., Jackson, H.J., Pantelis, C., Phillips, L.J., Yung, A.R., Anderson, V.A., and McGorry, P.D. (2005) Memory impairments identified in people at ultra-high risk for psychosis who later develop first-episode psychosis. *Am. J. Psychiatry* 162(1):71–78.

Brickman, A.M., Buchsbaum, M.S., Bloom, R., Bokhoven, P., Paul-Odouard, R., Haznedar, M.M., Dahlman, K.L., Hazlett, E., Aronowitz, J., Heath, D., and Shihabuddin, L. (2004) Neuropsychological functioning in first-break, never-medicated adolescents with psychosis. *J. Nerv. Men. Dis.* 192(9):615–622.

Bristol-Myers Squibb Company. (2004) Abilify (aripiprazole) tablets. *Physician's Desk Reference* 58th ed. Montvale, NJ: Thompson PDR, pp. 1034–1038.

Bymaster, F.P., Calligaro, D.O., Falcone, J.F., Marsh, R.D., Moore, N.A., Tye, N.C., Seeman, P., and Wong, D.T. (1996) Radioreceptor binding profile of the atypical antipsychotic olanzapine. *Neuropsychopharmacology* 14:87–96.

Cannon, T.D., Huttunen, M.O., Lonnqvist, J., Tuulio-Henriksson, A., Pirkola, T., Glahn, D., Finkelstein, J., Hietanen, M., Kaprio, J., and Koskenvuo, M. (2000) The inheritance of neuropsychological dysfunction in twins discordant for schizophrenia. *Am. J. Hum. Genet.* 67(2):369–382.

Carlsson, A., and Lindquist, L. (1963) Effect of chlorpromazine or haloperidol on formation of 3-methoxytyramine and normetanephrine in mouse brain. *Acta Pharmacol. Toxicol.* 20:140–145.

Carpenter, W.T., Jr., and Buchanan, R.W. (1994) Schizophrenia. *New Eng. J. Med.* 330:681–690.

Casey, D.E. (1996) Behavioral effects of sertindole, risperidone, clozapine and haloperidol in Cebus monkeys. *Psychopharmacology* 124:134–140.

Censits, D.M., Ragland, J.D., Gur, R.C., and Gur, R.E. (1997) Neuropsychological evidence supporting a neurodevelopmental model of schizophrenia: a longitudinal study. *Schizophr. Res.* 24(3):289–298.

Citrome, L., Josiassen, R., Bark, N., Salazar, D.E., and Mallikaarjun, S. (2005) Pharmacokinetics of aripiprazole and concomitant lithium and valproate. *J. Clin. Pharmacol.* 45(1):89–93.

Citrome, L., Macher, J.P., Salazar, D.E., Mallikaarjun, S., and Boulton, D.W. (2007) Pharmacokinetics of aripiprazole and concomitant carbamazepine. *J. Clin. Psychopharmacol.* 27(3):279–283.

Cohen, R.A., Kaplan, R.F., Zuffante, P., Moser, D.J., Jenkins, M.A., Salloway, S., and Wilkinson, H. (1999) Alteration of intention and self-initiated action associated with bilateral anterior cingulotomy. *J. Neuropsychiatry* 11(4):444–453.

Conley, R.R., Carpenter, W.T., Jr., and Tamminga, C.A. (1997) Time to clozapine response in a standardized trial. *Am. J. Psychiatry* 154:1243–1247.

Conley, R.R., Tamminga, C.A., and Beasley, C. (1997) Olanzapine versus chlorpromazine in therapy-refractory schizophrenia. *Schizophr. Res.* 24:190–202.

Cornblatt, B.A., and Erlenmeyer-Kimling, L. (1985) Global attentional deviance as a marker of risk for schizophrenia: specificity and predictive validity. *J. Abnorm. Psychol.* 94(4):470–486.

Coward, D.M. (1992) General pharmacology of clozapine [review]. *Br. J. Psychiatry* 17(Suppl):5–11.

Daniel, D.G., Potkin, S.G., Reeves, K.R., Swift, R.H., and Harrigan, E.P. (2001) Intramuscular (IM) ziprasidone 20 mg is effective in reducing acute agitation associated with psychosis: a double-blind, randomized trial. *Psychopharmacology (Berl.)* 155:128–134.

Daniel, D.G., Zimbroff, D.L., Potkin, S.G., Reeves, K.R., Harrigan, E.P., and Lakshminarayanan, M. (1999) Ziprasidone 80 mg/day and 160 mg/day in the acute exacerbation of schizophrenia and schizoaffective disorder: a 6-week placebo-controlled trial. Ziprasidone Study Group. *Neuropsychopharmacology* 20:491–505.

Davis, J.M. (1969) Review of antipsychotic drug literature. In: Klein, D.F., and Davis, J.M., eds. *Diagnosis and Drug Treatment of Psychiatric Disorders*. Baltimore: Williams & Wilkins, pp. 52–138.

Davis, J.M., Chen, N., and Glick, I.D. (2003) A meta-analysis of the efficacy of second-generation antipsychotics [see comment]. *Arch. Gen. Psychiatry* 60(6):553–564.

Delay, J., and Deniker, P. (1952) Le'traitement des psychoses par une methode neurolytique derivee de l'hibernotherapie. In: *Congres des Medecins Alienistes et Neurologistes de France*. Luxembourg, Belgium: pp. 497–502.

D'Esposito, M. (1998) Serotonin neurotoxicity: implications for cognitive neuroscience and neurology. *Neurology* 51(6):1529–1530.

Dickinson, D., Iannone, V.N., Wilk, C.M., and Gold, J.M. (2004) General and specific cognitive deficits in schizophrenia. *Biol. Psychiatry* 55(8):826–833.

Egan, M.F., Goldberg, T.E., Kolachana, B.S., Callicott, J.H., Mazzanti, C.M., Straub, R.E., Goldman, D., and Weinberger, D.R. (2001) Effect of COMT Val108/158 Met genotype on frontal lobe function and risk for schizophrenia. *Proc. Natl. Acad. Sci. USA* 98(12): 6917–6922.

Elvevag, B., Goldberg, T.E., Brown, G.D.A., Vousden, J.I., and McCormack, T. (2004) Identification of tone duration, line length, and letter position: an experimental approach to timing and working memory deficits in schizophrenia. *J. Abnorm. Psychol.* 113(4): 509–521.

Ereshefsky, L., and Lacombe, S. (1993) Pharmacological profile of risperidone. *Can. J. Psychiatry* 38(Suppl 3):S80–S88.

Farde, L., Mack, R.J., Nyberg, S., and Halldin, C. (1997) D2 occupancy, extrapyramidal side effects and antipsychotic drug treatment: a pilot study with sertindole in healthy subjects. *Int. Clin. Psychopharmacol.* 12(Suppl 1):S3–S7.

Farde, L., Nordstrom, A.L., Wiesel, F.A., Pauli, S., Halldin, C., and Sedvall, G. (1992) Positron emission tomographic analysis of central D1 and D2 dopamine receptor occupancy in patients treated with classical neuroleptics and clozapine. Relation to extrapyramidal side effects. *Arch. Gen. Psychiatry* 49:538–544.

Fink-Jensen, A., and Kristensen, P. (1994) Effects of typical and atypical neuroleptics on Fos protein expression in the rat forebrain. *Neurosci. Lett.* 182:115–118.

Fitzgerald, D., Lucas, S., Redoblado, M.A., Winter, V., Brennan, J., Anderson, J., and Harris, A. (2004) Cognitive functioning in young people with first episode psychosis: relationship to diagnosis and clinical characteristics. *Aust. N. Z. J. Psychiatry* 38:501–510.

Flashman, L.A., and Green, M.F. (2004) Review of cognition and brain structure in schizophrenia: profiles, longitudinal course, and effects of treatment. *Psychiatr. Clin. North Am.* 27(1):1–18, vii.

Freedman, R. (2003) Schizophrenia. *N. Eng. J. Med.* 349(18):1738–1749.

Friedman, J.I. (2004) Cholinergic targets for cognitive enhancement in schizophrenia: focus on cholinesterase inhibitors and muscarinic agonists. *Psychopharmacology* 174(1):45–53.

Gao, X.M., Sakai, K., Roberts, R.C., Conley, R.R., Dean, B., and Tamminga, C.A. (2000) Ionotropic glutamate receptors and expression of *N*-methyl-D-aspartate receptor subunits in subregions of human hippocampus: effects of schizophrenia. *Am. J. Psychiatry* 157(7):1141–1149.

Geddes, J., Mercer, G., Frith, C.D., MacMillan, F., Owens, D.G., and Johnstone, E.C. (1994) Prediction of outcome following a first episode of schizophrenia. A follow-up study of Northwick Park first episode study subjects. *Br. J. Psychiatry* 165:664–668.

Geyer, M.A., and Tamminga, C.A. (2007) MATRICS: Measurement and Treatment Research to Improve Cognition in Schizophrenia [Special Issue]. *Psychopharmacology* 174.

Glassman, A.H., and Bigger, J.T., Jr. (2001) Antipsychotic drugs: prolonged QTc interval, torsade de pointes, and sudden death. *Am. J. Psychiatry* 158:1774–1782.

Goldberg, T.E., and Weinberger, D.R. (1996) Effects of neuroleptic medications on the cognition of patients with schizophrenia: a review of recent studies. *J. Clin. Psychiatry* 57(Suppl 9):62–65.

Goldman-Rakic, P.S. (1994) Working memory dysfunction in schizophrenia. *J. Neuropsychiatry Clin. Neurosci.* 6(4):348–357.

Goldman-Rakic, P.S., Castner, S.A., Svensson, T.H., Siever, L.J., and Williams, G.V. (2004) Targeting the dopamine D1 receptor in schizophrenia: insights for cognitive dysfunction. *Psychopharmacology* 174(1):3–16.

Grace, A.A., Bunney, B.S., Moore, H., and Todd, C.L. (1997) Dopamine-cell depolarization block as a model for the therapeutic actions of antipsychotic drugs [review]. *Trends Neurosci.* 20: 31–37.

Green, M.F. (1996) What are the functional consequences of neurocognitive deficits in schizophrenia? *Am. J. Psychiatry* 153:321–330.

Green, M.F., Kern, R.S., Braff, D.L., and Mintz, J. (2000) Neurocognitive deficits and functional outcome in schizophrenia: are we measuring the "right stuff"? *Schizophr. Bull.* 26(1):119–136.

Gunne, L.M., Growdon, J., and Glaeser, B. (1982) Oral dyskinesia in rats following brain lesions and neuroleptic drug administration. *Psychopharmacology* 77:134–139.

Gur, R.C., Ragland, J.D., Moberg, P.J., Bilker, W.B., Kohler, C., Siegel, S.J., and Gur, R.E. (2001) Computerized neurocognitive scanning: II. The profile of schizophrenia. *Neuropsychopharmacology* 25(5):777–788.

Gur, R. E., Maany, V., Mozley, P. D., Swanson, C., Bilker, W., and Gur, R. C. (1998) Subcortical MRI volumes in neuroleptic-naive and treated patients with schizophrenia. *Am. J. Psychiatry* 155(12): 1711–1717.

Gur, R.E., Turetsky, B.I., Bilker, W.B., and Gur, R.C. (1999) Reduced gray matter volume in schizophrenia. *Arch. Gen. Psychiatry* 56(10):905–911.

Heinrichs, R.W., and Zakzanis, K.K. (1998) Neurocognitive deficit in schizophrenia: a quantitative review of the evidence. *Neuropsychology* 12(3):426–445.

Henderson, D.C., Cagliero, E., Gray, C., Nasrallah, R.A., Hayden, D.L., Schoenfeld, D.A., and Goff, D.C. (2000) Clozapine, diabetes mellitus, weight gain, and lipid abnormalities: a five-year naturalistic study. *Am. J. Psychiatry* 157:975–981.

Hill, S.K., Beers, S. R., Kmiec, J.A., Keshavan, M.S., and Sweeney, J.A. (2004) Impairment of verbal memory and learning in antipsychotic-naive patients with first-episode schizophrenia. *Schizophr. Res.* 68:127–136.

Hoff, A.L., Svetina, C., Maurizio, A.M., Crow, T.J., Spokes, K., and DeLisi, L.E. (2005) Familial cognitive deficits in schizophrenia. *Am. J. Med. Genet. Part B (Neuropsychiat. Genet.)* 133B:43–49.

Holcomb, H.H., Cascella, N.G., Thake, G.K., Medoff, D.R., Dannals, R.F., and Tamminga, C.A. (1996) Functional sites of neuroleptic drug action in the human brain: PET/FDG studies with and without haloperidol. *Am. J. Psychiatry* 153:41–49.

Hyman, S.E., and Fenton, W.S. (2003) MEDICINE: What are the right targets for psychopharmacology? *Science* 299(5605):350–351.

Inoue, A., Miki, S., Seto, M., Kikuchi, T., Morita, S., Ueda, H., Misu, Y., and Nakata, Y. (1997) Aripiprazole, a novel antipsychotic drug, inhibits quinpirole-evoked GTPase activity but does not up-regulate dopamine D2 receptor following repeated treatment in the rat striatum. *Eur. J. Pharmacol.* 321(1):105–111.

Jones, P.B., Barnes, T.R., Davies, L., Dunn, G., Lloyd, H., Hayhurst, K.P., Murray, R.M., Markwick, A., and Lewis, S.W. (2006) Randomized controlled trial of the effect on quality of life of second- vs first-generation antipsychotic drugs in schizophrenia: Cost Utility of the Latest Antipsychotic Drugs in Schizophrenia Study (CUtLASS 1). *Arch. Gen. Psychiatry* 63(10):1079–1087.

Jordan, S., Regardie, K., Johnson, J.L., Chen, R., Kambayashi, J., McQuade, R., Kitagawa, H., Tadori, Y., and Kikuchi, T. (2006) In vitro functional characteristics of dopamine D2 receptor partial agonists in second and third messenger-based assays of cloned human dopamine D2Long receptor signalling. *J. Psychopharmacol.* 21(6):620–627.

Kane, J., Canas, F., Kramer, M., Ford, L., Gassmann-Mayer, C., Lim, P., and Eerdekens, M. (2007) Treatment of schizophrenia with paliperidone extended-release tablets: a 6-week placebo-controlled trial. *Schizophr. Res.* 90(1-3):147–161.

Kane, J.M., Carson, W.H., Saha, A.R., McQuade, R.D., Ingenito, G.G., Zimbroff, D.L., and Ali, M.W. (2002) Efficacy and safety of aripiprazole and haloperidol versus placebo in patients with schizophrenia and schizoaffective disorder. *J. Clin. Psychiatry* 63(9):763–771.

Kane, J., Honigfeld, G., Singer, J., and Meltzer, H. (1988) Clozapine for the treatment-resistant schizophrenic. A double-blind comparison with chlorpromazine. *Arch. Gen. Psychiatry* 45:789–796.

Kane, J.M., Marder, S.R., Schooler, N.R., Wirshing, W.C., Umbricht, D., Baker, R.W., Wirshing, D.A., Safferman, A., Ganguli, R., McMeniman, M., and Borenstein, M. (2001) Clozapine and haloperidol in moderately refractory schizophrenia: a 6-month randomized and double-blind comparison. *Arch. Gen. Psychiatry* 58: 965–972.

Kane, J.M., and Smith, J.M. (1982) Tardive dyskinesia: prevalence and risk factors, 1959 to 1979. *Arch. Gen. Psychiatry* 39:473–481.

Kapur, S., Zipursky, R., Jones, C., Shammi, C.S., Remington, G., and Seeman, P. (2000) A positron emission tomography study of quetiapine in schizophrenia: a preliminary finding of an antipsychotic effect with only transiently high dopamine D2 receptor occupancy. *Arch. Gen. Psychiatry* 57:553–559.

Kapur, S., Zipursky, R.B., and Remington, G. (1999) Clinical and theoretical implications of 5-HT2 and D2 receptor occupancy of clozapine, risperidone, and olanzapine in schizophrenia. *Am. J. Psychiatry* 156:286–293.

Kapur, S., Zipursky, R.B., Remington, G., Jones, C., DaSilva, J., Wilson, A.A., and Houle, S. (1998) 5-HT2 and D2 receptor occupancy of olanzapine in schizophrenia: a PET investigation. *Am. J. Psychiatry* 155:921–928.

Karlsson, P., Farde, L., Halldin, C., and Sedvall, G. (2002) PET study of D(1) dopamine receptor binding in neuroleptic-naive patients with schizophrenia. *Am. J. Psychiatry* 159(5):761–767.

Kasper, S., Lerman, M.N., McQuade, R.D., Saha, A., Carson, W.H., Ali, M., Archibald, D., Ingenito, G., Marcus, R., and Pigott, T. (2003) Efficacy and safety of aripiprazole vs. haloperidol for long-term maintenance treatment following acute relapse of schizophrenia. *Int. J. Neuropsychopharmacol.* 6(4):325–337.

Kern, R.S., Green, M.F., Cornblatt, B.A., Owen, J.R., McQuade, R.D., Carson, W.H., Ali, M., and Marcus, R. (2006) The neurocognitive effects of aripiprazole: an open-label comparison with olanzapine. *Psychopharmacology (Berl.)* 187(3):312–320.

Kikuchi, T., Tottori, K., Uwahodo, Y., Hirose, T., Miwa, T., Oshiro, Y., and Morita, S. (1995) 7-(4-[4-(2,3-Dichlorophenyl)-1-piperazinyl] butyloxy)-3,4-dihydro-2(1H)-quinolinone (OPC-14597), a new putative antipsychotic drug with both presynaptic dopamine autoreceptor agonistic activity and postsynaptic D2 receptor antagonistic activity. *J. Pharmacol. Exp. Ther.* 274(1):329–336.

Kinon, B. (2007, April 1) *LY2140023, a metabotropic 2/3 agonist in schizophrenia.* Paper presented at the 10th International Congress on Schizophrenia Research, Colorado Springs, Colorado.

Kramer, M., Simpson, G., Maciulis, V., Kushner, S., Vijapurkar, U., Lim, P., and Eerdekens, M. (2007) Paliperidone extended-release tablets for prevention of symptom recurrence in patients with schizophrenia: a randomized, double-blind, placebo-controlled study. *J. Clin. Psychopharmacol.* 27(1):6–14.

Kravariti, E., Morris, R.G., Rabe-Hesketh, S., Murray, R.M., and Frangou, S. (2003) The Maudsley Early-Onset Schizophrenia Study: cognitive function in adolescent-onset schizophrenia. *Schizophr. Res.* 65:95–103.

Krystal, J.H., Karper, L.P., Seibyl, J.P., Freeman, G.K., Delaney, R., Bremner, D., Heninger, G.R., Bowers, M.B., and Charney, D.S. (1994) Subanesthetic effects of the noncompetitive NMDA antagonist, ketamine, in humans: psychotomimetic, perceptual, cognitive, and neuroendocrine responses. *Arch. Gen. Psychiatry* 51: 199–214.

Kurtz, M.M., Ragland, J.D., Bilker, W., Gur, R.C., and Gur, R.E. (2001) Comparison of the continuous performance test with and without working memory demands in healthy controls and patients with schizophrenia. *Schizophr. Res.* 48(2–3):307–316.

Lahti, A.C., Holcomb, H.H., Weiler, M.A., Medoff, D.R., and Tamminga, C.A. (2003) Functional effects of antipsychotic drugs: comparing clozapine with haloperidol. *Biol. Psychiatry* 53:601–668.

Lahti, A.C., Lahti, R.A., and Tamminga, C.A. (1996) New neuroleptics and experimental antipsychotics: future roles. In Breier, A., ed. *The New Pharmacotherapy of Schizophrenia.* Washington, DC: American Psychiatric Press, pp. 57–87.

Leucht, S., Wahlbeck, K., Hamann, J., and Kissling, W. (2003) New generation antipsychotics versus low-potency conventional antipsychotics: a systematic review and meta-analysis [see comment]. *Lancet* 361(9369):1581–1589.

Lewis, D.A., Volk, D.W., and Hashimoto, T. (2004) Selective alterations in prefrontal cortical GABA neurotransmission in schizophrenia: a novel target for the treatment of working memory dysfunction. *Psychopharmacology* 174(1):143–150.

Leysen, J.E., Janssen, P.M., Megens, A.A., and Schotte, A. (1994) Risperidone: a novel antipsychotic with balanced serotonin-dopamine antagonism, receptor occupancy profile, and pharmacologic activity. *J. Clin. Psychiatry* 55(Suppl):5–12.

Lieberman, J.A., Stroup, T. S., McEvoy, J.P., Swartz, M.S., Rosenheck, R.A., Perkins, D.O., Keefe, R.S.E., Davis, S.M., Davis, C.E., Lebowitz, B.D., Severe, J., Hsiao, J.K., and the Clinical Antipsychotic Trials of Intervention Effectiveness (CATIE) Investigators. (2005) Effectiveness of antipsychotic drugs in patients with chronic schizophrenia. *N. Eng. J. Med.* 353(12):1209–1223.

Love, R.C., Conley, R.R., Kelly, D.L., and Bartko, J.J. (1999) A dose-outcome analysis of risperidone. *J. Clin. Psychiatry* 60:771–775.

Marder, S.R., Kramer, M., Ford, L., Eerdekens, E., Lim, P., Eerdekens, M., and Lowy, A. (2007) Efficacy and safety of paliperidone extended-release tablets: results of a 6-week, randomized, placebo-controlled study. *Biol. Psychiatry* 6:1363–1370.

Marder, S.R., McQuade, R.D., Stock, E., Kaplita, S., Marcus, R., Safferman, A.Z., Saha, A., Ali, M., and Iwamoto, T. (2003) Aripiprazole in the treatment of schizophrenia: safety and tolerability in short-term, placebo-controlled trials. *Schizophr. Res.* 61(2/3):123–136.

Marder, S.R., and Meibach, R.C. (1994) Risperidone in the treatment of schizophrenia. *Am. J. Psychiatry* 151:825–835.

Martin, L.F., Kem, W.R., and Freedman, R. (2004) Alpha-7 nicotinic receptor agonists: potential new candidates for the treatment of schizophrenia. *Psychopharmacology* 174(1):54–64.

McEvoy, J.P., Lieberman, J.A., Stroup, T.S., Davis, S.M., Meltzer, H.Y., Rosenheck, R.A., Swartz, M.S., Perkins, D.O., Keefe, R.S.E., Davis, C.E., Severe, J., Hsiao, J.K., and for the CATIE

Investigators. (2006) Effectiveness of clozapine versus olanzapine, quetiapine, and risperidone in patients with chronic schizophrenia who did not respond to prior atypical antipsychotic treatment. *Am. J. Psychiatry* 163(4):600–610.

McGurk, S.R., Mueser, K.T., Feldman, K., Wolfe, R., and Pascaris, A. (2007) Cognitive training for supported employment: 2-3 year outcomes of a randomized controlled trial. *Am. J. Psychiatry* 164(3):437–441.

Meltzer, H.Y. (1995) Role of serotonin in the action of atypical antipsychotic drugs [review]. *Clin. Neurosci.* 3:64–75.

Moghaddam, B. (2004) Targeting metabotropic glutamate receptors for treatment of the cognitive symptoms of schizophrenia. *Psychopharmacology* 174(1):39–44.

Myles-Worsley, M., and Park, S. (2002) Spatial working memory deficits in schizophrenia patients and their first degree relatives from Palau, Micronesia. *Am. J. Med. Genet. (Neuropsychiat. Genet.)* 114:609–615.

Niendam, T.A., Bearden, C.E., Rosso, I.M., Sanchez, L.E., Hadley, T., Nuechterlein, K.H., and Cannon, T.D. (2003) A prospective study of childhood neurocognitive functioning in schizophrenic patients and their siblings. *Am. J. Psychiatry* 160(11):2060–2062.

Nuechterlein, K.H., Barch, D.M., Gold, J.M., Goldberg, T.E., Green, M.F., and Heaton, R.K. (2004) Identification of separate cognitive factors in schizophrenia. *Schizophr. Res.* 72(1):29–39.

Nyberg, S., Farde, L., Eriksson, L., Halldin, C., and Eriksson, B. (1993) 5-HT2 and D2 dopamine receptor occupancy in the living human brain. A PET study with risperidone. *Psychopharmacology (Berl.)* 110:265–272.

O'Carroll, R.E., Russell, H.H., Lawrie, S.M., Johnstone, E.C. (1999) Errorless learning and the cognitive rehabilitation of memory-impaired schizophrenic patients. *Psychol. Med.* 29:105–112,

Okubo, Y., Suhara, T., Suzuki, K., Kobayashi, K., Inoue, O., Terasaki, O., et al. (1997) Decreased prefrontal dopamine D1 receptors in schizophrenia revealed by PET. *Nature* 385:634–636.

Osser, D.N., Najarian, D.M., and Dufresne, R.L. (1999) Olanzapine increases weight and serum triglyceride levels. *J. Clin. Psychiatry* 60:767–770.

Penades, R., Boget, T., Lomena, F., Bernardo, M., Mateos, J.J., Laterza, C., Pavia, J., and Salamero, M. (2000) Brain perfusion and neuropsychological changes in schizophrenic patients after cognitive rehabilitation. *Psychiatry Res.* 98(2):127–132.

Potkin, S.G., Saha, A., Kujawa, M.J., Carson, W.H., Ali, M., Stock, E., Stringfellow, J., Ingenito, G., and Marder, S.R. (2003) Aripiprazole, an antipsychotic with a novel mechanism of action and risperidone vs placebo in patients with schizophrenia and schizoaffective disorder. *Arch. Gen. Psychiatry* 60(7):681–690.

Robertson, G.S., and Fibiger, H.C. (1996) Effects of olanzapine on regional c-fos expression in rat forebrain. *Neuropsychopharmacology* 14:105–110.

Robertson, G.S., Matsumura, H., and Fibiger, H.C. (1994) Induction patterns of Fos-like immunoreactivity in the forebrain as predictors of atypical antipsychotic activity. *J. Pharmacol. Exp. Ther.* 271:1058–1066.

Rosenheck, R., Cramer, J., Xu, W., Thomas, J., Henderson, W., Frisman, L., Fye, C., and Charney, D. (1997) A comparison of clozapine and haloperidol in hospitalized patients with refractory schizophrenia. Department of Veterans Affairs Cooperative Study Group on Clozapine in Refractory Schizophrenia. *N. Eng. J. Med.* 337(12):809–815.

Rosenheck, R.A., Leslie, D.L., Sindelar, J., Miller, E.A., Lin, H., Stroup, T.S., McEvoy, J., Davis, S.M., Keefe, R.S., Swartz, M., Perkins, D.O., Hsiao, J.K., and Lieberman, J. (2006) Cost-effectiveness of second-generation antipsychotics and perphenazine in a randomized trial of treatment for chronic schizophrenia. *Am. J. Psychiatry* 163(12):2080–2089.

Rosenheck, R., Perlick, D., Bingham, S., Liu-Mares, W., Collins, J., Warren, S., Leslie, D., Allan, E., Campbell, E.C., Caroff, S., Corwin, J., Davis, L., Douyon, R., Dunn, L., Evans, D., Frecska, E., Grabowski, J., Graeber, D., Herz, L., Kwon, K., Lawson, W., Mena, F., Sheikh, J., Smelson, D., and Smith-Gamble, V. (2003) Effectiveness and cost of olanzapine and haloperidol in the treatment of schizophrenia: a randomized controlled trial. *JAMA* 290(20): 2693–2702.

Roth, B.L., Hanizavareh, S.M., and Blum, A.E. (2004) Serotonin receptors represent highly favorable molecular targets for cognitive enhancement in schizophrenia and other disorders. *Psychopharmacology* 174(1):17–24.

Sakai, K., Gao, X.M., and Tamminga, C.A. (2001) Scopolamine fails to diminish chronic haloperidol-induced purposeless chewing in rats. *Psychopharmacology (Berl.)* 153:191–195.

Sakai, K., Gao, X.-M., Hashimoto, T., and Tamminga, C.A. (2001) Traditional and new antipsychotics differentially alter neurotransmission markers in basal ganglia-thalamocortical neural pathways. *Synapse* 39:152–160.

Saller, C.F., and Salama, A.I. (1993) Seroquel: biochemical profile of a potential atypical antipsychotic. *Psychopharmacology (Berl.)* 112:285–292.

Sartorius, N., Shapiro, R., and Jablensky, A. (1974) The international pilot study of schizophrenia. *Schizophr. Bull.* 11:21–34.

Saykin, A.J., Gur, R.C., Gur, R.E., Mozley, P.D., Mozley, L.H., Resnick, S.M., Kester, D.B., and Stafiniak, P. (1991) Neuropsychological function in schizophrenia. Selective impairment in memory and learning. *Arch. Gen. Psychiatry* 48(7):618–624.

Saykin, A.J., Shtasel, D.L., Gur, R.E., Kester, D.B., Mozley, L.H., Stafiniak, P., and Gur, R.C. (1994) Neuropsychological deficits in neuroleptic naive patients with first-episode schizophrenia. *Arch. Gen. Psychiatry* 51(2):124–131.

Seeger, T.F., Seymour, P.A., Schmidt, A.W., Zorn, S.H., Schulz, D.W., Lebel, L.A., McLean, S., Guanowsky, V., Howard, H.R., and Lowe, J.A., III (1995) Ziprasidone (CP-88,059): a new antipsychotic with combined dopamine and serotonin receptor antagonist activity. *J. Pharmacol. Exp. Ther.* 275:101–113.

Selemon, L.D., Rajkowska, G., and Goldman-Rakic, P.S. (1995) Abnormally high neuronal density in the schizophrenic cortex. A morphometric analysis of prefrontal area 9 and occipital area 17. *Arch. Gen. Psychiatry* 52(10):805–818.

Sharma, R.P., and Shapiro, L.E. (1996) The 5-HT1A receptor system: possible implications for schizophrenic negative symptomatology. *Psychiatr. Ann.* 26:88–92.

Shirakawa, O., and Tamminga, C.A. (1994) Basal ganglia GABAA and dopamine D1 binding site correlates of haloperidol-induced oral dyskinesias in rat. *Exp. Neurol.* 127:62–69.

Silverstein, S.M., Menditto, A.A., and Stuve, P. (2001) Shaping attention span: an operant conditioning procedure to improve neurocognition and functioning in schizophrenia. *Schizophr. Bull.* 27(2): 247–257.

Silverstone, T., Smith, G., and Goodall, E. (1988) Prevalence of obesity in patients receiving depot antipsychotics. *Br. J. Psychiatry* 153:214–217.

Skarsfeldt, T. (1995) Differential effects of repeated administration of novel antipsychotic drugs on the activity of midbrain dopamine neurons in the rat. *Eur. J. Pharmacol.* 281:662–668.

Stroup, T.S., Lieberman, J.A., McEvoy, J.P., Swartz, M.S., Davis, S.M., Rosenheck, R.A., Perkins, D.O., Keefe, R.S.E., Davis, C.E., Severe, Hsiao, J.K., and for the CATIE Investigators. (2006) Effectiveness of olanzapine, quetiapine, risperidone, and ziprasidone in patients with chronic schizophrenia following discontinuation of a previous atypical antipsychotic. *Am. J. Psychiatry* 163(4):611–622.

Sullivan, G., Bienroth, M., Jones, M., Millar, H., Ratna, L., and Taylor, D. (2007) Practical prescribing with aripiprazole in schizophrenia: consensus recommendations of a UK multidisciplinary panel. *Curr. Med. Res. Opin.* 23(7):1733–1744.

Tamminga, C.A. (1994) Development in somatic treatments: introduction. *Am. J. Psychiatry* 151:216–219.

Tamminga, C.A. (1997) Neuropsychiatric aspects of schizophrenia. In: Yudofsky, S.C., and Hales, R.E., eds. *The American Psychiatric Press Textbook of Neuropsychiatry*, 3rd ed. Washington, DC: American Psychiatric Press, pp. 855–882.

Tamminga, C. (1999) Glutamatergic aspects of schizophrenia. *Br. J. Psychiatry* 174(Suppl 37):12–15.

Tamminga, C.A. (2002) Partial agonists in the treatment of psychoses. *J. Neurol. Transm.* 109:411–420.

Tamminga, C.A., Dannals, R.F., Frost, J.J., Wong, D., and Wagner, H.N. (1993) Neuroreceptor and neurochemistry studies with positron emission tomography in psychiatric illness: promise and progress. In: Oldham, J.M., Riba, M.B., and Tasman, A., eds. *American Psychiatric Press Review of Psychiatry*. Washington, DC: American Psychiatric Press, pp. 487–510.

Tamminga, C.A., and Davis, J.M. (2007) The neuropharmacology of psychosis. *Schizophr. Bull.* 33(4):937–946.

Tamminga, C.A., and Holcomb, H.H. (2004) Phenotype of schizophrenia: a review and formulation. *Mol. Psychiatry* 10(1):27–39.

Tamminga, C.A., and Kane, J.M. (1997) Olanzapine (Zyprexa): characteristics of a new antipsychotic. *Expert Opin. Invest. Drugs* 6:1743–1752.

Tamminga, C.A., Thaker, G.K., Moran, M., Kakigi, T., and Gao, X.M. (1994) Clozapine in tardive dyskinesia: observations from human and animal model studies. *J. Clin. Psychiatry* 55(Suppl B):102–106.

Tohen, M., and Zarate, C.A., Jr. (1998) Antipsychotic agents and bipolar disorer. *J. Clin. Psychiatry* 59(Suppl 1):38–48.

Tollefson, G.D., Beasley, C.M., Jr., Tamura, R.N., Tran, P.V., and Potkin, J.H. (1997) Blind, controlled, long-term study of the comparative incidence of treatment-emergent tardive dyskinesia with olanzapine or haloperidol. *Am. J. Psychiatry* 154(9):1248–1254.

Tollefson, G.D., Beasley, C.M., Jr., Tran, P.V., Street, J.S., Krueger, J.A., Tamura, R.N., Graffeo, K.A., and Thieme, M.E. (1997) Olanzapine versus haloperidol in the treatment of schizophrenia and schizoaffective and schizophreniform disorders: results of an international collaborative trial. *Am. J. Psychiatry* 154:457–465.

Tsai, G., Passani, L.A., Slusher, B.S., Carter, R., Baer, L., Kleinman, J.E., and Coyle, J.T. (1995) Abnormal excitatory neurotransmitter metabolism in schizophrenic brains. *Arch. Gen. Psychiatry* 52(10):829–836.

Twamley, E.W., Jeste, D.V., and Lehman, A.F. (2003) Vocational rehabilitation in schizophrenia and other psychotic disorders: a literature review and meta-analysis of randomized controlled trials. *J. Nerv. Men. Dis.* 191(8):515–523.

VanPutten, T., Marder, S.R., Wirshing, W.C., Aravagiri, M., and Chabert, N. (1991) Neuroleptic plasma levels. *Schizophr. Bull.* 17:197–216.

Weiner, D.M., Meltzer, H.Y., Veinbergs, I., Donohue, E.M., Spalding, T.A., Smith, T.T., Mohell, N., Harvey, S.C., Lameh, J., Nash, N., Vanover, K.E., Olsson, R., Jayathilake, K., Lee, M., Levey, A.I., Hacksell, U., Burstein, E.S., Davis, R.E., and Brann, M.R. (2004) The role of M1 muscarinic receptor agonism of N-desmethylclozapine in the unique clinical effects of clozapine. *Psychopharmacology (Berl.)* 177(1/2):207–216.

Wexler, B.E., Anderson, M., Fulbright, R.K., and Gore, J.C. (2000) Preliminary evidence of improved verbal working memory performance and normalization of task-related frontal lobe activation in schizophrenia following cognitive exercises. *Am. J. Psychiatry* 157(10):1694–1697.

Wirshing, D.A., Wirshing, W.C., Kysar, L., Berisford, M.A., Goldstein, D., Pashdag, J., Mintz, J., and Marder, S.R. (1999) Novel antipsychotics: comparison of weight gain liabilities. *J. Clin. Psychiatry* 60:358–363.

Wykes, T., and van der Gaag, M. (2001) Is it time to develop a new cognitive therapy for psychosis—cognitive remediation therapy (CRT)? *Clin. Psychol. Rev.* 21(8):1227–1256.

Wykes, T., Brammer, M., Mellers, J., Bray, P., Reeder, C., Williams, C., and Corner, J. (2002) Effects on the brain of a psychological treatment: cognitive remediation therapy: functional magnetic resonance imaging in schizophrenia. *Br. J. Psychiatry* 181(2):144–152.

Zimbroff, D.L., Kane, J.M., Tamminga, C.A., Daniel, D.G., Mack, R.J., Wozniak, P.J., Sebree, T.B., Wallin, B.A., and Kashkin, K.B. (1997) A controlled, dose-response study of sertindole and haloperidol in schizophrenia. *Am. J. Psychiatry* 154:782–791.

IV MOOD DISORDERS

CHARLES B. NEMEROFF

VIRTUALLY all the field would agree that we have witnessed remarkable advances in psychiatry and neuroscience since publication of the second edition of this text, and no field has witnessed such advances more than affective disorders. The contributors to this section of the third edition, all leaders in mood disorders research, have provided a comprehensive description of the state of this field, with an appropriate emphasis on the newest findings. Below, I highlight the major contributions of these chapters.

Ghaemi and Goodwin provide a provocative discussion of nosology, preparing the reader for *Diagnostic and Statistical Manual of Mental Disorders*, 5th ed. (*DSM-V*), which is currently in the midst of intensive planning. The review of psychiatric genetics, with a focus on bipolar disorder, by Lohoff and Berrettini has been appropriately updated in view of the phenomenal advances in genetic research in psychiatry, as for example evidenced by the seminal work of Caspi and colleagues on the importance of the role of the serotonin transporter (SERT) polymorphism in mediating vulnerability to depression after exposure to child abuse. Clearly outlined are the essential steps necessary to link specific genetic polymorphisms with vulnerability to mood disorders. The summary of animal models by Sillaber, Holsboer, and Wotjak appropriately focuses on techniques of molecular neurobiology, namely, to change the expression of, and availability of, critical genes and their products, respectively, such as corticotropin releasing factor (CRF), glucocorticoids, and their receptors. Indeed, the available methodology has progressed from knockout models to the now almost routine ability to conditionally suppress or enhance specific gene expression in particular brain regions using viral vectors. However, the mismatch between our sophisticated understanding of mouse genetics and our relative ignorance of rat genetics, coupled with our relatively greater understanding of rat behavior compared with mouse behavior, remains a major impediment to progress in this field.

Catapano and colleagues contribute a state-of-the-art review of advances in cellular neurobiology that is of particular importance to mood disorders. For too long, investigators have focused almost exclusively on perturbations in monoamine transporter and receptor density and affinity, and on alterations in neurotransmitter availability as a potential substrate for major psychiatric illness. This group has redirected the field to manifold postreceptor signal transduction mechanisms including growth factors mediating neurogenesis and neuroprotection. Neurogenesis is one of the major topics covered by Duman in his updated review of the preclinical findings relevant to the neurochemistry of depression. He expands on his group's groundbreaking work indicating that all clinically effective antidepressant treatments increase hippocampal neurogenesis after chronic, but not acute, administration. This chapter is complementary to the chapter on animal models and the chapters on cellular neurobiology that precede it, as well as the chapter that follows by Dunlop, Garlow, and Nemeroff on the neurochemical pathology of mood disorders. The neuroendocrine and cerebrospinal fluid studies described in this chapter are largely congruent with the review by Drevets and colleagues of functional brain imaging studies and findings reviewed by Arango and Mann on postmortem studies of suicide victims. The former group of modalities has exhibited remarkable advances in the last few years. The resolution of new positron emission tomography imaging systems is now good enough, for example, to be able to visualize differences in the component nuclei of the amygdala, a brain region of great interest to investigators in mood disorders.

Berman and colleagues comprehensively review the pharmacological management of depression. They highlight our recent advances—for example, atypical antipsychotic augmentation of the therapy of selective serotonin reuptake inhibitor (SSRI) nonresponders—and remind us of our failures as well as describe novel treatments with novel mechanisms of action. This third edition is strengthened by the discussion of this very issue of new treatment development by Berton and Nestler, as well as the focus by Rubinow and his colleagues on the neurobiology of women's mood disorders, and the interface of depression and medical illness by Evans and his colleagues.

Clearly, impressive advances have occurred in our field since publication of the last edition of this book. Based on these comprehensive reviews, the next decade should be the setting for incremental advances, for example, in personalized psychiatry, that is, prediction of response to one or another treatment, as well as increasing our armamentarium for treatment refractory patients.

25 Diagnostic Classifications of Mood Disorders: Historical Context and Implications for Neurobiology

S. NASSIR GHAEMI AND FREDERICK K. GOODWIN

Mood disorders have been described since antiquity in the context of the phenomena of melancholia and mania. Melancholia and mania were well described in the Hippocratic era.

In the fifth and fourth centuries B.C., Hippocrates and his school described melancholia as a condition with changes in sleep, anger, restlessness, decreased appetite, and marked sadness (Jackson, 1986). The ancient Greeks also identified mania mainly as a state of high energy and euphoric happiness. Adding the diagnosis of "phrenitis" (similar to the modern conception of *delirium*), the Hippocratic nosology of mental illness comes together: melancholia, mania, and phrenitis—which is quite similar to modern nosology, if a category of nonaffective psychosis were added (Jouanna, 1999).

The relevance of Hippocratic nosology to modern psychiatry also plays out in the emphasis on the brain as the basis of behavior. In a now-famous passage, Hippocrates wrote: "Men ought to know that from the brain and from the brain only arrives our pleasures, joys, laughter and jests, as well as our sorrows, pains, griefs and tears . . . wherefore, I assert, the brain is the interpreter of consciousness" (Hippocrates, 1952, p. 159).

The Hippocratic school thus performed the first essential service toward scientific psychiatry: it argued that these were illnesses of the body, not of supernatural or magical spirits. The Hippocratic insight about the brain, however, was buried for over two millennia under other Greco-Roman theories about the physical nature of affective disorders. Melancholia, some held, was due to an excess of black bile, and mania an excess of yellow bile (Berrios and Porter, 1999; Angst and Marneros, 2001). Aristotle, the son of a physician, introduced the concept of a *predisposition to melancholia* by means of a relative excess of black bile. He also located the organ of melancholia in the heart, rather than the brain, and in this he was followed by many physicians (Berrios and Porter, 1999).

In the second century A.D., Aretaeus of Cappadocia appears to have been the first to suggest that mania was an end-stage of melancholia, a view that was to prevail for years to come (Angst and Marneros, 2001; F. Goodwin and Jamison, 2007). Aretaeus carefully described the spectrum of mania in the clearest detail. According to Aretaeus, the classical form of mania was the bipolar one: the patient who previously was gay, euphoric, and hyperactive suddenly "has a tendency to melancholy; he becomes, at the end of the attack, languid, sad, taciturn, he complaints that he is worried about his future, he feels ashamed." When the depressive phase is over, such patients go back to being gay, they laugh, they joke, they sing, "they show off in public with crowned heads as if they were returning victorious from the games; sometimes they laugh and dance all day and all night." In serious forms of mania, called furor, the patient "sometimes kills and slaughters the servants"; in less severe forms, he often exalts himself: "without being cultivated he says he is a philosopher . . . and the incompetent (say they are) good artisans . . . others yet are suspicious and they feel that they are being persecuted, for which reasons they are irascible" (F. Goodwin and Jamison, 2007, p. 32).

This descriptive approach to the diagnosis of mood disorders was lost throughout most of the Middle Ages, however, under the influence Galen's theory of humors. Instead of observing and describing the symptoms and course of mood conditions, as in the Hippocratic tradition, medieval physicians tended to speculate about the possible diagnoses that might be inferred from various alterations of the four humors (black bile, yellow bile, phlegm, and air) (Osler, 1921).

In general, this distinction between Hippocratic and Galenic approaches to medicine may be generalized to the nosology of mood disorders. Some have stayed close to clinical observation; others have tended to reason downward from accepted theory. It matters little whether those theories were Galenic humors, or Freudian psychoanalysis, or the latest neurobiological model.

Our view is that science progresses by staying close to clinical observation and diagnosis, and then working into the neurobiology of disease from that careful clinical starting point. The history of medicine teaches us that working in the other direction, from a theory, even one based on an advanced understanding of neurobiology, generally lead to dead ends.

THE NEO-HIPPOCRATIC REVIVAL

One might say that after the Galenic dark ages, the Enlightenment in medicine involved a revival of Hippocratic ideals of clinical observation and attentive diagnosis (Osler, 1921). Thomas Sydenham, called "the English Hippocrates," led this revival and established the signs and symptoms approach to establishing medical syndromes, which, to this day, remains the bread and butter of scientific medicine (Dewhurst, 1962). It is no accident that he was antagonistic to his contemporary William Harvey, who, instead of focusing on clinical presentations in patients, had turned his attention to laboratory-based research (Osler, 1921). Of course, the discoveries of both can now be seen, in retrospect, as complementary. Paraphrasing Kant (1998), one might say that neurobiology without careful clinical research is blind; clinical research without neurobiology is empty.

In the 19th century, the Hippocratic approach to diagnosis and treatment was advanced most strongly by Phillipe Pinel and his followers in France (Goldstein, 2002). Thus, it is no accident that they were the first to pick up where Aretaeus left off. The French school linked mania and melancholia together as one illness, not just two separate aspects of psychopathology (Goldstein, 2002). (They were preceded in this observation by Andres Piquer in Spain in the 17th century [Vieta and Barcia, 2000], and by Avicenna in Iran in the 10th century [Vakili and Gorji, 2006]; for instance, Avicenna held that "undoubtedly the material which is the effective producer of mania is of the same nature as that which produces melancholia.") However, the French school was the first to systematically advance the diagnosis of mania/melancholia as major mental illness. In 1854, Jules Falret, a student of Esquirol (the key disciple of Pinel), described a circular disorder (*la folie circulaire*), which for the first time expressly defined an illness in which "this succession of mania and melancholia manifests itself with continuity and in a manner almost regular." The same year, Baillarger described essentially the same thing (*la folie double forme*), emphasizing that the manic and depressive episodes were not different attacks but rather different stages of the same attack (Goldstein, 2002).

THE NEO-GALENIC REVIVAL IN GERMANY

At the same time as the French school took up the Hippocratic mantle, German academic psychiatry began to focus on neuropathology, neuroanatomy, experimental psychology, and other laboratory aspects of understanding the brain and mental function (Engstrom, 2004). The key leader of 19th-century German psychiatry, Wilhelm Griesinger, advanced the view that all mental illness is a disease of the brain. As a consequence, he, and his key followers Theodor Meynert and Carl Wernicke, maintained that understanding mental illness would depend on the ability to understand how abnormal brain function produced illness (Marx, 1970; Engstrom, 2004). Like Galen, though on more solid scientific grounds, they interpreted clinical aspects of mental illness based on their theory (their understanding of the brain) rather than based on pure clinical observation (as did the French school). In fact, Wernicke's (1906) textbook of psychiatry provides a quite extensive psychiatric nosology based on his understanding of the cerebral localization of mental function.

Kraepelin's Synthesis

Of course, today Wernicke's nosology has almost no relevance, whereas that of his contemporary Emil Kraepelin (1921) continues to have an impact. This is because Kraepelin realized that the French were more correct than his German colleagues, and further, although he subscribed to Griesinger's maxim about the brain and mental illness, he concluded that neurobiological knowledge was too rudimentary for any practical relevance to clinical nosology. Further, unlike the French, Kraepelin informed his nosology with the new ideas of the German school of experimental psychology (founded by one of his mentors, Wilhelm Wundt) (Berrios and Porter, 1999). He used Wundt's basic description of mental faculties as a triad of thought/feeling/will as a basis for much of his organization of the detailed clinical observations of the French school. Thus, like most seminal contributions in medicine, Kraepelin's originality lay in pulling together apparently disparate perspectives and showing that they could be combined creatively.

As a consequence, his nosology has stood the test of time, in clinical utility and in validation by clinical research (Kendler et al., 1998).

Kraepelin's Model of Manic-Depressive Insanity

Kraepelin's main idea, as developed in his mature nosology (from the sixth edition of his textbook in 1899

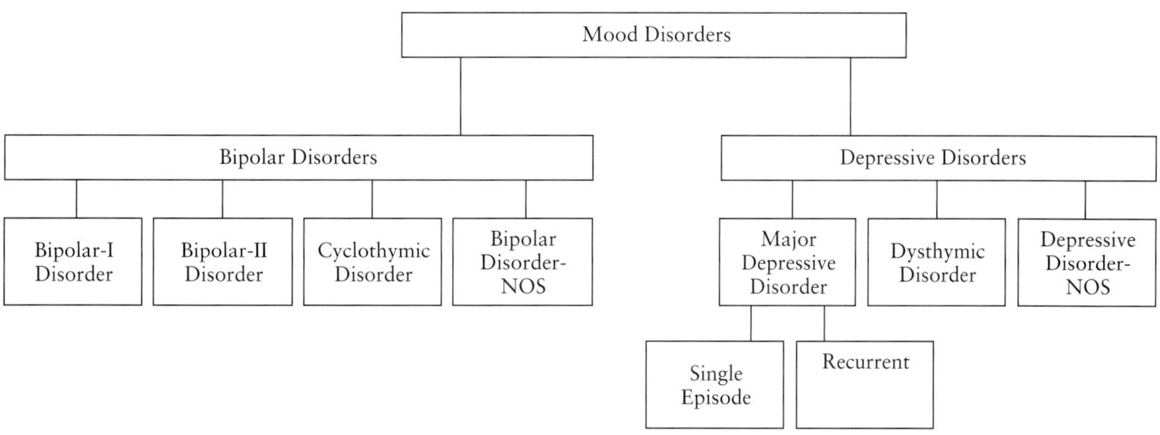

FIGURE 25.1 *DSM-IV* classification of mood disorders. NOS: not otherwise specified

onwards), was that *recurrence* was the key feature of manic-depressive insanity (MDI; see Fig. 25.1) (Trede et al., 2005; F. Goodwin and Jamison, 2007). Unlike the French school, he did not emphasize the clinical features of mania as being diagnostically distinctive; rather he saw the *course* of the illness, the cycling back and forth between mood episodes, as being the diagnostic essence of MDI.

Kraepelin replaced Griesinger's slogan with a new mantra: diagnosis is prognosis; the course identifies the disease (Shorter, 1997).

Besides being the first to identify recurrence, rather than polarity, as the fundamental defining characteristic of the illness, Kraepelin also had a very broad view: he did not think of MDI as an uncommon illness, restricted to euphoric mania. In fact, Kraepelin did not see melancholia as being diagnostically independent and subsumed it in his broad definition of recurrent mood disorder as MDI (Angst and Marneros, 2001; Akiskal, 2002). Thus, Kraepelin might legitimately be seen as the father of the "spectrum" concept, because for Kraepelin there was no bipolar/unipolar (BP/UP) distinction: it was all one spectrum of MDI (Akiskal, 2002).

Further, Kraepelin also described manic and depressive temperaments (Trede et al., 2005), the depressive being characterized by a "permanent gloomy emotional stress in all the experience of life," the manic characterized by a superficial understanding of life on the part of the individual, along with a "train of thought (that) is desultory, incoherent, aimless" and a mood that is "permanently exalted, careless, confident." By adding "slight colourings of mood" which "pass over without sharp boundary into the domain of personal predisposition," Kraepelin provided even more of a basis for the later development of spectrum concepts (Akiskal, 2000).

Criticism of Kraepelin's "Therapeutic Nihilism"

Unfortunately, Kraepelin and his colleagues did not possess many effective medical treatments for the two conditions they so painstakingly identified. Drug treatments for manic-depressive illness were not available, and the cure of psychosis seemed almost impossible. When Julius von Wagner-Jauregg, the chief of psychiatry at the University of Vienna, was able to cure some patients with psychosis, it was seen as such a major breakthrough at the time that he was the first and only psychiatrist ever to win the Nobel Prize (Shorter, 1997). It turned out that Wagner-Jaurregg's patients suffered from neurosyphilis, and his treatment, the injection of blood from patients with malaria into the patients with psychosis, led to improvement by producing intermittent fevers that would lead to a decline in the psychotic patients' spirochete counts. Penicillin obviously proved to be a more specific cure, but it was not available until the 1940s.

Given all these therapeutic difficulties, the Kraepelinian school was liable to being criticized as unhelpful in a practical sense. Manic-depressive illness could improve, but no treatments were available for it. Dementia praecox did not improve, and thus there was little to do. Working in Heidelberg just after Kraepelin had been chairman, Karl Jaspers (1986) remarked pithily: "We were therapeutically hopeless but kind." The psychoanalytic followers of Freud roundly criticized the therapeutic nihilism of the Kraepelinian tradition on this score (Menninger, 1963). It was not until the psychopharmacology revolution that a neo-Kraepelinian revival demonstrated the therapeutic utility of the traditional nosology (Shorter, 1997).

THE NEO-GALENIC RESTORATION: PSYCHOANALYSIS

Although most of Sigmund Freud's work focused on patients with hysteria, he also influenced psychiatric thinking about affective disorders (Roazen, 2002).

Partly in an attempt to preempt the original work of Victor Tausk (a young doctor with the bipolar form of manic-depressive illness who would commit suicide soon after Freud's rejection of him; Roazen, 1969) Freud's (1917) main direct work on affective disorders is present in his 1914 paper, *Mourning and Melancholia*. There he analogizes between the depressive feelings present during bereavement after the death of a parent, and the depressive feelings present in melancholia. Because the nature of the depressive symptoms appear to be similar in mourning as in melancholia, Freud postulated some possible similarities in their psychological bases. In mourning, Freud argued, we possess ambivalent feelings toward the dead parent. On the one hand, we loved the parent and thus feel bereft; on the other hand, there is often unresolved anger toward the parent. This mixture of frustration, anger, and sadness constitutes mourning. Freud wondered whether melancholia also involved ambivalent feelings toward a parent.

Freud's basic insight into the connection between mourning and melancholia was expanded by later psychoanalysts into the general notion that depression is related to feelings of hostility toward another person, often one's parents, and the introjection of these unacceptably hostile feelings inwards toward oneself rather than outwards toward others (Abraham, 1927). The empirical evidence in support of this view has been mixed.

Perhaps more important, about half of the 20th century was lost to a dogmatic veneration of Freudian doctrine. Mood disorders were no longer carefully observed and classified clinically, as in the French and German schools. Instead, diagnosis became almost irrelevant; theory was sufficient. Psychoanalysis allowed one to talk about mood disorders, as well as anything else, in terms of id, ego, superego, defense mechanisms, transference, and so on. Diagnostic clarity was viewed as unimportant (Shorter, 1997).

THE BIPOLAR/UNIPOLAR DISTINCTION

The recent return of Kraepelinian nosology has led many contemporary psychiatrists to underestimate other currents of nonpsychoanalytic thinking in Germany. The main competitor to Kraepelin's school was the neurobiology-based school of Wernicke and Meynert (Ungvari, 1993; Neumarker and Bartsch, 2003). That school never gave up the fight, despite Kraepelin's popularity in the early 20th century. Wernicke was succeeded by his disciple Kleist, who challenged Kraepelin by reasserting the importance of polarity as a basis for diagnosing mood disorders, mostly on theoretical grounds (Neumarker and Bartsch, 2003). Kleist's view was that the brain bases for mania and depression were different, and thus this difference was diagnostically important. Karl Leonhard, a student of Kleist (Leonhard, 1966; Franzek, 1990), took the next step and began to clinically study Kleist's proposal, an approach that gathered steam in the 1960s after genetic studies by Carlo Perris (1966) and epidemiological studies by Jules Angst (1966) produced evidence in support of the distinction between unipolar depression and bipolar disorder.

Nonetheless, perhaps these efforts would not have had too much impact if not for the rise of psychopharmacology. First antipsychotics, and soon thereafter antidepressants, were seen as being clinically specific: the former worked for mania and the latter for depression, and not vice versa (Healy, 2001). This therapeutic distinction seemed to support Kleist and Leonhard rather than Kraepelin.

DSM-III: NEO-KRAEPELINIAN?

Gerald Klerman famously coined the term "neo-Kraepelinian" (Klerman, 1986) to refer to an influential group of clinical researchers in psychiatry (centered at Washington University in St. Louis, Missouri) who provided empirical support for some of Kraepelin's views, which later became incorporated in *Diagnostic and Statistical Manual of Mental Disorders* (3rd ed.; *DSM-III*; American Psychiatric Association [APA], 1980) in 1980 (Shorter, 1997).

However, it is little understood that *DSM-III* was *not* Kraepelinian in any form in its description of mood disorders (though it did more directly apply Kraepelin's definition of *schizophrenia*). As for mood disorders, *DSM-III* is better termed Leonhardian, or Kleistian, or Wernickian (Ungvari, 1993); in other words, it supported a perspective that was more based on theory than on observation (though it was somewhat based on empirical research of Perris, 1966, and Angst, 1966).

Although the leaders of the *DSM-III* process often stated that they wanted future editions to evolve based on empirical research (Klerman et al., 1984; Spitzer, 1994), the BP/UP dichotomy has proven quite resistance to change (Andreasen, 2007). It has become so central to contemporary psychiatric practice that few practitioners even realize that before 1980, a completely different nosology existed based on MDI as an illness characterized by recurrent depressive episodes with or without mania (Fig. 25.2).

The genetic studies that seemed to support the BP/UP dichotomy are now much less clear; overlap between the two conditions seems extensive (Evans et al., 2005). Similarly, treatment studies clearly show much less diagnostic specificity for psychotropic medications than had been assumed in the 1970s (Healy, 2001). Lithium's prophylactic efficacy in bipolar disorder is matched by its ability to prevent highly recurrent unipolar depression (F. Goodwin and Jamison, 2007). Also, phenomenological research has revealed much more overlap in manic and depressive symptoms than had been assumed (Cassidy et al., 1998), and that variations of mixed states may be quite frequent (Benazzi, 2001).

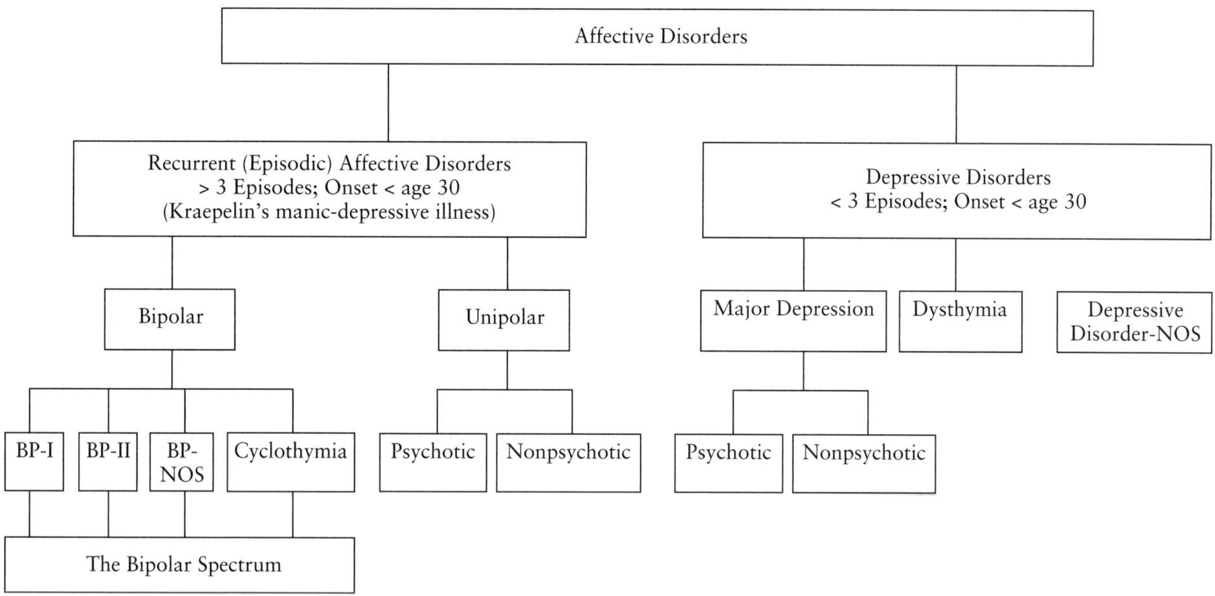

FIGURE 25.2 Affective disorders in *DSM-V*: A proposal. BP: bipolar; NOS: not otherwise specified.

All of this research tends to invalidate the phenomenology, genetic, and treatment basis for the BP/UP dichotomy (Koukopoulos et al., 2005), yet such findings have not had much impact on changing that nosology to date.

OUR CURRENT NOSOLOGY: PROMOTING MISDIAGNOSIS?

Bipolar disorder is frequently misdiagnosed, and common reasons cited include lack of insight into mania by patients (Ghaemi, 1997), poor clinical assessment of mania (Sprock, 1988), and stigma (Johnson and Orrell, 1995), among others. But a key issue is also that because our current polarity-based nosology requires the presence of mania to diagnose bipolar disorder even though depression is the main morbidity of this illness (Judd et al., 2002), our nosology almost guarantees a notable amount of misdiagnosis of bipolar disorder (F. Goodwin and Jamison, 2007). Many clinicians and patients tend to think of "depression" as being equivalent to unipolar depression, something fundamentally different from bipolar disorder (Ghaemi et al., 2000). Whether or not this proves to be the case biologically, certainly one can say that it is not the case clinically: both conditions are characterized by depression as their most common and prominent feature (Mitchell et al., 2001). It has now been well-established that depressive symptoms tend to last longer than manic symptoms (F. Goodwin and Jamison, 2007), and that patients with bipolar disorder spend about one-half of their lives depressed, versus only about one-tenth of their lives manic or hypomanic (Ghaemi et al., 2000; Judd et al., 2002). Unfortunately, many clinicians and patients jump from the recognition of a major depressive syndrome directly to a diagnosis of unipolar depression without carefully ruling out bipolar conditions (Ghaemi et al., 2000).

NEUROBIOLOGY OR CLINICAL DIAGNOSIS: WHICH COMES FIRST?

As future neurobiological research evolves, the complementary nature of clinical research and neurobiological research needs to be carefully appreciated: the historical example of the debate between Sydenham and Harvey should not be forgotten (Osler, 1921).

It would be a mistake, in our view, for neurobiological studies to be seen as a sufficient basis for nosological judgments. For example, in a neurobiologically driven nosology the diagnostic distinction between schizophrenia and bipolar psychosis would be undermined by observations of extensive neurobiological overlap between the two illnesses (Dutta et al., 2007). This view reflects what philosophers call a *category error*; it is important to differentiate between pathophysiology and etiology. Most neurobiological research involves pathophysiology—we can say that certain neurotransmitter systems, or other chemical changes in the brain or body, are involved when a person is acutely depressed, for example. This does not mean that those changes are the cause, or etiology, of the illness of major depressive disorder. The etiologies can be an environmental insult in pregnancy, or involve an infectious agent, or involve having certain genes, or some combination of these. These etiologies may eventually lead to depression through a mechanism that later entails changes in a neurotransmitter system. Varying etiologies can lead to the same clinical presentation via similar pathophysiological mechanisms called "final common pathways." The category mistake is this: to conclude, based on final common pathways of pathophysiology, that all the etiologies are the same is a mistake. If one further concludes that all those illnesses are the same, one is further mistaken (Ghaemi, 2003). This need not be the case. In fact, sometimes the reverse is the case: multiple diagnostic etiologies can produce a single pathophysiological mechanism, as with varied infectious causes of the same clinical syndrome (Nahmias et al., 2006).

In a nutshell, the neurobiology of pathogenesis is quite distinct from the neurobiology of ultimate etiology, and researchers should be aware of this distinction when considering nosological definitions (Ghaemi, 2003).

Further, diagnostic validity is not dependent on therapeutic specificity (Murray and Murphy, 1978). A disease is a disease, whether or not there is a treatment for it, and whether or not there are one or many treatments for it. For instance, coronary artery disease can be treated by a variety of different medications as well as different surgical interventions. Similarly, psychotropic medications may affect many different symptom complexes, possibly mediated by common neurobiological mechanisms (van Praag et al., 1990). It does not follow, logically or biologically, that such symptom complexes should replace our clinical diagnoses (van Praag et al., 1990), nor that the biological similarities of drug effects invalidate clinical diagnoses based on observation of symptoms, correlated with course of illness and genetic evidence (Stahl, 2005).

Clinical diagnosis should aid us in identifying etiologies of disease; as such work progresses, we may find that a single etiology leads to a single clinical syndrome, or that multiple etiologies lead to a single clinical syndrome, or that a single etiology leads to multiple clinical syndromes. The matter cannot be prejudged. And, those who would wish to replace clinical diagnoses, based on millennia of careful observation, with our neurobiological knowledge of today would do well to pay attention to the retardation of scientific progress when theory replaced observation in the Galenic era (Osler, 1921).

It would be harmful to the progress of neurobiology if the early state of our knowledge today led to premature theorization in place of continued careful contact with the reality of unbiased clinical observation (Jaspers, 1998). Otherwise, even the most up-to-date current neurobiologically based nosology is bound to be, sooner or later, as outdated as 19th-century brain-based models are today (Jaspers, 1998).

NEUROBIOLOGICAL IMPLICATIONS

The above discussion is relevant to future trends in neurobiology because the direction that neurobiological research takes partly depends on what kind of nosology we accept. In the case of contemporary nosology, which has been polarity based, neurobiological research has tended to focus on studies of the acute phases of mood disorders. Thus we have a large literature on the neurobiology of acute depression (Licinio and Wong, 2005), and a somewhat smaller literature on the neurobiology of acute mania (Soares and Gershon, 2000). These studies began by focusing on neurotransmitter systems and have extended to studies of abnormalities in other aspects of physiology, such as the hypothalamic pituitary adrenal (Gillespie and Nemeroff, 2005) or thyroid (Bauer et al., 2002) axes. Recent studies have further extended such studies into second-messenger and genetic changes in acute depression or mania (Gould et al., 2007). Although immensely useful, this is only one of two major approaches that could have been taken.

Neurobiological research could go in a completely different direction based on the other main perspective on the nosology of mood disorders: a recurrence-based nosology would direct research into the biology of recurrence (F.K. Goodwin, 1989), not the nature of acute phases. Mood cycling into and out of episodes would be the phenotype of interest, not the specific clinical features of the episodes. Such studies have begun to happen and have tended to occur mainly in the context of studies of circadian rhythms, sleep research, genetic studies, or long-term changes in neuroplasticity and neuronal circuits.

THE NEUROBIOLOGY OF RECURRENCE: THE KINDLING PARADIGM

As with all neurobiological research, theoretical models are needed to generate hypotheses for testing. These models include the kindling paradigm (Post et al., 1988), which builds on the physiological finding that intermittent subthreshold electrical or chemical stimuli produce increasingly strong neuronal depolarization in the brain, a process of sensitization that may possess temporal similarities to the episodic behavioral disturbances of recurrent mood disorders, with an emphasis on the bipolar subgroup (Post et al., 1988). As an explanatory model for these clinical phenomena, the kindling paradigm predicts that psychosocial stressors would be more frequent earlier in the course of illness, and that frequency of episodes would increase later in the course of illness (F. Goodwin and Jamison, 2007; Post, 2007). Post hypothesized that this process applies to at least a subgroup of patients with recurrent mood disorders (Post, 2007), though not necessarily all patients (S.R. Weiss and Post, 1994).

This literature has been reviewed in detail elsewhere (F. Goodwin and Jamison, 2007). In sum, the majority, but not all, of the studies that have examined the kindling hypothesis provide data that are consistent with the hypothesis. Although the issue is not settled, the accumulating empirical evidence suggests that the kindling hypothesis has had at least heuristic value in advancing our knowledge of the course of some forms of recurrent mood disorders, perhaps especially bipolar illness.

The kindling hypothesis dovetails with neurobiological research that demonstrates that stress can activate a cascade of changes in the brain that play out over progressively longer time frames. In animal studies of kindling, investigators have reported changes in genetic expression (of c-Fos and thyroid-releasing hormone genes), as well as effects on glucocorticoid receptor expression, as a result of repeated intermittent electrical and chemical stimulation (Clark et al., 1994; Kim et al., 1996).

These genetic changes are mediated by intermediary processes: the second-messenger systems that transmit information from the synapse to the cell nucleus. Many studies on the mechanisms of action of mood-altering drugs are now focusing on these postsynaptic changes (Manji, 1992; Manji et al., 1995; Bachmann et al., 2005; Gould and Manji, 2005; Gould et al., 2006; Gould et al., 2007) because it has long been noted that though the effects of treatments for mood disorders on neurotransmitters at the synaptic junction are immediate, the clinical effects on mood symptoms are delayed by weeks to months. In the investigation of these longer-acting and longer-lasting mechanisms, researchers have established a central role for G proteins and other second-messenger systems in mediating the effects of drugs, the most extensively studied of which is lithium (Bachmann et al., 2005; Gould and Manji, 2005; Gould et al., 2006; Gould et al., 2007).

THE NEUROBIOLOGY OF RECURRENCE: OTHER APPROACHES

The neurobiology of recurrence can also be approached through other fields such as circadian rhythm, genetic, and animal behavior studies.

Circadian rhythm research can be connected to some recent second-messenger research related to mechanisms of lithium action. Lithium has been shown to be a direct inhibitor of glycogen synthase kinase 3 (GSK3) (Gould and Manji, 2005), which has also been shown to be an essential component to the Drosophila circadian clock. Glycogen synthase kinase 3 knockout mice have a marked phase delay in their circadian rhythms, and an experimental study found that lithium produced a similar effect (Kaladchibachi et al., 2007).

Genetic studies have also tended to find that recurrence is a major predictor of increased genetic loading for mood disorders (Levinson, 2006). An example of genetic studies relevant to recurrence is a study in which a polymorphism in the human CLOCK gene, associated with diurnal preferences of human healthy participants, was observed at a significantly higher recurrence rate in homozygotes for the C variant (Benedetti et al., 2003).

Another approach would involve selective breeding for models of animal behavior that would reflect cycling into and out of animal models of depression and mania, rather than simply seeking to identify models of mania separately from models of depression. An example of potential for this kind of work has been published based on selective breeding of low as well as high motor activity in a swim test for rats (J.M. Weiss et al., 1998).

FUTURE NEEDS

Clinical work in the nosology of mood disorders needs to continue, and the profession needs to be open to incorporating this research into *DSM-V* and beyond. F. Goodwin and Jamison (2007) explicitly recommended that in *DSM-V* mood disorders should first be divided into those characterized by a significant degree of recurrence and those not so characterized. The UP/BP distinction would then be made among those with recurrent mood disorder (as was done in the original research supporting the UP–BP dichotomy). That is, the original meaning of *unipolar* was a type of recurrent mood disorder without mania/hypomania. In *DSM IV* (APA, 1994) *unipolar* has come to mean everything that is not bipolar. They also point out that the current *DSM-IV* definition of *recurrent unipolar depression* (more than one episode) is so broad as to be almost meaningless. Further, neurobiological research needs to be more flexible than our current nosology, with greater extension into a study of the neurobiology of recurrence. Also, premature theories based on the rapidly moving neurosciences should be avoided, and we should remain true to the Hippocratic tradition of the primacy of careful clinical observation for medical diagnosis.

The two lines of research should go hand in hand: clinical and neurobiological work, independent of each other but connected, need to progress together, or not at all.

REFERENCES

Abraham, K. (1927) Notes on the psychoanalytical investigation and treatment of manic-depressive insanity and allied conditions. In: Bryan, D., and Strachey, A., eds. *Selected Papers of Karl Abraham, M.D.* London: Hogarth, pp. 137–156.

Akiskal, H. (2000) Temperament and mood disorders. *Harv. Ment. Health Lett.* 16:5–6.

Akiskal, H. (2002) Classification, diagnosis and boundaries of bipolar disorders. In Maj, M., Akiskal, H., Lopez-Ibor, J., and Sartorius, N., eds. *Bipolar Disorder*. London: Wiley, pp. 1–52.

American Psychiatric Association. (1980) *Diagnostic and Statistical Manual of Mental Disorders*, 3rd ed. Washington, DC: Author.

American Psychiatric Association. (1994) *Diagnostic and Statistical Manual of Mental Disorders*, 4th ed. Washington, DC: Author.

Andreasen, N.C. (2007) DSM and the death of phenomenology in America: an example of unintended consequences. *Schizophr. Bull.* 33:108–112.

Angst, J. (1966) [On the etiology and nosology of endogenous depressive psychoses: A genetic, sociologic, and clinical study]. *Monogr. Gesamtgeb. Neurol. Psychiatr.* 112:1–118.

Angst, J., and Marneros, A. (2001) Bipolarity from ancient to modern times: conception, birth and rebirth. *J. Affect. Disord.* 67:3–19.

Bachmann, R.F., Schloesser, R.J., Gould, T.D., and Manji, H.K. (2005) Mood stabilizers target cellular plasticity and resilience cascades: implications for the development of novel therapeutics. *Mol. Neurobiol.* 32:173–202.

Bauer, M., Heinz, A., and Whybrow, P.C. (2002) Thyroid hormones, serotonin and mood: of synergy and significance in the adult brain. *Mol. Psychiatry* 7:140–156.

Benazzi, F. (2001) Depressive mixed state: testing different definitions. *Psychiatry Clin. Neurosci.* 55:647–652.

Benedetti, F., Serretti, A., Colombo, C., Barbini, B., Lorenzi, C., Campori, E., et al. (2003) Influence of CLOCK gene polymorphism on circadian mood fluctuation and illness recurrence in bipolar depression. *Am. J. Med. Genet. B Neuropsychiatr. Genet.* 123:23–26.

Berrios, G., and Porter, R. (Eds.). (1999) *A history of clinical psychiatry*. London: Athlone Press.

Calabrese, J.R., Keck, P.E., Jr., Macfadden, W., Minkwitz, M., Ketter, T.A., Weisler, R.H., et al. (2005) A randomized, double-blind, placebo-controlled trial of quetiapine in the treatment of bipolar I or II depression. *Am. J. Psychiatry* 162:1351–1360.

Cassidy, F., Murry, E., Forest, K., and Carroll, B.J. (1998) Signs and symptoms of mania in pure and mixed episodes. *J. Affect. Disord.* 50:187–201.

Clark, M., Smith, M.A., Weiss, S.R., and Post, R.M. (1994) Modulation of hippocampal glucocorticoid and mineralocorticoid receptor mRNA expression by amygdaloid kindling. *Neuroendocrinology* 59:451–456.

Davis, L.L., Bartolucci, A., and Petty, F. (2005) Divalproex in the treatment of bipolar depression: a placebo-controlled study. *J. Affect. Disord.* 85:259–266.

Dewhurst, K. (1962) Thomas Sydenham (1624-1689) reformer of clinical medicine. *Med. Hist.* 6:101–118.

Dutta, R., Greene, T., Addington, J., McKenzie, K., Phillips, M., and Murray, R.M. (2007) Biological, life course, and cross-cultural studies all point toward the value of dimensional and developmental ratings in the classification of psychosis. *Schizophr. Bull.* 33(4):868–876.

Engstrom, E. (2004) *Clinical Psychiatry in Imperial Germany*. Ithaca, NY: Cornell University Press.

Evans, L., Akiskal, H.S., Keck, P.E., Jr., McElroy, S.L., Sadovnick, A.D., Remick, R.A., et al. (2005) Familiality of temperament in bipolar disorder: support for a genetic spectrum. *J. Affect. Disord.* 85:153–168.

Franzek, E. (1990) Influence of Carl Wernicke on Karl Leonhard's nosology. *Psychopathology* 23:277–281.

Freud, S. (1917) *Mourning and Melancholia*. London: Hogarth.

Ghaemi, S. (1997) Insight and psychiatric disorders: a review of the literature, with a focus on its clinical relevance for bipolar disorder. *Psychiatric Annals* 27:782–790.

Ghaemi, S.N. (2003) *The Concepts of Psychiatry*. Baltimore: Johns Hopkins University Press.

Ghaemi, S.N., Boiman, E.E., and Goodwin, F.K. (2000) Diagnosing bipolar disorder and the effect of antidepressants: a naturalistic study. *J. Clin. Psychiatry* 61:804–808.

Gillespie, C.F., and Nemeroff, C.B. (2005) Hypercortisolemia and depression. *Psychosom. Med.* 67(Suppl 1):S26–S28.

Goldstein, S. (2002) *Console and Classify: The French Psychiatric Profession in the 19th Century*. Chicago: University of Chicago Press.

Goodwin, F.K. (1989) The biology of recurrence: new directions for the pharmacologic bridge. *J. Clin. Psychiatry* 50(Suppl):40–44; discussion 45–47.

Goodwin, F., and Jamison, K. (2007) *Manic Depressive Illness*, 2nd ed. New York: Oxford University Press.

Goodwin, G.M., Bowden, C.L., Calabrese, J.R., Grunze, H., Kasper, S., White, R., et al. (2004) A pooled analysis of 2 placebo controlled 18-month trials of lamotrigine and lithium maintenance in bipolar I disorder. *J. Clin. Psychiatry* 65:432–441.

Gould, T.D., Dow, E.R., O'Donnell, K.C., Chen, G., and Manji, H.K. (2007) Targeting signal transduction pathways in the treatment of mood disorders: recent insights into the relevance of the WNT pathway. *CNS Neurol. Disord. Drug Targets* 6:193–204.

Gould, T.D., and Manji, H.K. (2005) Glycogen synthase kinase-3: a putative molecular target for lithium mimetic drugs. *Neuropsychopharmacology* 30:1223–1237.

Gould, T.D., Picchini, A.M., Einat, H., and Manji, H.K. (2006) Targeting glycogen synthase kinase-3 in the CNS: implications for the development of new treatments for mood disorders. *Curr. Drug Targets* 7:1399–1409.

Healy, D. (2001) *The Creation of Psychopharmacology*. Cambridge, MA: Harvard University Press.

Hippocrates. (1952) On the sacred disease. In: Hutchins, R/M. ed. *Hippocratic Writings: Great Books of the Western World, Volume 10*. Chicago: Encyclopaedia Britanica, Inc, p. 159.

Jackson, S. (1986) *Melancholia and Depression: From Hippocratic Times to Modern Times*. New Haven, CT: Yale University Press.

Jaspers, K. (1986) An autobiographical account. In Ehrlich, E. L., and Pepper, G.B., eds. *Karl Jaspers: Basic Philosophical Writings*. Atlantic Highland, NJ: Humanities Press, p. 5.

Jaspers, K. (1998) *General Psychopathology*. Baltimore: Johns Hopkins University Press.

Johnson, S., and Orrell, M. (1995) Insight and psychosis: a social perspective. *Psychol. Med.* 25:515–520.

Jouanna, J. (1999) *Hippocrates*. Baltimore: Johns Hopkins University Press.

Judd, L.L., Akiskal, H.S., Schettler, P.J., Endicott, J., Maser, J., Solomon, D.A., et al. (2002) The long-term natural history of the weekly symptomatic status of bipolar I disorder. *Arch. Gen. Psychiatry* 59: 530–537.

Kaladchibachi, S.A., Doble, B., Anthopoulos, N., Woodgett, J.R., and Manoukian, A.S. (2007) Glycogen synthase kinase 3, circadian rhythms, and bipolar disorder: a molecular link in the therapeutic action of lithium. *J. Circadian Rhythms* 5:3.

Kant, I. (1998) *Critique of Pure Reason*. Cambridge, UK: Cambridge University Press. (Original work published 1781)

Kendler, K.S., Karkowski, L.M., and Walsh, D. (1998) The structure of psychosis. *Arch. Gen. Psychiatry* 55:492–499.

Kim, S.Y., Post, R.M., and Rosen, J.B. (1996) Differential regulation of basal and kindling-induced TRH mRNA expression by thyroid hormone in the hypothalamic and limbic structures. *Neuroendocrinology* 63:297–304.

Klerman, G. (1986) Historical perspectives on contemporary schools of psychopathology. In: Millon, T., and Klerman, G.L., eds. *Contemporary Directions in Psychopathology: Toward the DSM-IV*. New York: Guilford Press, pp. 3–28.

Klerman, G.L., Vaillant, G.E., Spitzer, R.L., and Michels, R. (1984) A debate on DSM-III. *Am. J. Psychiatry* 141:539–553.

Koukopoulos, A., Albert, M.J., Sani, G., Koukopoulos, A.E., and Girardi, P. (2005) Mixed depressive states: nosologic and therapeutic issues. *Int. Rev. Psychiatry* 17:21–37.

Kraepelin, E. (1921) *Manic-Depressive Insanity and Paranoia* (G. M. Robertson, Ed.). Edinburgh, UK: E and S Livingstone.

Leonhard, K. (1966) [Psychiatry on the clinical basis of Wernicke. In memory of Wernicke as a clinician on the occasion of the 60th anniversary of his death (June 15, 1905)]. *Psychiatr. Neurol. Med. Psychol. (Leipz)* 18:165–171.

Levinson, D. F. (2006) The genetics of depression: a review. *Biol. Psychiatry* 60:84–92.

Licinio, J., and Wong, M.-L. (Eds.). (2005) *Biology of Depression*. New York: John Wiley.

Manji, H.K. (1992) G proteins: implications for psychiatry. *Am. J. Psychiatry* 149:746–760.

Manji, H.K., Potter, W.Z., and Lenox, R.H. (1995) Signal transduction pathways: molecular targets for lithium's actions. *Arch. Gen. Psychiatry* 52:531–543.

Marx, O.M. (1970) Nineteenth-century medical psychology. Theoretical problems in the work of Griesinger, Meynert, and Wernicke. *Isis* 61:355–370.

Menninger, K. (1963) *The Vital Balance*. New York: Viking.

Mitchell, P.B., Wilhelm, K., Parker, G., Austin, M., Rutgers, P., and Malhi, G.S. (2001) The clinical features of bipolar depression: a comparison with matched major depressive disorder patients. *J. Clin. Psychiatry* 62:212–216.

Murray, R.M., and Murphy, D.L. (1978) Drug response and psychiatric nosology. *Psychol. Med.* 8:667–681.

Nahmias, A.J., Nahmias, S.B., and Danielsson, D. (2006) The possible role of transplacentally-acquired antibodies to infectious agents, with molecular mimicry to nervous system sialic acid epitopes, as causes of neuromental disorders: prevention and vaccine implications. *Clin. Dev. Immunol.* 13:167–183.

Neumarker, K.J., and Bartsch, A.J. (2003) Karl Kleist (1879-1960) - a pioneer of neuropsychiatry. *Hist. Psychiatry* 14:411–458.

Osler, W. (1921) *The Evolution of Modern Medicine*. New Haven, CT: Yale University Press.

Perris, C. (1966) A study of bipolar (manic-depressive) and unipolar recurrent depressive psychoses. *Acta Psychiatr. Scand.* 42(Suppl 194):58–67.

Post, R.M. (2007) Kindling and sensitization as models for affective episode recurrence, cyclicity, and tolerance phenomena. *Neurosci. Biobehav. Rev.* 31(6):858–873.

Post, R.M., Weiss, S.R., and Pert, A. (1988) Cocaine-induced behavioral sensitization and kindling: implications for the emergence of psychopathology and seizures. *Ann. N.Y. Acad. Sci.* 537:292–308.

Roazen, P. (1969) *Brother Animal: The Story of Freud and Tausk*. New York: Knopf.

Roazen, P. (2002) *The Trauma of Freud: Controversies in Psychoanalysis*. New Brunswick, NJ: Transaction Publishers.

Sachs, G., Chengappa, K., Suppes, T., Mullen, J., Brecher, M., Devine, N., et al. (2004) Quetiapine with lithium or divalproex for the treatment of bipolar mania: a randomized, double-blind, placebocontrolled study. *Bipolar Disord.* 6:213–223.

Sachs, G., Sanchez, R., Marcus, R., Stock, E., McQuade, R., Carson, W., et al. (2006) Aripiprazole in the treatment of acute manic or mixed episodes in patients with bipolar I disorder: a 3-week placebo-controlled study. *J. Psychopharmacol.* 20:536–546.

Shorter, E. (1997) *A History of Psychiatry*. New York: John Wiley and Sons.

Soares, J., and Gershon, S. (Eds.). (2000) *Bipolar Disorders: Basic Mechanisms and Therapeutic Implications*. Washington, DC: American Psychiatric Press.

Spitzer, M. (1994) The basis of psychiatric diagnosis. In: Sadler, J., Wiggins, O., and Schwartz, M., eds. *Philosophical Perspectives on Psychiatric Diagnostic Classification*. Baltimore: Johns Hopkins University Press, pp. 163–177.

Sprock, J. (1988) Classification of schizoaffective disorder. *Compr. Psychiatry* 29:55–71.

Stahl, S.M. (2005) *Essential Psychopharmacology*. Cambridge, UK: Cambridge University Press.

Trede, K., Salvatore, P., Baethge, C., Gerhard, A., Maggini, C., and Baldessarini, R. J. (2005) Manic-depressive illness: evolution in Kraepelin's textbook, 1883-1926. *Harv. Rev. Psychiatry* 13:155–178.

Ungvari, G. S. (1993) The Wernicke-Kleist-Leonhard school of psychiatry. *Biol. Psychiatry* 34:749–752.

Vakili, N., and Gorji, A. (2006) Psychiatry and psychology in medieval Persia. *J. Clin. Psychiatry* 67:1862–1869.

van Praag, H.M., Asnis, G.M., Kahn, R.S., Brown, S.L., Korn, M., Friedman, J.M., et al. (1990) Nosological tunnel vision in biological psychiatry. A plea for a functional psychopathology. *Ann. N.Y. Acad. Sci.* 600:501–510.

van Praag, H.M., Asnis, G.M., Kahn, R.S., Brown, S.L., Korn, M., Harkavy-Friedman, J.M., et al. (1990) Monamines and abnormal behavior: a multi-aminergic perspective. *Br. J. Psychiatry* 157: 723–734.

Vieta, E., and Barcia, D. (2000) *El Trastorno Bipolar en el Siglo XVIII* [Bipolar disorder in the eighteenth century]. Burdeos, Spain: Mra ediciones.

Weiss, J.M., Cierpial, M.A., and West, C.H. (1998) Selective breeding of rats for high and low motor activity in a swim test: toward a new animal model of depression. *Pharmacol. Biochem. Behav.* 61:49–66.

Weiss, S.R., and Post, R.M. (1994) Caveats in the use of the kindling model of affective disorders. *Toxicol. Ind. Health* 10:421–447.

Wernicke, C. (1906) *Grundriss der Psychiatrie in klinischen Vorlesungen* [Basic Lectures in Clinical Psychiatry]. Leipzig, Germany: Georg Thieme.

26 Genetics of Mood Disorders

FALK W. LOHOFF AND WADE H. BERRETTINI

The search for susceptibility genes for bipolar disorders (BPD) and recurrent unipolar disorders (RUP) is the subject of this chapter. Genetic factors play important roles for the development of BPD and to a lesser extend for RUP, as indicated by family, twin, and adoption studies. According to monozygotic and dizygotic twin studies of BPD, ~65%–80% of the risk for developing BPD is attributable to genetic factors (Berrettini, 2002). Bipolar disorder family studies reflect a degree of familial aggregation that is congruous with the twin studies: children of parents with BPD have approximately a ninefold increase in lifetime BPD risk, compared to the ~1% general population risk (Helzer and Winokur, 1974; James and Chapman, 1975; Johnson and Leeman, 1977; Angst et al., 1980; Baron et al., 1982; Gershon et al., 1982; Winokur et al., 1982; Weissman et al., 1984; Maier et al., 1993). For RUP, the lifetime prevalence is at least 10% (Moldin et al., 1991; Weissman et al., 1996; Tsuang et al., 2004) and twin studies suggest a heritability of 40%–50% (Torgersen, 1986; Kendler, Neale, et al., 1993; McGuffin et al., 1996; Bierut et al., 1999; Sullivan et al., 2000; Kendler et al., 2001). Family studies indicated a two- to threefold increase in lifetime risk to develop RUP for first-degree relatives (Gershon et al., 1982; Weissman et al., 1984; Maier et al., 1992). This degree of familial aggregation, coupled with the high heritability from twin studies, generated optimism that genetic linkage techniques (which have been so successful in identifying genes for Mendelian disorders) would reveal genes of substantial influence on BPD and RUP risks. Unfortunately, gene localization and identification has been a slow and labor intensive process. Genetic investigators have encountered similar frustrations with other common complex traits (such as asthma, hypertension, and diabetes mellitus).

The major impediments to mood disorders gene localization and identification are: (*1*) no single gene is necessary and sufficient for BPD or RUP; (*2*) each susceptibility gene contributes a small fraction of the total genetic risk; and (*3*) complex genetic heterogeneity, meaning that multiple, partially overlapping sets of susceptibility genes (which interact with the environment) can predispose to similar syndromes that are indistinguishable on clinical grounds.

Given that the inherited susceptibilities for BPD and RUP are explained by multiple genes of small effect, simulations indicate that universal confirmation of vulnerability genes cannot be expected due to power issues, sampling variation, and genetic heterogeneity. With this background, several valid linkages of BPD to genomic regions are reviewed, including some that may be shared with schizophrenia. These results suggest that nosology must be changed to reflect the genetic origins of the multiple disorders that are collectively described by the term *BPD*. The briefer history of RUP molecular linkage and linkage disequilibrium (LD) studies is reviewed.

GENETIC EPIDEMIOLOGY OF MOOD DISORDERS

Twin Studies

Evidence for a genetic component to mood disorders has been documented consistently using family, twin, and adoptions studies and is summarized in Table 26.1. The first genetic studies of mood disorders were conducted over 70 years ago and included assessment of concordance rates for monozygotic and dizygotic twins with mood disorders (Luxenberger, 1930; Rosanoff et al., 1935; Slater, 1936; Kallman, 1954; Allen et al., 1974; Harvald and Hauge, 1975; Bertelsen et al., 1977). The early studies did not distinguish between BPD and RUP; however, in nearly all these reports, RUP illness in the cotwin of a BPD index case was grounds for categorizing the twin pair as concordant. Bertelsen et al. (1977)

TABLE 26.1 *Genetic Epidemiology of Mood Disorders*

	Bipolar Disorder	*Unipolar Depression*
Lifetime prevalence (%)	2–3	10–15
Lifetime risk for first degree relatives (fold increase)	9–10	2–3
Proband-wise MZ twin concordance (%)	45–70	40–50
Heritability estimate (%)	65–80	33–42

and Allen et al. (1974) reported that ~20% of concordant monozygotic twin pairs were constituted by a BPD index twin and a RUP cotwin. These older results are quite consistent with the more recent studies of BPD (Kendler, Neale, et al., 1993; McGuffin et al., 2003) reporting significantly higher monozygotic twins' concordance rates, compared to those for dizygotic twins. A recent review of twin studies in RUP disorder estimated heritability at 37%, with a substantial component of unique individual environmental risk, but little shared environmental risk (Sullivan et al., 2000). These twin studies included four community-ascertained samples (Kendler, Pedersen, et al., 1995; Lyons et al., 1998; Bierut et al., 1999; Kendler and Prescott, 1999) and two clinically ascertained samples, one from the United Kingdom (McGuffin et al., 1996) and one from Sweden (Kendler, Pedersen, et al., 1995). The results are quite consistent in concluding that genetic influence is a significant factor in risk for RUP, independent of ascertainment and country or origin.

Family Studies

Family studies of BPD show that a spectrum of mood disorders is found among the first-degree relatives of BPD probands: BPI, BPII with major depression (hypomania and RUP illness in the same person), schizoaffective disorders, and RUP illness (Helzer and Winokur, 1974; James and Chapman, 1975; Johnson and Leeman, 1977; Angst et al., 1980; Tsuang et al., 1980; Baron et al., 1982; Gershon et al., 1982; Weissman et al., 1984; Maier et al., 1993; Taylor et al., 1993). The family studies suggest shared liability for BPD and RUP disorders. No BPD family study, conducted in an optimal manner, reports increased risk for schizophrenia (SZ) among relatives of BPD probands. Similarly, no SZ family study reports increased risk for BPD among relatives of SZ probands. However, several SZ family studies report increased risk for RUP and schizoaffective disorders among relatives of SZ probands (Gershon et al., 1988; Kendler, McGuire, et al., 1993; Maier et al., 1993; Taylor et al., 1993). These family studies are consistent with some degree of overlap in susceptibility to RUP and schizoaffective disorders for relatives of BPD probands and relatives of SZ probands. Kendler, McGuire, et al. (1993) specifically note an increase in risk for psychotic affective disorders among the relatives of SZ probands. Potash et al. reported that psychotic affective disorders cluster in families (Potash, Chiu, et al., 2003; Potash et al., 2001). Risk for psychotic affective disorders was significantly higher among the relatives of psychotic BPD probands, compared to the risk for relatives of nonpsychotic BPD probands. This raises the possibility that the partial overlap in risk for BPD and SZ nosological categories is due to a subset of BPD characterized by psychotic symptoms. This subset of BPD is probably quite common, as the majority of BPD probands from the Potash, Chiu, et al. (2003) study were psychotic.

Family studies of RUP show that first-degree relatives of RUP probands were at increased risk for RUP disorders, compared to first-degree relatives of control probands (Tsuang et al., 1980; Gershon et al., 1982; Weissman et al., 1984; Maier et al., 1993; Weissman et al., 1993). There was a two- to fourfold increased risk for RUP among the first-degree relatives of RUP probands. Characteristics of RUP disorders that yield a more heritable phenotype include early onset, for example, before age 30 (Cadoret et al., 1977; Mendlewicz and Baron, 1981; Bland et al., 1986; Weissman et al., 1986; Stancer et al., 1987; Kupfer et al., 1989; Weissman et al., 1993) and a high degree of recurrence (Bland et al., 1986; Gershon et al., 1986; Reich et al., 1987; Kendler et al., 1994; Kendler et al., 1999). A third characteristic that may identify a separate group of disorders is the presence of psychosis (Kendler, McGuire, et al., 1993). Additional genetic subtypes of RUP may be identified through examination of comorbidities with panic disorder and other anxiety disorders and with alcoholism (Winokur et al., 1971; Merikangas et al., 1994; Nurnberger et al., 2002).

Adoption Studies

Mendlewicz and Rainer (1977) reported a controlled adoption study of BPD probands, including a control group of probands with poliomyelitis (Mendlewicz and Rainer, 1977). The biological relatives of the BPD probands had a 31% risk for BPD or UP disorders, as opposed to 2% in the relatives of the control probands. The risk for affective disorder in biological relatives of adopted patients with BPD was similar to the risk in relatives of patients with BPD who were not adopted (26%). Adoptive relatives do not show increased risk compared to relatives of control probands. Wender et al. (1986) and Cadoret (1978) studied RUP and BPD probands. Although evidence for genetic susceptibility was found, adoptive relatives of affective probands had a tendency to more affective illness themselves, compared with the adoptive relatives of controls (Cadoret, 1978; Wender et al., 1986). Von Knorring et al. (1983) did not find concordance in psychopathology between adoptees and biological relatives when examining the records of 56 adoptees with RUP disorders.

LINKAGE STUDIES OF BIPOLAR DISORDERS

Because of the strong epidemiological evidence for a genetic component in particular for BPD, the field has hoped that the identification of genetic risk factors would have been straightforward. However, the search for susceptibility genes has been difficult and frustrating due to the complex mode of inheritance, multiple genes with small effects, and clinical sample heterogeneity. Although linkage studies have suggested several regions in the genome that might harbor risk alleles, there has been inconsistency in findings, and so far no established universal genetic risk factor or causative gene for mood disorders has been identified.

The term *linkage* refers to the observation that two genetic loci, found near one another on the same chromosome, tend to be inherited together more often than expected by chance within families. Two such loci are said to be *linked*. The key concept of *linkage* is that chromosomal fragments that might harbor vulnerability genes are inherited with an illness more often then expected by chance in families. LOD (the logarithm of the odds ratio) scores refer to the probability that observed cosegregation of alleles at two loci within a family has occurred because the two loci are linked. A LOD score > 3 is evidence (not proof) that two DNA sequences are linked. The numerical value of the LOD score is dependent on the proposed mode of inheritance (dominant, recessive, sex-linked) and penetrance. Because the LOD score is dependent on these parameters (mode of inheritance and penetrance), it is sometimes termed a *parametric* statistic. This dependence on inheritance mode and penetrance distinguishes the LOD score from nonparametric statistics (including affected sibling pair and affected pedigree member methods) because such statistics are not dependent on mode of inheritance or penetrance.

What level of statistical significance should be required for declaring linkage? A recommended level of statistical significance for an initial report ($p < \sim 0.00002$) is a stringent criterion, based on simulations that indicate that this level of significance would occur less than 5 times randomly in 100 genome scans for linkage (Lander and Kruglyak, 1995). This statistical criterion assumes that all the genetic information within the pedigrees studied would be extracted, an assumption that is not true in practice. Typically, no more than ~80% of the genetic information in a pedigree series is extracted through genotyping. As in any other area of science, however, no single report of linkage should be accepted as valid without independent confirmation. The requirement for independent confirmations (at $p \leq 0.01$) is not waived, no matter what level of statistical significance has been achieved in a single report. This confirmation requirement should be seen within the context that valid linkages will not be confirmed in some studies. Indeed, nonconfirmations should be expected, intuitively, because of population (ethnic) differences, sampling procedures, and genetic heterogeneity. Suarez et al. (1994) have examined the probability of confirmation in simulations.

Suarez et al. (1994) simulated a disorder caused by any one of six loci and determined that a large sample size and substantial time will be required for an initial linkage to be confirmed in a second sample. From his simulations, it is clear that consistent detection of a locus of moderate effect cannot be expected. Nonconfirmatory studies will always occur when an initially detected linkage is valid (Suarez et al., 1994).

One of the most critical issues in confirmation of reported linkages is power. Attempts at confirmation of a reported susceptibility locus should state what power has been achieved to detect the locus initially described. For example, if a locus increases risk for BPD by a factor of two, it may be necessary to study ~200 affected sibling pairs to have adequate (90%) power to detect such a locus (Hauser et al., 1996). Unfortunately, few studies address this key issue. If 200 affected sibling pairs are required to achieve adequate (90%) power to detect a previously described locus, then a publication with fewer than 150 sibling pairs does not address the central issue of confirmation. However, such power-limited publications may have an important role in meta-analyses, in that they identify invaluable sources of additional data.

Comprehensive scans of the human genome have been completed with sufficient numbers (for example, > 100) of individuals with BPD (Rice et al., 1997; Detera-Wadleigh et al., 1999; Cichon et al., 2001; Kelsoe et al., 2001; Bennett et al., 2002; Dick et al., 2003; Ekholm et al., 2003; J. Liu et al., 2003; McInnis et al., 2003). If a major locus (explaining > 50% of the risk in > 50% of persons with BPD) existed, it would have been detected in many of these studies. Thus, no such major locus exists for BPD. There are several confirmed reports of loci of smaller effect, which can be termed *susceptibility loci*. These loci are neither necessary nor sufficient for disease but increase risk for the disorder in a non-Mendelian manner.

Confirmed linkage loci are summarized in Table 26.2. From these genome scans and from additional, smaller studies, a picture has emerged in which there are several confirmed BPD linkage regions across the genome. It is highly probable that additional confirmed BPD linkages will be identified through future linkage studies. These BPD linkage regions are confirmed by virtue of at least one study with strong statistical significance ($p < 0.0001$) and at least two confirmatory studies ($p < 0.01$). As noted elsewhere (Berrettini, 2003), in some cases, these confirmed BPD linkage regions overlap with schizophrenia linkage reports, suggesting that the same loci may be involved in some aspects of both disorders.

In an attempt to further elucidate possible BPD linkage regions, two meta-analyses of BPD genome scans have been conducted (Badner and Gershon, 2002; Segurado et al., 2003). Badner and Gershon (2002) analyzed linkage results using a multiple scan probability approach, in which p values are combined across studies, after adjusting for the size of the linkage region. These authors concluded that two genomic regions, 13q32 and

TABLE 26.2 *Linkage Studies of Bipolar Disorder*

Location	*Primary Report*	*Independent Confirmations/Supportive Evidence*	*Evidence from Meta-analyses for Genome-wide Significance*
4q32	Ekholm et al., 2003	Adams et al., 1998; J. Liu et al., 2003; McInnis et al., 2003; Schumacher, Kaneva, et al., 2005	
4p15	Blackwood et al., 1996	Cichon et al., 2001; Detera-Wadleigh et al., 1999; Ewald et al., 2002; Ginns et al., 1998; Morissette et al., 1999	
6q16-24	Middleton et al., 2004	Dick et al., 2003; Ewald et al., 2002; Lambert et al., 2005; Pato et al., 2004; Rice et al., 1997; Schumacher, Kaneva, et al., 2005; Venken et al., 2005	McQueen et al., 2005
8q24	Cichon et al., 2001	Dick et al., 2003; Friddle et al., 2000; McInnis et al., 2003; Park et al., 2004; Segurado et al., 2003	McQueen et al., 2005
12q23	Morissette et al., 1999	Cassidy et al., 2007; Curtis et al., 2003; Dawson et al., 1995; Ekholm et al., 2003; Ewald et al., 2002; Maziade et al., 2001; Shink et al., 2005	
13q21-32	Detera-Wadleigh et al., 1999	Badenhop et al., 2001; Goes et al., 2007; Kelsoe et al., 2001; Liu et al., 2003; Potash, Zandi, et al., 2003	Badner and Gershon, 2002
16p12	Ewald et al., 2002	Dick et al., 2003; Ekholm et al., 2003; Savitz et al., 2007	
18p11.2	Berrettini et al., 1997	Bennett et al., 2002; M.W. Lin et al., 1997; Mukherjee et al., 2006; Nothen et al., 1999; Stine et al., 1995; Turecki et al., 1999a	
18q22	Stine et al., 1995	De bruyn et al., 1996; Fallin et al., 2004; Freimer et al., 1996; Lambert et al., 2005; McInnes et al., 1996; McInnis et al., 2003; McMahon et al., 1997	
21q22	Straub et al., 1994	Aita et al., 1999; Detera-Wadleigh et al., 1996; Kwok et al., 1999; Morissette et al., 1999; Smyth et al., 1996	
22q11-13	Kelsoe et al., 2001	Detera-Wadleigh et al., 1997; Detera-Wadleigh et al., 1999; Lachman et al., 1997	Badner and Gershon, 2002

Only primary linkage studies are shown with genome-wide significance according to Lander and Kruglyak (1995). Negative studies are not shown.

22q11-13, were the most promising loci for BPD. Segurado et al. (2003) used the method of Levinson et al. (2003), which ranks the *p* values across the genome of each study, then sums the rankings for each genomic "bin." In this approach, no genomic region reached genome-wide significance, although the regions which seemed most promising were 9p, 10q, 14q, and the pericentromeric region of chromosome 18 (Segurado et al, 2003).

A combined analysis of 11 previous linkage scans was carried out by McQueen et al. (2005). In contrast to the two previous meta-analyses, the authors used original genotyping data and showed genome-wide significant linkage for BPD on chromosomes 6q and 8q (McQueen et al., 2005). It is likely that several additional linkage loci will be identified in the future; in particular, when large enough sample sizes will allow the analyses of clinical subtypes like psychotic BPD, early onset of illness, or BPD with comorbid panic disorder. These subtypes have been suggested to have a strong heritable component to them (Potash et al., 2001; MacKinnon et al., 2002; Potash et al., 2003; P.I. Lin et al., 2005). Recent genome scans of psychotic BPD, for example, showed promising results to chromosome 9q31 and 8p21 (N. Park et al., 2004; Cheng et al., 2006) and 13q21-33 and 2p11-q14 (Goes et al., 2007). Interestingly, 8p21 and 13q overlap with SZ, further substantiating the concept of shared genomic regions that harbor shared susceptibility factors between BPD and SZ (Berrettini, 2004).

CANDIDATE GENE STUDIES OF BIPOLAR DISORDER

The human genome consists of ~3 billion base pairs of DNA (Venter et al., 2001). The recent completion of draft genomic sequences of the human genome (Venter et al., 2001) is consistent with ~35,000–40,000 genes. Physical distance along the linear sequence of DNA can be expressed in terms of base pairs of DNA. The most common sequence variation in the human genome is a single nucleotide polymorphism (SNP), where there are two different nucleotides (from the possible four, adenine [A], guanine [G], thymidine [T], and cytosine [C]) found among *homo sapiens* at the same position on different chromosomes. Single nucleotide polymorphisms (SNP) with a common minor allele (frequency of ~20%) occur every ~1000 base pairs of DNA (Venter et al., 2001). Analysis of closely spaced SNPs in outbred populations suggests a complex pattern of inheritance in which recombination is inhibited in a small region of DNA, such that blocks of DNA (containing multiple SNPs) tend to be inherited intact over many generations (Gabriel et al., 2002). Thus, blocks of DNA are shared among present-day individuals who may have had a common ancestor 10,000 generations ago. These blocks are variable in length and often contain multiple SNPs, but among outbred human populations, the block length rarely exceeds ~100,000 base pairs. Alleles of SNPs within a block form a haplotype (a set of alleles) that are usually inherited together across many generations. Such SNPs are said to be in strong linkage disequilibrium (LD) with each other. LD refers to the fact that two (or more) alleles can be found together in unrelated individuals more often than predicted by chance. The interested reader is referred to primary reports concerning LD (Gabriel et al., 2002).

LD is a useful tool to investigate the relatively small genomic regions that have been implicated in the genetic origins of BPD through linkage studies (see Table 26.2). In this process, SNPs spaced across genes in the linkage region are assessed in large groups (ideally several hundred at least) of ethnically matched cases and controls. Investigators compare allele and genotype frequencies among groups of cases and controls. If nominally significant differences in allele or genotype frequencies are found between groups, the investigators might conclude that the tested SNP or a variant in close proximity influences risk for BPD.

There have been a multitude of association studies in BPD over the past decade. Most studies have focused on neurotransmitter, neuroendocrine, neurotrophic, and cellular signaling systems. Unfortunately, the nearly complete absence of pathophysiologic data in BPD makes the process of rational candidate gene selection difficult. Additionally, these studies have typically involved smaller numbers of patients with BPD than is optimal, given that the effect size of individual alleles on risk must be small. Although the lack of adequate power of some studies might explain the high degree of nonreplication, other factors such as genetic heterogeneity and population differences further complicate matters. As indicated by the findings of multiple linkage loci, it is likely that there are several candidate genes that in combination contribute to the clinical phenotype of BPD. This paradigm is illustrated in Figure 26.1.

Assume that there are 20 risk alleles, each only contributing a small fraction to the overall risk. To develop BPD, let's suppose one needs five risk alleles. As shown, individual A and B have BPD but share only one risk allele. Individual C has also five risk alleles but shares one risk allele with individual A and one risk allele with individual B. Individual D has also BPD risk alleles but falls in the SZ continuum. This genetic heterogeneity can explain why it is difficult to find universal risk alleles. It is more likely that several sets of risk alleles will contribute to the clinical phenotype. The degree and amount of risk alleles might explain why we

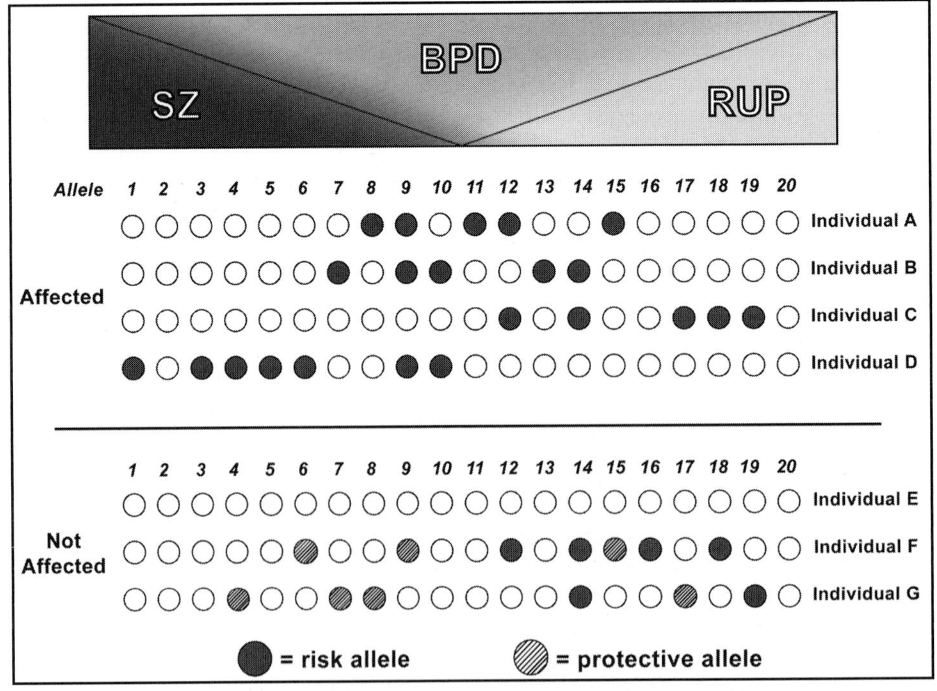

FIGURE 26.1 Model of risk and protective alleles involved in psychiatric disorders.

observe a continuum or spectrum of the bipolar disorders, or psychiatric disorders in general.

As shown for the unaffected group, there are several scenarios that could explain unaffected status. One simple explanation is the lack of risk alleles (individual E), but another possibility includes the presence of protective alleles (as shown for individual F and G in green). Although the majority of past studies have investigated risk alleles, it is becoming increasing clear that complex interactions of genetic risk and protective factors in concert with environmental stimuli contribute to the development of BPD. This observation has been made for example in cancer genetics, with the identification of oncogenes and tumor suppressor genes (Pierotti et al., 2000; B.H. Park and Vogelstein, 2003). Investigation of interaction of protective and susceptibility factors, in addition to complex gene–gene (epistatic) and gene–environment interactions, will be necessary to elucidate the genetic basis of complex behaviors (Feinberg, 2007). Furthermore, epigenetic regulation and mechanisms might influence gene expression without altering the genetic code and could mediate stable changes in brain function (Tsankova et al., 2007). Despite these difficulties and complexities, there are several candidate genes that deserve mention. On a general note, many candidate genes discussed here show also positive results for other psychiatric illnesses such as anxiety disorders, attention-deficit/hyperactivity disorder, psychotic disorders, and substance use disorders, supporting the concept of shared susceptibility factors and comorbidities across diagnostic categories (Fig. 26.1).

D-Amino Acid Oxidase Activator DAOA (G72)/G30

One promising candidate gene is the *G72/G30* locus on 13q32, the site of a confirmed linkage in BPD (see Table 26.2) and SZ (M.W. Lin et al., 1997; Blouin et al., 1998; Shaw et al., 1998; Brzustowicz et al., 1999; Camp et al., 2001; Cardno et al., 2001; Badner and Gershon, 2002; Faraone et al., 2002; Wijsman et al., 2003; Abecasis et al., 2004). *G72* is a primate-specific brain-expressed gene that activates D-amino acid oxidase (Chumakov et al., 2002) and was recently renamed *D-amino acid oxidase activator* (DAOA) (UCSC genome browser; Ensembl genome browser; National Center for Biotechnology Information, http://www.ncbi.nlm.nih.gov). D-amino acid oxidase may control levels of D-serine, which regulates glutamatergic receptors (Stevens et al., 2003), implicated in the pathophysiology of SZ and BPD.

Chumakov et al. (2002) identified a haplotype from *G72* SNPs (without obvious functional significance) that were in LD with SZ in a French Canadian sample. This has been confirmed in distinct SZ populations (Chumakov et al., 2002; Schumacher et al., 2004; Fallin et al., 2005; Williams et al., 2006), although different haplotypes have been associated in different ethnic populations. Similarly, in BPD there have been several positive findings with distinct haplotypes in different populations (Hattori et al., 2003; Chen et al., 2004; Schumacher et al., 2004; Fallin et al., 2005; Williams et al., 2006). A recent meta-analysis combined the published results at this locus and further substantiated the association of *G72/G30* with BPD and SZ (Detera-Wadleigh and McMahon, 2006). Although the *G72/G30* locus is arguably among the best replicated association findings in psychiatric genetics, no clear functional variants have been yet defined at this locus, and the biological relevance of this susceptibility locus remains elusive.

Brain-Derived Neurotrophic Factor (BDNF)

A second promising candidate gene is the *brain-derived neurotrophic factor* (*BDNF*). The *BDNF* gene is located on chromosome 11p13, a region of suggestive linkage for BPD (McInnes et al., 1996; Detera-Wadleigh et al., 1999). Two family-based association studies showed an overtransmission of Val-allele of the functional Val-66Met polymorphism (Neves-Pereira et al., 2002; Sklar et al., 2002). This finding was confirmed in a large case-control association study of unrelated participants with BPD from the National Institute of Mental Health (NIMH) Genetics Initiative (Lohoff et al., 2005). Additional evidence for an association of the Val66Met polymorphism was reported in three small childhood-onset samples: two using a family-based design (Geller et al., 2004; Strauss et al., 2005) and one employing a case-control approach (Strauss et al., 2004). Furthermore, two studies implicate the Val66Met polymorphism to be associated with rapid cycling (Green et al., 2006; Muller et al., 2006). However, there are also several negative findings (Hong et al., 2003; Nakata et al., 2003; Kunugi et al., 2004; Oswald et al., 2004; Skibinska et al., 2004; Neves-Pereira et al., 2005; Green et al., 2006; Surtees et al., 2007). Although some of these studies were likely underpowered, another explanation would be ethnic and clinical differences between samples. It should be also noted that most of the mentioned studies only investigated the Val66Met polymorphism. The *BDNF* gene structure is complex and might harbor several risk alleles in addition to haplotypes conferring risk as shown by Okada et al. (2006). These positive reports are promising because they involve a genetic variant with functional consequences. Egan et al. (2003) demonstrated allele-specific effects on intracellular trafficking and activity-dependent secretion of *BDNF* protein. Recent studies demonstrate a role of the *BDNF* Val66Met polymorphism in cognition (Egan et al., 2003; Hariri et al., 2003; Rybakowski et al., 2003; Rybakowski, Borkowska, Skibinska, and Hauser, 2006;

Rybakowski, Borkowska, Skibinska, Szczepankiewicz, et al., 2006), brain structures (Bueller et al., 2006), and *BDNF* serum levels (Tramontina et al., 2007). Growing evidence suggests that *BDNF* is involved in the etiology of mood disorders (K. Hashimoto et al., 2004; Post, 2007) and depressive personality traits (Lang et al., 2004). Serum levels of *BDNF* were decreased in patients who were depressed when compared to controls (Karege et al., 2002; Shimizu et al., 2003; Aydemir et al., 2005; Gonul et al., 2005) and postmortem brain studies in patients with BPD show decreased *BDNF* protein when compared to controls (Knable et al., 2004). The use of antidepressants, electroconvulsive therapy, and mood stabilizers such as lithium increase *BDNF* gene transcription (Nibuya et al., 1995; Fukumoto et al., 2001; R. Hashimoto et al., 2002), and infusion of *BDNF* into rat brain has a direct antidepressant effect in animal models of depression (Siuciak et al., 1997; Shirayama et al., 2002). Taken together, the convergent evidence from genetic, preclinical, and clinical studies makes *BDNF* a strong candidate for mood disorder.

Monoamine Oxidase A (MAO-A)

There have been numerous independent association studies of BPD and RUP and a Monoamine Oxidase A MAO-A (CA)n repeat polymorphism in European (Craddock et al., 1995; Lim et al., 1995; Nothen et al., 1995; Parsian and Todd, 1997; Furlong et al., 1999; Turecki et al., 1999b; Preisig et al., 2000; Syagailo et al., 2001; Serretti et al., 2002; Muller et al., 2007) and Asian populations (Kawada et al., 1995; Muramatsu et al., 1997; Kunugi et al., 1999).

Those studies reporting a positive association (Kawada et al., 1995; Lim et al., 1995; Furlong et al., 1999; Preisig et al., 2000; Muller et al., 2007) generally detect an overrepresentation of allele 5 or 6 of the MAO-A (CA)n repeat among patients with BPD, compared to controls, an observation that may be particularly evident among women (Deckert et al., 1999; S. Lin et al., 2000; Preisig et al., 2000; Schulze et al., 2000; Gutierrez et al., 2004). The effect size is small, the odds ratio being 1.49 (Preisig et al., 2000), and the sample size required for adequate power to detect is larger than most of the negative studies (Craddock et al., 1995; Lim et al., 1995; Nothen et al., 1995; Parsian and Todd, 1997; Furlong et al., 1999; Turecki et al., 1999b; Preisig et al., 2000; Syagailo et al., 2001; Serretti et al., 2002; Muller et al., 2007). There is also an MAO-A promoter polymorphism (Kunugi et al., 1999). These studies involve multiple ethnic groups, case-control methods, and family-based designs, with some studies having limited power to detect a small effect size. Thus, it is understandable that conflicting studies are reported.

Serotonin Transporter (5HTT)

Another intensively studied candidate gene is the *serotonin transporter* (*5HTT/SLC6A4*), a functional candidate gene for which multiple BPD LD studies have been published. The *5HTT* represents a logical candidate gene, as many antidepressants act through binding to the *5HTT* protein (Ramamoorthy et al., 1993). There are two variants of the *5HTT* that have been studied in BPD, and both have functional significance, based on in vitro analysis of these noncoding polymorphisms. The first variant is an insertion/deletion polymorphism in the promoter region (*5HTTLPR*). The shorter allele has much less transcriptional activity than the longer allele (Collier, Stober, et al., 1996; Heils et al., 1996). Moreover, the shorter allele has been associated with anxiety-related personality traits in humans (Lesch et al., 1996). The second variant is a variable number of tandem repeats (VNTR) polymorphism in intron 2. The two most common alleles are the 10 and 12 repeats, which confer differential transcriptional activity in an embryonic stem cell line (Fiskerstrand et al., 1999).

Collier et al. first reported that the *5HTT* intron 2 VNTR allele 12 was in LD with BPD among patients from the United Kingdom (Collier, Arranz, et al., 1996). Collier et al. also reported that the short allele of the *5HTT* promoter variant was more common among 454 European patients with BPD and patients with RUP, compared to 570 European controls, although the statistical significance was marginal ($p = 0.03$), emphasizing the small effect size involved (Collier, Stober, et al., 1996). Analysis by genotype suggested that homozygosity for the short allele was associated with BPD ($p < 0.05$) and RUP ($p < 0.01$). Since this initial report there have been numerous replication studies with positive (Kunugi et al., 1997; Rees et al., 1997; Bellivier et al., 1998; Vincent et al., 1999; Mynett-Johnson et al., 2000) and negative results (Kunugi et al., 1996; Bellivier et al., 1997; Gutierrez et al., 1998; Hoehe et al., 1998; Bocchetta et al., 1999; Kirov et al., 1999; Oliveira et al., 2000; Ospina-Duque et al., 2000; Saleem et al., 2000; Mendlewicz et al., 2004; Ikeda et al., 2006). Sampling variation and the small effect size coupled with limited power of this sample size are probable explanations for these mixed results.

Furlong et al. (1998) reported results of a meta-analysis for ~1400 individuals of European origin, including 772 controls, 375 patients with BPD, and 299 patients with UP. Although there was no evidence for LD with affective disorders for the VNTR, a marginally significant result was found for the short allele of the *5HTT* promoter polymorphism. This result is important because it suggests that samples in the thousands will be necessary to draw firm conclusions, due to the small effect sizes involved. In another large European study, Mendlewicz et al. (2004) examined the genetic contribution of the *5HTT* promoter polymorphism in a case-control sample, including 539 patients with RUP, 572 patients with BPD, and 821 controls. No evidence of LD was found for RUP or BPD, and subdividing the sample according to family history, suicidal attempts, or psychotic features did not reveal any role of the promoter variant in the genetic susceptibilities to these disorders.

A recent meta-analysis of published population-based and family-based association studies in BPD investigating the *5HTTLPR* and the VNTR polymorphism showed a small effect (odds ratio [OR] = 1.12) of both SNPs (Cho et al., 2005). Lasky-Su et al. (2005) performed a meta-analysis of these SNPs for BPD and RUP and could only document a small effect (OR = 1.13) of the insertion/deletion polymorphism with BPD (Lasky-Su et al., 2005). A recent large scale study of the *5HTTLPR* promoter polymorphism failed to show an association for neuroticism, major depression, or recurrent major depression (Willis-Owen et al., 2005). Taken together, these data suggest a small but significant effect of the 44-bp insertion/deletion polymorphism (*5HTTLPR*) in BPD, whereas the role in major depression remains unclear.

Other Genes and Whole-Genome Association Studies

Several other candidate genes have been investigated in BPD with some positive results for *COMT, DAT, HTR4, DRD4, DRD2, HTR2A, DISC1, P2RX7* (Craddock and Forty, 2006; Hayden and Nurnberger, 2006). Most of these candidate genes were selected based on a priori hypotheses regarding their neurobiological function. This approach of candidate gene selection has obvious limitations given our lack of understanding of the pathophysiology of mood disorders.

With the rapid development of technological advances in genomics, it is now possible to genotype 500,000–1,000,000 SNPs across the genome in cases and normal controls. This "whole-genome association" (WGA) study design has the advantage that no genes are preselected and robust findings might identify new pathways involved in mood disorders. Limitations of this approach are the immense large amount of data, costs, and issues regarding multiple testing. The stringent statistical correction for multiple testing might mask true signals from genes that confer only modest risk of disease (Clark et al., 2005; Jorgenson and Witte, 2006). The first WGA study in BPD using the DNA samples collected through the NIMH Genetic Initiative of Bipolar Disorder (www.nimhgenetics.org) and Germany was recently completed (Baum et al., 2007). The authors studied over 550,000 SNPs in two independent case-control samples of European origin. A total of 88 SNPs located in 80 different genes met criteria for association and replication in both samples. This large number of genes might still be an underestimation of the total number of genes involved in BPD, given the overall small effect size and stringent replication criteria. The strongest association signal was detected in an intron of the *diacylglycerol kinase eta* gene that encodes a key protein in the lithium-sensitive phosphatidyl inositol pathway. The results of the first WGA study in BPD confirm the polygenic nature of this complex trait and furthermore provide evidence for new genes and pathways involved in mood disorders. The recent completion of a WGA study by the Wellcome Trust Case Control Consortium using 14,000 participants with different diseases, including about 2,000 patients with BPD and 3,000 control subjects, confirmed the polygenic nature of a complex disease like BPD (Wellcome Trust Case Control Consortium, 2007). The strongest association signal was observed for an SNP on chromosome 16p12. With further advances in technology and larger sample sizes, it appears likely that some key genetic mechanism and pathways will be identified quite soon. Future studies will have to replicate findings and proof biological consequences, with ultimately improved drug development and patient care.

LINKAGE STUDIES OF RECURRENT UNIPOLAR DISORDERS

There have been relatively few RUP genome scans with > ~100 affected individuals, in contrast to BPD. Holmans et al. (2004) reported on the first phase of a multisite collaborative effort (Recurrent Early-Onset Depression [GenRED] sample). The sample consisted of 297 informative multiplex families (containing 685 informative affected relative pairs, 555 sibling pairs, and 130 other pair types). Affected cases had RUP with onset before age 31 for probands or 41 for other affected relatives; the mean age at onset was 18.5 and the mean number of depressive episodes was 7.3, indicating a highly recurrent form of illness. Families were excluded if there was a BPD first-degree or second-degree relative (Holmans et al., 2004). Linkage was observed on chromosome 15q25.3-26.2 (empirical genome-wide $p = 0.023$). The linkage was not sex specific. This was the sole significant linkage peak observed by this group. In the complete sample of 656 families, genome-wide suggestive linkage was confirmed on chromosome 15q and also observed on chromosomes 17p and 8p in a planned second analysis accounting for the sex of each pair of relatives (Holmans et al., 2007). Fine mapping of the 15q region demonstrated further evidence for linkage (Levinson et al., 2007).

Abkevich et al. (2003) reported a genome scan on 110 Utah pedigrees (each with at least four affected individuals), in which there were 784 individuals with

RUP, 161 persons with single-episode major depressive disorder, and 162 individuals with BPD, who were also considered affected. They observed a highly significant linkage signal at 12q23 (Abkevich et al., 2003), confirming a previously identified BPD locus (see Table 26.2). There were no other linkage peaks approaching statistical significance. It is probable that this study has detected the same BPD 12q23 locus, even though their families were ascertained from a RUP proband, because most kindreds probably did have at least one individual with BPD. These results confirm family and twin studies, suggesting genetic overlap between BPD and RUP disorders, and this study identifies the 12q23 region as a locus that increases risk for BPD and RUP disorders.

Camp et al. (2005) reanalyzed the large Utah pedigrees and excluded relatives with BPD. They considered three alternative phenotypes (major depressive disorder [MDD] age at onset before 31; MDD or anxiety; MDD and anxiety) and identified regions with at least suggestive genome-wide evidence for linkage on chromosomes 3centr, 7p, and 18q (Camp et al., 2005). Interestingly the region identified on 18q with MDD and anxiety is also a well-replicated linkage finding in BPD (see Table 26.2).

Zubenko et al. reported on a genome scan of 81 families ascertained through a proband with early-onset nonpsychotic RUP disorder (Zubenko, Maher, et al., 2003). They described a highly significant linkage ($p < 0.0001$) of this phenotype to 2q35 near marker *D2321*, which is near a candidate gene, *CREB1* (cyclic AMP-response element binding protein 1). Sequence variants in the CREB gene were found to segregate with RUP disorder among women in 2 of these 81 extended kindreds (Zubenko, Hughes, et al., 2003), thus nominating CREB as a RUP susceptibility gene. These intriguing results await independent confirmation.

Another recent genome-wide linkage scan was carried out using 497 sib pairs concordant for recurrent depression excluding BPD. The advantage of affected sib pair design is that it does not require knowledge of mode of inheritance and increased power under certain conditions. Suggestive evidence for linkage was observed on chromosome 1p36, 12q23.3-q24.11, and 13q31.1-q31.3 (McGuffin et al., 2005). The 12q locus has been previously implicated in linkage studies of UP (Abkevich et al., 2003) and BPDs (see Table 26.2 above) whereas the 13q peak lies within a region previously linked strongly to panic disorder (Hamilton et al., 2003).

CANDIDATE GENE STUDIES OF RECURRENT UNIPOLAR DISORDERS

Candidate gene studies of UP depression have received traditionally less attention in the past compared to BPD and SZ. Likely reasons for this discrepancy might be practical limitations given the much smaller expected effect size and a more heterogeneous clinical phenotype. However, with increasing sample sizes, the literature is developing rapidly. As with BPD, there is no universal susceptibility gene for RUP. It can be expected that multiple genes with small effect sizes contribute to RUP. Some of the candidate genes for BPD are also promising genes in RUP, including *BDNF* and *5HTT*. Similar to the search for BPD and SZ genes, whole genome scans for RUP are currently under way. Results are expected in the near future. Several candidate genes show promising preliminary results and are worthwhile mentioning.

Serotonin Transporter (*5HTT*)/Serotonin Receptor 2A (*HTR2A*)

The serotonin transporter gene and genes involved in the serotonergic system are logical candidate genes for susceptibility to depression, given that many antidepressant medications act on these systems. Several studies reported positive associations between variants in the *5HTT* gene and MDD (Collier, Stober, et al., 1996; Rees et al., 1997; W. Liu et al., 1999; Anguelova et al., 2003) whereas others could not confirm results (Kunugi et al., 1997; Bellivier et al., 1998; Furlong et al., 1998; Gutierrez et al., 1998; Hoehe et al., 1998; Oliveira et al., 2000; Minov et al., 2001; Anguelova et al., 2003). Case-control association studies of the *HTR2A* gene and major depression have yielded similar mixed results as for the *5HTT* gene (Anguelova et al., 2003). Because the *5HTT* gene encodes a direct target for antidepressant medications, there has been a great interest in correlating genetic variation to pharmacological treatment response (Malhotra et al., 2004; Serretti et al., 2005; Serretti et al., 2006; Smeraldi et al., 2006). A recent large scale study utilizing DNA samples from 1953 patients with MDD who were treated with citalopram in the Sequenced Treatment Alternatives for Depression (STAR*D) trial investigated genetic predictors for treatment response (McMahon et al., 2006). The authors could not find evidence for *5HTT* variation influencing treatment response; however, they report a significant effect with a marker in the serotonin receptor gene *HTR2A* and treatment outcome. As expected for a single gene, the clinical impact of *HTR2A* on treatment outcome is modest. Although these studies face similar complexities and obstacles as disease candidate gene studies and await replication, this pharmacogenetic approach will likely yield robust results in the near future.

Gene–environment interaction studies have received increasing attention in particular for MDD, given the robust correlation between stressful life events and risk for developing depressive symptoms (Kendler, Kessler, et al., 1995; Repetti et al., 2002; Leckman et al., 2004). In a recent population-based study, Caspi and colleagues noted that individuals with one or more copies of the short allele of the *5HTT* promoter variants were at increased risk for depression depending on the occurrence of adverse life events (Caspi et al., 2003). This article describes a plausible gene–environment interaction that may help explain the conflicting results for the *5HTT* promoter variant noted above. There have been positive (Kendler et al., 2005) and negative (Gillespie et al., 2005; Surtees et al., 2006) replication studies demonstrating the complexity of detecting these effects. Similar gene–environmental interactions have been demonstrated for variants in the *HTR2A* gene and childhood maternal nurturance and depressive symptoms in adulthood (Jokela et al., 2007). Future genetic studies of depression will have to pay close attention to these gene–environmental interactions.

BDNF

There is growing evidence suggesting an important role of *BDNF* in affective disorder (Nestler et al., 2002; Duman and Monteggia, 2006; Post, 2007). Preclinical animal studies have consistently documented a role of *BNDF* on neurogenesis (Duman, 2004), and animal models of depression further substantiate a role of *BNDF* in mood disorders. Decreased *BDNF* levels in hippocampus have been reported in animals exposed to chronic stress (Roceri et al., 2002; Zhang et al., 2002; Kuma et al., 2004; Roceri et al., 2004). Interestingly, administration of antidepressants increased hippocampal *BDNF*, preventing the stress-induced decrease (Nibuya et al., 1995). These findings are intriguing given the hippocampal volume loss observed in mood disorders (Bertolino et al., 2003; Blumberg et al., 2003; Monkul et al., 2003; Videbech and Ravnkilde, 2004). Several recent studies have shown that *BDNF* serum levels are decreased in individuals with mood disorders or depressive personality traits (Karege et al., 2002; Shimizu et al., 2003; Lang et al., 2004; Aydemir et al., 2005; Gonul et al., 2005). Based on these convergent preclinical and clinical data, the *BDNF* gene represents a logical target for genetic investigations of mood disorders.

Although there is stronger literature support for a genetic association between the Val66Met polymorphism in the *BDNF* gene and BPD (see above), several studies have also investigated this SNP in RUP. Results have been similarly mixed as with most other candidate genes for depression. Schumacher et al. (2005) examined 465 individuals with MDD but did not find a significant association with the Val66Met polymorphism. However, there was evidence for a haplotypic association. Surtees et al. (2007) failed to detect an association of the Val66Met polymorphism in 1214 individuals with a history of MDD, whereas studies of this polymorphism in Asian populations showed inconsistent results (Tsai et al., 2003; Hwang et al., 2006; Iga et al., 2007). Despite these mixed and negative results, interpretation of these data should be carried out with caution, given the complex structure of the gene (Okada et al., 2006) and the fact that most studies have only investigated the Val66Met SNP. It is likely that other variation in the *BDNF* gene might influence susceptibility to depression.

Tryptophan Hydroxylase (TPH2)

Tryptophan hydroxylase is the rate-limiting enzyme in brain serotonin synthesis. The discovery of a new brain-specific isoform of the *tryptophan hydroxylase* (*TPH2*) (Walther and Bader, 2003) has generated new interest in the connection between serotonergic systems and depression. The *TPH2* gene is located on chromosome 12q, a region implicated previously in linkage studies of BPD (Dawson et al., 1995; Ewald et al., 1998; Morissette et al., 1999).

Zill et al. (2004) reported first evidence for an association of variants in the *TPH2* gene and major depression. X. Zhang et al. (2005) identified a functional polymorphism (*Arg441His*) that results in approximately 80% loss of function in serotonin production when expressed in a cell system. The authors also reported that this rare mutation was not seen in 219 healthy controls but in 9 of 87 individuals with major depression (X. Zhang et al., 2005). However, subsequent replication attempts by other groups for this rare variant were negative (Garriock et al., 2005; Glatt et al., 2005; Van Den Bogaert et al., 2005; X. Zhang et al., 2005; Zhou, Peters, et al., 2005; Bicalho et al., 2006; Delorme et al., 2006). Haplotypic associations of sets of markers across the *TPH2* gene have yielded positive results (Van Den Bogaert et al., 2006), and interestingly variants were associated with suicidal behavior (De Luca et al., 2004; Zhou, Roy, et al., 2005; Ke et al., 2006; de Lara et al., 2007; Lopez et al., 2007). Deficits in brain serotonin synthesis secondary to genetic variation in the *TPH2* gene might represent an important risk factor for UP major depression.

CONCLUSIONS AND FUTURE DIRECTIONS

Family, twin, and adoption studies of BPD and RUP disorders were reviewed. They are, in general, consistent with substantial heritable components to risk, with the BPDs having higher heritability than the RUP disorders. Multiple regions of the genome (including 18p11, 18q22, 12q24, 21q21, 13q32, 4p15, 4q32, 16p12, 8q24, and 22q11) have been implicated by several independent groups in the genetic origins of BPD. It is likely that most of these regions will yield susceptibility genes within the near future, through the application of LD mapping methods and WGA studies to large sample sizes. LD approaches to candidate genes have yielded several promising candidate genes, including *G72* and *BDNF* for BPD. In addition, molecular genetic studies of various psychiatric phenotypes document shared genomic regions between disorders, indicating a continuum between diagnostic categories rather than dichotomy. Although the field of psychiatric genetics has been plagued by positive and negative replications, promising robust findings are now emerging with potential implications for future clinical practice.

REFERENCES

Abecasis, G.R., Burt, R.A., Hall, D., et al. (2004) Genomewide scan in families with schizophrenia from the founder population of Afrikaners reveals evidence for linkage and uniparental disomy on chromosome 1. *Am. J. Hum. Genet.* 74:403–417.

Abkevich, V., Camp, N.J., Hensel, C.H., et al. (2003) Predisposition locus for major depression at chromosome 12q22-12q23.2. *Am. J. Hum. Genet.* 73:1271–1281.

Adams, L.J., Mitchell, P.B., Fielder, S.L., Rosso, A., Donald, J.A., and Schofield, P.R. (1998) A susceptibility locus for bipolar affective disorder on chromosome 4q35. *Am. J. Hum. Genet.* 62:1084–1091.

Aita, V.M., Liu, J., Knowles, J.A., et al. (1999) A comprehensive linkage analysis of chromosome 21q22 supports prior evidence for a putative bipolar affective disorder locus. *Am. J. Hum. Genet.* 64:210–217.

Allen, M.G., Cohen, S., Pollin, W., and Greenspan, S.I. (1974) Affective illness in veteran twins: a diagnostic review. *Am. J. Psychiatry* 131:1234–1239.

Angst, J., Frey, R., Lohmeyer, B., and Zerbin-Rudin, E. (1980) Bipolar manic-depressive psychoses: results of a genetic investigation. *Hum. Genet.* 55:237–254.

Anguelova, M., Benkelfat, C., and Turecki, G. (2003) A systematic review of association studies investigating genes coding for serotonin receptors and the serotonin transporter: I. Affective disorders. *Mol. Psychiatry* 8:574–591.

Aydemir, O., Deveci, A., and Taneli, F. (2005) The effect of chronic antidepressant treatment on serum brain-derived neurotrophic factor levels in depressed patients: a preliminary study. *Prog. Neuropsychopharmacol. Biol. Psychiatry* 29:261–265.

Badenhop, R.F., Moses, M.J., Scimone, A., et al. (2001) A genome screen of a large bipolar affective disorder pedigree supports evidence for a susceptibility locus on chromosome 13q. *Mol. Psychiatry* 6:396–403.

Badner, J.A., and Gershon, E.S. (2002) Meta-analysis of whole-genome linkage scans of bipolar disorder and schizophrenia. *Mol. Psychiatry* 7:405–411.

Baron, M., Gruen, R., Asnis, L., and Kane, J. (1982) Schizoaffective illness, schizophrenia and affective disorders: morbidity risk and genetic transmission. *Acta Psychiatr. Scand.* 65:253–262.

Baum, A.E., Akula, N., Cabanero, M., et al. (2007) A genome-wide association study implicates diacylglycerol kinase eta (DGKH) and several other genes in the etiology of bipolar disorder. *Mol. Psychiatry* 13(2):197–207.

Bellivier, F., Henry, C., Szoke, A., et al. (1998) Serotonin transporter gene polymorphisms in patients with unipolar or bipolar depression. *Neurosci. Lett.* 255:143–146.

Bellivier, F., Laplanche, J.L., Leboyer, M., et al. (1997) Serotonin transporter gene and manic depressive illness: an association study. *Biol. Psychiatry* 41:750–752.

Bennett, P., Segurado, R., Jones, I., et al. (2002) The Wellcome Trust UK-Irish bipolar affective disorder sibling-pair genome screen: first stage report. *Mol. Psychiatry* 7:189–200.

Berrettini, W. (2002) Review of bipolar molecular linkage and association studies. *Curr. Psychiatry Rep.* 4:124–129.

Berrettini, W. (2003) Evidence for shared susceptibility in bipolar disorder and schizophrenia. *Am. J. Med. Genet.* 123C:59–64.

Berrettini, W. (2004) Bipolar disorder and schizophrenia: convergent molecular data. *Neuromolecular Med.* 5:109–117.

Berrettini, W.H., Ferraro, T.N., Goldin, L.R., et al. (1997) A linkage study of bipolar illness. *Arch. Gen. Psychiatry* 54:27–35.

Bertelsen, A., Harvald, B., and Hauge, M. (1977) A Danish twin study of manic-depressive disorders. *Br. J. Psychiatry* 130:330–351.

Bertolino, A., Frye, M., Callicott, J.H., Mattay, V.S., Rakow, R., Shelton-Repella, J., et al. (2003) Neuronal pathology in the hippocampal area of patients with bipolar disorder: a study with proton magnetic resonance spectroscopic imaging. *Biol. Psychiatry* 53:906–913.

Bicalho, M.A., Pimenta, G.J., Neves, F.S., et al. (2006) Genotyping of the G1463A (Arg441His) TPH2 polymorphism in a geriatric population of patients with major depression. *Mol. Psychiatry* 11:799–800.

Bierut, L.J., Heath, A.C., Bucholz, K.K., et al. (1999) Major depressive disorder in a community-based twin sample: are there different genetic and environmental contributions for men and women? *Arch. Gen. Psychiatry* 56:557–563.

Blackwood, D.H., He, L., Morris, S.W., et al. (1996) A locus for bipolar affective disorder on chromosome 4p. *Nat. Genet.* 12:427–430.

Bland, R.C., Newman, S.C., and Orn, H. (1986) Recurrent and nonrecurrent depression. A family study. *Arch. Gen. Psychiatry* 43:1085–1089.

Blouin, J.L., Dombroski, B.A., Nath, S.K., et al. (1998) Schizophrenia susceptibility loci on chromosomes 13q32 and 8p21. *Nat. Genet.* 20:70–73.

Blumberg, H.P., Kaugman, J., Martin, A., Whiteman, R., Zhang, J.H., Gore, J.C., et al. (2003) Amygdala and hippocampal volumes in adolescents and adults with bipolar disorder. *Arch. Gen. Psychiatry* 60:1201–1208.

Bocchetta, A., Piccardi, M.P., Palmas, M.A., Chillotti, C., Oi, A., and Del Zompo, M. (1999) Family-based association study between bipolar disorder and DRD2, DRD4, DAT, and SERT in Sardinia. *Am. J. Med. Genet.* 88:522–526.

Brzustowicz, L.M., Honer, W.G., Chow, E.W., et al. (1999) Linkage of familial schizophrenia to chromosome 13q32. *Am. J. Hum. Genet.* 65:1096–1103.

Bueller, J.A., Aftab, M., Sen, S., Gomez-Hassan, D., Burmeister, M., and Zubieta, J.K. (2006) BDNF Val66Met allele is associated with reduced hippocampal volume in healthy subjects. *Biol. Psychiatry* 59:812–815.

Cadoret, R.J. (1978) Evidence for genetic inheritance of primary affective disorder in adoptees. *Am. J. Psychiatry* 135:463–466.

Cadoret, R.J., Woolson, R., and Winokur, G. (1977) The relationship of age of onset in unipolar affective disorder to risk of alcoholism and depression in parents. *J. Psychiatr. Res.* 13:137–142.

Camp, N.J., Lowry, M.R., Richards, R.L., et al. (2005) Genomewide linkage analyses of extended Utah pedigrees identifies loci that influence recurrent, early-onset major depression and anxiety disorders. *Am. J. Med. Genet. B Neuropsychiatr. Genet.* 135:85–93.

Camp, N.J., Neuhausen, S.L., Tiobech, J., Polloi, A., Coon, H., and Myles-Worsley, M. (2001) Genomewide multipoint linkage analysis of seven extended Palauan pedigrees with schizophrenia, by a Markov-chain Monte Carlo method. *Am. J. Hum. Genet.* 69:1278–1289.

Cardno, A.G., Holmans, P.A., Rees, M.I., et al. (2001) A genomewide linkage study of age at onset in schizophrenia. *Am. J. Med. Genet.* 105:439–445.

Caspi, A., Sugden, K., Moffitt, T.E., et al. (2003) Influence of life stress on depression: moderation by a polymorphism in the 5-HTT gene. *Science* 301:386–389.

Cassidy, F., Zhao, C., Badger, J., et al. (2007) Genome-wide scan of bipolar disorder and investigation of population stratification effects on linkage: Support for susceptibility loci at 4q21, 7q36, 9p21, 12q24, 14q24, and 16p13. *Am. J. Med. Genet. B Neuropsychiatr. Genet.* 144:791–801.

Chen, Y.S., Akula, N., Detera-Wadleigh, S.D., et al. (2004) Findings in an independent sample support an association between bipolar affective disorder and the G72/G30 locus on chromosome 13q33. *Mol. Psychiatry* 9:87–92; image 5.

Cheng, R., Juo, S.H., Loth, J.E., et al. (2006) Genome-wide linkage scan in a large bipolar disorder sample from the National Institute of Mental Health genetics initiative suggests putative loci for bipolar disorder, psychosis, suicide, and panic disorder. *Mol. Psychiatry* 11:252–260.

Cho, H.J., Meira-Lima, I., Cordeiro, Q., et al. (2005) Population-based and family-based studies on the serotonin transporter gene polymorphisms and bipolar disorder: a systematic review and meta-analysis. *Mol. Psychiatry* 10:771–781.

Chumakov, I., Blumenfeld, M., Guerassimenko, O., et al. (2002) Genetic and physiological data implicating the new human gene G72 and the gene for D-amino acid oxidase in schizophrenia. *Proc. Natl. Acad. Sci. USA* 99:13675–13680.

Cichon, S., Schumacher, J., Muller, D.J., et al. (2001) A genome screen for genes predisposing to bipolar affective disorder detects a new susceptibility locus on 8q. *Hum. Mol. Genet.* 10:2933–2944.

Clark, A.G., Boerwinkle, E., Hixson, J., and Sing, C.F. (2005) Determinants of the success of whole-genome association testing. *Genome Res.* 15:1463–1467.

Collier, D.A., Arranz, M.J., Sham, P., et al. (1996) The serotonin transporter is a potential susceptibility factor for bipolar affective disorder. *Neuroreport* 7:1675–1679.

Collier, D.A., Stober, G., Li, T., et al. (1996) A novel functional polymorphism within the promoter of the serotonin transporter gene: possible role in susceptibility to affective disorders. *Mol. Psychiatry* 1:453–460.

Craddock, N., Daniels, J., Roberts, E., Rees, M., McGuffin, P., and Owen, M.J. (1995) No evidence for allelic association between bipolar disorder and monoamine oxidase A gene polymorphisms. *Am. J. Med. Genet.* 60:322–324.

Craddock, N., and Forty, L. (2006) Genetics of affective (mood) disorders. *Eur. J. Hum. Genet.* 14:660–668.

Curtis, D., Kalsi, G., Brynjolfsson, J., et al. (2003) Genome scan of pedigrees multiply affected with bipolar disorder provides further support for the presence of a susceptibility locus on chromosome 12q23-q24, and suggests the presence of additional loci on 1p and 1q. *Psychiatr. Genet.* 13:77–84.

Dawson, E., Parfitt, E., Roberts, Q., et al. (1995) Linkage studies of bipolar disorder in the region of the Darier's disease gene on chromosome 12q23-24.1. *Am. J. Med. Genet.* 60:94–102.

De bruyn, A., Souery, D., Mendelbaum, K., Mendlewicz, J., and Van Broeckhoven, C. (1996) Linkage analysis of families with bipolar illness and chromosome 18 markers. *Biol. Psychiatry* 39:679–688.

de Lara, C.L., Brezo, J., Rouleau, G., et al. (2007) Effect of tryptophan hydroxylase-2 gene variants on suicide risk in major depression. *Biol. Psychiatry* 62(1):72–80.

De Luca, V., Mueller, D.J., Tharmalingam, S., King, N., and Kennedy, J.L. (2004) Analysis of the novel TPH2 gene in bipolar disorder and suicidality. *Mol. Psychiatry* 9:896–897.

Deckert, J., Catalano, M., Syagailo, Y.V., et al. (1999) Excess of high activity monoamine oxidase A gene promoter alleles in female patients with panic disorder. *Hum. Mol. Genet.* 8:621–624.

Delorme, R., Durand, C.M., Betancur, C., et al. (2006) No human tryptophan hydroxylase-2 gene R441H mutation in a large cohort of psychiatric patients and control subjects. *Biol. Psychiatry* 60:202–203.

Detera-Wadleigh, S.D., Badner, J.A., Berrettini, W.H., et al. (1999) A high-density genome scan detects evidence for a bipolar-disorder susceptibility locus on 13q32 and other potential loci on 1q32 and 18p11.2. *Proc. Natl. Acad. Sci. USA* 96:5604–5609.

Detera-Wadleigh, S.D., Badner, J.A., Goldin, L.R., et al. (1996) Affected-sib-pair analyses reveal support of prior evidence for a susceptibility locus for bipolar disorder, on 21q. *Am. J. Hum. Genet.* 58:1279–1285.

Detera-Wadleigh, S.D., Badner, J.A., Yoshikawa, T., et al. (1997) Initial genome scan of the NIMH genetics initiative bipolar pedigrees: chromosomes 4, 7, 9, 18, 19, 20, and 21q. *Am. J. Med. Genet.* 74:254–262.

Detera-Wadleigh, S.D., and McMahon, F.J. (2006) G72/G30 in schizophrenia and bipolar disorder: review and meta-analysis. *Biol. Psychiatry* 60:106–114.

Dick, D.M., Foroud, T., Flury, L., et al. (2003) Genomewide linkage analyses of bipolar disorder: a new sample of 250 pedigrees from the National Institute of Mental Health Genetics Initiative. *Am. J. Hum. Genet.* 73:107–114.

Duman, R.S. (2004) Role of neurotrophic factors in the etiology and treatment of mood disorders. *Neuromolecular Med.* 5:11–25.

Duman, R.S., and Monteggia, L.M. (2006) A neurotrophic model for stress-related mood disorders. *Biol. Psychiatry* 59:1116–1127.

Egan, M.F., Kojima, M., Callicott, J.H., et al. (2003) The BDNF val66met polymorphism affects activity-dependent secretion of BDNF and human memory and hippocampal function. *Cell* 112:257–269.

Ekholm, J.M., Kieseppa, T., Hiekkalinna, T., et al. (2003) Evidence of susceptibility loci on 4q32 and 16p12 for bipolar disorder. *Hum. Mol. Genet.*12:1907–1915.

Ewald, H., Degn, B., Mors, O., and Kruse, T.A. (1998) Significant linkage between bipolar affective disorder and chromosome 12q24. *Psychiatr. Genet.* 8:131–140.

Ewald, H., Flint, T., Kruse, T.A., and Mors, O. (2002) A genome-wide scan shows significant linkage between bipolar disorder and chromosome 12q24.3 and suggestive linkage to chromosomes 1p22-21, 4p16, 6q14-22, 10q26 and 16p13.3. *Mol. Psychiatry* 7:734–744.

Fallin, M.D., Lasseter, V.K., Avramopoulos, D., et al. (2005) Bipolar I disorder and schizophrenia: a 440-single-nucleotide polymorphism screen of 64 candidate genes among Ashkenazi Jewish case-parent trios. *Am. J. Hum. Genet.* 77:918–936.

Fallin, M.D., Lasseter, V.K., Wolyniec, P.S., et al. (2004) Genome-wide linkage scan for bipolar-disorder susceptibility loci among Ashkenazi Jewish families. *Am. J. Hum. Genet.* 75:204–219.

Faraone, S.V., Skol, A.D., Tsuang, D.W., et al. (2002) Linkage of chromosome 13q32 to schizophrenia in a large veterans affairs cooperative study sample. *Am. J. Med. Genet.* 114:598–604.

Feinberg, A.P. (2007) Phenotypic plasticity and the epigenetics of human disease. *Nature* 447:433–440.

Fiskerstrand, C.E., Lovejoy, E.A., and Quinn, J.P. (1999) An intronic polymorphic domain often associated with susceptibility to affective disorders has allele dependent differential enhancer activity in embryonic stem cells. *FEBS Lett.* 458:171–174.

Freimer, N.B., Reus, V.I., Escamilla, M.A., et al. (1996) Genetic mapping using haplotype, association and linkage methods suggests a locus for severe bipolar disorder (BPI) at 18q22-q23. *Nat. Genet.* 12:436–441.

Friddle, C., Koskela, R., Ranade, K., et al. (2000) Full-genome scan for linkage in 50 families segregating the bipolar affective disease phenotype. *Am. J. Hum. Genet.* 66:205–215.

Fukumoto, T., Morinobu, S., Okamoto, Y., Kagaya, A., and Yamawaki, S. (2001) Chronic lithium treatment increases the expression of brain-derived neurotrophic factor in the rat brain. *Psychopharmacology (Berl)* 158:100–106.

Furlong, R.A., Ho, L., Rubinsztein, J.S., Walsh, C., Paykel, E.S., and Rubinsztein, D.C. (1999) Analysis of the monoamine oxidase A (MAOA) gene in bipolar affective disorder by association studies, meta-analyses, and sequencing of the promoter. *Am. J. Med. Genet.* 88:398–406.

Furlong, R.A., Ho, L., Walsh, C., et al. (1998) Analysis and meta-analysis of two serotonin transporter gene polymorphisms in bipolar and unipolar affective disorders. *Am. J. Med. Genet.* 81:58–63.

Gabriel, S.B., Schaffner, S.F., Nguyen, H., et al. (2002) The structure of haplotype blocks in the human genome. *Science* 296:2225–2229.

Garriock, H.A., Allen, J.J., Delgado, P., et al. (2005) Lack of association of TPH2 exon XI polymorphisms with major depression and treatment resistance. *Mol. Psychiatry* 10:976–977.

Geller, B., Badner, J.A., Tillman, R., Christian, S.L., Bolhofner, K., and Cook, E.H., Jr. (2004) Linkage disequilibrium of the brain-derived neurotrophic factor Val66Met polymorphism in children with a prepubertal and early adolescent bipolar disorder phenotype. *Am. J. Psychiatry* 161:1698–1700.

Gershon, E.S., DeLisi, L.E., Hamovit, J., et al. (1988) A controlled family study of chronic psychoses. Schizophrenia and schizoaffective disorder. *Arch. Gen. Psychiatry* 45:328–336.

Gershon, E.S., Hamovit, J., Guroff, J.J., et al. (1982) A family study of schizoaffective, bipolar I, bipolar II, unipolar, and normal control probands. *Arch. Gen. Psychiatry* 39:1157–1167.

Gershon, E.S., Weissman, M.M., Guroff, J.J., Prusoff, B.A., and Leckman, J.F. (1986) Validation of criteria for major depression through controlled family study. *J. Affect. Disord.* 11:125–131.

Gillespie, N.A., Whitfield, J.B., Williams, B., Heath, A.C., and Martin, N.G. (2005) The relationship between stressful life events, the serotonin transporter (5-HTTLPR) genotype and major depression. *Psychol. Med.* 35:101–111.

Ginns, E.I., St. Jean, P., Philibert, R.A., et al. (1998) A genome-wide search for chromosomal loci linked to mental health wellness in relatives at high risk for bipolar affective disorder among the Old Order Amish. *Proc. Natl. Acad. Sci. USA* 95:15531–15536.

Glatt, C.E., Carlson, E., Taylor, T.R., Risch, N., Reus, V.I., and Schaefer, C.A. (2005) Response to Zhang et al. (2005) loss-of-function mutation in tryptophan hydroxylase-2 identified in unipolar major depression. *Neuron* 45:11–16. *Neuron* 48:704–705; author reply 705–706.

Goes, F.S., Zandi, P.P., Miao, K., et al. (2007) Mood-incongruent psychotic features in bipolar disorder: familial aggregation and suggestive linkage to 2p11-q14 and 13q21-33. *Am. J. Psychiatry* 164:236–247.

Gonul, A.S., Akdeniz, F., Taneli, F., Donat, O., Eker, C., and Vahip, S. (2005) Effect of treatment on serum brain-derived neurotrophic factor levels in depressed patients. *Eur. Arch. Psychiatry Clin. Neurosci.* 255:381–386.

Green, E.K., Raybould, R., Macgregor, S., et al. (2006) Genetic variation of brain-derived neurotrophic factor (BDNF) in bipolar disorder: case-control study of over 3000 individuals from the UK. *Br. J. Psychiatry* 188:21–25.

Gutierrez, B., Arias, B., Gasto, C., et al. (2004) Association analysis between a functional polymorphism in the monoamine oxidase A gene promoter and severe mood disorders. *Psychiatr. Genet.* 14: 203–208.

Gutierrez, B., Arranz, M.J., Collier, D.A., et al. (1998) Serotonin transporter gene and risk for bipolar affective disorder: an association study in Spanish population. *Biol. Psychiatry* 43:843–847.

Hamilton, S.P., Fyer, A.J., Durner, M., et al. (2003) Further genetic evidence for a panic disorder syndrome mapping to chromosome 13q. *Proc. Natl. Acad. Sci. USA* 100:2550–2555.

Hariri, A.R., Goldberg, T.E., Mattay, V.S., et al. (2003) Brain-derived neurotrophic factor val66met polymorphism affects human memory-related hippocampal activity and predicts memory performance. *J. Neurosci.* 23:6690–6694.

Harvald, B., and Hauge, M. (1975) *Genetics and the Epidemiology of Chronic Diseases*, Vol. No. 1163. Washington, DC: PHS Publication.

Hashimoto, K., Shimizu, E., and Iyo, M. (2004) Critical role of brain-derived neurotrophic factor in mood disorders. *Brain Res. Brain Res. Rev.* 45:104–114.

Hashimoto, R., Takei, N., Shimazu, K., Christ, L., Lu, B., and Chuang, D.M. (2002) Lithium induces brain-derived neurotrophic factor and activates TrkB in rodent cortical neurons: an essential step for neuroprotection against glutamate excitotoxicity. *Neuropharmacology* 43:1173–1179.

Hattori, E., Liu, C., Badner, J.A., et al. (2003) Polymorphisms at the G72/G30 gene locus, on 13q33, are associated with bipolar disorder in two independent pedigree series. *Am. J. Hum. Genet.* 72:1131–1140.

Hauser, E.R., Boehnke, M., Guo, S.W., and Risch, N. (1996) Affected-sib-pair interval mapping and exclusion for complex genetic traits: sampling considerations. *Genet. Epidemiol.* 13:117–137.

Hayden, E.P., and Nurnberger, J.I. (2006) Molecular genetics of bipolar disorder. *Genes, Brain Behav.* 5:85–95.

Heils, A., Teufel, A., Petri, S., et al. (1996) Allelic variation of human serotonin transporter gene expression. *J. Neurochem.* 66:2621–2624.

Helzer, J.E., and Winokur, G. (1974) A family interview study of male manic depressives. *Arch. Gen. Psychiatry* 31:73–77.

Hoehe, M.R., Wendel, B., Grunewald, I., et al. (1998) Serotonin transporter (5-HTT) gene polymorphisms are not associated with susceptibility to mood disorders. *Am. J. Med. Genet.* 81:1–3.

Holmans, P., Weissman, M.M., Zubenko, G.S., et al. (2007) Genetics of recurrent early-onset major depression (GenRED) final genome scan report. *Am. J. Psychiatry* 164:248–258.

Holmans, P., Zubenko, G.S., Crowe, R.R., et al. (2004) Genomewide significant linkage to recurrent, early-onset major depressive disorder on chromosome 15q. *Am. J. Hum. Genet.* 74:1154–1167.

Hong, C.J., Huo, S.J., Yen, F.C., Tung, C.L., Pan, G.M., and Tsai, S.J. (2003) Association study of a brain-derived neurotrophic-factor genetic polymorphism and mood disorders, age of onset and suicidal behavior. *Neuropsychobiology* 48:186–189.

Hwang, J.P., Tsai, S.J., Hong, C.J., Yang, C.H., Lirng, J.F., and Yang, Y.M. (2006) The val66met polymorphism of the brain-derived neurotrophic-factor gene is associated with geriatric depression. *Neurobiol. Aging* 27:1834–1837.

Iga, J.I., Ueno, S.I., Yamauchi, K., et al. (2007) The val66met polymorphism of the brain-derived neurotrophic factor gene is associated with psychotic feature and suicidal behavior in Japanese major depressive patients. *Am. J. Med. Genet. B Neuropsychiatr. Genet.* 144(8):1003–1006.

Ikeda, M., Iwata, N., Suzuki, T., et al. (2006) No association of serotonin transporter gene (SLC6A4) with schizophrenia and bipolar disorder in Japanese patients: association analysis based on linkage disequilibrium. *J. Neural Transm.* 113:899–905.

James, N.M., and Chapman, C.J. (1975) A genetic study of bipolar affective disorder. *Br. J. Psychiatry* 126:449–456.

Johnson, G.F., and Leeman, M.M. (1977) Analysis of familial factors in bipolar affective illness. *Arch. Gen. Psychiatry* 34:1074–1083.

Jokela, M., Keltikangas-Jarvinen, L., Kivimaki, M., et al. (2007) Serotonin receptor 2a gene and the influence of childhood maternal nurturance on adulthood depressive symptoms. *Arch. Gen. Psychiatry* 64:356–360.

Jorgenson, E., and Witte, J.S. (2006) A gene-centric approach to genome-wide association studies. *Nat. Rev. Genet.* 7:885–891.

Kallman, F. (1954) *Depression*. New York: Grune and Stratton

Karege, F., Perret, G., Bondolfi, G., Schwald, M., Bertschy, G., and Aubry, J.M. (2002) Decreased serum brain-derived neurotrophic factor levels in major depressed patients. *Psychiatry Res.* 109:143–148.

Kawada, Y., Hattori, M., Dai, X.Y., and Nanko, S. (1995) Possible association between monoamine oxidase A gene and bipolar affective disorder. *Am. J. Hum. Genet.* 56:335–336.

Ke, L., Qi, Z.Y., Ping, Y., and Ren, C.Y. (2006) Effect of SNP at position 40237 in exon 7 of the TPH2 gene on susceptibility to suicide. *Brain Res.* 1122:24–26.

Kelsoe, J.R., Spence, M.A., Loetscher, E., et al. (2001) A genome survey indicates a possible susceptibility locus for bipolar disorder on chromosome 22. *Proc. Natl. Acad. Sci. USA* 98:585–590.

Kendler, K.S., Gardner, C.O., Neale, M.C., and Prescott, C.A. (2001) Genetic risk factors for major depression in men and women: similar or different heritabilities and same or partly distinct genes? *Psychol. Med.* 31:605–616.

Kendler, K.S., Gardner, C.O., and Prescott, C.A. (1999) Clinical characteristics of major depression that predict risk of depression in relatives. *Arch. Gen. Psychiatry* 56:322–327.

Kendler, K.S., Kessler, R.C., Walters, E.E., et al. (1995) Stressful life events, genetic liability, and onset of an episode of major depression in women. *Am. J. Psychiatry* 152:833–842.

Kendler, K.S., Kuhn, J.W., Vittum, J., Prescott, C.A., and Riley, B. (2005) The interaction of stressful life events and a serotonin transporter polymorphism in the prediction of episodes of major depression: a replication. *Arch. Gen. Psychiatry* 62:529–535.

Kendler, K.S., McGuire, M., Gruenberg, A.M., O'Hare, A., Spellman, M., and Walsh, D. (1993) The Roscommon Family Study. I. Methods, diagnosis of probands, and risk of schizophrenia in relatives. *Arch. Gen. Psychiatry* 50:527–540.

Kendler, K.S., Neale, M.C., Kessler, R.C., Heath, A.C., and Eaves, L.J. (1993) The lifetime history of major depression in women. Reliability of diagnosis and heritability. *Arch. Gen. Psychiatry* 50: 863–870.

Kendler, K.S., Neale, M.C., Kessler, R.C., Heath, A.C., and Eaves, L.J. (1994) The clinical characteristics of major depression as indices of the familial risk to illness. *Br. J. Psychiatry* 165:66–72.

Kendler, K.S., Pedersen, N.L., Neale, M.C., and Mathe, A.A. (1995) A pilot Swedish twin study of affective illness including hospital- and population-ascertained subsamples: results of model fitting. *Behav. Genet.* 25:217–232.

Kendler, K.S., and Prescott, C.A. (1999) A population-based twin study of lifetime major depression in men and women. *Arch. Gen. Psychiatry* 56:39–44.

Kirov, G., Rees, M., Jones, I., MacCandless, F., Owen, M.J., and Craddock, N. (1999) Bipolar disorder and the serotonin transporter gene: a family-based association study. *Psychol. Med.* 29: 1249–1254.

Knable, M.B., Barci, B.M., Webster, M.J., Meador-Woodruff, J., and Torrey, E.F. (2004) Molecular abnormalities of the hippocampus in severe psychiatric illness: postmortem findings from the Stanley Neuropathology Consortium. *Mol. Psychiatry* 9:609–620, 544.

Kuma, H., Miki, T., Matsumoto, Y., Gu, H., Li, H.P., Kusaka, T., et al. (2004) Early maternal deprivation induces alterations in brain-derived neurotrophic factor expression in the developing rat hippocampus. *Neurosci. Lett.* 372:68–73.

Kunugi, H., Hattori, M., Kato, T., et al. (1997) Serotonin transporter gene polymorphisms: ethnic difference and possible association with bipolar affective disorder. *Mol. Psychiatry* 2:457–462.

Kunugi, H., Iijima, Y., Tatsumi, M., et al. (2004) No association between the Val66Met polymorphism of the brain-derived neurotrophic factor gene and bipolar disorder in a Japanese population: a multicenter study. *Biol. Psychiatry* 56:376–378.

Kunugi, H., Ishida, S., Kato, T., et al. (1999) A functional polymorphism in the promoter region of monoamine oxidase-A gene and mood disorders. *Mol. Psychiatry* 4:393–395.

Kunugi, H., Tatsumi, M., Sakai, T., Hattori, M., and Nanko, S. (1996) Serotonin transporter gene polymorphism and affective disorder. *Lancet* 347:1340–1341.

Kupfer, D.J., Frank, E., Carpenter, L.L., and Neiswanger, K. (1989) Family history in recurrent depression. *J. Affect. Disord.* 17:113–119.

Kwok, J.B., Adams, L.J., Salmon, J.A., Donald, J.A., Mitchell, P.B., and Schofield, P.R. (1999) Nonparametric simulation-based statistical analyses for bipolar affective disorder locus on chromosome 21q22.3. *Am. J. Med. Genet.* 88:99–102.

Lachman, H.M., Kelsoe, J.R., Remick, R.A., et al. (1997) Linkage studies suggest a possible locus for bipolar disorder near the velo-cardio-facial syndrome region on chromosome 22. *Am. J. Med. Genet.* 74:121–128.

Lambert, D., Middle, F., Hamshere, M.L., et al. (2005) Stage 2 of the Wellcome Trust UK-Irish bipolar affective disorder sibling-pair genome screen: evidence for linkage on chromosomes 6q16-q21, 4q12-q21, 9p21, 10p14-p12 and 18q22. *Mol. Psychiatry* 10:831–841.

Lander, E., and Kruglyak, L. (1995) Genetic dissection of complex traits: guidelines for interpreting and reporting linkage results. *Nat. Genet.* 11:241–247.

Lang, U.E., Hellweg, R., and Gallinat, J. (2004) BDNF serum concentrations in healthy volunteers are associated with depression-related personality traits. *Neuropsychopharmacology* 29:795–798.

Lasky-Su, J.A., Faraone, S.V., Glatt, S.J., and Tsuang, M.T. (2005) Meta-analysis of the association between two polymorphisms in the serotonin transporter gene and affective disorders. *Am. J. Med. Genet. B Neuropsychiatr. Genet.* 133:110–115.

Leckman, J.F., Feldman, R., Swain, J.E., Eicher, V., Thompson, N., and Mayes, L.C. (2004) Primary parental preoccupation: circuits, genes, and the crucial role of the environment. *J. Neural Transm.* 111:753–771.

Lesch, K.P., Bengel, D., Heils, A., et al. (1996) Association of anxiety-related traits with a polymorphism in the serotonin transporter gene regulatory region. *Science* 274:1527–1531.

Levinson, D.F., Evgrafov, O.V., Knowles, J.A., et al. (2007) Genetics of recurrent early-onset major depression (GenRED) significant linkage on chromosome 15q25-q26 after fine mapping with single nucleotide polymorphism markers. *Am. J. Psychiatry* 164: 259–264.

Levinson, D.F., Levinson, M.D., Segurado, R., and Lewis, C.M. (2003) Genome scan meta-analysis of schizophrenia and bipolar disorder, part I: Methods and power analysis. *Am. J. Hum. Genet.* 73:17–33.

Lim, L.C., Powell, J., Sham, P., et al. (1995) Evidence for a genetic association between alleles of monoamine oxidase A gene and bipolar affective disorder. *Am. J. Med. Genet.* 60:325–331.

Lin, M.W., Sham, P., Hwu, H.G., Collier, D., Murray, R., and Powell, J.F. (1997) Suggestive evidence for linkage of schizophrenia to markers on chromosome 13 in Caucasian but not Oriental populations. *Hum. Genet.* 99:417–420.

Lin, P.I., McInnis, M.G., Potash, J.B., et al. (2005) Assessment of the effect of age at onset on linkage to bipolar disorder: evidence on chromosomes 18p and 21q. *Am. J. Hum. Genet.* 77:545–555.

Lin, S., Jiang, S., Wu, X., et al. (2000) Association analysis between mood disorder and monoamine oxidase gene. *Am. J. Med. Genet.* 96:12–14.

Liu, J., Juo, S.H., Dewan, A., et al. (2003) Evidence for a putative bipolar disorder locus on 2p13-16 and other potential loci on 4q31, 7q34, 8q13, 9q31, 10q21-24, 13q32, 14q21 and 17q11-12. *Mol. Psychiatry* 8:333–342.

Liu, W., Gu, N., Feng, G., et al. (1999) Tentative association of the serotonin transporter with schizophrenia and unipolar depression but not with bipolar disorder in Han Chinese. *Pharmacogenetics* 9:491–495.

Lohoff, F.W., Sander, T., Ferraro, T.N., Dahl, J.P., Gallinat, J., and Berrettini, W.H. (2005) Confirmation of association between the Val66Met polymorphism in the brain-derived neurotrophic factor (BDNF) gene and bipolar I disorder. *Am. J. Med. Genet. B Neuropsychiatr. Genet.* 139:51–53.

Lopez, V.A., Detera-Wadleigh, S., Cardona, I., Kassem, L., and McMahon, F.J. (2007) Nested association between genetic variation in tryptophan hydroxylase II, bipolar affective disorder, and suicide attempts. *Biol. Psychiatry* 61:181–186.

Luxenberger, H. (1930) Psychiatrisch-neurologische Zwillings pathologie. *Zentralblatt fur diagesamte Neurologie and Psychiatrie* 14: 145–180.

Lyons, M.J., Eisen, S.A., Goldberg, J., et al. (1998) A registry-based twin study of depression in men. *Arch. Gen. Psychiatry* 55:468–472.

MacKinnon, D.F., Zandi, P.P., Cooper, J., et al. (2002) Comorbid bipolar disorder and panic disorder in families with a high prevalence of bipolar disorder. *Am. J. Psychiatry* 159:30–35.

Maier, W., Lichtermann, D., Minges, J., et al. (1993) Continuity and discontinuity of affective disorders and schizophrenia. Results of a controlled family study. *Arch. Gen. Psychiatry* 50:871–883.

Maier, W., Lichtermann, D., Minges, J., Heun, R., Hallmayer, J., and Benkert, O. (1992) Schizoaffective disorder and affective disorders with mood-incongruent psychotic features: keep separate or combine? Evidence from a family study. *Am. J. Psychiatry* 149: 1666–1673.

Malhotra, A.K., Murphy, G.M., Jr., and Kennedy, J.L. (2004) Pharmacogenetics of Psychotropic Drug Response. *Am. J. Psychiatry* 161:780–796.

Maziade, M., Roy, M.A., Rouillard, E., et al. (2001) A search for specific and common susceptibility loci for schizophrenia and bipolar disorder: a linkage study in 13 target chromosomes. *Mol. Psychiatry* 6:684–693.

McGuffin, P., Katz, R., Watkins, S., and Rutherford, J. (1996) A hospital-based twin register of the heritability of DSM-IV unipolar depression. *Arch. Gen. Psychiatry* 53:129–136.

McGuffin, P., Knight, J., Breen, G., et al. (2005) Whole genome linkage scan of recurrent depressive disorder from the depression network study. *Hum. Mol. Genet.* 14:3337–3345.

McGuffin, P., Rijsdijk, F., Andrew, M., Sham, P., Katz, R., and Cardno, A. (2003) The heritability of bipolar affective disorder and the genetic relationship to unipolar depression. *Arch. Gen. Psychiatry* 60:497–502.

McInnes, L.A., Escamilla, M.A., Service, S.K., et al. (1996) A complete genome screen for genes predisposing to severe bipolar disorder in two Costa Rican pedigrees. *Proc. Natl. Acad. Sci. USA* 93:13060–13065.

McInnis, M.G., Lan, T.H., Willour, V.L., et al. (2003) Genome-wide scan of bipolar disorder in 65 pedigrees: supportive evidence for linkage at 8q24, 18q22, 4q32, 2p12, and 13q12. *Mol. Psychiatry* 8:288–298.

McMahon, F.J., Buervenich, S., Charney, D., et al. (2006) Variation in the gene encoding the serotonin 2A receptor is associated with outcome of antidepressant treatment. *Am. J. Hum. Genet.* 78:804–814.

McMahon, F.J., Hopkins, P.J., Xu, J., et al. (1997) Linkage of bipolar affective disorder to chromosome 18 markers in a new pedigree series. *Am. J. Hum. Genet.* 61:1397–1404.

McQueen, M.B., Devlin, B., Faraone, S.V., et al. (2005) Combined analysis from eleven linkage studies of bipolar disorder provides strong evidence of susceptibility loci on chromosomes 6q and 8q. *Am. J. Hum. Genet.* 77:582–595.

Mendlewicz, J., and Baron, M. (1981) Morbidity risks in subtypes of unipolar depressive illness: differences between early and late onset forms. *Br. J. Psychiatry* 139:463–466.

Mendlewicz, J., Massat, I., Souery, D., et al. (2004) Serotonin transporter 5HTTLPR polymorphism and affective disorders: no evidence of association in a large European multicenter study. *Eur. J. Hum. Genet.* 12:377–382.

Mendlewicz, J., and Rainer, J.D. (1977) Adoption study supporting genetic transmission in manic--depressive illness. *Nature* 268: 327–329.

Merikangas, K.R., Risch, N.J., and Weissman, M.M. (1994) Comorbidity and co-transmission of alcoholism, anxiety and depression. *Psychol. Med.* 24:69–80.

Middleton, F.A., Pato, M.T., Gentile, K.L., et al. (2004) Genome-wide linkage analysis of bipolar disorder by use of a high-density single-nucleotide-polymorphism (SNP) genotyping assay: a comparison with microsatellite marker assays and finding of significant linkage to chromosome 6q22. *Am. J. Hum. Genet.* 74:886–897.

Minov, C., Baghai, T.C., Schule, C., et al. (2001) Serotonin-2A-receptor and -transporter polymorphisms: lack of association in patients with major depression. *Neurosci. Lett.* 303:119–122.

Moldin, S.O., Reich, T., and Rice, J.P. (1991) Current perspectives on the genetics of unipolar depression. *Behav. Genet.* 21:211–242.

Monkul, E.S., Malhi, G.S., and Soares, J.C. (2003) Mood disorder—review of structural MRI studies. *Acta Neuropsychiatrica* 15: 368–380.

Morissette, J., Villeneuve, A., Bordeleau, L., et al. (1999) Genome-wide search for linkage of bipolar affective disorders in a very large pedigree derived from a homogeneous population in Quebec points to a locus of major effect on chromosome 12q23-q24. *Am. J. Med. Genet.* 88:567–587.

Mukherjee, O., Meera, P., Ghosh, S., et al. (2006) Evidence of linkage and association on 18p11.2 for psychosis. *Am. J. Med. Genet. B Neuropsychiatr. Genet.* 141B:868–873.

Muller, D.J., de Luca, V., Sicard, T., King, N., Strauss, J., and Kennedy, J.L. (2006) Brain-derived neurotrophic factor (BDNF) gene and rapid-cycling bipolar disorder: family-based association study. *Br. J. Psychiatry* 189:317–323.

Muller, D.J., Serretti, A., Sicard, T., et al. (2007) Further evidence of MAO-A gene variants associated with bipolar disorder. *Am. J. Med. Genet. B Neuropsychiatr. Genet.* 144:37–40.

Muramatsu, T., Matsushita, S., Kanba, S., et al. (1997) Monoamine oxidase genes polymorphisms and mood disorder. *Am. J. Med. Genet.* 74:494–496.

Mynett-Johnson, L., Kealey, C., Claffey, E., et al. (2000) Multimarkerhaplotypes within the serotonin transporter gene suggest evidence of an association with bipolar disorder. *Am. J. Med. Genet.* 96:845–849.

Nakata, K., Ujike, H., Sakai, A., et al. (2003) Association study of the brain-derived neurotrophic factor (BDNF) gene with bipolar disorder. *Neurosci. Lett.* 337:17–20.

Nestler, E.J., Barrot, M., DiLeone, R.J., Eisch, A.J., Gold, S.J., and Monteggia, L.M. (2002) Neurobiology of depression. *Neuron* 34:13–25.

Neves-Pereira, M., Cheung, J.K., Pasdar, A., et al. (2005) BDNF gene is a risk factor for schizophrenia in a Scottish population. *Mol. Psychiatry* 10:208–212.

Neves-Pereira, M., Mundo, E., Muglia, P., King, N., Macciardi, F., and Kennedy, J.L. (2002) The brain-derived neurotrophic factor gene confers susceptibility to bipolar disorder: evidence from a family-based association study. *Am. J. Hum. Genet.* 71:651–655.

Nibuya, M., Morinobu, S., and Duman, R.S. (1995) Regulation of BDNF and trkB mRNA in rat brain by chronic electroconvulsive seizure and antidepressant drug treatments. *J. Neurosci.* 15: 7539–7547.

Nothen, M.M., Cichon, S., Rohleder, H., et al. (1999) Evaluation of linkage of bipolar affective disorder to chromosome 18 in a sample of 57 German families. *Mol. Psychiatry* 4:76–84.

Nothen, M.M., Eggermann, K., Albus, M., et al. (1995) Association analysis of the monoamine oxidase A gene in bipolar affective disorder by using family-based internal controls. *Am. J. Hum. Genet.* 57:975–978.

Nurnberger, J.I., Jr., Foroud, T., Flury, L., Meyer, E.T., and Wiegand, R. (2002) Is there a genetic relationship between alcoholism and depression? *Alcohol Res. Health* 26:233–240.

Okada, T., Hashimoto, R., Numakawa, T., et al. (2006) A complex polymorphic region in the brain-derived neurotrophic factor (BDNF) gene confers susceptibility to bipolar disorder and affects transcriptional activity. *Mol. Psychiatry* 11:695–703.

Oliveira, J.R., Carvalho, D.R., Pontual, D., et al. (2000) Analysis of the serotonin transporter polymorphism (5-HTTLPR) in Brazilian patients affected by dysthymia, major depression and bipolar disorder. *Mol. Psychiatry* 5:348–349.

Ospina-Duque, J., Duque, C., Carvajal-Carmona, L., et al. (2000) An association study of bipolar mood disorder (type I) with the 5-HTTLPR serotonin transporter polymorphism in a human population isolate from Colombia. *Neurosci. Lett.* 292:199–202.

Oswald, P., Del-Favero, J., Massat, I., et al. (2004) Non-replication of the brain-derived neurotrophic factor (BDNF) association in bipolar affective disorder: a Belgian patient-control study. *Am. J. Med. Genet.* 129B:34–35.

Park, B.H., and Vogelstein, B. (2003) Tumor-suppressor genes. In: Kufe, D.W., Pollock, R.E., Weichselbaum, R.R., Bast, R.C., Jr., Gansler, T. S. eds. *Cancer Medicine*, 6th ed. Lewiston, NY: BC Decker, pp. 87–106.

Park, N., Juo, S.H., Cheng, R., et al. (2004) Linkage analysis of psychosis in bipolar pedigrees suggests novel putative loci for bipolar disorder and shared susceptibility with schizophrenia. *Mol. Psychiatry* 9:1091–1099.

Parsian, A., and Todd, R.D. (1997) Genetic association between monoamine oxidase and manic-depressive illness: comparison of relative risk and haplotype relative risk data. *Am. J. Med. Genet.* 74: 475–479.

Pato, C.N., Pato, M.T., Kirby, A., et al. (2004) Genome-wide scan in Portuguese Island families implicates multiple loci in bipolar disorder: fine mapping adds support on chromosomes 6 and 11. *Am. J. Med. Genet. B Neuropsychiatr. Genet.* 127:30–34.

Pierotti, N.S., Schichman, S.A., Sozzi, G., and Croce, C.M. (2000) *Oncogenes*. Hamilton, Canada: BC Decker Inc.

Post, R.M. (2007) Role of BDNF in bipolar and unipolar disorder: clinical and theoretical implications. *J. Psychiatr. Res.* 41(12): 979–990.

Potash, J.B., Chiu, Y.F., MacKinnon, D.F., et al. (2003) Familial aggregation of psychotic symptoms in a replication set of 69 bipolar disorder pedigrees. *Am. J. Med. Genet. B Neuropsychiatr. Genet.* 116:90–97.

Potash, J.B., Willour, V.L., Chiu, Y.F., et al. (2001) The familial aggregation of psychotic symptoms in bipolar disorder pedigrees. *Am. J. Psychiatry* 158:1258–1264.

Potash, J.B., Zandi, P.P., Willour, V.L., et al. (2003) Suggestive linkage to chromosomal regions 13q31 and 22q12 in families with psychotic bipolar disorder. *Am. J. Psychiatry* 160:680–686.

Preisig, M., Bellivier, F., Fenton, B.T., et al. (2000) Association between bipolar disorder and monoamine oxidase A gene polymorphisms: results of a multicenter study. *Am. J. Psychiatry* 157:948–955.

Ramamoorthy, S., Bauman, A.L., Moore, K.R., et al. (1993) Antidepressant- and cocaine-sensitive human serotonin transporter: molecular cloning, expression, and chromosomal localization. *Proc. Natl. Acad. Sci. USA* 90:2542–2546.

Rees, M., Norton, N., Jones, I., et al. (1997) Association studies of bipolar disorder at the human serotonin transporter gene (hSERT; 5HTT). *Mol. Psychiatry* 2:398–402.

Reich, T., Van Eerdewegh, P., Rice, J., Mullaney, J., Endicott, J., and Klerman, G.L. (1987) The familial transmission of primary major depressive disorder. *J. Psychiatr. Res.* 21:613–624.

Repetti, R.L., Taylor, S.E., and Seeman, T.E. (2002) Risky families: family social environments and the mental and physical health of offspring. *Psychol. Bull.* 128:330–366.

Rice, J.P., Goate, A., Williams, J.T., et al. (1997) Initial genome scan of the NIMH genetics initiative bipolar pedigrees: chromosomes 1, 6, 8, 10, and 12. *Am. J. Med. Genet.* 74:247–253.

Roceri, M., Cirulli, F., Pessina, C., Peretto, P., Racagni, G., and Riva, M.A. (2004) Postnatal repeated maternal deprivation produces age-dependent changes of brain-derived neurotrophic factor expression in selected rat brain regions. *Biol. Psychiatry* 55:708–714.

Roceri, M., Hendriks, W., Racagni, G., Ellenbroek, B.A., and Riva, M.A. (2002) Early maternal deprivation reduces the expression of BDNF and NMDA receptor subunits in rat hippoampus. *Mol. Psychiatry* 7:609–616.

Rosanoff, A.J., Handy, L., and Plesset, I.R. (1935) The etiology of manic-depressive syndromes with special reference to their occurrence in twins. *Am. J. Psychiatry* 91:725–762.

Rybakowski, J.K., Borkowska, A., Czerski, P.M., Skibinska, M., and Hauser, J. (2003) Polymorphism of the brain-derived neurotrophic factor gene and performance on a cognitive prefrontal test in bipolar patients. *Bipolar Disord.* 5:468–472.

Rybakowski, J.K., Borkowska, A., Skibinska, M., and Hauser, J. (2006) Illness-specific association of val66met BDNF polymorphism with performance on Wisconsin Card Sorting Test in bipolar mood disorder. *Mol. Psychiatry* 11:122–124.

Rybakowski, J.K., Borkowska, A., Skibinska, M., Szczepankiewicz, A., et al. (2006) Prefrontal cognition in schizophrenia and bipolar illness in relation to Val66Met polymorphism of the brain-derived neurotrophic factor gene. *Psychiatry Clin. Neurosci.* 60:70–76.

Saleem, Q., Ganesh, S., Vijaykumar, M., Reddy, Y.C., Brahmachari, S.K., and Jain, S. (2000) Association analysis of 5HT transporter gene in bipolar disorder in the Indian population. *Am. J. Med. Genet.* 96:170–172.

Savitz, J., Cupido, C.L., and Ramesar, R.K. (2007) Preliminary evidence for linkage to chromosome 1q31-32, 10q23.3, and 16p13.3 in a South African cohort with bipolar disorder. *Am. J. Med. Genet. B Neuropsychiatr. Genet.* 144:383–387.

Schulze, T.G., Muller, D.J., Krauss, H., et al. (2000) Association between a functional polymorphism in the monoamine oxidase A gene promoter and major depressive disorder. *Am. J. Med. Genet.* 96:801–803.

Schumacher, J., Jamra, R.A., Becker, T., et al. (2005) Evidence for a relationship between genetic variants at the brain-derived neurotrophic factor (BDNF) locus and major depression. *Biol. Psychiatry* 58:307–314.

Schumacher, J., Jamra, R.A., Freudenberg, J., et al. (2004) Examination of G72 and D-amino-acid oxidase as genetic risk factors for schizophrenia and bipolar affective disorder. *Mol. Psychiatry* 9:203–207.

Schumacher, J., Kaneva, R., Jamra, R.A., et al. (2005) Genomewide scan and fine-mapping linkage studies in four European samples with bipolar affective disorder suggest a new susceptibility locus on chromosome 1p35-p36 and provides further evidence of loci on chromosome 4q31 and 6q24. *Am. J. Hum. Genet.* 77:1102–1111.

Segurado, R., Detera-Wadleigh, S.D., Levinson, D.F., et al. (2003) Genome scan meta-analysis of schizophrenia and bipolar disorder, part III: Bipolar disorder. *Am. J. Hum. Genet.* 73:49–62.

Serretti, A., Benedetti, F., Zanardi, R., and Smeraldi, E. (2005) The influence of Serotonin Transporter Promoter Polymorphism (SERTPR) and other polymorphisms of the serotonin pathway on the efficacy of antidepressant treatments. *Prog. Neuropsychopharmacol. Biol. Psychiatry* 29:1074–1084.

Serretti, A., Cristina, S., Lilli, R., et al. (2002) Family-based association study of 5-HTTLPR, TPH, MAO-A, and DRD4 polymorphisms in mood disorders. *Am. J. Med. Genet.* 114:361–369.

Serretti, A., Cusin, C., Rausch, J.L., Bondy, B., and Smeraldi, E. (2006) Pooling pharmacogenetic studies on the serotonin transporter: a mega-analysis. *Psychiatry Res.* 145:61–65.

Shaw, S.H., Kelly, M., Smith, A.B., et al. (1998) A genome-wide search for schizophrenia susceptibility genes. *Am. J. Med. Genet.* 81:364–376.

Shimizu, E., Hashimoto, K., Okamura, N., et al. (2003) Alterations of serum levels of brain-derived neurotrophic factor (BDNF) in depressed patients with or without antidepressants. *Biol. Psychiatry* 54:70–75.

Shink, E., Morissette, J., Sherrington, R., and Barden, N. (2005) A genome-wide scan points to a susceptibility locus for bipolar disorder on chromosome 12. *Mol. Psychiatry* 10:545–552.

Shirayama, Y., Chen, A.C., Nakagawa, S., Russell, D.S., and Duman, R.S. (2002) Brain-derived neurotrophic factor produces antidepressant effects in behavioral models of depression. *J. Neurosci.* 22:3251–3261.

Siuciak, J.A., Lewis, D.R., Wiegand, S.J., and Lindsay, R.M. (1997) Antidepressant-like effect of brain-derived neurotrophic factor (BDNF). *Pharmacol. Biochem. Behav.* 56:131–137.

Skibinska, M., Hauser, J., Czerski, P.M., et al. (2004) Association analysis of brain-derived neurotrophic factor (BDNF) gene Val66Met polymorphism in schizophrenia and bipolar affective disorder. *World J. Biol. Psychiatry* 5:215–220.

Sklar, P., Gabriel, S.B., McInnis, M.G., et al. (2002) Family-based association study of 76 candidate genes in bipolar disorder: BDNF is a potential risk locus. Brain-derived neutrophic factor. *Mol. Psychiatry* 7:579–593.

Slater, E. (1936) The inheritance of manic-depressive insanity. *Proc. R. Soc. Med.* 29:981–990.

Smeraldi, E., Serretti, A., Artioli, P., Lorenzi, C., and Catalano, M. (2006) Serotonin transporter gene-linked polymorphic region: possible pharmacogenetic implications of rare variants. *Psychiatr. Genet.* 16:153–158.

Smith, M.A., Makino, S., Kvetnansky, R., and Post, R.M. (1995) Effects of stress on neurotrophic factor expression in the rat brain. *Ann. N.Y. Acad. Sci.* 771:234–239.

Smyth, C., Kalsi, G., Brynjolfsson, J., et al. (1996) Further tests for linkage of bipolar affective disorder to the tyrosine hydroxylase gene locus on chromosome 11p15 in a new series of multiplex British affective disorder pedigrees. *Am. J. Psychiatry* 153:271–274.

Stancer, H.C., Persad, E., Wagener, D.K., and Jorna, T. (1987) Evidence for homogeneity of major depression and bipolar affective disorder. *J. Psychiatr. Res.* 21:37–53.

Stevens, E.R., Esguerra, M., Kim, P.M., et al. (2003) D-serine and serine racemase are present in the vertebrate retina and contribute to the physiological activation of NMDA receptors. *Proc. Natl. Acad. Sci. USA* 100:6789–6794.

Stine, O.C., Xu, J., Koskela, R., et al. (1995) Evidence for linkage of bipolar disorder to chromosome 18 with a parent-of-origin effect. *Am. J. Hum. Genet.* 57:1384–1394.

Straub, R.E., Lehner, T., Luo, Y., et al. (1994) A possible vulnerability locus for bipolar affective disorder on chromosome 21q22.3. *Nat. Genet.* 8:291–296.

Strauss, J., Barr, C.L., George, C.J., et al. (2004) Association study of brain-derived neurotrophic factor in adults with a history of childhood onset mood disorder. *Am. J. Med. Genet.* 131B(1): 16–19.

Strauss, J., Barr, C.L., George, C.J., et al. (2005) Brain-derived neurotrophic factor variants are associated with childhood-onset mood disorder: confirmation in a Hungarian sample. *Mol. Psychiatry* 10:861–867.

Suarez, B.H., Hampe, C.L., and Van Eerdewegh, P. (1994) *Problems of replicating linkage claims in psychiatry*. Washington, DC: American Psychiatric Press.

Sullivan, P.F., Neale, M.C., and Kendler, K.S. (2000) Genetic epidemiology of major depression: review and meta-analysis. *Am. J. Psychiatry* 157:1552–1562.

Surtees, P.G., Wainwright, N.W., Willis-Owen, S.A., et al. (2007) No association between the BDNF Val66Met polymorphism and mood status in a non-clinical community sample of 7389 older adults. *J. Psychiatr. Res.* 41:404–409.

Surtees, P.G., Wainwright, N.W., Willis-Owen, S.A., Luben, R., Day, N.E., and Flint, J. (2006) Social adversity, the serotonin transporter (5-HTTLPR) polymorphism and major depressive disorder. *Biol. Psychiatry* 59:224–229.

Syagailo, Y.V., Stober, G., Grassle, M., et al. (2001) Association analysis of the functional monoamine oxidase A gene promoter polymorphism in psychiatric disorders. *Am. J. Med. Genet.* 105: 168–171.

Taylor, M.A., Berenbaum, S.A., Jampala, V.C., and Cloninger, C.R. (1993) Are schizophrenia and affective disorder related? preliminary data from a family study. *Am. J. Psychiatry* 150:278–285.

Torgersen, S. (1986) Genetic factors in moderately severe and mild affective disorders. *Arch. Gen. Psychiatry* 43:222–226.

Tramontina, J., Frey, B.N., Andreazza, A.C., Zandona, M., Santin, A., and Kapczinski, F. (2007) Val66met polymorphism and serum brain-derived neurotrophic factor levels in bipolar disorder. *Mol. Psychiatry* 12:230–231.

Tsai, S.J., Cheng, C.Y., Yu, Y.W., Chen, T.J., and Hong, C.J. (2003) Association study of a brain-derived neurotrophic-factor genetic polymorphism and major depressive disorders, symptomatology, and antidepressant response. *Am. J. Med. Genet. B Neuropsychiatr. Genet.* 123:19–22.

Tsankova, N., Renthal, W., Kumar, A., and Nestler, E.J. (2007) Epigenetic regulation in psychiatric disorders. *Nat. Rev. Neurosci.* 8:355–367.

Tsuang, M.T., Taylor, L., and Faraone, S.V. (2004) An overview of the genetics of psychotic mood disorders. *J. Psychiatr. Res.* 38:3–15.

Tsuang, M.T., Winokur, G., and Crowe, R.R. (1980) Morbidity risks of schizophrenia and affective disorders among first degree relatives of patients with schizophrenia, mania, depression and surgical conditions. *Br. J. Psychiatry* 137:497–504.

Turecki, G., Grof, P., Cavazzoni, P., et al. (1999a) Lithium responsive bipolar disorder, unilineality, and chromosome 18: A linkage study. *Am. J. Med. Genet.* 88:411–415.

Turecki, G., Grof, P., Cavazzoni, P., et al. (1999b) MAOA: association and linkage studies with lithium responsive bipolar disorder. *Psychiatr. Genet.* 9:13–16.

Van Den Bogaert, A., De Zutter, S., Heyrman, L., et al. (2005) Response to Zhang et al. (2005): loss-of-function mutation in tryptophan hydroxylase-2 identified in unipolar major depression. *Neuron* 48:704; author reply 705–706.

Van Den Bogaert, A., Sleegers, K., De Zutter, S., et al. (2006) Association of brain-specific tryptophan hydroxylase, TPH2, with unipolar and bipolar disorder in a Northern Swedish, isolated population. *Arch. Gen. Psychiatry* 63:1103–1110.

Venken, T., Claes, S., Sluijs, S., et al. (2005) Genomewide scan for affective disorder susceptibility Loci in families of a northern Swedish isolated population. *Am. J. Hum. Genet.* 76:237–248.

Venter, J.C., Adams, M.D., Myers, E.W., et al. (2001) The sequence of the human genome. *Science* 291:1304–1351.

Videbech, P., and Ravnkilde, B. (2004) Hippocampal volume and depression: a meta-analysis of MRI studies. *Am. J. Psychiatry* 161: 1957–1966.

Vincent, J.B., Masellis, M., Lawrence, J., et al. (1999) Genetic association analysis of serotonin system genes in bipolar affective disorder. *Am. J. Psychiatry* 156:136–138.

von Knorring, A.L., Cloninger, C.R., Bohman, M., and Sigvardsson, S. (1983) An adoption study of depressive disorders and substance abuse. *Arch. Gen. Psychiatry* 40:943–950.

Walther, D.J., and Bader, M. (2003) A unique central tryptophan hydroxylase isoform. *Biochem. Pharmacol.* 66:1673–1680.

Weissman, M.M., Bland, R.C., Canino, G.J., et al. (1996) Cross-national epidemiology of major depression and bipolar disorder. *JAMA* 276:293–299.

Weissman, M.M., Gershon, E.S., Kidd, K.K., et al. (1984) Psychiatric disorders in the relatives of probands with affective disorders. The Yale University—National Institute of Mental Health Collaborative Study. *Arch. Gen. Psychiatry* 41:13–21.

Weissman, M.M., Merikangas, K.R., Wickramaratne, P., et al. (1986) Understanding the clinical heterogeneity of major depression using family data. *Arch. Gen. Psychiatry* 43:430–434.

Weissman, M.M., Wickramaratne, P., Adams, P.B., et al. (1993) The relationship between panic disorder and major depression. A new family study. *Arch. Gen. Psychiatry* 50:767–780.

Wellcome Trust Case Control Consortium. (2007) Genome-wide association study of 14,000 cases of seven common diseases and 3,000 shared controls. *Nature* 447:661–678.

Wender, P.H., Kety, S.S., Rosenthal, D., Schulsinger, F., Ortmann, J., and Lunde, I. (1986) Psychiatric disorders in the biological and adoptive families of adopted individuals with affective disorders. *Arch. Gen. Psychiatry* 43:923–929.

Wijsman, E.M., Rosenthal, E.A., Hall, D., et al. (2003) Genome-wide scan in a large complex pedigree with predominantly male schizophrenics from the island of Kosrae: evidence for linkage to chromosome 2q. *Mol. Psychiatry* 8:695–705, 643.

Williams, N.M., Green, E.K., Macgregor, S., et al. (2006) Variation at the DAOA/G30 locus influences susceptibility to major mood episodes but not psychosis in schizophrenia and bipolar disorder. *Arch. Gen. Psychiatry* 63:366–373.

Willis-Owen, S.A., Turri, M.G., Munafo, M.R., et al. (2005) The serotonin transporter length polymorphism, neuroticism, and depression: a comprehensive assessment of association. *Biol. Psychiatry* 58:451–456.

Winokur, G., Cadoret, R., Dorzab, J., and Baker, M. (1971) Depressive disease: a genetic study. *Arch. Gen. Psychiatry* 24:135–144.

Winokur, G., Tsuang, M.T., and Crowe, R.R. (1982) The Iowa 500: affective disorder in relatives of manic and depressed patients. *Am. J. Psychiatry* 139:209–212.

Zhang, L.X., Levine, S., Dent, G., Zhan, Y., Xing, G., Okimoto, D., et al. (2002) Maternal deprivation increases cell death in the infant rat brain. *Brain Res.* 133:1–11

Zhang, X., Gainetdinov, R.R., Beaulieu, J.M., et al. (2005) Loss-of-function mutation in tryptophan hydroxylase-2 identified in unipolar major depression. *Neuron* 45:11–16.

Zhou, Z., Peters, E.J., Hamilton, S.P., et al. (2005) Response to Zhang et al. (2005) loss-of-function mutation in tryptophan hydroxylase-2 identified in unipolar major depression. *Neuron* 48:702–703; author reply 705–706.

Zhou, Z., Roy, A., Lipsky, R., et al. (2005) Haplotype-based linkage of tryptophan hydroxylase 2 to suicide attempt, major depression, and cerebrospinal fluid 5-hydroxyindoleacetic acid in 4 populations. *Arch. Gen. Psychiatry* 62:1109–1118.

Zill, P., Baghai, T.C., Zwanzger, P., et al. (2004) SNP and haplotype analysis of a novel tryptophan hydroxylase isoform (TPH2) gene provide evidence for association with major depression. *Mol. Psychiatry* 9:1030–1036.

Zubenko, G.S., Hughes, H.B., 3rd, Stiffler, J.S., et al. (2003) Sequence variations in CREB1 cosegregate with depressive disorders in women. *Mol. Psychiatry* 8:611–618.

Zubenko, G.S., Maher, B., Hughes, H.B., 3rd, et al. (2003) Genome-wide linkage survey for genetic loci that influence the development of depressive disorders in families with recurrent, early-onset, major depression. *Am. J. Med. Genet. B Neuropsychiatr. Genet.* 123:1–18.

27 Animal Models of Mood Disorders

INGE SILLABER, FLORIAN HOLSBOER,
AND CARSTEN T. WOTJAK

Animal models have proven to be indispensable tools for the advancement of medicine as a whole, and they are playing an increasingly important role as research tools in psychiatry. Ideally, the animal model created should mimic the human condition of interest with respect to its etiology (*etiological validity*), symptomatology (*face validity*), pharmacological treatment (*predictive validity*), and biological basis (*construct validity*; Fig. 27.1) (McKinney and Bunney, 1969). Clearly, meeting such requirements is difficult. This is particularly true for depression, where the presence of some of the cardinal features (for example, feelings of worthlessness and guilt and suicidal ideation) is defined by a subjective verbal report, something that can never be modelled in an animal. The presence of other features of depression can be defined operationally (for example, loss of appetite and weight, sleep disturbances, and psychomotor changes). However, a model that is limited to a decrease in appetite and psychomotor activity, for example, would be a very superficial reflection of the clinical condition of depression. Another difficulty in the development of animal models of depression stems from the way by which such models are generated. Most models using nonhuman primates or rodents are based on exposing healthy animals to adverse experience, in most cases a stressor, for prolonged periods of time. The resulting phenotype accounts only for experience-related behavioral changes bearing the resemblance to depression (Kalueff et al., 2007). In such models, the fact that the development of depression is strongly influenced by genetic factors is ignored.

In light of these difficulties, the development of a perfectly homologous model, reproducing as closely as possible all aspects of depression, seems out of reach. Instead, more pragmatic approaches are now being pursued, in which animal models are developed for distinct purposes: (*1*) as behavioral tests to screen for potential antidepressant effects of new pharmaceutical drugs and (2) as tools to investigate specific pathogenetic aspects of cardinal symptoms of depression. The traditional routes to animal models of depression have recently been expanded by the possibility of studying mice that have behavioral changes that are not experience related but rather are secondary to the insertion of a transgene or to a targeted disruption of a single gene.

This chapter starts with a brief overview of potential model organisms, followed by a description of depression-like symptoms that can be addressed in animal models and an introduction to stress paradigms used for inducing depression-like symptoms. A few representative examples of successfully established animal models are given, ending with an outlook on future requirements for animal models of depression.

MODEL ORGANISMS

Invertebrate model organisms such as fruit flies (*Drosophila melanogaster*) and maritime snails (*Aplysia californica*) turned out to be of inestimable value for our understanding of molecular mechanisms underlying synaptic plasticity and memory formation (Kandel, 2001; Margulies et al., 2005). However, they have their clear limitations if complex interactions between neuronal circuits, transmitter systems, hormones, and behavior have to be considered. Therefore, animal studies on mood disorders have to be performed in higher vertebrates with close homologies to humans in brain anatomy and physiology. Accordingly, most animal models of depression have been established with rodents and nonhuman primates. Among rodents, the rat (*Rattus norvegicus familiaris*) has been the preferred species for decades. With the advent of modern mouse genetics, however, a rapidly increasing number of studies employed mice (*Mus musculus*) (Cryan and Holmes, 2005). Today, there is a huge number of different rat and mouse strains available from commercial breeders. These strains can be roughly assigned to outbred or inbred strains. The former bear high genetic variability, whereas the latter are genetically homogeneous, as they are derived from brother–sister matings for more than 20 generations. Importantly, single strains not only display a characteristic behavioral phenotype under basal conditions, but also differ in their responsiveness to several manipulations, for example, stress or antidepressant treatment. Therefore, it is indispensable to distinguish between the

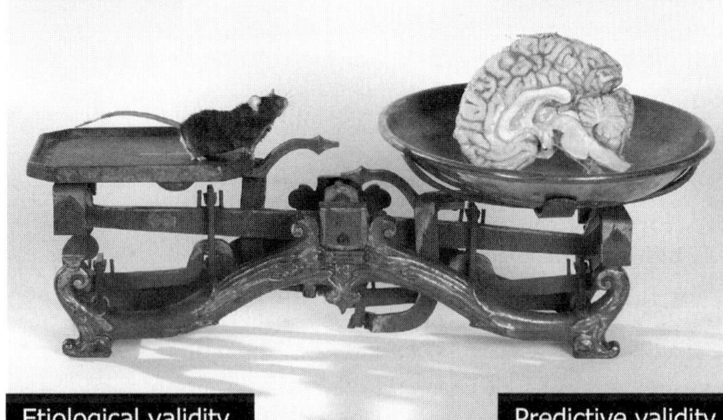

FIGURE 27.1 Criteria for an animal model of depression. Animal models cannot keep the balance with the complexity of human psychopathology (here illustrated with the balance used by Alois Alzheimer in Munich). However, different aspects of depression can be addressed in animals, and the validity of an animal model can be judged by a set of criteria, whereby it is not essential that all criteria are met at the same time.

different strains by strictly adhering to international recommendations of nomenclature (Wotjak, 2003).

In recent years a number of methods (for details, see Chapter 7 "Functional Genomics and Models of Mental Illness") have been established by which the mouse genome can be altered in a direct or reverse genetic manner, which opens up a new molecular approach to behavior. *Reverse genetics* refers to a set of techniques such as transgenesis and gene targeting in which a single cloned gene is used to generate a line of mice with an alteration specifically in that gene (Picciotto and Wickman, 1998). Genetically engineered mice were not originally generated to produce animal models with face validity for depression but rather to delineate the role of a specific gene product in bringing about the behavioral phenotype.

DEPRESSION-LIKE SYMPTOMS

As mentioned above, no animal model can reflect the complexity of depression, but certain key symptoms might be mimicked, including behavioral despair, anhedonia, sleep disturbances, dysregulation of the hypothalamic-pituitary-adrenal (HPA) axis, comorbidity with anxiety, altered brain morphology, and impaired cognitive performance (Fig. 27.1, Table 27.1). The following paragraphs illustrate how some of these symptoms might be addressed in animal experiments.

TABLE 27.1 *Experimental Access to Key Symptoms of Depression*

Symptoms	*Experimental Measures in Animal Models*
Despair	Increased immobility in forced swim and tail suspension tests
	"Learned helplessness"
Anhedonia	Decrease in intracranial self-stimulation
	Decreased sucrose preference
	Reduced sexual interest
Increased anxiety	Unconditioned and conditioned avoidance
	Suppression of punished responding
	Conditioned freezing
	Ultrasonic vocalization
Impaired cognition	Impairments in hippocampus-dependent learning tasks
Activity changes	Decreased home cage activity
	Decreased locomotion in novel environments
Sleep changes	Flattening of circadian rhythm (sleep/wakefulness)
	Increased rapid-eye-movement density
Changes in appetite	Hyperphagia / Hypophagia-anorexia
	Carbohydrate preference
Metabolic syndrome	Increased ratio of visceral and subcutaneous fat
	Altered glucose metabolism

Behavioral Despair

In rats and mice, behavioral despair is typically assessed by alterations in escape-oriented behavior in aversive situations, such as during exposure to water (Forced Swim Test), capture by the tail (Tail Suspension Test), and exposure to electric foot shocks (shuttle box avoidance).

Forced Swim Test (FST) and Tail Suspension Test (TST)

Both paradigms measure escape approaches and immobility responses in an unavoidable test situation (for comprehensive reviews, see Cryan and Mombereau, 2004; Cryan, Mombereau, and Vassout, 2005). In temporary versions of the FST (alias Porsolt's Test; Porsolt et al., 1977), mice or rats are forced to swim in a glass cylinder that is half-filled with water so that the animal cannot touch the bottom with its hind paws. The animal swims around attempting to escape, which is impossible, and eventually assumes an immobile posture called "floating." Over the course of the exposure and, in particular, in subsequent tests, the time spent immobile increases, indicating that the animals have learned that they cannot escape. This phenomenon was originally termed "behavioral despair," resembling the situation of "learned helplessness" (see below). More recent interpretations favor the view that immobility may also reflect a successful strategy, which involves memory processes aimed at conserving energy (West, 1990). Behavioral stress coping in the FST is affected by a variety of test modifications and biological parameters (Cryan and Mombereau, 2004; Petit-Demouliere et al., 2005), including single housing versus group housing and water temperature. In particular, the latter parameter gains importance if one considers that the test is typically performed at 21°C (rats) or 25°C (mice) water temperature, which causes a significant drop in core body temperature and brain temperature, which may partially account for the increase in floating time.

The TST is conceptually similar to the FST as both tests share a common theoretical basis and behavioral measure (Steru et al., 1985; Cryan, Valentino, and Lucki, 2005). In this test, mice are suspended by the tail to a bar, and as a consequence the animals engage in agitation-or escape-like behaviors, interrupted by periods of immobility. The immobile posture and its duration within a 5- or 6-minute test session are used as the measure of depression-like behavior, that is, behavioral despair or passive coping. Compared with the FST, the TST avoids confounding effects of hypothermia. Of disadvantage is that in particular the broadly used C57BL/6 strains fail to produce valid data in the TST as the animals climb their tail up to the bar (Mayorga and Lucki, 2001).

Many studies on effects of antidepressants of all major classes on behavioral performance in FST and TST reported an increase in escape-oriented behavior, resulting in a reduction of immobility. Specifically, inhibition of serotonin uptake reduces floating by promoting swimming behavior, whereas inhibition of noradrenaline uptake reduces immobility by promoting more vigorous escape attempts (that is, climbing and struggling; Cryan, Mombereau, and Vassout, 2005). One has to stress that in FST and TST drug effects are typically assessed after acute treatment, which is in contrast to the situation in human patients, where prolonged treatment with antidepressants is necessary to ameliorate depressive symptoms. It is conceivable that the acute drug effects relate to increased arousal in the animals due to acutely potentiated serotonergic and noradrenergic transmission.

Anhedonia

Another key symptom of depression is the inability to experience bliss and pleasure. In animal experiments, this symptom is assessed as a decrease in the value of otherwise rewarding stimuli by measuring voluntary consumption of saccharine or sucrose or by applying intracranial self-stimulation. Saccharine or sucrose consumption is typically assessed in a two-bottle choice test in the home cage, with one bottle containing tap water and the other saccharine or sucrose in concentrations from 1% to 10%. The amount of sweetened solution consumed will be set into relation to water consumption and serves as a measure of hedonic behavior.

For *intracranial self-stimulation*, an electrode is chronically implanted into brain structures belonging to the reward system of the brain (that is, primarily in the mesocorticolimbic dopaminergic system, which originates from the ventral tegmental area and projects to the nucleus accumbens and the prefrontal cortex). Animals can control electrical stimulation of the respective pathway by turning a wheel, nose-poking into a hole, or pressing a lever. A reduction in the respective behavioral parameter serves as a measure of anhedonia.

Hypothalamic-Pituitary-Adrenal (HPA) Axis Dysregulation

Changes in stress hormones and an aberrant regulation of the HPA axis functioning are often reported for patients with major depression: basal levels of cortisol are elevated and accompanied by a flattened diurnal variation in its secretion, cerebrospinal fluid (CSF) levels of corticotropin-releasing hormone (CRH, alias CRF) are increased, the response of adrenocorticotropic hormone (ACTH) to a challenge with exogenous CRH is blunted, and the negative feedback response to a synthetic glucocorticoid (dexamethasone [DEX]) is less effective (Holsboer, 1995; Plotsky et al., 1998; Holsboer, 2000; de Kloet et al., 2005). Bearing in mind that rats and mice are nocturnal animals, the regulation of the HPA axis under basal and stressful conditions is quite similar to the human situation. Importantly, in laboratory animals, molecular changes within the brain and pituitary and adrenal cortex can be determined in addition to measuring stress hormone levels in plasma.

Anxiety-Related Behavior

Depression is frequently associated with anxiety. Therefore, animal models of depression are typically tested for alterations in anxiety-related behavior as well. In humans as well as in laboratory animals, anxiety is not a unitary phenomenon as it includes innate (trait) anxiety and situation-evoked (state) or experience-related expression of anxiety, which are not separable from each other. Various test paradigms, often termed "animal models of anxiety," have been developed to assess behavioral parameters indicating anxiety (see Part V, Anxiety Disorders).

Altered Brain Morphology

Patients who are depressed often show a reduced size and neuronal integrity of hippocampus formation and prefrontal cortex, as assessed by magnetic resonance imaging (MRI) in combination with morphometry and/or magnetic resonance spectroscopy. These changes have been ascribed to long-lasting elevations of glucocorticoid levels. With the refinement of scanning methods, potentiation of the magnetic field and the adjustment of the setup for the use of small laboratory animals, MRI has only recently been adopted to animal models of depression (Czéh et al., 2001). The advantage of this method would be the possibility to perform longitudinal studies within the same experimental subject. So far, snapshots of morphological changes are obtained by Golgi impregnation of neurons in brain slices, followed by detailed analysis of dendritic profiles (for example, number of dendritic branches, maximal length of the dendrites, and number of dendritic spines). By means of this method, several studies compared the consequences of chronic stress on anxiety-like behavior and neuron morphology. For instance, rats showed a sustained increase in anxiety-like behavior following chronic immobilization stress that coincided with atrophy and debranching in pyramidal neurons in the CA3 region of the hippocampus (a brain structure likely to be involved in cognition and inhibitory control of hormonal stress responses), whereas pyramidal and stellate neurons exhibited enhanced dendritic arborization in the basolateral amygdala (a brain structure implicated in control of negative affects) (Vyas et al., 2002). Hence, it is conceivable that, if similar morphological changes occur in patients who are depressed, atrophy and hypotrophy of neurons in the hippocampus account for impairments in cognition, whereas hypertrophy in the amygdala would support the development of mood disturbances.

Impaired Neurogenesis

Neurogenesis exists in the mature brain of adult rats, mice, nonhuman primates, and even in humans, not only in the subventricular zone but also in the subgranular layer of the dentate gyrus (Lindsey and Tropepe, 2006). Today the molecular cascades underlying proliferation of progenitor cells and their differentiation into neurons start to emerge. However, our knowledge about the biological significance of these processes is still in its infancy. Surprisingly, a considerable number of animal models of depression displayed a reduction in neurogenesis in the dentate gyrus, whereas most of the antidepressants and antidepressive treatments turned out to increase neurogenesis (Duman, 2004). First evidence for a direct relationship between neurogenesis and depression-like symptoms came from a study on experimental inhibition of neurogenesis in mice by X-ray irradiation (Santarelli et al., 2003), which rendered the animals insensitive to anxiolytic effects of long-term antidepressant treatment. However, the exact nature of this relationship is far from being clear and its causality is questioned (Henn and Vollmayr, 2004).

Impaired Cognition

Severe human depressions are often accompanied by impaired cognitive functioning, primarily in hippocampus- or prefrontal cortex–dependent tasks. Accordingly, the behavioral analyses of animal models of depression often include tests of hippocampus-dependent learning, such as spatial learning along distal landmarks in dry mazes (for example, Barnes maze or radial maze) and wet mazes (for example, Morris water maze), passive avoidance tasks, and contextual fear conditioning (Sousa et al., 2006). To decide whether impairments in learning result from changes in synaptic plasticity rather than in performance and stress coping (see below), studies might include analyses of long-term potentiation or long-term depression preferably in the pathway to the CA1 region of the hippocampus.

ANIMAL MODELS OF DEPRESSION

In an attempt to understand the neurobiological basis of human depression and to predict successful treatment strategies, animal models for depression have been developed, whose depression-like symptoms have been assessed as described before. Existing models include pharmacological models (for example, depression-like

TABLE 27.2 *Animal Models of Depression (Selection)*

Strategy	*Description*
Lesions	Olfactory bulbectomy in rats (and mice)
Social stress	Tree shrews (*Tupaia belangeri*) exposed to a dominant conspecific undergo social defeat and subsequently develop depression-like symptoms
Selective breeding	Rats and mice have been selectively bred for extremes in depression-like symptoms
	• Learned helplessness-susceptible rats
	• Flinders Sensitive Line (FSL)
	• Wistar–Kyoto rats (WKY)
	• High anxiety (HAB) rats and mice
	• H/Rouen mice
	Several inbred and outbred mouse strains are commercially available that differ in their susceptibility for developing depression-like symptoms and in their responsiveness to antidepressants
Transgenic mice	Gain-of-function and loss-of-function mouse mutants, which, however, do not always fulfill the expectations in terms of depression-like symptoms (for details see text)

symptoms induced by withdrawal from psychostimulants or by monoamine depletion), the olfactory bulbectomy model, developmental models, and genetic models (Table 27.2). The following section exemplarily highlights a few of them.

Olfactory Bulbectomized Rats and Mice

Olfaction is the primary sensory system of rodents. Volatile odorants and pheromones are acquired and processed by the main and the accessory olfactory system, respectively. Bulbectomy in rats and mice leads to permanent destruction of these systems and, in consequence, to disinhibition of the amygdala, structural changes in hippocampus and prefrontal cortex, alterations in transmitter systems including serotonergic and noradrenergic transmission, and changes in a distinct set of behaviors (Song and Leonard, 2005). The latter includes increased exploratory behavior (likely because of impaired habituation) and impaired cognition. Although face and etiological validity of this model can be questioned, bulbectomized animals responded to the chronic administration of all types of therapeutically active antidepressants. They also responded to compounds not directly related to monoamine systems but with a different mechanism of action and potential antidepressant activity, for example, methyrapone or yohimbine (Song and Leonard, 2005) and might thus be useful for the screening of antidepressant drugs.

Developmental Animal Models of Depression

Stressful experiences have been reported to favor the evolution of depression (for review see Anisman and Matheson, 2005). Therefore most animal models of depression include stress paradigms for the induction of depression-like symptoms. In this context, various factors have been identified that influence the stress response of the animals. All in all, a stressor turns out to be particularly suitable for the induction of depression-like symptoms, if it is (*1*) long-lasting and/or intense, (*2*) uncontrollable, (*3*) unpredictable, and/or (*4*) uncertain in its occurrence (Anisman and Matheson, 2005). The efficiency of stress exposure depends on the genetic makeup of the individual. Moreover, there seem to be sensitive phases during development (for example, pre- and early postnatally, puberty/adolescence), during which stressors have a particular impact on the individual susceptibility for developing depression-like symptoms in later life.

Uncontrollable shock and learned helplessness models

The model using uncontrollable shock was introduced by Overmier and Seligman (1967). It is based on the observation that animals exposed to uncontrollable electric shocks developed behavioral deficits that were different from those seen in animals that were able to exert control over the shock. In a prototypic experiment, animals were tested in dyads with one animal being able to control the shock and the other not. To achieve this, the two animals were placed into two different shock chambers, which were connected to the same shock generator. Both chambers were equipped with a wheel, a nose-poke detector, or a lever. However, only the device from one of the chambers was connected with the shock generator. Accordingly, only the animal from that chamber could get operational control over the shock by turning the wheel, nose-poking into the hole, or pressing the lever, which switched off the shock. Importantly, the animal from the other chamber also had benefit from this, however, without the possibility to control the shock by itself. In other words, both animals received the same number of shocks, however, in a controllable or uncontrollable manner. Animals exposed to uncontrollable shock had decreased food and water intake and subsequent weight loss (Weiss, 1968, 1980), were more passive in the FST, and showed alterations in sleep patterns and a weakened response to previously rewarding brain stimulation (Anisman and Matheson, 2005). In addition, animals that had been exposed to uncontrollable shock were strongly impaired in an active avoidance task in a shuttle box compared to animals exposed to controllable stress. In this task, a foot shock is presented in a two-compartment chamber.

A tone or light signal precedes the foot shock, and the animals can avoid the foot shock if they move to the other compartment during presentation of the tone/light signal (pre-emptive response). Seligman and Beagley (1975) linked the behavioral consequences of uncontrollable shock in rats to the clinical condition of depression, and because patients with depression also have feelings of helplessness, the term "learned helplessness" was coined for this response in animals. Learned helplessness paradigms are limited by the fact that only a small proportion of the animals develop depression-like symptoms and that these symptoms persist for one or two days after induction only (Anisman and Matheson, 2005).

Chronic mild stress (CMS) models

Mice and rats rapidly habituate to a distinct stressor. To avoid this, complex protocols with exposure to different kinds of stressors have been established. For example, the chronic mild stress (CMS) model is generated by sequential applications of different unpredictable stressful conditions such as mild uncontrollable foot shock, forced swimming in cold water, changes in housing conditions, food and water deprivation, reversal of light/dark periods, and exposure to noise and bright light. After exposure to these stressors for 2 to 3 weeks, animals show a number of behavioral changes that are maintained for days (mice) or even weeks (rats) and that are reminiscent of depression-like symptoms. These changes include not only alterations in psychomotor behavior and sleep architecture, as evidenced by reduced open field activity and altered rapid eye movement sleep (REM sleep), but also a reduced sensitivity to rewards, such as a decrease in sucrose consumption, reduced intracranial self-stimulation, and the inability to associate rewards with a distinctive environment in a place conditioning. The stress protocol and the choice of rat or mouse strain might be very critical as some groups report failure to replicate the findings (for example, Nielsen et al., 2000). One strength of the CMS model is its predictive validity because only long-term treatment with various antidepressants causes a return to initial levels of sucrose intake (for comprehensive review see Willner, 2005).

Social and predator stress models

Acute or repeated exposures to dominant conspecifics (for example, to resident animals in social defeat paradigms) or to predators (for example, ferret or cat) have long-lasting consequences on vegetative, hormonal, and behavioral parameters in the test animals. For instance, exposure to predator stress in sensitive phases during development "primes" the individual susceptibility of rats to subsequent aversive encounters in terms of developing symptoms of posttraumatic depression or posttraumatic stress disorder (Tsoory et al., 2007). Of note, maternal influence (see next paragraph) and social hierarchies among cage mates can be regarded as special cases of social factors determining the individual susceptibility for developing depression-like symptoms. Submissive animals are prone to develop a depression-like phenotype (that is, anhedonia, passive stress coping, and anxiety-like behavior) following chronic stress, whereas dominant animals turn out to be resistant or even to display mania-like phenotypes (Malatynska and Knapp, 2005).

Applying a social stress paradigm to male tree shrews (*Tupaia belangeri*), Fuchs and colleagues collected an array of data showing a number of depression-like symptoms in the subordinate animal, which lives in visual and olfactory contact to a conspecific by which it has been defeated (Fuchs, 2005). The subordinate male showed not only behavioral changes and a reduction in body weight, but also changes in sleeping pattern, increased concentration of stress hormones, and structural changes in the hippocampus. The validity of this model is further supported by the finding that chronic treatment with antidepressants exerts a time-dependent restorative influence on most parameters affected by the stress paradigm including cell proliferation in the hippocampus (Fuchs et al., 1996, 2002; Czéh et al., 2006). The chronic psychosocial conflict in tree shrews may represent a natural and valid paradigm for studying behavioral, endocrine, and neurobiological changes underlying stress-related disorders such as depression in a species phylogenetically close to humans.

Early life stressors

Adverse experiences during development turned out to provide a fundamental factor for determining susceptibility to psychiatric disorders in adulthood. Many investigators have administered stressors to pregnant rats (prenatal stress) or newborn rats or mice (early postnatal stress) and studied their impact on behavior and hormonal stress coping in the offspring throughout adulthood. In a prototypical experiment employing postnatal stress, the litter will be separated from their mother for a certain amount of time, starting 2 days after birth. Duration and frequency of separations critically determine the success of the experiment (Macrì and Würbel, 2006; Millstein and Holmes, 2007). In fact, separation may just attract the interest of the mothers in their replaced litter, thus leading to intensive active grooming and licking. Such forms of maternal behavior, which can be seen also spontaneously without separation of the dams from their litter, influence the individual susceptibility of the offspring to stressors in later life. It could be shown that active nursing (that is, arched-back posture with frequent licking and grooming, Fig. 27.2) results in a "stress resistant" phenotype, whereas passive nursing behavior renders the offspring vulnerable for stress-induced depression-like symptoms (Champagne et al., 2003). These differences in stress susceptibility are accompanied by a variety of changes at the molecular level, including altered expression of neurotransmitter and hormone receptors (Champagne et al., 2003), at least in part due to epigenetic modifications at the level of the deoxyribonucleic acid (DNA) (Weaver et al., 2004).

A particular striking example for the role of pre- and postnatal factors is provided by the behavioral phenotype of two inbred mouse strains, C57BL/6J and BALB/c. Whereas C57BL/6J mice are good learners in the water maze task, BALB/c fail to do so, likely because of altered stress coping. In a cross-fostering experiment, however, BALB/c mice performed equally well as C57BL/6J mice, if reared by C57BL/6J mothers. Hence, the strain differences do not primarily relate to differences in the genetic makeup, but to strain-specific postnatal maternal factors. Interestingly, the good learning capabilities of C57BL/6J mice were unaffected if the animals had been reared by BALB/c mothers (Zaharia et al., 1996). As confirmed in an elegant embryo transfer and cross-fostering study (Francis et al., 2003), mice from this strain showed altered behavioral performance only if their development was influenced by BALB/c mothers pre- and postnatally (Fig. 27.2). These data demonstrate how epigenetic (that is, pre- and postnatal) factors during development on the basis of a distinct genetic

A Post-natal factors

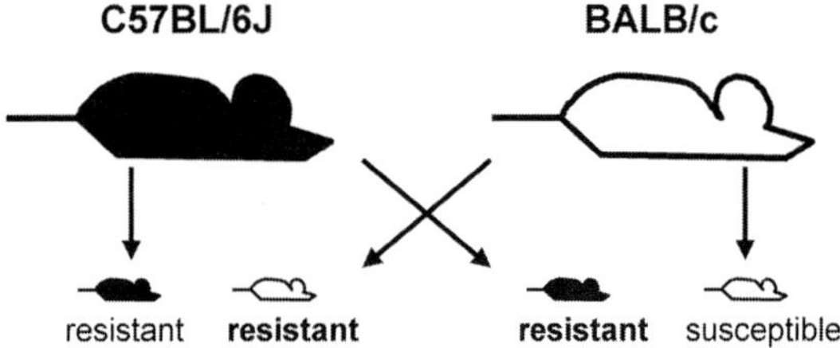

B Pre- and post-natal factors

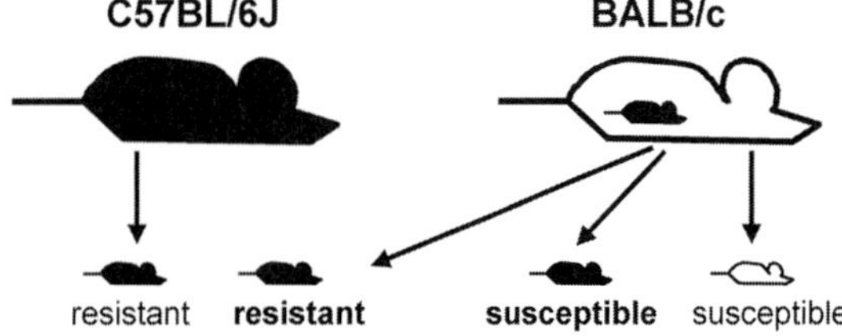

C Maternal behavior

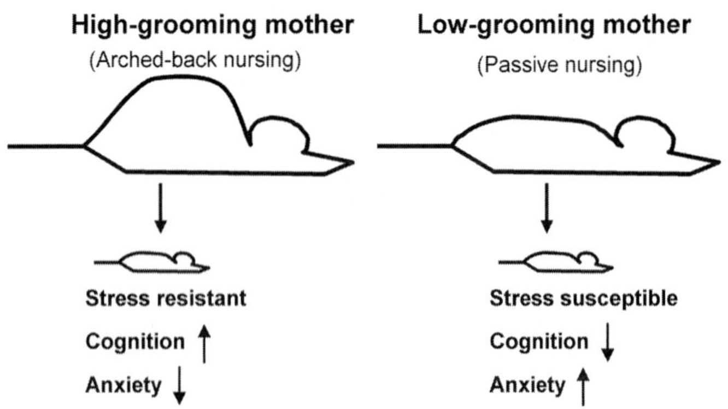

FIGURE 27.2 Developmental factors influencing the individual stress susceptibility in mice and rats. (*A*) Strain differences between two inbred mouse strains in terms of stress susceptibility can be overcome if offspring of mothers from the stress-susceptible strain (BALB/c) are reared by mothers from the stress-resistant strain (C57BL/6J). The same postnatal cross-fostering failed to affect stress resistance of C57BL/6J offspring, if reared by BALB/c mothers (Zaharia et al., 1996). (*B*) C57BL/6J offspring show increased stress susceptibility only following pre- (embryo transfer) and postnatal cross-fostering (Francis et al., 2003). (*C*) Maternal care has a strong impact on stress coping, cognition, and anxiety of the offspring of Long–Evans rats (Champagne et al., 2003).

makeup determine the stress susceptibility and most likely also the development of depression-like symptoms in adulthood.

Separation models are also used in nonhuman primates, species that due to the evolutionary proximity to humans seem to be particularly suited to providing insights into the biobehavioral underpinnings of depression. Infant monkeys respond to maternal separation with agitation, sleep disturbances, and screaming. After 1–2 days they become "despaired," a condition characterized in monkeys by a decrease in activity, appetite, and weight; play and social interaction; and the assumption of a hunched posture and "sad" facial expression (McKinney and Bunney, 1969; Hinde et al., 1978). Studies by many laboratories have also suggested that "depressive" responses during "despair" can be predicted by the amount of cortisol released immediately following separation. The link between the HPA system and depression-like behavior has been studied extensively by Kalin et al. (1989), who injected CRH into the central nervous system (CNS) of infant monkeys. The animals developed a phenotype similar to the "behavioral despair" produced by maternal separation. Furthermore, monkeys reared by mothers foraging under unpredictable conditions had a persistently elevated CSF concentration of CRH (Coplan et al., 1996). These findings lend support to the neuroendocrine hypothesis of depression, according to which depression can develop if the balance between stress-related elevation of CRH and corticosteroid-induced suppression is continously disturbed (Holsboer, 2000). If these animal models are applicable to humans, the conclusion can be drawn that early stressors such as neglect or abuse lead to persistent elevations of CRH, rendering an individual vulnerable to depression or anxiety, or both. The predictive value of "behavioral despair" in the context of drug treatment is not yet clear, but the few existing studies suggest that antidepressants can reduce at least some of the separation-induced deficits.

Genetic Animal Models of Depression

The previous sections of this chapter described the choice of the experimental models, how distinct symptoms of human depression can be studied in these animals, and how developmental and environmental factors contribute to the manifestation of depression-like symptoms. However, not the isolated entities by themselves, but their integration eventually results in an animal model of depression. In other words, genetic predisposition of the animals, environmental factors, and careful analysis of behavioral, hormonal, and morphological characteristics provide the basis for the study of depression-like symptoms in animals. The focus of interest dictates whether the animal model is used for studying molecular correlates and etiology of the behavioral alterations or for testing of novel pharmacotherapeutic strategies.

Genetic factors have been estimated to account for 40%–70% of the individual risk for developing major depression (Lesch, 2004). However, it is the interaction between genetic predisposition and environmental factors (Fig. 27.3) that results in a fully manifested disorder (Caspi et al., 2003). In recent years a rich methodological portfolio has been established that allows dissecting the genetic basis of behavior in animals (Fig. 27.4). Top-down or forward genetic approaches start with a certain behavioral phenotype. Natural variance in its expression due to strain differences, selective breeding, or spontaneous or randomly induced mutations (for example, by mutagenic compounds such as *N*-ethyl-*N*-nitroso-urea; Hotz Vitaterna et al., 2006) enable the characterization of candidate genes. This can be achieved

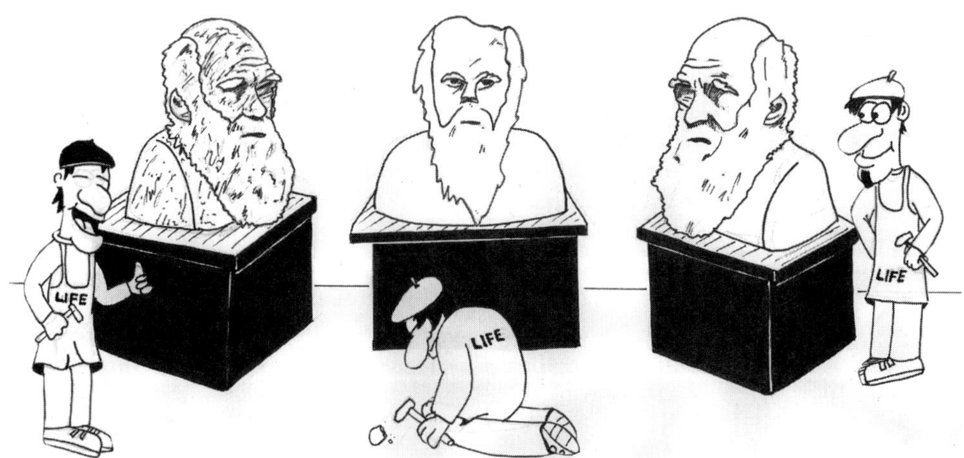

FIGURE 27.3 Gene-environment interaction. This cartoon illustrates that true masterpieces of art require outstanding quality of the artist (vulgo: life, environment or nurture) and of the raw material (vulgo: genetic makeup or nature; here sandstone for the left sculpture and marble for the middle and the right sculpture).

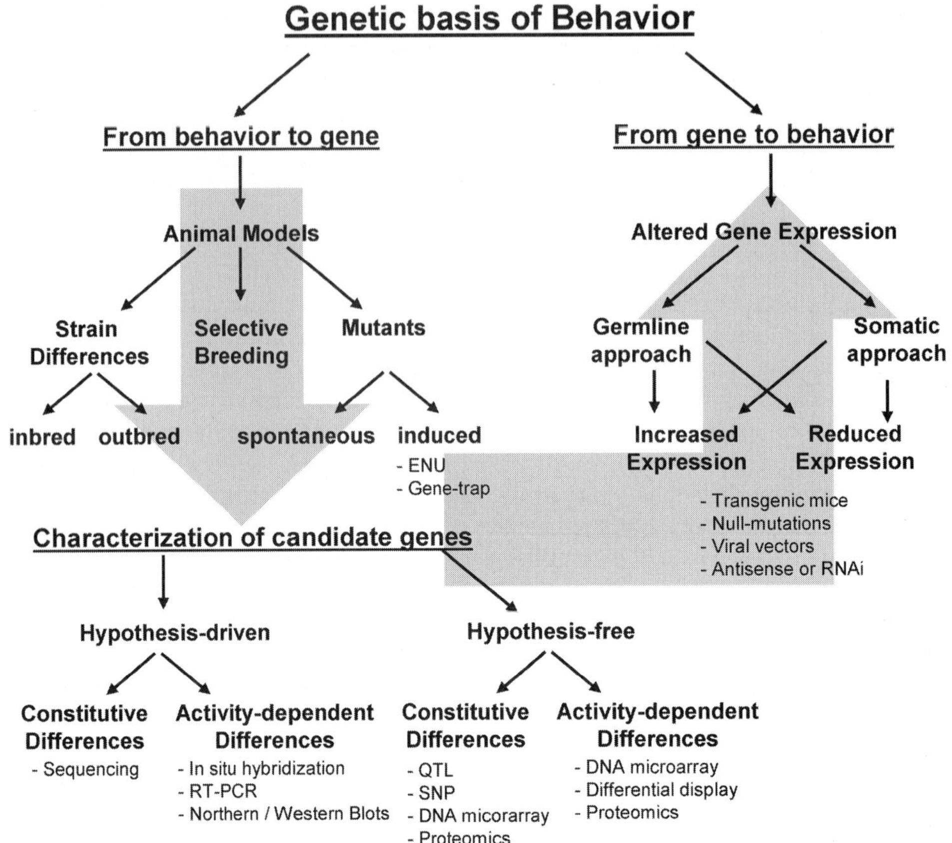

FIGURE 27.4 Strategic considerations for studying the genetic basis of behavior. Forward genetics tries to characterize candidate genes for a certain behavioral phenotype by starting with the respective animal model and ending with molecular biology. Reverse genetics, in turn, tries to demonstrate the causal involvement of a certain gene in the behavioral phenotype under study, thus starting with molecular biology and ending with behavioral analyses (modified from Wotjak, 2004). (ENU: N-ethyl-N-nitroso urea; RNAi: RNA interference; RT-PCR: reverse transcriptase polymerase chain reaction; QTL: quantitative trait loci analysis; SNP: single-nucleotide polymorphism; for further details, see text).

in a hypothesis-driven as well as in a hypothesis-free manner. In the latter case, methods such as quantitative trait loci analyses (QTL; Peters et al., 2007) or high-throughput approaches (for example, microarray analyses) are employed to identify genes or gene arrays that are associated with extremes in behavioral performance. The ultimate goal is to establish a causality between the candidate genes identified and the behavioral phenotype under study. This bottom-up approach or reverse route of behavioral genetics includes alterations in gene expression (gain-of-function or loss-of-function), which can be achieved by genetic modifications that will be germline transmitted (for example, transgenic or knockout mice) or by somatic recombinations (for example, by viral vectors that will be injected into a certain brain region, where they lead to expression of transgenes, short-interference ribonucleic acids [RNAs], or antisense oligonucleotides), and by subsequent behavioral phenotyping. The following examples illustrate the potential of some of these approaches.

Selective breeding for susceptibility to learned helplessness

Henn and colleagues (1985) selectively bred rats for susceptibility and resistance to behavioral deficits produced by uncontrollable shock. The "failure to escape" of susceptible rats can be attributed to psychomotor retardation and may thus reflect a depression-like symptom. After repeated testing and subsequent breeding of animals that showed "failure to escape" from uncontrollable shock for four generations, about one half of the animals showed the phenomenon, whereas none of the animals bred for rapid escape showed poor escape performance. The utility of this attractive model for studies of the neurobiological basis of depression can be assessed only if neuropathological and neurochemical characteristics of depression are better specified than is currently the case. Whereas this model has only limited construct validity (that is, it is not homologous to depression), it has considerable predictive validity, as both animals subjected to uncontrollable shock and those bred for susceptibility to the behavioral deficit ("failure to escape") respond to a variety of antidepressants.

The Flinders sensitive line (FSL)

Another model, based on genetic selection, makes use of two lines of rats that were bred to be either sensitive or resistant to pharmacological manipulation of cholinergic activity (Overstreet et al., 2005). This model was developed at Flinders University in Australia by selective breeding for differences in the effects of the cholinesterase inhibitor *diisopropylfluorophosphate* on body temperature, fluid intake, and body weight. Flinders sensitive line (FSL) rats are hypersensitive to cholinergic agonists and were proposed as an animal model of depression with good face validity because these rats exhibit (*1*) reduced locomotor activity, (*2*) reduced body weight, (*3*) increased REM sleep (a phenomenon frequently observed in patients who are depressed), and (*4*) a greater degree of anhedonic behavior after stress (Overstreet, 1993). However, the evidence that cholinergic hypersensitivity is the leading cause of depression is limited, and this hypothesis is further called into question by the therapeutic efficacy of new antidepressants lacking anticholinergic properties. In light of the behavioral phenomena observed following foot shocks and in the FST, it is of note that FSL rats show exaggerated immobility and that this behavior returns to normal after administration of antidepressants, including those without anticholinergic effects, which in turn is of interest in connection with reported changes in serotonergic activity in these animals (Zangen et al., 1997). More recently, this genetic animal model, together with the Wistar Kyoto rat line, has been proposed as putative genetic animal model of childhood depression (Malkesman et al., 2006).

Hyperanxious rat model

Increased anxiety is one cardinal symptom accompanying depression. According to current diagnostic standards, anxiety disorders and depression are classified as separate disorders; however, at some points they share a common pathophysiology. Animal models of high innate anxiety, gained by selective breeding, are valuable tools as those animals would exhibit pathological anxiety not because of the presentation of a stressor, but because it is an enduring feature of a strain or an individual, probably involving multiple genetic and environmental factors. One animal model meeting this criterion is the rat model of high (HAB) and low (LAB) anxiety-related behavior, developed by Landgraf and colleagues (Liebsch et al., 1998). These two rat lines differ not only in their inborn emotionality, but also in their stress-coping strategies and hormonal stress responses (Frank et al., 2006). Rats with high anxiety-related behavior seem to display deregulations of the HPA axis that are consistent with the neuroendocrine status of depressed patients. Importantly, the exaggerated corticosterone response in the dexamethasone/CRH test observed in these animals (Keck et al., 2002) disappeared following antidepressant treatment (Keck et al., 2003), similar to the situation in patients who were depressed. Using this rat model, the CRH type 1 receptor antagonist R121919—as a representative of a potential new class of antidepressants and which exerted antidepressive effects in human patients (Zobel et al., 2000)—was tested. Only in HAB rats was a significant dose-related reduction of anxiety-like behavior noted, while LAB rats showed no behavioral response (Keck, Welt, Wigger, et al., 2001). The two rat lines also differ in their reactivity to benzodiazepines (Liebsch et al., 1998), repetitive transcranial magnetic stimulation treatment (Keck, Welt, Post, et al., 2001), and chronic paroxetine treatment (Muigg et al., 2007). These results illustrate the predictive validity of this rat model. The consistency and stability of the observed high level of innate anxiety has been partially proven by studies in different laboratories. Recent data indicate that increased expression of vasopressin due to a single-nucleotide polymorphism (SNP) in regulatory structures of the vasopressin gene at least partially accounts for hyperanxiety and depression-like symptoms in these animals (for review see Landgraf et al., 2007).

Inbred and outbred mice

The high number of commercially available inbred and outbred strains provides an excellent tool for studying genetic differences in development and maintenance of depression-like symptoms. Such strain differences eventually resulted from genetic drift and accumulation of mutations (for example, absence of the gene encoding for α-synuclein specifically in C57BL/6JOlaHsd mice; Specht and Schoepfer, 2001; SNP in the tryptophan hydroxylase 2 gene in BALB/c and DBA/2 mice compared to C57BL/6 strains; Zhang et al., 2004). Strains may considerably differ in their FST and TST behavior, in their responsiveness to antidepressant treatment, and in stress-induced development of depression-like symptoms (for comprehensive review see Anisman and Matheson, 2005; Jacobson and Cryan, 2007). So far, only a few studies have tried to characterize the genetic basis of these differences using QTL analyses (Turri et al., 2001; Yoshikawa et al., 2002).

HAB and H/Rouen mice

Selective breeding of mice displaying specific behavioral traits is one starting point to develop genetic mouse models for depression. This concept was the basis for the development of the mouse version of the HAB rats mentioned above (Kromer et al., 2005). In a similar way the H/Rouen mice had been established (Vaugeois et al., 1997) by selective breeding of CD-1 mice for high and low immobility on the TST. After 10 generations, helpless (H/Rouen) and nonhelpless mice (NH/Rouen) were clearly distinguishable on the behavioral level. H/Rouen mice showed not only increased immobility in the TST and FST, but also reduced consumption of palatable sucrose solution, higher basal corticosterone levels, changes in the serotonin system, and alterations in sleep-wakefulness patterns that resemble those observed in patients who were depressed. Further characterization of this mouse line (Popa et al., 2006) validates the H/Rouen mice as a mouse model of particular interest for studying neurobiological mechanisms and, possibly, genetic substrates involved in sleep alterations in depression.

Mouse mutants

A different starting point for the generation of genetic mouse models is to target a specific gene putatively implicated in etiology and expression of depression. Today, there are three main hypotheses on the molecular and biochemical mechanisms underlying depression: the monoamine hypothesis, the HPA axis hypothesis, and the neurotrophin/neurogenesis hypothesis. Further, genetic studies in humans and animals come up with new candidate genes that might be involved in determining the vulnerability to develop depression or in mediating the effects of antidepressant action (e.g., Charney and Manji, 2004; Berton and Nestler, 2006; Ising and Holsboer, 2006; Lucae et al., 2006; Wong et al., 2006).

Targeting different components (for example, genes encoding transmitters, receptors, or transporters) of the systems involved in the above-mentioned hypotheses led to the generation of a number of mutant mouse lines, which have been systematically analyzed for alterations in depression-like symptoms (for comprehensive review see Urani et al., 2005). These mouse models do not only serve to validate a working hypothesis but also are of high value in terms of disentangling the role of single genes in highly complex frameworks such as, for example, the regulation of the HPA axis and the modulation of anxiety behavior by the CRH receptors 1 and 2 (Bale and Vale, 2004; Müller and Holsboer, 2006). In terms of representing animal models of depression, however, mutant mouse lines generated so far display clear limitations, and only few of them show depression-like behavior. In line with the neurotrophin/neurogenesis hypothesis of depression, a reduction of brain-derived neurotrophic factor (BDNF) should convey a depression-like phenotype. However, experiments with heterozygous BDNF knockout ($BDNF^{+/-}$) mice, which display a 50% reduction of BDNF, failed to reveal depression-like symptoms (Montkowski and Holsboer, 1997; Chourbaji et al., 2004). Moreover, in some mouse mutants the behavioral phenotype did not always meet the expectations, but rather the opposite was observed: serotonin transporter knockout mice (SERT KO), for instance, were supposed to show reduced anxiety but exhibited a more anxious phenotype (Holmes et al., 2003). To explain this one has to consider the strong influence of the genetic background and also that gene deletion eventually results in compensatory processes. Moreover, human studies imply that variants in many genes confer an individual's risk for mood disorders, and mutations found result in rather subtle changes in protein expression and function, which become overt under certain conditions only.

The ambition to develop new pharmacological treatments for patients who are depressed goes hand in hand with the attempt to learn more about the neurobiological basis of depression. Mouse mutants bearing a deficiency in gene products, which were so far not considered in the context of depression, represent an additional source for potential targets for new antidepressants. For instance, analyses of the behavioral phenotype of Kcnk2-knockout mice, which are deficient for the background potassium channel TREK-1, show a depression-resistant phenotype (Heurteaux et al., 2006). Compared to the wild-type, TREK-1 deficient mice showed reduced immobility in FST and TST, reduced conditioned suppression of motility, no increase in escape latencies after inescapable foot shocks, reduced latency in the novelty-suppressed feeding test, and no behavioral response to chronic treatment with the antidepressant paroxetine. This example illustrates the importance of including tests of depression-like behavior into standard screens for behavioral phenotyping of mouse mutants without apparent link to human depression.

FUTURE REQUIREMENTS

Despite the enormous progress in recent years, animal models of depression still bear limitations, which have to be overcome in the future:

1. Most tests of depression-like behavior (for example, FST, TST, anxiety tests) activate memory processes, which preclude their repeated application to one and the same animal. This renders it impossible to follow the progress of chronic antidepressant treatment and to study animal models with repeated depression-like episodes, for instance in the context of development of pharmacotolerance to antidepressants. Therefore, more attention has to be paid to read-outs, which can be repeatedly assessed (for example, by refined measurements of anhedonia).

2. Chronic antidepressant treatment should be initiated after, but not during, the induction of depression-like symptoms (for example, during chronic stress), if the therapeutic rather than preventive potential of the antidepressant is under study.

3. Depression-like episodes are often limited to a few days even after severe stress, which is in striking contrast to the situation in human patients. It appears to be necessary that animal models include developmental and genetic factors, for instance, by exposing animals with a certain genetic makeup (inbred strains, selectively bred animals, genetically modified mice) to uncontrollable, unpredictable and severe stressors, if possible during sensitive phases of development.

4. Even groups of inbred (that is, genetically identical) animals show considerable variability in their behavioral responses (Cohen and Zohar, 2004). Tests should be established that allow the identification of vulnerable and resilient individuals before induction of depression-like symptoms. Subsequent focusing on susceptible animals increases the power of pharmacological studies and enables, in comparison to resilient animals, the characterization of pathogenic versus salutogenic processes.

5. Results of behavioral studies need to be corroborated in complementary test paradigms. For instance, reduced consumption of sucrose solution not necessarily indicates anhedonia, because it might result from increased neophobia. Only a sustained reduction in sucrose intake over longer periods of time serves as a valid measure of anhedonia.

6. Animal models of depression too often lack reproducibility in other laboratories. This can be largely ascribed to differences in animal husbandry and in experimental conditions (Crabbe et al., 1999). Consequently, more effort has to be invested in the establishment of standard operating procedures, including the use of defined reference strains.

CONCLUSION

Depressive syndromes constitute a heterogeneous combination of symptoms, and these symptoms may vary considerably in type and severity. Thus, development of a "perfect" animal model of depression that meets all criteria is highly unlikely. A more pragmatic approach is to identify those behaviors and changes that frequently occur in the clinical condition and that can be confidently studied in animals. Such behaviors include anxiety, anhedonia, learning and memory retrieval, food consumption, sleep patterns, and the response to neuropsychopharmacological interventions. Models designed to simulate signs and symptoms prevalent in depression may be useful in detecting certain underlying pathologies, for example, aberrant HPA axis regulation as a causative factor for cognitive deficits. Until recently, available animal models of depression almost exclusively employed various stressors, and too little attention was paid to genetic and epigenetic factors. Although several neuroendocrine and behavioral phenomena that are characteristic for depression are consistent with the view that depression and inappropriate coping with stress have much in common, it must be noted that stressful life events per se are frequent, but not necessary, precipitators of depressive episodes in individuals that carry the genetic risk. Also, psychopathology following chronic stress does not mimic depression. To overcome the limitations associated with purely stress-derived animal models, more attention has to be paid to the increasing knowledge about genetic susceptibility. Future efforts will integrate molecular genetics, developmental factors, and behavioral research in such a way that animal models emerge that have a high overall validity for studies of complex clinical conditions such as mood disorders.

REFERENCES

Anisman, H., and Matheson, K. (2005) Stress, depression, and anhedonia: caveats concerning animal models. *Neurosci. Biobehav. Rev.* 29:525–546.

Bale, T.L., and Vale, W.W. (2004) CRF and CRF receptors: role in stress responsivity and other behaviors. *Annu. Rev. Pharmacol. Toxicol.* 44:525–557.

Berton, O., and Nestler, E.J. (2006) New approaches to antidepressant drug discovery: beyond monoamines. *Nat. Rev. Neurosci.* 7:137–151.

Caspi, A., Sugden, K., Moffitt, T.E., Taylor, A., Craig, I.W., Harrington, H., McClay, J., Mill, J., Martin, J., Braithwaite, A., and Poulton, R. (2003) Influence of life stress on depression: moderation by a polymorphism in the 5-HTT gene. *Science* 301:386–389.

Champagne, F.A., Francis, D.D., Mar, A., and Meaney, M.J. (2003) Variations in maternal care in the rat as a mediating influence for the effects of environment on development. *Physiol. Behav.* 79: 359–371.

Charney, D.S., and Manji, H.K. (2004) Life stress, genes, and depression: multiple pathways lead to increased risk and new opportunities for intervention. *Sci. STKE.* 2004(225):re5.

Chourbaji, S., Hellweg, R., Brandis, D., Zorner, B., Zacher, C., Lang, U.E., Henn, F.A., Hortnagl, H., and Gass, P. (2004) Mice with reduced brain-derived neurotrophic factor expression show decreased choline acetyltransferase activity, but regular brain monoamine levels and unaltered emotional behavior. *Brain Res. Mol. Brain Res.* 121:28–36.

Cohen, H., and Zohar, J. (2004) An animal model of posttraumatic stress disorder: the use of cut-off behavioral criteria. *Ann. N. Y. Acad. Sci.* 1032:167–178.

Coplan, J.D., Andrewa, M.W., Rosenblum, L.A., Owens, M.J., Freidman, S., Gorman, J.M., and Nemeroff, C.B. (1996) Persistent elevations of cerebrospinal fluid concentrations of corticotropin-releasing factor in adult nonhuman primates exposed to early-life stressors: implications for the pathophysiology of mood and anxiety disorders. *Proc. Natl. Acad. Sci. USA* 93:1619–1623.

Crabbe, J.C., Wahlsten, D., and Dudek, B.C. (1999) Genetics of mouse behavior: interactions with laboratory environment [see comments]. *Science* 284:1670–1672.

Cryan, J.F., and Holmes, A. (2005) The ascent of mouse: advances in modelling human depression and anxiety. *Nat. Rev. Drug Discov.* 4:775–790.

Cryan, J.F., and Mombereau, C. (2004) In search of a depressed mouse: utility of models for studying depression-related behavior in genetically modified mice. *Mol. Psychiatry* 9:326–357.

Cryan, J.F., Mombereau, C., and Vassout, A. (2005) The tail suspension test as a model for assessing antidepressant activity: review of pharmacological and genetic studies in mice. *Neurosci. Biobehav. Rev.* 29:571–625.

Cryan, J.F., Valentino, R.J., and Lucki, I. (2005) Assessing substrates underlying the behavioral effects of antidepressants using the modified rat forced swimming test. *Neurosci. Biobehav. Rev.* 29:547–569.

Czéh, B., Michaelis, T., Watanabe, T., Frahm, J., de Biurrun, G., van Kampen, M., Bartolomucci, A., and Fuchs, E. (2001) Stress-induced changes in cerebral metabolites, hippocampal volume, and cell proliferation are prevented by antidepressant treatment with tianeptine. *Proc. Natl. Acad. Sci. USA* 98:12796–12801.

Czéh, B., Simon, M., Schmelting, B., Hiemke, C., and Fuchs, E. (2006) Astroglial plasticity in the hippocampus is affected by chronic psychosocial stress and concomitant fluoxetine treatment. *Neuropsychopharmacology* 31:1616–1626.

de Kloet, E.R., Joels, M., and Holsboer, F. (2005) Stress and the brain: from adaptation to disease. *Nat. Rev. Neurosci.* 6:463–475.

Duman, R.S. (2004) Depression: a case of neuronal life and death? *Biol. Psychiatry* 56:140–145.

Francis, D.D., Szegda, K., Campbell, G., Martin, W.D., and Insel, T.R. (2003) Epigenetic sources of behavioral differences in mice. *Nat. Neurosci.* 6:445–446.

Frank, E., Salchner, P., Aldag, J.M., Salome, N., Singewald, N., Landgraf, R., and Wigger, A. (2006) Genetic predisposition to anxiety-related behavior determines coping style, neuroendocrine responses, and neuronal activation during social defeat. *Behav. Neurosci.* 120:60–71.

Fuchs, E. (2005) Social stress in tree shrews as an animal model of depression: an example of a behavioral model of a CNS disorder. *CNS Spectr.* 10:182–190.

Fuchs, E., Czeh, B., Michaelis, T., de Biurrun, G., Watanabe, T., and Frahm, J. (2002) Synaptic plasticity and tianeptine: structural regulation. *Eur. Psychiatry.* 17:311–317.

Fuchs, E., Kramer, M., Hermes, B., Netter, P., and Hiemke, C. (1996) Psychosocial stress in tree shrews: clomipramine counteracts behavioral and endocrine changes. *Pharmacol. Biochem. Behav.* 54: 219–228.

Henn, F.A., Johnson, J., Edwards, E., and Anderson, D. (1985) Melancholia in rodents: neurobiology and pharmacology. *Psychopharm. Bull.* 21:443–446.

Henn, F.A., and Vollmayr, B. (2004) Neurogenesis and depression: etiology or epiphenomenon? *Biol. Psychiatry* 56:146–150.

Heurteaux, C., Lucas, G., Guy, N., El Yacoubi, M., Thummler, S., Peng, X.D., Noble, F., Blondeau, N., Widmann, C., Borsotto, M., Gobbi, G., Vaugeois, J.M., Debonnel, G., and Lazdunski, M. (2006) Deletion of the background potassium channel TREK-1 results in a depression-resistant phenotype. *Nat. Neurosci.* 9:1134–1141.

Hinde, R.A., Leighton-Shapiro, M.E., and McGinnis, L. (1978) Effects of various types of separation experience on rhesus monkeys 5 months later. *J. Child Psychol. Psychiatry All. Disc.* 19: 199–211.

Holmes, A., Murphy, D.L., and Crawley, J.N. (2003) Abnormal behavioral phenotypes of serotonin transporter knockout mice: parallels with human anxiety and depression. *Biol. Psychiatry* 54: 953–959.

Holsboer, F. (1995) Neuroendocrinology of mood disorders. In: Bloom, F.E., and Kupfer, D.J., eds. *Psychopharmacology: The Fourth Generation of Progress.* New York: Raven Press, pp. 957–969.

Holsboer, F. (2000) The corticosteroid receptor hypothesis of depression. *Neuropsychopharmacology* 23:477–501.

Hotz Vitaterna, M., Pinto, L.H., and Takahashi, J.S. (2006) Large-scale mutagenesis and phenotypic screens for the nervous system and behavior in mice. *Trends Neurosci.* 29:233–240.

Ising, M., and Holsboer, F. (2006) Genetics of stress response and stress-related disorders. *Dialogues Clin. Neurosci.* 8:433–444.

Jacobson, L.H., and Cryan, J.F. (2007) Feeling strained? Influence of genetic background on depression-related behavior in mice: a review. *Behav. Genet.* 37:171–213.

Kalin, N.H., Shelton, S.E., and Barksdale, C.M. (1989) Behavioral and physiologic effects of CRH administration to infant primates undergoing maternal separation. *Neuropsychopharmacology* 2:97–104.

Kalueff, A.V., Wheaton, M., and Murphy, D.L. (2007) What's wrong with my mouse model? Advances and strategies in animal modeling of anxiety and depression. *Behav. Brain Res.* 179:1–18.

Kandel, E.R. (2001) The molecular biology of memory storage: a dialogue between genes and synapses. *Science* 294:1030–1038.

Keck, M.E., Welt, T., Müller, M.B., Uhr, M., Ohl, F., Wigger, A., Toschi, N., Holsboer, F., and Landgraf, R. (2003) Reduction of hypothalamic vasopressinergic hyperdrive contributes to clinically relevant behavioral and neuroendocrine effects of the antidepressant paroxetine in a psychopathological rat model. *Neuropsychopharmacology* 28:235–243.

Keck, M.E., Welt, T., Post, A., Müller, M.B., Toschi, N., Wigger, A., Landgraf, R., Holsboer, F., and Engelmann, M. (2001) Neuroendocrine and behavioral effects of repetitive transcranial magnetic stimulation in a psychopathological animal model are suggestive of antidepressant-like effects. *Neuropsychopharmacology* 24: 337–349.

Keck, M.E., Welt, T., Wigger, A., Renner, U., Engelmann, M., Holsboer, F., and Landgraf, R. (2001) The anxiolytic effect of the CRH1 receptor antagonist R121919 depends on innate emotionality in rats. *Eur. J. Neurosci.* 13:373–380.

Keck, M.E., Wigger, A., Welt, T., Muller, M.B., Gesing, A., Reul, J.M., Holsboer, F., Landgraf, R., and Neumann, I.D. (2002) Vasopressin mediates the response of the combined dexamethasone/CRH test in hyper-anxious rats: implications for pathogenesis of affective disorders. *Neuropsychopharmacology* 26:94–105.

Kromer, S.A., Kessler, M.S., Milfay, D., Birg, I.N., Bunck, M., Czibere, L., Panhuysen, M., Putz, B., Deussing, J.M., Holsboer, F., Landgraf, R., and Turck, C.W. (2005) Identification of glyoxalase-I as a protein marker in a mouse model of extremes in trait anxiety. *J. Neurosci.* 25:4375–4384.

Landgraf, R., Kessler, M.S., Bunck, M., Murgatroyd, C., Spengler, D., Zimbelmann, M., Nussbaumer, M., Czibere, L., Turck, C.W., Singewald, N., Rujescu, D., and Frank, E. (2007) Candidate genes of anxiety-related behavior in HAB/LAB rats and mice: focus on vasopressin and glyoxalase-I. *Neurosci. Biobehav. Rev.* 31:89–102.

Lesch, K.P. (2004) Gene-environment interaction and the genetics of depression. *J. Psychiatry Neurosci.* 29:174–184.

Liebsch, G., Linthorst, A.C.E., Neumann, I.D., Reul, J.M.H.M., Holsboer, F., and Landgraf, R. (1998) Behavioral, physiological, and neuroendocrine stress responses and differential sensitivity to diazepam in two Wistar rat lines selectively bred for high and low anxiety-related behavior. *Neuropsychopharmacology* 19:381–396.

Lindsey, B.W., and Tropepe, V. (2006) A comparative framework for understanding the biological principles of adult neurogenesis. *Prog. Neurobiol.* 80:281–307.

Lucae, S., Salyakina, D., Barden, N., Harvey, M., Gagne, B., Labbe, M., Binder, E.B., Uhr, M., Paez-Pereda, M., Sillaber, I., Ising, M., Bruckl, T., Lieb, R., Holsboer, F., and Muller-Myhsok, B. (2006) P2RX7, a gene coding for a purinergic ligand-gated ion channel, is associated with major depressive disorder. *Hum. Mol. Genet.* 15:2438–2445.

Macri, S., and Wurbel, H. (2006) Developmental plasticity of HPA and fear responses in rats: a critical review of the maternal mediation hypothesis. *Horm. Behav.* 50:667–680.

Malatynska, E., and Knapp, R.J. (2005) Dominant-submissive behavior as models of mania and depression. *Neurosci. Biobehav. Rev.* 29:715–737.

Malkesman, O., Braw, Y., Maayan, R., Weizman, A., Overstreet, D.H., Shabat-Simon, M., Kesner, Y., Touati-Werner, D., Yadid, G., and Weller, A. (2006) Two different putative genetic animal models of childhood depression. *Biol. Psychiatry*. 59:17–23.

Margulies, C., Tully, T., and Dubnau, J. (2005) Deconstructing memory in Drosophila. *Curr. Biol.* 15:R700–R713.

Mayorga, A.J., and Lucki, I. (2001) Limitations on the use of the C57BL/6 mouse in the tail suspension test. *Psychopharmacology* 155:110–112.

McKinney, W.T., Jr., and Bunney, W.E., Jr. (1969) Animal model of depression: I. Review of evidence: implications for research. *Arch. Gen. Psychiatry* 21:240–248.

Millstein, R.A., and Holmes, A. (2007) Effects of repeated maternal separation on anxiety- and depression-related phenotypes in different mouse strains. *Neurosci. Biobehav. Rev.* 31:3–17.

Montkowski, A., and Holsboer, F. (1997) Intact spatial learning and memory in transgenic mice with reduced BDNF. *Neuroreport* 8: 779–782.

Muigg, P., Hoelzl, U., Palfrader, K., Neumann, I., Wigger, A., Landgraf, R., and Singewald, N. (2007) Altered brain activation pattern associated with drug-induced attenuation of enhanced depression-like behavior in rats bred for high anxiety. *Biol. Psychiatry* 61: 782–796.

Müller, M.B., and Holsboer, F. (2006) Mice with mutations in the HPA-system as models for symptoms of depression. *Biol. Psychiatry* 59:1104–1115.

Nielsen, C.K., Arnt, J., and Sanchez, C. (2000) Intracranial self-stimulation and sucrose intake differ as hedonic measures following chronic mild stress: interstrain and interindividual differences. *Behav. Brain Res.* 107:21–33.

Overmier, J.B., and Seligman, M.E.P. (1967) Effects of inescapable shock upon subsequent escape and avoidance learning. *J. Comp. Physiol. Psychol.* 63:28–33.

Overstreet, D.H. (1993) The Flinders Sensitive Line rats: a genetic animal model of depression. *Neurosci. Biobehav. Rev.* 17:51–68.

Overstreet, D.H., Friedman, E., Mathe, A.A., and Yadid, G. (2005) The Flinders Sensitive Line rat: a selectively bred putative animal model of depression. *Neurosci. Biobehav. Rev.* 29:739–759.

Peters, L.L., Robledo, R.F., Bult, C.J., Churchill, G.A., Paigen, B.J., and Svenson, K.L. (2007) The mouse as a model for human biology: a resource guide for complex trait analysis. *Nat. Rev. Genet.* 8:58–69.

Petit-Demouliere, B., Chenu, F., and Bourin, M. (2005) Forced swimming test in mice: a review of antidepressant activity. *Psychopharmacology* 177:245–255.

Picciotto, M.R., and Wickman, K. (1998) Using knockout and transgenic mice to study neurophysiology and behavior. *Physiol. Rev.* 78:1131–1163.

Plotsky, P.M., Owens, M.J., and Nemeroff, C.B. (1998) Psychoneuroendocrinology of depression. Hypothalamic-pituitary-adrenal axis. *Psychiatr. Clin. North Am.* 21:293–307.

Popa, D., El Yacoubi, M., Vaugeois, J.M., Hamon, M., and Adrien, J. (2006) Homeostatic regulation of sleep in a genetic model of depression in the mouse: effects of muscarinic and 5-HT1A receptor activation. *Neuropsychopharmacology* 31:1637–1646.

Porsolt, R.D., Bertin, A., and Jalfre, M. (1977) Behavioral despair in mice: a primary screening test for antidepressants. *Arch. Int. Pharmacodyn. Ther.* 229:327–336.

Santarelli, L., Saxe, M., Gross, C., Surget, A., Battaglia, F., Dulawa, S., Weisstaubs, N., Lee, J., Duman, R., Arancio, O., Belzung, C., and Hen, R. (2003) Requirement of hippocampal neurogenesis for the behavioral effects of antidepressants. *Science* 301:805–809.

Seligman, M.E.P., and Beagley, G. (1975) Learned helplessness in the rat. *J. Comp. Physiol. Psychol.* 88:534–541.

Song, C., and Leonard, B.E. (2005) The olfactory bulbectomised rat as a model of depression. *Neurosci. Biobehav. Rev.* 29:627–647.

Sousa, N., Almeida, O.F., and Wotjak, C.T. (2006) A hitchhiker's guide to behavioral analysis in laboratory rodents. *Genes Brain Behav.* 5(Suppl 2):5–24.

Specht, C.G. and Schoepfer, R. (2001) Deletion of the alpha-synuclein locus in a subpopulation of C57BL/6J inbred mice. *BMC. Neurosci.* 2:11.

Steru, L., Chermat, R., Thierry, B., and Simon, P. (1985) The tail suspension test: a new method for screening antidepressants in mice. *Psychopharmacology* 85:367–370.

Tsoory, M., Cohen, H., and Richter-Levin, G. (2007) Juvenile stress induces a predisposition to either anxiety or depressive-like symptoms following stress in adulthood. *Eur. Neuropsychopharmacol.* 17:245–256.

Turri, M.G., Datta, S.R., DeFries, J., Henderson, N.D., and Flint, J. (2001) QTL analysis identifies multiple behavioral dimensions in ethological tests of anxiety in laboratory mice. *Curr. Biol.* 11: 725–734.

Urani, A., Chourbaji, S., and Gass, P. (2005) Mutant mouse models of depression: candidate genes and current mouse lines. *Neurosci. Biobehav. Rev.* 29:805–828.

Vaugeois, J.M., Passera, G., Zuccaro, F., and Costentin, J. (1997) Individual differences in response to imipramine in the mouse tail suspension test. *Psychopharmacology* 134:387–391.

Vyas, A., Mitra, R., Shankaranarayana Rao, B.S., and Chattarji, S. (2002) Chronic stress induces contrasting patterns of dendritic remodeling in hippocampal and amygdaloid neurons. *J. Neurosci.* 22:6810–6818.

Weaver, I.C., Cervoni, N., Champagne, F.A., D'Alessio, A.C., Sharma, S., Seckl, J.R., Dymov, S., Szyf, M., and Meaney, M.J. (2004) Epigenetic programming by maternal behavior. *Nat. Neurosci.* 7:847–854.

Weiss, J.M. (1968) Effects of coping responses on stress. *J. Comp. Physiol. Psychiol.* 65:251–260.

Weiss, J.M. (1980) Coping behavior: explaining behavioral depression following uncontrollable stressful events. *Behav. Res. Ther.* 18:485–504.

West, P.A. (1990) Neurobehavioral studies of forced swimming. The role of learning and memory in the forced swim test. *Progr. Neuropsychopharmacol. Biol. Psychiatry* 14:863–875.

Willner, P. (2005) Chronic mild stress (CMS) revisited: consistency and behavioural-neurobiological concordance in the effects of CMS. *Neuropsychobiology* 52:90–110.

Wong, M.L., Whelan, F., Deloukas, P., Whittaker, P., Delgado, M., Cantor, R.M., McCann, S.M., and Licinio J. (2006) Phosphodiesterase genes are associated with susceptibility to major depression and antidepressant treatment response. *Proc. Natl. Acad. Sci. USA* 103:15124–15129.

Wotjak, C.T. (2003) C57BLack/BOX? The importance of exact mouse strain nomenclature. *Trends Genet.* 19:183–184.

Wotjak, C.T. (2004) Of mice and men: potentials and caveats of behavioural experiments with mice. *B.I.F. FUTURA* 19:158–169.

Yoshikawa, T., Watanabe, A., Ishitsuka, Y., Nakaya, A., and Nakatani, N. (2002) Identification of multiple genetic loci linked to the propensity for "behavioral despair" in mice. *Genome Res.* 12: 357–366.

Zaharia, M.D., Kulczycki, J., Shanks, N., Meaney, M.J., and Anisman, H. (1996) The effects of early postnatal stimulation on Morris water-maze acquisition in adult mice: genetic and maternal factors. *Psychopharmacology* 128:227–239.

Zangen, A., Overstreet, D.H., and Yadid, G. (1997) High serotonin and 5-hydroxyindoleacetic acid levels in limbic brain regions in a rat model of depression: normalization by chronic antidepressant treatment. *J. Neurochem.* 69:2477–2483.

Zhang, X., Beaulieu, J.M., Sotnikova, T.D., Gainetdinov, R.R., and Caron, M.G. (2004) Tryptophan hydroxylase-2 controls brain serotonin synthesis. *Science* 305:217.

Zobel, A.W., Nickel, T., Kunzel, H.E., Ackl, N., Sonntag, A., Ising, M., and Holsboer, F. (2000) Effects of the high-affinity corticotropin-releasing hormone receptor 1 antagonist R121919 in major depression: the first 20 patients treated. *J. Psychiatr. Res.* 34:171–181.

28 Cellular Plasticity Cascades: Genes to Behavior Pathways in the Pathophysiology and Treatment of Bipolar Disorder

LISA A. CATAPANO, GUANG CHEN, JING DU, CARLOS A. ZARATE, JR., AND HUSSEINI K. MANJI

Bipolar disorder (BPD) is a complex illness, involving the dysregulation of mood, sleep, cognition, endocrine, and motor systems. A true understanding of the pathophysiology of this disorder must encompass these different systems, and the different physiologic levels at which the disease manifests: molecular, cellular, systems, and behavioral (Fig. 28.1). Building upon decades of research that has identified abnormalities in neurotransmitter systems in this disorder, there is a growing appreciation that signal transduction pathways play a pivotal role in mediating the dysfunction of multiple neurotransmitter systems and physiologic processes in bipolar illness. Complex signaling networks are undoubtedly involved in regulating such diverse functions as mood, appetite, and wakefulness and are therefore thought to be involved in the pathophysiology of mood and vegetative symptoms. Furthermore, there is clear evidence that signaling pathways are targets of the most effective pharmacologic treatments for BPD.

Neurobiological studies of mood disorders over the last 40 years have focused primarily on abnormalities of the monoaminergic neurotransmitter systems, characterizing alterations of individual neurotransmitters in disease states, and in response to mood stabilizer and antidepressant medications. The monoaminergic systems are extensively distributed throughout the network of limbic, striatal, and prefrontal cortical neuronal circuits thought to support the behavioral and visceral

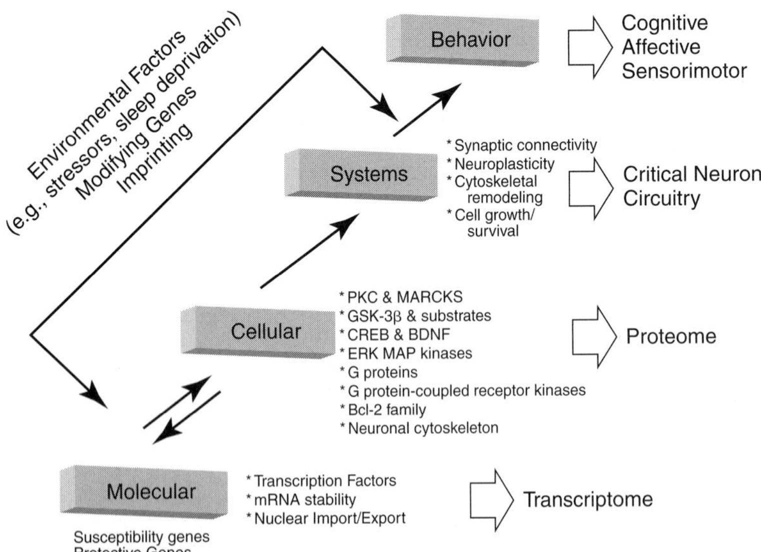

FIGURE 28.1 The pathophysiology of bipolar disorder. A complete understanding of the pathophysiology of bipolar disorder must address its neurobiology at different physiological levels: molecular, cellular, systems, and behavioral. PKC: protein kinase C; MARCKS: myristoylated alanine-rich C kinase substrate; GSK-3: glycogen synthase kinase-3; CREB: cyclic AMP response binding protein; BDNF: brain-derived neurotrophic factor; ERK MAP kinase: extracellular response kinase/mitogen-activated protein kinase; Bcl-2: B-cell leukemia/lymphoma; *transcriptome* refers to the population of cellular mRNA species and their expression level; *proteome* refers to the population of cellular protein species and their expression level. Modified and reproduced with (pending) permission from Manji and Lenox (2000a).

manifestations of mood disorders (Drevets, 2000). Assessments of cerebrospinal fluid (CSF) chemistry, neuroendocrine responses to pharmacological challenge, and neuroreceptor and transporter binding have demonstrated a number of abnormalities in monoaminergic neurotransmitter and neuropeptide systems in mood disorders (Table 28.1) (Goodwin and Jamison, 2007).

Unfortunately, these observations have not yet greatly advanced our understanding of the underlying biology of recurrent mood disorders, which must include an

TABLE 28.1 *Summary of Major Findings Implicating Multiple Systems in Bipolar Disorder*

Serotonergic system

- Reduced CSF 5-HIAA
- Blunted neuroendocrine and temperature responses to 5-HT agonists
- Reduced 5-HT_{1A} receptor binding in living brain and postmortem brain tissue
- Antidepressant efficacy of agents that increase intrasynaptic 5-HT
- Triggering of manic episodes by agents that increase intrasynaptic 5-HT
- Depressogenic effects of tryptophan depletion in patients treated with antidepressants
- Decrease 5-HT_{1A} and 5-HT_2 density and 5-HT turnover by antidepressants

Noradrenergic system

- Reduced CSF and urinary MHPG
- Elevated plasma NE
- Correlation between CSF NE levels and dysphoric symptoms and severity of illness
- Blunted neuroendocrine responses to clonidine
- Triggering of mania by agents that increase NE release or block reuptake
- Altered α_2-AR and β-AR density and responsivity in peripheral circulating cells
- Altered densities of α_2-AR and β-AR in areas of postmortem brain
- Antidepressant efficacy of agents that increase NE
- Reduction in NE turnover by most antidepressants
- Reduction β-AR density and/or function in limbic areas in response to antidepressants

Dopaminergic system

- Reduced CSF HVA
- Blunted neuroendocrine and temperature responses to DA agonists
- Antidepressant efficacy of agents whose biochemical effects include increasing DA
- Enhanced DA function by ECT
- Depressogenic effects of AMPT and reserpine in susceptible individuals
- Antimanic efficacy of antipsychotic medications (D_2 receptor blockers)
- Reduced internal jugular venoarterial DA metabolite concentration gradients
- Increased risk of depression in Parkinson's disease
- Prominent anhedonia and amotivation given role of DA in reward and motivation circuits

Cholinergic system

- Depressogenic and antimanic effects of cholinomimetics
- Enhanced cholinergic sensitivity
- Role in sleep EEG abnormalities

Glutamatergic system

- Key role of glutamate signaling in stress-induced atrophy
- Alterations of CSF, plasma, and platelet glutamate/glutamine levels
- Altered regional glutamate metabolism by positron emission tomography
- Facilitated glutamate reuptake, and protection against excitotoxicity, by lithium
- Regulation of hippocampal glutamate uptake capacity by valproate
- Attentuation of excess glutamate release by the mood stabilizer lamotrigine
- Downregulation of AMPA GluR1 synaptic expression by lithium and valproate
- Upregulation of AMPA GluR1 synaptic expression by antidepressants
- Regulation of NMDA receptor mRNA and binding by antidepressants
- Antidepressant effects of NMDA antagonists, including ketamine
- Attenuation of manic-like behavior in animals by AMPA antagonists

GABAergic system

- Altered CSF and plasma GABA in depressed and manic subjects
- Reduced occipital cortex GABA in unipolar (but not bipolar) depressed individuals
- Region-specific decrease in reelin (secreted by GABAergic interneurons)
- Region-specific decrease in GABA synthetic enzymes GAD_{65} and GAD_{67}
- Decreased GABA turnover in frontal cortex in response to mood stabilizers
- Increased GABA(B) receptors in hippocampus in response to mood stabilizers
- Genetic association of genes for GABA receptor α_3 and α_5 subunits with BPD

CRF and HPA axis

- Hypercortisolemia and resistance to feedback inhibition
- Adrenal and pituitary hypertrophy
- Increased CSF CRF, and reduced CRF receptors, in postmortem brain
- Depressogenic/anxiogenic effects of CRF agonists in preclinical models
- Hypercortisolemia normalized by successful antidepressant treatment

Peptides

- Anxiolytic/antidepressant properties of substance P receptor (NK-1) antagonists
- Reduced CSF NPY in depression, and increased NPY with lithium, antidepressants, and ECT
- Reduced somatostatin in CSF of patients with depression
- Abnormalities of vasopressin expression and receptor activity in depression

CSF: cerebrospinal fluid; 5-HIAA: 5-Hydroxyindoleacetic acid; MHPG: methoxy-hydroxy-phenyl-glycol; NE: norepinephrine; AR: adrenergic receptor; HVA: homovanillic acid; DA: dopamine; AMPT: alpha-methyl-p-tyrosine; EEG: electroencephalography; NMDA: *N*-methyl-D-aspartate; CRF: cortisol releasing factor; HPA: hypothalamic-pituitary axis; ECT: electroconvulsive therapy; NPY: Neuropeptide Y; AMPA: α-amino-3-hydroxy-5-methyl-4-isoxasdepropionic acid; mRNA: messenger ribonucleic acid; GABA: γ-aminobutyric acid; BPD: bipolar disorder.

explanation for the predilection to episodic and often profound mood disturbance that can become progressive over time. Bipolar disorder likely arises from the complex interaction of multiple susceptibility (and protective) genes and environmental factors, and the phenotypic expression of the disease includes not only mood disturbance, but also a constellation of cognitive, motoric, autonomic, endocrine, and sleep/wake abnormalities. Furthermore, though most antidepressants exert their initial effects by increasing intrasynaptic levels of serotonin and/or norepinephrine, their clinical antidepressant effects are observed only after chronic administration (over days to weeks), suggesting that a cascade of downstream events is ultimately responsible for their therapeutic effects. These observations have led to the idea that though dysfunction within the monoaminergic neurotransmitter systems is likely to play an important role in mediating some facets of the pathophysiology of BPD, it likely represents the downstream effects of other, more primary abnormalities in signaling pathways (Table 28.2) (Manji and Lenox, 2000a).

It is our hypothesis that BPD arises from abnormalities in cellular plasticity cascades, leading to aberrant information processing in synapses and circuits mediating affective, cognitive, motoric, and neurovegetative functions. Thus, these illnesses can be best conceptualized as genetically influenced disorders of synapses and circuits—rather than simply as deficits or excesses in individual neurotransmitters. Furthermore, many of these pathways play critical roles not only in synaptic (and therefore behavioral) plasticity, but also in long-term atrophic processes. Targeting these cascades in treatment may stabilize the underlying disease process by reducing the frequency and severity of the profound mood cycling that contributes to morbidity and mortality.

In this chapter, we focus upon the role of signaling cascades in the pathophysiology and treatment of BPD. The role of neurotransmitter and neuropeptide systems has been extensively covered elsewhere in recent publications (Goodwin and Jamison, 2007; Soares and Young, 2007) and is not covered here.

TABLE 28.2 *Putative Roles for Signaling Pathways in Mood Disorders*

- Amplify, attenuate, and integrate multiple signals that form the basis for intracellular circuits and cellular modules
- Regulate multiple neurotransmitter and peptide systems
- Play critical role in cellular memory and long-term neuroplasticity
- Regulate complex signaling networks that form the basis for higher-order brain function, mood, and cognition
- Act as major targets for many hormones implicated in mood disorders, including gonadal steroids, thyroid hormones, and glucocorticoids
- Act as targets for medications that are most effective in the treatment of mood disorders

SIGNALING NETWORKS: THE CELLULAR MACHINERY UNDERLYING INFORMATION PROCESSING AND LONG-TERM NEUROPLASTIC EVENTS

It is hardly surprising that abnormalities in multiple neurotransmitter systems and physiological processes have been found in a disorder as complex as BPD. Signal transduction pathways are in a pivotal position in the central nervous system (CNS), affecting the functional balance between multiple neurotransmitter systems, and therefore playing a role in mediating the more downstream abnormalities that likely underlie the pathophysiology of affective disorders (Fig. 28.2). Moreover, as we discuss below, recent research has clearly identified signaling pathways as therapeutically relevant targets for our most effective pharmacological treatments.

Multicomponent cellular signaling pathways interact at various levels, forming complex signaling networks that allow the cell to receive, process, and respond to information (Bhalla and Iyengar, 1999). Given their widespread and crucial role in the integration, regulation, amplification, and fine-tuning of physiological processes, it is not surprising that abnormalities in signaling pathways have now been identified in a variety of human diseases (Spiegel, 1998). Importantly, these diseases manifest relatively circumscribed symptomatology, despite widespread expression of the affected signaling proteins.

Although complex signaling networks are likely present in all eukaryotic cells and control various metabolic, humoral, and developmental functions, they may be especially important in the CNS, where they serve the critical roles of first amplifying and "weighting"

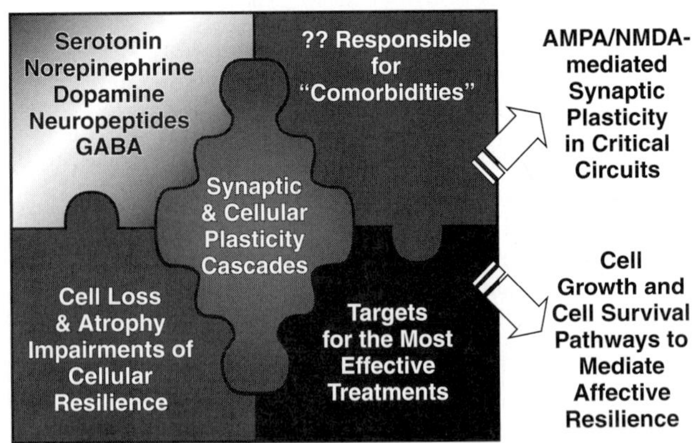

FIGURE 28.2 Signal transduction pathways provide good explanatory power for understanding the complex neurobiology of bipolar disorder. GABA: γ-aminobutyric acid; AMPA: AMPA-type glutamate receptor; NMDA: NMDA-type glutamate receptor.

numerous extracellularly generated signals, and then transmitting these integrated signals to effectors, thereby forming the basis for complex information processing. The high degree of complexity generated by these signaling networks may be one mechanism by which neurons acquire the flexibility for generating the wide range of responses observed in the nervous system. Recent studies provide evidence that impairments of signaling pathways play a role in the pathophysiology of BPD, and that mood stabilizers exert major effects on the signaling pathways that regulate neuroplasticity and cell survival. These data are reshaping views about the neurobiological underpinnings of BPD and generating exciting possibilities for the development of novel therapeutics.

ABNORMALITIES OF PLASTICITY AT THE SYNAPTIC AND/OR CELLULAR LEVEL IN MOOD DISORDERS

Evidence for Abnormalities of Synaptic/Cellular Plasticity in the Pathophysiology of Mood Disorders

Atrophic changes in recurrent mood disorders

Bipolar disorder is increasingly recognized as involving dysregulation of intracellular signaling cascades that produce not only functional but also morphological impairments. Several morphometric imaging and postmortem investigations have demonstrated abnormalities of brain structure that persist independent of mood state and may contribute to corresponding abnormalities in metabolic activity (Table 28.3) (Manji et al., 2001). Structural imaging studies have demonstrated reduced gray matter volumes in areas of the orbital and medial prefrontal cortex, ventral striatum, and hippocampus in patients with mood disorders (Drevets, 2001; Beyer and Krishnan, 2002; Strakowski et al., 2002). Also consistent is the presence of white matter hyperintensities in the brains of elderly depressed patients and patients with BPD, which may be associated with poor treatment response (Goodwin and Jamison, 2007).

Complementary to this neuroimaging evidence, postmortem brain studies have demonstrated reductions in regional CNS volume, cell number, and cell body size. Baumann et al. (1999) reported reduced volumes of the left nucleus accumbens, right putamen, and bilateral pallidum externum in postmortem brain samples from patients with major depressive disorder (MDD) or BPD. A number of morphometric analyses have revealed abnormal size and density of pyramidal and nonpyramidal neurons in dorsolateral prefrontal cortex (DLPFC), orbitofrontal cortex, anterior cingulate cortex, and hippocampus in patients with mood disorders, although not all studies have observed these findings (Goodwin and Jamison, 2007). Detailed studies from the Rajkowska laboratory have measured the density and size of

TABLE 28.3 *Postmortem Morphometric Brain Studies in Mood Disorders Demonstrating Cellular Atrophy and/or Loss*

Reduced volume
Cortical thickness of rostral orbitofrontal cortex in MDD
Laminar cortical thickness in layers III, V, and VI in subgenual anterior cingulate cortex in BPD
Volume of subgenual prefrontal cortex in MDD and BPD
Volumes of nucleus accumbens and basal ganglia in MDD and BPD
Parahippocampal cortex size in suicide
Reduced neuronal size and/or density
Neuronal size in layer V and VI in prefrontal cortex in MDD and BPD
Pyramidal neuronal density, layers III and V in dorsolateral prefrontal cortex in BPD and MDD
Neuronal density and size in layers II–VI in orbitofrontal cortex in MDD
Neuronal density in layers III, V, and VI in subgenual anterior cingulate cortex in BPD
Neuronal size in layer VI in anterior cingulate cortex in MDD
Layer-specific interneurons in anterior cingulate cortex in BPD and MDD
Nonpyramidal neuronal density in layer II in anterior cingulate cortex in BPD
Nonpyramidal neuronal density in the CA2 region in BPD
Reduced glia
Density/size of glia in dorsolateral prefrontal cortex and caudal orbitofrontal cortex in MDD and BPD
Glial cell density in layer V in prefrontal cortex in MDD
Glial number in subgenual prefrontal cortex in familial MDD and BPD
Glial cell density in layer VI in anterior cingulate cortex in MDD
Glial cell counts, glial density, and glia:neuron ratio in amygdala in MDD

MDD: major depressive disorder; BPD: bipolar disorder.

calbindin-immunoreactive neurons (presumed to be γ-aminobutyric acid [GABA]-ergic) in layers II and III of the DLPFC, revealing a 43% reduction in the density of these neurons in MDD compared with controls (Rajkowska, 2002). Of particular note, in the rostral orbitofrontal cortex, there was a trend toward a negative correlation between the duration of depression and the size of neuronal cell bodies, suggesting changes associated with disease progression (Rajkowska et al., 1999). In general, findings of decreased neuronal size have been more subtle in patients with BPD than in those with MDD. This difference may represent the long-term protective effects of mood stabilizers, as discussed below.

In addition to neuronal pathology, unexpected reductions in glial cell number and density have been found in postmortem brains of patients with MDD and BPD. In fact, observed glial changes have often been more dramatic than those of neurons. Layer-specific reductions in glial densities have been reported in prefrontal cortex in BPD and MDD (Öngür et al., 1998;

Rajkowska et al., 1999; Miguel-Hidalgo et al., 2000). Although the most prominent findings thus far have been from the frontal cortex, studies have also provided evidence for glial pathology in the hippocampus (Stockmeier et al., 2004), consistent with decreases in hippocampal volume noted by neuroimaging studies. Studies implicate astrocytic (Johnston-Wilson et al., 2000) and oligodendrocytic (Uranova et al., 2001; Tkachev et al., 2003; Aston et al., 2005) glial subtypes. These data are particularly intriguing in view of the growing appreciation of glia's roles in regulating synaptic glutamate concentrations and releasing trophic factors that participate in the development and maintenance of synaptic networks.

Increasing recent evidence supports the association between impaired neurogenesis and depression (Vollmayr et al., 2007). Several studies support the hypothesis that stress, which plays a major role in depression, reduces neurogenesis in the dentate gyrus, consistent with findings of reduced hippocampal volume in patients who are depressed. Studies suggest that altered neurogenesis is not necessary for depression-like states in animals (Vollmayr et al., 2007) but is nevertheless reversed by mood stabilizers and antidepressants, as discussed below. The precise nature of the relationship between neurogenesis and mood is still to be determined.

It must be acknowledged that it is not currently known if these impairments of structural plasticity (cell loss, cell atrophy, white matter changes) constitute developmental abnormalities conferring vulnerability to severe mood episodes, compensatory changes to other pathogenic processes, or the sequelae of recurrent affective episodes (Carlson et al., 2006). Indeed, data suggest that multiple factors may be operative. In support of a potential etiologic role of cellular plasticity cascades, some studies have observed reduced gray matter volumes and white matter hyperintensities in patients with mood disorders at first onset, and in children (Frazier et al., 2005). Reduced levels of *N*-acetylaspartate (NAA), generally regarded as a measure of neuronal viability and function (Tsai and Coyle, 1995), have also been found to be significantly reduced in the DLPFC of children with BPD (Sassi et al., 2005). Although these studies do not demonstrate that the changes precede illness onset, they are inconsistent with the theory that the changes represent the toxic sequelae of decades of illness. Consistent with these findings, a meta-analysis of imaging studies concluded that volumetric abnormalities in the subgenual prefrontal cortex, striatum, hippocampus, and amygdala are seen in first-episode patients with BPD, children with BPD, and unaffected siblings, raising the possibility that this endophenotype may constitute a heritable vulnerability factor in these patients (Hajek et al., 2005).

There are, however, also data to suggest that some brain changes may be associated with duration of illness and are the consequences of affective episodes per se. Sheline and colleagues measured hippocampal volumes of patients with a history of major depressive episodes and found that the degree of hippocampal volume reduction correlated with total duration of depression, and with duration of untreated depressive episodes (Sheline et al., 1996; Sheline et al., 2003). Another study found hippocampal volume reduction in patients with multiple depressive episodes, but not in first-episode patients (MacQueen et al., 2003). It is noteworthy that similar changes have not been reported in patients with BPD. This difference may reflect distinct pathophysiologies, or the neuroprotective effects of mood stabilizers (see below).

Overall, it seems likely that cell loss and atrophy represent both etiologic factors and the consequence of disease progression. There is almost no doubt that these atrophic brain changes contribute to illness pathophysiology by disrupting the circuits that mediate normal affective, cognitive, motoric and neurovegetative functioning. These findings suggest that neurotrophic effects of mood stabilizers—if they occur in humans—may be very relevant for the treatment of BPD.

Targeting Synaptic/Cellular Plasticity in the Treatment of Mood Disorders

Neurotrophic and neuroprotective actions of mood stabilizers

Numerous studies at the anatomic, cellular, and molecular levels, provide evidence for the neurotrophic and neuroprotective actions of mood stabilizers. As a complement to the findings of region-specific brain atrophy in BPD, many studies have found evidence that mood stabilizers promote neural viability in multiple preclinical paradigms. Moore and colleagues quantitated levels of NAA in a longitudinal clinical study using proton magnetic resonance spectroscopy (MRS) and found that chronic administration of the mood stabilizer lithium, at therapeutic doses, increases NAA (Moore, Bebchuk, Hasanat, et al., 2000). In follow-up studies, the authors examined brain tissue volumes using high-resolution three-dimensional magnetic resonance imaging (MRI) and demonstrated that chronic lithium administration significantly, and specifically, increased total gray matter content in the brains of patients with BPD (Moore, Bebchuk, Wilds, et al., 2000). A more recent MRI study reported increased hippocampal volume in patients who were treated with lithium (Yucel et al., 2007).

Providing evidence for the clinical significance of these findings, a longitudinal study using high-resolution volumetric MRI demonstrated significant regional volumetric differences between lithium responders and nonresponders (Moore et al., 2006). Only responders showed increases in gray matter in the prefrontal cortex and left subgenual prefrontal cortex, areas that are specifically implicated in the neuropathophysiology of BPD in various neuroimaging and postmortem neuropathology investigations.

At the cellular level, lithium has been shown to exert neuroprotective effects in a variety of preclinical paradigms (see Table 28.4). At therapeutically relevant concentrations, lithium has been demonstrated to protect against the deleterious effects of glutamate, *N*-methyl-D-aspartate (NMDA) receptor activation, aging, serum or growth factor deprivation, and other toxins in vitro (Manji and Lenox, 2000b). Lithium's neurotrophic and cytoprotective effects have also been demonstrated in rodent brain in vivo, in response to kainic acid infusion, forebrain cholinergic system lesions, middle cerebral artery occlusion, and cranial irradiation (Manji and Lenox, 2000b; Yazlovitskaya et al., 2006). Lithium prevents injury-induced degeneration and also promotes axon regeneration in retinal ganglion cells (Huang et al., 2003), presumably via up-regulation of Bcl-2 (discussed below).

A more direct recent study of synaptic plasticity has demonstrated that subchronic lithium, applied to hippocampal slices, resulted in increases in excitatory post-

TABLE 28.4 *Neurotrophic and Neuroprotective Effects of Lithium*

Protects (human and rodent) brain cells in vitro from
glutamate and NMDA toxicity
calcium toxicity
thapsigargin (which mobilizes MPP^+ and Ca^{2+}) toxicity
β-amyloid toxicity
aging-induced cell death
growth factor and serum deprivation
glucose deprivation
low K^+
C_2-ceramide
Ouabain
aluminum toxicity
HIV regulatory protein, Tat
Demonstrates following effects in rodent brain (in vivo)
enhanced hippocampal neurogenesis
protection against cholinergic lesions
protection against radiation injury
protection against medial cerebral artery occlusion (stroke model)
protection against quinolinic acid (Huntington's model)
Demonstrates following effects in human brain
increased gray matter volumes in lithium-treated bipolar patients
increased *N*-acetylaspartate (NAA) levels in lithium-treated bipolar patients
protection against reduced subgenual prefrontal cortex volumes
larger anterior cingulate volumes in lithium-treated bipolar patients
protection against reduced glial numbers or glia: neuron ratio in the amygdale

NMDA: *N*-methyl-D-asparate; HIV: human immuno-deficiency virus; MPP^+: 1-methyl-4-phenylpyridium.

synaptic responses, synaptic strength, and cell firing in dentate gyrus granule cells (Shim et al., 2007).

Although the mood stabilizer valproate has not been as extensively studied as lithium, a number of studies have found that it does indeed exert neuroprotective effects in injury paradigms such as thapsigargin and 1-methyl-4-phenylpyridinium (MPP^+) toxicity (Lai et al., 2006), excitotoxicity (Bruno et al., 1995), low K^+-induced apoptosis (Mora et al., 1999), and middle cerebral artery occlusion (Ren et al., 2004).

Neurotrophic and neuroprotective actions of antidepressants

Several studies demonstrate the neurotrophic-like effects of various classes of antidepressant medications (Goodwin and Jamison, 2007). One early study found that antidepressant treatment induced regeneration of catecholamine axon terminals in the cerebral cortex (Nakamura, 1990). Another study demonstrated that treatment with the atypical antidepressant tianeptine blocked the stress-induced atrophy of CA3 pyramidal neurons, measured as a blockade of the decrease in the number and length of apical dendrite branch points (Watanabe et al., 1992). In tree shrews subjected to chronic psychosocial stress, tianeptine was shown to reverse the stress-induced decreases in NAA, granule cell proliferation, and hippocampal volume (Czeh et al., 2001).

Regulation of hippocampal neurogenesis by mood stabilizers

Given lithium's neurotrophic and neuroprotective effects, the ability of lithium to promote neurogenesis has been of considerable interest. In the normal process of neurogenesis, a significant fraction of neural progenitor cells undergo programmed cell death, and the overexpression of anti-apoptotic Bcl-2 rescues these progenitors (Kuhn et al., 2005). As lithium has been shown to up-regulate Bcl-2 (as discussed below), the intriguing possibility that lithium might promote the survival of neural precursors has been investigated in a number of studies. In an early study, mice treated chronically with lithium were found to have an increase in recently dividing cells in the dentate gyrus (Chen et al., 2000), as identified with BrdU, a thymidine analog that is incorporated into deoxyribonucleic acid (DNA). Approximately two thirds of these BrdU-positive cells also stained with the neuronal marker NeuN, demonstrating their neuronal identity. These results have been replicated by others, in vitro and in vivo (Kim et al., 2004).

Valproate has also been shown to have neurogenic effects in at least one study. In cultured embryonic rat cortical cells and striatal primordial stem cells, valproate markedly increased the number and percentage of primarily GABAergic neurons, and increased neurite outgrowth (Laeng et al., 2004).

Regulation of hippocampal neurogenesis by antidepressants

Several studies have shown that antidepressant treatment increases neurogenesis of dentate gyrus granule cells (Vollmayr et al., 2007). These studies have found that chronic administration of different classes of antidepressants, including norepinephrine- and serotonin-selective reuptake inhibitors (SSRIs), and electroconvulsive shock (ECS; the animal model of electroconvulsive therapy, or ECT, which is an effective nonpharmacologic treatment for depression) increases the proliferation and survival of new neurons. Studies demonstrating that neurogenesis is increased by conditions that stimulate neuronal activity (for example, enriched environment, learning, exercise) suggest that this process is also positively regulated by, and may even be dependent on, neuronal plasticity (Kempermann, 2002).

In view of the opposite effects of stress and antidepressants on hippocampal neurogenesis, it is hypothesized that alterations in this process are fundamental to the clinical syndrome of depression. To investigate this, Hen and colleagues (Santarelli et al., 2003) conducted an important series of experiments in which mice were administered antidepressants and their responses on a novelty-suppressed feeding test measured. Antidepressant treatment was associated with an improvement in the speed of retrieving food or water, and a 60% increase in BrdU-positive cells in the dentate gyrus. To test whether hippocampal neurogenesis was necessary for the antidepressants' behavioral effects, mice were exposed to X-rays directed at the hippocampus, eliminating >80% of the BrdU-positive cells in the subgranular zone. In these mice, the previously noted antidepressant effects on the novelty-suppressed feeding test were not observed. These results suggest that the behavioral effects of chronic antidepressants may be mediated by new neuronal growth in the hippocampus, although further confirmation, using different behavioral paradigms, is necessary.

A problem to be addressed with the neurotrophic hypothesis of antidepressant drug action is the "tryptophan depletion conundrum." It is now well-established that patients successfully treated with SSRIs show a rapid depressive relapse following experimental procedures that deplete tryptophan and serotonin (Delgado et al., 1991; Aberg-Wistedt et al., 1998; Delgado et al., 1999). How are such rapid effects to be reconciled with the postulated neurotrophic actions of antidepressants? It is our contention that treatment of depression is attained by providing trophic and neurochemical support, such that the trophic support restores normal synaptic connectivity, allowing the chemical signal to reinstate the optimal functioning of critical circuits necessary for normal affective regulation. Furthermore, what is sometimes less well appreciated is the fact that the major function of brain-derived neurotrophic factor (BDNF), a major neurotrophin in the CNS, is its regulation of synaptic excitability/plasticity, not its cell growth/survival effects (Manji et al., 2003). Thus an antidepressant-induced neurotrophin increase would have effects on long-term cell trophic/survival pathways and also neurotransmitter function. The latter would, of course, be susceptible to rapid perturbations (for example, with tryptophan depletion).

AMPA- AND NMDA-TYPE GLUTAMATE RECEPTORS AND MOOD DISORDERS

Glutamate Receptors in the Pathophysiology of Mood Disorders

It is surprising that the glutamatergic system has only recently undergone extensive investigation with regard to its possible involvement in the pathophysiology of mood disorders, because it is the major excitatory neurotransmitter in the CNS and known to play a role in regulating the threshold for excitation of most other neurotransmitter systems. Although direct evidence for glutamatergic excitotoxicity in BPD is lacking, and the precise mechanisms underlying the cell atrophy and death that occur in recurrent mood disorders are unknown, considerable data have shown that impairments of the glutamatergic system play a major role in the morphometric changes observed with severe stresses (McEwen, 1999; Sapolsky, 2000).

It is now clear that modification of the levels of synaptic α-amino-3-hydroxy-5-methyl-4-isoxasolepropionic acid (AMPA)-type glutamate receptors, in particular by receptor subunit trafficking, insertion, and internalization, is a critically important mechanism for regulating various forms of synaptic plasticity and behavior. Recent studies have identified region-specific alterations in expression levels of AMPA and NMDA glutamate receptor subunits in patients with mood disorders (Beneyto et al., 2007). Supporting the suggestion that abnormalities in glutamate signaling may be involved in mood pathophysiology, AMPA receptors have been shown to regulate affective-like behaviors in rodents. Antagonists at the AMPA receptor have been demonstrated to attenuate amphetamine- and cocaine-induced hyperactivity, and psychostimulant-induced sensitization and hedonic behavior (Goodwin and Jamison, 2007).

Glutamate Receptors in the Treatment of Mood Disorders

Further evidence for the role of glutamate receptors in mood disorders comes from investigations of the mechanism of action of mood stabilizers and antidepressants. In postmortem human brain tissue, Künig et al. (1998) found that therapeutic levels of valproate decreased binding of AMPA to AMPA receptors, thus effectively blocking them. Chronic lithium and valproate (two structurally dissimilar mood stabilizers) have been shown to down-regulate synaptic expression of the AMPA receptor subunit GluR1 in hippocampus, in vitro and in vivo (Du et al., 2003). In cultured hippocampal neurons, lithium and valproate were found to attenuate surface GluR1 expression after long-term treatment. Furthermore, our group and the Greengard laboratory have found that antidepressants have the opposite effect of up-regulating AMPA synaptic strength in hippocampus (Svenningsson et al., 2002; Du et al., 2003). In addition to effects on AMPA receptor trafficking, valproate appears to block synaptic responses mediated by NMDA glutamate receptors (Loscher, 1999). Two independent studies (Ueda and Willmore, 2000; Hassel et al., 2001) showed that chronic valproate selectively altered glutamate transporter expression in hippocampus. Thus overall, chronic valproate likely decreases intrasynaptic glutamate levels through a variety of mechanisms. A growing body of data demonstrates that antidepressants also attenuate expression and/or function of NMDA receptor subunits (Goodwin and Jamison, 2007).

Building upon these preclinical data, recent clinical trials have investigated the clinical effects of glutamatergic agents in patients with mood disorders. Recent clinical studies have demonstrated effective and rapid antidepressant action of glutamatergic agents, including ketamine, an NMDA receptor antagonist, and riluzole, a glutamate release inhibitor (Zarate, Singh, and Manji, 2006; Sanacora et al., 2007). These and other data have led to the hypothesis that alterations in neural plasticity in critical limbic and reward circuits, mediated by increasing the postsynaptic AMPA to NMDA throughput, may represent a convergent mechanism for antidepressant action (Zarate, Singh, Carlson, et al., 2006). This line of research holds considerable promise for developing new treatments for depression and BPD.

THE G_S/CYCLIC ADENOSINE MONOPHOSPHATE (cAMP)-GENERATING SIGNALING PATHWAY IN THE PATHOPHYSIOLOGY AND TREATMENT OF MOOD DISORDERS

Evidence for the Role of the G_s/cAMP Pathway in the Pathophysiology of Mood Disorders

Several independent laboratories have now reported abnormalities in the G protein signaling cascade in mood disorders (Schreiber et al., 1991; Young et al., 1993; Manji et al., 1995; Garcia-Sevilla et al., 1997; Spleiss et al., 1998; Warsh et al., 2000). Postmortem brain studies have consistently reported increased levels of the stimulatory G protein ($G\alpha_s$) accompanied by increases in stimulated adenylate cyclase (AC) activity in BPD (Young et al., 1993; Warsh et al., 2000). These observations of elevated $G\alpha_s$ levels and/or function are further supported by the demonstration of increased agonist-activated [^{35}S]GTPγS binding to $G\alpha$ subunits in the frontal cortex of patients with BPD (Wang and Friedman, 1996). Several studies have also found elevated $G\alpha_s$ messenger ribonucleic acid (mRNA) and protein levels in peripheral circulating cells in BPD, although the dependency on clinical state remains unclear (Schreiber et al., 1991; Young et al., 1994; Manji et al., 1995; Spleiss et al., 1998). $G\alpha_{olf}$, which is highly homologous to $G\alpha_s$, is located in an area of chromosome 18 that has been identified as a potential site of BPD susceptibility loci. Heterozygous $G\alpha_{olf}$ knockout mice show a markedly abnormal behavioral response to psychostimulants (Corvol et al., 2001).

It should be emphasized that there is at present no evidence of mutations in the $G\alpha_s$ or $G\alpha_{olf}$ genes in mood disorders (Ram et al., 1997; Zill et al., 2003). There are numerous transcriptional and posttranscriptional mechanisms that regulate the levels of $G\alpha$ subunits, and elevated levels of $G\alpha_s$ could potentially represent the indirect sequelae of alterations in any one of these biochemical pathways (Manji and Chen, 2000). Overall, elevation of levels of the predominant subspecies of $G\alpha_s$ is a very consistent finding. Although it may appear unintuitive that disruption of such a ubiquitously expressed protein may lead to the relatively subtle abnormalities in brain function in mood disorders, there is precedent for clinical disorders with circumscribed clinical manifestations arising as a result of abnormalities in $G\alpha_s$ levels (Spiegel, 1998).

Considerable clinical research has focused on the activity of the cyclic adenosine monophosphate (cAMP)-generating system in readily accessible blood elements in patients with BPD. Overall, the preponderance of evidence demonstrates altered receptor and/or postreceptor sensitivity of the cAMP-generating system in the absence of consistent alterations in the number of receptors themselves (J.F. Wang et al., 1997; Warsh et al., 2000). Peripheral cell studies in patients with BPD have demonstrated increased protein kinase A (PKA) catalytic subunit levels, and increased cAMP-stimulated PKA activity (Perez et al., 1999; Tardito et al., 2003; Karege et al., 2004). Similarly, in a series of postmortem studies, Warsh and colleagues have found increased basal and stimulated PKA activity, and corresponding alterations in PKA regulatory and catalytic subunits in various brain areas in patients with BPD (Rahman et al., 1997; Fields et al., 1999; Chang et al., 2003). In addition, other studies have shown increased basal and stimulated AC activity in postmortem brain tissue of patients with BPD (Gould and Manji, 2002b).

Interestingly, quite distinct abnormalities have been observed in this signaling pathway in MDD compared to BPD. Peripheral cell studies have shown decreased cAMP levels and PKA activity in MDD (Mizrahi et al., 2004; Akin et al., 2005). Postmortem brain studies have shown increased levels of the inhibitory G protein ($G\alpha_i$) in the frontal cortex of antidepressant-free patients with MDD (Garcia-Sevilla et al., 1999), and decreased stimulated AC activity in the frontal cortex of victims of suicide (Cowburn et al., 1994; Lowther et al., 1996). These data suggest that MDD is associated with down-regulation of the cAMP pathway. This is consistent with data from studies investigating the mechanism of action of antidepressants and antimanic mood stabilizers, as discussed below.

A critical downstream target of the G_s/cAMP pathway, cAMP-response element binding protein (CREB), has also been implicated in mood disorders and suicide (Dwivedi et al., 2003; Yamada et al., 2003; Zubenko et al., 2003; Young et al., 2004). Markers near the CREB1 locus have been reported to cosegregate with MDD in women (Zubenko et al., 2003). By microarray analysis, CREB1 gene expression was found to be significantly reduced in postmortem orbitofrontal cortex from patients with BPD (Ryan et al., 2006). Induced CREB overexpression in the dentate gyrus resulted in an antidepressant-like effect in the learned helplessness paradigm and the Forced Swim Test in rats (A.C. Chen et al., 2001). Initial results suggesting an association between polymorphisms in CREB-regulated BDNF and BPD have not been confirmed (Kato, 2007). The effects of mood stabilizers and antidepressants on CREB and BDNF have generated much interest, as discussed below.

Evidence for the Role of the G_s/cAMP Pathway in the Treatment of Mood Disorders

Lithium

Although it appears that lithium, at therapeutic concentrations, does not directly affect G proteins, there is considerable evidence that chronic lithium administration indirectly affects G protein function (Risby et al., 1991; Mork et al., 1992; J.F. Wang et al., 1999). For G_s and G_i, lithium's major effects in humans and rodents are most compatible with stabilization of the heterotrimeric, undissociated, inactive $\alpha\beta\gamma$ conformation of the G protein (Manji et al., 1995; Li and El-Mallahk, 2000; Warsh et al., 2000). Lithium has been recently shown to promote membrane localization of G protein receptor kinase-3 (GRK-3), a serine-threonine kinase that regulates G protein–coupled receptor sensitivity (Ertley et al., 2007).

Lithium also exerts complex effects on the activity of AC, with the preponderance of the data demonstrating an elevation of basal AC activity but an attenuation of receptor-stimulated response in preclinical and clinical studies (Mork et al., 1992; J.F. Wang et al., 1997; Jope, 1999; Manji et al., 2000; Hahn et al., 2005). It has been postulated that these elevations of basal cAMP and dampening of receptor-mediated stimulated response play an important role in lithium's ability to prevent "excessive excursions from the norm" (Manji et al., 1995; Jope, 1999). These complex actions likely represent the net effects of direct inhibition of AC, up-regulation of certain AC subtypes, and effects on stimulatory and inhibitory G proteins (Manji and Lenox, 2000b).

Lithium's effects on the phosphorylation and activity of CREB have been examined in numerous preclinical studies, with conflicting results (Ozaki and Chuang, 1997; Einat et al., 2003; Tardito, Tiraboschi, et al., 2006). Postmortem studies have demonstrated decreased phosphorylated CREB in patients with BPD treated with lithium (Stewart et al., 2001; Young et al., 2004). As discussed below, CREB is also regulated by the mitogen-activated protein kinase (MAPK) signaling cascade, another target of lithium's actions. Thus, lithium's effects on CREB may be temporally and spatially specific, reflecting the relative contributions of these two major signaling pathways.

Valproate

Valproate is another major antimanic agent, but structurally dissimilar to lithium. Chronic valproate treatment has been shown to induce a significant reduction of β-adrenergic receptors (β-ARs), and even greater decrease in receptor- and postreceptor-mediated cAMP accumulation (G. Chen, Manji, et al., 1996), consistent with recent studies that show that valproate decreases receptor/G protein coupling (Hahn et al., 2005). In a recent microarray analysis, valproate treatment resulted in altered levels of several G protein subunits, a PKA catalytic subunit, and CREB (Bosetti et al., 2005).

Carbamazepine

Carbamazepine, an atypical anticonvulsant, is widely used in BPD as an alternative or adjunctive treatment to lithium. Carbamazepine exerts effects on G proteins that are largely, although not completely, in common with those of lithium. Like lithium, however, it has been recently found to regulate GRK-3, a regulator of G protein–coupled receptors (Ertley et al., 2007). Carbamazepine has been demonstrated in numerous studies to have significant effects on the cAMP signaling pathway. Carbamazepine has been shown to decrease basal concentrations of cAMP in mouse cerebral cortex and cerebellum and reduce pharmacologically induced cAMP production (Lewin and Bleck, 1977; Ferrendelli and Kinscherf, 1979; Palmer et al., 1979; van Calker et al., 1991). In patients, who were manic, carbamazepine decreased elevated CSF levels of cAMP (Post et al., 1982). At therapeutically relevant concentrations, carbamazepine was found to inhibit basal and stimulated cAMP production, an effect found also in AC extracts, suggesting that lithium acts directly on AC, or on closely associated factors that copurify with AC (G. Chen, Pan, et al., 1996).

Antidepressants

The cAMP signaling cascade appears to be a major target for the actions of chronic antidepressant treatments. Multiple lines of evidence support the up-regulation of the cAMP/PKA cascade by antidepressants (Fig. 28.3) (Tardito, Perez, et al., 2006). Duman and colleagues (2000) performed an elegant series of studies that first demonstrated antidepressant effects on CREB, an important downstream target of this cascade. Work from this group demonstrated increases in CREB mRNA, CREB protein, and CRE DNA binding activity in hippocampus in response to several different classes of antidepressants (Nibuya et al., 1996; Thome et al., 2000), as well as increases in the expression of two CREB-regulated genes that have been implicated in the pathophysiology of mood disorders: BDNF and its receptor, trkB (Nibuya et al., 1996), discussed further below.

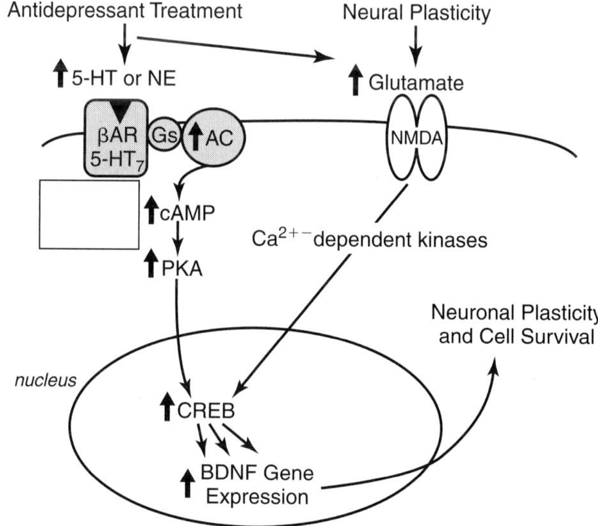

FIGURE 28.3 Influence of antidepressant treatment on the cAMP-CREB cascade. Antidepressant treatment increases synaptic levels of norepinephrine (NE) and serotonin (5-HT) by blocking the reuptake or breakdown of these monoamines, resulting in activation of intracellular signal transduction cascades, including the cAMP-CREB cascade. Chronic antidepressant treatment increases Gs coupling to adenylyl cyclase (AC), levels of cAMP-dependent PKA, and CREB. CREB is also phosphorylated by Ca^{2+}-dependent protein kinases, which can be activated by the phosphatidylinositol pathway (not shown) or by glutamate ionotropic receptors (for example, NMDA). Glutamate receptors and Ca^{2+}-dependent protein kinases are also involved in neural plasticity. One gene target of antidepressant treatment and the cAMP-CREB cascade is BDNF, which contributes to the cellular processes underlying neuronal plasticity and cell survival. AR: adrenergic receptor. cAMP: cyclic adenosine monophosphate; CREB: cAMP-response element binding; PKA: protein kinease A; BDNF: brain-derived neurotrophic factor; NMDA: *N*-methyl-D-aspartate. Reproduced with permission from Duman et al., (2000).

THE PI/PKC SIGNALING PATHWAY IN THE PATHOPHYSIOLOGY AND TREATMENT OF MOOD DISORDERS

Evidence for the Role of the Phosphoinositide (PI) Signaling Cascade in the Pathophysiology of Mood Disorders

Interest in the phosphoinositide (PI) signaling system in BPD was first generated by the seminal observation that lithium reduces brain levels of inositol (Allison and Stewart, 1971). The implication of this major second-messenger cascade was intriguing, given that several subtypes of adrenergic, cholinergic, and serotonergic receptors are coupled to this system. Further studies have supported the inositol signaling pathway (Fig. 28.4) as a target of lithium (see below), but evidence that disruptions in the PI/PKC (protein kinase C) signaling system play a role in the pathophysiology of mood disorders is less definitive.

Some evidence is provided by peripheral cell studies. Patients who were manic were found to have a significantly higher percentage of platelet membrane phosphoinositide 4,5-biphosphate (PIP_2) (Brown et al., 1993), a finding that was replicated in a follow-up study of medication-free patients with BPD who were depressed (Soares et al., 2001). Postmortem studies of patients with BPD have revealed lower free inositol levels in prefrontal cortex (Shimon et al., 1997) and reduced agonist-induced PI turnover in occipital cortex (Jope et al., 1996).

Importantly, a recent whole-genome association study of BPD has further implicated this pathway. Of the risk genes identified, that demonstrating by far the strongest association with BPD was diacylglycerol kinase eta (*DGKH*), an immediate regulator of PKC (Baum et al., 2008).

PKC in the Pathophysiology of Mood Disorders

There have been a limited number of studies directly examining PKC in BPD. In postmortem brain tissue from patients with BPD, there have been observations of an increase in PKC activity, PKC translocation, and cortical levels of specific PKC isozymes (H.Y. Wang and Friedman, 1996). Postmortem brains from patients with BPD were found to have increased association of PKC isozymes with the receptor for activated C kinase-1 (RACK1), which anchors PKC to the membrane (H.Y. Wang and

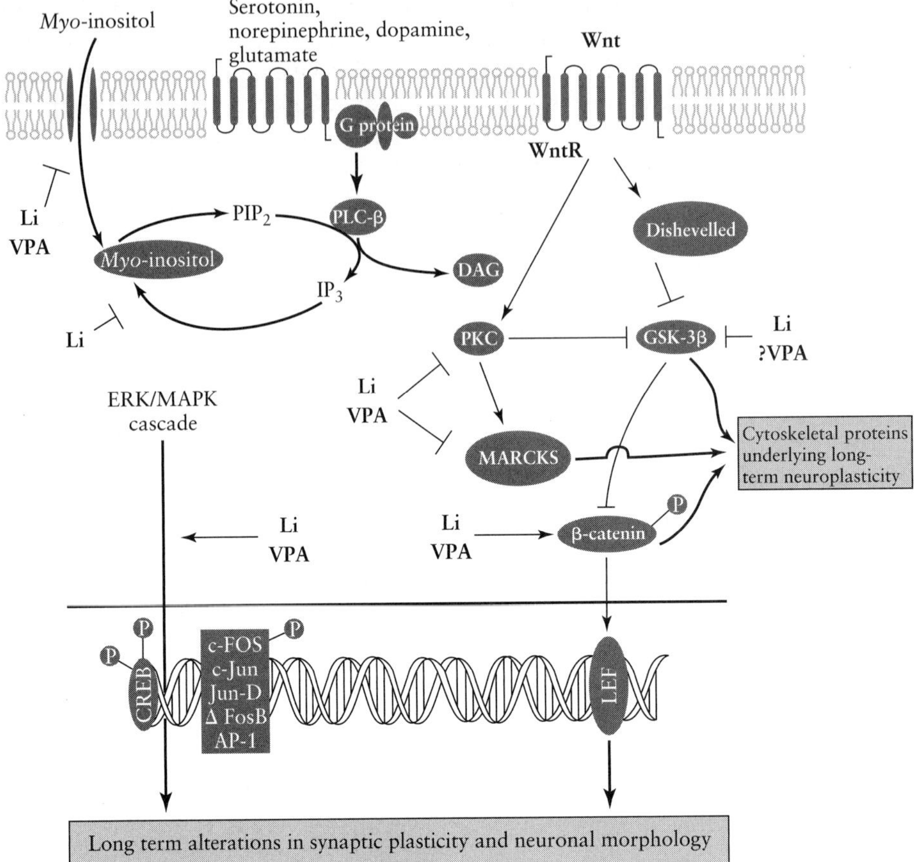

FIGURE 28.4 Intracellular signaling cascades involved in long-term stabilization of mood by Li and VPA. Activation of receptors coupled to PI hydrolysis results in the breakdown of PIP2 into two second messengers: IP3 and DAG, which is an endogenous activator of PKC. Li is an uncompetitive inhibitor of inositol monophosphatases, whereas Li and VPA, upon chronic administration, decrease myo-inositol uptake. These perturbations by mood stabilizers likely contribute to the reduction in PKC activity and the reduced levels of PKC-α, PKC-ε and MARCKS, a major PKC substrate in the CNS. In the Wnt signaling pathway, binding of the Wnt signal to the Wnt receptor (WntR) activates an intermediary protein, Dishevelled, which regulates GSK-3β. GSK-3β regulates cytoskeletal proteins and also has an important role in determining cell survival and cell death. Li (and possibly VPA) directly inhibit GSK-3β, which may underlie, at least in part, the increases in β-catenin that occur after chronic treatment with these agents. The ERK-MAP kinase cascade regulates several important transcription factors, most notably CREB and activator protein-1 (AP-1). Recent studies have demonstrated that Li and VPA activate the ERK MAP kinase cascade, which may contribute to the long-term changes in synaptic plasticity and morphology that follow chronic treatment. Together, the regulation of these signaling pathways brings about an enhancement of synaptic connectivity potentially necessary for long-term stabilization of mood. Li: lithium; VPA: valproic acid; PIP2: phosphoinositide 4,5-biphosphate; DAG: diacylglycerol; PKC: protein kinease C; MARCKS: myristoylated alanine-rich C kinase substrate; CNS: central nervous system; ERK: extracellular signal regulated kinases; MAP: mitogen-activated protein; CREB: cyclic adenosine monophosphate [AMP]-response element binding. Reproduced with permission from Coyle and Manji (2002).

Friedman, 2001). The same group also found elevated PKC activity in platelets from patients who were manic (Friedman et al., 1993). In contrast to these findings, other studies have reported evidence consistent with reduced PKC function in BPD from postmortem studies using [^{3}H]PDBu, a radioligand that binds to PKC, and one peripheral cell study using platelets from pediatric patients (Pandey et al., 1997; Coull et al., 2000; Pandey et al., 2007). Resolution of these apparent inconsistencies requires further study.

In animal models of mania, several studies have demonstrated that acute and chronic amphetamine produces an alteration in PKC activity, its relative cytosol to membrane distribution, and the phosphorylation of a major PKC substrate, GAP-43, which has been implicated in long-term alterations of neurotransmitter release (Giambalvo, 1992a, 1992b). Increased hedonistic drive and increased tendency to abuse drugs are well-known facets of manic behavior; notably, PKC inhibitors attenuate these important aspects of the manic-like syndrome in rodents (Einat and Manji, 2006; Einat et al., 2007). Importantly, recent preclinical studies have specifically investigated the antimanic effects of tamoxifen per se (because this is the only CNS-penetrant PKC inhibitor available for humans). These studies showed that tamoxifen significantly reduced amphetamine-induced hyperactivity and risk-taking behavior (Einat et al., 2007). Finally, with respect to cognitive dysfunction associated with mania, Birnbaum et al. (2004) demonstrated that excessive activation of PKC dramatically impaired the cognitive functions of the prefrontal cortex, and that inhibition of PKC protected cognitive function. In summary, preclinical biochemical and behavioral data support the notion that PKC activation may result in manic-like behaviors whereas PKC inhibition may be antimanic. These data have prompted clinical trials of tamoxifen for the treatment of mania (see below).

Abnormalities of Calcium Signaling in Mood Disorders

In response to the fact that calcium ions have been shown to regulate the synthesis and release of neurotransmitters, neuronal excitability, cytoskeletal remodeling, and long-term neuroplastic events, a large number of studies have investigated intracellular calcium in peripheral cells in BPD (Dubovsky et al., 1992; Emamghoreishi et al., 1997; J.F. Wang et al., 1997). Given the many caveats associated with studies of peripheral circulating cells, the consistency of the findings is remarkable. Studies have repeatedly revealed elevations in resting and stimulated intracellular calcium levels in platelets, lymphocytes, and neutrophils of patients with BPD. Whether these abnormalities are state- or trait-dependent is debated (Dubovsky et al., 1992; Emamghoreishi et al., 1997).

The regulation of free intracellular calcium is a complex multifaceted process involving extracellular entry, release from intracellular stores, uptake into organelles, and binding to specific proteins. Thus, the abnormalities observed in BPD could arise from dysfunction at a variety of levels, and studies suggest that the abnormality lies beyond the receptor (Hough et al., 1999). Recent evidence suggests altered regulation of calcium by PKC in patients with BPD (Akimoto et al., 2007). Linking abnormalities in the PI cascade to alterations in intracellular calcium, Warsh and colleagues (2000) demonstrated a correlation between altered IMPA2 (myo-inositol monophosphatase 2) mRNA levels and calcium levels in B lymphoblast cell lines from patients with BPD (Yoon et al., 2001).

The PI Signaling Cascade in the Treatment of Mood Disorders

The inositol depletion hypothesis posits that lithium, an uncompetitive inhibitor of inositol-monophosphatase (IMP), produces its therapeutic effects via a depletion of neuronal myo-inositol levels. Through this uncompetitive inhibition, lithium is proposed to selectively inhibit overactive components of the PI system without interfering with basal functioning (Berridge, 1989). Although this hypothesis has been of great heuristic value, studies that support this theory have often been small, inconsistent, and subject to numerous methodological differences (Jope and Williams, 1994).

Recent studies have investigated the possibility that lithium and other mood stabilizers regulate the PI system independently of IMPase. One interesting potential target is SMIT (sodium-dependent myo-inositol transporter). In an in vitro study, SMIT expression and activity were down-regulated in response to chronic lithium, valproate, or carbamazepine treatment (van Calker and Belmaker, 2000). In a follow-up in vivo study, neutrophils from untreated patients with BPD were found to have elevated SMIT levels, which were reduced by lithium or valproate treatment (Willmroth et al., 2007).

The effects of lithium on myo-inositol levels have also been documented by imaging studies. A number of studies have demonstrated lithium-induced reductions in myo-inositol levels in child and adult patients with BPD, in brain regions previously implicated in BPD (Moore et al., 1999; Davanzo et al., 2001; Yildiz et al., 2001). However, the time course of lithium's effect on inositol did not correlate with that of its therapeutic action, suggesting that the reduction of myo-inositol is not directly responsible for lithium's mood-stabilizing effects, but may instead initiate a cascade of secondary changes in the PKC signaling pathway and downstream gene expression.

PKC in the Treatment of Mood Disorders

Evidence from various laboratories has clearly demonstrated that lithium, at therapeutically relevant concentrations, exerts major effects on the PKC signaling cascade (Fig. 28.4) (Goodwin and Jamison, 2007). Data suggest that acute lithium exposure facilitates a number of PKC-mediated responses, whereas longer-term exposure results in an attenuation of phorbol ester-mediated responses accompanied by a down-regulation of specific PKC isozymes (Manji and Lenox, 1999). Studies in rodents have demonstrated that chronic lithium administration produces an isozyme-selective reduction in PKC α and ε in frontal cortex and hippocampus, and in immortalized hippocampal cells (Manji et al., 1993; G. Chen, Masana, and Manji, 2000). Chronic lithium administration has been demonstrated to dramatically reduce the hippocampal levels of MARCKS (myristoylated alanine–rich C kinase substrate), a major PKC substrate that has been implicated in the regulation of long-term neuroplastic events (Lenox et al., 1992). Further supporting the therapeutic relevance of these findings, studies have shown that the structurally dissimilar mood stabilizer valproate produces very similar effects on PKC α and ε isozymes and MARCKS (G. Chen et al., 1994; Watson et al., 1998). Interestingly, lithium and valproate appear to bring about their effects on the

PKC signaling pathway by distinct mechanisms (Manji and Lenox, 1999). These biochemical observations are consistent with the clinical observation that some patients show a preferential response to one of the two agents and that additive therapeutic effects are often observed when the two agents are coadministered.

These preclinical data, along with animal studies discussed above, have prompted clinical studies of PKC inhibitors and mood dysregulation. A number of small studies have found that tamoxifen, a nonsteroidal antiestrogen and a PKC inhibitor at high concentrations, possesses antimanic efficacy (Bebchuk et al., 2000; Kulkarni et al., 2006). Most recently, a double-blind, placebo controlled trial of tamoxifen in the treatment of acute mania was undertaken (Zarate et al., 2007). Patients on tamoxifen showed significant improvement in mania compared to placebo as early as 5 days, and the effect size for the drug difference was very large after 3 weeks.

Significant interest has been generated recently in the potential mood-stabilizing properties of another class of PKC inhibitors, omega-3 fatty acids (ω-3 FA). The predominant naturally occurring ω-3 FAs, docosahexaenoic acid (DHA) and eicosapentanoic acid (EPA), have been shown to inhibit PKC (Seung Kim et al., 2001), and a number of clinical trials have investigated these agents as monotherapy or adjunctive treatment for depression or BPD. Although many of these trials have demonstrated efficacy (Stoll et al., 1999; Nemets et al., 2002; Peet and Horrobin, 2002; Wozniak et al., 2007), others have not (Post et al., 2003; Keck et al., 2006). Thus, further evaluation of the efficacy of ω-3 FAs as monotherapy or adjunctive treatment in BPD or depression is warranted. Together with the emerging genetic evidence, these data suggest that PKC may play an important role in the pathophysiology and treatment of BPD.

GSK-3 AS A TARGET FOR TREATMENT IN BPD

Recently, considerable excitement has been generated by the identification of an unexpected and novel target for lithium: glycogen synthase kinase-3 (GSK-3). Glycogen synthase kinase-3 is a kinase that functions as an intermediary in numerous intracellular signaling pathways (Fig. 28.4) and is regulated by serotonin, dopamine, psychostimulants, and antidepressants (Gould and Manji, 2005). It is a major regulator of apoptosis and cellular plasticity/resilience, and this role has been postulated to be the target of lithium and valproate (Gould and Manji, 2002a; Li et al., 2002). Lithium is a direct inhibitor of GSK-3, via competition with magnesium for a binding site (Klein and Melton, 1996; Ryves and Harwood, 2001). In mice, GSK-3 has also been shown to be inhibited by valproate (G. Chen et al., 1999), and electroconvulsive therapy (ECT), a nonpharmacologic therapy for mood disorders (Roh et al., 2003).

Animal behavioral data from pharmacologic and genetic models have shown that manipulation of GSK-3 produces antidepressant and antimanic effects (Gould and Manji, 2005; Jope and Roh, 2006). To our knowledge, this is the only manipulation, other than that of lithium, that has been demonstrated to exert both such effects. Further studies have been carried out to identify the GSK-3 target most relevant to lithium's behavioral effects. Glycogen synthase kinase-3 inhibition results in a decrease in phosphorylation and degradation of its target β-catenin, and at therapeutically relevant concentrations, lithium increases β-catenin and Wnt-mediated gene expression in rodent brain. It was therefore hypothesized that transgenic mice that overexpress a constitutively active form of β-catenin would phenocopy lithium's behavioral effects. It was found that lithium-induced behaviors in wild-type mice are phenocopied by overexpression of β-catenin. Notably, lithium and β-catenin overexpression have mood-stabilizing-like actions in prototypical animal models of mania (D-amphetamine hyperlocomotion) and depression (Forced Swim Test) (Gould et al., 2007).

Interestingly, GSK-3 has been found to play a role in regulating circadian rhythm, in *Drosophila* (Martinek et al., 2001), and mice (Kaladchibachi et al., 2007). Patients with BPD often demonstrate circadian disturbances, and lithium has been shown to increase circadian period in many organisms including humans (Johnsson et al., 1979; Iwahana et al., 2004; Jolma et al., 2006), consistent with a decrease in GSK-3 activity.

Direct evidence for the role of GSK-3 in the etiology of BPD has not been reported, and genetic studies have not reproducibly found GSK-3 polymorphisms to be associated with the disease (reviewed in Kato, 2007). Therefore, it remains to be determined if bipolar pathophysiology involves abnormalities of GSK-3 itself, or of other signaling molecules regulated by GSK-3. Nevertheless, in view of the role of GSK-3 in neural plasticity, survival, and circadian rhythms, and its involvement in the action of mood stabilizers, development of GSK-3 inhibitors is actively under way by numerous pharmaceutical companies.

CELL SURVIVAL AND RESILIENCE PATHWAYS IN THE TREATMENT OF MOOD DISORDERS

Regulation of Cell Survival and Resilience Pathways by Mood Stabilizers

In conjunction with the body of data supporting mood stabilizers' effects on cell survival and plasticity at the cellular level, relevant intracellular signaling cascades have been shown to be regulated by these agents. The extracellular signal regulated kinases (ERK) MAPK-signaling cascade plays an important role in mediating neurotrophic and neuroplastic events (Segal and Greenberg, 1996). A series of studies investigating the effects of mood stabilizers on this signaling cascade showed that lithium and valproate, at therapeutically relevant concentrations, robustly activated the ERK MAPK cascade and promoted neurite outgrowth and growth cone formation in human neuroblastoma SH-SY5Y cells (Yuan et al., 2001). Furthermore, in vivo, chronic lithium and valproate robustly increased the levels of activated ERK in the frontal cortex and hippocampus, areas of brain that have been implicated in the pathophysiology and treatment of BPD (Einat et al., 2003).

Neurotrophic factors are known to promote cell survival by activating MAPKs to suppress intrinsic cellular apoptotic machinery (Thoenen, 1995; Pettmann and Henderson, 1998). A downstream target of the MAPK cascade, ribosomal S-6 kinase (Rsk), phosphorylates CREB, leading to expression of antiapoptotic Bcl-2 (Fig. 28.5). Studies by our group demonstrated that chronic treatment with lithium or valproate in rats produced a doubling of Bcl-2 levels in the frontal cortex, due primarily to a marked increase in the number of Bcl-2-immunoreactive cells in layers II and III of the frontal cortex (Manji et al., 2000). Chronic lithium also markedly increased the number of Bcl-2-immunoreactive cells in the dentate gyrus and striatum, and in cultured cells (R.W. Chen and Chuang, 1999; Manji et al., 2000). Lithium and valproate have also been shown to increase the expression of the Bcl-2-associated gene *BAG-1*. *BAG-1*

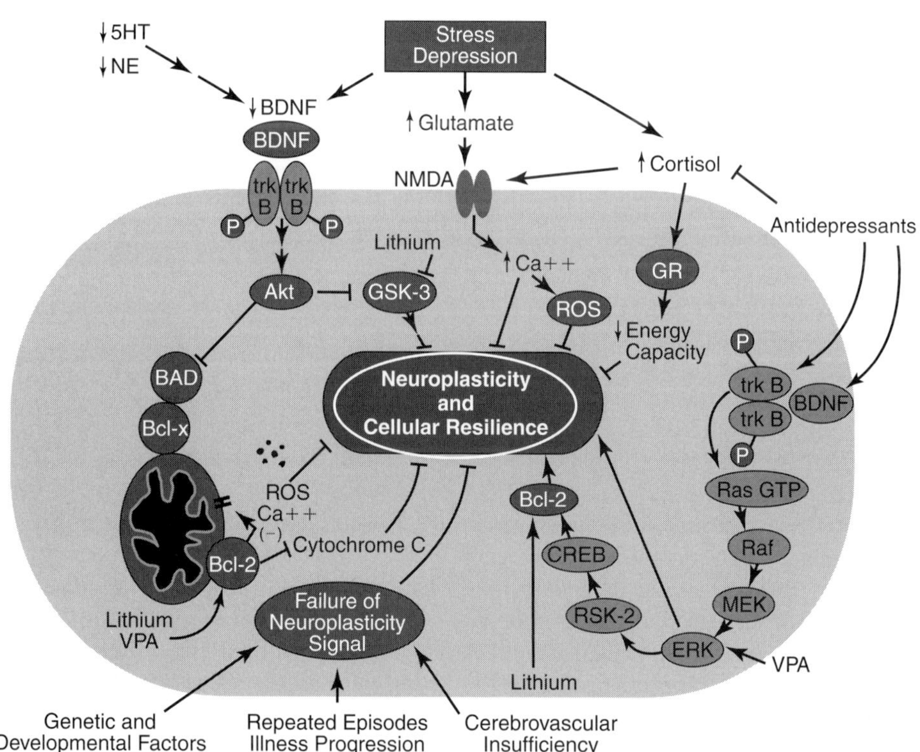

FIGURE 28.5 The multiple influences on neuroplasticity and cellular resilience in mood disorders. Genetic and neurodevelopmental factors, repeated affective episodes, and illness progression might all contribute to the impairments of cellular resilience, volumetric reductions, and cell death and atrophy observed in mood disorders. Stress and depression likely contribute to impairments of cellular resilience by a variety of mechanisms, including reductions in the levels of BDNF, facilitating glutamatergic transmission via NMDA and non-NMDA receptors, and reducing energy capacity of cells. Neurotrophic factors such as BDNF enhance cell survival by activating two distinct signaling pathways: the PI3-kinase pathway, and the ERK MAP kinase pathway. One of the major mechanisms by which BDNF promotes cell survival is by increasing the expression of the major cytoprotective protein, Bcl-2. Bcl-2 attenuates cell death through a variety of mechanisms, including impairment of the release of calcium and cytochrome c, sequestering of proforms of death-inducing caspase enzymes, and enhancement of mitochondrial calcium uptake. The chronic administration of a variety of antidepressants increases the expression of BDNF and its receptor TrkB. Lithium and valproic acid robustly upregulate the cytoprotective protein Bcl-2 and inhibit GSK-3β, both of which have neuroprotective results. Valproic acid also activates the ERK-MAP kinase pathway, which may play a major role in producing neurotrophic effects and neurite outgrowth. 5HT: serotonin; BAD and Bax: pro-apoptotic members of the Bcl-2 family; Bcl-2 and Bcl-x: anti-apoptotic members of the Bcl-2 family; BDNF: brain-derived neurotrophic receptor; NMDA: *N*-methyl-D-aspartate; ERK: extracellular signal regulated kinases; MAP: mitogen-activated protein; CREB: cyclic AMP-responsive element-binding protein; GR: glucocorticoid receptor; GSK-3: glycogen synthase kinase-3; NE: norepinephrine; NGF: nerve growth factor; ROS: reactive oxygen species; RSK-2: ribosomal S-6 kinase; VPA: valproic acid. Reprinted with permission from Manji et al. (2001).

attenuates glucocorticoid receptor (GR) nuclear translocation, activates MAPKs, and potentiates the anti-apoptotic functions of Bcl-2 (Zhou et al., 2005). Thus, lithium regulates a number of components of survival cascades, through which it may exert its neuroprotective effects.

Regulation of Cell Survival and Resilience Pathways by Antidepressants

As discussed above, many studies have demonstrated that antidepressant treatment up-regulates a key pathway involved in cell survival and plasticity, the cAMP–CREB cascade (Duman et al., 2000; Tardito, Perez, et al., 2006). A critical target of CREB gene regulation is the neurotrophic factor BDNF, and the effect of several different classes of antidepressants on BDNF expression has been demonstrated in a number of animal and human postmortem studies. ECT, a nonpharmacologic treatment for depression, has been consistently found to upregulate BDNF expression (Tardito, Perez, et al., 2006). In an elegant study from the Nestler laboratory, mice subjected to chronic social defeat stress exhibited adaptations in gene expression and chromatin remodeling of five BDNF splice variant mRNAs (I–V), including down-regulation of BDNF transcripts III and IV, and robustly increased repressive histone methylation at their corresponding promoters. Chronic imipramine (a tricyclic antidepressant) reversed this down-regulation and increased histone acetylation at these promoters (Tsankova et al., 2006). Other studies, however, have not shown antidepressant-induced BDNF expression; this lack of consistency may depend on experimental paradigm (Tardito, Perez, et al., 2006).

Further evidence to support the role of the cAMP–CREB cascade and BDNF in antidepressant action comes from studies using animal models of depression, in which up-regulation of these pathways results in an antidepressant-like effect (Duman et al., 2000; A.C. Chen, Shirayama, et al., 2001). Indirect human evidence comes from studies showing increased hippocampal BDNF expression in postmortem brain from patients treated with antidepressants at the time of death compared with untreated patients (B. Chen, Dowlatshahi, et al., 2001). In summary, there is strong evidence that the cAMP–CREB pathway, including CREB-regulated BDNF expression, is a major target of antidepressant action, but the precise nature of these actions is yet to be determined.

It is important to note that CREB is regulated by multiple upstream cascades. Although antidepressant induction of CREB activity has been primarily shown to be via the cAMP–PKA pathway, other signaling cascades, such as the calcium/calmodulin-dependent kinase (CaMK) and MAPK cascades, have been implicated in recent studies as possibly involved in the mechanism of antidepressant action (Tiraboschi et al., 2004; Tardito, Tiraboschi, et al., 2006).

NEUROTROPHIC SIGNALING-MEDIATED MITOCHONDRIAL FUNCTION IN BPD

Kato and Kato (2000) anticipated recent developments in the field when they first proposed that mitochondrial dysfunction plays an important role in the pathophysiology of BPD. In addition to critical roles in regulation of energy production via oxidative phosphorylation, regulation of intracellular Ca^{2+}, and mediation of apoptosis, increasing evidence suggests that mitochondrial calcium sequestration is integrally involved in regulating synaptic plasticity. Consistent with the growing appreciation of this role, a number of human neuroimaging and postmortem brain studies, as well as preclinical molecular and cellular biology studies, have implicated mitochondria in the impairments of plasticity and cellular resilience manifest in BPD.

As a point of clarification, it is not our contention that BPD is a classic mitochondrial disorder. Although individuals with mitochondrial dysfunction often manifest psychiatric symptoms, the vast majority of patients with BPD do not show the symptoms of classic mitochondrial disorders (Fadic and Johns, 1996). Nevertheless, these disorders may have a partially shared etiology: impaired regulation of Ca^{2+} cascades, and consequent toxic cell injury, is an essential component of the pathophysiology of classic mitochondriopathies, and has been the most reproducible biological measure of abnormalities described in research on BPD. In view of the growing body of evidence demonstrating the toxic effects of elevated intracellular Ca^{2+} on neurons and glia, Ca^{2+} dysregulation has been postulated to underlie aspects of the pathophysiology of BPD (Goodwin and Jamison, 2007).

Results from Kato's group (Kato et al., 2003) implicate the mitochondrial–endoplasmic reticulum (ER) calcium regulation system in the Ca^{2+} abnormalities seen in BPD. Building upon Kato's findings, a subsequent study (Kakiuchi et al., 2003) identified *XBP1*, a pivotal gene in the ER stress response, as contributing to the genetic risk for BPD. They identified a polymorphism (-116G/C) in the promoter region of *XBP1* that was associated with an increased risk for BPD. They showed that the polymorphism was associated with impaired induction of *XBP1* expression after ER stress, and that valproate rescued the impaired response by inducing *ATF6*, the gene upstream of *XBP1*.

An elegant series of postmortem brain microarray studies (Konradi et al., 2004) provided additional evidence for mitochondrial dysregulation in BPD. They found that nuclear mRNA coding for mitochondrial proteins that regulate oxidative phosphorylation and proteasome degradation was decreased in BPD. More recently, Benes et al. (2006) performed a post hoc analysis of an extant gene expression–profiling database obtained from the hippocampus. Postmortem brain tissue from patients with BPD showed a marked upregulation of several apoptosis genes, and a downregulation of antioxidant genes, suggesting that accumulation of free radicals might occur in the setting of a previously reported decrease of the electron transport chain in this disorder (Benes et al., 2006).

We outlined evidence to support the contention that neurotrophic signaling and its downstream effects on mitochondrial function are integral to many facets of BPD. This theory leads to the intriguing possibility that enhancing mitochondrial vigor may represent an important adjunctive strategy for the optimal long-term treatment of BPD.

CONCLUDING REMARKS

As we have demonstrated, there is a considerable body of evidence conceptually and experimentally to support abnormalities in the regulation of signaling as integral to the underlying neurobiology of BPD. Indeed, all of the highly significant associations in the recent bipolar whole-genome association study implicate signaling cascades (Baum et al., 2008). In fact, the contribution of these pathways to the pathophysiology of this illness must be reasonably robust, given the variability that might be expected in assessing such dynamic systems under the constraints in experimental design imposed upon such research. Figure 28.5 integrates many of the signaling pathways, and actions upon them by medications, presented in this chapter.

The role of cellular signaling cascades offers much explanatory power for understanding the complex neurobiology of BPD (Goodwin and Jamison, 2007). Signaling cascades regulate the multiple neurotransmitter and neuropeptide systems implicated in the disorder and are targets for the most effective treatments. Signaling pathways are also targets for hormones that have been implicated in the pathophysiology of BPD. The highly integrated monoamine and prominent neuropeptide pathways are known to originate and project heavily to limbic-related regions such as the hippocampus, hypothalamus, and brain stem that are likely associated with neurovegetative symptoms. Abnormalities in cellular signaling cascades that regulate diverse physiologic functions likely explain the tremendous medical comorbidity associated with the disorder.

Evidence also suggests that, somewhat akin to the treatment of conditions such as hypertension and diabetes, early and sustained treatment may be necessary to adequately prevent the deleterious long-term sequelae associated with mood disorders. Furthermore, for patients who are depressed and refractory to treatment, there may be a limited benefit to drugs that simply directly or indirectly alter neurotransmitter levels or bind to cell surface receptors. Such strategies implicitly assume that the target circuits are functionally intact and that altered synaptic activity will thus be transduced to modify the postsynaptic throughput of the system. However, the evidence presented here suggests that, in addition to neurochemical changes, many patients also have pronounced structural alterations (for example, neuropil reductions, reduced spine densities, neurite retraction) in critical neuronal circuits. Thus, optimal treatment may require more direct trophic support to enhance and maintain normal synaptic connectivity, thereby allowing the chemical signal to reinstate the optimal functioning of critical circuits necessary for normal affective regulation.

There are a number of pharmacologic "plasticity-enhancing" strategies that may be effective in the treatment of BPD. Indeed, this next generation of drugs, in addition to treating core mood symptoms, might be able to target other important aspects of the illness such as impaired cognition, epigenetic factors that may have a long-term negative impact of the course of illness (for example, histone deacetylase inhibitors), and medical comorbidities (for example, GSK inhibitors). The development of novel therapeutics holds much promise for the long-term treatment of severe mood disorders and for improving the lives of the many who suffer from them.

REFERENCES

Aberg-Wistedt, A., Hasselmark, L., Stain-Malmgren, R., Aperia, B., Kjellman, B.F., and Mathe, A.A. (1998) Serotonergic "vulnerability" in affective disorder: a study of the tryptophan depletion test and relationships between peripheral and central serotonin indexes in citalopram-responders. *Acta Psychiatr. Scand.* 97: 374–380.

Akimoto, T., Kusumi, I., Suzuki, K., and Koyama, T. (2007) Effects of calmodulin and protein kinase C modulators on transient Ca^{2+} increase and capacitative Ca^{2+} entry in human platelets: relevant to pathophysiology of bipolar disorder. *Prog. Neuropsychopharmacol. Biol. Psychiatry* 31:136–141.

Akin, D., Manier, D H., Sanders-Bush, E., and Shelton, R.C. (2005) Signal transduction abnormalities in melancholic depression. *Int. J. Neuropsychopharmacol.* 8:5–16.

Allison, J.H., and Stewart, M.A. (1971) Reduced brain inositol in lithium-treated rats. *Nat. New Biol.* 233:267–268.

Aston, C., Jiang, L., and Sokolov, B.P. (2005) Transcriptional profiling reveals evidence for signaling and oligodendroglial abnormalities in the temporal cortex from patients with major depressive disorder. *Mol. Psychiatry* 10:309–322.

Baum, A., Akula, N., Cabenero, M., Cardona, I., Corona, W., Klemens, B., Schulze, T.G., et al. (2008) A genome-wide association study implicates diacylglycerol kinase eta (DGKH) and several other genes in the etiology of bipolar disorder. *Mol. Psychiatry* 13(2):197–207.

Baumann, B., Danos, P., Krell, D., Diekmann, S., Wurthmann, C., Bielau, H., Bernstein, H.G., et al. (1999) Unipolar-bipolar dichotomy of mood disorders is supported by noradrenergic brainstem system morphology. *J. Affect. Disord.* 54:217–224.

Bebchuk, J.M., Arfken, C.L., Dolan-Manji, S., Murphy, J., Hasanat, K., and Manji, H.K. (2000) A preliminary investigation of a protein kinase C inhibitor in the treatment of acute mania. *Arch. Gen. Psychiatry* 57:95–97.

Benes, F.M., Matzilevich, D., Burke, R.E., and Walsh, J. (2006) The expression of proapoptosis genes is increased in bipolar disorder, but not in schizophrenia. *Mol. Psychiatry* 11:241–251.

Beneyto, M., Kristiansen, L.V., Oni-Orisan, A., McCullumsmith, R.E., and Meador-Woodruff, J H. (2007) Abnormal glutamate receptor expression in the medial temporal lobe in schizophrenia and mood disorders. *Neuropsychopharmacology* 32(9):1888–1902.

Berridge, M.J. (1989) The Albert Lasker Medical Awards. Inositol trisphosphate, calcium, lithium, and cell signaling. *JAMA* 262: 1834–1841.

Beyer, J.L., and Krishnan, K.R. (2002) Volumetric brain imaging findings in mood disorders. *Bipolar Disord.* 4:89–104.

Bhalla, U.S., and Iyengar, R. (1999) Emergent properties of networks of biological signaling pathways. *Science* 283:381–387.

Birnbaum, S.G., Yuan, P.X., Wang, M., Vijayraghavan, S., Bloom, A.K., Davis, D.J., Gobeske, K.T., et al. (2004) Protein kinase C overactivity impairs prefrontal cortical regulation of working memory. *Science* 306:882–884.

Bosetti, F., Bell, J.M., and Manickam, P. (2005) Microarray analysis of rat brain gene expression after chronic administration of sodium valproate. *Brain Res. Bull.* 65:331–338.

Brown, A.S., Mallinger, A.G., and Renbaum, L.C. (1993) Elevated platelet membrane phosphatidylinositol-4,5-bisphosphate in bipolar mania. *Am. J. Psychiatry* 150:1252–1254.

Bruno, V., Sortino, M.A., Scapagnini, U., Nicoletti, F., and Canonico, P.L. (1995) Antidegenerative effects of Mg(2+)-valproate in cultured cerebellar neurons. *Funct. Neurol.* 10:121–130.

Carlson, P.J., Singh, J.B., Zarate, C.A., Jr., Drevets, W.C., and Manji, H.K. (2006) Neural circuitry and neuroplasticity in mood disorders: insights for novel therapeutic targets. *NeuroRx* 3:22–41.

Chang, A., Li, P.P., and Warsh, J.J. (2003) Altered cAMP-dependent protein kinase subunit immunolabeling in post-mortem brain from patients with bipolar affective disorder. *J. Neurochem.* 84:781–791.

Chen, A.C., Shirayama, Y., Shin, K.H., Neve, R.L., and Duman, R.S. (2001) Expression of the cAMP response element binding protein (CREB) in hippocampus produces an antidepressant effect. *Biol. Psychiatry* 49:753–762.

Chen, B., Dowlatshahi, D., MacQueen, G.M., Wang, J.F., and Young, L.T. (2001) Increased hippocampal BDNF immunoreactivity in subjects treated with antidepressant medication. *Biol. Psychiatry* 50:260–265.

Chen, G., Huang, L.D., Jiang, Y.M., and Manji, H.K. (1999) The mood-stabilizing agent valproate inhibits the activity of glycogen synthase kinase-3. *J. Neurochem.* 72:1327–1330.

Chen, G., Manji, H.K., Hawver, D.B., Wright, C.B., and Potter, W.Z. (1994) Chronic sodium valproate selectively decreases protein kinase C alpha and epsilon in vitro. *J. Neurochem.* 63:2361–2364.

Chen, G., Manji, H.K., Wright, C.B., Hawver, D.B., and Potter, W.Z. (1996) Effects of valproic acid on beta-adrenergic receptors, G-proteins, and adenylyl cyclase in rat C6 glioma cells. *Neuropsychopharmacology* 15:271–280.

Chen, G., Masana, M.I., and Manji, H.K. (2000) Lithium regulates PKC-mediated intracellular cross-talk and gene expression in the CNS in vivo. *Bipolar Disord.* 2:217–236.

Chen, G., Pan, B., Hawver, D.B., Wright, C.B., Potter, W.Z., and Manji, H.K. (1996) Attenuation of cyclic AMP production by carbamazepine. *J. Neurochem.* 67:2079–2086.

Chen, G., Rajkowska, G., Du, F., Seraji-Bozorgzad, N., and Manji, H.K. (2000) Enhancement of hippocampal neurogenesis by lithium. *J. Neurochem.* 75:1729–1734.

Chen, R.W., and Chuang, D.M. (1999) Long term lithium treatment suppresses p53 and Bax expression but increases Bcl-2 expression. A prominent role in neuroprotection against excitotoxicity. *J. Biol. Chem.* 274:6039–6042.

Corvol, J.C., Studler, J.M., Schonn, J.S., Girault, J.A., and Herve, D. (2001) Galpha(olf) is necessary for coupling D1 and A2a receptors to adenylyl cyclase in the striatum. *J. Neurochem.* 76:1585–1588.

Coull, M.A., Lowther, S., Katona, C.L., and Horton, R.W. (2000) Altered brain protein kinase C in depression: a post-mortem study. *Eur. Neuropsychopharmacol.* 10:283–288.

Cowburn, R.F., Marcusson, J.O., Eriksson, A., Wiehager, B., and O'Neill, C. (1994) Adenylyl cyclase activity and G-protein subunit levels in postmortem frontal cortex of suicide victims. *Brain Res.* 633:297–304.

Coyle, J.T., and Manji, H.K. (2002) Getting balance: drugs for bipolar disorder share target. *Nat. Med.* 8:557–558.

Czeh, B., Michaelis, T., Watanabe, T., Frahm, J., de Biurrun, G., van Kampen, M., Bartolomucci, A., et al. (2001) Stress-induced changes in cerebral metabolites, hippocampal volume, and cell proliferation are prevented by antidepressant treatment with tianeptine. *Proc. Natl. Acad. Sci. USA* 98:12796–12801.

Davanzo, P., Thomas, M.A., Yue, K., Oshiro, T., Belin, T., Strober, M., and McCracken, J. (2001) Decreased anterior cingulate myo-inositol/creatine spectroscopy resonance with lithium treatment in children with bipolar disorder. *Neuropsychopharmacology* 24: 359–369.

Delgado, P.L., Miller, H.L., Salomon, R.M., Licinio, J., Krystal, J.H., Moreno, F.A., Heninger, G.R., et al. (1999) Tryptophan-depletion challenge in depressed patients treated with desipramine or fluoxetine: implications for the role of serotonin in the mechanism of antidepressant action. *Biol. Psychiatry* 46:212–220.

Delgado, P.L., Price, L.H., Miller, H.L., Salomon, R.M., Licinio, J., Krystal, J.H., Heninger, G.R., et al. (1991) Rapid serotonin depletion as a provocative challenge test for patients with major depression: relevance to antidepressant action and the neurobiology of depression. *Psychopharmacol. Bull.* 27:321–330.

Drevets, W.C. (2000) Neuroimaging studies of mood disorders. *Biol. Psychiatry* 48:813–829.

Drevets, W.C. (2001) Neuroimaging and neuropathological studies of depression: implications for the cognitive-emotional features of mood disorders. *Curr. Opin. Neurobiol.* 11:240–249.

Du, J., Gray, N.A., Falke, C., Yuan, P., Szabo, S., and Manji, H.K. (2003) Structurally dissimilar antimanic agents modulate synaptic plasticity by regulating AMPA glutamate receptor subunit GluR1 synaptic expression. *Ann. N.Y. Acad. Sci.* 1003:378–380.

Dubovsky, S.L., Murphy, J., Thomas, M., and Rademacher, J. (1992) Abnormal intracellular calcium ion concentration in platelets and lymphocytes of bipolar patients. *Am. J. Psychiatry* 149:118–120.

Duman, R.S., Malberg, J., Nakagawa, S., and D'Sa, C. (2000) Neuronal plasticity and survival in mood disorders. *Biol. Psychiatry* 48:732–739.

Dwivedi, Y., Rao, J.S., Rizavi, H.S., Kotowski, J., Conley, R.R., Roberts, R.C., Tamminga, C.A., et al. (2003) Abnormal expression and functional characteristics of cyclic adenosine monophosphate response element binding protein in postmortem brain of suicide subjects. *Arch. Gen. Psychiatry* 60:273–282.

Einat, H., and Manji, H.K. (2006) Cellular plasticity cascades: genes-to-behavior pathways in animal models of bipolar disorder. *Biol. Psychiatry* 59:1160–1171.

Einat, H., Yuan, P., Gould, T.D., Li, J., Du, J., Zhang, L., Manji, H.K., et al. (2003) The role of the extracellular signal-regulated kinase signaling pathway in mood modulation. *J. Neurosci.* 23:7311–7316.

Einat, H., Yuan, P., Szabo, S.T., Dogra, S., and Manji, H.K. (2007) Protein kinase C inhibition by tamoxifen antagonizes manic-like behavior in rats: implications for the development of novel therapeutics for bipolar disorder. *Neuropsychobiology* 55(3/4):123–131.

Emamghoreishi, M., Schlichter, L., Li, P.P., Parikh, S., Sen, J., Kamble, A., and Warsh, J.J. (1997) High intracellular calcium concentrations in transformed lymphoblasts from subjects with bipolar I disorder. *Am. J. Psychiatry* 154:976–982.

Ertley, R.N., Bazinet, R.P., Lee, H.J., Rapoport, S.I., and Rao, J.S. (2007) Chronic treatment with mood stabilizers increases membrane GRK3 in rat frontal cortex. *Biol. Psychiatry* 61:246–249.

Fadic, R., and Johns, D.R. (1996) Clinical spectrum of mitochondrial diseases. *Semin. Neurol.* 16:11–20.

Ferrendelli, J.A., and Kinscherf, D.A. (1979) Inhibitory effects of anticonvulsant drugs on cyclic nucleotide accumulation in brain. *Ann. Neurol.* 5:533–538.

Fields, A., Li, P.P., Kish, S.J., and Warsh, J.J. (1999) Increased cyclic AMP-dependent protein kinase activity in postmortem brain from patients with bipolar affective disorder. *J. Neurochem.* 73: 1704–1710.

Frazier, J.A., Ahn, M.S., DeJong, S., Bent, E.K., Breeze, J.L., and Giuliano, A.J. (2005) Magnetic resonance imaging studies in early-onset bipolar disorder: a critical review. *Harv. Rev. Psychiatry* 13:125–140.

Friedman, E., Hoau Yan, W., Levinson, D., Connell, T.A., and Singh, H. (1993) Altered platelet protein kinase C activity in bipolar affective disorder, manic episode. *Biol. Psychiatry* 33:520–525.

Garcia-Sevilla, J.A., Escriba, P.V., Ozaita, A., La Harpe, R., Walzer, C., Eytan, A., and Guimon, J. (1999) Up-regulation of immunolabeled alpha2A-adrenoceptors, Gi coupling proteins, and regulatory receptor kinases in the prefrontal cortex of depressed suicides. *J. Neurochem.* 72:282–291.

Garcia-Sevilla, J.A., Walzer, C., Busquets, X., Escriba, P.V., Balant, L., and Guimon, J. (1997) Density of guanine nucleotide-binding proteins in platelets of patients with major depression: increased abundance of the G alpha i2 subunit and down-regulation by antidepressant drug treatment. *Biol. Psychiatry* 42:704–712.

Giambalvo, C.T. (1992a) Protein kinase C and dopamine transport—1. Effects of amphetamine in vivo. *Neuropharmacology* 31:1201–1210.

Giambalvo, C.T. (1992b) Protein kinase C and dopamine transport—2. Effects of amphetamine in vitro. *Neuropharmacology* 31:1211–1222.

Goodwin, F.K., and Jamison, K.R. (2007) *Manic-Depressive Illness: Bipolar Disorders and Recurrent Depression.* New York: Oxford University Press.

Gould, T.D., Einat, H., O'Donnell, K.C., Picchini, A.M., Schloesser, R.J., and Manji, H.K. (2007) B-catenin overexpression in the mouse brain phenocopies lithium-sensitive behaviors. *Neuropsychopharmacology* 32:2173–83.

Gould, T.D., and Manji, H.K. (2002a) Signaling networks in the pathophysiology and treatment of mood disorders. *J. Psychosom. Res.* 53:687–697.

Gould, T.D., and Manji, H.K. (2002b) The WNT signaling pathway in bipolar disorder. *Neuroscientist* 8:497–511.

Gould, T.D., and Manji, H.K. (2005) Glycogen synthase kinase-3: a putative molecular target for lithium mimetic drugs. *Neuropsychopharmacology* 30:1223–1237.

Hahn, C.G., Umapathy, Wang, H.Y., Koneru, R., Levinson, D.F., and Friedman, E. (2005) Lithium and valproic acid treatments reduce PKC activation and receptor-G protein coupling in platelets of bipolar manic patients. *J. Psychiatr. Res.* 39:355–363.

Hajek, T., Carrey, N., and Alda, M. (2005) Neuroanatomical abnormalities as risk factors for bipolar disorder. *Bipolar Disord.* 7:393–403.

Hassel, B., Iversen, E.G., Gjerstad, L., and Tauboll, E. (2001) Up-regulation of hippocampal glutamate transport during chronic treatment with sodium valproate. *J. Neurochem.* 77:1285–1292.

Hough, C., Lu, S.J., Davis, C.L., Chuang, D.M., and Post, R.M. (1999) Elevated basal and thapsigargin-stimulated intracellular calcium of platelets and lymphocytes from bipolar affective disorder patients measured by a fluorometric microassay. *Biol. Psychiatry* 46:247–255.

Huang, X., Wu, D.Y., Chen, G., Manji, H., and Chen, D.F. (2003) Support of retinal ganglion cell survival and axon regeneration by lithium through a Bcl-2-dependent mechanism. *Invest. Ophthalmol. Vis. Sci.* 44:347–354.

Iwahana, E., Akiyama, M., Miyakawa, K., Uchida, A., Kasahara, J., Fukunaga, K., Hamada, T., et al. (2004) Effect of lithium on the circadian rhythms of locomotor activity and glycogen synthase kinase-3 protein expression in the mouse suprachiasmatic nuclei. *Eur. J. Neurosci.* 19:2281–2287.

Johnsson, A., Pflug, B., Engelmann, W., and Klemke, W. (1979) Effect of lithium carbonate on circadian periodicity in humans. *Pharmakopsychiatr. Neuropsychopharmakol.* 12:423–425.

Johnston-Wilson, N.L., Sims, C.D., Hofmann, J.P., Anderson, L., Shore, A.D., Torrey, E.F., and Yolken, R.H. (2000) Disease-specific alterations in frontal cortex brain proteins in schizophrenia, bipolar disorder, and major depressive disorder. The Stanley Neuropathology Consortium. *Mol. Psychiatry* 5:142–149.

Jolma, I.W., Falkeid, G., Bamerni, M., and Ruoff, P. (2006) Lithium leads to an increased FRQ protein stability and to a partial loss of temperature compensation in the Neurospora circadian clock. *J. Biol. Rhythms* 21:327–334.

Jope, R.S. (1999) A bimodal model of the mechanism of action of lithium. *Mol. Psychiatry* 4:21–25.

Jope, R.S., and Roh, M.S. (2006) Glycogen synthase kinase-3 (GSK3) in psychiatric diseases and therapeutic interventions. *Curr. Drug Targets* 7:1421–1434.

Jope, R.S., Song, L., Li, P.P., Young, L.T., Kish, S.J., Pacheco, M.A., and Warsh, J.J. (1996) The phosphoinositide signal transduction system is impaired in bipolar affective disorder brain. *J. Neurochem.* 66:2402–2409.

Jope, R.S., and Williams, M.B. (1994) Lithium and brain signal transduction systems. *Biochem. Pharmacol.* 47:429–441.

Kakiuchi, C., Iwamoto, K., Ishiwata, M., Bundo, M., Kasahara, T., Kusumi, I., Tsujita, T., et al. (2003) Impaired feedback regulation of XBP1 as a genetic risk factor for bipolar disorder. *Nat. Genet.* 35:171–175.

Kaladchibachi, S.A., Doble, B., Anthopoulos, N., Woodgett, J.R., and Manoukian, A.S. (2007) Glycogen synthase kinase 3, circadian rhythms, and bipolar disorder: a molecular link in the therapeutic action of lithium. *J. Circadian Rhythms* 5:3.

Karege, F., Schwald, M., Papadimitriou, P., Lachausse, C., and Cisse, M. (2004) The cAMP-dependent protein kinase A and brain-derived neurotrophic factor expression in lymphoblast cells of bipolar affective disorder. *J. Affect. Disord.* 79:187–192.

Kato, T. (2007) Molecular genetics of bipolar disorder and depression. *Psychiatry Clin. Neurosci.* 61:3–19.

Kato, T., Ishiwata, M., Mori, K., Washizuka, S., Tajima, O., Akiyama, T., and Kato, N. (2003) Mechanisms of altered Ca^{2+} signalling in transformed lymphoblastoid cells from patients with bipolar disorder. *Int. J. Neuropsychopharmacol* 6:379–389.

Kato, T., and Kato, N. (2000) Mitochondrial dysfunction in bipolar disorder. *Bipolar Disord.* 2:180–190.

Keck, P.E., Jr., Mintz, J., McElroy, S.L., Freeman, M.P., Suppes, T., Frye, M.A., Altshuler, L.L., et al. (2006) Double-blind, randomized, placebo-controlled trials of ethyl-eicosapentanoate in the treatment of bipolar depression and rapid cycling bipolar disorder. *Biol. Psychiatry* 60:1020–1022.

Kempermann, G. (2002) Why new neurons? Possible functions for adult hippocampal neurogenesis. *J. Neurosci.* 22:635–638.

Kim, J.S., Chang, M.Y., Yu, I.T., Kim, J.H., Lee, S.H., Lee, Y.S., and Son, H. (2004) Lithium selectively increases neuronal differentiation of hippocampal neural progenitor cells both in vitro and in vivo. *J. Neurochem.* 89:324–336.

Klein, P.S., and Melton, D.A. (1996) A molecular mechanism for the effect of lithium on development. *Proc. Natl. Acad. Sci. USA* 93: 8455–8459.

Konradi, C., Eaton, M., MacDonald, M.L., Walsh, J., Benes, F.M., and Heckers, S. (2004) Molecular evidence for mitochondrial dysfunction in bipolar disorder. *Arch. Gen. Psychiatry* 61:300–308.

Kuhn, H.G., Biebl, M., Wilhelm, D., Li, M., Friedlander, R.M., and Winkler, J. (2005) Increased generation of granule cells in adult Bcl-2-overexpressing mice: a role for cell death during continued hippocampal neurogenesis. *Eur. J. Neurosci.* 22:1907–1915.

Kulkarni, J., Garland, K.A., Scaffidi, A., Headey, B., Anderson, R., de Castella, A., Fitzgerald, P., et al. (2006) A pilot study of hormone modulation as a new treatment for mania in women with bipolar affective disorder. *Psychoneuroendocrinology* 31:543–547.

Künig, G., Niedermeyer, B., Deckert, J., Gsell, W., Ransmayr, G., and Riederer, P. (1998) Inhibition of [3H]alpha-amino-3-hydroxy-5-methyl-4-isoxazole-propionic acid [AMPA] binding by the anticonvulsant valproate in clinically relevant concentrations: an autoradiographic investigation in human hippocampus. *Epilepsy Res.* 31:153–157.

Laeng, P., Pitts, R.L., Lemire, A.L., Drabik, C.E., Weiner, A., Tang, H., Thyagarajan, R., et al. (2004) The mood stabilizer valproic acid stimulates GABA neurogenesis from rat forebrain stem cells. *J. Neurochem.* 91:238–251.

Lai, J.S., Zhao, C., Warsh, J.J., and Li, P.P. (2006) Cytoprotection by lithium and valproate varies between cell types and cellular stresses. *Eur. J. Pharmacol.* 539:18–26.

Lenox, R.H., Watson, D.G., Patel, J., and Ellis, J. (1992) Chronic lithium administration alters a prominent PKC substrate in rat hippocampus. *Brain Res.* 570:333–340.

Lewin, E., and Bleck, V. (1977) Cyclic AMP accumulation in cerebral cortical slices: effect of carbamazepine, phenobarbital, and phenytoin. *Epilepsia* 18:237–242.

Li, R., and El-Mallahk, R.S. (2000) A novel evidence of different mechanisms of lithium and valproate neuroprotective action on human SY5Y neuroblastoma cells: caspase-3 dependency. *Neurosci. Lett.* 294:147–150.

Li, X., Bijur, G.N., and Jope, R.S. (2002) Glycogen synthase kinase-3beta, mood stabilizers, and neuroprotection. *Bipolar Disord.* 4: 137–144.

Loscher, W. (1999) Valproate: a reappraisal of its pharmacodynamic properties and mechanisms of action. *Prog. Neurobiol.* 58:31–59.

Lowther, S., Crompton, M.R., Katona, C.L., and Horton, R.W. (1996) GTP gamma S and forskolin-stimulated adenylyl cyclase activity in post-mortem brain from depressed suicides and controls. *Mol. Psychiatry* 1:470–477.

MacQueen, G.M., Campbell, S., McEwen, B.S., Macdonald, K., Amano, S., Joffe, R. T., Nahmias, C., et al. (2003) Course of illness, hippocampal function, and hippocampal volume in major depression. *Proc. Natl. Acad. Sci. USA* 100:1387–1392.

Manji, H.K., and Chen, G. (2000) Post-receptor signaling pathways in the pathophysiology and treatment of mood disorders. *Curr. Psychiatry Rep.* 2:479–489.

Manji, H.K., Chen, G., Shimon, H., Hsiao, J.K., Potter, W.Z., and Belmaker, R.H. (1995) Guanine nucleotide-binding proteins in bipolar affective disorder. Effects of long-term lithium treatment. *Arch. Gen. Psychiatry* 52:135–144.

Manji, H.K., Drevets, W.C., and Charney, D.S. (2001) The cellular neurobiology of depression. *Nat. Med.* 7:541–547.

Manji, H.K., Etcheberrigaray, R., Chen, G., and Olds, J.L. (1993) Lithium decreases membrane-associated protein kinase C in hippocampus: selectivity for the alpha isozyme. *J. Neurochem.* 61: 2303–2310.

Manji, H.K., and Lenox, R.H. (1999) Ziskind-Somerfeld Research Award. Protein kinase C signaling in the brain: molecular transduction of mood stabilization in the treatment of manic-depressive illness. *Biol. Psychiatry* 46:1328–1351.

Manji, H. K., and Lenox, R.H. (2000a) The nature of bipolar disorder. *J. Clin. Psychiatry* 61(Supp 13):42–57.

Manji, H.K., and Lenox, R.H. (2000b) Signaling: cellular insights into the pathophysiology of bipolar disorder. *Biol. Psychiatry* 48: 518–530.

Manji, H.K., Moore, G.J., and Chen, G. (2000) Lithium up-regulates the cytoprotective protein Bcl-2 in the CNS in vivo: a role for neurotrophic and neuroprotective effects in manic depressive illness. *J. Clin. Psychiatry* 61(Suppl 9):82–96.

Manji, H.K., Quiroz, J.A., Sporn, J., Payne, J.L., Denicoff, K., Gray, A., Zarate, C. A., Jr., et al. (2003) Enhancing neuronal plasticity and cellular resilience to develop novel, improved therapeutics for difficult-to-treat depression. *Biol. Psychiatry* 53:707–742.

Martinek, S., Inonog, S., Manoukian, A.S., and Young, M.W. (2001) A role for the segment polarity gene shaggy/GSK-3 in the Drosophila circadian clock. *Cell* 105:769–779.

McEwen, B.S. (1999) Stress and hippocampal plasticity. *Annu. Rev. Neurosci.* 22:105–122.

Miguel-Hidalgo, J.J., Baucom, C., Dilley, G., Overholser, J.C., Meltzer, H.Y., Stockmeier, C.A., and Rajkowska, G. (2000) Glial fibrillary acidic protein immunoreactivity in the prefrontal cortex distinguishes younger from older adults in major depressive disorder. *Biol. Psychiatry* 48:861–873.

Mizrahi, C., Stojanovic, A., Urbina, M., Carreira, I., and Lima, L. (2004) Differential cAMP levels and serotonin effects in blood peripheral mononuclear cells and lymphocytes from major depression patients. *Int. Immunopharmacol.* 4:1125–1133.

Moore, C.M., Biederman, J., Wozniak, J., Mick, E., Aleardi, M., Wardrop, M., Dougherty, M., et al. (2006) Differences in brain chemistry in children and adolescents with attention deficit hyperactivity disorder with and without comorbid bipolar disorder: a proton magnetic resonance spectroscopy study. *Am. J. Psychiatry* 163:316–318.

Moore, G.J., Bebchuk, J.M., Hasanat, K., Chen, G., Seraji-Bozorgzad, N., Wilds, I.B., Faulk, M.W., et al. (2000) Lithium increases N-acetyl-aspartate in the human brain: in vivo evidence in support of bcl-2's neurotrophic effects? *Biol. Psychiatry* 48:1–8.

Moore, G.J., Bebchuk, J.M., Parrish, J.K., Faulk, M.W., Arfken, C.L., Strahl-Bevacqua, J., and Manji, H.K. (1999) Temporal dissociation between lithium-induced changes in frontal lobe myo-inositol and clinical response in manic-depressive illness. *Am. J. Psychiatry* 156:1902–1908.

Moore, G.J., Bebchuk, J.M., Wilds, I.B., Chen, G., and Manji, H.K. (2000) Lithium-induced increase in human brain grey matter. *Lancet* 356:1241–1242.

Mora, A., Gonzalez-Polo, R.A., Fuentes, J.M., Soler, G., and Centeno, F. (1999) Different mechanisms of protection against apoptosis by valproate and Li+. *Eur. J. Biochem.* 266:886–891.

Mork, A., Geisler, A., and Hollund, P. (1992) Effects of lithium on second messenger systems in the brain. *Pharmacol. Toxicol.* 71 (Suppl 1):4–17.

Nakamura, S. (1990) Antidepressants induce regeneration of catecholaminergic axon terminals in the rat cerebral cortex. *Neurosci. Lett.* 111:64–68.

Nemets, B., Stahl, Z., and Belmaker, R. H. (2002) Addition of omega-3 fatty acid to maintenance medication treatment for recurrent unipolar depressive disorder. *Am. J. Psychiatry* 159:477–479.

Nibuya, M., Nestler, E.J., and Duman, R.S. (1996) Chronic antidepressant administration increases the expression of cAMP response element binding protein (CREB) in rat hippocampus. *J. Neurosci.* 16:2365–2372.

Öngür, D., Drevets, W.C., and Price, J.L. (1998) Glial reduction in the subgenual prefrontal cortex in mood disorders. *Proc. Natl. Acad. Sci. USA* 95:13290–13295.

Ozaki, N., and Chuang, D.M. (1997) Lithium increases transcription factor binding to AP-1 and cyclic AMP-responsive element in cultured neurons and rat brain. *J. Neurochem.* 69:2336–2344.

Palmer, G.C., Jones, D.J., Medina, M.A., and Stavinoha, W.B. (1979) Anticonvulsant drug actions on in vitro and in vivo levels of cyclic AMP in the mouse brain. *Epilepsia* 20:95–104.

Pandey, G.N., Dwivedi, Y., Pandey, S.C., Conley, R.R., Roberts, R.C., and Tamminga, C.A. (1997) Protein kinase C in the postmortem brain of teenage suicide victims. *Neurosci. Lett.* 228:111–114.

Pandey, G.N., Ren, X., Dwivedi, Y., and Pavuluri, M.N. (2007) Decreased protein kinase C (PKC) in platelets of pediatric bipolar patients: Effect of treatment with mood stabilizing drugs. *J. Psychiatr. Res.* 42(2):106–116.

Peet, M., and Horrobin, D.F. (2002) A dose-ranging study of the effects of ethyl-eicosapentaenoate in patients with ongoing depression despite apparently adequate treatment with standard drugs. *Arch. Gen. Psychiatry* 59:913–919.

Perez, J., Tardito, D., Mori, S., Racagni, G., Smeraldi, E., and Zanardi, R. (1999) Abnormalities of cyclic adenosine monophosphate signaling in platelets from untreated patients with bipolar disorder. *Arch. Gen. Psychiatry* 56:248–253.

Pettmann, B., and Henderson, C.E. (1998) Neuronal cell death. *Neuron* 20:633–647.

Post, R.M., Ballenger, J.C., Uhde, T.W., Smith, C., Rubinow, D.R., and Bunney, W.E., Jr. (1982) Effect of carbamazepine on cyclic nucleotides in CSF of patients with affective illness. *Biol. Psychiatry* 17:1037–1045.

Post, R.M., Leverich, G.S., Altshuler, L.L., Frye, M.A., Suppes, T.M., Keck, P.E., Jr., McElroy, S.L., et al. (2003) An overview of recent findings of the Stanley Foundation Bipolar Network (Part I). *Bipolar Disord.* 5:310–319.

Rahman, S., Li, P.P., Young, L.T., Kofman, O., Kish, S.J., and Warsh, J.J. (1997) Reduced [3H]cyclic AMP binding in postmortem brain from subjects with bipolar affective disorder. *J. Neurochem.* 68: 297–304.

Rajkowska, G. (2002) Cell pathology in mood disorders. *Semin. Clin. Neuropsychiatry* 7:281–292.

Rajkowska, G., Miguel-Hidalgo, J.J., Wei, J., Dilley, G., Pittman, S.D., Meltzer, H.Y., Overholser, J.C., et al. (1999) Morphometric evidence for neuronal and glial prefrontal cell pathology in major depression. *Biol. Psychiatry* 45:1085–1098.

Ram, A., Guedj, F., Cravchik, A., Weinstein, L., Cao, Q., Badner, J.A., Goldin, L.R., et al. (1997) No abnormality in the gene for the G protein stimulatory alpha subunit in patients with bipolar disorder. *Arch. Gen. Psychiatry* 54:44–48.

Ren, M., Leng, Y., Jeong, M., Leeds, P.R., and Chuang, D.M. (2004) Valproic acid reduces brain damage induced by transient focal cerebral ischemia in rats: potential roles of histone deacetylase inhibition and heat shock protein induction. *J. Neurochem.* 89: 1358–1367.

Risby, E.D., Hsiao, J.K., Manji, H.K., Bitran, J., Moses, F., Zhou, D.F., and Potter, W.Z. (1991) The mechanisms of action of lithium. II. Effects on adenylate cyclase activity and beta-adrenergic receptor binding in normal subjects. *Arch. Gen. Psychiatry* 48:513–524.

Roh, M.S., Kang, U.G., Shin, S.Y., Lee, Y.H., Jung, H.Y., Juhnn, Y.S., and Kim, Y.S. (2003) Biphasic changes in the Ser-9 phosphorylation of glycogen synthase kinase-3beta after electroconvulsive shock in the rat brain. *Prog. Neuropsychopharmacol. Biol. Psychiatry* 27:1–5.

Ryan, M.M., Lockstone, H.E., Huffaker, S.J., Wayland, M.T., Webster, M.J., and Bahn, S. (2006) Gene expression analysis of bipolar disorder reveals downregulation of the ubiquitin cycle and alterations in synaptic genes. *Mol. Psychiatry* 11:965–978.

Ryves, W.J., and Harwood, A.J. (2001) Lithium inhibits glycogen synthase kinase-3 by competition for magnesium. *Biochem. Biophys. Res. Commun.* 280:720–725.

Sanacora, G., Kendell, S.F., Levin, Y., Simen, A.A., Fenton, L.R., Coric, V., and Krystal, J.H. (2007) Preliminary evidence of riluzole efficacy in antidepressant-treated patients with residual depressive symptoms. *Biol. Psychiatry* 61:822–825.

Santarelli, L., Saxe, M., Gross, C., Surget, A., Battaglia, F., Dulawa, S., Weisstaub, N., et al. (2003) Requirement of hippocampal neurogenesis for the behavioral effects of antidepressants. *Science* 301:805–809.

Sapolsky, R.M. (2000) Glucocorticoids and hippocampal atrophy in neuropsychiatric disorders. *Arch. Gen. Psychiatry* 57:925–935.

Sassi, R.B., Stanley, J.A., Axelson, D., Brambilla, P., Nicoletti, M.A., Keshavan, M.S., Ramos, R.T., et al. (2005) Reduced NAA levels in the dorsolateral prefrontal cortex of young bipolar patients. *Am. J. Psychiatry* 162:2109–2115.

Schreiber, G., Avissar, S., Danon, A., and Belmaker, R.H. (1991) Hyperfunctional G proteins in mononuclear leukocytes of patients with mania. *Biol. Psychiatry* 29:273–280.

Segal, R.A., and Greenberg, M.E. (1996) Intracellular signaling pathways activated by neurotrophic factors. *Annu. Rev. Neurosci.* 19:463–489.

Seung Kim, H.F., Weeber, E.J., Sweatt, J.D., Stoll, A.L., and Marangell, L.B. (2001) Inhibitory effects of omega-3 fatty acids on protein kinase C activity in vitro. *Mol. Psychiatry* 6:246–248.

Sheline, Y.I., Gado, M.H., and Kraemer, H.C. (2003) Untreated depression and hippocampal volume loss. *Am. J. Psychiatry* 160: 1516–1518.

Sheline, Y.I., Wang, P.W., Gado, M.H., Csernansky, J.G., and Vannier, M.W. (1996) Hippocampal atrophy in recurrent major depression. *Proc. Natl. Acad. Sci. USA* 93:3908–3913.

Shim, S.S., Hammonds, M.D., Ganocy, S.J., and Calabrese, J.R. (2007) Effects of sub-chronic lithium treatment on synaptic plasticity in the dentate gyrus of rat hippocampal slices. *Prog. Neuropsychopharmacol. Biol. Psychiatry* 31:343–347.

Shimon, H., Agam, G., Belmaker, R.H., Hyde, T.M., and Kleinman, J.E. (1997) Reduced frontal cortex inositol levels in postmortem brain of suicide victims and patients with bipolar disorder. *Am. J. Psychiatry* 154:1148–1150.

Soares, J.C., Dippold, C.S., Wells, K.F., Frank, E., Kupfer, D.J., and Mallinger, A.G. (2001) Increased platelet membrane phosphatidylinositol-4,5-bisphosphate in drug-free depressed bipolar patients. *Neurosci. Lett.* 299:150–152.

Soares, J.C., and Young, A. (2007) *Bipolar Disorder: Basic Mechanisms and Therapeutic Implications, 2nd edition.*. New York: Informa Healthcare.

Spiegel, A. (1998) *G Proteins, Receptors, and Disease*. Totowa, NJ: Humana Press.

Spleiss, O., van Calker, D., Scharer, L., Adamovic, K., Berger, M., and Gebicke-Haerter, P.J. (1998) Abnormal G protein alpha(s) - and alpha(i2)-subunit mRNA expression in bipolar affective disorder. *Mol. Psychiatry* 3:512–520.

Stewart, R.J., Chen, B., Dowlatshahi, D., MacQueen, G.M., and Young, L.T. (2001) Abnormalities in the cAMP signaling pathway in post-mortem brain tissue from the Stanley Neuropathology Consortium. *Brain Res. Bull.* 55:625–629.

Stockmeier, C.A., Mahajan, G.J., Konick, L.C., Overholser, J.C., Jurjus, G.J., Meltzer, H.Y., Uylings, H.B., et al. (2004) Cellular changes in the postmortem hippocampus in major depression. *Biol. Psychiatry* 56:640–650.

Stoll, A.L., Severus, W.E., Freeman, M.P., Rueter, S., Zboyan, H.A., Diamond, E., Cress, K.K., et al. (1999) Omega 3 fatty acids in bipolar disorder: a preliminary double-blind, placebo-controlled trial. *Arch. Gen. Psychiatry* 56:407–412.

Strakowski, S.M., Adler, C.M., and DelBello, M.P. (2002) Volumetric MRI studies of mood disorders: do they distinguish unipolar and bipolar disorder? *Bipolar Disord.* 4:80–88.

Svenningsson, P., Tzavara, E.T., Witkin, J.M., Fienberg, A.A., Nomikos, G.G., and Greengard, P. (2002) Involvement of striatal and extrastriatal DARPP-32 in biochemical and behavioral effects of fluoxetine (Prozac). *Proc. Natl. Acad. Sci. USA* 99:3182–3187.

Tardito, D., Mori, S., Racagni, G., Smeraldi, E., Zanardi, R., and Perez, J. (2003) Protein kinase A activity in platelets from patients with bipolar disorder. *J. Affect. Disord.* 76:249–253.

Tardito, D., Perez, J., Tiraboschi, E., Musazzi, L., Racagni, G., and Popoli, M. (2006) Signaling pathways regulating gene expression, neuroplasticity, and neurotrophic mechanisms in the action of antidepressants: a critical overview. *Pharmacol. Rev.* 58:115–134.

Tardito, D., Tiraboschi, E., Kasahara, J., Racagni, G., and Popoli, M. (2006) Reduced CREB phosphorylation after chronic lithium treatment is associated with down-regulation of CaM kinase IV in rat hippocampus. *Int. J. Neuropsychopharmacol.* 10(4):491–496.

Thoenen, H. (1995) Neurotrophins and neuronal plasticity. *Science* 270:593–598.

Thome, J., Sakai, N., Shin, K., Steffen, C., Zhang, Y.J., Impey, S., Storm, D., et al. (2000) cAMP response element-mediated gene transcription is upregulated by chronic antidepressant treatment. *J. Neurosci.* 20:4030–4036.

Tiraboschi, E., Tardito, D., Kasahara, J., Moraschi, S., Pruneri, P., Gennarelli, M., Racagni, G., et al. (2004) Selective phosphorylation of nuclear CREB by fluoxetine is linked to activation of CaM kinase IV and MAP kinase cascades. *Neuropsychopharmacology* 29:1831–1840.

Tkachev, D., Mimmack, M.L., Ryan, M.M., Wayland, M., Freeman, T., Jones, P.B., Starkey, M., et al. (2003) Oligodendrocyte dysfunction in schizophrenia and bipolar disorder. *Lancet* 362:798–805.

Tsai, G., and Coyle, J.T. (1995) *N*-acetylaspartate in neuropsychiatric disorders. *Prog. Neurobiol.* 46:531–540.

Tsankova, N.M., Berton, O., Renthal, W., Kumar, A., Neve, R.L., and Nestler, E.J. (2006) Sustained hippocampal chromatin regulation in a mouse model of depression and antidepressant action. *Nat. Neurosci.* 9:519–525.

Ueda, Y., and Willmore, L.J. (2000) Molecular regulation of glutamate and GABA transporter proteins by valproic acid in rat hippocampus during epileptogenesis. *Exp. Brain Res.* 133:334–339.

Uranova, N., Orlovskaya, D., Vikhreva, O., Zimina, I., Kolomeets, N., Vostrikov, V., and Rachmanova, V. (2001) Electron microscopy of oligodendroglia in severe mental illness. *Brain Res. Bull.* 55:597–610.

van Calker, D., and Belmaker, R.H. (2000) The high affinity inositol transport system--implications for the pathophysiology and treatment of bipolar disorder. *Bipolar Disord.* 2:102–107.

van Calker, D., Steber, R., Klotz, K.N., and Greil, W. (1991) Carbamazepine distinguishes between adenosine receptors that mediate different second messenger responses. *Eur. J. Pharmacol.* 206: 285–290.

Vollmayr, B., Mahlstedt, M.M., and Henn, F.A. (2007) Neurogenesis and depression: what animal models tell us about the link. *Eur. Arch. Psychiatry Clin. Neurosci.* 257(5):300–303.

Wang, H.Y., and Friedman, E. (1996) Enhanced protein kinase C activity and translocation in bipolar affective disorder brains. *Biol. Psychiatry* 40:568–575.

Wang, H.Y., and Friedman, E. (2001) Increased association of brain protein kinase C with the receptor for activated C kinase-1 (RACK1) in bipolar affective disorder. *Biol. Psychiatry* 50:364–370.

Wang, J.F., Asghari, V., Rockel, C., and Young, L.T. (1999) Cyclic AMP responsive element binding protein phosphorylation and DNA binding is decreased by chronic lithium but not valproate treatment of SH-SY5Y neuroblastoma cells. *Neuroscience* 91: 771–776.

Wang, J.-F., Young, L.T., Li, P.P., and Warsh, J.J. (1997) Signal transduction abnormalities in bipolar disorder. In: Joffe, R. T., ed. *Bipolar Disorder: Biological Models and Their Clinical Application.* New York: Dekker, pp. 41–79.

Warsh, J., Young, L., and Li, P. (2000) Guanine nucleotide binding (G) protein disturbances. In: Belmaker, R., ed. *Bipolar Affective Disorder in Bipolar Medications: Mechanisms of Action.* Washington, DC: American Psychiatric Press, pp. 299–329.

Watanabe, Y., Gould, E., Daniels, D.C., Cameron, H., and McEwen, B.S. (1992) Tianeptine attenuates stress-induced morphological changes in the hippocampus. *Eur. J. Pharmacol.* 222:157–162.

Watson, D.G., Watterson, J.M., and Lenox, R.H. (1998) Sodium valproate down-regulates the myristoylated alanine-rich C kinase substrate (MARCKS) in immortalized hippocampal cells: a property of protein kinase C-mediated mood stabilizers. *J. Pharmacol. Exp. Ther.* 285:307–316.

Willmroth, F., Drieling, T., Lamla, U., Marcushen, M., Wark, H.J., and van Calker, D. (2007) Sodium-myo-inositol co-transporter (SMIT-1) mRNA is increased in neutrophils of patients with bipolar 1 disorder and down-regulated under treatment with mood stabilizers. *Int. J. Neuropsychopharmacol.* 10:63–71.

Wozniak, J., Biederman, J., Mick, E., Waxmonsky, J., Hantsoo, L., Best, C., Cluette-Brown, J.E., et al. (2007) Omega-3 fatty acid monotherapy for pediatric bipolar disorder: A prospective open-label trial. *Eur. Neuropsychopharmacol.* 17:440–447.

Yamada, S., Yamamoto, M., Ozawa, H., Riederer, P., and Saito, T. (2003) Reduced phosphorylation of cyclic AMP-responsive element binding protein in the postmortem orbitofrontal cortex of patients with major depressive disorder. *J. Neural. Transm.* 110:671–680.

Yazlovitskaya, E.M., Edwards, E., Thotala, D., Fu, A., Osusky, K.L., Whetsell, W.O., Jr., Boone, B., et al. (2006) Lithium treatment prevents neurocognitive deficit resulting from cranial irradiation. *Cancer Res.* 66:11179–11186.

Yildiz, A., Demopulos, C.M., Moore, C.M., Renshaw, P.F., and Sachs, G.S. (2001) Effect of lithium on phosphoinositide metabolism in human brain: a proton decoupled (31)P magnetic resonance spectroscopy study. *Biol. Psychiatry* 50:3–7.

Yoon, I.S., Li, P.P., Siu, K.P., Kennedy, J.L., Cooke, R.G., Parikh, S. V., and Warsh, J.J. (2001) Altered IMPA2 gene expression and calcium homeostasis in bipolar disorder. *Mol. Psychiatry* 6:678–683.

Young, L.T., Bezchlibnyk, Y.B., Chen, B., Wang, J.F., and MacQueen, G.M. (2004) Amygdala cyclic adenosine monophosphate response element binding protein phosphorylation in patients with mood disorders: effects of diagnosis, suicide, and drug treatment. *Biol. Psychiatry* 55:570–577.

Young, L.T., Li, P.P., Kamble, A., Siu, K.P., and Warsh, J.J. (1994) Mononuclear leukocyte levels of G proteins in depressed patients with bipolar disorder or major depressive disorder. *Am. J. Psychiatry* 151:594–596.

Young, L.T., Li, P.P., Kish, S.J., Siu, K.P., Kamble, A., Hornykiewicz, O., and Warsh, J.J. (1993) Cerebral cortex Gs alpha protein levels and forskolin-stimulated cyclic AMP formation are increased in bipolar affective disorder. *J. Neurochem.* 61:890–898.

Yuan, P.X., Huang, L.D., Jiang, Y.M., Gutkind, J.S., Manji, H.K., and Chen, G. (2001) The mood stabilizer valproic acid activates mitogen-activated protein kinases and promotes neurite growth. *J. Biol. Chem.* 276:31674–31683.

Yucel, K., Taylor, V.H., McKinnon, M.C., Macdonald, K., Alda, M., Young, L.T., and Macqueen, G.M. (2007) Bilateral hippocampal volume increase in patients with bipolar disorder and short-term lithium treatment. *Neuropsychopharmacology* 33(2):361–367.

Zarate, C.A., Jr., Singh, J.B., Carlson, P.J., Brutsche, N.E., Ameli, R., Luckenbaugh, D.A., Charney, D.S., et al. (2006) A randomized trial of an *N*-methyl-D-aspartate antagonist in treatment-resistant major depression. *Arch. Gen. Psychiatry* 63:856–864.

Zarate, C.A., Jr., Singh, J.B., Carlson, P.J., Quiroz, J., Jolkovsky, L., Luckenbuagh, D., and Manji, H.K. (2007) Efficacy of a protein kinase c inhibitor (tamoxifen) in the treatment of acute mania: a pilot study. *Bipolar Disord.* 9(6):561–570.

Zarate, C.A., Jr., Singh, J., and Manji, H.K. (2006) Cellular plasticity cascades: targets for the development of novel therapeutics for bipolar disorder. *Biol. Psychiatry* 59:1006–1020.

Zhou, R., Gray, N.A., Yuan, P., Li, X., Chen, J., Chen, G., Damschroder-Williams, P., et al. (2005) The anti-apoptotic, glucocorticoid receptor cochaperone protein BAG-1 is a long-term target for the actions of mood stabilizers. *J. Neurosci.* 25:4493–4502.

Zill, P., Malitas, P.N., Bondy, B., Engel, R., Boufidou, F., Behrens, S., Alevizos, B.E., et al. (2003) Analysis of polymorphisms in the alpha-subunit of the olfactory G-protein Golf in lithium-treated bipolar patients. *Psychiatr. Genet.* 13:65–69.

Zubenko, G.S., Hughes, H.B., 3rd, Stiffler, J.S., Brechbiel, A., Zubenko, W.N., Maher, B.S., and Marazita, M.L. (2003) Sequence variations in CREB1 cosegregate with depressive disorders in women. *Mol. Psychiatry* 8:611–618.

29 Neurochemical Theories of Depression: Preclinical Studies

RONALD S. DUMAN

Preclinical and clinical studies suggest that the serotonin (5-HT) and norepinephrine (NE) neurotransmitter systems are involved in the treatment of depression. These studies have focused largely on levels of monoamines and their receptors and have led to several theories of depression, including the monoamine depletion and receptor sensitivity hypotheses. However, this work has not led to a unifying theory of antidepressant action. In addition, the pathophysiology of depression cannot be explained by simple dysregulation of 5-HT and/or NE neurotransmission. Recent advances in molecular and cellular neurobiology have provided new insights into the long-term adaptations that underlie the therapeutic actions of antidepressant treatments (Duman and Monteggia, 2006; Manji et al., 2001; Berton and Nestler, 2006). These studies have demonstrated that chronic antidepressant treatment regulates intracellular signal transduction pathways and expression of specific target genes. In combination with advances in our understanding of the neurobiology of stress, a primary cause of depression, this work is beginning to reveal potential molecular and anatomical sites that could contribute to the pathophysiology and treatment of depression.

This chapter provides a short review of basic and clinical work regarding the role of 5-HT and NE neurotransmission in depression. Then advances in molecular and cellular neurobiology that demonstrate a role for the cyclic adenosine monophosphate (cAMP) intracellular signal transduction pathway and regulation of specific target genes, particularly brain-derived neurotrophic factor (BDNF) in the actions of antidepressant treatment, as well as stress, are discussed. There are many other neurotransmitters and signal molecules that have been studied, as well as others not yet identified, for their role in mood disorders, and there is not sufficient space to cover all of this work in this chapter. However, taken together these studies support an emerging hypothesis of how stress and other environmental insults can induce neuronal atrophy and how antidepressant treatment can reverse or block these damaging effects.

MONOAMINES AND DEPRESSION

Monoamine Depletion and Depression

A role for 5-HT and NE in depression was first suggested by the observation that pharmacological manipulation of monoamine levels could either induce or alleviate the symptoms of depression. For example, early clinical studies demonstrated that treatment with reserpine, which interferes with storage and thereby depletes monoamine levels (Fig. 29.1), can cause depression in a small percentage of individuals. This led to the hypothesis that depression results from reduced availability of 5-HT and/or NE (Bunney and Davis, 1965; Schildkraut, 1965; Coppen, 1967). The monoamine depletion hypothesis was further supported by the discovery that the prototypical antidepressant drugs, the tricyclic and MAO inhibitor antidepressants, acutely increase synaptic levels of monoamines (Fig. 29.1). The tricyclic antidepressant drugs inhibit the transporter-mediated reuptake of 5-HT and NE, one of the primary mechanisms for removal and inactivation of monoamines. Selective 5-HT reuptake inhibitors, including fluoxetine and sertraline, have been developed that lack many of the side effects of the early tricyclic antidepressants. The MAO inhibitor antidepressants block one of the primary enzymes responsible for the degradation of 5-HT and NE and thereby increase levels of monoamines.

Although these observations suggest that monoamine levels are closely related to the cause and treatment of depression, additional paradigms for the depletion of 5-HT or NE suggest a more complex relationship (Shopsin et al., 1975; Delgado et al., 1994; Miller et al., 1996). Levels of 5-HT can be safely and significantly reduced by administration of an amino acid cocktail containing all essential amino acids except tryptophan, the precursor for 5-HT. Levels of NE can be reduced by administration of low doses of α-methyl-p-tyrosine (AMPT), a competitive inhibitor of tyrosine hydroxylase, the rate-limiting enzyme for the synthesis of NE. These paradigms have

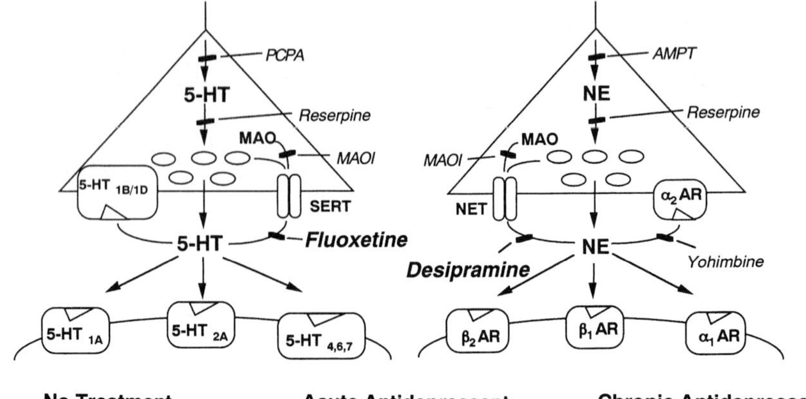

FIGURE 29.1 A model of the pre- and postsynaptic components of monoamine neurotransmission. 5-HT and NE neurotransmission is regulated at several levels, including the synthesis, storage, release, reuptake, and degradation of monoamines. Drugs that influence these sites can either decrease or increase synaptic levels of 5-HT and NE and can lead to depression, under certain conditions, or have antidepressant effects, respectively. The synthesis of 5-HT and NE can be inhibited by PCPA or AMPT, respectively. These agents act as competitive inhibitors of the 5-HT and NE limiting synthetic enzymes, tryptophan hydroxylase and tyrosine hydroxylase, respectively. The storage of monoamines in synaptic vesicles is disrupted by reserpine. Monoamines released into the synapse activate pre-and postsynaptic receptor binding sites. Postsynaptic 5-HT receptors include 5-HT_{1A}, 5-HT_{2A}, and 5-$HT_{4,6,7}$, and NE receptors include β_1AR, β_2AR, and α_1AR; this represents a partial list of the many 5-HT and NE receptor subtypes. Presynaptic autoreceptors, including 5-HT_{1A} and 5-HT_{1B} (5-HT_{1A} is localized to cell bodies and 5-HT_{1B} to terminals) and α_2AR, inhibit the firing rate of monoamine neurons. The human homologue of rodent 5-HT_{1B} is the 5-HT_{1D} receptor. Pindolol is an antagonist that has some selectivity for 5-HT_{1A} receptors located on 5-HT cell bodies. Yohimbine is an antagonist for the presynaptic α_2AR. Monoamine function is terminated by reuptake into neurons and glia and enzymatic neurotransmitter degradation. Reuptake is mediated by high affinity transporters for 5-HT (SERT) and NE (NET) that are inhibited by the antidepressants fluoxetine and desipramine, respectively. MAO, localized to mitochondrial membranes, catalyzes the degradation of 5-HT and NE, and is the site of action for the MAOI antidepressants. Degradation of monoamines is also catalyzed by COMT that has an extracellular location (not shown). 5HT: serontonin; NE: norepinephrine; PCPA: p-chlorophenylalanine; AMPT: α-methyl-para-tyrosine; MAO: Monoamine oxidase; MAOI: monoamine oxidase inhibitor; COMT: catechol-*O*-methyltransferase.

been used to examine the role of 5-HT and NE in normal patients and drug-remitted individuals who are depressed. The results are summarized as follows:

- Depression is not induced in normal patients upon depletion of either 5-HT and/or NE with these paradigms, including normal patients receiving antidepressant treatment.
- Patients who are depressed and being treated with 5-HT selective reuptake inhibitors (SSRIs), but not NE selective reuptake inhibitors (NSRIs), suffer a brief relapse upon depletion of 5-HT.
- Conversely, patients who are depressed being treated with NSRIs, but not SSRIs, suffer a brief relapse upon depletion of NE.
- Patients who are depressed, who are not medicated, are not made worse by depletion of either 5-HT or NE.

These studies indicate that monoamine depletion alone is not sufficient to cause depression in normal patients. However, when patients are successfully treated with either 5-HT or NE selective reuptake inhibitors they become vulnerable to depletion of the corresponding monoamine, suggesting that 5-HT and NE are involved in the maintenance of the antidepressant response.

Time Lag for the Therapeutic Action of Antidepressant Treatments

In addition to the depletion studies, the time course for the therapeutic action of antidepressant treatments provides additional evidence that there is a complex relationship between monoamines and depression. Although antidepressant drugs rapidly increase the levels of monoamines (that is, within days) the therapeutic action of these treatments is dependent on chronic administration (that is, several weeks or even months). One hypothesis to explain this delay is that the firing rate of monoamine neurons is reduced by inhibitory autoreceptors that become activated when levels of monoamines are increased by an antidepressant treatment. Electrophysiological studies in rodents support this possibility, demonstrating that the firing rate of 5-HT neurons is reduced by administration of certain antidepressants (Blier and de Montigny, 1994). In addition, inhibition of cell firing gradually diminishes with time, consistent with the time lag for the onset of the therapeutic actions of antidepressant treatment. Clinical studies suggest that treatment with a 5-HT_{1A} antagonist (for example, pindolol), which blocks the autoreceptor inhibition of cell firing, may hasten the response time to a 5-HT selective reuptake inhibitor (Artigas et al., 1994). However, inhibition of cell firing may only account for a fraction of the time lag. In addition, administration of tryptophan with a MAO inhibitor, a treatment known to rapidly elevate levels of 5-HT and induce a 5-HT behavioral syndrome, does not alleviate depressive symptoms (Price et al., 1985). Finally, administration of an α_2-adrenergic antagonist, which blocks NE autoreceptor inhibition of cell firing, has not proven effective in reducing the time lag for antidepressant drugs that influence this monoamine system (Heninger and Charney, 1987).

Neuroplasticity and Antidepressant Treatment

Another hypothesis to explain the delayed time course is that neuronal adaptations to the elevation of monoamines, which occurs over time, are required for the therapeutic action of antidepressants. Adaptation or neuroplasticity could also explain why the maintenance of antidepressant treatment, discussed above, is dependent on the presence of monoamines (for example, the antidepressant-induced neuronal adaptation could also mediate monoamine neurotransmission). Neuroplasticity has been studied in cellular and behavioral models of learning and memory but can also be viewed as a fundamental process that allows neuronal systems to respond to the constant influx of all types of stimuli, including environmental and endocrine, as well as pharmacological treatment (see Chapter 5). The mechanisms underlying neuroplasticity involve receptor-coupled intracellular signal transduction pathways and neuronal gene expression. Studies of these pathways have led to alternative theories of the mechanism of action of antidepressant treatment, as well as the pathophysiology of depression and are discussed in some detail below.

MONOAMINE RECEPTOR SENSITIVITY AND DEPRESSION

Release of 5-HT and NE into the synapse leads to activation of pre- and postsynaptic receptor subtypes (Fig. 29.1). Sustained release and/or elevation of monoamines by antidepressant treatment results in continued activation of these receptor sites. One proximal adaptive response to sustained activation is down-regulation of monoamine receptors. Indeed, antidepressant treatment is reported to down-regulate levels of several 5-HT and NE receptor subtypes. Listed below is a brief overview of the major monoamine receptor systems that are regulated by antidepressant treatment.

β-adrenergic receptor (βAR) Sensitivity and Depression

Chronic antidepressant treatment is known to down-regulate β-adrenergic receptor (β_1AR) ligand binding sites in limbic brain regions, such as cerebral cortex and hippocampus (Vetulani and Sulser, 1975; Banerjee et al., 1977). This led to the hypothesis that the therapeutic action of antidepressant treatment is mediated by down-regulation of βAR sites and that up-regulation of these receptors may lead to depression (Sulser et al., 1978; Charney et al., 1981). However, there are several problems with this hypothesis. First, levels of βAR ligand binding sites are not down-regulated by all antidepressants (Charney et al., 1981). This could mean that the action of different antidepressants is mediated by different receptors, or that other receptor sites are more relevant to the action of antidepressant treatments. Second, the time delay for down-regulation of βAR binding sites is more rapid than the therapeutic onset of these treatments (Riva and Creese, 1989). Third, inhibition of βARs by treatment with a selective antagonist is not an effective treatment for depression: in fact βAR antagonists are reported to produce depression in some individuals (Paykel et al., 1982; Avorn et al., 1986), and βAR agonists have antidepressant effects in behavioral models of depression (O'Donnell, 1993). Moreover, activation or facilitation of βAR function by administration of thyroid hormone or a specific receptor agonist can have antidepressant efficacy in some patients (Goodwin et al., 1982). Taken together, these findings indicate that βAR down-regulation does not mediate the therapeutic action of antidepressants. In fact, the results are more consistent with the possibility that inhibition or down-regulation of βAR may actually contribute to a depressive phenotype.

5-HT_{2A} Receptor-Sensitivity and Depression

Another monoamine receptor that is influenced by antidepressant treatment is the 5-HT_2 receptor (Peroutka and Snyder, 1980). There are two 5-HT_2 receptor subtypes expressed in brain, 5-HT_{2A} and 5-HT_{2C}. The 5-HT_{2A} receptor subtype is more widely distributed and is expressed at relatively higher levels in most limbic brain regions. The 5-HT_{2A} receptor subtype is also the primary receptor site for hallucinogenic compounds. Antidepressant treatments are reported to down-regulate the expression of 5-HT_{2A} receptors in rat brain, and brain-imaging studies demonstrate that levels of this receptor are altered in patients who are depressed (Heninger and Charney, 1987). In addition, several antidepressant drugs, including tricyclic antidepressants and the atypical antidepressant, mianserin, bind with relatively high affinity to 5-HT_{2A} receptor receptors. However, the 5-HT_{2A} receptor sensitivity hypothesis has many of the same problems as the βAR hypothesis: not all antidepressants decrease 5-HT_{2A} receptor binding; in fact, electroconvulsive seizures increase receptor levels; 5-HT_{2A} receptor binding is rapidly decreased after a few days of antidepressant treatment; and 5-HT_{2A} receptor antagonists when administered alone are not effective antidepressants (Heninger and Charney, 1987; Butler et al., 1993). However, recent studies demonstrate that administration of a 5-HT$_{2A}$ antagonist, such as risperidone or the atypical antipsychotics clozapine or olanzapine, to patients who are not responding to an SSRI can result in treatment response. Taken together these findings suggest that 5-HT$_{2A}$ receptor antagonism alone is not sufficient to produce an antidepressant response but can improve treatment response to a SSRI. In addition, a polymorphism in the *5-HT$_{2A}$* gene was associated with treatment outcome in the STAR*D study (McMahon et al., 2006).

5-HT$_{1A}$ Receptor Sensitivity and Depression

Studies of the 5-HT$_{1A}$ receptor have provided evidence that this receptor subtype also plays a role in the action of antidepressant treatments (Heninger and Charney, 1987; Butler et al., 1993). Results from electrophysiological studies indicate that chronic antidepressant treatment increases postsynaptic 5-HT$_{1A}$ receptor neurotransmission in the hippocampus. The proposed mechanisms for increased 5-HT$_{1A}$ receptor transmission differ for different classes of antidepressant drugs. For agents that inhibit MAO or selectively block 5-HT reuptake, the mechanism is thought to involve desensitization of presynaptic autoreceptors present on 5-HT neurons, leading to elevation of synaptic levels of 5-HT. The significance of presynaptic autoreceptor inhibition is supported by reports that administration of an autoreceptor antagonist can hasten the response to a SSRI. In contrast, chronic administration of a tricyclic antidepressant or electroconvulsive seizure increases the sensitivity of postsynaptic 5-HT$_{1A}$ receptors in hippocampus. A role for 5-HT$_{1A}$ receptors is also supported by studies of adult neurogenesis, which demonstrate that induction of adult neurogenesis by a 5-HT selective reuptake inhibitor is blocked in 5-HT$_{1A}$ null mice (Santarelli et al., 2003).

One problem with the 5-HT$_{1A}$ receptor hypothesis is that direct acting 5-HT$_{1A}$ receptor agonists are not very effective antidepressants. However, the drugs tested thus far are partial agonists (for example, buspirone), and it is possible that a full 5-HT$_{1A}$ receptor agonist would have better clinical efficacy. This hypothesis will require the testing of full 5-HT$_{1A}$ agonists. Another possibility is that increased 5-HT$_{1A}$ neurotransmission is necessary, but not sufficient, for antidepressant efficacy, and that activation of an additional 5-HT receptor(s) or other signaling factors are required.

An Alternative Hypothesis for Adaptation of Receptor Sensitivity

There are additional monoamine receptor subtypes that are regulated by antidepressant treatment. However, regulation of these receptors, as with the β_1AR, 5-HT$_{1A}$, and 5-HT$_{2A}$ receptors, cannot explain the therapeutic action of antidepressants. An alternative interpretation is that receptor regulation is an adaptation to elevated monoamine levels that is a cellular response to maintain homeostatic control of monoamine neurotransmission. In fact, down-regulation of receptors supports the possibility that these receptors remain activated during chronic antidepressant treatment. Indeed, levels of these receptors are reduced, not completely eliminated, by chronic antidepressant treatment, suggesting that there is a sufficient level of receptor remaining to respond to the elevated levels of 5-HT and NE (Fig. 29.2). In fact, in the presence of elevated monoamines, the functional output of a receptor may be increased, not decreased, during long-term treatment. This would suggest that there is a sustained activation of the intracellular signal transduction cascades regulated by these monoamine receptors. Intracellular pathways regulate the function and expression of many cellular proteins that may be targets of antidepressant treatment.

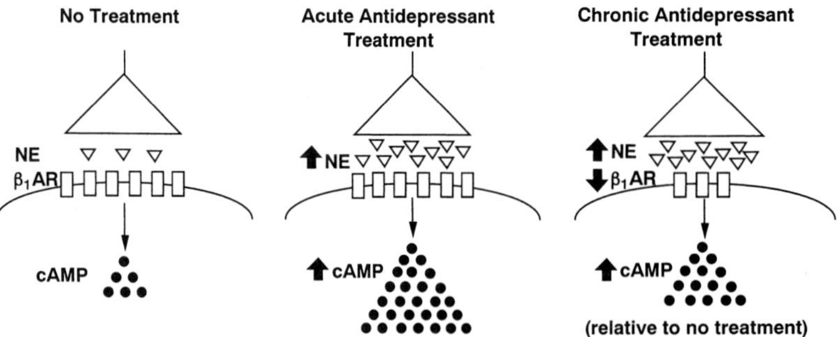

FIGURE 29.2 A model for regulation of the βAR-coupled cAMP system by acute and chronic antidepressant treatment. In the absence of antidepressant treatment, synaptic levels of NE stimulate βARs and thereby increase the formation of cAMP. Acute antidepressant treatment increases synaptic levels of NE and increases βAR-stimulation of cAMP formation. Chronic antidepressant treatment results in down-regulation of the number of βAR sites, and a reduction of cAMP formation relative to acute antidepressant treatment. However, because the level of NE remains elevated, the level of cAMP formation is greater than that in the absence of drug treatment. Although this hypothetical model requires testing, it is supported by studies demonstrating that antidepressant treatment increases the cAMP cascade and target genes of this second messenger pathway. cAMP: cyclic adenosine monophosphate; NE: norepinephrine.

NEUROPEPTIDE RECEPTORS AND DEPRESSION

In addition to the monoamine receptors, there are several neuropeptide receptors that have become the subject of intense investigation and interest as potential targets for antidepressant treatment. These include the corticortrophin releasing factor (CRF) and neurokinin (NK) receptors.

CRF Receptor System

Corticortrophin releasing factor was first characterized as a critical mediator of the stress response in the central nervous system. This neuropeptide is expressed prominently in the paraventricular nucleus of the hypothalamus and coordinates the stress-induced release of adrenocorticotrophin hormone (ACTH) from the anterior pituitary (Chalmers et al., 1996). Corticortrophin releasing factor is also found throughout the brain, and expression in several limbic structures, such as the amygdala, suggesting a role in anxiety and mood disorders. Support for this hypothesis was provided by studies demonstrating that levels of CRF are increased in the cerebrospinal fluid (CSF) of patients who are depressed or postmortem tissue of victims of suicide (Nemeroff et al., 1984). A large volume of work over several years has provided evidence that an antagonist of the CRF receptor could be efficacious for the treatment of psychiatric illnesses associated with stress (Holsboer, 1999; Owens and Nemeroff, 1999). Two CRF receptor subtypes, CRF-R_1 and CRF-R_2, have been identified and characterized in the brain. Although the CRF-R_1 receptor is more widely distributed in the brain, both receptor subtypes have been implicated in the response to stress. Preliminary clinical studies have been encouraging, but larger clinical trials have not been conducted due to toxicology problems. Development of safer agents will be required to confirm the therapeutic efficacy of CRF-R_1 antagonists. One of the concerns with these compounds is that they will also block the pituitary CRF receptor (R_1 subtype) and thereby interfere with the fine control of the hypothalamic-pituitary-adrenal (HPA) axis. However, preliminary studies in humans indicate that this may not be a problem.

NK_1 Receptor System

Early studies focused on the potential role of neurokinins (NKs), including substance P, in the control of pain, although subsequent work has not supported this hypothesis. However, recent studies have taken a broad overview of the possible function of NKs, resulting in clinical trials of a NK antagonist in depression. The first major clinical study demonstrated that treatment with a neurokinin-1 (NK_1) receptor antagonist was effective for the treatment of depression at a level that was comparable to a prototypical antidepressant agent (Kramer et al., 1998). Subsequent studies have not been as straightforward to interpret, highlighting a major problem in the development of novel antidepressant agents (that is, many clinical trials fail because of high placebo response rate or insufficient separation from comparator drugs). In the meantime, basic research studies in experimental animals indicate that NK_1 receptors are located on 5-HT terminals and can depress the activity of 5-HT neurons. Conversely, antagonist treatment blocks these receptors and thereby enhances 5-HT neurotransmission, suggesting that this may be the mechanism by which blockade of the NK_1 receptor produces an antidepressant response. Further studies will be necessary to test this hypothesis and to determine the possible role of other NK receptor subtypes in the treatment of mood disorders.

There are several other neuropeptide-receptor systems that have received attention, including 5-HT_4, vasopressin-1b, dynorphin, δ-opiate, and galanin receptor subtypes, to name a few. Preclinical studies provide evidence that drugs acting at these receptors can produce antidepressant responses in behavioral models and warrant the development and testing of agents in clinical trials.

INTRACELLULAR SIGNAL TRANSDUCTION PATHWAYS AND DEPRESSION

The intracellular signal transduction cascades that mediate the actions of monoamine receptors have been studied in some detail (see Chapters 4 and 5, and Nestler and Duman, 2006), making it possible to study the role of these pathways in the action of antidepressant treatment. The second-messenger signal transduction pathways (for example, cAMP, inositol triphosphate, Ca^{2+}, and diacyl glycerol) mediate the actions of many monoamine receptors, as well as many neuropeptide and amino acid receptors (Fig. 29.3). Receptor regulation of these pathways occurs via G proteins that couple neurotransmitter receptors to effectors, such as adenylyl cyclase and phospholipase C, that catalyze the formation of cAMP and inositol triphosphate, respectively. These second messengers, in turn, regulate the activity of second messenger–dependent protein kinases (Fig. 29.3). In addition to the second-messenger dependent pathways, neurotrophic factors influence cell function via another type of signal transduction cascade. Receptors for these factors contain a tyrosine kinase domain that is activated upon agonist binding to the receptor. This leads to the phosphorylation of tyrosine residues on other cellular proteins. The mitogen-associated protein kinase (MAPK) cascade is one pathway regulated by these receptors. There is also evidence for cross talk between the second messenger and neurotrophic factor–regulated tyrosine kinase pathways.

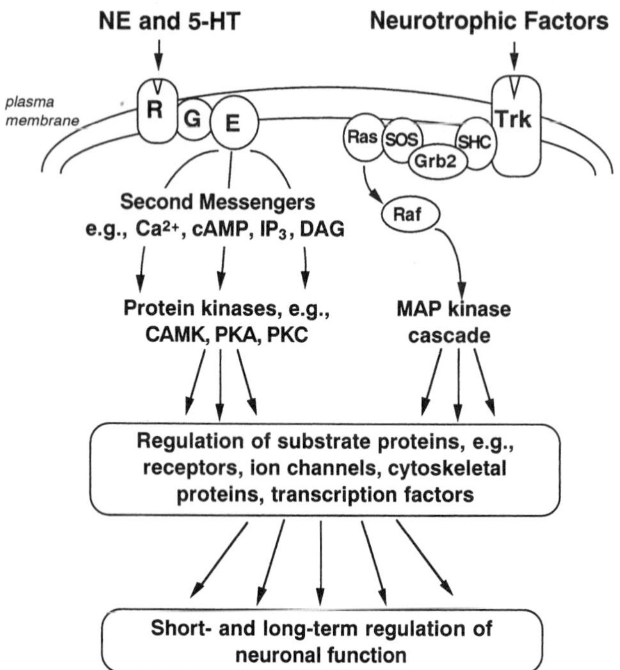

FIGURE 29.3 A model for monoamine and neurotrophic factor regulated intracellular signal transduction pathways. The actions of monoamines are mediated largely by activation of receptors (R) coupled to effectors (E) via G proteins (G). This leads to the formation of second messengers (for example, cAMP, IP_3, DAG, and Ca^{2+}) and then activation of second-messenger-dependent protein kinases (for example, Ca^{2+}/CAMK, PKA, and PKC). Neurotrophic factor signal transduction occurs via a different type of intracellular cascade. Binding of a neurotrophic factor to its receptor (Trk) results in activation of an intrinsic tyrosine kinase domain and autophosphorylation of intracellular receptor sites. This leads to binding to an adaptor protein in the Shc family. Shc becomes phosphorylated and binds to a Grb protein, such as Grb2. This complex of Shc and Grb2 then binds to Sos, a guanine nucleotide exchange factor. Sos then activates a small GTP binding protein, Ras, by enhancing the exchange of GDP for GTP. Ras then leads to activation of Raf, the first protein kinase in the MAP kinase cascade. The second-messenger-dependent protein kinases and the MAP kinase cascade result in phosphorylation and regulation of diverse cellular proteins that control all aspects of neuronal function. This includes the short- and long-term responses to psychotropic drugs, as well as neuroendocrine and environmental stimuli. cAMP: cyclic adenosine monophosphate; IP_3: inositol triphosphate; DAG: diacylglycerol; GDP: guanosine 5'-diphosphate; GTP: guanosine-5′ triphosphate; CAMK: calmodulin-dependent protein kinase; MAP: mitogen-activated protein; PKA: protein kinase A; PKC: protein kinase C.

These pathways control all aspects of neuronal function and ultimately underlie the ability of the brain to adapt and respond to pharmacological and environmental inputs. Some examples include increased or decreased synaptic efficacy in cellular models of learning and memory (Madison et al., 1991; Bliss and Collingridge, 1993; Kang and Schuman, 1995; Levine et al., 1995) and atrophy and growth of neurons in adults, as well as during development (Lindsay et al., 1994; Lindvall et al., 1994; Thoenen, 1995). These types of responses can be viewed as prototypical ways in which the brain adapts to environmental stimuli. It is likely that similar types of molecular and cellular adaptations occur in response to antidepressant treatment, and that dysfunction of this adaptive plasticity is involved in the pathophysiology of depression and other mood disorders. Although such adaptations are complicated and can be difficult to identify, their potential importance has stimulated a large number of studies to investigate the role of intracellular pathways and cellular adaptations in the pathophysiology and treatment of depression.

Cyclic AMP Signal Transduction and Depression

The cAMP cascade is one pathway that has been implicated in the action of antidepressant treatment (Fig. 29.2). Formation of cAMP can be regulated by direct coupling of receptors to adenylyl cyclase or indirectly by other second-messenger pathways. Receptors directly coupled to this pathway interact with either stimulatory (G_s) or inhibitory (G_i) G protein subtypes. This results in release of the α subunits of G_s or G_i and stimulation or inhibition, respectively, of adenylyl cyclase and cAMP formation. Indirect activation of certain forms of adenylyl cyclase occurs via elevation of Ca^{2+} and calmodulin, and is independent of G_s (Nestler and Duman, 2006). Elevation of cAMP leads to activation of protein kinase A (PKA), which in turn leads to regulation of cellular function by phosphorylation of specific proteins, including receptors, ion channels, G proteins, enzymes, and transcription factors. The cAMP-response element binding (CREB) protein is one transcription factor that can mediate the actions of the cAMP system (Meyer and Habener, 1993; Ghosh and Greenberg, 1995). The transcriptional activity of CREB is regulated primarily by phosphorylation of specific amino acid residues, although CREB function can also be influenced by increasing or decreasing the total amount of CREB protein (Widnell et al., 1994; Walker et al., 1995; Nibuya et al., 1996). In addition to PKA, other types of protein kinases are known to phosphorylate and activate CREB, including Ca^{2+}/calmodulin-dependent protein kinase and ribosomal S6 kinase, which is activated by the MAPK cascade (Russell and Duman, 2002).

The cAMP cascade and CREB could represent common downstream targets for 5-HT and NE neurotransmitter systems, as well as antidepressant treatment. There are several 5-HT and NE receptor subtypes that directly stimulate cAMP production (Fig. 29.4). β_1AR and β_2AR subtypes mediate NE-stimulated cAMP formation, and there are at least three 5-HT receptor subtypes that stimulate this second messenger system (that is, 5-HT_4, 5-HT_6, and 5-HT_7). A role for the β_1AR and 5-HT_7 receptor coupled regulation of the cAMP system is supported by reports that chronic antidepressant treatment down-regulates levels of βAR-stimulated cAMP forma-

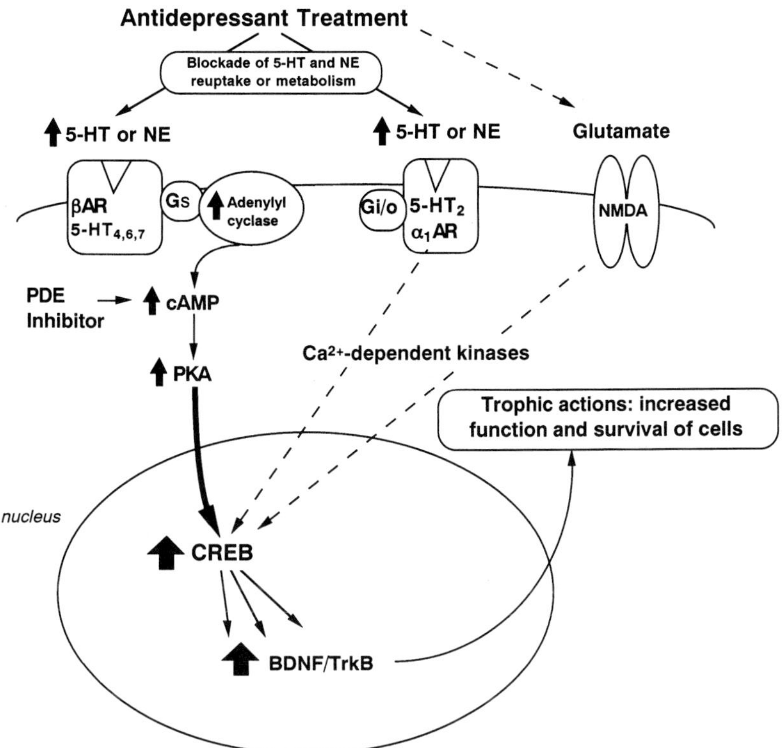

FIGURE 29.4 A model of the molecular actions of antidepressant treatment: adaptations of the cAMP-CREB cascade. Antidepressant treatment increases synaptic levels of 5-HT and NE via blockade of monoamine reuptake and degradation. This can lead to down-regulation of certain monoamine receptors (for example, β_1AR, 5-HT$_7$, 5-HT$_{2A}$). However, chronic antidepressant treatment results in up-regulation of the postreceptor components of the cAMP cascade, including levels of adenylyl cyclase enzyme activity, particulate levels of PKA, and expression of CREB. CREB is a common target for both 5-HT and NE and different types of antidepressants, because it is regulated by receptors coupled to the cAMP pathway (for example, β-AR, 5-HT$_{4,6,7}$) and receptors that activate Ca^{2+}-dependent protein kinases (for example, 5-HT$_{2A}$, α_1AR). In addition, the NMDA glutamate receptor complex can also influence CREB via activation of Ca^{2+}-dependent protein kinases, and chronic antidepressant treatment is reported to decrease the affinity of a modulatory glycine site on the NMDA receptor. Up-regulation of CREB increases the expression of target genes, such as BDNF and TrkB. BDNF and TrkB exert trophic actions on target neurons and thereby increase cell survival and function. 5-HT: serotonin: NE: norepinephrine; cAMP: cyclic adenosine monophosphate; PKA: protein kinase A; CREB: cAMP-response element binding; NMDA: *N*-methyl-D-aspartate; BDNF: brain-derived neurotrophic factor.

tion and decreases the level of 5-HT$_7$ receptor binding sites (Sleight et al., 1995). These findings indicate that there may be a sustained activation of the cAMP second-messenger system via these receptors (see Fig. 29.4). Recent studies also demonstrate that 5-HT$_4$ and 5-HT$_6$ receptors may be involved in the action of antidepressants. For example, activation of 5-HT$_4$ receptors located on 5-HT dorsal raphé nucleus neurons can increase the firing rate of these cells (Lucas and Debonnel, 2002). Moreover, this effect is maximal after only 3 days of treatment and is sustained with repeated treatment for up to 3 weeks (Lucas et al., 2005). Additional studies demonstrate antidepressant activity in cellular and behavioral models (Lucas et al., 2007). These studies suggest that 5-HT$_4$ receptor agonists may have a rapid response rate in patients who are depressed.

Studies of dopamine and cAMP-regulated phosphoprotein of 32 Kd molecular weight (DARPP-32) have implicated the 5-HT$_6$ receptor subtype in the actions of selective serotonin reuptake inhibitor (SSRI) antidepressants. The behavioral actions of fluoxetine in the forced swim test are mediated in part by phosphorylation of Thr34-DARPP-32 and Ser845-GluR1 (Svenningsson, Tzavara, Liu, et al., 2002). In vitro slice experiments have demonstrated that 5-HT-stimulated phosphorylation of Thr34-DARPP-32 and Ser845-GluR1 is mediated by 5-HT$_4$ and 5-HT$_6$ receptors, both of which are positively coupled to the cAMP–PKA pathway (Svenningsson, Tzavara, Witkin, et al., 2002). The distribution of 5-HT$_6$ receptors is localized to limbic structures that could influence various aspects of depression and antidepressant response (Hamon et al., 1999; Ballaz et al., 2007).

Another potential site of convergence for antidepressant treatments is CREB. In addition to regulation by the cAMP cascade, CREB can be activated by 5-HT or NE receptors that stimulate Ca^{2+}-dependent protein kinases (for example, 5-HT$_{2A}$, 5-HT$_{2C}$, α_1-adrenergic receptors) (Meyer and Habener, 1993; Ghosh and Greenberg,

1995). cAMP-response element binding can also be influenced by α-amino-3-hydroxy-5-methyl-4-isoxasole-propionic acid (AMPA) or N-methyl-D-aspartate (NMDA) type glutamate receptors, which form a ligand gated Ca^{2+} channel (Fig. 29.4) (Ghosh and Greenberg, 1995). N-methyl-D-aspartate receptor gating of Ca^{2+} is enhanced by a glycine modulatory site, and the affinity of glycine for this site is reduced by chronic antidepressant treatment (Paul et al., 1994). One interpretation of these results is that NMDA receptor function is reduced by antidepressant treatment. An alternative possibility is that this is an adaptive down-regulation of receptor affinity in response to sustained activation of receptor function, similar to that observed for the βAR (see Fig. 29.2). N-methyl-D-aspartate receptor activation alone can regulate cell function, but interaction of NMDA receptors with other neurotransmitters (for example, monoamines) and neurotrophic factors may be critical for maintaining the normal function and plasticity of neurons (A. McAllister et al., 1996). Additional studies are needed to determine the role of NMDA receptors in monoamine receptor function and the action of antidepressant treatment.

Adaptations of the cAMP Cascade by Antidepressant Treatment

The possibility that antidepressant treatment results in sustained activation of the cAMP second-messenger cascade is supported by studies of the postreceptor components of this system (Fig. 29.4). The level of adenylyl cyclase enzyme activity is increased by chronic administration of several different types of antidepressants (Menkes et al., 1983; Ozawa and Rasenick, 1991). This effect appears to result from enhanced coupling of G_s to the adenylyl cyclase catalytic subunit. In addition, chronic lithium treatment increases the expression of adenylyl cyclase types I and II in rat neocortex (Colin et al., 1991). Antidepressant treatment is also reported to increase levels of PKA enzyme activity in particulate fractions of rat neocortex (Fig. 29.4) (Nestler et al., 1989; Perez et al., 1989). Levels of PKA are increased in the nuclear fraction but decreased in the cytosolic fraction, suggesting that PKA is translocated to the nucleus in response to antidepressant treatments (Nestler et al., 1989; Tiraboschi et al., 2004). Although additional studies are required to confirm the cellular localization of this effect, the results indicate that PKA can be regulated by antidepressant treatments. However, nuclear localization analysis of several protein kinases indicates that PKA is less likely to account for the induction of gene transcriptin by CREB phosphorylation than CAMKIV and MAPK, although a role for PKA cannot be completely excluded (Tiraboschi et al., 2004).

Regulation of CREB by Antidepressant Treatment

Up-regulation of adenylyl cyclase and increased levels of PKA in the nucleus suggest that the function of CREB, as well as other transcription factors, is also regulated by antidepressant treatment. Regulation of CREB and expression of target genes may be particularly relevant to the action of antidepressant treatment because of the therapeutic time delay: altered expression of target genes and the cellular proteins they encode, as well as the transport and incorporation of these newly synthesized proteins into the cellular architecture, would be expected to require a time delay. In support of this possibility, the expression of CREB messenger ribonucleic acid (mRNA) and protein in rat hippocampus is increased by chronic antidepressant treatment (Nibuya et al., 1996; Conti et al., 2002). This could occur via regulation of a cAMP response element (CRE) in the promoter of the CREB gene (Walker et al., 1995; Nibuya et al., 1996). Up-regulation of CREB is observed with 5-HT or NE selective reuptake inhibitors, indicating that CREB is a target for both monoamine systems. Chronic antidepressant administration also increases the phosphorylation of CREB and CRE-mediated gene expression, demonstrating that CREB function is also increased by antidepressant treatment (Thome et al., 2000; Tiraboschi et al., 2004). Increased levels of CaMKIV and MAPK in nuclear fractions suggest that these kinases mediate the induction of CREB transcription activity (Tiraboschi et al., 2004).

Up-regulation of CREB suggests that genes containing CRE elements may be targets for antidepressant treatment. However, gene expression is regulated in a complex, region-specific manner, and not all CRE-regulated genes can be considered targets of antidepressant treatments. For example, in the locus coeruleus chronic antidepressant treatment decreases PKA activity and expression of tyrosine hydroxylase, which contains a CRE, suggesting that antidepressant treatment down-regulates CREB in this brain region (Melia et al., 1992). In addition, expression of a particular gene is dependent on the function and interaction of multiple transcription factors that either enhance or inhibit transcriptional activity. This indicates that even though antidepressant treatment regulates the cAMP cascade, the functional consequences of this regulation are region specific and are limited to a subset of target genes. Identification of the specific target genes will provide new insights into the therapeutic action of antidepressant treatments.

Behavioral Studies of CREB

A possible role for CREB in depression has gained additional support from behavioral studies in rodent models. One report demonstrates that overexpression of CREB in hippocampus produces an antidepressant-like effect in behavioral models of depression (Chen et al., 2001). In this study viral-mediated gene transfer was used to increase levels of CREB in the hippocampus, and animals were then tested in the forced swim and learned helplessness paradigms. In both paradigms, viral expression of CREB produced an effect similar to that observed with chemical antidepressant agents. These studies indicate that up-regulation of CREB in hippocampus is sufficient to produce an antidepressant response. However, studies of altered CREB expression in other brain regions and tests of CREB null mutant mice have reported different effects (that is, CREB is prodepressive) indicating that the actions of CREB are region specific (Pliakas et al., 2001; Newton et al., 2002). In particular, studies of the mesolimbic dopamine system demonstrate that in the nucleus accumbens, CREB serves a gating function between emotional stimuli and behavioral responding, such that increased CREB reduces and decreased CREB increases responding (Barrot et al., 2002). In addition, it is likely that the function of CREB is dependent on the timing and context in which the effect of overexpression on behavior is studied, as has been observed in models of learning and memory (that is, CREB is necessary for long-term memory, but not for short-term memory). Additional studies will be needed to fully understand the role of this transcription factor in the action of antidepressant treatment.

Clinical Studies of the cAMP-CREB Cascade

Studies of postmortem brain also provide evidence of altered CREB expression in patients who are depressed. cAMP-response element binding immunoreactivity is reported to be decreased in the temporal cortex of patients who are depressed relative to matched controls (Dowlatshahi et al., 1998; Odagaki et al., 2001; Dwivedi et al., 2003), and CREB phosphorylation is reduced in postmortem patients who are depressed (Yamada et al, 2003). Moreover, levels of CREB were significantly increased in patients who were depressed and who were being medicated with antidepressants at the time of death. Although these findings must be replicated, the results are consistent with the hypothesis that up-regulation of CREB could contribute to the action of antidepressant treatment and that decreased levels could play a role in the pathophysiology of depression. Dysfunction of other components of the cAMP cascade, including G proteins, adenylyl cyclase, and PKA subunits, have also been conducted in postmortem tissue (Dowlatshahi and Young, 2000). One of the most consistent findings in these studies is that levels of stimulated adenylyl cyclase enzyme activity are decreased in patients with depression. Studies of blood elements or fibroblasts also demonstrate a reduction in levels of PKA subunit immunoreactivity or enzyme activity (Manier et al., 1996; Perez et al., 2001). Taken together, these different lines of evidence suggest that the cAMP–CREB cascade is down-regulated in patients who are depressed.

Additional Signal Transduction Sites and Depression

Although studies of the cAMP–CREB cascade are highlighted in this chapter, it is likely that there are many other intracellular signaling cascades that also play a role in depression. For example, antidepressant treatment regulates monoamine receptors, including 5-HT_{2A} and β_1-AR, coupled to the phosphatidylinositol pathway and protein kinase C (PKC) (Charney et al., 1981; Heninger and Charney, 1987). Lithium also regulates PKC, and recent studies have identified glycogen-synthase kinase-3β as a novel target of this bipolar medication (Manji and Duman, 2001; Zarate et al., 2006). In addition to CREB, PKC could regulate distinct transcription factors, as well as other phosphoproteins.

Another study has found that P11, a member of the S100 family of small acidic proteins, is up-regulated by antidepressant treatment, is decreased by a behavioral model of stress and depression, and decreased in postmortem tissue of patients who are depressed (Svenningsson et al., 2006). P11 interacts with a variety of proteins, including 5-HT_{1B} receptors; notably, P11 increases the surface expression and function of 5-HT_{1B}, and P11 transgenic mice display an antidepressant phenotype in the tail suspension test.

The MAPK pathway, which is regulated by neurotrophic factors as well as other signaling pathways, has also been implicated in the actions of antidepressant treatment (Shirayama et al., 2002; Duman et al., 2007) (see also section on neurotrophic factors in this chapter). A role for glucocorticoid receptors, which regulate gene expression via binding to a glucocorticoid response element, in the treatment and etiology of depression has also been suggested (Barden et al., 1995). This most likely represents a partial listing of the signal transduction pathways and transcription factors that are involved in depression, and future studies will be necessary to fully characterize the relevant cellular adaptations.

NEURONAL ATROPHY AND LOSS IN ANIMAL MODELS OF DEPRESSION

Experimental studies have demonstrated that stress causes a loss of neurotrophic support in animal models. Moreover, several lines of evidence demonstrate that stress can lead to structural alterations in limbic brain regions. This includes atrophy of neurons and a reduction of neurogenesis in adult hippocampus. These deleterious effects of stress could contribute to the pathophysiology of depression. A brief overview of neurotrophic factors and the effects of stress on the hippocampus are reviewed in this section.

Neurotrophic Factors

There are several different families of neurotrophic factors that control the survival and growth of neurons during development but that also play a critical role in the survival and function of adult neurons. One of the best-characterized subgroups is the nerve growth factor (NGF) family, which includes nerve growth factor, brain-derived neurotrophic factor (BDNF), neurotrophin-3, and neurotrophin-4/5. The members of this family are expressed throughout the central nervous system and are known to have a wide range of effects on neuronal function (Thoenen, 1995; K. McAllister et al., 1999; Arancio and Chao, 2007). These neurotrophic factors produce cellular actions by binding to receptors, referred to as Trks A, B, and C for NGF, BDNF, and NT-3, respectively. The Trk receptors have intrinsic tyrosine kinase activity, and activation results in autophosphorylation and subsequent coupling to one of three effector systems: the MAPK cascade, phosphotidylinositol-3 kinase, and phospholipase Cγ (Russell and Duman, 2002; Tanis and Duman, 2007). Within this family of neurotrophic factors, BDNF is the most widely distributed and most abundant in brain. Preclinical studies of neurotrophic factors in the actions of stress and antidepressants have been conducted at the molecular, cellular, and behavioral levels. Taken together the results indicate that BDNF may be involved in the action of antidepressants, and that dysfunction of this or other neurotrophic factors could contribute to the pathophysiology of depression.

Stress Down-Regulates BDNF Expression in Hippocampus

Exposure to stressful conditions causes a rapid and long-lasting down-regulation of BDNF in rodent hippocampus (Nibuya et al., 1995; Smith et al., 1995). This effect is observed after short- (2 hours) and long-term (7 days) immobilization stress and is observed in the major subfields of the hippocampus (that is, the dentate gyrus granule cell layer, and CA1 and CA3 pyramidal cell layers). Down-regulation of BDNF is one of the most consistently reported effects of stress and is observed with many different paradigms, including unpredictable stress, foot shock, social isolation, social defeat, swim stress, and maternal deprivation (see Duman and Monteggia, 2006, for review). Glucocorticoid treatment causes a smaller, but significant, down-regulation of BDNF expression in hippocampus, indicating that adrenal steroids may contribute to this effect of stress. BDNF is also decreased upon reexposing animals to cues previously associated with foot shock (that is, conditioned response) (Rasmussen et al., 2002). This suggests that the recurrent memory of stressful or traumatic experiences could continue to result in down-regulation of BDNF long after the experience and thereby influence behavior.

In addition to BDNF, there is also evidence that other neurotrophic/growth factors are decreased by stress. One of the most interesting factors is vascular endothelial growth factor (VEGF). Vascular endothelial growth factor was first identified as an angiogenic factor and endothelial cell mitogen but has also been shown to increase the proliferation of neural progenitor cells in the hippocampus (Jin et al., 2004). Exposure to stress down-regulates the expression of VEGF in the hippocampus (Heine et al., 2005), and studies are currently under way to determine if decreased VEGF contributes to the reduction in neurogenesis resulting from stress (Heine et al., 2005).

Stress Induces Atrophy of Hippocampal Neurons in Experimental Animals

Chronic exposure of rodents to physical stress or exposure of nonhuman primates to psychosocial stress is reported to cause atrophy of CA3 pyramidal neurons in the hippocampus (Sapolsky et al., 1985; Uno et al., 1989; Sapolsky et al., 1990; Margarinos et al., 1996; also see Chapter 40 by McEwen). Chronic exposure to immobilization stress decreases the number and length of the CA3 pyramidal neuron apical dendrites. Atrophy of CA3 pyramidal neurons is also observed after chronic glucocorticoid treatment, indicating that activation of the HPA axis is sufficient to cause CA3 pyramidal cell atrophy (Wooley et al., 1990). It is also possible that down-regulation of BDNF could contribute to the stress-induced atrophy of CA3 neurons, and further studies are needed to test this hypothesis. In addition, atrophy may result from glucocorticoid enhancement of excitotoxicity, as well as reduced metabolic capacity of these neurons (Stein-Behrens et al., 1994). These effects of stress and elevated glucocorticoid levels could also make the CA3 pyramidal neurons more vulnerable to different types of neuronal insults, such as hypoxia and ischemia. The atrophy of neurons in response to corticosterone or stress has also been extended to pyramidal neurons of the prefrontal cortex (PFC) (Wellman, 2001; Radley et al., 2004), effects that could contribute to the atrophy observed in this brain region of patients who are depressed (see below). In contrast, stress is reported to cause hypertrophy of the pyramidal neurons of the amygdala, measured by an increase in spine density of pyramidal neurons in the basolateral nucleus of the amygdala, effects that could contribute to increased anxiety observed in response to stress (Mitra et al., 2005).

Stress Decreases Neurogenesis in Adult Hippocampus

In addition to causing atrophy of CA3 pyramidal neurons, stress also has profound effects on the dentate gyrus granule neurons in the hippocampus. The hippocampal dentate gyrus is one of the few brain structures (the other region is the subventricular zone) that retain the ability to generate new neurons throughout adult life (Gould et al., 1999; Gage, 2000). Adult neurogenesis has been observed in a variety of different animals, including humans, and occurs into old age. Progenitor cells located in the subgranular zone of the hippocampus proliferate, and many of the new cells migrate into the granule cell layer where they mature and make connections that are typical of adult granule cells. Moreover, the rate of proliferation and the survival of newborn cells are highly regulated by environmental and endocrine factors (Warner-Schmidt and Duman, 2006). For example, running, enriched environment, and hippocampal-dependent learning all increase proliferation and/or survival of newborn neurons. In contrast, stress, aging, and drugs of abuse decrease the proliferation of neurons in adult hippocampus (Gould et al., 1998; Warner-Schmidt and Duman, 2006). Decreased neurogenesis is observed after exposure to different types of stress, including predator odor, social stress, acute and chronic restraint, foot shock, and chronic mild stress (Duman, 2004). In addition, decreased neurogenesis is also associated with a depressive-like phenotype in an animal model of depression (Malberg and Duman, 2003). Administration of glucocorticoids also decreases adult neurogenesis, indicating that activation of the HPA axis is responsible for the down-regulation of neurogenesis by stress. Decreased neurogenesis could contribute to the reduction in hippocampal volume that is observed in patients who are depressed (see below).

EVIDENCE OF NEURONAL ATROPHY AND LOSS IN HUMAN BRAIN

Preclinical evidence demonstrating that stress decreases neurotrophic factor expression and causes the structural alterations in the brain has led to clinical investigations of morphological changes in patients who are depressed. A series of studies conducted in living patients (brain imaging) and in postmortem tissue demonstrates that there is also structural remodeling in patients with depression (also see Chapter 31).

Atrophy of Limbic Brain Regions in Depression and PTSD: Brain Imaging

The possibility that the morphology of hippocampal neurons is altered in depression is supported by clinical brain imaging reports. These studies demonstrate that the volume of hippocampus is reduced in patients with depression or posttraumatic disorder, suggesting that atrophy of hippocampus may be associated with these disorders (Bremner et al., 1995; Sapolsky, 1996; Sheline et al., 1996), although not all studies report a decrease in patients who are depressed (see Vythilingam et al., 2004). The magnitude of the change in hippocampal volume is directly proportional to the length of illness, suggesting that the reduction in hippocampal volume is a result, not cause, of depression (Sheline et al., 1999). However, it is possible that small structural changes occur prior to or coincident with onset of illness and could thereby contribute to the symptoms of depression. There is also a report that antidepressant treatment can reverse the reduced hippocampal volume in patients with post-traumatic stress disorder (PTSD) (Vermetten et al., 2003).

Evidence that the function of the hippocampus is altered in depression is also provided by studies of the feedback inhibition of the HPA axis. Glucocorticoids activate a fast feedback inhibitory pathway from the hippocampus to hypothalamus, and this pathway is down-regulated in patients who are depressed (Young et al., 1997). Atrophy and dysfunction of hippocampal neurons could also mediate other abnormalities observed in depression, including memory or cognitive deficits, which are controlled by this brain region. In addition, hippocampus has reciprocal connections with other brain structures that regulate mood and emotion (for example, amygdala and PFC) and could indirectly influence other symptoms of depression. Dysfunction of the hippocampus is also supported by studies demonstrating that patients who are depressed display deficits of declarative memory, a hippocampal-dependent behavior, and that antidepressant treatment improves memory (Vythilingham et al., 2004; Vermetten et al., 2003).

Neuronal Atrophy and Loss in Depression: Postmortem Analysis

Preclinical studies suggest that the reduction of hippocampal volume observed in patients who are depressed could result from atrophy or decreased neurogenesis of hippocampal neurons. There have been a few studies conducted to address this issue. There is one report that the number of nonpyramidal cells in the hippocampal CA2 region is decreased in patients with bipolar disorder (Benes et al., 1998). There was no difference in the number of pyramidal neurons, and analysis of granule neurons was not conducted in this study. Another study found no evidence for a reduction in the number of neurons or synaptic contacts in patients who are depressed or individuals treated with glucocorticoids (Muller et al., 2001). However, this was a semiquantitative study, and all of the patients in the depressed group were on antidepressant medication at the time of death, which could reverse or oppose neuronal atrophy (see below). A more recent study found that there is an increase in packing density in the granule cell layer, suggesting that there is a decrease in neuropil in patients who were depressed, but not a decrease in cell number (Stockmeier et al., 2004). Additional postmortem studies of the hippocampus will be necessary to determine the cellular mechanisms underlying the reduction in hippocampal volume reported in brain imaging studies.

Postmortem investigations of structural alterations have also been conducted in cortical brain regions implicated in depression. These studies report a reduction in the size of neurons and the number of glia in the orbital frontal cortex, subgenual PFC, and cingulate cortex (Ongur et al., 1998; Rajkowska et al., 1999; Cotter et al., 2001). Preclinical studies have also demonstrated that stress decreases the proliferation of glia in the PFC, which could underlie in part the decreases observed in patients who are depressed (Banasr et al., 2007). These results are consistent with brain imaging studies showing altered blood flow or metabolism in these cortical structures of patients who are depressed (Manji and Duman, 2001). Moreover, the alterations in cerebral cortex indicate that imbalances in the expression of neurotrophic factors and neuronal atrophy are not limited to the hippocampus.

NEUROTROPHIC ACTIONS OF ANTIDEPRESSANTS

In contrast to the atrophy and neuronal loss caused by stress, studies in rodents demonstrate that antidepressants produce effects that block or reverse the effects of stress. The clinical relevance of these findings is supported by studies of BDNF in patients who are depressed. A review of this literature is discussed in this section.

Antidepressant Treatment Increases BDNF Expression

The possibility that neurotrophic factors are involved in the action of antidepressants is supported by studies demonstrating that chronic antidepressant treatment increases the expression of BDNF in rat hippocampus (Nibuya et al., 1995; Nibuya et al., 1996; see Duman and Monteggia, 2006, for review). In addition, antidepressant pretreatment blocks the down-regulation of BDNF in response to stress (Nibuya et al., 1995). The antidepressants tested included 5-HT and NE selective reuptake inhibitors, MAO inhibitors, atypical antidepressants, and electroconvulsive seizures. In contrast, acute administration of antidepressant drugs or chronic administration of nonantidepressant psychotropic drugs, including morphine, cocaine, and haloperidol, does not increase the expression of BDNF in hippocampus. Although most studies have been positive, there are also studies that have not reported an up-regulation of BDNF in response to chronic antidepressant treatment (see Duman and Monteggia, 2006). Expression of BDNF is activity dependent and can therefore be influenced by a variety of external stimuli. This, as well as differences in drug treatment schedules (dose and length of treatment, as well as time after the last drug administration), could all contribute to the discrepancy in reports of antidepressant regulation of BDNF expression.

The time course and regional distribution of BDNF up-regulation is consistent with that for up-regulation of CREB by antidepressant treatment. In addition, chronic administration of a phosphodiesterase inhibitor increases the expression of BDNF and hastens the up-regulation of BDNF in response to a tricyclic antidepressant drug (Nibuya et al., 1996). The expression of BDNF in cultured cells is also up-regulated by activation of cAMP or Ca^{2+}-activated pathways (Condorelli et al., 1994; Ghosh et al., 1994), and a Ca^{2+}/CRE response element has been identified in the exon III promoter of the BDNF gene (Tao et al., 1998). A recent study also demonstrated that the regulation of BDNF by antidepressant treatment is mediated in part via regulation of histone remodeling (Tsankova et al., 2006). Taken together, these findings support the hypothesis that up-regulation of BDNF is mediated by activation of the cAMP cascade and chromatin remodeling and that BDNF is a target of antidepressant treatment.

BDNF and Antidepressant Treatment Enhance Neuronal Arborization and Survival

BDNF is reported to enhance the growth and survival of cortical neurons (Ghosh et al., 1994), as well as 5-HT and NE neurons (Mamounas et al., 1995; Sklair-Tavron and Nestler, 1995). This suggests that loss of BDNF support could adversely influence monoamine neurotransmission at pre- and postsynaptic sites. Antidepressant treatment is also reported to enhance the regeneration of catecholamine neurons in the cerebral cortex (Nakagawa et al., 2000), and chronic electroconvulsive shock (ECS) is reported to induce sprouting of dentate gyrus granule neurons in hippocampus (Vaidya et al., 1997). One study has demonstrated that administration of an atypical antidepressant, tianeptine, blocks the stress-induced atrophy of CA3 apical dendrites (Watanabe et al., 1992; McEwen, 2002). A more recent study has reported that antidepressant treatment increases the number of synapses, determined by electron microscopy (Hajszan et al., 2005). Studies of other antidepressants and additional stress paradigms (for example, psychosocial stress) are needed to determine if blockade of neuronal atrophy or enhanced neuronal growth are common actions of antidepressant treatments, and to determine if these effects are mediated by induction of BDNF.

BDNF Increases Synaptic Strength of Hippocampal Neurons

Antidepressant treatment and increased BDNF expression may also influence the strength of neuronal synapses, as well as the cognitive function of animals. The influence of BDNF and antidepressant treatment on synaptic strength has been assessed using a cellular model of learning and memory, long-term potentiation (LTP). Incubation with BDNF is reported to increase the synaptic efficacy of hippocampal neurons, and LTP is reduced in BDNF knockout mice expressing reduced levels of this neurotrophic factor (Kang and Schuman, 1995; Levine et al., 1995). Studies of antidepressant drugs have been mixed, with reports of enhanced and reduced LTP in hippocampus. However, these apparent discrepancies may be explained by the hippocampal circuits examined. Studies of granule cell LTP (stimulation of the perforant path) have reported that antidepressants enhance LTP (Stewart and Reid, 2000; Levkovitz et al., 2001), while studies of CA1 pyramidal cells (stimulation of the Schaffer collateral) report that LTP is suppressed (Massicotte et al., 1993; O'Connor et al., 1993; Von Frijtag et al., 2001).

There are also behavioral studies demonstrating that antidepressant treatment enhances learning and memory. There are reports that memory and cognitive function are enhanced in rodent models and in patients who are depressed by chronic antidepressant treatments (Allain et al., 1992; Yau et al., 1995). More recent studies have confirmed these effects, demonstrating that chronic administration of fluoxetine or venlafaxine, a mixed action reuptake inhibitor, improves performance in the Morris water maze, a spatial learning and memory model (Nowakowska et al., 2000, 2003; Nowakowska et al., 2006). There are also clinical studies reporting improvement in cognition and memory in response to chronic antidepressant treatment (Spring et al., 1992; Vermetten et al., 2003; Vythilingam et al., 2004). Together with the cellular LTP studies, these findings indicate that antidepressant treatment results in neuroplasticity-like responses. However, the actions of antidepressants are dependent on the type of drug tested, with reports that certain antidepressants worsen performance in learning and memory models (Yau et al., 2002; Naudon et al., 2007). Additional preclinical and clinical studies are needed to further examine the influence of antidepressants on behavioral models of memory and cognitive performance tasks in animals and humans.

BDNF Produces Antidepressant Effects in Behavioral Models of Depression

To determine if the induction of BDNF contributes to the actions of antidepressant treatment, the effects of BDNF in behavioral models of depression have been examined. These studies are consistent with the hypothesis that BDNF is sufficient to produce an antidepressant response and is required for the actions of antidepressants. Infusions of BDNF into the midbrain for 7 days produced an antidepressant-like effect in the forced swim and learned helplessness paradigms (Siuciak et al., 1997). The antidepressant effect of BDNF in this brain region could result from increased 5-HT neurotransmission, as indicated by increased levels of 5-HT and its metabolites in forebrain regions (Siuciak et al., 1994). The influence of BDNF applied in forebrain regions, where it is regulated by antidepressant treatment, has also been studied. Infusions of BDNF into the dentate gyrus or CA3 pyramidal cell layer, but not the CA1 layer, of hippocampus also produce antidepressant effects in the forced swim and learned helplessness paradigms (Shirayama et al., 2002). The effect of BDNF in hippocampus was notable because a single, local infusion into the hippocampal subfields was sufficient to produce an effect similar to that observed with repeated systemic administration of a chemical antidepressant. The actions of hippocampal BDNF are blocked by coadministration of a tyrosine kinase antagonist or by inhibition of the MAPK cascade, indicating that these pathways mediate the antidepressant effects of BDNF. More recent studies also demonstrate that blockade of the MAPK cascade results in a depressive phenotype in different models of depression (Duman et al., 2007). Infusion of BDNF into the lateral ventricle also produces an antidepressant response in the forced swim test (Hoshaw et al., 2005).

Studies of mutant mice have confirmed a role for BDNF and demonstrate that the actions of antidepressant treatment are dependent on BDNF-TrkB signaling. In transgenic mice that express a dominant negative form of TrkB (Saarelainen et al., 2003) or in BDNF conditional null mutant mice (Monteggia et al., 2004), the behavioral response to antidepressant treatment is blocked (see Duman and Monteggia, 2006, for review). Surprisingly, BDNF mutant mice do not have a depressive-like phenotype, although there is one report that female, but not male, conditional BDNF null mutant mice display behavioral despair and anhedonia (Monteggia et al., 2007). This suggests that reduction of BDNF is not always sufficient to produce a behavioral response, and that other environmental factors such as stress may be needed. This type of Gene × Environment interaction has been demonstrated in basic and clinical research studies (Kaufman et al., 2006; Duman et al., 2007).

Antidepressant Treatment Increases Neurogenesis

Interestingly, antidepressant treatment increases adult neurogenesis in the hippocampus (Malberg et al., 2000a;

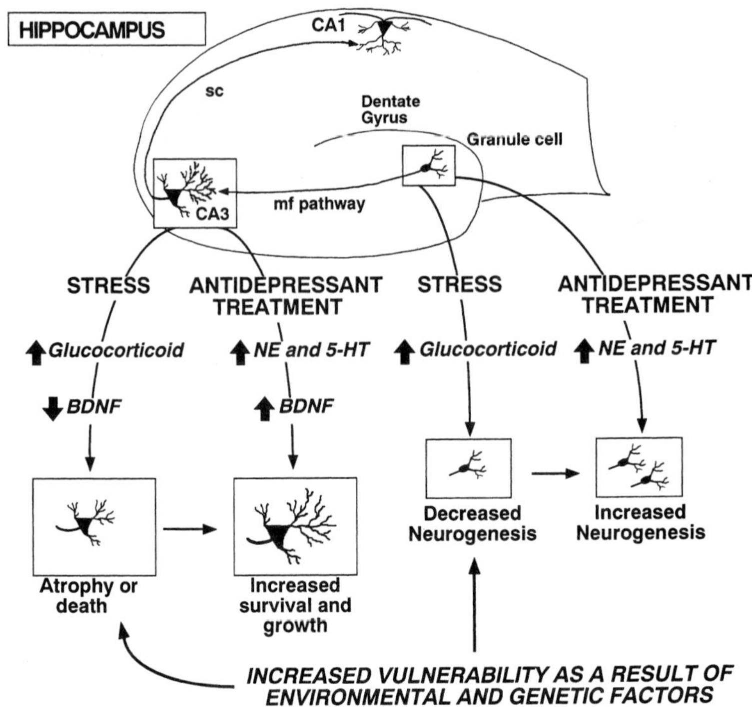

FIGURE 29.5 Neurotrophic actions of stress and antidepressants in the hippocampus. This model demonstrates the influence of stress and antidepressant treatments on subsets of neurons in the hippocampus. The major cell groups in the hippocampus include the dentate gyrus granule cells and CA3 and CA1 pyramidal cells. The mossy fiber (mf) pathway carries projections from the granule cell layer to CA3 neurons, which in turn project to CA1 neurons via the Schaffer collateral (sc) pathway. Chronic stress increases glucocorticoid levels and decreases BDNF and thereby causes atrophy of CA3 pyramidal neurons. CA3 neurons are also vulnerable to damage by other types of neuronal insult (for example, hypoxia-ischemia, hypoglycemia, neurotoxins, and viral infections). Genetic factors could also contribute to such selective vulnerability. Stress or glucocorticoid treatments also decrease neurogenesis of granule cells in adult hippocampus. In contrast, chronic antidepressant treatment increases the expression of BDNF and adult neurogenesis, and prevents the down-regulation of BDNF and neurogenesis in response to stress. These effects could reverse the atrophy of hippocampal neurons, as well as protect these neurons from further damage. Up-regulation of BDNF occurs via increased 5-HT and NE neurotransmission and up-regulation of the cAMP-CREB cascade. BDNF: brain-derived neurotrophic factor.

see Duman, 2004; Warner-Schmidt and Duman, 2006). The time course for induction of adult neurogenesis is consistent with the time course for the therapeutic response to antidepressants. Up-regulation of neurogenesis is observed with several different classes of antidepressants, indicating that this effect may be a common cellular mechanism of antidepressant action. Moreover, the down-regulation of adult neurogenesis caused by stress is blocked by antidepressant treatment (Malberg et al., 2000b; Czeh et al., 2001). Pharmacological and transgenic approaches also demonstrate that activation of the cAMP–CREB cascade increases adult neurogenesis (Nakagawa et al., 2002). Moreover, the induction of neurogenesis is required for the behavioral actions of antidepressant treatment (Santarelli et al., 2003). Blockade of neurogenesis by irradiation or in a mutant mouse model blocks the effects of chronic antidepressant treatment in two long-term behavioral models, chronic unpredictable stress and novelty suppressed feeding. These findings provide the first evidence that induction of neurogenesis has functional consequences related to the actions of antidepressants. However, it is likely that antidepressants also lead to additional effects (for example, altered plasticity, neuroprotection) in hippocampus as well as other brain regions that contribute to behavioral responding and the therapeutic actions of these agents.

A NEUROTROPHIC HYPOTHESIS OF DEPRESSION

The preclinical and clinical studies reviewed in this chapter form the basis of a neurotrophic theory of depression and antidepressant action (Fig. 29.5). Depression, particularly stress-associated cases, may result from atrophy, damage, or death of vulnerable neurons (that is, the CA3 pyramidal cells) or down-regulation of adult neurogenesis in the hippocampus. The atrophy, vulnerability, and reduced neurogenesis could result, at least in part, from the down-regulation of BDNF, as well as other trophic factors, in response to stress. In addition, sustained elevation of adrenal-glucocorticoids, often observed in patients who are depressed, could contribute to the atrophy of CA3 pyramidal neurons and down-regulation of neurogenesis. Antidepressant treatment could reverse the atrophy and reduced neurogenesis by up-regulating the cAMP-CREB cascade and expression of neurotrophic factors. This could lead to enhanced growth and function of hippocampal neurons, in conjunction with the antidepressant-induced increase in monoamine neurotransmission. The formation of new synaptic elements that are dependent on monoamine transmission could explain why patients who are depressed get worse upon the depletion of monoamines.

The neurotrophic hypothesis could also explain why stress leads to depression in some, but not all, individuals. Selective vulnerability of hippocampal neurons may be increased by prior exposure to neuronal insults, such as hypoxia-ischemia, hypoglycemia, neurotoxins, and viral infections, or there may be a genetic vulnerability. In these individuals the damage resulting from prior insult may not be sufficient to cause the behavioral abnormalities associated with depression. However, when exposed to a subsequent insult or stress, the atrophy or reduction in neurogenesis becomes sufficient to cause the hippocampal-dependent symptoms of depression. One example of this is the high incidence of depression in patients of stroke (Reding et al., 1986; Federoff et al., 1992; Stern and Bachmann, 1992). Another possibility is that genetic factors increase neuronal vulnerability to stress or other insults, a hypothesis also supported by recent studies of BDNF and stress or trauma (Kaufman et al., 2006; Duman et al., 2007). Subtle damage or genetic vulnerability could also reduce the fast feedback inhibition of the HPA axis. This would lead to increased levels of glucocorticoids and further damage to hippocampal neurons. This cycle of disinhibition and damage could have significant consequences on vulnerable hippocampal neurons.

This neurotrophic hypothesis provides a framework for future studies to characterize the pathophysiology and genetic basis of depression and other stress-related disorders. However, this model may be limited to certain types of depression associated with stress. Moreover, additional studies are required to determine if antidepressant treatment is neuroprotective and if it influences the atrophy or size of hippocampal neurons. Additional postmortem studies are also needed to determine if neuronal survival and dendritic arborization are associated with depression and reversed by antidepressant treatment.

NEUROANATOMICAL SUBSTRATES OF DEPRESSION

One of the major questions in depression research is what brain region underlies the endocrine, emotional, cognitive, and vegetative abnormalities associated with this disorder. The hippocampus, which has been the focus of many of the studies discussed in this review, is one of several regions that could contribute to many of these abnormalities. The hippocampus has been associated with learning and memory and therefore could also be involved in cognitive abnormalities of depression. Hippocampus is involved in feedback regulation of the HPA axis, and depression is associated with dysfunction of this neuroendocrine axis (Young et al., 1997). The hippocampus could also influence mood and emotion via indirect pathways to cortical brain regions. The results demonstrating atrophy and remodeling of hippocampal neurons in response to stress and in patients who are depressed indicate that altered function of this brain structure could contribute to certain symptoms of depression. However, there are several other limbic brain structures that also play a critical role in emotion and mood, including the PFC, amygdala, and nucleus accumbens, that are likely to be equally or even more important than hippocampus in understanding the neurobiological abnormalities that underlie mood disorders (Manji et al., 2001; Wong and Licinio, 2001; Nestler et al., 2002).

In the frontal cortex, glucose metabolism, blood flow, and electroencephalogram (EEG) activity are altered in unipolar and bipolar depression (Buchsbaum et al., 1986; Baxter et al., 1989; Drevets et al., 1992; Manji and Duman, 2001). Frontal cortex has been implicated in short-term, representational memory. Recent clinical and preclinical studies provide evidence of atrophy and cell loss of PFC, which extends the neurotrophic hypothesis (Ongur et al., 1998; Rajkowska et al., 1999; Cotter et al., 2001; Radley et al., 2004; Banasr et al., 2007). Based on these findings, it has been suggested that frontal cortex could mediate the ruminative ideation observed in depression.

The amygdala has been studied primarily in the regulation of fear and anxiety. This structure is associated with positive and aversive emotional stimuli. The amygdala appears to play a role in assigning affective significance to psychological and sensory stimuli (Nishijo et al., 1988; see Chapter 39). Evidence of increased blood flow and volume of the amygdala of patients who are depressive indicates a possible role of this structure in mood disorders (Drevets et al., 1992; Sheline et al., 1998; Manji and Duman, 2001). Experimental studies in animals also indicate a role for the amygdala in the pharmacological actions of antidepressant treatments (Gorka et al., 1979; Duncan et al., 1986; Ordway et al., 1991; Thome et al., 2000). Amygdala also sends and receives projections from the PFC, ventral striatum, and hippocampus, and interactions between these brain regions could underlie certain aspects of depressive behavior.

Dopaminergic brain reward regions have been implicated in certain aspects of depression, including anhedonia and anergy (Nestler et al., 2002). The mesolimbic dopamine system comprises dopamine cell bodies located in the ventral tegmental area and its major projection region, the nucleus accumbens. The anhedonia associated with depression can be studied in a behavioral model of depression that is based on the consumption of sweetened water (Muscat et al., 1990). Chronic stress is reported to reduce the consumption of sweetened water, and antidepressant treatment reverses this effect. Antidepressant treatment also enhances several aspects of dopamine neurotransmission in the nucleus accumbens (Serra et al., 1992). Interestingly, studies of the regional actions of CREB have provided evidence that this transcription factor produces opposite effects in the nucleus accumbens (that is, depressive-like behavior) compared to its actions in the hippocampus in behavioral models of depression (Pliakas et al., 2001; Newton et al., 2002; Conti et al., 2002). Further studies are required to characterize the molecular and cellular adaptations in the mesolimbic dopamine system that mediate the anhedonia and loss of motivation that are often seen as symptoms of depression.

Although it is possible that abnormal function of a single brain region underlies depression, it is more likely that dysfunction of multiple brain regions contribute to this disorder. Dysfunction of multiple brain regions could occur via independent mechanisms, or one region could lead to altered function of other brain regions connected to the first. Studies to further characterize the neuronal circuitry of the frontal cortex, hippocampus, amygdala, and nucleus accumbens, as well as other brain regions, will help elucidate the neuroanatomical substrates of depression.

NOVEL TARGETS FOR THERAPEUTIC INTERVENTION

The identification of intracellular signal transduction pathways and genes that mediate the action of antidepressant treatment will lead to novel targets for the development of faster acting and more efficacious therapeutic agents. Several possible targets that have been identified through these studies are discussed in this section.

Activation of Monoamine Receptors Directly Coupled to the cAMP Cascade

The hypothesis that the action of antidepressant treatment is mediated by up-regulation of the cAMP signal transduction cascade and increased expression of BDNF suggests several possible sites for intervention. First, agonist stimulation of 5-HT and NE receptors that are positively coupled to the cAMP system would lead to activation of CREB and increased expression of BDNF. Potential candidate receptors are the βAR and 5-$HT_{4,6,7}$ receptor subtypes, as well as other neurotransmitter or neuropeptide receptors coupled to cAMP or Ca^{2+}-activated cascades. One concern with direct-acting receptor agonists is that they may cause rapid desensitization of receptors and may not be more efficacious than currently available treatments. However, an advantage is that receptor agonists could have relatively specific effects in the hippocampus, depending on the distribution of the receptors targeted.

Activation of the cAMP Cascade

Another possibility would be to develop agents that directly influence the intracellular components of the cAMP pathway, for example, drugs that directly stimulate cAMP or Ca^{2+}-activated kinases, or that directly activate CREB. Blockade of cAMP metabolism, via inhibition of cAMP-specific phosphodiesterase type IV (PDE4) isozymes, is an additional possibility to consider. A concern with drugs acting at these intracellular targets is that they would influence cell systems in many brain regions, as well as tissues throughout the body. However, such agents have the promise of being more efficacious and faster acting than treatments that act on monoamine transporter systems as their primary site of action. It is difficult to predict the specificity and effectiveness of agents acting at intracellular sites. However, there are several currently used therapeutic agents that act in this manner. The best example of such an agent that is currently used for psychiatric illness is lithium, which inhibits several enzymatic steps in the phosphatidylinositol pathway and also inhibits glycogen synthase kinase-3β. Lithium is an effective treatment of bipolar disorder, although it does have side effects.

The possibility that PDE4 inhibitors may be effective for the treatment of depression is supported by basic research studies demonstrating that these agents increase the expression of CREB and BDNF and hasten the response time to other antidepressant drugs (Nibuya et al., 1996). Inhibitors of PDE4 have also been shown to be effective in animal models that predict antidepressant activity (Wachtel and Schneider, 1986; O'Donnell, 1993), and studies demonstrating an induction of adult neurogenesis (Nakagawa et al., 2002). The clinical utility of PDE inhibitors for the treatment of depression has been examined previously (Wachtel, 1983; Horowski and Sastre-Y-Hernandez, 1985). These early studies reported that rolipram, a relatively specific inhibitor of PDE4, had antidepressant effects in approximately two thirds of patients tested, similar to monoamine reuptake inhibitor antidepressants. However, rolipram also produced side effects, most notably nausea. Another possibility is that PDE4 inhibitors, at lower doses, may enhance or hasten the response to a typical antidepressant that blocks the reuptake or breakdown of 5-HT and NE. There is a preliminary report that cotreatment with a nonselective PDE inhibitor and an antidepressant drug resulted in a significant improvement of a drug resistant patient (Malison et al., 1997). Additional studies are needed to determine if PDE inhibitors may have general usefulness for enhancing the actions of antidepressant drugs.

It may also be possible to develop inhibitors that are selective for specific PDE isozymes. The PDE4 family includes four separate genes, each of which has multiple splice variants (Conti et al., 1995). Given this heterogeneity, it may be possible to identify a single PDE isozyme or splice variant, the inhibition of which may have antidepressant actions without unwanted side effects. Recent evidence suggests a possible role of the PDE4A and PDE4B isoforms (Takahashi et al., 1999), although PDE4D mutant mice also display an antidepressant-like behavioral phenotype, as would be predicted if this were a relevant isoform (Zhang et al., 2004). Further studies at the basic research level are needed to characterize the regional distribution and antidepressant regulation of the PDE isozymes, as well as isozymes for other intracellular signal transduction proteins, that may be targets for the development of antidepressant treatments.

CONCLUSIONS

The results and strategies discussed provide a framework for future studies, at the basic and clinical levels, to further characterize the pathophysiology and treatment of depression. Studies of intracellular signal transduction pathways provide new information about the action of antidepressant treatment that could not be determined from studies of monoamines or their receptors. Importantly, this work indicates that the cAMP system is increased, not decreased, by antidepressant treatments. In addition, identification of intracellular cascades provides new strategies for identification of target genes that are regulated by, and contribute to, the therapeutic action of antidepressant treatments. For example, the results of preclinical studies indicate that up-regulation of BDNF could serve to reverse the atrophy or damage of vulnerable neurons, or protect these neurons from further damage. Identification of these pathways and target genes will provide novel targets for the development of therapeutic agents. Moreover, dysfunction of intracellular signal transduction proteins and target genes could be closely related to the molecular determinants that underlie the pathophysiology of depression. In this case, decreased expression of BDNF could contribute to neuronal atrophy and depressed mood, especially when combined with stress or neuronal insult. This hypothesis could be tested at the basic research level using BDNF mutant mice that express altered levels of this neurotrophic factor. At the clinical level, additional postmortem studies will be needed to determine if there is a reduction in the size or number of hippocampal neurons in the brains of patients who are depressed, and if there is a relationship of these effects with the amount or function of CREB. Finally, a more complete understanding of depression will be dependent on critical, future studies to identify the additional intracellular pathways and target genes, and genetic polymorphisms that are involved in the etiology and treatment of this complex psychiatric disorder.

ACKNOWLEDGMENTS

This work is supported by U.S. Public Health Service grants MH45481, MH53199, and 2 PO1 MH25642 and by a Veterans Administration National Center Grant for PTSD at the West Haven Connecticut VA Medical Center.

REFERENCES

Allain, H., Lieury, A., Brunet-Bourgin, F., Mirabaud, C., Trebon, P., Le Coz, F., and Gandon, J.M. (1992) Antidepressants and cognition: comparative effects of moclobemide, viloxazine and maprotiline. *Psychopharmacology* 106:S56–S61.

Arancio, O., and Chao, M.V. (2007) Neurotrophins, synaptic plasticity and dementia. *Curr. Opin. Neurobiol.* 17:325–330.

Artigas, F., Perez, V., and Alvarez, E. (1994) Pindolol induces a rapid improvement of depressed patients treated with serotonin reuptake inhibitors. *Arch. Gen. Psychiatry* 51:248–251.

Avorn, J., Everitt, D.E., and Weiss, S (1986) Increased antidepressant use in patients prescribed b-blockers. *JAMA* 255:357–360.

Ballaz, S.J., Akil, H., and Watson, S.J. (2007) Analysis of 5-HT6 and 5-HT7 receptor gene expression in rats showing differences in novelty-seeing behavior. *Neurosci.* 247:428–438.

Banasr, M., Valentine, G.W., Li, X.Y., Gourley, S., Taylor, J., and Duman, R.S. (2007) Chronic stress decreases cell proliferation in adult cerebral cortex of rat: reversal by antidepressant treatment. *Biol. Psychiatry* 62:495–504.

Banerjee, S.P., Kung, L.S., Riggi, S.J., and Chanda, S.K. (1977) Development of b-adrenergic receptor subsensitivity by antidepressants. *Nature* 268:455–456.

Barden, N.R.J., Reul, J.M., and Holsboer, F. (1995) Do antidepressants stabilize mood through actions on the hypothalamic-pituitary-adrenocorticalo system? *Trends Neurosci.* 18(1):6–11.

Barrot, M., Olivier, J.D., Perrotti, L.I., DiLeone, R.J., Berton, O., Eisch, A.J., Impey, S., Storm, D.R., Neve, R.L., Yin, J.C., Zachariou, V., and Nestler, E.J. (2002) CREB activity in the nucleus accumbens shell controls gating of behavioral responses to emotional stimuli. *Proc. Natl. Acad. Sci. USA* 99:11435–11440.

Baxter, L., Schwartz, J.M., Phelps, M.E., Mazziota, J.C., Guze, B.H., Selin, C.R., Gerner, R.H., and Sumida, R.M. (1989) Reduction of prefrontal cortex glucose metabolism common to three types of depression. *Arch. Gen. Psychiatry* 46:243–250.

Benes, F., Kwok, E.W., Vincent, S.L., and Todtenkopf, M.S. (1998) A reduction of nonpyramidal cells in sector CA2 of schizophrenics and manic depressives. *Biol. Psychiatry* 15:88–97.

Berton, O., and Nestler, E. (2006) New approaches to antidepressant drug discovery: beyond monoamines. *Nat. Rev. Neurosci.* 7: 137–151.

Blier, P., and de Montigny, C. (1994) Current advances and trends in the treatment of depression. *Trends Pharmacol. Sci.* 15(7):220–226.

Bliss, T., and Collingridge, G. (1993) A synaptic model of memory: long-term potentiation in the hippocampus. *Nature* 361:31–39.

Bremner, J.D., Randall, P., Scott, T.M., Bronen, R.A., Seibyl, J.P., Southwick, S.M., Delaney, R.C., McCarthy, G., Charney, D.S., and Innis, R.B. (1995) MRI-based measurement of hippocampal volume in patients with combat-related posttraumatic stress disorder. *Am. J. Psychiatry* 152:973–981.

Buchsbaum, M., Wu, J., DeLisi, L.E., Holcomb, H., Kessler, R., Johnson, J., King, A.C., Hazlett, E., Langston, K., and Post, R.M. (1986) Frontal cortex and basal ganglia metabolic rates assisted by positron emission tomography with [18F]2-deoxyglucose in affective illness. *J. Affect. Disord.* 10:137–152.

Bunney, W., and Davis, J. (1965) Norepinephrine in depressive reactions: a review. *Arch. Gen. Psychiatry* 13:483–494.

Butler, M., Morinobu, S., and Duman, R.S. (1993) Chronic electrocovulsive seizures increase the expression of serotonin2 receptor mRNA in rat frontal cortex. *J. Neurochem.* 61:1270–1276.

Chalmers, D., Lovenberg, T.W., Grigoriadis, D.E., Behan, D.P., and DeSouza, E.B. (1996) Corticotrophin-releasing factor receptors: from molecular biology to drug design. *Trends Pharmacol. Sci* 17:166–172.

Charney, D.S., Menkes, D.B., and Heninger, G.R. (1981) Receptor sensitivity and the mechanism of action of antidepressant treatment. *Arch. Gen. Psychiatry* 38:1160–1173.

Chen, B., Dowlatshahi, D., MacQueen, G.M., Wang. J.-F., and Young, L.T. (2001) Increased hippocampal BDNF immunoreactivity in subjects treated with antidepressant medication. *Biol. Psychiatry* 50:260–265.

Colin, S., Chang, H.-C., Mollner, S., Pfeuffer, T., Reed, R.R., Duman, R.S., and Nestler, E.J. (1991) Chronic lithium regulates the expression of adenylate cyclase and Gi-protein alpha subunit in rat cerebral cortex. *Proc. Natl. Acad. Sci. USA* 88:10634–10637.

Condorelli, D., Dell'Albani, P., Mudo, G., Timmusk, T., and Belluardo, N. (1994) Expression of neurotrophins and their receptors in primary astroglial cultures: induction by cAMP elevating agents. *J. Neurochem.* 63:509–516.

Conti, A., Cryan, J.F., Dalvi, A., Lucki, L., and Blendy, J.A. (2002) CREB is essential for the upregulation of BDNF transcription, but not the behavioral or endocrine responses to antidepressant drugs. *J. Neurosci.* 22(8):3262–3268.

Conti, M., Nemoz, G., Sette, C., and Vicini, E. (1995) Recent progress in understanding the hormonal regulation of phosphodiesterases. *Endocr. Rev.* 16:370–389.

Coppen, A. (1967) The biochemistry of affective disorders. *Br. J. Psychiatry* 113:1237–1264.

Cotter, D., Mackay, D., Landau, S., Kerwin, R., and Everall, I. (2001) Reduced glial cell density and neuronal size in the anterior cingulate cortex in major depressive disorder. *Arch. Gen. Psychiatry* 58:545–553.

Czeh, B., Michaelis, T., Watanabe, T., Frahm, J., de Biurrun, G., van Kampen, M., Bartololomucci, A., and Fuchs, E. (2001) Stress-induced changes in cerebral metabolites, hippocampal volume, and cell proliferation are prevented by antidepressant treatment with tianeptine. *Proc. Natl. Acad. Sci. USA* 98(22):12796–12801.

Delgado, P., Price, L.H., Miller, H.L., Salomon, R.M., Aghajanian, G., Heninger, G.R., and Charney, D. (1994) Serotonin and the neurobiology of depression. *Arch. Gen. Psychiatry* 51:865–874.

Dowlatshahi, D., MacQueen, G.M., Wang, J.F., and Young, L.T. (1998) Increased temporal cortex CREB concentrations and antidepressant treatment in major depression. *Lancet* 352:1754–1755.

Dowlatshahi, D., and Young, L.T. (2000) Molecular abnormalities in brains of depressed patients. *Neuroscientist* 6:401–410.

Drevets, W., Videen, T.O., Price, J.L., Preskorn, S.H., Carmichael, S.T., and Raichle, M.E. (1992) A functional anatomical study of unipolar depression. *J. Neurosci.* 12:3628–3641.

Duman, C., Schlesinger, L., Kodama, M., Russell, D.S., and Duman, R.S. (2007) A role for MAPK signaling in behavioral models of depression and antidepressant treatment. *Biol. Psychiatry* 61(5): 660–670.

Duman, R. (2004) Depression: a case of neuronal life and death? *Biol. Psychiatry* 56:140–145.

Duman, R., Malberg, J., Nakagawa, S., and D'Sa, C. (2000) Neuronal plasticity and survival in mood disorders. *Biol. Psychiatry* 48: 732–739.

Duman, R., and Monteggia, L.M. (2006) A neurotrophic model for stress-related mood disorders. *Biol. Psychiatry* 59:1116–1127.

Duncan, G., Breese, G.R., Criswell, H., Stumpf, W.E., Mueller, R.A., and Covey, J.B. (1986) Effects of antidepressant drugs injected into the amygdala on behavioral responses of rats in the forced swim test. *J. Pharmacol. Exp. Ther.* 238:758–762.

Dwivedi, Y., Rao, J.S., Hooriyah, S.R., Kotowski, J., Conley, R.R., Roberts, R.C., Tamminga, C.A., and Pandey, G.N. (2003) Abnormal expression and functional characteristics of cyclic adenosine monophosphate response element binding protein in postmortem brain of suicide subjects. *Arch Gen. Psychiatry* 60: 273–282.

Federoff, J., Starkstein, S., and Forrester, A. (1992) Depression in patients with acute traumatic brain injury. *Am. J. Psychiatry* 149: 918–923.

Gage, F. (2000) Mammalian neural stem cells. *Science* 287:1433–1438.

Ghosh, A., Carnahan, J., and Greenberg, M.E. (1994) Requirement for BDNF in activity-dependent survival of cortical neurons. *Science* 263:1618–1623.

Ghosh, A., and Greenberg, M.E. (1995) Calcium signaling in neurons: molecular mechanisms and cellular consequences. *Science* 268:239–247.

Goodwin, F.K., Prange, A.J., Post, R.M., Muscettola, G., and Lipton, M.A (1982) Potentiation of antidepressant effect by triiodothyronine in tricyclic nonresponders. *Am. J. Psychiatry* 139:34–38.

Gorka, Z., Ossowska, K., and Stach, R. (1979) The effect of unilateral amygdala lesion on the imipramine action in behavioural despair in rats. *J. Pharm. Pharmacol.* 31:647–648.

Gould, E., Reeves, A.J., Graziano, M.S.A., and Gross, C.G. (1999) Neurogenesis in the neocortex of adult primates. *Science* 286:548–552.

Gould, E., Tanapat, P., McEwen, B.S., Flugge, G., and Fuchs, E. (1998) Proliferation of granule cell precursors in the dentate gyrus of adult monkeys is diminished by stress. *Proc. Natl. Acad. Sci. USA* 95:3168–3171.

Hajszan, T., Maclusky, N.J., and Leranth, C. (2005) Short-term treatment with the antidepressant fluoxetine triggers pyramidal dendritic spine synapse formation in rat hippocampus. *Eur. J. Neurosci.* 21:1299–1303.

Hamon, M., Doucet, E., Lefevre, K., Miquel, M.C., Lanfumey, L., Insausti, R., Frechilla, D., Del Rio, J., and Verge, D. (1999) Antibodies and antisense oligonucleotide for probing the distribution and putative functions of central 5-HT6 receptors. *Neuropsychopharmacology* 21:68S–76S.

Heine, V., Zareno, J., Maslam, S., Joels, M., and Lucassen, P.J. (2005) Chronic stress in the adult dentate gyrus reduces cell proliferation near the vasculature and VEGF and Flk-1 protein expression. *Eur. J. Neurosci.* 21:1304–1314.

Heninger, G.R., and Charney, D.S. (1987) *Mechanisms of Action of Antidepressant Treatments: Implications for the Etiology and Treatment of Depressive Disorders.* New York: Raven Press.

Holsboer, F. (1999) The rationale for corticotropoin-releasing hormone receptor (CRH-R) antagonists to treat depression and anxiety. *J. Psychiatric Res.* 33:181–214.

Horowski, R., and Sastre-Y-Hernandez, M. (1985) Clinical effects of the neurotrophic selective cAMP phosphodiesterase inhibitor rolipram in depressed patients: global evaluation of the preliminary reports. *Curr. Ther. Res.* 38:23–29.

Hoshaw, B., Malberg, J.E., and Lucki, I. (2005) Central administration of IGF-I and BDNF leads to long-lasting antidepressant-like effects. *Brain Res.* 1037:204–208.

Jin, K., Xie, L., Kim, S.H., Parmentier-Batteur, S., Sun, Y., Mao, X.O., Childs, J., and Greenberg, D.A. (2004) Defective adult neurogenesis in CB1 cannabinoid receptor knockout mice. *Mol. Pharmacol.* 66:204–208.

Kang, H., and Schuman, E.M. (1995) Long-lasting neurotrophin-induced enhancement of synaptic transmission in the adult hippocampus. *Science* 267:1658–1662.

Kaufman, J., Yang, B.Z., Douglas-Palumberi, H., Grasso, D., Lipschitz, D., Houshyar, S., Krystal, J.H., and Gelernter, J. (2006) Brain-derived neurotrophic factor-5-HTTLPR gene interactions and environmental modifiers of depression in children. *Biol. Psychiatry* 59:673–680.

Kramer, M., Cutler, N., Feighner, J., Shrivastava, R., Carman, J., Sramek, J.J., Reines, S.A., Liu, G., Snavely, D., Wyatt-Knowles, E., et al. (1998) Distinct mechanism for antidepressant activity by blockade of central substance P receptors. *Science* 281:1640–1645.

Levine, E., Dreyfus, C.F., Black, I.B., and Plummer, M.R. (1995) Brain-derived neuroprophic factor rapidly enhances synaptic transmission in hippocampal neurons via postsynaptic tyrosine kinase receptors. *Proc. Natl. Acad. Sci. USA* 92:8074–8077.

Levkovitz, Y., Grisaru, N., and Segal, N. (2001) Transcranial magnetic stimulation and antidepressive drugs share similar cellular effects in rat hippocampus. *Neuropsychopharmacology* 24: 608–616.

Lindsay, R.M., Wiegand, S.J., Altar, A., and DiStefano, P.S. (1994) Neurotrophic factors: from molecule to man. *Trends Neurosci.* 17:182–190.

Lindvall, O., Kokaia, Z., Bengzon, J., Elmer, E., and Kokaia, M. (1994) Neurotrophins and brain insults. *Trends Neurosci.* 17:490–496.

Lucas, G., Compran, V., Charnay, Y., Neve, R.L., Nestler, E.J., Bockaert, J., Barrot, M., and Debonnel, G. (2005) Frontocortical 5-HT4 receptors exert positive feedback on serotonergic activity: viral transfactions, subacute and chronic treatments with 5-HT4 agonists. *Biol. Psychiatry* 15:918–925.

Lucas, G., and Debonnel, G. (2002) 5-HT4 receptors exert a frenquency-related facilitatory control on dorsal raphe nucleus 5-HT neuronal activity. *Eur. J. Neurosci.* 16:817–822.

Lucas, G., Rymar, V.V., Du, J., Mnie-Filali, O., Bisgaard, C., Manta, S., Lambas-Senas, L., Wiborg, O., Haddjeri, N., Pineyro, G., Sadikot, A.F., and Debonnel, G. (2007) Serotonin (4) (5-HT (4)) receptor agonists are putative antidepressants with a rapid onset of action. *Neuron* 55:712–134.

Madison, D., Malenka, R.C., and Nicoll, R.A. (1991) Mechanisms underlying long-term potentiation of synaptic transmission. *Ann. Rev. Neurosci.* 14:379–399.

Malberg, J., and Duman, R.S. (2003) Cell proliferation in adult hippocmpus is decreased by inescapable stress: reversal by fluoxetine treatment. *Neuropsychopharmacology* 28:1562–1571.

Malberg, J., Eisch, A.J., Nestler, E.J., and Duman, R.S. (2000a) Chronic antidepressant treatment increases neurogenesis in adult hippocampus. *J. Neurosci.* 20:9104–9110.

Malberg, J., Eisch, A.J., Nestler, E.J., and Duman, R.S. (2000b) Effects of antidepressant treatment and learned helplessness training on hippocampal neurogenesis in adult rat. *Soc. Neurosci. Abstr.* 26:1044.

Malison, R., Price, L.H., Nestler, E.J., Heninger, G.R., and Duman, R.S. (1997) Efficacy of papaverine addition in treatment-refractory major depression. *Am. J. Psychiatry* 154:579–580.

Mamounas, L., Blue, M.E., Siuciak, J.A., and Anthony, A.C. (1995) BDNF promotes the survival and sprouting of serotonergic axons in the rat brain. *J. Neurosci.* 15:7929–7939.

Manier, D., Eiring, A., Shelton, R.C., and Sulser, F. (1996) b-Adrenoceptor-linked protein kinase A (PKA) activity in human fibroblasts from normal subjects and from patients with major depression. *Neuropsychopharmacology* 15:556–561.

Manji, H., Drevets, W.C., and Charney, D.S. (2001) The cellular neurobiology of depression. *Nat. Med.* 7:541–547.

Manji, H., and Duman, R.S. (2001) Impairments of neuroplasticity and cellular resilience in severe mood disorders: implications for the development of novel therapeutics. *Psychopharmacol. Bull.* 35:5–49.

Manji, H.K., Etcheberrigaray, R., Chen, G., and Olds, J.L. (1993) Lithium decreases membrane-associated protein kinase hippocampus selectivity for the alpha isozyme. *J. Neurosci.* 61:2303–2310.

Margarinos, A., McEwen, B.S., Flugge, G., and Fuchs, E. (1996) Chronic psychosocial stress causes apical dendritic atrophy of hippocampal CA3 pyramidal neurons in subordinate tree shrews. *J. Neurosci.* 16:3534–3540.

Massicotte, G., Bernard, J., and Ohayon, M. (1993) Chronic effects of trimipramine, an antidepressant, on hippocampal synaptic plasticity. *Behav. Neural Biol.* 59:100–106.

McAllister, A., Katz, L.C., and Lo, D.C. (1996) Neurotrophin regulation of cortical dendritic growth requires activity. *Neuron* 17: 1057–1064.

McAllister, K., Katz, L.C., and Lo, D.C. (1999) Neurotrophins and synaptic plasticity. *Ann. Rev. Neurosci.* 22:295–318.

McEwen, B. (2002) Sex, stress and the hippocampus: allostatic load and the aging process. *Neurobiol. Aging* 23:921–939.

McMahon, F., Buervenich, S., Charney, D., Lipsky, R., Rush, A.J., Wilson, A.F., Sorant, A.J., Papanicolaou, G.J., Laje, G., Fava, M., Trivedi, M.H., Wisniewski, S.R., and Manji, H. (2006) Variation in the gene encoding the serotonin 2A receptor is associated with outcome of antidepressant treatment. *Am. J. Hum. Genet.* 78:804–814.

Melia, K., Rasmussen, K., Haycock, J., Terwilliger, R.Z., Nestler, E.J., and Duman, R.S. (1992) Coordinate regulation of firing rate, tyrosine hydroxylase, and the cAMP system in rat locus coeruleus: effects of chronic stress and norepinephrine depleting agents. *J. Neurochem.* 58:494–502.

Menkes, D.B., Rasenick, M.M., Wheeler, M.A., and Bitensky, M.W. (1983) Guanosine triphosphate activation of brain adenylate cyclase: enhancement by long-term antidepressant treatment. *Science* 129:65–67.

Meyer, T., and Habener, J.F. (1993) Cyclic adenosine 3′,5′-monophosphate response element-binding protein (CREB) and related transcription-activating deoxyribonucleic acid-binding proteins. *Endocr. Rev.* 14:269–290.

Miller, H., Delgado, P.L., Salomon, R.M., Berman, R., Krystal, J.H., Heninger, G.R., and Charney, D.S. (1996) Clinical and biochemical effects of catecholamine depletion on antidepressant induced remission of depression: implications for monoamine hypothesis of antidepressant action. *Arch. Gen. Psychiatry* 53: 117–128.

Mitra, R., Jadhav, S., McEwen, B.S., Vyas, A., and Chattarji, S. (2005) Stress duration modulates the spatiotemporal patterns of spine formation in the basolateral amygdala. *Proc. Natl. Acad. Sci. USA* 102:9371–9376.

Monteggia, L., Barrot, M., Powell, C.M., Berton, O., Galanis, V., Gemelli, T., Meuth, S., Nagy, A., Greene, R.W., and Nestler, E.J. (2004) Essential role of brain-derived neurotrophic factor in adult hippocampal function. *Proc. Natl. Acad. Sci. USA* 101: 10827–10832.

Monteggia, L., Luikart, B., Barrot, M., Theobold, D., Malkovska, I., Nef, S., Parada, L.F., and Nestler, E.J. (2007) Brain-derived neurotrophic factor conditional knockouts show gender differences in depression-related behaviors. *Biol. Psychiatry* 61(2): 187–197.

Morinobu, S., Nibuya, M., and Duman, R.S. (1995) Chronic antidepressant treatment down-regulates the induction of c-fos mRNA in response to acute stress in rat frontal cortex. *Neuropsychopharmacology* 12:221–228.

Muller, M., Lucassen, P.J., Yassouridis, A., Hoogendijk, J.G., Holsboer, F., and Swabb, D.F. (2001) Neither major depression nor glucocorticoid treatment affects the cellular integrity of the human hippocampus. *Eur. J. Neurosci.* 14:1603–1612.

Muscat, R., Sampson, D., and Willner, P. (1990) Dopaminergic mechanism of imipramine action in an animal model of depression. *Biol. Psychiatry* 28:223–230.

Nakagawa, S., Kim, J.-E., Lee, R., Chen, J., and Duman, R.S. (2000) CREB plays a critical role in the survival of newborn cells in the adult hippocampus. *Soc. Neurosci. Abstr.* 26:2317.

Nakagawa, S., Kim, J.-E., Lee, R., Malberg, J.E., Chen, J., Steffen, C., Zhang, Y.-J., Nestler, E.J., and Duman, R.S. (2002) Regulation of neurogenesis in adult mouse hippocampus by cAMP and cAMP response element-binding protein. *J. Neurosci.* 22(9): 3673–3682.

Naudon, L., Hotte, M., and Jay, T.M. (2007) Effects of acute and chronic antidepressant treatment on memory performance: a comparison between paroxetine and imipramine. *Psychopharmacology (Berl)* 191:353–364.

Nemeroff, C., Widerlov, E., Bissette, G., Walleus, H., Karlsson, I., Eklund, K., Kilts, C.D., Loosen, P.T., and Vale, W. (1984) Elevated concentrations of CSF corticotropin-releasing factor-like immunoreactivity in depressed patients. *Science* 226:1342–1344.

Nestler, E., Barrot, M., DiLeone, R.J., Eisch, A.J., Gold, S.J., and Monteggia, L.M. (2002) Neurobiology of depression. *Neuron* 34:13–25.

Nestler, E., and Duman, R.S. (2006) *G Proteins*. New York: Elsevier.

Nestler, E., Terwilliger, R.Z., and Duman, R.S. (1989) Chronic antidepressant administration alters the subcellular distribution of cAMP-dependent protein kinase in rat frontal cortex. *J. Neurochem.* 53:1644–1647.

Newton, S., Thome, J., Wallace, T.L., Shirayama, Y., Schlesinger, L., Sakai, N., Chen, N., Neve, R., Nestler, E.J., and Duman, R.S. (2002) Inhibition of cAMP response element-binding protein or dynorphin in the nucleus accumbens produces an antidepressant-like effect. *J. Neurosci.* 24:10883–10890.

Nibuya, M., Morinobu,, S., and Duman, R.S. (1995) Regulation of BDNF and trkB mRNA in rat brain by chronic electroconvulsive seizure and antidepressant drug treatments. *J. Neurosci.* 15: 7539–7547.

Nibuya, M., Nestler, E.J., and Duman, R.S. (1996) Chronic antidepressant administration increases the expression of cAMP response element binding protein (CREB) in rat hippocampus. *J. Neurosci.* 16:2365–2372.

Nishijo, H., Ono, T., and Nishino, H. (1988) Single neuron responses in amygdala of alert monkey during complex sensory stimulation with affective significance. *J. Neurosci.* 8:3570–3583.

Nowakowska, E., Kus, K., Chodera, A., and Rybakowski, J. (2000) Behavioural effects of fluoxetine and tianeptine, two antidepressants with opposite action mechanisms, in rats. *Arzneimittelforschung* 50:5–10.

Nowakowska, E., Kus, K., Chodera, A., and Rybakowski, J. (2003) Comparison of behavioural effects of venlafaxine and imipramine in rats. *Arzneimittelforschung* 53:237–242.

Nowakowska, E., Kus, K., Florek, E., Czubak, A., and Jodynis-Liebert, J. (2006) The influence of tobacco smoke and nicotine on antidepressant and memory-improving effects of venlafaxine. *Hum. Exp. Toxicol.* 25:199–209.

O'Connor, J., Rowan, M.J., and Anwyl, R. (1993) Use-dependent effects of acute and chronic treatment with imipramine and buspirone on excitatory synaptic transmission in the rat hippocampus in vivo. *Naunyn Schmiedeberg's Arch. Pharmacol.* 348:158–163.

Odagaki, Y., Garcia-Sevilla, J.A., Huguelet, P., La Harpe, R., Koyama, T., Guimon, L (2001) Cyclic AMP-mediated signaling components are upregulated in the prefrontal cortex of depressed suicide cictims. *Brain Research* 898:224–231.

O'Donnell, J. (1993) Involvement of beta-1 and beta-2 adrenergic receptors in the antidepressant-like effects of centrally administered isoproterenol. *J. Pharm. Exp. Ther.* 271:246–254.

Ongur, D., Drevets, W.C., and Price, J.L. (1998) Glial reduction in the subgenual prefrontal cortex in mood disorders. *Proc. Natl. Acad. Sci. USA* 95:13290–13295.

Ordway, G., Gambarana, C., Tejani-Butt, S.M., Areso, P., Hauptmann, M., and Frazer, A. (1991) Preferential reduction of binding of 125I-Iodopindolol to beta-1-adrenoceptors in the amygdala of rat after antidepressant treatments. *J. Pharm. Exp. Ther.* 257:681–690.

Owens, M., and Nemeroff, C.B. (1999) Corticotropin-releasing factor antagonists in affective disorders. *Expert Opin. Invest. Drugs* 8:1849–1858.

Ozawa, H., and Rasenick, M.M. (1991) Chronic electroconvulsive treatment augments coupling of the GTP-binding protein Gs to the catalytic moiety of adenylyl cyclase in a manner similar to that seen with chronic antidepressant drugs. *J. Neurochem.* 56:330–338.

Paul, I., Nowak, G., Layer, R.T., Popik, P., and Skolnick, P. (1994) Adaptation of *N*-methyl-D-aspartate receptor complex following chronic antidepressant treatments. *J. Pharm. Exp. Ther.* 269:95–102.

Paykel, E.S., Fleminger, R., and Watson, J.P. (1982) Psychiatric side effects of antihypertensive drugs other than reserpine. *J. Clin. Psychopharmacol.* 2:14–39.

Perez, J., Tardito, D., Racagni, G., Smeraldi, E., and Zanardi, R. (2001) Protein kinase A and Rap1 levels in platelets of untreated patients with major depression. *Mol. Psychiatry* 6:44–49.

Perez, J., Tinelli, D., Brunello, N., and Racagni, G. (1989) cAMP-dependent phosphorylation of soluble and crude microtubule fractions of rat cerebral cortex after prolonged desmethylimipramine treatment. *Eur. J. Pharmacol.* 172:305–316.

Peroutka, S., and Snyder, S.H. (1980) Long-term antidepressant treatment decreases spiroperidol labeled serotonin receptor binding. *Science* 210:88–90.

Pliakas, A., Carlson, R.R., Neve, R.L., Konraki, C., Nestler, E.J., and Carlezon, W.A. (2001) Altered responsiveness to cocaine and increased immobility in the forced swim test associated with elevated CREB expression in the nucleus accumbens. *J. Neurosci.* 21:7397–7403.

Price, L., Charney, D.S., and Heninger, G.R. (1985) Effects of tranylcypromine treatment on neuroendocrine, behavioral, and autonomic responses to tryptophan in depressed patients. *Life Sci.* 37: 809–818.

Radley, J., Sisti, H.M., Hao, J., Rocher, A.B., McCall, T., Hof, P.R., McEwen, B.S., and Morrison, J.H. (2004) Chronic behavioral stress induces apical dendritic reorganization in pyramidal neurons of the medial prefrontal cortex. *Neurosci.* 125:1–6.

Rajkowska, G., Miguel-Hidalgo, J.J., Wei, J., Dilley, G., Pittman, S.D., Meltzer, H.Y., Overholser, J.C., Roth, B.L., and Stockmeier, C.A. (1999) Morphometric evidence for neuronal and glial prefrontal cell pathology in major depression. *Biol. Psychiatry* 45: 1085–1098.

Rasmussen, A., Shi, L., and Duman, R.S. (2002) Down-regulation of BDNF mRNA in the hippocampal dentate gyrus after reexposure to cues previously associated with footshock. *Neuropsychopharmacology* 27(2):133–142.

Reding, M., Orto, L.A., Winter, S.W., Firtuna, I.M., DiPoonte, P., and McDowell, F.H. (1986) Antidepressant therapy after stroke. *Arch. Neurol.* 43:763–765.

Riva, M., and Creese, I. (1989) Reevaluation of the regulation of b-adrenergic receptor binding by desipramine treatment. *Mol. Pharmacol.* 36:211–218.

Russell, D., and Duman, R.S. (2002) *Neurotrophic Factors and Intracellular Signal Transduction Pathways*. Philadelphia: Lippincott Williams and Wilkins.

Saarelainen, T., Hendolin, P., Lucas, G., Koponen, E., Sairanen, M., MacDonald, E., Agerman, K., Haapasalo, A., Nawa, H., Aloyz, R., Ernfors, P., and Castren, E. (2003) Activation of the trkB neurotrophin receptor is induced by antidepressant drugs and is required for antidepressant-induced behavioral effects. *J. Neurosci.* 23:349–357.

Santarelli, L., Saxe, M., Gross, C., Surget, A., Battaglia, F., Dulawa, S., Weisstaub, N., Lee, J., Duman, R., Aranico, O., Belzung, C., and Hen, R. (2003) Requirement of hippocampal neurogenisis for the behavioral effects of antidepressants. *Science* 301:805–809.

Sapolsky, R. (1996) Glucocorticoids and atrophy of the human hippocampus. *Science* 273:749–750.

Sapolsky, R., Krey, L.C., and McEwen, B.S. (1985) Prolonged glucocorticoid exposure reduces hippocampal neuron number: implications for aging. *J. Neurosci.* 5:1222–1227.

Sapolsky, R.M., Uno, H., Robert, C.S., and Finsh, C.E. (1990) Hippocampal damage associated with prolonged glucocorticoid exposure in primates. *J. Neurosci.* 10:2897–2902.

Schildkraut, J. (1965) The catecholamine hypothesis of affective disorders: a review of supporting evidence. *Am. J. Psychiatry* 122: 509–522.

Serra, G., Collu, M., D'Aquila, P.S., and Gessa, G.L. (1992) Role of the mesolimbic dopamine system in the mechanism of action of antidepressants. *Pharmol. Toxicol.* 71:72–85.

Sheline, Y., Gado, M.H., and Price, J.L. (1998) Amygdala core nuclei volumes are decreased in recurrent major depression. *Neuroreport* 9:2023–2028.

Sheline, Y., Sanghavi, M., Mintun, M.A., and Gado, M.H. (1999) Depression duration but not age predicts hippocampal volume loss in medically healthy women with recurrent major depression. *J. Neurosci.* 19:5034–5043.

Sheline, Y., Wany, P., Gado, M.H., Csernansky, J.G., and Vannier, M.W. (1996) Hippocampal atrophy in recurrent major depression. *Proc. Natl. Acad. Sci. USA* 93:3908–3913.

Shirayama, Y., Chen, A.C.-H., Nakagawa, S., Russell, R.S., and Duman, R.S. (2002) Brain derived neurotrophic factor produces antidepressant effects in behavioral models of depression. *J. Neurosci.* 22:3251–3261.

Shopsin, B., Gershon, S., Goldstein, M., Friedman, E., and Wilk, S. (1975) Use of synthesis inhibitors in defining a role for biogenic amines during imipramine treatment in depressed patients. *Psychopharmacol. Comm.* 1:239–249.

Siuciak. J., Altar, C.A., Wiegand, S.J., and Lindsay, R.M. (1994) Antinociceptive effect of brain-derived neurotrophic factor and neurotrophin-3. *Brain Res.* 633:326–330.

Siuciak, J.A., Lewis, D.R., Wiegand, S.J., and Lindsay, R. (1997) Antidepressant-like effect of brain derived neurotrophic factor (BDNF). *Pharmacol. Biochem. Beh.* 56:131–137.

Sklair-Tavron, L., and Nestler, E.J. (1995) Opposing effects of morphine and the neurotrophins, NT-3, NT-4, and BDNF, on locus coeruleus neurons in vitro. *Brain Res.* 702:117–125.

Sleight, A., Carolo, C., Petit, N., Zwingelstein, C., and Bourson, A. (1995) Identification of 5-hydroxytryptamine 7 receptor binding sites in rat hypothalamus: sensitivity to chronic antidepressant treatments. *Mol. Pharmacol.* 47:99–103.

Smith, M.A., Makino, S., Kvetnansky, R., and Post, R.M. (1995) Stress alters the express of brain-derived neurotrophic factor and neurotrophin-3 mRNAs in the hippocampus. *J. Neurosci.* 15:1768–1777.

Spring, B., Gelenberg, A.J., Garvin, R., and Thompson, S. (1992) Amitriptyline, clovoxamine and cognitive function: a placebo-controlled comparison in depressed outpatients. *Psychopharmacology* 108: 327–332.

Stein-Behrens, B., Mattson, M.P., Chang, I., Yeh, M., and Sapolsky, R. (1994) Stress exacerates neuron loss and cytoskeletal pathology in the hippocampus. *J. Neurosci.* 14:5373–5380.

Stern, R., and Bachmann, D.L. (1992) Depressive symptoms following stroke. *Am. J. Psychiatry* 148:351–356.

Stewart, C.A., and Reid, J.C. (2000) Repeated ECS and fluoxetine administration have equivalent effects on hippocampal synaptic plasticity. *Psychopharmacology* 48(3):217–123.

Stockmeier, C., Mahajan, G.J., Konick, L.C., Overholser, J.C., Jurjus, G.J., Meltzer, H.Y., Uylings, H.B.M., Friedman, L., and Rajkowska, G. (2004) Cellular changes in the postmortem hippocampus in major depression. *Biol. Psychiatry* 56:640–650.

Sulser, F., Vetulani, J., and Mobley, P. (1978) Mode of action of antidepressant drugs. *Biochem. Pharmacol.* 27:257–261.

Svenningsson, P., Chergui, K., Rachleff, I., Flajolet, M., Zhang, X., Le Jacobi, M., Vaugeois, J.M. Nomikos, G.G., and Greengard, P. (2006) Alterations in 5-HT1B receptor function by p11 in depression-like states. *Science* 311:77–80.

Svenningsson, P., Tzavara, E.T., Liu, F., Fienberg, A.A., Nomikos, G.G., and Greengard, P. (2002) DARPP-32 mediates serotonergic neurotransmission in the forebrain. *Proc. Natl. Acad. Sci. USA* 99:3188–3193.

Svenningsson, P., Tzavara, E.T., Witkin, J.M., Fienberg, A.A., Nomikos, G.G., and Greengard, P. (2002) Involvement of striatal and extrastriatal DARPP-32 in biochemical and behavioral effects of fluoxetine (Prozac). *Proc. Natl. Acad. Sci. USA* 99:3182–3187.

Takahashi, M., Terwilliger, R., Lane, S., Mezes, P.S., Conti, M., and Duman, R.S. (1999) Chronic antidepressant administration increases the expression of cAMP phosphodiesterase 4A and 4B isoforms. *J. Neurosci.* 19:610–618.

Tanis, K., and Duman, R.S. (2007) Intracellular signaling pathways pave roads to recovery for mood disorders. *Annals of Medicine* 39:531–544.

Tao, X., Finkbeiner, S., Arnold, D.B., Shaywitz, A.J., Greenberg, M.E. (1998) Ca2+ influx regulates BDNF transcription by a CREB family transcription factor-dependent mechanism. *Neuron* 20:709–726.

Tardito, D., Perez, J., Tiraboschhi, E., Musazzi, L., Racagni, G., Popoli, M. (2006) Signaling pathways regulating gene expression, neuroplasticity, and neurotrophic mechanisms in the action of antidepressants: a critical overview. *Pharmacol. Rev.* 58:115–134.

Thoenen, H. (1995) Neurotrophins and neuronal plasticity. *Science* 270:593–598.

Thome, J., Sakai, N., Shin, K.H., Steffen, C., Zhang, Y.-J., Impey, S., Storm, D.R., and Duman, R.S. (2000) cAMP response element-mediated gene transcription is upregulated by chronic antidepressant treatment. *J. Neurosci.* 20:4030–4036.

Tiraboschi, E., Tardito, D., Kasahara, J., Moraschi, S., Pruneri, P., Gennarelli, M., Racagni, G., and Popoli, M. (2004) Selective phosphorylation of nuclear CREB by fluoxetine is linked to activation of CaM kinase IV and MAP kinase cascades. *Neuropsychopharmacology* 29:1831–1840.

Tsankova, N., Berton, O., Renthal, W., Kumar, A., Neve, R., and Nestler, E.J. (2006) Sustained hippocampal chromatin regulation in a mouse model of depression and antidepressant action. *Nat. Neurosci.* 9:465–466.

Uno, H., Tarara,, R., Else, J.G., Suleman, M.A., and Sapolsky, R.M. (1989) Hippocampal damage associated with prolonged and fatal stress in primates. *J. Neurosci.* 9:1705–1711.

Vaidya, V., Marek, G.J., Aghajanian, G.A., and Duman, R.S. (1997) 5-HT2A receptor-mediated regulation of BDNF mRNA in the hippocampus and the neocortex. *J. Neurosci.* 17:2785–2795.

Vermetten, E., Vythilingam, M., Southwick, S.M., Charney, D.S., and Bremner, J.D. (2003) Long-term treatment with paroxetine increases verbal declarative memory and hippocampal volume in posttraumatic stress disorder. *Biol. Psychiatry* 54:693–702.

Vetulani, J., and Sulser, F. (1975) Action of various antidepressant treatments reduces reactivity of noradrenergic cAMP generating system in limbic forebrain. *Nature* 257:495–496.

Von Fritag, J., Kamal, A., Reijmers, L.G., Schrama, L.H., van den Bos, R., and Spruijt, B.M. (2001) Chronic imipramine treatment partially reverses the long-term changes of hippocampal synaptic plasticity in socially stressed rats. *Neurosci. Lett.* 309:153–156.

Vythilingam, M., Vermetten, E., Anderson, G.M., Luckenbaugh, D., Anderson, E.R., Snow, J., Staib, L.H., Charney, D.S., and Bremner, J.D. (2004) Hippocampal volume, memory, and cortisol status in major depressive disorder: effects of treatment. *Biol. Psychiatry* 56:101–112.

Wachtel, H. (1983) Potential antidepressant activity of rolipram and other selective cyclic adenosine 3′,5′-monophosphate phosphodiesterase inhibitors. *Neuropharmacology* 22:267–272.

Wachtel, T., and Schneider, H.D. (1986) Rolipram, a novel antidepressant drug, reverses the hypothermia and hypokinesia of monoamine-depleted mice by an action beyond postsynaptic monoamine receptors. *Neuropharmacology* 25:1119–1126.

Walker, W., Fucci, L., and Habener, J.F. (1995) Expression of the gene encoding transcription factor cAMP response element-binding protein (CREB): regulation by follicle stimulating hormone induced cAMP signaling in primary rat Sertoli cells. *Endocrinology* 136: 3534–3545.

Warner-Schmidt, J., and Duman, R.S. (2006) Hippocampal neurogenesis: opposing effects of stress and antidepressant treatment. *Hippocampus* 16:239–249.

Watanabe, Y., Gould, E., Daniels, D.C., Cameron, H., and McEwen, B.S (1992) Tianeptine attenuates stress-induced morphological changes in the hippocampus. *Eur. J. Pharmacol.* 222:157–162.

Wellman, C. (2001) Dendritic reorganization in pyramidal neurons in medial prefrontal cortex after chronic corticosterone administration. *J. Neurobiol.* 49:245–253.

Widnell, K., Russell, D., and Nestler, E.J. (1994) Regulation of cAMP response element binding protein in the locus coeruleus in vivo and in a locus coeruleus-like (CATH.a) cell line in vitro. *Proc. Natl. Acad. Sci. USA* 91:10947–10951.

Wong, M.-L., and Licinio, J. (2001) Research and treatment approaches to depression. *Nat. Rev./Neurosci.* 2:343–351.

Wooley, C.S., Gould, E., and McEwen, B.S. (1990) Exposure to excess glucocorticoids alters dendritic morphology of adult hippocampal pyramidal neurons. *Brain Res.* 531:225–231.

Yamada, S., Yamamoto, M., Ozawa, H., Riederer, P., and Saito, T. (2003) Reduced phosphorylation of cyclic AMP-responsive element binding protein in the postmortem orbitofrontal cortex of patients with major depressive disorder. *J. Neural Trans.* 110:671–680.

Yau, J., Noble, J., Hibberd, C., Rowe, W.B., Meaney, M.J., Morris, R.G.M., and Secki, J.R. (2002) Chronic treatment with the antidepressant amitriptyline prevents impairments in water maze learning in aging rats. *J. Neurosci.* 22:1436–1442.

Yau, J.L.W., Olsson, T., Morris, R.G.M., Meaney, M.J., and Seckl, J.R. (1995) Glucocorticoids, hippocampal corticosteroid receptor gene expression and antidepressant treatment: relationship with spatial learning in young and aged rats. *Neurosci.* 66:571–581.

Young, E., Haskett, R.F., Murphy-Weinberg, V., Watson, S.J., and Akil, H. (1997) Loss of glucocorticoid fast feedback in depression. *Arch. Gen. Psychiatry* 48:693–699.

Zarate, C., Singh, J., and Manji, H.K. (2006) Cellular plasticity cascades: targets for the development of novel therapeutics for bipolar disorder. *Biol. Psychiatry* 59:1006–1020.

Zhang, H.-T., Zhao, Y., Huang, Y., Dorairaj, N.R., Chandler, L.J., and O'Donnell, J.M. (2004) Inhibition of the phosphodiesterase 4 (PDE4) enzyme reverses memory deficits produced by infusion of the MEK inhibitor U0126 into the CAI subregion of the rat hippocampus. *Neuropsychopharmacology* 29:1432–1439.

30 The Neurochemistry of Depressive Disorders: Clinical Studies

BOADIE W. DUNLOP, STEVEN J. GARLOW, AND CHARLES B. NEMEROFF

Investigations into the neurochemical basis of psychiatric diseases began in the mid-1950s. This interest was largely stimulated by the identification of effective psychotherapeutic drugs, first chlorpromazine for the treatment of psychosis, followed later in the decade by the tricyclic antidepressants (TCAs) and monoamine oxidase inhibitors (MAOIs) for the treatment of depression. The earliest modern theories of the pathogenesis of psychiatric disorders were based in large part on the observable mechanisms of actions of these first effective psychopharmacological agents. The in vitro description of the mechanism of action of imipramine was one of the key observations in the development of the monoamine hypothesis of depression. A series of simple yet elegant experiments demonstrated that imipramine blocked the reuptake of norepinephrine (NE) into presynaptic neurons, and this action was considered to be the basis of its antidepressant activity (Glowinski et al., 1964; Glowinski and Axelrod, 1966; Glowinski and Iverson, 1966; Glowinski et al., 1966). The hypothesis that developed from these observations is that depression is due to a state of decreased NE availability in the synapse, a condition that is reversed by the actions of imipramine (Prange, 1964; Bunney and Davis, 1965; Schildkraut, 1965). This set the stage for a recurrent theme in the study of depression: to base theories of pathophysiology on the observed actions of antidepressants. In many ways, the introduction of efficacious noradrenergic (TCAs) and serotonergic (TCAs and selective serotonin reuptake inhibitors [SSRIs]) drugs has driven research and theory on the pathophysiology of depression. In particular, it has supported the idea that depression results from a relative deficiency of a particular neurotransmitter and that prolonging the transmitter's residence and/or concentration in the synapse, with reuptake inhibiting antidepressants, functionally reverses this deficiency.

METHODOLOGICAL CONSIDERATIONS

Studies seeking to elucidate the neurochemical pathology of depression have focused on the pre- and postsynaptic levels of neuronal functioning. Neurotransmitter release and availability are dependent on the functional state of the presynaptic neurons, and concentrations of neurotransmitters and their metabolites are considered to be reflective of presynaptic neuronal activity. Quantification of neurotransmitter and metabolite concentrations has been carried out in cerebrospinal fluid (CSF), blood, urine, and saliva. The underlying assumption of these studies is that the concentration of the transmitter or metabolite in the particular body fluid is directly proportional to its concentration in the synapse. Another approach to the study of presynaptic activity is neurotransmitter depletion studies. In these experiments, the central nervous system (CNS) availability of a particular transmitter is drastically and transiently depleted through either dietary or pharmacological manipulations. The impact of this depletion on mood (or anxiety) is then measured (Delgado et al., 1990; Delgado et al., 1994; Delgado et al., 1999).

Various measurements of neurotransmitter receptor and effector system activation are considered to reflect primarily postsynaptic neuronal activity. Postsynaptic mechanisms have been studied by direct postmortem measurement of particular receptors or effector systems in brains of patients who were depressed at the time of death. Often these studies are of victims of suicide in comparison to some nonpsychiatric control group. These experiments are frequently confounded by differences in postmortem interval prior to analysis and by agonal state, differences in handling and processing of tissues, and diagnostic uncertainties for the affected and control groups. With the development of positron emission tomography (PET) and other high-resolution neuroimaging techniques, studies previously possible only through postmortem analyses, such as neurotransmitter receptor-binding assays, can now be performed in living patients.

Another method used to study neurotransmitter systems in depression is neuroendocrine challenge assays, which use the neuroendocrine window strategy. This technique can measure pre- and postsynaptic mechanisms, depending on the assay employed. In these experiments, patients receive a pharmacological agent known to alter the secretion of an anterior pituitary or target gland hormone by an action on a particular neurotransmitter system. The underlying assumption is that the secretory response to the challenge agent is related to the functional state of that neurotransmitter system. Table 30.1 lists some of the commonly used agents, the systems they test, and the actual measurements (readout) made (Siever et al., 1982; Siever, Murphy, et al., 1984; Anand et al., 1994; Pitchot et al., 1995; Yatham et al., 1997; Whale et al., 2001).

A number of peripheral measures have been proposed as surrogates for their cognate systems in the CNS. The expression of neurotransmitter system components on blood cells has been posited to reflect these same systems in the CNS. In particular, platelets have been studied extensively in depression. The rationale for these studies is that the precursor cells from which platelets are derived, megakaryocytes, share embryological origins with 5-hydroxytryptamine (5-HT) neurons, and platelets contain serotonergic and adrenergic receptors, the serotonin transporter, and the inositol trisphosphate and adenylate cyclase second-messenger systems. Platelets concentrate 5-HT in and secrete it from secretory granules that resemble synaptic vesicles (Stahl, 1977; McBride et al., 1983; Da Prada et al., 1988; Wirz-Justice, 1988). Blood lymphocytes and skin fibroblasts are other peripheral cells that have also been studied in depression. Both of these cell types express a number of neurotransmitter receptors, glucocorticoid receptors, and second-messenger systems. The neurotransmitter receptors expressed on peripheral cells are indeed identical to those expressed in the CNS. The assumption that underlies the study of peripheral cell types is that the receptors, transporters, and second-messenger systems are subject to the same molecular regulation in the periphery as in the CNS and that peripheral alterations directly reflect changes in the CNS that occur in depression.

There are a large number of observations in major depression that have either not been replicated at all, have been replicated only in a minority of studies, or have yielded the opposite result from that initially reported. This could be due to a number of factors; the most prominent one is diagnostic heterogeneity. The diagnosis of major depression has evolved over the past 40 years, with progressively more precise definitions with each iteration of the *Diagnostic and Statistical Manual* (*DSM*); however, the interpretation of the *DSM* (and other diagnostic criteria) for depression is not standardized among all investigators and is quite broad in disease severity. The result is that it may not be possible to compare one study cohort to another, despite the efforts of investigators to employ standardized assessment and documentation instruments with their particular sample. Given the potential confounds, it is remarkable that changes in the serotonergic and noradrenergic systems have been so consistently documented in patients who are depressed, across many studies, from different investigators, with many different analytic techniques. This argues convincingly that these two systems play a central role in the pathophysiology of major depression.

TABLE 30.1 *Neuroendocrine Challenge Agents, Neurotransmitter System Tested, Specific Target, Synaptic Level, and Assay Readout*

Agent	*System*	*Target*	*Synaptic Level*	*Readout*
Intravenous tryptophan	5-HT	5-HT synthesis	Pre	Serum prolactin
Fenfluramine	5-HT	5-HT nerve terminals	Pre	Serum prolactin CNS metabolism by PET
Sumitriptan	5-HT	5-HT1D-R	Pre	Serum growth hormone
Zolmitriptan	5-HT	5-HT1D-R	Pre	Serum growth hormone
Citalopram	5-HT	SERT	Pre	Serum prolactin, cortisol
m-CPP	5-HT	5-HT_2 family	Post	Serum prolactin, growth hormone, cortisol
Clonidine	NE	A2-AR	Post	Serum growth hormone
Apomorphine	DA	DA-2-R	Post	Serum growth hormone

A_2-AR: a_2 adrenergic receptor; DA: dopamine; 5-HT: 5-hydroxytryptamine; 5-HTID-R: 5-HTID receptor; M-CPP: m-chlorophenylpiperidine; NE: norepinephrine; PET: positron emission tomography; SERT: serotonin transporter; CNS:central nervous system.

NEUROTRANSMITTER SYSTEMS

All of the major neurotransmitter systems, serotonin, NE, dopamine (DA), γ-aminobutyric acid (GABA), glutamate, many of the peptidergic systems, and many other systems have been scrutinized for a role in the pathogenesis of depressive disorders. A preponderance of evidence accumulated over four decades has consistently revealed alterations in the noradrenergic and serotonergic systems. Both of these systems appear to be central to the pathophysiology of depression, and one, the other, or both appear to be involved in the mechanism of action of most antidepressants. There are many other interesting yet less well studied findings in other neurotransmitter systems in depression, including the DA and corticotropin-releasing factor (CRF) circuits, that hint at the complexity and interrelatedness of these systems in the CNS and at the widespread impact that major depression has on the neurochemistry of the CNS.

Norepinephrine

The noradrenergic system was the first to be studied intensively in major depression. Early theories of the pathogenesis of depression focused on a relative deficiency of norepinephrine (NE) as the cause of depression (Prange, 1964; Bunney and Davis, 1965; Schildkraut, 1965). This was due in large part to the observed mechanisms of action of imipramine and other drugs. Theories of the mechanisms of action of antidepressants and of the pathophysiology of depression converged around the ability of TCAs to block uptake of NE into synaptic vesicles and the ability of the catecholamine-depleting agent *reserpine* to provoke symptoms of depression. The original catecholamine hypothesis of affective disorders proposed that depression was due to a relative deficiency of catecholamines, particularly NE, at important sites in the brain and that mania was due to relative NE excess. Key findings implicating dysfunction of the noradrenergic system in depression are summarized in Table 30.2.

The biochemical pathways that lead to production of catecholamines were described in exquisite detail as part of the effort to validate the catecholamine hypothesis. Norepinephrine, DA, and epinephrine contain the catechol ring structure or 1,2-dihydroxybenzene. The concentration of NE in bodily fluids is difficult to measure because the transmitter is rapidly catabolized, but the principal metabolite, 3-methoxy-4-hydroxyphenylglycol (MHPG), is stable, and its concentration has been proposed as a surrogate measure of NE levels. This metabolite can be measured in urine, and approximately 20% of urinary MHPG is derived from the CNS pool (Potter et al., 1984). The underlying assumption is that changes in urinary levels of MHPG are reflective of changes in the activity of NE neurons in the CNS. In early reports, urinary levels of MHPG were found to be significantly lower in patients who were depressed

TABLE 30.2 *Findings Implicating Noradrenergic Dysfunction in the Pathophysiology of Depression at Various Neuropharmacologic Levels of Action*

Level of Action	*Finding*	*Replicability*
Neurotransmitter synthesis	AMPT, inhibitor of tyrosine hydroxylase, results in depressive relapse in antidepressant-treated patients	++
Neurotransmitter storage	Long-term treatment with reserpine, which depletes monoamine stores, results in depressive symptoms in patients with a history of depression	++
Neurotransmitter reuptake	NE reuptake inhibitors are effective antidepressants TCAs block NE reuptake in vitro	+++
Neurotransmitter metabolism	MAOIs are effective antidepressants	+++
	Low NE metabolites in bipolar depression	++
	MAO-A levels elevated in depressed patients	+
Postsynaptic neurotransmitter receptors	α_2-Adrenergic receptor	
	• Increased B_{max} on platelets of depressed patients	++
	• Increased B_{max} in brains of suicide victims	+
	• Blunted GH response to clonidine challenge	+++
	β-Adrenergic receptor	
	• Increased B_{max} in brains of suicide victims	+++
	• Down-regulation in response to antidepressant treatment (patients)	+
	• Down-regulation in experimental animals systems	+++

AMPT: alpha-methyl-paratyrosine; MAOI: monoamine oxidase inhibitor; NE: norepinephrine; TCA: tricyclic antidepressant; GH: growth hormone; Replication key: +: one or no replication studies; ++: several replication studies; +++: highly replicated by more than two research groups.

compared to controls (Maas et al., 1972; Schildkraut, 1973). This finding has not, however, been consistently replicated, especially in patients with unipolar depression. Overall, urinary MHPG levels do not distinguish patients with unipolar depression from controls (Schildkraut et al., 1978; Schatzberg et al., 1982).

Subsequent research has attempted to classify subtypes of depression based on urinary catecholamine excretion. Because patients with unipolar depression display a wide range of urinary MHPG concentrations, attempts have been made to stratify these patients based on MHPG values as a means of analyzing symptom content and treatment response. Patients with unipolar depression have been classified as having low, intermediate, or high urinary MHPG values (Schatzberg et al., 1982; Schatzberg et al., 1989). Those patients in the low category are considered to have diminished activity of noradrenergic neurons resulting in low NE output and release, consistent with the original catecholamine hypothesis. These patients have been reported to respond to treatment with tricyclic and tetracyclic antidepressants and to fluoxetine, a specific serotonin reuptake inhibitor (Hollister et al., 1980; Schatzberg et al., 1981; Maas et al., 1984; Schatzberg, 1998). The nature of patients with unipolar depression with intermediate MHPG values remains obscure.

Patients with unipolar depression and high urinary MHPG are believed to have increased activity of presynaptic noradrenergic neurons. This may reflect dysfunction of one or more of the adrenergic receptors or an interaction with other transmitter systems. Patients in the high urinary MHPG group also tend to have high circulating plasma cortisol concentrations, to be nonsuppressors on the dexamethasone suppression test, and to be resistant to treatment with conventional antidepressants. These patients have been reported to respond poorly to TCAs and SSRIs.

Initial reports indicated that patients suffering from bipolar disorder (BPD) had the lowest urinary MHPG values during the depressed phase of the illness, lower than those of patients with unipolar depression and healthy controls. As the distinctions between bipolar types I and II have been realized, patients with type I bipolar disorder have been reported to have the lowest urinary MHPG values during the depressed phase. Patients with type II BPD have urinary MHPG values similar to those of patients with unipolar depression, which as a group are higher than those of patients who are depressed with type I BPD (Schatzberg et al., 1989). Some patients with unipolar depression also have low urinary MHPG values, similar to those with type I BPD. These patients may in fact have incipient type I BPD and have simply not yet suffered their first manic episode.

One obvious prediction from the reports that patients with type I BPD have the lowest concentrations of urinary MHPG during the depressed phase is that these same patients would have increased levels of MHPG during the manic phase. This prediction has been confirmed in several studies (Halaris, 1978). Patients with BPD during manic episodes have significantly higher plasma NE and epinephrine levels than when they are depressed or euthymic (Maj et al., 1984). Other investigators have reported that urinary MHPG and CSF NE levels are significantly higher in patients who are manic than in patients who are depressed or controls (Swann et al., 1987).

Measurement of NE and MHPG concentrations in blood and CSF has yielded equally confounding results. In a study that compared CSF MHPG levels between 99 hospitalized patients who were depressed, 14 patients who were manic, and 61 healthy controls, elevated CSF MHPG was observed in patients who were depressed with high levels of anxiety, agitation, somatization, and sleep disturbance (Redmond et al., 1986). This observation did not correlate to global severity of symptoms or to other symptom domains. In another study in which CSF was sampled hourly for 30 consecutive hours in patients with melancholic depression, patients had significantly elevated NE levels, across the entire circadian cycle, compared to controls (Wong et al., 2000). In a study of patients with nonbipolar, medication-refractory unipolar depression, venoarterial neurotransmitter gradients were determined by means of cannulas inserted into the internal jugular vein (Lambert et al., 2000). Venoarterial NE and DA gradients were reduced in the patients compared to the controls. Not only was the venoarterial NE gradient markedly reduced in the medication-refractory patients who were depressed, but similar results were also observed with the two major NE metabolites, MHPG and dihydroxyphenylglycol (DHPG). This is presumptive evidence of decreased activity of NE circuits in this sample of refractory patients who are depressed. In a different study comparing patients with posttraumatic stress disorder (PTSD), PTSD plus depression, depression, and normal controls, the group with PTSD alone had significantly elevated serum NE concentrations, while there were no differences in serum NE levels between the other three diagnostic groups (Yehuda et al., 1998).

A recent PET study using [^{11}C]harmine, a radioligand specific for the measurement of monoamine oxidase A (MAO-A) activity, demonstrated a dramatic 34% elevation in MAO-A in numerous brain regions of patients who were currently depressed versus controls (Meyer et al., 2006). MAO-A is responsible for catabolizing NE, serotonin. and, to a lesser extent, DA in the CNS, and elevated MAO-A levels may explain the reduced monoamine concentrations in major depression.

The cold-pressor test is one functional assay of NE system reactivity. In a comparison of patients with melancholic or psychotic depression, nonmelancholic depression, generalized anxiety disorder, and normal controls, the patients with melancholic/psychotic depression exhibited a significant decrease in NE response to cold-pressor compared with all of the other groups (Kelly and Cooper, 1998). This appears to be evidence for NE system under reactivity in melancholic/psychotic depression.

Clearly, the measurement of NE and its metabolites in peripheral samples has been invaluable historically in developing the disease concept of major depression. However, given the wide variance in levels of serum, CSF, and urinary NE and MHPG in unipolar depression, the original hypothesis that depression results from a deficiency of NE has not been validated by these methods. One of the original goals of these research efforts was to develop laboratory tests that would aid in the diagnosis of depression; however, measurement of peripheral NE or MHPG has never been validated as such a test. With the emergence of high-resolution functional neuroimaging methods with which to study catecholaminergic systems in the CNS, the peripheral measurement of catecholamine levels as an index of CNS function has now been superseded (Schatzberg and Schildkraut, 1995).

Even though the direct measurement of NE or MHPG has not yielded definitive evidence of catecholamine system dysfunction in depression, functional manipulation of the NE system does implicate this system in the pathophysiology of depression. Brief inhibition of tyrosine hydroxylase (TH) with α-methyl-para-tyrosine (AMPT) transiently depletes CNS NE and other catecholamine (DA and epinephrine) pools. Administration of AMPT to normal healthy patients with no history of depression does not produce mood symptoms (Salomon et al., 1997). Moreover, administration of AMPT to untreated patients who are depressed does not cause worsening of core symptoms of depression, but it does exacerbate some neurovegetative symptoms such as anergia (Miller et al., 1996b). In contrast, patients who are depressed treated with desipramine or mazindol, which are specific NE reuptake inhibitors, suffer a significant return of depressive symptoms when challenged with AMPT (Miller et al., 1996a; Berman et al., 1999). The AMPT-induced return of depressive symptoms in patients remitted from major depression during treatment with NE reuptake inhibitors is correlated with reduced brain metabolism in the dorsolateral prefrontal cortex (PFC), orbitofrontal cortex, and thalamus assessed by PET (Bremner et al., 2003). In contrast, patients treated with specific serotonin reuptake inhibitors (fluoxetine, sertraline) do not relapse when treated with AMPT. This implies parallel treatment response pathways that involve either NE or 5-HT systems and that manipulation of one or the other system is often adequate to cause resolution of depression (Heninger et al., 1996).

A number of different noradrenergic neurotransmitter receptors have been implicated in the pathophysiology of depression and in the mechanism of action of antidepressants (Duman and Nestler, 1995). The α_2-adrenergic and β-adrenergic receptors have been the focus of considerable research in the biology of depression. The expression and function of α_2 receptors on platelets have been studied on the assumption that the function of these receptors in platelets reflects that of those in the CNS. Increased density of α_2 receptors on platelets has been repeatedly reported in drug-free patients who were depressed (Garcia-Sevilla et al., 1987; Garcia-Sevilla et al., 1990; Piletz et al, 1990; Gurguis et al., 1999). The platelet α_2 receptor mediates platelet aggregation, and this response is exaggerated in patients who are depressed (Musselman et al., 1996). Platelet α_2 receptor density has been correlated with severity of depressive symptoms, as measured with the Hamilton Rating Scale for Depression (HRSD) (Marazziti et al., 2001). However, there are also reports that platelet α_2 receptor density is decreased in depression (Maes et al., 1999). Postmortem measurement of α_2 binding in the locus ceruleus in patients with major depression has been found to be elevated compared to controls (Ordway et al., 2003). Locus ceruleus α_2 receptors likely function as autoreceptors and act to inhibit noradrenergic cell firing. Although some investigators report increased postmortem B_{max} (maximum binding capacity) of α_2 receptors in the cerebral cortex of patients who were depressed versus controls (Meana et al., 1992), others have found no difference (Arango et al., 1993; Klimek et al., 1999). The findings of increased α_2 receptors in depression have been interpreted as reflecting increased sensitivity of this receptor, perhaps resulting in decreased activity of noradrenergic neurons and hence decreased CNS NE release in patients who are depressed, consistent with the original catecholamine hypothesis.

The clonidine challenge test is an indirect means of assessing the functional state of CNS α_2 receptors. Clonidine is an α_2 agonist that increases growth hormone (GH) release from the anterior pituitary gland, presumably through a postsynaptic mechanism. A blunted GH response to clonidine has been reported in patients who were depressed in several studies (Siever, Uhde, et al., 1984; Amsterdam et al., 1989). A blunted GH response to clonidine has been reported in patients who were acutely symptomatic depressed, in patients treated with antidepressants, and in those in remission (Mitchell et al., 1988; Siever et al., 1992). This suggests that the alteration in α_2 receptor function revealed by the clonidine challenge test might be a trait characteristic of some patients who are depressed. The clonidine challenge test does not discriminate between patients who are depressed and nonsuicidal and patients who are depressed and highly suicidal, which suggests that NE dysregulation is involved in the pathology of depression and not in suicide (Pitchot et al., 2001b). However, earlier studies did not adequately control for the presence of anxiety comorbid with depression. When patients who are depressed without anxiety were compared with patients who were not depressed and anxious or patients with mixed anxiety/depression, only those patients with some level of anxiety demonstrated reduced GH response to clonidine; those with depression without anxiety showed GH responses similar to healthy controls (Cameron et al., 2004). Nevertheless, drawing firm mechanistic conclusions from these results is difficult because many of the findings of increased α_2 receptor density in depression have not been consistently replicated or because the exact opposite has been observed.

β-Adrenergic receptors have also been postulated to contribute to the pathophysiology of depression and to the response to antidepressants. As with the α-adrenergic receptors, results with β-adrenergic receptors have been variable, contradictory, and difficult to interpret. There are reports of increased B_{max} for the β-adrenergic receptor in postmortem brain tissue of victims of suicide, but there are equally credible discrepant reports (Crow et al., 1984; Mann et al., 1986; De Paermentier et al., 1990, 1991). A number of different variables could account for the failure to replicate this finding, including diagnostic heterogeneity between studies, differences in antemortem antidepressant treatment, differences in processing of the postmortem tissue, and differences in analytical techniques. Similarly contradictory results have been reported for studies in which the B_{max} for β receptors on leukocytes was determined. There are reports of decreased B_{max} values for peripheral β receptors in patients who are depressed and studies that report no difference between patients who are depressed and healthy controls (Extein et al., 1979; Healy et al., 1985). Certainly, treatment with antidepressants can affect the B_{max} of β receptors, and much of the variability in these studies could be accounted for by differences in the type, duration, and intensity of antidepressant treatment.

Down-regulation of β receptors has been postulated to be integral to antidepressant action (Banarjee et al., 1977). In animal models, one consistent action of many antidepressants is to decrease the numbers of β receptors and uncouple the receptors from their second-messenger systems. These effects occur after chronic but not acute treatment, corresponding to the temporal response to these agents in clinical practice. However, studies with primarily serotonergic agents have found no effect on β adrenoreceptors (Ordway et al., 1991).

Serotonin

There is considerable evidence for dysfunction of the serotonergic system in major depression, which has culminated in the serotonin hypothesis of depression (Meltzer and Lowy, 1987; Maes and Meltzer, 1995). Alterations in serotonergic function have been observed at pre- and postsynaptic levels in patients who are depressed. There are voluminous treatment response data implicating the serotonergic system as a principal target for the action of antidepressants (Owens, 1997). Whether serotonergic dysfunction is sufficient to cause depression or is a necessary risk factor remains an open question. Key findings implicating dysfunction of serotonergic circuits in depression are summarized in Table 30.3.

All of the serotonin in the CNS is synthesized in raphé nuclei neurons. Serotonin synthesized in the periphery does not enter the CNS. Disruption of 5-HT synthesis in the CNS has been hypothesized as a major pathophysiological mechanism leading to major depression. Serotonin is synthesized from the essential amino acid l-tryptophan (l-TRP), and the availability of l-TRP determines the amount of serotonin synthesized (Maes et al., 1990). Plasma l-TRP concentrations determine the amount of l-TRP that crosses the blood-brain barrier, and hence the amount of 5-HT synthesized and available in the CNS. There is evidence that the concentration of plasma l-TRP is lower in patients who are depressed than in controls. This may be due at least partly to increased clearance of l-TRP via hepatic biotransformation. Peak plasma concentrations of l-TRP are lower in patients who are depressed than in controls after oral or intravenous l-TRP loading doses, perhaps due to induction of the hepatic metabolic pathway responsible for the processing of l-TRP (Maes et al., 1987).

Dietary depletion of l-TRP decreases the serum concentration of l-TRP, which in turn results in a transient fall in CNS 5-HT availability. In normal controls, lowering plasma l-TRP via dietary manipulation can produce a transient depressed mood (S.N. Young et al., 1985); this may represent a trait vulnerability factor for depression. The occurrence of depression and dysphoria following l-TRP depletion occurs much more prominently in normal patients with first-degree relatives who suffer from depression than in healthy patients with no family history of depression (Benkelfat et al., 1994; Ellenbogen et al., 1996).

The mood-altering effect of l-TRP depletion is dramatically demonstrated in patients who are depressed with recent remission (Heninger et al., 1992; Smith et al., 1997). These patients display a remarkably rapid return of depressed mood, and the attendant cognitive and neurovegetative symptoms, with l-TRP depletion. Patients treated with SSRIs are much more sensitive to this manipulation than patients treated with antidepressants that act on noradrenergic neurons. This response has not been universally replicated, but the failure to replicate may be due to differences in severity of depression, intensity of treatment, or the presence of suicidal ideation between different study cohorts. In at least one study that did not find an effect of l-TRP de-

TABLE 30.3 *Findings Implicating Serotonergic Dysfunction in the Pathophysiology of Depression at Various Neuropharmacologic Levels of Action*

Level of Action	*Finding*	*Replicability*
Precursor availability	Plasma TRP is lower in subgroups of depressed patients	+/−
	Depletion of plasma TRP results in depressive relapse in antidepressant-treated patients	++
	Depletion of plasma TRP causes dysphoria in first-degree relatives of depressed patients	++
Neurotransmitter synthesis	PCPA, inhibitor of TRP hydroxylase, results in depressive relapse in antidepressant-treated patients	+
Neurotransmitter storage	Long-term treatment with reserpine, which depletes monoamine stores, results in depressive symptoms in patients with a history of depression	++
Neurotransmitter release	Fenfluramine and MDMA, which increase synaptic 5-HT, cause mild euphoria and a sense of well-being	+
	Lithium, which enhances 5-HT release, augments antidepressant action	+++
	Prolactin release in response to intravenous TRP blunted in depressed patients	++
	Prolactin release in response to fenfluramine challenge blunted in depressed patients	+++
	Cerebral glucose use reaction blunted in response to fenfluramine challenge in depressed patients	+
	Prolactin release in response to citalopram challenge blunted	+
Presynaptic autoreceptor function	5-HT_{1A} agonists (gepirone, buspirone) may have antidepressant properties	++
Neurotransmitter reuptake	5-HT reuptake inhibitors are effective antidepressants	+++
	Decreased platelet 5-HT reuptake sites in depressed patients	+++
	Decreased 5-HT reuptake sites in postmortem brains of depressed patients	+/−
	5-HT reuptake site down-regulated in response to antidepressants (patients)	+/−
	5-HT reuptake sites down-regulated in response to antidepressants (experimental animals)	++
Neurotransmitter metabolism	MAOIs are effective antidepressants	+++
	Low 5-HT metabolites in subgroups of depressed patients	+/−
	Low 5-HT metabolites in CSF of patients prone to violent suicide	+++
	MAO-A levels elevated in depressed patients	+
Postsynaptic neurotransmitter receptors	5-HT_{1A} receptor	
	Increased B_{max} in brains of suicide victims	+/−
	5-HT_{1D} receptor	
	Blunted GH response to sumatriptan/zolmitriptan	++
	5-HT_2 receptor	
	Increased B_{max} in brains of suicide victims	++/−
	Increased B_{max} on platelets of depressed patients	+++
	Antagonists (trazodone, nefazodone, mianserin) are antidepressants	+++
	Down-regulation in response to antidepressant treatment (patients)	+
	Down-regulation in experimental animal systems	+++

CSF: cerebral spinal fluid; 5-HT: serotonin; MAOI: monoamine oxidase inhibitor; MDMA: 3,4-methlenedioxymethamphetamine; PCPA: parachloropheny-lalanine; TCA: tricyclic antidepressant; TRP: tryptophan; GH; growth hormone.

Replication key: +: one or no replication studies; ++: several replication studies; +++: highly replicated by more than two research groups; +/−: mixed or inconsistent results.

pletion, patients who were considered at risk for suicide or self-destructive behavior were excluded (Leyton et al., 1997). A study of patients who were depressed and subsequently treated with antidepressants to the point of remission suggests there is a threshold effect, wherein insufficient tryptophan depletion does not provoke depressive relapse but more thorough depletion does (Spillmann et al., 2001). Such "low dose" depletion can produce changes in emotion processing and cognitive functioning without detectable reduction in mood (Hayward et al., 2005). This finding is consistent with findings from patients with Alzheimer's dementia, in which l-TRP depletion can worsen the cognitive performance without causing symptoms of depression (Porter et al., 2000).

Interestingly, untreated patients who were depressed do not worsen in response to l-TRP depletion. Patients who were depressed and without thoughts of suicide who had been successfully treated with antidepressants, to the point of euthymia and discontinuation of medication, were more resistant to the mood-altering effects of l-TRP depletion than patients with recent remission (Leyton et al., 1997). Tryptophan depletion has been shown, with $[^{15}O]H_2O$ PET, to cause diminished neural activity in the ventral anterior cingulate, orbitofrontal cortex, and caudate nucleus in recently remitted patients who were depressed (Smith et al., 1999). A subsequent PET study using $[^{18}F]$fluorodeoxyglucose (FDG) found similar reductions in metabolism in orbital frontal cortex, ventral striatum, cingulate cortex, and thalamus (Neumeister et al., 2004). However, this study did not identify differences in cerebral metabolism between those patients who did or did not have a return of depressive symptoms, suggesting that the abnormal metabolism may reflect a trait abnormality associated with major depression. More recently, serum concentrations of brain-derived neurotrophic factor (BDNF) have been shown to differ between patients who were depressed and controls exposed to l-TRP depletion, with normal controls demonstrating an increase in BDNF, but patients who were depressed showing no such change (Neumeister et al., 2005). Brain-derived neurotrophic factor has been shown to be crucial for the normal function of serotonergic and neurotrophic systems. Taken together, these findings suggest that l-TRP availability may be decreased in some patients who are depressed, leading to decreased serotonin synthesis in the CNS. Moreover, available l-TRP and, by extension, CNS serotonin likely plays a role in the treatment response to antidepressants, in particular for the SSRIs.

Additional evidence for dysfunction of presynaptic serotonergic neurons in major depression is provided by a number of different neuroendocrine challenge paradigms. Prolactin is released from the anterior pituitary gland upon activation of 5HT-2a and -2c receptors (Coccaro et al., 1996). Intravenous infusion of tryptophan causes an acute increase in serotonergic transmission associated with an increase in serum prolactin levels (Price et al., 1991). Patients who were depressed demonstrate a blunted prolactin response to l-TRP infusion compared to controls (Cappiello et al., 1996). The appetite suppressant fenfluramine causes a rapid release of serotonin from presynaptic neurons and increases serum prolactin levels. Patients who were depressed have been shown repeatedly to exhibit a blunted prolactin response to fenfluramine challenge (Mitchell and Smythe, 1990; O'Keane and Dinan, 1991; Malone et al., 1993; Shapira et al., 1993), though discrepant reports have appeared (Kavoussi et al., 1998). There is evidence that the blunted prolactin response may be a marker of suicidality or impulsivity and not depression (Correa et al., 2000). Studies of the effect of antidepressant treatment on prolactin response to fenfluramine challenge are highly conflicting, with increases, decreases, and no changes reported in the literature (Kavoussi et al., 1999; Dulchin et al., 2001). A novel variation of the fenfluramine challenge test measures cerebral glucose utilization with PET imaging instead of prolactin release in response to the fenfluramine challenge (Mann et al., 1996). Consistent with the prolactin results obtained, patients who were depressed displayed reduced cerebral glucose use in response to fenfluramine challenge. Interestingly, prolactin responses to fenfluramine challenge are also blunted in bipolar patients who are acutely manic (Thakore et al., 1996). This has been interpreted as indicative of a general serotonergic dysfunction in mood disorders, in BPD and in unipolar depression.

Another neuroendocrine assay of presynaptic serotonergic function uses sumatriptan as the challenge agent. This antimigraine compound is an agonist at the 5-HT_{1D} receptor, the nerve terminal autoreceptor on serotonergic neurons. Sumatriptan administration results in an increase in plasma GH concentrations. The GH response to sumatriptan in patients who are depressed is blunted compared to that of normal controls or patients with bipolar mania (Yatham et al., 1997; Cleare et al., 1998). A similar result has been reported for patients with melancholic depression challenged with the related compound zolmitriptan (Whale et al., 2001). Citalopram, an SSRI, which is a specific serotonin transporter antagonist, has also been used as a challenge agent to study presynaptic serotonergic function. Patients who were depressed had a significantly blunted prolactin response to a challenge dose of citalopram compared with controls (Kapitany et al., 1999).

That the abnormalities in response to the neuroendocrine challenge tests observed in patients who are depressed are caused by dysfunction of presynaptic serotonergic neurons is suggested by the results of the m-chlorophenylpiperazine (m-CPP) challenge test (Anand et al., 1994). This agent has mixed pharmacodynamic actions at postsynaptic serotonin receptors, principally the 5-HT_2 receptor family. There are no differences in neuroendocrine measures between patients who were depressed and controls in response to intravenous infusion of m-CPP (Anand et al., 1994; Price et al., 1997). Concatenation of the results of these many neuroendocrine challenge assays is consistent with and very supportive of the hypothesis that major depression is characterized by significant dysfunction of presynaptic serotonergic neurons.

Synaptic activity of serotonergic neurons frequently has been estimated by measuring the CSF concentration of the major serotonin metabolite 5-hydroxyindoleacetic acid (5-HIAA). Although consistent evidence for serotonergic hypofunction in depression in general has not emerged from these studies, the most reproducible finding is of reduced CSF 5-HIAA concentrations, presumably a measure of reduced CNS serotonergic function, in patients who attempted or committed suicide. The finding of low CSF 5-HIAA concentrations is particularly robust in patients who used violent means to commit suicide (Asberg et al., 1976; Gibbons and Davis, 1986; Roy et al., 1989), independent of psychiatric diagnosis (Traskman et al., 1981; Van Praag, 1982). There are also reports linking low CSF 5-HIAA concentrations with poor impulse control in violent criminal offenders and arsonists (Virkkunen et al., 1994; Virkkunen et al., 1995; Virkkunen et al., 1996). In all of these patient samples, the strongest relationship appears to be between low CSF 5-HIAA concentrations and violent, impulsive behavior (Linnoila and Virkkunen, 1992). This behavioral spectrum is quite distinct from the constellation of symptoms that constitute major depression, but it does appear to intersect with the depressive syndrome. One hypothesis is that depression in combination with low CNS serotonin availability, as demonstrated by low CSF 5-HIAA concentrations, is a prominent risk factor for impulsive and highly lethal suicide attempts. A corollary to this hypothesis is that there may be separate pathological processes that distinguish depression and suicide, and that suicide may be associated with a distinct pathophysiology.

Another measure of presynaptic serotonergic function that has received a great deal of research attention is serotonin transporter (SERT) binding. In the CNS, the SERT is expressed exclusively in serotonergic perikarya and subsequently transported to and localized on the 5HT-containing nerve terminals. Serotonergic neurotransmission is terminated by the SERT, which clears 5-HT from the synapse, pumping it back into the presynaptic terminal. The efficiency or availability of this transporter directly controls the concentration of 5-HT in the synapse. The hypothesis that has emerged is that changes in the activity state or number of SERT sites may play a preeminent role in major depression (Owens and Nemeroff, 1994, 1997). The SERT is also expressed on platelets, where it concentrates 5-HT from plasma, eventually in secretory granules. The SERT is transcribed from a single copy gene, and therefore the transporters expressed on platelets and in the CNS are identical. Because the SERT is identical in both cell types, and because blood platelets are much easier to study than CNS neurons, platelet SERT indices have been exploited as surrogate measures of CNS SERT function. The transport kinetics of serotonin in human cortical brain synaptosomes and platelets have been shown to be highly correlated, suggesting that studies of platelet SERT do reflect CNS SERT function (Rausch et al., 2005). The underlying (and not yet proven) assumption is that the SERT gene is subject to identical regulation in both tissues so that changes measured in platelets mirror changes in the CNS (Lesch et al., 1993).

The concentration of the SERT on platelets has been measured with [^{3}H]-imipramine binding and [^{3}H]-paroxetine binding. Although there have been some discrepant reports that failed to detect differences in the B_{max} for the platelet SERT between patients who are depressed and controls, the vast majority report a decrease in the platelet SERT B_{max} between patients who were depressed and a variety of comparison groups (Briley et al., 1979; Briley et al., 1980). A comprehensive meta-analysis of the worldwide platelet [^{3}H]-imipramine binding data identified 70 independent studies that included data on approximately 1900 patients who were depressed and slightly fewer controls (Ellis and Salmond, 1994). The meta-analysis revealed that the lower B_{max} value for platelet [^{3}H]-imipramine binding is a highly significant finding in major depression. This appears to be a state marker for depression because the B_{max} tends to normalize with treatment and syndrome resolution.

The B_{max} of the SERT has also been measured in postmortem brain tissue of victims of suicide. These studies are not nearly as consistent as the platelet studies; some reported decreased B_{max} for the SERT in the frontal cortices of victims of suicide when compared to controls, and others reported no such differences (Perry et al., 1983; Gross-Isseroff et al., 1989; Lawrence et al., 1990; Leake et al., 1991; Bligh-Glover et al., 2000). There are methodological issues related to these postmortem studies. The first is that the number of patients is low, especially compared to the platelet data; the second is that the postmortem processing of the tissue varies between different centers and studies; and the third is that different analytical techniques were employed by the different research groups.

PET and single photon emission computed tomography (SPECT) ligands relatively specific for the SERT have been used to assess SERT binding in patients with major depression. In one study, drug-free patients who were depressed were compared to healthy controls using the SERT ligand [^{123}I]-β-CIT, imaged with SPECT (Malison et al., 1998). This study revealed a significant reduction in SERT binding in the raphé nuclei in the patients who were depressed compared to the controls. This is interpreted as indicating fewer SERT sites in the brain stem of the patients who were depressed. Interestingly, there were no differences in platelet [^{3}H]-paroxetine binding between the depressed and control groups, suggesting that central and peripheral regulation of the SERT may in fact be different.

A tri-allelic functional genetic polymorphism has been described in the promoter of the SERT gene (Heils et al., 1996; Hu et al., 2004). Initially only two alleles, the short (S) and long (L) forms, were described, though subsequent work identified two functional variants of the long form: L_A, which results in greater SERT experession than the S form, and L_G, which expresses the SERT comparably to the S form. Differences in promoter strength could be one molecular mechanism that causes differences in the SERT B_{max}. Association and linkage studies have produced contradictory results, with some reporting an overrepresentation of the S allele in patients who are depressed and others finding no association between SERT promoter alleles and depression. This inconsistency may stem partly from variations in ethnicity between sampled populations, as the effects of SERT promoter polymorphism on measures of CNS serotonin function have been shown to vary by race in healthy patients (Williams et al., 2003). Positron emission tomography studies of SERT density have found a lower binding potential in patients who were depressed versus controls (Malison et al., 1998; Parsey, Hastings, et al., 2006) though correlations with SERT promoter polymorphisms have not been made, and one study found no difference (Meyer et al., 2004). Similarly, postmortem analyses have found that the SERT B_{max} in the CNS is decreased in depression, but independently from promoter genotype (Mann et al., 2000; Ordway, 2000).

The most consistent finding from studies of the SERT polymorphisms is that the S and L_G forms convey increased risk for the development of major depression following stressful life events (Caspi et al., 2003; Kendler et al., 2005; Zalsman et al., 2006). In fact of 20 studies identified, 17 confirmed the finding (Zammit and Owen, 2006). Healthy S-allele carriers have been found by functional magnetic resonance imaging (MRI) to have increased amygdala reactivity to fearful or angry facial expressions, and to have impaired functional connectivity between the amygdala and anterior cingulate regulatory regions, which may represent a risk factor for depression in the face of stress (Hariri et al., 2005; Pezawas et al., 2005). Patients in remission from major depression who carry at least one copy of the L_A allele have greater worsening of depressive symptoms, and increased cortical metabolism as assessed by PET in the amygdala, subgenual cingulate cortex, and hippocampus, than do patients with two copies of the S allele when undergoing tryptophan depletion (Neumeister et al., 2006).

There are at least 14 distinct 5-HT receptor subtypes (Glennon and Dukat, 1995; Saxena, 1995). The advent of low-stringency polymerase chain reaction (PCR) cloning strategies has revealed the existence of a large number of previously unknown and unpredicted 5-HT receptors. These receptors are grouped into seven different families based on their molecular structure, which also determines their other characteristics such as ligand affinities, second-messenger coupling, and so on. The 5-HT_3 receptor is a ligand-gated ion channel, whereas all of the others are seven-transmembrane, G protein–coupled receptors. Prior to the discovery of the "new" serotonin receptors, the 5-HT_{1A} and 5-HT_{2A} receptors were the subject of the majority of 5-HT receptor research in depression. The contribution of the newly discovered 5-HT receptors to the pathophysiology of depression and the mechanism of action of antidepressants have yet to be determined.

The 5-HT_{2A} receptor is positively coupled to phospholipase C and the mobilization of intracellular calcium, whereas the 5-HT_{1A} receptor is negatively coupled to adenylate cyclase (AC) activity. The 5-HT_{1A} and 5-HT_{2A} receptors are postsynaptic in location, though the 5-HT_{1A} receptor is the predominant 5-HT receptor on the serotonergic perikarya in the raphé nuclei, therefore controlling the firing rate of the serotonergic neurons. The 5-HT_{2A} receptor is located on a number of different cell types in the CNS, on platelets, smooth muscle cells, cells in the immune system, skin fibroblasts, and a number of other peripheral cell types. The 5-HT_{1A} receptor is found predominantly in the CNS but also on lymphocytes in the periphery. The promoter region of the gene for the 5-HT_{1A} receptor has a functional single nucleotide polymorphism (SNP) (C[-1019]G 5-HT_{1A}), in which a guanine (G) is substituted for a cytosine (C) residue. The G allele results in greater 5-HT_{1A} autoreceptor expression and consequently greater inhibition of basal raphé neuronal activity (Lemonde et al., 2003). The G allele has been reported to be twice as frequent in patients who were depressed versus controls, and 4 times more common in persons who completed suicide. Individuals with a G/G genotype at this polymorphism have been shown to exhibit increased expression of 5-HT_{1A} autoreceptors (Parsey, Oquendo, et al., 2006)

The platelet 5-HT_{2A} receptor has been the focus of considerable scrutiny in depression, with at least 12 independent studies published in which the B_{max} for the platelet 5-HT_{2A} receptor in major depression was measured (Biegon et al., 1987; Cowen et al., 1987; Arora and Meltzer, 1989a; Biegon, Essar, et al., 1990; Biegon, Grinspoon, et al., 1990; Pandey et al., 1990, 1995; Mann et al., 1992; Arora and Meltzer, 1993; McBride et al., 1994; Hrdina et al., 1995, 1997; Sheline et al., 1995). One of these studies reported no difference between patients who were depressed and controls. The others all reported a significant increase in the B_{max} for the platelet 5-HT_{2A} receptor for patients who were depressed or suicidal. Several of the studies reported that the increased B_{max} is related to suicidality, while others suggested that it is related to the syndromal diagnosis of depression. Initially, this finding was considered a state marker of depression because the B_{max} was reported to normalize with recovery from depression. One group has, however, reported that the increased B_{max} does not normalize with successful treatment, raising the question of whether this may be a trait marker for vulnerability to depression (Bakish et al., 1997). There are several other studies that have inferred changes in the B_{max} for the platelet 5-HT_{2A} receptor by a number of secondary measures of receptor function including platelet shape change, phosphatidyl inositol (PI) hydrolysis, and calcium mobilization.

There are at least 10 publications in which the B_{max} for the 5-HT_{2A} receptor has been measured in the CNS of victims of suicide (Owen et al., 1983; Stanley and Mann, 1983; Crow et al., 1984; Mann et al., 1986; Owen et al., 1986; McKeith et al., 1987; Cheetham et al., 1988; Arora and Meltzer, 1989b; Arango et al., 1990; Hrdina et al., 1993; Lowther et al., 1994). The results of these analyses are considerably more variable than those of the platelet studies. Approximately half of the publications report an increase in the B_{max} for the 5-HT_{2A} receptor in the brains of victims of suicide, and the other half report no difference. As in other postmortem studies, the variability in these results could be due to a number of technical and artifactual factors. Based on postmortem analysis, it is not clear whether the B_{max} for the 5-HT_{2A} receptor is altered in the CNS of individuals who were depressed.

The 5-HT_{1A} receptor controls the rate of firing of the serotonergic neurons and hence the availability of 5-HT in the synapse. Changes in the numbers or responsiveness of the 5-HT_{1A} receptor might affect the firing rate of the serotonergic neurons, which in turn could lead to symptoms of depression. There is at least one report of increased B_{max} of the 5-HT_{1A} receptor in the frontal cortex of patients who committed suicide via nonviolent means versus those who used violent means or nonsuicidal controls (Matsubara et al., 1991). Discordant reports have also appeared (Cheetham et al., 1990). In one postmortem study of victims of suicide with a "firm" retrospective diagnosis of depression, no differences in 5-HT_{1A} B_{max} were detected in all brain regions analyzed, and there was no relationship between B_{max} and method of suicide or antidepressant exposure (Lowther et al., 1997).

The development of PET ligands specific to the 5-HT_{1A} and 5-HT_{2A} receptors has allowed these receptors to be studied in vivo (Fujita et al., 2000). The ligand [^{11}C] WAY100635 has been consistently used to image the 5-HT_{1A} receptor in PET studies. Two studies comparing patients with familial depression versus controls have reported reduced 5-HT_{1A} receptor binding in midbrain raphé, frontal cortex, and mesiotemporal cortex (Drevets et al., 1999; Sargent et al., 2000). More recently, patients with temporal lobe epilepsy (TLE) and major depression were found to have a greater reduction in 5-HT_{1A} receptor binding in limbic regions than patients with TLE without depression (Hasler et al., 2007). However, another study found significantly greater 5-HT_{1A} binding in antidepressant naïve patients who were depressed versus controls, but previously treated patients who were depressed did not differ from controls (Parsey, Oquendo, et al., 2006). Previously treated men remitted from major depression were found to have a persistent 17% decrease in cortical 5-HT_{1A} receptor binding potential compared to controls in another study (Bhagwagar et al., 2004). Taken together, these findings leave unresolved the question of whether reduced 5-HT_{1A} expression is a trait marker for major depression but do provide some support for the theory that antidepressant use may have long-term effects on the 5-HT_{1A} receptor.

The results with 5-HT_{2A} specific ligands are also variable, likely due to methodological variability in the specific radioligand employed and use of psychotropic medications in temporal proximity to the scanning. One study compared 14 patients who were depressed to 19 healthy controls and found no differences in ligand binding between the two groups (Meyer et al., 1999). These investigators attempted to study the 5-HT_{2A} receptor in depression, independent of suicidality, by excluding patients with a history of suicide attempt within 5 years of the study. In another study of 8 drug-free patients who were depressed compared to 22 healthy controls, there was a significant reduction in the 5-HT_{2A} binding in the right posterolateral orbitofrontal cortex and anterior cingulate cortex of the patients who were depressed (Biver et al., 1997). A study of 20 unmedicated patients who were depressed compared to 20 healthy controls yielded a similar result, that is, reduced 5-HT_{2A} binding in frontal, temporal, parietal, and occipital cortex (Yatham et al., 2000). In a PET study of patients with late-life depression, there was no difference between those who were depressed and controls in 5-HT_{2A} labeling, but there was a dramatic decrease in 5-HT_{2A} signal in patients with dementia (Meltzer et al., 1999). The largest study to date, comparing 46 patients who were depressed with 29 controls, found patients who were depressed to have 29% lower 5-HT_{2A} receptor binding in the hippocampus, and nonsignificantly reduced binding in several other brain regions (Mintun et al., 2004). Recently, increased 5-HT_{2A} receptor binding in frontal, parietal, and occipital cortical regions was demonstrated using PET in 20 unmedicated patients remitted from a major depressive episode compared to 20 controls (Bhagwagar et al., 2006).

Results of PET studies of 5-HT_{2A} binding in patients who were depressed who had been treated with antidepressants have been even more variable. In a study of patients who were depressed treated with the TCA clomipramine, there was a significant reduction in cortical 5-HT_{2A} binding density (Attar-Levy et al., 1999). These authors reported no relationship between measures of depression severity and the intensity of labeling of the 5-HT_{2A} receptor in the treated group. A similar result was reported in a study of 10 patients who were depressed treated with desipramine (Yatham et al., 1999). In this study, 8 of the 10 patients exhibited a significant antidepressant response, as revealed by a 50% reduction in the Hamilton Depression Rating Scale (HDRS), but all of the patients demonstrated a reduction in 5-HT_{2A} binding bilaterally throughout the cortex, regardless of the antidepressant response. However, as in the previous study, there was no relationship between measures of depression severity and change in 5-HT_{2A} labeling. The opposite result has also been reported (Massou et al., 1997). In this study of six patients who were depressed treated with SSRIs, there was an increase in cortical 5-HT_{2A} labeling compared to untreated patients who were depressed. Clearly, no firm conclusions can be drawn from these results about the impact of antidepressants on CNS 5-HT_{2A} binding kinetics.

There is an abundance of data implicating the serotonergic system in the pathophysiology of major depression. Although one specific causal pathological change has not been found, multiple perturbations of the serotonergic system, pre- and postsynaptic, have been documented in major depression. Many different antidepressants have pharmacodynamic targets within the serotonergic system, and many, if not all, act in part by modifying the activity of serotonergic circuits. Future research into the function of 5-HT systems will surely address the molecular mechanisms that result in the observed changes in depression and in response to antidepressants.

Dopamine

Historically, dopamine (DA) has not received the attention accorded 5-HT and NE in theories of the pathophysiology of depression. The DA systems were largely considered to have little or no importance in the biology of mood disorders, with the exception of a central role in psychotic depression (Schatzberg et al., 1985). Several lines of evidence are consistent with a role for DA systems in the pathophysiology of depression, including evidence of altered DA function in patients who are depressed, pathological mood symptoms in patients suffering from other diseases that affect DA systems (principally Parkinson's disease), and the effects on mood of psychopharmacological agents that alter DA neurotransmission (Dunlop and Nemeroff, 2007). Moreover, some antidepressants appear to enhance and may even predominantly act via a dopaminergic action. Key findings implicating dysfunction of the dopaminergic system in depression are summarized in Table 30.4.

Dopamine neurotransmission is frequently estimated by measuring its major metabolite, homovanillic acid (HVA), in bodily fluids. The concentration of HVA is directly related to the extracellular concentration of DA, and therefore the concentration of HVA is thought to reflect the activity state of presynaptic DA neurons. The majority of studies examining CSF HVA concentrations in major depression have found lower concentrations in patients who are depressed compared to controls, particularly in patients with psychomotor retardation (Kapur and Mann, 1992). Careful matching for age between patients who are depressed and controls is necessary as there is a functionally significant and progressive loss of DA activity with advancing age, largely due to a loss of DA neurons. In a unique study employing internal jugular venous sampling, medication-free treatment-resistant patients with unipolar depression were found to exhibit reduced concentrations of NE and its metabolites, and HVA, but not 5-HIAA, compared to healthy controls (Lambert et al., 2000). In this study, estimates of brain DA turnover were inversely correlated with the severity of depressive illness.

Low CSF HVA concentrations are not specific to major depression because this finding has also been reported in Parkinson's and Alzheimer's diseases (Van Praag et al., 1975; Wolfe et al., 1990). There are also reports of increased CSF HVA in patients who are agitated and manic (Willner, 1983), providing further evidence that CSF HVA levels and hence DA neurotransmission may be more a marker for psychomotor activity than for mood state.

Dopamine metabolites are detectable in urine and have been measured in cohorts of patients who are depressed compared to various control groups. In one study of 28 patients who were depressed and 25 controls, the urinary concentration of 3,4-dihydroxyphenyl acetic acid (DOPAC), another DA metabolite, was significantly lower in the patients who were depressed compared to the controls (Roy et al., 1986). In another study in which the 24-hour urinary excretion of a number of DA metabolites was measured, patients with depression and a suicide attempt had lower DA metabolite concentrations than patients with depression and no suicide attempts (Roy et al., 1992).

TABLE 30.4 *Findings Implicating Dopaminergic Dysfunction in the Pathophysiology of Depression at Various Neuropharmacologic Levels of Action*

Level of Action	*Finding*	*Replicability*
Neurotransmitter storage	Long-term treatment with reserpine, which depletes monoamine stores, results in depressive symptoms in patients with a history of depression	++
	Depression comorbid with Parkinson's disease	+++
Neurotransmitter release	L-DOPA relieves mood symptoms in Parkinson's disease patients	++
Neurotransmitter reuptake	Stimulants (amphetamine, methylphenidate) elevate mood in depressed and nondepressed individuals	+++
	"Novel" antidepressants block dopamine reuptake; for example, nomifensine, amineptine	++
Neurotransmitter metabolism	MAOIs are effective antidepressants	+++
	Low CSF HVA in subgroups of depressed patients	+
	Increased CSF HVA in manic patients	++
	MAO-A levels elevated in depressed patients	+
Postsynaptic neurotransmitter receptors	Typical antipsychotics (D_2 antagonists) induce apathy, anhedonia, and avolition	++

CSF: cerebrospinal fluid; L-DOPA: L-dihydroxyphenylalanine; MAOI: monoamine oxidase inhibitor; HVA: homovanillic acid (dopamine metabolite).
Replication key: +: one or no replication studies; ++: several replication studies, +++: highly replicated by more than two research groups.

Another line of evidence that supports a role for DA system dysfunction in depressive syndromes is suggested by the mood symptoms that occur in patients with Parkinson's disease. The incidence of major depression in community samples of Parkinson's disease patients is 5%–10%, with an additional 10%–30% experiencing subsyndromal depressive symptoms (Tandberg et al., 1996). Depressive symptoms in these patients often precede the development of the physical manifestations of the disorder (Van Praag et al., 1975; Guze and Barrio, 1991). The symptoms of depression in patients with Parkinson's disease do not appear to be related to the severity of disability resulting from the disease itself (Murray, 1996). Treatment of patients with Parkinson's disease with L-dihydroxyphenylalanine (L-DOPA) is often associated with antidepressant effects that can precede the improvement in the physical symptoms of the disease (Murphy, 1972).

Results of functional neuroimaging studies of DA function in patients who are depressed have been informative, though the D_2 receptor binding studies in major depressive disorder (MDD) have been inconsistent (Table 30.2). Early studies examining striatal D_2 binding found elevated levels in inpatients who were depressed, either in whole group samples (D'haenen and Bossuyt, 1994; Shah et al., 1997), or when limited to a psychomotor retarded group (Ebert et al., 1996). Elevated D_2 receptor binding may reflect increased numbers of D_2 receptors in depression (possibly reflecting presynaptic hypofunction), an increase in affinity of the receptor for the ligand, or a decrease in availability of synaptic DA (which competes with the radiolabeled ligand, albeit weakly, for D_2 binding). Two later studies failed to confirm these findings, though one study used a nonhealthy control group and the other studied outpatients (Klimke et al., 1999; Parsey et al., 2001). A major confound across the studies was the medication status of the patients, as most were either on antidepressant therapy or had only a 7-day washout prior to the imaging procedure. Variability in the level of anxiety may also confound the results, as anxiety has been associated with reduced D_2 receptor expression (Schneier et al., 2000).

In the two studies comparing D_2 binding pre- and postantidepressant treatment for depression, clinical improvement was noted with either an increase or decrease in D_2 receptor binding, perhaps due to the differing mechanism of action of the drugs employed (Ebert et al., 1996; Klimke et al., 1999). Studies of dopamine transporter (DAT) expression have also found conflicting results, though the most comprehensive PET study observed reduced DAT binding in depression (Meyer et al., 2001). In a PET study assessing DA neuronal function by measuring [^{18}F]-fluoro-DOPA uptake in the striatum, patients who were depressed with psychomotor retardation exhibited reduced striatal uptake of the radioligand compared to inpatients who were anxious and depressed and healthy volunteers (Martinot et al., 2001).

Anhedonia is a core symptom of depression that has been posited to be particularly related to DA transmission because DA neurotransmission has long been known to be critical to a wide variety of pleasurable experiences and reward. Severity of depression has been found to correlate highly with the magnitude of reward experienced after oral d-amphetamine, which increases DA availability by a variety of mechanisms (Tremblay et al., 2002). In particular, medication-free patients who were severely depressed experienced greater reward than controls, while those with milder forms of depression did not differ from the control group. In an fMRI study extending these findings, patients who were severely depressed demonstrated a markedly greater behavioral response to the rewarding effects of the psychostimulant than controls, and had altered brain activation of the ventrolateral prefrontal cortex, orbitofrontal cortex, caudate, and putamen (Tremblay et al., 2005). Glucocorticoids selectively facilitate DA transmission in the nucleus accumbens, thereby providing a potential link between the findings of hypercortisolemia and altered reward experience in severe depression (Marinelli and Piazza, 2002).

Another important link between glucocorticoids and DA function may be present in psychotic depression. Increased DA neurotransmission is considered to be central to the production of psychotic symptoms in schizophrenia, stimulant-induced psychoses, and major depression with psychotic features. Patients with psychotic depression have increased serum levels of DA and HVA compared to patients with nonpsychotic depression (Devanand et al., 1985; Schatzberg et al., 1985). The increased levels of glucocorticoids routinely observed in psychotic depression may drive the increase in DA activity (Rothschild et al., 1984). This has led to the hypothesis that increased glucocorticoid secretion in patients who are depressed produces increased DA neurotransmission, which in turn leads to the development of psychotic symptoms (Schatzberg and Rothschild, 1992; Posener et al., 1999).

Results of neuroendocrine challenge tests have been used to explore DA dysfunction in depression. Apomorphine is an agonist at D_2/D_3 DA receptors and causes increased secretion of GH via binding to postsynaptic DA receptors in the arcuate nucleus of the hypothalamus. The majority of studies have found no difference in GH response to apomorphine between patients who were depressed and healthy controls (McPherson et al., 2003). Results from this paradigm in patients who were actively manic were equivocal and did not directly support the hypothesis of excessive DA activity in mania (Ansseau et al., 1987). The GH response to apomorphine also does not differ between subjects with panic disorder and controls. The apomorphine challenge test may be a marker for suicidality in patients who are depressed because there are reported differences in GH response between patients who are depressed who make suicide attempts or commit suicide and those with no history of suicide attempts (Pitchot et al., 2001a, 2001b).

Postmortem studies of the DA system in patients who are depressed are relatively few and have provided conflicting results. Dopamine concentrations in the brains of victims of suicide are unchanged compared to controls (Moses and Robins, 1975; Bowden, Cheetham, et al., 1997). In victims of suicide, HVA concentrations in the frontal cortex have been found to be elevated (Beskow et al., 1976; Ohmori et al., 1992), or unaltered (Crow et al., 1984), and unaltered in the basal ganglia (Beskow et al., 1976; Bowden, Cheetham, et al., 1997). Cerebrospinal fluid HVA concentrations from those who attempted suicide have been found to be lower than those of controls (Engstrom et al., 1999), but not different between those who were high- versus low-lethality attempters (Mann and Malone, 1997). Concentrations of DA metabolites in the caudate, putamen, and nucleus accumbens were reduced in antidepressant-free patients who were depressed who died by suicide compared to controls (Bowden, Theodorou, et al., 1997). A postmortem study comparing psychiatrically normal controls with patients who were depressed using immunohistochemical and autoradiographic methods found reduced DAT density and elevated D_2/D_3 receptor binding in the central and basal nuclei of the amygdala in the patients who were depressed (Klimek et al., 2002). A second study using different methods and larger brain regions found no difference in D_2 receptor number or affinity (Bowden, Theodorou, et al., 1997). No studies have reported a difference in D_1 receptor binding between patients who were depressed who died by suicide and controls.

The actions of a number of different drugs suggest that increasing DA transmission is associated with improvement in depressive symptoms. The psychostimulants d-amphetamine and methylphenidate increase DA release, with resultant increased energy, activation, and elevated mood. Although these drugs cause transient mood elevations in individuals who are depressed and euthymic (Jacobs and Silverstone, 1988; Little, 1988), they are ineffective as antidepressants, at least as monotherapy. They may be effective as adjuncts to SSRIs and other antidepressants in nonresponders (Fawcett and Busch, 1998). Several individual studies have found an inverse association between CSF HVA concentrations and the magnitude of clinical response to agents with relatively specific effects on DA, including L-DOPA, piribedil, and nomifensine (van Praag et al., 1975; Post et al., 1978; van Scheyen et al., 1977). The atypical antidepressants bupropion (Ascher et al., 1995) and amineptine (Garattini, 1997) have been suggested to be antagonists of the DA transporter, but in vitro and in vivo data on the former are not persuasive. Remarkably, the high potency of sertraline as a DA transporter antagonist has been largely overlooked (Owens et al., 1997a, 1997b). Pramipexole, a nonergot DA agonist used in the treatment of Parkinson's disease and restless legs syndrome, exhibits marked selectivity for D_2-like receptors, particularly the D_3 receptor. In a neuroimaging study of baboons, pramipexole reduced cerebral blood flow in the orbitofrontal cortex, subgenual anterior cingulate cortex, and insula, all regions thought to contribute significantly to mood regulation (Black et al., 2002). Pramipexole has demonstrated efficacy for depressive symptoms in two double-blind, placebo-controlled studies of patients with bipolar depression on mood stabilizer therapy (Goldberg et al., 2004; Zarate et al., 2004), and in a monotherapy study in unipolar major depression (Corrigan et al., 2000). Ropinirole, another D_2/D_3 agonist, has also demonstrated antidepressant efficacy (Cassano et al., 2005). In contrast, typical antipsychotic drugs are potent antagonists of multiple DA receptors. A syndrome that resembles depression often results from treatment with these agents, with symptoms that include anhedonia, anergia, and dysphoria (Belmaker and Wald, 1977).

GABA

Gamma (γ)-aminobutyric acid (GABA) is the predominant inhibitory neurotransmitter in the CNS, with GABAergic neurons constituting 20%–40% of all neurons in the cortex and more than three fourths of all striatal neurons (Hendry et al., 1987; Tepper et al., 2004). Most GABAergic cells in the brain are interneurons, with short axons that form synapses within a few hundred microns of their cell body, connecting different neurons together and coordinating neuronal activity within local brain regions. GABA neurons provide tonic inhibition of raphé nuclei neurons, and 5HT-containing neurons from the raphé project to the cortex and preferentially synapse on GABA interneurons (more so than pyramidal neurons), increasing their firing rate. Cerebrospinal fluid and plasma GABA concentrations have been demonstrated to be lower in patients who were depressed than controls, with persistence of low plasma GABA levels up to 4 years after remission, suggesting that low plasma GABA levels may be a trait marker for depression (Gold et al., 1980). Support for this hypothesis emerged from the finding that plasma GABA levels are lower in individuals who were not depressed who have a first-degree relative with a history of major depression than in those without such a family history (Bjork et al., 2001). The source of plasma GABA remains obscure and may not be the CNS. Moreover, recent studies employing magnetic resonance spectroscopy found that reduced cortical GABA concentrations present in the acutely depressed state resolved after successful treatment with medication or electro-convulsive therapy (ECT) (Sanacora et al., 2002, 2003; Hasler et al., 2005). Reductions in GABA concentrations are not specific to depression, having also been demonstrated in alcohol dependence and mania (Petty, 1994). Further evidence of reduced GABAergic tone in patients who are depressed is suggested by lower resting-state levels of cortical inhibition as assessed by transcranial magnetic stimulation (Bajbouj et al., 2006).

Neuropeptides

Many different peptide neurotransmitter systems have been scrutinized in major depression. In particular, those peptides that regulate the hypothalamic-pituitary-adrenal (HPA) and the hypothalamic-pituitary-thyroid (HPT) axes have been hypothesized to play a significant role in the pathophysiology of mood disorders (Plotsky et al., 1995). The changes in neuroendocrine function that have been repeatedly documented in major depression support the proposition that the peptide systems that regulate the neuroendocrine axes are intimately involved in depression and may even be one of the primary substrates in the pathophysiology of depression. Corticotropin-releasing factor (CRF), which regulates the activity of the HPA axis; somatostatin, which regulates the secretion of GH from somatotrophs; and thyrotropin-releasing hormone (TRH), which regulates the HPT axis, have all been intensively studied in mood disorders. Key findings implicating dysfunction of these three neuropeptide systems in depression are summarized in Table 30.5.

Corticotropin-releasing Factor

Corticotropin-releasing factor (CRF) is the major secretogogue controlling the release of adrenocorticotropic hormone (ACTH) from the corticotrophs in the anterior pituitary and is also a neurotransmitter in extrahypothalamic brain regions. There is considerable evidence that the extrahypothalamic CRF system orchestrates the stress responses, coordinating endocrine, autonomic, immune, and behavioral outputs. Given the global role of CRF in coordinating stress responsivity, hyperactivity of this system has been hypothesized to be central to the pathophysiology of depression (Nemeroff, 1996; Arborelius et al., 1999).

The CSF concentration of CRF in untreated patients who are depressed has been demonstrated to be increased compared to healthy controls in several studies (Hartline et al., 1996). Intracisternally collected CSF concentrations of CRF have been found to be elevated in victims of suicide, who presumably were suffering from depression at the time of death (Arato et al., 1989). Higher plasma concentrations of CRF have been reported in patients who were depressed compared to controls (Catalan et al., 1998). The increase in CRF in major depression appears to be due to up-regulated production and release because there is increased expression of the messenger ribonucleic acid (mRNA) that encodes CRF in the hypothalamus of victims of suicide

TABLE 30.5 *Findings Implicating Three Neuropeptide Systems in the Pathophysiology of Depression*

Neuropeptide	*Finding*	*Replicability*
Corticotrophin releasing factor (CRF)	Increased concentration in CSF of depressed patients	+++
	CSF level normalizes with treatment	++
	Increased CRF mRNA in postmortem brains of suicides	+
CRF receptors	Decreased B_{max} in postmortem brains of suicides	+
	Blunted ACTH release in response to CRF challenge	+++
	ACTH response normalizes with treatment	+
Somatostatin	Decreased CSF concentration in unipolar and bipolar depression	+++
	"State" marker, normalizes with treatment	++
	Not specific to depression; also decreased in Alzheimer's disease, Parkinson's disease, multiple sclerosis	++
Thyrotropin-releasing hormone (TRH)	Increased CSF concentration in depressed patients	++
	25%–30% of euthyroid depressed patients have blunted TSH response to TRH challenge	+++
	25%–30% of euthyroid depressed patients have abnormal T_3/T_4 levels	+

ACTH: adrenocorticotropic hormone; CSF: cerebral spinal fluid; TSH: thyroid stimulating hormone; T_3/T_4: thyroid hormones; mRNA: messenger ribonucleic acid.

Replication key: +: one or no replication studies; ++: several replication studies; +++: highly replicated by more than two research groups.

who were depressed (Raadsheer et al., 1995) and an increase in the number of CRF immunopositive neurons. Similar findings have been observed in other brain regions including the cerebral cortex and locus ceruleus (Bissette et al., 2003; Merali et al., 2004).

The CSF concentration of CRF has also been shown to be elevated in patients with anorexia nervosa (Kaye et al., 1987). In these patients, CSF CRF levels normalize with restoration of normal weight. The relationship, if any, between the regulation of CRF expression in depression and anorexia nervosa remains obscure. Two studies have reported elevated CSF CRF concentrations in patients with PTSD (Bremner et al., 1997; Baker et al., 1999). The increased CSF CRF levels appear to be relatively specific for depression, PTSD, and anorexia nervosa because they have not been observed in patients with schizophrenia, neurological disorders, dementia, or in those with mania, panic disorder, or other psychiatric diagnoses, unless they also suffered from comorbid depression.

The CSF CRF concentration in depression appears to be a state-dependent measure because the levels normalize after treatment with ECT, fluoxetine, and other antidepressants (Nemeroff et al., 1991; DeBellis et al., 1993). In a cohort of elderly individuals who were depressed and treated with amitriptyline, CSF CRF concentrations decreased in those who responded to treatment (Heuser et al., 1998). In a control cohort, also treated with amitriptyline, there was a nonsignificant decrease in CSF CRF concentrations. This suggests a general reduction of CRF secretion in response to antidepressant treatment. Normalization of the CSF CRF concentration may be predictive of long-term remission, while failure to normalize may predict early relapse (Banki et al., 1992).

In two studies, we observed decreased B_{max} values for CRF receptors in the frontal cortex of victims of suicide who were depressed (Nemeroff et al., 1988). This finding has been confirmed in an elegant study using sensitive polymerase chain reaction (PCR) methods to assess CRF-1 mRNA expression (Merali et al., 2006). However, there is one discrepant report of no differences in CRF receptor B_{max} values in depression (Hucks et al., 1997). In this study of victims of suicide with a "firm" antemortem diagnosis of depression, there were no differences in CRF receptor density, nor did exposure to antidepressants or method of suicide correlate with CRF receptor B_{max}.

One interpretation of the finding of decreased CRF receptor B_{max} is down-regulation of CRF receptors in response to the chronic hypersecretion of CRF in depression. Concordant with this are results of the CRF stimulation test, in which the ACTH response to a standard intravenous dose of CRF is measured. In patients who are depressed, there is blunting of the ACTH response to intravenously administered CRF compared to controls (Holsboer et al., 1987; E.A. Young et al., 1990). The ACTH response to CRF challenge in patients who are depressed has been reported to normalize with treatment and syndrome resolution (Amsterdam et al., 1988). More recently a combination of the dexamethasone suppression test (DST) and the CRF stimulation test, the so-called Dex-CRF test, has been developed and is arguably the most sensitive measure of the HPA axis activity (von Bardeleben and Holsboer, 1989). It is markedly abnormal in many patients who are depressed.

Based on the CRF hypersecretion model, antagonists of the CRF_1 receptor subtype have been scrutinized as potential antidepressants. Proof-of-concept studies suggest that blocking this receptor does relieve symptoms of depression (Zobel et al., 2001). These agents do demonstrate an antidepressant profile in animal models.

A confluence of data, neurochemical, postmortem, and pharmacological, is concordant with the CRF hypersecretion hypothesis of major depression. What remains obscure is whether the CRF system is subject to a higher level of regulation that is also altered in depression, by 5-HT or NE systems, for example, or whether the dysfunction of the CRF system is the primary pathophysiological alteration in major depression.

Somatostatin and the Growth Hormone Axis

Somatostatin is a tetradecapeptide that inhibits the secretion of GH from the anterior pituitary. This peptide is also referred to as GH-release inhibiting hormone (GHRF) or somatotropin release-inhibiting factor (SRIF). Like CRF, SRIF has been clearly demonstrated to be a neurotransmitter, with a heterogeneous distribution outside of the hypothalamus. At least four different SRIF receptor subtypes have been cloned, with overlapping affinities and effector couplings. Somatostatin has been shown to affect sleep, ingestive behaviors, activity state, memory and cognition, and nociception. Growth hormone secretion is blunted in major depression in the clonidine, sumatriptan/zolmitriptan, and apomorphine challenge assays. These are probes of the NE, 5-HT, and DA systems, respectively, which suggests possible dysfunction of the somatostatin–GH axis in major depression, revealed by each of these neuroendocrine challenge assays. The GH response to SRIF is also blunted in patients who are depressed in most but not all studies. The GH response to SRIF is blunted in children who are depressed and in children at high risk for depression due to familial loading, suggestive of a trait marker (Birmaher et al., 2000; Dahl et al., 2000).

The CSF concentration of SRIF is decreased in major depression (Gerner and Yamada, 1982; Rubinow et al., 1983; Bissette et al., 1986; Rubinow, 1986). Levels of CSF SRIF are decreased in unipolar depression and in BPD during the depressed phase of the illness. Levels of CSF SRIF appear to be a state marker of depression because they normalize with successful treatment and symptom resolution. This has been observed in patients with unipolar and bipolar depression. Concentrations of CSF SRIF are not altered in schizophrenia, anorexia nervosa, euthymic BPD, or remitted depression. Remarkably, CSF SRIF levels are also increased in patients with obsessive-compulsive disorder (Altemus et al., 1993).

The finding of decreased CSF somatostatin concentrations is not specific to major depression. The same finding has been reported in a number of neurological diseases without prominent comorbid psychiatric symptoms. Thus, decreased CSF SRIF levels have been reported in dementing diseases including Alzheimer's disease, Parkinson's disease, and multiple sclerosis. In contrast, increased levels of CSF SRIF have been reported in traumatic or inflammatory neurological processes including compression injuries, meningitis, and encephalopathies. Although a decreased CSF SRIF concentration represents a state-dependent marker of depression, it appears to be relatively nonspecific, as it occurs in a number of unrelated nonpsychiatric conditions. Whether the decreased somatostatin level plays a role in the pathophysiology of depression, or is an epiphenomenon of the generalized HPA dysfunction that has been hypothesized by some investigators to occur in depression, remains to be determined.

Hypothalamic-Pituitary-Thyroid Axis

The manifestations of hypothyroidism can appear indistinguishable from those of major depression, with symptoms of depressed mood, impaired cognition, and multiple neurovegetative symptoms in both conditions. For this reason, the HPT axis has been intensively scrutinized in major depression. Approximately 20%–30% of patients with major depression have discernible HPT dysfunction. Secretion of thyroid-stimulating hormone (TSH) from the anterior pituitary gland is primarily regulated by thyrotropin-releasing hormone (TRH), a tripeptide that is released into the hypothalamic-hypophyseal portal system from hypothalamic neurons that project to the median eminence. Thyroid-stimulating hormone induces the secretion of l-triiodothyronine (T_3) and thyroxine (T_4) from the thyroid gland.

As with other peptide neurotransmitters, the CSF concentration of TRH has been measured in patients with major depression. Two studies reported that the concentration of TRH was increased in patients who were depressed compared to neurological and nondepressed controls (Kirkegaard et al., 1979; Banki et al., 1988). A negative study has also appeared (Roy et al., 1994). The CSF concentration of TRH has been reported to be unaltered in Alzheimer's disease, anxiety disorders, and alcoholism. The CSF concentration of transthyretin has been reported to be decreased in major depression (Sullivan et al., 1999), and a recent replication of this finding found a strong inverse correlation between transthyretin levels and suicidal ideation (Sullivan et al., 2006). Transthyretin transports and distributes thyroid hormones in the CNS. Decreased availability of this molecule in the CNS could result in a hypometabolic state in the neurons of individuals who are affected. This finding could account for observations of "normal" concentrations of thyroid hormones in depression, as well as the utility of thyroid hormone augmentation in nonresponders to antidepressants. Decreased transthyretin would functionally result in hypothyroidism within the CNS.

A number of peripheral thyroid indices have been measured in major depression. Red blood cell T_3 uptake is increased in major depression, and changes in this marker in response to antidepressants may predict a further treatment response (Moreau et al., 2000). In another study, pretreatment plasma T_3 and T_4 levels did not correlate to Rush/Thase stage of treatment resistance (Joffe, 1999). In a naturalistic study of patients with unipolar depression treated by "clinician choice" to the point of remission, serum T_3 levels were inversely related to time to relapse after initial remission (Joffe and Marriott, 2000). Higher T_3 levels appear to be protective against relapse. Interestingly, treatment of patients who are severely depressed with the SSRI paroxetine was noted to cause an 11.2% reduction in circulating T_4, whereas 24 weeks of sertraline treatment in 15 inpatient women who were depressed increased T_3 levels by 24% but did not affect T_4 levels (Konig et al., 2000; Sagud et al., 2002).

The TRH stimulation test is generally considered to be one of the most sensitive measures of HPT axis function. In this test, plasma TSH concentrations are measured at baseline and at 30-minute intervals for at least 2 hours after a challenge dose of TRH. This test has been administered to a large number of patients who were depressed and controls in many independent studies (Kastin et al., 1972; Prange et al., 1972). Across all of these studies, 25%–30% of the patients who were depressed exhibit a blunted TSH response to TRH challenge. This is apparently not due to primary hyperthyroidism because these patients who were depressed were euthyroid at the time of assessment. In one study, patients were specifically identified as being depressed but having "high-normal" baseline circulating TSH levels (Kraus et al., 1997). In this particular cohort of patients who were depressed, 38% demonstrated exaggerated TSH secretion in response to TRH challenge. The magnitude of the TSH response was not related to the baseline TSH value. The authors of this study suggest that there may be a subset of patients who are depressed who are in fact hypothyroid, a condition that is revealed only by the TRH challenge assay. In a related study, 26% of patients who were depressed were reported to have abnormal concentrations of circulating thyroid hormones (T_3 and/or T_4), which normalized with treatment and syndrome resolution (Shelton et al., 1993).

One possible explanation for the blunted TSH response to TRH challenge is down-regulation of TRH receptors in the pituitary in response to increased secretion of TRH into the hypophyseal-portal circulation. This has been tested in a cohort of 15 patients who were depressed who had pretreatment measurement of CSF TRH followed by a TRH stimulation test (Frye et al., 1999). There was no relationship between CSF TRH levels and TSH response to TRH in these patients. These authors also reported no correlation between CSF TRH concentrations and severity of depression. However these results are in contrast to those of Adinoff et al. (1991), who found a very significant correlation between CSF TRH concentrations and the TSH response to TRH in patients who were alcoholic. The significance of alteration of the HPT axis in the pathogenesis of depression remains to be elucidated. Certainly, one could postulate a subtype of depression (or hypothyroidism) in which there was disruption of the HPT axis revealed only by the TRH challenge test. Whether this represents a distinct disease entity has not been determined, nor is it clear that the patients with depression and altered TRH challenge respond preferentially to any particular treatment regimen. Potentially relevant to these findings are studies that have demonstrated the efficacy of T_3 in accelerating the response to older antidepressants and in converting antidepressant partial responders into full responders (Altshuler et al., 2001; Aronson et al., 1996). Whether addition of T_3 improves the speed and rate of response with SSRIs remains uncertain. A placebo-controlled study with paroxetine found no benefit on outcome with T_3 supplementation (Appelhof et al., 2004), but a similar study combining sertraline with T_3 did show improved response and remission rates (Cooper-Kazaz et al., 2007).

Thyroid hormones may contribute to the biology of major depression through the effects of T_3 on serotonin function. T_3, alone and in combination with fluoxetine, reduces transcription of the 5-HT_{1A} and 5-HT_{1B} receptors (Lifschytz et al., 2006). Down-regulation of the 5-HT_{1A} autoreceptor may be an important mechanism of action of antidepressants. The ability of T_3 augmentation to enhance this down-regulation may provide benefits, in the speed and overall response, when used to augment an antidepressant.

One intriguing observation that suggests a role for HPT system dysfunction in major depression comes from the antidepressant actions of TRH. In two small studies reported by the same research group, TRH appeared to have antidepressant actions in patients with treatment-refractory depression (Callahan et al., 1997; Marangell et al., 1997). In one report, two patients responded to intravenous and intrathecal administration of TRH, though tolerance developed to the intravenous route. In a second study by the same group, eight patients with treatment-refractory depression were treated with intrathecal TRH in a double-blind trial. Five of the eight patients had a 50% or greater reduction in HDRS, but the responses were transient. These results are clearly preliminary, but they further support a role for the TRH system in the biology of major depression and may point the way to a novel treatment strategy.

CONCLUSIONS

Despite 40 years of concerted research, the primary neurochemical pathology of major depression has not been identified. Dysfunction of many different neurotransmitter systems has been documented in depression, yet no one system or one perturbation has clearly emerged as the fundamental pathology in major depression. Reconciling the clinical manifestations of depression with the described neurochemical manifestations of depressed patients is one of the great challenges facing psychiatric researchers in the future.

There is clearly a great deal of redundancy and functional reserve within the CNS, such that pathological changes that result in depression would be quickly and diffusely compensated for by other neurochemical systems. In fact, many of the neurochemical changes documented above could be manifestations of adaptive responses to depression and not at all related to the primary pathological process. Thus, it is not surprising that the primary defect in depression has not been identified. A disease such as major depression that manifests symptoms in many different neurobehavioral domains, including mood and emotion, cognition, perception, autonomic function, homeostatic function, and stress responsiveness, would be expected to cause disruption of the neurochemical systems that regulate these diverse processes.

There are many avenues for future research into the pathophysiology of major depression. With the emergence of functional neuroimaging modalities, the opportunity to study patients across the course of their illness is now available. The development of well-characterized and consistently acquired banks of postmortem tissues will further allow the study of the changes that major depression causes in the CNS. The other major intellectual resource that will illuminate the search for the etiopathology of depression is the rapidly evolving human genome initiative. As knowledge of the molecular genetics of the nervous system advances and new technologies such as high-density microarray systems become available, new insights into the function and dysfunction of the brain will increase our knowledge of the pathophysiology of major depression.

ACKNOWLEDGMENTS

Boadie W. Dunlop is supported by a K-12 grant from the National Institutes of Health (NIH) Center for Research Resources, K12 RR 017643. Charles B. Nemeroff is supported by NIH Grants MH-42088, MH-39415, MH–77083 and MH-69056, and MH-58922, an American Foundation for Suicide Prevention Distinguished Investigator Award, and a National Alliance for Research on Schizophrenia and Depression (NARSAD) Established Investigator Award.

REFERENCES

Adinoff, B., Nemeroff, C.B., et al. (1991) Inverse relationship between CSF TRH concentrations and the TSH response to TRH in abstinent alcohol-dependent patients. *Am. J. Psychiatry* 148: 1586–1588.

Altemus, M., Pigott, T., et al. (1993) CSF somatostatin in obsessive-compulsive disorder. *Am. J. Psychiatry* 150(3):460–464.

Altshuler, L.L., Bauer, M., et al. (2001) Does thyroid supplementation accelerate tricyclic antidepressant response? A review and meta-analysis of the literature. *Am. J. Psychiatry* 158:1617–1622.

Amsterdam, J.D., Maislin, G., et al. (1988) The oCRH test before and after clinical recovery from depression. *J. Affect. Disord.* 14: 213–222.

Amsterdam, J.D., Maislin, G., et al. (1989) Multiple hormone responses to clonidine administration in depressed patients and healthy volunteers. *Biol. Psychiatry* 26(3):265–278.

Anand, A., Charney, D.S., et al. (1994) Neuroendocrine and behavioral responses to intravenous m-chlorophenylpiperazine (m-CPP) in depressed patients and healthy comparison subjects. *Am. J. Psychiatry* 151(11):1626–1630.

Ansseau, M., von Frenckell, R., et al. (1987) Neuroendocrine evaluation of catecholamine neurotransmission in mania. *Psychiatry Res.* 22(3):193–206.

Appelhof, B.C., Brouwer, J.P., et al. (2004) Triiodothyronine addition to paroxetine in the treatment of major depressive disorder. *J. Clin. Endocrinol. Metab.* 89(12):6271–6276.

Arango, V., Ernsberger, P., et al. (1990) Autoradiographic demonstration of increased serotonin 5-HT2 and b-adrenergic receptor binding sites in the brain of suicide victims. *Arch. Gen. Psychiatry* 47:1038–1047.

Arango, V., Ernsberger, P., et al. (1993) Quantitative autoradiography of a1 and a2 adrenergic receptors in the cerebral cortex of controls and suicide victims. *Brain Res.* 630:271–282.

Arato, M., Banki, C.M., et al. (1989) Elevated CSF CRF in suicide victims. *Biol. Psychiatry* 25:355–359.

Arborelius, L., Owens, M.J., et al. (1999) The role of corticotropin-releasing factor in depression and anxiety disorders. *J. Endocrinol.* 160(1):1–12.

Aronson, R., Offman, H.J., et al. (1996) Triiodothyronine augmentation in the treatment of refractory depression. A meta-analysis. *Arch. Gen. Psychiatry* 53(9):842–848.

Arora, R.C., and Meltzer, H.Y. (1989a) Increased serotonin2 (5-HT2) receptor binding as measured by 3H-lysergic diethylamide (3H-LSD) in the blood platelets of depressed patients. *Life Sci.* 44: 725–734.

Arora, R.C., and Meltzer, H.Y. (1989b) Serotonergic measures in the brains of suicide victims: 5-HT_2 binding sites in the frontal cortex of suicide victims and control subjects. *Am. J. Psychiatry* 146(6):730–736.

Arora, R.C., and Meltzer, H.Y. (1993) $Serotonin_2$ receptor binding in blood platelets of schizophrenic patients. *Psychol. Res.* 47: 111–119.

Asberg, M., Traskman, L., et al. (1976) 5-HIAA in the cerebrospinal fluid: a biochemical suicide predictor? *Arch. Gen. Psychiatry* 33: 1193–1197.

Ascher, J.A., Cole, J.O., et al. (1995) Bupropion: a review of its mechanism of antidepressant activity. *J. Clin. Psychiatry* 56(9):395–401.

Attar-Levy, D., Martinot, J.L., et al. (1999) The cortical serotonin2 receptors studied with positron-emission tomography and [^{18}F]-setoperone during depressive illness and antidepressant treatment with clomipramine. *Biol. Psychiatry* 45(2):180–186.

Bajbouj, M., Lisanby, S.H., et al. (2006) Evidence for impaired cortical inhibition in patients with unipolar major depression. *Biol. Psychiatry* 59:395–400.

Baker, D.G., West, S.A., et al. (1999) Serial CSF corticotropin-releasing hormone levels and adrenocortical activity in combat veterans with posttraumatic stress disorder. *Am. J. Psychiatry* 156(4):585–588.

Bakish, D., Cavazzoni, P., et al. (1997) Effects of selective serotonin reuptake inhibitors on platelet serotonin parameters in major depressive disorders. *Biol. Psychiatry* 41(2):184–190.

Banarjee, S.P., Kung, L.S., et al. (1977) Development of ß adrenergic receptor subsensitivity by antidepressants. *Nature* 268:455–456.

Banki, C.M., Bissette, G., et al. (1988) Elevation of immunoreactive CSF TRH in depressed patients. *Am. J. Psychiatry* 145:1526–1531.

Banki, C.M., Karmacsi, L., et al. (1992) CSF corticotropin-releasing hormone and somatostatin in major depression: response to antidepressant treatment and relapse. *Eur. Neuropsychopharmacol.* 2: 107–113.

Belmaker, R.H., and Wald, D. (1977) Haloperidol in normals. *Br. J. Psychiatry* 131:222–223.

Benkelfat, C., Ellenbogen, M.A., et al. (1994) Mood-lowering effect of tryptophan depletion. Enhanced susceptibility in young men at genetic risk for major affective disorders. *Arch. Gen. Psychiatry* 51(9):687–697.

Berman, R.M., Narasimhan, M., et al. (1999) Transient depressive relapse induced by catecholamine depletion: potential phenotypic vulnerability marker? *Arch. Gen. Psychiatry* 56(5):395–403.

Beskow, J., Gotffries, C.G., et al. (1976) Determination of monoamine and monoamine metabolites in the human brain: postmortem studies in a group of suicides and in a control group. *Acta Psychiatr. Scand.* 53:7–20.

Bhagwagar, Z., Hinz, R., et al. (2006) Increased 5-HT_{2A} receptor binding in euthymic medication-free patients recovered from depression: a positron emission study with [^{11}C] MDL 100,907. *Am. J. Psychiatry* 163:1580–1587.

Bhagwagar, Z., Rabiner, E.A., et al. (2004) Persistent reduction in brain $serotonin_{1A}$ receptor binding in recovered depressed men measured by positron emission tomography with [^{11}C]WAY-100635. *Mol. Psychiatry* 9:386–392.

Biegon, A., Essar, N., et al. (1990) Serotonin 5-HT2 receptor binding on blood platelets as a state dependant marker in major affective disorder. *Psychopharmacology* 102:73–75.

Biegon, A., Grinspoon, A., et al. (1990) Increased serotonin 5-HT2 receptor binding on blood platelets of suicidal men. *Psychopharmacology* 100:165–167.

Biegon, A., Weizman, A., et al. (1987) Serotonin 5-HT2 receptor binding on blood platelets—a peripheral marker for depression? *Life Sci.* 41:2485–2492.

Birmaher, B., Dahl, R.E., et al. (2000) Growth hormone secretion in children and adolescents at high risk for major depressive disorder. *Arch. Gen. Psychiatry* 57(9):867–872.

Bissette, G., Klimek, V., et al. (2003) Elevated concentrations of CRF in the locus coeruleus of depressed subjects. *Neuropsychopharmacology* 28:1328–1335.

Bissette, G., Widerlov, E., et al. (1986) Alterations in cerebrospinal fluid somatostatin-like immunoreactivity in neuropsychiatric disorders. *Arch. Gen. Psychiatry* 43(12):1148–1151.

Biver, F., Wikler, D., et al. (1997) Serotonin 5-HT2 receptor imaging in major depression: focal changes in orbito-insular cortex. *Br. J. Psychiatry* 171:444–448.

Bjork, J.M., Moeller, F.G., et al. (2001) Plasma GABA levels correlate with aggressiveness in relatives of patients with unipolar depressive disorder. *Psychiatry Res.* 101:131–136.

Black, K.J., Hershey, T., et al. (2002) A possible substrate for dopamine-related changes in mood and behavior: prefrontal and limbic effects of a D3-preferring dopamine agonist. *Proc. Natl. Acad. Sci. USA* 99:17113–17118.

Bligh-Glover, W., Kolli, T.N., et al. (2000) The serotonin transporter in midbrain suicide victims with major depression. *Biol. Psychiatry* 47(12):1015–1024.

Bowden, C., Cheetham, S.C., et al. (1997) Reduced dopamine turnover in the basal ganglia of depressed suicides. *Brain Res.* 769:135–140.

Bowden, C., Theodorou, A.E., et al. (1997) Dopamine D1 and D2 receptor binding sites in brain samples form depressed suicides and controls. *Brain Res.* 752:227–233.

Bremner, J.D., Licinio, J., et al. (1997) Elevated CSF corticotropin-releasing factor concentrations in posttraumatic stress disorder. *Am. J. Psychiatry* 154(5):624–629.

Bremner, J.D., Vythilingam, M., et al. (2003) Regional brain metabolic correlates of alpha-methylparatyrosine-induced depressive symptoms: Implications for the neural circuitry of depression. *JAMA* 289:3125–3134.

Briley, M.S., Langer, S.Z., et al. (1980) Tritiated imipramine binding sites are decreased in platelets of untreated depressed patients. *Science* 209:303–305.

Briley, M.S., Raisman, R., et al. (1979) Human platelets possess high affinity binding sites for ^{3}H-imipramine. *Eur. J. Pharmacol.* 58: 347–348.

Bunney, W.E., and Davis, M. (1965) Norepinephrine in depressive reactions. *Arch. Gen. Psychiatry* 13:137–152.

Callahan, A.M., Frye, M.A., et al. (1997) Comparative antidepressant effects of intravenous and intrathecal thyrotropin-releasing hormone: confounding effects of tolerance and implications for therapeutics. *Biol. Psychiatry* 41(3):264–272.

Cameron, O.G., Abelson, J.L., et al., (2004) Anxious and depressive disorders and their comorbidity: effect on central nervous system noradrenergic function. *Biol. Psychiatry* 56:875–883.

Cappiello, A., Malison, R.T., et al. (1996) Seasonal variation in neuroendocrine and mood response to iv L-tryptophan in depressed patients and healthy subjects. *Neuropsychopharmacology* 15(5): 475–483.

Caspi, A., Sugden, K., et al. (2003) Influence of life stress on depression: moderation by a polymorphism in the 5-HTT gene. *Science* 301:386–389.

Cassano, P., Lattanzi, L., et al. (2005) Ropinirole in treatment-resistant depression: a 16-week pilot study. *Can. J. Psychiatry* 50:357–360.

Catalan, R., Gallart, J.M., et al. (1998) Plasma corticotropin-releasing factor in depressive disorders. *Biol. Psychiatry* 44(1):15–20.

Cheetham, S.C., Crompton, M., et al. (1988) Brain 5-HT2 receptor binding sites in depressed suicide victims. *Brain Res.* 443:272–280.

Cheetham, S.C., Crompton, M.R., et al. (1990) Brain 5-HT1 binding sites in depressed suicides. *Psychopharmacology* 102:544–548.

Cleare, A.J., Murray, R.M., et al. (1998) Abnormal 5-HT1D receptor function in major depression: a neuropharmacological challenge study using sumatriptan. *Psychol. Med.* 28(2):295–300.

Coccaro, E.F., Kavoussi, R.J., et al. (1996) 5-HT2a/2c receptor blockade by amesergide fully attenuates prolactin response to d-fenfluramine challenge in physically healthy human subjects. *Psychopharmacology (Berl)* 126:24–30.

Cooper-Kazaz, R., Apter, J.T., et al. (2007) Combined treatment with sertraline and liothyronine in major depression. *Arch. Gen. Psychiatry* 64:679–688.

Correa, H., Duval, F., et al. (2000) Prolactin response to D-fenfluramine and suicidal behavior in depressed patients. *Psychiatry Res.* 93(3):189–199.

Corrigan M.H., Denahan, A.Q., et al. (2000) Comparison of pramipexole, fluoxetine, and placebo in patients with major depression. *Depress. Anxiety* 11:58–65.

Cowen, P., Charig, E., et al. (1987) Platelet 5-HT receptor binding during depressive illness and tricyclic antidepressant treatment. *J. Affect. Disord.* 13:45–50.

Crow, T., Cross, A., et al. (1984) Neurotransmitter receptors and monoamine metabolites in the brains of patients with Alzheimer-type dementia and depression, and suicides. *Neuropharmacology* 23(12B):1561–1569.

D'haenen, H.A., and Bossuyt, A. (1994) Dopamine D2 receptors in depression measured with single photon emission computed tomography. *Biol. Psychiatry* 35(2):128–132.

Da Prada, M., Cesura, A.M., et al. (1988) Platelets as model for neurones. *Experentia* 44:115–126.

Dahl, R.E., Birmaher, B., et al. (2000) Low growth hormone response to growth hormone-releasing hormone in child depression. *Biol. Psychiatry* 48(10):981–988.

DeBellis, M.D., Gold, P.W., et al. (1993) Fluoxetine significantly reduces CSF CRH and AVP concentrations in patients with major depression. *Am. J. Psychiatry* 150:656–657.

Delgado, P.L., Charney, D.S., et al. (1990) Neuroendocrine and behavioral effects of dietary tryptophan restriction in healthy subjects. *Life Sci.* 45:2323–2332.

Delgado, P.L., Miller, H.L., et al. (1999) Tryptophan-depletion challenge in depressed patients treated with desipramine or fluoxetine: implications for the role of serotonin in the mechanism of antidepressant action. *Biol. Psychiatry* 46(2):212–220.

Delgado, P.L., Price, L.H., et al. (1994) Serotonin and the neurobiology of depression. Effects of tryptophan depletion in drug-free depressed patients. *Arch. Gen. Psychiatry* 51(11):865–874.

De Paermentier, F., Cheetham, S.C., et al. (1990) Brain beta-adrenoceptor binding sites in antidepressant-free depressed suicide victims. *Brain Res.* 525(1):71–77.

De Paermentier, F., Cheetham, S.C., et al. (1991) Brain beta-adrenoceptor binding sites in depressed suicide victims: effects of antidepressant treatment. *Psychopharmacology* 105(2):283–288.

Devanand, D.P., Bowers, M.B., et al. (1985) Elevated plasma homovanillic acid in depressed females with melancholia and psychosis. *Psychiatry Res.* 15(1):1–4.

Drevets, W.C., Frank, E., et al. (1999) PET imaging of serotonin 1A receptor binding in depression. *Biol. Psychiatry* 46(10):1375–1387.

Dulchin, M.C., Oquendo, M.A., et al. (2001) Prolactin response to dl-fenfluramine challenge before and after treatment with paroxetine. *Neuropsychopharmacology* 25:395–401.

Duman, R.S., and Nestler, E.J. (1995) Signal transduction pathways for catecholamine receptors. In: Bloom, F.E., and Kupfer, D.J., eds. *Psychopharmacology: The Fourth Generation of Progress.* New York: Raven Press, pp. 303–320.

Dunlop, B.W., and Nemeroff, C.B. (2007) The role of dopamine in the pathophysiology of depression. *Arch. Gen. Psychiatry* 64:327–337.

Ebert, D., Feistel, H., et al. (1996) Dopamine and depression – Striatal dopamine D2 receptor SPECT before and after antidepressant therapy. *Psychopharmacology* 126:91–94.

Ellenbogen, M.A., Young, S.N., et al. (1996) Mood response to acute tryptophan depletion in healthy volunteers: sex differences and temporal stability. *Neuropsychopharmacology* 15(5):465–474.

Ellis, P.M., and Salmond, C. (1994) Is platelet imipramine binding reduced in depression? A meta-analysis. *Biol. Psychiatry* 36:292–299.

Engstrom, G., Alling, C., et al. (1999) Reduced cerebrospinal HVA concentration and HVA/5-HIAA ratios in suicide attempters. *Eur. Neuropsychopharmacol.* 9:399–405.

Extein, I., Tallman, J., et al. (1979) Changes in lymphocyte beta-adrenergic receptors in depression and mania. *Psychiatry Res.* 1(2):191–197.

Fawcett, J., and Busch, K.A. (1998) Stimulants in psychiatry. In: Schatzberg, A.F., and Nemeroff, C.B., eds. *Textbook of Psychopharmacology*, 2nd ed. Washington, DC: American Psychiatric Press, pp. 503–522.

Frye, M.A., Dunn, R.T., et al. (1999) Lack of correlation between cerebrospinal fluid thyrotropin-releasing hormone (TRH) and TRH stimulated thyroid-stimulating hormone in patients with depression. *Biol. Psychiatry* 45(8):1049–1052.

Fujita, M., Charney, D.S., et al. (2000) Imaging serotonergic neurotransmission in depression: hippocampal pathophysiology may mirror global brain alterations. *Biol. Psychiatry* 48(8):801–812.

Garattini, S. (1997) Pharmacology of amineptine, an antidepressant agent acting on the dopaminergic system: a review. *Int. Clin. Psychopharmacol.* 12(Suppl 3):S15–S19.

Garcia-Sevilla, J.A., Padro, D., et al. (1990) Alpha 2-adrenoceptor-mediated inhibition of platelet adenylate cyclase and induction of aggregation in major depression. Effect of long-term cyclic antidepressant drug treatment. *Arch. Gen. Psychiatry* 47(2):125–132.

Garcia-Sevilla, J.A., Udina, C., et al. (1987) Enhanced binding of [^{3}H]-adrenaline to platelets of depressed patients with melacholia: effect of long-term clomipramine treatment. *Acta Psychiatr. Scand.* 75(2):150–157.

Gerner, R.H., and Yamada, T. (1982) Altered neuropeptide concentrations in cerebrospinal fluid of psychiatric patients. *Brain Res.* 238:298–302.

Gibbons, R.D., and Davis, J.M. (1986) Consistent evidence for a biological subtype of depression characterized by low CSF monoamine levels. *Acta Psychiatr. Scand.* 74:8–12.

Glennon, R.A., and Dukat, M. (1995) Serotonin receptor subtypes. In: Bloom, F.E., and Kupfer, D.J., eds. *Psychopharmacology: The Fourth Generation of Progress.* New York: Raven Press, pp. 415–429.

Glowinski, J., and Axelrod, J. (1966) Effects of drugs on the disposition of H-3-norepinephrine in the rat brain. *Pharmacol. Rev.* 18(1): 775–785.

Glowinski, J., Axelrod, J., et al. (1964) Physiological disposition of ^{3}H-norepinephrine in the developing rat. *J. Pharmacol. Exp. Ther.* 146:48–53.

Glowinski, J., and Iverson, L.L. (1966) Regional studies of catecholamines in the rat brain. *J. Neurochem.* 13:665–669.

Glowinski, J., Snyder, S., et al. (1966) Subcellular localization of H3-norepinephrine in the rat brain and the effect of drugs. *J. Pharmacol. Exp. Ther.* 152(2):282–292.

Gold, B.I., Bowers, M.B., et al. (1980) GABA levels in CSF of patients with psychiatric disorders. *Am. J. Psychiatry* 137:362–364.

Goldberg. J.F., Burdick, K.E., et al. (2004) Preliminary randomized, double-blind, placebo-controlled trial of pramipexole added to mood stabilizers for treatment-resistant bipolar depression. *Am. J. Psychiatry* 161:564–566.

Gross-Isseroff, R., Israeli, M., et al. (1989) Autoradiographic analysis of tritiated imipramine binding in the human brain postmortem: effects of suicide. *Arch. Gen. Psychiatry* 46:237–241.

Gurguis, G.N., Vo, S.P., et al. (1999) Platelet alpha2A-adrenoceptor function in major depression: Gi coupling, effects of imipramine and relationship to treatment outcome. *Psychiatry Res.* 89(2): 73–95.

Guze, B.H., and Barrio, J.C. (1991) The etiology of depression in Parkinson's disease patients. *Psychosomatics* 32:390–394.

Halaris, A. (1978) 3-Methoxy-4-hydroxyphenyl-glycol in manic psychosis. *Am. J. Psychiatry* 135:493–494.

Hariri, A.R., Drabant, E.M., et al. (2005) A susceptibility gene for affective disorders and the response of the human amygdala. *Arch. Gen. Psychiatry* 62:146–152.

Hartline, K.M., Owens, M.J., et al. (1996) Postmortem and cerebrospinal fluid studies of corticotropin-releasing factor in humans. *Ann. N. Y. Acad. Sci.* 780:96–105.

Hasler, G., Bonwetsch, R., et al. (2007) 5-HT1A receptor binding in temporal lobe epilepsy patients with and without major depression. *Biol. Psychiatry* 62(11):1258–1264..

Hasler, G., Neumeister A., et al. (2005) Normal prefrontal gamma-aminobutyric acid levels in remitted depressed subjects determined by proton magnetic resonance spectroscopy. *Biol. Psychiatry* 58:969–973.

Hayward, G., Goodwin, G.M., et al. (2005) Low-dose tryptophan depletion in recovered depressed patients induces changes in cognitive processing without depressive symptoms. *Biol. Psychiatry* 57:517–552.

Healy, D., Carney, P.A., et al. (1985) Peripheral adrenoceptors and serotonin receptors in depression. Changes associated with response to treatment with trazodone or amitriptyline. *J. Affect. Disord.* 9(3):285–296.

Heils, A., Teufel, A., et al. (1996) Allelic variation of human serotonin transporter gene expression. *J. Neurochem.* 66:2621–2624.

Hendry, S.H., Schwark, H.D., et al. (1987) Numbers and proportions of GABA-immunoreactive neurons in different areas of monkey cerebral cortex. *J. Neurosci.* 7:1503–1509.

Heninger, G.R., Delgado, P.L., et al. (1992) Tryptophan-deficient diet and amino acid drink deplete plasma tryptophan and induce a relapse of depression in susceptible patients. *J. Chem. Neuroanat.* 5:347–348.

Heninger, G.R., Delgado, P.L., et al. (1996) The revised monoamine theory of depression: a modulatory role for monoamines, based on new findings from monoamine depletion experiments in humans. *Pharmacopsychiatry* 29(1):2–11.

Heuser, I., Bissette, G., et al. (1998) Cerebrospinal fluid concentrations of corticotropin-releasing hormone, vasopressin, and somatostatin in depressed patients and healthy controls: response to amitriptyline treatment. *Depress. Anxiety* 8(2):71–79.

Hollister, L.E., David, K.L., et al. (1980) Subtypes of depression based on excretion of MHPG and response to nortriptyline. *Arch. Gen. Psychiatry* 37:1107–1110.

Holsboer, F., Gerken, A., et al. (1987) Blunted aldosterone and ACTH release after human corticotropin-releasing factor administration in depressed patients. *Am. J. Psychiatry* 144:229–231.

Hrdina, P.D., Bakish, M.D., et al. (1995) Serotonergic markers in platelets of patients with major depression: upregulation of 5-HT_2 receptors. *J. Psychiatr. Neurosci.* 20(1):11–19.

Hrdina, P.D., Bakish, D., et al. (1997) Platelet serotonergic indices in major depression: up-regulation of 5-HT_{2A} receptors unchanged by antidepressant treatment. *Psychiatry Res.* 66:73–85.

Hrdina, P.D., Demeter, E., et al. (1993) 5-HT uptake sites and 5-HT_2 receptors in brain of antidepressant-free suicide victims/depressives: increase in 5-HT_2 sites in cortex and amygdala. *Brain Res.* 614:37–44.

Hu, X., Zhu, G., et al. (2004) HTTLPR allele expression is codominant, correlating with gene effects on fMRI and SPECT imaging intermediate phenotypes, and behavior (abstract). *Biol. Psychiatry* 55 (Suppl 1):191S.

Hucks, D., Lowther, S., et al. (1997) Corticotropin-releasing factor binding sites in cortex of depressed suicides. *Psychopharmacology* 134(2):174–178.

Jacobs, D., and Silverstone, T. (1988) Dextroamphetamine arousal in human subjects as a model for mania. *Psychol. Med.* 16:323–329.

Joffe, R.T. (1999) Peripheral thyroid hormone levels in treatment resistant depression. *Biol. Psychiatry* 45(8):1053–1055.

Joffe, R.T., and Marriott, M. (2000) Thyroid hormone levels and recurrence of major depression. *Am. J. Psychiatry* 157:1689–1691.

Kapitany, T., Schindl, M., et al. (1999) The citalopram challenge test in patients with major depression and in healthy controls. *Psychiatry Res.* 88(2):75–88.

Kapur, S., and Mann, J.J. (1992) Role of the dopaminergic system in depression. *Biol. Psychiatry* 32:1–17.

Kastin, A.J., Ehrensing, R.H., et al. (1972) Improvement in mental depression with decreased thyrotropin response after administration of thyrotropin-releasing hormone. *Lancet* 2(780):740–742.

Kavoussi, R.J., Hauger, R.L., et al. (1999) Prolactin response to d-fenfluramine in major depression before and after treatment with serotonin reuptake inhibitors. *Biol. Psychiatry* 45(3):295–299.

Kavoussi, R.J., Kramer, J., et al. (1998) Prolactin response to D-fenfluramine in outpatients with major depression. *Psychiatry Res.* 79(3):199–205.

Kaye, W.H., Gwirtsman, H.E., et al. (1987) Elevated cerebrospinal fluid levels of immunoreactive corticotropin-releasing hormone in anorexia nervosa: relation to state of nutrition, adrenal function, and intensity of depression. *J. Clin. Endocrinol. Metab.* 64(2): 203–208.

Kelly, C.B., and Cooper, S.J. (1998) Plasma norepinephrine response to a cold pressor test in subtypes of depressive illness. *Psychiatry Res.* 81(1):39–50.

Kendler, K.S., Kuhn, J.W., et al. (2005) The interaction of stressful life events and a serotonin transporter polymorphism in the prediction of episodes of major depression. *Arch. Gen. Psychiatry* 62:529–535.

Kirkegaard, C., Faber, J., et al. (1979) Increased levels of TRH in cerebrospinal fluid from patients with endogenous depression. *Psychoneuroendocrinology* 4:227–235.

Klimek, V., Rajkowska, G., et al. (1999) Brain noradrenergic receptors in major depression and schizophrenia. *Neuropsychopharmacology* 21:69–81.

Klimek, V., Schenck, J.E., et al. (2002) Dopaminergic abnormalities in amygdaloid nucleus in major depression: a postmortem study. *Biol. Psychiatry* 52:740–748.

Klimke, A., Larisch, R., et al. (1999) Dopamine D2 receptor binding before and after treatment of major depression measured by [^{123}I]IZBM SPECT. *Psychiatry Res.* 90:91–101.

Konig, F., Hauger, B., et al. (2000) Effect of paroxetine on thyroid hormone levels in severely depressed patients. *Neuropsychobiology* 42(3):135–138.

Kraus, R.P., Phoenix, E., et al. (1997) Exaggerated TSH responses to TRH in depressed patients with normal baseline. *J. Clin. Psychiatry* 58(6):266–270.

Lambert, G., Johansson, M., et al. (2000) Reduced brain norepinephrine and dopamine release in treatment-refractory depressive illness: evidence in support of the catecholamine hypothesis of mood disorders. *Arch. Gen. Psychiatry* 57(8):787–793.

Lawrence, K.M., DePaermentier, F., et al. (1990) Brain 5-HT uptake sites, labelled with [^{3}H]paroxetine, in antidepressant-free depressed suicides. *Brain Res.* 526:17–22.

Leake, A., Fairbairn, A.F., et al. (1991) Studies on the serotonin uptake binding site in major depressive disorder and control postmortem brain: neurochemical and clinical correlates. *Psychiatry Res.* 39:155–165.

Lemonde, S., Turecki, G., et al. (2003) Impaired repression at a 5-hydroxytryptamine 1A receptor gene polymorphism associated with major depression and suicide. *J. Neurosci.* 23:8788–8799.

Lesch, K.P., Wolozin, B.L., et al. (1993) Primary structure of the human platelet serotonin uptake site: identity with the brain serotonin transporter. *J. Neurochem.* 60:2319–2322.

Leyton, M., Young, S.N., et al. (1997) The effect of tryptophan depletion on mood in medication-free, former patients with major affective disorder. *Neuropsychopharmacology* 16(4):294–297.

Lifschytz, T., Segman, R., et al. (2006) Basic mechanisms of augmentation of antidepressant effects with thyroid hormone. *Curr. Drug Targets* 7:203–210.

Linnoila, M., and Virkkunen, M. (1992) Aggression, suicidality and serotonin. *J. Clin. Psychiatry* 53(Suppl):46–51.

Little, K.Y. (1988) Amphetamine, but not methylphenidate, predicts antidepressant response. *J. Clin. Psychopharmacol.* 8:177–183.

Lowther, S., De Paermentier, F., et al. (1994) Brain 5-HT2 receptors in suicide victims: violence of death, depression and effects of antidepressant treatment. *Brain Res.* 642:281–289.

Lowther, S., De Paermentier, F., et al. (1997) 5-HT1A receptor binding sites in post-mortem brain samples from depressed suicides and controls. *J. Affect. Disord.* 42(2–3):199–207.

Maas, J.W., Fawcett, J.A., et al. (1972) Catecholamine metabolism, depressive illness and drug response. *Arch. Gen. Psychiatry* 26: 252–262.

Maas, J.W., Koslow, S.H., et al. (1984) Pretreatment neurotransmitter metabolite levels and response to tricyclic antidepressant drugs. *Am. J. Psychiatry* 141(10):1159–1171.

Maes, M., De Ruyter, M., et al. (1987) The renal excretion of xanthurenic acid following L-tryptophan loading in depressed patients. *Hum. Psychopharmacol.* 2:231–235.

Maes, M., Jacobs, M.-P., et al. (1990) Suppressant effects of dexamethasone on the availability of plasma L-tryptophan and tyrosine in healthy controls and depressed patients. *Acta Psychiatr. Scand.* 81:19–23.

Maes, M., and Meltzer, H.Y. (1995) The serotonin hypothesis of major depression. In: Bloom, F.E., and Kupfer, D.J., eds. *Psychopharmacology: The Fourth Generation of Progress.* New York: Raven Press, pp. 933–944.

Maes, M., Van Gastel, A., et al. (1999) Decreased platelet alpha-2 adrenoceptor density in major depression: effects of tricyclic antidepressants and fluoxetine. *Biol. Psychiatry* 45(3):278–284.

Maj, M., Ariano, M.G., et al. (1984) Plasma cortisol, catecholamine and cyclic AMP levels, response to dexamethasone suppression test and platelet MAO activity in manic-depressive patients. A longitudinal study. *Neuropsychobiology* 11(3):168–173.

Malison, R.T., Price, L.H., et al. (1998) Reduced brain serotonin transporter availability in major depression as measured by [^{123}I]-2-beta-carbomethoxy-3 beta-(4-iodophenyl)tropane and single photon emission computed tomography. *Biol. Psychiatry* 44(11): 1090–1098.

Malone, K.M., Thase, M.E., et al. (1993) Fenfluramine challenge test as predictor of outcome in major depression. *Psychopharmacol. Bull.* 29(2):155–161.

Mann, J., McBride, P., et al. (1992) Relationship between central and peripheral serotonin indexes in depressed and suicidal psychiatric inpatients. *Arch. Gen. Psychiatry* 49:442–446.

Mann, J., Stanley, M., et al. (1986) Increased serotonin2 and b-adrenergic receptor binding in the frontal cortices of suicide victims. *Arch. Gen. Psychiatry* 43:954–959.

Mann, J.J., Huang, Y., et al. (2000) A serotonin transporter gene promoter polymorphism (5-HTTLPR) and prefrontal cortical binding in major depression and suicide. *Arch. Gen. Psychiatry* 57: 729–738.

Mann, J.J., and Malone, K.M. (1997) Cerebrospinal fluid amines and higher-lethality suicide attempts in depressed inpatients. *Biol. Psychiatry* 41:162–171.

Mann, J.J., Malone, K.M., et al. (1996) Demonstration in vivo of reduced serotonin responsivity in the brain of untreated depressed patients. *Am. J. Psychiatry* 153(2):174–182.

Marangell, L.B., George, M.S., et al. (1997) Effects of intrathecal thyrotropin-releasing hormone (protirelin) in refractory depressed patients. *Arch. Gen. Psychiatry* 54(3):214–222.

Marazziti, D., Baroni, S., et al. (2001) Correlation between platelet alpha (2)-adrenoceptors and symptom severity in major depression. *Neuropsychobiology* 44(3):122–125.

Marinelli, M., and Piazza, P.V. (2002) Interaction between glucocorticoid hormones, stress and psychostimulant drugs. *Eur. J. Neurosci.* 16:387–394.

Martinot, M., Bragulat, V., et al. (2001) Decreased presynaptic dopaminergic function in the left caudate of depressed patients with affective flattening and psychomotor retardation. *Am. J. Psychiatry* 158(2):314–316.

Massou, J.M., Trichard, C., et al. (1997) Frontal 5-HT2A receptors studied in depressive patients during chronic treatment by selective serotonin reuptake inhibitors. *Psychopharmacology* 133(1): 99–101.

Matsubara, S., Arora, R.C., et al. (1991) Serotonergic measures in suicide brain: 5-HT1A binding sites in frontal cortex of suicide victims. *J. Neural Transm.* 85:181–194.

McBride, P.A., Brown, R., et al. (1994) The relationship of platelet 5-HT2 receptor indices to major depressive disorder, personality traits, and suicidal behavior. *Biol. Psychiatry* 35:295–308.

McBride, P.A., Mann, J.J., et al. (1983) Characterization of serotonin binding sites on human platelets. *Life Sci.* 33:2033–2041.

McKeith, I., Marshall, E., et al. (1987) 5-HT receptor binding in post-mortem brain from patients with affective disorder. *J. Affect. Disord.* 13:67–74.

McPherson, H., Walsh, A., et al. (2003) Growth hormone and prolactin response to apomorphine in bipolar and unipolar depression. *J. Affect. Disord.* 76:121–125.

Meana, J.J., Barturen, F., et al. (1992) Alpha 2-adrenoceptors in the brain of suicide victims: increased receptor density associated with major depression. *Biol. Psychiatry* 31(5):471–490.

Meltzer, C.C., Price, J.C., et al. (1999) PET imaging of serotonin type 2 receptors in late-life neuropsychiatric disorders. *Am. J. Psychiatry* 156(12):1871–1878.

Meltzer, H.Y., and Lowy, M.T. (1987) The serotonin hypothesis of depression. In: Meltzer, H.Y., ed. *Psychopharmacology: The Third Generation of Progress*. New York: Raven Press, pp. 513–526.

Merali, Z., Du, L., et al. (2004) Dysregulation in the suicide brain: mRNA expression of corticotropin-releasing hormone receptors and GABA(A) receptor subunits in frontal cortical brain region. *J. Neurosci.* 24:1478–1485.

Merali, Z., Kent, P., et al. (2006) Corticotropin-releasing hormone, arginine vasopressin, gastrin-releasing peptide, and neuromedin B alterations in stress-relevant brain regions of suicides and control subjects. *Biol. Psychiatry* 59:594–602.

Meyer, J.H, Ginovart, N., et al. (2006) Elevated monoamine oxidase A levels in the brain. *Arch. Gen. Psychiatry* 63:1209–1216.

Meyer, J.H., Houle, S., et al. (2004) Brain serotonin transporter binding potential measured with carbon 11-labeled DASB positron emission tomography. *Arch. Gen. Psychiatry* 61:1271–1279.

Meyer, J.H., Kapur, S., et al. (1999) Prefrontal cortex 5-HT2 receptors in depression: an [^{18}F]setoperone PET imaging study. *Am. J. Psychiatry* 156(7):1029–1034.

Meyer, J.H., Kruger, S., et al. (2001) Lower dopamine transporter binding potential in striatum during depression. *Neuroreport* 12: 4121–4125.

Miller, H.L., Delgado, P.L., et al. (1996a) Clinical and biochemical effects of catecholamine depletion on antidepressant-induced remission of depression. *Arch. Gen. Psychiatry* 53(2):117–128.

Miller, H.L., Delgado, P.L., et al. (1996b) Effects of alpha-methyl-paratyrosine (AMPT) in drug-free depressed patients. *Neuropsychopharmacology* 14(3):151–157.

Mintun, M.A., Sheline, Y.I., et al. (2004) Decreased hippocampal 5-HT_{2A} receptor binding in major depressive disorder: in vivo measurement with [^{18}F]altanserin positron emission tomography. *Biol. Psychiatry* 55:217–224.

Mitchell, P.B., Bearn, J.A., et al. (1988) Growth hormone response to clonidine after recovery in patients with endogenous depression. *Br. J. Psychiatry* 152:34–38.

Mitchell, P.B., and Smythe, G. (1990) Hormonal responses to fenfluramine in depressed and control subjects. *J. Affect. Disord.* 19(1): 43–51.

Moreau, X., Azorin, J.M., et al. (2000) Red blood cell triiodothyronine uptake in unipolar major depression: effect of a chronic antidepressant treatment. *Prog. Neuro-Psychopharm. Biol. Psychiatry* 24(1):23–35.

Moses, S.G., and Robins, E. (1975) Regional distribution of norepinephrine and dopamine in brains of depressive suicides and alcoholic suicides. *Psychopharmacol. Commun.* 1:327–337.

Murphy, D.L. (1972) L-DOPA, behavioral activation and psychopathology. *Res. Publ. Ass. Res. Nerv. Ment. Dis.* 50:430–437.

Murray, J.B. (1996) Depression in Parkinson's disease. *J. Psychol.* 130(6):659–667.

Musselman, D.L., Tomer, A., et al. (1996) Exaggerated platelet reactivity in major depression. *Am. J. Psychiatry* 153(10):1313–1317.

Nemeroff, C.B. (1996) The corticotropin-releasing factor (CRF) hypothesis of depression: new findings and new directions. *Mol. Psychiatry* 1(4):336–342.

Nemeroff, C.B., Bissette, G., et al. (1991) Neuropeptide concentrations in cerebrospinal fluid of depressed patients treated with electroconvulsive therapy: corticotropin-releasing factor, B-endorphin and somatostatin. *Br. J. Psychiatry* 158:59–63.

Nemeroff, C.B., Owens, M.J., et al. (1988) Reduced corticotropin releasing factor binding sites in the frontal cortex of suicide victims. *Arch. Gen. Psychiatry* 45(6):577–579.

Neumeister, A., Hu, X.Z., et al. (2006) Differential effects of 5-HTTLPR genotypes on the behavioral and neural responses to tryptophan depletion in patients with major depression and controls. *Arch. Gen. Psychiatry* 63:978–986.

Neumeister, A., Nugent, A.C., et al. (2004) Neural and behavioral responses to tryptophan depletion in unmedicated patients with remitted major depressive disorder and controls. *Arch. Gen. Psychiatry* 61:765–773.

Neumeister, A., Yuan, P., et al. (2005) Effects of tryptophan depletion on serum levels of brain-derived neurotrophic factor in unmedicated patients with remitted depression and healthy subjects. *Am. J. Psychiatry* 162:805–807.

O'Keane, V., and Dinan, T.G. (1991) Prolactin and cortisol responses to d-fenfluramine in major depression: evidence of diminished responsivity of central serotonergic function. *Am. J. Psychiatry* 148(8): 1009–1015.

Ohmori, T., Arora, R.C., et al. (1992) Serotonergic measures in suicide brain: the concentration of 5-HIAA, HVA and tryptophan in frontal cortex of suicide victims. *Biol. Psychiatry* 32:57–71.

Ordway, G. (2000) Searching for the chicken's egg in transporter gene polymorphisms. *Arch. Gen. Psychiatry* 57(8):739–740.

Ordway, G., Schenk, J., et al., (2003) Elevated agonist binding to a2-adrenoreceptors in the locus ceruleus in major depression. *Biol. Psychiatry* 53:315–323.

Ordway, G.A., Gambarana, C., et al. (1991) Preferential reduction of binding of ^{125}I-iodopindolol to beta-1 adrenoceptors in the amygdala of rat after antidepressant treatments. *J. Pharmacol. Exp. Ther.* 257:681–690

Owen, F., Chambers, D., et al. (1986) Serotonergic mechanisms in brains of suicide victims. *Brain Res.* 362:185–188.

Owen, F., Cross, A.J., et al. (1983) Brain 5-HT2 receptors and suicide. *Lancet* 2(8361):1256.

Owens, M.J. (1997) Molecular and cellular mechanisms of antidepressant drugs. *Depress. Anxiety* 4:153–159.

Owens, M.J., Morgan, W.N., et al. (1997a) Neurotransmitter receptor binding profile of antidepressants. *J. Pharm. Exp. Ther.* 283(3): 1305–1322.

Owens, M.J., Morgan, W.N., et al. (1997b) Receptor binding profile of monoamine transporter antagonist antidepressants and their metabolites. *J. Pharm. Exp. Ther.* 283(3):1305–1322.

Owens, M.J., and Nemeroff, C.B. (1994) Role of serotonin in the pathophysiology of depression: focus on the serotonin transporter. *Clin. Chem.* 40:288–295.

Owens, M.J., and Nemeroff, C.B. (1997) The serotonin transporter and depression. *Depress. Anxiety* 8(Suppl 1):5–12.

Pandey, G.N., Pandey, S.C., et al. (1990) Platelet serotonin-2 receptor binding sites in depression and suicide. *Biol. Psychiatry* 28: 215–222.

Pandey, G.N., Pandey, S.C., et al. (1995) Platelet serotonin-2A receptors: a potential biological marker for suicidal behavior. *Am. J. Psychiatry* 152(6):850–855.

Parsey, R.V., Hastings, R.S., et al. (2006) Lower serotonin transporter binding potential in the human brain during major depressive episodes. *Am. J. Psychiatry* 163:52–58.

Parsey, R.V., Oquendo, M.A., et al. (2001) Dopamine D2 receptor availability and amephetamine-induced dopamine release in unipolar depression. *Biol. Psychiatry* 50:313-322.

Parsey, R.V., Oquendo, M.A., et al. (2006) Altered serotonin 1A binding in major depression: a [carbonyl-C-11]WAY100635 positron emission tomography study. *Biol. Psychiatry* 59:106-113.

Perry, E.K., Marshall, E.F., et al. (1983) Decreased imipramine binding in the brains of patients with depressive illness. *Br. J. Psychiatry* 142:188–192.

Petty, F. (1994) Plasma concentrations of GABA and mood disorders: a blood test for manic depressive disease? *Clin. Chem.* 40:296–302.

Pezawas, L., Meyer-Lindenberg, A., et al. (2005) 5-HTTLPR polymorphism impacts human cingulate-amygdala interactions: a genetic susceptibility mechanism for depression. *Nat. Neurosci.* 8: 828–834.

Piletz, J.E., Halaris, A.S., et al. (1990) Elevated -3H-para-aminoclonidine binding to platelet purified plasma membranes from depressed patients. *Neuropsychopharmacology* 3(3):201-210.

Pitchot, W., Hansenne, M., et al. (1995) Growth hormone response to apomorphine in panic disorder: comparison to major depression and normal controls. *Eur. Arch. Psych. Clin. Neurosci.* 245(6): 306–308.

Pitchot, W., Hansenne, M., et al. (2001a) Alpha-2-adrenoceptors in depressed suicide attempters: relationship to medical lethality of the attempt. *Neuropsychobiology* 44(2):91–94.

Pitchot, W., Hansenne, M., et al. (2001b) Reduced dopamine function in depressed patients is related to suicidal behavior but not its lethality. *Psychoneuroendocrinology* 26(7):689–696.

Plotsky, P.M., Owens, M.J., et al. (1995) Neuropeptide alterations in mood disorders. In: Bloom, F.E., and Kupfer, D.J., eds. *Psychopharmacology: The Fourth Generation of Progress.* New York: Raven Press, pp. 971–981.

Porter, R.J., Lunn, B.S., et al. (2000) Cognitive deficit induced by acute tryptophan depletion in patients with Alzheimer's disease. *Am. J. Psychiatry* 157(4):638–640.

Posener, J.A., Schatzberg, A.F., et al. (1999) Hypothalamic-pituitary-adrenal axis effects on plasma homovanillic acid in man. *Biol. Psychiatry* 45(2):222–228.

Post, R.M., Gerner, R.H., et al. (1978) Effects of a dopamine agonist piribedil in depressed patients. *Arch. Gen. Psychiatry* 35: 609–615.

Potter, W.Z., Karoum, F., et al. (1984) Common mechanisms of action of biochemically specific antidepressants. *Prog. Neuropsychopharmacol. Biol. Psychiatry* 8:153–161.

Prange, A.J. (1964) The pharmacology and biochemistry of depression. *Dis. Central Nerv. Syst.* 25:217–221.

Prange, A.J., Lara, P.P., et al. (1972) Effects of thyrotropin-releasing hormone in depression. *Lancet* 2(785):999–1002.

Price, L.H., Charney, D.S., et al. (1991) Serotonin function and depression: neuroendocrine and mood responses to intravenous L-tryptophan in depressed patients and healthy comparison subjects. *Am. J. Psychiatry* 148(11):1518–1525.

Price, L.H., Malison, R.T., et al. (1997) Neurobiology of tryptophan depletion in depression: effects of m-chlorophenypiperazine (mCPP). *Neuropsychopharmacology* 17(5):342–350.

Raadsheer, F.C., van Heerikhuize, J.J., et al. (1995) Corticotropin-releasing hormone mRNA levels in paraventricular nucleus of patients with Alzheimer's disease and depression. *Am. J. Psychiatry* 152(9):1372–1379.

Rausch, J.L., Johnson, M.E., et al. (2005) Serotonin transport kinetics correlated between human platelets and brain synaptosomes. *Psychopharmacology* 180:391–398.

Redmond, D.E., Kratz, M.M., et al. (1986) Cerebrospinal fluid amine metabolites. Relationships with behavioral measurements in depressed, manic and healthy control subjects. *Arch. Gen. Psychiatry* 43(10):938–947.

Rothschild, A.J., Langlais, P.J., et al. (1984) Dexamethasone increases plasma free dopamine in man. *J. Psychiatr. Res.* 18(3):217–223.

Roy, A., DeJong, J., et al. (1989) Cerebrospinal fluid monoamine metabolites and suicidal behavior in depressed patients. A 5-year follow-up study. *Arch. Gen. Psychiatry* 46(7):609–612.

Roy, A., Karoum, F., et al. (1992) Marked reduction in indexes of dopamine transmission among patients with depression who attempted suicide. *Arch. Gen. Psychiatry* 49:447–450.

Roy, A., Pickar, D., et al. (1986) Urinary monoamines and monoamine metabolites in subtypes of unipolar depressive disorder and normal controls. *Psychol. Med.* 16(3):541–546.

Roy, A., Wolkowitz, O.M., et al. (1994) Differences in CSF concentrations of thyrotropin-releasing hormone in depressed patients and normal subjects: negative findings. *Am. J. Psychiatry* 151(4): 600–602.

Rubinow, D.R. (1986) Cerebrospinal fluid somatostatin and psychiatric illness. *Biol. Psychiatry* 21:341–365.

Rubinow, D.R., Gold, P.W., et al. (1983) CSF somatostatin in affective illness. *Arch. Gen. Psychiatry* 40:409–412.

Sagud, M., Pivac, N., et al. (2002) Effects of sertraline treatment on plasma cortisol, prolactin and thyroid hormones in female depressed patients. *Neuropsychobiology* 45:139–143.

Salomon, R.M., Miller, H.L., et al. (1997) Lack of behavioral effects of monoamine depletion in healthy subjects. *Biol. Psychiatry* 41(1): 58–64.

Sanacora, G., Mason, G.F., et al (2003) Increased cortical GABA concentrations in depressed patients receiving ECT. *Am. J. Psychiatry* 160:577–579.

Sanacora, G., Mason, G.F., et al. (2002) Increased occipital cortex GABA concentrations in depressed patients after therapy with selective serotonin reuptake inhibitors. *Am. J. Psychiatry* 159:663–665.

Sargent, P.A., Kjaer, K.H., et al. (2000) Brain serotonin 1A receptor binding measured by positron emission tomography with [^{11}C]WAY-100635: effects of depression and antidepressant treatment. *Arch. Gen. Psychiatry* 57(2):174–180.

Saxena, P.R. (1995) Serotonin receptors: subtypes, functional responses, and therapeutic relevance. *Pharmacol. Ther.* 66:339–368.

Schatzberg, A.F. (1998) Noradrenergic versus serotonergic antidepressants: Predictors of treatment response. *J. Clin Psychiatry* 59 (Suppl 14):15–18.

Schatzberg, A.F., Orsulak, P.J., et al. (1982) Toward a biochemical classification of depressive disorders, V: heterogeneity of unipolar depressions. *Am. J. Psychiatry* 139(4):471–475.

Schatzberg, A.F., Rosenbaum, A.H., et al. (1981) Toward a biochemical classification of depressive disorders, III: pretreatment urinary MHPG levels as predictors of response to treatment with maprotiline. *Psychopharmacology* 75:34–38.

Schatzberg, A.F., and Rothschild, A.J. (1992) Psychotic (delusional) major depression: should it be included as a distinct syndrome in DSM-IV? *Am. J. Psychiatry* 149:733–745.

Schatzberg, A.F., Rothschild, A.J., et al. (1985) A corticosteroid/dopamine hypothesis for psychotic depression and related states. *J. Psychiatr. Res.* 19(1):57–64.

Schatzberg, A.F., Samson, J.A., et al. (1989) Toward a biochemical classification of depressive disorders, X: urinary catecholamines, their metabolites, and D-type scores in subgroups of depressive disorders. *Arch. Gen. Psychiatry* 46(3):260–268.

Schatzberg, A.F., and Schildkraut, J.J. (1995) Recent studies on norepinephrine systems in mood disorders. In: Bloom, F.E., and Kupfer, D.J., eds. *Psychopharmacology: The Fourth Generation of Progress.* New York: Raven Press, pp. 911–920.

Schildkraut, J.J. (1965) The catecholamine hypothesis of affective disorders: a review of supporting evidence. *Am. J. Psychiatry* 122: 509–522.

Schildkraut, J.J. (1973) Norepinephrine metabolites as biochemical criteria for classifying depressive disorders and predicting response to treatment. Preliminary findings. *Am. J. Psychiatry* 130:695–699.

Schildkraut, J.J., Orsulak, P.J., et al. (1978) Toward a biochemical classification of depressive disorders, I: differences in urinary excretion of MHPG and other catecholamine metabolites in clinically defined subtypes of depression. *Arch. Gen. Psychiatry* 35(12): 1427–1433.

Schneier, F.R.,, Liebowitz, M.R., et al. (2000) Low dopamine D(2) receptor binding potential in social phobia. *Am. J. Psychiatry* 157:457–459.

Shah, P.J., Ogilvie, A.D., et al. (1997) Clinical and psychometric correlates of dopamine D2 binding in depression. *Psychol. Med.* 27(6):1247–1256.

Shapira, B., Cohen, J., et al. (1993) Prolactin response to fenfluramine and placebo challenge following maintenance pharmacotherapy withdrawal in remitted depressed patients. *Biol. Psychiatry* 33(7):531–535.

Sheline, Y., Bargett, M., et al. (1995) Platelet serotonin markers and depressive symptomatology. *Biol. Psychiatry* 37:442–447.

Shelton, R.C., Winn, S., et al. (1993) The effects of antidepressants on the thyroid axis in depression. *Biol. Psychiatry* 33:120–126.

Siever, L.J., Murphy, D.L., et al. (1984) Plasma prolactin changes following fenfluramine in depressed patients compared to controls: an evaluation of central serotonergic responsivity in depression. *Life Sci.* 34(11):1029–1039.

Siever, L.J., Trestmen, R.L., et al. (1992) The growth hormone response to clonidine in acute and remitted depressed male patients. *Neuropsychopharmacology* 6(3):165–177.

Siever, L.J., Uhde, T.W., et al. (1982) Growth hormone response to clonidine as a probe of noradrenergic receptor responsiveness in affective disorder patients and controls. *Psychiatry Res.* 7(2): 139–144.

Siever, L.J., Uhde, T.W., et al. (1984) Differential inhibitory noradrenergic responses to clonidine in 25 depressed patients and 25 normal control subjects. *Am. J. Psychiatry* 141(6):733–741.

Smith, K.A., Fairburn, C.G., et al. (1997) Relapse of depression after rapid depletion of tryptophan. *Lancet* 349:915–919.

Smith, K.A., Morris, J.S., et al. (1999) Brain mechanisms associated with depressive relapse and associated cognitive impairment following acute tryptophan depletion. *Br. J. Psychiatry* 174:525–529.

Spillmann, M.K., Van der Does, A.J., et al. (2001) Tryptophan depletion in SSRI-recovered depressed outpatients. *Psychopharmacologia* 155(2):123–127.

Stahl, S. (1977) The human platelet. *Arch. Gen. Psychiatry* 34: 509–516.

Stanley, M., and Mann, J.J. (1983) Increased serotonin-2 binding sites in frontal cortex of suicide victims. *Lancet* 1:214–216.

Sullivan, G.M., Hatterer, J.A., et al. (1999) Low levels of transthyretin in CSF of depressed patients. *Am. J. Psychiatry* 156(5):710–715.

Sullivan, M., Mann, J.J., et al. (2006) Low cerebral spinal fluid transthyretin levels in depression: correlations with suicidal ideation and low serotonin function. *Biol. Psychiatry* 60:500–506.

Swann, A.C., Koslow, S.H., et al. (1987) Lithium carbonate treatment of mania. *Arch. Gen. Psychiatry* 44(4):345–354.

Tandberg, E., Larsen J.P., et al. (1996) The occurrence of depression in Parkinson's disease. *Arch. Neurol.* 53:175–179.

Tepper, J.M., Koos, T., et al. (2004) GABAergic microcircuits in the neostriatum. *Trends Neurosci.* 11:662–669.

Thakore, J.H., O'Keane, V., et al. (1996) d-Fenfluramine-induced prolactin responses in mania: evidence for serotonergic subsensitivity. *Am. J. Psychiatry* 153(11):1460–1463.

Traskman, L., Asberg, M., et al. (1981) Monoamine metabolites in CSF and suicidal behavior. *Arch. Gen. Psychiatry* 38(6):631–636.

Tremblay, L.K., Naranjo, C.A., et al. (2002) Probing brain reward system function in major depressive disorder: altered response to dextroamphetamine. *Arch. Gen. Psychiatry* 59:409–416.

Tremblay, L.K., Naranjo, C.A., et al. (2005) Functional neuroanatomical substrates of altered reward processing in major depressive disorder revealed by a dopaminergic probe. *Arch. Gen. Psychiatry* 62:1228–1236.

Van Praag, H.M. (1982) Depression, suicide, and the metabolites of serotonin in the brain. *J. Affect. Disord.* 4:21–29.

Van Praag, H.M., Korf, J., et al. (1975) Dopamine metabolism in depressions, psychoses and Parkinson's disease: the problem of the specificity of biological variables in behavior disorders. *Psychol. Med.* 5:138–146.

Van Scheyen, J.D., Van Praag, H.M., et al. (1977) Controlled study comparing nomifensine and clomipramine in unipolar depression, using the probenecid technique. *Br. J. Clin. Pharmacol.* 4:179S–184S.

Virkkunen, M., Eggert, M., et al. (1996) A prospective follow-up study of violent offenders and fire setters. *Arch. Gen. Psychiatry* 53(6):523–529.

Virkkunen, M., Goldman, D., et al. (1995) Low brain serotonin turnover rate (low CSF 5-HIAA) and impulsive violence. *J. Psychiatry Neurosci.* 20(4):271–275.

Virkkunen, M., Rawlings, R., et al. (1994) CSF biochemistries, glucose metabolism, and diurnal activity rhythms in alcoholic, violent offenders, fire setters, and healthy volunteers. *Arch. Gen. Psychiatry* 51(1):20–27.

Von Bardeleben, U., and Holsboer, F. (1989) Cortisol response to a combined dexamethasone-human corticotropin-releasing hormone (CRH) challenge in patients with major depression. *J. Neuroendocrinol.* 1:485–488.

Whale, R., Clifford, E.M., et al. (2001) Decreased sensitivity of 5-HT1D receptors in melancholic depression. *Br. J. Psychiatry* 178: 454–457.

Williams, R.B., Marchuk, D.A., et al. (2003) Serotonin-related gene polymorphisms and central nervous system function. *Neuropsychopharmacology* 28:533–541.

Willner, P. (1983) Dopamine and depression: a review of recent evidence. *Brain Res. Rev.* 6:211–246.

Wirz-Justice, A. (1988) Platelet research in psychiatry. *Experientia* 44:145–152.

Wolfe, N., Katz, D.I., et al. (1990) Neuropsychological profile linked to low dopamine: in Alzheimer's disease, major depression, and Parkinson's disease. *J. Neurol. Neurosurg. Psychiatry* 53(10): 915–917.

Wong, M.L., Kling, M.A., et al. (2000) Pronounced and sustained central hypernoradrenergic function in major depression with melacholic features: relation to hypercortisolism and corticotropin-releasing hormone. *Proc. Natl. Acad. Sci. USA* 97(1):325–330.

Yatham, L.N., Liddle, P.F., et al. (1999) Decrease in brain serotonin 2 receptor binding in patients with major depression following desipramine treatment. *Arch. Gen. Psychiatry* 56:705–711.

Yatham, L.N., Liddle, P.F., et al. (2000) Brain serotonin2 receptors in major depression: a positron emission tomography study. *Arch. Gen. Psychiatry* 57(9):850–858.

Yatham, L.N., Zis, A.P., et al. (1997) Sumatriptan-induced growth hormone release in patients with major depression, mania, and normal controls. *Neuropsychopharmacology* 17(4):258–263.

Yehuda, R., Siever, L.J., et al. (1998) Plasma norepinephrine and 3-methoxy-4-hydroxylglycol concentrations and severity of depression in combat posttraumatic stress disorder and major depressive disorder. *Biol. Psychiatry* 44(1):56–63.

Young, E.A., Watson, S.J., et al. (1990) Beta-lipotropin-beta-endorphin response to low-dose ovine corticotropin releasing factor in endogenous depression. *Arch. Gen. Psychiatry* 47(5):449–457.

Young, S.N., Smith, S.E., et al. (1985) Tryptophan depletion causes a rapid lowering of mood in normal males. *Psychopharmacology* 87:173–177.

Zalsman, G., Yung-yu, H., et al. (2006) Association of a triallelic serotonin transporter gene promoter region (5-HTTLPR) polymorphism with stressful life events and severity of depression. *Am. J. Psychiatry* 163:1588–1593.

Zammit, S., and Owen M.J. (2006) Stressful life events, 5-HTT genotype and risk of depression. *Br. J. Psychiatry* 188:199–201.

Zarate, C.A., Payne, J.L., et al. (2004) Pramipexole for bipolar II depression: a placebo-controlled proof of concept study. *Biol. Psychiatry* 56:54–60.

Zobel, A.W., Nickel, T., et al. (2001) Effects of high-affinity corticotropin-releasing hormone receptor 1 antagonist R121919 in major depression: the first 20 patients. *J. Psychiatric Res.* 34(3): 171–181.

31 Neuroimaging Studies of Mood Disorders

WAYNE C. DREVETS, KISHORE M. GADDE,
AND K. RANGA R. KRISHNAN

The application of neuroimaging technology in clinical neuroscience research holds the potential to transport psychiatry into an era in which pathophysiology, rather than signs and symptoms, guides the nosology of psychiatric disorders. The past two decades of imaging technology development have produced a variety of techniques that make possible noninvasive examination of brain structure, function, and chemistry. These tools are being applied to elucidate the anatomical correlates of normal and pathological emotional states and the physiological correlates of antidepressant and mood stabilizing treatments in humans. The results of such studies are guiding the clinical neuroscience field toward models of depression in which functional and structural factors play roles in the pathogenesis of mood disorders.

STRUCTURAL NEUROIMAGING STUDIES OF MOOD DISORDERS

Structural imaging technologies for evaluating morphology and elements of tissue composition in vivo became available in the late 1970s with the advent of computed tomography (CT), and shortly thereafter, magnetic resonance imaging (MRI). These techniques revolutionized clinical diagnostic evaluation by affording the ability to visualize gross neuropathology in vivo. They also enabled noninvasive investigation of brain structure without the limitations of postmortem studies, such as the requirement for excised brain tissue and the uncertain adjustment for the variable changes in brain volume occurring with tissue fixation.

In the evaluation of mood disorders, structural imaging technology is used clinically to facilitate differential diagnosis in cases where depressive or manic syndromes are suspected of arising secondary to lesions or degenerative processes. However, structural imaging has played more direct and pivotal roles in quantitative neuromorphological and neuromorphometric studies of depression (assessment of the appearance and volume of brain structure, respectively), where such research has demonstrated the existence of white matter pathology and abnormalities of brain structure volume in some mood disorder subtypes. This chapter reviews these findings in mood-disordered samples and discusses their specificity with respect to diagnostic subtype and other neuropsychiatric conditions.

Technical Issues Relevant to the Interpretation of Structural Brain Images

The sensitivity of structural imaging assessments depends upon a variety of technical factors related to the imaging modality, the spatial resolution of the images, and the tissue contrast resolution (that is, discrimination between lesions, grey matter, white matter, and cerebrospinal fluid [CSF]). Although CT and MRI permit detection of neuromorphological abnormalities and assessment of cerebral volumes, MRI is superior for these purposes in psychiatric research. Relative to CT, MRI provides greater spatial resolution (0.5 mm for newer scanners) and higher contrast resolution for delimiting neuroanatomical structures and depicting white matter pathology. Magnetic resonance imaging also allows greater flexibility of acquisition parameters for varying tissue contrast and image plane orientation. In contrast, CT images have low-contrast resolution between gray and white matter, are susceptible to artifacts near bony surfaces (obscuring visualization of the brain stem, basotemporal cortex, and posterior fossa), and are limited to acquisition in the axial orientation. Finally, though CT involves exposure to ionizing radiation, there are no known biological risks associated with the magnetic field strengths currently employed for MRI studies (unless metallic objects or pacemaker devices are present inside the body).

Neuromorphometric assessments generally are performed by segmenting MRI images using manual or semiautomated techniques. The reliability of such measures has progressively increased with improvements in MR signal homogeneity and reductions in image-slice thickness.

However, the reliability and validity of such measures are also influenced by the reproducibility of anatomical rules for delimiting target structures, the tissue contrast resolution, and the effects of partial volume averaging (which diminish as either spatial resolution or structure size increase).

These issues limit the structures that can be reliably assessed by volumetric MRI (vMRI). For example, of regions that participate in emotional processing, cerebral cortical regions, mesiotemporal lobe structures such as the amygdala and hippocampus, and basal ganglia structures such as the caudate and putamen have been examined in vMRI studies. In contrast, structures such as the hypothalamus, the periaqueductal gray (PAG) matter, and brainstem monoaminergic nuclei, which have also been implicated in depression, are less tractable to neuroimaging approaches because of their small size and lack of clear demarcation from adjacent grey matter structures in MRI images.

Clinical differences between depressive samples related to current age, age at illness-onset, and capacity for developing mania or psychosis also affect structural imaging measures. Differences in control samples may also influence study results, as some groups selected controls who were not depressed who underwent MRI as part of an evaluation for headaches or seizures, whereas others limited controls to participants who are healthy. Finally, because the magnitude of the differences between participants who are depressed and controls is subtle relative to the variability of structural imaging measures, vMRI abnormalities are not evident in individual participants, and relatively large samples are needed to ensure adequate statistical sensitivity.

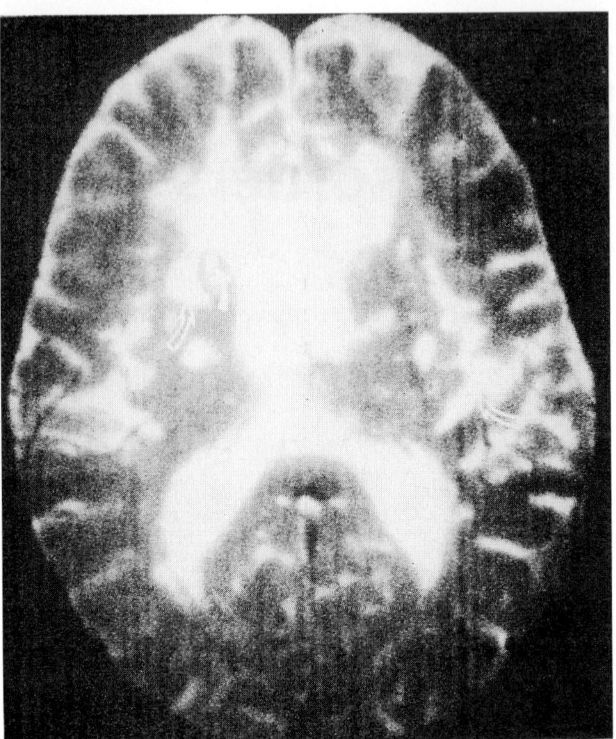

FIGURE 31.1 Brain MRI, axial view through base of lateral ventricles showing large, confluent, deep white matter hyperintensities (open arrows) and hyperintensity in the right caudate head (closed arrow) in an elderly depressed subject. MRI: magnetic resonance imaging. Reproduced with permission from Drevets (1993).

Neuromorphological Imaging Studies of Mood Disorders

The most robust finding from structural imaging studies of mood disorders has been the elevated prevalence of MR signal hyperintensities in the deep and periventricular white matter of elderly participants with major depressive disorder (MDD; that is, "unipolar depression") (Table 31.1). These abnormalities are predominantly seen in subjects who experienced their initial major depressive episode (MDE) in late life. As discussed below, the implications of these structural imaging findings with respect to the pathogenesis of late-life-onset depression is beginning to set this mood disorder subtype apart phenomenologically as a type of depression that may arise secondarily to cerebrovascular disease (Krishnan et al, 1993).

MR Signal Hyperintensities: Clinical and Neuropathological Correlates

The improved sensitivity of MRI technology to tissue contrasts and white matter pathology led to the observation that many individuals who otherwise appear neurologically healthy have lesions, seen as hyperintense foci of the MR signal, in the deep white matter, periventricular white matter, basal ganglia, and pons (Fig. 31.1). Although the correlates of such signal abnormalities occasionally were evident in CT scans (initially termed *leukoaraiosis*), their extent and frequency are more clearly visualized using MRI. In MRI images, white matter hyperintensities (WMH) were initially referred to as "unidentified bright objects" or "leukoencephalopathy," but these lesions now are descriptively classified as either WMH or lacunae, and graded by their size and location in T_2-weighted MRI scans.

In elderly participants without known white matter disease such as multiple sclerosis (which presents with transient, focal areas of WMH that reflect a distinct neuropathological process), postmortem assessment of brain tissue where WMH were evident in MRI images antemortem indicate that "patches" and "caps" of signal hyperintensity in the deep and periventricular white matter generally correspond to areas affected by cerebrovascular disease (Awad, Johnson, et al., 1986; Chimowitz et al., 1992). Histopathological characterization of such patches demonstrates myelin pallor, gliosis, dilated perivascular spaces, white matter necrosis, and/or axonal loss within the cap- or patch-like areas of signal hyperintensity, and these findings are absent in the surrounding tissue where the MRI signal appeared normal (Chimowitz et al., 1992). Consistent with the interpretation that these histopathological changes reflect cerebrovascular disease, functional imaging studies find local reductions in blood flow in the areas where WMH are apparent in MRI scans from the same participants (Fazekas, 1989; Herholz et al., 1990; Kobari et al., 1990).

Lacunae also are more prevalent in MRI images from participants with late-onset depression than in age-matched controls without depression, a finding that further supports the hypothesis that cerebrovascular disease increases the risk for depression. Lacunae appear in MRI images within grey matter as irregularly shaped, signal hyperintensities >5 mm in T2-weighted images, and as signal hypointensities in T1-weighted images. Such lesions reflect areas where infarcted tissue has been replaced by CSF. Lacunae are distinguished from Virchow–Robin spaces, which are small, punctate foci evident on T2-weighted MR images that reflect dilated perivascular spaces.

The hypothesis that the pathogenesis of late-life depression involves cerebrovascular disease also is supported by epidemiological evidence. The risk factors for developing WMH also constitute risk factors for atherosclerotic cerebrovascular disease, namely advancing age, hypertension, diabetes, and ischemic stroke (Awad, Johnson, et al., 1986; Awad, Spetzler, et al., 1986; Gerard and Weisberg, 1986; Fazekas, 1989; Coffey et al., 1990; Chimowitz et al., 1992). For example, Fazekas (1989) reported that the proportion of participants having subcortical or deep WMH ranged from 11% of participants scanned between age 40 and 49 to 83% of participants age 70 and older, and was highest in participants with known risk factors for cerebrovascular disease.

Incidence of MR Signal Hyperintensities in Late-Life Depression

The elevated prevalence of signal hyperintensities in T2-weighted MRI scans from elderly participants with depression was initially observed in uncontrolled studies. Krishnan et al. (1988) reported patchy white matter lesions in 72% of a depressive sample (n = 35) with illness-onset after age 45, and Coffey et al. (1988) noted "moderate-to-severe" WMH in 66% of a sample of predominantly elderly participants with depression (n = 67) referred for electroconvulsive therapy. That these prevalence rates are higher than the corresponding rates in age-matched, healthy controls was subsequently established in controlled studies (Table 31.1). Coffey et al. (1990) reported that the incidence of moderate-to-severe signal hyperintensities (graded by size) is increased in

TABLE 31.1 *Deep White Matter (DWMH) and Periventricular (PVH) Hyperintensities on MRI Scans in Patients with Affective Disorders - Controlled Studies*

Year	*Investigators*	*Patients*	*Controls*	*Results*
Studies in unipolar depression				
1990	Coffey et al.	51 elderly	22	More DWMHs and PVHs in patients over controls
1990	Zubenko et al.	67	44	More cortical and white matter hyperintensities in patients
1991	Lesser et al.	14 (psychotic)	72	More DWMHs and PVHs in patients over controls
1991	Rabins et al.	21 elderly	14	More cortical and white matter hyperintensities in patients
1993	Krishnan et al.	25 elderly	20	More DWMHs and PVHs in patients over controls
1995	Dupont et al.	30	26	No difference in abnormal white matter
1996	O'Brien, Desmond, et al.	60	39	More DWMHs in patients
1998	Greenwald et al.	35 elderly	31	More left frontal DWMHs in patients
Studies in bipolar disorder				
1987	Dupont et al.	14	8	More DWMHs and PVHs in patients over controls
1990	Dupont et al.	19	10	More DWMHs and PVHs in patients over controls
1990	Swayze et al.	48	47	More DWMHs and PVHs in patients over controls
1991	McDonald et al.	12 late-onset	12	More large subcortical hyperintensities in patients
1991	Figiel, Krishnan, Rao, et al.	18	18	More DWMHs and PVHs in patients over controls
1992	Brown et al.	22	154	No differences
1993	Strakowski et al.	17 first mania	16	No differences
1994	Aylward et al.	30	30	More DWMHs in patients (mostly frontal) in patients
1995	Dupont et al.	36	26	More abnormal white matter in patients

elderly participants who are depressed relative to age-matched controls in the periventricular (62% vs. 23%, respectively) and deep white matter (55% vs. 14%) and in the thalamus/ basal ganglia (51% vs. 5%). Similarly, Iidaka et al. (1996) found hyperintensities in the putamen and the globus pallidus in 57% of elderly participants with depression versus 27% of controls. Greenwald et al. (1996; Greenwald et al., 1998) localized the areas where such lesions predominate in participants with depression versus controls to the left frontal lobe and left striatum—the same areas where cerebral infarctions increased risk for poststroke MDE (Starkstein and Robinson, 1989). In an extension of these findings, MacFall et al. (2001) found that within the left orbitofrontal cortex (OFC) was the specific cortical area where WMH were associated with an increased risk for MDE. These data converge with evidence from functional imaging studies of early- and mid-life depression indicating that the left OFC plays a modulatory role over depressive symptoms, and that dysfunction of this region from various etiologies increases risk for depression (reviewed below).

The increased prevalence of MR signal hyperintensities in elderly depression appears to be largely attributable to participants with a late-life-onset of MDD. Figiel, Krisnan, Doraiswamy, et al. (1991) initially observed that 6 of 10 participants with late-onset depression (first MDE after age 60) but only 1 of 9 age-matched, early-onset cases (first MDE before age 60) had WMH larger than 1 cm in diameter, and that the same proportions of each subsample had basal ganglia lesions. Krishnan et al. (1993) later demonstrated that elderly participants with depression (n = 25) had an increased frequency of subcortical hyperintensities, smaller caudate nuclei, and smaller putamenal complexes than age-matched controls and noted that these findings were all more pronounced in the late-onset subset.

This association between the extent of MR signal hyperintensities and the age at which participants suffer their first MDE has been confirmed in several studies. Hickie et al. (1995) showed that in hospitalized participants with depression (n = 39, ages 28–86), the occurrence of WMH correlated with onset of MDD after age 50. Lesser et al. (1996) reported that the frequency of more severe WMH was higher in participants with depression whose first MDE occurred after age 50 (n = 60) relative to participants with depression with a first MDE before age 35 (n = 35) and to controls with other neuropsychiatric disorders (n = 165). Lesser et al. (1991) also observed that 50% of participants with depression who developed psychotic features after age 45 (n = 14) had combined periventricular and deep WMH volume of greater than 3 cm^3 compared with less than 10% of healthy controls (n = 72). Finally, Fujikawa et al. (1993), showed that of depressives studied in mid- to late life (n = 205), participants aged 50–65 years who had their first MDE after age 50 had a higher incidence of WMH meeting criteria for "silent cerebral infarction" (see below) than participants with earlier-onset depression. This study also showed that among participants with depression aged 65 or older, 94% of participants with their first MDE occurring after age 65 had such lesions compared with 66% of participants whose first MDE occurred between ages 50 and 65.

These findings suggest that cerebrovascular disease plays a major role in the pathogenesis of MDE arising in late life, extending evidence from studies of poststroke depression (Starkstein and Robinson, 1989; Krishnan et al., 1993). Consistent with this hypothesis, elderly participants with depression with WMH meeting criteria for putative cerebral infarction were less likely to have a family history of a mood disorder (the major risk factor for early-onset depression) but more likely to have a family history of hypertension (Fujikawa et al., 1994). One group argued that the term *silent cerebral ischemia* should be applied to areas of MR signal hyperintensity greater than 5 mm in size (in T2-weighted images) in participants without a history of neurological signs of cerebrovascular infarction (Fujikawa et al., 1993). Nevertheless, though such lesions may not be associated with motor, sensory, or cognitive impairment, their association with depression implies that they are not clinically "silent." In participants with late-onset depression with MRI evidence of cerebrovascular lesions, the depressive syndrome itself may reflect a neuropsychiatric sequela of cerebral dysfunction involving the brain structures that modulate emotional processing (Krishnan et al., 1993; Drevets and Todd, 1997). The clinical impact of such lesions is evidenced further by the poorer clinical response to treatment, the higher likelihood of treatment-related adverse reactions (for example, delirium), and the more prominent cognitive impairment found in elderly participants with depression with moderate-to-severe WMH and/or lacunae relative to elderly participants with depression without such lesions (Figiel et al., 1989; Figiel et al., 1990; Fujikawa et al., 1996; Lesser et al., 1996).

MR Signal Hyperintensities in Bipolar Disorder

The incidence of MR signal hyperintensities also appears elevated in bipolar disorder (BPD). Dupont et al. (1987; Dupont et al., 1990) reported deep or periventricular WMH in 8 of 14 participants with BPD and subcortical hyperintensities in 9 of 19 participants with BPD compared with none of the controls. In bipolar cases with subcortical WMH reimaged one year later, the lesions persisted. Dupont et al. (1995) later compared 30 participants with MDD, 36 participants with BPD, and 26 controls with no depression and found that the mean volume of abnormal white matter was larger in the participants with BPD than the participants with MDD and participants who were healthy (who did not differ from each other). However, in similar or larger samples sizes of participants with BPD, other investigators found much smaller rates of participants with MR signal hyperintensities that did not differ significantly from controls in incidence or size (Swayze et al., 1990; Brown et al., 1992; Strakowski et al., 1993). The age-at-onset of BPD may prove relevant for studies assessing MR signal hyperintensities in BPD, as McDonald et al. (1991) observed that participants with BPD with an age-of illness-onset after age 50 were more likely to have large subcortical hyperintensities.

Incidence of MR Signal Hyperintensities in Dementia

Magnetic resonance imaging evidence of WMH is not specific to mood disorders and also is common in multi-infarct and Alzheimer's-type dementia (O'Brien, Ames, and Schwietzer, 1996). Zubenko et al. (1990) found that the incidence of lacunae, cortical infarction, and deep or periventricular WMH were similar in participants with dementia (n = 61) and age-matched, participants with depression (n = 67), although cortical atrophy was more prominent in dementia (all of these abnormalities were more common in the participants with depression and dementia relative to an age-matched, healthy sample: n = 44). Similarly, Rabins et al. (1991) found no differences in the rates of WMH and lacunae between participants with dementia of the Alzheimer type (n = 16) and elderly patients with depression (n = 21), both of whom had a greater size and frequency of basal ganglia lesions than age-matched, healthy controls (n = 14). Finally, in a study comparing MRI scans of 61 participants with Alzheimer's-type dementia, 60 participants with MDD and 39 controls, O'Brien, Desmond, et al. (1996) found that deep WMH were more common in the participants with depression (especially in those with late-life onset) whereas periventricular WMH were more common in the participants with dementia.

Neuromorphometric Studies of Mood Disorders

Cerebral ventricles

More than 30 studies have examined ventricular size in depression using CT or MRI. The methods for measuring ventricle-to-brain ratio (VBR) vary across studies, with most groups obtaining linear or areal measures from the axial slice where the ventricles appear largest and others using dimensional measures of ventricular volume (Coffey et al., 1993; Drevets and Botteron, 1997). Enlargement of the lateral ventricles was consistently found in participants with MDD who were elderly, particular in those with late-life-onset MDD (in whom ventricular enlargement likely signify *ex vacuo* changes associated with ischemic neuropathology), and less consistently found in participants with delusional depression (reviewed in Elkis et al., 1995; Drevets and Botteron, 1997). In contrast, enlargement of the lateral ventricles has generally not been present in MRI studies of samples limited to midlife, nondelusional, participants with MDD, and to older participants with MDD with an early age-onset of MDD. In some studies, the increased VBR in participants with depression samples was shown to correlate with cognitive impairment, cortisol hypersecretion, hypothyroidism, or reduced CSF concentrations of the serotonin metabolite *5-HIAA*.

Enlargement of the third ventricle has been found in most studies of BPD (reviewed in Drevets and Botteron, 1997; Pearlson et al., 1997). In contrast, third ventricle enlargement was less consistently found in MDD (Drevets and Botteron, 1997). The brain structures where tissue loss may result in third ventricle enlargement in BPD have not been identified but may involve structures that line the third ventricle, such as the medial thalamus, hypothalamus, or habenula. The magnitude of ventricular enlargement in BPD generally is similar to that found in schizophrenia.

Frontal lobe structures

Although total cerebral volume generally has not differed between participants with depression and healthy samples, neuromorphometric abnormalities have been reported in specific frontal lobe, temporal lobe, and basal ganglia structures. Krishnan et al. (1992) reported decreased width of the frontal lobe, and Coffey et al. (1993) reported decreased frontal lobe volume (by 7%) in MRI studies of participants with mid- and late-life depression relative to age-matched, healthy controls. Similarly, Kumar et al. (1997) found the prefrontal cortex (PFC) volume smaller in participants with late-life "minor depression" compared with age-matched controls.

More pronounced reductions of grey matter volume were found in MDD and BPD in specific subregions of the PFC. In the anterior cingulate cortex (ACC) ventral to the genu of the corpus callosum (that is, subgenual), left-lateralized reductions (20%–40%) of grey matter volume were evident in participants with familial MDD, participants with familial BPD, and participants with MDD with psychotic features (Drevets et al., 1997, Hirayasu et al., 1999; Botteron et al., 2002; Coryell et al. 2005; Fig. 31.2; see also COLOR FIGURE 31.2 in separate insert). This finding has been confirmed by postmortem studies of clinically similar samples (Öngür et al., 1998). This reduction in volume exists early in the illness in familial BPD (Hirayasu et al., 1999) and MDD (Botteron et al., 2002). Although effective treatment with selective serotonin reuptake inhibitors (SSRIs) did not alter the subgenual PFC volume in MDD (Drevets et al., 1997), this cortex appeared larger in participants

A

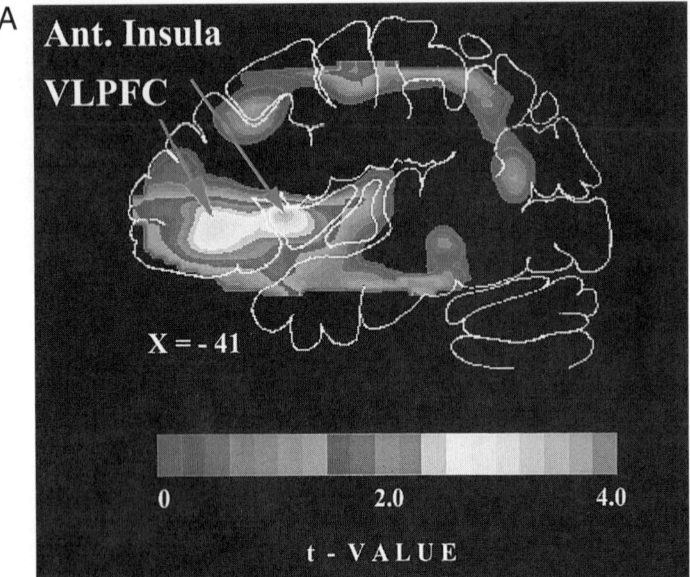

B

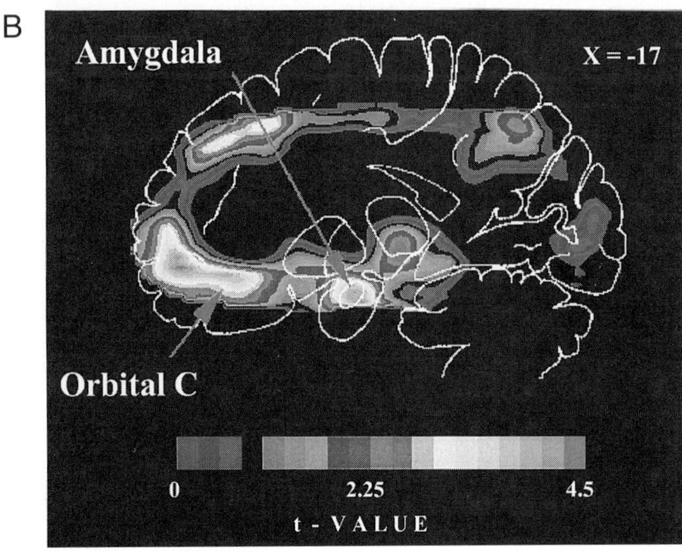

FIGURE 31.2 (*A-B*) Areas of abnormally increased blood flow in patients with major depressive disorder. The image sections shown are from an image of t-values, produced by a voxel-by-voxel computation of the unpaired t-statistic to compare regional CBF between a depressed sample selected according to criteria for familial pure depressive disease (n = 13) and a healthy control sample (n = 33) (Drevets et al., 1992). The positive t-values shown correspond to areas where flow is increased in the depressives relative to the controls. The abnormal activity in these regions was replicated using glucose metabolism imaging in independent subject samples (Drevets, Spitznagel, and Raichle, 1995; Drevets, Bogers and Raichle, 2002; Drevets, Price, et al., 2002). (*A*) Sagittal section at 17 mm left of midline illustrating areas of increased CBF in depression in the amygdala and orbital cortex. (*B*) This area of increased flow extended through the lateral orbital cortex (C) to the ventrolateral prefrontal cortex (VLPFC) and anterior (Ant) insula (Drevets et al., 1992; Drevets, Bogers and Raichle, 2002). The x coordinate locates sagittal sections in mm to the left of midline. (*A-B*) The PET images from which the t-image was generated have been stereotaxically transformed to the coordinate system of Talairach and Tournoux (*Co-Planar Stereotaxic Atlas of the Human Brain*, Stuttgart, Thieme, 1988), from which the corresponding atlas outline is shown. Anterior is left. Illustration *A* is modified from Price et al. (1996) and *B* is reproduced from Drevets (1994) with permission. CBF: cerebral blood flow; PET: positron emission tomography

with BPD medicated with lithium compared to participants with BPD who were unmedicated, compatible with evidence that chronic administration of these mood stabilizers increases expression of the neuroprotective protein, Bcl-2, in the frontal cortex of experimental animals (Moore et al., 2004).

In the lateral orbital cortex, volume has also been found reduced in vMRI studies of MDD (Lai et al., 2000) and BPD (Lyoo et al., 2004; Nugent et al. 2006), as well as in postmortem neuropathological studies of MDD (Rajkowska et al., 1999).

Temporal lobe structures

The volume of the entire temporal lobe was reportedly decreased in participants with BPD versus healthy controls by Hauser et al. (1989) and Altschuler et al. (1991). However, this finding was not replicated by Johnstone et al. (1989), Swayze et al. (1992), or Pearlson et al. (1997) in BPD, or by Coffey et al. (1993) in a predominantly MDD sample. An abnormal degree of temporal lobe asymmetry (right larger than left) was noted in four studies of MDD and one study of BPD. Another study found reduced grey matter in the superior temporal gyrus in participants with BPD versus controls (Nugent et al., 2006).

Morphometric MRI studies of medial temporal lobe structures have reported significant reductions in hippocampal volume in MDD, with the magnitudes of difference ranging from 8% to 19% versus healthy controls (Bremner et al., 2000; Mervaala et al., 2000; Steffens et al., 2000). The reduction in hippocampal volume in MDD persists into remission (Neumeister et al., 2005). Sheline et al. (1996) reported that the hippocampal volume correlated inversely with the estimated total time spent depressed in MDD. Nevertheless, many groups found no significant differences between MDD and control samples (Hauser et al., 1989; Axelson et al., 1993; Pantel et al., 1997; P.J. Shah et al., 1998; Ashtari et al., 1999; Vakili et al., 2000; von Gunten et al., 2000), possibly reflecting biological heterogeneity across MDD samples. For example, Vythilingam et al. (2002) reported that the hippocampal volume was abnormally decreased in women with depression who also had suffered early-life trauma, but not in women with depression without early-life trauma.

In BPD, reduced hippocampal volume was reported by Noga et al. (2001) and Swayze et al. (1992) relative to healthy controls, but Pearlson et al. (1997) found no differences between BPD and control samples. Notably, postmortem studies of BPD found histopathological changes in the hippocampus may be more limited to the subiculum (e.g., Eastwood and Harrison, 2000).

Two studies reported abnormalities of the hippocampal T1 MR signal in MDD. Krishnan, Doraiswamy, Figiel, et al. (1991) observed that the T1 relaxation time was reduced in the hippocampus, but not in the entire temporal lobe, in participants with MDD relative to healthy controls, and Sheline et al. (1996) observed that elderly participants with MDD had a higher number of areas showing low MR signal than age-matched controls in T1-weighted images. The significance of such abnormalities remains unclear.

Finally, the volume of the amygdala has been reported to be decreased, increased (e.g., Frodl et al., 2004), or not different (e.g., Mervaala et al., 2000) in participants with MDD relative to healthy controls. Similarly in BPD amygdala volume was reported to be increased (e.g., Altshuler et al., 1998; Strakowski et al., 1999), decreased (Pearlson et al., 1997; Blumberg et al., 2003; DelBello et al., 2004), or not different (Swayze et al., 1992) relative to healthy controls. The disagreements in the results across studies may be attributable to technical factors, as the amygdala's small size and proximity to other grey matter structures limits the validity and reliability for delimiting amygdala boundaries in images acquired using MRI scanners of ≤1.5 Tesla field strength.

Basal ganglia

Some MRI studies reported that volumes of basal ganglia structures also are abnormal in MDD (Table 31.2). Husain et al. (1991) reported that the putamen was smaller in depressives (mean age = 55) versus controls, and Krishnan et al. (1992) found a smaller caudate volume in participants with depression (mean age = 48) than controls. In elderly participants with depression, Krishnan et al. (1993) reported smaller volumes of putamen and caudate relative to age-matched controls. These findings were consistent with the postmortem study of Baumann et al. (1999), which found that smaller caudate and accumbens area volumes in participants with MDD than controls. However, Dupont et al. (1995) and Lenz et al. (2000) found no significant differences in caudate or lenticular nucleus (putamen plus globus pallidus) volumes between younger participants with MDD (mean age = 39) and controls.

Volumetric MRI studies of BPD have not found significant differences in the volumes of basal ganglia structures

TABLE 31.2 *Basal Ganglia Pathology in Affective Disorders—Controlled MRI Studies*

Year	*Investigators*	*Patients*	*Controls*	*Results*
Studies in unipolar depression				
1990	Coffey et al.	51 elderly	22	More basal ganglia lesions in patients
1991	Rabins et al.	21 elderly	14	More basal ganglia lesions in patients
1991	Husain et al.	41	44	Smaller putamen in patients
1992	Krishnan et al.	50	50	Smaller caudate in patients
1993	Krishnan et al.	25 elderly	20	Smaller caudate and putamen in patients
1995	Dupont et al.	30	26	No significant differences in caudate and lenticular volumes (decreased thalamic volume in patients)
1996	Greenwald et al.	48 elderly	39	More severe hyperintensities in the subcortical gray matter in patients
1996	Iidaka et al.	30 elderly	30	More hyperintensities in the putamen and globus pallidus in patients
1998	Greenwald et al.	35	31	More left putaminal hyperintensities in patients
Studies in bipolar disorder				
1992	Swayze et al.	48	47	No significant differences
1994	Aylward et al.	30	30	Larger caudate volume in patients
1994	Harvey et al.	26	34	Subcortical tissue volume estimated; no differences
1995	Dupont et al.	36	26	No significant differences in caudate and lenticular volumes (larger thalamic volume in patients)

relative to controls (reviewed in Drevets and Botteron, 1997). However, one postmortem study reported reduced caudate and accumbens area volumes in participants with BPD versus controls (Baumann et al., 1999). It remains unclear whether the discrepant results across studies may be accounted for by differences in the age or age at depression onset of their participants.

Other cerebral structures

Other brain structures have been less often studied in mood disorders. Of vMRI studies of the thalamus, Dupont et al. (1995) found reduced thalamic volume in participants with MDD versus controls, whereas Krishnan et al. (Krishnan, Doraiswamy, Figiel, et al., 1991; Krishnan et al., 1993) found no difference between participants with depression and controls. Studies of thalamic volume in BPD also reported conflicting results. In the posterior cingulate cortex, Nugent et al. (2006) reported reduced grey matter in BPD. In the cerebellum, some studies found reduced vermal volume in participants with depression versus controls (S.A. Shah et al., 1992; Escalona et al., 1993) whereas others did not.

Endocrine glands

Consistent with evidence that cortisol hypersecretion and hypothalamic-pituitary-adrenal (HPA) axis dysfunction exists in some participants with depression, a substantial proportion of participants with MDD showed enlargement of the adrenal and pituitary glands. Amsterdam et al. (1987) reported that 8 of 16 participants with depression who underwent abdominal CT were judged by radiologist's clinical reading to have enlarged adrenal glands. Similarly, Nemeroff et al. (1992) found that the abdominal CT films of 11 of 38 participants with depression but 0 of 11 healthy controls were clinically reported as showing adrenal enlargement, with the mean adrenal volume of the participants with depression exceeding that of the controls by 57%. Rubin et al. (1995) similarly reported that the median adrenal volume was increased 68% in participants with depression (n = 11) versus controls (n = 11) using abdominal MRI, but that the median adrenal volume of the participants with depression decreased approximately to that of controls following remission. In a subsequent study, Rubin et al. (1996) showed that the mean adrenal volume was 38% larger in participants with depression (n = 35) than controls (n = 35), and that the magnitude of the enlargement did not correlate with the severity or duration of the index MDE or the lifetime number of episodes. The results of these imaging studies are consistent with the finding that the mean adrenal gland weight is abnormally increased in victims of suicide (Zis and Zis, 1987). The cause of adrenal enlargement is putatively related to the hypersecretion of corticotrophin-releasing hormone and/or other adrenocorticotropic hormone (ACTH) secretagogues in depression, as chronic stimulation by ACTH results in hypertrophy of the adrenal cortex.

Pituitary size is also enlarged in MRI studies of depression. Krishnan, Doraiswamy, Lurie, et al. (1991) showed that MRI-based measures of the cross-sectional area and the volume of the pituitary were increased (by 34% and 41%, respectively) in participants with depression (n = 19) relative to controls (n =19).

Diffusion Tensor Imaging

Magnetic resonance diffusion tensor imaging (DTI) is a noninvasive in vivo method for characterizing the integrity of anatomical connections and white matter circuitry and provides a quantitative assessment of the brain's white matter microstructure. Hyperintensities showed more abnormalities than normal regions thus suggesting that hyperintensities reflect a pathophysiological process that damages the structure of brain tissue (Taylor et al., 2001). Microstructural changes in the frontal lobe also are associated with late-life depression (Taylor et al., 2004). This has been shown in young and elderly participants with depression (Li et al., 2007). Microstructural changes in the white matter of the OFC appear to be associated with BPD using DTI (Beyer et al., 2005).

FUNCTIONAL NEUROIMAGING: APPLICATIONS IN MOOD DISORDERS RESEARCH

Functional imaging research also holds great promise for elucidating the pathophysiology of mood disorders because neurochemical and neuroendocrine data indicate that these conditions are associated with disruptions of brain function, yet with the exception of late-onset MDD, structural imaging and postmortem studies have shown that the corresponding brain morphology largely is intact. The episodic nature and responsiveness to treatment of mood disorders permit imaging in symptomatic and asymptomatic states so that the physiological correlates of depressive symptoms can be distinguished from the pathophysiological changes underlying the tendency to develop depressive episodes. Moreover, because depressive symptoms reflect distortions of emotional states that can be expressed by participants without depression, the nature of neurophysiological changes related to the depressed state can be explored by imaging hemodynamic changes in participants who are healthy during experimentally induced states of sadness or anxiety, or during the processing of emotionally valenced stimuli. Finally, imaging techniques for quantifying neuroreceptor binding and neurotransmitter function enable in vivo characterization of the neurochemical abnormalities in mood disorders. The data offered from such studies are being used to localize specific brain regions for histopathological assessment, to investigate treatment mechanisms, and to guide genetic and treatment-outcome studies.

In contrast to their utility in research, the clinical capabilities of functional imaging techniques for determining diagnosis or guiding treatment selection have not been established. The abnormalities identified thus far in depression have had relatively small effect sizes, and the sensitivity and specificity have not been characterized sufficiently to support clinical application.

Significance of Cerebral Blood Flow and Glucose Metabolism

Local cerebral blood flow (CBF) and glucose metabolism predominantly reflect a summation of the metabolic activity associated with terminal field synaptic transmission within each image volume element, or voxel (Raichle, 1987; DiRocco et al., 1989). Altered regional CBF and metabolism thus may signify corresponding changes in neurotransmission from afferent projections arising from within the same structure or from a distal structure (Raichle, 1987; DiRocco et al., 1989). Dynamic brain images thus provide maps of regional neural function associated with ongoing mental activity. Metabolic and CBF images also are affected by the integrity of the cerebrovascular system, the amount of viable grey matter within an image voxel, and other factors that may be abnormal in mood disorders.

Differences in CBF or metabolism between participants with depression and controls thus may reflect neurophysiological correlates of emotional, behavioral, or cognitive symptoms of MDE, mood-congruent biases on neural processing in depression, pathophysiological changes that predispose to or result from affective disease, or compensatory mechanisms invoked to modulate or inhibit pathological processes. The physiological correlates of depressive symptoms and behaviors putatively appear as baseline abnormalities of local CBF or metabolism that normalize following effective treatment and that may, to some extent, be reproduced in participants who are healthy imaged while performing tasks that mimic the corresponding depressive manifestation. In contrast, neuroimaging abnormalities that reflect pathophysiological changes in synaptic transmission associated with altered neurotransmitter function, receptor sensitivity/density, or neuronal arborization (e.g., Wooten and Collins, 1981; Ågren et al., 1993) may persist whether participants are symptomatic or asymptomatic (Drevets et al., 1992). Irreversible abnormalities in CBF and metabolism also may be associated with grey matter volume reductions in familial mood disorders, or cerebrovascular disease in elderly participants with depression with a late-age of depression-onset (see below; Fig. 31.1; Drevets et al., 1997; Krishnan et al., 1993.

Technical Issues Relevant to the Interpretation of Functional Brain Images

The functional imaging literature reflects some disagreement in the results across studies. Many inconsistencies within this literature likely reflect limitations of statistical power for replicating findings across studies because the sample sizes employed have been small and the effect sizes of the abnormalities found to date also are small. Other apparent discrepancies across studies may be resolved by considering issues related to participant selection, image acquisition, and image analysis. Nevertheless, some of the variability within the literature is likely accounted for by the biological heterogeneity encompassed within the *Diagnostic and Statistical Manual of Mental Disorders–4th ed.* (*DSM-IV*: American Psychiatric Association, 1994) diagnostic categories for mood disorders.

Issues related to image acquisition and analysis

Understanding the neuroimaging literature requires critical assessment of a few key aspects of experimental design and analysis. The precision of anatomical localization in functional images has benefited from progressive improvements in spatial resolution (to 4 mm for the newest generation of positron emission tomography [PET] camera and < 1mm for high resolution functional MRI [fMRI]) and development of PET-MRI image coregistration techniques and of voxel-wise analysis approaches capable of identifying inherent differences between groups (Drevets and Botteron, 1997; Figs. 31.2 and 31.3; see also COLOR FIGURE 31.3 in separate insert). However, older studies applied techniques that were more severely constrained with respect to sensitivity and spatial resolution (Drevets and Botteron, 1997; Raichle, 1987). For example, images acquired using single photon emission computed tomography (SPECT) or nontomographic systems during ^{133}Xe administration provided CBF measures limited to the cortical grey matter lying near the scalp, precluding measures from limbic, basal ganglia, and ventral and medial frontal and temporal lobe structures (Raichle, 1987). Moreover, perfusion measures obtained using SPECT and either ^{99m}Tc-HMPAO or ^{133}I-iodoamphetamine, agents that are not freely diffusable across the blood-brain-barrier, were relatively insensitive to CBF increases within the physiological range. Moreover, though PET affords relatively higher spatial resolution and sensitivity for deep structures, in most PET studies the images have been blurred to much lower spatial resolutions prior to analysis to reduce the effects of anatomical variability across participants.

Another image processing issue that influences specificity and sensitivity involves "normalization" of regional data by dividing local-by-global measures. Because of the small sample sizes involved in imaging studies,

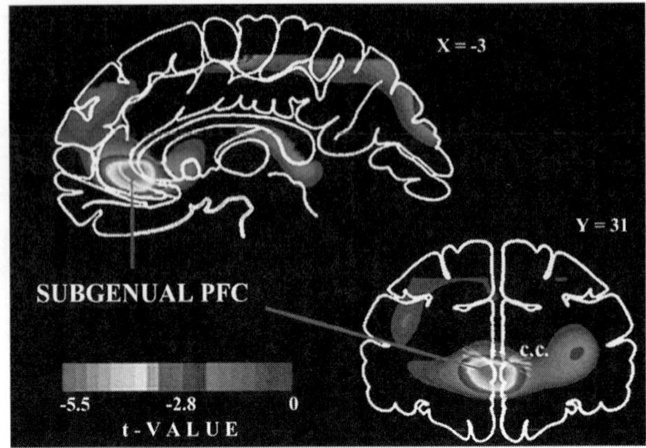

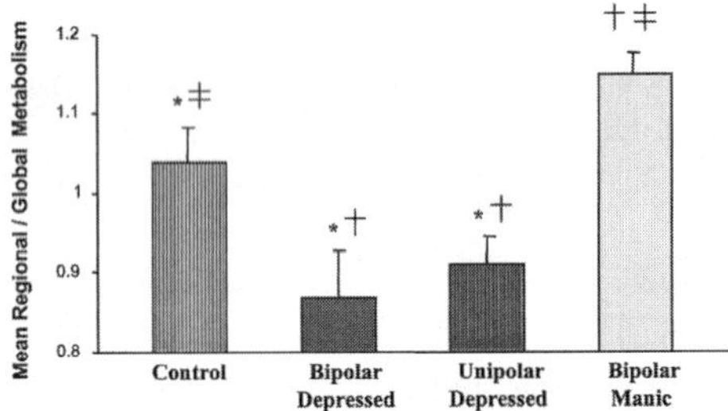

FIGURE 31.3 Altered metabolism in PFC ventral to the genu of the corpus callosum (that is, subgenual PFC) in mood disorders. The top panel shows negative voxel t-values where glucose metabolism is decreased in depressives relative to controls in coronal (31 mm anterior to the anterior commissure, or y = 31) and sagittal (3 mm left of midline, or x = −3) planes of a statistical parametric image that compares depressives to controls (Drevets et al., 1997). This image localized an abnormality in the subgenual portion of the ACC (subgenual ACC; Drevets et al., 1997), which was subsequently shown to be accounted for by a corresponding reduction in cortex volume on the left side (see text). Anterior or left is to left. The bar histogram in the lower panel shows mean, normalized, glucose metabolic values for the left subgenual ACC measured using MRI-based region-of-interest analysis. Metabolism is decreased in depressed patients with either BD or MDD relative to healthy controls. In contrast, subjects scanned in the manic phase of BD have higher metabolism than either depressed or control patients in this region. Asterisk: difference between controls and bipolar depressives significant at $p < 0.025$; cross: difference between depressed and manic significant at $p < 0.01$; double cross: difference between control and manic significant at $p < 0.05$. Although none of these patients were involved in the study that generated the images shown in Figure 31.2, the mean glucose metabolism in this independent sample of depressed patients and controls also confirmed the areas of abnormally increased activity in the depressed patients in the amygdala, lateral orbital cortex, ventrolateral PFC, and medial thalamus (not shown in the t-image section in the figure, which only illustrates negative t-values corresponding to hypometabolic areas in the patients who were depressed). Reproduced with permission from Drevets et al. (1997) (upper panel) and Drevets (2001) (lower panel). PFC: prefrontal cortex; ACC: anterior cingulate cortex; MRI: magnetic resonance imaging; BD: bipolar depressed; MDD: unipolar depressed.

normalization is usually required to reduce the variability of regional values so that intergroup differences can be detected. In most studies of unmedicated, midlife participants with depression the whole-brain CBF and glucose metabolism have not differed significantly between participants with depression and controls, so whole-brain activity serves as a useful denominator for factoring out nonspecific global effects (e.g., Baxter et al., 1985; Silfverskiöld and Risberg, 1989; Bench et al., 1993; Drevets et al., 1997, Kimbrell et al., 2002). In contrast, normalization of regional values by measurements confined to another region can prove more difficult to interpret. For example, early SPECT studies of depression normalized regional perfusion by flow in the cerebellum, a practice that confounded results because PET studies showed that medial cerebellar flow was abnormally increased in MDD (normalization to cerebellar flow thus artifactually decreased ratios obtained for other brain regions; Philpot et al., 1993). Nevertheless, whole-brain CBF and metabolism can be reduced by benzodiazepines, antipsychotic drugs, or cerebrovascular disease (Silfverskiöld and Risberg, 1989; Maes et al., 1993; Lesser et al., 1994), potentially confounding the interpretation of absolute and normalized values, so such issues merit specific consideration in experimental design.

Image analysis approaches for detecting differences in regional physiology between participants with depression and controls also influence the sensitivity for detecting differences. The most anatomically precise technique involves MRI-based region-of-interest (ROI) analysis in which ROI is predefined on each participant's own anatomical MRI scan and then transferred to coregistered, lower resolution functional images. This approach can nevertheless mislocalize the peak difference or excessively dilute differences if the ROI defined is too large (Mazziotta et al., 1981; Drevets, Price, et al., 2002). Voxel-wise approaches (for example, Statistical Parametric Mapping, or SPM) thus were developed to survey entire data sets and localize peak, inherent differences between conditions. These approaches nevertheless reduce sensitivity for detecting abnormalities in structures that are either small or characterized by a high degree of anatomical variability (e.g., Drevets, Bogers, et al., 2002) because they depend upon spatial transformation of the primary tomographs into a standardized stereotaxic space using algorithms that do not precisely align small structures or variable anatomy across participants. To reduce the effects of this misalignment error, images are blurred ("filtered") to lower spatial resolutions. One approach that has proven useful is to iteratively apply MRI-based ROI analysis and voxel-wise analysis to exploit the strengths and address the limitations inherent in each method (e.g., Drevets et al., 1997).

To increase sensitivity for detecting abnormalities (that is, reduce Type II error), most studies compared image data between participants with depression and controls either in large numbers of predefined ROI or using voxel-wise approaches. Voxel-wise approaches compute tens of thousands of independent statistical comparisons per image set, however, so the probability that an apparent difference between groups reflects multiple comparison artifact is high. Studies applying such approaches must therefore establish the significance of findings by replication in independent samples or by applying appropriate corrections of *p* values for multiple comparisons (Drevets et al., 1992; Drevets et al., 1997; Poline et al., 1997).

Clinical sources of variability in image data from depressed samples

Medication effects comprise an important source of variability in functional imaging studies, as regional physiology and chemistry of the brain areas of interest in depression can be altered by antidepressant, antipsychotic, and antianxiety drugs (e.g., Silfverskiöld and Risberg, 1989; Maes et al., 1993; Drevets and Botteron, 1997). These agents also affect the behavioral and hemodynamic responses to emotionally valenced sensory stimuli employed as neurocognitive probes in fMRI studies. Image data acquired in participants medicated with these drugs thus are difficult to interpret unless scans in the unmedicated condition also are available. Nevertheless, most published studies of depression report data confounded by medication effects, potentially introducing artifactual differences or obscuring true biological differences between participants with depression and controls. Notably, studies of participants with depression confounded by medication effects generally fail to detect the areas of abnormally elevated metabolism seen in unmedicated participants and instead often report regional reductions in flow or metabolism that cannot be replicated in unmedicated samples (reviewed in Drevets and Botteron, 1997).

The clinical heterogeneity reflected within mood disorders introduces another source of variability, as diverse signs and symptoms may have distinct neurophysiological correlates (Drevets and Todd, 1997). For example, clinical features such as psychomotor slowing have been reported to influence neurophysiological and receptor pharmacological measures (see below). Few studies have had sufficiently large samples to characterize the imaging correlates of distinct clinical features, however, so the extent to which differing symptom profiles across depressed samples have contributed to differences in the results across studies remains unclear.

A related challenge for imaging studies is the likelihood that the diagnostic criteria for MDD and BPD encompass groups of disorders that are heterogenous with respect to pathophysiology and etiology. Biological heterogeneity is evidenced by the variety of antecedents to MDE (genetic, medical, psychosocial), the diversity of responses to somatic or psychological therapies, and the variable presence of neuroendocrine, neurochemical, and circadian rhythm disturbances in depressive samples (Drevets and Todd, 1997). If depression is associated with multiple pathophysiologic states, it also may be characterized by an assortment of distinct functional imaging abnormalities.

Consistent with this hypothesis, the reproducibility of some imaging findings in depression depends upon subtyping participants with depression. For example, participants with MDD with familial pure depressive disease (FPDD) were more likely to show imaging abnormalities such as elevated CBF and metabolism in the amygdala (see below). This subgroup also was more likely to show neuroendocrine and other types of biological abnormalities relative to other depressive subtypes (reviewed in Drevets, Price, et al., 2002). This MDD subtype thus may be more often associated with pathophysiologically linked abnormalities (for example, through interactions between the amygdala and CRF/glucocorticoid secretion). Nevertheless, it remains unclear whether subtyping strategies that increase sensitivity for detecting regional abnormalities in depression identify pathophysiologically distinct phenotypes of MDD or more generally "enrich" samples with participants likely to have biological markers for depression.

Effects of structural abnormalities in functional brain images

The vMRI abnormalities seen in some regions in depression can profoundly influence functional imaging measures. Tissue reductions decrease the magnitude of functional or receptor imaging measures from the corresponding regions via "partial volume averaging" effects (Mazziotta et al., 1981). Because of the low spatial resolution of PET and SPECT images, reductions in the proportion of grey matter relative to CSF and/or white matter within corresponding image voxels reduces the measured CBF or metabolism via the partial volume effect of averaging in more CSF, which is metabolically inactive, and white matter, which is one fourth as metabolically active as grey matter, relative to the diminished contribution of grey matter (Mazziotta et al., 1981). Because the ventricular and sulcal enlargement evident in late-onset depression is not apparent in participants with nondelusional MDD with a young age-of-onset, image data from these latter groups constitute a benchmark against which physiological imaging measures in other depressive subtypes are compared (Drevets and Botteron, 1997). Nevertheless, evidence that focal areas of reduced grey matter volume exist even in young participants with nondelusional MDD emphasizes the importance of evaluating areas where CBF and metabolism are irreversibly decreased in participants with depression relative to controls using vMRI and postmortem histopathological studies (Fig. 31.3; Drevets et al., 1997; Öngür et al., 1998.

The WMH patches and lacunae evident in MRI images from participants with late-onset depression present an even greater problem for functional imaging studies because these abnormalities putatively reflect arteriosclerotic or ischemic disease. In vivo imaging studies demonstrate that elderly participants with depression with WMH have decreased CBF and metabolism in the frontal cortex and other areas where WMH are seen relative to age-matched participants with depression without WMH (Lesser et al., 1994). Moreover, because the relationship between regional BF, metabolism, and local synaptic transmission are altered by cerebrovascular disease, functional imaging studies of elderly participants with depression are difficult to interpret unless participants with prominent or diffuse MRI signal hyperintensities have not been excluded.

Effect of behavioral state on flow and metabolism

Because of the sensitivity of CBF and metabolism to changes in neural activity, the behavioral state in which participants are imaged profoundly influences neurophysiological image data. The pattern of physiological imaging abnormalities seen in depression thus depends on the behavioral state under which image data are acquired. For example, limbic and paralimbic areas such as the amygdala, ventral ACC, ventrolateral PFC/lateral orbital cortex, and posterior cingulate cortices normally deactivate during the performance of attentionally demanding tasks (Drevets and Raichle, 1998; Drevets, Bogers, and Raichle, 2002). Presumably because of this phenomenon, the elevations of CBF and metabolism seen in these areas in participants who are depressed scanned while resting with eyes closed have usually not been evident in images acquired as participants are engaged in attentionally demanding tasks.

NEUROPHYSIOLOGICAL IMAGING ABNORMALITIES IN DEPRESSION

Functional imaging studies have begun to characterize the neuroanatomical correlates of MDE, the neurophysiological effects of antidepressant treatments, and the trait-like abnormalities that persist into remission. These studies have identified CBF and metabolic differences between participants with depression and healthy controls in multiple regions, consistent with the expectation that the emotional, cognitive, psychomotor, neurovegetative, neuroendocrine, and neurochemical disturbances associated with depression implicate extended anatomical networks. The ensuing review highlights major findings from studies of unmedicated depressed samples.

Abnormalities within the Prefrontal Cortex (PFC)

Within the PFC, depression is associated with decreased physiological activity in some regions, together with increased activity in others (Drevets and Raichle, 1998). Interpreting this complex pattern requires consideration both of the reductions in tissue volume described above, and also of the principles derived from brain-mapping and lesion analysis studies. Brain-mapping studies show that regional hemodynamic activity increases in patterns specific to the mental operations demanded by a particular cognitive-behavioral state, and that simultaneously hemodynamic activity decreases in some other regions, presumably to facilitate task performance via suppression of unattended, potentially competing background processes (Drevets, Burton et al., 1995; Drevets and Raichle, 1998). For example, the functional image data converge with evidence from anatomical, electrophysiological, and lesion analysis studies to implicate areas within the orbital and medial PFC (OMPFC) in the integration of sensory processing and emotional salience, decision-making pertaining to reward contingencies, modulation of emotional experience and expression, and experience of internally generated emotion and thought (reviewed in Drevets and Raichle, 1998; Öngür et al., 2003).

Ventral anterior cingulate cortex (ACC)

The ACC situated ventral and anterior to the genu of the corpus callosum (termed *subgenual* and *pregenual*, respectively) has been consistently implicated in the pathophysiology of MDD and BPD. In the subgenual PFC, a complex relationship between CBF, metabolism, and illness state exists that appears accounted for by the volumetric reduction of the corresponding cortex described above. In recurrent BPD and MDD, the baseline subgenual ACC CBF and metabolism appear abnormally decreased in PET images during MDE (Drevets et al., 1997), and correlated inversely with the number of lifetime depressive episodes (Kimbrell et al., 2002). However, computer simulations that correct PET data for the partial volume effect of reduced grey matter volume conclude the "actual" metabolic activity in the remaining subgenual PFC tissue is increased in participants with depression relative to controls.

This hypothesis appears compatible with the observation that effective antidepressant pharmacotherapy results in a decrease in metabolic activity in this region in MDD (Buchsbaum et al., 1997; Mayberg et al., 1999; Drevets, Bogers, and Raichle, 2002; Drevets, Thase, et al., 2002). Computer simulations that correct posttreatment image data from MDD samples for spatial resolution (partial volume) effects find that actual metabolism (that is, corrected for the effect of the volumetric reduction in this region on PET measures) decreases to normative levels during effective treatment. Furthermore, these data are consistent with indications that during depressive episodes, metabolism shows a positive relationship with depression severity (Osuch et al., 2000; Drevets,

Bogers, and Raichle, 2002). This mood state-dependency of subgenual ACC metabolism thus appears consistent with PET studies showing that flow increases in this region in healthy humans who are not depressed during sadness internally induced via contemplation of sad thoughts or memories (M.S. George et al., 1995; Mayberg et al., 1999). Notably, Mayberg et al. (2005) showed that deep brain stimulation within the subgenual ACC at frequencies expected to inhibit local neuronal function exerts antidepressant effects in treatment refractory cases.

Neuroimaging measures obtained from the subgenual ACC have been associated with treatment outcome. Siegle et al. (2006) reported that decreased pretreatment reactivity to negative words in the subgenual ACC and increased pretreatment reactivity in the amygdala predicted stronger recovery with cognitive-behavioral therapy in participants who had depression. In addition, Chen et al. (2007) reported that the rate of clinical improvement after 8 weeks of fluoxetine treatment was positively predicted by the grey matter volume and the hemodymanic responsiveness to sad faces in the subgenual and pregenual ACC.

In the pregenual ACC, Drevets et al. (1992) initially found increased CBF in MDD. Although other laboratories also reported abnormalities of CBF and metabolism in this area during depression, these data have been inconsistent (Table 31.3). The variability of these results may have clinical relevance, as several studies report relationships between pregenual ACC activity and subsequent antidepressant treatment outcome. Wu et al. (1992) reported that participants who are depressed whose mood improved during sleep deprivation showed elevated metabolism in the pregenual ACC and amygdala in their pretreatment scans. Mayberg et al. (1997) reported that though metabolism in the pregenual ACC was abnormally increased in participants with depression who subsequently responded to antidepressant drugs, metabolism was decreased in participants with depression who later had poor treatment response. Finally, in a tomographic electroencephalogram (EEG) analysis, Pizzagalli et al. (2001) reported that participants with depression who ultimately showed the best response to nortriptyline showed hyperactivity (higher theta activity) in the pregenual ACC at baseline, as compared to participants showing the poorer response.

The effects of treatment on pregenual ACC flow and metabolism also have differed across studies, with activity decreasing in some but increasing in others in post- relative to pretreatment scans (Table 31.4). Positron emission tomography studies of chronic SSRI treatment have been more consistent, showing reductions in pregenual ACC metabolism in post- relative to pretreatment scans in all but one study (Table 31.4).The extent to which these discrepant findings are explained by differential effects across subregions of this area remains unclear. The pregenual ACC shows elevated CBF during a greater variety of emotional conditions elicited in healthy humans or humans with anxiety disorders (reviewed in Drevets and Raichle, 1998). Electrical stimulation of this region elicits fear, panic, or a sense of foreboding in humans, and vocalization in experimental animals (reviewed in Price et al., 1996).

Postmortem assessment of the subgenual ACC (part of BA 24) demonstrated this abnormal reduction in grey matter was associated with a reduction in glia, no equivalent loss of neurons, and increased neuronal density in MDD and BPD relative to control samples (Öngür et al., 1998). In a tissue section that appeared to correspond to Brodmann area 24 cortex of the pregenual ACC, Cotter et al. (2002) found that glial density was significantly reduced in layer VI from participants with MDD or schizophrenia, but not in participants with BPD (most of whom were receiving mood stabilizers that appear to exert neurotrophic/neuroprotective effects). The mean size of neurons was also reported to be reduced in the deep layers of participants with MDD. In BPD, Benes et al. (2001) found reductions in nonpyramidal cells in the pregenual ACC. The volumetric abnormality in the subgenual PFC most likely reflects a reduction of neuropil rather than in the number of cell bodies. The neuropil (the fibrous layers comprising dendrites and axons) occupies most of the cortex volume and can be remodeled by dendritic atrophy during repeated stress (McEwen, 1999).

In rodents and nonhuman primates the cortex that appears homologous to human subgenual and pregenual ACC has extensive reciprocal connections with areas implicated in the expression of behavioral, autonomic, and endocrine responses to stressors, aversive stimuli and rewarding stimuli, such as the hypothalamus, amygdala, accumbens, subiculum, ventral tegmental area, raphé, locus coeruleus, PAG, and nucleus tractus solitarius (NTS) (reviewed in Drevets et al., 1998, Öngür et al, 2003). Humans with lesions that include the ventral ACC show abnormal autonomic responses to emotionally provocative stimuli, inability to experience emotion related to concepts that ordinarily evoke emotion, and inability to use information regarding the likelihood of punishment and reward in guiding social behavior (Damasio, 1994). In rats, bilateral or right-lateralized lesions of the infralimbic, prelimbic and ventral ACC cortex attenuate sympathetic autonomic responses, stress-induced corticosterone secretion, and gastric stress pathology during restraint stress or exposure to fear-conditioned stimuli (reviewed in Drevets et al., 1998). In contrast, left-sided lesions of this area increase sympathetic autonomic arousal and corticosterone responses to restraint stress (Sullivan and Gratton, 1999). These data suggest the hypothesis that the right subgenual PFC facilitates expression of visceral responses during emotional processing, while the left subgenual PFC modulates such responses

TABLE 31.3 *Functional Imaging Results in Prefrontal Cortex (PFC) for Studies Limited to Unmedicated, Primary, Unipolar Depressives*[a] *Imaged in the Resting Condition*

Authors	*Sample Size*		*Imaging Technique*	*Blood Flow or Glucose Metabolism in DEP Relative to CON*	
	DEP	*CON*		*Ventral PFC*	*Dorsal PFC*
Baxter et al., 1987	14	14	PET, ^{18}FDG	↑ medial orbital C (BL)[b]	N/A
Baxter et al., 1989	10	12	PET, ^{18}FDG	N/A	↓ dorsal anterolateral(BL)
Bench et al., 1992	33[c]	23	PET, $H_2{}^{15}O$	N/A[d]	↓ dorsolateral (L) ↓ dorsal ant. cingulate
Biver et al., 1994	12	12	PET, ^{18}FDG	↑ medial and lateral orbital(BL)	↓ dorsolateral (L)
Brody et al., 2001	24	16	PET, ^{18}FDG	↑ ventrolateral PFC, lateral orbital C	n.s. dorsolateral
Buchsbaum et al., 1997	39	28	PET, ^{18}FDG	↑ pregenual ACC ↓ subgenual ACC/ ventromedial PFC[e]	↓ dorsal medial n.s. dorsolateral
Drevets et al., 1992	13	33	PET, $H_2{}^{15}O$	↑ L. ventrolateral PFC, lateral orbital ↑ pregenual ACC	n.s.
Drevets, Spitznagel, & Raichle, 1995	31	17	PET, ^{18}FDG	↑ ventrolateral PFC, lat. orbital (BL)[g] ↓ subgenual ACC[f]	N/A
Drevets, Bogers, & Raichle, 2002	27	14	PET, ^{18}FDG	↑ lateral orbital C, ↓ ventrolateral PFC (BL)	↓ dorsomedial/ dorsal anterolateral (BL)
Ebert et al., 1991	10	8	SPET,^{99m}TcHMPAO	↑ orbital C (BL)[g]	↓ dorsal anterolateral (L)
Kennedy et al., 2001	13	24	PET, ^{18}FDG	↑ pregenual ACC	↓ dorsolateral (L)
Mayberg et al., 1997	18[i]	15	PET, ^{18}FDG	↑ pregenual ACC in treatment-responsive but ↓ in treatment-resistant; n.s. orbital[i]	↓ dorsolateral (BL)
Nofzinger et al., 1999	6	10	PET, ^{18}FDG	↑ L. medial orbital C ↑ R. lateral orbital C	↓ dorsolateral (L)

Postalache et al., 2002	15	15	PET, ^{18}FDG	↑ ventrolateral PFC, lateral orbital C	n.s.
Saxena et al., 2002	27	17	PET, ^{18}FDG	n.s. (trend to↑ ventrolateral PFC, BL)	n.s.
Silfverskiöld & Risberg, 1989	31	31	Multidetector Probes, ^{133}Xe[j]	n.s. (trend to↑ L ventrolateral PFC)	n.s.
Uytdenhoef et al., 1983	16	20	Multidetector Probes, ^{133}Xe[j]	↑ left "frontal ratio" (which included ventrolateral PFC)	↑ superior frontal g (L)
Wu et al., 1992	15	15	PET, ^{18}FDG	↑ ACC[g]; orbital C N/A	N/A

ACC: anterior cingulate cortex; BL: bilateral; C: cortex; CON: controls; DEP: depressed patients; ^{18}FDG: ^{18}F-fluorodeoxyglucose; g: gyrus; $H_2{}^{15}O$; oxygen-15 water; L: left; PFC: prefrontal cortex; R: right; ^{99m}Tc-HMPAO: technetium-99 HMPAO; ^{133}Xe (xenon-133) used to measure blood flow; n.s: difference assessed and not significant; N/A: region not assessed; ↑ and ↓ indicate increases and decreases, respectively, in the depressed patients; relative to the controls.

a. Image data from studies that are uninterpretable due to confounding medication effects are not reviewed unless data were separately assessed for the unmedicated subsample. Data from studies of "secondary" depression and bipolar depression are addressed separately (see text). Some of these studies included bipolar patients in their depressed samples, but only the results from the unipolar subsample are reported here (unless data were not presented separately for bipolar and unipolar patients). The descriptive terms used to locate regions vary across study, and in some cases distinct terms may be used to describe the same area. Conversely, studies using the same term may be describing different cortical areas (e.g., the "dorsolateral PFC" spans several cm^2 and encompasses thousands of independent resolution elements).

b. This paper compared regional metabolism between patients with obsessive-compulsive disorder and patients with either primary unipolar depression or healthy controls. While the difference between depressed patients and controls was not statistically assessed in this paper, the published values for the orbital-to-hemisphere ratio in the depressives (n = 14; right: 1.17 ± 0.06, left: 1.14 ± 0.05) and the controls (n = 13; right: 1.11 ± 0.08, left: 1.09 ± 0.06) showed differences that were similar in magnitude and variability to the differences found in other studies using images of similar resolution, and would be significant by t test (right: $p < 0.05$, left: $p < 0.02$) (from Table 3 of Baxter et al., 1987).

c. Nineteen of the depressed patients were imaged while receiving various medications. The reported abnormalities were initially identified using image data from the entire depressed sample (n = 33), but the difference between DEP and CON was also confirmed in the unmedicated subsample (n = 14) *post hoc*.

d. This study identified abnormalities using a statistical image that excluded pixels in the orbital cortex, because the images acquired did not extend into this ventral structure for all subjects (Dolan, personal communication).

e. Abnormally reduced metabolism was found in predefined regions-of-interest in ventral ACC and "rectal gyrus" lying within the same horizontal image plane, implying these ventromedial PFC areas were likely located in subgenual ACC.

f. Abnormalities significant in subgroup meeting criteria for familial pure depressive disease, but not for subgroup with familial loading for alcoholism.

g. Abnormality found only in subgroup who proved responsive to sleep deprivation.

h. Reflects the sample size for the unmedicated patients only, who were independently compared to controls and to another 13 benzodiazepine-treated patients.

i. Five of these patients had been subchronically treated with antidepressant drugs prior to scanning. It is unclear whether subchronic antidepressant drug therapy has the same effect of decreasing orbital metabolism as does chronic treatment (Table 31.4).

j. Blood flow is only measured near the scalp using this technique, so results are unavailable for the orbital or cingulate cortices (see text).

TABLE 31.4 *Antidepressant Treatment Effects Upon Ventral Prefrontal Cortical Blood Flow and Metabolism in Major Depression*[a]

Authors	*Treatment Modality*	*Change in CBF or Glucose Metabolism Post- vs. Pretreatment Scans*
Bonne et al., 1996	ECT	↑ pregenual ACC in responders
Brody et al., 2001	paroxetine	↓ pregenual ACC and ventrolateral PFC
	interpersonal therapy	↓ pregenual ACC, ↑ left anterior insula
Buchsbaum et al., 1997	sertraline	↓ pregenual ACC, ↓ ventromedial PFC (see Table 31.3, note e)
Cohen et al., 1992	phototherapy	↓ medial orbital C[b]
Drevets & Raichle, 1992	desipramine	↓ left ventrolateral PFC/ lateral orbital C
Drevets, Bogers, & Raichle, 2002	sertraline	↓ subgenual ACC
Drevets, Thase, et al., 2002	citalopram	↓ ventrolateral PFC/ lateral orbital C (BL) ↓ subgenual and pregenual ACC, ↓ anterior insula (BL)
Ebert et al., 1991	sleep deprivation	↓ orbital C in responders[b]
Goodwin et al., 1993	various drug treatments	↑ anterior cingulate, n.s. ventral anterolateral
Kennedy et al., 2001	paroxetine	↓ anterior insula (BL) ↑ pregenual ACC
Mayberg et al., 1999, Mayberg et al., 2000	fluoxetine	↓ anterior insula ↓ subgenual ACC ↑ left ventrolateral PFC
Nobler et al., 1994	ECT	↓ left ventrolateral PFC in responders[c]
Nobler et al., 2000	nortriptyline or sertraline	↓ left ventrolateral PFC in responders[c]
Nobler et al., 2001	ECT	↓ left ventrolateral PFC ↓ subgenual PFC
Saxena et al., 2002	paroxetine	↓ left ventrolateral PFC ↓ orbital C (BL)
Smith et al., 1999	sleep deprivation	↓ right ventrolateral PFC ↓ pregenual ACC,
Wu et al., 1992	sleep deprivation	↓ ACC in responders

ACC, anterior cingulate cortex; BL, bilateral; C, cortex; CBF: cerebral blood flow; ECT, electroconvulsive therapy; PFC, prefrontal cortex; RTMS, repeated transcranial magnetic stimulation; ↑, ↓, and n.s. indicate increases, decreases, or no significant changes, respectively, in the treated relative to the untreated state for regions assessed. Not all studies examined the same regions, and the absence of a listed result for a specific region indicates that no image data were provided for that region.

a. The changes in these ventral PFC regions show similar results to studies of antidepressant drug treatment in obsessive compulsive disordered samples. In contrast to these ventral prefrontal changes in depression, CBF and metabolism in the dorsal anterior cingulate and the dorsolateral PFC have been shown to increase in some studies of depression (e.g., Baxter et al., 1989; Bonne et al., 1996), but to decrease in others (Nobler et al., 1994; Nobler et al., 2001) following effective treatment.

b. The treatment-associated change reported in this study was not shown by paired statistical tests but rather by the observation that in the treatment responders, the abnormal increase that was evident pretreatment was not present posttreatment.

c. These studies were performed using the radiotracer xenon-133, which only provides CBF measures near the scalp. Thus results were not available for the orbital or the cingulate cortices (see text).

(Sullivan and Gratton, 1999). If so, then the left-lateralized grey matter reduction of the ventral ACC in MDD and BPD may contribute to dysregulation of neuroendocrine and autonomic function in depression.

The subgenual ACC and adjacent ventromedial PFC also participates in evaluating the reward-related significance of stimuli (Elliott et al., 2000). These areas send efferent projections to the ventral tegmental area (VTA) and substantia nigra and receive dense dopaminergic innervation from VTA (reviewed in Drevets et al., 1998). In rats, electrical or glutamatergic stimulation of the medial PFC areas elicits burst firing patterns from DA cells in the VTA and increases DA release in the accumbens (reviewed in Drevets et al., 1998).

Because these phasic, burst-firing patterns of DA neurons are thought to encode information regarding stimuli that predict reward and deviations between such predictions and occurrence of reward, ventral ACC dysfunction may conceivably contribute to disturbances of hedonic perception and motivated behavior in mood disorders. In this regard, the magnitude of abnormal metabolic activity in the subgenual PFC may relate to switches between depression and mania, as even in the presence of reduced volume, apparent subgenual PFC activity appears abnormally increased in small samples of participants with mania (e.g., Drevets et al., 1997).

Dorsomedial/dorsal anterolateral PFC

Many studies reported decreased CBF and metabolism in areas of the dorsolateral and dorsomedial PFC in participants with MDD and BPD relative to controls (Table 31.3). The dorsomedial region where flow and metabolism are decreased in MDD appears to include the dorsal ACC (Bench et al., 1992) and an area rostral to the dorsal ACC involving cortex on the medial and lateral surface of the superior frontal gyrus (approximately corresponding to Brodmann area 9) (Baxter et al., 1989; Drevets, Bogers, and Raichle, 2002). Postmortem studies of MDD and BPD have found abnormal reductions in the size of neurons and/or the density of glia in this portion of BA 9 (Rajkowska et al., 1999; Cotter et al., 2002). The reduction in metabolism in this region in the unmedicated depressed condition may thus reflect these histopathological changes and account for the failure of antidepressant drug treatment to alter metabolism in these areas (Drevets, Bogers, and Raichle, 2002). Nevertheless, currently remitted participants with MDD who experience depressive relapse during tryptophan depletion show increased metabolic activity within these areas in the depressed versus the remitted conditions (Neumeister et al., 2004), similar to other structures where histopathological and grey matter volume changes exist in MDD.

Flow normally increases in the vicinity of this dorsomedial/dorsal anterolateral PFC in healthy humans as they perform tasks that elicit emotional responses or require emotional evaluations (Dolan et al., 1996; Reiman et al., 1997). In primates the BA 9 cortex sends efferent projections to the lateral PAG and the dorsal hypothalamus through which it may modulate cardiovascular responses associated with emotional behavior (Öngür et al, 2003). Dysfunction of the dorsomedial/dorsal anterolateral PFC may also impair the ability to modulate emotional responses in mood disorders.

In contrast, the reduction in CBF in the dorsal ACC has been associated with impaired mnemonic and attentional processing derived from neuropsychological test scores obtained near the time of scanning (Dolan et al., 1994). This area has been implicated in selective attentional processing during cognitive tasks, and Drevets and Raichle (1998) demonstrated that hemodynamic activity decreases in the same area in participants who are healthy in whom anxiety is induced via fear of electrical shock. The reciprocal pattern of activation/deactivation in this region during cognitive versus emotional processing may conceivably relate to the neuropsychological manifestations of depression (Drevets and Raichle, 1998).

In other areas of the dorsolateral PFC the spatial locations of reported differences between participants with depression and controls have varied widely across studies, and new studies performed in independent participant samples have had difficulty replicating the originally described abnormalities (e.g., see Brody et al., 2001; Saxena et al. 2002). In a more posterior area of the dorsolateral PFC, Bench et al. (1992) also reported an area where flow was abnormally reduced in MDD. Dolan et al. (1993) subsequently observed that the reductions in CBF in this area correlated with ratings of impoverished speech in participants with depression and schizophrenia and proposed that this abnormality reflected a correlate of slowed cognitive processing.

Lateral orbital/ventrolateral PFC

In the lateral orbital cortex, ventrolateral PFC, and anterior insula, CBF and metabolism have been abnormally increased in most studies of unmedicated participants with primary MDD scanned while resting with eyes closed (Table 31.3). In contrast, image data acquired as participants who are either medicated or are engaging in attentionally demanding tasks during scanning (Kimbrell et al., 2002) have usually not detected this abnormality. The elevated activity in these areas in MDD appears mood-state dependent (Drevets et al., 1992). Flow and metabolism also increase in these areas during induced sadness and anxiety in participants who are healthy and induced anxiety and obsessional states in participants with anxiety disorders (reviewed in Drevets and Raichle, 1998; Charney and Drevets, 2002). Many studies also report that flow or metabolism decrease during antidepressant treatment in the orbital cortex, ventrolateral PFC, and/or anterior insula (Table 31.4).

A complex relationship exists between depression severity and physiological activity in the orbital cortex and ventrolateral PFC. Although CBF and metabolism increase in these areas in participants who are depressed relative to the remitted phase of MDD, the magnitude of these measures correlates inversely with ratings of depressive ideation and severity (Drevets et al., 1992; Drevets, Spitznagel, and Raichle, 1995). Moreover, though metabolic activity is abnormally increased in these areas in treatment-responsive participants with MDD and BPD, more severely ill or treatment refractory samples show CBF and metabolic values that were lower than or not different from those of controls (Mayberg et al., 1997). This inverse relationship between orbital cortex/ventrolateral PFC activity and depression severity appears compatible with similar assessments in other conditions. Posterior orbital cortex flow also increases in participants with obsessive-compulsive disorder (OCD) and animal phobias during exposure to phobic stimuli and in participants who are healthy during induced sadness (Rauch, et al., 1994; Drevets, Simpson, and Raichle, 1995; Schneider et al., 1995), and the change in posterior orbital CBF correlated inversely with changes in obsessive thinking, anxiety, and sadness, respectively.

Some OFC regions modulate the behavioral, endocrine, and autonomic responses associated with defensive, fear, and reward-directed behavior via anatomical projections to the amygdala, striatum, hypothalamus, PAG, hippocampal subiculum, and other limbic and brainstem structures (Rolls, 1995; Öngür et al., 2003). The orbital cortex and amygdala send overlapping projections to each of these structures as well as to each other through which they appear to modulate each other's neural transmission (Timms, 1977; Öngür et al., 2003). Activation of the orbital cortex during depression may thus reflect endogenous attempts to attenuate emotional expression or interrupt unreinforced aversive thought and emotion.

Consistent with this hypothesis, cerebrovascular lesions and tumors involving the frontal lobe increase the risk for developing major depression (e.g., Starkstein and Robinson, 1989), with the orbital cortex having been more specifically implicated as the area where such lesions induce depression (MacFall et al., 2001). Finally, serotonin depletion (Bremner et al., 1997; Hasler et al. 2008) and Parkinson's disease appear to impair orbital cortex function (Mayberg et al., 1990; Ring et al., 1994), suggesting other mechanisms through which deficits in orbital cortex function may increase risk for depression. These observations further suggest that the abnormal reduction in grey matter in the lateral OFC (Rajkowska et al., 1999) contributes to the perseverative or persistent nature of depressive mood and ideation.

The reduction of CBF and metabolism in the orbital cortex and ventrolateral PFC seen during antidepressant drugs treatment (Table 31.4) may, therefore, not be a primary mechanism through which such agents ameliorate depressive symptoms. Instead, direct inhibition of pathological limbic activity in areas such as the amygdala and ventral ACC may be more essential for correcting the pathophysiology associated with the production of mood symptoms (Drevets, Bogers, and Raichle, 2002). The orbital cortex neurons may thus be able to "relax," as reflected by the reduction of metabolism to normal levels, as antidepressant drug therapy attenuates the pathological limbic activity to which these neurons respond.

Notably, other OFC regions participate in integrating experiential stimuli with emotional salience and in associating reward-directed behavioral responses with the outcome of such responses, allowing redirection of behavior as reinforcement contingencies change (Rolls, 1995). Thus OFC dysfunction in mood disorders also may contribute to the attenuation of motivated behavior and reward salience during depression.

The Amygdala

In the amygdala, neurophysiological activity at rest and during exposure to emotionally valenced stimuli is altered in some depressive subgroups. Resting CBF and metabolism are elevated in subgroups with mood disorders who meet criteria for either FPDD (Fig. 31.2; Drevets et al., 1992; Drevets, Spitznagel, and Raichle, 1995; Drevets, Bogers, and Raichle, 2002; Drevets, Price, et al., 2002), MDD-melancholic subtype (Nofzinger et al., 1999), Type II BPD or nonpsychotic, Type I BPD (Ketter et al., 2001; Drevets, Price, et al., 2002), or who prove responsive to sleep deprivation (Wu et al., 1992). In contrast, metabolism has not been found to be abnormal in participants with MDD meeting criteria for depression spectrum disease (Drevets, Spitznagel, and Raichle, 1995; Drevets, Price, et al., 2002), or in depressed samples who meet *DSM* criteria for MDD as the only entrance criterion (Abercrombie et al., 1998; Brody et al., 2001; Saxena et al., 2002). Nevertheless, the extent to which such nonreplications reflect technical limitations related to the small size of the amygdala remains unclear (discussed in Drevets, Price, et al., 2002).

In FPDD the magnitude of the abnormal elevation of flow and metabolism ranges averages about 6% with state-of-the-art PET cameras (Fig. 31.4). When corrected for spatial resolution effects, this difference would reflect an increase in the actual CBF and metabolism of about 70% (Drevets et al., 1992). These magnitudes are in the physiological range.

The elevation of resting amygdala CBF/metabolism appears relatively specific for primary mood disorders, insofar as this abnormality has not been reported in OCD, panic disorder, phobic disorders, or schizophrenia (Charney and Drevets, 2002). In participants with these conditions and in healthy humans, the amygdala CBF generally increases during exposure to emotionally salient sensory stimuli, but not during anxiety or sadness states elicited by internally generated thoughts (reviewed in Charney and Drevets, 2002. In contrast, amygdala metabolism is abnormally elevated in MDD during resting wakefulness and during sleep, as Nofzinger et al. (1999) reported that though amygdala metabolism was increased in participants with depression versus controls during wakefulness, the increase in metabolism occurring in the amygdaloid complex during rapid-eye-movement (REM) sleep also was greater in participants with depression than controls. These data imply that amygdala hypermetabolism exists in MDD even when stressors are not being consciously processed.

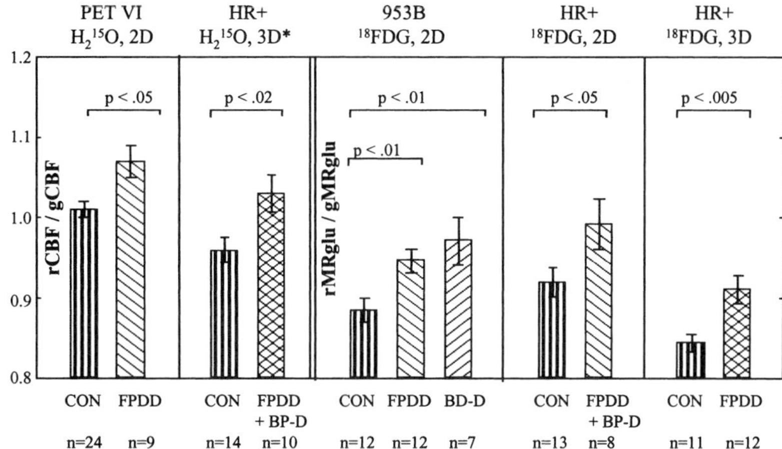

FIGURE 31.4 Elevation of mean normalized physiological activity (± SEM) in the left amygdala, measured in terms of CBF or glucose metabolism, in mid-life depressed subjects relative to healthy controls. The five consecutive studies obtained using different PET cameras (PETT VI, HR+ and 953B are PET scanner model numbers—the latter two manufactured by Siemens/CTI; *2D* and *3D* refer to distinct image acquisition modes) in different laboratories in independent subject samples are summarized in Drevets et al. (1992; Drevets, Spitznagel, and Raichle, 1995; Drevets et al., 1999; Drevets, Bogers, and Raichle, 2002; Drevets, Price, et al., 2002). Because the first glucose metabolism study (center) showed that FPDD and BD-D samples significantly differed from controls, but not from each other, patients from these categories were combined for two subsequent studies (panels 2 and 4). SEM: standard error of mean; CBF: cerebral blood flow; PET: positron emission tomography; rCBF/gCBF: regional-to-global CBF ratio; rMRglu/gMRglu: ratio of regional-to-global metabolic rates for glucose; CON: healthy controls; FPDD: familial pure depressive disease; BD-D: depressed phase of bipolar disorder.

During antidepressant treatment that ameliorates depressive symptoms and prophylaxes against relapse, amygdala metabolism decreases toward normal in MDD (Drevets, Bogers, and Raichle, 2002). Similarly, a preliminary study of BPD showed that mean amygdala metabolism in remitted participants taking mood stabilizers was lower than in remitted participants taking mood-stabilizing drugs and not different from healthy controls (Drevets, Price, et al., 2002). Compatible with these observations, antidepressant-medicated, remitted participants with MDD who did not relapse during tryptophan depletion (which putatively decreases CNS serotonin concentrations) had a lower baseline amygdala metabolism (that is, prior to depletion) than remitted participants with MDD who did relapse (Bremner et al., 1997). Finally, Sheline et al. (2001) showed that the left amygdala's hemodynamic response to emotionally valenced stimuli was attenuated in participants with MDD following chronic sertraline treatment.

Functional imaging data acquired as participants view emotionally valenced stimuli that normally activate the amygdala also demonstrate altered physiological responses in MDD. In the left amygdala, the hemodynamic response to viewing fearful faces (relative to viewing either smiling or neutral faces) was blunted in children with depression (Thomas et al., 2001). This finding was consistent with the elevation of basal CBF and metabolism in the left amygdala in such cases because tissue that is physiologically activated is expected to show an attenuation of further rises in the hemodynamic/metabolic signal in response to tasks that normally engage the same tissue. Nevertheless, Sheline et al. (2001) reported that hemodynamic responses were exaggerated in participants with MDD exposed to fearful or smiling faces that were displayed briefly (40 msec) and then masked by faces with "neutral" expressions, so that participants were unaware of having seen the emotional faces. Similarly, the hemodynamic response of the amygdala to happy or fearful faces was increased in participants with depression with BPD relative to healthy controls (Yurgelun-Todd et al., 2000; Lawrence et al., 2004; Blumberg et al., 2005).

The duration of the amygdala response to emotionally valenced stimuli also is abnormal in depression. Drevets et al. (2001) observed that although the initial amydgala blood-flow response to sad faces was similar to that of controls, the response habituated during repeated exposures to the same stimuli in controls, but not in participants with depression. Moreover, Siegle et al. (2002) reported that the increase in hemodynamic activity occurring in the amygdala during exposure to negatively valenced words in participants with depression and controls was sustained for a longer time in the participants with depression.

The observation of Siegle et al. (2002) is particularly noteworthy in light of neuroimaging, electrophysiological, and lesion analysis studies in humans and experimental animals that demonstrate the amygdala is involved in the acquisition and recall of emotional or arousing memories (Ferry et al., 1999; Canli et al., 2000). In humans, bursts of EEG activity occur in the amygdala during recollection of specific emotional events, and electrical stimulation of the amygdala can evoke emotional experiences (fear, anxiety, dysphoria) and recall of emotionally charged, life events from remote memory (reviewed in Drevets, 2003). Taken together with the finding of elevated amygdala metabolism in MDD, these observations suggest the hypothesis that excessive amygdala stimulation of cortical structures involved in declarative memory may account for the tendency of participants with depression to ruminate about memories of emotionally aversive or guilt-provoking life events.

Amygdala dysfunction also may conceivably alter the initial evaluation and memory consolidation related to social or sensory stimuli with respect to their emotional significance in mood disorders (Drevets, 2003). The amygdala is involved in recognizing sadness and fear in facial expression and fear and anger in spoken language (reviewed in Drevets, 2003). Norepinephrine (NE) release in the amygdala plays a critical role in at least some types of emotional learning, and the activation of NE release is facilitated by glucocorticoid secretion (Ferry et al., 1999). At least some participants with depression have abnormally elevated secretion of NE and cortisol, which in the presence of amygdala activation may conceivably increase the likelihood that sensory or social stimuli are perceived or remembered as emotionally arousing or aversive (reviewed in Drevets, 2003).

The amygdala also plays an important role in organizing other emotional, behavioral, neuroendocrine, and autonomic aspects of emotional/ stress responses as well, potentially compatible with reports that amygdala CBF and metabolism correlate positively with ratings of depression severity that score emotional and neurovegetative aspects of the major depressive syndrome (Drevets et al., 1992; Drevets, Spitsnagel, and Raichle, 1995; Abercrombie et al., 1998; Drevets, Price, et al., 2002). For example, the amygdala facilitates stress-related corticotropin-releasing hormone (CRH) release (Herman and Cullinan, 1997) and electrical stimulation of the amygdala in humans increases cortisol secretion (Rubin et al., 1966), suggesting a mechanism via which excessive amygdala activity may play a role in inducing CRH hypersecretion in MDD (see Chapter 30 by Dunlop, Garlow, and Nemeroff). In PET studies of MDD and BPD, CBF and glucose metabolism in the left amygdala correlated positively with stressed plasma cortisol secretion, which may conceivably reflect either the effect of amygdala activity on CRH secretion or the effect of cortisol on amygdala function (Drevets, Price, et al., 2002).

Abnormalities in Anatomically Related Limbic and Subcortical Structures

The ventrolateral PFC, ACC, and OFC areas where metabolism is abnormal in depression share extensive interconnections with the amygdala, mediodorsal nucleus of the thalamus, and the ventromedial striatum (Öngür et al, 2003; Price et al., 1996). In the medial thalamus and ventral striatum, CBF and metabolism are abnormally increased in MDD and BPD depression and decrease during antidepressant drug treatment (Drevets et al., 1992; Drevets, Spitznagel, and Raichle, 1995; Videbech et al., 2001; Drevets, Thase, et al., 2002; Saxena et al., 2002; Wilson et al., 2002). In the dorsal caudate, in contrast, some depressed samples have shown abnormally decreased resting activity (Baxter et al., 1985; Schwartz et al., 1987; Drevets et al., 1992), while others showed abnormally increased activity (Brody et al., 2001). Finally, during exposure to positive or rewarding stimuli, participants with depression have shown blunted hemodynamic responses relative to controls in the ventral striatum (Tremblay et al., 2005; Epstein et al., 2006).

Other Brain Areas

Several groups reported abnormally increased CBF in the posterior cingulate cortex in MDD (e.g., Bench et al., 1993; Buchsbaum et al., 1997; Drevets, Bogers, and Raichle, 2002), and some showed that posterior cingulate flow and metabolism decreased during antidepressant treatment (Buchsbaum et al., 1997). Bench et al. (1993) specifically reported that the posterior cingulate flow in participants with depression correlated positively with anxiety ratings. Exposure to aversive stimuli of various types results in increased physiological activity in the posterior cingulate cortex (reviewed in Charney and Drevets, 2002). Nevertheless, Mayberg et al. (1999) reported that script-driven sadness resulted in decreased activity in participants who are healthy in the dorsal posterior cingulate cortex, and that flow also was decreased in the depressed relative to the remitted phase of MDD, raising the possibility that this large region is functionally heterogenous with respect to emotional processing. The posterior cingulate cortex appears to serve as a sensory association cortex and may participate in processing the affective salience of sensory stimuli. The posterior cingulate cortex sends major anatomical projections to the ACC, through which it may relay such information into the limbic circuitry (Öngür et al., 2003).

Abnormally increased CBF has also been consistently reported in the medial cerebellum in MDD (e.g., Bench et al., 1992; Videbech et al., 2001). Flow increases in this region in experimentally induced anxiety or sadness in participants who are healthy and in participants with anxiety disorders (reviewed in George et al., 1995; Charney and Drevets, 2002). Activation of this structure during depression and anxiety may conceivably reflect either the activation of established anatomical loops between the cortex and cerebellum or the role of the paleocerebellum in modulating autonomic function.

Regional CBF and metabolic abnormalities in other structures have been less consistently replicated. In the lateral temporal and inferior parietal cortex, some studies found reduced regional CBF and metabolism (e.g., Cohen et al., 1992; Drevets et al., 1992; Philpot et al., 1993; Biver et al., 1994). Some of these areas have been implicated in processing sensory information. Although the significance of reduced activity in such areas in depression remains unclear, it may conceivably relate to neuropsychological impairments associated with depression (Drevets and Raichle, 1998).

Implications for Anatomical Circuits Related to Depression

Because alterations in regional CBF and metabolism primarily reflect changes in local synaptic activity, interpreting the regional abnormalities in depression requires consideration of anatomical connectivity (Raichle, 1987; Drevets et al., 1992). The functional and structural imaging data in primary depression converge with evidence from lesion analysis studies to implicate circuits involving parts of the frontal and temporal lobes along with related parts of the striatum, pallidum, and thalamus in the pathophysiology of depression. For example, the findings in participants with MDD of abnormally increased CBF and metabolism in the ventrolateral and orbital PFC, ventral ACC, amygdala, ventral striatum, and medial thalamus implicate two interconnected circuits in the pathophysiology of depression: a limbic-thalamo-cortical circuit involving the amygdala, mediodorsal nucleus of the thalamus (in the medial thalamus), and OMPFC; and a limbic-striatal-pallidal-thalamic (LCSPT) circuit involving related parts of the striatum and ventral pallidum as well as the components of the other circuit (Drevets et al., 1992). The amygdala and OMPFC are connected by excitatory projections with each other and with the mediodorsal nucleus of the thalamus, so increased metabolic activity in these structures would presumably reflect increased synaptic transmission through the limbic-thalamo-cortical circuit. It is noteworthy that neurosurgical procedures and deep brain stimulation that ameliorate treatment-resistant depression interrupt projections within these circuits (reviewed in Drevets et al., 1992; Mayberg et al., 2005).

Within the LCSPT circuitry, the volumetric and histopathological changes found in the subgenual and pregenual ACC, lateral OFC, hippocampal subiculum, amygdala, and ventral striatum in MDD and BPD include a reduction in glial cells with no equivalent loss of neurons, loss of synaptic markers or proteins, elevated neuronal density, and reduced neuronal size, findings that would be consistent with a reduction in neuropil (Öngür et al., 1998; Baumann et al., 1999; Rajkowska et al., 1999; Cotter et al., 2002; Eastwood and Harrison, 2000; Bowley et al., 2002). Although the pathogenesis of these changes has not been established, notably the dendritic arbors that form the neuropil can, in some limbic and medial PFC structures, undergo atrophy or "remodeling" during exposure to stress-induced elevations in excitatory amino acid (EAA) neurotransmitters and glucocorticoid secretion (McEwen, 1999). The targeted nature of the grey matter volume reductions to specific areas of the limbic-thalamo-cortical (LTC) and LCSPT circuits that show increased glucose metabolism is noteworthy because the glucose metabolic signal is dominated by glutamatergic transmission (Shulman et al., 2004). The reduction in metabolism in these regions during chronic antidepressant drug treatment may thus signal the attenuation of elevated glutamatergic transmission through this circuit. Notably, chronic antidepressant drug administration and repeated electroconvulsive shocks also desensitize *N*-methyl-D-aspartate (NMDA)-glutamatergic receptors in the rat frontal cortex (Paul and Skolnick, 2003) and increase expression of neurotrophic and neuroprotective factors that may protect the cortex from continuing loss of neuropil (Manji et al., 2001).

Functional Imaging Studies of Secondary Depression

Transmission through these circuits may differ across depressive subtypes because the lesions involving the PFC (that is, tumors or infarctions) and the diseases of the basal ganglia (for example, Parkinson's or Huntington's disease) that are associated with increased risk for depression result in dysfunction at distinct points within these circuits that affect synaptic transmission in diverse ways (Table 31.5; reviewed in Starkstein and Robinson, 1989; Drevets and Todd, 1997). Consistent with this hypothesis, imaging studies of depressive syndromes arising secondary to neurological disorders have generally shown results that differ from those reported for primary mood disorders. For example, in contrast to the findings of increased CBF or metabolism in parts of the orbital cortex in primary participants with depression (Table 31.3), orbital cortex flow is reportedly decreased or not significantly different in participants with depressive syndromes arising secondary to Parkinson's disease, Huntington's disease, or basal ganglia infarction relative to participants with no depressive syndromes with the same illnesses (Table 31.5). Moreover, CBF and metabolism in the dorsolateral PFC generally have not differed between participants who are depressed with the above mentioned neurological conditions and nondepressed controls with the same conditions.

Studies of the physiological correlates of depressive symptoms in participants who have primary psychiatric disorders other than mood disorders have generally reported abnormalities resembling those found in primary participants with depression. In bulimia nervosa, Andreason et al. (1992) reported a negative correlation between metabolism in the dorsolateral PFC and depression ratings (as reported in primary MDD by Baxter et al., 1989) while metabolism in the orbital

TABLE 31.5 *Regional Blood Flow and Metabolic Abnormalities in the Ventral Prefrontal Cortex in Primary and Secondary Neuropsychiatric Syndromes*[a]

	Primary	*Secondary*	*Authors (and Primary Diagnosis)*
		$\Downarrow$	Mayberg et al., 1990 (Parkinson's D)[c]
Unipolar major depression			Mayberg et al., 1992 (Huntington's D)[c]
			Ring et al., 1994 (Parkinson's D)[c]
	$\Uparrow$[b]		
		n.s.	Mayberg et al., 1991 (basal ganglia infarction)[c]
		$\Downarrow$	LaPlane et al., 1989 (basal ganglia lesions)[e]
Obsessive-compulsive disorder	$\Uparrow$[d]		
		n.s.	George et al., 1992 (Tourette's syndrome)[f]

D: disease; n.s: difference not significant.

a. Additional studies of patients who had depressive symptoms but did not meet criteria for the major depressive syndrome are reviewed in the text.

b. Cerebral blood flow (CBF) and metabolism generally increased in unmedicated, primary depressed patients vs. controls (Table 31.3).

c. Comparison between depressed and nondepressed patients with the same illness.

d. CBF and metabolism generally increased in unmedicated patients with primary obsessive-compulsive disorder relative to controls (Baxter et al., 1987; chap. 44).

e. Patients with secondary obsessive-compulsive syndrome compared to healthy controls.

f. Comparison between Tourette's patients who manifest obsessions and compulsions vs. Tourette's patients without such features.

cortex was abnormally elevated and inversely correlated with obsessive-compulsive ratings (similar to the relationships between posterior orbital CBF and obsession ratings in primary OCD; Rauch et al., 1994) and between orbital metabolism and depressive ideation ratings in primary MDD (Drevets, Spitznagel, and Raichle, 1995). In participants who were cocaine dependent and scanned within the first week of cocaine withdrawal as they experienced depressive symptoms and cocaine craving, glucose metabolism was elevated in the medial orbital cortex and basal ganglia relative to healthy controls (Volkow et al., 1991).

Primary and secondary depressive syndromes may thus involve the same neural network, although the direction of the physiological abnormalities within individual structures may differ across conditions. This observation supports a circuitry-based model in which mood disorders are associated with dysfunctional interactions within limbic-cortical-striatal-pallidal-thalamic circuits, rather than increased or decreased activity within a single structure (Drevets and Todd, 1997). A common substrate in these cases may be the dysfunction of frontal-striatal modulation of limbic and visceral functions. The idiopathic, neuropathological changes evident in the OMPFC and ventral striatum in primary mood disorders (see above) and the degenerative processes found in conditions that can induce depressive syndromes (see above) have in common the disturbance of function within the OMPFC and striatum.

This model also has relevance for considering the pathophysiology of neuropsychiatric syndromes that occur comorbidly with major depression. For example, neuroimaging studies implicate the same neural circuits in the pathophysiology of OCD, providing insights into the common coincidence of depressive and obsessional syndromes (Drevets and Todd, 1997). Notably the differences found in the OFC between primary and secondary depression parallel the findings in primary and secondary obsessive-compulsive syndromes, in which OFC metabolism is increased in the former but decreased or unchanged in the latter (Table 31.5).

NEURORECEPTOR IMAGING STUDIES OF DEPRESSION

The development of neuroreceptor radioligands is providing expanding capabilities for noninvasive quantitation of in vivo receptor binding and dynamic neurotransmitter function. Such data complement neuropharmacological assessments performed postmortem. Although this area is expected to become an increasingly common application for PET and SPECT technology, studies conducted in mood disorders largely remain limited to assessments of monoaminergic receptor systems.

Dopamine Receptor Imaging

Neuroimaging studies have discovered abnormalities involving multiple aspects of the central dopaminergic system in depression, which converge with other types of evidence to implicate this system in the pathophysiology of mood disorders. With respect to dopamine (DA) D_1 receptors, Suhara et al. (1992) reported that the binding of [^{11}C]SCH-23990 was decreased in the frontal cortex of participants with BPD. In participants with MDD with anger attacks, Dougherty et al. (2006) found decreased striatal D_1 receptor binding to [^{11}C]SCH 23390. Both findings await replication using D_1 receptor ligands that are more amenable to quantitation.

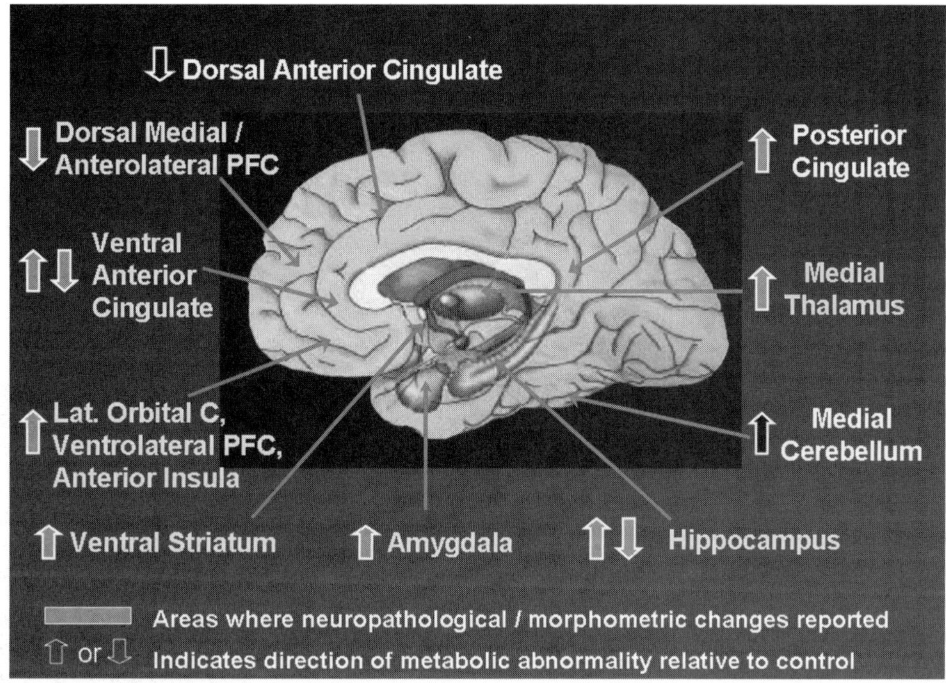

FIGURE 31.5 Summary of neuroimaging abnormalities in early-onset, primary MDD. Regions where physiological imaging abnormalities have been replicated in unmedicated MDD samples are listed and approximately shown on this midsagittal brain diagram in which subcortical structures are highlighted onto the medial surface. Because only the medial wall of the cortex is shown, the location of the lateral orbital/ventrolateral PFC/anterior insular region is better illustrated in Figure 31.2B. The "ventral anterior cingulate" region refers to pregenual and subgenual portions (see text and Figure 31.3). The arrows in front of each region name indicate the direction of resting state abnormalities in glucose metabolism in unmedicated, depressed MDD samples relative to healthy control samples. In some cases abnormalities in both directions have been reported that may depend either on the specific region involved or on the clinical state (for example, treatment responsive vs. nonresponsive—see text). The shaded regions have been shown to have histopathological and/or grey matter volumetric abnormalities in postmortem studies of primary mood disorders. PFC: prefrontal cortex; MDD: major depressive disorder.

Abnormal DA D_2/D_3 receptor binding also was reported in depression. Pearlson et al. (1995) showed that psychotic participants with BPD had increased striatal uptake of the DA D_2/D_3 receptor ligand, [^{11}C]-*N*-methylspiperone, relative to healthy controls and nonpsychotic participants with BPD. In MDD, SPECT studies performed using ^{123}I-iodobenzamide (IBZM), a DA D_2/D_3 receptor ligand that is sensitive to endogenous DA concentrations, found increased striatal uptake during the depressed phase (D'haenen and Bossuyt, 1994; P.J. Shah et al., 1997), which potentially may reflect a reduction in endogenous DA release. Ebert et al. (1996) also found increased striatal DA D_2/D_3 receptor availability in participants with depression with psychomotor slowing, and Shah et al. (1997) reported that striatal [^{123}I]-IBZM binding correlated inversely with movement speed and verbal fluency measures.

Other preliminary PET data appear compatible with the hypothesis that DA release is reduced in MDD. Meyer et al. (2001) found decreased DA transporter binding in participants with MDD versus controls, which may reflect a compensatory response to reduced DA release. Moreover, Ågren et al. (1993) found abnormally reduced brain uptake of the catecholamine precursor [^{11}C]*L*-DOPA in MDD, suggesting that DA synthesis is reduced in depression, consistent with observations that CSF homovanillic acid concentrations are reduced in MDD (Fig. 31.5).

Serotonin Receptor Imaging

Within the serotonin system, the pre- and postsynaptic serotonin type 1A (5-HT_{1A}) receptor binding is abnormally decreased in most, but not all, studies of MDD and BPD, and in participants with depression with temporal lobe epilepsy (Drevets et al., 2007). The reduction in 5-HT_{1A} receptor binding was demonstrated using PET and [*carbonyl*-^{11}C]WAY-100635 in the raphé, hippocampus, amygdala, temporopolar cortex, insula, anterior and posterior cingulate cortex, and left OFC (Drevets et al., 1999; Drevets et al., 2007) (Fig. 31.6). The magnitudes of these differences have been similar to those found postmortem in studies of primary MDD samples or depressed, nonalcoholic victims of suicides. These data also were compatible with evidence that unmedicated participants with MDD show blunted thermic and endocrine responses to 5-HT_{1A} receptor agonist challenge (reviewed in Drevets et al., 1999). Treatment with SSRI did not alter the changes in 5-HT_{1A} receptor BP in any area (reviewed in Drevets et al., 2007).

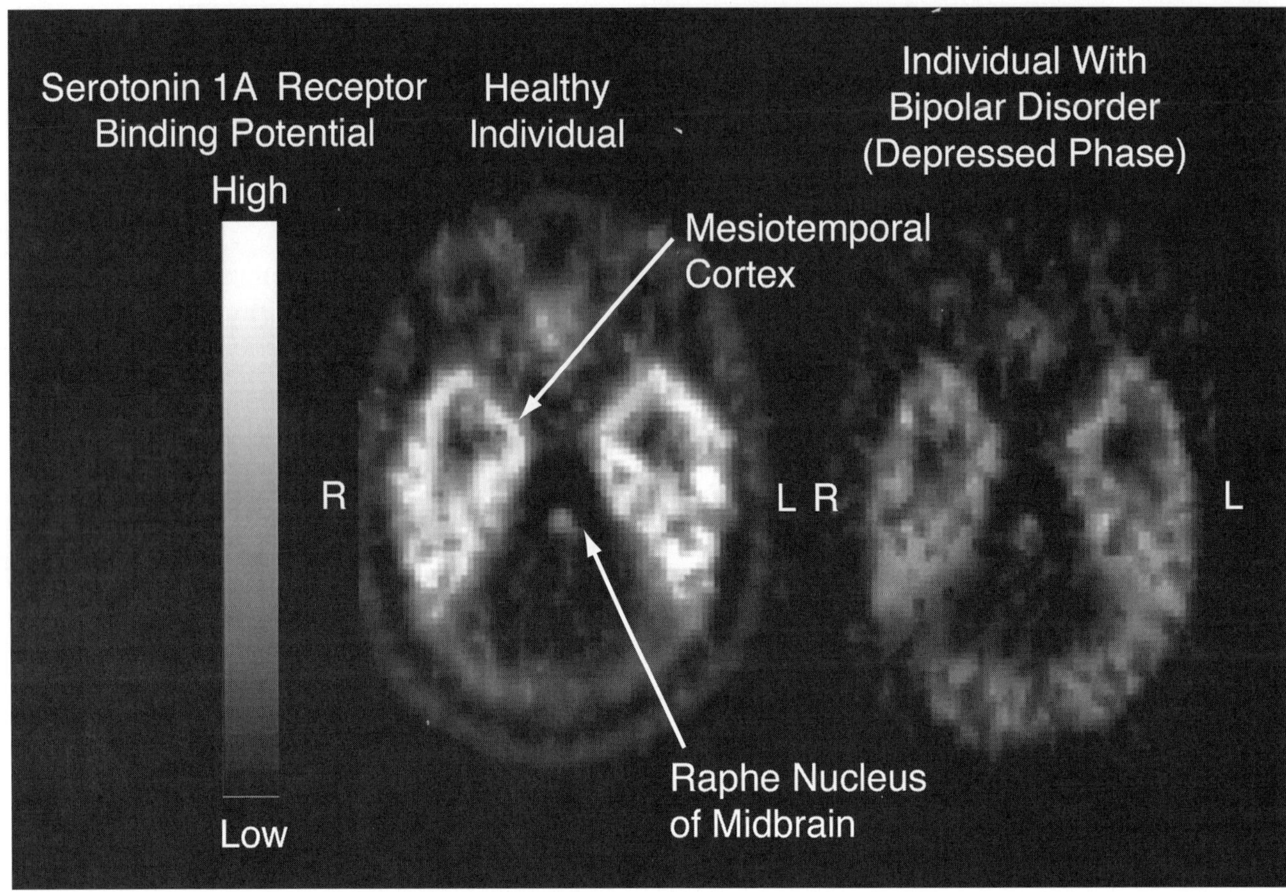

FIGURE 31.6 Transverse images of 5-HT type 1A receptor binding potential obtained using PET and [carbonyl-11C]WAY100635 in a young male with bipolar disorder and a healthy control male (see text). The full study for which these images were obtained demonstrated reduced 5-HT_{1A} receptor binding in depressed patients versus controls in brain regions where these receptors are expressed postsynaptically (for example, mesiotemporal cortex) and presynaptically (for example, raphé) (Drevets et al., 1999). PET: positron emission tomography. Reproduced from *Journal of the American Medical Association* 287(14):1787–1788.

Neuroimaging studies of other 5-HT binding sites found less consistent differences in depression. One study reported reduced 5-HT_{2A} receptor binding in the hippocampus in depressed participants with MDD versus controls (Sheline et al., 2004), although other studies found no significant difference between participants with depression and controls when age effects were controlled (Meltzer et al., 1999; Meyer et al., 1999). In contrast, several studies conducted postmortem in victims of suicide reported increases in 5-HT_{2A} receptor binding relative to nonsuicide controls (reviewed in Stockmeier, 2003).

Neuroreceptor imaging and postmortem histochemical studies also reported abnormalities of 5-HTT binding in mood disorders (Stockmeier, 2003). Studies performed using 5-HTT radioligands with high selectivity for 5-HTT sites, such as [^{11}C]DASB, reported abnormally increased 5-HTT binding in the striatum, thalamus, insula, and ACC in participants with early-onset MDD (Cannon et al., 2007) and/or in participants with MDD with negativistic attitudes (Meyer et al., 2004). Similarly depressed participants with BPD showed elevated 5-HTT binding in the striatum, thalamus, and insula, along with reduced binding in the vicinity of the pontine raphé. Of studies that used the less selective 5-HTT radioligands, [^{11}C](+)McN5652 or [^{123}I]βCIT, some also found abnormally increased 5-HTT binding in the thalamus (Ichimiya et al., 2002), PFC, and ACC (Reivich et al., 2004), but others found reduced 5-HTT binding in the amygdala and/or midbrain in MDD (Malison et al., 1998; Parsey et al., 2006), or reduced binding in thalamus, midbrain, putamen, amygdala, hippocampus, and ACC in BPD (Oquendo et al., 2007). Whether differences in the selectivity of these radiotracers accounts for the discrepant findings across studies remains unclear.

CONCLUDING REMARKS

The convergent results from studies of mood disorders conducted using neuroimaging, lesion analysis, and postmortem techniques support a model in which the signs and symptoms of major depression emanate from dysfunction within circuits involving the OMPFC, temporal lobe, striatum, and brain stem that normally modulate emotional behavior. Antidepressant therapies may compensate for this dysfunction by attenuating the pathological limbic activity that mediates such symptoms (Drevets, Bogers, and Raichle, 2002; Drevets, Thase, et al., 2002), and by increasing genetic transmission of neurotrophic factors that exert neuroplastic effects within the pathways modulating emotional expression (Manji et al., 2001).

REFERENCES

Abercrombie, H.C., Schaefer, S.M., Larson, C.L., Oakes, T.R., Lindgren, K.A., Holden, J.E., Perlman, S.B., Turski, P.A., Krahn, D.D., Benca, R.M., and Davidson, R.J. (1998) Metabolic rate in the right amygdala predicts negative affect in depressed patients. *Neuroreport* 9(14):3301–3307.

Ågren, H., Reibring, L., Hartvig, P., Tedroff, J., Bjurling, P., Lundqvist, H., and Långström, B. (1993) Monoamine metabolism in human prefrontal cortex and basal ganglia. PET studies using [^{11}C]*L*-hydroxytryptophan and [^{11}C]*L*-DOPA in healthy volunteers and patients with unipolar depression. *Depression* 1:71–81.

Altschuler, L.L., Bartzokis, G., Thomas, G., Curran, J., and Mintz, J. (1998) Amygdala enlargement in bipolar disorder and hippocampal reduction in schizophrenia: an MRI study demonstrating neuroanatomic specificity. *Arch. Gen. Psychiatry* 55:663–664.

Altschuler, L.L., Conrad, A., Hauser, P., et al. (1991) Reduction of temporal lobe volume in bipolar disorder: a preliminary report of magnetic resonance imaging. *Arch. Gen. Psychiatry* 48:482–483.

American Psychiatric Association. (1994) *Diagnostic and Statistical Manual of Mental Disorders*, 4th ed. Washington, DC: Author.

Amsterdam, J.D., Marinelli, D.L., Arger, P., et al. (1987) Assessment of adrenal gland volume by computed tomography in depressed patients and healthy volunteers: a pilot study. *Psychiatry Res.* 21:3 84–387.

Andreason, P.J., Altemus, M.S., Zametkin, A.J., King, A.C., Lucinio, J., and Cohen, R.M. (1992) Regional cerebral glucose metabolism in bulimia nervosa. *Am. J. Psychiatry* 149:1506–1513.

Ashtari, M., Greenwald, B.S., Kramer-Ginsberg, E., Hu, J., Wu, H., Patel, M., Aupperle, P., and Pollack, S. (1999) Hippocampal/amygdala volumes in geriatric depression. *Psychol. Med.* 29: 629–638.

Awad, I.A., Johnson, P.C., Spetzler, R.J., et al. (1986) Incidental subcortical lesions identified on magnetic resonance imaging in the elderly, II: Postmortem pathological correlations. *Stroke* 17:1090–1097.

Awad, I.A., Spetzler, R.F., Hodak, J.A., et al. (1986) Incidental subcortical lesion identified on magnetic resonance imaging in the elderly: I. Correlation with age and cerebrovascular risk factor. *Stroke* 17:1084–1089.

Axelson, D., Doraiswamy, P.M., McDonald, W.M., et al. (1993) Hypercortisolemia and amygdala hippocampal changes in depression. *Psychiatry Res.* 47:167–173.

Aylward, E.H., Roberts-Twillie, J.V., Barta, P.E., et al. (1994) Basal ganglia volumes and white matter hyperintensities in patients with bipolar disorder. *Am. J. Psychiatry* 151:687–693.

Baumann, B., Danos, P., Krell, D., Diekmann, S., Leschinger, A., Stauch, R., Wurthman, C., Bernstein, H.-G., and Bogerts, B. (1999) Reduced volume of limbic system-affiliated basal ganglia in mood disorders: preliminary data from a post mortem study. *J. Neuropsych. Clin. Neurosci.* 11(1):71–78.

Baxter, L.R., Phelps, M.E., Mazziotta, J.C., Guze, B.H., Schwartz, J.M., and Selin, C.E. (1987) Local cerebral glucose metabolic rates in obsessive-compulsive disorder. *Arch. Gen. Psychiatry* 44: 211–218.

Baxter, L.R., Phelps, M.E., Mazziotta, J.C., Schwartz, J.M., Gerner, R.H., Selin, C.E., and Sumida, R.M. (1985) Cerebral metabolic rates for glucose in mood disorders. *Arch. Gen. Psychiatry* 42: 441–447.

Baxter, L.R., Schwartz, J.M., Phelps, M.E., Mazziota, J.C., Guze, B.H., Selin, C.E., Gerner, R.H., and Sumida, R.M. (1989) Reduction of prefrontal cortex glucose metabolism common to three types of depression. *Arch. Gen. Psychiatry* 46:243–250.

Bench, C.J., Friston, K.J., Brown, R.G., Frackowiak, R.S., and Dolan, R.J. (1993) Regional cerebral blood flow in depression measured by positron emission tomography: the relationship with clinical dimensions. *Psychol. Med.* 23:579–590.

Bench, C.J., Friston, K.J., Brown, R.G., Scott, L.C., Frackowiak, S.J., and Dolan, R.J. (1992) The anatomy of melancholia - focal abnormalities of cerebral blood flow in major depression. *Psychol. Med.* 22:607–615.

Benes, F.M., Vincent, S.L., and Todtenkopf, M. (2001) The density of pyramidal and nonpyramidal neurons in anterior cingulate cortex of schizophrenic and bipolar subjects. *Biol. Psychiatry* 50(6): 395–406.

Beyer, J.L., Taylor, W.D., MacFall, J.R., Kuchibhatla, M., Payne, M.E., Provenzale, J.M., Cassidy, F., and Krishnan, K.R. (2005) Cortical white matter microstructural abnormalities in bipolar disorder. *Neuropsychopharmacology* 30(12):2225–2229.

Biver, F., Goldman, S., Delvenne, V., Luxen, A., DeMaertelaer, V., Hubain, P., Mendlewicz, J., and Lotstra, F. (1994) Frontal and parietal metabolic disturbances in unipolar depression. *Biol. Psychiatry* 36:381–388.

Blumberg, H.P., Donegan, N.H., et al. (2005) Preliminary evidence for medication effects on functional abnormalities in the amygdala and anterior cingulate in bipolar disorder. *Psychopharmacology (Berl)* 183(3):308–313.

Blumberg, H.P., Kaufman, J., Martin, A., Whiteman, R., Zhang, J.H., Gore, J.C., Charney, D.S., Krystal, J.H., and Peterson, B.S. (2003) Amygdala and hippocampal volumes in adolescents and adults with bipolar disorder. *Arch. Gen. Psychiatry* 60(12):1201–1208.

Bonne, O., Krausz, Y., Shapira, B., Bocher, M., Karger, H., Gorfine, M., Chisin, R., and Lerer, B. (1996) Increased cerebral blood flow in depressed patients responding to electroconvulsive therapy. *J. Nucl. Med.* 37:1075–1080.

Botteron, K.N., Raichle, M.E., Drevets, W.C., Heath, A.C., and Todd, R.D. (2002) Volumetric reduction in left subgenual prefrontal cortex in early onset depression. *Biol. Psychiatry* 51(4):342–344.

Bowley, M.P., Drevets, W.C., Öngür, D., and Price, J.L. (2002) Low glial numbers in the amygdala in mood disorders. *Biol. Psychiatry* 52(5): 404–41.

Bremner, J.D., Innis, R.B., Salomon, R.M., Staib, L.H., Ng, C.K., Miller, H.L., et al. (1997) Positron emission tomography measurement of cerebral metabolic correlates of tryptophan depletion-induced depressive relapse. *Arch. Gen. Psychiatry* 54:364–374.

Bremner, J.D., Narayan, M., Anderson, E.R., Staib, L.H., Miller, H.L., and Charney, D.S. (2000) Hippocampal volume reduction in major depression. *Am. J. Psychiatry* 157:115–118.

Brody, A.L., Saxena, S., Stoessel, P., Gillies, L.A., Fairbanks, L.A., Alborzian, S., Phelps, M.E., Huang, S.C., Wu, H.M., Ho, M.L., Ho, M.K., Au, S.C., Maidment, K., and Baxter, L.R. (2001) Regional brain metabolic changes in patients major depressive disorder from pre- to post-treatment with paroxetine. *Arch. Gen. Psychiatry* 58:631–640.

Brown, F.W., Lewine, R.J., Hudgins, P.A., et al. (1992) White matter hyperintensity signals in psychiatric and nonpsychiatric subjects. *Am. J. Psychiatry* 149:620–625.

Buchsbaum, M.S., Wu, J., Siegel, B.V., Hackett, E., Trenary, M., Abel, L., and Reynolds, C. (1997) Effect of sertraline on regional metabolic rate in patients with affective disorder. *Biol. Psychiatry* 41: 15–22.

Canli, T., Zhao, Z., Brewer, J., Gabrieli, J.D., and Cahill, L. (2000) Event-related activation in the human amygdala associates with later memory for individual emotional experience. *J. Neurosci.* 20:RC99.

Cannon, D.M., Ichise, M., Rollis, D., Klaver, J.M., Gandhi, S.K., Charney, D.S., Manji, H.K., and Drevets, W.C. (2007) Elevated serotonin transporter binding in major depressive disorder assessed using [11C]DASB and positron emission tomography: comparison with bipolar disorder. *Biol. Psychiatry* 62(8):870–877.

Charney, D.S., and Drevets, W.C. (2002) The neurobiological basis of anxiety disorders. In: Davis, K., Charney, D.S., Coyle, J., Nemeroff, C.B. eds. *The Fifth Generation of Progress. Psychopharmacology.* New York: Lippencott, Williams and Wilkins, pp. 901–930.

Chen, C.H., Ridler, K., et al. (2007) Brain imaging correlates of depressive symptom severity and predictors of symptom improvement after antidepressant treatment. *Biol. Psychiatry 62*(5):407–414.

Chimowitz, M.I., Estes, M.L., Furlan, A.J., et al. (1992) Further observations on the pathology, 1992 of subcortical lesions identified on magnetic resonance imaging. *Arch. Neurol.* 49:747–752.

Coffey, C.E., Figiel, G.S., Djang, W.T., et al. (1988) Leukoencephalopathy in elderly depressed patients referred for ECT. *Biol. Psy chiatry* 24:143–161.

Coffey, C.E., Figiel, G.S., Djang, W.T., et al. (1990) Subcortical hyperintensity on magnetic resonance imaging: a comparison of normal and depressed elderly subjects. *Am. J. Psychiatry* 147:187–189.

Coffey, C.E., Wilkinson, W.E., Weiner, R.D., et al. (1993) Quantitative cerebral anatomy in depression. A controlled magnetic resonance imaging study. *Arch. Gen. Psychiatry* 50:7–16.

Cohen, R.M., Gross, M., Nordahl, T.E., Semple, W.E., Oren, D.A., and Rosenthal, N. (1992) Preliminary data on the metabolic brain pattern of patients with winter seasonal affective disorder. *Arch. Gen. Psychiatry* 49:545–552.

Coryell, W., Nopoulos, P., Drevets, W.C., and Andreasen, N.C. (2005) Subgenual PFC volumes in MDD and schizophrenia: diagnostic specificity and prognostic implications. *Am. J. Psychiatry* 162:1706–1712.

Cotter, D., Mackay, D., Chana, G., Beasley, C., Landau, S., and Everall, I. (2002) Reduced neuronal size and glial cell density in Area 9 of the dorsolateral prefrontal cortex in subjects with major depressive disorder. *Cereb. Cortex* 12:386–394.

Damasio, A.R. (1994) *Descarte's Error: Emotion, Reason, and the Human Brain.* New York: G.P. Putnam.

DelBello, M.P., Zimmerman, M.E., Mills, N.P., Getz, G.E., and Strakowski, S.M. (2004) Magnetic resonance imaging analysis of amygdala and other subcortical brain regions in adolescents with bipolar disorder. *Bipolar Disord.* 6:43–52.

D'haenen, H.A., and Bossuyt, A. (1994) Dopamine D_2 receptors in depression measured with single photon emission computed tomography. *Biol. Psychiatry* 35:128–132.

DiRocco, R.J., et al. (1989) The relationship between CNS metabolism and cytoarchitecture: a review of ^{14}C-deoxyglucose studies with correlation to cytochrome oxidase histochemistry. *Comput. Med. Imaging Graph.* 13:81–92.

Dolan, R.J., Bench, C.J., Brown, R.G., Scott, L.C., and Frackowiak, R.S.J. (1994) Neuropsychological dysfunction in depression: the relationship to regional cerebral BF. *Psychol. Med.* 24:849–857.

Dolan, R.J., Bench, C.J., Liddle, P.F., et al. (1993) Dorsolateral prefrontal cortex dysfunction in the major psychoses: symptom or disease specificity? *J. Neurol. Neurosurg. Psychiatry* 56:1290–1294.

Dolan, R.J., Fletcher, P., Morris, J., Kapur, N., Deakin, J.F., and Frith, C.D. (1996) Neural activation during covert processing of positive emotional facial expressions. *Neuroimage.* 4(3 Pt 1):194–200.

Dougherty, D.D., et al. (2006) Decreased striatal D1 binding as measured using PET and [11C]SCH 23,390 in patients with major depression with anger attacks. *Depress. Anxiety* 23(3):175–177.

Drevets, W.C. (1993) Brain imaging in psychiatry. In: Sierles, F.S., ed. *Behavioral Science for Medical Students.* Baltimore: Williams and Wilkins, pp. 212–235.

Drevets, W.C. (1994) Geriatric depression: brain imaging correlates and pharmacologic considerations. *J. Clin. Psychiatry* 55:71–81.

Drevets, W.C. (2001) Neuroimaging and neuropathologial studies of depression: implications for the cognitive emotional manifestations of mood disorders. *Curr. Opin. Neurobiol.* 11:240–249.

Drevets, W.C. (2003) Neuroimaging abnormalities in the amygdala in mood disorders. In: *The Amygdala in Brain Function: Basic and Clinical Approaches.* Annals of the New York Academy of Sciences. New York: New York Academy of Sciences, pp. 959–967.

Drevets, W.C., Bogers, W., and Raichle, M.E. (2002) Functional anatomical correlates of antidepressant drug treatment assessed using PET measures of regional glucose metabolism. *Eur. J. Neuropharmacol.* 12(6):527–544.

Drevets, W.C., and Botteron, K. (1997) Neuroimaging in psychiatry. In: Guze, S.B., ed.. *Adult Psychiatry.* St. Louis, MO: Mosby Press, pp. 53–81.

Drevets, W.C., Burton, H., Simpson, J.R., Videen, T.O., Snyder, A.Z., and Raichle, M.E. (1995) Blood flow changes in human somatosensory cortex during anticipated stimulation. *Nature* 373:249–252.

Drevets, W.C., Frank, E., Price, J.C., Kupfer, D.J., Holt, D., Greer, P.J., Huang, H., Gautier, C., and Mathis, C. (1999) PET imaging of serotonin 1A receptor binding in depression. *Biol. Psychiatry* 46(10):1375–1387.

Drevets, W.C., Gautier, C., Lowry, T., Bogers, W., Greer, P., and Kupfer, D.J. (2001) Abnormal hemodynamic responses to facially expressed emotion in major depression. *Soc. Neurosci. Abstr.* 31.

Drevets, W.C., Öngür, D., and Price, J.L. (1998) Neuroimaging abnormalities in the subgenual prefrontal cortex: implications for pathophysiology of familial mood disorders. *Mol. Psychiatry* 3(3):220–226.

Drevets, W.C., Price, J.L., Bardgett, M.E., Reich, T., Todd, R., and Raichle, M.E. (2002) Glucose metabolism in the amygdala in depression: relationship to diagnostic subtype and stressed plasma cortisol levels. *Pharmacol. Biochem. Behav.* 71:431–447.

Drevets, W.C., Price, J.L., Simpson, J.R., Todd, R.D., Reich, T., Vannier, M., and Raichle, M.E. (1997) Subgenual prefrontal cortex abnormalities in mood disorders. *Nature* 386:824–827.

Drevets, W.C., and Raichle, M.E. (1992) Neuroanatomical circuits in depression: implications for treatment mechanisms. *Psychopharm. Bull.* 28:261–274.

Drevets, W.C., and Raichle, M.E. (1998) Reciprocal suppression of regional cerebral blood flow during emotional versus higher cognitive processes: implications for interactions between emotion and cognition. *Cognition and Emotion* 12(3):353–385.

Drevets, W.C., Simpson, J.R., and Raichle, M.E. (1995) Regional blood flow changes in response to phobic anxiety and habituation. *J. Cereb. Blood Flow Metab.* 15(1):S856.

Drevets, W.C., Spitznagel, E., and Raichle, M.E. (1995) Functional anatomical differences between major depressive subtypes. *J. Cereb. Blood Flow Metab.* 15(1):S93.

Drevets, W.C., Thase, M., Moses-Kolko, E., Price, J.C., Frank, E., Kupfer, D.J., and Mathis, C.A. (2007) Serotonin-1A receptor imaging in recurrent depression: replication and literature review. *Nuc. Med. Biol.* 34(7):865–878.

Drevets, W.C., Thase, M., Price, J.C., Bogers, W., Greer, P.J., and Kupfer, D.K. (2002) Antidepressant drug effects on regional glucose metabolism in major depression. *Soc. Neurosci. Abstr.* 32.

Drevets, W.C., and Todd, R.D. (1997) Depression, mania and related disorders. In: Guze, S.B., ed. *Adult Psychiatry.* St. Louis, MO: Mosby Press, pp. 99–141.

Drevets, W.C., Videen, T.O., Price, J.L., Preskorn, S.H., Carmichael, S.T., and Raichle, M.E. (1992) A functional anatomical study of unipolar depression. *J. Neuroscience* 12:3628–3641.

Dupont, R.M., Jernigan, T.L., Butters, N., et al. (1990) Subcortical abnormalities detected in bipolar affective disorder using magnetic resonance imaging: clinical and neuropsychological significance. *Arch. Gen. Psychiatry* 47:55–59.

Dupont, R.M., Jernigan, T.L., Gillin, J.C., et al. (1987) Subcortical signal hyperintensities in bipolar patients detected by MRI. *Psychiatry Res.* 21:357–358.

Dupont, R.M., Jernigan, T.L., Heindel, W., et al. (1995) Magnetic resonance imaging and mood disorders - Localization of white matter and other subcortical abnormalities. *Arch. Gen. Psychiatry* 52:747–755.

Eastwood, S.L., and Harrison, P.J. (2000): Hippocampal synaptic pathology in schizophrenia, bipolar disorder, and major depression: a study of complexin mRNAs. *Mol. Psychiatry* 5:425–432.

Ebert, D., Feistel, H., and Barocka, A. (1991) Effects of sleep deprivation on the limbic system and the frontal lobes in affective disorders: a study with Pc-99m-HMPAO SPECT. *Psychiatry Res. Neuroimaging* 40:247–251.

Ebert, D., Feistel, H., Loew, T., and Pirner, A. (1996): Dopamine and depression-striatal dopamine D2 receptor SPECT before and after antidepressant therapy. *Psychopharmacology* 126:91–94.

Elkis, H., Friedman, L., Wise, A., et al. (1995) Meta-analyses of studies of ventricular enlargement and cortical sulcal prominence in mood disorders - Comparisons with controls or patients with schizophrenia. *Arch. Gen. Psychiatry* 52:735–746.

Elliott, R., Friston, K. J., et al. (2000) Dissociable neural responses in human reward systems. *J. Neurosci.* 20(16):6159–6165.

Epstein, J., Pan, H., et al. (2006) Lack of ventral striatal response to positive stimuli in depressed versus normal subjects. *Am. J. Psychiatry* 163(10):1784–1790.

Escalona, P.R., McDonald, W.M., Doraiswamy, P.M., et al. (1993) Reduction of cerebellar volume in major depression: a controlled MRI study. *Depression* 1:156–158.

Fazekas, F. (1989) Magnetic resonance signal abnormalities in asymptomatic individuals: their incidence and functional correlates. *Eur. Neurol.* 29:164–168.

Ferry, B., Roozendaal, B., and McGaugh, J.L. (1999) Role of norepinephrine in mediating stress hormone regulation of long- term memory storage: a critical involvement of the amygdala. *Biol. Psychiatry* 46:1140–1152.

Figiel, G.S., Coffey, C.E., Djang, W.T., et al. (1990) Brain magnetic resonance imaging findings in ECT induced delirium. *J. Neuropsychiatry* 2:53–58.

Figiel, G.S., Krishnan, K.R.R., Breitner, J.C., et al. (1989) Radiologic correlates of antidepressant induced delirium: the possible significance of basal ganglia lesion. *J. Neuropsychiatry* 1:188–190.

Figiel, G.S., Krishnan, K.R.R., Doraiswamy, P.M., et al. (1991) Subcortical hyperintensities on brain magnetic resonance imaging: a comparison between late age onset and early onset elderly depressed subjects. *Neurobiol. of Aging* 26:245–247.

Frodl, T., Meisenzahl, E.M., Zetzsche, T., Hohne, T., Banac, S., Schorr, C., et al. (2004) Hippocampal and amygdala changes in patients with major depressive disorder and healthy controls during a 1-year follow-up. *J. Clin. Psychiatry* 65:492–499.

Fujikawa, T., Yamawaki, S., and Touhouda, Y. (1993) Incidence of silent cerebral infarction in patients with major depression. *Stroke* 24:1631–1634.

Fujikawa, T., Yamawaki, S., and Touhouda, Y. (1994) Background factors and clinical symptoms of major depression with silent cerebral infarction. *Stroke* 25:798–801.

Fujikawa, T., Yokota, N., Muraoka, M., et al. (1996) Response of patients with major depression and silent cerebral infarction to antidepressant drug therapy, with emphasis on central nervous system adverse effects. *Stroke* 27:2040–2042.

George, M.S., Ketter, T.A., Parekh, P.I., Horwitz, B., Herscovitch, P., and Post, R.M. (1995) Brain activity during transient sadness and happiness in healthy women. *Am. J. Psychiatry* 152:341–351.

George, M.S., Trimble, M.R., Costa, D.C., Robertson, M.M., Ring, H.A., and Ell, P.J. (1992) Elevated frontal CBF in Gilles de la Tourette syndrome: a ^{99}Tc^{m}-HMPAO SPECT study. *Psychiatry Res.* 45:143–151.

Gerard, G., and Weisberg, L.A. (1986) MRI periventricular lesions in adults. *Neurology* 36:998–1001.

Goodwin, G.M., Austin, M.P., Dougall, N., Ross, M., Murray, C., O'Carroll, R.E., Moffoot, A., Prentice, N., and Ebmeier, K.P. (1993) State changes in brain activity shown by the uptake of ^{99m}Tc-exametazine with SPET in major depression before and after treatment. *J. Affect. Disord.* 29:243–253.

Greenwald, B.S., et al. (1998) Neuroanatomic localization of magnetic resonance imaging signal hyperintensities in geriatric depression. *Stroke* 29(3):613–617.

Greenwald, B.S., Kramerginsberg, E., Krishnan, K.R.R., et al. (1996) MRI signal hyperintensities in geriatric depression. *Am. J. Psychiatry* 153:1212–1215.

Harvey, I., Persaud, R., Ron, M.A., and Murray, R.M. (1994) Volumetric MRI measurements in bipolars compared with schizophrenics and healthy controls. *Psychol. Med.* 24(3):689–699.

Hasler, G., Fromm, S., Carlson, P.J., Luckenbaugh, D.A., Waldeck, T., Geraci, M., Roiser, J.P., Neumeister, A., Meyers, N., Charney, D.S., and Drevets, W.C. (2008) Neural response to catecholamine depletion in unmedicated, remitted subjects with major depressive disorder and healthy subjects. *Archives of General Psychiatry*, in press.

Hauser, P., Altschuler, L.L., Berrettini, W., et al. (1989) Temporal lobe measurement in primary affective disorder by magnetic resonance imaging. *J. Neuropsychiatry Clin. Neurosci.* 1:128–134.

Herholz, K., Heindel, W., Rackl, A., et al. (1990) Regional cerebral blood in patients with leuko-araiosis and atherosclerotic carotid artery disease. *Arch. Neurol.* 47:392–396.

Herman, J.P., and Cullinan, W.E. (1997) Neurocircuitry of stress: central control of the hypothalamo-pituitary-adrenocortical axis. *Trends Neurosci.* 20(2):78–84.

Hickie, I., Scott, E., Mitchell, P., et al. (1995) Subcortical hyperintensities on magnetic resonance imaging: clinical correlates and prognostic significance in patients with severe depression. *Biol. Psychiatry* 37:151–160.

Hirayasu, Y., Shenton, M.E., Salisbury, D.F., Kwon, J.S., Wible, C.G., Fischer, I.A., Yurgelun-Todd, D., Zarate, C., Kikinis, R., Jolesz, F.A., and McCarley, R.W. (1999) Subgenual cingulate cortex volume in first-episode psychosis. *Am. J. Psychiatry* 156:1091–1093.

Husain, M.M., McDonald, W.M., Doraiswamy, P.M., et al. (1991) A magnetic resonance imaging study of putamen nuclei in major depression. *Psychiatry Res.* 40:95–99.

Ichimiya, T., Suhara, T., Sudo, Y., Okubo, Y., Nakayama, K., Nankai, M., et al. (2002) Serotonin transporter binding in patients with mood disorders: a PET study with [11C](+)McN5652. *Biol. Psychiatry* 51:715–722.

Iidaka, T., Nakajima, T., Kawamoto, K., et al. (1996) Signal hyperintensities on brain magnetic resonance imaging in elderly depressed patients. *Eur. Neurol.* 36:293–299.

Johnstone, E.C., Owens, D.G., Crow, T.J., et al. (1989) Temporal lobe structure as determined by nuclear magnetic resonance in schizophrenia and bipolar affective disorder. *J. Neurol. Neurosurg. Psychiatry* 52:736–741.

Kennedy, S.H., Evans, K.R., Kruger, S., Mayberg, H.S., Meyer, J.H., McCann, S., Arifuzzman, A.I., Houle, S., and Vaccarino, F.J. (2001) Changes in regional brain glucose metabolism measured with PET after paroxetine treatment of major depression. *Am. J. Psychiatry* 158:899–905.

Ketter, T.A., Kimbrell, T.A., George, M.S., Dunn, R.T., Speer, A.M., Benson, B.E., et al. (2001) Effects of mood and subtype on cerebral glucose metabolism in treatment-resistant bipolar disorder. *Biol. Psychiatry* 49:97–109.

Kimbrell, T.A., Ketter, T.A., George, M.S., Little, J.T., Benson, B.E., Willis, M.W., Herscovitch, P., and Post, R.M. (2002) Regional cerebral glucose utilization in patients with a range of severities of unipolar depression. *Biol. Psychiatry* 51:237–252.

Kobari, M., Meyer, J.S., and Ichijo, M. (1990) Leuko-araiosis, cerebral atrophy, and cerebral perfusion in normal aging. *Arch. Neurol.* 47:161–165.

Krishnan, K.R.R., Doraiswamy, P.M., Figiel, G.S., et al. (1991) Hippocampal abnormalities in depression. *J. Neuropsychiatry Clin. Neurosci.* 3:387–391.

Krishnan, K.R.R., Doraiswamy, P.M., Lurie, S.N., et al. (1991) Pituitary size in depression. *J. Clin. Endocrinol. Metab.* 72:256–259.

Krishnan, K.R.R., Goli, V., Ellinwood, E.H., et al. (1988) Leukoencephalopathy in patients diagnosed as major depressive. *Biol. Psychiatry* 23:519–522.

Krishnan, K.R.R., McDonald, W.M., Doraiswamy, P.M., et al. (1993) Neuroanatomical substrates of depression in the elderly. *Eur. Arch. Psychiatry Neurosci.* 243:41–46.

Krishnan, K.R.R., McDonald, W.M., Escalona, P.R., et al. (1992) Magnetic resonanace imaging of the caudate nuclei in depression: Preliminary observations *Arch. Gen. Psychiatry* 49:553–557.

Kumar, A., Schweizer, E., Jin, Z.S., et al. (1997) Neuroanatomical substrates of late-life minor depression - A quantitative magnetic resonance imaging study. *Arch. Neurology* 54:613–617.

Lai, T., Payne, M.E., Byrum, C.E., Steffens, D.C., and Krishnan, K.R. (2000) Reduction of orbital frontal cortex volume in geriatric depression. *Biol. Psychiatry* 48(10):971–975.

LaPlane, D., Levasseur, M., Pillon, B., Dubois, B., Baulac, M., Mazoyer, B., Tran Dinh, S., Sette, G., Danze, F., and Baron, J.C. (1989) Obsessive-compulsive and other behavioral changes with bilateral basal ganglia lesions. *Brain* 112:699–725.

Lawrence, N.S., Williams, A. M., et al. (2004) Subcortical and ventral prefrontal cortical neural responses to facial expressions distinguish patients with bipolar disorder and major depression. *Biol. Psychiatry* 55(6):578–587.

Lesser, I.M., Boone, K.B., Mehringer, C.M., et al. (1996) Cognition and white matter hyperintensities in older depressed patients. *Am. J. Psychiatry* 153:1280–1287.

Lesser, I.M., Mena, I., Boone, K.B., Miller, B.L., Mehringer, C.M., and Mohl, M. (1994) Reduction of cerebral blood flow in older depressed patients. *Arch. Gen. Psychiatry* 51:677–686.

Lesser, I.M., Miller, B.L., Boone, K.B., et al. (1991) Brain injury and cognitive function in late-onset psychotic depression. *J. Neuropsychiatry Clin. Neurosci.* 3:33–40.

Li, L., Ma, N., Li, Z., Tan, L., Liu, J., Gong, G., Shu, N., He, Z., Jiang, T., and Xu, L. (2007) Prefrontal white matter abnormalities in young adult with major depressive disorder: A diffusion tensor imaging study. *Brain Res.* 1168:124–128.

Lyoo, I. K., et al. (2004) Frontal lobe gray matter density decreases in bipolar I disorder. *Biol. Psychiatry* 55:648–651.

MacFall, J.R., Payne, M.E., Provenzale, J.E., and Krishnan, K.R.R. (2001) Medial orbital frontal lesions in late onset depression. *Biol. Psychiatry* 49:803–806.

Maes, M., Dierckx, R., Meltzer, H., Ingels, M., Schotte, C., Vandewoude, M., Calabrese, J., and Cosyns, P. (1993) Regional cerebral blood flow in unipolar depression measured with Tc-99m-HMPAO SPECT: negative findings. *Psychiatry Res./Neuroimaging* 50:77–88.

Malison, R.T., Price, L.H., Berman, R., van Dyck, C.H., Pelton, G.H., Carpenter, L., et al. (1998) Reduced brain serotonin transporter availability in major depression as measured by [123I]-2 beta-carbomethoxy-3 beta-(4-iodophenyl)tropane and single photon emission computed tomography. *Biol. Psychiatry* 44:1090–1098.

Manji, H., Drevets, W.C., and Charney, D. (2001) The cellular neurobiology of depression. *Nat. Medi.* 7(5):541–547.

Mayberg, H.S., Brannan, S.K., Mahurin, R.K., Jerabek, P.A., Brickman, J.S., Tekell, J.L., Silva, J.A., McGinnis, S., Glass, T.G., Martin, C.C., and Fox, P.T. (1997) Cingulate function in depression: a potential predictor of treatment response. *Neuroreport* 8:1057–1061.

Mayberg, H.S., Brannan, S.K., Tekell, J.L., Silva, J.A., Mahurin, R.K., McGinnis, S., and Jerabek, P.A. (2000) Regional metabolic effects of fluoxetine in major depression: serial changes and relationship to clinical response. *Biol. Psychiatry* 48:830–843.

Mayberg, H.S., Liotti, M., Brannan, S.K., McGinnis, B.S., Mahurin, R.K., Jerabek, P.A., et al. (1999) Reciprocal limbic-cortical function and negative mood: converging PET findings in depression and normal sadness. *Am. J. Psychiatry* 156:675–682.

Mayberg, H.S., Lozano, A.M., Voon, V., McNeeley, H.E., Seminowicz, D., Hamani, C., Schwalb, J. M., and Kennedy, S.H. (2005) Deep brain stimulation for treatment-resistant depression. *Neuron* 45: 651–660.

Mayberg, H.S., Starkstein, S.E., Morris, P.L., et al. (1991) Remote cortical hypometabolism following focal basal ganglia injury: relationship to secondary changes in mood. *Neurology* 41(Suppl): 266.

Mayberg, H.S., Starkstein, S.E., Peyser, C.E., Brandt, J., Dannals, R.F., and Folstein, S.E. (1992) Paralimbic frontal lobe hypometabolism in depression associated with Huntington's disease. *Neurology* 42:1791–1797.

Mayberg, H.S., Starkstein, S.E., Sadzot, B., Preziosi, T., Andrezejewski, P.L., Dannals, R.F., Wanger, H.N., Jr., and Robinson, R.G. (1990) Selective hypometabolism in the inferior frontal lobe in depressed patients with Parkinson's disease. *Ann. Neurol.* 28:57–64.

Mazziotta, J.C., Phelps, M.E., Plummer, D., and Kuhl, D.E. (1981) Quantitation in positron emission computed tomography. 5. Physical-anatomical effects. *J. Comput. Assist. Tomogr.* 5:734–743.

McDonald, W.M., Krishnan, K.R.R., Doraiswamy, P.M., et al. (1991) Occurrence of subcortical hyperintensities in elderly subjects with mania. *Psychiatry Res.* 40:211–220.

McEwen, B.S. (1999) Stress and hippocampal plasticity. *Ann. Rev. Neurosci.* 22:105–122.

Meltzer, C.C., Price, J.C., Mathis, C.A., Greer, P.J., Cantwell, M.N., Houck, P.R., Mulsant, B.H., Ben-Eliezer, D., Lopresti, B., DeKosky S.T., and Reynolds, C.F. III. (1999) PET imaging of serotonin type 2A receptors in late-life neuropsychiatric disorders. *Am. J. Psychiatry* 156:1871–1878.

Mervaala, E., Fohr, J., Kononen, M., Valkonen-Korhonen, M., Vainio, P., Partanen, K., et al. (2000) Quantitative MRI of the hippocampus and amygdala in severe depression. *Psychol. Med.* 30:117–125.

Meyer, J.H., Houle, S., Sagrati, S., Carella, A., Hussey, D.F., Ginovart, N., et al. (2004) Brain serotonin transporter binding potential measured with carbon 11-labeled DASB positron emission tomography: effects of major depressive episodes and severity of dysfunctional attitudes. *Arch. Gen. Psychiatry* 61:1271–1279.

Meyer, J.H., Kapur, S., Houle, S., DaSilva, J., Owczarek, B., Brown, G.M., Wilson, A.A., and Kennedy, S.H. (1999) Prefrontal cortex 5-HT2 receptors in depression: An [^{18}F] Setoperone PET imaging study. *Am. J. Psychiatry* 156(7):1029–1034.

Meyer, J.H., Kruger, S., Wilson, A.A., Christensen, B.K., Goulding, V.S., Schaffer, A., Minifie, C., Houle, S., and Kennedy, S.H. (2001) Lower dopamine transporter binding potential in striatum during depression. *Neuroreport* 12(18):4121–4125.

Moore, G., Cortese, B., Glitz, D., Zajac-Benitez, C., Keenan, P., Drevets, W.C., and Manji, H.K. (2004) Chronic lithium increases prefrontal and subgenual prefrontal gray matter in patients with bipolar disorder: a longitudinal high resolution volumetric MRI study. *Soc. Neurosci. Abstr.*

Nemeroff, C.B., Krishnan, K.R.R., Reed, D., et al. (1992) Adrenal gland enlargement in major depression: a computed tomographic study. *Arch. Gen. Psychiatry* 49:384–387.

Neumeister, A., Nugent, A.C., Waldeck, T., Geraci, M., Schwarz, M., Bonne, O., Luckenbaugh, D., Herscovitch, P., Charney, D.S., and Drevets, W.C. (2004) Behavioral and neural responses to tryptophan depletion in unmedicated remitted patients with major depressive disorder and controls. *Arch. Gen. Psychiatry* 61: 765–773.

Neumeister, A., Wood, S., Bonne, O., Nugent, A.C., Luckenbaugh, D.A., Young, T., Bain, E.E., Charney, D.S., and Drevets, W.C. (2005) Reduced hippocampal volume in unmedicated, remitted patients with major depressive disorder versus control subjects. *Biol. Psychiatry* 58(8):935–937.

Nobler, M.S., Oquendo, M.A., Kegeles, L.S., Malone, K.M., Campbell, C., Sackeim, H.A., and Mann, J.J. (2001) Decreased regional brain metabolism after ECT. *Am. J. Psychiatry* 158:305–308.

Nobler, M.S., Roose, S., Prohovnik, I., Moeller, J.R., Louie, J., Van Heertum, R.L., and Sackeim, H.A. (2000) Regional cerebral blood flow in mood disorders, V. Effects of antidepressant medication in late-life depression. *Am. J. Geriatr. Psychiatry* 8:289–296.

Nobler, M.S., Sackeim, H.A., Prohovnik, I., Moeller, J.R., Mukherjee, S., Schnur, D.B., Prudic, J., and Devanand, D.P. (1994) Regional cerebral BF in mood disorders, III. Treatment and clinical response. *Arch. Gen. Psychiatry* 51:884–897.

Nofzinger, E.F., Nichols, T.E., Meltzer, C.C., Price, J., Steppe, D.A., Miewald, J.M., Kupfer, D.J., and Moore, R.Y. (1999) Changes in forebrain function from waking to REM sleep in depression: preliminary analyses of [^{18}F]FDG PET studies. *Psychiatry Res. Neuroimaging* 91:59–78.

Noga, J.T., Vladar, K., Torrey, E.F. (2001) A volumetric magnetic resonance imaging study of monozygotic twins discordant for bipolar disorder. *Psychiatry Res* 106:25–34.

Nugent, A. C., et al. (2006) Cortical abnormalities in bipolar disorder investigated with MRI and voxel-based morphometry. *Neuroimage* 30(2):485–497.

O'Brien, J.T., Ames, D., and Schwietzer, I. (1996) White matter changes in depression and Alzheimer's disease: a review of magnetic resonance imaging studies. *Int. J. Geriatric Psychiatry* 11:681–694.

O'Brien, J.T., Desmond, P., Ames, D., et al. (1996) Magnetic resonance imaging study of white matter lesions in depression and Alzheimer's disease. *Br. J. Psychiatry* 168:477–485.

Öngür, D., Drevets, W.C., and Price, J.L. (1998) Glial reduction in the subgenual prefrontal cortex in mood disorders. *Proceedings of the National Academy of Science* 95:13290–13295.

Öngür, D., Ferry, A. T., and Price, J.L. (2003) Architectonic subdivision of the human orbital and medial prefrontal cortex. *J. Comp. Neurol.* 460:425–449.

Oquendo, M.A., Hastings, R.S., Huang, Y.Y., Simpson, N., Ogden, R.T., Hu, X.Z., et al. (2007) Brain serotonin transporter binding in depressed patients with bipolar disorder using positron emission tomography. *Arch. Gen. Psychiatry* 64:201–208.

Osuch, E.A., Ketter, T.A., Kimbrell, T.A., George, M.S., Benson, B.E., Willis, M.W., Herscovitch, P., and Post, R.M. (2000) Regional cerebral metabolism associated with anxiety symptoms in affective disorder patients. *Biol. Psychiatry* 48(10):1020–1023.

Pantel, J., Schroder, J., Essig, M., et al. (1997) Quantitative magnetic resonance imaging in geriatric depression and primary degenerative dementia. *J. Affect. Disord.* 42:69–83.

Parsey, R.V., Hastings, R.S., Oquendo, M.A., Huang, Y.Y., Simpson, N., Arcement, J., et al. (2006) Lower serotonin transporter binding potential in the human brain during major depressive episodes. *Am. J. Psychiatry* 163:52–58.

Paul, I. A., and Skolnick, P. (2003) Glutamate and depression: clinical and preclinical studies. *Ann. N. Y. Acad. Sci.* 1003:250–272.

Pearlson, G.D., Barta, P.E., Powers, R.E., Menon, R.R., Richards, S.S., Aylward, E.H., Federman, E.B., Chase, G.A., Petty, R.G., and Tien, A.Y. (1997) Medial and superior temporal gyral volumes and cerebral asymmetry in schizophrenia versus bipolar disorder. *Biol. Psychiatry* 41:1–14.

Pearlson, G.D., Wong, D.F., Tune, L.E., et al. (1995) In vivo D_2 dopamine receptor density in psychotic and nonpsychotic patients with bipolar disorder. *Arch. Gen. Psychiatry* 52:471–477.

Philpot, M.P., Banerjee, S., Needham-Bennett, H., Costa, D.C., and Ell, P.J. (1993) ^{99mm}Tc-HMPAO single photon emission tomography in late life depression: a pilot study of regional cerebral blood flow at rest and during a verbal fluency task. *J. Affect. Disord.* 28:233–240.

Pizzagalli, D., Pascual-Marqui, R.D., Nitschke, J.B., Oakes, T.R., Larson, C.L., Abercrombie, H.C., Schaefer, S.M., Koger, J.V., Benca, R.M., and Davidson, R.J. (2001) Anterior cingulate activity as a predictor of degree of treatment response in major depression: evidence from brain electrical tomography analysis. *Am. J. Psychiatry* 158(3):405–415.

Poline, J.B., Holmes, A., Worsley, K., and Friston, K.J. (1997) Making statistical inferences. In: Frackowiak, R., Friston, K.J., Frith, C.D., Dolan, R.J., and Mazziotta J.C., eds. *Human Brain Function*. London: Academic Press, pp. 85–106.

Postalache, T.T., Matthews, J.R., Turner, E.H., Benson, B.E., Guzman, A., Rosenthal, N.E., and Drevets, W.C. (2002, June 13-15) Cerebral blood flow in depressed individuals with seasonal affective disorder as compared to matched controls. *Soc. Light Treatment Bio Rhythms Abstracts*, 14:23.

Price, J.L., Carmichael, S.T., and Drevets, W.C. (1996) Networks related to the orbital and medial prefrontal cortex: a substrate for emotional behavior? *Prog. Brain Res.* 107:523–536.

Rabins, P.V., Pearlson, G.D., Aylward, E., et al. (1991) Cortical magnetic imaging changes in elderly inpatients with major depression. *Am. J. Psychiatry* 148:617–620.

Raichle, M.E. (1987) Circulatory and metabolic correlates of brain function in normal humans. In: Brookhart, J.M., and Mountcastle, V.B., ed. *Handbook of Physiology - the Nervous System V*. Baltimore: Williams and Wilkins, pp. 643–674.

Rajkowska, G., Miguel-Hidalgo, J.J., Wei, J., Dilley, G., Pittman, S.D., Meltzer, H.Y., Overholser, J.C., Roth, B.L., and Stockmeier, C.A. (1999) Morphometric evidence for neuronal and glial prefrontal cell pathology in major depression. *Biol. Psychiatry* 45(9): 1085–1098

Rauch, S.L., Jenike, M.A., Alpert, N.M., Baer, L., Breiter, H., Savage, C.R., and Fischman, A.J. (1994) Regional cerebral blood flow measured during symptom provocation in obsessive-compulsive disorder using oxygen 15-labeled carbon dioxide and positron emission tomography. *Arch. Gen. Psychiatry* 51:62–70

Reiman, E.M., Lane, R.D., Ahern, G.L., Schwartz, G.E., Davidson, R.J., Friston, K.J., Yun, L.S., and Chen, K. (1997) Neuroanatomical correlates of externally and internally generated human emotion. *Am. J. Psychiatry* 154(7):918–925

Reivich, M., Amsterdam, J.D., Brunswick, D.J., and Shiue, C.Y. (2004) PET brain imaging with [^{11}C](+)McN5652 shows increased serotonin transporter availability in major depression. *J. Affect. Disord.* 82:321–327.

Ring, H.A., Bench, C.J., Trimble, M.R., Brooks, D.J., Frackowiak, R.S.J., and Dolan, R.J. (1994) Depression in Parkinson's disease: a positron emission study. *Br. J. Psychiatry* 165:333–339.

Rolls, E.T. (1995) A theory of emotion and consciousness, and its application to understanding the neural basis of emotion. In: Gazzaniga M, ed. *The Cognitive Neurosciences*. Cambridge, MA: MIT Press, pp. 1091–1106.

Rubin, R.T., Mandell, A.J., and Crandall, P.H. (1966) Corticosteroid responses to limbic stimulation in man: localization of stimulus sites. *Science* 153:767–768.

Rubin, R.T., Phillips, J.J., McCracken, J.T., Sadow, T.F. (1996) Adrenal gland volume in major depression: relationship to basal and stimulated pituitary-adrenal cortical axis function. *Biol. Psychiatry* 40(2):89–97

Rubin, R.T., Phillips, J.J., Sadow, T.F., et al. (1995) Adrenal gland volume in major depression: increase during the depressive episode and decrease with successful treatment. *Arch. Gen. Psychiatry* 52:213–218.

Saxena, S., Brody, A.L., Ho, M.L., Alborzian, S., Maidment, K., Zohrabi, N., Ho, M.K., Huang, S.C., Wu, H.M., and Baxter, L.R. (2002) Differential cerebral metabolic changes with paroxetine treatment of obsessive-compulsive disorder vs major depression. *Arch. Gen. Psychiatry* 59:250–261.

Schneider, F., Gur, R.E., Alavi, A., Mozley, L.H., Smith, R.J., Mozley, P.D., Censits, D.M., and Gur, R.C. (1995) Mood effects on limbic blood flow correlate with emotion self-rating: a PET study with oxygen-15 labeled water. *Psychiatry Res. Neuroimaging* 61: 265–283.

Schwartz, J.M., Baxter, L.R., Mazziota, J.C., Gerner, R.H., and Phelps, M.E. (1987) The differential diagnosis of depression: Relevance of positron emission tomography studies of cerebral glucose metabolism to the bipolar-unipolar dichotomy. *JAMA* 258:1368–1373.

Shah, P.J., Ebmeier, K.P., Glabus, M.F., and Goodwin, G.M. (1998) Cortical grey matter reductions associated with treatment-resistant chronic unipolar depression. Controlled magnetic resonance imaging study. *Br. J. Psychiatry* 172:527–532.

Shah, P.J., Ogilvie, A.D., Goodwin, G.M., and Ebmeier, K.P. (1997) Clinical and psychometric correlates of dopamine D2 binding in depression. *Psychol. Med.* 27:1247–1256

Shah, S.A., Doraiswamy, P.M., Husain, M.M., et al. (1992) Posterior fossa abnormalities in major depression: a controlled magnetic resonance imaging study. *Acta Psychiatr. Scand.* 85:474–479.

Sheline, Y.I., Barch, D.M., Donnelly, J.M., Ollinger, J.M., Snyder, A.Z., and Mintun, M.A. (2001) Increased amygdala response to masked emotional faces in depressed subjects resolves with antidepressant treatment: an fMRI study. *Biol. Psychiatry* 50:651–658.

Sheline, Y.I., Gado, M.H., and Price, J.L. (1998) Amygdala core nuclei volumes are decreased in recurrent major depression. *Neuroreport* 9(9):2023–2028.

Sheline, Y.I., Mintun, M.A., Barch, D.M., Wilkins, C., Snyder, A.Z., and Moerlein, S.M. (2004) Decreased hippocampal 5-HT(2A) receptor binding in older depressed patients using [18F]altanserin positron emission tomography. *Neuropsychopharmacology* 29(12): 2235–2241.

Sheline, Y.I., Wang, P.W., Gado, M.H., Csernansky, J.G., and Vannier, M.W. (1996) Hippocampal atrophy in recurrent major depression. *Proc. Natl. Acad. Sci. USA* 93:3908–3913.

Shulman, R.G., Rothman, D.L., Behar, K.L. and Hyder, F. (2004) Energetic basis of brain activity: implications for neuroimaging. *Trends Neurosci.* 27:489–495.

Siegle, G.J., Carter, C. S., et al. (2006) Use of FMRI to predict recovery from unipolar depression with cognitive behavior therapy. *Am. J. Psychiatry* 163(4):735–738.

Siegle, G.J., Steinhauer, S.R., Thase, M.E., Stenger, V.A., and Carter, C.C. (2002) Can't shake that feeling: event-related fMRI assessment of sustained amygdala activity in response to emotional information in depressed individuals. *Biol. Psychiatry* 51:693–707.

Silfverskiöld, P., and Risberg, J. (1989) Regional blood flow in depression and mania. *Arch. Gen. Psychiatry* 46:253–259.

Smith, G.S., Reynolds, C.F., Pollock, B., Derbyshire, S., Nofzinger, E., Dew, M.A., Houck, P.A., Milko, D., Meltzer, C.C., and Kupfer, D.J. (1999) Cerebral glucose metabolic response to combined total sleep deprivation and antidepressant treatment in geriatric depression. *Am. J. Psychiatry* 156:683–689.

Starkstein, S.E., and Robinson, R.G. (1989) Affective disorders and cerebral vascular disease. *Br. J. Psychiatry* 154:170–182.

Steffens, D.C., Byrum, C.E., McQuoid, D.R., Greenberg, D.L., Payne, M.E., Blitchington, T.F., MacFall, J.R., and Krishnan, K.R. (2000) Hippocampal volume in geriatric depression. *Biol. Psychiatry* 48:301–309.

Stockmeier, C.A. (2003) Involvement of serotonin in depression: evidence from postmortem and imaging studies of serotonin receptors and the serotonin transporter. *J. Psychiatry Res.* 37:357–373.

Strakowski, S.M., DelBello, M.P., Sax, K.W., Zimmerman, M.E., Shear, P.K., Hawkins, J.M., and Larson, E.R. (1999) Brain magnetic resonance imaging of structural abnormalities in bipolar disorder. *Arch. Gen. Psychiatry* 56:254–260.

Strakowski, S.M., Wilson, D.R., Tohen, M., et al. (1993) Structural brain abnormalities in first-episode mania. *Biol. Psychiatry* 33: 602–609.

Suhara, T., Nakayama, K., Inoue, O., Fukuda, H., Shimizu, M., Mori, A., and Tateno, Y. (1992) D1 dopamine receptor binding in mood disorders measured by PET. *Psychopharmacology* 106:14–18.

Sullivan, R.M., and Gratton, A. (1999) Lateralized effects of medial prefrontal cortex lesions on neuroendocrine and autonomic stress responses in rats. *J. Neurosci.* 19:2834–2840

Swayze, V.W., Andreasen, N.C., Alliger, R.J., et al. (1990) Structural brain abnormalties in bipolar affective disorder. Ventricular enlargement and focal signal hyperintensities. *Arch. Gen. Psychiatry* 47:1054–1059.

Swayze, V.W., 2nd, Andreasen, N.C., Alliger, R.J., Yuh, W.T., and Ehrhardt, J.C. (1992) Subcortical and temporal structures in affective disorder and schizophrenia: a magnetic resonance imaging study. *Biol. Psychiatry* 31(3):221–240

Taylor, W.D., MacFall, J.R., Payne, M.E., McQuoid, D.R., Provenzale, J.M., Steffens, D.C., and Krishnan, K.R. (2004) Late-life depression and microstructural abnormalities in dorsolateral prefrontal cortex. *Am. J. Psychiatry* 161(7):1293–1296.

Taylor, W.D., Payne, M.E., Krishnan, K.R., Wagner, H.R., Provenzale, J.M., Steffens, D.C., and MacFall, J.R. (2001) Evidence of white matter tract disruption in MRI hyperintensities. *Biol. Psychiatry* 50(3):179–183.

Thomas, K.M., Drevets, W.C., Dahl, R.E., Ryan, N.D., Birmaher, B., Eccard, C.H., Axelson, D., Whalen, P.J., and Casey, B.J. (2001) Abnormal amygdala response to faces in anxious and depressed children. *Arch. Gen. Psychiatry* 58:1057–1063.

Timms, R.J. (1977) Cortical inhibition and facilitation of the defence reaction. *J. Physiol. Lond.* 266:98P–99P.

Tremblay, L.K., Naranjo, C.A., et al. (2005) Functional neuroanatomical substrates of altered reward processing in major depressive disorder revealed by a dopaminergic probe. *Arch. Gen. Psychiatry* 62(11):1228–1236.

Uytdenhoef, P., Portelange, P., Jacquy, J., Charles, G., Linkowski, P., and Mendlewicz, J. (1983) Regional cerebral blood flow and lateralized hemispheric dysfunction in depression. *Br. J. Psychiatry* 143:128–132.

Vakili, K., Pillay, S.S., Lafer, B., Fava, M., Renshaw, P.F., and Bonello-Cintron, C.M. (2000) Hippocampal volume in primary unipolar major depression: a magnetic resonance imaging study. *Biol. Psychiatry* 47:1087–1090.

Videbech, P., Ravnkilde, B., Pedersen, A.R., Egander, A., Landbo, B., Rasmussen, N.A., Andersen, F., Stodkilde-Jorgensen, H., Gjedde, A., and Rosenberg, R. (2001) The Danish PET/depression project: PET findings in patients with major depression. *Psychol. Med.* 31: 1147–1158.

Volkow, N.D., Fowler, J.S., Wolf, A.P., Hitzemann, R., Dewey, S., Bendriem, B., Alpert, R., and Hoff, A. (1991) Changes in brain glucose metabolism in cocaine dependence and withdrawal. *Am. J. Psychiatry* 148:621–626.

von Gunten, A., Fox, N.C., Cipolotti, L., and Ron, M.A. (2000) A volumetric study of hippocampus and amygdala in depressed patients with subjective memory problems. *J. Neuropsychiatry Clin. Neurosci.* 12:493–498.

Vythilingam, M., Heim, C., Newport, J., Miller, A.H., Anderson, E., Bronen, R., et al. (2002) Childhood trauma associated with smaller hippocampal volume in women with major depression. *Am. J. Psychiatry* 159:2072–2080.

Wilson, J., Kupfer, D.J., Thase, M., Bogers, W., Greer, P., and Drevets, W.C. (2002) Ventral striatal metabolism is increased in depression, and decreases with treatment. *Biol. Psychiatry* 51:122S.

Wooten, G.F., and Collins, R.C. (1981) Metabolic effects of unilateral lesion of the substantia nigra. *J. Neurosci.* 1:285–291.

Wu, J.C., Gillin, J.C., Buchsbaum, M.S., Hershey, T., Johnson, J.C., Bunney, W.E. (1992) Effect of sleep deprivation on brain metabolism of depressed patients. *Am. J. Psychiatry* 149:538–543.

Yurgelun-Todd, D.A., Gruber, S.A., Kanayama, G., Killgore, W.D., Baird, A.A., and Young, A.D. (2000) fMRI during affect discrimination in bipolar affective disorder. *Bipolar Disord.* 2: 237–248.

Zis, K.D., and Zis, A.P. (1987) Increased adrenal weight in victims of violent suicide. *Am. J. Psychiatry* 144:1214–1215.

Zubenko, G.S., Sullivan, P., Nelson, J.P., et al. (1990) Brain imaging abnormalities in mental disorders of late life. *Arch. Neurol.* 47: 1107–1113.

32 Principles of the Pharmacotherapy of Depression

ROBERT M. BERMAN,* JONATHAN SPORN*, DENNIS S. CHARNEY, AND SANJAY J. MATHEW

Serendipitous discoveries in the 1950s led to the development of the first antidepressant agents, iproniazid (Crane, 1956; Kline, 1970) and imipramine (Kuhn, 1958). These agents were strategically developed as potential treatments for tuberculosis and psychosis, respectively. The observations that these agents improved mood and boosted psychomotoric activity led to their testing in clinical trials for the treatment of depression. Further investigation revealed their pharmacological activity on monoamine systems, subsequently leading to the development of over two dozen medications with demonstrated antidepressant properties. In the 1960s, knowledge that tricyclic antidepressants inhibited uptake of not only the catecholamine *norepinephrine* but also *serotonin* led to a search for specific serotonin reuptake inhibitors (SSRIs). This culminated in the derivation of the first SSRI, zimelidine, which was withdrawn due to an idiosyncratic side effect. In addition, observation of decreased serotonin levels in postmortem and cerebrospinal fluid (CSF) studies of depression provided further stimulus for a search for specific SSRIs, culminating in the discovery of the landmark SSRI, fluoxetine (Blardi et al., 2002). Clinical development of new agents has been limited by the lack of homogeneity within diagnostically defined entities and by the limited validity and sensitivity of rating instruments for testing change. As well, patients treated in antidepressant trials represent only a subset of individuals, and results may not be fully generalizable with regard to effectiveness in the field (Zimmerman et al., 2002).

Rational use of these medications requires an understanding of their pharmacological properties and clinical effects in varied patient populations. Despite appropriate use of medications, for a long time it has been thought only 40%–50% of patients with depression can expect timely remission with antidepressant treatment (Frank et al., 1993). However, the recent large-scale STAR*D study noted even lower remission rates (circa 30%) with acute citalopram treatment (Trivedi, Rush, et al., 2006). Some 10%–20% of care-seeking patients with depression remain significantly symptomatic after 2 years (Keller et al., 1982).

THE ANTIDEPRESSANTS

For clinical purposes, a useful classification system for antidepressants is based on known receptor affinities—specifically, affinities thought to be related to their mechanism of action. Such a categorization belies the structural diversity of the members of each class; hence, the members of each category may not resemble each other in terms of pharmacokinetics, metabolism, or toxicity (Table 32.1). However, most antidepressants have pharmacological action on the metabolism and at the receptors for the monoamine neurotransmitters *norepinephrine* (NE), *serotonin*, and *dopamine* (DA). In addition, multiple classes of antidepressant agents augment intracellular cyclic adenosine monophosphate (cAMP) and levels of neurotrophic and transcription factors such as cAMP-response element binding protein (CREB) and brain-derived neurotrophic factor (BDNF). Antidepressants may also modulate excitatory transmission by decreasing binding at *N*-methyl-D-aspartate (NMDA) receptors or by inducing changes at other excitatory receptors such as the α-amino-3-hydroxy-5-methyl-4-isoxasolepropionic acid (AMPA) receptor. Last, there are novel antidepressants that in part may exert effects on melatonin receptors.

Tricyclic Antidepressants

The standard tricyclic antidepressant, imipramine, a dibenzazepine drug, is similar in structure to the phenothiazines. Kuhn (1958) determined that it lacked the capacity to

* Contributed equally to the writing of this chapter.

TABLE 32.1 *Functionally Relevant Receptor Antagonism and Associated Side Effects*[a]

Antidepressant	*Histamine-1 (Sedation, Weight Gain, Hypotension, Potentiation of CNS Depressants)*	*Muscarinic (Tachycardia, Memory Impairment, Constipation, Urinary Retention, Blurred Vision, Dry Mouth)*	*α_1-Adrenergic (Hypotension, Tachycardia)*
Tricyclic agents			
Amitriptyline	1111	111	1111
Doxepine	1111	111	1111
Imipramine	111	11	1111
Protripyline	111	111	1111
Trimipramine	1111	11	1111
Desipramine	11/111	11	111
Nortripyline	111	11	111
SSRIs			
Fluoxetine	1	1	1
Sertraline	1	1	11
Paroxetine	1	1	1
Fluvoxamine	1	1	1
Citalopram	1	1	1
Other agents			
Mirtazapine	1111	1	11
Venlafaxine	1	1	1
Duloxetine	1	1	1
Nefazodone	1	1	111
Trazodone	1	1	1111
Bupropion	1	1	1

CNS: central nervous system; SSRI: specific serotonin reuptake inhibitor.
a. Negligible (1), mild (11), moderate (111), and high (1111) affinities. Receptor-mediated side effects are more likely with higher-affinity agents.
Source: Adapted from Richelson (1991).

calm patients who were agitated but observed robust positive effects in patients who were depressed.

Tricyclic antidepressants (TCAs)—so labeled because of a core structure consisting of three rings—also include imipramine, amitriptyline, trimipramine, doxepin, desipramine, nortriptyline, and protriptyline. Tricyclics antidepressants that are either secondary amines or the *N*-demethylated (nor) metabolites of tertiary-amine structures (for example, amoxapine, desipramine, and nortriptyline) have relative selectivity for the inhibition of noradrenaline uptake, whereas the older tertiary-amine tricyclics additionally inhibit the reuptake and inactivation of serotonin while maintaining NE reuptake inhibition vis-à-vis their metabolites. Amoxapine additionally is a DA_2 antagonist and thus has neuroleptic properties that are important in the treatment of psychotic depression; however, it may lead to extrapyramidal side effects, especially in patients with Parkinson's disease (Richelson, 1991). Within a narrow dose range, and typically at therapeutic doses, these antidepressants are active at multiple nonmonoamine receptors, resulting in a complex set of adaptive processes from the level of the receptor to that of genomic regulatory factors. Augmentation of α_1-receptor activity, desensitization of α_2-receptors, and possibly desensitization of D_2 autoreceptors may facilitate serotonin, NE, and DA signaling. Subsequently, 5-HT_1 autoreceptors and 5-HT_2 receptors postsynaptically may be down-regulated and involved in generating an antidepressant signal. As indicated in Table 32.1, such high affinity for other receptors leads to bothersome side effects. Blockade of muscarinic acetylcholine receptors may cause dry mouth, blurred vision, constipation, urinary retention, memory impairment, and tachycardia. Blockade of histamine-1 receptors may cause sedation, weight gain, hypotension, and the potentiation of other central nervous system (CNS) depressants. Blockade of α_1-adrenergic receptors may cause postural hypotension, reflex tachycardia, and perhaps sedation. Via unclear mechanisms, TCAs, especially clomipramine and amoxapine, are associated with a 0.1%–0.5% rate of seizures (Skowron and Stimmel, 1992), likely occurring early in treatment or during periods of acute dose escalation. After its release, maprotiline—a tetracyclic compound—was associated with higher rates of seizures probably due to too rapid a dosage escalation (Dessain et al., 1986). Revision of the recommended dosing schedule appeared to decrease the risk substantially.

When given in doses up to one order of magnitude greater than typical therapeutic doses, TCAs may be lethal, causing fatal arrhythmias. At these doses, conduction abnormalities may emerge, such as prolonged PR, QRS, or QTc intervals, as well as flattening or inversion of T waves. Also, slowing of depolarization may lead to atrioventricular or bundle branch block, as well as premature ventricular contractions. Some TCAs may also decrease heart rate variability, which is a risk factor for sudden cardiac death. Nevertheless, at standard doses, clinically significant cardiac abnormalities are not common (Nelson, 1997a). An important consideration is that drugs that inhibit the cytochrome CYP-2D6 isozyme may lead to potentially dangerous increases in TCA blood levels that can be problematic for patients who are elderly.

Once the mainstay of antidepressant treatment, TCAs have been replaced by newer agents with more favorable side-effect and safety profiles. Despite their resulting diminished popularity, the tolerability of TCAs may well be underestimated by most clinicians (Nelson, 1997a). They are still commonly used for patients with chronic pain.

Monoamine Oxidase Inhibitors

Monoamine oxidase inhibitors (MAOIs) used to treat depression can be irreversible inhibitors (for example, phenelzine and tranylcypromine) or short acting and reversible, such as the MAOI-A, moclobemide. They are either of the hydrazine class, such as phenalzine and isocarboxazide, or unrelated to the hydrazines and related to the CNS stimulants such as tranylcypromine. Reversible MAOIs such as moclobemide have a moderate degree of antidepressant activity (Davidson, 1992). The older agents in this class irreversibly inhibit the MAO isozymes A and B, whereas moclobemide competitively inhibits MAO-A. Increased MAO-A activity in brain has recently been reported using positron emission tomography (PET) imaging (Meyer et al, 2006). Antidepressant activity of these agents has been attributed to their ability to inhibit MAO-A, which metabolizes noradrenaline and serotonin because oral agents that specifically inhibit MAO-B, such as deprenyl, have limited antidepressant efficacy (Mann et al., 1989). However, transdermal deprenyl does appear effective (Feighner et al., 2006) and is safer than other orally available MAOIs. It is now on the U.S. market. Preclinical data indicate that when administered transdermally the agent is a potent inhibitor of central MAO-A and MAO-B activity (Wecker et al., 2003).

The older MAOIs became unpopular in clinical practice because of side effects and potential toxicity. The MAOIs may cause acute, severe elevations in blood pressure (that is, hypertensive crises) with ingestion of tyramine-containing foods and sympathomimetic medications. Other symptoms of this syndrome include headache, nausea, sweating, pallor, and vomiting. Fatalities secondary to intracranial hemorrhage have been reported. Patients must adhere to dietary restrictions aimed at eliminating foods rich in tyramine, such as aged cheeses, soy sauce, sauerkraut, air-dried sausage, pickled herring, concentrated yeast extract, and fava beans. Tyramine, ordinarily metabolized by gastrointestinal MAO, acts as a direct and/or indirect pressor agent when absorbed by patients on MAOIs. Rare cases of hypertensive crisis without demonstrable dietary indiscretions have also been reported. However, clinicians should be aware that recent studies of food tyramine content indicate that a simple, limited list of absolutely restricted foods can be developed and that a user-friendly MAOI diet may enhance patient compliance and physician comfort with this important class of agents (Gardner et al., 1996; Walker et al., 1996). Patients must also be diligent about avoiding dangerous medication interactions with MAOIs. Drugs that increase synaptic monoamine effects should be eliminated, such as tricyclics, SSRIs, cocaine, stimulants, and many over-the-counter flu medications. Furthermore, idiosyncratic hyperthermic reactions with certain medications such as pethidine and meperidine, as well as other opiates, can be lethal. Due to such dramatic toxic effects, irreversible MAOIs are best reserved for cases when multiple previous treatment trials have been unsuccessful.

Moclobemide and brofaromine represented a newer generation of MAOIs that were distinguished by their reversible inhibition of MAO. Consequently, these agents had less interaction with dietary tyramine to cause hypertensive crises. Nevertheless, drug interactions with SSRIs or SNRIs could cause a serotonin syndrome. U.S. trials with these agents were not as robust as European studies, and their development has been on hold in the United States.

Selective Serotonin Reuptake Inhibitors

The SSRIs generally have affinity for the serotonin transporter that is one to two orders of magnitude greater than their affinity for the noradrenergic transporter (Table 32.2) (Richelson, 1991). At typical therapeutic doses, they generally inhibit about 80% of serotonin transporter activity (Meyer et al., 2001). Increased serotonin levels at the synapse stimulate a large number of serotonin receptor subtypes and are putatively related to the antidepressant effect and many of the side effects of these agents. Increased serotonin availability occurs following desensitization of dendritic 5-HT_{1A} receptors and terminal 5-HT_{1D} receptors. Down-regulation of postsynaptic 5-HT_{2A} receptors may also be impor-

TABLE 32.2 *Potency of Selected Antidepressants to Inhibit Monoamine Reuptake*[a]

	IC_{50} Values (nM)	
Antidepressant	*Norepinephrine*	*Serotonin*
Tricyclic agents		
Amitriptyline	25	100
Doxepine	150	2,000
Imipramine	25	50
Protriptyline	10	250
Trimipramine	5,000	10,000
Desipramine	2	300
Nortriptyline	6	200
SSRIs		
Fluoxetine	200	15
Sertraline	300	4
Paroxetine	70	1
Fluvoxamine	500	5
Citalopram	3,900	3
Other agents		
Mirtazapine	2,000	5,000
Venlafaxine	300	50
Duloxetine	9	3
Nefazodone	600	150
Trazodone	20,000	750
Bupropion	2,500	15,000
Reboxetine	8	1,070

SSRI: specific serotonin reuptake inhibitor.

a. The depicted inhibitory constants reflect the concentration of antidepressant that blocks one half of the reuptake of monoamines, serotonin, and norepinephrine by their respective transporters.

Source: Frazer (1997).

tant in generating an antidepressant signal. Beyond the receptor, fluoxetine, via the cAMP-dependent protein kinase A (PKA) pathway in frontal cortex and hippocampus, has been observed to regulate the phosphorylation state of DA- and cAMP-regulated phosophoprotein of M_r 32,000 (DARPP-32) (Svenningsson et al., 2002). DARPP-32 mediates changes in the phosphorylation state and activity of AMPA, a glutamate receptor that is a therapeutic target in depression. Ease of use made the SSRIs the standard first-line treatment for major depression by most practitioners. Available SSRIs worldwide include fluoxetine, paroxetine, sertraline, fluvoxamine, citalopram, and escitalopram (the enantiomer of citalopram). The agents in this class may be distinguished by their half-lives. Fluoxetine and its metabolite have respective half-lives of approximately 2 and 7 days. Plasma levels for fluoxetine reach their peak 30 days after starting the drug. Platelet serotonin level decreases and increases in plasma serotonin are also greatest after 30 days (Blardi et al., 2002). Nevertheless, common practice is once-daily dosing of fluoxetine as well as most other SSRIs. Fluvoxamine, approved in the United States for obsessive compulsive disorder but not major depression, is distinguished by having the shortest half-life (approximately 16 hours), which requires twice daily dosing, and by being the least protein bound. The SSRIs are very rarely associated with fatalities when large doses are ingested unless other agents are also taken. The SSRIs may be safe in pregnancy if absolutely necessary, with the most observational retrospective data available for fluoxetine and sertraline. There are reports of possible subtle motoric effects with late pregnancy exposure to SSRIs (Casper et al., 2003).

Proliferation and increased use of SSRIs has necessitated a keen awareness of potentially lethal interactions involving drug metabolism (Nemeroff et al., 1996). The cytochrome P450 enzymes are a superfamily of heme-thiolate proteins, and blockade or polymorphisms of these enzymes result in altered drug metabolism. Inhibition of the hepatic isozyme CYP-2D6 can lead to significant elevations in blood levels of TCAs and neuroleptics. Although fluoxetine and paroxetine most potently inhibit this isozyme and are, therefore, more commonly associated with related interactions, sertraline can also cause clinically relevant isozyme inhibition. About 70 single-nucleotide polymorphisms have been found for CYP-2D6, and a relatively common genetic polymorphism may profoundly reduce the activity of this isozyme in up to 10% of Caucasians as well as 2% of Asians and Blacks (Kroemer and Eichelbaum, 1995). Given the prevalence of such poor metabolizers, the clinician should be aware of potential interactions involving CYP-2D6 isozymes even when using agents such as sertraline. However, a recent pharmacogenetic study of paroxetine in geriatric patients with depression did not observe increased dropouts due to adverse events in slow metabolizers (Murphy et al., 2003).

Fluvoxamine is a potent inhibitor of CYP-3A4 and hence may lead to dangerous cardiotoxic elevations related to the metabolism of terfenadine, astemizole, and cisapride. The prudent clinician must take heed of potentially expectable interactions, and careful monitoring is necessary when a patient is concurrently taking medications with a narrow therapeutic index (Nemeroff et al., 1996). The newer antidepressants have less inhibition of clinically important CYPs with the exception of nefazadone, a potent inhibitor of CYP-3A4.

A possible lethal interaction involves the use of SSRIs with MAOIs or other agents that may potentiate serotonergic transmission. A resultant serotonin syndrome may emerge, consisting of hyperpyrexia, cardiogenic shock, abdominal pain, agitation, delirium, myoclonus, and/or hypertension (Lane and Baldwin, 1997).

The SSRIs, as a class, have been associated with a common set of side effects; consequently, these effects may potentially be mediated via serotonin receptors. Sexual dysfunction consisting of anorgasmia and impotence may be present in one-third or more of patients. Specific receptors associated with this phenomenon have yet to be elucidated but may involve 5-HT_2 receptors. Sildenafil may be effective in some patients for as-needed treatment of SSRI-induced erectile dysfunction (Nurnberg et al., 2001), and bupropion may modestly be helpful for increasing drive or interest even though a small controlled trial failed to show an effect (DeBattista et al., 2005). Nausea may be mediated via 5-HT_3 receptor stimulation and may be blocked by agents with 5-HT3 antagonists such as mirtazapine.

Nefazodone and Trazodone

Nefazodone and trazodone are potent inhibitors of 5-HT_{2A} receptors. They may have weak affinity for serotonin reuptake sites; however, this activity may have little clinical significance. Nefazadone and trazodone improve sleep continuity, and 5-HT_2 antagonists increase delta or slow-wave sleep. Significant histaminergic and α_1-adrenergic antagonist activities are responsible for the common side effects of sedation and orthostatic hypotension—less problematic for nefazodone than trazodone. Additionally, arrhythmias have been reported with trazodone in patients with preexisting premature ventricular contractions or mitral valve prolapse (Lippman et al., 1983). Although these agents do not cause impotence or anorgasmia, trazodone is associated with priapism, a rare emergency requiring immediate attention. Nefazadone was associated with hepatic toxicity and liver failure in a very small percentage of patients, and this led the original manufacturer to cease production. It is available as a generic. Hepatic toxicity has been observed with trazodone as well.

Mirtazapine

Mirtazapine has potent affinity for the 5-HT_{2A} (K_i of about 10 nM) and α_2-adrenoceptors (K_i of about 100 nm) (Frazer, 1997). Adrenergic blockade may lead to enhanced noradrenergic neurotransmission, via autoreceptor blockade, and enhanced serotonergic neurotransmission, via release of heterologous α_2-mediated inhibition and potentiation of the α_1-mediated serotonin cell firing rate. Additionally, significant histaminergic antagonism may contribute to this medication's potential side effects of sedation, dry mouth, weight gain, and constipation. Cardiac side effects have not been reported. Rare idiosyncratic cases of agranulocytosis or neutropenia have been reported. Furthermore, preliminary experience with this drug worldwide suggests that it has a high therapeutic index, and no known deaths due to overdose have been cited to date (Preskorn, 1997, Waring et al., 2007). Mirtazapine is effective in acute treatment of major depression as well as in relapse prevention with continuation therapy. In the United States, it has become commonly used for geriatric patients.

Bupropion

The mechanism of action of bupropion remains unclear but likely acts via effects on NE neurons and augmentation of NE release (Dong and Blier, 2001). In preclinical studies, bupropion is a potent inhibitor of DA, but the lack of decrease in CSF levels of homovanillic acid after bupropion use suggests that its efficacy in vivo is not related to changes in DA reuptake; however, clinical studies suggest that it has more potent activity on noradrenergic function, as evidenced by its effects on monoamine metabolite levels (Golden et al., 1988). It is approved in smoking cessation. Bupropion rarely causes orthostatic hypotension, sexual dysfunction, daytime drowsiness, or weight gain. Common side effects include headache, insomnia, nausea, and restlessness. At daily doses below 450 mg, there is a 0.4% incidence of seizures. At daily doses between 450 and 600 mg, a 2.4% seizure rate was observed (Johnston et al., 1991), but this side effect is less problematic with more slowly released formulations. An extended release formulation of bupropion received regulatory approval in 2006 in the U.S. for the prevention of recurrence of major depressive episodes in patients with seasonal affective disorder.

Fourth-Generation Antidepressants: Selective Serotonin and Noradrenaline Reuptake Inhibitors (SNRIs): Venlafaxine, Duloxetine, and Milnacipran

Venlafaxine

Venlafaxine is a newly introduced antidepressant agent with selectively high affinity for the noradrenergic and serotonergic reuptake sites in vitro. However, its NE reuptake inhibition becomes evident only at higher doses, usually above 150–200 mg/day. Low affinity for histaminergic, cholinergic, and adrenergic receptors is corroborated by venlafaxine's side-effect profile. Furthermore, venlafaxine is only 30% protein bound and thus does not displace highly protein-bound drugs, and because it does not block hepatic cytochrome P450 activity, it is not likely to interfere with hepatic metabolism of other drugs (Holliday and Benfield, 1995).

Venlafaxine's dual mechanism of action is likely responsible for the high rates of remission of depression compared to SSRIs (Thase, Entsuah, et al., 2001) and may contribute to its efficacy in generalized anxiety disorder as well (Allgulander et al., 2001). This agent is generally well tolerated when prescribed in its extended-release form and shares a side-effect profile similar to that of SSRIs in that both can be associated with increased sweating and sedation. In patients treated with over 200 mg daily, 5.5% were observed to have clinically significant blood pressure elevations. Such increases were defined as a diastolic blood pressure greater than 105 mmHg and a minimum 15 mmHg increase that was sustained on recordings over three consecutive visits. Nevertheless, this incidence does not differ from that of TCAs, as seen in comparator trials (Feighner, 1995). At doses of over 300 mg daily of immediate release venlafaxine, the incidence of hypertension increases to 13%. Infrequently, increases in serum lipids are observed. Also, rapid discontinuation of venlafaxine, or even missed doses, may result in rebound hypotension, nausea, dizziness, and other withdrawal symptoms. Venlafaxine may be associated with a higher incidence of toxicity in overdose than the SSRIs. Desvenlafaxine, the major active metabolite of venlafaxine, was approved in 2008 for major depressive disorder at a dose of 50mg/day.

Duloxetine

Duloxetine, in contrast to venlafaxine, has a relatively balanced ratio of serotonergic to noradrenergic reuptake inhibition. Its SNRI profile may account for its perceived robust efficacy. The agent is approved for the treatment of diabetic peripheral neuropathy and has been reported to be effective in fibromyalgia. In addition to major depressive disorder, the agent is approved for generalized anxiety disorder, diabetic peripheral neuropathy, and fibromyalgia.

Milnacipran

Milnacipran is an SNRI not available in the United States that is equal in efficacy to TCAs and may be superior to SSRIs, especially in patients who are severely ill and agitated with insomnia. Urological side effects can occur (Fukuchi and Kanemoto, 2002). The drug is being developed in the United States for treatment of fibromyalgia.

Reboxetine

Reboxetine is an NRI approved in Europe and other regions, but it is not approved by the U.S. Food and Drug Administration (FDA) for the treatment of major depression due to equivocal Phase III efficacy results. Reboxetine alters noradrenergic neuronal activity by blocking NE transporters. It appears to increase ventral tegmental neuronal activity and consequently increases prefrontal cortex (PFC) DA levels as well (Linner et al., 2001). It has observed efficacy in some short- and long-term studies and may have advantages in improving social function over SSRIs (Kasper et al., 2000). Reboxetine is effective on the Hamilton Depression Rating Scale (HAM-D) psychomotor retardation, anxiety, and cognitive clusters of symptoms, with possibly less efficacy for insomnia (Ferguson et al., 2002). It may also be effective in panic disorder and possibly in attention deficit disorder. Urinary hesitancy, sedation, and noradrenergic/anticholinergic side effects such as dry mouth and tachycardia can occur. Reboxetine does not cause prominent sexual side effects in doses below 8 mg and has limited potential for pharmacokinetic interactions, but levels can be effected by inhibitors of CYP-3A4 (Herman et al., 1999).

CHOICE OF ANTIDEPRESSANT

Given the wide variety of antidepressants, how does the clinician rationally choose a treatment option? Although most patients will eventually respond to treatment, there are no (or only nominally useful) predictors for the initial selection of a specific agent, although there are some budding pharmacogenetic leads. Initial treatment is typically chosen on the basis of side effects, safety, cost, and convenience; differential efficacy plays little role in selecting an antidepressant (Table 32.3).

INITIAL CLINICAL ASSESSMENT: ESTABLISHING DIAGNOSIS INITIATING ACUTE THERAPY

Assessment of the patient with depression must include a thorough medical as well as psychiatric evaluation. The presence and severity of functional impairment should be carefully evaluated, including interpersonal relationships and work. Patients should be encouraged not to make drastic or irreversible decisions while in a major depression and may require problem-solving assistance and support to adjust their responsibilities and schedules until improvement in functioning occurs. A medical evaluation will be useful to exclude underlying medical conditions that are associated with depressive symptoms and conditions that should be the focus of intervention. In one study, approximately one half of tertiary care patients were found to have previously undiagnosed general medical illnesses upon thorough medical assessment (Hall et al., 1981). Treating these illnesses significantly alleviated their depressive symptoms. Furthermore, occult general medical illness may diminish responsiveness to treatment (Akiskal, 1982). Drugs of abuse or even prescription medications may generate or exacerbate depressive symptoms. Clinicians need to inquire about their patients' use of recreational substances of abuse, noting

TABLE 32.3 *Clinical and Medical Guides to Treatment Choice*

Characteristic	*Comment*
Uncomplicated unipolar	All antidepressants have similar efficacy
	More severe depression or depression with agitation may respond better to SNRIs
	Choice based on side effects, tolerability, cost, convenience
Psychotic	Requires concurrent antipsychotic and antidepressant therapy or ECT
Melancholic/endogenous	Requires somatic treatment; poor response to placebo treatment
Atypical	Moderately increased responsiveness to MAOIs and perhaps SSRIs
Seasonal	Responsive to phototherapy
Anxiety	Increased risk of suicide; consider agents with high therapeutic index
Panic	Use agents known to be effective for panic (e.g., SSRIs, MAOIs, TCAs)
	Modestly reduced response rate
Bipolar	Observe for induction of "manic switch"; need to consider lithium, anticonvulsants, and atypical antipsychotics, especially for bipolar I disorder
Dysthymia	Responsive to treatment
Geriatric	Avoid agents with anticholinergic side effects if possible
	Start at low doses and increase dose gradually as needed
	Consider complicating medical illnesses (see text)

ECT: electroconvulsive therapy; MAOI: monoamine oxidase inhibitor; SNRI: selective serotonin and norepinephrine reuptake inhibitor; SSRI: selective serotonin reuptake inhibitors; TCA: tricyclic antidepressants.

Source: Bymaster et al. (2001).

that even modest use may diminish treatment responsiveness—as may be the case for alcohol. Few studies have adequately examined the impact of subsyndromal substance use on depression. During treatment, it is important to carefully monitor the patient's mental status for the presence of self-destructive thoughts or other dangerous impulses, and for the emergence of mania as well as drug-induced side effects characteristic of the prescribed agent. The risk of converting from a unipolar course to a bipolar course of illness should be considered. Overall, 5%–10% of patients initially characterized as unipolar will eventually develop mania, and subsyndromal levels of hypomania are common. In a young cohort of patients who were hospitalized and thus severely depressed (especially with psychotic features), almost one half will eventually experience a manic or hypomanic episode if followed longitudinally (Goldberg et al., 2001). A high suspicion of bipolar disorder (BPD) is also important in women presenting with postpartum depression. Education of the patient and family about depression and treatment options may alleviate guilt, hopelessness, and criticism by emphasizing that depression is a real illness with effective treatments. A family history of psychiatric illness and suicide should be acquired, and corroborative information from intimates is often helpful. The importance of adherence to treatment should be emphasized from the start of therapy, and frequent visits early on may combat demoralization and allow for dose adjustment for efficacy and side effects. Adjunctive psychotherapy may be helpful in ensuring compliance and may be more effective than medication alone; in one study, patients with chronic depression had a significantly better outcome with nefazadone plus cognitive-behavioral psychotherapy than with either treatment alone (Keller et al., 2000). If at least moderate improvement is not observed by 4 weeks of treatment, reassessment for adjustment of therapy should occur (patients with more chronic depression may respond more slowly to therapy). Maximizing therapy, switching therapy, and adjunctive therapy are options discussed below under "Treatment-Resistant Depression."

Clinical Factors Influencing Choice of Treatment

Despite decades of vigorous research, there remains a lack of consensus on useful predictors of response to specific treatments in depressed populations. Nevertheless, some clinical factors merit consideration.

Psychotic Depression

Psychotic depression has been thought to respond poorly to monotherapy with either antidepressants (particularly in the early TCA studies) or antipsychotics, with response rates ranging from 20%–40% (Chan et al., 1987). Additionally, mood-incongruent psychosis may confer a poorer prognosis than mood-congruent psychosis (Coryell et al., 1982). Italian investigators have argued that some SSRIs can be effective in monotherapy (Zanardi et al., 1996), an observation questioned by others. Electro-convulsive therapy (ECT) studies point to high response rates (Prudic et al., 2004), but to a relatively rapid and moderate loss of response (Prudic et al., 2004). Antidepressant-refractory patients with depression with psychotic features were found to respond readily when antipsychotic medication was added to the treatment regimen (Spiker et al., 1985). Typical antipsychotics as well as atypical agents such as olanzapine are effective in combination with antidepressants (Rothschild et al., 2004). Patients with "near"-psychotic symptoms (for example, highly overvalued ideas focusing on depressive themes) may also respond preferentially to combination treatment (Nelson et al., 1994).

Melancholic/Endogenous Severe Major Depression

Historically, patients with melancholic or endogenous depression have been thought to be particularly unresponsive to placebo treatment (Pesclow et al., 1992) and, hence, to have a significantly greater differential response (that is, response rate to medication compared to placebo) to medication treatment. Although some controversy exists as to whether SSRIs are as effective as TCAs in the treatment of melancholic depression, multiple studies have shown equivalent effectiveness in varied depressed populations, including severely depressed, inpatient, and melancholic samples. Furthermore, TCA-refractory melancholia may respond to subsequent SSRI treatment (e.g., Amsterdam et al., 1994). Nevertheless, in the subgroup of melancholic in-patients with depression, European studies suggested that one TCA, *clomipramine,* was more efficacious than were SSRIs and coupled with U.S. experience this has led some to argue SSRIs are less effective in this subgroup (Danish University Antidepressant Study Group, 1990; Roose et al., 1994). The significance of this subgroup remains unclear. Some evidence suggests that venlafaxine and escitalopram have differential efficacy in a severely ill population (Clerc et al., 1994; Montgomery et al., 2007). Further work is necessary to clarify the role of newer antidepressants in the treatment of melancholic or severe major depression.

Atypical Depression

Definitions of *atypical depression* (now predominantly characterized by mood reactivity, hypersomnia, hyperphagia, leaden paralysis, and rejection sensitivity) have evolved over the past four decades (West and Dally, 1959), although the correlation among the atypical symptoms is modest (Posternak and Zimmerman, 2002). Patients with atypical depression may respond better to MAOIs than to TCAs or placebo, as demonstrated in one series (e.g., Quitkin et al., 1991); however, the advantage may have modest clinical relevance (Joyce and Paykel, 1989). The SSRIs may be preferable first-line agents in these patients (Roose, 1994). Patients with atypical depression may be more likely to have a history of symptoms of hypomania than patients with a typical pattern of symptoms. In contrast with melancholic and psychotic depression, preliminary data have suggested that atypical depression may be associated with exaggerated negative feedback control of the hypothalamic-pituitary-adrenal (HPA) axis (Levitan et al., 2002).

Seasonal Depression

Seasonal or "winter" depression (SAD) is distinguished among depressive subpopulations by its differential response to treatment. Decreased levels of DA transporter in the striatum have been reported in SAD, and remitted patients relapse when challenged with the catecholamine depleter *α-methyl-para-tyrosine* (AMPT) (Lam et al., 2001). Genetic polymorphism variation in the 5-HT_{2A} receptor gene may be associated with SAD (Arias et al., 2001). Specifically, several studies support the rapid efficacy of phototherapy for this depressive subtype. Furthermore, hypersomnia and carbohydrate cravings may predict responsiveness to light therapy (Berman et al., 1997). Antidepressants can also be a very effective treatment.

Comorbid Anxiety Symptoms and Panic Disorder

Common neuropathological and neuroendocrine features may lead to anxiety and depressive disorders, and comorbidity is common. Nonspecific anxiety symptoms in depression do not suggest differential antidepressant efficacy or nonresponsiveness (Nelson et al., 1994). Meta-analysis suggests, however, that addition of a benzodiazepine may improve the outcome and decrease dropout rates in patients with depression with anxiety compared to administration of an antidepressant alone. The benefit of adjunctive benzodiazepine treatment must be balanced against the risks of dependence and accident proneness (Furukawa et al., 2001). Approximately one third of patients with depression may experience concurrent panic attacks (Clayton, 1990). Because comorbid panic attacks are associated with a worse acute and long-term prognosis (Coryell et al., 1988), such dually diagnosed patients should be prescribed agents with known antipanic efficacy—such as MAOIs, TCAs, SSRIs, or venlafaxine. In patients with comorbid anxiety disorder and major depression, the SSRIs and venlafaxine are generally considered first-line therapies. A history of panic attacks may predict a poor treatment outcome and a greater number of treatments and side effects in the acute treatment of BPD (Feske et al., 2000). In STAR*D, patients who were anxious and depressed who failed to respond in Phase I to citalopram did very poorly in subsequent phases (Fava et al., 2008). Optimal strategies for refractory depressives with anxiety are needed.

Bipolar Depression

Patients with bipolar depression may respond less consistently to standard antidepressants and commonly develop treatment-resistant depression. They also may have a higher rate of psychotic depression, and early-onset psychotic depression may be a form fruste of BPD. High depression scores during mania predict subsequent depression, and 16% of patients treated for a first episode of mania will cycle into depression over the following 2 years (Zarate et al., 2001). The efficacy of standard marketed antidepressants in BPD is, surprisingly, not well established (reviewed in Thase and Sachs, 2000). None of the available antidepressants have demonstrated efficacy in two well-powered and controlled trials, and the FDA has never approved an antidepressant specifically for depression BPD, although lamotrigine was recently approved for the long-term maintenance treatment of bipolar I to delay the onset of recurrent mood episodes, and olanzapine–fluoxetine combination (Tohen et al., 2003) is now approved for bipolar depression. Bipolar disorder is associated with autoimmune thyroiditis, and low or low-normal thyroid function may be a marker of a poor response to antidepressants in BPD (Cole et al., 2002). The appropriate duration of antidepressant therapy in bipolar depression has not been established. Especially for individuals with bipolar I, mood stabilizers are necessary to protect against dangerous manic switching, and addition of a second mood stabilizer is often as effective as addition of marketed antidepressants, though prone to induce intolerable side effects in some patients. Quetiapine (300–600 mg/day) has been reported to be significantly more effective than placebo in patients with bipolar I and II depression (Thase et al., 2006) and is now FDA approved for that use. Lithium has proven efficacy in bipolar depression and protective properties against suicide, and carbamazepine (and, by extension, possibly oxcarbazepine) has modest antidepressant properties. The SSRIs are considered first-rank antidepressants for episodes of bipolar depression and can be robustly effective in some patients with limited mania induction if patients are maintained on mood stabilizers (this may not always be necessary in patients with bipolar II). The SSRIs are generally favored in terms of efficacy over tricyclics (Bauer et al., 1999), which also have a high propensity to induce mania; however, a recent randomized study failed to find a difference between placebo and imipramine or paroxetine, except post hoc in the low lithium-level subgroup (Nemeroff et al., 2001). The SSRIs are generally safe in combination with lithium, but several cases of serotonin syndrome have been reported. Metabolic effects are of concern for atypical antipsychotics. Bupropion is favored by experts in BPD, and its noradrenergic properties may be helpful in treating the severe anergy, reversed vegetative symptoms, and psychomotor retardation often seen in bipolar depression. It also is not prone to cause the weight gain and sexual side effects that can be induced by concomitant medications and may have a lower rate of manic switch than TCAs (Sachs et al., 1994). Venlafaxine was associated with a much higher switch rate into hypomanic or mania than bupropion in a recent multicenter study (Leverich et al., 2006). Nefazadone and mirtazapine, by virtue of their sleep-enhancing properties, may also have a place in the treatment of bipolar depression.

Limited evidence suggests that some patients with bipolar (especially those with depressions characterized by anergia, psychomotor retardation, and hypersomnia) may be more responsive to MAOIs (in particular tranylcypromine) than TCAs (Himmelhoch et al., 1972; Thase et al., 1992) Response rates to MAOIs in bipolar depression are estimated overall to be 50%–60% (Malinger et al., 1999), and MAOIs may be an alternative to ECT for refractory patients. Lamotrigine is an antiglutamatergic agent that decreases presynatic release of excitatory neurotransmitters and is the most promising new treatment for BPD based on a large, uncontrolled database and published double-blind study (Calabrese et al., 1999). It has putative efficacy in bipolar depression and decreases the subsequent relapse rate in rapidly cycling bipolar patients. Several studies suggest that the anticonvulsant carbamazepine also has antidepressant properties (Post et al., 1997). Controlled trials do not support the efficacy of gabapentin, though its sleep-promoting and anxiolytic properties may be useful in selected individuals. Electroconvulsive therapy is highly effective in unipolar and bipolar depression and may be particularly effective in patients who are delusional. Patients characterized as bipolar may have more rapid improvement and require fewer treatments than patients characterized as unipolar (Daly et al., 2001).

Although almost all antidepressants have been associated with induction of a manic switch in patients who were bipolar depressed, evidence suggests that bupropion and the SSRIs may be less likely to cause this phenomenon than TCAs or MAOIs (Peet, 1994; Leverich et al., 2006). Antidepressant medication in the patient with bipolar may lead to cycle acceleration (Post and Weiss, 1995) or mania induction, but the risk of mania or hypomania induction in patients maintained on mood stabilizer therapy is probably less than 10% during the acute phase of treatment (Thase and Sachs, 2000). Given the severe morbidity of bipolar illness and the striking paucity of clinical trials, this subtype of affective illness should become a prime agenda for future research and drug development.

Geriatric Depression

Depression that recurs or first emerges late in life may be underappreciated and undertreated (Lebowitz et al., 1997). Relatively few controlled trials of antidepressants have been conducted in depressed populations older than age 65 years (Roose and Schatzberg, 2005). Available evidence suggests that TCAs and SSRIs are likely equivalent in efficacy (Schneider, 1996). However, there is a paucity of positive data on SSRIs or SNRIs being more effective than placebo. Large-scale trials have at times been needed to demonstrate statistical superiority over placebo (Tollefson et al., 1995). In one recent trial, venlafaxine, fluoxetine, and placebo all produced high response rates (Schatzberg and Roose, 2006).

Too few studies in the very old who are depressed (that is, older than age 85 years) have been conducted to draw conclusions concerning antidepressant efficacy. In one recent trial, Roose and colleagues (2004) failed to observe statistical superiority of citalopram over placebo.

Infirmity may reduce responsiveness in the elderly and make them more prone to side effects. The effects of TCAs on cardiac conduction, cognition, and blood pressure may limit their use in geriatric populations with cardiac disease, cognitive decline, and/or proneness to falling. Nevertheless, given that TCAs can be quite effective in the elderly (Roose, Glassman, et al., 1994), occasions may arise to prescribe such agents. Desipramine and nortriptyline may be the preferred tricyclic agents because they have fewer anticholinergic, sedative, and cardiovascular effects than the other agents. The clinician must be aware that SSRIs may alter metabolism of other drugs, such as β-adrenergic blockers, and displace highly protein-bound drugs, such as coumadin. Among the least protein-bound antidepressants, venlafaxine may be an advantageous choice for patients who are taking coumadin. Bupropion may also be efficacious in elderly patients (Branconnier et al., 1983). Additionally, stimulants may be effective in geriatric patients who are medically ill with depressive symptoms characterized by apathy (Satel and Nelson, 1989). Further considerations on how medical illnesses may influence treatment choice are reviewed below.

Dysthymia

Dysthymia is responsive to a variety of antidepressants, including TCAs, MAOIs, and SSRIs (e.g., Thase et al., 1996). The reversible inhibitor of MAO-A, moclobemide, at high doses has efficacy comparable to that of imipramine and is superior to placebo (Versiani et al., 1997). Interpretation of studies in this area is limited by the variability of diagnostic criteria and the use of heterogeneous patient populations (inclusion of patients with comorbid major depression). The relationship of dysthymia to major depression remains unclear; however, it is well established that patients who are dysthymic are at significantly greater risk for development of major depression. In elderly males, dysthymia may relate to a hypogonadal state with low testosterone levels (Seidman et al., 2002). Fluoxetine has been reported to be of limited efficacy in geriatric dysthymic patients (Devanand et al., 2005).

Biological Predictors of Response

Considerable research over the past three decades has focused on elucidating the pathophysiology of depression and the mechanism of antidepressant action. Despite clear-cut advances in this endeavor, efforts to identify biological predictors of response to antidepressants have been largely unsuccessful. Biological assays have had limited clinical utility in the pharmacotherapy of depression (Joyce and Paykel, 1989), although pharmacogenetics offer great promise.

Monoamine Markers

Many groups have examined the correlation of varied monoamine markers with antidepressant response. Several have reported that low urinary levels of 3-methoxy-4-hydroxyphenylglycol (MHPG), a noradrenaline metabolite, predict responsiveness to noradrenergic TCAs—imipramine, nortryptiline, maprotiline treatment; however, some findings contradict this. The significance of this association is questionable, as MHPG levels may not reliably predict the response to other antidepressant treatments. Consistency of results may be confounded by variance in circadian rhythm, diet, stress, psychomotor activity, and activation of neurotransmitter systems that indirectly influence catecholamine activity. In a unique invasive small-*n* study of NE and DA release via internal jugular sampling in refractory unipolar depression, deficits in brain NE and DA levels were observed compared to healthy controls (Lambert et al., 2000).

Although multiple clinical markers of serotonergic alteration exist in drug-free patients with depression, the ability to correlate treatment response to these biological markers reliably also does not exist.

Dexamethasone Suppression Test as a Marker

An abnormal response to the dexamethasone suppression test (DST) is found in less than one half of patients with depression and is most frequent in individuals who are psychotically depressed or very severely depressed (Nelson and Davis, 1997) and least frequent in outpatients who are mildly ill. Nonsuppression does not correlate with response to medication treatment; however, nonsuppression was associated with a much lower rate of response to placebo treatment. In a meta-analysis of 412 patients, DST nonsuppressers responded much more poorly to placebo treatment than did DST suppressers (that is, 14% vs. 36%, respectively) (Ribeiro et al., 1993). These findings underscore the increased relative benefit of antidepressant medication in DST nonsuppressers. Some studies suggest that pretreatment DST nonsuppression may be associated with a poor long-term outcome, specifically an increased risk of significant suicidal behaviors (e.g., Coryell, 1990). Nonsuppression appears to increase the risk of subsequent suicide tenfold (Coryell and Schlesser, 2001). Also, nonsupression after a course of treatment has been associated with higher rates of recurrence on longer term follow-up (Ribeiro et al., 1993). Despite early hopes, the DST has not proven clinically useful in predicting the differential response to treatment. However, an exaggerated cortisol response using the dexamethasone/corticotpropin-releasing hormone (CRH) test may be predictive of subsequent relapse in treatment responders (Zobel et al., 2001). One study found a reduced skin vasoconstrictor response to the corticosteroid *beclamethasone* in depression compared with controls, suggesting subsensitivity of skin glucocorticoid receptor (GR) signal transduction, that was not correlated with DST results (Cotter et al., 2002). Thus, pituitary-level GR function may not reflect other tissue-specific changes in depression.

Sleep Studies

Patients with depression commonly manifest sleep abnormalities, many of which have been assessed for the ability to predict responsiveness to treatment. These include decreased sleep continuity, decreased slow-wave sleep, and reduced rapid-eye-movement (REM) latency and may be more prominent in patients with recurrent and hence more virulent depressive illness (Jindal et al., 2002). Agents that block 5-HT_2 receptors, such as nefazadone and mirtazapine, may increase slow-wave sleep toward normal in depression (Sharpley et al., 1994). Reduced REM latency reliably correlates with a favorable response to acute treatment with TCAs and ECT (Joyce, 1992). Subsequently, reduced REM latency did not predict responsiveness to fluoxetine but did predict a poor response to placebo (Heiligenstein et al., 1994). Pretreatment-reduced REM latency may also be associated with higher rates of relapse (Giles et al., 1987). Overall, these findings underscore the value of medication treatment in patients with reduced REM latency but do not provide a rationale for predicting specific responses.

In sum, biological markers do not suggest specific antidepressant choice. However, abnormalities on the DST and shortened REM latency reliably indicate better response with antidepressant medications than placebo treatment. Furthermore, these markers may have relevance to long-term prognosis. Although these tests are not used in common practice, it remains to be tested whether they can be exploited to effectively guide long-term clinical management.

Pharmacogenetics

Pharmacogenetics offer an opportunity to develop customized therapies for patients with depression. Data indicate that Caucasian patients with the short/short (s/s) form of the serotonin transporter respond poorly to SSRIs (Smeraldi et al., 1998; Zanardi et al., 2000; Hu et al., 2007). In contrast, Asians with the s/s genotype respond better to SSRIs than do those with the long form (Kim et al., 2006). Others have reported that s/s patients actually experience greater dropout rates due to adverse events, and that may explain the poorer responses observed by others (Perlis et al., 2003; Murphy et al., 2004). In addition, genetic variants for the serotonin 2_A receptor have been reported to predict positive responses or side effects with SSRIs (Murphy et al., 2003; McMahon et al., 2006). A recent report (Perlis et al., 2007) suggests alleles for CREB protein may predict those male patients who experience suicidal ideation with SSRIs.

Medical Factors in Antidepressant Selection

Careful medical assessment remains crucial in guiding the safe selection of antidepressant treatment.

Cardiovascular disease

Depression is associated with reduced heart rate variability that may reflect abnormal autonomic nervous system modulation. Furthermore, clinical depression is a risk factor for coronary artery disease and diabetes and is associated with higher rates of mortality after a myocardial infarction (MI). Most SSRIs (for example, sertraline, paroxetine, and fluoxetine) and bupropion have minimal effects on heart rate, cardiac conduction, and blood pressure. Hence, they are good first choices for patients with cardiovascular disease. The SSRIs have been associated with a rare incidence of severe sinus node slowing (Glassman et al., 1993). Further experience with these drugs in cardiac patients is warranted before their safety is firmly established, but observational data suggest that SSRIs may have a protective effect against MI (Sauer et al., 2001).

Although TCAs have been safely employed in patients with cardiovascular disease, their effects on blood pressure and cardiac conduction should limit their common use as a first-line agent. The TCAs have conduction effects similar to those of class I anti-arrhythmic agents. In large-scale clinical trials, these latter agents have been associated with increased mortality when administered chronically to patients with ventricular arrhythmias following MI and with atrial fibrillation. Potentially, TCAs confer similar risks in this cardiac population (Glassman et al., 1993). More studies are required to assess the safety of antidepressant medications in patients with underlying conduction abnormalities and ischemic heart disease.

Caution regarding hypertension needed to be exercised particularly when administering high doses of immediate release (i.r.) venlafaxine. Approximately one in eight patients experienced blood pressure elevation when prescribed 300 mg or more daily of the i.r. compound. The extended release formulation appears to be less problematic in part because of the prolonged release as well as lower doses used. Duloxetine has not produced a significant increase in blood pressure. Conversely, trazodone and nefazodone have been associated with significant decreases in blood pressure.

Neurological diseases

Seizures due to antidepressants are generally dose-dependent and can occur in patients with a genetically or environmentally reduced seizure threshold. Medications to be potentially avoided in patients with a history of seizure disorder include maprotiline, clomipramine, and bupropion (in head injury patients in particular); phenelzine, tranylcypromine, fluoxetine, paroxetine, sertraline, venlafaxine, and trazadone have a relatively low risk of seizure (Rosenstein et al., 1993; Charney et al., 1998; Pisani et al., 2002). Poststroke depression occurs in about one third of patients and affects cognition and survival at 1 and 2 years. Recent review of the literature indicates that poststroke depression is not specific to patients with specific neuroanatomical lesions (that is, left frontal lesions). Fluoxetine has been found to effectively treat poststroke depression, and the SSRIs as a class may be safer and induce fewer side effects than older agents, although according to Robinson et al. (2001), nortriptyline may have superior efficacy than fluoxetine and may be a noradrenergic alternative to the SSRI class in this population (Gainotti and Marra, 2002). Head injury is associated with increased risk of major depression for decades afterward (Holsinger et al., 2002). Patients with Parkinson's disease have a high rate of depression as well as treatment-induced psychotic symptoms.

Other illnesses

The pharmacological effects of some antidepressants that lead to bothersome side effects may be exploited positively. For example, the antihistaminergic activity of mirtazapine and many TCAs may be useful for increasing weight gain in anorectic patients (for example, secondary to cancer or other systemic illnesses) or for patients with common allergies. Conversely, these agents may best be avoided in patients who are morbidly obese. For patients with premorbid sexual dysfunction, bupropion, nefazodone, and trazodone may be the most benign agents. Most others classes of drugs are associated with impotence or anorgasmia. Anticholinergic properties of the TCAs may complicate prostatic hypertrophy or narrow-angle glaucoma. Treatment of chronic active hepatitis and malignancies with interferon-a immunotherapy induces depression via putative activation of proinflammatory cytokine networks that may affect serotonin metabolism and can be effectively treated with SSRIs (Dieperink et al., 2000; Bonaccorso et al., 2002) or even prevented with them (Musselman et al., 2001). However, the SSRIs tend to treat the mood symptoms (such as suicidal ideation) but may be less effective against vegetative symptoms such as fatigue.

Targeting Response and Duration of Treatment

Little attention has been given to developing a clinically useful definition of an adequate treatment response. Definitions abound in the literature (Prien et al., 1991). Most studies have defined response as a 50% decrease in the HAM-D score or some other measure of the symptom state. Limits on maximum absolute scores may also be employed. Although the use of standardized scales is essential to the study of depression, the vast majority of clinicians have not found such instruments useful. Rating instruments, upon which most of what we know about depression is based, may not characterize key dimensions of patients' depression: overall severity, social/occupational adjustment, and quality of life. Social adjustment improves with greater responses or remission (Miller et al., 1998).

Furthermore, patients fulfilling categorical definitions of response may still have residual symptoms that are significant. For example, partial responders may have an increased risk for suicide, impaired occupational function, and markedly greater rates of relapse (Fawcett, 1994; Paykel et al., 1995). These phenomena underscore the fact that depression is a chronic illness, typified by periods of full and partial remission alternating with depressive episodes. Further work is needed to assess whether more aggressive antidepressant therapy is warranted in patients with minor residual symptoms.

Although depression is an enduring illness, little direct evidence is available to guide the clinician as to how long a patient should be medicated. Ten to 15 years after an index first depressive episode, approximately 80%–90% of patients can be expected to experience a recurrence (e.g., Kiloh et al., 1988; Lee and Murray, 1988). Studies of maintenance treatment have typically lasted up to 1 year, reliably suggesting that continued treatment reduces the risk of relapse. In one 3-year maintenance study, 20% of patients relapsed on full-dose imipramine, whereas 80% relapsed on placebo (Frank et al., 1990).

The most well established predictor of a recurrence or relapse of major depression is a history of multiple previous episodes (Lee and Murray, 1988; Winokur et al., 1993). Keller and colleagues (1982) found that patients with a history of three or more prior depressive episodes had approximately a 1.5-fold greater risk of relapse after 1 year than patients with two or fewer prior episodes.

Given these considerations, the duration of treatment is a clinical decision that should be based on individual patient factors: presence of continued depressive symptoms, number of previous episodes, potential impairment predicted from a recurrence, and medication tolerance (Charney et al., 1998).

Treatment-resistant depression

Historically, 40%–50% of patients with depression who are prescribed antidepressants do not experience a full response in a timely manner (Frank et al., 1993). Treatment resistance is defined by failure to respond for an adequate period (6–8 weeks) to a maximal dosage (or blood level) with an adequate decrease in depression ratings to one antidepressant or two antidepressants from different classes. Augmentation strategies may be preferable in patients labeled as partial responders to treatment. Management of this apparently treatment-refractory group must be methodical (Berman et al., 1997). Potential factors contributing to nonresponse must be considered: inadequacy of the trial, medication intolerance, noncompliance, underlying medical illness, and comorbid psychiatric conditions or substance use. Once true treatment resistance has been established, there are multiple treatment options that fall into four main categories: optimization/maximization, switching, combination, and augmentation (Table 32.4). Treatment with antidepressants that have a dual mechanism of action via inhibition of serotonin and NE uptake (SNRIs) may have an advantage in terms of improved rate of remission over SSRIs (Thase, Entsuah et al., 2001). Thus, venlafaxine and possibly duloxetine or milnacipran may be of value in treating patients nonresponsive to SSRI therapy. This may be due in part to increasing activity in the PKA-related second-messenger system pathway. As well, SSRIs decrease burst firing in the locus coeruleus and agents that block NE reuptake increase burst firing and may thus increase alertness and decrease depression through this mechanism (Szabo and Blier, 2001).

TABLE 32.4 *Management of Treatment-Resistant Depression*

	Efficacy[a]	*Replicability*[b]
Lithium augmentation	111	111
ECT (bilateral or high-intensity unilateral)	111	111
Interclass switching	11/111	111
Thyroid augmentation	11/111	11
Stimulant augmentation	1/11	11
SSRI/TCA combination	11	1
Buspirone augmentation	11	1
High-dose MAOI	11	1
Estrogen in postmenopausal women	11	1
Antiglucocorticoid therapy	1/11	1
Pindolol augmentation	1	1
Bupropion/SSRI combination	1/11	1
Intraclass switching	11	1
Transcranial magnetic stimulation	1	1
SSRI/mirtazapine combination	11	1
Pramipexole augmentation	1	1
Olanzapine augmentation of fluoxetine	11	11
Reboxetine augmentation of SSRI	1	1
SSRI/nefazodone combination	1	1
Adjunctive gabapentin	1	1
Adjunctive aripiprazole	11	11

ECT: electroconvulsive therapy; MAOI: monoamine oxidase inhibitor; SSRI: selective serotonin reuptake inhibitor; TCA: tricyclic antidepressant.

a. Efficacy was rated as modest (1), moderate (11), or very (111) effective.

b. Replicability was rated as follows: (1) open studies; (11) controlled studies and/or multiple open studies; (111) multiple controlled studies.

Source: Charney et al. (1998).

Optimization/maximization

When a patient does not respond fully to an initial dose of an antidepressant, the clinician may improve the response by 20%–30% simply by increasing the dose and/or duration of the trial. However, it is important to first consider whether the patient has fully complied with treatment because poor adherence to therapy may account for as many as 20% of treatment-resistant cases. Discrepancy exists in defining an optimal dose. For nortriptyline, desipramine, and imipramine, blood levels of these agents and metabolites may best guide the clinician. As tolerated, gradual dose escalation up to the highest recommended doses (for example, as indicated in the *Physicians Desk Reference* [PDR]) may ensure that therapeutic drug levels are attained. Conversely, there have been reports on the effective use of "megadoses" of TCAs (Garvey et al., 1991) and MAOIs (Amsterdam, 1991), doses higher than those maximally suggested by the *PDR*. The unclear medical risks of using such doses should limit their use to highly refractory patients. Although most trials are recommended to last at least up to 6 weeks—as supported by available research—a subset of patients may respond especially slowly (Georgotas and McCue, 1989; Thase and Rush, 1995); therefore, extending a trial beyond 6 weeks may be useful in some patients. It is recommended that this strategy be reserved for patients demonstrating at least a mild to moderate response to an ongoing treatment regimen by 5 or 6 weeks.

Switching

Monotherapy offers the advantages of improved compliance, lower cost, and fewer side effects. For these practical reasons, many clinicians choose to discontinue one medicine and initiate another when a patient fails to respond. Switching response rates generally range from 40%–60% over various classes of antidepressants.

Interclass switching. Interclass switching has been the logical first choice, as it represents a shifting of pharmacological strategies. Thus, although overall response rates with SSRIs and SNRIs are similar, different subgroups of patients may respond preferentially to one drug versus another. Although limited empirical work has assessed which class of antidepressant should best follow a failed trial, a pharmacological rationale could be made to use agents with significantly differing mechanisms of action (for example, move from SSRIs to agents with significant noradrenergic activity such as TCAs, venlafaxine, bupropion, MAOIs, or mirtazapine). Multiple studies suggest a range of response rates to interclass switching—with approximately one half of the patients adequately responding (Nelson, 1997b; Thase and Rush, 1995). Thus, approximately 50% of patients with chronic depression responded when switched from imipramine to sertraline or vice versa (Thase et al., 2002). STAR*D assessed switching from citalopram to one of three agents—venlafaxine, bupropion, or sertraline. The three yielded similar response rates (Rush et al., 2006).

Intraclass switching. Intraclass switching has been only modestly successful with the TCAs (Nelson, 1997b). Available studies on intraclass switching with the SSRIs are generally limited by the use of mixed patient populations consisting of patients who exhibited resistance and intolerance. Although preliminary open data suggest that response rates, for instance in switching from fluoxetine to citalopram or from sertraline to fluoxetine, may be substantial (Thase et al., 1997; Thase, Feighner, et al., 2001), the response rate of switching from citalopram to either venlafaxine or sertraline was not impressive (Rush et al., 2006).

Electroconvulsive therapy

For patients who are severely or psychotically depressed, and for patients with prominent suicidality or who are refusing food and hydration, a switch from pharmacological management to ECT should be considered. Approximately one half of TCA-resistant patients with depression may be expected to demonstrate a response (Prudic et al., 1990). Although the likelihood of response is diminished in patients who have failed multiple medication trials, are female, and have severe depression, an ECT trial merits strong consideration. High-dosage right unilateral and bilateral ECT appears to produce equivalent response rates and is twice as effective as low- or moderate-dose unilateral ECT (Sackeim et al., 2000). However, bilateral ECT results in greater cognitive impairment. Indeed, a recent community-based trial pointed to considerable memory effects (Sackeim et al., 2007). Without maintenance therapy, the majority of patients will relapse 6 months after an ECT response (Sackeim et al., 2001). At 2 years, one half of patients relapse after ECT plus maintenance antidepressant therapy, whereas over 90% are relapse free if they receive maintenance ECT treatment over the same period (Gagne et al., 2000).

Combination therapy

Combination strategies involve the use of multiple antidepressant medications from different classes. This approach represents a broadening of pharmacological targets, an approach that may be particularly attractive when a patient has already demonstrated a modest response and the clinician wants to minimize the risk of losing these gains. The large permutations of such possible combinations have prevented systematic study of many newer medication combinations. Favorable anecdotal reports need to be followed up with controlled trials. Combinations supported by a preclinical rationale should also be pursued. For example, the a_2-adrenergic antagonism of mirtazapine may potentiate SSRI-mediated serotonergic neurotransmission via blockade of heterologous autoreceptors.

Tricyclic antidepressant–monoamine oxidase inhibitor combinations. Initial successes with TCA-MAOI combinations in case series with over 200 patients suggest that over one half of TCA nonresponders may respond to the addition of MAOIs (Charney et al., 1998). The abundance of safer treatment options that do not risk hypertensive crises should make this strategy avoidable.

Tricyclic antidepressant–selective serotonin reuptake inhibitor combinations. TCA-SSRI combinations may be a useful strategy. A case series of 30 refractory patients, predominantly on TCAs, demonstrated an 87% response rate when fluoxetine was added (Weilburg et al., 1989). Such combinations have also been used successfully in geriatric populations (Seth et al., 1992). Furthermore, preliminary evidence suggests that a desipramine–fluoxetine combination may hasten the treatment response in newly treated patients (Nelson et al., 1991). Case reports suggest that reboxetine plus citalopram may also be effective in refractory depression (Dursun and Devarajan, 2001).

Bupropion–selective serotonin reuptake inhibitor combinations. Bupropion-SSRI combinations were described early on in approximately 50 refractory patients with depression in two case series (Boyer and Feighner, 1995; Bodkin et al., 1997). Twenty seven, or approximately one half, demonstrated improvement. Twelve patients discontinued therapy because of side effects. The recent STAR*D indicated approximately 30% of patients who had failed to respond to citalopram remitted when bupropion was added (Trivedi, Fava, et al., 2006).

Augmentation

Augmentation involves the addition of an agent that is not intrinsically a full antidepressant to an ongoing antidepressant treatment for the purposes of potentiating the activity of the antidepressant.

Lithium augmentation. Lithium augmentation is a strategy based on preclinical observations that lithium potentiates TCA-mediated serotonergic neurotransmission (De Montigny et al., 1981). Numerous case series and seven of nine placebo-controlled trials established the efficacy of lithium in the treatment of refractory depression (Charney et al., 1998), with response rates typically between 30% and 70%. This support made lithium augmentation the most proven treatment strategy in refractory depression. Although a fraction of patients will demonstrate dramatic responses within 1 week of adding lithium, more commonly the response is gradual, evident after 3 weeks. Unclear issues in the management of these patients include how long lithium should be continued. Lithium augmentation is probably effective in patients treated with SSRIs, but the data are not as compelling as those related to TCAs. Indeed in STAR*D, lithium augmentation resulted in remission in less than 20% of patients (Nierenberg et al., 2006).

Mirtazapine augmentation. Open and randomized pilot data suggest that mirtazapine augmentation of SSRIs and possibly other antidepressants may result in about a 60% response rate in refractory patients (Carpenter et al., 2002).

Atypical antipsychotic augmentation. Combining atypical antipsychotic medications with SSRIs may increase levels of DA and/or NE in the PFC, resulting in an improved antidepressant response. Apathy has also been observed as a side effect of SSRIs and may be reduced by addition of an atypical antipsychotic such as olanzapine. Blockade of 5-HT_{2A} and 5-HT_{2C} receptors may also decrease some SSRI-induced side effects, but blockade of 5-HT_{2C} receptors may also be responsible for some of the weight gain potential of this class of drug. Pilot test data suggested that addition of olanzapine to SSRIs was effective and rapidly acting (Shelton et al., 2001), particularly in more severely refractory patients. Olanzapine–fluoxetine combination has been demonstrated to be effective in refractory depressives (Thase et al., 2007). The atypical agent *quetiapine* has been shown to attenuate the stress-induced decrease in BDNF expression in the hippocampus (Xu et al., 2002), which could protect against stress-related neuroplastic changes in affective and anxiety disorders. Aripiprazole augmentation appears to convert SSRI nonresponders to responders and is now approved by the FDA. There are also positive data for risperidone augmentation.

Thyroid hormone augmentation. Initial open-label reports on the addition of thyroid hormone (specifically triiodothyronine) to antidepressant regimens suggested that it may hasten and potentiate the response. Systematic studies have yielded mixed results, both supporting (Goodwin et al., 1982; Joffe et al., 1993) and refuting (Gitlin et al., 1987; Thase et al., 1989) its efficacy. In one placebo-controlled study (Joffe et al., 1993), 59% (10/17) versus 19% (3/19) of triiodothyronine- and placebo-treated patients, respectively, demonstrated a response. In STAR*D, triiodothyronine appeared if anything more effective than lithium (Nierenberg et al., 2006). The safety and tolerability of thyroid augmentation make it an alternative to consider.

Stimulant augmentation. Addition of stimulants to an ongoing antidepressant regimen would expectably enhance monoamine neurotransmission. The use of stimulant augmentation in over 60 patients in combination with TCAs, MAOIs, and SSRIs has been described in published case series (Nelson, 1997b). Stimulant augmentation was moderately effective and not associated with tolerance problems. These agents have been found to be relatively safe, with a low incidence of dangerous cardiac side effects (Satel and Nelson, 1989). Abuse potential has limited the popularity of this combination. Furthermore, controlled studies have not been reported.

Serotonin-1A augmentation. Prevailing theories of antidepressant action suggest that efficacy derives from enhanced postsynaptic 5-HT_{1A}-mediated neurotransmission and that the delay in efficacy may be due to the timing of presynaptic 5-HT_{1A} receptor desensitization. Stimulation of $5HT_{1A}$ receptors increases levels of BDNF, which may be associated with antidepressant activity, and knocking out the gene for the 5-HT_{1A} receptor decreases the responses to antidepressants in animal models of depression such as the Forced Swim Test. Augmentation with buspirone, a partial agonist at this receptor, has been tested in an open-label manner in treatment-resistant depression (Nelson, 1997b). Up to two thirds of patients remitted. In STAR*D, buspirone was about as efficacious as bupropion as an augmentator (Trivedi, Fava, et al., 2006). Pindolol is a β-adrenergic antagonist and a 5-HT_{1A} antagonist putatively selective for presynaptic sites. In two open-label studies with a total of 25 medication-refractory patients with depression, pindolol augmentation (2.5 mg thrice daily) was associated with a complete remission in approximately two thirds of the sample, achieved within 1 week (Artigas et al., 1994; Blier and Bergeron, 1995). A subsequent controlled trial in 10 SSRI-refractory patients failed to demonstrate its efficacy over placebo augmentation (Moreno et al., 1997). Most investigators currently believe pindolol is a better facilitator of response—particularly in patients who are more mildly ill in primary care settings—than it is an augmentation.

Estrogen augmentation. Despite a half-century's investigation of the role of estrogen in the treatment of depression, a clear understanding has not emerged. Discovery of a second estrogen receptor with high concentrations in the CNS (the β-estrogen receptor) has led to speculation that with stimulation, complex interactions between the canonical α-estrogen receptor and the β-estrogen receptor may give rise to observed hormonal effects on cognition and mood. Evidence suggests that the recently discovered β-estrogen receptor may stimulate increased serotonin levels via transcriptional effects in the raphé nucleus, and estrogen may increase BDNF levels and inhibit MAO-A activity (Gibbs, 1999; Bethea et al., 2000; Gundlah et al., 2001, 2002). Mixed results were found in treatment trials using estrogen as monotherapy in pre- and postmenopausal women, and estrogen does not appear to be useful in preventing postpartum depression. Observations in the literature suggest that estrogen may be an effective augmenting agent (Shapira et al., 1985; Charney et al., 1998; Schneider et al., 1997). For example, postmenopausal women were more than twice as likely to respond to fluoxetine (that is, 40% vs. 17% response rates) if they were concurrently undergoing estrogen replacement therapy (Schneider et al., 1997). In a short 2-week controlled trial, estrogen augmentation of 11 patients who were imipramine resistant was associated with one case of clinical remission and another case of a manic switch. These observations suggest that longer controlled trials of estrogen augmentation in treatment-refractory postmenopausal women are warranted. Recent studies suggest that perimenopausal depression is effectively treated with transdermal estrogen (Schmidt et al., 2000; Soares et al., 2001). This treatment option should be explored only with gynecological consultation, as the effects of long-term estrogen replacement therapy have not been definitively determined. Novel tissue-specific and estrogen β-receptor-specific agents such as raloxifene may be tested in the future as augmentation agents for SSRIs because they affect serotonin neuron function in the raphé.

NEW DIRECTIONS

Over the past three decades, a proliferation of antidepressant drugs has made the pharmacotherapy of depression effective and well tolerated. Nevertheless, several important limitations remain.

1. Forty to 50% of patients with depression do not experience a timely remission upon initial medication treatment.
2. Although patients may respond to subsequent treatment options, there are no useful clinical or biological predictors of these subsequent treatments.
3. Furthermore, the antidepressant response typically lags weeks behind the institution of treatment.
4. Some patients cannot tolerate therapeutic doses of many medications, and many patients choose to discontinue effective regimens because of significant side effects.
5. Few studies are available to guide the clinician in the long-term pharmacotherapy of depression, the choice of pharmacological strategies in cases of treatment resistant depression, or the management of bipolar depressions.

Much remains to be understood about the mechanism of antidepressant action and the pathophysiology of depression. Effort focused beyond the monoamine systems may lead to new classes of agents that will effectively treat depression and, ideally, prevent its emergence.

Major depression may be associated with blunted cAMP signaling, and studies have demonstrated that antidepressant treatment results in increased activation of the cAMP second-messenger system. In turn, this increased activation would be expected to set in motion a cascade of intracellular events that would regulate specific target genes, genes that are known to include the transcription factor CREB and BDNF, along with its receptor, trkB. Staining of BDNF in postmortem samples is greater in the hippocampus of psychiatric patients treated with antidepressants compared with those not treated with antidepressants prior to death (Chen et al., 2001). Enhanced levels of BDNF may modify the function of neuronal elements crucial in mood regulation (Duman et al., 1997). Levels of BDNF may be increased by exercise, dietary restriction, estrogen, glutamate AMPA receptor agonists, and cAMP phosphodiesterase-4 inhibitors, as well as by antidepressants. Agents that increase cAMP levels (that is, rolipram and papaverine) have modest antidepressant efficacy when given alone or when added to an ongoing antidepressant regimen (Malison et al., 1997). Compelling preclinical evidence combined with somewhat favorable efficacy studies warrants the development of specific phosphodiesterase-4 inhibitors with potential antidepressant properties for augmentation therapy. Other pharmacological strategies could target other sites along this hypothesized intracellular cascade of events (for example, BDNF agonists and agents that stimulate transcription factors or directly stimulate cAMP or Ca^{21}-activated kinases).

Modulation of Neuropeptide and Glucocorticoid Receptors

The potential importance of neuropeptides and glucocorticoid signaling for the regulation of behavior and cognition is the result of many decades of research. However, only now are small molecules for neuropeptide receptors and safe antiglucocorticoids becoming available for clinical trials. Substance P, also known as neurokinin, was discovered in 1931. Initial evidence on the successful use of a substance P antagonist in the treatment of major depression (Kramer et al., 1998) was followed by five failed or negative trials (Keller et al., 2006).

Substance P antagonists, similar to imipramine, increased locus coeruleus firing rates, and knockout of the neurokinin-1 receptor for substance P produces adapative changes in 5-HT_{1A} receptors that mimicked antidepressant-induced desensitization (Froger et al., 2001; Maubach et al., 2002). Two trials with substance P antagonists have been positive, but negative trials have also been reported. Further side effects and other neuropeptide-related antidepressant strategies may be developed. Well-established abnormalities in the HPA axis in patients with depression may reflect underlying abnormalities in CRH function. Supporting evidence, summarized elsewhere (Musselman and Nemeroff, 1993), includes findings that CRH causes depressive-like symptoms in animals when injected intracerebroventricularly. As well, early-life administration of CRH reduces memory function, as well as progressive loss of hippocampal neurons and up-regulation of CRH production in the hippocampus (Brunson et al., 2001). Chronic antidepressant treatment appears to reduce stress-induced release and synthesis of CRH but not basal levels (Stout et al., 2002). Furthermore, patients with depression have been found to have elevated levels of CSF CRH. Compelling findings such as these have motivated the development of nonpeptide small-molecule CRH antagonists for testing as antidepressants and anxiolytics. Data indicate that the CRH system may be intricately involved in regulating serotonin output and raphé nucleus firing rate such that antagonists of CRH could have antidepressant effects by augmenting serotonin levels (Penalva et al., 2002). Zobel et al. (2000) and Kunzel et al. (2003) reported on use of CRH antagonist in an open-label inpatient trial although a recent negative placebo-controlled trial was published (Binneman et al., 2008). In a related strategy, the use of steroid synthesis inhibitors or steroid antagonists has been shown to have modest efficacy in lowering depressive symptoms (Murphy, 1997). Data with the antiglucocorticoid mifepristone (RU-486) indicate that it may be rapidly effective in treating psychotic symptoms in delusional forms of depression, which has the highest rate of HPA axis hyperactivity (Belanoff et al., 2001; DeBattista et al., 2006), although there are failed trials as well. Young et al. (2004) have reported positive benefit of mifepristone on cognition in bipolar depression. Agomelatine—a melatonin receptor, 1 and 2 agonist, and a $5HT_2$ antagonist—appears effective in major depression (Kennedy and Emsley, 2006). Last, there are efforts to develop compounds with novel effects—β_3 agonism, NK-2 antagonism, and so on.

Modulation of Excitatory Neurotransmitter Activity

Glutamate and aspartate signal through a variety of receptors. The NMDA receptor is a ligand-gated ion channel critically involved in excitatory neurotransmission. Aberrant NMDA activity may be of pathophysiological importance in neurodegenerative diseases and depression, where decreased neuronal size and loss of glial cells have been observed postmortem. Long-term exposure to antidepressants may alter NMDA receptor subunit expression and function. The efficacy of lamotrigine in bipolar depression and the known effects of many antidepressants on NMDA glutamate receptor binding have led to increased interest in the importance of the excitatory and inhibitory neurotransmitter balance in depression. Ketamine has been reported to have a rapid antidepressant effect in at least two studies (Berman et al., 2000; Zarate, Singh, Carlson, et al., 2006) although memantine had little antidepressant effect (Zarate, Singh, Quiroz, et al., 2006). This is also supported by some evidence of a decrease in CNS γ-aminobutyric acid (GABA)ergic activity in depression. Agents that inhibit glutamatergic activity may also be neuroprotective and affect neurotrophic activity. Preliminary evidence indicates that lamotrigine has substantial efficacy in bipolar depression but not in unipolar depression. However, this may be a function of the greater heterogeneity of unipolar disorder, and a subset of patients characterized as unipolar may be identified as responsive with future research. Other agents with antiglutamatergic mechanisms of action are under investigation. Drugs that affect the activity or membrane cycling of AMPA glutamate receptors may also be good candidates for antidepressant trials, and "AMPAkines" are in early testing in affective illness, as well as for cognitive enhancement in patients with mild cognitive impairment and against negative symptoms in schizophrenia. Tianeptine is a French antidepressant that, in contrast to SSRIs, may increase serotonin uptake. In preclinical studies, it has been found to be neuroprotective against stress-induced limbic damage to the hippocampus. It is just as effective as fluoxetine, imipramine, and paroxetine and has demonstrated efficacy compared to placebo (Waintraub et al., 2002). Its mechanism of action may be related to decreasing NMDA glutamate receptor signaling.

Dopamine agonists such as the D_3 agonist pramipexole have observed efficacy that, in one large trial, was equivalent to that of an SSRI, and pilot data suggest its efficacy in bipolar depression (Zarate et al., 2004) and in treatment-resistant depression. Pramipexole may also be protective against activation of apoptotic cell death pathways and may be neuroprotective. Agents with a similar profile may see further development for depression (Sporn et al., 2000). Alternative or complementary strategies have also been explored in pilot add-on studies using omega-3 fatty acids in treatment-resistant and breakthrough unipolar and BPD. Epidemiological data suggest that high consumption of fish oils is protective against depression and heart disease. In recurrent unipolar disorder, eicosapentaenoic acid was effective compared to placebo after 2 weeks, with improvement in core depressive symptoms (Nemets et al.,

2002). In a bipolar study, time to relapse was longer in the omega-3-treated group compared to the placebo group (Stoll et al., 1999). Other complementary agents such as chromium, trace minerals, and isoflavones may be tested in the future for their anxiolytic and antidepressant activity.

Until recently, there has been almost no capacity to exploit clinically our emerging understanding of the neuroanatomy of major depression. Developed over the past decade, the technique of transcranial magnetic stimulation (TMS) can now be used to affect brain circuitry directly. In this technique, a rapidly generated magnetic field is applied over specific scalp and brain regions. The magnetic field, if of sufficient strength, can alter neuronal firing patterns over a quarter-sized area of cortex. In controlled studies of patients who were treatment resistant, TMS, when applied over the left dorsolateral PFC, has been associated with significant reductions in depressive symptoms compared to sham TMS treatment (Pascual-Leone et al., 1996; George et al., 1997). This innovative modality represents a radical frameshift in the treatment of depression, based on directly altering underlying neurocircuitry, but it may only produce transient improvement and does not appear to approach the efficacy of ECT. Transcranial magnetic stimulation is only able to affect cortical tissue, whereas depression may involve deeper limbic structures not directly accessible via TMS. A recent controlled trial pointed to efficacy in mildly refractory patients (O'Reardon et al., 2007).

In sum, advances in neuroscience over the past three decades have led to the development of dozens of antidepressant agents, almost all of which target monoamine systems. A significant number of new and novel agents are in either early clinical development or are under study preclinically for depression. Our present understanding of the pathophysiology of depressive illness suggests many other biological treatment strategies. The next three decades promise radically novel approaches to the current treatment armamentarium. Targeting neuropeptide receptors may lead to effective antidepressants with fewer adverse effects. Targeting DA receptors, signal transduction pathways (for example with phoshodiesterase inhibitors), immunoreceptors, and glutamate and GABA receptors are also future strategies of interest. Neuroprotective strategies and approaches that improve neuroplasticity are also actively being pursued.

UPDATES

Paroxetine and Pregnancy

In 2005, the U.S. Food and Drug Administration (FDA) issued a public health advisory regarding the risks of paroxetine and pregnancy, based on preliminary analyses of two epidemiological studies (http://www.fda.gov/cder/drug/advisory/paroxetine). A U.S. epidemiologic study of major malformations following first trimester maternal exposure to antidepressants showed a trend towards a 1.5-fold increased risk for cardiovascular malformations for paroxetine specifically. There was also a statistically significant increased overall risk of major congenital malformations in infants exposed to paroxetine compared to other antidepressants. A second, independent retrospective epidemiological analysis utilizing the Swedish national registry database reported a twofold increased risk of cardiac defects in infants exposed to paroxetine, compared with the general population (Källén et al., 2007). These reports resulted in a change of paroxetine's classification from Pregnancy Category C to D.

Bipolar Depression

A large NIH-funded effectiveness study of bipolar depression found that adjunctive antidepressant medication did not show increased efficacy relative to mood stabilizer alone, but also was not associated with an increased risk of treatment-emergent affective switch (Sachs et al., 2007).

REFERENCES

Akiskal, H. (1982) Factors associated with incomplete recovery in primary depressive illness. *J. Clin. Psychiatry* 43:266–271.

Allgulander, C., Hackett, D., et al. (2001) Venlafaxine extended release (ER) in the treatment of generalised anxiety disorder: twenty-four-week placebo-controlled dose-ranging study. *Br. J. Psychiatry* 179:15–22.

Amsterdam, I. (1991) Use of high dose tranylcypromine in resistant depression. In: Amsterdam, J.E., ed. *Advances in Neuropsychiatry and Psychopharmacology*. New York: Raven Press, pp. 123–129.

Amsterdam, I., Maislin, G., and Potter, L. (1994) Fluoxetine efficacy in treatment resistant depression. *Prog. Neuropsychopharmacol. Biol. Psychiatry* 18:243–261.

Arias, B., Gutierrez, B., et al. (2001) Variability in the 5-HT(2A) receptor gene is associated with seasonal pattern in major depression. *Mol. Psychiatry* 6(2):239–242.

Arnold, L.M., Pritchett, Y.L., D'Souza, D.N., Kajdasz, D.K., Ivengar, S., and Wernicke, J.F. (2007) Duloxetine for the treatment of fibromyalgia in women: pooled results from two randomized, placebo-controlled clinical trials. *J. Women's Health (Larchmt)* 16(8):1145–1156.

Artigas, F., Perez, V., and Alvarez, E. (1994) Pindolol induces a rapid improvement of depressed patients treated with serotonin reuptake inhibitors. *Arch. Gen. Psychiatry* 51:248–251.

Bauer, M., Zaninelli, R., et al. (1999) Paroxetine and amitriptyline augmentation of lithium in the treatment of major depression: a double-blind study. *J. Clin. Psychopharmacol.* 19(2):164–171.

Belanoff, J.K., Flores, B.H., et al. (2001) Rapid reversal of psychotic depression using mifepristone. *J. Clin. Psychopharmacol.* 21(5): 516–521.

Berman, R.M., Cappiello, A., Anand, A., Oren, D.A., Heninger, G.R., Charney, D.S., and Krystal, J.H. (2000) Antidepressant effects of ketamine in depressed patients. *Biol. Psychiatry* 47(4):351–354.

Berman, R.M., Narasimhan, M., and Charney, D.S. (1997) Treatment-refractory depression: definitions and characteristics. *Depress. Anxiety* 5(4):154–164.

Bethea, C.L., Gundlah, C., et al. (2000) Ovarian steroid action in the serotonin neural system of macaques. *Novartis Found. Symp.* 230:112–130; discussion:130–133.

Binneman, B., Feltner, D., et al. (2008) A 6-week randomized, placebo-controlled trial of CP-316,311 (a selective CRH_1 antagonist) in the treatment of major depression. *Am. J. Psychiatry* 165(5):617–620.

Blardi, P., De Lalla, A., et al. (2002) Serotonin and fluoxetine levels in plasma and platelets after fluoxetine treatment in depressive patients. *J. Clin. Psychopharmacol.* 22(2):131–136.

Blier, P., and Bergeron, P. (1995) Effectiveness of pindolol with selected antidepressant drugs in the treatment of major depression. *J. Clin. Psychopharmacol.* 15:217–222.

Bodkin, I.A., Lasser, R.A., Wines, I.D., Gardner, D.M., and Baldessarini, R.I. (1997) Combining serotonin reuptake inhibitors and bupropion in partial responders to antidepressant monotherapy. *J. Clin. Psychiatry* 58:137–145.

Bonaccorso, S., Marino, V., et al. (2002) Increased depressive ratings in patients with hepatitis C receiving interferon-alpha-based immunotherapy are related to interferon-alpha-induced changes in the serotonergic system. *J. Clin. Psychopharmacol.* 22(1):86–90.

Boyer, W.F., and Feighner, I.P. (1995, May 27) *The combined use of fluoxetine and bupropion.* Presented at the annual meeting of the American Psychiatric Association, Miami, FL.

Branconnier, R.J., Cole, J.O., Ghazvinian, S., Spera, K.F., Oxenkrug, G.F., and Bass, I.L. (1983) Clinical pharmacology of bupropion and imipramine in elderly depressives. *J. Clin. Psychiatry* 44(5, Sec. 2):130–133.

Brunson, K.L., Eghbal-Ahmadi, M., et al. (2001) Long-term, progressive hippocampal cell loss and dysfunction induced by early-life administration of corticotropin-releasing hormone reproduce the effects of early-life stress. *Proc. Natl. Acad. Sci. USA* 98(15):8856–8861.

Bymaster, F.P., Dreshfield-Ahmad, L.J., Threlkeld, P.G., Shaw, J.L., Thompson, L., Nelson, D.L., Hemrick-Luecke, S.K., and Wong, D.T. (2001) Comparative affinity of duloxetine and venlafaxine for serotonin and norepinephrine transporters in vitro and in vivo, human serotonin receptor subtypes, and other neuronal receptors. *Neuropsychopharmacology* 25(6):871–880.

Calabrese, J.R., Bowden, C.L., et al. (1999) A double-blind placebo-controlled study of lamotrigine monotherapy in outpatients with bipolar I depression. Lamictal 602 Study Group. *J. Clin. Psychiatry* 60(2):79–88.

Carpenter, L.L., Yasmin, S., et al. (2002) A double-blind, placebo-controlled study of antidepressant augmentation with mirtazapine. *Biol. Psychiatry* 51(2):183–188.

Casper, R.C., Fleisher, B.E., Lee-Ancajas, J.C., Gilles, A., Gaylor, E., DeBattista, A., and Hoyme, H.E. (2003) Follow-up of children of depressed mothers exposed or not exposed to antidepressant drugs during pregnancy. *J. Pediatr.* 142(4):402–408.

Chan, C.H., Janicak, P.G., Davis, J.M., Altman, E., Andriukaitis, S., and Hedecker, D. (1987) Response of psychotic and nonpsychotic depressed patients to tricyclic antidepressants. *J. Clin. Psychiatry* 47:197–200.

Charney, D.S., Berman, R.M., and Miller, H.L. (1998). Treatment of depression. In: Schatzberg, A., and Nemeroff, A.C., eds. *The American Psychiatric Association Textbook of Psychiatry*, 2nd ed. Washington, DC: American Psychiatric Press, pp. 705–733.

Chen, B., Dowlatshahi, D., et al. (2001) Increased hippocampal BDNF immunoreactivity in subjects treated with antidepressant medication. *Biol. Psychiatry* 50(4):260–265.

Clayton, P.J. (1990) The comorbidity factor: establishing the primary diagnosis in patients with mixed symptoms of anxiety and depression. *J. Clin. Psychiatry* 51(11, Suppl):35–39.

Clerc, G., Ruimy, P., and Verdeau-Pailles, J. (1994) A double-blind comparison of venlafaxine and fluoxetine in patients hospitalized for major depression and melancholia. *Int. Clin. Psychopharmacol.* 9:139–143.

Cole, D.P., Thase, M.E., et al. (2002) Slower treatment response in bipolar depression predicted by lower pretreatment thyroid function. *Am. J. Psychiatry* 159(1):116–121.

Coryell, W. (1990) DST abnormality as a predictor of course in major depression. *J. Affect. Disord.* 19:163–169.

Coryell, W., Endicott, I., Andreasen, N., Keller, M., Clayton, P., Hirschfeld, R., Scheftner, W., and Winokur, G. (1988) Depression and panic attacks: the significance of overlap as reflected in follow-up and family study data. *Am. J. Psychiatry* 145:293–300.

Coryell, W., and Schlesser, M. (2001) The dexamethasone suppression test and suicide prediction. *Am. J. Psychiatry* 158(5):748–753.

Coryell, W., Tsuang, M., and McDaniel, J. (1982) Psychotic features in major depression: is mood congruence important? *J. Affect. Disord.* 4:227–236.

Cotter, P.A., Mulligan, O.F., et al. (2002) Vasoconstrictor response to topical beclomethasone in major depression. *Psychoneuroendocrinology* 27(4):475–487.

Crane, G.E. (1956) The psychiatric side-effects of iproniazid. *Am. J. Psychiatry* 112:494–501.

Daly, J.J., Prudic, J., et al. (2001) ECT in bipolar and unipolar depression: differences in speed of response. *Bipolar Disord.* 3(2): 95–104.

Danish University Antidepressant Study Group. (1990) Paroxetine: a selective serotonin reuptake inhibitor showing better tolerance, but weaker antidepressant effect than clomipramine in a controlled multicenter study. *J. Affect. Disord.* 18:289–299.

Davidson, R.T. (1992). Monoamine oxidase inhibitors. In: Paykel, E.S., ed. *Handbook of Affective Disorders*. New York: Churchill Livingstone, pp. 345–358.

De Montigny, C., Grunberg, F., Mayer, A., and Deschenes, J.P. (1981) Lithium induces rapid relief of depression in tricyclic antidepressant drug non-responders. *Br. J. Psychiatry* 138:252–256.

DeBattista, C., Belanoff, J., Glass, S., Khan, A., Horne, R.L., Blasey, C., Carpenter, L.L., and Alva, G. (2006) Mifepristone versus placebo in the treatment of psychosis in patients with psychotic major depression. *Biol. Psychiatry* 60(12):1343–1349.

DeBattista, C., Solvason, B., Poirier, J., Kendrick, E., and Loraas, E. (2005) A placebo-controlled, randomized, double-blind study of adjunctive bupropion sustained release in the treatment of SSRI-induced sexual dysfunction. *J. Clin. Psychiatry* 66(7):844–848.

Dessain, E.C., Schatzberg, A.F., Woods, B.T., and Cole, J.O. (1986) Maprotiline treatment in depression. A perspective on seizures. *Arch. Gen. Psychiatry* 43(1):86–90.

Devanand, D.P., Nobler, M.S., Cheng, J., Turret, N., Pelton, G.H., Roose, S.P., and Sackeim, H.A. (2005) Randomized, double-blind, placebo-controlled trial of fluoxetine treatment for elderly patients with dysthymic disorder. *Am. J. Geriatr. Psychiatry* 13(1):59–68.

Dieperink, E., Willenbring, M., et al. (2000) Neuropsychiatric symptoms associated with hepatitis C and interferon alpha: a review. *Am. J. Psychiatry* 157(6):867–876.

Dong, J., and Blier, P. (2001) Modification of norepinephrine and serotonin, but not dopamine, neuron firing by sustained bupropion treatment. *Psychopharmacology (Berl.)* 155(1):52–57.

Duman, R., Heninger, G., and Nestler, E. (1997) A molecular and cellular theory of depression. *Arch. Gen. Psychiatry* 54:597–606.

Dursun, S.M., and Devarajan, S. (2001) Reboxetine plus citalopram for refractory depression not responding to venlafaxine: possible mechanisms. *Psychopharmacology (Berl.)* 153(4):497–498.

Fava, M., Rush, A.J., Alpert, J.E., Alasubramani, G.K., Wisniewski, S.R., Carmin, C.N., Biggs, M.M., Zisook, S., Leuchter, A., Howland, R., Warden, D., and Trivedi, M.H. (2008) Difference in treatment outcome in outpatients with anxious versus nonanxious depression: a STAR*D report. *Am. J. Psychiatry* 165:342–351.

Fawcett, I. (1994) Antidepressants: partial response in chronic depression. *Br. J. Psychiatry* 165:37–41.

Feighner, A.D., Rickels, K., Rynn, M.A., Zimbroff, D.L., and Robinson, D.S. (2006) Selegiline transdermal system for the treatment of major depression disorder: an 8-week, double-blind, placebo-controlled, flexible-dose titration trial. *J. Clin. Psychiatry* 67(9):1354–1361.

Feighner, J. (1995) Cardiovascular safety in depressed patients: focus on venlafaxine. *J. Clin. Psychiatry* 56:574–579.

Ferguson, J.M., Mendels, J., et al. (2002) Effects of reboxetine on Hamilton Depression Rating Scale factors from randomized, placebo-controlled trials in major depression. *Int. Clin. Psychopharmacol.* 17(2):45–51.

Feske, U., Frank, E., et al. (2000) Anxiety as a correlate of response to the acute treatment of bipolar I disorder. *Am. J. Psychiatry* 157(6):956–962.

Frank, E., Karp, I., and Rush, A. (1993) Efficacy of treatments for major depression. *Psychopharmacol. Bull.* 29:457–475.

Frank, E., Kupfer, D., Perel, I., Comes, C., Jarret, D., Mallinger, A., Thase, M., McEachran, A., and Grochocinski, V. (1990) Three-year outcomes for maintenance therapies in recurrent depression. *Arch. Gen. Psychiatry* 47:1093–1099.

Frazer, A. (1997) Antidepressants. *J. Clin. Psychiatry* 58(Suppl. 6):9–25.

Froger, N., Gardier, A.M., et al. (2001) 5-Hydroxytryptamine (5-HT)1A autoreceptor adaptive changes in substance P (neurokinin 1) receptor knock-out mice mimic antidepressant-induced desensitization. *J. Neurosci.* 21(20):8188–8197.

Fukuchi, T., and Kanemoto, K. (2002) Differential effects of milnacipran and fluvoxamine, especially in patients with severe depression and agitated depression: a case-control study. *Int. Clin. Psychopharmacol.* 17(2):53–58.

Furukawa, T.A., Streiner, D.L., et al. (2001) Is antidepressant-benzodiazepine combination therapy clinically more useful? A meta-analytic study. *J. Affect. Disord.* 65(2):173–177.

Gagne, G.G., Jr., Furman, M.J., et al. (2000) Efficacy of continuation ECT and antidepressant drugs compared to long-term antidepressants alone in depressed patients. *Am. J. Psychiatry* 157(12): 1960–1965.

Gainotti, G., and Marra, C. (2002) Determinants and consequences of post-stroke depression. *Curr. Opin. Neurol.* 15(1):85–89.

Gardner, D.M., Shulman, K.I., et al. (1996) The making of a user friendly MAOI diet. *J. Clin. Psychiatry* 57(3):99–104.

Garvey, M., DeRubeis, R., Hollon, S., Evans, M., and Tuason, V. (1991) Response of depression to very high plasma levels of imipramine plus desipramine. *Biol. Psychiatry* 30:57–62.

George, M.S., Wassermann, E.M., Kimbrell, T.A., and Little, I.T. (1997) Mood improvement following daily left prefrontal repetitive transcranial magnetic stimulation in patients with depression—a placebo-controlled crossover trial. *Am. J. Psychiatry* 154: 1752–1756.

Georgotas, A., and McCue, A. (1989) Factors affecting the delay of antidepressant effect in responders to nortriptyline and phenelzine. *Psychiatry Res.* 28:1–9.

Gibbs, R.B. (1999) Treatment with estrogen and progesterone affects relative levels of brain-derived neurotrophic factor mRNA and protein in different regions of the adult rat brain. *Brain Res.* 844(1/2):20–27.

Giles, D.E., Jarrett, R.B., Roffwarg, H.P., and Rush, A.I. (1987) Reduced rapid eye movement latency. A predictor of recurrence in depression. *Neuropsychopharmacology* 1:33–39.

Gitlin, M.I., Weiner, H., Fairbanks, L., Hershman, I.M., and Friedfeld, N. (1987) Failure of T3 to potentiate tricyclic antidepressant response. *J. Affect. Disord.* 13:267–272.

Glassman, A.H., Roose, S.P., and Bigger, I.T., Jr. (1993) The safety of tricyclic antidepressants in cardiac patients: risk-benefit reconsidered. *JAMA* 269:2673–2675.

Goldberg, J.F., Harrow, M., et al. (2001) Risk for bipolar illness in patients initially hospitalized for unipolar depression. *Am. J. Psychiatry* 158(8):1265–1270.

Golden, R.N., DeVane, C.L., Laizure, S.C., Rudorfer, M.V., Sherer M.A., and Potter, W.Z. (1988) Bupropion in depression, II: the role of metabolites in clinical outcome. *Arch. Gen. Psychiatry* 45:145–149.

Goodwin, F.K., Prange, A.I., Jr., Post, R.M., Muscettola, G., and Lipton, M.A. (1982) Potentiation of antidepressant effects by 1-triiodothyronine in tricyclic nonresponders. *Am. J. Psychiatry* 139: 34–38.

Gundlah, C., Lu, N.Z., et al. (2001) Estrogen receptor beta (ERbeta) mRNA and protein in serotonin neurons of macaques. *Brain Res. Mol. Brain Res.* 91(1/2):14–22.

Gundlah, C., Lu, N.Z., et al. (2002) Ovarian steroid regulation of monoamine oxidase-A and B mRNAs in the macaque dorsal raphe and hypothalamic nuclei. *Psychopharmacology (Berl.)* 160(3): 271–282.

Hall, C., Gardner, E., Popkin, M., Lecann, A., and Stickney, S. (1981) Unrecognized physical illness prompting psychiatric admission: a prospective study. *Am. J. Psychiatry* 138:629–635.

Heiligenstein, I., Raries, D., Rush, I., Andersen, I., Pande, A., Roff-Warg, H., Dunner, D., Gillin, I., James, S., Lahmeyer, H., Zajecka, I., Tollefson, G., and Gardner, D. (1994) Latency to rapid eye movement sleep as a predictor of treatment response to fluoxetine and placebo in nonpsychotic depressed outpatients. *Psychiatry Res.* 52:327–339.

Herman, B.D., Fleishaker, J.C., et al. (1999) Ketoconazole inhibits the clearance of the enantiomers of the antidepressant reboxetine in humans. *Clin. Pharmacol. Ther.* 66(4):374–379.

Himmelhoch, J.M., Detre, T., Kupfer, D.J., Swartzburg, M., and Byck, R. (1972) Treatment of previously intractable depressions with tranylcypromine and lithium. *J. Nerv. Ment. Dis.* 155:216–220.

Holliday, S.M., and Benfield, P. (1995) Venlafaxine. A review of its pharmacology and therapeutic potential in depression. *Drugs* 49(2): 280–294.

Holsinger, T., Steffens, D.C., et al. (2002) Head injury in early adulthood and the lifetime risk of depression. *Arch. Gen. Psychiatry* 59(1):17–22.

Hu, X.Z., Rush, A.J., Charney, D., Wilson, A.F., Sorant, A.J., Papanicolaou, G.J., Fava, M., Trivedi, M.H., Wisniewski, S.R., Laje, G., Paddock, S., McMahon, F.J., Manji, H., and Lipsky, R.H. (2007) Association between a functional serotonin transporter promoter polymorphism and citalopram treatment in adult outpatients with major depression. *Arch. Gen. Psychiatry* 65(7):783–792.

Jindal, R.D., Thase, M.E., et al. (2002) Electroencephalographic sleep profiles in single-episode and recurrent unipolar forms of major depression: II. comparison during remission. *Biol. Psychiatry* 51(3): 230–236.

Joffe, R.T., Singer, W., Levitt, A.J., and MacDonald, C. (1993) A placebo-controlled comparison of lithium and triiodothyronine augmentation of tricyclic antidepressants in unipolar refractory depression. *Arch. Gen. Psychiatry* 50:387–393.

Johnston, J.A., Lineberry, C.G., Ascher, I.A., Davidson, I., Khayrallah, M.A., Feighner, I.P., and Stark, P. (1991) A 102-center prospective study of seizure in association with bupropion. *J. Clin. Psychiatry* 52:450–456.

Joyce, P.R. (1992). Prediction of treatment response. In: Paykel, E. S., ed. *Handbook of Affective Disorders*. New York: Churchill Livingston, pp. 453–462.

Joyce, P.R., and Paykel, E.S. (1989) Predictors of drug response in depression (review). *Arch. Gen. Psychiatry* 46:89–99.

Källén, B.A., Otterblad Olausson, P. (2007) Maternal use of selective serotonin re-uptake inhibitors in early pregnancy and infant congenital malformations. *Birth Defects Res. A. Clin. Mol. Teratol.* 79(4):301–308.

Kasper, S., el Giamal, N., et al. (2000) Reboxetine: the first selective noradrenaline re-uptake inhibitor. *Expert Opin. Pharmacother.* 1(4):771–782.

Keller, M., Montgomery, S., Ball, W., Morrison, M., Snavely, D., Liu, G., Hargreaves, R., Hietala, J., Lines, C., Beebe, K., and Reines, S. (2006) Lack of efficacy of the substance ρ (neirokinin1 receptor) antagonist aprepitant in the treatment of major depressive disorder. *Biol. Psychiatry* 59(3):216–223.

Keller, M.B., McCullough, J.P., et al. (2000) A comparison of nefazodone, the cognitive behavioral-analysis system of psychotherapy, and their combination for the treatment of chronic depression. *N. Engl. J. Med.* 342(20):1462–1470.

Keller, M.B., Shapiro, R.W., Lavori, P.W., and Wolfe, N. (1982) Recovery in major depressive disorder: analysis with the life table and regression models. *Arch. Gen. Psychiatry* 39:905–910.

Kennedy, S.H., and Emsley, R. (2006) Placebo-controlled trial of agomelatine in the treatment of major depressive disorder. *Eur. Neuropsychopharmacol.* 16(2):93–100.

Kiloh, L., Andrews, G., and Neilson, M. (1988) The long-term outcome of depressive illness. *Br. J. Psychiatry* 153:752–757.

Kim, H., Lim, S.W., Kim, S., Kim, J.W., Chang, Y.H., Carroll, B.J., and Kim, D.K. (2006) Monoamine transporter gene polymorphisms and antidepressant response in Koreans with late-life depression. *JAMA* 296(13):1609–1618.

Kline, N.S. (1970). Monoamine oxidase inhibitors: an unfinished picaresque tale. In: Ayd, F.J., and Blackwell, B., eds. *Discoveries in Biological Psychiatry*. Philadelphia: J.B. Lippincott, pp. 194–204.

Kramer, M.S., Cutler, N., Feighner, J., Shrivastava, R., Carman, J., Sramek, J.J., Reines, S.A., Liu, G., Snavely, D., Wyatt-Knowles, E., Hale, J.J., Mills, S.G., MacCoss, M., Swain, C.J., Harrison, T., Hill, R.G., Hefti, F., Scolnick, E.M., Casciéri, M.A., Chichi, C.G., Sadowski, S., Williams, A.R., Hewson, L., Smith, D., Carlson, E.J. Hargreaves, R.J., and Rupniak, N.M.J. (1998) Distinct mechanism for antidepressant activity by blockade of central substance p receptors. *Science* 281:1640–1645.

Kroemer, H.K., and Eichelbaum, M. (1995) "It's the genes, stupid": molecular basis and clinical consequences of genetic cytochrome P450 2D6 polymorphism. *Life Sci.* 56:2285–2298.

Kuhn, R. (1958) The treatment of depressive states with G22355 (imipramine) hydrochloride. *Am. J. Psychiatry* 115:459–464.

Künzel, H.E., Zobel, A.W., Nickel, T., Ackl, N., Uhr, M., Sonntag, A., Ising, M., and Holsboer, F. (2003) Treatment of depression with the CRH-1-receptor antagonist R121919: endocrine changes and side effects. *J. Psychiatry Res.* 37(6):525–533.

Lam, R.W., Tam, E.M., et al. (2001) Effects of alpha-methyl-para-tyrosine-induced catecholamine depletion in patients with seasonal affective disorder in summer remission. *Neuropsychopharmacology* 25(5 Suppl):S97–S101.

Lambert, G., Johansson, M., et al. (2000) Reduced brain norepinephrine and dopamine release in treatment-refractory depressive illness: evidence in support of the catecholamine hypothesis of mood disorders. *Arch. Gen. Psychiatry* 57(8):787–793.

Lane, R., and Baldwin, D. (1997) Serotonin syndrome and drug combinations: selective serotonin reuptake. *Eur. Arch. Psychiatry Clin. Neurosci.* 247:113–119.

Lebowitz, B.D., Pearson, I.L., Schneider, L.S., Reynolds, C.F. III, Alexopoulos, G.S., Bruce, M.L., Conwell, Y., Katz, I.R., Meyers, B.S., Morrison, M.F., Mossey, I., Niederehe, G., and Parmelee, P. (1997) Diagnosis and treatment of depression in late life. Consensus statement update. *JAMA* 278:1186–1190.

Lee, A., and Murray, R. (1988) The long-term outcome of Maudsley Depressives. *Br. J. Psychiatry* 153:741–753.

Leverich, G.S., Atshuler, L.L., Frye, M.A., Suppes, T., McElroy, S.L., Keck, P.E., Jr., Kupka, R.W., Denicoff, K.D., Nolen, W.A., Grunze, H., Marinez, M.I, and Post, R.M. (2006) Risk of switch in mood polarity to hypomania or mania in patients with bipolar depression during acute and continuation trials of venlafaxine, sertraline, and bupropion as adjuncts to mood stabilizers. *Am. J. Psychiatry* 163(2):232–239.

Levitan, R.D., Vaccarino, F.J., et al. (2002) Low-dose dexamethasone challenge in women with atypical major depression: pilot study. *J. Psychiatry Neurosci.* 27(1):47–51.

Linner, L., Endersz, H., et al. (2001) Reboxetine modulates the firing pattern of dopamine cells in the ventral tegmental area and selectively increases dopamine availability in the prefrontal cortex. *J. Pharmacol. Exp. Ther.* 297(2):540–546.

Lippman, S., Bedford, P., Manshadi, M., and Mather, S. (1983) Trazodone cardiotoxicity. *Am. J. Psychiatry* 140:1383.

Malinger, A.G., Frank, E., et al. (1999). *Effectiveness of Traditional Antidepressants Is Suboptimal in the Depressed Phase of Bipolar Disorder*. Boca Raton, FL: New Clinical Drug Evaluation Unit Program.

Malison, R., Price, L., Nestler, E., Heninger, G., and Duman, R. (1997) Efficacy of papaverine addition for treatment-refractory major depression. *Am. J. Psychiatry* 154:579–580.

Mann, J.J., Aarons, S.F., Wilner, P.J., Keilp, J.G., Sweeney, J.A., Pearlstein, T., Frances, A.J., Kocsis, J.H., and Brown, R.P. (1989) A controlled study of the antidepressant efficacy and side-effects of (2)-deprenyl: a selective monoamine oxidase inhibitor. *Arch. Gen. Psychiatry* 46:45–50.

Maubach, K.A., Martin, K., et al. (2002) Chronic substance P (NK1) receptor antagonist and conventional antidepressant treatment increases burst firing of monoamine neurones in the locus coeruleus. *Neuroscience* 109(3):609–617.

McMahon, F.J., Buervenich, S., Charney, D., Lipsky, R., Rush, A.J., Wilson, A.F., Sorant, A.J., Papanicolaou, G.J., Laje, G., Fava, M., Trivedi, M.H., Wisniewski, S.R., and Manji, H. (2006) Variation in the gene encoding the serotonin 2A receptor is associated with outcome of antidepressant treatment. *Am. J. Hum. Genet.* 78(3):804–814.

Meyer, J.H., Ginovart, N., Boovariwala, A., Sagrati, S., Hussey, D., Garcia, A., Young, T., Praschak-Rieder, N., Wilson, A.A., and Houle, S. (2006) Elevated monoamine oxidase a levels in the brain: an explanation for the monoamine imbalance of major depression. *Arch. Gen. Psychiatry* 63(11):1209–1213.

Meyer, J.H., Wilson, A.A., et al. (2001) Occupancy of serotonin transporters by paroxetine and citalopram during treatment of depression: a [(11)C]DASB PET imaging study. *Am. J. Psychiatry* 158(11):1843–1849.

Miller, I.W., Keitner, G.I., Schatzberg, A.F., Klein, D.N., Thase, M.E., Rush, A.J., Markowitz, J.C., Schlager, D.S., Kornstein, S.G., Davis, S.M., Harrison, W.M., and Keller, M.B. (1998) The treatment of chronic depression, part 3: psychosocial functioning before and after treatment with sertraline or imipramine. *J. Clin. Psychiatry* 59(11):608–619.

Montgomery, S.A., Baldwin, D.S., Blier, P., Fineberg, N.A., Kasper, S., Lader, M., Lam, R.W., Lépine, J.P., Möller, H.J., Nutt, D.J., Rouillon, F., Schatzberg, A.F., and Thase, M.E. (2007) Which antidepressants have demonstrated superior efficacy? A review of the evidence. *Int. Clin. Psychopharmacol.* 22(6):323–329.

Moreno, F.A., Gelenberg, A.J., Bachar, K., and Delgado, P.L. (1997) Pindolol augmentation of treatment-resistant depressed patients. *J. Clin. Psychiatry* 58:437–439.

Murphy, B. (1997) Antiglucocorticoid therapies in major depression—a review. *Psychoneuroendocrinology* 22(Suppl 1):125–132.

Murphy, G.M., Jr., Hollander, S.B., Rodrigues, H.E., Kremer, C, and Schatzberg, A.F. (2004) Effects of the serotonin transporter gene promoter polymorphism on mirtazapine and paroxetine efficacy and adverse events in geriatric major depression. *Arch. Gen. Psychiatry* 61(11):1163–1169.

Murphy, G.M., Jr., Kemer, C., Rodrigues, H.E., and Schatzberg, A.F. (2003) Pharmacogenetics of antidepressant medication intolerance. *Am. J. Psychiatry* 160(10):1830-1835.

Musselman, D., and Nemeroff, C. (1993) The role of corticotropin-releasing factor in the pathophysiology of psychiatric disorders. *Psychiatr. Ann.* 23:676–681.

Musselman, D.L., Lawson, D.H., Gumnick, J.F., Manatunga, A.K., Penna, S., Goodkin, R.S., Greiner, K., Nemeroff, C.B., and Miller,

A.H. (2001) Paroxetine for the prevention of depression induced by high-dose interferon alfa. *N. Engl. J. Med.* 344(13):961–966.

Nelson, J.C. (1997a) Safety and tolerability of the new antidepressants (review). *J. Clin. Psychiatry* 6:26–31.

Nelson, J.C. (1997b) Treatment of refractory depression. *Depress. Anxiety* 5(4):165–174.

Nelson, J.C., and Davis, J.M. (1997) DST studies in psychotic depression: a meta-analysis. *Am. J. Psychiatry* 154(11):1497–1503.

Nelson, J.C., Mazure, C.M., Bowers, M.B., Jr., and Jatlow, P.I. (1991) A preliminary, open study of the combination of fluoxetine and desipramine for rapid treatment of major depression. *Arch. Gen. Psychiatry* 48:303–307.

Nelson, J.C., Mazure, C.M., and Jatlow, P.I. (1994) Characteristics of desipramine refractory depression. *J. Clin. Psychiatry* 55:12–19.

Nemeroff, C.B., DeVane, C.L., Pollock, B.G., Hilton, S.E., Maradit, H., and Moller, H.I. (1996) Newer antidepressants and the cytochrome P450 system (see comments). *Am. J. Psychiatry* 153: 311–320.

Nemeroff, C.B., Evans, D.L., Gyulai, L., Sachs, G.S., Bowden, C.L., Gergel, I.P., Oakes, R., and Pitts, C.D. (2001). Double-blind, placebo-controlled comparison of imipramine and paroxetine in the treatment of bipolar depression. *Am. J. Psychiatry* 158(6): 906–912.

Nemets, B., Stahl, Z., et al. (2002) Addition of omega-3 fatty acid to maintenance medication treatment for recurrent unipolar depressive disorder. *Am. J. Psychiatry* 159(3):477–479.

Nierenberg, A.A., Fava, M., Trivedi, M.H., Wisniewski, S.R., Thase, M.E., McGrath, P.J., Alpert, J.E., Warden, D., Luther, J.F., Niederehe, G., Lebowitz, B., Shores-Wilson, K., and Rush, A.J. (2006) A comparison of lithium and T(3) augmentation following two failed medication treatments for depression: a STAR*D report. *Am. J. Psychiatry* 163(9):1519–1530.

Nurnberg, H.G., Gelenberg, A., et al. (2001) Efficacy of sildenafil citrate for the treatment of erectile dysfunction in men taking serotonin reuptake inhibitors. *Am. J. Psychiatry* 158(11):1926–1928.

O'Reardon, J.P., Solvason, H.B., Janicak, P.G., Sampson, S., Isenberg, K.E., Nahas, Z., McDonald, W.M., Avery, D., Fitzgerald, P.B., Loo, C., Demitrack, M.A., George, M.S., and Sackeim, H.A. (2007) Efficacy and safety of transcranial magnetic stimulation in the acute treatment of major depression: a multisite randomized controlled trial. *Biol. Psychiatry* 62(11):1208–1216.

Pascual-Leone, A., Rubio, B., Pallardo, F., Catala, M.D., George, M.S., Wassermann, E.M., Williams, W.A., Callahan, A., Ketter, T.A., and Basser, P. (1996) Rapid-rate transcranial magnetic stimulation of left dorsolateral prefrontal cortex in drug-resistant depression (see comments). *Lancet* 348:233–237.

Paykel, E., Ramana, R., Cooper, Z., Hayhurst, H., Kerr, I., and Barocka, A. (1995) Residual symptoms after partial remission: an important outcome in depression. *Psychol. Med.* 25:1171–1180.

Peet, M. (1994) Induction of mania with selective serotonin reuptake inhibitors. *Int. Clin. Psychopharmacol.* 1:49–53.

Penalva, R.G., Flachskamm, C., et al. (2002) Corticotropin-releasing hormone receptor type 1-deficiency enhances hippocampal serotonergic neurotransmission: an in vivo microdialysis study in mutant mice. *Neuroscience* 109(2):253–266.

Perlis, R.H., Purcell, S., Fava, M., Fagerness, J., Rush, A.J., Trivedi, M.H., and Smoller, J.W. (2007) Association between treatment-emergent suicidal ideation with citalopram and polymorphisms near cyclic adenosine monophosphate response element binding protein in the STAR*D study. *Arch. Gen. Psychiatry* 64(6):689–697.

Perlis, R.H., Mischoulon, D., Smoller, J.W., Wan, Y.J., Lamon-Fava, S., Lin, K.M., Rosenbaum, J.F., and Fava, M. (2003) Serotonin transporter polymorphisms and adverse effects with fluoxetine treatment. *Biol. Psychiatry* 54(9):879-883.

Peselow, E., Sanfilipo, M., Difiglia, C., and Fieve, R. (1992) Melancholic/endogenous depression and response to somatic treatment and placebo. *Am. J. Psychiatry* 149:1324–1334.

Pisani, F., Oteri, G., et al. (2002) Effects of psychotropic drugs on seizure threshold. *Drug Saf.* 25(2):91–110.

Post, R., and Weiss, S. (1995). The neurobiology of treatment-resistant mood disorders. In: Bloom, F.E., and Kupfer, D.J., eds. *Psychopharmacology: The Fourth Generation of Progress*. New York: Raven Press, pp. 1155–1170.

Post, R.M., Leverich, G.S., Denicoff, K.D., Frye, M.A., Kimbrell, T.A., and Dunn, R. (1997) Alternative approaches to refractory depression in bipolar illness. *Depress. Anxiety* 5(4):175–189.

Posternak, M.A., and Zimmerman, M. (2002) Partial validation of the atypical features subtype of major depressive disorder. *Arch. Gen. Psychiatry* 59(1):70–76.

Preskorn, S.H. (1997) Selection of an antidepressant: mirtazapine (review). *J. Clin. Psychiatry* 6(17):3–8.

Prien, R., Carpenter, L., and Kupfer, D. (1991) The definition and operational criteria for treatment outcome of major depressive disorder: a review of the current research literature. *Arch. Gen. Psychiatry* 48:796–800.

Prudic, I., Sackeim, H.A., and Devanand, D.P. (1990) Medication resistance and clinical response to electroconvulsive therapy. *Psychiatry Res.* 31:287–296.

Prudic, J., Olfson, M., Marcus, S.C., Fuller, R.B., and Sackeim, H.A. (2004) Effectiveness of electroconvulsive therapy in community settings. *Biol. Psychiatry* 55(3):301–312.

Quitkin, F.M., Harrison, W., Stewart, J.W., McGrath, P.J., Tricamo, E., Ocepek-Welikson, K., Rabkin, J.G., Wager, S.G., Nunes, E., and Klein, D.F. (1991) Response to pheneizine and imipramine in placebo nonresponders with atypical depression. *Arch. Gen. Psychiatry* 48:319–323.

Ribeiro, S., Tandon, R., Grunhaus, L., and Greden, I. (1993) The DST as a predictor of outcome in depression: a meta-analysis. *Am. J. Psychiatry* 150:1618–1629.

Richelson, E. (1991) Biological basis of depression and therapeutic relevance *J. Clin. Psychiatry* 52(6, Suppl):4–10.

Robinson, R.G., Schultz, S.K., Castillo, C., Koppel, T., Kosier, J.T., Newman, R.M., Curdue, K., Petracca, G., and Starkstein, S.E. (2001) Nortriptyline versus fluoxetine in the treatment of depression and in short-term recovery after stroke: a placebo-controlled, double-blind study. *Am J. Psychiatry* 158(4):351-359.

Roose, S. (1994). Selective serotonin reuptake inhibitors in refractory depression. In: Nolen, W.A., Zohar, J., Roose, S.I., and Amsterdam, J.D., eds. *Refractory Depression: Current Strategies and Future Directions*. New York: Wiley, pp. 37–46.

Roose, S., Glassman, A., Attia, E., and Woodring, S. (1994) Comparative efficacy of selective serotonin reuptake inhibitors and tricyclics in the treatment of melancholia. *Am. J. Psychiatry* 151: 1735–1739.

Roose, S.P., Sackeim, H.A., Krishnan, K.R., Pollock, B.G., Alexopoulos, G., Lavretsky, H., Katz, I.R., Hakkarainen, H., Old-Old Depression Study Group. (2004) Antidepressant pharmacotherapy in the treatment of depression in the very old: a randomized, placebo-controlled trial. *Am. J. Psychiatry* 161(11):2050–2059.

Roose, S.P., and Schatzberg, A.F. (2005) The efficacy of antidepressants in the treatment of late-life depression. *J. Clin. Psychopharmacol.* 25(4 Suppl 1):S1–S7.

Rosenstein, D., Nelson, I., and Jacobs, S. (1993) Seizures associated with antidepressants: a review. *J. Clin. Psychiatry* 54:289–299.

Rothschild, A.J., Williamson, D.J., Tohen, M.F., Schatzberg, A.F., Anderson, S.W., Van Campen, L.E., Sanger, T.M., and Tollefson, G.D. (2004) A double-blind, randomized study of olanzapine and olanzapine/fluoxetine combination for major depression with psychotic features. *J. Clin. Psychopharmacol.* 24(4):365–373.

Rush, A.J., Trivedi, M.H., Wisniewski, S.R., Stewart, J.W., Nierenberg, A.A., Thase, M.E., Ritz, L., Biggs, M.M., Warden, D., Luther, J. F., Shores-Wilson, K., Niederehe, G., Fava, M.; STAR*D Study Team. (2006) Bupropion-SR, sertraline, or venlafaxine-XR after failure of SSRIs for depression. *N. Engl. J. Med.* 354(12):1231–1242.

Sachs, G.S., Lafer, B., et al. (1994) A double-blind trial of bupropion versus desipramine for bipolar depression. *J. Clin. Psychiatry* 55(9): 391–393.

Sachs, G.S., Nierenberg, A.A., et al. (2007) Effectiveness of adjunctive antidepressant treatment for bipolar depression. *N. Engl. J. Med.* 356(17):1711–1722.

Sackeim, H.A., Haskett, R.F., et al. (2001) Continuation pharmacotherapy in the prevention of relapse following electroconvulsive therapy: a randomized controlled trial. *JAMA* 285(10):1299–1307.

Sackeim, H.A., Prudic, J., Devanand, D.P., et al. (2000) A prospective, randomized, double-blind comparison of bilateral and right unilateral electroconvulsive therapy at different stimulus intensities. *Arch. Gen. Psychiatry* 57(5):425–434.

Sackeim, H.A., Prudic, J., Fuller, R., Keilp, J., Lavor, P.W., and Olfson, M. (2007) The cognitive effects of electroconvulsive therapy in community settings. *Neuropsychopharmacology* 32(1):244–254.

Satel, S., and Nelson, J. (1989) Stimulants in the treatment of depression: a critical overview. *J. Clin. Psychiatry* 50:241–249.

Sauer, W.H., Berlin, J.A., et al. (2001) Selective serotonin reuptake inhibitors and myocardial infarction. *Circulation* 104(16): 1894–1898.

Schatzberg, A.F., and Roose, S. (2006) A double-blind, placebo-controlled study of venlafaxine and fluoxetine in geriatric outpatients with major depression. *Am. J. Geriatr. Psychiatry* 14(4): 361–370.

Schmidt, P.J., Nieman, L., et al. (2000) Estrogen replacement in perimenopause-related depression: a preliminary report. *Am. J. Obstet. Gynecol.* 183(2):414–420.

Schneider, L.S. (1996) Pharmacological considerations in the treatment of late life depression. *Am. J. Geriatr. Psychiatry* 4(Suppl 1):S51–S65.

Schneider, L.S., Small, G.W., Hamilton, S.H., Bystritsky, A., Nemeroff, C.B., and Meyers, A.B. (1997) Estrogen replacement and response to fluoxetine in a multicenter geriatric depression trial. Fluoxetine Collaborative Study Group. *Am. J. Geriatr. Psychiatry* 5:97–106.

Seidman, S.N., Araujo, A.B., et al. (2002) Low testosterone levels in elderly men with dysthymic disorder. *Am. J. Psychiatry* 159(3): 456–449.

Seth, R., Jennings, A.L., Bindman, I., Phillips, I., and Bergmann, K. (1992) Combination treatment with noradrenaline and serotonin reuptake inhibitors in resistant depression. *Br. J. Psychiatry* 161: 562–565.

Shapira, B., Oppenheim, G., Zohar, I., Segal, M., Malach, D., and Belmaker, R.H. (1985) Lack of efficacy of estrogen supplementation to imipramine in resistant female depressives. *Biol. Psychiatry* 20:576–579.

Sharpley, A.L., Elliott, J.M., et al. (1994) Slow wave sleep in humans: role of 5-HT2A and 5-HT2C receptors. *Neuropharmacology* 33(3/4):467–471.

Shelton, R.C., Tollefson, G.D., et al. (2001) A novel augmentation strategy for treating resistant major depression. *Am. J. Psychiatry* 158(1):131–134.

Skowron, D.M., and Stimmel, G.L. (1992) Antidepressant and the risk of seizures. *Pharmacotherapy* 12:18–22.

Smeraldi, E., Zanardi, R., Benedetti, F., Di Bella, D., Perez, J., and Catalano, M. (1998) Polymorphism within the promoter of the serotonin transporter gene and antidepressant efficacy of fluvoxamine. *Mol. Psychiatry* 3(6):508–511.

Soares, C.N., Almeida, O.P., et al. (2001) Efficacy of estradiol for the treatment of depressive disorders in perimenopausal women: a double-blind, randomized, placebo-controlled trial. *Arch. Gen. Psychiatry* 58(6):529–534.

Spiker, D.G., Weiss, J.C., Dealy, R.S., Griffin, S.J., Hanin, I., Neil, J. F., Perel, J.M., Rossi, A.J., and Soloff, P.H. (1985) The pharmacologic treatment of delusional depression. *Am. J. Psychiatry* 142: 430–436.

Sporn, J., Ghaemi, S.N., et al. (2000) Pramipexole augmentation in the treatment of unipolar and bipolar depression: a retrospective chart review. *Ann. Clin. Psychiatry* 12(3):137–140.

Stoll, A.L., Severus, W.E., et al. (1999) Omega 3 fatty acids in bipolar disorder: a preliminary double-blind, placebo-controlled trial [see comments]. *Arch. Gen. Psychiatry* 56(5):407–412.

Stout, S.C., Owens, M.J., et al. (2002) Regulation of corticotropin-releasing factor neuronal systems and hypothalamic-pituitary-adrenal axis activity by stress and chronic antidepressant treatment. *J. Pharmacol. Exp. Ther.* 300(3):1085–1092.

Svenningsson, P., Tzavara, E.T., et al. (2002) Involvement of striatal and extrastriatal DARPP-32 in biochemical and behavioral effects of fluoxetine (Prozac). *Proc. Natl. Acad. Sci. USA* 99(5): 3182–3187.

Szabo, S.T., and Blier, P. (2001) Functional and pharmacological characterization of the modulatory role of serotonin on the firing activity of locus coeruleus norepinephrine neurons. *Brain Res.* 922(1): 9–20.

Thase, M.E., Blomgren, S.L., et al. (1997) Fluoxetine treatment of patients with major depressive disorder who failed initial treatment with sertraline. *J. Clin. Psychiatry* 58(1):16–21.

Thase, M.E., Corya, S.A., Osuntokun, O., Case, M., Henley, D.B., Sanger, T.M., Watson, S.B., and Dubé, S. (2007) A randomized, double-blind comparison of olanzapine/fluoxetine combination, olanzapine, and fluoxetine in treatment-resistant major depressive disorder. *J. Clin. Psychiatry* 68(2):224–236.

Thase, M.E., Entsuah, A.R., et al. (2001) Remission rates during treatment with venlafaxine or selective serotonin reuptake inhibitors. *Br. J. Psychiatry* 178:234–241.

Thase, M.E., Fava, M., Halbreich, U., Kocsis, I., Koran, L., Davidson, I., Rosenbaum, I., and Harrison, W. (1996) A placebo-controlled, randomized clinical trial comparing sertraline and imipramine for the treatment of dysthymia. *Arch. Gen. Psychiatry* 53:777–784.

Thase, M.E., Feighner, J.P., et al. (2001) Citalopram treatment of fluoxetine nonresponders. *J. Clin. Psychiatry* 62(9):683–687.

Thase, M.E., Kupfer, D.J., and Jarrett, D.B. (1989) Treatment of imipramine-resistant recurrent depression: I. An open clinical trial of adjunctive 1-triiodothyronine. *J. Clin. Psychiatry* 50:385–388.

Thase, M.E., Macfadden, W., Weisler, R.H., Chang, W., Paulsson, B., Khan, A., Calabrese, J.R.; Bolder II Study Group. (2006) Efficacy of quetiapine monotherapy in bipolar I and II depression: a double-blind, placebo-controlled study (the BOLDER II study). *J. Clin. Psychopharmacol.* 26(6):600–609.

Thase, M.E., Mallinger, A.G., et al. (1992) Treatment of imipramine-resistant recurrent depression, IV: A double-blind crossover study of tranylcypromine for anergic bipolar depression. *Am. J. Psychiatry* 149(2):195–198.

Thase, M.E., and Rush, A. (1995). Treatment-resistant depression. In: Bloom, F.E., and Kupfer, D.F., eds. *Psychopharmacology: The Fourth Generation of Progress*. New York: Raven Press, pp. 1081–1097.

Thase, M.E., Rush, A.J., et al. (2002) Double-blind switch study of imipramine or sertraline treatment of antidepressant-resistant chronic depression. *Arch. Gen. Psychiatry* 59(3):233–239.

Thase, M.E., and Sachs, G.S. (2000) Bipolar depression: pharmacotherapy and related therapeutic strategies. *Biol. Psychiatry* 48(6): 558–572.

Tohen, M., Vieta, E., Calabrese, J., Ketter, T.A., Sachs, G., Bowden, C., Mitchell, P.B., Centorrino, F., Risser, R., Baker, R.W., Evans, A.R., Beymer, K., Dube, S., Tollefson, G.D., and Breier, A. (2003) Efficacy of olanzapine and olanzapine-fluoxetine combination in the treatment of bipolar I depression. *Arch. Gen. Psychiatry* 60(11): 1079–1088.

Tollefson, G.D., Bosomworth, J.C., Heiligenstein, J.H., Potvin, J.H., and Holman, S. (1995) A double-blind, placebo-controlled clinical trial of fluoxetine in geriatric patients with major depression.

The Fluoxetine Collaborative Study Group. *Int. Psychogeriatr.* 7(1):89–104.

Trivedi, M.H., Fava, M., Wisniewski, S.R., Thase, M.E., Quitkin, F., Warden, D., Ritz, L., Nierenberg, A.A., Lebowitz, B.D., Biggs, M.M., Luther, J.F., Shores-Wilson, K., Rush, A.J.; STAR*D Study Team. (2006) Medication augmentation after the failure of SSRIs for depression. *N. Engl. J. Med.* 354(12):1243–1252.

Trivedi, M.H., Rush, A.J., Wisniewski, S.R., Nierenberg, A.A., Warden, D., Ritz, L., Norquist, G., Howland, R.H., Lebowitz, B.D., McGrath, P.J., Shores-Wilson, K., Biggs, M.M., Balasubramani, G.K., Fava, M.; STAR*D Study Team. (2006) Evaluation of outcomes with citalopram for depression using measurement-based care in STAR*D: implications for clinical practice. *Am. J. Psychiatry* 163(1):28–40.

Versiani, M., Amrein, R., et al. (1997) Moclobemide and imipramine in chronic depression (dysthymia): an international double-blind, placebo-controlled trial. International Collaborative Study Group. *Int. Clin. Psychopharmacol.* 12(4):183–193.

Waintraub, L., Septien, L., et al. (2002) Efficacy and safety of tianeptine in major depression: evidence from a 3-month controlled clinical trial versus paroxetine. *CNS Drugs* 16(1):65–75.

Walker, S.E., Shulman, K.I., et al. (1996) Tyramine content of previously restricted foods in monoamine oxidase inhibitor diets. *J. Clin. Psychopharmacol.* 16(5):383–388.

Waring, W.S., Good, A.M., Bateman, D.N. (2007) Lack of significant toxicity after mirtazapine overdose: a five-year review of cases admitted to a regional toxicology unit. *Clin. Toxicol. (Phila)* 45(1):45–50.

Wecker, L., James, S., Copeland, N., and Pacheco, M.A. (2003) Transdermal selegiline: targeted effects on monoamine oxidases in the brain. *Biol. Psychiatry* 54(10):1099–1104.

Weilburg, J.B., Rosenbaum, J.F., Biederman, I., Sachs, G.S., Pollack, M.H., and Kelly, K. (1989) Fluoxetine added to non-MAOI antidepressants converts nonresponders to responders: a preliminary report. *J. Clin. Psychiatry* 50:447–449.

Wernicke, J.F., Pritchett, Y.L., D'Souza, D.N., Waninger, A., Tran, P., Ivengar, S., and Raskin, J. (2006) A randomized controlled trial of duloxetine in diabetic peripheral neuropathic pain. *Neurology* 67(8):1411–1420.

West, D., and Dally, P. (1959) Effect of iproniazid in depressive syndromes. *Br. Med. J.* 1:1491–1494.

Winokur, G., Coryell, W., Keller, M., Endicott, I., and Akiskal, H. (1993) A prospective follow-up of patients with bipolar and primary unipolar affective disorder. *Arch. Gen. Psychiatry* 50:457–465.

Xu, H., Qing, H., et al. (2002) Quetiapine attenuates the immobilization stress-induced decrease of brain-derived neurotrophic factor expression in rat hippocampus. *Neurosci. Lett.* 321(1/2): 65–68.

Young, A.H., Gallagher, P., Watson, S., Del-Estal, D., Owen, B.M., and Ferrer, I.N. (2004) Improvements in neurocognitive function and mood following adjunctive treatment with mifepristone (RU-486) in bipolar disorder. *Neuropsychopharmacology* 29(8): 1538–1545.

Zanardi, R., Benedetti, F., De Bella, D., Catalano, M., and Smeraldi, E. (2000) Efficacy of paroxetine in depression is influenced by a functional polymorphism within the promoter of the serotonin transporter gene. *J. Clin. Psychopharmacol.* 20(1):105–107.

Zanardi, R., Franchini, L., Gasperini, M., Perez, J., and Smeraldi, E. (1996) Double-blind controlled trial of sertraline versus paroxetine in the treatment of delusional depression. *Am. J. Psychiatry* 153(12):1631–1633.

Zarate, C.A., Jr., Payne, J.L., Singh, J., Quiroz, J.A., Luckenbaugh, D.A., Denicoff, K.D., Charney, D.S., and Manji, H.K. (2004) Pramipexole for bipolar II depression: a placebo-controlled proof of concept study. *Biol. Psychiatry* 56(1):54–60.

Zarate, C.A., Jr., Singh, J., Carlson, P.J., Brutsche, N.E., Ameli, R., Luckenbaugh, D.A., Charney, D.S., and Manji, H.K. (2006) A randomized trial of *N*-methy-D-asparate antagonist in treatment-resistant major depression. *Arch. Gen. Psychiatry* 63(8):856–864.

Zarate, C.A., Jr., Singh, J., Quiroz, J.A., DeJesus, G., Denicoff, K.K., Luckenbaugh, D.A., Manji, H.K. and Charney, D.S. (2006) A double-blind, placebo-controlled study of memantine in the treatment of major depression. *Am. J. Psychiatry* 163(1):153–155.

Zarate, C.A., Jr., Tohen, M., et al. (2001) Cycling into depression from a first episode of mania: a case-comparison study. *Am. J. Psychiatry* 158(9):1524–1526.

Zimmerman, M., Mattia, J.I., et al. (2002) Are subjects in pharmacological treatment trials of depression representative of patients in routine clinical practice? *Am. J. Psychiatry* 159(3):469–473.

Zobel, A.W., Nickel, T., Künzel, H.E., Ackl, N., Sonntag, A., Ising, M., and Holsboer, F. (2000) Effects of the high-affinity corticotrophin-releasing hormone receptor 1 antagonist R121919 in major depression: the first 20 patients treated. *J. Psychiatr. Res.* 34(3):171–181.

Zobel, A.W., Nickel, T., Sonntag, A., et al. (2001) Cortisol response in the combined dexamethasone/CRH test as predictor of relapse in patients with remitted depression. a prospective study. *J. Psychiatr. Res.* 35(2):83–94.

33 Abnormalities of Brain Structure and Function in Mood Disorders

VICTORIA ARANGO AND J. JOHN MANN

This chapter describes our current knowledge of brain structure and function in mood disorders based on postmortem brain studies and should be read in conjunction with other chapters on in vivo imaging and neurochemistry studies. A confluence of structural and functional imaging studies have suggested that the prefrontal cortex (PFC) is reduced in size and/or function in major depression. Altered indices of noradrenergic (NA) and serotonergic function have been found in major depression, and their molecular components and the anatomical location have been identified. In addition, associated second-messenger systems in cortical target regions are affected, raising questions over whether the primary abnormalities are in the monoamine source neurons or in target cortical or subcortical neurons. It is important to determine which abnormalities detected in postmortem studies are related specifically to the pathogenesis of mood disorders and which changes are related to nonspecific effects of stress, the most common cause of death in such studies of persons with depression, namely suicide, homeostatic mechanisms, or other comorbid psychopathology. We discuss these alternative possibilities throughout this chapter.

POSTMORTEM STUDIES OF THE SEROTONERGIC SYSTEM IN DEPRESSION

Of all the neurotransmitter systems altered in mood disorders and suicide, the serotonergic system is most consistently affected (Stanley et al., 1982; Arango and Mann, 1992; Arango et al., 1995; Pandey et al., 2002; Stockmeier, 2003). Major depressive disorder (MDD; Coccaro et al., 1989; Delgado et al., 1990; O'Keane and Dinan, 1991; Price et al., 1991; Mann et al., 1992; Mann et al., 1995; Flory et al., 1998; Arango et al., 2002; Stockmeier, 2003) and suicidal behavior (Arango and Mann, 1992; Arango et al., 1995; Arango and Underwood, 1997; Mann et al., 2000; Arango et al., 2002; Mann, 2002; Pandey et al., 2002; Mann, 2003) are independently correlated with direct indicators of altered serotonergic function in the brain and indirectly through measures in the cerebrospinal fluid (CSF; Mann, 1998; Mann et al., 2000). This dysfunction of the serotonergic system appears to be a trait as patients with remitted mood disorder continue to demonstrate an impairment of serotonergic function (Delgado et al., 1990; Delgado et al., 1994; Flory et al., 1998).

Moreover, individuals with major depression who have died by suicide or made more lethal suicide attempts have an additional deficiency in serotonergic function over and above the abnormality associated with depression (Shaw et al., 1967; Bourne et al., 1968; Pare et al., 1969; Lloyd et al., 1974; Åsberg et al., 1976; Beskow et al., 1976; Agren, 1980; Brown et al., 1982; Malone et al., 1996; Mann, Malone, et al., 1996; Mann and Malone, 1997), consistent with the hypothesis that reduced serotonergic activity is associated with suicide risk. In individuals who attempt suicide, there appears to be a biological trait involving impaired serotonergic function that can predict risk of future suicide (Nordström et al., 1994; Mann et al., 2006). Genetics and early-life environment can both influence serotonergic function in a manner that can affect adult behavior and that may explain such traits as impulsive aggressive behaviors in adulthood as well as the development of recurrent mood disorders. Given evidence that serotonergic function is under substantial genetic regulation (Higley et al., 1993; Fairbanks et al., 2004; Rogers et al., 2004), we have proposed that the genetic factors causing recurrent mood disorders and regulating the risk of suicidal behavior may be at least partly mediated by the serotonergic system and its impact on development of mood disorders and on impulse regulation via executive function (Mann et al., 2001; Arango, Huang, et al., 2003; Mann et al., 2005). It is in this context that studies of the serotonergic system in major depression and violent suicides and controls are best understood. We emphasize suicide because many individuals with major depression that come to autopsy have died by suicide, and thus most postmortem studies of patients with depression include a very high proportion of suicides. There are fewer postmortem studies of patients with depression dying of natural causes or accidents, and it is difficult to obtain suitable cases of patients with major depression dying from causes other than suicide. For example, some studies of individuals with mood disorder who died from natural causes may be compromised by inclusion of patients in remission at the time of death, and/or receiving antidepressant medications that down-regulate 5-hydroxytryptophan (5-HT; serotonin)$_{1A}$ or 5-HT$_{2A}$ receptors and thereby reverse any potential increase in these receptors due to depression.

Ferrier et al. (1986) found lower cortical 5-hydroxyindole acetic acid (5-HIAA) and a trend for more 5-HT$_{2A}$ binding in patients who were depressed but not on antidepressants in the month prior to death. A subsequent study by the same group reported higher 5-HT$_{2A}$ binding (Yates et al., 1990). A study by McKeith et al. (1987) found greater ^{3}H-ketanserin (^{3}H-KET) binding to 5-HT$_{2A}$ receptors in the cortex of the frontal pole (Brodmann area [BA] 10) of patients with depression dying from causes other than suicide compared to controls, despite the fact that only four of the nine patients with major depression were off antidepressants for at least one month prior to death. Owen et al. (1986) reported on patients with depression, not all of whom were depressed at time of death, and some of whom were on antidepressants, and found no differences in frontal cortical or hypothalamic levels of 5-HIAA; however, the postmortem delay was over 40 hours, which can lead to degradation of this metabolite. In addition, they reported no change in 5-HT$_{2A}$ binding in the same brain samples. Yates and Ferrier (1990) found less 5-HT$_{1A}$ binding in frontal cortex of medicated patients with depression compared with euthymic unmedicated patients and suggested down-regulation by antidepressants as an explanation for less binding. Perry et al. (1983) found lower imipramine binding in occipital cortex. Imipramine binds to the serotonin transporter (SERT), but also to nontransporter sites. Thus, this study suggests there are fewer SERT sites but cannot rule out a contribution by nontransporter sites. We published the largest postmortem study to date, assaying PFC tissue samples from 159 individuals for SERT binding (^{3}H-cyanoimipramine; Arango et al., 1995), by quantitative receptor autoradiography (Mann et al., 2000). Clinical information, including *Diagnostic and Statistical Manual of Mental Disorders*-3rd ed. revised (*DSM-III-R*; American Psychiatric Association, 1987) axis I and axis II diagnoses, was obtained by psychological autopsy (Kelly and Mann, 1996). Serotonin transporter binding in individuals with a history of major depression was lower throughout all prefrontal cortical areas studied. This contrasted with the finding that suicide was associated with less SERT binding only in the ventral prefrontal and anterior cingulate cortex (Arango et al., 2002).

In summary, studies in patients with depression dying from causes other than suicide have found more 5-HT$_{2A}$ binding and less SERT binding, changes that are in the same direction as those seen in individuals who die by suicide regardless of diagnosis. Mapping studies of SERT binding suggest that mood disorders involve a widespread alteration in the PFC, whereas suicide involves a localized change in serotonin function confined to the ventral PFC. Clearly, more data are required on the serotonergic system in the brain of patients with depression to determine the qualitative or quantitative differences in the serotonergic system associated with mood disorders as distinct from suicide.

POSTMORTEM STUDIES OF THE SEROTONERGIC SYSTEM IN SUICIDES

An association between serotonin and suicidal behavior is one of the most consistent findings in biological psychiatry (Mann, 2003; Mann and Currier, 2007). Numerous studies have reported less postmortem SERT binding in ventromedial PFC related to suicide independent of psychiatric diagnosis, and an independent deficiency in transporter binding across most of the PFC related to major depression (Mann et al., 2000; Arango et al., 2002). Similarly, we have reported higher postmortem postsynaptic 5-HT$_{1A}$ binding in ventral PFC related to suicide but not to major depression (Arango et al., 1995). Therefore, serotonin-related factors may hold important clues to the etiology of suicidal behavior, particularly that aspect that cannot be explained by the presence of psychiatric illness alone.

Early neurochemical studies of 5-HT or 5-HIAA in the brainstem of suicides found small differences of 10%–20% in brain stem, but not in cortex, in suicides compared to controls (reviewed in Mann et al., 1989; Arango and Mann, 1992; Mann, Underwood, and Arango, 1996). Korpi et al. (1986) found lower hypothalamic 5-HT in suicides without schizophrenia, but not in suicides with schizophrenia. The brain stem differences were of similar magnitude in suicides with a depressive illness (about 60% of all suicides in most studies have a major depression at the time of suicide; Mann et al., 1989), compared with suicides with other psychiatric diagnoses, suggesting that lower brain stem 5-HT and 5-HIAA levels are primarily associated with suicidal behavior rather than with major depression (Mann et al., 1989).

Levels of 5-HT or 5-HIAA postmortem are only a crude index of presynaptic serotonergic function because 5-HT and 5-HIAA concentrations decline rapidly after death and the removal of the brain from the calvarium, and also because 5-HT is found in a fast and in a slow turnover pool that cannot be distinguished by tissue assay even though the pools have different functions. Postsynaptic receptors and transporter sites, and membrane-bound proteins, are more stable postmortem indicators of altered function and have proven valuable in the localization of abnormalities in the brain.

We and others reviewed elsewhere postmortem brain serotonin receptor studies in suicides (Arango and Mann, 1992; Mann, Underwood, and Arango, 1996; Stockmeier, 2003). In summary, 9 of 18 studies found an increase in 5-HT_{2A} binding. The discrepant results appear to be due to a combination of ligand specificity, agonist versus antagonist, and region-specific or agonal effects (Lewis, 2002). A separate body of studies (Biegon et al., 1990; Pandey et al., 1990; McBride et al., 1994; Pandey et al., 1995; Hrdina and Du, 2001) have found more platelet 5-HT_{2A} receptors in association with suicidal behavior, lending further support to the conclusion that 5-HT_{2A} receptor binding may be altered in suicide. Our original finding in dorsolateral PFC, where specific 5-HT_{2A} binding was defined by mianserin (Mann et al., 1986), may have included binding to non-5-HT_{2A} receptor populations. The majority of earlier studies of 5-HT_{2A} receptors, including ours, used ^{3}H-spiroperidol or ^{125}I-LSD in membrane preparations from dorsolateral PFC. Six of 11 studies found more 5-HT_{2A} binding sites. Using the agonist ^{125}I-LSD and ketanserin as a displacer for autoradiography (Arango et al., 1990), we found more 5-HT_{2A} sites in dorsolateral PFC, a finding replicated in homogenates using the same ligand (Pandey et al., 2001). Moreover, Pandey et al. (2002) found more 5-HT_{2A} protein and gene expression in PFC of adolescent suicides, suggesting that at least part of the explanation of more binding lay in more gene expression. Our most recent autoradiography study using the selective 5-HT_{2A} antagonist ligand ^{3}H-ketanserin throughout the pregenual PFC indicates an increase in 5-HT_{2A} binding that appears most pronounced in ventral PFC (Fig. 33.1A), although using the same ligand, a study in homogenates revealed higher B_{max} in dorsal PFC (Turecki et al., 1999). A recent study by our group (Underwood et al., 2004) showed that adult suicides (> 25 years) who were alcoholic had higher binding than controls in ventrolateral PFC (BA 45 and 46). In the younger age group (≤ 25 years), nonalcoholic suicides had more binding than controls in orbital cortex (BA 47, 11 and 12). A shift in the ratio of high- and low-affinity binding sites can explain some discrepancies in the literature because only agonists detect the difference in binding affinity.

We also reported higher 5-HT_{1A} binding localized to the ventrolateral PFC (Arango et al., 1995, Fig. 33.1B). The 5-HT_{1A} receptor appears to be involved in the actions of anxiolytic and antidepressant drugs. Overall, three (Matsubara et al., 1991; Joyce et al., 1993; Arango et al., 1995) of seven studies have found increased 5-HT_{1A} binding in localized brain regions in suicides. Negative studies (Dillon et al., 1991; Arranz et al., 1994; Lowther et al., 1997; Stockmeier et al., 1997) did not study multiple areas by autoradiography and may have missed regions of change or included tissue from patients on medications at the time of death. Using quantitative autoradiography we studied 5-HT_{1A} binding in nine pregenual cortical Brodmann areas (11, 12, 32, 24, 8, 9, 46, 45, and 47) in large coronal sections of the PFC of suicides and controls. The suicide group had higher 5-HT_{1A} binding compared with the control group in ventral PFC (BA 45 and 46) with differences ranging from 17%–30% (Fig. 33.2; Arango et al., 1995), a finding we replicated with almost double the sample size (Arango et al., 1998; Arango et al., 2004, Figs. 33.1B and 33.2). Females have higher 5-HT_{1A} binding than males in some of the PFC areas studied (Arango et al., 1995). Some studies of 5-HT_{1A} receptors in the hippocampus report an increase in suicides (Joyce et al., 1993), but most do not (Dillon et al., 1991; Lowther et al., 1997; Stockmeier et al., 1997).

Conflicting reports exist in the literature as to whether binding to the SERT on serotonin nerve terminals is lower in cortical regions of suicides (Arango and Mann, 1992; Stockmeier, 2003). Serotonin transporter binding is an index of serotonin nerve terminals. Early studies used ligands that did not distinguish high-affinity SERT binding from a very similar non-SERT binding site that has no known functional role (Mann, Henteleff, et al., 1996). Presynaptic imipramine binding density in the frontal cortex and hypothalamus of suicides was lower compared to controls (Stanley et al., 1982; Paul et al., 1984). Other later studies failed to find fewer imipramine or paroxetine binding sites in PFC (Meyerson et al., 1982; Crow et al., 1984; Owen et al., 1986; Gross-Isseroff et al., 1989; Lawrence et al., 1990; Arora and Meltzer, 1991). In summary, 7 of 17 studies report less SERT binding associated with suicide.

In our autoradiography studies (Arango et al., 1995; Mann et al., 2000; Arango et al., 2002, Fig. 33.1C), SERT binding was 15%–27% lower in the ventral PFC of suicides compared with controls. We found no difference in dorsolateral PFC in suicides where most other investigators focused, but we did find binding to be lower in that brain region in major depression, suggesting brain region and diagnosis associated with suicide are crucial (Lewis, 2002). We also reported that nontransporter (non-SERT), defined by independence from sodium concentration, paroxetine binding is lower in dorsolateral PFC (Mann, Henteleff, et al., 1996). Because ^{3}H-imipramine binds with high affinity to the SERT and non-SERT sites, the finding of lower ^{3}H-imipramine binding in dorsolateral PFC is probably due to non-SERT sites.

In contrast to suicides, SERT binding in individuals with a history of major depression who died by natural causes or accident was lower throughout all prefrontal

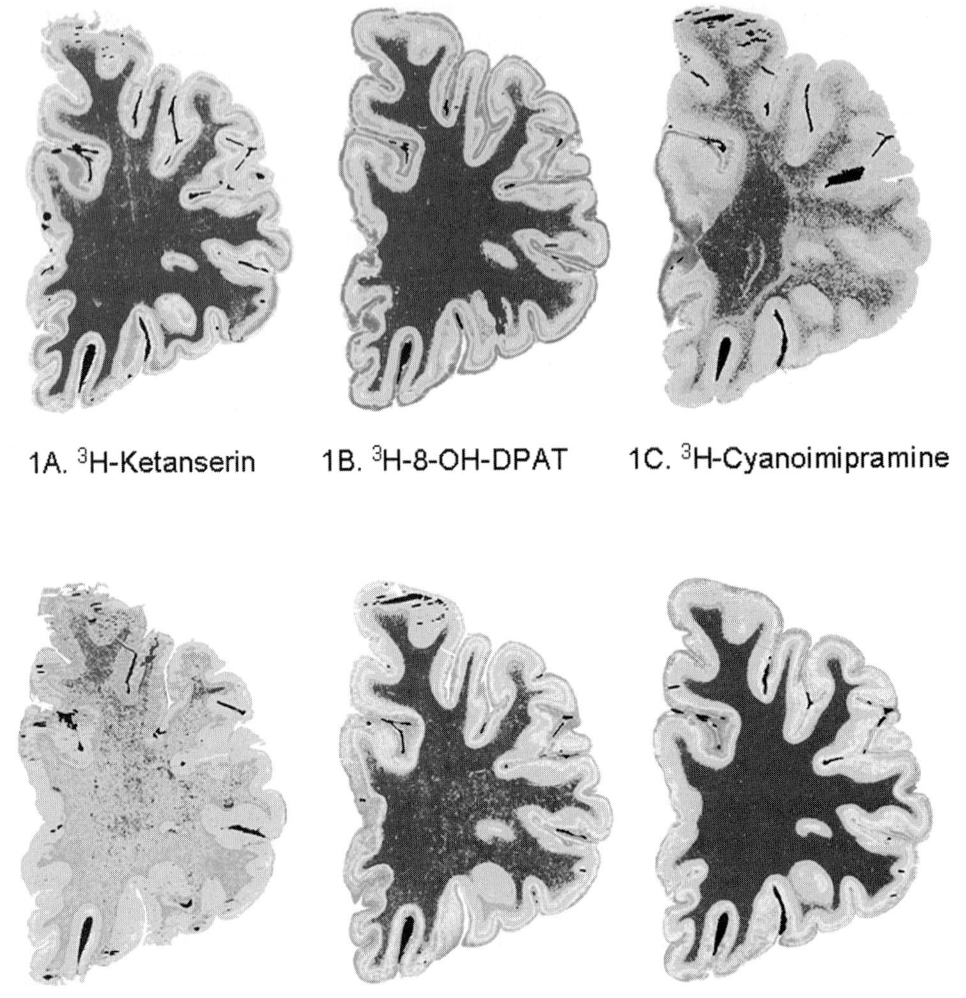

FIGURE 33.1 Upper panel: Serotonin receptors. Pseudocolor images of subtracted autoradiograms representing total specific 5-HT_{2A} (*A*), 5-HT_{1A} (*B*), and serotonin transporter (*C*) binding sites in adjacent coronal sections of the prefrontal cortex of the human. Lower panel: Adrenergic receptors. Pseudocolor images of subtracted autoradiograms representing total specific β_1-adrenergic (high-affinity) (*D*), α_1-adrenergic (*E*), and α_2-adrenergic (*F*) binding. Note that each receptor has a different lamination within the cortex and varies dorso-ventrally with ventral cortical areas having more binding.

cortical areas studied (Mann et al., 2000; Arango et al., 2002). Thus, SERT binding revealed what appear to be regionally distinct neurobiological correlates of major depression and suicide. Levels of 5-HT and 5-HIAA did not correlate with SERT binding, but 5-HT_{1A} binding and SERT binding correlated negatively in controls and suicides in the same brain region.

THE DORSAL RAPHÉ NUCLEUS

In nonhuman primates, serotonergic innervation of the cerebral cortex and much of the forebrain is derived from serotonin-synthesizing neurons in the dorsal (DRN) and median raphé nucleus (MRN; Törk, 1990). In the human, the DRN is a large group of neurons embedded in the ventral part of the central gray matter of caudal mesencephalon and rostral pons. Based on topographic and cytoarchitectonic characteristics in Nissl-stained material, the DRN has been subdivided into distinct subnuclei (Baker et al., 1990). These subdivisions correspond to those observed in tissue immunoreacted with antiphenylalanine hydroxylase sera (Törk, 1990; Törk and Hornung, 1990), which also revealed an additional component (the ventral subnucleus) not recognized in Nissl material. The subnuclei are median (or interfascicular), ventrolateral, dorsal, lateral, and caudal.

At present it is not possible to verify the cortical targets of the various DRN nuclear subdivisions in the human. The projection from the DRN to cortical targets in the monkey exhibits a coarse rostrocaudal topographic relationship, as opposed to the MRN projections that are not separated rostrocaudally (Wilson and Molliver, 1991). The serotonergic projection to the PFC

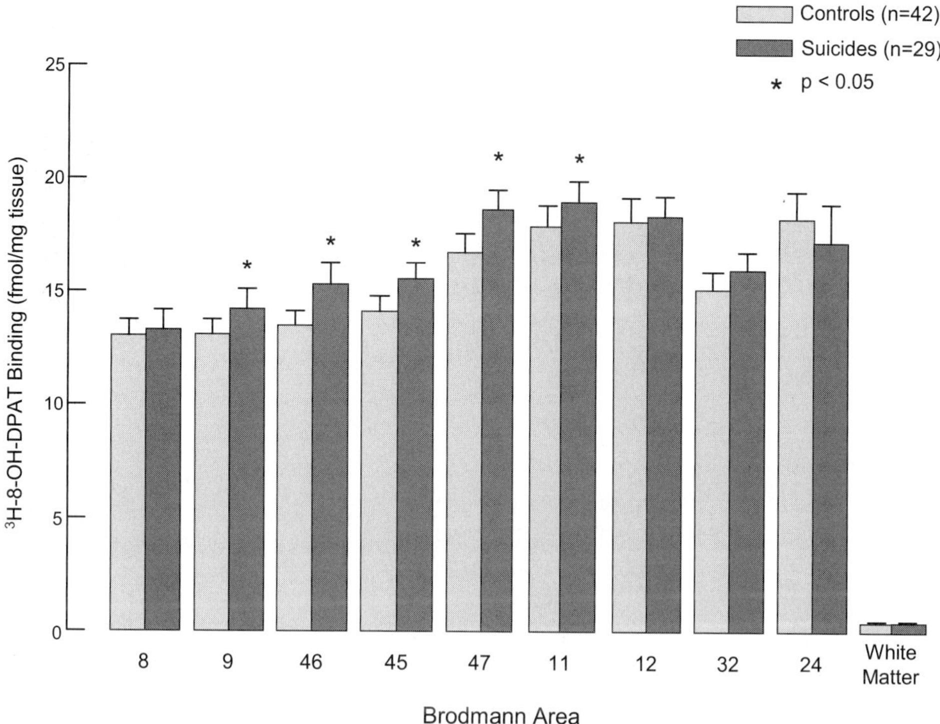

FIGURE 33.2 Binding to the 5-HT_{1A} receptor in sulci of the prefrontal cortex in controls and suicides. The coronal section was taken at a level just anterior to the genu of the corpus callosum and includes dorsal Brodmann areas (BA) 8 and 9, lateral (BA 46) orbital (BA 45, 47, and 11) and medial (BA 12, 32, and 24). Note that binding is higher in orbital regions and that suicides had more binding than controls in dorsolateral and orbital regions.

has a substantial component arising from cells in the rostral part of the DRN. Regarding cortical innervation by serotonin projections in the primate, density is highest in layer I, except in sensory areas where the highest density is in layer IV. The serotonergic target cells in the cortex are mostly GAD-IR, indicating that they are γ-aminobutyric acid (GABA)ergic inhibitory neurons, but in some brain regions, such as in the pyriform cortex, the target neurons are pyramidal cells (Sheldon and Aghajanian, 1990).

One possible simple explanation for impaired serotonergic neurotransmission in depression and/or suicide may be that there are fewer serotonergic neurons in the DRN resulting in a compensatory increase in 5-HT_{2A} and 5-HT_{1A} postsynaptic receptors in the PFC, and associated with fewer presynaptic SERT sites. Using a specific tryptophan hydroxylase antibody to identify only serotonergic neurons, we ruled out the possibility that the serotonergic deficiency is due to fewer serotonin-synthesizing neurons in the DRN where we found more rather than fewer 5-HT neurons in suicides with depression (Underwood et al., 1999, Fig. 33.3). A replication of this study by the Gundersen group (Dorph-Petersen et al., 2001) also found that suicides did not have fewer cell numbers in the DRN. We then counted the number of Nissl-stained neurons in suicides and controls and found no differences. However, when the TPH-IR neurons were expressed as a percent of the total number of DRN neurons, approximately 54% of DRN neurons in controls were serotonergic compared to 78% of the neurons in suicides, indicating a change in the phenotype (Arango, Underwood, et al., 2003, Fig. 33.4). Thus, not only are there more serotonergic neurons in the suicides, there is evidence of more TPH2 protein (Underwood et al., 1999; Boldrini et al., 2005), and more TPH2 messenger ribonucleic acids (mRNA) (Bach-Mizrachi et al., 2006) in the DRN of suicides, a condition predicting more, not less, 5-HT transmitter synthesis. However, not all groups find these differences in the DRN of suicides (Bonkale et al., 2004), but they report higher levels of TPH protein in the DRN of alcohol dependent individuals with depression (Bonkale et al., 2006). The presence of TPH does not necessarily indicate functional capacity. Such superfluous expression of TPH may explain our observation of increased enzyme, presumably with reduced 5-HT synthesis, release, and turnover. However, it remains unclear whether it is at the transcriptional level or at the translational level that TPH is aberrantly regulated.

Studies using quantitative reverse transcription polymerase chain reaction (RT-PCR) report low levels of TPH2 transcript in the terminal fields of 5-HT neurons in human postmortem tissue (De Luca et al., 2005; Zill et al., 2007), with the level of TPH2 mRNA in the

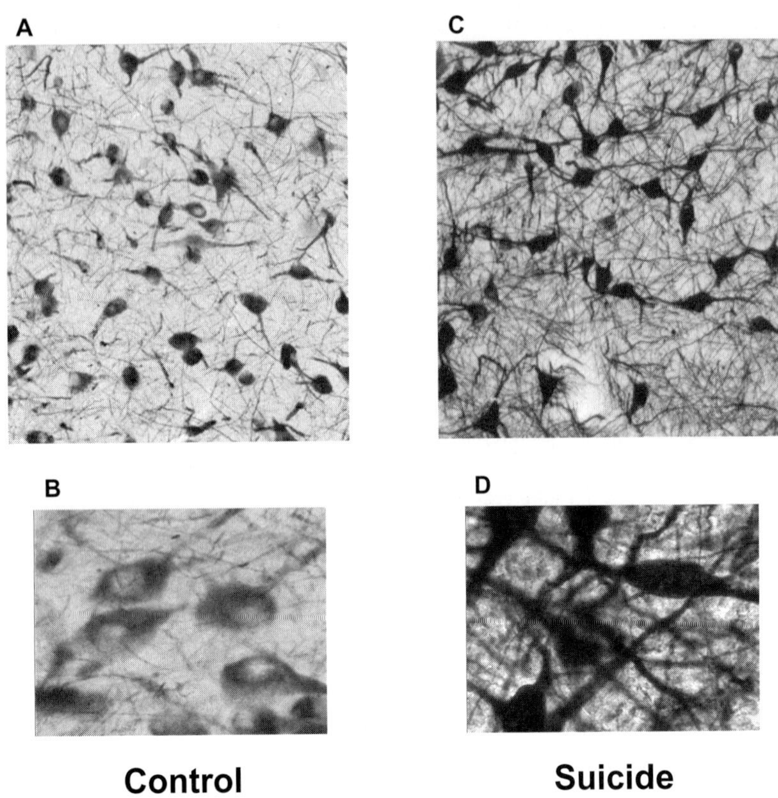

FIGURE 33.3 TPH immunoreactivity in the DRN in a representative control (*A* & *B*) and suicide (C & *D*) at medium (400X, *A* & C) and high (1000X, *B* & *D*) magnification. TPH was labeled using an antibody to phenylalanine hydroxylase, as described in the text. The photomicrographs were taken from the ventrolateral subnucleus. Note that the intensity of staining is greater in the DRN of the suicide victim. The increase in staining extends to neuronal processes. TPH: tryptophan hydroxylase; DRN: dorsal raphé nucleus.

DRN being tenfold higher than in the cortex (Zill et al., 2007). One study examined TPH2 mRNA levels in the PFC of suicides (De Luca et al., 2006) and found no significant differences between groups. TPH mRNA was reported to be higher in PFC of patients with bipolar disorder, but not in patients with schizophrenia, compared to controls (De Luca et al., 2005), an alteration not present in the parietal cortex (Shamir et al., 2005). TPH2 protein is very abundant in cortex as measured with Western Blots, but no differences were detected between suicides and controls (Ono et al., 2002).

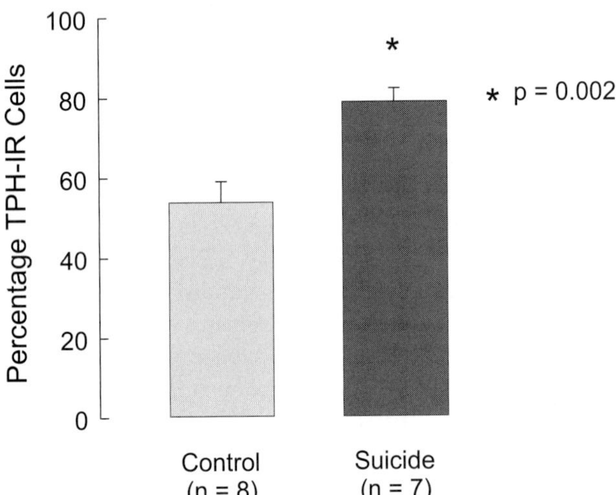

FIGURE 33.4 The percentage of DRN neurons that are tryptophan hydroxylase-immunoreactive in controls (left, light gray) and suicides (right, dark gray). Note that, while the number of neurons (stained for Nissl substance) is not different between groups, the number of serotonergic neurons is higher in the DRN of suicide victims. DRN: dorsal raphé nucleus.

Within the raphé nuclei, serotonin neuron firing and therefore serotonin release are negatively regulated by 5-HT_{1A} somatodendritic inhibitory autoreceptors (see review by Sibille and Hen, 2001). Altered autoinhibition at the 5-HT_{1A} receptor in the brain-stem raphé nuclei might be a contributing mechanism to reduced serotonergic neurotransmission in PFC in suicides and patients with depression. Initial in vivo positron emission tomography (PET) studies report lower brainstem 5-HT_{1A} receptor binding in depression (Drevets et al., 1999; Sargent et al., 2000), an effect that is likely to enhance serotonergic activity through reduced autoinhibition, perhaps as a homeostatic mechanism. Using PET, our group recently demonstrated that there is no difference in the binding potential of patients with MDD versus controls, although patients that were medication naïve had higher 5-HT_{1A} receptor binding potential than those exposed to antidepressants and normal controls (Parsey et al., 2006) in cortical regions and in the brain stem. The patients with MDD were more likely to possess the higher expressing G allele of the C-1019G 5-HT_{1A} receptor gene promoter polymorphism than controls, which may have contributed to higher levels of 5-HT_{1A} receptor BP. Although we studied suicides with MDD, not MDD per se, the in vivo findings in the brain stem appear to counter our postmortem findings, as suicides have fourfold higher GG genotypes compared to controls (Lemonde et al., 2003), yet we report a reduction in total binding in the DRN of suicides (Arango, Underwood, Boldrini, et al., 2001; Boldrini et al., 2007). In contrast to our findings, 5-HT_{1A} autoreceptor levels were reported to be elevated in the midbrain of suicides (Stockmeier et al., 1998). These discrepant findings were reconciled in our recent work (Boldrini et al., 2007) showing more 5-HT_{1A} receptors in the rostral part of the DRN in suicides and lower binding in the remaining caudal 15 mm (~75% of the DRN), for a net decrease in binding throughout the DRN. Stockmeier et al. (1998) examined the most rostral 5 mm of the DRN and, like our study (Boldrini et al., 2007), found an increase in binding. Another determining factor may be found in the sex composition of the study cohorts. We find that females have significantly higher 5-HT_{1A} binding than males (Arango, Underwood, Boldrini, et al., 2001), a finding replicated by our group in vivo with PET (Parsey et al., 2002).

POSTMORTEM NORADRENERGIC CORRELATES OF SUICIDE AND DEPRESSION

The catecholamine hypothesis of depression proposes impaired NA transmission as the basic neurochemical defect. There is a paucity of data on the NA system in brain of patients with depression (Birkmayer and Riederer, 1975). We have reported higher β-adrenergic binding (without distinguishing β_1 and β_2 subtypes) in the frontal cortex of violent suicides (Arango et al., 1990). Based on psychological autopsy, approximately 60% of suicides in our sample have a major depression around the time of suicide. Biegon and Israeli (1988) also found higher B_{max} and no change in K_D in β-adrenergic binding in multiple brain regions of suicides, whereas De Paermentier et al. (1990) and others (Stockmeier and Meltzer, 1991) did not find higher β_1-adrenergic binding. Little et al. (1993) found less ^{125}I-pindolol binding in suicides. More recently we found less high-affinity β_1-adrenoreceptor binding in localized areas of the PFC (Fig. 33.1D), and hypothesize that the previously reported increase in nonselective β-adrenergic binding may be due to the β_2-subtype, although this remains to be directly tested. As most studies do not separately report on patients with major depression, it is not clear whether observed changes in β-adrenergic binding are associated with major depression or suicide. However, less high-affinity β_1-adrenergic receptor binding could contribute to reduced NA transmission if the receptor change is primary and would be consistent with the catecholamine hypothesis of depression. An alternative formulation is that β_1-adrenergic binding is reduced because of down-regulation due to NA overactivity, a potential consequence of increased norepinephrine (NE) release in response to stress. Animal studies report that maternal deprivation can heighten stress responses in adulthood as evidenced by higher cortisol and NE release (Barr et al., 2004; Pryce et al., 2004; Levine, 2005).

We found elevated α_1-adrenergic binding (Fig. 33.1E) in a layer of dorsolateral PFC (Arango, Ernsberger, et al., 1993). Consistent with Gross-Isseroff et al. (1990), who found less binding in presumably other cortical areas in suicides, we also found that binding appears lower in ventral PFC. In contrast, we previously found less α_2-binding by autoradiography of the dorsolateral PFC (Fig. 33.1F), but this requires confirmation in a larger series of cases (Arango, Ernsberger, et al., 1993). However, others (Klimek et al., 1999) found no differences, whereas García-Sevilla's group (Meana and García-Sevilla, 1987) reported greater α_2-adrenergic homogenate binding from an unspecified area of frontal cortex, emphasizing the need for comparing results from similar brain regions using the same ligands. They also examined α_2-adrenoreceptor protein immunolabeling and mRNA expression in suicides and showed that the immunolabeling of α_2-receptor in the PFC was higher in suicides (Garcia-Sevilla et al., 1999). A subsequent publication (Escriba et al., 2004) reported higher mRNA levels for α_2-receptors in the PFC of suicides and found a correlation between α_2-receptor mRNA and the protein measured by immunolabeling, suggesting that higher protein is related to increased transcription. Ordway et al. (Ordway, Widdowson, et al., 1994) found elevated α_2-adrenergic agonist binding to autoreceptors in the locus coeruleus (LC) of suicides. This may be secondary up-regulation due to deficient NE release from the LC because less autoreceptor binding would favor higher firing rates and more NE release. Studies, largely confined to nonviolent suicides, have reported no change in NE levels (Bourne et al., 1968; Pare et al., 1969), but we found increased NE levels in the PFC of violent suicides (Arango et al., 1990). This finding must be considered in the context of reports of more tyrosine hydroxylase (TH) immunoreactivity and more α_2-binding in the LC of suicides with depression (Ordway, Smith, et al., 1994) and less NE transporter (NET; Ordway, Widdowson, et al., 1994; Klimek et al., 1997; Ordway et al., 1997). The Ordway group also reported higher TH-immunoreactivity along the rostro-caudal axis of the LC of suicides compared to controls (Zhu et al., 1999). Others report less TH immunoreactivity in the LC neurons in suicides, as measured by optical density (Biegon and Fieldust, 1992) and in depressed, nonsuicide cases (Baumann, Danos, Diekmann, et al., 1999). When comparing suicides with bipolar and unipolar depression, we find less TH-IR in the bipolar group, compared to unipolar suicides and controls (Wiste et al.,

2008). All bipolar suicides in this study, except one, died during the depressed phase of the illness, and the patients who were manic at the time of death had much higher TH-IR than any other patient (Wiste et al., in press). Contrary reports notwithstanding, the possible scenario of greater TH enzyme activity and fewer NET sites suggests increased NA activity and may be a consequence of an excess NE release leading to deficiency or depletion. A deficiency in NA activity may be the consequence of previous excessive NA output, as seen in stress models in adult rodent studies, particularly after adverse childhood-rearing experiences. Other cortical measures are consistent with a recent increase in NA activity, such as secondary cortical β_1-adrenoreceptor and perhaps α_2-adrenoreceptor down-regulation. However, the attribution of changes in the NA system to suicide versus a depressive illness remains to be determined. The studies by Ordway and colleagues (Ordway, Smith, and Haycock, 1994) have largely been in suicides with major depression. Most other studies have not distinguished between suicides with and without a recent episode of major depression. Hence, it is not possible to distinguish biochemical changes associated with major depression from those associated with suicide.

In summary, there is evidence of NA overactivity, based on higher cortical NE levels and less high affinity β-adrenergic receptor binding. More α_1- and less α_2-adrenergic binding will also affect NA transmission in the cortex. Depletion of LC stores of NE may trigger a compensatory increase in NE synthesis and reduction in LC NET sites. The presence of fewer NA neurons may mean that the functional reserve of the NA system is lower in suicide and/or major depression; therefore, there is greater likelihood of NA depletion in the face of severe or prolonged stress. The cause of this increase in NA activity is unknown, but it could be a response to the stress of the depressive illness. Moreover, in the case of suicides with depression there is the additional stress of feeling suicidal. The NA response to stress may be greater in those with an adverse experience in childhood who are then at greater risk in adulthood for major depression (Heim and Nemeroff, 2001) and suicidal acts (Brodsky et al., 2001).

MORPHOMETRIC STUDIES OF THE LOCUS COERULEUS

We found 23% fewer LC neurons and 38% lower density of pigmented LC neurons in suicides with depression (Arango et al., 1996) compared with controls (Fig. 33.5). The difference in neuron number was localized to the rostral two thirds of the LC. Neither the LC length nor the LC volume in suicides with depression differed from controls. Altered brain NA neurotransmission in suicides with depression appears associated with fewer NA neurons in the LC. These neurons may be hyperactive in response to the stress of major depression or suicidal feelings (Ordway, Smith, and Haycock, 1994; Ordway, Widdowson, et al., 1994; Ordway, 1997). Further studies are needed to determine whether this NA neuron deficit is associated with an underlying major depression or specifically with suicidal behavior. Subtype of mood disorder may be relevant. For example, Baumann, Danos, Krell, et al. (1999) found that patients with bipolar disorder had significantly more LC neurons, compared with patients with unipolar depression, suggesting that polarity of affective illness may have an impact on brain-stem morphology. Morphometric studies should be combined with receptor and biochemical assays (Ordway, Smith, and Haycock, 1994) as the latter greatly enhance the available information regarding functional status.

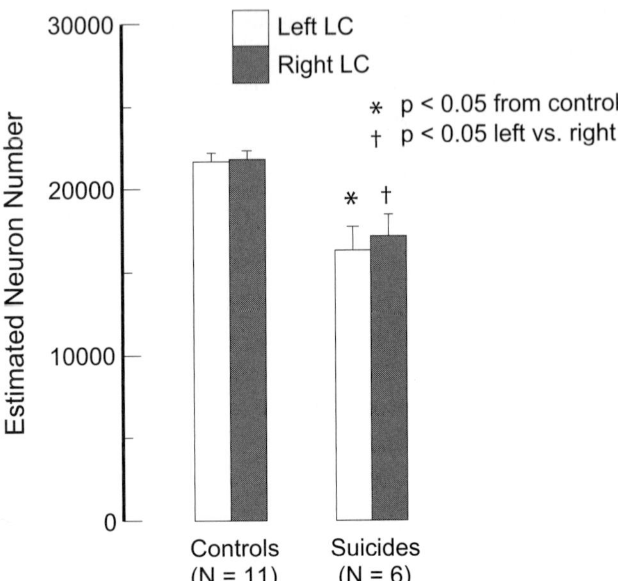

FIGURE 33.5 Estimated total number of pigmented neurons in the left and right locus coeruleus (LC) in controls and suicide victims. Note that the total number of pigmented neurons was significantly reduced in the suicide group. The number of LC neurons was symmetrical in the left and right LC of controls. In suicides, however, there were significantly fewer pigmented neurons in the left than right LC.

Morphological Studies of the Cerebral Cortex

Reports indicate that there is an increased density of neurons and reduced neuropil in the PFC of individuals with schizophrenia (Selemon et al., 1995; Rajkowska et al., 1998). Before examining the integrity of cortical neurons and glia in mood disorders, Dr. Goldman-Rakic and colleagues pioneered morphometric studies in normal cortex (Rajkowska and Goldman-Rakic, 1995a, 1995b), providing a guide for structural and functional in vivo imaging studies by producing a detailed mapping of PFC (BA 9 and 46) in Talairach space (Talairach and Tournoux, 1988). Rajkowska's group (Rajkowska et al., 1999) reported neuronal and glial alterations in the orbitofrontal cortex of individuals with MDD, mostly restricted to the rostral aspect (BA10). They found a 12% reduction in cortical thickness, accompanied by an overall reduction in glial density and a 20%–60% reduction in the density of "large" cortical neurons (reviewed in Rajkowska, 2002). The same group reported a 30% reduction in packing density of pyramidal neurons in the orbital cortex of elderly depressed (Rajkowska et al., 2005).

To investigate possible cytoarchitectonic alterations that may explain the changes in receptor binding in the ventral PFC observed in suicide, we used three-dimensional unbiased stereology to estimate the density of neurons in the same areas where the receptor binding was measured (Arango, Underwood, Le, et al., 2001; Arango et al., 2002). Combining receptor binding and neuron density, we calculated an index of receptor binding per neuron: (fmol/mg tissue)/(neurons/mm^3). Ventral PFC (right hemisphere) was analyzed in 15 pairs of matched suicides and controls, all psychiatrically characterized. We found neuron density to be lower in suicides with depression.

A review of structural imaging data found that results suggest smaller volume of the PFC in major depression (Soares and Mann, 1997a). Functional imaging data are even more convincing regarding hypofunction of the PFC (Rubin et al., 1995; Drevets et al., 1997; Mayberg, 1997; Drevets, 2000; Milak et al., 2005). Therefore, it is of particular importance to pursue the morphometric studies of the PFC. No functional imaging method can match the image resolution of postmortem light microscopy, electron microscopy and film-based autoradiography of receptor binding, and in situ hybridization histochemistry. Studies of this kind should include individuals with major depression dying from causes other than suicide to clearly distinguish the neurochemistry of major depression. Such studies are rarely performed and are a priority.

Hypothalamic-Pituitary-Adrenal Axis

A great deal of work on depression and suicide has focused on the hypothalamic-pituitary-adrenal (HPA) axis (Bunney et al., 1969; Carroll et al., 1981; Nemeroff et al., 1988; Mann and Currier, 2006). Hypercortisolism is a well-documented abnormality in mood disorders (Carroll, Curtis, Davies, et al., 1976; Carroll, Curtis, and Mendels, 1976; Coryell et al., 2006). Suicides have heavier adrenal glands than individuals who die by other causes (Szigethy et al., 1994), higher levels of corticotropin-releasing hormone (CRH) in the CSF (Arato et al., 1989) and fewer CRH receptors in the cortex (Nemeroff et al., 1988; Nemeroff et al., 1992). Patients with major depression also show adrenal gland hypertrophy by computerized tomography (Nemeroff et al., 1992) and more CRH-synthesizing neurons and mRNA in the paraventricular hypothalamic nucleus (Raadsheer et al., 1994; Raadsheer et al., 1995).

A hypothesized breakdown in cortisol feedback on CRH secretion at the level of the hypothalamus, perhaps due to hippocampal damage, has little direct experimental data support. Structural magnetic resonance imaging (MRI) studies of reduced hippocampal volume in individuals with major depression are suggestive (Sheline et al., 1996; Sheline et al., 1999; Bremner et al., 2000; Sheline, 2000), especially following traumatic brain injury (Jorge et al., 2007), but not conclusive (see Soares and Mann, 1997b; Sala et al., 2004). Studies in elderly individuals with depression showed that the hippocampal volume reduction seen in this population was not associated with increased cortisol level, but correlated with memory deficits (O'Brien et al., 2004). Lyons and colleagues (2001) examined the effects of early life stressors and inherited variation in hippocampal volume of monkeys. They concluded that small hippocami were more the result of an inherited characteristic than the result of cortisol-induced volume loss. Postmortem studies in individuals with depression have demonstrated atrophy of the PFC and hippocampus, as indicated by fewer neurons and glia, smaller size and/or lower cell density and dendritic length (Sheline et al., 1996; Benes et al., 1998; Öngür et al., 1998; Rajkowska et al., 1999; Sheline et al., 1999; Rajkowska, 2000; Sapolsky, 2000; Arango et al., 2002).

Extra Hypothalamic CRH System

Corticotropin-releasing hormone neurons are localized in brain areas other than the hypothalamus in several species (Fischman and Moldow, 1982; Cote et al., 1983), including nonhuman primates (Foote and Cha, 1988; Lewis et al., 1989), and humans (Pammer et al., 1990; Austin et al., 1995). We were the first to describe a group of CRH immunoreactive neurons in the peduculo pontine tegmental nucleus and laterodorsal complex in the brain stem of the human that also expressed CRH mRNA (Arango, Rice, et al., 1993; Austin et al., 1995). These neurons are in a position close to the LC, the DRN and MRN, and the substantia nigra, all monoaminergic nuclei that are differentially innervated by CRH axons (Austin et al., 1995; Austin et al., 1997; Ruggiero et al., 1999). The specificity of this anatomical localization may dictate the differential influence that CRH may exert on a specific neurotransmitter system. No studies have quantified these brain-stem CRH neurons. Light microscopy immunocytochemical studies suggest that CRH neuronal processes terminate on DRN serotonergic neurons and on NA neurons (Arango, Rice, et al., 1993; Austin et al., 1997; Ruggiero et al., 1999) and, if so, are uniquely situated to modulate monoaminergic function. These studies will help complete the picture in terms of this major neurohumoral stress–response system.

CONCLUSIONS

Considerable new information has emerged from postmortem brain studies implicating altered serotonergic, NA, and HPA function in major depression and suicide. These findings should be considered in the context of in vivo studies of these systems in patients who are depressed and remitted. In vivo studies suggest that serotonergic abnormalities may be a stable trait reflecting the vulnerability to recurrent episodes of major depression, whereas NA changes are at least partly mood state-dependent. HPA axis dysfunction is also partly state-dependent, although enlargement of the pituitary and adrenal glands, and hippocampal atrophy, may persist between episodes and originate in childhood adversity. Functional and structural imaging studies will be able to bridge postmortem brain studies and in vivo studies involving cerebrospinal fluid and neuroendocrine challenge techniques by allowing quantitative imaging of neurotransmitter systems in vivo. This kind of approach will allow determination of state- and trait-dependent changes related to the pathogenesis of mood disorders. Monitoring of effects of antidepressant treatments will permit identification of actions critical for a clinical response, and thereby aid the clinician, as well as assist in the design of better treatments. Because the data generated by postmortem studies evaluate the brain at one point in time (namely at death), the data offer a high-resolution picture of brain structure and function that cannot distinguish between state and trait, pathogenesis, or treatment effects. Hence, these studies must be interpreted in the context of data from in vivo longitudinal studies that can make these distinctions.

ACKNOWLEDGMENTS
This work was supported by NIMH grants MH40210, MH62185 and NIAAA grant AA09004.

REFERENCES

Agren, H. (1980) Symptom patterns in unipolar and bipolar depression correlating with monoamine metabolites in the cerebrospinal fluid: II. Suicide. *Psychiatry Res.* 3:225–236.

American Psychiatric Association. (1987) *Diagnostic and Statistical Manual of Mental Disorders*, 3rd ed., rev. Washington, DC: American Psychiatric Association.

Arango, V., Ernsberger, P., Marzuk, P.M., Chen, J.S., Tierney, H., Stanley, M., Reis, D.J., and Mann, J.J. (1990) Autoradiographic demonstration of increased serotonin 5-HT2 and beta-adrenergic receptor binding sites in the brain of suicide victims. *Arch. Gen. Psychiatry* 47:1038–1047.

Arango, V., Ernsberger, P., Sved, A.F., and Mann, J.J. (1993) Quantitative autoradiography of alpha 1- and alpha 2-adrenergic receptors in the cerebral cortex of controls and suicide victims. *Brain Res.* 630:271–282.

Arango, V., Huang, Y.Y., Underwood, M.D., and Mann, J.J. (2003) Genetics of the serotonergic system in suicidal behavior. *J. Psychiatry Res.* 37:375–386.

Arango, V., and Mann, J.J. (1992) Relevance of serotonergic postmortem studies to suicidal behavior. *Int. Rev. Psychiatry* 4:131–140.

Arango, V., Rice, P.M., Smith, R.W., Austin, M.C., and Mann, J.J. (1993) Immunocytochemical localization of corticotropin-releasing factor in the human brainstem. *Society for Neuroscience Abstracts* 19:1148.

Arango, V., and Underwood, M.D. (1997) Serotonin chemistry in the brain of suicide victims. In: Maris, R., Silverman, M., Canetto, S., eds. *Review of Suicidology*. New York: Guilford Press, pp. 237–250.

Arango, V., Underwood, M.D., Bakalian, M.J., Kassir, S.A., Ellis, S.P., and Mann, J.J. (2004) Widespread 5-HT1A binding increase in suicide but not in major depression or alcoholism. *Society for Neuroscience Abstracts*.

Arango, V., Underwood, M.D., Boldrini, M., Tamir, H., Kassir, S.A., Hsiung, S., Chen, J.J.X., and Mann, J.J. (2001) Serotonin 1A receptors, serotonin transporter binding and serotonin transporter mRNA expression in the brainstem of depressed suicide victims. *Neuropsychopharmacology* 25:892–903.

Arango, V., Underwood, M.D., Gubbi, A.V., and Mann, J.J. (1995) Localized alterations in pre- and postsynaptic serotonin binding sites in the ventrolateral prefrontal cortex of suicide victims. *Brain Res.* 688:121–133.

Arango, V., Underwood, M.D., Kassir, S.A., Bakalian, M.J., Ellis, S.P., Oppenheim, S., and Mann, J.J. (1998, Dec 14–18) *Revisiting serotonin 5-HT$_{1A}$ binding in prefrontal cortex of suicide victims.* Paper presented at the ACNP 37th Annual Meeting, Las Croabas, Puerto Rico.

Arango, V., Underwood, M.D., Le, E., Johnson, V.L., Kassir, S.A., and Mann, J.J. (2001, Dec 9–13) *Suicide victims have lower neuronal density, decreased 5-HT innervation and higher 5-HT$_{1A}$ and 5-HT$_{2A}$ receptor binding per neuron than controls in orbital prefrontal cortex.* Paper presented at the ACNP 40th Annual Meeting, Waikoloa, Hawaii.

Arango, V., Underwood, M.D., and Mann, J.J. (1996) Fewer pigmented locus coeruleus neurons in suicide victims: preliminary results. *Biol. Psychiatry* 39:112–120.

Arango, V., Underwood, M.D., and Mann, J.J. (2002) Serotonin brain circuits involved in major depression and suicide. In: Azmitia, E.C., DeFelipe, J., Jones, E.G., Rakic, P., Ribak, C.E., ed. *Changing Views of Cajal's Neuron*. Amsterdam: Elsevier, pp. 443–453.

Arango, V., Underwood, M.D., and Mann, J.J. (2003, Dec 7–11) *Serotonin and neuropeptide circuitry in depression and suicide.* Paper presented at the ACNP 42nd Annual Meeting, San Juan, Puerto Rico.

Arato, M., Banki, C.M., Bissette, G., and Nemeroff, C.B. (1989) Elevated CSF CRF in suicide victims. *Biol. Psychiatry* 25:355–359.

Arora, R.C., and Meltzer, H.Y. (1991) Laterality and 3H-imipramine binding: studies in the frontal cortex of normal controls and suicide victims. *Biol. Psychiatry* 29:1016–1022.

Arranz, B., Eriksson, A., Mellerup, E., Plenge, P., and Marcusson, J. (1994) Brain 5-HT1A, 5-HT1D, and 5-HT2 receptors in suicide victims. *Biol. Psychiatry* 35:457–463.

Åsberg, M., Träskman, L., and Thorén, P. (1976) 5-HIAA in the cerebrospinal fluid. A biochemical suicide predictor? *Arch. Gen. Psychiatry* 33:1193–1197.

Austin, M.C., Rhodes, J.L., and Lewis, D.A. (1997) Differential distribution of corticotropin-releasing hormone immunoreactive axons in monoaminergic nuclei of the human brainstem. *Neuropsychopharmacology* 17:326–341.

Austin, M.C., Rice, P.M., Mann, J.J., and Arango, V. (1995) Localization of corticotropin-releasing hormone in the human locus coeruleus and pedunculopontine tegmental nucleus: an immunocytochemical and in situ hybridization study. *Neuroscience* 64: 713–727.

Bach-Mizrachi, H., Underwood, M.D., Kassir, S.A., Bakalian, M.J., Sibille, E., Tamir, H., Mann, J.J., and Arango, V. (2006) Neuronal tryptophan hydroxylase mRNA expression in the human dorsal and median raphe nuclei: major depression and suicide. *Neuropsychopharmacology* 31:814–824.

Baker, K.G., Halliday, G.M., and Tork, I. (1990) Cytoarchitecture of the human dorsal raphe nucleus. *J. Comp. Neurol.* 301:147–161.

Barr, C.S., Newman, T.K., Lindell, S., Becker, M.L., Shannon, C., Champoux, M., Suomi, S.J., and Higley, J.D. (2004) Early experience and sex interact to influence limbic-hypothalamic-pituitary-adrenal-axis function after acute alcohol administration in rhesus macaques (Macaca mulatta). *Alcohol Clin. Exp. Res.* 28: 1114–1119.

Baumann, B., Danos, P., Diekmann, S., Krell, D., Bielau, H., Geretsegger, C., Wurthmann, C., Bernstein, H.-G., and Bogerts, B. (1999) Tyrosine hydroxylase immunoreactivity in the locus coeruleus is reduced in depressed non-suicidal patients but normal in depressed suicide patients. *Eur. Arch. Psychiatry Clin. Neurosci.* 249:212–219.

Baumann, B., Danos, P., Krell, D., Diekmann, S., Wurthmann, C., Bielau, H., Bernstein, H.G., and Bogerts, B. (1999) Unipolar-bipolar dichotomy of mood disorders is supported by noradrenergic brainstem system morphology. *J. Affect. Disord.* 54:217–224.

Benes, F.M., Kwok, E.W., Vincent, S.L., and Todtenkopf, M.S. (1998) A reduction of nonpyramidal cells in sector CA2 of schizophrenics and manic depressives. *Biol. Psychiatry* 44:88–97.

Beskow, J., Gottfries, C.G., Roos, B.E., and Winblad, B. (1976) Determination of monoamine and monoamine metabolites in the human brain: post mortem studies in a group of suicides and in a control group. *Acta Psychiatr. Scand.* 53:7–20.

Biegon, A., and Fieldust, S. (1992) Reduced tyrosine hydroxylase immunoreactivity in locus coeruleus of suicide victims. *Synapse* 10:79–82.

Biegon, A., Grinspoon, A., Blumenfeld, B., Bleich, A., Apter, A., and Mester, R. (1990) Increased serotonin 5-HT2 receptor binding on blood platelets of suicidal men. *Psychopharmacology (Berl)* 100:165–167.

Biegon, A., and Israeli, M. (1988) Regionally selective increases in beta-adrenergic receptor density in the brains of suicide victims. *Brain Res.* 442:199–203.

Birkmayer, W., and Riederer, P. (1975) Biochemical postmortem findings in depressed patients. *J. Neural Transm.* 37:95–109.

Boldrini, M., Underwood, M.D., Mann, J.J., and Arango, V. (2005) More tryptophan hydroxylase in the brainstem dorsal raphe nucleus in depressed suicides. *Brain Res.* 1041:19–28.

Boldrini, M., Underwood, M.D., Mann, J.J., and Arango, V. (2007) Serotonin-1A autoreceptor binding in the dorsal raphe nucleus of depressed suicides. *Psychiatry Res.* 42(6):433–442.

Bonkale, W.L., Murdock, S., Janosky, J.E., and Austin, M.C. (2004) Normal levels of tryptophan hydroxylase immunoreactivity in the dorsal raphe of depressed suicide victims. *J. Neurochem.* 88: 958–964.

Bonkale, W.L., Turecki, G., and Austin, M.C. (2006) Increased tryptophan hydroxylase immunoreactivity in the dorsal raphe nucleus of alcohol-dependent, depressed suicide subjects is restricted to the dorsal subnucleus. *Synapse* 60:81–85.

Bourne, H.R., Bunney, W.E., Jr., Colburn, R.W., Davis, J.M., Shaw, D.M., and Coppen, A.J. (1968) Noradrenaline, 5-hydroxytryptamine, and 5-hydroxyindoleacetic acid in hindbrains of suicidal patients. *Lancet* 2(7572):805–808.

Bremner, J.D., Narayan, M., Anderson, E.R., Staib, L.H., Miller, H.L., and Charney, D.S. (2000) Hippocampal volume reduction in major depression. *Am. J. Psychiatry* 157:115–118.

Brodsky, B.S., Oquendo, M.A., Ellis, S.P., Haas, G.L., Malone, K.M., and Mann, J.J. (2001) The relationship of childhood abuse to impulsivity and suicidal behavior in adults with major depression. *Am. J. Psychiatry* 158:1871–1877.

Brown, G.L., Goodwin, F.K., and Bunney, W.E., Jr. (1982) Human aggression and suicide: their relationship to neuropsychiatric diagnoses and serotonin metabolism. *Adv. Biochem. Psychopharmacol.* 34:287–307.

Bunney, W.E., Jr., Fawcett, J.A., Davis, J.M., and Gifford, S. (1969) Further evaluation of urinary 17-hydroxycorticosteroids in suicidal patients. *Arch. Gen. Psychiatry* 21:138–150.

Carroll, B.J., Curtis, G.C., Davies, B.M., Mendels, J., and Sugerman, A.A. (1976) Urinary free cortisol excretion in depression. *Psychol. Med.* 6:43–50.

Carroll, B.J., Curtis, G.C., and Mendels, J. (1976) Cerebrospinal fluid and plasma free cortisol concentrations in depression. *Psychol. Med.* 6:235–244.

Carroll, B.J., Greden, J.F., and Feinberg, M. (1981) Suicide, neuroendocrine dysfunction and CSF 5-H1AA concentrations in depression. In: Angris, B., ed. *Recent Advances in Neuropsychopharmacology: Selected Papers from the 12th Congress of the Collegium Internationale Neuro-Psychopharmacologicum, Ghoteborg, Sweden, 22-26 June 1980.* New York: Pergamon Press Oxford, pp. 307–313.

Coccaro, E.F., Siever, L.J., Klar, H.M., Maurer, G., Cochrane, K., Cooper, T.B., Mohs, R.C., and Davis, K.L. (1989) Serotonergic studies in patients with affective and personality disorders. Correlates with suicidal and impulsive aggressive behavior. *Arch. Gen. Psychiatry* 46:587–599.

Coryell, W., Young, E., and Carroll, B. (2006) Hyperactivity of the hypothalamic-pituitary-adrenal axis and mortality in major depressive disorder. *Psychiatry Res.* 142:99–104.

Cote, J., Lefevre, G., Labrie, F., and Barden, N. (1983) Distribution of corticotropin-releasing factor in ovine brain determined by radioimmunoassay. *Regl. Pept.* 5:189–195.

Crow, T.J., Cross, A.J., Cooper, S.J., Deakin, J.F.W., Ferrier, I.N., Johnson, J.A., Joseph, M.H., Owen, F., Poulter, M., Lofthouse, R., Corsellis, J.A.N., Chambers, D.R., Blessed, G., Perry, E.K., Perry, R.H., and Tomlinson, B.E. (1984) Neurotransmitter receptors and monoamine metabolites in the brains of patients with Alzheimer-type dementia and depression, and suicides. *Neuropharmacology* 23:1561–1569.

De Luca, V., Likhodi, O., Van Tol, H.H., Kennedy, J.L., and Wong, A.H. (2005) Tryptophan hydroxylase 2 gene expression and promoter polymorphisms in bipolar disorder and schizophrenia. *Psychopharmacology (Berl)* 183(3):378–382.

De Luca, V., Likhodi, O., Van Tol, H.H., Kennedy, J.L., and Wong, A.H. (2006) Gene expression of tryptophan hydroxylase 2 in postmortem brain of suicide subjects. *Int. J. Neuropsychopharmacol.* 9(1):21–25.

De Paermentier, F., Cheetham, S.C., Crompton, M.R., Katona, C.L.E., and Horton, R.W. (1990) Brain b-adrenoceptor binding sites in antidepressant-free depressed suicide victims. *Brain Res.* 525: 71–77.

Delgado, P.L., Charney, D.S., Price, L.H., Aghajanian, G.K., Landis, H., and Heninger, G.R. (1990) Serotonin function and the mechanism of antidepressant action. Reversal of antidepressant-induced remission by rapid depletion of plasma tryptophan. *Arch. Gen. Psychiatry* 47:411–418.

Delgado, P.L., Price, L.H., Miller, H.L., Salomon, R.M., Aghajanian, G.K., Heninger, G.R., and Charney, D.S. (1994) Serotonin and the neurobiology of depression. Effects of tryptophan depletion in drug-free depressed patients. *Arch. Gen. Psychiatry* 51:865–874.

Dillon, K.A., Gross-Isseroff, R., Israeli, M., and Biegon, A. (1991) Autoradiographic analysis of serotonin 5-HT_{1A} receptor binding in the human brain postmortem: Effects of age and alcohol. *Brain Res.* 554:56–64.

Dorph-Petersen, K.-A., Nyengaard, J.R., Rosenberg, R., and Gundersen, H.J.G. (2001) No change in serotonergic neuron number and volume in the human dorsal raphe in depression but observation of a pronounced sexual dismorphism - A stereological study using unbiased principles. *Society for Neuroscience Abstracts*. 27.

Drevets, W.C. (2000) Neuroimaging studies of mood disorders. *Biol. Psychiatry* 48:813–829.

Drevets, W.C., Frank, E., Price, J.C., Kupfer, D.J., Holt, D., Greer, P.J., Huang, Y., Gautier, C., and Mathis, C. (1999) PET imaging of serotonin 1A receptor binding in depression. *Biol. Psychiatry* 46:1375–1387.

Drevets, W.C., Price, J.L., Simpson, J.R., Jr., Todd, R.D., Reich, T., Vannier, M., and Raichle, M.E. (1997) Subgenual prefrontal cortex abnormalities in mood disorders. *Nature* 386:824–827.

Escriba, P.V., Ozaita, A., and Garcia-Sevilla, J.A. (2004) Increased mRNA expression of alpha2A-adrenoceptors, serotonin receptors and mu-opioid receptors in the brains of suicide victims. *Neuropsychopharmacology* 29:1512–1521.

Fairbanks, L.A., Jorgensen, M.J., Huff, A., Blau, K., Hung, Y.Y., and Mann, J.J. (2004) Adolescent impulsivity predicts adult dominance attainment in male vervet monkeys. *Am. J. Primatol.* 64: 1–17.

Ferrier, I.N., McKeith, I.G., Cross, A.J., Perry, E.K., Candy, J.M., and Perry, R.H. (1986) Postmortem neurochemical studies in depression. *Ann. N. Y. Acad. Sci.* 487:128–142.

Fischman, A.J., and Moldow, R.L. (1982) Extrahypothalamic distribution of CRF-like immunoreactivity in the rat brain. *Peptides* 1:149–153.

Flory, J.D., Mann, J.J., Manuck, S.B., and Muldoon, M.F. (1998) Recovery from major depression is not associated with normalization of serotonergic function. *Biol. Psychiatry* 43:320–326.

Foote, S.L., and Cha, C.I. (1988) Distribution of corticotropin-releasing-factor-like immunoreactivity in brainstem of two monkey species (*Saimiri sciureus and Macaca fascicularis*): An immunohistochemical study. *J. Comp. Neurol.* 276:239–264.

Garcia-Sevilla, J.A., Escriba, P.V., Ozaita, A., La Harpe, R., Walzer, C., Eytan, A., and Guimon, J. (1999) Up-regulation of immunolabeled alpha2A-adrenoceptors, Gi coupling proteins, and regulatory receptor kinases in the prefrontal cortex of depressed suicides. *J. Neurochem.* 72:282–291.

Gross-Isseroff, R., Dillon, K.A., Fieldust, S.J., and Biegon. A. (1990) Autoradiographic analysis of a_1-noradrenergic receptors in the human brain postmortem. *Arch. Gen. Psychiatry* 47:1049–1053.

Gross-Isseroff, R., Israeli, M., and Biegon, A. (1989) Autoradiographic analysis of tritiated imipramine binding in the human brain post mortem: effects of suicide. *Arch. Gen. Psychiatry* 46:237–241.

Heim, C., and Nemeroff, C.B. (2001) The role of childhood trauma in the neurobiology of mood and anxiety disorders: preclinical and clinical studies. *Biol. Psychiatry* 49:1023–1039.

Higley, J.D., Thompson, W.W., Champoux, M., Goldman, D., Hasert, M.F., Kraemer, G.W., Scanlan, J.M., Suomi, S.J., and Linnoila, M. (1993) Paternal and maternal genetic and environmental contributions to cerebrospinal fluid monoamine metabolites in Rhesus monkeys (Macaca mulatta). *Arch. Gen. Psychiatry* 50:615–623.

Hrdina, P.D., and Du, L. (2001) Levels of serotonin receptor 2A higher in suicide victims? *Am. J. Psychiatry* 158:147–148.

Jorge, R.E., Acion, L., Starkstein, S.E., and Magnotta, V. (2007) Hippocampal volume and mood disorders after traumatic brain injury. *Biol. Psychiatry* 62:332–338.

Joyce, J.N., Shane, A., Lexow, N., Winokur, A., Casanova, M.F., and Kleinman, J.E. (1993) Serotonin uptake sites and serotonin receptors are altered in the limbic system of schizophrenics. *Neuropsychopharmacology* 8:315–336.

Kelly, T.M., and Mann, J.J. (1996) Validity of DSM-III-R diagnosis by psychological autopsy: a comparison with clinician ante-mortem diagnosis. *Acta Psychiatr. Scand.* 94:337–343.

Klimek, V., Rajkowska, G., Luker, S.N., Dilley, G., Meltzer, H.Y., Overholser, J.C., Stockmeier, C.A., and Ordway, G.A. (1999) Brain noradrenergic receptors in major depression and schizophrenia. *Neuropsychopharmacology* 21:69–81.

Klimek, V., Stockmeier, C.A., Overholser, J., Meltzer, H.Y., Kalka, S., Dilley, G., and Ordway, G.A. (1997) Reduced levels of norepinephrine transporters in the locus coeruleus in major depression. *J. Neurosci.* 17:8451–8458.

Korpi, E.R., Kleinman, J., Goodman, S.I., Phillips, I., DeLisi, L.E., Linnoila, M., and Wyatt, R.J. (1986) Serotonin and 5-hydroxyindoleacetic acid in brains of suicide victims. Comparison in chronic schizophrenic patients with suicide as cause of death. *Arch. Gen. Psychiatry* 43:594–600.

Lawrence, K.M., De Paermentier, F., Cheetham, S.C., Crompton, M.R., Katona, C.L.E., and Horton, R.W. (1990) Symmetrical hemispheric distribution of ^{3}H-paroxetine binding sites in postmortem human brain from controls and suicides. *Biol. Psychiatry* 28: 544–546.

Lemonde, S., Turecki, G., Bakish, D., Du, L., Hrdina, P.D., Bown, C.D., Sequeira, A., Kushwaha, N., Morris, S.J., Basak, A., Ou, X.M., and Albert, P.R. (2003) Impaired repression at a 5-hydroxytryptamine 1A receptor gene polymorphism associated with major depression and suicide. *J. Neurosci.* 23:8788–8799.

Levine, S. (2005) Developmental determinants of sensitivity and resistance to stress. *Psychoneuroendocrinology* 30:939–946.

Lewis, D.A. (2002) The human brain revisited. Opportunities and challenges in postmortem studies of psychiatric disorders. *Neuropsychopharmacology* 26:143–154.

Lewis, D.A., Foote, S.L., and Cha, C.I. (1989) Corticotropin-releasing factor immunoreactivity in monkey neocortex: An immunohistochemical analysis. *J. Comp. Neurol.* 290:599–613.

Little, K.Y., Clark, T.B., Ranc, J., and Duncan, G.E. (1993) b-Adrenergic receptor binding in frontal cortex from suicide victims. *Biol. Psychiatry* 34:596–605.

Lloyd, K.G., Farley, I.J., Deck, J.H.N., and Hornykiewicz, O. (1974) Serotonin and 5-hydroxyindoleacetic acid in discrete areas of the brainstem of suicide victims and control patients. *Adv. Biochem. Psychopharmacol.* 11:387–397.

Lowther, S., De Paermentier, F., Cheetham, S.C., Crompton, M.R., Katona, C.L., and Horton, R.W. (1997) 5-HT1A receptor binding sites in post-mortem brain samples from depressed suicides and controls. *J. Affect. Disord.* 42:199–207.

Lyons, D.M., Yang, C., Sawyer-Glover, A.M., Moseley, M.E., and Schatzberg, A.F. (2001) Early life stress and inherited variation in monkey hippocampal volumes. *Arch. Gen. Psychiatry* 58: 1145–1151.

Malone, K.M., Corbitt, E.M., Li, S, and Mann, J.J. (1996) Prolactin response to fenfluramine and suicide attempt lethality in major depression. *Br. J. Psychiatry* 168:324–329.

Mann, J.J. (1998) The neurobiology of suicide. *Nat. Med.* 4:25–30.

Mann, J.J. (2002) A current perspective of suicide and attempted suicide. *Ann. Intern. Med.* 136:302–311.

Mann, J.J. (2003) Neurobiology of suicidal behaviour. *Nat. Rev. Neurosci.* 4:819–828.

Mann, J.J., Arango, V., Marzuk, P.M., Theccanat, S., and Reis, D.J. (1989) Evidence for the 5-HT hypothesis of suicide. A review of post-mortem studies. *Br. J. Psychiatry Suppl* 155 (Suppl 8):7–14.

Mann, J.J., Bortinger, J., Oquendo, M.A., Currier, D., Li, S., and Brent, D.A. (2005) Family history of suicidal behavior and mood disorders in probands with mood disorders. *Am. J. Psychiatry* 162:1672–1679.

Mann, J.J., Brent, D.A., and Arango, V. (2001) The neurobiology and genetics of suicide and attempted suicide: a focus on the serotonergic system. *Neuropsychopharmacology* 24:467–477.

Mann, J.J., and Currier, D. (2006) Effects of genes and stress on the neurobiology of depression. *Int. Rev. Neurobiol.* 73:153–189.

Mann, J.J., and Currier, D. (2007) A review of prospective studies of biologic predictors of suicidal behavior in mood disorders. *Arch. Suicide Res.* 11:3–16.

Mann, J.J., Currier, D., Stanley, B., Oquendo, M.A., Amsel, L.V., and Ellis, S.P. (2006) Can biological tests assist prediction of suicide in mood disorders? *Int. J. Neuropsychopharmacol.* 9:465–474.

Mann, J.J., Henteleff, R.A., Lagattuta, T.F., Perper, J.A., Li, S., and Arango, V. (1996) Lower 3H-paroxetine binding in cerebral cortex of suicide victims is partly due to fewer high affinity, non-transporter sites. *J. Neural Transm.* 103:1337–1350.

Mann, J.J., Huang, Y.Y., Underwood, M.D., Kassir, S.A., Oppenheim, S., Kelly, T.M., Dwork, A.J., and Arango, V. (2000) A serotonin transporter gene promoter polymorphism (5-HTTLPR) and prefrontal cortical binding in major depression and suicide. *Arch. Gen. Psychiatry* 57:729–738.

Mann, J.J., and Malone, K.M. (1997) Cerebrospinal fluid amines and higher-lethality suicide attempts in depressed inpatients. *Biol. Psychiatry* 41:162–171.

Mann, J.J., Malone, K.M., Sweeney, J.A., Brown, R.P., Linnoila, M., Stanley, B., and Stanley, M. (1996) Attempted suicide characteristics and cerebrospinal fluid amine metabolites in depressed inpatients. *Neuropsychopharmacology* 15:576–586.

Mann, J.J., McBride, P.A., Brown, R.P., Linnoila, M., Leon, A.C., DeMeo, M., Mieczkowski, T., Myers, J.E., and Stanley, M. (1992) Relationship between central and peripheral serotonin indexes in depressed and suicidal psychiatric inpatients. *Arch. Gen. Psychiatry* 49:442–446.

Mann, J.J., McBride, P.A., Malone, K.M., DeMeo, M.D., and Keilp, J.G. (1995) Blunted serotonergic responsivity in depressed patients. *Neuropsychopharmacology* 13:53–64.

Mann, J.J., Stanley, M., McBride, P.A., and McEwen, B.S. (1986) Increased serotonin2 and beta-adrenergic receptor binding in the frontal cortices of suicide victims. *Arch. Gen. Psychiatry* 43:954–959.

Mann, J.J., Underwood, M.D., and Arango, V. (1996) Postmortem studies of suicide victims. In: Watson, S.J., ed. *Biology of Schizophrenia and Affective Disease*. Washington, DC: American Psychiatric Press, pp. 197–220.

Matsubara, S., Arora, R.C., and Meltzer, H.Y. (1991) Serotonergic measures in suicide brain: 5-HT1A binding sites in frontal cortex of suicide victims. *J. Neural Transm. Gen. Sect.* 85:181–194.

Mayberg, H.S. (1997) Limbic-cortical dysregulation: a proposed model of depression. *J. Neuropsychiatry Clin. Neurosci.* 9:471–481.

McBride, P.A., Brown, R.P., DeMeo, M., Keilp, J., Mieczkowski, T., and Mann, J.J. (1994) The relationship of platelet 5-HT2 receptor indices to major depressive disorder, personality traits, and suicidal behavior. *Biol. Psychiatry* 35:295–308.

McKeith, I.G., Marshall, E.F., Ferrier, I.N., Armstrong, M.M., Kennedy, W.N., Perry, E.K., and Eccleston, D. (1987) 5-HT receptor binding in post-mortem brain from patients with affective disorder. *J. Affect. Disord.* 13:67–74.

Meana, J.J., and García-Sevilla, J.A. (1987) Increased a_2-adrenoceptor density in the frontal cortex of depressed suicide victims. *J. Neural Transm.* 70:377–381.

Meyerson, L.R., Wennogle, L.P., Abel, M.S., Coupet, J., Lippa, A.S., Rauh, C.E., and Beer, B. (1982) Human brain receptor alterations in suicide victims. *Pharmacol. Biochem. Behav.* 17:159–163.

Milak, M.S., Parsey, R.V., Keilp, J., Oquendo, M.A., Malone, K.M, and Mann, J.J. (2005) Neuroanatomic correlates of psychopathologic components of major depressive disorder. *Arch. Gen. Psychiatry* 62:397–408.

Nemeroff, C.B., Krishnan, K.R., Reed, D., Leder, R., Beam, C., and Dunnick, N.R. (1992) Adrenal gland enlargement in major depression. A computed tomographic study. *Arch. Gen. Psychiatry* 49:384–387.

Nemeroff, C.B., Owens, M.J., Bissette, G., Andorn, A.C., and Stanley, M. (1988) Reduced corticotropin releasing factor binding sites in the frontal cortex of suicide victims. *Arch. Gen. Psychiatry* 45: 577–579.

Nordström, P., Samuelsson, M., Åsberg, M., Träskman-Bendz, L., Aberg-Wistedt, A., Nordin, C., and Bertilsson, L. (1994) CSF 5-HIAA predicts suicide risk after attempted suicide. *Suicide Life Threat. Behav.* 24:1–9.

O'Brien, J.T., Lloyd, A., McKeith, I., Gholkar, A., and Ferrier, N. (2004) A longitudinal study of hippocampal volume, cortisol levels, and cognition in older depressed subjects. *Am. J. Psychiatry* 161:2081–2090.

O'Keane, V., and Dinan, T.G. (1991) Prolactin and cortisol responses to *d*-fenfluramine in major depression: Evidence for diminished responsivity of central serotonergic function. *Am. J. Psychiatry* 148:1009–1015.

Öngür, D., Drevets, W.C., and Price, J.L. (1998) Glial reduction in the subgenual prefrontal cortex in mood disorders. *Proc. Natl. Acad. Sci. USA* 95:13290–13295.

Ono, H., Shirakawa, O., Kitamura, N., Hashimoto, T., Nishiguchi, N., Nishimura, A., Nushida, H., Ueno, Y., and Maeda, K. (2002) Tryptophan hydroxylase immunoreactivity is altered by the genetic variation in postmortem brain samples of both suicide victims and controls. *Mol. Psychiatry* 7:1127–1132.

Ordway, G.A. (1997) Pathophysiology of the locus coeruleus in suicide. *Ann. N. Y. Acad. Sci.* 836:233–252.

Ordway, G.A., Smith, K.S., and Haycock, J.W. (1994) Elevated tyrosine hydroxylase in the locus coeruleus of suicide victims. *J. Neurochem* 62:680–685.

Ordway, G.A., Stockmeier, C.A., Cason, G.W., and Klimek, V. (1997) Pharmacology and distribution of norepinephrine transporters in the human locus coeruleus and raphe nuclei. *J. Neurosci.* 17: 1710–1719.

Ordway, G.A., Widdowson, P.S., Smith, K.S., and Halaris, A. (1994) Agonist binding to a_2-adrenoceptors is elevated in the locus coeruleus from victims of suicide. *J. Neurochem.* 63:617–624.

Owen, F., Chambers, D.R., Cooper, S.J., Crow, T.J., Johnson, J.A., Lofthouse, R., and Poulter, M. (1986) Serotonergic mechanisms in brains of suicide victims. *Brain Res.* 362:185–188.

Pammer, C., Gorcs, T.J., and Palkovits, M. (1990) Peptidergic innervation of the locus coeruleus cells in the human brain. *Brain Res.* 515:247–255.

Pandey, G.N., Dwivedi, Y., Ren, X., Robert, R.C., Conley, R., and Tamminga, C. (2001) Increased 5HT2A receptors and impaired phosphoinositide siginaling in the postmortem brain of suicide victims. In: Miyoshi, K., Shapiro, C.M., Gaviria, M., Morita, Y., eds. *Contemporary Neuropsychiatry*. Tokyo: Springer-Verlag, pp. 314–321.

Pandey, G.N., Dwivedi, Y., Rizavi, H.S., Ren, X., Pandey, S.C., Pesold, C., Roberts, R.C., Conley, R.R., and Tamminga, C.A. (2002) Higher expression of serotonin 5-HT(2A) receptors in the postmortem brains of teenage suicide victims. *Am. J. Psychiatry* 159:419–429.

Pandey, G.N., Pandey, S.C., Dwivedi, Y., Sharma, R.P., Janicak, P.G., and Davis, J.M. (1995) Platelet serotonin-2A receptors: a potential biological marker for suicidal behavior. *Am. J. Psychiatry* 152:850–855.

Pandey, G.N., Pandey, S.C., Janicak, P.G., Marks, R.C., and Davis, J.M. (1990) Platelet serotonin-2 receptor binding sites in depression and suicide. *Biol. Psychiatry* 28:215–222.

Pare, C.M.B., Yeung, D.P.H., Price, K., and Stacey, R.S. (1969) 5-Hydroxytryptamine, noradrenaline, and dopamine in brainstem, hypothalamus, and caudate nucleus of controls and of patients committing suicide by coal-gas poisoning. *Lancet* 2(7612): 133–135.

Parsey, R.V., Oquendo, M.A., Ogden, R.T., Olvet, D.M., Simpson, N., Huang, Y.Y., Van Heertum, R.L., Arango, V., and Mann, J.J. (2006) Altered serotonin 1A binding in major depression: a [carbonyl-C-11]WAY100635 positron emission tomography study. *Biol. Psychiatry* 59:106–113.

Parsey, R.V., Oquendo, M.A., Simpson, N.R., Ogden, R.T., Van Heertum, R., Arango, V., and Mann, J.J. (2002) Effects of sex, age, and aggressive traits in man on brain serotonin 5- HT(1A) receptor binding potential measured by PET using [C-11]WAY-100635. *Brain Res.* 954:173–182.

Paul, S.M., Rehavi, M., Skolnick, P., and Goodwin, F.K. (1984) High affinity binding of antidepressants to a biogenic amine transport site in human brain and platelet; studies in depression. In: Post,

R.M., Bellinger, C.J., eds. *Neurobiology of Mood Disorders*. Baltimore: Williams and Wilkins, pp. 846–853.

Perry, E.K., Marshall, E.F., Blessed, G., Tomlinson, B.E., and Perry, R.H. (1983) Decreased imipramine binding in the brains of patients with depressive illness. *Br. J. Psychiatry* 142:188–192.

Price, L.H., Charney, D.S., Delgado, P.L., and Heninger, G.R. (1991) Serotonin function and depression: neuroendocrine and mood responses to intravenous L-tryptophan in depressed patients and healthy comparison subjects. *Am. J. Psychiatry* 148:1518–1525.

Pryce, C.R., Dettling, A., Spengler, M., Spaete, C., and Feldon, J. (2004) Evidence for altered monoamine activity and emotional and cognitive disturbance in marmoset monkeys exposed to early life stress. *Ann. N. Y. Acad. Sci.* 1032:245–249.

Raadsheer, F.C., Hoogendijk, W.J.G., Stam, F.C., Tilders, F.J.H., and Swaab, D.F. (1994) Increased numbers of corticotropin-releasing hormone expressing neurons in the hypothalamic paraventricular nucleus of depressed patients. *Neuroendocrinology* 60:436–444.

Raadsheer, F.C., Van Heerikhuize, J.J., Lucassen, P.J., Hoogendijk, W.J.G., Tilders, F.J.H., and Swaab, D.F. (1995) Corticotropin-releasing hormone mRNA levels in the paraventricular nucleus of patients with Alzheimer's disease and depression. *Am. J. Psychiatry* 152:1372–1376.

Rajkowska, G. (2000) Postmortem studies in mood disorders indicate altered numbers of neurons and glial cells [Dysfunction in neural circuits involved in the pathophysiology of mood disorders]. *Biol. Psychiatry* 48:766–777.

Rajkowska, G. (2002) Cell pathology in mood disorders. *Semin. Clin. Neuropsychiatry* 7:281–292.

Rajkowska, G., and Goldman-Rakic, P.S. (1995a) Cytoarchitectonic definition of prefrontal areas in the normal human cortex: I. Remapping of areas 9 and 46 using quantitative criteria. *Cereb. Cortex* 5:307–322.

Rajkowska, G., and Goldman-Rakic, P.S. (1995b) Cytoarchitectonic definition of prefrontal areas in the normal human cortex: II. Variability in locations of areas 9 and 46 and relationship to the Talairach Coordinate System. *Cereb. Cortex* 5:323–337.

Rajkowska, G., Miguel-Hidalgo, J.J., Dubey, P., Stockmeier, C.A., and Krishnan, K.R. (2005) Prominent reduction in pyramidal neurons density in the orbitofrontal cortex of elderly depressed patients. *Biol. Psychiatry* 58:297–306.

Rajkowska, G., Miguel-Hidalgo, J.J., Wei, J., Dilley, G., Pittman, S.D., Meltzer, H.Y., Overholser, J.C., Roth, B.L., and Stockmeier, C.A. (1999) Morphometric evidence for neuronal and glial prefrontal cell pathology in major depression. *Biol. Psychiatry* 45:1085–1098.

Rajkowska, G., Selemon, L.D., and Goldman-Rakic, P.S. (1998) Neuronal and glial somal size in the prefrontal cortex. A postmortem morphometric study of schizophrenia and Huntington disease. *Arch. Gen. Psychiatry* 55:215–224.

Rogers, J., Martin, L.J., Comuzzie, A.G., Mann, J.J., Manuck, S.B., Leland, M., and Kaplan, J.R. (2004) Genetics of monoamine metabolites in baboons: overlapping sets of genes influence levels of 5-hydroxyindolacetic acid, 3-hydroxy-4-methoxyphenylglycol, and homovanillic acid. *Biol. Psychiatry* 55:739–744.

Rubin, E., Sackeim, H.A., Prohovnik, I., Moeller, J.R., Schnur, D.B., and Mukherjee, S. (1995) Regional cerebral blood flow in mood disorders: IV. Comparison of mania and depression. *Psychiatry Res.* 61:1–10.

Ruggiero, D.A., Underwood, M.D., Rice, P.M., Mann, J.J., and Arango, V. (1999) Corticotropic-releasing hormone and serotonin interact in the human brainstem: behavioral implications. *Neuroscience* 91:1343–1354.

Sala, M., Perez, J., Soloff, P., Ucelli di Nemi, S., Caverzasi, E., Soares, J.C., and Brambilla, P. (2004) Stress and hippocampal abnormalities in psychiatric disorders. *Eur. Neuropsychopharmacol.* 14: 393–405.

Sapolsky, R.M. (2000) The possibility of neurotoxicity in the hippocampus in major depression: a primer on neuron death. *Biol. Psychiatry* 48:755–765.

Sargent, P.A., Kjaer, K.H., Bench, C.J., Rabiner, E.A., Messa, C., Meyer, J., Gunn, R.N., Grasby, P.M., and Cowen, P.J. (2000) Brain serotonin 1A receptor binding measured by positron emission tomography with [11C]WAY-100635: effects of depression and antidepressant treatment. *Arch. Gen. Psychiatry* 57:174–180.

Selemon, L.D., Rajkowska, G., and Goldman-Rakic, P.S. (1995) Abnormally high neuronal density in the schizophrenic cortex - A morphometric analysis of prefrontal area 9 and occipital area 17. *Arch. Gen. Psychiatry* 52:805–818.

Shamir, A., Shaltiel, G., Levi, I., Belmaker, R.H., and Agam, G. (2005) Postmortem parietal cortex TPH2 expression is not altered in schizophrenic, unipolar-depressed, and bipolar patients vs control subjects. *J. Mol. Neurosci.* 26:33–37.

Shaw, D.M., Camps, F.E., and Eccleston, E.G. (1967) 5-Hydroxytryptamine in the hind-brain of depressive suicides. *Br. J. Psychiatry* 113:1407–1411.

Sheldon, P.W., and Aghajanian, G.K. (1990) Serotonin (5-HT) induces IPSPs in pyramidal layer cells of rat piriform cortex: evidence for the involvement of a 5-HT2-activated interneuron. *Brain Res.* 506: 62–69.

Sheline, Y.I. (2000) 3D MRI studies of neuroanatomic changes in unipolar major depression: the role of stress and medical comorbidity. *Biol. Psychiatry* 48:791–800.

Sheline, Y.I., Sanghavi, M., Mintun, M.A., and Gado, M.H. (1999) Depression duration but not age predicts hippocampal volume loss in medically healthy women with recurrent major depression. *J. Neurosci.* 19:5034–5043.

Sheline, Y.I., Wang, P.W., Gado, M.H., Csernansky, J.G., and Vannier, M.W. (1996) Hippocampal atrophy in recurrent major depression. *Proc. Natl. Acad. Sci. USA* 93:3908–3913.

Sibille, E., and Hen, R. (2001) Serotonin(1A) receptors in mood disorders: a combined genetic and genomic approach. *Behav. Pharmacol.* 12:429–438.

Soares, J.C., and Mann, J.J. (1997a) The anatomy of mood disorders—review of structural neuroimaging studies. *Biol. Psychiatry* 41:86–106.

Soares, J.C., and Mann, J.J. (1997b) The functional neuroanatomy of mood disorders. *J. Psychiatr. Res.* 31:393–432.

Stanley, M., Virgilio, J., and Gershon, S. (1982) Tritiated imipramine binding sites are decreased in the frontal cortex of suicides. *Science* 216:1337–1339.

Stockmeier, C.A. (2003) Involvement of serotonin in depression: evidence from postmortem and imaging studies of serotonin receptors and the serotonin transporter. *J. Psychiat. Res.* 37:357–373.

Stockmeier, C.A., Dilley, G.E., Shapiro, L.A., Overholser, J.C., Thompson, P.A., and Meltzer, H.Y. (1997) Serotonin receptors in suicide victims with major depression. *Neuropsychopharmacology* 16:162–173.

Stockmeier, C.A., and Meltzer, H.Y. (1991) b-Adrenergic receptor binding in frontal cortex of suicide victims. *Biol. Psychiatry* 29: 183–191.

Stockmeier, C.A., Shapiro, L.A., Dilley, G.E., Kolli, T.N., Friedman, L., and Rajkowska, G. (1998) Increase in serotonin-1A autoreceptors in the midbrain of suicide victims with major depression-postmortem evidence for decreased serotonin activity. *J. Neurosci.* 18:7394–7401.

Szigethy, E., Conwell, Y., Forbes, N.T., Cox, C., and Caine, E.D. (1994) Adrenal weight and morphology in victims of completed suicide. *Biol. Psychiatry* 36:374–380.

Talairach, J., and Tournoux, P. (1988) *Co-Planar Stereotaxic Atlas of the Human Brain. Dimensional Proportional System: An Approach to Cerebral Imaging*. New York: Thieme Medical Publishers, Inc.

Törk, I. (1990) Anatomy of the serotonergic system. *Ann. N. Y. Acad. Sci.* 600:9–35.

Törk, I., and Hornung, J.-P. (1990) Raphe nuclei and the serotonergic system. In: Paxinos, G., edr. *The Human Nervous System*. San Diego: Academic Press, pp. 1001–1022.

Turecki, G., Briere, R., Dewar, K., Antonetti, T., Lesage, A.D., Seguin, M., Chawky, N., Vanier, C., Alda, M., Joober, R., Benkelfat, C., and Rouleau, G.A. (1999) Prediction of level of serotonin 2A receptor binding by serotonin receptor 2A genetic variation in postmortem brain samples from subjects who did or did not commit suicide. *Am. J. Psychiatry* 156:1456–1458.

Underwood, M.D., Khaibulina, A.A., Ellis, S.P., Moran, A., Rice, P.M., Mann, J.J., and Arango, V. (1999) Morphometry of the dorsal raphe nucleus serotonergic neurons in suicide victims. *Biol. Psychiatry* 46:473–483.

Underwood, M.D., Mann, J.J., and Arango, V. (2004) Serotonergic and noradrenergic neurobiology of alcoholic suicide. *Alcohol Clin. Exp. Res.* 28:57S–69S.

Wilson, M.A., and Molliver, M.E. (1991) The organization of serotonergic projections to cerebral cortex in primates: retrograde transport studies. *Neuroscience* 44:555–570.

Wiste, A.K., Arango, V., Ellis, S.P., Mann, J.J., and Underwood, M.D. (2008) Norepinephrine and serotonin imbalance in the locus coeruleus in bipolar disorder. *Bipolar Disord.* 10:349–359.

Yates, M., and Ferrier, I.N. (1990) 5-HT_{1A} receptors in major depression. *J. Psychopharmacol.* 4:69–74.

Yates, M., Leake, A., Candy, J.M., Fairbairn, A.F., McKeith, I.G., and Ferrier, I.N. (1990) 5HT2 receptor changes in major depression. *Biol. Psychiatry* 27:489–496.

Zhu, M.Y., Klimek, V., Dilley, G.E., Haycock, J.W., Stockmeier, C.A., Overholser, J.C., Meltzer, H.Y., and Ordway, G.A. (1999) Elevated levels of tyrosine hydroxylase in the locus coeruleus in major depression. *Biol. Psychiatry* 46:1275–1286.

Zill, P., Buttner, A., Eisenmenger, W., Moller, H.J., Ackenheil, M., and Bondy, B. (2007) Analysis of tryptophan hydroxylase I and II mRNA expression in the human brain: A post-mortem study. *J. Psychiat. Res.* 41:168–173.

34 Novel Targets for Antidepressant Treatments

OLIVIER BERTON AND ERIC J. NESTLER

Despite our still limited knowledge of the etiology and pathophysiology of depression, there are many effective treatments for depressive disorders. These are described in other chapters of this text (Nestler et al., 2002; Berton and Nestler, 2006). However, there is still substantial room for faster acting, safer, and more effective treatments (Agid et al., 2007). All currently available treatments must be administered for weeks or months to see maximum clinical benefits, and side effects are still a major problem, even with newer medications. Moreover, roughly one half of all patients with depression never show full remission with optimized treatment.

From the point of view of market analysts, antidepressants have always been profitable, even though the market has consistently been one of the most crowded, since around 1960, when antidepressants were first commercialized. The successive generations of drugs that have emerged since the 1960s have been more "new" than "novel." Virtually all such drugs are based on a version of the same mechanistic template: increasing the synaptic levels of monoamines (Wermuth, 2006). Tricyclic antidepressants are believed to act by inhibiting the plasma membrane transporters for serotonin and/or norepinephrine (NE), whereas monoamine oxidase inhibitors (MAOIs) reduce the enzymatic breakdown of serotonin, NE, or dopamine (DA) (depending on which MAO isoform—A or B—they target). The serotonin-selective reuptake inhibitors (SSRIs) and norepinephrine reuptake inhibitors (NRIs) developed since the 1980s work by selectively inhibiting the reuptake of their respective monoaminergic targets, whereas serotonin and norepinephrine reuptake inhibitors (SNRIs) and the triple reuptake inhibitors (TRIs) now in development purposely target multiple monoamine transporters (Shaw et al., 2007). Although there have been claims that TRIs may offer advantages in efficacy, such as addressing a broader array of symptoms, this remains highly speculative.

Despite an impressive accumulation of knowledge about nonmonoamine systems that might contribute to the pathophysiology of depression (Manji et al., 2001; Duman and Monteggia, 2006), none of these relatively recent discoveries has yet been translated into a new bona fide treatment for depression. There are several reasons. First, it is not known whether the preclinical screens (essentially behavioral models in rodents), which have been designed to accurately predict antidepressant action for monoamine-based drugs, efficiently detect antidepressants with different mechanisms. Indeed, there is so far no non-monoamine-based compound adequately validated in humans to be used as a reference drug in these animal models (Pacher and Kecskemeti, 2004; Agid et al., 2007). Second, antidepressant efficacy studies are extremely expensive (they involve chronic treatment of large numbers of patients) and notoriously risky (large placebo responses cause many trials to fail). This increases the threshold for a pharmaceutical or biotech company to embark on a trial of any antidepressant, especially one with a non-monoamine-based (and hence riskier) mechanism. Third, to increase their confidence level in a non-monoamine-based drug, many groups have looked for effects of such drugs on serotonin and NE systems. According to this view, if one can show that a non-monoamine-based drug enhances, for example, serotonergic neurotransmission, this would increase the cache of that drug. But this approach destines us to not develop drugs with truly novel mechanisms of action. Finally, profits from monoamine-based drugs are still extremely strong, and small alterations added upon existing scaffolds have been sufficient to keep them growing.

However, most experts agree that antidepressant drug discovery is now at a crossroads. With the large majority of today's monoaminergic-based drugs facing loss of patent around 2010, molecules with mechanisms truly distinct from the compounds available as generics may gain stronger appeal for the pharmaceutical industry. The \$16 billion/year antidepressant market should provide a strong enough incentive for the industry to take the risks involved in developing drugs with non-monoamine-based actions. A search of the database maintained by the International Federation of Pharmaceutical Manufacturers and Associations (http://clinicaltrials.ifpma.org), which keeps a worldwide inventory of active clinical trials, indicates that in May 2007 approximately two thirds of the current phase 2 and 3 trials for depression are being conducted with non-monoamine-based drugs. This is an interesting trend, which suggests that the tide may be turning.

Although some efforts to find better monoaminergic agents are still under way with some promising leads, these are addressed in other chapters of this text and are not discussed here. Rather, we focus on some of the best hopes for non-monoamine-based drugs for the treatment of depression. Given space limitations, this review is not comprehensive. We only highlight some examples of current nonmonoamine approaches to antidepressant drug discovery, with some additional, more preliminary examples given in Table 34.1.

STRESS HORMONES AND NEUROPEPTIDES

A prominent line of antidepressant targets comprises a variety of ligands for stress hormone and neuropeptide receptors. The physiological systems targeted with this approach are directly involved in the neuroendocrine and behavioral components of stress responses. The rationale for the development of such molecules, which often block acute stress responses, is the assumption that depression results from an overactivation of these stress systems. Although the characterization of these systems started in some cases more than 50 years ago, the first leads with therapeutic potential are just coming out of pharmaceutical pipelines. Results of the first

TABLE 34.1 *Example of Other Antidepressant Drug Discovery Strategies*

Mechanism	*Brief Summary of Evidence*
κ opioid antagonists	Stress causes a CREB-mediated induction of the opioid peptide dynorphin in the nucleus accumbens. Dynorphin induction in this region causes certain depression-like behaviors (e.g., anhedonia). Accordingly, administration of κ antagonists, which block dynorphin action, either systemically or into the nucleus accumbens, have been shown to decrease depression-like behavior in rodents.
CB_1 agonists or antagonists	Manipulation of the CB_1 receptor, the major target for cannabinoids in brain, causes potent effects on anxiety and stress-related behaviors in rodents. This suggests that ligands for the CB_1 receptor, or drugs that affect the production of endogenous ligands for the receptor, may be antidepressant. However, results to date are inconsistent, with agents that promote and attenuate CB_1 activity reported to be beneficial in animal models.
Cytokines	Sickness behavior, which is mediated by proinflammatory cytokines (e.g., interleukins IL1 and IL6, tumor necrosis factor-α, or interferon-γ), resembles symptoms of depression (e.g., anhedonia, reduced social interactions, and fatigue). Moreover, interferon-γ, when used to treat hepatitis C, causes a high incidence of depression, and several cytokines are regulated in brain by stress and antidepressant treatments. This has raised the potential of exploiting cytokine-regulated pathways in the development of novel antidepressants.
HDAC inhibitors	Histone deacetylation by HDACs represses gene transcription. HDAC inhibitors reportedly promote synaptic plasticity and enhance memory, addiction, and other forms of behavioral adaptation. The potential utility of HDAC inhibitors in the treatment of mood disorders comes from the observations that: (*1*) valproic acid (an antimanic agent), among many other actions, is a weak HDAC inhibitor, (*2*) antidepressant treatments regulate histone acetylation in brain, and (*3*) imipramine selectively decreases levels of one form of HDAC ($HDAC_5$) in hippocampus, and this effect is required for its antidepressant efficacy in a social defeat model of depression. The brain regions involved in these actions are not known with certainty. Histone and DNA methylation may also be involved in stress and antidepressant responses. Although clearly in very early stages of development, drugs that affect chromatin structure deserve further consideration in depression research.
Par-4	This protein, initially described in apoptotic prostate cancer cells, was recently identified as a partner, and an important endogenous modulator, of dopamine D_2 receptor signal transduction. Genetic impairment of Par-4 mediated modulation of D_2 function, at dopaminergic synapses in the striatum, results in a depression-like syndrome in mice.
p11	p11 (also named S100A10) interacts with the serotonin $5\text{-}HT_{1B}$ receptor and increases localization of the receptor at the cell surface. p11 is increased in rodent brains by antidepressants or electroconvulsive seizures, and decreased in an animal model of depression and in brain tissue from depressed patients. Overexpression of p11 increases $5\text{-}HT_{1B}$ receptor function in cells and recapitulates certain behaviors seen after antidepressant treatment in mice. p11 knockout mice exhibit a depression-like phenotype and have reduced responsiveness to $5\text{-}HT_{1B}$ receptor agonists and to an antidepressant.
TREK-1	TREK-1 is a two-pore-domain K^+ channel important in shaping the overall excitability of individual neurons. Its genetic disruption produces animals with an increased efficacy of 5-HT neurotransmission, reduced stress reactivity, and a resistance to depression in several behavioral models, suggesting that a blocker of this particular K^+ channel may be a potential target for new antidepressants.

CREB: cyclic adenosine monophosphate (cAMP)-response element binding; NPY: neuropeptide Y; HDAC: histone deacetylase; DNA: deoxyribonucleic acid. See: Berton and Nestler (2006), Tsankova et al. (2007), Park et al. (2005), Svenningsson et al. (2006), and Heurteaux et al. (2006).

phase 2 and 3 trials for some of the best neuropeptide and neuroendocrine targets are now available and should keep coming over the next several years. These results are highly anticipated. In addition to being among the best hopes for patients and clinicians, these trials also will constitute a test for the generally accepted theoretical framework in which mood disorder research is currently conducted.

The Hypothalamic-Pituitary-Adrenal (HPA) Axis

Glucocorticoid release is controlled by the hypothalamic-pituitary-adrenal (HPA) axis, where corticotropin releasing factor (CRF) released by the paraventricular nucleus of the hypothalamus stimulates the release of adrenocorticotropic hormone (ACTH) from the anterior pituitary, which in turn stimulates glucocorticoid secretion from the adrenal cortex. The HPA axis is an essential component of an individual's capacity to cope with stress. However, excessive stimulation of the axis has been implicated in depression. Hyperactivity of the HPA axis is observed in a majority of patients with depression, as manifested by increased expression of CRF in hypothalamus, increased levels of CRF in cerebrospinal fluid (CSF), and reduced feedback inhibition of the axis by CRF and glucocorticoids (Sapolsky, 2000; Pariante and Miller, 2001; Barden, 2004; de Kloet et al., 2005; Gillespie and Nemeroff, 2005; Korte et al., 2005). Although the molecular basis of these derangements in the HPA axis remains unknown, numerous clinical studies suggest that normalization of the axis may be a necessary step for stable remission of depressive symptoms. In animal models, hypercortisolemia can potentiate excitotoxicity of hippocampal pyramidal neurons, as evidenced by dendritic atrophy and spine loss, and possibly cell death, as well as inhibit the birth of new granule cell neurons in the hippocampal dendate gyrus, and many of these changes can be prevented by antidepressant treatment (Drew and Hen, 2007; Tanis et al., 2007). Excessive glucocorticoids could, therefore, be a causative factor for the small reductions in hippocampal volume seen in patients with depression or post-traumatic stress disorder, although this finding remains controversial (Manji et al., 2001).

Besides its role in the HPA axis, CRF also serves as a neurotransmitter in several brain areas outside the hypothalamus, in particular, the central nucleus of the amygdala (Pare et al., 2004; Charmandari et al., 2005). These amygdala neurons send wide projections to forebrain and brain stem and have a crucial role in negative emotional memory (for example, as measured by fear conditioning), as well as in the generation of anxiety-like behavior and in mediating negative emotional symptoms of drug withdrawal states (Heinrichs and Koob, 2004). Elevated levels of CRF have been found in some of these target regions (for example, locus coeruleus) of patients with depression. This impressive literature has directed intense interest in the CRF and glucocorticoid systems as targets for the development of novel antidepressants.

CRF antagonists

Overexpression of CRF in transgenic mice, or CRF administration into the central nervous system (CNS), causes several depression-like symptoms, including hypercortisolemia, increased anxiety and arousal, decreased appetite and weight loss, and decreased sexual behavior (Bale and Vale, 2004; de Kloet et al., 2005; Keck et al., 2005; Keck, 2006). These symptoms are presumably induced via increased CRF function in the HPA axis and amygdala and related circuits. Physiological actions of CRF are mediated through two receptors, CRF_1 and CRF_2, both of which are coupled to the G_s subunit of G proteins—the subunit that can stimulate adenylyl cylcase to increase cyclic adenosine monophosphate (cAMP) synthesis. CRF_1 receptors are the predominant subtype: they are enriched in pituitary where they regulate the HPA axis and are also highly expressed throughout limbic brain regions where their selective deletion attenuates behavioral responses to stress (Keck, 2006). These data have supported a massive effort to develop CRF_1 antagonists as anxiolytic and antidepressant medications. Such compounds dramatically reduce anxiety-like behavior and fear conditioning in rodents (Li et al., 2005; Kehne, 2007) and also antagonize a range of depression-like symptoms seen during withdrawal from several drugs of abuse (Heinrichs and Koob, 2004). On the other hand, CRF_1 antagonists have not demonstrated consistent activity in standard antidepressant screens (Kehne, 2007). Open-label clinical trials found that a nonpeptidic CRF_1 antagonist is effective in reducing psychosocial stress and depressive symptoms and in improving sleep in patients suffering from major depression (Ising et al., 2007). No serious side effects and no significant disruption of endocrine systems, including the HPA axis, thyroid hormone, gonadal steriods, prolactin, and vasopressin, were found. However, no well controlled study has yet verified these findings. Unfortunately, pharmacokinetic and hepatoxicity issues have led to the discontinuation of numerous CRF_1 antagonists, an all-too-common occurrence for drugs aimed at neuropeptide receptors. The failure to obtain clear proof of concept of the CRF_1 antagonist mechanism as anxiolytic or antidepressant in humans, despite decades of research, is a major disappointment and frustration for the field.

CRF_2 receptors show more restricted expression in brain, and their role in regulating complex behavior is still under investigation (Hillhouse and Grammatopoulos,

2006; Fekete and Zorrilla, 2007). CRF_2 knockout mice show normal anxiety-like behavior, but CRF_2 antagonists show anxiolytic properties in animal models, and some, but not all, show significant efficacy in the learned helplessness and chronic mild stress depression paradigms as well (Bale and Vale, 2004). Recent results indicate that the endogenous ligands for CRF_2 receptors, in addition to CRF, may be the urocortin peptides, which promote adaptive responses to stress (Hillhouse and Grammatopoulos, 2006; Fekete and Zorrilla, 2007). There remains considerable interest in the clinical development of CRF_2 antagonists, particularly because they are less likely than CRF_1 antagonists to cause side effects via the HPA axis.

Vasopressin antagonists

The neuropeptide *vasopressin*, synthesized in the paraventricular and supraoptic hypothalamic nuclei, is well known for its role in fluid metabolism. It also regulates the HPA axis: stress stimulates the release of vasopressin that then potentiates the effects of CRF on ACTH release. Vasopressin is found outside the hypothalamus as well, notably in the amygdala and bed nucleus of the stria terminalis, and is believed to exert effects throughout the limbic system via activation of V_{1a} and V_{1b} receptors. Vasopressin levels are reportedly increased in some patients with depression (Bao et al., 2007). Nonpeptide V_{1b} antagonists exhibit antidepressant-like effects in rodents partly via amygdala-dependent mechanisms (Keck et al., 2003). This is in contrast to V_{1b} knockout mice, which display normal stress responses (Lolait et al., 2007). Vasopressin antagonists have yet to be evaluated in humans.

Glucocorticoids: agonists or antagonists?

Glucocorticoids diffuse passively through cellular membranes and bind to intracellular glucocorticoid receptors (GR) causing their translocation into the nucleus. Within the nucleus, these ligand-activated transcription factors bind to specific DNA response elements, or to other transcription factors, and alter gene expression. In the brain, glucocorticoid-regulated genes affect many aspects of neuronal function, including metabolism, structure, and synaptic transmission. Glucocorticoids also promote the termination of stress reactions through complex feedback loops, in part mediated through the hippocampus, ultimately leading to the repression of target genes implicated in stress responses, such as CRF (Hillhouse and Grammatopoulos, 2006).

As mentioned earlier, insufficient feedback suppression of the HPA axis by CRF and glucocorticoids is seen in a large subset of patients with depression (de Kloet et al., 2005). This neuroendocrine abnormality was reproduced recently in adult mice with selective deletion of GR in forebrain (Boyle et al., 2004; Boyle et al., 2005). Interestingly, this mutation also resulted in a robust depression-like phenotype normalized after chronic treatment with tricyclic antidepressants. Conversely, transgenic mice overexpressing GR in the forebrain are more sensitive to the acute effects of antidepressants (Wei et al., 2004). These findings raise the possibility that enhanced GR activity in the forebrain might be antidepressant. Most antidepressant treatments can restore efficient negative feedback of the HPA axis and increase the expression of GR in forebrain regions such as the hippocampus (de Kloet et al., 2005). Some patients with depression carry a polymorphism in the FKBP5 gene (which encodes a cochaperone of heat shock protein 90) that results in higher affinity of GR for cortisol (Binder et al., 2004; Gillespie and Nemeroff, 2005). These individuals reportedly respond much faster to antidepressants than a group without this mutation.

These findings are paradoxical, given the evidence, cited above, that hypercortisolemia may contribute to the pathophysiology of depression, but the two sets of results could be reconciled in the following way. Deficient inhibitory feedback of the HPA axis might result from excessive activation of GR in the hippocampus and subsequent damage to this region (Sapolsky, 2000; Korte et al., 2005). Recently, viral vectors have been used to deliver chimeric GR receptors into the hippocampus that combined the ligand-binding domain of GR with the DNA-binding domain of estrogen receptors, thereby converting the glucocorticoid signal into an estrogen-like effect (Kaufer et al., 2004; Akama and McEwen, 2005). The expression of the chimeric receptor potently reduced hippocampal damage and rendered excess glucocorticoids protective rather than destructive. The behavioral effects of such genetically altered GR receptors have not yet been reported in animal models of depression.

In the clinic, preliminary evidence indicates that some symptoms of psychotic depression might be rapidly ameliorated by GR antagonists (Flores et al., 2006). The GR antagonist *mifepristone*, which is also a progesterone receptor antagonist and approved as a "morning after" pill, is currently in phase 3 clinical trials for psychotic major depression. In March 2007, the results of the third phase 3 trial (443 patients randomized, double-blind, placebo-controlled study) were communicated by Corcept Therapeutics. Although the effect of the treatment did not achieve overall statistical significance, the company reported a statistically significant correlation between plasma drug levels and clinical outcome achieved during treatment. At higher plasma levels, patients did respond to the treatment when compared to placebo. This result confirmed a similar finding obtained in a previous phase 3 trial completed in 2006, suggesting that the drug can produce desired clinical effects within a week when dosages are tailored to achieve an optimal plasma level. A point to emphasize here is that the primary endpoint set in the study was a 50% improvement in the severity of positive symptoms, which are the psychotic rather than the depressive features of the disease. Several other large multicenter trials are currently under way and will confirm whether the medication is useful for the treatment of psychotic depression.

Galanin

The discovery of the neuropeptide galanin was first reported in the early 1980s after its extraction from the intestine. Galanin has attracted interest in the field in view of its anatomical distribution and the physiological functions it mediates (Lu, Mazarati, et al., 2005; Karlsson and Holmes, 2006; Ogren et al., 2006; Lu et al., 2007). Despite a wide distribution in rodent brain, the neuropeptide has a particularly high level of expression in the brain stem, where it is strongly colocalized with NE and serotonin. Galanin acts through three G protein–coupled receptors, Gal_1, Gal_2, and Gal_3, which are also enriched in brain regions containing monoaminergic cell bodies and terminals (Hawes and Picciotto, 2004; Lu, Mazarati, et al., 2005). The Gal_1 and Gal_3 receptors are coupled to Gi and exert an inhibitory influence on cell excitability and adenylyl cyclase, whereas Gal_2 receptors are Gq coupled and lead to the activation of phospholipase C (PLC) (Lu, Lundstrom, et al., 2005).

Upon intracerebroventricular (ICV) administration, galanin exerts potent neurobehavioral effects, including modulation of seizure activity, pain-processing, feeding, sexual behavior, fear-related behaviors, and cognitive functions. The contribution of each receptor subtype to this complex profile remains unclear, due to the unavailability, until recently, of selective galanin receptor ligands (Holmes and Picciotto, 2006). In depression models, synthetic galanin receptor agonists, galnon and galmic (which act on Gal_1 and Gal_2), were found to reduce immobility time in the rat Forced Swim Test (FST) when given systemically, indicating an antidepressant-like effect, likely mediated through Gal_2 receptor. Galanin transcripts were found to increase almost twofold in the dorsal raphé and locus coeruleus after subchronic fluoxetine treatment, whereas Galanin (2-11) binding (which reflects primarily Gal_2 binding capacity) also showed a 50% increase in dorsal raphé (Yoshitake et al., 2003; Lu, Barr, et al., 2005). Interestingly, M40, a peptidic nonselective Gal_1/Gal_2 receptor antagonist, has been shown to attenuate the antidepressant-like effects of fluoxetine in the FST. Together, these results suggest that acute galanin signaling through Gal_2 receptors may mediate an antidepressant-like response and may provide one mechanism through which fluoxetine acts in rodent models. These results are reinforced by a recent clinical study, which demonstrated a potent antidepressant effect of galanin upon acute intravenous administration in patients with depression (Murck et al., 2004).

In 2005, the characterization of the first nonpeptide antagonists for the Gal_3 receptor (SNAP37889 and SNAP398299) was published by Lundbeck (Swanson et al., 2005). This report demonstrated potent anxiolytic- and antidepressant-like properties of Gal_3 antagonists in several social behavior–based models in rats and guinea pigs, as well as more classical tests such as the forced swimming and stress induced-hyperthermia in mice. Interestingly, like with Gal_2 receptor agonist, these antidepressant-like effects were observed after acute administration of the drug and did not desensitize after chronic administration. Electrophysiological and microdialysis studies indicate that these anxiolytic- and antidepressant-like effects of Gal_3 antagonists could possibly result from an attenuation of the inhibitory influence of galanin, released during stress, on serotonergic transmission at the level of the dorsal raphé. Another interesting property of galanin is its action as a trophic factor during development and in adult brain after injury. Galanin and galanin receptor expression have been identified in the proliferative zones of adult and postnatal brain. In cultured neurospheres, galanin decreases cell proliferation, an effect blocked by the nonselective antagonist M35. Nevertheless, much further work is needed to validate galanin-based drugs as effective agents in humans.

Neurokinins

The neuropeptides known as neurokinins were discovered over 70 years ago, but compounds that antagonize their action at specific receptors were only developed during the past decade. They are products of two genes that code for substance P (SP), the most abundant in the CNS, neurokinin A, and neurokinin B. Three subtypes of neurokinin receptors have been identified and designated as NK_1, NK_2, and NK_3. Substance P is the preferred endogenous agonist for NK_1 receptors, which are coupled to G_q and stimulate phospholipase C, whereas neurokinin A exhibits the highest affinity for the NK_2 receptor and neurokinin B for the NK_3 receptor (Pennefather et al., 2004).

Substance P has been studied primarily for its role as a central mediator of pain, an indication for which nonpeptidic NK_1 antagonists were initially developed. The rationale for considering NK_1 antagonists in depression was based on the expression of SP and NK_1 receptors in fear- and anxiety-related circuits, the release of SP in animals in response to fearful stimuli, and the strong colocalization of SP with serotonin and NE or their receptors in human brain. Reciprocally, local application of SP agonists was shown to induce a range of neural, behavioral, and cardiovascular changes characteristic of defensive responses, including increased firing of the locus coeruleus, place aversion, distress vocalizations, escape behavior, and cardiovascular activation. Moreover, some effects of stress can be blocked by systemic administration of NK_1 receptor antagonists. These effects have since been confirmed by the anxiolytic- and antidepressant-like phenotype of SP and NK_1 receptor knockout mice (Rupniak et al., 2001).

Kramer et al. published in 1998 the first evidence that chronic treatment with a nonpeptidic NK_1 receptor antagonist might be antidepressant in humans. This report was greeted with great enthusiasm, but it has been difficult to replicate its findings, such that the validity of NK_1 antagonism as an effective antidepressant strategy is now questioned (Chahl, 2006). Indeed, several pharmaceutical companies have discontinued their NK_1 antagonist programs in yet another major disappointment for the field.

Although NK_1 antagonists were initially claimed to act through a completely novel mechanism of action, subsequent studies have suggested that their therapeutic action, if any, could be secondary to changes in monoaminergic systems. NK_1 antagonists have a delayed onset of action similar to monoamine-based antidepressants, and their chronic administration causes increased firing of serotonergic neurons—a change also observed in NK_1 knockout mice (Blier et al., 2004). In addition, genetic or pharmacological blockade of NK_1 receptors induces some of the same long-term effects in the brain as bona fide antidepressants on cell signaling proteins, such as brain-derived neurotrophic factor (BDNF), and hippocampal neurogenesis (Musazzi et al., 2005). These results raise the possibility that NK_1 antagonists could conceivably be used as augmentation agents in combination with a traditional antidepressant.

Following the lack of success of NK_1 receptor antagonists, some companies have shifted their focus toward antagonists at other NK receptors. There are indications from preclinical studies that NK_2 antagonists may have more consistent anxiolytic and antidepressant effects than NK_1 antagonists. For example, saredutant (SR48968) is an NK_2 antagonist currently in phase 3 clinical trials. Saredutant is also being tested for the treatment of generalized anxiety disorder.

Hypothalamic Feeding Peptides

There have been explosive advances over the past decade in understanding hypothalamic peptides that regulate feeding behavior. Recent work has begun to draw connections between these hypothalamic feeding peptides and depression (Nestler and Carlezon, 2006). Of particular note is melanin-concentrating hormone (MCH), a major orexigenic (proappetite) peptide expressed in a subset of lateral hypothalamic neurons. The MCH_1 receptor, the only subtype expressed in rodents, is coupled to G_i and shows remarkable enrichment in the nucleus accumbens. Direct administration of MCH into this region stimulates feeding behavior, whereas blockade of the MCH_1 receptor decreases feeding (Georgescu et al., 2005). Intracerebroventricular or intrahypothalamic MCH administration has similar effects. Moreover, several MCH_1 receptor antagonists, including nonpeptidic small molecule antagonists, administered systemically or directly into the nucleus accumbens, exert antidepressant-like effects in the FST (Shimazaki et al., 2006). A similar antidepressant-like phenotype is observed in mice lacking MCH or the MCH_1 receptor, while a prodepressant-like phenotype is seen in MCH-overexpressing animals. Taken together, these data provide a strong case that MCH antagonists, by disrupting MCH signaling to the nucleus accumbens, might provide a highly novel mechanism for antidepressant medications. These drugs would also reduce weight, which could be particularly useful in the subset of patients with depression who show weight gain. Evaluating these agents in humans is now the major obstacle.

Several other hypothalamic feeding peptides have also attracted attention in the depression field. These include anorexigenic peptides, such as melanocortin (αMSH) and cocaine- and amphetamine-regulated transcript (CART), and orexigenic peptides, such as orexin (hypocretin), agouti-related peptide (ARP), and neuropeptide Y (NPY). Many of these peptides have been shown to not only regulate feeding, but to also alter reward mechanisms, which suggests possible effects on anhedonia-related symptoms (Nestler and Carlezon, 2006).

This is the case of NPY, which has attracted particular attention as a possible antidepressant target, because of its pattern of expression and regulation, well beyond the hypothalamus, in limbic brain circuits (Karl and Herzog, 2007). The role of NPY in the regulation of stress responses has been widely investigated in human and animal investigations. Several studies have demonstrated down-regulation of NPY levels in CSF, plasma, and prefrontal cortex (PFC) of patients with depression and victims of suicide. Similar alterations of NPY gene expression and peptide content have been reported in animal models of depression, including stress-induced anhedonia and the learned helplessness. Several lines of evidence suggest that stimulation of NPY neurotransmission may bear antidepressant properties. In rodents, central administration of NPY has been shown to elicit dose-dependent anxiolytic and antidepressant-like effects in several animal models, including the FST, in rats and mice. Up to now, two of the six NPY receptors (Y_1–Y_6) have received significant attention as possible mediators of NPY antidepressant-like activity. The Y_1 receptor is mainly located postsynaptically and is enriched in the cerebral cortex and hippocampus. Intracerebroventricular administration of the Y_1 selective peptidic agonist [Leu31;Pro34]PYY reduced the immobility time of rats in the FST. More recently, selective Y_1 nonpeptidic antagonists, BIBP3226 and BIBO3304, were shown to block the effect of NPY (Ishida et al., 2007).

Due to their function as inhibitory presynaptic auto- and hetero-receptors in human and rat CNS, NPY Y_2 receptors are also interesting targets (Tschenett et al., 2003). Deletion or blockade of these receptors results in enhanced release of NPY, as well as other transmitters such as γ-aminobutyric acid (GABA) and dopamine (DA). Y_2 receptor knockout mice display an anxiolytic- and antidepressant-like phenotype. A similar profile was observed after administration of the potent and selective Y_2 receptor antagonist BIIE0246 (Bacchi et al., 2006). Several clinical trials of NPY-based compounds are being conducted for obesity, but to our knowledge no clinical study of the aforementioned compounds has yet been carried out for depression.

NEUROTROPHIC FACTORS AND RELATED TRANSDUCTION PATHWAYS

A host of fundamentally new targets has emerged as a result of open-ended molecular and cellular approaches. In some cases, these targets were previously studied for their role in seemingly unrelated biological functions. In most cases, their role in normal brain function and in the pathophysiology of depression is not currently understood. However, these molecules appear as effective as monoaminergic reference compounds in several animal models.

BDNF and TrkB signaling

The neurotrophic hypothesis of depression and antidepressant action was based originally on findings in rodents that acute or chronic stress decreases expression of BDNF in hippocampus and that diverse classes of antidepressant treatments produce the opposite effect and prevent the actions of stress (R.S. Duman and Monteggia, 2006). These observations led to the suggestion (still unproven) that perhaps such changes in BDNF could in part mediate the structural damage and reduced neurogenesis seen in hippocampus after stress and the prevention of these effects by antidepressant treatments (see above). Importantly, reduced BDNF levels in the hippocampus have been reported in some patients with depression on autopsy, an abnormality not seen in those patients treated with antidepressants. Up-regulation of hippocampal BDNF expression by numerous types of pharmacological and nonpharmacological clinically effective antidepressant interventions is now a highly replicated result (Conti et al., 2007).

Together, these data support the possibility that drugs that activate BDNF signaling in hippocampus might be antidepressant. Direct evidence for this hypothesis comes from experiments where injection of BDNF into the rodent hippocampus exerts antidepressant-like effects in the FST and learned helplessness test (Shirayama et al., 2002; Tanis et al., 2007). Conversely, inducible knockout of BDNF from the hippocampus and other forebrain regions prevents the antidepressant effects of drugs that activate BDNF (Monteggia et al., 2004).

Although a great deal of work remains to validate this hypothesis, the main challenge from a drug discovery point of view is that BDNF is not an easy drug target. A range of compounds have been designed to modulate BDNF signaling through various mechanisms, such as direct or indirect tyrosine kinase receptor (TrkB) receptor agonists and neurotrophin potentiators or releasers. Several clinical trials have failed, due to problems in delivery and unforeseen severe side effects of neurotrophic factors. Nevertheless, a small subset of the compounds, acting on intracellular signaling pathways downstream of TrkB receptors, shows promise. Indeed, BDNF activation of TrkB leads to diverse physiological effects by regulating a complex cascade of postreceptor pathways, which involve PI3K-Akt, PLCγ, and Ras-Raf-Erk, each of which represents a putative drug target.

Inhibition of extracellular signal regulated kinases (ERK) has, for example, been shown to block the activity of antidepressants in animal models (C.H. Duman et al., 2007). This raises the possibility that drugs that stimulate ERK signaling, such as inhibitors of dual-specificity phosphatases (enzymes that dephosphorylate and inactivate ERK), may be used to potentiate antidepressant activity (Tanis et al., 2007). Activation of TrkB receptors can also be induced by ligands at G protein–coupled receptors in the absence of neurotrophins. Adenosine and pituitary adenylyl cyclase-activating peptide (PACAP), for example, have been shown to induce Trk activation through their respective G protein–coupled receptors and the subsequent activation of Src family kinases to promote cell survival. Transactivation of Trks by G protein–coupled receptors is emerging as a new strategy to transactivate trophic activities and could potentially reveal novel drug targets (Jeanneteau and Chao, 2006). In theory, numerous other proteins might be targeted for antidepressant development; however, several obstacles remain: first, we do not yet know which of these pathways are most crucial for the antidepressant actions of BDNF in animal models; second, most of these signaling proteins are broadly expressed throughout the brain and peripheral tissues, which heightens concerns about toxicity of any drug directed against them; and third, the lack of availability of small molecule agonists for most of these signaling proteins means that their potential antidepressant activity cannot easily be assessed.

Another complication is that, although BDNF might exert antidepressant-like effects at the level of the hippocampus, its actions might be different, or even the opposite, in other neural circuits. The best example is the ventral tegmental area-nucleus accumbens reward circuit, in which chronic stress increases BDNF expression, local BDNF infusion exerts a pro-depression-like effect in the FST, and blockade of BDNF function exerts an antidepressant-like effect (Eisch et al., 2003). A more recent study found a similar antidepressant-like effect upon viral-mediated local knockout of BDNF from the ventral tegmental area in a social defeat paradigm (Berton et al., 2006). These findings raise caution about the goal of developing an antidepressant based on BDNF because a drug that promotes BDNF function might produce competing effects in different brain regions.

In addition to BDNF, other neurotrophic factors warrant consideration as potential leads for antidepressant development. A recent DNA microarray study of the human hippocampus found that several genes in the fibroblast growth factor (FGF) family—FGF and some of its receptors—are down-regulated in the hippocampus of patients with depression (Turner et al., 2006). This is interesting in light of the knowledge that FGF seems to be an important endogenous regulator of neurogenesis in the adult rat hippocampus. Another candidate of interest is vascular endothelial growth factor (VEGF), which was initially characterized for its role in angiogenesis but also exerts direct mitogenic effects on neural progenitors in vitro. Results from a recent study demonstrate that VEGF is induced by multiple classes of antidepressants at time points consistent with the induction of cell proliferation and therapeutic action of these treatments. Vascular endothelial growth factor signaling through the Flk-1 receptor seems to be required for antidepressant-induced cell proliferation and behavioral responses to chronic antidepressants (Warner-Schmidt and Duman, 2007). Still other neurotrophic factors are known to be regulated in the hippocampus by stress and antidepressant treatments, which are currently being evaluated in depression models (Tanis et al., 2007).

Although studies of neurotrophic mechanisms in depression and antidepressant action have provided important heuristic models for the field, it may be difficult to translate these discoveries into new treatment approaches for depression due to the complex biology of these systems.

PHOSPHODIESTERASE INHIBITORS

Phosphodiesterases (PDEs) catalyze the degradation of cAMP and cyclic guanosine monophosphate (cGMP). The potential antidepressant activity of PDE inhibitors dates back decades to the notion that these drugs would be expected to promote the actions of NE at β-adrenergic receptors, which were hypothesized at the time to partly mediate antidepressant responses. Indeed, there were early indications that rolipram, a nonselective PDE4 inhibitor, might be antidepressant in small clinical trials (see R.S. Duman et al., 1997; R.S. Duman, 2004). These early trials failed because of intense nausea and vomiting induced by rolipram and related PDE4 inhibitors.

Renewed interest in PDE4 inhibitors as antidepressants has come from the findings that they induce BDNF expression in hippocampus. This effect might be mediated by activation of the cAMP pathway, which leads to the activation of the transcription factor cAMP-response element (CRE) binding protein (CREB) and to the direct induction of the BDNF gene via a CRE site in its promoter. Induction of CREB itself in the hippocampus exerts an antidepressant-like effect in the FST (R.S. Duman, 2004). Thus, PDE4 inhibitors might provide an indirect way to promote CREB and BDNF function and exert an antidepressant effect. Meanwhile, there is intense interest in PDE4 inhibitors as cognitive enhancers, a possibility that is also based on the role of CREB in the hippocampus in mediating important forms of learning and memory.

The major challenge, however, remains side effects: is it possible to inhibit PDE4 in the hippocampus and exert antidepressant and cognitive enhancing effects without inhibiting PDE4 in brain-stem regions which causes nausea and vomiting? A second major challenge is that inhibition of PDE isoforms might not be antidepressant or cognitive enhancing in all brain regions. There is growing evidence that stimulation of the cAMP pathway and CREB in nucleus accumbens is prodepressant. Thus, mechanisms to oppose, rather than to enhance, activity of this pathway might be more suitable for antidepressant drug discovery efforts (Carlezon et al., 2005). Similarly, stimulation of the cAMP pathway in frontal cortical regions can inhibit cognitive function in aged animals, which again highlights potential problems of targeting PDE isoforms that are widely expressed in the brain. On the positive side, there are four subtypes of PDE4, PDE4A through PDE4D, each encoded by a different gene, with multiple splice variants of each subtype. It is conceivable that a particular subtype enriched in hippocampus could be targeted for antidepressant and cognition-enhancing effects, although this remains conjectural. In addition, there are many other PDE isoforms, some of which show highly restricted patterns of expression in the brain. For example, PDE10A is highly enriched in the striatum. It, too, could potentially be targeted for antidepressant development. A recent study pointed to the PDE4B isoform as a choice candidate by showing that mutation in DISC1 (disrupted in schizophrenia 1), a specific binding partner of PDE4B, results in lower PDE4B activity, a depressive phenotype in mice, and a selective resistance to the antidepressant effect of rolipram (Clapcote et al., 2007).

Moreover, there are many other families of signaling proteins that modulate G protein-adenylyl cyclase activity, such as regulators of G protein signaling (RGS) proteins, subtypes of which show restricted expression patterns in the brain. These proteins too represent potential drug targets.

GLUTAMATE ACTING DRUGS

The link between glutamatergic neurotransmission and the pathophysiology of depression has been increasingly demonstrated since the 1950s, when the mood-elevating properties of anti-infectious agents with some *N*-methyl-D-aspartate (NMDA) glutamate receptor antagonist activity (for example, D-cycloserine and amantadine) were first reported (Paul and Skolnick, 2003; Sanacora et al., 2003). A rapid and sustained antidepressant effect of a single IV bolus of ketamine, a dissociative anesthetic and NMDA receptor antagonist, was subsequently demonstrated in a placebo-controlled trial (Zarate, Singh, Carlson, et al., 2006). The application of ketamine and related drugs as antidepressants is obviously limited by their severe psychotomimetic effects. However, recent clinical trials have been assessing the antidepressant potential of the weaker NMDA antagonist *memantine* and the glutamate release inhibitor, riluzole, both of which have been approved by the U.S. Federal Drug Administration (FDA) for cognitive enhancement and neuroprotection, respectively. Although memantine proved devoid of antidepressant activity in a double-blind, placebo-controlled study (Zarate, Singh, Quiroz, et al., 2006), recent work suggests the efficacy of riluzole as an augmentation strategy for treatment-resistant depression (Sanacora et al., 2007). Although clinical evidence that supports the antidepressant efficacy of NMDA antagonists is still relatively weak, preclinical research increasingly suggests that reduced NMDA receptor function is antidepressant-like in several animal models and prevents stress-induced alterations in hippocampal neuronal morphology, and that chronic treatment with bona fide antidepressants down-regulates NMDA receptors or reduces glutamate release via presynaptic mechanisms (Pittenger et al., 2007).

In parallel, it has been reported that activation of α-amino-3-hydroxy-5-methyl-4-isoxasolepropionic acid (AMPA) glutamate receptors increases BDNF expression and rapidly stimulates neurogenesis and neuronal sprouting, in the hippocampus. Based on these observations, AMPA receptor potentiators have been evaluated in models of depression (Bleakman et al., 2007). Positive allosteric modulators, which avoid the rapid desensitization of AMPA receptors seen with full agonists, were reported to have similar activity as tricyclic and SSRI antidepressants in the FST and tail suspension test. Interestingly, AMPA receptor potentiators were also active in reducing rat submissive behavior (a behavioral model that responds selectively to chronic antidepressant treatment) with a shorter onset of action than an SSRI. There are also some indications that monoamine-based antidepressants promote AMPA receptor function. Given the dominant role of ionotropic glutamate receptors in synaptic activity and plasticity throughout the brain, including cognition-, emotion-, and reward-related circuits, it is not surprising that agents that affect these receptors could exert antidepressant activity. It remains to be seen whether such drugs could have the selectivity and safety required. One proposed strategy would be to target any of several metabotropic (or G protein–coupled) glutamate receptors, which seem to differentially modulate the activity of the ionotropic receptors and might thereby mediate safer and more selective effects. mGlu receptors indeed modulate glutamatergic neuronal excitation and plasticity via presynaptic, postsynaptic, and glial mechanisms. In particular, compounds that antagonize mGluR2, mGluR3, and/or mGluR5 receptors have shown antidepressant-like activity in rodent models (Witkin et al., 2007).

CIRCADIAN GENE PRODUCTS

Several observations link mood disorders and circadian rhythms. Prominent alterations of circadian rhythms have long been described in depression and other mood disorders (see McClung, 2007). Many patients with depression report their most serious symptoms in the morning with some improvement as the day progresses. This might represent an exaggeration of diurnal fluctuations in mood, motivation, energy level, and responses to rewarding stimuli that are seen commonly in the healthy population. The molecular basis for these rhythms seen under normal and pathological conditions is poorly understood.

Most of the treatments that are currently employed to treat mood disorders are known to alter the circadian clock. This is obviously the case of total sleep deprivation (TSD) and bright light therapy, but there are data supporting the idea that many chemical mood stabilizers and antidepressants also derive at least some of their therapeutic efficacy by affecting the circadian clock. For example, the mood stabilizers *lithium* and *valproate* have been shown to alter the circadian period, leading to a longer period in *Drosophila*, rodents, nonhuman primates, and humans. This effect on circadian rhythms could involve the inhibition of glycogen synthase kinase 3 β (GSK3β) that modifies multiple members of the molecular clock. It is proposed that this action of lithium on the circadian clock is important in its therapeutic efficacy. Similarly, the antidepressant *fluoxetine* also affects circadian output by producing a phase advance in the firing of suprachiasmatic nucleus (SCN) neurons.

The biology that underlies the association between circadian rhythms and mood disorders is still unknown but may come from the influence of the molecular clock on certain neurotransmitters and their receptors. Indeed, some of the neurotransmitters that have been implicated in mood regulation, including serotonin, NE, and dopamine, have a circadian rhythm in their levels, release, and synthesis-related enzymes or in the expression and activity of several of their receptors. How these circuits are controlled in a circadian fashion is still uncertain, but molecular mechanisms are starting to be unraveled.

Most research on circadian rhythms has focused on the SCN of the hypothalamus, which is considered the master circadian pacemaker of the brain (Reppert and Weaver, 2002; Takahashi, 2004). Here, circadian rhythms are generated at the molecular level by Clock (a Pas domain containing transcription factor), which dimerizes with Bmal; and the dimer induces the expression of Per (Period) and Cry (Cryptochrome) genes, which in turn feedback to repress Clock-Bmal activity. In addition, Clock-Bmal, Per, and Cry regulate the expression of many other genes, which presumably drive the many circadian variations in cell function. This molecular cycle in the SCN is entrained by light and appears to be essential for matching circadian rhythms with the light–dark cycle. More recent research, however, has indicated that control of circadian rhythms is far more complicated than this simple model. Clock, Bmal, Per, and Cry genes, as well as several related genes, are expressed broadly throughout the brain, including limbic regions implicated in mood regulation, although little is known about their function outside the SCN.

Behavioral studies aimed at investigating the role of individual circadian genes in mood regulation are just beginning. Interestingly, transgenic mice overexpressing the circadian modulator, GSK3β, are hyperactive and have reduced immobility in the FST, indicative of less depression-like behavior, and an increased startle response (Prickaerts et al., 2006). A similar manic- or antidepressant-like-phenotype has also been observed in mice lacking functional Clock protein (King et al., 1997). Their behavioral phenotype includes an antidepressant-like profile in the FST and learned helplessness test, and reduced anxiety or increased risk-taking behavior in several assays. These mice also display an increase in the rewarding effects of cocaine, sucrose, and intracranial self-stimulation (Roybal et al., 2007). Interestingly, in vivo recordings have demonstrated increased in vivo firing of dopaminergic neurons in the ventral tegmental area of the Clock mutant mice. These neurons express Clock, which regulates several genes that are important in dopaminergic transmission (McClung et al., 2005). A major influence of the Clock gene in the ventral tegmental area on emotional behavior is further emphasized by the partial rescue of the manic-like phenotype in Clock mutant mice upon overexpression of Clock protein selectively in this brain region (Roybal et al., 2007). Interestingly, antidepressant treatments also increase Clock expression in hippocampus (Uz et al., 2005; Manev and Uz, 2006). Additional behavioral studies with mice lacking other circadian genes are ongoing. There has been interest in a Clock-like protein, termed *neuronal Pas domain protein-2* (NPAS2), which dimerizes with Bmal to regulate the circadian expression of Per, Cry, and many other genes (Garcia et al., 2000). Interestingly, NPAS2 is not expressed in the SCN but is found at high levels in several limbic regions, particularly the nucleus accumbens. NPAS2 knockout mice show deficits in the ability to entrain to nonlight stimuli, such as food. It has been suggested that NPAS2 is a crucial mediator of circadian rhythms in an individual's emotional state via actions in nucleus accumbens and other limbic regions.

Taken together, these early studies support the hypothesis that circadian genes may function abnormally in depression and other mood disorders. This work also suggests that drugs aimed at influencing particular target genes for these circadian transcription factors, which are expressed within distinct brain circuits, deserve attention as targets for possible new treatment agents for depression.

Melatonin, the main secretory product of the pineal gland, which contributes to circadian rhythm synchronization, has also triggered significant interest as a possible antidepressant target. Because initial attempts to demonstrate antidepressant activity of melatonin were unsuccessful, the hypothesis was tested that melatonin receptor agonists could improve psychomotor tone in patients with depression. This was confirmed with agomelatine, an agonist of the MT_1 and MT_2 melatonin receptors; the drug is also an antagonist at the serotonin $5\text{-}HT_{2C}$ receptor (Bourin et al., 2004). The compound has proven to be highly effective in animal models of depression, including induction of hippocampal neurogenesis, and reported to have significant activity in human depression trials (den Boer et al., 2006). Agomelatine also seems to produce fewer adverse side effects than some other antidepressant medications, and it alleviates many of the sleep problems associated with depression that can be exacerbated by SSRI treatment, making it a potentially valuable new treatment for depression (Fuchs et al., 2006). As expected by its pharmacologic profile, agomelatine has been shown to resynchronize circadian rhythms in body temperature, cortisol, and other hormones in animal models and in humans, which may underlie some of its therapeutic effects. On the other hand, there have been negative trials of agomelatine in depression such that its efficacy will require further investigation. The contribution of $5\text{-}HT_{2C}$ antagonism to agomelatine's actions remains unknown.

FUTURE DIRECTIONS

Antidepressant drug discovery is at a crossroads. Available medications with monoamine-based mechanisms will be going off patent in the next decade, while proof of concept studies for some of the best neuropeptide and neuroendocrine targets (for example, CRF, SP, and glucocorticoid receptors), which are based largely on stress models, should at long last be available within the next few years. At the same time, a host of fundamentally new targets has emerged as a result of more open-ended molecular and cellular approaches in concert with improving, albeit still imperfect, animal models of stress. Progress with some of these targets (for example, BDNF) has been hampered by the difficult chemistry involved. Nevertheless, this research has suggested numerous biomarkers or endophenotypes for depression, for example, BDNF expression, hippocampal neurogenesis, neuronal morphology, CREB activity, to name just a few, but all of these remain inaccessible in living patients.

A major leap forward in the field will require identification of genes that confer risk for depression in humans, and understanding how specific types of environmental factors interact synergistically with that genetic vulnerability. This will make it possible to develop more valid animal models of human depression. Important advances will also require the development of ever more penetrating brain imaging methodologies to enable the detection of molecular and cellular biomarkers in living patients. Such discoveries should make it possible at long last to delineate bona fide subtypes of depression, which will likely show distinct etiological and pathophysiological mechanisms.

Ultimately, translation of these discoveries into improved treatments, with fundamentally novel mechanisms of action, may require such advances, so that a particular treatment can be matched to a particular genotype or endophenotype. More invasive treatments may also become feasible for individuals who are severely ill, including deep brain stimulation or even viral-mediated gene transfer, to correct abnormalities observed in particular patients. Of course, all this remains a promissory note. Given past failures to develop non-monoamine-based antidepressants, it is possible that there is something unique about prolonged enhancement of serotonergic or noradrenergic function that causes palliative improvement in a wide range of stress-related disorders including depression and many other conditions. But we reject this nihilistic view based on the extraordinary advances in neurobiology and molecular therapeutics, which make it difficult for us to fully anticipate today improvements that might occur decades from now in psychiatric treatments. We believe that the difficulty of developing non-monoamine-based antidepressants must not obfuscate the importance and eventual feasibility of the goal, given the great clinical need.

REFERENCES

Agid, Y., Buzsaki, G., Diamond, D.M., Frackowiak, R., Giedd, J., Girault, J.A., Grace, A., Lambert, J.J., Manji, H., Mayberg, H., Popoli, M., Prochiantz, A., Richter-Levin, G., Somogyi, P., Spedding, M., Svenningsson, P., and Weinberger, D. (2007) How can drug discovery for psychiatric disorders be improved? *Nat. Rev. Drug Discov.* 6:189–201.

Akama, K.T., and McEwen, B.S. (2005) Gene therapy to bet on: protecting neurons from stress hormones 1. *Trends Pharmacol. Sci.* 26:169–172.

Bacchi, F., Mathe, A.A., Jimenez, P., Stasi, L., Arban, R., Gerrard, P., and Caberlotto, L. (2006) Anxiolytic-like effect of the selective neuropeptide Y Y2 receptor antagonist BIIE0246 in the elevated plus-maze. *Peptides* 27:3202–3207.

Bale, T.L., and Vale, W.W. (2004) CRF and CRF receptors: role in stress responsivity and other behaviors. *Ann. Rev. Pharmacol. Toxicol.* 44:525–557.

Bao, A.M., Meynen, G., and Swaab, D.F. (2007) The stress system in depression and neurodegeneration: focus on the human hypothalamus. *Brain Res. Rev.* Epub ahead of print.

Barden, N. (2004) Implication of the hypothalamic-pituitary-adrenal axis in the physiopathology of depression. *J. Psychiatr. Neurosci.* 29:185–193.

Berton, O., McClung, C.A., Dileone, R.J., Krishnan, V., Renthal, W., Russo, S.J., Graham, D., Tsankova, N.M., Bolanos, C.A., Rios, M., Monteggia, L.M., Self, D.W., and Nestler, E.J. (2006) Essential role of BDNF in the mesolimbic dopamine pathway in social defeat stress. *Science* 311:864–868.

Berton, O., and Nestler, E.J. (2006) New approaches to antidepressant drug discovery: beyond monoamines. *Nat. Rev. Neurosci.* 7:137–151.

Binder, E.B., Salyakina, D., Lichtner, P., Wochnik, G.M., Ising, M., Putz, B., et al. (2004) Polymorphisms in FKBP5 are associated with increased recurrence of depressive episodes and rapid response to antidepressant treatment. *Nature Gen.* 36:1319–1325.

Bleakman, D., Alt, A., and Witkin, J.M. (2007) AMPA receptors in the therapeutic management of depression. *CNS Neurol. Disord. Drug Targets* 6:117–126.

Blier, P., Gobbi, G., Haddjeri, N., Santarelli, L., Mathew, G., and Hen, R. (2004) Impact of substance P receptor antagonism on the serotonin and norepinephrine systems: relevance to the antidepressant/anxiolytic response 18. *J. Psychiatr. Neurosci.* 29:208–218.

Bourin, M., Mocaer, E., and Porsolt, R. (2004) Antidepressant-like activity of S 20098 (agomelatine) in the forced swimming test in rodents: involvement of melatonin and serotonin receptors. *J. Psychiatry Neurosci.* 29:126–133.

Boyle, M.P., Brewer, J.A., Funatsu, M., Wozniak, D F., Tsien, J.Z., Izumi, Y., and Muglia, L.J. (2005) Acquired deficit of forebrain glucocorticoid receptor produces depression-like changes in adrenal axis regulation and behavior. *Proc. Natl. Acad. Sci. USA* 102:473–478.

Boyle, M.P., Brewer, J.A., Vogt, S.K., Wozniak, D.F., and Muglia, L.J. (2004) Genetic dissection of stress response pathways in vivo. *Endocr. Res.* 30:859–863.

Carlezon, W.A., Jr., Duman, R.S., and Nestler, E.J. (2005) The many faces of CREB. *Trends Neurosci.* 28:436–445.

Chahl, L.A. (2006) Tachykinins and neuropsychiatric disorders. *Curr. Drug Targets* 7:993–1003.

Charmandari, E., Tsigos, C., and Chrousos, G. (2005) Endocrinology of the stress response 1. *Ann. Rev. Physiol.* 67:259–284.

Clapcote, S.J., Lipina, T.V., Millar, J.K., Mackie, S., Christie, S., Ogawa, F., Lerch, J.P., Trimble, K., Uchiyama, M., Sakuraba, Y., Kaneda, H., Shiroishi, T., Houslay, M.D., Henkelman, R.M., Sled, J.G., Gondo, Y., Porteous, D.J., and Roder, J.C. (2007) Behavioral phenotypes of Disc1 missense mutations in mice. *Neuron* 54:387–402.

Conti, B., Maier, R., Barr, A.M., Morale, M.C., Lu, X., Sanna, P.P., Bilbe, G., Hoyer, D., and Bartfai, T. (2007) Region-specific transcriptional changes following the three antidepressant treatments electro convulsive therapy, sleep deprivation and fluoxetine. *Mol. Psychiatry* 12:167–189.

de Kloet, E.R., Joels, M., and Holsboer, F. (2005) Stress and the brain: from adaptation to disease. *Nat. Rev. Neurosci.* 6:463–475.

den Boer, J.A., Bosker, F.J., and Meesters, Y. (2006) Clinical efficacy of agomelatine in depression: the evidence. *Int. Clin. Psychopharmacol.* 21(Suppl 1):S21–S24.

Drew, M.R., and Hen, R. (2007) Adult hippocampal neurogenesis as target for the treatment of depression. *CNS Neurol. Disord. Drug Targets* 6:205–218.

Duman, C.H., Schlesinger, L., Kodama, M., Russell, D.S., and Duman, R.S. (2007) A role for MAP kinase signaling in behavioral models of depression and antidepressant treatment. *Biol. Psychiatry* 61: 661–670.

Duman, R.S. (2004) Role of neurotrophic factors in the etiology and treatment of mood disorders. *Neuromolecular Med.* 5:11–25.

Duman, R. S., Heninger, G.R., and Nestler, E.J. (1997) A molecular and cellular theory of depression. *Arch. Gen. Psychiatr.* 54:597–606.

Duman, R.S., and Monteggia, L.M. (2006) A neurotrophic model for stress-related mood disorders. *Biol. Psychiatry* 59:1116–1127.

Eisch, A.J., Bolanos, C.A., de Wit, J., Simonak, R.D., Pudiak, C.M., Barrot, M., Verhaagen, J., and Nestler, E.J. (2003) Brain-derived neurotrophic factor in the ventral midbrain-nucleus accumbens pathway: a role in depression. *Biol. Psychiatry* 54:994–1005.

Fekete, E.M., and Zorrilla, E.P. (2007) Physiology, pharmacology, and therapeutic relevance of urocortins in mammals: ancient CRF paralogs. *Front. Neuroendocrinol.* 28:1–27.

Flores, B.H., Kenna, H., Keller, J., Solvason, H.B., and Schatzberg, A.F. (2006) Clinical and biological effects of mifepristone treatment for psychotic depression. *Neuropsychopharmacology* 31:628–636.

Fuchs, E., Simon, M., and Schmelting, B. (2006) Pharmacology of a new antidepressant: benefit of the implication of the melatonergic system. *Int. Clin. Psychopharmacol.* 21(Suppl 1):S17–S20.

Garcia, J.A., Zhang, D., Estill, S.J., Michnoff, C., Rutter, J., Reick, M., Scott, K., Diaz-Arrastia, R., and McKnight, S.L. (2000) Impaired cued and contextual memory in NPAS2-deficient mice. *Science* 288:2226–2230.

Georgescu, D., Sears, R.M., Hommel, J.D., Barrot, M., Bolanos, C.A., Marsh, D.J., Bednarek, M.A., Bibb, J.A., Maratos-Flier, E., Nestler, E.J., and DiLeone, R.J. (2005) The hypothalamic neuropeptide melanin-concentrating hormone acts in the nucleus accumbens to modulate feeding behavior and forced-swim performance. *J. Neurosci.* 25:2933–2940.

Gillespie, C. F., and Nemeroff, C.B. (2005) Hypercortisolemia and depression. *Psychosom. Med.* 67(Suppl 1):S26–S28.

Hawes, J.J., and Picciotto, M.R. (2004) Characterization of GalR1, GalR2, and GalR3 immunoreactivity in catecholaminergic nuclei of the mouse brain. *J. Comp. Neurol.* 479:410–423.

Heinrichs, S.C., and Koob, G.F. (2004) Corticotropin-releasing factor in brain: a role in activation, arousal, and affect regulation. *J. Pharmacol. Exp. Ther.* 311:427–440.

Heurteaux, C., Lucas, G., Guy, N., El Yacoubi, M., Thummler, S., Peng, X.D., Noble, F., Blondeau, N., Widmann, C., Borsotto, M., Gobbi, G., Vaugeois, J. M., Debonnel, G., and Lazdunski, M. (2006) Deletion of the background potassium channel TREK-1 results in a depression-resistant phenotype. *Nat. Neurosci.* 9:1134–1141.

Hillhouse, E.W., and Grammatopoulos, D.K. (2006) The molecular mechanisms underlying the regulation of the biological activity of corticotropin-releasing hormone receptors: implications for physiology and pathophysiology. *Endocr. Rev.* 27:260–286.

Holmes, A., and Picciotto, M.R. (2006) Galanin: a novel therapeutic target for depression, anxiety disorders and drug addiction? *CNS Neurol. Disord. Drug Targets* 5:225–232.

Ishida, H., Shirayama, Y., Iwata, M., Katayama, S., Yamamoto, A., Kawahara, R., and Nakagome, K. (2007) Infusion of neuropeptide Y into CA3 region of hippocampus produces antidepressant-like effect via Y1 receptor. *Hippocampus* 17:271–280.

Ising, M., Zimmermann, U.S., Kunzel, H.E., Uhr, M., Foster, A.C., Learned-Coughlin, S.M., Holsboer, F., and Grigoriadis, D.E. (2007) High-affinity CRF(1) receptor antagonist NBI-34041: preclinical and clinical data suggest safety and efficacy in attenuating elevated stress response. *Neuropsychopharmacology* 32(9):1941–1949.

Jeanneteau, F., and Chao, M.V. (2006) Promoting neurotrophic effects by GPCR ligands. *Novartis Found. Symp.* 276:181–189; discussion 189–192, 233–187, 275–181.

Karl, T., and Herzog, H. (2007) Behavioral profiling of NPY in aggression and neuropsychiatric diseases. *Peptides* 28:326–333.

Karlsson, R.M., and Holmes, A. (2006) Galanin as a modulator of anxiety and depression and a therapeutic target for affective disease. *Amino Acids* 31:231–239.

Kaufer, D., Ogle, W.O., Pincus, Z.S., Clark, K.L., Nicholas, A.C., Dinkel, K.M., Dumas, T.C., Ferguson, D., Lee, A.L., Winters, M.A., and Sapolsky, R.M. (2004) Restructuring the neuronal stress response with anti-glucocorticoid gene delivery. *Nat. Neurosci.* 7: 947–953.

Keck, M.E. (2006) Corticotropin-releasing factor, vasopressin and receptor systems in depression and anxiety. *Amino Acids* 31:241–250.

Keck, M.E., Ohl, F., Holsboer, F., and Muller, M.B. (2005) Listening to mutant mice: a spotlight on the role of CRF/CRF receptor systems in affective disorders. *Neurosci. Biobehav. Rev.* 29:867–889.

Keck, M.E., Welt, T., Muller, M.B., Uhr, M., Ohl, F., Wigger, A., Toschi, N., Holsboer, F., and Landgraf, R. (2003) Reduction of hypothalamic vasopressinergic hyperdrive contributes to clinically relevant behavioral and neuroendocrine effects of chronic paroxetine treatment in a psychopathological rat model. *Neuropsychopharmacology* 28:235–243.

Kehne, J.H. (2007) The CRF1 receptor, a novel target for the treatment of depression, anxiety, and stress-related disorders. *CNS Neurol. Disord. Drug Targets* 6:163–182.

King, D.P., Zhao, Y., Sangoram, A.M., Wilsbacher, L.D., Tanaka, M., Antoch, M.P., Steeves, T.D., Vitaterna, M.H., Kornhauser, J.M., Lowrey, P.L., Turek, F.W., and Takahashi, J.S. (1997) Positional cloning of the mouse circadian clock gene. *Cell* 89:641–653.

Korte, S.M., Koolhaas, J.M., Wingfield, J.C., and McEwen, B.S. (2005) The Darwinian concept of stress: benefits of allostasis and costs of allostatic load and the trade-offs in health and disease 17. *Neurosci. Biobehav. Rev.* 29:3–38.

Kramer, M.S., Cutler, N., Feighner, J., Shrivastava, R., Carman, J., Sramek, J.J., Reines, S.A., Liu, G.H., Snavely, D., Wyatt-Knowles, E., Hale, J.J., Mills, S.G., MacCoss, M., Swain, C.J., Harrison, T., Hill, R.G., Hefti, F., Scolnick, E.M., Cascieri, M.A., Chicchi, G.G., Sadowski, S., Williams, A.R., Hewson, L., Smith, D., Carlson, E.J., Hargreaves, R.J., and Rupniak, N.M.J. (1998) Distinct mechanism for antidepressant activity by blockade of central substance P receptors 50. *Science* 281:1640–1645.

Li, Y.W., Fitzgerald, L., Wong, H., Lelas, S., Zhang, G., Lindner, M.D., Wallace, T., McElroy, J., Lodge, N.J., Gilligan, P., and Zaczek, R. (2005) The pharmacology of DMP696 and DMP904, non-peptidergic CRF1 receptor antagonists. *CNS Drug Rev.* 11: 21–52.

Lolait, S.J., Stewart, L.Q., Jessop, D.S., Young, W.S., 3rd, and O'Carroll, A.M. (2007) The hypothalamic-pituitary-adrenal axis response to stress in mice lacking functional vasopressin V1b receptors. *Endocrinology* 148:849–856.

Lu, X., Barr, A.M., Kinney, J.W., Sanna, P., Conti, B., Behrens, M.M., and Bartfai, T. (2005) A role for galanin in antidepressant actions with a focus on the dorsal raphe nucleus. *Proc. Natl. Acad. Sci. USA* 102:874–879.

Lu, X., Lundstrom, L., Langel, U., and Bartfai, T. (2005) Galanin receptor ligands. *Neuropeptides* 39:143–146.

Lu, X., Mazarati, A., Sanna, P., Shinmei, S., and Bartfai, T. (2005) Distribution and differential regulation of galanin receptor subtypes in rat brain: effects of seizure activity. *Neuropeptides* 39: 147–152.

Lu, X., Sharkey, L., and Bartfai, T. (2007) The brain galanin receptors: targets for novel antidepressant drugs. *CNS Neurol. Disord. Drug Targets* 6:183–192.

Manev, H., and Uz, T. (2006) Clock genes: influencing and being influenced by psychoactive drugs. *Trends Pharmacol. Sci.* 27:186–189.

Manji, H.K., Drevets, W.C., and Charney, D.S. (2001) The cellular neurobiology of depression. *Nat. Med.* 7:541–547.

McClung, C.A. (2007) Circadian genes, rhythms and the biology of mood disorders. *Pharmacol. Ther.* 114:222–232.

McClung, C.A., Sidiropoulou, K., Vitaterna, M., Takahashi, J.S., White, F.J., Cooper, D.C., and Nestler, E.J. (2005) Regulation of dopaminergic transmission and cocaine reward by the Clock gene. *Proc. Natl. Acad. Sci. USA* 102:9377–9381.

Monteggia, L.M., Barrot, M., Powell, C.M., Berton, O., Galanis, V., Gemelli, T., Meuth, S., Nagy, A., Greene, R.W., and Nestler, E.J. (2004) Essential role of brain-derived neurotrophic factor in adult hippocampal function. *Proc. Natl. Acad. Sci. USA* 101:10827–10832.

Murck, H., Held, K., Ziegenbein, M., Kunzel, H., Holsboer, F., and Steiger, A. (2004) Intravenous administration of the neuropeptide galanin has fast antidepressant efficacy and affects the sleep EEG. *Psychoneuroendocrinology* 29:1205–1211.

Musazzi, L., Perez, J., Hunt, S.P., Racagni, G., and Popoli, M. (2005) Changes in signaling pathways regulating neuroplasticity induced by neurokinin 1 receptor knockout. *Eur. J. Neurosci.* 21:1370–1378.

Nestler, E.J., Barrot, M., DiLeone, R.J., Eisch, A.J., Gold, S.J., and Monteggia, L.M. (2002) Neurobiology of depression. *Neuron* 34: 13–25.

Nestler, E.J., and Carlezon, W.A., Jr. (2006) The mesolimbic dopamine reward circuit in depression. *Biol. Psychiatry* 59:1151–1159.

Ogren, S.O., Kuteeva, E., Hokfelt, T., and Kehr, J. (2006) Galanin receptor antagonists: a potential novel pharmacological treatment for mood disorders. *CNS Drugs* 20:633–654.

Pacher, P., and Kecskemeti, V. (2004) Trends in the development of new antidepressants. Is there a light at the end of the tunnel? *Curr. Med. Chem.* 11:925–943.

Pare, D., Quirk, G.J., and Ledoux, J.E. (2004) New vistas on amygdala networks in conditioned fear. *J. Neurophysiol.* 92:1–9.

Pariante, C.M., and Miller, A.H. (2001) Glucocorticoid receptors in major depression: Relevance to pathophysiology and treatment 1. *Biol. Psychiatry* 49:391–404.

Park, S.K., Nguyen, M.D., Fischer, A., Luke, M.P., Affar el, B., Dieffenbach, P.B., Tseng, H.C., Shi, Y., and Tsai, L.H. (2005) Par-4 links dopamine signaling and depression. *Cell* 122:275–287.

Paul, I.A., and Skolnick, P. (2003) Glutamate and depression: clinical and preclinical studies. *Ann. N. Y. Acad. Sci.* 1003:250–272.

Pennefather, J.N., Lecci, A., Candenas, M.L., Patak, E., Pinto, F.M., and Maggi, C.A. (2004) Tachykinins and tachykinin receptors: a growing family. *Life Sci.* 74:1445–1463.

Pittenger, C., Sanacora, G., and Krystal, J.H. (2007) The NMDA receptor as a therapeutic target in major depressive disorder. *CNS Neurol. Disord. Drug Targets* 6:101–115.

Prickaerts, J., Moechars, D., Cryns, K., Lenaerts, I., van Craenendonck, H., Goris, I., Daneels, G., Bouwknecht, J.A., and Steckler, T. (2006) Transgenic mice overexpressing glycogen synthase kinase 3beta: a putative model of hyperactivity and mania. *J. Neurosci.* 26: 9022–9029.

Reppert, S.M., and Weaver, D.R. (2002) Coordination of circadian timing in mammals. *Nature* 418:935–941.

Roybal, K., Theobold, D., Graham, A., DiNieri, J.A., Russo, S.J., Krishnan, V., Chakravarty, S., Peevey, J., Oehrlein, N., Birnbaum, S., Vitaterna, M.H., Orsulak, P., Takahashi, J.S., Nestler, E.J., Carlezon, W.A., Jr., and McClung, C.A. (2007) Mania-like behavior induced by disruption of CLOCK. *Proc. Natl. Acad. Sci. USA* 104:6406–6411.

Rupniak, N.M.J., Carlson, E.J., Webb, J.K., Harrison, T., Porsolt, R.D., Roux, S., de Felipe, C., Hunt, S.P., Oates, B., and Wheeldon, A. (2001) Comparison of the phenotype of NK1R–/– mice with pharmacological blockade of the substance P (NK1) receptor in assays for antidepressant and anxiolytic drugs. *Behav. Pharmacol.* 12: 497–508.

Sanacora, G., Kendell, S.F., Levin, Y., Simen, A.A., Fenton, L.R., Coric, V., and Krystal, J.H. (2007) Preliminary evidence of riluzole efficacy in antidepressant-treated patients with residual depressive symptoms. *Biol. Psychiatry* 61:822–825.

Sanacora, G., Rothman, D.L., Mason, G., and Krystal, J.H. (2003) Clinical studies implementing glutamate neurotransmission in mood disorders. *Ann. N. Y. Acad. Sci.* 1003:292–308.

Sapolsky, R.M. (2000) Stress hormones: Good and bad.. *Neurobiol. Dis.* 7:540–542.

Shaw, A.M., Boules, M., Zhang, Y., Williams, K., Robinson, J., Carlier, P.R., and Richelson, E. (2007) Antidepressant-like effects of novel triple reuptake inhibitors, PRC025 and PRC050. *Eur. J. Pharmacol.* 555:30–36.

Shimazaki, T., Yoshimizu, T., and Chaki, S. (2006) Melanin-concentrating hormone MCH1 receptor antagonists: a potential new approach to the treatment of depression and anxiety disorders. *CNS Drugs* 20:801–811.

Shirayama, Y., Chen, A.C., Nakagawa, S., Russell, D.S., and Duman, R.S. (2002) Brain-derived neurotrophic factor produces antidepressant effects in behavioral models of depression. *J. Neurosci.* 22:3251–3261.

Svenningsson, P., Chergui, K., Rachleff, I., Flajolet, M., Zhang, X., El Yacoubi, M., Vaugeois, J.M., Nomikos, G.G., and Greengard, P. (2006) Alterations in 5-HT1B receptor function by p11 in depression-like states. *Science* 311:77–80.

Swanson, C.J., Blackburn, T.P., Zhang, X., Zheng, K., Xu, Z.Q., Hokfelt, T., Wolinsky, T.D., Konkel, M.J., Chen, H., Zhong, H., Walker, M.W., Craig, D.A., Gerald, C.P., and Branchek, T.A. (2005) Anxiolytic- and antidepressant-like profiles of the galanin-3 receptor (Gal3) antagonists SNAP 37889 and SNAP 398299. *Proc. Natl. Acad. Sci. USA* 102:17489–17494.

Takahashi, J.S. (2004) Finding new clock components: past and future. *J. Biol. Rhythms* 19:339–347.

Tanis, K.Q., Newton, S.S., and Duman, R.S. (2007) Targeting neurotrophic/growth factor expression and signaling for antidepressant drug development. *CNS Neurol. Disord. Drug Targets* 6: 151–160.

Tsankova, N., Renthal, W., Kumar, A., and Nestler, E.J. (2007) Epigenetic regulation in psychiatric disorders. *Nature Rev. Neurosci.* 8:355–367.

Tschenett, A., Singewald, N., Carli, M., Balducci, C., Salchner, P., Vezzani, A., Herzog, H., and Sperk, G. (2003) Reduced anxiety and improved stress coping ability in mice lacking NPY-Y2 receptors. *Eur. J. Neurosci.* 18:143–148.

Turner, C.A., Akil, H., Watson, S.J., and Evans, S.J. (2006) The fibroblast growth factor system and mood disorders. *Biol. Psychiatry* 59:1128–1135.

Uz, T., Ahmed, R., Akhisaroglu, M., Kurtuncu, M., Imbesi, M., Dirim Arslan, A., and Manev, H. (2005) Effect of fluoxetine and cocaine on the expression of clock genes in the mouse hippocampus and striatum. *Neuroscience* 134:1309–1316.

Warner-Schmidt, J.L., and Duman, R.S. (2007) VEGF is an essential mediator of the neurogenic and behavioral actions of antidepressants. *Proc. Natl. Acad. Sci. USA* 104:4647–4652.

Wei, Q., Lu, X.Y., Liu, L., Schafer, G., Shieh, K.R., Burke, S., Robinson, T.E., Watson, S.J., Seasholtz, A.F., and Akil, H. (2004) Glucocorticoid receptor overexpression in forebrain: a mouse model of increased emotional lability. *Proc. Natl. Acad. Sci. USA* 101:11851–11856.

Wermuth, C.G. (2006) Similarity in drugs: reflections on analogue design. *Drug Discov. Today* 11:348–354.

Witkin, J.M., Marek, G.J., Johnson, B.G., and Schoepp, D.D. (2007) Metabotropic glutamate receptors in the control of mood disorders. *CNS Neurol. Disord. Drug Targets* 6:87–100.

Yoshitake, T., Reenila, I., Ogren, S.O., Hokfelt, T., and Kehr, J. (2003) Galanin attenuates basal and antidepressant drug-induced increase of extracellular serotonin and noradrenaline levels in the rat hippocampus. *Neurosci. Lett.* 339:239–242.

Zarate, C.A., Jr., Singh, J.B., Carlson, P.J., Brutsche, N.E., Ameli, R., Luckenbaugh, D.A., Charney, D.S., and Manji, H.K. (2006) A randomized trial of an *N*-methyl-D-aspartate antagonist in treatment-resistant major depression. *Arch. Gen. Psychiatry* 63:856–864.

Zarate, C.A., Jr., Singh, J.B., Quiroz, J.A., De Jesus, G., Denicoff, K.K., Luckenbaugh, D.A., Manji, H.K., and Charney, D.S. (2006) A double-blind, placebo-controlled study of memantine in the treatment of major depression. *Am. J. Psychiatry* 163:153–155.

35 The Neurobiology of Menstrual Cycle-Related Mood Disorders

DAVID R. RUBINOW, PETER J. SCHMIDT, SAMANTHA MELTZER-BRODY, AND VERONICA HARSH

Reproductive endocrine-related mood disorders are affective disturbances that appear in concert with changes in reproductive endocrine activity. They include psychiatric disturbances occurring during menarche, pregnancy or postpartum, the perimenopause, or the menstrual cycle. Also included are disturbances consequent to manipulation of gonadal steroids or reproductive status (for example, hormone replacement therapy or gonadal suppression). *Menstrual cycle–related mood disorders* refer to disturbances of mood and behavior that are observed in a menstrual-cycle-phase specific fashion. These include disturbances that appear de novo during a given menstrual cycle phase (for example, during the luteal phase) as well as menstrual cycle modulation of the appearance or symptom severity of a preexisting psychiatric disorder. In this chapter, we focus on the former, that is, mood disorders appearing de novo during the luteal phase (hereafter referred to as MRMD). By posing and answering a series of questions, we organize recently obtained data that will help to define the effects of gonadal steroids on the brain and the contribution of gonadal steroids to the underlying neurobiology of MRMD.

NEUROMODULATORY EFFECTS OF GONADAL STEROIDS

The best support for the neuromodulatory effects of gonadal steroids is found in their dramatic and widely ranging cellular actions. In fact, gonadal steroids have been shown to play a role in all stages of neural development, including neurogenesis, synaptogenesis, neural migration, growth, differentiation, survival, and death (Pilgrim and Hutchison, 1994). These effects occur largely as a consequence of the ability of gonadal steroids to modulate genomic transcription. As transcriptional regulators, the receptors for gonadal steroids direct or modulate the synthesis of the synthetic and metabolic enzymes as well as receptor proteins for many neurotransmitters and neuropeptides (Ciocca and Roig, 1995). The advances of the past 15 years, however, have demonstrated that the cellular effects of gonadal steroids are far more complex, powerful, and comprehensive than suggested by their originally described genomic actions. First, as the mechanics of transcription became elucidated, it became clear that activated steroid receptors influence transcription not as solitary agents but in combination with other intracellular proteins (Halachmi et al., 1994). These protein–protein interactions were such that an activated receptor might enhance, reduce, initiate, or terminate transcription of a particular gene solely as a function of the specific proteins with which it interacted (and the ability of these proteins to enhance or hinder the recruitment of the general transcription factor apparatus). The expression or activation state of these proteins—coregulators (coactivators or corepressors)—proved to be tissue specific, thus suggesting the means by which a hormone receptor modulator (for example, tamoxifen) could act like an (estrogen) agonist in some tissues (for example, bone) and like an (estrogen) antagonist in others (for example, breast) (Jackson et al., 1997; C.L. Smith et al., 1997; Hall and McDonnell, 2005). Another group of intracellular proteins, the cointegrators, provided a means by which classical hormone receptors could bind to and regulate sites other than hormone response elements (for example, estrogen receptor [ER] or glucocorticoid receptor [GR] binding cyclic AMP-response element binding [CREB] protein [CBP] and, subsequently, the AP1 binding site) (Uht et al., 1997), and competition for cointegrator or other transcriptional regulatory proteins was demonstrated as a mechanism by which even ligand-free hormone receptors could influence (for example, squelch or interfere with) the transcriptional efficacy of other activated hormone receptors (Meyer et al., 1989). Thus, the intracellular hormone receptor environment as well as the extracellular hormone environment might dictate the response to hormone receptor activation.

Second, the hormone receptors were found to exist in different forms. For example, isoforms of the progesterone receptor, PRA and PRB (the latter of which contains a 164 amino acid N-terminal extension), have different distributions and biological actions (Chalbos and Galtier, 1994), and two separate forms of the estrogen receptor, ER_{α} and ER_{β}, are encoded on different chromosomes (6 and 14, respectively), have different patterns of distribution in the brain, different affinity patterns for certain ligands, and a range of different actions (including those created by estrogen receptor heterodimers; Paech et al., 1997; Shughrue et al., 1997; Kuiper et al., 1998). Further, a variant of ER_{β}, $ER_{\beta2}$, is expressed in the brain, where it can heterodimerize with the ER_{α} or ER_{β} receptors (J.T. Moore et al., 1998) and inhibit their transcriptional actions (Maruyama et al., 1998).

Third, a variety of substances (for example, nerve growth factor, insulin) are capable of activating a steroid receptor even in the absence of ligand (Ignar-Trowbridge et al., 1992; Aronica et al., 1994). This crosstalk is exemplified by the ability of dopamine to induce lordosis by activating the progesterone receptor (Power et al., 1991; Mani et al., 1994).

Fourth, the relatively slow, genomic effects of gonadal steroids have been expanded in two dimensions: time, with a variety of rapid (seconds to minutes) effects observed; and targets, which now include ion channels and a variety of second-messenger systems. Several lines of evidence indicate that the rapid effects of E_2 are not likely to be the consequence of nuclear events but rather must be related to events occurring at the cell surface (Karkanias and Etgen, 1993; Black et al., 1994; Kelly and Wagner, 1999; Collins and Webb, 1999;Toran-Allerand et al., 1999; Singh et al., 2000; Kato, 2001; Wyckoff et al., 2001; Razandi et al., 2002; Qiu et al., 2003). Both classical and unique ERs exist in the caveolae or caveolar-like microdomains of membranes where they link to scaffolding proteins (for example, caveolin-1, flotillin; Toran-Allerand et al., 2002) and multiple signaling molecules, particularly the G proteins, which then activate a wide array of signal transduction systems, including adenylate cyclase/protein kinase A (PKA; Szego and Davis, 1967; Aronica et al., 1994; Gu and Moss, 1996; Qiu et al., 2003), phospholipase C/phosphotidylinositol/diacylglycerol (Le Mellay et al., 1997; Simoncini et al., 2000; Qiu et al., 2003), nitric oxide synthase (Simoncini et al., 2000), protein kinase B (Akt) (L. Zhang et al., 2001), and mitogen-activated protein kinase (MAPK) (Black et al., 1994; Collins and Webb, 1999; Toran-Allerand et al., 1999; Singh et al., 2000; Kato, 2001; Razandi et al., 2003). Through alterations in signal transduction or by direct binding, E_2 can also regulate ion channel activity (for example, calcium and potassium channels) and hence, cellular activation (Qiu et al., 2003; Razandi et al., 2003; Zhang et al., 2005). Finally, the activity of membrane receptors is acutely modulated by gonadal steroids (for example, glutamate receptors by estradiol and γ-aminobutyric acid [GABA] receptors by the 5-alpha reduced metabolite of progesterone, *allopregnanolone*) (Majewska et al., 1986; Wong and Moss, 1992). Adding to the complexity of the effects described above is their tissue- and even cell-specific nature (for example, estradiol increases MAPK in neurons but decreases it in astrocytes) (Watters et al., 1997; L. Zhang et al., 2002).

Fifth, gonadal steroids regulate cell survival. Neuroprotective effects of E_2 have been described in neurons grown in serum-free media or those exposed to glutamate, amyloid-β, hydrogen peroxide, ischemia, or glucose deprivation (McEwen and Alves, 1999; Dubal and Wise, 2002). Some of these effects appear to lack stereospecificity (that is, are not classical receptor mediated) and may be attributable to the antioxidant properties of E_2 (Mooradian, 1993; Behl et al., 1997), although data from one report are consistent with a receptor-mediated effect (Singer et al., 1996). Gonadal steroids may also modulate cell survival through effects on cell survival proteins (for example, Bcl-2, BAX), MAPK, Akt, or even amyloid precursor protein and Aβ metabolism (Black et al., 1994; Garcia-Segura et al., 1998; Gouras et al., 2000; L. Zhang et al., 2002).

Sixth, some actions of gonadal steroids on brain appear to be context and developmental stage dependent. Toran-Allerand (1994) showed that estrogen displays reciprocal interactions with growth factors and their receptors (for example, p51 and trk A, neurotrophins) in such a way as to regulate, throughout development, the response to estrogen stimulation: estrogen stimulates its own receptor early in development, inhibits it during adulthood, and stimulates it again in the context of brain injury. Additionally, we demonstrated that the ability to modulate serotonin receptor subtype and GABA receptor subunit transcription in rat brain with exogenous administration of gonadal steroids or gonadal steroid receptor blockade is largely dependent on the developmental stage (for example, last prenatal week vs. fourth postnatal week) during which the intervention occurs (L. Zhang et al., 1999).

Finally, the effects of gonadal steroids do not occur in isolation but, rather, in exquisite interaction with the environment. Juraska (1990), for example, demonstrated that the rearing environment (enriched vs. impoverished) dramatically influences sex differences in dendritic branching in the rat cortex and hippocampus. Further, the size of the spinal nucleus of the bulbocavernosus and the degree of adult male sexual behavior in rats is in part regulated by the amount of anogenital licking they receive as pups from their mothers, an activity that is elicited from the dams by the androgen the pups secrete in their urine (C.L. Moore et al., 1992). These environmental influences may include diet and medication, as short-chain fatty acids (including valproic acid) dramatically increase cellular sensitivity to gonadal steroids by amplifying their transcriptional potency through inhibition of histonic deacetylase and stimulation of MAPK (Jansen et al., 2004).

The vicissitudes of gonadal steroids and their receptors, therefore, direct neural architecture and provide the means by which the response of the CNS to incoming stimuli may be altered. The extent to which these effects underlie or contribute to differential pharmacologic efficacy or behavioral differences observed across individuals is unclear but is of considerable potential relevance for MRMD and other reproductive endocrine-related mood disorders.

THE VALIDITY OF MENSTRUAL CYCLE–RELATED MOOD DISORDERS AS A DIAGNOSIS

Unlike other diagnoses in medicine, MRMD is a time-oriented and not a symptom-oriented diagnosis. The symptoms are relatively nonspecific; rather it is their exclusive appearance during the luteal phase that defines the disorder. As such, the diagnosis cannot be made based on history but instead requires a prospective demonstration that symptoms are confined to the luteal phase, disappearing at or soon after the onset of menses. Although many variations on this theme may potentially exist, use of a more restrictive definition has been necessary to ensure the homogeneity of samples across studies necessary for comparison and generalization of results obtained. Employment of diagnostic guidelines (National Institute of Mental Health, 1983; American Psychiatric Association, 1994; Pincus et al., 2007) has demonstrated the existence of MRMD and permitted resolution of many (but not all) of the controversies in the literature regarding the neurobiological basis of MRMD.

LUTEAL PHASE–SPECIFIC PHYSIOLOGIC ABNORMALITIES AND MRMD

Given the temporal coincidence of symptoms and the luteal phase in women with MRMD, early investigators sought, as an etiology, a disturbance in reproductive endocrine function. Comparisons of basal plasma hormone levels in women with MRMD and controls have revealed no consistent diagnosis-related differences. Specifically, we observed no diagnosis-related differences in the plasma levels, areas under the curve, or patterns of hormone secretion for estradiol, progesterone, follicle stimulating hormone (FSH), or luteinizing hormone (LH) (Rubinow et al., 1988), findings in concert with those of Backstrom et al. (1983) comparing patients with high and low degrees of cyclical mood change.

Findings from subsequent studies of estradiol, progesterone, testosterone, and LH pulsatility also have been inconsistent (Backstrom and Aakvaag, 1981; Facchinetti et al., 1990; Eriksson et al., 1992; Reame et al., 1992; Facchinetti et al., 1993; Redei and Freeman, 1995; Wang et al., 1996; Bloch et al., 1998), suggesting that MRMD is not characterized by abnormal circulating plasma levels of gonadal steroids or gonadotropins or by hypothalamic-pituitary-ovarian axis dysfunction. Several studies do, however, suggest that levels of estrogen, progesterone, or "neurosteroids" (for example, pregnenolone sulfate) may be correlated with symptom severity in women with MRMD (Halbreich et al., 1986; Schechter et al., 1996; Wang et al., 1996).

Studies of a variety of other endocrine factors in patients with MRMD have been similarly unrevealing. In general, no differences have been observed in basal plasma cortisol levels, urinary free cortisol, the circadian pattern of plasma cortisol secretion, or basal plasma adrenocorticotropic hormone (ACTH) levels (Rubinow and Schmidt, 1995). (Decreased ACTH levels in MRMD patients across the menstrual cycle and no differences from controls have been reported; Redei and Freeman, 1993; Rosenstein et al., 1996; Bloch et al., 1998.) We did observe a significantly greater cortisol (but not ACTH) response to ovine corticotropin releasing hormone (CRH) in patients with MRMD compared with controls; the exaggerated response appeared to reflect lower baseline plasma cortisol values and appeared in the follicular and luteal phases (Rabin et al., 1990). In contrast, the ACTH and cortisol responses to the serotonin$_{2C}$ (5-HT$_{2C}$) agonist/5-HT$_{2A}$ antagonist m-chlorophenylpiperazine (m-CPP) were blunted in patients with MRMD during both menstrual cycle phases (with the difference in cortisol reaching statistical significance in the luteal phase only) (Su et al., 1997). Despite the appearance of abnormal baseline thyroid function in 10% of our patients and abnormal (blunted and exaggerated) thyroid stimulating hormone (TSH) response to thyroid releasing hormone (TRH) in 30% of our patients, the vast majority of patients with MRMD have normal hypothalamic-pituitary-thyroid axis function (Schmidt et al., 1993). Luteal phase decreases in plasma beta endorphin (Chuong et al., 1985; Facchinetti et al., 1987) and platelet serotonin uptake (Ashby et al., 1988) have been reported in MRMD; neither the diagnostic group–related decreases nor their confinement to the luteal phase are consistently observed (Malmgren et al., 1987; Tulenheimo et al., 1987; Hamilton and Gallant, 1988; Veeninga and Westenberg, 1992; Bloch et al., 1998). Finally, neither diagnostic nor cycle-related (with the exception of 3-methoxy-4-hydroxyphenylglycol [MHPG]) differences were observed in two studies of cerebrospinal fluid (Parry et al., 1991; Eriksson et al., 1994).

In conclusion, there are no clearly demonstrated endocrine or other biological abnormalities in MRMD. Further, for the overwhelming majority of biologic factors for which diagnostic group–related differences have been suggested or demonstrated, the difference is not confined to the luteal phase but rather appears in follicular and luteal phases. These differences include increased prevalence of abnormal TSH response to TRH (Roy-Byrne et al., 1987), decreased slow-wave sleep (Lee et al., 1990), increased brain-stem auditory–evoked response latencies (Howard et al., 1992), phase advanced temperature minima and offset of melatonin secretion (Parry et al., 1989; Parry et al., 1990), decreased red blood cell magnesium level (Sherwood et al., 1986; Rosenstein et al., 1994), decreased arginine vasopressin (AVP) level (Prange et al., 1977), blunted growth hormone and cortisol response to L-tryptophan (Bancroft et al., 1991), blunted ACTH response to m-CPP (Su et al., 1997), decreased evening basal plasma cortisol (Rabin et al., 1990), decreased (or increased) free testosterone (Eriksson et al., 1992; Bloch et al., 1998), and increased cortisol response to CRH infusion (Rabin et al., 1990). Even if these differences are confirmed, their persistence across the menstrual cycle would appear to argue against their direct role in the expression of a disorder confined to the luteal phase. Presently, then, there is no clearly demonstrated luteal phase–specific physiologic abnormality in MRMD.

LUTEAL PHASE OVARIAN STEROIDS AND THE SYMPTOMS OF MRMD

Given the absence of basal or stimulated reproductive endocrine abnormalities or luteal phase–specific biological abnormalities in MRMD, one could reasonably ask whether the luteal phase is required for the expression of MRMD. We (Schmidt et al., 1991) answered this question by blinding women with MRMD to menstrual cycle phase with the progesterone antagonist mifepristone (RU-486) combined with either human chorionic gonadotropin (hCG) or placebo. Mifepristone administered alone 7 days after the midcycle LH surge precipitated menses and the premature termination of the luteal phase, while the addition of hCG preserved the luteal phase even after the mifepristone-induced menses. Consequently, following the mifepristone-induced menses, patients did not know whether they were in the follicular phase of a new cycle (mifepristone alone) or in the preserved luteal phase of the first cycle (mifepristone plus hCG). We observed that women with MRMD experienced their characteristic premenstrual mood state after the mifepristone-induced menses in both groups, despite the presence of an experimentally induced follicular phase in the women receiving mifepristone alone. The mid to late luteal phase, then, is clearly not required for the appearance of MRMD symptoms. It, nonetheless, remained possible that symptoms could be triggered by hormonal events prior to the mid to late luteal phase, consistent with reports that the suppression of ovulation results in a remission of MRMD symptoms (Muse et al., 1984; Casson et al., 1990).

IS OVARIAN ACTIVITY REQUIRED FOR THE EXPRESSION OF MRMD?

Studies that employ different methods to suppress or eliminate ovarian function (for example, gonadotropin releasing hormone [GnRH] agonists, the synthetic androgen danazol, or oophorectomy) consistently demonstrate the therapeutic efficacy of ovarian suppression in MRMD. It is, however, difficult to ascribe the efficacy to ovarian suppression per se, given the lack of efficacy of oral contraceptives (which inhibit ovulation) (Graham and Sherwin, 1992) and the reported efficacy of danazol when administered after ovulation (Sarno et al., 1987), thereby leaving unclear the mechanisms of its efficacy. We (Schmidt et al., 1998) confirmed the efficacy shown by others of GnRH agonists (for example, leuprolide acetate [Lupron] in the treatment of MRMD; Muse et al., 1984; Glazener et al., 1985; Bancroft et al., 1987; Mortola et al., 1991; Mezrow et al., 1994). Consistent with Bancroft et al.'s (1987) earlier observations, a therapeutic response was not observed in all patients despite the consistent reduction of gonadal steroid levels to hypogonadal levels. Although the majority of study participants did show a therapeutic response (10/18), the mechanism of action remained unclear (for example, low plasma gonadal steroid levels, consistent gonadal steroid levels, anovulation, suppression of follicular development). This uncertainty was in part addressed by the double-blind, placebo-controlled reintroduction of estradiol (0.1 mg estraderm patch) or progesterone (200 mg BID by suppository) in the study participants in whom Lupron displayed efficacy. The results unequivocally demonstrated the precipitation of a wide range of characteristic symptoms of MRMD during estrogen and progesterone addback but not during placebo addback (Fig. 35.1). Muse (1989) and Mortola et al. (1991) previously described the return of symptoms during 1-month trials of estrogen, progestin, or placebo, although symptom return was not seen by Mortola et al. (1991) with the combination of estrogen and progestin. Despite the questions raised by Mortola's study (for example, why was placebo as able to induce the return of behavioral symptoms as were the gonadal steroids, and why did solitary gonadal steroids precipitate the return of symptoms but sequential administration fail to stim-

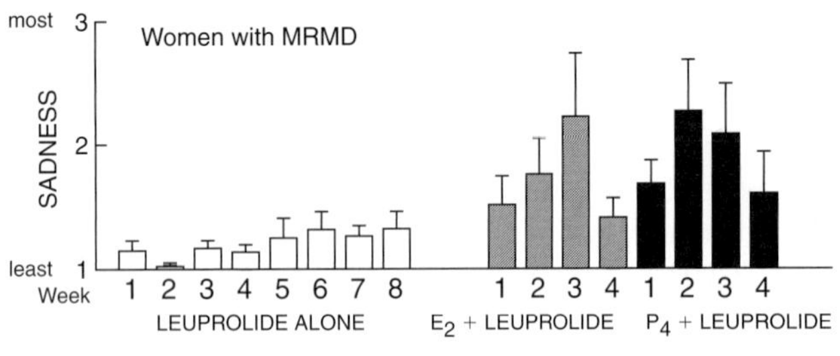

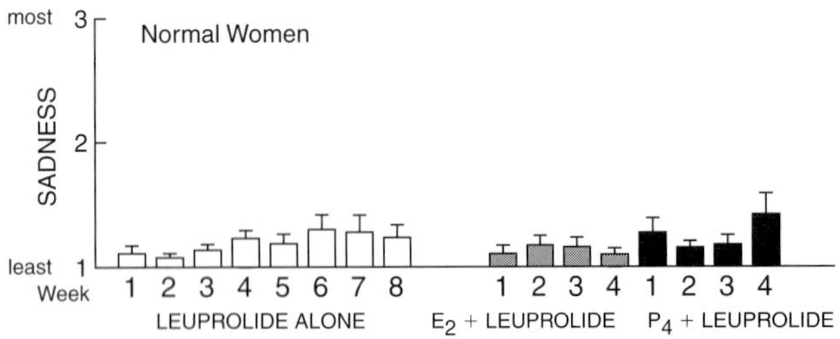

FIGURE 35.1 Ten women with MRMD and 15 controls had minimal mood and behavioral symptoms during Lupron. In contrast, women with MRMD but not the controls had a significant increase in sadness during either estradiol (E2) or progesterone (P4) administration. Histograms represent the mean (+/– SE) of the seven daily scores on the daily rating form sadness scale for each of the 8 weeks preceding hormone replacement (Lupron alone) and during the 4 weeks of Lupron plus E2 and Lupron plus P4 replacement. A score of one indicates that the symptom was not present and a score of six indicates that it was present in the extreme. MRMD: menstrual cycle–related mood disorders; SE: standard error. (Schmidt et al., 1998).

ulate symptom return?), the combined results from our study and those of Muse (1989) and Mortola et al. (1991) strongly suggest the role of gonadal steroids in the occurrence of MRMD symptoms. Particularly striking, however, is the observation that controls lacking a history of MRMD and going through the same protocol (that is, Lupron-induced hypogonadism followed by gonadal steroid addback) showed no perturbation of mood during hypogonadism and no mood disturbance during hormonal addback (Fig. 35.1). It would appear, therefore, that women with a history of MRMD are differentially sensitive to the mood-perturbing effects of gonadal steroids, as similar steroid manipulations in women without a history of MRMD are without effect. This differential sensitivity may also be consistent with the observations mentioned earlier that MRMD symptoms are correlated with progesterone levels in women with MRMD despite mean levels in patients that are not different from those in controls.

TRIGGER AND SUSCEPTIBILITY

If gonadal steroids trigger MRMD in some women, how do they do so and why not in all women?

Trigger

To determine whether the steroid-induced mood disturbances in women with MRMD are caused by the change in hormone levels (with reintroduction representing permissive—but not sufficient— effects of elevated hormone levels interacting with an infradian driver), we recently administered Lupron followed by 3 months of continuous estradiol and progesterone replacement. This paradigm demonstrated that it is the change in gonadal steroids that triggers the mood disturbance; that is, reintroduction of gonadal steroids precipitated a self-limited episode with no subsequent dysphoria over the remainder of the 3 months. These findings suggest that continuous administration of oral contraceptives might, after the first precipitated episode, effectively prevent the recurrence of all other symptoms (due to the stable hormone levels). Possibly consistent with this hypothesis is the recent demonstration of the efficacy of oral contraceptives when administered with a reduced pill-free interval (Yonkers et al., 2005).

Susceptibility

An obvious source of differences in response phenotype is found in possible genotypic differences. Known polymorphisms in gonadal steroid receptors have been shown to alter receptor transcriptional efficiency (for example, CAG repeat in exon 1 of the androgen receptor; progins insertion in intron 7 of the progesterone receptor) and to be associated with differential illness risk (that is, prostate cancer, breast cancer; Giovannucci et al., 1997; Beilin et al., 1999; Wang-Gohrke et al., 2000; J.X. Zhang et al., 2004). Additionally, the susceptibility to the disruptive effects of estradiol on reproductive development differs enormously (up to a hundredfold) between mouse strains, with genotype contributing more to the variance than the dose of estradiol employed (Spearow et al., 1999). There is precedent, then, for inferring that polymorphisms in genes involved in the gonadal steroid signaling pathway or in gonadal steroid-regulated genes may alter the nature or strength of the steroid signal as well as the phenotype. Although some earlier candidate gene studies did not find significant associations with MRMD (Melke et al., 2003), we have recently identified a region of the estrogen receptor ER_{α} gene (*ESR1*) containing multiple polymorphic alleles that are associated with MRMD (Huo et al., 2007). Further, this association was significant only in those women with the Val Val genotype of the COMT Val158Met polymorphism, thus lending support to the idea that the effects of multiple genes may interact in creating a dysphoric behavioral response to normal gonadal steroid levels.

Demonstration of a relationship between genetic variations in *ESR1* and MRMD is very promising for several reasons. First, ER alpha plays a major role in arousal

(Garey et al., 2003), the dysfunction of which could underlie somatic, cognitive, and affective symptoms of MRMD. Second, ER_α regulates the signaling of neurotransmitter systems implicated in the etiopathogenesis and treatment of MRMD. For example, extensive links exist between estrogen and serotonin function, with the latter involved in mood regulation and the selective therapeutic effects of selective serotonin reuptake inhibitors (SSRIs) in MRMD (Rubinow et al., 1998). At least some of the effects of estradiol are mediated through serotonin 1A receptors, which are up-regulated through nuclear factor-kappa B (NF-κB) by ER_α but not ER_β (Wissink et al., 2001). Third, the estrogen receptor has clear physiologic relevance in MRMD as the receptor for a hormone that can trigger the onset of symptoms of the disorder (Schmidt et al., 1998).

OTHER NEUROBIOLOGIC SYSTEMS IMPLICATED IN THE PATHOPHYSIOLOGY OF MRMD

Serotonin

A variety of observations implicate dysfunction of serotonergic neurons in MRMD. Although investigations utilizing pharmacologic probes to test 5-HT system function in women with MRMD have yielded inconsistent results (Bancroft et al., 1991; Veeninga and Westenberg, 1992), treatment studies consistently demonstrate the therapeutic efficacy of serotonin-enhancing agents (for example, clomipramine and fluoxetine) for many women with MRMD (Dimmock et al., 2000). Nonserotonin selective antidepressants appear inferior in efficacy to the SSRIs (Eriksson et al., 1995). Further, acute tryptophan depletion, mediated by a dietary manipulation, was reported in one study (Menkes et al., 1994) to exacerbate symptoms in women with MRMD during follicular and luteal phases of the menstrual cycle. Additionally, we observed an acute therapeutic response in women with MRMD following oral administration of the 5-HT_{2C} agonist/$5HT_{2A}$ antagonist, m-CPP, as well as a delayed (24 hours) reversal of the efficacy of fluoxetine by the serotonin receptor "antagonist" *metergoline* (Su et al., 1997; Roca et al., 2002). These data converge to strongly suggest the role of the serotonin system in the pathophysiology of MRMD. As the majority of abnormalities in neuroendocrine response to serotonergic agents in MRMD are observed in both phases of the cycle (and because approximately 40% of women with MRMD do not respond to SSRIs), serotonergic dysfunction cannot be implicated as a direct cause of MRMD. It may, however, convey a vulnerability to mood destabilization in association with changes in gonadal steroids seen during the menstrual cycle, a particularly intriguing possibility given the multiple reciprocal interactions that exist throughout development between gonadal steroids and serotonin (Rubinow et al., 1998).

Neurosteroids

A second potential source of susceptibility is the conversion of progesterone to its neurosteroid metabolites. Observations central to these speculations include the following:

1. The GABA receptor (the presumed mediator of anxiolysis) is positively modulated by the 5-alpha and -beta reduced metabolites of progesterone (allopregnanolone and pregnanolone, respectively) (Majewska et al., 1986) and is remodeled by these metabolites (Li and O'Malley, 2003; Shen et al., 2005; Maguire and Mody, 2007).
2. Withdrawal of progesterone in rats produces anxiety and insensitivity to benzodiazepines due to withdrawal of allopregnanolone, with consequent induction of $GABA_A$ alpha-4 subunit levels, and inhibition of GABA currents (S.S. Smith, Gong, Hsu, et al., 1998; S.S. Smith, Gong, Li, et al., 1998).
3. Allopregnanolone displays anxiolytic effects in several animal anxiety models (Kellner et al., 1983; Bitran et al., 1991; Wieland et al., 1991) and may be involved in the stress response (Purdy et al., 1991).
4. Decreased plasma allopregnanolone levels are seen in major depressive disorder and in depression associated with alcohol withdrawal, with an increase in levels seen in plasma and cerebrospinal fluid (CSF) following successful antidepressant treatment (Romeo et al., 1996; Romeo et al., 1998; Uzunova et al., 1998; Ströhle et al., 1999; although see Eser et al., 2006).
5. Antidepressants may promote the reductive activity of one of the neurosteroid synthetic enzymes (3 alpha-hydroxysteroid oxidoreductase), thus favoring the formation of allopregnanolone (Griffin and Mellon, 1999).
6. Cerebral cortical inhibition increases during the luteal phase, a presumed effect of increased allopregnanolone levels and a finding absent in women with MRMD (M.J. Smith et al., 2002; M.J. Smith et al., 2003; Maguire et al., 2005).
7. Patients with MRMD show differences in pregnanolone-modulated saccadic eye velocity (SEV) and sedation in the luteal phase compared with controls (Sundstrom and Backstrom, 1998b) (although the reported differences seem attributable to an SEV response to vehicle in those with MRMD and a blunted sedation response in the follicular phase in controls).
8. Patients with high severity MRMD show blunted SEV and sedation responses to $GABA_A$ receptor agonists—pregnanolone (Sundstrom and Backstrom, 1998a) or midazolam (Sundstrom et al., 1997)—compared with patients with low severity MRMD.
9. Women with MRMD have blunted allopregnanolone responses to stress and evidence of altered metabo-

lism of progesterone to allopregnanolone (Girdler et al., 2001; Klatzkin et al., 2006).

Studies to date fail to demonstrate any consistent diagnosis-related differences in allopregnanolone or pregnanolone (Schmidt et al., 1994; Wang et al., 1996; Girdler et al., 2001) nor any difference in pregnanolone levels in women with MRMD before and after successful treatment with antidepressants (Sundstrom and Backstrom, 1998a). Nonetheless, a recent study by Shen et al. (2007) demonstrated that changes in the GABA receptor induced by decreases in allopregnanolone can reverse the effects of allopregnanolone on the receptor and exaggerate anxiolytic responses to stressors in the absence of basal changes in anxiety. Consequently, changes in neurosteroid levels remain intriguing as possible contributors to the triggering of or susceptibility to MRMD.

HYPOTHALAMIC-PITUITARY-ADRENAL (HPA) AXIS

Disturbances of the hypothalamic-pituitary-adrenal (HPA) axis function are implicated in the pathophysiology of affective disorder, and it is, therefore, tempting to speculate that similar dysregulation of the stress response may contribute to the susceptibility to affective disturbance seen in women with MRMD. Observations of abnormal HPA axis activity in depression and numerous reciprocal regulatory interactions between the stress and reproductive axes suggested that MRMD might be characterized by disturbances in the HPA axis. As mentioned above, studies of basal plasma measures of the HPA axis have been largely unrevealing. Nonetheless, studies of stimulated HPA axis activity provide evidence of the involvement of this neuroendocrine axis in MRMD. Roca et al. (2003) showed a differential HPA axis response to exercise stimulation in women with MRMD compared with controls. Women with MRMD fail to show the luteal phase increase in stimulated AVP, ACTH, and cortisol seen in normal women and additionally display adrenal hyporesponsivity. As it is progesterone rather than estradiol that enhances exercise-stimulated HPA activity (Roca et al., 2003), women with MRMD display an abnormal response to progesterone. A variety of data support these observations. In a prior study (Su et al., 1997), we showed that m-CPP stimulated cortisol was significantly blunted in the luteal (but not the follicular) phase in women with MRMD, consistent with the current findings as well as with data from Girdler et al. (2001) showing decreased luteal phase–stimulated cortisol in women with MRMD. Additionally, blunted or absent cortisol response to CRH or naloxone, respectively, was observed in the luteal phase in women with MRMD (Facchinetti et al., 1994). In a separate earlier study (Rabin et al., 1990), we showed that women with MRMD display low evening cortisol levels across the menstrual cycle, seen as well by Parry et al. (2000) and Odber et al. (1998) and consistent with either adrenal hyposensitivity or altered circadian cortisol dynamics (although, see Steiner et al., 1984; Parry et al., 1994). Bancroft et al. (1991) identified blunted levels across the menstrual cycle of tryptophan-stimulated cortisol secretion in women with MRMD. Finally, an abnormal response to (presumed) luteal phase progesterone in women with MRMD was also seen in their failure to manifest the normal luteal phase alteration in the timing of the cortisol acrophase (Parry et al., 2000). These data, then, suggest the following: stimulated cortisol (albeit paradigm specific) is decreased in women with MRMD relative to controls during the luteal phase; the adrenal response to ACTH may be blunted in women with MRMD; women with MRMD manifest an abnormal HPA axis (and mood) response to progesterone; women with MRMD display disturbances of the HPA axis that are markedly different from those identified in major depression. Although the determinants of these observations are unclear, they provide another compelling example of differential response to gonadal steroids in women with MRMD and suggest an additional potential source of vulnerability to affective disturbance.

CONCLUSIONS

To identify what the study of MRMD may contribute to our understanding of the effects of gonadal steroids on brain and behavior, several observations must be integrated. First, there does not appear to be a disturbance of reproductive endocrine function that underlies MRMD. Second, changes in levels of estrogen and progesterone appear to be capable of triggering mood disturbances in a susceptible population; that is, some preexisting vulnerability must explain the capacity of the same biologic stimulus (for example, gonadal steroids) to elicit a differential behavioral response across groups of people. Third, perturbations of nonreproductive endocrine systems appear capable of precipitating MRMD. Menstrual cycle–related mood disorders may appear in the context of hypothyroidism (with symptoms responsive to thyroid hormone replacement; Schmidt et al., 1990), and provocative (Bancroft, 1993; Su et al., 1997) and especially treatment studies (Stone et al., 1990) suggest the relevance of the serotonin system to MRMD. Menstrual cycle–related mood disorders, then, may represent a behavioral state that is triggered by a reproductive endocrine stimulus in those who may be rendered susceptible to behavioral state changes by antecedent experiential events (for example, history of major depression; DeJong et al., 1985) or physical or sexual abuse (Paddison et al., 1990) or biological conditions (for example, hypothyroidism; Schmidt et al., 1990). Treatment can, therefore, be directed to either eliminating the trigger (for example, ovarian suppression) or correcting the "vulnerability" (for example, serotonergic antidepressants; Stone et al., 1990). Although the means by which alterations in gonadal steroids trigger changes in behavioral state in certain individuals are unclear, it is nonetheless striking that, in contrast to the pathological function of other endocrine systems (for example, adrenal, thyroid) seen in association with mood disorders, gonadal steroids may precipitate mood disturbances in the context of normal ovarian function. This suggests that further study of the interactions between gonadal steroids and other neuroactive systems may help elucidate general mechanisms underlying affective regulation as well as the physiologic substrate that predisposes certain people to experience reproductive endocrine-related mood disorders.

REFERENCES

American Psychiatric Association. (1994) *Diagnostic and Statistical Manual of Mental Disorders,* 4th ed. Washington, DC: Author.

Aronica, S.M., Kraus, W.L., and Katzenellenbogen, B.S. (1994) Estrogen action via the cAMP signaling pathway: stimulation of adenylate cyclase and cAMP-regulated gene transcription. *Proc. Natl. Acad. Sci. USA* 91(18):8517–8521.

Ashby, C.R., Jr., Carr, L.A., Cook, C.L., Steptoe, M.M., and Franks, D.D. (1988) Alteration of platelet serotonergic mechanisms and monoamine oxidase activity in premenstrual syndrome. *Biol. Psychiatry* 24(2):225–233.

Backstrom, T., and Aakvaag, A. (1981) Plasma prolactin and testosterone during the luteal phase in women with premenstrual tension syndrome. *Psychoneuroendocrinology* 6(3):245–251.

Backstrom, T., Sanders, D., Leask, R., Davidson, D., Warner, P., and Bancroft, J. (1983) Mood, sexuality, hormones, and the menstrual cycle: II. Hormone levels and their relationship to the premenstrual syndrome. *Psychosom. Med.* 45(6):503–507.

Bancroft, J. (1993) The premenstrual syndrome—a reappraisal of the concept and the evidence. *Psychol. Med.* (Suppl 24):1–47.

Bancroft, J., Boyle, H., Warner, P., and Fraser, H.M. (1987) The use of an LHRH agonist, buserelin, in the long-term management of premenstrual syndromes. *Clin. Endocrinol.* 27(2):171–182.

Bancroft, J., Cook, A., Davidson, D., Bennie, J., and Goodwin, G. (1991) Blunting of neuroendocrine responses to infusion of L-tryptophan in women with perimenstrual mood change. *Psychol. Med.* 21(2):305–312.

Behl, C., et al. (1997) Neuroprotection against oxidative stress by estrogens: structure-activity relationship. *Mol. Pharmacol.* 51(4): 535–541.

Beilin, J., and Zajac, J.D. (1999) Function of the human androgen receptor varies according to CAG repeat number within the normal range. *Proceedings of the 81st Annual Meeting of the Endocrine Society* 500(abstr.).

Bitran, D., Hilvers, R.J., and Kellogg, C.K. (1991) Anxiolytic effects of 3a-hydroxy-5a[b]-pregnan-20-one: endogenous metabolites of progesterone that are active at the $GABA_A$ receptor. *Brain Res.* 561:157–161.

Black, L.J., et al. (1994) Raloxifene (LY139481 HCI) prevents bone loss and reduces serum cholesterol without causing uterine hypertrophy in ovariectomized rats. *J. Clin. Invest.* 93(1):63–69.

Bloch, M., Schmidt, P.J., Su, T.-P., Tobin, M.B., and Rubinow, D.R. (1998) Pituitary-adrenal hormones and testosterone across the menstrual cycle in women with premenstrual syndrome and controls. *Biol. Psychiatry* 43(12):897–903.

Casson, P., Hahn, P.M., VanVugt, D.A., and Reid, R.L. (1990) Lasting response to ovariectomy in severe intractable premenstrual syndrome. *Am. J. Obstet. Gynecol.* 162(1):99–105.

Chalbos, D., and Galtier, F. (1994) Differential effect of forms A and B of human progesterone receptor on estradiol-dependent transcription. *J. Biol. Chem.* 269(37):23007–23012.

Chuong, C.J., Coulam, C.B., Kao, P.C., Bergstralh, E., and Go, V.L. (1985) Neuropeptide levels in premenstrual syndrome. *Fert. Steril.* 44(6):760–765.

Ciocca, D.R., and Roig, L.M. (1995) Estrogen receptors in human nontarget tissues: biological and clinical implications. *Endocr. Rev.* 16(1):35–62.

Collins, P., and Webb, C. (1999) Estrogen hits the surface. *Nat. Med.* 5(12):1130–1131.

DeJong, R., Rubinow, D.R., Roy-Byrne, P.P., Hoban, M.C., Grover, G.N., and Post, R.M. (1985) Premenstrual mood disorder and psychiatric illness. *Am. J. Psychiatry* 142:1359–1361.

Dimmock, P.W., Wyatt, K.M., Jones, P.W., and O'Brien, P.M.S. (2000) Efficacy of selective serotonin-reuptake inhibitors in premenstrual syndrome: a systematic review. *Lancet* 356(9236):1131–1136.

Dubal, D.B., and Wise, P.M. (2002) Estrogen and neuroprotection: from clinical observations to molecular mechanisms. *Dialogues Clin. Neurosci.* 4:149–162.

Eriksson, E., Alling, C., Andersch, B., Andersson, K., and Berggren, U. (1994) Cerebrospinal fluid levels of monoamine metabolites: a preliminary study of their relation to menstrual cycle phase, sex steroids, and pituitary hormones in healthy women and in women with premenstrual syndrome. *Neuropsychopharmacology* 11(3):201–213.

Eriksson, E., Hedberg, M.A., Andersch, B., and Sundblad, C. (1995) The serotonin reuptake inhibitor paroxetine is superior to the noradrenaline reuptake inhibitor maprotiline in the treatment of premenstrual syndrome. *Neuropsychopharmacology* 12(2):167–176.

Eriksson, E., Sundblad, C., Lisjo, P., Modigh, K., and Andersch, B. (1992) Serum levels of androgens are higher in women with premenstrual irritability and dysphoria than in controls. *Psychoneuroendocrinology* 17(2/3):195–204.

Eser, D., Schule, C., Baghai, T.C., Romeo, E., and Rupprecht, R. (2006) Neuroactive steroids in depression and anxiety disorders: clinical studies. *Neuroendocrinology* 84:244–254.

Facchinetti, F., Fioroni, L., Martignoni, E., Sances, G., Costa, A., and Genazzani, A.R. (1994) Changes of opioid modulation of the hypothalamo-pituitary-adrenal axis in patients with severe premenstrual syndrome. *Psychosomatic Med.* 56(5):418–422.

Facchinetti, F., Genazzani, A.D., Martignoni, E., Fioroni, L., Nappi, G., and Genazzani, A.R. (1993) Neuroendocrine changes in luteal function in patients with premenstrual syndrome. *J. Clin. Endocrinol. Metab.* 76(5):1123–1127.

Facchinetti, F., Genazzani, A.D., Martignoni, E., Fioroni, L., Sances, G., and Genazzani, A.R. (1990) Neuroendocrine correlates of premenstrual syndrome: changes in the pulsatile pattern of plasma LH. *Psychoneuroendocrinology* 15(4):269–277.

Facchinetti, F., Martignoni, E., Petraglia, F., Sances, M., Nappi, G., and Genazzani, A. (1987) Premenstrual fall of plasma B-endorphin in patients with premenstrual syndrome. *Fertil. Steril.* 47(4): 570–573.

Garcia-Segura, L.M., Cardona-Gomez, P., Naftolin, F., and Chowen, J.A. (1998) Estradiol upregulates Bcl-2 expression in adult brain neurons. *Neuroreport* 9(4):593–597.

Garey, J., et al. (2003) Genetic contributions to generalized arousal of brain and behavior. *Proc. Natl. Acad. Sci. USA* 100(19):11019–11022.

Giovannucci, E., et al. (1997) The CAG repeat within the androgen receptor gene and its relationship to prostate cancer. *Proc. Natl. Acad. Sci. USA* 94(7):3320–3323.

Girdler, S.S., Straneva, P.A., Light, K.C., Pedersen, C.A., and Morrow, A.L. (2001) Allopregnanolone levels and reactivity to mental stress in premenstrual dysphoric disorder. *Biol. Psychiatry* 49(9):788–797.

Glazener, C.M.A., Bailey, I., and Hull, M.G.R. (1985) Effectiveness of vaginal administration of progesterone. *Br. J. Obstet. Gynaecol.* 92(4):364–368.

Gouras, G.K., et al. (2000) Testosterone reduces neuronal secretion of Alzheimer's beta-amyloid peptides. *Proc. Natl. Acad. Sci. USA* 97(3):1202–1205.

Graham, C.A., and Sherwin, B.B. (1992) A prospective treatment study of premenstrual symptoms using a triphasic oral contraceptive. *J. Psychosom. Res.* 36(3):257–266.

Griffin, L.D., and Mellon, S.H. (1999) Selective serotonin reuptake inhibitors directly alter activity of neurosteroidogenic enzymes. *Proc. Natl. Acad. Sci. USA* 96(23):13512–13517.

Gu, Q., and Moss, R.L. (1996) 17 beta-estradiol potentiates kainate-induced currents via activation of the cAMP cascade. *J. Neurosci.* 16(11):3620–3629.

Halachmi, S., Marden, E., Martin, G., MacKay, H., Abbondanza, C., and Brown, M. (1994) Estrogen receptor-associated proteins: possible mediators of hormone-induced transcription. *Science* 264(5164):1455–1458.

Halbreich, U., Endicott, J., Goldstein, S., and Nee, J. (1986) Premenstrual changes and changes in gonadal hormones. *Acta Psychiatr. Scand.* 74:576–586.

Hall, J.M., and McDonnell, D.P. (2005) Coregulators in nuclear estrogen receptor action. *Mol. Interv.* 5(6):343–356.

Hamilton, J.A., and Gallant, S. (1988) Premenstrual symptom changes and plasma b-endorphin/b-lipotropin throughout the menstrual cycle. *Psychoneuroendocrinology* 13:505–514.

Howard, R., Mason, P., Taghavi, E., and Spears, G. (1992) Brainstem auditory evoked responses (BAERs) during the menstrual cycle in women with and without premenstrual syndrome. *Biol. Psychiatry* 32(8):682–690.

Huo, L., et al. (2007) Risk for premenstrual dysphoric disorder is associated with genetic vatiation in ESR1, the estrogen receptor alpha gene. *Biol. Psychiatry* 62(8):925–933.

Ignar-Trowbridge, D.M., et al. (1992) Coupling of dual signaling pathways: epidermal growth factor action involves the estrogen receptor. *Proc. Natl. Acad. Sci USA* 89(10):4658–4662.

Jackson, T.A., Richer, J.K., Bain, D.L., Takimoto, G.S., Tung, L., and Horwitz, K.B. (1997) The partial agonist activity of antagonist-occupied steroid receptors is controlled by a novel hinge domain-binding co-activator L7/SPA and the corepressors N-COR or SMRT. *Mol. Endocrinol.* 11:693–705.

Jansen, M., Nagal, S., Miranda, P., Lobenhofer, E., Afshari, C., and McDonnell, D.P. (2004) Short-chain fatty acids enhance nuclear receptor activity through mitogen-activated protein kinase activation and histone deacetylase inhibition. *Proc. Natl. Acad. Sci. USA* 101(18):7199–7204.

Juraska, J.M. (1990). The structure of the rat cerebral cortex: effects of gender and the environment. In: Kolb, B., and Tees, R.C., eds. *The Cerebral Cortex of the Rat.* Cambridge, MA: MIT Press, pp. 483–505.

Karkanias, G.B., and Etgen, A.M. (1993) Estradiol attenuates alpha 2-adrenoceptor-mediated inhibition of hypothalamic norepinephrine release. *J. Neuroscience* 13(8):3448–3455.

Kato, S. (2001) Estrogen receptor-mediated cross-talk with growth factor signaling pathways. *Breast Cancer* 8(1):3–9.

Kellner, C.H., Rakita, R.M., Rubinow, D.R., Gold, P.W., Ballenger, J.C., and Post, R.M. (1983) Tetrahydrobiopterin levels in cerebrospinal fluid of affectively ill patients [letter]. *Lancet* 2(8340):55–56.

Kelly, M.J., and Wagner, E.J. (1999) Estrogen modulation of G-protein-coupled receptors. *Trends Endocrin. Metab.* 10:369–374.

Klatzkin, R.R., Morrow, A.L., Light, K.C., Pedersen, C., and Girdler, S.S. (2006) Histories of depression, allopregnanolone responses to stress, and premenstrual symptoms in women. *Biol. Psychol.* 116(1):2–11.

Kuiper, G.G.J.M., Shughrue, P.J., Merchenthaler, I., and Gustafsson, J.-A. (1998) The estrogen receptor b subtype: a novel mediator of estrogen action in neuroendocrine systems. *Front. Neuroendocrinol.* 19:253–286.

Le Mellay, V., Grosse, B., and Lieberherr, M. (1997) Phospholipase C beta and membrane action of calcitriol and estradiol. *J. Biol. Chem.* 272(18):11902–11907.

Lee, K.A., Shaver, J.F., Giblin, E.C., and Woods, N.F. (1990) Sleep patterns related to menstrual cycle phase and premenstrual affective symptoms. Sleep 13(5):403–409.

Li, X., and O'Malley, B.W. (2003) Unfolding the action of progesterone receptors. *J. Biol. Chem.* 278(41):39261–39264.

Maguire, J.L., and Mody, I. (2007) Neurosteroid synthesis-mediated regulation of GABA(a) receptors: relevance to the ovarian cycle stress. *J. Neurosci.* 27(9):2155–2162.

Maguire, J.L., Stell, B.M., Rafizadeh, M., and Mody, I. (2005) Ovarian cycle-linked changes in GABAA receptors mediating tonic inhibition after seizure susceptibility and anxiety. *Nat. Neurosci.* 8(6):797–804.

Majewska, M.D., Harrison, N.L., Schwartz, R.D., Barker, J.L., and Paul, S.M. (1986) Steroid hormone metabolites are barbiturate-like modulators of the GABA receptor. *Science* 232(4753): 1004–1007.

Malmgren, R., Collins, A., and Nilsson, C.G. (1987) Platelet serotonin uptake and effects of vitamin B6-treatment in premenstrual tension. *Neuropsychobiology* 18(2):83–88.

Mani, S.K., Blaustein, J.D., Allen, J.M.C., Law, S.W., O'Malley, B.W., and Clark, J.H. (1994) Inhibition of rat sexual behavior by antisense oligonucleotides to the progesterone receptor. *Endocrinology* 135(4):1409–1414.

Maruyama, K., et al. (1998) A novel isoform of rat estrogen receptor b with 18 amino acid insertion in the ligand binding domain as a putative dominant negative regular of estrogen action. *Biochem. Biophys. Res. Comm.* 246:142–147.

McEwen, B.S., and Alves, S.E. (1999) Estrogen actions in the central nervous system. *Endocr. Rev.* 20:279–307.

Melke, J., et al. (2003) Serotonin transporter gene polymorphisms and platelet [^{3}H]paroxetine binding in premenstrual dysphoria. *Psychoneuroendocrinology* 28(3):446–458.

Menkes, D.B., Coates, D.C., and Fawcett, J.P. (1994) Acute tryptophan depletion aggravates premenstrual syndrome. *J. Affect. Disord.* 32(1):37–44.

Meyer, M.-E., Gronemeyer, H., Turcott, B., Bocquel, M.-T., Tasset, D., and Chambon, P. (1989) Steroid hormone receptors compete for factors that mediate their enhancer function. *Cell* 57(3):433–442.

Mezrow, G., Shoupe, D., Spicer, D., Lobo, R., Leung, B., and Pike, M. (1994) Depot leuprolide acetate with estrogen and progestin add-back for long-term treatment of premenstrual syndrome. *Fertil. Steril.* 62(5):932–937.

Mooradian, A.D. (1993) Antioxidant properties of steroids. *J. Steroid Biochem. Mol. Biol.* 45:509–511.

Moore, C.L., Dou, H., and Juraska, J.M. (1992) Maternal stimulation affects the number of motor neurons in a sexually dimorphic nucleus of the lumbar spinal cord. *Brain Res.* 572(1/2): 52–56.

Moore, J.T., et al. (1998) Cloning and characterization of human estrogen receptor b isoforms. *Biochem. Biophys. Res. Comm.* 247: 75–78.

Mortola, J.F., Girton, L., and Fischer, U. (1991) Successful treatment of severe premenstrual syndrome by combined use of gonadotropin-releasing hormone agonist and estrogen/progestin. *J. Clin. Endocrinol. Metab.*72(2):252A–252F.

Muse, K. (1989) Gonadotropin-releasing hormone agonist-suppressed premenstrual syndrome (PMS): PMS symptom induction by estrogen, progestin, or both. *Abstracts of the Society for Gynecologic Investigation* 4:118.

Muse, K.N., Cetel, N.S., Futterman, L.A., and Yen, S.S.C. (1984) The premenstrual syndrome: effects of "medical ovariectomy." *New Eng. J. Med.* 311(21):1345–1349.

National Institute of Mental Health. (1983). *NIMH Premenstrual Syndrome Workshop Guidelines*. NIMH 6001 Executive Blvd., Room 8235, MSC9669 Bethesda, MD, 20892.

Odber, J., Cawood, E.H.H., and Bancroft, J. (1998) Salivary cortisol in women with and without premenstrual mood changes. *J. Psychosom. Res.* 45(6):557–568.

Paddison, P.L., Gise, L.H., Lebovits, A., Strain, J.J., Cirasole, D.M., and Levine, J.P. (1990) Sexual abuse and premenstrual syndrome: comparison between a lower and higher socioeconomic group. *Psychosomatics* 31(3):265–272.

Paech, K., et al. (1997) Differential ligand activation of estrogen receptors ERa and ERb at AP1 sites. *Science* 277:1508–1510.

Parry, B.L., et al. (1990) Altered waveform of plasma nocturnal melatonin secretion in premenstrual syndrome. *Arch. Gen. Psychiatry* 47(12):1139–1146.

Parry, B.L., et al. (1991) CSF and endocrine studies of premenstrual syndrome. *Neuropsychopharmacology* 5(2):127–137.

Parry, B.L., et al. (1994) Neuroendocrine effects of light therapy in late luteal phase dysphoric disorder. *Biol. Psychiatry* 36(6):356–364.

Parry, B.L., Javeed, S., Laughlin, G.A., Hauger, R., and Clopton, P. (2000) Cortisol circadian rhythms during the menstrual cycle and with sleep deprivation in premenstrual dysphoric disorder and normal control subjects. *Biol. Psychiatry* 48(9):920–931.

Parry, B.L., Mendelson, W.B., Duncan, W.B., Sack, D.A., and Wehr, T.A. (1989) Longitudinal sleep EEG, temperature, and activity measurements across the menstrual cycle in patients with premenstrual depression and in age-matched controls. *Psychiatry Res.* 30(3):285–303.

Pilgrim, C., and Hutchison, J.B. (1994) Developmental regulation of sex differences in the brain: can the role of gonadal steroids be redefined? *Neuroscience* 60(4):843–855.

Pincus, S.M., Schmidt, P.J., Palladino-Negro, P., and Rubinow, D.R. (2007) Differentiation of women with premenstrual dysphoric disorder, recurrent brief depression, and healthy controls by daily mood rating dynamics. *J. Psychiatric Res.* 42(5):337–347.

Power, R.F., Mani, S.K., Codina, J., Conneely, O.M., and O'Malley, B.W. (1991) Dopaminergic and ligand-independent activation of steroid hormone receptors. *Science* 254(5038):1636–1639.

Prange, A.J., Jr., Lipton, M.A., Nemeroff, C.B., and Wilson, I.C. (1977) The role of hormones in depression. *Life Sci.* 20(8):1305–1318.

Purdy, R.H., Morrow, A.L., Moore, P.H., Jr., and Paul, S.M. (1991) Stress-induced elevations of gamma-aminobutyric acid type A receptor-active steroids in the rat brain. *Proc. Natl. Acad. Sci. USA* 88(10):4553–4557.

Qiu, J., et al. (2003) Rapid signaling of estrogen in hypothalamic neurons involves a novel G-protein-coupled estrogen receptor that activates protein kinase C. *J. Neurosci.* 23(29):9529–9540.

Rabin, D.S., et al. (1990) Hypothalamic-pituitary-adrenal function in patients with the premenstrual syndrome. *J. Clin. Endocrinol. Metab.* 75(5):1158–1162.

Razandi, M., Oh, P., Pedram, A., Schnitzer, J., and Levin, E.R. (2002) ERs associate with and regulate the production of caveolin: implications for signaling and cellular actions. *Mol. Endocrinology* 16(1):100–115.

Razandi, M., Pedram, A., Park, S.T., and Levin, E.R. (2003) Proximal events in signaling by plasma membrane estrogen receptors. *J. Biol. Chem.* 278(4):2701–2712.

Reame, N.E., Marshall, J.C., and Kelch, R.P. (1992) Pulsatile LH secretion in women with premenstrual syndrome (PMS): evidence for normal neuroregulation of the menstrual cycle. *Psychoneuroendocrinology* 17(2/3):205–213.

Redei, E., and Freeman, E.W. (1993) Preliminary evidence for plasma adrenocorticotropin levels as biological correlates of premenstrual symptoms. *Acta Endocrinol. (Copenh)* 128(6):536–542.

Redei, E., and Freeman, E.W. (1995) Daily plasma estradiol and progesterone levels over the menstrual cycle and their relation to premenstrual symptoms. *Psychoneuroendocrinology* 20(3):259–267.

Roca, C.A., et al. (2003) Differential menstrual cycle regulation of hypothalamic-pituitary-adrenal axis in women with premenstrual syndrome and controls. *J. Clin. Endocrinol. Metab.* 88(7):3057–3063.

Roca, C.A., Schmidt, P.J., Smith, M.J., Danaceau, M.A., Murphy, D.L., and Rubinow, D.R. (2002) Effects of metergoline on symptoms in women with premenstrual dysphoric disorder. *Am. J. Psychiatry* 159(11):1876–1881.

Romeo, E., et al. (1996) Marked decrease of plasma neuroactive steroids during alcohol withdrawal. *Clin. Neuropharmacol.* 19(4): 366–369.

Romeo, E., et al. (1998) Effects of antidepressant treatment on neuroactive steroids in major depression. *Am. J. Psychiatry* 155(7): 910–913.

Rosenstein, D.L., Elin, R.J., Hosseini, J.M., Grover, G., and Rubinow, D.R. (1994) Magnesium measures across the menstrual cycle in premenstrual syndrome. *Biol. Psychiatry* 35(8):557–561.

Rosenstein, D.L., Kalogeras, K.T., Kalafut, M., Malley, J., and Rubinow, D.R. (1996) Peripheral measures of arginine vasopressin, atrial natriuretic peptide and adrenocorticotropic hormone in premenstrual syndrome. *Psychoneuroendocrinology* 21(3):347–359.

Roy-Byrne, P.P., Rubinow, D.R., Hoban, M.C., Grover, G.N., and Blank, D. (1987) TSH and prolactin responses to TRH in patients with premenstrual syndrome. *Am. J. Psychiatry* 144(4):480–484.

Rubinow, D.R., et al. (1988) Changes in plasma hormones across the menstrual cycle in patients with menstrually related mood disorder and in control subjects. *Am. J. Obstet. Gynecol.* 158(1): 5–11.

Rubinow, D.R., and Schmidt, P.J. (1995) The neuroendocrinology of menstrual cycle mood disorders. *Ann. N. Y. Acad. Sci.*771:648–659.

Rubinow, D.R., Schmidt, P.J., and Roca, C.A. (1998) Estrogen-serotonin interactions: implications for affective regulation. *Biol. Psychiatry* 44(9):839–850.

Sarno, A.P., Miller, E.J., Jr., and Lundblad, E.G. (1987) Premenstrual syndrome: beneficial effects of periodic, low-dose danazol. *Obstet. Gynecol.* 70(1):33–36.

Schechter, D., Strasser, T.J., Endicott, J., Petkova, E., and Nee, J. (1996) Role of ovarian steroids in modulating mood in premenstrual syndrome. *Abstracts of the Society of Biological Psychiatry 51st Annual Meeting* 39:646.

Schmidt, P.J., Grover, G.N., Roy-Byrne, P.P., and Rubinow, D.R. (1993) Thyroid function in women with premenstrual syndrome. *J. Clin. Endocrinol. Metab.* 76(3):671–674.

Schmidt, P.J., Nieman, L.K., Danaceau, M.A., Adams, L.F., and Rubinow, D.R. (1998) Differential behavioral effects of gonadal steroids in women with and in those without premenstrual syndrome. *N. Eng. J. Med.* 338(4):209–216.

Schmidt, P.J., Nieman, L.K., Grover, G.N., Muller, K.L., Merriam, G.R., and Rubinow, D.R. (1991) Lack of effect of induced menses on symptoms in women with premenstrual syndrome. *N. Eng. J. Med.* 324(17):1174–1179.

Schmidt, P.J., Purdy, R.H., Moore, P.H., Jr., Paul, S.M., and Rubinow, D.R. (1994) Circulating levels of anxiolytic steroids in the luteal phase in women with premenstrual syndrome and in control subjects. *J. Clin. Endocrinol. Metab.* 79(5):1256–1260.

Schmidt, P.J., Rosenfeld, D., Muller, K.L., Grover, G.N., and Rubinow, D.R. (1990) A case of autoimmune thyroiditis presenting as menstrual related mood disorder. *J. Clin. Psychiatry* 51(1): 434–436.

Shen, H., et al. (2007) Reversal of neurosteroid effects at a4ß2d GABAa receptors triggers anxiety at puberty. *Nat. Neurosci.* 10(4):469–477.

Shen, H., Gong, Q.H., Yuan, M., and Smith, S.S. (2005) Short-term steroid treatment increases delta GABA(A) receptor subunit expression in rat CA1 hippocampus: pharmacological and behavioral effects. *Neuropharmacology* 49(5):573–586.

Sherwood, R.A., Rocks, B.F., Stewart, A., and Saxton, R.S. (1986) Magnesium and the premenstrual syndrome. *Ann. Clin. Biochem.* 23:667–670.

Shughrue, P.J., Lane, M.V., and Merchenthaler, I. (1997) Comparative distribution of estrogen receptor-a and -b mRNA in the rat central nervous system. *J. Comp. Neurol.* 388:507–525.

Simoncini, T., Hafezi-Moghadam, A., Brazil, D.P., Ley, K., Chin, W.W., and Liao, J.K. (2000) Interaction of oestrogen receptor with the regulatory subunit of phyosphatidylinositol-3-OH-kinase. *Nature* 407(6803):538–541.

Singer, C.A., Rogers, K.L., Strickland, T.M., and Dorsa, D.M. (1996) Estrogen protects primary cortical neurons from glutamate toxicity. *Neurosci. Lett.* 212(1):13–16.

Singh, M., Setalo, G., Jr., Guan, X., Frail, D.E., and Toran-Allerand, C.D. (2000) Estrogen-induced activation of the mitogen-activated protein kinase cascade in the cerebral cortex of estrogen receptor-alpha knock-out mice. *J. Neurosci.* 20(5):1694–1700.

Smith, C.L., Nauaz, Z., and O'Malley, B.W. (1997) Co-activator and co-repressor regulation of the agonist/antagonist activity of the mixed antiestrogen, 4-hydroxytamoxifen. *Mol. Endocrinol.* 11(6):657–666.

Smith, M.J., Adams, L.F., Schmidt, P.J., Rubinow, D.R., and Wassermann, E.M. (2002) Effects of ovarian hormone on human cortical excitability. *Ann. Neurol.* 51(5):599–603.

Smith, M.J., Adams, L.F., Schmidt, P.J., Rubinow, D.R., and Wassermann, E.M. (2003) Abnormal luteal phase excitability of the motor cortex in women with premenstrual syndrome. *Biol. Psychiatry* 54(7):757–762.

Smith, S.S., Gong, Q.H., Hsu, F.-C., Markowitz, R.S., French-Mullen, J.M.H., and Li, X. (1998) $GABA_A$ receptor alpha-4 subunit suppression prevents withdrawal properties of an endogenous steroid. *Nature* 392(6679):926–930.

Smith, S.S., Gong, Q.H., Li, X., et al. (1998) Withdrawal from 3a-OH-5a-pregnan-20-one using a pseudopregnancy model alters the kinetics of hippocampal $GABA_A$-gated current and increases the $GABA_A$ receptor a4 subunit in association with increased anxiety. *J. Neurosci.* 18(14):5275–5284.

Spearow, J.L., Doemeny, P., Sera, R., Leffler, R., and Barkley, M. (1999) Genetic variation in susceptibility to endocrine disruption by estrogen in mice. *Science* 285(5431):1259–1261.

Steiner, M., Haskett, R.F., Carroll, B.J., Hays, S.E., and Rubin, R.T. (1984) Plasma prolactin and severe premenstrual tension. *Psychoneuroendocrinology* 9(1):29–35.

Stone, A.B., Pearlstein, T.B., and Brown, W.A. (1990) Fluoxetine in the treatment of premenstrual syndrome. *Psychopharmacol. Bull.* 26:331–335.

Ströhle, A., et al. (1999) Concentrations of 3 alpha-reduced neuroactive steroids and their precursors in plasma of patients with major depression and after clinical recovery. *Biol. Psychiatry* 45(3):274–277.

Su, T.-P., Schmidt, P.J., Danaceau, M., Murphy, D.L., and Rubinow, D.R. (1997) Effect of menstrual cycle phase on neuroendocrine and behavioral responses to the serotonin agonist m-chlorophenylpiperazine in women with premenstrual syndrome and controls. *J. Clin. Endocrinol. Metab.* 82(4):1220–1228.

Sundstrom, I., and Backstrom, T. (1998a) Citalopram increases pregnanolone sensitivity in patients with premenstrual syndrome: an open trial. *Psychoneuroendocrinology* 23(1):73–88.

Sundstrom, I., and Backstrom, T. (1998b) Patients with premenstrual syndrome have decreased saccadic eye velocity compared to control subjects. *Biol. Psychiatry* 44(8):755–764.

Sundstrom, I., Nyberg, S., and Backstrom, T. (1997) Patients with premenstrual syndrome have reduced sensitivity to midazolam compared to control subjects. *Neuropsychopharmacology* 17(6): 370–381.

Szego, C.M., and Davis, J.S. (1967) Adenosine 3', 5'-monophosphate in rat uterus: acute elevation by estrogen. *Proc. Natl. Acad. Sci. USA* 58:1711–1718.

Toran-Allerand, C.D. (1994). Developmental interactions of estrogens with the neurotrophins and their receptors. In: Micevych, P., and Hammer, R.P., eds. *Neurobiological Effects of Sex Steroid Hormones*. Cambridge, UK: Cambridge University Press, pp. 391–411.

Toran-Allerand, C.D., et al. (2002) ER-X: a novel, plasma membrane-associated, putative estrogen receptor that is regulated during development and after ischemic brain injury. *J. Neurosci.* 22(19):8391–8401.

Toran-Allerand, C.D., Singh, M., and Setalo, G., Jr. (1999) Novel mechanisms of estrogen action in the brain: new players in an old story. *Front. Neuroendocrinol.* 20(2):97–121.

Tulenheimo, A., Laatikainen, T., and Salminen, K. (1987) Plasma b-endorphin immunoreactivity in premenstrual tension. *Br. J. Obstet. Gynaecol.* 94(1):26–29.

Uht, R.M., Anderson, C.M., Webb, P., and Kushner, P.J. (1997) Transcriptional activities of estrogen and glucocorticoid receptors are functionally integrated at the AP-1 response element. *Endocrinology* 138(7):2900–2908.

Uzunova, V., et al. (1998) Increase in the cerebrospinal fluid content of neurosteroids in patients with unipolar major depression who are receiving fluoxetine or fluvoxamine. *Proc. Natl. Acad. Sci. USA* 95:3239–3244.

Veeninga, A.T., and Westenberg, H.G.M. (1992) Serotonergic function and late luteal phase dysphoric disorder. *Psychopharmacology (Berl)* 108(1/2):153–158.

Wang, M., Seippel, L., Purdy, R.H., and Bäckström, T. (1996) Relationship between symptom severity and steroid variation in women with premenstrual syndrome: study on serum pregnenolone, pregnenolone sulfate, 5a-pregnane-3,20-dione and 3a-hydroxy-5a-pregnan-20-one. *J. Clin. Endocrinol. Metab.* 81:1076–1082.

Wang-Gohrke, S., Chang-Claude, J., Becher, H., Kieback, D.G., and Runnebaum, I.B. (2000) Progesterone receptor gene polymorphism is associated with decreased risk for breast cancer by age 50. *Cancer Res.* 60(9):2348–2350.

Watters, J.J., Campbell, J.S., Cunningham, M.J., Krebs, E.G., and Dorsa D.M. (1997) Rapid membrane effects of steroids in neuroblastoma cells: effects of estrogen on mitogen activated protein kinase signaling cascade and c-fos immediate early gene transcription. *Endocrinology* 138:4030–4033.

Wieland, S., Lan, N.C., Mirasedeghi, S., and Gee, K.W. (1991) Anxiolytic activity of the progesterone metabolite 5a-pregnan-3a-ol-one. *Brain Res.* 27:263–268.

Wissink, S., van der Burg, B., Katzenellenbogen, B.S., and van der Saag, P.T. (2001) Synergistic activation of the serotonin-1A receptor by nuclear factor-kappaB and estrogen. *Mol. Endocrinol.* 15(4):543–552.

Wong, M., and Moss, R.L. (1992) Long-term and short-term electrophysiological effects of estrogen on the synaptic properties of hippocampal CA1 neurons. *J. Neurosci.* 12(8):3217–3225.

Wyckoff, M.H., et al. (2001) Plasma membrane estrogen receptors are coupled to endothelial nitric-oxide synthase through Ga_i. *J. Biol. Chem.* 279(29):27071–27076.

Yonkers, K.A., Brown, C., Pearlstein, T.B., Foegh, M., Sampson-Landers, C., and Rapkin, A. (2005) Efficacy of a new low-dose oral contraceptive with drospirenone in premenstrual dysphoric disorder. *Obstet. Gynecol.* 106(3):492–501.

Zhang, J.X., Labaree, D.C., Mor, G., and Hochberg, R.B. (2004) Estrogen to antiestrogen with a single methylene group resulting in an unusual steroidal selective estrogen receptor modulator. *J. Clin. Endocrinol. Metab.* 89:3527–3535.

Zhang, L., et al. (2001) Estrogen protects against beta-amyloid-induced neurotoxicity in rat hippocampal neurons by activation of Akt. *Neuroreport* 12(9):1919–1923.

Zhang, L., et al. (2002) Sex-related differences in MAPKs activationin rat astrocytes: effects of estrogen on cell death. *Mol. Brain Res.* 103(1/2):1–11.

Zhang, L., et al. (2005) Direct binding of estradiol enhances Slack (sequence like a calcium-activated potassium channel) channels' activity. *Neuroscience* 131(2):275–282.

Zhang, L., Ma, W., Barker, J.L., and Rubinow, D.R. (1999) Sex differences in expression of serotonin receptors (subtypes 1A and 2A) in rat brain: a possible role of testosterone. *Neuroscience* 94(1):251–259.

36 Depression and Medical Illness

TAMI D. BENTON, PAUL CRITS-CHRISTOPH, BENOIT DUBÉ, AND DWIGHT L. EVANS

Depression continues to threaten the health and wellbeing of individuals worldwide. Current prevalence estimates of major depressive disorder and dysthymia suggest that 16.6% of individuals will experience a depressive episode during their lifetimes (Kessler et al., 2005). The World Health Organization projected that depression will remain a leading cause of disability by the year 2020, second only to cardiovascular disease (Michaud et al., 2001).

Depression is much more prevalent among those with medical conditions when compared to the general population of the United States (Patten, 2001; Egede, 2007) and is associated with higher health care costs, adverse health behaviors, significant functional impairment, lost work productivity, occupational disability, and increased health care utilization (Katon, 2003). Moreover, a growing body of evidence suggests that depression may be a cause or consequence of some medical illnesses, such as cardiovascular disease, human immunodeficiency virus/acquired immunodeficiency syndrome (HIV/AIDS), cancer, epilepsy, and stroke (Evans and Charney, 2003). Depression makes everything worse.

Increased efforts to understand the comorbidity between medical illnesses and depression have now prompted investigators to search for potential shared etiological mechanisms that might explain the higher comorbidity between medical illnesses and depression (Evans et al., 2005). This research has identified the potential role of inflammatory responses in the pathophysiology of depression, finding higher levels of pro-inflammatory cytokines, acute phase proteins, chemokines, and cellular adhesion molecules (Raison et al., 2006).

In this chapter, we provide an overview of the relevant recent research linking depression and medical illness. We first present an overview of the link between depression and medical illness in general, beginning with epidemiological studies. This is followed by review of research on the possible mechanism for the connection between depression and medical illness, highlighting the role of the immune system and research on sickness behaviors. The nature of the connection between depression and several specific medical illnesses in humans (cardiac disease, cancer, HIV/AIDS) is then explored. We then outline basics of the assessment of depression in the context of medical illness. We conclude with a presentation of treatment considerations for depression in specific medically ill populations.

PREVALENCE OF DEPRESSION IN THE MEDICALLY ILL

Major depressive disorder (MDD) is a common medical disorder with an average lifetime prevalence of about 16.6% of the U.S. population and is 2 times more prevalent in women when compared to men (Kessler et al., 2005; Wang et al., 2005). Depressive disorders are even more prevalent among the medically ill when compared to the general population of the United States (Egede, 2007). The prevalence of depression among individuals who are medically ill increases as one moves along the continuum from community settings (3%–5%) to primary care settings (5%–10%) to inpatient medical settings (10%–14%) (Katon, 2003). Prevalence estimates for depressive disorders among those populations with specific medical conditions are even higher, ranging from 20%–55% (Evans et al., 2005).

Mechanisms of Comorbidity

Although a considerable body of evidence supports the relationship between depression and medical illnesses, the mechanisms mediating these relationships remain unclear. Recent research efforts, prompted in part by the high prevalence of depression among medically ill populations such as those with diabetes, cancer, and cardiovascular disease (Table 36.1), have sought to link the known inflammatory processes underlying these disorders to that of major depression. In fact, recent evidence suggests that depressive disorders may be characterized as conditions of immune activation (Wellens and Ridker, 2004; Wellens and Hotamisligil, 2005). These theories have been based upon the observations that the treatment of patients with cytokines can produce symptoms of depression, that immune system activation is present in some individuals with depression, and that depression occurs more frequently in those indi-

TABLE 36.1 *Depression in Patients with Comorbid Medical Illness*

Comorbid Medical Illness	*Prevalence Rate (%)*
Cardiac disease	17–27 (Rudisch and Nemeroff, 2003)
Cerebrovascular disease	14–19 (Robinson, 2003)
Alzheimer's disease	30–50 (H.B. Lee and Lyketsos, 2003)
Parkinson's disease	4–75 (McDonald et al., 2003)
Epilepsy	
Recurrent	20–55 (Kanner, 2003)
Controlled	3–9 (Kanner, 2003)
Diabetes	
Self-reported	26 (Anderson et al., 2001)
Diagnostic interview	9 (Anderson et al., 2001)
Cancer	22–29 (Raison and Miller, 2003)
HIV/AIDS	5–20 (Cruess et al., 2003)
Pain	30–54 (Campbell et al., 2003)
Obesity	20–30
General population	10.3 (Kessler et al., 1994)

AIDS = acquired immunodeficiency syndrome; HIV = human immunodeficiency virus.

Adapted from Evans et al., 2005, with permission.

viduals with medical disorders associated with immune dysfunction. Furthermore, immune activation can be induced in animals by the administration of specific endotoxins and cytokines, producing a sickness behavior in animals that resembles that of humans with major depression, and chronic antidepressant treatment can inhibit sickness behaviors in humans who are depressed. Additionally, certain cytokines activate cerebral noradernergic and serotonergic systems that have been implicated in major depressive illness and its treatment (Dunn et al., 2005).

Recent investigations of inflammatory processes as potential contributors to the pathogenesis of major depression represent a significant shift in the conceptualization of depression. Central to these theories is the role of cytokines. Cytokines are proteins and glycoproteins secreted by immune cells that function as signals among and between immune cells. Cytokines are the hormones of the immune system. They can be secreted by immune and nonimmune cells and can affect cells outside of the immune system. They function locally and systemically to modulate and regulate immune functions throughout the body, including those of the central nervous system.

The role of cytokines in the pathogenesis of depression has been suggested by clinical and experimental observations. Cytokines have been shown to be effective in the treatment of certain cancers, hepatitis C, viral infections, and multiple sclerosis. Moreover, individuals treated with cytokines for the treatment of infectious diseases or cancer have been observed to develop a behavioral syndrome referred to as the "sickness syndrome" that is very similar to major depression. This syndrome is characterized by anhedonia, cognitive dysfunction, anxiety, irritability, psychomotor slowing, anergia, fatigue, anorexia, sleep alterations, and increased sensitivity to pain (Dunn et al., 1999; Yirmiya et al., 1999; de Beaurepaire et al., 2005). Although the exact prevalence is unknown, studies suggest that the incidence of depression associated with cytokine therapy ranges from 0%–45%, depending upon the medical conditions and study designs. Moreover, the behavioral syndrome induced by cytokine treatment has been shown to be responsive to treatment with standard antidepressant medications, suggesting that the behaviors described as the "sickness syndrome" are related to major depression. However, antidepressant treatment has been noted to be more effective on the mood symptoms than on neurovegetative symptoms (Miyoka et al., 1999; Musselman, Lawson, et al., 2001; Capuron et al., 2002).

Sickness Behaviors in Animals

Investigators have sought to understand the observed immune abnormalities in individuals with depression for more than 30 years (Weisse, 1992). Some early studies suggested increased immune activation in individuals with depression (Kronfol, 2002). The observations by investigators using animal models that immune challenge produced a syndrome in animals similar to depression in adults provided further evidence for a relationship between depression and immunity. These behavioral observations in animals, called "sickness behaviors," are characterized by decreases in feeding, exploration and sexual activities, and increases in sleep and body temperature. These changes were thought to be protective, to facilitate recovery, and to protect the animal during illness. It was also recognized that sickness behavior could be induced in animals by administering endotoxin and interleukin-1 (IL-1) (Hart, 1988), suggesting that these symptoms might be effectively treated with cytokine antagonists (Kent et al., 1992).

R.S. Smith (1991) posited a macrophage theory of depression in an attempt to explain the relationship between sickness behavior and depression, suggesting that the IL-1 secreted by macrophages caused depression. These early efforts to link theories of depression and inflammation have stimulated much investigation and information about sickness behaviors in animals and depression in humans. Although the analogies between sickness behaviors and depression are not perfect, they are informative and useful for understanding the potential relationships between inflammation and depression (R.S. Smith, 1991; Maes et al., 1993).

Studies utilizing animal models to test the effect of cytokines on behavior using IL-1 and the endotoxin lipopolysaccharide (LPS), a potent stimulator of the pro-inflammatory cytokines IL1, IL6, tumor necrosis factor alpha (TNF-) and interferon gamma (IFN-γ), have yielded the following results:

1. IL1 and LPS induce sickness behaviors (Kent et al., 1992; Dantzer, 2001; Larson and Dunn, 2001).
2. IFN-α produces some mild behavioral changes but not sickness syndrome, fever or hypothalamic-pituitary-adrenal (HPA) axis activation (Valentine et al., 1998).
3. LPS and IL-1 induce a hypersensitivity to pain (Watkins et al., 1994).
4. IL-1, LPS, and infections decrease feeding and result in weight loss (Swiergiel et al., 1997).
5. IL1 and LPS increase slow-wave sleep time (Krueger et al., 2003).

The suggested similarities between sickness behaviors and depression are further supported by reported efficacy of antidepressants in the treatments of sickness behaviors in animals. Yirmiya (1996), using rats, studied the effects of LPS-induced sickness behavior and its response to antidepressant treatment. In an experiment designed to test depression using anhedonia as a proxy, a saccharin solution was used as a reward each time the animals pressed a bar. The rats in this experiment pressed the bar for the release of the reward (saccharin) much less frequently after administration of LPS. The same rats were then treated for 3–5 weeks with imipramine, resulting in the inhibition of anhedonia in the LPS-treated rats (Yirmiya, 1996). These results were replicated by other investigators using desmethylimipramine (Shen et al., 1999) and fluoxetine (Yirmiya et al., 2001), although the fluoxetine effect was less robust. Studies using paroxetine and venlafaxine have not demonstrated the same effect (Shen et al., 1999). These same experiments were carried out with mice; however, similar effects were not evident in mice (Yirmiya et al., 1999; Dunn and Swiergel, 2001). These studies suggest that the effects of chronic antidepressant treatments are observed most often with LPS and less so with IL1 in rats, but not in mice.

Cytokine Theory of Depression

The hypothesis that pro-inflammatory cytokines play a key role in depression has been generated by the above findings and others suggesting that immune abnormalities might contribute to depression. Several studies comparing cytokines in people with MDD have found increases in certain cytokines compared to people without MDD (Anisman et al., 2005; K.M. Lee and Kim, 2006; Pavon et al., 2006). Although association does not mean causality, there are many reasons to believe that the abnormalities of inflammation found in depression may contribute to its pathology. Patients who are medically ill who exhibit immune activation or inflammation secondary to infections, autoimmune diseases (Minden and Schiffer, 1990; Dickens et al., 2002), and neoplastic diseases demonstrate higher rates of depression. Additionally, the use of cytokines for treatments of infections or neoplasms induces behavioral changes, including a depressive syndrome.

Cytokines have also been found to influence all of the pathophysiologic domains relevant to depression. Cytokines have been shown to cause alterations in the metabolism of monoamine neurotransmitters relevant to depression, specifically serotonin, dopamine (DA), and norepinephrine (NE) (Szabo et al., 2004); to have stimulatory effects on HPA axis functioning through activation of corticotropin-releasing hormone (CRH) in the amygdala and the hypothalamus; to induce resistance of nervous, endocrine, and immune system tissues to circulating glucocorticoid hormones stimulating the glucocorticoid resistance found in patients with depression; to induce enzymes that metabolize tryptophan, the primary precursor of serotonin, and may inhibit pathways involved in thyroid hormone metabolism and to activate NF-κB, a transcription factor that signals the inflammatory cascade, in the brain (Irwin and Miller, 2007).

DEPRESSION IN MEDICAL ILLNESS

Early investigations suggested the presence of defective immune functioning in individuals with depression (Weisse, 1992), and that the defects might place them at risk for certain medical illnesses. Additionally, several large epidemiologic studies suggest that prior episodes of major depression may be an important risk factor for the development of some medical illnesses such as coronary artery disease and diabetes (Eaton et al., 1996). Recent theories suggest that individuals with depression and who are medically healthy have activated inflammatory pathways manifested by increased pro-inflammatory cytokines, increased acute phase proteins, increased chemokines, and adhesion molecules (Danner et al., 2003; Tiemeier et al., 2003; Alesci et al., 2005). This association between depression and inflammation remains evident even in the context of mild depressive symptoms (Suarez et al., 2004).

If, as suggested, immune activation is the direct cause of depression, then depression should be more prevalent in disease states characterized by chronic inflammation. Indeed, depression has been reported to be more common in some inflammatory illnesses such as multiple sclerosis (MS) (Minden and Schiffer, 1990), allergy (Marshall and Colon, 1993), and rheumatoid arthritis (Dickens et al., 2002). Depression and depressive symptoms have also been associated with inflammatory markers in cardiovascular disease (Lesperance et al., 2004; Miller et al., 2005) and cancer (Musselman, Miller, et al., 2001; Bower et al., 2002; Meyers et al., 2005).

TABLE 36.2 *Screening Tools Used for Depression in Patients Who Are Medically Ill*

Instrument	*Description*	*Advantage/Disadvantage*
Center for Epidemiological Studies Depression Scale (CES-D; Radloff, 1977)	20-item self-report instrument of which only four are somatic; recommended cutoff score of 17	Wide use in patients who are medically ill High sensitivity and specificity Lack of consensus on optimal cut scores Positive predictive value low
The Hospital Anxiety and Depression Scale (HADS; Zigmond and Snaith, 1983)	14-item self-report with separate 7-item subscale for depression and anxiety Cutoff scores range from 7–21	Brief and highly acceptable to patients Not extensively validated as a screen Lack of consensus about utility of cutoff scores
Beck Depression Inventory–II (BDI-II; Beck et al., 1996)	21-item self-report measure Cutoff scores: 10 - mild; 20 - moderate; 30 - severe	Validated as an accurate self-report measure in patients who are medically ill Less acceptable to patients due to forced-choice format and complex response alternatives Sensitivity and specificity high and positive predictive value high
The Patient Health Questionnaire–9 (PHQ-9; Kroenke et al., 2002)	9-item self-report depression module of the PHQ Cutoff Scores: 5 - mild; 10 - moderate; 15 - moderately severe; 20 - severe	Full PHQ well validated in primary care/medical specialty clinics in United States, Europe, and China Good sensitivity and specificity
Zung Self-Rating Scale for Depression (Zung, 1965)	20-item self-report Likert-type scale scores 1–4 with highest possible score of 80 Cutoff scores: > 50 for depression	Validated as an accurate self-report measure in patients who are medically ill Good sensitivity and specificity
Hamilton Depression Rating Scale (Hamilton, 1960)	17-item scale; Clinician administered Cutoff: 10–13 mild; 14–17 moderate; >17 severe	Validated as an accurate measure in patients who are medically ill Good treatment change measure High specificity and sensitivity

Although a relatively large evidence base supports the idea that dysregulation of the immune system may contribute to the pathogenesis of major depression, other studies have found conflicting results or no association between depression and immune parameters or inflammation (Haack et al., 1999; Steptoe et al., 2003; Whooley et al., 2007). As suggested by Glassman and Miller (2007), some negative studies are to be expected and those negative studies do not cancel out multiple positive ones. Another factor that might explain variation between studies is the type of immune system variable or inflammatory marker examined. Along these lines, Pike and Irwin (2006) found that, among patients with MDD relative to controls, there was evidence for decreases in NK cell activity (indicating impairment in the immune system) and higher levels of IL-6 (indicating immune activation). Furthermore, changes in NK cell activity were uncorrelated with levels of IL-6. Thus, depression may have independent effects on these different aspects of the immune system.

Cardiac Disease

A relatively large body of literature has established that there is an intimate connection between depression and cardiovascular disease. Prevalence rates of depression among individuals with coronary artery disease (CAD) (including those with unstable angina, acute myocardial infarction, congestive heart failure, and coronary artery bypass graft surgery) are significantly higher than in the general population, ranging from 17%–27% (Rudish and Nemeroff, 2003). When depressive symptoms are present, the risk for onset of CAD is increased by 1.64-fold (95% confidence interval [CI], 1.41–1.90) (Wulsin, 2004). If an episode of MDD occurs in the 3–4 months following a myocardial infarction (MI), the likelihood of dying in the next year is more than 3 times greater than that observed when no episode of MDD has occurred (Lett et al., 2004).

The connection between depression and cardiac disease does not appear to be due to the association between depression and other known risk factors (for example, smoking, history of MI).Thus, depression appears to be an independent cardiac risk factor. For example, depression has been found to be a significant predictor of mortality 6 and 18 months following MI, even after adjusting for other risk factors such as left ventricular dysfunction and previous MI (Frasure-Smith et al., 1993, 1995).

Depression also affects the outcome of cardiac surgery. In the one year following coronary artery bypass graft (CABG), the presence of depression is associated with recurrence of cardiac events (Connerney et al., 2001). Another study found that moderate to severe depressive symptoms on the day prior to surgery, or mild depression persisting from baseline to 6-month follow-up after surgery, were associated with increased mortality rates over the next 5 years.

Mechanisms of comorbidity

Emerging evidence points to several possible mechanisms linking depression to cardiovascular diseases. These include hypothalamic-pituitary-adrenocortical and sympathomedullary hyperactivity, platelet mechanisms, inflammation, and reduced heart rate variability (HRV) (Musselman et al., 1998; Skala et al., 2006).

Early studies documented HPA axis dysregulation in depression (Nemeroff, 1996; Wulsin, 2004). It is also well known that the administration of corticosteroids is associated with increases in cardiovascular disease risk factors, including hypercholesterolemia, hypertriglyceridemia, and hypertension (Musselman et al., 1998). Consistent with this potential mechanism, elevated plasma cortisol has been found to be associated with moderate to severe coronary atherosclerosis in young and middle-aged men (Troxler et al., 1977).

Sympathoadrenal hyperactivity may also influence platelets. Individuals with depression show increased levels of plasma NE in response to cold or orthostatic challenge (Roy et al., 1987), and such stressors may enhance platelet activity (Markovitz and Matthews, 1991; Anfossi and Tovati, 1996). Increased platelet activity has been found in those with MDD (Musselman et al., 1996). Moreover, patients with depression and with ischemic heart disease show elevated platelet factor 4 and plasma β-thromboglobulin levels (Laghrissi-Thode et al., 1997; Kuipers et al., 2002).

We reviewed in the previous section on depression and medical illness the literature proposing inflammatory processes, particularly the role of cytokines, as potential contributors to the pathogenesis of MDD. But inflammatory cytokines have also been found to be elevated in patients with CAD, and the extent of elevation of specific markers such as IL-6, TNF-α and C reactive protein (CRP), are directly associated with coronary and cerebrovascular disease events and progression of heart failure (Cesari et al., 2003; Shapiro, 2005). Increases in circulating levels of IL-6 and CRP are also found in depression (Miller et al., 2002).

Two recent studies have provided further pieces of the puzzle linking inflammation, depression, and CAD. In one small, carefully controlled study examining the relationships between depression and inflammation, Kling and colleagues (2007) examined CRP and serum amyloid A (SAA) in a group of 18 unmedicated women with major depression in remission compared to 18 body mass index (BMI) matched healthy controls. Serum amyloid A was increased significantly and on average by 86% in the remitted unmedicated groups, and serum CRP was increased significantly and by an average of almost threefold when compared to controls. Their findings suggest a sustained pro-inflammatory state in women who have clinically recovered and who no longer take antidepressant medications. The authors suggest that the persistence of this pro-inflammatory state might contribute to the increased CAD risk associated with MDD.

In the second recent study examining the relationship between depression and coronary events, Frasure-Smith and colleagues (Frasure-Smith, et al., 2007) assessed 702 individuals (602 men) for depression and inflammatory markers (CRP), IL-6, and soluble adhesion molecules at 2 months postdischarge for an acute coronary syndrome, and then followed them for 2 years for major adverse cardiac events defined as cardiac death, survived MI or cardiac arrest, and nonelective revascularization. Of this sample, 102 individuals (78 men) experienced at least one major adverse cardiac event. Elevated scores on the Beck Depression Inventory–II > 14 (BDI-II) and current major depression were significantly related to major adverse coronary events over 2 years, and this association was stronger in men than women. The study also found an association between elevated depressive symptoms, CRP, and soluble intercellular adhesion molecules (sICAM-1), but not IL-6, providing support for the association of depression and inflammation (Frasure-Smith et al., 2007).

Another possible mechanism linking depression and CAD may be HRV, a measure of the balance between sympathetic and parasympathetic inputs to the cardiac conduction system. In healthy individuals with good cardiac function, a high degree of HRV is typically observed. Patients with severe CAD or heart failure often have significantly decreased HRV (Richardson et al., 1996). Reduced HRV has been found to contribute to ventricular arrhythmias and sudden cardiac death (Dekker et al., 2000). Studies that found diminished HRV in depression raised the possibility that HRV might be the link between depression and CAD (Rechlin et al., 1994; Stein et al., 2000; Nahsoni et al., 2004; van der Kooy et al., 2006). Indeed, a recent study found that HRV partially mediates the relation between depression and increased risk for mortality after acute myocardial infarction (Carney et al., 2005). Heart rate variability has also been recently found to be associated with increased markers of inflammation in patients with heart failure and acute coronary syndromes (Aronson et al., 2001; Malave et al., 2003; Lanza et al., 2006).

In addition to its direct impact on CAD, depression also appears to worsen the impact of other cardiac risk factors. For example, this appears to be true for premature ventricular contractions. A meta-analysis of psychosocial risks for cardiac mortality found that the highest death rate (60%) for patients at 18 months post-MI was in a subgroup with elevated depressive symptoms and high levels of premature ventricular contractions (PVCs) (Frasure-Smith et al., 1995).

Depression can also indirectly increase the risk of CAD. The pessimism and low energy often found in clinical depression can lead individuals to be less adherent to exercise programs, smoking cessation programs, dietary changes, and pharmacological interventions for CAD (Blumenthal et al., 1982; Camacho et al., 1991; Glazer et al., 2002; Wang et al., 2002; Skala et al., 2006). The lack of adequately addressing these other risk factors will then put the individual with depression at even greater risk for a future cardiac event.

Cancer

The prevalence of depression is higher among those with cancer than in the general population, potentially substantially so (Evans et al., 1986; Carr et al., 2002; Raison and Miller, 2003). Prevalence estimates, however, vary across malignancy types and disease severity (Raison and Miller, 2003; Evans et al., 2005). Small sample sizes and nonstandardized definitions of *depression* have also hindered research in this area (Evans et al., 2005). The general range of prevalence estimates for MDD among patients with cancer has been reported to be 1.5%–50% across studies, with an overall rate of 24% (McDaniel et al., 1995).

The presence of depression has been associated with a poorer prognosis and increased mortality in patients with cancer (Hermann-Lingen et al., 2001; Faller and Bulzebruck, 2002; Evans et al., 2005). However, like with other medical illnesses, the bidirectionality of the relationship between the medical condition and depression needs to be considered. A number of cancer-related factors, such as stress related to the cancer diagnosis and treatment, cancer medications, nutritional or endocrine disturbances, or brain metastasis, may contribute to the onset of depression (Raison and Nemeroff, 2000; Massie and Greenberg, 2005). Furthermore, as discussed with cardiac disease, patients with depression and cancer might be poorly adherent to treatment regimens or might engage in adverse health behaviors.

The other direction of influence—the impact of depression on the course of cancer—has been an increasing focus of research. Although early studies reported depression was associated with immunosuppression, which might increase cancer risk in susceptible individuals (Evans et al., 1992; Herbert and Cohen, 1993; Evans et al., 2005), recent studies suggest that the inflammation associated with the illness may be associated with the onset of depressive symptoms. Recent evidence suggests that release of pro-inflammatory cytokines during tissue damage and destruction and its associated inflammation can have a substantial impact on neurotransmitter function, neuroendocrine function, and behavior resulting in the "sickness syndrome."

The observation that a significant percentage of patients with cancer treated with the cytokine IFN-α develops a behavioral syndrome with similarities to major depression has been an impetus for the recent investigations in this area. Cytokine therapies are well known to cause neurobehavioral symptoms including major depression in up to 50% of patients with cancer undergoing cytokine treatment with IFN-α (Musselman, Lawson, et al., 2001; Capuron et al., 2002) and IL-2 (Capuron et al., 2004). Among patients with cancer, patients with depression and cancer were found to have significantly higher levels of IL-6 compared to patients with cancer and no depression and healthy controls (Musselman, Miller, et al., 2001). More recent studies have found associations between specific depressive symptoms and elevated cytokines; for example, some investigators have found elevated IL-6 concentrations in patients with cancer presenting with fatigue and impaired executive functioning (Collado-Hidalgo et al., 2006).

Capuron and colleagues (Capuron et al., 2002; Capuron et al., 2004) and Musselman, Lawson, et al. (2001) have described two distinct behavioral syndromes that occur in individuals who become depressed with cytokine therapies. One syndrome is characterized by depressed mood, anxiety, irritability, and memory and attentional disturbances. This syndrome is reported to occur within the first 3 months of therapy in susceptible individuals (Musselman, Lawson, et al., 2001; Capuron et al., 2002; Capuron et al., 2004). The other syndrome, characterized by the neurovegetative symptoms of fatigue, psychomotor slowing, anorexia, and altered sleep patterns, occurs within the first few weeks of IFN-α therapy and persists at later stages of therapy (Capuron et al., 2002). These two different syndromes are thought to have different responsiveness to antidepressant treatment. The mood and cognitive symptoms were responsive to pretreatment with paroxetine (Capuron et al., 2002) whereas the neurovegetative symptoms were not, suggesting that these systems may have different pathophysiologic pathways.

Although depressive symptoms are very responsive to antidepressant treatment, the neurovegetative symptoms described in the "sickness syndrome" have been less responsive to antidepressant treatments, perhaps requiring a different treatment approach (Capuron et al., 2002; Raison and Miller, 2003).

HIV/AIDS

Early studies of prevalence rates of depression among individuals with HIV/AIDS showed wide variability across studies due to varying methods of assessment of depression, regional variations, and small sample sizes (Smith et al., 1996). In general, however, meta-analyses of these early studies revealed that those with HIV were nearly twice as likely to have a diagnosis of major depression compared to individuals who were HIV-negative (Ciesla and Roberts, 2001). Subsequent studies have provided better prevalence estimates, overcoming the limitations of earlier studies. A large-scale study using a national representative probability sample in the United States found that, among individuals who were HIV-positive receiving medical care for HIV, 35% screened positive for MDD and 26.5% screened positive for dysthymia (21% screened positive for both) (Lyketsos et al., 1993). As these diagnoses were based on a brief screening interview, a subsequent article examined only the subset of individuals who had received a full diagnostic interview and reported prevalence rates of 22% for MDD and 5% for dysthymia (Orlando et al., 2002). These rates are still substantially higher than the rates of depressive disorders found in the general population. Rates for men and women who are HIV-positive did not differ in this national study (Lyketsos et al., 1993), although other studies have found that women who were HIV-positive may be particularly susceptible to MDD, with rates of current MDD about 4 times higher in women who are HIV-positive (19.4%) compared to women who were HIV-negative (4.8%) (Morrison et al., 2002). Large-scale studies of depressive disorders among children who are HIV-positive are lacking, but meta-analyses of available small studies estimated the prevalence of a *Diagnostic and Statistical Manual of Mental Disorders* (*DSM-IV*; American Psychiatric Association, 1994) depressive disorder in this population at 25% (Scharko, 2006).

The impact of depression on the course and treatment of HIV/AIDS is striking. Clinical depression, elevated levels of depressive symptoms, or general psychological stress are associated with poor adherence to antiretroviral treatment, deterioration in psychosocial functioning, more rapid progression of HIV/AIDS, and higher mortality (Burack et al., 1993; Lyketsos et al., 1993; Evans et al., 1995; Mayne et al., 1996; Page-Shafer et al., 1996; Patterson et al., 1996; Ickovics et al., 2001; Leserman et al., 2002; Evans et al., 2005). One study of over 2000 women who were HIV-positive followed for 7½ years found that those with chronic depression had 1.7 times greater odds of dying compared to women without depression (Cook et al., 2004). The impact of depression on mortality remained even after controlling for antiretroviral therapy use, mental health treatment, medication adherence, substance abuse, clinical indicators (baseline CD4 count, baseline viral load, baseline HIV symptoms), and demographic factors.

It is important to note that the impact of depression on the progression of HIV/AIDS needs to be assessed over a relatively long period of time given the long latency period between infection with the HIV virus and the progression of AIDS. Indeed, studies that examined the impact of depression on HIV over relatively shorter periods of time (6 months to 2 years) have sometimes failed to document an influence (Rabkin et al., 1991; Vedhara et al., 1999).

Mechanisms of HIV effect and depression

Although there is evidence supporting a relationship between depression and HIV disease progression, little is known about the mechanisms underlying this relationship. It is possible that poor health habits might explain the relationship between depression and course of HIV/AIDS, but support for the impact of poor health habits on this relationship is lacking (Page-Shafer et al., 1996; Ickovics et al., 2001; Leserman et al., 2002; Leserman, 2003).

Disruption of the HPA axis has been investigated as a possible mediator of the depression–immune status relationship in animal and human studies (Friedman and Irwin, 1997; Cupps and Fauci, 2002). Levels of cortisol have been linked to stress and depression in HIV (Gorman et al., 1991), and it is hypothesized that cortisol may influence immune response by altering the profiles of cytokines secreted (Clerici et al., 1997). In addition, NE has been shown to affect HIV replication (Cole et al., 1998). Another possible mediator is the neuropeptide substance P. Studies have found plasma levels of substance P to be higher in persons with HIV, and elevated substance P levels associated with decreased NK cell populations (Ho et al., 1996; Douglas et al., 2001). Depression might affect HIV disease progression by altering the functioning of killer lymphocytes (NK and cytotoxic T-lymphocytes) thereby diminishing host defenses against HIV infection (Ironson et al., 2001; Evans et al., 2002; Leserman, 2003). Consistent with this hypothesis, stressful life events, poor social support, and chronic depression have all been associated with more rapid declines in CD4 lymphocyte counts (Burack et al., 1993; Kemeny and Dean, 1995; Kemeny et al., 1995) and progression to AIDS (Ickovics et al., 2001; Leserman et al., 2002; Leserman, 2003).

Depression also has an affect on adherence to HIV treatment regimens. Patients with HIV and depressive disorders have greater difficulty in accessing antiretroviral therapy and adhering to treatment once accessed (Fairfield et al., 1999; Gordillo et al., 1999; Li et al., 2005).

ASSESSMENT OF DEPRESSION IN MEDICAL ILLNESS

Many psychological and physical factors can make the diagnosis of depression among those with medical illness challenging for the clinician. The classic signs and symptoms of depressive disorders such as depressed mood, dysphoric affect, fatigue, pain, psychomotor retardation, anorexia, weight loss, cognitive impairment, and insomnia can represent demoralization or the medical illness itself. Thoughts of death or a hastened desire for death is not a reliable sign for depressive disorders in this population but may represent demoralization (Radloff, 1977; Kissane et al., 2001). The loss of ability to experience pleasure in many activities may be the result of physical suffering or disability and not a symptom of depression. Some medical conditions that are progressive, such as cancers and neurological conditions, have depressive symptoms that may change over time due to the illness or treatments for the illness. No standardized approach exists currently for diagnosing depression among the individuals who are medically ill. We continue to rely on the mental status examination and *DSM-IV* criteria for depression (Evans et al., 2005). Investigators have examined the utility of excluding symptoms that can occur as part of the medical condition and the depressive condition (exclusive approach) versus the more favored inclusive approach that counts all symptoms when making a diagnosis of depression, but the findings have been inconclusive (Newport and Nemeroff, 1998; Raison and Miller, 2003). Fortunately, several well-validated instruments are available to assist the clinician in making the diagnosis of depression in the presence of medical symptoms and in monitoring treatment response (Table 36.2).

TREATMENT OF DEPRESSION IN MEDICAL ILLNESS

There are a growing number of well-controlled trials examining the efficacy of antidepressant treatments among individuals who are medically ill. This growing body of evidence provides strong support for the effective use of antidepressant medications for the treatment of mood disorders in these populations. The challenge for the clinician is to identify an effective agent and dosing regimen, whose mechanism of action and side-effect profile will not exacerbate the coexisting medical condition.

In addition to studies of cardiac disease, HIV/AIDS, and cancer (reviewed below), double-blind, randomized controlled trials have demonstrated the effectiveness of antidepressants in the treatment of depression in individuals with stroke (Anderson and Lauritzen, 1994; Rasmussen et al., 2003), Alzheimer's disease (Karlsson et al., 2000; Lyketsos et al., 2000), diabetes (Lustman et al., 2000), and MS (Mohr et al., 2001). There is increasing evidence that selective serotonin reuptake inhibitors (SSRIs) in particular not only improve depressive symptoms but also may result in positive effects on the co-occurring medical illness. For example, fluoxetine has been shown to improve glycemic control in patients with diabetes mellitus (Lustman et al., 2000).

One caution in the use of SSRI or serotonin norepinephrine reuptake inhibitors (SNRIs) is that under certain circumstances the side effects of these medications may add to the existing physical problems associated with the medical condition. Potentially serious side effects of SSRIs include the syndrome of inappropriate antidiuretic hormone secretion (SIADH) and platelet dysfunction that can lead to bleeding problems (Turner et al., 2007). There is also some evidence that the motor symptoms in Parkinson's disease can be exacerbated by SSRIs (Richard et al., 1999).

An even greater concern is the potential for drug interactions. Patients with serious medical conditions, particularly the elderly, often are receiving multiple medications for their illnesses, elevating the risk of drug interactions. The presence of hepatic disease, for example, may affect metabolism and excretion of SSRIs and significantly alter their pharmacokinetics (Beliles and Stoudemire, 1998). Tricyclic antidepressants (TCAs) are effective in the treatment of depression, and their safety and side-effect profiles are well known. Despite evidence of their efficacy in the treatment of depression among patients with cerebrovascular disease, Alzheimer's disease, Parkinson's disease, cancer, HIV/AIDS, epilepsy, chronic pain, and diabetes (Evans et al., 2005), the widespread use of SSRIs and SNRIs has substantially reduced the clinical use of TCAs. Moreover, because TCAs are strong antagonists of cholinergic, histaminic, and α-adrenergic receptors and can affect cardiac conduction, there are concerns about the use of TCAs with some co-occurring medical conditions. Tricyclic antidepressant discontinuation rates as high as one third have been observed in patients who were medically ill because of adverse effects (Popkin et al., 1985; Rabkin, Rabkin, Harrison, and Wagner, 1994).

Like TCAs, monoamine oxidase inhibitors (MAOIs) are effective in the treatment of depression but are now less commonly used. The MAOIs, phenelzine and tranyclcypromine, can produce hypertensive reactions following the ingestion of foods containing high levels of tyramine, over-the-counter sympathomimetics, and stimulants. A potentially fatal serotonin syndrome may occur when SSRIs or SNRIs are combined with MAOIs (Bernstein, 1994).

Psychostimulants (methylphenidate and dextroamphetamine) have also been used to treat depression in patients with various medical conditions. Limited data, however, support their use in patients who are medically ill. These agents may be useful due to their rapid onset of action in elevating mood, increasing appetite, and diminishing fatigue (Masand, Pickett, and Murray, 1991).

ANTIDEPRESSANT TREATMENTS FOR DEPRESSION IN CARDIAC DISEASE, CANCER, AND HIV

Cardiac Disease

The treatment of depression in the context of cardiac disease has been an area of great interest due to the well-established relationships between CAD, depression, and mortality. Four randomized controlled trials (RCTs) have established the efficacy and safety of antidepressants in the treatment of patients with cardiac disease with depression. In the Sertraline Antidepressant Heart Attack Trial (SADHART) trial (Glassman et al., 2002), 369 patients with major depression after hospitalization for unstable angina or acute MI were randomized to double-blind treatment with sertraline or placebo. The primary goal of the study was to examine the effects of sertraline on depressive symptoms in this population; the trial was not powered to determine effects on morbidity and mortality (that is, only seven deaths occurred during the follow-up period). The results indicated that sertraline was safe and effective for the treatment of depression in patients who were post-MI (Glassman et al., 2002). In addition, sertraline was superior in absolute numerical terms to placebo in the rate of recurrent MI, mortality, heart failure, and angina. Limited data from the SADHART study also suggests a potential cardioprotective effect of sertraline in the treatment of this population, although these data require confirmation by larger prospective trials (Glassman et al., 2002).

The second major trial examining antidepressants in cardiac disease was the Enhancing Recovery in Coronary Heart Disease (ENRICHD) trial. In this trial, 2481 patients who were post-MI with depression or low perceived social support were randomized to a 6-month course of either cognitive-behavioral therapy (CBT) or usual care, both of which were supplemented with an SSRI antidepressant (typically sertraline) when indicated. Primary outcomes in these trials were reinfarction rates and mortality; secondary outcomes were measures of depression and social support. No treatment effects were seen in regard to mortality or recurrence of MI. However, the CBT intervention had significantly greater improvements in depression and social support compared to those in the usual care group. There was some evidence that antidepressant treatment had an impact on mortality, but because there was no randomization to antidepressant treatment in this study this effect must be interpreted with caution (Writing Committee for the ENRICHD Investigators, 2003).

The third study, the Myocardial Infarction and Depression Intervention Trial (MIND-IT), examined the antidepressant efficacy of an SNRI (mirtazapine) in patients (N = 91) with post-MI depressive disorder. Although no significant difference between drug and placebo was evident on the primary measure of depressive symptoms, there was evidence of a drug effect on several secondary depression measures and global improvement (Honig et al., 2007).

The fourth study was the Canadian Cardiac Randomized Evaluation of Antidepressant and Psychotherapy Efficacy (CREATE) project (Lesperance et al., 2007). In a 2 × 2 design, patients (N = 284) with CAD and depression were randomly assigned to receive 12 weekly sessions of interpersonal psychotherapy (IPT) plus clinical management or clinical management only, and also randomly assigned to the SSRI citalopram or placebo. Citalopram was superior to placebo on the primary measure of depression. There was no evidence of a benefit of IPT over clinical management alone. Taken in total, these trials provide considerable evidence that SSRIs are efficacious in the treatment of depression among those with cardiac disease. However, a positive impact of such depression treatment on the course of cardiac disease has not been clearly established.

Cancer

A number of antidepressant treatment trials in patients with depression with cancer have demonstrated the effectiveness of TCAs and SSRIs (Evans et al., 1988; Razavi et al., 1996; Holland et al., 1998; Pezella et al., 2001; Roscoe et al., 2005). One small study of major depression among women with breast cancer compared the efficacy of an SSRI (paroxetine) to a TCA (desipramine) but found no difference in efficacy (Musselman et al., 2006). As with the treatment of depression in patients with no cancer, SSRIs are generally preferred over TCAs because of fewer sedative and autonomic side effects. In addition to the SSRIs and TCAs, mirtazapine and mianserin have shown promising results in open trials (Costa et al., 1985; Van Heeringen and Zivkov, 1996; Theobald et al., 2002). Mirtazapine can cause weight gain, which might actually be advantageous in anorexic-cachectic patients with cancer but may be a concern in those already gaining weight from steroids or from chemotherapy (Theobald et al., 2002). SSRIs and the SNRI venlafaxine have been shown to reduce the number and intensity of hot flashes and night sweats in women without depression who become menopausal after chemotherapy for breast cancer or who have a recurrence of vasomotor symptoms when they discontinue hormone replacement therapy (Duffy et al., 1999; Stearns et al., 2000; Loberiza et al., 2002).

Psychostimulants (methylphenidate, dextroamphetamine) also are used with patients with cancer to promote a sense of well being, treat depression, decrease fatigue, and improve cognitive function (Rozans et al., 2002) In addition, psychostimulants may be used as adjuvants to potentiate the analgesic effects of opioids and to counteract their sedative effects (Rozans et al., 2002). Another consideration in patients with cancer is depression that can result from certain cancer treatments that activate the immune system. In particular, treatment with IFN-α can cause the onset of new depressive episodes or trigger a recurrence of a recent episode. In one study, patients with advanced melanoma who received 12 months of IL-α developed fatigue, anxiety, insomnia, and depression (Kirkwood et al., 2002). In a placebo-controlled trial, the use of an antidepressant (paroxetine) at the time of IFN-α treatment was found to reduce the incidence of depressive episodes and reduce the rate of discontinuation of IFN-α treatment (Musselman, Lawson, et al., 2001). Despite this finding, prophylactic use of antidepressants for patients with cancer is not currently recommended.

HIV/AIDS

Numerous well-designed studies have supported the effectiveness of TCAs and SSRIs for treating depression in adults with HIV (Rabkin, Rabkin, Harrison, and Wagner, 1994; Rabkin, Rabkin, and Wagner, 1994; Rabkin, Wagner, and Rabkin, 1994; Ferrando et al., 1997; Grassi et al., 1997; Elliot et al., 1998; Zisook et al, 1998; Ferrando et al., 1999; Cruess et al., 2003; Caballero and Nahata, 2005). Head-to-head studies comparing TCAs and SSRIs have shown equal efficacy for both, but, as expected, a less favorable side-effect profile for TCAs. For example, in one placebo-controlled study comparing imipramine, paroxetine, and placebo in 75 individuals who were HIV-positive, the two antidepressants were found to be equally effective when compared to placebo, but the dropout rates due to anticholinergic side effects with imipramine were 48%, compared to 20% with paroxetine and 24% with placebo (Elliot et al., 1998). One small open-label study evaluated the efficacy of three SSRIs (paroxetine, fluoxetine, and sertraline) in individuals who were HIV-seropositive (Ferrando et al., 1997). A substantial (83%) number of individuals reported improvements in depression and somatic symptoms related to HIV disease, but the dropout rate (27%) in this 6-week study was high. Because of the small sample size, the comparative effects of the three SSRIs could not be evaluated. Another small noncontrolled study found that paroxetine improved depressive symptoms among individuals who were HIV-positive with clinical depression (Grassi et al., 1997). Overall, these studies are suggestive of the effectiveness of SSRIs in reducing depressive symptoms in individuals who are HIV-seropositive, although larger placebo-controlled studies are needed.

Open trials have also suggested that sustained-release bupropion (Theobald et al., 2002) and mirtazapine (Currier et al., 2003) may be useful for the treatment of depression in individuals who are HIV-seropositive. Although no studies have yet examined duloxetine in patients who are HIV-positive, this medication has shown efficacy for the treatment of certain pain conditions, including diabetic peripheral neuropathic pain (Wernicke et al., 2006). It is possible that duloxetine might therefore be helpful with the polyneuropathy that occurs in HIV/AIDS, although this hypothesis awaits empirical support.

Psychostimulants (methylphenidate and dextroamphetamine) have also been studied in placebo-controlled trials in patients with depression and HIV. There have been two small uncontrolled studies of psychostimulants in the treatment of depression in HIV/AIDS (Fernandez et al., 1995; Wagner et al., 1997), and one small, placebo-controlled study that showed efficacy (Wagner and Rabkin, 2000). Reductions in depressive symptoms as early as 2 weeks after initiating treatment have been reported (Wagner et al., 1997). In another study, among patients who were HIV-positive who also had significant levels of fatigue, methylphenidate and pemoline (another psychostimulant) were found to be significantly superior to placebo in decreasing fatigue, and improvement in fatigue was significantly associated with improved quality of life and decreased levels of depression (Breitbart et al., 2001).

Reductions in testosterone levels among individuals with HIV/AIDS can be associated with changes in mood, appetite, and sexual function (Rabkin, Wagner, and Rabkin, 2000). Testosterone supplementation has therefore been examined as one way to improve mood, energy, and sexual function. In one study enrolling symptomatic patients who were HIV-positive, testosterone was significantly better than placebo at restoring libido and energy, alleviating depressed mood, and increasing muscle mass (Rabkin, Ferrando, et al., 2000). The adrenal steroid dehydroepiandrosterone (DHEA) has also been evaluated in an uncontrolled pilot study and appears promising (Rabkin, Wagner, and Rabkin, 2000).

As with other medical and nonmedical populations, the choice of an antidepressant agent in patients with HIV must be guided by the potential for drug–drug interactions and potential positive or negative interactions between drug and disease.

CONCLUSIONS

Depressive disorders are prevalent among those with chronic medical conditions and have been shown to increase symptom burden and functional disability, adversely affect self-care, decrease adherence to treatment, and to decrease quality of life. A considerable body of evidence suggests that depression is associated with immune suppression and immune activation. Depression-associated cellular immune suppression may be a mechanism whereby depression may have an adverse effect on immune-based diseases such as cancer and AIDS. On the other hand, depression-associated immune activation may be a mechanism whereby depression may have an adverse effect on diseases such as cardiovascular disease and diabetes.

Antidepressant treatments have been effective in the treatment of many of the symptoms of depression in individuals who are medically ill, and the presence of depression should be aggressively identified and targeted, Larger-scale studies are needed to determine if the treatment of depression in individuals who are medically ill might improve overall medical outcomes or prevent disease progression. Further studies may also shed light on the immune mechanisms underlying depression and comorbid medical illness.

REFERENCES

Alesci, S., Martinez, P.E., Kelkar, S., Ilias, I., Ronsaville, D.S., Listwak, S.J., Licinio, J., Gold, H.K.,Chrousos, G.P., Gold, P.W., and Kling, M.A. (2005) Major depression is associated with significant diurnal elevations in plasma interleukin-6 levels, a shift of its circadian rhythm and loss of physiological complexity in its secretion: clinical implications. *J. Clin. Endocrinol. Metab.* 90: 1279–1283.

American Psychiatric Association. (1994) *Diagnostic and Statistical Manual of Mental Disorders*, 4th ed. Washington, DC: APPI.

Anderson, G.B.K., and Lauritzen, L. (1994) Effective treatment of poststroke depression with the selective serotonin reuptake inhibitor citalopram. *Stroke* 25:1099–1104.

Anderson, R.L., Clouse, R.E., Freedland, K.E., and Lustman, P.J. (2001) The prevalence of comorbid depression in adults with diabetes; A meta-analysis. *Diabetes* 24:1069–1078.

Anfossi, G., and Tovati, M. (1996) Role of catecholamines in platelet function: pathophysiological and clinical significance. *Eur. J. Clin. Invest.* 32:643–648.

Anisman, H., Merali, Z., Poulter, M.O., and Hayley, S. (2005) Cytokines as a precipitant of depressive illness: animal and human studies. *Curr. Pharm. Des.* 11:963–972.

Aronson, D., Mittleman, M.A., and Burger, A.J. (2001) Interleukin-6 levels are inversely correlated with heart rate variability in patients with decompensated heart failure, *J. Cardiovasc. Electrophysiol.* 12:294–300.

Banki, C.M., Bissette, G., Arato, M., O'Connor, L., Nemeroff, C.B. (1987) Cerebrospinal fluid corticotropin-releasing factor-like immunoreactivity in depression and schizophrenia. *Am. J. Psychiatry* 144:873–877.

Barron, L., and Shapiro, M. (2001) Psychiatric disorders and drug use among human immunodeficiency virus-infected adults in the United States. *Archi. Gen. Psychiatry* 58:721–728

Beck, A.T., Steer, R., and Brown, G.K. (1996) *Manual for the Beck Depression Inventory-II*. San Antonio, TX: Psychological Corporation.

Beliles, K., and Stoudemire, A. (1998) Psychopharmacologic treatment of depression in the medically ill. *Psychosomatics* 39:S2–S19.

Bernstein, J.G. (1994) *Handbook of Drug Therapy in Psychiatry*. St. Louis, MO: Mosby Yearbook Inc.

Blumenthal, J.A., Williams, R.S., Wallace, A.G., Williams, R.B., Jr., and Needles, T.L. (1982) Physiological and psychological variables predict compliance to prescribed exercise therapy in patients recovering from myocardial infarction. *Psychosom. Med.* 44:519–527.

Bower, J.E., Ganz, P.A., Najib, A., and Fahey, J.L. (2002) Fatigue and proinflammatory cytokines activity in breast cancer survivors. *Psychosom. Med.* 64:604–611.

Breitbart, W., Rosenfeld, B., Kaim, M., and Funesti-Esch, J. (2001) A randomized, double-blind, placebo-controlled trial of psychostimulants for the treatment of fatigue in ambulatory patients with human immunodeficiency virus disease. *Arch. Intl. Med.* 161:411–420.

Burack, J.H., Barrett, D.C., Stall, R.D., Chesney, M.A., Ekstrand, M.L., and Coates, T.J. (1993) Depressive symptoms and CD4 lymphocyte decline among HIV-infected men. *JAMA* 270:2568–2573.

Caballero, J., and Nahata, M.C. (2005) Use of selective serotonin-reuptake inhibitors in the treatment of depression in adults with HIV. *Ann. Pharmacother.* 39:141–145.

Camacho, T.C., Roberts, R.E., Lazarus, N.B., Kaplan, G.A., and Cohen, R.D. (1991) Physical activity and depression: evidence from the Alameda County Study. *Am. J. Epidemiol.* 134:220–231.

Campbell, L.C., Claum, D.J., and Keefe, F.J. (2003) Persistent pain and depression: a biopsychosocial perspective. *Biol. Psychiatry* 54:399–409.

Capuron, L., Gumnick, J.F., Musselman, D.C., Lawson, D.H., Reemsnydira, A., Nemeroff, C.B., and Miller, A.H. (2002) Neurobehavioral effects of interferon-alpha in cancer patients: phenomenology and paroxetine responsiveness of symptom dimensions. *Neuropsychopharmacology* 26:643–652.

Capuron, L., Raison, C.L., Musselman, D.L., Lawson, D.H., Nemeroff, C.B., and Miller, A.H. (2003) Association of HPA axis response to initial injection of interferon-alpha. *Am. J. Psychiatry* 160:1342–1345.

Capuron, L., Ravaud, A., Miller, A.H., and Dantzer, R. (2004) Baseline mood and psychosocial characteristics of patients developing depressive symptoms during interleukin-2 and/or interferon-alpha cancer therapy. *Brain Behav. Immun.* 18:205–213.

Carney, R.M., Blumenthal, J.A., Freedland, K.E., Stein, P.K., Howells, W.B., Berkman, L.F., Watkins, L.L., Czajkowski, S.M., Hayana, J., Domitrovich, P.P., and Jaffe, A.S. (2005) Low heart rate variability and the effect of depression on post-myocardial infarction mortality. *Arch. Int. Med.* 165:1486–1491.

Carr, D., Goudas, L., Lawrence, D., Pirl, W., Lau, J., DeVine, D., Litt, M., Kupelnick, B., and Miller, K. (2002) *Management of Cancer Symptoms: Pain, Depression and Fatigue* (Agency for Healthcare Research and Quality: Evidence Report/Technology Assessment Number 61). Agency for Healthcare Research and Quality, Rockville, MD.

Cesari, M., Penninx, B.W.J.H., Newman, A.B., Kritchevsky, S.B., Nieklas, B.J., Sutton-Tyrell, K., Rubin, S.M., Ding, J.Z., Simmonsick, E.M., Harris, T.B., and Pahon, M. (2003) Inflammatory markers and onset of cardiovascular events: results from the health ABC study. *Circulation* 108:2317–2322.

Ciesla, J.A., and Roberts, J.E. (2001) Meta-analysis of the relationship between HIV infection and risk for depressive disorders. *Am. J. Psychiatry* 158:725–730.

Clerici, M., Trabattoni, D., Piconi, S., Fusi, M.L., Ruzzante, S., Clerici, C., and Villa, M.L. (1997) A possible role for the cortisol/anticortisols imbalance in the progression of human immunodeficiency virus. *Psychoneuroendocrinology* 22:S27–S31.

Cole, S.W., Korin, Y.D., Fahey, J.L., and Zack, J.A. (1998) Norepinephrine accelerates HIV replication via protein kinase A dependent effects on cytokine production. *J. Immunol.* 161:610–616.

Collado-Hidalgo, A., Bower, J.E., Ganz, P.A., Cole, S.W., and Irwin, M.R. (2006) Inflammatory biomarkers for persistent fatigue in breast cancer survivors. *Clin. Cancer Res.* 12:2759–2766.

Connerney, I., Shapiro, P.A., McLaughlin, J.S., Bagiella, E., and Sloan, R.P. (2001) Relation between depression after coronary artery bypass surgery and 12-month outcome: a prospective study. *Lancet* 358:1766–1771.

Cook, J.A., Grey, D., Burke, J., Cohen, M.H., Gurtman, A.C., Richardson, J.L., Wilson, T.E., Young, M.A., and Hessol, N.A. (2004) Depressive symptoms and AIDS-related mortality among a multisite cohort of HIV positive women. *Am. J. Pub. Health* 94:1133–1140.

Costa, D., Mogos, I., and Toma, T. (1985) Efficacy and safety of mianserin in the treatment of depression in women with cancer. *Acta Psychiatr. Scand.* 320:85–92.

Cruess, D.G., Evans, D.L., Repetto, M.J., Gettes, D., Douglas, S.D., and Petitto, J.M. (2003) Prevalence, diagnosis and pharmacological treatment of mood disorders in HIV disease. *Biol. Psychiatry* 54:307–316.

Cupps, T.R., and Fauci, A.S. (2002) Cortiscosteroid-mediated immunoregulation in man. *Immunol. Rev.* 65:133–155.

Currier, M.B., Molina, G., and Kato, M.A. (2003) A prospective trial of sustained buproprion for depression in HIV-seropositive and AIDS patients. *Psychosomatics* 44:120–125.

Danner, M., Stanislav, V., Abramson, J., and Vaccarino, V. (2003) Association between depression and elevated C-reactive protein. *Psychosom. Med.* 65:347–356.

Dantzer, R. (2001) Cytokine-induced sickness behavior: where do we stand? *Brain Behav. Immun.* 15:7–24.

De Beaurepaire, R., Swiergiel, A.H., and Dunn, A.J. (2005) Neuroimmune mediators: are cytokines mediators of depression? In: Licinio, J., and Wong, M.-L., eds. *Biology of Depression: From Novel Insights to Therapeutic Strategies*. Weinheim, Germany: Wiley-VCH, pp. 557–581.

Dekker, J.M., Crow, R.S., Folsom, A.R., Hannan, P.J., Liao, D., Swenne, C.A., and Shouten, E.G. (2000) Low heart rate variability in a 2-minute rhythm strip predicts risk of coronary heart disease and mortality from several causes: the ARIC Study. Atherosclerosis Risk in Communities. *Circulation* 102(11):1239–1244.

Dickens, C., McGowan, L., Clark-Carter, D., and Creed, F. (2002) Depression in rheumatoid arthritis: a systematic review of the literature with meta-analysis. *Psychosom. Med.* 64:52–60.

Douglas, S.D., Ho, W.Z., Gettes, D.R., Cnaan, A., Zuao, H.G., Leserman, J., Petitto, J.M., Golden, R.N., and Evans, D.L. (2001) Elevated substance P levels in HIV-infected men. *AIDS* 15:2043–2045.

Duffy, L.S., Greenberg, D.B., Younger, J., and Ferraro, M.G. (1999) Iatrogenic acute estrogen deficiency and psychiatric syndromes in breast cancer patients. *Psychosomatics* 40:304–308.

Dunn, A.J., and Swiergiel, A.H. (2001) The reductions in sweetened milk intake induced by interleukin-1 and endotoxin are not prevented by chronic antidepressant treatment. *Neuroimmunomodulation* 9:163.

Dunn, A.J., Swiergiel, A.H., and de Beaurepaire, R. (2005) Cytokines as mediators of depression: what can we learn from animal studies? *Neurosci. Biobehav. Rev.* 29:891–909.

Dunn, A.J., Wang, J., and Ando, T. (1999) Effects of cytokines on cerebral neurotransmission. Comparison with the effects of stress. *Adv. Exp. Med. Biol.* 461:117–127.

Eaton, W., Armenian, H., Gallo, J., Pratt, L., and Ford, D.E. (1996) Depression and risk for onset of type II diabetes. A prospective population based study. *Diabetes Care* 19:1097–2002.

Egede, L.E. (2007) Major depression in individuals with chronic medical disorders: prevalence, correlates and association with health utilization, lost productivity and functional disability. *Gen. Hosp. Psychiatry* 29:409–416.

Elliot, A.J., Uldall, K.K., Bergam, K., Russo, J., Claypoole, K., and Roy-Bryne, P.P. (1998) Randomized placebo-controlled trial of paroxetine versus imipramine in depressed HIV-positive outpatients. *Am. J. Psychiatry* 155:367–372.

Evans, D.L., and Charney, D.S. (2003) Mood disorders and medical illness: a major public health problem. *Biol. Psychiatry* 54:177–180.

Evans, D.L., Charney, D.S., Lewis, L., Golden, R.N., Gorman, J.M., Krishnan, K.R.R., Nemeroff, C.B., Bremner, J.D., Carney, R.M., Coyne, J.C., Delong, M.R., Frasure-Smith, N., Glassman, A.H., Gold, P.W., Grant, I., Gwyther, L., Ironson, G., Johnson, R.L., Kanner, A.M., Katon, W.J., Kaufmann, P.G., Keefe, F.J., Ketter, T., Laughren, T.P., Leserman, J., Lyketsos, C.G., McDonald, W.M., McEwen, B.S., Miller, A.H., Musselman, D., O'Connor, C., Petitto, J.M., Pollock, B.G., Robinson, R.G., Roose, S.P., Rowland, J., Sheline, Y., Sheps, D.S., Simon, G., Spiegel, D., Stunkard, A., Sunderland, T., Tibbits, P., and Valvo, W.J. (2005) Mood disorders in the medically ill: scientific review and recommendations. *Biol. Psychiatry* 58:175–189.

Evans, D.L., Leserman, J., Perkins, D.O., Stern, R.A., Murphy, C., Tamul, K., Liao, D.P., Vanderhost, C.M., Hall, C.D., Folds, J.D., Golden, R.N., and Petitto, J.M. (1995) Stress associated reductions of cytoxic T lymphocytes and natural killer cells in asymptomatic HIV infection. *Am. J. Psychiatry* 152:543–550.

Evans, D.L., McCartney, C.F., Haggerty, J.J., Nemeroff, C.B., Golden, R.N., Simon, J.B., Quade, D., Holmes, V., Droba, M., Mason, G.A., Fowler, W.C., and Raft, D. (1988) Treatment of depression in cancer patients is associated with better life adaptation: a pilot study. *Psychosom. Med.* 50:72–76.

Evans, D.L., McCartney, C.F., Nemeroff, C.B., Raft, D., Quade, D., and Golden, R.N., Haggerty, J.J., Holmes, V., Simon, J.S., Droba, M., Mason, G.A., and Fowler, W.C. (1986) Depression in women treated for gynecological cancer: clinical and neuroendocrine assessment. *Am. J. Psychiatry* 143:447–452.

Evans, D.L., Petitto, J.M., Golden, R.N., Pederson, C.A., Corrigan, M., Gilmore, J.H., Silva, S.G., Quade, D., and Ozer, H. (1992) Circulating natural killer cell phenotypes in men and women with major depression: relation to cytotoxic activity and severity of depression. *Arch. Gen. Psychiatry* 49:388–395.

Evans, D.L., Ten Have, T., Douglas, S.D., Gettes, D.R., Morrison, M., Chiappini, M.S., Brinker-Spence, P., Job, C., Mercer, D.E., Wang, Y.L., Cruess, D., Dube, B., Dalen, E.A., Brown, T., Bauer, R., and Petitto, J.M. (2002) Association of depression with viral load, CD8 T lymphocytes, and natural killer cells in women with HIV infection. *Am. J. Psychiatry* 159:1752–1759.

Fairfield, K.M., Libman, H., Davis, R.B., Eisenberg, D.M., and Phillips, R.S. (1999) Delays in protease inhibitor use in clinical practice. *J. Gen. Intl. Med.* 14:395–401.

Faller, H., and Bulzebruck, H. (2002) Coping and survival in lung cancer: A 10-year follow-up. *Am. J. Psychiatry* 159:2105–2107.

Fernandez, F., Levy, J.K., Samley, H.R., Pirozzolo, F.J., Lachar, D., Crowley, J., Adams, S., Ross, B., and Ruiz, P. (1995) Effects of methylphenidate in HIV-related depression: a comparative trial with Desipramine. *Int. J. Psychiat. Med.* 25:53–67.

Ferrando, S.J., Goldman, J.D., and Charness, W. (1997) Selective serotonin reuptake inhibitor treatment of depression in symptomatic HIV infection and AIDS: improvement in affective and somatic symptoms. *Gen. Hosp. Psychiatry* 19:89–97.

Ferrando, S.J., Rabkin, J.G., de Moore, G.M., and Rabkin, R. (1999) Antidepressant treatment of depression in HIV-seropositive women. *J. Clin. Psychiatry* 60:741–746.

Frasure-Smith, N., Irwin, M.R., Suave, C., Lesperance, J., and Theroux, P. (2007) Depression, C-reactive protein and two-year major adverse cardiac events in men after acute coronary syndromes. *Biol. Psychiatry* 62:302–308.

Frasure-Smith, N., Lesperance, F., and Talajic, M. (1993) Depression following myocardial infarction: impact on 6-month survival. *JAMA* 270:1819–1825.

Frasure-Smith, N., Lesperance, F., and Talajic, M. (1995) Depression and 18 month prognosis after myocardial infarction. *Circulation* 91:999–1005.

Friedman, E.M., and Irwin, M.R. (1997) Modulation of immune cell function by the autonomic nervous system. *Pharmacol. Thera.* 74:27–38.

Glassman, A.H., Califf, R.M., and Swedberg, K. (2002) Sertraline treatment of major depression in patients with acute MI or unstable angina. *JAMA* 288:701–709.

Glassman, A.H., and Miller, G.E. (2007) Where there is depression, there is inflammation ... sometimes! *Biol. Psychiatry* 62:280–281.

Glazer, K.M., Emery, C.F., Frid, D.J., and Banyasz, R.E. (2002) Psychological predictors of adherence and outcomes among patients in cardiac rehabilitation. *J. Cardiopulm. Rehab.* 22:40–46.

Gordillo, V., del Amo, J., Soriano, V., and Gonzalez-Lahorz, J. (1999) Sociodemographic and psychological variables influencing adherence to antiretroviral therapy. *AIDS* 13:1763–1769.

Gorman, J.M., Kertzner, R., Cooper, T., Goetz, R.R., Lagomasino, I., Novacenko, H., Williams, J.B.W., Stern, Y., Mayeux, R., and Ehrhardt, A.A. (1991) Glucocorticoid level and neuropsychiatric symptoms in homosexual men with HIV infection. *Am. J. Psychiatry* 148:42–45.

Grassi, B., Gambini, O., and Graghentini, I. (1997) Efficacy of paroxetine for treatment of depression in the context of HIV infection. *Pharmacotherapy* 30:70–71.

Haack, M., Hinze-Selch, D., Fenzel, T., Kraus, T., Kuhn, M., Schuld, A., and Pollmacher, T. (1999) Plasma levels of cytokines and soluble cytokine receptors in psychiatric patients upon hospital admission: effects of confounding factors and diagnosis. *J. Psychiatric Res.* 33:407–418.

Hamilton, M. (1960) A rating scale for depression. *J. Neurol Neurosurg Psychiatry* 23:56–62.

Hart, B.L. (1988) Biological basis of behavior of sick animals. *Neurosci. Behav. Rev.* 12:123–137.

Herbert, T.B., and Cohen, S. (1993) Depression and immunity: A meta-analytic review. *Psychol. Bull.* 113:472–486.

Herrmann-Lingen, C., Klemme, H., and Meyer, T. (2001) Depressed mood, physician-rated prognosis, and comorbidity as independent predictors of 1-year mortality in consecutive medical inpatients. *J. Psychosom. Res.* 50:295–301.

Ho, W.Z., Cnaan, A., Li, Y.H., Zhao, H.Q., Lee, H.R., Song, L., and Douglas, S.D. (1996) Substance P modulates human immunodeficiency virus replication in human peripheral blood monocyte-derived macrophages. *Aids Res. Human Retrov.* 12:195–198.

Holland, J.C., Romano, S.J., Heiligenstein, J.H., Tepner, R.G., and Wilson, M.G. (1998) A controlled trial of fluoxetine and desipramine in depressed women with advanced cancer. *Psycho-Oncology* 7:291–300.

Honig, A., Kuyper, A.M.G., Schene, A.H., Van Melle, J.P., DeJonge, P., Tulner, D.M., Schins, A., Crijns, H.J.G.M., Kuijpers, P.M.J.C., Vossen, H., Lousbereg, R., and Ormel, J. (2007) Treatment of post-myocardial infarction depressive disorder: a randomized, placebo-controlled trial with mirtazapine. *Psychosom. Med.* 69:606–613.

Ickovics, J.R., Hamburger, M.E., Vlahov, D., Schoenbaum, E.E., Schuman, P., Boland, R.J., Moore, J., HIV Epidemiology Research Study. (2001) CD4 cell count decline and depressive symptoms among HIV seropositive women: longitudinal analysis from the HIV Epidemiology Research study. *JAMA* 285:1466–1474.

Ironson, G., Balbin, E., Solomon, G., Fahey, J., Klimas, N., Schneiderman, N., and Fletcher, M.A. (2001) Relative preservation of natural killer cell cytoxicity and number in healthy AIDS patients with low CD4 counts. *AIDS* 15:2065–2073.

Irwin, M.R., and Miller, A.H. (2007) Depressive disorders and immunity: 20 years of progress and discovery. *Brain, Behav. Immun.* 21(4):374–383.

Kanner, A. (2003) Depression in epilepsy: prevalence, clinical semiology, pathogenic mechanisms and treatment. *Biol. Psychiatry* 54:388–298.

Karlsson, I., Goddaris, J., Lima, G.A.D., Nygaard, H., Simanyi, M., Taal, M., and Eglin, M. (2000) A randomized double blind comparison of the efficacy and safety of citalopram compared to mianserin in elderly, depressed patients with or without mild to moderate dementia. *Int. J. Geriat. Psychiatry* 15:295–305.

Katon, W.J. (2003) Clinical and health services relationships between major depression, depressive symptoms and general medical illness. *Biol. Psychiatry* 54:216–226.

Kemeny, M.E., and Dean, L. (1995) Effects of AIDS-related bereavement on HIV progression among New York City gay men. *AIDS Educ. Prev.* 7(Supp):36–47.

Kemeny, M.E., Weiner, H., Duran, R., Taylor, S.E., Visscher, B., and Fahey, J.L. (1995) Immune system changes after the death of a partner in HIV-positive gay men. *Psychosom. Med.* 57:547–554.

Kent, S., Bluthe, R.M., Kelley, K.W., and Dantzer, R. (1992) Sickness behavior as a new target for drug development. *Trends Pharmacol. Sci.* 13:24–28.

Kessler, R.C., Berglund, P., Demler, O., Jin, R., Merikangas, K.R., and Walters, E.E. (2005) Lifetime prevalence and age-of-onset distributions of DSM-IV disorders in the National Comorbidity Survey Replication. *Arch. Gen. Psychiatry* 62:593–602.

Kessler, R.C., McGonagle, K.A., Zhao, S.Y., Nelson, C.B., Huges, M., Eshleman, S., Wittchin, H.U., and Kendler, K.S. (1994) Lifetime and 12-month prevalence of DSM-III-R psychiatric disorders in the United States: results from the National Comorbidity Survey. *Arch. Gen. Psychiatry* 51:8–19.

Kirkwood, J.M., Bender, C., Agarwala, S., Tarhini, A., Shipe-Spotloe, J., Smelko, B., Donnely, S., and Stover, L. (2002) Mechanisms and management of toxicities associated with high-dose interferon alfa-2b therapy. *J. Clin. Oncology* 20:3703–3718.

Kissane, D., Clarke, D.M., and Street, A.F. (2001) Demoralization syndrome: a relevant psychiatric diagnosis for palliative care. *J. Palliat. Care* 17:12–21.

Kling, M.A., Alesci, S., Csako, G., Costello, R., Luckenbaugh, D.A., Bonne, O., Duncko, R., Drevets, W.C., Manji, H.K., Charney, D.S., Gold, P.W., and Neumeister, A. (2007) Sustained low-grade pro-inflammatory state in unmedicated, remitted women with major depressive disorder as evidenced by elevated serum levels of the acute phase proteins C-reactive protein and serum amyloid A. *Biol. Psychiatry* 62:309–313.

Kroenke, K., Spritzer, R.L., and Williams, J.B. (2002) The PHQ-9: a new depression diagnostic and severity measure. *Psychiatric Annals* 32:509–515.

Kronfol, Z. (2002) Immune dysregulation in major depression: a critical review of existing evidence. *Int. J. Neuropsychopharmacol.* 5:333–343.

Krueger, R.F., Chentsova-Dutton, Y.E., Markon, K.E., Goldberg, D., and Ormel, J. (2003) A cross-cultural study of the structure of comorbidity among common psychopathological syndromes in the general health care setting. *J. Abnorm. Psychol.* 112:437–447.

Kuipers, P.M., Hamulyuk, K., Strik, J.J., Wellens, H.J., and Honig, A. (2002) Beta-thromboglobulin and platelet factor 4 levels in post- myocardial infarction patients with major depression. *Psychiatry Res.* 109:207–210.

Laghrissi-Thode, F., Wagner, W.R., Pollack, B.G., Johnson, P.C., and Finkel, M.S. (1997) Elevated platelet factor 4 and beta-thromboglobulin plasma levels in depressed patients with ischemic heart disease. *Biol. Psychiatry* 42:290–295.

Lanza, G.A., Sgueglia, G.A., Cianflone, D., Rebuzz, A.G., Angeloni, G., Sestito, A., Infusino, F., Crea, F., and Maseri, A. (2006) Relation of heart rate variability to serum levels of C-reactive protein in patients with unstable angina pectoris. *Am. J. Cardiology* 97: 1702–1706.

Larson, S.J., and Dunn, A.J. (2001) Behavioral effects of cytokines. *Brain Beh. Immun.* 15:371–387.

Lee, H.B., and Lyketsos, C.G. (2003) Depression in Alzheimer's disease: heterogeneity and related issues. *Biol. Psychiatry* 54:353–362.

Lee, K.M., and Kim, Y.K. (2006) The role of IL-12 and TGF-beta1 in the pathophysiology of major depressive disorder. *Int. Immunopharmacol.* 6:298–1304.

Leserman, J. (2003) HIV disease progression: Depression, stress, and possible mechanisms. *Biol. Psychiatry* 54:295–306.

Leserman, J., Petitto, M., Gu, H., Gaynes, B.N., Barroso, J., Golden, R.N., Perkins, D.O., Folds, J.D., and Evans, D.L. (2002) Progression to AIDS, a clinical AIDS condition and mortality: Psychosocial and physiological predictors. *Psychol. Med.* 32:1059–1073.

Lesperance, F., Frasure-Smith, N., Koszycki, D., Laliberte, M.A., Van Zyl, L.T., Baker, B., Swenson, J.R., Ghatavi, K., Abramson, B.L., Dorian, P., and Guertain, M.C. (2007) Effects of citalopram and interpersonal psychotherapy on depression in patients with coronary artery disease: the Canadian Cardiac Randomized Evaluation of Antidepressant and Psychotherapy Efficacy (CREATE) trial. *JAMA* 297:367–379.

Lesperance, F., Frasure-Smith, N., Theroux, P., and Irwin, M. (2004) The association between major depression and levels of soluble intercellular adhesion molecule 1, interleukin-6, and C-reactive protein in patients with recent acute coronary syndromes. *Am. J. Psychiatry* 161:271–277.

Lett, H.S., Blumenthal, J.A., Babyak, M.A., Sherwood, A., Strauman, T., Robins, C., and Newman, M.F. (2004) Depression as a risk factor for coronary artery disease: evidence, mechanisms, and treatment. *Psychosom. Med.* 66:305–315.

Li, A., Withoff, S., and Verma, I.M. (2005) Inflammation-associated cancer: NF-kappaB is the lynchpin. *Trends Immunol.* 26:318–325.

Loberiza, F.R., Jr., Rizzo, J.D., Bredeson, Cn., Antin, J.H., Horowitz, M.M., Weeks, J.C., and Lee, S.J. (2002) Association of depressive syndrome and early deaths among patients after stem-cell transplantation for malignant diseases. *J. Clin. Oncology* 20: 2118–2126.

Lustman, P.J., Freedland, K.E., Griffith, L.S., and Clouse, R.E. (2000) Fluoxetine for depression in diabetes: a randomized double-blind placebo controlled trial. *Diabetes Care* 23:618–623.

Lyketsos, C.G., Hoover, D.R., Guccione, M., Senterfitt, W., Dew, M.A., Wesch, J., Vanraden, M.J., Treisman, G.J., and Morgenstern, H. (1993) Depressive symptoms as predictors of medical outcomes in HIV infection. *JAMA* 270:2563–2567.

Lyketsos, C.G., Sheppard, J.M.E., Steele, C.D., Kopunek, S., Steinberg, M., Baker, A.S., Brandt, J., and Rabins, P.V. (2000) Randomized placebo-controlled double blind clinical trial of sertraline in the treatment of depression complicating Alzheimer's disease: initial results from the depression in Alzheimer's disease study. *Am. J. Psychiatry* 157:1686–1689.

Maes, M., Bosmans, E., Meltzer, H.Y., Sharpe, S., and Suy, E. (1993) Interleukin-1β: A putative mediator of HPA axis hyperactivity in major depression? *Am. J. Psychiatry* 150:1189–1193.

Malave, H.A., Taylor, A.A., Nattama, J., Deswal, A., and Mann, D. L. (2003) Circulating levels of tumor necrosis factor correlate with indexes of depressed heart rate variability: a study in patients with mild-to-moderate heart failure. *Chest* 123:716–724.

Markovitz, J.H., and Matthews, K.A. (1991) Platelets and coronary heart disease: potential psychophysiologic mechanisms. *Psychosom. Med.* 53:643–668.

Marshall, P., and Colon, E. (1993) Effects of allergy season on mood and cognitive function. *Ann. Allergy* 71:251–258.

Masand, P., Pickett, P., and Murray, G.B. (1991) Psychostimulants for secondary depression in medical illness. *Psychosomatics* 32: 203–208.

Massie, M.J., and Greenberg, D.B.L. (2005) Oncology. In: Levenson, J., ed. *Textbook of Psychosomatic Medicine*. Washington, DC: American Psychiatric Publishing, pp. 517–534.

Mayne, T.J., Vittinghoff, E., Chesney, M.A., Barrett, D.C., and Coates, T.J. (1996) Depressive affect and survival among gay and bisexual men infected with HIV. *Arch. Int. Med.* 156:2233–2238.

McDaniel, J.S., Musselman, D.L., Porter, M.R., Reed, D.A., and Nemeroff, C.B. (1995) Depression in patients with cancer: diagnosis, biology, and treatment. *Arch. Gen. Psychiatry* 52:89–99.

McDonald, W.M., Richards, I.H., and DeLong, M.R. (2003) The prevalence, etiology and treatment of depression in Parkinson's disease. *Biol. Psychiatry* 54:363–375.

Meyers, C.A., Albitar, M., and Estey, E. (2005) Cognitive impairment, fatigue and cytokine levels in patients with acute myelogenous leukemia or myelodysplastic syndrome. *Cancer* 104:788–793.

Michaud, C.M., Murray, M.C., and Bloom, B.R. (2001) Burden of disease: implications for future research. *JAMA* 285:535–539.

Miller, G.E., Freedland, K.E., Duntley, S., and Carney, R.M. (2005) Relation of depressive symptoms to C reactive protein and pathogen burden cytomegalovirus, herpes simplex virus, Epstein Barr virus: in patients with earlier acute coronary syndromes. *Am. J. Cardiol.* 95:317–321.

Miller, G.E., Stetler, C.A., Carney, R.M., Freedland, K.E., and Banks, W.A. (2002) Clinical depression and inflammatory risk markers for coronary heart disease. *Am. J. Cardiol.* 90:1279–1283.

Minden, S.L., and Schiffer, R.B. (1990) Affective disorders in multiple sclerosis: review and recommendations for clinical research. *Arch. Neurol.* 47:98–104.

Miyoka, H., Otsubo, T., Kamijima, K., Ishii, M., Onuki, M., and Mitamura, K. (1999) Depression from interferon therapy in patients with hepatitis C. *Am. J. Psychiatry* 156:1120.

Mohr, D.C., Boudewyn, A.C., Goodkin, D.E., Bostrom, A., and Epstein, L. (2001) Comparative outcomes for individual cognitive-behavior therapy, supportive-expressive group psychotherapy and sertraline for the treatment of depression in multiple sclerosis. *J. Consult. Clin. Psychol.* 69:942–949.

Morrison, M.F., Petitto, J.M., Ten Have, T., Gettes, D.R., Chiappini, M.S., Weber, A.L., Brinker-Spence, P., Bauer, R.M., Douglas, S.D., and Evans, D.L. (2002) Depressive and anxiety disorders in women with HIV infection. *Am. J. Psychiatry* 159:789–796.

Musselman, D.L., Evans, D.L., and Nemeroff, C.B. (1998) The relationship of depression to cardiovascular disease. *Arch. Gen. Psychiatry* 55:580–592.

Musselman, D.L., Lawson, D.H., Gumnick, J.F., Manatunga, A.K., Penna, S., Goodkin, R.S., Greiner, K., Nemeroff, C.B., and Miller, A.H. (2001) Paroxetine for the prevention of depression induced by high-dose interferon alpha. *N. Eng. J. Med.* 344:961–966.

Musselman, D.L., Miller, A.H., Porter, M.R., Manatunga, A., Gao, F., Penna, S., Landry, J., Glover, S., McDaniel, J.S., and Nemeroff, C.B. (2001) Higher than normal plasma interleukin-6 concentrations in cancer patients with depression: preliminary findings. *Am. J. Psychiatry* 158:1252–1257.

Musselman, D.L., Somerset, W.I., Guo, Y., Manatunga, A.K., Porter, M., Penna, S., Lewison, B., Goodkin, R., Lawson, K., Lawson, D., Evans, D.L., and Nemeroff, C.B. (2006) A double-blind, multicenter, parallel group study of paroxetine, desipramine, or placebo in breast cancer patients (stages I, II, III, and IV) with major depression. *J. Clin. Psychiatry* 67:288–296.

Musselman, D.L., Tomer, A., Manatunga, A.K., Knight, B.T., Porter, M.R., Kasey, S., Marzec, U., Harker, L.A., and Nemeroff, C.B. (1996) Exaggerated platelet reactivity in major depressive disorder. *Am. J. Psychiatry* 153:1313–1317.

Nahshoni, E., Aravat, D., Aizenberg, D., Sigler, M., Zalsman, G., Strasberg, B., Imbar, S., Adler, E., and Weizman, A. (2004) Heart rate variability in patients with major depression. *Psychosomatics* 45:129–134.

Nemeroff, C.B. (1996) The corticotrophin-releasing factor (CRF) hypothesis of depression: new findings and new directions. *Mol. Psychiatry* 1:336–342.

Newport, D.J., and Nemeroff, C.F. (1998) Assessment and treatment of depression in cancer treatment. *J. Psychosom. Res.* 45:215–237.

Orlando, M., Burnam, M.A., Beckman, R., Morton, S.C., London, A.S., Bing, E.G., and Fleishman, J.A. (2002) Re-estimating the prevalence of psychiatric disorders in a nationally representative sample of persons receiving care for HIV: results from the HIV Cost and Services Utilization Study. *Int. J. Meth. Psychiatric Res.* 11:75–82.

Page-Shafer, K., Delorenze, G.N., Satariano, W.A., and Winkelstein, W., Jr. (1996) Comorbidity and survival in HIV-infected men in the San Francisco Men's Health Survey. *Ann. Epidemiol.* 6:420–430.

Patten, S. (2001) Long-term medical conditions and major depression in a Canadian population study at waves 1 and 2. *J. Affect. Disord.* 63:35–41.

Patterson, T.L., Shaw, W.S., Semple, S.J., Cherner, M., McCutchan, J.A., Atkinson, J.H., Grant, I., and Nannis, E. (1996) Relationship of psychosocial factors to HIV disease progression. *Ann. Behav. Med.* 18:30–39.

Pavon, L., Sandoval-Lopez, G., Eugenia Hernandez, M., Loria, F., Estrada, I., Perez, M., Moreno, J., Avila, U., Leff, P., Anton, B., and Heinze, G. (2006) Th2 cytokine response in major depressive disorder patients before treatment. *J. Neuroimmunol.* 172: 156–165.

Pezella, G., Moslinger-Gehmayr, R., and Contu, A. (2001) Treatment of depression in patients with breast cancer: a comparison between paroxetine and amitriptyline. *Breast Cancer Res. Treat.* 70:1–10.

Pike, J.L., and Irwin, M.R. (2006) Dissociation of inflammatory markers and natural killer cell activity in major depressive disorder. *Brain Behav. Immun.* 20(2):169–174.

Popkin, M.K., Callies, A.L., and Mackenzie, T.B. (1985) The outcome of antidepressant use in the medically ill. *Arch. Gen. Psychiatry* 42:1160–1163.

Rabkin, J.G., Ferrando, S.J., Wagner, G.J., and Rabkin, R. (2000) DHEA treatment for HIV+ patients: effects on mood, androgenic and anabolic parameters. *Psychoneuroendocrinology* 25:53–68.

Rabkin, J.G., Rabkin, R., Harrison, W., and Wagner, G. (1994) Effect of imipramine on mood and enumerative measures of immune status in depressed patients with HIV illness. *Am. J. Psychiatry* 151:516–523.

Rabkin, J.G., Rabkin, R., and Wagner, G. (1994) Effect of fluoxetine on mood and immune status in depressed patients with HIV illness. *J. Clin. Psychiatry* 55:92–97.

Rabkin, J.G., Wagner, G.J., and Rabkin, R. (1994) Effects of sertraline on mood and immune status in patients with major depression and HIV illness: an open trial. *J. Clin. Psychiatry* 55:433–439.

Rabkin, J.G., Wagner, G.J., and Rabkin, R. (2000) A double-blind, placebo-controlled trial of testosterone for HIV-positive men with hypogonadal symptoms. *Arch. Gen. Psychiatry* 57:141–147.

Rabkin, J.G., Williams, J.B., Remien, R.H., Goetz, R., Kertzner, R., and Gorman, J.M. (1991) Depression, distress, lymphocyte subsets, and human immunodeficiency virus symptoms on two occasions in HIV-positive homosexual men. *Arch. Gen. Psychiatry* 48:111–119.

Radloff, L.S. (1977) The CES-D: a self report depression scale for research in the general population. *Applied Psychological Measures* 3:385–401.

Raison, C.L., Capuron, L., and Miller, A. (2006) Cytokines sing the blues: inflammation and the pathogenesis of depression. *Trends Immunol.* 27:24–31.

Raison, C.L., and Miller, A.H. (2003) Depression in cancer: new developments regarding diagnosis and treatment. *Biol. Psychiatry* 54:283–294.

Raison, C.L., and Nemeroff, C.B. (2000) Cancer and depression: prevalence, diagnosis, and treatment. *Home Health Care Consult.* 7:34–41.

Rasmussen, A., Lunde, M., Poulsen, D.L., Sorensen, K., Qvitzau, S., and Bech, P. (2003) A double-blind, placebo-controlled study of sertraline in the prevention of depression in stroke patients. *Psychosomatics* 44:216–221.

Razavi, D., Allilaire, J.F., Smith, M., Salimpour, A., Verra, M., Desclaux, B., Saltel, P., Piollet, I., Gauvain Piquard, A., Trichard, C., Cordier, B., Fresco, R., Guillibert, E., Sechter, D., Orth, J.P., Bouhassira, M., Mesters, P., and Blin, P. (1996) The effect of fluoxetine on anxiety and depression symptoms in cancer patients. *Acta Psychiatr. Scand.* 94:205–210.

Rechlin, T., Weis, M., Spitzer, A., and Kaschka, W.P. (1994) Are affective disorders associated with alterations of heart rate variability? *J. Affect. Disord.* 32:271–275.

Richard, I.H., Maughan, A., and Kurlan, R. (1999) Do serotonin reuptake inhibitor antidepressants worsen Parkinson's disease? A retrospective case series. *Movement Disord.* 14:155–157.

Richardson, P., Mckenna, W., Bristow, M., Maisch, B., Mautner, B., O'Connell, J., Olson, E., Thiene, G., Goodwin, J., Gyarfas, I., Martin, I., Nordet, P. (1996) Report of the 1995 World Health Organization/International Society and Federation of Cardiology Task Force on the definition and classification of cardiomyopathies. *Circulation* 93(5):1043–1065.

Robinson, R.G. (2003) Post-stroke depression: prevalence, diagnosis, treatment and disease progression. *Biol. Psychiatry* 54:376–387.

Roscoe, J.A., Morrow, G.R., Hickock, J.T., Mustian, K.M., Griggs, J.J., Matteson, S.E., Bushunow, P., Qazi, R., and Smith, B. (2005) Effect of paroxetine hydrochloride (paxil) on fatigue and depression in breast cancer patients receiving chemotherapy. *Breast Cancer Res. Treat.* 89:243–249.

Roy, A., Guthrie, S., and Pickar, D. (1987) Plasma norepinephrine responses to cold challenge in depressed patients and normal controls. *Psychiatry Res.* 21:161–168.

Rozans, M., Dreisbach, A., Lertora, J.J., and Kahn, M.J. (2002) Palliative uses of methylphenidate in patients with cancer: a review. *J. Clin. Oncology* 20:335–339.

Rudish, B., and Nemeroff, C.B. (2003) Epidemiology of comorbid coronary artery disease and depression. *Biol. Psychiatry* 54:227–240.

Scharko, A.M. (2006) DSM psychiatric disorders in the context of pediatric HIV/AIDS. *AIDS Care* 18:441–445.

Shapiro, A.P. (2005) Heart disease. In: Levenson, J., ed. *Textbook of Psychosomatic Medicine*. Washington, DC: America Psychiatric Publishing, pp. 423–444.

Shen, W.W., Swartz, C.M., and Calhoun, J.W. (1999) Is inhibition of nitric oxide synthase a mechanism for SSRI-induced bleeding? *Psychosomatics* 40:268–269.

Skala, J.A., Freedland, K.E., and Carney, R.M. (2006) Coronary heart disease and depression: a review of recent mechanistic research. *Can. J. Psychiatry* 51:738–745.

Smith, D.K., Warren, D., Solomon, L., Schuman, P., Stein, M., Greenburg, B., and Moore, J. (1996) The design, participants and selected early findings of the HIV Epidemiology Research study. In: O'Leary, A., Jemmott, L.S., eds. *Women and AIDS: Coping and Care*. New York: Plenum Press, pp. 185–206.

Smith, R.S. (1991) The macrophage theory of depression. *Medical Hypotheses* 35:298–306.

Stearns, V., Isaacs, C., Rowland, J., Crawford, J., Ellis, M.J., and Kramer, R. (2000) A pilot trial assessing the efficacy of paroxetine hydrochloride (paxil) in controlling for hot flashes in breast cancer survivors. *Ann. Oncology* 11:17–22.

Stein, P.K., Carney, R.M., Freedland, K.E., Skala, J.A., Jaffe, A.S., Kleiger, R.E., and Rottman, J.N. (2000) Heart rate variability is related to the severity of depression in patients with coronary heart disease. *J. Psychosom. Res.* 48:493–500.

Steptoe, A., Kunz-Ebrecht, S.R., and Owen, N. (2003) Lack of association between depressive symptoms and markers of immune and vascular inflammation in middle-aged men and women. *Psychol. Med.* 33:667–674.

Suarez, E.C., Lewis, J.G., Krishnan, R.R., and Young, K.H. (2004) Enhanced expression of cytokines and chemokines by blood monocytes to in vitro and lipopolysaccharide stimulation are associated with hostility and severity of depressive symptoms in healthy women. *Psychoneuroendocrinology* 29:1119–1128.

Swiergiel, A.H., Smagin, G.N., and Dunn, A.J. (1997) Influenza virus infection of mice induces anorexia: comparison with endotoxin and interleukin-1 and the effects of indomethacin. *Pharmacol. Biochem. Behav.* 57:389–396.

Szabo, S.T., Gould, T.D., and Manji, H.K. (2004) Neurotransmitters, receptors, signal transduction, and second messengers in psychiatric disorders. In: Schatzberg, A.F., and Nemeroff, C.B., eds. *Textbook of Psychopharmacology*, 3rd ed. Arlington, VA: American Psychiatric Publishing, Inc., pp. 3–52.

Theobald, D.E., Kirsch, K.L., Holtsclaw, E., Donaghy, K., and Passik, S.D. (2002) An open label, crossover trial of Mirtazapine (15 and 30 mg) in cancer patients with pain and other distressing symptoms. *J. Pain Sympt. Mgmt.* 23:442–227.

Tiemeier, H., Hofman, A., van Tujil, H.R., Kiliaan, A.J., Meijer, J., and Breteler, M.M. (2003) Inflammatory proteins and depression in the elderly. *Epidemiology* 14:103–107.

Troxler, R.G., Sprague, E.A., Albanese, R.A., Fuchs, R., and Thompson, A.J. (1977) The association of elevated plasma cortisol and early atherosclerosis as demonstrated by coronary angiography. *Atherosclerosis* 26:151–162.

Turner, M.S., May, D.B., Arthur, R.R., and Xiong, G.L. (2007) Clinical impact of selective serotonin reuptake inhibitors therapy with bleeding risks. *J. Int. Med.* 261:205–213.

Valentine, A.D., Meyers, C.A., Kling, M.A., Richelson, E., and Hauser, P. (1998) Mood and cognitive side effects of interferon-alpha therapy. *Semin. Oncology* 25:39–47.

Van der Kooy, K.G., Van Hout, H.P., Van Marwijk, H.W., De Haan, M., Stehouwer, C.D., and Beekman, A.T. (2006) Differences in heart rate variability between depressed and non-depressed elderly. *Int. J. Geriat. Psychiatry* 21:147–150.

Van Heeringen, K., and Zivkov, M. (1996) Pharmacological treatment of depression in cancer patients: a placebo controlled study of mianserin. *Br. J. Psychiatry* 169:440–443.

Vedhara, K., Schifitto, G., and McDermott, M. (1999) Disease progression in HIV-positive women with moderate to severe immunosupression: the role of depression. Dana Consortium on Therapy for HIV Dementia and Related Cognitive Disorders. *Behav. Med.* 25:43–47.

Wagner, G.J., Rabkin, J., and Rabkin, R. (1997) Dextroamphetamine as a treatment for depression and low energy in AIDS patients: a pilot study. *J. Psychosom. Res.* 42:407–411.

Wagner, G.J., and Rabkin, R. (2000) Effects of dextramphetamine on depression and fatigue inn men with HIV: a double-blind, placebo-controlled trial. *J. Clin. Psychiatry* 61:436–440.

Wang, P.S., Bong, R., Knight, E., Glynn, R.J., Mogun, H., and Avorn, J. (2002) Noncompliance with antihypertensive medications: the impact of depressive symptoms and psychosocial factors. *J. Gen. Int. Med.* 17:504–511.

Wang, P.S., Lane, M., Olfson, M., Pincus, H.A., Wells, K.B., and Kessler, R.C. (2005) Twelve-month use of mental health services in the United States. Results from the National Comorbidity Survey Replication. *Arch. Gen. Psychiatry* 62:629–640.

Watkins, L.F., Weirtelak, E.P., Goehler, L.E., Smith, K.P., Martin, D., Maier, S.F. (1994) Characterization of cytokine induced hyperalgesia. *Brain Res.*654:15–26.

Weisse, C.S. (1992) Depression and immunocompetence, a review of the literature. *Psychol. Bull.* 111:475–489.

Wellens, J.T., and Ridker, P.M. (2004) Inflammation as a cardiovascular risk factor. *Circulation* 109:2–10.

Wellens, K.E., and Hotamisligil, G.S. (2005) Inflammation, stress and diabetes. *J. Clin. Invest.* 115:1111–1119.

Wernicke, J.F., Pritchett, Y.L., D'Souza, D.N., Waninger, A., Tran, P., Iyengar, S., and Raskin, J. (2006) A randomized controlled trial of duloxetine in diabetic peripheral neuropathic pain. *Neurology* 67:1411–1420.

Whooley, M.A., Caska, C.M., Hendrickson, B.E., Rourke, M.A., Ho, J., and Ali, S. (2007) Depression and inflammation in patients with coronary heart disease: findings from the Heart and Soul Study. *Biol. Psychiatry* 62:314–320.

Williams, L.S., Kroenke, K., Bakas, T., Plue, L.D., Brizendine, E., Tu, W.Z., and Hendrie, H. (2007) Care management of post-stroke depression: a randomized, controlled trial. *Stroke* 38:998–1003.

Writing Committee for the ENRICHD Investigators. (2003) Effects of treating depression and low perceived social support on clinical events after myocardial infarction: the enhancing recovery in coronary heart disease patients (ENRICHD). *JAMA* 289:3106–3116.

Wulsin, L.R., (2004) Is depression a major risk factor for coronary disease? A systematic review of the epidemiologic evidence. *Harv. Rev. Psychiatry* 12:79–95.

Wulsin, L.R., Viewig, W.V., and Fernandez, A. (2004) Treating depression in patients with cardiovascular disease. *Curr. Psychiatry* 3:20–34.

Yirmiya, R. (1996) Endotoxin produces a depressive-like episode in rats. *Brain Res.* 711:163–174.

Yirmiya, R., Pollack, Y., Barak, O., Avitsur, R., Ovadia, H., Bette, M., Weihe, E., and Weidenfeld, J. (2001) Effects of antidepressant drugs on the behavioral and physiological responses to lipopolysaccharide (LPS) in rodents. *Neuropsychopharmacology* 24: 531–543.

Yirmiya, R., Weidenfeld, J., Pollak, Y., Morag, M., Morag, A., Avitsur, R., Barak, O., Reichenberg, A., Cohen, E., Shavit, Y., and Ovadia, H. (1999) Cytokines, 'depression due to general medical condition' and antidepressant drugs. *Adv. Exper. Med. Biol.* 461:283–316.

Zigmond, A.S., and Snaith, R.P. (1983) The Hospital Anxiety and Depression Scale. *Acta Psychiatr. Scand.* 67:361–370.

Zisook, S., Peterkin, J., Goggin, K.J., Sledge, P., Atkinson, J.H., and Grant, I. (1998) Treatment of major depression in HIV-seropositive men. *J. Clin. Psychiatry* 59:217–224.

Zung, W.W. (1965) A self-rating scale for depression. *Arch. Gen. Psychiatry* 12:63–70.

V ANXIETY DISORDERS

ANTONIA S. NEW AND DENNIS S. CHARNEY

THE chapters in this section reflect the advances in preclinical and clinical neuroscience that have enhanced our understanding of the diagnosis, pathophysiology, and treatment of anxiety disorders. This progress has the potential to revolutionize the means by which anxiety disorders are diagnosed. The major limitation of current diagnostic classification systems is that they are not based on etiology, pathophysiology, or treatment response. Stein and Bienvenu (Chapter 37) provide a comprehensive review of the current and future classification systems for anxiety disorders. They review the empirical evidence for and against alternative classification systems to *Diagnostic and Statistical Manual of Mental Disorders*, 4th ed. (*DSM-IV*; American Psychiatric Association, 1994), including a model that considers anxiety disorders to emerge from a single core-pathological process, and a related dimensional model for anxiety disorders. They argue that neurobiological evidence in anxiety disorder is growing very rapidly and that any classification that does not take into account, over the coming years, the relationship between genotype, anxiety phenotype (including specific neurocircuitry), and environmental influences will be unsatisfying and temporary (Caspi and Moffitt, 2006).

It is imperative to discover specific genes that relate to vulnerability to anxiety disorders if we are to make fundamental progress in improving diagnostic precision, understanding pathophysiology, and identifying new molecular targets for drug development. Hamilton and Fyer (Chapter 38) review evidence for heritability as well as studies that have implicated specific genes for a number of anxiety disorders, including panic disorder, phobias, generalized anxiety disorder, obsessive-compulsive disorder (OCD), and anxiety personality traits. All of these disorders carry rather high heritability, with 20%–40% of the phenotypic variance accounted for by additive genetic effects. They review the complexity of identifying specific genes or haplotypes for these disorders. For example, a number of different chromosomal locations have been discovered in pedigrees replete with panic disorder (Crowe et al., 2001; Gelernter et al., 2001; Thorgeirsson et al., 2003; Fyer et al., 2006), raising the possibility of genetic heterogeneity across different populations. They also review preclinical investigations using "knockout" and "knockin" technology, which have implicated specific genes in anxiety disorders. These techniques have demonstrated a critical role for the 5-hydroxytryptamine-1A (5-HT_{1A}) receptor in anxiety, supported by findings in 5-HT_{1A} knockout mice indicating that altered function of 5-HT_{1A} receptors early in life can produce long-term abnormalities in the regulation of anxiety behaviors (Gross et al., 2002) and by evidence that the overexpression of 5-HT_{1A} results in lower levels of "anxiety-like" behavior (Kusserow et al., 2004). Preclinical studies have also demonstrated a role for different subtypes of the corticotrophin releasing hormone (CRH-R1, CRH-R2) and the possible interplay between these two subtypes in mediating stress responsiveness (Bale and Vale, 2004).

Important clues to the pathogenesis of anxiety disorders come from the work by McEwen (Chapter 40). The results from these preclinical investigations have had a major influence on the focus of current clinical investigations of anxiety disorders. Animal models of anxiety disorders have been very useful in identifying, with a surprising degree of specificity, the effects of psychological stress on brain structure and function. Among the prominent examples are the observations that a variety of stressors in different animal species suppress neurogenesis and reduce hippocampal volume and that specific pharmacological agents such as glutamate release inhibitors, glucocorticoid receptor antagonists, standard antidepressants, and putative antidepressants such as substance P antagonists may reverse or prevent these effects. This line of research has produced a number of hypotheses that may lead to novel therapeutic approaches to stress-related anxiety disorders. Elegant work by McEwen and colleagues has emphasized the role of allostasis and allostatic load as important principles when considering the acute adaptive and maladaptive responses of the brain and body to stress. This work has implications for preventive approaches to stress-related psychopathology and the psychobiological mechanisms of resilience and vulnerability to extreme psychological stress (Charney, 2004).

The neural circuits and associated neural mechanisms that may relate to the signs and symptoms of anxiety disorders are the subject of intensive preclinical investigation. Sullivan and colleagues (Chapter 39) review the adaptive value of fear and anxiety and present models for how the neural systems underlying these normal behaviors might go awry in pathological anxiety disorders. They review the evidence for the roles for brain structures such as the amygdala, hippocampus, locus coeruleus, bed nucleus of the stria terminalis, and cortical regions in fear conditioning, extinction, sensitization, and the consolidation and reconsolidation of emotional memories. The neurochemical modulation of these brain structures by neuromodulators such as cortisol, corticotropin releasing hormone (CRH), glutamate, and norepinephrine have provided important clues to prevent, attenuate, or reverse the effects of traumatic and fear-inducing stimuli on the symptoms associated with fear conditioning and the impact of memories on psychological and physiological functions. Finally, they introduce a multimodal model for acquired adaptation to stress through "stress inoculation" in squirrel monkeys (Lyons and Parker, 2007).

These neural mechanisms and associated brain structures have proven to be related to the pathophysiology and treatment of anxiety disorders as described by Kent and Rauch (Chapter 43) and Swedo and Grant (Chapter 42). Neuroimaging studies in patients with post-traumatic stress disorder (PTSD) have largely been consistent with preclinical studies and have revealed abnormalities in a neural fear circuit featuring the amygdala, hippocampus, and prefrontal cortex. Reductions in hippocampal volume have repeatedly been identified in patients with PTSD. Neuroreceptor imaging studies have begun to identify alterations in receptor systems implicated in anxiety and fear regulation. Functional imaging findings in panic disorder, though less conclusive than that of some of the other anxiety disorders, point to abnormalities in the hippocampal/parahippocampal region at rest. During symptom provocation, patients with panic disorder exhibit activation of insular and motor striatal regions, whereas reductions are seen in widespread cortical regions, including the prefrontal cortex. Magnetic resonance spectroscopy (MRS) findings suggest that patients with panic disorder exhibit an exaggerated hemodynamic response to hypocapnea, which is manifest as relatively greater global vasoconstriction. Likewise, receptor binding studies suggest widespread abnormalities in the γ-aminobutyric acid (GABA)ergic/benzodiazepine system. Neuroimaging studies in OCD differ substantially from that of other anxiety disorders because of evidence of specific frontocortical-striatal inefficiency in conjunction with orbitofrontal hyperactivity.

Swedo and Grant consider current hypotheses regarding the etiology and pathophysiology of OCD. It appears highly likely that OCD, as currently defined, probably reflects several different disease entities whose psychopathology ranges from neuroimmune dysfunction to abnormalities in neurotransmitters and neuropeptides. This chapter reviews recent evidence of specific molecular targets for the immune response that underlies pediatric autoimmune neuropsychiatric disorders associated with streptococcal infections (PANDAS). In addition, recent clinical trials in OCD are reviewed.

In the next to last chapter in this section, Mathew and colleagues (Chapter 44) review novel pharmacology in the treatment of anxiety disorders. Selective serotonin reuptake inhibitors (SSRIs) are the first-line treatment for a number of anxiety disorders, due to their favorable side-effect profile, although tricyclic antidepressants and monoamine oxidase inhibitors continue to have a role. This chapter also reviews recent head-to-head trials of SSRIs and selective noradrenergic reuptake inhibitors (SNRIs) and demonstrates comparable efficacy for these agents. Finally, the authors point to disappointing results in the treatment of PTSD, with a recent report from the Institute of Medicine as evidence of the inadequacy of determining efficacy in the treatment of PTSD.

REFERENCES

American Psychiatric Association. (1994) *Diagnostic and Statistical Manual of Mental Disorders,* 4th ed. Washington, DC: Author.

Bale, T.L., and Vale, W.W. (2004) CRF and CRF receptors: role in stress responsivity and other behaviors. *Ann. Rev. Pharmacol. Toxicol.* 44:525–557.

Caspi, A., and Moffitt, T.E. (2006) Gene-environment interactions in psychiatry: joining forces with neuroscience. *Nat. Rev. Neurosci.* 7:583–590.

Charney, D.S. (2004) Psychobiological mechanisms of resilience and vulnerability: implications for successful adaptation to extreme stress. *Am. J. Psychiatry* 161:195–216.

Crowe, R.R., Goedken, R., Samuelson, S., et al. (2001) Genomewide survey of panic disorder. *Am. J. Med. Genet.* 105:105–109.

Fyer, A.J., Hamilton, S.P., Durner, M., et al. (2006) A third-pass genome scan in panic disorder: evidence for multiple susceptibility loci. *Biol. Psychiatry* 60:388–401.

Gelernter, J., Bonvicini, K., Page, G., et al. (2001) Linkage genome scan for loci predisposing to panic disorder or agoraphobia. *Am. J. Med. Genet.* 105:548–557.

Gross, C., Zhuang, X., Stark, K., et al. (2002) Serotonin1A receptor acts during development to establish normal anxiety-like behaviour in the adult. *Nature* 416:396–400.

Kusserow, H., Davies, B., Hortnagl, H., et al. (2004) Reduced anxiety-related behaviour in transgenic mice overexpressing serotonin 1A receptors. *Brain Res. Mol. Brain Res.* 129:104–116.

Lyons, D.M., Parker, K.J. (2007) Stress inoculation-induced indications of resilience in monkeys. *J. Trauma Stress* 20:423–433.

Thorgeirsson, T.E., Oskarsson, H., Desnica, N., et al. (2003) Anxiety with panic disorder linked to chromosome 9q in Iceland. *Am. J. Hum. Genet.* 72:1221–1230.

37 Diagnostic Classification of Anxiety Disorders: *DSM-V* and Beyond

MURRAY B. STEIN AND O. JOSEPH BIENVENU

The goal of this chapter is to provide a synthetic overview of current and future classification systems for anxiety disorders. In so doing, we intend to familiarize the reader with the historical origins of our current nosology, as a preface for showing how these have evolved to their present state. We touch on some of the current controversies in the diagnosis of anxiety disorders and comment on how these may be reflected in future changes to the diagnostic criteria. Much of the content of this chapter focuses on alternative models for diagnostic classification of the anxiety disorders. Prominent among these models is the specification that the anxiety disorders might be more parsimoniously represented by a core pathological process that underlies them all (for example, neurosis). The empirical evidence for and against this notion will be reviewed. Finally, we propose future approaches to diagnostic classification that take into account the neurobiology of the conditions, and perhaps even their etiologic origins.

BACK TO THE FUTURE

It has been said that those who do not remember the past are doomed to repeat it. In an effort to prevent this from happening, we believe that a backward look at the evolution of the anxiety disorder diagnostic criteria is in order. This retrospective viewpoint provides a framework from which to speculate about how future versions of the *Diagnostic and Statistical Manual of Mental Disorders (DSM)* (*DSM-V* and beyond) might be configured, and on what basis.

DSM-II (and International Classification of Diseases [ICD]-8) included what we now call the anxiety disorders in the "neuroses" category. Anxiety neurosis subsumed panic disorder and generalized anxiety disorder (GAD); phobic neurosis included agoraphobia, social phobia, specific phobia, and separation anxiety disorder; and obsessive-compulsive neurosis equates to obsessive-compulsive disorder (OCD). (Traumatic neurosis, though not codified in *DSM-II*, was used in the literature of the era and fits with what we now term *posttraumatic stress disorder*.) *DSM-III* came along in 1980 and made some radical changes to the diagnostic criteria, most notably the separation of the neuroses along the diagnostic lines we now recognize. *DSM-III* dropped the "neurosis" category in large part, it seems, to prevent clinicians from inferring that a psychodynamic etiologic process was being named (as *DSM-III* was furtively and consistently an atheoretical, descriptive document). But it also took note that panic disorder and GAD, in particular, were different entities with different family history, course, and perhaps response to treatment (American Psychiatric Association [APA], 1980).

Centrality of Panic to Diagnostic Classification

The idea that panic attacks (and panic disorder) are distinguishable from other forms of background anxiety has been one of the major (if not the major) organizing principles in the classification of anxiety disorders for the past two decades. From *DSM-III* through *DSM-III-R* and *DSM-IV*, epidemiologic studies have been guided by the construct of panic attacks and panic disorder as distinct from other forms of anxiety (Markowitz et al., 1989; Klerman et al., 1991; Horwath et al., 1993; Eaton et al., 1994; Fyer et al., 1996). Influenced strongly by the seminal observations of Donald F. Klein and colleagues that panic attacks responded to imipramine, whereas anticipatory anxiety did not (Klein et al., 1978), this position has proved instrumental in the way we approach anxiety disorder classification, particularly in North America.

Agoraphobia Without Panic: The Exception to a Rule?

It is beyond the scope of this chapter to review the evidence for and against considering panic disorder (distinguished by the presence of uncued, or spontaneous panic attacks) as distinct from other forms of anxiety where panic attacks also occur but are less likely to be spontaneous (that is, any of the phobic disorders, where paroxysms of anxiety and physical symptoms may occur upon exposure to the phobic stimulus). Suffice it to say that there is ample evidence, though this has not gone unchallenged. Most contentious has been the idea that agoraphobia is virtually always a consequence of panic disorder. Many epidemiological studies have reported a high prevalence of "agoraphobia without panic" (Robins et al., 1984; Eaton et al., 1994; Wittchen et al., 1998), the existence of which runs contrary to the dogma that agoraphobia develops only as a complication of unbridled panic attacks (Katerndahl, 2000). Although some cases of agoraphobia without panic undoubtedly reflect the limitations of large-scale diagnostic interviews that miss some cases of preexisting spontaneous panic while picking up the more current agoraphobia, and which misclassify some cases of specific phobia as agoraphobia (Horwath et al., 1993), there are inarguably many cases of agoraphobia where panic was never present (Wittchen et al., 1998; Hayward et al., 2003). Some of these cases are probably pseudo-agoraphobia associated with limitations attributable to medical illness (for example, phobic limitations associated with the postural instability of vestibular dysfunction) (Marks, 1981; Stein et al., 1994), some are better considered specific phobias (Wittchen et al., 1998; Bienvenu et al., 2006), and others are more classic agoraphobia where panic is truly absent.

Furthermore, whereas panic disorder is thought to develop from panic attacks that occur "out of the blue," there is evidence that persons prone to panic have prodromal symptoms (some of which can be thought of as agoraphobic symptoms) that can antedate the panic by many years (Fava et al., 1988; Lelliott et al., 1989). Bienvenu and colleagues (2006) examined prospective data from the Baltimore Epidemiologic Catchment Area (ECA) site wherein a sample of 1920 adults were assessed with the Diagnostic Interview Schedule (DIS) in 1981 and again approximately 13 years later. As expected, baseline DIS/*DSM-III* panic disorder strongly predicted first incidence of *DSM-III-R* agoraphobia; however, baseline agoraphobia without spontaneous panic attacks also robustly predicted first incidence of panic disorder, even when possible diagnostic misclassification of agoraphobia was taken into account using clinical reappraisal methods. These data strongly suggest that the implied one-way causal relationship between spontaneous panic attacks and agoraphobia in *DSM-IV* is incorrect. Observations such as these have called into question the primacy of panic for our diagnostic classification system, but the idea is sufficiently ensconced that resistance to change may be substantial.

Generalized Anxiety Disorder: Worrying About Worries and Duration

Since *DSM-III*, nosologists have attempted to reliably and validly define GAD. Over time, the diagnostic construct has been narrowed and may be more reliable, but several investigators have cast doubt on its ultimate utility. For example, in *DSM-III-R*, the minimum duration criterion was increased from 1 month to 6 months, with little empirical support for this change (Breslau & Davis, 1985). Kendler et al. (1992a) found that, if anything, 1-month GAD was more heritable than 6-month GAD, thus disputing the notion that shorter-duration symptoms are more likely to be environmentally mediated transient stress reactions. We divided community participants into five mutually exclusive symptom categories: (*1*) *DSM-III-R* GAD, (*2*) 6 months of worry or anxiety with 6 associated symptoms, (*3*) 1 month of anxiety with or (*4*) without 6 associated symptoms, and (*5*) no anxiety, and investigated their demographic and comorbidity profiles as external construct validators. The first three groups were homogeneous with regard to these validators, but their profiles differed from those of participants with fewer than six symptoms or no anxiety. Thus, requiring six symptoms produced a group with a particular epidemiologic profile. Neither the nature of the participants' worries nor the duration of symptoms influenced this profile (Bienvenu et al., 1998).

Other groups have used external construct validators to address the GAD duration criterion. Kessler and colleagues (2005) examined data from the U.S. National Comorbidity Survey Replication (NCS-R), a U.S. household survey carried out during 2001–2003. There were few differences between cases with episodes of 1–5 months and those with episodes of ≥ 6 months in onset, persistence, impairment, comorbidity, parental GAD, or sociodemographic correlates. The authors concluded that, given the relative comparability of persons with a GAD-like syndrome with episodes of < 6 months duration to those with 6 or more months duration, little basis could be provided for excluding the former group from a diagnosis (Kessler et al., 2005). Angst et al. (2006) conducted a similar analysis using data from the Zurich Cohort Study. The authors defined generalized anxiety syndromes with varying duration criteria (2 weeks, 1 month, 3 months, and 6 months) and found no significant differences in family history of anxiety, work impairment, distress, treatment rates, or comorbidity with major depressive episodes, bipolar disorder, or suicide attempts. Only social impairment related to the length of episodes. Importantly, the 6-month criterion of *DSM-III-R* and *DSM-IV* GAD would preclude this diagnosis in about one half of the participants treated for generalized anxiety syndromes. The authors concluded that GAD syndromes of varying duration form a continuum with comparable clinical relevance.

DSM-IV considers "excessive" worry to be paramount for a GAD diagnosis, but this requirement is absent in ICD-10. Again analyzing data from the NCS-R, Ruscio et al. (2005) compared (*1*) nonexcessive worriers meeting all other *DSM-IV* criteria for GAD with (*2*) respondents who met full GAD criteria, and (*3*) other survey respondents to consider the implications of removing the excessiveness requirement. When the "excessiveness" requirement was removed, the lifetime prevalence of GAD increased by approximately 40%. Interestingly, there were some important differences between GAD with and without "excessive" worry: the latter had an earlier age at onset and greater chronicity, symptom severity, and psychiatric co-morbidity. However, cases not meeting the "excessive" requirement still had substantial impairment and treatment seeking compared to respondents without GAD, suggesting that they represented a less severely affected group than the "excessive" cases. It is reasonable to conclude from these data that the "excessive" requirement, while having the impact of identifying more severe cases of GAD, does not seem to distinguish a qualitatively distinct group of individuals. In that sense, it could be argued that retaining the "excessive" requirement is somewhat arbitrary but perhaps establishes a clinically reasonable threshold for severity that warrants particular attention. The authors concluded that the findings challenge the validity of the excessiveness requirement and highlight the need for further research into the optimal definition of GAD (Ruscio et al., 2005).

In conclusion, among the anxiety disorders, the diagnostic criteria for GAD have fluxed the most in the various iterations of *DSM*—perhaps for good reason, as better empirical data emerge to challenge current criteria—and may do so again in *DSM-V* (see below).

PROPHESIZING CHANGES TO *DSM*

There are several areas where changes to the diagnostic criteria may occur in *DSM-V*. In making these prognostications, we must emphasize that expressed here are the opinions of the authors, based largely on our knowledge of discussions that ensued during the preparation of the *DSM-IV*, text revision (*DSM-IV TR*; APA, 2000) and published information relevant to *DSM-V* (Regier, 2007). But they do not represent any official position on the part of the DSM-V Task Force and may or may not be acted upon.

Joining MDD and GAD at the Hip?

One proposal being considered for *DSM-V* is to add GAD to the mood disorders category. The rationale for this proposal is that GAD and major depressive disorder (MDD) overlap substantially, cross-sectionally and longitudinally (Kessler et al., 2001). There are also data suggesting that genetic risk factors for GAD and MDD are substantially overlapping (Kendler et al., 1992b; Hettema, Prescott, and Kendler, 2001), lending further credence to the notion that these two disorders belong in the same category. Interestingly, although both these disorders are associated with high neuroticism, much of the genetic covariance between GAD and MDD is not shared with genetic factors that influence neuroticism (Kendler et al., 2007; Hettema et al., 2006). The proposal to put MDD and GAD in the same category raises interesting, fundamental questions about what constitutes a "category" of mental disorders, and what shared factors would warrant mutual categorization of disorders. Another interesting question is what impact moving a disorder from one category to another will have on research, clinical practice, and health policy. If this proposal moves forward in *DSM-V*, we may find out.

Should OCD Go its Own Way?

Some in the field argue that OCD and related conditions should have their own diagnostic grouping, separate from the rest of the conditions traditionally categorized as anxiety disorders (Bartz & Hollander, 2006); at least one workgroup has met to discuss this notion for *DSM-V* (Regier, 2007). Several arguments have been put forth for this separation, including evidence that the functional neurocircuitry implicated in OCD appears to differ, to some extent, from that of other anxiety disorders; these arguments have varying levels of empirical support and are not uncontroversial (Bartz and Hollander, 2006). Mataix-Cols et al. (2007) found that 40% of 187 OCD experts surveyed felt that OCD should not be removed from the supraordinate category of anxiety disorders. This position was particularly common among nonpsychiatrists, and the main reasons for this position were that OCD and anxiety disorders tend to co-occur and respond to similar treatments. The authors concluded that there is insufficient consensus at this time to decide whether or not OCD should be removed from the anxiety disorders (Mataix-Cols et al., 2007)

Categorizing the Response to Trauma

The history of PTSD as a diagnostic entity is uniquely informative as a case in point of how accrued scientific knowledge has influenced classification decisions. Known variously in the literature as traumatic neurosis, shell shock, or war neurosis, PTSD first appeared in *DSM-III* to describe a syndrome that occurred following a psychologically traumatic event "that is generally outside the range of usual human experience" (APA, 1980). When viewed from this perspective, PTSD was a fairly uncommon disorder (Helzer et al., 1987). Subsequent epidemiologic research revealed, however, that many forms of serious, potentially deleterious psychological trauma were unfortunately not outside the range of usual human experience (Breslau et al., 1991), leading to a refinement and broadening of the criteria in *DSM-IV* to their present form that specify the "potentially life-threatening" characteristics of the trauma (Breslau & Kessler, 2001). A PTSD symptom was shuffled among categories between *DSM-III* and *DSM-III-R* (physiologic reactivity upon exposure to reminders of the event moved from the hyperarousal to the reexperiencing cluster) when it was shown that it clustered with other symptoms in that category. And a new diagnostic entity, acute stress disorder (ASD), was introduced into the diagnostic nomenclature in *DSM-IV*. This entity was created to account for persons who have significant symptoms in the immediate (within 1 month) aftermath of serious trauma, before PTSD can have developed (by definition, PTSD is only diagnosed 1 month after trauma).

The PTSD and ASD criteria seem ripe for change. First, it has often (though not always) (Breslau et al., 2004) been noted that the *DSM-IV* criteria for PTSD are too restrictive in that they fail to identify many persons with PTSD symptoms and clinically significant impairment and/or distress in the aftermath of trauma (Stein et al., 1997; Marshall et al., 2001). This observation has led to the widespread convention in the literature of identifying (and often lumping together with full syndromal PTSD) persons with "subthreshold" or "partial" PTSD. These are persons who have experienced significant trauma and yet fall one or two symptoms short of meeting the full *DSM-IV* criteria. Most investigators have acknowledged that reexperiencing (cluster B) symptoms are integral to the diagnosis of PTSD and required that these symptoms be present for a subthreshold diagnosis, while permitting fewer than the required (that is, by *DSM-IV*) number of avoidance or numbing (cluster C) or hyperarousal (cluster D) symptoms. Adding to the confusion is the requirement in the *DSM* that PTSD symptoms be spread across the three diagnostic clusters in a stereotyped fashion, a custom that has little empirical support. Simplified approaches to diagnosis (for example, doing away with specific cluster C or D requirements), which have the virtue of being easier to remember and therefore more likely to be appropriately applied in clinical settings, are currently being tested (Norman et al., 2007). For these reasons, the diagnostic criteria for PTSD may see refinement in *DSM-V*.

The ASD diagnostic category has also seen its share of controversy in its short existence. It emphasizes the presence of dissociative symptoms to a much greater extent than its slightly later-occurring counterpart, PTSD. The rationale for the emphasis on dissociative symptoms is the finding in many studies that the presence of peritraumatic dissociative symptoms predicts later PTSD symptoms over and above the variance accounted for by other (that is, reexperiencing, avoidance and numbing, and hyperarousal) acute stress symptoms (Classen et al., 1998; Ehlers et al., 1998; Murray et al., 2002). However, some studies have failed to find that dissociative symptoms provide any unique predictive utility for subsequent PTSD (Brewin et al., 1999), supporting an argument against requiring dissociative symptoms as a core feature of ASD (Marshall et al., 1999). Although the controversy is far from settled, it is clear that the current ASD criteria—though perhaps offering good positive predictive value for subsequent PTSD—fail to account for many (more than one half, in some studies) (Murray et al., 2002) of the individuals who go on to develop PTSD (that is, despite not having *DSM-IV* ASD as a forerunner). Some investigators have found that an ASD definition that does not necessitate the presence of dissociative symptoms ("subthreshold ASD") is equally predictive of later PTSD (Harvey and Bryant, 1999). It is also arguable that the ASD is part of a continuum of the response to traumatic stress, and that it merges with time into acute and then chronic PTSD (Shalev, 2002). If this is true, and there are no clear demarcations between ASD and PTSD other than chronology, then it is in fact reasonable to wonder if there is merit to retaining the ASD diagnosis at all (Brewin et al., 2003), or if it would be more parsimonious to identify stages of one disorder—PTSD. For all these reasons, the ASD diagnostic criteria are prime candidates for revision—or serious consideration as to the merits of excising the diagnosis altogether—in *DSM-V*.

Spinning Psychopathology on its Axes: Tilting at Windmills?

Another area where changes relevant to *DSM* anxiety disorders might be anticipated is in the overlap between certain Axis I and Axis II (that is, personality) disorders. It is well-recognized, and has been for some time (Holt et al., 1992; Widiger, 1992), that the generalized form of social anxiety disorder (GSAD) on Axis I and avoidant personality disorder (APD) on Axis II are substantially (50%–90% of cases) overlapping (van Velzen et al., 2000; Tillfors et al., 2001). Although *DSM-IV* explicitly directs attention to this extensive overlap in the diagnostic criteria for social anxiety disorder, it did nothing to resolve the apparent redundancy of this bi-axial representation for what is almost certainly the same set of phenomena (Chavira and Stein, 2002). This particular issue exemplifies one of the problems that beleaguer the Axis I versus Axis II distinction, namely, that some so-called Axis I disorders have characteristics typically ascribed to an Axis II disorder: onset in childhood and characteristic of the individual's long-term functioning. Persons with GSAD usually have the onset of the disorder very early in life and, in fact, often start off with a behaviorally inhibited temperament that merges imperceptibly into the social phobia once the individual is old enough to express symptoms that meet diagnostic criteria (Biederman et al., 2001; Stein et al., 2001). In this regard, this particular Axis I disorder often has the look and feel of a personality disorder. What, then, is the additional information contained in additionally applying an Axis II diagnosis, APD, to so many of these individuals?

One might argue that applying the Axis II diagnosis would be warranted if it told us something useful about the course or prognosis of such persons. In a large naturalistic 5-year follow-up study of patients with anxiety disorders, the presence of APD was found to predict a 41% lower likelihood of remission from social anxiety disorder, compared to those without APD (Massion et al., 2002). In that study, Global Assessment Scale scores at baseline clearly demonstrated that patients with APD, who made up approximately 35% of the sample, were more severely impaired than those without APD. If APD is predictive of poorer outcomes only because it denotes a more severe form of the illness, then this fact could easily be conveyed without invoking the need for an additional diagnosis on a separate axis. For this reason, as foreshadowed in the *DSM-IV TR* (APA, 2000), we expect APD to go the way of the dinosaur in *DSM-V*. This is not to imply, however, that personality is unimportant in GSAD (or, indeed, in other forms of psychopathology). It is merely intended to underscore the notion that abnormal personality characteristics are implicitly embedded within certain Axis I disorder definitions—GSAD being a case in point—and that future versions of our classificatory system would do well to eliminate this nosological redundancy. However, before we consign APD to the diagnostic scrap heap, we must address the somewhat unexpected finding in some surveys (e.g., Grant et al., 2005) that there are substantial numbers of individuals in the community who meet diagnostic criteria for APD but not for social anxiety disorder.

ALTERNATIVE MODELS FOR DIAGNOSTIC CLASSIFICATION OF ANXIETY DISORDERS

DSM is a categorical nosology wherein you either have a disorder or you don't. An alternative to the categorical approach to classification is a dimensional approach (Kessler, 2002), which some would call a spectrum approach (Maser and Patterson, 2002). There are pros and cons to each of these classificatory approaches. A categorical approach to diagnosis has the advantage of yielding a picture of a classic patient, from which deviations are to be expected. This may be easier to teach and might be expected to yield more reliable diagnoses (though this claim is unproven). A dimensional approach lets you see an individual from various perspectives, thereby reducing the need to pigeonhole people (or rely heavily on "not otherwise specified [NOS]" diagnoses). A dimensional approach also has the advantage of strictly limiting the tendency for persons to acquire more and more diagnoses with each subsequent edition of *DSM*. The current and lifetime prevalence of additional (that is, comorbid) Axis I disorders in principal anxiety and mood disorders among patients in an anxiety disorders outpatient clinic was found to be 57% and 81%, respectively (Brown et al., 2001). This comorbidity conundrum, surely an artifact of *DSM*'s categorical imperative, would not occur (or would be markedly attenuated) with a dimensional approach to diagnosis: Each individual would have only one diagnosis (or perhaps only one diagnosis in the mood–anxiety spectrum, though he or she might carry another in the substance-use spectrum, for example), but the variegation in his or her psychopathology would be expressed along dimensional lines. To the extent that simplification can be seen as a virtue in and of itself, the reduction in comorbidity that would be associated with a move to a dimensional approach is appealing.

Are there other considerations? At first glance, it might seem that a categorical approach would do a better job than a dimensional approach at enabling the separation of normal from pathological. But this is illusory, as we see from the flurry of publications about the high prevalence of "subthreshold" anxiety disorders (for example, subthreshold panic disorder; Batelaan et al., 2007), and the difficulty (or futility) of separating them from "full" anxiety disorders (Davidson et al., 1994; Olfson et al., 1996; Bienvenu et al., 1998; Stein et al., 2000; Marshall et al., 2001). *DSM* with its categorical nosology implies that if you have less than the "disorder," you have nothing. Yet empirical research and common sense indicate that this is surely not the case. A better solution might be to identify dimensions of psychopathology that afflict an individual and then independently assess the aggregate extent to which that individual is impaired by his or her symptoms. It is this latter assessment that would determine presence of a mental disorder and the trappings thereof (for example, eligibility for treatment, possibility of disability determination). In contrast, awareness of the patient's symptom dimensions could guide treatment with an eye toward including therapeutic elements empirically proven for that symptom cluster. For example, if the patient suffered from obsessive–compulsive and depressive symptoms, it might be possible to prioritize these on the basis of severity, and then sequentially institute cognitive-behavioral modules targeted at the symptoms. Farther in the future, if dimensional approaches to psychopathology are more successful than have been our current diagnostic approaches at elucidating differential neurobiologies (Maser and Patterson, 2002), it might be possible to similarly choose among neural system–specific treatments in an equally rational fashion.

Personality theorists seem to be leaning toward instituting a dimensional approach to personality disorder diagnosis in *DSM-V* (Livesley and Jang, 1998; Widiger and Samuel, 2005). Applying a dimensional nosology to anxiety disorders, for many of the same reasons, has considerable appeal. Let us consider several possible approaches to this venture.

Neurosis Revisited: Splitters Unite!

Neurosis is a concept that has been present since the beginning of modern psychiatric classification. Though initially considered a single condition (Tyrer, 1985), it has gradually been divided into many supposedly distinct entities, as influenced by clinicians such as Carter (1853), Freud (1895/1924), Janet (1908), Kraepelin (1921), Lewis (1934), and Klein (1964). In *DSM-II*, there were phobic, anxiety, obsessive–compulsive, hysterical, depressive, and neurasthenic neuroses. In *DSM-III*, the anxiety disorders were reconstructed as above, hysterical neuroses were classified as either somatoform or dissociative disorders, depressive neuroses were classified as affective disorders, and neurasthenic neurosis was eliminated.

One argument for the utility of the neurosis construct is that there is such extensive "comorbidity" among the various neurotic conditions, especially if one takes a lifetime perspective. High comorbidity among anxiety and depressive disorders is a consistent finding in clinical and community studies (Maser and Cloninger, 1990; Kessler, 1995; Merikangas et al., 1996). It may be that, by focusing on what is distinct about each condition, we have paid too little attention to what they have in common. That is, there may be a "core psychopathological process" that relates these conditions (Krueger, 1999a).

What accounts for the high comorbidity among neurotic conditions? Slater and Slater (1944) proposed a theory of neurosis in which constitutional predisposing factors, including personality, influence the likelihood of neurotic symptoms in the context of environmental stressors. Hans Eysenck believed that the combination of personality traits, high neuroticism (one's tendency to experience negative emotions and cope poorly), and low extraversion (one's quantity and intensity of interpersonal interactions and positive emotions) predisposed persons to neurotic conditions (Eysenck and Rachman, 1965). This combination of personality traits is also referred to as "trait anxiety" (Gray, 1970) and "harm avoidance" (Cloninger et al., 1993) and is highly related to mood and anxiety disorders, as is its related construct, neuroticism (also referred to as "negative affect"; Clark et al., 1994). However, in the context of the current nomenclature of anxiety and depressive disorders, neither extraversion nor one of its aspects, "positive affect," appear to be associated with all of these conditions, though low extraversion is associated with social phobia and agoraphobia (Solyom et al., 1986; Brown et al., 1998; Bienvenu et al., 2001; Bienvenu et al., 2007). Bievenu and colleagues (2001) found that elevated neuroticism, and, to a lesser extent, reduced extraversion, accounted for a substantial portion of anxiety and depressive disorder comorbidity in a community sample.

It should be noted that it remains unclear how personality traits are related to anxiety disorders, as this area has not been investigated nearly as much as has the relationship between high neuroticism and major depression. High neuroticism appears to be a predisposing factor for, a complication of, a negative prognostic factor in, and a result of common genetic and environmental determinants with major depression (Kendler et al., 1993; Clark et al., 1994). A few studies suggest that high neuroticism or its analogues predict the onset of anxiety disorders (Angst and Vollrath, 1991; Krueger, 1999a). Cross-sectional twin analyses suggest that there is substantial overlap between the genetic factors that influence individual variation in neuroticism and those that increase liability for a variety of anxiety disorders (Hettema et al., 2006). Extraversion has received less attention, though we recently found that the genetic factors that influence (low) extraversion also appear to influence liability to social phobia and agoraphobia (Bienvenu et al., 2007).

A Fear-Phobia-Anxiety Dimension?

Alternate systems for dimensional classification have recently been proposed. These have been empirically derived by examining the co-aggregation of symptoms elicited by *DSM-III-R* or *DSM-IV*–based diagnostic interviews. Krueger (1999b) conducted a confirmatory factor analysis of common mental disorders in the community-based National Comorbidity Survey. He found that two factors—"internalizing" (represented as one higher-order factor with two lower-order, highly intercorrelated factors, "anxious-misery" and "fear") and "externalizing" (encompassing *DSM-III-R* diagnoses of antisocial personality disorder, alcohol and drug dependence) emerged. The internalizing factor covered all of the anxiety (and mood) disorders. Krueger and colleagues (1998) further argued that if so many disorders have "comorbidity," then maybe this is the signal rather than the noise, and that the true structure of mental disorders is represented by these latent constructs. In looking in detail at the internalizing factor that includes the anxiety and unipolar mood diagnoses, Krueger and Finger (2001) also found that higher scores along this factor are associated with higher social costs, "a phenomenon not well captured by the 'comorbidity' concept" (p. 140). They concluded that the field would benefit from the development of measures that permit the assessment of the full range of the internalizing factor in a graded, continuous fashion.

With similar goals in mind, Vollebergh and colleagues (2001) analyzed the underlying latent structure of 12-month *DSM-III-R* diagnoses of nine common disorders in a large ($N = 7076$) Dutch general population sample. They tried to establish stability across a 1-year period ("structural stability") and to evaluate individual differences in mental disorders at the levels of the latent dimensions (differential stability). They found that a three-dimensional model provided the best fit to the observed data: (*1*) alcohol, drug dependence; (*2*) mood disorders (MDD, dysthymia)—including GAD; and (*3*) phobic disorders and panic. The authors concluded that their findings "underline the argument for focusing on core psychopathological processes rather than on their manifestation as distinguished disorders in future population studies on common mental disorders" (Vollebergh et al., 2001, p. 597).

Both of the aforementioned studies are constrained in having limited their questions to those already instrumental to the *DSM-III-R* and *DSM-IV* definitions. It might not be surprising, then, that certain *DSM* disorders fit neatly into the latent structure underlying such a system. Future epidemiologic studies that ask respondents about a much broader range of symptoms may or may not find a similar latent structure; this remains to be determined. Despite this limitation, however, the take-home message from these studies is that nature does not feel compelled to follow the rules of our current *DSM*. If this is true, we must seriously wonder about the futility of conducting research (epidemiologic, neurobiologic, and outcomes) that adheres so carefully to the *DSM* nosology. Future studies in our field should strongly consider measuring at least some of these dimensional aspects, even if the primary focus is on more "traditional" *DSM*-based diagnoses. As a case in point, a recent population-based twin study showed that whereas genetic correlations between neuroticism and each of the "internalizing disorders" were high, there was a neuroticism-independent genetic factor that significantly increased risk for MDD, GAD, and panic disorder (Hettema et al., 2006). In contrast, there was no evidence of personality-independent genetic factors for social phobia or agoraphobia (Bienvenu et al., 2007). This type of approach demonstrates the complexities of diagnostic categorization, as well as the heuristic value of using a multimodel approach to research of this genre.

A FEAR FOR ALL REASONS: A DIMENSIONAL OR QUANTITATIVE TRAIT APPROACH

The neurosis construct, as outlined above, attempts to inclusively describe core features that cut across most of what we recognize as anxiety and related conditions. The attempt there is to model key characteristics of anxiety within a single domain, thereby explaining much of the variance in what separates normality from anxiety-based psychopathology. The neurosis model has as one of its very appealing properties the ability to boil down multiple anxiety-related behaviors into a single construct. This might be thought of as a higher-order factor that is typical of all or most persons with anxiety disorders.

An alternative, though conceptually related notion, would be to identify and quantify the presence of anxiety-related psychopathology along a variety of dimensions. For example, one might identify a panic–agoraphobic spectrum, a social phobia–shyness spectrum, and an obsessive–compulsive spectrum, as has recently been espoused (Cassano et al., 1997; Dell'Osso et al., 2002; Maser and Patterson, 2002; Nestadt et al., 2002). This approach could, we suppose, be integrated with the concept of neurosis. Just as neurosis can be viewed as a higher-order factor underlying the symptoms of most anxiety-related conditions (Andrews et al., 1990), these more disorder-specific dimensions could be viewed as more differentiated (lower-order) factors. This model, it should be noted, is consistent with genetic modeling of the heritability of phobias: There appear to exist common genes that convey a general vulnerability for "phobia proneness" (Kendler et al., 1999), as well as other genes that convey unique (or disorder-specific) vulnerability (Hettema, Neale, and Kendler, 2001). From a clinical perspective, we might note that an individual has a "neurotic disorder," and then specify the characteristics of that person's neurotic disorder along dimensional lines. An example might be: neurotic disorder with predominantly social anxiety-related features.

A New "*DSM*": A "Dimensional Symptoms Manual"

What are the practical implications of considering a move to a dimensional system of anxiety (and perhaps mood) disorder nosology? First, we can expect an outcry from practitioners and researchers alike questioning the need to change the status quo. Any dramatic change to our classificatory system, a mere 20-plus years after the introduction of *DSM-III*, is bound to elicit cries of incredulity, "What, not again!" This outcry would be warranted, as there are presently insufficient data to support this sea change in our approach to diagnosis. Before a wholesale switch from discrete to dimensional diagnosis could be recommended, a plethora of studies comparing and contrasting the strengths or weaknesses of each approach in a variety of settings (for example, community, cross-cultural, primary care, specialty outpatient clinic, hospital-based) would be necessary. We should not expect these changes to come swiftly (if at all). They will surely not be a part of *DSM-V* but may see the light of day in future generations of this venerable tome.

Farther into the Future

Ultimately, scientific support will accrue for moving from a symptom-based classification system to an etiologically based diagnostic system for anxiety disorders. Although our understanding of the neurobiology of anxiety disorders is growing in leaps and bounds, we are not there yet. If forced to speculate, we could envision the trajectory of current research eventually (5 to 10 years down the road) leading to a genetically based classification system (for example, disorders associated with abnormal serotonin transporter function) (Lesch et al., 1996; Jorm et al., 2000) or a system that recognizes interactions between life stress and genetic susceptibility (for example, disorders associated with childhood maltreatment and abnormal serotonin transporter function) (Caspi and Moffitt, 2006; Stein et al., 2008). Alternative—although by no means mutually exclusive—systems could group disorders based on shared abnormalities in function within specific brain regions (for example, the amygdala) (Etkin and Wager, 2007; Stein et al., 2007; Tillfors et al., 2002; Phan et al., 2006) or alterations in corticolimbic connectivity (Shin et al., 2005) (which may, at least in part, be genetically mediated; Pezawas et al., 2005). Prefaced on a solid understanding of the neurobiological basis of anxiety, the development of an etiologically based diagnostic system is our field's holy grail. We must recognize that anything short of that is bound to be inadequate, certain to be ephemeral, but nonetheless clinically and heuristically useful as we strive toward that goal.

REFERENCES

American Psychiatric Association. (1980) *Diagnostic and Statistical Manual of Mental Disorders*, 3rd ed. Washington, DC: Author.

American Psychiatric Association. (2000) *Diagnostic and Statistical Manual of Mental Disorders*, 4th ed., text rev. Washington, DC: Author.

Andrews, G., Stewart, G., Morris-Yates, A., Holt, P., and Henderson, S. (1990) Evidence for a general neurotic syndrome. *B. J. Psychiatry* 157:6–12.

Angst, J., Gamma, A., Joseph, B.O., Eaton, W.W., Ajdacic, V., Eich, D., et al. (2006) Varying temporal criteria for generalized anxiety disorder: prevalence and clinical characteristics in a young age cohort. *Psychol. Med.* 36:1283–1292.

Angst, J., and Vollrath, M. (1991) The natural history of anxiety disorders. *Acta Psychiatr. Scand.* 84:446–452.

Bartz, J.A., and Hollander, E. (2006) Is obsessive-compulsive disorder an anxiety disorder? *Prog. Neuropsychopharmacol. Biol. Psychiatry* 30:338–352.

Batelaan, N., de Graaf, R., Van Balkom, A., Vollebergh, W., and Beekman, A. (2007) Thresholds for health and thresholds for illness: panic disorder versus subthreshold panic disorder. *Psychol. Med.* 37:247–256.

Biederman, J., Hirshfeld-Becker, D.R., Rosenbaum, J.F., Hérot, C., Friedman, D., Snidman, N., et al. (2001) Further evidence of association between behavioral inhibition and social anxiety in children. *Am. J. Psychiatry* 158:1673–1679.

Bienvenu, O.J., Brown, C., Samuels, J.F., et al. (2001) Normal personality traits and comorbidity among phobic, panic, and major depressive disorders. *Psychiatry Res.* 102:73–85.

Bienvenu, O.J., Hettema, J.M., Neale, M.C., Prescott, C.A., and Kendler, K.S. (2007) Low extraversion and high neuroticism as indices of genetic and environmental risk for social phobia, agoraphobia, and animal phobia. *Am. J. Psychiatry* 164(11): 1714–1721.

Bienvenu, O.J., Nestadt, G., and Eaton, W.W. (1998) Characterizing generalized anxiety: temporal and symptomatic thresholds. *J. Nerv. Ment. Dis.* 186:51–56.

Bienvenu, O.J., Nestadt, G., Samuels, J.F., Howard, W.T., Costa, P. T., Jr., and Eaton, W.W. (2001) Phobic, panic, and major depressive disorders and the five-factor model of personality. *J. Nerv. Ment. Dis.* 189:154–161.

Bienvenu, O.J., Onyike, C.U., Stein, M.B., Chen, L.S., Samuels, J., Nestadt, G., et al. (2006) Agoraphobia in adults: incidence and longitudinal relationship with panic. *Br. J. Psychiatry* 188:432–438.

Breslau, N., and Davis, G.C. (1985) *DSM-III* generalized anxiety disorder: an empirical investigation of more stringent criteria. *Psychiatry Res.* 14:231–238.

Breslau, N., Davis, G.C., Andreski, P., and Peterson, E.L. (1991) Traumatic events and posttraumatic stress disorder in an urban population of young adults. *Arch. Gen. Psychiatry* 48:216–222.

Breslau, N., and Kessler, R.C. (2001) The stressor criterion in DSM-IV posttraumatic stress disorder: an empirical investigation. *Biol. Psychiatry* 50:699–704.

Breslau, N., Lucia, V.C., and Davis, G.C. (2004) Partial PTSD versus full PTSD: an empirical examination of associated impairment. *Psychol. Med.* 34:1205–1214.

Brewin, C.R., Andrews, B., and Rose, S. (2003) Diagnostic overlap between acute stress disorder and PTSD in victims of violent crime. *Am. J. Psychiatry* 160:783–785.

Brewin, C.R., Andrews, B., Rose, S., and Kirk, M. (1999) Acute stress disorder and posttraumatic stress disorder in victims of violent crime. *Am. J. Psychiatry* 156:360–366.

Brown, T.A., Campbell, L.A., Lehman, C.L., Grisham, J.R., and Mancill, R.B. (2001) Current and lifetime comorbidity of the DSM-IV anxiety and mood disorders in a large clinical sample. *J. Abnorm. Psychol.* 110:585–599.

Brown, T.A., Chorpita, B.F., and Barlow, D.H. (1998) Structural relationships among dimensions of the DSM-IV anxiety and mood disorders and dimensions of negative affect, positive affect, and autonomic arousal. *J. Abnorm. Psychol.* 107:179–192.

Carter, R.B. (1853) *On the Pathology and Treatment of Hysteria.* London: Churchill.

Caspi, A., and Moffitt, T.E. (2006) Gene-environment interactions in psychiatry: joining forces with neuroscience. *Nat. Rev. Neurosci.* 7:583–590.

Cassano, G.B., Michelini, S., Shear, M.K., Coli, E., Maser, J.D., and Frank, E. (1997) The panic agoraphobic spectrum: a descriptive approach to the assessment and treatment of subtle symptoms. *Am. J. Psychiatry* 154:27–38.

Chavira, D.A., and Stein, M.B. (2002) Phenomenology of social phobia. In: Stein, D.J., and Hollander, E., eds. *The American Psychiatric Publishing Textbook of Anxiety Disorders.* Washington, DC: American Psychiatric Publishing, pp. 289–300.

Clark, L.A., Watson, D., and Mineka, S. (1994) Temperament, personality, and the mood and anxiety disorders. *J. Abnorm. Psychol.* 103:103–116.

Classen, C., Koopman, C., Hales, R., and Spiegel, D. (1998) Acute stress disorder as a predictor of posttraumatic stress symptoms. *Am. J. Psychiatry* 155:620–624.

Cloninger, C.R., Svrakic, N.M., and Przybeck, T.R. (1993) A psychobiological model of temperament and character. *Arch. Gen. Psychiatry* 50:975–990.

Davidson, J.R., Hughes, D.C., George, L.K., & Blazer, D.G. (1994) The boundary of social phobia. Exploring the threshold. *Arch. Gen. Psychiatry* 51:975–983.

Dell'Osso, L., Rucci, P., Cassano, G.B., Maser, J.D., Endicott, J., Shear, M.K., et al. (2002) Measuring social anxiety and obsessive-compulsive spectra: Comparison of interviews and self-report instruments. *Compre. Psychiatry* 43:81–87.

Eaton, W.W., Kessler, R.C., Wittchen, H.-U., and Magee, W.J. (1994) Panic and panic disorder in the United States. *Am. J. Psychiatry* 151:413–420.

Ehlers, A., Mayou, R.A., and Bryant, B. (1998) Psychological predictors of chronic posttraumatic stress disorder after motor vehicle accidents. *J. Abnorm. Psychol.* 107:508–519.

Etkin, A., and Wager, T.D. (2007) Functional neuroimaging of anxiety: A meta-analysis of emotional processing in PTSD, Social Anxiety Disorder, and Specific Phobia. *Am. J. Psychiatry* 164:1476–1488.

Eysenck, H.J., and Rachman, S. (1965) *The Causes and Cures of Neurosis*. San Diego, CA: Robert R. Knapp.

Fava, G. A., Grandi, S., and Canestrari, R. (1988) Prodromal symptoms in panic disorder with agoraphobia. *Am. J. Psychiatry,* 145: 1564–1567.

Freud, S. (1895) The justification for detaching from neurasthenia a particular syndrome: the anxiety neurosis. In: J. Strachey, trans. and ed. *Standard Edition of the Complete Psychological Works of Sigmund Freud, volume 3*. London: Hogarth Press, pp. 90–116. (Original work published 1924)

Fyer, A.J., Katon, W., Hollifield, M., Rassnick, H., Mannuzza, S., Chapman, T., et al. (1996) The DSM-IV Panic Disorder Field Trial: Panic attack frequency and functional disability. *Anxiety* 2:157–166.

Grant, B.F., Hasin, D.S., Blanco, C., Stinson, F.S., Chou, S.P., Goldstein, R.B., et al. (2005) The epidemiology of social anxiety disorder in the United States: results from the National Epidemiologic Survey on Alcohol and Related Conditions. *J. Clin. Psychiatry* 66:1351–1361.

Gray, J.A. (1970) The psychophysiological basis of introversion-extraversion. *Behav. Res. Ther.* 8:249–266.

Harvey, A.G., and Bryant, R.A. (1999) The relationship between acute stress disorder and posttraumatic stress disorder: a 2-year prospective evaluation. *J. Consult. Clin. Psychol.* 67:985–988.

Hayward, C., Killen, J.D., and Taylor, C.B. (2003) The relationship between agoraphobia symptoms and panic disorder in a non-clinical sample of adolescents. *Psychol. Med.* 33:733–738.

Helzer, J., Robins, L., and McEvoy, L. (1987) Post-traumatic stress disorder in the general population: findings of the Epidemiologic Catchment Area survey. *New Engl. J. Med.* 317:1630–1634.

Hettema, J.M., Neale, M.C., and Kendler, K.S. (2001) A review and meta-analysis of the genetic epidemiology of anxiety disorders. *Am. J. Psychiatry* 158:1568–1578.

Hettema, J.M., Neale, M.C., Myers, J.M., Prescott, C.A., and Kendler, K.S. (2006) A population-based twin study of the relationship between neuroticism and internalizing disorders. *Am. J. Psychiatry* 163:857–864.

Hettema, J.M., Prescott, C.A., and Kendler, K.S. (2001) A population-based twin study of generalized anxiety disorder in men and women. *J. Nerv. Ment. Dis.* 189:413–420.

Holt, C.S., Heimberg, R.G., and Hope, D.A. (1992) Avoidant personality disorder and the generalized subtype of social phobia. *J. Abnorm. Psycho.* 101:318–325.

Horwath, E., Lish, J.D., Johnson, J., Hornig, C.D., and Weissman, M. M. (1993) Agoraphobia without panic: clinical reappraisal of an epidemologic finding. *Am. J. Psychiatry* 150:1496–1501.

Janet, P. (1908) *Obsessions and Psychasthenia*. Paris: Alcan.

Jorm, A.F., Prior, M., Sanson, A., Smart, D., Zhang, Y., and Easteal, S. (2000) Association of a functional polymorphism of the serotonin transporter gene with anxiety-related temperament and behavior problems in children: a longitudinal study from infancy to the mid-teens. *Mol. Psychiatry* 5:542–547.

Katerndahl, D.A. (2000) Predictors of the development of phobic avoidance. *J. Clin. Psychiatry* 61:618–623.

Kendler, K.S., Gardner, C.O., Gatz, M., and Pedersen, N.L. (2006) The sources of co-morbidity between major depression and generalized anxiety disorder in a Swedish national twin sample. *Psychol. Med.* 37(3):453–462.

Kendler, K.S., Karkowski, L.M., and Prescott, C.A. (1999) Fears and phobias: reliability and heritability. *Psychol. Med.* 29:539–553.

Kendler, K.S., Neale, M.C., Kessler, R.C., Heath, A.C., and Eaves, L.J. (1992a) Generalized anxiety disorder in women: a population-based twin study. *Arch. Gen. Psychiatry* 49:267–272.

Kendler, K.S., Neale, M.C., Kessler, R.C., Heath, A.C., and Eaves, L.J. (1992b) Major depression and generalized anxiety disorder: same genes, (partly) different environments? *Arch. Gen. Psychiatry* 49:716–722.

Kendler, K.S., Neale, M.C., Kessler, R.C., Heath, A.C., Martin, N. G., and Eaves, L. J. (1993) A longitudinal twin study of personality and major depression in women. *Arch. Gen. Psychiatry* 50: 853–862.

Kessler, R.C. (1995) Epidemiology of psychiatric comorbidity. In: Tsuang, M.T., Tohen, M., and Zahner, G.E.P., eds. *Textbook in Psychiatric Epidemiology*. New York: John Wiley and Sons, pp. 179–197.

Kessler, R.C. (2002) The categorical versus dimensional assessment controversy in the sociology of mental illness. *J. Health Soc. Behav.* 43:171–188.

Kessler, R.C., Brandenburg, N., Lane, M., Roy-Byrne, P., Stang, P. D., Stein, D.J., et al. (2005) Rethinking the duration requirement for generalized anxiety disorder: evidence from the National Comorbidity Survey Replication. *Psychol. Med.* 35:1073–1082.

Kessler, R.C., Keller, M.B., and Wittchen, H.-U. (2001) The epidemiology of generalized anxiety disorder. *Psychiatr. Clin. North Am.* 24:19–37.

Klein, D.F. (1964) Delineation of two drug-responsive anxiety syndromes. *Psychopharmacology* 5:397–408.

Klein, D.F., Zitrin, C.M., and Woerner, M.G. (1978) Antidepressants, anxiety, panic and phobia. In Lipton, M.A., DiMascio, A., and Killam, K.F., eds. *Psychopharmacology: A Generation of Progress*. New York: Raven Press, pp. 1401–1410.

Klerman, G.L., Weissman, M.M., Ouellette, R., Johnson, J., and Greenwald, S. (1991) Panic attacks in the community: Social morbidity and health care utilization. *JAMA* 265:742–746.

Kraepelin, E. (1921) *Manic-Depressive Insanity and Paranoia*. Edinburgh, UK: Livingstone Press.

Krueger, R.F. (1999a) Personality traits in late adolescence predict mental disorders in early adulthood: a prospective-epidemiological study. *J. Pers.* 67:39–65.

Krueger, R.F. (1999b) The structure of common mental disorders. *Arch. Gen. Psychiatry* 56:921–926.

Krueger, R.F., Caspi, A., Moffitt, T.E., and Silva, P.A. (1998) The structure and stability of common mental disorders (DSM-III-R): a longitudinal-epidemiological study. *J. Abnorm. Psychol.* 107: 216–227.

Krueger, R.F., and Finger, M.S. (2001) Using item response theory to understand comorbidity among anxiety and unipolar mood disorders. *Psychol. Assess.* 13:140–151.

Lelliott, P., Marks, I., McNamee, G., and Tobena, A. (1989) Onset of panic disorder with agoraphobia. Toward an integrated model. *Arch. Gen. Psychiatry* 46:1000–1004.

Lesch, K.-P., Bengel, D., Heils, A., Sabol, S.A., Greenberg, B.D., Petri, S., et al. (1996) Association of anxiety-related traits with a polymorphism in the serotonin transporter gene regulatory region. *Science* 274:1527–1531.

Lewis, A.J. (1934) Melancholia: a historical review. *J. Ment. Sci.* 80:1–42.

Livesley, W.J., and Jang, K.L. (1998) Toward an empirically based classification of personality disorder. *J. Personal. Disord.* 14:137–151.

Markowitz, J.S., Weissman, M.M., Ouellette, R., Lish, J.D., and Klerman, G.L. (1989) Quality of life in panic disorder. *Arch. Gen. Psychiatry* 46:984–992.

Marks, I.M. (1981) Space "phobia": a pseudo-agoraphobic syndrome. *J. Neurol. Neurosurg. Psychiatry* 44:387–391.

Marshall, R.D., Olfson, M., Hellman, F., Blanco, C., Guardino, M., and Struening, E. (2001) Comorbidity, impairment, and suicidality in subthreshold PTSD. *Am. J. Psychiatry* 158:1467–1473.

Marshall, R.D., Spitzer, R.L., and Liebowitz, M.R. (1999) Review and critique of the new DSM-IV diagnosis of Acute Stress Disorder. *Am. J. Psychiatry* 156:1677–1685.

Maser, J.D., and Cloninger, C.R. (1990) Comorbidity of anxiety and mood disorders: introduction and overview. In: Maser, J.D., and Cloninger, C. R., eds. *Comorbidity of Mood and Anxiety Disorders*. Washington, DC: American Psychiatric Press, pp. 3–12.

Maser, J.D., and Patterson, T. (2002) Spectrum and nosology: implications for DSM-V. *Psychiatr. Clin. North Am.* 25(4):855–885.

Massion, A.O., Dyck, I., Shea, M.T., Phillips, K.A., Warshaw, M.G., and Keller, M.B. (2002) Personality disorders and time to remission in generalized anxiety disorder, social phobia, and panic disorder. *Arch. Gen. Psychiatry* 59:434–440.

Mataix-Cols, D., Pertusa, A., and Leckman, J.F. (2007) Issues for DSM-V: how should obsessive-compulsive and related disorders be classified? *Am. J. Psychiatry* 164:1313–1314.

Merikangas, K.R., Angst, J., Eaton, W.W., Canino, G., Rubio-Stipec, M., Wacker, H., et al. (1996) Comorbidity and boundaries of affective disorders with anxiety disorders and substance misuse: results of an international task force. *Br. J. Psychiatry* 168: 58–67.

Murray, J., Ehlers, A., and Mayou, R.A. (2002) Dissociation and post-traumatic stress disorder: two prospective studies of road traffic accident survivors. *Br. J. Psychiatry* 180:363–368.

Nestadt, G., Samuels, J.F., Riddle, M.A., Bienvenu, O.J., Liang, K.-Y., Grados, M., et al. (2002) OCD: Defining the phenotype. *Journal of Clinical Psychiatry* 63(Suppl 6):5–7.

Norman, S.B., Stein, M.B., and Davidson, J.R. (2007) Profiling posttraumatic functional impairment. *J. Nerv. Ment. Dis.* 195: 48–53.

Olfson, M., Broadhead, W.E., Weissman, M.M., Leon, A.C., Farber, L., Hoven, C., et al. (1996) Subthreshold psychiatric symptoms in a primary care group practice. *Arch. Gen. Psychiatry* 53:880–886.

Pezawas, L., Meyer-Lindenberg, A., Drabant, E.M., Verchinski, B. A., Munoz, K.E., Kolachana, B.S., et al. (2005) 5-HTTLPR polymorphism impacts human cingulate-amygdala interactions: a genetic susceptibility mechanism for depression. *Nat. Neurosci.* 8: 828–834.

Phan, K.L., Britton, J.C., Taylor, S.F., Fig, L.M., and Liberzon, I. (2006) Corticolimbic blood flow during nontraumatic emotional processing in posttraumatic stress disorder. *Arch. Gen. Psychiatry* 63:184–192.

Regier, D.A. (2007) Obsessive-compulsive behavior spectrum: refining the research agenda for the DSM-V. *CNS. Spectr.* 12:343–344.

Robins, L.N., Helzer, J.E., Weissman, M.M., Orvaschel, H., Gruenber, E., Burke, J.D., et al. (1984) Lifetime prevalence of specific psychiatric disorders in three sites. *Arch. Gen. Psychiatry* 41:949–958.

Ruscio, A.M., Lane, M., Roy-Byrne, P., Stang, P.E., Stein, D.J., Wittchen, H.U., et al. (2005) Should excessive worry be required for a diagnosis of generalized anxiety disorder? Results from the US National Comorbidity Survey Replication. *Psychol. Med.* 35: 1761–1772.

Shalev, A.Y. (2002) Acute stress reactions in adults. *Biol. Psychiatry* 51:532–543.

Shin, L.M., Wright, C.I., Cannistraro, P.A., Wedig, M.M., McMullin, K., Martis, B., et al. (2005) A functional magnetic resonance imaging study of amygdala and medial prefrontal cortex responses to overtly presented fearful faces in posttraumatic stress disorder. *Arch. Gen. Psychiatry* 62:273–281.

Slater, E., and Slater, P. (1944) A heuristic theory of neurosis. *J. Neurol. Neurosurg. Psychiatry* 7:49–55.

Solyom, L., Ledwidge, B., and Solyom, C. (1986) Delineating social phobia. *Br. J. Psychiatry* 149:464–470.

Stein, M.B., Asmundson, G.J.G., Ireland, D., and Walker, J.R. (1994) Panic disorder in patients attending a clinic for vestibular disorders. *Am. J. Psychiatry* 151:1697–1700.

Stein, M.B., Chavira, D.A., and Jang, K.L. (2001) Bringing up bashful baby: Developmental pathways to social phobia. *Psychiatr. Clin. North Am.* 24:661–675.

Stein, M.B., Schork, N.J., and Gelernter, J. (2008) Gene-by-environment (serotonin transporter and childhood maltreatment) interaction for anxiety sensitivity, an intermediate phenotype for anxiety disorders. *Neuropsychopharmacology* 33:312–319.

Stein, M.B., Simmons, A., Feinstein, J.S., and Paulus, M.P. (2007) Increased amygdala and insula activation during emotion processing in anxiety-prone subjects. *Am. J. Psychiatry* 164:318–327.

Stein, M.B., Torgrud, L.J., and Walker, J.R. (2000) Social phobia symptoms, subtypes and severity: findings from a community survey. *Arch. Gen. Psychiatry* 57:1046–1052.

Stein, M.B., Walker, J.R., Hazen, A.L., and Forde, D.R. (1997) Full and partial posttraumatic stress disorder: findings from a community survey. *Am. J. Psychiatry* 154:1114–1119.

Tillfors, M., Furmark, T., Ekselius, L., and Fredrikson, M. (2001) Social phobia and avoidant personality disorder as related to parental history of social anxiety: a general population study. *Behav. Res. Ther.* 39:289–298.

Tillfors, M., Furmark, T., Marteinsdottir, I., and Fredrikson, M. (2002) Cerebral blood flow during anticipation of public speaking in social phobia: a PET study. *Biol. Psychiatry* 52:1113–1119.

Tyrer, P. (1985) Neurosis divisible? *Lancet* 1:685–688.

van Velzen, C.J.M., Emmelkamp, P.M.G., and Scholing, A. (2000) Generalized social phobia versus avoidant personality disorder: Differences in psychopathology, personality traits, and social and occupational functioning. *J. Anx. Disord.* 14:395–411.

Vollebergh, W.A.M., Iedema, J., Bijl, R.V., de Graaf, R., Smit, F., and Ormel, J. (2001) The structure and stability of common mental disorders: The NEMESIS study. *Arch. Gen. Psychiatry* 58: 597–603.

Widiger, T.A. (1992) Generalized social phobia versus avoidant personality disorder: a commentary on three studies. *J. Abnorm. Psychol.* 101:340–343.

Widiger, T.A., and Samuel, D.B. (2005) Diagnostic categories or dimensions? A question for the Diagnostic and Statistical Manual of Mental Disorders--fifth edition. *J. Abnorm. Psychol.* 114: 494–504.

Wittchen, H.-U., Reed, V., and Kessler, R.C. (1998) The relationship of agoraphobia and panic in a community sample of adolescents and young adults. *Arch. Gen. Psychiatry* 55:1017–1024.

38 The Molecular Genetics of Anxiety Disorders

STEVEN P. HAMILTON AND ABBY J. FYER

Anxiety disorders are the most common type of mental disorder. The lifetime incidence of *Diagnostic and Statistical Manual of Mental Disorders*, 4th ed. (*DSM-IV*; American Psychiatric Association [APA], 1994) anxiety disorders is estimated to be 28.8% among 9282 participants in the National Comorbidity Survey Replication (Kessler, Berglund, et al., 2005). This face-to-face fully structured survey additionally found that the average age of onset of anxiety disorders was 11 years. Among the anxiety disorders studied, the lifetime prevalence rates were 4.7% for panic disorder (PD), 12.5% for specific phobia, 12.1% for social anxiety disorder (SAD), 5.7% for generalized anxiety disorder (GAD), and 1.6% for obsessive–compulsive disorder (OCD). Data from the same survey found that the 12-month prevalence of *DSM-IV* anxiety disorders was estimated to be 18.1%, nearly twice that of mood disorders (Kessler, Chiu, et al., 2005). For specific disorders, 12-month prevalence rates were 2.7% for PD, 8.7% for specific phobia, 6.8% for SAD, 3.1% for GAD, and 1.0% for OCD. A striking observation among anxiety disorders involves the marked imbalance in the ratio of female-to-male cases of these disorders. Females show a 1.6-fold higher risk for an anxiety disorder than do males (Kessler, Berglund, et al., 2005).

For much of the 20th century, anxiety disorders (subsumed under neuroses) were conceptualized as psychogenic conditions related to intrapsychic conflict. Contemporary biological psychiatry builds a case for a more prominent role for dysfunction of key neural circuits involved with emotional regulation and fear processing. Much of this argument relies on empirical psychopharmacological observations in humans (Klein, 1964), as well as experimental data from nonhuman model systems (Shekhar et al., 2001). In addition to acquired alterations in the distributed networks involved with anxiety, it is possible that an inherited biological predisposition to anxiety disorders may account for a substantial proportion of the likelihood for developing such disorders. Several decades of epidemiologically oriented research in human populations has shown that anxiety disorders consistently exhibit aggregation in families, and that the source of this aggregation is likely due to genetic factors. Meta-analysis of family studies, in which the risk of having a disorder in relatives of a proband affected with the disorder is calculated and compared to relatives of persons without the disorder, has been carried out for major anxiety disorders. This assessment showed that PD, specific phobia, SAD, GAD, and OCD all showed significant levels of familial aggregation (Hettema, Neale, and Kendler, 2001). Twin studies, in which differences in disease concordance rates between monozygotic and dizygotic twins are used to support a genetic component to a trait, suggest a strong contribution from genes in the liability to PD, specific phobia, SAD, and GAD. The lack of twin studies for OCD for meta-analysis precluded adequate assessment of heritability (Hettema, Neale, and Kendler, 2001). Further exploration of twin data using multivariate structural equation modeling led to the conclusion that though there are prevalence differences between genders, it appears that genetic and environmental risk factors underlying anxiety disorders do not differ between males and females (Hettema et al., 2005).

GENETIC EPIDEMIOLOGY AND MOLECULAR GENETICS OF ANXIETY DISORDERS

Panic Disorder

Genetic epidemiology

Panic disorder (PD) is characterized by panic attacks, defined as the experience of spontaneous intense anxiety associated with an array of psychological and somatic symptoms. The diagnosis of PD requires recurrent panic attacks, accompanied by anticipatory anxiety, worry about the implications of the attacks, or significant attack-related behavior changes for at least one month (APA, 1994). As a disorder, PD is a relatively recent clinical concept, deriving from observations of the pharmacologic dissection of anxiety syndromes (Klein, 1964) as well as the development of operational criteria for the syndrome in *DSM-III* (APA, 1980).

As noted above, the 12-month prevalence of PD is 2.7% (Kessler, Chiu, et al., 2005). This recent estimate is similar to previous estimates from an international epidemiologic study involving 40,000 participants, in whom the lifetime prevalence of PD was reported to be between 1.4% and 2.9% (Weissman et al., 1997). On Taiwan, where the reported rates of psychiatric disorders are generally lower than other countries, there was an outlier with a rate of 0.4%. Twice as many females are affected as males (Eaton et al., 1994). The mean age of onset is 24 years, with the span between 25 and 44 years of age being the period of highest risk for the disorder (Robins et al., 1984).

Early descriptions of syndromes corresponding to PD have noted a familial pattern (Oppenheimer and Rothschild, 1918; Cohen et al., 1951). The use of direct interviews of probands and their relatives using operationalized criteria led to rigorous family studies. Crowe et al. found that depending on the clinical definition, the relative risk for first-degree relatives of panic probands was 7.8–10.7, suggesting prominent familial aggregation (Crowe et al., 1980; Crowe et al., 1983). These studies showed that compared with male relatives, the risk was double for female relatives. These initial observations have been confirmed in a series of family studies from a variety of research groups (Noyes et al., 1986; Hopper et al., 1987; Maier et al., 1993; Mendlewicz et al., 1993; Weissman, 1993; Fyer et al., 1995). A review of adequately designed studies reports that familial aggregation studies demonstrate a relative risk of 7.8 (range 2.6–20) to first-degree relatives of persons with PD (Knowles and Weissman, 1995). Extension of the analyses to second-degree relatives of probands with PD using the family history approach showed a relative risk of 6.8, with 9.5% of second-degree relatives of panic probands compared to 1.4% among relatives of controls, again with female relatives being at higher risk (Pauls, Noyes, and Crowe, 1979). The family study method has also been used to identify interesting clinical patterns that appear to have a familial component. For example, one study found an increased relative risk of PD in first-degree relatives of PD probands with early (< 20 years) versus later onset panic (Goldstein et al., 1997). Similar approaches have used theoretical and clinical observations about PD, namely the "false suffocation alarm" hypothesis of PD (Klein, 1993), to test for familial transmission of symptom complexes. Using smothering symptoms as a probe, it was found that the first-degree relatives of probands with panic accompanied by smothering symptoms had a 2.7-fold higher risk for panic and a 5.7-fold higher risk for panic with smothering symptoms when compared to the first-degree relatives of panic probands who did not experience smothering symptoms (Horwath et al., 1997).

Although family studies demonstrate a familial pattern of PD aggregation, other epidemiological designs, such as twin studies, are required to show that the pattern is a result of genetic factors. Prior to the use of rigorous diagnostic criteria, early twin studies using vaguely defined syndromes, such as "neurosis," showed higher concordance rates in monozygotic twins when compared to dizygotic twins, suggesting a genetic etiology (Slater and Shields, 1969). Studies using *DSM* criteria also supported a genetic component for PD, first in smaller samples (Torgersen, 1983; Skre et al., 1993; Perna et al., 1997), and then in much larger twin registry samples (Kendler et al., 1993b; Scherrer et al., 2000). A meta-analysis combining family study and twin data found that the observed data best fit a model consisting of additive genetic factors and individual environmental factors, with a heritability of 0.48 (Hettema, Neale, and Kendler, 2001). Family and twin studies thus support a modest genetic contribution to PD.

Despite this observation, it is not apparent how genetic transmission occurs in PD; an initial study using *DSM* criteria proposed a single-gene dominant model (Pauls, Crowe, and Noyes, 1979; Pauls et al., 1980), a model subsequently modified as showing that neither dominant nor polygenic modes of inheritance could be ruled out (Crowe et al., 1983). Later segregation analyses argued that recessive and dominant models were equally likely (Vieland et al., 1993), and predicted known twin concordance rates (Vieland et al., 1996). Although segregation analyses accept a genetic component to PD, they have not determined the mode of inheritance.

The co-occurrence of PD with other psychiatric conditions has led to hypotheses about genetic determinants common to more than one disorder. For example, one study of families demonstrated that by itself PD was not associated with increased risk of depression in relatives, yet comorbid depression and panic increased the risk that relatives would have either condition by itself, or as comorbid panic and depression (Weissman et al., 1993). These data argue for panic and depression being separable conditions. Nonetheless, it has been observed that children of parents with depression show high rates of anxiety disorders in general (Weissman et al., 2005), although not necessarily PD (Biederman et al., 2001). Studies of bipolar disorder (BPD) pedigrees have resulted in the observation of segregation of PD in particular families. In one study, investigators documented that approximately 18% of persons with BPD in their pedigrees had comorbid PD, and that only 5 of 41 persons with PD did not also have BPD (MacKinnon et al., 1997), providing support for a subgroup of families with a heritable susceptibility to BPD and/or PD (MacKinnon et al., 2002). This research group determined that the genetic linkage signal previously detected on chromosome 18 with their entire family set (Stine et al., 1995) could be further narrowed to the group of families in which the index BPD proband had PD (MacKinnon et al., 1998). Clinically, mania is notable for rapid mood switching in the presence of familiar PD (MacKinnon et al., 2003). More evidence for the possibility that both disorders share a common genetic mechanism would come from a reciprocal assessment of BPD in pedigrees selected for the segregation of PD.

There is now a large literature indicating that infused lactate, inhaled carbon dioxide (CO_2), or other "panicogens" precipitate panic attacks in individuals with PD, but not in healthy controls (Gorman et al., 1990). More recently, several groups have investigated whether this vulnerability may be related to a heritable risk factor that predisposes to PD. The two studies investigating lactate vulnerability are inconclusive. One found that participants with high rates of anxiety disorders among their first-degree family members were more likely to exhibit panic attacks in response to the infusion of lactate (Balon et al., 1989). The other found no differences in rates of panic or any other anxiety disorders in relatives of patients with PD who panicked during lactate infusion versus relatives of patients with PD who did not panic during the infusion (Reschke et al., 1995). More extensive exploration of heritability has been done with carbon dioxide (CO_2) challenges. The observations that panic attacks in response to 35% CO_2 challenge are significantly more common among healthy relatives of PD probands than among similarly healthy first-degree relatives of controls has been replicated by three investigator groups (Perna et al., 1995; Coryell, 1997; van Beek and Griez, 2000). Panic to CO_2 has also been associated with a higher familial risk for PD (Perna et al., 1996) and a community-based twin study found concordance for a panic attack after CO_2 inhalation to be 4 times higher in monozygotic twins compared to dizygotic twins, suggesting a genetic component (Bellodi et al., 1998). A second twin study, using mathematical modeling, found an additive genetic contribution to panic symptoms following CO_2 challenge with moderate heritability estimate (that is, 0.4–0.5) (Battaglia et al., 2007). One exception to these findings is the lack of the response in children with a parent with PD (Pine et al., 2005). It remains to be seen if the genetic factors underlying CO_2 and lactate sensitivity contribute to the genetic risk of PD.

Molecular genetics

Guided by suggestive family study and twin data, efforts have been mounted over the past two decades to identify genes for PD. Prior to the use of deoxyribonucleic acid (DNA)-based microsatellite markers, genetic linkage analysis in 26 pedigrees segregating PD with polymorphic blood cell markers and DNA markers near those loci were not positive (Crowe et al., 1987; Crowe et al., 1990). Twenty-three of these same families underwent a genome scan, with modest evidence for linkage (logarithm of odds ratio [LOD] score = 2.23) on chromosome 7p12 (Crowe et al., 2001). A second group ascertained families with multiple individuals with PD (Fyer and Weissman, 1999) and carried out a genome scan in 23 families that resulted in modest linkage also in the chromosome 7p15 region (Knowles et al., 1998). Expansion of this sample to 120 families showed diminished support for this region but identified two loci, on chromosomes 15q and 2q, exhibiting genome-wide statistical significance (Fyer et al., 2006). A third group performed genetic linkage analysis of a genome scan in 20 pedigrees, reporting modest evidence for linkage on chromosome 1q (Gelernter et al., 2001), a region not identified in previous scans. An additional 25 Icelandic families underwent genome scanning using a complex phenotype including PD, phobias, GAD, and somatoform pain, with a reported LOD score of 4.18 in the region of chromosome 9q31, again a region not seen in previous scans (Thorgeirsson et al., 2003). The discrepancy between these findings may suggest genetic heterogeneity in that differing samples from differing populations may harbor different combinations of risk alleles.

Given the rich research literature in the biology of fear and anxiety, there are numerous plausible candidate genes potentially involved in PD susceptibility. Attempts to associate variants on these genes with PD have proven inconclusive (Gratacos et al., 2007). Genes representing most components of putative panic-related physiology, including receptors for γ-aminobutyric acid (GABA), monoamines, and neuropeptides, have been studied. Two genes stand out from these studies: the adenosine 2A receptor and catechol-*O*-methyltransferase (*COMT*). Two studies in Caucasian populations investigating the adenosine 2A receptor reported association or linkage (Deckert et al., 1998; Hamilton et al., 2004); however, two Asian studies did not report a similar association (Yamada et al., 2001; Lam et al., 2005). Catechol-*O*-methyltransferase is notable in that atleast five studies support the role of this gene in PD (Hamilton et al., 2002; Woo et al., 2002; Domschke et al., 2004; Woo et al., 2004; Rothe et al., 2006) in Caucasian and Asian populations. Several reasons may explain the typically negative or conflicting findings, most notably (*1*) low statistical power due to limited sample sizes, (*2*) population heterogeneity at the genetic level, (*3*) low prior probability compounding by multiple comparisons issues, and (*4*) heterogeneity in phenotype.

In summary, linkage studies have not provided strong evidence of genomic regions that are highly likely to be related to PD, possibly reflective of the lower sensitivity of parametric linkage studies in diseases of uncertain mode of inheritance and in which multiple genes of small effect may be operative. This last point has also hampered candidate gene-oriented studies. It is hoped that the current use of genome-wide association methods in large clinical samples will provide novel insights into PD genetics.

Phobias

Specific phobia and SAD constitute the most common anxiety disorders. Specific phobia is notable for an unreasonable and persistent fear of objects or situations. The phobic stimulus rapidly elicits intense anxiety accompanied by physiological symptoms of arousal, leading to avoidance of the stimulus. Social anxiety disorder (formerly social phobia) is characterized by marked fear of social or performance situations. Again, these stimuli provoke intense anxiety, often panic attacks, and result in avoidance behaviors. There are fewer family studies of phobia, but they support familial aggregation of these disorders. For specific phobia, rates of the disorder among first-degree relatives of probands was 31%, compared to 9% in relatives of nonphobic controls, resulting in a four-fold increase in risk (Fyer et al., 1995). Studies focusing on familial aggregation of generalized social phobia also document elevated rates in families of probands compared to controls (Fyer et al., 1993; Mannuzza et al., 1995; Stein, Chartier, Hazen, et al., 1998). Twin studies also support a genetic contribution to phobias, suggesting moderate genetic heritability in the range of 0.3–0.4 across phobia types. Interestingly, the residual risk has little contribution from shared environment and instead derives from environmental factors unique to the individual (Hettema, Neale, and Kendler, 2001). The strongest evidence derives from investigation of over 2000 twin pairs in the population-based Virginia Twin Registry (Kendler et al., 1992b, 1993a; Hettema et al., 2005) using a *DSM*-based instrument that identified social phobia and the animal and situational subtypes of specific phobia. The multivariate genetic model that best fit the observed data suggested a shared genetic liability between phobias, amounting to 30%–40% of the risk, as well as individual-specific environmental factors (Kendler et al., 1992b; Kendler et al., 2001) Specific heritabilities were estimated at 0.51, 0.47, and 0.46 for social phobia, and the animal and situational subtypes of specific phobia, respectively. More recently, twin studies of preadolescent children in which parents were interviewed about fears and phobias in their children showed high heritability and a more prominent contribution from family environment (that is shared environment) (Lichtenstein and Annas, 2000; Bolton et al., 2006).

Other twin studies have focused on determining the heritability of a broader nonclinical definition of irrational fears (Torgersen, 1979; Rose and Ditto, 1983; Phillips et al., 1987; Sundet et al., 2003). These studies identify participants who have specific irrational fears, but some will also have *DSM* phobia, whereas some will not meet full criteria. For example, two studies using the Fear Survey Schedule (Geer, 1965), which includes 51 common fears were carried out in a substantial number of twins (Phillips et al., 1987; Sundet et al., 2003). Both studies found that specific genetic factors account for substantial liability for fears that are commonly seen in specific phobia, such as small animals or situations (water, heights, enclosed spaces), with moderate heritability, ranging from 20%–47%.

Molecular genetics

Despite its high prevalence, specific phobia has not been the focus of molecular genetic investigations. No linkage studies in pedigrees identified through specific phobia probands have been carried out. One study focusing on specific phobia as a phenotype utilized a pedigree sample collected using PD probands (Gelernter et al., 2003). Fourteen of the available pedigrees contained more than one participant with *DSM-III-R* specific phobia, with natural environment and situational phobias predominating, with most having onset prior to age 20. Parametric analysis of a microsatellite genomic screen showed a peak on chromosome 14 at 36.7cM, with a LOD score = 3.17 under a dominant genetic model. Correlation of phobia subtypes with linkage results suggests that the observed chromosome 14 region was identified in families enriched for nonsituational phobia subtypes.

Using a similar approach in their PD pedigrees, Gelernter et al. (2004) performed analyses focusing on SAD. A nonparametric linkage score of 3.4 occurred at 62cM on chromosome 16, while a parametric LOD score of 2.22 was observed at 71cM, also on chromosome 16 (Gelernter et al., 2004). This same group subsequently broadened their anxiety phenotype and utilized a novel statistical method implementing "fuzzy clustering" methodology (Kaabi et al., 2006). The phenotypes of specific phobia, SAD, PD, and agoraphobia were examined in 19 pedigrees, assuming that all of these disorders were expression of a single underlying genetic trait. This analysis resulted in a genome-wide significant linkage to chromosome 4q31-q34, near the neuropeptide Y1 receptor gene (*NPY1R*), which encodes a protein that plays a role in experimental anxiety (Sorensen et al., 2004). A similar approach was carried out in Icelandic pedigrees by combining anxiety disorder phenotypes in 62 pedigrees in which 33% and 50% of participants with anxiety disorder had specific phobia and SAD, respectively. A maximum allele-sharing LOD score of 2.0 was reported for chromosome 9q at 104cM for the broad anxiety phenotype, increasing to 4.18 when examining a smaller group of 25 families that had one or more individuals with PD

(Thorgeirsson et al., 2003). There are no reported candidate gene studies of specific phobia. Two negative candidate gene studies of SAD, looking at dopamine and serotonin genes (Stein, Chartier, Kozak, et al., 1998; Kennedy et al., 2001) have been reported.

Generalized Anxiety Disorder

Genetic epidemiology

Generalized anxiety disorder (GAD) is characterized by persistent and excessive worry about several aspects of everyday life (for example, work, relationships) that is present "more days than not" for at least 6 months (*DSM-IV*) and is accompanied by two or more symptoms of arousal (for example, irritability, muscle tension, sleep disturbance). The lifetime prevalence of GAD is estimated at 5%–6% (Kessler, Berglund, et al., 2005) using the 6-month *DSM-IV* duration criterion and 9% if this requirement is reduced to 1 month (Ruscio et al., 2007). Generalized anxiety disorder is more common in women, and as many as 80% of individuals have comorbid anxiety or depression (Kessler, Chiu, et al., 2005). The genetic epidemiology of GAD has been a subject of interest in recent years, particularly in connection with attempts to clarify the diagnosis and its relationship to depression. As part of these efforts the criteria have changed a great deal over the past 30 years so that the relevance of earlier findings to the current *DSM-IV* definition may require additional verification.

There are three reported direct interview family studies of GAD. Two were conducted in clinical populations (Noyes et al., 1987; Mendlewicz et al., 1993) and the third in a population based community sample (Newman and Bland, 2006). Results are generally consistent with familial aggregation of GAD but vary in the strength. Noyes et al. (1987) found significant familial aggregation of GAD in relatives of GAD probands versus relatives of well controls (19.5% vs. 3.5%; $p < 001$). The Mendlewicz et al. (1993) study included four proband groups (major depressive disorder [MDD], panic disorder [PD], GAD, and well controls). Although the morbidity risk for GAD in relatives of GAD probands was higher than that in relatives of controls (8.9 vs. 1.9) this difference did not reach the 0.05 level of significance in the four-way comparison. Newman and Bland (2006) found that relatives of GAD probands were 1½ to 2 times as likely to have GAD as relatives of controls.

Molecular genetics

Results of two large registry-based twin studies (Roy et al., 1995; Kendler, 1996; Hettema, Prescott, and Kendler, 2001; Mackintosh et al., 2006) indicate a modest to moderate genetic contributions to GAD with heritabilities in the range of 15%–40%. The residual heritability for GAD comes from specific environmental events, with no evidence of influence from family (common) environment. Analyses by Kendler and colleagues in both of these twin registries (Virginia, Sweden) also indicate that there is complete overlap in the genetic factors that contribute to risk for GAD and major depression. According to this model, environmental factors specific to the individual determine whether the clinical syndrome is expressed as GAD or MDD (Kendler et al., 1992a; Roy et al., 1995; Kendler, 1996; Kendler et al., 2007). There are no published linkage studies or replicated candidate gene findings for GAD, although two small studies of a mixture of individuals with anxiety disorder found an association between the monoamine oxidase A gene (MAO-A) and GAD, although using different genetic markers (Tadic et al., 2003; Samochowiec et al., 2004).

Obsessive–Compulsive Disorder

Genetic epidemiology

In obsessive–compulsive disorder (OCD), patients report obsessions, or persistent intrusive thoughts, usually focused on checking, symmetry, or contamination. Compulsions, or ritualistic tasks interfering with normal functioning, are also characteristic of OCD. Obsessive–compulsive disorder was thought to be relatively uncommon, with a prevalence of about 0.05%, before the methodological improvements seen in the large epidemiologic studies of the 1980s (Rasmussen and Eisen, 1992). The Epidemiologic Catchment Area (ECA) study, using some 9500 participants in early reports (Robins et al., 1984), and then 18,500 persons in later analyses (Karno et al., 1988), reported lifetime prevalence of *DSM-III* OCD ranging from 1.3% to 3.0%, in line with the 1.9% to 2.5% rates of the Cross National Collaborative Group (Weissman et al., 1994) and the more recent estimate of lifetime prevalence of 1.6% in the National Comorbidity Survey replication (Kessler, Berglund, et al., 2005). Estimates of prevalence over 6 months in the ECA sample were 1.3%–2.0% (Myers et al., 1984), although there has been some question about the stability of the diagnosis (Nelson and Rice, 1997).

Like most anxiety disorders, OCD is more common in females, although this difference is slight, with some reports prior to 1970 of a slight excess (51% female vs. 49% male) (Black, 1974), although more recent studies suggest a female to male ratio of about 1.2–1.6 to one (Weissman et al., 1994). The typical age at onset of OCD is 19.5 years for males and 22.0 years for females, which represents a significant difference (Rasmussen and Eisen, 1992). This difference appears to be reflected in the difference in OCD gender ratios for prepubertal childhood onset (3:1, male:female) and postpubertal adolescent onset (~1:1, male:female). It has been observed that early-onset OCD in males is associated with more frequent birth complications as well as severe and sustained symptomatology (Flament et al., 1990; Lensi et al., 1996). Obsessive–compulsive disorder has been closely studied in children and adolescents, where the disorder can be particularly impairing. As mentioned above, one provocative finding in children is the reversal of the gender ratio (Hollingsworth et al., 1980; Swedo, Rapoport, Leonard, et al., 1989), although the sex ratio observed in adolescent OCD is more characteristic of that in adults (Flament et al., 1988).

Family studies prior to the use of operationalized diagnostic criteria suggested familial aggregation of obsessional states (Lewis, 1936; Brown, 1942). A large number of studies carried out starting in the 1970s, despite prominent methodological heterogeneity, also documented higher risk of OCD in first-degree relatives of OCD probands. For example, a review of 11 OCD family studies found rates of OCD in first-degree relatives to be 9.5%–25% for child probands and 0%–20% in adult probands (Sobin and Karayiorgou, 2000). Rates were higher for studies using direct interviews as opposed to family histories. The data also suggest that early-onset OCD may represent a more heritable form of the disorder (Pauls et al., 1995; Nestadt, Samuels, et al., 2000; Hanna, Himle, et al., 2005), though this finding is not universal (Black et al., 1992; Fyer et al., 2005), and suggests that there may exist heterogeneity in OCD with regard to familial aggregation.

Twin studies are not common for OCD, and there are no adoption studies. Several early studies, utilizing a total of 328 dizygotic twin pairs and 233 monozygotic twin pairs, found marginal evidence for a genetic component for OCD based on twin concordance, and usually only when OCD was grouped with other psychopathology (Carey and Gottesman, 1981; Torgersen, 1983; Andrews et al., 1990). For example, when considering a clustering of disorders comprised of dysthymia, MDD, GAD, PD, and OCD, monozygotic concordance rates were 10.2% in 186 pairs, compared to 9.6% in 260 dizygotic pairs, an insignificant difference (Andrews et al., 1990). Assessment of *DSM-IV* OCD at age 6 with a much larger collection of twins supports a more substantial genetic influence (Bolton et al., 2007). An alternative approach has been to use twin studies for the analysis of the heritability of obsessive–compulsive symptoms, instead of the categorical disorder. An investigation of 10,110 twin pairs from the Netherlands and the United States, composed only of children, found that there was a strong additive genetic influence (~55%) for obsessive–compulsive symptoms, with the remainder influenced by unique environmental factors (Hudziak et al., 2004). Similar studies in adults are generally supportive of this estimate, although they tend to be somewhat smaller (Clifford et al., 1984; Jonnal et al., 2000; Van Grootheest et al., 2007). The heterogenous experimental methodologies in the OCD twin literature add complexity to interpreting the data, especially given the lack of unbiased epidemiologically based samples. Because of these differences, meta-analysis of the extant twin studies has not been possible (Hettema, Neale, and Kendler, 2001). Yet the overall implication of these studies is that OCD has a genetic component, particularly when assessed in childhood (Van Grootheest et al., 2005).

Efforts to define the mode of inheritance of OCD, as with PD, are not supportive of a simple pattern of genetic transmission. Although some studies of segregation suggest a simple genetic model (Cavallini et al., 1999; Nestadt, Lan, et al., 2000; Hanna, Fingerlin, et al., 2005), others are unable to discern a precise mode of inheritance (Alsobrook et al., 1999). Given the phenotypic heterogeneity of OCD, it would be surprising if a single major locus influences the predisposition to OCD, and it may be prudent to consider the possibility that multiple genes may be involved.

Careful investigation of early-onset OCD has generated intriguing observations relating to broader categories of psychopathology (Leonard et al., 1999). For example, early-onset OCD appears to cluster in families (do Rosario-Campos et al., 2005) and is often associated with Tourette's disorder and tics (Pauls et al., 1986; Leonard et al., 1992; Pauls et al., 1995), whereas by themselves tics are more common in families segregating OCD (Grados et al., 2001). The presence of obsessive–compulsive symptoms in disorders such as autism has been used to subset families for genetic studies (Buxbaum et al., 2004; McCauley et al., 2004) and has been proposed as a way to focus gene-finding efforts (Miguel et al., 2004). A striking example of this approach stems from the observation of high rates of obsessive–compulsive symptoms in children with the post-streptococcal autoimmune syndrome Sydenham's chorea (Swedo, Rapoport, Cheslow, et al., 1989), leading to description of pediatric autoimmune neuropsychiatric disorder associated with streptococcal infections (PANDAS) (Swedo et al., 1998). Subsequent research showed that children with PANDAS, Sydenham's chorea, and Tourette's disorder were positive for D8/17, a monoclonal antibody, significantly more often than controls (Murphy et al., 1997; Swedo et al., 1997). The fact that first-degree relatives of PANDAS probands have higher rates of OCD when compared to the population suggests a potential genetic component to this interesting phenotype (Lougee et al., 2000).

Molecular genetics

Seven families were analyzed in the first OCD genome scan and were ascertained through pediatric-onset probands (Hanna et al., 2002). The authors observed a maximum multipoint linkage score of 2.25 on chromosome 9p, which was to 1.97 when additional samples and markers were added. When an additional 26 families were added, support for linkage in this region dissipated, while a separate peak on chromosome 10p emerged (Hanna et al., 2007). Another group, using 41 affected sibling pairs, also observed linkage in the region of chromosome 9p described above, reporting a parametric heterogeneity LOD score of 2.26 (Willour et al., 2004). When this latter sample was expanded to 219 families, a genome scan was performed, this region was not prominent. Instead, the investigators observed their strongest finding to be a multipoint nonparametric analysis (p = 0.0003) on chromosome 3q, with less support for regions on chromosomes 1, 7, and 15 (Shugart et al., 2006). These same families have been used to analyze obsessive–compulsive symptoms as endophenotypes, with some evidence for linkage (p = 0.0001) of chromosome 14 to hoarding symptoms in families with two or more relatives with hoarding obsessions or compulsions (Samuels et al., 2007), which have been found to cluster in families (Hasler et al., 2007) and show moderate heritability (Mathews et al., 2007).

Candidate gene association studies in OCD are driven primarily by clinical observations and pharmacologic data (Goodman et al., 1990), with serotonin pathway genes under the most initial focus. For example, serotonin transporter function in blood and brain in patients with OCD is altered (Delorme et al., 2005; Hesse et al., 2005; Hasselbalch et al., 2007), and early studies of the coding sequence of the gene showed it to be unaltered in patients with OCD (Altemus et al., 1996; Di Bella et al., 1996). A number of family-based and case-control association studies have been reported, with conflicting results. Some groups report associations with particular variants within the gene (Ozaki et al., 2003; Hu et al., 2006). The largest studies do not support an association to the repeat polymorphism (5-HTTLPR) in the promoter region of the gene (Wendland et al., 2007), and meta-analysis suggests very minimal association (Dickel et al., 2007; Lin, 2007). The investigation of other candidate genes, including those encoding serotonin receptors and dopamine system proteins, have likewise shown inconclusive findings (Hemmings and Stein, 2006). Another gene gaining much attention with OCD is *COMT*, which is involved in the enzymatic metabolism of monoamine neurotransmitters. Analysis of a polymorphism leading to a valine to methionine substitution in the protein that results in alterations in activity initially suggested an association between the lower activity allele in male patients with OCD (Karayiorgou et al., 1997), which was confirmed in a subsequent study using family samples (Karayiorgou et al., 1999). Subsequent studies and a meta-analysis of extant literature (Azzam and Mathews, 2003) suggest that this gene likely has a small effect on OCD, which may be concentrated in males (Denys et al., 2006; Pooley et al., 2007). Researchers have capitalized on the positional cloning efforts in OCD described in the previous section by identifying in the chromosome 9p region a reasonable candidate gene, *SLC1A1*, which encodes the neuronal and epithelial high-affinity glutamate transporter EAAC1. Initial sequencing of the coding sequence of this gene revealed no functional polymorphisms or mutations (Veenstra-VanderWeele et al., 2001). Two later studies with a combined total of 228 families used family-based analyses of nine markers in each study, with five overlapping between studies. One study reported three single nucleotide polymorphisms (SNPs) being associated with OCD, with the signal primarily coming from males (Arnold et al., 2006). The second study reported two SNPs being associated with OCD, with one of those being associated in male samples (Dickel et al., 2006). Interestingly, these two SNPs were also genotyped in the first study but were not associated with OCD.

As with PD, linkage analysis has not identified strong regions of linkage to OCD, a common experience with complex disorders. Given the modest samples used for hypothesis-based candidate gene testing, it is not surprising that results are equivocal. Similarly, the limited understanding of the biological substrates for OCD has led to analysis of sensible candidates, albeit with a very low a priori likelihood of success (Sullivan et al., 2001; Sullivan, 2007).

Genetic Studies of Anxious Personality Traits

As a tendency toward negative affective states, neuroticism is a personality trait included in most all models of personality (Cloninger, 1987). For example, in the five-factor model, neuroticism is characterized by traits corresponding to anxiety, depression, impulsiveness, and self-consciousness (Ebstein, 2006). Genes likely play a prominent role in neuroticism, as a study of nearly 46,000 twins found that a simple genetic model was sufficient to explain familial correlation of neuroticism, and that there was little evidence of nongenetic origins for intrafamily resemblance (Lake et al., 2000). This and other studies suggest neuroticism to be more than moderately heritable (for example, heritability [h^2] = 0.5–0.6) (Jang et al., 1996; Rettew et al., 2006).

Most studies in clinical and community populations have also noted a strong association between neuroticism and anxiety and depression. For example, higher neuroticism scores are correlated with levels of depression and anxiety symptoms as measured by the Eysenck Personality Inventory and the Beck Depression Scale (Jylha and Isometsa, 2006). In a survey of some 731 participants from the general U.S. population, elevated neuroticism was associated with the diagnosis of depression, as well as all anxiety disorders that were examined, including specific phobia, SAD, agoraphobia, PD, GAD, and OCD (Bienvenu et al., 2004). In a smaller subsample from the same population, neuroticism was associated with comorbidity between many of these same disorders (Bienvenu et al., 2001), a finding also observed in psychiatric outpatients (Cuijpers et al., 2005). These data suggest that it might prove beneficial to consider personality traits such as neuroticism to share an underlying genetic architecture with anxiety disorders. Using structural equation modeling in a sample of 9270 twins, Hettema et al. (2006) sought to examine this possibility of looking at the correlation between neuroticism and a group of "internalizing" disorders, including depression, PD, agoraphobia, SAD, GAD, and two subtypes of specific phobias (situational, animal). They found that neuroticism shared significant genetic risk with these disorders (Hettema et al., 2006). When examining GAD alone, the genetic overlap between GAD and neuroticism was nearly complete, with a correlation of 0.8 (Hettema et al., 2004). Twin studies also suggest a substantial genetic correlation between major depression and neuroticism (Kendler et al., 2006).

The observations above have prompted attempts to identify the genetic determinants of personality traits such as neuroticism. Given the relative ease in acquiring personality data via self-administered instruments, large samples are often feasible for genetic studies of personality traits. For example, one group used information gathered from nearly 35,000 sibling pairs, allowing them to select pairs discordant for measures of neuroticism, as well as pairs concordant for high scores or low scores, resulting in 629 sibling pairs for analysis (Fullerton et al., 2003). A genome screen reported significant linkage to neuroticism, or quantitative trait loci (QTL), on chromosomes 1q, 4q, 7p, 12q, and 13q. The authors further observed that the findings on chromosomes 1, 12, and 13 were specific to females. A study with a similar design, selecting 757 individuals in 297 sibships out of a total of over 34,000 individuals, was used to examine a phenotype based on factor analysis involving neuroticism scores combined with subscales of anxiety and mood questionnaires. A genome screen in these families revealed modestly elevated LOD scores on chromosomes 1p and 6p, also with a gender effect (Nash et al., 2004). A study carried out in 129 sibling pairs collected on the basis of nicotine dependence, in which personality measures were taken, was also subjected to a genome screen, which found elevated, but not significant at the genome-wide level, LOD scores in the 1p and 11q regions (Neale et al., 2005), which were also present in the analysis of Fullerton et al. (2003). A final study utilizes a genome-wide association approach, in which hundreds of thousands of SNPs are genotyped simultaneously on a microarray. These markers, roughly spaced across the genome, allow a test of association between the marker and a phenotype, typically by comparing the magnitude of allele frequency differences for each marker between cases and matched controls (Christensen and Murray, 2007). In the first such study of this kind with neuroticism, 2054 individuals were selected from over 88,000 participants for their extreme high and low neuroticism scores (Shifman et al., 2008). Given the prohibitive cost of individually genotyping the samples, the investigators pooled DNA samples for genotyping. They obtained data on about 450,000 SNPs and found that none of the markers met statistical significance using a threshold taking into account the large number of tests carried out. They genotyped the 19 best SNPs in a replication sample of 1534 individuals in the top or bottom 10% of the neuroticism distribution taken from their original 88,000 participants. Only one SNP, in the cyclic adenosine monophosphate (cAMP)-specific phosphodiesterase 4D gene (*PDE4D*), met their criteria for replicating the association seen in their initial sample. Unfortunately, this finding was not seen in three additional external replication groups the investigators genotyped, totaling 2199 individuals. The authors did not observe association signals in the previously reported linkage regions mentioned above. These results raise the possibility that much larger samples may be required to detect small genetic influences on neuroticism.

Genetic association studies have also been used to look at the possible role of specific genes in neuroticism. These genes are typically chosen based on biological hypotheses regarding mood and anxiety. For example, the serotonin transporter has been studied, with an association reported in a sample of 505 participants (Lesch et al., 1996), as well as in a meta-analysis of a number of small studies (Sen et al., 2004). This finding did not stand up in a larger single study of 4800 participants (Willis-Owen et al., 2005), nor in other recent large samples (Middeldorp et al., 2007).

Animal Studies of Anxiety

Much work has been carried out using rodents to understand the neurophysiology, neuropharmacology, and neuroanatomy of anxiety. The slow progress in identifying genes conferring risk for anxiety disorder has led to great interest in pursuing genetic approaches in animal model systems. Two genetic approaches have been extensively utilized in rodents to advance the understanding of anxiety biology. First, genome screens for linkage to anxiety-related traits make use of standard behavior paradigms and the ability to cross large numbers of mice efficiently. Behaviors that are analogous to human anxiety can be identified, and animals can be bred and selected for extremes of these traits such that they are homozygous across the genome. Interbreeding of these inbred and phenotypically divergent strains results in animals (F1 generation) each harboring a copy from each parent (for example, high trait vs. low trait) for each chromosome pair. These F1 mice are then interbred, and the resulting F2 generation tested for their behavioral trait of interest. This random mixing of genomes facilitates mapping of QTLs, by looking for regions of the genome most resembling the high-trait line in F2 animals with the highest trait scores (Flint et al., 2005). One example of this approach involves an analysis of behavior of mice on the elevated plus maze, a measure of anxiety-related behavior. This model uses the observation that rodents tend to avoid open and well-lit areas where they may be visible to predators. Paradigms like the elevated plus measure the frequency in which animals will explore these open spaces, presumably testing a balance between exploratory behavior and fear-based behavior. Investigators have further refined analysis of such behaviors, including activity on the maze and defecation, conceptualizing them as measures of "emotionality." One such group genotyped 879 F2 mice progeny of two strains selected to have high and low levels of activity on the elevated plus maze. Behavioral testing carried out on these F2 mice showed strong evidence of linkage between three chromosomal regions and emotionality (Flint et al., 1995). Subsequent work with larger numbers of animals and more anxiety phenotypes has confirmed many of these findings (Turri et al., 1999; Turri, Datta, et al., 2001; Turri, Henderson, et al., 2001; Turri et al., 2004), as have other investigators (Gershenfeld et al., 1997; Gershenfeld and Paul, 1997), yet the actual identification of a gene that serves as the QTL has proven elusive and suggests substantial complexity underlying anxiety-related traits in mice (Willis-Owen and Flint, 2006). Other anxiety-related traits, such as contextual fear conditioning, have been used to discover QTLs (Caldarone et al., 1997; Wehner et al., 1997; Fernandez-Teruel et al., 2002). Although genes identified in this manner will be examined in human behaviors, there are challenges in interpreting these studies with regard to human pathology. The applicability of these ethological paradigms is itself problematic, particularly when extrapolating from adaptive behavior in rodents to maladaptive behavior in humans (Overall, 2000; Shekhar et al., 2001). The resolution of mapping in F2 generations is low, making it necessary to pursue large genomic regions or to use outbred mice in follow-up studies (Talbot et al., 1999). Finally, the genetic architecture of the trait may require innovative statistical approaches (Mott et al., 2000).

The second major approach for using genetics to address similarities between anxiety in animal systems and anxiety disorders in humans involves gene targeting studies. These studies typically delete a gene or components of a gene in vitro on a length of DNA identical to the genomic region in vivo. This is done in such a way that the gene is rendered inactive and not transcribed or translated. This engineered targeting construct is introduced into embryonic stem cells, where it replaces the normal copy of the gene through homologous recombination. Clones of embryonic stem cells bearing the mutated gene are selected, typically through the use of a toxic drug that can only be deactivated by a drug-resistance gene that is one module of the targeting construct. These recombinant embryonic stem cells are then injected into mouse embryos that are 3 to 4 days of age, followed by implantation into foster mothers. The embryos develop into "chimeras" derived from the embryo and the embryonic stem cells; thus some fraction of the mouse will consist of cells bearing the introduced mutation, with the hope that the germ cell line will contain mutant cells to allow transmission of the mutation. These mice are bred to normal mice, and the offspring are tested for the presence of the altered gene. Mice carrying the introduced "null" allele can be interbred to generate animals homozygous for that allele. Dosage effects can be examined when the deletion or "knock-out" is heterozygous or homozygous, and technical innovations allow temporal and spatial precision to the inactivation of the gene target (Tecott, 2003). Mice can then be examined for gross defects and also subjected to behavioral testing paradigms such as the open field or elevated plus maze, as described above. It is possible to also introduce constitutively active or over-active versions of genes. This approach can similarly be used to introduce specific versions of human gene, such as those carrying particular mutations or polymorphisms seen in human genes (Chen et al., 2006).

This approach has been used to examine the effects of gene deletion for a large array of genes thought to play a role in anxiety. These genes include components of the serotonergic pathway (serotonin transporter, serotonin receptors), monoamine-related genes (MAO-A, *COMT*, dopamine receptors), GABA and glutamate pathways, and corticotropin releasing hormone-related genes (Holmes, 2001). Beyond these genes, deletion (or overexpression) of any of a lengthy list of other genes involved in various central nervous system has been noted to result in alterations in anxiety-related behaviors. These include genes as obscure as those encoding α1,3-fucosyltransferase IX, the cellular prion protein, or transient receptor potential vanilloid type 1 channel, to more obvious genes for norepinephrine and vasopressin receptors.

One of the most well studied genes in this manner involves the serotonin 1A ($5\text{-}HT_{1A}$) receptor. The near simultaneous reports of successful deletion of this gene by three groups all described mice who spent significantly less time in the center of an open field or entered open arms of an elevated maze when compared to their wild-type littermates (Heisler et al., 1998; Parks et al., 1998; Ramboz et al., 1998). A dosage effect was noted, with mice heterozygous for the null allele showing an intermediate phenotype and approximately half the expression of the $5\text{-}HT_{1A}$ protein compared to wild type (Ramboz et al., 1998). Subsequent work using conditional knockout methods showed that a normal phenotype could be "rescued" when $5\text{-}HT_{1A}$ was expressed selectively in knockout mice in the hippocampus and cortex (but not in the raphé nuclei) and during the postnatal (but not adult) period (Gross et al., 2002). Interestingly, mice engineered to overexpress $5\text{-}HT_{1A}$ exhibit less anxiety-like behavior than control animals (Kusserow et al., 2004). These observations provide support for the contention that dysfunction of the $5\text{-}HT_{1A}$ receptor may lead to elevated serotonin levels, resulting in excess anxiety. This hypothesis has led to much subsequent investigation into the role that this interesting receptor may play in mood and anxiety states (Santarelli et al., 2003; Klemenhagen et al., 2005) and provides rationale for candidate gene studies in human anxiety disorders such as PD, where a common promoter SNP in HTR1A was found to be associated (Rothe et al., 2004).

One molecular component of the stress response is corticotropin releasing hormone (CRH), whose release from the hypothalamus stimulates adrenocorticotropic hormone (ACTH) release from cells of the anterior pituitary, leading to adrenal gland release of glucocorticoids to elicit blood glucose mobilization. Several lines of research suggest that CRH function is dysregulated in mood and anxiety disorders (Britton et al., 1986; Butler et al., 1990), leading to a rationale for using CRH antagonists for treatment of these disorders (Arborelius et al., 1999). Not surprisingly, gene-targeting studies in mice have been used to examine the role of CRH-related genes in anxiety and other phenotypes. Overexpression of the protein CRH itself showed elevated anxiety, as measured on the elevated plus, which was reversed with administration of a CRH antagonist (Stenzel-Poore et al., 1994). Surprisingly, deletion of this gene does not result in a discernible anxiety phenotype (Weninger et al., 1999). There are two CRH receptors, termed *types 1* and *2*. Both have different distributions in the central nervous system, and both bind to CRH as well as the anxiogenic neuropeptide *urocortin* (Moreau et al., 1997). Each of the genes encoding these receptors has been deleted in mice. Deletion of *CRHR1*, which is expressed in the amygdala, hippocampus, anterior pituitary, neocortex, and cerebellum, led to mice that exhibited less anxiety-like behavior in standard experimental paradigms (Smith et al., 1998; Timpl et al., 1998). These results are in keeping with the known anxiolytic effect of *CRHR1* antagonists (Zorrilla et al., 2002). Given the known pharmacology of the *CRHR2* receptor, it would be expected that deletion of the *CRHR2* gene would have similar effects to *CRHR1*. It turns out that removal of *CRHR2* resulted in increased anxiety-related behaviors in three separate strains of mice (Bale et al., 2000; Coste et al., 2000; Kishimoto et al., 2000). Each of the three strains differed slightly in the extent of their anxiety phenotypes, suggesting parental strain effects. These results suggest a scenario in which *CRHR1* and *CRHR2* act to balance responsiveness to stress, with *CRHR1* mediating CRH signals increasing anxiety, and *CRHR2* dampening anxiety via urocortin or related peptides (Bale and Vale, 2004).

CONCLUSION

The anxiety disorders discussed in this chapter are all moderately heritable, with 20%–40% of the phenotypic variance explained by additive genetic effects. The standard methods of the past two decades for mapping genes for complex disorders, linkage analysis in pedigrees or candidate gene association studies, while providing important leads, are being supplanted by methods made possible by several developments in the field. First, the Human Genome Project and International HapMap Project have provided the raw material for studies examining dense maps of informative markers across the genome. Second, technological advances in array-based genotyping have facilitated the simultaneous, and relatively inexpensive, analysis of hundreds of thousands of SNPs in a single assay. Finally, the recognition that very large samples will be needed to recognize subtle genetic effects has led to increased efforts to ascertain sizable (that is, 1000 to 2000 cases) population-based samples and has fostered collaboration between research groups. Numerous successful applications of this genome-wide association approach have surfaced since 2005 (Klein et al., 2005; Scott et al., 2007; Wellcome Trust Case Control Consortium, 2007), with the promise of such studies for psychiatric disorders becoming a reality. Challenges for this approach involve the reliance on assumptions regarding the genetic model for anxiety disorders, as well as how to differentiate authentic genetic associations in the midst of hundreds of thousands or even millions of statistical tests involving billions of genotypes. An example of the former problem involves debate about whether risk variants for any particular disorder are common in a chosen population, versus the possibility that risk at any gene is determined by a collection of uncommon or rare variants. The latter challenge derives from the fundamental problem of assessing statistical significance of any particular association between a DNA variant and a phenotype. For example, at least 25,000 markers in a genome scan of 500,000 markers would be expected to meet traditional criteria ($p = 0.05$) for statistical significance, by chance. Yet correction for every test ignores the realities of marker-to-marker correlation, as well as the possibility that multiple variants may be associated with the phenotype. Many of these debates may be resolved when reported associations are replicated in independent samples or in meta-analyses. Although animal studies have provided hints at the identity of genes that may influence anxiety disorders in humans, it is hoped that the unbiased genome-wide approaches described here will foster new discoveries of new genes or known genes not considered to be related to anxiety disorders and their many manifestations. Such discoveries are likely to generate focused genetic analyses in human anxiety disorder populations and to foster new directions for animal model studies.

REFERENCES

Alsobrook, J.P. II, Leckman, J.F., Goodman, W.K., Rasmussen, S.A., and Pauls, D.L. (1999) Segregation analysis of obsessive-compulsive disorder using symptom- based factor scores. *Am. J. Med. Genet.* 88:669–675.

Altemus, M., Murphy, D.L., Greenberg, B., and Lesch, K.-P. (1996) Intact coding region of the serotonin transporter gene in obsessive-compulsive disorder. *Am. J. Med. Genet.* 67:409–411.

American Psychiatric Association. (1980) *Diagnostic and Statistical Manual of Mental Disorders*, 3rd ed. Washington, DC: American Psychiatric Association.

American Psychiatric Association. (1994) *Diagnostic and Statistical Manual of Mental Disorders*, 4th ed. Washington, DC: American Psychiatric Association.

Andrews, G., Stewart, G., Allen, R., and Henderson, A.S. (1990) The genetics of six neurotic disorders: a twin study. *J. Affect. Disord.* 19:23–29.

Arborelius, L., Owens, M.J., Plotsky, P.M., and Nemeroff, C.B. (1999) The role of corticotropin-releasing factor in depression and anxiety disorders. *J. Endocrinol.* 160:1–12.

Arnold, P.D., Sicard, T., Burroughs, E., Richter, M.A., and Kennedy, J.L. (2006) Glutamate transporter gene SLC1A1 associated with obsessive-compulsive disorder. *Arch. Gen. Psychiatry* 63:769–776.

Azzam, A., and Mathews, C.A. (2003) Meta-analysis of the association between the catecholamine-O-methyl-transferase gene and obsessive-compulsive disorder. *Am. J. Med. Genet. B Neuropsychiatr. Genet.* 123:64–69.

Bale, T.L., Contarino, A., Smith, G.W., Chan, R., Gold, L.H., Sawchenko, P.E., Koob, G.F., Vale, W.W., and Lee, K.F. (2000) Mice deficient for corticotropin-releasing hormone receptor-2 display anxiety-like behaviour and are hypersensitive to stress. *Nat. Genet.* 24:410–414.

Bale, T.L., and Vale, W.W. (2004) CRF and CRF receptors: role in stress responsivity and other behaviors. *Ann. Rev. Pharmacol. Toxicol.* 44: 525–557.

Balon, R., Jordan, M., Pohl, R., and Yeragani, V.K. (1989) Family history of anxiety disorders in control subjects with lactate-induced panic attacks. *Am. J. Psychiatry* 146:1304–1306.

Battaglia, M., Ogliari, A., Harris, J., Spatola, C.A.M., Pesenti-Gritti, P., Reichborn-Kjennerud, T., Torgersen, S., Kringlen, E., and Tambs, K. (2007) A genetic study of the acute anxious response to carbon dioxide stimulation in man. *J. Psychiatric Res.* 41:906–917.

Bellodi, L., Perna, G., Caldirola, D., Arancio, C., Bertani, A., and Di Bella, D. (1998) CO2-induced panic attacks: a twin study. *Am. J. Psychiatry* 155:1184–1188.

Biederman, J., Faraone, S.V., Hirshfeld-Becker, D.R., Friedman, D., Robin, J.A., and Rosenbaum, J.F. (2001) Patterns of psychopathology and dysfunction in high-risk children of parents with panic disorder and major depression. *Am. J. Psychiatry* 158: 49–57.

Bienvenu, O.J., Brown, C., Samuels, J.F., Liang, K.Y., Costa, P.T., Eaton, W.W., and Nestadt, G. (2001) Normal personality traits and comorbidity among phobic, panic and major depressive disorders. *Psychiatry Res.* 102:73–85.

Bienvenu, O.J., Samuels, J.F., Costa, P.T., Reti, I.M., Eaton, W.W., and Nestadt, G. (2004) Anxiety and depressive disorders and the five-factor model of personality: a higher- and lower-order personality trait investigation in a community sample. *Depress. Anxiety* 20:92–97.

Black, A. (1974) The natural history of obsessional neurosis. In: Beech, H.R., ed. *Obsessional States*. London: Methuen, pp. 19–54.

Black, D.W., Noyes, R., Jr., Goldstein, R.B., and Blum, N. (1992) A family study of obsessive-compulsive disorder. *Arch. Gen. Psychiatry* 49:362–368.

Bolton, D., Eley, T.C., O'Connor, T.G., Perrin, S., Rabe-Hesketh, S., Rijsdijk, F., and Smith, P. (2006) Prevalence and genetic and environmental influences on anxiety disorders in 6-year-old twins. *Psychol. Med.* 36:335–344.

Bolton, D., Rijsdijk, F., O'Connor, T.G., Perrin, S., and Eley, T.C. (2007) Obsessive-compulsive disorder, tics and anxiety in 6-year-old twins. *Psychol. Med.* 37:39–48.

Britton, K.T., Lee, G., Vale, W., Rivier, J., and Koob, G.F. (1986) Corticotropin releasing factor (CRF) receptor antagonist blocks activating and "anxiogenic" actions of CRF in the rat. *Brain Res.* 369:303–306.

Brown, F.W. (1942) Heredity in the psychoneuroses. *Proc. Royal Soc. Med.* 35:785–790.

Butler, P.D., Weiss, J.M., Stout, J.C., and Nemeroff, C.B. (1990) Corticotropin-releasing factor produces fear-enhancing and behavioral activating effects following infusion into the locus coeruleus. *J. Neuroscience* 10:176–183.

Buxbaum, J.D., Silverman, J., Keddache, M., Smith, C.J., Hollander, E., Ramoz, N., and Reichert, J.G. (2004) Linkage analysis for autism in a subset families with obsessive-compulsive behaviors: evidence for an autism susceptibility gene on chromosome 1 and further support for susceptibility genes on chromosome 6 and 19. *Mol. Psychiatry* 9:144–150.

Caldarone, B., Saavedra, C., Tartaglia, K., Wehner, J.M., Dudek, B. C., and Flaherty, L. (1997) Quantitative trait loci analysis affecting contextual conditioning in mice. *Nat. Genet.* 17:335–337.

Carey, G., and Gottesman, I.I. (1981) Twin and family studies of anxiety, phobic, and obsessive disorders. In: Klein, D.F., and Rabkin, J.D., eds. *Anxiety: New Research and Changing Concepts*. New York: Raven Press, pp. 117–136.

Cavallini, M.C., Pasquale, L., Bellodi, L., and Smeraldi, E. (1999) Complex segregation analysis for obsessive compulsive disorder and related disorders. *Am. J. Med. Genet.* 88:38–43.

Chen, Z.Y., Jing, D., Bath, K.G., Ieraci, A., Khan, T., Siao, C.J., Herrera, D.G., Toth, M., Yang, C., McEwen, B.S., Hempstead, B.L., and Lee, F.S. (2006) Genetic variant BDNF (Val66Met) polymorphism alters anxiety-related behavior. *Science* 314:140–143.

Christensen, K., and Murray, J.C. (2007) What genome-wide association studies can do for medicine. *New Engl. J. Med.* 356:1094–1097.

Clifford, C.A., Murray, R.M., and Fulker, D.W. (1984) Genetic and environmental influences on obsessional traits and symptoms. *Psychol. Med.* 14:791–800.

Cloninger, C.R. (1987) A systematic method for clinical description and classification of personality variants. A proposal. *Arch. Gen. Psychiatry* 44:573–588.

Cohen, M.E., Badal, D.W., Kilpatrick, A., Reed, E.W., and White, P. D. (1951) The high familial prevalence of neurocirculatory asthenia (anxiety neurosis, effort syndrome) *Am. J. Hum. Genet.* 3:126–158.

Coryell, W. (1997) Hypersensitivity to carbon dioxide as a disease-specific trait marker. *Biol. Psychiatry* 41:259–263.

Coste, S.C., Kesterson, R.A., Heldwein, K.A., Stevens, S.L., Heard, A.D., Hollis, J.H., Murray, S.E., Hill, J.K., Pantely, G.A., Hohimer, A.R., Hatton, D.C., Phillips, T.J., Finn, D.A., Low, M.J., Rittenberg, M.B., Stenzel, P., and Stenzel-Poore, M.P. (2000) Abnormal adaptations to stress and impaired cardiovascular function in mice lacking corticotropin-releasing hormone receptor-2. *Nat. Genet.* 24:403–409.

Crowe, R.C., Pauls, D.L., Slymen, D.J., and Noyes, R. (1980) A family study of anxiety neurosis. Morbidity risk in families of patients with and without mitral valve prolapse. *Arch. Gen. Psychiatry* 37:77–79.

Crowe, R.R., Goedken, R., Wilson, R., Samuelson, S., Nelson, J., and Noyes, R., Jr. (2001) A genome-wide survey of panic disorder. *Am. J. Med. Genet. (Neuropsychiatr. Genet.)* 105:105–109.

Crowe, R.R., Noyes, R., Jr., Pauls, D.L., and Slymen, D. (1983) A family study of panic disorder. *Arch. Gen. Psychiatry* 40:1065–1069.

Crowe, R.R., Noyes, R., Jr., Samuelson, S., Wesner, R., and Wilson, R. (1990) Close linkage between panic disorder and alpha-haptoglobin excluded in 10 families. *Arch. Gen. Psychiatry* 47: 377–380.

Crowe, R.R., Noyes, R., Jr., Wilson, A.F., Elston, R.C., and Ward, L.J. (1987) A linkage study of panic disorder. *Arch. Gen. Psychiatry* 44:933–937.

Cuijpers, P., van Straten, A., and Donker, M. (2005) Personality traits of patients with mood and anxiety disorders. *Psychiatry Res.* 133:229–237.

Deckert, J., Nothen, M.M., Franke, P., Delmo, C., Fritze, J., Knapp, M., Maier, W., Beckmann, H., and Propping, P. (1998) Systematic mutation screening and association study of the A1 and A2a adenosine receptor genes in panic disorder suggest a contribution of the A2a gene to the development of disease. *Mol. Psychiatry* 3:81–85.

Delorme, R., Betancur, C., Callebert, J., Chabane, N., Laplanche, J.L., Mouren-Simeoni, M.C., Launay, J.M., and Leboyer, M. (2005) Platelet serotonergic markers as endophenotypes for obsessive-compulsive disorder. *Neuropsychopharmacology* 30:1539–1547.

Denys, D., Van Nieuwerburgh, F., Deforce, D., and Westenberg, H. (2006) Association between the dopamine D2 receptor TaqI A2 allele and low activity COMT allele with obsessive-compulsive disorder in males. *Eur. Neuropsychopharmacology* 16:446–450.

Di Bella, D., Catalano, M., Balling, U., Smeraldi, E., and Lesch, K.P. (1996) Systematic screening for mutations in the coding region of the human serotonin transporter (5-HTT) gene using PCR and DGGE. *Am. J. Med. Genet.* 67:541–545.

Dickel, D.E., Veenstra-VanderWeele, J., Bivens, N.C., Wu, X., Fischer, D.J., Van Etten-Lee, M., Himle, J.A., Leventhal, B.L., Cook, J., and Hanna, G.L. (2007) Association studies of serotonin system candidate genes in early-onset obsessive-compulsive disorder. *Biol. Psychiatry* 61:322–329.

Dickel, D.E., Veenstra-VanderWeele, J., Cox, N.J., Wu, X., Fischer, D.J., Van Etten-Lee, M., Himle, J.A., Leventhal, B.L., Cook, E. H., Jr., and Hanna, G.L. (2006) Association testing of the positional and functional candidate gene SLC1A1/EAAC1 in early-onset obsessive-compulsive disorder. *Arch. Gen. Psychiatry* 63: 778–785.

do Rosario-Campos, M.C., Leckman, J.F., Curi, M., Quatrano, S., Katsovitch, L., Miguel, E.C., and Pauls, D.L. (2005) A family study of early-onset obsessive-compulsive disorder. *Am. J. Med. Genet. B Neuropsychiatr. Genet.* 136:92–97.

Domschke, K., Freitag, C.M., Kuhlenbaumer, G., Schirmacher, A., Sand, P., Nyhuis, P., Jacob, C., Fritze, J., Franke, P., Rietschel, M., Garritsen, H.S., Fimmers, R., Nothen, M.M., Lesch, K.P., Stogbauer, F., and Deckert, J. (2004) Association of the functional V158M catechol-O-methyl-transferase polymorphism with panic disorder in women. *Int. J. Neuropsychopharmacol.* 7:183–188.

Eaton, W.W., Kessler, R.C., Wittchen, H.U., and Magee, W.J. (1994) Panic and panic disorder in the United States. *Am. J. Psychiatry* 151:413–420.

Ebstein, R.P. (2006) The molecular genetic architecture of human personality: beyond self-report questionnaires. *Mol. Psychiatry* 11:427–445.

Fernandez-Teruel, A., Escorihuela, R.M., Gray, J.A., Aguilar, R., Gil, L., Gimenez-Llort, L., Tobena, A., Bhomra, A., Nicod, A., Mott, R., Driscoll, P., Dawson, G.R., and Flint, J. (2002) A quantitative trait locus influencing anxiety in the laboratory rat. *Genome Res.* 12:618–626.

Flament, M.F., Koby, E., Rapoport, J.L., Berg, C.J., Zahn, T., Cox, C., Denckla, M., and Lenane, M. (1990) Childhood obsessive-compulsive disorder: a prospective follow-up study. *J. Child Psychol. Psychiatry* 31:363–380.

Flament, M.F., Whitaker, A., Rapoport, J.L., Davies, M., Berg, C.Z., Kalikow, K., Sceery, W., and Shaffer, D. (1988) Obsessive compulsive disorder in adolescence: an epidemiological study. *J. Am. Acad. Child Adolesc. Psychiatry* 27:764–771.

Flint, J., Corley, R., DeFries, J.C., Fulker, D.W., Gray, J.A., Miller, S., and Collins, A.C. (1995) A simple genetic basis for a complex psychological trait in laboratory mice. *Science* 269:1432–1435.

Flint, J., Valdar, W., Shifman, S., and Mott, R. (2005) Strategies for mapping and cloning quantitative trait genes in rodents. *Nat. Rev. Genet.* 6:271–286.

Fullerton, J., Cubin, M., Tiwari, H., Wang, C., Bomhra, A., Davidson, S., Miller, S., Fairburn, C., Goodwin, G., Neale, M.C., Fiddy, S., Mott, R., Allison, D.B., and Flint, J. (2003) Linkage analysis of extremely discordant and concordant sibling pairs identifies quantitative-trait loci that influence variation in the human personality trait neuroticism. *Am. J. Hum. Genet.* 72:879–890.

Fyer, A.J., Hamilton, S.P., Durner, M., Haghighi, F., Heiman, G.A., Costa, R., Evgrafov, O., Adams, P., de Leon, A.B., Taveras, N., Klein, D.F., Hodge, S.E., Weissman, M.M., and Knowles, J.A. (2006) A third-pass genome scan in panic disorder: evidence for multiple susceptibility loci. *Biol. Psychiatry* 60:388–401.

Fyer, A.J., Lipsitz, J.D., Mannuzza, S., Aronowitz, B., and Chapman, T.F. (2005) A direct interview family study of obsessive-compulsive disorder. I. *Psychol. Med.* 35:1611–1621.

Fyer, A.J., Mannuzza, S., Chapman, T.F., Liebowitz, M.R., and Klein, D.F. (1993) A direct interview family study of social phobia. *Arch. Gen. Psychiatry* 50:286–293.

Fyer, A.J., Mannuzza, S., Chapman, T.F., Martin, L.Y., and Klein, D.F. (1995) Specificity in familial aggregation of phobic disorders. *Arch. Gen. Psychiatry* 52:564–573.

Fyer, A.J., and Weissman, M.M. (1999) Genetic linkage study of panic: clinical methodology and description of pedigrees. *Am. J. Med. Genet. (Neuropsychiatr. Genet.)* 88:173–181.

Geer, J.H. (1965) The development of a scale to measure fear. *Behav. Res. Ther.* 3:45–53.

Gelernter, J., Bonvicini, K., Page, G., Woods, S.W., Goddard, A.W., Kruger, S., Pauls, D.L., and Goodson, S. (2001) Linkage genome scan for loci predisposing to panic disorder or agoraphobia. *Am. J. Med. Genet.* 105:548–557.

Gelernter, J., Page, G.P., Bonvicini, K., Woods, S.W., Pauls, D.L., and Kruger, S. (2003) A chromosome 14 risk locus for simple phobia: results from a genomewide linkage scan. *Mol. Psychiatry* 8:71–82.

Gelernter, J., Page, G.P., Stein, M.B., and Woods, S.W. (2004) Genome-wide linkage scan for loci predisposing to social phobia: evidence for a chromosome 16 risk locus. *Am. J. Psychiatry* 161: 59–66.

Gershenfeld, H.K., Neumann, P.E., Mathis, C., Crawley, J.N., Li, X., and Paul, S.M. (1997) Mapping quantitative trait loci for open-field behavior in mice. *Behav. Genet.* 27:201–210.

Gershenfeld, H.K., and Paul, S.M. (1997) Mapping quantitative trait loci for fear-like behaviors in mice. *Genomics* 46:1–8.

Goldstein, R.B., Wickramaratne, P.J., Horwath, E., and Weissman, M.M. (1997) Familial aggregation and phenomenology of "early-onset" (at or before age 20 years) panic disorder. *Arch. Gen. Psychiatry* 54:271–278.

Goodman, W.K., McDougle, C.J., Price, L.H., Riddle, M.A., Pauls, D.L., and Leckman, J.F. (1990) Beyond the serotonin hypothesis: a role for dopamine in some forms of obsessive compulsive disorder? *J. Clin. Psychiatry* 51(Suppl 8):36–43.

Gorman, J.M., Papp, L.A., Martinez, J., Goetz, R.R., Hollander, E., Liebowitz, M.R., and Jordan, F. (1990) High-dose carbon dioxide challenge test in anxiety disorder patients. *Biol. Psychiatry* 28:743–757.

Grados, M.A., Riddle, M.A., Samuels, J.F., Liang, K.Y., Hoehn-Saric, R., Bienvenu, O.J., Walkup, J.T., Song, D., and Nestadt, G. (2001) The familial phenotype of obsessive-compulsive disorder in relation to tic disorders: the Hopkins OCD family study. *Biol. Psychiatry* 50:559–565.

Gratacos, M., Sahun, I., Gallego, X., Mador-Arjona, A., Estivill, X., and Dierssen, M. (2007) Candidate genes for panic disorder: insight from human and mouse genetic studies. *Genes Brain Behav.* 6:2–23.

Gross, C., Zhuang, X., Stark, K., Ramboz, S., Oosting, R., Kirby, L., Santarelli, L., Beck, S., and Hen, R. (2002) Serotonin1A receptor acts during development to establish normal anxiety-like behaviour in the adult. *Nature* 416:396–400.

Hamilton, S.P., Slager, S.L., De Leon, A.B., Heiman, G.A., Klein, D. F., Hodge, S.E., Weissman, M.M., Fyer, A.J., and Knowles, J.A. (2004) Evidence for genetic linkage between a polymorphism in the adenosine 2A receptor and panic disorder. *Neuropsychopharmacology* 29:558–565.

Hamilton, S.P., Slager, S.L., Heiman, G.A., Deng, Z., Haghighi, F., Klein, D.F., Hodge, S.E., Weissman, M.M., Fyer, A.J., and Knowles, J.A. (2002) Evidence for a susceptibility locus for panic disorder near the catechol-O-methyltransferase gene on chromosome 22. *Biol. Psychiatry* 51:591–601.

Hanna, G.L., Fingerlin, T.E., Himle, J.A., and Boehnke, M. (2005) Complex segregation analysis of obsessive-compulsive disorder in families with pediatric probands. *Hum. Hered.* 60:1–9.

Hanna, G.L., Himle, J.A., Curtis, G.C., and Gillespie, B.W. (2005) A family study of obsessive-compulsive disorder with pediatric probands. *Am. J. Med. Genet. B Neuropsychiatr. Genet.* 134:13–19.

Hanna, G.L., Veenstra-VanderWeele, J., Cox, N.J., Boehnke, M., Himle, J.A., Curtis, G.C., Leventhal, B.L., and Cook, E.H., Jr. (2002) Genome-wide linkage analysis of families with obsessive-compulsive disorder ascertained through pediatric probands. *Am. J. Med. Genet.* 114:541–552.

Hanna, G.L., Veenstra-VanderWeele, J., Cox, N.J., Van Etten, M., Fischer, D.J., Himle, J.A., Bivens, N.C., Wu, X., Roe, C.A., Hennessy, K.A., Dickel, D.E., Leventhal, B.L., and Cook, E.H., Jr. (2007) Evidence for a susceptibility locus on chromosome 10p15 in early-onset obsessive-compulsive disorder. *Biol. Psychiatry* 62 (8):831–832.

Hasler, G., Pinto, A., Greenberg, B.D., Samuels, J., Fyer, A.J., Pauls, D., Knowles, J.A., McCracken, J.T., Piacentini, J., Riddle, M.A., Rauch, S.L., Rasmussen, S.A., Willour, V.L., Grados, M.A., Cullen, B., Bienvenu, O.J., Shugart, Y.Y., Liang, K.Y., Hoehn-Saric, R., Wang, Y., Ronquillo, J., Nestadt, G., and Murphy, D.L. (2007) Familiality of factor analysis-derived YBOCS dimensions in OCD-affected sibling pairs from the OCD Collaborative Genetics Study. *Biol. Psychiatry* 61:617–625.

Hasselbalch, S.G., Hansen, E.S., Jakobsen, T.B., Pinborg, L.H., Lonborg, J.H., and Bolwig, T.G. (2007) Reduced midbrain-pons serotonin transporter binding in patients with obsessive-compulsive disorder. *Acta Psychiatr. Scand.* 115:388–394.

Heisler, L.K., Chu, H.M., Brennan, T.J., Danao, J.A., Bajwa, P., Parsons, L.H., and Tecott, L.H. (1998) Elevated anxiety and antidepressant-like responses in serotonin 5-HT1A receptor mutant mice. *Proc. Natl. Acad Sci. USA* 95:15049–15054.

Hemmings, S.M., and Stein, D.J. (2006) The current status of association studies in obsessive-compulsive disorder. *Psychiatry Clin. North Am.* 29:411–444.

Hesse, S., Muller, U., Lincke, T., Barthel, H., Villmann, T., Angermeyer, M.C., Sabri, O., and Stengler-Wenzke, K. (2005) Serotonin and dopamine transporter imaging in patients with obsessive-compulsive disorder. *Psychiatry Res. Neuroimaging* 140:63–72.

Hettema, J.M., Neale, M.C., and Kendler, K.S. (2001) A review and meta-analysis of the genetic epidemiology of anxiety disorders. *Am. J. Psychiatry* 158:1568–1578.

Hettema, J.M., Neale, M.C., Myers, J.M., Prescott, C.A., and Kendler, K.S. (2006) A population-based twin study of the relationship between neuroticism and internalizing disorders. *Am. J. Psychiatry* 163:857–864.

Hettema, J.M., Prescott, C.A., and Kendler, K.S. (2001) A population-based twin study of generalized anxiety disorder in men and women. *J. Nerv. Ment. Dis.* 189:413–420.

Hettema, J.M., Prescott, C.A., and Kendler, K.S. (2004) Genetic and environmental sources of covariation between generalized anxiety disorder and neuroticism. *Am. J. Psychiatry* 161:1581–1587.

Hettema, J.M., Prescott, C.A., Myers, J.M., Neale, M.C., and Kendler, K.S. (2005) The structure of genetic and environmental risk factors for anxiety disorders in men and women. *Arch. Gen. Psychiatry* 62:182–189.

Hollingsworth, C.E., Tanguay, P.E., Grossman, L., and Pabst, P. (1980) Long-term outcome of obsessive-compulsive disorder in childhood. *J. Am. Acad. Child Adolesc. Psychiatry* 19:134–144.

Holmes, A. (2001) Targeted gene mutation approaches to the study of anxiety-like behavior in mice. *Neurosci. Biobehav. Rev.* 25: 261–273.

Hopper, J.L., Judd, F.K., Derrick, P.L., and Burrows, G.D. (1987) A family study of panic disorder. *Genet. Epidemiol.* 4:33–41.

Horwath, E., Adams, P., Wickramaratne, P., Pine, D., and Weissman, M.M. (1997) Panic disorder with smothering symptoms: evidence for increased risk in first-degree relatives. *Depress. Anxiety* 6:147–153.

Hu, X.Z., Lipsky, R.H., Zhu, G., Akhtar, L.A., Taubman, J., Greenberg, B.D., Xu, K., Arnold, P.D., Richter, M.A., Kennedy, J.L., Murphy, D.L., and Goldman, D. (2006) Serotonin transporter promoter gain-of-function genotypes are linked to obsessive-compulsive disorder. *Am. J. Hum. Genet.* 78:815–826.

Hudziak, J.J., van Beijsterveldt, C.E.M., Althoff, R.R., Stanger, C., Rettew, D.C., Nelson, E.C., Todd, R.D., Bartels, M., and Boomsma, D.I. (2004) Genetic and environmental contributions to the Child Behavior Checklist Obsessive-Compulsive Scale: A cross-cultural twin study. *Arch. Gen. Psychiatry* 61:608–616.

Jang, K.L., Livesley, W.J., and Vernon, P.A. (1996) Heritability of the big five personality dimensions and their facets: a twin study. *J. Pers.* 64:577–591.

Jonnal, A.H., Gardner, C.O., Prescott, C.A., and Kendler, K.S. (2000) Obsessive and compulsive symptoms in a general population sample of female twins. *Am. J. Med. Genet.* 96:791–796.

Jylha, P., and Isometsa, E. (2006) The relationship of neuroticism and extraversion to symptoms of anxiety and depression in the general population. *Depress. Anxiety* 23:281–289.

Kaabi, B., Gelernter, J., Woods, S.W., Goddard, A., Page, G.P., and Elston, R.C. (2006) Genome scan for loci predisposing to anxiety disorders using a novel multivariate approach: strong evidence for a chromosome 4 risk locus. *Am. J. Hum. Genet.* 78:543–553.

Karayiorgou, M., Altemus, M., Galke, B.L., Goldman, D., Murphy, D.L., Ott, J., and Gogos, J.A. (1997) Genotype determining low catechol-O-methyltransferase activity as a risk factor for obsessivecompulsive disorder. *Proc. Natl. Acad. Sci. USA* 94:4572–4575.

Karayiorgou, M., Sobin, C., Blundell, M.L., Galke, B.L., Malinova, L., Goldberg, P., Ott, J., and Gogos, J.A. (1999) Family-based association studies support a sexually dimorphic effect of COMT and MAOA on genetic susceptibility to obsessive-compulsive disorder. *Biol. Psychiatry* 45:1178–1189.

Karno, M., Golding, J.M., Sorenson, S.B., and Burnam, M.A. (1988) The epidemiology of obsessive-compulsive disorder in five US communities. *Arch. Gen. Psychiatry* 45:1094–1099.

Kendler, K.S. (1996) Major depression and generalised anxiety disorder. Same genes, (partly) different environments—revisited. *Br. J. Psychiatry* 30(Suppl):68–75.

Kendler, K.S., Gardner, C.O., Gatz, M., and Pedersen, N.L. (2007) The sources of co-morbidity between major depression and generalized anxiety disorder in a Swedish national twin sample. *Psychol. Med.* 37:453–462.

Kendler, K.S., Gatz, M., Gardner, C.O., and Pedersen, N.L. (2006) Personality and major depression: a Swedish longitudinal, population-based twin study. *Arch. Gen. Psychiatry* 63:1113–1120.

Kendler, K.S., Myers, J., Prescott, C.A., and Neale, M.C. (2001) The genetic epidemiology of irrational fears and phobias in men. *Arch. Gen. Psychiatry* 58:257–265.

Kendler, K.S., Neale, M.C., Kessler, R.C., Heath, A.C., and Eaves, L.J. (1992a) Major depression and generalized anxiety disorder. Same genes, (partly) different environments? *Arch. Gen. Psychiatry* 49:716–722.

Kendler, K.S., Neale, M.C., Kessler, R.C., Heath, A.C., and Eaves, L.J. (1992b) The genetic epidemiology of phobias in women. The interrelationship of agoraphobia, social phobia, situational phobia, and simple phobia. *Arch. Gen. Psychiatry* 49:273–281.

Kendler, K.S., Neale, M.C., Kessler, R.C., Heath, A.C., and Eaves, L.J. (1993a) Major depression and phobias: the genetic and environmental sources of comorbidity. *Psychol. Med.* 23:361–371.

Kendler, K.S., Neale, M.C., Kessler, R.C., Heath, A.C., and Eaves, L.J. (1993b) Panic disorder in women: a population-based twin study. *Psychol. Med.* 23:397–406.

Kennedy, J.L., Neves-Pereira, M., King, N., Lizak, M.V., Basile, V.S., Chartier, M.J., and Stein, M.B. (2001) Dopamine system genes not linked to social phobia. *Psychiatr. Genet.* 11:213–217.

Kessler, R.C., Berglund, P., Demler, O., Jin, R., Merikangas, K.R., and Walters, E.E. (2005) Lifetime prevalence and age-of-onset distributions of DSM-IV disorders in the National Comorbidity Survey Replication. *Arch. Gen. Psychiatry* 62:593–602.

Kessler, R.C., Chiu, W.T., Demler, O., and Walters, E.E. (2005) Prevalence, severity, and comorbidity of 12-month DSM-IV disorders in the National Comorbidity Survey Replication. *Arch. Gen. Psychiatry* 62:617–627.

Kishimoto, T., Radulovic, J., Radulovic, M., Lin, C.R., Schrick, C., Hooshmand, F., Hermanson, O., Rosenfeld, M.G., and Spiess, J. (2000) Deletion of crhr2 reveals an anxiolytic role for corticotropin- releasing hormone receptor-2. *Nat. Genet.* 24:415–419.

Klein, D.F. (1964) Delineation of two drug-responsive anxiety syndromes. *Psychopharmacology* 5:397–408.

Klein, D.F. (1993) False suffocation alarms, spontaneous panics, and related conditions. An integrative hypothesis. *Arch. Gen. Psychiatry* 50:306–317.

Klein, R.J., Zeiss, C., Chew, E.Y., Tsai, J.Y., Sackler, R.S., Haynes, C., Henning, A.K., SanGiovanni, J.P., Mane, S.M., Mayne, S.T., Bracken, M.B., Ferris, F.L., Ott, J., Barnstable, C., and Hoh, J. (2005) Complement factor H polymorphism in age-related macular degeneration. *Science* 308:385–389.

Klemenhagen, K.C., Gordon, J.A., David, D.J., Hen, R., and Gross, C.T. (2005) Increased fear response to contextual cues in mice lacking the 5-HT1A receptor. *Neuropsychopharmacology* 31: 101–111.

Knowles, J.A., Fyer, A.J., Vieland, V.J., Weissman, M.M., Hodge, S.E., Heiman, G.A., Haghighi, F., de Jesus, G.M., Rassnick, H., Preud'homme-Rivelli, X., Austin, T., Cunjak, J., Mick, S., Fine, L.D., Woodley, K.A., Das, K., Maier, W., Adams, P.B., Freimer, N.B., Klein, D.F., and Gilliam, T.C. (1998) Results of a genome-wide genetic screen for panic disorder. *Am. J. Med. Genet. (Neuropsychiatr. Genet.)* 81:139–147.

Knowles, J.A., and Weissman, M.M. (1995) Panic disorder and agoraphobia. In: Oldham, J.M., and Riba, M.B., eds. *Review of Psychiatry, Volume 14*. Washington, DC: American Psychiatric Press, pp. 383–404.

Kusserow, H., Davies, B., Hortnagl, H., Voigt, I., Stroh, T., Bert, B., Deng, D.R., Fink, H., Veh, R.W., and Theuring, F. (2004) Reduced anxiety-related behaviour in transgenic mice overexpressing serotonin1A receptors. *Mol. Brain Res.* 129:104–116.

Lake, R.I., Eaves, L.J., Maes, H.H., Heath, A.C., and Martin, N.G. (2000) Further evidence against the environmental transmission of individual differences in neuroticism from a collaborative study of 45,850 twins and relatives on two continents. *Behav. Genet.* 30:223–233.

Lam, P., Hong, C.J., and Tsai, S.J. (2005) Association study of A2a adenosine receptor genetic polymorphism in panic disorder. *Neurosci. Lett.* 378:98–101.

Lensi, P., Cassano, G.B., Correddu, G., Ravagli, S., Kunovac, J.L., and Akiskal, H.S. (1996) Obsessive-compulsive disorder. Familial-developmental history, symptomatology, comorbidity and course with special reference to gender- related differences. *Br. J. Psychiatry* 169:101–107.

Leonard, H.L., Lenane, M.C., Swedo, S.E., Rettew, D.C., Gershon, E.S., and Rapoport, J.L. (1992) Tics and Tourette's disorder: a 2- to 7-year follow-up of 54 obsessive- compulsive children. *Am. J. Psychiatry* 149:1244–1251.

Leonard, H.L., Swedo, S.E., Garvey, M., Beer, D., Perlmutter, S., Lougee, L., Karitani, M., and Dubbert, B. (1999) Postinfectious and other forms of obsessive-compulsive disorder. *Child Adolesc. Psychiatry Clin. N. Am.* 8:497–511.

Lesch, K.-P., Bengel, D., Heils, A., Sabol, S.Z., Greenberg, B.D., Petri, S., Benjamin, J., Müller, C.R., Hamer, D.H., and Murphy, D. L. (1996) Association of anxiety-related traits with a polymorphism in the serotonin transporter gene regulatory region. *Science* 274:1527–1531.

Lewis, A. (1936) Problems of obsessional illness. *Proc. Royal Soc. Med.* 29:325–336.

Lichtenstein, P., and Annas, P. (2000) Heritability and prevalence of specific fears and phobias in childhood. *J. Child Psychol. Psychiatry* 41:927–937.

Lin, P.Y. (2007) Meta-analysis of the association of serotonin transporter gene polymorphism with obsessive-compulsive disorder. *Prog. Neuro-Psychopharm. Biol. Psychiatry* 31:683–689.

Lougee, L., Perlmutter, S.J., Nicolson, R., Garvey, M.A., and Swedo, S.E. (2000) Psychiatric disorders in first-degree relatives of children with pediatric autoimmune neuropsychiatric disorders associated with streptococcal infections (PANDAS). *J. Am. Acad. Child Adolesc. Psychiatry* 39:1120–1126.

MacKinnon, D.F., McMahon, F.J., Simpson, S.G., McInnis, M.G., and DePaulo, J.R. (1997) Panic disorder with familial bipolar disorder. *Biol. Psychiatry* 42:90–95.

MacKinnon, D.F., Xu, J., McMahon, F.J., Simpson, S.G., Stine, O.C., McInnis, M.G., and DePaulo, J.R. (1998) Bipolar disorder and panic disorder in families: an analysis of chromosome 18 data. *Am. J. Psychiatry* 155:829–831.

MacKinnon, D.F., Zandi, P.P., Cooper, J., Potash, J.B., Simpson, S. G., Gershon, E., Nurnberger, J., Reich, T., and DePaulo, J.R. (2002) Comorbid bipolar disorder and panic disorder in families with a high prevalence of bipolar disorder. *Am. J. Psychiatry* 159: 30–35.

MacKinnon, D.F., Zandi, P.P., Gershon, E.S., Nurnberger, J.I., Jr., and DePaulo, J.R., Jr. (2003) Association of rapid mood switching with panic disorder and familial panic risk in familial bipolar disorder. *Am. J. Psychiatry* 160:1696–1698.

Mackintosh, M.A., Gatz, M., Wetherell, J.L., and Pedersen, N.L. (2006) A twin study of lifetime generalized anxiety disorder (GAD) in older adults: genetic and environmental influences shared by neuroticism and GAD. *Twin Res. Hum. Genet.* 9:30–37.

Maier, W., Lichtermann, D., Minges, J., Oehrlein, A., and Franke, P. (1993) A controlled family study in panic disorder. *J. Psychiatry Res.* 27:79–87.

Mannuzza, S., Schneier, F.R., Chapman, T.F., Liebowitz, M.R., Klein, D.F., and Fyer, A.J. (1995) Generalized social phobia. Reliability and validity. *Arch. Gen. Psychiatry* 52:230–237.

Mathews, C.A., Nievergelt, C.M., Azzam, A., Garrido, H., Chavira, D.A., Wessel, J., Bagnarello, M., Reus, V.I., and Schork, N.J. (2007) Heritability and clinical features of multigenerational families with obsessive-compulsive disorder and hoarding. *Am. J. Med. Genet. B Neuropsychiatr. Genet.* 144:174–182.

McCauley, J.L., Olson, L.M., Dowd, M., Amin, T., Steele, A., Blakely, R.D., Folstein, S.E., Haines, J.L., and Sutcliffe, J.S. (2004) Linkage and association analysis at the serotonin transporter (SLC 6A4) locus in a rigid-compulsive subset of autism. *Am. J. Med. Genet. B Neuropsychiatr. Genet.* 127:104–112.

Mendlewicz, J., Papadimitriou, G., and Wilmotte, J. (1993) Family study of panic disorder: comparison with generalized anxiety disorder, major depression and normal subjects. *Psychiatry Genet.* 3:73–78.

Middeldorp, C.M., de Geus, E.J., Beem, A.L., Lakenberg, N., Hottenga, J.J., Slagboom, P.E., and Boomsma, D.I. (2007) Family based association analyses between the serotonin transporter gene polymorphism (5-HTTLPR) and neuroticism, anxiety and depression. *Behav. Genet.* 37:294–301.

Miguel, E.C., Leckman, J.F., Rauch, S., do Rosario-Campos, M.C., Hounie, A.G., Mercadante, M.T., Chacon, P., and Pauls, D.L. (2004) Obsessive-compulsive disorder phenotypes: implications for genetic studies. *Mol. Psychiatry* 10:258–275.

Moreau, J.L., Kilpatrick, G., and Jenck, F. (1997) Urocortin, a novel neuropeptide with anxiogenic-like properties. *Neuroreport* 8: 1697–1701.

Mott, R., Talbot, C.J., Turri, M.G., Collins, A.C., and Flint, J. (2000) A method for fine mapping quantitative trait loci in outbred animal stocks. *Proc. Natl. Acad. Sci. USA* 97:12649–12654.

Murphy, T.K., Goodman, W.K., Fudge, M.W., Williams, R.C., Jr., Ayoub, E.M., Dalal, M., Lewis, M.H., and Zabriskie, J.B. (1997) B lymphocyte antigen D8/17: a peripheral marker for childhood-onset obsessive-compulsive disorder and Tourette's syndrome? *Am. J. Psychiatry* 154:402–407.

Myers, J.K., Weissman, M.M., Tischler, G.L., Holzer, C.E. III, Leaf, P.J., Orvaschel, H., Anthony, J.C., Boyd, J.H., Burke, J.D., Jr., and Kramer, M. (1984) Six-month prevalence of psychiatric disorders in three communities 1980 to 1982. *Arch. Gen. Psychiatry* 41:959–967.

Nash, M.W., Huezo-Diaz, P., Williamson, R.J., Sterne, A., Purcell, S., Hoda, F., Cherny, S.S., Abecasis, G.R., Prince, M., Gray, J.A., Ball, D., Asherson, P., Mann, A., Goldberg, D., McGuffin, P., Farmer, A., Plomin, R., Craig, I.W., and Sham, P.C. (2004) Genome-wide linkage analysis of a composite index of neuroticism and mood-related scales in extreme selected sibships. *Hum. Mol. Genet.* 13:2173–2182.

Neale, B.M., Sullivan, P.F., and Kendler, K.S. (2005) A genome scan of neuroticism in nicotine dependent smokers. *Am. J. Med. Genet. B Neuropsychiatr. Genet.* 132:65–69.

Nelson, E. and Rice, J. (1997) Stability of diagnosis of obsessive-compulsive disorder in the Epidemiologic Catchment Area Study. *Am. J. Psychiatry* 154:826–831.

Nestadt, G., Lan, T., Samuels, J., Riddle, M., Bienvenu, O.J. III, Liang, K.Y., Hoehn-Saric, R., Cullen, B., Grados, M., Beaty, T. H., and Shugart, Y.Y. (2000) Complex segregation analysis provides compelling evidence for a major gene underlying obsessive-compulsive disorder and for heterogeneity by sex. *Am. J. Hum. Genet.* 67:1611–1616.

Nestadt, G., Samuels, J., Riddle, M., Bienvenu, O.J. III, Liang, K.Y., LaBuda, M., Walkup, J., Grados, M., and Hoehn-Saric, R. (2000) A family study of obsessive-compulsive disorder. *Arch. Gen. Psychiatry* 57:358–363.

Newman, S.C., and Bland, R.C. (2006) A population-based family study of DSM-III generalized anxiety disorder. *Psychol. Med.* 36: 1275–1281.

Noyes, R., Jr., Clarkson, C., Crowe, R.R., Yates, W.R., and McChesney, C.M. (1987) A family study of generalized anxiety disorder. *Am. J. Psychiatry* 144:1019–1024.

Noyes, R., Jr., Crowe, R.R., Harris, E.L., Hamra, B.J., McChesney, C.M., and Chaudhry, D.R. (1986) Relationship between panic disorder and agoraphobia. A family study. *Arch. Gen. Psychiatry* 43:227–232.

Oppenheimer, B.S., and Rothschild, M.A. (1918) The psychoneurotic factor in the irritable heart of soldiers. *JAMA* 70:1919–1922.

Overall, K.L. (2000) Natural animal models of human psychiatric conditions: assessment of mechanism and validity. *Prog. Neuropsychopharmacol. Biol. Psychiatry* 24:727–776.

Ozaki, N., Goldman, D., Kaye, W.H., Plotnicov, K., Greenberg, B. D., Lappalainen, J., Rudnick, G., and Murphy, D.L. (2003) Serotonin transporter missense mutation associated with a complex neuropsychiatric phenotype. *Mol. Psychiatry* 8:933–936.

Parks, C.L., Robinson, P.S., Sibille, E., Shenk, T., and Toth, M. (1998) Increased anxiety of mice lacking the serotonin1A receptor. *Proc. Natl. Acad. Sci. USA* 95:10734–10739.

Pauls, D.L., Alsobrook, J.P., Goodman, W., Rasmussen, S., and Leckman, J.F. (1995) A family study of obsessive-compulsive disorder. *Am. J. Psychiatry* 152:76–84.

Pauls, D.L., Bucher, K.D., Crowe, R.R., and Noyes, R., Jr. (1980) A genetic study of panic disorder pedigrees. *Am. J. Hum. Genet.* 32:639–644.

Pauls, D.L., Crowe, R.R., and Noyes, R., Jr. (1979) Distribution of ancestral secondary cases in anxiety neurosis (panic disorder). *J. Affect. Disord.* 1:387–390.

Pauls, D.L., Noyes, R., Jr., and Crowe, R.R. (1979) The familial prevalence in second-degree relatives of patients with anxiety neurosis (panic disorder). *J. Affect. Disord.* 1:279–285.

Pauls, D.L., Towbin, K.E., Leckman, J.F., Zahner, G.E., and Cohen, D.J. (1986) Gilles de la Tourette's syndrome and obsessive-compulsive disorder. Evidence supporting a genetic relationship. *Arch. Gen. Psychiatry* 43:1180–1182.

Perna, G., Bertani, A., Caldirola, D., and Bellodi, L. (1996) Family history of panic disorder and hypersensitivity to CO2 in patients with panic disorder. *Am. J. Psychiatry* 153: 1060–1064.

Perna, G., Caldirola, D., Arancio, C., and Bellodi, L. (1997) Panic attacks: a twin study. *Psychiatry Res.* 66:69–71.

Perna, G., Cocchi, S., Bertani, A., Arancio, C., and Bellodi, L. (1995) Sensitivity to 35% CO2 in healthy first-degree relatives of patients with panic disorder. *Am. J. Psychiatry* 152:623–625.

Phillips, K., Fulker, D.W., and Rose, R.J. (1987) Path analysis of seven fear factors in adult twin and sibling pairs and their parents. *Genet. Epidemiol.* 4:345–355.

Pine, D.S., Klein, R.G., Roberson-Nay, R., Mannuzza, S., Moulton, J.L. III, Woldehawariat, G., and Guardino, M. (2005) Response to 5% carbon dioxide in children and adolescents: relationship to panic disorder in parents and anxiety disorders in subjects. *Arch. Gen. Psychiatry* 62:73–80.

Pooley, E.C., Fineberg, N., and Harrison, P.J. (2007) The met158 allele of catechol-O-methyltransferase (COMT) is associated with obsessive-compulsive disorder in men: case-control study and meta-analysis. *Mol. Psychiatry* 12:556–561.

Ramboz, S., Oosting, R., Amara, D.A., Kung, H.F., Blier, P., Mendelsohn, M., Mann, J.J., Brunner, D., and Hen, R. (1998) Serotonin receptor 1A knockout: an animal model of anxiety-related disorder. *Proc. Natl. Acad. Sci USA* 95:14476–14481.

Rasmussen, S.A., and Eisen, J.L. (1992) The epidemiology and clinical features of obsessive compulsive disorder. *Psychiatry Clin. North Am.* 15:743–758.

Reschke, A.H., Mannuzza, S., Chapman, T.F., Lipsitz, J.D., Liebowitz, M.R., Gorman, J.M., Klein, D.F., and Fyer, A.J. (1995) Sodium lactate response and familial risk for panic disorder. *Am. J. Psychiatry* 152:277–279.

Rettew, D.C., Vink, J.M., Willemsen, G., Doyle, A., Hudziak, J.J., and Boomsma, D.I. (2006) The genetic architecture of neuroticism in 3301 Dutch adolescent twins as a function of age and sex: a study from the Dutch twin register. *Twin Res. Hum. Genet.* 9:24–29.

Robins, L.N., Helzer, J.E., Weissman, M.M., Orvaschel, H., Gruenberg, E., Burke, J.D., Jr., and Regier, D.A. (1984) Lifetime prevalence of specific psychiatric disorders in three sites. *Arch. Gen. Psychiatry* 41:949–958.

Rose, R.J., and Ditto, W.B. (1983) A developmental-genetic analysis of common fears from early adolescence to early adulthood. *Child Dev.* 54:361–368.

Rothe, C., Gutknecht, L., Freitag, C., Tauber, R., Mossner, R., Franke, P., Fritze, J., Wagner, G., Peikert, G., Wenda, B., Sand, P., Jacob, C., Rietschel, M., Nothen, M.M., Garritsen, H., Fimmers, R., Deckert, J., and Lesch, K.P. (2004) Association of a functional 1019C>G 5-HT1A receptor gene polymorphism with panic disorder with agoraphobia. *Int. J. Neuropsychopharmacol.* 7:189–192.

Rothe, C., Koszycki, D., Bradwejn, J., King, N., Deluca, V., Tharmalingam, S., Macciardi, F., Deckert, J., and Kennedy, J.L. (2006) Association of the Val158Met catechol o-methyltransferase genetic polymorphism with panic disorder. *Neuropsychopharmacol.* 10:2237–2242

Roy, M.A., Neale, M.C., Pedersen, N.L., Mathe, A.A., and Kendler, K.S. (1995) A twin study of generalized anxiety disorder and major depression. *Psychol. Med.* 25:1037–1049.

Ruscio, A.M., Chiu, W.T., Roy-Byrne, P., Stang, P.E., Stein, D.J., Wittchen, H.U., and Kessler, R.C. (2007) Broadening the definition of generalized anxiety disorder: Effects on prevalence and associations with other disorders in the National Comorbidity Survey Replication. *J. Anxiety Disord.* 21:662–676.

Samochowiec, J., Hajduk, A., Samochowiec, A., Horodnicki, J., Stepien, G., Grzywacz, A., and Kucharska-Mazur, J. (2004) Association studies of MAO-A, COMT, and 5-HTT genes polymorphisms in patients with anxiety disorders of the phobic spectrum. *Psychiatry Res.* 128: 21–26.

Samuels, J., Shugart, Y.Y., Grados, M.A., Willour, V.L., Bienvenu, O.J., Greenberg, B.D., Knowles, J.A., McCracken, J.T., Rauch, S.L., Murphy, D.L., Wang, Y., Pinto, A., Fyer, A.J., Piacentini, J., Pauls, D.L., Cullen, B., Rasmussen, S.A., Hoehn-Saric, R., Valle, D., Liang, K.Y., Riddle, M.A., and Nestadt, G. (2007) Significant linkage to compulsive hoarding on chromosome 14 in families with obsessive-compulsive disorder: results from the OCD Collaborative Genetics Study. *Am. J. Psychiatry* 164:493–499.

Santarelli, L., Saxe, M., Gross, C., Surget, A., Battaglia, F., Dulawa, S., Weisstaub, N., Lee, J., Duman, R., Arancio, O., Belzung, C., and Hen, R. (2003) Requirement of hippocampal neurogenesis for the behavioral effects of antidepressants. *Science* 301:805–809.

Scherrer, J.F., True, W.R., Xian, H., Lyons, M.J., Eisen, S.A., Goldberg, J., Lin, N., and Tsuang, M.T. (2000) Evidence for genetic influences common and specific to symptoms of generalized anxiety and panic. *J. Affect. Disord.* 57:25–35.

Scott, L.J., Mohlke, K.L., Bonnycastle, L.L., Willer, C.J., Li, Y., Duren, W.L., Erdos, M.R., Stringham, H.M., Chines, P.S., Jackson, A. U., Prokunina-Olsson, L., Ding, C.J., Swift, A.J., Narisu, N., Hu, T., Pruim, R., Xiao, R., Li, X.Y., Conneely, K.N., Riebow, N.L., Sprau, A.G., Tong, M., White, P.P., Hetrick, K.N., Barnhart, M. W., Bark, C.W., Goldstein, J.L., Watkins, L., Xiang, F., Saramies, J., Buchanan, T.A., Watanabe, R.M., Valle, T.T., Kinnunen, L., Abecasis, G.R., Pugh, E.W., Doheny, K.F., Bergman, R.N., Tuomilehto, J., Collins, F.S., and Boehnke, M. (2007) A genome-wide association study of type 2 diabetes in Finns detects multiple susceptibility variants. *Science* 316:1341–1345.

Sen, S., Burmeister, M., and Ghosh, D. (2004) Meta-analysis of the association between a serotonin transporter promoter polymorphism (5-HTTLPR) and anxiety-related personality traits. *Am. J. Med. Genet. B Neuropsychiatr. Genet.* 127:85–89.

Shekhar, A., McCann, U.D., Meaney, M.J., Blanchard, D.C., Davis, M., Frey, K.A., Liberzon, I., Overall, K.L., Shear, M.K., Tecott, L.H., and Winsky, L. (2001) Summary of a National Institute of Mental Health workshop: developing animal models of anxiety disorders. *Psychopharmacology (Berl)* 157:327–339.

Shifman, S., Bhomra, A., Smiley, S., Wray, N.R., James, M.R., Martin, N.G., Hettema, J.M., An, S.S., Neale, M.C., van den Oord, E.J.C.G., Kendler, K.S., Chen, X., Boomsma, D.I., Middeldorp, C.M., Hottenga, J.J., Slagboom, P.E., and Flint, J. (2008) A whole genome association study of neuroticism using DNA pooling. *Mol. Psychiatry* 13(3):302–312.

Shugart, Y.Y., Samuels, J., Willour, V.L., Grados, M.A., Greenberg, B.D., Knowles, J.A., McCracken, J.T., Rauch, S.L., Murphy, D. L., Wang, Y., Pinto, A., Fyer, A.J., Piacentini, J., Pauls, D.L., Cullen, B., Page, J., Rasmussen, S.A., Bienvenu, O.J., Hoehn-Saric, R., Valle, D., Liang, K.Y., Riddle, M.A., and Nestadt, G. (2006) Genomewide linkage scan for obsessive-compulsive disorder: evidence for susceptibility loci on chromosomes 3q, 7p, 1q, 15q, and 6q. *Mol. Psychiatry* 11:763–770.

Skre, I., Onstad, S., Torgersen, S., Lygren, S., and Kringlen, E. (1993) A twin study of DSM-III-R anxiety disorders. *Acta Psychiatr. Scand.* 88:85–92.

Slater, E., and Shields, J. (1969) Genetical aspects of anxiety. In Lader, M.H., ed. *Studies of Anxiety*. Ashford, UK: Headly Brothers, pp. 62–71.

Smith, G.W., Aubry, J.M., Dellu, F., Contarino, A., Bilezikjian, L. M., Gold, L.H., Chen, R., Marchuk, Y., Hauser, C., Bentley, C.A., Sawchenko, P.E., Koob, G.F., Vale, W., and Lee, K.F. (1998) Corticotropin releasing factor receptor 1-deficient mice display decreased anxiety, impaired stress response, and aberrant neuroendocrine development. *Neuron* 20:1093–1102.

Sobin, C., and Karayiorgou, M. (2000) The genetic basis and neurobiological characteristics of obsessive-compulsive disorder. In: Pfaff, D.W., Berrettini, W.H., Joh, T.H., and Maxson, S.C., eds. *Genetic Influences on Neural and Behavioral Functions*. Boca Raton: CRC Press, pp. 83–104.

Sorensen, G., Lindberg, C., Wortwein, G., Bolwig, T.G., and Woldbye, D.P. (2004) Differential roles for neuropeptide Y Y1 and Y5 receptors in anxiety and sedation. *J. Neurosci. Res.* 77:723–729.

Stein, B., Chartier, J., Kozak, M.V., King, N., and Kennedy, J.L. (1998) Genetic linkage to the serotonin transporter protein and 5HT2A receptor genes excluded in generalized social phobia. *Psychiatry Res.* 81:283–291.

Stein, M.B., Chartier, M.J., Hazen, A.L., Kozak, M.V., Tancer, M.E., Lander, S., Furer, P., Chubaty, D., and Walker, J.R. (1998) A direct-interview family study of generalized social phobia. *Am. J. Psychiatry* 155:90–97.

Stenzel-Poore, M.P., Heinrichs, S.C., Rivest, S., Koob, G.F., and Vale, W.W. (1994) Overproduction of corticotropin-releasing factor in transgenic mice: a genetic model of anxiogenic behavior. *J. Neuroscience* 14:2579–2584.

Stine, O.C., Xu, J., Koskela, R., McMahon, F.J., Gschwend, M., Friddle, C., Clark, C.D., McInnis, M.G., Simpson, S.G., and Breschel, T.S. (1995) Evidence for linkage of bipolar disorder to chromosome 18 with a parent- of-origin effect. *Am. J. Hum. Genet.* 57:1384–1394.

Sullivan, P.F. (2007) Spurious genetic associations. *Biol. Psychiatry* 61:1121–1126.

Sullivan, P.F., Eaves, L.J., Kendler, K.S., and Neale, M.C. (2001) Genetic case-control association studies in neuropsychiatry. *Arch. Gen. Psychiatry* 58:1015–1024.

Sundet, J.M., Skre, I., Okkenhaug, J.J., and Tambs, K. (2003) Genetic and environmental causes of the interrelationships between self-reported fears. A study of a non-clinical sample of Norwegian identical twins and their families. *Scand. J. Psychology* 44:97–106.

Swedo, S.E., Leonard, H.L., Garvey, M., Mittleman, B., Allen, A.J., Perlmutter, S., Lougee, L., Dow, S., Zamkoff, J., and Dubbert, B.K. (1998) Pediatric autoimmune neuropsychiatric disorders associated with streptococcal infections: clinical description of the first 50 cases. *Am. J. Psychiatry* 155:264–271.

Swedo, S.E., Leonard, H.L., Mittleman, B.B., Allen, A.J., Rapoport, J.L., Dow, S.P., Kanter, M.E., Chapman, F., and Zabriskie, J. (1997) Identification of children with pediatric autoimmune neuropsychiatric disorders associated with streptococcal infections by a marker associated with rheumatic fever [see comments]. *Am. J. Psychiatry* 154:110–112.

Swedo, S.E., Rapoport, J.L., Cheslow, D.L., Leonard, H.L., Ayoub, E.M., Hosier, D.M., and Wald, E.R. (1989) High prevalence of obsessive-compulsive symptoms in patients with Sydenham's chorea. *Am. J. Psychiatry* 146:246–249.

Swedo, S.E., Rapoport, J.L., Leonard, H., Lenane, M., and Cheslow, D. (1989) Obsessive-compulsive disorder in children and adolescents. Clinical phenomenology of 70 consecutive cases. *Arch. Gen. Psychiatry* 46:335–341.

Tadic, A., Rujescu, D., Szegedi, A., Giegling, I., Singer, P., Moller, H.J., and Dahmen, N. (2003) Association of a MAOA gene variant with generalized anxiety disorder, but not with panic disorder or major depression. *Am. J. Med. Genet. B Neuropsychiatr. Genet.* 117:1–6.

Talbot, C.J., Nicod, A., Cherny, S.S., Fulker, D.W., Collins, A.C., and Flint, J. (1999) High-resolution mapping of quantitative trait loci in outbred mice. *Nat. Genet.* 21:305–308.

Tecott, L.H. (2003) The genes and brains of mice and men. *Am. J. Psychiatry* 160:646–656.

Thorgeirsson, T.E., Oskarsson, H., Desnica, N., Kostic, J.P., Stefansson, J.G., Kolbeinsson, H., Lindal, E., Gagunashvili, N., Frigge, M.L., Kong, A., Stefansson, K., and Gulcher, J.R. (2003) Anxiety with panic disorder linked to chromosome 9q in Iceland. *Am. J. Hum. Genet.* 72:1221–1230.

Timpl, P., Spanagel, R., Sillaber, I., Kresse, A., Reul, J.M., Stalla, G. K., Blanquet, V., Steckler, T., Holsboer, F., and Wurst, W. (1998) Impaired stress response and reduced anxiety in mice lacking a functional corticotropin-releasing hormone receptor 1. *Nat. Genet.* 19: 162–166.

Torgersen, S. (1979) The nature and origin of common phobic fears. *Br. J. Psychiatry* 134:343–351.

Torgersen, S. (1983) Genetic factors in anxiety disorders. *Arch. Gen. Psychiatry* 40:1085–1089.

Turri, M.G., Datta, S.R., DeFries, J., Henderson, N.D., and Flint, J. (2001) QTL analysis identifies multiple behavioral dimensions in ethological tests of anxiety in laboratory mice. *Curr. Biol.* 11: 725–734.

Turri, M.G., DeFries, J.C., Henderson, N.D., and Flint, J. (2004) Multivariate analysis of quantitative trait loci influencing variation in anxiety-related behavior in laboratory mice. *Mamm. Genome* 15:69–76.

Turri, M.G., Henderson, N.D., DeFries, J.C., and Flint, J. (2001) Quantitative trait locus mapping in laboratory mice derived from a replicated selection experiment for open-field activity. *Genetics* 158:1217–1226.

Turri, M.G., Talbot, C.J., Radcliffe, R.A., Wehner, J.M., and Flint, J. (1999) High-resolution mapping of quantitative trait loci for emotionality in selected strains of mice. *Mamm. Genome* 10: 1098–1101.

van Beek, N., and Griez, E. (2000) Reactivity to a 35% CO_2 challenge in healthy first-degree relatives of patients with panic disorder. *Biol. Psychiatry* 47:830–835.

Van Grootheest, D.S., Cath, D.C., Beekman, A.T., and Boomsma, D.I. (2005) Twin studies on obsessive-compulsive disorder: a review. *Twin Res. Hum. Genet.* 8:450–458.

Van Grootheest, D.S., Cath, D.C., Beekman, A.T., and Boomsma, D.I. (2007) Genetic and environmental influences on obsessive-compulsive symptoms in adults: a population-based twin-family study. *Psychol. Med.* 11:1635–1644.

Veenstra-VanderWeele, J., Kim, S.J., Gonen, D., Hanna, G.L., Leventhal, B.L., and Cook, E.H., Jr. (2001) Genomic organization of the SLC1A1/EAAC1 gene and mutation screening in early-onset obsessive-compulsive disorder. *Mol. Psychiatry* 6:160–167.

Vieland, V.J., Goodman, D.W., Chapman, T., and Fyer, A.J. (1996) New segregation analysis of panic disorder. *Am. J. Med. Genet.* 67:147–153.

Vieland, V.J., Hodge, S.E., Lish, J.D., Adams, P., and Weissman, M.M. (1993) Segregation analysis of panic disorder. *Psychiatry Genet.* 3:63–71.

Wehner, J.M., Radcliffe, R.A., Rosmann, S.T., Christensen, S.C., Rasmussen, D.L., Fulker, D.W., and Wiles, M. (1997) Quantitative trait locus analysis of contextual fear conditioning in mice. *Nat. Genet.* 17:331–334.

Weissman, M.M. (1993) Family genetic studies of panic disorder. *J. Psychiatry Res.* 27:69–78.

Weissman, M.M., Bland, R.C., Canino, G.J., Faravelli, C., Greenwald, S., Hwu, H.-G., Joyce, P.R., Karam, E.G., Lee, C.-K., Lellouch, J., Lépine, J.-P., Newman, S.C., Oakley-Browne, M.A., Rubio-Stipec, M., Wells, J.E., Wickramaratne, P.J., Wittchen, H.-U., and Yeh, E.-K. (1997) The cross-national epidemiology of panic disorder. *Arch. Gen. Psychiatry* 54:305–309.

Weissman, M.M., Bland, R.C., Canino, G.J., Greenwald, S., Hwu, H.G., Lee, C.K., Newman, S.C., Oakley-Browne, M.A., Rubio-Stipec, M., and Wickramaratne, P.J. (1994) The cross national epidemiology of obsessive compulsive disorder. The Cross National Collaborative Group. *J. Clin. Psychiatry* 55(Suppl): 5–10.

Weissman, M.M., Wickramaratne, P.J., Adams, P.B., Lish, J.D., Horwath, E., Charney, D., Woods, S.W., Leeman, E., and Frosch, E. (1993) The relationship between panic disorder and major depression. *Arch. Gen. Psychiatry* 50:767–780.

Weissman, M.M., Wickramaratne, P., Nomura, Y., Warner, V., Verdeli, H., Pilowsky, D.J., Grillon, C., and Bruder, G. (2005) Families at high and low risk for depression: a 3-generation study. *Arch. Gen. Psychiatry* 62:29–36.

Wellcome Trust Case Control Consortium. (2007) Genome-wide association study of 14,000 cases of seven common diseases and 3,000 shared controls. *Nature* 447:661–678.

Wendland, J.R., Kruse, M.R., Cromer, K.C., and Murphy, D.L. (2007) A large case-control study of common functional SLC6A4 and BDNF variants in obsessive-compulsive disorder. *Neuropsychopharmacology* 32:2543–2551.

Weninger, S.C., Dunn, A.J., Muglia, L.J., Dikkes, P., Miczek, K.A., Swiergiel, A.H., Berridge, C.W., and Majzoub, J.A. (1999) Stress-induced behaviors require the corticotropin-releasing hormone (CRH) receptor, but not CRH. *Proc. Natl. Acad. Sci. USA* 96: 8283–8288.

Willis-Owen, S.A., and Flint, J. (2006) The genetic basis of emotional behaviour in mice. *Eur. J. Hum. Genet.* 14:721–728.

Willis-Owen, S.A.G., Turri, M.G., Munafo, M.R., Surtees, P.G., Wainwright, N.W.J., Brixey, R.D., and Flint, J. (2005) The serotonin transporter length polymorphism, neuroticism, and depression: a comprehensive assessment of association. *Biol. Psychiatry* 58: 451–456.

Willour, V.L., Yao, S.Y., Samuels, J., Grados, M., Cullen, B., Bienvenu, O.J. III, Wang, Y., Liang, K.Y., Valle, D., Hoehn-Saric, R., Riddle, M., and Nestadt, G. (2004) Replication study supports evidence for linkage to 9p24 in obsessive-compulsive disorder. *Am. J. Hum. Genet.* 75:508–513.

Woo, J.M., Yoon, K.S., Choi, Y.H., Oh, K.S., Lee, Y.S., and Yu, B.H. (2004) The association between panic disorder and the L/L genotype of catechol-O-methyltransferase. *J. Psychiatric Res.* 38: 365–370.

Woo, J.M., Yoon, K.S., and Yu, B.H. (2002) Catechol O-methyltransferase genetic polymorphism in panic disorder. *Am. J. Psychiatry* 159:1785–1787.

Yamada, K., Hattori, E., Shimizu, M., Sugaya, A., Shibuya, H., and Yoshikawa, T. (2001) Association studies of the cholecystokinin B receptor and A2a adenosine receptor genes in panic disorder. *J. Neural Transm.* 108:837–848.

Zorrilla, E.P., Valdez, G.R., Nozulak, J., Koob, G.F., and Markou, A. (2002) Effects of antalarmin, a CRF type 1 receptor antagonist, on anxiety-like behavior and motor activation in the rat. *Brain Res.* 952:188–199.

39 The Neurobiology of Fear and Anxiety: Contributions of Animal Models to Current Understanding

GREGORY M. SULLIVAN, JACEK DEBIEC, DAVID E.A. BUSH, DAVID M. LYONS, AND JOSEPH E. LEDOUX

Animal models have played an essential role in elucidating the pathophysiology of a broad range of human diseases. The yield from animal work in the behavioral sciences is becoming increasingly realized, especially in anxiety and other psychiatric disorders. Animal models offer unparalleled access to the biochemical pathways, cellular mechanisms, synaptic changes, and neuronal circuits that mediate the physiological and behavioral responses of fear, anxiety, and avoidance. There has been a broader appreciation of the relevance of many decades of neuroscience studies for elucidating the neurobiology mediating anxious behaviors. Notable progress has been especially made in understanding innate and learned fear.

Recent years have seen more cross-disciplinary communication and collaborations between clinical researchers of the anxiety disorders and neuroscientists focused on the underpinnings of emotional behaviors. Greater emphasis has been placed on the translational potential of animal models for the development of novel therapeutic approaches to pathological anxiety, and the fruits of these labors are beginning to emerge. Although there is no ideal or comprehensive model for any particular anxiety disorder, there has been the reciprocal development of more clinically informed animal models. To this end, adaptations of existing animal models of anxiety allow an improved ability to investigate key aspects of psychopathology. This chapter focuses on the fundamental contributions of animal models to the emerging understanding of fearful and anxious behaviors and the neuropathologies that underlie the anxiety disorders.

WHAT IS FEAR?

Imagine this. You step into the street. Without a thought, you jump back, barely avoiding being struck down. You find yourself back on the curb trembling, breaking out in a sweat; your heart is racing, you can barely catch your breath; the "feeling of adrenaline" is spreading throughout your body, you feel nauseated, confused; the environment seems unreal. Only after do you realize a car was moving directly toward you at high speed. Knowing that you escaped fate, your reaction quickly subsides. You feel back to yourself in the next few minutes. What happened? Simply put, you just witnessed the operation of one of the most basic emotion systems of the brain: the fear system. This system, which evolved to cope with sudden dangers, was activated more or less unconsciously by the sensory input coming though your visual system. It saved you from harm.

Fear occurs when one encounters stimuli that predict danger. It is a normal and adaptive response to a threatening situation. Activation of the fear system results in a coordinated and rapid array of behavioral, autonomic, and endocrine changes that enhance the likelihood of the organism's survival. Yet we often refer to fear as if it were solely a subjective state of consciousness. William James (1884) pointed out over a century ago that the conscious feeling of fear that a human experiences when confronted with a threat is but one outcome of an array of responses rather than the essence of the underlying emotion, and that, contrary to popular opinion, behavioral and physiological responses during emotion do not depend on conscious processing. Indeed, all animals have the ability to detect danger and respond physiologically in such a way as to enhance the probability of survival, regardless of whether they are able to consciously experience fear (LeDoux, 1996, 2000). When you jumped back from the speeding car, you were unconsciously responding to the threat. A conscious feeling of fear played no role. Recent human studies support the idea that conscious awareness of fear-inducing stimuli is not requisite for the production of emotional responses (Ohman and Mineka, 2001; Whalen et al., 2004; Phelps, 2006).

The defensive behavioral responses to adverse challenge are often termed "freeze, fight, or flight" behaviors. The concurrent physiological changes generally support these motor responses by increasing availability of energy and shifting blood supply to body systems necessary for immediate defense, namely the brain and musculoskeletal system. Included are changes in the autonomic nervous system and the release of stress hormones. These are components of Selye's (1950) general adaptation system. In the short run, they support behavioral responses that increase survival, such as enhancement of learning and memory (McGaugh and Roozendaal, 2002). Over time, however, they can lead to maladaptive consequences, including impairments in memory and other cognitive functions and physical well-being (McEwen, 2004).

Converging evidence has shown that despite the great differences in the sensory, cognitive, and behavioral capacities of the human brain compared with those of other animal species (Kalueff and Tuohimaa, 2004), the systems that have evolved in all animals to detect danger and regulate the fear response involve similar molecular, cellular, and circuitry mechanisms (LeDoux, 1996, 2000; Maren, 2001; Kalin et al. 2004; Phelps, 2004; Sotres-Bayon et al., 2004; Phelps and LeDoux, 2005; Quirk and Beer, 2006). In humans, monkeys, and rodents, a temporal lobe region known as the amygdala plays a key role in threat processing, the medial prefrontal cortex (PFC) plays a key role in fear regulation, and the hippocampus plays a key role in providing information about the context in which a threatening challenge is occurring (Figure 39.1). Therefore, regardless of whether other animals have conscious feelings of emotion similar to those experienced by humans, the fundamental similarities in the evolutionarily conserved fear networks form the basis for exploring the mechanisms underlying the behavioral and physiological responses associated with fear using animal models. Nonhuman primate models play a vital role in bridging the gap between rodent models and clinical studies in humans, particularly with regard to elucidating the functional neuroanatomy of brain regions such as PFC in which the prospects for rodent research are limited by phylogeny.

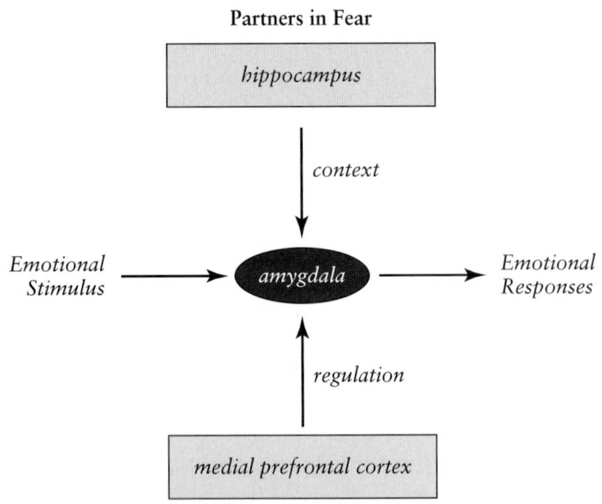

FIGURE 39.1 Partners in fear—amygdala, hippocampus, vmPFC. vmPFC: ventromedial prefrontal cortex.

THE CONTRAST BETWEEN FEAR AND ANXIETY

Like fear, anxiety is a normal and adaptive response that ensures dangers are either avoided or reduced through preparation and vigilance. Well-defined threatening stimuli that are immediately present or imminent in the environment elicit a fear response. When the threat is more poorly defined and temporally remote, such as anticipation of a future adverse or threatening circumstance, the behavioral state it elicits is typically referred to as anxiety. From this perspective, an operational distinction between fear and anxiety is that fear is a sensory-driven and time-limited response to potential adversity, whereas anxiety is a preparatory state activated by cognitive processes predicting more distant future adversity. This activated state may be time limited or self-sustaining. It may also be reinforced further by the arousal of the fear system by external stimuli, internal stimuli (somatic sensations of the fear response itself), or cognitive processes ruminating on potential adversity, whether real or imagined, and whether the threat is possible and likely or physically impossible, at least as we understand the world (alien abduction).

A distinction between state anxiety and trait anxiety in humans has often been emphasized (Spielberger et al., 1970). State anxiety is considered a transient response elicited by a particular stimulus or situation. Trait anxiety is considered an enduring or chronic anxious condition that is present across multiple situations. Trait anxiety is not necessarily pathological, as it may improve survival depending on the environmental challenges encountered. For example, in chimpanzees the level of maternal vigilance for ensuring the safety of their dependent offspring from outside predation, as well as danger from conspecifics, members of their own species, is an adaptive anxious trait (Kutsukake, 2006). Only when such traits lead to behaviors that are counterproductive to a healthy or adaptive lifestyle does a disorder exist.

PATHOLOGICAL FEAR AND ANXIETY

Fear and anxiety become pathological when they are exaggerated in form, are nonadaptive with respect to environmental challenges, and result in marked disability and/or maladaptive avoidance. As we just noted, under some conditions hypervigilance is adaptive. However, it is also a common symptom of posttraumatic stress disorder (PTSD) and is considered pathological in this anxiety disorder because it is activated by situations or contexts in which threat is unlikely to be present.

Pathological anxiety is not unique to humans. A common example occurs in certain breeds of dogs that exhibit objective physiological and behavioral responses remarkably similar to several clinical anxiety syndromes in humans including separation anxiety, specific phobias (thunder, loud or noxious noises), panic-like attacks, posttraumatic stress responses, and compulsive behaviors (Overall, 2000). Moreover, there are a number of rodent and nonhuman primate models of pathological fear and anxiety that have been developed for neurobiological study in the laboratory. Despite our inability to gauge the conscious experience of the afflicted animal, the pathological anxiety syndromes observed in animals represent convincing models for pathological states of anxiety in humans. Support for the notion of common underlying neurobiological substrates is provided by the fact that the same classes of pharmacological treatments and behavioral interventions shown to be efficacious in human anxiety disorders also relieve the signs of pathological anxiety in monkeys, dogs, and rodents (Kalin et al., 1991; Overall, 1997; Huot et al., 2001; Burghardt et al., 2004).

The term *anxiety* is often used as if it describes one basic emotional state. Yet the term is employed clinically and colloquially to label a number of quite diverse psychic and physical symptoms. Table 39.1 lists common symptoms of anxiety, divided into broader categories of psychic, somatic, and motoric anxiety symptoms. Because most of these symptoms require self-report, it might appear untenable to elucidate the underlying brain mechanisms by use of animal models. Yet the current diagnostic method in psychiatry involves a patient interview regarding the behavioral and physiological symptoms experienced over time, and, to a lesser extent, anxious behaviors observed by the clinician during the interview. In other words, the patient is asked to provide a retrospective report from the perspective of an observer of the symptoms that lead to seeking treatment. One could imagine an alternative method, albeit impractical, in which instead the clinician trailed the patient for some period of time, scoring different behaviors and measuring physiological responses manifested upon the variety of daily challenges of life. From this perspective, investigating the mediators of the defensive behaviors and the physiological responses within controlled environmental conditions in animal models of anxiety is a reasonable approach for revealing the neurobiology underlying the expression of anxiety signs and symptoms that occur naturalistically in humans.

TABLE 39.1 *Examples of the Wide Array of Symptoms Encompassed by the Term Anxiety*

Psychic
Ruminative inappropriate worry
Catastrophic misappraisals
Feelings of unreality (derealization)
Feeling outside one's self (depersonalization)
Overwhelming urge to flee
Somatic
Shortness of breath
Chest pressure, pains, or tightness
Palpitations or heart pounding
Sweating or hot flushes
Chills
Dry mouth
Choking sensation
Nausea or abdominal discomfort
Urinary urgency
Hyperesthesia
Numbness or tingling
Motoric
Feeling "jittery" or "keyed up"
Muscular tension
Fidgeting or pacing
Akisthisia-like agitation

Human anxiety disorders are currently diagnosed using the categorical system of the American Psychiatric Association's *Diagnostic and Statistical Manual of Mental Disorders* (*DSM*). Most of the anxiety disorders included in the current edition (*DSM-IV-TR*) are characterized by extreme symptoms of fear, anxiety, and avoidance that, by definition, have been significantly impairing to the individual's psychosocial function (American Psychiatric Association, 2000). They are grouped into the diagnostic class of anxiety disorders based on subjective criterion of shared phenomenological features. It is the unique constellations of these features that distinguish the anxiety disorders diagnostically.

In the *DSM-V*, due to be completed in a few years, there will be greater emphasis on categorizing mood and anxiety conditions within an empirically based structure that reflects inherent similarities among disorders (Watson, 2005). Underlying factor analytic structural dimensions, supported by genotypic evidence, point to a reclassification of panic disorder, agoraphobia, social phobia, and specific phobia as within the dimension of "fear disorders," whereas generalized anxiety disorder would be reclassified within the dimension of "distress disorders" along with major depressive disorder and dysthymic disorder. Posttraumatic stress disorder poses a bigger quandary as the current symptom constellation includes elements of the distress disorders such as diminished interests in activities as well as those of fear disorders such as avoidance and hyperarousal. It is likely that such a new categorization system will work better with animal models of anxiety, as the measurable behaviors in the models parallel the common underlying dimensions more than the currently employed phenomenological clusterings.

ANIMAL MODELS OF FEAR AND ANXIETY

Below, we start by summarizing several key features of animal models that help in understanding the value of a particular animal model. Then, we turn to animal models of fear and anxiety. We argue that most animal models reflect normal fear and anxiety—that is, the kinds of fear and anxiety responses that occur in the daily life of a species—rather than reflecting pathological fear and anxiety. Of the various models of normal fear and anxiety, we will focus on Pavlovian fear conditioning because it is the model most amenable to a neurobiological analysis. We then consider several variations or manipulations that, when added to fear conditioning, provide ways of pursuing the underlying mechanisms of pathological anxiety.

Features of Animal Models

Animal models do not typically mimic the *DSM* anxiety syndromes, but, rather, they can be adapted to specify and study key behavioral and physiological components or symptoms of the clinical syndromes. For example, greater or prolonged physiological responses to perceived threats are often observed in most anxiety disorders, such as changes in autonomic responses or facilitated startle responses (Hoehn-Saric et al., 1991; Roth, 2005; Cornwell et al., 2006). Similarly, rodent behavioral paradigms of Pavlovian fear conditioning and fear-potentiated startle elicit autonomic and startle responses, and they are therefore used as models of these components of anxiety (Davis, 2006).

The last several decades have seen the introduction of a host of animal models, predominantly involving rodents, which are proposed to measure different aspects of anxiety. The behavioral parameters measured in these models are quite varied. Examples include the degree of spontaneous avoidance of environmental stimuli (bright lighting, open spaces, heights), social avoidance of conspecifics, response to predators or predator odors, learned responses to aversive stimuli, and behavioral responses to conflict between appetitive behaviors and avoidance of fear-inducing stimuli. Measurements may also be made of the physiological responses to the challenges posed by the paradigm. Table 39.2 lists some examples of commonly measured behavioral and physiological parameters in anxiety models.

TABLE 39.2 *Examples of Commonly Measured Behavioral and Physiological Parameters in Anxiety Models*

Behavioral		
	Motor behaviors	Types
		Intensities
		Frequencies
		Latencies
	Vocalizations	
Physiological		
	Neuroendocrine	ACTH
		Corticosterone (rodent)
		Cortisol (primate)
		Adrenaline
	Autonomic	Blood pressure
		Heart rate
		Respiration
		Temperature
	Incontinence	Urinary
		Fecal
Electrophysiological		
	Single neurons	
	Field potentials	
Microdialysis		
	Chemical milieu	Neurotransmitter release
Histopathology		
	Central	Molecular, cellular, structural
		Confirmation of electrode, cannulae, or lesion placement
	Peripheral	Stomach ulceration
		Immune organs and function

ACTH = adrenocorticotrophic hormone.

Animal models of anxiety permit the acquisition of prospective data on a short-term and long-term basis under controlled conditions. Much of this critical work cannot be performed in humans for ethical and practical reasons. The anxiety models allow exploration of interventions that attenuate or enhance particular responses as well as studies that elucidate underlying neurobiological mechanisms of anxious behaviors. Importantly, adaptations of the basic anxiety models are playing a critical role in many of the advances in the elucidation of the neuropathologies of the various anxiety disorders.

The validity of a model is the degree to which a model is useful for some purpose. *Face validity* refers to the phenomenological similarities between the model and the human psychiatric condition. As originally proposed by McKinney and Bunney (1969), animal models of psychiatric disorders have a high degree of face validity when the model is produced by etiological factors known to produce the human disorder; the model resembles the behavioral manifestations and symptoms of the human disorder; the model has an underlying physiology similar to the human disorder; and the model responds to therapeutic treatments known to be effective in human patients. How these criteria are evaluated and established in animal models of psychiatric disorders is clearly discussed elsewhere in detail (Weiss and Kilts, 1998; McKinney, 2001).

Construct validity refers to the theoretical rational for linking a process in a model to a process hypothesized to produce in humans a key symptom of a given disorder. To establish construct validity, a theory for understanding a process in the human disorder is mapped or shown to be equivalent to the process being studied in an animal model (Sarter and Bruno, 2002). Due to the shared aspects of the phylogenetic histories, humans and other animals are often homologous at molecular, cellular, synaptic, and circuitry levels of analysis.

A model is considered to have good *predictive validity* based on the ability to make accurate predictions about the human phenomenon of interest. More specifically in the realm of drug development, predictive validity is the ability of the model to identify drugs of therapeutic efficacy in humans. Here, the goal is often to screen many drugs to identify the few that alter a behavior in a similar manner to an existing set of drugs such as a particular class of anxiolytics. The measured behavior need not resemble a behavior of human anxiety conditions.

Models for Pursuing the Neurobiology of "Normal" Fear and Anxiety

As noted, most models of fear and anxiety are models of perfectly natural states of fear or anxiety that occur in the daily lives of animals rather than models of pathological fear or anxiety. Models of "normal" fear and anxiety can be broadly divided into those that do not require learning (unlearned) and those that are based on conditioning (learned). Table 39.3A lists some examples of unlearned behavioral paradigms including the open field test, the elevated plus-maze (EPM), the light–dark box exploration test, predator exposure, and the social interaction test. Because little or no training is involved in such paradigms, they are often described as tests of innate fear. However, it is not possible to rule out prior experiences that contribute to the way an animal performs under these conditions. In contrast, learned fear tasks are variations on fear conditioning, instrumental avoidance conditioning, or conflict tests in which an aversive stimulus must be endured to obtain an appetitive reward. Table 39.3B lists examples of learned behavioral paradigms including Pavlovian fear conditioning (to a cue or a context), fear-potentiated startle, instrumental avoidance (active and passive), and punishment-induced conflict.

Behavioral models of anxiety generally provide for two main avenues of pursuit. One is the rapid screening of compounds for therapeutic potential. The other is the elucidation of the underlying neurobiology. What constitutes a good animal model for fearful, anxious, or avoidant behaviors depends to a large degree on which avenue is being pursued. For the purpose of screening drugs for activity on particular behavioral measures, the model should have good predictive validity, be easy to execute, be cost effective, and produce consistent and stable results. For these reasons, the unlearned models are especially useful for drug screening. However, some learned conflict paradigms have also been notably useful in the identification and testing of novel agents (McCown et al., 1983; Millan and Brocco, 2003). It is important to note that most of the antianxiety drugs that have been developed and screened using animal models have employed tests of normal fear and anxiety rather than models of pathological fear or anxiety.

For pursuing the underlying neural mechanisms of normal and pathological anxiety, choosing a behavioral paradigm in which the circuitry is well-defined assumes greater importance. A model may prove to have excellent face and predictive validity, yet it may also be unmanageable for pursuing specific underlying mechanisms. For example, the EPM is a popular model for drug discovery that includes the measurement of spontaneous avoidance of the open arms and has good predictive validity for anxiolytic and anxiogenic agents that alter time spent in the open arms (relative to total time spent in open and closed arms). The model allows for rapid drug screening without behavioral training or other more involved procedures. Yet very little is understood about the neural substrates that mediate these behaviors, and therefore this model is not amenable to circuit analysis. Given that circuit analysis is a critical early step in the detailed pursuit of neuronal, synaptic, molecular, and genetic mechanisms in the brain (J.A. Gray, 1983; Lister, 1990; Willner, 1991; Shekhar et al., 2001), inability to pursue the circuitry is a significant drawback of the EPM and other unlearned models.

In fact, many of the commonly employed animal models of fear and anxiety are not very suitable for circuit analyses due to the lack of specificity of either the conditions eliciting the behavior or of the behavioral responses themselves. Pavlovian fear conditioning is a noteworthy exception, as it has turned out to be highly

TABLE 39.3A *Examples of Unlearned/Unconditioned Anxiety Models*

Animal Model	*Related Disorders/ Human Analogue*	*Key References*
Ethological conflict tests		
Open field test (± appetitive stimuli)	GAD, panic w/agoraphobia	General: (Hall, 1934; Prut and Belzung, 2003) Amygdala: (Wallace et al., 2004; Heldt and Ressler, 2006) Hippocampus: (Kostowski et al., 1989) Lateral Septum: (Henry et al., 2006)
Elevated plus-maze	GAD, panic w/agoraphobia, fear of heights	General: (Pellow and File, 1986; Treit and Menard, 1997) Amygdala: (Helfer et al., 1996; Akwa et al., 1999; Moller et al., 1999; Wallace et al., 2004; Kokare et al., 2005); but see (Decker et al., 1995; Gonzalez et al., 1996; Moller et al., 1997) Hippocampus: (Kostowski et al., 1989; Cheeta et al., 2000; Degroot et al., 2001; Degroot and Treit, 2002) Septum: (Pesold and Treit, 1992; Cheeta et al., 2000; Degroot et al., 2001) Medial prefrontal cortex: (Shah and Treit, 2004) Dorsal periaqueductal gray (Aguiar and Brandao, 1996; Matheus and Guimaraes, 1997; Kask et al., 1998; Netto and Guimaraes, 2004)
Light-dark box exploration test	GAD	General: (Costall et al., 1989; Bourin and Hascoet, 2003) Amygdala: (de la Mora et al., 2005) Lateral Septum: (Henry et al., 2006)
Holeboard (nose pokes)		(File and Wardill, 1975)
Social interaction test	Social anxiety disorder; fear of crowds, GAD	General: (File and Seth, 2003) Amygdala: (Gonzalez et al., 1996; Helfer et al., 1996) Hippocampus and Lateral Septum: (Cheeta et al., 2000)
Neophobia (to novel objects)	Behavioral inhibition	(Griebel et al., 1993)
Hyponeophagia (latency to start eating)		(Shephard and Broadhurst, 1982)
Aversion tests		
Defensive burying/shock probe	GAD, active coping	General: (Treit et al., 1981; Treit and Menard, 1997) Hippocampus: (Degroot et al., 2001; Degroot and Treit, 2002) Septum: (Degroot et al., 2001) mPFC: (Shah and Treit, 2004)
Predator exposure (actual or odor)	Traumatic experience, fear of predators of humans (lions, coyotes)	General: (D.C. Blanchard et al., 2003; Adamec et al., 2005) Amygdala: (L.K. Takahashi et al., 2007) Hippocampus: (Diamond et al., 2006) Bed Nucleus of the Stria Terminalis: (Fendt et al., 2005) PFC: (Beekman et al., 2005)
Underwater immersion	PTSD	(Richter-Levin, 1998; Datta and Tipton, 2006)

GAD: generalized anxiety disorder; PTSD: posttraumatic stress disorder.

amenable to pursuing neural mechanisms. As is reviewed below, studies of fear conditioning have already characterized the fear system at the level of the circuits, neurons, synapses, genes, and molecules involved. Moreover, the circuits underlying the acquisition, expression, and extinction of conditioned fear have been shown to be similar in humans and rodents (Phelps and LeDoux, 2005). This has not been possible for most other anxiety paradigms not only because of the poorly defined circuitry, but also the human behavioral equivalents are not obvious for the apparent species-specific behaviors found in paradigms such as those measured in

TABLE 39.3B *Examples of Learned Anxiety Models*

Animal Model	*Related Disorders/ Human Analogue*	*Key References*
Conditioned fear to cues		
Directly elicited:		
Fear conditioning (cued)	PTSD, specific phobias, panic attacks	(Phillips and LeDoux, 1992)
Suppression of instrumental behavior:		
Conditioned suppression (bar pressing to CS)	GAD, conflict	(Thiebot et al., 1980; Moller et al., 1997; Akwa et al., 1999; Moller et al., 1999; Repa et al., 2001; Anglada-Figueroa and Quirk, 2005)
Reflex potentiation:		
Fear-potentiated acoustic startle	PTSD, specific phobias, increased startle reflex	(Liang et al., 1992; Davis et al., 1993; M. Kim and Davis, 1993; D.L. Walker et al., 2003)
Conditioned fear to context		
Fear conditioning (context)	PTSD, specific phobias, panic disorder with agoraphobia	(J.J. Kim and Fanselow, 1992; Phillips and LeDoux, 1992; Nader et al., 2001)
Conditioned place-aversion/drug discrimination	Substance use disorders	General: (Cunningham et al., 2006)
Fear-motivated instrumental responses		
Instrumental escape/avoidance tasks		(Nation and Matheny, 1980)
Passive avoidance	PTSD, GAD	(Quirarte et al., 1997; Roozendaal and McGaugh, 1997; Treit and Menard, 1997; Roozendaal et al., 1999)
Active avoidance		(Miyamoto et al., 1985; Nordby et al., 2006)
Escape from fear (EFF)	PTSD, GAD, panic disorder with agoraphobia, active coping	General and Amygdala: (Amorapanth et al., 2000)
Punishment-induced conflict		
Geller–Seifter Test (frequency of conditioned response coincidental to shock)	Conflict	(Iversen, 1980)
Vogel Lick Test (frequency of conditioned licking coincidental to shock)	Conflict	(Vogel et al., 1971)

PTSD: posttraumatic stress disorder; GAD: generalized anxiety disorder.

the EPM, the open field test, or shock probe burying. The value of fear conditioning–based models is also highlighted by the observation that learned fear is an important component of most, if not all, anxiety disorders (Rosen and Schulkin, 1998; Shekhar et al., 2005). Therefore, there is reason to suspect that information processing through, or dependent upon, the brain's fear system may be different in individuals suffering from pathological anxiety. We therefore review in detail much of what has been learned about fear conditioning, from the circuitry down to the molecular mediators. We then discuss several ways in which the fear conditioning model for anxiety may be adapted to form hybrid models that offer improved opportunities for identifying the neuropathological correlates of the anxiety disorders.

Pavlovian Fear Conditioning as a Model for Pursuing the Neural Mechanisms Underlying Normal Fear

Much of the current understanding of the neurobiology of fear and anxiety has come from studies of fear conditioning. Below, we first summarize behavioral aspects of fear conditioning; we next turn to the neural pathways underlying the acquisition, expression, and storage of fear memory, and circuits of fear regulation and extinction; and finally, we describe the cellular, synaptic, and molecular mechanisms involved.

Behavioral aspects of fear conditioning

Pavlov first described how an initially neutral, innocuous stimulus, termed the *conditioned stimulus* (CS), could acquire emotional properties if it was perceived simultaneously with a biologically salient event, termed the *unconditioned stimulus* (US) (Pavlov and Anrep, 1927). The hardwired response to the US is termed the *unconditioned response* (UR), and the acquired response to the CS is the *conditioned response* (CR). For example, in classical fear conditioning a rat is exposed to a tone, and, before the tone ceases, it also receives a mild electric shock to the feet. As a result it learns that the CS predicts threat. Now the physiological and behavioral responses that are hard wired for response to the US have also come under the control of the CS. However, it should also be mentioned that the UR and CR are not identical. Certain UR behaviors, such as jumping and vocalization, are elicited by the foot shock US but are not elicited by the tone CS alone.

In general, after as few as one CS–US pairing, it can be demonstrated that the animal has learned to respond to the tone alone with an array of stereotyped elements that make up a fear response. These measurable responses include defensive postures (freezing), autonomic changes (heart rate, blood pressure, respiration), decreased pain sensitivity (hypoalgesia), potentiation of reflexes (for example, fear-potentiated startle and eyeblink response), and endocrine activation (corticosteroid and adrenaline release). Figure 39.2 presents a schematic diagram of fear conditioning. Although the characteristics of the individual elements tend to be species specific, the array of responses is common to many species including humans, monkeys, and rodents.

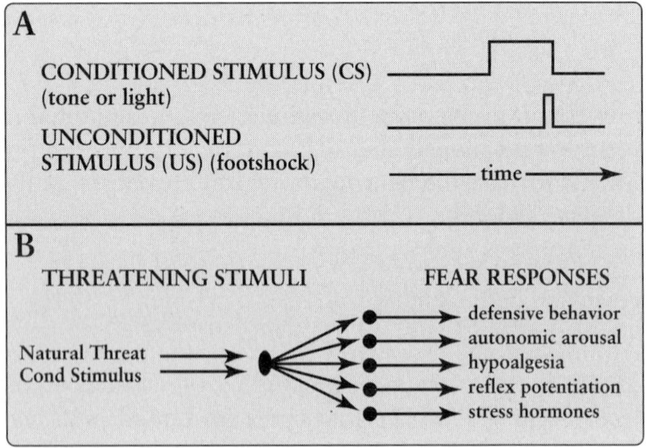

FIGURE 39.2 Schematic diagram of fear conditioning.

It is also possible to establish conditioned fear associations through "higher order conditioning." Here a distinct stimulus (CS2) is paired with an established fear CS (CS1), which endows the CS2 with fear-eliciting properties indirectly through its association with CS1 (Gewirtz and Davis, 2000). In addition, it has been shown in monkeys that simply observing a fearful response, such as to a snake, in a conspecific can result in a CR in the observer when later exposed to the stimulus (Mineka and Cook, 1993). Recent work in humans indicates observational conditioning also can occur in humans (Olsson and Phelps, 2004).

Neural mechanisms of acquisition, storage, and expression of conditioned fear

The neurocircuitry of Pavlovian fear conditioning is well established, with general agreement that the amygdala is essential for the acquisition and expression of conditioned fear responses (Davis, 1992; Kapp et al., 1992; LeDoux, 1992; Fanselow, 1994). The amygdala is composed of several structurally and functionally heterogeneous nuclei residing in the medial temporal lobe. It is within the amygdala that information about the CS and the US converge, and efferent pathways from the amygdala control, in parallel, the autonomic, endocrine, and behavioral responses. The nuclei of the amygdala identified as relevant to fear conditioning are the lateral (LA), basal (B), accessory basal (AB), and central (CE) nuclei. Sometimes the adjacent LA and B nuclei are referred to together as the basolateral nucleus (BLA). Studies in several species including rats, cats, and monkeys are in general agreement about the interconnections between LA, B, AB, and CE (Amaral et al., 1992; Pare et al., 1995; Pitkänen et al., 1997; Cassell et al., 1999). Although LA and CE participate in fear conditioning (LeDoux, 2000; Maren, 2001; Davis, 2006), some debate exists about the role of each and the manner in which they interact (Cardinal et al., 2002; Pare et al., 2004; Balleine and Killcross, 2006; Wilensky et al., 2006). Other brain regions to which the amygdala sends projections mediate the individual components of the fear response.

The circuit crucial to auditory fear conditioning involves tone CS information that is received via the sensory apparatus of the ear and is relayed through brain stem to the auditory portion of thalamus (LeDoux, 1996, 2000; Sigurdsson et al., 2007). Auditory thalamus relays the CS information via at least two distinct pathways. Electrophysiological studies have demonstrated a rapid, monosynaptic thalamo-amygdala pathway (12 msec) and a slower, polysynaptic thalamo-cortico-amygdala pathway (30–40 msec). Both pathways, which transmit information via ionotropic glutamatergic synapses, converge on neurons in LA. The thalamo-amygdala pathway is believed to provide for a rapid response to threatening environmental stimuli, but the representation of the environmental stimuli is considered crude. In contrast, the thalamo-cortico-amygdala pathway may provide a more complex representation due to processing through sensory cortex, providing for a more appropriate, albeit slower, response to the perceived stimuli. This arrangement allows the response to danger to begin before there is conscious appreciation of the stimulus. See Figure 39.3 for a diagram of the neural circuits identified through auditory fear conditioning.

The transmission of US information (representing the mild foot shock) is less well understood but is thought in part to involve a relay via the spinothalamic tract to thalamic areas projecting to LA (LeDoux et al., 1987; LeDoux et al., 1990). An electrophysiological response of neurons in LA is recorded when pain receptors are stimulated, and some of these cells have also been demonstrated to respond to the auditory CS (Romanski et al., 1993). As well, other sensory modalities have pathways with nerve terminals that synapse mainly in LA (LeDoux et al., 1990; Amaral et al., 1992; Mascagni et al., 1993; McDonald, 1998).

The central nucleus is often referred to as the main output station of the amygdala because it is critical for the expression of the conditioned fear response (LeDoux et al., 1988; Davis, 1992; Kapp et al., 1992; Maren and Fanselow, 1996). More recent work suggests CE may also play a role in fear acquisition and memory consolidation (Pare et al., 2004; Samson and Pare, 2005; Wilensky et al., 2006). The central nucleus sends projections to diverse brain regions that mediate the specific components of a fear response. For example, CE projections to the periaqueductal gray are involved in freezing behavior and pain modulation; those through the bed nucleus of the stria terminalis (BNST) and preoptic area, as well as sparse projections directly from CE to the paraventricular nucleus of the hypothalamus, appear to modulate hypothalamic-pituitary-adrenal (HPA) axis activity; and those to the parabrachial nucleus, lateral hypothalamus, and dorsal motor nucleus of the vagus are involved in autonomic responses such as cardiovascular and respiratory alterations (LeDoux et al., 1988; Van de Kar et al., 1991; Davis, 1992; Manning, 1998) (see Fig. 39.3). Another view is that CE mediates different learned fear responses than those mediated by the LA (Cardinal et al., 2002; Balleine and Killcross, 2006).

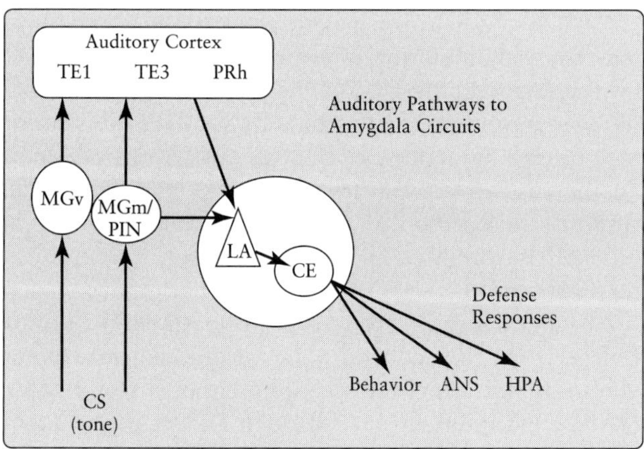

FIGURE 39.3 Diagram of neural circuits identified through auditory fear conditioning.

Contextual fear conditioning is similar to fear conditioning to a cue CS, such as a tone, in that an association can rapidly be learned between a foot shock and a representation of the environment (the context) in which the foot shock was received. When simply placed back in that environment in which it had previously received a foot shock, the animal will respond with the same stereotyped array of responses described for auditory fear conditioning. The pathways that mediate this association appear to differ from conditioning to a simple cue in that conditioning to the context depends not only on the amygdala nuclei involved in auditory fear conditioning, but also on the hippocampus (R.J. Blanchard et al., 1970; J.J. Kim and Fanselow, 1992; Phillips and LeDoux, 1992; Maren et al., 1997; Frankland et al., 1998). Similar to auditory fear conditioning, intra-amygdala processing of contextual information predicting danger ultimately results in output pathways from amygdala to particular brain areas mediating components of the fear response.

Different amygdala nuclei appear to mediate independent fear learning systems. For example, rats can be trained on an operant conditioning paradigm known as the escape from fear (EFF) task in which the CS reinforces an escape motor response that terminates the CS. Whereas CE lesion blocks conditioned freezing but not EFF behavior, lesions of B block EFF but not conditioned freezing (Amorapanth et al., 2000). Lateral nucleus lesions interfere with both responses, suggesting plasticity there contributes to both. A related paradigm involves the ability to learn avoidance of a CS-paired shock that was contingent upon a lever press (Killcross et al., 1997). Lesions of BLA but not CE block the avoidance learning. In these paradigms, LA relays information to B, which processes the CS as a learned incentive. This processing in turn may activate motor circuits of striatum.

The amygdala has also been shown to have a modulatory influence for implicit learning systems that do not involve fear. For example, intra-amygdala amphetamine administration enhances memory for a spatial, hippocampus-dependent memory task as well as for a motor learning, caudate-dependent task (Packard and Teather, 1998). Inhibitory avoidance, for example, is a complex task that depends on the hippocampus and other structures. In this task, an animal must learn to avoid entering a context that was previously paired with a foot shock. Neurochemical activity in the amygdala has been shown to contribute to the efficacy of this complex form of learning (for reviews see McGaugh, 2004, 2006). However, the amygdala does not seem to perform this modulatory function for fear conditioning because inactivation of the amygdala immediately posttraining does not affect the strength of the memory stored (Wilensky et al., 1999, 2000).

Neural systems of fear regulation and extinction

The PFC also plays a critical role in the normal expression and extinction of fear responses (Morgan et al., 1993; Morgan and LeDoux, 1995, 1999; Morgan et al., 2003; Quirk and Beer, 2006). Extinction is the form of learning whereby the CR to a repeatedly presented CS (in a previously conditioned animal) diminishes over repetitions of the CS. Importantly, extinction of a previously consolidated fear memory does not typically erase the learned association between the CS and the US. Rather, extinction involves new learning that regulates fear expression. However, recent study suggests that extinction training administered shortly after an aversive experience, when the fear memories are not yet consolidated, may engage mechanisms resembling "unlearning" processes (Myers et al., 2006). Furthermore, another report demonstrates that the efficacy of early extinction depends on the level of fear present during the extinction trial intervention (Maren and Chang, 2006).

Lesion studies suggest that the ventromedial PFC (vmPFC), which in rat includes the prelimbic and infralimbic cortex, plays a role in the consolidation and/or expression of extinction (Morgan et al., 1993; Quirk et al., 2000). However, the initial acquisition of extinction appears to critically involve *N*-methyl-D-aspartate (NMDA) receptor activation in the LA/B (Sotres-Bayon et al., 2007). Hippocampal inputs to vmPFC appear to perform a gating function for expression of extinction, with the hippocampus-vmPFC circuit likely providing contextual information (Sotres-Bayon et al., 2004). Projections from vmPFC to γ-aminobutyric acid (GABA) ergic interneurons of amygdala, known as intercalated cells (ITC), appear to be inhibitory for CE output, and ITC activity may be modulated by D_1-dopaminergic, μ-opioid, and oxytocin receptors. Prefrontal cortex dopamine has been specifically implicated in the expression and extinction of conditioned fear responses (Pezze and Feldon, 2004).

Although infralimbic cortex has an inhibitory role in fear expression, the more dorsally located prelimbic cortex has been shown to be excitatory. Human functional magnetic resonance imaging (fMRI) studies support a role for vmPFC in the expression of extinction learning, with recent evidence suggesting the human homologues of infralimbic and prelimbic cortex, the subgenual (BA25) and dorsal anterior cingulate cortex (dACC; BA32), respectively, play opposing roles in modulation of response to conditioned fear stimuli (Quirk and Beer, 2006). Expression of extinction learning in humans has been shown to activate vmPFC and hippocampus in a context-dependent manner, implicating the hippocampal-vmPFC circuit in fear regulation after extinction (Kalisch et al., 2006). Anxiety disorders such as PTSD may involve fear system hyperactivity as a result of deficient function in the hippocampal-vmPFC circuit, with impairment in extinction recall and its modulation by context (Rauch et al., 2006). Current psychotherapies for PTSD such as prolonged exposure (to the individual's own trauma story) may work by encouraging extinction of cue and contextual fear memories associated with the trauma rather than sustaining the typical avoidance pattern to such stimuli. Because the prelimbic cortex has been found to be excitatory for fear expression, localized disruption of its homologue in humans, the dACC, via deep brain stimulation (DBS) may offer a therapeutic approach for particular anxiety conditions similar to the use of DBS in refractory depression (Mayberg et al., 2005).

Synaptic and modulatory mechanisms of fear acquisition, expression, and extinction

Neurotransmission through the aforementioned fear circuits is largely carried out through glutamatergic neurons that transmit across synapses via rapid, ion-channel-dependent mechanisms. Several classes of neurochemicals released at synaptic boutons by other types of neurons have been shown to be modulators of the fearful and anxious responses mediated by such glutamatergic neurons. These include the amino acid transmitter GABA; monoamines such as serotonin, noradrenaline, and dopamine; and neuropeptides such as corticotropin-releasing factor (CRF).

GABAergic neurons make up the main braking system for glutamatergic neurotransmission, also transmitting through ion-channel receptors. Indeed, removal of tonic inhibition in amygdala by local administration of a GABA antagonist to BLA in awake rats results in an increase in anxiety-like behaviors and autonomic response (Sanders et al., 1995), and this effect can be blocked by preinfusion of glutamatergic receptor antagonists into BLA (Sajdyk and Shekhar, 1997).

Monoaminergic (serotonergic, dopaminergic, noradrenergic) neurons generally play a modulatory role on glutamatergic neurotransmission, either directly or via GABAergic interneurons, through slower postsynaptic mechanisms involving G protein–coupled receptors. For example, within LA serotonin appears to inhibit ionotropic glutamatergic neurotransmission via activation of GABAergic interneurons, a process that depends on presence of the stress hormone *corticosterone* (Stutzmann et al., 1998; Stutzmann and LeDoux, 1999). Noradrenaline enhances consolidation of inhibitory avoidance through activation of β-adrenergic receptors in BLA (Ferry et al., 1999). Although there is much evidence showing the enhancing effect of norepinephrine (NE) on fear learning (McGaugh, 2006), the exact role of noradrenergic transmission in LA in the acquisition (Bush et al., in prep), consolidation (Kobayashi and Kobayashi, 2001; H.J. Lee et al., 2001; Debiec and Ledoux, 2004; Murchison et al., 2004; Bush et al., 2007) and retrieval (Murchison et al., 2004) of fear conditioning requires further studies. Recent data demonstrate that postretrieval noradrenergic blockade in LA using β-adrenergic receptor antagonist *propranolol* disrupts reconsolidation processes and results in lasting attenuation of learned fear responses (Debiec and LeDoux, 2004).

There are also glutamatergic neurons that form slower, metabotropic, glutamatergic synapses that also modulate ionotropic glutamatergic neurotransmission. The group I metabotropic glutamate receptor subtype 5 (mGluR5) is requisite for acquisition of fear memory (Fendt and Schmid, 2002; Rodrigues et al., 2002), whereas the mGluR1 is essential for extinction of learned fear but not acquisition (J. Kim et al., 2007).

Corticotrophin-releasing factor is a 41-amino acid polypeptide first isolated from hypothalamus that was shown to activate the HPA axis (Vale et al., 1981). The amygdala is a major extra-hypothalamic source of CRF-secreting neurons and has significant expression of the two major types of CRF receptors (De Souza et al., 1985; Perrin et al., 1993; Chalmers et al., 1995; Smagin et al., 1996; Dieterich et al., 1997; Rominger et al., 1998). Stressful challenge results in CRF release in amygdala (Roozendaal et al., 2002). Direct stimulation of CRF receptors in BLA increases anxiety-related behaviors (Sajdyk et al., 1999). In fact, CRF agonists generally enhance anxious responding on diverse anxiety paradigms, including facilitation of conditioned fear acquisition, facilitation of acoustic startle, suppression of exploration on the EPM, enhancement of place aversion, and enhancement of defensive burying. Corticotrophin-releasing factor antagonists generally reduce these same behaviors (Swiergiel et al., 1992; Menzaghi et al., 1994; T.S. Gray and Bingaman, 1996; Smagin et al., 1996; Koob, 1999; Koob and Heinrichs, 1999; Martins et al., 2000). The enhancement of acoustic startle by intraventricular CRF is blocked by chemical lesion of BNST, indicating another important site of action for CRF in an anxiety-related behavior (Y. Lee and Davis, 1997). Also, CRF-expressing neurons project from CE to locus coeruleus (Van de Kar et al., 1991) and modulate output of noradrenaline in forebrain (Bouret et al., 2003).

Molecular mediators of learning and memory in the fear system

New learning implies lasting changes in brain so that what has been learned may be retrieved in the future. Memory consolidation is the process whereby short-term memory is transformed into long-term memory, and much work indicates this is a process dependent on new protein synthesis (for review see Rodrigues et al., 2004). Studies using targeted pharmacological manipulations have characterized the role of LA in the acquisition, consolidation and storage of auditory fear conditioning in rodents (Fanselow and LeDoux, 1999; Maren, 2001; Schafe et al., 2001; Rodrigues et al., 2004; Dityatev and Bolshakov, 2005; Faber et al., 2005; Pape et al., 2005). Interference or enhancement of the molecular pathways involved in aversive learning in LA modulates retention of conditioned fear responses. A growing body of data suggests that retrieval of consolidated fear memories, by presentation of a learned cue, triggers a reconsolidation process in LA that renders the retrieved memories susceptible to pharmacological disruption (Nader et al., 2000).

One widely studied model for the establishment of stable memories is long-term potentiation (LTP). In LTP, application of a high-frequency stimulation of afferent fibers to a synapse can result in long-lasting increase in the efficiency of neurotransmission through the synapse (Bliss and Lomo, 1973). In the case of fear learning, LTP-like changes occur in the auditory thalamo-amygdala pathway after fear conditioning to tone (Rogan et al., 1997). Stimulation of this glutamatergic pathway has been shown to result in LTP of synapses in LA through a mechanism dependent on activation of voltage-gated calcium ion channels on the postsynaptic neuron (Weisskopf et al., 1999). Known inhibitors of LTP, including inhibition of protein synthesis, protein kinase A (PKA), and extracellular signal regulated kinases/mitogen-activated protein (ERK/MAP) kinase activity (Huang et al., 1996; Huang and Kandel, 1998; Huang et al., 2000), have also been shown to disrupt fear memory consolidation given by systemic injection and local amygdala infusion, yet they leave short-term memory intact (Schafe et al., 1999; Schafe et al., 2000; Schafe and LeDoux, 2000) (see Figure 39.4a-e).

The long-term changes that support stable fear memory appear to occur through plastic changes in the synapses within amygdala. Coincident activation of postsynaptic neurons in amygdala by presynaptic afferents separately carrying the CS and US sensory information sets in motion a molecular cascade of synaptic events that involve activation of postsynaptic receptors, ion flow through membrane channels, action potentials, activation of second-messenger systems, activation of transcriptional factors, new protein synthesis, and, ultimately, microstructural changes in the microanatomy of

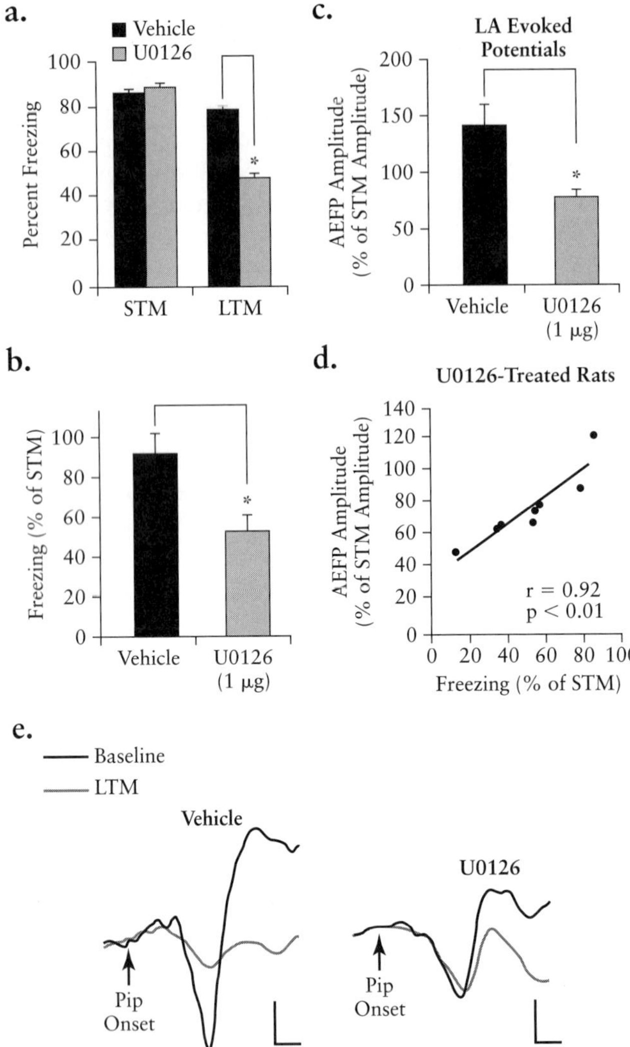

FIGURE 39.4 Map kinase inhibitor on short-term memory/long-term memory (STM/LTM).

the synapse. Within the more dorsal region of the dorsal portion of LA (LAd) there are neurons with converging sensory inputs that demonstrate transient plastic changes, termed *trigger cells* (Repa et al., 2001). Neurons in the more ventral region of LAd demonstrate long-lasting plastic changes, termed *storage cells.* It appears that the storage cells of LAd relay information to the medial portion of LA, and from there information is relayed to CE.

One of the three main types of postsynaptic ionotropic receptors for glutamate is termed the *NMDA receptor*. Within BLA, NMDA-dependent and NMDA-independent forms of LTP have been identified (Weisskopf et al., 1999; Bauer et al., 2002). One of the peptide subunits that make up this receptor is termed the *NR2B subunit*. It has been shown using an inhibitor of the NR2B subunit that it is involved in acquisition but not consolidation of fear memory (Rodrigues et al., 2001), and the subunit is requisite for LTP in amygdala (Bauer et al., 2002). This suggests the NR2B subunit is involved in the short-term form of synaptic memory required for transient changes in neurotransmission that occur during fear learning, but not in the protein synthesis–dependent changes that occur over hours that mediate development of long-term synaptic plasticity.

Corticotrophin-releasing factor receptors have been implicated in the long-lasting changes that occur within the amygdala associated with pathological anxiety responses (Sajdyk et al., 1999). Acute activation of CRF receptors in BLA in vitro has been shown to increase the excitability of BLA neurons through effects on the slow after hyperpolarizing potential (Rainnie et al., 1992). Moreover, the CRF-induced behavioral syndrome correlates with cellular mechanisms of neuronal plasticity, suggesting a mechanism by which stressful challenges result in lasting changes in response to future adversity (Rainnie et al., 2004).

Homologous to the amygdala's role in fear memory consolidation, the vmPFC appears to be key to extinction-related plasticity. Local administration of inhibitors of protein synthesis and protein kinases in vmPFC does not affect short-term expression of extinction but does impair consolidation of extinction (Quirk and Beer, 2006). However, the vmPFC contribution to the consolidation of fear extinction may depend on learning mechanisms that first take place in the amygdala, because infusion of ifenprodil, an antagonist for NR2B-containing NMDA receptors, directly into the amygdala disrupts the initial acquisition of fear extinction (Sotres-Bayon et al, 2007). A model for fear extinction has proposed that the amygdala is crucial for the acquisition of extinction, and that plasticity in the vmPFC is important for gating the later expression of extinction (Sotres-Bayon et al., 2004).

Animal model work on consolidation of fear memories and extinction has directly led to several potential modes of therapeutic intervention for anxiety conditions with presumed fear system hyperactivity. For example, there have been trials of amnestic agents to block memory consolidation (Pitman and Delahanty, 2005) or reconsolidation (Nader et al., 2000; Debiec and LeDoux, 2004; Brunet et al., 2008) to reduce anxiety-provoking intrusive memories in trauma and PTSD. Also, there has been employment of the antibiotic *d*-cycloserine to enhance extinction in exposure therapy, based on this molecule's partial NMDA antagonist properties (Walker et al., 2002; Ressler et al., 2004; Davis et al., 2006).

Use of fear conditioning as a biological probe

The breadth of molecular, synaptic, cellular, and circuitry information on fear conditioning make this anxiety paradigm ideal to serve as a biological probe of the roles of the individual components of the fear network, in particular anxious behaviors and anxiety disorders (Cannistraro and Rauch, 2003). Thus, not only may contributions of intra-amygdala processes for anxious responding be investigated, but those of other mediators of the fear circuitry such as hippocampus and regions of PFC may be detected and pursued at many levels within the fear conditioning model.

Functional imaging in humans may be used to verify the applicability of fear conditioning models, dissect distinguishing loci of abnormal activity between anxiety disorders, and study the neurobiological effects of therapeutic interventions. For example, PTSD and panic involve exaggerated amygdala responses to a conditioned fear stimulus (Bremner, 2004). However, activity in hippocampus and PFC regions may separate PTSD and panic. One might predict that PTSD may have a muted hippocampal response to context, given that such patients often respond to threats in inappropriate contexts. Patients with panic, on the other hand, may have heightened hippocampal activity due to their exaggerated concern about contexts in which panic may be evoked.

Although the central role of the amygdala in fear conditioning is well established, it should be noted that the amygdala's role in anxiety has been debated. Gray and McNaughton's behavioral inhibition model of anxiety places emphasis on the role of the septo-hippocampal system (McNaughton and Gray, 2000; McNaughton, 2006), and Davis has described a key role for BNST in anxiety as opposed to fear (Davis et al., 1997; Walker et al., 2003). Yet the behavioral paradigms on which these theories are based involve tasks that require the processing of fear-inducing contextual information. Given that the BNST (G.M. Sullivan et al., 2004) and hippocampus (J.J. Kim and Fanselow, 1992; Phillips and LeDoux, 1992; Maren et al., 1997; Fanselow, 2000; Liu et al., 2004) are requisite for contextual fear conditioning and are densely interconnected (Herman et al., 2005), it is important to distinguish the roles of these regions in contextual processing from a specialized role in anxiety. Anxiety does appear to engage cognitive processes to a greater extent than fear, which is consistent with key roles for hippocampus and BNST. But imaging studies in healthy volunteers have demonstrated an increase in amygdala signal upon induction of anxiety (Phelps et al., 2001). Moreover, there are several examples of abnormally enhanced amygdala signal in several of the anxiety disorders (Stein et al., 2002; Protopopescu et al., 2005; Shin et al., 2005; Straube et al., 2005), suggesting a role for the amygdala in anxiety as well as fear.

Multimodal Models for Understanding Pathological Anxiety and the Anxiety Disorders

The aforementioned animal models generally involve healthy animals in which measurements are made of the fearful and anxious responses to the environmental challenges posed by the paradigms (Lister, 1990). Due to the relatively poor reliability of an individual's performance between tasks, it is suggested that most models, especially those in normal animals with limited genetic variability, measure state fear and anxiety to a greater degree than trait fear and anxiety (Andreatini and Bacellar, 2000). This is not analogous to human anxiety disorders in which pathological anxiety is commonly an enduring feature, and a large degree of the variability in symptoms is accounted for by genetic predisposition. In other words, individuals with anxiety disorders are not simply reacting to the environmental conditions (Hidalgo and Davidson, 2000) but, rather, appear to have a greater predisposition or susceptibility. Therefore, for the purpose of uncovering the neurobiology of pathological anxiety and the anxiety disorders, a paradigm should instead reveal a condition present in the animal through a measurable response. The basic anxiety paradigms may be better adapted through various manipulations to better model the pathological behavioral symptoms characteristic of particular anxiety disorders. In this section we look beyond models of normal fear and anxiety to consider hybrid models that explicitly examine factors that are thought to contribute to psychopathology.

An approach to modeling anxiety disorders that shows much promise for understanding pathological anxiety is combining fear conditioning with other experimental manipulations that enhance the predictive, face, and/or construct validity of the model. Table 39.3C lists some examples of hybrid models that may be more relevant to trait anxiety and the pathological anxiety found in the anxiety disorders. Although hybrid anxiety models may utilize other anxiety paradigms, including the unlearned types, fear conditioning offers the advantage of the well-described circuitry and cellular biology. The manipulations we briefly discuss fall into a few general categories: physiological interventions, usually involving systemic or localized administration of drugs with known physiological effects; stressful interventions during development or in adulthood; and genetic alterations, such as those produced by selective breeding or by modification of deoxyribonucleic acid (DNA). We also discuss a novel route of selection by phenotype or trait.

Physiological models have been used to assess the effects of altering function in fear circuits on subsequent fearful and anxious behaviors. This has involved generation of hyperexcitability of specific brain regions such as BLA and hypothalamus by administration of chemicals or induction of partial kindling (Sanders et al., 1995; Keim and Shekhar, 1996; Rosen et al., 1996; Sajdyk et al., 1999). Models considered relevant to panic disorder include treatments with drugs that produce panic attacks in humans, including lactate (Shekhar et al.,

TABLE 39.3C *Examples of Hybrid (Learned/Unlearned) Models of Trait Anxiety*

Animal Model	*Related Disorders/ Human Analogue*	*Key References*
Pathophysiological models		
Periaqueductal gray stimulation	Panic disorder, GAD	(Graeff et al., 1993)
Lactate and social interaction	Panic disorder	Amygdala (BLA): (Sajdyk et al., 1999) Hypothalamus (dorsomedial): (Shekhar et al., 1996)
Doxapram and fear conditioning	Panic with agoraphobia	(G.M. Sullivan et al., 2003)
Bicuculline	Aversive memory consolidation	(Brioni and McGaugh, 1988; Castellano and McGaugh, 1990)
Stress models		
Developmental stress		
Stress in altricial neonate		(R. Sullivan et al., 2006)
Maternal separation/handling		(Plotsky et al., 2005)
Ultrasonic vocalization (abrupt isolation from nest)		(Hofer, 1996)
Variable foraging demand (bonnet macaque)	PTSD, panic disorder, GAD, social anxiety disorder	(Rosenblum and Paully, 1984; Coplan et al., 1992; Rosenblum and Andrews, 1994; Coplan et al., 1998; Coplan et al., 2001)
Stress inoculation (squirrel monkey)	No PTSD subsequent to trauma (resilience)	(Parker et al., 2004; Lyons and Parker, 2007)
Adult stress		
Single prolonged stress	PTSD	(Liberzon et al., 1999)
Fear-potentiated behavior on the elevated plus-maze	GAD, PTSD	(Adamec et al., 2004; also see Mechiel Korte and De Boer, 2003)
Genetic models		
Selective breeding		
Roman rat; Lewis rats		(Driscoll et al., 1998; Cohen et al., 2006)
Transgenic and knock-out models		(Finn et al., 2003)
5-HT system		(Heisler et al., 1998; Parks et al., 1998; Ramboz et al., 1998)
CRF system		(Heinrichs et al., 1997)
GABA system		(Kash et al., 1999)
Trait selection models		
Selection based on behavioral phenotype	PTSD	(Bush et al., 2007)

GAD: generalized anxiety disorder; PTSD: posttraumatic stress disorder; BLA: basolateral amygdala; CRF: corticotrophin releasing factor; GABA: γ-aminobutyric acid.

1996) or doxapram (G.M. Sullivan et al., 2003), and testing for enhancement of fear and anxiety on unlearned and learned tests such as the open field test, the social interaction test, and fear conditioning. An example of a physiological intervention is the combination of fear conditioning with administration of the respiratory stimulant *doxapram*, a drug that elicits a panic attack in most patients with panic disorder (Y.J. Lee et al., 1993). Doxapram enhances acquisition of conditioned fear memory (G.M. Sullivan et al., 2003), and, at the same dose, enhances CRF release in CE but not in BNST or hypothalamus (Choi et al., 2005). Doxapram is known to induce hyperventilation via activation of carotid body chemoreceptors, thereby producing a (false) visceral signal to brain indicating poor air. Because the circuitry of conditioned fear is well described, it is possible to test the hypothesis that this visceral signal induces panic-like symptoms by altering the threat processing of internal or external events through CE.

Developmental models have assessed the effects of stress in early life on fearful and anxious behaviors manifested later in life (Rosenblum and Paully, 1984; Coplan et al., 1992; Levine, 1994; Shanks et al., 1995;

Hofer, 1996; Meaney et al., 1996; Heim et al., 1997; Francis et al., 1999; Francis and Meaney, 1999; Graham et al., 1999; Meaney et al., 2000; R. Sullivan, 2003; Moriceau et al., 2004; Imanaka et al., 2006; R. Sullivan et al., 2006; Tsoory and Richter-Levin, 2006). In rodents, for example, early exposure to maternal deprivation permanently alters central CRF systems and related behavioral and hormonal responses to subsequent stressors throughout life (Plotsky et al., 2005). Ecologically informed studies of maternal availability have likewise identified similar outcomes in nonhuman primates. Bonnet macaque monkeys raised by their mothers in variable-foraging demand conditions respond to novel situations with increased anxiety compared to age-matched monkeys raised as low-foraging demand controls (Rosenblum and Andrews, 1994). As adults, these same monkeys exhibit significant differences in cerebrospinal fluid levels of monoamines, somatostatin, and CRF (Coplan et al., 1998; Coplan et al., 2001). These findings agree with evidence from humans that early exposure to severe forms of stress is a risk factor for the development of mood and anxiety disorders (Davidson et al., 2004; Heim et al., 2004). Far less researched, but of equal importance, are indications that early life stressors may also foster resilience. Ongoing studies of squirrel monkeys suggest that early exposure to stressful events that are not overwhelming but challenging enough to elicit emotional activation and cognitive processing may make subsequent coping efforts more efficient, and therefore easier and more likely to be used later in life (Lyons and Parker, 2007). Figures 39.5A and 39.5B show the behavioral and neuroendocrine differences, respectively, of such "stress inoculation."

Behavioral manipulations in adulthood that affect structure and function of fear circuits often involve exposure to acute or chronic stressors (Cohen and Zohar, 2004; Miller and McEwen, 2006). Examples include restraint or immobilization, cold exposure, electric shock, predator exposure, and underwater submersion (Rittenhouse et al., 1992; Richter-Levin, 1998; Mechiel Korte and De Boer, 2003; Cohen et al., 2004; Morilak et al., 2005; Rau et al., 2005; Adamec et al., 2006). Repeated exposure to these stressors in adulthood increases fear and aggression, alters contextual fear responses, affects performance on the EPM, and attenuates spatial memory. Restraint stress also facilitates fear conditioning, results in dendritic atrophy in hippocampus and medial PFC, suppresses neurogenesis in the dentate gyrus, and induces dendritic hypertrophy and sprouting of new synapses in the amygdala (Miller and McEwen, 2006). These stress-induced aspects of neural plasticity suggest a putative link between remodeling of fear circuits and the development of anxiety as modeled in adult rodents. Chronic stress and underwater submersion have also been used in rodent research to mimic the requisite stressful events of traumatic anxiety disorders such as PTSD (Servatius et al., 1995; Richter-Levin, 1998; Cohen et al., 1999; Adamec et al., 2004; Cohen and Zohar, 2004; Pitman and Delahanty, 2005; Matar et al., 2006; T. Takahashi et al., 2006).

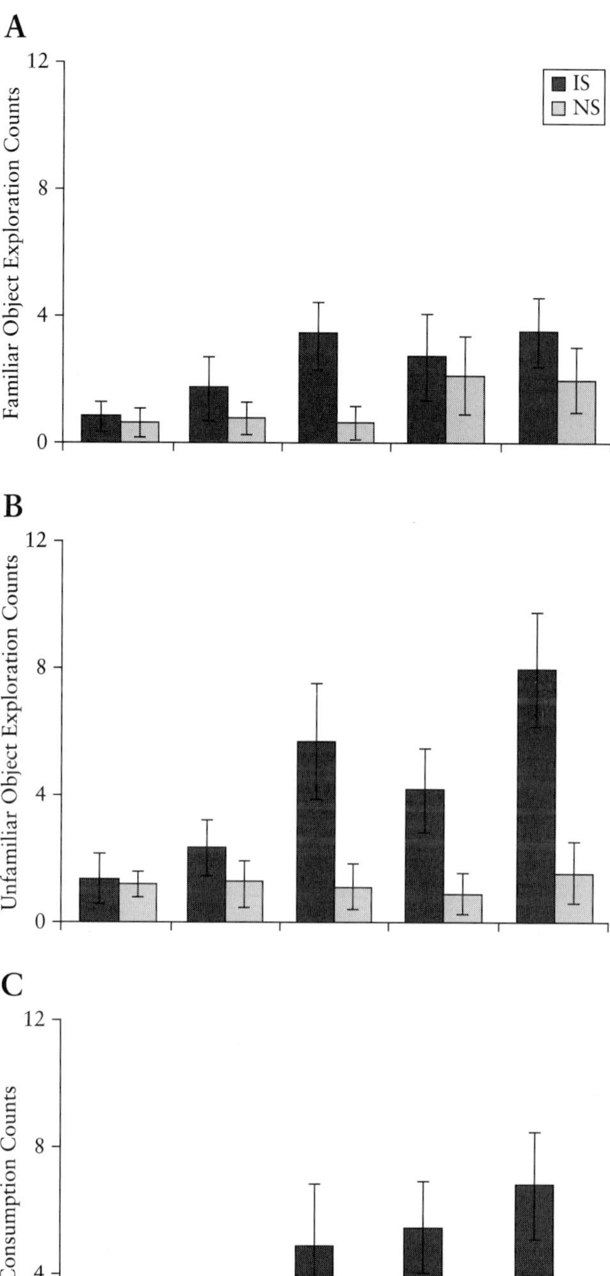

FIGURE 39.5A Measures of behavior in monkeys exposed to intermittent stress inoculation (IS) compared to no-stress (NS) condition (adapted from Parker et al., 2004).

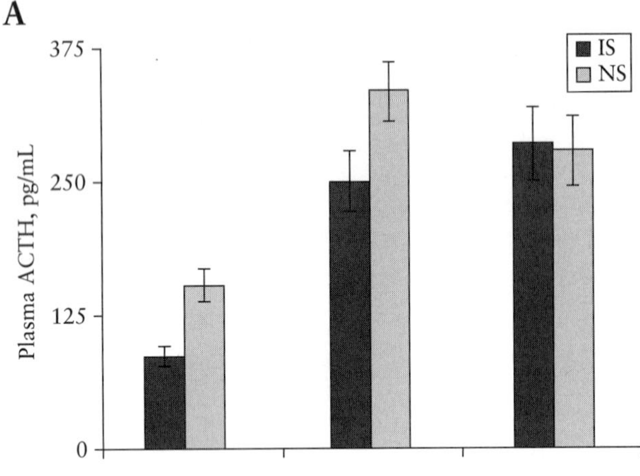

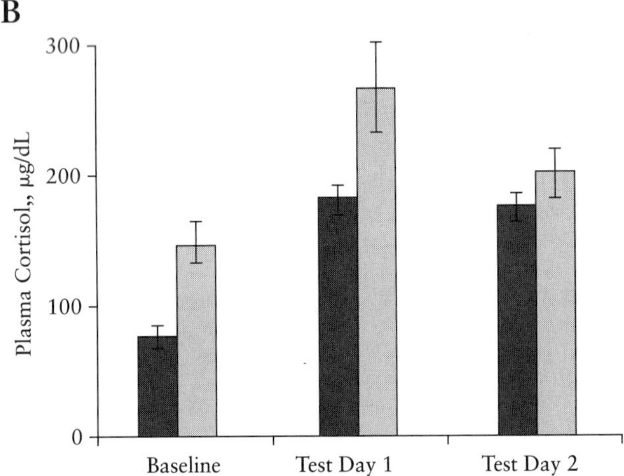

FIGURE 39.5B Plasma levels of hormones in monkeys exposed to intermittent stress inoculation (IS) compared to a no-stress (NS) condition (adapted from Parker et al., 2004).

Genetic manipulations before behavioral assessments of fear and anxiety in rodent models have generally been achieved by two main methods. One is selective breeding of rat strains with the goal of enhancing or attenuating particular measures of fear and anxiety (C.D. Walker et al., 1989; Ferrel et al., 1995; Escorihuela et al., 1997; Wehner et al., 1997; Escorihuela et al., 1999; Pisula and Osinski, 2000; Paterson et al., 2001; Yilmazer-Hanker et al., 2002; Steimer and Driscoll, 2003; Aguilar et al., 2004; Morilak et al., 2005). The other is creation of transgenic mice that have altered expression of particular genes that code for proteins in brain circuits of interest, and testing for changes in behavioral performance on anxiety-inducing paradigms (Heisler et al., 1998; Tecott et al., 1998; Low et al., 2000; Tecott, 2000; Sibille and Hen, 2001; Gross and Hen, 2004; Leonardo and Hen, 2006). An example of the latter approach comes from studies of fear conditioning in the 5-HT_{1A} knockout mouse. When previously context-conditioned 5-HT_{1A}-null mice are tested in the same context but with novel cues added, they do not exhibit the normal decrement in fear response seen in wild-type mice (Klemenhagen et al., 2006). This difference in sensitivity to novel stimuli has been likened to a memory bias for threatening cues in an otherwise neutral environment as may occur in human patients with panic disorder and PTSD. Given the well-described role of hippocampus in providing a representation of context to amygdala, focused investigation of hippocampal-amygdala interactions involving the 5-HT_{1A} receptor is suggested.

The serotonin system has also been implicated in the discovery of associations between anxiety and naturally occurring genetic polymorphisms. In particular, an insertion/deletion event in the serotonin transporter–linked polymorphic region (5HTTLPR) is known to produce long (l) and short (s) alleles in humans and rhesus monkeys (Lesch et al., 1997). The short allele decreases transcriptional efficiency and is thought to diminish expression of the serotonin transporter that

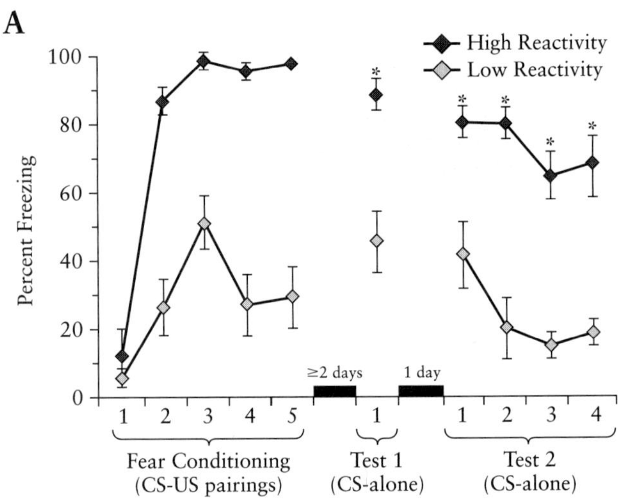

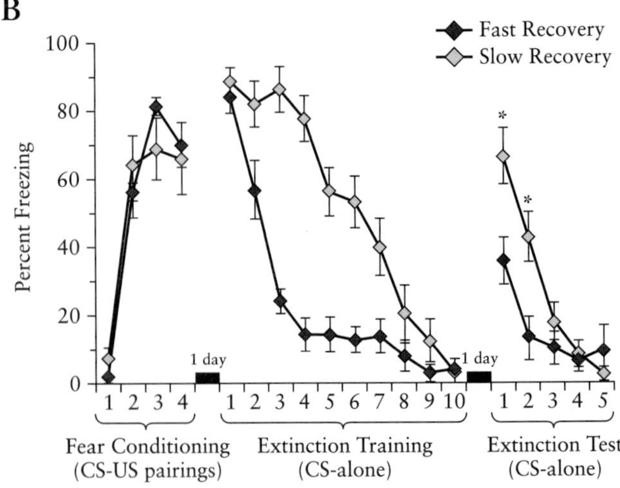

FIGURE 39.6 Phenotype selection for fear reactivity and recovery.

disrupts control of extracellular concentrations of serotonin in neural circuits. Humans homozygous for the short allele (s/s) are more anxious and display greater muscle tension, increased shyness, and more harm avoidance compared to humans that are homozygous (l/l) or heterozygous (l/s) for the long allele. Similar associations have been reported for infant and adult rhesus monkeys (Champoux et al., 2002; Barr et al., 2004; Bethea et al., 2004).

It has been proposed that consideration be given to individual differences in susceptibility and resilience in animal models of anxiety disorders (Charney, 2004). This is particularly important in models for PTSD, as it is well documented that similar levels of exposure to a horrific trauma results in development of PTSD in a relatively small proportion of those exposed (Charney, 2004; Yehuda, 2004). Of note, phenotypic variability in most animal models of fear and anxiety is obscured by the usual practice of reporting the variation around the mean. Recent work shows that fear reactivity scores in conditioned animals are normally distributed in unselected Sprague–Dawley rats (Bush et al., 2007). When given fear extinction training, rats that show similarly high levels of fear reactivity can also be separated into fast and slow fear recovery groups. Figures 39.6A and 39.6B show the phenotypic differences in fear reactivity and fear recovery of these selected groups. The slow-extinguishing group is proposed to have relevance for PTSD, the psychopathology of which involves a failure to recover from trauma (Yehuda, 2004). Similar to microarray analyses of gene expression in selectively bred rats (Zhang et al., 2005; Pearson et al., 2006), these trait-selected rats offer opportunities to correlate gene expression with fearful and anxious phenotypic expression. Thus, models that consider individual phenotypic differences in fearful and anxious responding will likely be among the more effective for modeling the anxiety disorders (Cohen et al., 2004; Bush et al., 2007).

CONCLUSIONS

A variety of animal models have been developed for fear and anxiety. Much of the current conceptualization of the underlying neurobiology of the anxiety disorders has been derived from neuroscience research employing rodent and nonhuman primate models. Some models apply to normal fearful and anxious responses in humans, whereas others are more applicable to anxiety disorders. Because each of the *DSM*-defined anxiety disorders has a unique symptom profile, it is especially important to carefully attend to behavioral details of the models to provide insights into specific disorders. Behavioral models that induce fear and anxiety symptoms in normal animals can be combined with other manipulations to emulate anxiety disorders. Some models such as fear conditioning apply to many disorders (learning in anxiety disorders) whereas others focus on specific disorders. In addition to face, predictive, and construct validity, consideration needs to be given to the value of the model for pursuing underlying neural mechanisms. Fear conditioning is particularly good in this category because of the extensively defined molecular, cellular, synaptic, and circuitry foundations. Brain regions involved in conditioned fear acquisition, expression, and regulation such as amygdala, hippocampus, and vmPFC have been implicated in a variety of anxiety disorders; therefore fear conditioning can be utilized as a bioassay to assess different functional changes that may occur in these areas in different disorders. Basic neuroscience research on animal models is providing hypotheses that can be tested in patients with anxiety disorders, with functional imaging technologies now offering a heretofore unavailable window on the correlates of regional activity in the human brain. Future research will likely offer many additional and perhaps more powerful applications of findings from animal models to our emerging understanding of anxiety disorders.

REFERENCES

Adamec, R.E., Blundell, J., et al. (2005) Neural circuit changes mediating lasting brain and behavioral response to predator stress. *Neurosci. Biobehav. Rev.* 29(8):1225–1241.

Adamec, R.E., Blundell, J., et al. (2006) Relationship of the predatory attack experience to neural plasticity, pCREB expression and neuroendocrine response. *Neurosci. Biobehav. Rev.* 30(3):356–375.

Adamec, R., Walling, S., et al. (2004) Long-lasting, selective, anxiogenic effects of feline predator stress in mice. *Physiol. Behav.* 83(3):401–410.

Aguiar, M.S., and Brandao, M.L. (1996) Effects of microinjections of the neuropeptide substance P in the dorsal periaqueductal gray on the behaviour of rats in the plus-maze test. *Physiol. Behav.* 60(4):1183–1186.

Aguilar, R., Gil, L., et al. (2004) Genetically-based behavioral traits influence the effects of Shuttle Box avoidance overtraining and extinction upon intertrial responding: a study with the Roman rat strains. *Behav. Processes* 66(1):63–72.

Akwa, Y., Purdy, R.H., et al. (1999) The amygdala mediates the anxiolytic-like effect of the neurosteroid allopregnanolone in rat. *Behav. Brain Res.* 106(1-2):119–125.

Amaral, D.G., Price, J.L., et al. (1992) Anatomical organization of the primate amygdaloid complex. In: Aggleton, J.P., ed. *The Amygdala: Neurobiological Aspects of Emotion, Memory, and Mental Dysfunction*. New York: Wiley-Liss, Inc., pp. 1–66.

American Psychiatric Association. (2000) *Diagnostic and Statistical Manual of Mental Disorders*, text rev.. Washington, DC: Author.

Amorapanth, P., LeDoux, J.E., et al. (2000) Different lateral amygdala outputs mediate reactions and actions elicited by a fear-arousing stimulus. *Nat. Neurosci.* 3(1):74–79.

Andreatini, R., and Bacellar, L.F. (2000) Animal models: trait or state measure? The test-retest reliability of the elevated plus-maze and behavioral despair. *Prog. Neuropsychopharmacol. Biol. Psychiatry* 24(4):549–560.

Anglada-Figueroa, D., and Quirk, G.J. (2005) Lesions of the basal amygdala block expression of conditioned fear but not extinction. *J. Neurosci.* 25(42):9680–9685.

Balleine, B.W., and Killcross, S. (2006) Parallel incentive processing: an integrated view of amygdala function. *Trends Neurosci.* 29(5): 272–279.

Barr, C. S., T. K. Newman, et al. (2004) Sexual dichotomy of an interaction between early adversity and the serotonin transporter gene promoter variant in rhesus macaques. *Proc. Natl. Acad. Sci. USA* 101(33):12358–12363.

Bauer, E. P., Schafe, G.E., et al. (2002) NMDA receptors and L-type voltage-gated calcium channels contribute to long-term potentiation and different components of fear memory formation in the lateral amygdala. *J. Neurosci.* 22(12):5239–5249.

Beekman, M., Flachskamm, C., et al. (2005) Effects of exposure to a predator on behaviour and serotonergic neurotransmission in different brain regions of C57bl/6N mice. *Eur. J. Neurosci.* 21(10): 2825–2836.

Bethea, C.L., Streicher, J.M., et al. (2004) Anxious behavior and fenfluramine-induced prolactin secretion in young rhesus macaques with different alleles of the serotonin reuptake transporter polymorphism (5HTTLPR). *Behav. Genet.* 34(3):295–307.

Blanchard, D.C., Griebel, G., et al. (2003) Conditioning and residual emotionality effects of predator stimuli: some reflections on stress and emotion. *Prog. Neuropsychopharmacol. Biol. Psychiatry* 27(8):1177–1185.

Blanchard, R.J., Blanchard, D.C., et al. (1970) Hippocampal lesions in rats and their effect on activity, avoidance, and aggression. *J. Comp. Physiol. Psychol.* 71(1):92–101.

Bliss, T.V., and Lomo, T. (1973) Long-lasting potentiation of synaptic transmission in the dentate area of the anaesthetized rabbit following stimulation of the perforant path. *J. Physiol.* 232(2): 331–356.

Bouret, S., Duvel, A., et al. (2003) Phasic activation of locus ceruleus neurons by the central nucleus of the amygdala. *J. Neurosci.* 23(8):3491–3497.

Bourin, M., and Hascoet, M. (2003) The mouse light/dark box test. *Eur. J. Pharmacol.* 463(1/3):55–65.

Bremner, J.D. (2004) Brain imaging in anxiety disorders. *Expert Rev. Neurother.* 4(2):275–284.

Brioni, J.D., and McGaugh, J.L. (1988) Post-training administration of GABAergic antagonists enhances retention of aversively motivated tasks. *Psychopharmacology (Berl)* 96(4):505–510.

Brunet, A., Orr, S.P., Tremblay, J., Robertson, K., Nader, K., Pitman, R.K. (2008) Effect of post-retrieval propranolol on psychophysiologic responding during subsequent script-driven traumatic imagery in post-traumatic stress disorder. *J. Psychiatry Res.* 42(6): 503–506.

Burghardt, N.S., Sullivan, G.M., et al. (2004) The selective serotonin reuptake inhibitor citalopram increases fear after acute treatment but reduces fear with chronic treatment: a comparison with tianeptine. *Biol. Psychiatry* 55(12):1171–1178.

Bush, D.E.A., Sotres-Bayon, F., et al. (2007) Individual differences in fear: isolating fear reactivity and fear recovery phenotypes. *J. Trauma Stress* 20(4):413–422.

Cannistraro, P.A., and Rauch, S.L. (2003) Neural circuitry of anxiety: evidence from structural and functional neuroimaging studies. *Psychopharmacol. Bull.* 37(4):8–25.

Cardinal, R.N., Parkinson, J.A., et al. (2002) Effects of selective excitotoxic lesions of the nucleus accumbens core, anterior cingulate cortex, and central nucleus of the amygdala on autoshaping performance in rats. *Behav. Neurosci.* 116(4):553–567.

Cassell, M.D., Freedman, L.J., et al. (1999) The intrinsic organization of the central extended amygdala. *Ann. N. Y. Acad. Sci.* 877:217–241.

Castellano, C., and McGaugh, J.L. (1990) Effects of post-training bicuculline and muscimol on retention: lack of state dependency. *Behav. Neural Biol.* 54(2):156–164.

Chalmers, D.T., Lovenberg, T.W., et al. (1995) Localization of novel corticotropin-releasing factor receptor (CRF2) mRNA expression to specific subcortical nuclei in rat brain: comparison with CRF1 receptor mRNA expression. *J. Neurosci.* 15(10):6340–6350.

Champoux, M., Bennett, A., et al. (2002) Serotonin transporter gene polymorphism, differential early rearing, and behavior in rhesus monkey neonates. *Mol. Psychiatry* 7(10):1058–1063.

Charney, D.S. (2004) Psychobiological mechanisms of resilience and vulnerability: implications for successful adaptation to extreme stress. *Am. J. Psychiatry* 161(2):195–216.

Cheeta, S., Kenny, P.J., et al. (2000) Hippocampal and septal injections of nicotine and 8-OH-DPAT distinguish among different animal tests of anxiety. *Prog. Neuropsychopharmacol. Biol. Psychiatry* 24(7):1053–1067.

Choi, S.H., Kim, S.J., et al. (2005) Doxapram increases corticotropin-releasing factor immunoreactivity and mRNA expression in the rat central nucleus of the amygdala. *Peptides* 26(11):2246–2251.

Cohen, H., and Zohar, J. (2004) An animal model of posttraumatic stress disorder: the use of cut-off behavioral criteria. *Ann. N. Y. Acad. Sci.* 1032:167–178.

Cohen, H., Zohar, J., et al. (2004) Setting apart the affected: the use of behavioral criteria in animal models of post traumatic stress disorder. *Neuropsychopharmacology* 29(11):1962–1970.

Cohen, H., Zohar, J., et al. (2006) Blunted HPA axis response to stress influences susceptibility to posttraumatic stress response in rats. *Biol. Psychiatry* 59(12):1208–1218.

Cohen, H., Kaplan, Z., et al. (1999) CCK-antagonists in a rat exposed to acute stress: implication for anxiety associated with posttraumatic stress disorder. *Depress. Anxiety* 10(1):8–17.

Coplan, J.D., Rosenblum, L.A., et al. (1992) Behavioral effects of oral yohimbine in differentially reared nonhuman primates. *Neuropsychopharmacology* 6(1):31–37.

Coplan, J.D., Smith, E.L., et al. (2001) Variable foraging demand rearing: sustained elevations in cisternal cerebrospinal fluid corticotropin-releasing factor concentrations in adult primates. *Biol. Psychiatry* 50(3):200–204.

Coplan, J.D., Trost, R.C., et al. (1998) Cerebrospinal fluid concentrations of somatostatin and biogenic amines in grown primates reared by mothers exposed to manipulated foraging conditions. *Arch. Gen. Psychiatry* 55(5):473–477.

Cornwell, B.R., Johnson, L., et al. (2006) Anticipation of public speaking in virtual reality reveals a relationship between trait social anxiety and startle reactivity. *Biol. Psychiatry* 59(7):664–666.

Costall, B., Jones, B.J., et al. (1989) Exploration of mice in a black and white test box: validation as a model of anxiety. *Pharmacol. Biochem. Behav.* 32(3):777–785.

Cunningham, C.L., Gremel, C.M., et al. (2006) Drug-induced conditioned place preference and aversion in mice. *Nat. Protoc.* 1(4): 1662–1670.

Datta, A., and Tipton, M. (2006) Respiratory responses to cold water immersion: neural pathways, interactions, and clinical consequences awake and asleep. *J. Appl. Physiol.* 100(6):2057–2064.

Davidson, J.R., Stein, D.J., et al. (2004) Posttraumatic stress disorder: acquisition, recognition, course, and treatment. *J. Neuropsychiatry Clin. Neurosci.* 16(2):135–147.

Davis, M. (1992) The role of the amygdala in fear and anxiety. *Annu. Rev. Neurosci.* 15:353–375.

Davis, M. (2006) Neural systems involved in fear and anxiety measured with fear-potentiated startle. *Am. Psychol.* 61(8):741–756.

Davis, M., Falls, W.A., et al. (1993) Fear-potentiated startle: a neural and pharmacological analysis. *Behav. Brain Res.* 58(1/2):175–198.

Davis, M., Ressler, K., et al. (2006) Effects of D-cycloserine on extinction: translation from preclinical to clinical work. *Biol. Psychiatry* 60(4):369–375.

Davis, M., Walker, D.L., et al. (1997) Roles of the amygdala and bed nucleus of the stria terminalis in fear and anxiety measured with the acoustic startle reflex. Possible relevance to PTSD. *Ann. N. Y. Acad. Sci.* 821:305–331.

de la Mora, M.P., Cardenas-Cachon, L., et al. (2005) Anxiolytic effects of intra-amygdaloid injection of the D1 antagonist SCH 23390 in the rat. *Neurosci. Lett.* 377(2):101–105.

De Souza, E.B., Insel, T.R., et al. (1985) Corticotropin-releasing factor receptors are widely distributed within the rat central nervous system: an autoradiographic study. *J. Neurosci.* 5(12):3189–3203.

Debiec, J., and LeDoux, J.E. (2004) Disruption of reconsolidation but not consolidation of auditory fear conditioning by noradrenergic blockade in the amygdala. *Neuroscience* 129(2):267–272.

Decker, M.W., Curzon, P., et al. (1995) Influence of separate and combined septal and amygdala lesions on memory, acoustic startle, anxiety, and locomotor activity in rats. *Neurobiol. Learn. Mem.* 64(2):156–168.

Degroot, A., Kashluba, S., et al. (2001) Septal GABAergic and hippocampal cholinergic systems modulate anxiety in the plus-maze and shock-probe tests. *Pharmacol. Biochem. Behav.* 69(3-4):391–399.

Degroot, A., and Treit, D. (2002) Dorsal and ventral hippocampal cholinergic systems modulate anxiety in the plus-maze and shock-probe tests. *Brain Res.* 949(1-2):60–70.

Diamond, D.M., Campbell, A.M., et al. (2006) Influence of predator stress on the consolidation versus retrieval of long-term spatial memory and hippocampal spinogenesis. *Hippocampus* 16(7): 571–576.

Dieterich, K.D., Lehnert. H., et al. (1997) Corticotropin-releasing factor receptors: an overview. *Exp. Clin. Endocrinol. Diabetes* 105(2):65–82.

Dityatev, A.E., and Bolshakov, V.Y. (2005) Amygdala, long-term potentiation, and fear conditioning. *Neuroscientist* 11(1):75–88.

Driscoll, P., Escorihuela, R.M., et al. (1998) Genetic selection and differential stress responses. The Roman lines/strains of rats. *Ann. N. Y. Acad. Sci.* 851:501–510.

Escorihuela, R.M., Fernandez-Teruel, A., et al. (1997) Labyrinth exploration, emotional reactivity, and conditioned fear in young Roman/Verh inbred rats. *Behav. Genet.* 27(6):573–578.

Escorihuela, R.M., Fernandez-Teruel, A., et al. (1999) Inbred Roman high- and low-avoidance rats: differences in anxiety, novelty-seeking, and shuttlebox behaviors. *Physiol. Behav.* 67(1):19–26.

Faber, E.S., Delaney, A.J., et al. (2005) SK channels regulate excitatory synaptic transmission and plasticity in the lateral amygdala. *Nat. Neurosci.* 8(5):635–641.

Fanselow, M.S. (1994) Neural organization of the defensive behavior system responsible for fear. *Psychonom. Bull. Rev.* 1:429–438.

Fanselow, M.S. (2000) Contextual fear, gestalt memories, and the hippocampus. *Behav. Brain Res.* 110(1-2):73–81.

Fanselow, M.S., and LeDoux, J.E. (1999) Why we think plasticity underlying Pavlovian fear conditioning occurs in the basolateral amygdala. *Neuron* 23(2):229–232.

Fendt, M., and Schmid, S. (2002) Metabotropic glutamate receptors are involved in amygdaloid plasticity. *Eur. J. Neurosci.* 15(9): 1535–1541.

Fendt, M., Siegl, S., et al. (2005) Noradrenaline transmission within the ventral bed nucleus of the stria terminalis is critical for fear behavior induced by trimethylthiazoline, a component of fox odor. *J. Neurosci.* 25(25):5998–6004.

Ferre, P., Fernandez-Teruel, A., et al. (1995) Behavior of the Roman/Verh high- and low-avoidance rat lines in anxiety tests: relationship with defecation and self-grooming. *Physiol. Behav.* 58(6): 1209–1213.

Ferry, B., Roozendaal, B., et al. (1999) Role of norepinephrine in mediating stress hormone regulation of long-term memory storage: a critical involvement of the amygdala. *Biol. Psychiatry* 46(9): 1140–1152.

File, S.E., and Seth, P. (2003) A review of 25 years of the social interaction test. *Eur. J. Pharmacol.* 463(1/3):35–53.

File, S.E., and Wardill, A.G. (1975) Validity of head-dipping as a measure of exploration in a modified hole-board. *Psychopharmacologia* 44(1):53–59.

Finn, D.A., Rutledge-Gorman, M.T., et al. (2003) Genetic animal models of anxiety. *Neurogenetics* 4(3):109–135.

Francis, D.D., Caldji, C., et al. (1999) The role of corticotropin-releasing factor--norepinephrine systems in mediating the effects of early experience on the development of behavioral and endocrine responses to stress. *Biol. Psychiatry* 46(9):1153–1166.

Francis, D.D., and Meaney, M.J. (1999) Maternal care and the development of stress responses. *Curr. Opin. Neurobiol.* 9(1): 128–134.

Frankland, P.W., Cestari, V., et al. (1998) The dorsal hippocampus is essential for context discrimination but not for contextual conditioning. *Behav. Neurosci.* 112(4):863–874.

Gewirtz, J.C., and Davis, M. (2000) Using pavlovian higher-order conditioning paradigms to investigate the neural substrates of emotional learning and memory. *Learn. Mem.* 7(5):257–266.

Gonzalez, L.E., Andrews, N., et al. (1996) 5-HT1A and benzodiazepine receptors in the basolateral amygdala modulate anxiety in the social interaction test, but not in the elevated plus-maze. *Brain Res.* 732(1/2):145–153.

Graeff, F.G., Silveira, M.C., et al. (1993) Role of the amygdala and periaqueductal gray in anxiety and panic. *Behav. Brain Res.* 58 (1-2):123–131.

Graham, Y.P., Heim, C., et al. (1999) The effects of neonatal stress on brain development: implications for psychopathology. *Dev. Psychopathol.* 11(3):545–565.

Gray, J.A. (1983) A theory of anxiety: the role of the limbic system. *Encephale.* 9(4 Suppl 2):161B–166B.

Gray, T.S., and Bingaman, E.W. (1996) The amygdala: corticotropin-releasing factor, steroids, and stress. *Crit. Rev. Neurobiol.* 10(2): 155–168.

Griebel, G., Belzung, C., et al. (1993) The free-exploratory paradigm: an effective method for measuring neophobic behaviour in mice and testing potential neophobia-reducing drugs. *Behav. Pharmacol.* 4(6):637–644.

Gross, C., and Hen, R. (2004) The developmental origins of anxiety. *Nat. Rev. Neurosci.* 5(7):545–552.

Hall, C.S. (1934) Emotional behavior in the rat. I. Defecation and urination as measures of individual differences in emotionality. *J. Comp. Psychology* 18(3):385–403.

Heim, C., Owens, M.J., et al. (1997) Persistent changes in corticotropin-releasing factor systems due to early life stress: relationship to the pathophysiology of major depression and post-traumatic stress disorder. *Psychopharmacol. Bull.* 33(2):185–192.

Heim, C., Plotsky, P.M., et al. (2004) Importance of studying the contributions of early adverse experience to neurobiological findings in depression. *Neuropsychopharmacology* 29(4):641–648.

Heinrichs, S.C., Lapsansky, J., et al. (1997) Corticotropin-releasing factor CRF1, but not CRF2, receptors mediate anxiogenic-like behavior. *Regul. Pept.* 71(1):15–21.

Heisler, L.K., Chu, H.M., et al. (1998) Elevated anxiety and antidepressant-like responses in serotonin 5-HT1A receptor mutant mice. *Proc. Natl. Acad. Sci. USA* 95(25):15049–15054.

Heldt, S.A., and Ressler, K.J. (2006) Localized injections of midazolam into the amygdala and hippocampus induce differential changes in anxiolytic-like motor activity in mice. *Behav. Pharmacol.* 17(4):349–356.

Helfer, V., Deransart, C., et al. (1996) Amygdala kindling in the rat: anxiogenic-like consequences. *Neuroscience* 73(4):971–978.

Henry, B., Vale, W., et al. (2006) The effect of lateral septum corticotropin-releasing factor receptor 2 activation on anxiety is modulated by stress. *J. Neurosci.* 26(36):9142–9152.

Herman, J.P., Ostrander, M.M., et al. (2005) Limbic system mechanisms of stress regulation: hypothalamo-pituitary-adrenocortical axis. *Prog. Neuropsychopharmacol. Biol. Psychiatry* 29(8): 1201–1213.

Hidalgo, R.B., and Davidson, J.R. (2000) Posttraumatic stress disorder: epidemiology and health-related considerations. *J. Clin. Psychiatry* 61(Suppl 7):5–13.

Hoehn-Saric, R., McLeod, D.R., et al. (1991) Psychophysiological response patterns in panic disorder. *Acta Psychiatr. Scand.* 83(1):4–11.

Hofer, M.A. (1996) Multiple regulators of ultrasonic vocalization in the infant rat. *Psychoneuroendocrinology* 21(2):203–217.

Huang, Y.Y., and Kandel, E.R. (1998) Postsynaptic induction and PKA-dependent expression of LTP in the lateral amygdala. *Neuron* 21(1):169–178.

Huang, Y.Y., Martin, K.C., et al. (2000) Both protein kinase A and mitogen-activated protein kinase are required in the amygdala for the macromolecular synthesis-dependent late phase of long-term potentiation. *J. Neurosci.* 20(17):6317–6325.

Huang, Y.Y., Nguyen, P.V., et al. (1996) Long-lasting forms of synaptic potentiation in the mammalian hippocampus. *Learn. Mem.* 3(2/3):74–85.

Huot, R.L., Thrivikraman, K.V., et al. (2001) Development of adult ethanol preference and anxiety as a consequence of neonatal maternal separation in Long Evans rats and reversal with antidepressant treatment. *Psychopharmacology (Berl)* 158(4):366–373.

Imanaka, A., Morinobu, S., et al. (2006) Importance of early environment in the development of post-traumatic stress disorder-like behaviors. *Behav. Brain Res.* 173(1):129–137.

Iversen, S.D. (1980) Animal models of anxiety and benzodiazepine actions. *Arzneimittelforschung* 30(5a):862–868.

James, W. (1884) What is an emotion? *Mind* 9:188–205.

Kalin, N.H., Shelton, S.E., et al. (1991) Effects of alprazolam on fear-related behavioral, hormonal, and catecholamine responses in infant rhesus monkeys. *Life Sci.* 49(26):2031–2044.

Kalin, N.H., Shelton, S.E., et al. (2004) The role of the central nucleus of the amygdala in mediating fear and anxiety in the primate. *J. Neurosci.* 24(24):5506–5515.

Kalisch, R., Korenfeld, E., et al. (2006) Context-dependent human extinction memory is mediated by a ventromedial prefrontal and hippocampal network. *J. Neurosci.* 26(37):9503–9511.

Kalueff, A.V., and Tuohimaa, P. (2004) Experimental modeling of anxiety and depression. *Acta Neurobiol. Exp. (Wars)* 64(4):439–448.

Kapp, B.S., Whalen, P.J., et al. (1992) Amygdaloid contributions to conditioned arousal and sensory information processing. In: Aggleton, J.P., ed. *The Amygdala: Neurobiological Aspects of Emotion, Memory, and Mental Dysfunction.*. New York: Wiley-Liss, pp. 229–254.

Kash, S.F., Tecott, L.H., et al. (1999) Increased anxiety and altered responses to anxiolytics in mice deficient in the 65-kDa isoform of glutamic acid decarboxylase. *Proc. Natl. Acad. Sci. USA* 96(4): 1698–1703.

Kask, A., Rago, L., et al. (1998) Anxiogenic-like effect of the NPY Y1 receptor antagonist BIBP3226 administered into the dorsal periaqueductal gray matter in rats. *Regul. Pept.* 75-76:255–262.

Keim, S.R., and Shekhar, A. (1996) The effects of GABAA receptor blockade in the dorsomedial hypothalamic nucleus on corticotrophin (ACTH) and corticosterone secretion in male rats. *Brain Res.* 739(1/2):46–51.

Killcross, S., Robbins, T.W., et al. (1997) Different types of fear-conditioned behaviour mediated by separate nuclei within amygdala. *Nature* 388(6640):377–380.

Kim, J.J., and Fanselow, M.S. (1992) Modality-specific retrograde amnesia of fear. *Science* 256(5057):675–677.

Kim, J., Lee, S., et al. (2007) Blockade of amygdala metabotropic glutamate receptor subtype 1 impairs fear extinction. *Biochem. Biophys. Res. Commun.* 355(1):188–193.

Kim, M., and Davis, M. (1993) Electrolytic lesions of the amygdala block acquisition and expression of fear-potentiated startle even with extensive training but do not prevent reacquisition. *Behav. Neurosci.* 107(4):580–595.

Klemenhagen, K.C., Gordon, J.A., et al. (2006) Increased fear response to contextual cues in mice lacking the 5-HT1A receptor. *Neuropsychopharmacology* 31(1):101–111.

Kobayashi, K., and Kobayashi, T. (2001) Genetic evidence for noradrenergic control of long-term memory consolidation. *Brain Dev.* 23(Suppl 1):S16–S23.

Kokare, D.M., Dandekar, M.P., et al. (2005) Interaction between neuropeptide Y and alpha-melanocyte stimulating hormone in amygdala regulates anxiety in rats. *Brain Res.* 1043(1/2):107–114.

Koob, G.F. (1999) Corticotropin-releasing factor, norepinephrine, and stress. *Biol. Psychiatry* 46(9):1167–1180.

Koob, G.F., and Heinrichs, S.C. (1999) A role for corticotropin releasing factor and urocortin in behavioral responses to stressors. *Brain Res.* 848(1/2):141–152.

Kostowski, W., Plaznik, A., et al. (1989) Intra-hippocampal buspirone in animal models of anxiety. *Eur. J. Pharmacol.* 168(3):393–396.

Kutsukake, N. (2006) The context and quality of social relationships affect vigilence behavior in wild chimpanzees. *Ethology* 112 (6):581–591.

LeDoux, J.E. (1992) Emotion and the amygdala. In: Aggleton, J.P., ed. *The Amygdala: Neurobiological Aspects of Emotion, Memory, and Mental Dysfunction.* New York: Wiley-Liss, Inc., pp. 339–351.

LeDoux, J.E. (1996) *The Emotional Brain: the Mysterious Underpinnings of Emotional Life.* New York: Simon & Schuster.

LeDoux, J.E. (2000) Emotion circuits in the brain. *Annu. Rev. Neurosci.* 23:155–184.

LeDoux, J.E., Farb, C., et al. (1990) Topographic organization of neurons in the acoustic thalamus that project to the amygdala. *J. Neurosci.* 10(4):1043–1054.

LeDoux, J.E., Ruggiero, D.A., et al. (1987) Topographic organization of convergent projections to the thalamus from the inferior colliculus and spinal cord in the rat. *J. Comp. Neurol.* 264(1): 123–146.

LeDoux, J.E., Iwata, J., et al. (1988) Different projections of the central amygdaloid nucleus mediate autonomic and behavioral correlates of conditioned fear. *J. Neurosci.* 8(7):2517–2529.

LeDoux, J.E., Cicchetti, P., et al. (1990) The lateral amygdaloid nucleus: sensory interface of the amygdala in fear conditioning. *J. Neurosci.* 10(4):1062–1069.

Lee, H.J., Berger, S.Y., et al. (2001) Post-training injections of catecholaminergic drugs do not modulate fear conditioning in rats and mice. *Neurosci. Lett.* 303(2):123–126.

Lee, Y., and Davis, M. (1997) Role of the hippocampus, the bed nucleus of the stria terminalis, and the amygdala in the excitatory effect of corticotropin-releasing hormone on the acoustic startle reflex. *J. Neurosci.* 17(16):6434–6446.

Lee, Y.J., Curtis, G.C., et al. (1993) Panic attacks induced by doxapram. *Biol. Psychiatry* 33(4):295–297.

Leonardo, E.D., and Hen, R. (2006) Genetics of affective and anxiety disorders. *Annu. Rev. Psychol.* 57:117–137.

Lesch, K.P., Meyer, J., et al. (1997) The 5-HT transporter gene-linked polymorphic region (5-HTTLPR) in evolutionary perspective: alternative biallelic variation in rhesus monkeys. Rapid communication. *J. Neural Transm.* 104(11/12):1259–1266.

Levine, S. (1994) The ontogeny of the hypothalamic-pituitary-adrenal axis. The influence of maternal factors. *Ann. N. Y. Acad. Sci.* 746:275–288; discussion 289–293.

Liang, K.C., Melia, K.R., et al. (1992) Lesions of the central nucleus of the amygdala, but not the paraventricular nucleus of the hypothalamus, block the excitatory effects of corticotropin-releasing factor on the acoustic startle reflex. *J. Neurosci.* 12(6):2313–2320.

Liberzon, I., Lopez, J.F., et al. (1999) Differential regulation of hippocampal glucocorticoid receptors mRNA and fast feedback: relevance to post-traumatic stress disorder. *J. Neuroendocrinol.* 11(1): 11–17.

Lister, R.G. (1990) Ethologically-based animal models of anxiety disorders. *Pharmacol. Ther.* 46(3):321–340.

Liu, I.Y., Lyons, W.E., et al. (2004) Brain-derived neurotrophic factor plays a critical role in contextual fear conditioning. *J. Neurosci.* 24(36):7958–7963.

Low, K., Crestani, F., et al. (2000) Molecular and neuronal substrate for the selective attenuation of anxiety. *Science* 290(5489):131–134.

Lyons, D.M., and Parker, K.J. (2007) Stress inoculation-induced indications of resilience in monkeys. *J. Traum. Stress* 24(4):423–433.

Manning, B.H. (1998) A lateralized deficit in morphine antinociception after unilateral inactivation of the central amygdala. *J. Neurosci.* 18(22):9453–9470.

Maren, S. (2001) Neurobiology of Pavlovian fear conditioning. *Annu. Rev. Neurosci.* 24:897–931.

Maren, S., and Chang, C.H. (2006) Recent fear is resistant to extinction. *Proc. Natl. Acad. Sci. USA* 103(47):18020–18025.

Maren, S., and Fanselow, M.S. (1996) The amygdala and fear conditioning: has the nut been cracked? *Neuron* 16(2):237–240.

Maren, S., Aharonov, G., et al. (1997) Neurotoxic lesions of the dorsal hippocampus and Pavlovian fear conditioning in rats. *Behav. Brain Res.* 88(2):261–274.

Martins, A.P., Marras, R.A., et al. (2000) Anxiolytic effect of a CRH receptor antagonist in the dorsal periaqueductal gray. *Depress. Anxiety* 12(2):99–101.

Mascagni, F., McDonald, A.J., et al. (1993) Corticoamygdaloid and corticocortical projections of the rat temporal cortex: a Phaseolus vulgaris leucoagglutinin study. *Neuroscience* 57(3):697–715.

Matar, M.A., Cohen, H., et al. (2006) The effect of early poststressor intervention with sertraline on behavioral responses in an animal model of post-traumatic stress disorder. *Neuropsychopharmacology* 31(12):2610–2618.

Matheus, M.G., and Guimaraes, F.S. (1997) Antagonism of non-NMDA receptors in the dorsal periaqueductal grey induces anxiolytic effect in the elevated plus maze. *Psychopharmacology (Berl)* 132(1):14–18.

Mayberg, H.S., Lozano, A.M., et al. (2005) Deep brain stimulation for treatment-resistant depression. *Neuron* 45(5):651–660.

McCown, T.J., Vogel, R.A., et al. (1983) An efficient chronic conflict paradigm: lick suppression by incremental footshock. *Pharmacol. Biochem. Behav.* 18(2):277–279.

McDonald, A.J. (1998) Cortical pathways to the mammalian amygdala. *Prog. Neurobiol.* 55(3):257–332.

McEwen, B.S. (2004) Protection and damage from acute and chronic stress: allostasis and allostatic overload and relevance to the pathophysiology of psychiatric disorders. *Ann. N. Y. Acad. Sci.* 1032:1–7.

McGaugh, J.L. (2004) The amygdala modulates the consolidation of memories of emotionally arousing experiences. *Annu. Rev. Neurosci.* 27:1–28.

McGaugh, J.L. (2006) Make mild moments memorable: add a little arousal. *Trends Cogn. Sci.* 10(8):345–347.

McGaugh, J.L., and Roozendaal, B. (2002) Role of adrenal stress hormones in forming lasting memories in the brain. *Curr. Opin. Neurobiol.* 12(2):205–210.

McKinney, W.T. (2001) Overview of the past contributions of animal models and their changing place in psychiatry. *Semin. Clin. Neuropsychiatry* 6(1):68–78.

McKinney, W.T., Jr., and Bunney, W.E., Jr. (1969) Animal model of depression. I. Review of evidence: implications for research. *Arch. Gen. Psychiatry* 21(2):240–248.

McNaughton, N. (2006) The role of the subiculum within the behavioural inhibition system. *Behav. Brain Res.* 174(2):232–250.

McNaughton, N., and Gray, J.A. (2000) Anxiolytic action on the behavioural inhibition system implies multiple types of arousal contribute to anxiety. *J. Affect. Disord.* 61(3):161–176.

Meaney, M.J., Diorio, J., et al. (1996) Early environmental regulation of forebrain glucocorticoid receptor gene expression: implications for adrenocortical responses to stress. *Dev. Neurosci.* 18 (1/2):49–72.

Meaney, M.J., Diorio, J., et al. (2000) Postnatal handling increases the expression of cAMP-inducible transcription factors in the rat hippocampus: the effects of thyroid hormones and serotonin. *J. Neurosci.* 20(10):3926–3935.

Mechiel Korte, S., and De Boer, S.F. (2003) A robust animal model of state anxiety: fear-potentiated behaviour in the elevated plus-maze. *Eur. J. Pharmacol.* 463(1/3):163–175.

Menzaghi, F., Howard, R.L., et al. (1994) Characterization of a novel and potent corticotropin-releasing factor antagonist in rats. *J. Pharmacol. Exp. Ther.* 269(2):564–572.

Millan, M.J., and Brocco, M. (2003) The Vogel conflict test: procedural aspects, gamma-aminobutyric acid, glutamate and monoamines. *Eur. J. Pharmacol.* 463(1/3):67–96.

Miller, M.M., and McEwen, B.S. (2006) Establishing an agenda for translational research on PTSD. *Ann. N. Y. Acad. Sci.* 1071:294–312.

Mineka, S., and Cook, M. (1993) Mechanisms involved in the observational conditioning of fear. *J. Exp. Psychol. Gen.* 122(1): 23–38.

Miyamoto, M., Shintani, M., et al. (1985) Lesioning of the rat basal forebrain leads to memory impairments in passive and active avoidance tasks. *Brain Res.* 328(1):97–104.

Moller, C., Wiklund, L., et al. (1997) Decreased experimental anxiety and voluntary ethanol consumption in rats following central but not basolateral amygdala lesions. *Brain Res.* 760(1-2):94–101.

Moller, C., Sommer, W., et al. (1999) Anxiogenic-like action of galanin after intra-amygdala administration in the rat. *Neuropsychopharmacology* 21(4):507–512.

Morgan, M.A., and LeDoux, J.E. (1995) Differential contribution of dorsal and ventral medial prefrontal cortex to the acquisition and extinction of conditioned fear in rats. *Behav. Neurosci.* 109 (4):681–688.

Morgan, M.A., and LeDoux, J.E. (1999) Contribution of ventrolateral prefrontal cortex to the acquisition and extinction of conditioned fear in rats. *Neurobiol. Learn. Mem.* 72(3):244–251.

Morgan, M.A., Schulkin, J., et al. (2003) Ventral medial prefrontal cortex and emotional perseveration: the memory for prior extinction training. *Behav. Brain Res.* 146(1/2):121–130.

Morgan, M.A., Romanski, L.M., et al. (1993) Extinction of emotional learning: contribution of medial prefrontal cortex. *Neurosci. Lett.* 163(1):109–113.

Moriceau, S., Roth, T.L., et al. (2004) Corticosterone controls the developmental emergence of fear and amygdala function to predator odors in infant rat pups. *Int. J. Dev. Neurosci.* 22(5/6): 415–422.

Morilak, D.A., Barrera, G., et al. (2005) Role of brain norepinephrine in the behavioral response to stress. *Prog. Neuropsychopharmacol. Biol. Psychiatry* 29(8):1214–1224.

Murchison, C.F., Zhang, X.Y., et al. (2004) A distinct role for norepinephrine in memory retrieval. *Cell* 117(1):131–143.

Myers, K.M., Ressler, K.J., et al. (2006) Different mechanisms of fear extinction dependent on length of time since fear acquisition. *Learn. Mem.* 13(2):216–223.

Nader, K., Schafe, G.E., et al. (2000) Fear memories require protein synthesis in the amygdala for reconsolidation after retrieval. *Nature* 406(6797):722–726.

Nader, K., Majidishad, P., et al. (2001) Damage to the lateral and central, but not other, amygdaloid nuclei prevents the acquisition of auditory fear conditioning. *Learn. Mem.* 8(3):156–163.

Nation, J.R., and Matheny, J.L. (1980) Instrumental escape responding after passive avoidance training: support for an incompatible response account of learned helplessness. *Am. J. Psychol.* 93(2): 299–308.

Netto, C.F., and Guimaraes, F.S. (2004) Anxiogenic effect of cholecystokinin in the dorsal periaqueductal gray. *Neuropsychopharmacology* 29(1):101–107.

Nordby, T., Torras-Garcia, M., et al. (2006) Posttraining epinephrine treatment reduces the need for extensive training. *Physiol. Behav.* 89(5):718–723.

Ohman, A., and Mineka, S. (2001) Fears, phobias, and preparedness: toward an evolved module of fear and fear learning. *Psychol. Rev.* 108(3):483–522.

Olsson, A., and Phelps, E.A. (2004) Learned fear of "unseen" faces after Pavlovian, observational, and instructed fear. *Psychol. Sci.* 15(12):822–828.

Overall, K.L. (1997) *Clinical Behavioral Medicine for Small Animals*. St. Louis, MO: Mosby, Inc.

Overall, K.L. (2000) Natural animal models of human psychiatric conditions: assessment of mechanism and validity. *Prog. Neuropsychopharmacol. Biol. Psychiatry* 24(5):727–776.

Packard, M.G., and Teather, L.A. (1998) Amygdala modulation of multiple memory systems: hippocampus and caudate-putamen. *Neurobiol. Learn. Mem.* 69(2):163–203.

Pape, H.C., Narayanan, R.T., et al. (2005) Theta activity in neurons and networks of the amygdala related to long-term fear memory. *Hippocampus* 15(7):874–880.

Pare, D., Quirk, G.J., et al. (2004) New vistas on amygdala networks in conditioned fear. *J. Neurophysiol.* 92(1):1–9.

Pare, D., Smith, Y., et al. (1995) Intra-amygdaloid projections of the basolateral and basomedial nuclei in the cat: Phaseolus vulgaris-leucoagglutinin anterograde tracing at the light and electron microscopic level. *Neuroscience* 69(2):567–583.

Parker, K.J., Buckmaster, C.L., et al. (2004) Prospective investigation of stress inoculation in young monkeys. *Arch. Gen. Psychiatry* 61(9):933–941.

Parks, C.L., Robinson, P.S., et al. (1998) Increased anxiety of mice lacking the serotonin1A receptor. *Proc. Natl. Acad. Sci. USA* 95 (18):10734–10739.

Paterson, A., Whiting, P.J., et al. (2001) Lack of consistent behavioural effects of Maudsley reactive and non-reactive rats in a number of animal tests of anxiety and activity. *Psychopharmacology (Berl)* 154(4):336–342.

Pavlov, I.P., and Anrep, G.V. (1927) *Conditioned reflexes; an investigation of the physiological activity of the cerebral cortex*. London: Oxford University Press: Humphrey Milford.

Pearson, K.A., Stephen, A., et al. (2006) Identifying genes in monoamine nuclei that may determine stress vulnerability and depressive behavior in Wistar-Kyoto rats. *Neuropsychopharmacology* 31(11):2449–2461.

Pellow, S., and File, S.E. (1986) Anxiolytic and anxiogenic drug effects on exploratory activity in an elevated plus-maze: a novel test of anxiety in the rat. *Pharmacol. Biochem. Behav.* 24(3):525–529.

Perrin, M.H., Donaldson, C.J., et al. (1993) Cloning and functional expression of a rat brain corticotropin releasing factor (CRF) receptor. *Endocrinology* 133(6):3058–3061.

Pesold, C., and Treit, D. (1992) Excitotoxic lesions of the septum produce anxiolytic effects in the elevated plus-maze and the shock-probe burying tests. *Physiol. Behav.* 52(1):37–47.

Pezze, M.A., and Feldon, J. (2004) Mesolimbic dopaminergic pathways in fear conditioning. *Prog. Neurobiol.* 74(5):301–320.

Phelps, E.A. (2004) Human emotion and memory: interactions of the amygdala and hippocampal complex. *Curr. Opin. Neurobiol.* 14(2):198–202.

Phelps, E.A. (2006) Emotion and cognition: insights from studies of the human amygdala. *Annu. Rev. Psychol.* 57:27–53.

Phelps, E.A., and LeDoux, J.E. (2005) Contributions of the amygdala to emotion processing: from animal models to human behavior. *Neuron* 48(2):175–187.

Phelps, E.A., O'Connor, K.J., et al. (2001) Activation of the left amygdala to a cognitive representation of fear. *Nat. Neurosci.* 4(4): 437–441.

Phillips, R.G., and LeDoux, J.E. (1992) Differential contribution of amygdala and hippocampus to cued and contextual fear conditioning. *Behav. Neurosci.* 106(2):274–285.

Pisula, W., and Osinski, J.T. (2000) A comparative study of the behavioral patterns of RLA/Verh and RHA/Verh rats in the exploration box. *Behav. Genet.* 30(5):375–384.

Pitkänen, A., Savander, V., et al. (1997) Organization of intra-amygdaloid circuitries: an emerging framework for understanding functions of the amygdala. *Trends Neurosci.* 20(11):517–523.

Pitman, R.K., and Delahanty, D.L. (2005) Conceptually driven pharmacologic approaches to acute trauma. *CNS Spectr.* 10(2):99–106.

Plotsky, P.M., Thrivikraman, K.V., et al. (2005) Long-term consequences of neonatal rearing on central corticotropin-releasing factor systems in adult male rat offspring. *Neuropsychopharmacology* 30(12):2192–2204.

Protopopescu, X., Pan, H., et al. (2005) Differential time courses and specificity of amygdala activity in posttraumatic stress disorder subjects and normal control subjects. *Biol. Psychiatry* 57(5): 464–473.

Prut, L., and Belzung, C. (2003) The open field as a paradigm to measure the effects of drugs on anxiety-like behaviors: a review. *Eur. J. Pharmacol.* 463(1/3):3–33.

Quirarte, G.L., Roozendaal, B., et al. (1997) Glucocorticoid enhancement of memory storage involves noradrenergic activation in the basolateral amygdala. *Proc. Natl. Acad. Sci. USA* 94(25):14048–14053.

Quirk, G.J., and Beer, J.S. (2006) Prefrontal involvement in the regulation of emotion: convergence of rat and human studies. *Curr. Opin. Neurobiol.* 16(6):723–727.

Quirk, G.J., Russo, G.K., et al. (2000) The role of ventromedial prefrontal cortex in the recovery of extinguished fear. *J. Neurosci.* 20(16):6225–6231.

Rainnie, D.G., Fernhout, B.J., et al. (1992) Differential actions of corticotropin releasing factor on basolateral and central amygdaloid neurones, in vitro. *J. Pharmacol. Exp. Ther.* 263(2):846–858.

Rainnie, D.G., Bergeron, R., et al. (2004) Corticotrophin releasing factor-induced synaptic plasticity in the amygdala translates stress into emotional disorders. *J. Neurosci.* 24(14):3471–3479.

Ramboz, S., Oosting, R., et al. (1998) Serotonin receptor 1A knockout: an animal model of anxiety-related disorder. *Proc. Natl. Acad. Sci. USA* 95(24):14476–14481.

Rau, V., DeCola, J.P., et al. (2005) Stress-induced enhancement of fear learning: an animal model of posttraumatic stress disorder. *Neurosci. Biobehav. Rev.* 29(8):1207–1223.

Rauch, S.L., Shin, L.M., et al. (2006) Neurocircuitry models of posttraumatic stress disorder and extinction: human neuroimaging research--past, present, and future. *Biol. Psychiatry* 60(4):376–382.

Repa, J.C., Muller, J., et al. (2001) Two different lateral amygdala cell populations contribute to the initiation and storage of memory. *Nat. Neurosci.* 4(7):724–731.

Ressler, K.J., Rothbaum, B.O., et al. (2004) Cognitive enhancers as adjuncts to psychotherapy: use of D-cycloserine in phobic individuals to facilitate extinction of fear. *Arch. Gen. Psychiatry* 61(11): 1136–1144.

Richter-Levin, G. (1998) Acute and long-term behavioral correlates of underwater trauma—potential relevance to stress and post-stress syndromes. *Psychiatry Res.* 79(1):73–83.

Rittenhouse, P.A., Bakkum, E.A., et al. (1992) Comparison of neuroendocrine and behavioral effects of ipsapirone, a 5-HT1A agonist, in three stress paradigms: immobilization, forced swim and conditioned fear. *Brain Res.* 580(1/2):205–214.

Rodrigues, S.M., Bauer, E.P., et al. (2002) The group I metabotropic glutamate receptor mGluR5 is required for fear memory formation and long-term potentiation in the lateral amygdala. *J. Neurosci.* 22(12):5219–5229.

Rodrigues, S.M., Schafe, G.E., et al. (2001) Intra-amygdala blockade of the NR2B subunit of the NMDA receptor disrupts the acquisition but not the expression of fear conditioning. *J. Neurosci.* 21(17):6889–6896.

Rodrigues, S.M., Schafe, G.E., et al. (2004) Molecular mechanisms underlying emotional learning and memory in the lateral amygdala. *Neuron* 44(1):75–91.

Rogan, M.T., Staubli, U.V., et al. (1997) Fear conditioning induces associative long-term potentiation in the amygdala. *Nature* 390 (6660):604–607.

Romanski, L.M., Clugnet, M.C., et al. (1993) Somatosensory and auditory convergence in the lateral nucleus of the amygdala. *Behav. Neurosci.* 107(3):444–450.

Rominger, D.H., Rominger, C.M., et al. (1998) Characterization of [125I]sauvagine binding to CRH2 receptors: membrane homogenate and autoradiographic studies. *J. Pharmacol. Exp. Ther.* 286 (1):459–468.

Roozendaal, B., and McGaugh, J.L. (1997) Basolateral amygdala lesions block the memory-enhancing effect of glucocorticoid administration in the dorsal hippocampus of rats. *Eur. J. Neurosci.* 9(1):76–83.

Roozendaal, B., Nguyen, B.T., et al. (1999) Basolateral amygdala noradrenergic influence enables enhancement of memory consolidation induced by hippocampal glucocorticoid receptor activation. *Proc. Natl. Acad. Sci. USA* 96(20):11642–11647.

Roozendaal, B., Brunson, K.L., et al. (2002) Involvement of stress-released corticotropin-releasing hormone in the basolateral amygdala in regulating memory consolidation. *Proc. Natl. Acad. Sci. USA* 99(21):13908–13913.

Rosen, J.B., and Schulkin, J. (1998) From normal fear to pathological anxiety. *Psychol. Rev.* 105(2):325–350.

Rosen, J.B., Hamerman, E., et al. (1996) Hyperexcitability: exaggerated fear-potentiated startle produced by partial amygdala kindling. *Behav. Neurosci.* 110(1):43–50.

Rosenblum, L.A., and Andrews, M.W. (1994) Influences of environmental demand on maternal behavior and infant development. *Acta Paediatr.* (Suppl 397):57–63.

Rosenblum, L.A., and Paully, G.S. (1984) The effects of varying environmental demands on maternal and infant behavior. *Child Dev.* 55(1):305–314.

Roth, W.T. (2005) Physiological markers for anxiety: panic disorder and phobias. *Int. J. Psychophysiol.* 58(2/3):190–198.

Sajdyk, T.J., and Shekhar, A. (1997) Excitatory amino acid receptor antagonists block the cardiovascular and anxiety responses elicited by gamma-aminobutyric acidA receptor blockade in the basolateral amygdala of rats. *J. Pharmacol. Exp. Ther.* 283(2):969–977.

Sajdyk, T.J., Schober, D.A., et al. (1999) Role of corticotropin-releasing factor and urocortin within the basolateral amygdala of rats in anxiety and panic responses. *Behav. Brain Res.* 100(1/2): 207–215.

Samson, R.D., and Pare, D. (2005) Activity-dependent synaptic plasticity in the central nucleus of the amygdala. *J. Neurosci.* 25(7):1847–1855.

Sanders, S.K., Morzorati, S.L., et al. (1995) Priming of experimental anxiety by repeated subthreshold GABA blockade in the rat amygdala. *Brain Res.* 699(2):250–259.

Sarter, M., and Bruno, J.P. (2002) Animal models in biological psychiatry. In: D'haenen, H., den Boer, J.A., and Willner, P., eds. *Biological Psychiatry*. New York: John Wiley & Sons Ltd., pp. 1–8.

Schafe, G.E., Atkins, C.M., et al. (2000) Activation of ERK/MAP kinase in the amygdala is required for memory consolidation of Pavlovian fear conditioning. *J. Neurosci.* 20(21):8177–8187.

Schafe, G.E., and LeDoux, J.E. (2000) Memory consolidation of auditory Pavlovian fear conditioning requires protein synthesis and protein kinase A in the amygdala. *J. Neurosci.* 20(18):RC96.

Schafe, G.E., Nadel, N.V., et al. (1999) Memory consolidation for contextual and auditory fear conditioning is dependent on protein synthesis, PKA, and MAP kinase. *Learn. Mem.* 6(2):97–110.

Schafe, G.E., Nader, K., et al. (2001) Memory consolidation of Pavlovian fear conditioning: a cellular and molecular perspective. *Trends Neurosci.* 24(9):540–546.

Selye, H. (1950) *The Physiology and Pathology of Exposure to Stress.* Montreal, Canada: Acta, Inc.

Servatius, R.J., Ottenweller, J.E., et al. (1995) Delayed startle sensitization distinguishes rats exposed to one or three stress sessions: further evidence toward an animal model of PTSD. *Biol. Psychiatry* 38(8):539–546.

Shah, A.A., and Treit, D. (2004) Infusions of midazolam into the medial prefrontal cortex produce anxiolytic effects in the elevated plus-maze and shock-probe burying tests. *Brain Res.* 996 (1):31–40.

Shanks, N., Larocque, S., et al. (1995) Neonatal endotoxin exposure alters the development of the hypothalamic-pituitary-adrenal axis: early illness and later responsivity to stress. *J. Neurosci.* 15(1 Pt 1): 376–384.

Shekhar, A., Keim, S.R., et al. (1996) Dorsomedial hypothalamic GABA dysfunction produces physiological arousal following sodium lactate infusions. *Pharmacol. Biochem. Behav.* 55(2):249–256.

Shekhar, A., McCann, U.D., et al. (2001) Summary of a National Institute of Mental Health workshop: developing animal models of anxiety disorders. *Psychopharmacology (Berl)* 157(4):327–339.

Shekhar, A., Truitt, W., et al. (2005) Role of stress, corticotrophin releasing factor (CRF) and amygdala plasticity in chronic anxiety. *Stress* 8(4):209–219.

Shephard, R.A., and Broadhurst, P.L. (1982) Hyponeophagia and arousal in rats: effects of diazepam, 5-methoxy-N,N-dimethyltryptamine, d-amphetamine and food deprivation. *Psychopharmacology (Berl)* 78(4):368–372.

Shin, L.M., Wright, C.I., et al. (2005) A functional magnetic resonance imaging study of amygdala and medial prefrontal cortex responses to overtly presented fearful faces in posttraumatic stress disorder. *Arch. Gen. Psychiatry* 62(3):273–281.

Sibille, E., and Hen, R. (2001) Combining genetic and genomic approaches to study mood disorders. *Eur. Neuropsychopharmacol.* 11(6):413–421.

Sigurdsson, T., Doyere, V., et al. (2007) Long-term potentiation in the amygdala: a cellular mechanism of fear learning and memory. *Neuropharmacology* 52(1):215–227.

Smagin, G.N., Harris, R.B., et al. (1996) Corticotropin-releasing factor receptor antagonist infused into the locus coeruleus attenuates immobilization stress-induced defensive withdrawal in rats. *Neurosci. Lett.* 220(3):167–170.

Sotres-Bayon, F., Bush, D.E.A. et al. (2007) Acquisition of fear extinction requires activation of NR2B-containing NMDA receptors in the lateral amygdala. *Neuropsychopharmacology* 32(9): 1929–1940.

Sotres-Bayon, F., Bush, D.E.A., et al. (2004) Emotional perseveration: an update on prefrontal-amygdala interactions in fear extinction. *Learn. Mem.* 11(5):525–535.

Spielberger, C.D., Gorsuch, R.C., et al. (1970) *Manual for the Stait Trait Anxiety Inventory*. Palo Alto, CA: Consulting Psychologists Press.

Steimer, T., and Driscoll, P. (2003) Divergent stress responses and coping styles in psychogenetically selected Roman high-(RHA) and low-(RLA) avoidance rats: behavioural, neuroendocrine and developmental aspects. *Stress* 6(2):87–100.

Stein, M.B., Goldin, P.R., et al. (2002) Increased amygdala activation to angry and contemptuous faces in generalized social phobia. *Arch. Gen. Psychiatry* 59(11):1027–1034.

Straube, T., Mentzel, H.J., et al. (2005) Common and distinct brain activation to threat and safety signals in social phobia. *Neuropsychobiology* 52(3):163–168.

Stutzmann, G.E., and LeDoux, J.E. (1999) GABAergic antagonists block the inhibitory effects of serotonin in the lateral amygdala: a mechanism for modulation of sensory inputs related to fear conditioning. *J. Neurosci.* 19(11):RC8.

Stutzmann, G.E., McEwen, B.S., et al. (1998) Serotonin modulation of sensory inputs to the lateral amygdala: dependency on corticosterone. *J. Neurosci.* 18(22):9529–9538.

Sullivan, G.M., Apergis, J., et al. (2003) Rodent doxapram model of panic: behavioral effects and c-Fos immunoreactivity in the amygdala. *Biol. Psychiatry* 53(10):863–870.

Sullivan, G.M., Apergis, J., et al. (2004) Lesions in the bed nucleus of the stria terminalis disrupt corticosterone and freezing responses elicited by a contextual but not by a specific cue-conditioned fear stimulus. *Neuroscience* 128(1):7–14.

Sullivan, R.M. (2003) Developing a sense of safety: the neurobiology of neonatal attachment. *Ann. N. Y. Acad. Sci.* 1008:122–131.

Sullivan, R., Wilson, D.A., et al. (2006) The International Society for Developmental Psychobiology Annual Meeting Symposium: Impact of early life experiences on brain and behavioral development. *Dev. Psychobiol.* 48(7):583–602.

Swiergiel, A.H., Takahashi, L.K., et al. (1992) Antagonism of corticotropin-releasing factor receptors in the locus coeruleus attenuates shock-induced freezing in rats. *Brain Res.* 587(2):263–268.

Takahashi, L.K., Hubbard, D.T., et al. (2007) Predator odor-induced conditioned fear involves the basolateral and medial amygdala. *Behav. Neurosci.* 121(1):100–110.

Takahashi, T., Morinobu, S., et al. (2006) Effect of paroxetine on enhanced contextual fear induced by single prolonged stress in rats. *Psychopharmacology (Berl)* 189(2):165–173.

Tecott, L.H. (2000) Designer genes and anti-anxiety drugs. *Nat. Neurosci.* 3(6):529–530.

Tecott, L.H., Logue, S.F., et al. (1998) Perturbed dentate gyrus function in serotonin 5-HT2C receptor mutant mice. *Proc. Natl. Acad. Sci. USA* 95(25):15026–15031.

Thiebot, M.H., Jobert, A., et al. (1980) Conditioned suppression of behavior: its reversal by intra raphe microinjection of chlordiazepoxide and GABA. *Neurosci. Lett.* 16(2):213–217.

Treit, D., and Menard, J. (1997) Dissociations among the anxiolytic effects of septal, hippocampal, and amygdaloid lesions. *Behav. Neurosci.* 111(3):653–658.

Treit, D., Pinel, J.P., et al. (1981) Conditioned defensive burying: a new paradigm for the study of anxiolytic agents. *Pharmacol. Biochem. Behav.* 15(4):619–626.

Tsoory, M., and Richter-Levin, G. (2006) Learning under stress in the adult rat is differentially affected by "juvenile" or "adolescent" stress. *Int. J. Neuropsychopharmacol.* 9(6):713–728.

Vale, W., Spiess, J., et al. (1981) Characterization of a 41-residue ovine hypothalamic peptide that stimulates secretion of corticotropin and beta-endorphin. *Science* 213(4514):1394–1397.

Van de Kar, L.D., Piechowski, R.A., et al. (1991) Amygdaloid lesions: differential effect on conditioned stress and immobilization-induced increases in corticosterone and renin secretion. *Neuroendocrinology* 54(2):89–95.

Vogel, J.R., Beer, B., et al. (1971) A simple and reliable conflict procedure for testing anti-anxiety agents. *Psychopharmacologia* 21(1):1–7.

Walker, C.D., Rivest, R.W., et al. (1989) Differential activation of the pituitary-adrenocortical axis after stress in the rat: use of two genetically selected lines (Roman low- and high-avoidance rats) as a model. *J. Endocrinol.* 123(3):477–485.

Walker, D.L., Toufexis, D.J., et al. (2003) Role of the bed nucleus of the stria terminalis versus the amygdala in fear, stress, and anxiety. *Eur. J. Pharmacol.* 463(1–3):199–216.

Walker, D.L., Ressler, K.J., et al. (2002) Facilitation of conditioned fear extinction by systemic administration or intra-amygdala infusions of D-cycloserine as assessed with fear-potentiated startle in rats. *J. Neurosci.* 22(6):2343–2351.

Wallace, T.L., Stellitano, K.E., et al. (2004) Effects of cyclic adenosine monophosphate response element binding protein overexpression in the basolateral amygdala on behavioral models of depression and anxiety. *Biol. Psychiatry* 56(3):151–160.

Watson, D. (2005) Rethinking the mood and anxiety disorders: a quantitative hierarchical model for DSM-V. *J. Abnorm. Psychol.* 114(4):522–536.

Wehner, J.M., Radcliffe, R.A., et al. (1997) Quantitative trait locus analysis of contextual fear conditioning in mice. *Nat. Genet.* 17(3):331–334.

Weiss, J.M., and Kilts, C.D. (1998) Animal models of depression and schizophrenia. In: Schatzberg, A.F., and Nemeroff, C.B., eds. *Textbook of Psychopharmacology*. Washington, DC: American Psychiatric Press, pp. 89–131.

Weisskopf, M.G., Bauer, E.P., et al. (1999) L-type voltage-gated calcium channels mediate NMDA-independent associative long-term potentiation at thalamic input synapses to the amygdala. *J. Neurosci.* 19(23):10512–10519.

Whalen, P.J., Kagan, J., et al. (2004) Human amygdala responsivity to masked fearful eye whites. *Science* 306(5704):2061.

Wilensky, A.E., Schafe, G.E., et al. (1999) Functional inactivation of the amygdala before but not after auditory fear conditioning prevents memory formation. *J. Neurosci.* 19(24):RC48.

Wilensky, A.E., Schafe, G.E., et al. (2000) The amygdala modulates memory consolidation of fear-motivated inhibitory avoidance learning but not classical fear conditioning. *J. Neurosci.* 20(18):7059–7066.

Wilensky, A.E., Schafe, G.E., et al. (2006) Rethinking the fear circuit: the central nucleus of the amygdala is required for the acquisition, consolidation, and expression of Pavlovian fear conditioning. *J. Neurosci.* 26(48):12387–12396.

Willner, P. (1991) Animal models as simulations of depression. *Trends Pharmacol. Sci.* 12(4):131–136.

Yehuda, R. (2004) Risk and resilience in posttraumatic stress disorder. *J. Clin. Psychiatry* 65(Suppl 1):29–36.

Yilmazer-Hanke, D.M., Faber-Zuschratter, H., et al. (2002) Contribution of amygdala neurons containing peptides and calcium-binding proteins to fear-potentiated startle and exploration-related anxiety in inbred Roman high- and low-avoidance rats. *Eur. J. Neurosci.* 15(7):1206–1218.

Zhang, S., Amstein, T., et al. (2005) Molecular correlates of emotional learning using genetically selected rat lines. *Genes Brain Behav.* 4(2):99–109.

40 Stress-Induced Structural and Functional Plasticity in the Brain: Protection, Damage, and Brain–Body Communication

BRUCE S. McEWEN

There is increasing evidence that the adult brain possesses a remarkable ability to adapt and change with experience. Long regarded as a rather static and unchanging organ, except for electrophysiological responsivity, such as long-term potentiation (LTP) (Bliss and Lomo, 1973), the brain has gradually been recognized as capable of undergoing rewiring after brain damage (Parnavelas et al., 1974) and also able to grow and change in terms of dendritic branching, angiogenesis, and glial cell proliferation during cumulated experience (Greenough and Bailey, 1988). More specific physiological changes in synaptic connectivity have also been recognized in relation to hormone action in the spinal cord (Arnold and Breedlove, 1985), and in environmentally directed plasticity of the adult songbird brain (DeVoogd and Nottebohm, 1981). Seasonally varying neurogenesis of restricted areas of the adult songbird brain is recognized as a part of this plasticity (Rasika et al., 1994; Rasika et al., 1999). Rather than being isolated examples of plasticity in certain species, there are increasing indications that structural change—neuronal replacement, remodeling of dendrites, turnover of synapses—is a feature of the adult brain's response to what happens to the individual. Nowhere is this better illustrated in the mammalian brain than in the hippocampus, where all three types of structural plasticity have been recently recognized and investigated using a combination of morphological, molecular, pharmacological, electrophysiological, and behavioral approaches.

The hippocampal formation is an important brain structure in episodic, declarative, contextual, and spatial learning, as well as a component of the control of a variety of vegetative functions such as adrenocorticotropic hormone (ACTH) secretion (Jacobson and Sapolsky, 1991; Eichenbaum and Otto, 1992; Phillips and LeDoux, 1992). It is also a plastic and vulnerable brain structure that is damaged by stroke and head trauma and is susceptible to damage during aging and repeated stress (Sapolsky, 1992). In 1968, we showed that hippocampal neurons express receptors for circulating adrenal steroids (McEwen et al., 1968), and subsequent work in many laboratories has shown that the hippocampus has two types of adrenal steroid receptors that mediate a variety of effects on neuronal excitability, neurochemistry, and structural plasticity (De Kloet et al., 1996). Hippocampal neurons also possess receptors for estrogens (Loy et al., 1988; DonCarlos et al., 1991; Weiland, Orikasa, et al., 1997) and androgens (J.E. Kerr et al., 1995) and show plasticity during sexual differentiation and in adult life in responses to gonadal steroids (Gould, Westlind-Danielsson, et al., 1990; Roof, 1993).

Recent work has revealed that adrenal and gonadal steroids are involved in four types of plasticity in the hippocampal formation. First, they reversibly and biphasically modulate excitability of hippocampal neurons and influence the magnitude of LTP, as well as producing long-term depression (Pavlides et al., 1994; Pavlides, Kimura, et al., 1995; Pavlides, Watanabe, et al., 1995; Pavlides et al., 1996). These effects may be involved in biphasic effects of adrenal secretion on excitability and cognitive function and memory during the diurnal rhythm and after stress (Barnes et al., 1977; Dana and Martinez, 1984; Diamond et al., 1992; Diamond et al., 1996). Second, adrenal steroids participate along with excitatory amino acids in regulating neurogenesis and neuronal replacement of dentate gyrus granule neurons, in which acute stressful experiences can suppress the ongoing neurogenesis (Cameron and Gould, 1996a). It is likely that these effects may be involved in fear-related learning and memory because of the anatomical connections between the dentate gyrus and the amygdala, a brain area important in memory of aversive and fear-producing experiences (LeDoux, 1995). Third, ovarian steroids regulated synaptic turnover in the hippocampus by a mechanism involving excitatory amino acids (McEwen et al., 2001; McEwen, Gould, et al., 1995). These effects may underlie the impairment of hippocampal-dependent memory functions in women after loss or suppression of ovarian function.

Finally, adrenal steroids participate along with excitatory amino acids in stress-induced remodeling of dendrites in the CA3 region of hippocampus, a process that affects only the apical dendrites and results in cognitive impairment in the learning of spatial and short-term memory tasks (McEwen, 1999). Besides atrophy of neuronal processes, severe and prolonged stress causes neuronal loss (Rozovsky et al., 2002), and the relationship between reversible atrophy and permanent damage is an important issue that is relevant to recent reports that the human hippocampus undergoes shrinkage in Cushing's syndrome, normal aging, dementia, recurrent depressive illness, schizophrenia, and posttraumatic stress disorder (PTSD). There is also stress-induced remodeling in amygdala and prefrontal cortex (PFC).

This chapter summarizes these various types of plasticity and discusses them in the broader context of how the brain responds to environmental demands, including those related to stressful life events. It is likely that the pathophysiological aspects of the adaptation to prolonged stress involves a loss of plasticity and an increased vulnerability to damage. This is discussed in relation to human psychiatric illness, aging, and comorbidities associated with them.

ROLE OF THE HIPPOCAMPUS IN BEHAVIORAL AND NEUROENDOCRINE ADAPTATION

The hippocampus and amygdala are key limbic brain structures that process experiences by interfacing with lower vegetative brain areas and higher cortical centers, particularly the PFC. They also help to interpret, on the basis of current and past experiences, whether an event is threatening or otherwise stressful and help to determine the behavioral, neuroendocrine, and autonomic responses. The amygdala is an essential neural component in the memory of fearful and emotionally laden events, whereas the hippocampus is concerned with determining the context in which such events take place, as well as other aspects of episodic and declarative memory (Squire and Zola-Morgan, 1991; Eichenbaum and Otto, 1992; Phillips and LeDoux, 1992). Whereas lesions of the central or lateral amygdala will abolish conditioning of the freezing response of an animal to tone paired with shock, a hippocampal lesion has no such effect; on the other hand, the hippocampal lesion will abolish conditioning of the freezing response to the "context," that is, to the environment of a particular conditioning chamber (Phillips and LeDoux, 1992).

The amygdala and hippocampus are also linked to each other anatomically and functionally (Knigge, 1961; Pitkanen et al., 2000). For example, lesions of the basolateral amygdaloid nucleus reduce LTP in the dentate gyrus, and stimulation of this nucleus facilitates dentate gyrus LTP (Ikegaya et al., 1994, 1995). The hippocampus and amygdala also have a regulatory role in the hypothalamic-pituitary-adrenal (HPA) axis activity, with the hippocampus in general being inhibitory and the amygdala acting as a facilitator of the HPA stress response (Knigge, 1961; McEwen, 1977; Jacobson and Sapolsky, 1991; Herman et al., 1996). However, this statement oversimplifies a great deal of complexity. For example, within the hippocampus, certain sites respond to electrical stimulation by increasing HPA activity (Dunn and Orr, 1984). Moreover, other brain areas are involved: for example, a recent brain lesion and steroid implant study indicates that the medial PFC plays an important role in containing the HPA response to psychological (for example, restraint), but not to ether stress (Diorio et al., 1993).

Glucocorticoid implants into the medial PFC reduce the magnitude of the HPA response to stress, as well as reducing plasma insulin levels (Diorio et al., 1993; Akana et al., 2001). These findings point to the important topic of steroid feedback, in general, and sites outside of the hippocampus and hypothalamus in the control of HPA activity. It is important to note that the HPA axis is dynamically regulated, and that steroid feedback operates at several levels in relation to neural control of the turning on and shutting off of the stress response (Akana et al., 1988; Jacobson et al., 1988). Besides rate-sensitive and level-sensitive feedback, delayed feedback may be viewed as a thermostat (steroid elevation turning down ACTH release) and a modulation by neural activity, which can be inhibitory (perhaps via the γ-aminobutyric acid [GABA] system), as well as excitatory upon the paraventricular nucleus (PVN), corticotrophin releasing factor (CRF), and arginine vasopressin (AVP) neurons (Herman et al., 1996). The bed nucleus of the stria terminalis is reported to have inhibitory and excitatory pathways to the PVN that regulate limbic system inputs to the HPA axis (Spano et al., 2007). The demonstration that constant steroid feedback via corticosterone (CORT) pellets implanted into rats with an adrenalectomy (ADX rats) normalizes ACTH levels but allows for sustained ACTH secretion after stress highlights the importance of neural control in the shut-off of the HPA stress response (Akana et al., 1988; Jacobson et al., 1988). The fact that in the same study, diurnal exposure to corticosterone (CORT) in the drinking water also normalized ACTH levels in ADX rats but allowed for a more rapid termination of the HPA stress response, even when no steroid was present, further highlights the importance of understanding the role of adrenal steroids in priming neural mechanisms that subserve shut-off of the HPA axis (Akana et al., 1988; Jacobson et al., 1988). A further aspect of feedback regulation of HPA function is the ability of energy sources, such as sucrose, to reduce ACTH secretion independently of adrenal steroids (Laugero et al., 2001).

Because of these two interrelated roles of the hippocampus (see Fig. 40.1), a role in aspects of memory and regulation of HPA activity, impairment of hippocampal function through changes in either excitability, reversible plasticity, or permanent damage may be expected to have two effects: The first is to impair hippocampal involvement in episodic, declarative, contextual, and spatial memory; impairments of these functions are likely to debilitate an individual's ability to process information in new situations and to make decisions about how to deal with new challenges. The second effect is to impair the hippocampal role in regulating HPA activity, particularly the shut-off of the stress response, leading to elevated HPA activity and further exacerbating the actions of adrenal steroids in the long-term effects of repeated stress. This concept, first called the glucocorticoid cascade hypothesis of hippocampal aging (Sapolsky et al., 1986), stands at the center of the notion of "allostasis" and "allostatic load" that are discussed at the conclusion of this chapter.

In summary, the amygdala, PFC, and hippocampus are brain structures that play a key role in turning on and shutting off the HPA axis during stress, acting at least in part through the bed nucleus of the stria terminalis and its projections to the paraventricular nuclei where corticotrophin releasing factor (CRF) is produced that drives ACTH secretion. Negative feedback by glucocorticoids is one aspect of a more complex process of neurally mediated regulation of HPA axis activity in which adrenal steroids play a regulatory role.

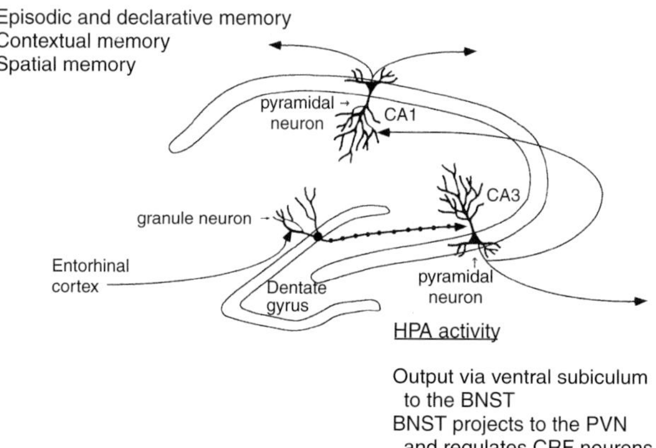

FIGURE 40.1 Hippocampal circuitry showing the two main functions of the hippocampal formation, cognitive function, and influencing hypothalamo-pituitary-adrenal (HPA) activity.

ADAPTIVE PLASTICITY OF THE HIPPOCAMPUS

The hippocampus expresses receptors for circulating adrenal steroids, as well as gonadal steroids; this remarkable property has made this brain structure a focal point for understanding the central nervous system (CNS) actions of circulating stress and gonadal hormones. As part of the cognitive and the vegetative aspects of the response to stressful events, the hippocampus is itself a very dynamic structure and is capable of changes in neuronal morphology and function that are modulated by circulating adrenal steroids acting through Type I (mineralocorticoid) and Type II (glucocorticoid) receptors (McEwen et al., 1968). Such receptors are expressed together in principal neurons of the Ammon's horn and dentate gyrus. The hippocampus also has receptors for gonadal steroids, with androgen receptors having been found in CA1 pyramidal neurons (J.E. Kerr et al., 1995) and estrogen receptors (ERs) in scattered interneurons in CA1 and dentate gyrus (Loy et al., 1988; DonCarlos et al., 1991; Weiland, Orikasa, et al., 1997). The hippocampus undergoes sexual differentiation and displays neuroanatomical sex differences as a result of the developmental actions of testosterone (Gould, Westlind-Danielsson, et al., 1990; Roof, 1993). Below, several types of plasticity are summarized, starting with a discussion of rapid plasticity related to excitability changes and then followed by a summary of structural plasticity in which changes in synapse formation, dendritic remodelling, and neuronal turnover are found in the adult hippocampus.

Rapid Plasticity of Excitability and Long-Term Potentiation

Adrenal steroids modulate the excitability of hippocampal neurons, as illustrated by the phenomenon of LTP (Bliss and Lomo, 1973) (see Fig. 40.2). A single burst of high-frequency stimulation to hippocampal afferents immediately alters the responsiveness of neurons to subsequent acute stimulation, an effect lasting over many hours to days. A number of recent studies have demonstrated in the hippocampal CA1 field and the dentate gyrus that acute stress and acute glucocorticoid elevation produces an impairment in LTP or its close relative, primed-burst potentiation, PBP (Diamond et al., 1992; Pavlides et al., 1993; Diamond et al., 1994). There is a *U*-shaped dose-response curve, with low levels of CORT facilitating PBP and high levels inhibiting PBP in the CA1 region (Diamond et al., 1992). In the dentate gyrus and CA1 and CA3 fields, LTP can be modulated rapidly (within 1 hour) and biphasically by

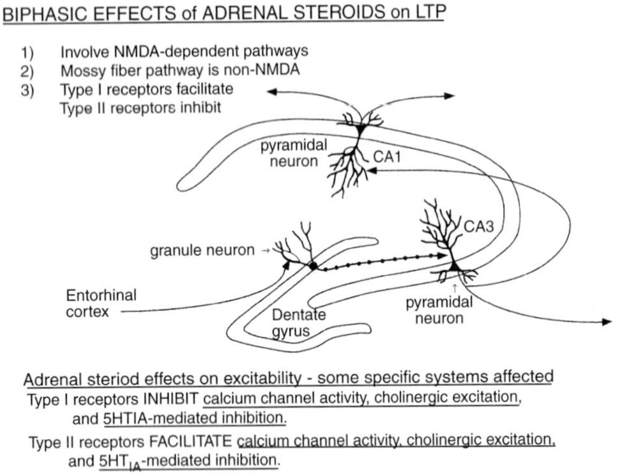

BIPHASIC EFFECTS of ADRENAL STEROIDS on LTP

1) Involve NMDA-dependent pathways
2) Mossy fiber pathway is non-NMDA
3) Type I receptors facilitate
Type II receptors inhibit

pyramidal neuron
CA1
CA3
granule neuron
Entorhinal cortex
Dentate gyrus
pyramidal neuron

Adrenal steriod effects on excitability - some specific systems affected
Type I receptors INHIBIT calcium channel activity, cholinergic excitation, and 5HTIA-mediated inhibition.
Type II receptors FACILITATE calcium channel activity, cholinergic excitation, and $5HT_{IA}$-mediated inhibition.

FIGURE 40.2 Hippocampal 3-cell circuitry. Adrenal steroids had biphasic effects on long-term potentiation in *N*-methyl-D-aspartate (NMDA)-dependent pathways. Type I (mineralocorticoid) and Type II (glucocorticoid) receptors have opposite effects on calcium channel activity, cholinergic excitation, and $5HT_{1A}$-receptor mediated inhibition.

adrenal steroids acting, respectively, via Type I and Type II receptors (Pavlides, Kimura, et al., 1995; Pavlides, Watanabe, et al., 1995; Pavlides et al., 1996). Moreover, in awake, freely moving ADX rats, the enhancement of LTP by the Type I receptor agonist, aldosterone, lasts for at least 24 hours, at which time it is still markedly higher than ADX rats given only vehicle treatment before LTP induction (Pavlides et al., 1994).

Mineralocorticoid receptors (MR or Type I) have an unusual role, namely, that, as determined by genetic deletion of the MR, they are essential for a rapid nongenomic effect of CORT in the mouse hippocampus that increases excitatory postsynaptic potentials (Karst et al., 2005). A similar rapid CORT effect on glutamate levels has been reported for the rat hippocampus, and this action is not blocked by RU-486 and hence does not appear to be mediated by the glucocorticoid receptors (GR or Type II) (Venero and Borrell, 1999).

Regarding how these biphasic effects come about, it is very likely that principal neurons in dentate gyrus and Ammon's horn contain both types of receptors, considering the distribution of messenger ribonucleic acid (mRNA), immunocytochemical reactivity, and binding for Type I and Type II adrenal steroid receptor subtypes (De Kloet et al., 1996). In studies on pyramidal neurons of the CA1 region, adrenal steroids have been shown to act via Type I and Type II adrenal steroid receptors to maintain and modulate excitability of hippocampal neurons (Beck et al., 1994; Joels and De Kloet, 1994; Birnstiel and Beck, 1995). Type I receptor activation in hippocampus from ADX rats is associated with reduced calcium currents through voltage-gated channels, reduced responses to serotonin via 5-HT_{1A} receptors and to carbachol via muscarinic receptors, and stable responses to synaptic inputs involving excitatory and inhibitory amino acids (Hesen and Joels, 1996a, 1996b). Additional activation of Type II receptors causes increased calcium currents and enhanced responses to excitatory amino acids, serotonin, and carbachol (Joels and De Kloet, 1994; Joels, 1997), and very high levels of Type II receptor activation markedly increase calcium currents (D. Kerr and Campbell, 1992) and also leads to increased *N*-methyl-D-aspartate (NMDA) receptor expression on hippocampal neurons (Weiland et al., 1995). Acute stress also increases NMDA R1 mRNA but decreases α-amino-3-hydroxy-5-methyl-4-isoxasole-propionic acid (AMPA) receptor subunit A mRNA levels without affecting mRNA levels of subunits B and C (Bartanusz et al., 1995). Kainate receptor mRNA levels were also affected by acute CORT treatment, with low-dose occupancy of Type I receptors increasing mRNA levels for kainate receptor 1 and 2 and also for the GluR7 subunit of the AMPA receptor and high-dose occupancy of Type II, as well as Type I receptors reversing this effect (Joels et al., 1996). Besides these effects, specific Type I and Type II agonists given to ADX rats produce a variety of other effects on various aspects of gene expression in hippocampus associated with neurotransmission (Lupien and McEwen, 1997).

Taken together with effects on hippocampal neuronal excitability described in the next section, what is surprising about these nonoverlapping actions of Type I and Type II receptors on gene products in hippocampus is that they defy the classical model of adrenal steroid receptor action via a common glucocorticoid response element (GRE) (Evans and Arriza, 1989) and point to a different and possibly more complex mode of MR and glucocorticoid regulation of gene expression (Miner and Yamamoto, 1991; Reichardt and Schutz, 1998). It should be noted that the regulation of preprotachykinin A gene mRNA levels in rat forebrain regions does follow the predictions of the classic GRE in that Type I and Type II agonist treatments of ADX rats elevate mRNA levels for this neuropeptide (Pompei et al., 1995). However, many other responses to glucocorticoids follow a pattern independent of the GRE because deletion of the deoxyribonucleic acid (DNA) binding domain of the glucocorticoid receptors still allows certain actions of glucocorticoids to occur (Reichardt and Schutz, 1998).

The fact that Type I and Type II adrenal steroid receptor activation has been characterized separately in ADX rats using selective agonists raises the question of what happens when both receptors are activated simultaneously over the physiological range of CORT. Under such conditions it is necessary to consider Type I/Type II receptor heterodimers (Trapp et al., 1994), as well as other comodulators of steroid-regulated gene expression such as immediate early genes (see below). This is important because we have noted that hippocampal neurons in Ammon's horn and dentate gyrus express both types of receptors, and it remains to be seen how different the consequences of combined receptor activation are from the information summarized using selective Type I and Type II receptor agonists and antagonists. Another issue to be resolved is the extent to which pyramidal neurons and granule neurons show similar molecular responses to adrenal steroid actions on excitability. From the standpoint of LTP, the biphasic actions of adrenal steroids in dentate gyrus and Ammon's horn occur in pathways using NMDA receptors and not in the mossy fiber non-NMDA pathway (Pavlides and McEwen, 1999). The commonality of adrenal steroid effects on NMDA receptor expression, on calcium channel activity, and on the sensitivity to carbachol and to serotonin via $5HT_{1A}$ receptors is, therefore, an important issue when looking at different hippocampal fields.

Behavioral actions can be attributed to Type I (MR) or Type II (GR) activation (Korte, 2001). At low concentrations that occupy Type I receptors, CORT exerts a permissive effect on acute freezing behavior and acute fear-related plus maze behavior. At high circulating levels that occupy Type II as well as Type I receptors, CORT enhances acquisition, conditioning, and consolidation of an inescapable stressful experience. High corticosteroid levels also potentiate fear but at the same time appear to play a role in the extinction of active avoidance.

In summary, adrenal steroids play a regulatory role on excitability in the hippocampus by acting through Type I (mineralocorticoid) and Type II (glucocorticoid) receptors that are present in neurons of Ammon's horn and the dentate gyrus. There are parallel effects on behavior and excitability of neurons that suggest an inverted *U*-shaped dose-response relationship, with low-to-moderate corticosteroid levels enhancing function and high stress levels having the opposite effect. Type I receptors also determine the ability of glucocorticoids to rapidly enhance excitatory transmission through a nongenomic mechanism.

Hormones, Neurotransmitters, and Neuronal Birth and Death in Dentate Gyrus

Removal of adrenal steroids

Granule neurons of the adult dentate gyrus depend on adrenal steroids for their survival, and adrenalectomy (ADX) of an adult rat increases the rate of granule neuron death (Sloviter et al., 1989; Gould, Woolley, et al., 1990). Three months after ADX, some rats showed an almost total loss of dentate gyrus granule neurons (Sloviter et al., 1989), and this finding at the time conflicted with the prevailing view that adrenal steroids cause neuronal death in Ammon's horn (see below), and it was puzzling because only some ADX rats showed the loss of the entire dentate gyrus. It now appears that a unique property of adult dentate granule neurons, not shared by cerebellar or olfactory bulb granule neurons, is for bilateral ADX to cause apoptotic death within 3–7 days (Gould, Woolley, et al., 1990). Besides apoptosis, the lack of adrenal steroids leads to a decreased branching of dendrites of dentate gyrus granule cells (Gould, Woolley, et al., 1990; Wossink et al., 2001).

The enhanced expression after ADX of the neuropeptide, calcitonin gene-related peptide (CGRP), in the inner molecular layer of the dentate gyrus may be related to the adaptation of the surrounding tissue to the rapid loss of neurons (Bulloch et al., 1996). The loss of the entire dentate gyrus occurs only in some rats and may well be explained by the absence of accessory adrenal tissue in those rats. When not removed at the time of ADX, this tissue can supply enough adrenal steroids to prevent neuronal loss, and we have found that very low levels of adrenal steroids, sufficient to occupy Type I adrenal steroid receptors, block dentate gyrus neuronal loss (Woolley et al., 1991). Although this is the case for adult hippocampus, Type II adrenal steroid receptors appear to be involved in inhibiting apoptosis in the neonatal hippocampus (Gould, Tanapat, and McEwen, 1997). This latter finding helps explain how massive apoptosis in the dentate gyrus occurs around postnatal day 6, in spite of glucocorticoid levels that are sufficient to occupy Type I receptors around this age (Meaney, Viau, et al., 1988).

Cell proliferation in the dentate gyrus of rats and other mammals

In adult rats, granule cell birth is accelerated by ADX (Gould and McEwen, 1993) (see Fig. 40.3). Newly born neurons, staining for neuron-specific enolase, arise in the hilus of the adult rat dentate gyrus, very close to the granule cell layer, and then migrate into the granule cell layer, presumably along a vimentin-staining radial glial network that is also enhanced by ADX (Gould and McEwen, 1993; Cameron and Gould, 1996a,1996b). The precursors for the newly generated cells appear to be related to astrocytes that express glial fibrillary acidic protein (GFAP) (Seri et al., 2001). Although Type I adrenal steroid receptors suppress neuronal turnover in adult dentate gyrus, most neuroblasts labeled with $[^3H]$ thymidine lack Type I and Type II adrenal steroid receptors (Cameron and Gould, 1996a), indicating steroidal regulation occurs via messengers from unidentified steroid-sensitive cells. The possibility that other trophic factors may be involved is currently under investigation by Gould and her colleagues.

Is the neurogenesis seen in rat and vole dentate gyrus an isolated phenomenon for those species or a broader phenomenon applicable to a select group of neurons in

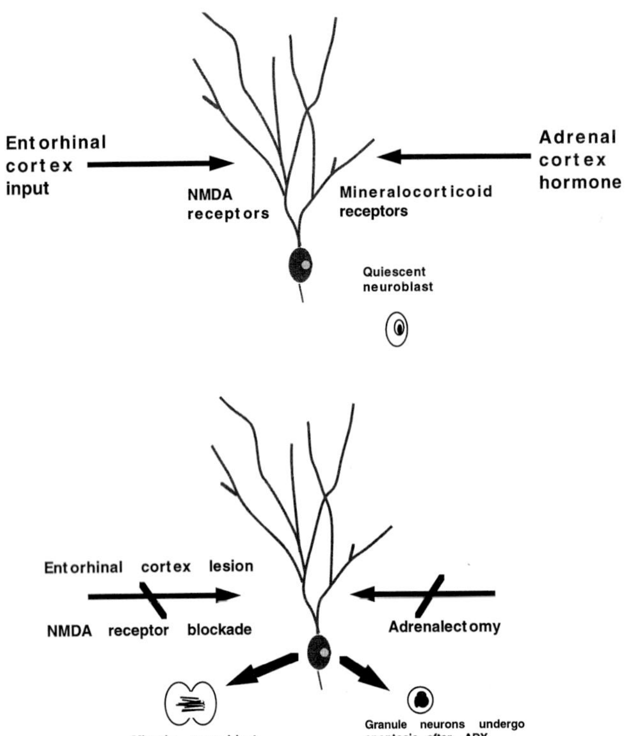

FIGURE 40.3 Entorhinal cortex input to the dentate gyrus and circulating adrenal steroids regulate turnover of granule neurons in the adult rat brain. Adrenalectomy increases the rates of cell birth and cell death, whereas entorhinal cortex lesions or blockade of *N*-methyl-D-aspartate (NMDA) receptors increase neurogenesis without affecting the number of dying granule neurons. As a result of NMDA receptor blockade, the size of the adult dentate gyrus increases.

the adult vertebrate brain? Studies of neurogenesis in songbird brain in relation to season of the year support the broader view (Rasika et al. 1994), but previous studies of neurogenesis in adult primate and human brain have produced largely negative results (Rakic, 1985). However, the dentate gyrus has not been a primary focus, and there have been no attempts to increase neurogenesis using either NMDA receptor blockade or ADX. Recent studies of the tree shrew, an insectovore, indicate that adult neurogenesis does occur in the dentate gyrus, and that it increases after acute NMDA receptor blockade and decreases after acute psychosocial stress (Gould, McEwen, et al., 1997). Dentate gyrus neurogenesis also has been shown to occur in the marmoset (Gould et al., 1998), a new-world primate, as well as in an old-world primate species, the rhesus monkey (Fuchs and Gould, 2000; Gould et al., 2001) and in the adult human dentate gyrus (Eriksson et al., 1998). In the human brain, it should also be noted that acute adrenocortical insufficiency, analogous to ADX, has been reported to result in dentate gyrus granule neuron death (Maehlen and Torvik, 1990).

Concerning the impairment of hippocampal function that may accompany adrenocortical insufficiency, several reports have indicated that long-term ADX rats that have damage to the dentate gyrus, like that described by Sloviter et al., (1989), show modest deficits in spatial memory (Armstrong et al., 1993; Conrad and Roy, 1995). It is particularly interesting that the spatial memory deficits after 42 days of ADX cannot be reversed by either glucocorticoid treatment or the antidepressant fluoxetine (Gong et al., 2007), which, in non-ADX animals, is able to increase neurogenesis (Duman et al., 2001). It is of further interest in relation to antidepressant actions that serotonin modulates the ability of CORT to suppress neurogenesis (Huang and Herbert, 2005) and that the ability of selective serotonin reuptake inhibitors (SSRIs) such as fluoxetine to increase neurogenesis requires the normal diurnal rhythm of HPA activity (Huang and Herbert, 2006).

Regulators of neurogenesis

There are negative and positive regulators of neurogenesis. Among the most important negative regulators discovered thus far are the excitatory amino acids. Blockade of NMDA receptors or removal of excitatory entorhinal cortical input to dentate gyrus markedly accelerates neurogenesis (see Fig. 40.3). *N*-methyl-D-aspartate receptor blockade also increases total dentate granule neuron number because it does not change the rate of granule neuron death (Cameron et al., 1995) until several weeks later when there is an elimination of cells that have not established connections (Nacher and McEwen, 2006). Application of NMDA has the opposite effect, namely, to suppress neuronal birth (Cameron et al., 1995). Like the story with Type I (MR) receptors, newly born granule neurons do not express NMDA R1 receptors, and so there must be another NMDA-responsive, as well as steroid-sensitive, cell type involved.

Certain types of acute and chronic stress inhibit neurogenesis. Acute stress involving the odor of a natural predator, the fox, inhibits neurogenesis in the adult rat (Galea et al., 1996). Acute psychosocial stress in the adult tree shrew, involving largely visual cues, inhibits neurogenesis (Gould, McEwen, et al., 1997). Inhibition of neurogenesis is also seen in the dentate gyrus of the marmoset after acute psychosocial stress (Gould et al., 1998). However, acute restraint stress does not inhibit neurogenesis, although chronic restraint stress for 21 days does inhibit dentate gyrus neurogenesis (Pham et al., 2003), and the learning of a contextual fear conditioning task is accompanied by suppression of dentate gyrus cell proliferation (Pham et al., 2003).

Granule neuron birth is accelerated by seizure-like activity (Parent et al., 1997), and the stimulus for this neurogenesis is likely to be apoptotic cell death because seizures kill granule neurons (Bengzon et al., 1997) and local increases in apoptosis simulate local neurogenesis (Cameron and Gould, 1996b). Granule neuron birth is also accelerated by blocking NMDA receptors or lesioning the excitatory perforant pathway input from the entorhinal cortex (Cameron et al., 1995). Unlike ADX, these treatments do not increase granule neuron apoptosis acutely, but only after a lag of several weeks, and a single dose of an NMDA-blocking drug results in a 20% increase in dentate gyrus neuron number several weeks later (Cameron et al., 1995; Nacher et al., 2001). Thus, although increased apoptosis leads to increased neurogenesis (Gould and Tanapat, 1997), the two processes occur in different regions of the granule cell layer and can be uncoupled from each other. Nevertheless, the adrenal steroid suppression of neurogenesis is through an NMDA-receptor mechanism (Gould, Tanapat, and Cameron, 1997; Noguchi et al., 1990).

As noted earlier, serotonin is a positive signal for neurogenesis in the adult dentate gyrus (Brezun and Daszuta, 1999, 2000). Treatment with the serotonin-releasing drug d fenfluramine increased neurogenesis (Gould, 1999). Likewise, the 5-HT_{1A} agonist 8 hydroxy DPAT stimulated neurogenesis, whereas blockade of 5-HT_{1A} receptors had the opposite effect and prevented the effect of d fenfluramine treatment (Gould, 1999), as well as preventing increased neurogenesis caused by pilocarpine-induced seizures (Radley and Jacobs, 2002). Various chronic antidepressant treatments also increase dentate gyrus cell proliferation in the absence of applied stress (Malberg et al., 2000). One antidepressant has been shown to prevent the suppression of neurogenesis by psychosocial stress in the tree shrew (Czeh et al., 2001).

Estrogen treatment acutely enhances dentate gyrus cell proliferation (Tanapat et al., 1999). The mechanism for this enhancement may well involve serotonin because serotonin depletion by P-chlorophenylalanine (PCPA) abolishes the stimulatory effect of estradiol in ovariectomized female rats (Brezun and Daszuta, 1999). Interestingly, the enhancement of polysialated neural cell adhesion molecule (PSA-NCAM) expression by estrogen is not prevented by serotonin depletion.

Circulating insulin-like growth factor (IGF-1) is another stimulator of neurogenesis (Aberg et al., 2000; O'Kusky et al., 2000). IGF-1 is a 7.5kDa protein and, yet, it is taken up into cerebrospinal fluid (CSF) by a process that is independent of IGF receptors or binding proteins (Pulford and Ishii, 2001). In rats, voluntary running in a running wheel has been reported to increase neurogenesis in the dentate gyrus (van Praag et al., 1999). Such exercise increases the uptake of IGF-1 from the blood and activates c-Fos expression in dentate gyrus and other brain regions in a manner that is mimicked by IGF-1 administration into the circulation (Carro et al., 2000). Moreover, immunoneutralization of IGF-1 blocks the effects of exercise to enhance neurogenesis (Trejo et al., 2001). Receptors for IGF-1, IGF-2, and insulin are expressed in the hippocampus (Dore, Kar, Rowe, et al., 1997), with IGF-1 receptors undergoing a decrease after adrenalectomy (Islam et al., 1998). Although IGF-1, IGF-2, and insulin binding do not decrease with age in the rat hippocampus (Dore, Kar, Rowe, et al., 1997), the level of IGF-1 mRNA undergoes a small but selective decrease in some hippocampal fields (Lai et al., 2000). Exogenous IGF-1 ameliorates memory deficits in aging rats (Markowska et al., 1998) and enhances glucose uptake in the aging hippocampus (Lynch et al., 2001) as well as having neuroprotective actions (Dore, Kar, and Quirion, 1997; Takadera et al., 1999; Gleichmann et al., 2000).

Adaptive value of neuronal turnover in the dentate gyrus

Adult neurogenesis in the dentate gyrus and cerebral cortex results in neurons that eventually turn over and are replaced by other neurons (Gould et al., 2001). Naturalistic stimuli, such as the odor of a predator to a rat, or a psychosocial stress encounter for a tree shrew, turn off ongoing neurogenesis (Gould, McEwen, et al., 1997; Parent et al., 1998). Chronic psychosocial stress in the tree shrew results in a more substantial inhibition of neurogenesis than after a single acute stressful encounter; moreover, the dentate gyrus is 30% smaller in the chronically stressed tree shrew, although granule neuron number only shows a trend for reduction (Gould and Fuchs, unpublished observations). This finding suggests that there may be other changes such as remodeling of dendritic branching to account for the decrease in dentate gyrus volume, and, indeed, recent studies on dendritic remodeling caused by glucocorticiods and also by repeated stress indicate that dentate gyrus dendrites undergo dendritic remodeling along with dendrites in CA3 and CA1 pyramidal neurons (Sousa et al., 2000).

Thus the ability of the dentate gyrus to expand and contract its neuronal population may be a natural event in the life of an adult rat and tree shrew. What other uses could there be for this mechanism? One explanation for why the dentate gyrus makes new cells in adult life, as well as gets rid of them, is to process spatial information and related aspects of memory (Sherry et al., 1992). Birds that use space around them to hide and locate food, and voles as well as deer mice that traverse large distances to find mates, have larger hippocampal volumes than closely related species that do not; moreover, there are indications that hippocampal volume may change during the breeding season (Sherry et al., 1992; Galea et al., 1994). Indeed, the rate of neurogenesis in the male and female prairie vole varies according to the breeding season (Galea and McEwen, 1998). Recent data on voles suggests that it is the dentate gyrus that exhibits this plasticity (Galea and McEwen, 1999).

The hippocampus also appears to affect the survival of newly formed dentate granule neurons. When rats were trained in a task involving the hippocampus, the survival of previously labelled granule neurons was prolonged (Gould et al., 1999). In contrast, an enriched environment has been found to increase dentate gyrus volume in mice by increasing neuronal survival without altering the rate of neurogenesis (Kempermann et al., 1997). In the enriched environment studies (Kempermann et al., 1997), increased dentate gyrus volume was accompanied by better performance on spatial learning tasks. In contrast, decreased dentate gyrus volume in chronically stressed tree shrews is paralleled by impaired spatial learning and memory (Ohl and Fuchs, 1999), although this might be as much due to atrophy of dendrites of CA3 pyramidal neurons and dentate granule neurons (see above) as to reduced dentate gyrus neurogenesis. Thus there are several ways to maintain the balance between neuronal apoptosis and neurogenesis.

There is an ongoing debate regarding the function of newly generated neurons in learning and memory and other functions of the hippocampus (Leuner et al., 2006). For example, there is evidence that behavioral tasks that involve the hippocampus prolong survival of newly generated neurons. Ablation of newly generated neurons by chemical means or X irradiation impairs some but not all hippocampal functions.

In summary, neurogenesis and neuronal replacement occurs in the dentate gyrus of the hippocampal formation. It is increased by exercise and by a number of antidepressant treatments and decreased by certain types of stress (Malberg et al., 2000; Leuner et al., 2006; Saxe et al., 2006). Learning tasks that involve the hippocampus appear to increase survival of recently generated neurons, and ablation of newly generated neurons impairs some hippocampal dependent memory tasks (Leuner et al., 2006; Saxe et al., 2006).

Formation and Breakdown of Synapses

Hippocampal pyramidal neurons demonstrate a reversible synaptogenesis in CA1 pyramidal neurons that is regulated by ovarian steroids and excitatory amino acids via NMDA receptors in female rats (McEwen, Gould, et al., 1995). The CA1 synaptic plasticity is a rapid event, occurring during the female rats' 5-day estrous cycle, with the synapses taking several days to be induced under the influence of estrogens and endogenous glutamic acid, and then disappearing within 12 hours under the influence of the proestrus surge of progesterone (McEwen, Gould, et al., 1995).

Even though the hippocampus expresses few estrogen and progestin receptors, this structure displays a robust response to estrogen and progestin treatment and to endogenous ovarian steroids during the natural estrous cycle. This first became evident with the finding of cyclic variations in the threshold of the dorsal hippocampus to elicitation of seizures, with the greatest sensitivity occurring on proestrus (Terasawa and Timiras, 1968). But, does the hippocampus contain ERs? Mapping studies of [^{3}H]estradiol uptake in hippocampus (Loy et al., 1988), and then by immunocytochemistry (DonCarlos et al., 1991; Weiland et al., 1996), showed a sparse distribution of cells containing intracellular ERs in what appear to be interneurons in the CA1 region, as well as other regions of Ammon's horn (Loy et al., 1988). There was also an indication that the CA1 region of hippocampus contains some estrogen-inducible progesterone receptors, albeit at much lower levels than in the hypothalamus (Parsons et al., 1982), although it has been impossible thus far to localize them in the hippocampus using immunocytochemistry (Waters et al., in press). However, data from in situ hybridization revealed the presence of low levels of progestin receptor mRNA in the CA1 and CA3 regions of Ammon's horn (Hagihara et al., 1992).

None of the receptor localization data suggested that the hippocampus would be a major target for estrogen or progesterone action, compared to brain regions such as the hypothalamus. The picture changed when morphological studies demonstrated that estrogen treatment induces dendritic spines and new synapses not only in the ventromedial hypothalamus of the female rat but also increases density of dendritic spines on pyramidal neurons in the hippocampus (for review, see McEwen and Woolley, 1994). Estrogen effects on dendritic spines were found only in the CA1 region and not in the CA3 region or in dentate gyrus. Moreover, spine density changed cyclically during the estrus cycle of the female rat. There were also parallel changes in synapse density on dendritic spines revealed by electron microscopy, strongly supporting the notion that new synapses are induced by estradiol. Taken together, these morphological studies indicate that synapses are formed and broken down rapidly during the natural reproductive cycle of the rat.

The critical involvement of progesterone was indicated by the fact that progesterone administration rapidly potentiated estrogen-induced spine formation but then triggered the down-regulation of spines on CA1 neurons. The down-regulation of dendritic spines occurred slowly when estrogen was withdrawn but took place within 8–12 hours when progesterone was administered; moreover, the natural down-regulation of dendritic spines between the proestrus peak and the trough on the day of estrus was blocked by the progesterone antagonist RU38486 (Woolley and McEwen, 1993).

Antagonism of the progesterone effect by RU38486 is consistent with the involvement of intracellular progestin receptors and is compatible with the finding, noted above, of estrogen-inducible progestin receptors in the CA1 region of hippocampus (Parsons et al., 1982).

However, there is another important factor, namely, the fact that estrogen induction of new spine synapses on CA1 pyramidal neurons is blocked by concurrent administration of NMDA receptor antagonists but not by antagonists of cholinergic and AMPA-kainate receptors (Woolley and McEwen, 1994). Spine synapses are excitatory, and it is likely that NMDA receptors occur on them; one of the long-term effects of estradiol is to induce NMDA receptor binding sites in the CA1 region of the hippocampus (Weiland, 1992a) and to increase immunoreactivity for the NMDA R1 subunit in the cell bodies and dendrites of CA1 pyramidal neurons, while not altering NMDA R1 mRNA levels measured by in situ hybridization (Gazzaley et al., 1996) (see Fig. 40.4). Thus, it may be that activation of NMDA receptors themselves could lead to induction of new synapses, in which case estrogen induction of NMDA receptors would then become a primary event leading to synapse formation. As discussed by Woolley and McEwen (1994), NMDA receptors gate calcium ions, and this may be an important factor in the extension and retraction of dendritic spines: for example, NMDA receptor activation promotes dephosphorylation of mitogen-activated protein (MAP2) and alters the interaction of this cytoskeletal protein with actin and tubulin.

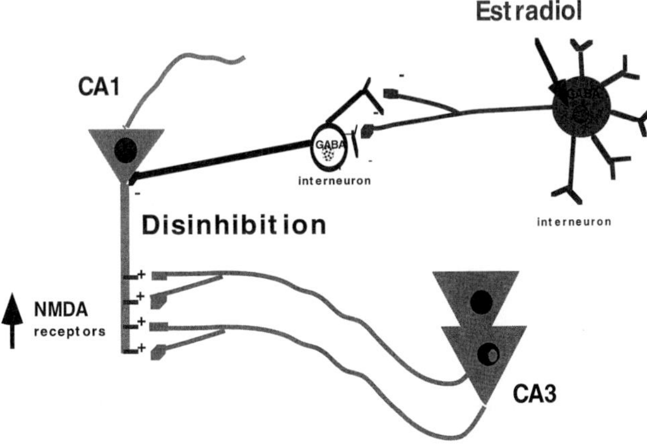

FIGURE 40.4 Estradiol regulates synaptogenesis on CA1 pyramidal neurons in the adult female rat hippocampus. Blocking *N*-methyl-D-aspartate (NMDA) receptors prevents the estrogen effect, and estrogen treatment increases expression of NMDA receptor protein on CA1 neurons. Estrogen-receptor immunoreactivity is found in interneurons, which are likely to be inhibitory. We speculate in this figure that these interneurons may synapse on other inhibitory interneurons and thus produce a disinhibition on the CA1 pyramidal neurons.

As to the possible significance of the presence of ERs in inhibitory interneurons and not in CA1 pyramidal neurons in which spine formation takes place, estradiol treatment induced glutamic acid decarboxylase (GAD) mRNA in inhibitory interneurons within the CA1 pyramidal cell layer (Weiland, 1992b). This would potentially increase inhibitory activity within these neurons, although it is not clear where they exert their inhibitory effect, on the pyramidal neurons themselves or on other inhibitory interneurons (see Fig. 40.4). In this connection, there are studies pointing to estrogen effects that excite hippocampal CA1 pyramidal neurons, possibly through disinhibition. One explanation is that estrogen actions on inhibitory interneurons might in some manner disinhibit the pyramidal neurons, allowing for removal of the magnesium blockade and activation of NMDA receptors (see Woolley and McEwen, 1994, for discussion).

Recent data on embryonic hippocampal neurons in cell culture have shown that estradiol induces spines over a time course of 24–48 hours by a process that is blocked by the antiestrogen *tamoxifen* and by the NMDA antagonist APV but not by the AMPA/kainate antagonist DNQX (D.D. Murphy and Segal, 1996). The phosphorylation of cyclic adenosine monophosphate (cAMP)-response element binding (CREB) has been implicated in this process (D.D. Murphy and Segal, 1997), and a decrease in brain-derived neurotrophic factor (BDNF) and inhibitory GABA transmission are also implicated (D.D. Murphy, Cole, Greenberger, et al., 1998; D.D. Murphy, Cole, and Segal, 1998). In vivo data also support a role for a transient estrogen-induced inhibition of GABA levels in inhibitory interneurons in the CA1 region (Rudick and Woolley, 2001).

Besides cell nuclear ER, there is increasing evidence for nonnuclear ER that interact with second-messenger pathways. A seminal study reported that transfection of ERα and ERβ into Chinese hamster ovarian cells resulted in expression of both ERs in a form that couples to second-messenger systems that are stimulated by estrogen and blocked at least partially by nonsteroidal estrogen antagonists (Razandi et al., 1999). Previous studies had indicated that nonnuclear ERs can be seen at the light microscopic level in cultured cells (Clarke et al., 2000) and also at the electron microscopic (EM) level in hypothalamus (Blaustein et al., 1992). The proliferation of articles on nonnuclear actions of estrogen via membrane ER and membrane-associated ER (e.g., Kelly and Levin, 2001; see above) has reinforced the importance of investigating nonnuclear actions of estrogens in the hippocampus.

Stimulated by this evidence, we used electron microscopy to examine ERα localization in rat hippocampal formation (Milner et al., 2001). We were able to see at the EM level the cell nuclear labelling seen by light microscopy in some GABA interneurons. In addition, some pyramidal and granule neuron perikarya have small amounts of ERα immunoreactive (IR) in the nuclear membrane, which is consistent with a recent report that 125 I estradiol labels a small number of estrogen binding sites in cell nuclei of hippocampal principal cells (Shughrue and Merchenthaler, 2000). In stratum radiatum of CA1, we found half of the total ERα-IR in unmyelinated axons and axon terminals containing small synaptic vesicles. This is of potential functional relevance, given findings that estrogen can influence neurotransmitter release (see McEwen et al., 2001, for references). The synaptic ERα-IR was found in terminals that formed asymmetric and symmetric synapses on dendritic shafts and spines, suggesting that excitatory and inhibitory transmitter systems are associated with ERα (Milner et al., 2001). Around 25% of the ERα-IR was found in dendritic spines of principal cells, where it was often associated with spine apparati and/or postsynaptic densities, suggesting that estrogen might act locally to regulate calcium availability, phosphorylation, or protein synthesis. Finally, the remaining 25% of ERα-IR was found in astrocytic profiles, often located near the spines of principal cells.

The close association between the ERα-IR and dendritic spines supports a possible local, nongenomic role for this ER in regulation of dendritic spine density via second-messenger systems. Initial in vivo and in vitro studies in the hippocampus of one second-messenger pathway, the phosphorylation of CREB, have indicated that estrogen has rapid effects that are evident within as little as 15 minutes to increase phosphoCREB immunoreactivity in cell nuclei of hippocampal pyramidal neurons (Lee et al., 2000). One pathway by which CREB phosphorylation may occur involves phosphoinositol-3 (PI3) kinase, or Akt, system (Datta et al., 1999). Studies are under way to try to connect these events together in the early actions of estrogen on hippocampal neurons that precede the induction of synapse formation. We next consider how nonnuclear and nuclear actions of ER may be coordinated in regulating synapse formation.

How can nuclear and nonnuclear actions of estrogen work together in the hippocampus? There is strong evidence in vivo and in vitro supporting an indirect GABAergic mediation of estrogen actions on synapse formation involving the ERα-containing inhibitory interneurons (D.D. Murphy, Cole, Greenberger, et al., 1998; Rudick and Woolley, 2000). The in vitro evidence comes from in vitro studies of E-induced synapse formation, in which estrogen induces spines on dendrites of dissociated hippocampal neurons by a process that is blocked by an NMDA receptor antagonist and not by an AMPA/kainate receptor blocker (D.D. Murphy and Segal, 1996). Furthermore, estrogen treatment was found to increase expression of phosphorylated CREB, and a specific antisense to CREB prevented the formation of dendritic spines and the elevation in phosphoCREB IR (D.D. Murphy and Segal, 1997). The cellular location of ERα in the cultures, resembling the in vivo localization, was in putative inhibitory interneurons, that is, GAD-immunoreactive cells that constituted around 20% of total neuronal population. Estrogen treatment caused decreases in GAD content and the number of neurons expressing GAD, and mimicking this decrease with an inhibitor of GABA synthesis, mercaptopropionic acid, caused an up-regulation of dendritic spine density, paralleling the effects of estrogen (D.D. Murphy, Cole, Greenberger, et al., 1998). Thus, estrogen-induced synapse formation may involve the suppression of GABA inhibitory input to the pyramidal neurons where the synapses are being generated.

An additional role of estrogen is to mobilize the movement of synaptic vesicles in ERα-containing presynaptic boutons of inhibitory interneurons that have the cholecystokinin neurochemical phenotype and which also express neuropeptide Y (NPY), a modulator that inhibits excitatory activity (Het and Wolf, 2007). Estrogen treatment has also been shown to increase expression of NPY in a subset of inhibitory interneurons in hippocampus (Nakamura and McEwen, 2005). Estrogen treatment may exert effects on NPY expression via BDNF (Franklin and Perrot-Sinal, 2006). These effects of estrogen via NPY may be relevant not only to synapse formation but also to the neuroprotective effects of estrogens in relation to stroke (Wise et al., 2005).

Thus, nuclear ER in interneurons plays a role in regulating the inhibitory tone upon pyramidal cells that, on the one hand, helps to regulate synapse formation and, on the other hand, may reduce neuronal excitability in relation to seizures and seizure-related damage. Concurrently, ER in dendritic spines may be associated with the activation of messenger ribonucleic acid (mRNA) translation from polyribosomes (Tiedge et al., 2001) or endomembrane structures found in spines (Pierce et al., 2000). In addition, other second-messenger signaling effects might include the phosphorylation of neurotransmitter receptors or ion channels. Estrogen receptor in certain presynaptic terminals might modulate neurotransmitter release or reuptake (see McEwen et al., 2001, for references). Moreover, ER-mediated activation of second-messenger systems in dendritic spines and presynaptic endings might lead to retrograde signal transduction back to the cell nucleus, perhaps via Akt or CREB, providing another pathway through which estrogen could regulate gene expression.

In summary, estradiol exerts important regulatory effects on synapse formation in the hippocampus by acting via nongenomic and genomic ERs found in diverse locations: inhibitory interneurons, cholinergic synapses, dendrites, and spines of excitatory neurons. Besides enhancing aspects of cognitive function (Sherwin, 2003), estrogen effects also include neuroprotection in relation to stroke.

Rapid Plasticity of Dendrites During Hibernation and Recovery

Hibernating ground squirrels and hamsters show a rapid atrophy or retraction of apical dendrites of CA3 pyramidal neurons that develops as fast as the hibernating state and can be reversed rapidly within several hours (Popov and Bocharova, 1992; Popov, Bocharova, and Bragin, 1992; Magarinos et al., 2006; Spanswick et al., 2007). This plasticity is seen on apical dendrites of CA3 pyramidal neurons that receive a powerful synaptic input from the dentate gyrus. Although anatomically similar to the stress-induced atrophy in rats and tree shrews (see below), it is not yet clear if this process involves the same mechanisms; however, if this is the case, the question becomes what factors make the atrophy rapid in hibernation and slow in relation to repeated stress.

Delayed Remodeling of Dendrites

Prolonged or repeated stress or glucocorticoid exposure causes atrophy of apical dendrites of CA3 pyramidal neurons, which resembles at least superficially what is seen in hibernation. In the hibernation and stress studies, dendritic length and branching are assessed by morphometry after silver staining neurons with the single-section Golgi technique. More recently, electron microscopy has revealed that stress and glucocorticoids alter morphology of presynaptic mossy fiber terminals in the stratum lucidum region of CA3 (Magarinos et al., 1997). Initially, atrophy of apical dendrites of CA3 pyramidal neurons, and not dentate granule neurons or CA1 pyramidal neurons, was found after 21 days of daily CORT exposure and also after 21 days of 6 hours/day repeated restraint stress (reviewed in McEwen, Albeck, et al., 1995). Psychosocial stress also causes apical dendrites of CA3 pyramidal neurons to atrophy in rats (McKittrick et al., 2000) and in an insectivore, the tree shrew (Magarinos et al., 1996).

Stress- and CORT-induced atrophy were prevented by the antiepileptic drug, phenytoin (Dilantin), thus implicating the release and actions of excitatory amino acids because phenytoin blocks glutamate release and antagonizes sodium channels and T-type calcium channels that are activated during glutamate-induced excitation (Taylor and Meldrum, 1995). This result is consistent with evidence that stress induces release of glutamate in hippocampus and other brain regions by a process dependent on the presence of the adrenal glands (see Magarinos et al., 1996; McEwen, Albeck, et al., 1995). Indeed, NMDA receptor blockade is also effective in preventing stress-induced dendritic atrophy (see McEwen, Albeck, et al., 1995).

A model of the cellular and neurochemical interactions involved in dendritic atrophy is presented in Figure 40.5, and it emphasizes the interactions among neurons and neurotransmitters. The role of adrenal steroids is discussed below. Besides glutamate, other participating neurotransmitters include GABA and serotonin. Inhibitory interneurons have a significant role in controlling hippocampal neuronal excitability (Freund and Buzsaki, 1996), and involvement of the GABA-benzodiazepine receptor system is strongly suggested by the ability of a benzodiazepine, adinazolam, to block dendritic atrophy (Magarinos et al., 1999). As for serotonin, repeated restraint stress in rats and psychosocial stress causes changes in the hippocampal formation that include not only atrophy of dendrites of CA3c pyramidal neurons but also suppression of 5-HT_{1A} receptor binding (McEwen, Albeck, et al., 1995; McKittrick et al., 2000).

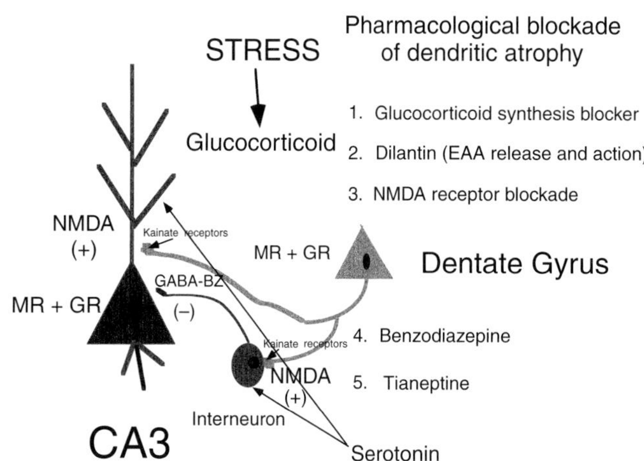

FIGURE 40.5 Stress causes atrophy, or remodelling, of apical dendrites of CA3 pyramidal neurons. Pharmacological blockade of dendritic atrophy indicates that glucocorticoid secretion is involved and that the final common path involves excitatory amino acid release via *N*-methyl-D-aspartate (NMDA) receptors. The mossy fiber terminals on the base of the apical dendrites appears to play the primary role in initiating the atrophy, and presynaptic kainate receptors on mossy fiber endings are likely to play an important role. However, serotonin release also appears to play a role because a serotonin reuptake enhancer, tianeptine, prevents atrophy (see text). Benzodiazepine treatment also prevents atrophy, presumably by enhancing the inhibitory input on interneurons. GR: glucocorticoid receptor; MR: mineralocorticoid receptor.

Serotonin is released by stressors and tianeptine, an atypical tricyclic antidepressant that enhances serotonin reuptake and thus reduces extracellular 5-HT levels, preventing stress- and CORT-induced dendritic atrophy of CA3c pyramidal neurons (Watanabe et al., 1992). In contrast, several inhibitors of serotonin reupake—fluoxetine, fluvoxamine, and desipramine, an inhibitor of noradrenaline uptake—failed to block atrophy (Magarinos et al., 1999). Thus the effect of tianeptine on CA3 pyramidal neuron morphology is not likely to be due to its reported effects to reduce CORT secretion (Delbende et al., 1991) but may instead be related to its reported effects to enhance the reuptake of serotonin within the hippocampus (Whitton et al., 1991). Further evidence for serotonin involvement in dendritic atrophy comes from studies of psychosocial stress in rats, in that dominant and subordinant rats show both dendritic atrophy as well as down-regulation of 5-HT transporter expression in the CA3 region, indicating either a reduced density of serotonin terminals or a reduced expression of the transporter (McKittrick et al., 2000). However, dominant rats show a greater reduction in 5-HT transporter sites than subordinants, and dominants also show a greater dendritic atrophy (McKittrick et al., 2000).

Because CORT- and stress-induced atrophy of CA3 pyramidal neurons is blocked by phenytoin as well as by tianeptine (see McEwen, Albeck, et al., 1995), serotonin released by stress or CORT may interact pre- or postsynaptically with glutamate released by stress or CORT, and the final common path may involve interactive effects between serotonin and glutamate receptors on the dendrites of CA3 neurons innervated by mossy fibers from the dentate gyrus. There is evidence for interactions between serotonin and NMDA receptors, indicating that serotonin potentiates NMDA receptor binding as well as activity of NMDA receptors and may do so via 5-HT_2 receptors (Mennini and Miari, 1991; Rahmann and Neumann, 1993).

Glucocorticoid treatment causes dendritic atrophy, and stress-induced atrophy is blocked by treatment with an adrenal steroid synthesis blocker, cyanoketone (see Magarinos and McEwen, 1995a, 1995b). What is the role of adrenal steroids in relation to the neurotransmitter involvement cited above? A primary site of action is the release of glutamate, because ADX markedly reduces the magnitude of the excitatory amino acid (EAA) release evoked by restraint stress (Lowy et al., 1993; Moghaddam et al., 1994). In this connection, mossy fiber terminals from dentate granule neurons in the stratum lucidum of CA3 apical dendrites show morphological alterations as a result of chronic stress (Magarinos et al., 1997). These changes involve reorganization of synaptic vesicles in the synaptic terminal, with a higher density occurring in regions adjacent to active synaptic zones.

The stratum lucidum zone of CA3 contains high levels of kainate receptors, as demonstrated by quantitative autoradiography, and, as noted above, these receptors are decreased in density by ADX and restored to normal by CORT replacement (Watanabe et al., 1995). Because kainate receptors are feed-forward autoreceptors for EAAs on presynaptic mossy fiber nerve endings (see Fig. 40.5), the effects of adrenal steroids are consistent with the dependence of stress-induced glutamate release on the presence of the adrenal glands (Lowy et al., 1993; Moghaddam et al., 1994).

Another possibility is that CORT or stress alters CA3 neuronal atrophy through regulation of GABAergic synaptic inhibition (see Fig. 40.5). In support of this notion, low levels of CORT alter mRNA levels for specific subunits of GABA-A receptors in CA3 and the dentate gyrus of ADX rats (Orchinik et al., 1994), whereas stress levels of CORT have produced different effects on GABA-A receptor subunit mRNA levels and receptor binding in hippocampal subregions, including CA3 (Orchinik et al., 2001). Therefore, it appears that CORT may alter the excitability of hippocampal neurons through regulation of GABA-A receptor expression, but it remains to be seen if the corticosteroid effects on neuronal morphology involve changes in the number or pharmacological properties of GABA-A receptors.

Stress and glucocorticoid treatment cause enhanced expression of NMDA receptors in hippocampus (Bartanusz et al., 1995; Weiland, Orchinik, and Tanapat, 1997), and this is another potential mechanism by which adrenal steroids are involved in dendritic atrophy (see Fig. 40.5). It is puzzling, however, that NMDA receptors are not expressed in the stratum lucidum where mossy fibers terminate (Monaghan et al., 1983), given the evidence cited above for the importance of this innervation for dendritic atrophy. The presence of NMDA receptors on the more distal aspects of CA3 dendrites suggests that the mossy fiber activation of glutamate release triggers a much more widespread activity of EAAs affecting the entire dendritic tree of the CA3 pyramidal neurons.

Following upon the widespread activation of NMDA receptors, the increased levels of intracellular calcium may make the dendritic cytoskeleton become depolymerized or undergo proteolysis (see McEwen, Albeck, et al., 1995, for discussion). Stress is also reported to alter the expression of the neurotrophins, BDNF and Neurotrophin-3 (NT-3), in hippocampus (Smith et al., 1995). Very little is known about the adrenal steroid receptor types involved in these effects, or the localization of stress and adrenal steroid effects on neurotrophin expression within the hippocampus and their relationship to the conditions of repeated stress that bring about morphological changes. However, conditions that cause dendritic atrophy, such as repeated restraint stress or psychosocial stress, do not appear to change neurotrophin expression in hippocampus (Kuroda and McEwen, 1998), indicating that neurotrophins are probably not directly involved in the mechanism of dendritic atrophy.

In summary, stress and application of glucocorticoids cause a remodeling of dendrites of neurons in the hippocampus, primarily those of pyramidal cells in the CA3 region but also granule neurons of the dentate gyrus. This process is reversible with termination of the stressor or excess glucocorticoid, and it is blocked by inhibitors of EAA neurotransmission. Thus, as is also the case, with E-induced synapse formation, the stress-induced remodeling is not due to steroid hormones acting alone but rather in combination with EAA neurotransmission.

Remodeling of Neurons in Amygdala and Hippocampus

Acute and repeated stress (21 days of chronic restraint stress [CRS]) also cause functional and structural changes in other brain regions such as the PFC and amygdala. Chronic restraint stress and chronic immobilization caused dendritic shortening in medial PFC (Sousa et al., 2000; Wellman, 2001; Vyas et al., 2002; Cook and Wellman, 2004; Kreibich and Blendy, 2004; Radley et al., 2004; Brown et al., 2005; Radley et al., 2005; Radley et al., 2006) but produced dendritic growth in neurons in amygdala (Vyas et al., 2002), as well as in orbitofrontal cortex (OFC) (Liston et al., 2006). These actions of stress are reminiscent of recent work on experimenter versus self-administered morphine and amphetamine, in which different, and sometimes opposite, effects were seen on dendritic spine density in OFC, medial PFC, and hippocampus CA1 (Robinson and Kolb, 1997). For example, amphetamine self-administration increased spine density on pyramidal neurons in the medial PFC and decreased spine density on OFC pyramidal neurons (Crombag et al., 2005).

Along with many other brain regions, the amygdala and PFC also contain adrenal steroid receptors (Ahima and Harlan, 1990; Ahima et al., 1991); however, the role of adrenal steroids, EAAs, and other mediators has not yet been studied in detail in these brain regions, in contrast to the hippocampus. Nevertheless, glucocorticoids do appear to play a role because 3 weeks of chronic CORT treatment was shown to produce retraction of dendrites in medial PFC (Wellman, 2001), although with subtle differences in the qualitative nature of the effect from what has been described after CRS (Radley et al., 2004). Another study determined the effect of ADX or either chronic treatment for 4 weeks with CORT or dexamethasone on volume and neuron number in the PFC (Cerqueira et al., 2005). Dexamethasone treatment at a dose that may have been high enough to enter the brain (although this was not directly measured) caused a loss of neurons in Layer II of the infralimbic, prelimbic, and cingulate cortex, whereas CORT treatment reduced the volume but not the neuron number of these cortical regions (Cerqueira et al., 2005). The dexamethasone treatment was particularly effective in impairing working memory and cognitive flexibility using working memory task in a Morris water maze (Cerqueira et al., 2005). Effects of chronic stress were not investigated in this study. These data notwithstanding, the cautions expressed above concerning differences between chronic stress and chronic glucocorticoid treatment must be kept in mind for the PFC, as well as the amygdala, that has not been studied yet in this regard.

Behavioral correlates of CRS-induced remodeling in the PFC include impairment in attention set shifting, possibly reflecting structural remodeling in the medial PFC (Liston et al., 2006). Attention set shifting is a task in which a rat first learns that either odor or the digging medium in a pair of bowls predicts where food reward is to be found; then new cues are introduced, and the rat needs to learn which ones predict the location of food (Birrell and Brown, 2000). There is also a report that CRS impairs extinction of a fear conditioning task (Miracle et al., 2006). This is an important lead because the PFC is involved in extinction, a type of learning (Santini et al., 2004), but much more research is needed to explore the complex relationship between stress, fear conditioning, extinction, and possible morphological remodeling that may well accompany each of these experiences.

Regarding the amygdala, chronic stress for 21 days or longer not only impairs hippocampal-dependent cognitive function (McEwen, 1999), but also enhances amygdala-dependent unlearned fear and fear conditioning (Conrad et al., 1999) that are consistent with the opposite effects of stress on hippocampal and amygdala structure. Chronic stress also increases aggression between animals living in the same cage, and this is likely to reflect another aspect of hyperactivity of the amygdala (Wood et al., 2003). Moreover, chronic CORT treatment in the drinking water produces an anxiogenic effect in mice (Ardayfio and Kim, 2006), an effect that could be due to the glucocorticoid enhancement of corticotrophin releasing factor (CRF) activity in the amygdala (Corodimas et al., 1994; Makino et al., 1994).

As for mechanism of remodeling, besides the possible role of glucocorticoids and EAAs, tissue plasminogen activator (tPA) is required for acute stress to not only activate indices of structural plasticity but also to enhance anxiety (Melchor et al., 2003). These effects occur in the medial and central amygdala and not in basolateral amygdala, and the release of CRF acting via CRF-1 receptors appears to be responsible (Matys et al., 2004). Nothing is yet known about the role of tPA, if any, in the PFC, although tPA does appear to play a role in stress-induced reductions of spine synapse number in the CA1 region of the mouse hippocampus (Pawlak et al., 2005), as noted earlier.

Brain-derived neurotrophic factor may also play a role in amygdala because overexpression of BDNF, without any applied stressor, enhances anxiety in an elevated plus maze and increases spine density on basolateral amygdala neurons, and this occludes the effect of immobilization stress on anxiety and spine density (Govindarajan et al., 2006). As noted above for hippocampus, BDNF overexpressing mice also show reduced behavioral depression in the Porsolt forced-swim task and show protection against stress-induced shortening of dendrites in the CA3 region (Govindarajan et al., 2006).

In summary, repeated stress causes dendrites in the basolateral amygdala and OFC to expand and increases the density of excitatory spine synapse, whereas repeated stress causes dendrites and spines in the medial PFC to undergo shortening and retraction. Although the role of glucocorticoids and EAAs is likely, but so far unexplored, there is evidence in amygdala for the participation of other mediators such as BDNF and tPA.

Interactions between amygdala, prefrontal cortex, and hippocampus

The PFC, amygdala, and hippocampus are interconnected and influence each other via direct and indirect neural activity (McDonald, 1987; McDonald et al., 1996; Akirav and Richter-Levin, 1999; Petrovich et al., 2001; Ghashghaei and Barbas, 2002). For example, inactivation of the amygdala blocks stress-induced impairment of hippocampal LTP and spatial memory (Kim et al., 2005), and stimulation of basolateral amygdala enhances dentate gyrus field potentials (Ikegaya et al., 1996), whereas stimulation of medial PFC decreases responsiveness of central amygdala output neurons (Quirk et al., 2003). The processing of emotional memories with contextual information requires amygdala–hippocampal interactions (Phillips and LeDoux, 1992; Richardson et al., 2004) whereas the PFC, with its powerful influence on amygdala activity (Quirk et al., 2003), plays an important role in fear extinction (Milad and Quirk, 2002; Morgan and LeDoux, 1995). Because of these interactions, future studies need to address their possible role in the morphological and functional changes produced by single and repeated stress.

HIPPOCAMPAL NEURONAL DAMAGE RESULTING FROM CHRONIC STRESS AND AGING

Neuroanatomical Findings

An important issue is the relationship between the remodeling of CA3 neurons induced by repeated doses of CORT or by CRS and the thinning and apparent loss of pyramidal neurons that has been reported after 12 weeks of CORT treatment in rats and prolonged, severe psychosocial stress in vervet monkeys (see Sapolsky, 1992). As noted above, we have seen that chronic psychosocial stress in tree shrews causes remodeling of CA3 pyramidal neurons, much as restraint stress does in rats (Magarinos et al., 1996). However, we have also noted that the remodeling produced by stress in rats is reversible, within 7–14 days after the termination of stress. A possible link may be the fate of inhibitory interneurons that receive intense innervation from mossy fibers of dentate gyrus granule neurons and which are especially vulnerable to a variety of insults (Hsu and Buzsaki, 1993). If some of these neurons were to die as a result of repeated restraint stress, then there might be a cumulative effect over time, in which repeated bouts of stress might progressively deplete the dentate gyrus of the buffering action that these inhibitory neurons appear to provide.

However, there is a big gap in our understanding between neuronal remodeling and permanent cell loss either of interneurons or of pyramidal neurons, and one of the most surprising and puzzling findings concerning glucocorticoids and neuronal damage in the hippocampus was the morphological changes resulting from prolonged exposure to stress or stress hormones that were interpreted as indicating neuronal damage and pyramidal cell loss. Adrenocorticotrophic hormone or cortisone administration was reported to mature guinea pigs, causing neurons in hippocampus and other forebrain regions to stain darkly and appear necrotic, as if undergoing remodeling, then perhaps also dying (AusDerMuhlen and Ockenfels, 1969). Other investigators have described the appearance of "darkly stained" CA3 pyramidal neurons following repeated cold swim stress in rats (Mizoguchi et al., 1992) and psychosocial stress in tree shrews (Fuchs et al., 1995).

Although the interpretation of these findings may be questioned in light of the report that darkly stained neurons can develop artifactually from physical trauma in fixing brains for histological analysis (Cammermeyer, 1978), the findings in the guinea pig were instrumental in stimulating the work of Landfield and colleagues that showed that aging in the rat results in thinning of the pyramidal cell layer in hippocampus and that this change was retarded by ADX in midlife (Landfield, 1987). Robert Sapolsky (1992) then demonstrated that 12 weeks of daily CORT injections into young adult rats mimicked the pyramidal neuron thinning seen in aging, and subsequent work on subordinant vervet monkeys revealed a thinning and apparent necrosis of CA3 pyramidal neurons that implied some kind of stress-related hippocampal damage.

However, dying cells are rarely seen because they disappear rapidly, and the evidence for neuronal loss depends on counting of cells in histological material. This issue has been raised recently (Rasmussen et al., 1996), using revised stereological procedures for estimated neuronal number, showing that aging rats that are cognitively impaired do not necessarily show reduced hippocampal neuron number. A similar conclusion was reached for cognitively impaired middle-aged rats without the use of elaborate neuronal counting methods (Issa et al., 1990), and a recent study on rats with age-related spatial memory impairment has revealed altered expression of markers of glial hypertrophy and oxidative stress that are interpreted as evidence for synaptic and dendritic pruning rather than neuronal loss (Sugaya et al., 1996). However, none of these studies have directly looked for dendritic remodeling or synapse loss, and such studies are urgently needed. Moreover, there is not sufficient evidence presently to exclude neuronal loss as a later stage of the aging process, and some of the evidence mentioned above can be interpreted either way.

Furthermore, the work of Sapolsky alluded to above first showed thinning of pyramidal neuron number in aging rats and rats treated for 12 weeks with daily CORT injections; Sapolsky then demonstrated that EAAs play an important role in the cell loss by showing, first, that glucocorticoids exacerbate kainic acid–induced damage to hippocampus, as well as ischemic damage; and, second, that glucocorticoids potentiate EAA killing of hippocampal neurons in culture (Sapolsky, 1992). Recent work (Lowy et al., 1995) has brought this issue full circle by demonstrating using intracerebral microdialysis in hippocampus that restraint stress-induced glutamate release is not only exacerbated in aging rats but that it continues for some time after stress is terminated. Although this mechanism is consistent with enhanced dendritic remodeling and synapse loss in the aging hippocampus, it is also consistent with the possibility of enhanced rates of neuronal damage and loss by the same mechanisms that are implicated in ischemia- and trauma-induced hippocampal neuronal destruction (Choi, 1988; Siesjo and Bengtsson, 1989; Sapolsky, 1992).

In summary, the aging hippocampus appears to lose functional capacity more rapidly in some individuals than in others. Rather than being the result of outright neuron loss, these changes appear to reflect loss of synaptic connectivity and dendritic pruning resulting from increased oxidative stress in which excitatory amino acid activity and glucocorticoids very likely play a role.

LIFELONG IMPLICATIONS OF STRESSFUL EXPERIENCES

Long-term stress also accelerates a number of biological markers of aging in rats, including increasing the excitability of CA1 pyramidal neurons via a calcium-dependent mechanism and causing loss of hippocampal pyramidal neurons (S. Kerr et al., 1991). An important factor may be the enhancement by glucocorticoids of calcium currents in hippocampus (D. Kerr and Campbell, 1992) (see also Table 40.1), in view of the key role of calcium ions in destructive, as well as plastic processes in hippocampal neurons. It will be important to learn how regional neural activity is altered in such conditions as traumatic stress and recurrent depressive illness and how long-term changes in neural activity may alter structure and function of neurons, particularly in the hippocampus.

Another aspect of stressful experiences is the developmental influence of early stress and of neonatal handling on the life course of aging and age-related cognitive impairment. As discussed elsewhere (Meaney, Aitken, et al., 1988; Meaney et al., 1994), such early experiences can either increase or decrease the rate of brain aging through a mechanism in which the activity of the HPA axis appears to be involved. The early experiences are believed to set the level of responsiveness of the HPA axis and autonomic nervous system in such a way that these systems either overreact in animals subject to early unpredictable stress or underreact in animals exposed to the neonatal handling procedure.

TABLE 40.1 *Atrophy of the Human Hippocampus*

Situation or Condition	*References*
Recurrent depressive illness	(Sheline et al., 1996; Sheline et al., 1999)
PTSD	(Bremner et al., 1995; Gurvits et al., 1996)
Aging, preceding dementia	(Golomb et al., 1994; Zhuang et al., 1999)
Dementia	(Quirk and Armony, 1997)
Cushing's syndrome	(Starkman et al., 1999; Snyder et al., 2001)
Schizophrenia	(Bogerts et al., 1993; Fukuzako et al., 1996)

For another summary of hippocampal atrophy in the human brain, see Sapolsky (1996).

PTSD: posttraumatic stress disorder.

TRANSLATION TO THE HUMAN BRAIN

Much of the impetus for studying the effects of stress on the structure of the human brain has come from the animal studies summarized thus far. Although there is very little evidence regarding the effects of ordinary life stressors on brain structure, there are indications from functional imaging of individuals undergoing ordinary stressors, such as counting backwards, that there are lasting changes in neural activity (Wang et al., 2005). Moreover, the study of depressive illness and anxiety disorders has also provided some insights. Life events are known to precipitate depressive illness in individuals with certain genetic predispositions (Kessler, 1997; Kendler, 1998; Caspi et al., 2003). Moreover, brain regions such as the hippocampus, amygdala, and PFC show altered patterns of activity in positron emission tomography (PET) and functional magnetic resonance imaging (fMRI) and also demonstrate changes in volume of these structures with recurrent depression: decreased volume of hippocampus and PFC and amygdala (Drevets et al., 1997; Sheline et al., 1999; Sheline et al., 2003). Interestingly, amygdala volume has been reported to increase in the first episode of depression, whereas hippocampal volume is not decreased (Frodl et al., 2003; MacQueen et al., 2003). It has been known for some time that stress hormones, such as cortisol, are involved in psychopathology, reflecting emotional arousal and psychic disorganization rather than the specific disorder per se (Sachar et al., 1973). We now know that adrenocortical hormones enter the brain and produce a wide range of effects upon it.

In Cushing's disease, there are depressive symptoms that can be relieved by surgical correction of the hypercortisolemia (B.E.P. Murphy, 1991; Starkman and Schteingart, 1981). Major depression and Cushing's disease are associated with chronic elevation of cortisol that results in gradual loss of minerals from bone and abdominal obesity. In major depressive illness, as well as in Cushing's disease, the duration of the illness and not the age of the patients predicts a progressive reduction in volume of the hippocampus, determined by structural MRI (Starkman et al., 1992; Sheline et al., 1999). Moreover, there are a variety of other anxiety-related disorders, such as PTSD (Pitman, 2001; Bremner, 2002) and borderline personality disorder (Driessen et al., 2000), in which atrophy of the hippocampus has been reported, suggesting that this is a common process reflecting chronic imbalance in the activity of adaptive systems, such as the HPA axis, but also including endogenous neurotransmitters, such as glutamate.

Another important factor in hippocampal volume and function is glucose regulation. Poor glucose regulation is associated with smaller hippocampal volume and poorer memory function in individuals in their sixties and seventies who have "mild cognitive impairment" (MCI) (Convit et al., 2003), and MCI and Type 2, as well as Type 1, diabetes are recognized as risk factors for dementia (Ott et al., 1996; de Leon et al., 2001; Haan, 2006). That the hippocampus and possibly other brain regions is responsive to glucose and insulin, as well as other metabolic hormones, makes it imperative to consider broader aspects of brain–body relationships in relation to acute and chronic stress.

STRESSFUL EXPERIENCE AND DISEASE

What is Lacking in the Current Discussion of Stress

Having noted the effects of stress on the brain, and particularly on the hippocampus, we now turn to the broader topic of stress, that is, how individuals interpret and respond to potentially stressful events, and how this may lead to disease. The problem with the concept of *stress* is that it does not do justice to the many situations in an individual's life that are more pervasive and long-lasting than a stressful life event, such as those related to living environment, interpersonal relationships, and employment. Moreover, the stress concept does not adequately reconcile the paradox between the body's adaptive mechanisms and how these same mechanisms may become involved in pathophysiological processes. As an alternative to talking about stress, we discuss below two concepts: "allostasis" (Sterling and Eyer, 1988) and "allostatic load" (McEwen and Stellar, 1993), which pertain to adaptation and the cost of adaptation for the body and brain, respectively. The sensitivity and vulnerability of the hippocampus discussed above, as manifested in the interactions between EAAs, serotonin, and glucocorticoids, is an especially good example of the notion of *allostasis* and *allostatic load*, in that the release of these neuromodulators is an adaptive response (allostasis) to a potentially stressful event, whereas the long-term consequences of this allostasis is an atrophy of neuronal processes that compromises hippocampal function (allostatic load). Moreover, the role of the hippocampus in interpreting and responding to potential stressors plays an important role in determining the level of "allostatic load" that an individual will experience because selective attention to cues and use of contextual information based upon prior experiences may improve the discriminative capability and allow the individual to respond to a potential stressor in a way that minimizes the allostatic load.

Allostasis and Allostatic Load

What is *allostasis*? The body has systems that respond to the body state (like waking, sleeping, lying, standing, exercising) and to the external environment and that promote adaptation to activities such as locomotion and to aversive stimuli—like noise and crowding, hostility, fatigue, isolation, hunger, excessive heat or cold—and threats to safety. These systems include the HPA axis; the autonomic nervous system; the metabolic systems—thyroid axis, insulin, glucagon and the gut; and the immune system. They are closely coupled to the psychological make-up of the individual, in that those people who are fearful and reactive will have more reactive physiological responses, whereas those individuals who have proactive planning skills and psychological buffers will have less reactive responses and more stability in their physiology.

Adversity, including interpersonal conflict and social instability, accelerate pathophysiological processes and result in increased incidence of morbidity and mortality. The cardiovascular system is one of the most susceptible. For example, blood pressure increases are a sensitive index of job stress in factory workers and other repetitive jobs with time pressures (Melin et al., 1999) and of job instability in British civil service departments undergoing privitization (Ferrie et al., 2002), and cardiovascular disease is a primary reason for the increased death rate in Eastern Europe in the social collapse following the fall of communism (Bobak and Marmot, 1996). It should be noted that blood pressure surges are linked to accelerated atherosclerosis (Kaplan et al., 1991), as well as increased risk for myocardial infarction (Muller et al., 1989). Besides the cardiovascular system, there are indications that metabolic disorders and abdominal obesity are increased at the lower end of the socioeconomic status gradient in Swedish males (Larsson et al., 1989). Immune system function is also a likely target (Cohen et al., 1992), with increased vulnerability to infections and possibly even to cancer, but there is far less evidence on this point.

We have noted throughout this chapter that individuals respond in different ways to adversity and threats (real or implied) to their safety and homeostasis. Physiological responses of the autonomic nervous system, HPA axis, cardiovascular, metabolic, and immune systems lead to protection and adaptation of the organism to these challenges. This process, referred to as allostasis, is an essential component of maintaining homeostasis. However, adaptation to adversity has a price, and we have come to define the cost of adaptation as allostatic load (McEwen and Stellar, 1993). Much of our ability to make a breakthrough in understanding the linkage between behavior, brain function, and health depends on our making progress in defining and operationalizing the concept of *allostatic load*. Allostatic load is the wear and tear on the body and brain resulting from chronic overactivity or inactivity of physiological systems that are normally involved in adaptation to environmental challenge. Although it is true that physiological parameters such as blood oxygen and pH are maintained in a narrow range (homeostasis), the cardiovascular system, metabolic machinery, immune system, and central nervous system all show a large range of activity as a function of the time of day and in response to external and internal demands (allostasis). These systems are involved in coping and adaptation, and, as a general rule, they are most useful when they can be rapidly mobilized and then turned down in their activity again when not needed. It is when they are not turned off or turned down that these systems become dangerous for health. Moreover, the inability to turn on these systems when needed also produces a load on the body because the normal protection afforded by these systems is lacking.

An important aspect of allostasis and allostatic load is the notion of anticipation (Schulkin et al., 1994). Although originally introduced in relation to explaining the reflex that prevents us from blacking out when we get out of bed in the morning (Sterling and Eyer, 1988), anticipation also implies psychological states, such as worry and anxiety, as well as cognitive preparation for a coming event. Because anticipation can drive the output of mediators (this is particularly true of hormones such as ACTH, cortisol, and adrenalin), it is likely that states of prolonged anxiety and anticipation can result in allostatic load (Schulkin et al., 1994). However, this is one of many notions that need experimental testing.

Other important aspects of individual responses in relation to allostasis and allostatic load are the health-damaging and health-promoting behaviors such as smoking, drinking, choice of diet, and exercise. These may be regarded as part of the overall notion of allostasis—that is, how individuals attempt to cope with a challenge—and they also contribute in some ways that are known to allostatic load (for example, a rich diet accelerates atherosclerosis and progression to Type II diabetes; smoking exacerbates blood pressure and atherogenesis; exercise has an ameliorative effect).

Types of allostatic load

There are three types of physiological response that make up allostatic load. The first type is simply due to frequent stressors; for example, blood pressure surges not only trigger myocardial infarction (MI) in susceptible individuals, but their repetition also accelerates atherosclerosis and primes the risk for MI. Here, it is the frequency and intensity of the "hits" or events that determine how much allostatic load of this type, although frequent stress may lead into the other types described below as the body responds to repeated events by either failing to shut off neural and endocrine responses or failing to respond adequately. Posttraumatic stress disorder is an example of how an acute traumatic event leads to an HPA axis that may not respond adequately to acute challenge (Yehuda et al., 1991).

The second type of allostatic load involved failure to turn off adaptive autonomic and neuroendocrine responses, for example, blood pressure elevations in repetitive, time-pressured work (Lundberg et al., 1989) and the fact that glucocorticoids accelerate obesity and Type II diabetes. Moreover, we have seen above that persistent glucocorticoid elevation and/or excitatory activity in brain causes dendritic remodeling and neuronal death in hippocampus.

The third type of allostatic load is the failure to respond adequately to a challenge, for example, autoimmunity and inflammation that is associated with inadequate endogenous glucocorticoid responses, as in the Lewis rat (Sternberg et al., 1989) and possibly also in chronic fatigue syndrome and fibromyalgia (Griep et al., 1993; Crofford et al., 1994; Demitrack, 1996). In this situation, other systems—such as inflammatory cytokines—show elevated activity, and this respect shows an allostatic load because of the inadequate HPA activity, which normally "contains" their activity.

Individuals showing these patterns are likely to be distributed differently across gradients of socioeconomic status but not confined exclusively to one part of the gradient. Thus it is important to distinguish between characteristics of groups and the vulnerability of individuals. It is necessary to study the biology–behavior interface to understand the forms of allostatic load and their relationship to diseases in individuals, while developing tools for recognizing how these traits are distributed and what aspects of the various communities in which they live may contribute to their occurrence.

Measurement of allostatic load

One of the major challenges is how to measure allostatic load. An initial attempt in this direction (Seeman et al., 1997; McEwen and Seeman, 1999) used data from the MacArthur Successful Aging study to follow 10 measures of increased activity of allostatic systems between 1988 and 1991. Individuals were classified as to whether they were in the most extreme quartile (highest in systolic blood pressure; overnight urinary cortisol, catecholamines; waist/hip ratio; glycosylated hemoglobin; ratio cholesterol:high density lipoprotein [HDL]; lowest in dehydroepiandrosterone [DHEA]-sulfate and HDL cholesterol). The analysis indicated that individuals who were high functioning in 1988 had lower allostatic load scores than individuals who were lower functioning; moreover, those people who were higher functioning in 1988 who had the highest allostatic load scores (most extreme quartile in at least one or more allostatic load measures) had the highest probability of showing cardiovascular disease in 1991 and also showed the greatest decline in cognitive measures and measures of physical functioning (Seeman et al., 1997; Seeman et al., 2001). The cognitive decline was unexpected on the basis of traditional thinking about the allostatic load measures and risk for disease, but it is quite consistent with the picture that is painted in the present review and in other chapters in this volume. Clearly, this is just the beginning of this type of analysis, and much more needs to be done to test and operationalize the utility of allostatic load measures, as well as to broaden them to include immune system related disorders and the three types of allostatic load described above.

How and why do allostatic systems malfunction and lead to allostatic load?

Allostatic load refers to an imbalance in systems that promote adaptation. As noted above, this imbalance can simply be the result of too much repeated stress, but it also can be the result of adaptive systems that are out of balance and fail to shut off or, alternatively, systems that fail to turn on adequately. How does such imbalance arise? One possibility is that repeated stress causes systems to wear out or become exhausted, leading either to the failure of shut-off or failure to respond. As proposed by Sapolsky in the glucocorticoid cascade hypothesis of stress and aging (Sapolsky et al., 1986; Sapolsky, 1992), the wearing out of the mechanism that keeps HPA activity contained is likely to involve, at least in part, dysfunction of the hippocampus. Evidence to support this has been obtained in studies of aging rats by finding that there are age-impaired animals with HPA hyperactivity and cognitive impairment (Meaney, Aitken, et al., 1988; Issa et al., 1990; Meaney et al., 1994). On the other extreme, we have noted the failure to mount an adequate HPA response is a feature of the Lewis rat that results in increased vulnerability to autoimmune and inflammatory disturbances (Sternberg et al., 1989; Sternberg et al., 1996). Such a hyporesponsive state may be induced by severe stress because we have found a stress-induced state of HPA hyporesponsiveness among rats that become subordinate in a psychosocial living situation called the "visible burrow system" (VBS) (Blanchard et al., 1993; Albeck et al., 1997). In these rats, there is a very limited HPA response to experimenter-applied stressors, and hypothalamic CRF mRNA levels are abnormally low (Albeck et al., 1997), and this is a condition that develops gradually during the 14-day VBS exposure, indicating that it is brought about in response to the severity of the stress and the individual responses to the stress.

In summary, the same mediators that help the body and brain adapt to acute stressors (allostasis) are also involved in processes that impair function and exacerbate disease processes (allostatic load).

POSITIVE AFFECT, SELF-ESTEEM, AND SOCIAL SUPPORT

Not all stressful experiences are bad, and there are factors in the social environment and personalities of individuals that provide some buffering and resilience in the face of stressors. Having a positive outlook on life and good self-esteem appear to have long-lasting health consequences (Pressman and Cohen, 2005), and good social support is also a positive influence on the measures of allostatic load (Seeman et al., 2002). Positive affect, assessed by aggregating momentary experiences throughout a working or leisure day, was found to be associated with lower cortisol production and higher heart rate variability (showing higher parasympathetic activity), as well as a lower fibrinogen response to a mental stress test (Steptoe et al., 2005).

On the other hand, poor self-esteem has been shown to cause recurrent increases in cortisol levels during a repetition of a public-speaking challenge in which those individuals with good self-esteem are able to habituate, that is, attenuate their cortisol response after the first speech (Kirschbaum et al., 1995). Furthermore, poor self-esteem and low internal locus of control have been related to 12%–13% smaller volume of the hippocampus, as well as higher cortisol levels during a mental arithmetic stressor (Pruessner et al., 1999; Pruessner et al., 2005).

Related to positive affect and self-esteem is the role of friends and social interactions in maintaining a healthy outlook on life. Loneliness, often found in people with low self-esteem, has been associated with larger cortisol responses to wakening in the morning and higher fibrinogen and natural killer cell responses to a mental stress test, as well as sleep problems (Steptoe et al., 2004). On the other hand, having three or more regular social contacts, as opposed to none to two such contacts, is associated with lower allostatic load scores (Seeman et al., 2002).

CONCLUSIONS

The main thesis of this chapter is that the adult brain is a plastic and malleable organ and that changes brought about by the environment are largely beneficial to the individual. The hippocampus is a brain region in which this plasticity has been seen in various forms, ranging from replacement of neurons of the dentate gyrus, to synapse turnover in the estrous cycle of the female rat, to remodelling of dendrites in hibernation and after repeated psychosocial stress. We suspect that, although the hippocampus is exceptionally sensitive and vulnerable, the plasticity seen in the hippocampus is representative of plasticity going on to various extents in other brain regions as well. We have also seen that structural plasticity with stress goes on in the amygdala and regions of the PFC, with increases in dendritic branching and synapse density occurring in some regions and decreases in others.

We have seen that the various forms of hippocampal plasticity occur as a result of an interaction between circulating hormones and endogenous neurotransmitters, especially, EAAs. This means that neural activity, and therefore the neural responses to experience, and the circulating hormonal environment that is also sensitive to experience are important regulators of adult plasticity. The existence of multiple regulators of this plasticity allows for a greater range of outcomes.

N-methyl-D-aspartate receptors play a key role in regulating neurogenesis in dentate gyrus, synapse turnover on CA1 pyramidal neurons, and dendritic remodelling of CA3 neurons. Yet that is not all, and NMDA receptors are also involved in the developing nervous system as facilitators of neuronal migration (Komuro and Rakic, 1995). However, there is a noteworthy paradox, in that NMDA receptors are implicated in the developing visual system in reducing synaptic contact in the developing retinal axon arbors (Yen et al., 1995) and NMDA receptor blockade results in rapid acquisition of dendritic spines by visual thalamic neurons (J.E. Kerr et al., 1995). It seems that hippocampus and visual system neurons respond in opposite ways to NMDA receptors because a recent report on embryonic hippocampal neurons in culture indicated that NMDA receptor blockade prevents E-induced synaptogenesis (D.D. Murphy and Segal, 1996).

Besides discussing plasticity, we have also noted the potentially damaging aspects of stressful experience and we have described two concepts: allostasis, the process of adaptation that maintains homeostasis, and allostatic load, the price the body pays for having to adapt to various challenges. The gradual wear and tear on tissues and organs of the body resulting from allostatic load is postulated to be a major factor in accelerating disease processes for which there is either a pathogen or a genetic predisposition. Allostatic load provides a more physiological conceptualization of the consequences of "chronic stress."

One of the implications of allostatic load is that the wear and tear is a form of "premature aging." One of the features of the aging process is the loss of plasticity, and this has been reported for stress responsiveness of the aging HPA axis (reviewed in McEwen, 1992). Is this in fact the case for the types of plasticity described at the beginning of this article? In several cases we can say that there is a loss of plasticity with age. For example, the aging dentate gyrus loses the ability to replace granule neurons (Seki and Arai, 1995; Kuhn et al., 1996), although this suppression is reversed by ADX (Cameron and McKay, 1999) and, at least partially, by blocking NMDA receptors (Nacher et al., 2001).

We also know that the ability of repeated stress to down-regulate GRs in the rat hippocampus is lost in aging rats, with the emergence of stress-induced neuronal thinning in the pyramidal cell layer (Landfield and Eldridge, 1994). We do not yet know whether aging increases or decreases stress-induced dendritic remodeling, and the answer to this question will help us know if atrophy and remodelling of dendrites of CA3 pyramidal neurons is the first step to damage or a protective mechanism. Because the atrophy does not affect the whole neuron, and is reversible, we believe that it represents a physiological adaptive mechanism to severe and recurrent stress. However, it is unclear if atrophy is the first stage that leads to neuronal death or a mechanism that protects neurons at the expense of some cognitive function. Insofar as the atrophy seen in CA3 pyramidal neurons is the tip of the iceberg, so to speak, and represents atrophy occurring throughout the hippocampus, this model is relevant to the atrophy of the human hippocampus that has been described in Cushing's syndrome, normal aging, dementia, recurrent depressive illness, schizophrenia, and PTSD. In these cases, the problem is to distinguish between reversible atrophy and permanent cell loss because the former situation is potentially treatable at the time that the atrophy is discovered, whereas the latter may be preventable with earlier intervention at the time the initial trauma is taking place.

REFERENCES

Aberg, M.A.I., Aberg, N.D., Hedbacker, H., Oscarsson, J., and Eriksson, P.S. (2000) Peripheral infusion of IGF-1 selectively induces neurogenesis in the adult rat hippocampus. *J. Neurosci.* 20:2896–2903.

Ahima, R., Krozowski, Z., and Harlan, R. (1991) Type I corticosteroid receptor-like immunoreactivity in the rat CNS: distribution and regulation by corticosteroids. *J. Comp. Neurol.* 313:522–538.

Ahima, R.S., and Harlan, R.E. (1990) Charting of type II glucocorticoid receptor-like immunoreactivity in the rat central nervous system. *Neuroscience* 39:579–604.

Akana, S., Jacobson, L., Cascio, C., Shinsako, J., and Dallman, M. (1988) Constant corticosterone replacement normalizes basal adrenocorticotropin (ACTH) but permits sustained ACTH hypersecretion after stress in adrenalectomized rats. *Endocrinology* 122: 1337–1342.

Akana, S.F., Chu, A., Soriano, L., and Dallman, M.F. (2001) Corticosterone exerts site-specific and state-dependent effects in prefrontal cortex and amygdala on regulation of adrenocorticotropic hormone, insulin and fat depots. *J. Neuroendocrin.* 13: 625–637.

Akirav, I., and Richter-Levin, G. (1999) Biphasic modulation of hippocampal plasticity by behavioral stress and basolateral amygdala stimulation in the rat. *J. Neurosci.* 19:10530–10535.

Albeck, D.S., McKittrick, C.R., Blanchard, D.C., Blanchard, R.J., Nikulina, J., McEwen, B.S., and Sakai, R.R. (1997) Chronic social stress alters expression of corticotrophin releasing factor and arginine vasopressin mRNA expression in rat brain. *J. Neurosci.* 17:4895–4903.

Ardayfio, P., and Kim, K.-S. (2006) Anxiogenic-like effect of chronic corticosterone in the light-dark emergency task in mice. *Behav. Neurosci.* 120:249–256.

Armstrong, J.D., McIntyre, D.C., Neubort, S., and Sloviter, R.S. (1993) Learning and memory after adrenalectomy-induced hippocampal dentate granule cell degeneration in the rat. *Hippocampus* 3:359–371.

Arnold, A., and Breedlove, S. (1985) Organizational and activational effects of sex steroids on brain and behavior: a reanalysis. *Horm. Behav.* 19:469–498.

AusDerMuhlen, K., and Ockenfels, H. (1969) Morphologische veranderungen im diencephalon und telencephalon: storungen des regelkreises adenohypophysenebennierenrinde [Morphological alterations in the diencephalons and telencephalon: disturbance of the HPA axis]. *Mikrosck. Anat.* 93:126–141.

Barnes, C., McNaughton, B., Goddard, G., Douglas, R., and Adamec, R. (1977) Circadian rhythm of synaptic excitability in rat and monkey central nervous system. *Science* 197:91–92.

Bartanusz, V., Aubry, J.M., Pagliusi, S., Jezova, D., Baffi, J., and Kiss, J.Z. (1995) Stress-induced changes in messenger RNA levels of N-methyl-D-aspartate and Ampa receptor subunits in selected regions of the rat hippocampus and hypothalamus. *Neuroscience* 66:247–252.

Beck, S.G., List, T.J., and Choi, K.C. (1994) Long- and short- term administration of corticosterone alters CA1 hippocampal neuronal properties. *Neuroendocrinology* 60:261–272.

Bengzon, J., Kokaia, Z., Elmer, E., Nanobashvili, A., Kokaia, M., and Lindvall, O. (1997) Apoptosis and proliferation of dentate gyrus neurons after single and intermittent limbic seizures. *Proc. Natl. Acad. Sci. USA* 94:10432–10437.

Birnstiel, S., and Beck, S.G. (1995) Modulation of the 5-hydroxytryptamine-4 receptor-mediated response by short-term and long-term administration of corticosterone in rat CA1 hippocampal pyramidal neurons. *J. Pharm. Exp. Ther.* 273:1132–1138.

Birrell, J.M., and Brown, V.J. (2000) Medial frontal cortex mediates perceptual attentional set shifting in the rat. *J. Neurosci.* 20: 4320–4324.

Blanchard, D.C., Sakai, R.R., McEwen, B.S., Weiss, S.M., and Blanchard, R.J. (1993) Subordination stress: behavioral, brain and neuroendocrine correlates. *Behav. Brain Res.* 58:113–121.

Blaustein, J.D., Lehman, M.N., Turcotte, J.C., and Greene, G. (1992) Estrogen receptors in dendrites and axon terminals in guinea pig hypothalamus. *Endocrinology* 131:281–290.

Bliss, T.V.P., and Lomo, T. (1973) Long-lasting potentiation of synaptic transmission in the dentate area of the anaesthetized rabbit following stimulation of the perforant path. *J. Physiology* 232: 331–356.

Bobak, M., and Marmot, M. (1996) East-West mortality divide and its potential explanations: proposed research agenda. *BMJ* 312: 421–425.

Bogerts, B., Lieberman, J.A., Ashtair, M., Bilder, R.M., De Greef, G., Lerner, G., Johns, C., and Masiar, S. (1993) Hippocampus-amygdala volumes and psychopathology in chronic schizophrenia. *Biol. Psychiatry* 33:236–246.

Bremner, J.D. (2002) Neuroimaging studies in post-traumatic stress disorder. *Curr. Psychiatry Reports* 4:254–263.

Bremner, J.D., Randall, P., Scott, T.M., Bronen, R.A., Seibyl, J.P., Southwick, S.M., Delaney, R.C., McCarthy, G., Charney, D.S., and Innis, R.B. (1995) MRI-based measurement of hippocampal volume in patients with combat-related posttraumatic stress disorder. *Am. J. Psychiatry* 152:973–981.

Brezun, J.M., and Daszuta, A. (1999) Depletion in serotonin decreases neurogenesis in the dentate gyrus and the subventricular zone of adult rats. *Neuroscience* 89:999–1002.

Brezun, J.M., and Daszuta, A. (2000) Serotonin may stimulate granule cell proliferation in the adult hippocampus, as observed in rats grafted with foetal raphe neurons. *Eur. J. Neurosci.* 12:391–396.

Brown, S.M., Henning, S., and Wellman, C.L. (2005) Mild, short-term stress alters dendritic morphology in rat medial prefrontal cortex. *Cereb. Cortex* 30:1–9.

Bulloch, K., Prasad, A., Conrad, C.D., McEwen, B.S., and Milner, T.A. (1996) Calcitonin gene-related peptide level in the rat dentate gyrus increases after damage. *Neuroreport* 7:1036–1040.

Cameron, H.A., and Gould, E. (1996a) The control of neuronal birth and survival. In: Shaw, C.A., ed. *Receptor Dynamics in Neural Development.* New York: CRC Press, pp. 141–157.

Cameron, H.A., and Gould, E. (1996b) Distinct populations of cells in the adult dentate gyrus undergo mitosis or apoptosis in response to adrenalectomy. *J. Comp. Neurol.* 369:56–63.

Cameron, H.A., McEwen, B.S., and Gould, E. (1995) Regulation of adult neurogenesis by excitatory input and NMDA receptor activation in the dentate gyrus. *J. Neurosci.* 15:4687–4692.

Cameron, H.A., and McKay, R.D.G. (1999) Restoring production of hippocampal neurons in old age. *Nat. Neurosci.* 2:894–897.

Cammermeyer, J. (1978) Is the solitary dark neuron a manifestation of postmortem trauma to the brain inadequately fixed by perfusion? *Histochemistry* 56:97–115.

Carro, E., Nunez, A., Busiguina, S., and Torres-Aleman, I. (2000) Circulating insulin-like growth factor I mediates effects of exercise on the brain. *J. Neurosci.* 20:2926–2933.

Caspi, A., Sugden, K., Moffitt, T.E., Taylor, A., Craig, I.W., Harrington, H., McClay, J., Mill, J., Martin, J., Braithwaite, A., and Poulton, R. (2003) Influence of life stress on depression: moderation by a polymorphism in the 5-HTT gene. *Science* 301:386–389.

Cerqueira, J.J., Pego, J.M., Taipa, R., Bessa, J.M., Almeida, O.F.X., and Sousa, N. (2005) Morphological correlates of corticosteroid-induced changes in prefrontal cortex-dependent behaviors. *J. Neurosci.* 25:7792–7800.

Choi, D.W. (1988) Glutamate neurotoxicity and diseases of the nervous system. *Neuron* 1:623–634.

Clarke, C.H., Norfleet, A.M., Clarke, M.S.F., Watson, C.S., Cunningham, K.A., and Thomas, M.L. (2000) Perimembrane localization of the estrogen receptor protein in neuronal processes of cultured hippocampal neurons. *Neuroendocrinology* 71:34–42.

Cohen, S., Kaplan, J.R., Cunnick, J.E., Manuck, S.B., and Rabin, B. S. (1992) Chronic social stress, affiliation and cellular immune response in nonhuman primates. *Psychol. Sci.* 3:301–304.

Conrad, C.D., Magarinos, A.M., LeDoux, J.E., and McEwen, B.S. (1999) Repeated restraint stress facilitates fear conditioning independently of causing hippocampal CA3 dendritic atrophy. *Behav. Neurosci.* 113:902–913.

Conrad, C.D., Magarinos, A.M., LeDoux, J.E., and McEwen, B.S. (1999) Repeated restraint stress facilitates fear conditioning independently of causing hippocampal CA3 dendritic atrophy. *Behav. Neurosci.* 113:902–913.

Conrad, C.D., and Roy, E.J. (1995) Dentate gyrus destruction and spatial learning impairment after corticosteroid removal in young and middle-aged rats. *Hippocampus* 5:1–15.

Convit, A., Wolf, O.T., Tarshish, C., and de Leon, M.J. (2003) Reduced glucose tolerance is associated with poor memory performance and hippocampal atrophy among normal elderly. *Proc. Natl. Acad. Sci. USA* 100:2019–2022.

Cook, S.C., and Wellman, C.L. (2004) Chronic stress alters dendritic morphology in rat medial prefrontal cortex. *J. Neurobiol.* 60:236–248.

Corodimas, K.P., LeDoux, J.E., Gold, P.W., and Schulkin, J. (1994) Corticosterone potentiation of learned fear. *Ann. N. Y. Acad. Sci.* 746:392.

Crofford, L.J., Pillemer, S.R., Kalogeras, K., Cash, J.M., Michelson, D., Kling, M.A., Sternberg, E.M., Gold, P.W., Chrousos, G.P., and Wilder, R.L. (1994) Hypothalamic-pituitary-adrenal axis perturbations in patients with fibromyalgia. *Arthritis Rheum.* 37: 1583–1592.

Crombag, H.S., Gorny, G., Li, Y., Kolb, B., and Robinson, T.E. (2005) Opposite effects of amphetamine self-administration experience on dendritic spines in the medial and orbital prefrontal cortex. *Cereb. Cortex* 15:341–348.

Czeh, B., Michaelis, T., Watanabe, T., Frahm, J., de Biurrun, G., van Kampen, M., Bartolomucci, A., and Fuchs, E. (2001) Stress-induced changes in cerebral metabolites, hippocampal volume and cell proliferation are prevented by antidepressant treatment with tianeptine. *Proc. Natl. Acad. Sci. USA* 98:12796–12801.

Dana, R.C., and Martinez, J.L. (1984) Effect of adrenalectomy on the circadian rhythm of LTP. *Brain Res.* 308:392–395.

Datta, S.R., Brunet, A., and Greenberg, M.E. (1999) Cellular survival: a play in three Akts. *Genes & Devel.* 13:2905–2927.

De Kloet, E.R., Azmitia, E.C., and Landfield, P.W. (1996) Brain corticosteroid receptors: studies on the mechanism, function, and neurotoxicity of corticosteroid action. *Ann. N. Y. Acad. Sci.* 746: 1–499.

de Leon, M.J., Convit, A., Wolf, O.T., Tarshish, C.Y., DeSanti, S., Rusinek, H., Tsui, W., Kandil, E., Scherer, A.J., Roche, A., Imossi, A., Thorn, E., Bobinski, M., Caraos, C., Lesbre, P., Schlyer, D., Poirier, J., Reisberg, B., and Fowler, J. (2001) Prediction of cognitive decline in normal elderly subjects with 2-[^{18}F]fluoro-2-deoxy-D-glucose/positron-emission tomography (FDG/PET). *Proc. Natl. Acad. Sci. USA* 98:10966–10971.

Delbende, C., Contesse, V., Mocaer, E., Kamoun, A., and Vaudry, H. (1991) The novel antidepressant, tianeptine, reduces stress-evoked stimulation of the hypothalamo-pituitary-adrenal axis. *Eur. J. Pharmacol.* 202:391–396.

Demitrack, M.A. (1996) Neuroendocrine research strategies in chronic fatigue syndrome. In: Goodnick, P.J., and Klimas, N.G., eds. *Chronic Fatigue and Related Immune Deficiency Syndromes*. Washington, DC: American Psychiatric Press, Inc, pp. 45–66.

DeVoogd, T., and Nottebohm, F. (1981) Gonadal hormones induce dendritic growth in the adult avian brain. *Science* 214:202–204.

Diamond, D.M., Bennett, M.C., Fleshner, M., and Rose, G.M. (1992) Inverted-U relationship between the level of peripheral corticosterone and the magnitude of hippocampal primed burst potentiation. *Hippocampus* 2:421–430.

Diamond, D.M., Fleshner, M., Ingersoll, N., and Rose, G.M. (1996) Psychological stress impairs spatial working memory: relevance to electrophysiological studies of hippocampal function. *Behav. Neurosci.* 110:661–672.

Diamond, D.M., Fleshner, M., and Rose, G.M. (1994) Psychological stress repeatedly blocks hippocampal primed burst potentiation in behaving rats. *Behav. Brain Res.* 62:1–9.

Diorio, D., Viau, V., and Meaney, M.J. (1993) The role of the medial prefrontal cortex (cingulate gyrus) in the regulation of hypothalamic-pituitary-adrenal responses to stress. *J. Neurosci.* 13: 3839–3847.

DonCarlos, L.L., Monroy, E., and Morrell, J.I. (1991) Distribution of estrogen receptor-immunoreactive cells in the forebrain of the female guinea pig. *J. Comp. Neurol.* 305:591–612.

Dore, S., Kar, S., and Quirion, R. (1997) Insulin-like growth factor I protects and rescues hippocampal neurons against beta-amyloid and human amylin-induced toxicity. *Proc. Natl. Acad. Sci. USA* 94:4772–4777.

Dore, S., Kar, S., Rowe, W., and Quirion, R. (1997) Distribution and levels of [^{125}I]IGF-I, [^{125}I]IGF-II and [^{125}I]insulin receptor binding sites in the hippocampus of aged memory-unimpaired and -impaired rats. *Neurosci.* 80:1033–1040.

Drevets, W.C., Price, J.L., Simpson, J.R. Jr, Todd, R.D., Reich, T., Vannier, M., and Raichle, M.E. (1997) Subgenual prefrontal cortex abnormalities in mood disorders. *Nature* 386:824–827.

Driessen, M., Hermann, J., Stahl, K., Zwaan, M., Meier, S., Hill, A., Osterheider, M., and Petersen, D. (2000) Magnetic resonance imaging volumes of the hippocampus and the amygdala in women with borderline personality disorder and early traumatization. *Arch. Gen. Psychiatry* 57:1115–1122.

Duman, R.S., Nakagawa, S., and Malberg, J. (2001) Regulation of adult neurogenesis by antidepressant treatment. *Neuropsychopharmacology* 25:836–844.

Dunn, J., and Orr, S. (1984) Differential plasma corticosterone responses to hippocampal stimulation. *Exp. Brain Res.* 54:1–6.

Eichenbaum, H., and Otto, T. (1992) The hippocampus - what does it do? *Behav. Neural. Biol.* 57:2–36.

Eriksson, P.S., Permlieva, E., Bjork-Eriksson, T., Alborn, A.-M., Nordborg, C., Peterson, D.A., and Gage, F.H. (1998) Neurogenesis in the adult human hippocampus. *Nat. Med.* 4:1313–1317.

Evans, R.M., and Arriza, J.L. (1989) A molecular framework for the actions of glucocorticoid hormones in the nervous system. *Neuron* 2:1105–1112.

Ferrie, J.E., Shipley, M.J., Stansfeld, S.A., and Marmot, M.G. (2002) Effects of chronic job insecurity and change in job security on self reported health, minor psychiatric morbidity, physiological measures, and health related behaviours in British civil servants: the Whitehall II study. *J. Epidemiol. Community Health* 56:450–454.

Franklin, T.B., and Perrot-Sinal, T.S. (2006) Sex and ovarian steroids modulate brain-derived neurotrophic factor (BDNF) protein levels in rat hippocampus under stressful and non-stressful conditions. *Psychoneuroendocrinology* 31:38–48.

Freund, T.F., and Buzsaki, G. (1996) Interneurons of the hippocampus. *Hippocampus* 6:345–470.

Frodl, T., Meisenzahl, E.M., Zetzsche, T., Born, C., Jager, M., Groll, C., Bottlender, R., Leinsinger, G., and Moller, H.-J. (2003) Larger amygdala volumes in first depressive episode as compared to recurrent major depression and healthy control subjects. *Biol. Psychiatry* 53:338–344.

Fuchs, E., and Gould, E. (2000) Mini-review: in vivo neurogenesis in the adult brain: regulation and functional implications. *Eur. J. Neurosci.* 12:2211–2214.

Fuchs, E., Uno, H., and Flugge, G. (1995) Chronic psychosocial stress induces morphological alterations in hippocampal pyramidal neurons of the tree shrew. *Brain Res.* 673:275–282.

Fukuzako, H., Fukuzako, T., Hashiguchi, T., Hokazono, Y., Takeuchi, K., Hirakawa, K., Ueyama, K., Takigawa, M., Kajiya, Y., Nakajo, M., and Fujimoto, T. (1996) Reduction in hippocampal formation volume is caused mainly by its shortening in chronic schizophrenia: Assessment by MRI. *Biol. Psychiatry* 39:938–945.

Galea, L.A.M., Kavaliers, M., Ossenkopp, K.-P., Innes, D., and Hargreaves, E.L. (1994) Sexually dimorphic spatial learning varies seasonally in two populations of deer mice. *Brain Res.* 635:18–26.

Galea, L.A.M., and McEwen, B.S. (1999) Sex and seasonal differences in the rate of cell proliferation in the dentate gyrus of adult wild meadow voles. *Neuroscience* 89:955–964.

Galea, L.A.M., Tanapat, P., and Gould, E. (1996) Exposure to predator odor suppresses cell proliferation in the dentate gyrus of adult rats via a cholinergic mechanism. *Abstract, Soc. Neurosci.* 22:474.8.

Gazzaley, A.H., Weiland, N.G., McEwen, B.S., and Morrison, J.H. (1996) Differential regulation of NMDAR1 mRNA and protein by estradiol in the RAt hippocampus. *J. Neurosci.* 16:6830–6838.

Ghashghaei, H.T., and Barbas, H. (2002) Pathways for emotion: Interactions of prefrontal and anterior temporal pathways in the amygdala of the Rhesus monkey. *Neuroscience* 115:1261–1279.

Gleichmann, M., Weller, M., and Schulz, J.B. (2000) Insulin-like growth factor-1 mediated protection from neuronal apoptosis is linked to phosphorylation of the pro-apoptotic protein BAD but not to inhibition of cytochrome c translocation in rat cerebellar neurons. *Neurosci. Lett.* 282:69–72.

Golomb, J., DeLeon, M.J., George, A.E., Kluger, A., Convit, A., Rusinek, H., DeSanti, S., Litt, A., Foo, S.H., and Ferris, S.H. (1994) Hippocampal atrophy correlates with severe cognitive impairment in elderly patients with suspected normal pressure hydrocephalus. *J. Neurol. Neurosurg. Psychiatry* 57:590–593.

Gong, C., Wang, T.-W., Huang, H.S., and Parent, J.M. (2007) Reelin regulates neuronal progenitor migration in intact and epileptic hippocampus. *J. Neurosci.* 27:1803–1811.

Gould, E. (1999) Serotonin and hippocampal neurogenesis. *Neuropsychopharmacology* 21:46S–51S.

Gould, E., Beylin, A., Tanapat, P., Reeves, A., and Shors, T.J. (1999) Learning enhances adult neurogenesis in the hippocampal formation. *Nat. Neurosci.* 2:260–265.

Gould, E., and McEwen, B.S. (1993) Neuronal birth and death. *Curr. Opin. Neurobiol.* 3:676–682.

Gould, E., McEwen, B.S., Tanapat, P., Galea, L.A.M., and Fuchs, E. (1997) Neurogenesis in the dentate gyrus of the adult tree shrew is regulated by psychosocial stress and NMDA receptor activation. *J. Neurosci.* 17:2492–2498.

Gould, E., and Tanapat, P. (1997) Lesion-induced proliferation of neuronal progenitors in the dentate gyrus of the adult rat. *Neuroscience* 80:427–436.

Gould, E., Tanapat, P., and Cameron, H.A. (1997) Adrenal steroids suppress granule cell death in the developing dentate gyrus through an NMDA receptor-dependent mechanism. *Devel. Brain Res.* 103:91–93.

Gould, E., Tanapat, P., and McEwen, B.S. (1997) Activation of the type 2 adrenal steroid receptor can rescue granule cells from death during development. *Devel. Brain Res.* 101:265–268.

Gould, E., Tanapat, P., McEwen, B.S., Flugge, G., and Fuchs, E. (1998) Proliferation of granule cell precursors in the dentate gyrus of adult monkeys is diminished by stress. *Proc. Natl. Acad. Sci. USA* 95:3168–3171.

Gould, E., Vail, N., Wagers, M., and Gross, C.G. (2001) Adult-generated hippocampal and neocortical neurons in macaques have a transient existence. *Proc. Natl. Acad. Sci. USA* 98:10910–10917.

Gould, E., Westlind-Danielsson, A., Frankfurt, M., and McEwen, B.S. (1990) Sex differences and thyroid hormone sensitivity of hippocampal pyramidal neurons. *J. Neurosci.* 10:996–1003.

Gould, E., Woolley, C., and McEwen, B.S. (1990) Short-term glucocorticoid manipulations affect neuronal morphology and survival in the adult dentate gyrus. *Neuroscience* 37:367–375.

Govindarajan, A., Rao, B.S.S., Nair, D., Trinh, M., Mawjee, N., Tonegawa, S., and Chattarji, S. (2006) Transgenic brain-derived neurotrophic factor expression causes both anxiogenic and antidepressant effects. *Proc. Natl. Acad. Sci. USA* 103:13208–13213.

Greenough, W.T., and Bailey, C.H. (1988) The anatomy of a memory: convergence of results across a diversity of tests. *Trends Neurosci.* 11:142–147.

Griep, E.N., Boersma, J.W., and De Kloet, E.R. (1993) Altered reactivity of the hypothalamic-pituitary-adrenal axis in the primary fibromyalgia syndrome. *J. Rheumatol.* 20:469–474.

Gurvits, T.V., Shenton, M.E., Hokama, H., Ohta, H., Lasko, N.B., Gilbertson, M.W., Orr, S.P., Kikinis, R., Jolesz, F.A., McCarley, R.W., and Pitman, R.K. (1996) Magnetic resonance imaging study of hippocampal volume in chronic, combat-related posttraumatic stress disorder. *Biol. Psychiatry* 40:1091–1099.

Haan, M.N. (2006) Therapy insight: type 2 diabetes mellitus and the risk of late-onset Alzheimer's disease. *Nat. Clin. Prac. Neurol.* 2: 159–166.

Hagihara, K., Hirata, S., Osada, T., Hirai, M., and Kato, J. (1992) Distribution of cells containing progesterone receptor mRNA in the female rat di- and telencephalon: an in situ hybridization study. *Mol. Brain Res.* 14:239–249.

Herman, J.P., Prewitt, C.M.F., and Cullinan, W.E. (1996) Neuronal circuit regulation of the hypothalamo-pituitary-adrenocortical stress axis. *Crit. Rev. Neurobiol.* 10:371–394.

Hesen, W., and Joels, M. (1996a) Carbachol responsiveness of rat CA1 hippocampal neurons in vitro: Modulation by corticosterone and stress. *Stress* 1:63–72.

Hesen, W., and Joels, M. (1996b) Modulation of $5HT_{1A}$ responsiveness in CA1 pyramidal neurons by in vivo activation of corticosteroid receptors. *J. Neuroendocrinol.* 8:433–438.

Het, S., and Wolf, O.T. (2007) Mood changes in response to psychosocial stress in healthy young women: effects of pretreatment with cortisol. *Behav. Neurosci.* 121:11–20.

Hsu, M., and Buzsaki, G. (1993) Vulnerability of mossy fiber targets in the rat hippocampus to forebrain ischemia. *J. Neurosci.* 13: 3964–3979.

Huang, G.-J., and Herbert, J. (2005) Serotonin modulates the suppressive effects of corticosterone on proliferating progenitor cells in the dentate gyrus of the hippocampus in the adult rat. *Neuropsychopharmacology* 30:231–241.

Huang, G.-J., and Herbert, J. (2006) Stimulation of neurogenesis in the hippocampus of the adult rat by fluoxetine requires rhythmic change in corticosterone. *Biol. Psychiatry* 59:619–624.

Ikegaya, Y., Saito, H., and Abe, K. (1994) Attenuated hippocampal long-term potentiation in basolateral amygdala-lesioned rats. *Brain Res.* 656:157–164.

Ikegaya, Y., Saito, H., and Abe, K. (1995) High-frequency stimulation of the basolateral amygdala facilitates the induction of long-term potentiation in the dentate gyrus in vivo. *Neurosci. Res.* 22:203–207.

Ikegaya, Y., Saito, H., and Abe, K. (1996) Dentate gyrus field potentials evoked by stimulation of the basolateral amygdaloid nucleus in anesthetized rats. *Brain Res.* 718:53–60.

Islam, A., Ayer-LeLievre, C., Heigenskold, C., Bogdanovic, N., Winblad, B., and Adem, A. (1998) Changes in IGF-1 receptors in the hippocampus of adult rats after long-term adrenalectomy: receptor autoradiography and in situ hybridization histochemistry. *Brain Res.* 797:342–346.

Issa, A., Rowe, W., Gauthier, S., and Meaney, M. (1990) Hypothalamic-pituitary-adrenal activity in aged, cognitively impaired and cognitively unimpaired rats. *J. Neurosci.* 10:3247–3254.

Jacobson, L., Akana, S.F., Cascio, C.S., Shinsako, J., and Dallman, M.F. (1988) Circadian variations in plasma corticosterone permit normal termination of adrenocorticotropin responses to stress. *Endocrinology* 122:1343–1348.

Jacobson, L., and Sapolsky, R. (1991) The role of the hippocampus in feedback regulation of the hypothalamic-pituitary-adrenocortical axis. *Endocr. Rev.* 12:118–134.

Joels, M. (1997) Steroid hormones and excitability in the mammalian brain. Front. *Neuroendocrinol.* 18:2–48.

Joels, M., Bosma, A., Hendriksen, H., Diegenbach, P., and Kamphuis, W. (1996) Corticosteroid actions on the expression of kainate receptor subunit mRNAs in rat hippocampus. *Mol. Brain Res.* 37: 15–20.

Joels, M., and De Kloet, E.R. (1994) Mineralocorticoid and glucocorticoid receptors in the brain. Implications for ion permeability and transmitter systems. *Progr. Neurobiol.* 43:1–36.

Kaplan, J.R., Pettersson, K., Manuck, S.B., and Olsson, G. (1991) Role of sympathoadrenal medullary activation in the initiation and progression of atherosclerosis. *Circulation* 84(Suppl 6):VI23–VI32.

Karst, H., Berger, S., Turiault, M., Tronche, F., Schutz, G., and Joels, M. (2005) Mineralocorticoid receptors are indispensable for nongenomic modulation of hippocampal glutamate transmission by corticosterone. *Proc. Natl. Acad. Sci. USA* 102:19204–19207.

Kelly, M.J., and Levin, E.R. (2001) Rapid actions of plasma membrane estrogen receptors. *Trends Endo. Metab.* 12:152–156.

Kempermann, G., Kuhn, H.G., and Gage, F.H. (1997) More hippocampal neurons in adult mice living in an enriched environment. *Nature* 586:493–495.

Kendler, K.S. (1998) Major depression and the environment: a psychiatric genetic perspective. *Pharmacopsychiatry* 31:5–9.

Kerr, D., and Campbell, L. (1992) Hippocampal glucocorticoid receptor activation enhances voltage-dependent calcium conductances: relevance to brain aging. *Proc. Natl. Acad. Sci. USA* 89: 8527–8531.

Kerr, J.E., Allore, R.J., Beck, S.G., and Handa, R.J. (1995) Distribution and hormonal regulation of androgen receptor (AR) and AR messenger ribonucleic acid in the rat hippocampus. *Endocrinology* 136:3213–3221.

Kerr, S., Campbell, L., Applegate, M., Brodish, A., and Landfield, P. (1991) Chronic stress-induced acceleration of electrophysiologic and morphometric biomarkers of hippocampal aging. *J. Neurosci.* 11:1316–1324.

Kessler, R.C. (1997) The effects of stressful life events on depression. *Annu. Rev. Psychol.* 48:191–214.

Kim, J.J., Koo, J.W., Lee, H.J., and Han, J.-S. (2005) Amygdalar inactivation blocks stress-induced impairments in hippocampal long-term potentiation and spatial memory. *J. Neurosci.* 25:1532–1539.

Kirschbaum, C., Prussner, J.C., Stone, A.A., Federenko, I., Gaab, J., Lintz, D., Schommer, N., and Hellhammer, D.H. (1995) Persistent high cortisol responses to repeated psychological stress in a subpopulation of healthy men. *Psychosom. Med.* 57:468–474.

Knigge, K. (1961) Adrenocortical response to stress in rats with lesions in hippocampus and amygdala. *Proc. Soc. Exp. Biol. Med.* 180:18–20.

Komuro, H., and Rakic, P. (1995) Modulation of neuronal migration by NMDA receptors. *Science* 260:95–97.

Korte, S.M. (2001) Corticosteroids in relation to fear, anxiety and psychopathology. *Neurosci. & Biobehav. Rev.* 25:117–142.

Kreibich, A.S., and Blendy, J.A. (2004) cAMP response element-binding protein is required for stress but not cocaine-induced reinstatement. *J. Neurosci.* 24:6686–6692.

Kuhn, G.H., Dickinson-Anson, H., and Gage, F.H. (1996) Neurogenesis in the dentate gyrus of the adult rat: age-related decrease of neuronal progenitor proliferation. *J. Neurosci.* 16:2027–2033.

Kuroda, Y., and McEwen, B.S. (1998) Effect of chronic restraint stress and tianeptine on growth factors, GAP-43 and MAP2 mRNA expression in the rat hippocampus. *Mol. Brain Res.* 59: 35–39.

Lai, M., Hibberd, C.J., Gluckman, P.D., and Seckl, J.R. (2000) Reduced expression of insulin-like growth factor 1 messenger RNA in the hippocampus of aged rats. *Neurosci. Lett.* 288:66–70.

Landfield, P. (1987) Modulation of brain aging correlates by long-term alterations of adrenal steroids and neurally-active peptides. *Prog. Brain Res.* 72:279–300.

Landfield, P.W., and Eldridge, J.C. (1994) Evolving aspects of the glucocorticoid hypothesis of brain aging: hormonal modulation of neuronal calcium homeostasis. *Neurobiol. Aging* 15:579–588.

Larsson, B., Seidell, J., Svardsudd, K., Welin, L., Tibblin, G., Wilhelmesen, L., and Bjorntorp, P. (1989) Obesity, adipose tissue distribution and health in men-the study of men born in 1913. *Appetite* 13:37–44.

Laugero, K.D., Bell, M.E., Bhatnagar, S., Soriano, L., and Dallman, M.F. (2001) Sucrose ingestion normalizes central expression of corticotropin-releasing-factor messenger ribonucleic acid and energy balance in adrenalectomized rats: a glucocorticoid-metabolic-brain axis? *Endocrinology* 142:2796–2804.

LeDoux, J.E. (1995) In search of an emotional system in the brain: leaping from fear to emotion and consciousness. In: Gazzaniga M, ed. *The Cognitive Neurosciences.* Cambridge, MA: MIT Press, pp. 1049–1061.

Lee, S.J., Dunlop, J.C., Alves, S.E., Brake, W.G., and McEwen, B.S. (2000) PCREB immunoreactivity in the rat hippocampus following estrogen treatment: In vivo and in vitro studies. *Abstracts Soc. Neurosci.* 26:294.

Leuner, B., Gould, E., and Shors, T.J. (2006) Is there a link between adult neurogenesis and learning? *Hippocampus* 26:216–224.

Liston, C., Miller, M.M., Goldwater, D.S., Radley, J.J., Rocher, A.B., Hof, P.R., Morrison, J.H., and McEwen, B.S. (2006) Stress-induced alterations in prefrontal cortical dendritic morphology predict selective impairments in perceptual attentional set-shifting. *J. Neurosci.* 26:7870–7874.

Lowy, M.T., Gault, L., and Yamamoto, B.K. (1993) Adrenalectomy attenuates stress-induced elevations in extracellular glutamate concentrations in the hippocampus. *J. Neurochem.* 61:1957–1960.

Lowy, M.T., Wittenberg, L., and Yamamoto, B.K. (1995) Effect of acute stress on hippocampal glutamate levels and spectrin proteolysis in young and aged rats. *J. Neurochem.* 65:268–274.

Loy, R., Gerlach, J., and McEwen, B.S. (1988) Autoradiographic localization of estradiol-binding neurons in rat hippocampal formation and entorhinal cortex. *Dev. Brain Res.* 39:245–251.

Lundberg, U., Granqvist, M., Hansson, T., Magnusson, M., and Wallin, L. (1989) Psychological and physiological stress responses during repetitive work at an assembly line. *Work & Stress* 3: 143–153.

Lupien, S.J., and McEwen, B.S. (1997) The acute effects of corticosteroids on cognition: integration of animal and human model studies. *Brain Res. Rev.* 24:1–27.

Lynch, C.D., Lyons, D., Khan, A., Bennett, S.A., and Sonntag, W.E. (2001) Insulin-like growth factor-1 selectively increases glucose utilization in brains of aged animals. *Endocrinology* 142:506–509.

MacQueen, G.M., Campbell, S., McEwen, B.S., Macdonald, K., Amano, S., Joffe, R.T., Nahmias, C., and Young, L.T. (2003) Course of illness, hippocampal function, and hippocampal volume in major depression. *Proc. Natl. Acad. Sci. USA* 100:1387–1392.

Maehlen, J., and Torvik, A. (1990) Necrosis of granule cells of hippocampus in adrenocortical failure. *Acta Neuropathol.* 80: 85–87.

Magarinos, A.M., Deslandes, A., and McEwen, B.S. (1999) Effects of antidepressants and benzodiazepine treatments on the dendritic structure of CA3 pyramidal neurons after chronic stress. *Eur. J. Pharm.* 371:113–122.

Magarinos, A.M., and McEwen, B.S. (1995a) Stress-induced atrophy of apical dendrites of hippocampal CA3c neurons: comparison of stressors. *Neuroscience* 69:83–88.

Magarinos, A.M., and McEwen, B.S. (1995b) Stress-induced atrophy of apical dendrites of hippocampal CA3c neurons: involvement of glucocorticoid secretion and excitatory amino acid receptors. *Neuroscience* 69:89–98.

Magarinos, A.M., McEwen, B.S., Flugge, G., and Fuchs, E. (1996) Chronic psychosocial stress causes apical dendritic atrophy of hippocampal CA3 pyramidal neurons in subordinate tree shrews. *J. Neurosci.* 16:3534–3540.

Magarinos, A.M., McEwen, B.S., Saboureau, M., and Pevet, P. (2006) Rapid and reversible changes in intrahippocampal connectivity during the course of hibernation in European hamsters. *Proc. Natl. Acad. Sci. USA* 49:18775–18780.

Magarinos, A.M., Verdugo Garcia, J.M., and McEwen, B.S. (1997) Chronic restraint stress alters synaptic terminal structure in hippocampus. *Proc. Natl. Acad. Sci. USA* 94:14002–14008.

Makino, S., Gold, P.W., and Schulkin, J. (1994) Corticosterone effects on corticotropin-releasing hormone mRNA in the central nucleus of the amygdala and the parvocellular region of the paraventricular nucleus of the hypothalamus. *Brain Res.* 640:105–112.

Malberg, J.E., Eisch, A.J., Nestler, E.J., and Duman, R.S. (2000) Chronic antidepressant treatment increases neurogenesis in adult rat hippocampus. *J. Neurosci.* 20:9104–9110.

Markowska, A.L., Mooney, M., and Sonntag, W.E. (1998) Insulin-like growth factor-1 ameliorates age-related behavioral deficits. *Neuroscience* 87:559–569.

Matys, T., Pawlak, R., Matys, E., Pavlides, C., McEwen, B.S., and Strickland, S. (2004) Tissue plasminogen activator promotes the effects of corticotropin releasing factor on the amygdala and anxiety-like behavior. *Proc. Natl. Acad. Sci. USA* 101:16345–16350.

McDonald, A.J. (1987) Organization of amygdaloid projections to the mediodorsal thalamus and prefrontal cortex: a fluorescence retrograde transport study in the rat. *J. Comp. Neurol.* 262:46–58.

McDonald, A.J., Mascagni, F., and Guo, L. (1996) Projections of the medial and lateral prefrontal cortices to the amygdala: a Phaseolus vulgaris leucoagglutinin study in the rat. *Neuroscience* 71:55–75.

McEwen, B.S. (1977) Adrenal steroid feedback on neuroendocrine tissues. *Ann. N.Y. Acad. Sci.* 297:568–579.

McEwen, B.S. (1992) Re-examination of the glucocorticoid cascade hypothesis of stress and aging. In: Swaab, D., Hoffman, M., Mirmiran, R., Ravid, F., van Leeuwen, F., eds. *Progress in Brain Research*. Amsterdam: Elsevier, pp. 365–383.

McEwen, B.S. (1999) Stress and hippocampal plasticity. *Annu. Rev. Neurosci.* 22:105–122.

McEwen, B.S., Akama, K., Alves, S., Brake, W.G., Bulloch, K., Lee, S., Li, C., Yuen, G., and Milner, T.A. (2001) Tracking the estrogen receptor in neurons: implications for estrogen-induced synapse formation. *Proc. Natl. Acad. Sci. USA* 98:7093–7100.

McEwen, B.S., Albeck, D., Cameron, H., Chao, H.M., Gould, E., Hastings, N., Kuroda, Y., Luine, V., Magarinos, A.M., McKittrick, C.R., Orchinik, M., Pavlides, C., Vaher, P., Watanabe, Y., and Weiland, N. (1995) Stress and the brain: a paradoxical role for adrenal steroids. In: Litwack, G.D., ed. *Vitamins and Hormones*. Academic Press, Inc., pp. 371–402.

McEwen, B.S., Gould, E., Orchinik, M., Weiland, N.G., and Woolley, C.S. (1995) Oestrogens and the structural and functional plasticity of neurons: implications for memory, ageing and neurodegenerative processes. In: Goode, J., ed. *Ciba Foundation Symposium #191 The Non-reproductive Actions of Sex Steroids*. London: CIBA Foundation, pp. 52–73.

McEwen, B.S., and Seeman, T. (1999) Protective and damaging effects of mediators of stress: elaborating and testing the concepts of allostasis and allostatic load. *Ann. N.Y. Acad. Sci.* 896:30–47.

McEwen, B.S., and Stellar, E. (1993) Stress and the individual: mechanisms leading to disease. *Arch. Int. Med.* 153:2093–2101.

McEwen, B.S., Weiss, J., and Schwartz, L. (1968) Selective retention of corticosterone by limbic structures in rat brain. *Nature* 220: 911–912.

McEwen, B.S., and Woolley, C.S. (1994) Estradiol and progesterone regulate neuronal structure and synaptic connectivity in adult as well as developing brain. *Exp. Gerontol.* 29:431–436.

McKittrick, C.R., Magarinos, A.M., Blanchard, D.C., Blanchard, R.J., McEwen, B.S., and Sakai, R.R. (2000) Chronic social stress reduces dendritic arbors in CA3 of hippocampus and decreases binding to serotonin transporter sites. *Synapse* 36:85–94.

Meaney, M., Aitken, D., Berkel, H., Bhatnagar, S., and Sapolsky, R. (1988) Effect of neonatal handling of age-related impairments associated with the hippocampus. *Science* 239:766–768.

Meaney, M., Viau, V., Aitken, D., and Bhatnagar, S. (1988) Stress-induced occupancy and translocation of hippocampal glucocorticoid receptors. *Brain Res.* 445:198–203.

Meaney, M.J., Tannenbaum, B., Francis, D., Bhatnagar, S., Shanks, N., Viau, V., O'Donnell, D., and Plotsky, P.M. (1994) Early environmental programming hypothalamic-pituitary-adrenal responses to stress. *Sem. Neurosci.* 6:247–259.

Melchor, J.P., Pawlak, R., and Strickland, S. (2003) The tissue plasminogen activator - plasminogen proteolytic cascade accelerates amyloid-β (Aβ) degradation and inhibits Aβ-induced neurodegeneration. *J. Neurosci.* 23:8867–8871.

Melin, B., Lundberg, U., Soderlund, J., and Granqvist, M. (1999) Psychological and physiological stress reactions of male and female assembly workers: a comparison between two different forms of work organization. *J. Organiz. Behav.* 20: 47–61.

Mennini, T., and Miari, A. (1991) Modulation of (3H) glutamate binding by seratonin in the rat hippocampus: an autoradiographic study. *Life Sci.* 49:283–292.

Milad, M.R., and Quirk, G.J. (2002) Neurons in medial prefrontal cortex signal memory for fear extinction. *Nature* 420:70–74.

Milner, T.A., McEwen, B.S., Hayashi, S., Li, C.J., Reagen, L., and Alves, S.E. (2001) Ultrastructural evidence that hippocampal alpha estrogen receptors are located at extranuclear sites. *J. Comp. Neurol.* 429:355–371.

Miner, J.N., and Yamamoto, K.R. (1991) Regulatory crosstalk at composite response elements. *Trends Biochem. Sci.* 16:423–426.

Miracle, A.D., Brace, M.F., Huyck, K.D., Singler, S.A., and Wellman, C.L. (2006) Chronic stress impairs recall of extinction of conditioned fear. *Neurobiol. Learn. Mem.* 85:213–218.

Mizoguchi, K., Kunishita, T., Chui, D.H., and Tabira, T. (1992) Stress induces neuronal death in the hippocampus of castrated rats. *Neurosci. Letts.* 138:157–160.

Moghaddam, B., Boliano, M.L., Stein-Behrens, B., and Sapolsky, R. (1994) Glucocorticoids mediate the stress-induced extracellular accumulation of glutamate. *Brain Res.* 655:251–254.

Monaghan, D.T., Holets, V.R., Toy, D.W., and Cotman, C.W. (1983) Anatomical distributions of four pharmacologically distinct 3H-L-glutamate binding sites. *Nature* 306:176–179.

Morgan, M.A., and LeDoux, J.E. (1995) Differential contribution of dorsal and ventral medial prefrontal cortex to the acquisition and extinction of conditioned fear in rats. *Behav. Neurosci.* 109: 681–688.

Muller, J.E., Tofler, G., and Stone, P. (1989) Circadian variation and triggers of onset of acute caridovascular disease. *Circulation* 79:733–743.

Murphy, B.E.P. (1991) Treatment of major depression with steroid suppressive drugs. *J. Steroid Biochem. Molec. Biol.* 39:239–244.

Murphy, D.D., Cole, N.B., Greenberger, V., and Segal, M. (1998) Estradiol increases dendritic spine density by reducing GABA neurotransmission in hippocampal neurons. *J. Neurosci.* 18: 2550–2559.

Murphy, D.D., Cole, N.B., and Segal, M. (1998) Brain-derived neurotrophic factor mediates estradiol-induced dendritic spine formation in hippocampal neurons. *Proc. Natl. Acad. Sci. USA* 95: 11412–11417.

Murphy, D.D., and Segal, M. (1996) Regulation of dendritic spine density in cultured rat hippocampal neurons by steroid hormones. *J. Neurosci.* 16:4059–4068.

Murphy, D.D., and Segal, M. (1997) Morphological plasticity of dendritic spines in central neurons is mediated by activation of cAMP response element binding protein. *Proc. Natl. Acad. Sci. USA* 94:1482–1487.

Nacher, J., and McEwen, B.S. (2006) The role of *N*-methyl-D-aspartate receptors in neurogenesis. *Hippocampus* 16:267–270.

Nacher, J., Rosell, D.R., Alonso-Llosa, G., and McEwen, B.S. (2001) NMDA receptor antagonist treatment induces a long-lasting increase in the number of proliferating cells, PSA-NCAM-immunoreactive granule neurons and radial glia in the adult rat dentate gyrus. *Eur. J. Neurosci.* 13:512–520.

Nakamura, N.H., and McEwen, B.S. (2005) Changes in interneuronal phenotypes regulated by estradiol in the adult rat hippocampus: A potential role for neuropeptide Y. *Neuroscience* 136:357–369.

Noguchi, S., Higashi, K., and Kawamura, M. (1990) A posssible role of the α-subunit of (Na,K)-ATPase in facilitating correct assembly of the β-subunit into the membrane. *J. Biol. Chem.* 265: 5991–5995.

Ohl, F., and Fuchs, E. (1999) Differential effects of chronic stress on memory processes in the tree shrew. *Cog. Brain Res.* 7:379–387.

O'Kusky, J.R., Ye, P., and D'Ercole, A.J. (2000) Insulin-like growth factor-1 promotes neurogenesis and synaptogenesis in the hippocampal dentate gyrus during postnatal development. *J. Neurosci.* 20:8435–8442.

Orchinik, M., Carroll, S.S., Li, Y.-H., McEwen, B.S., and Weiland, N.G. (2001) Heterogeneity of hippocampal $GABA_A$ receptors: regulation by corticosterone. *J. Neurosci.* 21:330–339.

Orchinik, M., Weiland, N.G., and McEwen, B.S. (1994) Adrenalectomy selectively regulates GABAa receptor subunit expression in the hippocampus. *Mol. Cell. Neurosci.* 5:451–458.

Ott, A., Stolk, R.P., Hofman, A., van Harskamp, F., Grobbee, D.E., and Breteler, M.M.B. (1996) Association of diabetes mellitus and dementia: The Rotterdam study. *Diabetologia* 39:1392–1397.

Parent, J.M., Janumpalli, S., McNamara, J.O., and Lowenstein, D.H. (1998) Increased dentate granule cell neurogenesis following amygdala kindling in the adult rat. *Neurosci. Lett.* 247:9–12.

Parent, J.M., Yu, T.W., Leibowitz, R.T., Geschwind, D.H., Sloviter, R.S., and Lowenstein, D.H. (1997) Dentate granule cell neurogenesis is increased by seizures and contributes to aberrant network reorganization in the adult rat hippocampus. *J. Neurosci.* 17:3727–3738.

Parnavelas, J., Lynch, G., Brecha, N., Cotman, C., and Globus, A. (1974) Spine loss and regrowth in hippocampus following deafferentation. *Nature* 248:71–73.

Parsons, B., Rainbow, T.C., MacLusky, N., and McEwen, B.S. (1982) Progestin receptor levels in rat hypothalamic and limbic nuclei. *J. Neurosci.* 2:1446–1452.

Pavlides, C., Kimura, A., Magarinos, A.M., and McEwen, B.S. (1994) Type I adrenal steroid receptors prolong hippocampal long-term potentiation. *Neuroreport* 5:2673–2677.

Pavlides, C., Kimura, A., Magarinos, A.M., and McEwen, B.S. (1995) Hippocampal homosynaptic long-term depression/depotentiation induced by adrenal steroids. *Neuroscience* 68:379–385.

Pavlides, C., and McEwen, B.S. (1999) Effects of mineralocorticoid and glucocorticoid receptors on long-term potentiation in the CA3 hippocampal field. *Brain Res.* 851:204–214.

Pavlides, C., Ogawa, S., Kimura, A., and McEwen, B. (1996) Role of adrenal steroid mineralocorticoid and glucocorticoid receptors in long-term potentiation in the CA1 field of hippocampal slices. *Brain Res.* 738:229–235.

Pavlides, C., Watanabe, Y., Magarinos, A.M., and McEwen, B.S. (1995) Opposing role of adrenal steroid Type I and Type II receptors in hippocampal long-term potentiation. *Neuroscience* 68: 387–394.

Pavlides, C., Watanabe, Y., and McEwen, B.S. (1993) Effects of glucocorticoids on hippocampal long-term potentiation. *Hippocampus* 3:183–192.

Pawlak, R., Rao, B.S.S., Melchor, J.P., Chattarji, S., McEwen, B., and Strickland, S. (2005) Tissue plasminogen activator and plasminogen mediate stress-induced decline of neuronal and cognitive functions in the mouse hippocampus. *Proc. Natl. Acad. Sci. USA* 102:18201–18206.

Petrovich, G.D., Canteras, N.S., and Swanson, L.W. (2001) Combinatorial amygdalar inputs to hippocampal domains and hypothalamic behavior systems. *Brain Res. Rev.* 38:247–289.

Pham, K., Nacher, J., Hof, P.R., and McEwen, B.S. (2003) Repeated, but not acute, restraint stress suppresses proliferation of neural precursor cells and increases PSA-NCAM expression in the adult rat dentate gyrus. *J. Neurosci.* 17:879–886.

Phillips, R.G., and LeDoux, J.E. (1992) Differential contribution of amygdala and hippocampus to cued and contextual fear conditioning. *Behav. Neurosci.* 106:274–285.

Pierce, J.P., van Leyen, K., and McCarthy, J.B. (2000) Translocation machinery for synthesis of integral membrane and secretory proteins in dendritic spines. *Nat. Neurosci.* 3:311–313.

Pitkanen, A., Pikkarainen, M., Nurminen, N., and Ylinen, A. (2000) Reciprocal connections between the amygdala and the hippocampal formation, perirhinal cortex, and postrhinal cortex in rat. *Ann. N.Y. Acad. Sci.* 911:369–391.

Pitman, R.K. (2001) Hippocampal diminution in PTSD: More (or less?) than meets the eye. *Hippocampus* 11:73–74.

Pompei, P., Riftina, F., and McEwen, B.S. (1995) Effect of adrenal steroids on prepreneurokinin-A gene expression in discrete regions of the rat brain. *Mol. Brain Res.* 33:209–216.

Popov, V.I., and Bocharova, L.S. (1992) Hibernation-induced structural changes in synaptic contacts between mossy fibres and hippocampal pyramidal neurons. *Neuroscience* 48:53–62.

Popov, V.I., Bocharova, L.S., and Bragin, A.G. (1992) Repeated changes of dendritic morphology in the hippocampus of ground squirrels in the course of hibernation. *Neuroscience* 48:45–51.

Pressman, S.D., and Cohen, S. (2005) Does positive affect influence health? *Psychol. Bull.* 131:925–971.

Pruessner, J.C., Baldwin, M.W., Dedovic, K., Renwick, R.M.N.K., Lord, C., Meaney, M., and Lupien, S. (2005) Self-esteem, locus of control, hippocampal volume, and cortisol regulation in young and old adulthood. *NeuroImage* 28:815–826.

Pruessner, J.C., Hellhammer, D.H., and Kirschbaum, C. (1999) Low self-esteem, induced failure and the adrenocortical stress response. *Personality and Individual Differences* 27:477–489.

Pulford, B.E., and Ishii, D.N. (2001) Uptake of circulating insulin-like growth factors (IGFs) into cerebrospinal fluid appears to be independent of the IGF receptors as well as IGF-binding proteins. *Endocrinology* 142:213–220.

Quirk, G.J., and Armony, J.L. (1997) Fear conditioning enhances different temporal components of tone-evoked spike trains in auditory cortex and lateral amygdala. *Neuron* 19:613–624.

Quirk, G.J., Likhtik, E., Pelletier, J.G., and Pare, D. (2003) Stimulation of medial prefrontal cortex decreases the responsiveness of central amygdala output neurons. *J. Neurosci.* 23:8800–8807.

Radley, J.J., and Jacobs, B.L. (2002) 5-HT1A receptor antagonist administration decreases cell proliferation in the dentate gyrus. *Brain Res.* 955:264–267.

Radley, J.J., Sisti, H.M., Hao, J., Rocher, A.B., McCall, T., Hof, P.R., McEwen, B.S., and Morrison, J.H. (2004) Chronic behavioral stress induces apical dendritic reorganization in pyramidal neurons of the medial prefrontal cortex. *Neuroscience* 125:1–6.

Radley, J.J., Rocher, A.B., Janssen, W.G.M., Hof, P.R., McEwen, B.S., and Morrison, J.H. (2005) Reversibility of apical dendritic retraction in the rat medial prefrontal cortex following repeated stress. *Exp. Neurol.* 196:199–203.

Radley, J.J., Rocher, A.B., Miller, M., Janssen, W.G.M., Liston, C., Hof, P.R., McEwen, B.S., and Morrison, J.H. (2006) Repeated stress induces dendritic spine loss in the rat medial prefrontal cortex. *Cereb. Cortex* 16:313–320.

Rahmann, S., and Neumann, R.S. (1993) Activation of 5-HT2 receptors facilitates depolarization of neocortical neurons by N-methyl-D-aspartate. *Eur. J. Pharmacol.* 231:347–354.

Rakic, P. (1985) Limits of neurogenesis in primates. *Science* 227: 1054–1056.

Rasika, S., Alvarez-Buylla, A., and Nottebohm, F. (1999) BDNF mediates the effects of testosterone on the survival of new neurons in an adult brain. *Neuron* 22:53–62.

Rasika, S., Nottebohm, F., and Alvarez-Buylla, A. (1994) Testosterone increases the recruitment and/or survival of new high vocal center neurons in adult female canaries. *Proc. Natl. Acad. Sci. USA* 91:7854–7858.

Rasmussen, T., Schliemann, T., Sorensen, J.C., Zimmer, J., and West, M.J. (1996) Memory impaired aged rats: no loss of principal hippocampal and subicular neurons. *Neurobiol. Aging* 14:143–147.

Razandi, M., Pedram, A., Greene, G.L., and Levin, E.R. (1999) Cell membrane and nuclear estrogen receptors (ERs) originate from a single transcript: Studies of ERα and ERβ expressed in Chinese hamster ovary cells. *Mol. Endocrinol.* 13:307–319.

Reichardt, H.M., and Schutz, G. (1998) Glucocorticoid signalling - multiple variations of a common theme. *Mol. Cell. Endocrinol.* 146:1–6.

Richardson, M.P., Strange, B.A., and Dolan, R.J. (2004) Encoding of emotional memories depends on amygdala and hippocampus and their interactions. *Nat. Neurosci.* 7:278–285.

Robinson, T.E., and Kolb, B. (1997) Persistent structural modifications in nucleus accumbens and prefrontal cortex neurons produced by previous experience with amphetamine. *J. Neurosci.* 17:8491–8497.

Roof, R.L. (1993) The dentate gyrus is sexually dimorphic in prepubescent rats: testosterone plays a significant role. *Brain Res.* 610: 148–151.

Rozovsky, I., Wei, M., Stone, D.J., Zanjani, H., Anderson, C.P., Morgan, T.E., and Finch, C.E. (2002) Estradiol (E2) enhances neurite outgrowth by repressing glial fibrillary acidic protein expression and reorganizing laminin. *Endocrinology* 143:636–646.

Rudick, C.N., and Woolley, C.S. (2000) Estradiol induces a phasic Fos response in the hippocampal CA1 and CA3 regions of adult female rats. *Hippocampus* 10:274–283.

Rudick, C.N., and Woolley, C.S. (2001) Estrogen regulates functional inhibition of hippocampal CA1 pyramidal cells in the adult female rat. *J. Neurosci.* 21:6532–6543.

Sachar, E.J., Hellman, L., Roffwarg, H.P., Halpern, F.S., Fukushima, D.K., and Gallagher, T.F. (1973) Disrupted 24-hour patterns of cortisol secretion in psychotic depression. *Arch. Gen. Psychiatry* 28:19–24.

Santini, E., Ge, H., Ren, K., Pena de Ortiz, S., and Quirk, G.J. (2004) Consolidation of fear extinction requires protein synthesis in the medial prefrontal cortex. *J. Neurosci.* 24:5704–5710.

Sapolsky, R. (1992) *Stress, the Aging Brain and the Mechanisms of Neuron Death*. Cambridge, MA: MIT Press.

Sapolsky, R.M. (1996) Why stress is bad for your brain. *Science* 273:749–750.

Sapolsky, R., Krey, L., and McEwen, B.S. (1986) The neuroendocrinology of stress and aging: the glucocorticoid cascade hypothesis. *Endocr. Rev.* 7:284–301.

Saxe, M.D., Battaglia, F., Wang, J.-W., Malleret, G., David, D.J., Monckton, J.E., Garcia, A.D.R., Sofroniew, M.V., Kandel, E.R., Santarelli, L., Hen, R., and Drew, M.R. (2006) Ablation of hippocampal neurogenesis impairs contextual fear conditioning and synaptic plasticity in the dentate gyrus. *Proc. Natl. Acad. Sci. USA* 103:17501–17506.

Schulkin, J., McEwen, B.S., and Gold, P.W. (1994) Allostasis, amygdala, and anticipatory angst. *Neurosci. Biobehav. Rev.* 18:385–396.

Seeman, T.E., McEwen, B.S., Rowe, J.W., and Singer, B.H. (2001) Allostatic load as a marker of cumulative biological risk: MacArthur Studies of Successful Aging. *Proc. Natl. Acad. Sci. USA* 98: 4770–4775.

Seeman, T.E., Singer, B.H., Rowe, J.W., Horwitz, R.I., and McEwen, B.S. (1997) Price of adaptation--allostatic load and its health consequences: MacArthur studies of successful aging. *Arch. Intern. Med.* 157:2259–2268.

Seeman, T.E., Singer, B.H., Ryff, C.D., Dienberg, G., and Levy-Storms, L. (2002) Social relationships, gender, and allostatic load across two age cohorts. *Psychosom. Med.* 64:395–406.

Seki, T., and Arai, Y. (1995) Age-related production of new granule cells in the adult dentate gyrus. *Neuroreport* 6:2479–2482.

Seri, B., Garcia-Verdugo, J.M., McEwen, B.S., and Alvarez-Buylla, A. (2001) Astrocytes give rise to new neurons in the adult mammalian hippocampus. *J. Neurosci.* 21:7153–7160.

Sheline, Y.I., Gado, M.H., and Kraemer, H.C. (2003) Untreated depression and hippocampal volume loss. *Am. J. Psychiatry* 160: 1516–1518.

Sheline, Y.I., Sanghavi, M., Mintun, M.A., and Gado, M.H. (1999) Depression duration but not age predicts hippocampal volume loss in medically healthy women with recurrent major depression. *J. Neurosci.* 19:5034–5043.

Sheline, Y.I., Wang, P.W., Gado, M.H., Csernansky, J.C., and Vannier, M.W. (1996) Hippocampal atrophy in recurrent major depression. *Proc. Natl. Acad. Sci. USA* 93:3908–3913.

Sherry, D.F., Jacobs, L.F., and Gaulin, S.J. (1992) Spatial memory and adaptive specialization of the hippocampus. *Trends Neurosci.* 15:298–303.

Sherwin, B.B. (2003) Estrogen and cognitive functioning in women. *Endocrine Rev.* 24:133–151.

Shughrue, P.J., and Merchenthaler, I. (2000) Evidence for novel estrogen binding sites in the rat hippocampus. *Neuroscience* 99: 605–612.

Siesjo, B., and Bengtsson, F. (1989) Calcium fluxes, calcium antagonists and calcium-related pathology in brain ischemia, hypoglycemia and spreading depression: a unifying hypothesis. *J. Cereb. Blood Flow Metab.* 9:127–140.

Sloviter, R., Valiquette, G., Abrams, G., Ronk, E., Sollas, A., Paul, L., and Neubort, S. (1989) Selective loss of hippocampal granule cells in the mature rat brain after adrenalectomy. *Science* 243: 535–538.

Smith, M.A., Makino, S., Kvetnansky, R., and Post, R.M. (1995) Stress and glucocorticoids affect the expression of brain-derived neurotrophic factor and neurotrophin-3 mRNAs in the hippocampus. *J. Neurosci.* 15:1768–1777.

Snyder, J.S., Kee, N., and Wojtowicz, J.M. (2001) Effects of adult neurogenesis on synaptic plasticity in the rat dentate gyrus. *J. Neurophysiol.* 85:2423–2431.

Sousa, N., Lukoyanov, N.V., Madeira, M.D., Almeida, O.F.X., and Paula-Barbosa, M.M. (2000) Reorganization of the morphology of hippocampal neurites and synapses after stress-induced damage correlates with behavioral improvement. *Neuroscience* 97: 253–266.

Spano, M.S., Ellgren, M., Wang, X., and Hurd, Y.L. (2007) Prenatal cannabis exposure increases heroin seeking with allostatic changes in limbic enkephalin systems in adulthood. *Biol. Psychiatry* 61: 554–563.

Spanswick, S.C., Epp, J.R., Keith, J.R., and Sutherland, R.J. (2007) Adrenalectomy-induced granule cell degeneration in the hippocampus causes spatial memory deficits that are not reversed by chronic treatment with corticosterone or fluoxetine. *Hippocampus* 17:137–146.

Squire, L.R., and Zola-Morgan, S. (1991) The medial temporal lob memory system. *Science* 253:1380–1386.

Starkman, M.N., Gebarski, S.S., Berent, S., and Schteingart, D.E. (1992) Hippocampal formation volume, memory dysfunction, and cortisol levels in patients with Cushing's syndrome. *Biol. Psychiatry* 32:756–765.

Starkman, M.N., Giordani, B., Gebrski, S.S., Berent, S., Schork, M.A., and Schteingart, D.E. (1999) Decrease in cortisol reverses human hippocampal atrophy following treatment of Cushing's disease. *Biol. Psychiatry* 46:1595–1602.

Starkman, M.N., and Schteingart, D.E. (1981) Neuropsychiatric manifestations of patients with Cushing's syndrome. *Arch. Intern. Med.* 141:215–219.

Steptoe, A., Owen, N., Kunz-Ebrecht, S.R., and Brydon, L. (2004) Loneliness and neuroendocrine, cardiovascular, and inflammatory stress responses in middle-aged men and women. *Psychoneuroendocrinology* 29:593–611.

Steptoe, A., Wardle, J., and Marmot, M. (2005) Positive affect and health-related neuroendocrine, cardiovascular, and inflammatory processes. *Proc. Natl. Acad. Sci. USA* 102:6508–6512.

Sterling, P., and Eyer, J. (1988) Allostasis: A new paradigm to explain arousal pathology. In: Fisher, S., and Reason, J., eds. *Handbook of Life Stress, Cognition and Health*. New York: John Wiley & Sons, pp. 629–649.

Sternberg, E., Young, S.I., Bernardini, R., Calogero, A., Chrousos, G., Gold, P., and Wilder, R. (1989) A central nervous system defect in biosynthesis of corticotropin-releasing hormone is associated with susceptibility to streptococcal cell wall-induced arthritis in Lewis rats. *Proc. Natl. Acad. Sci. USA* 86:4771–4775.

Sternberg, E.M., Hill, J.M., and Chrousos, G.P. (1996) Inflammatory mediator-induced hypothalamic-pituitary-adrenal axis activation is defective in streptococcal cell wall arthritis susceptible Lewis rats. *Proc. Natl. Acad. Sci. USA* 86:2374–2378.

Sternberg, E.M., Young, W.S., Bernardini, R., Calogero, A.E., Chrousos, G.P., Gold, P.W., and Wilder, R.L. (1989) A central nervous system defect in biosynthesis of corticotropin-releasing hormone is associated with susceptibility to streptococcal cell wall-induced arthritis in Lewis rats. *Proc. Natl. Acad. Sci. USA* 86:4771–4775.

Sugaya, K., Chouinard, M., Greene, R., Robbins, M., Personett, D., Kent, C., Gallagher, M., and McKinney, M. (1996) Molecular indices of neuronal and glial plasticity in the hippocampal formation in a rodent model of age-induced spatial learning impairment. *J. Neurosci.* 16:3427–3443.

Takadera, T., Matsuda, I., and Ohyashiki, T. (1999) Apoptotic cell death and caspase-3 activation induced by N-methyl-D-aspartate receptor antagonists and their prevention by insulin-like growth factor I. *J. Neurochem.* 73:548–556.

Tanapat, P., Hastings, N.B., Reeves, A.J., and Gould, E. (1999) Estrogen stimulates a transient increase in the number of new neurons in the dentate gyrus of the adult female rat. *J. Neurosci.* 19:5792–5801.

Taylor, C.P., and Meldrum, B.S. (1995) Na^+ channels as targets for neuroprotective drugs. *Trends Neurosci.* 16:309–316.

Terasawa. E., and Timiras, P. (1968) Electrical activity during the estrous cycle of the rat: cyclic changes in limbic structures. *Endocrinology* 83:207N216.

Tiedge, H., Bloom, F.E., and Richter, D. (2001) Colloquium: Molecular kinesis in cellular function and plasticity. *Proc. Natl. Acad. Sci. USA* 98:6997–7106.

Trapp, T., Rupprecht, R., Castren, M., Reul, J.M.H.M., and Holsboer, F. (1994) Heterodimerization between mineralocorticoid and glucocorticoid receptor: A new principle of glucocorticoid action in the CNS. *Neuron* 13:1457–1462.

Trejo, J.L., Carro, E., and Torres-Aleman, I. (2001) Circulating insulin-like growth factor I mediates exercise-induced increases in the number of new neurons in the adult hippocampus. *J. Neurosci.* 21:1628–1634.

van Praag, H., Kempermann, G., and Gage, F.H. (1999) Running increases cell proliferation and neurogenesis in the adult mouse dentate gyrus. *Nat. Neurosci.* 2:266–270.

Venero, C., and Borrell, J. (1999) Rapid glucocorticoid effects on excitatory amino acid levels in the hippocampus: a microdialysis study in freely moving rats. *Eur. J. Neurosci.* 1:2465–2473.

Vyas, A., Mitra, R., Rao, B.S.S., and Chattarji, S. (2002) Chronic stress induces contrasting patterns of dendritic remodeling in hippocampal and amygdaloid neurons. *J. Neurosci.* 22:6810–6818.

Wang, J., Rao, H., Wetmore, G.S., Furlan, P.M., Korczykowski, M., Dinges, D.F., and Detre, J.A. (2005) Perfusion functional MRI reveals cerebral blood flow pattern under psychological stress. *Proc. Natl. Acad. Sci. USA* 102:17804–17809.

Watanabe, Y., Gould, E., Daniels, D., Cameron, H., and McEwen, B.S. (1992) Tianeptine attenuates stress-induced morphological changes in the hippocampus. *Eur. J. Pharm.* 222:157–162.

Watanabe, Y., Weiland, N.G., and McEwen, B.S. (1995) Effects of adrenal steroid manipulations and repeated restraint stress on dynorphin mRNA levels and excitatory amino acid receptor binding in hippocampus. *Brain Res.* 680:217–225.

Waters, E.M., Torres-Reveron, A., McEwen, B.S., Milner, T.A. (in press) Ultrastructural localization of extranuclear progestin receptors in the rat hippocampal formation. *J. Comp. Neurol.* in press

Weiland, N.G. (1992a) Estradiol selectively regulates agonist binding sites on the *N*-methyl-D-aspartate receptor complex in the CA1 region of the hippocampus. *Endocrinology* 131:662–668.

Weiland, N.G. (1992b) Glutamic acid decarboxylase messenger ribonucleic acid is regulated by estradiol and progesterone in the hippocampus. *Endocrinology* 131:2697–2702.

Weiland, N.G., Orchinik, M., and McEwen, B.S. (1995) Corticosterone regulates mRNA levels of specific subunits of the NMDA receptor in the hippocampus but not in cortex of rats. *Abstracts, Soc. Neurosci.* 21:207.12.

Weiland, N.G., Orchinik, M., and Tanapat, P. (1997) Chronic corticosterone treatment induces parallel changes in N-methyl-D-aspartate receptor subunit messenger RNA levels and antagonist binding sites in the hippocampus. *Neuroscience* 78:653–662.

Weiland N.G., Orikasa, C., Hayashi, S., and McEwen, B.S. (1996) Localization of estrogen receptors in the hippocampus of male and female rats. *Soc. Neurosci. Abstr.* 22:618.

Weiland, N.G., Orikasa, C., Hayashi, S., and McEwen, B.S. (1997) Distribution and hormone regulation of estrogen receptor immunoreactive cells in the hippocampus of male and female rats. *J. Comp. Neurol.* 388:603–612.

Wellman, C.L. (2001) Dendritic reorganization in pyramidal neurons in medial prefrontal cortex after chronic corticosterone administration. *J. Neurobiol.* 49:245–253.

Whitton, P.S., Sarna, G.S., O'Connell, M.T.O., and Curzon, G. (1991) The effect of the novel antidepressant tianeptine on the concentration of 5-hydroxytryptamine in rat hippocampal dialysates in vivo. *Neuropharmacology* 30:1–4.

Wise, P.M., Dubal, D.B., Rau, S.W., Brown, C.M., and Suzuki, S. (2005) Are estrogens protective or risk factors in brain injury and neurodegeneration? Reevaluation after the women's health initiative. *Endocrine Rev.* 26:308–312.

Wood, G.E., Young, L.T., Reagan, L.P., and McEwen, B.S. (2003) Acute and chronic restraint stress alter the incidence of social conflict in male rats. *Horm. & Behav.* 43:205–213.

Woolley, C., Gould, E., Sakai, R., Spencer, R., and McEwen, B.S. (1991) Effects of aldosterone or RU28362 treatment on adrenalectomy-induced cell death in the dentate gyrus of the adult rat. *Brain Res.* 554:312–315.

Woolley, C., and McEwen, B.S. (1993) Roles of estradiol and progesterone in regulation of hippocampal dendritic spine density during the estrous cycle in the rat. *J. Comp. Neurol.* 336: 293–306.

Woolley, C., and McEwen, B.S. (1994) Estradiol regulates hippocampal dendritic spine density via an N-methyl-D-aspartate receptor dependent mechanism. *J. Neuroscience* 108:263–272.

Wossink, J., Karst, H., Mayboroda, O., and Joels, M. (2001) Morphological and functional properties of rat dentate granule cells after adrenalectomy. *Neuroscience* 108:263–272.

Yehuda, R., Giller, E., Southwick, S., Lowy, M., and Mason, J. (1991) Hypothalamic-pituitary-adrenal dysfunction in posttraumatic stress disorder. *Biol. Psychiatry* 30:1031–1048.

Yen, L., Sibley, J.T., and Constantine-Paton, M. (1995) Analysis of synaptic distribution within single retinal axonal arbors after chronic NMDA treatment. *J. Neurosci.* 15:4712–4725.

Zhuang, X., Gross, C., Santarelli, L., Compan, V., Trillat, A.-C., and Hen, R. (1999) Altered emotional states in knockout mice lacking 5-HT1A or 5-HT1B receptors. *Neuropsychopharmacology* 21:52S–60S.

41 The Neurobiology of Anxiety Disorders

AMIR GARAKANI, JAMES W. MURROUGH, DENNIS S. CHARNEY, AND J. DOUGLAS BREMNER

There is continuing expansion in our knowledge of the neurobiological and neurochemical bases of fear and anxiety. Specific neurochemical and neuropeptide systems have been demonstrated to play important roles in the behaviors associated with fear and anxiety-producing stimuli. Long-term dysregulation of these systems appear to contribute to the development of anxiety disorders, including panic disorder, posttraumatic stress disorder (PTSD), and social anxiety disorder. These neurochemical and neuropeptide systems have been shown to have effects on distinct cortical and subcortical brain areas that are relevant to the mediation of the symptoms associated with anxiety disorders. These areas include the amygdala, prefrontal cortex (PFC), hippocampus, anterior cingulate cortex (ACC), and the insula. Advances in functional neuroimaging have allowed for the intensive investigation of how these regions contribute to anxiety states. Moreover, advances in molecular genetics portend the identification of the genes underlying the neurobiological disturbances that increase the vulnerability to anxiety disorders. This chapter reviews preclinical and clinical research pertinent to the neurobiological basis of anxiety disorders. The implications of this synthesis for the discovery of anxiety disorder vulnerability genes and novel psychopharmacological approaches is also discussed.

NEURAL MECHANISMS OF FEAR AND ANXIETY

Classical Fear Conditioning

The concept of classical conditioning was set forth in the famous experiment of Ivan Pavlov (1927). He began by describing how a dog, when presented with food, salivates. The food represents an unconditioned stimulus (US) creating an unconditioned response (UR). He then rang a bell, a neutral stimulus, while presenting the food, thereby linking the US to the ringing. After several trials of ringing the bell while presenting the food (learning), he then removed the food, and rang the bell only. This caused the dog to salivate, a conditioned response (CR) to a new conditioned stimulus (CS). In summary, classical conditioning is a process by which a neutral stimulus becomes a CS.

Pavlovian conditioning can also be applied to the model of fear learning. In nature, animals need to be able to recognize and respond appropriately to threats (Blair et al., 2001); therefore, fear is a highly useful adaptive trait meant to protect us from potential danger. When certain environmental cues, traumas, persistent stress, or other stimuli trigger persistent aversive responses, fear can develop into anxiety. A notable example was the Little Albert experiment (J.B. Watson and Raynor, 1920). In their experiment, an 11-year-old boy was given a rat with which to play and had no fear reaction. The rat was presented again, but this time coupled with a long banging noise (an US), causing Albert to cry (UR). After several trials, Albert was shown the rat (CS) without the noise but still cried (CR). He had the same reaction when he was presented with a piece of fur that resembled the color and shape of the rat, which is an example of how his fear had generalized. In addition to being unethical, this experiment illustrates how an aversive stimulus (US) can continue to cause a CR, whereas nonaversive cues will not cause a CR if they are continually presented without the US. This process is called *extinction* and is discussed later (see also Garakani et al., 2006, for a review of classical conditioning).

Neuroanatomy of Anxiety

A comprehensive review of this area is covered in Chapter 39. G.M. Sullivan and others discuss in detail the pathway by which fear stimuli are translated into the expression of anxiety symptoms. A brief overview follows now.

The amygdala has a prominent role in the etiology of anxiety disorders (Pare et al., 2004). It has been shown to be involved in the acquisition of fearful stimuli, and a part of the "fear loop pathway." Studies of humans with damage to their amygdala have shown that they have impairment in their ability to acquire fear responses (Adolphs et al., 2005). The amygdala, which is found in the medial temporal lobes, consists of 13 nuclei, with the basal amygdala, lateral amygdala, and central nucleus of the amygdala (CEA) playing a role in the fear response (Rosen, 2004). The pathway begins when fear-related conditioned stimuli are transmitted to the thalamus by external and visceral pathways. Afferents then reach the lateral amygdala via two parallel circuits: a rapid subcortical path directly from the dorsal (sensory) thalamus and a slower regulatory cortical pathway encompassing primary somatosensory cortices, the insula, and anterior cingulate/PFC. Contextual CSs are projected to the lateral amygdala from the hippocampus and perhaps the bed nucleus of the stria terminalis (BNST). The long loop pathway indicates that sensory information relayed to the amygdala undergoes substantial higher-level processing, thereby enabling assignment of significance, based upon prior experience, to complex stimuli. Cortical involvement in fear conditioning is clinically relevant because it provides a mechanism by which cognitive factors will influence whether symptoms are experienced or not following stress exposure (LeDoux, 2000; Sotres-Bayon et al., 2006).

During the expression of fear-related behaviors, the lateral amygdala engages the CEA, which as the principal output nucleus projects to areas of the hypothalamus and brain stem that mediate the autonomic, endocrine, and behavioral responses associated with fear and anxiety (Schafe et al., 2001). The molecular and cellular mechanisms that underlie synaptic plasticity in amygdala-dependent learned fear are an area of very active investigation (Shumyatsky et al., 2002; Schroeder and Shinnick-Gallagher, 2004). Long-term potentiation (LTP) in the lateral amygdala (LA) appears to be a critical mechanism for storing memories of the CS–US association (Chapman et al., 1990; Blair et al., 2001). A variety of behavioral and electrophysiological data have led LeDoux and colleagues to propose a model to explain how neural responses to the CS and US in the LA could influence LTP-like changes that store memories during fear conditioning. This model proposes that calcium entry through *N*-methyl-D-aspartate (NMDA) receptors and voltage-gated calcium channels (VGCCs) initiates the molecular processes to consolidate synaptic changes into long-term memory (Blair et al., 2001). Short-term memory requires calcium entry only through NMDA receptors.

This hypothesis leads to several predictions that may have relevance to the discovery of novel therapeutics for anxiety disorders. It suggests that blocking NMDA receptors in the amygdala during learning should impair short- and long-term fear memory. It has been demonstrated in rodents that NMDA antagonists such as D,L-2-amino-5-phosphonovaleric acid (AP5) can block fear acquisition (Rodrigues et al., 2001; Goosens and Maren, 2004; Matus-Amat et al., 2007), whereas some studies have shown that expression is blocked as well (Maren et al., 1996; Jasnow et al., 2004). Studies of NMDA receptor antagonists for anxiety in humans have been limited. Blockade of VGCCs appears to block long-term but not short-term memory (Bauer et al., 2002; Cain et al., 2002; McKinney and Murphy, 2006). This would suggest that clinically available calcium channel blockers such as verapamil and nimodipine may be helpful in diminishing the intensity and impact of recently acquired fear memory. There are, however, a limited number of studies of these agents for anxiety disorders (Balon and Ramesh, 1996). A more promising area is the investigation of agents such as gabapentin and pregabalin that act as alpha2delta ligands to calcium channels (Stahl, 2004). See Mula et al. (2007) for a recent comprehensive review of anticonvulsants in anxiety disorders.

Consolidation

The process of consolidation refers to the transfer of short-term memory into long-term memory (McGaugh, 2002). This process requires protein synthesis, which is thought to occur in the hippocampus each time a memory is retrieved (Rossato et al., 2007). After retrieval, memory traces are unstable and require another consolidation, known as reconsolidation, to become formed (see below). Protein synthesis inhibitors such as anisomycin have been used to block memory consolidation (Lin et al, 2003; Santini et al., 2004), by a proposed mechanism of regulating transcription of brain-derived neurotrophic factor (BDNF) (Ou and Gean, 2007). Anisomycin has been shown to have anxiolytic properties in an animal model of predator stress (Adamec, Strasser, et al., 2006), and to reduce PTSD symptoms in rats (Cohen et al., 2006).

Studies using inhibitory avoidance learning procedures have been used to support the view that the amygdala is not the sole site for fear learning but, in addition, can modulate the strength of memory storage in other brain structures (McGaugh and Roozendaal, 2002). Specific drugs and neurotransmitters infused into the basolateral amygdala (BLA) influence consolidation of memory for inhibitory avoidance training. Posttraining peripheral or intraamygdala infusions of drugs affecting γ-aminobutyric acid (GABA), opioid, glucocorticoid, and muscarinic acetylcholine receptors have dose- and time-dependent effects on memory consolidation (McGaugh, 2002). Norepinephrine (NE) infused directly into the BLA after inhibitory avoidance training enhances memory consolidation, indicating that the degree of activation of the noradrenergic system within the amygdala by an aversive experience may predict the extent of the long-term memory for the experience (McIntyre et al., 2002).

Interactions among corticotropin releasing hormone (CRH), cortisol, and NE have very important effects on memory consolidation, which is likely to be relevant to the effects of traumatic stress on memory. Extensive evidence indicates that glucocorticoids influence long-term memory consolidation via stimulation of glucocorticoid receptors (GR). The glucocorticoid effects on memory consolidation require activation of the BLA, and lesions of the BLA block retention enhancement of intrahippocampal infusions of a GR agonist. Additionally, the BLA is a critical locus of interaction between glucocorticoids and NE in modulating memory consolidation (McGaugh and Roozendaal, 2002; Roozendaal, Okuda, et al., 2006).

There is extensive evidence consistent with a role for CRH in mediating stress effects on memory consolidation. Activation of CRH receptors in the BLA by CRH released from the CEA facilitates stress effects on memory consolidation. Memory enhancement produced by CRH infusions in the hippocampus is blocked by propranolol, suggesting that CRH, through a presynaptic mechanism, stimulates NE release in the hippocampus (Roozendaal et al., 2002; Roozendaal, Hui, et al., 2006).

Excessive stress-induced release of CRH, cortisol, and NE are likely to lead to development of indelible traumatic memories and associated reexperiencing symptoms. Administration of CRH antagonists, GR antagonists, and β-adrenergic receptor antagonists may prevent these effects in vulnerable individuals. A preclinical trial with mice showed that corticosterone, a glucocorticoid, administered after contextual fear reactivation, can block memory recall (Cai et al., 2006). This effect on memory has been found in human investigations as well (de Quervain et al., 2000; de Quervain et al., 2003). A double-blind, placebo-controlled, crossover trial by de Quervain's group (Aerni et al., 2004) reported that 3-month treatment with low-dose cortisol resulted in a reduction in PTSD symptoms as rated by the Clinician Administered PTSD Scale (CAPS). More recently, cortisol or placebo was administered to patients with spider phobia and social phobia. In two separate trials, they found that cortisol reduced fear in response to a Trier Social Stress Test, and in individuals with spider phobia, to a photographic stimulus (Soravia et al., 2006). There is also some support for the use of glucocorticoids to prevent PTSD after trauma (de Quervain, 2008). In summary, these results support the concept that CRH, via an interaction with glucocorticoids, interacts with the noradrenergic system to consolidate traumatic memories. Drugs that target this pathway may provide novel therapeutics for anxiety disorders such as PTSD and phobia.

Reconsolidation

The process by which old, reactivated memories undergo another round of consolidation is called *reconsolidation* (Dębiec et al., 2002; Myers and Davis, 2002). The process of reconsolidation is relevant to vulnerability and resilience to the effects of extreme stress. It is the rule rather than the exception that memories are reactivated by cues associated with the original trauma. Repeated reactivation of these memories may serve to strengthen the memories and facilitate long-term consolidation (Przbyslawski et al., 1999; Sara, 2000). Each time a traumatic memory is retrieved, it is integrated into an ongoing perceptual and emotional experience and becomes part of a new memory. It is also worth noting that traumatic memories have been shown to mask a neutral one. For example, stimuli that are emotionally laden are more likely to cause amnesia to preceding words, when compared to neutral stimuli (Kern et al., 2005).

Moreover, recent preclinical studies indicate that consolidated memories for auditory fear conditioning, which are stored in the amygdala (Jin et al., 2007), hippocampal-dependent contextual fear memory (Fischer et al., 2004), and hippocampal-dependent memory associated with inhibitory avoidance (Milekic and Alberini, 2002) are sensitive to disruption upon reactivation, by administration with a protein synthesis inhibitor directly into the amygdala and hippocampus. The reconsolidation process, which has enormous clinical implications, results in a reactivated memory trace that returns to a state of lability and must undergo consolidation once more if it is to remain in long-term storage. Some controversies remain regarding the temporal persistence of systems reconsolidation. Dębiec and colleagues (2002) found that intrahippocampal infusions of anisomycin caused amnesia for a consolidated hippocampal-dependent memory if the memory was reactivated even up to 45 days after training. Milekic and Alberini (2002), however, found that the ability of an intrahippocampal infusion of anisomycin to produce amnesia for an inhibitory avoidance task was evident only when the memory was recent (up to 7 days). Duvarci and Nader (2004) showed that there was no recovery of the anisomycin-induced reconsolidation deficit over 24 days. Other studies have shown that after hippocampal injections of anisomycin, there are no immediate deficits, but in some cases amnesia was present at 48 hours (Power et al., 2006; Canal and Gold, 2007; Canal et al., 2007). Further work is needed in this area to clarify these findings, and their applicability to clinical treatment (Rudy et al., 2006).

The reconsolidation process involves NMDA receptors, β-adrenergic receptors, and requires cyclic adenosine monophosphate (cAMP) response-element binding protein (CREB) induction. The CREB requirement suggests that nuclear protein synthesis is necessary (Kida et al., 2002, Wagatsuma et al., 2006). This remarkable lability of a memory trace, which permits reorganization of an existing memory in a retrieval environment, provides a theoretical basis for psychotherapeutic and pharmatherapeutic intervention for traumatic stress exposure as well as other anxiety disorders. Preclinical studies have shown that NMDA receptor antagonists impair reconsolidation (Przbyslawski and Sara, 1997; J.L. Lee et al., 2006). There are also studies under way investigating the use of glucocorticoids to block reconsolidation of fear memories. Recently, it was shown that RU 28486 (mifepristone) impairs retrieval of traumatic memories during an inhibitory avoidance procedure using foot shock (Tronel and Alberini, 2007).

Propranolol, a beta-receptor antagonist, also act, to block reconsolidation but does not impair integration of new memories (Dębiec and Ledoux, 2004). It can exert these central effects because it crosses the blood-brain-barrier (BBB), in contrast to peripherally acting beta blockers (Van Stegeren et al., 1998). Propranolol has been shown to block reconsolidation of emotional stimuli in animal studies (Przybyslawski et al., 1999; Dębiec and Ledoux, 2004; Diergaarde et al., 2006), and impaired recall and retention of emotional memories in humans (Cahill et al., 1994; Van Stegeren et al., 1998; Strange et al., 2003; Hurlemann et al., 2005; Van Stegeren et al., 2005). Grillon et al. (2004) showed that in healthy volunteers receiving propranolol versus placebo, those on propranolol had a reduction contextual fear conditioning, but no effect on cue conditioning, as measured by skin conductance and subjective arousal levels. A study by Pitman's group, however, could not confirm this finding using skin conductance measures in patients with PTSD (Orr et al., 2006).

The implication of these preliminary findings is that administration of a beta-receptor antagonist shortly after trauma exposure or after reactivation of memory associated with the anxiety-inducing event may reduce the strength of the original memory. Indeed, there have been studies using these agents immediately after trauma and in patients with PTSD. Pitman et al. (2002) were the first to conduct a randomized, double-blind placebo-controlled trial of propranolol administered 6 hours after exposure to a trauma, for up to 10 days, to determine if it was effective in preventing PTSD. The results were not statistically significant due to a small sample size. A recently published trial studied adult men and women admitted to a trauma service, and in a randomized, double-blind fashion, administered within 48 hours either propranolol, gabapentin, or placebo for 14 days, and followed the patients over 8 months. In spite of a large number of eligible subjects (n=569), only a small number (n=48) enrolled in one of the three study arms, in large part due to patient refusal. Overall, the investigation failed to show that the medications differed from placebo. Other antiadrenergic agents have been studied as potential treatments for PTSD, by reducing NE. Two studies have reported that guanfacine, an α-2 agonist, was not effective in reducing symptoms (Davis et al., 2008). Conversely, prazosin, an α-1 antagonist that has been used off-label for treatment of nightmares in PTSD, was shown in replication to reduce nightmares (Raskind et al., 2003; Raskind et al., 2007) and to reduce daytime symptoms, as evidenced by attenuated distress from verbal trauma cues on an emotional Stroop paradigm (Taylor et al., 2006).

It is important to note that there have been ethical concerns raised about the use of these agents when their mechanism of action in reducing symptoms is not fully understood (Henry et al., 2007). Nonetheless, drugs like propranolol do not "erase" or "block" memories but instead merely attenuate their "overconsolidation" and excessive recall. Further research will hopefully help elucidate the importance of this work in the treatment and possible prevention of PTSD.

Extinction

The process of extinction occurs when the CS is presented repeatedly in the absence of the US, thereby reducing the conditioned fear response (for example, the dog in Pavlov's experiments stops salivating after several trials of hearing the bell but seeing no food). Extinction represents a new form of learning and is not simply an erasing of old memories (Quirk, 2002). It forms the rational for exposure-based psychotherapies for the treatment of anxiety disorders characterized by exaggerated fear responses. Individuals who have the ability to quickly attenuate learned fear through a powerful and efficient extinction process are likely to function more effectively under dangerous conditions.

Extinction is characterized by many of the same neural mechanisms that occur in fear acquisition. The pathway begins with a reduction in neuronal firing in the LA in response to the fear stimulus. The lateral amygdala then interacts with the CEA and basal nuclei, either directly or through intercalated cell masses (ICM) (Sotres-Bayon et al., 2006). The hippocampus modulates contextual fear processing. It is important to note the integral role of the medial prefrontal cortex (mPFC) in regulating fear extinction by inhibition of the amygdala. It has been shown that the consolidation of extinction most likely involves potentiation of inputs into the mPFC by means of NMDA-dependent plasticity (Burgos-Robles et al., 2007). The BLA sends direct excitatory inputs to the mPFC, and NMDA antagonists infused into the BLA blocks extinction (Feltenstein and See, 2007; Yang et al., 2007). The ability of the mPFC to modulate fear behaviors is probably related to projections from the mPFC via GABA interneurons to the BLA (Royer et al., 2000). Infralimbic neurons, which are part of the mPFC, fire only when rats are recalling extinction; greater firing correlates with reduced fear behaviors (Milad and Quirk, 2002). Some studies have shown that lesions in the mPFC, in particular the infralimbic nucleus (M.A. Morgan et al., 1993; Quirk et al., 2000; Milad and Quirk, 2002), or injection with protein synthesis inhibitors (Santini et al., 2004), block extinction, indicating that the mPFC might store long-term extinction memory. There have, however, been inconsistent findings in other studies (Farinelli et al., 2006; Garcia et al., 2006). More research is needed to clarify the exact mechanism of interaction of the mPFC with other structures in the fear loop (Myers and Davis, 2007).

Failure to achieve an adequate level of activation of the mPFC after extinction might lead to persistent fear responses (Herry and Garcia, 2002). Animal models have shown that acute or chronic stress adversely affect fear extinction in the mPFC (Miracle et al., 2006), by a mechanism of dendritic retraction (Cook and Wellman, 2004; Radley et al., 2004; Izquierdo et al., 2006). Individuals with the capacity to function well following states of high fear may have potent mPFC inhibition of amygdala responsiveness. In contrast, patients with PTSD exhibit depressed ventral mPFC activity that correlates with increased autonomic arousal after exposure to traumatic reminders (Bremner et al., 1999; Williams et al., 2006). Consistent with this hypothesis, it has been shown that patients with PTSD had increased amygdala activation during fear acquisition and decreased mPFC/anterior cingulate activity during extinction (Bremner et al., 2005; Williams et al., 2006).

Activation of amygdala NMDA receptors by glutamate (Glu) is essential to extinction (Myers and Davis, 2007), and L-type VGCCs also contribute to extinction plasticity (Cain et al., 2002; Cain et al., 2005). *N*-methyl-D-aspartate receptor antagonists have been shown to block extinction, whereas an NMDA receptor partial agonist, d-cycloserine (DCS), had the opposite effect (J.L. Lee et al., 2006; Tomilenko and Dubrovina, 2007). Preclinical studies found that DCS injected into the amygdala reduced fear startle and may facilitate the extinction process when DCS is given in combination with behavioral therapy in patients with anxiety disorders (Davis, 2002). There have been several human studies using DCS in anxiety disorders. In a pilot double-blind, placebo-controlled trial of patients with PTSD, DCS was not effective as a stand-alone treatment (Heresco-Levy et al., 2002). Studies have focused on the effect of DCS on enhancing response to exposure therapy. To date, it has been reported that augmentation of exposure therapy with DCS is effective in reducing fear in patients with acrophobia, a specific phobia (Ressler et al., 2004), and social phobia (Hofmann et al., 2006; Guastella et al., 2008), although it had no statistically significant effect in a study of spider phobia (Guastella et al., 2007). These preclinical and clinical investigations suggest that clinical research paradigms capable of evaluating the mechanisms of fear conditioning in clinical populations would be of great value. As these mechanisms become better understood, potential therapeutic interventions will emerge as well.

THE NEUROCHEMICAL BASIS OF FEAR AND ANXIETY

Specific neurotransmitters and neuropeptides act on brain areas noted above in the mediation of fear and anxiety responses. These neurochemicals are released during stress, and chronic stress results in long-term alterations in the function of these systems. Stress axis neurochemical systems prepare the organism for threat in multiple ways: through increased attention and vigilance, modulation of memory (to maximize the use of prior experience), planning, and preparation for action. In addition, these systems have peripheral effects, which include increased heart rate and blood pressure (catecholamines) and rapid modulation of the body's use of energy (cortisol). The neurobiological responses to threat and severe stress are clearly adaptive and have survival value, but they also can have maladaptive consequences when they become chronically activated. Examination of the preclinical data concerning neurochemical substrates of the stress response, the long-term impact of early life exposure to stress, and possible stress-induced neurotoxicity provides a context to consider clinical investigations of the pathophysiology of the anxiety disorders.

Noradrenergic System

Stressful stimuli of many types produce marked increases in brain noradrenergic function. Stress produces regional selective increases in NE turnover in the locus coeruleus (LC), limbic regions (hypothalamus, hippocampus, and amygdala), and cerebral cortex. These changes can be elicited with immobilization stress, foot shock stress, tail-pinch stress, and conditioned fear. Exposure to stressors from which the animal cannot escape results in behavioral deficits termed *learned helplessness*. The learned helplessness state is associated with depletion of NE, probably reflecting the point at which synthesis cannot keep up with demand. These studies have been reviewed elsewhere in detail (Bremner et al., 1996a, 1996b).

Neurons in the LC are activated in association with fear and anxiety states (Abercrombie and Jacobs, 1987; Redmond, 1987), and the limbic and cortical regions innervated by the LC are involved in the elaboration of adaptive responses to stress (Foote et al., 1983; Morilak et al., 2005). Most types of sensory stimuli result in a brief activation of NE neurons, whereas a wide array of stressful stimuli, such as electric shock, immobilization, loud noise, or forced swim, result in a more robust, prolonged activation. Norepinephrine has been shown to specifically modulate the behavioral component of the stress response in animals, and anxiety-like behaviors are increased by drugs that potentiate NE transmission (Charney et al., 1987a). Locus coeruleus NE neurons in freely moving cats were activated twofold to threefold by confrontation with either a dog or an aggressive cat, although exposure to other novel stimuli (such as a nonaggressive cat) did not increase the firing rate (Levine et al., 1990). Although the integrity of NE neurons is necessary for certain types of fear-related behaviors, normal patterns of non-fear-related ambulatory activity are not necessarily disrupted by chemical lesions of the NE system in rats (Murrough et al., 2000).

A series of investigations have shown that certain stressors elicit increased responsiveness of LC neurons to excitatory stimulation, which is in part mediated by α-2 adrenoreceptors (AR). α-2-ARs are a heterogeneous group of inhibitory G protein–coupled receptors in the central nervous system (CNS) that are found as autoreceptors on the somas of NE-containing neurons and serve an important role in providing negative feedback and containment of the NE response. Antagonism of α-2-ARs with idazoxan or yohimbine increases the response of LC neurons to excitatory stimuli without altering their baseline firing rate (Simson and Weiss, 1988). Acute cold restraint stress results in decreased density of α-2-ARs in the hippocampus and amygdala (Torda et al., 1984). Further, in chronically cold-stressed rats, the release of NE produced by yohimbine (Nisenbaum and Abercrombie, 1993) or repeated stress (Nisenbaum et al., 1991) in the hippocampus is enhanced. It has been hypothesized that a functional blockade of α-2-ARs is a consequence of NE depletion with inescapable stress, resulting in enhancement of LC neurons responsiveness to stimuli (Simson and Weiss, 1988). In addition, α-2-AR knockout mice exhibit increases in autonomic activity and anxiety-related behaviors (Lähdesmäki et al., 2002), enhanced startle response and deficiencies in prepulse inhibition (Sallinen et al., 1998; Lähdesmäki et al., 2004), and enhanced physiological and behavioral alterations resulting from administration of D-amphetamine (Lähdesmäki et al., 2004).

An important recent study in healthy humans demonstrated the effects of an α-2C-AR polymorphism on NE activity at rest and in response to a yohimbine challenge (Neumeister et al., 2005). The α-2C-Del322-325 polymorphism is an in-frame deletion of homologous repeats at codons 322–325 of the α-2C-AR subtype and has been associated with impaired feedback and enhanced NE release in animals. African American carriers of the α-2C-Del322-325 polymorphisms have an elevated risk of congestive heart failure, perhaps due to chronic higher levels of circulating peripheral NE. The study by Neumeister and colleagues (2005) found that individuals homozygous for the α-2C-Del322-325 polymorphism had higher levels of NE at rest and more sustained increases in NE, heart rate, and anxiety in response to a yohimbine challenge compared to noncarriers of the polymorphism. A second study of the polymorphism in patients with remitted major depressive disorder (MDD) demonstrated differential recruitment of cortical and limbic brain regions in carriers, suggesting a direct impact of the α-2C-Del322-325 polymorphism on brain function relevant to emotional processing (Neumeister et al., 2006).

There is strong evidence that the brain noradrenergic system is involved in mediating fear conditioning (Rasmussen et al., 1986; Charney and Deutch, 1996). Neutral stimuli paired with shock (CS) produce increases in brain NE metabolism and behavioral deficits similar to those elicited by the shock alone (Cassens et al., 1981), as well as increased firing of cells in the LC (Rasmussen et al., 1986). An intact noradrenergic system appears to be necessary for the acquisition of fear-conditioned responses (Cose and Robbins, 1987), and NE activation in the amygdala was recently demonstrated to be necessary for glucocorticoid-mediated enhancement of memory (Roozendaal, Okuda, et al., 2006).

Chronic symptoms experienced by patients with an anxiety disorder, such as panic attacks, insomnia, startle, and autonomic hyperarousal, are characteristic of increased noradrenergic function (Charney et al., 1984; Charney et al., 1987a). Potential drugs of abuse, such as alcohol, opiates, and benzodiazepines (but not cocaine), decrease firing of noradrenergic neurons. Increases in the abuse of these substances parallel increased anxiety symptoms, providing evidence for self-medication of these symptoms that is explainable based on animal studies of noradrenergic function. In addition, patients with anxiety disorders frequently report significant improvement of symptoms of hyperarousal and intrusive memories with alcohol, benzodiazepines, and opiates, which decreases LC firing, but worsening of these symptoms with cocaine, which increases LC firing.

Many patients with anxiety disorders demonstrate an increased susceptibility to psychosocial stress. Behavioral sensitization may account for these clinical phenomena. In the laboratory model of sensitization, single or repeated exposure to physical stimuli or pharmacological agents sensitizes an animal to subsequent stressors (reviewed in Charney et al., 1993). For example, in animals with a history of prior stress, there is a potentiated release of NE in the hippocampus with subsequent exposure to stressors (Nisenbaum et al., 1991). Similar findings were observed in mPFC (Finlay and Abercrombie, 1991). The hypothesis that sensitization is the underlying neural mechanism contributing to the course of anxiety disorders is supported by clinical studies demonstrating that repeated exposure to traumatic stress is an important risk factor for the development of anxiety disorders, particularly PTSD (Table 41.1).

There is compelling evidence that NE plays a role in the pathophysiology of PTSD. Well-designed psychophysiological studies have documented heightened autonomic or sympathetic nervous system arousal in combat veterans with chronic PTSD (Prins et al., 1995). Because central noradrenergic and peripheral sympathetic systems function in concert (Aston-Jones et al., 1991), the data from these psychophysiological investigations are consistent with the hypothesis that noradrenergic hyperreactivity in patients with PTSD may be associated with the conditioned or sensitized responses to specific traumatic stimuli.

TABLE 41.1 *Neural Mechanisms Related to Pathophysiology and Treatment of Anxiety Disorders*

Mechanism	*Neurochemical Systems*	*Brain Regions*	*Pathophysiology*	*Treatment Development*
Pavlovian (cue-specific) fear conditioning	Glutamate, NMDA receptors, VGCCs	Medial prefrontal cortex, cingulate, dorsal thalamus, lateral amygdala, central nucleus of amygdala	May account for common clinical observation in panic disorder and PTSD that sensory and cognitive stimuli associated with or resembling the frightening experience elicit panic attacks, flashbacks, and autonomic symptoms	Treatment with NMDA receptor antagonist and VGCC antagonist may attenuate acquisition of fear
Inhibitory avoidance (contextual fear)	Norepinephrine/β-adrenergic receptor, cortisol/glucocorticoid receptor, CRH, GABA, opioids, acetylcholine	Medial prefrontal cortex, basolateral amygdala, hippocampus, BNST, entorhinal cortex	Excessive stress-mediated release of CRH, cortisol, development of indelible fear memories. Chronic anxiety and phobic symptoms may result from excessive contextual fear conditioning	CRH antagonists and β-adrenergic receptor agonists and NE may have preventive effects
Reconsolidation	Glutamate, NMDA receptors, norepinephrine, β-adrenergic receptors, CREB	Amygdala, hippocampus	Repeated reactivation and reconsolidation may further strengthen the memory trace and lead to persistence of trauma and phobia-related symptoms	Treatment with NMDA receptor and β-adrenergic receptor antagonists after memory reactivation may reduce the strength of the original anxiety-provoking memory
Extinction	Glutamate, NMDA receptors, VGCCs, NE, DA, GABA	Medial prefrontal sensory cortex, amygdala	Failure in neural mechanisms of extinction may relate to persistent traumatic memories, reexperiencing symptoms, autonomic hyperarousal, and phobic behaviors	Psychotherapies need to be developed that facilitate extinction through the use of conditioned inhibitors and the learning of new memories. The combination of extinction-based psychotherapy and D-cycloserine may be a particularly effective treatment.
Sensitization	Dopaminergic, noradrenergic NMDA receptors	Nucleus accumbens, amygdala, striatum, hypothalamus	May explain the adverse effects of early-life trauma on subsequent responses to stressful life events. May play a role in the chronic course of evolution of the many anxiety disorders and, in some cases, the worsening of the illness over time	Suggests that the efficacy of treatment may vary according to the state of evolution of the disease process. Emphasizes the importance of early intervention.

BNST: bed nucleus of the stria terminalis; CREB: cyclic adenosine monophosphate response element binding protein; CRH: corticotropin releasing hormone; GABA: γ-aminobutyric acid; NE: norepinephrine; NMDA: *N*-methyl-D-aspartate; PAG: periaqueductal gray; VGCC: voltage gated calcium channels; PTSD: posttraumatic stress disorder; DA: dopamine.

Evaluation of plasma and urinary NE concentrations have generally, but not entirely, supported the idea of exaggerated NE activity in patients with PTSD. Yehuda and colleagues found elevated plasma NE levels in combat veterans with PTSD compared to patients with MDD (Yehuda et al., 1998), and elevated 24-hour urinary NE and epinephrine among a group of inpatients with PTSD compared to healthy controls (Yehuda et al., 1992). Plasma levels of NE were found to be elevated throughout a 24-hour collection period in another study (Yehuda et al., 1995), as were cerebrospinal fluid (CSF) levels of NE in patients with PTSD (D.G. Baker et al., 1997). Exposure to traumatic reminders in the form of combat films results in increased epinephrine (McFall et al., 1992) and NE (Blanchard et al., 1991) release. However, some studies have demonstrated no difference in plasma NE levels between patients with PTSD and healthy controls (Southwick et al., 1993), or in urinary 24-hour concentrations (Mellman et al., 1995). Women with PTSD secondary to childhood sexual abuse did have significantly elevated levels of NE, epinephrine, and cortisol in 24-hour urine samples (Lemieux and Coe, 1995), and girls who were sexually abused excreted significantly greater amounts of catecholamine metabolites, metanephrine, vanillylmandelic acid, and homovanillic acid than girls who were not sexually abused (DeBellis et al., 1994).

A more recent investigation of CSF NE in patients with PTSD found a positive association between severity of PTSD symptoms and CSF NE level (Geracioti et al., 2001). A second study by this group found that CSF NE levels correlated with mean systolic blood pressure in healthy controls but not in patients with PTSD, further suggesting an uncoupling of central and peripheral NE function in patients with PTSD (Strawn et al., 2004).

Studies of peripheral NE function have demonstrated alterations in α-2-AR function and the cAMP signal transduction system in patients with PTSD. Decreases in platelet α-2-AR number (Perry et al., 1987), platelet basal adenosine, isoproterenol, forskolin-stimulated cAMP signal transduction (Lerer et al., 1987), and basal platelet monoamine oxidase (MAO) activity (Davidson et al., 1985) have been found in PTSD. These findings may reflect chronic high levels of NE release that would lead to compensatory receptor down-regulation and decreased responsiveness. Patients with combat-related PTSD compared to healthy controls had enhanced behavioral, biochemical, and cardiovascular responses to the α-2-AR antagonist yohimbine, which stimulates central NE release (Southwick et al., 1993; Southwick et al., 1997). Moreover, a positron emission tomography (PET) study demonstrated that patients with PTSD have a cerebral metabolic response to yohimbine consistent with increased NE release (Bremner, Innis, et al., 1997).

There is considerable evidence that abnormal regulation of brain noradrenergic systems is also involved in the pathophysiology of panic disorder. Patients with panic disorder are very sensitive to the anxiogenic effects of yohimbine in addition to having exaggerated plasma 3-methoxy-4 hydroxyphenylethylene glycol (MHPG), cortisol, and cardiovascular responses (Charney et al., 1984; Charney et al., 1987a; Gurguis and Uhde, 1990; Albus et al., 1992; Charney et al., 1992; Yeragani et al., 1992). Children with a variety of anxiety disorders exhibit greater anxiogenic responses to yohimbine than normal comparison children (Sallee et al., 2000). The responses to the α-2-AR agonist clonidine are also abnormal in patients with panic disorder. Clonidine administration caused greater hypotension, greater decreases in plasma MHPG, and less sedation in patients with panic than in controls (Uhde et al., 1988; Nutt, 1989; Coplan, Papp, et al., 1995; Coplan, Pine, et al., 1995; Marshall et al., 2002).

Few studies have examined noradrenergic function in patients with phobic disorders. In patients with specific phobias, increases in subjective anxiety and increased heart rate, blood pressure, plasma NE, and epinephrine have been associated with exposure to the phobic stimulus (Nesse et al., 1985). This finding may be of interest from the standpoint of the model of conditioned fear, reviewed above, in which a potentiated release of NE occurs in response to a reexposure to the original stressful stimulus. Patients with social phobia have been found to have greater increases in plasma NE than healthy controls and patients with panic disorder (Stein et al., 1992). In contrast to patients with panic disorder, the density of lymphocyte α-2-AR is normal in patients with social phobia (Stein et al., 1993). The growth hormone response to intravenous clonidine (a marker of central α2-receptor function) is blunted in patients with social phobia (Tancer et al., 1990) (Table 41.2).

Hypothalamic-Pituitary-Adrenal (HPA) Axis

There is consistent evidence that many forms of psychological stress increase the synthesis and release of cortisol. Cortisol serves to mobilize and replenish energy stores and contributes to increased arousal, vigilance, focused attention, and memory formation, as well as inhibition of the growth and reproductive systems and containment of the immune response. Cortisol has important regulatory effects on brain regions important for fear and anxiety including the hippocampus, amygdala, and PFC. Glucocorticoids can enhance amygdala activity, increase CRH messenger ribonucleic acid (mRNA) concentrations in the CEA (Makino et al., 1994, 1995; Shepard et al., 2000), increase the effects of CRH on conditioned fear, and facilitate the encoding of emotion-related memory (Roozendaal, 2000).

TABLE 41.2 *Evidence for Altered Catecholaminergic Function in Anxiety Disorders*

	PTSD	*Panic Disorder*
Increased resting heart rate and blood pressure at rest	+/–	+/–
Increased heart rate and blood pressure response to traumatic reminders/panic attacks	+++	++
Increased resting urinary NE and E	+	+/–
Increased resting plasma NE or MHPG	++	–
Increased plasma NE with traumatic reminders/panic attacks	+	+/–
Decreased binding to platelet α_2 receptors	+	+/–
Decrease in basal and stimulated activity of cAMP	+/–	–
Decrease in platelet MAO activity	–	NS
Increased symptoms, heart rate, and plasma MHPG with yohimbine noradrenergic challenge	++	+++
Differential brain metabolic response to yohimbine	+	+

–, one or more studies did not support this finding (with no positive studies) or the majority of studies do not support this finding; +/–, an equal number of studies do and do not support this finding; +, at least one study supports this finding and no studies do not support the finding or the majority of studies support the finding; ++, two or more studies support this finding and no studies do not support the finding; +++, three or more studies support this finding, and no studies do not support the finding.

PTSD: posttraumatic stress disorder; NE: norepinephrine; E: epinephrine; MHPG: 3-methosy-4-hydroxyphenylglycol; cAMP: cyclic adenosine 39,59-monophosphate; MAO: monoamine oxidase; NS: not studied.

Interestingly, this glucocorticoid enhancement of emotional memory has recently been shown to be dependent on arousal-induced endogenous activation of NE in the amygdala (Roozendal, Hui, et al., 2006; Roozendal, Okuda, et al., 2006). Adrenal steroids such as cortisol have biphasic effects on hippocampal excitability and cognitive function and memory (Diamond et al., 1996). These effects contribute to adaptive alterations in behaviors induced by cortisol during the acute response to stress.

It is key, however, that the stress-induced increases in cortisol ultimately be constrained through an elaborate negative feedback system involving GR and mineralocorticoid receptors (MR). The hippocampus has a very high concentration of corticosteroid receptors and plays an important role in GR-mediated negative feedback of the HPA axis. Excessive, sustained cortisol secretion can have serious adverse effects on the body including hypertension, osteoporosis, immunosuppression, insulin resistance, dyslipidemia, dyscoagulation, and, ultimately, atherosclerosis and cardiovascular disease (Karlamangla et al., 2002). In the brain, a sustained increase in glucocorticoid levels negatively affects multiple aspects of neural cell structure and function in the hippocampus, including impaired cell survival, altered metabolism, and changes in cell morphology, and adversely affects hippocampal-dependent cognitive and memory function (McEwen, 2000). Antidepressants have demonstrated the ability to decease the negative effects of stress-related glucocorticoid elevations on hippocampal structure and function, at least in part by promoting neurogenesis and/or reducing apoptosis (Malberg et al., 2000).

Alterations in the HPA axis and the hippocampus have been demonstrated in patients with PTSD. Studies of baseline peripheral cortisol levels using 24-hour measurement have yielded mixed results, although the preponderance of data suggest either normal or lower levels of cortisol, contrary to original expectations (Rasmusson et al., 2001; Yehuda, 2006). However, a recent study did demonstrate elevated CSF concentrations of cortisol in eight patients with PTSD, suggesting a dissociation between peripheral and CNS cortisol levels (D.G. Baker et al., 2005). Patients with chronic PTSD consistently demonstrate increased suppression of cortisol with low-dose dexamethasone, the opposite pattern to that of major depression. Using a cognitive challenge paradigm, Bremner and colleagues (2003) demonstrated increased cortisol levels during a prestress anticipatory anxiety period and in response to the stressor in patients with PTSD, although low baseline 24 hour cortisol during a resting period, compared to controls. Patients with PTSD may also have an increased number of GRs on peripheral lymphocytes. An increase in GR function in central brain structures such as the hypothalamus or hippocampus may result in enhanced suppression of cortisol feedback and therefore decreased peripheral cortisol levels (Yehuda, 2002, 2006). Overall, the character of the HPA axis in PTSD appears to be one of decreased peripheral cortisol and increased central feedback sensitivity, although the clinical significance of these findings remains to be determined. Consistent with preclinical evidence of stress- and glucocorticoid-mediated hippocampal impairments, several studies have now replicated the original finding of reduced hippocampal volume in patients with PTSD (Bremner, 2006). Please see Chapter 43 of this volume for a complete discussion of neuroanatomical and neuroimaging findings in PTSD.

Studies of HPA axis function in patients with panic disorder have been inconsistent, although an increased "central drive" is suggested. Blunted adrenocorticotropic hormone (ACTH) responses to CRH have been reported in some studies (Roy-Byrne, Uhde, Post, et al., 1986; Holsboer et al., 1987) but not in others (Rapaport et al., 1989). Normal and elevated rates of cortisol nonsuppression following dexamethasone (DEX) administration have been reported (Coryell and Noyes, 1988).

The responsiveness of the HPA system to a combined DEX-CRH challenge test was found to be higher in patients with panic disorder than in healthy controls but lower than in patients with depression (Roy-Byrne, Uhde, Post, et al., 1986; Rapaport et al., 1989). Urinary-free cortisol test results have been inconsistent (Kathol et al., 1988; Uhde et al., 1988). In a study of 24-hour secretion of ACTH and cortisol in panic disorder, only subtle abnormalities were seen. Patients had elevated overnight cortisol secretion and greater amplitude of ultraradian secretory episodes (Abelson and Curtis, 1996). Patients with more severe panic disorder symptoms may be more likely to have elevated cortisol secretion (Bandelow et al., 2000). Interestingly, a study of cognitive intervention in patients with panic disorder and healthy controls found that the intervention was able to significantly reduce the elevation of cortisol and ACTH by pentagastrin challenge, although it had no effect on panic symptoms (Abelson et al., 2005). In a recent review of their own data utilizing circadian and challenge paradigms, Abelson et al. (2007) argued that panic disorder is associated with HPA axis hypersensitivity to environmental contextual cues such as novelty, rather than baseline hyperactivity per se (Table 41.3).

Corticotropin Releasing Hormone

Corticotropin releasing hormone is one of the most important mediators of the stress response, coordinating the adaptive behavioral and physiological changes that occur during stress (Grammatopoulos and Chrousos, 2002). Mounting preclinical and clinic evidence implicates CRH dysregulation in human anxiety disorders and depression. Hypothalamic levels of CRH are increased by stress, resulting in activation of the HPA axis and increased release of cortisol and dehydroepiandrosterone (DHEA). Equally important are the extrahypothalamic effects of CRH. Neurons containing CRH are located throughout the brain, including the prefrontal and cingulate cortices, central nucleus of the amygdala, BNST, nucleus accumbens, periaqueductal gray (PAG), and brain-stem nuclei such as the major NE-containing nucleus, the LC, and the serotonin nuclei in the dorsal and median raphé (Steckler and Holsboer, 1999).

Increased activity of CRH-containing neurons in the amygdala is associated with fear-related behaviors, whereas cortical CRH may reduce reward expectation. In animals, CRH inhibits a variety of appetitive functions such as food intake, sexual activity, and endocrine programs for growth and reproduction, whereas administration of CRH antagonists increases appetitive and sexual behaviors. It appears that early-life stress can produce long-term elevation of brain CRH activity, and that the individual response to heightened CRH function may depend upon the social environment, past trauma history, and behavioral dominance (Brunson et al., 2001; Strome et al., 2002). Persistent elevation of hypothalamic and extrahypothalamic CRH contributes greatly to the psychobiological allostatic load.

CRH-1 and CRH-2 receptors are found in the pituitary gland and throughout the neocortex (especially in prefrontal, cingulate, striate, and insular cortices), amygdala, and hippocampal formation in the primate brain. The presence of CRH-1 (but not CRH-2) receptors within the LC, nucleus of the solitary tract, thalamus, and striatum, and the presence of CRH-2 (but not CRH-1) receptors in the choroid plexus, certain hypothalamic nuclei, the nucleus prepositus, and BNST suggest that each receptor subtype has distinct roles within the primate brain (Sanchez et al., 1999).

Mice deficient in CRH-1 display decreased anxiety-like behavior and an impaired stress response (Bale et al., 2002). In contrast, CRH-2-deficient mice display increased anxiety-like behavior and are hypersensitive to stress (Bale et al., 2000; Coste et al., 2000). Thus, evidence exists in favor of opposite functional roles for the two known CRH receptors; activation of CRH-1 receptors may be responsible for increased anxiety-like responses, and stimulation of CRH-2 receptors may produce anxiolytic-like responses. Regulation of the relative contributions of the two CRH receptor subtypes to brain CRH pathways may be essential to coordinating psychological and physiological responses to stressors (Bale et al., 2002). Thus far, it has not been possible

TABLE 41.3 *Evidence for Alterations in CRF-HPA Axis Function in Anxiety Disorders*

	PTSD	*Panic Disorder*
Alterations in urinary cortisol	+/–[a]	+/–
Altered plasma cortisol with 24-hour sampling	++ (dec.)	+ (inc.)
Supersuppression with DST	+++	NS
Blunted ACTH response to CRF	+/–	+/–
Elevated CRF in CSF	++	–
Increased lymphocyte glucocorticoid receptors	++	NS

–, one or more studies did not support this finding (with no positive studies) or the majority of studies do not support this finding; +/–, an equal number of studies do and do not support this finding; +, at least one study supports this finding and no studies do not support the finding or the majority of studies support the finding; ++, two or more studies support this finding and no studies do not support the finding; +++, three or more studies support this finding, and no studies do not support the finding.

[a]Findings of decreased urinary cortisol in older male combat veterans and Holocaust survivors and increased cortisol in younger female abuse survivors may be explainable by differences in gender, age, trauma type, or developmental epoch at the time of the trauma.

ACTH: adrenocorticotropic hormone; CRF: corticotropin releasing factor; CSF: cerebrospinal fluid; dec.: decrease; DST: dihydrostreptomycin; HPA: hypothalamic-pituitary-adrenal axis; inc.: increase; NS: not studied; PTSD: posttraumatic stress disorder.

to evaluate CRH-1 and CRH-2 receptors in living humans, although efforts are ongoing to develop CRH receptor PET ligands. Given the evidence for anxiogenic effects of CRH-1 receptor stimulation, the development of CRH-1 antagonists constitutes a promising future pharmacotherapy for anxiety disorders, and clinical investigations in humans are currently under way for PTSD, as well as major depression (Risbrough and Stein, 2006; Valdez, 2006).

Most studies of the CRH system in humans have focused on major depression and suggest excessive CRH activity. Available evidence also points to increased CRH activity in PTSD. It was recently reported that patients with PTSD had higher plasma CRH levels compared to traumatized veterans without PTSD and healthy volunteers (de Kloet, Vermetten, Geuze, Lentjes et al., 2008). Bremner, Licinio, and colleagues (1997) found increased levels of CRH in the CSF in patients with combat-related chronic PTSD based upon a single lumbar puncture determination. D.G. Baker and associates (1997) found elevations of CSF CRH throughout a 24-hour period. These findings are important to consider in the context of preclinical studies demonstrating that basal CSF CRH is elevated in primates that have experienced early life stress (Coplan et al., 1996); that the effects of CRH on behavior occur in a context-dependent manner (Strome et al., 2002); and that early-life exposure of the hippocampus to elevated levels of CRH is associated with hippocampal damage later in life (Brunson et al., 2001). Intracerebroventricular injection of CRH produces an increase in hippocampal MR levels, suggesting that CRH is an important regulator of HPA axis regulation. A single nucleotide polymorphism (SNP) in the CRH gene has recently been associated with behavioral inhibition, a childhood trait that predicts adult anxiety, although the functional impact of the SNP on CRH has yet to be determined (Smoller et al., 2003; Smoller et al., 2005).

The findings of elevated CRH in PTSD may be related to the clinical observation that early-life stress increases the risk of developing PTSD following traumatic stress exposure later in life. Whether elevated CRH is a trait vulnerability for the development PTSD, or is a state-dependent marker of PTSD, is an important question that has yet to be resolved. Elevated CRH in the hippocampus may relate to the mechanism responsible for reduced hippocampal volume observed in PTSD. Finally, the ability of CRH to increase MR density may provide an explanation for the elevated CRH and normal-to-low cortisol levels found in some patients with PTSD (Table 41.3).

Neurosteroids

Certain steroids are considered neuroactive steroids, or neurosteroids, by their influence on neuronal function. This occurs by their binding to intracellular receptors, which may act as transcription factors in the regulation of gene expression (Rupprecht, 2003). Several neurosteroids, particularly 3α-reduced metabolites of progesterone and deoxycorticosterone, modulate ligand-gated channels via nongenomic mechanisms (Strömberg et al., 2006). They are positive modulators of GABA-A receptors through the central nucleus of the amygdala, in a process involving NMDA receptors (Wang et al., 2007). Thus, they have been shown to have anxiolytic effects in animal models (Vanover et al., 2000). They counteract the anxiogenic effects of CRH and reduce CRH gene expression (Rupprecht, 2003).

In challenge studies of patients with panic disorder, cholecystokinin-4 (CCK-4) and lactate-induced panic attacks are associated with a decrease in the metabolites 3α, 5α-tetrahydroprogesterone (THP) (allopregnanolone, ALLO), 3, 5β-THP (pregnanolone), and an increase in 3B, 5α-THP in patients with panic disorder, suggesting that a decrease in GABA tone that does not occur in healthy subjects (Ströhle et al., 2003; Zwanzger et al., 2004; Eser et al., 2005). Interestingly, Eser et al. (2005) did find an increase in 3α, 5α-tetrahydrodeoxycorticosterone (THDOC) after CCK-4-induced panic in healthy volunteers.

Progesterone has been shown to have anxiolytic effects in animal models, which was shown to be a result of the increase in ALLO (Bitran et al., 1993; Reddy et al., 2005). Studies of neurosteroid levels in patients with social phobia and GAD have been inconsistent, with some showing decreased pregnenolone plasma levels, but no significant change in other steroids such as ALLO (Semeniuk et al., 2001; Heydari and Le Mellédo, 2002), and others showing no difference between groups (Laufer et al., 2005). Rasmusson et al. (2006) found decreased CSF ALLO in premenopausal women with PTSD. Studies in panic disorder have found elevated progesterone levels in female patients with panic disorder during the mid-luteal and premenstrual phase, a finding suggesting that 3α-reduced neurosteroids may serve as a counterregulatory mechanism against spontaneous panic attacks (Brambilla et al., 2003). Consistent with the increase in progesterone during pregnancy, it has been shown in animal studies that anxiety behaviors decrease as well, an effect that is reversed by finasteride (de Brito Faturi et al., 2006; Mann, 2006). A study of pregnant women found an improvement in baseline anxiety scores in healthy subjects (Paoletti et al., 2006) and those with preexisting panic disorder (Hertzberg and Wahlbeck, 1999), correlated with increased levels of ALLO and THDOC.

Finally, neurosteroids may play a role in the antidepressant and anxiolytic mechanism of selective serotonin reuptake inhibitors (SSRIs). Animal models of induced stress have shown that agents such as fluoxetine increase brain ALLO or normalize decreased brain

ALLO, by a nonserotonergic mechanism (Pinna et al., 2006; Matsumoto et al., 2007). To date, the development of neurosteroids as potential treatment of anxiety disorders has been limited. The availability of synthetic analogues of 3α-reduced neuroactive steroids (for example, ganaxolone) can test the concept that such compounds might have anxiolytic efficacy (Eser at al., 2006).

Arginine Vasopressin

CRH and arginine vasopressin (AVP) are the major secretagogues of the HPA/stress system. However, AVP has been studied much less than CRH, and our knowledge of the functional activity and pharmacology of AVP and its receptors in the regulation of HPA activity rests largely on studies conducted in rodents. Arginine vasopressin has ACTH-releasing properties when administered alone in humans, a response that may be dependant on the ambient endogenous CRH level. Following the combination of AVP and CRH, a much greater ACTH response is seen, and both peptides are required for maximal pituitary-adrenal stimulation. The sensitivity of CRH and AVP transcription to glucocorticoid feedback apparently differs, and AVP-stimulated ACTH secretion may be refractory to glucocorticoid feedback (Tilbrook and Clarke, 2006). Vasopressinergic regulation of the HPA axis may therefore be critical for sustaining corticotrophic responsiveness in the presence of high-circulating glucocorticoid levels during chronic stress (Makara et al., 2004). S. Watson et al. (2006) found elevated AVP in subjects with bipolar and depression disorders after a DEX suppression test. In animals deficient for the CRH-1 receptor, selective compensatory activation of the hypothalamic AVP system occurs, which maintains basal ACTH secretion and HPA activity (Müller et al., 2000). Similar response patterns have been observed following chronic stress, leading to the hypothesis that CRH plays a predominantly permissive role in HPA regulation but that AVP represents the dynamic mediator of ACTH release (Aguilera and Rabadan-Diehl, 2000).

Arginine vasopressin is produced by the parvocellular neurons of the paraventricular nucleus and is secreted into the pituitary portal circulation from axon terminals projecting to the external zone of the median eminence (Engelman et al., 2004). It is primarily released following a variety of stimuli including increasing plasma osmolality, hypovolemia, hypotension, and hypoglycemia. In addition to its role in fluid metabolism regulation, AVP has been implicated in learning and memory processes, pain sensitivity, synchronization of biological rhythms, and the timing and quality of rapid eye movement sleep. Extrahypothalamic AVP-containing neurons have also been characterized in the rat, notably in the medial amygdala, that innervate limbic structures such as the lateral septum and the ventral hippocampus. In these latter structures, AVP was suggested to act as a neurotransmitter, exerting its action by binding to specific G protein–coupled receptors, that is, V1A and V1B, which are widely distributed in the CNS, including the septum, cortex, and hippocampus (Hernando et al., 2001). Studies have shown V1A receptor knockout mice to have reduced anxiety behaviors in tasks such as the elevated plus maze and forced swim, suggesting a significant role of AVP in social recognition (Bielsky et al., 2004; Egashira et al., 2007). In addition, overexpression of V1A caused increased anxiety behaviors (Bielsky et al., 2005). In recent years, AVP V1B antagonists, in particular SSR 149415, have exhibited significant anxioloytic and antidepressant effects in various classical animal models (Griebel et al., 2002; Salomé et al., 2006; Shimazaki et al., 2006; Hodgson et al., 2007). There is work under way to develop these agents as antidepressants and anxiolytics (Serradeil-Le Gal et al., 2005).

In the first reported AVP-related study conducted in patients with anxiety disorder (Maes et al., 1999), increased serum prolyl endopeptidase (an AVP-degradating enzyme) activity was found in PTSD, suggesting a lower AVP concentration in PTSD, leading to decreased HPA axis activity in this disorder. This finding is of particular interest given the discrepant findings of increased CSF CRH levels and normal-low cortisol reported for PTSD. Also, a recent study found elevated plasma AVP in male veterans with PTSD, compared to veterans without PTSD and healthy controls (de Kloet, Vermetten, Geuze, Wiegant et al., 2008). Therefore, AVP may play a pivotal role in PTSD. In a study using intransal AVP administration to healthy men and women (aged 17–24), Thompson and others (2006) reported that AVP, versus placebo, attenuated heart rate and skin conductance responses to angry faces. There was also a sex difference in regards to the effects of AVP versus placebo on social recognition, with men having greater agonistic facial muscle response and decreased perception of friendliness to unfamiliar male faces, whereas women had the opposite response when presented with unfamiliar female faces. Sex differences have been found in animal studies as well and were hypothesized to be related to testosterone (Toufexis et al., 2005). Additional studies of AVP function in other anxiety disorders are indicated.

Neuropeptide Y

Neuropeptide Y (NPY) is a highly conserved 36 amino acid peptide and is among the most abundant peptides found in the mammalian brain. To date, a total of seven NPY receptor subtypes (Y1–Y7) have been identified, with only Y1–Y5 being found in mammals. There are four brain areas in which neurons containing NPY are densely concentrated: the LC (Makino et al., 2000), paraventricular nucleus of the hypothalamus (R.A. Baker and Herkenham, 1995), septohippocampal neurons (Risold and Swanson, 1997), and nucleus of solitary tract and ventrolateral medulla (Pieribone et al., 1992). Moderate levels are found in the amygdala, hippocampus, cerebral cortex, basal ganglia, and the thalamus (Allen et al., 1983).

Evidence suggesting the involvement of the amygdala in the anxiolytic effects of NPY is robust and probably occurs via the NPY-Y1 receptor (Heilig et al., 1993; Heilig, 1995; Sajdyk, Vandergriff, et al., 1999). Microinjection of NPY into the central nucleus of the amygdala reduces anxious behaviors. The up-regulation of amygdala NPY mRNA levels following chronic stress suggests that NPY may be involved in the adaptive responses to stress exposure (Thorsell et al., 1999). Primeaux et al. (2005) showed in rats that NPY overexpression, accomplished by a Herpes virus vector, caused increased amygdalar NPY, and increased time in open arms of mazes, as compared to rats with reduced amygdalar NPY. Their study also showed that injection of an NPY-1 antagonist bilaterally into the amygdala had a reduction of time in the open maze (a sign of increased anxiety behavior), compared to rats receiving saline. Treatment of rats exposed to maternal separation with acupuncture increased NPY expression in the BLA reduced anxiety-like behaviors (Park et al., 2005). In addition, NPY may be involved in the consolidation of fear memories; injection of NPY into the amygdala impairs memory retention in a foot shock avoidance paradigm (Flood et al., 1989). It is thought that NPY exerts its anxiolytic effects via modulation of the glutamatergic system, as evidenced by changes in NPY mRNA after administration of Glu receptor agonists (Wierońska et al., 2005). The anxiolytic effects of NPY also involve the LC, possibly via the NPY-Y2 receptor. Also, NPY reduces the firing of LC neurons (Illes et al., 1993). Finally, NPY has behaviorally relevant effects on the hippocampus. Transgenic rats with hippocampal NPY overexpression have attenuated sensitivity to the behavioral consequences of stress and impaired spatial learning (Thorsell et al., 2000). Intrahippocampal injection of NPY into rats had an anxiolytic effect via Glu receptor ligands, which was blocked by injection of Y1 and Y2 antagonists (Smiałowska et al., 2007).

There are important functional interactions between NPY and CRH (Heilig et al., 1994; Britton et al., 2000). Neuropeptide Y counteracts the anxiogenic effects of CRH, and a CRH antagonist blocks the anxiogenic effects of an NPY-Y1 antagonist (Kask et al., 1997). The antagonistic interaction has been shown to be related to bidirectional synaptic GABAergic transmission in the BNST (Kash and Winder, 2006). Thus, it has been suggested that the balance between NPY and CRH neurotransmission is important to the emotional responses to stress (Heilig et al., 1994). In general, brain regions that express CRH and CRH receptors also contain NPY and NPY receptors, and their functional effects are often opposite (Kask et al., 2002) especially at the level of the LC (Smagin et al., 1996; Kask et al., 1998a), amygdala (Sajdyk, Vandergriff, et al., 1999; Sheriff et al., 2001), and PAG (Kask et al., 1998b; Martins et al., 2001).

These data suggest an important role for the NPY system in the psychobiology of resilience and vulnerability to stress. Neuropeptide Y has counterregulatory effects on CRH and LC-NE systems at brain sites that are important in the expression of anxiety, fear, and depression. Preliminary studies in special operations soldiers under extreme training stress indicate that high NPY levels are associated with better performance (C.A. Morgan et al., 2000; C.A. Morgan et al., 2002). Patients with PTSD have been shown to have reduced plasma NPY levels and a blunted yohimbine-induced NPY increase (Rasmusson et al., 2000). A study comparing plasma NPY levels in combat veterans with PTSD, healthy combat veterans, and healthy noncombat veterans found that the combat veterans had lower plasma NPY, while there was no difference between the veterans with and without PTSD (C.A. Morgan et al., 2003). This suggests that trauma exposure itself, independent of the development of PTSD, has a role in regulating stress and peptide levels. Liberzon et al. (2007) reported a similar finding in opioid peptide receptors (see below). A recent study of patients recovered from PTSD showed that they had increased plasma NPY (Yehuda et al., 2006). Studies of NPY levels in other anxiety disorders are limited. Rasmusson et al. (1998) showed an increase in plasma NPY in subjects receiving the panicogen yohimbine, compared to saline placebo. One trial failed to show a difference in plasma NPY levels among patients with panic disorder, social phobia, and normal controls (Stein et al., 1996).

To date, there are no published studies of NPY for the treatment of anxiety disorders. Antoninjevic et al. (2000) administered NPY intravenously to healthy volunteers and found it to increase sleep, by a mechanism of HPA axis inhibition. It has been shown that NPY can be administered safely via an intranasal route and rapidly cross the BBB (Born et al., 2002). Intranasal NPY has been studied in healthy volunteers to evaluate its systemic effects (Lacroix et al., 1996; Hallschmid et al., 2003). Further investigations of this unique mode of administration are currently under way, with the hope to apply these findings to develop novel therapeutics for mood and anxiety disorders.

Galanin

Galanin is a peptide that, in humans, contains 30 amino acids. It has been demonstrated to be involved in a number of physiological and behavioral functions including learning and cognition, pain control, food intake, neuroendocrine control, cardiovascular regulation, and, more recently, depression, and anxiety (Karlsson and Holmes, 2006).

Approximately 80% of noradrenergic cells in the LC coexpress galanin. A dense galanin immunoreactive fiber system originating in the LC innervates forebrain and midbrain structures including the hippocampus, hypothalamus, amygdala, and PFC (Gentleman et al., 1989; P.V. Holmes and Crawley, 1995; Perez et al., 2001; Hawes and Picciotto, 2004). Neurophysiological studies have shown that galanin reduces the firing rate of the LC, possibly by stimulating the galanin-1 receptor (Gal-R1) (Sevcik et al., 1993; Xu et al., 2001; Hawes et al., 2005).The mechanism by which galanin reduces NE release at LC projections to the amygdala, hypothalamus, and PFC may be via a direct action of galanin on these brain regions via galanin-synthesizing neurons or by stimulating galanin receptors in these regions (Khoshbouei, Cecchi, Dove, et al., 2002; Xu et al., 2001). Of the three known galanin receptor subtypes (Gal-R1, Gal-R2, Gal-R3), Gal-1 has also been shown to play a role in fear processes, Gal-R1 receptor mRNA levels are high in the amygdala, hypothalamus, and BNST (Gustafson et al., 1996), and Gal-R1-deficient mice show increased anxiety-like behavior (A. Holmes, Kinney, et al., 2003). Gottsch and others (2005) reported that Gal-R2 receptor knockout mice were found to have no behavioral or physiological changes in response to contextual fear conditioning or stress-induced hypothermia, whereas K.R. Bailey et al. (2007) found anxiogenic-like phenotype to the elevated-plus maze (EPM) task only.

Galanin-overexpressing transgenic mice do not exhibit an anxiety-like phenotype when tested under baseline (nonchallenged) conditions. However, these mice are unresponsive to the anxiogenic effects of the α-2 receptor antagonist, yohimbine (A. Holmes, Yang, and Crawley, 2002). Consistent with this observation, galanin administered directly into the CEA blocks the anxiogenic effects of stress, which is associated with increased NE release in the CEA. Yohimbine increases galanin release in the CEA (Khoshbouei, Cecchi, Dove, et al., 2002; Barrera et al., 2006). Galanin administration and galanin overexpression in the hippocampus result in deficits in fear conditioning (Kinney et al., 2002).

Studies in rats have shown that galanin administered centrally modulates anxiety-related behaviors, exhibiting effects that were either anxiolytic (Bing et al., 1993; Karlsson et al., 2005) or anxiogenic (Moller et al., 1999; Khoshbouei, Cecchi, and Morilak, 2002). Recently, Rajarao and others (2007) reported that galnon, a galanin receptor agonist, had anxiolytic-like properties that were reversible when M35, a galanin receptor antagonist, was injected. A similar finding was reported on a Forced Swim Test with rats, suggesting an antidepressant effect of galanin as well (Kuteeva et al., 2007). It should be noted, however, that Gal-R3 antagonists, SNAP 37889 and SNAP 398299, were found to have anxiolytic and antidepressant properties in several animal models, such as forced swim and stress-induced hyperthermia (Swanson et al., 2005). This study suggests that the galanin exerts this effect by demonstrating a diminishing of inhibition of 5-HT receptors in the hippocampus.

The study of galanin function in persons with psychiatric illness has been limited. A study of postmenopausal women compared to women of normal menstruation reported lower serum galanin levels in postmenopausal women with climacteric symptoms and ratings of subjective nervousness (Słopieć et al., 2004). To date, there is only one known study of galanin in anxiety disorders. Unschuld et al. (2008) conducted a genetic study of men and women with panic disorder, investigating six SNPs of the galanin gene. They reported a statistically significant association between severity of symptoms and two haplotypes, but only in the female patients. This finding, taken with the preclinical studies, should provide the impetus for the use of galanin receptor agonists as novel targets for antianxiety drug development (Karlsson and Holmes, 2006).

Dopaminergic System

In animals, acute stress influences dopamine (DA) release and metabolism in a number of specific brain areas important in affective behavior, including the basolateral nucleus of the amygdala, the nucleus accumbens and the mPFC. Dopamine innervation of the mPFC appears to be particularly vulnerable to stress; low-intensity stress (such as that associated with conditioned fear) or brief exposure to stress increases DA release and metabolism in the PFC in the absence of overt changes in other mesotelencephalic DA regions. Low-intensity electric foot shock increases in vivo tyrosine hydroxylase and DA turnover in the mPFC, but not in the nucleus accumbens or striatum. Stress can enhance DA release and metabolism in other areas receiving DA innervation, provided that greater-intensity or longer-duration stress is used. Thus, mPFC DA innervation is preferentially activated by stress compared to mesolimbic and nigrostriatal systems, and the mesolimbic DA innervation appears to be more sensitive to stress than the striatal DA innervation (Deutch and Young, 1995).

Uncontrollable stress activates mPFC DA release (Ventura et al., 2002) and inhibits nucleus accumbens DA release (Cabib and Puglisi-Allegra, 1996; Cabib et al., 2002), which may reflect reciprocal interactions between cortical and subcortical DA targets. Lesions of the amygdala before and after training in a CS model block stress-induced mPFC DA metabolic activation, suggesting amygdala control of stress-induced DA activation and a role for integrating the behavioral and neuroendocrine components of the stress response (Goldstein et al., 1996). There is preclinical evidence that the susceptibility of the mesocortical DA system to stress activation may be in part genetically determined. It has been suggested that excessive mesocortical DA release by stressful events may represent a vulnerability to depression and favor helpless reactions through an inhibition of subcortical DA transmission (Cabib et al., 2002; Ventura et al., 2002). These observations may be due to the effect of DA on reward mechanisms.

On the other hand, lesions of mPFC DA neurons delay extinction of the conditioned fear stress response (no effect on acquisition), indicating that prefrontal DA neurons are involved in facilitating extinction of the fear response. This suggests that reduced prefrontal cortical DA results in the preservation of fear produced by a conditioned stressor, a situation hypothesized to occur in PTSD (Morrow et al., 1999). One way to reconcile these two sets of data is to suggest that there is an optimal range for stress-induced increases in mPFC cortical DA release to facilitate adaptive behavioral responses. Too much mPFC cortical DA release produces cognitive impairment, and an inhibition in nucleus accumbens DA activity results in abnormalities in motivation and reward mechanisms. Insufficient prefrontal cortical DA release delays extinction of conditioned fear.

Several clinical investigations have reported increased urinary and plasma DA concentrations (Hamner and Diamond, 1993; Lemieux and Coe, 1995) in PTSD. Two candidate genes in the DA system that have been investigated to date in PTSD are the gene for the DA D2 receptor (*DRD2*) and the dopamine transporter gene (*DAT*) (Broekman et al., 2007). *DRD2* has been previously implicated in substance abuse, attention-deficit/hyperactivity disorder (ADHD), and Tourette's syndrome. Although an associated between the *DRD2* A1 allele and PTSD was initially reported (Comings et al., 1996), this was not replicated by a subsequent study (Gelernter et al., 1999). A later study found an association between the *DRD2* A1 allele and PTSD, but only in individuals with significant comorbid alcohol abuse (Young et al., 2002). The only study to date of the *DAT* gene in PTSD did find an association between the *DAT* SLC6A3 3'-variable number tandem repeat (VNTR) and DA reactivity in patients with PTSD. The clinical significance of this finding remains to be determined.

Roy-Byrne, Uhde, Post, et al. (1986) found a higher concentration of the DA metabolite homovanillic acid in plasma in patients with panic disorder with high levels of anxiety and frequent panic attacks. Patients with panic disorder were shown to have a greater growth hormone response to the DA agonist *apomorphine* than patients with depression (Pichot et al., 1992). However, Eriksson et al. (1991) found no alteration in CSF homovanillic acid levels in patients with panic disorder and no correlations with anxiety severity or panic attacks. Catechol-O-methyltransferase (COMT) catalyzes the degradation of DA and the Val158Met polymorphism demonstrated an association with phobic anxiety in a large group of healthy woman (McGrath et al., 2004). A recent meta-analysis of six case-control studies of COMT Val158Met in panic disorder found no overall association but did find a significant association of the 158Val allele in Caucasian populations, and on the other hand, a trend towards association of the 158Met allele in Asian populations (Domschke et al., 2007). There is preliminary evidence that a reduced density of the DA transporter and D_2 receptor density exists in patients with social anxiety disorders (Tiihonen et al., 1997; Schneier et al., 2000).

Serotonin

Different types of acute stress result in increased serotonin (5-HT) turnover in the PFC, nucleus accumbens, amygdala, and lateral hypothalamus (Kent et al., 2002; Briones-Aranda et al., 2005). Serotonin release may have anxiogenic and anxiolytic effects, depending upon the region of the forebrain involved and the receptor subtype activated. According to the hypothesis of Deakin and Graeff (1991), serotonin, released from the dorsal raphé nucleus, has a dual role in anxiety: acting via the amygdala and PFC to regulate defensive responses to threats and anticipatory anxiety (as seen in GAD); and, activating the dorsal periaqueductal gray (dPAG), thereby inhibiting defensive behaviors such as fight or flight (associated with panic disorder). For example, anxiogenic effects are mediated via the 5-HT_{2A} receptor, whereas stimulation of 5-HT_{1A} receptors is anxiolytic and may even relate to adaptive responses to aversive events (Charney and Drevets, 2002; Graeff, 2004).

Understanding the function of the 5-HT_{1A} receptor is probably most pertinent to the current review. The 5-HT_{1A} receptors are found in the superficial cortical layers, hippocampus, amygdala, and raphé nucleus (primarily presynaptic) (Hamon et al., 1990; Varnas et al., 2004). The behavioral phenotype of 5-HT_{1A} knockout mice includes increases in anxiety-like behaviors (Parks et al., 1998; Klemenhagen et al., 2006), whereas in mice overexpressing the 5-HT receptor these traits are reduced (Kusserow et al., 2004). These behaviors are mediated by postsynaptic 5-HT_{1A} receptors in the hippocampus, amygdala, and cortex (Gross et al., 2002; Mehta et al., 2007). Of great interest is the finding that embryonic and early postnatal shutdown of 5-HT_{1A} receptor expression produces an anxiety phenotype that cannot be rescued with restoration of 5-HT_{1A} receptors

(Gross et al., 2002). However, when 5-HT_{1A} receptor expression is reduced in adulthood and then reinstated, the anxiety phenotype is no longer present. These results suggest that altered function of 5-HT_{1A} receptors early in life can produce long-term abnormalities in the regulation of anxiety behaviors (Gross et al., 2002). This has been shown in animal studies using the stress model of maternal separation (Gartside et al., 2003; Vicentic et al., 2006).

There may also be important functional interactions between the 5-HT_{1A} and benzodiazepine receptors. In one study of 5-HT_{1A} knockout mice, down-regulation of benzodiazepine GABA α-1 and α-2 receptor subunits as well as benzodiazepine-resistant anxiety in the EPM was reported (Sibille et al., 2000; S.J. Bailey and Toth, 2004). However, a subsequent study did not replicate these results using mice with a different genetic background (Pattij et al., 2002), raising the possibility that genetic background can affect the functional interplay between 5-HT_{1A} and benzodiazepine systems (Bruening et al., 2006).

These results suggest a scenario in which early-life stress is postulated to increase CRH and cortisol levels, which in turn down-regulate 5-HT_{1A} receptors, resulting in lower threshold for anxiogenic stressful life events (van Riel et al., 2004). Alternatively, 5-HT_{1A} receptors may be decreased on a genetic basis. The density of 5-HT_{1A} receptors is reduced in patients with depression when they are depressed as well as in remission (Drevets et al., 1999; Bhagwagar et al., 2004; Moses-Kolko et al., 2007). Examination in patients with anxiety disorders, compared to healthy controls, have shown a reduction of 5-HT_{1A} receptor binding in certain brain regions such as the amygdala, anterior cingulate, and raphé nucleus, in patients with panic disorder (Neumeister et al., 2004) and social anxiety disorder (Lanzenberger et al., 2007). There was no change in 5-HT_{1A} receptor binding after exposure to stress in PTSD (Bonne et al., 2005).

Another important area of investigation has been the serotonin transporter (5-HTT) and its gene (*SCL6A4*). Polymorphisms of promoter region of *SCL6A4* (5-HTTLPR), with a short (s) and long (l) allele coded on chromosome 17q11.2, have been linked to mood and anxiety disorders (Hariri et al., 2005). In particular, carriers of one (ls, heterozygotes) or two (ss, homozygotes) of the s allele have been shown to have lower 5-HTT expression and decreased 5-HT reuptake (Lesch et al., 1996). Preclinical trials have reported greater anxiety-like behaviors in rodents with altered 5-HT transporters, either by 5-HTT knockout mutation (Holmes, Lit, et al., 2003; Adamec, Burton, et al., 2006), or blockade of 5-HTT with SSRIs (Ansorge et al., 2004). In humans, studies of healthy volunteers, with no psychiatric history, showed, using blood oxygen level dependent (BOLD) functional magnetic resonance imaging (fMRI), that carriers of the s allele had higher reactivity in the amygdala to fearful faces, without apparent gender differences (Hariri et al., 2002; Hariri et al., 2005). A PET investigation of healthy volunteers showed that individuals heterozygous (sl) or homozygous (ss) for the 5-HTTLPR s allele had lower 5-HT_{1A} receptor binding than individuals homozygous (ll) for the l allele (David et al., 2005). A study of children with homozygous s alleles had higher rates of shyness, a potential predictor of anxiety disorders later in life (Battaglia et al., 2005; Hayden et al., 2007). Early-life stresses, in combination with the presence of the s allele, confer greater susceptibility to depression or behavioral inhibition in children (Kaufman et al., 2004; Fox et al., 2005) or later-life depression (Caspi et al., 2003). These above studies suggest a strong interplay between genes and environment. There are, however, ample numbers of trials failing to show an association between the s allele and fear behaviors as they relate to life stress in children and adults (Lang et al., 2004; Becker et al., 2007), whereas meta-analyses reveal a heterogeneity of results (Munafo et al., 2003; Sen et al., 2004). In addition, studies of the 5-HRRLPR in anxiety disorders have been inconsistent. Smaller-scale studies have found an association between serotonin transporter promoter polymorphism and susceptibility to PTSD (H.J. Lee et al., 2005), symptom severity in social phobia (Furmark et al., 2004), and response to SSRI in social phobia (Stein et al., 2006). A recent meta-analysis found a lack of association between 5-HTTLPR and panic disorder (Blaya et al., 2007).

Clinical studies of 5-HT function in anxiety disorders have had similarly mixed results. Platelet imipramine binding (a marker of the serotonin reuptake site), which is generally reduced in depression, has been found to be normal in panic disorder (Innis et al., 1987; Uhde et al., 1987), whereas platelet 5-HT uptake in panic disorder has been reported to be elevated (Norman et al., 1986), normal (Balon et al., 1987), or reduced (Pecknold et al., 1988). Dell'Osso et al. (2004) found that patients with panic disorder had reduced responsiveness to 5-HT in platelets due to dysfunction in the cAMP pathway, an effect that was reversed with treatment with paroxetine. One study found that patients with panic disorder had lower levels of circulating 5-HT than controls (Schneider et al., 1987). Thus, no clear pattern of abnormality in 5-HT function in panic disorder has emerged from analysis of peripheral blood elements. Interestingly, a recent study did show increased turnover of 5-HT (taken from a jugular venous blood sample) in patients with panic disorder, but not during a panic attack, and that this turnover was reversed by an SSRI and was not related to the serotonin transporter genotype (Esler et al., 2007).

To date, pharmacological challenge studies of 5-HT in panic disorder have also been unable to establish a definite role for 5-HT in the pathophysiology of panic

(Maron and Shlik, 2006). Challenges with the 5-HT precursors l-tryptophan (Charney and Heninger, 1986) and 5-hydroxytryptophan (5-HTP) (DenBoer and Westenberg, 1990; Schruers et al., 2002) did not discriminate between panic disorder and controls on neuroendocrine measures. Conversely, tryptophan depletion (TD) was not anxiogenic in unmedicated patients with panic disorder (Goddard et al., 1994). Tryptophan depletion has also been shown to acutely lower brain 5-HT levels, with some studies showing an enhanced response to panicogens such as carbon dioxide (Schruers et al., 2000), and a reversal of the antipanic effects of paroxetine using flumazenil (C. Bell et al., 2002). Another study failed to demonstrate such an effect after CCK-4 challenge in patients with panic disorder successfully treated with citalopram (Tõru et al., 2006). Challenge with the 5-HT releasing agent *fenfluramine* has been reported to be anxiogenic and to produce greater increases in plasma prolactin and cortisol in patients with panic disorder compared to controls (Targum and Marshall, 1989). Studies with the 5-HT agonist *m-chloromethylpiperazine* (mCPP), a probe of postsynaptic 5-HT_2 receptor function, have produced equivocal findings. Increases in anxiety and plasma cortisol in patients with panic disorder compared to controls have been reported with oral (Kahn et al., 1988) but not intravenous administration of mCPP (Charney et al., 1987b), although van der Wee et al. (2004) did show greater behavioral effects of intravenous mCPP in patients with panic disorder versus controls. Overall, it remains unclear whether the etiology of panic disorder is related to an excess of 5-HT or is instead due to a deficit of serotonin (Maron and Shlik, 2006). It is likely that serotonin exerts an inhibitory effect on panic through its interactions with other neurotransmitters.

Challenge studies in other anxiety disorders have been limited. In one study, 5 of 14 patients with PTSD had a panic attack and four had a flashback following mCPP administration. In contrast, no patient had a panic attack and one patient experienced a flashback following the infusion of placebo saline. Thus, a subgroup of patients with PTSD exhibited a marked behavioral sensitivity to serotonergic provocation, raising the possibility of pathophysiologic subtypes among traumatized combat veterans (Southwick et al., 1997) (Table 41.4). An investigation of 14 patients with social anxiety disorder treated with either paroxetine or citalopram found that TD caused an increase in behavioral anxiety on the challenge day, suggesting that the efficacy of SSRI is dependent on 5-HT availability (Argyropoulos et al., 2004). In addition, patients with panic and social anxiety disorders undergoing treatment with SSRI or cognitive-behavioral therapy (CBT) were shown that TD caused a greater psychological and cardiovascular reactivity to stress, compared to sham depletion (Davies et al., 2006) (Table 41.4).

TABLE 41.4 *Evidence for Alterations in Other Neurotransmitter Systems in Anxiety Disorders*

	PTSD	*Panic Disorder*
Benzodiazepine		
Increased symptomatology with benzodiazepine antagonist	–	++
Decreased number of benzodiazepine receptors	+	++
Opiate		
Naloxone-reversible analgesia	+	NS
Increased plasma b-endorphin response to exercise	+	NS
Elevated levels of CSFendorphin	+	–
Serotonin		
Decreased serotonin reuptake site binding in platelets	++	+/–
Decreased serotonin transmitter in platelets	–	+/–
Blunted prolactin response to 5-HT_{1A} probe	–	+
Altered serotonin effect on cAMP in platelets (5-HT_{1A} probe)	–	NS
Increased anxiogenic responses to 5-HT agonists	+	+/–
Thyroid		
Increased baseline indices of thyroid function	+	–
Increased TSH response to TRH	+	–
Somatostatin		
Increased somatostatin levels at baseline in CSF	+	–
Cholecystokinin		
Increased anxiogenic responses to CCK agonists	+	+++

–, one or more studies did not support this finding (with no positive studies) or the majority of studies do not support this finding; +/–, an equal number of studies do and do not support this finding; +, at least one study supports this finding and no studies do not support the finding or the majority of studies support the finding; ++, two or more studies support this finding and no studies do not support the finding; +++, three or more studies support this finding, and no studies do not support the finding.

cAMP: cyclic adenosine 39,59-monophosphate; CCK: cholecystokinin; CSF: cerebrospinal fluid; 5-HT: serotonin; NS: not studied; PTSD: posttraumatic stress disorder; SPECT: single photon emission computed tomography; TSH: thyroid stimulating hormone; TRH: thyrotropin releasing hormone.

Benzodiazepine System

γ-amino butyric acid (GABA), the primary inhibitory neurotransmitter in the brain, consists of GABA-A, fast-acting, chloride-gated ligand receptors, and GABA-B, slower-acting G protein–coupled potassium ligand receptors. GABA-A, a heteropentameric receptor, is made up of five protein subunits and at least seven families (α 1–6; β 1–3; α 1–3; δ; ρ 1–3; ε; θ), with the majority of GABA complexes consisting of α-1 (Mohler, 2006). Agents such as benzodiazepines, barbiturates, ethanol, anticonvulsants, and neurosteroids are positive allosteric modulators of GABA-A receptors. In addition to GABA receptor, benzodiazepine receptors are also present throughout the brain, with the highest concentration in cortical gray matter. Central benzodiazepine receptors and GABA-A receptors are part of the same macromolecular complex. These receptors have distinct binding sites, although they are functionally coupled and regulate each other in an allosteric manner. Interestingly, the presence of these endogenous benzodiazepine receptors has led to speculation about the existence of naturally occurring benzodiazepines (Sand et al., 2000).

γ-amino butyric acid has been known to play an important role in the pathophysiology and treatment of anxiety disorders (Nemeroff, 2003). Preclinical studies have contributed to the understanding of the nature of this role. Administration of inverse agonists of benzodiazepine receptors, such as b-carboline-3-carboxylic acid ethyl ester (b-CCE), result in behavioral and biological effects similar to those seen in anxiety and stress, including increases in heart rate, blood pressure, plasma cortisol, and catecholamines (Braestrup et al., 1982). Administration of the b-carboline FG 7142 results in an increase in local cerebral glucose use in brain structures involved in memory, including the lateral septal nucleus, mammillary bodies, and anterior thalamic nuclei (Ableitner and Herz, 1987). The effects of the b-carbolines are blocked by administration of benzodiazepines (Ninan et al., 1982).

Recent investigations using anxiogenic inverse agonists (Atack et al., 2005), anxiolytic selective agonists (Dias et al., 2005), or behavioral paradigms (Morris et al., 2006), have suggested that α-2 and α-3 subunits are both critical in mediating anxiety processes. Studies of mixed selective α-2/α-3 agonists such as have shown them to have potential anxiolytic properties in animal studies (see review by Rupprecht et al., 2006). One partial α-2/α-3 agonist, TPA-23, was shown to be an effective nonsedating anxiolytic in rodents and primates, an effect thought to be due to its antagonism of α-1/α-5 (Atack et al., 2006). In addition to its sedating effects, the α-1 subunit is also involved in the amnestic effects of benzodiazepines, as demonstrated in studies of learning and memory (Savić, Obradović, Uresić, Cook, Sarma, et al., 2005; Savić, Obradović, Uresić, Cook, Yin, et al., 2005). A recent study found a reduction in expression of the GABA-A α-2 subunit 6 hours after fear conditioning (Mei et al., 2005).

Studies using uncontrollable stress as an animal model for the anxiety disorders found evidence for alterations in benzodiazepine receptor function. Animals exposed to acute inescapable stress in the form of cold swim or foot shock develop a decrease in benzodiazepine receptor binding in frontal cortex, with mixed results for cerebral cortex, hippocampus, and hypothalamus and no change in occipital cortex, striatum, midbrain, thalamus, cerebellum, and pons (Weizman et al., 1990). Chronic stress in the form of foot shock or cold swim resulted in decreases in benzodiazepine receptor binding in cerebral cortex, frontal cortex, hippocampus, and hypothalamus, with mixed results for cerebellum, midbrain, and striatum, and no changes in occipital cortex or pons (Drugan et al., 1989; Weizman et al., 1989, 1990). Decreases in benzodiazepine receptor binding are associated with alterations in memory manifested by deficits in maze escape behaviors (Drugan et al., 1989; Weizman et al., 1989). A decrease in benzodiazepine receptor binding (B_{max}) has been demonstrated in the so-called Maudsley genetically fearful strain of rat in comparison to nonfearful rats in several brain structures including the hippocampus (Robertson et al., 1978). Rat pups exposed to prenatal stress showed decreased numbers of benzodiazepine receptors in the central nucleus of the amygdala and the hippocampus and increased anxiety-like behaviors during an EPM (Barros et al., 2006). A study of the genetic effects of chronic stress on the GABA system did not show a change in expression of the GABA-A subunits (Verkuyl et al., 2004).

Despite preclinical support for the involvement of benzodiazepine systems in stress, clinical investigations of the function of this system in patients with anxiety disorders have been limited. The inability to identify measurable variables *in vivo* in humans that reflect central benzodiazepine system function has contributed to the paucity of research in this area. However, evidence from clinical studies performed to date suggests a possible role for alterations in benzodiazepine receptor function in disorders of anxiety and stress.

Pharmacological challenge studies support a role for benzodiazepine function in anxiety in normal humans. The benzodiazepine receptor inverse agonist FG 7142 induces severe anxiety resembling panic attacks and biological characteristics of anxiety in healthy individuals (Dorow et al., 1983). This observation raises the question of whether there exist endogenous equivalents to FG 7142 that might be released to provoke panic attacks. One candidate for such an endogenous ligand is diazepam-binding inhibitor (DBI). However, CSF levels of DBI are normal in patients with panic disorder (Payeur et al., 1992). Interestingly, a recent genetic study showed a higher rate of a polymorphism of the DBI gene in persons with anxiety disorders with panic attack, as compared to controls (Thoeringer et al., 2007). Administration of the benzodiazepine receptor antagonist flumazenil to patients with panic disorder results in an increase in panic attacks and subjective anxiety in comparison to controls (Nutt et al., 1990; Woods et al., 1991). Oral (Woods et al., 1991) and intravenous flumazenil (Nutt et al., 1990) have been shown to produce panic in a subgroup of patients with panic disorder but not in healthy individuals (Zedkova et al., 2003; E.C. Bell et al., 2004). Benzodiazepine-induced changes in sedation and cortisol levels, as well as in saccadic eye movement velocity, have been suggested to be indicative of benzodiazepine receptor–mediated actions. Patients with panic disorder were found to be less sensitive than controls to diazepam using saccadic eye movement velocity as a dependent measure, suggesting a functional subsensitivity of the GABA-benzodiazepine supramolecular complex in brain-stem regions controlling saccadic eye movements (Roy-Byrne et al., 1996). Other evidence for alterations in benzodiazepine receptor function in patients with panic disorder includes a diminished sensitivity to suppression of plasma NE, epinephrine, and pulse following administration of diazepam in comparison to controls (Roy-Byrne et al., 1989).

Neuroimaging studies reveal reduced cortical and subcortical benzodiazepine receptor binding in patients with panic disorder (Bremner, Innis, White, et al., 2000) and PTSD (Bremner, Innis, Southwick, et al., 2000), although Fujita et al. (2004) was unable to replicate this finding in a subsequent study of patients with PTSD. Imaging studies comparing patients with panic disorder to controls have reported reduced GABA levels in the occipital cortex (Goddard et al., 2001) and the anterior cingulate and basal ganglia (Ham et al., 2007). Using magnetic resonance spectroscopy (MRS), Goddard et al. (2004) also showed in a small sample that patients with panic disorder had a decreased GABA neural response to acute benzodiazepine administration, and decreased cortical GABA with chronic treatment. In addition, a recent PET study showed a reduction in GABA-A binding in the insula of patients with panic disorder (Cameron et al., 2007). These findings could be related to a down-regulation of benzodiazepine receptor binding following exposure to the stress. Other possible explanations are that stress results in changes in receptor affinity, changes in an endogenous benzodiazepine ligand (the existence of which is controversial), or stress-related alterations in GABAergic transmission or neurosteroids that affect benzodiazepine receptor binding. A preexisting low level of benzodiazepine receptor density may be a genetic risk factor for the development of stress-related anxiety disorders (Table 41.4). Vaiva et al. (2004) studied victims of motor vehicle accidents, measuring plasma GABA immediately after the accident, and reported that individuals who developed PTSD 6 weeks later had lower plasma GABA, compared to those who did not develop PTSD. At one year, the PTSD group continued to have lower plasma GABA than the non-PTSD group, but those with plasma GABA levels above 0.2 mmol no longer had symptoms of PTSD (Vaiva et al., 2006).

The last two decades have seen a shift away from the practice of indiscriminate prescribing of benzodiazepines, due to concerns relating to long-term effects on cognition and the abuse liability (Rosenbaum, 2005). In turn, other GABA agonists, in particular the new class of anticonvulsants, have been studied as a safer option. Pregabalin has been shown in several double-blind, placebo-controlled trials to be effective and safe for the treatment of GAD (Rickels et al., 2005; Montgomery et al., 2006; Feltner et al., 2008) and social phobia (Pande et al., 2004). Tiagabine, a GABA reuptake inhibitor, was shown in a study of patients with GAD to reduced symptoms versus placebo in one analysis but not another (Pollack et al., 2005), and in a study of PTSD patients, was shown to not be statistically significant from placebo (Davidson et al., 2007). Larger trials need to be done to determine if these agents are effective as a stand-alone treatment for various anxiety disorders.

Cholecystokinin

Cholecystokinin (CCK) is an anxiogenic neuropeptide present in the gastrointestinal tract as well as in the brain that has recently been suggested as a neural substrate for human anxiety (Harro, 2006). Neurons containing CCK are found with high density in the cerebral cortex, amygdala, and hippocampus. They are also found in the midbrain including the PAG, substantia nigra, and raphé nuclei. Iontophoretic administration of CCK has depolarizing effects on pyramidal neurons, suggesting that CCK it may serve as an excitatory neurotransmitter. Cholecystokinin-4-8 has stimulatory effects on action potentials in the dentate gyrus of the hippocampus. Activation of hippocampal neurons is suppressed by low-dose benzodiazepines. Cholecystokinin agonists are anxiogenic in a variety of animal models of anxiety, while CCK antagonists have anxiolytic effects in these tests (Hano et al., 1993; Bourin and Dailly, 2004). Several studies have shown that the panicogenic effect of CCK-4 on the dorsolateral PAG was blocked when rats were pretreated with a CCK-2 antagonist (Netto and Guimaraes, 2004; Zanoveli et al., 2004; Bertoglio and Zangrossi, 2005; Bertoglio et al., 2007). One study of patients with panic disorder found them to be more sensitive to the anxiogenic effects of CCK-4 and a closely related peptide, pentagastrin, and these effects were blocked by L-365,260, a CCK antagonist (Bradwejn, Koszycki, Couetoux du Tetre, et al., 1994). CCK-4 was found to not have anxiogenic effects in a small sample of patients with social phobia and obsessive–compulsive disorder (OCD) (Katzman et al., 2004). In a small sample of patients with PTSD, CCK-4 had enhanced anxiogenic effects compared to responses in healthy subjects (Kellner et al., 2000). Imipramine also antagonizes the panicogenic effects of CCK-4 in patients with panic disorder (Bradwejn and Koszycki, 1994). The mechanism is unclear but may relate to the ability of imipramine to down-regulate β-adrenergic receptors because propranolol antagonizes the anxiogenic actions of CCK-4 (Bradwejn and Koszycki, 1994). Levels of CCK in the CSF are lower in patients with panic disorder than in controls, raising the possibility of enhanced function of CCK receptors (Lydiard et al., 1992). The mechanism responsible for the enhanced sensitivity to CCK-4 has not been elucidated. Patients may have elevated production or turnover of CCK or increased sensitivity of CCK receptors. There is also evidence of CCK-B gene polymorphisms in patients with panic disorder, suggesting a possible genetic vulnerability (Hösing et al., 2004).

All of this evidence has prompted the study of CCK-B receptor antagonists as potential antianxiety drugs, but placebo-controlled trials have consistently shown these agents to not be effective in panic and GAD (Adams et al., 1995; Goddard et al., 1999) and panic disorder (Kramer et al., 1995; van Megen et al., 1997; Pande et al., 1999). Neuroimaging research should further elucidate the role of CCK in anxiety and help identify potential targets for treatment.

Opioid Peptides

One of the primary behavioral effects of uncontrollable stress is analgesia, which results from the release of endogenous opiates, which include beta-endorphin, enkephalin, and dynorphin. Significant analgesia is observed following uncontrollable but not controllable stress and also is seen following presentation of neutral stimuli previously paired with aversive stimuli (Fanselow, 1986). Stress-induced analgesia was also found to be correlated with the development of PTSD hyperarousal in women who were battered 3 months after the index trauma (Nishith, et al., 2002). There is also evidence that sensitization occurs because reexposure to less intense shock in rats previously exposed to uncontrollable shock also results in analgesia (Maier, 1986). These effects are likely to be mediated, in part, by a stress-induced release of endogenous opiates in the brain stem. Moreover, opioid peptides are elevated after acute uncontrollable shock (Madden et al., 1977), and uncontrollable but not controllable shock decreases the density of m-opiate receptors (Stuckey et al., 1989). It is thought that opioid peptides play a role in Pavlovian fear conditioning, in particular extinction (McNally et al., 2004). McNally and others (McNally and Cole, 2006; Cole and McNally, 2007) have shown that mu-opioid receptors in the ventrolateral PAG are involved in predicting errors during fear learning in rats, using electric foot shock. Their studies have also shown that opioid receptor antagonists, such as naloxone, block this learning. These opioid peptides may also exert an effect on fear learning and cognition through an antagonistic interaction with CCK (see review by Hebb et al., 2005). Given these facts, it is reasonable to study opiate systems in the anxiety disorders.

Only a few studies have looked at opiate function in PTSD. Hoffman et al. (1989) reported significantly lower morning and evening plasma beta-endorphin levels in 21 patients with PTSD compared to 20 controls. The results were viewed as support for van der Kolk's (1981) hypothesis that patients with PTSD have a chronic depletion of endogenous opiates, which causes them to seek out recurrent stressors to increase opiate release. Another study found no differences in plasma levels of methionine-enkephalin between patients with PTSD and controls, although the degradation half-life was significantly higher in the PTSD group (Wolf, 1991). In a pharmacological challenge of the opiate system, patients with PTSD showed reduced pain sensitivity compared to veterans without PTSD following exposure to a combat film. This reaction was reversible by the opiate antagonist *naloxone*. These findings could be explained by increased release of endogenous opiates with stress in PTSD (Pitman et al., 1990). This conclusion is supported by a report of elevated levels of CSF beta-endorphin in PTSD (D.G. Baker et al., 1997).

Whether alterations in endogenous opiates contribute to the core symptoms seen in PTSD is not clear. It has been hypothesized that symptoms of avoidance and numbing are related to a dysregulation of opioid systems in PTSD (Charney et al., 1993). Further, it has been suggested that the use of opiates in chronic PTSD may represent a form of self-medication. Consistent with this, Bremner, Southwick, Darnell, and Charney (1996) found, in structured interviews, that a significant number of patients with combat-related PTSD reported that opiates reduced their symptoms of hyperarousal. Animal studies have shown that opiates are powerful suppressants of central and peripheral noradrenergic activity. If, as suggested earlier in this chapter, some PTSD symptomatology is mediated by noradrenergic hyperactivity, then opiates may serve to "treat" or reduce that hypersensitivity and accompanying symptoms. On the other hand, during opiate withdrawal, when opiates are decreased and noradrenergic activity is increased, PTSD symptoms may become acutely exacerbated. In fact, many symptoms of PTSD are similar to those seen during opiate withdrawal. Liberzon et al. (2007) conducted a PET imaging study of combat and noncombat subjects with and without PTSD, versus healthy volunteers, to study mu-opioid receptor binding potential (BP) in relevant cortical and limbic areas. They reported that in combat individuals, with and without PTSD, there was a decrease in mu-opioid receptor BP in the mPFC, insula, and dorsal ACC, and higher BP in the orbitofrontal cortex and subgenual ACC, compared to controls. This difference was greater in the combat

PTSD group compared to the non-PTSD combat group. These findings may be due to adaptive increase in endogenous opioid after trauma exposure, though leads to a down-regulation of opioid receptors, or may be the result of a decrease in inhibitory interneurons (Liberzon et al., 2007). Studies of trauma in children indicate that opiates, such as morphine, given in the hospital after the event, may prevent the development of PTSD, by reduction of separation anxiety (Saxe et al., 2001; Saxe et al., 2006). Conversely, opioid antagonists, such as naloxone, naltrexone, and nalmefene, have been shown, in a few small-scale pilot studies, to have efficacy in treating hyperarousal symptoms in patients with preexisting PTSD (Glover, 1993; Lubin et al., 2002; Petrakis et al., 2007). Additional studies of opiate receptor function and its functional interaction with other neurotransmitter and peptide systems in anxiety disorders are indicated (Zubieta et al., 2003) (Table 41.4).

Respiratory System Dysfunction in Panic Disorder

The original observation that an intravenous infusion of lactate produces panic anxiety in susceptible individuals but not in normal individuals was made by Pitts and McClure (1967). Subsequently, the reliability of panic provocation by sodium lactate was well established (reviewed in Papp et al., 1993). The lactate response appears to be specific for panic disorder compared with other anxiety disorders and psychiatric conditions.

The panicogenic mechanism of lactate has not been established. One theory is based upon the fact that systemic alkalosis causes vasoconstriction of cerebral vessels, which in turn induces cerebral ischemia, with a rise in the intracellular lactate:pyruvate ratio. Further, infused lactate results in a rapid passive elevation in the lactate:pyruvate ratio in localized brain regions outside the blood-brain-barrier, such as the chemoreceptor zones. These two mechanisms lower the intracellular pH in medullary chemoreceptors. The theory suggests that in patients with panic there is dysregulation (greater sensitivity to alterations in pH) in this region; thus, a panic response is triggered. This theory predicts that panic could be triggered in any patient if the medullary pH is changed sufficiently.

The limitations of the model include the fact that it is not yet known whether the pH changes in the local circulation are mirrored intracellularly. Recent evidence on the physiological effects of sodium bicarbonate has revealed a paradoxical intracellular acidosis, so the same may be true of lactate. Still, there is no clear evidence that intracellular acidosis will initiate neural activity, as the theory requires. The model predicts that hypoxia is a profound stimulus for chemoreceptor stimulation, and hyperventilation is belied by experiments in which removal of CO_2 from inspired air leads to loss of consciousness without anxiety or air hunger.

A second major hypothesis of lactate's panicogenic effect asserts that it occurs via the induction of a metabolic alkalosis. Infused lactate is metabolized to bicarbonate. Bicarbonate is further metabolized to CO_2, which quickly permeates the CNS. This central buildup of CO_2 increases the ventilatory rate via a direct stimulation of ventral medullary chemoreceptors. Increasing the brain pCO_2 concentration has been shown to be a profound stimulus for LC activation, which could cause panic via central noradrenergic activation (Gorman et al., 1989).

Although the lactate-CO_2 theory has considerable appeal, there is a suggestion from initial studies with the isomer d-lactate that this may not be the whole explanation. There is a preliminary report that this isomer also is panicogenic (Gorman et al., 1990) but is not metabolized to CO_2. The behavioral effects of lactate and bicarbonate infusion have been compared (Gorman et al., 1989). Both substances provoke panic in susceptible patients; however, bicarbonate is somewhat less anxiogenic than lactate. This finding argues against alkalosis alone being the panicogenic stimulus. Gorman and colleagues (1989) concluded that stimulation of respiratory centers to produce increased ventilation, hypocapnia, and respiratory alkalosis were common effects produced by bicarbonate and lactate.

Panic can also be provoked by increases in pCO_2 (hypercapnia). This can be done slowly, such as by rebreathing air or by breathing 5%–7% CO_2 in air (Gorman et al., 1988; Gorman et al., 1989). Alternatively, panic attacks can be provoked by taking only one or two deep breaths of 35% CO_2 (van Den Hout and Griez, 1984; Griez et al., 1987). The CO_2 studies have revealed abnormalities in ventilatory physiology in children and adults with panic disorder (Pine et al., 1998)

Hyperventilation and increased CO_2 hypersensitivity have also been posited as an explanation for symptoms of panic disorder (Papp et al., 1993). According to the model, elevated levels of pCO_2 lead to activation of the vagus nerve, which, through the nucleus tractus solitarius, stimulates the LC and provokes hyperventilation. Increased tidal volume drives down pCO_2, with increased respiratory alkalosis and symptoms of panic. Hyperactive chemoreceptors lead to hyperventilation to reduce pCO_2, which results in panic symptomatology. A corollary model to the hyperventilation hypothesis (Klein, 1993) states that patients with panic disorder suffer from a physiological misinterpretation of a suffocation monitor that evokes a suffocation alarm system. This produces sudden respiratory distress, quickly followed by hyperventilation, panic, and an urge to flee. This model posits that hypersensitivity to CO_2 is due to the deranged suffocation alarm system. The neuroanatomical site for such a dysfunction in respiratory control could involve a number of structures including activation of the rostral and ventral anterior cingulate cortices, hippocampus, amygdala, insula, and fusiform gyrus, and deactivation of anterior and dorsal cingulate cortices and PFC (Brannan et al., 2001). More recent investigations have used different agents to induce panic. Doxapram, a carotid body stimulant, has been shown to reliably induce panic symptoms in patients with panic disorder but not healthy controls (Abelson, Nesse, et al., 1996). Imaging studies have reliably used doxapram to cause physiological symptoms of panic, such as increased respiration and heart rate, including one study that obtained PET images of patients during a doxapram challenge versus saline placebo (Garakani et al., 2007).

CONCLUDING REMARKS

This chapter began with a description of the neuroanatomical and neurochemical bases of classical fear conditioning, a model based on findings from abundant animal studies. The task of finding correlates in humans has been more of a challenge. Most research done in healthy volunteers has demonstrated the role of the amygdala in fear pathways but has also shown the critical importance of other areas, such as the anterior cingulate cortex, PFC, and hippocampus. Using functional neuroimaging, combined with emotional faces paradigms, emotional Stroop, and memory and learning tasks, several neuroimaging studies of patients with PTSD, social phobia, and panic disorder have shown, in addition to amygdalar activation, increased signal in areas such as the anterior cingulate cortex, and reduced activity in the medial PFC. Recent work has also begun to shed light on the insula, and how altered function in this brain region contributes to exaggerated interoceptive responses in individuals who are anxiety prone. This has been supported by recent findings of altered insular function in patients with panic disorder (Cameron et al., 2007), PTSD, and social phobia (Lanzenberger et al., 2007; Sareen et al., 2007); please see Chapter 43 on Neuroimaging Studies of Anxiety Disorders for further discussion of this topic.

Various neurochemicals and neuropeptides are implicated in the etiology of anxiety disorders. Although originally thought to involve primarily norepinephrine, it is apparent now that the manifestation of anxiety symptoms involves a complex interplay of compounds in the CNS and periphery. A good example is the manner in which neurosteroids such as allopregnanolone can modulate the activity of GABA-A receptors, an effect that can be reversed by administration of fluoxetine, a serotonergic agent (Matsumoto et al., 2007). Although the significance of substances such as galanin and NPY in human anxiety remains unclear, further investigations will continue to shed light in this area. Other compounds such as oxytocin (Kirsch et al., 2005; Meinlschmidt and Heim, 2007) and substance P have shown a potential role in the etiology of anxiety and thereby are potential targets of novel therapeutics. For instance, there was a study showing that a substance P-neurokinin-1 receptor antagonist alleviated symptoms of social phobia, when compared with placebo (Furmark et al., 2005). A large Phase II investigation of this drug in the treatment of PTSD is under way.

Work is commencing to examine the genetic basis of the neural mechanisms of fear conditioning. There have been several recent advances in understanding the genetic contribution and molecular machinery related to amygdala-dependent learned fear. A gene encoding gastrin-releasing peptide (Grp) has been identified in the lateral amygdala. The Grp receptor (GRPR) is expressed in GABAergic interneurons and mediates their inhibition of principal neurons. In GRPR knockout mice, this inhibition is reduced and LTP is enhanced. These mice have enhanced and prolonged fear memory for auditory and contextual cues, indicating that the Grp signaling pathway may serve as an inhibitory feedback constraint on learned fear (Bédard et al., 2007). Gastrin-releasing peptide antagonists have been shown to have anxiolytic effects in animal models (Bastaki et al., 2003). The work further supports the role of GABA in fear and anxiety states (Goddard et al., 2001) and suggests that the genetic basis of vulnerability to anxiety may relate to Grp, GRPR, and GABA (Ishikawa-Brush et al., 1997). In addition, there continues to be investigation of other genetic polymorphisms, such as the 5-HTTLPR, CRH gene, diazepam binding inhibitor, and COMT Val-158Met, to determine more conclusively whether these genetic alterations are associated with and/or confer susceptibility to anxiety disorders. Multidisciplinary studies that use neurochemical, neuroimaging, and genetic approaches have the potential to clarify the complex relationships among genotype, phe-notype, and psychobiological responses to stress.

REFERENCES

Abelson, J.L., and Curtis, G.C. (1996) Hypothalamic-pituitary-adrenal axis activity in panic disorder. *Arch. Gen. Psychiatry* 53:323–332.

Abelson, J.L., Khan, S., Liberzon, I., and Young, E.A. (2007) HPA axis activity in patients with panic disorder: review and synthesis of four studies. *Depress. Anxiety* 24:66–76.

Abelson, J.L., Liberzon, I., Young, E.A., and Khan, S. (2005) Cognitive modulation of the endocrine stress response to a pharmacological challenge in normal and panic disorder subjects. *Arch. Gen. Psychiatry* 62:668–675.

Abelson, J.L., Nesse, R.M., Weg, J.G., and Curtis, G.C. (1996) Respiratory psychophysiology and anxiety: cognitive intervention in the doxapram model of panic. *Psychosom. Med.* 58:302–313.

Abercrombie, E.D., and Jacobs, B.L (1987) Single-unit response of noradrenergic neurons in the locus coeruleus of freely moving cats, I: acutely presented stressful and nonstressful stimuli. *J. Neurosci.* 7:2837–2843.

Ableitner, A., and Herz, A. (1987) Changes in local cerebral glucose utilization induced by the a-carbolines FG 7142 and DMCM reveal brain structures involved in the control of anxiety and seizure activity. *J. Neurosci.* 7:1047–1055.

Adamec, R., Burton, P., Blundell, J., Murphy, D.L., and Holmes, A. (2006) Vulnerability to mild predator stress in serotonin transporter knockout mice. *Behav. Brain Res.* 170(1):126–140.

Adamec, R., Strasser, K., Blundell, J., Burton, P., and McKay, D.W. (2006) Protein synthesis and the mechanisms of lasting change in anxiety induced by severe stress. *Behav. Brain Res.* 167:270–286.

Adams, J.B., Pyke, R.E., Costa, J., Cutler, N.R., Schweizer, E., Wilcox, C.S., Wisselink, P.G., Greiner, M., Pierce, M.W., and Pande, A.C. (1995) A double-blind, placebo-controlled study of a CCK-B receptor antagonist, CI-988, in patients with generalized anxiety disorder. *J. Clin. Psychopharmacol.* 15:428–434.

Adolphs, R., Gosselin, F., Buchanan, T.W., Tranel, D., Schyns, P., and Damasio, A.R. (2005) A mechanism for impaired fear recognition after amygdala damage. *Nature* 433:68–72.

Aerni, A., Traber, R., Hock, C., Roozendaal, B., Schelling, G., Papassotiropoulos, A., Nitsch, R.M., Schnyder, U., and de Quervain, D.J. (2004) Low-dose cortisol for symptoms of posttraumatic stress disorder. *Am. J. Psychiatry* 161:1488–1490.

Aguilera, G., and Rabadan-Diehl, C. (2000) Vasopressinergic regulation of the hypothalamic-pituitary-adrenal axis: implications for stress adaptation. *Regul. Pept.* 96:23–29.

Albus, M., Zahn, T.P., and Brier, A. (1992) Anxiogenic properties of yohimbine: behavioral, physiological and biochemical measures. *Eur. Arch. Psychiatry* 241:337–344.

Allen, Y.S., Adrian, T.E., Allen, J.M., Tatemoto, K., Crow, T.J., Bloom, S.R., and Polak, J.M. (1983) Neuropeptide Y distribution in the rat brain. *Science* 221:877–879.

Ansorge, M.S., Zhou, M., Lira, A., Hen, R., and Gingrich, J.A. (2004) Early-life blockade of the 5-HT transporter alters emotional behavior in adult mice. *Science* 306:879–881.

Antonijevic, I.A., Murck, H., Bohlhalter, S., Frieboes, R.M., Holsboer, F., and Steiger, A. (2000) Neuropeptide Y promotes sleep and inhibits ACTH and cortisol release in young men. *Neuropharmacology* 39:1474–1481.

Argyropoulos, S.V., Hood, S.D., Adrover, M., Bell, C.J., Rich, A.S., Nash, J.R., Rich, N.C., Witchel, H.J., and Nutt, D.J. (2004) Tryptophan depletion reverses the therapeutic effect of selective serotonin reuptake inhibitors in social anxiety disorder. *Biol. Psychiatry* 56:503–509.

Aston-Jones, G., Shipley, M.T., Chouvet, G., Ennis, M., VanBockstaele, E.J., Pieribone, V., and Shiekhattar, R. (1991) Afferent regulation of locus coeruleus neurons: anatomy, physiology and pharmacology. *Progr. Brain Res.* 88:47–75.

Atack, J.R., Hutson, P.H., Collinson, N., Marshall, G., Bentley, G., Moyes, C., Cook, S.M., Collins, I., Wafford, K., McKernan, R. M., and Dawson, G.R. (2005) Anxiogenic properties of an inverse agonist selective for alpha3 subunit-containing GABA A receptors. *Br. J. Pharmacol.* 144:357–366.

Atack, J.R., Wafford, K.A., Tye, S.J., Cook, S.M., Sohal, B., Pike, A., Sur, C., Melillo, D., Bristow, L., Bromidge, F., Ragan, I., Kerby, J., Street, L., Carling, R., Castro, J.L., Whiting, P., Dawson, G. R., and McKernan, R.M. (2006) TPA023 [7-(1,1-dimethylethyl)-6-(2-ethyl-2H-1,2,4-triazol-3-ylmethoxy)-3-(2-fluorophenyl)-1,2,4-triazolo[4,3-b]pyridazine], an agonist selective for alpha2- and alpha3-containing GABAA receptors, is a nonsedating anxiolytic in rodents and primates. *J. Pharmacol. Exp. Ther.* 316: 410–422.

Bailey, K.R., Pavlova, M.N., Rohde, A.D., Hohmann, J.G., and Crawley, J.N. (2007) Galanin receptor subtype 2 (GalR2) null mutant mice display an anxiogenic-like phenotype specific to the elevated plus-maze. *Pharmacol. Biochem. Behav.* 86:8–20.

Bailey, S.J., and Toth, M. (2004) Variability in the benzodiazepine response of serotonin 5-HT1A receptor null mice displaying anxiety-like phenotype: evidence for genetic modifiers in the 5-HT-mediated regulation of GABA(A) receptors. *J. Neurosci.* 24:6343–6351.

Baker, D.G., Ekhator, N.N., Kasckow, J.W., Dashevsky, B., Horn, P.S., Bednarik, L., and Geracioti, T.D., Jr. (2005) Higher levels of basal serial CSF cortisol in combat veterans with posttraumatic stress disorder. *Am. J. Psychiatry* 162:992–994.

Baker, D.G., West, S.A., Orth, D.N., Hill, K.K., Nicholson, W.E., Ekhator, N.N., Bruce, A.B., Wortman, M.D., Keck, P.E., and Geracioti, J.D. (1997) Cerebrospinal fluid and plasma beta endorphin in combat veterans with posttraumatic stress disorder. *Psychoneuroendocrinology* 22:517–529.

Baker, R.A., and Herkenham, M. (1995) Arcuate nucleus neurons that project to the hypothalamic paraventricular nucleus: neuropeptidergic identity and consequences of adrenalectomy on mRNA levels in the rat. *J. Comp. Neurol.* 358:518–530.

Bale, T.L., Contarino, A., Smith, G.W., Chan, R., Gold, L.H., Sawchenko, P.E., Koob, G.F., Vale, W.W., and Lee, K.F. (2000) Mice deficient for corticotrophin-releasing hormone receptor-2 display anxiety-like behavior and are hypersensitive to stress. *Nature Genet.* 24:410–414.

Bale, T.L., Picetti, R., Contarino, A., Koob, G.F., Vale, W.W., and Kuo-Fen, L. (2002) Mice deficient for both corticotrophin-releasing factor receptor 1 (CRFR1) and CRFR2 have an impaired stress response and display sexually dichotomous anxiety-like behavior. *J. Neurosci.* 22:193–199.

Balon, R., Poh, R., Yeragani, V., Rainey, J., and Oxenkrug, G.F. (1987) Platelet serotonin levels in panic disorder. *Acta Psychiatr. Scand.* 75:315.

Balon, R., and Ramesh, C. (1996) Calcium channel blockers for anxiety disorders? *Ann. Clin. Psychiatry* 8:215–220.

Bandelow, B., Wedekind, D., Sandvoss, V., Broocks, A., Hajak, G., Pauls, J., Peter, H., and Ruther, E. (2000) Diurnal variation of cortisol in panic disorder. *Psychiatry Res.* 95:245–250.

Barrera, G., Hernandez, A., Poulin, J.F., Laforest, S., Drolet, G., and Morilak, D.A. (2006) Galanin-mediated anxiolytic effect in rat central amygdala is not a result of corelease from noradrenergic terminals. *Synapse* 59:27–40.

Barros, V.G., Rodriguez, P., Martijena, I.D., Perez, A., Molina, V.A., and Antonelli, M.C. (2006) Prenatal stress and early adoption effects on benzodiazepine receptors and anxiogenic behavior in the adult rat brain. *Synapse* 60:609–618.

Bastaki, S.M., Hasan, M.Y., Chandranath, S.I., Schmassmann, A., and Garner, A. (2003) PD-136,450: a CCK2 (gastrin) receptor antagonist with antisecretory, anxiolytic and antiulcer activity. *Mol. Cell Biochem.* 252:83–90.

Battaglia, M., Ogliari, A., Zanoni, A., Citterio, A., Pozzoli, U., Giorda, R., Maffei, C., and Marino, C. (2005) Influence of the serotonin transporter promoter gene and shyness on children's cerebral responses to facial expressions. *Arch. Gen. Psychiatry* 62:85–94.

Bauer, E.P., Schafe, G.E., and LeDoux, J.E. (2002) NMDA receptors and L-type voltage-gated calcium channels contribute to long-term potentiation and different components of fear memory formation in the lateral amygdala. *J. Neurosci.* 22:5239–5249.

Becker, K., El-Faddagh, M., Schmidt, M.H., and Laucht, M. (2007) Is the serotonin transporter polymorphism (5-HTTLPR) associated with harm avoidance and internalising problems in childhood and adolescence? *J. Neural Transm.* 114:395–402.

Bédard, T., Mountney, C., Kent, P., Anisman, H., and Merali, Z. (2007) Role of gastrin-releasing peptide and neuromedin B in anxiety and fear-related behavior. *Behav. Brain Res.* 179:133–140.

Bell, C., Forshall, S., Adrover, M., Nash, J., Hood, S., Argyropoulos, S., Rich, A., and Nutt, D.J. (2002) Does 5-HT restrain panic? A tryptophan depletion study in panic disorder patients recovered on paroxetine. *J. Psychopharmacol.* 16:5–14.

Bell, E.C., Baker, G.B., Poag, C., Bellavance, F., Khudabux, J., and Le Melledo, J.M. (2004) Response to flumazenil in the late luteal phase and follicular phase of the menstrual cycle in healthy control females. *Psychopharmacology (Berl)* 172:248–254.

Bertoglio, L.J., de Bortoli, V.C., and Zangrossi, H., Jr. (2007) Cholecystokinin-2 receptors modulate freezing and escape behaviors evoked by the electrical stimulation of the rat dorsolateral periaqueductal gray. *Brain Res.* 1156:133–138.

Bertoglio, L.J., and Zangrossi, H., Jr. (2005) Involvement of dorsolateral periaqueductal gray cholecystokinin-2 receptors in the regulation of a panic-related behavior in rats. *Brain Res.* 1059: 46–51.

Bhagwagar, Z., Rabiner, E.A., Sargent, P.A., Grasby, P.M., and Cowen, P.J. (2004) Persistent reduction in brain serotonin1A receptor binding in recovered depressed men measured by positron emission tomography with [11C]WAY-100635. *Mol. Psychiatry* 9: 386–392.

Bielsky, I.F., Hu, S.B., Ren, X., Terwilliger, E.F., and Young, L.J. (2005) The V1a vasopressin receptor is necessary and sufficient for normal social recognition: a gene replacement study. Neuron 47:503–513.

Bielsky, I.F., Hu, S.B., Szegda, K.L., Westphal, H., and Young, L.J. (2004) Profound impairment in social recognition and reduction in anxiety-like behavior in vasopressin V1a receptor knockout mice. *Neuropsychopharmacology* 29:483–493.

Bing, O., Moller, C., Engel, J.A., Soderpal, B., and Heilig, M. (1993) Anxiolytic-like action of centrally administered galanin. *Neurosci. Lett.* 164:17–20.

Bitran, D., Purdy, R.H., and Kellogg, C.K. (1993) Anxiolytic effect of progesterone is associated with increases in cortical allopregnanolone and GABA A receptor function. *Pharmacol. Biochem. Behav.* 45:423–428.

Blair, H.T., Schafe, G.E., Bauer, E.P., Rodrigues, S.M., and LeDoux, J.E. (2001) Synaptic plasticity in the lateral amygdala: a cellular hypothesis of fear conditioning. *Learn. Mem.* 8:229–242.

Blanchard, E.B., Kolb, L.C., Prins, A., Gates, S., and McCoy, G.C. (1991) Changes in plasma norepinephrine to combat-related stimuli among Vietnam veterans with posttraumatic stress disorder. *J. Nerv. Ment. Dis.* 179:371–373.

Blaya, C., Salum, G.A., Lima, M.S., Leistner-Segal, S., and Manfro, G.G. (2007) Lack of association between the serotonin transporter promoter polymorphism (5-HTTLPR) and panic disorder: a systematic review and meta-analysis. *Behav. Brain Funct.* 3:41.

Bonne, O., Bain, E., Neumeister, A., Nugent, A.C., Vythilingam, M., Carson, R.E., Luckenbaugh, D.A., Eckelman, W., Herscovitch, P., Drevets, W.C., and Charney, D.S. (2005) No change in serotonin type 1A receptor binding in patients with posttraumatic stress disorder. *Am. J. Psychiatry* 162:383–385.

Born, J., Lange, T., Kern, W., McGregor, G.P., Bickel, U., and Fehm, H.L. (2002) Sniffing neuropeptides: a transnasal approach to the human brain. *Nat. Neuroscience* 5:514–516.

Bourin, M., and Dailly, E. (2004) Cholecystokinin and panic disorder. *Acta Neuropsychiatr.* 16:85–93.

Bradwejn, J., and Koszycki, D. (1994) Imipramine antagonism of the panicogenic effects of CCK-4 in panic disorder patients. *Am. J. Psychiatry* 151:261–263.

Bradwejn, J., Koszycki, D., Couetoux du Tetre, A., van Megen, H., den boer, J., Westenberg, H., and Annable, L. (1994) The panicogenic effects of CCK-4 are antagonized by L-365-260, a CCK receptor antagonist, in patients with panic disorder. *Arch. Gen. Psychiatry* 51:486–493.

Braestrup, C., Schmiechen, R., Neef, G., Nielsen, M., and Petersen, E.N. (1982) Interaction of convulsive ligands with benzodiazepine receptors. *Science* 216:1241–1243.

Brambilla, F., Biggio, G., Pisu, M.G., Bellodi, L., Perna, G., Bogdanovich-Djukic, V., Purdy, R.H., and Serra, M. (2003) Neurosteroid secretion in panic disorder. *Psychiatry Res.* 118:107–116.

Brannan, S., Liotti, M., Egan, G., Shade, R., Masdden, L., Robillard, R., Stofer, K., Denton, D., and Fox, P.T. (2001) Neuroimaging of cerebral activations and deactivations associated with hypercapnia and hunger for air. *Proc. Natl. Acad. Sci. USA* 98:2029–2034.

Bremner, J.D. (2006) Stress and brain atrophy. *CNS Neurol. Disord. Drug Targets* 5:503–512.

Bremner, J.D., et al. (1999) Neural correlates of exposure to traumatic pictures and sound in Vietnam combat veterans with and without posttraumatic stress disorder: a positron emission tomography study. *Biol. Psychiatry* 45:806–816.

Bremner, J.D., Innis, R.B., Ng, C.K., Staib, L., Duncan, J., Bronen, R., Zubal, G., Rich, D., Krystal, J.H., Dey, H., Soufer, R., and Charney, D.S. (1997) PET measurement of central metabolic correlates of yohimbine administration in posttraumatic stress disorder. *Arch. Gen. Psychiatry* 54:246–256.

Bremner, J.D., Innis, R.B., Southwick, S.M., Staib, L., Zoghbi, S., and Charney, D.S. (2000) Decreased benzodiazepine receptor binding in prefrontal cortex in combat-related posttraumatic stress disorder. *Am. J. Psychiatry* 157:1120–1126.

Bremner, J.D., Innis, R.B., White, T., Fujita, M., Silbersweig, D., Goddard, A.W., Staib, L., Stern, E., Cappiello, A., Woods, S., Baldwin, R., and Charney, D.S. (2000) SPECT [I-123] iomazenil measurement of the benzodiazepine receptor in panic disorder. *Biol. Psychiatry* 47:96–106.

Bremner, J.D., Krystal, J.H., Southwick, S.M., and Charney, D.S. (1996a) Noradrenergic mechanisms in stress and anxiety: I. Preclinical studies. *Synapse* 23:28–38.

Bremner, J.D., Krystal, J.H., Southwick, S.M., and Charney, D.S. (1996b) Noradrenergic mechanisms in stress and anxiety: II. Clinical studies. *Synapse* 23:39–51.

Bremner, J.D., Licinio, J., Darnell, A., Krystal, J.H., Owens, M., Southwick, S.M., Nemeroff, C.B., and Charney, D.S. (1997) Elevated CSF corticotropin-releasing factor concentrations in posttraumatic stress disorder. *Am. J. Psychiatry* 154:624–629.

Bremner, J.D., Southwick, S.M., Darnell, A., and Charney, D.S. (1996) Chronic PTSD in Vietnam combat veterans: course of illness and substance abuse. *Am. J. Psychiatry* 153:369–375.

Bremner, J.D., Vermetten, E., Schmahl, C., Vaccarino, V., Vythilingam, M., Afzal, N., Grillon, C., and Charney, D.S. (2005) Positron emission tomographic imaging of neural correlates of a fear acquisition and extinction paradigm in women with childhood sexual-abuse-related post-traumatic stress disorder. *Psychol. Med.* 35: 791–806.

Bremner, J.D., Vythilingam, M., Vermetten, E., Adil, J., Khan, S., Nazeer, A., Afzal, N., McGlashan, T., Elzinga, B., Anderson, G.M., Heninger, G., Southwick, S.M., and Charney, D.S. (2003) Cortisol response to a cognitive stress challenge in posttraumatic stress disorder (PTSD) related to childhood abuse. *Psychoneuroendocrinology* 28:733–750.

Briones-Aranda, A., Rocha, L., and Picazo, O. (2005) Influence of forced swimming stress on 5-HT1A receptors and serotonin levels in mouse brain. *Prog. Neuropsychopharmacol. Biol. Psychiatry* 29:275–281.

Britton, K.T., Akwa, Y., Spina, M.G., and Koob, G.F. (2000) Neuropeptide Y blocks anxiogenic-like behavioral action of corticotrophin-releasing factor in an operant conflict test and elevated plus maze. *Peptides* 21:37–44.

Broekman, B.F., Olff, M., and Boer, F. (2007) The genetic background to PTSD. *Neurosci. Biobehav. Rev.* 31:348–362.

Bruening, S., Oh, E., Hetzenauer, A., Escobar-Alvarez, S., Westphalen, R.I., Hemmings, H.C., Jr., Singewald, N., Shippenberg, T., and Toth, M. (2006) The anxiety-like phenotype of 5-HT receptor null mice is associated with genetic background-specific perturbations in the prefrontal cortex GABA-glutamate system. *J. Neurochem.* 99:892–899.

Brunson, K.L., Eghbal-Ahmadi, M., Bender, R., Chen, Y., and Baram, T.Z. (2001) Long-term, progressive hippocampal cell loss and dysfunction induced by early-life administration of corticotrophin-releasing hormone reproduce the effects of early-life stress. *Proc. Natl. Acad. Sci. USA* 98:8856–8861.

Burgos-Robles, A., Vidal-Gonzalez, I., Santini, E., and Quirk, G.J. (2007) Consolidation of fear extinction requires NMDA receptor-dependent bursting in the ventromedial prefrontal cortex. *Neuron* 53:871–880.

Cabib, S., and Puglisi-Allegra, S. (1996) Different effects of repeated stressful experiences on mesocortical and mesolimbic dopamine metabolism. *Neuroscience* 73:375–380.

Cabib, S., Ventgura, R., and Puglisi-Allegra, S. (2002) Opposite imbalances between mesocortical and mesoaccumbens dopamine responses to stress by the same genotype depending on living conditions. *Behav. Brain Res.* 129:179–185.

Cahill, L., Prins, B., Weber, M., and McGaugh, J.L. (1994) Beta-adrenergic activation and memory for emotional events. *Nature* 371:702–704.

Cai, W.H., Blundell, J., Han, J., Greene, R.W., and Powell, C.M. (2006) Postreactivation glucocorticoids impair recall of established fear memory. *J. Neurosci.* 26:9560–9566.

Cain, C., Blouin, A., and Barad, M.G. (2002) L-type voltage-gated calcium channels are required for extinction but not for acquisition or expression, of conditional fear in mice. *J. Neurosci.* 22: 9113–9121.

Cain, C.K., Godsil, B.P., Jami, S., and Barad, M. (2005) The L-type calcium channel blocker nifedipine impairs extinction, but not reduced contingency effects, in mice. *Learn. Mem.* 12: 277–284.

Cameron, O.G., Huang, G.C., Nichols, T., Koeppe, R.A., Minoshima, S., Rose, D., and Frey, K.A. (2007) Reduced gamma-aminobutyric acid(A)-benzodiazepine binding sites in insular cortex of individuals with panic disorder. *Arch. Gen. Psychiatry* 64:793–800.

Canal, C.E., Chang, Q., and Gold, P.E. (2007) Amnesia produced by altered release of neurotransmitters after intraamygdala injections of a protein synthesis inhibitor. *Proc. Natl. Acad. Sci. USA* 104:12500–12505.

Canal, C.E., and Gold, P.E. (2007) Different temporal profiles of amnesia after intra-hippocampus and intra-amygdala infusions of anisomycin. *Behav. Neurosci.* 121:732–741.

Caspi, A., Sugden, K., Moffitt, T.E., Taylor, A., Craig, I.W., Harrington, H., McClay, J., Mill, J., Martin, J., Braithwaite, A., and Poulton, R. (2003) Influence of life stress on depression: moderation by a polymorphism in the 5-HTT gene. *Science* 301: 386–389.

Cassens, G., Kuruc, A., Roffman, M., Orsulak, P., and Schildkraut, J.J. (1981) Alterations in brain norepinephrine metabolism and behavior induced by environmental stimuli previously paired with inescapable shock. *Behav. Brain Res.* 2:387–407.

Chapman, P.F., Kairiss, E.W., Keenan, C.L., and Brown, T.H. (1990) Long-term synaptic potentiation in the amygdala. *Synapse* 6:271–278.

Charney, D.S. and Deutch, A.Y. (1996) A functional neuroanatomy of anxiety and fear: implications for the pathophysiology and treatment of anxiety disorders. *Crit. Rev. Neurobiol.* 10:419–446.

Charney, D.S., Deutch, A.Y., Krystal, J.H., Southwick, S.M., and Davis, M. (1993) Psychobiologic mechanisms of posttraumatic stress disorder. *Arch. Gen. Psychiatry* 50:294–299.

Charney, D.S., and Drevets, W.D. (2002) Neurobiological basis of anxiety disorders. In: Davis, K.L., Charney, D., Coyle, J.T., and Nemeroff, C., eds. *Neuropsychopharmacology: The Fifth Generation of Progress*. Baltimore: Lippincott Williams & Wilkins, pp. 901–930.

Charney, D.S., and Heninger, G.R. (1986) Serotonin function in panic disorders. The effects of intravenous tryptophan in healthy subjects and panic disorder patients before and after alprazolam treatment. *Arch. Gen. Psychiatry* 43:1059–1065.

Charney, D.S., Heninger, G.R., and Breier, A. (1984) Noradrenergic function in panic anxiety: effects of yohimbine in healthy subjects and patients with agoraphobia and panic disorder. *Arch. Gen. Psychiatry* 41:751–763.

Charney, D.S., Woods, S.W., Goodman, W.K., and Heninger, G.R. (1987a) Neurobiological mechanisms of panic anxiety: biochemical and behavioral correlates of yohimbine-induced panic attacks. *Am. J. Psychiatry* 144:1030–1036.

Charney, D.S., Woods, S.W., Goodman, W.K., and Heninger, G.R. (1987b) Serotonin function in anxiety. II. Effects of the serotonin agonist MCPP in panic disorder patients and healthy subjects. *Psychopharmacology* 92:14–24.

Charney, D.S., Woods, S.W., Krystal, J.H., Nagy, L.M., and Heninger, G.R. (1992) Noradrenergic neuronal dysregulation in panic disorder: the effects of intravenous yohimbine and clonidine in panic disorder patients. *Acta Psychiatr. Scand.* 86:273–282.

Cohen, H., Kaplan, Z., Matar, M.A., Loewenthal, U., Kozlovsky, N., and Zohar, J. (2006) Anisomycin, a protein synthesis inhibitor, disrupts traumatic memory consolidation and attenuates posttraumatic stress response in rats. *Biol. Psychiatry* 60:767–776.

Cole, S., and McNally, G.P. (2007) Opioid receptors mediate direct predictive fear learning: evidence from one-trial blocking. *Learn. Mem.* 14:229–235.

Comings, D.E., Muhleman, D., and Gysin, R. (1996) Dopamine D2 receptor (DRD2) gene and susceptibility to posttraumatic stress disorder: a study and replication. *Biol. Psychiatry* 40:368–372.

Cook, S.C., and Wellman, C.L. (2004) Chronic stress alters dendritic morphology in rat medial prefrontal cortex. *J. Neurobiol.* 60:236–248.

Coplan, J.D., Andrews, M.W., Rosenblum, L.A., Owens, M.J., Friedman, S., Gorman, J.M., and Nemeroff, C.B. (1996) Persistent elevations of cerebrospinal fluid concentrations of corticotropin-releasing factor in adult nonhuman primates exposed to early-life stressors: implications for the pathophysiology of mood and anxiety disorders. *Proc. Natl. Acad. Sci. USA* 93:1619–1623.

Coplan, J.D., Papp, L.A., Martinez, M.A., Pine, P., Rosenblum, L. A., Cooper, T., Liebowitz, M.R., and Gorman, J.M. (1995) Persistence of blunted human growth hormone response to clonidine in fluoxetine-treated patients with panic disorder. *Am. J. Psychiatry* 152:619–622.

Coplan, J.D., Pine, D., Papp, L., Martinez, J., Cooper, T., Rosenblum, L.A., and Gorman, J.M. (1995) Uncoupling of the noradrenergic-hypothalamic-pituitary adrenal axis in panic disorder patients. *Neuropsychopharmacology* 13:65–73.

Coryell, W., and Noyes, R. (1988) HPA axis disturbance and treatment outcome in panic disorder. *Biol. Psychiatry* 24:762–766.

Cose, B.J., and Robbins, T.W. (1987) Dissociable effects of lesions to dorsal and ventral noradrenergic bundle on the acquisition, performance, and extinction of aversive conditioning. *Behav. Neurosci.* 101:476–488.

Coste, S.C., Kesterson, R.A., Heldwein, K.A., Stevens, S.L., Heard, A.D., Hollis, J.H., Murray, S.E., Hill, J.K., Pantely, G.A., Hohimer, A.R., Hatton, D.C., Phillips, T.J., Finn, D.A., Low, M.J., Rittenberg, M.B., Stenzel, P., and Stenzel-Poore, M.P. (2000) Abnormal adaptations to stress and impaired cardiovascular function in mice lacking corticotrophin-releasing hormone receptor-2. *Nature Genet.* 24:403–409.

David, S.P., Murthy, N.V., Rabiner, E.A., Munafo, M.R., Johnstone, E.C., Jacob, R., Walton, R.T., and Grasby, P.M. (2005) A functional genetic variation of the serotonin (5-HT) transporter affects 5-HT1A receptor binding in humans. *J. Neurosci.* 25:2586–2590.

Davidson, J., Lipper, S., Kilts, C.D., Mahorney, S., and Hammett, E. (1985) Platelet MAO activity in posttraumatic stress disorder. *Am. J. Psychiatry* 142:1341–1343.

Davidson, J.R., Brady, K., Mellman, T.A., Stein, M.B., and Pollack, M.H. (2007) The efficacy and tolerability of tiagabine in adult patients with post-traumatic stress disorder. *J. Clin. Psychopharmacol.* 27:85–88.

Davies, S.J., Hood, S.D., Argyropoulos, S.V., Morris, K., Bell, C., Witchel, H.J., Jackson, P.R., Nutt, D.J., and Potokar, J.P. (2006) Depleting serotonin enhances both cardiovascular and psychological stress reactivity in recovered patients with anxiety disorders. *J. Clin. Psychopharmacol.* 26:414–418.

Davis, L.L., Ward, C., Rasmusson, A., Newell, J.M., Frazier, E., Southwick, S.M. (2008) A placebo-controlled trial of guanfacine for the treatment of posttraumatic stress disorder in veterans. *Psychopharmacol. Bull.* 41:8–18.

Davis, M. (2002) The role of NMDA receptors and MAP kinase in the amygdala in extinction of fear: clinical implications for exposure therapy. *Eur. J. Neurosci.* 16:395–398.

DeBellis, M.D., Lefter, L., Trickett, P.K., and Putnam, F.W. (1994) Urinary catecholamine excretion in sexually abused girls. *J. Am. Acad. Child Adolesc. Psychiatry* 33:320–327.

Dębiec, J., and Ledoux, J.E. (2004) Disruption of reconsolidation but not consolidation of auditory fear conditioning by noradrenergic blockade in the amygdala. *Neuroscience* 129:267–272.

Dębiec, J., LeDoux, J.E., and Nader, K. (2002) Cellular and systems reconsolidation in the hippocampus. *Neuron* 36:527–538.

de Brito Faturi, C., Teixeira-Silva, F., and Leite, J.R. (2006) The anxiolytic effect of pregnancy in rats is reversed by finasteride. *Pharmacol. Biochem. Behav.* 85:569–574.

de Kloet, C.S., Vermetten, E., Geuze, E., Lentjes, E.G., Heijnen, C.J., Stalla, G.K., and Westenberg, H.G. (2008) Elevated plasma corticotrophin-releasing hormone levels in veterans with posttraumatic stress disorder. *Prog. Brain Res.* 167:287– 291.

de Kloet, C.S., Vermetten, E., Geuze, E., Wiegant, V.M., and Westenberg, H.G. (2008) Elevated plasma arginine vasopressin levels in veterans with posttraumatic stress disorder. *J. Psychiatr. Res.* 42:192–198.

Dell'Osso, L., Carmassi, C., Palego, L., Trincavelli, M.L., Tuscano, D., Montali, M., Sbrana, S., Ciapparelli, A., Lucacchini, A., Cassano, G.B., and Martini, C. (2004) Serotonin-mediated cyclic AMP inhibitory pathway in platelets of patients affected by panic disorder. *Neuropsychobiology* 50:28–36.

DenBoer, J.A., and Westenberg, H.G.M. (1990) Behavioral, neuroendocrine, and biochemical effects of 5-hydroxytryptophan administration in panic disorder. *Psychiatry Res.* 31:367–378.

de Quervain, D.J. (2008) Glucocorticoid-induced reduction of traumatic memories: implications for the treatment of PTSD. *Prog. Brain Res.* 167:239–247.

de Quervain, D.J., Henke, K., Aerni, A., Treyer, V., McGaugh, J.L., Berthold, T., Nitsch, R.M., Buck, A., Roozendaal, B., and Hock, C. (2003) Glucocorticoid-induced impairment of declarative memory retrieval is associated with reduced blood flow in the medial temporal lobe. *Eur. J. Neurosci.* 17:1296–302.

de Quervain, D.J., Roozendaal, B., Nitsch, R.M., McGaugh, J.L., and Hock, C. (2000) Acute cortisone administration impairs retrieval of long-term declarative memory in humans. *Nat. Neurosci.* 3:313–314.

Deutch, A.Y., and Young, C.D. (1995) A model of the stress-induced activation of prefrontal cortical dopamine systems: coping and the development of post-traumatic stress disorder. In: Friedman, M.J., Charney, D.S., and Deutch, A.Y., eds. *Neurobiological and Clinical Consequences of Stress.* Philadelphia: Lippincott-Raven, pp. 163–175.

Diamond, D.M., Fleshner, M., Ingersoll, N., and Rose, G.M. (1996) Psychological stress impairs spatial working memory: relevance to electrophysiological studies of hippocampal function. *Behav. Neurosci.* 110:661–672.

Dias, R., Sheppard, W.F., Fradley, R.L., Garrett, E.M., Stanley, J.L., Tye, S.J., Goodacre, S., Lincoln, R.J., Cook, S.M., Conley, R., Hallett, D., Humphries, A.C., Thompson, S.A., Wafford, K.A., Street, L.J., Castro, J.L., Whiting, P.J., Rosahl, T.W., Atack, J.R., McKernan, R.M., Dawson, G.R., and Reynolds, D.S. (2005) Evidence for a significant role of alpha 3-containing GABAA receptors in mediating the anxiolytic effects of benzodiazepines. *J. Neurosci.* 25:10682–10688.

Diergaarde, L., Schoffelmeer, A.N., and De Vries, T.J. (2006) Beta-adrenoceptor mediated inhibition of long-term reward-related memory reconsolidation. *Behav. Brain Res.* 170:333–336.

Domschke, K., Deckert, J., O'donovan, M.C., and Glatt, S.J. (2007) Meta-analysis of COMT val158met in panic disorder: ethnic heterogeneity and gender specificity. *Am. J. Med. Genet.* 144: 667–673.

Dorow, R., Horowski, R., Paschelke, G., Amin, M., and Braestrup, C. (1983) Severe anxiety induced by FG7142, a beta-carboline ligand for benzodiazepine receptors. *Lancet* 2:98–99.

Drevets, W.C., Frank, J.C., Kupfer, D.J., Holt, D., Greer, P.J., Huang, Y., Gautier, C., and Mathis C. (1999) PET imaging of serotonin 1A receptor binding in depression. *Biol. Psychiatry* 46:1375–1387.

Drugan, R.C., Morrow, A.L., Weizman, R., Weizman, A., Deutsch, S.I., Crawley, J.N., and Paul, S.M. (1989) Stress-induced behavioral depression in the rat is associated with a decrease in GABA receptor-mediated chloride ion flux and brain benzodiazepine receptor occupancy. *Brain Res.* 487:45–51.

Duvarci, S., and Nader, K. (2004) Characterization of fear memory reconsolidation. *J. Neurosci.* 24:9269–9275.

Egashira, N., Tanoue, A., Matsuda, T., Koushi, E., Harada, S., Takano, Y., Tsujimoto, G., Mishima, K., Iwasaki, K., and Fujiwara, M. (2007) Impaired social interaction and reduced anxiety-related behavior in vasopressin V1a receptor knockout mice. *Behav. Brain Res.* 178:123–127.

Engelmann, M., Landgraf, R., Wotjak, C.T. (2004) The hypothalamic-neurohypophysial system regulates the hypothalamic-pituitary-adrenal axis under stress: an old concept revisited. *Front. Neuroendocrinol.* 25:132–149.

Eriksson, E., Westberg, P., Alling, C., Thuresson, K., and Modigh, K. (1991) Cerebrospinal fluid levels of monoamine metabolites in panic disorder. *Psychiatry Res.* 36:243–251.

Eser, D., di Michele, F., Zwanzger, P., Pasini, A., Baghai, T.C., Schule, C., Rupprecht, R., and Romeo, E. (2005) Panic induction with cholecystokinin-tetrapeptide (CCK-4) Increases plasma concentrations of the neuroactive steroid 3alpha, 5alpha tetrahydrodeoxycorticosterone (3alpha, 5alpha-THDOC) in healthy volunteers. *Neuropsychopharmacology* 30:192–195.

Eser, D., Schule, C., Baghai, T.C., Romeo, E., and Rupprecht, R. (2006) Neuroactive steroids in depression and anxiety disorders: clinical studies. *Neuroendocrinology* 84:244–254.

Esler, M., Lambert, E., Alvarenga, M., Socratous, F., Richards, J., Barton, D., Pier, C., Brenchley, C., Dawood, T., Hastings, J., Guo, L., Haikerwal, D., Kaye, D., Jennings, G., Kalff, V., Kelly, M., Wiesner, G., and Lambert, G. (2007) Increased brain serotonin turnover in panic disorder patients in the absence of a panic attack: reduction by a selective serotonin reuptake inhibitor. *Stress* 10:295–304.

Fanselow, M.S. (1986) Conditioned fear-induced opiate analgesia: a competing motivational state theory of stress analgesia. *Ann. N.Y. Acad. Sci.* 467:40–54.

Farinelli, M., Deschaux, O., Hugues, S., Thevenet, A., and Garcia, R. (2006) Hippocampal train stimulation modulates recall of fear extinction independently of prefrontal cortex synaptic plasticity and lesions. *Learn. Mem.* 13:329–334.

Feltenstein, M.W., and See, R.E. (2007) NMDA receptor blockade in the basolateral amygdala disrupts consolidation of stimulus-reward memory and extinction learning during reinstatement of cocaine-seeking in an animal model of relapse. *Neurobiol. Learn. Mem.* 88:435–444.

Feltner, D., Wittchen, H.U., Kavoussi, R., Brock, J., Baldinetti, F., and Pande, A.C. (2008) Long-term efficacy of pregabalin in generalized anxiety disorder. *Int. Clin. Psychopharmacol.* 23:18–28.

Finlay, J.M., and Abercrombie, E.D. (1991) Stress induced sensitization of norepinephrine release in the medial prefrontal cortex. *Soc. Neurosci. Abstr.* 17:151.

Fischer, A., Sananbenesi, F., Schrick, C., Spiess, J., and Radulovic, J. (2004) Distinct roles of hippocampal de novo protein synthesis and actin rearrangement in extinction of contextual fear. *J. Neurosci.* 24:1962–1966.

Flood, J.F., Baker, M.L., Hernandez, E.N., and Morley, J.E. (1989) Modulation of memory processing by neuropeptide Y varies with brain injection site. *Brain Res.* 503:73–82.

Foote, S.L., Bloom, F.E., and Aston-Jones, G. (1983) Nucleus locus coeruleus: new evidence for anatomical and physiological specificity. *Physiol. Rev.* 63:844–914.

Fox, N.A., Nichols, K.E., Henderson, H.A., Rubin, K., Schmidt, L., Hamer, D., Ernst, M., and Pine, D.S. (2005) Evidence for a gene-environment interaction in predicting behavioral inhibition in middle childhood. *Psychol. Sci.* 16:921–926.

Fujita, M., Southwick, S.M., Denucci, C.C., Zoghbi, S.S, Dillon, M.S., Baldwin, R.M., Bozkurt, A., Kugaya, A., Verhoeff, N.P., Seibyl, J.P., and Innis, R.B. (2004) Central type benzodiazepine receptors in Gulf War veterans with posttraumatic stress disorder. *Biol. Psychiatry* 56:95–100.

Furmark, T., Appel, L., Michelgard, A., Wahlstedt, K., Ahs, F., Zancan, S., Jacobsson, E., Flyckt, K., Grohp, M., Bergstrom, M., Pich, E. M., Nilsson, L.G., Bani, M., Langstrom, B., and Fredrikson, M. (2005) Cerebral blood flow changes after treatment of social phobia with the neurokinin-1 antagonist GR205171, citalopram, or placebo. *Biol. Psychiatry* 58(2):132–142.

Furmark, T., Tillfors, M., Garpenstrand, H., Marteinsdottir, I., Långström, B., Oreland, L., and Fredrikson, M. (2004) Serotonin transporter polymorphism related to amygdala excitability and symptom severity in patients with social phobia. *Neurosci. Lett.* 362: 189–192.

Garakani, A., Buchsbaum, M.S., Newmark, R.E., Goodman, C., Aaronson, C.J., Martinez, J.M., Torosjan, Y., Chu, K.W., and Gorman, J.M. (2007) The effect of doxapram on brain imaging in patients with panic disorder. *Eur. Neuropsychopharmacol.* 17: 672–686.

Garakani, A., Mathew, S.J., and Charney, D.S. (2006) Neurobiology of anxiety disorders and implications for treatment. *Mt. Sinai J. Med.* 73:941–949.

Garcia, R., Chang, C.H., and Maren, S. (2006) Electrolytic lesions of the medial prefrontal cortex do not interfere with long-term memory of extinction of conditioned fear. *Learn. Mem.* 13: 14–17.

Gartside, S.E., Johnson, D.A., Leitch, M.M., Troakes, C., and Ingram, C.D. (2003) Early life adversity programs changes in central 5-HT neuronal function in adulthood. *Eur. J. Neurosci.* 17: 2401–2408.

Gelernter, J., Southwick, S., Goodson, S., Morgan, A., Nagy, L., and Charney, D.S. (1999) No association between D2 dopamine receptor (DRD2) "A" system alleles or DRD2 haplotypes and posttraumatic stress disorder. *Biol. Psychiatry* 45:620–625.

Gentleman, S.M., Falkai, P., Bogerts, B., Herrero, M.T., Polak, J.M., and Roberts, G.W. (1989) Distribution of galanin-like immunoreactivity in the human brain. *Brain Res.* 505:311–315.

Geracioti, T.D., Jr., Baker, D.G., Ekhator, N.N., West, S.A., Hill, K.K., Bruce, A.B., Schmidt, D., Rounds-Kugler, B., Yehuda, R., Keck, P.E., Jr., and Kasckow, J.W. (2001) CSF norepinephrine concentrations in posttraumatic stress disorder. *Am. J. Psychiatry* 158:1227–1230.

Glover, H. (1993) A preliminary trial of nalmefene for the treatment of emotional numbing in combat veterans with post-traumatic stress disorder. *Isr. J. Psychiatry Relat. Sci.* 30:255–263.

Goddard, A.W., Mason, G.F., Almai, A., Rothman, D.L., Behar, K.L., Petroff, O.A., Charney, D.S., and Krystal, J.H. (2001) Reductions in occipital cortex GABA levels in panic disorder detected with 1h-magnetic resonance spectroscopy. *Arch. Gen. Psychiatry* 58:556–561.

Goddard, A.W., Mason, G.F., Appel, M., Rothman, D.L., Gueorguieva, R., Behar, K.L., and Krystal, J.H. (2004) Impaired GABA neuronal response to acute benzodiazepine administration in panic disorder. *Am. J. Psychiatry* 161:2186–2193.

Goddard, A.W., Sholomskas, D.E., Augeri, F.M., Walton, K.E., Charney, D.S., Heninger, G.R., Goodman, W.K. and Price, L.H. (1994) Effects of tryptophan depletion in panic disorders. *Biol. Psychiatry* 36:775–777.

Goddard, A.W., Woods, S.W., Money, R., Pande, A.C., Charney, D.S., Goodman, W.K., Heninger, G.R., and Price, L.H. (1999) Effects of the CCK(B) antagonist CI-988 on responses to mCPP in generalized anxiety disorder. *Psychiatry Res.* 85:225–240.

Goldstein, L.E., Rasmusson, A.M., Bunney, B.S., and Roth, R.H. (1996) Role of the amygdala in the coordination of behavioral, neuroendocrine, and prefrontal cortical monoamine responses to psychological stress in the rat. *J. Neurosci.* 16:4787–4798.

Goosens, K.A., and Maren, S. (2004) NMDA receptors are essential for the acquisition, but not expression, of conditional fear and associative spike firing in the lateral amygdala. *Eur. J. Neurosci.* 20:537–548.

Gorman, J.M., Battista, D., Goetz, R., et al. (1989) A comparison of sodium bicarbonate and sodium lactate infusion in the induction of panic attacks. *Arch. Gen. Psychiatry* 46:145–150.

Gorman, J.M., Fyer, M.R., Goetz, R., Askanazi, J., Liebowitz, M.R., Fyer, A.J., and Klein, D.F. (1988) Ventilatory physiology of patients with panic disorder. *Arch. Gen. Psychiatry* 45:31–39.

Gorman, J.M., Goetz, R.R., Dillon, D., et al. (1990) Sodium d-lactate infusion in panic disorder patients. *Neuropsychopharmacology* 3:181–190.

Gottsch, M.L., Zeng, H., Hohmann, J.G., Weinshenker, D., Clifton, D.K., and Steiner, R.A. (2005) Phenotypic analysis of mice deficient in the type 2 galanin receptor (GALR2). *Mol. Cell Biol.* 25:4804–4811.

Graeff, F.G. (2004) Serotonin, the periaqueductal gray and panic. *Neurosci. Biobehav. Rev.* 28:239–259.

Grammatopoulos, D.K., and Chrousos, G.P. (2002) Functional characteristics of CRH receptors and potential clinical applications of CRH-receptor antagonists. *Trends Endocrinol. Metab.* 13:436–444.

Griebel, G., Simiand, J., Serrradeil-Le Gal, L.C., Wagnon, J., Pascal, M., Scatton, B., Maffrand, J.P., and Soubrie, P. (2002) Anxiolytic-and antidepressant-like effects of the non-peptide vasopressin V1b receptor antagonist, SSR149415, suggest an innovative approach for the treatment of stress-related disorders. *Proc. Natl. Acad. Sci. USA* 99(9):6370–6375.

Griez, E., Lousberg, H., Van Den Hout, M.A., and van der Molen, G.M. (1987) Carbon dioxide vulnerability in panic disorder. *Psychiatry Res.* 20:87–95.

Grillon, C., Cordova, J., Morgan, C.A., Charney, D.S., and Davis, M. (2004) Effects of the beta-blocker propranolol on cued and contextual fear conditioning in humans. *Psychopharmacology (Berl)* 175:342–352.

Gross, C., Zhuang, X., Stark, K., Ramboz, S., Oosting, R., Kirby, L., et al. (2002) Serotonin 1A receptor acts during development to establish normal anxiety-like behavior in the adult. *Nature* 416:396–400.

Guastella, A.J., Richardson, R., Lovibond, P.F., Rapee, R.M., Gaston, J.E., Mitchell, P., and Dadds, M.R. (2008) A randomized controlled trial of D-cycloserine enhancement of exposure therapy for social anxiety disorder. *Biol. Psychiatry* 63:544–549.

Guastella, A.J., Dadds, M.R., Lovibond, P.F., Mitchell, P., and Richardson, R. (2007) A randomized controlled trial of the effect of d-cycloserine on exposure therapy for spider fear. *J. Psychiatry Res.* 41:466–471.

Gurguis, G.N.M., and Uhde, T.W. (1990) Plasma 3-methoxy-4 hydroxyphenylethylene glycol (MHPG) and growth hormone responses in panic disorder patients and normal controls. *Psychoneuroendocrinology* 15:217–224.

Gustafson, E.L., Smith, K.E., Durkin, M.M., Gerald, C., and Branchek, T.A. (1996) Distribution of a rat galanin receptor mRNA in rat brain. *Neuroreport* 7:953–957.

Hallschmid, M., Gais, S., Meinert, S., and Born, J. (2003) NPY attenuates positive cortical DC-potential shift upon food intake in man. *Psychoneuroendocrinology* 28:529–539.

Ham, B.J., Sung, Y., Kim, N., Kim, S.J., Kim, J.E., Kim, D.J., Lee, J. Y., Kim, J.H., Yoon, S.J., and Lyoo, I.K. (2007) Decreased GABA levels in anterior cingulate and basal ganglia in medicated subjects with panic disorder: a proton magnetic resonance spectroscopy (1H-MRS) study. *Prog. Neuropsychopharmacol. Biol. Psychiatry* 31:403–411.

Hamner, M.B., and Diamond, B.I. (1993) Elevated plasma dopamine in posttraumatic stress disorder: a preliminary report. *Biol. Psychiatry* 33:304–306.

Hamon, M., Gozlan, H., El Mestikawy, S., Emerit, M., Bolanos, F., and Schechter, L. (1990) The central 5-HT1a receptors: pharmacological biochemical, functional, and regulatory properties. *Ann. NY Acad. Sci.* 600:114–129.

Hano, J., Vasar, E., and Bradwejn, J. (1993) Cholecystokinm in animal and human research on anxiety. *Trends Pharmacol. Sci.* 14: 244–249.

Hariri A.R., Drabant, E.M., Munoz, K.E., Kolachana, B.S., Mattay, V.S., Egan, M.F., and Weinberger, D.R. (2005) A susceptibility gene for affective disorders and the response of the human amygdala. *Arch. Gen. Psychiatry* 62:146–152.

Hariri, A.R., Mattay, V.S., Tessitore, A., Kolachana, B., Fera, F., Goldman, D., Egan, M.F., and Weinberger, D.R. (2002) Serotonin transporter genetic variation and the response of the human amygdala. *Science* 297:400–403.

Harro, J. (2006) CCK and NPY as anti-anxiety treatment targets: promises, pitfalls, and strategies. *Amino Acids* 31:215–230.

Hawes, J.J., Brunzell, D.H., Wynick, D., Zachariou, V., and Picciotto, M.R. (2005) GalR1, but not GalR2 or GalR3, levels are regulated by galanin signaling in the locus coeruleus through a cyclic AMP-dependent mechanism. *J. Neurochem.* 93:1168–1176.

Hawes, J.J., and Picciotto, M.R. (2004) Characterization of GalR1, GalR2, and GalR3 immunoreactivity in catecholaminergic nuclei of the mouse brain. *J. Comp. Neurol.* 479(4):410–423.

Hayden, E.P., Dougherty, L.R., Maloney, B., Emily Durbin, C., Olino, T.M., Nurnberger, J.I., Jr., Lahiri, D.K., and Klein, D.N. (2007) Temperamental fearfulness in childhood and the serotonin transporter promoter region polymorphism: a multimethod association study. *Psychiatr. Genet.* 17:135–142.

Hebb, A.L., Poulin, J.F., Roach, S.P., Zacharko, R.M., and Drolet, G. (2005) Cholecystokinin and endogenous opioid peptides: interactive influence on pain, cognition, and emotion. *Prog. Neuropsychopharmacol. Biol. Psychiatry* 29:1225–1238.

Heilig, M. (1995) Antisense inhibition of neuropeptide Y (NPY)-Y1 receptor expression blocks the anxiolytic-like action of NPY in amygdala and paradoxically increases feeding. *Regul. Pept.* 59: 201–205.

Heilig, M., Koob, G.F., Ekman, R., and Britton, K.T. (1994) Corticotropin-releasing factor and neuropeptide Y: role in emotional integration. *Trends Neurosci.* 17:80–85.

Heilig, M., McLeod, S., Brot, M., Heinrichs, S.C., Menzaghi, F., Koob, G.F., and Britton, K.T. (1993) Anxiolytic-like action of neuropeptide Y: mediation by Y1 receptors in amygdala, and dissociation from food intake effects. *Neuropsychopharmacology* 8: 357–363.

Henry, M., Fishman, J.R., and Youngner, S.J. (2007) Propranolol and the prevention of post-traumatic stress disorder: is it wrong to erase the "sting" of bad memories? *Am. J. Bioeth.* 7:12–20.

Heresco-Levy, U., Kremer, I., Javitt, D.C., Goichman, R., Reshef, A., Blanaru, M., and Cohen, T. (2002) Pilot-controlled trial of D-cycloserine for the treatment of post-traumatic stress disorder. *Int. J. Neuropsychopharmacol.* 5:301–307.

Hernando, F., Schoots, O., Lolait, S.J., and Burbach, J.P. (2001) Immunohistochemical localization of the vasopressin V1b receptor in the rat brain and pituitary gland: anatomical support for its involvement in the central effects of vasopressin. *Endocrinology* 142:1659–1668.

Herry, C., and Garcia, R. (2002) Prefrontal cortex long-term potentiation but not long-term depression is associated with maintenance of extinction of learned fear in mice. *J. Neurosci.* 22:577–583.

Hertzberg, T., and Wahlbeck, K. (1999) The impact of pregnancy and puerperium on panic disorder: a review. *J. Psychsom. Obstet. Gynaecol.* 20:59–64.

Heydari, B., and Le Mellédo, J.M. (2002) Low pregnenolone sulphate plasma concentrations in patients with generalized social phobia. *Psychol. Med.* 32:929–933.

Hodgson, R.A., Higgins, G.A., Guthrie, D.H., Lu, S.X., Pond, A.J., Mullins, D.E., Guzzi, M.F., Parker, E.M., and Varty, G.B. (2007) Comparison of the V1b antagonist, SSR149415, and the CRF1 antagonist, CP-154,526, in rodent models of anxiety and depression. *Pharmacol. Biochem. Behav.* 86:431–440.

Hoffman, L., Watsgon, P.D., Wilson, G., and Montgomery, J. (1989) Low plasma endorphin in posttraumatic stress disorder. *Aust. N.Z. J. Psychiatry* 23:268–273.

Hofmann, S.G., Meuret, A.E., Smits, J.A., Simon, N.M., Pollack, M.H., Eisenmenger, K., Shiekh, M., and Otto, M.W. (2006) Augmentation of exposure therapy with D-cycloserine for social anxiety disorder. *Arch. Gen. Psychiatry* 63:298–304.

Holmes, A., Kinney, J.W., Wrenn, C.C., Li, Q., Yang, R.J., Ma, L., Vishwanath, J., Saavedra, M., Innerfield, C.E., Jacoby, A.S., Shine, J., Iismaa, T.P., and Crawley, J.N. (2003) Galanin GAL-R1 receptor null mutant mice display increased anxiety-like behavior specific to the elevated plus-maze. *Neuropsychopharmacology* 28: 1031–1044.

Holmes, A., Lit, Q., Murphy, D.L., Gold, E., and Crawley, J.N. (2003) Abnormal anxiety-related behavior in serotonin transporter null mutant mice: the influence of genetic background. *Genes Brain Behav.* 2:365–380.

Holmes, A., Yang, R.J., and Crawley, J.N. (2002) Evaluation of an anxiety-related phenotype in galanin overexpressing transgenic mice. *J. Mol. Neurosci.* 18:151–165.

Holmes, A., Yang, R.J., Murphy, D.L., and Crawley, J.N. (2002) Evaluation of antidepressant-related behavioral responses to mice lacking the serotonin transporter. *Neuropsychopharmacology* 27: 914–923.

Holmes, P.V., and Crawley, J.N. (1995) Coexisting neurotransmitters in central noradrenergic neurons. In: Bloom, F.E., and Kupfer, D.J., eds. *Psychopharmacology: The Fourth Generation of Progress*. New York: Raven Press, pp. 347–353.

Holsboer, F., von Bardeleben, U., Buller, R., Heuser, I., and Steiger, A. (1987) Stimulation response to corticotropin-releasing hormone (CRH) in patients with depression, alcoholism and panic disorder. *Horm. Metab. Res.* 16(Suppl.):80–88.

Hösing, V.G., Schirmacher, A., Kuhlenbäumer, G., Freitag, C., Sand, P., Schlesiger, C., Jacob, C., Fritze, J., Franke, P., Rietschel, M., Garritsen, H., Nöthen, M.M., Fimmers, R., Stögbauer, F., and Deckert, J. (2004) Cholecystokinin- and cholecystokinin-B-receptor gene polymorphisms in panic disorder. *J. Neural Transm.* (Suppl. 68):147–156.

Hurlemann, R., Hawellek, B., Matusch, A., Kolsch, H., Wollersen, H., Madea, B., Vogeley, K., Maier, W., and Dolan, R.J. (2005) Noradrenergic modulation of emotion-induced forgetting and remembering. *J. Neurosci.* 25:6343–6349.

Illes, P., Finta, E.P., and Nieber, K. (1993) Neuropeptide Y potentiates via Y2-receptors: the inhibitory effect of noradrenaline in rat locus coeruleus neurons. *Nauyn Schmiedebergs Arch. Pharmacol.* 348:546–548.

Innis, R.B., Charney, D.S., and Heninger, G.R. (1987) Differential 3H imipramine platelet binding in patients with panic disorder and depression. *Psychiatry Res.* 21:33–41.

Ishikawa-Brush, Y., Powell, J.F., Bolton, P., Miller, A.P., Francis, F., Willard, H.F., Lehrach, H., and Monaco, A.P. (1997) Autism and multiple exostoses associated with an X-8 translocation occurring within the GRPR gene and 39 to the SDC2 gene. *Hum. Mol. Genet.* 6:1241–1250.

Izquierdo, A., Wellman, C.L., and Holmes, A. (2006) Brief uncontrollable stress causes dendritic retraction in infralimbic cortex and resistance to fear extinction in mice. *J. Neurosci.* 26:5733–5738.

Jasnow, A.M., Cooper, M.A., and Huhman, K.L. (2004) *N*-methyl-D-aspartate receptors in the amygdala are necessary for the acquisition and expression of conditioned defeat. *Neuroscience* 123: 625–634.

Jin, X.C., Lu, Y.F., Yang, X.F., Ma, L., and Li, B.M. (2007) Glucocorticoid receptors in the basolateral nucleus of amygdala are required for postreactivation reconsolidation of auditory fear memory. *Eur. J. Neurosci.* 25:3702–3712.

Kahn, R.S., Asnis, G.M., Wetzler, S., Asnis, G.M., and Barr, G. (1988) Serotonin and anxiety revisited. *Biol. Psychiatry* 23:189–208.

Karlamangla, A.S., Singer, B.H., McEwen, B.S., Rowe, J.W., and Seeman, T.E. (2002) Allostatic load as a predictor of functional decline: MacArthur studies of successful aging. *J. Clin. Epidemiol.* 55:696–710.

Karlsson, R.M., and Holmes, A. (2006) Galanin as a modulator of anxiety and depression and a therapeutic target for affective disease. *Amino Acids* 31:231–239.

Karlsson, R.M., Holmes, A., Heilig, M., and Crawley, J.N. (2005) Anxiolytic-like actions of centrally-administered neuropeptide Y, but not galanin, in C57BL/6J mice. *Pharmacol. Biochem. Behav.* 80:427–436.

Kash, T.L., and Winder, D.G. (2006) Neuropeptide Y and corticotropin-releasing factor bi-directionally modulate inhibitory synaptic transmission in the bed nucleus of the stria terminalis. *Neuropharmacology* 51:1013–1022.

Kask, A., Harro, J., von Horsten, S., Redrobe, J.P., Dumont, Y., and Quiron, R. (2002) The neurocircuitry and receptor subtypes mediating anxiolytic-like effects of neuropeptide Y. *Neurosci. Behav. Rev.* 26:259–283.

Kask, A., Rago, L., and Harro, J. (1997) Alpha-lhelical CRF (9-41) prevents anxiogenic-like effect on NPY Y1 receptor antagonist BIBP3226 in rats. *Neuroreport* 8:3645–3647.

Kask, A., Rago, L., and Harro, J. (1998a) Anxiolytic-like effect of neuropeptide Y (NPY) and NPY 13-36 microinjected into vicinity of locus coeruleus in rats. *Brain Res.* 788:345–348.

Kask, A., Rago, L., and Harro, J. (1998b) NPY Y1 receptors in the dorsal periaqueductal gray matter regulate anxiety in the social interaction test. *Neuroreport* 9:2713–2716.

Kathol, R.G., Anton, R., Noyes, R., Lopez, A.L., and Reich, J.H. (1988) Relationship of urinary free cortisol levels in patients with panic disorder to symptoms of depression and agoraphobia. *Psychiatry Res.* 24:211–221.

Katzman, M.A., Koszycki, D., and Bradwejn, J. (2004) Effects of CCK-tetrapeptide in patients with social phobia and obsessive-compulsive disorder. *Depress. Anxiety* 20:51–58.

Kaufman, J., Yang, B.Z., Douglas-Palumberi, H., Houshyar, S., Lipschitz, D., Krystal, J.H., and Gelernter, J. (2004) Social supports and serotonin transporter gene moderate depression in maltreated children. *Proc. Natl. Acad. Sci. USA* 101:17316–17321.

Kellner, M., Wiedemann, K., Yassouridis, A., Levengood, R., Guo, L.S., Holsboer, F., and Yehuda, R. (2000) Behavioral and endocrine response to cholecystokinin tetrapeptide in patients with posttraumatic stress disorder. *Biol. Psychiatry* 47:107–111.

Kent, J.M., Mathew, S.J., and Gorman, J.M. (2002) Molecular targets in the treatment of anxiety. *Biol. Psychiatry* 52:1008–1030.

Kern, R.P., Libkuman, T.M., Otani, H., and Holmes, K. (2005) Emotional stimuli, divided attention, and memory. *Emotion* 5:408–417.

Khoshbouei, H., Cecchi, M., Dove, S., Javors, M., and Morilak, D.A. (2002) Behavioral reactivity to stress: Amplification of stress-induced noradrenergic activation elicits a galanin-mediated anxiolytic effect in central amygdala. *Pharmacol. Biochem. Behav.* 71:407–417.

Khoshbouei, H., Cecchi, M., and Morilak, D.A. (2002) Modulatory effects of galanin in the lateral bed nucleus of the stria terminalis on behavioral and neuroendocrine responses to acute stress. *Neuropsychopharmacology* 27:25–34.

Kida, S., Josselyn, S.A., de Ortiz, S.P., Kogan, J.H., Chevere, I., Masushige, S., and Silva, A.J. (2002) CREB required for the stability of new and reactivated fear memories. *Nature Neurosci.* 4:348–355.

Kim, J.J., and Diamond, D.M. (2002) The stressed hippocampus, synaptic plasticity and lost memories. *Nat. Rev. Neurosci.* 3:453–462.

Kinney, J.W., Starosta, G., Holmes, A., Wrenn, C.C., Yang, R.J., Harris, A.P., Long, K.C., and Crawley, J.N. (2002) Deficits in trace cued fear conditioning in galanin-treated rats and galanin-overexpressing transgenic mice. *Learn. Mem.* 9:178–190.

Kirsch, P., Esslinger, C., Chen, Q., Mier, D., Lis, S., Siddhanti, S., Gruppe, H., Mattay, V.S., Gallhofer, B., and Meyer-Lindenberg, A. (2005) Oxytocin modulates neural circuitry for social cognition and fear in humans. *J. Neurosci.* 25:11489–11493.

Klein, D.F. (1993) False suffocation alarms, spontaneous panics, and related conditions. *Arch. Gen. Psychiatry* 50:306–317.

Klemenhagen, K.C., Gordon, J.A., David, D.J., Hen, R., and Gross, C.T. (2006) Increased fear response to contextual cues in mice lacking the 5-HT1A receptor. *Neuropsychopharmacology* 31:101–111.

Kramer, M.S., Cutler, N.R., Ballenger, J.C., Patterson, W.M., Mendels, J., Chenault, A., Shrivastava, R., Matzura-Wolfe, D., Lines, C., and Reines, S. (1995) A placebo-controlled trial of L-365,260, a CCKB antagonist, in panic disorder. *Biol. Psychiatry* 37:462–466.

Kusserow, H., Davies, B., Hörtnagl, H., Voigt, I., Stroh, T., Bert, B., Deng, D.R., Fink, H., Veh, R.W., and Theuring, F. (2004) Reduced anxiety-related behaviour in transgenic mice overexpressing serotonin 1A receptors. *Brain Res. Mol. Brain Res.* 129:104–116.

Kuteeva, E., Wardi, T., Hokfelt, T., and Ogren, S.O. (2007) Galanin enhances and a galanin antagonist attenuates depression-like behaviour in the rat. *Eur. Neuropsychopharmacol.* 17:64–69.

Lacroix, J.S., Ricchetti, A.P., Morel, D., Mossimann, B., Waeber, B., and Grouzmann, E. (1996) Intranasal administration of neuropeptide Y in man: systemic absorption and functional effects. *Br. J. Pharmacol.* 118:2079–2084.

Lähdesmäki, J., Sallinen, J., MacDonald, E., Kobilka, B.K., Fagerholm, V., and Scheinin, M. (2002) Behavioral and neurochemical characterization of alpha(2A)-adrenergic receptor knockout mice. *Neuroscience* 113:289–299.

Lähdesmäki, J., Sallinen, J., MacDonald, E., and Scheinin, M. (2004) Alpha2A-adrenoceptors are important modulators of the effects of D-amphetamine on startle reactivity and brain monoamines. *Neuropsychopharmacology* 29:1282–1293.

Lang, U.E., Bajbouj, M., Wernicke, C., Rommelspacher, H., Danker-Hopfe, H., and Gallinat, J. (2004) No association of a functional polymorphism in the serotonin transporter gene promoter and anxiety-related personality traits. *Neuropsychobiology* 49:182–184.

Lanzenberger, R.R., Mitterhauser, M., Spindelegger, C., Wadsak, W., Klein, N., Mien, L.K., Holik, A., Attarbaschi, T., Mossaheb, N., Sacher, J., Geiss-Granadia, T., Kletter, K., Kasper, S., and Tauscher, J. (2007) Reduced serotonin-1A receptor binding in social anxiety disorder. *Biol. Psychiatry* 61:1081–1089.

Laufer, N., Maayan, R., Hermesh, H., Marom, S., Gilad, R., Strous, R., and Weizman, A. (2005) Involvement of GABA-A receptor modulating neuroactive steroids in patients with social phobia. *Psychiatry Res.* 137:131–136.

LeDoux, J.E. (2000) Emotion circuits in the brain. *Annu. Rev. Neurosci.* 23:155–184.

Lee, H.J., Lee, M.S., Kang, R.H., Kim, H., Kim, S.D., Kee, B.S., Kim, Y.H., Kim, Y.K., Kim, J.B., Yeon, B.K., Oh, K.S., Oh, B.H., Yoon, J.S., Lee, C., Jung, H.Y., Chee, I.S., and Paik, I.H. (2005) Influence of the serotonin transporter promoter gene polymorphism on susceptibility to posttraumatic stress disorder. *Depress. Anxiety* 21:135–139.

Lee, J.L., Milton, A.L., and Everitt, B.J. (2006) Reconsolidation and extinction of conditioned fear: inhibition and potentiation. *J. Neurosci.* 26:10051–10056.

Lee, Y., Schulkin, J., and Davis, M. (1994) Effect of corticosterone on the enhancement of the acoustic startle reflex by corticotrophin releasing factor (CRF). *Brain Res.* 666:93–98.

Lemieux, A.M., and Coe, C.L. (1995) Abuse-related PTSD: evidence for chronic neuroendocrine activation in women. *Psychosom. Med.* 57:105–115.

Lerer, B., Ebstein, R.P., Shestatsky, M., Shemesh, Z., and Greenberg, D. (1987) Cyclic AMP signal transduction in posttraumatic stress disorder. *Am. J. Psychiatry* 144:1324–1327.

Lesch, K.P., Bengel, D., Heils, A., Sabol, S.Z., Greenberg, B.D., Petri, S., Benjamin, J., Muller, C.R., Hamer, D.H., and Murphy, D. L. (1996) Association of anxiety-related traits with a polymorphism in the serotonin transporter gene regulatory region. *Science* 274:1527–1531.

Levine, E.S., Litto, W.J., and Jacobs, B.L. (1990) Activity of cat locus coeruleus noradrenergic neurons during the defense reaction. *Brain Res.* 531:189–195.

Liberzon, I., Taylor, S.F., Phan, K.L., Britton, J.C., Fig, L.M., Bueller, J.A., Koeppe, R.A., and Zubieta, J.K. (2007) Altered central micro-opioid receptor binding after psychological trauma. *Biol. Psychiatry* 61:1030–1038.

Lin, C.H., Yeh, S.H., Lu, H.Y., and Gean, P.W. (2003) The similarities and diversities of signal pathways leading to consolidation of conditioning and consolidation of extinction of fear memory. *J. Neurosci.* 23:8310–8317.

Lubin, G., Weizman, A., Shmushkevitz, M., and Valevski, A. (2002) Short-term treatment of post-traumatic stress disorder with naltrexone: An open-label preliminary study. *Hum. Psychopharmacol.* 17:181–185.

Lydiard, R.B., Ballenger, J.C., Laraia, M.T., Fossey, M.D., and Beinfeld, M.C. (1992) CSF cholecystokinin concentrations in patients with panic disorder and normal comparison subjects. *Am. J. Psychiatry* 149:691–693.

Madden, J., Akil, H., Patrick, R.L., and Barchas, J.D. (1977) Stress induced parallel changes in central opioid levels and pain responsiveness in the rat. *Nature* 265:358–360.

Maes, M., Lin, A.H., Delmeire, L., Van Gastael, A., Kenis, G., De Jongh, R., and Bosmans, E. (1999) Elevated serum interleukin-6 (IL-6) and IL-6 receptor concentrations in posttraumatic stress disorder following accidental man-made traumatic events. *Biol. Psychiatry* 45(7):833–839.

Maier, S.F. (1986) Stressor controllability and stress induced analgesia. *Ann. N.Y. Acad. Sci.* 467:55–72.

Makara, G.B., Mergl, Z., and Zelena, D. (2004) The role of vasopressin in hypothalamo-pituitary-adrenal axis activation during stress: an assessment of the evidence. *Ann. N. Y. Acad. Sci.* 1018:151–161.

Makino, S., Baker, R.A., Smith, M.A., and Gold, P.W. (2000) Differential regulation of neuropeptide Y mRNA expression in the accurate nucleus and locus coeruleus by stress and antidepressants. *J. Neuroendocrinol.* 12:387–395.

Makino, S., Gold, P.W., and Schulkin, J. (1994) Effects of corticosterone on CRH mRNA and content in the bed nucleus of the stria terminalis; comparison with the effects in the central nucleus of the amygdala and the paraventricular nucleus of the hypothalamus. *Brain Res.* 675:141–149.

Makino, S., Gold, P.W., and Schulkin, J. (1995) Corticosterone effects on corticotrophin-releasing hormone mRNA in the central nucleus of the amygdala and the parvocellular region of the paraventricular nucleus of the hypothalamus. *Brain Res.* 640:105–112.

Malberg, J.E., Eisch, A.J., Nestler, E.J., and Duman, R.S. (2000) Chronic antidepressant treatment increases neurogenesis in adult rat hippocampus. *J. Neurosci.* 20:9104–9110.

Mann, P.E. (2006) Finasteride delays the onset of maternal behavior in primigravid rats. *Physiol. Behav.* 88:333–338.

Maren, S., Aharonov, G., Stote, D.L., and Fanselow, M.S. (1996) *N*-methyl-D-aspartate receptors in the basolateral amygdala are required for both acquisition and expression of conditional fear in rats. *Behav. Neurosci.* 110:1365–1374.

Maron, E., and Shlik, J. (2006) Serotonin function in panic disorder: important, but why? *Neuropsychopharmacology* 31:1–11.

Marshall, R.D., Blanco, C., Printz, D., Liebowitz, M.R., Klein, D.F., and Coplan, J. (2002) A pilot study of noradrenergic and HPA axis functioning in PTS vs. panic disorder. *Psychiatry Res.* 110: 219–230.

Martins, A.P., Maras, R.A., and Guimaraes, F.S. (2001) Anxiolytic effect of a CRH receptor antagonist in the dorsal periaqueductal gray. *Depress. Anxiety* 12:99–101.

Matsumoto, K., Puia, G., Dong, E., and Pinna, G. (2007) GABA(A) receptor neurotransmission dysfunction in a mouse model of social isolation-induced stress: possible insights into a non-serotonergic mechanism of action of SSRIs in mood and anxiety disorders. *Stress* 10:3–12.

Matus-Amat, P., Higgins, E.A., Sprunger, D., Wright-Hardesty, K., and Rudy, J.W. (2007) The role of dorsal hippocampus and basolateral amygdala NMDA receptors in the acquisition and retrieval of context and contextual fear memories. *Behav. Neurosci.* 121:721–731.

McEwen B.S. (2000) Effects of adverse experiences for brain structure and function. *Biol. Psychiatry* 48:721–731.

McFall, M.E., Veith, R.C., and Murburg, M.M. (1992) Basal sympathoadrenal function in posttraumatic stress disorder. *Biol. Psychiatry* 31:1050–1056.

McGaugh, J.L. (2002) Memory consolidation and the amygdala: a systems perspective. *Trends Neurosci.* 25:456–461.

McGaugh, J.L., and Roozendaal, B. (2002) Role of adrenal stress hormones in forming lasting memory in the brain. *Curr. Opin. Neurobiol.* 12:205–210.

McGrath, M., Kawachi, I., Ascherio, A., Colditz, G.A., Hunter, D. J., and De Vivo, I. (2004) Association between catechol-O-methyltransferase and phobic anxiety. *Am. J. Psychiatry* 161:1703–1705.

McIntyre, C.K., Hatfield, T., and McGaugh, J.L. (2002) Amygdala norepinephrine levels after training predict inhibitory avoidance retention performance in rats. *Eur. J. Neurosci.* 16:1223–1226.

McKinney, B.C., and Murphy, G.G. (2006) The L-type voltage-gated calcium channel Cav1.3 mediates consolidation, but not extinction, of contextually conditioned fear in mice. *Learn. Mem.* 13: 584–589.

McNally, G.P. and Cole, S. (2006) Opioid receptors in the midbrain periaqueductal gray regulate prediction errors during Pavlovian fear conditioning. *Behav. Neurosci.* 120:313–323.

McNally, G.P., Pigg, M., and Weidemann, G. (2004) Opioid receptors in the midbrain periaqueductal gray regulate extinction of pavlovian fear conditioning. *J. Neurosci.* 24:6912–6919.

Mehta, M., Ahmed, Z., Fernando, S.S., Cano-Sanchez, P., Adayev, T., Ziemnicka, D., Wieraszko, A., and Banerjee, P. (2007) Plasticity of 5-HT 1A receptor-mediated signaling during early postnatal brain development. *J. Neurochem.* 101:918–928.

Mei, B., Li, C., Dong, S., Jiang, C.H., Wang, H., and Hu, Y. (2005) Distinct gene expression profiles in hippocampus and amygdala after fear conditioning. *Brain Res. Bull.* 67:1–12.

Meinlschmidt, G., and Heim, C. (2007) Sensitivity to intranasal oxytocin in adult men with early parental separation. *Biol. Psychiatry* 61:1109–1111.

Mellman, T.A., Kumar, A., Kulick-Bell, R., Kumar, M., and Nolan, B. (1995) Nocturnal/daytime urine norepinephrine measures and sleep in combat-related PTSD. *Biol. Psychiatry* 38:174–179.

Milad, M.R., and Quirk, G.J. (2002) Neurons in medial prefrontal cortex signal memory for fear extinction. *Nature* 420:70–74.

Milekic, M.H., and Alberini, C.M. (2002) Temporally graded requirement for protein synthesis following memory reactivation. *Neuron* 36:521–525.

Miracle, A.D., Brace, M.F., Huyck, K.D., Singler, S.A., and Wellman, C.L. (2006) Chronic stress impairs recall of extinction of conditioned fear. *Neurobiol. Learn. Mem.* 85:213–218.

Möhler, H. (2006) GABAA receptors in central nervous system disease: anxiety, epilepsy, and insomnia. *J. Recept. Signal Transduct. Res.* 26:731–740.

Moller, C., Sommer, W., Thorsell, A., and Heilig, M. (1999) Anxiogenic-like action of galanin after intra-amygdala administration in the rat. *Neuropsychopharmacology* 21:507–512.

Montgomery, S.A., Tobias, K., Zornberg, G.L., Kasper, S., and Pande, A.C. (2006) Efficacy and safety of pregabalin in the treatment of generalized anxiety disorder: a 6-week, multicenter, randomized, double-blind, placebo-controlled comparison of pregabalin and venlafaxine. *J. Clin. Psychiatry* 67:771–782.

Morgan, C.A., Rasmusson, A.M., Wang, S., Hoyt, G., Hauger, R.L., and Hazlett, G. (2002) Neuropeptide-Y, cortisol, and subjective distress in humans exposed to acute stress: replication and extension of previous report. *Biol. Psychiatry* 52:136–142.

Morgan, C.A., Rasmusson, A.M., Winters, B., Hauger, R.L., Morgan, J., Hazlett, G., and Southwick, S. (2003) Trauma exposure rather than posttraumatic stress disorder is associated with reduced baseline plasma neuropeptide-Y levels. *Biol. Psychiatry* 54:1087–1091.

Morgan, C.A., Wang, S., Mason, J., Southwick, S.M., Fox, P., Hazlett, G., Charney, D.S., and Greenfield, G. (2000) Hormone profiles in humans experiencing military survival training. *Biol. Psychiatry* 47:891–901.

Morgan, M.A., Romanski, L.M., and LeDoux, J.E. (1993) Extinction of emotional learning: contribution of medial prefrontal cortex. *Neurosci. Lett.* 163:109–113.

Morilak, D.A., Barrera, G., Echevarria, D.J., Garcia, A.S., Hernandez, A., Ma, S., and Petre, C.O. (2005) Role of brain norepinephrine in the behavioral response to stress. *Prog. Neuropsychopharmacol. Biol. Psychiatry* 29:1214–1224.

Morris, H.V., Dawson, G.R., Reynolds, D.S., Atack, J.R., and Stephens, D.N. (2006) Both alpha2 and alpha3 GABAA receptor subtypes mediate the anxiolytic properties of benzodiazepine site ligands in the conditioned emotional response paradigm. *Eur. J. Neurosci.* 23:2495–504.

Morrow, B.A., Elsworth, J.D., Rasmusson, A.M., and Roth, R.H. (1999) The role of mesoprefrontal dopamine neurons in the acquisition and expression of conditioned fear in the rat. *Neuroscience* 92(2):553–564.

Moses-Kolko, E.L., Price, J.C., Thase, M.E., Meltzer, C.C., Kupfer, D.J., Mathis, C.A., Bogers, W.D., Berman, S.R., Houck, P.R., Schneider, T.N., and Drevets, W.C. (2007) Measurement of 5-HT1A receptor binding in depressed adults before and after antidepressant drug treatment using positron emission tomography and [11C]WAY-100635. *Synapse* 61:523–530.

Mula, M., Pini, S., and Cassano, G.B. (2007) The role of anticonvulsant drugs in anxiety disorders: a critical review of the evidence. *J. Clin. Psychopharmacol.* 27:263–272.

Müller, M.B., Landgraf, R., Preil, J., Sillaber, I., Kresse, A.E., Keck, M.E., Zimmermann, S., Holsboer, F., and Wurst, W. (2000) Selective activation of the hypothalamic vasopressinergic system in mice deficient for the corticotropin-releasing hormone receptor 1 is dependent on glucocorticoids. *Endocrinology* 141:4262–4269.

Munafo, M.R., Clarke, T.G., Moore, L.R, Payne, E., Walton, R., and Flint, J. (2003) Genetic polymorphisms and personality in healthy adults: a systematic review and meta-analysis. *Mol. Psychiatry* 8:471–484.

Murrough, J.W., Boss-Williams, K.A., Emery, M.S., Bonsall, R.W., and Weiss, J.M. (2000) Depletion of brain norepinephrine does not reduce spontaneous ambulatory activity of rats in the home cage. *Brain Res.* 883:125–130.

Myers, K.M., and Davis, M. (2002) Systems-level reconsolidation: re-engagement of the hippocampus with memory reactivation. *Neuron* 36:340–343.

Myers, K.M., and Davis, M. (2007) Mechanisms of fear extinction. *Mol. Psychiatry* 12:120–150.

Nemeroff, C.B. (2003) The role of GABA in the pathophysiology and treatment of anxiety disorders. *Psychopharmacol. Bull.* 37: 133–146.

Nesse, R.M., Curtis, G.C., Thyer, B.A., McCann, D.S., Huber-Smith, M.J., and Knopf, R.F. (1985) Endocrine and cardiovascular responses during phobic anxiety. *Psychosom. Med.* 47:320–327.

Netto, C.F., and Guimaraes, F.S. (2004) Anxiogenic effect of cholecystokinin in the dorsal periaqueductal gray. *Neuropsychopharmacology* 29:101–107.

Neumeister, A., Bain, E., Nugent, A.C., Carson, R.E., Bonne, O., Luckenbaugh, D.A., Eckelman, W., Herscovitch, P., Charney, D. S., and Drevets, W.C. (2004) Reduced serotonin type 1A receptor binding in panic disorder. *J. Neurosci.* 24:589–591.

Neumeister, A., Charney, D.S., Belfer, I., Geraci, M., Holmes, C., Sharabi, Y., Alim, T., Bonne, O., Luckenbaugh, D.A., Manji, H., Goldman, D., and Goldstein, D.S. (2005) Sympathoneural and adrenomedullary functional effects of alpha2C-adrenoreceptor gene polymorphism in healthy humans. *Pharmacogenet. Genomics* 15:143–149.

Neumeister, A., Drevets, W.C., Belfer, I., Luckenbaugh, D.A., Henry, S., Bonne, O., Herscovitch, P., Goldman, D., and Charney, D.S. (2006) Effects of a alpha 2C-adrenoreceptor gene polymorphism on neural responses to facial expressions in depression. *Neuropsychopharmacology* 31:1750–1756.

Neylan, T.C., Lenoci, M., Samuelson, K.W., Metzler, T.J., Henn-Haase, C., Hierholzer, R.W., Lindley, S.E., Otte, C., Schoenfeld, F.B., Yesavage, J.A., and Marmar, C.R. (2006) No improvement of posttraumatic stress disorder symptoms with guanfacine treatment. *Am. J. Psychiatry* 163:2186–2188.

Ninan, P.T., Insel, T.M., Cohen, R.M., Cook, J.M., Skolnick, P., and Paul, S.M. (1982) Benzodiazepine receptor-mediated experimental "anxiety" in primates. *Science* 218:1332–1334.

Nisenbaum, L.K., and Abercrombie, E.D. (1993) Presynaptic alterations associated with enhancement of evoked release and synthesis of NE in hippocampus of chemically cold stressed rats. *Brain Res.* 608:280–287.

Nisenbaum, L.K., Zigmund, M.J., Sved, A.F., and Abercrombie, E. D. (1991) Prior exposure to chronic stress results in enhanced synthesis and release of hippocampal norepinephrine in response to a novel stressor. *J. Neurosci.* 11:1473–1484.

Nishith, P., Griffin, M.G., and Poth, T.L. (2002) Stress-induced analgesia: prediction of posttraumatic stress symptoms in battered versus nonbattered women. *Biol. Psychiatry* 51:867–874.

Norman, T.R., Judd, F.K., Gregory, M., James, R.H., Kimber, N.M., McIntyre, I.M., and Burrows, G.D. (1986) Platelet serotonin uptake in panic disorder. *J. Affect. Disord.* 11:69–72.

Nutt, D.J. (1989) Altered alpha$_2$-adrenoceptor sensitivity in panic disorder. *Arch. Gen. Psychiatry* 46:165–169.

Nutt, D.J., Glue, P., Lawson, C., and Wilson, S. (1990) Flumazenil provocation of panic attacks: evidence for altered benzodiazepine receptor sensitivity in panic disorder. *Arch. Gen. Psychiatry* 47: 917–925.

Orr, S.P., Milad, M.R., Metzger, L.J., Lasko, N.B., Gilbertson, M. W., and Pitman, R.K. (2006) Effects of beta blockade, PTSD diagnosis, and explicit threat on the extinction and retention of an aversively conditioned response. *Biol. Psychol.* 73:262–771.

Ou, L.C., and Gean, P.W. (2007) Transcriptional regulation of brain-derived neurotrophic factor in the amygdala during consolidation of fear memory. *Mol. Pharmacol.* 72:350–358.

Pande, A.C., Feltner, D.E., Jefferson, J.W., Davidson, J.R., Pollack, M., Stein, M.B., Lydiard, R.B., Futterer, R., Robinson, P., Slomkowski, M., DuBoff, E., Phelps, M., Janney, C.A., and Werth, J.L. (2004) Efficacy of the novel anxiolytic pregabalin in social anxiety disorder: a placebo-controlled, multicenter study. *J. Clin. Psychopharmacol.* 24:141–149.

Pande, A.C., Greiner, M., Adams, J.B., Lydiard, R.B., and Pierce, M.W. (1999) Placebo-controlled trial of the CCK-B antagonist, CI-988, in panic disorder. *Biol. Psychiatry* 46:860–862.

Paoletti, A.M., Romagnino, S., Contu, R., Orrù, M.M., Marotto, M.F., Zedda, P., Lello, S., Biggio, G., Concas, A., and Melis, G.B. (2006) Observational study on the stability of the psychological status during normal pregnancy and increased blood levels of neuroactive steroids with GABA-A receptor agonist activity. *Psychoneuroendocrinology* 31:485–492.

Papp, L.A., Klein, D.F., and Gorman, J.M. (1993) Carbon dioxide hypersensitivity, hyperventilation, and panic disorder. *Am. J. Psychiatry* 150:1149–1155.

Pare, D., Quirk, G.J., and Ledoux, J.E. (2004) New vistas on amygdala networks in conditioned fear. *J. Neurophysiol.* 92:1–9.

Park, H.J., Chae, Y., Jang, J., Shim, I., Lee, H., and Lim, S. (2005) The effect of acupuncture on anxiety and neuropeptide Y expression in the basolateral amygdala of maternally separated rats. *Neurosci. Lett.* 377:179–184.

Parks, C., Robinson, P., Sibille, E., Shenk, T., and Toth, M. (1998) Increased anxiety of mice lacking the serotonin 1A receptor. *Proc. Natl. Acad. Sci. USA* 95:10734–10739.

Pattij, T., Groenink, L., Oosting, R.S., van der Gugten, J., Maes, R.A.A., and Olivier, B. (2002) $GABA_A$-benzodiazepine receptor complex sensitivity in 5-HT1A receptor knockout mice on a 129/Sv background. *Eur. J. Pharmacol.* 447:67–74.

Pavlov, I.P. (1927) *Conditioned Reflexes*. London: Oxford University Press.

Payeur, R., Lydiard, R.B., Ballenger, J.C., Laraia, M.T., Fossey, M.D., and Zealberg, J. (1992) CSF diazepam-binding inhibitor concentrations in panic disorder. *Biol. Psychol.* 32:712–716.

Pecknold, J.C., Suranyi-Cadotte, B., Chang, H., and Nait, N.P.V. (1988) Serotonin uptake in panic disorder and agoraphobia. *Neuropsychopharmacology* 1:173–176.

Perez, S.E., Wynic, D., Steiner, R.A., and Mufson, E.J. (2001) Distribution of galaninergic immunoreactivity in the brain of the mouse. *J. Comp. Neurol.* 434:158–185.

Perry, B.D., Giller, E.L., and Southwick, S.M. (1987) Altered platelet $alpha_2$ adrenergic binding sites in posttraumatic stress disorder. *Am. J. Psychiatry* 144:1511–1512.

Petrakis, I., Ralevski, E., Nich, C., Levinson, C., Carroll K, Poling, J., Rounsaville, B., and VA VISN I MIRECC Study Group. (2007) Naltrexone and disulfiram in patients with alcohol dependence and current depression. *J. Clin. Psychopharmacol.* 27:160–165.

Pichot, W., Annsseau, M., Moreno, A.G., Hansenne, M., and Von Frenckell, R. (1992) Dopaminergic function in panic disorder: comparison with major and minor depression. *Biol. Psychiatry* 32:1004–1011.

Pieribone, V.A., Brodin, L., Friberg, K., Dahlstrand, J., Soderberg, C., Larhammar, D., and Hokfelt, T. (1992) Differential expression of mRNAs for neuropeptide Y-related peptides in rat nervous tissues: possible evolutionary conservation. *J. Neurosci.* 12: 3361–3371.

Pine, D.S., Coplan, J.D., Lazlo, A.P., Klein, R.G., Martinez, J.M., Kovalenko, P., Tancer, N., Moreau, D., Dummit, E.S., Shaffer, D., Klein, D.F., and Gorman, J.M. (1998) Ventilatory physiology of children and adolescents with anxiety disorders. *Arch. Gen. Psychiatry* 55:123–129.

Pinna, G., Costa, E., and Guidotti, A. (2006) Fluoxetine and norfluoxetine stereospecifically and selectively increase brain neurosteroid content at doses that are inactive on 5-HT reuptake. *Psychopharmacology* 186:362–372.

Pitman, R.K., Sanders, K.M., Zusman, R.M., Healy, A.R., Cheema, F., Lasko, N.B., Cahill, L., and Orr, S.P. (2002) Pilot study of secondary prevention of posttraumatic stress disorder with propranolol. *Biol. Psychiatry* 51:189–192.

Pitman, R.K., van der Kolk, B.A., Orr, S.P., and Greenberg, M.S. (1990) Naloxone reversible analgesic response to combat-related stimuli in posttraumatic stress disorder. *Arch. Gen. Psychiatry* 47:541–544.

Pitts, L.N., and McClure, J.N. (1967) Lactate metabolism in anxiety neuroses. *N. Engl. J. Med.* 277:1329–1336.

Pollack, M.H., Roy-Byrne, P.P., Van Ameringen, M., Snyder, H., Brown, C., Ondrasik, J., and Rickels, K. (2005) The selective GABA reuptake inhibitor tiagabine for the treatment of generalized anxiety disorder: results of a placebo-controlled study. *J. Clin. Psychiatry* 66:1401–1408.

Power, A.E., Berlau, D.J., McGaugh, J.L., and Steward, O. (2006) Anisomycin infused into the hippocampus fails to block "reconsolidation" but impairs extinction: the role of re-exposure duration. *Learn. Mem.* 13:27–34.

Primeaux, S.D., Wilson, S.P., Cusick, M.C., York, D.A., and Wilson, M.A. (2005) Effects of altered amygdalar neuropeptide Y expression on anxiety-related behaviors. *Neuropsychopharmacology* 30:1589–1597.

Prins, A., Kaloupek, D.G., and Keane, T.M. (1995) Psychophysiological evidence for autonomic arousal and startle in traumatized adult populations. In: Friedman, M.J., Charney, D.S., and Deutch, A.Y., eds. *Neurobiological and Clinical Consequences of Stress: From Normal Adaptation to PTSD*. New York: Raven Press, pp. 291–314.

Przybyslawski, J., Roullet, P., and Sara, S.J. (1999) Attenuation of emotional and nonemotional memories after their reactivation: role of b-adrenergic receptors. *J. Neurosci.* 19:6623–6628.

Przybyslawski, J., and Sara, S.J. (1997) Reconsolidation of memory after its reactivation. *Behav. Brain Res.* 84:241–246.

Quirk, G.J. (2002) Memory for extinction of conditioned fear is long-lasting and persists following spontaneous recovery. *Learn. Mem.* 9:402–407.

Quirk, G.J., Russo, G.K., Barron, J.L., and Lebron, K. (2000) The role of ventral medial prefrontal cortex in the recovery of extinguished fear. *J. Neurosci.* 20:6225–6231.

Radley, J.J., Sisti, H.M., Hao, J., Rocher, A.B., McCall, T., Hof, P.R., McEwen, B.S., and Morrison, J.H. (2004) Chronic behavioral stress induces apical dendritic reorganization in pyramidal neurons of the medial prefrontal cortex. *Neuroscience* 125:1–6.

Rajarao, S.J., Platt, B., Sukoff, S.J., Lin, Q., Bender, C.N., Nieuwenhuijsen, B.W., Ring, R.H., Schechter, L.E., Rosenzweig-Lipson, S., and Beyer, C.E. (2007) Anxiolytic-like activity of the non-selective galanin receptor agonist, galnon. *Neuropeptides* 41:307–320.

Rapaport, M.H., Risch, S.C., Golshan, S., and Gillin, J.C. (1989) Neuroendocrine effects of ovine corticotropin-releasing hormone in panic disorder patients. *Biol. Psychiatry* 26:344–348.

Raskind, M.A., Peskind, E.R., Hoff, D.J., Hart, K.L., Holmes, H.A., Warren, D., Shofer, J., O'Connell, J., Taylor, F., Gross, C., Rohde, K., and McFall, M.E. (2007) A parallel group placebo controlled study of prazosin for trauma nightmares and sleep disturbance in combat veterans with post-traumatic stress disorder. *Biol. Psychiatry* 61:928–934.

Raskind, M.A., Peskind, E.R., Kanter, E.D., Petrie, E.C., Radant, A., Thompson, C.E., Dobie, D.J., Hoff, D., Rein, R.J., Straits-Troster, K., Thomas, R.G., and McFall, M.M. (2003) Reduction of nightmares and other PTSD symptoms in combat veterans by prazosin: a placebo-controlled study. *Am. J. Psychiatry* 160:371–373.

Rasmusson, A.M., Southwick, S.M., Hauger, R.L., and Charney, D.S. (1998) Plasma neuropeptide Y (NPY) increases in humans in response to the alpha 2 antagonist yohimbine. *Neuropsychopharmacology* 19:95–98.

Rasmusson, A.M., Hauger, R.I., Morgan, C.A., Bremner, J.D., Charney, D.S., and Southwick, S.M. (2000) Low baseline and yohimbine-stimulated plasma neuropeptide Y (NPY) levels in combat-related PTSD. *Biol. Psychiatry* 47:526–539.

Rasmusson, A.M., Lipschitz, D.S., Wang, S., Hu, S., Vojvoda, D., Bremner, J.D., Southwick, S.M., and Charney, D.S. (2001) Increased pituitary and adrenal reactivity in premenopausal women with posttraumatic stress disorder. *Biol. Psychiatry* 50:965–977.

Rasmusson, A.M., Pinna, G., Paliwal, P., Weisman, D., Gottschalk, C., Charney, D., Krystal, J., and Guidotti, A. (2006) Decreased cerebrospinal fluid allopregnanolone levels in women with posttraumatic stress disorder. *Biol. Psychiatry* 60:704–713.

Rasmussen, K., Marilak, D.A., and Jacobs, B.L. (1986) Single unit activity of the locus coeruleus in the freely moving cat. I: during naturalistic behaviors and in response to simple and complex stimuli. *Brain Res.* 371:324–334.

Reddy, D.S., O'Malley, B.W., and Rogawski, M.A. (2005) Anxiolytic activity of progesterone in progesterone receptor knockout mice. *Neuropharmacology* 48:14–24.

Redmond, D.E., Jr. (1987) Studies of the nucleus locus coeruleus in monkeys and hypotheses for neuropsychopharmacology. In: Meltzer, H.Y., ed. *Psychopharmacology: The Third Generation of Progress.* New York: Raven Press, pp. 967–975.

Ressler, K.J., Rothbaum, B.O., Tannenbaum, L., Anderson, P., Graap, K., Zimand, E., Hodges, L., and Davis, M. (2004) Cognitive enhancers as adjuncts to psychotherapy: use of D-cycloserine in phobic individuals to facilitate extinction of fear. *Arch. Gen. Psychiatry* 61:1136–1144.

Rickels, K., Pollack, M.H., Feltner, D.E., Lydiard, R.B., Zimbroff, D.L., Bielski, R.J., Tobias, K., Brock, J.D., Zornberg, G.L., and Pande, A.C. (2005) Pregabalin for treatment of generalized anxiety disorder: a 4-week, multicenter, double-blind, placebo-controlled trial of pregabalin and alprazolam. *Arch. Gen. Psychiatry* 62:1022–1030.

Risbrough, V.B., and Stein, M.B. (2006) Role of corticotropin releasing factor in anxiety disorders: a translational research perspective. *Horm. Behavior* 50:550–561.

Risold, P.Y., and Swanson, L.W. (1997) Chemoarchitecture of the rat lateral septal nucleus. *Brain Res. Rev.* 24:91–113.

Robertson, H.A., Martin, I.L., and Candy, J.M. (1978) Differences in benzodiazepine receptor binding in Maudsley-reactive and nonreactive rats. *Eur. J. Pharmacol.* 50:455–457.

Rodrigues, S.M., Schafe, G.E., and LeDoux, J.E. (2001) Intra-amygdala blockade of the NR2B subunit of the NMDA receptor disrupts the acquisition but not the expression of fear conditioning. *J. Neurosci.* 21:6889–6896.

Roozendaal, B. (2000) Glucocorticoids and the regulation of memory consolidation. *Psychoneuroendocrinology* 25:213–238.

Roozendaal, B., Brunson, K.L., Holloway, B.L., McGaugh, J.L., and Baram, T.Z. (2002) Involvement of stress-released corticotrophin-releasing hormone in the basolateral amygdala in regulating memory consolidation. *Proc. Natl. Acad. Sci. USA* 99:13908–13913.

Roozendaal, B., Hui, G.K., Hui, I.R., Berlau, D.J., McGaugh, J.L., and Weinberger, N.M. (2006) Basolateral amygdala noradrenergic activity mediates corticosterone-induced enhancement of auditory fear conditioning. *Neurobiol. Learn. Mem.* 86:249–255.

Roozendaal, B., Okuda, S., Van der Zee, E.A., and McGaugh, J.L. (2006) Glucocorticoid enhancement of memory requires arousal-induced noradrenergic activation in the basolateral amygdala. *Proc. Natl. Acad. Sci. USA* 103:6741–6746.

Rosen, J.B. (2004) The neurobiology of conditioned and unconditioned fear: a neurobehavioral system analysis of the amygdala. *Behav. Cogn. Neurosci. Rev.* 3:23–41.

Rosenbaum, J.F. (2005) Attitudes toward benzodiazepines over the years. *J. Clin. Psychiatry* 66 (Suppl 2):4–8.

Rossato, J.I., Bevilaqua, L.R., Myskiw, J.C., Medina, J.H., Izquierdo, I., and Cammarota, M. (2007) On the role of hippocampal protein synthesis in the consolidation and reconsolidation of object recognition memory. *Learn. Mem.* 14:36–46.

Roy-Byrne, P.P., Lewis, N., Villacres, E., Diem, H., Greenblatt, D.J., Shader, R.I., and Veith, R. (1989) Preliminary evidence of benzodiazepine subsensitivity in panic disorder. *Biol. Psychiatry* 26: 744–748.

Roy-Byrne, P.P., Uhde, T.W., Post, R.M., Gallucci, W., Chrousos, G.P., and Gold, P.W. (1986) The corticotropin-releasing hormone stimulation test in patients with panic disorder. *Am. J. Psychiatry* 143:896–899.

Roy-Byrne, P.P., Wingerson, D.K., Radant, A., Greenblatt, D.J., and Cowley, D.S. (1996) Reduced benzodiazepine sensitivity in patients with panic disorder: comparison with patients with obsessive-compulsive disorder and normal subjects. *Am. J. Psychol.* 153:1444–1449.

Royer, S., Martina, M., and Paré, D. (2000) Polarized synaptic interactions between intercalated neurons of the amygdala. *J. Neurophysiol.* 83:3509–3518.

Rudy, J.W., Biedenkapp, J.C., Moineau, J., and Bolding, K. (2006) Anisomycin and the reconsolidation hypothesis. *Learn. Mem.* 13:1–3.

Rupprecht, R. (2003) Neuroactive steroids: mechanism of action and neuropharmacological properties. *Psychoneuroendocrinology* 28: 139–168.

Rupprecht, R., Eser, D., Zwanzger, P., and Moller, H.J. (2006) GABAA receptors as targets for novel anxiolytic drugs. *World J. Biol. Psychiatry* 7:231–237.

Sajdyk, T.J., Vandergriff, M.G., and Gehlert, D.R. (1999) Amygdala neuropeptide Y Y1 receptors mediate the anxiolytic-like actions of neuropeptide Y in the social interaction test. *Eur. J. Pharmacol.* 368:143–147.

Sallee, F.R., Sethuraman, G., Sine, L., and Liu, H. (2000) Yohimbine challenge in children with anxiety disorders. *Am. J. Psychiatry* 157:1236–1242.

Sallinen, J., Haapalinna, A., Viitamaa, T., Kobilka, B.K., and Scheinin, M. (1998) Adrenergic alpha2C-receptors modulate the acoustic startle reflex, prepulse inhibition, and aggression in mice. *J. Neurosci.* 18:3035–3042.

Salomé, N., Stemmelin, J., Cohen, C., and Griebel, G. (2006) Differential roles of amygdaloid nuclei in the anxiolytic- and antidepressant-like effects of the V1b receptor antagonist, SSR149415, in rats. *Psychopharmacology (Berl)* 187:237–244.

Samson, R.D., and Pare, D. (2005) Activity-dependent synaptic plasticity in the central nucleus of the amygdala. *J. Neurosci.* 25:1847–1855.

Sanchez, M.M., Young, L.J., Plotsky, P.M., and Insel, T.R. (1999) Autoradiographic and in situ hybridization localization of corticotrophin-releasing factor 1 and 2 receptors in nonhuman primate brain. *J. Comp. Neurol.* 408:365–377.

Sand, P., Kavvadias, D., Feineis, D., Riederer, P., Schreier, P., Kleinschnitz, M., Czygan, F.C., Abou-Mandour, A., Bringmann, G., and Beckmann, H. (2000) Naturally occurring benzodiazepines: current status of research and clinical implications. *Eur. Arch. Psychiatry Clin. Neurosci.* 250:194–202.

Santini, E., Ge, H., Ren, K., Peña de Ortiz, S., and Quirk, G.J. (2004) Consolidation of fear extinction requires protein synthesis in the medial prefrontal cortex. *J. Neurosci.* 24:5704–5410.

Sara, S.J. (2000) Retrieval and reconsolidation: toward a neurobiology of remembering. *Learn. Mem.* 7:73–84.

Sareen, J., Campbell, D.W., Leslie, W.D., Malisza, K.L., Stein, M.B., Paulus, M.P., Kravetsky, L.B, Kjernisted, K.D., Walker, J.R., and Reiss, J.P. (2007) Striatal function in generalized social phobia: a functional magnetic resonance imaging study. *Biol. Psychiatry* 61: 396–404.

Savić, M.M., Obradović, D.I., Ugresić, N.D., Cook, J.M., Sarma, P.V., and Bokonjić, D.R. (2005) Bidirectional effects of benzodiazepine binding site ligands on active avoidance acquisition and retention: differential antagonism by flumazenil and beta-CCt. *Psychopharmacology (Berl)* 180:455–465.

Savić, M.M., Obradović, D.I., Ugresić, N.D., Cook, J.M., Yin, W., and Bokonjić, D.R. (2005) Bidirectional effects of benzodiazepine binding site ligands in the passive avoidance task: differential antagonism by flumazenil and beta-CCt. *Behav. Brain Res.* 158:293–300.

Saxe, G., Geary, M., Bedard, K., Bosquet, M., Miller, A., Koenen, K., Stoddard, F., and Moulton, S. (2006) Separation anxiety as a mediator between acute morphine administration and PTSD symptoms in injured children. *Ann. N.Y. Acad. Sci.* 1071:41–45.

Saxe, G., Stoddard, F., Courtney, D., Cunningham, K., Chawla, N., Sheridan, R., King, D., and King, L. (2001) Relationship between acute morphine and the course of PTSD in children with burns. *J. Am. Acad. Child. Adolesc. Psychiatry* 40:915–921.

Schafe, G.E., Nader, K., Blair, H.T., and LeDoux, J.E. (2001) Memory consolidation of Pavlovian fear conditioning: a cellular and molecular perspective. *Trends Neurosci.* 24:540–546.

Schneider, L.S., Munjack, D., Severson, J.A., and Palmer, R. (1987) Platelet H3 imipramine binding in generalized anxiety disorder, panic disorder, and agoraphobia with panic attacks. *Biol. Psychiatry* 21:3–41.

Schneier, F.R., Liebowitz, M.R., Abi-Dargham, A., Zea-Ponce, Y., Lin, S.H., and Laruelle, M. (2000) Low dopamine D2 receptor binding in social phobia. *Amer. J. Psychiatry* 157:457–459.

Schroeder, B.W., and Shinnick-Gallagher, P. (2004) Fear memories induce a switch in stimulus response and signaling mechanisms for long-term potentiation in the lateral amygdala. *Eur. J. Neurosci.* 20:549–556.

Schruers, K., Klaassen, T., Pols, H., Overbeek, T., Deutz, N.E., and Griez, E. (2000) Effects of tryptophan depletion on carbon dioxide provoked panic in panic disorder patients. *Psychiatry Res.* 93:179–187.

Schruers, K., vanDiest, R., Nicolson, N., and Griez, E. (2002) L-5-Hydroxytryptophan induced increase in salivary cortisol in panic disorder patients and healthy volunteers. *Psychopharmacology* 161:365–369.

Semeniuk, T., Jhangri, G.S., and Le Mellédo, J.M. (2001) Neuroactive steroid levels in patients with generalized anxiety disorder. *J. Neuropsychiatry Clin. Neurosci.* 13:396–398.

Sen, S., Burmeister, M., and Ghosh, D. (2004) Meta-analysis of the association between a serotonin transporter promoter polymorphism (5-HTTLPR) and anxiety-related personality traits. *Am. J. Med. Genet. B. Neuropsychiatr. Genet.* 127:85–89.

Serradeil-Le Gal, C., Wagnon, J. 3rd, Tonnerre, B., Roux, R., Garcia, G., Griebel, G., and Aulombard, A. (2005) An overview of SSR149415, a selective nonpeptide vasopressin V(1b) receptor antagonist for the treatment of stress-related disorders. *CNS Drug Rev.* 11:53–68.

Sevcik, J., Finta, E.P., and Illes, P. (1993) Galanin receptors inhibit the spontaneous firing of locus coeruleus neurons and interact with mu-opioid receptors. *Eur. J. Pharmacol.* 230:223–230.

Shepard, J.D., Barron, K.W., and Myers, D.A. (2000) Corticosterone delivery to the amygdala increases corticotrophin-releasing factor mRNA in the central amygdaloid nucleus and anxiety-like behavior. *Brain Res.* 861:288–295.

Sheriff, S., Dautzenberg, F.M., Mulchahey, J.J., Pisarska, M., Hauger, R.L., Chance, W.T., Balasubramaniam, A., and Kasckow, J.W. (2001) Interaction of neuropeptide Y and corticotrophin-releasing factor signaling pathways in AR-5 amygdalar cells. *Peptides* 22 (12):2083–2089.

Shimazaki, T., Iijima, M., and Chaki, S. (2006) The pituitary mediates the anxiolytic-like effects of the vasopressin V1B receptor antagonist, SSR149415, in a social interaction test in rats. *Eur. J. Pharmacol.* 543:63–67.

Shumyatsky, G., Tsvetkov, E., Malleret, G., Vronskaya, S., Horton, M., Hampton, L., Battey, J.F., Dulac, C., Kandel, E.R., and Bolshakov, V.Y. (2002) Identification of a signaling network in lateral nucleus of amygdala important for inhibiting memory specifically related to learned fear. *Cell* 111:905–918.

Sibille, E., Pavlides, C., Benke, D., and Thth, M. (2000) Genetic inactivation of the serotonin 1A receptor in mice results in downregulation of major GABA-A receptor a subunits, reduction of GABA-A receptor binding, and benzodiazepine-resistant anxiety. *J. Neurosci.* 20:2758–2765.

Simson, P.E., and Weiss, J.M. (1988) Altered activity of the locus coeruleus in an animal model of depression. *Neuropsychopharmacology* 1:287–295.

Słopieć, R., Meczekalski, B., and Warenik-Szymankiewicz, A. (2004) Relationship between climacteric symptoms and serum galanin levels in post menopausal women. *J. Endocrinol. Invest.* 27: RC21–23.

Smagin, G.N., Harris, R.B., and Ryan, D.H. (1996) Corticotropin-releasing factor receptor antagonist infused into the locus coeruleus attenuates immobilization stress-induced defensive withdrawal in rats. *Neurosci. Lett.* 220:167–170.

Smiałowska, M., Wierośska, J.M., Domin, H., and Zieba, B. (2007) The effect of intrahippocampal injection of group II and III metobotropic glutamate receptor agonists on anxiety; the role of neuropeptide Y. *Neuropsychopharmacology* 32:1242–1250.

Smoller, J.W., Rosenbaum, J.F., Biederman, J., Kennedy, J., Dai, D., Racette, S.R., Laird, N.M., Kagan, J., Snidman, N., Hirshfeld-Becker, D., Tsuang, M.T., Sklar, P.B., and Slaugenhaupt, S.A. (2003) Association of a genetic marker at the corticotropin-releasing hormon locus with behavioral inhibition. *Biol. Psychiatry* 54:1376–1381.

Smoller, J.W., Yamaki, L.H., Fagerness, J.A., Biederman, J., Racette, S., Laird, N.M., Sklar, P.B., Kagan, J., Snidman, N., Faraone, S. V., and Hirshfeld-Baker, D. (2005) The corticotropin-releasing hormone gene and behavioral inhibition in children at risk for panic disorder. *Biol. Psychiatry* 57:1485–1492.

Soravia, L.M., Heinrichs, M., Aerni, A., Maroni, C., Schelling, G., Ehlert, U., Roozendaal, B., de Quervain, D.J. (2006) Glucocorticoids reduce phobic fear in humans. *Proc. Natl. Acad. Sci. USA* 103:5585–5590.

Sotres-Bayon, F., Cain, C.K., and LeDoux, J.E. (2006) Brain mechanisms of fear extinction: historical perspectives on the contribution of prefrontal cortex. *Biol. Psychiatry* 60:329–336.

Southwick, S.M., Krystal, J.H., Bremner, J.D., Morgan, C.A., Nicolaou, A., Nagy, L.M., Johnson, D.R., Heninger, G.R., and Charney, D.S. (1997) Noradrenergic and serotonergic function in posttraumatic stress disorder. *Arch. Gen. Psychiatry* 54:749–758.

Southwick, S.M., Krystal, J.H., Morgan, C.A., Johnson, D., Nagy, L.M., Nicolaou, A., Heninger, G.R., and Charney, D.S. (1993) Abnormal noradrenergic function in posttraumatic stress disorder. *Arch. Gen. Psychiatry* 50:266–274.

Stahl, S.M. (2004) Mechanism of action of alpha2delta ligands: voltage sensitive calcium channel (VSCC) modulators. *J. Clin. Psychiatry* 65:1033–1034.

Steckler, T., and Holsboer, F. (1999) Corticotropin-releasing hormone receptor subtypes and emotion. *Biol. Psychiatry* 46:1480–1508.

Stein, M.B., Hauger, R.L., Dhalla, K.S., Chartier, M.J., and Asmundson, G.J. (1996) Plasma neuropeptide Y in anxiety disorders: findings in panic disorder and social phobia. *Psychiatry Res.* 59:183–188.

Stein, M.B., Huzel, L.L., and Delaney, S.M. (1993) Lymphocyte b-adrenoceptors in social phobia. *Biol. Psychiatry* 34:45–50.

Stein, M.B., Seedat, S., and Gelernter, J. (2006) Serotonin transporter gene promoter polymorphism predicts SSRI response in generalized social anxiety disorder. *Psychopharmacology (Berl)* 187:68–72.

Stein, M.B., Tancer, M.E., and Uhde, T.W. (1992) Heart rate and plasma norepinephrine responsivity to orthostatic challenge in anxiety disorders. Comparison of patients with panic disorder and social phobia and normal control subjects. *Arch. Gen. Psychiatry* 49:311–317.

Strange, B.A., Hurlemann, R., and Dolan, R.J. (2003) An emotion-induced retrograde amnesia in humans is amygdala- and beta-adrenergic-dependent. *Proc. Natl. Acad. Sci. USA* 100:13626–13631.

Strawn, J.R., Ekhator, N.N., Horn, P.S., Baker, D.G., and Geracioti, T.D., Jr. (2004) Blood pressure and cerebrospinal fluid norepinephrine in combat-related posttraumatic stress disorder. *Psychosom. Med.* 66:757–759.

Ströhle, A., Romeo, E., DiMichele, F., Pasini, A., Herman, B., Gajewsky, G., Holsboer, F., and Rupprecht, R. (2003) Induced panic attacks shift g-aminobutyric acid type A receptor modulatory neuroactive steroid composition in patients with panic disorder. *Arch. Gen. Psychiatry* 60:161–168.

Strömberg, J., Haage, D., Taube, M., Bäckström, T., and Lundgren, P. (2006) Neurosteroid modulation of allopregnanolone and GABA effect on the GABA-A receptor. *Neuroscience* 143:73–81.

Strome, E.M., Trevor, G.H.W., Higley, J.D., Liriaux, D.L., Suomi, S. J., and Doudet, D.J. (2002) Intracerebroventricular corticotrophin-releasing factor increased limbic glucose metabolism and has social context dependent behavioral effects in nonhuman primates. *Proc. Natl. Acad. Sci. USA* 99:15749–15754.

Stuckey, J., Marra, S., Minor, T., and Insel, T.R. (1989) Changes in m opiate receptors following inescapable shock. *Brain Res.* 476: 167–169.

Swanson, C.J., Blackburn, T.P., Zhang, X., Zheng, K., Xu, Z.Q., Hokfelt, T., Wolinsky, T.D., Konkel, M.J., Chen, H., Zhong, H., Walker, M.W., Craig, D.A., Gerald, C.P., and Branchek, T.A. (2005) Anxiolytic- and antidepressant-like profiles of the galanin-3 receptor (Gal3) antagonists SNAP 37889 and SNAP 398299. *Proc. Natl. Acad. Sci. USA* 102:17489–7494.

Tancer, M.E., Stein, M.B., and Uhde, T.W. (1990) Effects of thyrotropin-releasing hormone on blood pressure and heart rate in phobic and panic patients: a pilot study. *Biol. Psychiatry* 27:781–783.

Targum, S.D., and Marshall, L.E. (1989) Fenfluramine provocation of anxiety in patients with panic disorder. *Psychiatry Res.* 28: 295–306.

Taylor, F.B., Lowe, K., Thompson, C., McFall, M.M., Peskind, E.R., Kanter, E.D., Allison, N., Williams, J., Martin, P., and Raskind, M.A. (2006) Daytime prazosin reduces psychological distress to trauma specific cues in civilian trauma posttraumatic stress disorder. *Biol. Psychiatry* 59:577–581.

Thoeringer, C.K., Binder, E.B., Salyakina, D., Erhardt, A., Ising, M, Unschuld, P.G., Kern, N., Lucae, S., Brueckl, T.M., Mueller, M. B., Fuchs, B., Puetz, B., Lieb, R., Uhr, M., Holsboer, F., Mueller-Myhsok, B., and Keck, M.E. (2007) Association of a Met88Val diazepam binding inhibitor (DBI) gene polymorphism and anxiety disorders with panic attacks. *J. Psychiatry Res.* 41:579–584.

Thompson, R.R., George, K., Walton, J.C., Orr, S.P., and Benson, J. (2006) Sex-specific influences of vasopressin on human social communication. *Proc. Natl. Acad. Sci. USA* 103:7889–7894.

Thorsell, A., Carlsson, K., Ekman, R., and Heilig, M. (1999) Behavioral and endocrine adaptation, and up-regulation of NPY expression in rat amygdala following repeated restraint stress. *Neuroreport* 10:3003–3007.

Thorsell, A., Michalkiewicz, M., Dumont, Y., Quirion, R., Caberlotto, L., Rimondini, R., Mathe, A.A., and Helig, M. (2000) Behavioral insensitivity to restraint stress, absent fear suppression of behavior and impaired spatial learning in transgenic rats with hippocampal neuropeptide Y overexpression. *Proc. Natl. Acad. Sci. USA* 97:12852–12857.

Tiihonen, J., Kuikka, J., Bergstrom, K., Lepola, U., Koponen, H., and Leinonen, E. (1997) Dopamine reuptake site densities in patients with social phobia. *Am. J. Psychiatry* 154:239–242.

Tilbrook, A.J., and Clarke, I.J. (2006) Neuroendocrine mechanisms of innate states of attenuated responsiveness of the hypothalamo-pituitary adrenal axis to stress. *Front. Neuroendocrinol.* 27:285–307.

Tomilenko, R.A., and Dubrovina, N.I. (2007) Effects of activation and blockade of NMDA receptors on the extinction of a conditioned passive avoidance response in mice with different levels of anxiety. *Neurosci. Behav. Physiol.* 37:509–515.

Torda, T., Kvetnansky, R., and Petrikova, M. (1984) Effect of repeated immobilization stress on rat central and peripheral adrenoceptors. In: Usdin, E., Kvetnansky, R., and Axelrod, J., eds. *Stress: The Role of Catecholamines and Other Neurotransmitters.* New York: Gordon & Breach, pp. 691–701.

Tõru, I., Shlik, J., Maron, E., Vasar, V., and Nutt, D.J. (2006) Tryptophan depletion does not modify response to CCK-4 challenge in patients with panic disorder after treatment with citalopram. *Psychopharmacology (Berl)* 186:107–112.

Toufexis, D., Davis, C., Hammond, A., and Davis, M. (2005) Sex differences in hormonal modulation of anxiety measured with light-enhanced startle: possible role for arginine vasopressin in the male. *J. Neurosci.* 25:9010–9016.

Tronel, S., and Alberini, C.M. (2007) Persistent disruption of a traumatic memory by postretrieval inactivation of glucocorticoid receptors in the amygdala. *Biol. Psychiatry* 62:33–39.

Uhde, T.W., Berrettini, W.H., Roy-Byrne, P.P., Boulenger, J.P., and Post, R.M. (1987) Platelet 3H-imipramine binding in patients with panic disorder. *Biol. Psychiatry* 22:52–58.

Uhde, T.W., Joffe, R.T., Jimerson, D.C., and Post, R.M. (1988) Normal urinary free cortisol and plasma MHPG in panic disorder: clinical and theoretical implications. *Biol. Psychiatry* 23:575–585.

Unschuld, P.G., Ising, M., Erhardt, A., Lucae, S., Kohli, M., Kloiber, S., Salyakina, D., Thoeringer, C.K., Kern, N., Lieb, R., Uhr, M., Binder, E.B., Müller-Myhsok, B., Holsboer, F., and Keck, M.E. (2008) Polymorphisms in the galanin gene are associated with symptom-severity in female patients suffering from panic disorder. *J. Affect. Disord.* 105:177–184.

Vaiva, G., Boss, V., Ducrocq, F., Fontaine, M., Devos, P., Brunet, A., Laffargue, P., Goudemand, M., and Thomas, P. (2006) Relationship between posttrauma GABA plasma levels and PTSD at 1-year follow-up. *Am. J. Psychiatry* 163:1446–1448.

Vaiva, G., Thomas, P., Ducrocq, F., Fontaine, M., Boss, V., Devos, P., Rascle, C., Cottencin, O., Brunet, A., Laffargue, P., and Goudemand, M. (2004) Low posttrauma GABA plasma levels as a predictive factor in the development of acute posttraumatic stress disorder. *Biol. Psychiatry* 55:250–254.

Valdez, G.R. (2006) Development of CRF1 receptor antagonists as antidepressants and anxiolytics. *CNS Drugs* 20:887–896.

van Den Hout, M.A., and Griez, E. (1984) Panic symptoms after inhalation of carbon dioxide. *Br. J. Psychiatry* 144:503–507.

van der Kolk, B.A., Greenberg, M.S., Orr, S.P., et al. (1981) Endogenous opioids, stress induced analgesia and posttraumatic stress disorder. *Psychopharmacol. Bull.* 25:417–421.

van der Wee, N.J., Fiselier, J., van Megen, H.J., and Westenberg, H.G. (2004) Behavioural effects of rapid intravenous administration of meta-chlorophenylpiperazine in patients with panic disorder and controls. *Eur. Neuropsychopharmacol.* 14:413–417.

van Megen, H.J., Westenberg, H.G., den Boer, J.A., Slaap, B., van Es-Radhakishun, F., and Pande, A.C. (1997) The cholecystokinin-B receptor antagonist CI-988 failed to affect CCK-4 induced symptoms in panic disorder patients. *Psychopharmacology (Berl)* 129:243–248.

van Riel, E., van Gemert, N.G., Meijer, O.C., and Joels, M. (2004) Effect of early life stress on serotonin responses in the hippocampus of young adult rats. *Synapse* 53:11–19.

Van Stegeren, A.H., Everaerd, W., Cahill, L., McGaugh, J.L., and Gooren, L.J. (1998) Memory for emotional events: differential effects of centrally versus peripherally acting beta-blocking agents. *Psychopharmacology (Berl)* 138:305–310.

Van Stegeren, A.H., Goekoop, R., Everaerd, W., Scheltens, P., Barkhof, F., Kuijer, J.P., and Rombouts, S.A. (2005) Noradrenaline mediates amygdala activation in men and women during encoding of emotional material. *NeuroImage* 24:898–909.

Vanover, K.E., Rosenzweig-Lipson, S., Hawkinson, J.E., Lan, N.C., Belluzzi, J.D., Stein, L., Barrett, J.E., Wood, P.L., and Carter, R. B. (2000) Characterization of the anxiolytic properties of a novel neuroactive steroid, Co 2-6749 (GMA-839; WAY-141839; 3alpha, 21-dihydroxy-3beta-trifluoromethyl-19-nor-5beta-pregnan-20-one), a selective modulator of gamma-aminobutyric acid(A) receptors. *J. Pharmacol. Exp. Ther.* 295:337–345.

Varnas, K., Halldin, C., and Hall, H. (2004) Autoradiographic distribution of serotonin transporters and receptor subtypes in human brain. *Hum. Brain Mapp.* 22:246–260.

Ventura, R., Cabib, S., and Puglisi-Allegra, S. (2002) Genetic susceptibility of mesocortical dopamine to stress determines liability to inhibition of mesoaccumbens dopamine and to behavioral despair in a mouse model of depression. *Neuroscience* 115:99–1007.

Verkuyl, J.M., Hemby, S.E., and Joëls, M. (2004) Chronic stress attenuates GABAergic inhibition and alters gene expression of parvocellular neurons in rat hypothalamus. *Eur. J. Neurosci.* 20: 1665–1673.

Vicentic, A., Francis, D., Moffett, M., Lakatos, A., Rogge, G., Hubert, G.W., Harley, J., and Kuhar, M.J. (2006) Maternal separation alters serotonergic transporter densities and serotonergic 1A receptors in rat brain. *Neuroscience* 140:355–365.

Wagatsuma, A., Azami, S., Sakura, M., Hatakeyama, D., Aonuma, H., and Ito, E. (2006) De Novo synthesis of CREB in a presynaptic neuron is required for synaptic enhancement involved in memory consolidation. *J. Neurosci. Res.* 84:954–960.

Wang, C., Marx, C.E., Morrow, A.L., Wilson, W.A., and Moore, S.D. (2007) Neurosteroid modulation of GABAergic neurotransmission in the central amygdala: a role for NMDA receptors. *Neurosci. Lett.* 415:118–123.

Watson, J.B., and Raynor, R. (1920) Conditioned emotional reactions. *J. Exp. Psychol.* 3:1–14.

Watson, S., Gallagher, P., Ferrier, I.N., and Young, A.H. (2006) Post-dexamethasone arginine vasopressin levels in patients with severe mood disorders. *J. Psychiatry Res.* 40:353–359.

Weizman, A., Weizman, R., Kook, K.A., Vocci, F., Deutsch, S.I., and Paul, S.M. (1990) Adrenalectomy prevents the stress-induced decrease in in vivo [^{3}H]Ro 15-1788 binding to GABAA benzodiazepine receptors in the mouse. *Brain Res.* 519:347–350.

Weizman, R., Weizman, A., Kook, K.A., Vocci, F., Deutsch, S.I., and Paul, S.M. (1989) Repeated swim stress alters brain benzodiazepine receptors measured in vivo. *J. Pharmacol. Exp. Ther.* 249: 701–707.

Wierońska, J.M., Szewczyk, B., Pałucha, A., Brański, P., Zieba, B., and Smiałowska, M. (2005) Anxiolytic action of group II and III metabotropic glutamate receptors agonists involves neuropeptide Y in the amygdala. *Pharmacol. Rep.* 57:734–743.

Williams, L.M., Kemp. A.H., Felmingham, K., Barton, M., Olivieri, G., Peduto, A., Gordon, E., and Bryant, R.A. (2006) Trauma modulates amygdala and medial prefrontal responses to consciously attended fear. *Neuroimage* 29:347–357.

Wolf, M. (1991) Plasma methionine enkephalin in PTSD. *Biol. Psychiatry* 29:295–308.

Woods, S.W., Charney, D.S., Silver, J.M., Krystal, J.H., and Heninger, G.R. (1991) Behavioral, biochemical and cardiovascular responses to the benzodiazepine receptor antagonist flumazenil in panic disorder. *Psychiatry Res.* 36:115–124.

Xu, Z.Q., Tong, Y.G., and Hokfelt, T. (2001) Galanin enhances noradrenaline-induced outward current on locus coeruleus noradrenergic neurons. *Neuroreport* 12:1179–1182.

Yang, Y.L., Chao, P.K., Ro, L.S., Wo, Y.Y., and Lu, K.T. (2007) Glutamate NMDA receptors within the amygdala participate in the modulatory effect of glucocorticoids on extinction of conditioned fear in rats. *Neuropsychopharmacology* 32:1042–1051.

Yehuda, R. (2002) Posttraumatic stress disorder. *N. Engl. J. Med.* 346:108–114.

Yehuda, R. (2006) Advances in understanding neuroendocrine alterations in PTSD and their therapeutic implications. *Ann. N. Y. Acad. Sci.* 1071:137–166.

Yehuda, R., Boisoneau, D., Lowy, M.T., and Giller, E.L., Jr. (1995) Dose response changes in plasma cortisol and lymphocyte glucocorticoid receptors following dexamethasone administration in combat veterans with and without posttraumatic stress disorder. *Arch. Gen. Psychiatry* 52:583–593.

Yehuda, R., Brand, S., and Yang, R.K. (2006) Plasma neuropeptide Y concentrations in combat exposed veterans: relationship to trauma exposure, recovery from PTSD, and coping. *Biol. Psychiatry* 59:660–663.

Yehuda, R., Siever, L.J., and Teicher, M.H. (1998) Plasma norepinephrine and 3-methoxy-4-hydroxyphenylglycol concentrations and severity of depression in combat posttraumatic stress disorder and major depressive disorder. *Biol. Psychiatry* 44:56–63.

Yehuda, R., Southwick, S., Giller, E.L., Ma, X., and Mason, J.W. (1992) Urinary catecholamine excretion and severity of PTSD symptoms in Vietnam combat veterans. *J. Nerv. Ment. Dis.* 180: 321-325.

Yeragani, V.K., Berger, R., Pohl, R., Srinivasan, K., Balon, R., Ramesh, C., Weinberg, P., and Berchou, R. (1992) Effects of yohimbine on heart rate variability in panic disorder patients and normal controls. *J. Cardiovasc. Pharmacol.* 20:609–618.

Young, B.R., Lawford, E.P., Noble, B., Kann, A., Wilkie, T., Ritchie, L., Shadforth, A., and Shadforth, S. (2002) Harmful drinking in military veterans with post-traumatic stress disorder: association with the D2 dopamine receptor A1 allele. *Alcohol and Alcoholism* 37:451–456.

Zanoveli, J.M., Netto, C.F., Guimarães, F.S., and Zangrossi, H., Jr. (2004) Systemic and intra-dorsal periaqueductal gray injections of cholecystokinin sulfated octapeptide (CCK-8s) induce a panic-like response in rats submitted to the elevated T-maze. *Peptides* 25:1935–1941.

Zedkova, L., Coupland, N.J., Man, G.C., Dinsa, G., and Sanghera, G. (2003) Panic-related responses to pentagastrin, flumazenil, and thyrotropin-releasing hormone in healthy volunteers. *Depress. Anxiety* 17:78–87.

Zubieta, J.K., Heitzeg, M.M., Smith, Y.R., Bueller, J.A., Xu, K., Xu, Y., Koeppe, R.A., Stohler, C.S., and Goldamn, D. (2003) COMT val met genotype affects m-opioid neurotransmitter response to a pain stressor. *Science* 299:1240–1243.

Zwanzger, P., Eser, D., Padberg, F., Baghai, T.C., Schule, C., Rupprecht, R., di Michele, F., Romeo, E., Pasini, A., and Strohle, A. (2004) Neuroactive steroids are not affected by panic induction with 50 microg cholecystokinin-tetrapeptide (CCK-4) in healthy volunteers. *J. Psychiatry Res.* 38:215–217.

42 The Neurobiology and Treatment of Obsessive–Compulsive Disorder

SUSAN E. SWEDO AND PAUL GRANT

Obsessive–compulsive disorder (OCD) is defined in *Diagnostic and Statistical Manual of Mental Disorders* (*DSM-IV*) by the presence of repetitive, intrusive thoughts and/or compulsions that are felt to be unreasonable or irrational and that interfere significantly with function or cause marked distress (American Psychiatric Association [APA], 1994). There is currently debate over some aspects of the diagnostic criteria—including whether obsessions are inevitably present and what degree of insight is required concerning the irrationality of symptoms. The *DSM-IV* states that compulsions are designed to neutralize or prevent some dreaded event, yet over one third of adults and about 40% of children deny that their compulsions are driven by an obsessive thought (Karno et al., 1988; Swedo et al., 1989). The degree of insight needed for the diagnosis is also in dispute, as some adult patients believe their obsessions, at least some of the time (Insel and Akiskal, 1986; Kozak and Foa, 1994). Eisen and colleagues (1998) developed the Brown Assessment of Beliefs Scale (BABS) to assess insight among patients with OCD and found that 30% had limited insight into their obsessions. The current definition of OCD allows the diagnosis to be made "with poor insight" for an individual who "for most of the time in the current episode, does not recognize that the obsessions or compulsions are excessive or unreasonable" (APA, 1994, p. 419). Children are particularly likely to lack insight into the irrationality of their symptoms, as noted in the *DSM-IV* criteria, which allow the diagnosis to be made in pediatric patients despite a lack of awareness of the irrationality of the symptoms (APA, 1994).

Obsessions commonly involve a preoccupation with contamination, doubting, symmetry, religious or sexual themes, or a premonition that a bad outcome will result if a specific ritual is not executed. Compulsions consist of ritualized behaviors such as washing, cleaning, checking, repeating, counting, arranging, and hoarding. Although compulsions usually involve a physical action, they may also take the form of a mental ritual, such as repeating specific thoughts or prayers. The compulsions may also be tic-like in character and require repetition until the person experiences the "just right" feeling of having eliminated a feeling of disquiet. The "just right" characteristic is one of several symptom clusters that Leckman and colleagues (1997) use to divide OCD into four phenomenological subtypes. The Yale-Brown Obsessive-Compulsive Scale (Y-BOCS) (Goodman et al., 1989) is a useful tool in assessing the presence and severity of obsessions and compulsions, not only because it provides a means of systematic assessment, but also because many patients find it reassuring to see their "crazy" obsessive–compulsive symptoms listed and categorized.

EPIDEMIOLOGY

Obsessive–compulsive disorder was once considered rare, but advances in diagnosis and treatment have led to recognition that the disorder is a major worldwide health problem (Weissman et al., 1994). The Epidemiological Catchment Area (ECA) study of over 18,500 adults at five different sites in the United States (New Haven, Connecticut; Baltimore, Maryland; St. Louis, Missouri; Durham, North Carolina; and Los Angeles, California) was the first large-scale epidemiological study to include OCD as a separate category and to provide information about the incidence and prevalence of the disorder (Robins et al., 1981). Using the Diagnostic Interview Schedule (DIS), a structured interview designed for lay interviewers, lifetime prevalence rates ranging from 1.9%–3.3% were demonstrated at the various sites. Even when other disorders were excluded, the rates were 1.2%–2.4%, approximately 25–60 times greater than had been estimated on the basis of clinical populations (Karno et al., 1988). A recent study conducted in northern Germany found that the lifetime prevalence of OCD in adults aged 18–64 was 0.5% (Grabe et al., 2000). The discrepancy between earlier and more recent estimates is discussed in a report based on Australian National Survey of Mental Heath and Well-Being

(Crino et al., 2005). In that epidemiological survey, the 12-month prevalence of adult OCD was 0.6%, a number attributed to employing *DSM-IV* criteria, rather than the *DSM-III* criteria of earlier surveys. The mean age of onset in the ECA study ranged from 20 to 25 years, with nearly one half of the patients reporting that their symptoms had begun during childhood or adolescence (Karno and Golding, 1990). Subsequent epidemiological studies of children and adolescents have confirmed that the disorder is common in the pediatric population as well, with reported prevalence rates ranging from 0.5% (Wittchen et al., 1998) to 4.0% (Douglass et al., 1995). Several authors have reported the prevalence of OCD among adolescents to be approximately 2%, consistent with adults' reports of symptom onset during childhood or adolescence (reviewed in A.H. Zohar, 1999.)

COMORBIDITY

Comorbid psychopathology is common among patients with OCD. In a recently published study of a large health maintenance organization population in northern California, three fourths of the adults were found to have at least one comorbid psychiatric diagnosis (Fireman et al., 2001). The secondary disorders included major depression (56%), other anxiety disorders (26%; particularly panic disorder, 14%, and generalized anxiety disorder, 14%), and adjustment disorder (12%). Comorbidity was also common among the pediatric patients with OCD, with attention-deficit/hyperactivity disorder (ADHD) occurring most commonly (34%), closely followed by major depression (33%), Tourette syndrome (18%), oppositional defiant disorder (17%), and overanxious disorder (16%) (Fireman et al., 2001). This pattern of comorbidity was similar to that previously observed in the National Institute of Mental Health (NIMH) pediatric OCD cohort, where only 26% of the pediatric patients had OCD as a single diagnosis (Swedo et al., 1989). Tic disorders (30%), major depression (26%), and specific developmental disabilities (24%) were the most common comorbidities found. Rates were also increased for simple phobias (17%), overanxious disorder (16%), adjustment disorder with depressed mood (13%), oppositional disorder (11%), attention deficit disorder (10%), conduct disorder (7%), separation anxiety disorder (7%), and enuresis/encopresis (4%) (Swedo et al., 1989).

It is quite likely that an early onset of OCD is associated with particular phenotypic differences. For example, higher rates of tic-like compulsions and of tics may be seen in adult OCD when the onset was in childhood (Rosario-Campos et al., 2001).

Early investigations suggested that obsessive–compulsive personality disorder (OCPD) might serve as a temperamental predisposition for OCD (Black et al., 1993) or as an alternative manifestation of the disorder (Rasmussen and Tsuang, 1986). These conclusions were brought into question by subsequent studies reporting that the prevalence of compulsive personality disorder in adult patients with OCD was not higher than expected in the community (reviewed by Attiullah et al., 2000.) Baer and colleagues (1990) used the Structured Interview for the DSM-III Personality Disorders (SID-P) to assess personality traits among patients with OCD and found that dependent (12%) and histrionic (9%) personality disorders occurred more frequently than OCPD (6%) among patients with OCD. Further, when individual factors of OCPD were considered, patients with OCD were found to have difficulties with perfectionism (82%) and indecisiveness (70%) more frequently than did healthy controls, but not other OCPD characteristics, such as restricted ability to express warmth (32%), rigidity (32%), and excessive devotion to work (18%) (as cited in Attiullah et al., 2000). A more recent longitudinal study revealed that three of the eight OCPD criteria were significantly more frequent among patients with OCD (n = 89) than among patients without OCD (n = 540 with major depression and/or anxiety disorders) (Eisen et al., 2006). The possibility has been raised that OCPD may develop as a secondary or adaptive response to OCD. Evidence supporting this postulate comes from follow-up evaluations of adolescents diagnosed with OCD in a community survey, a significant proportion of whom no longer met criteria for OCD but did have features of OCPD: rigidity, excessive attention to details, and social isolation, among others (Berg et al., 1989). A study conducted by Ricciardi and colleagues at Harvard (1992) provides additional support for the concept that OCPD may occur as a consequence of OCD rather than as a predictor of disease, as features of OCPD remitted in 9 of 10 patients successfully treated for OCD. This suggests that there may be unique associations between OCD and OCPD symptoms, as compared to other anxiety disorders or to major depression. On the other hand, Albert and colleagues (2004) did not find a specific increase in OCPD among patients with OCD, as those with panic disorder had similarly elevated rates (23% and 17%, respectively), in comparison with healthy controls (3%).

NEUROBIOLOGY

Basal Ganglia Dysfunction

Systematic research over the past two decades has demonstrated that OCD is associated with dysfunction of the corticostriato-thalamocortical circuitry, particularly in the orbitofrontal cortex and caudate nucleus (see Saxena and Rauch, 2000, for review). As shown in Figure 42.1, dysfunction at several different points in the corticostriato-thalamocortical circuit might produce similar neuropsychiatric symptoms.

Evidence for basal ganglia dysfunction is provided by neuroimaging studies (reviewed in Chapter 43) and by the association of OCD with neurological disorders known to involve basal ganglia structures, including Tourette syndrome (TS), Sydenham's chorea (SC; discussed below), and Huntington's chorea (Cummings and Cunningham, 1992). The first description of neurologically based OCD comes from Constantin von Economo's treatise (1931) on postencephalitic Parkinson's disease, wherein patients suffered basal ganglia destruction as a result of severe influenza infections. Von Economo noted the "compulsory nature" of the motor tics and ritual-like behaviors that his patients exhibited. Von Economo's patients, like patients with OCD, described "having to" act, while not "wanting to"—that is, they experienced a neurologically based loss of volitional control.

Motor and vocal tics, including TS, occur frequently in association with OCD. The relationship between tics and OCD is complex, as motor tics often have a behavioral component suggestive of compulsive rituals, whereas OCD compulsions may lack accompanying obsessive thoughts, making them look like tics if the rituals are simple, repetitive behaviors such as touching or tapping. The overlap between tics and OCD is most apparent in pediatric patient populations, where up to two thirds of children with OCD are observed to have comorbid tics (Leonard et al., 1992) and 20%–80% of children with TS report obsessive–compulsive symptoms (Leckman et al., 1997). It is unknown just how the pattern and severity of obsessive–compulsive symptoms differ between patients with TS and those with primary OCD, but preliminary impressions suggest that the compulsions associated with TS may be less severe than those in nontic OCD and more likely to involve symmetry, rubbing, touching, staring, or blinking rituals than washing and cleaning (Leckman et al., 1997).

Indirect evidence for basal ganglia involvement in OCD is provided by the efficacy of psychosurgical lesions that disconnect the basal ganglia from the frontal cortex, particularly capsulotomy (Mindus, 1991) and cingulectomy (Dougherty et al., 2002). In capsulotomy, bilateral basal lesions are made in the anterior limb of the internal capsule to interrupt frontal-cingulate projections; however, the surgical target lies within the striatum, near the caudate nuclei. To perform a cingulectomy, the anterior portion of the cingulate gyrus is lesioned, interrupting tracks between the cingulate gyrus and the frontal lobes and destroying all of the efferent projections of the anterior cingulate cortex. Both procedures result in significant reduction of obsessions and compulsions. The success of psychosurgery is, of course, not conclusive evidence of a basal ganglia defect in OCD, as the lesions could be anywhere upstream from the site of treatment (Fig. 41.1), but it does focus interest on frontal-striatal tracts (for review, see Greenberg et al., 2000).

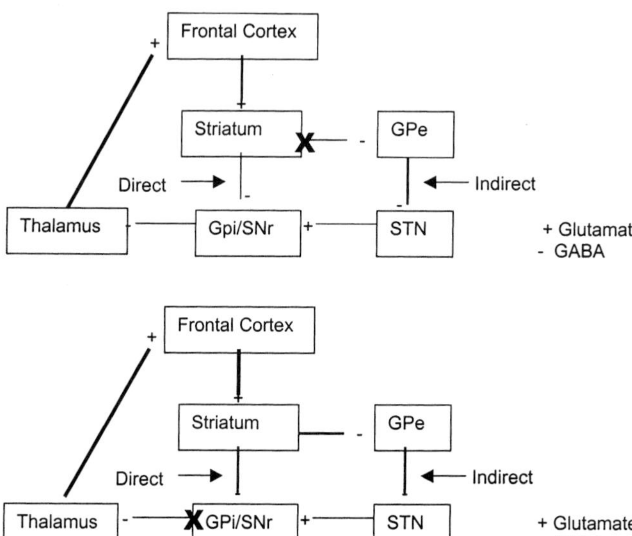

FIGURE 42.1 Models of basal ganglia dysfunction in obsessive–compulsive disorder. A. In this model, the primary area of dysfunction is in the striatum, reducing its inhibition of the globus pallidus externa (GPe) (indirect pathway), which causes the GPe to increase its inhibition of the subthalamic nucleus (STN), thus reducing the STN's stimulation of the globus pallidus interna/substantia nigra (Gpi/SNr) (pars reticulata). This causes a reduction in GPi/SNr inhibition of the thalamus, which then can increase its stimulation of the frontal cortex. B. In this alternative construct, the GPi is the primary site of pathology. Without the GPi's inhibition, the thalamus increases its stimulation of the frontal cortex, which could produce symptoms directly, or through increased stimulation of the striatum.

Neuroimmune Dysfunction

Parallels between SC, the neurological manifestation of rheumatic fever, and childhood-onset OCD suggest that the two disorders may have a shared etiopathogenesis (Garvey et al., 1998). The disorders have similar regional localization, with evidence of dysfunction of the orbitofrontal-striatal circuitry in OCD and SC. Further, over 70% of children with SC report that they experienced an abrupt onset of repetitive, unwanted thoughts and behaviors 2 to 4 weeks prior to the onset of their chorea (Swedo et al., 1993). The obsessions and compulsions peak in intensity concomitantly with the chorea and wane slowly over the ensuing months. A subgroup of patients with childhood-onset OCD was noted to have a similar symptom course. The OCD exacerbations occurred following group A beta-hemolytic streptococcal (GABHS) infections, accompanied by a cluster of comorbid symptoms, including emotional lability, separation anxiety, and attentional difficulties (Swedo et al., 1998). The children were young (6–7 years old at symptom onset), predominantly male, and often had comorbid tics. To indicate their shared clinical features (and presumed etiopathogenesis), the subgroup was identified by the acronym PANDAS—pediatric autoimmune neuropsychiatric disorders associated with streptococcal infections (Swedo et al., 1998).

The major distinguishing feature of the PANDAS subgroup is the temporal association between neuropsychiatric symptom exacerbations and GABHS infections—that is, positive (or rising) antistreptococcal antibody titers or a positive throat culture during neuropsychiatric symptom relapses and evidence of GABHS negativity during periods of remission (Perlmutter et al., 1998). This one-to-one correlation is necessary to distinguish GABHS-triggered exacerbations of the PANDAS subgroup from the more typical waxing and waning course seen in TS and some cases of childhood-onset OCD. The temporal association between GABHS infections and neuropsychiatric symptom exacerbations suggested that prevention of the infections might result in decreased severity of the obsessive-compulsive symptoms. An 8-month-long placebo-controlled crossover trial of penicillin prophylaxis was undertaken (4 months of penicillin followed by 4 months of placebo or vice versa) (Garvey et al., 1999). The penicillin prophylaxis failed to achieve the primary objective of significantly reducing GABHS infections (14 of 35 infections occurred during the penicillin phase), so it was not surprising that there were no between-phase differences in OCD or tic severity. Poor compliance appeared to have contributed to penicillin's lack of effectiveness because missed doses were frequent. This problem was addressed in a trial comparing the effectiveness of penicillin and azithromycin as prophylactic agents, in which data demonstrated a reduction in the number of GABHS infections and neuropsychiatric symptom exacerbations during the study period (Snider et al., 2005).

The role of the immune system in the etiology of OCD and tic disorders is unclear, but clinical observations suggest that symptoms result from a combination of local, regional, and systemic abnormalities (Hamilton et al., 2001). The striking effectiveness of immunomodulatory therapies, such as therapeutic plasma exchange and intravenous immunoglobulin (IVIG), suggests that there is systemic involvement, at least in individuals who are severely affected (Perlmutter et al., 1999). Magnetic resonance imaging (MRI) scans reveal enlargements of the caudate, putamen, and globus pallidus, which points to regional inflammatory changes (Giedd et al., 1996; Giedd et al., 2000), whereas local autoimmune reactions are suggested by the presence of serum antibodies that cross-react with neurons of the caudate, putamen, and globus pallidus (Kiessling et al., 1994). Husby and colleagues (1976) were the first to describe cross-reactive antibodies in SC. Although the antibodies were labeled antineuronal, they noted that the antibodies must have been raised against epitopes on the GABHS bacteria, and then cross-reacted with cells of the caudate nucleus and subthalamus. It was the cross-reactivity that distinguished the antibodies found in the patients with SC from antineuronal antibodies found in patients with lupus erythematosus and other neurological disorders (Husby et al., 1976). Several groups have subsequently reported the presence of antineuronal antibodies in patients with childhood-onset OCD and/or tic disorders (Kiessling et al., 1994; Singer et al., 1998; Morshed et al., 2001). A more specific autoimmune effect has been demonstrated recently. Antibodies found in patients with acute SC reacted with neuronal cells and induced calcium calmodulin–dependent protein kinase II, raising tyrosine hydroxylase, and leading to dopamine (DA) release, possibly accounting for the movement disorder in that syndrome (Kirvan et al., 2006). In the same laboratory, serum from children in the PANDAS subgroup reacted with *N*-acetylglucosamine from GABHS and with human lysoganglioside in a manner parallel to that seen in SC.

The most compelling evidence for a role for immunological dysfunction in the PANDAS subgroup comes from results of a randomized, placebo-controlled trial of IVIG and plasma exchange (Perlmutter et al., 1999). Both immunomodulatory therapies produced significant improvements in neuropsychiatric symptom severity. Placebo IVIG administration had no demonstrable effect on obsessive–compulsive symptoms at 1-month follow-up, whereas IVIG and plasma exchange treatments produced mean symptom reductions of 45% and 58%, respectively. One-year follow-up revealed that 14 of 17 children (82%) continued to be "much" or "very much" improved from baseline (Perlmutter et al., 1999). The effectiveness of the immunomodulatory therapies suggests that circulating immune factors play a role in the pathophysiology of the symptoms, but no specific hypotheses can be formulated on the basis of the treatment response because of the broad spectrum of action of IVIG and plasma exchange.

Neurotransmitter Abnormalities

Serotonin

The serotonergic hypothesis of OCD is based on the selective efficacy of drugs with specific serotonergic activity (Ananth et al., 1981; Insel et al., 1985; DeVeaugh-Geiss et al., 1989) and on challenge tests with serotonergic agonists. Challenges with sumatriptin (Bastani et al., 1990) and metachlorophenylpiperazine (mCPP) (J. Zohar et al., 1987; J. Zohar et al., 1988; Pigott et al., 1991) show that OCD symptoms are exacerbated by these serotonin agonists. In contrast, metergoline, a serotonin antagonist, has been shown to protect against mCPP's behavioral effects (Pigott et al., 1991). Medications that block serotonin reuptake, such as clomipramine and the selective serotonin reuptake inhibitors (SSRIs), fluoxetine, fluvoxamine, sertraline, paroxetine, and citalopram, have been shown to be the most effective pharmacological treatments for OCD (see "Pharmacotherapy"). Clomipramine is a tricyclic antidepressant that is a relatively selective and potent inhibitor of active serotonin uptake in the brain (it also blocks histamine H_2 receptors, and cholinergic and adrenergic receptors and has antidopaminergic properties). Its metabolite, desmethylclomipramine, is also effective in blocking serotonin reuptake (and reuptake of noradrenaline) (Vythilingum et al., 2000). The response of OCD symptoms to clomipramine, and not to the equally effective antidepressant *desipramine* (Ananth et al., 1981; Insel et al., 1985; Leonard et al., 1989), indicates a remarkable specificity of effect of the serotonin uptake inhibitors for OCD. No unselected group of patients with depression, for example, would show such a differential response.

Additional evidence for the serotonergic hypothesis is provided by several studies in children and adolescents with OCD. The first, conducted by Flament et al. (1985; Flament et al., 1987), demonstrated that response to clomipramine correlated with the pretreatment platelet serotonin concentration. A high pretreatment level of serotonin was a strong predictor of a clinical response, and, within this sample, platelet serotonin concentrations were lower in the patients who are more severely ill. However, there were no differences in serotonin concentration from age-/sex-matched controls. A study of cerebrospinal fluid (CSF) monoamines in 43 children and adolescents with OCD revealed that 5-hydroxyindoleacetic acid, the major metabolite of serotonin, correlated most strongly with the response to clomipramine therapy; that is, the most successful responders had the highest levels of 5-hydroxyindoleacetic acid in the CSF (Swedo et al., 1992). A more recent study, employing positron emission tomography (PET) and serotonergic ligands, found evidence for decreased serotonin synthesis in the ventral prefrontal cortex and caudate nucleus in treatment-naive patients with OCD 8 to 13 years of age (Rosenberg et al., 1998). The latter study provides support for the serotonergic hypothesis of OCD and for dysfunction within the basal ganglia–frontal cortex circuitry.

The serotonergic hypothesis is undoubtedly too simple to account for the complexity of OCD (Delgado and Moreno, 1998; Greist and Jefferson, 1998). If the defect were limited to serotonergic dysfunction, clomipramine and the SSRIs would be effective in eliminating symptoms in all patients; unfortunately, this is not the case. Partial treatment response is common in OCD, and up to 40% of patients fail to improve significantly with SSRI administration (Hollander et al., 2000). Individual patients also have variable patterns of response to the different SSRIs, suggesting that the nonserotonergic properties of the medication may also play key roles, and that the antiobsessional effect may actually result from an alteration in the balance of serotonin and other monoamines, and/or changes in receptor functions (Murphy et al., 1989). Support for this hypothesis is provided by the results of meta-analyses demonstrating that clomipramine (a relatively "dirty" drug) is significantly more effective than the SSRIs, fluoxetine, fluvoxamine, and sertraline, in the treatment of OCD (Greist et al., 1995). A meta-analysis of studies of pharmacologic treatment of OCD in children has demonstrated a similar effect (Geller et al., 2003).

Dopamine and other neurotransmitters

Dopaminergic dysfunction in OCD is suggested not only by the obsessive–compulsive symptoms in patients with basal ganglia disorders (discussed above), but also by the increase in obsessive–compulsive symptoms following high-dose stimulant administration (Frye and Arnold, 1981) and by occasional amelioration of symptoms following the use of DA blocking agents (Goodman et al., 1990; McDougle, 1997; Stein et al., 1997). High-dose stimulant administration has been thought to produce simple stereotypies, rather than more complex compulsive or obsessive behavior; however, compulsive symptoms have been observed in children with attention deficit disorder and hyperactivity during treatment with high-dose amphetamines (1 mg/kg d-amphetamine or 2 mg/kg methylphenidate) (Borcherding et al., 1990). For example, a 7-year-old boy spent several hours each evening vacuuming the carpet in his home and another played with Lego blocks for 2 days, stopping only to eat and sleep. As in OCD, the children also became overly concerned with details and produced holes in their papers with repeated erasing, trying to get a single letter perfectly shaped. However, no psychological distress accompanied the obsessive–compulsive behaviors in the stimulant-induced cases, leading to speculation that repetitive thoughts and behaviors (obsessions and compulsions) may result from dopaminergic overactivity and that serotonin dysregulation is required for ego-dystonicity. Observations in TS appear to provide support for this hypothesis. In TS, motor and vocal tics are not reported to be ego-dystonic (although they may become physically uncomfortable) and appear to result from dopaminergic overactivity overcoming serotonergic inhibition. Some direct support is found in one study in which single photon emission computed tomography (SPECT) scans demonstrated increased DA transporter in left caudate and left putamen nuclei in adult drug-naïve patients with OCD (van der Wee et al., 2004). In contrast, OCD is primarily a serotonergic defect. Here, a primary lack of serotonin results in an inability to inhibit normal dopaminergic activity, and fixed action patterns (obsessions and compulsions) are inappropriately released. Ego-dystonicity could then be related to the primary serotonin defect or could be secondary to the loss of volitional control (Swedo and Rapoport, 1990).

Glutamate, the primary excitatory neurotransmitter in the brain, plays a key role at several points in the frontostriatal-thalamocortical circuit. Glutamatergic excess (relative or absolute) could contribute to OCD symptomatology through a variety of mechanisms. Evidence for a glutamatergic excess in the pathophysiology of OCD is found in a recent report in which CSF had significantly higher glutamate levels in drug-naïve adult patients with clinically significant OCD compared to controls (Chakrabarty et al., 2005). Additional support is provided by an open label trial of riluzole, a relative glutamate antagonist, which demonstrated benefits for five of 13 patients with OCD (Coric et al., 2005). These therapeutic effects in OCD are postulated to result from a reduction in frontal cortical (excitatory) output to the striatum, which would reduce the striatal inhibition of the globus pallidus and substantia nigra, and allow greater inhibition of the thalamus and less cortical excitation. McGrath and colleagues (2000) postulated effectiveness of similar compounds in a mouse model of TS and OCD.

Neuroendocrine Dysfunction

Although most OCD investigations concentrate on hormonal aberrations as secondary rather than primary to the disorder, case reports and anecdotal experience suggest that hormonal dysfunction and OCD may be etiologically related (Swedo, 1989). Symptoms of OCD often begin during early puberty, and some female patients experience an increase in obsessive thoughts and rituals immediately before their menses. Other hints at an influence of gonadal steroid on obsessive–compulsive symptomatology include the increased frequency of OCD during the postpartum period (Rasmussen and Eisen, 1992) and reports of successful antiandrogen therapy for obsessive–compulsive symptoms (Casas et al., 1986). In the latter study, five of five patients with OCD experienced a remission in their symptoms following treatment with cyproterone acetate, a potent antiandrogen. At the NIMH, two boys (aged 8 and 15) and a 14-year-old girl were treated with spironolactone, a peripheral antiandrogen, with antitesterone effects and testolactone, a peripheral antiestrogen medication. All experienced a temporary reduction of obsessions and compulsions but relapsed within 3–4 months (Salzberg and Swedo, 1992).

Leckman and colleagues (1994) suggested that oxytocin abnormalities may be involved in OCD. These investigators cited oxytocin-mediated mating behaviors in animals as a possible model for some OCD symptoms (Leckman and Mayes, 1999) and found abnormal concentrations of CSF oxytocin among a small group of children with OCD and tic disorders. In a larger group of 43 children and adolescents studied at the NIMH (Swedo et al., 1992; Altemus et al., 1994), CSF oxytocin levels were not significantly correlated with OCD severity but were correlated with depressive symptoms. Interestingly, arginine vasopressin (AVP) concentrations were inversely related to OCD severity (Swedo et al., 1992) but decreased following treatment with clomipramine (Altemus et al., 1994). Altemus et al. (1992) found significantly increased CSF AVP concentrations at baseline among adult patients with OCD and noted that patients secreted significantly more AVP into plasma in response to hypertonic saline than did controls. The latter results are in keeping with Barton's (1987) observations of OCD among patients with diabetes insipidus, a disorder with elevated central AVP concentrations.

At present, there is not sufficient evidence to implicate hormonal dysfunction as a direct cause of OCD. However, some intriguing data build a circumstantial case for an association between OCD and growth hormone abnormalities, perhaps through the serotonergic system. In an epidemiological study of OCD among high school students (Flament et al., 1988), males with OCD were noted to be smaller and thinner than the community normal controls and males with other psychiatric illnesses (Hamburger et al., 1989). There were no reductions in the height or weight of the adolescent girls with OCD. The small size of the OCD males could be due to an effective lack of growth hormone or to a delay in the pubertal growth spurt, although, of course, no causality is demonstrated by the relationship. To address the issue of causality, future research might employ direct assays, hormonal challenges, or therapeutic interventions.

TREATMENT OF OBSESSIVE–COMPULSIVE DISORDER

The treatment of OCD requires an integrated approach, as it is unusual for patients to respond fully to either cognitive-behavior therapy (CBT) or medications. A combination of behavioral and pharmacological approaches provides the maximum benefit for most patients. Obsessive–compulsive disorder is a chronic condition, and long-term therapy is often required, although lower medication doses may suffice (Ravizza et al., 1998). Discontinuation studies have shown that 80% of patients relapsed by the 2-year follow-up (Dolberg et al., 1996), although the rate was somewhat lower among patients receiving concomitant CBT (Stanley and Turner, 1995). When discontinuation is attempted, tapering should be gradual, usually over several weeks. Long-term (that is, indefinite) drug maintenance is suggested after two to four relapses.

Cognitive-Behavioral Therapy

Cognitive-behavioral therapy for OCD encompasses three treatment types: (*1*) exposure and response prevention (ERP), (*2*) cognitive therapy, and (*3*) relaxation training. Of the three, only ERP has been shown to be consistently effective in reducing OCD symptom severity (Baer and Greist, 1997; Marks, 1997; Shafran, 1998). Cognitive therapy (for example, changing false beliefs regarding risk and responsibility, challenging the reality of obsessions and the necessity for compulsions; Emmelkamp and Beens, 1991) is generally viewed as ineffective if used as the sole treatment for OCD, but it may be helpful for patients with overvalued ideation (Neziroglu et al., 2000), and if it facilitates participation in ERP (Shafron and Somers, 1998). Relaxation therapy is used mainly to manage anxiety during exposure (March, 1995), but it has no direct benefits for the obsessive–compulsive symptoms.

Exposure and response prevention for OCD involves (*1*) daily exposure to cues avoided because of their inducing discomfort and rituals and (*2*) maintaining exposure and not ritualizing for at least an hour or until the discomfort slowly subsides (March, 1995; Greist, 1996). A minimal trial of ERP consists of 10–20 hours of treatment with ERP (Baer and Greist, 1997), with in vivo exposure being preferred over imaginal exposure (Foa et al., 1985). The strategies employed must be tailored to the patient's symptoms. For example, contamination fears, symmetry rituals, counting/repeating, hoarding, and aggressive urges are amenable to ERP, but the technique is not generally appropriate for pathological doubting or pure obsessions such as scrupulosity or violent images. Obsessional slowness is difficult to treat with either behavioral therapy or medications (Wolff and Rapoport, 1988). Exposure with response prevention can have lasting benefits and long-term symptom remissions are possible, particularly when booster sessions are used to address migration of symptoms and relapses brought on by stress (Greist, 1996).

Therapist-directed ERP has been shown to be the most effective means of treating OCD (Abramowitz, 1998). However, the shortage of trained therapists and the expense of therapist-directed ERP have mandated the development of alternative strategies. Several self-help programs for behavior therapy have been developed, including computer- and telephone-administered programs (e.g., Baer and Greist, 1997; Clark et al., 1998). Manualized approaches have also proven successful for adults (Van Noppen et al., 1997) and pediatric patients (March et al., 1994; March and Mulle, 1998). Cognitive behavioral group therapy has also been demonstrated to be effective (Sousa et al., 2006). In general, ERP appears to confer similar benefits in the pediatric population as it does for adults (March et al., 2001). The child must be old enough to understand fully the goals and requirements of treatment and to tolerate the discomforts inherent to exposure (see March et al., 2001, for more details.) There is recent evidence that the combination of CBT and medication may have greater clinical efficacy in adults and children (March et al., 2004; O'Connor et al., 2006).

Pharmacotherapy

A serotonin reuptake inhibitor (SRI), most often an SSRI, is the drug treatment of choice for OCD. If there is an insufficient response to the SSRI at 10–12 weeks, another SSRI may be tried. Although only 50%–60% of patients respond to initial SSRI treatment, approximately 70%–80% will have at least a partial response to at least one of the SSRIs. To date, no baseline predictors of treatment response have been identified. Augmentation with other agents may be helpful for partial responders, particularly when comorbid tics are present (McDougle, 1997).

Serotonin reuptake inhibitors

Clomipramine was the first SRI antidepressant to be shown to be effective for OCD (Clomipramine Collaborative Study Group, 1991), with subsequent controlled trials documenting antiobsessional effects of the SSRIs (in order of increasing selectivity: fluoxetine, fluvoxamine, sertraline, paroxetine, and citalopram). All have been shown to be effective in multicenter double-blind trials (see Vythilingum et al., 2000, for a review of adult studies; Rapoport and Inoff-Germain, 2000, for a review of pediatric studies.)

Table 42.1 gives the dosage ranges of the SRIs for treatment of adult and pediatric patients, as well as the half-life of the compounds (Montgomery et al., 2001). To avoid difficulties with adverse effects, it is advisable to "start low, go slow," initiating therapy with low dosages and titrating upward slowly over a period of a few weeks. Patients should be warned that the medications take time to work and that an adequate trial is usually at least 10 weeks in duration (at the maximally tolerated dosage). Patients should also be told that trials of more than one agent or use of augmenting agents may be required.

Recent research in adults (e.g., Sallee et al., 1998), including one placebo-controlled study (Fallon et al., 1998), indicates that intravenous administration of clomipramine speeds the initial response and increases response rates (even among previously nonresponsive patients). The hypothesized mechanism involves the greater bioavailability of the more serotonergic parent

TABLE 42.1 *Serotonin Reuptake Inhibitor Treatment of Obsessive–Compulsive Disorder*

Drug	*Adult Dosage*	*Child/Adolescent Dosage*	*Half-Life*
Clomipramine 24 hours	Up to 250 mg/day	Controlled trials for patients aged 6 years 3 mg/kg (max. 250 mg)	12–
Fluoxetine 96 hours	Up to 80 mg/day (NorFLX, 7–10 days)	Controlled trials for patients aged 8 years 2.5–80 mg	48–
Fluvoxamine 24 hours	Up to 300 mg/day	Indicated for patients aged 8 years 50–200 mg/day	12–
Sertraline 24 hours	Up to 200 mg/day	Indicated for patients aged 6 years 25–200 mg/day	12–
Paroxetine hours	Up to 60 mg/day	Open trial in 8- to 17-year-olds No pediatric indications	24
Citalopram hours	Up to 60 mg/day (indicated for open trial in 9- to 18-year-olds treatment of depression, not OCD)	No pediatric indications	35

OCD: Obsessive–compulsive disorder.

compound, clomipramine, versus the more noradrenergic metabolite, desmethylclomipramine, as a result of bypassing first-pass hepatoenteric metabolism. Following the initial intravenous infusion, clomipramine therapy is maintained orally. Experience in pediatric patients is limited, but two open trials and two placebo-controlled cases suggest that intravenous clomipramine may offer therapeutic benefits to children as well (Sallee et al., 1998).

Other medications

Clonazepam is a benzodiazepine with anxiolytic properties and serotonergic effects (Pigott, L'Heureux, Rubenstein, et al., 1992; Park et al., 1997). Pigott, L'Heureux, Rubenstein, and colleagues (1992) found significant improvement on one of three ratings of OCD severity when clonazepam (3–4 mg/day) was added to ongoing fluoxetine or clomipramine therapy. A case report of pediatric efficacy has also been published (Leonard et al., 1994).

Venlafaxine, a serotonin-norepinephrine reuptake inhibitor, has demonstrated efficacy equal to that of the SRI paroxetine in a double-blind comparison with 75 patients in each arm of the study (Denys et al., 2003).

Buspirone is a partial agonist of the 5-hydroxytryptamine-1A (5-HT_{1A}) receptor and appears to enhance serotonergic neurotransmission. Open trials had suggested benefit from buspirone augmentation of SSRIs, but placebo-controlled trials failed to demonstrate significant benefits when buspirone was added to clomipramine (Pigott, L'Heureux, Hill, et al., 1992), fluvoxamine (McDougle et al., 1993), or fluoxetine therapy (Grady et al., 1993).

Neuroleptics, such as haloperidol, have been shown to be useful as augmenting agents, particularly in cases with comorbid tic disorders. McDougle and colleagues (1994) demonstrated significant improvements when haloperidol (mean dose 6.2 +/–3.0 mg/day) was added to fluvoxamine therapy. Eleven of 17 (65%) patients randomized to receive haloperidol responded to therapy, while none of the 17 patients receiving placebo had significant treatment gains. Further, eight of eight patients with comorbid tics had a significant reduction in OCD symptom severity (McDougle et al., 1994). Pediatric experience with haloperidol has been limited in OCD, although it is used frequently in children and adolescents with tic disorders (Leckman et al., 1997). Pimozide was noted to be of significant benefit among 9 of 17 patients previously nonresponsive to fluvoxamine therapy (McDougle et al., 1990). Because of the long-term risks of tardive dyskinesias occurring with neuroleptic administration, these drugs should be considered only if atypical antipsychotics are ineffective.

Risperidone is an atypical antipsychotic medication with demonstrated benefits as an augmenting agent in OCD. Saxena and colleagues (1996) treated 16 patients with a combination of risperidone and SSRI and found that 14 (87%) had a significant reduction in OCD severity within 3 weeks of the addition of risperidone. Of particular interest, given the treatment-refractory nature of violent obsessive images, patients with this symptom were most likely to respond and to demonstrate significant benefits after only a few days of augmentation

(Saxena et al., 1996). Lombroso and colleagues (1995) found that risperidone augmentation of paroxetine or sertraline was effective for pediatric patients with comorbid OCD and tic disorders.

Riluzole was used successfully to augment other pharmacotherapy in an adult patient who had failed treatment with prior regimens for his severe and refractory OCD and major depressive disorder (Coric et al., 2003). There have also been case reports of benefit of riluzole for a patient with chronic skin-picking as well as an eating disorder (Sasso et al., 2006) and in a patient with self-injurious behavior (Pittenger et al., 2005). To our knowledge, there have been no reports of the use of riluzole for the treatment of children and adolescents with OCD. But in an open-label study in our own laboratory, six young people (ages 8–16) took riluzole up to 60 mg twice a day for 12 weeks. Four patients were considered "responders" and have elected to discontinue other medications and continue taking riluzole (Grant et al., 2007) Two other patients did not have significant symptom improvement but have elected to remain on riluzole therapy. Of the two nonresponders, one was female—of possible importance, given the recent finding of significant association of a gene, which codes for an excitatory amino acid carrier, with early onset OCD in male (but not female) patients (Arnold et al., 2006; Dickel et al., 2006).

A number of other drugs (namely, *N*-acetylcysteine, psilocin, morphine, inositol, sumatriptan) have seemed to show promise in individual cases, but published controlled trials are not yet available.

SUMMARY

Obsessive–compulsive disorder is a chronic disabling condition that often has its onset during childhood. The neurobiological basis for the disorder is unknown but appears to involve dysregulation of frontostriatal-thalamocortical circuitry and the serotonergic system. Cognitive-behavior therapy and serotonin-reuptake inhibiting medications have been shown to be effective treatments for OCD, particularly when used in combination. Further research is needed to better define the clinical characteristics of OCD, as well as to delineate its etiology and pathophysiology.

REFERENCES

Abramowitz, J.S. (1998) Does cognitive-behavioral therapy cure obsessive-compulsive disorder? A meta-analytic evaluation of clinical significance. *Behav. Ther.* 29:339–355.

Albert, U., Maina, G., Forner, F., and Bogetto, F. (2004) DSM-IV obsessive-compulsive personality disorder: prevalence in patients with anxiety disorders and in healthy comparison subjects. *Compr. Psychiatry* 45:325–332.

Altemus, M., Pigott, T., Kalogeras, K.T., Demitrack, M., Dubbert, B., Murphy, D.L., and Gold, P.W. (1992) Abnormalities in the regulation of vasopressin and corticotropin releasing factor secretion in obsessive-compulsive disorder. *Arch. Gen. Psychiatry* 49:9–20.

Altemus, M., Swedo, S.E., Leonard, H.L., Richter, D., Rubinow, D.R., Potter, W.Z., and Rapoport, J.L. (1994) Changes in cerebrospinal fluid neurochemistry during treatment of obsessive-compulsive disorder with clomipramine. *Arch. Gen. Psychiatry* 51:794–803.

American Psychiatric Association. (1994) *Diagnostic and Statistical Manual of Mental Disorders*, 4th ed. Washington, DC: Author.

Ananth, J., Pecknold, J., van Den Steen, N., and Engelsmann, F. (1981) Double-blind comparative study of clomipramine and amitryptyline in obsessive neurosis. *Prog. Neuropsychopharmacol. Biol. Psychiatry* 5:257–262.

Arnold, P.D., Sicard, T., Burrougs, E., Richter, M.A., and Kennedy, J.L. (2006) Glutamate transporter gene slc1a1 associated with obsessive-compulsive disorder. *Arch. Gen. Psychiatry* 63:769–776.

Attiullah, N., Eisen, J.L., and Rasmussen, S.A. (2000) Clinical features of obsessive-compulsive disorder. *Psychiatr. Clin. North Am.* 23(3):469–491.

Baer L., and Greist, J.H. (1997) An interactive computer-administered self-assessment and self-help program for behavior therapy. *J. Clin. Psychiatry* 58(Suppl 12):23–28.

Baer, L., Jenike, M.A., Ricciardi, J.N., et al. (1990) Standardized assessment of personality disorders in obsessive-compulsive disorder. *Arch. Gen. Psychiatry* 47:826–830.

Barton, R. (1987) Diabetes insipidus and obsessional neurosis. *Adv. Biochem. Psychopharmacol.* 43:347–349.

Bastani, B., Nash, J.F., and Meltzer, H.Y. (1990) Prolactin and cortisol responses to MK-212, a serotonin agonist, in obsessive-compulsive disorder. *Arch. Gen. Psychiatry* 47:833–839.

Berg, C.Z., Rapoport, J.L., Whitaker, A., Davies, M., Leonard, H., Swedo, S.E., et al. (1989) Childhood obsessive compulsive disorder: a two-year prospective follow-up of a community sample. *J. Am. Acad. Child Adolesc. Psychiatry* 28:528–533.

Black, D., Noyes, R., Pfohl, B., et al. (1993) Personality disorder in obsessive-compulsive volunteers, well comparison subjects and their first-degree relatives. *Am. J. Psychiatry* 150:1226–1232.

Borcherding, B., Keysor, C., Rapoport, J.L., Elia, J., and Amass, J. (1990) Motor vocal tics and compulsive behaviors on stimulant drugs: is there a common vulnerability? *Psychiatry Res.* 33: 83–94.

Casas, M.E., Alvarez, P., Duro, C., Garcia Ribera, C., Udina, C., Velat, A., et al. (1986) Antiandrogenic treatment of obsessive compulsive disorder neurosis. *Acta Psychiatr. Scand.* 73:221–222.

Chakrabarty, K., Bhattacharyya, S., Khanna, S., and Christopher, R. (2005) Glutamatergic dysfunction on OCD. *Neuropsychopharmacology* 30:1735–1740.

Clark, A., Kirby, K.C., Daniels, B.A., and Marks, I.M. (1998) A pilot study of computer-aided vicarious exposure for obsessive-compulsive disorder. *Aust. NZ J. Psychiatry* 32:268–275.

Clomipramine Collaborative Study Group. (1991) Clomipramine in the treatment of patients with obsessive-compulsive disorder. *Arch. Gen. Psychiatry* 43:730–738.

Coric, V., Milanovic, S., Wasylink, S., Patel, P., Malison, R., Krystal, J.H. (2003) Beneficial effects of the antiglutamatergic agent riluzole in a patient diagnosed with obsessive-compulsive disorder and major depressive disorder. *Psychopharmacology* 167:219–220.

Coric, V., Taskiran, S., Pittenger, C., Wasylink, S., Mathalon, D.H., Valentine, G., Saksa, J., Wu, Y., Gueorguieva, R., Sanacora, G., Malison, R., and Krystal, J.H. (2005) Riluzole augmentation in treatment-resistant obsessive-compulsive disorder: an open-label trial. *Biol. Psychiatry* 58:424–428.

Crino, R., Slade, T., and Andrews, G. (2005) The changing prevalence and severity of obsessive-compulsive disorder criteria from DSM-III to DSM-IV. *Am. J. Psychiatry* 162:876–882.

Cummings, J.L., and Cunningham, K. (1992) Obsessive-compulsive disorder in Huntington's disease. *Biol. Psychiatry* 31:263–270.

Delgado, P.L., and Moreno, F.A. (1998) Different roles for serotonin in anti-obsessional drug action and the pathophysiology of obsessive-compulsive disorder. *Br. J. Psychiatry* 173(Suppl 35):21–25.

Denys, D.A., van der Wee, N., Van Megen, H.J., and Westenberg, H.M. (2003) A double blind comparison of venlafaxine and paroxetine in obsessive-compulsive disorder. *J. Clin. Psychopharmacology* 23:568–575.

DeVeaugh-Geiss, J., Landau, P., and Katz, R. (1989) Treatment of obsessive-compulsive disorder with clomipramine. *Psychiatry Ann.* 19:97–101.

Dickel, D.E., Veenstr-Vanderweele, J., Cox, N.J., Wu, X., Fischer, D.J., Van Etten-Lee, M., Himle, J.A., Leventhal, B.L., Cook, J.E., Hanna, G.L. (2006) Association testing of the positional and functional candidate gene slc1a1/eaac1 in early-onset obsessive-compulsive disorder. *Arch. Gen. Psychiatry* 63:778–785.

Dolberg, O.T., Iancu, I., and Zohar, J. (1996) Treatment duration of obsessive compulsive disorder. *Eur. Psychiatry* 11:403–406.

Dougherty, D.D., Baer, L., Cosgrove, G.R., Cassem, E.H., Price, B.H., Nierenberg, A.A., Jenike, M.A., and Rauch, S.L. (2002) Prospective long-term follow-up of 44 patients who received cingulotomy for treatment refractory obsessive-compulsive disorder. *Am. J. Psychiatry* 159(2):269–275.

Douglass, H.M., Moffitt, T.E., Dar, R., et al. (1995) Obsessive-compulsive disorder in a birth cohort of 18 year olds: prevalence and predictors. *J. Am. Acad. Child Adolesc. Psychiatry* 34:1424–1431.

Eisen, J.L., Coles, M.E., Shea, M.T., Pagano, M.E., Stout, R.L., Yen, S., Grilo, C.M., and Rasmussen, S.A. (2006) Clarifying the convergence between obsessive-compulsive personality disorder criteria and obsessive-compulsive disorder. *J. Personality Disord.* 20:294–305.

Eisen, J.L., Phillips, K.A., Rasmussen, S.A., et al. (1998) The Brown Assessment of Beliefs Scale (BABS): reliability and validity. *Am. J. Psychiatry* 155:102–108.

Emmelkamp, P.M., and Beens, H. (1991) Cognitive therapy with obsessive-compulsive disorder: a comparative evaluation. *Behav. Res. Ther.* 29:293–300.

Fallon, B.A., Liebowitz, M.R., Campeas, R., Schneier, F.R., Marshall, R., Davies, S., et al. (1998) Intravenous clomipramine for obsessive-compulsive disorder refractory to oral clomipramine. A placebo controlled study. *Arch. Gen. Psychiatry* 55:918–924.

Fireman, B., Koran, L.M., Leventhal, J.L., and Jacobson, A. (2001) The prevalence of clinically recognized obsessive-compulsive disorder in a large health maintenance organization. *Am. J. Psychiatry* 158:1904–1910.

Flament, M.F., Rapoport, J.L., Berg, C.J., Sceery, W., Kilts, C., Mellstrom, B., et al. (1985) Clomipramine treatment of childhood compulsive disorder: a double-blind controlled study. *Arch. Gen. Psychiatry* 42:977–983.

Flament, M.F., Rapoport, J.L., Murphy, D.L., Berg, C.J., and Lake, R. (1987) Biochemical changes during clomipramine treatment of childhood obsessive compulsive disorder. *Arch. Gen. Psychiatry* 44:219–225.

Flament, M.F., Whitaker, A., Rapoport, J., Davis, M., Berg, C.Z., Kalikow, K., et al. (1988) Obsessive compulsive disorder in adolescence: an epidemiological study. *J. Am. Acad. Child Adolesc. Psychiatry* 27:764–771.

Foa, E.B., Steketee, G.S., and Grayson, J.B. (1985) Imaginal and in vivo exposure: a comparison with obsessive-compulsive checkers. *Behav. Ther.* 16:292–303.

Frye, P., and Arnold, L. (1981) Persistent amphetamine-induced compulsive rituals: response to pyridoxine (B_6). *Biol. Psychiatry* 16:583–587.

Garvey, M.A., Giedd, J., and Swedo, S.E. (1998) PANDAS: the search for environmental triggers of pediatric neuropsychiatric disorders. Lessons from rheumatic fever. *J. Child. Neurol.* 13(9): 413–423.

Garvey, M.A., Perlmutter, S.J., Allen, A.J., Hamburger, S., Lougee, L., Leonard, H.L., Witowski, M.E., Dubbert, B., and Swedo, S.E. (1999) A pilot study of penicillin prophylaxis for neuropsychiatric exacerbations triggered by streptococcal infections. *Biol. Psychiatry* 45:1564–1571.

Geller, D., Biederman, J., Stewart, S.E., Mullen, B., Martin, A., Spencer, T., and Faraone, S.V. (2003) Which SSRI? a meta-analysis of pharmacotherapy trials in pediatric obsessive-compulsive disorder. *Am. J. Psychiatry* 160:1919–1928.

Giedd, J.N., Rapoport, J.L., Garvey, M.A., Perlmutter, S., and Swedo, S.E. (2000) MRI assessment of children with obsessive-compulsive disorder or tics associated with streptococcal infection. *Am. J. Psychiatry* 157:281–283.

Giedd, J.N., Rapoport, J.L., Leonard, H.L., Richter, D., and Swedo, S.E. (1996) Case study: acute basal ganglia enlargement and obsessive-compulsive symptoms in an adolescent boy. *J. Am. Acad. Child Adolesc. Psychiatry* 35:913–915.

Goodman, W.K., McDougle, C.J., Price, L.H., Riddle, M.A., Pauls, D.L., and Leckman, J.F. (1990) Beyond the serotonin hypothesis: a role for dopamine in some forms of obsessive compulsive disorder? *J. Clin. Psychiatry* 51(Suppl):36–43.

Goodman, W.K., Price, L.H., Rasmussen, S.A., et al. (1989) The Yale-Brown Obsessive-Compulsive Scale: I. Development, use and reliability. *Arch. Gen. Psychiatry* 46:1006–1011.

Grabe, H.J., Meyer, C.H., Hapke, U., et al. (2000) Prevalence, quality of life and psychosocial function in obsessive-compulsive disorder and subclinical obsessive-compulsive disorder in northern Germany. *Eur. Arch. Psychiatry Clin. Neurosci.* 250:262–268.

Grady, T.A., Pigott, T.A., L'Heureux, F., Hill, J.L., Bernstein, S.E., and Murphy, D.L. (1993) Double-blind study of adjuvant buspirone for fluoxetine-treated patients with obsessive-compulsive disorder. *Am. J. Psychiatry* 150:819–821.

Grant, P., Lougee L., Hirschtritt, M., and Swedo, S.E. (2007) An open-label trial of riluzole, a glutamate antagonist, in children with treatment-resistant obsessive-compulsive disorder. *J. Child Adolesc. Psychopharmacology* 17(6): 761–767.

Greenberg, B.D., Murphy, D.L., and Rasmussen, S.A. (2000) Neuroanatomically based approaches to obsessive-compulsive disorder. *Psychiatry Clin. North Am.* 23(3):671–686.

Greist, J.H. (1996) New developments in behaviour therapy for obsessive-compulsive disorder. *Int. Clin. Psychopharmacol.* 11(Suppl 5): 63–73.

Greist, J.H., and Jefferson, J.W. (1998) Pharmacotherapy for obsessive-compulsive disorder. *Br. J. Psychiatry* 173(Suppl 35):64–70.

Greist, J.H., Jefferson, J.W., Kobak, K.A., et al. (1995) Efficacy and tolerability of serotonin transport inhibitors in obsessive-compulsive disorder: a meta-analysis. *Arch. Gen. Psychiatry* 52:53–60.

Hamburger, S.D., Swedo, S., Whitaker, A., Davies, M., and Rapoport, J.L. (1989) Growth rate in adolescents with obsessive-compulsive disorder. *Am. J. Psychiatry* 146:652–655.

Hamilton, C.S., Garvey, M.A., and Swedo, S.E. (2001) Therapeutic implications of immunology for tics and obsessive-compulsive disorder. In: Cohen, D.J., Goetz, C.G., and Jankovic, J., eds. *Tourette Syndrome*. Philadelphia: Lippincott, Williams & Wilkins, pp. 311–318.

Hollander, E., Kaplan, A., Allen, A., and Cartwright, C. (2000) Pharmacotherapy for obsessive-compulsive disorder. *Psychiatr. Clin. North Am.* 23(3):643–656.

Husby, G., Van de Rijn, I., Zabriskie, J.B., Abdin, Z.H., and Williams, R.C. (1976) Antibodies reacting with cytoplasm of subthalamic and caudate nuclei neurons in chorea and acute rheumatic fever. *J. Exp. Med.* 144:1094–1110.

Insel, T.R., and Akiskal, H.S. (1986) Obsessive-compulsive disorder with psychotic features: a phenomenologic analysis. *Am. J. Psychiatry* 143:1527–1533.

Insel, T.R., Mueller, E.A., Alterman, I., Linnoila, M.M., and Murphy, D.L. (1985) Obsessive-compulsive disorder and serotonin: is there a connection? *Biol. Psychiatry* 20:1174–1188.

Karno, M., and Golding, J. (1990) Obsessive compulsive disorder. In: Robins, L., and Regier D.A., eds. *Psychiatric Disorders in America: The Epidemiological Catchment Area Study*. New York: Free Press, pp. 204-209.

Karno, M., Golding, J., Sorenson, S., and Burnam, A. (1988) The epidemiology of obsessive compulsive disorder in five U.S. communities. *Arch. Gen. Psychiatry* 45:1094–1099.

Kiessling, L.S., Marcotte, A.C., and Culpepper, L. (1994) Antineuronal antibodies: tics and obsessive-compulsive symptoms. *J. Dev. Behav. Pediatr.* 15:421–425.

Kirvan, C.A., Swedo, S., Kurahara, D., and Cunningham, M.W. (2006) Streptococcal mimicry and antibody-mediated cell signaling in the pathogenesis of Sydenham's chorea. *Autoimmunity* 39:21–29.

Kozak, M.J., and Foa, E.B. (1994) Obsessions, overvalued ideas and delusions in obsessive-compulsive disorder. *Behav. Res. Ther.* 32:343–353.

Leckman, J.F., and Mayes, L.C. (1999) Preoccupations and behaviors associated with romantic and Parental love: Perspectives on the origin of obsessive-compulsive disorder. *Child Adolesc. Psychiatr. Clin. North Am.* 8(3):635–665.

Leckman, J.F., Goodman, W.K., North, W.G., Chappell, P.B., Price, L.H., Pauls, D.L., et al. (1994) The role of central oxytocin in obsessive compulsive disorder and related normal behavior. *Psychoneuroendocrinology* 19:723–749.

Leckman, J.F., Grice, D.E., Boardman, J., Zhang, H., Vitale, A., Bondi, C., et al. (1997) Symptoms of obsessive-compulsive disorder. *Am. J. Psychiatry* 154(7):911–917.

Leonard, H.L., Lenane, M.C., Swedo, S.E., Rettew, D.C., Gershon, E.S., and Rapoport, J.L. (1992) Tics and Tourette's disorder: a 2-to 7-year follow-up of 54 obsessive-compulsive children. *Am. J. Psychiatry* 149:1244–1251.

Leonard, H.L., Swedo, S., Rapoport, J., Koby, E., Lenane, M., Cheslow, D., et al. (1989) Treatment of childhood obsessive compulsive disorder with clomipramine and desmethylimipramine: a double-blind crossover comparison. *Arch. Gen. Psychiatry* 46: 1088–1092.

Leonard, H.L., Topol, D., Bukstein, O., Hindmarsh, D., Allen, A.J., and Swedo, S.E. (1994) Clonazepam as an augmenting agent in the treatment of childhood-onset obsessive-compulsive disorder. *J. Am. Acad. Child Adolesc. Psychiatry* 33:792–794.

Lombroso, P.J., Scahill, L., King, R.A., Lynch, K.A., Chappell, P.B., Peterson, B.S., et al. (1995) Risperidone treatment of children and adolescents with chronic tic disorders: a preliminary report. *J. Am. Acad. Child Adolesc. Psychiatry* 34:1147–1152.

March, J., et al. (2004) Cognitive-behavioral therapy, sertraline, and their combination for children and adolescents with obsessive-compulsive disorder. the POTS Randomized Controlled Trial. *JAMA* 292:1969–1976.

March, J.S. (1995) Cognitive-behavioral psychotherapy for children and adolescents with OCD: a review and recommendations for treatment. *J. Am. Acad. Child Adolesc. Psychiatry* 34:7–18.

March, J.S., Franklin, M., Nelson, A., and Foa, E. (2001) Cognitive-behavioral psychotherapy for pediatric obsessive-compulsive disorder. *J. Clin. Child Psychol.* 30(1):8–18.

March, J.S., and Mulle, K. (1998) *OCD in Children and Adolescents. A Cognitive-Behavioral Treatment Manual*. New York: Guilford Press.

March, J.S., Mulle, K., and Herbel, B. (1994) Behavioral psychotherapy for children and adolescents with obsessive-compulsive disorder: an open trial of a new protocol-driven treatment package. *J. Am. Acad. Child Adolesc. Psychiatry* 33:333–341.

Marks, I. (1997) Behavior therapy for obsessive-compulsive disorder. A decade of progress. *Can. J. Psychiatry* 42:1021–1026.

McDougle, C.J. (1997) Update on pharmacologic management of OCD: agents and augmentation. *J. Clin. Psychiatry* 58(Suppl 12):11–17.

McDougle, C.J., Goodman, W.K., Leckman, J.F., Holzer, J.C., Barr, L.C., McCance-Katz, E.F., Heninger, G.R., and Price, L.H. (1993) Limited therapeutic effect of addition of buspirone to fluvoxamine-refractory obsessive compulsive disorder. *Am. J. Psychiatry* 150:647–649.

McDougle, C.J., Goodman, W.K., Leckman, J.F., Lee, N.C., Heninger, G.R., and Price, L.H. (1994) Haloperidol addition in fluvoxamine-refractory obsessive-compulsive disorder—a double-blind, placebo-controlled study in patients with and without tics. *Arch. Gen. Psychiatry* 51:302–308.

McDougle, C.J., Goodman, W.K., Price, L.H., Delgado, P.L., Krystal, J.H., Charney, D.S., and Heninger, G.R. (1990) Neuroleptic addition in fluvoxamine-refractory obsessive-compulsive disorder. *Am. J. Psychiatry* 147:652–654.

McGrath, M.J., Campbell, K.M., Parks, C.R.I., and Burton, F.H. (2000) Glutamatergic drugs exacerbate symptomatic behavior in a transgenic model of comorbid Tourette's syndrome and obsessive-compulsive disorder. *Brain Res.* 877:23–30.

Mindus, P. (1991) *Capsulotomy in Anxiety Disorders: A Multidisciplinary Study*. Stockholm: Karolinska Institute Press.

Montgomery, S.A., Kasper, S., Stein, D.J., Bang Hedgaard, K., and Lemming, O.M. (2001) Citalopram 20 mg, 40 mg, and 60 mg are all effective and well tolerated compared with placebo in obsessive-compulsive disorder. *Int. Clin. Psychopharmacol.* 16(2): 75–86.

Morshed, S.A., Parveen, S., Leckman, J.F., Mercadante, M.T., Bittencourt Kiss, M.H., Miguel, E.C., et al. (2001) Antibodies against neural, nuclear, cytoskeletal, and streptococcal epitopes in children and adults with Tourette's syndrome, Sydenham's chorea, and autoimmune disorders. *Biol. Psychiatry* 50(8):566–577.

Murphy, D., Zohar, J., Pato, M., Pigott, T., and Insel, T. (1989) Obsessive compulsive disorder as a 5-HT subsystem behavioral disorder. *Br. J. Psychiatry* 155(Suppl):15–24.

Neziroglu, F., Hsia, C., and Yaryura-Tobias, J.A. (2000) Behavioral, cognitive, and family therapy for obsessive-compulsive and related disorders. *Psychiatry Clin. North Am.* 23(3):657–670.

O'Connor, K.P., Aardema, F., Robillard, S., Guay, S., Pelissier, M.C., Todorov, C., Borgeat, F., Leblanc, V., Grenier, S., and Doucet, P. (2006) Cognitive behaviour therapy and medication in the treatment of obsessive-compulsive disorder. *Acta Psychiatr. Scand.* 113:408–419.

Park, L.T., Jefferson, J.W., and Greist, J.H. (1997) Obsessive-compulsive disorder. Treatment options. *CNS Drugs* 7:187–202.

Perlmutter, S.J., Garvey, M.A., Castellanos, X., Mittleman, B.B., Giedd, J., Rapoport, J.L., and Swedo, S.E. (1998) A case of pediatric autoimmune neuropsychiatric disorders associated with stretpcoccal infections (PANDAS). *Am. J. Psychiatry* 155(11): 1592–1598.

Perlmutter, S.J., Leitman, S.F., Garvey, M.A., Hamburger, S., Feldman, E., Leonard, H.L., et al. (1999) Therapeutic plasma exchange and intravenous immunoglobulin for obsessive compulsive disorder and tic disorders in childhood. *Lancet* 354: 1153–1158.

Pigott, T.A., L'Heureux, F., Hill, J.L., Bihari, K., Bernstein, S.E., and Murphy, D.L. (1992) A double-blind study of adjuvant buspirone hydrochloride in clomipramine-treated patients with obsessive-compulsive disorder. *J. Clin. Psychopharmacol.* 12:11–18.

Pigott, T.A., L'Heureux, F., Rubenstein, C.S., Hill, J.L., and Murphy, D.L. (1992) A controlled trial of clonazepam augmentation in OCD patients tested with clomipramine or fluoxetine [Abstract no. 144]. In: *New Research Program and Abstracts of the 145th Annual Meeting of the American Psychiatric Association*. Washington, DC: American Psychiatric Association, p. 82.

Pigott, T.A., Zohar, J., Hill, J.L., Berstein, S.E., Grover, G.N., Zohar-Kadouch, R.C., and Murphy, D.L. (1991) Metergoline blocks the behavioral and neuroendocrine effects of orally administered m-CPP in patients with OCD. *Biol. Psychiatry* 29:418–426.

Pittenger, C., Krystal, J.H., and Coric, V. (2005) Initial evidence of the benefits of glutamate modulating agents in the treatment of self-injurious behavior associated with borderline personality disorder. *J. Clinical Psychiatry* 66:1492–1493.

Rapoport, J.L., and Inoff-Germain, G. (2000) Treatment of obsessive-compulsive disorder in children and adolescents. *J. Child Psychol. Psychiatry* 41(4):419–431.

Rasmussen, S.A., and Eisen, J.L. (1992) The epidemiology and differential diagnosis of obsessive-compulsive disorder. *J. Clin. Psychiatry* 53(Suppl):4–10.

Rasmussen, S.A., and Tsuang, M.T. (1986) DSM-III obsessive-compulsive disorder: clinical characteristics and family history. *Am. J. Psychiatry* 143:317–322.

Ravizza, L., Maina, G., Bogetto, F., Albert, U., Barzega, G., and Bellino, S. (1998) Long term treatment of obsessive-compulsive disorder. *CNS Drugs* 10:247–255.

Ricciardi, J.N., Baer, L., Jenike, M.A., et al. (1992) Changes in DSM-III-R axis II diagnoses following treatment of obsessive-compulsive disorder. *Am. J. Psychiatry* 149:829–831.

Robins, L., Helzer, J., Crougham, J., and Ratcliffe, K. (1981) The NIMH Epidemiological Catchment Area study. *Arch. Gen. Psychiatry* 38:381–389.

Rosario-Campos, M., Leckman, J.F., Mercadante, M.T., Shavitt, R.G., Silva, D.A., Prado, H., Sada, P., Zamignani, D., and Miguel, E.C. (2001) Adults with early-onset obsessive-compulsive disorder. *Am. J. Psychiatry* 158:1899–1903.

Rosenberg, D.R., Chugani, D.C., Muzik, O., et al. (1998) Altered serotonin synthesis in fronto-striatal circuitry in pediatric obsessive-compulsive disorder. *Biol. Psychiatry* 43(8 Suppl 1): 245.

Sallee, F.R., Koran, L.M., Pallanti, S., Carson, S.W., and Sethuraman, G. (1998) Intravenous clomipramine challenge in obsessive-compulsive disorder: predicting response to oral therapy at eight weeks. *Biol. Psychiatry* 44:220–227.

Salzberg, A., and Swedo, S.E. (1992) Oxytocin and vasopressin in obsessive-compulsive disorder. *Am. J. Psychiatry* 149:713–714.

Sasso, D.A., Kalanithi, P.S.A., Trueblood, K.V., Pittenger, C., Kelmendi, B., Wayslink, S., Malison, R.T., Krystal, J.H., and Coric, V. (2006) Beneficial effects of the glutamate-modulating agent riluzole on disordered eating and pathological skin-picking behaviors. *J. Clin. Psychopharmacol.* 26:685–686.

Saxena, S., and Rauch, S.L. (2000) Functional neuroimaging and the neuroanatomy of obsessive-compulsive disorder. *Psychiatr. Clin. North Am.* 23(3):563–586.

Saxena, S., Wang, D., Bystritsky, A., and Baxter, L.R., Jr. (1996) Risperidone augmentation of SRI treatment for refractory obsessive-compulsive disorder. *J. Clin. Psychiatry* 57:303–306.

Shafran, R. (1998) Childhood obsessive-compulsive disorder. In: Graham, P., ed. *Cognitive Behavior Therapy for Children and Families*. Cambridge, UK: Cambridge University Press, pp. 45–73.

Shafron, N.A., and Somers, J. (1998) Treating adolescent obsessive-compulsive disorder: applications of the cognitive theory. *Behav. Res. Ther.* 36:93–97.

Singer, H.S., Giuliano, J.D., Hansen, B.H., et al. (1998) Antibodies against human putamen in children with Tourette syndrome. *Neurology* 50:1618–1624.

Snider, L.A., Lougee, L., Slattery, M., Grant, P., and Swedo, S.E. (2005) Anatibiotic prophylaxis with azithromycin or penicillin in childhood-onset neuropsychiatric disorders. *Biol. Psychiatry* 57: 788–792.

Sousa, M.B., Isolan, L.R., Oliveira, R.R., Manfro, G.G., Cordioli, A. (2006) A randomized clinical trial of cognitive-behavioral group therapy and sertraline in the treatment of obsessive-compulsive disorder. *J. Clin. Psychiatry* 67:1133–1139.

Stanley, M.A., and Turner, S.M. (1995) Current status of pharmacological and behavioral treatment of obsessive-compulsive disorder. *Behav. Ther.* 26:163–186.

Stein, D.J., Bouwer, C., Hawkridge, S., and Emsley, R.A. (1997) Risperidone augmentation of serotonin reuptake inhibitors in obsessive-compulsive and related disorders. *J. Clin. Psychiatry* 58: 119–122.

Swedo, S., and Rapoport, J.L. (1990) Neurochemical and neuroendocrine consideration of obsessive-compulsive disorders in childhood. In: Deutsch, S.I., Weizman, A., and Weizman, R., eds. *Application of Basic Neurosciences to Child Psychiatry*. New York: Plenum Medical Books, pp. 275–284.

Swedo, S., Leonard, H.L., Kruesi, M.J.P., Rettew, D., Listwak, S.J., Berrettini, W., et al. (1992) Cerebrospinal fluid neurochemistry of children and adolescents with obsessive compulsive disorder. *Arch. Gen. Psychiatry* 49:29–36.

Swedo, S., Rapoport, J.L., Leonard, H.L., Lenane, M., and Cheslow, D. (1989) Obsessive compulsive disorder in children and adolescents: clinical phenomenology of 70 consecutive cases. *Arch. Gen. Psychiatry* 46:335–341.

Swedo, S.E. (1989) Rituals and releasers: an ethological model of OCD. In: Rapoport, J.L., ed. *Obsessive Compulsive Disorder in Children and Adolescents*. Washington, DC: American Psychiatric Press, pp. 269–288.

Swedo, S.E., Leonard, H.L., Garvey, M., Mittleman, B., Allen, A.J., Perlmutter, S., et al. (1998) Pediatric autoimmune neuropsychiatric disorders associated with streptococcal infections (PANDAS): clinical description of the first 50 cases. *Am. J. Psychiatry* 155: 264–271.

Swedo, S.E., Leonard, H.L., Schapiro, M.B., Casey, B.J., Mannheim, G.B., Lenane, M.C., et al. (1993) Sydenham's chorea: physical and psychological symptoms of St. Vitus dance. *Pediatrics* 91: 706–713.

van der Wee, N., Stevens, H., Hardeman, J.A., Mandl, R.C., Denys, D.A., Van Megen, H.J., Kahn, R.S., and Westenberg, H.M. (2004) Enhanced dopamine transporter density in psychotropic-naive patients with obsessive-compulsive disorder shown by [^{123}i]b-cit spect. *Am. J. Psychiatry* 161:2201–2206.

Van Noppen, B., Skeketee, G., McCorkle, B., et al. (1997) Group and multifamily behavioral treatment for obsessive compulsive disorder: a pilot study. *J. Anxiety Disord.* 11:431–446.

Von Economo, C. (1931) *Encephalitis Lethargica: Its Sequelae and Treatment*. London: Oxford University Press.

Vythilingum, B., Cartwright, C., and Hollander, E. (2000) Pharmacotherapy of obsessive-compulsive disorder: experience with the selective serotonin reuptake inhibitors. *Int. Clin. Psychopharmacol.* 15(Suppl 2):S7–S13.

Weissman, M.M., Bland, R.C., Canino, G.J., Greenwald, S., Hwu, H-G., Lee, C.K., et al. (1994) The cross-national epidemiology of obsessive-compulsive disorder. *J. Clin. Psychiatry* 55(Suppl 3):5–10.

Wittchen, H.U., Nelson, C.B., and Lachner, G. (1998) Prevalence of mental disorders and psychosocial impairments in adolescents and young adults. *Psychol. Med.* 28:109–126.

Wolff, R., and Rapoport, J.L. (1988) Behavioral treatment of childhood obsessive compulsive disorder. *Behav. Modif.* 12:252–256.

Zohar, A.H. (1999) The epidemiology of obsessive-compulsive disorder in children and adolescents. *Child Adolesc. Psychiatr. Clin. North Am.* 8(3):445–460.

Zohar, J., Insel, T., and Zohar-Kadouch, R. (1988) Serotonergic responsivity in obsessive-compulsive effects of chronic clomipramine treatment. *Arch. Gen. Psychiatry* 45:167–172.

Zohar, J., Mueller, E.A., Insel, T.R., Zohar-Kadouch, R., and Murphy, D. (1987) Serotonergic responsivity in obsessive-compulsive disorder: comparison with patients and healthy controls. *Arch. Gen. Psychiatry* 44:946–951.

43 Neuroimaging Studies of Anxiety Disorders

JUSTINE M. KENT AND SCOTT L. RAUCH

A virtual explosion in neuroimaging research has marked the past decade, with convergent data from various imaging studies informing our neurobiological models of the anxiety disorders. Within the field of anxiety disorders research, neuroimaging techniques are being used to investigate the structure, function, and neurochemistry of the brain in vivo. In this chapter, we discuss the burgeoning field of neuroimaging research in the context of neurocircuitry models of the anxiety disorders. This chapter necessarily extends previous reviews that we have written, together with our colleagues, on the neurobiology of anxiety (Rauch and Baxter, 1998; Rauch, Shin, Whalen, et al., 1998; Rauch, Whalen, et al., 1998; Kent et al., 2000; Saxena and Rauch, 2000; Kent, Sullivan, Rauch, et al., 2002; Cannistraro and Rauch, 2003; Phillips et al., 2003; Deckersbach et al., 2006; Rauch et al., 2006; Shin et al., 2006).

ANXIETY AND THE ANXIETY DISORDERS

Although anxiety and fear are normal human emotional states, the anxiety disorders are characterized by maladaptive fearful responding and distressing psychic and somatic symptoms, which result in significant functional impairment. Obsessive–compulsive disorder (OCD) is characterized by intrusive, unwanted thoughts (that is, obsessions) and ritualized, repetitive behaviors (that is, compulsions). Obsessions are typically accompanied by anxiety that drives the compulsions. The compulsions are performed to neutralize the obsessions and associated anxiety. Posttraumatic stress disorder (PTSD) is one of few psychiatric conditions for which an etiology is clearly defined. It is characterized by significant anxiety symptoms following an emotionally severely traumatic event. The main features of PTSD include reexperiencing phenomena (for example, flashbacks), avoidance (for example, avoiding situations that remind the individual of the traumatic event), and hyperarousal (for example, an exaggerated startle response). Phobias are characterized by consistently heightened anxiety responses to innocuous stimuli or situations. Social phobia (or social anxiety disorder) is characterized by excessive, often-paralyzing anxiety in response to a range of different social and performance situations. Specific phobias involve phobic responses to any of various stimuli or situations (for example, heights, insects, snakes, enclosed spaces). Finally, panic disorder (PD) is characterized by recurrent panic attacks, often occurring spontaneously, without overt precipitants, and the presence of anticipatory anxiety and phobic avoidance. During panic attacks, the individual experiences an acute crescendo of fear and anxiety, accompanied by physical symptoms such as shortness of breath, racing heart, palpitations, sweating, and dizziness, as well as emotional and cognitive symptoms such as an intense feeling of dread and the desire to escape the given situation/surroundings. Unreasonable avoidance of places or situations where the individual believes panic attacks are more likely to occur is a common result of repeated panic episodes.

A common factor of the anxiety disorders is exaggerated fear in response to relatively innocuous stimuli (for example, phobias) or spontaneous fear responses in the absence of true threat (for example, PD). Thus, normal fear responding has been examined as a potential model for the neuroanatomical basis of maladaptive anxiety. Current neurobiological models of anxiety are based primarily on patterns of dysfunction within the so-called fear neurocircuitry, largely established through preclinical models of stress responding and fear conditioning (LeDoux et al., 1988; Davis, 1992).

NEUROANATOMY RELEVANT TO ANXIETY AND FEAR

Sensory information processing is critical to threat assessment and occurs via pathways running through the anterior thalamus to the amygdala (LeDoux et al., 1990). The amygdala, located in the anterior part of the medial temporal lobe, is the central node for the coordination of autonomic and behavioral fear responding. Thus, the amygdala is critical in preliminary threat assessment, and in preparation for action in response to threat via its ascending projections to motor areas and descending projections to brain stem nuclei that control autonomic responses and arousal. Importantly, the amygdala also facilitates the acquisition of additional information regarding the specific threat via reciprocal projections to subcortical and limbic cortical regions (Aggleton, 1992; LeDoux, 1996). Brain regions providing important feedback to the amygdala include (*1*) medial frontal cortex, (*2*) the hippocampus, and (*3*) cortico-striato-thalamic circuits that mediate gating at the level of the thalamus, thereby regulating the flow of incoming information that reaches the amygdala. Medial frontal cortex, including anterior cingulate and medial and orbitofrontal cortex (OFC), is believed to provide critical top-down governance over the amygdala, suppressing the fear response once danger has passed or when the meaning of a potentially threatening stimulus has changed. The hippocampus provides information about the context of a situation and may call on information about the environment retrieved from explicit memory stores. Dysfunction of the hippocampus has been shown to result in poor contextual stimulus discrimination, which may be related to the overgeneralization of fear responding seen in anxiety disorders.

In addition, neurochemical modulators may affect the activity within each of these various brain areas and at nodes of the entire neurocircuitry system outlined above. Ascending projections from the raphé nuclei (serotonin) and the locus ceruleus (norepinephrine) are prime modulators of activity (Salzman et al., 1993; Charney et al., 1995; Kent et al., 1998). Recently, there has been increasing interest in the role of glutamate in anxiety disorders, as numerous preclinical studies have shown that chronic stress increases the activity of this potentially neurotoxic excitatory amino acid. Theoretical models now link stress to increased glucocorticoid activity, to hippocampal damage, and to anxiety and depression. It has been proposed that glucocorticoids may actually affect the suppression of neurogenesis in the hippocampus via their action on excitatory glutamate pathways (Cameron et al., 1998). In addition, chronically raised cortisol levels facilitate hippocampal neuronal death, leading to further dysregulation of the hypothalamic-pituitary axis (Sapolsky, 1986, 2000). Although this area is somewhat controversial, it has nevertheless led to attempts to treat anxiety with corticotropin releasing factor (CRF) antagonists (Holsboer, 1999), in addition to traditional anxiolytic medications targeting the serotonergic, noradrenergic, and γ-aminobutyric acid (GABA) ergic systems.

In this chapter, we discuss modern neuroimaging techniques employed in investigating structural, functional, and neurochemical aspects of anxiety. Morphometric magnetic resonance imaging (mMRI) has replaced computed axial tomography (CAT scanning) as the current approach to structural neuroimaging. Contemporary mMRI typically entails semiautomated or fully automated schemes for segmenting defined brain structures so that corresponding volumes can be precisely calculated. Strategies for parcellating cortical territories, as well as subdividing subcortical nuclei, are being implemented to provide more exact volumetric data. Magnetic resonance diffusion tensor imaging (DTI) is a complementary neuroimaging technique used for assessing regional white matter tract orientation and connectivity in vivo. Fiber tract orientation and tissue anisotropy are estimated with DTI, then algorithms are employed in three dimensions to determine white matter tract orientations (Jones et al., 1999). Methods for inferring regional connectivity from diffusion data are being implemented to create directional maps (Poupon et al., 2001; Sato et al., 2001). Thus, this noninvasive technique is a potential means of assessing alterations in orientation and connectivity within white matter tracks and of evaluating progressive changes in connectivity over time in psychiatric, neurological, and developmental disorders. Functional imaging methods include positron emission tomography (PET) with tracers that measure blood flow (for example, oxygen-15-labeled carbon dioxide or oxygen-15-labeled water) or glucose metabolism (that is, F-18-labeled fluorodeoxyglucose [FDG]); single photon emission computed tomography (SPECT) with tracers that measure correlates of blood flow (for example, technetium-99-labeled hexamethyl propylene amine oxime [TcHMPAO]); and functional magnetic resonance imaging (fMRI) to measure blood oxygenation level-dependent (BOLD) signal changes. Patterns reflecting regional brain activity are generated with each of these techniques.

The resultant brain activity maps from functional imaging studies are sensitive to the state of the subject at the time of tracer distribution or image acquisition. Therefore, functional imaging paradigms are categorized by the type of state manipulations employed. In neutral state paradigms, subjects are studied during a nominal resting state or while performing a nonspecific continuous task. Between-group comparisons are then made to test hypotheses regarding group differences in regional brain activity, without particular attention to state variables. In symptom provocation paradigms, subjects are typically scanned during a neutral (control) state, and then scanned in a symptomatic state in which anxiety is intentionally induced through the use of specific pharmacological and/or behavioral stimuli. Within-group comparisons are made to test hypotheses regarding the anatomy underlying the symptomatic state, whereas group × condition interactions identify differing responses in patient versus control groups. In cognitive activation paradigms, subjects are studied while performing specially designed cognitive-behavioral tasks.

This approach aims to increase sensitivity by employing tasks that specifically activate brain regions or systems of interest. Again, group × condition interactions are sought to test the functional integrity of specific brain systems in patients versus healthy controls. In treatment paradigms, patients are scanned in the context of a treatment protocol, usually before and after a pharmacological or behavioral therapy treatment trial. Within-group comparisons are then made to test hypotheses regarding changes in patterns of brain activity associated with symptomatic improvement. Also, correlational analyses can be performed to identify pretreatment brain activity predictive of treatment response.

Imaging studies of neurochemistry have employed PET and SPECT methods in conjunction with radiolabeled high-affinity ligands to characterize regional receptor number and or affinity in vivo (that is, neuroreceptor characterization studies). Proton magnetic resonance spectroscopy (^{1}H MRS) is a brain-imaging technique that permits a noninvasive means of quantifying endogenous brain chemistry and examining regional cellular energetics and function in vivo. Employing the physical principles used in MRI, several chemical species are routinely measured by ^{1}H MRS, including *N*-acetylaspartate (NAA), cytosolic choline (Cho), myoinositol (mI), and creatine (Cr). In addition, particular ^{1}H MRS editing techniques (Rothman et al., 1993) now allow for investigation of amino acid concentrations of glutamate, glutamine, and GABA (Sanacora et al., 1999). *N*-acetylaspartate is a cell marker, the concentration of which correlates with neuronal density (Barker, 2001). Another MRS-visible compound, the Cho resonance, reflects a pool of choline composed of acetylcholine and the by-products of phosphatidylcholine hydrolysis, phosphocholine, and glycerophosphocholine. Abnormalities in the Cho resonance have been linked to abnormalities in myelination, cerebral oxidative metabolism, and alterations in intraneuronal signaling (Jung et al., 2002). The Cr resonance reflects systemic energy use and storage. The Cr signal is considered a valid internal standard in ratio analyses commonly used in measuring neurometabolic change due to its stability within individuals over time (Moats et al., 1994; Ross and Michaelis, 1994).

These various neuroimaging techniques should be viewed as complementary, providing convergent information about structural, functional, and neurochemical integrity in brain systems of interest.

OBSESSIVE–COMPULSIVE DISORDER

Neuroanatomical Model of Obsessive–Compulsive Disorder (Cortico-Striatal Model)

Aberrant functioning within the cortico-striato-thalamocortical circuitry is the foundation of current models of OCD (see Rauch, Whalen, et al., 1998; Saxena and Rauch, 2000, for review). Within the context of this model, one view is that striatal pathology (specifically within the caudate nucleus) leads to inefficient gating at the level of the thalamus, which results in hyperactivity within orbitofrontal and anterior cingulate cortices (Fig. 43.1). The symptomatic expression of hyperactivity within orbitofronal cortex may manifest as intrusive thoughts, whereas hyperactivity within the anterior cingulate cortex (ACC) may be associated with generalized anxiety. In this model, compulsions are viewed as repetitive behaviors that are performed to recruit the inefficient striatum so as to ultimately achieve thalamic gating and thereby neutralize unwelcome thoughts and attendant anxiety.

Structural Imaging Findings

Volumetric MRI studies in OCD have focused on brain structures identified in functional neuroimaging studies as key areas of aberrant activity. These brain regions include the striatum, thalamus, amygdala, and OFC. Studies of adult patients with OCD examining the striatum with modern mMRI techniques have reported inconsistent findings. Results from three of these investigations suggest volumetric abnormalities in OCD involving the caudate nucleus (Scarone et al., 1992;

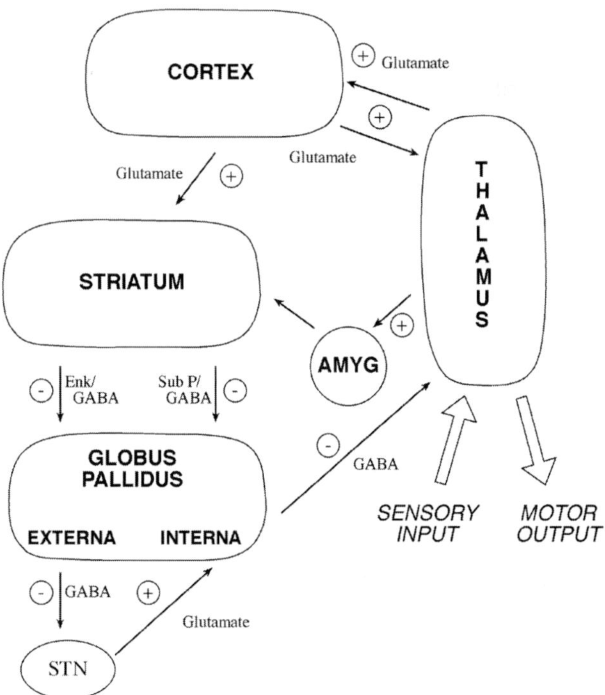

FIGURE 43.1 Schematized neuroanatomical model of obsessive–compulsive disorder indicating direct and indirect (via the STN) pathways of the cortico-striato-thalamo-cortical circuit. AMYG: amygdala; GABA: γ-aminobutyric acid; STN: subthalamic nucleus.

Robinson et al., 1995; Jenike et al., 1996), with other studies reporting no significant differences in caudate volumes versus controls groups (Aylward et al., 1996; J.-J. Kim et al., 2001; Riffkin et al., 2005). Magnetic resonance imaging has also demonstrated abnormal thalamus volumes in several studies (Gilbert et al., 2000; Rosenberg, Benazon, et al., 2000; J.-J. Kim et al., 2001)

Perhaps more consistent is the report of reduced volume of the orbitofrontal cortices in OCD (Szeszko et al., 1999; Choi et al., 2004; Kang et al., 2004; Pujol et al., 2004; Atmaca et al., 2006; Atmaca et al., 2007). Of note, using a voxel-based analysis of segmented gray matter images, J.-J. Kim and colleagues (2001) reported increased gray matter volume in the OFC of patients with OCD. Thus, despite potentially overall reduced volume, increased gray matter density in the orbitofrontal region suggests hyperconnectivity, consistent with the hypermetabolism seen in the frontal-subcortical circuitry implicated as being aberrant in OCD. In this context, of particular interest is a report using mMRI techniques to examine changes in subcortical structures following lesioning of the anterior cingulate in nine patients with treatment-resistant OCD (Rauch, Kim, et al., 2000). Significant reductions in the caudate nucleus postcingulotomy were found, with the degree of reduction correlating positively with the extent of lesioning. These findings confirm the important connectivity between the anterior cingulate and the caudate and suggest that changes in structures distant from the site of lesioning may be responsible for clinical improvement.

Studies examining amygdala volumes in OCD have yielded contradictory results, with one study reporting decreased amygdala volume bilaterally in patients with OCD compared with healthy controls (Szesko et al., 1999), whereas another study reported increased left amygdala volume and reduced hippocampal volume bilaterally (Kwon et al., 2003).

Several pediatric studies have focused on brain regional volumetric changes in OCD. Rosenberg et al. (1997) performed the first mMRI study in treatment-naïve pediatric patients, examining 19 patients with OCD and 19 case-matched, psychiatrically healthy comparisons. They found reduced striatal volumes in the OCD group versus the control group, with volume inversely related to OCD symptom severity. Several years later, Szeszko and colleagues (2004) reported similar findings in a study of 23 drug-naïve pediatric patients with OCD when compared with 27 healthy controls. Patients with OCD had smaller globus pallidus volumes than healthy volunteers, although there were no volumetric differences between the two groups for the caudate or putamen.

Two studies have focused on children with streptococcal infection-associated OCD. In a study by Giedd et al. (2000) of 34 children with OCD and/or chronic tics associated with group A b-hemolytic streptococcal (GABHS) infection compared to 82 matched healthy controls, average basal ganglia size (caudate, putamen, globus pallidus) was increased in the OCD group. No difference was reported in basal ganglia size between the 18 children with a primary diagnosis of OCD and the 16 children with a primary diagnosis of chronic tic disorder, although there was much overlap in symptomatology across the two groups. Because of the significant comorbidity of OCD, tic disorders, and attention-deficit/hyperactivity disorder (ADHD), Peterson and colleagues (2000) attempted to clarify the association between diagnosis, GABHS infection, and basal ganglia enlargement. They studied a primarily pediatric sample, consisting of patients with OCD, chronic tic disorder, or ADHD ranging in age from 7 to 55 years. High anti-GABHS antibody titers were associated with a diagnosis of ADHD, while increasing titers of GABHS antibodies were associated with enlargement of putamen and globus pallidus volumes in the ADHD and OCD diagnostic groups. The finding of elevated titers associated with ADHD raises the question of whether outcomes in previous studies reporting associations between elevated antibodies and OCD may have been affected by the presence of comorbid ADHD.

Pursuing an interest in investigating potential volumetric abnormalities related to limbic-hypothalamic-pituitary-adrenal axis abnormalities in OCD, MacMaster and colleagues (2006) used mMRI to investigate pituitary volumes in pediatric patients with OCD versus healthy controls. They found smaller pituitary volume in boys with OCD versus healthy boys, which was inversely correlated with compulsive behavior severity.

Two studies have examined the effect of treatment on thalamic volumes in children with OCD. Gilbert and colleagues (2000) reported enlarged thalamic volumes in 21 drug-naïve children with OCD when compared to 21 case-matched controls, consistent with the group's earlier report with a smaller sample (Rosenberg et al., 1997). Ten of these 21 patients with OCD underwent repeat mMRI studies posttreatment with 12 weeks of paroxetine monotherapy. Paroxetine treatment was associated with a significant decrease in thalamic volume (19%) and was associated with improvement in OCD symptoms. In a study by the same group (Rosenberg, Benazon, et al., 2000) employing cognitive-behavioral therapy (CBT) as the treatment in a similar 12-week design, 11 drug-naïve children with OCD, aged 8–17, underwent mMRI studies before and after treatment. Although these children demonstrated significant overall improvement in their OCD symptoms (30% reduction), unlike the investigators' earlier study employing paroxetine treatment, the authors did not find a positive response to CBT to be associated with significant change in thalamic volume. This suggests that reductions in thalamic size in response to treatment may be specific to selective serotonin reuptake inhibitor (SSRI) treatment and not necessarily directly related to treatment response.

In summary, although there has been a recent growth in the number of structural brain imaging studies in OCD, these studies have not consistently demonstrated volumetric differences which could be considered pathognomonic for OCD. Differing results may be due to methodology (region-of-interest [ROI] vs. voxel-based morphometry [VBM] ROI vs. VBM approaches) and/or heterogeneity in OCD samples.

Functional Imaging Findings

A convergence of data from a majority, but not all (Crespo-Facorro et al., 1999), neutral-state paradigm studies employing PET and SPECT indicates that patients with OCD exhibit elevated regional brain activity within OFC and ACC in comparison with normal controls (Baxter et al., 1987; Baxter et al., 1988; Nordahl et al., 1989; Swedo et al., 1989; Machlin et al., 1991; Rubin et al., 1992; Alpetkin et al., 2001); however, decreased activity has been reported in the dorsal posterior cingulate cortex (Saxena et al., 2004). A meta-analysis reconciled these apparently inconsistent findings with regard to OFC results in OCD (Milad and Rauch, 2007); specifically, elevated OFC activity is consistently observed in anterior and lateral portions of OFC whereas findings of decreased OFC activity have been confined to posteromedial regions. This is consistent with a model whereby anterolateral OFC mediates negative cognitions (obsessions), whereas the posteromedial OFC plays a critical role in extinction capacity (see Milad and Rauch, 2007) Increased activity in the thalamus has also been reported in several neutral-state studies (Swedo et al., 1989; Perani et al., 1995; Alpetkin et al., 2001; Saxena et al., 2001). Observed differences in regional activity within the caudate nucleus have been less consistent (Baxter et al., 1987; Baxter et al., 1988; Rubin et al., 1992).

Findings from functional imaging studies focusing on treatment effects (Benkelfat et al., 1990; Hoehn-Saric et al., 1991; Baxter et al., 1992; Swedo et al., 1992; Perani et al., 1995; J.M. Schwartz et al., 1996; Saxena et al., 1999; Hoehn-Saric et al., 2001; Hansen et al., 2002; Saxena et al., 2002; Diler et al., 2004; Ho Pian et al., 2005) suggest that attenuation of abnormal regional brain activity within OFC, ACC, and caudate nucleus is associated with symptomatic improvement. Interestingly, similar changes have been observed with pharmacological and behavioral therapies (e.g., Baxter et al., 1992; J.M. Schwartz et al., 1996).

Of note, the magnitude of frontal cortical activity prior to treatment has been found to predict the treatment response, with lower pretreatment OFC metabolism associated with better serotonin reuptake inhibitor (SRI) response (Swedo et al., 1992; Brody et al., 1998; Saxena et al., 1999; Rauch et al., 2002). Decreased regional brain activity in the right caudate (Baxter et al., 1992; J.M. Schwartz et al., 1996; Saxena et al., 1999; Saxena et al., 2002; Diler et al., 2004) and the thalamus (Baxter et al., 1992; Saxena et al., 2002; Ho Pian et al., 2005) have also been associated with treatment response in OCD. In summary, the brain changes best correlated with OCD treatment response are attenuation of activity in the OFC, right caudate, and thalamus.

Given the explosion of functional imaging studies in OCD utilizing symptom provocation and emotional stimuli techniques, a complete review of these studies is outside of the scope of this chapter. Results of these studies are briefly summarized in Table 43.1. Overall, functional imaging studies employing symptom provocation have fairly consistently reported increased brain activity within anterior/lateral OFC, thalamus, and caudate. This includes studies employing PET (McGuire et al., 1994; Rauch et al., 1994) as well as functional MRI (Breiter et al., 1996; Adler et al., 2000; Chen et al., 2004; Mataix-Cols et al., 2004) techniques. Response to symptom provocation in the cingulate cortex varies across studies. About half of studies have reported increased cingulate activation in OCD versus healthy control subjects during symptom provocation. Comparison of these results with those from studies of other anxiety disorders suggests that anterior/lateral orbitofrontal and caudate activation is relatively specific to OCD, whereas activation of posteromedial orbitofrontal and ACC may be a nonspecific marker of anxiety, often observed in other anxiety disorders and in normal anxiety states (Rauch and Baxter, 1998).

Various cognitive activation paradigms have also been employed in the study of OCD, with the intention of targeting specific brain regions of interest. These cognitive activation paradigms have focused in two areas: memory/learning and response inhibition. Rauch and colleagues (Rauch et al., 1997a; Rauch, Whalen, Curran, et al., 2001) employed an implicit (that is, nonconscious) learning paradigm shown to reliably recruit striatum (Rauch, Savage, Brown, et al., 1995; Rauch, Whalen, Savage, et al., 1997). Findings from the first study using PET (Rauch et al., 1997a) were later replicated in a second study using fMRI (Rauch, Whalen, Curran, et al., 2001). Consistent across these two studies was a failure of patients with OCD to normally recruit striatum, instead activating medial temporal regions typically associated with conscious information processing. This occurred despite normal performance by the patients with OCD on the learning task, suggesting that temporal cortex activation is actively compensating for deficits within the frontal cortical-striato-thalamo-frontal cortical circuitry. Following on these first studies, other groups have also demonstrated fail-

TABLE 43.1 *Summary of Functional Neuroimaging Findings in OCD*

Paradigm Employed	*Identified Areas of Elevated Metabolism, CBF or BOLD Signal*	*Identified Areas of Decreased Metabolism, CBF or BOLD Signal*	*References*
Neutral state	OFC, ACC		Alpetkin et al., 2001 Baxter et al., 1987; Baxter et al., 1988 Diler et al., 2004 Machlin et al., 1991 Nordahl et al., 1989 Perani et al., 1995 Rubin et al., 1992 Swedo et al., 1989
	thalamus		Alpetkin et al., 2001 Perani et al., 1995 Saxena et al., 2001 Swedo et al., 1989
Symptom provocation	OFC, caudate, thalamus		Adler et al., 2000 Breiter et al., 1996 Chen et al., 2004 Mataix-Cols et al., 2004 McGuire et al., 1994 Rauch et al., 1994 Shapira et al., 2003
Cognitive tasks:			
• Implicit learning paradigm	Medial temporal cortex	Lack of normal striatal activation	Rauch, Savage, et al., 1997; Rauch, Whalen, Curran, et al., 2001
• Word generation	OFC	Lack of OFC suppression at rest	Pujol et al., 1999
• Tower of Hanoi		Lack of L caudate activation	Fernandez et al., 2003
• Response-conflict task	ACC		Ursu et al., 2003
• Spatial N-back task	ACC		Van der Wee et al., 2003
• Interference task	Rostral ACC		Fitzgerald et al., 2005
• Go/No-Go task	Rostral & caudal ACC, OFC		Maltby et al., 2005
• Stroop task		ACC, R caudate	Nakao et al., 2005
• Tower of London task	ACC	DLPFC, caudate	Van der Heuvel et al., 2005a
• Stroop task	Amygdala, L hypothalamus		Van der Heuvel et al., 2005b
• Conflict task	ACC, L parietal		Viard et al., 2005

OFC: orbitofrontal cortex; ACC: anterior cingulate gyrus; AMCC: anterior-medial cingulate gyrus; PCC: posterior cingulate gyrus; DLPFC: dorsolateral prefrontal cortex; CBF: cerebral blood flow; BOLD: blood oxygen level dependent; OCD: obsessive-compulsive disorder.

ure of activation of the striatum in patients with OCD during tasks of learning and memory involving planning and sequencing (A. Fernandez et al., 2003; Van den Heuvel et al., 2005b). Other groups have employed cognitive paradigms and fMRI to study cognitive interference and response inhibition in OCD. Results of these studies suggest that overactivity in the anterior-medial cingulate cortex in patients with OCD may reflect heightened error monitoring and heightened conflict monitoring in this population (Ursu et al., 2003; Fitzgerald et al., 2005; Maltby et al., 2005; Viard et al., 2005). In a study employing emotional and color Stroop tasks, van den Heuvel and colleagues (2005a) demonstrated that greater interference by OCD-related words was associated with increased activity in the dorsal anterior cingulate in patients with OCD versus healthy controls. In addition, OCD-related word naming elicited greater amygdalar and hypothalamic activation in the OCD group when contrasted with neutral words.

Imaging Studies of Neurochemistry, Neurotransmitter, and Neuroreceptor Imaging

Magnetic resonance spectroscopy studies in OCD have reported neurochemical abnormalities in several of the brain regions central to neuroanatomical models of

OCD: striatum, thalamus, and ACC. Ebert and colleagues (1997) reported relatively reduced NAA resonance (a marker of healthy neuronal density) in right striatum and ACC in 12 patients with OCD in comparison with 6 healthy controls. Similarly, Bartha and colleagues (1998) found reduced left striatal NAA concentrations in 13 patients with OCD versus 13 matched controls. Rosenberg et al. (2001) studied 11 children, aged 8–15, with OCD and 11 healthy case-matched controls using MRS. They found a significant bilateral increase in cytosolic Cho in the medial thalami of the children with OCD versus the control group, with no between-group differences in NAA or Cr signals in this region. Russell and colleagues (2003) reported abnormalities in NAA and Cr in the dorsolateral PFC. Results of the adult studies of MRS-NAA are convergent with those from mMRI studies; reduced NAA is consistent with primary pathology within the striatum associated with subtle volumetric abnormalities or reductions in measures of healthy neuronal density.

Several studies have reported the reduction of elevated glutamate and glutamine (Glx) in the caudate in response to SRI treatment (Moore et al., 1998; Rosenberg, MacMaster, et al., 2000; Bolton et al., 2001), whereas CBT did not result in Glx reductions (Benazon et al., 2003). These findings are consistent with the model of OCD suggesting orbitofrontal hyperactivity, mirrored by elevated glutamate at the site of glutamatergic projections from OFC to the striatum, which is attenuated by successful SRI treatment.

Studies in OCD examining neurotransmitter and receptor dysfunction have focused on the serotonin and dopamine (DA) systems. Results have been somewhat contradictory, with some (Stengler-Wenzke et al., 2004; Hesse et al., 2005), but not all (Simpson et al., 2003), studies reporting decreased serotonin transporter availability in the brain stem and midbrain in patients with OCD versus healthy controls. Adams and colleagues (2005) reported increased 5-HT_{2A} receptor binding in the caudate in patients with OCD. Results from studies of the DA system in OCD have also been contradictory. To date, studies have reported increased DA transporter (DAT) density (C.-H. Kim et al., 2003; van der Wee et al., 2004), and decreased DAT density (Hesse et al., 2005) in the basal ganglia of patients with OCD. Reduced D_2 receptor binding has been reported in the caudate in OCD (Denys et al., 2005).

Summary

Dysregulation of activity in the orbitofrontal-caudate pathway within the cortico-striato-thalamo-cortical circuitry has been identified in OCD and appears to be specific to this disorder. In particular, elevated activity in anterolateral OFC may be central to obsessions. It should be noted that abnormal activity of the paralimbic cortex, including ACC, has been implicated in several anxiety disorders, and these regions are believed to mediate nonspecific aspects of the anxious state. Likewise, diminished activity in posteromedial OFC may be a common feature of anxiety disorders. Primary striatal pathology is also suggested in OCD by results from mMRI studies showing reduced striatal volume, as well as MRS results of reduced striatal NAA signal. In the provoked symptomatic state, hyperactivity within OFC is consistently identified in OCD. In addition, in normal patients, the performance of repetitive motor routines does facilitate striatal recruitment in the service of thalamic gating, a pattern that does not occur in patients with OCD. In summary, data from structural, functional, and neurochemical imaging studies support a working model of striatal pathology and striato-thalamic inefficiency, together with anterolateral orbitofrontal hyperactivity. And of possible clinical relevance, the magnitude of orbitofrontal hyperactivity in OCD predicts response to treatment, with lesser activity correlated with a better response to SRIs.

POSTTRAUMATIC STRESS DISORDER

Neuroanatomical Model of Posttraumatic Stress Disorder (Amygdalocentric Model)

Here we briefly summarize a neurocircuitry model of PTSD (Rauch, Shin, Whalen, et al., 1998; Rauch et al., 2006) that emphasizes the amygdala's central role in directing an individual's response to perceived danger through its reciprocal connections with the hippocampus, medial prefrontal cortex (PFC), and other cortical areas associated with higher cognitive functions. This model hypothesizes hyperresponsivity within the amygdala to threat-related stimuli, with inadequate top-down governance over the amygdala by ventral/medial PFC (including the rostral ACC, medial PFC, subcallosal cortex, and OFC) and the hippocampus (Fig. 43.2). This hyperresponsivity of the amygdala mediates symptoms of hyperarousal and may explain the indelible quality of the emotional memory of the traumatic event. Activity in the ventral/medial PFC has been linked to habituation to repetitive stimuli in which there is no imminent threat. Inadequate influence by ventral/medial PFC on the amygdala is believed to be responsible for the lack of habituation that characterizes PTSD, as well as the capacity to suppress attention and response to trauma-related stimuli. Another hallmark of PTSD, the overgeneralization of fear responding to nonthreatening stimuli, is associated with decreased hippocampal function. Abnormal hippocampal input is thus believed to result in deficits in identifying safe versus threatening contexts, as well as accompanying explicit memory difficulties (Bremner et al., 1995). Functional

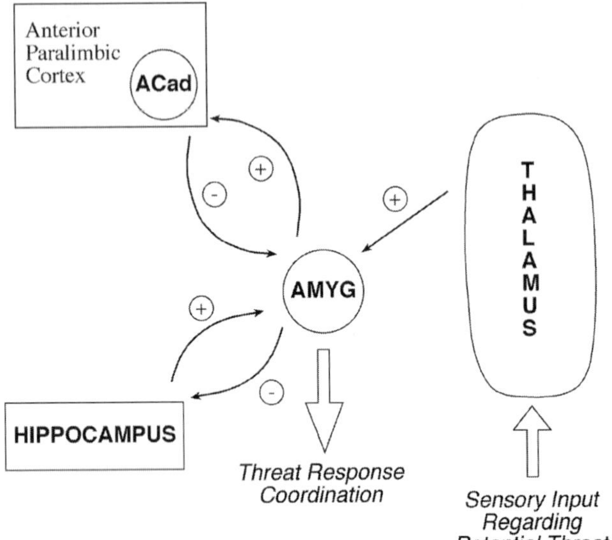

FIGURE 43.2 Schematized neuroanatomical model of posttraumatic stress disorder indicating critical pathways in threat assessment and responding. ACad: affective division of the anterior cingulate; AMYG: amygdala.

neuroimaging findings in PTSD also suggest that in threatening situations, patients with PTSD reallocate neural resources to regions that mediate fear responding at the expense of cortical areas mediating higher cognitive functions.

This model might be viewed as fear conditioning gone awry, with a lack of appropriate habituation and extinction and a lack of contextual discrimination. The pathogenesis of PTSD can be conceptualized as a fear conditioning process that is superimposed on some diathesis, which might involve a predisposition to amygdala hyperresponsivity, lack of sufficient functional connectivity between the anterior cingulate and the amygdala, hippocampal deficiency, and/or exaggerated susceptibility to stress. In fact, current theories suggest that damage to or sensitization of this system may be a consequence of prior exposure to stress. In this model, chronic PTSD is a result of progressive deterioration of function within this amygdala-based system.

Structural Imaging Findings

The focus of mMRI studies of PTSD has been primarily the hippocampus, a brain structure known to be susceptible to stress-induced damage via the action of glucocorticoids and excitatory amino acids. In the first study to examine relative hippocampal volumes in PTSD using mMRI techniques, Bremner and colleagues (1995) studied 26 Vietnam combat veterans with PTSD and 22 civilian comparison subjects. They found that right hippocampal volumes were 8% smaller in the PTSD group than in the control group, and this difference persisted when years of education and alcohol abuse were considered as covariates. Of note, the mean left hippocampal volume was also smaller (3.8%) in the PTSD group versus the comparison group, although this difference did not achieve statistical significance. On a task measuring verbal performance, the patients with PTSD performed more poorly than the controls, and their percent retention scores on this test directly correlated with right hippocampal volume (that is, lower scores were associated with smaller right hippocampal volumes). Pavic and colleagues (2007) reported similar findings of reduced right hippocampal volumes in patients with PTSD versus healthy controls in a group of 15 war veterans with combat-related chronic PTSD.

To compare the relative contribution of combat exposure to hippocampal structural change, Gurvits and colleagues (1996) studied three groups of individuals using mMRI: seven Vietnam combat veterans with PTSD, seven Vietnam combat veterans without PTSD, and eight nonveterans without PTSD. They found significantly smaller hippocampal volumes bilaterally in the PTSD group compared with the combat-exposed and civilian control cohorts. These findings withstood adjustments for age, total brain volume, and lifetime alcohol consumption. There were no significant differences in hippocampal volume between the two control groups. Interestingly, when the 14 combat-exposed veterans were examined together, total hippocampal volume was inversely correlated with the extent of combat exposure and PTSD symptom severity. In a carefully controlled study examining pairs of Vietnam combat veterans and their noncombat-exposed identical twins, Pitman and colleagues (2006) attempted to tease out whether decreased hippocampal volume represents a preexisting vulnerability to develop PTSD or whether it results from trauma exposure. They reported that decreased hippocampal volume and the presence of abnormal cavum septum pellucidum were present in combat veteran twins with PTSD and their unexposed twins, compared to combat veterans without PTSD and their unexposed twins, suggesting that these structural abnormalities represent vulnerability factors for the development of PTSD.

Similar to the negative results of mMRI studies of children and adolescents with OCD, results of pediatric studies of PTSD differed from those of adult trauma studies in that investigators failed to find differences in hippocampal volumes between patients with PTSD and healthy controls. Four recent studies investigated potential brain alterations in children and adolescents with PTSD (De Bellis et al., 1999; De Bellis et al., 2001; De Bellis et al., 2002; Carrion et al., 2001). In a cross-sectional study, De Bellis et al. (1999) measured hippocampal volumes in 44 children who were maltreated and adolescents with PTSD and in 61 age-matched controls. The children with PTSD did not show significant differences in hippocampal volume compared with healthy controls; however, the patients with PTSD had smaller total brain and cerebral volumes. Of note, brain volume correlated positively with age of onset of PTSD trauma, with the children who experienced traumatic stress at the youngest ages exhibiting the smallest brain volumes. In addition, brain volume was negatively correlated with duration of abuse.

Because hippocampal volume is known to increase in children before puberty and then decrease in the postpubertal period, De Bellis and colleagues (2001) conducted a second study to longitudinally examine brain volume changes in nine prepubertal patients with maltreatment-related PTSD and in an equal number of matched healthy controls who were yoked to the patients with PTSD on several variables including age, Tanner developmental stage, and length of time between scans. Subjects underwent mMRI at baseline (prepuberty) and at least 2 years later (late stages of puberty). The investigators hypothesized that childhood trauma would affect hippocampal growth during puberty, and that as a result, the PTSD groups would show greater reductions in hippocampal volume over time than the matched controls. However, they found no significant differences in hippocampal, amygdala, or temporal lobe volumes either at baseline or at follow-up, and there were no differences in volumes between groups across time and pubertal development.

Carrion et al. (2001) used mMRI to measure brain volumes in a sample of 24 children and adolescents with a history of trauma and PTSD symptoms (50% of the sample had a formal diagnosis of current PTSD). The MRI scans of these 24 children were compared to 24 age- and gender-matched controls' MRI scans from an archived sample of children with no psychopathology and normal development. The children with a history of trauma exposure had smaller total brain and cerebral volumes than the control group. Of note, the PTSD group did not demonstrate the typical frontal lobe asymmetry (right/left) seen in the control group, instead manifesting symmetrical frontal lobes. Although hippocampal volume was reduced in the PTSD group, this finding was not significant when corrected for total brain volume.

Directed by findings of superior temporal gyrus event–related potential abnormalities in adult patients with PTSD, De Bellis and colleagues (2002) performed a volumetric study of this region, implicated in verbal and nonverbal auditory processing, in a pediatric sample with PTSD. The comparison of 43 children and adolescents who were maltreated with PTSD with 61 healthy controls demonstrated larger superior temporal gyrus volumes in the patients with PTSD associated with a loss of the normal asymmetry pattern. The authors concluded that these alterations may be due to abnormal developmental changes in this maltreated sample with pediatric PTSD. Other studies' findings support the idea that, in children, trauma exposure and the development of PTSD may hinder the normal development of the cerebellum, which is known to play a role in cognitive development. In a study of children with maltreatment-related PTSD, right, left, and total cerebellar volumes were smaller in patients with PTSD than in the control groups of children with generalized anxiety disorder and healthy children who were nonabused (De Bellis and Kuchibhatla, 2006).

Overall, the sum of the findings from these pediatric PTSD studies suggests a more generalized effect of traumatic stress in early development, affecting not just hippocampal, but also total brain volume. One potential area of exception, where a specific effect has been demonstrated, is within the superior temporal gyrus.

Contrary to the pediatric findings, in mMRI studies of adults with PTSD resulting from childhood abuse, investigators have reported hippocampal volumetric differences similar to those found in studies examining samples with PTSD resulting from traumatic exposure in adulthood. Bremner and colleagues (1997) studied 17 adult survivors of childhood sexual and/or physical abuse with PTSD and 21 healthy comparisons with no reported history of childhood abuse. The patients with PTSD had 12% smaller left hippocampal volumes than the control group. Stein and colleagues (1997) studied hippocampal volume in 21 adult survivors of childhood sexual abuse (most of whom had PTSD) and a control group of 21 adults who reported no childhood history of abuse. They reported 5% smaller left hippocampal volumes in the abused cohort. Of note, total hippocampal volume in patients with PTSD was negatively correlated with PTSD symptom severity. In a related study, Driessen et al. (2000) measured hippocampal and amygdala volumes in 21 women with borderline personality disorder (BPD), most of whom had reported histories of early trauma, and in 21 healthy women with no psychiatric histories. They found that the patients with BPD had smaller hippocampal and amygdalar volumes than the control group. Interestingly, hippocampal volume was negatively correlated with the degree and duration of early trauma only when the patients with BPD and controls were examined together.

A meta-analysis of structural brain abnormalities in PTSD (Karl et al., 2006) confirmed that patients with PTSD have significantly smaller hippocampal volumes compared to controls with and without a history of trauma exposure. The authors highlighted that several factors influence outcome in structural neuroimaging studies, including imaging methodology, symptom severity, medication exposure, and age and gender. Results of this meta-analysis suggest that hippocampal volume differences correlate with PTSD severity, and that these differences may not be evident until adulthood.

Other areas of structural investigation in PTSD include the ACC, caudate, and cerebellum. Rauch and colleagues (2003) reported selective reductions in the rostral ACC and subcallosal cortex in trauma-exposed women with PTSD when compared with trauma-exposed women without PTSD, supporting the importance of these structures in prevailing neurocircuitry models of PTSD. Cohen and colleagues (2006) reported that exposure to traumatic adverse childhood events among adults without psychopathology correlated with reduced anterior cingulate and caudate volumes, which may represent the effects of early life stress on brain development. Interestingly, one study reported possible shape differences in the anterior cingulate in PTSD (Corbo et al., 2005). In addition, PTSD severity has been found to be inversely correlated with anterior cingulate volume (Yamasue et al., 2003; Woodward et al., 2006).

In response to several functional neuroimaging studies demonstrating involvement of the cerebellar vermis in PTSD, Levitt and colleagues (2006) examined the volume of the cerebellar vermis using mMRI in a group of veterans discordant for combat exposure in Vietnam. They found no significant structural differences of the cerebellar vermis in veterans with combat-related PTSD versus veterans with no PTSD.

In summary, most but not all (Jatzko et al., 2006) studies of adult patients with PTSD with either childhood or adult traumatic exposure support an association between reduced hippocampal volume and PTSD. However, the negative findings reported in pediatric studies suggest that hippocampal atrophy may develop progressively over time. In support of the hypothesis that the maintenance of chronic PTSD symptoms is required to affect hippocampal volumes, studies of patients with new-onset PTSD have not reported reduced hippocampal volumes (Bonne et al., 2001, Notestine et al., 2002). Several studies have reported decreased frontal cortex volumes in PTSD, with the anterior cingulate in particular noted to be reduced in patients with PTSD when compared to trauma-exposed controls. However, lingering questions regarding the effects of acute versus prolonged exposure to trauma and the age at which trauma exposure occurs remain to be answered.

Functional Imaging Findings

The literature reporting on functional imaging in PTSD is rapidly expanding (see Lanius et al., 2005; Liberzon and Martis, 2006; Shin et al., 2006, for reviews). Although there is some heterogeneity in these reports, certain findings are fairly consistent and point to many of the same areas implicated in neuroanatomical models of anxiety based on fear conditioning: the amygdala, hippocampus, anterior cingulate and orbitofrontal cortices, and related frontal cortical areas. Functional imaging studies in PTSD have been conducted during resting, so-called neutral states, and by employing several different provocation paradigms: (*1*) external trauma reminders, (*2*) script-driven imagery, (*3*) pharmacological challenge, (*4*) cognitive tasks, and (*5*) auditory performance tasks.

In the first study to employ a script-drive imagery paradigm to induce PTSD symptoms while acquiring functional images, Rauch and colleagues (1996) studied a mixed-gender cohort of patients with PTSD using PET under neutral versus provoked conditions. Patients with PTSD exhibited increased regional cerebral blood flow (rCBF) within right orbitofrontal, insular, anterior temporal, and visual cortex, as well as ACC and the right amygdala in response to symptom provocation. Decreases in rCBF were observed within left inferior frontal (Broca's area) and left middle temporal cortex. Although conclusions from this study are limited by the lack of a comparison group, the areas of increased versus decreased activity during symptom provocation are consistent with the model of shunting of CBF to limbic areas involved in fight/flight responding at the expense of cortical areas mediating higher cognitive functions. The need for controlled studies was emphasized by Fischer and colleagues (1996), who studied individuals exposed to the emotional stress of an armed bank robbery who did not go on to develop PTSD. Using PET, rCBF measurements were made during a provoked condition, while individuals watched an actual security videotape of the robbery, and during a control condition, while they watched a neutral videotape of park scenes. In the exposure versus control contrast, the authors also found rCBF increases within orbitofrontal and visual cortex, as well as within posterior cingulate cortex. In addition, rCBF decreases were noted in a variety of regions, including Broca's area. Results of this study suggest that individuals with PTSD and psychiatrically healthy controls may demonstrate similar patterns of brain activity in response to stimuli reminiscent of emotionally traumatic events. This early work established the groundwork for the more formal, controlled comparisons to follow.

Since the time of these initial studies, a growing body of controlled functional imaging studies in PTSD has been reported. The major findings of these studies are highlighted in Table 43.2.

Among studies employing symptom provocation paradigms, brain areas demonstrating the greatest relative differences in PTSD versus controls are the amygdala, anterior cingulate, and areas of the frontal cortex (Bremner et al., 1997; Bremner, Narayan, et al., 1999; Bremner, Staib, et al., 1999; Britton et al., 2005; Liberzon et al., 1999; Zubieta et al., 1999; Pissiota et al., 2002; Rauch et al., 1996; Shin et al., 1997; Shin et al., 1999; Lanius et al., 2001; Osuch et al., 2001; Lanius et al., 2002; Lanius et al., 2003; Shin et al., 2004; Phan, Britton, et al., 2006).

TABLE 43.2 *Summary of Functional Neuroimaging Findings in PTSD*

Paradigm Employed	*Identified Areas of Elevated Metabolism, CBF or BOLD Signal*	*Identified Areas of Decreased Metabolism, CBF or BOLD Signal*	*References*
Combat script-driven imagery or external trauma reminders	amygdala, sensorimotor cortex, periaqueductal gray	ACC, inferior frontal gyrus (Broca's area), medial PFC hippocampus	Rauch et al., 1996 Shin et al., 1997 Liberzon et al., 1999 Bremner, Narayan, et al., 1999a Pissiota et al., 2002 Shin et al., 2004 Britton et al., 2005
Noncombat script-driven imagery or external trauma reminders	PCC, orbitofrontal cortex, amygdala	ACC, thalamus, hippocampus Medial PFC, inferior frontal gyrus (Broca's area)	Bremner, Staib, et al., 1999b Lanius et al., 2001 Shin et al., 1999 Gilboa et al., 2004 Protopopescu et al., 2005
Symptom provocation (Pharmacologic challenge)		hippocampus, PFC	Bremner et al., 1997
Cognitive task		ACC	Shin et al., 2001
Non-trauma-related emotional image processing		Medial PFC	Phan et al., 2006
Emotional facial expressions: Fearful vs. happy (masked)	Amygdala		Rauch, Whalen, Shin et al., 2000 Armony et al., 2005
Fearful vs. neutral (explicit)	Left amygdala	ACC, Medial PFC	Williams et al., 2006
Fearful vs. happy (explicit)	Amygdala	Medial PFC	Shin et al., 2005

OFC: orbitofrontal cortex; ACC: anterior cingulate gyrus; PCC: posterior cingulate gyrus; PFC: prefrontal cortex; CBF: cerebral blood flow; BOLD: blood oxygen level dependent.

Heightened amygdala activity has been reported in patients with PTSD in response to symptom provocation using various script-driven and trauma cue paradigms (Rauch et al., 1996; Shin et al., 1997; Liberzon et al., 1999; Pissiota et al., 2002; Shin et al., 2004; Protopopescu et al., 2005).

Shin and colleagues (1997) studied patients with combat-related PTSD and matched trauma-exposed controls without PTSD in a PET cognitive activation paradigm. Subjects were required to make judgments about pictures from three categories: neutral, general negative, and combat-related. The paradigm also entailed two types of tasks: one involved responding while actually seeing the pictures (perception), and the other involved responding while recalling the pictures (imagery). The PTSD group showed several areas of significant rCBF change not seen in the controls: increased rCBF was found within the right amygdala and ACC during the combat imagery versus comparison conditions, and decreased rCBF was found within left inferior frontal cortex (Broca's area) for the combat perception versus negative perception contrast. These findings closely paralleled results from the PTSD symptom provocation study of Rauch et al. (1996). In a PET-CBF study of seven patients with PTSD resulting from trauma experienced in wars within the past decade, Pissiota et al. (2002) used traumatic war-related sounds to provoke symptoms of PTSD during scanning. When contrasting traumatic and neutral sound exposure, the investigators demonstrated greater activation in the right amygdala, right sensorimotor areas/sensory cortex, primary and supplementary motor cortices, cerebellar vermis, and periaqueductal gray during the traumatic condition. Activation of these motor and sensorimotor areas, the cerebellum, the amygdala, and the PAG is consistent with a functional circuitry coordinating motor preparedness in response to threatening emotional sensory inputs.

Using fMRI techniques, Rauch, Whalen, Shin, et al. (2000) studied eight men with combat-related PTSD and the same number of combat-exposed controls using a backward-masking technique employing exposure to fearful, neutral, and happy facial expressions. In comparison to the control group, the patients with PTSD exhibited significantly greater activation of the amygdala during the masked-fearful versus masked-happy exposures. In addition, fMRI signal intensity change in the amygdala in response to the fearful versus happy contrast correlated with the severity of PTSD symptoms as measured by the Clinician Administered PTSD Scale (CAPS). Lack of significant medial prefrontal recruitment during this task suggests that amygdalar differences between the groups were occurring independently of frontal cortical input.

Although the findings are not completely consistent, the majority of neuroimaging studies in PTSD have reported no significant response or diminished activation in the ACC (Bremner, Narayan, et al., 1999; Bremner, Staib, et al., 1999; Shin et al., 1999; Semple et al., 2000; Shin et al., 2001; Britton et al., 2005). Attenuation of the ACC and ventral prefrontal cortical areas has been shown in patients with PTSD traumatized by sexual abuse (Bremner, Narayan, et al., 1999; Shin et al., 1999) and by combat exposure (Bremner, Staib, et al., 1999).

Shin and colleagues (2001) designed a study to specifically test the functional integrity of the ACC in patients with PTSD using an Emotional Counting Stroop task, a reliable means of recruiting the anterior cingulate in healthy, nonpsychiatric patients. Eight combat veterans with PTSD and eight combat-exposed veterans were studied with fMRI under three separate conditions in which they counted combat-related, generally negative, and neutral words. The PTSD group failed to activate rostral ACC in the combat versus general negative word conditions, while the non-PTSD group exhibited significant rostral ACC activation. Whalen, Bush, and colleagues (1998) proposed that activation of rostral anterior cingulate may play a regulatory role in processing emotional stimuli so as not to impair competing task performance. Similar results were recently reported by Lanius and colleagues (2001) using fMRI and a high field strength (4 Tesla) magnet with superior resolution. Using a symptom provocation paradigm with scripted imagery to study patients with noncombat-related PTSD, they found brain activation to be lower in the PTSD group versus the control group in the anterior cingulate, medial frontal cortex (BA 11), and thalamus. The authors hypothesized that the differential thalamic activation may be related to disruption in sensory processing at the level of the thalamus and/or disruption of the relay of sensory information from the thalamus to other subcortical structures.

Although the majority of studies have found that PTSD patients fail to recruit anterior cingulate during provoked conditions, this finding is not completely consistent. In the Pissiota study described above, the investigators found no significant difference in anterior cingulate activity between the neutral and provocation conditions (Pissiota et al., 2002). Liberzon and colleagues (1999) used SPECT to study Vietnam veterans with and without PTSD, as well as a group of controls with no history of combat exposure. They contrasted the brain activation profiles associated with exposure to auditory combat stimuli versus white noise. Although all three groups showed increased rCBF in anterior cingulate and middle prefrontal gyrus, only the PTSD group exhibited significant activation of the left amygdala/nucleus accumbens region.

Osuch and colleagues (2001) suggested that some of the differences in reported findings in symptom provocation studies in PTSD may be attributable to the presence or absence of flashbacks, episodes of intense reexperiencing of trauma imagery. They used PET to study a mixed-gender cohort of 12 treatment-unresponsive patients with PTSD at rest and after exposure to individually tailored trauma scripts. All patients were taking stable doses of antidepressants and/or benzodiazepines at the time of scanning. Eight patients, who had adequate data and reported experiencing flashbacks during the scanning, were included in the rCBF analyses. Positive correlations were reported between flashback intensity and left hippocampal, left inferior frontal, left somatosenory, and cerebellar cortices, brain stem, right insula, and right putamen. Flashback intensity was inversely correlated with bilateral superior frontal, fusiform, and medial temporal cortices. These results are consistent with several other studies showing relatively decreased superior frontal rCBF in PTSD versus control groups in response to symptom provocation paradigms (Rauch et al., 1996; Liberzon et al., 1999; Shin et al., 1999).

Another approach to examining the functional neurocircuitry of PTSD is the use of trauma-unrelated affective stimuli such as emotional facial expressions. In response to fearful facial expressions, patients with PTSD show exaggerated responses in the amygdala (Rauch, Whalen, Shin, et al., 2000; Shin et al., 2005; Williams et al., 2006). Neutral auditory oddball paradigms and continuous performance tasks have also elicited exaggerated amygdalar activation in patients with PTSD versus healthy controls (Bryant et al., 2005; Semple et al., 2000).

In summary, amygdalar hyperactivity and anterior cingulate hyporesponsivity have been identified as key features of the functional neurocircuitry of PTSD. Amygdala responsivity has been found to be positively correlated with PTSD symptom severity, whereas medial PFC responsivity has been shown to be inversely correlated.

Imaging Studies of Neurochemistry

In a preliminary study, Schuff and colleagues (1997) measured NAA using proton MRS imaging in seven veterans with PTSD and an equal number of nonveteran controls. Although they found a nonsignificantly smaller volume of the right hippocampus (6%) in the PTSD group versus the control group with mMRI, they found a more marked 18% reduction in right hippocampal NAA with MRS. This study did not, however, control for level of alcohol abuse, a factor known to affect the volume of certain brain structures. To clarify the potential contribution of alcohol exposure, Schuff et al. (2001) conducted a second, larger study of 18 men with combat-related PTSD and 19 male comparisons. An attempt was made to control for alcohol exposure by including only men with no reported alcohol or drug abuse during the 5 years prior to scanning. In this larger sample, no significant difference in hippocampal volume was found between the groups; however, a bilateral reduction in NAA averaging 23% was reported in the men with PTSD compared to the controls. Creatine-containing compounds were also reduced in the right hippocampus of the men with PTSD. Two recent studies lend support to the hypothesis that hippocampal neuronal function may be compromised in PTSD. In a study of 26 subway fire survivors with PTSD compared with 25 age- and sex-matched controls, NAA levels were reduced in the bilateral hippocampi, as measured by proton MRS (Ham et al., 2007). *N*-acetylasparate (NAA) levels were negatively correlated with reports of reexperiencing symptoms of the traumatic event in the PTSD group. In another study examining the results of traumatic exposure to a major fire, Li and colleagues (2006) studied 12 patients with PTSD compared with 12 subjects exposed to the same trauma without developing PTSD. Using proton MRS, the NAA/Cr ratio was reduced in the left hippocampus of those patients with PTSD compared to those without. These metabolic changes suggest that aberrations in hippocampal neurochemistry may be present, affecting function, regardless of hippocampal volume loss in patients with PTSD.

Following functional imaging studies implicating the ACC in the pathophysiology of PTSD, De Bellis et al. (2000) measured NAA concentration using proton MRS in the anterior cingulate of 11 children and adolescents with maltreatment-related PTSD and an equal number of matched comparisons. They found that the PTSD cohort exhibited relatively lower NAA/Cr ratios than the control group, concluding that neuronal integrity in the anterior cingulate may be altered in childhood PTSD. Ham and colleagues (2007) reported a similar finding of reduced NAA levels in the ACC of patients with PTSD surviving a subway fire, again suggesting reduced neuronal function in the ACC. In a study of women reporting a history of intimate partner violence and PTSD, an increase in Cho/Cr ratio in the ACC, suggestive of glial alterations, was found (Seedat et al., 2005).

A limited number of investigations of neuroreceptor function in PTSD have been reported, focusing on the benzodiazepine/GABA and serotonin receptor systems. Bremner, Innis, Southwick, et al. (2000) measured benzodiazepine receptor binding in 13 patients with combat-related PTSD and 13 case-matched controls. Subjects were studied with the radioligand [^{123}I]iomazenil using SPECT, with distribution volume, a benzodiazepine receptor binding measure, as the outcome measure. Patients with PTSD showed a significant reduction (41%) in distribution volume in the PFC (BA 9) compared to healthy controls. No other brain regions demonstrated group differences of either increased or decreased binding. Although the finding of lower benzodiazepine binding in frontal cortex is consistent with animal studies showing decreased benzodiazepine binding in the same region in response to stress, it should be noted that a subsequent study also examining combat veterans failed to replicate this finding (Fujita et al., 2004). Bonne and colleagues (2005) examined the serotonin 5-HT$_{1A}$ receptor in PTSD using PET and found no significant differences in the 5-HT$_{1A}$ volume of distribution or binding potential between the PTSD and healthy comparison groups in any brain region. Lack of a finding for the 5-HT$_{1A}$ receptor in PTSD differs from studies in panic disorder and social anxiety disorder (SAD), where reductions in 5-HT$_{1A}$ binding have been reported (Neumeister et al., 2004; Lanzenberger et al., 2007).

Summary

Taken together, imaging data from various studies support the current neurocircuitry model of PTSD that emphasizes the functional relationship between a triad of brain structures: the amygdala, hippocampus, and ventral/medial PFC. Morphometric MRI studies show decreased hippocampal volume, which is convergent with MRS findings of decreased NAA in the hippocampus. Functional studies indicate a rightward shift in hippocampal activity at rest. When exposed to reminders of traumatic events, patients most consistently appear to recruit anterior paralimbic regions as well as the amygdala, while exhibiting decreased activity within other heteromodal cortical areas. In comparison with controls, however, patients with PTSD exhibit diminished anterior cingulate activation, and morphometric MRI studies suggest that anterior cingulate volume may be reduced in PTSD.

PANIC DISORDER

Neuroanatomical Models of Panic Disorder

Pathophysiological models of PD are as disparate as the methods used to provoke panic attacks in neurobiological challenge studies (Coplan and Lydiard, 1998). Proposed models have emphasized a number of widely varied factors including dysregulated ascending noradrenergic and/or serotonergic systems, abnormal responsivity to CO_2 at the level of brain stem (so-called false suffocation alarm), global cerebral abnormalities in lactate metabolism, and abnormalities in the hippocampal-amygdalar circuitry. Perhaps the greatest challenge to investigators has been to provide a satisfactory model to explain the occurrence of spontaneous panic attacks. By contrast, the behavioral sequelae of recurrent panic attacks, such as agoraphobic avoidance, are more readily explained by learning theory and the fear conditioning model.

Abnormal regulation of homeostasis in the fear neurocircuitry, due to either aberrant modulation by monoamine systems or aberrant processing of sensory and/or biochemical information, might lead to spontaneous recruitment of the normal anxiety/fear circuitry, resulting in a spontaneous panic attack as an aberrant event. Another possibility is that panic attacks evolve in the context of what should be minor anxiety episodes because of failures in constraint by systems responsible for limiting anxiety responding. Similar to the previously discussed model of PTSD, hippocampal deficits might underlie such a mechanism in the case of PD. Finally, panic episodes that are described as spontaneous, without an identifiable precipitant, might in fact be anxiety responses to unconscious stimuli, and therefore the anxiety circuitry is being recruited without conscious awareness. Because it is now established that activation of the subcortical amygdalar circuit described by LeDoux (1996) occurs in the absence of conscious awareness that a threat-related stimulus has been presented (e.g., Whalen, Rauch, et al., 1998), this is another possible explanation for the occurrence of spontaneous panic episodes (Fig. 43.3). In summary, PD might be characterized by fundamental amygdala hyperresponsivity to subtle (even unconscious) environmental cues, triggering full-scale, threat-related responding with insufficient top-down governance.

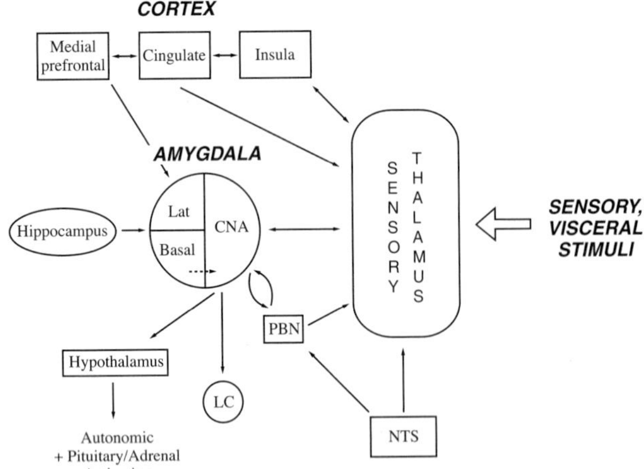

FIGURE 43.3 Pathways critical in fear conditioning, with relevance to preliminary models in panic disorder and social anxiety disorder. CNA: central nucleus of the amygdala; LC: locus ceruleus; NTS: nucleus of the solitary tract.

Structural Imaging Findings

Of the structural imaging studies reported in PD, an early qualitative study by Fontaine and colleagues (1990) examined the MRI scans of 31 consecutive patients with PD and 20 matched healthy controls. They found a higher frequency of gross structural abnormalities in the PD group (40%) compared with the control group (10%), with the most striking focal findings in the PD group being abnormal signal or asymmetric atrophy of the right temporal lobe. Vythilingam and colleagues (2000) published a quantitative mMRI study focusing on the temporal lobe and hippocampus of 13 patients with PD and 14 healthy comparisons. They found a significantly smaller mean volume of the temporal lobes in the PD group versus the comparison group, while finding no significant differences in hippocampal volume between the groups. In a more recent voxel-based morphometric study, patients with PD demonstrated significantly increased gray matter volume in the midbrain and brain-stem rostral pons in comparison to healthy controls, and a trend for decreased PFC volume (Protopopescu et al., 2006). These results support earlier proposed neuroanatomical models of panic disorder, hypothesizing panic attacks originating in brain-stem loci (Gorman et al., 1989; Gorman et al., 2000).

Functional Imaging Findings

Two studies have examined rCBF in patients with PD at rest. In an early neutral-state PET study, Reiman and colleagues (1986) studied 16 patients with PD and 25 normal controls. Of the 16 patients with PD, 8 had previously been determined to be sensitive to lactate-induced panic. This subset of patients with PD had abnormally low left/right ratios of parahippocampal blood flow at rest. Several years later, De Cristofaro et al. (1993) used SPECT to measure rCBF at rest in seven treatment-naive patients with PD and five age-matched healthy comparisons. The investigators found that the patients with PD exhibited greater rCBF in left occipital cortex and lower rCBF in the hippocampal area compared to the control group.

In studies examining regional cerebral glucose metabolic rate (rCMRglu in patients with PD in neutral (unprovoked) states, Nordahl et al. (1990) used PET-FDG methods to measure (rCMRglu) in 12 patients with PD and 30 normal controls while they engaged in an auditory continuous performance task. The PD group exhibited a lower left/right hippocampal ratio compared to the healthy comparisons. In a later study including female subjects only, Bisaga et al. (1998) used PET-FDG to study six patients with PD and an equal number of

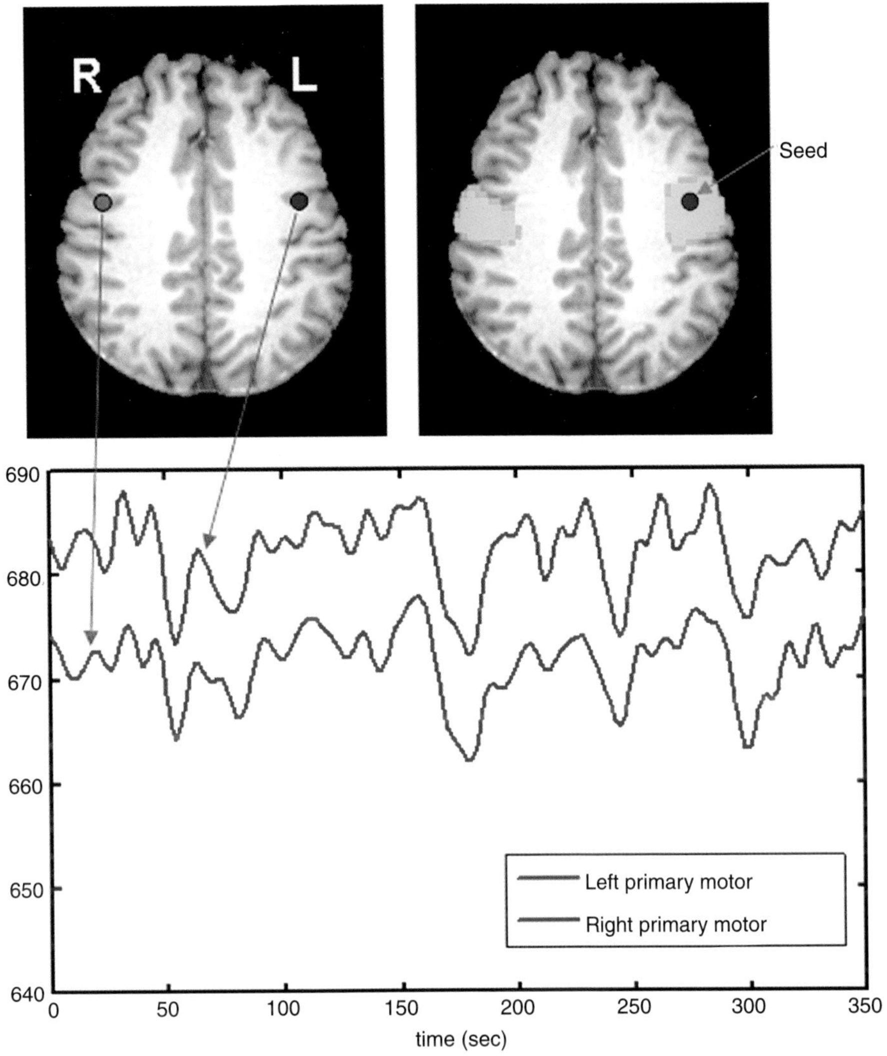

COLOR FIGURE 13.3 Functional magnetic resonance imaging (fMRI) signals at rest (bottom) from the left and right primary sensorimotor cortices (upper left), and functional connectivity map (upper right) obtained from cross-correlation analysis using the left sensorimotor cortex as a reference.

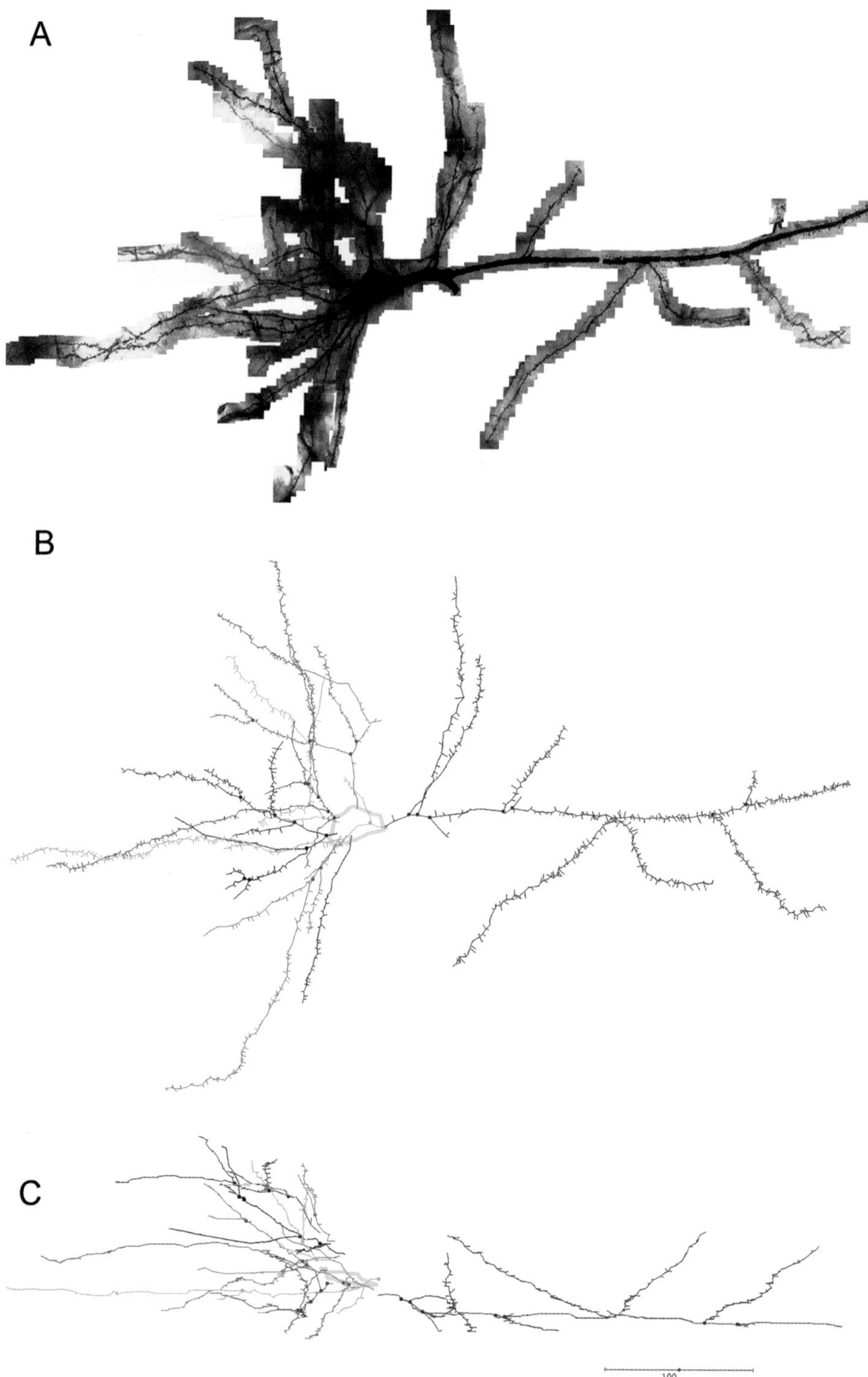

COLOR FIGURE 21.3 (*A*) Photomontage and (*B*) computer-recorded tracing of Golgi stain (on unfixed autopsy specimen) of a subicular pyramidal neuron. (*C*) Rotation of tracing perpendicular to the plane of section demonstrates that several dendrites, including the main shaft of the apical dendrite, were truncated at the cut surface of the 200 micron-thick section. Scale bar = 100 microns. (Thanks to Tatiana Schnieder.)

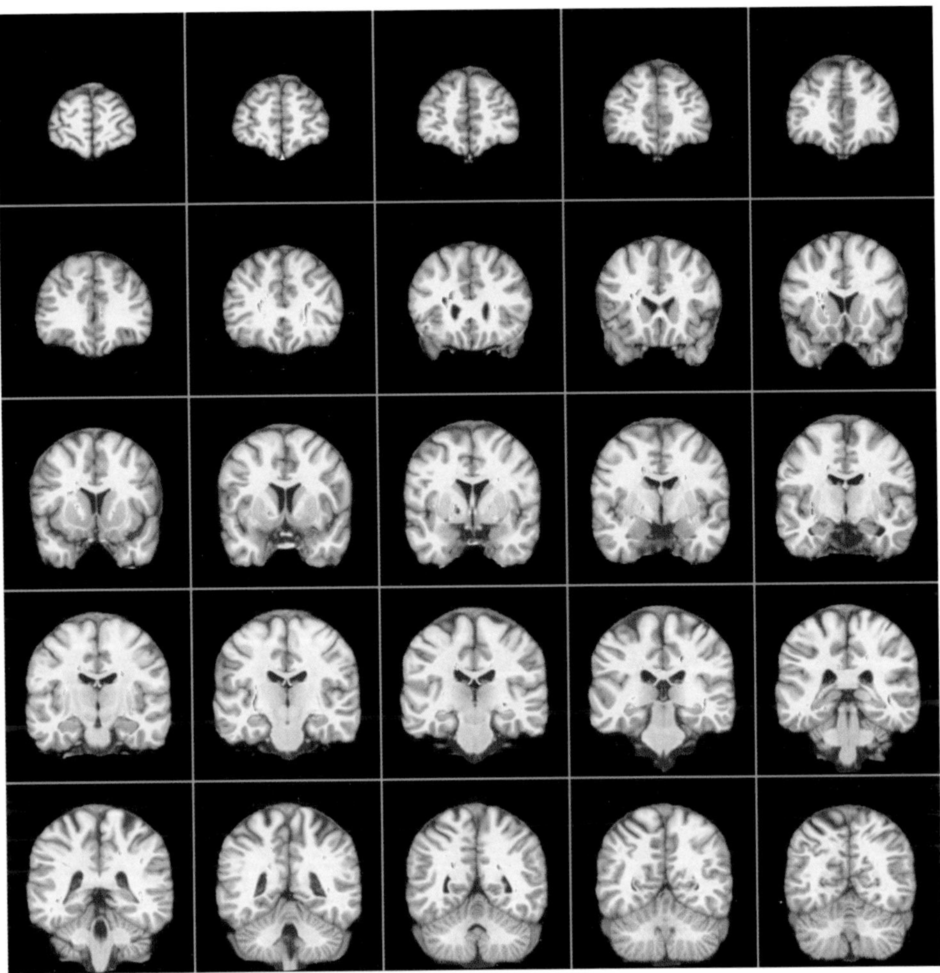

COLOR FIGURE 21.4 Widespread differences in white matter fractional anisotropy (FA) between 43 subjects with schizophrenia or schizoaffective disorder and 47 healthy comparison subjects. Yellow = areas in which FA is higher in controls, Blue = areas in which FA is higher in subjects. Images are thresholded at $p = .0065$ (false discovery rate $q = .05$), with a 50mm^3 extent threshold. Every fifth coronal millimeter is shown, from anterior to posterior.

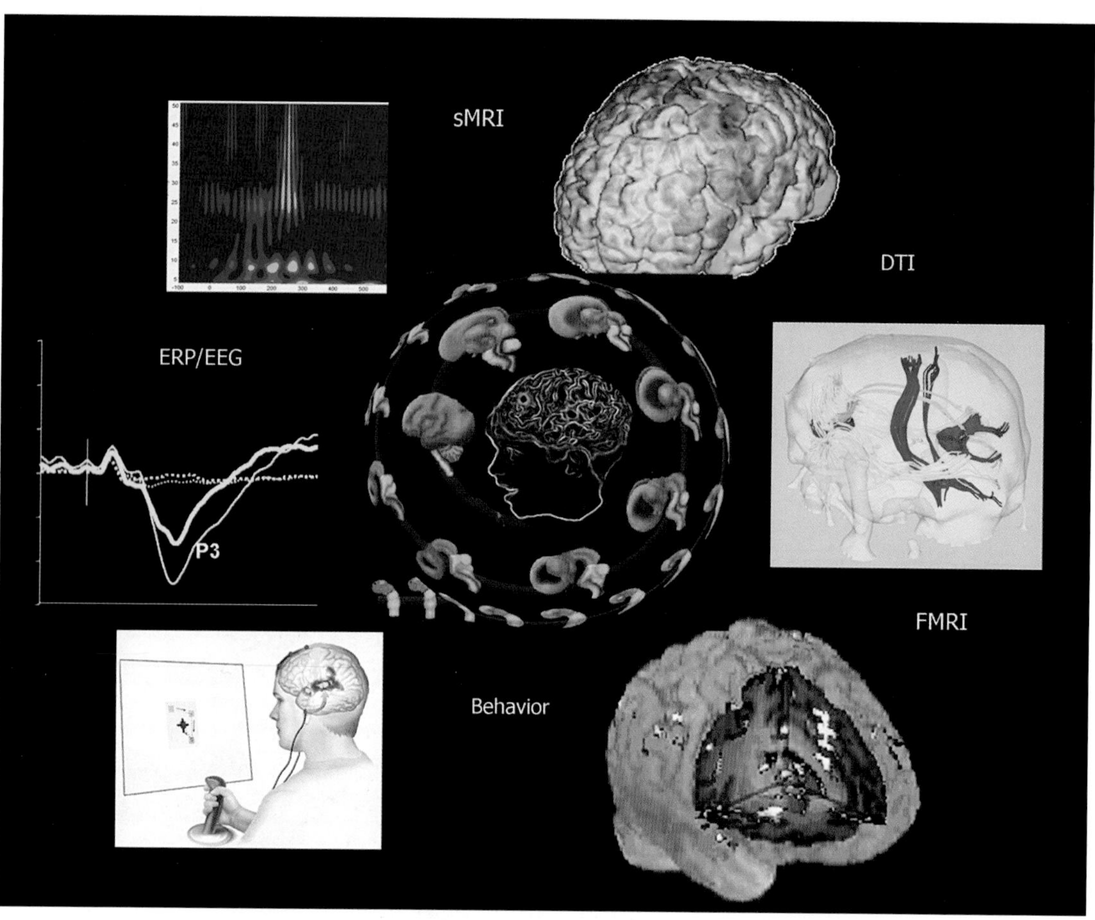

COLOR FIGURE 22.1 Representation of converging methods and techniques typically used by cognitive neuroscientists to study behaviors, associated brain functions, and their underlying neuroanatomy. Many of these methods are non-invasive, and can be implemented repeated times to enable longitudinal assessments to track disease progression and treatment effects.

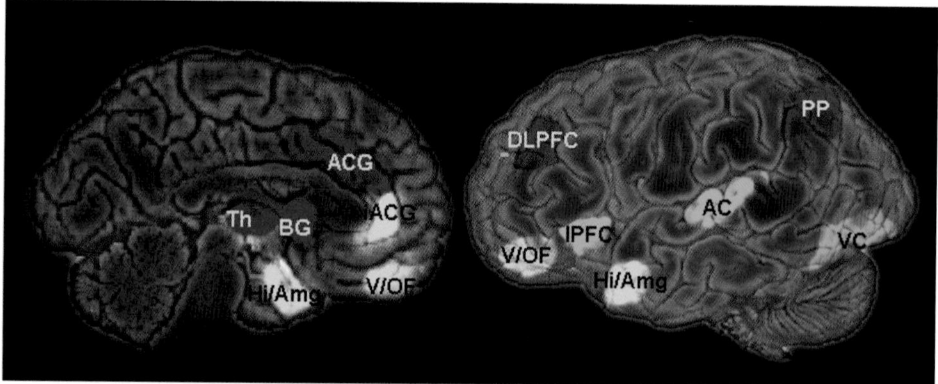

COLOR FIGURE 22.2 Neural circuits associated with the three primary domains of information processing deficits in schizophrenia: green: sensory cortices; red: fronto-striate and fronto-parietal executive and attention control regions; yellow: fronto-limbic affective processing and episodic memory regions.

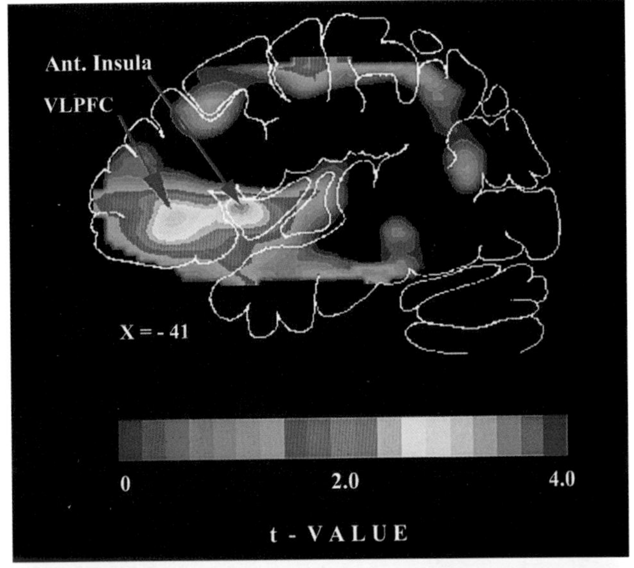

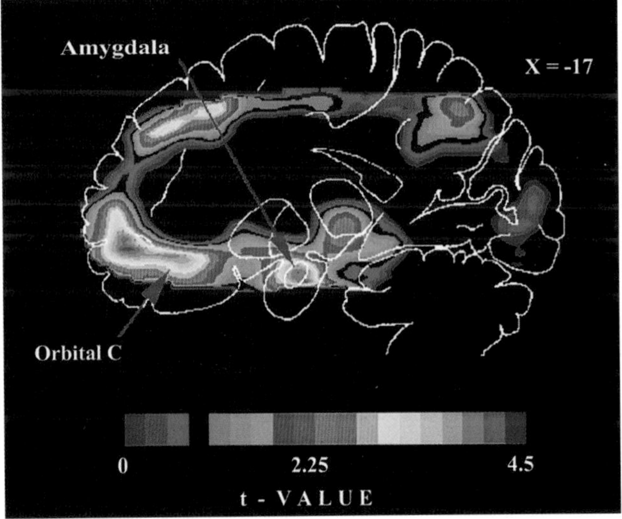

COLOR FIGURE 31.2 (*A-B*). Areas of abnormally increased blood flow in patients with major depressive disorder. The image sections shown are from an image of t-values, produced by a voxel-by-voxel computation of the unpaired t-statistic to compare regional CBF between a depressed sample selected according to criteria for familial pure depressive disease (n = 13) and a healthy control sample (n = 33) (Drevets et al., 1992). The positive t-values shown correspond to areas where flow is increased in the depressives relative to the controls. The abnormal activity in these regions was replicated using glucose metabolism imaging in independent subject samples (Drevets, Spitznagel, and Raichle, 1995; Drevets, Bogers, and Raichle, 2002; Drevets, Price, et al., 2002). (*A*) Sagittal section at 17 mm left of midline illustrating areas of increased CBF in depression in the amygdala and orbital cortex. (*B*) This area of increased flow extended through the lateral orbital cortex (C) to the ventrolateral prefrontal cortex (VLPFC) and anterior (Ant) insula (Drevets et al., 1992; Drevets, Bogers, and Raichle, 2002). The x coordinate locates sagittal sections in mm to the left of midline. (*A-B*). The PET images from which the t-image was generated have been stereotaxically transformed to the coordinate system of Talairach and Tournoux (*Co-Planar Stereotaxic Atlas of the Human Brain*, Stuttgart, Thieme, 1988), from which the corresponding atlas outline is shown. Anterior is left. Illustration *A* is modified from Price et al. (1996) and *B* is reproduced from Drevets (1994) with permission. CBF: cerebral blood flow; PET: positron emission tomography

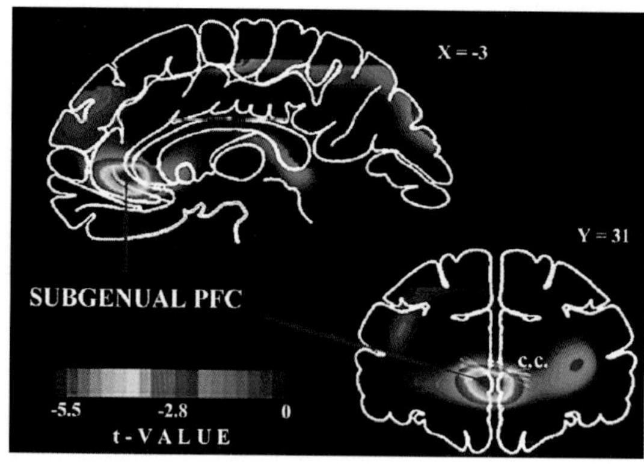

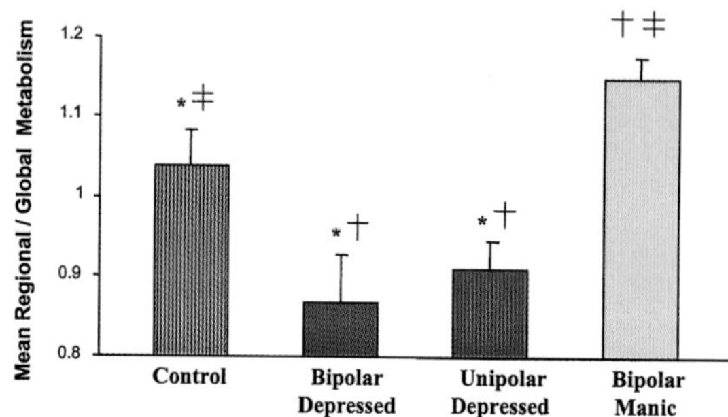

COLOR FIGURE 31.3 Altered metabolism in PFC ventral to the genu of the corpus callosum (that is, subgenual PFC) in mood disorders. The top panel shows negative voxel t-values where glucose metabolism is decreased in depressives relative to controls in coronal (31 mm anterior to the anterior commissure, or y = 31) and sagittal (3 mm left of midline, or x = −3) planes of a statistical parametric image that compares depressives relative to controls (Drevets et al., 1997). This image localized an abnormality in the subgenual portion of the ACC (subgenual ACC; Drevets et al., 1997), which was subsequently shown to be accounted for by a corresponding reduction in cortex volume on the left side (see text). Anterior or left is to left. The bar histogram in the lower panel shows mean, normalized, glucose metabolic values for the left subgenual ACC measured using MRI-based region-of-interest analysis. Metabolism is decreased in depressed patients with either BD or MDD relative to healthy controls. In contrast, subjects scanned in the manic phase of BD have higher metabolism than either depressed or control patients in this region. Asterisk: difference between controls and bipolar depressives significant at $p < 0.025$; cross: difference between depressed and manic significant at $p < 0.01$; double cross: difference between control and manic significant at $p < 0.05$. Although none of these patients were involved in the study that generated the images shown in Figure 31.2, the mean glucose metabolism in this independent sample of depressed patients and controls also confirmed the areas of abnormally increased activity in the depressed patients in the amygdala, lateral orbital cortex, ventrolateral PFC, and medial thalamus (not shown in the t-image section in the figure, which only illustrates negative t-values corresponding to hypometabolic areas in the patients who were depressed). Reproduced with permission from Drevets et al. (1997) (upper panel) and Drevets (2001) (lower panel). PFC: prefrontal cortex; ACC: anterior cingulate cortex; MRI: magnetic resonance imaging; BD: bipolar depressed; MDD: unipolar depressed.

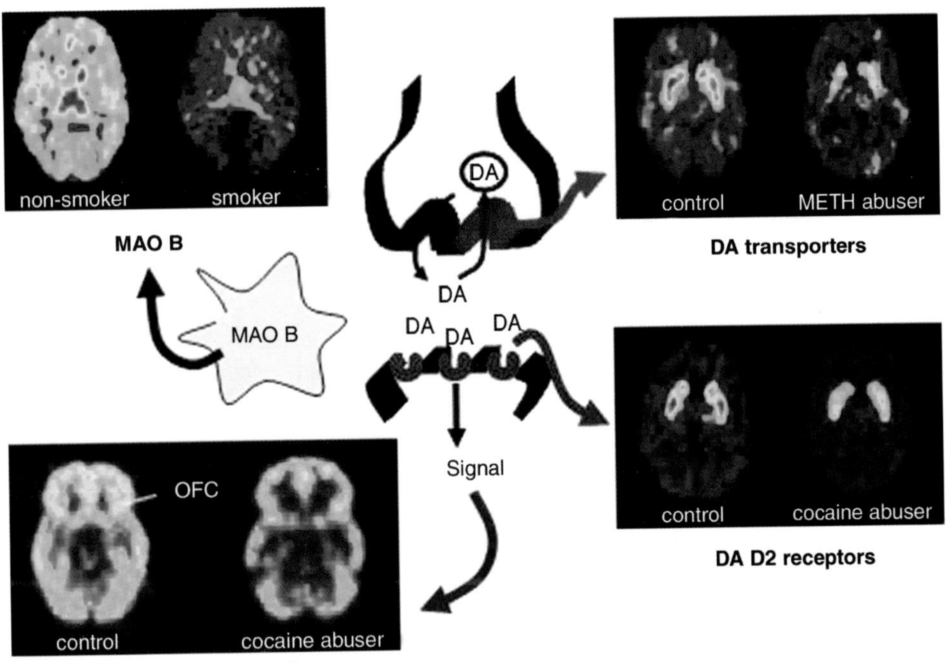

COLOR FIGURE 49.1 Simplified diagram of a dopamine synapse showing the dopamine transporter (red), dopamine receptors (blue) and MAO-B (in glia cells). PET images of the human brain (clockwise from upper left) show brain MAO-B inhibition in a smoker measured with [^{11}C]L-deprenyl-D2 , reduced dopamine transporter availability in an abuser of methamphetamine (measured with [^{11}C]d-threo-methylphenidate), reduced dopamine D_2/D_3 receptors in an abuser of cocaine (measured with [^{11}C]raclopride) and reduced glucose metabolism in the orbitofrontal cortex in a cocaine abuser (measured with 18FDG). A rainbow color scale is used where red is highest activity and blue is lowest. MOA-B: monoamine oxidase B; PET: positron emission tomography.

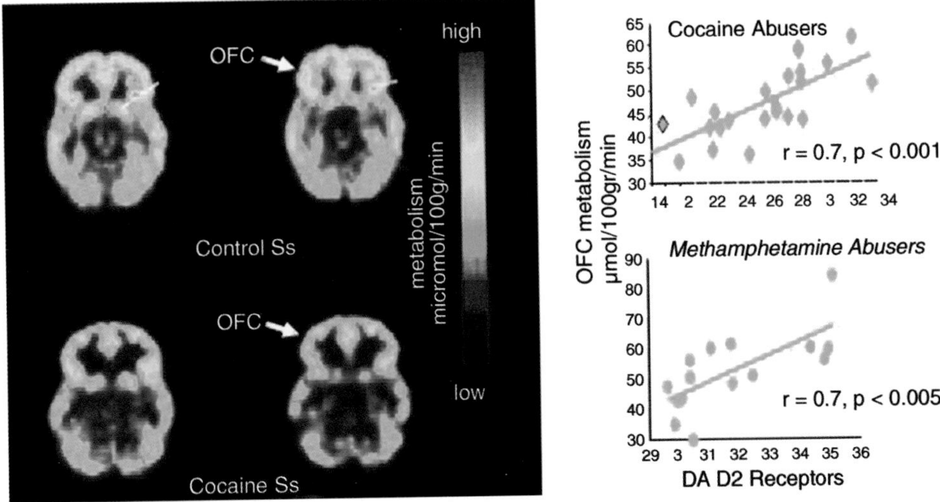

COLOR FIGURE 49.2 The left shows images of brain glucose metabolism in a control and in an abuser of cocaine at the level where the OFC is located. The right side of the figure shows the regression slopes between the availability of dopamine D_2 receptors and metabolism in OFC for a group of abusers of cocaine and for a group of abusers of methamphetamine. Note that the lower the D_2 receptor availability, the lower the metabolism in OFC. Modified from Volkow et al., 2004. OFC: orbitofrontal cortex.

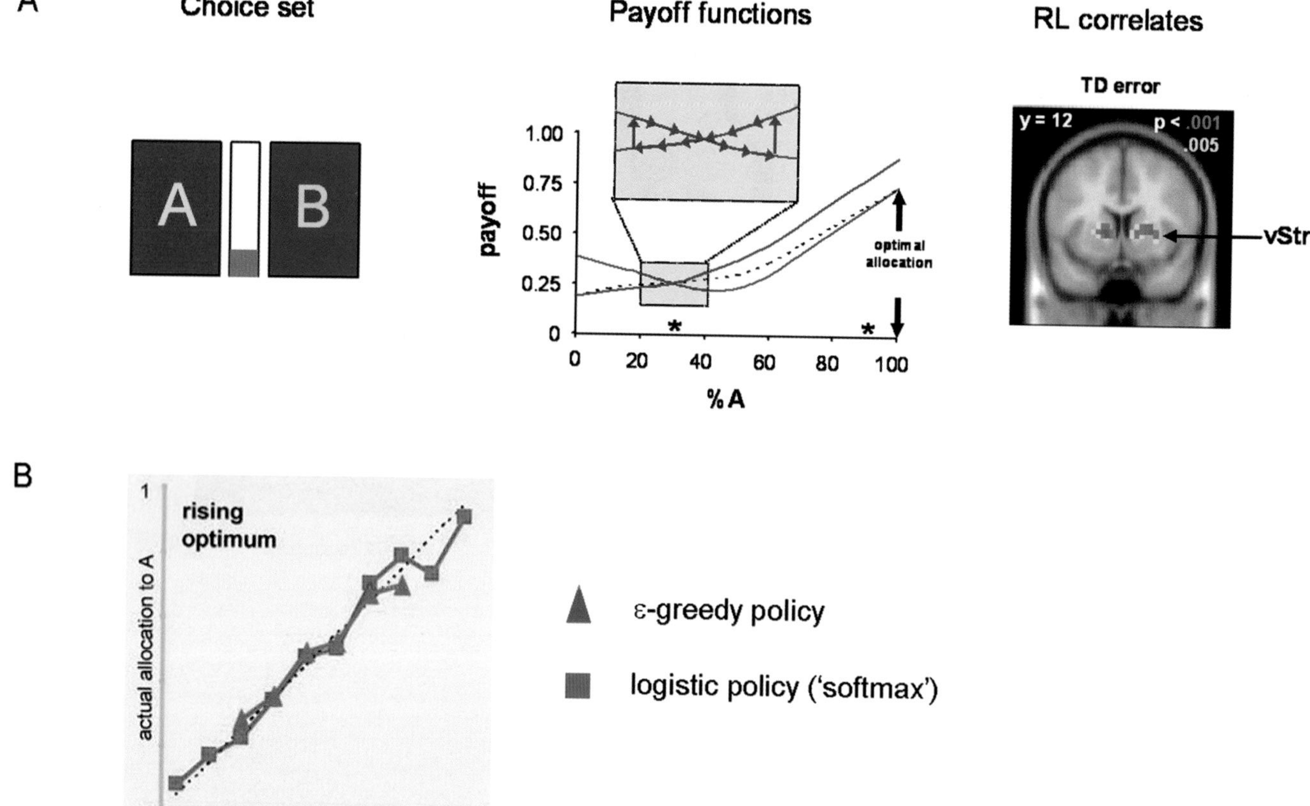

COLOR FIGURE 50.5 Actor–critic signals during sequential two-choice decision task. (*A*) Neural correlate of reward prediction error during sequential choice task. (Left) Two-choice task with returns encoded by centrally placed slider bar. (Middle) Inset shows the average behavior of a temporal difference (TD)-error-driven actor–critic model near the crossing point in the reward function. The colored arrows show what happens when red (A) or blue (B) is chosen, and they indicate the direction that the participants move along the *x* axis. The inset shows how these functions model one typical real-world occurrence for simple choices—choosing to sample A (red) tends to decrease returns from A while the unsampled returns from B increase, like flowers refilling with nectar while they are not being sampled. An actor–critic model will tend to stick near crossing points (explained in Montague and Berns, 2002). (Right) The hemodynamic correlate of a TD error signal throughout the entire 250 choices in this task is shown at two levels of significance (.001 and .005 [random effect]; $N = 46$; y = 12mm). This payoff functions for this task are modified from a task originally proposed by Herrnstein and Prelec (1991) to test a theory of choice called *melioration* (adapted almost verbatim from Li et al., 2006). (*B*) Actor–critic model captures choice behavior. Participant decisions were predicted using a reinforcement learning model with two different methods to determine the probability to choose an action (ε-greedy method and sigmoid method). For both methods, we assume that participants maintained independent estimates of the reward expected for each choice, A and B, and updated these values based on experienced rewards using a choice-dependent TD-error (that is, the Rescorla-Wagner learning algorithm). Choices were assumed to be (*1*) probabilistically related to choice values according to a sigmoid function (softmax method, green curve) or (*2*) have a fixed probability of $1\text{-}\varepsilon/2$ for choice associated with bigger weight (ε-greedy method, pink curve). Decisions were binned (*x* axis) based on predicted likelihood that subjects would choose A. Y values indicate the actual average allocation to A for all choices within each bin. Linear regression shows there is a strong correlation between predicted and actual choices. (MS: $r = 0.97$, RO: $r = 0.99$, FR: $r = 0.97$, PR: $r = 0.97$ for softmax method; MS: $r = 0.97$, RO: $r = 0.99$, FR: $r = 0.95$, PR: $r = 0.99$ for ε-greedy method). (Adapted almost verbatim from Li et al., 2006.) MS: Matching Shoulder; RO: Rising Optimum: FR: Flat Return; PR: Pseudorandom.

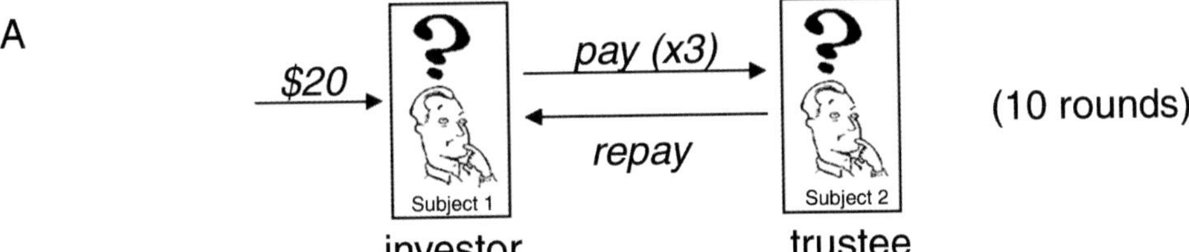

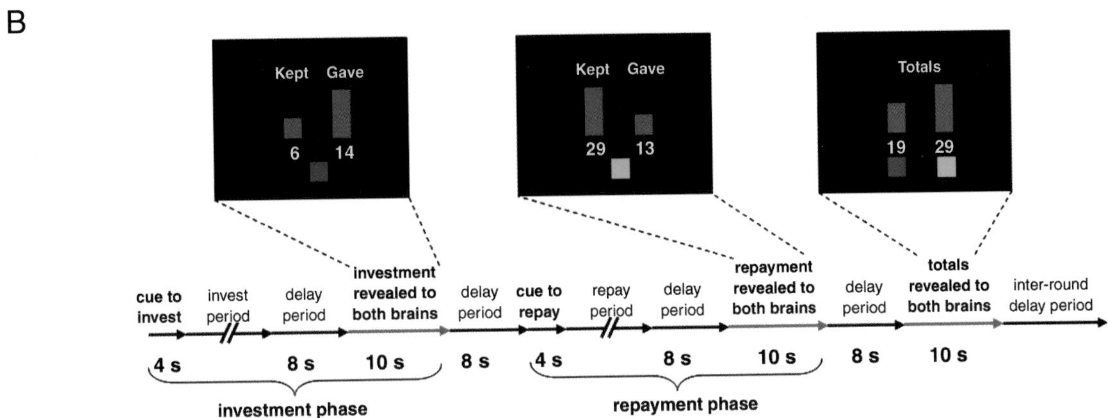

COLOR FIGURE 50.9 Multiround trust game: harvesting rewards from other humans. (*A*) On each round, one player called the *investor* is endowed with $20 and can send ("trust") the other player (called the *trustee*) any fraction of this amount. The amount sent is tripled en route to the trustee who then decides what fraction of the tripled amount to repay. Players execute 10 rounds of this pay–repay cycle. Players maintain their respective roles throughout the entire task permitting the development of reputations with one another. (*B*) Timeline for events in the multiround trust game. Outcome screens are revealed simultaneously to both players; both interacting brains were scanned simultaneously (see King-Casas et al., 2005; multiround trust game is a variation on the game proposed by Camerer and Weigelt, 1988; Berg et al., 1995).

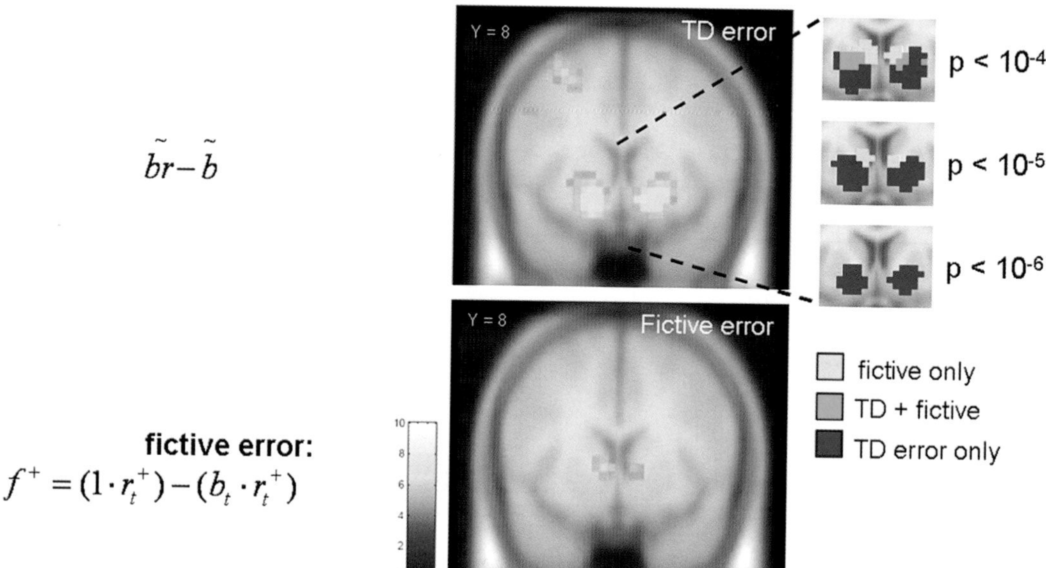

COLOR FIGURE 50.14 Separable neural responses for reward prediction error and fictive error. The fictive error signal (Figs. 50.12, 50.13) and the experiential error signal (version of a temporal difference (TD) error signal) are sometimes colinear and must be mathematically separated. This figure shows those activations (at the prescribed statistical threshold) associated with the TD error alone, the fictive error alone, and both. The fictive error is computed as explained in Figure 50.13. At each decision, the experiential error is taken as the difference between the z-scored bet $\tilde{b}$ (proxy for expected value of return) and the actual return $\tilde{b}r_t$. Here, r_t is the market as defined in Figure 50.13 (relative fractional change in the price; adapted from Lohrenz et al., 2007; also see Montague et al., 2006; Chiu et al., 2008).

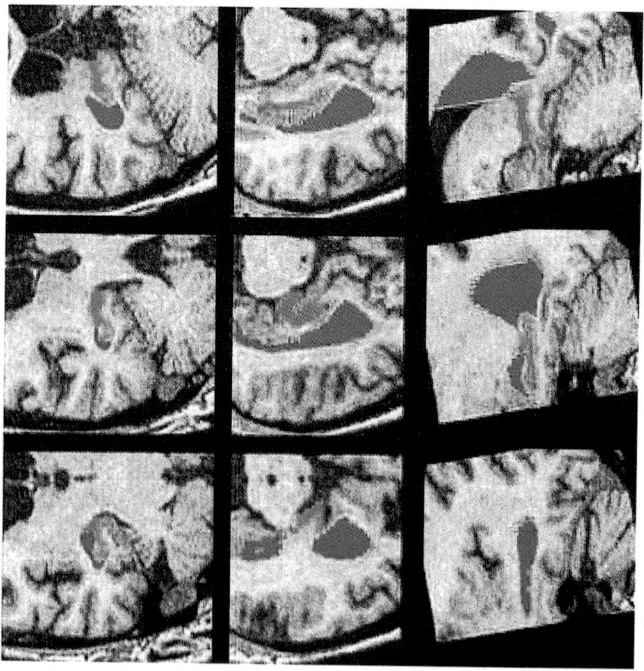

COLOR FIGURE 57.3B The magnetic resonance imaging scans were obtained on a General Electric Advantage 1.5T imager using a spoiled gradient echo sequence of 35/9/1 (TR/TE/excitations), a 60 degree flip angle, an 18 cm field of view, and a 256 × 128 acquisition matrix. We obtained 124 contiguous coronal images with a slice thickness of 1.3 mm. On 56 of these images, using a twofold image magnification to aid in region drawing (pixel size = 0.35 mm), we outlined and coded in yellow the hippocampal fissures. Also, the cerebrospinal fluid (CSF) of the lateral ventricle was outlined and coded in red. The top panel shows 3 of the 56 slices coded. All 56 coronal images and the coded regions were reformatted and displayed as 5 mm contiguous slices in a negative angulation axial plane (middle panel) and in a sagittal plane (bottom panel). The reformatted axial images and sagittal images depict the anatomical relationship of the two CSF compartments.

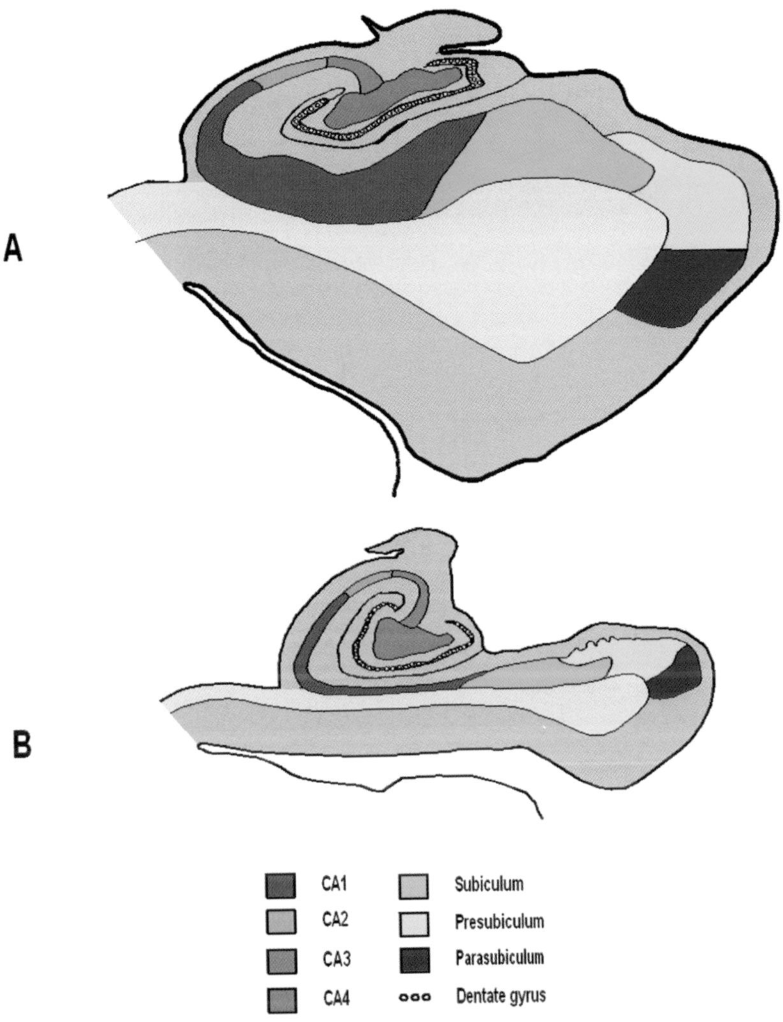

COLOR FIGURE 57.4 Schematic drawings of histologically derived volumes of the hippocampus and subicular complex. (*A*) is the average normal control and (*B*) is the average Alzheimer's disease (AD) patient.

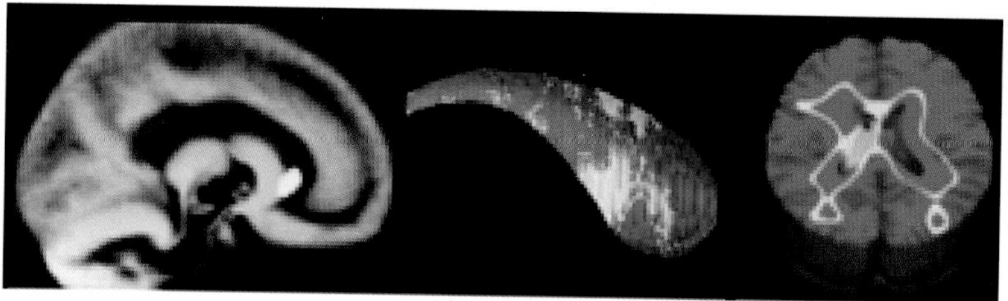

COLOR FIGURE 67.1 Increased caudate size as measured by voxel-based morphometry (left), surface based mapping (middle) and tensor-based morphometry (right) (Lee et al., 2007).

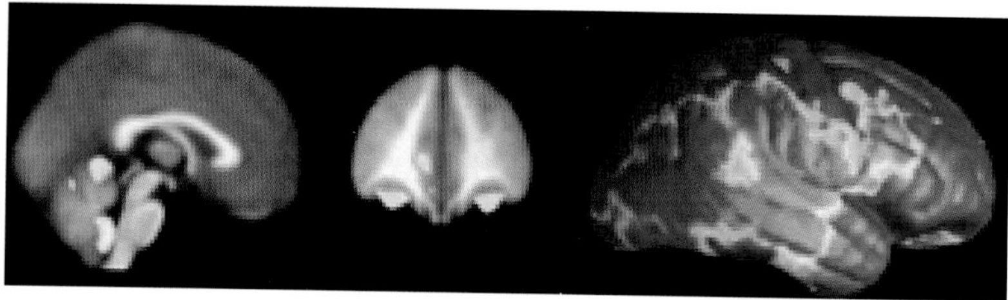

COLOR FIGURE 67.3 Structural abnormalities in individuals with Williams syndrome: increased cerebellar vermis and orbito-frontal region as measured by voxel-based morphometry (left); and increased cortical thickness including superior temporal gyrus (STG) (Gaser et al., 2006).

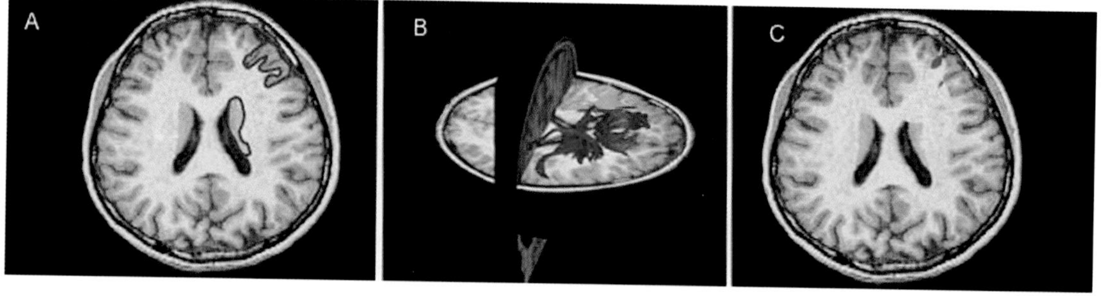

COLOR FIGURE 68.1 Structural magnetic resonance imaging (MRI) is used to produce structural images of the brain useful for anatomical and morphometric studies (Panel A), diffusion tensor imaging (DTI) measures fiber tracts between anatomical structures (Panel B), and functional MRI (fMRI) measures patterns of brain activity within those structures (Panel C). From Casey et al. (2002).

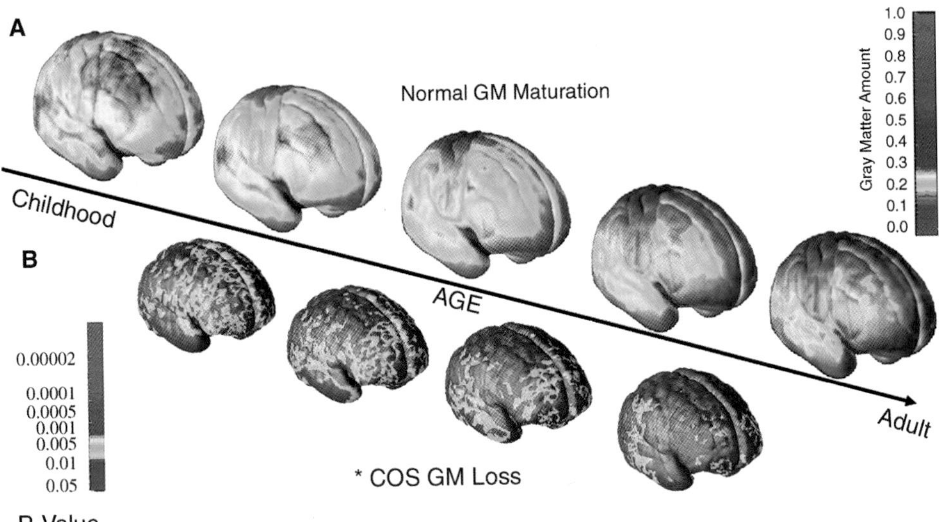

COLOR FIGURE 76.1 Comparison of the patterns of cortical gray matter (GM) loss in childhood-onset schizophrenia (COS) (between ages 12 and 16) to that seen in normal cortical maturation (between ages 4 to 22). (*A*) Right lateral view of the dynamic sequences of cortical GM maturation in healthy children between ages 4 and 22 (n = 13; 54 scans; upper panel) rescanned every 2 years. Scale bar shows GM amount at each of the 65,536 cortical points across the entire cortex represented using a color scale (Red to Pink – More GM; Blue – GM Loss). Cortical GM maturation appears to progress in a "back to front" (parieto-temporal) manner. (*B*) Right lateral view of the dynamic sequence of cortical GM maturation in COS between ages 12 to 16 compared with age- and sex-matched healthy controls (n = 12, 36 scans in each group), where children are rescanned every 2 years. Dynamic maps represent p values for the difference in GM amount between COS and controls at each of the 65,536 cortical points, and p values are represented using a color scale (for example, Pink $p <$ 0.00002). Cortical GM loss in COS also appears to follow in a "back to front" direction on the lateral surface, thus suggesting that the COS pattern is an exaggeration of the normal GM maturation.
*Data on Childhood Schizophrenia only age 12 to 16.

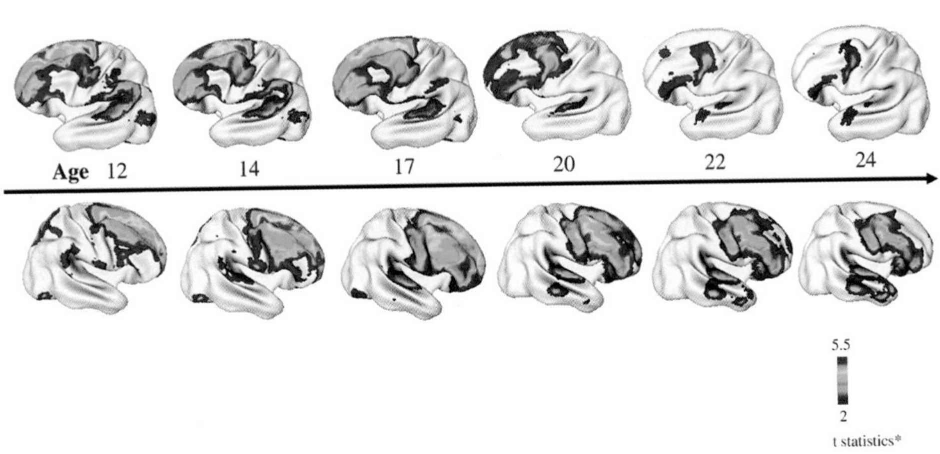

COLOR FIGURE 76.2 Progression of cortical gray matter (GM) loss in childhood-onset schizophrenia (COS) (n = 70, 162 scans) relative to age-, sex-, and scan interval–matched healthy controls (n = 72, 168 scans) from adolescence to young adulthood (age 12 to 24). Analyses were done using mixed model regression statistics and covaried for mean cortical thickness. Side bar shows t statistic with threshold to control for multiple comparisons using the false discovery rate (FDR) procedure with q = .05. Differences are from mixed model regression with age centered at approximate 3-year intervals for middle 80% of the age range and colors represent areas of statistically significant thinning in COS.

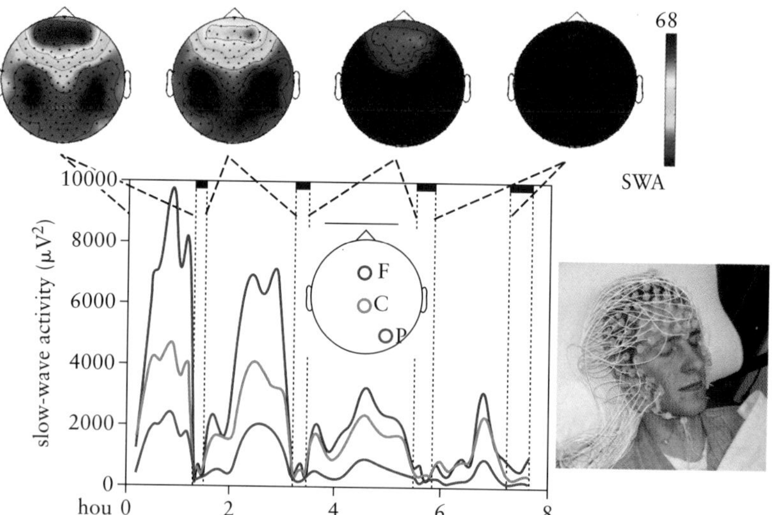

COLOR FIGURE 85.4 Sleep slow waves as a marker of sleep pressure. Bottom panel: During early sleep, at the end of a day of wakefulness, sleep pressure is maximal. This is reflected in frequent and large sleep slow waves, measured here as slow wave activity (power in the 0.5–4 Hz band, in red for a frontal electroencephalogram (EEG) channel, green for a central channel, and blue for an occipital channel). During sleep slow-wave activity decreases exponentially, reflecting a reduction of sleep pressure. The transitory drops in slow-wave activity correspond to episodes of rapid-eye-movement (REM) sleep. Top panel: topographic display of slow-wave activity over the scalp for the four sleep cycles. Notice the frontal predominance and the progressive decline in the course of the night.

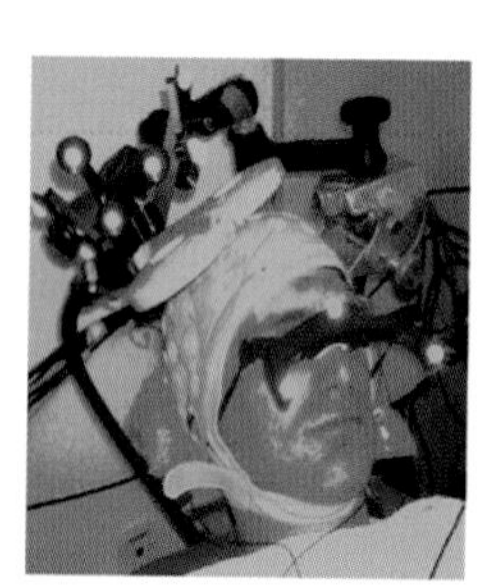

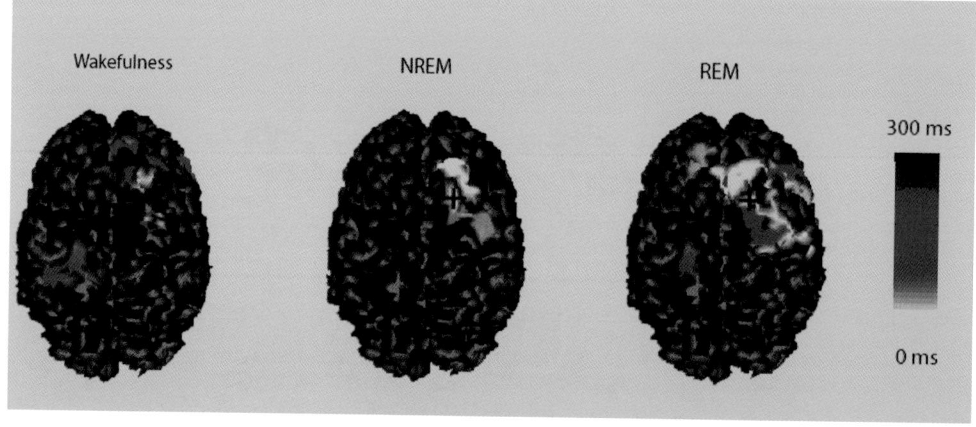

COLOR FIGURE 85.7 Spatiotemporal cortical current maps of transcranial magnetic stimulation (TMS)-induced activity during wakefulness, non-rapid-eye-movement (NREM), and rapid-eye-movement (REM) sleep. On the left is the setup for TMS/EEG. From the electroencephalogram (EEG) data, maximum current sources corresponding to periods of significant activations were plotted and color-coded according to their latency of activation (light blue, 0 ms; red, 300 ms). The yellow cross marks the TMS target on the cortical surface. Note the rapidly changing patterns of activation during wakefulness, lasting up to 300 ms and involving several different areas; the brief activation that remains localized to the area of stimulation during NREM sleep; and an intermediate pattern of activation during REM sleep. From Massimini and Tononi, 2005).

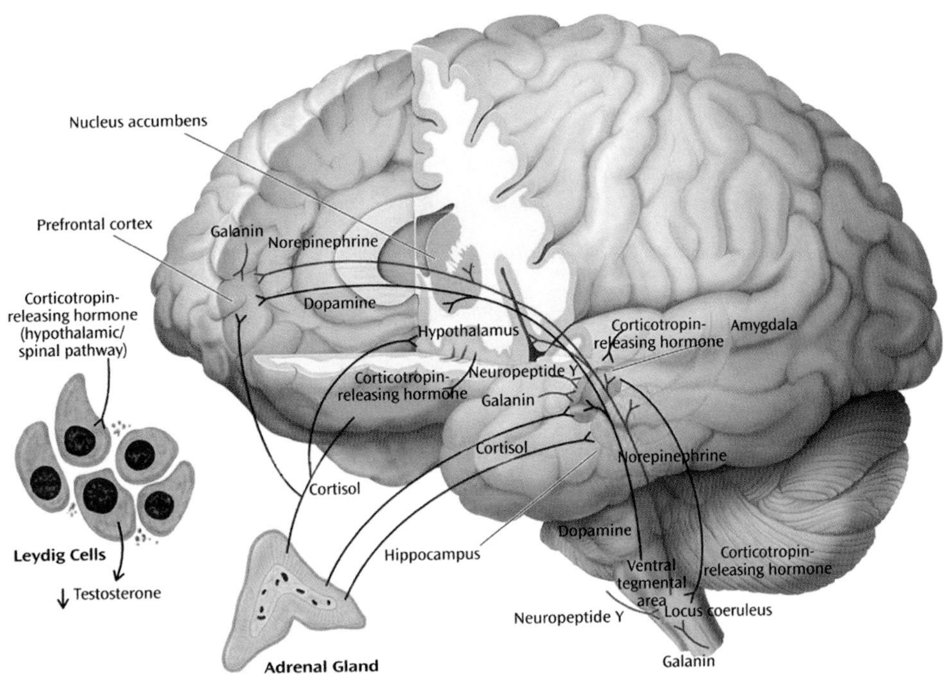

COLOR FIGURE 86.1 Neurochemical response patterns to acute stress. This figure illustrates some of the key brain structures involved in the neurochemical response patterns following acute psychological stress. The functional interactions among the different neurotransmitters, neuropeptides, and hormones are emphasized. The functional status of brain regions such as the amygdala (neuropeptide Y, galanin, corticotropin releasing hormone [CRH], cortisol, and norepinephrine), hippocampus (cortisol and norepinephrine), locus coeruleus (neuropeptide Y, galanin, and CRH), and prefrontal cortex (dopamine, norepinephrine, galanin, and cortisol) depends upon the balance among multiple inhibitory and excitatory neurochemical inputs. Functional effects may vary depending on the brain region. For example, cortisol increases CRH concentrations in the amygdala and decreases concentrations in the paraventricular nucleus of the hypothalamus. As described in the text, these neurochemical response patterns may relate to resilience and vulnerability to the effects of extreme psychological stress. (Modified and reprinted with permission from Cambridge University Press, 2007).

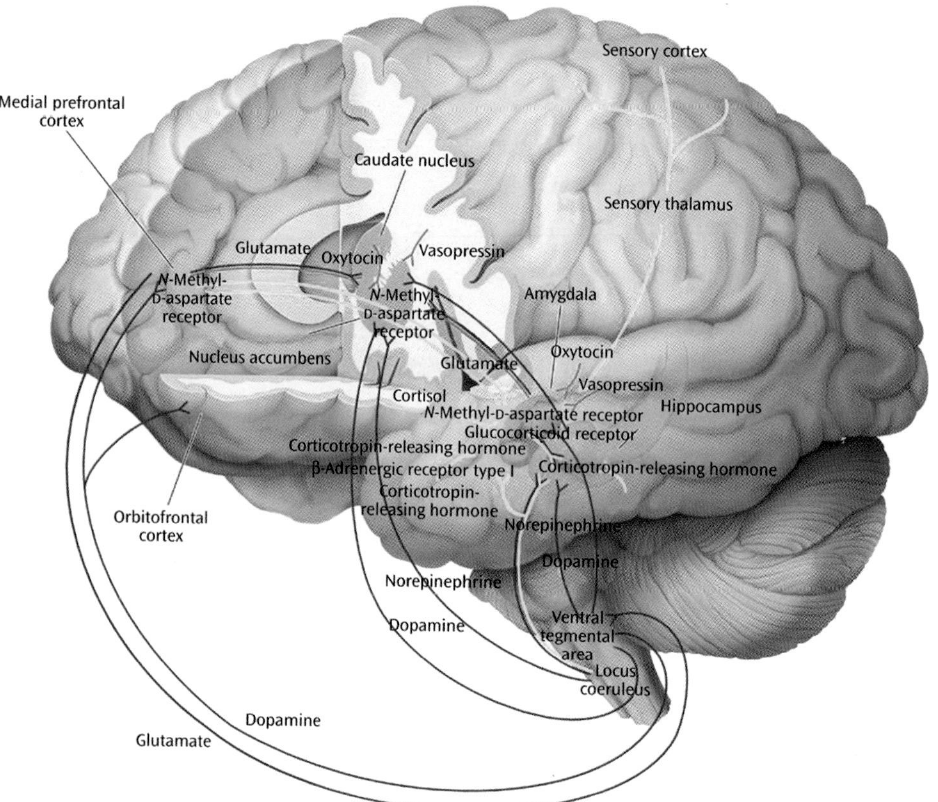

COLOR FIGURE 86.2. Neural circuits associated with reward, fear conditioning, and social behavior. The figure depicts a simplified summary of some of the brain structures and relevant neurochemistry mediating the neural mechanisms of reward (purple paths), fear conditioning, and extinction (yellow paths), and social behaviors (blue paths). Only a subset of the many known interconnections among these various regions is shown, and relevant interneurons are not illustrated, yet it can be seen there is considerable overlap in the brain structures associated with these neural mechanisms. This suggests that there may be clinically relevant functional interactions among the circuits. For example, a properly functioning reward circuit may be necessary for the reinforcement of positive social behaviors. An overly responsive fear circuit or impaired extinction process may negatively influence functioning of the reward system. The assessment of these neural mechanisms must be considered in the context of their neurochemical regulation. Alterations in one neurotransmitter, neuropeptide, or hormone system will affect more than one circuit. Several receptors that may be targeted by new anti-anxiety and antidepressant drugs are illustrated. The functional status of these circuits has important influences on stress-related psychopathology and the discovery of novel therapeutics (see text). (Modified and reprinted with permission from Cambridge University Press, 2007).

matched controls. Differing from earlier studies, which found lower left-sided activity, the patients with PD in this study displayed elevated rCMRglu in the left hippocampus and parahippocampal area. In addition, the patients with PD demonstrated reduced rCMRglu in right inferior parietal and right superior temporal cortex.

Four symptom provocation studies of PD have been published, three of which employed pharmacological challenges while the fourth employed anxiety situation imagery exposure. In an early provocation study, Stewart et al. (1988) used the xenon inhalation method in conjunction with SPECT to measure CBF in superficial cortical areas during lactate-induced panic. Ten patients with PD and five normal controls were studied during sodium lactate infusion and during saline infusion as a control measure. Six of the patients with PD and none of the controls experienced panic attacks in response to lactate infusion. The patients with PD who experienced lactate-induced panic attacks displayed global cortical decreases in CBF, while the patients with PD and healthy controls who did not panic exhibited global cortical increases in CBF during lactate infusions, the normal expected physiological response to an osmotic load. In another pharmacological challenge study employing yohimbine and SPECT, Woods et al. (1988) studied six patients with PD and an equal number of normal controls. Yohimbine administration increased anxiety and decreased rCBF in bilateral frontal cortex in the patients with PD versus the controls. In another study, Reiman et al. (1989) used PET methods to measure rCBF in 17 patients with PD and 15 normal controls during lactate infusions. The eight patients who panicked to lactate infusion exhibited rCBF increases in bilateral temporopolar cortex and bilateral insular cortex/claustrum/putamen relative to the normal controls and to the patients with PD who did not experience lactate-induced panic attacks. The finding of increased rCBF in the temporal poles was later attributed to extracranial artifact from muscular contractions (Drevets et al., 1992; Benkelfat et al., 1995). In the only published symptom provocation study using fMRI, directed imagery in neutral and high-anxiety situations was individually tailored for six patients with PD and six healthy controls. Imaging during exposure blocks revealed increased activity during high-anxiety versus neutral anxiety imagery in the patients with PD, but not the controls in the inferior frontal cortex, OFC, hippocampus, and anterior and posterior cingulate (Bystritsky et al., 2001).

In a published case report, Fischer and colleagues (1998) captured a spontaneous panic attack during PET imaging. The neuroimaging profile revealed decreased rCBF in right orbitofrontal, prelimbic (area 25), anterior cingulate, and anterior temporal cortex during the acute event.

Of relevance are two studies in medically healthy, nonpsychiatric subjects examining the brain rCBF response to the panicogen, cholecystokinin tetrapeptide (CCK-4). Benkelfat and colleagues (1995) used CCK-4 infusions to produce a reliable panic response and normal saline infusions as a control condition. Subjects were also studied in an anticipatory anxiety condition during which they expected to receive CCK-4 but were actually injected with saline. During anticipatory anxiety, rCBF increased in the left OFC and cerebellum. Anxiety induced by CCK-4 was associated with rCBF increases in ACC, cerebellum, and a bilateral region spanning the insula, claustrum, and amygdala. Following this study, Javenmard and colleagues (1999) examined rCBF during CCK-4-induced panic attacks at two different time points (the first minute or the second minute after CCK-4 bolus injection). Early phase changes in rCBF occurred in the hypothalamus region, while late phase changes included rCBF increases in the claustrum-insular region. Consistent with findings of decreased frontal cortical blood flow in patients with PD during panic episodes, early and late phases in this study were associated with rCBF decreases in the medial frontal region. However, in contrast to results of the group's previous study, an anticipatory anxiety condition was associated with rCBF increases in ACC and decreases in visual cortex.

In a study examining the effects of imipramine treatment on rCMRglu in patients with PD using PET-FDG, Nordahl and colleagues (1998) found a rightward shift in symmetry within hippocampus and posterior inferior frontal cortex, consistent with their previously reported findings in untreated patients with PD (Nordahl et al., 1990). In addition, compared with the untreated group, the imipramine-treated group exhibited rCMRglu decreases in posterior OFC similar to the changes observed in OCD following successful treatment (e.g., Baxter et al., 1992). More recently, the effect of CBT on regional brain glucose utilization in PD was examined using the 18-FDG PET technique (Sakai et al., 2006). Treatment responders (11 of 12) demonstrated attenuation of glucose utilization in the right hippocampus, left ACC, left cerebellum, and pons. In addition, increased glucose utilization was found in the medial PFC bilaterally, supporting the idea of an adaptive increase in top-down governance via prefrontal cortical inhibition of limbic circuitry.

In a PET imaging study using an agonist challenge to alter serotonin neurotransmission, Meyer and colleagues (2000) measured rCBF before and after an intravenous infusion of d-fenfluramine (an inducer of serotonin release) in a sample of women with PD. Nine patients with PD and 18 healthy comparisons underwent PET scans, pre- and post-fenfluramine injection. The patients with PD demonstrated relatively lower baseline rCBF in the cingulate and the left posterior parietal-superior temporal region compared to the nonanxious controls. In response to the fenfluramine challenge, patients with PD demonstrated increased rCBF in the cingulate and left dorsolateral PFC and decreased rCBF in the posterior temporal cortex (also seen in the control group). Differences in fenfluramine-related changes were found between patients and controls, with a significantly greater increase in rCBF occurring in the women with PD in the left posterior inferior parietal-superior temporal cortex compared to the healthy controls.

Imaging Studies of Neurochemistry

Dager and colleagues have used MRS methods in three successive studies focusing on brain lactate levels in PD (Dager et al., 1995; Dager et al., 1999; Friedman et al., 2000). In a 1995 report, the group measured brain lactate levels during hyperventilation in seven treatment-responsive patients with PD and an equal number of healthy controls. Although no significant differences were found in brain lactate levels at rest, the PD group showed a significantly greater rise in brain lactate in response to the same level of hyperventilation compared to the control group. Notably, there were no significant between-group differences in blood lactate levels either before or after hyperventilation. Dager and colleagues hypothesized that patients with PD might develop higher levels of brain lactate during hyperventilation as a consequence of an exaggerated rCBF vasoconstrictive response to hypocapnia. In their second study, Dager et al. (1999) used MRS to measure brain lactate levels during lactate infusions in 15 patients with PD and 10 healthy comparison subjects. Compared to the healthy controls, the PD group showed significantly higher brain lactate levels during lactate infusion, suggesting reduced clearance rather than higher production of lactate in PD. The fact that this effect was global, rather than regional, is consistent with a potential widespread abnormality in cerebral vascular regulation in PD. In a third study, the investigators examined brain tissue versus the cerebrospinal fluid (CSF) compartment lactate response to metabolic challenge with lactate infusion in four patients with PD (Friedman et al., 2000). Through this study, they were able to confirm their hypothesis that the differentially greater rise in brain lactate in patients with PD postlactate infusion demonstrated in their first two studies is the result of tissue-based changes and is not attributable to CSF changes. The group went on to examine whether excessive brain lactate and delayed end-tidal CO_2 recovery was a result of aberrant brain acid-base regulation in PD (Friedman et al., 2006). Nine patients with PD and 11 healthy controls were compared during regulated hyperventilation and recovery, using phosphorous spectroscopy to measure brain pH. Patients with PD demonstrated greater hypocapnia during hyperventilation, but in comparison with healthy controls, their pH response was blunted. The authors hypothesized that this exaggerated buffering seen in patients with PD might be accounted for by increased lactate levels.

Owing to the popular use of the SRIs as first-line treatments for PD, there has been interest in investigating potential abnormalities in serotonergic transmission in the pathophysiology of PD. Preclinical models of chronic anxiety have implicated the 5-HT_{1A} receptor (Fedotova et al., 2004). In a study aimed at investigating the relevance of the 5-HT_{1A} receptor binding properties to panic anxiety, Neumeister et al. (2004) used PET and the [^{18}F]-FCWAY radioligand to measure central 5-HT_{1A} receptor binding in 16 unmedicated patients with PD (7 with comorbid depression) and 15 matched healthy controls. The PD group, regardless of comorbid depression status, demonstrated lower volumes of distribution in the anterior and posterior cingulate and the raphé, implicating the 5-HT_{1A} receptor in the pathophysiology of PD.

The hypothesized involvement of the benzodiazepine receptor in stress and anxiety has prompted several investigators to measure benzodiazepine receptor binding in patients with PD. Because some of these studies suffer from various methodological problems, (including lack of a medically healthy, nonanxious control group), only those studies with an adequate control group and medication-free patients are discussed below. Using SPECT with [^{123}I]iomazenil, Kuikka et al. (1995) measured benzodiazepine receptor uptake in 17 patients with PD and an equal number of matched healthy comparisons. Compared to the control group, the patients with PD exhibited a greater left/right ratio in benzodiazepine receptor uptake, which was most prominent in PFC. Malizia et al. (1998) used PET and carbon-11-labeled flumazenil to measure benzodiazepine receptor binding in 7 patients with PD and 8 healthy comparisons. They reported global reductions in benzodiazepine receptor binding in the patients with PD versus the controls, which was greatest in the right orbitofrontal and right insular cortices. Bremner, Innis, White, and colleagues (2000) used SPECT and [^{123}I] iomazenil to measure benzodiazepine receptor density in 13 patients with PD and 16 healthy controls. Decreased benzodiazepine receptor binding was found in the left hippocampus and precuneus in the patients with PD relative to the controls. Although the authors did not find between-group differences in binding in PFC overall, they did report a negative correlation between binding in the PFC and panic attack symptoms in the patients with PD. This finding suggests that the decrease in prefrontal benzodiazepine binding may be a state-specific rather than a trait finding.

In addition to benzodiazepine receptor binding abnormalities, reductions in cortical GABA levels have also been demonstrated in patients with PD compared to healthy controls. Goddard et al. (2004) examined whether patients with PD might also have an abnormal GABA response to the administration of a benzodiazepine. Using a proton MRS technique, they studied occipital GABA levels before and after clonazepam administration in 10 patients with PD and 9 healthy controls. Patients with PD demonstrated a minimal reduction in occipital GABA levels in response to acute clonazepam administration compared to the expected significant reduction measured in healthy comparisons. The authors hypothesize that the blunted, deficient response to benzodiazepine administration in patients with PD may be related to an abnormality in gene expression or function of the GABA synthetic enzyme *glutamate decarboxylase 65* (GAD65).

In summary, the majority (Malizia et al., 1998; Bremner, Innis, White, et al., 2000) but not all (Brandt et al., 1998) of benzodiazepine receptor binding studies have demonstrated decreased binding in frontal and insular cortex, areas important in modulating the amygdala-centered fear circuitry.

Summary

The body of neuroimaging data on PD is less conclusive than that of some of the other anxiety disorders. Overall, together with mMRI findings, functional abnormalities in the hippocampal/parahippocampal region appear to be a marker at rest. During symptom provocation, patients with PD exhibit activation of insular and motor striatal regions, while reductions are seen in widespread cortical regions, including the PFC. Dager and colleagues' MRS studies of brain lactate suggest that patients with PD exhibit an exaggerated hemodynamic response to hypocapnia, manifest as relatively greater vasoconstriction, which appears to be global. Likewise, receptor binding studies suggest widespread abnormalities in the GABAergic/benzodiazepine system. These findings are also most pronounced in hippocampal, insular, and prefrontal regions; however, they should be interpreted with caution, considering the potential effects of prior exposure to psychotropic medications. Neurobiological models of PD have proposed aberrant monoaminergic neurotransmitter modulation, originating in the corresponding brain stem nuclei, as a key factor underlying the abnormalities of metabolism, hemodynamics, and chemistry found in widespread cortical areas. Although limited, data implicate medial temporal lobe structures in PD, suggesting a potential role for hippocampal or amygdala dysfunction in this disorder.

SOCIAL AND SPECIFIC PHOBIAS

Neuroanatomical Models of Phobias

If one accepts the premise that all phobias are learned, they can be viewed as another example of fear conditioning to specific stimuli or situations. However, evidence exists indicating that phobias develop principally in the absence of an initial threatening exposure. Researchers have suggested that modeling of fearful responding by others underlies the appearance of phobias in the absence of direct experience. However, another possibility is that phobias represent dysfunction within systems specific to archetypal varieties of potentially threatening stimuli or situations. For instance, if humans have evolved one neural network specifically designed to assess social cues for threatening content and another to assess threat from small animals, and so on, aberrant functioning in these pathways might represent the pathophysiology underlying phobias. Currently, neuroanatomically based models for the phobias remain in the early stages of development (Fyer, 1998; Stein, 1998; Mathew et al., 2001), with neuroimaging studies of the type described below informing such models.

Structural Imaging Findings

Despite the high prevalence of specific and social phobias, there are surprisingly few neuroimaging studies in these areas. Using mMRI methods, Rauch and colleagues (2004) demonstrated increased cortical thicknesses in the insular, rostral anterior cingulate and posterior cingulate along with the left visual cortex in a group of patients with specific phobia (animal type) compared with a nonphobic control group. A single volumetric study has been reported in social phobia (Potts et al., 1994); however, no significant between-group differences were found in any of the brain regions examined.

Functional Imaging Findings

Studies employing functional imaging in combination with symptom provocation paradigms in patients with specific phobias have reported varying results. In an initial study by Mountz and colleagues (1989), patients with small-animal phobias responded to feared stimuli with increases in heart rate and respiratory rates, and with subjective reports of increasing anxiety during exposure. However, no changes in rCBF measurements were observed with PET imaging. Review of this study suggests that the negative findings may have been a result of the data analytic methods employed.

In a series of studies of specific phobias from another laboratory, exposure to fearful stimuli resulted in fairly uniform results. In the earliest study, Wik and colleagues (1993) measured rCBF in patients with snake phobias during exposure to videotapes of neutral, generally aversive, and snake-related scenes. During the phobic condition, they found significant increases in rCBF within secondary visual cortex, while rCBF decreases were noted within PFC, posterior cingulate cortex, anterior temporopolar cortex, and hippocampus.

In two other studies, including an analogous study of patients with spider phobias, these findings were largely replicated (Fredrikson et al., 1993; Fredrikson et al., 1995). Rauch, Savage, Alpert, and colleagues (1995), using PET, employed a different paradigm from the studies described above, exposing a sample of patients with a variety of small-animal phobias to phobia-related and control stimuli in vivo and acquired images with the patients' eyes closed, as opposed to the eyes-open method employed in previous studies. This difference resulted in a lack of visual cortical activation, which, interestingly, appeared to be replaced by somatosensory cortical activation, suggesting that the patients may have been involved in tactile imagery, as indeed they reported fears of coming into contact with the feared animal. Besides the somatosensory cortex, the main areas exhibiting rCBF increases in response to the feared stimuli included multiple anterior paralimbic territories (that is, right anterior cingulate, right anterior temporal pole, left posterior OFC, and left insular cortex), left somatosensory cortex, and left thalamus. Scheinle and colleagues (2005) reported similar results in a group of patients with spider phobias and were the first group to demonstrate activation of the amygdala during exposure to feared stimuli when compared with healthy controls. Later, Straube, Mentzel, and colleagues (2006) examined brain activation patterns to phobia-related (spiders) versus neutral pictures during a direct viewing task and a distraction task. They found greater amygdalar activation in patients with phobias versus healthy controls in both tasks but found that the right amygdala was activated only during the distraction task, suggesting its role may be in automatic processing of potentially threatening stimuli.

Although regional brain activation changes had been found in response to treatment in other anxiety disorders, Paquette et al. (2003) were the first group to study the regional brain changes resulting from treatment of specific phobia with CBT. They studied 12 patients with spider phobias using fMRI, before and after CBT during the viewing of an emotional activation task involving viewing films of spiders. Prior to treatment, the right dorsolateral PFC and parahippocampal gyrus were activated, which was significantly attenuated postsuccessful CBT treatment. In a similar study, patients with spider phobias were randomly assigned to treatment with CBT or to a waiting list (control group) (Straube, Glauer, et al., 2006). Attenuation of hyperactivity in the insula and ACC correlated with reduction in phobic symptoms in response to CBT treatment.

The number of functional imaging studies in social phobia continues to expand, with cognitive activation studies performed in conjunction with fMRI yielding informative results (Table 43.3). Patients with social phobia demonstrate specific areas of enhanced regional brain activity when exposed to social threat signaled by viewing negative facial expressions. Functional MRI studies have shown that patients with social phobia demonstrate greater amygdala activation than healthy comparisons to angry (Stein et al., 2002; Straube et al., 2004; Phan, Fitzgerald, et al., 2006) and neutral facial expressions (Birbaumer et al., 1998; Viet et al., 2002; Cooney et al., 2006). Patients with social phobia also demonstrate increased insula activation to faces displaying anger or disgust versus neutral faces when compared to controls (Straube et al., 2004; Amir et al., 2005; Straube et al., 2005). The ACC also shows greater activation in patients with social phobia than in healthy controls during exposure to negative facial expressions (Straube et al., 2004; Amir et al., 2005) In addition to these regions, an area implicated in the processing of emotional facial content is the fusiform gyrus, located in the extrastriatal visual cortex. Patients with social phobia show greater activation in the fusiform during the processing of facial expressions, regardless of valence, suggesting enhanced processing of human facial expressions in social phobia (Straube et al., 2005).

Although enhanced activity within the regions of the amygdala, insula, and ACC in response to cues suggesting social disapproval or threat is predicted based on neurocircuitry models of fear, there is evidence that patients with social phobia are more likely to interpret neutral or ambiguous facial expressions negatively (Winton et al., 1995). Several studies have demonstrated enhanced amygdala activation in patients with social phobia versus controls when viewing neutral faces alone (Cooney et al., 2006) or paired with aversive stimuli (Birbaumer et al., 1998; Schneider et al., 1999; Viet et al., 2002). Functional MRI techniques have also been used to demonstrate that amygdala reactivity in patients with generalized social phobia increases in relationship to the emotional intensity of the faces presented (Yoon et al., 2007).

Public speaking, a prominent performance fear in patients with social phobia, has been effective as a means of provoking anxiety during neuroimaging. In a symptom provocation study that required subjects to speak in front of an audience (public speaking task) versus alone (private speaking task), Tillfors and colleagues (2001) studied the rCBF response of 18 patients with social phobia and 6 nonanxious, healthy comparisons using PET. Patients with social phobia demonstrated a significantly greater rCBF response in the right amygdala and periamygdaloid cortex compared to controls in response to the public versus private speaking task. In addition, rCBF decreased in patients with social phobia in the orbitofrontal and insular cortices and the temporal pole, while healthy comparisons demonstrated increases in rCBF in these same areas. In a similar study, Loberbaum and colleagues (2004) used fMRI to image brain activity while eight patients with generalized so-

TABLE 43.3 *Summary of Functional Neuroimaging Findings in Social Phobia*

Paradigm Employed	*Identified Areas of Elevated Metabolism, CBF or BOLD Signal in Patients with Social Phobia versus Healthy Controls*	*References*
Emotional facial expressions:		
Neutral (explicit)	Amygdala	Birbaumer et al., 1998 Cooney et al., 2006
Neutral (conditioned using aversive odor	Amygdala and hippocampus	Schneider et al., 1999
Neutral (conditioned using painful stimulus)	Orbitofrontal cortex, R insula, ACC, R amygdala, L dorsolateral PFC	Veit et al., 2002
Angry vs. happy (implicit)	Amygdala, parahippocampal gyrus, uncus, Medial PFC, sup and inf frontal gyri	Stein et al., 2002
Angry vs. neutral (implicit)	Amygdala, parahippocampal gyrus, fusiform Gyrus, sup temportal sulcus	Straube et al., 2004
Angry (explicit)	R amygdala, fusiform gyrus	Straube et al., 2005
Contempt vs. happy (implicit)	Amygdala, parahippocampal gyrus, uncus, Medial PFC, sup and inf frontal gyri	Stein et al., 2002
Harsh vs. happy (implicit)	Dorsal medial PFC, L inf frontal gyrus, R sup frontal gyrus, L amygdala, uncus L parahippocampal gyrus	Stein et al., 2002
Harsh vs. happy (explicit)	R amygdala	Phan, Fitzgerald et al., 2006
Disgust vs. neutral (explicit)	ACC, caudate, insula, inf and mid frontal gyri, Mid and sup frontal gyri, sup occipital gyrus	Amir et al., 2005
Happy (explicit)	R amygdala, fusiform	Straube et al., 2005
Faces of varying emotional intensity	Amygdala, L insula, R sup parietal gyrus, R mid frontal gyrus, R lingual gyrus	Yoon et al., 2007
Public speaking:		
Public vs. private speaking	R amygdaloid complex	Tillfors et al., 2001
Anticipation of public speaking	L amygdaloid complex, L insula, L temporal pole, L pons, L striatum	Loberman et al., 2004

OFC: orbitofrontal cortex; ACC: anterior cingulate gyrus; PCC: posterior cingulate gyrus; PFC: prefrontal cortex; CBF: Cerebral blood flow; BOLD: blood oxygen level dependent; SAD: social anxiety disorder.

cial phobia and six healthy controls anticipated making public speeches. When brain activity during the rest period was subtracted from the anticipation period, patients with social phobia demonstrated greater subcortical, limbic, and lateral paralimbic activity (including the amygdala, parahippocampal gyrus, and insula), while showing decreases in the PFC compared to healthy controls.

Thus, there is a relatively consistent response pattern across social phobia provocation studies. This pattern consists of increased subcortical/limbic activity accompanied by relatively decreased frontal cortical activity. This shift in brain activity likely reflects a failure of cortical processing and activation of the phylogenetically older subcortical fear circuitry. Thus, in response to exposure to either human face stimuli or the stress of public speaking, patients with social phobia display exaggerated activity within key structures in fear responding, such as the amygdala and medial temporal areas at the expense of activity in prefrontal cortical regions.

There are two reported imaging studies examining the effects of treatment on regional brain activity in social phobia. Van der Linden et al. (2000) examined the effects of pharmacotherapy with the SSRI citalopram on rCBF with SPECT. Fifteen patients with social phobia underwent scanning before and after 8 weeks of treatment with citalopram. Because no control group was studied, baseline differences in rCBF were not reported; nonetheless, in response to treatment, reductions in rCBF were noted in the anterolateral left temporal cortex, left cingulate, and left midfrontal cortex. Those patients judged as nonresponders to treatment demonstrated greater rCBF at baseline in the anterolateral left temporal cortex and the lateral left midfrontal cortex compared to responders. Interpretation of the results of this study is limited by the fact that several patients had other comorbid anxiety disorders and two patients were taking additional psychotropic medications at the time of scanning.

Another study examined the effects of two different anxiety treatments, pharmacotherapy with an SSRI and CBT, on rCBF in patients with social phobia. In a randomized design, 18 patients were scanned using PET techniques during a public speaking task (Furmark et al., 2002). Patients were divided into three groups: citalopram treatment, CBT, or waiting list (control group). Regional CBF was measured before and after 9 weeks of treatment or 9 weeks on the waiting list. Results demonstrated similar changes in rCBF in responders of both treatment groups in response to public speaking: bilateral decreases in rCBF in the amygdala, hippocampus, and related periamygdaloid, perihippocampal, and rhinal cortices, while no significant changes in rCBF were observed in the waiting list control group. These findings suggest that pharmacotherapy and CBT, in reducing social anxiety symptoms, attenuate activity in brain regions associated with the neural network identified as underlying danger perception and fear responding. Change in rCBF followed improvement and was not specific to treatment modality.

Imaging Studies of Neurochemistry

The DA and serotonin systems have been the focus of investigation in imaging studies of neurochemistry in social phobia. Tiihonen et al. (1997) used the radiotracer I-123-labeled-2b-carbomethoxy-3b-(4-iodophenyl) (bCIT) with SPECT to measure the density of DA reuptake sites in 11 patients with social phobia and 28 healthy comparisons. They reported significantly reduced striatal DA reuptake binding site density in the social phobia group compared to the control group. Subsequent to this report of low DAT density in social phobia, Schneier et al. (2000) measured DA D_2 receptor binding in the striatums of 10 patients with social phobia and 10 matched healthy comparisons using the radiotracer [^{123}I]iodobenzamide with SPECT. The patients with social phobia demonstrated significantly decreased D_2 receptor binding, with a trend (p = .07) toward a negative correlation of binding potential and score on the Liebowitz Social Anxiety Scale.

Using PET techniques, Kent, Coplan, Lombardo, et. al. (2002) examined paroxetine occupancy of the serotonin reuptake transporter (SERT) in patients with social phobia during treatment at typical antianxiety doses (20–40mg/day). After 3 to 6 months of continuous treatment, paroxetine achieved very high occupancy levels at the SERT in all brain regions measured. In a PET study examining 5-HT_{1A} receptor binding potential in social phobia (Lanzenberger et al., 2007), several brain areas implicated in the fear circuitry were identified as having significantly lower 5-HT_{1A} binding potential in patients with social phobia, including the amygdala, insula, and dorsal raphe. These studies lend support to the validity of the SERT and 5-HT_{1A} receptors as targets in the treatment of social anxiety.

Summary

The sum of imaging findings in specific phobia suggests that activation of anterior paralimbic regions, in addition to activation of the sensory cortex mediating input of the phobic stimulus, is associated with excessive fearful responding on stimulus exposure. It is promising that there are now several convergent findings in the social phobia literature. In response to exposure either to human face stimuli or to the stress of public speaking, patients with social phobia demonstrate exaggerated activity in the amygdala and related medial temporal lobe areas. Patients with social phobia also show abnormal activity within medial temporal lobe structures during aversive conditioning with human face stimuli, consistent with aberrant assignment of threat to human faces. Evidence supporting deficits in DA function in social phobia has now been reported in two studies, consistent with theories implicating the DA system in social reward (Stein, 1998). In addition to the DA system, results of imaging studies support the targeting of the serotonin system in treatment.

CONCLUSIONS AND FUTURE DIRECTIONS

Neurobiological models of the anxiety disorders are evolving as a result of significant input from findings of neuroimaging studies related to the structure, function, and neurochemistry of the brain. These findings suggest that the anxiety disorders share certain mediating anatomy such as the anterior paralimibic cortex, sensory cortex, amygdala, hippocampus, and striatum. However, imaging techniques have also begun to delineate signature abnormalities of brain structure and/or function specific to the individual anxiety disorders. Overall, this work holds the promise of pathophysiology-based diagnosis, which, in turn, will lead to more targeted and effective treatments.

Neuroimaging studies of OCD have demonstrated dysfunction within the cortico-striato-thalamo-cortical circuitry. Future investigations will likely focus on these structures and on the interactions among the nodes that constitute this system. Theories about the neurobiology of PTSD have been informed by animal studies of fear conditioning implicating the amygdala and related limbic cortical structures. Neuroimaging studies of PTSD have provided an initial means for testing the relevance of this neurocircuitry in patients. A convergence of evidence from these studies supports prevailing models of PTSD focusing on the amygdala and its relationship with the hippocampus and medial PFC (particularly anterior cingulate dysfunction). Although less neuroimaging research pertaining to the phobias exists in the literature, there is preliminary evidence of increased activity within sensory pathways and anterior paralimbic regions in specific phobias, which may reflect a hypersensitivity within systems evolved for assessing specific archetypal classes of potentially threatening stimuli (for example, animals, heights). In social phobia, exaggerated amygdalar responsivity to human face stimuli is likewise consistent with hypersensitivity within a specialized system to a discrete class of stimuli. For PD, neuroimaging research has identified a wide range of possible neural substrates underlying this anxiety disorder. Regional abnormalities within the temporal lobe may reflect fundamental deficits in threat assessment similar to those found in social phobia and PTSD. However, more global abnormalities in homeostatic mechanisms related to lactate metabolism and vascular responses to CO_2, as well as widespread abnormalities in benzodiazepine receptor binding, may prove specific to PD.

Clearly, an issue in all neuroimaging research in anxiety disorders is the presence of other comorbid anxiety disorders, substance abuse, and varying degrees of comorbid depression. Future studies should begin to include psychiatric comparison groups in addition to healthy controls, and to consider the contributing role of substance abuse and depressive symptoms to neurobiological findings. This is necessary to establish the specificity of findings versus their generalizability across classes of psychopathology. As evidenced by the mounting evidence in OCD, longitudinal studies with a developmental perspective will be critical in understanding the pathophysiology of anxiety disorders. For example, the relationship between early temperament and the development of social phobia (C.E. Schwartz et al., 1999) calls for studies beginning in childhood, as do OCD and related disorders that have an early onset. Also, proneness to developing PTSD and how brain changes evolve following trauma exposure is best addressed with studies that acquire data prior to trauma exposure and follow patients over time.

As morphometric and functional imaging methods improve with advances in technology, neurochemical methods will continue to evolve. As new radioligands with greater specificity and sensitivity are developed, it will become possible to investigate receptor population changes at critical nodes within the relevant neurocircuitry and answer questions regarding neuropharmacology. Magnetic resonance spectroscopy is enabling measurement of metabolic markers in specific brain regions in vivo, as well as the change in neurochemical balance associated with specific pharmacological interventions.

In summary, neuroimaging data are being used to help advance neurobiological models of the anxiety disorders. Convergent data have provided relatively cohesive models of OCD and PTSD, whereas the data for phobias and PD do not yet provide as clear a picture. The potential of neuroimaging to help delineate the pathophysiology of the anxiety disorders is now being realized, and future research in this domain will likely also lead to enhanced treatments for people suffering from these disorders.

REFERENCES

Adams, K.H., Hansen, E.S., Pinborg, L.H., et al. (2005) Patients with obsessive-compulsive disorder have increased 5-HT2a receptor binding in the caudate nuclei. *Int. J. Neuropsychopharmacol.* 8:1–11.

Adler, C.M., McDonough-Ryan, P., Sax, K.W., Holland, S.K., Arndt, S., and Strakowski, S.M. (2000) fMRI of neuronal activation with symptom provocation in unmedicated patients with obsessive compulsive disorder. *J. Psychiatr. Res.* 34:317–324.

Aggleton, J.P., ed. (1992) *The Amygdala: Neurobiological Aspects of Emotion, Memory and Mental Dysfunction.* New York: Wiley-Liss.

Alptekin, K., Degirmenci, B., Kivircik, B., Durak, H., Yemez, B., Derebek, E., and Tunca, Z. (2001) Tc-99m HMPAO brain perfusion SPECT in drug-free obsessive-compulsive patients without depression. *Psychiatry Res.* 107:51–56.

Amir, N., Klumpp, H., Elias, J., et al. (2005) Increased activation of the anterior cingulate cortex during processing of disgust faces in individuals with social phobia. *Biol. Psychiatry* 57:975–981.

Armony, J.L., Corbo, V., Clement, M.H., et al. (2005) Amygdala response in patients with acute PTSD to masked and unmasked emotional facial expressions. *Am. J. Psychiatry* 162:1961–1963.

Atmaca, M., Yildirim, B.H., Ozdemir, B.H., et al. (2006) Volumetric MRI assessment of brain regions in patients with refractory obsessive-compulsive disorder. *Prog. Neuropsychopharmacol. Biol. Psychiatry* 30:1051–1057.

Atmaca, M., Yildirim, H., Ozdemir, H., et al. (2007) Volumetric MRI study of key brain regions implicated in obsessive-compulsive disorder. *Prog. Neuropsychopharmacol. Biol. Psychiatry* 31: 46–52.

Aylward, E.H., Harris, G.J., Hoehn-Saric, R., et al. (1996) Normal caudate nucleus in obsessive-compulsive disorder assessed by quantitative neuroimaging. *Arch. Gen. Psychiatry* 53:577–584.

Barker, P.B. (2001) N-acetyl aspartate—a neuronal marker? *Ann. Neurol.* 49(4):423–424.

Bartha, R., Stein, M.B., Williamson, P.C., et al. (1998) A short echo ^{1}H spectroscopy and volumetric MRI study of the corpus striatum in patients with obsessive-compulsive disorder and comparison subjects. *Am. J. Psychiatry* 155(11):1584–1591.

Baxter, L.R., Phelps, M.E., Mazziotta, J.C., et al. (1987) Local cerebral glucose metabolic rates in obsessive compulsive disorder: a comparison with rates in unipolar depression and in normal controls. *Arch. Gen. Psychiatry* 44:211–218.

Baxter, L.R., Jr., Schwartz, J.M., Bergman, K.S., et al. (1992) Caudate glucose metabolic rate changes with both drug and behavior therapy for obsessive-compulsive disorder. *Arch. Gen. Psychiatry* 49:681–689.

Baxter, L.R., Schwartz, J.M., Mazziotta, J.C., et al. (1988) Cerebral glucose metabolic rates in nondepressed patients with obsessive-compulsive disorder. *Am. J. Psychiatry* 145:1560–1563.

Benazon, N.R., Moore, G.J., and Rosenberg, D.R. (2003) Neurochemical analyses in pediatric obsessive-compulsive disorder in patients treated with cognitive behavioral therapy. *J. Am. Acad. Child Adoles. Psychiatry* 42:1279–1285.

Benkelfat, C., Bradwejn, J., Meyer, E., et al. (1995) Functional neuroanatomy of CCK_4-induced anxiety in normal healthy volunteers. *Am. J. Psychiatry* 152:1180–1184.

Benkelfat, C., Nordahl, T.E., Semple, W.E., et al. (1990) Local cerebral glucose metabolic rates in obsessive-compulsive disorder: patients treated with clomipramine. *Arch. Gen. Psychiatry* 47: 840–848.

Birbaumer, N., Grodd, W., Diedrich, O., et al. (1998) fMRI reveals amygdala activation to human faces in social phobics. *Neuroreport* 9(6):1223–1226.

Bisaga, A., Katz, J.L., Antonini, A., et al. (1998) Cerebral glucose metabolism in women with panic disorder. *Am. J. Psychiatry* 155: 1178–1183.

Bolton, J., Moore, G.J., MacMillan, S., et al. (2001) Case study: caudate glutamaterigc changes with paroxetine persist after medication discontinuation in pediatric OCD. *J. Am. Acad. Child Adoles. Psychiatry* 40:903–906.

Bonne, O., Baine, E., Neumeister, A., et al. (2005) No change in serotonin type 1A receptor binding in patients with posttraumatic stress disorder. *Am. J. Psychiatry* 162:383–385.

Bonne, O., Brandes, D., Gilboa, A., Bomori, J.M., Shenton, M.E., Pitman, R.K., and Shalev, A.Y. (2001) Longitudinal MRI study of hippocampal volume in trauma survivors with PTSD. *Am. J. Psychiatry* 158:1248–1251.

Brandt, C.A., Meller, J., Keweloh, L., et al. (1998) Increased benzodiazepine receptor density in the prefrontal cortex in patients with panic disorder. *J. Neural Transm.* 105:1325–1333.

Breiter, H.C., Rauch, S.L., Kwong, K.K., et al. (1996) Functional magnetic resonance imaging of symptom provocation in obsessive compulsive disorder. *Arch. Gen. Psychiatry* 53:595–606.

Bremner, J.D., Innis, R.B., Southwick, S.M., Staib, L., Zoghbi, S., and Charney, D.S. (2000) Decreased benzodiazepine receptor binding in prefrontal cortex in combat-related posttraumatic stress disorder. *Am. J. Psychiatry* 157:1120–1126.

Bremner, J.D., Innis, R.B., White, T., Fujita, M., Silbersweig, D., Goddard, A.W., Staib, L., Stern, E., Cappiello, A., Woods, S., Baldwin, R., and Charney, D.S. (2000) SPECT [I-123]Iomazenil measurement of the benzodiazepine receptor in panic disorder. *Biol. Psychiatry* 47:96–106.

Bremner, J.D., Narayan, M., Staib, L.H., Southwick, S.M., McGlashum, T., and Charney, D.S. (1999) Neural correlates of memories of childhood sexual abuse in women with and without posttraumatic stress disorder. *Am. J. Psychiatry* 156:1787–1795.

Bremner, J.D., Randall, P., Scott, T.M., et al. (1995) MRI-based measurement of hippocampal volume in patients with combat-related posttraumatic stress disorder. *Am. J. Psychiatry* 152:973–981.

Bremner, J.D., Randall, P., Vermetten, E., et al. (1997) Magnetic resonance imaging–based measurement of hippocampal volume in posttraumatic stress disorder related to childhood physical and sexual abuse—a preliminary report. *Biol. Psychiatry* 41:23–32.

Bremner, J.D., Staib, L.H., Kaloupek, D., et al. (1999) Neural correlates of exposure to traumatic pictures and sound in Vietnam combat veterans with and without posttraumatic stress disorder: a positron emission tomography study. *Biol. Psychiatry* 45:806–816.

Britton, J.C., Phan, K.L., Taylor, S.F., et al. (2005) Corticolimbic blood flow in posttraumatic stress disorder during script-driven imagery. *Biol. Psychiatry* 57:832–840.

Brody, A.L., Saxena, S., Schwartz, J.M., et al. (1998) FDG-PET predictors of response to behavioral therapy versus pharmacotherapy in obsessive-compulsive disorder. *Psychiatry Res. Neuroimag.* 84:1–6.

Bryant, R.A., Felmingham, K.L., Kempt, A.H., et al. (2005) Neural networks of information processing in posttraumatic stress disorder: a functional magnetic resonance imaging study. *Biol. Psychiatry* 58:111–118.

Bystritsky, A., Pontillo, D., Powers, M., Sabb, F.W., Craske, M.G., and Bookheimer, S.Y. (2001) Functional MRI changes during panic anticipation and imagery exposure. *Neuroreport* 12:3953–3957.

Cameron, H.A., Hazel, T.G., and McKay, R.D. (1998) Regulation of neurogenesis by growth factors and neurotransmitters. *J. Neurobiol.* 36(2):287–306.

Cannistraro, P.A., and Rauch, S.L. (2003) Neural circuitry of anxiety: evidence from structural and functional neuroimaging studies. *Psychopharmacol. Bull.* 37:8–25.

Carrion, V.G., Weems, C.F., Eliez, S., Patwardhan, A., Brown, W., Ray, R.D., and Reiss, A.L. (2001) Attenuation of frontal asymmetry in pediatric posttraumatic stress disorder. *Biol. Psychiatry* 50:943–951.

Charney, D.S., Bremner, J.D., and Redmond, D.E. (1995) Noradrenergic neural substrates for anxiety and fear: clinical associations based on pre-clinical research. In: Bloom, F.E., and Kupfer, D.J., eds. *Psychopharmacology: The Fourth Generation of Progress.* New York: Raven Press, pp. 387–396.

Chen, X.L., Xiet, J.X., Han, H.B., et al. (2004) MR perfusion-weighted imaging and quantitative analysis of cerebral hemodynamics with symptom provocation in unmedicated patients with obsessive-compulsive disorder. *Neurosci. Lett.* 370:206–211.

Choi, J.S., Kang, D.H., Kim, J.J., et al. (2004) Left anterior subregion of orbitofrontal cortex volume reduction and impaired organizational strategies in obsessive-compulsive disorder. *J. Psychiatr. Res.* 38:193–199.

Cohen, R.A., Grieve, S., Hoth, K.F., et al. (2006) Early life stress and morphometry of the adult anterior cingulate cortex and caudate nuclei. *Biol. Psychiatry* 59:975–982.

Cooney, R.E., Atlas, L.Y., Joormann, J. et al. (2006) Amygdala activation in the processing of neutral faces in social anxiety disorder: is neutral really neutral? *Psychiatry Res. Neuroimag.* 148: 55–59.

Coplan, J.D., and Lydiard, R.B. (1998) Brain circuits in panic disorder. *Biol. Psychiatry* 44:1264–1276.

Corbo, V., Clement, M.H., Armony, J.L., et al. (2005) Size versus shape differences: contrasting voxel-based and volumetric analyses of the anterior cingulate cortex in individuals with acute posttraumtic stress disorder. *Biol. Psychiatry* 58:119–124.

Crespo-Facorro, B., Cabranes, J.A., Lopez-Ibor Alcocer, M.I., Paya, B., Fernandez Perez, C., Encinas, M., Ayuso Mateos, J.L., and Lopez Ibor, J.J., Jr. (1999) Regional cerebral blood flow in obsessive-compulsive patients with and without a chronic tic disorder. A SPECT study. *Eur. Arch. Psychiatry Clin. Neurosci.* 249:156–161.

Dager, S.R., Friedman, S.D., Heide, A., Layton, M.E., Richards, T., Artru, A., Strauss, W., Hayes, C., and Posse, S. (1999) Two-dimensional proton echo-planar spectroscopic imaging of brain metabolic changes during lactate-induced panic. *Arch. Gen. Psychiatry* 56(1):70–77.

Dager, S.R., Strauss, W.L., Marro, K.I., Richards, T.L., Metzger, G.D., and Artru, A.A. (1995) Proton magnetic resonance spectroscopy investigation of hyperventilation in subjects with panic disorder and comparison subjects. *Am. J. Psychiatry* 152(5):666–672.

Davis, M. (1992) The role of the amygdala in fear and anxiety. *Annu. Rev. Neurosci.* 58(Suppl 2):26–28.

De Bellis, M.D., Hall, J., Boring, A.M., Frustaci, K., and Moritz, G. (2001) A pilot longitudinal study of hippocampal volumes in pediatric maltreatment-related posttraumatic stress disorder. *Biol. Psychiatry* 50:305–309.

De Bellis, M.D., Keshavan, M.S., Clark, D.B., Case, B.J., Giedd, J.N., Boring, A.M., Frustaci, K., and Ryan, N.C. (1999) A.E. Bennett Research Award. Developmental traumatology. Part II: Brain development. *Biol. Psychiatry* 45:1271–1284.

De Bellis, M.D., Keshavan, M.S., Frustaci, K., Shifflett, H., Iyengar, S., Beers, S.R., and Hall, J. (2002) Superior temporal gyrus volumes in maltreated children and adolescents with PTSD. *Biol. Psychiatry* 51:544–552.

De Bellis, M.D., Keshavan, M.S., Spencer, S., and Hall, J. (2000) N-acetylaspartate concentration in the anterior cingulate of maltreated children and adolescents with PTSD. *Am. J. Psychiatry* 157:1175–1177.

De Bellis, M.D., and Kuchibhatla, M. (2006) Cerebellar volumes in pediatric maltreatment-related posttraumatic stress disorder. *Biol. Psychiatry* 60:697–703.

Deckersbach, T., Dougherty, D.D., and Rauch, S.L. (2006) Functional imaging of mood and anxiety disorders. *Neuroimaging* 16: 1–10.

De Cristofaro, M.T., Sessarego, A., Pupi, A., Biondi, F., and Faravelli, C. (1993) Brain perfusion abnormalities in drug-naive, lactate-sensitive panic patients: a SPECT study. *Biol. Psychiatry* 33(7): 505–512.

Denys, D., van der Wee, N.J., Janssen, J., et al. (2005) Low level of dopaminergic D2 receptor binding in obsessive-compulsive disorder. *Biol. Psychiatry* 55:1041–1045.

Diler, R.S., Kibar, M., and Avci, A. (2004) Pharmacotherapy and regional cerebral blood flow in children with obsessive-compulsive disorder. *Yonsei Medical Journal* 45:90–99.

Drevets, W.C., Videen, T.O., MacLeod, A.K., et al. (1992) PET images of blood flow changes during anxiety: a correction. *Science* 256:1696.

Driessen, M., Herrmann, J., Stahl, K., Zwaan, M., Meier, S., Hill, A., Osterheider, M., and Petersen, D. (2000) Magnetic resonance imaging volumes of the hippocampus and amygdala in women with borderline personality disorder and early traumatization. *Arch. Gen. Psychiatry* 57:1115–1122.

Ebert, D., Speck, O., Konig, A., Berger, M., Hennig, J., and Hohagen, F. (1997) ^{1}H-magnetic resonance spectroscopy in obsessive-compulsive disorder: evidence for neuronal loss in the cingulate gyrus and the right striatum. *Psychiatry Res.* 74(3):173–176.

Fedotova, J.O., Hartmann, G., Lenard, L., et al. (2004) Effects of 5-HT1A receptor agonist and antagonist on anxiety in intact and ovariectomized female rats. *Acta Physiol. Hung.* 91:175–184.

Fernandez, A., Pino Alonso, M., Matix-Cols, D., et al. (2003) Neuroactivation o f the Tower of Hanoi in patients with obsessive-compulsive disorder and healthy volunteers. Rev. *Esp. Med. Nuc.* 22:376–385.

Fischer, H., Andersson, J.L., Furmark, T., and Fredrikson, M. (1998) Brain correlates of an unexpected panic attack: a human positron emission tomographic study. *Neurosci. Lett.* 251(2):137–140.

Fischer, H., Wik, G., and Fredrikson, M. (1996) Functional neuroanatomy of robbery re-experience: affective memories studied with PET. *Neuroreport* 7:2081–2086.

Fitzgerald, K.D., Welsh, R.C., Gehring, W.J., et al. (2005) Error-related hyperactivity of the anterior cingulate cortex in obsessive-compulsive disorder. *Biol. Psychiatry* 57:287–294.

Fontaine, R., Breton, G., Dery, R., Fontaine, S., and Elie, R. (1990) Temporal lobe abnormalities in panic disorder: an MRI study. *Biol. Psychiatry* 27(3):304–310.

Fredrikson, M., Wik, G., Annas, P., et al. (1995) Functional neuroanatomy of visually elicited simple phobic fear: additional data and theoretical analysis. *Psychophysiology* 32:43–48.

Fredrikson, M., Wik, G., Greitz, T., et al. (1993) Regional cerebral blood flow during experimental fear. *Psychophysiology* 30:126–130.

Friedman, S.D., Dager, S.R., Richards, T.L., Petropoulos, H., and Posse, S. (2000) Modeling brain compartmental lactate response to metabolic challenge: a feasibility study. *Psychiatry Res.* 98: 55–66.

Friedman, S.D., Mathis, C.M., Hayes, C., Renshaw, P., and Dager, S.R. (2006) Brain pH response to hyperventilation in panic disorder: preliminary evidence for altered acid-base regulation. *Am. J. Psychiatry* 163:710–715.

Fujita, M., Southwick, S.M., Denucci, C.C., et al. (2004) Central type benzodiazepine receptors in gulf War veterans with posttraumatic stress disorder. *Biol. Psychiatry* 56:95–100.

Furmark, T., Tillfors, M., Marteinsdottir, I., Fischer, H., Pissiota, A., Langstrom, B., and Fredrikson M. (2002) Common changes in cerebral blood flow in patients with social phobia treated with citalopram or cognitive-behavioral therapy. *Arch. Gen. Psychiatry* 59:425–433.

Fyer, A.J. (1998) Current approaches to etiology and pathophysiology of specific phobia. *Biol. Psychiatry* 44:1295–1304.

Giedd, J.N., Rapoport, J.L., Garvey, M.A., Perlmutter, S., and Swedo, S.E. (2000) MRI assessment of children with obsessive-compulsive disorder or tics associated with streptococcal infection. *Am. J. Psychiatry* 157:281–283.

Gilbert, A.R., Moore, G.J., Keshavan, M.S., Paulson, L.A.D., Narula, V., MacMaster, F.P., Stewart, C.M., and Rosenberg, D.R. (2000) Decrease in thalamic volumes of pediatric patients with obsessive-compulsive disorder who are taking paroxetine. *Arch. Gen. Psychiatry* 57:449–456.

Gilboa, A., Shalev, A.Y., Laor, L., et al. (2004) Functional connectivity of the prefrontal cortex and the amygdala in posttraumatic stress disorder. *Biol. Psychiatry* 55:263–272.

Goddard, A.W., Mason, G.F., Appel, M., et al. (2004) Impaired GABA neuronal response to acute benzodiazepine administration in panic disorder. *Am. J. Psychiatry* 161:2186–2193.

Gorman, J.M., Kent, J.M., Sullivan, G.M., et al. (2000) Neuroanatomical hypothesis of panic disorder, revised. *Am. J. Psychiatry* 157:493–505.

Gorman, J.M., Lietowitz, M.R., Fyer, A.J., et al. (1989) A neuroantomical hypothesis for panic disorder. *Am. J. Psychiatry* 146: 148–161.

Gurvits, T.V., Shenton, M.E., Hokama, H., et al. (1996) Magnetic resonance imaging study of hippocampal volume in chronic, combat-related posttraumatic stress disorder. *Biol. Psychiatry* 40:1091–1099.

Ham, B.J., Chey, J., Yoon, S.J., et al. (2007) Decreased N-acetyl-aspartate levels in anterior cingulate and hippocampus in subjects with post-traumatic stress disorder: a proton magnetic resonance spectroscopy study. *Eur. J. Neurosci.* 25:324–329.

Hansen, E.S., Hasselbach, S., Law, I., et al. (2002) The caudate nucleus in obsessive-compulsive disorder. Reduced metabolism following treatment with paroxetine: a PET study. *Int. J. Neuropsychopharmacol.* 5:1–10.

Hesse, S., Muller, U., Lincke, T., et al. (2005) Serotonin and dopamine transporter imaging in patients with obsessive-compulsive disorder. *Psychiatry Res.* 30:63–72.

Hoehn-Saric, R., Pearlson, G.D., Harris, G.J., et al. (1991) Effects of fluoxetine on regional cerebral blood flow in obsessive-compulsive patients. *Am. J. Psychiatry* 148:1243–1245.

Hoehn-Saric, R., Schlaepfer, T.E., Greenberg, B.D., et al. (2001) Cerebral blood flow in obsessive-compulsive patients with major depression: effect of treatment with sertraline or desipramine on treatment responders and non-responders. *Psychiatry Res.* 108: 89–100.

Holsboer, F. (1999) The rationale for corticotropin-releasing hormone receptor (CRH-R) antagonists to treat depression and anxiety. *J. Psychiatr. Res.* 33:181–214.

Ho Pian, K.L., van Megan, H.J.G.M., Ramsy, N.F., et al. (2005) Decreased thalamic blood flow in obsessive-compulsive disorder patients responding to fluvoxamine. *Psychiatry Res: Neuroimag.* 138: 89–97.

Jatzko, A., Rothenhofer, S., Schmitt, A., et al. (2006) Hippocampal volume in chronic posttraumatic stress disorder (PTSD): MRI study using two different evaluation methods. *J. Affect. Disord.* 94:121–126.

Javanmard, M., Shlik, J., Kennedy, S.H., Vaccarino, F.J., Houle, S., and Bradwejn, J. (1999) Neuroanatomic correlates of CCK-4-induced panic attacks in healthy humans: a comparison of two time points. *Biol. Psychiatry* 45(7):872–882.

Jenike, M.A., Breiter, H.C., Baer, L., et al. (1996) Cerebral structural abnormalities in obsessive-compulsive disorder: a quantitative morphometric magnetic resonance imaging study. *Arch. Gen. Psychiatry* 53:625–632.

Jones, D.K., Simmons, A., Williams, S.C., and Horsfield, M.A. (1999) Non-invasive assessment of axonal fiber connectivity in the human brain via diffusion tensor MRI. *Magn. Reson. Med.* 42: 37–41.

Jung, R.E., Yeo, R.A., Love, T.M., Petropoulos, H., Sibbitt, W.L., and Brooks, W.M. (2002) Biochemical markers of mood: a proton MR spectroscopy study of normal human brain. *Biol. Psychiatry* 51:224–229.

Kang, D.H., Kim, J.J., Choi, J.S., et al. (2004) Volumetric investigation of the frontal-subcortical circuitry in patients with obsessive-compulsive disorder. *J. Neuropsychiatry Clin. Neurosci.* 16: 342–349.

Karl, A., Schaefer, M., Malta, L.S., et al. (2006) A meta-analysis of structural brain abnormalities in PTSD. *Neurosci. Biobehav. Rev.* 30:1004–1031.

Kent, J.M., Coplan, J.D., and Gorman, J.M. (1998) Clinical utility of the selective serotonin reuptake inhibitors in the spectrum of anxiety. *Biol. Psychiatry* 44:812–824.

Kent, J.M., Coplan, J.D., Lombardo, I., et al. (2002) Occupancy of brain serotonin transporters during treatment with paroxetine in patients with social phobia: a positron emission tomography study with 11C McN 5652. *Psychopharmacology (Berl)* 164:341–348.

Kent, J.M., Sullivan, G.S., and Rauch, S.L. (2000) The neurobiology of fear: relevance to panic disorder and posttraumatic stress disorder. *Psychiatr. Ann.* 30:733–742.

Kent, J.M., Sullivan, G.S., and Rauch, S.L. (2002) Neural circuitry and signaling in anxiety. In: Kaplan, G.B., and Hammer, R.P., eds. *Brain Circuitry and Signaling in Psychiatry*. Washington, DC: American Psychiatric Press, pp. 125–152.

Kim, C.-H., Koo, M.-S., Cheon, K.-A., et al. (2003) Dopamine transporter density of basal ganglia assessed [123I] IPT SPET in obsessive-compulsive disorder. *Eur. J Nucl. Med. Molecular Imaging* 30:1637–1643.

Kim, J.-J., Lee, M.C., Kim, J., Kim, I.Y., Kim, S.I., Han, M.H., Chang, K.-H., and Kwon, J.S. (2001) Grey matter abnormalities in obsessive-compulsive disorder. *Br. J. Psychiatry* 179:330–334.

Kuikka, J.T., Pitkanen, A., Lepola, U., et al. (1995) Abnormal regional benzodiazepine receptor uptake in the prefrontal cortex in patients with panic disorder. *Nucl. Med. Commun.* 16(4):273–280.

Kwon, J.S., Shin, Y.W., Kim, C.W., et al. (2003) Similarity and disparity of obsessive-compulsive disorder and schizophrenia in MR volumetric abnormalities of the hippocampus-amygdala complex. *J. Neurol. Neurosurg. Psychiatry* 74:962–964.

Lanius, R.A., Williamson, P.C., Bluhm, R.L, et al. (2005) Functional connectivity of dissociative responses in posttraumatic stress disorder: a functional magnetic resonance imaging investigation. *Biol. Psychiatry* 57:873–884.

Lanius, R.A., Williamson, P.C., Boksman, K., et al. (2002) Brain activation during script-driven imagery induced dissociative responses in PTSD: a functional MRI investigation. *Biol. Psychiatry* 52:305–311.

Lanius, R.A., Williamson, P.C., Densmore, M., Boksman, K., Gupta, M.A., Neufeld, R.W., Gati, J.S., and Menon, R.S. (2001) Neural correlates of traumatic memories in posttraumatic stress disorder: a functional MRI investigation. *Am. J. Psychiatry* 158:1920–1922.

Lanius, R.A., Williamson, P.C., Hopper, J., et al. (2003) Recall of emotional states in posttraumatic stress disorder: an fMRI investigation. *Biol. Psychiatry* 53:204–210.

Lanzenberger, R.R., Mitterhauser, M., Spindelegger, C., et al. (2007) Reduced serotonin-1A receptor binding in social anxiety disorder. *Biol. Psychiatry* 61:1081–1089.

LeDoux, J.E. (1996) *The Emotional Brain*. New York: Simon & Schuster.

LeDoux, J.E., Cicchetti, P., Xagoraris, A., et al. (1990) The lateral amygdaloid nucleus: sensory interface of the amygdala in fear conditioning. *J. Neurosci.* 10:1062–1069.

LeDoux, J.E., Iwata, J., Cicchetti, P., et al. (1988) Different projections of the central amygdaloid nucleus mediate autonomic and behavioral correlates of conditioned fear. *J. Neurosci.* 8:2517–2519.

Levitt, J.J., Chen, Q.C., May, F.S., et al. (2006) Volume of cerebellar vermis in monozygotic twins discordant for combat exposure: lack of relationship to post-traumatic stress disorder. *Psychiatry Res.* 148:143–149.

Li, L., Chen, S., Liu, J., Zhang, J., He, Z., and Lin, X. (2006) Magnetic resonance imaging and magnetic resonance spectroscopy study of deficits in hippocampal structure in fire victims with recent-onset posttraumatic stress disorder. *Can. J. Psychiatry* 51:431–437.

Liberzon, I., and Martis, B. (2006) Neuroimaging studies of emotional responses in PTSD. *Ann. N.Y. Acad. Sci.* 1071:87–109.

Liberzon, I., Taylor, S.F., Amdur, R., et al. (1999) Brain activation in PTSD in response to trauma-related stimuli. *Biol. Psychiatry* 45: 817–826.

Loberbaum, J.P., Kose, S., Johnson, M.R., et al. (2004) Neural correlates of speech anticipatory anxiety in generalized social phobia. *Neuroreport* 15:2701–2705.

Machlin, S.R., Harris, G.J., Pearlson, G.D., et al. (1991) Elevated medial-frontal cerebral blood flow in obsessive-compulsive patients: a SPECT study. *Am. J. Psychiatry* 148:1240–1242.

MacMaster, F.P., Russell, A., Mirza, Y., et al. (2006) Pituitary volume in pediatric obsessive-compulsive disorder. *Biol. Psychiatry* 59:252–257.

Malizia, A.L., Cunningham, V.J., Bell, C.J., Liddle, P.F., Jones, T., and Nutt, D.J. (1998) Decreased brain GABA(A)-benzodiazepine receptor binding in panic disorder: preliminary results from a quantitative PET study. *Arch. Gen. Psychiatry* 55:715–720.

Maltby, N., Tolin, D.F., Worhunsky, P., et al. (2005) Dysfunctional action monitoring hyperactivates frontal-striatal circuits in obsessive-compulsive disorder: an event-related fMRI study. *NeuroImage* 24:495–503.

Mataix-Cols, D., Wooderson, S., Lawrence, N., et al. (2004) Distinct neural correlates of washing, checking, and hoarding symptom dimensions in obsessive-compulsive disorder. *Arch. Gen. Psychiatry* 61:564–576.

Mathew, S.J., Coplan, J.D., and Gorman, J.M. (2001) Neurobiological mechanisms of social anxiety disorder. *Am. J. Psychiatry* 158: 1558–1567.

McGuire, P.K., Bench, C.J., Frith, C.D., et al. (1994) Functional anatomy of obsessive-compulsive phenomena. *Br. J. Psychiatry* 164: 459–468.

Meyer, J.H., Swinson, R., Kennedy, S.H., Houle, S., and Brown, G.M. (2000) Increased left posterior parietal-temporal cortex activation after d-fenfluramine in women with panic disorder. *Psychiatry Res.* 98:133–143.

Milad, M.R., Rauch S.L. (2007) The role of the orbitofrontal cortex in anxiety disorders. *Ann. N.Y. Acad. Sci.* Dec;1121:546–561. Epub 2007 Aug 14.

Moats, R., Ernst, T., Shonk, R., and Ross, B. (1994) Abnormal cerebral metabolite concentrations in patients with probable Alzheimer disease. *Magn. Reson. Med.* 32:110–115.

Moore, G.J., MacMaster, F.P., Stewart, C., and Rosenberg, D.R. (1998) Case study: caudate glutamatergic changes with paroxetine therapy for pediatric obsessive-compulsive disorder. *Am. Acad. Child Adolesc. Psychiatry* 37(6):663–667.

Mountz, J.M., Modell, J.G., Wilson, M.W., et al. (1989) Positron emission tomographic evaluation of cerebral blood flow during state anxiety in simple phobia. *Arch. Gen. Psychiatry* 46:501–504.

Nakao, T., Nakagawa, A., Yoshiura, T., et al. (2005) A functional MRI comparison of patients with obsessive-compulsive disorder and normal controls during a Chinese character Stroop task. *Psychiatry Res.* 139:101–114.

Neumeister, A., Bain, E., Nugent, A.C., et al. (2004) Reduced serotonin type 1A receptor binding in panic disorder. *J. Neurosci.* 24:589–591.

Nordahl, T.E., Benkelfat, C., Semple, W., et al. (1989) Cerebral glucose metabolic rates in obsessive-compulsive disorder. *Neuropsychopharmacology* 2:23–28.

Nordahl, T.E., Semple, W.E., Gross, M., et al. (1990) Cerebral glucose metabolic differences in patients with panic disorder. *Neuropsychopharmacology* 3:261–272.

Nordahl, T.E., Stein, M.B., Benkelfat, C., et al. (1998) Regional cerebral metabolic asymmetries replicated in an independent group of patients with panic disorders. *Biol. Psychiatry* 44(10):998–1006.

Notestine C.F., Stein M.B., Kennedy, C.M., et al. (2002) Brain morphometry in female victims of intimate partner violence with and without posttraumatic stress disorder. *Biol. Psychiatry* 51:1089–1101.

Osuch, E.A., Benson, B., Geraci, M., Podell, D., Herscovitch, P., McCann, U.D., and Post, R.M. (2001) Regional cerebral blood flow correlated with flashback intensity in patients with posttraumatic stress disorder. *Biol. Psychiatry* 50:246–253.

Paquette, V., Lavesque, J., Mensour, B, et al. (2003) "Change the mind and you change the brain": effects of cognitive-behavioral therapy on the neural correlatos of spider phobia. *NeuroImage* 18:401–409.

Pavic, L., Gregurek, R., Rados, M., et al. (2007) Smaller right hippocampus in war veterans with posttraumatic stress disorder. *Psychiatry Res.* 154:191–198.

Perani, D., Colombo, C., Bressi, S., et al. (1995) FDG PET study in obsessive-compulsive disorder: a clinical metabolic correlation study after treatment. *Br. J. Psychiatry* 166:244–250.

Peterson, B.S., Leckman, J.F., Tucker, D., Scahill, L., Staib, L., Zhang, H., King, R., Cohen, D.J., Gore, J.C., and Lombroso, P. (2000) Preliminary findings of antistreptococcal antibody titers and basal ganglia volumes in tic, obsessive-compulsive, and attention-deficit/hyperactivity disorders. *Arch. Gen. Psychiatry* 57: 364–372.

Phan, K.L., Britton, J.C., Taylor, S.F., et al. (2006) Corticolimbic flood flow during nontraumatic emotional processing in posttraumatic stress disorder. *Arch. Gen. Psychiatry* 63:184–192.

Phan, K.L., Fitzgerald, D.A., Nathan P.J., and Tancer, M.E. (2006) Association between amygdala hyperactivity to harsh faces and severity of social anxiety in generalized social phobia. *Biol. Psychiatry* 59:424–429.

Phillips, M.L., Drevets, W.C., Rauch, S.L., et al. (2003) Neurobiology of emotion perception II: Implications for major psychiatric disorders. *Biol. Psychiatry* 54:515–528.

Pillay S.S., Rogowska, J., Gruber, S.A., Simpson, N., and Yurgelun-Todd, D.A. (2007) Recognition of happy facial affect in panic disorder: An fMRI study. *J. Anxiety Disord.* 21:38–93.

Pissiota, A., Frans, O., Fernandez, M., von Knorring, L., Fischer, H., and Fredrikson, M. (2002) Neurofunctional correlates of posttraumatic stress disorder: a PET symptom provocation study. *Eur. Arch. Psychiatry Clin. Neurosci.* 252:68–75.

Pitman, R.K., Gilbertson, M.W., Gurvits, T.V., et al. (2006) Clarifying the origin of biological abnormalities in PTSD through the study of identical twins discordant for combat exposure. *Ann. N.Y. Acad. Sci.* 1071:242–254.

Potts, N.L., Davidson, J.R., Krishnan, K.R., and Doraiswamy, P.M. (1994) Magnetic resonance imaging in social phobia. *Psychiatry Res.* 52(1):35–42.

Poupon, P., Mangin, J., Clark, C.A., Frouin, V., Regis, J., Le Bihan, D., and Bloch, I. (2001) Towards inference of human brain connectivity from MR diffusion tensor data. *Med. Image Anal.* 5: 1–15.

Protopopescu, X., Pan, H., Tuescher, O., et al. (2005) Differential time courses and specificity of amygdala activity in posttraumatic stress disorder subjects and normal control subjects. *Biol. Psychiatry* 57:464–473.

Protopopescu, X., Pan, H., Tuescher, O., et al. (2006) Increased brain stem volume in panic disorder: a voxel-based morphometric study. *Neuroreport* 17:361–363.

Pujol, J., Soriano-Mas, C., Alonso, P., et al. (2004) Mapping structural brain alterations in obsessive-compulsive disorder. *Arch. Gen. Psychiatry* 61:720–730.

Pujol, J., Torres, L., Deus, J., et al. (1999) Functional magnetic resonance imaging study of frontal lobe activation during word generation in obsessive-compulsive disorder. *Biol. Psychiatry* 45:891–897.

Rauch, S.L., and Baxter, L.R. (1998) Neuroimaging of OCD and related disorders. In: Jenike, M.A., Baer, L., Minichiello, W.E., eds. *Obsessive-Compulsive Disorders: Theory and Management*. Boston: Mosby, pp. 289–317.

Rauch, S.L., Jenike, M.A., Alpert, N.M., et al. (1994) Regional cerebral blood flow measured during symptom provocation in obsessive-compulsive disorder using ^{15}O-labeled CO_2 and positron emission tomography. *Arch. Gen. Psychiatry* 51:62–70.

Rauch, S.L., Kim, H., Makris, N., Cosgrove, G.R., Cassem, E.H., Savage, C.R., Price, B., Nierenberg, A.A., Shera, D., Baer, L., Buchbinder, B., Caviness, V., Jenike, M.A., and Kennedy, D.N. (2000) Volume reduction in caudate nucleus following stereotactic lesions of anterior cingulate cortex in humans: a morphometric magnetic resonance imaging study. *J. Neurosurg.* 93:1019–1025.

Rauch, S.L., Savage, C.R., Alpert, N.M., et al. (1995) A positron emission tomographic study of simple phobic symptom provocation. *Arch. Gen. Psychiatry* 52:20–28.

Rauch, S.L., Savage, C.R., Alpert, N.M., et al. (1997) The functional neuroanatomy of anxiety: a study of three disorders using PET and symptom provocation. *Biol. Psychiatry* 42:446–452.

Rauch, S.L., Savage, C.R., Brown, H.D., et al. (1995) A PET investigation of implicit and explicit sequence learning. *Hum. Brain Mapp.* 3:271–286.

Rauch, S.L., Shin, L.M., and Phelps, E.A. (2006) Neurocircuitry models of posttraumatic stress disorder and extinction: human neuroimaging research—past, present, and future. *Biol. Psychiatry* 60:376–382.

Rauch, S.L., Shin, L.M., Dougherty, D.D., et al. (2002) Predictors of fluvoxamine response in contamination-related obsessive-compulsive disorder: a PET symptom provocation study. *Neuropsychopharmacology* 27:782–791.

Rauch, S.L, Shin, L.M., Segal, E., et al. (2003) Selectively reduced regional cortical volumes in post-traumatic stress disorder. *Neuroreport* 14:913–916.

Rauch, S.L., Shin, L.M., Whalen, P.J., and Pitman, R.K. (1998) Neuroimaging and the neuroanatomy of PTSD. *CNS Spectrums* 3(Suppl 2):30–41.

Rauch, S.L., van der Kolk, B.A., Fisler, R.E., et al. (1996) A symptom provocation study of posttraumatic stress disorder using positron emission tomography and script-driven imagery. *Arch. Gen. Psychiatry* 53:380–387.

Rauch, S.L., Whalen, P.J., Curran, T., Shin, L.M., Coffey, B.J., Savage, C.R., McInerney, S.C., Baer, L., and Jenike, M.A. (2001) Probing striato-thalamic function in OCD and TS using neuroimaging methods. In: Cohen, D.J., Jankovic, J., and Goetz, C.G., eds. *Tourette Syndrome*. Philadelphia: Lippincott, Williams & Wilkins, pp. 207–224.

Rauch, S.L., Whalen, P.J., Dougherty, D.D., and Jenike, M.A. (1998) Neurobiological models of obsessive compulsive disorders. In: Jenike, M.A., Baer, L., and Minichiello, W.E., eds. *Obsessive-Compulsive Disorders: Practical Management*. Boston: Mosby, pp. 222–253.

Rauch, S.L., Whalen, P.J., Savage, C.R., et al. (1997) Striatal recruitment during an implicit sequence learning task as measured by functional magnetic resonance imaging. *Hum. Brain Mapp.* 5: 124–132.

Rauch, S.L., Whalen, P.J., Shin, L.M., McInerney, S.C., Macklin, M.L., Lasko, N.B., Orr, S.P., and Pittman, R.K. (2000) Exaggerated amygdala response to masked facial stimuli in posttraumatic stress disorder: a functional MRI study. *Biol. Psychiatry* 47:769–776.

Rauch, S.L, Wright, C.I., Martix, B., et al. (2004) A magnetic resonance imaging study of cortical thickness in animal phobia. *Biol. Psychiatry* 55:946–952.

Reiman, E.M., Raichle, M.E., Robins, E., et al. (1986) The application of positron emission tomography to the study of panic disorder. *Am. J. Psychiatry* 143:469–477.

Reiman, E.M., Raichle, M.E., Robins, E., et al. (1989) Neuroanatomical correlates of a lactate-induced anxiety attack. *Arch. Gen. Psychiatry* 46:493–500.

Riffkin J., Yacel, M., Maruff, P., et al. (2005) A manual and automated MRI study of anterior cingulate and orbito-frontal cortices and caudate nucleus in obsessive-compulsive disorder: comparison with healthy controls and patients with schizophrenia. *Psychiatry Res.* 138:99–113.

Robinson, D., Wu, H., Munne, R.A., et al. (1995) Reduced caudate nucleus volume in obsessive-compulsive disorder. *Arch. Gen. Psychiatry* 52:393–398.

Rosenberg, D.R., Amponsah, A., Sullivan, A., MacMillan, S., and Moore, G.J. (2001) Increased medial thalamic choline in pediatric obsessive-compulsive disorder as detected by quantitative in vivo spectroscopic imaging. *J. Child Neurol.* 16:636–641.

Rosenberg, D.R., Benazon, N.R., Gilbert, A., Sullivan, A., and Moore, G.J. (2000) Thalamic volume in pediatric obsessive-compulsive disorder patients before and after cognitive behavioral therapy. *Biol. Psychiatry* 48:294–300.

Rosenberg, D.R., Keshevan, M.S., O'Hearn, K.M., et al. (1997) Frontostriatal measurement in treatment-naive children with obsessive-compulsive disorder. *Arch. Gen. Psychiatry* 554: 824–830.

Rosenberg, D.R., MacMaster, F.P., Keshavan, M., et al. (2000) Decrease in caudate glutamate concentrations in pediatric obsessive-compulsive disorder patients taking paroxetine. *J. Am. Acad. Child Adoles. Psychiatry* 39:1096–1103.

Ross, B.D., and Michaelis, T. (1994) Clinical applications of magnetic resonance spectroscopy. *Magn. Reson. Q.* 10:191–247.

Rothman, D.L., Petroff, O.A.C., Behar, K.L., and Mattson, R.H. (1993) Localized H NMR measurements of g-aminobutyric acid in human brain in vivo. *Proc. Natl. Acad. Sci. USA* 90:5662–5666.

Rubin, R.T., Villaneuva-Myer, J., Ananth, J., et al. (1992) Regional xenon-133 cerebral blood flow and cerebral technetium 99m HMPAO uptake in unmedicated patients with obsessive-compulsive disorder and matched normal control subjects. *Arch. Gen. Psychiatry* 49:695–702.

Russell, A., Cortese, B., Lorch, E., et al. (2003) Localized functional neurochemical marker abnormalities in dorsolateral prefrontal cortex in pediatric obsessive-compulsive disorder. *J. Chil. Adolesc. Psychopharmacol.* 13 Suppl 1:S31–38.

Sakai, Y., Kumano, H., Nishikawa, M., et al. (2006) Changes in cerebral glucose utilization in patients with panic disorder treated with cognitive behavioral therapy. *NeuroImage* 33: 218–226.

Salzman, C., Miyawaki, E.K., le Bars, P., and Kerrihard, T.N. (1993) Neurobiologic basis of anxiety and its treatment. *Harv. Rev. Psychiatry* 1:197–206.

Sanacora, G., Mason, G.F., Rothman, D.L., Behar, K.L., Hyder, F., Petroff, O.A.C., Berman, R.M., Charney, D.S., and Krystal, J.H. (1999) Reduced cortical g-aminobutyric acid levels in depressed patients by proton magnetic spectroscopy. *Arch. Gen. Psychiatry* 56:1043–1047.

Sapolsky, R.M. (1986) Glucocorticoid toxicity in the hippocampus. Temporal aspects of synergy with kainic acid. *Neuroendocrinology* 43(3):440–444.

Sapolsky, R.M. (2000) Glucocorticoids and hippocampal atrophy in neuropsychiatric disorders. *Arch. Gen. Psychiatry* 57:825–835.

Sato, T., Hasan, K., Alexander, A.L., and Minato, K. (2001) Structural connectivity in white matter using the projected diffusion-tensor distance. *Medinfo* 10(Pt 2):929–932.

Saxena, S., and Rauch, S.L. (2000) Functional neuroimaging and the neuroanatomy of obsessive-compulsive disorder. *Psychiatr. Clin. North Am.* 23:563–584.

Saxena, S., Brody, A.L., Ho, M.L., Alborzian, S., Ho, M.K., Maidment, K.M., Huang, S.-C., Wu, H.-M., Au, S.C., and Baxter, L.R. (2001) Cerebral metabolism in major depression and obsessive-compulsive disorder occurring separately and concurrently. *Biol. Psychiatry* 50:159–170.

Saxena, S., Brody, A.L., Ho, M.L., Alborzian, S., Maidment, K.M., Zohrabi, S., Ho, M.K., Huang, S.-C., Wu, H.-M., and Baxter, L. R. (2002) Differential cerebral metabolic changes with paroxetine treatment of obsessive-compulsive disorder vs major depression. *Arch. Gen. Psychiatry* 59:250–261.

Saxena, S., Brody, A.L., Maidment, K.M., et al. (2004) Cerebral glucose metabolism in obsessive-compulsive hoarding. *Am. J. Psychiatry* 161:1038–1048.

Saxena, S., Brody, A.L., Maidment, K.M., Dunkin, J.J., Colgan, M., Alborzian, S., Phelps, M.E., and Baxter, L.R. (1999) Localized orbitofrontal and subcortical metabolic changes and predictors of response to paroxetine treatment in obsessive-compulsive disorder. *Neuropsychopharmacology* 21:683–693.

Scarone, S., Colombo, C., Livian, S., et al. (1992) Increased right caudate nucleus size in obsessive compulsive disorder: detection with magnetic resonance imaging. *Psychiatry Res. Neuroimag.* 45:115–121.

Schienle, A., Schaufer, A., Walter, B., et al. (2005) Brain activation of spider phobics towards disorder-relevant, generally disgust- and fear-inducing pictures. *Neurosci. Lett.* 388:1–6.

Schneider, F., Weiss, U., Kessler, C., et al. (1999) Subcortical correlates of differential classical conditioning of aversive emotional reactions in social phobia. *Biol. Psychiatry* 45:863–871.

Schneier, F.R., Liebowitz, M.R., Abi-Dargham, A., Zea-Ponce, Y., Shu-Hsing, L., and Laruelle, M. (2000) Low dopamine D_2 receptor binding potential in social phobia. *Am. J. Psychiatry* 157:457–459.

Schuff, N., Marmar, C.R., Weiss, D.S., et al. (1997) Reduced hippocampal volume and N-acetyl aspartate in posttraumatic stress disorder. In: Yehuda, R., and McFarlane, A.C., eds. *Psychobiology of Posttraumatic Stress Disorder*, Vol. 821. New York: New York Academy of Sciences, pp. 516–520.

Schuff, N., Neylan, T.C., Lenoci, M.A., Du, A.-T., Weiss, D.S., Marmar, C.R., and Weiner, M.W. (2001) Decreased hippocampal N-acetylaspartate in the absence of atrophy in posttraumatic stress disorder. *Biol. Psychiatry* 50:952–959.

Schunck, T., Erb, G., Mathis A., et al. (2006) Functional magnetic resonance imaging characterization of CCK-4 –induced panic attack and subsequent anticipatory anxiety. *NeuroImage* 31:1197–1208.

Schwartz, C.E., Snidman, N., and Kagan, J. (1999) Adolescent social anxiety as an outcome of inhibited temperament in childhood. *J. Am. Acad. Child Adolesc. Psychiatry* 38:1008–1015.

Schwartz, J.M., Stoessel, P.W., Baxter, L.R., et al. (1996) Systematic changes in cerebral glucose metabolic rate after successful behavior modification. *Arch. Gen. Psychiatry* 53:109–113.

Seedat, S., Videen, J.S., Kennedy, C.M., and Stein, M.B. (2005) Single voxel proton magnetic resonance spectroscopy in women with and without intimate partner violence-related posttraumatic stress disorder. *Psychiatry Res.* 139:249–258.

Semple, W.E., Goyer, P.F., McCormick, R., Donovan, B., Muzic, R.F., Jr., Rugle, L., McCutcheon, K., Lewis, C., Liebling, D., Kowaliw, S., Vapenik, K., Semple, M.A., Flener, C.R., and Schulz, S.C. (2000) Higher brain blood flow at amygdala and lower frontal cortex blood flow in PTSD patients with comorbid cocaine and alcohol abuse compared with normals. *Psychiatry* 63:65–74.

Shapira, N.A., Liu, Y., He, A.G., et al. (2003) Brain activation by disgust-inducing pictures in obsessive-compulsive disorder. 54: 751–756.

Shin, L.M., Kosslyn, S.M., McNally, R.J., et al. (1997) Visual imagery and perception in posttraumatic stress disorder: a positron emission tomographic investigation. *Arch. Gen. Psychiatry* 54: 233–241.

Shin, L.M., McNally, R.J., Kosslyn, S.M., et al. (1999) Regional cerebral blood flow during script-driven imagery in childhood sexual abuse–related posttraumatic stress disorder: a PET investigation. *Am. J. Psychiatry* 156:575–584.

Shin, L.M., Orr, S.P., Carson, M.A., et al. (2004) Regional cerebral blood flow in the amygdala and medial prefrontal cortex during traumatic imagery in male and female Vietnam veterans with PTSD. *Arch. Gen. Psychiatry* 61:168–176.

Shin, L.M., Rauch, R.L., and Pitman, R.K. (2006) Amygdala, medial prefrontal cortex and hippocampal function in PTSD. *Ann. N.Y. Acad. Sci.* 1071:67–79.

Shin, L.M., Whalen, P.J., Pitman, R.K., Bush, G., Macklin, M.L., Lasko, N.B., Orr, S.P., McInerney, S.C., and Rauch, S.L. (2001) An fMRI study of anterior cingulate function in posttraumatic stress disorder. *Biol. Psychiatry* 50:932–942.

Shin, L.M., Wright, C.I., Cannistraro, P.A., et al. (2005) A functional magnetic resonance imaging study of amygdala and medial prefrontal cortex responses to overtly presented fearful faces in posttraumatic stress disorder. *Arch. Gen. Psychiatry* 62: 273–281.

Simpson, H.B., Lombardo, I., Slifstein, M., et al. (2003) Serotonin transporters in obsessive-compulsive disorder: A positron emission tomography study with [11-C]McN 5652. *Biol. Psychiatry* 54:1414–1421.

Stein, M.B. (1998) Neurobiological perspectives on social phobia: from affiliation to zoology. *Biol. Psychiatry* 44:1277–1285.

Stein, M.B., Goldin, P.R., Sareen, J, et al. (2002) Increased amygdala activation to angry and contemptuous faces in generalized social phobia. *Arch. Gen. Psychiatry* 59:1027–1034.

Stein, M.B., Koverola, C., Hanna, C., et al. (1997) Hippocampal volume in women victimized by childhood sexual abuse. *Psychol. Med.* 27:951–960.

Stengler-Wenzke, K., Muller, U., Angermeyer, M.C., et al. (2004) Reduced serotonin transporter availability in obsessive-compulsive disorder. *Eur. Arch. Clin. Neurosci.* 254:252–255.

Stewart, R.S., Devous, M.D. Sr., Rush, A.J., Lane, L., and Bonte, F.J. (1988) Cerebral blood flow changes during sodium-lactate-induced panic attacks. *Am. J. Psychiatry* 145(4):442–449.

Straube, T., Glauer, M., Dilger, S., et al. (2006) Effects of cognitive-behavioral therapy on brain activation in specific phobia. *NeuroImage* 29:125–135.

Straube, T., Kolassa, I-T., Glauer, M., et al. (2004) Effect of task conditions on brain responses to threatening faces in social phobics: an event-related functional magnetic resonance imaging study. *Biol. Psychiatry* 56:921–930.

Straube, T., Mentzel, H.J., and Miltner, W.H. (2005) Common and distinct brain activation to threat and safety signals in social phobia. *Neuropsychobiology* 52:163–168.

Straube, T., Mentzel, H.J., and Miltner, W.H. (2006) Neural mechanisms of automatic and direct processing of phobogenic stimuli in specific phobia. *Biol. Psychiatry* 59:162–170.

Swedo, S.E., Pietrini, P., Leonard, H.L., et al. (1992) Cerebral glucose metabolism in childhood-onset obsessive-compulsive disorder: revisualization during pharmacotherapy. *Arch. Gen. Psychiatry* 49:690–694.

Swedo, S.E., Shapiro, M.B., Grady, C.L., et al. (1989) Cerebral glucose metabolism in childhood-onset obsessive-compulsive disorder. *Arch. Gen. Psychiatry* 46:518–523.

Szeszko, P.R., MacMillan, S., McMeniman, M., et al. (2004) Brain structural abnormalities in psychotropic drug-naïve pediatric obsessive compulsive disorder. *Am. J. Psychiatry* 161:1049–1056.

Szeszko, P.R., Robinson, D., Alvir, J.M., et al. (1999) Orbital frontal and amygala volume reductions in obsessive-compulsive disorder. *Arch. Gen. Psychiatry* 56:913–919.

Tiihonen, J., Kuikka, J., Bergstrom, K., Lepola, U., Koponen, H., and Leinonen, E. (1997) Dopamine reuptake site densities in patients with social phobia. *Am. J. Psychiatry* 154(2):239–242.

Tillfors, M., Furmark, T., Marteinsdottir, I., Fischer, H., Pissiota, A., Langstrom, B., and Fredrikson, M. (2001) Cerebral blood flow in subjects with social phobia during stressful speaking tasks: a PET study. *Am. J. Psychiatry* 158:1220–1226.

Ursu, S., Stenger, V.A., Shear, M.K., et al. (2003) Overactive action monitoring in obsessive-compulsive disorder: evidence from functional magnetic resonance imaging. *Psychological Sci.* 14: 347–353.

van den Heuvel, O.A., Veltman, D.J., Groenewegen, H.J., et al. (2005a) Disorder-specific neuroanatomical correlates of attentional bias in obsessive-compulsive disorder, panic disorder, and hypochondriasis. *Arch. Gen. Psychiatry* 62:922–933.

van den Heuvel, O.A., Veltman, D.J., Groenenwegen, H.J., et al. (2005b) Frontal striatal dysfunction during planning in obsessive-compulsive disorder. *Arch. Gen. Psychiatry* 62:301–310.

Van der Linden, G., van Heerden, B., Warwick, J., Wessels, C., van Kradenburg, J., Zungu-Dirwayi, N., and Stein, D.J. (2000) Functional brain imaging and pharmacotherapy in social phobia: single photon emission computed tomography before and after treatment with the selective serotonin reuptake inhibitor citalopram. *Prog. Neuro-Psychopharmacol. Biol. Psychiatry* 24:419–438.

van der Wee, N.J., Stevens, H., Hardeman, J.A., et al. (2004) Enhanced dopamine transporter density in psychotropic-naive patients with obsessive-compulsive disorder shown by [123-I]β-CIT SPECT. *Am. J. Psychiatry* 161:2201–2206.

Whalen, P.J., Bush, G., McNally, R.J., et al. (1998) The emotional counting Stroop paradigm: an fMRI probe of the anterior cingulate affective division. *Biol. Psychiatry* 44:1219–1228.

Whalen, P.J., Rauch, S.L., Etcoff, N.L., McInerney, S., Lee, M.B., and Jenike, M.A. (1998) Masked presentations of emotional facial expressions modulate amygdala activity without explicit knowledge. *J. Neurosci.* 18:411–418.

Viard, A., Flament, M.F., Artiges, E., et al. (2005) Cognitive control in childhood-onset obsessive-compulsive disorder: a functional MRI study. *Psychol. Med.* 35:1007–1017.

Viet, R., Flor, H., Erb, M., et al. (2002) Brain circuits involved in emotional learning in antisocial behavior and social phobia in humans. *Neurosci. Lett.* 328:233–236.

Vythilingam, M., Anderson, E.R., Goddard, A., Woods, S.W., Staib, L.H., Charney, D.S., and Bremner, J.D. (2000) Temporal lobe volume in panic disorder—a quantitative magnetic resonance imaging study. *Psychiatry Res.* 99:75–82.

Wik, G., Fredrikson, M., Ericson, K., et al. (1993) A functional cerebral response to frightening visual stimulation. *Psychiatry Res. Neuroimag.* 50:15–24.

Williams, L.M., Kempt, A.H., Felmingham, K., et al. (2006) Trauma modulates amygdala and medial prefrontal responses to consciously attended fear. *NeuroImage* 29:347–357.

Winton, E.C., Clark, D.M., and Edelmann, R.J. (1995) Social anxiety, fear or negative evaluation and the detection of negative emotion in others. *Behaviour Res. Ther.* 33:193–196.

Woods, S.W., Koster, K., Krystal, J.K., et al. (1988) Yohimbine alters regional cerebral blood flow in panic disorder. *Lancet* 2:678.

Woodward, S.H., Kaloupek, D.F., Streeter, C.C., et al. (2006) Decreased anterior cingulate volume in combat-related PTSD. *Biol. Psychiatry* 59:582–587.

Yamasue, H., Kasai, K., Iwanami, A., et al. (2003) Voxel-based analysis of MRI reveals anterior cingulate gray-matter volume reduction in posttraumatic stress disorder due to terrorism. *Proc. Natl. Acad. Sci.* 1000:9039–9043.

Yoon, K.L., Fitzgerald, D.A., Angstadt, M. et al. (2007) Amygdala reactivity to emotional faces at high and low intensity in generalized social phobia: a 4-Tesla functional MRI study. *Psychiatry Res: Neuroimag.* 154:93–98.

Zubieta, J.K., Chinitz, J.A., Lombardi, U., et al. (1999) Medial frontal cortex involvement in PTSD symptoms: a SPECT study. *J. Psychiatric Res.* 33:259–264.

44 Pharmacotherapy of Anxiety Disorders

SANJAY J. MATHEW, ELLEN J. HOFFMAN, AND DENNIS S. CHARNEY

This chapter reviews pharmacological treatments for patients with anxiety disorders, focusing on the published randomized controlled trial (RCT) literature (pharmacological treatment of obsessive–compulsive disorder (OCD) is discussed elsewhere in this volume (see Chapter 42). The anxiety disorders with the greatest evidence for the efficacy of pharmacotherapy are generalized anxiety disorder (GAD), panic disorder (PD), and social anxiety disorder (SAD); accordingly, the chapter is primarily devoted to these three disorders. The medication classes most commonly used for these disorders, the selective serotonin reuptake inhibitors (SSRIs) and serotonin and norepinephrine reuptake inhibitors (SNRIs), are first presented, and then other commonly utilized pharmacotherapy approaches such as the benzodiazepines, anticonvulsants, and atypical antipsychotics are reviewed. We conclude with recommendations for areas of future investigation and limitations of current approaches.

Due to space limitations (and publication bias), we undoubtedly have failed to review every RCT conducted in the anxiety disorders as of July 2007, including those therapies categorized under complementary and alternative medicine. With new clinical trials data emerging in this therapeutic area at a rapid pace, the evidence base is a constantly moving target. Thus, in making informed decisions regarding an individual medication's efficacy, it is imperative for clinicians and researchers to consult several sources for up-to-date safety and efficacy information. First, drug manufacturer websites are encouraged to maintain registries of all clinical trials conducted on a compound, regardless of publication status, in which key methodological details of clinical trials are available (however, for older generic medications this data is unavailable). Second, all clinical trials initiated after 2005 must be formally registered on www.clinicaltrials.gov, which summarizes the major end points and trial design for new studies. For a reasonably updated collection of evidence-based guidelines for anxiety and related conditions, including post-traumatic stress disorder (PTSD), the reader is encouraged to evaluate summaries of clinical trials data from several independent, web-accessible sources that include published and unpublished drug manufacturer data: (*1*) National Institute for Health and Clinical Excellence (NICE) guidelines (www.nice.org.uk) and (*2*) Cochrane Reviews, specifically Cochrane Depression, Anxiety & Neurosis Group (CCDAN) Controlled Trials Register (www.cochrane.org), and for PTSD, the International Psychopharmacology Algorithm Project (www.ipap.org).

SELECTIVE SEROTONIN REUPTAKE INHIBITORS (SSRIs)

Selective serotonin reuptake inhibitors are considered first-line medications for the treatment of the anxiety disorders, including GAD, PD, SAD, and PTSD (Davidson 2006; Katon, 2006; D.J. Stein, Ipser, et al. 2006; Mathew and Hoffman, in press). Table 44.1 shows the SSRIs that have received U.S. Food and Drug Administration (FDA) approval for the treatment of these disorders. Although older classes of antidepressant medications, such as the tricyclic antidepressants (TCAs) and monoamine oxidase inhibitors (MAOIs) have been shown to be effective for many anxiety and mood disorders, SSRIs are the most commonly prescribed due to their more favorable side-effect profile. In addition, in contrast to the benzodiazepines (BZDs), SSRIs have the critical advantage of treating comorbid mood disorders, whereas long-term administration is not associated with physiological dependence or abuse liability.

SSRIs in Generalized Anxiety Disorder

In the treatment of GAD, multiple randomized, double-blind, placebo-controlled clinical trials using large multicenter sample sizes in the range of approximately 300 to 600 have demonstrated the efficacy of several SSRIs (Mathew and Hoffman, in press). Of the SSRIs, paroxetine and escitalopram are FDA-approved for GAD.

TABLE 44.1 *FDA-Approved Medications for the Anxiety Disorders[a] in Adults*

Medication	*GAD*	*PD*	*PTSD*	*SAD*	*Anxiety Disorders[b]*	*Year of Initial FDA Approval*	*Daily Dose Range*	*Other Approved Psychiatric Indications*
SSRIs								
Escitalopram (Lexapro)	Y	-	-	-	-	2002	10–20 mg	MDD
Fluoxetine (Prozac)	-	Y	-	-	-	1987	20–60 mg	MDD, OCD, PMDD Bulimia Nervosa
Paroxetine (Paxil)	Y	Y	Y	Y	-	1992	PD: 10–60 mg SAD: 20–60 mg GAD, PTSD: 20–50 mg	MDD, OCD
Paroxetine CR (Paxil CR)	-	Y	-	Y	-	2002	PD: 12.5–75 mg SAD: 12.5–37.5 mg	MDD, PMDD
Sertraline (Zoloft)	-	Y	Y	Y	-	1991	50–200 mg	MDD, OCD, PMDD
SNRIs								
Duloxetine (Cymbalta)	Y	-	-	-	-	2004	30–120 mg	MDD
Venlafaxine XR (Effexor XR)	Y	Y	-	Y	-	1997	37.5–225 mg	MDD
Azapirone								
Buspirone (BuSpar)	Y[c]	-	-	-	Y	1986	15–60 mg	Short-term relief of anxiety sx.
Benzodiazepines								
Alprazolam (Xanax)	Y[c]	Y	-	-	Y	1981	0.75–4 mg	Short-term relief of anxiety sx; Anxiety assoc. w/ depression
Alprazolam XR (Xanax XR)	-	Y	-	-	-	2003	3–6 mg (suggested) 1–10 mg (used in clinical trials)	None
Chlordiazepoxide (Librium)	-	-	-	-	Y	1960	15–100 mg	Short-term relief of anxiety sx; ETOH w/d; preoperative anxiety
Clonazepam (Klonopin)	-	Y	-	-	-	1975	0.5–4 mg	None
Clorazepate (Tranxene)	-	-	-	-	Y	1972	15–60 mg	Short-term relief of anxiety sx.; ETOH w/d
Diazepam (Valium)	-	-	-	-	Y	1963	4–40 mg	Short-term relief of anxiety sx.; ETOH w/d
Lorazepam (Ativan)	-	-	-	-	Y	1977	1–10 mg	Short-term relief of anxiety sx; anxiety assoc. w/ depression
Oxazepam (Serax)	-	-	-	-	Y	1965	30–120 mg	Short-term relief of anxiety sx; anxiety assoc. w/depression; anxiety in older patients; ETOH w/d

SSRI: selective serotonin reuptake inhibitor; SNRI: serotonin an norepinephrine reuptake inhibitor; GAD: generalized anxiety disorder; PD: panic disorder; PTSD: posttraumatic stress disorder; SAD: social anxiety disorder; MDD: major depressive disorder; PMDD: premenstrual dysphoric disorder; OCD: obsessive–compulsive disorder; ETOH: alcohol; FDA: U.S. Food and Drug Administration.

[a] Table includes *DSM-IV-TR* anxiety disorders, except OCD.

[b] No individual disorder specified.

[c] Approved for anxiety disorders that correspond most closely to GAD as described in *DSM-III*.

Two 8-week studies found that paroxetine, in fixed or flexible doses, led to significant reductions in the Hamilton Rating Scale for Anxiety (HAM-A) in GAD compared to placebo (Pollack et al., 2001; Rickels et al., 2003). Rickels et al. (2003) documented that 62% and 68% of patients with GAD receiving paroxetine (20 mg or 40 mg/day, respectively) were responders on the Clinical Global Impression–Improvement (CGI-I) scale (obtaining scores of 1 or 2) after 2 months, compared to 46% of patients receiving placebo. In addition, a significant percentage of patients in the paroxetine groups (30% and 36% in the 20 mg, 40 mg groups, respectively) achieved remission (defined as HAM-A ≤ 7) versus placebo (20%) (Rickels et al., 2003). A flexible dose study of paroxetine (20–50 mg/day) found a significant decrease in the anxious mood item on the HAM-A, which includes "worrying" and "anticipating the worst," by the first week of treatment. Significant overall rates of response (62% vs. 47%), defined as CGI-I of 1 or 2, and remission (36% vs. 23%), defined as HAM-A ≤ 7, versus placebo, were found after 8 weeks (Pollack et al., 2001).

Escitalopram (10–20 mg/day) was found to result in significant reductions in total and psychic anxiety subscale scores on HAM-A beginning in the first week of treatment, with significant rates of CGI-I response versus placebo (58% vs. 38%) in the last observation carried forward (LOCF) analysis, and remission (36% vs. 16%, in completers) at the conclusion of the 8-week trial (Davidson, Bose, et al. 2004). Davidson et al. (2005) demonstrated the long-term efficacy of escitalopram in GAD, in a 6-month, open-label extension study for completers of three 8-week, double-blind, controlled escitalopram trials (*N* = 521, intent-to-treat). This study showed ongoing improvement in HAM-A and quality-of-life scores in the open-label phase, such that 76% of patients were responders and 49% were remitters in the LOCF analysis (Davidson et al., 2005).

Longer-term continuation studies have also shown that escitalopram and paroxetine are effective in preventing relapse in GAD (Stocchi et al., 2003; Allgulander et al., 2005). Compared to patients who continued to receive escitalopram or paroxetine for 6 months, the risk of relapse was approximately 4 or 5 times greater, respectively, in the placebo groups (Stocchi et al., 2003; Allgulander et al., 2005). In a head-to-head study of these two SSRIs in GAD (see Table 44.2 for an overview of head-to-head studies in GAD), Bielski et al. (2005) showed that both medications led to improvement in quality of life and similar reductions in HAM-A scores after 6 months, though escitalopram resulted in fewer dropouts due to adverse events (AEs) than paroxetine.

Although not FDA-approved, sertraline has also been shown to be effective in GAD (Allgulander, Dahl, et al., 2004; Dahl et al., 2005). Allgulander, Dahl, et al. (2004) identified similar response and remission rates for sertraline (50–150 mg/day) after 3 months as those described in the paroxetine studies, with significant reductions in HAM-A scores occurring after 1 month of treatment. One head-to-head study found that sertraline (25–100 mg/day) and paroxetine (10–40 mg/day) resulted in comparable response and remission rates, as well as improvement in quality of life scores, after 2 months (Ball et al., 2005; see Table 44.2). Although there is evidence that the other SSRIs (citalopram, fluoxetine, fluvoxamine) treat anxiety symptoms in patients with depression, to our knowledge there are no published RCTs of these medications specifically for GAD.

A meta-analysis of 8 RCTs of antidepressants, including imipramine, venlafaxine, and paroxetine, in adults with GAD without comorbid Axis I diagnoses (*N* = 2058), found that antidepressants were more effective than placebo, with a number-needed-to-treat (NNT) of 5.15 (Kapczinski et al., 2003). Dropout rates were not different among the different antidepressants (Kapczinski et al., 2003).

SSRIs in Panic Disorder

The goals of PD treatment with SSRIs, according to the Working Group on Panic Disorder (1998), are to decrease the frequency and intensity of panic attacks, decrease anticipatory anxiety, and treat associated depressive symptoms. The safety and overall tolerability of the SSRIs has led to the recommendation of these medications as first-line agents in PD, though SSRIs, TCAs, and BZDs have been shown to be equally effective in the treatment of PD and associated anxiety symptoms (Heuer et al., in press). As patients with PD may be particularly sensitive to medication side effects, starting SSRIs at low doses with slow titration is recommended to minimize adverse effects that may occur early in treatment, including nausea, anxiety, tremors, jitteriness, anorexia, insomnia, and sexual dysfunction (Katon, 2006; Heuer et al., in press). If a patient with PD does not respond to initial treatment with an SSRI, then a trial of another SSRI should be attempted; if an adequate response is not obtained, then switching to a different medication class, such as the SNRIs, TCAs, or BZDs, is recommended (Heuer et al., in press).

Meta-analyses support the efficacy of SSRIs in treating PD and have found similar effect sizes of SSRIs compared to older agents, including TCAs and BZDs (Otto et al., 2001; Mitte, 2005). Mitte (2005) performed a meta-analysis of 124 studies examining psychotherapy and pharmacotherapy in PD, finding that though pharmacotherapy was superior to placebo, cognitive-behavioral and behavioral therapies were at least as effective as pharmacotherapy. In addition, there were similar, moderate effect sizes for anxiety reduction (Hedges' $g \approx 0.40$), and similar attrition rates among

TABLE 44.2 *Head-to-Head Trials of SSRIs and SNRIs in the Anxiety Disorders*[a]

Author, Study Funding Source	*Design, Weeks*	*Medication(s) Studied, mg/Day*	*n*	*Primary Outcome Measures*[b]	*Secondary Outcome Measures*[b]	*Remission Rates %*[b]	*Tolerability*[b]	*Comment*
GENERALIZED ANXIETY DISORDER								
Ball et al. (2005), Pfizer, Inc.	Randomized, double-blind, flexible-dose, 8	Paroxetine 10–40 Sertraline 25–100	25 28	% Reduction in HAM-A: 57.3 55.9 % Responders (≥50% HAM-A reduction from baseline): 68 61	No significant difference in reductions on IU-GAMS and BAI scores, or improvement of Q-LES-Q between 2 groups.	CGI-S = 1 (normal): 40% 46%	No significant difference between groups in posttreatment SAFTEE scores.	No significant difference between two groups. No placebo arm.
Bielski et al. (2005), Forest Laboratories, Inc.	Randomized, double-blind flexible-dose 24	Paroxetine 20–50 Escitalopram 10–20	61 60	Mean reduction in HAM-A: −13.3 −15.3 % CGI-I ≤ 2 by 24 weeks: 62.3 78.3	Both medications led to improvements over time in CGI-I, CGI-S, quality of life.	NA	Withdrew due to AE [Sign.]: 22.6% 6.6%	No placebo arm.
Kim et al. (2006), Korean Health 21 R&D Project	Randomized, open-label, flexible-dose, 8	Venlafaxine XR 37.5–225 Paroxetine 10–40	21 25	% Responders (≥50% HAM-A reduction from baseline): 90.5 92.0	Significant improvement in CGI-S over time, but no group or time x group interactions found.	33.3 36.0	Paroxetine resulted in a significant weight gain compared to venlafaxine, (though no patient had weight gain ≥7% baseline body weight); venlafaxine XR led to significant increases in BP compared to paroxetine.	No placebo. There were significant decreases in HAM-A and CGI-S in both groups, though no significant differences between groups.
Hartford et al. (2007), Eli Lilly and Company, Boehringer Ingelheim	Randomized, double-blind, Placebo-controlled, flexible, 10	Duloxetine 60–120 Venlafaxine XR 75–225 (as active comparator) Placebo	162 164 161	Mean change in HAM-A: −11.80[c] −12.40[c] −9.19 % Responders (≥50% HAM-A reduction from baseline): 47	Both medications led to significant improvements vs. placebo on CGI-I, PGI-I, SDS, HADS anxiety and depression subscales.	% HAM-A ≤ 7: 23 30[c] 19	% Discontinuation due to AE: 14.2[c] 11.0[c] 1.9 % DEAEs: 19.4 26.9[c] 15.8	No statistical comparisons made between medication groups. Duloxetine and venlafaxine XR led to significant decreases in HAM-A beginning at weeks 1 and 2, respectively, vs. placebo. Discontinuation rates overall were not different among three groups.

				54[c] 37 % Responders (CGI-I ≤ 2): 55.7[c] 60.4[c] 41.8				
PANIC DISORDER								
Perna et al. (2001), None	Randomized, single-blind, flexible, 8.6	Citalopram 20–50 Paroxetine 20–50	27 25	% No agoraphobia: 70 62 % No anticipatory anxiety: 85 84	Significant decrease in mean PASS scores over time (from beginning to study end), that is, significant "time" effect, for both citalopram and paroxetine, in post-hoc comparison.	NA	No significant differences in AE between groups.	Single-blind study. No placebo. Analyses only included completers.
Stahl et al. (2003), Forest Laboratories, Inc.	Randomized, double-blind, Placebo-controlled, flexible, 10	Escitalopram 10–20 Citalopram 20–40 Placebo	128 119 119	Panic attack frequency: −1.61[c] −1.43 −1.32	% Panic free: 50 ($p = 0.051$) 39 38	NA	Discontinuation rates due to AE: 6.3% 8.4% 7.6%	Both escitalopram and citalopram led to significant changes vs. PBO on PAS and CGI-I.
Bandelow et al. (2004), Pfizer, Inc.	Randomized, double-blind, flexible, 12	Paroxetine 40–60 Sertraline 50–150	113 115	PAS total score: −12.7 −13.5	Panic attack frequency: −2.13 −1.82 CGI-I: −2.4 2.2	NA	More patients discontinued due to AE in paroxetine group, but NS; Significantly higher weight gain in paroxetine group.	No placebo. During 3-week taper, significantly more patients in sertraline group were panic free vs. paroxetine group.
Pollack et al. (2007), Wyeth Research	Randomized, double-blind, placebo-controlled, fixed, 12	Venlafaxine XR 75 Venlafaxine XR 150 Paroxetine 40 Placebo	158 159 161 156	% Panic-free (full symptom attacks) on PAS: 54.4[c] 59.7[c] 60.9[c] 35.3	Significant decrease in PASS total score and PAAS full symptom panic attack frequency, in all medication groups beginning by week 4. Significant improvements in all	CGI-S ≤ 2 and no full panic attacks on PASS: 43.0[c] 43.4[c] 44.4[c] 23.7	% ≥1 AE: 74 71 75 67 % Taper AE: 37 43	No significant differences in efficacy between the two venlafaxine XR groups or the venlafaxine and paroxetine groups. Significant % attained remission vs. placebo by week 6 in both venlafaxine XR groups and by week 8 in the paroxetine group.

(Continued)

TABLE 44.2 *Head-to-Head Trials of SSRIs and SNRIs in the Anxiety Disorders*[a] *(Continued)*

Author, Study Funding Source	*Design, Weeks*	*Medication(s) Studied, mg/Day*	*n*	*Primary Outcome Measures*[b]	*Secondary Outcome Measures*[b]	*Remission Rates %*[b]	*Tolerability*[b]	*Comment*
				% Responders (CGI-I ≤ 2):	medication groups on SDS.		43	
							17	
				76.6[c]				
				79.2[c]				
				80.6[c]				
				55.8				
SOCIAL ANXIETY DISORDER								
Allgulander, Mangano et al. (2004),	Randomized,			Change in LSAS:	Significant improvement on SPIN scores and CGI-S in both venlafaxine XR and paroxetine groups vs. placebo.	LSAS ≤ 30:	% TEAEs:	Significant reductions in LSAS total scores in venlafaxine XR and paroxetine groups vs. placebo beginning at week 3.
Wyeth Research	double-blind,	Venlafaxine XR 75–225	129	−36.0[c]		38[c]	90	
	placebo-controlled,	Paroxetine 20–50	128	−35.4[c]		29[c]	89	
	flexible,	Placebo	132	−19.1		13	82	
	12			% Responders (week 12) (CGI-I ≤ 2):			Significant increases in total and HDL cholesterol in both medication groups vs. placebo; greater mean increases in heart rate in paroxetine vs. venlafaxine XR groups. Significant increase in weight from baseline in venlafaxine XR group.	
				69[c]				
				66[c]				
				36				
Lader et al. (2004),	Randomized,	Escitalopram 5	167	Change in LSAS (week 12):	All medication groups with significant reductions on CGI-S vs. placebo at weeks 12 and 24, (observed cases)	NA	% TEAEs (week 24):	LOCF data only given for primary efficacy measure at week 12. LSAS improvement in escitalopram 20 mg group significantly greater than in paroxetine 20 mg group in observed cases by week 16.
H. Lundbeck A/S	double-blind,	Escitalopram 10	167	−38.7[c]			68.9	
	placebo-controlled,	Escitalopram 20	170	−34.6			72.5	
	fixed,	Paroxetine 20 (active comparator)	169	−39.8[c]			78.2	
	12 and 24	Placebo	166	−39.3[c]			79.3	
				−29.5			60.8	
				% Responders (week 12) (CGI-I ≤ 2) (Observed Cases):				

				69[c] 66[c] 71[c] 72[c] 50 % Responders (week 24) (CGI-I ≤ 2) (Observed Cases): 79[c] 76 88[c] 80[c] 66				
Liebowitz, Gelenberg et al. (2005), Wyeth Research	Randomized, double-blind, placebo-controlled, flexible, 12	Venlafaxine XR 75–225 Paroxetine 20–50 Placebo	146 147 147	Change in LSAS (week 12): –35.00[c] –39.20[c] –22.20 % Responders (week 12) (CGI-I ≤ 2): 58.6[c] 62.5[c] 36.1	Both medication groups with significant improvement vs. placebo on Social Phobia Inventory and CGI-S by study end. No significant differences observed between medication groups.	NA	%TEAEs: 95.7 91.5 85.6 Significant increases in diastolic and systolic blood pressure, total cholesterol, and HDL vs. placebo observed in both medication groups. Significant decrease in weight noted in venlafaxine XR vs. placebo and paroxetine groups.	Significant differences in LSAS between venlafaxine XR and placebo beginning at week 1, and paroxetine and placebo beginning at week 3. No significant differences in LSAS between medication groups.

[a] Table includes *DSM-IV-TR* Anxiety Disorders (except OCD and PTSD). LOCF data given unless otherwise noted.

[b] Differences between medication groups were *not significant* unless otherwise noted.

[c] : Significant vs. placebo

AE: adverse events; BAI: Beck Anxiety Inventory; CGI-I: Clinical Global Impressions-Improvement scale; CGI-S: Clinical Global Impressions-Severity of Illness; DEAE: Discontinuation-emergent adverse events; HADS: Hospital Anxiety and Depression Scale; HAM-A: Hamilton Rating Scale for Anxiety; IU-GAMS: Indiana University Generalized Anxiety Measurement Scale; LSAS: Liebowitz Social Anxiety Scale; NA: not available; NS: not significant; PAS: Panic and Agoraphobia Scale; PASS: Panic Associated Symptoms Scale; PBO: placebo; PGI-I: Patient Global Impression of Improvement; Q-LES-Q: Quality of Life Enjoyment and Satisfaction Questionnaire; SAFTEE: Systematic Assessment for Treatment Emergent Events; SDS: Sheehan Disability Scale; [Sign.]: significant; SNRI: serotonin-norepinephrine reuptake inhibitor; SPIN: Social Phobia Inventory; SSRI: selective serotonin reuptake inhibitor; TEAEs: treatment-emergent adverse events; BP: blood pressure; HDL: high-density lipoprotein; LOCF: last observation carried forword; OCD: obsessive–compulsive disorder; PTSD: posttraumatic stress disorder.

SSRIs (17 trials), TCAs (23 trials), and BZDs (25 trials) (Mitte, 2005). Otto et al. (2001) analyzed 12 placebo-controlled trials of SSRIs in PD and likewise noted no significant differences in effect size or tolerability between SSRIs and older antidepressants, with a mean study effect size of 0.55 for SSRIs. A meta-analysis by the Cochrane Collaboration reviewed 23 randomized comparisons of combined psychotherapy and antidepressants in PD (Furukawa et al., 2007). This meta-analysis also found that SSRIs (7 trials) and TCAs (14 trials) were similarly effective (Furukawa et al., 2007). Additionally, the authors concluded that in the first 2–4 months of treatment, combination psychotherapy and pharmacotherapy was more effective than either antidepressant treatment or psychotherapy alone. In the long-term (6–24 months), however, though combination therapy continued to be superior to antidepressant medication alone, it was not superior to psychotherapy alone, though there was no disadvantage of long-term combination treatment (Furukawa et al., 2007).

Randomized controlled trials have supported the efficacy of most SSRIs, including the four that are FDA-approved (paroxetine, paroxetine CR, sertraline, and fluoxetine; Table 44.1), as well as fluvoxamine, citalopram, and escitalopram. Paroxetine was the first SSRI to obtain the FDA indication for PD. Placebo-controlled studies, using clomipramine as an active comparator agent, demonstrated that paroxetine's efficacy in PD after 12 and 36 weeks (Lecrubier, Bakker, et al. 1997, Lecrubier and Judge, 1997). In a 10-week RCT, Ballenger et al. (1998) compared three fixed doses of paroxetine (10, 20, or 40 mg/day) and demonstrated that only the group receiving 40 mg/day of paroxetine was significantly free of panic attacks during the 2 weeks prior to the end of the study (86% of patients) and showed significant reductions in total number of panic attacks by week 4. In a pooled analysis of three 10-week RCTs, controlled-release paroxetine (paroxetine CR) was determined to be significantly more effective than placebo with respect to the percentage of patients who were free of panic attacks in the 2 weeks prior to study end point (63% vs. 53% in the LOCF analysis; 73% vs. 60% of completers) (Sheehan et al., 2005). In addition, paroxetine CR resulted in a significant reduction in the number of full panic attacks by the last 2 weeks of the study, and there was a significant difference in CGI-I response in the paroxetine CR group beginning at week 3 (Sheehan et al., 2005).

RCTs have also demonstrated the efficacy of sertraline in PD (Pohl et al., 1998; Pollack et al., 1998; Rapaport et al., 2001). Pohl et al. (1998) provided evidence that treatment with sertraline (50–200 mg/day) was associated with a decrease in number of panic attacks after 10 weeks (77% in the sertraline group vs. 51% for placebo). The authors described a significant decrease in the number of panic attacks per week compared to placebo by week 3 (observed cases analysis), and significantly more patients in the sertraline group (62%) were panic free by study end point, compared to 46% in the placebo group (Pohl et al., 1998). Also, Pollack et al. (1998) showed that after 10 weeks, sertraline (50–200 mg/day) led to significant reductions compared to placebo in the frequency of panic attacks and in scores on the Panic Disorder Severity Scale (PDSS), which measures the frequency and severity of panic and agoraphobic symptoms. In a 28-week discontinuation RCT, Rapaport et al. (2001) showed that significantly more patients in the placebo group (33%), compared to those continued on sertraline after 1 year of open-label treatment (13%), experienced exacerbation of PD symptoms ($p = 0.005$), though the difference in full relapse rates between the two groups was not statistically significant.

In a 10-week RCT of two fixed doses of fluoxetine (10 or 20 mg/day), the higher dose resulted in significant improvements on more outcome variables than the lower dose (for example, CGI-I, overall functioning), though only the 10-mg dose resulted in a significant reduction in total panic attack frequency compared to placebo beginning at week 4 (LOCF analysis) (Michelson et al. 1998). In a 24-week continuation phase of this trial, greater numbers of those receiving fluoxetine, compared to those switched to or continuing on placebo, showed ongoing improvement on CGI-I, although this was not a statistically significant difference at end point (Michelson et al., 1998). Michelson et al. (2001) conducted a 12-week RCT of fluoxetine (20 mg/day, increased to a maximum of 60 mg/day after 6 weeks in patients who did not respond sufficiently) and found a statistically significant reduction in PDSS overall scores and a significant increase in the proportion of patients who were panic attack free after 6 and 12 weeks of treatment.

There is also controlled evidence for fluvoxamine (Hoehn-Saric et al., 1993; Black et al., 1993; Asnis et al., 2001), escitalopram (Stahl et al., 2003), and citalopram (Wade et al., 1997; Lepola et al., 1998) in PD. Stahl et al. (2003) conducted a 10-week RCT comparing escitalopram (10–20 mg/day), citalopram (20–40 mg/day), and placebo and found that escitalopram, but not citalopram, led to a significant decrease in panic attack frequency by study end point, though the proportion of patients who were panic free was significant only at the trend level for the escitalopram group ($p = 0.051$) (see Table 44.2). Both active medication groups demonstrated significant improvements by study end point on the Panic and Agoraphobia Scale (PAS) as well as CGI-I (Stahl et al., 2003). Two published double-blind studies (8 weeks of acute treatment, followed by 1 year of continuation treatment) found that citalopram or clomipramine was effective compared to placebo (Wade et al., 1997; Lepola et al., 1998). Of note, these studies identified citalopram 20–30 mg/day to be more effective than higher citalopram doses (40–60 mg/day) (Wade et al., 1997; Lepola et al., 1998). Another head-to-head randomized, relatively small single-blind randomized study found that after 60 days, citalopram (20–50 mg/day) and paroxetine (20–50 mg/day) resulted in similar reductions in Panic Associated Symptoms Scale (PASS) scores, which includes panic attack frequency, anticipatory anxiety, and phobic avoidance. No significant difference was observed between the two medication groups; however, only completer analyses are reported (Perna et al., 2001). A head-to-head study of sertraline (50–150 mg/day) and paroxetine (40–60 mg/day), found that both medications led to similar reductions in the PASS after 12 weeks, though sertraline resulted in less weight gain and had fewer dropouts due to AEs (Bandelow et al., 2004).

SSRIs in Social Anxiety Disorder

The SSRIs that are FDA approved for SAD are paroxetine, paroxetine CR, and sertraline (Table 44.1). In SAD, SSRIs are typically initiated at one-half of the usual effective dose and increased after the first week of treatment (Schneier, 2006). Although many patients improve within the first few weeks of treatment, it has been suggested that initial SSRI trials should last 12 weeks, as at least 25% of patients who do not respond by week 8 may respond during the ensuing 4 weeks at the same medication dose (Schneier, 2006). Consensus guidelines support the use of continuation pharmacotherapy for those patients who respond during 12 weeks of treatment to decrease the risk of relapse (Schneier, 2006).

Meta-analytic studies support the use of SSRIs in SAD. One meta-analysis of 15 published RCTs of SSRIs (with an average duration of 13–14 weeks), found the following averaged *d* scores for the Liebowitz Social Anxiety Scale (LSAS): paroxetine, 0.526 (5 trials), fluvoxamine, 0.581 (3 trials), sertraline, 0.345 (2 trials), and fluoxetine, –0.029 (1 trial) (Hedges et al., 2007). The between-group differences were not significant, though the authors noted a significant Q statistic, suggesting heterogeneity, or lower level of agreement, in the paroxetine trials for LSAS (Hedges et al., 2007). Effect sizes (ES) for LSAS ranged from –0.029 to 1.214 for all studies, with a significant Q statistic (Hedges et al., 2007). For CGI-I, the average *d* score for all studies, which included fluoxetine, fluvoxamine, fluvoxamine CR, paroxetine, paroxetine CR, sertraline, and escitalopram, was 0.986 (Hedges et al., 2007). Another meta-analysis of placebo-controlled studies of SSRIs and non-SSRIs in SAD found an ES for LSAS of 0.65 for six SSRI trials, which included fluvoxamine, paroxetine, and sertraline, with no heterogeneity identified in the SSRI studies (Blanco et al., 2003). No statistically significant differences were found between medications or medication classes, which included phenelzine (ES = 1.02), clonazepam (0.97), gabapentin (0.78), and brofaromine (0.66), with ES heterogeneity in the phenelzine group (Blanco et al., 2003). Effect sizes for responders (defined as CGI-I $\leq$ 2) was 4.10 for SSRIs, 5.53 for phenelzine, and 16.61 for BDZs, though there was heterogeneity in the SSRI (due to one study) and phenelzine groups (Blanco et al., 2003). Blanco et al. (2003) supported SSRIs as first-line treatments in SAD due to their tolerability, ability to treat comorbid conditions, and the stability of the ES.

The Cochrane Collaboration reviewed 37 RCTs of either SSRIs (paroxetine, sertraline, fluoxetine, fluvoxamine, and escitalopram), MAOIs, reversible inhibitors of monoamine oxidase (RIMAs), and other medications (including BDZs, buspirone, gabapentin) in SAD (D.J. Stein et al., 2000). The authors found that patients who received any medication were less likely than those given placebo to be nonresponders (D.J. Stein et al., 2000). On LSAS and Clinical Global Impression-Severity of Illness (CGI-S), SSRIs were found to reduce symptom severity, while MAOIs (on LSAS) and RIMAs (on CGI-S) did not (D.J. Stein et al., 2000). Selective serotonin reuptake inhibitors were the only class of medications found to significantly reduce depressive symptoms. The authors also described similar dropout rates for the medication versus placebo groups (D.J. Stein et al., 2000). They suggest that publication bias was likely based on a CGI-I funnel plot, indicating that there might be more variation in medication responses in SAD than in the trials included in the meta-analysis (D.J. Stein et al., 2000). However, maintenance trials included in the meta-analysis demonstrated decreased relapse risk of medication versus placebo (D.J. Stein et al., 2000). In another meta-analysis of 25 published SSRI trials in SAD, which included 8 RCTs, the authors reported that SSRIs are effective in SAD, as the number of patients responding to medication was approximately 2 times that of the placebo responders (van der Linden et al., 2000). In this report, ES for LSAS in the RCTs ranged from 0.3 to 2.2 (van der Linden et al., 2000).

Another meta-analysis compared psychological interventions, including cognitive restructuring and exposure, with pharmacological treatments of SAD, including SSRIs, BZDs, and MAOIs, in trials of approximately 11 weeks (Fedoroff and Taylor, 2001). This meta-analysis included nonblind and uncontrolled studies, as the ESs were similar to those in the double-blind and controlled trials (Fedoroff and Taylor, 2001). On self-report measures, SSRIs and BZDs were found to be equally effective, with the largest mean ESs compared to psychological and other pharmacological treatments (ES for SSRIs = 1.697, BZDs = 2.095) and their confidence intervals overlapped. A trend favored BZDs overall, which outperformed MAOIs and the psychological treatments, though SSRIs did not (Fedoroff and Taylor, 2001). On observer-rated measures, which included data from only a small number of trials, all of the treatments, including BZDs, SSRIs, MAOIs, and exposure with cognitive restructuring, were similarly effective, and superior to placebo or wait-list control (Fedoroff and Taylor, 2001).

Paroxetine was the first medication approved for the treatment of SAD (Davidson et al., 2006). Two flexibly dosed, 12-week, multicenter RCTs of paroxetine 20–50 mg/day demonstrated that paroxetine was more effective than placebo in SAD (M.B. Stein et al., 1998; Baldwin et al., 1999). In one study, there were a significant number of CGI-I responders in the paroxetine versus placebo groups (55% vs. 24% by study end point), beginning at week 4 (M.B. Stein et al., 1998). This study also found that paroxetine resulted in a significant reduction in LSAS compared to placebo beginning at week 2 (M.B. Stein et al., 1998). Another study found that there was a significant reduction in LSAS total score and a significant percentage of CGI-I responders (approximately 66% vs. 32%) in the paroxetine compared to the placebo groups by study end, beginning at week 4 (Baldwin et al., 1999). In a 12-week, placebo-controlled trial of three fixed doses of paroxetine (20, 40, and 60 mg), the 20-mg dose resulted in a significant decrease in LSAS total scores by study end, beginning at week 8, while the number of responders on CGI-I in the 40-mg group (46.6%) was significant compared to placebo (28.3%) by study end and at week 6 (Liebowitz et al., 2002).

Paroxetine CR (12.5–37.5 mg/day) has also been shown to be more effective than placebo in SAD in a 12-week RCT (Lepola et al., 2004). Reduction in LSAS total score in the paroxetine CR group was significantly greater than in the placebo group beginning at week 6, and 57% of patients treated with paroxetine CR compared to about 30% of those receiving placebo were responders on CGI-I by study end (Lepola et al., 2004). Also, 28% of patients in the paroxetine CR group achieved CGI-I scores of 1, indicating remission, which was significantly greater than 12% in the placebo group (Lepola et al., 2004).

In a 12-week, flexibly dosed RCT of sertraline (50–200 mg/day) in SAD, significant reductions in LSAS were observed in the sertraline group versus placebo beginning at week 6, with an effect size for LSAS change of 0.43 (Liebowitz et al., 2003). Also, 47% of patients treated with sertraline were CGI-I responders by study end compared to 26% in the placebo group (Liebowitz et al., 2003). Another flexibly dosed, multicenter RCT of sertraline (50–200 mg/day) in SAD also found significant CGI-I response versus placebo by study end (53% vs. 29%) (Van Ameringen et al., 2001). Significantly more patients receiving sertraline (40%) achieved CGI-I scores of 1 by study end, compared to 13% of those receiving placebo (Van Ameringen et al., 2001). Sertraline also resulted in significant reductions on the Marks Fear Questionnaire Social Phobia subscale and the Brief Social Phobia Scale (BSPS) (Van Ameringen et al., 2001).

One RCT compared the efficacy of sertraline monotherapy (50–150 mg/day), exposure therapy, and combination therapy versus placebo or general medical care during 24 weeks in patients with SAD (Blomhoff et al., 2001). Blomhoff et al. (2001) reported a greater percentage of responders (defined as ≥ 50% reduction of Social Phobia Scale [SPS] symptoms, CGI–Social Phobia [CGI-SP] severity score ≤ 3 and improvement score ≤ 2) in the groups receiving sertraline compared to the nonsertraline groups. Combination therapy and sertraline alone led to significantly greater response compared to placebo (Blomhoff et al., 2001). However, there were more responders in the combination therapy group beginning at week 12, while sertraline alone resulted in a significant percentage of responders by study end point (Blomhoff et al., 2001). In a 1-year follow-up of the patients in the Blomhoff et al. (2001) study, all groups (sertraline alone, exposure alone, combination therapy, and placebo) demonstrated a significant reduction in CGI-SP scores compared to baseline (Haug et al., 2003). This study also found that in the 28 weeks following the conclusion of the 24-week trial, there was a significant reduction in CGI-SP severity scores in the exposure and placebo groups, and a slight nonsignificant deterioration in CGI-SP severity and SPS scores in the sertraline groups (Haug et al., 2003). It should be noted, however, that during the follow-up period, approximately 15%–20% of the patients in each of the groups received treatment with SSRIs, and some patients had been offered exposure therapy or referred to a psychologist or psychiatrist (Haug et al., 2003).

Escitalopram (10–20 mg) was also shown in a flexibly dosed, 12-week, multinational RCT to result in significant reductions in LSAS total score and a significant percentage of CGI-I responders (54% vs. 39%) compared to placebo by study end (Kasper et al., 2005). In one 2-site RCT comparing fluoxetine (titrated to 40–60 mg/day), group comprehensive cognitive-behavioral therapy (CCBT), the combination of fluoxetine and CCBT, and CCBT plus placebo versus placebo alone, CGI-I response rates and BSPS scores for all treatment groups were significantly greater than placebo after 14 weeks, though no differences between the active treatments were described (Davidson, Foa, et al., 2004). There are two published negative RCTs of fluoxetine in SAD, however (Koback et al., 2002; Clark et al., 2003). Clark et al. (2003) found that cognitive therapy was superior to fluoxetine (20–60 mg/day) plus self-exposure on social phobia measures after 16 weeks. A relatively small, single-site, 14-week RCT of fluoxetine (20 mg/day for the first 8 weeks, then up to 60 mg/day), found significant difference versus placebo on LSAS or CGI-I (Kobak et al., 2002). There is evidence from RCTs for the efficacy of fluvoxamine in SAD. One 12-

week multicenter study showed that fluvoxamine (50–300 mg/day) led to a significant percentage of CGI-I responders by study end, and significant reductions in LSAS beginning at week 6 (M.B. Stein et al., 1999). Fluvoxamine (150 or 300 mg/day) resulted in a significant improvement compared to placebo in LSAS-Japanese Version total score and CGI-I after 10 weeks in a RCT in Japan (Asakura et al., 2007). Also, two multisite, 12-week RCTs of fluvoxamine CR found that it was superior to placebo in SAD, resulting in significant reductions in LSAS by week 4 at doses ranging from 100–300 mg/day (Davidson, Yaryura, et al., 2004; Westenberg et al., 2004). However, a 12-week extension of one of the 12-week multicenter RCTs of fluvoxamine CR (100–300 mg/day) in SAD found that reductions in LSAS total scores only at trend level significance ($p = 0.074$) from baseline to the 24-week end point, with a nonsignificant trend towards more CGI-I responders and remitters in the fluvoxamine CR group versus placebo (D.J. Stein et al., 2003).

Lader et al. (2004) conducted a 24-week head-to-head study comparing escitalopram at fixed doses of 5, 10, or 20 mg/day, paroxetine 20 mg/day, and placebo in SAD (see Table 44.2). Escitalopram 5 and 20 mg and paroxetine 20 mg produced significant LSAS reductions compared to placebo after 12 weeks in the LOCF analysis (Lader et al., 2004). The efficacy analyses in this study, however, were primarily based on data from observed cases (OC), as LOCF data were not provided (Lader et al., 2004). In the OC sample, all three escitalopram groups and the paroxetine group resulted in significant LSAS reductions by weeks 12 and 24, and a significant percentage of CGI-I responders by week 24 compared to placebo (Lader et al., 2004). Escitalopram 20 mg resulted in significantly greater reductions than paroxetine 20 mg in LSAS mean score by week 16 (Lader et al., 2004).

Longer-term relapse-prevention studies of paroxetine, sertraline, and escitalopram in SAD have been conducted. In a 24-week, randomized, double-blind maintenance phase following 12 weeks of single-blind treatment with paroxetine (20–50 mg/day) in a multicenter study, 14% of patients receiving paroxetine relapsed compared to 39% of those receiving placebo ($p < 0.001$) (D.J. Stein, Versiani, et al., 2002). In addition, patients who received paroxetine in the maintenance phase experienced significant improvements on CGI-I and LSAS by study end point compared to those switched to placebo (D.J. Stein, Versiani, et al., 2002). A small double-blind study ($N = 65$) randomly assigned patients with SAD who responded to sertraline (50–200 mg/day) in a 20-week RCT to continue sertraline or switch to placebo for 24 weeks; placebo-responders from the initial trial were continued on placebo (Walker et al., 2000). This study reported a relative risk of relapse of about 10 for patients who switched to placebo compared to those continued on sertraline, though the number of completers was small ($N = 38$). Although there was no significant difference in CGI-I response between the sertraline-continuation and placebo-switch groups, there were significant differences between the groups on CGI-S and Duke BSPS from baseline to study end, with those continuing on sertraline experiencing reductions in these scores, while the scores of those switched to placebo increased; scores of those in the placebo-responder group also increased (Walker et al., 2000). In a multinational RCT, patients who responded to escitalopram (10–20 mg/day) during a 12-week, open-label phase were randomly assigned either to continue receiving the same dose of escitalopram or to switch to placebo for 24 weeks (Montgomery et al., 2005). This study reported an approximately 3 times greater risk of relapse for those patients switched to placebo compared to those continuing on escitalopram (Montgomery et al., 2005). In the escitalopram group, 22% of patients relapsed compared to 50% in the placebo group, and the median time to relapse was 407 versus 144 days, respectively (Montgomery et al., 2005).

SSRIs in Post-Traumatic Stress Disorder

Although there are two FDA-approved medications for PTSD (paroxetine and sertraline), ESs have been modest for short-term trials, and superiority of drug over placebo in all three clusters of illness (avoidance/numbing, reexperiencing, and hyperarousal) have only been observed for paroxetine (Marshall et al., 2001; Tucker et al., 2001). A major limitation in the literature to date is the paucity of long-term studies of pharmacotherapy in PTSD (see Cochrane Review of PTSD; D.J. Stein, Ipser, et al., 2006). In view of the limited efficacy of RCT pharmacotherapy data for PTSD and more robust evidence for exposure-based psychotherapies, NICE guidelines have suggested that pharmacotherapy should not be used as a routine first-line treatment for adults in preference to a trauma-focused psychological therapy.

SEROTONIN AND NOREPINEPHRINE REUPTAKE INHIBITORS (SNRIs)

Serotonin and norepinephrine reuptake inhibitors have emerged as first-line medications along with the SSRIs for the treatment of anxiety disorders. Venlafaxine XR is approved by the FDA for the treatment of GAD, PD, and SAD, and duloxetine recently received FDA approval for GAD (see Table 44.1).

SNRIs in Generalized Anxiety Disorder

Short- and long-term RCTs have shown that venlafaxine XR is effective in GAD. Regarding long-term studies, two multicenter, 6-month RCTs demonstrated the efficacy of venlafaxine XR over placebo in patients with

GAD (Gelenberg et al., 2000; Allgulander et al., 2001). In a fixed-dose, 24-week RCT, venlafaxine XR (37.5, 75, or 150 mg/day) resulted in significant reductions in HAM-A total scores by study end compared to placebo (Allgulander et al., 2001). All three doses led to significant improvements on HAM-A and CGI-I versus placebo from week 2 onwards except for the venlafaxine XR 37.5-mg group at week 8 (Allgulander et al., 2001). This study provided evidence for a dose-response relationship, as higher doses of venlafaxine XR (75 and 150 mg/day) resulted in greater response rates and relatively faster onset of action on a number of variables assessing anxiety compared to venlafaxine XR 37.5 mg/day (Allgulander et al., 2001). Another 6-month RCT found that flexibly dosed venlafaxine XR (75–225 mg/day) resulted in significant response rates (defined as ≥ 40% reduction in HAM-A scores or CGI-I ≤ 2) by week 1, with response rates of ≥ 69% beginning at week 6, compared to rates of 42%–46% in the placebo group (Gelenberg et al., 2000).

Short-term studies of venlafaxine XR in GAD include four separate 8-week, multicenter RCTs (Davidson et al., 1999; Rickels et al., 2000; Hackett et al., 2003; Nimatoudis et al., 2004). Rickels et al. (2000) studied venlafaxine XR (75 mg, 150 mg, or 225 mg/day), and found that only venlafaxine XR 225 mg/day resulted in significant reductions in HAM-A and CGI-I scores compared to placebo after 8 weeks. Davidson et al. (1999) compared venlafaxine XR (75 mg or 150 mg/day), buspirone (30 mg/day, dosed 10 mg three times per day [TID]), and placebo, and reported that by study end point, CGI-I scores, but not total HAM-A scores, significantly improved in the venlafaxine XR 75 mg/day and buspirone groups only compared to placebo (Davidson et al., 1999). In a small RCT (*N* = 46), Nimatoudis et al. (2004) reported that HAM-A scores were reduced by ≥ 50% in 92% of patients receiving venlafaxine XR (75–150 mg/day) compared to 27% for placebo. This study also identified a significant remission rate (63%) in the venlafaxine XR group (Nimatoudis et al., 2004). Another 8-week, placebo-controlled study compared venlafaxine XR (75 or 150 mg/day) with diazepam (15 mg/day) and found no significant differences in HAM-A or CGI-I scores between the medication and placebo groups. A secondary analysis that omitted study centers where there was no difference between diazepam and placebo showed significant HAM-A and CGI-I reductions in both venlafaxine XR groups versus placebo (Hackett et al., 2003).

Regarding head-to-head studies, a small (*N* = 46), open-label study compared venlafaxine XR (37.5–225 mg/day) and paroxetine (10–40 mg/day) in GAD (Kim et al., 2006) (see Table 44.2). Both medications resulted in significant reductions in HAM-A and CGI-S after 8 weeks, though there were no significant differences in efficacy between the two groups (Kim et al., 2006). However, paroxetine resulted in significantly more weight gain than venlafaxine XR, while venlafaxine XR led to significant increases in systolic and diastolic blood pressure compared to paroxetine by study end point (Kim et al., 2006).

The efficacy of duloxetine in GAD was demonstrated two 10-week, multicenter RCTs (Hartford et al., 2007; Rynn et al., 2007). Duloxetine (60–120 mg/day, progressively titrated) resulted in a significant decrease in HAM-A total scores compared to placebo, beginning at week 2, in a mixed-effects repeated measures (MMRM) analysis, with response rates of 40% compared to 32% in the placebo group after 10 weeks (Rynn et al., 2007). There were no significant differences in remission rates, however (Rynn et al., 2007). Also, there were significant increases in heart rate, blood pressure, and some liver measures in the duloxetine group compared to placebo, but the magnitude of the changes was not considered clinically relevant (Rynn et al., 2007). Hartford et al. (2007) conducted a placebo-controlled, head-to-head RCT, in which duloxetine (60–120 mg/day) was compared to venlafaxine XR (75–225 mg/day) (see Table 44.2). After 10 weeks, HAM-A total scores decreased significantly in both active treatment groups compared to placebo (Hartford et al., 2007). Mixed-effect repeated measure analysis showed that there were significant reductions in HAM-A beginning in week 1 for the duloxetine group and week 2 for the venlafaxine group (Hartford et al., 2007). However, the percentage of patients achieving response (defined as ≥ 50% reduction in HAM-A) and remission (HAM-A total score ≤ 7) by study end was only significant in the venlafaxine XR group versus placebo, though both medications led to a significant percentage of responders on CGI-I (Hartford et al., 2007). There were more discontinuation-emergent AEs during a tapering period for venlafaxine XR versus placebo compared to duloxetine versus placebo (Hartford et al., 2007).

SNRIs in Panic Disorder

There are two multicenter, double-blind RCTs of venlafaxine XR in PD (Bradwejn et al., 2005, Pollack et al., 2006). In a 10-week trial, venlafaxine XR (75–225 mg/day) resulted in a significant reduction in the frequency of full-symptom panic attacks compared to placebo by study end (Bradwejn et al., 2005). Although venlafaxine XR did not result in a significantly greater number of patients who were panic free by study end point, there was a significant percentage of CGI-I responders and remitters in the venlafaxine XR group versus placebo beginning at weeks 3 and 6, respectively (Bradwejn et al., 2005). There was a significant increase in heart rate in the venlafaxine XR group (change from baseline in supine pulse rate = 2.18 beats/min) (Bradwejn et al., 2005). Another placebo-controlled, double-blind

RCT compared venlafaxine XR (75 or 150 mg/day) and paroxetine 40 mg/day in PD (see Table 44.2) (Pollack et al., 2007). After 12 weeks, both doses of venlafaxine XR and paroxetine resulted in a significant percentage of patients who were free of full-symptom panic attacks, as assessed by the Panic and Anticipatory Anxiety Scale (PAAS), compared to placebo (Pollack et al., 2007). There were no significant differences in comparisons on most efficacy measures between the two venlafaxine XR arms or the venlafaxine XR and paroxetine study arms. All three active medication groups resulted in a significant percentage of CGI-I responders, ranging from approximately 77 to 81%, compared to the placebo response of 56%, by study end point (Pollack et al., 2007). Significantly more patients attained remission (defined as panic free and CGI-S ≤ 2) in the venlafaxine XR and paroxetine groups versus placebo by weeks 6 and 8, respectively (Pollack et al., 2007).

A multinational relapse prevention study, in which patients who responded to 12 weeks of open-label treatment with venlafaxine XR (75–225 mg/day) were randomly assigned to continue receiving venlafaxine XR or switch to placebo for a 26-week double-blind phase, showed that venlafaxine XR was significantly better than placebo in preventing relapse (Ferguson et al., 2007). The relapse rate in the placebo group was 50% compared to 22.5% in the venlafaxine XR group, and the percentage of patients who were panic free by study end was 55% versus 76.4% in the two groups, respectively (Ferguson et al., 2007). As of this writing (July 2007), there are no published RCTs of duloxetine in PD.

SNRIs in Social Anxiety Disorder

There are RCTs to support the efficacy of venlafaxine XR in generalized SAD. Two 12-week, multicenter RCTs of SAD found that venlafaxine XR (75–225 mg/day) led to significantly greater reductions on LSAS than placebo, beginning at week 4 (Rickels et al., 2004) or week 6 (Liebowitz, Mangano, et al., 2005). Rickels et al. (2004) identified 50% of patients as CGI-I responders in the venlafaxine XR group by study end, which was significantly greater than 34% in the placebo group. Liebowitz, Mangano, et al. (2005) also reported a significantly greater percentage of responders in the venlafaxine XR group (44%) compared to placebo (30%), as well as remitters (20% vs. 7%, with remission defined as LSAS ≤ 30) by study end point. Of note, both studies described small but significant increases in supine systolic (~0.5-2.3 mmHg) and diastolic (~0.25-2.6 mmHg) blood pressure, supine pulse rate (~1.3-4.9 beats/min), and cholesterol levels (~0.3 mmol/L) compared to placebo (Rickels et al., 2004; Liebowitz, Mangano, et al., 2005). In a 6-month, multicenter RCT, fixed low-dose venlafaxine XR (75 mg/day) was compared to flexible higher doses (150–225 mg/day) (M.B. Stein et al., 2005). The low- and high-dose venlafaxine XR groups resulted in significant reductions in LSAS compared to placebo beginning at week 4, and significant response (CGI-I ≤ 2) and remission (defined as LSAS ≤ 30) rates versus placebo by study end (M.B. Stein et al. 2005). There were no significant differences in response and remission rates between the two venlafaxine XR groups (M.B. Stein et al., 2005).

There are two head-to-head, placebo-controlled, randomized, 12-week trials comparing venlafaxine XR (75–225 mg/day) and paroxetine (20–50 mg/day) in SAD (see Table 44.2). Both studies found that the active treatment groups resulted in significant reductions in LSAS and significant response rates compared to placebo, though no significant differences in efficacy were noted between the venlafaxine XR and paroxetine groups by the end point of the studies (Allgulander, Mangano, et al., 2004; Liebowitz, Gelenberg, et al., 2005). At this time (July 2007), there are no published RCTs of duloxetine in SAD.

SNRIs in Post-Traumatic Stress Disorder

Venlafaxine ER was investigated in a 6-month flexible dose (37.5–300 mg/day) RCT conducted primarily in European study sites (Davidson, Baldwin, et al., 2006). Remission rates, indexed by Clinician-Administered PTSD Scale (CAPS) scores of 20 or lower, were 50.9% for venlafaxine ER and 37.5% for placebo, and improvements were found for reexperiencing and avoidance/numbing symptoms, but not for hyperarousal (Davidson, 2006). Despite the overall efficacy compared to placebo, the ES for CAPS was 0.31, representing a small effect, with a number NNT for remission of eight. A 12-week multicenter RCT with placebo and sertraline control arms also found efficacy of venlafaxine ER in PTSD (Davidson, Rothbaum, et al., 2006), although the ES for venlafaxine versus placebo was only 0.266. Importantly, both studies used a maximum daily dosage of venlaxine higher than its FDA-approved labeling for its other indications (GAD, SAD, PD, and major depressive disorder).

TRICYCLIC ANTIDEPRESSANTS

Tricyclic antidepressants have a long history of use in anxiety and related conditions, though their overall poorer tolerability compared to the SSRIs and SNRIs has limited their use. Tricyclic antidepressants are effective treatments for GAD, although few studies have investigated TCAs in *Diagnostic and Statistical Manual of Mental Disorders*, 4th ed. (*DSM-IV*; American Psychiatric Association [APA], 1994) defined GAD (Mathew and Hoffman, in press). Rickels et al. (1993)

conducted an 8-week double-blind, placebo-controlled trial comparing imipramine, diazepam, and trazodone in the treatment of patients with *DSM-III* (APA, 1980) GAD, in which diazepam resulted in the greatest improvement during the first 2 weeks, after which imipramine was significantly more effective in reducing total HAM-A scores (reviewed in Baldwin and Polkinghorn, 2005); all three treatment groups were found to be effective in reducing anxiety symptoms by study end point (reviewed in Lydiard and Monnier, 2004).

Meta-analyses have demonstrated similar effect sizes of SSRIs and TCAs in PD (see previous SSRIs section for details) (Mitte, 2005; Furukawa et al., 2007). There is support from RCTs for the use of TCAs in the treatment of PD. Barlow et al. (2000) conducted a randomized, placebo-controlled trial in which patients with PD with mild or no agoraphobia were treated with either imipramine alone (up to 300 mg/day), cognitive-behavioral therapy (CBT) alone, CBT and imipramine, or CBT and placebo for 3 months (acute phase), and responders were then followed for 6 months (maintenance phase), and another 6 months after discontinuing treatment. In the acute and maintenance phases, imipramine and CBT were each statistically superior to placebo on PDSS, and on CGI-I in the maintenance phase (Barlow et al., 2000). There were no significant differences in efficacy between imipramine alone and CBT alone, though response quality, as assessed by PDSS average scores, was higher in the imipramine group versus the CBT group in the acute phase (Barlow et al., 2000). Also, in the acute and maintenance phases, CBT plus imipramine produced a higher quality of responses compared to CBT alone (Barlow et al., 2000). In the acute phase, CBT plus imipramine was not superior to CBT plus placebo, but in the maintenance phase, combined treatment produced a significant change in PDSS average score compared to CBT plus placebo (Barlow et al., 2000). At 6-month follow-up, only the CBT groups continued to demonstrate some efficacy versus placebo (Barlow et al., 2000). There is also short- and long-term evidence of clomipramine in PD (Lecrubier and Judge, 1997; Lecrubier et al., 1997). There is no RCT evidence to support the use of TCAs in generalized SAD.

MONOAMINE OXIDASE INHIBITORS (MAOIs) AND REVERSIBLE INHIBITORS OF MONOAMINE OXIDASE (RIMAs)

There is evidence for the efficacy of MAOIs in PD, SAD, and PTSD (Liebowitz, Hollander, et al., 1990). The use of MAOIs in these disorders is limited by their poorer tolerability, risks of toxicity, and the requirement for patients taking them to follow a low tyramine diet to prevent hypertensive crisis (Davidson, 2006). The RIMAs are less likely to cause hypertensive crisis, though this class of medications is not approved for use in the United States (Davidson, 2006). In PD, two studies (8 and 24 weeks) found no difference in the efficacy of SSRIs and RIMAs (fluoxetine vs. moclobemide, fluvoxamine vs. brofaromine), after 8 and 24 weeks, respectively, though there were no placebo comparison groups (van Vliet et al., 1996; Tiller et al., 1999). A small, 12-week study found that brofaromine did not result in significant improvement versus placebo in PD (van Vliet et al., 1993). In SAD, some meta-analyses have shown that MAOIs and SSRIs are similarly effective (Fedoroff and Taylor, 2001; Blanco et al., 2003). However, the Cochrane Collaboration reported in their meta-analysis that though all medication groups were superior to placebo in SAD, SSRIs were more effective than RIMAs (see SSRIs section for details) (D.J. Stein et al., 2000). Phenelzine, a nonselective, irreversible MAOI, was found to be significantly more effective in *DSM-III* SAD than atenolol or placebo in 4- and 8-week RCTs (Liebowitz, Schneier, et al., 1990; Liebowitz et al., 1992). Another RCT found that phenelzine and cognitive-behavioral group therapy (CBGT) each led to similar, significant improvements in SAD versus control conditions after 12 weeks, though phenelzine led to better performance on some measures than CBGT (Heimberg et al., 1998), and continued to do so in a 1-year extension of this study for responders to phenelzine or CBGT (Liebowitz et al., 1999). The extension study found no difference in relapse and drop-out rates between the two groups in a 6-month maintenance phase, though there was a trend toward greater relapse in the phenelzine group in a 6-month treatment-free follow-up phase (Liebowitz et al., 1999). Some RCTs found that the RIMAs are effective in the short-and long-term in SAD (International et al., 1997; Lott et al., 1997; D.J. Stein, Cameron, et al., 2002; Prasko et al., 2006), whereas other short-term RCTs did not (Noyes et al., 1997; Schneier et al., 1998). There are no RCTs to our knowledge support the use of MAOIs or RIMAs in GAD.

ANTICONVULSANTS

A number of antiepileptic drugs (AEDs) have been investigated in anxiety disorders, though the strongest evidence to date is for pregabalin in GAD (Mula et al., 2007). Pregabalin, which acts by binding to the $\alpha_2\gamma$ subunit of voltage-gated calcium channel, is FDA approved in 4 conditions: diabetic peripheral neuropathy, postherpetic neuralgia, adjunctive treatment for partial seizures, and most recently, fibromylagia. Randomized controlled trials in GAD have demonstrated short-term efficacy, although no continuation or relapse prevention studies have been published. Pande et al. (2003)

demonstrated significant baseline-to-end point reductions in HAM-A in patients receiving pregabalin (150 or 600 mg/day) or lorazepam (6 mg/day) versus placebo after 4 weeks, and the magnitude of the HAM-A reductions did not differ significantly between treatment groups. However, significantly more patients in the pregabalin 600 mg/day (46%) and lorazepam groups (61%) were HAM-A responders (≥ 50% reduction in HAM-A) compared to the pregabalin 150 mg/day and placebo (27%) groups (Pande et al., 2003). In a randomized, double-blind, placebo-controlled study by Pohl et al. (2005), pregabalin (200 mg/day divided twice a day (BID), 400 mg/day div. BID, or 450 mg/day div. TID) resulted in significantly greater HAM-A response rates (53%–56% vs. 34%) after 6 weeks. Of note, all 3 pregabalin doses resulted in significant reductions in HAM-A compared to placebo beginning at week 1 (Pohl et al., 2005). Rickels et al. (2005) conducted a 4-week, placebo-controlled trial of pregabalin (300, 450, or 600 mg/day div. TID), with alprazolam (1.5 mg/day) as an active comparator. There were significant reductions in HAM-A scores in all three pregabalin groups and the alprazolam group versus placebo by study end point, but only pregabalin 300 mg/day and 600 mg/day resulted in a significant percentage of HAM-A and CGI-I responders compared to placebo (Rickels et al., 2005). There was suggestion of rapidity of onset, as all doses of pregabalin and alprazolam significantly decreased HAM-A scores compared to placebo at week 1 in an observed case analysis (Rickels et al., 2005). Another multicenter, 4-week RCT found that pregabalin 600 mg/day div. TID and lorazepam (6 mg/day div. TID), but not pregabalin 150 mg/day div. TID, resulted in significant reductions in HAM-A scores versus placebo by study end point. This study, however, did not find significant differences in CGI-I and HAM-A response rates, a secondary outcome measure, for any of the treatment groups (Feltner et al., 2003). Montgomery et al. (2006) conducted a 6-week, randomized, placebo-controlled trial comparing pregabalin (400 or 600 mg/day div. BID) and venlafaxine (75 mg/day div. BID) in GAD and found that both pregabalin doses and venlafaxine resulted in significant HAM-A reductions versus placebo by end point (Montgomery et al., 2006). There was significant improvement compared to placebo in HAM-A scores beginning at week 1 in both pregabalin groups and at week 2 in the venlafaxine group (Montgomery et al., 2006). The most commonly reported side effects of pregabalin in these studies were somnolence and dizziness, and patients taking the higher doses of pregabalin experienced weight gain of almost 2 kg. Pande et al. (2003) found no significant difference in Physician Withdrawal Checklist (PWC) scores for pregabalin versus placebo, unlike lorazepam, during discontinuation, whereas other studies reported some significant increases in PWC scores for pregabalin versus placebo, though these changes were not considered clinically significant (Feltner et al., 2003; Pohl et al., 2005; Rickels et al., 2005). It has been noted that larger PWC changes than those observed for pregabalin were described in studies of long-term benzodiazepine withdrawal (Feltner et al., 2003), though long-term studies of pregabalin in GAD are needed.

As of July 2007, there was only one published multicenter RCT of pregabalin in SAD. Pande et al. (2004) conducted a 10-week, placebo-controlled trial of pregabalin (150 mg/day or 600 mg/day, div. TID), and found that pregabalin 600 mg/day resulted in significant LSAS reductions beginning at week 1, while pregabalin 150 mg/day did not lead to improvements in any efficacy measures (Pande et al., 2004). In the pregabalin 600 mg/day group, 43% of patients were CGI-I responders, which was significantly greater than in the placebo group (22%), though the percentage of LSAS responders was not significant (Pande et al., 2004). There are no published RCTs of pregabalin in PD or PTSD to date.

Gabapentin, an older anticonvulsant medication FDA approved for partial seizures, neuropathic pain, and postherpetic neuralgia, has been extensively used "off-label" in anxiety disorders, although RCT data has only demonstrated modest benefit. Pande et al. (1999) conducted a 14-week RCT ($N = 69$) in SAD. Gabapentin (900–3600 mg/day, div. TID) resulted in significant reductions versus placebo in LSAS, BSPS, Social Phobia Inventory, and CGI-I by study end point (Pande et al., 1999). However, LSAS response rate was only 32% in the gabapentin group versus 14% in the placebo group for the ITT population ($p = 0.08$) (Pande et al., 1999). There is one RCT ($N = 103$) of gabapentin in PD, which found that there was no significant difference on PAS between the gabapentin (600–3600 mg/day) and placebo groups after 8 weeks (Pande et al., 2000). In a post-hoc analysis, gabapentin resulted in significant PAS improvement versus placebo in patients with more severe symptoms (PAS ≥ 20), though there was no significant difference versus placebo in the percentage of PAS responders (≥ 50% decrease in PAS from baseline to end point) (Pande et al., 2000). Although case reports have suggested that gabapentin may be an effective adjunctive treatment in GAD and PTSD, there are no published RCTs of gabapentin in these conditions (reviewed in Mula et al., 2007).

Although lamotrigine is extensively used in mood disorders, and is FDA approved for maintenance therapy for bipolar disorder, there is minimal data supporting its efficacy in primary anxiety disorders. A preliminary, small ($N = 15$), 12-week RCT of lamotrigine in PTSD suggested some benefit (Hertzberg et al., 1999). Lamotrigine (slowly titrated over 8 weeks from 25 mg/day to a maximum dose of 500 mg/day) led to response on the Duke Global Rating for PTSD Scale-Improvement in 5 of 10 patients, versus 1 of 4 patients treated with placebo (Hertzberg et al., 1999). Improvement in reexperiencing and avoidance/numbing symptoms was described in the lamotrigine group, but not the placebo group (Hertzberg et al., 1999). Surprisingly, there are no published studies of lamotrigine in GAD, PD, or SAD (reviewed in Mula et al., 2007).

There is one RCT of topiramate, an FDA-approved medication for migraine prophylaxis and seizures, in PTSD (Tucker et al., 2007). This 12-week study of 38 patients with non-combat-related PTSD found that there was no statistically significant difference in CAPS scores between the topiramate (25 mg/day titrated to 400 mg/day or maximum tolerated dose, div. BID) and placebo groups by study end point, though there were significant reductions in the topiramate group in the reexperiencing subscale score on CAPS and in Treatment Outcome PTSD Scale, but not in the other secondary efficacy measures (Tucker et al., 2007). There have been two small open-label studies of topiramate as an adjunctive treatment or monotherapy in PTSD (Berlant and van Kammen, 2002; Berlant, 2004) and one in SAD (van Ameringen et al., 2004) suggesting efficacy, though with notable limitations (reviewed in Mula et al., 2007). There are no other published RCTs of topiramate in the non-OCD anxiety disorders.

Another anticonvulsant *tiagabine*, a γ-aminobutyric acid (GABA) reuptake inhibitor, has been studied most extensively for GAD. In a multicenter, 8-week RCT, Pollack et al. (2005) found no significant difference in response rates between tiagabine (titrated from 4 mg/day to a maximum of 16 mg/day, div. BID) and placebo in the LOCF analysis, though reduction of anxiety symptoms was noted in the tiagabine group in secondary statistical analyses (observed case and MMRM analyses). A small (N = 40), randomized, open-label trial of tiagabine (4–16 mg/day, div. BID) versus paroxetine (20–60 mg/day) in GAD demonstrated that both medications significantly reduced anxiety symptoms per HAM-A after 10 weeks, though this study did not include a placebo arm (Rosenthal, 2003). Davidson et al. (2007) conducted a multicenter, 12-week RCT of tiagabine in PTSD and found no significant differences between the tiagabine (4–16 mg/day) and placebo groups on CAPS or other outcome measures by study end point. A small (N = 29), open-label study of tiagabine in PTSD suggested improvement in the open-label phase, but in a double-blind discontinuation phase, there was no difference in relapse between the tiagabine and placebo groups (Connor et al., 2006). A small (N = 54), open-label study of tiagabine in SAD suggested initial promise (Dunlop et al., 2007). Regarding side effects, post-marketing reports found an association with seizures and status epilepticus in patients without epilepsy; since this addition to the package labelling in February 2005, the off-label use of this medication for anxiety has decreased significantly.

A small, 7-week, RCT (N = 19) of the AED levetiracetam was conducted in SAD (Zhang et al., 2005), which found no significant difference in BSPS or LSAS scores between the levetiracetam (500–3000 mg/day) and placebo groups. The calculated effect size was 0.33 for BSPS and 0.5 for LSAS (Zhang et al., 2005). There are no other RCTs of levetiracetam in the non-OCD anxiety disorders (reviewed in Mula et al., 2007). Small, open-label studies of levetiracetam suggesting some efficacy in SAD (Simon et al., 2004), and in PD (Papp, 2006), and a small, retrospective case analysis suggested efficacy of levetiracetam as an adjunctive medication in treatment-refractory PTSD (Kinrys et al., 2006).

Regarding the commonly used AEDs *carbamazepine* and *valproate*, there is also limited data supporting its efficacy in primary anxiety disorders. There is a negative RCT of carbamazepine in 14 patients with PD (Uhde et al., 1988). There are three small, open-label studies, two of which did not use standardized measures, and a large retrospective study suggesting some benefit of carbamazepine in PTSD, and an open-label study suggesting possible efficacy in PD (reviewed in Mula et al., 2007). Several open-label studies have suggested efficacy of valproate in PTSD and PD, and one in SAD, and one negative open-label study of valproate monotherapy in PTSD (reviewed in Mula et al., 2007).

Evidence for the efficacy of additional AEDs in anxiety disorders, such as oxcarbazepine, phenytoin, and vigabatrin, is low, with no published RCTs of these medications in GAD, PD, SAD, or PTSD to date.

BENZODIAZEPINES AND AZAPIRONES

Multiple RCTs have demonstrated the short- and long-term efficacy of BZDs in GAD, PD, and SAD (Davidson, 2006; Katon, 2006; Mathew and Hoffman, in press). The principal advantages of BZDs are their rapid onset of action and their ability to be used on a PRN or "as needed" basis for acute panic/anxiety. However, the well-noted disadvantages of BZDs include the risk of physiological dependence with long-term use (O'Brien, 2005), and their lack of antidepressant effects. Table 44.1 shows the U.S. FDA approved BZDs for anxiety disorders, and Table 44.3 reviews the clinical pharmacology and available preparations of commonly used BZDs. Due to their rapid onset of action, BZDs are commonly used in clinical practice as adjunctive agents for stabilization during initiation of an SSRI/SNRI. Longer-acting BZDs (for example, clonazepam, alprazolam XR) may be utilized to decrease breakthrough anxiety (reviewed in Katon, 2006).

Randomized controlled trials have demonstrated that BZDs are efficacious in the acute treatment of GAD, with a rapid onset of action (Rickels et al., 1993, Rocca et al., 1997). However, long-term use of BZDs in GAD is problematic, as very few patients achieve and sustain remission with BZD monotherapy (Mathew and Hoffman, in press). Rickels et al. (1993) and Rocca et al. (1997) noted that BZDs affected mostly somatic symptoms in GAD (for example, muscle tension, gastrointestinal symptoms), whereas psychic symptoms (for example, worry, rumination) were preferentially responsive to antidepressants (imipramine, trazodone). There is evidence from RCTs that BZDs are effective in PD as well (Tesar et al., 1991; Cross-National and S. Group, 1992; Schweizer et al., 1993; Ballenger et al., 1988).

TABLE 44.3 *Characteristics of Commonly Used Benzodiazepines*

Generic Name (Brand name)	*Routes of Administration*	*Oral Dose Equivalency (mg)*	*Approved Oral Dose Range (mg)*	*Rate of Onset after Oral Dose*	*Elimination Half-Life (hr)*	*Active Metabolites*	*Strengths (mg)/ Available Preparations*
Alprazolam (Xanax)	PO	0.5	0.75–4 Alprazolam XR: 3–6(suggested) 1–0 (used in clinical trials)	Intermediate	6–20	-	0.25, 0.5, 1, 2 *Alprazolam Intensol (concentrate solution)*: 1 mg/ml *Alprazolam XR*: 0.5, 1, 2, 3 *Niravam (alprazolam orally disintegrating)*: 0.25, 0.5, 1, 2
Chlordiazepoxide (Librium)	PO	10.0	15–100	Intermediate	30–100	+	5, 10, 25
Clonazepam (Klonopin)	PO	0.25	0.5–4	Intermediate	18–40	-	0.5, 1, 2 *Klonopin Wafers*: 0.125, 0.25, 0.5, 1, 2
Clorazepate (Tranxene)	PO	7.5	15–60 Tranxene SD: 11.25–5	Rapid	30–100	+	*Tranxene T-tab*: 3.75, 7.5, 15 *Tranxene SD*: 11.25, 22.5
Diazepam (Valium)	PO, PR, IM, IV	5.0	4–40	Rapid	30–100	+	2, 5, 10 *Solution*: 5 mg/5 ml *Intensol*: 5 mg/ml *Diastat (diazepam rectal)*: 2.5 gel; *AcuDial gel*: 10, 20 IM, IV
Lorazepam (Ativan)	PO, IM, IV	1.0	1–10	Intermediate	10–20	-	0.5, 1, 2 *Conc.*: 2 mg/ml IM, IV
Oxazepam (Serax)	PO	15.0	30–120	Intermediate-Slow	8–12	-	10, 15, 30
Temazepam (Restoril)	PO	30.0	7.5–30	Intermediate	8–20	-	7.5, 15, 30
Triazolam (Halcion)	PO	0.25	0.125–0.5	Intermediate	2–5	-	0.125, 0.25

Source: Adapted from Rosenbaum et al. (2005), Goddard et al. (2002).
PO: by mouth; PR: per rectum; IM: intramuscular; IV: intervenous.

Several RCTs have addressed the practical question of the utility of combination SSRI/benzodiazepine for acute treatment of PD. In a RCT in PD ($N = 47$), Goddard et al. (2001) compared responses of patients with PD to sertraline (open-label, target dose, 100 mg/day) given in combination with either the BZD clonazepam (0.5 mg TID) or placebo, during the first 4 of 12 weeks of treatment, after which clonazepam was tapered over 3 weeks and discontinued. There was a significantly greater number of responders ($p = 0.003$) at the end of week 1 in the combined sertraline/clonazepam group (41%) versus sertraline/placebo (4%) (Goddard et al., 2001). At week 3, there was a between-group difference ($p = 0.05$) favoring the sertraline/clonazepam group, though there were no group differences in response after 4 or 12 weeks, or at other time points during the trial (Goddard et al., 2001). Pollack et al. (2003) conducted a 12-week RCT of patients with PD ($N = 60$, 34 completers), comparing three treatment arms: paroxetine (mean dose = 39 mg/day)/placebo, paroxetine (mean dose = 37 mg/day)/clonazepam (mean dose = 1.6 mg/day), followed by a taper of clonazepam (over 3 weeks, beginning at week 4), or ongoing combination treatment (mean dose paroxetine = 38.6 mg/day, clonazepam = 1.5 mg/day by study end). Similar to the Goddard et al. (2001) report, there was significant improvement on PDSS early in treatment (generally from weeks 1–5) in the two groups receiving combination treatment versus paroxetine monotherapy, but that all three groups exhibited a significant improvement on PDSS from baseline to end point, and there was no significant difference in outcome among the three groups by study end point (Pollack et al., 2003).

There is also evidence to support the use of BZDs in SAD in patients resistant to or unable to tolerate SSRIs (Davidson, 2006; Schneier, 2006). However, in a small RCT of 28 patients with SAD treated with open-label paroxetine (20–40 mg/day) and either clonazepam (1–2 mg/day, div. BID) or placebo for 10 weeks, no significant differences between the two groups were noted early or later in treatment (Seedat and Stein, 2004).

To date, there are no published large RCTs of BZDs in adequately characterized samples of PTSD.

The azapirone *buspirone*, a serotonin 1A (5-HT_{1A}) agonist, is approved by the FDA for treating "anxiety disorders," which correspond most closely to GAD as described in *DSM-III*. A retrospective analysis of pooled data from eight studies of buspirone versus placebo in GAD found that buspirone resulted in significant improvement on HAM-A versus placebo ($p \leq 0.001$) (Gammans et al., 1992). Advantages of the serotonin 1A partial and full agonists include their overall tolerability, lack of addictive potential, and minimal sexual dysfunction or blood pressure effects (reviewed in Mathew and Hoffman, in press), though an important limitation of the azapirones is evidence of decreased efficacy in patients with past benzodiazepine use (DeMartinis et al., 2000). Randomized controlled trials have not found buspirone to be effective in treating PD (Pohl et al., 1989; Sheehan et al., 1990; Sheehan et al., 1993), or SAD (van Vliet et al., 1997).

ATYPICAL ANTIPSYCHOTICS

Due to their broad neurochemical effects on postsynaptic 5-HT_2 receptors and modulation of 5-HT_{1A}, atypical antipsychotics have been tested for their anxiolytic potential. Two small RCTs have investigated olanzapine and risperidone as adjunctive agents to the SSRIs in GAD (Brawman-Mintzer et al., 2005; Pollack et al., 2006). Pollack et al. (2006) reported in a small ($N = 24$), single-site RCT that in patients with GAD who did not respond to fluoxetine (20 mg/day) after 6 weeks, olanzapine (mean dose = 8.7 mg/day) versus placebo augmentation resulted in a significant number of responders on HAM-A and CGI-S after 6 weeks. There were no other significant findings on other outcome measures and olanzapine resulted in sedation and significant weight gain (11.0 ± 5.1 lbs. on average, range 2–16 lbs.). In another small ($N = 39$) RCT, risperidone (0.5–1.5 mg/day) was used as an adjunctive treatment in patients with GAD who did not respond to at least 4 weeks of another medication, either an SSRI, SNRI, benzodiazepine, or other anxiolytic or antidepressant (Brawman-Mintzer et al., 2005). After 5 weeks of adjunctive treatment with risperidone or placebo, there were statistically significant reductions in HAM-A total and psychic anxiety scores in the risperidone versus the placebo augmentation group, but CGI-S reductions and CGI-I response rates were not significant (Brawman-Mintzer et al., 2005). Risperidone was well-tolerated overall, though side effects included somnolence, dizziness, and blurred vision (Brawman-Mintzer et al., 2005). Olanzapine (5–20 mg/day) was also investigated as monotherapy for SAD in a very small ($N = 12$, 7 completers), 8-week RCT, in which there was significant improvement on the BSPS and Social Phobia Inventory, but not on LSAS and CGI-I, in the olanzapine versus placebo groups (Barnett et al., 2002).

Risperidone adjunctive therapy was found to have some efficacy in combat-related PTSD (reviewed in Gao et al., 2006). Bartzokis et al. (2004) found that in male patients with chronic, combat-related PTSD, risperidone (titrated to a maximum of 3 mg/day in most patients), added to a stable psychotropic medication regimen (in 92% of patients), including antidepressants, anxiolytics, and/or hypnotics, resulted in significant improvement versus placebo on the CAPS after 16 weeks of treatment, which included an initial Veterans Administration (VA) residential psychosocial program for 5 weeks. Hamner et al. (2003) found that in combat veterans with chronic PTSD and psychotic symptoms, adjunctive risperidone (1–6 mg/day) resulted in significant improvement in psychotic symptoms, but not on the CAPS, compared to placebo after 5 weeks. In a 12-week pilot study of 20 women with PTSD related to sexual assault and domestic abuse, Padala et al. (2006) report that risperidone monotherapy (mean dose = 2.62 mg/day) resulted in a significant decline in Treatment Outcomes PTSD Scale-8 scores from baseline, whereas no difference was observed from baseline to visit in the placebo group. Overall, RCTs of olanzapine in PTSD have been inconsistent, as a small ($N = 15$) RCT of olanzapine monotherapy (5–20 mg/day) in PTSD found no effect after 10 weeks (Butterfield et al., 2001), whereas an 8-week RCT of olanzapine (mean dose = 15 mg/day) or placebo augmentation of SSRIs in 19 patients with combat-related PTSD found that olanzapine resulted in significant reductions in CAPS total scores, as well as depressive symptoms and sleep disturbance, but not in the percentage of CGI-I responders (M.B. Stein, Kline, et al., 2002). As of July 2007, to our knowledge, there were no published RCTs of quetiapine, aripiprazole, or ziprasidone in the anxiety disorders.

SUMMARY AND FUTURE DIRECTIONS

SSRIs and SNRIs will continue to be the primary pharmacotherapy treatments for anxiety disorders for the immediate future, given their overall better tolerability than older antidepressants. In the next decade, further refinements of these monoaminergic-based drugs, including triple reuptake inhibitors will be introduced. Innovations in the development of novel drugs, such as glutamate-modulators, corticotrophin releasing factor CRF antagonists, and neurokinin receptor 1 (NK1) receptor antagonists, as well as anxiety applications for newer anticonvulsants such as pregabalin, may turn out to be valuable alternatives to the benzodiazepines for the induction of rapid anxiolysis. Several areas for further study are recommended.

Placebo Responsivity of Anxiety Disorders

Randomized controlled trials of anxiety disorders have been plagued by high placebo responsivity, with notable differences across anxiety disorders in the magnitude of placebo responses (Huppert et al., 2004). Identifying moderators and predictors of placebo response in RCTs of anxiety disorders is critical, but very few clinical or demographic characteristics associated with placebo response have been identified (D.J. Stein, Baldwin, et al., 2006). Somewhat surprisingly, trials of PTSD are beleaguered by high placebo responsivity; as a recent example, a multicenter study of venlafaxine XR in chronic PTSD yielded placebo response rates of > 60% at 12 weeks (Davidson, Baldwin, et al., 2006). These extraordinarily high rates of placebo responsivity may result from the therapeutic "exposure" and extensive time requirements inherent to the major outcome instrument used in pivotal FDA regulatory studies, the CAPS. Briefer instruments, including self-report inventories, should be used in FDA-pivotal clinical trials, as suggested by Davidson, Baldwin, et al. (2006). Given the very high expected rates of placebo response, placebo arms remain an essential design feature for head-to-head drug comparison studies, although industry-supported trials generally have avoided three-arm designs (two comparison drugs and placebo).

Head-to-Head Comparisons of Medications

The vast majority of comparative pharmacological studies in anxiety disorders is inconclusive (Table 44.2) and offer little guidance to clinicians in choice of agent. With a few noteworthy exceptions (for example, the Eli Lilly-funded head-to-head study of duloxetine and effexor XR), industry-funded clinical trials have found equivalence, or more commonly, noninferiority, of newer agents to older drugs in similar classes. Large-scale National Institute of Mental Health (NIMH) and/or foundation-sponsored comparative effectiveness trials (including psychotherapy arms) are needed in adult anxiety disorders, as has been performed for major depression, bipolar disorder, schizophrenia, and attention-deficit disorder, among other conditions. However, a search of the National Institutes of Health database of funded studies in 2007 (CRISP-Computer Retrieval of Information on Scientific Projects) did not find a single pharmacological clinical trial in any anxiety disorder using the R01 or Center Grant funding mechanisms, suggesting that major gaps in our knowledge base will continue.

Analytic Methods

As seen in Table 44.2, multiple analytic methods have been used (LOCF, MMRM, OC, completer), often without justification. Journal editors must serve as important arbiters of reporting standards for clinical trials for the anxiety disorders. The recent requirement of posting methodological details of RCTs on www.clinicaltrials.gov is an important step towards transparency. It has been proposed that RCTs in psychiatry should report, in addition to p values, the NNT and success rate difference (SRD) with its standard error and confidence interval (Kraemer and Kupfer, 2006).

Assessment of Acute and Long-Term Response in RCTs

The ACNP Task Force on Response and Remission for major depressive disorder has recommended that response criteria be met for 3 consecutive weeks to account for unstable symptomatic fluctuations and measurement error (Rush et al., 2006). Reliance on a single time point evaluation for 8- or 12-week RCTs in anxiety disorders as the primary outcome measure hinders analyses of durable and clinically meaningful drug–placebo differences. FDA pivotal RCTs in anxiety disorders also rarely assess the durability of acute pharmacotherapy. In contrast, it is standard for psychotherapy trials in anxiety disorders to report long-term outcome (3–6 months or 1 year).

Areas of Critical Need

Despite the high prevalence and morbidity associated with PTSD, there are currently only two FDA-approved medications for PTSD (sertraline and paroxetine). However, both these medications have ESs below 0.5. Many placebo-controlled trials of other medications in PTSD have failed, and even recent studies of approved medications (for example, sertraline) have failed to show efficacy in specific subgroups of patients with PTSD such as combat veterans (Friedman et al., 2007).

REFERENCES

Allgulander, C., Dahl, A.A., Austin, et al. (2004) Efficacy of sertraline in a 12-week trial for generalized anxiety disorder. *Am. J. Psychiatry* 161(9):1642–1649.

Allgulander, C., Florea, I., et al. (2005) Prevention of relapse in generalized anxiety disorder by escitalopram treatment. *Int. J. Neuropsychopharm.* 9:1–11.

Allgulander, C., Hackett, D., and Salinas, E. (2001) Venlafaxine extended release (ER) in the treatment of generalised anxiety disorder: twenty-four-week placebo-controlled dose-ranging study. *Br. J. Psychiatry* 179:15–22.

Allgulander, C., Mangano, R., et al. (2004) Efficacy of venlafaxine ER in patients with social anxiety disorder: a double-blind, placebo-controlled, parallel-group comparison with paroxetine. *Hum. Psychopharmacol.* 19:387–396.

American Psychiatric Association (1980) *Diagnostic and Statistical Manual of Mental Disorders*, 3rd ed. Washington, DC: Author.

American Psychiatric Association. (1994) *Diagnostic and Statistical Manual of Mental Disorders*, 4th ed. Washington, DC: Author.

Asakura, S., Tajima, O., and Koyama, T. (2007) Fluvoxamine treatment of generalized social anxiety disorder in Japan: a randomized double-blind, placebo-controlled study. *Int. J. Neuropsychopharm.* 10(2):263–274.

Asnis, G.M., Hameedi, F.A., et al. (2001) Fluvoxamine in the treatment of panic disorder: a multi-center, double-blind, placebo-controlled study in outpatients. *Psychiatry Res.* 103:1–14.

Baldwin, D., Bobes, J., et al. (1999) Paroxetine in social phobia/social anxiety disorder. Randomised, double-blind, placebo-controlled study. Paroxetine Study Group. *Br. J. Psychiatry* 175:120–126.

Baldwin, D.S., and Polkinghorn, C. (2005) Evidence-based pharmacotherapy of generalized anxiety disorder. *Int. J. of Neuropsychopharm.* 8:293–302.

Ball, S.G., Kuhn, A., et al. (2005) Selective serotonin reuptake inhibitor treatment for generalized anxiety disorder: a double-blind, prospective comparison between paroxetine and sertraline. *J. Clin. Psychiatry* 66(1):94–99.

Ballenger, J.C., Burrows, G.D., et al. (1988) Alprazolam in panic disorder and agoraphobia: results from a multicenter trial. I. Efficacy in short-term treatment. *Arch. Gen. Psychiatry* 45(5):413–422.

Ballenger, J.C., Wheadon, D.E., et al. (1998) Double-blind, fixed-dose, placebo-controlled study of paroxetine in the treatment of panic disorder. *Am. J. Psychiatry* 155(1):36–42.

Bandelow, B., Behnke, K., et al. (2004) Sertraline versus paroxetine in the treatment of panic disorder: an acute, double-blind noninferiority comparison. *J. Clin. Psychiatry* 65:405–413.

Barlow, D.H., Gorman, J.M., et al. (2000) Cognitive-behavioral therapy, imipramine, or their combination for panic disorder: A randomized controlled trial. *JAMA* 283(19):2529–2536.

Barnett, S.D., Kramer, M.L., et al. (2002) Efficacy of olanzapine in social anxiety disorder: a pilot study. *J. Psychopharmacol.* 16(4):365–368.

Bartzokis, G., Lu, P.H., et al. (2004) Adjunctive risperidone in the treatment of chronic combat-related posttraumatic stress disorder. *Biol. Psychiatry* 57:474–479.

Berlant, J., and van Kammen, D.P. (2002) Open-label topiramate as primary or adjunctive therapy in chronic civilian posttraumatic stress disorder: a preliminary report. *J. Clin. Psychiatry* 6(1):15–20.

Berlant, J.L. (2004) Prospective open-label study of add-on and monotherapy topiramate in civilians with chronic nonhallucinatory posttraumatic stress disorder. *BMC Psychiatry* 18(4):24.

Bielski, R.J., Bose, A., et al. (2005) A double-blind comparison of escitalopram and paroxetine in the long-term treatment of generalized anxiety disorder. *Ann. Clin. Psychiatry* 17(2):65–69.

Black, D.W., Wesner, R., et al. (1993) A comparison of fluvoxamine, cognitive therapy, and placebo in the treatment of panic disorder. *Arch. Gen. Psychiatry* 50 (1):44–50.

Blanco, C., Schneier, F.R., et al. (2003) Pharmacological treatment of social anxiety disorder: a meta-analysis. *Depress. Anxiety* 18:29–40.

Blomhoff, S., Haug, T.T., et al. (2001) Randomised controlled general practice trial of sertraline, exposure therapy and combined treatment in generalised social phobia. *Br. J. Psychiatry* 179:23–30.

Bradwejn, J., Ahokas, A., et al. (2005) Venlafaxine extended-release capsules in panic disorder: flexible-dose, double-blind, placebo-controlled study. *Br. J. Psychiatry* 187:352–359.

Brawman-Mintzer, O., Knapp, R.G., and Nietert, P.J. (2005) Adjunctive risperidone in generalized anxiety disorder: a double-blind, placebo-controlled study. *J. Clin. Psychiatry* 66(10):1321–1325.

Butterfield, M.I., Becker, M.E., et al. (2001) Olanzapine in the treatment of post-traumatic stress disorder: a pilot study. *Int. Clin. Psychopharmacol.* 16:197–203.

Clark, D.M., Ehlers, A., et al. (2003) Cognitive therapy versus floxetine in generalized social phobia: a randomized placebo-controlled trial. *J. Consult. Clin. Psychology* 71(6):1058–1067.

Connor, K.M., Davidson, J.R., et al. (2006) Tiagabine for post-traumatic stress disorder: effects of open-label and double-blind discontinuation treatment. *Psychopharmacol. (Berl)* 184(1):21–25.

Cross-National Collaborative Panic Study, Second Phase Investigators (1992) Drug treatment of panic disorder. Comparative efficacy of alprazolam, imipramine, and placebo. *Br. J. Psychiatry* 160:191–202; discussion 202–205.

Dahl, A.A., Ravindran, A., et al. (2005) Sertraline in generalized anxiety disorder: efficacy in treating the psychic and somatic anxiety factors. *Acta. Psychiatr. Scand.* 111:429–435.

Davidson, J., Baldwin, D., Stein, D.J., Kuper, E., Benattia, I., Ahmed, S., Pedersen, R., and Musgnung, J. (2006) Treatment of posttraumatic stress disorder with venlafaxine extended release: a 6-month randomized controlled trial. *Arch. Gen. Psychiatry* 63:1158–1165.

Davidson, J., Rothbaum, B.O., Tucker, P., Asnis, G., Benattia, I., and Musgnung, J.J. (2006) Venlafaxine extended release in posttraumatic stress disorder: A sertraline- and placebo-controlled study. *J Clin Psychopharmacol.* 26 (3): 259–267.

Davidson, J., Yaryura, T., et al. (2004) Fluvoxamine-controlled release formulation for the treatment of generalized social anxiety disorder. *J. Clin. Psychopharm.* 24(2):118–125.

Davidson, J.R.T. (2006) Pharmacotherapy of social anxiety disorder: what does the evidence tell us? *J. Clin. Psychiatry* 67 (Suppl 12):20–26.

Davidson, J.R.T., Bose, A., et al. (2004) Escitalopram in the treatment of generalized anxiety disorder: double-blind, placebo controlled, flexible-dose study. *Depress. Anxiety* 19:234–240.

Davidson, J.R.T., Bose, A., et al. (2005) Safety and efficacy of escitalopram in the long term treatment of generalized anxiety disorder. *J. Clin. Psychiatry* 66(11):1441–1446.

Davidson, J.R.T., Brady, K., et al. (2007) The efficacy and tolerability of tiagabine in adult patients with post-traumatic stress disorder. *J. Clin. Psychopharmacol.* 27(1):85–88.

Davidson, J.R.T., DuPont, R.L., et al. (1999) Efficacy, safety, and tolerability of venlafaxine extended release and buspirone in outpatients with generalized anxiety disorder. *J. Clin. Psychiatry* 60(8): 528–535.

Davidson, J.R.T., Foa, E.B., et al. (2004) Fluoxetine, comprehensive cognitive behavioral therapy, and placebo in generalized social phobia. *Arch. Gen. Psychiatry* 61:1005–1013.

DeMartinis, N., Rynn, M., et al. (2000) Prior benzodiazepine use and buspirone response in the treatment of generalized anxiety disorder. *J. Clin. Psychiatry* 62(8):657–658.

Dunlop, B.W., Papp, L., et al. (2007) Tiagabine for social anxiety disorder. *Hum. Psychopharmacol.* 22(4):241–244.

Federoff, I.C., and Taylor, S. (2001) Psychological and pharmacological treatments of social phobia: a meta-analysis. *J. Clin. Psychopharmacol.* 21(3):311–324.

Feltner, D.E., Crockatt, J.G., et al. (2003) A randomized, double-blind, placebo-controlled, fixed-dose, multicenter study of pregabalin in patients with generalized anxiety disorder. *J. Clin. Psychopharm.* 223(3):240–249.

Ferguson, J.M., Khan, A., et al. (2007) Relapse prevention of panic disorder in adult outpatient responders to treatment with venlafaxine extended release. *J. Clin. Psychiatry* 68(1):58–68.

Friedman, M.J., Marmar, C.R., et al. (2007) Randomized, double-blind comparison of sertraline and placebo for posttraumatic stress disorder in a Department of Veterans Affairs setting. *J. Clin. Psychiatry* 68 (5):711–720.

Furukawa, T.A., Watanabe, N., et al. (2007) Combined psychotherapy plus antidepressants for panic disorder with or without agoraphobia. *Cochrane Database of Systematic Reviews* Issue 1. Art. No.: CD004364. DOI: 10.1002/14651858.CD004364.pub2.

Gammans, R.E., Stringfellow, J.C., et al. (1992) Use of buspirone in patients with generalized anxiety disorder and coexisting depressive symptoms. A meta-analysis of eight, randomized, controlled studies. *Neuropsychobiology* 25(4):193–201.

Gao, K., Muzina, D., et al. (2006) Efficacy of typical and atypical antipsychotics for primary and comorbid anxiety symptoms or disorders: a review. *J. Clin. Psychiatry* 67:1327–1340.

Gellenberg, A.J., Lydiard, R.B., et al. (2000) Efficacy of venlafaxine extended-release capsules in nondepressed outpatients with generalized anxiety disorder: a 6-month randomized controlled trial. *JAMA* 283(23):3082–3088.

Goddard, A.W., Brouette, T., et al. (2001) Early coadministration of clonazepam with sertraline for panic disorder. *Arch. Gen. Psychiatry* 58:681–686.

Goddard, A.W., Coplan, J.D., et al. (2002) Principles of pharmacotherapy for the anxiety disorders. In: Charney, D.S., ed. *Neurobiology of Mental Illness*, 2nd ed. New York: Oxford University Press.

Hackett, D., Haudiquet, V., and Salinas, E. (2003) A method for controlling for a high placebo response rate in a comparison of venlafaxine XR and diazepam in the short-term treatment of patients with generalised anxiety disorder. *Eur. Psychiatry* 18:182–187.

Hamner, M.B., Faldowski, R.A., et al. (2003) Adjunctive risperidone treatment in post-traumatic stress disorder: a preliminary controlled trial of effects on comorbid psychotic symptoms. *Int. Clin. Psychopharmacol.* 18:1–8.

Hartford, J., Kornstein, S., et al. (2007) Duloxetine as an SNRI treatment for generalized anxiety disorder: results from a placebo and active-controlled trial. *Int. Clin. Psychopharmacol.* 22:167–174.

Haug, T.T., Blomhoff, S., et al. (2003) Exposure therapy and sertraline in social phobia: 1-year follow-up of a randomised controlled trial. *Br. J. Psychiatry* 182:312–318.

Hedges, D.W., Brown, B.L., et al. (2007) The efficacy of selective serotonin reuptake inhibitors in adult social anxiety disorder: a meta-analysis of double-blind, placebo-controlled trials. *J. Psychopharmacol.* 21(1):102–111.

Heimberg, R.G., Liebowitz, M.R., et al. (1998) Cognitive behavioral group therapy vs. phenelzine therapy for social phobia: 12-week outcome. *Arch. Gen. Psychiatry* 55(12):1133–1141.

Hertzberg, M.A., Butterfield, M.I., et al. (1999) A preliminary study of lamotrigine for the treatment of posttraumatic stress disorder. *Biol. Psychiatry* 45(9):1226–1229.

Heuer, L., Mathew, S.J., and Charney, D.S. (in press) Panic disorder. In: Squire, L., Albright, T., Bloom, F., Gage, F., Spitzer, N., eds. *New Encyclopedia of Neuroscience.* Oxford, UK: Elsevier Ltd.

Hoehn-Saric, R., McLeod, D.R., and Hipsley, P.A. (1993) Effect of fluvoxamine on panic disorder. *J. Clin. Psychopharmacol.* 13(5): 321–326.

Huppert, J.D., Schultz, L.T., Foa, E.B., Barlow, D.H., Davidson, J.R.T., Gorman, J.M., Shear, M.K., Simpson, H.B., and Woods, S.W. (2004) Differential response to placebo among patients with social phobia, panic disorder, and obsessive-compulsive disorder. *Am. J. Psychiatry* 161:1485–1487.

International Multicenter Clinical Trial Group on Moclobemide in Social Phobia (1997) The International Multicenter Clinical Trial Group on Moclobemide in Social Phobia. A double-blind, placebo-controlled clinical study. *Eur. Arch. Psychiatry Clin. Neurosci.* 247(2):71–80.

Kapczinski, F., Lima, M.S., et al. (2003) Antidepressants for generalized anxiety disorder. *Cochrane Database of Systematic Reviews* Issue 2. Art. No.: CD003592. DOI: 10.1002/14651858. CD003592.

Kasper, S., Stein, D.J., et al. (2005) Escitalopram in the treatment of social anxiety disorder. *Br. J. Psychiatry* 186:222–226.

Katon, W.J. (2006) Panic disorder. *N. Engl. J. Med.* 354(22):2360–2367.

Kim, T.-S., Pae, C.-U., et al. (2006) Comparison of venlafaxine extended release versus paroxetine for treatment of patients with generalized anxiety disorder. *Psychiatry Clin. Neurosci.* 60:347–351.

Kinrys, G., Wygant, L.E., et al. (2006) Levetiracetam for treatment-refractory posttraumatic stress disorder. *J. Clin. Psychiatry* 67: 211–214.

Kobak, K.A., Greist, J.H., et al. (2002) Fluoxetine in social phobia: a double-blind, placebo-controlled pilot study. *J. Clin. Psychopharmacol.* 22:257–262.

Kraemer, H.C., and Kupfer, D.J. (2006) Size of treatment effects and their importance to clinical research and practice. *Biol. Psychiatry* 59(11):990–996.

Lader, M., Stender, K., et al. (2004) The efficacy and tolerability of escitalopram in the short- and long-term treatment of social anxiety disorder: a randomized, double-blind, placebo-controlled, fixed-dose study. *Depress. Anxiety* 19:241–248.

Lecrubier, Y., Bakker, A., et al. (1997) A comparison of paroxetine, clomipramine and placebo in the treatment of panic disorder. Collaborative Paroxetine Panic Study Investigators. *Acta Psychiatr. Scand.* 95(2):145–152.

Lecrubier, Y., and Judge R. (1997) Long-term evaluation of paroxetine, clomipramine and placebo in panic disorder. Collaborative Paroxetine Panic Study Investigators. *Acta Psychiatr. Scand.* 95(2): 153–60.

Lcopola, U.M., Wade, A.G., et al. (1998) A controlled, prospective, 1-year trial of citalopram in the treatment of panic disorder. *J. Clin. Psychiatry* 59(10):528–534.

Lepola, U., Bergtholdt, B., et al. (2004) Controlled-release paroxetine in the treatment of patients with social anxiety disorder. *J. Clin. Psychiatry* 65:222–229.

Liebowitz, M.R., DeMartinis, N.A., et al. (2003) Efficacy of sertraline in severe generalized social anxiety disorder: results of a double-blind, placebo-controlled study. *J. Clin. Psychiatry* 64(7): 785–792.

Liebowitz, M.R., Gelenberg, A.J., and Munjack, D. (2005) Venlafaxine extended release vs. placebo and paroxetime in social anxiety disorder. *Arch. Gen. Psychiatry* 62:190–198.

Liebowitz, M.R., Heimberg, R.G. et al. (1999) Cognitive-behavioral group therapy versus phenelzine in social phobia: long-term outcome. *Depress. Anxiety* 10(3):89–98.

Liebowitz, M.R., Hollander, E., et al. (1990) Reversible and irreversible monoamine oxidase inhibitors in other psychiatric disorders. *Acta Psychiatr. Scand.* (Suppl. 360):29–34.

Liebowitz, M.R., Mangano, R.M., et al. (2005) A randomized controlled trial of venlafaxine extended release in generalized social anxiety disorder. *J. Clin. Psychiatry* 66(2):238–247.

Liebowitz, M.R., Schneier, F., et al. (1990) Phenelzine and atenolol in social phobia. *Psychopharmacol. Bull.* 26(1):123–125.

Liebowitz, M.R., Schneier, F., et al. (1992) Phenelzine vs. atenolol in social phobia. A placebo-controlled comparison. *Arch. Gen. Psychiatry* 49(4):290–300.

Liebowitz, M.R., Stein, M.B., Tancer, M., et al. (2002) A randomized, double-blind, fixed-dose comparison of paroxetine and placebo in the treatment of generalized social anxiety disorder. *J. Clin. Psychiatry* 63:66–74.

Lott, M., Greist, J.H., et al. (1997) Brofaromine for social phobia: a multicenter, placebo-controlled, double-blind study. *J. Clin. Psychopharmacol.* 17(4):255–260.

Lydiard, R.B., and Monnier, J. (2004) Pharmacological treatment. In Heimberg, R.C., Turk, C.L., Mannin, D.S., eds. *Generalized Anxiety Disorder: Advances in Research and Practice*. New York: Guilford Press, pp. 351–379.

Marshall, R.D., Beebe, K.L., Oldham, M., and Zaninelli, R. (2001) Efficacy and safety of paroxetine treatment for chronic PTSD: a fixed-dose, placebo-controlled study. *Am. J. Psychiatry* 158:1982–1988.

Mathew, S.J., and Hoffman, E.J. (in press) Pharmacotherapy of generalized anxiety disorder. In: Antony, M., and Stein, M., eds. *Oxford Handbook of Anxiety and Anxiety Disorders*. New York: Oxford University Press.

Michelson, D., Allgulander, K., et al. (2001) Efficacy of usual antidepressant dosing regimens of fluoxetine in panic disorder. *Br. J. Psychiatry* 179:514–518.

Michelson, D., Lydiard, R.B., et al. (1998) Outcome assessment and clinical improvement in panic disorder: evidence from a randomized controlled trial of fluoxetine and placebo. *Am. J. Psychiatry* 155(11):1570–1577.

Mitte, K. (2005) A meta-analysis of the efficacy of psycho- and pharmacotherapy in panic disorder with and without agoraphobia. *J. Affect. Disord.* 88:27–45.

Montgomery, S.A., Nil, R., et al. (2005) A 24-week randomized, double-blind, placebo-controlled study of escitalopram for the prevention of generalized social anxiety disorder. *J. Clin. Psychiatry* 66:1270–1278.

Montgomery, S.A., Tobias, K., et al. (2006) Efficacy and safety of pregabalin in the treatment of generalized anxiety disorder: a 6-week, multicenter, randomized, double-blind placebo-controlled comparison of pregabalin and venlafaxine. *J. Clin. Psychiatry* 67: 771–782.

Mula, M., Pini, S., and Cassano, G.B. (2007) The role of anticonvulsant drugs in anxiety disorders: a critical review of the evidence. *J. Clin. Psychopharmacol.* 27(3):263–272.

Nimatoudis, I., Zissis, N.P., et al. (2004) Remission rates with venlafaxine extended release in Greek outpatients with generalized anxiety disorder. A double-blind, randomized, placebo controlled study. *Int. Clin. Psychopharmacol.* 19:331–336.

Noyes, R., Moroz, G., et al. (1997) Moclobemide in social phobia: a controlled dose-response trial. *J. Clin. Psychopharmacol.* 17(4): 247–254.

O'Brien, C.P. (2005) Benzodiazepine use, abuse, and dependence. *J. Clin. Psychiatry* 66(Suppl 2):28–33.

Otto, M. W., Tuby, K.S., et al. (2001) An effect-size analysis of the relative efficacy and tolerability of serotonin selective reuptake inhibitors for panic disorder. *Am. J. Psychiatry* 158:1989–1992.

Padala, P.R., Madison, J., et al. (2006) Risperidone monotherapy for post-traumatic stress disorder related to sexual assault and domestic abuse in women. *Int. Clin. Psychopharmacol.* 21:275–280.

Pande, A.C., Crockatt, J.G., et al. (2003) Pregabalin in generalized anxiety disorder: a placebo-controlled trial. *Am J. Psychiatry* 160(3):533–540.

Pande, A.C., Davidson, J.R.T., et al. (1999) Treatment of social phobia with gabapentin: a placebo-controlled study. *J. Clin. Psychopharmacol.* 19(4):341–348.

Pande, A.C., Feltner, D.E., et al. (2004) Efficacy of the novel anxiolytic pregabalin in social anxiety disorder: a placebo-controlled, multicenter study. *J. Clin. Psychopharmacol.* 24(2):141–149.

Pande, A.C., Pollack, M.H., et al. (2000) Placebo-controlled study of gabapentin treatment of panic disorder. *J. Clin. Psychopharmacol.* 20(4):467–471.

Papp, L.A. (2006) Safety and efficacy of levetiracetam for patients with panic disorder: results of an open-label, fixed-flexible dose study. *J. Clin. Psychiatry* 67(10):1573–1576.

Perna, G., Bertani, A., et al. (2001) A comparison of citalopram and paroxetine in the treatment of panic disorder: a randomized, single-blind study. *Pharmacopsychiatry* 34:85–90.

Pohl, R., Balon, R., et al. (1989) Serotonergic anxiolytics in the treatment of panic disorder: a controlled study with buspirone. *Psychopathology* 22(Suppl 1):60–67.

Pohl, R.B., Feltner, D.E., et al. (2005) Efficacy of pregabalin in the treatment of generalized anxiety disorder. *J. Clin. Psychopharm.* 25(2):151–158.

Pohl, R.B., Wolkow, R.M., et al. (1998) Sertraline in the treatment of panic disorder: a double-blind multicenter trial. *Am. J. Psychiatry* 155(9):1189–1195.

Pollack, M.H., Lepola, U., et al. (2007) A double-blind study of the efficacy of venlafaxine extended-release, paroxetine, and placebo in the treatment of panic disorder. *Depress. Anxiety* 24:1–14.

Pollack, M.H., Otto, M.W., et al. (1998) Sertraline in the treatment of panic disorder. *Arch. Gen. Psychiatry* 55:1010–1016.

Pollack, M.H., Roy-Byrne, P.P., et al. (2005) The selective GABA reuptake inhibitor tiagabine for the treatment of generalized anxiety disorder: results of a placebo-controlled study. *J. Clin. Psychiatry* 66(11):1401–1408.

Pollack, M.H., Simon, N.M., et al. (2003) Combined paroxetine and clonazepam treatment strategies compared to paroxetine monotherapy for panic disorder. *J. Psychopharmacol.* 17(3):276–282.

Pollack, M.H., Zaninelli, R., et al. (2001) Paroxetine in the treatment of generalized anxiety disorder: results of a placebo-controlled, flexible-dosage trial. *J. Clin. Psychiatry* 62(5):350–357.

Pollack, M.H., Simon, N.M., et al. (2006) Olanzapine augmentation of fluoxetine for refractory generalized anxiety disorder: a placebo controlled study. *Biol. Psychiatry* 59:211–215.

Prasko, J., Dockery C., et al. (2006) Moclobemide and cognitive behavioral therapy in the treatment of social phobia. A six-month controlled study and 24 months of follow up. *Neuro. Endocrinol. Lett.* 27(4):473–481.

Rapaport, M.H., Wolkow, R., et al. (2001) Sertraline treatment of panic disorder: results of a long-term study *Acta Psychiatr. Scand.* 104:289–298.

Rickels, K., Downing, R., et al. (1993) Antidepressants for the treatment of generalized anxiety disorder: a placebo-controlled comparison of imipramine, trazodone, and diazepam. *Arch. Gen. Psychiatry* 50:884–895.

Rickels, K., Mangano, R., and Khan, A. (2004) A double-blind, placebo-controlled study of a flexible dose of venlafaxine ER in adult outpatients with generalized social anxiety disorder. *J. Clin. Psychopharm.* 24(5):488–496.

Rickels, K., Pollack, M.H., et al. (2000) Efficacy of extended-release venlafaxine in nondepressed outpatients with generalized anxiety disorder. *Am. J. Psychiatry* 157(6):968–974.

Rickels, K., Pollack, M.H., et al. (2005) Pregabalin for treatment of generalized anxiety disorder: a 4-week, multicenter, double-blind, placebo-controlled trial of pregabalin and alprazolam. *Arch. Gen. Psychiatry* 62:1022–1030.

Rickels, K., Zaninelli, R., et al. (2003) Paroxetine treatment of generalized anxiety disorder: a double-blind, placebo-controlled study. *Am. J. Psychiatry* 160(4):749–756.

Rocca, P., Fonzo, V., et al. (1997) Paroxetine efficacy in the treatment of generalized anxiety disorder. *Acta Psychiatr Scand.* 95(5): 444–450.

Rosenbaum, J.F., Arana, G.W., et al. (2005) *Handbook of Psychiatric Drug Therapy*, 5th ed. Philadelphia: Lippincott Williams & Wilkins.

Rosenthal, M. (2003) Tiagabine for the treatment of generalized anxiety disorder: a randomized, open-label clinical trial with paroxetine as a positive control. *J. Clin. Psychiatry* 64(10):1245–1249.

Rush, A.J., Kraemer, H.C., et al. (2006) Report by the ACNP Task Force on Response and remission in major depressive disorder. *Neuropsychopharmacology* 31 (9):1841–1853.

Rynn, M., Russell, J., et al. (2007) Efficacy and safety of duloxetine in the treatment of generalized anxiety disorder: a flexible-dose, progressive-titration, placebo-controlled trial. *Depress. Anxiety* 0:1–8.

Schneier, F.R. (2006) Social anxiety disorder. *N. Engl. J. Med.* 355(10): 1029–1036.

Schneier, F.R., Goetz, D., et al. (1998) Placebo-controlled trial of moclobemide in social phobia. *Br. J. Psychiatry* 172:70–77.

Schweizer, E., Rickels, K., et al. (1993) Maintenance drug treatment of panic disorder. I. Results of a prospective, placebo-controlled comparison of alprazolam and imipramine. *Arch. Gen. Psychiatry* 50(1):51–60.

Seedat, S., and Stein, M.B. (2004) Double-blind placebo-controlled assessment of combined clonazepam with paroxetine compared with paroxetine monotherapy for generalized social anxiety disorder. *J. Clin. Psychiatry* 65(2):244–248.

Sheehan, D.V., Burnham, D.B., et al. (2005) Efficacy and tolerability of controlled-release paroxetine in the treatment of panic disorder. *J. Clin. Psychiatry* 66(1):34–40.

Sheehan, D.V., Raj, A.B., et al. (1990) Is buspirone effective for panic disorder? *J. Clin. Psychopharmacol.* 10(1):3–11.

Sheehan, D.V., Raj, A.B., et al. (1993) The relative efficacy of high dose buspirone and alprazolam in the treatment of panic disorder: a double-blind placebo-controlled study. *Acta Psychiatr. Scand.* 88(1):1–11.

Simon, N.M., Worthington, J.J., et al. (2004) An open-label study of levetiracetam for the treatment of social anxiety disorder. *J. Clin. Psychiatry* 65:1219–1222.

Stahl, S.M., Gergel, I., and Li, D. (2003) Escitalopram in the treatment of panic disorder: a randomized, double-blind, placebo-controlled trial. *J. Clin. Psychiatry* 64:1322–1327.

Stein, D.J., Baldwin, D.S., Dolberg, O.T., Despiegel, N., and Bandelow, B. (2006) Which factors predict placebo response in anxiety disorders and major depression? An analysis of placebo-controlled studies of escitalopram. *J. Clin. Psychiatry* 67(11):1741–1746.

Stein, D.J., Cameron, A., et al. (2002) Moclobemide is effective and well tolerated in the long-term pharmacotherapy of social anxiety disorder with or without comorbid anxiety disorder. *Int. Clin. Psychopharmacol.* 17 (4):161–170.

Stein, D.J., Ipser, J.C., and van Balkom A.J. (2000) Pharmacotherapy for social anxiety disorder. *Cochrane Database of Systematic Reviews* Issue 4. Art. No.: CD001206. DOI: 10.1002/14651858.CD001206.pub2.

Stein, D.J., Ipser J.C., et al. (2006) Pharmacotherapy for post traumatic stress disorder (PTSD). *Cochrane Database Syst. Rev.* Issue 1: CD002795.

Stein, D.J., Versiani, M., et al. (2002) Efficacy of paroxetine for relapse prevention in social anxiety disorder: a 24-week study. *Arch. Gen. Psychiatry* 59:1111–1118.

Stein, D.J., Westenberg, H.G.M., et al. (2003) Fluvoxamine CR in the long-term treatment of social anxiety disorder: the 12- to 24-week extension phase of a multicentre, randomized, placebo-controlled trial. *Int. J. Neuropsychopharm.* 6(4):317–323.

Stein, M.B., Fyer, A.J., et al. (1999) Fluvoxamine treatment of social phobia (social anxiety disorder): a double-blind, placebo-controlled study. *Am. J. Psychiatry* 156:756–760.

Stein, M.B., Kline, N.A., and Matloff, J.L. (2002) Adjunctive olanzapine for SSRI-resistant combat-related PTSD: a double-blind, placebo-controlled study. *Am. J. Psychiatry* 159:1777–1779.

Stein, M.B., Liebowitz, M.R., et al. (1998) Paroxetine treatment of generalized social phobia (social anxiety disorder): a randomized controlled trial. *JAMA* 280(8):708–713.

Stein, M.B., Pollack, M.H., et al. (2005) Efficacy of low and higher dose extended-release venlafaxine in generalized social anxiety disorder: a 6-month randomized controlled trial. *Psychopharmacol.* 177:280–288.

Stocchi, F., Nordera, G., et al. for the Paroxetine Generalized Anxiety Disorder Study Team. (2003) Efficacy and tolerability of paroxetine for the long-term treatment of generalized anxiety disorder. *J. Clin. Psychiatry* 64(3):250–258.

Tesar, G.E., Rosenbaum, J.F., et al. (1991) Double-blind, placebo-controlled comparisons of clonzaepam and alprazolam for panic disorder. *J. Clin. Psychiatry* 52(2):69–76.

Tiller, J.W., Bouwer, C., and Behnke, K. (1999) Moclobemide and fluoxetine for panic disorder. International Panic Disorder Study Group. *Eur. Arch. Psychiatry Clin. Neurosci.* 249(Suppl 1):S7–S10.

Tucker, P., Trautman, R.P., et al. (2007) Efficacy and safety of topiramate monotherapy in civilian post-traumatic stress disorder: a randomized, double-blind, placebo-controlled study. *J. Clin. Psychiatry* 68:201–206.

Tucker, P., Zaninelli, R., Yehuda, R., Ruggiero, L., Dillingham, K., Pitts, C.D. (2001) Paroxetine in the treatment of chronic post-traumatic disorder: results of a placebo-controlled, flexible-dosage trial. *J. Clin. Psychiatry* 62:860–868.

Uhde, T.W., Stein, M.B., and Post, R.M. (1988) Lack of efficacy of carbamazepine in the treatment of panic disorder. *Am. J. Psychiatry* 145(9):1104–1109.

Van Ameringen, M., Mancini, C., et al. (2004) An open trial of topiramate in the treatment of generalized social phobia. *J. Clin. Psychiatry* 65(12):1674–1678.

Van Ameringen, M.A., Lane, R.M., et al. (2001) Sertraline treatment of generalized social phobia: a 20-week, double-blind, placebo-controlled study. *Am. J. Psychiatry* 158(2):275–281.

Van der Linden, G.J., Stein, D.J., and van Balkom, A.J. (2000) The efficacy of the selective serotonin reuptake inhibitors for social anxiety disorder (social phobia): a meta-analysis of randomized controlled trials. *Int. Clin. Psychopharmacol.* 15(Suppl 2):S15–S23.

van Vliet, I.M., den Boer, J.A., et al. (1996) A double-blind comparative study of brofaromine and fluvoxamine in outpatients with panic disorder. *J. Clin. Psychopharmacol.* 16(4):299–306.

van Vliet, I.M., den Boer, J.A., et al. (1997) Clinical effects of buspirone in social phobia: a double-blind placebo-controlled study. *J. Clin. Psychiatry* 58(4):164–168.

van Vliet, I.M., Westenberg, H.G., and Den Boer, J.A. (1993) MAO inhibitors in panic disorder: clinical effects of treatment with brofaromine. A double blind placebo controlled study. 112(4):483–489.

Wade, A.G., Lepola, U., et al. (1997) The effect of citalopram in panic disorder. *Br. J. Psychiatry* 170:549–553.

Walker, J.R., Van Ameringen, M.A., et al. (2000) Prevention of relapse in generalized social phobia: results of a 24-week study in responders to 20 weeks of sertraline treatment. *J. Clin. Psychopharm.* 20(6):636–644.

Westenberg, G.M., Stein, D.J., et al. (2004) A double-blind placebo-controlled study of controlled release fluvoxamine for the treatment of generalized social anxiety disorder. *J. Clin. Psychopharm.* 24(1):49–55.

Working Group on Panic Disorder. (1998) Practice guideline for the treatment of patients with panic disorder. *Am. J. Psychiatry* 155 (Suppl):1–34.

Zhang, W., Connor, K.M., and Davidson, J.R. (2005) Levetiracetam in social phobia: a placebo controlled pilot study. *J. Psychopharmacol.* 19(5):551–553.

VI SUBSTANCE ABUSE DISORDERS

STEVEN E. HYMAN

Abuse of and addiction to nicotine, alcohol, psychostimulants, opiates, and marijuana result in profoundly negative effects on public health and more broadly on societies. The negative effects on health result from the direct pharmacological effects of abused drugs and from the ways in which they are used—for example, smoked or injected using nonsterile needles. Disorders that all too commonly result from drug use include lung cancer, cirrhosis, hepatitis B and C, human immunodeficiency virus, and depression. Drug-related illness and lives focused on obtaining, using, and recovering from drugs entail enormous social costs in terms of lost educational opportunities, lost productivity, and failure in myriad life roles. As a result of direct pharmacological effects and illegal drug trafficking, these substances are also a major cause of violence and crime.

The chapters that follow discuss recent progress in neuroscience, behavioral neuroscience, and clinical investigation that sheds light on a very complex series of disorders and their treatment. During the past decade, progress in neuroscience at the molecular and cellular levels has accelerated rapidly (Chapter 46), and the powerful tools of modern genomics and genetics have been brought to bear on the problems of drug abuse and addiction (Chapter 47). The application of genetic engineering to mouse models has brought an important synthesis between behavioral neuroscience and more reductionist approaches (Chapter 45). More recently, mechanistic studies of brain function in animal models has informed (and been informed by) human neurobiology through the application of noninvasive neuroimaging to drugs of abuse and addictive disorders as well as to natural rewards (Chapters 49 and 50).

The search for genetic variants that contribute to the human risk of substance abuse disorders (Chapter 47) has proven extremely challenging given the difficulty of defining phenotypes and the complexity of the genetic and nongenetic contributions to risk. The combination of increasingly sophisticated genetic epidemiology with methods derived from modern genomics will likely result, in the coming decade, in the identification of multiple genetic loci that modify risk. Such discoveries will have important implications for early intervention and prevention. Even more significant, perhaps, such discoveries will provide critical tools for understanding the pathophysiology of addiction and for the identification of new protein targets in the brain for the development of pharmacological therapies. The need to develop such therapies is clear. While incremental progress continues, the development of broadly effective treatments still lags, especially for psychostimulant addiction. There is, nonetheless, a growing base of convincing data to guide treatment (Chapter 51).

The impact of drugs of abuse on the developing fetus can be dire—and all too prevalent (Chapter 48). The challenges facing investigators in this field are enormous. Although the core of research on addiction can focus on known brain reward pathways, research on the developmental effects of drugs must examine the whole brain. The relationship between the human situation and animal models is also quite complex because pregnant human drug abusers are rarely exposed only to a single drug in pure form but often expose themselves and their unborn children to multiple agents, often impure, as well as to malnutrition, high levels of stress, disturbed cycles of sleep, and other problems. Thus, using animal models that are truly informative requires that investigators think through a whole host of issues, including not only the myriad complicating factors just enumerated but also the relevance of different species to human neurobiology, the timing of drug administration during gestation, and when, during subsequent development, to look for behavioral or anatomical abnormalities.

Despite the challenges, understanding of the pathophysiology of drug abuse and addiction is further advanced than that of most other psychiatric disorders. The basis for this progress is knowledge of the initial molecular targets for virtually all classes of addictive drugs, of the neural pathways that underlie the rewarding effects of addictive drugs, and availability of useful animal models. As described by Gardner and Wise (Chapter 45) and by Nestler (Chapter 46), the major shared substrate of the reinforcing properties of addictive drugs is the dopaminergic projection that extends from the ventral tegmental area (VTA) of the midbrain to the nucleus accumbens and several regions of frontal cortex. The complex inputs and outputs of this mesoaccumbens/mesocortical brain reward pathway and drug-induced changes in the structure and function of these neurons have been critical foci of investigation for more than a decade. Although there is no standard or even fully valid animal model of addiction, the models that we do have are more compelling in terms of their face validity than models we have of essentially any other behavioral disorder. Armed with an anatomical locus and with at least partially successful animal models, a great deal of pharmacological and neurobiological investigation has been possible at a level of detail that has not been feasible for many other disease categories described in this book.

By knowing where in the brain to look, and by having the drugs that initiate behaviors of interest, it has been possible to deepen our knowledge of the short- and long-term effects of drugs of abuse on the brain (Chapter 46). This knowledge has also served to focus the neuroimaging research that can be performed on humans on relevant circuits and relevant neurochemical systems—again, an advantage compared with research on most other disease classes described in this book. Thus, Montague and Chiu can study the role of the mesoaccumbens reward circuit in regulating responses to natural rewards (Chapter 50), while Fowler and Volkow are in a position (Chapter 49) to describe not only adaptations that occur in response to drugs of abuse but also potential vulnerability factors related to brain dopamine systems. Importantly, hypotheses suggested by human imaging experiments can be applied to animal models to investigate underlying mechanisms.

Advances in neurobiology have even provided a platform for thinking about therapeutic development. The use of naltrexone and other long-acting opiate antagonists for the treatment of alcoholism follows from our increasing scientific understanding of neural adaptations to drugs of abuse and of neural circuitry contributing to reinforcement.

It is important, however, not to underestimate the remaining challenges for our basic scientific understandings and for treatment. For example, we should recognize that our existing treatment armamentarium for adults, let alone for children exposed to drugs in utero, is far from satisfactory. Overcoming the hurdles relating brain mechanisms to behavior, for example, will require increasing discourse among scientists working at different levels of analysis. In some sense, the challenges now facing the addiction research and treatment development communities presage the challenges that will face researchers on mood disorders and schizophrenia as better animal models emerge.

45 Animal Models of Addiction

ELIOT L. GARDNER AND ROY A. WISE

Most of our knowledge of the neurobiology of addiction comes from animal models. Inasmuch as addiction is a uniquely human phenomenon (animals only become truly addicted with human help), each animal model is an approximation that captures some but not all of the characteristics of the human condition. The most troublesome fact for the development of animal models is that there is no generally accepted definition of *addiction*. *Addiction* is a term usually used to describe a drug self-administration habit, but there is no single criterion that distinguishes habits that qualify as addictions from habits that do not. Thus, there are major differences of opinion as to which drugs are truly addictive. Moreover, there is no single "official" animal model of addiction. Rather, there are several animal models, each of which reflects some real or presumed aspect of the habit-forming properties of addictive drugs. Although the models differ fundamentally, both at the operational and at the theoretical levels, they each tend to identify the same major drugs, the same dose ranges, the same sites of action, and the same routes of administration as being associated with addiction liability (Wise, 1989). The most strongly addictive substances are effective in each of the several models. Because each model seems, on the surface at least, to reflect a different aspect of the habit-forming actions of addictive drugs, the most balanced picture of the abuse liability of a given drug comes from an integrated consideration of the drug's actions across the full range of models.

THEORETICAL PARADIGMS OF HABIT AND CONDITIONING

The critical property of addictive drugs is that they are habit forming. Habit has long been studied as one of the central topics of experimental psychology. Three legendary figures have established two broad paradigms for the study of habit formation and habit maintenance. The central process in theories of habit formation is the process of reinforcement. The first to identify the process that would later be given this name was Thorndike, who discussed habit formation as involving the "stamping in" of associations between responses and environmental stimuli. In his formulation of the "law of effect," Thorndike held that those actions (responses) regularly followed by a satisfying state of affairs would have their association with a given situation (stimulus) strengthened. Thorndike and Skinner eventually came to use Pavlov's term *reinforcement* to refer to the increase in response probability that accompanies the response-contingent presentation of a reward or "reinforcer." Drug rewards, like food rewards, serve as a reinforcer in the Thorndikean or Skinnerian sense; each, when presented in a response-contingent manner, increases the probability of the response habits that precede its delivery. This form of reinforcement, termed *instrumental* or *operant* reinforcement, is thought to be a core attribute of habit-forming drugs; indeed, instrumental reinforcement is seen by many as the primary, but not the only, contribution to the habits formed by drugs.

The instrumental (or operant) paradigm is focused on the behavior of an animal just prior to the presentation of the reinforcer. The reinforcer is presented if and only if the animal meets some arbitrary response criterion, such as pressing a certain lever with a certain force or running down a certain arm of a runway. The experimenter waits patiently for the animal to make the required response and, when the response is made, presents the reinforcing "stimulus." The dependent variable is the rate or probability of responding, which increases as a habit is established or "learned." This paradigm has the most obvious face validity; it most clearly represents the acquisition of a drug-seeking habit in laboratory animals.

However, it was Pavlov who first used the term and articulated the concept of *reinforcement*; Pavlov used it to refer to the stamping in of associations between unconditioned and conditioned stimuli rather than between stimuli and responses. Habit-forming drugs are reinforcers in Pavlov's as well as Skinner's sense; they establish learned preferences for various stimuli that are associated with their presentation.

In the Pavlovian paradigm, the reinforcer is given independent of the animal's behavior. The reinforcer is the unconditioned stimulus in the Pavlovian paradigm, and it is given in association with an initially neutral stimulus that comes to have significance to the animal only because of its learned association with the reinforcer.

The initially neutral stimulus comes to have significance as a "conditioned stimulus" or "conditioned reinforcer" as the association between it and the drug state develops. Skinner acknowledged Pavlov's form of reinforcement as *respondent reinforcement* and distinguished it from the instrumental (operant) reinforcement that was his and Thorndike's main interest. Skinner was the first to assert that Pavlovian and instrumental reinforcement reflected fundamentally different principles and properties.

Laboratory Models

The drug self-administration paradigm offers the most obvious animal model of addiction. Laboratory animals will self-administer several classes of addictive drugs by the oral, intragastric, intraperitoneal, intravenous, or even intracranial routes and will do so, in some cases, to the point of physiological dependence. Oral self-administration of ethanol and intravenous self-administration of heroin represent obvious analogues of human drug seeking, though physical dependence is readily demonstrated in the latter but not so readily demonstrated in the former case. In the strongest version of the model, the animal is required to work for access to the drug and not merely to ingest it. This is an instrumental conditioning paradigm, reflecting response learning, inasmuch as the drug is given in a response-contingent manner. Because the animal gets the drug if and only if it makes some arbitrary response, the injection is more reliably associated with the internal feedback from action than with any of the external stimuli that are present. In the case where the animal lever-presses for presentation of the drug, the lever-pressing is termed the *instrumental* response and the ingesting of the drug is termed the *consummatory* response. The term *consummatory* reflects the fact that the ingestive response consummates the instrumental sequence; it applies to the terminal acts in all instrumental sequences, not just to ingestion (consider, for example, the consummation of marriage). In the case where the animal lever-presses for injection of the drug, the lever-press qualifies as an instrumental and a consummatory act.

Although the drug self-administration model is most often used with fixed-ratio reinforcement contingencies, an interesting variant is one in which progressive-ratio reinforcement is used (Richardson and Roberts, 1996). In progressive-ratio drug self-administration, a progressively increasing workload is imposed upon the animal to receive a drug injection. For example, the workload may increase in a steeply incremental fashion: one lever press required for the first injection, two for the second injection, four for the third, eight for the fourth, and so on. Although typically the workload is not incremented so steeply, in every progressive-ratio drug self-administration session, a point is reached at which the animal's responding falls below some criterion level (often, an abrupt cessation of responding)—the progressive-ratio "break-point." This break-point is taken as a measure of reinforcing efficacy. Although originally developed to measure the "reward strength" of sweetened milk solutions (Hodos, 1961), progressive-ratio reinforcement schedules have since been widely used to measure the rewarding efficacy of a wide variety of addictive drugs in several animal species. Rather different estimates of drug-induced reward efficacy are obtained when progressive-ratio break-point is used in different manners—for example, incremental increases in response cost immediately following reinforcement versus incremental increases in response cost at the beginning of a discrete trial or daily test session. Psychostimulants respond preferentially to the former, opiates to the latter—evidence surely that the progressive-ratio reinforcement paradigm cannot be uniformly implemented across drug groups, and evidence perhaps that the motivation to self-administer psychostimulants versus opiates is qualitatively different (Arnold and Roberts, 1997). When implemented astutely, progressive-ratio break-point estimates of the rewarding efficacy of different classes of addictive drugs in animals parallel quite closely the verbal rank orderings of appetitiveness for different classes of addictive drugs given by experienced poly-drug abusing humans (Gardner, 2000).

The conditioned place preference paradigm reflects the ability of neutral stimuli to take on conditioned importance for the animal because of their repeated presence in the environment where intoxication is experienced. In the conditioned place preference model, the animals are given drug injections and then confined to one part of the testing apparatus on some days, whereas they are given vehicle injections then confined to another part of the testing apparatus on other days. On test days, the animals are given free choice between the two regions of the test apparatus, and the time spent in each region is measured. Drug reinforcement is reflected in an increase in the time spent in the drug-associated portion of the environment. The conditioned place preference paradigm is a Pavlovian paradigm, reflecting stimulus learning, because the drug is given in a response-independent manner, such that no particular act of the animal is consistently associated with the injection. Rather, it is a particular set of environmental stimuli that becomes associated with drug intoxication.

Several models utilize hybrid paradigms, involving instrumental and Pavlovian conditioning. The conditioned reinforcement paradigm involves animals responding instrumentally for a stimulus that has reinforcing value because of its Pavlovian association with drug reward. In the most frequently reported version of this paradigm, the animal is trained to self-administer intravenous drugs with a light flash associated with each injection. The animals are then tested in extinction conditions, where the drug reinforcer is no longer available. Here, animals given response-contingent presentations of the light stimulus will respond longer in the absence of any drug reinforcement than will animals in the absence of the light stimulus. A more convincing demonstration of conditioned reinforcement involves animals that passively receive random (response-independent) drug injections that are associated with a light stimulus. In this case, conditioned reinforcement can be demonstrated by the learning of a new instrumental response that is reinforced by the light alone. This is a hybrid paradigm because the conditioned reinforcer is established through Pavlovian conditioning but is demonstrated through instrumental responding.

An example of the conditioned reinforcement paradigm is the so-called second-order drug self-administration reinforcement schedule (Everitt and Robbins, 2000). Originally used to study the reinforcing properties of natural rewards, second-order reinforcement schedules were developed into useful tools for studying drug-induced reward in the early 1970s (e.g., Goldberg, 1973). Under a second-order reinforcement schedule, a lengthy response sequence is maintained by intermittent reinforcement by a conditioned stimulus (for example, a light flash) that has acquired reinforcing properties by virtue of previous pairing with a primary reinforcer (for example, drug). A typical second-order reinforcement schedule might, for example, require an animal to emit 50 responses to receive a light flash conditioned stimulus, with the drug primary reinforcer being given following the 10th response emitted after an hour of responding has elapsed. The obvious virtue of such reinforcement schedules is that responding for drug reinforcement can be maintained for prolonged periods prior to the actual delivery of the drug. Arguably, such responding can be termed *drug-seeking* behavior (Goldberg and Tang, 1977) rather than the "drug-taking" behavior measured by more common ratio or interval reinforcement schedules and is uncontaminated by cumulative drug effects. Under such second-order schedules, responding for drug reward has been shown to be linearly related to dose: the higher the dose, the greater the number of responses (Goldberg and Tang, 1977). This is quite different from the inverted *U*-shaped dose-response curve generated by more common reinforcement schedules, where higher doses satiate reward substrates in the brain or recruit response-inhibiting (for example, motoric) artifacts.

Of clear value to studies of addictive processes, second-order schedules have been used to dissociate neural mechanisms subserving drug-cue-controlled drug seeking from those subserving drug reward itself. Thus, lesions of the basolateral amygdala prevent the learning of cocaine self-administration under second-order reinforcement but not the learning of cocaine self-administration under continuous reinforcement (Whitelaw et al., 1996), suggesting that the basolateral amygdala is not involved in cocaine's primary rewarding effects but is critically involved in the neural processes by which cocaine-associated environmental cues drive drug-seeking behavior. Compellingly, identical conclusions about the involvement of the basolateral amygdala in cocaine-seeking behavior versus cocaine-induced primary reward were reached (Grimm and See, 2000) using the reinstatement paradigm (see below). Also seemingly clear is the value of the second-order reinforcement paradigm for studying drugs with putative therapeutic utility against cue-evoked drug-seeking behavior. Thus, BP897—an experimental drug with dopamine (DA) D_3 receptor antagonist properties (Wood et al., 2000; Wicke and Garcia-Ladona, 2001)—selectively reduces cocaine-seeking behavior as measured by second-order reinforcement but does not modify cocaine self-administration under continuous reinforcement (Pilla et al., 1999).

The cue-induced *reinstatement paradigm* is a second hybrid paradigm. In this paradigm, the animal is trained to self-administer a drug, usually intravenously, and is then subjected to extinction—that is, it is tested under conditions of nonreinforcement until the response habit appears to be "extinguished" (also a term first coined by Pavlov, who used it to describe the loss of a conditioned response when elicited repeatedly by the conditioned stimulus alone, without the "reinforcement" of the unconditioned stimulus). When the animal reaches some criterion of unresponsiveness to the instrumental manipulandum (usually the lever), various stimuli are presented and the behavior of the animal is noted. A stimulus is said to "reinstate" the drug-seeking habit if it causes renewed responding despite the absence of any further response-contingent drug reward. When the stimulus is a drug-associated conditioned stimulus, this is a hybrid paradigm because the animal is trained in the instrumental manner, with response-contingent reinforcement, but is tested in the Pavlovian manner, with potential priming stimuli presented independent of the animal's behavior. In this paradigm, effective stimuli for reinstatement of seemingly extinguished drug-seeking habits are the stimuli associated with unearned injections of the drug. Such injections are termed *priming* injections because, like the priming of a pump, they reestablish the normal, but temporarily absent, response. Also effective at reinstating seemingly extinguished drug-seeking habits in this paradigm are stress and environmental cues previously associated with the drug-taking habit (Shalev et al., 2002).

Many significant contributions to understanding the neuroanatomical substrates of relapse to drug-seeking behavior have recently been achieved using the reinstatement paradigm. The nucleus accumbens and the neurotransmitter DA appear to be essential substrates for drug triggered relapse in the reinstatement paradigm (Grimm and See, 2000; Shalev et al., 2002). The basolateral amygdala and the neurotransmitter glutamate appear to be essential substrates for cue-triggered relapse in the reinstatement paradigm (Grimm and See, 2000; Hayes et al., 2003). The central nucleus of the amygdala, bed nucleus of the stria terminalis, the lateral tegmental noradrenergic projection system, and the corticotrophin-releasing factor (CRF) projection pathways from the central nucleus of the amygdala to the bed nucleus of the stria terminalis and from an unknown origin to the ventral tegmental area appear to be substrates for stress-triggered relapse in the reinstatement paradigm (Shalev et al., 2002; Wang et al., 2005).

The brain stimulation reward paradigm can also be used to assess the reward-relevant properties of drugs of abuse; it is also, in this context, a hybrid paradigm. Most drugs of abuse have not only rewarding actions of their own but also tend to potentiate or summate with the rewarding actions of other substances or events. Cannabis is said to enhance the enjoyment of music and sex, and cannabis and alcohol are said to enhance the taste of food. Alcohol and caffeine are said to enhance the enjoyment of nicotine. The brain stimulation reward paradigm models the enhancement of a non-drug reward by a drug reward. In this paradigm, the animals are trained to respond for electrical stimulation of certain brain regions. If response-contingent stimulation is given at a variety of frequencies or intensities, response rate can be assessed as a function of these "dose" parameters, and rate-frequency or rate-intensity functions—analogues of dose-response functions in pharmacology—can be determined. A variety of drugs of abuse cause leftward shifts in these functions, suggesting summation or synergism between the reward provided by the stimulation and some related action of the drug. Inasmuch as only drugs, doses, and central sites of administration known to be rewarding in their own right cause such leftward shifts, it is assumed that it is the rewarding properties of the drugs that summate with the rewarding property of the stimulation (Wise, 1996).

The brain stimulation reward paradigm is particularly useful because the effectiveness of various doses of various drugs can be compared on a logarithmic scale that offers a yardstick of the reward-relevant efficacy of the drugs and doses. It is a hybrid paradigm because the animals respond instrumentally for the brain stimulation but receive the drug in a response-independent manner. The brain stimulation reward paradigm has characteristics that differ from drug-induced reward paradigms. For example, the pattern of responding produced by brain stimulation reward differs from the pattern of responding produced by drug reward. Similarly, extinction patterns differ markedly between the two paradigms. Also, pharmacological antagonism of reinforcement produces an initial compensatory increase in responding for drug reward but an almost immediate decrease in responding for electrical brain stimulation reward. To test the hypothesis that these differences between paradigms reflect differences in the kinetics of drug reward and electrical brain stimulation reward, Lepore and Franklin (1992) developed an interesting variant of the brain stimulation reward paradigm, using frequency-modulated trains of electrical brain stimulation that they labeled "self-administration of self-stimulation." Using this variant of the brain stimulation reward paradigm, they showed that when the kinetics of rewarding electrical brain stimulation are adjusted to emulate the kinetics of rewarding drugs, differences between brain stimulation reward and drug-induced reward essentially disappear (Lepore and Franklin, 1992).

THEORETICAL MODELS OF ADDICTION

There are, broadly speaking, two theoretical models of addiction; they are, more generally speaking, two models of motivation. The two models are polar opposites: one involves the striving for pleasure, euphoria, or some other supra-normal condition, whereas the other involves the striving to alleviate pain or discomfort or to satisfy a homeostatic need. The terms describing the motivational extremes are familiar: pleasure versus pain, reward versus punishment, the stick versus the carrot, drive versus incentive. In the first model, termed the *positive reinforcement* model, the animal is seen as striving for a treat—something special that elevates the animal's mood above the ordinary. In the subjective terms that accompany addiction theory, the drug is seen in this view as being habit forming because it produces euphoria. In the second model, termed the *negative reinforcement* model, the drug is seen as reinforcing because it terminates an aversive state, relieving the pain of injury, illness, social isolation, poverty, depression, or relieving its own withdrawal distress, and returning the animal's mood to normal.

The strength of the positive reinforcement model is that it needs no outside agent to account for the acquisition of a drug habit. The drug is viewed as a treat, something that satisfies no need of the individual but rather, like sexual gratification, is simply a source of enjoyment. If a drug serves as a positive reinforcer, that fact alone is sufficient to explain response acquisition. Indeed, response acquisition is the phenomenon that positive (instrumental) reinforcement was intended to explain. Positive reinforcement is sufficient, theoretically, to explain why an animal learns a drug-seeking habit and also why an animal maintains such a habit once it is acquired. It also is sufficient to explain why drug habits are quickly reacquired when detoxified patients are returned to situations where they have learned how to earn drugs. The weakness of the positive reinforcement model, if it has a weakness, is that it does not seem, on the surface at least, to explain why drug-seeking habits that once seemed marginal become, eventually, compulsive. The positive reinforcement theorist would answer that this is a potential characteristic of all habits involving strong reinforcement, and that even such seemingly trivial habits as not stepping on cracks can become compulsive with sufficient repetition.

The negative reinforcement model suggests that some abnormal negative state must be present before drug-seeking habits become compulsive: that the compulsivity of drug seeking in addiction results from the increasing need for the drug just to feel normal. The pure version of this model holds that it is the physiological adaptation to the drug itself that produces the need, that the need is an acquired need analogous, except for the fact that it is acquired, to the need for food. From the perspective of the negative reinforcement model, drug taking is seen as a case of self-medication: self-medication of withdrawal distress in the simple version, or, alternatively, self-medication of some preexisting problem such as illness, estrangement, grief, depression, or poverty. The weakness of the negative reinforcement model is that, unless some preexisting problem like depression, disability, or situational stress is invoked, the model requires an external explanation of how the drug-seeking habit is established. If the relief of withdrawal distress were the only explanation of drug reinforcement, then animals would never take drugs to the point of physiological dependence. A second weakness of the negative reinforcement model is that it offers little explanation of the reinstatement of drug-seeking habits when withdrawal symptoms have abated and preexisting problems have been alleviated.

Substrates of Positive Reinforcement

Portions of the neural substrates of positive reinforcement have been tentatively identified from converging evidence involving each of these models of addiction and also involving natural rewards such as food and water and the laboratory reward of direct electrical brain stimulation. The most clearly identified elements of brain reward circuitry are the mesolimbic DA system and its primary target neurons, the medium spiny neurons of nucleus accumbens and olfactory tubercle. The first evidence to implicate monoamine systems in reward function came from studies of the pharmacological modulation of brain stimulation reward: the catecholamine agonist *amphetamine* increased lever pressing for brain stimulation reward, whereas the catecholamine antagonist *chlorpromazine* and the catecholamine depleter *reserpine* each decreased it (Stein, 1962). Subsequent studies with more selective drugs implicated DA rather than the initial suspect, noradrenaline, as the critical transmitter. Selective DA blockers blocked the rewarding effects of hypothalamic brain stimulation while selective noradrenergic blockers did not (Wise, 1989). Selective DA antagonists also proved to block the rewarding effects of intravenous amphetamine (Yokel and Wise, 1975) and cocaine (de Wit and Wise, 1977) as well as the rewarding effects of food and water (Wise, 1982). Subsequent work with cocaine and other catecholamine uptake inhibitors confirms that it is the affinity for the DA transporter rather than the noradrenaline or serotonin transporter that predicts the rewarding effectiveness of these drugs in normal animals (Ritz et al., 1987).

That it is the mesolimbic and not the nigro-striatal or the mesocortical branch of the DA system that plays the most important role is suggested by several findings. First, DA-selective lesions of nucleus accumbens, the principal target of the mesolimbic system, block or attenuate the rewarding effects of cocaine and amphetamine. Second, the selective DA antagonist *spiroperidol* blocks intravenous cocaine reinforcement when injected locally in the nucleus accumbens. Although the neurotoxin-induced lesions of nucleus accumbens may have disrupted the mesocortical as well as the mesolimbic DA system, nucleus accumbens injections of spiroperidol would not. Moreover, direct injections of amphetamine into nucleus accumbens are rewarding as reflected in intracranial self-administration, in conditioned place preference, and in the ability of amphetamine to potentiate hypothalamic brain stimulation reward (for a review, see Wise, 1989).

Although the nucleus accumbens has figured strongly in the drug abuse literature, it is not the only reward-relevant DA terminal field. Cocaine is readily self-administered into the medial prefrontal cortex (Goeders and Smith, 1983), the major projection of the mesocortical DA system, and is not readily self-administered into the core of nucleus accumbens (Goeders and Smith, 1983; Carlezon et al., 1995). On the other hand, it is self-administered into the shell of nucleus accumbens (Carlezon et al., 1995) and is even more readily self-administered into the medial olfactory tubercle, an even more ventral portion of the ventral striatum (Ikemoto and Wise, 2004). Thus, it is clear that more than one DA terminal field can serve as a trigger zone for the rewarding effects of addictive drugs.

When rats are allowed to control their own intake of fixed doses of intravenous amphetamine or cocaine by lever pressing, they learn to adjust their response rate to defend their hourly amphetamine or cocaine intake (Pickens and Thompson, 1971). If the dose per injection is varied within sessions, the latency to the next response is proportional to the size of the previous dose, and if supplemental drug is slowly infused, the animals adjust their response rate in such a way as to compensate accurately (Gerber and Wise, 1989). In the case of *d*-amphetamine, the animals respond for more drug whenever their blood levels fall to 0.2 μg/ml (Yokel and Pickens, 1974). It seems unlikely that the animals are regulating these drugs independently; rather, it seems likely that they are regulating some common consequence of cocaine and amphetamine in the blood, such as nucleus accumbens DA levels. Indeed, nucleus accumbens DA levels are elevated during intravenous cocaine self-administration, and nucleus accumbens DA levels—which, of course, are correlated with intravenous cocaine levels—appear to be regulated as well (Wise et al., 1995).

Opiates also activate the mesolimbic DA system, and, again, each of the animal models points to habit-forming actions involving the activation of the mesolimbic system—opiates disinhibit the DA neurons—or direct inhibition of the medium spiny neurons of nucleus accumbens (which are similarly inhibited by DA).

Rewarding opiate actions in the ventral tegmental area have been demonstrated by intracranial morphine and mu and delta opioid self-administration, by conditioned place preference, and by potentiation of brain stimulation reward; ventral tegmental injections of mu and delta opioids also potentiate feeding (see Wise and Bozarth, 1987). The mu opioid (D-Ala^2, N-Me-Phe^4-Gly^5-ol)-enkephalin (DAMGO) is 100 times more potent as a reinforcer than is the delta opioid (D-Pen^2, D-Pen^5)-enkephalin (DPDPE) (Devine and Wise, 1994); similarly, DAMGO is 100 times more potent in potentiating brain stimulation reward, feeding, and, as measured by nucleus accumbens microdialysis, DA release (Devine et al., 1993). Moreover, ventral tegmental injections of opioid antagonists attenuate the rewarding efficacy of intravenous heroin (Bozarth and Wise, 1986). The habit-forming actions of ventral tegmental opiates appear to involve the disinhibition of dopaminergic cell firing; mu opioids act to inhibit γ-aminobutyric acid (GABA)ergic neurons that normally provide tonic inhibition of their dopaminergic neighbors (Johnson and North, 1992).

Opiates also have habit-forming effects in nuclus accumbens itself. Morphine is self-administered directly into this nucleus (Olds, 1982), and morphine injections into this nucleus cause conditioned place preference (van der Kooy et al., 1982). Mu and delta opioids injected into this nucleus also potentiate the rewarding effects of lateral hypothalamic brain stimulation, and opioid antagonists injected into this nucleus can attenuate the rewarding effects of intravenous heroin (Vaccarino et al., 1985). The rewarding actions of opiates in nucleus accumbens appear to be due to the direct inhibition of medium spiny neurons; mu and delta opiates infused into nucleus accumbens itself do not alter local DA levels, whereas kappa agonists decrease local DA levels (Spanagel et al., 1990).

It is not clear whether it is the ventral tegmental area or the nucleus accumbens that plays the more dominant role in the rewarding effects of intravenous heroin, but it is clear that self-administered intravenous heroin is sufficient to elevate nucleus accumbens DA (Devine et al., 1993). As with the case of intravenous cocaine self-administration (Wise et al., 1995), intravenous heroin self-administration is initiated when DA levels fall to some critical "trigger point" that is well above normal resting DA levels.

Nucleus accumbens medium spiny neurons also seem important for the habit-forming effects of phencyclidine. Phencyclidine is self-administered directly into nucleus accumbens (Carlezon and Wise, 1996a), where it also facilitates the rewarding effects of lateral hypothalamic brain stimulation (Carlezon and Wise, 1996b). Despite the fact that phencyclidine is, like cocaine and nomifensine, a DA uptake inhibitor, the rewarding effects of nucleus accumbens injections of phencyclidine are, unlike the rewarding effects of nucleus accumbens nomifensine, unaffected by coadministration of the DA antagonist *sulpiride* (Carlezon and Wise, 1996a). Moreover, the habit-forming effects of phencyclidine are shared by dizocilpine and (±)-3-2-carboxypiperazin-4-yl propyl-1-phosphonic acid (CPP), drugs that block *N*-methyl-D-aspartate (NMDA) receptors, as does phencyclidine, but that do not share with phencyclidine the ability to block DA uptake. Thus, the habit-forming effects of phencyclidine appear to be DA independent and depend instead on the blockade of NMDA-type glutamate receptors. Nucleus accumbens medium spiny neurons receive glutamatergic input from a variety of sites, and glutamate normally excites medium spiny neurons. Thus, NMDA antagonists have the same net effect on the output of nucleus accumbens output neurons as do elevated DA levels; whereas DA decreases nucleus accumbens output by inhibiting medium spiny neuron firing, NMDA antagonists appear to do so by blocking tonic excitatory input to the medium spiny neurons.

The mesolimbic DA system is also activated by nicotine and ethanol; although the mechanism of ethanol's action is not known, nicotine receptors are known to be localized to mesolimbic DA neurons (Clarke and Pert, 1985). Ventral tegmental injections of a nicotinic agonist cause conditioned place preferences (Museo and Wise, 1994). Blockade of ventral tegmental nicotinic receptors does not itself alter brain stimulation reward, but it blocks the ability of nicotine to do so (Wise et al., 1998). Cannabis, too, enhances brain stimulation reward (Gardner et al., 1988) and elevates nucleus accumbens DA (Chen et al., 1990), and may be habit forming for this reason. Conditioned place preference for cannabinoid-paired environments has been reported (Lepore et al., 1995; Valjent and Maldonado, 2000; Braida et al., 2001), although contrary findings exist (for a review, see Gardner, 2002). Cannabinoid self-administration in laboratory animals has also recently been reported (Martellotta et al., 1998; Ledent et al., 1999; Tanda et al., 2000; Justinova et al., 2003; for a review, see Justinova, Goldberg, et al., 2005), as has self-administration of the endogenous cannabinoid anandamide (Justinova, Solinas, et al., 2005).

There has been considerable recent attention to the fact that subregions of the ventral striatum have different afferent and efferent connections. The core of nucleus accumbens is similar in this regard to the overlying caudate, whereas the shell of the nucleus accumbens and the olfactory tubercle have similarities to the central amygdala and have been identified as part of the "extended" amygdala. Intracranial self-administration of phencyclidine, dizocilpine, CPP, and nomifensine occurs preferentially with shell and not core injections of the drugs (Carlezon et al., 1995; Carlezon and Wise, 1996a), and intracranial self-administration of cocaine occurs preferentially with olfactory tubercle and, to a lesser extent, shell injections (Ikemoto, 2003).

The medial prefrontal cortex also appears to play a role in drug reward. In addition to cocaine (Goeders and Smith, 1983), phencyclidine, dizocilpine, and CPP are self-administered into this region (Carlezon and Wise, 1996a). The mechanism of action has not yet been identified.

Substrates of Physical Dependence

It has long been assumed that the compulsive drug self-administration accompanying true addiction results from adaptations in the nervous system resulting from chronic drug exposure. These adaptations are evident during intoxication only insomuch as they reduce the effectiveness of the drug that produces them; they are drug-opposite adaptations and thus the theories of addiction in which such adaptations figure prominently are termed *opponent-process* theories. This phrase was coined by Solomon and Corbit (1974), but it applies to all of the classic theories of drug dependence.

The most dramatic dependence signs accompany withdrawal from predominantly depressant drugs like opiates, alcohol, barbiturates, and benzodiazepines. The drug-opposite withdrawal symptoms in these cases are signs of hyperexcitability; animals withdrawn from these drugs are agitated and hyperactive, and they are abnormally susceptible to epileptic seizures. Although this hyperexcitable state is not pleasant and can be alleviated by self-administration of the responsible drug, it seems unlikely that the distress of these signs is a powerful source of the motivation to compulsively self-administer drug. Indeed, the experimental manipulations that maximize the classic alcohol withdrawal syndrome are manipulations that minimize voluntary alcohol consumption in laboratory animals, and the manipulations that maximize voluntary consumption are incompatible with physiological dependence (Wise, 1974). Moreover, the brain sites (and, indeed, peripheral autonomic sites) at which opiates induce the neuroadaptations associated with classic withdrawal signs are anatomically distant from the sites at which opiates trigger their habit-forming consequences (Bozarth and Wise, 1984). Finally, the psychomotor activation associated with opiate, alcohol, barbiturate, and benzodiazepine withdrawal result from neuroadaptations opposite in fundamental nature to the psychomotor depression associated with cocaine and amphetamine withdrawal. Thus, the classic autonomic and central signs of withdrawal from depressant drugs do not offer a unifying hypothesis of addiction (Wise and Bozarth, 1987).

Dependence theory does not necessarily rest, however, on classic withdrawal symptoms. Any one of the multiple neuroadaptations resulting from chronic drug use could serve as a predisposing factor in the compulsive drug craving of addicts. Recent interest has focused on drug-opposite changes in the brain pathways that mediate the rewarding effects of drugs of abuse. Even depressant drugs such as opiates, alcohol, barbiturates, and benzodiazepines have psychomotor stimulant properties that are associated with drug reward (Wise and Bozarth, 1987). Rebound depression of the reward pathways appears to reflect neuroadaptations to chronic intoxication of much greater relevance to drug self-administration than are the traditional withdrawal symptoms of classic addiction theory (Koob and Bloom, 1988).

The notion that the reward systems of the brain undergo rebound depression after treatment with addictive drugs was first articulated by Leith and Barrett (1976), who found that brain stimulation reward thresholds were elevated following chronic dosing with amphetamine. Similarly, brain stimulation reward thresholds are elevated following withdrawal from chronic cocaine treatment, and such elevations can be demonstrated after self-administered doses of cocaine (Markou and Koob, 1991). Moreover, similar elevations can be demonstrated during spontaneous or precipitated opiate withdrawal states. Thus, depression of brain reward mechanisms offers a possible common denominator bridging the withdrawal symptoms associated with the opiates and the less dramatic signs of dependence associated with the psychomotor stimulants.

A number of neurochemical correlates of stimulant and opiate withdrawal have been identified. Among the first to be suggested was DA depletion. Although it was depletion of intracellular DA that was first posited by Dackis and Gold (1985) as a correlate of withdrawal from chronic cocaine treatment, it is depletion of extracellular DA that has been reported following withdrawal of chronic cocaine, amphetamine, morphine, and alcohol. In addition, a number of intracellular changes have been identified in the mesolimbic DA system and in the medium spiny neurons of nucleus accumbens during withdrawal from cocaine, opiates, and alcohol (Self and Nestler, 1995). These changes are associated with alterations of intracellular signaling functions and go beyond the up- or down-regulation of receptors once hypothesized as the basis for changes in drug sensitivity during the development of tolerance and dependence and are more consistent with hypotheses involving enzyme and second-messenger alterations (Goldstein and Goldstein, 1961; Collier, 1980). In each case, the anatomical locus of the changes under current investigation is the diencephalic reward circuitry associated with the rewarding effects of the drugs.

Contributions to Knowledge from Animal Models

The study of animal models of addiction has contributed a number of insights into the nature of the human condition. First, it reveals that all mammalian species are probably susceptible to the habit-forming effects of opiates and psychomotor stimulants. Thus, it suggests that recreational use of these agents offers a significant risk for most if not all individuals. Given in strong doses and by rapid routes of administration, these drugs have robust actions on biologically primitive circuitry in the brain, and their self-administration is likely to lead to compulsive drug-seeking habits. The animal literature makes it clear that craving is a conditioned response because the drug solution has no distal sensory properties that are evident to the animal (it is usually neither visible nor detectable by smell). Thus, the significance of the place in the environment where the drug is experienced and of the manipulandum that allows the animal to earn injections or drug presentations must be learned by association with the drug state and not with the external stimulus properties of the drug. The instrumental response (for example, lever pressing) that delivers the drug must be learned, and it can be reinstated by the stimulus properties of the drug itself or by stimuli that have been paired with the drug as well as by some forms of stress (Shaham and Stewart, 1995). Animal self-administration studies have made it clear that physiological dependence is not a necessary condition for compulsive drug-seeking behavior, even in the case of drugs like opiates that are associated with a clear and robust dependence syndrome (Bozarth and Wise, 1984). Animal studies have shown, however, that drug-opposite neuroadaptations occur—within the reward pathways themselves—as a result of self-administered doses of addictive drugs. The effects of each of these neuroadaptations on the rewarding impact of the drugs that produce them remain to be fully identified.

Animal studies also reveal that there are individual differences in the likelihood of initiation of drug self-administration, and they suggest that deprivation states and environmental choices can influence the amount of drug self-administration. Such studies underscore the obvious fact that these differences and influences are most evident when marginal doses (for example, ED_{50}) and routes of administration (for example, oral) are offered.

Use of Animal Models in the Search for Effective Treatments for Addiction

As useful as animal models have been and continue to be in elucidating the neurobiological substrates of addiction, they have also in recent years been put to a more classically pragmatic and practical use in medicine—as screening tools in the search for effective treatments for drug addiction. We illustrate this utility by citing the recent and continuing use of animal models in the identification and development of possible pharmacotherapies for addiction based on three different pharmacotherapeutic strategies.

The development of slow-onset long-acting DA transporter blockers is one such strategy. It is based on the hypothesis that vulnerability to addictive drugs may derive, at least in part, from a pathological hypofunctionality of DA neurons in the reward-related meso-accumbens dopaminergic projection system (for reviews, see Gardner, 1999, and Volkow, Fowler, and Wang, 1999; see also Nestler, 1993; Volkow, Wang, et al. 1999; Volkow et al., 2001). On the basis of this hypothesis, a number of approaches have been taken to the discovery and development of selective and potent DA transporter blockers that may serve as developmental templates for anticocaine-addiction pharmacotherapeutic agents (Rothman and Glowa, 1995). A wide variety of structural classes have served as such chemical templates for the development of potential therapeutic agents for cocaine addiction, including cocaine analogues (Carroll et al., 1992), tropanes (Madras et al., 1989), benzotropines (Meltzer et al., 1994; Newman et al., 1994), mazindol (Aeberli et al., 1975; Berger et al., 1989), substituted piperazines (Andersen, 1987; Berger et al., 1985; Bonnet et al., 1986; Hsin et al., 2002), indanamines (Froimowitz et al., 2000), and trans-aminotetralines (Welch et al., 1984; Froimowitz et al., 2000).

The rapidity with which an addictive drug reaches the brain and elevates nucleus accumbens DA levels appears to correlate positively with addictive potency (Oldendorf, 1992; Volkow et al., 1995). Conversely, slow onset or prolonged duration appears to confer lower reinforcing efficacy. Thus, the cocaine analogue 2β-propanoyl-3β-(4-tolyl)-tropane (PTT), a selective DA reuptake blocker with a slower onset and much longer duration of action than cocaine, does not support intravenous self-administration under fixed-interval reinforcement in rhesus monkeys (Nader et al., 1997). Congruently, the phenyltropane analog 3β-(4-chlorophenyl)tropane-2β-carboxylic acid phenyl ester (RTI-113), which has a cocaine-like rapid onset but a much longer duration of action, supports much lower intravenous self-administration in monkeys than does cocaine, despite markedly higher DA receptor occupancy by RTI-113 (99%) than by cocaine (65%) (Howell et al., 2000). In addition, several benzotropine analogues with slower pharmacokinetic properties than cocaine maintain only low rates of intravenous self-administration in rhesus monkeys even though the compounds have substantially higher affinities than cocaine at the DA transporter (Woolverton et al., 2000). Therefore, a major emphasis in the slow-onset long-acting DA transporter blocker medication discovery and development strategy has been on the development of compounds producing slow enhancement of nucleus accumbens DA, having long duration, and showing a slow deactivation profile.

Animal models have proven useful in the preclinical screening and development of such compounds. Thus, PTT decreases intravenous cocaine self-administration in rhesus monkeys on a fixed-interval cocaine reinforcement schedule, assessed in terms of decreased response rates and decreased total cocaine intake per test session (Nader et al., 1997). Congruently, 1-[2-[bis(4-fluorophenyl-)methoxy]ethyl]-4-(3-phenylpropyl)piperazine (GBR-12909) dose-dependently decreases cocaine self-administration in rhesus monkeys under multiple fixed-ratio schedules of cocaine and food reinforcement (Glowa, Wojnicki, Matecka, Bacher, et al., 1995), with significant reductions in cocaine self-administration obtained at GBR-12909 doses that had little or no effect on food self-administration (Villemange et al., 1999; Schenk, 2002). However, GBR-12909's selectivity for reducing cocaine self-administration versus food self-administration was seen only at low unit doses of cocaine (Glowa, Wojnicki, Matecka, Bacher, et al., 1995). On the other hand, repeated treatment with lower GBR-12909 doses appears to sustain the selective suppression of cocaine self-administration versus food self-administration (Glowa, Wojnicki, Matecka, Rice, and Rothman, 1995). Taken with the report that GBR-12909 attenuates cocaine-induced meso-accumbens extracellular DA enhancement in rats (Baumann et al., 1994), the suggestion that development of long-acting GBR-12909 analogues may yield useful compounds for treating cocaine addiction appears rational. This line of development has yielded several long-acting piperazine analogues (including decanoate ester depot formulations) that decrease cocaine self-administration in selective and sustained fashion in monkeys and augment extracellular nucleus accumbens DA in slow-onset, sustained fashion in laboratory rats (Glowa et al., 1996; Lewis et al., 1999; Hsin et al., 2002; see review by Howell and Wilcox, 2001).

Illustrating the use of second-order schedules to infer "drug-seeking" behavior in such medication development schemes, the long-acting phenyltropane analogue RTI-113 has been reported to decrease cocaine self-administration in squirrel monkeys under second-order reinforcement (Howell et al., 2000). Indanamine analogues have also been developed as potential anti-addiction medications using some of the animal models discussed in this chapter (Froimowitz et al., 2000). Thus, several slow-onset, long-acting indanamine analogue DA transporter blockers have been shown to enhance nucleus accumbens in slow-onset long-duration fashion (Gardner et al., 2006), enhance electrical brain-stimulation reward (Gardner et al., 2006), and decrease intravenous cocaine self-administration (Gardner et al., 2006) in laboratory rats, while being devoid of the ability to sustain self-administration themselves (Gardner et al., 2006). Provocatively, the protective effects of at least some of these indanamine analogues against intravenous cocaine self-administration may be most pronounced in genetic strains of rats most prone to high levels of cocaine self-administration (Froimowitz et al., 1999). Trans-aminotetraline derivatives have also been tested using animal models discussed in this chapter, with preliminarily promising results. Slow-onset long-duration enhancement of extracellular nucleus accumbens DA, electrical brain-stimulation reward, and dose-dependent reductions in cocaine self-administration have all been observed (Peng et al., 2005; Peng et al., 2006).

The development of GABAmimetic compounds acting specifically at the $GABA_B$ receptor is another such strategy. It is based on the following facts: (*1*) GABAergic afferents heavily innervate and modulate neural tone within the ventral tegmental area (Kalivas et al., 1990; Klitenick et al., 1992; Kalivas et al., 1993; Sesack and Pickel, 1995) and nucleus accumbens (Christie et al., 1987; Kiyatkin and Rebec, 1999; Meredith, 1999; Yan, 1999; Ward et al., 2000); (*2*) the GABAergic medium spiny output neurons from the accumbens have been proposed to constitute a brain reward final common output path (Carlezon and Wise, 1996a); (*3*) pharmacological modulation of GABAergic tone can affect mesoaccumbens brain-reward functions (Nazzaro and Gardner, 1980); (*4*) microinjections of the $GABA_B$ receptor agonist baclofen into the ventral tegmental area block mu opiate-agonist-induced enhancement of DA release in nucleus accumbens (Kalivas et al., 1990), suggesting that activation of $GABA_B$ receptors on DA perikarya inhibits mesoaccumbens dopaminergic reward functions; and (*5*) acquisition and expression of a conditioned emotional response are accompanied by increased nucleus accumbens GABA levels, and hippocampal lesions attenuate both the enhanced accumbens GABA levels and the expression of the conditioned emotional response (Saul'skaya and Gorbachevskaya, 1999).

On the basis of these kinds of data, several of the animal models discussed in this chapter have been used to investigate the possibility that GABAmimetic compounds (especially those targeted at the $GABA_B$ receptor) may have potential as antiaddiction pharmacotherapies. Some of this work has focused on the irreversible GABA transaminase inhibitor gamma-vinyl-GABA (GVG). Gamma-aminobutyric acid transaminase is the primary enzyme involved in the metabolic catabolism of GABA. Gamma-vinyl-GABA, by interfering with this process, significantly enhances brain GABA levels (Jung et al., 1977). As the enhanced GABA is stored within axon terminals and only released during synaptic transmission, GVG preferentially enhances physiologically relevant brain GABA levels (Mattson et al., 1995). GVG dose-dependently attenuates the enhanced nucleus accumbens DA overflow produced by cocaine (Dewey et al., 1997; Dewey et al., 1998; Morgan and Dewey, 1998), nicotine (Dewey et al., 1999; Schiffer et al., 2000), methamphetamine (Gerasimov et al., 1999), heroin (Gerasimov et al., 1999; Xi and Stein, 2000), ethanol (Gerasimov et al., 1999), or a cocaine/heroin ("speedball") combination (Gerasimov and Dewey, 1999).

The effects of GVG on cocaine-enhanced nucleus accumbens DA are mimicked by GVG's cyclized analogue (a competitive reversible GABA transaminase inhibitor) and by the GABA reuptake inhibitor NNC-711 (Gerasimov et al., 2000). Provocatively, GVG also antagonizes the augmented nucleus accumbens DA produced by environmental cues previously associated with cocaine administration (Gerasimov et al., 2001). When GVG is coadministered intravenously with heroin or microinjected into either the ventral tegmental area or nucleus accumbens, it dose-dependently reduces heroin's reinforcing efficacy, as indicated by compensatory increases in unit heroin self-administration (Xi and Stein, 2000). At higher doses of GVG, a complete blockade of intravenous heroin (Knapp et al., 1999; Xi and Stein, 2000) or cocaine (Kushner et al., 1999) self-administration is seen. Similar effects on heroin self-administration are produced by the reversible GABA transaminase inhibitors aminooxy-acetic acid (AOAA) or ethanolamine-O-sulfate (EOS), and the GABA reuptake inhibitors (±)-nipecotic acid or NO-711 (Xi and Stein, 2000). Gamma-vinyl-GABA also lowers the progressive-ratio break point for intravenous cocaine self-administration (Kushner et al., 1999). Gamma-vinyl-GABA also attenuates cocaine's enhancement of electrical brain-stimulation reward (Kushner et al., 1997). Gamma-vinyl-GABA's inhibition of cocaine-induced DA elevations in the nucleus accumbens is antagonized by the selective $GABA_B$ antagonist SCH-50911 (Ashby et al., 1999), implicating the $GABA_B$ receptor in GVG's potential antiaddiction effects. Recently, GVG has been shown to inhibit cocaine-triggered relapse to drug-seeking behavior using the reinstatement model (Peng et al., 2004; Peng et al., 2006; Peng et al., in press; Filip et al., 2007) but fails to inhibit cocaine's discriminative stimulus effects (Barrett et al., 2005). Provocatively, local nucleus accumbens microinjections of $GABA_A$ or $GABA_B$ receptor agonists, but not GABA itself, inhibit extracellular nucleus accumbens DA and glutamate (Xi and Stein, 1998, 1999; Xi et al., 2003) and similarly inhibit cocaine or heroin self-administration and reinstatement of drug-seeking behavior (Xi and Stein, 1999; McFarland et al., 2003), raising questions about the neural substrates underlying GVG's demonstrated actions in animal models. Nonetheless, GVG has moved forward to preliminary clinical trials in humans with promising results (Brodie, Figueroa, and Dewey, 2003; Brodie, Figueroa, Laska, and Dewey 2003), a step that would have been of very low probability without the preceding extensive preclinical investigations using animal models.

Similar work has focused on the selective $GABA_B$ agonist baclofen. Baclofen produces a dose-dependent reduction in progressive ratio break points for intravenous cocaine self-administration (Roberts et al., 1996; Brebner et al., 2000). Baclofen's protective effect against cocaine self-administration was also examined using a discrete trials procedure, which permits measurements of circadian patterns of self-administration (Roberts and Andrews, 1997). Regardless of the time of light onset, maximum cocaine intake occurred during the final 6 hours of the dark period and was followed by a period of relative abstinence from cocaine self-administration during the light phase. This highly predictable behavioral pattern of self-administration allowed observation of baclofen's effect on initiation of cocaine self-administration. Baclofen treatment suppressed cocaine self-administration for at least 4 hours without having any significant effect on operant responding for food self-administration (Roberts and Andrews, 1997). When cocaine was self-administered on a simple fixed ratio (FR1) reinforcement schedule, baclofen suppressed intake of low but not high unit doses of cocaine (Brebner et al., 2000). The baclofen-induced suppression of low-dose cocaine intake was characterized by long pauses in the cocaine self-administration pattern—in contrast to DA antagonist-induced suppression of cocaine self-administration, which is characterized by altered distribution of interinfusion intervals for cocaine. Recently, baclofen pretreatment has been shown to dose-dependently reduce cocaine-enhanced extracellular nucleus accumbens DA (Fada et al., 2003), cocaine-enhanced electrical brain-stimulation reward (Slattery et al., 2005), cocaine-seeking behavior under second-order reinforcement (Di Ciano and Everitt, 2003), and cocaine-triggered relapse to drug-seeking behavior in the reinstatement model (Campbell et al., 1999; Weerts et al., 2007).

The novel and highly selective $GABA_B$ agonist CGP-44532 shows a baclofen-like profile of protection against cocaine self-administration, that is, a dose-dependent decrease in progressive ratio break point for cocaine self-administration, a dose-dependent suppression of initiation of cocaine intake in the discrete trials procedure, and a failure to disrupt operant responding for food (Brebner et al., 1999). Baclofen also appears to protect against opiate self-administration (Xi and Stein, 1999). Baclofen coadministration with intravenous heroin inhibits development of heroin self-administration in drug-naïve rats, and maintenance of heroin self-administration behavior in heroin-experienced rats. In addition, microinjections of baclofen into the ventral tegmental area reduce heroin-induced enhancement of extracellular DA in the nucleus accumbens (Xi and Stein, 1999). This effect was significantly attenuated by microinjections of the $GABA_B$ antagonist 2-hydroxysaclofen into the ventral tegmental area. On the basis of such findings with animal models, augmentation of brain GABA-ergic function—mediated through the $GABA_B$ receptor—may be a rational strategy to pursue at the human level for the pharmacotherapeutic treatment of drug addiction. Preliminary recent clinical trials of baclofen in human patients appear promising (Ling et al., 1998; Shoptaw et al., 2003; Haney et al., 2006; but see Lile et al., 2004).

A third medication development strategy for possible addiction treatment that owes its existence to the animal models discussed in this chapter is that of DA D_3 receptor antagonists. This strategy is based on the following: (*1*) the hypothesis that mesoaccumbens dopaminergic hypofunctionality may contribute to addiction vulnerability; (*2*) the fact that the DA D_3 receptor shows preferential localization in the mesocorticolimbic system (Levant, 1998; Suzuki et al., 1998); (*3*) the suggestion that D_3 receptor inhibition may activate the mesoaccumbens DA system (Nissbrandt et al., 1995; Ashby et al., 2000); and (*4*) the suggestion that the D_3 receptor plays a role in emotional, motivational, and reinforcement functions, including the reinforcement produced by addictive drugs (Caine and Koob, 1993; Parsons et al., 1996; Pilla et al., 1999). These considerations have prompted the study of compounds acting on the DA D_3 receptor system in animal models of addiction. Such studies were initially hampered by lack of D_3-selective compounds, until the development of trans-N-[4-[2-(6-cyano-1,2,3,4-tetrahydroisoquinolin-2-yl) ethyl]cyclohexyl]-4-quinolininecarboxamide (SB-277011A), a novel brain-penetrant, highly selective D_3 receptor antagonist (Reavill et al., 2000; Stemp et al., 2000). SB-277011A has high affinity for human and rat D_3 receptors, with an 80- to 100-fold selectivity over DA D_2 receptors and 180 other central nervous system receptors, enzymes, and ion channels (Reavill et al., 2000; Heidbreder et al., 2005; C.A. Heidbreder et al., 2007, unpublished data). Also, SB-277011A readily enters the brain after systemic administration in laboratory rodents (Reavill et al., 2000; Stemp et al., 2000).

In preclinical animal tests with many of the addiction models described in this chapter, SB-277011A shows a highly promising profile (see review by Heidbreder et al., 2005). Specifically, SB-277011A attenuates cocaine- or methamphetamine-enhanced electrical brain-stimulation reward (Vorel et al., 2002; Spiller et al., 2008); dose-dependently attenuates acquisition and expression of cocaine-induced conditioned place preference (Vorel et al., 2002); attenuates the acquisition and expression of heroin-induced conditioned place preference (Ashby et al., 2003); produces a pronounced down-shift in the break point (that is, reduces motivation) for intravenous cocaine or methamphetamine self-administration under progressive-ratio reinforcement conditions (Xi et al., 2005; Higley et al., 2007); attenuates cocaine-seeking behavior under second-order reinforcement conditions (Everitt et al., 2001; Di Ciano et al.,

2003); dose-dependently attenuates cocaine-triggered, stress-triggered, or environmental cue-triggered relapse to cocaine-seeking behavior in the reinstatement paradigm (Vorel et al., 2002; Cervo et al., 2003; Xi et al., 2004; Gilbert et al., 2005; Gál and Gyertyán, 2006); attenuates incubation of cocaine craving (Xi et al., 2007); attenuates nicotine-enhanced electrical brain-stimulation reward (Pak et al., 2006); attenuates nicotine-induced conditioned place preference (Pak et al., 2006); attenuates nicotine-paired environmental cue-induced locomotor activation (Pak et al., 2006); and attenuates ethanol self-administration in laboratory rats (Thanos et al., 2005) and mice (Heidbreder et al., 2007). Corroborative evidence that SB-277011A's remarkably broad profile of antiaddiction properties in such a wide variety of preclinical animal models is due to its DA D_3 receptor antagonist properties, rather than to some other idiosyncratic pharmacological property, is based upon the similar pattern of animal model findings from another highly selective DA D_3 receptor antagonist—NGB-2904 (see, e.g., Xi et al., 2006; for review, see Xi and Gardner, 2007). Arguably, SB-277011A has been shown to have a promising antiaddiction profile in a broader range of addiction-related animal models than any other putative pharmacotherapeutic agent in the history of addiction medicine (for reviews, see Heidbreder et al., 2004; Heidbreder et al., 2005), although GVG and baclofen have also been screened in a broad array of animal models (see above). On a cautionary note, SB-277011A does not attenuate intravenous cocaine self-administration under low-effort (that is, low fixed-ratio reinforcement) or high payoff (large amounts of cocaine per reinforcement) conditions (Vorel et al., 2002; Gál and Gyertyán, 2003; Xi et al., 2005). Despite this caution, the overall profile of SB-277011A's effects in the animal models of addiction in which it has been tested is highly suggestive of potential utility for DA D_3 antagonists as anti-addiction pharmacotherapies. Further development of SB-277011A itself has been halted due to unexpectedly poor bioavailability and short half-life in primates (Austin et al., 2001; Remington and Kapur, 2001). However, the preclinical animal model evidence for presumptive antiaddiction efficacy of high-affinity high-selectivity DA D_3 receptor antagonists is so extensive that development of other D_3-selective antagonists with better bioavailability and more promising pharmacokinetic profiles continues (see, e.g., Newman et al., 2005).

Caveats Regarding Animal Models

What animal studies do not reveal, except by contrast, is the importance of language and cultural influences in human drug self-administration. One animal apparently cannot learn from another's death that recreational drug use can be dangerous; they cannot be told that "speed kills." Nor are singly caged animals influenced by peer pressure, advertising, or warnings from the surgeon general. These aspects of human drug experience are not modeled in animal studies, though they and human intelligence play an important role in human drug self-administration. What animal models can tell us about is our common biological heritage, and about the pharmacological impact of addictive substances on the mammalian species that share that heritage. Thus, they are useful tools of construct validity in the study of the underlying mechanisms—neurobiological and psychological—of addictive processes. To the extent that animal models may also have either face or predictive validity to human addiction, they may also be useful in the search for new and effective treatments for addiction at the human level, and are routinely so used in present-day addiction medicine research.

ACKNOWLEDGMENTS

Preparation of this chapter was supported by the Intramural Research Program, National Institute on Drug Abuse, National Institutes of Health.

REFERENCES

Aeberli, P., Eden, P., Gogerty, J.H., Houlihan, W.J., and Penberthy, C. (1975) 5-Aryl-2,3-dihydro-5*H*-imidazo[2,1-*a*]isoindol-5-ols. A novel class of anorectic agents. *J. Med. Chem.* 18:177–182.

Andersen, P.H. (1987) Biochemical and pharmacological characterization of [^{3}H]GBR-12935 binding in vitro to rat striatal membranes: labeling of the dopamine uptake complex. *J. Neurochem.* 48:1887–1896.

Arnold, J.M., and Roberts, D.C.S. (1997) A critique of fixed and progressive ratio schedules used to examine the neural substrates of drug reinforcement. *Pharmacol. Biochem. Behav.* 57:441–447.

Ashby, C.R., Jr., Minabe, Y., Stemp, G., Hagan, J.J., and Middlemiss, D.N. (2000) Acute and chronic administration of the selective D_3 receptor antagonist SB-277011-A alters activity of midbrain dopamine neurons in rats: an in vivo electrophysiological study. *J. Pharmacol. Exp. Ther.* 294:1166–1174.

Ashby, C.R., Jr., Paul, M., Gardner, E.L., Heidbreder, C.A., and Hagan, J.J. (2003) Acute administration of the selective D_3 receptor antagonist SB-277011A blocks the acquisition and expression of the conditioned place preference response to heroin in male rats. *Synapse* 48:154–156.

Ashby, C.R., Jr., Rohatgi, R., Ngosuwan, J., Borda, T., Gerasimov, M.R., Morgan, A.E., Kushner, S., Brodie, J.D., and Dewey, S.L. (1999) Implication of the $GABA_B$ receptor in gamma vinyl-GABA's inhibition of cocaine-induced increases in nucleus accumbens dopamine. *Synapse* 31:151–153.

Austin, N.E., Baldwin, S.J., Cutler, L., Deeks, N., Kelly, P.J., Nash, M., Shardlow, C.E., Stemp, G., Thewlis, K.M., Ayrton, A., and Jeffrey, P. (2001) Pharmacokinetics of the novel, high-affinity and selective dopamine D3 receptor antagonist SB-277011 in rat, dog and monkey: *in vitro/in vivo* correlation and the role of aldehyde oxidase. *Xenobiotica* 31:677–686.

Barrett, A.C., Negus, S.S., Mello, N.K., and Caine S.B. (2005) Effect of GABA agonists and GABA-A receptor modulators on cocaine- and food-maintained responding and cocaine discrimination in rats. *J. Pharmacol. Exp. Ther.* 315:858–871.

Baumann, M.H., Char, G.U., de Costa, B.R., Rice, K.C., and Rothman, R.B. (1994) GBR 12909 attenuates cocaine-induced activation of mesolimbic dopamine neurons in the rat. *J. Pharmacol. Exp. Ther.* 271:1216–1222.

Berger, P., Gawin, F., and Kosten, T.R. (1989) Treatment of cocaine abuse with mazindol. *Lancet* 1:283.

Berger, P., Janowsky, A., Vocci, F., Skolnick, P., Schweri, M., and Paul, S.M. (1985) [^{3}H]GBR-12935: a specific high affinity ligand for labeling the dopamine transport complex. *Eur. J. Pharmacol.* 107:289–290.

Bonnet, J.J., Protais, P., Chagraoui, A., and Costentin, J. (1986) High affinity [^{3}H]GBR 12783 binding to a specific site associated with the neuronal dopamine uptake complex in the central nervous system. *Eur. J. Pharmacol.* 126:211–222.

Bozarth, M.A., and Wise, R.A. (1984) Anatomically distinct opiate receptor fields mediate reward and physical dependence. *Science* 224:516–518.

Bozarth, M.A., and Wise, R.A. (1986) Involvement of the ventral tegmental dopamine system in opioid and psychomotor stimulant reinforcement. *NIDA Res. Monogr.* 67:190–196.

Braida, D., Pozzi, M., Cavallini, R., and Sala, M. (2001) Conditioned place preference induced by the cannabinoid agonist CP 55,940: interaction with the opioid system. *Neuroscience* 104:923–926.

Brebner, K., Froestl, W., Andrews, M., Phelan, R., and Roberts, D. C.S. (1999) The $GABA_B$ agonist CGP 44532 decreases cocaine self-administration in rats: demonstration using a progressive ratio and a discrete trials procedure. *Neuropharmacology* 38:1797–1804.

Brebner, K., Phelan, R., and Roberts, D.C.S. (2000) Effects of baclofen on cocaine self-administration in rats reinforced under fixed-ratio 1 and progressive-ratio schedules. *Psychopharmacology* 148:314–321.

Brodie, J.D., Figueroa, E., and Dewey S.L. (2003) Treating cocaine addiction: from preclinical to clinical trial experience with γ-vinyl GABA. *Synapse* 50:261–265.

Brodie, J.D., Figueroa, E., Laska, E.M., and Dewey S.L. (2003) Safety and efficacy of γ-vinyl GABA (GVG) for the treatment of methamphetamine and/or cocaine addiction. *Synapse* 55:122–125.

Caine, S.B., and Koob, G.F. (1993) Modulation of cocaine self-administration in the rat through D-3 dopamine receptors. *Science* 260:1814–1816.

Campbell, U.C., Lac, S.T., and Carroll, M.E. (1999) Effects of baclofen on maintenance and reinstatement of intravenous cocaine self-administration in rats. *Psychopharmacology* 143:209–214.

Carlezon, W.A., Jr., Devine, D.P., and Wise, R.A. (1995) Habit-forming actions of nomifensine in nucleus accumbens. *Psychopharmacology* 122:194–197.

Carlezon, W.A., Jr., and Wise, R.A. (1996a) Rewarding actions of phencyclidine and related drugs in nucleus accumbens shell and frontal cortex. *J. Neurosci.* 16:3112–3122.

Carlezon, W.A., Jr., and Wise, R.A. (1996b) Microinjections of phencyclidine (PCP) and related drugs into nucleus accumbens shell potentiate medial forebrain bundle brain stimulation reward. *Psychopharmacology* 128:413–420.

Carroll, F.I., Lewin, A.H., Boja, J.W., and Kuhar, M.J. (1992) Cocaine receptor: biochemical characterization and structure-activity relationships of cocaine analogues at the dopamine transporter. *J. Med. Chem.* 35:969–981.

Cervo, L., Carnovali, F., Stark, J.A., and Mennini, T. (2003) Cocaine-seeking behavior in response to drug-associated stimuli in rats: involvement of D_3 and D_2 dopamine receptors. *Neuropsychopharmacology* 28:1150–1159.

Chen, J., Paredes, W., Li, J., Smith, D., Lowinson, J., and Gardner, E. L. (1990) Δ^9-Tetrahydrocannabinol produces naloxone-blockable enhancement of presynaptic basal dopamine efflux in nucleus accumbens of conscious, freely-moving rats as measured by intracerebral microdialysis. *Psychopharmacology* 102:156–162.

Christie, M.J., Summers, R.J., Stephenson, J.A., Cook, C.J., and Beart, P.M. (1987) Excitatory amino acid projections to the nucleus accumbens septi in the rat: a retrograde transport study utilizing D[^{3}H]aspartate and [^{3}H]GABA. *Neuroscience* 22:425–439.

Clarke, P.B.S., and Pert, A. (1985) Autoradiographic evidence for nicotine receptors on nigrostriatal and mesolimbic dopaminergic neurons. *Brain Res.* 348:355–358.

Collier, H.O.J. (1980) Cellular site of opiate dependence. *Nature* 283:625–629.

Dackis, C.A., and Gold, M.S. (1985) New concepts in cocaine addiction: the dopamine depletion hypothesis. *Neurosci. Biobehav. Rev.* 9:469–477.

Devine, D.P., Leone, P., Pocock, D., and Wise, R.A. (1993) Differential involvement of ventral tegmental *mu*, *delta* and *kappa* opioid receptors in modulation of basal mesolimbic dopamine release: *in vivo* microdialysis studies. *J. Pharmacol. Exp. Ther.* 266:1236–1246.

Devine, D.P., and Wise, R.A. (1994) Self-administration of morphine, DAMGO, and DPDPE into the ventral tegmental area of rats. *J. Neurosci.* 14:1978–1984.

Dewey, S.L., Brodie, J.D., Gerasimov, M., Horan, B., Gardner, E.L., and Ashby, C.R., Jr. (1999) A pharmacologic strategy for the treatment of nicotine addiction. *Synapse* 31:76–86.

Dewey, S.L., Chaurasia, C.S., Chen, C.-E., Volkow, N.D., Clarkson, F.A., Porter, S.P., Straughter-Moore, R.M., Alexoff, D.L., Tedeschi, D., Russo, N.B., Fowler, J.S., and Brodie, J.D. (1997) GABAergic attenuation of cocaine-induced dopamine release and locomotor activity. *Synapse* 25:393–398.

Dewey, S.L., Morgan, A.E., Ashby, C.R., Jr., Horan, B., Kushner, S.A., Logan, J., Volkow, N.D., Fowler, J.S., Gardner, E.L., and Brodie, J.D. (1998) A novel strategy for the treatment of cocaine addiction. *Synapse* 30:119–129.

de Wit, H., and Wise, R.A. (1977) Blockade of cocaine reinforcement in rats with the dopamine receptor blocker pimozide but not with the noradrenergic blockers phentolamine or phenoxybenzamine. *Can. J. Psychol.* 31:195–203.

Di Ciano, P., and Everitt, B.J. (2003) The $GABA_B$ receptor agonist baclofen attenuates cocaine- and heroin-seeking behavior by rats. *Neuropsychopharmacology* 28:510–518.

Di Ciano, P., Underwood, R.J., Hagan, J.J., and Everitt, B.J. (2003) Attenuation of cue-controlled cocaine-seeking by a selective D_3 dopamine receptor antagonist SB-277011-A. *Neuropsychopharmacology* 28:329–338.

Everitt, B.J., Di Ciano, P., Underwood, R., and Hagan, J. (2001) Attenuation of drug-seeking by a selective D3 dopamine receptor antagonist. *Soc. Neurosci. Abstr.* 27:1711.

Everitt, B.J., and Robbins, T.W. (2000) Second-order schedules of drug reinforcement in rats and monkeys: measurement of reinforcing efficacy and drug-seeking behaviour. *Psychopharmacology* 153:17–30.

Fada, P., Scherma, M., Fresu, A., Collu, M., and Fratta, W. (2003) Baclofen antagonizes nicotine-, cocaine-, and morphine-induced dopamine release in the nucleus accumbens of rat. *Synapse* 50: 1–6.

Filip, M., Frankowska, M., Zaniewska, M. Golda, A., Przegaliński, E., and Vetulani, J. (2007) Diverse effects of GABA-mimetic drugs on cocaine-evoked self-administration and discriminative stimulus effects in rats. *Psychopharmacology* 192:17–26.

Froimowitz, M., Wu, K.-M., Liu, X., Spector, J., Hayes, R., Vorel, S.R., Paredes, W., Ashby, C.R., Jr., and Gardner, E.L. (1999) Slow-onset, long-lasting prodrugs as potential medications for cocaine addiction: intravenous cocaine self-administration studies in rat strains with different vulnerabilities to drug-seeking behavior. *Soc. Neurosci. Abstr.* 25:1574.

Froimowitz, M., Wu, K.-M., Moussa, A., Haidar, R.M., Jurayi, J., George, C., and Gardner, E.L. (2000) Slow-onset, long-duration 3-(3',4'-dichlorophenyl)-1-indanamine monoamine reuptake blockers as potential medications to treat cocaine abuse. *J. Med. Chem.* 43:4981–4992.

Gál, K., and Gyertyán, I. (2003) Targeting the dopamine D_3 receptor cannot influence continuous reinforcement cocaine self-administration in rats. *Brain Res. Bull.* 61:595–601.

Gál, K., and Gyertyán, I. (2006) Dopamine D3 as well as D2 receptor ligands attenuate the cue-induced cocaine-seeking in a relapse model in rats. *Drug Alcohol Depend.* 81:63–70.

Gardner, E.L. (1999) The neurobiology and genetics of addiction: implications of the "reward deficiency syndrome" for therapeutic strategies in chemical dependency. In: Elster, J., ed. *Addiction: Entries and Exits.* New York: Russell Sage, pp. 57–119.

Gardner, E.L. (2000) What we have learned about addiction from animal models of drug self-administration. *Am. J. Addict.* 9:285–313.

Gardner, E.L. (2002) Marijuana addiction and CNS reward-related events. In: Onaivi, E., ed. *Biology of Marijuana: From Gene to Behaviour.* London: Taylor & Francis, pp. 75–109.

Gardner, E.L., Liu, X., Paredes, W., Giordano, A., Spector, J., Lepore, M., Wu, K.-M., and Froimowitz, M. (2006) A slow-onset, long-duration indanamine monoamine reuptake inhibitor as a potential maintenance pharmacotherapy for psychostimulant abuse: effects in laboratory rat models relating to addiction. *Neuropharmacology* 51:993–1003.

Gardner, E.L., Paredes, W., Smith, D., Donner, A., Milling, C., Cohen, D., and Morrison, D. (1988) Facilitation of brain stimulation reward by Δ^9-tetrahydrocannabinol. *Psychopharmacology* 96:142–144.

Gerasimov, M.R., Ashby, C.R., Jr., Gardner, E.L., Mills, M.J., Brodie, J.D., and Dewey, S.L. (1999) Gamma-vinyl GABA inhibits methamphetamine, heroin, or ethanol-induced increases in nucleus accumbens dopamine. *Synapse* 34:1–19.

Gerasimov, M.R., and Dewey, S.L. (1999) Gamma-vinyl γ-aminobutyric acid attenuates the synergistic elevations of nucleus accumbens dopamine produced by a cocaine/heroin (speedball) challenge. *Eur. J. Pharmacol.* 380:1–4.

Gerasimov, M.R., Schiffer, W.K., Brodie, J.D., Lennon, I.C., Taylor, S.J., and Dewey, S.L. (2000) γ-Aminobutyric acid mimetic drugs differentially inhibit the dopaminergic response to cocaine. *Eur. J. Pharmacol.* 395:129–135.

Gerasimov, M.R., Schiffer, W.K., Gardner, E.L., Marsteller, D.A., Lennon, I.C., Taylor, S.J., Brodie, J.D., Ashby, C.R., Jr., and Dewey, S.L. (2001) GABAergic blockade of cocaine-associated cue-induced increases in nucleus accumbens dopamine. *Eur. J. Pharmacol.* 414:205–209.

Gerber, G.J., and Wise, R.A. (1989) Pharmacological regulation of intravenous cocaine and heroin self-administration in rats: a variable dose paradigm. *Pharmacol. Biochem. Behav.* 32:527–531.

Gilbert, J.G., Newman, A.H., Gardner, E.L., Ashby, C.R., Jr., Heidbreder, C.A., Pak, A.C., Peng, X.-Q., and Xi, Z.-X. (2005) Acute administration of SB-277011A, NGB 2904, or BP 897 inhibits cocaine cue-induced reinstatement of drug-seeking behavior in rats: role of dopamine D_3 receptors. *Synapse* 57:17–28.

Glowa, J.R., Fantegrossi, W.F., Lewis, D.B., Matecka, D., Rice, K.C., and Rothman, R.B. (1996) Sustained decrease in cocaine-maintained responding in rhesus monkeys with 1-[2-[bis(4-fluorophenyl)methyoxy]ethyl]-4-(3-hydroxy-3-phenylpropyl) piperazinyl decanoate, a long-acting ester derivative of GBR 12909. *J. Med. Chem.* 39:4689–4691.

Glowa, J.R., Wojnicki, F.H.E., Matecka, D., Bacher, J.D., Mansbach, R.S., Balster, R.L., and Rice, K.C. (1995) Effects of dopamine reuptake inhibitors on food- and cocaine-maintained responding: I. Dependence on unit dose of cocaine. *Exp. Clin. Psychopharmacol.* 3:219–231.

Glowa, J.R., Wojnicki, F.H.E., Matecka, D., Rice, K., and Rothman, R.B. (1995) Effects of dopamine reuptake inhibitors on food- and cocaine-maintained responding: II. Comparisons with other drugs and repeated administrations. *Exp. Clin. Psychopharmacol.* 3:232–239.

Goeders, N.E., and Smith, J.E. (1983) Cortical dopaminergic involvement in cocaine reinforcement. *Science* 221:773–775.

Goeders, N.E., and Smith, J.E. (1993) Intracranial cocaine self-administration into the medial prefrontal cortex increases dopamine turnover in the nucleus accumbens. *J. Pharmacol. Exp. Ther.* 265:592–600.

Goldberg, S.R. (1973) Comparable behavior maintained under fixed-ratio and second-order schedules of food presentation, cocaine injection or *d*-amphetamine injection in the squirrel monkey. *J. Pharmacol. Exp. Ther.* 186:18–30.

Goldberg, S.R., and Tang, A.H. (1977) Behavior maintained under second-order schedules of intravenous morphine injection in squirrel and rhesus monkeys. *Psychopharmacology* 51:235–242.

Goldstein, D.B., and Goldstein, A. (1961) Possible role of enzyme inhibition and repression in drug tolerance and addiction. *Biochem. Pharmacol.* 8:48.

Grimm, J.W., and See, R.E. (2000) Dissociation of primary and secondary reward-relevant limbic nuclei in an animal model of relapse. *Neuropsychopharmacology* 22:473–479.

Haney, M., Hart, C.L., and Foltin, R.W. (2006) Effects of baclofen on cocaine self-administration: opioid- and nonopioid-dependent volunteers. *Neuropsychopharmacology* 31:1814–1821.

Hayes, R.J., Vorel, S.R., Spector, J., Liu, X., and Gardner, E.L. (2003) Electrical and chemical stimulation of the basolateral complex of the amygdala reinstates cocaine-seeking behavior. *Psychopharmacology* 168:75–83.

Heidbreder, C.A., Andreoli, M., Marcon, C., Hutcheson, D.M., Gardner, E.L., and Ashby, C.R., Jr. (2007) Evidence for the role of dopamine D_3 receptors in oral operant alcohol self-administration and reinstatement of alcohol-seeking behavior in mice. *Addict. Biol.* 12:35–50.

Heidbreder, C.A., Andreoli, M., Marcon, C., Thanos, P.K., Ashby, C.R., Jr., and Gardner, E.L. (2004) Role of dopamine D_3 receptors in the addictive properties of ethanol. *Drugs Today* 40:355–365.

Heidbreder, C.A., Gardner, E.L., Xi, Z.-X., Thanos, P.K., Mugnaini, M., Hagan, J.J., and Ashby, C.R., Jr. (2005) The role of central dopamine D_3 receptors in drug addiction: a review of pharmacological evidence. *Brain Res. Rev.* 49:77–105.

Higley, A., Li, X., Dillon, C., Ashby, C.R., Jr., Heidbreder, C.A., Gaál, J., Xi, Z.-X., and Gardner, E.L. (2007) *The dopamine D3 receptor antagonist SB277011A inhibits methamphetamine self-administration under a progressive-ratio reinforcement schedule.* Paper presented at the 37th annual meeting of the Society for Neuroscience, San Diego, CA, Abstract 814.1.

Hodos, W. (1961) Progressive ratio as a measure of reward strength. *Science* 134:943–944.

Howell, L.L., Czoty, P.W., Kuhar, M.J., and Carroll, F.I. (2000) Comparative behavioral pharmacology of cocaine and the selective dopamine uptake inhibitor RTI-113 in the squirrel monkey. *J. Pharmacol. Exp. Ther.* 292:521–529.

Howell, L.L., and Wilcox, K.M. (2001) The dopamine transporter and cocaine medication development: drug self-administration in nonhuman primates. *J. Pharmacol. Exp. Ther.* 298:1–6.

Hsin, L.-W., Dersch, C.M., Baumann, M.H., Stafford, D., Glowa, J.R., Rothman, R.B., Jacobson, A.E., and Rice, K.C. (2002) Development of long-acting dopamine transporter ligands as potential cocaine-abuse therapeutic agents: chiral hydroxyl-containing derivatives of 1-[2-[bis(4-fluorophenyl)methoxy]ethyl]-4-(3-phenyl propyl) piperazine and 1-[2-(diphenylmethoxy)ethyl]-4-(3-phenyl propyl) piperazine. *J. Med. Chem.* 45:1321–1329.

Ikemoto, S. (2003) Involvement of the olfactory tubercle in cocaine reward. *J. Neurosci.* 23:9305–9311.

Ikemoto, S., and Wise, R.A. (2004) Mapping of chemical trigger zones for reward. *Neuropharmacology* 47:190–201.

Johnson, S.W., and North, R.A. (1992) Opioids excite dopamine neurons by hyperpolarization of local interneurons. *J. Neurosci.* 12:483–488.

Jung, M.J., Lippert, B., Metcalf, B.W., Bohlen, P., and Schechter, P.J. (1977) γ-Vinyl GABA (4-amino-hex-5-enoic acid), a new selective inhibitor of GABA-T: effects on brain GABA metabolism in mice. *J. Neurochem.* 29:797–802.

Justinova, Z., Goldberg, S.R., Heishman, S.J., and Tanda, G. (2005) Self-administration of cannabinoids by experimental animals and human marijuana smokers. *Pharmacol. Biochem. Behav.* 81: 285–299.

Justinova, Z., Solinas, M., Tanda, G., Redhi, G.H., and Goldberg, S.R. (2005) The endogenous cannabinoid anandamide and its synthetic analog *R*(+)-methanandamide are intravenously self-administered by squirrel monkeys. *J. Neurosci.* 25:5645–5650.

Justinova, Z., Tanda, G., Redhi, G.H., and Goldberg, S.R. (2003) Self-administration of Δ^9-tetrahydrocannabinol (THC) by drug naïve squirrel monkeys. *Psychopharmacology* 169:135–140.

Kalivas, P.W., Churchill, L., and Klitenick, M.A. (1993) GABA and enkephalin projection from the nucleus accumbens and ventral pallidum to the ventral tegmental area. *Neuroscience* 57:1047–1060.

Kalivas, P.W., Duffy, P., and Eberhardt, H. (1990) Modulation of A10 dopamine neurons by γ-aminobutyric acid agonists. *J. Pharmacol. Exp. Ther.* 253:858–866.

Kiyatkin, E.A., and Rebec, G.V. (1999) Modulation of striatal neuronal activity by glutamate and GABA: iontophoresis in awake, unrestrained rats. *Brain Res.* 822:88–106.

Klitenick, M.A., DeWitte, P., and Kalivas, P.W. (1992) Regulation of somatodendritic dopamine release in the ventral tegmental area by opioids and GABA: an in vivo microdialysis study. *J. Neurosci.* 12:2623–2632.

Knapp, C.M., Cottam, N., Dewey, S.L., and Kornetsky, C. (1999) The GABA transaminase inhibitor, vigabatrin, reduces responding for heroin self-administration. *Soc. Neurosci. Abstr.* 25:558.

Koob, G.F., and Bloom, F.E. (1988) Cellular and molecular mechanisms of drug dependence. *Science* 242:715–723.

Kushner, S.A., Dewey, S.L., and Kornetsky, C. (1997) Gamma-vinyl GABA attenuates cocaine-induced lowering of brain stimulation reward thresholds. *Psychopharmacology* 133:383–388.

Kushner, S.A., Dewey, S.L., and Kornetsky, C. (1999) The irreversible γ-aminobutyric acid (GABA) transaminase inhibitor γ-vinyl-GABA blocks cocaine self-administration in rats. *J. Pharmacol. Exp. Ther.* 290:797–802.

Ledent, C., Valverde, O., Cossu, G., Petitet, F., Aubert, J.-F., Beslot, F., Böhme, G.A., Imperato, A., Pedrazzini, T., Roques, B.P., Vassart, G., Fratta, W., and Parmentier, M. (1999) Unresponsiveness to cannabinoids and reduced addictive effects of opiates in CB_1 receptor knockout mice. *Science* 283:401–404.

Leith, N.J., and Barrett, R.J. (1976) Amphetamine and the reward system: evidence for tolerance and post-drug depression. *Psychopharmacologia* 46, 19–25.

Lepore, M., and Franklin, K.B.J. (1992) Modelling drug kinetics with brain stimulation: dopamine antagonists increase self-stimulation. *Pharmacol. Biochem. Behav.* 41:489–496.

Lepore, M., Vorel, S.R., Lowinson, J., and Gardner, E.L. (1995) Conditioned place preference induced by Δ^9-tetrahydrocannabinol: comparison with cocaine, morphine, and food reward. *Life Sci.* 56:2073–2080.

Levant, B. (1998) Differential distribution of D_3 dopamine receptors in the brains of several mammalian species. *Brain Res.* 800:269–274.

Lewis, D.B., Matecka, D., Zhang, Y., Hsin, L.-W., Dersch, C.M., Stafford, D., Glowa, J.R., Rothman, R.B., and Rice, K.C. (1999) Oxygenated analogues of 1-[2-(diphenylmethoxy)ethyl]- and 1-[2-[bis(4-fluorophenyl)methyoxy]ethyl]-4-(3-phenylpropyl) piperazines (GBR 12935 and GBR 12909) as potential extended-action cocaine-abuse therapeutic agents. *J. Med. Chem.* 42:5029–5042.

Lile, J.A., Stoops, W.W., Allen, T.S., Glaser, P.E., Hays, L.R., and Rush, C.R. (2004) Baclofen does not alter the reinforcing, subject-related or cardiovascular effects of intranasal cocaine in humans. *Psychopharmacology* 171:441–449.

Ling, W., Shoptaw, S., and Majewska, D. (1998) Baclofen as a cocaine anti-craving medication: a preliminary clinical study. *Neuropsychopharmacology* 18:403–404.

Madras, B.K., Spealman, R.D., Fahey, M.A., Neumeyer, J.L., Saha, J.K., and Milius, R.A. (1989) Cocaine receptors labeled by $[^3H]2\beta$-carbomethoxy-3β-(fluorophenyl)tropane. *Mol. Pharmacol.* 36:518–524.

Markou, A., and Koob, G.F. (1991) Postcocaine anhedonia: an animal model of cocaine withdrawal. *Neuropsychopharmacology* 4:17–26.

Martellotta, M.C., Cossu, G., Fattore, L., Gessa, G.L., and Fratta, W. (1998) Self-administration of the cannabinoid receptor agonist WIN 55,212-2 in drug-naive mice. *Neuroscience* 85:327–330.

Mattson, R.H., Petroff, O.A., Rothman, D., and Behar, K. (1995) Vigabatrin: effect on brain GABA levels measured by nuclear magnetic resonance spectroscopy. *Acta Neurol. Scand. Suppl.* 162:27–30.

McFarland, K., Lapish, C.C., and Kalivas, P.W. (2003) Prefrontal glutamate release into the core of the nucleus accumbens mediates cocaine-induced reinstatement of drug-seeking behavior. *J. Neurosci.* 23:3531–3537.

Meltzer, P.C., Liang, A.Y., and Madras, B.K. (1994) The discovery of an unusually selective and novel cocaine analogue: difluoropine. Synthesis and inhibition of binding at cocaine recognition sites. *J. Med. Chem.* 37:2001–2010.

Meredith, G.E. (1999) The synaptic framework for chemical signaling in nucleus accumbens. *Ann. N.Y. Acad. Sci.* 877:140–156.

Morgan, A.E., and Dewey, S.L. (1998) Effects of pharmacologic increases in brain GABA levels on cocaine-induced changes in extracellular dopamine. *Synapse* 28:60–65.

Museo, E., and Wise, R.A. (1994) Place preference conditioning with ventral tegmental injections of cytisine. *Life Sci.* 55:1179–1186.

Nader, M.A., Grant, K.A., Davies, M.L.H., Mach, R.H., and Childers, S.R. (1997) The reinforcing and discriminative stimulus effects of a novel cocaine analog 2β-propanoyl-3β-(4-tolyl)-tropane in rhesus monkeys. *J. Pharmacol. Exp. Ther.* 280:541–550.

Nazzaro, J.M., and Gardner, E.L. (1980) GABA antagonism lowers self-stimulation thresholds in the ventral tegmental area. *Brain Res.* 189:279–283.

Nestler, E.J. (1993) Molecular mechanisms of drug addiction in the mesolimbic dopamine pathway. *Sem. Neurosci.* 5:369–376.

Newman, A.H., Allen, A.C., Izenwasser, S., and Katz, J.L. (1994) Novel 3α-(diphenylmethoxy)tropane analogues: potent dopamine uptake inhibitors without cocaine-like behavioral profiles. *J. Med. Chem.* 37:2258–2261.

Newman, A.H., Grundt, P., and Nader, M.A. (2005) Dopamine D_3 receptor partial agonists and antagonists as potential drug abuse therapeutic agents. *J. Med. Chem.* 48:3663–3679.

Nissbrandt, H., Ekman, A., Eriksson, E., and Heilig, M. (1995) Dopamine D3 receptor antisense influences dopamine synthesis in rat brain. *Neuroreport* 6:573–576.

Oldendorf, W.H. (1992) Some relationships between addiction and drug delivery to the brain. *NIDA Res. Monogr.* 120:13–25.

Olds, M.E. (1982) Reinforcing effects of morphine in the nucleus accumbens. *Brain Res.* 237:429–440.

Pak, A.C., Ashby, C.R., Jr., Heidbreder, C.A., Pilla, M., Gilbert, J., Xi, Z.-X., and Gardner, E.L. (2006) The selective dopamine D_3 receptor antagonist SB-277011A reduces nicotine-enhanced brain reward and nicotine-paired environmental cue functions. *Int. J. Neuropsychopharmacol.* 9:585–602.

Parsons, L.H., Caine, S.B., Sokoloff, P., Schwartz, J.-C., Koob, G.F., and Weiss, F. (1996) Neurochemical evidence that postsynaptic nucleus accumbens D3 receptor stimulation enhances cocaine reinforcement. *J. Neurochem.* 67:1078–1089.

Peng, X.-Q., Li, X., Gilbert, J.G., Pak, A.C., Ashby, C.R., Jr., Brodie, J.D., Dewey, S.L., Gardner, E.L., and Xi, Z.-X. (in press) Gamma-vinyl GABA inhibits cocaine-triggered reinstatement of drug-seeking behavior in rats by a non-dopaminergic mechanism. *Drug Alcohol Depend.*

Peng, X.-Q., Xi, Z.-X., Gilbert, J., Campos, A., Dewey, S.L., Schiffer, W.K., Brodie, J.D., Ashby, C.R., Jr., and Gardner, E.L. (2004) *Gamma-vinyl GABA, but not gabapentin, inhibits cocaine-triggered reinstatement of drug-seeking behavior in the rat.* Paper presented at the 34th annual meeting of the Society for Neuroscience, San Diego, CA, Abstract 691.8.

Peng, X.-Q., Xi, Z.-X., Gilbert, J.G., Pak, A.C., Kleitz, H., Gardner, E.L., Gu, Y., and Froimowitz, M. (2005) *Behavioral and neurochemical effects of CTDP-31,345, a novel slow-onset and long-duration dopamine transporter inhibitor: alone and in combination with cocaine.* Paper presented at the 35th annual meeting of the Society for Neuroscience, Washington, DC, Abstract 227.10.

Peng, X.-Q., Xi, Z.-X., Li, X., Gilbert, J., Pak, A., Froimowitz, M., and Gardner, E.L. (2006) *Methadone pretreatment attenuates heroin's rewarding effects and heroin-induced dopamine release in the nucleus accumbens: comparison to the effects of CTDP-31,345, a long-lasting dopamine transporter inhibitor.* Paper presented at the 36th annual meeting of the Society for Neuroscience, Atlanta, GA, Abstract 591.8.

Pickens, R., and Thompson, T. (1971) Characteristics of stimulant reinforcement. In: Thompson, T., and Pickens, R., eds. *Stimulus Properties of Drugs.* New York: Appleton-Century-Crofts, pp. 177–192.

Pilla, M., Perachon, S., Sautel, F., Garrido, F., Mann, A., Wermuth, C.G., Schwartz, J.-C., Everitt, B.J., and Sokoloff, P. (1999) Selective inhibition of cocaine-seeking behaviour by a partial dopamine D_3 receptor agonist. *Nature* 400:371–375.

Reavill, C., Taylor, S.G., Wood, M.D., Ashmeade, T., Austin, N.E., Avenell, K.Y., Boyfield, I., Branch, C.L., Cilia, J., Coldwell, M.C., Hadley, M.S., Hunter, A.J., Jeffrey, P., Jewitt, F., Johnson, C.N., Jones, D.N.C., Medhurst, A.D., Middlemiss, D.N., Nash, D.J., Riley, G.J., Routledge, C., Stemp, G., Thewlis, K.M., Trail, B., Vong, A.K.K., and Hagan, J.J. (2000) Pharmacological actions of a novel, high-affinity, and selective human dopamine D_3 receptor antagonist, SB-277011-A. *J. Pharmacol. Exp. Ther.* 294: 1154–1165.

Remington, G., and Kapur, S. (2001) SB-277011 GlaxoSmithKline. *Curr. Opin. Invest. Drugs* 2:946–949.

Richardson, N.R., and Roberts D.C.S. (1996) Progressive ratio schedules in drug self-administration studies in rats: a method to evaluate reinforcing efficacy. *J. Neurosci. Meth.* 66:1–11.

Ritz, M.C., Lamb, R.J., Goldberg, S.R., and Kuhar, M.J. (1987) Cocaine receptors on dopamine transporters are related to self-administration of cocaine. *Science* 237:1219–1223.

Roberts, D.C.S., and Andrews, M.M. (1997) Baclofen suppression of cocaine self-administration: demonstration using a discrete trials procedure. *Psychopharmacology* 131:271–277.

Roberts, D.C.S., Andrews, M.M., and Vickers, G.J. (1996) Baclofen attenuates the reinforcing effects of cocaine. *Neuropsychopharmacology* 15:417–423.

Rothman, R.B., and Glowa, J.R. (1995) A review of the effects of dopaminergic agents on humans, animals, and drug-seeking behavior, and its implications for medication development—focus on GBR-12909. *Mol. Neurobiol.* 11:1–19.

Saul'skaya, N.B., and Gorbachevskaya, A.I. (1999) The role of the hippocampal formation in controlling GABA release in the nucleus accumbens during an emotional conditioned response. *Neurosci. Behav. Physiol.* 29:461–466.

Schenk, S. (2002) Effects of GBR 12909, WIN 35,428 and indatraline on cocaine self-administration and cocaine seeking in rats. *Psychopharmacology* 160:263–270.

Schiffer, W.K., Gerasimov, M.R., Bermel, R.A., Brodie, J.D., and Dewey, S.L. (2000) Stereoselective inhibition of dopaminergic activity by gamma vinyl-GABA following a nicotine or cocaine challenge: a PET/microdialysis study. *Life Sci.* 66:PL169–PL173.

Self, D.W., and Nestler, E.J. (1995) Molecular mechanisms of drug reinforcement and addiction. *Annu. Rev. Neurosci.* 18:463–495.

Sesack, S.R., and Pickel, V.M. (1995) Ultrastructural relationships between terminals immunoreactive for enkephalin, GABA, or both transmitters in the rat ventral tegmental area. *Brain Res.* 672:261–275.

Shaham, Y., and Stewart, J. (1995) Stress reinstates heroin-seeking in drug-free animals: an effect mimicking heroin, not withdrawal. *Psychopharmacology* 119:334–341.

Shalev, U., Grimm, J.W., and Shaham, Y. (2002) Neurobiology of relapse to heroin and cocaine seeking: a review. *Pharmacol. Rev.* 54:1–42.

Shoptaw, S., Yang, X., Rotheram-Fuller, E.J., Hsieh, Y.C., Kintaudi, P.C., Charuvastra, V.C., and Ling, W. (2003) Randomized placebo-controlled trial of baclofen for cocaine dependence: preliminary effects for individuals with chronic patterns of cocaine use. *J. Clin. Psychiatry* 64:1440–1448.

Slattery, D.A., Markou, A., Froestl, W., and Cryan, J.F. (2005) The $GABA_B$ receptor-positive modulator GS39783 and the $GABA_B$ receptor agonist baclofen attenuate the reward-facilitating effects of cocaine: intracranial self-stimulation studies in the rat. *Neuropsychopharmacology* 30:2065–2072.

Solomon, R.L., and Corbit, J.D. (1974) An opponent-process theory of motivation: I. Temporal dynamics of affect. *Psychol. Rev.* 81: 119–145.

Spanagel, R., Herz, A., and Shippenberg, T.S. (1990) The effects of opioid peptides on dopamine release in nucleus accumbens: an in vivo microdialysis study. *J. Neurochem.* 55:1734–1740.

Spiller, K., Xi, Z.-X., Peng, X.-Q., Newman, A.H., Ashby, C.R., Jr., Heidbreder, C., Gaál, J., and Gardner E.L. (2008) The putative dopamine D_3 receptor antagonists SB-277011A and NGB 2904 and the putative partial D_3 receptor agonist BP 897 attenuate methamphetamine-enhanced brain stimulation reward in rats. *Psychopharmacology* 196:533–542.

Stein, L. (1962) Effects and interactions of imipramine, chlorpromazine, reserpine and amphetamine on self-stimulation: possible neurophysiological basis of depression. In: Wortis, J., ed. *Recent Advances in Biological Psychiatry.* New York: Plenum, pp. 288–308.

Stemp, G., Ashmeade, T., Branch, C.L., Hadley, M.S., Hunter, A.J., Johnson, C.N., Nash, D.J., Thewlis, K.M., Vong, A.K.K., Austin, N.E., Jeffrey, P., Avenell, K.Y., Boyfield, I., Hagan, J.J., Middlemiss, D.N., Reavill, C., Riley, G.J., Routledge, C., and Wood, M. (2000) Design and synthesis of *trans*-N-[4-[2-(6-cyano-1,2,3,4-tetrahydroisoquinolin-2-yl)ethyl]cyclohexyl]-4-quinolinecarboxamide (SB-277011): a potent and selective dopamine D_3 receptor antagonist with high oral availability and CNS penetration in the rat. *J. Med. Chem.* 43:1878–1885.

Suzuki, M., Hurd, Y.L., Sokoloff, P., Schwartz, J.-C., and Sedvall, G. (1998) D_3 dopamine receptor mRNA is widely expressed in the human brain. *Brain Res.* 779:58–74.

Tanda, G., Munzar, P., and Goldberg, S.R. (2000) Self-administration behavior is maintained by the psychoactive ingredient of marijuana in squirrel monkeys. *Nat. Neurosci.* 3:1073–1074.

Thanos, P.K., Katana, J.M., Ashby, C.R., Jr., Michaelides, M., Gardner, E.L., Heidbreder, C.A., and Volkow, N.D. (2005) The selective dopamine D3 receptor antagonist SB-277011-A attenuates ethanol consumption in ethanol preferring (P) and non-preferring (NP) rats. *Pharmacol. Biochem. Behav.* 81:190–197.

Vaccarino, F.J., Bloom, F.E., and Koob, G.F. (1985) Blockade of nucleus accumbens opiate receptors attenuates intravenous heroin reward in the rat. *Psychopharmacology* 86:7–42.

Valjent, E., and Maldonado, R. (2000) A behavioural model to reveal place preference to Δ^9-tetrahydrocannabinol in mice. *Psychopharmacology* 147:436–438.

van der Kooy, D., Mucha, R.F., O'Shaughnessy, M., and Bucenieks, P. (1982) Reinforcing effects of brain microinjections of morphine revealed by conditioned place preference. *Brain Res.* 243:107–117.

Villemange, V.L., Rothman, R.B., Yokoi, F., Rice, K.C., Matecka, D., Dannals, R.F., and Wong, D.F. (1999) Doses of GBR12909 that suppress cocaine self-administration in non-human primates substantially occupy dopamine transporters as measured by [^{11}C] WIN35,428 PET scans. *Synapse* 32:44–50.

Volkow, N.D., Chang, L., Wang, G.-J., Fowler, J.S., Ding, Y.-S., Sedler, M., Logan, J., Franceschi, D., Gatley, S.J., Hitzemann, R., Gifford, A., Wong, C., and Pappas, N. (2001) Low level of brain dopamine D_2 receptors in methamphetamine abusers: association with metabolism in the orbitofrontal cortex. *Am. J. Psychiatry* 158:2015–2021.

Volkow, N.D., Ding, Y.-S., Fowler, J.S., Wang, G.-J., Logan, J., Gatley, J.S., Dewey, S., Ashby, C., Liebermann, J., Hitzemann, R., and Wolf, A.P. (1995) Is methylphenidate like cocaine? Studies on their pharmacokinetics and distribution in the human brain. *Arch. Gen. Psychiatry* 52:456–463.

Volkow, N.D., Fowler, J.S., and Wang, G.-J. (1999) Imaging studies on the role of dopamine in cocaine reinforcement and addiction in humans. *J. Psychopharmacol.* 13:337–345.

Volkow, N.D., Wang, G.-J., Fowler, J.S., Logan, J., Gatley, S.J., Gifford, A., Hitzemann, R., Ding, Y.-S., and Pappas, N. (1999) Prediction of reinforcing responses to psychostimulants in humans by brain dopamine D_2 receptor levels. *Am. J. Psychiatry* 156: 1440–1443.

Vorel, S.R., Ashby, C.R., Jr., Paul, M., Liu, X., Hayes, R., Hagan, J.J., Middlemiss, D.N., and Gardner, E.L. (2002) Dopamine D_3 receptor antagonism inhibits cocaine-seeking and cocaine-enhanced brain reward in rats. *J. Neurosci.* 22:9595–9603.

Wang, B., Shaham, Y., Zitzman, D., Azari, S., Wise, R.A., and You, Z.-B. (2005) Cocaine experience establishes control of midbrain glutamate and dopamine by corticotropin-releasing factor: a role in stress-induced relapse to drug seeking. *J. Neurosci.* 25: 5389–5396.

Ward, B.O., Somerville, E.M., and Clifton, P.G. (2000) Intraaccumbens baclofen selectively enhances feeding behavior in the rat. *Physiol. Behav.* 68:463–468.

Weerts, E.M., Froestl, W., Kaminski, B.J., and Griffiths, R.R. (2007) Attenuation of cocaine-seeking by $GABA_B$ receptor agonists baclofen and CGP44532 but not the GABA reuptake inhibitor tiagabine in baboons. *Drug Alcohol Depend.* 89:206–213.

Welch, W.M., Kraska, A.R., Sarges, R., and Koe, B.K. (1984) Nontricyclic antidepressant agents derived from the *cis*- and *trans*-1-amino-4-aryltetralins. *J. Med. Chem.* 27:1508–1515.

Whitelaw, R.B., Markou, A., Robbins, T.W., and Everitt, B.J. (1996) Excitotoxic lesions of the basolateral amygdala impair the acquisition of cocaine-seeking behaviour under a second-order schedule of reinforcement. *Psychopharmacology* 127:213–224.

Wicke, K., and Garcia-Ladona, J. (2001) The dopamine D3 receptor partial agonist, BP 897, is an antagonist at human dopamine D3 receptors and at rat somatodendritic dopamine D3 receptors. *Eur. J. Pharmacol.* 424:85–90.

Wise, R.A. (1974) Maximization of ethanol intake in the rat. In: Gross, M.M., ed. *Alcohol Intoxication and Withdrawal*, 2nd ed. New York: Plenum, pp. 279–294.

Wise, R.A. (1982) Neuroleptics and operant behavior: the anhedonia hypothesis. *Behav. Brain Sci.* 5:39–87.

Wise, R.A. (1989) The brain and reward. In: Liebman, J.M., and Cooper, S.J., ed. *The Neuropharmacological Basis of Reward*. Oxford, UK: Oxford University Press, pp. 377–424.

Wise, R.A. (1996) Addictive drugs and brain stimulation reward. *Annu. Rev. Neurosci.* 19:319–340.

Wise, R.A., and Bozarth, M.A. (1987) A psychomotor stimulant theory of addiction. *Psychol. Rev.* 94:469–492.

Wise, R.A., Marcangione, C., and Bauco, P. (1998) Blockade of the reward-potentiating effects of nicotine on lateral hypothalamic brain stimulation by chlorisondamine. *Synapse* 29:72–79.

Wise, R.A., Newton, P., Leeb, K., Burnette, B., Pocock, D., and Justice, J.B., Jr. (1995) Fluctuations in nucleus accumbens dopamine concentration during intravenous cocaine self-administration in rats. *Psychopharmacology* 120:10–20.

Wood, M.D., Boyfield, I., Nash, D.J., Jewitt, F.R., Avenell, K.Y., and Riley, G.J. (2000) Evidence for antagonist activity of the dopamine D3 receptor partial agonist, BP 897, at human dopamine D3 receptor. *Eur. J. Pharmacol.* 407:47–51.

Woolverton, W.L., Rowlett, J.K., Wilcox, K.M., Paul, I.A., Kline, R.H., Newman, A.H., and Katz, J.L. (2000) 3'- and 4'-Chloro-substituted analogs of benztropine: intravenous self-administration and *in vitro* radioligand bindings studies in rhesus monkeys. *Psychopharmacology* 147:426–435.

Xi, Z.-X., and Gardner, E.L. (2007) Pharmacological actions of NGB 2904, a selective dopamine D_3 receptor antagonist, in animal models of drug addiction. *CNS Drug Rev.* 2:240–259.

Xi, Z.-X., Gilbert, J.G., Campos, A.C., Kline, N., Ashby, C.R., Jr., Hagan, J.J., Heidbreder, C.A., and Gardner, E.L. (2004) Blockade of mesolimbic dopamine D_3 receptors inhibits stress-induced reinstatement of cocaine-seeking in rats. *Psychopharmacology* 176:57–65.

Xi, Z.-X., Gilbert, J.G., Pak, A.C., Ashby, C.R., Jr., Heidbreder, C. A., and Gardner, E.L. (2005) Selective dopamine D_3 receptor antagonism by SB-277011A attenuates cocaine reinforcementas assessed by progressive-ratio and variable-ratio—variable-payoff fixed-ratio cocaine self-administration in rats. *Eur. J. Neurosci.* 21:3427–3438.

Xi, Z.-X., Gilbert, J.G., Peng, X.-Q., Ashby, C.R., Jr., Heidbreder, C.A., and Gardner, E.L. (2007) *Blockade of dopamine D_3 receptors by SB-277011A inhibits incubation of craving for cocaine in rats.* Paper presented at the 69th annual meeting of the College on Problems of Drug Dependence, Quebec City, Canada.

Xi, Z.-X., Newman, A.H., Gilbert, J.G., Pak, A.C., Peng, X.-Q., Ashby, C.R. Jr., Gitajn, L., and Gardner, E.L. (2006) The novel dopamine D_3 receptor antagonist NGB 2904 inhibits cocaine's rewarding effects and cocaine-induced reinstatement of drug-seeking behavior in rats. *Neuropsychopharmacology* 31:1393–1405.

Xi, Z.-X., Ramamoorthy, S., Shen, H., Lake, R., Samuvel, D.J., and Kalivas, P.W. (2003) GABA-transmission in the nucleus accumbens is altered after withdrawal from repeated cocaine. *J. Neurosci.* 23:3498–3505.

Xi, Z.-X., and Stein, E.A. (1998) Nucleus accumbens dopamine release modulation by mesolimbic $GABA_A$ receptors—an in vivo electrochemical study. *Brain Res.* 798:156–165.

Xi, Z.-X., and Stein, E.A. (1999) Baclofen inhibits heroin self-administration behavior and mesolimbic dopamine release. *J. Pharmacol. Exp. Ther.* 290:1369–1374.

Xi, Z.-X., and Stein, E.A. (2000) Increased mesolimbic GABA concentration blocks heroin self-administration in the rat. *J. Pharmacol. Exp. Ther.* 294:613–619.

Yan, Q.-S. (1999) Focal bicuculline increases extracellular dopamine concentration in the nucleus accumbens of freely moving rats as measured by in vivo microdialysis. *Eur. J. Pharmacol.* 385:7–13.

Yokel, R.A., and Pickens, R. (1974) Drug level of *d* and *l*-amphetamine during intravenous self-administration. *Psychopharmacologia* 34: 255–264.

Yokel, R.A., and Wise, R.A. (1975) Increased lever-pressing for amphetamine after pimozide in rats: implications for a dopamine theory of reward. *Science* 187:547–549.

46 Cellular and Molecular Mechanisms of Drug Addiction

ERIC J. NESTLER

This chapter provides an overview of recent progress made in understanding the molecular basis of drug addiction. After terms commonly used in the field are defined, a brief description of the mechanisms by which drugs of abuse influence synaptic transmission after an acute exposure is provided. Next described are the types of gradually developing, progressive changes that repeated exposure to drugs of abuse can induce in specific brain regions that appear to underlie aspects of addiction.

DEFINITION OF TERMS

Drug addiction is often defined by the pharmacological terms *tolerance, sensitization, dependence,* and *withdrawal. Tolerance* refers to the situation where repeated administration of a drug at the same dose elicits a diminishing effect or the need for an increasing drug dose to produce the same effect. *Sensitization*, or "reverse tolerance," refers to the opposite situation where repeated administration of the same drug dose elicits an escalating effect. The same drug can elicit simultaneously tolerance and sensitization to its many different effects. *Dependence* is defined as the need for continued drug exposure to avoid a withdrawal syndrome, characterized by physical or emotional disturbances when the drug is withdrawn. Each of these responses to repeated drug exposure is presumably caused by molecular and cellular adaptations that the drug produces in specific brain regions. It is important to emphasize that tolerance, sensitization, dependence, and withdrawal are not associated uniquely with drugs of abuse; many medications used clinically that are not addicting (for example, clonidine, propranolol, and tricyclic antidepressants, to name a few) can also produce these effects.

Drugs of abuse are unique, however, in terms of their reinforcing properties, described in greater detail in Chapter 45. A drug is classified as a reinforcer if the probability of a drug-seeking response is increased when the response is temporally paired with drug exposure. Upon acute exposure, most abused drugs function as positive reinforcers; this probably involves positive affective responses (for example, euphoria) to the drug, although reinforcement per se may well be distinct from euphoria. Rapid and powerful associations between a drug reinforcer and a drug-seeking response reflect the drug's ability to directly modulate preexisting brain reinforcement mechanisms, which normally mediate the reinforcement produced by natural reinforcers such as food, sex, and social interaction (Wise, 1998; Koob and LeMoal, 2001; Everitt and Wolf, 2002; Kelley and Berridge, 2002; Hyman et al., 2006).

Chronic exposure to reinforcing drugs can lead to drug addiction, best defined as the compulsive seeking (drug craving) and administration of a drug despite grave adverse consequences or as a loss of control over drug intake. The drug-seeking behavior that characterizes drug addiction is different from that seen with acute drug reinforcement, in that addicted individuals exhibit a sustained increase in drug-seeking behavior even when the drug is absent or withdrawn for prolonged periods of time. In this chronic context, a drug may serve not only as a positive reinforcer but also as a negative reinforcer by reducing negative emotional symptoms that can persist long after drug taking ceases.

Addictive disorders are often defined clinically as a state of dependence, for example, in the *Diagnostic and Statistical Manual of Mental Disorders* (published by the American Psychiatric Association). However, it is important to emphasize that in more precise pharmacological terms, we do not yet know the types of neurobiological changes that are responsible for the compulsive drug-seeking behavior that is the clinical hallmark of an addictive disorder. There is evidence that drug craving involves adaptations that underlie the aversive motivational symptoms (for example, dysphoria, anxiety) associated with drug dependence and withdrawal. There also is evidence that drug craving involves adaptations that underlie tolerance to a drug's reinforcing effects, which might be expected to contribute to the pattern of escalating drug intake often seen clinically. In addition, considerable evidence suggests that drug craving involves adaptations that underlie sensitization to the acute reinforcing effects of a drug and to the priming effects of a drug or its conditioned cues. These various mechanisms are not mutually exclusive, as complex combinations of them are likely to account for drug addiction.

THE SYNAPSE AS THE ACUTE TARGET OF DRUGS OF ABUSE

Our understanding of the pharmacological effects of drugs of abuse on the brain has focused on the synapse as the acute target of drug action. All drugs of abuse affect the brain initially by influencing the amount of a neurotransmitter present at the synapse or by interacting with specific neurotransmitter receptors. Table 46.1 lists examples of such acute pharmacological actions of some commonly used drugs of abuse. Opiates are agonists at μ and δ opioid receptors. Cocaine increases synaptic levels of dopamine (DA), serotonin, and norepinephrine (NE) by inhibiting the presynaptic (reuptake) transporters for these monoamines. Amphetamine and its derivatives also increase synaptic levels of the monoamines, but via a distinct mechanism: by increasing monoamine release. Amphetamine itself serves as a substrate for all three monoamine transporters and is transported into monoaminergic nerve terminals, where it disrupts the storage of the monoamine neurotransmitters. This leads to an increase in extravesicular levels of the monoamines and to the reverse transport of the monoamine into the synaptic cleft via the transporters.

TABLE 46.1 *Examples of Acute Pharmacological Actions of Drugs of Abuse*

Drug	*Action*
Opiates	Agonist at μ, δ, and κ opioid receptors[a]
Cocaine	Inhibits dopamine reuptake transporters[b]
Amphetamine	Stimulates dopamine release[b]
Ethanol	Facilitates GABA-$_A$ receptor function and inhibits NMDA glutamate receptor function[c]
Nicotine	Agonist at nicotinic acetylcholine receptors
Cannabinoids[a]	Agonist at cannabinoid receptors[d]
Hallucinogens	Partial agonist at 5-HT$_{2A}$ serotonin receptors
Phencyclidine (PCP)	Antagonist at NMDA glutamate receptors
Inhalants	Unknown

[a]Activity at μ and δ receptors mediates the reinforcing actions of opiates; activity at κ receptors can produce aversion.

[b]Cocaine and amphetamine exert analogous actions on serotonergic and noradrenergic systems, which may also contribute to the reinforcing effects of these drugs.

[c]Ethanol affects several other ligand-gated channels and, at higher concentrations, voltage-gated channels as well. In addition, ethanol is reported to influence many other neurotransmitter systems, including serotonergic, opioidergic, and dopaminergic systems. It is not known whether these effects are direct or achieved indirectly via actions on various ligand-gated channels.

[d]Activity at CB_1 receptors mediates the reinforcing actions of cannabinoids. Proposed endogenous ligands for the CB_1 receptor include the arachidonic acid metabolites, anandamide and 2-arachidonylglycerol.

$GABA_A$: γ-aminobutyric acid-A; 5-HT$_{2A}$: 5-hydroxytryptamine-2A; NMDA: *N*-methyl-D-aspartate.

The best established acute action of ethanol is its ability to facilitate activation of the γ-aminobutyric acid-A (GABA-A) receptor by GABA. This action is similar to that of the benzodiazepines and all other sedative-hypnotic drugs. The GABA-A receptor is a heteromeric complex (see Chapters 2 and 3); the ability of ethanol and sedative hypnotics to facilitate receptor function depends on the actual subunit composition of the receptor, which differs markedly throughout the brain. Although these drugs interact with the GABA-A receptor at apparently distinct sites, the fact that they converge on the functioning of the same protein complex no doubt explains the long-appreciated cross-tolerance and cross-dependence exhibited by these drugs. Ethanol, unlike other sedative-hypnotics, also exerts potent effects on the *N*-methyl-D-aspartate (NMDA) glutamate receptor. Ethanol inhibits the functioning of the receptor, again, not by blocking the glutamate binding site but via a more complex allosteric effect on the receptor complex, which results in diminished glutamate-induced Na^+ and Ca^{2+} flux through the receptor *ionophore*. Ethanol antagonism of the NMDA receptor appears to contribute to the intoxicating effects of ethanol and perhaps to the dissociative effects seen in people with high ethanol blood levels. Whether ethanol antagonism of the NMDA receptor also contributes to its reinforcing effects remains to be established. At still higher doses, ethanol can exert more general inhibitory effects on other ligand-gated channels as well as on voltage-gated ion channels, particularly Na^+ and Ca^{2+} channels. These actions occur only at the extremely high concentrations seen clinically and therefore do not appear to be involved in the reinforcing actions of ethanol, although they may contribute to the severe nervous system depression, and even coma, seen at these blood levels.

The fact that drugs of abuse initially influence different neurotransmitter and receptor systems in the brain explains the very different actions produced by these drugs acutely. This is illustrated in Figure 46.1. For example, the presence of very high levels of opioid receptors in the brain stem and spinal cord explains why opiates can exert such profound effects on respiration, level of consciousness, and nociception. In contrast, the importance of noradrenergic mechanisms in the regulation of cardiac function explains why cocaine can exert such profound cardiotoxic effects.

In contrast to the many disparate acute actions of drugs of abuse, the drugs do appear to exert some common behavioral effects: as discussed above, they are all positively reinforcing after acute exposure. This suggests that there are certain regions of the brain where

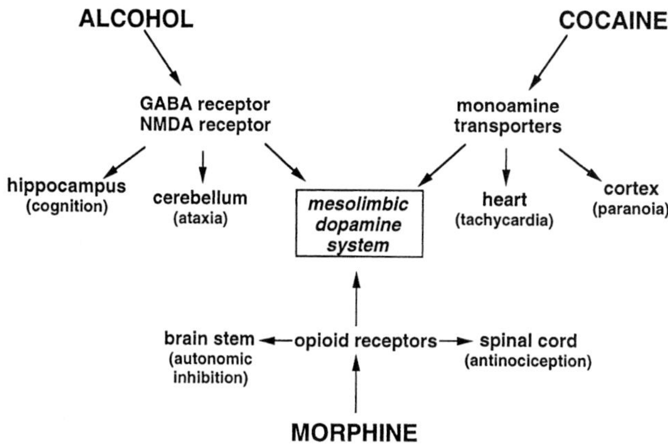

FIGURE 46.1 Scheme illustrating how initial divergent actions of drugs of abuse can converge on a common neural substrate. Opiates, cocaine, and ethanol act on different initial protein targets. As a result, the drugs elicit very different effects after acute administration because the targets are distributed differentially throughout the central nervous system. However, the targets are each present in the mesolimbic dopamine system, and drug action on the targets results in common functional effects within this system (that is, drug reinforcement). GABA: γ-aminobutyric acid; NMDA: *N*-methyl-D-aspartate.

the distinct, acute pharmacological actions of the drugs converge in producing the common effect of reinforcement (Fig. 46.1). That is, in certain regions of the brain, which are discussed below, activation of opioid receptors (by opiates), inhibition of monoamine reuptake (by cocaine), or facilitation of GABAergic and inhibition of NMDA glutamatergic neurotransmission (by ethanol) appear to elicit some common responses that mediate drug reinforcement.

MOLECULAR AND CELLULAR ADAPTATIONS TO DRUGS OF ABUSE

The acute pharmacological actions of a drug of abuse do not per se explain the long-term effects of repeated drug exposure such as addiction. To understand such long-term effects, it is necessary to consider postreceptor intracellular messenger pathways and a neuron's long-term adaptations to repeated perturbations (see Chapters 4–6). This means that, despite the initial actions of drugs of abuse on extracellular aspects of synaptic function (receptors, transporters, neurotransmitter levels, etc.), the many actions that the drugs exert on brain function are achieved ultimately through the complex network of intracellular messenger pathways that mediates these extracellular mechanisms. Moreover, repeated exposure to drugs of abuse would be expected to produce repeated perturbation of these intracellular pathways, which presumably triggers the many types of molecular and cellular adaptations throughout the brain responsible for tolerance, sensitization, dependence, withdrawal, and, ultimately, addiction.

A major advantage of the drug abuse field, as opposed to studies of other mental disorders, is that a great deal is known about the neural circuits in the brain responsible for the behavioral abnormalities that characterize addictive disorders. This knowledge has resulted from the availability of increasingly sophisticated animal models of addiction, described in Chapter 45, which replicate many key features of drug addiction seen clinically. The development of such animal models, in turn, has been facilitated by the fact that drugs of abuse are clear etiological factors in drug addiction, whereas etiological factors for other mental disorders are not yet known with certainty. One of the most important neural circuits involved in addiction is the mesolimbic DA system, which is composed of dopaminergic neurons in the ventral tegmental area (VTA) of the midbrain and the limbic forebrain regions to which these neurons project, most notably the nucleus accumbens (NAc; also called ventral striatum) (Wise, 1998; Koob and LeMoal, 2001). There is now a wealth of evidence that the VTA–NAc pathway is a crucial substrate for the acute rewarding effects of virtually all drugs of abuse and for the derangements in reward mechanisms that contribute to drug addiction. The amygdala appears particularly important in mediating the cue-conditioning effects of drugs of abuse, whereby drug-associated cues elicit powerful drug craving or withdrawal-like symptoms even after prolonged abstinence (Everitt et al., 2001). Another memory-associated brain region, the hippocampus, likely also contributes to the powerful memories of addiction that drive drug seeking and relapse. Regions of frontal cortex, for example, orbitofrontal cortex or medial prefrontal cortex, which normally mediate executive function, are also affected by drugs of abuse: reduced function of these regions is thought to mediate the increased impulsivity and compulsivity associated with addictive states (Kalivas et al., 2005). All of these brain structures, and many others, operate as functionally interconnected circuits, in which drug-induced alterations in their functioning mediate a state of addiction (Hyman et al., 2006).

Based on this impressive knowledge of the neural substrates of drug abuse and addiction, it has been possible to focus efforts on identifying drug-induced changes, at the molecular and cellular levels, within these specific brain regions that underlie the behavioral abnormalities used to define addiction-like behavior in animal models. The remainder of this chapter discusses the types of molecular and cellular adaptations in reward-related brain regions that have been shown to play important roles in animal models of drug addiction. This chapter cannot be comprehensive due to space limitations. Rather, the sections that follow outline examples of some of the most characterized adaptations implicated in drug addiction. An interesting outcome of this research is that several types of drugs of abuse produce some common molecular and cellular adaptations within reward-related brain regions, which has suggested common general mechanisms of drug addiction (Fig. 46.2) in addition to numerous adaptations specific for each addictive substance (Nestler, 2005).

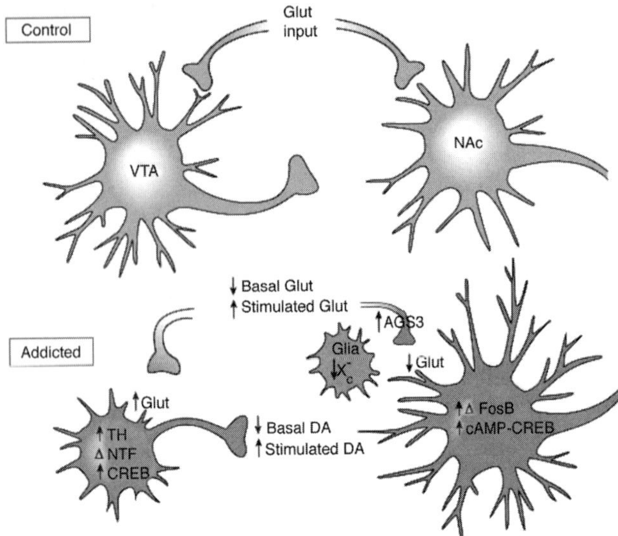

FIGURE 46.2 Highly simplified scheme of some common, chronic actions of drugs of abuse on the VTA-NAc circuit. The top panel (Control) shows a VTA neuron innervating a NAc neuron, and cortical glutamatergic inputs to the VTA and NAc neurons, under normal conditions. After chronic drug administration, several adaptations occur. In the VTA, drug exposure induces TH and increases AMPA glutamatergic responses (Glut), possibly via induction of GluR1 and altered trafficking of AMPA receptors. Also, VTA dopamine neurons decrease in size, an effect demonstrated thus far with chronic opiates only, but presumed for other drugs of abuse due to common associated biochemical adaptations (for example, reduced levels of neurofilament proteins). Induction of CREB activity, and alterations in NTF signaling may partly mediate these various effects. In the NAc, all drugs of abuse induce the transcription factor ΔFosB, which may then mediate some of the shared aspects of addiction via regulation of numerous target genes. Several, but not all, drugs of abuse also induce CREB activity in this region, which may be mediated via up-regulation of the cAMP pathway. Several additional changes have been found for stimulant exposure; it is not yet known whether they generalize to other drugs. Stimulants decrease AMPA glutamatergic responses in NAc neurons, possibly mediated via induction of GluR2 or repression of several postsynaptic density proteins (for example, PSD95, Homer-1). These changes in postsynaptic glutamate responses are associated with complex changes in glutamatergic innervation of the NAc, including reduced glutamatergic transmission at baseline and in response to normal rewards, but enhanced transmission in response to cocaine and associated cues, effects possibly mediated in part via up-regulation of AGS3 (activator of G protein signaling) in cortical neurons and down-regulation of the cystine-glutamate transporter (system xc-) in glia. Stimulants and nicotine also induce dendritic outgrowth of NAc neurons, although opiates are reported to produce the opposite action. The net effect of this complex dysregulation in glutamate function and synaptic structure is not yet known. From Nestler, 2005. VTA: ventral tegmental area; NAc: nucleus accumbens; TH: tyrosine hydroxylase; AMPA: α-amino-3-hydroxy-5-methyl-4-isoxasolepropionic acid; CREB: cyclic adenosine monophosphate [cAMP]-response element binding; NTF: neurotrophic factor.

Up-regulation of the cAMP-CREB Pathway in the VTA-NAc

One of the best-established molecular mechanisms of drug tolerance and dependence is up-regulation of the cAMP (cyclic adenosine monophosphate) second-messenger and protein phosphorylation pathway (Nestler and Aghajanian, 1997). As reviewed in Chapter 4, this pathway mediates the effects of numerous G protein–coupled receptors, including opioid, DA, and cannabinoid receptors, on neuronal function. According to this hypothesis, depicted in Figure 46.3, prolonged exposure to a drug of abuse, which activates receptors that inhibit the cAMP pathway, triggers compensatory adaptations that oppose this inhibition and restores cAMP pathway function to normal levels. For example, the affected cells make more adenylyl cyclase (the enzyme that catalyzes the synthesis of cAMP) and more protein kinase A (PKA; the enzyme that mediates most of the effects of cAMP on cell function). In the continued presence of the drug, such adaptations mediate tolerance. Upon removal of the drug, the up-regulated cAMP pathway becomes fully functional and mediates aspects of dependence and withdrawal.

Such up-regulation of the cAMP pathway, first demonstrated in cultured cells and later characterized more

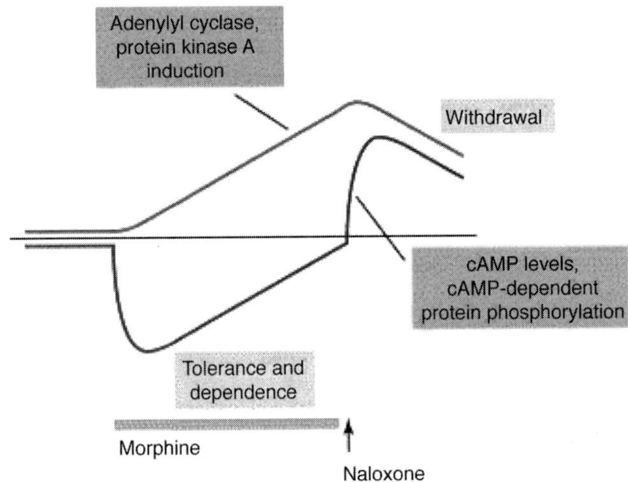

FIGURE 46.3 Up-regulation of the cAMP pathway as a mechanism of opiate tolerance and dependence. Opiates acutely inhibit the functional activity of the cAMP pathway (indicated by cellular levels of cAMP and cAMP-dependent protein phosphorylation). With continued opiate exposure, functional activity of the cAMP pathway gradually recovers and increases far above control levels following removal of the opiate (for example, by administration of the opioid receptor antagonist *naloxone*). These changes in the functional state of the cAMP pathway are mediated via the induction of adenylyl cyclase and PKA in response to chronic administration of opiates. Induction of these enzymes accounts for the gradual recovery in the functional activity of the cAMP pathway that occurs during chronic opiate exposure (tolerance) and activation of the cAMP pathway observed upon removal of opiate (dependence and withdrawal). From Nestler, 2004. cAMP: cyclic adenosine monophosphate; PKA: protein kinase A.

fully in noradrenergic neurons of the locus coeruleus, has now been found in diverse neuronal cell types in the central and peripheral nervous systems in response to chronic exposure to any of several drugs of abuse (Nestler, 2004). Accordingly, this adaptation mediates diverse aspects of drug addiction, depending on the neurons affected (Table 46.2). In the locus coeruleus, for example, up-regulation of the cAMP pathway, seen in response to chronic opiate administration, mediates aspects of physical opiate dependence and withdrawal, while in the NAc, up-regulation of the cAMP pathway in response to chronic opiate, cocaine, amphetamine, or ethanol administration mediates tolerance and dependence in reward mechanisms and is, therefore, an example of a common mechanism of drug addiction mentioned earlier (Fig. 46.2).

Drug-induced up-regulation of the cAMP pathway is mediated, in part, via the transcription factor CREB (cAMP response element binding protein). Thus, opiate or stimulant exposure activates CREB in several brain regions, where it serves, among other actions, to increase expression of adenylyl cyclase or PKA isoforms (Nestler and Aghajanian, 1997). Drug regulation of CREB was first discovered in the locus coeruleus and shown, like the up-regulated cAMP pathway, to mediate opiate physical dependence and withdrawal. In contrast, CREB activation in the NAc, in response to opiates or stimulants, mediates tolerance and dependence in drug reward.

Drug regulation of CREB in the NAc has received particular attention as a common mechanism of addiction, where its role in the addiction process has been characterized by use of advanced molecular biology tools discussed in Chapter 7. Overexpression of CREB in the NAc, by use of viral-mediated gene transfer or of inducible bitransgenic mice, which mimics drug activation of the protein in this region, decreases an animal's

TABLE 46.2 *Upregulation of the cAMP Pathway in Opiate Addiction*

Site of Up-regulation	*Functional Consequence*
Locus coeruleus	Physical dependence and withdrawal
Ventral tegmental area	Dysphoria during early withdrawal periods
Periaqueductal gray	Dysphoria during early withdrawal periods, and physical dependence and withdrawal
Nucleus accumbens	Dysphoria during early withdrawal periods
Amygdala	Conditioned aspects of addiction
Dorsal horn of spinal cord	Tolerance to opiate-induced analgesia
Myenteric plexus of gut	Tolerance to opiate-induced reductions in intestinal motilityand increases in motility during withdrawal

From Nestler, 2004.

sensitivity to the rewarding effects of drugs of abuse (Nestler, 2004; Carlezon et al., 2005). Conversely, blockade of CREB function in this brain region, by overexpression of a dominant negative mutant of CREB (termed *mCREB*), has the opposite effect. Studies of constitutive CREB knockout mice generally support these overexpression findings (Walters and Blendy, 2001). Together, these investigations substantiate a role for CREB as a homeostatic feedback mechanism that decreases an animal's responses to subsequent drug exposure. Activation of CREB also induces a negative emotional state, characterized by anhedonia-like symptoms (decreased responses to natural rewards) and increased depression-like behavior in animal models. These findings support the view that CREB activation by drugs of abuse contributes to aversive symptoms that characterize drug withdrawal states. A recent study has shown that this emotional state induced by CREB contributes to increased drug self-administration, presumably as an effort to overcome the aversive symptoms (Choi et al., 2006).

One of the target genes through which CREB, in the NAc, decreases drug reward and produces negative emotional symptoms is the opioid peptide *dynorphin* (Carlezon et al., 2005). Dynorphin is expressed by a subset of NAc medium spiny neurons. When released, dynorphin activates μ opioid receptors present on VTA DA neuron terminals, where it inhibits DA release (Kreek, 1996; Shippenberg et al., 2001). Dynorphin is therefore part of a feedback loop, which dampens further DA-mediated reward. Activation of CREB in the NAc leads to induction of the dynorphin gene, which increases the gain on this feedback loop and thereby reduces drug reward and induces a negative emotional state. These findings have led to the suggestion that μ opioid antagonists might be of use in treating drug withdrawal states and may also represent a novel treatment for depression (McLaughlin et al., 2003; Carlezon et al., 2005).

Chronic exposure to opiates, cocaine, or nicotine induces CREB in the VTA as well, where the behavioral effects are more complex (Olson et al., 2005; Walters et al., 2005). Here, CREB activation can either promote or oppose drug reward mechanisms based on the subregion of the VTA involved. Work is under way to identify target genes for CREB in this region that mediate these effects.

Regulation of Opioid and Dopamine Receptor Sensitivity in the VTA–NAc

A mechanism of drug tolerance, which has gained increasing attention in recent years, is drug-induced alteration of the physiological responsiveness of opioid, DA, or other G protein–coupled receptors in the VTA–NAc circuit (Fig. 46.4). Chronic exposure to certain opiate drugs down-regulates opioid receptors, and prolonged activation of DA receptors (for example, as seen after cocaine or amphetamine administration) leads to their down-regulation as well. The best-established mechanism of such receptor tolerance involves the functional uncoupling of the receptors from their G proteins via their phosphorylation by G protein–coupled receptor kinase (GRKs). According to this mechanism, the binding of an agonist to a G protein–coupled receptor induces a conformational change in the receptors that render them good substrates for these kinases (Chavkin et al., 2001; von Zastrow et al., 2003). The phosphorylated receptors then bind arrestin, which triggers internalization of the receptor-arrestin complex via a dynamin-dependent pathway (Chapter 5). Another proposed mechanism of receptor tolerance involves drug-induced down-regulation of G protein subunits (for example, G αi), which has been observed in several neuronal cell types. A related possibility is that drugs regulate a newly characterized class of signaling protein, regulators of G protein–signaling proteins (RGSs), which regulate the guanosine triphosphate (GTP)ase activity of G protein α subunits and, consequently, the efficacy of receptor signaling (Zachariou et al., 2003). It will be important for future studies to establish the functional role played by these various types of adaptations in receptor signaling within the mesolimbic DA system

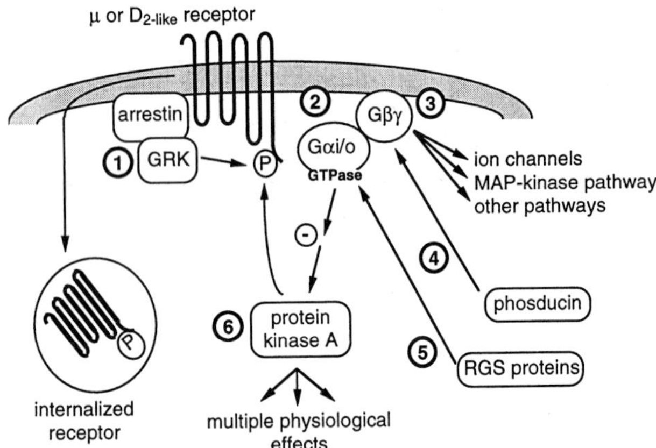

FIGURE 46.4 Scheme illustrating possible mechanisms of drug-induced changes in opioid or D_2-like dopamine receptor sensitivity. Drug-induced adaptations in the efficacy of receptor-Gi/o coupling could contribute to aspects of drug tolerance or sensitization. One possible mechanism is adaptations in processes that mediate acute desensitization of receptor function, such as receptor phosphorylation GRKs and subsequent receptor internalization (1). Other possible mechanisms include alterations in levels of G protein a (2) or bg (3) subunits or of other proteins (for example, phosducin [4]; RGS proteins [5]) that modulate G protein function. Phosphorylation of the receptor by PKA does not mediate acute receptor desensitization (because receptor activation leads to inhibition of the kinase). However, up-regulation of the kinase (6) after chronic drug administration (Fig. 46.3) could phosphorylate and regulate receptor function during withdrawal states. From Nestler and Aghajanian (1997). GRKs: G protein–receptor kinases; RGS: regulators of G protein signaling; PKA: protein kinase A; MAP: mitogen-activated protein.

and other reward-related brain regions in drug abuse models in vivo.

Synaptic Plasticity and Regulation of Glutamatergic Systems in the VTA–NAc

Although a great deal of attention has focused on drug regulation of DA neurotransmission from the VTA to the NAc, a major advance over the past decade has been an increased appreciation of the importance of glutamatergic innervation to both of these brain regions and the regulation of this excitatory transmission by drugs of abuse. Major glutamatergic inputs to the VTA arise from frontal regions of cerebral cortex and from the peduncular pontine tegmentum and lateral dorsal tegmentum. Major glutamatergic inputs to the NAc arise from frontal cortex, hippocampus, and amygdala. An exciting finding is that virtually any type of drug of abuse induces a long-term potentiation (LTP)–like phenomenon at glutamatergic synapses in the VTA, while cocaine and other stimulants induce long-term depression (LTD)–like changes in the NAc (Thomas and Malenka, 2003; Kauer, 2004).

Recent work has focused on the molecular mechanisms by which drugs induce these examples of synaptic plasticity in the VTA–NAc circuit. In the VTA, where drugs enhanced glutamatergic transmission, there is evidence that chronic exposure to drugs of abuse promotes the insertion of AMPA glutamate receptors into active postsynaptic sites of DA neurons in this brain region. There is also evidence that drugs induce the expression of certain α-amino-3-hydroxy-5-methyl-4-isoxasolepropionic acid (AMPA) receptor subunits, for example, GluR1 (Carlezon and Nestler, 2002). Indeed, this induction may be mediated via CREB.

The situation is more complicated in the NAc, where drugs are reported to dampen glutamatergic-dependent synaptic plasticity (Wolf, 1998; Sutton et al., 2003; Kalivas, 2004). Here, there remains controversy in the literature concerning whether chronic drug exposure enhances or diminishes glutamatergic neurotransmission, with increases and decreases in glutamate receptor subunits reported. Moreover, there is evidence for increased insertion of AMPA receptors into postsynaptic sites, which is correlated with sensitized behavioral responses to drug (Boudreau and Wolf, 2005). As well, drugs of abuse have been shown to alter the expression of an array of modulatory proteins, located at postsynaptic sites in the NAc, which regulate the activity, stability, or localization of AMPA and NMDA receptors. Some of the drug-induced changes in glutamate receptor subunit expression have been related to induction of CREB or another transcription factor, ΔFosB, as is discussed in the next section.

It is likely that drugs also alter glutamergic transmission, and mechanisms of synaptic plasticity in many other brain regions, such as frontal cortex, amygdala, and hippocampus, to name a few (see below), although these changes are not as well characterized as similar mechanisms in the VTA–NAc.

Induction of ΔFosB in the NAc

ΔFosB is a member of the Fos family of transcription factors, which dimerize with a Jun family member to form an active AP-1 (activator protein-1) transcription factor complex. Acute exposure to virtually any drug of abuse rapidly induces c-Fos and all other Fos family members in the NAc and dorsal striatum, with maximal induction seen 2–4 hours after drug administration. Due to the instability of these proteins and their messenger ribonucleic acids (mRNAs), this induction is highly transient, with levels of the transcription factors returning to basal levels within 8–12 hours. ΔFosB shows dramatically different temporal properties of induction. Like the other Fos family members, it is induced rapidly in response to an acute drug exposure, but only to a slight degree (see Fig. 6.7 in Chapter 6). However, unlike all other Fos family proteins, ΔFosB is unusually stable. As a result, during a course of chronic drug administration, ΔFosB protein levels gradually accumulate to high levels in NAc and dorsal striatal neurons and become by far the predominant Fos family protein present (Nestler et al., 2001; McClung et al., 2004). ΔFosB's stability also means that it persists in these neurons long after cessation of drug intake. ΔFosB thereby provides a novel mechanism by which chronic exposure to drugs of abuse produces long-lasting changes in gene expression even after prolonged withdrawal.

The unusual stability of ΔFosB is due to at least two recently discovered mechanisms. ΔFosB is derived from the *FosB* gene via alternative splicing. Another product of the gene is full-length *FosB*, which behaves like other Fos family members. The only difference between ΔFosB and *FosB* is that ΔFosB lacks the terminal 101 amino acids present in the C-terminal end of *FosB*. Recent work has shown that this C-terminal domain contains two degrons that target full-length *FosB* to rapid degradation via proteosomal and nonproteosomal mechanisms (Carle et al., 2007). All other Fos family proteins possess similar degrons domains, which are lacking uniquely in ΔFosB. As well, ΔFosB is further stabilized by its phoshorylation at its N-terminus by casein kinase 2 (CK2) and perhaps other protein kinases (Ulery et al., 2006). These biochemical properties offer unique ways to possibly intervene to disrupt the prolonged effects of ΔFosB, for example, CK2 inhibitors, as potential treatments for drug addiction.

There is now substantial evidence that induction of ΔFosB in the NAc by drugs of abuse mediates a sensitized state: increased sensitivity to the rewarding effects of drugs of abuse as well as increased incentive motivation to self-administer the drugs (Kelz et al., 1999; Colby et al., 2003; McClung et al., 2004; Zachariou et al., 2006). ΔFosB similarly enhances motivation for natural rewards, such as wheel running and sucrose. A great deal of effort has been expended to identify the target genes through which ΔFosB produces this interesting behavioral state. Early estimates are that ΔFosB may account for more than 25% of all the genes whose expression is altered by chronic cocaine administration (McClung and Nestler, 2003). One target gene is cyclin-dependent kinase 5 (*Cdk5*): its induction by cocaine and ΔFosB appears to be one mechanism underlying cocaine's regulation of NAc neuronal morphology (see next section). Another target gene is the AMPA glutamate receptor *GluR*: its regulation may be part of the molecular mechanisms involved in drug regulation of glutamatergic transmission as outlined earlier.

Neurotrophic Mechanisms, Regulation of Neuronal Morphology in the VTA–NAc

Recent models of neural plasticity have increasingly implicated changes in neural morphology and synaptic structure in functional adaptations in the nervous system. As just one example, LTP has been associated with increases in the density of dendritic spines on hippocampal neurons (Yuste and Bonhoeffer, 2001). It is not surprising, then, that neurotrophic mechanisms and morphological adaptations have also been implicated in the neural plasticity associated with drug addiction. For example, chronic administration of morphine decreases the size of VTA DA neuron cell bodies as well as axonal transport from the VTA to the NAc (Sklair-Tavron et al., 1996; Russo et al., 2007). These changes are associated with decreased levels of neurofilament proteins and increased levels of glial fibrillary acidic protein (GFAP) in the VTA. Decreased levels of neurofilaments and increased levels of GFAP are often a sign of neural insult or injury, consistent with the morphological changes seen in VTA DA neurons in the drug-treated state (Fig. 46.2). Recent evidence suggests that the reduction in DA cell size in response to chronic morphine is a mechanism of drug tolerance (Russo et al., 2007).

Morphological changes have also been observed in the NAc. Chronic administration of several types of stimulants, for example, cocaine, amphetamine, or nicotine increases the density of dendritic spines of NAc medium spiny neurons (Robinson and Kolb, 2004). These changes are similar to those observed in hippocampal neurons in concert with LTP, with one important difference: the changes associated with LTP are relatively short lived, whereas the changes induced by stimulants persist for at least 1 month after drug withdrawal. Although direct evidence linking drug-induced dendritic spine increases in the NAc to altered physiological function of the neurons is lacking, it is tempting to speculate that such morphological changes might contribute to sensitized responses to drug exposure (Fig. 46.5). Moreover, there is evidence that stimulants induce dendritic outgrowth in NAc neurons via induction of ΔFosB and via ΔFosB's induction of *Cdk5* (Norrholm et al., 2003; Lee et al., 2006). Thus, prolonged induction of dendritic spines after chronic cocaine occurs in ΔFosB+ cells and can be prevented by local infusion of a *Cdk5* inhibitor. However, the connection between increased dendritic spine density and sensitization remains less certain, given that fact that opiates reportedly decrease dendritic outgrowth in the NAc despite the fact that they clearly induce sensitization (Robinson and Kolb, 2004), and inhibition of *Cdk5*, while it blocks cocaine's effects on dendritic spines and increases rather than decreases behavioral responses to the drug (Taylor et al., 2007). Thus, further work is needed to understand the functional consequences of drug-induced morphological changes in the NAc.

Identification of drug-induced morphological changes in the VTA and NAc raises the critical question of the underlying molecular mechanisms involved. Possible mediators of these effects are various neurotrophic factors. Although such factors were studied originally for their role in neural growth and differentiation during development, they are now known to regulate signal transduction and neuronal viability in the fully differentiated adult brain (see Chapters 2 and 4). Indeed, there is now direct evidence that several types of neurotrophic factors, including brain-derived neurotrophic factor (BDNF), glial cell line–derived neurotrophic factors (GDNF), and fibroblast growth factor (FGF), among others, acting at the level of the VTA or NAc, can modify an animal's molecular, cellular, and behavioral responses to drugs of abuse, and that chronic drug exposure can modify these neurotrophic factors or their signaling pathways (see Pierce and Bari, 2001; Bolaños and Nestler, 2004). For example, the ability of morphine to decrease the size of VTA DA neurons has been demonstrated recently to be mediated via morphine-induced downregulation of one of the main signaling pathways for BDNF: the insulin receptor substrate (IRS)-phosphatidylinositol-3-kinase (PI-3-kinase)-protein kinase B (Akt) pathway (Russo et al., 2007). Although further work is clearly needed to better delineate the relationship between drugs of abuse and neurotrophic factors, this line of investigation has provided new information concerning the mechanisms underlying drug addiction and has suggested novel ways to approach its treatment.

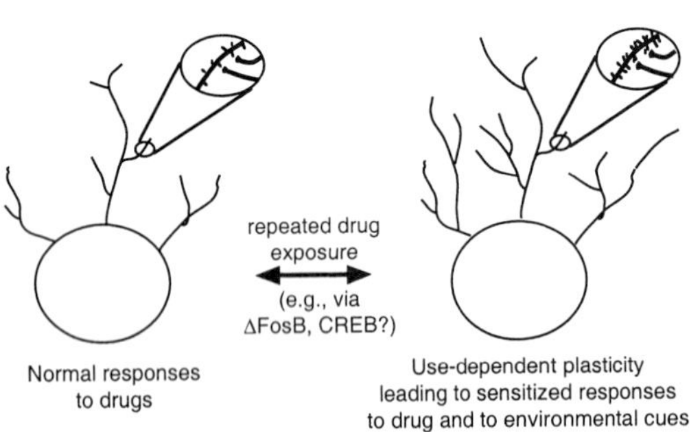

FIGURE 46.5 Regulation of dendritic structure by drugs of abuse. The figure shows the expansion of a neuron's dendritic tree after chronic exposure to a drug of abuse, as has been observed in the NAc and prefrontal cortex for cocaine and related psychostimulants. The areas of magnification show an increase in dendritic spines, which is postulated to occur in conjunction with activated nerve terminals. Such alterations in dendritic structure, which are similar to those observed in some learning models (for example, LTP), could mediate long-lived sensitized responses to drugs of abuse or environmental cues. There is evidence that, in the NAc, the cocaine-induced increase in dendritic spines may be mediated via ΔFosB and its induction of Cdk5. NAc: nucleus accumbens; LTP: long-term potentiation; Cdk5: cyclin-dependent kinase-5.

Regulation of Chromatin Remodeling Mechanisms

Recent years have brought explosive increases in our knowledge of how changes in gene expression are associated with changes in chromatin structure. Most of this work has come from the cancer and developmental biology fields and only recently has been applied to neural plasticity in the adult brain (Tsankova et al., 2007). Chromatin remodeling, discussed in greater detail in Chapter 8, refers to posttranslational modifications of histones (for example, acetylation, phosphorylation, and many others), as well as methylation of deoxyribonucleic acid (DNA) itself, which is associated with activation or repression of a given gene. Studies of chromatin remodeling is a high priority for the drug abuse field for two reasons. First, chromatin remodeling, studied with chromatin immunoprecipitation (ChIP) assays, offers the first-ever window into mechanisms of gene regulation within the brain in vivo. For example, this work has made it possible for the first time to study directly whether a particular gene is activated or repressed in the NAc in vivo in addiction models and to identify associated transcription factors. In contrast, before ChIP, it was possible to identify changes in steady state mRNA levels in vivo, but then all studies of mechanisms relied on in vitro investigations. This has been a huge inherent weakness in the field. Second, certain changes in chromatin structure are particularly long lived and hence provide an attractive mechanism by which drugs of abuse cause long-lasting changes in gene expression and, consequently, behavior.

To date, a small number of studies have implicated chromatin remodeling in drug abuse models. Acute or chronic administration of cocaine has been shown to increase global levels of histone acetylation (a marker of gene activation) in striatum, with selective increases demonstrated at several specific genes of interest, including c-Fos, FosB, *Cdk5*, and BDNF (Brami-Cherrier et al., 2005; Kumar et al., 2005; Levine et al., 2005). Such ChIP studies have confirmed a role for ΔFosB in directly activating the *Cdk5* gene, as inferred from earlier studies (see above). Binge cocaine exposure to adolescent rats causes increased sensitivity to cocaine in adults, which is associated with reduced global levels of histone methylation in frontal cortex (Black et al., 2006). In addition, chromatin remodeling mechanisms have been implicated directly in addiction-related behavior, with modification of histone acetylation altering behavioral responses to cocaine (Kumar et al., 2005; Levine et al., 2005).

An exciting innovation is to utilize so-called ChIP on chip assays (ChIP followed by analysis on promoter arrays) to gain a genome-wide view of alterations in chromatin structure and transcription factor binding in brain reward regions after chronic drug exposure. It would be interesting to overlay such information on to DNA expression arrays (e.g., Freeman et al., 2001; McClung and Nestler, 2003; Yao et al., 2004; Yuferov et al., 2005) to obtain a more reliable determination of the genomic effects of drugs of abuse on the brain and to gain initial insight into the underlying mechanisms involved.

Although these various studies of chromatin remodeling are clearly in early stages of development, this line of investigation in drug abuse models promises new insight into the molecular mechanisms of drug addiction.

Drug-Induced Adaptations in Other Reinforcement-Related Brain Regions

The preceding discussion focused on the VTA and NAc as the major sites in the brain of drug-induced adaptations that underlie addiction. Although these regions are no doubt important—indeed, they may be critical—it is also clear that many other brain regions contribute to addiction. As mentioned earlier, there is increasing evidence to indicate the importance of the amygdala, frontal cortical regions, and hippocampus, as well as still other brain areas such as the periaqueductal gray, serotonergic raphé nuclei, and hypothalamus.

Considerable work in rodents and humans has shown reduced functional activity of frontal cortical regions as a consequence of chronic drug exposure, and these changes have been related directly to the increased impulsivity and compulsivity seen in addicted states (Volkow and Fowler, 2000). Although the molecular basis of this "hypofrontality" remains incompletely understood, there have been recent advances. The basal activity of cortical glutamatergic pyramidal neurons appears to be reduced at baseline after chronic exposure to cocaine, whereas an acute challenge with cocaine elicits enhanced activation of these neurons. Chronic cocaine use also has been reported to decrease levels of the cystine–glutamate transporter in glial cells in the NAc; this transporter promotes release of glutamate from prefrontal cortical glutamatergic nerve terminals, perhaps further exaggerating glutamatergic transmission to the NAc when the cell bodies fire in response to cocaine and associated cues (Kalivas et al., 2005) (Fig. 46.2). This has raised the interesting possibility that ligands that regulate this transporter might be of benefit in the treatment of cocaine addiction. Clearly, these changes are complex, and interact with the postsynaptic adaptations in glutamate receptor function in NAc neurons discussed earlier, in ways that remain incompletely understood. Nevertheless, these important findings now highlight the need to characterize the effects of other drugs of abuse, as well as natural rewards, on these same end points.

Another interesting outcome of research on these other reward-related brain areas is the finding that many of the drug-induced adaptations characterized in the VTA and NAc are also seen in some of these other brain regions. Drug-induced up-regulation of the cAMP pathway and activation of CREB have been observed not only in the VTA–NAc, as stated above, but also in the amygdala, periaqueductal gray, frontal cortex, and elsewhere (Nestler, 2004, 2005). ΔFosB is induced by chronic drug exposure in prefrontal and orbitofrontal cortex and amygdala as well as in the NAc. In fact, induction seen in the orbitofrontal cortex is much greater in animals that self-administer drug as opposed to those that receive drug passively. This finding suggests particular relevance of ΔFosB induction in orbitofrontal cortex in regulating motivational aspects of addiction, although this remains speculative. The expansion of dendritic spines, observed as a consequence of chronic stimulant exposure in the NAc, is also seen in prefrontal cortex (Robinson and Kolb, 2004). As the roles played by these various brain regions in addiction are established, it will be increasingly possible to relate specific molecular adaptations in these regions to particular functional aspects of addiction.

CONCLUSIONS

The availability of animal models that increasingly reproduce important features of drug addiction in humans has made it possible to identify specific regions in the brain that play an important role in addictive disorders. The mesolimbic DA system, and related neural circuits involving the amygdala, frontal regions of cerebral cortex, and hippocampus, among several others, are integrally involved in drug reward and in derangements in drug reward mechanisms that are the essential feature of drug addiction clinically. Basic neurobiological investigations are beginning to provide an understanding of the adaptations at the molecular and cellular levels that occur in these various brain regions that are responsible for behavioral features of drug addiction. This chapter focused on drug-induced adaptations in the cAMP pathway, in G protein–coupled receptors, in glutamatergic neurotransmission and synaptic plasticity, in neurotrophic factors and their signaling cascades, and in several transcription factors (for example, CREB and ΔFosB) and associated changes in chromatin structure. Some of these molecular and cellular adaptations have been related to drug-induced morphological changes in neurons located within several reward-related brain regions. However, these adaptations, though important, are merely illustrative of modifications in numerous additional neurotransmitters, neurotrophic factors, intracellular signaling pathways, and transcriptional mechanisms induced within these various brain reward regions. As the pathophysiological mechanisms underlying drug addiction become increasingly understood, it will be possible to develop more efficacious pharmacotherapies for the treatment of addictive disorders.

REFERENCES

Black, Y.D., Maclaren, F.R., Naydenov, A.V., Carlezon, W.A., Jr., Baxter, M.G., and Konradi, C. (2006) Altered attention and prefrontal cortex gene expression in rats after binge-like exposure to cocaine during adolescence. *J. Neurosci.* 26:9656–9665.

Bolaños, C.A., and Nestler, E.J. (2004) Neurotrophic mechanisms in drug addiction. *J. Neuromol. Med.* 5:69–83.

Boudreau, A.C., and Wolf, M.E. (2005) Behavioral sensitization to cocaine is associated with increased AMPA receptor surface expression in the nucleus accumbens. *J. Neurosci.* 25:9144–9151.

Brami-Cherrier, K., Valjent, E., Herve, D., Darragh, J., Corvol, J.C., Pages, C., Arthur, S.J., Girault, J.A., and Caboche, J. (2005) Parsing molecular and behavioral effects of cocaine in mitogen- and stress-activated protein kinase-1 deficient mice. *J. Neurosci.* 25: 11444–11454.

Carle, T.L., Ohnishi. Y.N., Ohnishi, Y.H., Alibhai, I.N., Wilkinson, M.B., Kumar, A., and Nestler, E.J. (2007) Absence of conserved C-terminal degron domain contributes to ΔFosB's unique stability. *Eur. J. Neurosci.* 25:3009–3019.

Carlezon, W.A., Jr., Duman, R.S., and Nestler, E.J. (2005) The many faces of CREB. *Trends Neurosci.* 28:436–445.

Carlezon, W.A., Jr., and Nestler, E.J. (2002) Elevated levels of GluR1 in the midbrain: a trigger for sensitization to drugs of abuse? *Trends Neurosci.* 25:610–615.

Chavkin, C., McLaughlin, J.P., and Celver, J.P. (2001) Regulation of opioid receptor function by chronic agonist exposure: constitutive activity and desensitization. *Mol. Pharmacol.* 60:20–25.

Choi, K.H., Whisler, K., Graham, D.L., and Self, D.W. (2006) Antisense-induced reduction in nucleus accumbens cyclic AMP response element binding protein attenuates cocaine reinforcement. *Neuroscience* 137:373–383.

Colby, C.R., Whisler, K., Steffen, C., Nestler, E.J., and Self, D.W. (2003) ΔFosB enhances incentive for cocaine. *J. Neurosci.* 23:2488–2493.

Everitt, B.J., Dickinson, A., and Robbins, T.W. (2001) The neuropsychological basis of addictive behaviour. *Brain Res. Rev.* 36:129–138.

Everitt, B.J., and Wolf, M.E. (2002) Psychomotor stimulant addiction: a neural systems perspective. *J. Neurosci.* 22:3312–3320.

Flores, C., Samaha, A.N., and Stewart, J. (2000) Requirement of endogenous basic fibroblast growth factor for sensitization to amphetamine. *J. Neurosci.* 20:RC55.

Freeman, W.M., Nader, M.A., Nader, S.H., Robertson, D.J., Gioia, L., Mitchell, S.M., Daunais, J.B., Porrino, L.J., Friedman, D.P., and Vrana, K.E. (2001) Chronic cocaine-mediated changes in non-human primate nucleus accumbens gene expression. *J. Neurochem.* 77:542–549.

Hyman, S.E., Malenka, R.C., and Nestler, E.J. (2006) Neural mechanisms of addiction: the role of reward-related learning and memory. *Annu. Rev. Neurosci.* 29:565–598.

Kalivas, P.W. (2004) Glutamate systems in cocaine addiction. *Curr. Opin. Pharmacol.* 4:23–29.

Kalivas, P.W., Volkow, N., and Seamans, J. (2005) Unmanageable motivation in addiction: a pathology in prefrontal-accumbens glutamate transmission. *Neuron* 45:647–650.

Kauer, J.A. (2004) Learning mechanisms in addiction: synaptic plasticity in the ventral tegmental area as a result of exposure to drugs of abuse. *Annu. Rev. Physiol.* 66:447–475.

Kelley, A.E. and Berridge, K.C. (2002) The neuroscience of natural rewards: Relevance to addictive drugs. *J. Neurosci.* 22:3306–3311.

Kelz, M.B., Chen, J.S., Carlezon, W.A., Whisler, K., Gilden, L., Beckmann, A.M., Steffen, C., Zhang, Y.-J., Marotti, L., Self, D.W., Tkatch, R., Baranauskas, G., Surmeier, D.J., Neve, R.L., Duman, R.S., Picciotto, M.R., and Nestler, E.J. (1999) Expression of the transcription factor ΔFosB in the brain controls sensitivity to cocaine. *Nature* 401:272–276.

Koob, G.F., and Le Moal, M. (2001) Drug addiction, dysregulation of reward, and allostasis. *Neuropsychopharmacology* 24:97–129.

Kreek, M.J. (1996) Cocaine, dopamine and the endogenous opioid system. *J. Addict. Dis.* 15:73–96.

Kumar, A., Choi, K.-H., Renthal, W., Tsankova, N.M., Theobald, D.E.H., Truong, H.-T., Russo, S.J., LaPlant, Q., Sasaki, T.S., Whistler, K.N., Neve, R.L., Self, D.W., and Nestler, E.J. (2005) Chromatin remodeling is a key mechanism underlying cocaine-induced plasticity in striatum. *Neuron* 48:303–314.

Lee, K.W., Kim, Y., Kim, A.M., Helmin, K., Nairn, A.C., and Greengard, P. (2006) Cocaine-induced dendritic spine formation in D1 and D2 dopamine receptor-containing medium spiny neurons in nucleus accumbens. *Proc. Natl. Acad. Sci. USA* 103: 3399–3404.

Levine, A.A., Guan, Z., Barco, A., Xu, S., Kandel, E.R., and Schwartz, J.H. (2005) CREB-binding protein controls response to cocaine by acetylating histones at the fosB promoter in the mouse striatum. *Proc. Natl. Acad. Sci. USA* 102:19186–19191.

McClung, C.A., and Nestler, E.J. (2003) Regulation of gene expression and cocaine reward by CREB and ΔFosB. *Nat. Neurosci.* 11:1208–1215.

McClung, C.A., Ulery, P.G., Perrotti, L.I., Zachariou, V., Berton, O., and Nestler, E.J. (2004) ΔFosB: A molecular switch for long-term adaptation in the brain. *Mol. Brain Res.* 132:146–154.

McLaughlin, J.P., Marton-Popovici, M., and Chavkin, C. (2003) Kappa opioid receptor antagonism and prodynorphin gene disruption block stress-induced behavioral responses. *J. Neurosci.* 23:5674–5683.

Nestler, E.J. (2004) Historical review: molecular and cellular mechanisms of opiate and cocaine addiction. *Trends Pharmacol. Sci.* 25:210–218.

Nestler, E.J. (2005) Is there a common molecular pathway for addiction? *Nat. Neurosci.* 8:1445–1449.

Nestler, E.J., and Aghajanian, G.K. (1997) Molecular and cellular basis of addiction. *Science* 278:58–63.

Nestler, E.J., Barrot, M., and Self, S.W. (2001) ΔFosB: a molecular switch for addiction. *Proc. Natl. Acad. Sci. USA* 98:11042–11046.

Norrholm, S.D., Bibb, J.A., Nestler, E.J., Ouimet, C.C., Taylor, J.R., and Greengard, P. (2003) Cocaine-induced proliferation of dendritic spines in nucleus accumbens is dependent on the activity of the neuronal kinase Cdk5. *Neuroscience* 116:19–22.

Olson, V.G., Zabetian, C.P., Bolaños, C.A., Edwards, S., Barrot, M., Eisch, A.J., Hughes, T., Self, D.W., Neve, R.L., and Nestler, E.J. (2005) Regulation of drug reward by CREB: evidence for two functionally distinct subregions of the ventral tegmental area. *J. Neurosci.* 25:5553–5562.

Pierce, R.C., and Bari, A.A. (2001) The role of neurotrophic factors in psychostimulant-induced behavioral and neuronal plasticity. *Rev. Neurosci.* 12:95–110.

Robinson, T.E., and Kolb, B. (2004) Structural plasticity associated with exposure to drugs of abuse. *Neuropharmacology* 47:S33–S46.

Russo, S.J., Bolanos, C.A., Theobald, D.E., DeCarolis, N., Kumar, A., Self, D.W., Russell, D.S., Neve, R.L., Eisch, A.J., and Nestler, E.J. (2007) Insulin receptor substrate-2 in midbrain dopaminergic neurons regulates behavioral and cellular responses to opiates. *Nat. Neurosci.* 10:93–99.

Self, D.W., Genova, L.M., Hope, B.T., Barnhart, W.J., Spencer, J.J., and Nestler, E.J. (1998) Involvement of cAMP-dependent protein kinase in the nucleus accumbens in cocaine self-administration and relapse of cocaine-seeking behavior. *J. Neurosci.* 18:1848–1859.

Shippenberg, T.S., Chefer, V.I., Zapata, A., and Heidbreder, C.A. (2001) Modulation of the behavioral and neurochemical effects of psychostimulants by kappa-opioid receptor systems. *Ann. N.Y. Acad. Sci.* 937:50–73.

Sklair-Tavron, L., Shi, W.-X., Lane, S.B., Harris, H.W., Bunney, B.S., and Nestler, E.J. (1996) Chronic morphine induces visible changes in the morphology of mesolimbic dopamine neurons. *Proc. Natl. Acad. Sci. USA* 93:11202–11207.

Sutton, M.A., Schmidt, E.F., Choi, K.H., Schad, C.A., Whisler, K., Simmons, D., Karanian, D.A., Monteggia, L.M., Neve, R.L., and Self, D.W. (2003) Extinction-induced upregulation in AMPA receptors reduces cocaine-seeking behaviour. *Nature* 421:70–75.

Taylor, J.R., Lynch, W.J., Sanchez, H., Olausson, P., Nestler, E.J., and Bibb, J.A. (2007) Inhibition of Cdk5 in the nucleus accumbens enhances the locomotor activating and incentive motivational effects of cocaine. *Proc. Natl. Acad. Sci. USA* 104:4147–4152.

Thomas, M.J., and Malenka, R.C. (2003) Synaptic plasticity in the mesolimbic dopamine system. *Philos. Trans. R. Soc. Lond. B Biol. Sci.* 358:815–819.

Tsankova, N., Renthal, W., Kumar, A., and Nestler, E.J. (2007) Epigenetic regulation in psychiatric disorders. *Nat. Rev. Neurosci.* 8:355–367.

Ulery, P.G., Rudenko, G., and Nestler, E.J. (2006) Regulation of ΔFosB stability by phosphorylation. *J. Neurosci.* 26:5131–5142.

Volkow, N.D., and Fowler, J.S. (2000) Addiction, a disease of compulsion and drive: involvement of the orbitofrontal cortex. *Cereb. Cortex* 10:318–325.

von Zastrow, M., Svingos, A., Haberstock-Debic, H., and Evans, C. (2003) Regulated endocytosis of opioid receptors: cellular mechanisms and proposed roles in physiological adaptation to opiate drugs. *Curr. Opin. Chem. Biol.* 13:348–353.

Walters, C.L., and Blendy, J.A. (2001) Different requirements for cAMP response element binding protein in positive and negative reinforcing properties of drugs of abuse. *J. Neurosci.* 21:9438–9444.

Walters, C.L., Cleck, J.N., Kuo, Y.C., and Blendy, J.A. (2005) Mu-opioid receptor and CREB activation are required for nicotine reward. *Neuron* 46:933–943.

Wise, R.A. (1998) Drug-activation of brain reward pathways. *Drug Alcohol Depend.* 51:13–22.

Wolf, M.E. (1998) The role of excitatory amino acids in behavioral sensitization to psychomotor stimulants. *Prog. Neurobiol.* 54:679–720.

Yao, W.D., Gainetdinov, R.R., Arbuckle, M.I., Sotnikova, T.D., Cyr, M., Beaulieu, J.M., Torres, G.E., Grant, S.G., and Caron, M.G. (2004) Identification of PSD-95 as a regulator of dopamine-mediated synaptic and behavioral plasticity. *Neuron* 41:625–638.

Yuferov, V., Nielsen, D., Butelman, E., and Kreek, M.J. (2005) Microarray studies of psychostimulant-induced changes in gene expression. *Addict. Biol.* 10:101–118.

Yuste, R., and Bonhoeffer, T. (2001) Morphological changes in dendritic spines associated with long-term synaptic plasticity. *Annu. Rev. Neurosci.* 24:1071–1089.

Zachariou, V., Bolanos, C.A., Selley, D.E., Theobald, D., Cassidy, M.P., Kelz, M.B., Shaw-Lutchman, T., Berton, O., Sim-Selley, L.J., DiLeone, R.J., Kumar, A., and Nestler, E.J. (2006) ΔFosB: an essential role for ΔFosB in the nucleus accumbens in morphine action. *Nat. Neurosci.* 9:205–211.

Zachariou, V., Georgescu, D., Sanchez, N., Rahman, Z., DiLeone, R., Berton, O., Simon, M., Neve, R.L., Sim-Selley, L.J., Selley, D.E., Gold, S.J., and Nestler, E.J. (2003) Essential role for RGS9 in opiate action. *Proc. Natl. Acad. Sci. USA* 100:13656–13661.

47 Genetic Epidemiology of Substance Use Disorders

KATHLEEN R. MERIKANGAS AND KEVIN P. CONWAY*

Substance abuse is one of the most pervasive psychiatric disorders in contemporary society. Of people sampled in the National Comorbidity Survey Replication (NCS-R), a recently completed nationwide survey of Americans aged 18 and older, 14.6% had a lifetime history of a substance use disorder (SUD; that is, abuse or dependence) (Kessler et al., 2005). In addition, data from the Monitoring the Future study (MTFS), a large-scale study of American high-school students, show high prevalence rates of substance use, which increase steadily with age. According to this study, past-month rates of any illicit drug use were 8.5% among 8th graders, 17.3% for 10th graders, and 23.1% for 12th graders (Johnston et al., 2006).

A strikingly high number of people develop addictions to substances. Further, children are exposed to substances frequently and at a young age. These high prevalence and exposure rates highlight the need to better understand the etiology of SUDs. Although the majority of people who engage in recreational and/or experimental substance use will not develop drug abuse or dependence, it is important to understand the factors that determine the progression from drug use to dependence. Indeed, a recent survey reveals that Americans view drug abuse as one of the most serious public health problems facing the United States (ICR, 1996).

Despite the dramatic advances generated by the sequencing of human genes (Human Genome Project) and progress in molecular biology in gene expression, the identification of specific genetic vulnerability factors for the development of SUDs will require a further complex series of studies of multiple domains influencing susceptibility to drug abuse/dependence. Unlike Mendelian diseases where a specific gene mutation is directly associated with susceptibility to a particular disease, substance abuse/dependence is a multifactorial disorder, which requires environmental exposure to a particular drug as well as several different classes of genes involved in the metabolism, and direct and indirect central nervous system (CNS) effects of drugs. Although socioenvironmental factors appear to play a key role in the initial use of a substance, an interaction between individual biological, physiological, psychological, and environmental processes is associated with the progression to more problematic use.

The goals of this chapter are (*1*) to summarize evidence regarding the genetic epidemiology of SUDs, (*2*) to review sources of complexity in the etiology of SUDs, and (*3*) to review current research on the genetic influences in the development of SUDs.

GENETIC EPIDEMIOLOGIC STUDIES

Family Studies

The family-study design has been useful in illustrating the magnitude of aggregation of SUDs within families as well as the patterns of transmission of SUDs. The family-study method has long been used to show whether a disorder "runs in families," which often indicates that a disorder has a genetic component. The family-study method compares the prevalence of a disorder in first-degree relatives of cases to the prevalence of the disorder in first-degree relatives of controls, who are frequently matched to cases on key characteristics such as age, gender, and psychiatric diagnosis. The familial aggregation of alcoholism has been well-established through decades of comprehensive study (for reviews of alcoholism, see Merikangas, 1990; McGue, 1994). Although there has been less systematic research on the familial aggregation of drug use disorders, available empirical evidence demonstrates that drug use disorders also tend to aggregate within families. The results of many family-history and uncontrolled family studies (Hill et al., 1977; Croughan, 1985; Gfroerer, 1987; Meller et al., 1988; Mirin et al., 1988; Mirin et al., 1991; Rounsaville et al., 1991; Compton et al., 2002), and controlled stud-

* The views and opinions expressed in this report are those of the authors and should not be construed to represent the views of any of the sponsoring agencies or the United States government.

ies of first-degree relatives of substance abusers (Bierut et al., 1998; Merikangas, Stolar, et al., 1998; Nurnberger et al., 2004) show elevated rates of SUDs among relatives of drug abusers compared to rates of SUDs in controls. The family study of Merikangas, Stolar, et al. (1998) found an eightfold increased risk of drug use disorders among relatives of probands with drug use disorders as compared to relatives of people with psychiatric disorders and to unaffected controls (Merikangas, Stolar, et al., 1998).

High-Risk Studies

Studies of offspring of parents with substance abuse disorders are a subset of family studies that provides information on the order of onset and patterns of transitions across drug categories, as well as on premorbid risk factors for the development of substance abuse. Although there have been several high-risk studies of children of alcoholics (Johnson et al., 1989; Chassin et al., 1991; Sher et al., 1991; Hill and Hruska, 1992; Reich et al., 1993; Merikangas, Dierker, et al., 1998; Shuckit and Smith, 1996), there have been very few controlled studies of the offspring of drug abusers. Available studies have yielded consistent findings regarding an increased risk of SUDs among offspring of parents with substance abuse or dependence when compared to those of nonsubstance abusers (Martin et al., 1994; Moss et al., 1994; Merikangas, Dierker, and Szatmari, 1998). In an 8-year follow-up study, offspring of substance abusers were at a twofold increased risk for any SUD and a threefold increased risk for alcohol and marijuana abuse or dependence compared to offspring of control parents (Merikangas and Avenevoli, 2000). Hopfer et al. (2003) also reported parent–child transmission for marijuana use, abuse, and dependence. Some studies have reported specificity for substance use, such that adolescents are particularly likely to use the same illicit drug as their parents (Andrews et al., 1997; Hoffman and Cerbone, 2002; Merikangas and Avenevoli, 2000).

High-risk studies are particularly informative for prevention efforts as they aid in the identification of premorbid vulnerability factors that serve as sources of identification for children at risk for particular disorders. One candidate risk factor for SUDs is behavioral disinhibition, a trait-like dysfunction in the ability to control behavior that is socially undesirable or has adverse consequences (Gorenstein and Newman, 1980). Multivariate analysis of a community sample of Colorado twins showed that the considerable covariation among behavior disorders and drug use was accounted for almost entirely by behavioral disinhibition, which is highly heritable and only weakly influenced by shared environmental influences (Young et al., 2000). Recent analyses of family-study data by Tarter and colleagues similarly support a common neurobehavioral disinhibition factor underlying the risk for drug abuse and dependence, which includes a prominent component of impaired executive decision making in youth at risk for drug abuse (Tarter et al., 2003; Tarter et al., 2004). Parents may increase their offspring's risk of developing substance abuse in numerous ways. Parents increase offspring's risk by serving as negative role models for the use/abuse of drugs and by using drugs as a coping mechanism (Brook et al., 1986). Additionally, positive expectancies of the effects of substances (Conway et al., 2003) and availability and tolerance of substance use in the home (Hawkins et al., 1992) increase a child's risk for the development of a SUD. Further, adolescents with a family history of substance abuse are more likely to associate with deviant peers than those without a familial loading (Kandel and Andrews, 1987), indicating interplay between familial and peer influences.

Likewise, nearly all of the high-risk studies reveal that different risk factors may be involved across the different "stages" of development of SUDs. Whereas individual characteristics and peer influences strongly influence exposure to and initial patterns of use of alcohol and drugs, family history and psychopathology play a more salient role in the transition to problematic alcohol use and dependence (Cadoret et al., 1986). A more comprehensive review of the literature on family risk and protective factors related to the etiology and progression of SUDs is available elsewhere (Avenevoli et. al., 2005).

Twin Studies

Although family studies have been helpful in showing that genes may be involved in the development of a SUD, twin studies can provide actual estimates of heritability. Twin studies are informative because identical (monozygotic; MZ) twins share 100% of their genes whereas fraternal (dizygotic; DZ) twins share, on average, 50% of their genes. If genetic factors play an important role in substance use and disorders, then studies of twins should find greater similarity between MZ than DZ twins, assuming that the influence of familial environment on drug use outcomes is equal for MZ and DZ twins. The aggregate twin study data are remarkably consistent in demonstrating that genetic factors play a far greater role in the etiology of more severe patterns of drug use, particularly those which meet diagnostic criteria for abuse or dependence, than initial use or early stages of use, which appear to be more strongly determined by environmental influences (Tsuang et al., 1996; Kendler and Prescott, 1998b; Rhee et al., 2003; Fowler et al., 2007). Studies have examined drug use, abuse, and dependence in general (Grove et al., 1990; Pickens et al., 1991; Jang et al., 1995; Kendler et al.,

2000), as well as a diverse range of specific drugs including nicotine, caffeine, tranquilizers, sedatives, cannabis, cocaine, stimulants, hallucinogens, and opiates (Claridge, Ross, and Hume, 1978; Pedersen, 1981; Gurling et al., 1985; Heath et al., 1993; Heath and Madden, 1995; Heath et al., 1997; True et al., 1997; Kendler and Prescott, 1998a, 1998b; Tsuang et al., 1998; Kendler, Karkowski, and Prescott, 1999; True et al., 1999; Kendler et al., 2000).

Table 47.1 gives a summary of recent population-based twin studies of drug dependence. The tetrachoric correlations shown in Table 47.1 reflect the correlations in the inferred underlying liability for the development of drug abuse. The results of these studies have been highly consistent in demonstrating the role of genetic factors in the etiology of drug use disorders. However, the extent of genetic influence differs according to the trait definition employed, and the age, sex, and source of the sample. The studies reviewed in Table 47.1 demonstrate a wide range of heritability estimates ranging from 0% to 87% in males and 0% to 77% in females, with a median of 53% and 55% for males and females, respectively. The approximately twofold larger correlation between MZ compared to DZ twins reflects the contributions of genetic factors to the specific drug phenotype. Surprisingly, common environmental influences are low in most studies, whereas unique environmental factors play a major role in drug abuse/dependence in these samples. These studies demonstrate the complex interplay (interactions and correlations) between genetic and environmental factors in the etiology of drug abuse.

Adoption Studies

The classic adoption studies of Cadoret and colleagues (Cadoret et al., 1986; Cadoret, 1992; Cadoret et al., 1995, 1996) have also been highly informative in elucidating the role of genetic factors in the development of drug use and abuse. Although data on biologic parents are often limited with respect to specific patterns of drug use and abuse, Cadoret et al.'s studies provide the strongest evidence to date that genetic factors play an important role in the development of drug abuse. These studies identify two major biologic/genetic pathways to the development of drug abuse in adoptees. The first pathway links substance abuse in the biological parent to drug abuse and dependence in the adoptee. The second pathway appears to be an expression of underlying aggressivity in the adoptee and relates to antisocial personality disorder (ASPD) in the biologic parent (Cadoret et al., 1995, 1996). Moreover, adopted-away offspring of fathers who are antisocial addicts (compared to either antisocial or addicted) are at especially elevated risk for substance abuse (Langbehn et al., 2003).

SOURCES OF COMPLEXITY OF GENETICS OF SUBSTANCE USE DISORDERS

Demographic Correlates

Sex differences

Substance use disorders are more common in males than in females. Based on the rates from the Epidemiologic Catchment Area Study, men are 5 times more likely to have an alcohol use disorder and 2 to 3 times more likely to have a drug use disorder than women (Anthony and Helzer, 1995). Likewise, the NCS (Kessler et al., 1997), National Longitudinal Alcohol Epidemiologic Survey (NLAES), and National Epidemiologic Survey on Alcohol and Related Conditions (NESARC) found that SUDs were more prevalent among men than women (Grant et al., 2004; Compton et al., 2007).

Findings from family and twin studies that have observed the effect of sex on transmission of SUDs have been inconsistent. Whereas some studies show that the relatives of females with alcoholism have a lower threshold for manifestation of alcoholism than those of males with alcoholism, other studies found no difference in the familial aggregation of alcoholism among men and women. For example, one study found that alcohol abuse and dependence were familial among females, whereas only dependence aggregated among the relatives of males with alcohol dependence (Merikangas, Stolar, et al., 1998). Sex differences in transmission of SUDs also emerged in the clinical twin study of van den Bree et al. (1998), who found that the heritability estimates for males were much higher than for females across a broad spectrum of drug use disorders. In contrast, data from the Australian Twin Registry indicate no significant sex differences in estimates of heritability or environmental influence for cannabis dependence (Lynskey et al., 2002) or nicotine withdrawal (Pergadia et al., 2006). The similarity in heritability estimates for males and females shown in Table 47.1 provides further evidence that there are few sex differences in the transmission of SUDs in population-based samples.

Age/developmental stage. Twin studies have also begun to examine the role of genetic factors in the development of SUDs in prospective samples of children and adolescents. These studies may inform our understanding of the influence of age and developmental level in the etiology of SUDs. For example, McGue (1994) revealed far greater heritability of drug use disorders among males with early age of onset compared to either those with later age of onset or females. These data suggest that different factors may exert influence at different stages of development, and/or that certain developmental periods are more sensitive than others. Because exposure to drugs generally occurs during early adolescence, the above-cited data derived from adult

TABLE 47.1 *Population-Based Twin Studies of Abuse/Dependence of Specific Drugs Conducted in the Last 10 Years*

				Tetrachoric Correlations				*Components of Variance*					
				Monozygotic		*Dizygotic*		*Addictive Genetic*		*Common Environment*		*Unique Environ/ Error*	
Substance	*Author(s) and Year*	*Sample*[a]	*DX Interview*[b]	*Male*	*Female*	*Male*	*Female*	*Male*	*Female*	*Male*	*Female*	*Male*	*Female*
Alcohol	Prescott & Kendler, 1999	VETR	SCID-111-R & SSAGA	0.53	—	0.18	—	0.51	—	—	—	0.49	—
	Heath et al., 1997[d]	ANH&MRC	SSAGA	0.68	0.58	0.20	0.29	0.64	0.64	0.03	0.01	0.33	0.35
	True, Xian, et al., 1999	VETR	DIS-111-R	0.55	—	0.29	—	0.55	—	—	—	0.45	—
	True, Heath, et al., 1999[c]	VETR	DIS-111-R	—	—	—	—	0.45	—	0.12	—	0.44	—
Tobacco	Pergadia et al., 2006[c, f, h, j]	ATR	SSAGA	—	—	—	—	0.61	0.61	0.01	0.01	0.38	0.38
	Kendler, Neale, et al., 1999[c, k]	VETR	FTQ	—	0.47	—	0.30	—	0.30	—	0.20	—	0.50
	True, Xian, et al., 1999[c]	VETR	DIS-111-R	0.61	—	0.31	—	0.60	—	—	—	0.40	—
Marijuana	Agrawal et al., 2005	VATSPSUD	SCID-111-R	—	—	—	—	0.31	0.36	0.00	0.00	0.69	0.65
	Agrawal et al., 2007	ATR	SSAGA	—	—	—	—	0.68	0.55	0.14	0.16	0.18	0.29
	Kendler et al., 2006[b]	NIPHTP	M-CIDI	0.77	0.77	0.31	0.31	0.77	0.77	0.00	0.00	0.23	0.23
	Lynskey et al., 2002[c]	ATR	SSAGA	0.70	0.59	0.35	0.51	0.56	0.21	0.13	0.39	0.31	0.40
	Kendler et al., 2000	VTR	SCID-111-R	0.59	—	0.20	—	0.58	—	0.00	—	0.42	—
	Kendler & Prescott, 1998[a]	VETR	SCID-111-R	—	0.58	—	0.41	—	0.62	—	0.00	—	0.38
	True, Heath, et al., 1999[c]	VETR	DIS-111-R	—	—	—	—	0.44	—	0.21	—	0.36	—
	Tsuang et al., 1996	VETR	DIS-111-R	0.62	—	0.46	—	0.33	—	0.29	—	0.38	—

TABLE 47.1 *Population-Based Twin Studies of Abuse/Dependence of Specific Drugs Conducted in the Last 10 Years (Continued)*

				Tetrachoric Correlations				*Components of Variance*					
				Monozygotic		*Dizygotic*		*Addictive Genetic*		*Common Environment*		*Unique Environ/ Error*	
Substance	*Author(s) and Year*	*Sample*[a]	*DX Interviewb*	*Male*	*Female*	*Male*	*Female*	*Male*	*Female*	*Male*	*Female*	*Male*	*Female*
Stimulants	Agrawal et al., 2005	VATSPSUD	SCID-111-R	—	—	—	—	0.53	0.00	0.00	0.99	0.47	0.01
	Lynskey et al., 2007[h]	ATR	SSAGA	—	—	—	—	0.65	0.65	0.08	0.08	0.28	0.28
	Kendler et al., 2000	VTR	SCID-111-R	0.43	—	0.34	—	0.00	—	0.39	—	0.61	—
	Tsuang et al., 1996[j]	VETR	DIS-111-R	0.53	—	0.24	—	0.44	—	0.00	—	0.49	—
Sedatives	Agrawal et al., 2005	VATSPSUD	SCID-111-R	—	—	—	—	0.08	0.38	0.00	0.00	0.92	0.62
	Kendler et al., 2000	VETR	SCID-111-R	0.83	—	0.00	—	0.87	—	0.00	—	0.13	—
	Tsuang et al., 1996	VETR	DIS-111-R	0.44	—	0.25	—	0.38	—	0.06	—	0.56	—
Psychedelics	Kendler et al., 2000	VETR	SCID-111-R	0.00	—	0.00	—	0.79	—	0.00	—	0.21	—
	Tsuang et al., 1996	VETR	DIS-111-R	0.44	—	0.32	—	0.25	—	0.19	—	0.56	—
Cocaine	Agrawal et al., 2005	VATSPSUD	SCID-111-R	—	—	—	—	0.08	0.38	0.00	0.00	0.92	0.62
	Kendler et al., 2000	VETR	SCID-111-R	0.77	—	0.37	—	0.79	—	0.00	—	0.21	—
	Kendler & Prescott, 1998[b/c]	VETR	SCID-111-R	—	0.68	—	0.08	—	0.65	—	0.00	—	0.35
Opiates	Tsuang et al., 1996[j]	VETR	DIS-111-R	0.67	—	0.29	—	0.43	—	0.00	—	0.31	—

[a] VATSPSUD: Virginia Adult Twin Study of Psychoactive and Substance Use Disorders; VTR: Virginia Twin Registry; VETR, Vietnam Era Twin Registry; ANH & MRC: Australian National Health and Medical Research Council; ATR: Australian Twin Register; MTS: Minnesota Twin Study; NIPHTP: Norwegian Institute of Public Health Twin Panel.

[b] SCID: Structured Clinical Interview for *DSM-111-R*; SSAGA: Semi-Structured Assessment for the Genetics of Alcoholism; DIS-111-R: Diagnostic Interview Schedule Version 111 Revised; FTQ: Fagerstrom Tolerance Questionnaire; DIS-111: Diagnostic Interview Schedule Version 111; M-CIDI: Munich-Composite International Diagnostic Interview.

[c] Study examines dependence without abuse.

[d] Sample also included 754 unlike-sex pairs.

[e] Sample also included 655 unlike-sex pairs and 753 (377 female and 376 male) single twins.

[f] Sample also included 559 unlike-sex pairs.

[g] Sample also included 338 unlike-sex pairs.

[h] Best-fitting model was obtained when components of variance were constrained to equality across the sexes, thus sex-specific estimates reported here are identical.

[i] *DSM-IV* nicotine withdrawal was the phenotype.

[j] Non-additive genetic effects were reported for stimulants (0.07) and opiates (0.26).

[k] Study reports Pearson's *r*, rather than the tetrachoric correlation. *DSM*: *Diagnostic and Statistical Manual of Mental Disorders*.

samples are necessarily susceptible to the biases of all retrospective studies. A study of adolescent twins from the Netherlands (Boomsma et al., 1994) yielded evidence to suggest that the heritability of alcohol use increased with age, whereas shared environmental factors had a stronger impact in early adolescence. Similarly, relying on retrospective reports from adults, Gillespie and colleagues (2007) reported an overall increase in genetic influence and a decline in shared environmental influence from ages 8 to 25. Follow-up studies of this topic will increase understanding of the joint influences of genetic, environmental, and developmental factors on occurrence and persistence of dependence as individuals pass through the risk period for the development of substance dependence.

Cohort and generation effects. One key source of complexity in studying the familial transmission of drug abuse is the dramatic changes in patterns of drug use in the general population, as well as within specific subgroups. Rapid shifts in the availability of specific drugs and cultural and geographic patterns of drug use complicate traditional inspection of vertical patterns of concordance for drug use and dependence. Whereas alcohol has been readily available during the past several decades, and cannabis use has been somewhat stable as well, crack cocaine and ecstasy have only been widely available during the past decade, and the misuse of prescription drugs has dramatically increased in very recent years. Conversely, nicotine use has been decreasing rapidly in more recent cohorts. These differences in availability and cultural norms contribute to the difficulty in discriminating exposed but unaffected relatives from those who were never exposed to a particular drug, an issue that poses major methodological challenges (Neal et al., 2006). Within-generation comparisons are therefore more likely to control for exposure to specific substances. Siblings, however, are often responsible for the initiation of other siblings to drugs, which could lead to an overestimation in the heritability of drug use. The association between cohort effects and heritability is largely unexplored. One study found that though prevalence rates for psychoactive substance use differed substantially across three cohorts, there was no systematic relationship between heritability and prevalence of psychoactive substance use (Kendler et al., 2005), suggesting that evolving patterns of drug accessibility and consumption do not significantly affect rates of heritability.

Spouse concordance. Several studies have shown spouse concordance for drug use (Vanyukov et al., 1996; Merikangas et al., 1992). This tendency for spouses to be concordant for substance use is another issue that must be integrated into the evaluation of genetic evidence (Grant et al., 2007). Merikangas et al. (1992) reported that more than 90% of interviewed opioid-dependent proband spouses had a history of opioid dependence themselves. Furthermore, these investigations showed a strong association between rates of drug abuse in adult siblings of opioid abusers and the number of their parents with substance abuse. It is therefore critical that spouse concordance be incorporated in genetic analyses of substance abuse.

Phenotype Definition

One of the major impediments to genetic studies of SUDs is that these conditions are the net result of a series of complex processes that are difficult to capture using currently available methods of measurement. Although analysis requires the drawing of thresholds between different stages of progression of drug use to distinguish drug abuse and dependence from patterns of use, such divisions have limited our ability to characterize the drug use disorder phenotype. A dimensional rating, which depicts progression across a continuum, may better represent the development of addictions. Aggregation of the findings across genetic epidemiologic studies of drug use and drug use disorders is difficult because of the wide variability in the measures employed in these studies, ranging from a few items regarding substance use on self-reported questionnaires to longitudinal characterization of patterns of progression. For example, twin studies of smoking have examined diverse components of smoking, including use, frequency, quantity, age at onset, continued use, current use, current frequency, dependence, severity, and ability to quit (Heath and Madden, 1995); however, the consistency of these measures varies greatly by study. Table 47.2 presents a summary of the range of phenotypes that have been investigated in linkage and association studies of substance use and SUDs. Studies of smoking have employed a full range of components of smoking behaviors, whereas those of illicit drugs, such as those of opioids or cocaine, have generally only assessed dependence.

Genetic epidemiologic studies have contributed to our understanding of substance use/abuse phenotypes through systematic investigation of the familiality or heritability of different components of drug use trajectories. For example, the results of several twin studies reveal that genetic factors have greater influence on the development of alcohol dependence and persistence than on initiation and early stages of alcohol use (Whitfield et al., 2004; Sartor et al., 2007). Likewise, family studies have shown that familial factors are more influential in transitions at the more severe end of the drinking spectrum (Bucholz et al., 2000).

Polysubstance Use

Another important consideration in examining the role of genetic factors in drug use disorders is the tendency

TABLE 47.2 *Candidate Genes for Substance Use and Disorders*

Genes	*Protein*	*Smoking*	*Alcohol*	*Cocaine*	*Opioids*	*Polysubstance*
Alcohol metabolism						
ALDH1B	Alcohol dehydrogenase 1B		X			
ALDH2	Alcohol dehydrogenase 1C		X			
ADH1A	Aldehyde dehydrogenase		X			
ADH1B	Aldehyde dehydrogenase		X			
ADH4	Aldehyde dehydrogenase		X			
Cannabinoid system						
CNR1	Cannabinoid Receptor 1				X	X
Cholinergic system						
CHRNA4	Muscarinic acetylcholine receptor α-4	X				
CHRM2	Muscarinic acetylcholine receptor μ-2			X	X	
Dopaminergic system						
DRD2	Dopamine receptor 2	X		X	X	X
DRD3	Dopamine receptor 3			X	X	
DRD4	Dopamine receptor 4				X	
DβH	Dopamine beta-hydroxylase			X		
DAT(1) SLC6A3	Dopamine Transporter				X	X
COMT	Catechol-O-methyltransferase	X			X	
Gabaergic system						
GABRA1	GABA receptor subunit α_1		X			
GABRA2	GABA receptor subunit α_2		X			
GABRB1	GABA receptor subunit β_1		X			
Nicotine metabolism						
CYP2A6	Cytochrome P450	X			X	X
CYP2D6					X	X
Opioid system						
OPRM	μ-opioid receptor	X	X	X	X	X
OPRD1	κ-opioid receptor				X	X
OPRD1	δ-opioid receptor		X		X	
PENK	Proenkephalin				X	X
PDYN	Prodynorphin			X		
Serotonergic system						
Metabolism						
TPH1	Tryptophan hydroxylase	X	X	X		
HTR1$_B$	Serotonin receptor 1_B		X		X	
COMT	Catechol-O-methyltransferase				X	
SLC6A4	Serotonin Transporter	X	X	X		

GABA: γ-aminobutyric acid.

for substance abusers to misuse multiple substances, simultaneously as well as longitudinally (Mirin et al., 1991; Merikangas, Dierker, et al., 1998). Most uncontrolled family studies suggest that alcohol and drug dependence aggregate independently in families (Hill et al., 1977; Meller et al., 1988; Mirin et al., 1991; Rounsaville et al., 1991; Luthar and Rounsaville, 1993), although controlled family studies and family-history studies report an increased risk of alcoholism among relatives of drug abusers (or the converse) (Bierut et al., 1998; Merikangas, Stolar, et al., 1998; Compton et al., 2002). Likewise, one twin study revealed a moderate degree of heritability for the frequency of use and the tendency to use numerous illicit substances (h^2 = .32; Jang et al., 1995).

The specificity of familial aggregation of particular types of substance dependence has been examined in family and twin studies (Bierut et al., 1998; Merikangas, Stolar, et al., 1998; Nurnberger et al., 2004; Tsuang et al., 1998). The results of these studies suggest that the genetic factors underlying drug use disorders are common and specific across different drug use disorders (Vanyukov and Tarter, 2000; Volk et al., 2007). Data from the Yale Family Study of Comorbidity of Substance Abuse and Psychopathology examined the specificity of familial aggregation of the predominant drug of abuse among adult relatives of probands with similar classification. The results revealed a remarkable degree of specificity for familial aggregation of opiates, cannabis, and alcohol, and to a lesser extent, cocaine (Merikangas, Stolar, et al., 1998). On this issue, twin data have been especially useful through the application of biometrical modeling techniques that permit the quantification and comparison of genetic (common and drug-specific) and environmental (shared and nonshared) influences across a range of illicit drugs of abuse (Rhee et al., 2003). Findings from several twin studies show that specific and common factors influence the risk for the different drug use disorders, with increasing consensus for a common vulnerability model (Tsuang et al., 1998; Karkowski et al., 2000; Kendler et al., 2003; Agrawal et al., 2004; Maes et al., 2006; Young et al., 2006; Agrawal et al., 2007). In summary, the aggregate findings of the twin and family studies provide evidence for common familial and genetic factors underlying SUDs in general, as well as substantial components that are unique for specific drugs.

Comorbidity with Psychopathology

Another phenomenon that has complicated phenotypic definitions of SUDs is the widespread comorbidity between substance use and psychiatric disorders. Some of the largest and most consistent findings have been reported between drug use disorders and ASPD, mood disorders, anxiety disorders, and attention deficit disorder (Quitkin et al., 1972; Rounsaville et al., 1982; Khantzian, 1983; Mirin et al., 1984; Khantzian and Treece, 1985; Weiss and Mirin, et al., 1985; Mirin et al., 1988; Regier et al., 1990; Kessler et al., 1996; Conway et al., 2006). Ross et al. (1988) found that 78% of their treatment sample of patients with SUDs met *Diagnostic and Statistical Manual of Mental Disorders*, 3rd ed. (*DSM-III*; American Psychiatric Association, 1980) criteria for a lifetime comorbid psychiatric disorder.

Several family studies of drug-dependent probands have examined the effects of comorbid disorders on familial aggregation of SUDs and other psychiatric disorders. Most of the family studies have found increased rates of all major disorders among relatives of substance abusers; however, most have been uncontrolled, and few have accounted for comorbid disorders within the probands (Mirin et al., 1984; Croughan, 1985; Rounsaville et al., 1991). The results of the family studies have demonstrated consistently that there is independent familial aggregation of ASPD and drug use disorders (Rounsaville et al., 1991).

Twin studies may provide information on the extent to which familial correlations between disorders result from shared genetic or familial factors. For example, Lin et al. (1996) compared the familial versus nonfamilial links between major depression with alcohol use disorders and drug use disorders. They concluded that whereas comorbidity between major depression and alcohol use disorders resulted from common familial factors, comorbidity with drug use disorders was attributable to nonfamilial factors.

Environmental Influences

Because environmental exposure to a drug is inherent to the development of SUDs, studies of the genetics of SUDs must account for gene–environment interaction as a major source of complexity of this phenotype. There are numerous environmental factors related to drug exposure, including family dynamics, peer interaction, temperament features, socioeconomic related factors, and cultural norms. These factors interact with the individual's genetic makeup to influence phenotypic expression (Brook et al., 1986; Simcha-Figan and Schwartz, 1986; Brown, 1989; Brook et al., 1990; Avenevoli et al., 2005). However, because of the overlap in the role of genetic and environmental factors underlying vulnerability to SUDs, it may not be fruitful to devote substantial effort to determining whether risk factors fall on either the environmental or the genetic side of the risk equation. For example, an individual's genotype may influence his or her use of drugs (gene–environment correlation), and many putative environmental factors, such as exposure to family violence, may actually result from genetic factors common to disinhibition, aggression, and substance abuse.

Cross-national comparisons and migration studies are useful in identifying environmental and cultural risk factors. Several studies have shown that despite tremendous international variation in rates of SUDs, international patterns of comorbidity are nearly identical. This suggests that the links between SUDs and mental and behavioral disorders may result from biologic factors involved in drug preference, response, and metabolism (Merikangas et al., 1998). Likewise, cross-national comparisons in twin concordance reveal similar heritability estimates despite large differences in prevalence estimates (for example, Norway [low illicit drug use] vs. United States and Australia [high illicit drug use]), thereby suggesting that heritability is unaffected by drug availability (Kendler et al., 2006).

The migrant study design is one of the most powerful approaches for identifying cultural and environmental risk factors for a disease. Studies of Asian immigrants to the United States have been used to demonstrate strong environmental contributions to many forms of cancer and heart disease (Kolonel et al., 2004). Recent findings from a migration study of adolescent offspring of Puerto Rican migrant parents compared to nonmigrant parents revealed greater rates of alcohol use among the island Puerto Ricans as compared to the mainland Puerto Rican children (47.7% vs. 28.9%, respectively), whereas the use of illicit drugs was far greater among mainland compared to island Puerto Rican youth (that is, 15.0 vs. 6.9%, respectively; Conway et al., 2007). Investigation of the explanations for greater illicit drug use among migrant youth may yield information on the environmental factors that contribute to substance use and abuse. These findings highlight the importance of country or culture-specific influences on patterns of substance use.

GENETIC INFLUENCES

Advances in molecular and human genetics have led to the identification of nearly all of the genes underlying Mendelian diseases (that is, those with clear-cut adherence to Mendelian law such as autosomal dominant, autosomal recessive, or X-linked). This progress has been revolutionary in terms of prediction of disease risk (for example, Huntington's disease; Langbehn et al., 2004), and understanding of pathogenesis (for example, familial hemiplegic migraine; and Alzheimer's disease, Hardy and Selkoe, 2002). The rapid success in identifying genes for Mendelian diseases generated the expectation that the same research strategies would eventually be successful in identifying genes for complex diseases, such as heart disease, obesity, cancer, diabetes, and many psychiatric conditions, but identification of genes for other complex disorders has proven far more difficult. Recent successes, however, have renewed hopes that replicable candidate genes will be identified in psychiatry in the future.

Linkage Studies

The traditional approach for locating a disease gene in humans is *linkage analysis*, which tests the association between deoxyribonucleic acid (DNA) polymorphic markers and affected status within families. After linkage is detected with an initial marker, many other markers nearby may also be examined. Markers showing the strongest correlation with disease in families are assumed to be closest to the disease locus. Linkage analysis uses DNA sequences with high variability (that is, polymorphisms) to increase the power to identify markers that are associated with a disease within families. Historically, different methodological approaches have been applied. Earlier linkage studies employed restriction fragment length polymorphisms (RFLPs), whereas subsequent studies examined short tandem repeat markers, or "microsatellites," DNA sequences that show considerable variability among people but whose variability has no functional consequences. More recently, linkage and association studies have examined single nucleotide polymorphisms (SNPs) to track diseases in families.

Markers in the candidate region identified by linkage analysis can be used to narrow the location of the disease gene through *linkage disequilibrium analysis*. Linkage disequilibrium is a population association between two alleles at different loci and occurs when the same founder mutation exists in a large proportion of individuals who are affected in the population studied. Usually, the closer the marker is to the disease locus, the greater the proportion of individuals who are affected who carry the identical allele at the marker (Risch, 2000). However, in measuring the strength of linkage disequilibrium for a given marker, it is also important to select unaffected control individuals from the same population because an allele shared among individuals who are affected may also be common in the general population and thus shared by chance rather than due to proximity to the disease locus (Risch, 2000).

For complex human diseases, a simple mode of genetic inheritance is not apparent, and indeed, multiple contributing genetic loci are likely to be involved. Study designs that do not depend on the particular mode of inheritance are required for linkage analysis. Because relatives who are affected provide most of the information for such analyses, studies that focus on searching for increased sharing of marker alleles above chance expectation among relatives who are affected may be employed. The simplest of such studies involves sibships who are affected, where allele sharing in excess of 50% (the expectation when there is no linkage) is sought.

Association Studies

Association studies generally employ a case-control design to compare candidate genes among individuals affected to those among unrelated unaffected controls.

Failure to equate cases and controls may lead to confounding (that is, a spurious association due to an unmeasured factor that is associated with the candidate gene and the disease). In genetic case-control studies, the most likely source of confounding is ethnicity because of differential gene and disease frequencies in different ethnic subgroups.

The association study design also generally employs a candidate gene approach to identify susceptibility genes for a particular disorder. The candidate gene approach has enjoyed only limited success because few of the genes that have been identified have withstood the test of replication (Altmuller et al., 2001; Ioannidis et al., 2001; Hirschhorn et al., 2002; Hirschhorn and Daly, 2005). The chief obstacles to identifying genes for complex diseases with the candidate gene approach include the lack of validity of phenotype characterization, biased sampling, inadequate controls, failure to correct for multiple tests, high false-positive rate due to low a priori probability, use of an overly liberal alpha value, and the lack of adequate power of gene searching approaches (Risch, 2000; Glazier et al., 2002; Wacholder et al., 2004; Todd, 2006). In addition, there is a strong publication bias against reports of negative association studies (Ioannidis et al., 2001; Ott, 2004). To offset the high false-positive rate that has plagued the literature on complex disease genetics, journals in nearly all fields of medicine have published editorials about these high rates of false positives or have adopted publication policies that take into account the potential for false positives when reviewing articles (Begg, 2005).

Genome-Wide Association Studies

Because of the lack of replication of association studies of candidate genes, the genome-wide association method has been proposed as the most promising approach to gene identification in future studies of complex diseases (Botstein and Risch, 2003; Hirschhorn and Daly, 2005). The genome-wide association method, which is based on a systematic search of equally spaced genetic markers across the genome among cases and controls, was demonstrated to have greater power than linkage (within-family associations between genetic markers and disease) and association studies, which evaluate associations of prespecified candidate genes and diseases between sibling pairs or between cases and controls (Risch and Merikangas, 1996). The identification of a large set of common SNPs, which explains much of the common variation in the human genome, by the International HapMap Consortium (2005) and the advent of high throughput genotyping chips that can survey over 500,000 of these SNPs at a single pass, have increased the feasibility of mapping individual genome variation quickly, which allows for the comparison of large numbers of cases and controls. Because of these advances, it is possible to conduct whole genome association studies that could link common SNPs as well as copy number variations to vulnerability to complex disorders.

Recent successes using this approach include the identification of genes for macular degeneration (Edwards et al., 2005; Haines et al., 2005; Klein et al., 2005) and several other complex disorders including inflammatory bowel diseases (Crohn's disease and ulcerative colitis; Duerr et al., 2006), diabetes (Groves et al., 2006; Field et al., 2007; Grant et al., 2006; Sladek et al., 2007), and prostate cancer (Amundadottir et al., 2006; Freedman et al., 2006). Although independent replications have confirmed the potential fruitfulness of this approach, it has not yet been successfully applied to gene identification for psychiatric disorders (Couzin and Kaiser, 2007).

Gene Identification Studies in Psychiatry

Based on the dramatic advances in molecular genetics during the past 20 years, as described above, there has been a major shift in the focus of psychiatric genetic investigations during the past decade from elucidating patterns of familial transmission to localizing genes underlying mental disorders using linkage studies and association studies. Although there remains controversy regarding the constitution of replications of genetic findings for several mental disorders, there are several recent, promising findings in psychiatric genetics. The increasing tendency for collaborative efforts on genetics studies within psychiatry may yield greater power to detect genes of small effect. The emergence of an international consensus on standards for replication (Chanock et al., 2007) and the application of new approaches for identifying genes may lead to an understanding of the etiology of psychiatric disorders such as already exists for numerous other complex diseases.

Selection of candidate genes for substance use and disorders has been based either on drug metabolism (pharmacokinetics) or drug response (pharmacodynamics) in the CNS or periphery (Saxon et al., 2007). The brain reward pathway is the system that has been studied most extensively in identifying genetic factors underlying drug abuse. Candidate genes for substance use and disorders have been summarized for smoking by Ho and Tyndale (2007), for opioids and cocaine by Saxon et al. (2007), for alcoholism (Edenberg and Faroud, 2006), and for general vulnerability factors by Kreek et al. (2005). The reader can refer to http://geneticassociationdb.nih.gov for a complete and updated list of the status of findings on specific candidate genes. A summary of candidate genes that have been investigated for one or more of these substances is presented in Table 47.2. With the exception of the alcohol metabolism genes, most of the genes have been investigated in only a few studies, and replications have not been forthcoming.

One area that has received widespread attention in the drug abuse field has been the translation of findings regarding susceptibility genes to clinical settings and to public health as a whole. Because of the multiple levels of influence on drug availability—including macro-influences such as government, health care, industry, and the education system, as well as environment—it has been proposed that the identification of genes underlying drug use may have less of a contribution to the prevention of drug abuse and dependence than the institution of policy measures that reduce drug exposure (Merikangas and Risch, 2003; Hall, 2005). On the other hand, identification of the genetic factors involved in conferring increased biological vulnerability to drug abuse and dependence as well as cessation may advance our understanding of the pathogenesis of drug abuse and inform efforts to block the effects of drugs and to enhance the effects of treatment. The most compelling potential benefit of gene identification would be the development of medications that block relevant metabolic enzymes to reduce dependence on a particular drug (Saxon et al., 2007). The use of genetic testing for drug abuse vulnerability is far less feasible because of ethical concerns engendered by the potential danger of labeling such individuals as well as the potential for increasing drug use among those who lack a susceptibility marker (Merikangas and Risch, 2003; Hall, 2005; Saxon et al., 2007).

SUMMARY AND FUTURE DIRECTIONS

Substance use is a complex phenomenon, inherently characterized by a gene–environment interaction because exposure to an exogenous substance is necessary for its expression. This phenotype is ideally suited for investigation using the tools of epidemiology, which can examine the interactions between individual vulnerability factors and environmental exposure. Additional large-scale community epidemiological studies from diverse populations are critical for elucidating the role of genetic and environmental factors in the transmission of substance abuse, validating phenotypic definitions of substance use/abuse, and identifying sources of heterogeneity in the etiology of substance abuse, particularly with respect to the role of comorbid psychiatric disorders and polysubstance abuse. The information gleaned from these studies will ultimately lead to more effective gene identification.

This chapter summarized the results of family, twin, adoption, and high-risk studies that concur in concluding that drug use and abuse/dependence are highly familial. The results of twin and adoption studies demonstrate that genetic factors underlie a substantial component of the familial clustering of drug use disorders. Although these human genetic studies have been helpful in looking at patterns of transmission, possible degrees of genetic heritability, and environmental catalysts, there are numerous phenomena that complicate the application of the traditional tools of genetics in identifying the specific genes underlying these conditions. Additional research is necessary for the refinement of the definitions and phenotypic descriptions of substance use and progression. Likewise, discrimination of risk factors common to drug use versus those unique to the use of a particular substance, as well as those related to use versus progression and dependence, will be critical in identifying genetic sources of variance.

Progress in identifying genes for substance use and disorders through linkage and association studies of candidate genes have generated few findings that meet the standards of external replication. Nevertheless, there is a number of promising candidate genes that may prove to contribute to drug abuse phenotypes as the results of the genome-wide approaches in large samples from collaborative efforts among investigators begin to emerge. These studies may also identify new candidate genes that could advance our understanding of the complex pathways that lead to drug abuse.

REFERENCES

Agrawal, A., Lynskey, M.T., Bucholz, K.K., Martin, N.G., Madden, P.A., and Heath, A.C. (2007) Contrasting models of genetic comorbidity for cannabis and other illicit drugs in adult Australian twins. *Psychol. Med.* 37(1):49–60.

Agrawal, A., Neale, M.C., Jacobson, K.C., Prescott, C.A., and Kendler, K.S. (2005) Illicit drug use and abuse/dependence: modeling of two-stage variables using the CCC approach. *Addict. Behav.* 30:1043–1048.

Agrawal, A., Neale, M.C., Prescott, C.A., and Kendler, K.S. (2004) Cannabis and other illicit drugs: comorbid use and abuse/dependence in males and females. *Behav. Genet.* 34:217–228.

Altmuller, J., Palmer, L.J., Fischer, G., Scherb, H., and Wjst, M. (2001) Genomewide scans of complex human diseases: true linkage is hard to find. *Am. J. Hum. Genet.* 69(5):936–950.

American Psychiatric Association. (1980) *Diagnostic and Statistical Manual of Mental Disorders*, 3rd ed. Washington, DC: Author.

Amundadottir, L.T., et al. (2006) A common variant associated with prostate cancer in European and African populations. *Nat. Genet.* 38:652–658.

Andrews, J.A., Hops, H., and Duncan, S.C. (1997) Adolescent modeling of partent substance use: the moderating effect of the relationship with the parent. *J. Fam. Psychol.* 11:259–270.

Anthony, J.C., and Helzer, J.E. (1995) Epidemiology of drug dependence. In: Tsuang, M.T., Tohen, M., Zahner, G.E.P., eds. *Textbook in Psychiatric Epidemiology*. New York: John Wiley & Sons, pp. 1364–1365.

Avenevoli, S., Conway, K.P., and Merikangas, K.R. (2005) Familial risk factors for substance use disorders. In: Hudson, J.L., and Rapee, R.M., eds. *Current Thinking on Psychopathology and the Family*. Boston: Elsevier, pp. 167–192.

Begg, C.B. (2005) Reflections on publication criteria for genetic association studies. *Cancer Epidemiol. Biomarkers Prev.* 14:1364–1365.

Bierut, L.J., Dinwiddie, S.H., Begleiter, H., Crowe, R.R., Hesselbrock, V., Nurnberger, J.I., Jr., Porjesz, B., Schuckit, M.A., and Reich, T. (1998) Familial transmission of substance dependence: alcohol, marijuana, cocaine, and habitual smoking: a report from the Collaborative Study on the Genetics of Alcoholism. *Arch. Gen. Psychiatry* 55(11):982–988.

Boomsma, D.I., Koopmans, J.R., Van Doornen, L.J.P., and Orlebeke, J.F. (1994) Genetic and social influences on starting to smoke: A study of Dutch adolescent twins and their parents. *Addiction* 89: 219–226.

Botstein, D., and Risch, N. (2003) Discovering genotypes underlying human phenotypes: past successes for Mendelian disease, future approaches for complex disease. *Nat. Gen.*33(Suppl):228–237.

Brook, J.S., Brook, D.W., Gordon, A.S., Whiteman, M., and Cohen, P. (1990) The psychosocial etiology of adolescent drug use: a family interactional approach. *Genet. Soc. Gen. Psychol. Monogr.* 116:111–267.

Brook, J.S., Whiteman, M., Gordon, A.S., and Cohen, P. (1986) Some model mechanisms for explaining the impact of maternal and adolescent characteristics on adolescent stage of drug use. *Dev. Psychology* 22:460–467.

Brown, S.A. (1989) Life events of adolescents in relation to personal and parental substance abuse. *Am. J. Psychiatry* 146:484–489.

Bucholz, K.K., Heath, A.C., and Madden, P.A. (2000) Transitions in drinking in adolescent females: evidence from the Missouri adolescent female twin study. *Alcohol Clin. Exp. Res.* 4(6):914–923.

Cadoret, R.J. (1992) Genetic and environmental factors in initiation of drug use and the transition to abuse. In: Glantx, M., and Pickens, R., eds. *Vulnerability to Drug Abuse*. Washington, DC: American Psychological Association, pp. 99–113.

Cadoret, R.J., Troughton, E., O'Gorman, T., and Heywood, E. (1986) An adoption study of genetic and environmental factors in drug abuse. *Arch. Gen. Psychiatry* 43:1131–1136.

Cadoret, R.J., Yates, W.R., Troughton, E., Woodworth, G., and Stewart, M.A. (1995) Adoption study demonstrating two genetic pathways to drug abuse. *Arch. Gen. Psychiatry* 52:42–52.

Cadoret, R.J., Yates, W.R., Troughton, E., Woodworth, G., and Stewart, M.A. (1996) An adoption study of drug abuse/dependence in females. *Compr. Psychiatry* 37:88–94.

Chanock, S.J., et al. (2007) Replicating genotype-phenotype associations. *Nature* 447(7145):655–660.

Chassin, L., Rogosch, F., and Barera, M. (1991) Substance use and symptomatology among adolescent children of alcoholics. *J. Abnorm. Psychol.* 100(4):449–463.

Claridge, G., Ross, E., and Hume, W.I. (1978) *Sedative Drug Tolerance in Twins*. Oxford, UK: Pergamon Press.

Compton, W.M., Cottler, L.B., Ridenour, T., Ben-Abdallah, A., and Spitznagel, E.L. (2002) The specificity of family history of alcohol and drug abuse in cocaine abusers. *Am. J. Addict.* 11(2):85–94.

Compton, W.M., Thomas, Y.F., Stinson, F.S., and Grant, B.F. (2007) Prevalence, correlates, disability, and comorbidity of *DSM-IV* drug abuse and dependence in the United States: results from the national epidemiologic survey on alcohol and related conditions. *Arch. Gen. Psychiatry* 64(5):566–576.

Conway, K.P., Compton, W.M., Stinson, F.S., & Grant, B.F. (2006) Lifetime comorbidity of DSM-IV mood and anxiety disorders and specific drug use disorders: results from the National Epidemiologic Survey on Alcohol and Related Conditions. *J. Clin. Psychiatry* 67:247–257.

Conway, K.P., Swendsen, J.D., Dierker, L., Canino, G., and Merikangas, K.R. (2007) Psychiatric comorbidity and acculturation stress among Puerto Rican substance abusers. *Am. J. Prev. Med.* 32: S219–S225.

Conway, K.P., Swendsen, J.D., and Merikangas, K.R. (2003) Expectancies, alcohol consumption, and problem drinking: the importance of family history. *Addict. Behav.* 28:823–836.

Couzin, J., and Kaiser, J. (2007) Genome wide association studies: closing the net on complex disease genes. *Science* 64:820–822.

Croughan, J.L. (1985) The contributions of family studies to understanding drug abuse. In: Robins, L., ed. *Studying Drug Abuse*. New Brunswick, NJ: Rutgers University Press, pp. 240–264.

Duerr, R.H., Taylor, K.D., Brant, S.R., Rioux, J.D., Silverberg, M.S., Daly, M.J., Steinhart, A.H., Abraham, C., Regueiro, M., Griffiths, A., Dassopoulos, T., Bitton, A., Yang, H., Targan, S., Datta, L.W., Kistner, E.O., Schumm, L.P., Lee, A.T., Gregersen, P.K., Barmada, M.M., Rotter, J.I., Nicolae, D.L., and Cho, J.H. (2006) A genome-wide association study identifies IL23R as an inflammatory bowel disease gene. *Science* 314:1461–1463.

Edenberg, H.J., and Faroud, T. (2006) The genetics of alcoholism: Identifying specific genes through family studies. *Addiction Biol.* 11:386–396.

Edwards, A., Ritter, R., and Abel, K. (2005) Complement factor H polymorphism and age-related macular degeneration. *Science* 308: 421–424.

Field, S.F., Howson, J.M., Smyth, D.J., Walker, N.M., Dunger, D.B., and Todd, J.A. (2007) Analysis of the type 2 diabetes gene, TCF7L2, in 13,795 type 1 diabetes cases and control subjects. *Diabetologia* 50:212–213.

Fowler, T., Lifford, K., Shelton, K., Rice, F., Thapar, A., Neale, M.C., McBride, A., and van den Bree, M.B. (2007) Exploring the relationship between genetic and environmental influences on initiation and progression of substance use. *Addiction* 102(3):413–422.

Freedman, M.L., Haiman, C.A., Patterson, N., McDonald, G.J., Tandon, A., Waliszewska, A., Penney, K., Steen, R.G., Ardlie, K., John, E.M., Oakley-Girvan, I., Whittemore, A.S., Cooney, K.A., Ingles, S.A., Altshuler, D., Henderson, B.E., and Reich, D. (2006) Admixture mapping identifies 8q24 as a prostate cancer risk locus in African-American men. *Proc. Natl. Acad. Sci. USA* 103: 14068–14073.

Gfroerer, J. (1987) Correlation between drug use by teenagers and drug use by older family members. *Am. J. Drug Alcohol Abuse* 13:95–108.

Gillespie, N.A., Kendler, K.S., Prescott, C.A., Aggen, S.H., Gardner, C.O., Jacobson, K., and Neale, M.C. (2007) Longitudinal modeling of genetic and environmental influences on self-reported availability of psychoactive substances: alcohol, cigarettes, marijuana, cocaine, and stimulants. *Psychol. Med.* 37(7):947–959.

Glazier, A.M., Nadeau, J.H., and Aitman, T.J. (2002) Finding genes that underlie complex traits. *Science* 298(5602):2345–2349.

Gorenstein, E.E., and Newman, J.P. (1980) Disinhibitory psychopathology: a new perspective and a model for research. *Psychol. Rev.* 87(3):301–315.

Grant, B.F., Dawson, D.A., Stinson, F.S., Chou, S.P., Dufour, M.C., and Pickering, R.P. (2004) The 12-month prevalence and trends in DSM-IV alcohol abuse and dependence: United States, 1991–1992 and 2001–2002. *Drug Alcohol Depend.* 74(3):223–234.

Grant, J.D., Heath, A.C., Bucholz, K.K., Madden, P.A., Agrawal, A., Statham, D.J., and Margin, N.G. (2007) Spousal concordance for alcohol dependence: evidence for assortative mating or spousal interaction effects? *Alcohol Clin. Exp. Res.* 31(5):717–728.

Grant, S.F., et al. (2006) Variant of transcription factor 7-like 2 (TCF7L2) gene confers risk of type 2 diabetes. *Nat. Genet* 38: 320–323.

Grove, W., Eckert, E., Heston, L., Bouchard, T., Segal, N., and Lykken, D. (1990) Heritability of substance abuse and antisocial behavior: A study of monozygotic twins reared apart. *Biol. Psychiatry* 27:1293–1304.

Groves, C.J., et al. (2006) Association analysis of 6,736 U.K. subjects provides replication and confirms TCF7L2 as a type 2 diabetes susceptibility gene with a substantial effect on individual risk. *Diabetes* 55:2640–2644.

Gurling, H., Grant, S., and Dangl, J. (1985) The genetic and cultural transmission of alcohol use, alcoholism, cigarette smoking and coffee drinking: a review and an example using a log linear cultural transmission model. *Br. J. Addict.* 80:269–279.

Haines, J., Hauser, M., Schmidt, S., et al. (2005) Complement factor H variant increases the risk of age-related macular degeneration. *Science* 308:419–421.

Hall, W.D. (2005) Will nicotine genetics and a nicotine vaccine prevent cigarette smoking and smoking-related diseases? *PLoS Med.* 2:860–863.

Hardy, J., and Selkoe, D.J. (2002) The amyloid hypothesis of Alzheimer's disease: progress and problems on the road to therapeutics. *Science* 297:353–356.

Hawkins, J.D., Catalano, R.F., and Miller, J.Y. (1992) Risk and protective factors for alcohol and other drug problems in adolescence and early adulthood: implications for substance abuse prevention. *Psychol. Bull.* 112:64–105.

Heath, A.C., Bulchoz, K.K., Madden, P., Dinwiddie, S.H., Slutske, W.S., Bierut, L.J., Statham, D.J., Dunne, M.P., Whitfield, J.B., and Martin, N.G. (1997) Genetic and environmental contributions to alcohol dependence risk in a national twin sample: consistency of findings in women and men. *Psychol. Med.* 27:1381–1396.

Heath, A.C., Cates, R., Martin, N.G., Meyer, J., Hewitt, J.K., Neale, M.C., and Eaves, L.J. (1993) Genetic contribution to risk of smoking initiation: Comparisons across birth cohorts and across cultures. *J. Subst. Abuse* 5:221–246.

Heath, A.C., and Madden, P.A.F. (1995) Genetic influences on smoking behavior. In: Turner, J.R., Cardon, L.R., and Hewitt, J.K., eds. *Behavior Genetic Approaches in Behavioral Medicine*. New York: Plenum Press, pp. 45–63.

Hill, S.Y., Cloninger, C.R., and Ayre, A.B. (1977) Independent familial transmission of alcoholism and opiate abuse. *Alcohol Clin. Exp. Res.* 1:335–342.

Hill, S.Y., and Hruska, D.R. (1992) Childhood psychopathology in families with multigenerational alcoholism. *J. Am. Acad. Child Adolesc. Psychiatry* 31(6):1024–1030.

Hirschhorn, J.N., and Daly, M.J. (2005) Genome-wide association studies for common diseases and complex traits. *Nat. Rev. Genet.* 6:95–108.

Hirschhorn, J.N., Lohmueller, K., Byrne, E., and Hirschhorn, K. (2002) A comprehensive review of genetic association studies. *Genet. Med.* 4:45–61.

Ho, M.K., and Tyndale, R.F. (2007) Overview of the pharmacogenomics of cigarette smoking. *Pharmacogenomics J.* 7:81–98.

Hoffman, J.P., and Cerbone, F.G. (2002) Parental substance use disorder and the risk of adolescent drug abuse: an event history analysis. *Drug Alcohol Depend.* 66:255–264.

Hopfer, C.J., Crowlery, T.J., and Hewitt, J.K. (2003) Review of twin and adoption studies of adolescent substance use. *J. Am. Acad. Child Adolesc. Psychiatary* 42:710–719.

ICR/International Communications Research. (1996) *Public Health Survey*. Harvard School of Public Health and the Robert Wood Johnson Foundation.

International HapMap Consortium. (2005) A haplotype map of the human genome. *Nature* 437:1299–1320.

Ioannidis, J.P., Ntzani, E.E., Trikalinos, T.A., and Contopoulos-Ioannidis, D.G. (2001) Replication validity of genetic association studies. *Nat. Genet.* 29:306–309.

Jang, K.L., Livesley, W.J., and Vermon, P.A. (1995) Alcohol and drug problems: a multivariate behavioral genetic analysis of comorbidity. *Addiction* 90:1213–1221.

Johnson, S., Leonard, K.E., and Jacob, T. (1989) Drinking, drinking styles and drug use in children of alcoholics, depressives and controls. *J. Stud. Alcohol* 50(5):427–431.

Johnston, L.D., O'Malley, P.M., Bachman, J.G., and Schulenberg, J.E. (2006) *Monitoring the Future national survey results on drug use, 1975–2005*. Volume I, Secondary school students (NIH Publication No. 06-5883). Bethesda, MD: National Institute on Drug Abuse.

Joutel, A., Bousser, M.G., Biousse, V., et al. (1993) A gene for familial hemiplegic migraine maps to chromosome 19. *Nat. Genet.* 5:40–45.

Kandel, D.B., and Andrews, K. (1987) Processes of adolescent socialization by parents and peers. *Int. J. Add.* 22:319–342.

Karkowski, L.M., Prescott, C.A., and Kendler, K.S. (2000) Multivariate assessment of factors influencing illicit substance use in twins from female-female pairs. *Am. J. Med. Genet.* 96:665–670.

Kendler, K., Aggen, S., Tambs, K., and Reichborn-Kjennerud, T. (2006) Illicit psychoactive substance use, abuse and dependence in a population-based sample of Norwegian twins. *Psychol. Med.* 36(7): 955–962.

Kendler, K.S., Gardner, C., Jacobson, K., Neale, M., and Prescott, C. (2005) Genetic and environmental influences on illicit drug use and tobacco use across birth cohorts. *Psychol. Med.* 35(9):1349–1356.

Kendler, K.S., Jacobsdon, K.C., Prescott, C.A., and Neale, M.C. (2003) Specificity of genetic and environmental risk factors for use and abuse/dependence of cannabis, cocaine, hallucinogens, sedatives, stimulants, and opiates in male twins. *Amer. J. Psychiatry* 160: 687–695.

Kendler, K.S., Karkowski, L.M., Neale, M.C., and Prescott, C.A. (2000) Illicit psychoactive substance use, heavy use, abuse and dependence in a US population-based sample of male twins. *Arch. Gen. Psychiatry* 57:261–269.

Kendler, K.S., Karkowski, L.M., and Prescott, C.A. (1999) Hallucinogen, opiate, sedative and stimulant use and abuse in a population-based sample of female twins. *Acta Psychiatr. Scand.* 99: 368–376.

Kendler, K.S., Neale, M.C., Sullivan, P., Corey, L.A., Gardner, C.O., and Prescott, C.A. (1999) A population-based twin study in women of smoking initiation and nicotine dependence. *Psychol. Med.* 29:299–308.

Kendler, K.S., and Prescott, C.A. (1998a) Cannabis use, abuse and dependence in a population-based sample of female twins. *Am. J. Psychiatry* 155:1016–1022.

Kendler, K.S., and Prescott, C.A. (1998b) Cocaine use, abuse and dependence in a population based sample of female twins. *Br. J. Psychiatry* 173:345–350.

Kessler, R.C., Berglund, P., Demler, O., Jin, R., Merikangas, K.R., and Walters, E.E. (2005) Lifetime prevalence and age-of-onset distributions of *DSM-IV* disorders in the national comorbidity survey replication. *Arch. Gen. Psychiatry* 62(6):593–602.

Kessler, R.C., Crum, R.M., Warner, L.A., Nelson, C.B., Schulenberg, J., and Anthony, J.C. (1997) Lifetime co-occurrence of DSM-III-R alcohol abuse and dependence with other psychiatric disorders in the National Comorbidity Survey. *Arch. Gen. Psychiatry* 54: 313–321.

Kessler, R.C., Nelson, C.B., McGonagle, K.A., Edlund, M.J., Frank, R.G., and Leaf, P.J. (1996) The epidemiology of co-occurring addictive and mental disorders: implications for prevention and service utilization. *Am. J. Orthopsychiatry* 66:17–31.

Khantzian, E.J. (1983) An extreme case of cocaine dependence and marked improvement with methylphenidate treatment. *Am. J. Psychiatry* 140:784–785.

Khantzian, E.J., and Treece, C. (1985) *DSM-III* psychiatric diagnosis of narcotic addicts: recent findings. *Arch. Gen. Psychiatry* 42: 1067–1077.

Kleber, H.D., and Riordan, C.E. (1982) The treatment of narcotic withdrawal: a historical review. *J Clin. Psychiatry* 43(6):30–34.

Klein, R., Zeiss, C., Chew, E., et al. (2005) Complement factor H polymorphism in age-related macular degeneration. *Science* 308: 385–389.

Kolonel, L.N., Altshuler, D., and Henderson, B.E. (2004) The multiethnic cohort study: exploring genes, lifestyle and cancer risk. *Nat. Rev. Cancer* 4:519–527.

Kreek, M.J., Nielsen, D.A., Butelman, E.R., and LaForge, K.S. (2005) Genetic influences on impulsivity, risk taking, stress responsivity and vulnerability to drug abuse and addiction. *Nat. Neurosci.* 8(11):1450–1457.

Langbehn, D.R., Brinkman, R.R., Falush, D., et al. (2004) A new model for prediction of the age of onset and penetrance for Huntington's disease based on CAG length. *Clin. Genet.* 65(4):267–277.

Langbehn, D.R., Cadoret, R.J., Caspers, K., Troughton, E.P., and Yucuis, R. (2003) Genetic and environmental risk factors for the onset of drug use and problems in adoptees. *Drug Alcohol Depend.* 69(2):151–167.

Lin, N., Eisen, S.A., Scherrer, J.F., Goldberg, J., True, W.R., Lyons, M.J., and Tsuang, M.T. (1996) The influence of familial and nonfamilial factors on the association between major depression and substance abuse/dependence in 1874 monozygotic male twin pairs. *Drug Alcohol Depend.* 43(1/2):49–55.

Luthar, S.S., and Rounsaville, B.J. (1993) Substance misuse and comorbid psychopathology in a high-risk group: a study of siblings of cocaine misusers. *Int. J. Addict.* 28:415–434.

Lynskey, M.T., Grant, J.D., Li, L., Nelson, E.C., Bucholz, K.K., Madden, P.A., Statham, D., Martin, N.G., and Heath, A.C. (2007) Stimulant use and symptoms of abuse/dependence: epidemiology and associations with cqannabis use—a twin study. *Drug Alcohol Depend.* 86(2–3):147–153.

Lynskey, M.T., Heath, A.C., Nelson, E.C., Bucholz, K.K., Madden, P.A.F., Slutske, W.S., Statham, D.J., and Martin, N.G. (2002) Genetic and environmental contributions to cannabis dependence in a national young adult twin sample. *Psychol. Med.* 32:195–207.

Maes, H.H., Neale, M.C., Kendler, K.S., Martin, N.G., Heath, A.C., and Eaves, L.J. (2006) Genetic and cultural transmission of smoking initiation: an extended trwin kinship model. *Behav. Genet.* 36(3):795–808.

Martin, C.S., Earleywine, M., Blackson, T.C., Vanyukov, M.M., Moss, H.B., and Tarter, R.E. (1994) Aggressivity, inattention, hyperactivity, and impulsivity in boys at high and low risk for substance abuse. *J. Abnorm. Child Psychol.* 22(2):177–203.

McGue, M (1994) Genes, environment, and the etiology of alcoholism. In: Zucker, R., Boyd, G., and Howard, J. eds. *The Development of Alcohol Problems: Exploring the Biopsychosocial Matrix* (Research Monograph No. 26). Rockville, MD: U.S. Department of Health and Human Services.

Meller, W.H., Rinehart, R., Cadoret, R.J., and Troughton, E. (1988) Specific familial transmission in substance abuse. *Int. J. Addict.* 23:1029–1039.

Merikangas, K.R. (1990) The genetic epidemiology of alcoholism. *Psychol. Med.* 20:11–22.

Merikangas, K.R., and Avenevoli, S. (2000) Implications of genetic epidemiology for the prevention of substance use disorders. *Addict. Behav.* 256:807–820.

Merikangas, K.R., Dierker, L.C., and Szatmari, P. (1998) Psychopathology among offspring of parents with substance abuse and/or anxiety: a high risk study. *J. Child Psychol. Psychiatry* 39(5): 711–720.

Merikangas, K.R., and Risch, N. (2003) Genomic priorities and public health. *Science* 24:599–601.

Merikangas, D.R., Rounsaville, B.J., and Prusoff, B.A. (1992) Familial factors in vulnerability to substance abuse. In: Glantz, M.D., and Pickens, R.W., eds. *Vulnerability to Drug Abuse*. Washington, DC: American Psychological Association, pp. 75–98.

Merikangas, K.R., Stolar, M., Stevens, D.E., Goulet, J., Preisig, M., Fenton, B., O'Malley, S., and Rounsaville, B.J. (1998) Familial transmission of substance use disorders. *Arch. Gen. Psychiatry* 55(11): 973–979.

Mirin, S.M., Weiss, R.D., Griffin, M.L., and Michael, J.L. (1991) Psychopathology in drug abusers and their families. *Compr. Psychiatry* 32:36–51.

Mirin, S.M., Weiss, R.D., and Michael, J.L. (1988) Pyschopathology in substance abusers: diagnosis and treatment. *Am. J. Drug Alcohol Abuse* 14:139–157.

Mirin, S.M., Weiss, R.D., Sollogub, A., and Michael, J.L. (1984) *Affective Illness in Substance Abusers, in Substance Abuse and Psychopathology*. Washington, DC: American Psychiatric Press, pp. 58–77.

Moss, H.B., Majumder, P.P., and Vanyukov, M. (1994) Familial resemblance for psychoactive substance use disorders: behavioral profile of high risk boys. *Addict. Behav.* 19(2):199–208.

NCI-NHGRI Working Group on Replication in Association Studies, Chanock, S.J., Manolio, T., Boehnke, M., Boerwinkle, E., Hunter, D.J., Thomas, G., Hirschhorn, J.N., Abecasis, G., Altshuler, D., Bailey-Wilson, J.E., Brooks, L.D., Cardon, L.R., Daly, M., Donnelly, P., Fraumeni, J.F., Jr., Freimer, N.B., Gerhard, D.S., Gunter, C., Guttmacher, A.E., Guyer, M.S., Harris, E.L., Hoh, J., Hoover, R., Kong, C.A., Merikangas, K.R., Morton, C.C., Palmer, L.J., Phimister, E.G., Rice, J.P., Roberts, J., Rotimi, C., Tucker, M.A., Vogan, K.J., Wacholder, S., Wijsman, E.M., Winn, D.M., and Collins, F.S. (2007) Replicating genotype-phenotype associations. *Nature* 447(7145):655–660.

Neal, M.C., Aggen, S.H., Maes, H.H., Kubarych, T.S., and Scmitt, J.E. (2006) Methodological issures in the assessment of substance use phenotypes. *Addict. Behav.* 31(6):1010–1034.

Nurnberger, J.I., Wiegand, R., Bucholz, K., O'Connor, S., Meyer, E. T., Reich, T., Rice, J., Schuckit, M., King, L., Petti, T., Bierut, L., Hinrichs, A.L., Kuperman, S., Hesselbrock, V., and Porjesz, B. (2004) A family study of alcohol dependence: coaggregation of multiple disorders in relatives of alcohol-dependent probands. *Arch. Gen. Psychiatry* 61(12):1246–1256.

Ott, J. (2004) Association of genetic loci: replication or not, that is the question. *Neurology* 63:955–958.

Pedersen, N. (1981) Twin similarity for usage of common drugs. *Prog. Clin. Biol. Res.* 69:53–59.

Pergadia, M.L, Heath, A., Martin, N., and Madden, P. (2006) Genetic analyses of *DSM-IV* nicotine withdrawal in adult twins. *Psychol. Med.* 36(7):963–972.

Pickens, R., Svikis, D., McGue, M., Lykken, D., Heston, L., and Clayton, P. (1991) Heterogeneity in the inheritance of alcoholism: a study of male and female twins. *Arch. Gen. Psychiatry* 48:19–28.

Prescott, C.A., and Kendler, K.S. (1999) Genetic and environmental contributions to alcohol abuse and dependence in a population-based sample of male twins. *Am. J. Psychiatry* 156:34–40.

Quitkin, F.M., Rifkin, A., Kaplan, J., and Klein, D.F. (1972) Phobic anxiety syndrome complicated by drug dependence and addiction. *Arch. Gen. Psychiatry* 27(2):159–162.

Regier, D., Farmer, M.E., Rae, D.S., Locke, B.Z., Keith, S.J., Judd, L.L., et al. (1990) Comorbidity of mental disorders with alchohol and other drug abuse: results from the Epidemiologic Catchment Area (ECA) Study. *JAMA* 264:2511–2518.

Reich, W., Earls, F., Frankel, O., and Shayka, J.J. (1993) Psychopathology in children of alcoholics. *J. Am. Acad. Child Adolesc. Psychiatry* 32:955–1002.

Rhee, S.H., Hewitt, J.D., Young, S.E., Corley, R.P., Crowley, T.J., and Stallings, M.C. (2003) Genetic and environmental influences on substance initiation, use, and problem use in adolescents. *Arch. Gen. Psychiatry* 60:1256–1264.

Risch, N. (2000) Searching for genetic determinants in the new millennium. *Nature* 405:847–856.

Risch, N., and Merikangas, K.R. (1996) The future of genetic studies of complex human diseases. *Science* 273:1516–1517.

Ross, H.E., Glaser, F.B., and Germanson, T. (1988) The prevalence of psychiatric disorders in patients with alcohol and other drug problems. *Arch. Gen. Psychiatry* 45:1023–1032.

Rounsaville, B.J., Kosten, T.R., Weissman, M.M., Prosoff, B., Pauls, D., Anton, S.F., and Merikangas, K.R. (1991) Psychiatric disorders in relatives of probands with opiate addiction. *Arch. Gen. Psychiatry* 48:33–42.

Rounsaville, B.J., Weissman, M.M., Kleber, H., and Wilber, C. (1982) Heterogeneity of psychiatric diagnosis in treated opiate addicts. *Arch. Gen. Psychiatry* 39(2):161–166.

Sartor, C.E., Lynskey, M.T., Heath, A.C., Jacob, T., and True, W. (2007) The role of childhood risk factors in initiation of alcohol use and progression to alcohol dependence. *Addiction* 102(2):216–225.

Saxon, A.J., Oreskovich, M.R., and Brkanac, Z. (2007) Genetic determinants of addiction to opioids and cocaine. *Harv. Rev. Psychiatry* 13(4):218–232.

Sher, K.J., Walitzer, K.S., Wood, P.K., and Brent, E.E. (1991) Characteristics of children of alcoholics: putative risk factors, substance use and abuse, and psychopathology. *J. Abnorm. Child Psychol.* 100:427–448.

Simcha-Fagagn, O., and Schwartz, J. (1986) Neighborhood and delinquency: an assessment of contextual effects. *Criminology* 24: 667–703.

Sladek, R., Rocheleau, G., Rung, J., et al. (2007) A genome wide association study identifies novel risk loci for type 2 diabetes. *Nature* 22:881–885.

Tarter, R.E., Kirisci, L., Habeych, M., Reynolds, M., and Vanyukov, M.M. (2004) Neurobehavior disinhibition in childhood predisposes boys to substance use disorder by young adulthood: direct and mediated etiologic pathways. *Drug Alcohol Depend.* 73:121–132.

Tarter, R.E., Kirisci, L., Mezzich, A., Cornelius, J.R., Pajer, K., Vanyukov, M.M., et al. (2003) Neurobehavioral disinhibition in childhood predicts early age at onset of substance use disorder. *Am. J. Psychiatry* 160:1078–1085.

Todd, J.A. (2006) Statistical false positive or true disease pathway? *Nat. Genet.* 38:731–733.

True, W.R., Heath, A.C., Scherrer, J.F., Waterman, B., Goldberg, J., Lin, N., Eisen, S.A., Lyons, M.J., and Tsuang, M.T. (1997) Genetic and environmental contributions to smoking. *Addiction* 92:1277–1287.

True, W.R., Heath, A.C., Scherrer, J.F., Xian, H., Lin, N., Eisen, S.A., Lyons, M.J., Goldberg, J., and Tsuang, M.T. (1999) Interrelationship of genetic and environmental influences on conduct disosrder and alcohol and marijuana dependence symptoms. *Am. J. Med. Genet.* 88(4):391–397.

True, W.R., Xian, H., Scherrer, J.F., Madden, P., Bucholz, K.K., Heath, A.C., Eisen, S.A., Lyons, M.J., Goldberg, J., and Tsuang, M. (1999) Common genetic vulnerability for nicotine and alcohol dependence in men. *Arch. Gen. Psychiatry* 56:655–661.

Tsuang, M.T., Lyons, M.J., Eisen, S.A., Goldberg, J., True, W., Lin, N., Meyer, J.M., Toomey, R., Farone, S.V., and Eaves, L. (1996) Genetic influences on *DSM-III-R* drug abuse and dependence: a study of 3,372 twin pairs. *Am. J. Med. Genet.* 67:473–477.

Tsuang, M.T., Lyons, M.J., Meyer, J.M., Doyle, T., Eisen, S.A., Goldberg, J., True, W., Lin, N., Toomey, R., and Eaves, L. (1998) Co-occurrence of abuse of different drugs in men: the role of drug-specific and shared vulnerabilities. *Arch. Gen. Psychiatry* 55: 967–972.

Van den Bree, M.B., Johnson, E.O., Neale, M.C., and Pickens, R.W. (1998) Genetic and environmental influences on drug use and abuse/dependence in male and female twins. *Drug Alcohol Depend.* 52:231–241.

Vanyukov, M.M., Neale, M.C., Moss, H.B., and Tarter, R.E. (1996) Mating assortment and the liability to substance abuse. *Drug Alcohol Depend.* 42(1):1–10.

Vanyukov, M.M., and Tarter, R.E. (2002) Genetic studies of substance abuse. *Drug Alcohol Depend.* 59:101–123.

Volk, H.E., Scherrer, J.F., Bucholz, K.K., Todorov, A., Heath, A.C., Jacob, T., and True, W.R. (2007) Evidence for specificity of transmission of alcohol and nicotine dependence in a offspring of twins design. *Drug Alcohol Depend.* 87(2–3):225–232.

Wacholder, S., Chanock, S., Garcia-Closas, M., El Ghormli, L., and Rothman, N. (2004) Assessing the probability that a positive report is false: an approach for molecular epidemiology studies. *J. Natl. Cancer Inst.* 96:434–442.

Weiss, R.D., and Mirin, S.M. (1985) Treatment of chronic cocaine abuse and attention deficit disorder, residual type with magnesium pemoline. *Drug Alcohol Depend.* 15:69–72.

Whitfield, J.B., Zhu, G., Madden, P.A., Neale, M.C., Heath, A.C., and Martin, N.G. (2004) The genetics of alcohol intake and of alcohol dependence. *Alcohol Clin. Exp. Res.* 28(8):1153–1160.

Young, S.E., Rhee, S., Stallings, M., Corley, r., and Hewitt, J. (2006) Genetic and environmental vulnerabilities underlying adolescent substance use and problem use: general or specific? *Behav. Genet.* 36(4):603–615.

Young, S.E., Stallings, M.C., Corley, R.P., Krauter, K.S., and Hewitt, J.K. (2000) Genetic and environmental influences on behavioral dishinhibition. *Am. J. Med. Genet.* 96:684–695.

48 Effects of Drugs of Abuse on Brain Development

BARRY M. LESTER AND BARRY E. KOSOFSKY

The most recent National Household Survey on Drug Abuse estimated that in 2004–2005, 3.9% of pregnant mothers used illicit drugs, including cocaine, in the past month (SAMHSA, 2005a). Even more alarming, the prevalence rate of illegal drug use was higher for pregnant women in the 15- to 18-year age range (12.3%) than for women 18–25 years old (7%). Moreover, the women who abuse illicit drugs often use licit drugs: An estimated 32% of those using one illicit drug during pregnancy also use alcohol and cigarettes. This national survey was based on self-report and thus is likely to underestimate the scope of the problem. Even with these conservative estimates, however, it is safe to say that gestational exposure to licit drugs of abuse such as alcohol and cigarettes and illicit drugs of abuse such as marijuana, cocaine, methamphetamine, and opiates is the single largest preventable cause of in utero developmental compromise of infants in the United States today.

PROGRAMS UNDERLYING BRAIN DEVELOPMENT

Central nervous system (CNS) development requires a complex orchestration of genetic factors and environmental forces that direct brain maturation and shape infant development in a reproducible yet individualized manner. The protracted timetable of CNS maturation affords a continuum of biologic vulnerability to the developing brain, which starts by 28 days postconception, when the template for brain development is established, and continues throughout gestation, infancy, and childhood. Moreover, the developmental consequences of a toxic CNS insult relate critically to the gestational timing of that exposure and at a given time during fetal development may vary from one brain region to another. Two general classes of CNS developmental disorders can be distinguished: those occurring in the first half of gestation that affect cytogenesis and histogenesis, and those occurring during the second half of gestation that affect brain growth and differentiation. During the organizational phase in the second half of gestation, progressive events (neuroblast proliferation and migration, axonal projection, and synaptogenesis) and regressive events (programmed cell death and selective elimination of processes) critically shape the maturation of brain circuitry. Toxic influences during this period may dramatically alter brain development but may also alter the regressive events that underlie the capacity of the developing brain to compensate for injury. A pattern of molecular, biochemical, and metabolic maturation must parallel normal brain development and may impose regional stage-specific developmental requirements and vulnerabilities for maldevelopment. An understanding of basic mechanisms of drug action on the mother and the fetus following transplacental administration is crucially important for appreciating how such substances mediate their toxic effects in utero. Likewise, a deeper understanding of mechanisms operative during fetal brain development will form the basis for an improved understanding of how programs for brain development can be altered following in utero drug exposures with lasting consequence for brain structure and function.

BEHAVIORAL TERATOLOGY

This chapter reviews current thinking on the extent to which drugs of abuse may act as behavioral teratogens—drugs capable of altering brain development and subsequent function. Behavioral teratogens can alter internal fetal brain structure and function without any external changes, such as dysmorphic features. To determine whether drugs of abuse are behavioral teratogens requires consideration at four levels of analysis (Grimm, 1987):

1. Behavioral/cognitive level: Are there specific behavioral or cognitive deficits evident in subsets of infants and children who are exposed to drugs?
2. Systems level: Can alterations in particular brain structures and neurochemical systems that underlie the behavioral or cognitive deficits be identified?

3. Developmental level: At which specific time(s) during fetal development is the brain susceptible to the actions of drugs of abuse?

4. Pharmacological/physiological level: What are the mechanisms by which particular drugs of abuse mediate their actions in utero?

Part of the difficulty in establishing drugs of abuse as behavioral teratogens is that the behavioral consequences of gestational exposure to such drugs may not be evident at birth but may appear as the behavioral repertoire of the developing child matures. Therefore, one strives to identify antecedents of the behavioral abnormality. One also strives to identify predictive markers (clinical, neuroanatomical, neurophysiological, or neurochemical) of the subsequent expression of the behavioral anomaly. Implicit in this approach is a consideration of the role of genetic and environmental factors that may alter the susceptibility to, or expression of, a teratogenic effect. Over the last 20 years, there has been a tremendous effort to identify in the clinical setting and in preclinical models the extent to which drugs of abuse may act as behavioral teratogens. In general, experimental studies in animals have pursued a "bottom-up" approach towards establishing a causal role for drugs of abuse in altering programs for brain development, moving from (*4*) the pharmacological/physiological level to (*3*) the developmental level, with the goal of modeling the relevant "clinical deficits" consequent to specific drug exposures at the (*2*) systems and (*1*) behavioral/cognitive levels. Clinical research has progressed in a more "top-down" approach, with the goal of defining at (*1*) the behavioral/cognitive level and ideally at (*2*) the systems level, some of the phenotypic consequences in humans exposed to drugs of abuse, with efforts to reach towards (*3*) the developmental and (*4*) the pharmacological/physiological levels regarding the mechanistic basis of gestational drug exposure in contributing to that phenotype. One goal for future research would be to bridge across all four levels in preclinical models and clinical studies; although those bridges are most easily constructed in preclinical models, where confounding variables can be controlled (see below), it is often the case that some of the behaviors that one would like to model (for example, selective language delay) may not be accessible to modeling through preclinical experimental animal research programs.

BEHAVIORAL AND MOLECULAR MALFORMATION VERSUS DEFORMATION

The effects of drug abuse on the adult brain should be distinguished from the effects of maternal drug abuse on the developing brain in the womb of a pregnant drug abuser. Current progress in substance abuse research identifies that the brain is plastic and that there are adaptations at the level of neurochemical systems, gene expression, and associated behaviors as a consequence of chronic drug abuse in adults. The repetitive use of drugs leads to alterations in "homeostatic" mechanisms controlling certain central brain structures and chemical systems that have been subverted by virtue of the chronic and recurrent exposure to drugs of abuse. In an effort to adapt to drug-induced alterations in neuronal communication and function, the brain of the drug addict undergoes certain functional neurochemical and molecular maladaptations, which may have behavioral correlates. These maladaptive changes in brain function can be considered a form of "molecular deformation": the brain was normally formed before drug abuse and was subsequently altered or deformed as a consequence of continued drug administration.

It is important to contrast this with the effects of exposing the developing brain to drugs of abuse. The pregnant woman who abuses drugs may in turn perturb fetal neurochemical systems and neuronal communication during critical developmental periods when normal brain structure, circuitry, and biochemical and molecular features are being established. Altered brain function that may ensue can be considered a form of "molecular malformation": In such infants, the brain is prevented from forming normally. The postnatal consequences of altering genetic and molecular programs for brain development may be sustained for years to come and may be evidenced as altered brain growth, delayed developmental milestones, or altered cognitive, linguistic, or behavioral maturation. As mentioned above, the specific developmental programs affected, and brain structures and systems altered, are likely to depend on the specific pattern of drug abuse as well as the gestational period during which drug exposure occurred. This distinction, that the brain of the infant exposed to drugs of abuse in utero may be malformed, not deformed, is an important extension of a principle of teratogenesis, which has implications regarding appropriate intervention and amelioration of gestational drug-induced disability. One of the critical goals of future clinical research will be to determine the extent to which individual drugs may cause specific molecular malformations, to identify what the behavioral and clinical correlates of such malformations are, and to identify the extent to which particular prenatal interventions may prevent, and specific postnatal therapeutics may correct, compensate, or modify, the expression of such malformations and their behavioral correlates.

METHODOLOGICAL COMPLEXITIES AND CONFOUNDING ASPECTS OF CLINICAL STUDIES

Some of the limitations of conducting and interpreting clinical research in this area include the multitude of confounding environmental factors that are associated with maternal (licit and illicit) drug abuse that may affect fetal and infant development including, but not limited to, altered socioeconomic status (SES); restricted access or limited use of prenatal care; exposure to sexually transmitted diseases; violent and abusive domestic relationships; and chaotic home environments, which may include multiple out-of-home placements, and lifestyles with a lack of adequate and appropriate social supports for mothers or infants. In collecting clinical data to relate in utero drug exposure to altered postnatal development, there are additional methodological complexities: selection biases of health care workers in terms of who is screened, identified, and studied; difficulty with longitudinal follow-up of mothers and infants; problems with the validity of self report versus laboratory testing (for example, of blood, urine, hair, or meconium) to define exposed versus control infants, and with quantitating exposure to one, or more commonly multiple drugs (that is, polypharmacy); and difficulty in conducting prospective longitudinal studies of exposed infants. Identifying the independent effects of in utero exposure to drugs in altering developmental outcomes poses some additional analytical problems (Table 48.1). If a child born to a woman who abuses drugs has altered development postnatally, as compared with control children not exposed to drugs of abuse in utero, are those alterations in development and behavioral maturation:

1. a consequence of inheriting an altered genetic predisposition from one or both parents, which contributed to (maternal) substance-abusing behaviors during pregnancy?

TABLE 48.1 *Determinants of Behavioral Outcomes in Drug-Exposed Children*

- Genetic predisposition
  - Novelty seeking, risk taking
  - Inattention, impulsivity, hyperactivity, learning disabilities
  - Personality disorders, psychiatric diagnoses
- Prenatal environment
  - Inadequate prenatal medical care
  - Poverty/malnutrition
  - Sexually transmitted diseases/intrauterine infection
- In utero drug exposure
  - Pattern of drug use: Quantity/frequency/route
  - Gestational timing of drug use during pregnancy
  - Concurrent use of multiple drugs of abuse
- Postnatal environment
  - Impaired parental–infant interaction
  - Inadequate social supports/chaotic lifestyle
  - Poverty/malnutrition
  - Depression/abuse

2. a consequence of an altered postnatal home environment that is often chaotic, due to continued drug-seeking behaviors and substance abuse by the parents, which can alter parent–infant interaction and thereby affect subsequent development?

3. or are they truly a consequence of gestational exposure to drugs of abuse and to the effects that those drugs exert in altering programs for brain development and subsequent behavioral maturation?

To some extent, rigorously designed and executed prospective longitudinal clinical studies can control for some of these prenatal and postnatal factors in an effort to correlate gestational exposure to drugs of abuse with altered postnatal outcomes. However, the interpretation of such data is further complicated by the fact that any child who sustains an in utero insult is more sensitive to the quality of the postnatal environment and thereby more vulnerable for developmental impairment when raised in a compromised setting. As with other gestational factors that compromise in utero development, such as prenatal malnutrition, prematurity, infection, or asphyxia, the infant at risk for developmental compromise by virtue of such gestational exposures has a deficit that is contextual: The richer the environment postnatally, the less likely the in utero exposure will be of developmental consequence. Therefore, the child born to a mother who abuses drugs may be at potential risk for "double trouble" resulting from the biological exposure in utero compounded by the effects of a potentially suboptimal postnatal environment, which may accentuate the expression of that insult.

In addition, the kinds of behaviors that may be impaired in infants exposed to drugs of abuse in utero may be very subtle alterations in affect, attention, arousal, and action, which are difficult to assess in adults and may be even harder to characterize in developing children or to quantitate in ways that facilitate analytic efforts to identify drug-induced alterations in such behaviors. Having outlined these complexities, a selective review of the literature can highlight how some of the best-designed studies have identified specific prenatal risks that are associated with particular alterations in postnatal outcomes and the extent to which there are markers, either in the perinatal or early postnatal period, that define antecedents of developmental compromise.

ALCOHOL

Although alcohol teratogenicity, the adverse consequences of excessive drinking by pregnant women on infant outcome, had been established in biblical times, it was not until the thalidomide epidemic of the 1950s that investigators started thinking more critically about the potential role of alcohol and other drugs of abuse as teratogens. Over 30 years ago, clinical investigators reported a constellation of abnormalities evident in infants born to women who abused alcohol. In 1973, investigators identified a clinical syndrome comprising prenatal growth retardation, specific dysmorphic facial features, and CNS compromise and labeled this triad *fetal alcohol syndrome* (Jones et al., 1973). The incidence of fetal alcohol syndrome (FAS) is approximately one per thousand in the general population but may be somewhat higher in certain ethnic groups. The term *fetal alcohol effects* (FAE) has been developed to describe children exposed to alcohol in utero with less significant compromise of one or more components of the triad mentioned above (D.W. Smith, 1981). Fetal alcohol effects are probably 3 to 5 times more common than FAS, though there has been much discussion about the definition and use of this terminology and descriptors (for review, see Aase et al., 1995). An alternative proposal for nomenclature followed from an Institute of Medicine report on FAS released in 1996 (Stratton et al., 1996) that identified five categories of diagnostic consequence resulting from fetal exposure to alcohol:

1. FAS with confirmed maternal alcohol exposure
2. FAS without confirmed maternal alcohol exposure
3. Partial FAS with confirmed maternal alcohol exposure
4. Alcohol-related birth defects (ARBD)
5. Alcohol-related neurodevelopmental disorder (ARND)

Categories 4 and 5 can coexist and are considered to be "possible prenatal alcohol-related effects," though categories 1, 2, and 3 are by definition mutually exclusive. Others consider these outcomes as a continuum, lumped under the heading of fetal alcohol spectrum disorder (FASD). Whichever diagnostic categories prove to be most useful and become most widely adopted is less important than an appreciation of the biological complexities involved in attributing specific clinical deficits to gestational exposure to alcohol. Even with a clear phenotype, including the dysmorphic facial appearance associated with FAS, it is often difficult to identify FAS and to attribute the syndrome to maternal alcohol consumption. For reasons including those mentioned above, to confirm the maternal history of a pattern of substantial regular or excessive alcohol intake or of heavy episodic drinking can be problematic either because children are in foster or adoptive care and not accompanied by their biological mothers at clinic visits or because biological mothers are "in denial" or at risk for legal consequences if they define the specifics of their drinking and/or drug habits during pregnancy. Moreover, the fact that certain other gestational toxins can produce facial features consistent with fetal alcohol facies (including anticonvulsant embryopathy, fetal toluene exposure, infants born to mothers with phenylketonuria [PKU], Noonan's syndrome, and velocardiofacial syndrome) combined with other reasons for failure to diagnose FAS at birth (including lack of recognition of the syndrome, reluctance to identify or label women as users, and difficulty making the diagnosis in newborns) has led to imprecise surveillance and identification of the syndrome. It would appear that FAS is correlated with maternal drinking habits that continue despite intervention and can be associated with an early age of onset of drinking, a family history of drinking (especially in female relatives), alcohol-related medical problems, alcohol dependence criteria, and a host of alcohol-related behaviors. However, even with these maternal historic correlates of alcoholism, it is clear that not all fetuses exposed to high levels of alcohol will be affected: Only 4.3% of offspring of "heavy" drinkers (defined as greater than five drinks per occasion, or two drinks per day) demonstrate FAS, and only an estimated 30%–50% of fetuses born to alcoholics show evidence of FAE. Observations that the incidence of FAS and FAE varies considerably in different ethnic groups may relate to variations in the frequency of particular isozymes of enzymes required for alcohol metabolism (that confer protection vs. vulnerability to the teratogenic effects of alcohol), which may be altered in their distribution among particular ethnic populations. It may also be the case that the cultural acceptability and pattern of drinking varies within certain ethnic groups, and together with socioeconomic factors may contribute to an increased incidence of FAS in certain populations. In particular, lower SES is associated with an approximately 10-fold increased risk for FAS than is seen in middle to higher socioeconomic groups.

Mechanisms of Alcohol-Induced Brain Maldevelopment

Over the last 15 years, molecular and cellular mechanisms underlying the effects of alcohol on the adult and developing brain have been elucidated, identifying specific neural systems and signal transduction pathways that mediate aspects of alcohol's effects. Ethanol intoxication occurs at mmol/L concentrations, which are high enough to perturb hydrophobic regions of cell membranes and the lipids and proteins that constitute them (Deitrich et al., 1989). In addition to these nonspecific membrane effects, a subset of receptor-mediated signaling mechanisms is altered by acute ethanol exposure. The receptor for γ-aminobutyric acid (GABA) and the associated chloride channel have been implicated as one of the central sites at which ethanol acts. The long isoform of the γ_2 subunit (2L) of the GABA-A receptor is required for modulation of chloride currents by benzodiazepines and ethanol (Wafford et al., 1991). This common site of action for both drugs via altered GABAergic neurotransmission is supported by clinical data (Charness, 1992): Benzodiazepine administration and ethanol intoxication share similar features, there is cross tolerance between these drugs when chronically administered, and ethanol withdrawal is partially suppressed by benzodiazepines (whose chief action is to augment GABAergic neurotransmission). Ethanol causes a dose-dependent potentiation of 5-HT_3 currents (the serotonin-gated ion channel) in NCB-20 neuroblastoma cells (Lovinger and White, 1991). Because serotonergic systems are implicated in affect and motivation, one can speculate that the rewarding as well as intoxicating properties of alcohol may in part be related to its action at 5-HT receptors. Ethanol inhibits *N*-methyl-D-aspartate (NMDA)-gated chloride currents in a dose-dependent manner in the nmol range of concentrations (Lovinger et al., 1989) and is associated with postreceptor changes in calcium and cyclic guanosine monophosphate (cGMP). Alterations in memory in alcoholics (such as alcohol blackouts) could conceivably be related to changes in the efficacy of signals transduced via the NMDA receptor. Ethanol has been found to modify opioid systems and signaling, including opioid peptide concentration, release, and binding (Charness, 1992). Some of alcohol's effects on opiates are mediated by μ-opioid receptor blockade. Ethanol can selectively block adenosine uptake through the nucleoside transporter (Nagy et al., 1990) and may be involved in the adaptive responses to ethanol via second-messenger pathway (cyclic adenosine monophosphate [cAMP]) stimulation. These and additional mechanisms may be operative in compromising the developing fetus.

The following factors have been suggested and potentially implicated in contributing to the FAE and FAS phenotype in alcohol-exposed infants: nutritional factors, socioeconomic factors, genetic susceptibility to alcohol effects including alcohol dehydrogenase (ADH) and aldehyde dehydrogenase (ALDH) polymorphisims, acetaldehyde and fatty acid ethyl ester metabolism, ethanol inhibition of retinoic acid synthesis, alteration of insulin-like growth factor action, alcohol-induced hypoxia and alcohol-induced free radical production, inhibition of cell adhesion mediated by the human L1 gene, and release of L-glutamate by ethanol (for review, see Stoler et al., 1998). Which, if any, of these mechanisms contribute to altered brain growth and differentiation by alcohol has not been clearly established, and additional mechanisms may be operative, with specific consequences on brain maturation. For example, researchers have determined that exposure of developing mouse brain to alcohol alters cell-cycle kinetics (Burchfield et al., 1991), which in turn alters maturation of glial cells (Miller and Robertson, 1993), which is associated with failure of neuroblasts to migrate to their proper targets (Gressens, Lammens, et al., 1992). These investigators suggest that alcohol-induced impairment of neurogenesis and neuronal migration alters brain size and cortical architecture. Other mechanisms "downstream" of alcohol-induced receptor mediated changes described above may be operative during CNS maldevelopment. For example, interference with cAMP-dependent kinase activity may account for alcohol-induced growth retardation (Pennington, 1990). Recent studies have emphasized the relevance of prenatal alcohol-induced apoptotic neurodegeneration mediated by glutamatergic antagonism at the NMDA receptor and GABAmimetic actions at the GABA-A receptor as contributing to the impaired brain growth and development seen in FAE and FAS (Ikonomidou et al., 2000). These and many additional animal experiments have clearly documented that ethanol damages developing organisms and that the developing nervous system is particularly vulnerable to these effects (for review, see Driscoll et al., 1990).

The Alcohol-Affected Phenotype(s)

In the spectrum of alcohol-related effects, FAS is on the most affected end, whereas FAE is a milder phenotype, though even lesser effects may be seen in some subset of infants who are impaired. In a fully affected case, FAS may have the following features (Streissguth et al., 1996):

1. growth retardation including low birth weight, microcephaly, decreased adipose tissue, and failure to thrive
2. A pattern of craniofacial anomalies with the most discriminant features being midface hypoplasia, evident as small palpebral fissures, a flat indistinct philtrum, a thin vermilion border, epicanthal folds, and a depressed nasal bridge

3a. neurological effects which in younger children can include fine and gross motor delays, hypotonia, and tremor

3b. neurological effects which in older children can include impaired IQ (with a mean IQ of 68 for FAS); learning disabilities with impaired cognition, dysfunctional language, deficits in verbal learning and memory, and difficulty dealing with multiple sensory inputs, particularly auditory information; and a specific pattern of behavioral effects including impulsivity, decreased attention span, hyperactivity, difficulty establishing normal peer relationships, lack of remorse, failure to learn from mistakes, lack of judgment, and aggressiveness.

As opposed to the alcohol-related growth retardation mentioned above, which is most evident in the newborn and perinatal period, some of the other features of FAE and FAS, in particular the dysmorphic facial appearance and evidence of neurological compromise, are often and easily missed in newborns. During adolescence, the continued growth of alcohol-exposed children may lead to height that overlaps with low normal values for the general population and weight that may normalize or may become obese in some cases.

Microcephaly often persists, but the change in facial features associated with puberty may mask dysmorphic features that define the fetal alcohol facies. It has been noted that there are increased adverse effects seen in subsequent offspring of alcoholic mothers and an increased association of FAE and FAS with mothers older than 30 years of age, independent of drinking levels (J.L. Jacobson et al., 1996). This suggests that in addition to the worsened drinking habits that are often associated with the progression of alcoholism, there may be other biological factors associated with increased maternal age that puts the fetus at increased risk for adverse effects. Such factors may also contribute to the complexity of quantifying the relationship between exposure and outcome: clear thresholds or dose-response relationships between amount of alcohol consumed and effects on the offspring have never been established. However, the pattern of drinking seems to contribute to outcome in an important way: Daily maternal drinking is not necessary for adverse effects, as binge drinking (greater than five drinks at a sitting) has been associated with learning problems such as impaired academic skills, memory, and attention in exposed offspring. Efforts to relate the timing of the worst alcohol drinking with developmental consequences have suggested, but not clearly confirmed, that alcohol exposure during all three trimesters is associated with worsened growth retardation, an increased incidence of craniofacial abnormalities, and more profound CNS compromise (Autti-Ramo et al., 1992). What has also been shown is that the performance on sequential simultaneous mental composite achievement tests and nonverbal scores in those infants born to women who never drank was better than in those born to mothers who stopped drinking during pregnancy, which in turn was better than in those infants born to mothers who continued to drink (Coles et al., 1991). What the additional burden of other substances commonly used with alcohol in polypharmacy have been raised and considered including whether such effects may be has been considered, including whether such effects may be additive or synergistic.

Socialization and Adaptation

Alterations in specific postnatal developmental outcomes that have been reported following in utero alcohol exposure include neuropathological, neurophysiological, linguistic, and social and adaptive consequences. In animal studies, ethanol-induced impairment in behavioral performance occurs in ways that parallel several outcome measures from clinical studies (Driscoll et al., 1990). In nonhuman primates, prenatal ethanol exposure results in deficits in object permanence, increased distractibility, and delays in gross motor development (Clarren et al., 1988; Clarren et al., 1992). In rodent models, increases in basal activity (Abel and Berman, 1994) and deficits in habituation to new environments are observed, which have been interpreted as an impairment of inhibitory systems (Driscoll et al., 1990). Specific deficits in classical (Westergren et al., 1996) and operant conditioning (Clausing et al., 1995; Furuya et al., 1996) have also been reported with gestational ethanol administration in a dose-dependent fashion in adult rats. In clinical studies, the particular impairment of adaptive skills and social judgment in children and teenagers with FAS seems to be out of proportion to intellectual impairment and may be associated with an inability of such individuals to become fully integrated and functional members of society. In a follow-up of 415 patients with FAS and FAE, ages 6 to 51, Streissguth et al. (1996) noted that the most common problems encountered by this population include school difficulties (with a dropout or suspension rate of over 60% by the time children reach 12 years of age); difficulty with the law in 60% of children who are affected by their 12th birthday; mental health problems in approximately 90% of children who are exposed; alcohol and/or drug problems in over 30% of children before 12 years of age; homelessness; confinement, with in-patient treatment for mental health, drug abuse, or criminality in over 50% of those reaching 21 years of age; inappropriate sexual behavior in over 50% of individuals who are affected; dependent living in over 80% who have reached the age of 21; and problems with employment in over 80% who have reached the age of 21. The complexities associated with impaired adaptation and socialization that precluded full societal integration was seen in as significant a fraction of those with FAE as with FAS. In that same study (Streissguth et al., 1996), it was reported that males had a higher rate of school difficulties, were more likely to have been in trouble with the law, and more commonly demonstrated an IQ versus adaptive behavior discrepancy that was associated with a greater incidence of dependent living situations. Of note, in that study the protective factors included living in a stable and nurturing home for more than 70% of the child's life; diagnoses at younger than age 6 years; no history of physical abuse; a stable living situation for more than 2.8 years; a good-quality home between the years of 8 and 12; eligibility for division of developmental disabilities (that is, support services); and having FAS versus FAE. These data do not imply that having FAS is more protective than FAE. Rather, it may reflect that children with the full-blown syndrome, once identified by virtue of more significant compromise, may be more carefully watched and supervised, with less risk for the secondary disabilities mentioned above.

Summary of Alcohol's Clinical Effects

As reviewed above, during the preschool period some children with FAE and FAS demonstrate deficits that may include hyperactivity, language delay, and perceptual motor problems. During school years, attention deficit and behavioral problems often emerge. It is important to note that the extent of CNS compromise parallels the degree of dysmorphism, as the individuals with FAS demonstrate the greatest deficits. Other studies incorporating infants exposed to lower amounts of alcohol in utero have demonstrated normal Brazelton Neonatal Behavioral Assessment Scale (NBAS) scores, normal language development at 1, 2, and 3 years, and normal cognition and sustained attention in children who are exposed. This may partially reflect differences in study design, patient ascertainment, and biological exposure. One resolution to these discrepancies is suggested by some of the principles of teratology; there may be many outcomes, with the most profound alterations induced by exposures of greater amount over increased gestational time. For all of these reasons, counseling pregnant women about alcohol exposure and its risks to the fetus is problematic because no lower threshold exists regarding the amount of exposure that is safe, no pattern of drinking seems to be safe, all three trimesters of pregnancy have been implicated as vulnerable times, and the concomitant use of other substances can only aggravate the alcohol effects. Emphasizing the importance of cessation of drinking and its potential benefits to the fetus is the clearest message that can be delivered to pregnant women. Delivering this message to women considering pregnancy, or in their early stages of pregnancy, is an important goal. So is the ability to reinforce this message to alcoholics even during the later stages of pregnancy, when they can be more readily identified and engaged in coordinate efforts to optimize prenatal health care. Efforts in the treatment community to utilize a "stages of change" model (Prochaska and DiClemente, 1992) have tried to use pregnancy as a motivating force to engage pregnant women in therapeutic efforts to decrease drug use and abuse during pregnancy. Implicit in this and other approaches is that by decreasing the incidence and severity of maternal drug abuse, there will be decreased developmental compromise of their offspring, resulting in better outcomes for all.

COCAINE

The gestational consequences of exposing the fetal brain to cocaine are not yet as clearly understood or characterized as those for alcohol. Reasons for this include

1. There is no observable dysmorphic phenotype that can be attributed to gestational cocaine exposure.
2. Almost every woman who abuses cocaine also uses other substances including alcohol, tobacco, and to a lesser extent marijuana, requiring complex statistical design to look for interactive effects, or multivariate-regression analyses to determine the additional burden that cocaine imparts on the developing brain beyond that imparted by alcohol.
3. Evaluation of children born to women who were part of the crack epidemic, which peaked in the late 1980s, is not "as far advanced" as the study of the alcohol-exposed population. Cocaine-exposed children, who are now populating middle schools and high schools in greater numbers in many urban centers, are just having their complex academic needs and behavioral problems better defined, and the independent contribution of cocaine exposure to those problems is being ascertained.

In the 1980s, the "war on drugs" associated with the crack-cocaine epidemic focused national attention on the relationship between drug use and social and economic problems in society. Early reports on prenatal cocaine effects created a public frenzy and the myth about "unfit to parent" women and their damaged "crack babies." This affected legal activities by states on policy decisions affecting women who use illegal drugs during pregnancy. The later studies have failed to support significant associations between prenatal cocaine exposure and increased prevalence of serious newborn congenital malformations and medical complications at birth. Longitudinal follow-up studies of the behavior and development of these children suggest that cocaine effects are apparent but more subtle than originally feared. A number of reviews have described inconsistencies in the cocaine literature (Lester et al., 1998; Frank et al., 2001) due to methodological issues including small sample size, confounding of cocaine exposure with exposure to other drugs, lack of biochemical verification for exposure status and levels, lack of adequate control for demographic variables as prenatal care, SES, and out-of-home placement.

Current thinking has evolved towards a more balanced position that appreciates that not every child exposed to cocaine in utero has developmental problems but that exposure to cocaine, especially at high doses, in some subset of infants places them at risk for developmental compromise. As with other gestational toxins that have been studied, the expression of that insult depends on the context in which the child is raised. As with alcohol, there does not appear to be one outcome but a spectrum of outcomes, which may relate to the genetics of the mother and infant, to the postnatal environment, and to the specifics of the gestational exposure, including route, dosing, timing, and frequency of drug administration with respect to trimester of fetal development. Moreover, the fact that certain outcomes can be a consequence of gestational cocaine or alcohol exposure (such as microcephaly) makes it very difficult to design and interpret the results of clinical studies and to espouse causality to cocaine and/or alcohol in independently contributing to adverse outcomes. In an effort to meet these challenges, the second generation of clinical research on infants who were exposed to drugs has striven to quantitate the exposure to alcohol and cocaine during pregnancy and relate them to the degree and nature of altered postnatal outcomes (see Table 48.2). These more recent studies have investigated whether the timing and amount of cocaine and alcohol used during pregnancy identify which exposures are most likely contributing to which sets of outcomes. Many of these current studies demonstrate greater sophistication in study design and statistical analysis, affording a more rich and complex appreciation of the biology underlying the effects of cocaine and other gestational toxins on the developing brain.

The National Institutes of Health (NIH) Maternal Lifestyle Study (MLS) is the largest study of prenatal cocaine exposure and was developed against the backdrop of debate and controversy about the effects on prenatal cocaine exposure on child outcome to address many of these methodological issues. Maternal Lifestyle Study recruited mother/child dyads from 1993 to 1995 at four sites: Wayne State University, the University of Tennessee at Memphis, the University of Miami, and Brown University. The longitudinal sample included 658 children who were exposed, with 730 comparisons group matched on prematurity, race and sex was selected from a larger initial pool of 11,811 children of which 10% were prenatally exposed to cocaine. The exposed group included cocaine and/or opiate use during the pregnancy determined by self-report and/or meconium toxicology. Inclusion in the unexposed group required denial of cocaine or opiate use during pregnancy and negative toxicology results. Other substances known to be associated with cocaine and opiate use (alcohol, marijuana, and tobacco) were included in both groups.

TABLE 48.2 *Clinical Studies of* In Utero *Drug Effects: The Second Generation*

- Better study design
  - Improved controls
  - Multivariate design and analysis
  - Longer study period of parent–infant interaction
  - More sensitive instruments
- Quantitating exposure
  - Dose-related vs. threshold effects
  - High-dose vs. low-dose effects
  - Polypharmacy (? independent effects)
- Analysis of specific though subtle effects
  - Effect size may be small, requiring larger numbers of participants
  - Need to relate exposure(s) to outcome(s)
  - Must analyze drug-specific effects

Mechanisms of Cocaine-Induced Brain Maldevelopment

The primary action of cocaine is mediated by blocking the reuptake of the catecholamine neurotransmitters *norepinephrine* (NE) and *dopamine* (DA) and the indoleamine *serotonin*, thereby potentiating their action at nerve terminals. The peripheral effects of cocaine are a catecholamine-induced increase in sympathetic drive leading to vasoconstriction, hypertension, and tachycardia. The central effects of cocaine derive from increased central aminergic drive leading to CNS stimulation. Numerous investigators have suggested additional mechanisms by which gestational cocaine exposure may alter brain development following acute or chronic (recurrent) drug exposure (see Wilkins et al., 1998). It has been suggested that prenatal cocaine exposure may induce injury to developing tissues (including the brain) by fetal arterial vasoconstriction with resulting alterations in perfusion of vascular territories, perhaps mediated by ischemia/reperfusion injury (Fantel et al., 1992). Cocaine, which crosses the placenta in all species examined, including humans, primates, sheep, rats, and mice, may act directly on fetal tissues, perhaps as a local anesthetic, thereby altering ion permeability in the CNS. One transplacental mechanism by which maternal cocaine exposure may compromise fetal well-being has been suggested by physiologic studies in pregnant sheep. In the model of the fetal ewe (Woods et al., 1987), intravenous injection of cocaine into the pregnant mother (at a dose of cocaine of 1 mg/kg, comparable to commonly abused doses) results in maternal hypertension, with a 34% decrease in uterine blood flow from catecholamine-mediated vasoconstriction of the uterine arteries evident. In that model, the fetal consequences of decreased uterine blood flow are reduced oxygen delivery (hypoxemia), fetal hypertension, and tachycardia (Woods et al., 1987). One of the fetal responses to hypoxemia is release of endogenous catecholamines. The fetal catecholamines and maternal catecholamines, which are transmitted to fetus via the placenta, are circulating in high quantities in the fetus because cocaine, which diffuses to the fetal circulation, prevents their reuptake. These animal studies point to the following classes of potential mechanisms whereby maternal cocaine abuse can compromise fetal brain development:

Indirect (maternal): Via catecholamine-mediated placental vascular compromise with consequent fetal hypoxemia and/or ischemic injury

Direct (fetal) peripheral: Via catecholamine-mediated effects on fetal vasculature

Direct (fetal) central: Via direct actions of cocaine on fetal brain (for example, as a local anesthetic)

Direct (fetal) central: Via aminergic mechanisms:

1. Altering the fidelity of aminergic signals, which may subserve a trophic role in CNS maturation
2. Altering the integrity of aminergic transmitter systems secondary to developmental perturbation of amine concentration and distribution in fetal brain.

In support of the relevance of aminergic mechanisms in contributing to cocaine-induced brain maldevelopment, several preclinical studies have identified alterations in the maturation of aminergic systems consequent to prenatal cocaine exposure. These include a persistent elevation of dopaminergic innervation in rat cortex and hippocampus (Akbari and Azmitia, 1992); a hyperinnervation of serotonin fibers in adult rat striatum (Snyder-Keller and Keller, 1993); alterations in the state of phosphorylation of tyrosine hydroxylase (TH) in postnatal rats (Meyer and Dupont, 1993); an altered density of DA uptake pumps (the site of cocaine binding) in postnatal rats (Stadlin and Keller., 1994); alterations in fetal monkey brain including *(1)* decreased TH in the substantia nigra and (2) increased D_1, D_2, and D_5 receptor messenger ribonucleic acids (mRNA) and binding in the striatum and forebrain (Ronnekleiv and Naylor, 1995); impaired DA-mediated signal transduction as evidenced by impaired G_S coupling, cocaine-induced c-Fos activation, and DA release in postnatal rabbits (Friedman et al., 1993); neurophysiological data suggesting that the basal firing rate of midbrain dopaminergic neurons is altered (Wang and Pitts, 1994); and altered levels of monoamines in rat brain (Keller et al., 1994). Thus, there is increasing evidence from various structural, neurochemical, and neurophysiological studies that young and adult offspring exhibit deficits consistent with an altered "aminergic repertoire" that is associated with transplacental cocaine exposure. Investigators using preclinical models have demonstrated alterations in additional features of brain structure and function: The density of opiate receptors in striatum is altered in the brains of animals exposed to cocaine in utero (Clow et al., 1991); there are long-lived changes in the metabolic rate of limbic brain structures in adults exposed to cocaine in utero (Dow-Edwards et al., 1990); and there is altered precision of cortical cytoarchitectonics in the brains of mice (Gressens, Kosofsky, et al., 1992; see Figure 48.1); and primates (Lidow, 1995) exposed to cocaine in utero. In vitro studies of human fetal brain–derived neural precursor cells treated with cocaine showed marked inhibition of proliferation, migratory response, and cell differentiation. These results point towards existence of several molecular and cellular mechanisms triggered by exposure to cocaine that could adversely affect the fetal brain, with long-term implications (Linares et al., 2006). It is likely, though not proven, that similar mechanisms are relevant in clinical settings (for review, see Spear, 1995).

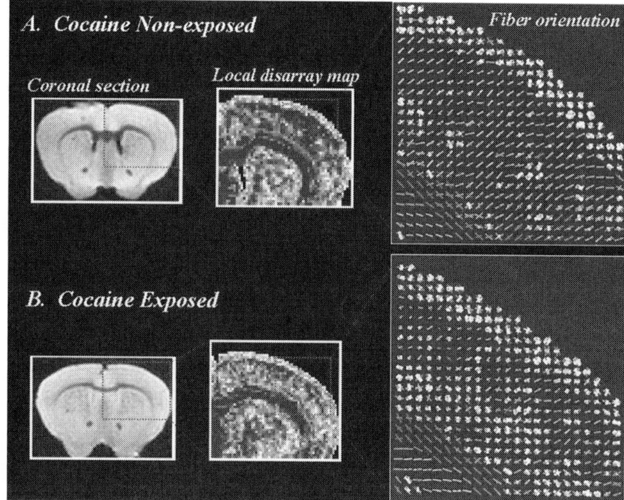

FIGURE 48.1 Images of rat brain from animals exposed to saline (left side) or cocaine (right side) in utero (20 mg/kg, subcutaneously, twice a day, from E8 to E17 inclusive), reared to adulthood, sacrificed by perfusion, and imaged on a 11.7T Bruker spectrometer (TR/TE = 800ms/32ms). Magnetic resonance imaging microscopy demonstrates that prenatal exposure to cocaine compromises brain growth, reflected as less neocortical area and an abnormal periventricular signal in striatum in these horizontal images (courtesy of Dr. Russ Jacobs and Dr. Scott Fraser, Beckman Institute, Biological Imaging Center, California Institute of Technology).

The Cocaine-Affected Phenotype

Maternal cocaine use during pregnancy is a major public health problem, resulting in perinatal and neonatal complications of enormous cost to society as well as mothers and infants. Some of the alterations in specific postnatal developmental outcomes that have been reported following in utero cocaine exposure will be reviewed by the topic below.

Prenatal effects

Clinical evidence suggests that cocaine independently contributes to impairment in brain growth that is prenatal in origin and exhibits an inverse dose–response relationship (Mirochnick et al., 1995; Bateman and Chiriboga, 2000). The selective impairment of brain growth demonstrated in a significant subset of infants exposed to cocaine in utero, which is beyond that resulting from the malnutrition associated with maternal cocaine use or with the sociodemographic attributes that characterize pregnant mothers who use cocaine (Zuckerman et al., 1989), is in contrast to the infants exposed to marijuana studied in that same cohort who showed evidence of asymmestric growth retardation with relative "head sparing." The symmetric growth retardation (that is, brain growth impairments that are coordinate with body growth compromise) evident following in utero cocaine (and alcohol) exposure suggests that these drugs are selectively neurotoxic and directly alter fetal brain growth. An interesting and a plausible explanation for the microcephaly seen with cocaine exposure was put forth by Chiroboga (1998): *in utero* exposure to cocaine results in excess accumulation of postsynaptic monoamines, attributable to the property of cocaine to block the uptake of monoamines. The resulting imbalance of monoamines leads to abnormal growth of the neural cone and dendritic arborization; these events may result in cortical dysgenesis and impaired neuropil growth that in turn could ultimately contribute to microcephaly (Chiriboga, 1998). Consistent with this formulation, some investigators have reported that here is an increased incidence of seizures in neonates exposed to cocaine.

In addition to the studies identifying impaired prenatal brain growth, many studies have shown effects of prenatal cocaine use on fetal and neonatal outcomes, including decreases in gestational age, birth weight, and birth length (Oro and Dixon, 1987; Fulroth et al., 1989; Zuckerman et al., 1989). In the MLS, medical complications of mothers in the exposed group were more common but still rare (< 5%; Bauer et al., 2002). Previously reported congenital anomalies identified using head ultrasound were not found in the MLS cohort (Bauer et al., 2005). In contrast, there were some effects on physical growth and central/autonomic nervous system (CNS/ANS) signs (Bada, Das, et al., 2002; Shankaran et al., 2003), though perhaps in part attributable to polydrug use: cocaine-using MLS mothers were 49 times more likely to use other drugs (Lester et al., 2001).

Perinatal behavior

The results reported from the MLS cohort, as well as others, identifies that cocaine appears to affect dimensions of arousal and reactivity, including greater excitability, poor state regulation, more rapid changes in arousal with stimulation, increased arousal from sleep, and increased physiological lability (Gingras et al., 1990; DiPietro et al., 1995; Mayes et al., 1995; Regalado et al., 1995; Mayes and Carroll, 1996; Regalado et al., 1996; Bendersky and Lewis, 1998; Gingras and O'Donnell, 1998). Numerous investigators have employed the Brazelton NBAS to study habituation, orientation, motor performance, range of state, regulation of state, autonomic regulation, and reflexes in infants exposed to cocaine during the perinatal period. In some studies, cluster-score comparisons between infants exposed to cocaine and control populations demonstrate significant impairment of orientation, motor ability, state regulation, and a number of abnormal reflexes, though there have been some evident inconsistencies (for review, see Lester et al., 1996). One factor contributing to the variability may relate to the amount of in utero cocaine exposure because impaired regulation of state and motor performance, as reflected by NBAS cluster scores, demonstrates a dose-response relationship with cocaine metabolites (Delaney-Black et al., 1996). Studies of the MLS cohort have confirmed (Bauer et al., 2002) and extended through at least one month of life (Lester et al., 2003) observations that prenatal cocaine exposure affected arousal, hypertonicity, excitability, and acoustic cry characteristics in newborns. Of note, mothers in the cocaine group are less engaged during feeding interaction (LaGasse et al., 2003). Early effects on the trajectory of motor development are additionally evident (Miller-Loncar et al., 2005).

A variant of the NBAS specifically developed to evaluate high-risk infants exposed to drugs, termed the *Neonatal Intensive Care Unit (NICU) Network Neurodevelopmental Scale (NNNS)*, may provide increased sensitivity to detect altered neonatal behaviors, as evidenced by an ability to discriminate newborn neurobehavioral patterns of excitability versus lethargy (Napiorkowski et al., 1996). Such alternative behavioral states may reflect direct versus indirect drug action (Napiorkowski et al., 1996). This formulation is supported by data collected with a version of the NBAS modified to study 3-week-old infants (Tronick et al., 1996) that demonstrates a persistence of dose-related effects of cocaine, particularly on the regulation of arousal. Infants exposed to cocaine show more negative affect during face-to-face interaction at 3 months of age in a mother–infant interaction test (Tronick et al., 2005) and at 18 months showed more insecure attachment (Seifer et al., 2004). Infant behavior in this high-risk sample is also affected by factors such as postpartum maternal depression (Salisbury et al., 2007) and parenting stress (Sheinkopf et al., 2005).

Neurological development

Investigators have defined a syndrome of "hypertonic tetraparesis," an increase in muscle tone evident in all four extremities, in almost two thirds of the examined infants born to mothers who were abusing cocaine, which was associated with smaller head size at birth (Chiriboga et al., 1995). Most of the affected children in this cohort grew out of their hypertonic tetraparesis by 12–18 months of age, though within the cocaine-exposed group there was an association between those infants who were initially hypertonic with those children who were subsequently developmentally delayed, as assessed by the Bayley Scales of Infant Development (BSID) through 12 months of age (Chiriboga et al., 1995). Although the motor impairments of newborns exposed to cocaine are dose-dependent (Chiriboga et al., 1999), the lasting effects of such exposure on motor function, as measured with the psychomotor development index of the BSID, appear not to be related to level of prenatal exposure (Frank et al., 2001). Recent studies of 2-year old toddlers exposed to cocaine have suggested that motor but not cognitive outcomes may be better than originally anticipated (Singer et al., 2004) and that the motor effects of gestational drug exposure may be significantly ameliorated by early intervention (Frank et al., 2002).

The syndrome of hypertonic tetraparesis may distinguish those infants who sustain significant in utero exposure to cocaine versus alcohol, as infants with FAE/FAS often demonstrate decreased muscle tone (that is, "floppiness") as compared with the increased muscle tone (that is, "stiffness") reported in infants exposed to cocaine. Hypertonia is also reported in some infants exposed to opiates in utero. The neuropathophysiological basis for the hypertonia in infants exposed to cocaine, and the extent to which it is a sign of spasticity (that is, implying corticospinal involvement) verses rigidity (that is, implying extrapyramidal involvement) constitutes an important topic for subsequent clinical and preclinical research.

As infants who are prenatally exposed to cocaine get older, motor developmental delays and cognitive deficits have been reported, in addition to abnormalities in physical growth (Zuckerman et al., 1989; McCalla et al., 1991; Bateman and Chiriboga, 2000; Behnke et al., 2002; Minnes et al., 2006; Lumeng et al., 2007). Imaging studies showed structural brain abnormalities including periventricular hemorrhages, subependymal and periventricular cysts have been found in children exposed to cocaine in utero (Dixon and Bejar, 1989; Sims, Walther, et al., 1989; Cohen et al., 1994; Singer et al., 1994). Occasional anomalies like cortical infarcts, pachygyria, and schizencephaly have been noted more frequently in association with prenatal cocaine exposure, on computed tomography (CT) and magnetic resonance imaging (MRI) studies (Heier et al., 1991; Gieron-Korthals et al., 1994; Gomez-Anson and Ramsey, 1994). However, prospective controlled studies showed no concrete association of cocaine exposure with cranial anomalies (Behnke et al., 1998; L.M. Smith et al., 2001a; Warner et al., 2006).

Language development

To address whether selective alterations in expressive language skills were a consequence of in utero cocaine exposure or a consequence of an impoverished postnatal environment, investigators compared 23 infants who were exposed to cocaine in foster care with 23 infants who were not exposed to cocaine in foster care. On the average, children exposed to cocaine demonstrated a 6-month delay in expressive speech at 2 years of age as compared with the unexposed foster-care control population (Nulman et al., 1994). That study additionally determined that the children exposed to cocaine had statistically significant impairments in postnatal brain growth through 2 years of age, which likewise suggests that despite proper nutrition and a nurturing postnatal environment, the foster-care cohort exposed to cocaine demonstrated postnatal brain growth retardation. However, investigators have also demonstrated significant deficits in total language acquisition through 7 years of age that are independent of the effects of cocaine on head circumference in a large, well-controlled sample of children exposed to cocaine (Bandstra et al., 2002). Several reports on cocaine literature support moderate language deficits and delay in children exposed to cocaine (Lester et al., 1998; Mentis, 1998; Bandstra et al., 2002; Lewis et al., 2004). Other investigators (Mentis and Lundgren, 1995) employed more sophisticated analyses of the pragmatics of language and reported that the population exposed to cocaine is deficient in some of these more subtle, yet crucially important, features of expressive language maturation. As with FAS, the small head at birth may serve as a "marker" of the child who was exposed to cocaine in utero, and impaired postnatal brain growth may additionally distinguish those children in whom gestational exposure to cocaine has altered programs for brain development in a significant way. However, as with some patients with FAE following in utero cocaine exposure, there may be adverse consequences on language and cognitive development independent of effects on prenatal or postnatal brain growth.

Intelligence, learning, and academic performance

Follow-up studies through school age show that children exposed to cocaine show small deficits in intelligence (Lester et al., 1998; Richardson, 1998; Bennett et al., 2002; Arendt et al., 2004; Singer et al., 2004). Further, children exposed to cocaine show deficits in component academic skills including poor sustained attention, visual motor integration and visuospatial memory, more disorganization, and less abstract thinking (Loebstein et al., 1997; Delaney-Black et al., 1998; Richardson, 1998; Leech et al., 1999; Delaney-Black et al., 2000; Bandstra et al., 2001; Arendt et al., 2004; Schroder et al., 2004; Noland et al., 2005). In MLS reports, there were no effects due to prenatal cocaine exposure on mental development at ages 1–3 (Messinger et al., 2004). However, effects on IQ emerged at age 4 and increased through age 7 (Lester et al., 2003). This could suggest that cocaine may affect some areas of the brain that are more "transparent" until children reach school age. In the same study (Lester et al., 2003), children exposed to cocaine were 1.5 times more likely to be referred for special education services at age 7.

Affect, attention, arousal

The MLS investigators have focused on the "four A's"—affect, attention, arousal, and action—as being those areas most at risk for compromise in infants exposed to drugs. Theoretically, primary compromise in the domain of arousal regulation, with its consequences on attentional mechanisms and thereby on executive functioning directly and socialization indirectly, may predict the cognitive and behavioral abnormalities observed in children exposed to cocaine in utero (Mayes, 2002). Although it is a significant challenge to assess affect, attention, and arousal in infants and children younger than 5 years of age, researchers have developed paradigms to assess visual habituation, response to novelty, social attachments, and infant attention. Alterations of state control (Delaney-Black et al., 1996), arousal (Tronick et al., 1996), and habituation evident in some neonates exposed to cocaine, especially those who sustained the most significant in utero exposures, may persist through infancy (Mayes et al., 1995), early childhood (S.W. Jacobson et al., 1996), and beyond (Richardson et al., 1997). Prospective studies reporting such changes have demonstrated differences in response to novelty, but not information processing, in some 3-month-olds exposed to cocaine (Mayes et al., 1995), reflected as a decreased likelihood to start a habituation procedure, and for those who did, an increased likelihood to react with irritability early in the procedure. A dose-response relationship relating the offspring of heavy cocaine users to faster responsiveness on an infant visual expectancy test but to poorer novelty preference performance during their first year of life has been established (S.W. Jacobson et al., 1996). School-age children born to mothers who reported light to moderate cocaine use during pregnancy exhibited deficits in their ability to sustain attention on a computerized vigilance task (Richardson et al., 1997).

Problem behavior and externalizing and internalizing behavior have also been reported in children exposed to cocaine through age 7 (Delaney-Black et al., 1998; Delaney-Black et al., 2000; Covington et al., 2001; Accornero et al., 2002; Linares et al., 2006; Bada et al., 2007). In MLS, high prenatal cocaine exposure was associated with higher internalizing, externalizing, and total behavior problems scores on the Child Behavior Checklist (CBCL) from 3 to 7 years of age (Bada et al., 2007). It is anticipated that the use of these and other instruments that are designed to assess more subtle impairments of attention, vigilance, responsivity, and behavioral dysregulation, combined with quantitative assessments of gestational drug exposures, will facilitate an improved understanding of the relationship of in utero drug exposure with alterations in these subtle, but profoundly important, outcomes.

Summary of Cocaine's Clinical Effects

In summary, the data outlined regarding transplacental cocaine exposure suggest:

1. Many infants born to mothers who abuse cocaine during gestation demonstrate impaired fetal growth. This appears to be mediated through an indirect effect of poor maternal nutrition and a direct effect of cocaine. The independent contribution of cocaine is a 0.43 cm decrement in head circumference of the newborn (Zuckerman et al., 1989).
2. Some newborns of mothers who abuse cocaine during gestation (including women who limit their cocaine habits to the first trimester) demonstrate altered behavior, as evidenced by abnormalities in state control (abnormalities on the NBAS and the NNNS), with the most pronounced difficulties in orientation, alertness, and arousal.
3. A neurological syndrome of increased tone termed *hypertonic tetraparesis* is seen in a subset of children exposed to cocaine in utero. This motor system abnormality is transient and resolves in most infants who are affected by 18 months of age.
4. Neurophysiological studies suggest that some newborns exposed to cocaine in utero may evidence CNS dysmaturation; that is, they characterize such infants exposed to cocaine as being younger than chronological age by demonstration of more immature patterns of electrophysiological activity. Normalization of neurophysiological testing (as with neurological examination) occurs in most of the infants who are affected during the first 12–18 months of life.
5. Persistent deficits may be evident in children exposed to cocaine as they get older, including delayed language acquisition, cognitive impairment, or behavioral abnormalities, including difficulty modulating attention, impulsivity, and responsivity, which are challenged in classroom settings.

Conclusions regarding the effects of cocaine on the developing human brain are less definite than for the effects of alcohol: The resulting deficits appear to be more subtle, and as with alcohol, only a subset of exposed infants and children exhibit lasting deficits. What is emerging, as was evident in children exposed to alcohol, is that some of the more subtle behaviors that are felt to be at risk in these infants as they grow older are important for socialization, educability, and the adaptive skills that are required for individuals to become enfranchised in schools, communities, and society. Future research will bring a clearer characterization of the deficits evident in these children, of the extent and role that in utero cocaine exposure contributes to these deficits, and of the impact of postnatal interventions to ameliorate such deficits. Whether some children exposed to cocaine will grow up to have other behavioral, learning, and emotional deficits as defined in the section above for alcohol remains to be determined. What is very clear is that clinicians, educators, and biological and adoptive parents should be vigilant regarding the special needs of such children as they enter school and beyond.

METHAMPHETAMINE

The abuse of methamphetamine (METH) in the United States has been well documented. Methamphetamine is the most widely abused amphetamine and, along with other amphetamines, has been categorized as a Schedule II stimulant since 1971 because of its high potential for abuse (Lukas, 1997). In 1999, the number of Americans who had tried METH in their lifetime was 9.4 million (SAMHSA, 2002), double from what it was in 1994 (SAMHSA, 1995). By 2004, the number had reached nearly 12 million (SAMHSA, 2005a). Treatment Episode Data Set (TEDS; based on treatment admissions for substance abuse) recorded a 307% increase in admissions due to METH between 1993 and 2003 (SAMHSA, 2005b), with the highest rates in the Pacific, Mountain, and West North Central states, reflecting the well-known regional concentration of METH use. Although there is controversy about the nature and extent of the METH problem in the United States, including exaggerations reminiscent of the cocaine "epidemic," there is little argument that METH is a dangerous drug that substantially challenges policy makers, health care professionals, social service providers, and the law enforcement community (King, 2006). There is little information about METH use by pregnant women (Wouldes et al., 2004), further complicated by methodological issues such as definitions of use, sampling methods, and drug use detection procedures (Smeriglio, 1999). The National Pregnancy and Health Survey (National Institute on Drug Abuse [NIDA], 1996) conducted in 1993, was designed to provide a nationally representative sample of live births. This study is based on self-report but includes a subsample with toxicological verification and showed less than 1% METH use by pregnant women. The most recent estimate from the National Survey on Drug Use and Health, based on self-report data from the 2004 survey (SAMHSA, 2005a) showed that, for women of childbearing age, 0.4% of nonpregnant women and 0.1% of pregnant women used METH. The 2003 TEDS database showed a 6.4% prevalence rate for pregnant METH users.

Pharmacology

Methamphetamine is a CNS stimulant of the sympathetic nervous system with neurotoxic potential for developing monoaminergic systems. As the "first cousin" of amphetamine with the addition of the methyl radical, METH exerts its action by releasing DA and serotonin, blocking monoamine reuptake mechanisms, and inhibiting monoamine oxidase (Heller, 2000). The mechanism of action most likely occurs by increasing the synaptic concentrations of the neurotransmitters DA and NE (Heller, 2000) either by direct release from storage vesicles or by inhibition of reuptake (Karch, 1993; Catanzarite and Stein, 1995). Methamphetamine may enhance synaptic catecholamine levels by inhibiting monoamine oxidase, the enzyme responsible for the oxidation of NE and serotonin (Bennett et al., 1993). Amphetamines are considered noncatecholamine sympathomimetics because they lack catecholamine structure yet have sympathomimetic actions (Plessinger, 1998). The structural characteristics are important because they account for the wide distribution and long duration of action of amphetamine. Methamphetamine also has vasoconstrictive effects (Burchfield et al., 1991; Stek et al., 1993) resulting in decreased uteroplacental blood flow and fetal hypoxia (Stek et al., 1995). In addition, METH has anorexic effects on the mother. These maternal/placental effects could affect fetal development to the above monoaminergic effects. Weight control may also help explain the popularity of METH with women, including pregnant women.

Preclinical Studies

Administration of METH to laboratory animals results in profound and long-lasting toxicity to the brain. In rodents, METH is toxic to dopaminergic and serotonergic neurons (Fuller and Hemrick-Leucke, 1992; Pu and Voorhees, 1993). Damage to DA terminals (Seiden and Sabol, 1996; Gibb et al., 1997) is thought to reflect irreversible terminal degeneration (Ricaurte and McCann, 1992). Neurotoxic effects of prenatal METH exposure on serotogenetic neurons produce neurochemical alternations in the CNS (Cabrera et al., 1993; Weissman and Caldecott-Hazard, 1995) thought to be associated with learning impairment, behavioral deficits (Weissman and Caldecott-Hazard, 1995), increased motor activity (Acuff-Smith et al., 1992), enhanced conditioned avoidance responses (Cho et al., 1991), and postural motor movements (Slamberova et al., 2006) seen in METH-exposed animals. Rhesus monkeys show reduced brain monoamines 4 years after the last drug exposure (Woolverton et al., 1989).

Administration of METH to laboratory animals also results in motor (Wallace et al., 1999) and learning and memory impairment (Itoh et al., 1991). Studies with rats have shown a range of physical, motor, neurotransmitter, and behavioral effects in offspring exposed to METH. These include increased maternal and offspring mortality, retinal eye defects (Acuff-Smith et al.,

1992; Yamamoto et al., 1992; Acuff-Smith et al., 1996), cleft palate and rib malformations (Yamamoto et al., 1992), and decreased rate of physical growth and delayed motor development (Cho et al., 1991; Acuff-Smith et al., 1996). Methamphetamine exposure to pregnant dams showed effects on spatial learning in their adult offspring (Slamberova et al., 2006). Spatial learning and attenuated corticosterone response was found in rats with prenatal METH exposure (Williams et al., 2003). In pregnant mice, METH caused dopaminergic nerve terminal degeneration and long-term motor deficits in offspring (Jeng et al., 2005).

Clinical Studies—Adult Brain Imaging

There is an emerging literature on METH effects on the structure and chemistry of the human brain. Neuroimaging studies of adult METH abusers showed potential neurotoxic effects in subcortical brain structures, including DA transporters, brain metabolism, and perfusion (Ernst et al., 2000; Volkow et al., 2001; Chang et al., 2002). In studies using positron emission tomography (PET), METH abusers show lower levels of DA transporters in the striatum (McCann et al., 1998; Volkow et al., 2001; Sekine et al., 2003) and prefrontal cortex (Sekine et al., 2003), and differences in regional glucose metabolism (Volkow et al., 2001; London et al., 2004). Other imaging studies of METH abusers have reported alterations in perfusion (Chang et al., 2002), levels of neuronal metabolites (Ernst et al., 2000), and cortical activation (Paulus et al., 2002).

There are also relations between imaging and behavior findings. In one study, DA transmitter loss reported in METH abusers (24%–30%) was associated with reduced motor speed and impaired verbal learning (Volkow et al., 2001). Also, in this study the lower DA transporter levels were even seen in patients detoxified for at least 1 year, suggesting that METH effects on the brain may be long lasting. Positron emission tomography studies have shown inhibitory control related to glucose metabolism in the orbitofrontal gyrus in patients who were recovering from METH dependence (Goldstein et al., 2002) and to anterior cingulate, insular, and amygdalar regions of cortex that were correlated with self-report of negative affective states (London et al., 2004). Thompson and associates (Thompson et al., 2004) found gray-matter deficits in the cingulate, limbic, and paralimbic corticies; smaller hippocampal volumes; and white matter hypertrophy in chronic METH users with the hippocampal deficits correlated with memory performance.

Clinical Studies—Child Brain Imaging

A study of 12 children exposed to METH and 14 controls using magnetic resonance spectroscopy (Smith et al., 2001b) found increased creatine in the striatum of the METH exposure group suggesting an abnormality in energy metabolism. In an MRI study of brain morphometry, these children also exhibited smaller subcortical volumes in the putamen, globus pallidus, and hippocampus (Chang et al., 2004). They also showed neurocognitive deficits in visual motor integration (Beery Test), sustained attention (TOVA), verbal memory, and long-term spatial memory, but no differences in IQ. The deficits in sustained attention and verbal memory, were correlated with reduction in brain structures (Chang et al., 2004).

Prenatal exposure

There are few studies of the effects of prenatal METH exposure. These studies have many of the methodological problems of the early cocaine literature, including small sample size, confounding with other variables especially other drugs, and problems with the detection of METH exposure status (Billing et al., 1980; Oro and Dixon, 1987; Dixon and Bejar, 1989; Struthers and Hansen, 1992; Hansen et al., 1993; Plessinger, 1998; L. Smith et al., 2003).

Medical Outcomes

Retrospective studies showed increased incidence of small for gestational age (SGA; Oro and Dixon, 1987; L. Smith et al., 2003) and decreased birth weight and head circumference (Oro and Dixon, 1987). These findings could be due to the vasoconstrictive effects of METH that induced increases in maternal blood pressure, restriction of nutritional substrate, increases in fetal blood pressure, decreases in fetal oxy-hemoglobin saturation, and arterial pH in the fetal ovine model (Burchfield et al., 1991; Stek et al., 1995). Some of METH effects reported in animal studies have also been found in human infants exposed to METH. These include clefting, cardiac anomalies, and fetal growth retardation (Plessinger, 1998). A high rate (35%) of cranial abnormalities was reported in a group of infants prenatally exposed to METH and cocaine (Dixon and Bejar, 1989).

Behavioral Outcomes

In work by Struthers and associates (Struthers and Hansen, 1992; Hansen et al., 1993), infants who were exposed to METH and/or cocaine at 6 months and 1 year were compared with unexposed controls on the Fagan Test of Infant Intelligence and showed lower visual recognition memory and differences on attention and distractibility and activity level. The most extensive work on prenatal METH exposure is from a series of studies from Sweden with a sample of 66 children exposed to amphetamine who were followed to the age of 14 (Cernerud et al., 1996). Initial findings (Billing et al., 1985) included drowsiness during the first few months, emotional signs of autism, speech problems, and signs of wariness of strangers at 1 year, if the mother continued to use throughout pregnancy. At age 4 (Billing et al., 1985), there were no differences in physical growth or health. IQ was lower than a separately selected control group from the population, and the amphetamine group had more disturbed or problem children if the mother was still addicted. Also at age 4 (Billing et al., 1988), child adjustment was predicted by maternal alcohol and drug use, maternal stress, and paternal criminal convictions. At age 8 (Billing et al., 1994), the extent of prenatal exposure predicted psychometric outcome, aggression, peer problems, adjustment, and general assessment. Alcohol also correlated with outcome, as did pregnancy attitudes. Maternal psychiatric treatment, alcohol abuse, and number of custodians correlated with aggressive behavior and general assessment. These children had problems with advancement in school due to delays in math and language and at age 14, they had difficulties with physical fitness activities (Cernerud et al., 1996). The limitations of this work include lack of a control group, small sample size, and confounding with other prenatal drug use (30% used heroin, 81% used alcohol with one third meeting criteria for alcohol abuse, and 80% smoked more than 10 cigarettes/day). The study is also based on self-report and the route of administration of amphetamine was injection, which is less common today in the United States. Therefore, although these findings are limited, they do suggest that these children are at risk for poor child outcome due to drug and psychosocial risk factors.

Clearly, we are at the very beginning of our understanding of the effects of prenatal METH exposure on child development (Wouldes et al., 2004) The scant literature that is available is beset by methodological problems. This sentiment was summarized in a 2005 Expert Panel (National Toxicology Program, 2005), which concluded that in terms of the potential adverse reproductive and developmental effects of METH exposure, "studies that focused upon humans were uninterpretable due to such factors as a lack of control of potential confounding factors" (p. 177). Mindful of these limitations and of the "rush to judgment" that followed early cocaine findings, the NIH (NIDA) Infant Development, Environment and Lifestyle (IDEAL) longitudinal study of the effects of prenatal was established in four sites among the hardest hit areas in the United States with regard to rates of METH use: DeMoines, IA; Tulsa, OK; Los Angeles, CA; and Honolulu, HI (for details of the study design, see Arria et al., 2006). IDEAL participants were recruited following delivery and before discharge in 2002–2004. Methamphetamine exposure was determined through mothers' self-reported use of METH and/or GC/MS confirmation of METH in meconium. Unexposed participants denied METH use during pregnancy and had a negative METH screen. Initial findings, based on the first 1,632 participants (Arria et al., 2006) showed a 5.2% prevalence rate for METH. Smoking was the most common route of administration (79%), and the average age of first METH use was 19 years (range 8 to 38 years).

For the longitudinal follow-up, 204 infants exposed to METH were matched with unexposed infants on maternal race, infant birth weight, type of medical insurance, and maternal education. Mothers who used alcohol, tobacco, or marijuana during pregnancy were included in both groups. Methamphetamine use was related to polydrug use, poverty, delayed prenatal care, and increased out-of-home placement of their infant (Grant et al., 2004). These mothers reported lower maternal perceptions on quality of life, greater likelihood of substance use among family and friends, increased risk for ongoing legal difficulties, and a markedly increased likelihood of developing a substance abuse disorder (Derauf et al., 2007). They also reported high levels of exposure to family violence during their own childhood and scored higher on the Child Abuse Potential Inventory (Newman et al., 2007)

There were effects of METH on the infant. Infants exposed to METH were 3.5 times more likely to be SGA. Although most infants were full term, the average birth weight was 204 gm less in the METH group than in the comparison group (L.M. Smith et al., 2006). On the NNNS, exposure to METH was associated with lower arousal and increased physiological stress. First trimester METH use was related to greater stress/abstinence signs including CNS stress and physiological stress. Third trimester use was related to poorer quality of movement and greater physiological stress. Higher level of amphetamine metabolites in meconium was associated with poorer quality of movement, increased CNS stress, and poorer regulation (L.M. Smith et al., 2008) Acoustical analysis of the infants' cry showed prenatal METH exposure related to cry characteristics indicative of CNS reactivity, poorer respiratory control, and neural control of the vocal track (LaGasse et al., 2004). NNNS and cry effects are similar to findings reported in infants exposed to cocaine suggesting neurotoxic effects to the developing fetus.

OPIATES

Mechanisms of Opioid-Induced Brain Maldevelopment

Opiates act through three separate and distinct receptor subtypes, μ, δ, and κ, which have been molecularly cloned and pharmacologically well-characterized. These receptors have different anatomical distributions in the CNS and cellular mechanisms of action employing different second-messenger systems. μ and δ-receptors act through inhibition of adenylyl cyclase (Duman et al., 1988) and activation of outward potassium currents (North et al., 1987) via inhibitory (G_i/G_O) G proteins; κ-receptors act through inhibition of calcium currents, primarily but not exclusively at presynaptic terminals. The differences between the most commonly abused opiate narcotic, heroin (3,6-diacetylmorphine), the common drug of choice for the treatment of opioid dependence, methadone, and morphine are pharmacokinetic, not pharmacodynamic: all three act as at least partially-selective μ-receptor agonists, whereas heroin, more lipophilic than morphine, more readily crosses the blood–brain barrier, and methadone has a significantly longer elimination half-life (Jaffe and Martin, 1985). Like cocaine, the anatomical and physiological substrate for the rewarding properties of the opiates lie in the dopaminergic mesolimbic and mesocortical projections from the ventral tegmental area (VTA) to the basal forebrain (Koob and Le Moal, 1997; Nestler, 1997). In the case of the opiates, however, enhancement of dopaminergic tone is not a direct action on the nucleus accumbens (NAc) and other forebrain targets but rather occurs through disinhibition of VTA dopaminergic neurons through inhibition of GABAergic inhibitory interneurons intrinsic to the VTA (Johnson and North, 1992). Opiate narcotics therefore utilize the existing enkephalinergic circuitry within the VTA, which acts to increase VTA activity and subsequently enhance dopaminergic transmission to the NAc and other sites within the basal forebrain (Johnson and North, 1992). Many of the experimental findings on the role of DA in the basal forebrain on reward and reinforcement, therefore, are relevant to the mechanism of drug-craving and drug-consuming behavior for the opiates, as well. At a molecular level, the reinforcing actions of the opiates are dependent largely, if not entirely, on their activity at μ-receptors, as μ-receptor knockout mice do not experience the analgesic effects of morphine, do not respond to morphine as if it were rewarding, and do not become physically dependent with chronic administration (Matthes et al., 1996).

In preclinical studies, exposure to opiates in utero results in transient and persistent structural and behavioral changes in animal offspring. Morphine treatment of pregnant dams results in changes in the packing density of neurons and their morphology in rat pups: cortical density of neurons is decreased and neuronal processes (for example, dendritic arborization, axonal branching) are significantly smaller compared to controls (Hammer et al., 1989). Conversely, prenatal exposure to the opiate antagonist *naloxone* results in a significant increase in neuronal packing in the cortex and an increase in neuronal process length and extension (Zagon and McLaughlin, 1986; Hauser et al., 1987), raising the interesting possibility that endogenous opioid systems play a morphogenetic role in the normal development of the brain. From this standpoint, the toxicity of gestational opiates could be viewed as an impact on normal modulatory, in this instance inhibitory, influences in the normal developmental program of cortical structures. Neurochemical studies of the effects of prenatal opiate exposure on several neurotransmitter systems have yielded mixed results (Fried, 1992). Increases and decreases in opioid receptors have been reported with gestational opiate exposure. Similarly, changes in brain content of the different monoamine neurotransmitters and acetylcholine have been reported by different laboratories to increase, decrease, or remain unchanged. A more consistent finding has been that gestational opiate exposure results in a decrease in nucleic acid synthesis and protein production in the fetal brain. Although studies focusing more specifically on brain reward circuitry have found that G protein–coupled cAMP production is critical to opiate self-administration (Self et al., 1994), that changes in this signal transduction pathway occur with chronic opiate administration in the NAc and VTA of adult animals (Bandstra et al., 2001), and that the change in these neurons is associated with immediate-early gene expression and subsequent target gene regulation (Nestler, 1997), similar studies have not been undertaken in animals who were gestationally exposed to opiates.

The Opioid-Affected Phenotype(s)

Although the preclinical literature on effects of gestational opiate exposure has described differing findings, perhaps due to different animal species using widely differing doses and scheduling of different opiates (Fried, 1992), a few consistent findings across studies have emerged. Most studies in young animals have shown a decrease in exploratory behavior and an increased latency in response to noxious stimuli after fetal exposure to opiates. Interestingly, similar to results with fetal cocaine exposure, gestational morphine exposure results in increased self-administration of heroin and cocaine (Ramsey et al., 1993) and enhances place preference to morphine (Gagin et al., 1997) in adult animals. Furthermore, prenatal cocaine exposure appears to sensitize rat pups to the pharmacological effects of opiates (Goodwin et al., 1993), lending further support to the idea that drugs of abuse not only act but also exert their developmental toxicities through actions on brain reward systems, and that this toxicity may consist in part of an increased sensitivity of the gestationally drug-exposed brain to novel or reinforcing stimuli.

In human studies, as with other drugs of abuse, measurement of the precise effects of gestational opiate exposure on neurodevelopment in the absence of the confounding effects of other prenatal and postnatal variables presents a significant challenge to clinical investigators.

Nonetheless, several small, well-controlled studies have revealed a set of developmental and behavioral abnormalities in these children that appear to be relatively specific to opiate exposure in utero. For example, 1-year-old infants of mothers who were on methadone maintainance showed more disorganized and avoidant behavior when assessed for maternal attachment than infants of mothers who were not abusing drugs matched for age, parity, and socioeconomic factors including educational level and marital status (Goodman et al., 1999). Neonates exposed to opiates scored with the NBAS consistently demonstrate higher levels of arousal at baseline but poorer consolability and poorer motor control, decreased alertness and orientation to stimuli, and decreased habituation to repetitive stimuli than nonexposed controls across several studies (Hans, 1992). Measuring developmental progress with either the Griffith's Developmental Scale (GDS) or the BSID, 12- to 18-month-old infants of mothers who were addicted to opiates and on methadone-maintainance have been found to have significantly lower scores than age-matched controls (Rosen and Johnson, 1982; Bunikowski et al., 1998); interestingly, one study (Bunikowski et al., 1998) showed no significant difference between the children of mothers who were on methadone maintainance and mothers who continued to abuse illicit opiates (that is, heroin) during pregnancy. Although studies have shown that children exposed to opiates demonstrate later problems with socialization and inattention and may be more impulsive than children who are not exposed (Wilson, 1989; Hans, 1992; Suess et al., 1997), these findings, like those in children exposed to cocaine, are subtle, and the relative contribution of drug exposure per se remains unclear.

CANNABIS

Mechanisms of Cannabinoid-Induced Brain Maldevelopment

Among the drugs of abuse, cannabinoids were the last for which endogenous receptors (Devane et al., 1988; Matsuda et al., 1990) and ligands (Devane et al., 1992) were identified, and until recently had defied attempts at animal modeling through self-administration (Martellotta et al., 1998). However, it is now appreciated that like all drugs of abuse, delta-9-tetrahydrocannabinol (Δ-9-THC, the primary pharmacologically active alkaloid extract from marijuana) exerts its effects in part through facilitation of dopaminergic transmission from the VTA to the forebrain, and that this mechanism involves activation of endogenous opioid systems in the VTA (Tanda et al., 1997). Ironically, changes in brain dopaminergic function with prenatal cannabinoid exposure were recognized prior to the demonstration of THC action on mesoaccumbal DA systems: cortical and striatal D_1 and D_2 receptor binding and TH activity (the rate-limiting enzyme in DA biosynthesis) are persistently decreased in animals who are gestationally exposed to cannabinoid (Walters and Carr, 1986; Rodriguez de Fonseca et al., 1991). Changes are evident among other neurotransmitter systems relevant to the brain reward system, as well. For example, neither GABA content nor the activity of its synthetic enzyme, glutamic acid decarboxylase (GAD), are altered by prenatal Δ-9-THC exposure; however, motor inhibition induced by administration of the GABA-B receptor agonist baclofen, but not by the GABA-A receptor agonist muscimol, was greater in rats which were gestationally exposed to cannabinoid than in controls (Garcia et al., 1996). More often than with other drugs of abuse, sexually dimorphic effects of prenatal cannabinoid exposure are evident in animal studies: measurement of regional brain serotonin levels in newborn rat pups exposed to Δ-9-THC in utero show decreased 5-HT in diencephalic structures in males, but not in females (Molina-Holgado et al., 1996). Adult male rats exposed to Δ-9-THC in utero demonstrate decreased μ-opioid receptor binding in the striatum and amygdala, whereas adult females show increased μ-opioid receptor binding in the prefrontal cortex, the amygdala, and the VTA (Vela et al., 1998). Conversely, proenkephalin expression in the striatum of exposed females is decreased, while males are unaffected (Corchero et al., 1998). These and other studies have suggested a functional, and possibly developmental, interrelatedness between the endogenous opioid and cannabinoid systems (Manzanares et al., 1999; Fernandez-Ruiz et al., 2000). At this time, it remains unclear whether these sexually dimorphic effects of prenatal exposure are due to cannabinoid interactions with developing brain monoamine systems, their actions on the developing hypothalamic-pituitary-adrenal axis (Dalterio et al., 1984; Dalterio et al., 1986), or both.

The Cannabinoid-Affected Phenotype(s)

Although relatively fewer animal studies have looked in detail at behavioral outcomes, increases in grooming behavior, alterations in habituation to novel environments, and interestingly, enhanced sensitization to the reinforcing effects of morphine have been observed in adult animals following gestational cannabinoid exposure (Navarro et al., 1994; Navarro et al., 1995). Inhibition of open-field motor behavior by a D_1-selective antagonist, SCH 23390, but not by a D_2-selective antagonist, sulpiride, was less marked in adult rats exposed to Δ-9-THC than in controls (Garcia et al., 1996). Sexually dimorphic effects of prenatal cannabinoid exposure are also evident in behavioral experiments in adult animals: female rats exposed to Δ-9-THC in utero demonstrate an increased rate of morphine self-administration compared to controls, whereas males do not (Vela et al., 1998). Conversely, males exposed to Δ-9-THC demonstrate an increased baseline pain threshold and increased tolerance to the analgesic effects of morphine in a tail-flick assay, whereas females do not (Vela et al., 1995). Taken together, these preclinical biochemical and behavioral results suggest that one consequence of prenatal cannabinoid exposure may be that in females the endogenous opioid system is down-regulated, resulting in a relatively sensitized state, while in males this system is up-regulated, resulting in a relatively tolerant, or desensitized, state.

Much of the clinical data on cognitive and behavioral outcomes following prenatal exposure to marijuana comes from two ongoing long-term longitudinal studies of large cohorts of at-risk children: The Ottawa Prenatal Prospective Study (OPPS) and the Maternal Health Practices and Child Development Study (MHPCD). The primary differences between the patient populations in these two cohorts are that the majority of women in the OPPS are Caucasian and of middle-class SES, whereas the majority of women in the MHPCD are of lower SES and are evenly distributed between Caucasian and African American ethnicities. Nonetheless, the findings of studies of these two cohorts are in significant agreement. On neurological examination, neonates born to mothers using marijuana during pregnancy resemble neonates undergoing mild narcotic withdrawal in that they exhibit more jitteriness and have an exaggerated startle response compared to normal infants (Fried et al., 1987). As toddlers, children exposed to marijuana demonstrate poorer language development than nonexposed age-mates, but not to the same extent as children of mothers who smoked cigarettes during pregnancy; children exposed to marijuana also show more specific impairments in verbal memory (Fried and Watkinson, 1990). A more recent study of a larger cohort using a maternal self-reporting survey (Faden and Graubard, 2000) showed that toddlers that were exposed to marijuana are less socially engaging; once engaged, play for shorter periods of time; and are more fearful than their nonexposed, alcohol-exposed, or cigarette-exposed age-mates. In 6-year-old children, prenatal marijuana exposure appears to result in increased inattention and impulsivity as measured by parent–teacher reporting through a modified Conner's Rating Scale and by testing in a continuous performance task (Leech et al., 1999; Bandstra et al., 2001). This same cohort of children continue to demonstrate poor impulse control, diminished attention span, poor visuospatial reasoning skills, and poor hypothesis testing that persists into adolescence (Fried et al., 1998; Cornelius et al., 2000; Bandstra et al., 2001), suggesting that taken together, the effects of prenatal marijuana exposure may be related more to selective impairment of executive functioning than to overall delay in global development (Bandstra et al., 2001).

NICOTINE

Mechanisms of Nicotine-Induced Brain Maldevelopment

The alkaloid nicotine was for many decades thought to exert its pharmacological effects solely through its activity at peripheral autonomic ganglia. Only recently has it come to be fully appreciated that not only does nicotine act at CNS acetylcholine receptors, but also that it is the central actions of nicotine that lead to the physical dependence characteristic of its use. The neural substrate for its addictive properties has been identified as the mesocorticolimbic dopaminergic system (Pich et al., 1997), common to other drugs of abuse. Pharmacologically, it has been clearly demonstrated in animal studies that nicotine stimulates dopaminergic neurotransmission from the VTA to the NAc (Pontieri et al., 1996; Pidoplichko et al., 1997), the sine qua non of brain reward processing in general and of responses to drugs of abuse in particular. Nicotine acts at nicotinic cholinoceptors (nAChR), which are ligand-gated ion channels that mediate excitatory cellular responses and for which the endogenous ligand is the classical neurotransmitter acetylcholine. Like most other ligand-gated ion channels, it is a heteromeric, or multisubunit, assembly with binding sites on different protein subunit types. At the molecular level, it has been demonstrated that one particular nAChR subunit, β_2, is necessary for the reinforcing effects of nicotine, as β_2-subunit deficient knockout mice will not self-administer nicotine (Picciotto et al., 1998). Preclinical studies have demonstrated the effects of fetal nicotine exposure on brain and body growth parameters and have shown changes in several neurochemical systems, particularly NE (Slotkin, 1992). For example, in young adult animals exposed to nicotine in utero, basal NE content and nicotine-stimulated NE release were decreased compared to controls (Seidler et al., 1992). Animal studies have also demonstrated changes in other monoamine systems with gestational nicotine exposure. Dopamine synthesis and turnover is decreased in the forebrain and brain stem (Muneoka et al., 1997; Muneoka et al., 1999), striatal and VTA dopamine content is reduced, and striatal D_2 receptor binding is decreased in rats exposed to nicotine (Richardson and Tizabi, 1994). Serotonin synthesis and turnover are likewise decreased in the forebrain and brain stem of exposed rats (Muneoka et al., 1997); in addition, serotonin transporter density is increased in brain stem and decreased in forebrain regions with prenatal nicotine exposure (Xu et al., 2001). Prenatal in the neocortex: decreases in somatosensory cortical thickness and neuronal size were observed in rats who were gestationally exposed to nicotine (Roy and Sabherwal, 1994), suggesting a delay in neocortical neuronal maturation and/or migration similar to that observed in mice who were gestationally exposed to cocaine (Gressens, Kosofsky et al., 1992; Kosofsky et al., 1994).

The Nicotine-Affected Phenotype

Many preclinical studies have demonstrated clearly that prenatal exposure to nicotine is associated with hyperactivity in young animals that persists into adulthood, measured as increases in open-field exploratory behavior, vertical rearing, and stereotypical movements (Ajarem and Ahmad, 1998; Newman et al., 1999; Richardson and Tizabi, 1994; Shacka et al., 1997; Tizabi et al., 2000). Clinical studies have demonstrated the risks of tobacco smoking on fetal outcome, most notably on spontaneous abortion, birth weight, and other growth measures, including head circumference (Fried et al., 1999; Bandstra et al., 2001). The two large prospective studies of the OPPS and MHPCD cohorts have followed the behavioral and cognitive development of children of mothers who smoked cigarettes from birth through adolescence. In addition, a more recent multicenter survey of a large cohort of children who were exposed to marijuana, alcohol, and/or tobacco (Faden and Graubard, 2000) has corroborated these findings in toddlers. Three-year-old children exposed to nicotine appear to have poorer overall language development than toddlers exposed to marijuana during gestation and their age-matched unexposed peers (Fried and Watkinson, 1990; Faden and Graubard, 2000). Their specific language delays are persistent and are reflected in lower scores on verbal subtests of the Weschler Intelligence Scale for Children–III (WISC-III) administered in early adolescence (Fried et al., 1998). Toddlers exposed to nicotine also appear to be more impulsive and more active than nonexposed playmates, and engage in significantly more oppositional behavior with caregivers than age-matched controls (Cornelius et al., 2000; Faden and Graubard, 2000). Later in development, school-age children exposed to tobacco demonstrate a reduced attention span (Fried, 1992; Leech et al., 1999) that persists into adolescence (Fried and Watkinson, 2001). An additional behavioral outcome that has been relatively less studied is the incidence of substance abuse in offspring of mothers who abused drugs during their pregnancy. Although difficult to examine prospectively as yet in children who were exposed to cocaine or opiates, as most cohorts of these children under study are still younger than the typical age of onset of substance experimentation and abuse, a recent investigation (Cornelius et al., 2000) of 10-year-old children exposed to tobacco suggests that prenatal nicotine exposure is an independent risk factor for early experimentation with cigarette smoking, confirming previous findings regarding increased incidence of smoking in offspring exposed to nicotine in utero (Kandel et al., 1994).

SYNTHESIS: DRUGS OF ABUSE

The literature reviewed above suggests that there are some significant similarities in the way that drugs of abuse with widely different cellular mechanisms of action affect the developing brain. First and foremost, alcohol, cocaine, and tobacco can lead to brain growth retardation. The microcephaly observed at the extreme of the FAS and in a statistically significant percentage of infants exposed to cocaine or tobacco speaks to the selective toxicity of these agents in developing brain. With all three agents, it appears as if the larger the dose of drug and the longer the time of exposure, the more profound the effect. However, the majority of infants exposed to cocaine and/or alcohol and/or tobacco do not have microcephaly. A central question is whether the brains in those children are in fact normal: Is there a continuum of brain vulnerability that only at its extreme results in microcephaly? Can brains be normal in size but not normal in architecture nor normal in function? Are the brains that are smaller necessarily aberrant in structure or function (that is, are the right elements there, just too few of them)? It is interesting that at the neuropathological level, there is evidence that all of these agents exert their teratogenic effects as brain growth retardation, albeit at the higher levels of drug exposures, but is the microcephaly induced by cocaine the same as the microcephaly induced by alcohol or tobacco? Are the mechanisms by which brain growth is compromised following cocaine exposure the same as those following alcohol or tobacco exposure? Are the correlates at the molecular, cellular, and systems level of brain growth retardation the same in individuals within an exposure group or when comparing exposures to different drugs of abuse? Most important, how do the cognitive, language, affective, or attentional deficits evidenced in some of these patients relate to the gross or microscopic changes in their brains?

It is of particular interest to note the overlap of behaviors that may be compromised in some individuals exposed to different drugs of abuse. Neonates exposed to alcohol, cocaine, or opiates may demonstrate impaired state regulation as evidenced by altered cluster scores on the NBAS (and more recently, the NNNS). Developmental delay as assessed by the BSID may be evident during the first 2 years of life in individuals exposed to alcohol, cocaine, or opiates. There is some suggestion of compromise of antecedents of language and normal language maturation in 2- to 7-year-olds exposed to either alcohol, cocaine, or marijuana, and more compelling evidence in children exposed to tobacco.

Impaired attention, impulsive or aggressive behavior, and hyperactivity are observed to some extent in children exposed to cocaine, alcohol, or opiates, and to a greater extent in those exposed to cannabinoids or nicotine. In young adults with FAS, a persistence of cognitive deficits but particular compromise of socialization and communication skills is evident, which is similar to deficits seen in children exposed to nicotine. Whether this overlap reflects the fact that there are restricted final common pathways reflecting brain compromise or whether this is an artifact of the limited measures with which we can assess neurodevelopmental, cognitive, affective, and language attributes in infants and children should become clearer as more sensitive instruments and more rigorous analyses of larger numbers of exposed infants achieve maturity (see Table 48.2). Alternatively, some have suggested that the common features that characterize drug-exposed infants may be a reflection of a compromised postnatal environment where the mother who abused drugs interacts less and suboptimally with her child, resulting in a child who is less adaptive and socially inappropriate. The limited data on infants who were exposed who have been foster raised, many of whom have similar deficits to those who stay in the biological parent's household, imply that environment is not wholly responsible for the persistent deficits (Nulman et al., 1994).

Developmental Model

The model shown in Figure 48.2 (Lester et al., 2004) describes three types of consequences of maternal drug use on child outcome: (*1*) immediate drug effects (*2*) latent drug effects, and (*3*) postnatal environment effects. *Immediate drug effects* refer to the direct teratogenic consequences of prenatal drug exposure. Such immediate effects emerge during the first year before postnatal environmental effects become increasingly salient. These effects may be transient, such as catch-up in physical growth, or more long lasting, such as behavioral dysregulation that is observed in infancy and persists through school age. *Latent drug effects* also refer to direct teratogenic effects, but these effects reflect brain function that becomes relevant later in development. Two kinds of latent effects can be described. First, drugs may affect brain function that does not manifest until children are older such as executive function, antisocial behavior, psychopathology, and substance use onset. Second, drugs may affect the brain by causing a predisposition for dependence on drugs. These conditions would be activated during school age when opportunities to use drugs arise, leading to early substance use onset and the gateway hypothesis, that use of licit drugs opens the door to experimentation with illicit drugs. *Postnatal environment effects* include general environmental factors that include risk and protective factors. Environmental risk factors such as poverty that occur in drug-using and non-drug-using populations are well-established correlates of poor child outcomes. There are also specific aspects of the caregiving environment unique to mothers who use drugs, such as the "children of alcoholics" (COA) effects. Passive exposure to cigarette smoke is a direct teratogenic environmental effect. The model acknowledges the role of genetic factors that may have immediate or latent effects or be transmitted through the caregiving environment. Protective factors can be naturally occurring (connectedness to others) as well as services and interventions.

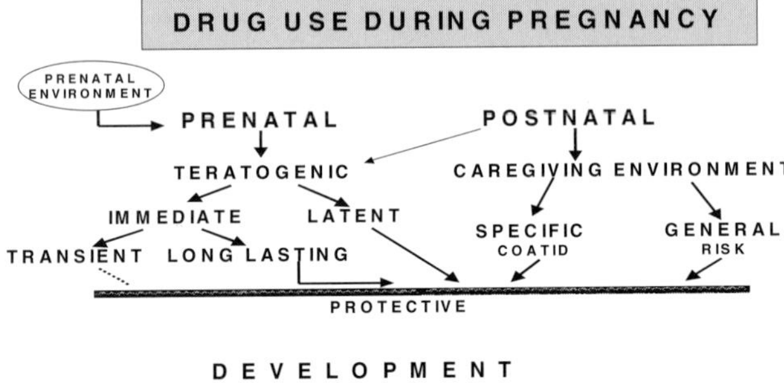

FIGURE 48.2 The model shown in the figure describes three types of consequences of maternal drug use on child outcome: (*1*) immediate drug effects, (*2*) latent drug effects, and (*3*) postnatal environment effects. Immediate drug effects refer to the direct teratogenic consequences of prenatal drug exposure. From Lester et al., 2004.

AN AMINERGIC PERSPECTIVE

One possibility is that certain chemical systems within the brain subserving particular functions are compromised after exposure to drugs of abuse in utero. One hypothesis is that the affective behaviors that seem to be compromised in some of the drug-exposed population affect behavioral development with primary and secondary consequences. If affect, or the systems subserving affect, are compromised in the neonate, one would observe altered alerting, orientation, and state control. Altered affect in infancy can alter parent–infant interaction and subsequent socialization. One possibility is that compromise of the "affective repertoire" of the neonate prevents and precludes the normal maturation of language: That is, the prevocalization skills including turn taking, face recognition, and imitation require intact affective behaviors. Compromise of those systems may compromise the development of the normal antecedents of language and subsequently the definitive ontogeny of language skills.

Additionally, there can be interactions between systems subserving different functions. For example, aminergic systems are thought to play a central role in arousal, attention, and affect, as well as motivation and the perception of reward, which are crucial in establishing reinforcement. It is possible that the neurotransmitter systems that store and release the amines (NE, DA, and serotonin) are not normally functioning in some infants exposed to drugs of abuse. As a consequence, cortical and subcortical circuits and targets that require discrete and differential aminergic control as the basis for selective attention may not develop or function normally. Alternatively, or additionally, those cortical and subcortical targets may be abnormal as an independent consequence of the toxic exposure.

FUTURE DIRECTIONS

These hypotheses can be tested in scientific and clinical domains. It is important to make no assumptions about the relevance of particular neurotransmitter systems or preconceptions about the anatomic or chemical localization of particular skills or behaviors or their antecedents. However, it is important to think about the ontogeny of behavior with respect to its morphological and functional correlates. Traditional clinical assessments of the structure and function of developing brain are restricted to noninvasive measures: head ultrasound, CT scans, and MRI morphometry to look at brain structure; evoked potentials to measure CNS conduction times; electroencephalogram (EEG) to assess electrophysiological function; and assessments of behavior, cognition, language, and temperament. For example, clinical developments in magnetic resonance spectroscopy are now being applied to children exposed to drugs of abuse in utero and suggest that there may be regional changes in energy metabolism in the brains of these children in the absence of frank structural abnormalities (L.M. Smith, et al., 2001a, 2001b). Similarly, functional MRI techniques are becoming more widely employed at many clinical centers and increasingly in pediatric populations, which will ultimately allow investigators to ask questions regarding regional differences in brain activation and blood flow using specific attentional, cognitive, and behavioral tasks. These clinical measures are evolving, and at a first approximation, they afford an opportunity to test hypotheses.

One goal for future research is to establish (or refute) relationships between gestational exposures to drugs of abuse and alterations in developmental outcomes. This will allow us to differentiate among the abstract hypotheses we can consider and to frame our subsequent experiments in more direct scientific and clinical initiatives. Most important, it will in an unbiased fashion provide greater biological understanding of the effects of drugs of abuse on the developing brain. In so doing, our attention can be focused on relevant interventions, prenatally and postnatally, with the goal of improving outcomes. In considering such future directions for research, clinical questions can be formulated at the four levels of analysis previously discussed (Grimm, 1987):

1. Pharmacological/physiological level: What are the mechanisms by which drugs of abuse can exert toxic effect on the developing brain?
2. Developmental level: What are the factors that influence the individual susceptibility and timing of biological vulnerability of developing brain to the toxic effects of drugs of abuse?
3. Systems level: What are the brain structures and neurochemical systems that subserve the behavioral or cognitive deficits?
4. Behavioral/cognitive level: What behavioral and cognitive deficits are evident in children exposed to drugs of abuse in utero? When do these deficits become evident? What tests are available or can be developed to assess these deficits, and to identify their antecedents? What role do postnatal environmental factors play in the expression of these deficits? To what extent can allocation of appropriate interventions and resources improve the outcomes of infants who are exposed?

One challenge for the next phase of clinical research on the effects of drugs of abuse on the developing brain is to design studies that will provide meaningful answers to these questions at each level of analysis.

REFERENCES

Aase, J.M., Jones, K.L., et al. (1995) Do we need the term "FAE"? *Pediatrics* 95:428–430.

Abel, E.L., and Berman, R.F. (1994) Long-term behavioral effects of prenatal alcohol exposure in rats. *Neurotoxicol. Teratol.* 16(5): 467–470.

Accornero, V.H., Morrow, C.E., et al. (2002) Behavioral outcome of preschoolers exposed prenatally to cocaine: role of maternal behavioral health. *J. Pediatrl. Psychol.* 27(3):259–269.

Acuff-Smith, K.D., George, M., et al. (1992) Preliminary evidence for methamphetamine-induced behavioral and ocular effects in rat offspring following exposure during early organogenesis. *Psychopharmacology (Berl)* 109(3):255–263.

Acuff-Smith, K.D., Schilling, M.A., et al. (1996) Stage-specific effects of prenatal d-methamphetamine exposure on behavioral and eye development in rats. *Neurotoxicol. Teratol.* 18(2):199–215.

Ajarem, J.S., and Ahmad M. (1998) Prenatal nicotine exposure modifies behavior of mice through early development. *Pharmacol. Biochem. Behav.* 59(2):313–318.

Akbari, H.M., and Azmitia, E.C. (1992) Increased tyrosine hydroxylase immunoreactivity in the rat cortex following prenatal cocaine exposure. *Developmental Brain Res.* 66:277–281.

Arendt, R.E., Short, E.J., et al. (2004) Children prenatally exposed to cocaine: developmental outcomes and environmental risks at seven years of age. *J. Dev. Behav. Pediatr.* 25(2): 83–90.

Arria, A.M., Derauf, C., et al. (2006) Methamphetamine and other substance use during pregnancy: preliminary estimates from the Infant Development, Environment and Lifestyles (IDEAL) Study. *Matern. Child Health J.* 10(3):293–302.

Autti-Ramo, I., Korkman, M., et al. (1992) Mental development of 2-year-old children exposed to alcohol in utero. *J. Pediatr.* 120: 740–746.

Bada, H.S., Bauer, C.R., et al. (2002) Central and autonomic system signs with in utero drug exposure. *Arch. Dis. Child Fetal Neonatal. Ed.* 87(2):F106–F112.

Bada, H.S., Das, A., et al. (2002) Gestational cocaine exposure and intrauterine growth: maternal lifestyle study. *Obstet. Gynecol.* 100(5 Pt 1):916–924.

Bada, H.S., Das, A., et al. (2007) Impact of prenatal cocaine exposure on child behavior problems through school age. *Pediatrics* 119(2) 348–359.

Bandstra, E.S., Morrow, C.E., et al. (2001) Longitudinal investigation of task persistence and sustained attention in children with prenatal cocaine exposure. *Neurotoxicol. Teratol.* 23(6):545–559.

Bandstra, E.S., Morrow, C.E., et al. (2002) Longitudinal influence of prenatal cocaine exposure on child language functioning. *Neurotoxicol. Teratol.* 24(3):297–308.

Bateman, D.A., and Chiriboga, C.A. (2000) Dose-response effect of cocaine on newborn head circumference. *Pediatrics* 106(3):E33.

Bauer, C.R., Langer, J.C., et al. (2005) Acute neonatal effects of cocaine exposure during pregnancy. *Arch. Pediatr. Adolesc. Med.* 159(9):824–834.

Bauer, C.R., Shankaran, S., et al. (2002) The Maternal Lifestyle Study: drug exposure during pregnancy and short-term maternal outcomes. *Am. J. Obstet. Gynecol.* 186(3):487–495.

Behnke, M., Davis Eyler, F., et al. (1998) Incidence and description of structural brain abnormalities in newborns exposed to cocaine. *J. Pediatr.* 132(2):291–294.

Behnke, M., Eyler, F.D. et al. (2002) Cocaine exposure and developmental outcome from birth to 6 months. *Neurotoxicol. Teratol.* 24(3):283–295.

Bendersky, M., and Lewis, M. (1998) Arousal modulation in cocaine-exposed infants. *Dev. Psychol.* 34(3):555–564.

Bennett, D.S., Bendersky, M., et al. (2002) Children's intellectual and emotional-behavioral adjustment at 4 years as a function of cocaine exposure, maternal characteristics, and environmental risk. *Dev. Psychol.* 38(5):648–658.

Bennett, S., Hyde, J., et al. (1993) Differing neurotoxic potencies of methamphetamine, mazinol, and cocaine in mesencephalic cultures. *J. Neurochem.* 60(4):1444–1452.

Billing, L., Eriksson, M., et al. (1980) Amphetamine addiction and pregnancy: III. One year follow-up of the children. Psychosocial and pediatric aspects. *Acta Paediatr. Scand.* 69(5):675–680.

Billing, L., Eriksson, M., et al. (1985) Pre-school children of amphetamine-addicted mothers: I. Somatic and psychomotor development. *Acta Paediatr. Scand.* 74(2):179–184.

Billing, L., Eriksson, M., et al. (1988) Predictive indicators for adjustment in 4-year-old children whose mothers used amphetamine during pregnancy. *Child Abuse Negl.* 12(4):503–507.

Billing, L., Eriksson, M., et al. (1994) The influence of environmental factors on behavioural problems in 8-year-old children exposed to amphetamine during fetal life. *Child Abuse Negl.* 18(1):3–9.

Bunikowski, R., Grimmer, I., et al. (1998) Neurodevelopmental outcome after prenatal exposure to opiates. *Eur. J. Pediatr.* 157(9): 724–730.

Burchfield, D.J., Lucas, V.W., et al. (1991) Disposition and pharmacodynamics of methamphetamine administration in sheep. *JAMA* 265:1968–1973.

Cabrera, T.M., Levy, A.D., et al. (1993) Prenatal methamphetamine attenuates serotonin mediated renin secretion in male and female rat progeny: evidence for selective long-term dysfunction of serotonin pathways in brain. *Synapse* 15(3):198–208.

Catanzarite, V.A., and Stein, D.A. (1995) "Crystal" and pregnancy--methamphetamine-associated maternal deaths. *West J. Med.* 162(5): 454–458.

Cernerud, L., Eriksson, M., et al. (1996) Amphetamine addiction during pregnancy: 14-year follow-up of growth and school performance. *Acta Paediatr.* 85(2):204–208.

Chang, L., Ernst, T., et al. (2002) Perfusion MRI abnormalities and computerized cognitive deficits in abstinent methamphetamine users. *Psychiatry Res.: Neuroimaging* 114(2):65–79.

Chang, L., Smith, L.M., et al. (2004) Smaller subcortical volumes and cognitive deficits in children with prenatal methamphetamine exposure. *Psychiatry Res.* 132(2):95–106.

Charness, M.E. (1992) Molecular mechanisms of ethanol intoxication, tolerance, and physical dependence. In: Mendelson J.H., and Mello, N.K., ed. *Medical Diagnosis and Treatment of Alcoholism,* 3rd ed. New York: McGraw-Hill, pp. 155–200.

Chiriboga, C.A. (1998) Neurological correlates of fetal cocaine exposure. *Ann. N.Y. Acad. Sci.* 846:109–125.

Chiriboga, C.A., Brust, J.C., et al. (1999) Dose-response effect of fetal cocaine exposure on newborn neurologic function. *Pediatrics* 103(1):79–85.

Chiriboga, C.A., Vibbert, M., et al. (1995) Neurological correlates of fetal cocaine exposure: transient hypertonia of infancy and early childhood. *Pediatrics* 96(6):1070–1077.

Cho, D.H., Lyu, H.M., et al. (1991) Behavioral teratogenicity of methamphetamine. *J. Toxicol.* 16(Suppl 1):37–49.

Clarren, S.K., Astley, S. J., et al. (1988) Physical anomalies and developmental delays in nonhuman primate infants exposed to weekly doses of ethanol during gestation. *Teratology* 37(6): 561–569.

Clarren, S.K., Astley, S.J., et al. (1992) Cognitive and behavioral deficits in nonhuman primates associated with very early embryonic binge exposures to ethanol. *J. Pediatr.* 121(5 Pt 1):789–796.

Clausing, P., Ferguson S.A., et al. (1995) Prenatal ethanol exposure in rats: long-lasting effects on learning. *Neurotoxicol. Teratol.* 17(5):545–552.

Clow, D.W., Hammer, R.P., Jr., et al. (1991) Gestational cocaine exposure increases opiate receptor binding in weanling offspring. *Developmental Brain Res.* 59:179–185.

Cohen, H.L., Sloves, J.H., et al. (1994) Neurosonographic findings in full-term infants born to maternal cocaine abusers: visualization of subependymal and periventricular cysts. *J. Clin. Ultrasound.* 22(5):327–333.

Coles, C.D., Brown, R.T., et al. (1991) Effects of prenatal alcohol exposure at 6 years: I. Physical and cognitive development. *Neurotoxicology* 13:1–11.

Corchero, J., Garcia-Gil, L., et al. (1998) Perinatal delta9-tetrahydrocannabinol exposure reduces proenkephalin gene expression in the caudate-putamen of adult female rats. *Life Sci.* 63(10): 843–850.

Cornelius M.D., Leech S.L., et al. (2000) Prenatal tobacco exposure: is it a risk factor for early tobacco experimentation? *Nicot. Tob. Res.* 2(1):45–52.

Covington, C., Nordstrom-Klee, B., et al. (2001) Development of an instrument to assess problem behavior in first grade students prenatally exposed to cocaine: II. Validation. *J. Subst. Abuse* 22(4):217–233.

Dalterio, S., Steger R., et al. (1984) Early cannabinoid exposure influences neuroendocrine and reproductive functions in male mice: I. Prenatal exposure. *Pharmacol. Biochem. Behav.* 20(1):107–113.

Dalterio, S.L., Michael S.D., et al. (1986) Perinatal cannabinoid exposure: demasculinization in male mice. *Neurobehav. Toxicol. Teratol.* 8(4):391–397.

Deitrich, R.A., Dunwiddie, T.V., et al. (1989) Mechanism action of ethanol: initial central nervous system actions. *Pharmacologic Rev.* 41:489–537.

Delaney-Black, V., Covington, C., et al. (1996) Prenatal cocaine and neonatal outcome: evaluation of dose-response relationship. *Pediatrics* 98:735–740.

Delaney-Black, V., Covington, C., et al. (1998) Prenatal cocaine exposure and child behavior. *Pediatrics* 102(4 Pt 1):945–950.

Delaney-Black, V., Covington, C., et al. (2000) Teacher-assessed behavior of children prenatally exposed to cocaine. *Pediatrics* 106(4): 782–791.

Derauf, C., LaGasse, L.L., et al. (2007) Demographic and psychosocial characteristics of mothers using methamphetamine during pregnancy: preliminary results of the Infant Development, Environment and Lifestyle Study (IDEAL). *Am. J. Drug Alcohol Abuse* 33(81):189.

Devane, W.A., Dysarz, F.A., et al. (1988) Determination and characterization of a cannabinoid receptor in rat brain. *Mol. Pharmacol.* 34(5):605–613.

Devane, W.A., Hanus, L., et al. (1992) Isolation and structure of a brain constituent that binds to the cannabinoid receptor [see comments]. *Science* 258(5090):1946–1949.

DiPietro, J.A., Suess, P.E., et al. (1995) Reactivity and regulation in cocaine-exposed neonates. *Infant Behav. Dev.* 18:407–414.

Dixon, S.D., and Bejar, R. (1989) Echoencephalographic findings in neonates associated with maternal cocaine and methamphetamine use: incidence and clinical correlates. *J. Pediatr.* 115:770–778.

Dow-Edwards, D.L., Freed, L.A., et al. (1990) Structural and functional effects of prenatal cocaine exposure in adult rat brain. *Developmental Brain Res.* 57:263–268.

Driscoll, C.D., Streissguth, A.P., et al. (1990) Prenatal alcohol exposure: comparability of effects in humans and animal models. *Neurotox. Teratol.* 12:231–237.

Duman, R.S., Tallman, J.F., et al. (1988) Acute and chronic opiate-regulation of adenylate cyclase in brain: specific effects in locus coeruleus. *J. Pharmacol. Exp. Ther.* 246(3):1033–1039.

Ernst, T., Chang, L., et al. (2000) Evidence for long-term neurotoxicity associated with methamphetamine abuse: a 1H MRS study. *Neurology* 54(6):1344–1349.

Faden, V.B., and Graubard, B.I. (2000) Maternal substance use during pregnancy and developmental outcome at age three. *J. Subst. Abuse* 12(4):329–340.

Fantel, A.G., Barber, C.V., et al. (1992) Studies of the role of ischemia/reperfusion and superoxide anion radical production in the teratogenicity of cocaine. *Neurotox. Teratology* 46(3):293–300.

Fernandez-Ruiz, J., Berrendero F., et al. (2000) The endogenous cannabinoid system and brain development. *Trends Neurosci.* 23(1):14–20.

Frank, D.A., Augustyn, M., et al. (2001) Growth, development, and behavior in early childhood following prenatal cocaine exposure: a systematic review. *JAMA* 285(12):1613–1625.

Frank, D.A., Jacobs, R.R., et al. (2002) Level of prenatal cocaine exposure and scores on the Bayley Scales of Infant Development: modifying effects of caregiver, early intervention, and birth weight. *Pediatrics* 110(6):1143–1152.

Fried, P.A. (1992) Clinical implications of smoking: determination of long-term teratogenicity. In: Zagon, I.S., and Slotkin, T.A., eds. *Maternal Substance Abuse and the Developing Nervous System.* San Diego, CA: Academic Press, pp. 77–76.

Fried, P.A., and Watkinson, B. (1990) 36- and 48-month neurobehavioral follow-up of children prenatally exposed to marijuana, cigarettes, and alcohol. *J. Dev. Behav. Pediatr.* 11(2):49–58.

Fried, P.A., and Watkinson, B. (2001) Differential effects on facets of attention in adolescents prenatally exposed to cigarettes and marihuana. *Neurotoxicol. Teratol.* 23(5):421–430.

Fried, P.A., Watkinson, B., et al. (1987) Neonatal neurological status in a low-risk population after prenatal exposure to cigarettes, marijuana, and alcohol. *J. Dev. Behav. Pediatr.* 8(6):318–326.

Fried, P.A., Watkinson, B., et al. (1998) Differential effects on cognitive functioning in 9- to 12-year olds prenatally exposed to cigarettes and marijuana. *Neurotoxicol. Teratol.* 20(3):293–306.

Fried, P.A., Watkinson B., et al. (1999) Growth from birth to early adolescence in offspring prenatally exposed to cigarettes and marijuana. *Neurotoxicol. Teratol.* 21(5):513–525.

Friedman, E., Butkerait, P., et al. (1993) Analysis of receptor-stimulated and basal guanine nucleotide binding to membrane G proteins by sodium dodecyl sulfate—polyacrylamide gel electrophoresis. *Anal. Biochem.* 214:171–178.

Fuller, R.W., and Hemrick-Leucke, S.K. (1992) Further studies on the long-term depletion of striatal dopamine in iprindole-treated rats by amphetamine. *Neuropharmocology* 21(5):433–438.

Fulroth, R., Phillips, B., et al. (1989) Perinatal outcome of infants exposed to cocaine and/or heroin in utero. *Am. J. Dis. Child* 143(8):905–910.

Furuya, H., Aikawa, H., et al. (1996) Effects of ethyl alcohol administration to THA rat dams during their gestation period on learning behavior and on levels of monoamines and metabolites in the brain of pups after birth. *Alcohol. Clin. Exp. Res.* 20(9 Suppl):305A–310A.

Gagin, R., Kook, N., et al. (1997) Prenatal morphine enhances morphine-conditioned place preference in adult rats. *Pharmacol. Biochem. Behav.* 58(2):525–528.

Garcia, L., de Miguel, R., et al. (1996) Perinatal delta 9-tetrahydrocannabinol exposure in rats modifies the responsiveness of midbrain dopaminergic neurons in adulthood to a variety of challenges with dopaminergic drugs. *Drug Alcohol Depend.* 42(3):155–166.

Gibb, J.W., Johnson, M., et al. (1997) Neurotoxicity of amphetamines and their metabolites. *NIDA Res. Monogr.* 173:128–145.

Gieron-Korthals, M.A., Helal, A., Martinez, C. R. (1994) Expanding spectrum of cocaine induced central nervous system malformations. *Brain Dev.* 16(3):253–256.

Gingras, J.L., and O'Donnell, K.J. (1998) State control in the substance-exposed fetus: I. The fetal neurobehavioral profile: an assessment of fetal state, arousal, and regulation competency. *Ann. NY Acad. Sci.* 846:262–276.

Gingras, J.L., O'Donnell, K.J., et al. (1990) Maternal cocaine addiction and fetal behavioral state: I. A human model for the study of sudden infant death syndrome. *Med. Hypotheses* 33(4):227–230.

Goldstein, R.Z., Volkow, N.D., et al. (2002) The orbitofrontal cortex in methamphetamine addiction: involvement in fear. *Neuroreport* 13(17):2253–2257.

Gomez-Anson, B., and Ramsey, R.G. (1994) Pachygyria in a neonate with prenatal cocaine exposure: MR features. *J Comput. Assist. Tomogr.* 18(4):637–639.

Goodman, G., Hans, S.L., et al. (1999) Attachment behavior and its antecedents in offspring born to methadone-maintained women. *J. Clin. Child Psychol.* 28(1):58–69.

Goodwin, G.A., Moody, C.A., et al. (1993) Prenatal cocaine exposure increases the behavioral sensitivity of neonatal rat pups to ligands active at opiate receptors. *Neurotoxicol. Teratol.* 15(6):425–431.

Grant, P., LaGasse, L., et al. (2004) Prenatal methamphetamine use and maternal health care characteristics: preliminary results from the Infant Development, Environment, and Lifestyle Study (IDEAL). *Ped. Res.* 55(4 Part 2):72A.

Gressens, P., Kosofsky, B.E., et al. (1992) Cocaine-induced disturbances of corticogenesis in the developing murine brain. *Neurosci. Lett.* 140:113–116.

Gressens, P., Lammens, M., et al. (1992) Ethanol-induced disturbances of gliogenesis and neuronogenesis in the developing murine brain: an in vitro and in vivo immunohistochemical and ultrastructural study. *Alcohol.* 27(3):219–226.

Grimm, V.E. (1987) Effect of teratogenic exposure on the developing brain: research strategies and possible mechanisms. *Dev. Pharmacol. Ther.* 10:328–345.

Hammer, R.P., Jr., Ricalde, A.A., et al. (1989) Effects of opiates on brain development. *Neurotoxicology* 10(3):475–483.

Hans, S.L. (1992) Maternal opioid drug use and child development. In: Zagon, I.S., and Slotkin, T.A., eds. *Maternal Substance Abuse and the Developing Nervous System.* San Diego, CA: Academic Press, pp. 177–213.

Hansen, R.L., Struthers, J.M., et al. (1993) Visual evoked potentials and visual processing in stimulant drug-exposed infants. *Dev. Med. Child Neurol.* 35(9):798–805.

Hauser, K.F., McLaughlin P.J., et al. (1987) Endogenous opioids regulate dendritic growth and spine formation in developing rat brain. *Brain Res.* 416(1):157–161.

Heller, A. (2000) *Neurotoxicology and Developmental Effects of Meth and MDMA: Effects of in Utero Exposure to Methamphetamines*. Bethesda, MD: National Institute on Drug Abuse.

Heier, L.A., Carpanzano, C.R., et al. (1991) Maternal cocaine abuse: the spectrum of radiologic abnormalities in the neonatal CNS. *Am. J. Neuroradiol.* 12(5):951–956.

Ikonomidou, C., Bittigau, P., et al. (2000) Ethanol-induced apoptotic neurodegeneration and fetal alcohol syndrome. *Science* 287(5455): 1056–1060.

Itoh, J., Nabeshima, T., et al. (1991) Utility of an elevated plus-maze for dissociation of amnesic and behavioral effects of drugs in mice. *Eur. J. Pharmacol.* 194(1):71–76.

Jacobson, J.L., Jacobson, S.W., et al. (1996) Increased vulnerability to alcohol-related birth defects in the offspring of mothers over 30. *Alcohol Clin. Exp. Res.* 20:359–363.

Jacobson, S.W., Jacobson, J.L., et al. (1996) New evidence for neurobehavioral effects of in utero cocaine exposure. *J. Pediatrics* 129:581–589.

Jaffe, J.H., and Martin, W.R. (1985) Opioid analgesics and antagonists. In: Gilman, A.G., Goodman, L.S., Rall, T.W., and Murad, F., eds. *The Pharmacological Basis of Therapeutics* (7th ed.). New York: Macmillan, pp. 491–531.

Jeng, W., Wong, A.W., et al. (2005) Methamphetamine-enhanced embryonic oxidative DNA damage and neurodevelopmental deficits. *Free Radic. Biol. Med.* 39(3):317–326.

Johnson, S.W., and North, R.A. (1992) Opioids excite dopamine neurons by hyperpolarization of local interneurons. *J. Neurosci.* 12(2):483–488.

Jones, K.L., Smith, D.W., et al. (1973) Pattern of malformation in offspring of chronic alcoholic mothers. *Lancet* 1:1267–1271.

Kandel, D.B., Wu, P., et al. (1994) Maternal smoking during pregnancy and smoking by adolescent daughters. *Am. J. Pub. Health* 84(9):1407–1413.

Karch, S. (1993) *The Pathology of Drug Abuse*. Boca Raton, FL: CRC Press.

Keller, R.W., Jr., Maisonneuve, I.M., et al. (1994) Effects of prenatal cocaine exposure on the nigrostriatal dopamine system: an in vivo microdialysis study in the rat. *Brain Res.* 634:266–274.

King, R. (2006) The next big thing: methamphetamine in the United States. The Sentencing Project: research and advocacy for reform. Washington, DC: pp. 1–41.

Koob, G.F., and Le Moal, M. (1997) Drug abuse: hedonic homeostatic dysregulation. *Science* 278(5335):52–58.

Kosofsky, B.E., Wilkins, A.S., et al. (1994) Transplacental cocaine exposure: a mouse model demonstrating neuroanatomic and behavioral abnormalities. *J. Child Neurol.* 9:234–241.

LaGasse, L., Derauf, C., et al. (2004) Prenatal methamphetamine exposure and neonatal cry acoustic analysis: preliminary results from the Infant Development, Environment, and Lifestyle Study (IDEAL). *Ped. Res.* 55(4, Part 2):72A.

LaGasse, L., Messinger, D., et al. (2003) Prenatal drug exposure and maternal and infant feeding behavior. *Arch. Dis. Child.* 88:F391–F399.

Leech, S.L., Richardson G.A., et al. (1999) Prenatal substance exposure: effects on attention and impulsivity of 6-year-olds. *Neurotoxicol. Teratol.* 21(2):109–118.

Lester, B.M., Das, A., et al. (2003) Prenatal cocaine exposure and 7-year outcome: IQ and special education. *Pediatric Research* (53): 534A.

Lester, B.M., El Sohly, M., et al. (2001) The Maternal Lifestyle Study: drug use by meconium toxicology and maternal self-report. *Pediatrics* 107(2):309–317.

Lester, B.M., LaGasse, L., et al. (1996) Studies of cocaine-exposed human infants. *NIDA Research Monograph*. 164:175–210.

Lester, B.M., LaGasse, L.L., et al. (1998) Cocaine exposure and children: the meaning of subtle effects. *Science* 282(5389):633–634.

Lester, B.M., LaGasse, L., et al. (2003) The Maternal Lifestyle Study (MLS): Effects of prenatal cocaine and/or opiate exposure on auditory brain response at one month. *J. Pediatrics* 142(3):279–285.

Lester, B.M., and Tronick, E.Z. (2004) History and description of the Neonatal Intensive Care Unit Network Neurobehavioral Scale. *Pediatrics* 113(3 Pt 2):634–640.

Lewis, B.A., Singer, L.T., et al. (2004) Four-year language outcomes of children exposed to cocaine in utero. *Neurotoxicol. Teratol.* 26(5) 617–627.

Lidow, M.S. (1995) Prenatal cocaine exposure adversely affects development of the cerebral cortex. *Synapse* 21(4):332–341.

Linares, T.J., Singer, L.T., et al. (2006) Mental health outcomes of cocaine-exposed children at 6 years of age. *J. Pediatr. Psychol.* 31(1):85–97.

Loebstein, R., Koren, G., et al. (1997) Pregnancy outcome and neurodevelopment of children exposed in utero to psychoactive drugs: the Motherisk experience. *J. Psychiatry Neurosci.* 22(3): 192–196.

London, E.D., Simon, S.I., et al. (2004) Regional cerebral dysfunction associated with mood disturbances in abstinent methamphetamine abusers. *Arch. Gen. Psychiatry* 61:73–84.

Lovinger, D.M., and White, G. (1991) Ethanol potentiation of 5-HT3 receptor-mediated ion currents in neuroblastoma cells and isolated adult mammalian neurons. *Mol. Pharmacol.* 40:263–273.

Lovinger, D.M., White, G., et al. (1989) Ethanol inhibits NMDA-activated ion currents in hippocampal neurons. *Science* 243:1721.

Lukas, S. (1997) *Proceedings of the National Consensus Meeting on the Use, Abuse, and Sequelae of Methamphetamine with Implications for Prevention, Treatment, and Research*. Washington, DC: Center for Substance Abuse Treatment.

Lumeng, J.C., Cabral, H.J., et al. (2007) Pre-natal exposures to cocaine and alcohol and physical growth patterns to age 8 years. *Neurotoxicol. Teratol.* 29(4):446–457.

Manzanares, J., Corchero, J., et al. (1999) Pharmacological and biochemical interactions between opioids and cannabinoids. *Trends Pharmacol. Sci.* 20(7):287–294.

Martellotta, M.C., Cossu, G., et al. (1998) Self-administration of the cannabinoid receptor agonist WIN 55,212-2 in drug-naive mice. *Neuroscience* 85(2):327–330.

Matsuda, L.A., Lolait, S.J., et al. (1990) Structure of a cannabinoid receptor and functional expression of the cloned cDNA [see comments]. *Nature* 346(6284):561–564.

Matthes, H.W., Maldonado, R., et al. (1996) Loss of morphine-induced analgesia, reward effect and withdrawal symptoms in mice lacking the mu-opioid-receptor gene [see comments]. *Nature* 383(6603):819–823.

Mayes, L.C. (2002) A behavioral teratogenic model of the impact of prenatal cocaine exposure on arousal regulatory systems. *Neurotoxicol. Teratol.* 24(3):385–395.

Mayes, L.C., Bornstein, M.H., et al. (1995) Information processing and developmental assessments in 3-month-old infants exposed prenatally to cocaine. *Pediatrics* 95(4):539–545.

Mayes, L.C., and Carroll, K.M. (1996) Neonatal withdrawal syndrome in infants exposed to cocaine and methadone. *Subst. Use Misuse* 31(2):241–253.

McCalla, S., Minkoff, H.L., et al. (1991) The biologic and social consequences of perinatal cocaine use in an inner-city population: results of an anonymous cross-sectional study. *Am. J. Obstet. Gynecol.* 164 (2):625–630.

McCann, U.D., Wong, D.F., et al. (1998) Reduced striatal dopamine transporter density in abstinent methamphetamine and methcathinone users: evidence from positron emission tomography studies with [^{11}C]WIN-35,428. *J. Neurosci.* 18:8417–8422.

Mentis, M. (1998) In utero cocaine exposure and language development. *Semin. Speech Lang.* 19(2):147–164.

Mentis, M., and Lundgren, K. (1995) Effects of prenatal exposure to cocaine and associated risk factors on language development. *J. Speech Hear. Res.* 38:1303–1318.

Messinger, D.S., Bauer, C.R., et al. (2004) The maternal lifestyle study: cognitive, motor, and behavioral outcomes of cocaine-exposed and opiate-exposed infants through three years of age. *Pediatrics* 113(6):1677–1685.

Meyer, J.S., and Dupont, S.A. (1993) Prenatal cocaine administration stimulates fetal brain tyrosine hydroxylase activity. *Brain Res.* 608:129–137.

Miller, M.W., and Robertson, S. (1993) Prenatal exposure to ethanol alters the postnatal development and transformation of radial glia to astrocytes in the cortex. *J. Comp. Neurol.* 337(2): 253–266.

Miller-Loncar, C., Lester, B.M., et al. (2005) Predictors of motor development in children prenatally exposed to cocaine. *Neurotoxicol. Teratol.* 27(2):213–220.

Minnes, S., Robin, N.H. et al. (2006) Dysmorphic and anthropometric outcomes in 6-year-old prenatally cocaine-exposed children. *Neurotoxicol. Teratol.* 28(1):28–38.

Mirochnick, M., Frank, D.A., et al. (1995) Relation between meconium concentration of the cocaine metabolite benzoylecgonine and fetal growth. *J. Pediatrics* 126:636–638.

Molina-Holgado, F., Amaro, A., et al. (1996) Effect of maternal delta 9-tetrahydrocannabinol on developing serotonergic system. *Eur. J. Pharmacol.* 316(1):39–42.

Muneoka, K., Nakatsu T., et al. (1999) Prenatal administration of nicotine results in dopaminergic alterations in the neocortex. *Neurotoxicol. Teratol.* 21(5):603–609.

Muneoka, K., Ogawa T., et al. (1997) Prenatal nicotine exposure affects the development of the central serotonergic system as well as the dopaminergic system in rat offspring: involvement of route of drug administrations. *Brain Res. Dev. Brain Res.* 102(1): 117–126.

Nagy, L.E., Diamond, I., et al. (1990) Ethanol increases extracellular adenosine by inhibiting adenosine uptake via the nucleoside transporter. *J. Biol. Chem.* 265:1946–1951.

Napiorkowski, B.S., Lester, B.M., et al. (1996) Effects of in utero substance exposure on infant neurobehavior. *Pediatrics* 98:71–75.

National Institute on Drug Abuse. (1996) *National Pregnancy & Health Survey*. Rockville, MD: National Institutes of Health.

National Toxicology Program. (2005) NTP-CERHR, Expert Panel Report on the Reproductive and Developmental Toxicity of Amphetamine and Methamphetamine. Page 177. http://cerhr.niehs.nih.gov/chemicals/stimulants/amphetamines/Amphetamine_final.pdf.

Navarro, M., Rubio P., et al. (1994) Sex-dimorphic psychomotor activation after perinatal exposure to (-)-delta 9-tetrahydrocannabinol. An ontogenic study in Wistar rats. *Psychopharmacology (Berl)* 116(4):414–422.

Navarro, M., Rubio P., et al. (1995) Behavioural consequences of maternal exposure to natural cannabinoids in rats. *Psychopharmacology (Berl)* 122(1):1–14.

Nestler, E.J. (1997) Molecular mechanisms of opiate and cocaine addiction. *Curr. Opin. Neurobiol.* 7(5):713–719.

Newman, E., Risch, E.C., et al. (2007, June 6–9) *Methamphetamine abuse, trauma history and child abuse potential.* Poster presented at 10th European Conference on Traumatic Stress (ECOTS), Opatija, Croatia.

Newman, M.B., Shytle R.D., et al. (1999) Locomotor behavioral effects of prenatal and postnatal nicotine exposure in rat offspring. *Behav. Pharmacol.* 10(6–7):699–706.

Noland, J.S., Singer, L.T. et al. (2005) Prenatal drug exposure and selective attention in preschoolers. *Neurotoxicol. Teratol.* 27(3): 429–438.

North, R.A., Williams, J.T., et al. (1987) Mu and delta receptors belong to a family of receptors that are coupled to potassium channels. *Proc. Natl. Acad. Sci. USA* 84(15):5487–5491.

Nulman, I., Rovet, J., et al. (1994) Neurodevelopment of adopted children exposed in utero to cocaine. *Can. Med. Assoc. J.* 151: 1592–1597.

Oro, A.S., and Dixon, S.D. (1987) Perinatal cocaine and methamphetamine exposure: maternal and neonatal correlates. *J. Pediatr.* 111(4):571–578.

Paulus, M.P., Hozack, N.E., et al. (2002) Behavioral and functional neuroimaging evidence for prefrontal dysfunction in methamphetamine-dependent subjects. *Neuropsychopharmacology* 26(1): 53–63.

Pennington, S.N. (1990) Molecular changes associated with ethanol-induced growth suppression in the chick embryo. *Alcohol Clin. Exp. Res.* 14:832.

Picciotto, M.R., Zoli, M., et al. (1998) Acetylcholine receptors containing the beta2 subunit are involved in the reinforcing properties of nicotine. *Nature* 391(6663):173–177.

Pich, E.M., Pagliusi, S.R., et al. (1997) Common neural substrates for the addictive properties of nicotine and cocaine. *Science* 275 (5296):83–86.

Pidoplichko, V.I., DeBiasi M., et al. (1997) Nicotine activates and desensitizes midbrain dopamine neurons. *Nature* 390:401–404.

Plessinger, M.A. (1998) Prenatal exposure to amphetamines. Risks and adverse outcomes in pregnancy. *Obstet. Gynecol. Clin. North Am.* 25(1):119–138.

Pontieri, F.E., Tanda G., et al. (1996) Effects of nicotine on the nucleus accumbens and similarity to those of addictive drugs. *Nature* 382:255–257.

Prochaska, J.O., and DiClemente, C.C. (1992) Stages of change in the modification of problem behaviors. In: Hersen, M., Eisler, R., Miller, P., eds. *Progress in Behavior Modification*. New York: Sycamore, pp. 183–218.

Pu, C., and Voorhees, C.V. (1993) Developmental dissociation of methamphetamine-induced depletion of dopaminergic terminals and astrocyte reaction in rat striatum. *Brain Res. Dev. Brain Res.* 72(2):325–328.

Ramsey, N.F., Niesink, R.J., et al. (1993) Prenatal exposure to morphine enhances cocaine and heroin self-administration in drug-naive rats. *Drug Alcohol Depend.* 33(1):41–51.

Regalado, M.G., Schechtman, V.L., et al. (1995) Sleep disorganization in cocaine-exposed neonates. *Infant Beh. Dev.* 18(3):319–327.

Regalado, M.G., Schechtman, V.L., et al. (1996) Cardiac and respiratory patterns during sleep in cocaine-exposed neonates. *Early Hum. Dev.* 44(3):187–200.

Ricaurte, G.A., and McCann, U.D. (1992) Neurotoxic amphetamine analogues: effects in monkeys and implications for humans. *Ann. NY Acad. Sci.* 648:371–382.

Richardson, G.A., Conroy, M.L., et al. (1997) Prenatal cocaine exposure: effects on the development of school-age children. *Neurotox. Teratol.* 18:627–634.

Richardson, S.A., and Tizabi, Y. (1994) Hyperactivity in the offspring of nicotine-treated rats: role of the mesolimbic and nigrostriatal dopaminergic pathways. *Pharmacol. Biochem. Behav.* 47(2): 331–337.

Richardson, G.A. (1998) Prenatal cocaine exposure. A longitudinal study of development. *Ann. NY Acad. Sci.* 846:144–152.

Rodriguez de Fonseca, F., Cebeira M., et al. (1991) Effects of pre- and perinatal exposure to hashish extracts on the ontogeny of brain dopaminergic neurons. *Neuroscience* 43(2–3):713–723.

Ronnekleiv, O.K., and Naylor, B.R. (1995) Chronic cocaine exposure in the fetal rhesus monkey: consequences for early development of dopamine neurons. *J. Neurosci.* 15:7330–7343.

Rosen, T.S., and Johnson, H.L. (1982) Children of maintained mothers: Follow up at 18 months of age. *J. Pediatr.* 101:192–196.

Roy, T.S., and Sabherwal, U. (1994) Effects of prenatal nicotine exposure on the morphogenesis of somatosensory cortex. *Neurotoxicol. Teratol.* 16(4):411–421.

Salisbury, A.L., Lester, B., et al. (2007) Prenatal cocaine use and maternal depression: effects on infant neurobehavior. *Neurotoxicol. Teratol.* 29(3):331–340.

Substance Abuse and Mental Health Services Administration (SAMHSA). (1995) *National Household Survey on Drug Abuse #18*. Rockville, MD: Author

SAMHSA. (2002) *Summary of Findings from the 1999–2000 National Household Survey on Drug Abuse*. Rockville, MD: Author.

SAMHSA. (2005a) *Results from the 2004 National Survey on Drug Use and Health: National Findings*. Rockville, MD: Author.

SAMHSA. (2005b) *Treatment Episode Data Set (TEDS) 1993–2003: National Admissions to Substance Abuse Treatment Services for the Department of Health and Human Services*. Rockville, MD: Author.

Schroder, M.D., Snyder, P.J., et al. (2004) Impaired performance of children exposed in utero to cocaine on a novel test of visuospatial working memory. *Brain Cogn.* 55(2):409–412.

Seiden, L., and Sabol, K.E. (1996) Methamphetamine and methylenedioxymethamphetamine neurotoxicity: possible mechanisms of cell destruction. *NIDA Res. Monogr.* 163:251–276.

Seidler, F.J., Levin, E.D., et al. (1992) Fetal nicotine exposure ablates the ability of postnatal nicotine challenge to release norepinephrine from rat brain regions. *Brain Res. Dev. Brain Res.* 69(2):288–291.

Seifer, R., LaGasse, L.L., et al. (2004) Attachment status in children prenatally exposed to cocaine and other substances. *Child Dev.* 75(3):850–868.

Sekine, Y., Minabe, Y., et al. (2003) Association of dopamine transporter loss in the orbitofrontal and dorsolateral prefrontal cortices with methamphetamine-related psychiatric symptoms. *Am. J. Psychiatry* 160(9):1699–1701.

Self, D.W., Terwilliger, R.Z., et al. (1994) Inactivation of Gi and G(o) proteins in nucleus accumbens reduces both cocaine and heroin reinforcement. *J. Neurosci.* 14(10):6239–6247.

Shacka, J.J., Fennell, O.B., et al. (1997) Prenatal nicotine sex-dependently alters agonist-induced locomotion and stereotypy. *Neurotoxicol. Teratol.* 19(6):467–476.

Shankaran, S., Bauer, C.R., et al. (2003) Health-care utilization among mothers and infants following cocaine exposure. *J. Perinatol.* 23(5):361–367.

Sheinkopf, S.J., Lester, B., et al. (2005) Neonatal irritability, prenatal substance exposure, and later parenting stress. *J. Pediatr. Psychol.* 31:27–40.

Sims, M.E., Walther, F.J., et al. (1989) Neonatal ultrasound casebook. Antenatal brain injury and maternal cocaine use. *J. Perinatol.* 9(3):349–350.

Singer, L.T., Minnes, S., et al. (2004) Cognitive outcomes of preschool children with prenatal cocaine exposure. *JAMA* 291(20):2448–2456.

Singer, L.T., Yamashita, T. S., et al. (1994) Increased incidence of intraventricular hemorrhage and developmental delay in cocaine-exposed, very low birth weight infants. *J. Pediatr.* 124(5 Pt 1):765–771.

Slamberova, R., Pometlova, M., et al. (2006) Postnatal development of rat pups is altered by prenatal methamphetamine exposure. *Prog. Neuropsychopharmacol. Biol. Psychiatry* 30(1):82–88.

Slotkin, T.A. (1992) What can we learn from animal models? In: Zagon, I.S., Slotkin, T.A., eds. *Maternal Substance Abuse and the Developing Nervous System*. San Diego, CA: Academic Press, pp. 97–124.

Smeriglio, V.L. (1999) Prenatal drug exposure and child outcome. Past, present, future. *Clin. Perinatol.* 26(1):1–16.

Smith, D.W. (1981) Fetal alcohol syndrome and fetal alcohol effects. *Neurobehav. Toxicol. Teratol.* 3:127.

Smith, L., Yonekura, M.L., et al. (2003) Effects of prenatal methamphetamine exposure on fetal growth and drug withdrawal symptoms in infants born at term. *J. Dev. Behav. Pediatr.* 24(1):17–23.

Smith, L.M., Chang, L., et al. (2001a) Brain proton magnetic resonance spectroscopy and imaging in children exposed to cocaine in utero. *Pediatrics* 107:227–231.

Smith, L.M., Chang, L., et al. (2001b) Brain proton magnetic resonance spectroscopy in children exposed to methamphetamine in utero. *Neurology* 57(2):255–260.

Smith, L.M., LaGasse, L.L., et al. (2008) Prenatal methamphetamine use and neonatal neurobehavioral outcome. *Neurotoxicol. Teratol.* 30:20–28.

Smith, L.M., LaGasse, L.L., et al. (2006) The infant development, environment, and lifestyle study: effects of prenatal methamphetamine exposure, polydrug exposure, and poverty on intrauterine growth. *Pediatrics* 118(3):1149–1156.

Snyder-Keller, A.M., and Keller, R.W., Jr. (1993) Prenatal cocaine increases striatal serotonin innervation without altering the patch/matrix organization of intrinsic cell types. *Dev. Brain Res.* 74:261–267.

Spear, L.P. (1995) Neurobehavioral consequences of gestational cocaine exposure: a comparative analysis. In: Rovee-Collier, C., and Lipsitt, L.P., eds. *Advances in Infancy Research*, Vol. 9. Norwood, NJ: Ablex, pp. 55–105.

Stadlin, A., Choi, H.L., et al. (1994) Postnatal changes in [^{3}H] mazindol-labelled dopamine uptake sites in the rat striatum following prenatal cocaine exposure. *Brain Res.* 637:345–348.

Stek, A.M., Baker, R.S., et al. (1995) Fetal responses to maternal and fetal methamphetamine administration in sheep. *Am. J. Obstet. Gynecol.* 173(5):1592–1598.

Stek, A.M., Fisher, B.K., et al. (1993) Maternal and fetal cardiovascular responses to methamphetamine in the pregnant sheep. *Am. J. Obstet. Gynecol.* 169(4):888–897.

Stoler, J.M., Huntington K.S., et al. (1998) The prenatal detection of significant alcohol exposure with maternal blood markers. *J. Pediatr.* 133(3):346–352.

Stratton, K., Howe, C., et al. (1996) *Fetal Alcohol Syndrome*. Washington, DC: National Academy Press.

Streissguth, A.P., Barr, H.M., et al. (1996) *Understanding the Occurence of Secondary Disabilities in Clients with Fetal Alcohol Syndrome and Fetal Alcohol Effects*. Seattle: University of Washington Press.

Struthers, J.M., and Hansen, R.L. (1992) Visual recognition memory in drug-exposed infants. *J. Dev. Behav. Pediatr.* 13(2):108–111.

Suess, P.E., Newlin D.B., et al. (1997) Motivation, sustained attention, and autonomic regulation in school-age boys exposed in utero to opiates and alcohol. *Exp. Clin. Psychopharmacol.* 5(4):375–387.

Tanda, G., Pontieri, F.E., et al. (1997) Cannabinoid and heroin activation of mesolimbic dopamine transmission by a common mu1 opioid receptor mechanism [see comments]. *Science* 276(5321):2048–2050.

Thompson, P.M., Hayashi, K.M., et al. (2004) Structural abnormalities in the brains of human subjects who use methamphetamine. *J. Neurosci.* 24(26):6028–6036.

Tizabi, Y., Russell L.T., et al. (2000) Prenatal nicotine exposure: effects on locomotor activity and central [125I]alpha-BT binding in rats. *Pharmacol. Biochem. Behav.* 66(3):495–500.

Tronick, E.Z., Frank, D.A., et al. (1996) Late dose-response effects of prenatal cocaine exposure on newborn behavioral performance. *Pediatrics* 98:76–83.

Tronick, E.Z., Messinger, D.S., et al. (2005) Cocaine exposure is associated with subtle compromises of infants' and mothers' social emotional behavior and dyadic features of their interaction in the face-to-face still-face paradigm. *Dev. Psychol.* 41(5):711–722.

Vela, G., Fuentes, J.A., et al. (1995) Perinatal exposure to delta 9-tetrahydrocannabinol (delta 9-THC) leads to changes in opioid-related behavioral patterns in rats. *Brain Res.* 680(1/2):142–147.

Vela, G., Martin S., et al. (1998) Maternal exposure to delta9-tetrahydrocannabinol facilitates morphine self-administration behavior and changes regional binding to central mu opioid receptors in adult offspring female rats. *Brain Res.* 807(1–2):101–109.

Volkow, N.D., Chang, L., et al. (2001) Dopamine transporter losses in methamphetamine abusers are associated with psychomotor impairment. *Am. J. Psychiatry* 158:377–382.

Wafford, K.A., Burnett, D.M., et al. (1991) Ethanol sensitivity of the GABA-A receptor expressed in xenopus oocytes requires 8 amino acids contained in the gamma 2L subunit. *Neuron* 7:1–20.

Wallace, T.L., Gudelsky, G.A., et al. (1999) Methamphetamine-induced neurotoxicity alters locomotor activity, stereotypic behavior, and stimulated dopamine release in the rat. *J. Neurosci.* 19(20):9141–9148.

Walters, D.E. and Carr, L.A. (1986) Changes in brain catecholamine mechanisms following perinatal exposure to marijuana. *Pharmacol. Biochem. Behav.* 25(4):763–768.

Wang, L., and Pitts, D.K. (1994) Perinatal cocaine exposure decreases the number of spontaneously active midbrain dopamine neurons in neonatal rats. *Synapse* 17:275–277.

Warner, T.D., Behnke, M., et al. (2006) Diffusion tensor imaging of frontal white matter and executive functioning in cocaine-exposed children. *Pediatrics* 118(5):2014–2024.

Weissman, A.D., and Caldecott-Hazard, S. (1995) Developmental neurotoxicity to methamphetamines. *Clin. Exp. Pharmacol. Physiol.* 22(5):372–374.

Westergren, S., Rydenhag, B., et al. (1996) Effects of prenatal alcohol exposure on activity and learning in Sprague-Dawley rats. *Pharmacol. Biochem. Behav.* 55(4):515–520.

Wilkins, A.S., Jones K., et al. (1998) Transplacental cocaine exposure. 2: Effects of cocaine dose and gestational timing. *Neurotoxicol. Teratol.* 20(3):227–238.

Williams, M.T., Blankenmeyer, T.L., et al. (2003) Long-term effects of neonatal methamphetamine exposure in rats on spatial learning in the Barnes maze and on cliff avoidance, corticosterone release, and neurotoxicity in adulthood. *Brain Res. Dev. Brain Res.* 147(1-2):163–175.

Wilson, G. S. (1989) Clinical studies of infants and children exposed prenatally to heroin. *Ann. NY Acad. Sci.* 562:183–194.

Woods, J.R., Plessinger, M.A., et al. (1987) Effect of cocaine on uterine blood flow and fetal oxygenation. *JAMA* 257:957–961.

Woolverton, W.L., Ricaurte, G.A., et al. (1989) Long-term effects of chronic methamphetamine administration in rhesus monkeys. *Brain Res.* 486(1):73–78.

Wouldes, T., LaGasse, L., et al. (2004) Maternal methamphetamine use during pregnancy and child outcome: what do we know? *N.Z. Med. J.* 117(1206):U1180.

Xu, Z., Seidler F.J., et al. (2001) Fetal and adolescent nicotine administration: effects on CNS serotonergic systems. *Brain Res.* 914(1–2):166–178.

Yamamoto, Y., Yamamoto, K., et al. (1992) Teratogenic effects of methamphetamine in mice. *Nihon Hoigaku Zasshi* 46(2):126–131.

Zagon, I.S., and McLaughlin, P.J. (1986) Opioid antagonist-induced modulation of cerebral and hippocampal development: histological and morphometric studies. *Brain Res.* 393(2):233–246.

Zuckerman, B., Frank, D.A., et al. (1989) Effects of maternal marijuana and cocaine use on fetal growth. *N. Engl. J. Med.* 320(12): 762–768.

49 PET and SPECT Imaging in Substance Abuse Research

JOANNA S. FOWLER AND NORA D. VOLKOW

The addiction to legal and illegal drugs poses one of the most medically, socially, and economically devastating public health problems facing modern society. Yet resources dedicated to the prevention and treatment of the addictions lags behind other medical problems. Although the perception of addiction as a lack of willpower or a moral weakness rather than a disease of the brain still persists, modern imaging technologies developed over the last 30 years have documented that drugs of abuse produce measurable changes on the human brain and that many factors including individual biology and genetics, environmental factors, and the characteristics of the drug and the route or vehicle for its administration all play a role.

In this chapter we describe positron emission tomography (PET) and single photon emission computed tomography (SPECT) technology that are the main brain imaging methods that have been used in the study of drug addiction. We highlight some of the insights on the effects of drugs of abuse on the human brain that have been gained through the use of brain imaging in humans. We note that there is an increasing trend to use combinations of different radiotracers and imaging methods along with behavioral and drug challenge strategies to probe the complex relationship of pharmacological and functional factors and addictive behaviors. This carries with it the need for large-scale statistical analyses of imaging data sets to extract correlations that will provide mechanistic information of relationships between brain chemistry and behavior. In addition, preclinical studies in animals have been valuable in elucidating mechanisms and in providing deeper insights into results gained from human studies. This chapter is intended to be an update since 2002 (Fowler and Volkow, 2004). We note that a number of recent review articles have appeared on the topic of neuroimaging and addiction (Volkow et al., 2004; Gatley et al., 2005; Lingford-Hughes, 2005; Chang and Haning, 2006).

PET AND SPECT TECHNOLOGY

Modern brain imaging instruments have provided mechanistic information on how the brain works and how drugs of abuse affect the brain. These properties include (*1*) brain anatomy and tissue composition, (*2*) neurochemical processes, (*3*) physiological and functional processes that provide information on brain energy utilization and blood flow and hence can be used to assess regional brain function, and (*4*) drug distribution and kinetics that provide information uptake, regional distribution, and residence time in the brain. Although we focus on PET and SPECT that are nuclear imaging methods, we note that the use of magnetic resonance imaging (MRI) in addiction research continues to increase and complement the nuclear imaging studies by providing information on brain anatomy and tissue composition as well as brain activation through the use of anatomical MRI, magnetic resonance spectroscopy (MRS), and functional magnetic resonance imaging (fMRI) (Lecchi et al., 2007).

Positron emission tomography and SPECT are unique relative to other currently available imaging techniques because they have the highest sensitivity to detect very small concentrations of cellular elements (Fowler et al., 2003; Kung et al., 2003). This property enables the measurement of cellular elements involved with neurotransmission such as receptors, transporters, and enzymes involved with synthesis or metabolism of neurotransmitters (Volkow et al., 2003). There are different radiotracers that can be used to visualize different elements (usually proteins) of the cell. In a PET or SPECT study, a radioactive molecule (radiotracer) is injected into the bloodstream. The energy emitted by the decay of the radioisotope penetrates the body barrier, and thus its location and movement into and out of the brain can be visualized from outside the body using a PET or SPECT scanner.

Positron emission tomography and SPECT instruments differ in several aspects including the characteristics of the instrumentation, the isotopes used, and the availability of the technology. Generally speaking, the resolution and sensitivity of PET instruments exceeds that of SPECT instruments. The use of positron-emitting isotopes with PET offers advantage because positrons interact with electrons generating photons that are liberated 180 degrees apart from each other, which enables their detection without the need of collimators as required with single photon emitter isotopes used with SPECT, and that decrease sensitivity.

Positron emission tomography studies are carried out with compounds labeled with positron (β+) emitting radioisotopes that are very short lived. There are positron emitting isotopes for the natural elements of life: carbon-11 ($t_{1/2}$: 20.4 minutes), oxygen-15 ($t_{1/2}$: 2 minutes), and nitrogen-13 ($t_{1/2}$: 10 minutes). There is also a positron emitting isotope of fluorine, fluorine–18(($t_{1/2}$: 110 minutes and that can often be used to substitute for hydrogen or oxygen). Thus, organic compounds (including drugs) can be labeled without changing the properties of the parent molecule by substituting carbon–11 for stable carbon (carbon–12) in the molecule. Positron emission tomography can therefore be uniquely used to determine how much drug penetrates the brain, where a drug binds in the brain, and how fast it moves into and out of the brain (Fowler et al., 1999). This information is crucial because the rate at which a drug enters the brain is known to be a powerful determinant of reinforcement. Positron emission tomography is also unique in the availability of 2-deoxy-2-[^{18}F]fluoro-D-glucose (^{18}FDG, a radiotracer for glucose) can be used to assess glucose metabolism in brain that is of major importance because glucose is the major source of energy for the human brain (Fowler and Ido, 2002).

Single photon emission computed tomography radiotracers are labeled with single photon emitting radioisotopes that are significantly longer lived than PET radiotracers. Single photon emission computed tomography radiotracers are usually labeled with iodine-123 ($t_{1/2}$: 13.3 hours) or technetium-99m ($t_{1/2}$: 6.5 hours). These isotopes cannot be incorporated into a drug molecule because these elements are not found in drugs. Nonetheless, many radioiodine-substituted radiotracers have been developed that have high biological selectivity and affinity for specific proteins in the cell (Kung et al., 2003), and Tc-99m labeled radiotracers such as Tc-99m-HMPAO are widely used to measure brain blood flow. There is no SPECT counterpart to ^{18}FDG for measuring brain glucose metabolism.

Positron emission tomography and SPECT can be used as tracer techniques, that is, the radiolabeled compounds are administered in a very tiny chemical quantity so that there is no pharmacological effect. The use of PET and SPECT radiotracers that have specificity for important cellular elements provides high biochemical specificity and sensitivity to changes produced by drugs or by disease. For example, these radiotracers can be used to differentiate dopamine (DA) transporters that are molecules located in presynaptic terminals from receptors that are mostly located in postsynaptic cells, despite the fact that the transporters and receptors are 20–50 nanometers apart.

COCAINE

Cocaine binds to DA, norepinephrine (NE), and serotonin transporters (SERTs) with micromolar to submicromolar affinity (Ritz et al., 1987). There is mounting evidence that the binding of cocaine to the DA transporter (DAT) with its rapid ensuing elevation of DA dominates its powerful behavioral effects in humans (Volkow et al., 2003). Cocaine addiction is also typically associated with intense drug craving stimulated by internal (pharmacological) or by environmental cues associated with past drug experience that are likely to be strong contributing factors to relapse that is typical in cocaine treatment approaches. Imaging studies have addressed cocaine abuse from its pharmacokinetic and pharmacodynamic perspectives (Volkow et al., 2003).

When a behaviorally active dose of cocaine is administered intravenously along with [^{11}C]cocaine in current cocaine abusers, there is very high and very rapid brain uptake and clearance of the drug in the striatum that contains the reward center (nucleus accumbens). The movement of cocaine into and out of the brain parallels the time course of the intense behavioral "high" measured in the same individuals. Rapid kinetics is consistent with the intense but short-lived "high" and the binge-like pattern of cocaine use in the individual who is addicted. In these same studies, it was determined that a DAT occupancy in excess of 60% is required for a "high" to be perceived (Volkow, Wang, Fischman, et al., 1997). Interestingly, behaviorally active doses of cocaine occupy > 60% of the DATs irrespective of the route of administration (intravenous vs. smoked vs. snorted). However, the time course of the behavioral response was significantly different with the "high" appearing most rapidly with the smoked >intravenous >> intranasal (Volkow et al., 2000). This study provides the first evidence in humans that differences in the reinforcing effects of cocaine as a function of the route of administration are not due to differences in DAT occupancy. It also highlights the importance of the rate of cocaine's delivery into the brain on its reinforcing effects and corroborates the landmark studies of Balster and Schuster, who pointed this out more than 30 years ago (Balster and Schuster, 1973).

Positron emission tomography studies measuring DA D_2 receptors with [^{11}C]raclopride and other radiotracers have consistently shown long-lasting decreases in DA D_2 receptors in cocaine abusers when compared with controls (Fig. 49.1; see also COLOR FIGURE 49.1 in separate insert) (Volkow et al., 2003). Reductions in DA D_2 receptors occur across striatal subdivisions in individuals who are cocaine dependent relative to healthy controls (Martinez et al., 2004). Cocaine abusers also showed significant reductions in DA release in response to a challenge dose of the stimulant drug *methylphenidate* relative to a control group (Volkow, Wang, Fowler, et al., 1997). Decreased DA release is consistent with the hypothesis that the decreases in DA D_2 receptors coupled with the decreases in DA release would result in a decreased sensitivity of reward circuits to stimulation by natural reinforcers such as food because the reinforcing effects of food also appear to involve DA release and stimulation of DA D_2 receptors (Volkow, Wang, Fowler, et al., 2002). This would be predicted to lead to a decrease in motivational salience for day-to-day environmental stimuli, which would put individuals at greater risk for seeking drug stimulation as a means to temporarily activate these reward circuits.

Brain glucose metabolism as measured with ^{18}FDG has been used to identify brain regions that differ as a result of chronic cocaine exposure as well as identifying the brain regions that are activated in response to pharmacological challenge or to cocaine cues. For example, brain glucose metabolism measured in this same group of cocaine abusers in whom DA D_2 receptors was measured previously revealed that the reductions in DA D_2 receptors were associated with decreased activity in anterior cingulate gyrus (CG) and orbitofrontal cortex (OFC) (Figs. 49.1 and 49.2; see also COLOR FIGURE 49.2 in separate insert) (reviewed in Volkow et al., 2003). These associations could either reflect a disruption of these cortical brain regions secondary to the changes in DA activity or alternatively, it could be interpreted as indicating a disruption of frontal regions, which then deregulate DA cell activity.

In contrast to the decrements in metabolic activity observed in detoxified cocaine abusers, the OFC was hypermetabolic in active cocaine abusers in proportion to the intensity of the craving (Volkow et al., 1991). Metabolism also increases in the OFC in the cocaine abusers in response to intravenous administration of the stimulant drug methylphenidate in the abusers reporting intense craving (Volkow, Wang, et al., 1999). This and a more recent study comparing the regional metabolic response to an intravenous dose of methylphenidate identified the right medial prefrontal cortex as a region that is uniquely activated in individuals who are addicted and decreased in controls (Volkow et

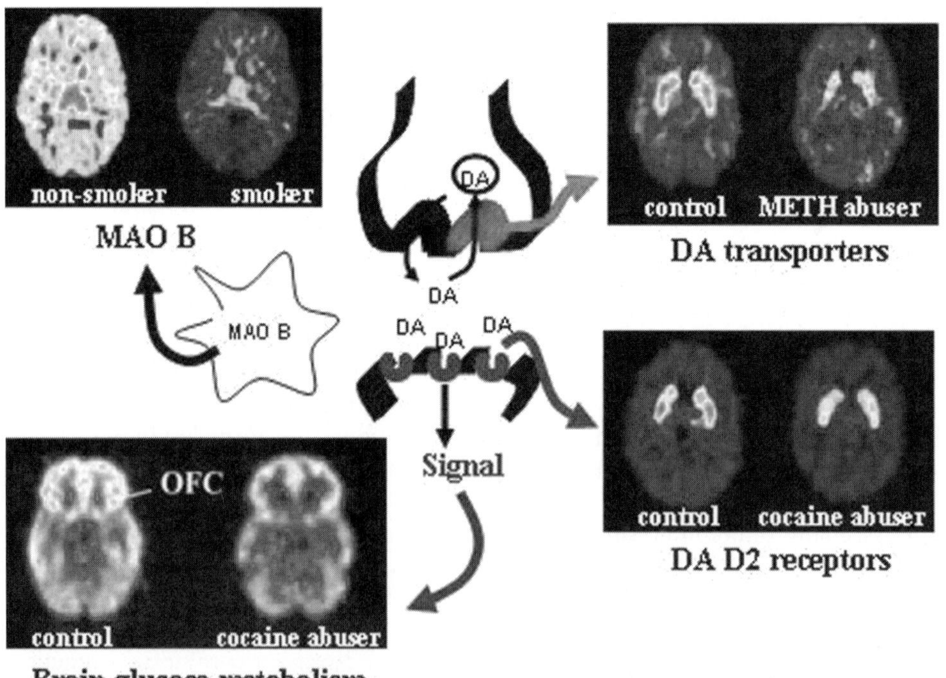

FIGURE 49.1 Simplified diagram of a dopamine synapse showing the dopamine transporter, dopamine receptors, and MAO-B (in glia cells). PET images of the human brain (clockwise from upper left) show brain MAO-B inhibition in a smoker measured with [^{11}C]L-deprenyl-D2, reduced dopamine transporter availability in an abuser of methamphetamine (measured with [^{11}C]d-threo-methylphenidate), reduced dopamine D_2/D_3 receptors in an abuser of cocaine (measured with [^{11}C]raclopride) and reduced glucose metabolism in the orbitofrontal cortex (OFC) in a cocaine abuser (measured with ^{18}FDG). MAO-B: monoamine oxidase B; PET: positron emission tomography.

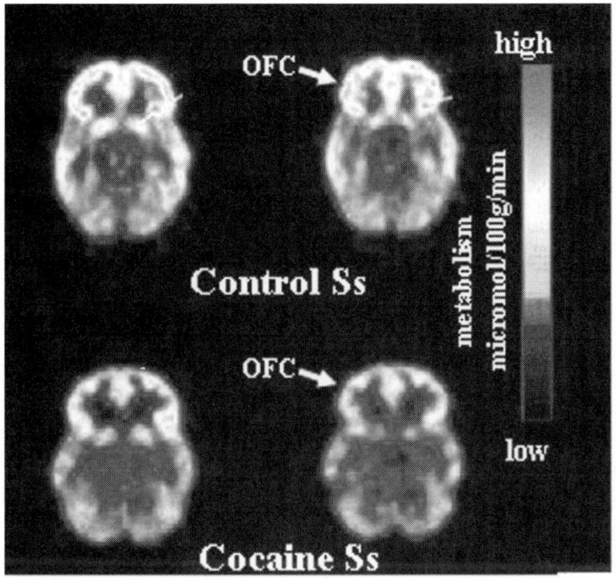

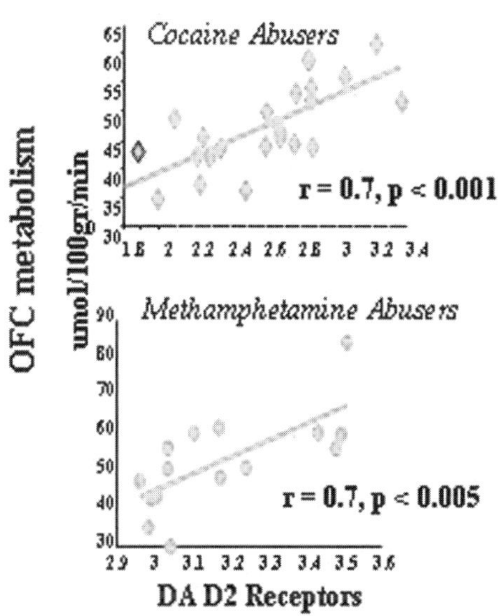

FIGURE 49.2 The left shows images of brain glucose metabolism in a control and in an abuser of cocaine at the level where the OFC is located. The right side of the figure shows the regression slopes between the availability of dopamine D_2 receptors and metabolism in OFC for a group of abusers of cocaine and for a group of abusers of methamphetamine. Note that the lower the D_2 receptor availability, the lower the metabolism in OFC. Modified from Volkow et al., 2004. OFC: orbitofrontal cortex.

al., 2005). These findings suggest that enhanced sensitivity of right medial orbital prefrontal cortex in individuals who are addicted to cocaine may underlie the strong emotional response to the drug and the intense desire to procure it that results in craving and compulsive drug intake. The OFC is involved with learning stimulus–reinforcement associations and with conditioned responses (Rolls, 2000) and could therefore participate in cues or drug-induced craving. Activation of the OFC has also been shown in drug abusers during craving elicited by viewing a video of drug paraphernalia (Grant et al., 1996; Childress et al., 1999) and by recalling previous drug experiences (Wang et al., 1999).

Preclinical studies have shown that with repeated drug exposure, neutral stimuli paired with the drug (conditioned stimuli) start to increase DA by themselves, which is an effect that could underlie drug-seeking behavior (P.E. Phillips et al., 2003). Recent studies using [^{11}C]raclopride have shown that the presentation of cocaine cues to the cocaine abuser results in a measurable change in [^{11}C]raclopride binding in the dorsal striatum, indicating that the cocaine cue alone is sufficient to change brain DA levels. Moreover, the magnitude of the DA elevation is associated with the degree of craving that is elicited by these cues (Volkow, Wang, Telang, et al., 2006; Wong et al., 2006). These studies provide evidence that DA in the dorsal striatum (region implicated in habit learning and in action initiation) is involved with craving and is a fundamental component of addiction. Because craving is a key contributor to relapse, strategies aimed at inhibiting DA increases from conditioned responses are likely to be therapeutically beneficial in cocaine addiction.

The endogenous opioid system has also been implicated in cocaine dependence and craving. Brain mu-opioid binding was increased in cocaine addicts studied 1–4 days after their last use of cocaine using PET and [^{11}C]carfentanil, a radioligand with specificity for the mu-opioid receptor. Increased binding persisted for 4 weeks and was positively correlated with the severity of cocaine craving (Zubieta et al., 1996). In another study extending the experimental period to 12 weeks, mu-opioid receptor binding was found to be elevated in the frontal, anterior cingulate, and lateral temporal cortex after 1 day of abstinence. Mu-opioid receptor binding potential remained elevated in the first two regions after 1 week and in the anterior cingulate and anterior frontal cortex after 12 weeks. Increased binding in some regions at 1 day and 1 week was positively correlated with self-reported cocaine craving, suggesting that chronic cocaine use influences endogenous opioid systems in the human brain and might explain mechanisms of cocaine craving and reinforcement (Gorelick et al., 2005).

The role of the brain serotonin system in the chronic neural adaptations to cocaine dependence was studied in 15 individuals who were cocaine dependent during acute abstinence using [^{123}I]β-CIT (Jacobsen et al., 2000) a SPECT tracer for measuring SERT availability and showed significant increases in diencephalic and brain-stem SERT binding, suggesting serotonergic dysfunction during acute cocaine abstinence.

METHAMPHETAMINE

Methamphetamine (METH) is a highly addictive stimulant drug. Its principle pharmacological action is the release of DA and other neurotransmitters through the individual neurotransmitter transporters on the presynaptic neurons and on intracellular vesicles (Barr et al., 2006). Methamphetamine has been shown to be neurotoxic to laboratory animals at doses that are self-administered in human abusers (Zhu et al., 2006, and references therein), and studies in abusers of METH have documented significant losses in DAT postmortem (Wilson et al., 1996). Among other causes, oxidative stress, excitotoxicity, and mitochondrial dysfunction appear to play a major role in the neurotoxicity produced by METH and other substituted amphetamines (Quinton and Yamamoto, 2006).

Neuroimaging studies have addressed the effects of chronic METH abuse on the brain glucose metabolism and on DATs and DA receptors in the METH abuser. In one of these studies, recently abstinent abusers of METH (< 6 months) were scanned with ^{18}FDG, [^{11}C]raclopride (to measure DA D_2/D_3 receptors) and [^{11}C]d-threo-methylphenidate to measure DATs (reviewed in Volkow et al., 2003) and were evaluated for cognitive and motor performance. Methamphetamine abusers showed losses in DAT that were associated with reduced motor speed and impaired verbal learning (Fig. 49.1). Dopamine D_2 receptors were also lower than in the comparison group, and these reductions were associated with reduced glucose metabolism in the OFC (Fig. 49.2). This association is similar to the correlation between DA D_2 receptors and brain glucose metabolism observed in cocaine abusers, suggesting that D_2 receptor-mediated dysregulation of the OFC could be a common mechanism underlying loss of control and compulsive drug intake (Volkow and Fowler, 2000).

Positron emission tomography studies with ^{18}FDG have assessed regional brain function in recently abstinent METH abusers and its relationship to executive function, cognitive deficits, and mood disturbances. One of these studies in abusers who were abstinent with METH reported persistent hypometabolism in the frontal white matter and impairment in frontal executive function that was more prominent in men than in women (Kim et al., 2005). Another study in abusers who were recently abstaining from METH (4–7 days) reported abnormalities in limbic and paralimbic regions that were related to self-reports of depression and anxiety, suggesting that these regions are involved in affective dysregulation and may be an important target of intervention for methamphetamine dependence (London et al., 2004). A combined PET-^{18}FDG/MRI study examining the links between METH-induced deficits in regional brain metabolism and cognitive deficits reported that abusers who were recently abstaining from METH (4–7 days) have cognitive, metabolic, and structural deficits in limbic and paralimbic cortices, and reduced hippocampal volume and that dysfunction in the cingulate and insular cortices contribute to impaired vigilance and other cognitive functions requiring sustained attention (London et al., 2005).

The question of whether DAT, brain glucose metabolism, and motor and cognitive function recovers after protracted abstinence (12–17 months) has been addressed in some abusers of METH who had been scanned during early detoxification. Although these studies showed recovery of DAT levels, clinical improvement was not significant (Volkow, Chang, Wang, Fowler, Franceschi, Sedler, Gatley, Miller, et al., 2001). Another PET study in male abusers of METH provided evidence that longer use of METH may cause more severe psychiatric symptoms and greater reduction of DAT (as measured with [^{11}C]WIN 35428) and that the decrease in DAT persists even when METH use ceases (Sekine et al., 2001). A more recent study in this same group of individuals reported that DAT level in the PFC was significantly associated with duration of METH use and severity of psychiatric symptoms (Sekine et al., 2003).

The recovery of brain function (as measured with ^{18}FDG) in abusers of METH after protracted withdrawal has also been assessed. During early abstinence, abusers of METH showed changes in metabolism in DA and non-DA brain regions when compared to a control group (Volkow, Chang, Wang, Fowler, Franceschi, Sedler, Gatley, Hitzemann, et al., 2001). Whole brain metabolism in the abusers of METH was 14% higher than that of control, with differences most prominent in the parietal cortex (+20%), a region devoid of DA innervation (Volkow, Chang, Wang, Fowler, Franceschi, Sedler, Gatley, Hitzemann, et al., 2001). Metabolic deficits in the striatum and the thalamus were also observed. Follow-up studies in some of these abusers showed significant metabolic recovery in the thalamus that was associated with improvements in motor and verbal memory tests, whereas decrements in striatal metabolism persisted, possibly accounting for the amotivation and anhedonia in these abusers (Wang et al., 2004). These results suggest that, though protracted abstinence may reverse some of the METH-induced alterations in brain function, other deficits persist.

The documentation of METH-induced neurotoxicity in serotonin neurons and associated aggression in animals stimulated a recent investigation of the effects of METH abuse on SERTs in humans and relationships to clinical phenotypes (Sekine et al., 2006). This study with [^{11}C](+)McN-5652 revealed that the SERT density in global brain regions (for example, the midbrain, thalamus, caudate, putamen, cerebral cortex, and cerebellum) was significantly lower in abusers of METH than in controls, and this reduction was inversely correlated with the duration of METH use. Furthermore, statistical parametric mapping analyses indicated that the density in the orbitofrontal, temporal, and anterior cingulate areas was closely associated with the magnitude of aggression in abusers of METH. The authors concluded that protracted abuse of METH may reduce the density of the SERT in the brain, leading to elevated aggression, even in abusers who are currently abstinent.

METHYLENEDIOXYMETHAMPHETAMINE (MDMA)

Methylenedioxymethamphetamine (MDMA; also called ecstasy) is a popular recreational drug that is toxic to serotonin neurons in laboratory animals (Ricaurte et al., 1988; McCann et al., 2001). It potently releases serotonin and DA from their vesicular storage sites (for review, see Huether et al., 1997). Similar to METH and other substituted amphetamines, excitotoxicity and oxidative stress may account in part for its neurotoxicity (Quinton and Yamamoto, 2006). Due to its increased use and the potential for neurotoxicity, neuroimaging studies in users of MDMA have been used to evaluate toxicity in the human MDMA user. There are several recent reviews of neuroimaging studies of MDMA (Reneman et al., 2006; Thomasius et al., 2006; Cowan, 2007). The controversies, gaps in knowledge, and methodological challenges associated with PET studies to determine whether or not MDMA is neurotoxic in humans have been discussed (Lyvers, 2006).

Most PET studies have been directed to understanding its potential for damaging serotonergic neurons. Positron emission tomography-^{18}FDG studies to examine changes in brain function after long-term use of MDMA report a global reduction in ^{18}FDG uptake rates that is most pronounced in the striatum. Reductions tended to be correlated with cumulative MDMA doses, suggesting that younger MDMA users may be more vulnerable to MDMA-induced neurotoxicity (Obrocki et al., 2002). Early studies using [^{11}C]McN5652 to examine SERT density in users of MDMA reported that heavy use of MDMA is associated with neurotoxic effects on serotonin neurons, that women may be more susceptible than men, and that MDMA-induced changes in several brain regions of female ex-MDMA users are reversible (Reneman et al., 2001). More recent studies have confirmed reductions in SERTs in MDMA users during early abstinence in 30 current MDMA users, 29 former MDMA users, 29 drug-naïve comparisons, and 29 polydrug users (Buchert et al., 2004). In the users of MDMA, SERT availability as assessed by [^{11}C]McN5652 was significantly reduced in the mesencephalon, thalamus, left caudate, hippocampus, occipital cortex, temporal lobes, and posterior cingulate gyrus. Reduction was more pronounced in female than in male users, and there was no significant difference between the MDMA users and the other groups. These findings support the hypothesis of MDMA-induced protracted alterations of the serotonergic system and indicate that the reduced availability of SERT, as measured by PET, might be reversible. Similar findings were reported in another study in which two different radiotracers, [^{11}C]McN5652 and [^{11}C]DASB, were compared in 23 abstinent users of MDMA and 19 non-MDMA controls (McCann et al., 2005). Comparisons in 15 regions of interest demonstrated that the two different tracers gave comparable results showing that reductions occurred in selected cortical and subcortical structures. Exploratory correlational analyses suggested that SERT measures recover with time, and that loss of the SERTs is directly associated with MDMA use intensity.

The possibility that decreases in SERT levels are an artifact of tracer kinetic model used for [^{11}C]McN5652 was evaluated in 30 current, 29 former users of ecstasy, 29 drug-naïve comparisons, and 28 polydrug controls using a model that is less sensitive to the effect of statistical noise (Buchert et al., 2006). The equilibrium specific-to-nonspecific partition coefficient V3 was obtained voxel-wise by application of the simplified reference tissue method (SRTM), showed SERT reductions in the striatum and in the thalamus in current users of ecstasy. This was corroborated by volume-of-interest–based analysis confirming previous reports and indicating that reduced SERT binding potential is not an artifact of tracer kinetic modeling. However, SRTM analysis did not confirm previous finding of SERT reductions in neocortical brain areas.

ALCOHOL

The neurochemical mechanisms by which alcohol produces its acute and chronic effects are complex and not well understood. However, there is evidence that alcohol reinforcement is mediated by an activation of γ-aminobutyric acid (GABA)-A receptors, release of opioid peptides, release of DA, inhibition of glutamate receptors, and interaction with serotonin systems, making these systems of special relevance in understanding the effects of alcohol on the brain (Koob et al., 1998). Many different radiotracers including ^{18}FDG as well as others with specificity for different neurotransmitter systems have been used to examine the acute and chronic effects of alcohol on brain metabolism and brain neurotransmitter activity in normal individuals, individuals with an alcohol addiction, and individuals at risk (reviewed in Volkow et al., 2003). Neuroimaging has also been used to study alcohol toxicity (reviewed in Mann et al., 2001).

Positron emission tomography measures of brain glucose metabolism using ^{18}FDG have shown that individuals with an alcohol addiction and individuals who are not addicted respond differently to an alcohol challenge. Individuals with an alcohol addiction show a smaller behavioral response and a larger metabolic response than normal individuals (reviewed in Volkow et al., 2003). Different responsivity between individuals with an alcohol addiction and a comparison group was also seen for the lorazepam (a benzodiazepine drug that, like alcohol, also enhances GABA transmission) challenge, indicating altered GABA-BZR function in individuals with an alcohol addiction (reviewed in Volkow et al., 2003).

The effects of an acute challenge with an intoxicating dose of alcohol (0.75 g/kg) on brain glucose metabolism were measured in normal healthy individuals with ^{18}FDG and PET and produced substantial decreases in occipital cortex and increases in left temporal cortex similar to previous studies with lorazepam (Volkow, Wang, Overall, et al., 1997) that has been interpreted to reflect alcohol-induced decreases on brain GABA-BZR activity. Building on evidence that alcohol has effects on the GABA, PET and SPECT imaging have shown decreased benzodiazepine receptor levels in individuals with an alcohol addiction and in controls with [^{11}C]flumazenil (Gilman et al., 1996) and [^{123}I]iomazenil (Abi-Dargham, et al., 1998). A recent study designed to test the hypothesis that alcohol dependence is associated with reduced benzodiazepine receptor function showed that although alcohol dependence is associated with decreased midazolam-induced time asleep, there is no difference in receptor occupancy by midazolam (as measured with [^{11}C]flumazenil) in individuals who were dependent upon alcohol relative to a control group. This was not predicted and may be accounted for by a difference in GABA-BDZ subunit profile (Lingford-Hughes et al., 2005).

Gender has also been studied as a variable in the acute effects of alcohol by comparing changes in brain glucose metabolism during alcohol intoxication (0.75 g/kg) in healthy male and female controls (Wang et al., 2003). The magnitude of the alcohol-induced change in brain metabolism was significantly larger in male ($-25 \pm 6\%$) than in female ($-14 \pm 11\%$; $p < .005$) individuals; in contrast, the self-reports for the perception of intoxication were significantly greater in females than in males. This study shows a markedly blunted sensitivity to the effects of acute alcohol on brain glucose metabolism in females. Blunted metabolic responses could reflect other effects of alcohol, for which the regional metabolic signal may be hidden within the large decrements in metabolism that occur during alcohol intoxication.

In a recent study in normal healthy individuals, two relatively low doses of alcohol (0.25 g/kg and 0.5 g/kg, or 5–10 mM in total body water) significantly decreased whole-brain glucose metabolism (10% and 23%, respectively) while not affecting cognitive performance (Volkow, Wang, Franceschi, et al., 2006). This contrasts with previous results showing that a 13% reduction in brain metabolism by lorazepam was associated with significant cognitive impairment. This seemingly paradoxical finding where the same degree of metabolic decrease produces cognitive impairment for lorazepam and not for alcohol raises the possibility that the large brain metabolic decrements during alcohol intoxication could reflect a shift in the substrate for energy utilization. In-fact there is new evidence that blood-borne acetate, which is markedly increased during intoxication, is a substrate for energy production by the brain (Waniewski and Martin, 1998).

Imaging studies have also examined the relationship of gender and chronic alcohol toxicity, following up on the general belief that women are more vulnerable to alcohol's toxic effects than men. However, whereas males with an alcohol addiction have consistently shown reductions in brain glucose metabolism relative to comparison subjects, a PET study with ^{18}FDG in 10 recently detoxified females with an alcohol addiction reported no differences between individuals with an alcohol addiction and female controls (Wang et al., 1998). These results do not support a higher toxicity for the effects of alcohol in the female brain, as assessed with regional brain glucose metabolism. However, the authors point out that the severity of alcohol use in these females with an alcohol addiction was less than that of the males with an alcohol addiction previously investigated in PET studies. Another study comparing males and females with an alcohol addiction suggests that alcohol has a differential effect on GABA-BZR in men and women (Lingford-Hughes et al., 2000).

Postmortem studies have also documented significant reductions in D_2 receptors in the nucleus accumbens and amygdala in individuals with an alcohol addiction when compared with controls (Tupala et al., 2001; Tupala et al., 2003). Dopamine D_2 receptor measurements as assessed with PET predominantly reflect postsynaptic receptors (Volkow et al., 1996), which are mostly located in GABA cells, suggesting involvement of these cells in the ventral striatum of individuals with an alcohol addiction. The DA D_2 receptor is one of the DA receptor subtypes involved in transmitting DA's reinforcing signals (Nowak et al., 2000). This has been documented in a variety of ways. For example, D_2 receptor antagonist drugs decrease reinforcing responses to alcohol in rodents (Pfeffer and Samson, 1986) and in humans (Ahlenius et al., 1973). Also, studies have shown differences in D_2 receptor levels between rat strains that differ in their preferences for alcohol (Stefanini et al., 1992; McBride et al., 1993), and D_2 receptor knockout mice exhibit reduced reinforcing responses to alcohol (T.J. Phillips et al., 1998). Moreover, overexpression of D_2 receptor in NAc markedly reduces alcohol intake (Thanos et al., 2001), even in selectively bred P rats who prefer alcohol (Thanos et al., 2004).

A recent PET/[^{11}C]raclopride study comparing DA D_2 receptor levels in subregions of the striatum in individuals with an alcohol addiction versus a control group provides evidence for reduced receptor levels throughout the different subregions of the human striatum (limbic [ventral], sensorimotor, and associative) (Martinez et al., 2005). This same study also reported a decrease in amphetamine-induced DA release in ventral striatum in individuals with an alcohol addiction compared to a control group further supporting decrements in brain DA activity in individuals with an alcohol addiction. These findings replicate previous studies documenting lower DA D_2 receptors in ventral striatum in individuals with an alcohol addiction than in controls (Heinz et al., 2004; Martinez et al., 2005). For one of these studies, the low D_2 receptors in ventral striatum were associated with alcohol craving (Heinz et al., 2004).

A simultaneous assay by PET of pre- and postsynaptic markers of DA neurotransmission (with 6-[^{18}F]fluoro-DOPA as a marker of dopamine synthesis and [^{18}F]des methoxyfallypride to map DA D_2/D_3 receptors) in the same individuals indicated that a striatal DA deficit correlated with alcohol craving, which was associated with a high relapse risk in a 6-month follow-up of these patients (Heinz, Siessmeier, et al., 2005). In humans, differences in D_2 receptor availability in individuals with no alcohol addiction are associated with differences in sensitivity to the intoxicating effects of alcohol (Yoder et al., 2005). Thus, the low D_2 receptor availability in ventral striatum in individuals with an alcohol addiction in conjunction with reduced DA release and synthesis could compound their vulnerability for alcohol abuse.

We note that the literature contains inconsistencies with imaging and postmortem studies reporting on measures of baseline D_2 receptors in striatum in individuals with an alcohol addiction, with some studies showing no changes (Guardia et al., 2000; Kuikka et al., 2000; Repo et al., 1999) whereas others (including our laboratory) reporting decreases (Hietala et al., 1994; Volkow et al., 1996; Volkow, Wang, Maynard, et al., 2002; Tupala et al., 2003; Heinz et al., 2004; Martinez et al., 2005). The discrepancy could reflect, among others, the fact that many of the earlier imaging studies, including our own, did not distinguish the dorsal from the ventral striatum and reported the averaged values of both regions. Alternatively, differences could reflect patient characteristics such as age of patients, chronicity of drinking, early- versus late-onset alcoholism, stage of withdrawal, ethnicity, gender, and comorbidity with smoking.

An early SPECT study with [^{123}I]β-CIT (a nonselective radiotracer that measures SERT concentration in the brain stem) reported a 30% decrease in availability of brain-stem SERTs in individuals with an alcohol addiction (Heinz et al., 1998). However, a recent PET study with [^{11}C]DASB, a selective radiotracer for the SERT, showed no difference in transporter availability between individuals with an alcohol addiction (parsed into a group of aggressive and nonaggressive sybtypes) and a control group (Brown et al., 2007).

A recent PET study highlighting the relationship between alcohol dependence and the endogenous opioid system used the mu-opioid receptor subtype selective radiotracer [^{11}C]carfentanil to show a strong functional relationship between alcohol craving, mood, and mu-OR binding in specific brain regions (right dorsal lateral PFC, right anterior frontal cortex, and right parietal cortex) in men who were dependent upon alcohol (Bencherif et al., 2004). Similarly, another study with [^{11}C]carfentanil in patients who were abstaining from alcohol reported an increase in mu-opiate receptors in the ventral striatum, including the nucleus accumbens, which correlated with the severity of alcohol craving (Heinz, Reimold, et al., 2005). These findings are consistent with the moderate effectiveness of mu-opiate receptor active drug naltrexone in reducing the risk of relapse among some individuals with an alcohol addiction (Soyka and Roesner, 2006).

^{18}FDG and other PET tracers have been used to probe the recovery of brain function and brain neurotransmitter activity in individuals with an alcohol addiction after alcohol withdrawal. Decrements in brain glucose metabolism were reported to partially recover in individuals with an alcohol addiction, particularly during the first 16–30 days after withdrawal (Volkow et al., 1994). Dopamine transporter levels, though reported in one study to be lower in individuals with an alcohol addiction than in controls, have been reported to recover to near-normal levels after abstinence as determined with SPECT and [^{123}I]β-CIT (Laine et al., 1999). However a PET study reported normal DAT levels in individuals with an alcohol addiction (Volkow et al, 1996). The discrepancy may relate to the time interval between the study and the last use of alcohol because the DATs are subject to rapid up- and down-regulation in response to drug challenge (Zahniser and Doolen, 2001). Positron emission tomography with [^{11}C]raclopride measuring DA D_2 receptor levels in individuals with an alcohol addiction tested within 6 weeks of detoxification and then retested 1–4 months later while alcohol free showed the absence of significant recovery during alcohol detoxification (Volkow, Wang, Franceschi, et al., 2002). These findings suggest that low DA D_2 receptor availability in individuals with an alcohol addiction is not due to alcohol withdrawal and may reflect a predisposing factor. In another PET study, [^{11}C]dihydrotetrabenazine, a radiotracer for the type 2 vesicular monoamine transporter (VMAT2) that has been reported to be insensitive to up- and down-regulation (Vander Borght et al., 1995), was reported to be reduced in males with a severe alcohol addiction (Gilman et al., 1998). This indicates that nigrostriatal monoaminergic terminals are reduced and suggests that the damaging effects of severe chronic alcoholism on the central nervous system are more extensive than previously considered.

NICOTINE AND TOBACCO SMOKE

The effects of nicotine and tobacco smoke on brain function, blood flow, and neurochemistry have been studied using a variety of imaging techniques (reviewed in Volkow et al., 2003; McClernon and Gilbert, 2004). The pharmacokinetics of nicotine itself have been measured using [^{11}C]nicotine in humans revealing rapid uptake into the brain reaching peak uptake at 2–4 minutes after intravenous injection and clearing with a half-life between 22 minutes for thalamus and 36 minutes for temporal cortex (reviewed in Volkow, Fowler, et al., 1999). This is consistent with the rapid onset of its pharmacological effects in humans and the frequency of cigarette smoking. However, there is growing appreciation for the role of the nonnicotine chemical components of tobacco and the reinforcing sensory stimulation provided by smoking a cigarette that contribute to smoking behavior and addiction (Rose, 2006).

Although [^{11}C]nicotine provides valuable information on nicotine pharmacokinetics, its uptake is dominated by nonspecific binding. This has led to the development of radiotracers such as 2- and 6-[^{18}F]fluoro A85380 and [125I]5-iodo A 85380 based on $\alpha_4\beta_2$ agonist A 85380 that binds predominantly to the $\alpha_4\beta_2$ nicotinic acetylcholine receptor subtype (Ding and Fowler, 2005; Horti and Villemagne, 2006) and to the initiation of measures of neuronal nicotinic receptor (nAChR) occupancy by smoking one or more cigarettes and nAChR levels in smokers who were recently abstinent. Smoking a full cigarette (or more) resulted in more than 88% receptor occupancy and was accompanied by a reduction in cigarette craving. Thus, daily smoking almost completely saturates the nAChR throughout the day, suggesting that smoking may alleviate withdrawal symptoms by maintaining nAChRs in the desensitized state (Brody et al., 2006). A SPECT study with [^{125}I]5-iodo-A 85380 recently documented abnormally high levels of $\alpha_4\beta_2$ in the brains of smokers during early abstinence (6.8 ± 1.9 days) (Staley et al., 2006), consistent with the observation of elevated $\alpha_4\beta_2$ nAChR in smokers' brains postmortem (Perry et al., 1999). Neuronal nicotinic receptor levels correlated with the days since last cigarette and the urge to smoke to relieve withdrawal symptoms may affect the ability of smokers to maintain abstinence.

The hypothesis that some of the effects of smoking cigarettes in humans are mediated through nicotine activation of opioid, and DA neurotransmission has also been investigated using the radiotracers [^{11}C]carfentanil and [^{11}C]raclopride, which label mu-opioid and DA D2 receptors, respectively (D.J. Scott et al., 2007) under conditions where the radiotracer was injected and individuals smoked two denicotinized cigarettes followed by two nicotinized cigarettes. Smokers had significantly lower baseline mu-opioid receptor levels than nonsmokers during the denicotinized cigarette part of the study. Parametric maps corresponding to low and high nicotine smoking periods showed that smoking an average cigarette was associated with the activation of DA D_2 and mu-opioid release as evidenced by the reductions of DA D_2 and mu-opioid receptor availability from the denicotinized to the nicotinized conditions. There were no differences in DA D_2 receptor levels between nonsmokers and smokers that is similar to a recent PET study with [^{123}I]-IBZM (Yang et al., 2006). The ability of cigarette smoking to cause DA release was also documented in another study with [^{11}C]raclopride that showed that the magnitude of the release was comparable to that found in studies that used similar methods to examine the effects of other addictive drugs (Brody et al., 2004).

Positron emission tomography studies were the first to document low brain monoamine oxidase A and B (MAO-A and -B) in smokers relative to nonsmokers and former smokers (Fig. 49.1) (reviewed in Fowler et al., 2005). The average reductions in MAO-A and -B are 30% and 40%, respectively. Positron emission tomography studies confirmed early reports that nicotine does not inhibit MAO, that smoking a single cigarette does not produce a measurable change in brain MAO-B in nonsmokers, and that an overnight cigarette abstinence for smokers does not produce a measurable recovery of brain MAO activity (Fowler et al., 2005, and references therein). Low brain MAO in smokers may be one of the mechanisms by which smoking contributes to some of the behavioral and epidemiological features of smoking, including the decreased risk of Parkinson's disease in smokers (W.K. Scott et al., 2005) and an increased rate of smoking in patients with psychiatric and substance use disorders (Kalman et al., 2005). Reduced brain MAO activity would be predicted to spare biogenic amines such as DA, serotonin, and NE and to reduce the production of hydrogen peroxide, a by-product from MAO-catalyzed oxidation and a potential source of free radicals. Both of these effects would be predicted to have therapeutic benefit in neurological and psychiatric disorders. Thus, there is biochemical rationale for the neuroprotective effect of tobacco smoke and for the self-medication hypothesis. Recently, L-deprenyl showed efficacy in smoking cessation (George et al., 2003). In addition, a nonselective MAO inhibitor, 2,3,6-trimethylbenzoquinone, has been isolated from flue-cured tobacco leaves (Khalil et al., 2000) and shown to possess neuroprotective properties (Castagnoli et al., 2003).

Positron emission tomography studies of brain function, as measured with ^{18}FDG, documented reversible changes in brain metabolism during different stages of nicotine dependence (overnight abstinence vs. 2-week exposure to denicotinized cigarettes + nicotine patches vs. 2 weeks after returning to the regular cigarette) and highlight the likely role of thalamic gating and striatal reward and corticolimbic regulatory pathways in maintaining cigarette addiction (Rose et al., 2007). Similarly, recent measures of the effects of smoking on cerebral blood flow with O-15 water revealed that smoking affects regional cerebral blood flow (rCBF) not only in areas of the brain rich in nicotinic cholinergic receptors but also in areas implicated in the rewarding effects of drugs of abuse (Zubieta et al., 2005). In this same study, the craving for a cigarette in chronic smokers has been correlated with elevation in regional metabolism in the right hippocampus, an area involved in associating environmental cues with drugs, and in the left dorsal anterior cingulate, which has been implicated in drug craving and relapse to drug-seeking behavior, similar to an earlier study with FDG (Brody et al., 2002). These regional brain activations and associations with craving are similar to findings with other addictive substances. An interesting study recently reported that the administration of patch nicotine *decreased* gender differences in brain metabolism between men and women performing a continuous performance task or a competition and retaliation task (Fallon et al., 2005).

OPIATES

Mu, delta, and kappa opioid receptors are the physiological targets of endogenous and exogenous opioids. There are a number of PET radiotracers for imaging and quantifying these receptors (Lever, 2007). [^{11}C]carfentanil that is selective for the mu subtype is the most widely used, specifically in studies of the opioid receptors. Others such as [^{11}C]diprenorphine (nonselective) and [^{18}F]cyclofoxy (nonselective) are also available for studies of receptor availability, and other subtype selective opioid receptor radiotracers are under development (Lever, 2007). We also note that a large fraction of the PET research on opioid receptors is related to studies of the neurobiology of pain (Sprenger et al., 2005). Although neuroimaging has not been applied to studies of abuse of prescription pain medications per se, we note that abuse of pain medications, most notably the opiates, is one of the most rapidly growing areas of drug abuse.

Over the past several years, PET has been used to study opiate abuse in current heroin abusers, in individuals treated with opiate agonists such as methadone, and in those undergoing opiate withdrawal. Parameters measured include brain metabolism in abusers of opiates, neuroanatomical correlates of craving, opiate receptor occupancy with treatment drugs and during withdrawal, and DA receptor levels. Briefly, these studies showed that, similar to other addictions, abusers of opiates have lower DA D_2 receptors relative to a control group; that individuals addicted to opiates have a blunted response to prototypical human rewards; and that craving is associated with activations of blood flow in the prefrontal cortical regions (reviewed in Volkow et al., 2003).

Methadone substitution is one of the main ways to treat opiate addiction, and it has been shown that its use improves health and social outcome. However, little is known about methadone pharmacology, including the degree to which it occupies opioid receptors at the doses required to suppress withdrawal symptoms. A recent study examined the relationship between methadone dose and occupation of brain opioid receptors using [^{11}C]diprenorphine and PET, comparing a group of eight individuals who were dependent on opioids and stable on their substitute methadone (18–90 mg daily) and eight healthy controls (Melichar et al., 2005). Surprisingly, no difference in [^{11}C]diprenorphine binding was found between the groups, and there was no relationship between methadone dose and receptor occupancy. Methadone also did not block [^{11}C]diprenorphine binding in rats. This report contrasts to an earlier study with [^{18}F]cyclofoxy showing that methadone administration modestly but significantly (19%–32%) reduces the uptake of [^{18}F]cyclofoxy (Kling et al., 2000). Potential reasons for this discrepancy were discussed (Melichar et al., 2005) and include differences in radiotracer characteristics, possible receptor internalization, and up-regulation of opioid receptors after chronic dosing. The authors suggested that the lack of a measurable occupancy of opioid receptor by methadone is evidence that efficacy occurs at very low levels of opioid receptor occupancy.

Buprenorphine is a relatively new and effective treatment of opioid dependence. Following earlier studies showing occupancy of mu-opioid receptors by buprenorphine (Zubieta et al., 2000), a recent PET study with [^{11}C]carfentanil examined the duration of receptor occupancy by buprenorphine, measuring occupancy at different times after buprenorphine administration. Plasma buprenorphine concentration, withdrawal symptoms, and blockade of the effects of hydromorphone were also recorded. Relative to placebo, mu-opioid receptor occupancy was 30%, 54%, 67%, and 82% at 4, 28, 52, and 76 hours, respectively, after buprenorphine. Moreover mu-opioid receptor availability correlated with plasma buprenorphine levels, withdrawal symptoms, and hydromorphone blockade. Together with a previous study (Greenwald et al., 2003), this study showed that mu-opiate receptor occupancy by buprenorphine is long lasting, that receptor availability as measured with PET predicts changes in pharmacokinetic and pharmacodynamic measures and that buprenorphine (unlike methadone) occupies about 50%–60% or the mu-opioid receptors at doses required to suppress withdrawal symptoms.

Nalmefene is a long-acting opioid antagonist that is used in the treatment of alcoholism and other disorders (Mason et al., 1999). Similar to the study with buprenorphine, [^{11}C]carfentanil was used to determine the relationship between nalmefene plasma concentration and central mu-opioid receptor occupancy. Central mu-opioid receptor occupancy was measured at four time points (3, 26, 50, 74 hours) after a clinically effective dose (20 mg, orally) either as a single dose or after repeated dosing over 7 days (Ingman et al., 2005). Both nalmefene dosings resulted in a very high occupancy at mu-opioid receptors (87%–100%), and the decline in the brain receptor occupancy was similar after both dosings but clearly slower than the decline in the plasma concentration of nalmefene or metabolites. High nalmefene occupancy (83%–100%) persisted at 26 hours after the dosings, consistent with slow dissociation of the drug from mu-opioid receptors. This study supports the rationale of administering nalmefene when needed and suggests that once-daily dosing is sufficient to achieve a high mu-opioid receptor occupancy.

MARIJUANA

Marijuana is the most widely used illegal substance in the United States, and thus the nature of its effects on the brain is of major importance. However, there are surprisingly few studies applying neuroimaging methods to the effects of marijuana abuse on the human brain (for reviews, see Lindsey et al., 2003; Volkow et al., 2003; Quickfall and Crockford, 2006). The main psychoactive substance of marijuana is delta9-tetrahydrocannibinol (THC), which has been postulated to exert its psychoactive effects through interactions with cannabinoid receptors that are highly localized in the cerebellum and hippocampus (Herkenham et al., 1990). A SPECT ligand for the cannabinoid receptor (Gatley et al., 1998) has recently been labeled with ^{124}I for PET studies in a patient with schizophrenia, though the long half-life of ^{124}I (4.17 days) is limiting because of radiation exposure (Berding et al., 2006). A number of PET radiotracers have been synthesized and evaluated and though most have not demonstrated sufficient brain uptake and specificity for translation to humans, [^{18}F]MK-9470, a selective high-affinity inverse agonist, has recently been evaluated and shows promise in human studies (Burns et al., 2007). There is a clear need to make advances in this area not only because of the intrinsic importance of this abundant receptor in the brain that is the target of the most widely abused drug but also because the central cannabinoid receptor is an important target for drug research and development, including drugs to treat obesity.

Marijuana smoking increases brain blood flow in a number of paralimbic brain regions (for example, orbital frontal lobes, insula, temporal poles) and in anterior cingulate and cerebellum. In contrast, rCBF decreased in temporal regions that are sensitive to auditory attention effects. This is consistent with speculation that the intoxicating and mood-related effects of marijuana may be mediated by brain regions showing increases in rCBF, whereas impaired cognitive function during intoxication may be associated with brain regions showing decreases in rCBF (O'Leary et al., 2000). Studies on the effects of marijuana intoxication on regional brain glucose metabolism reported differences in the patterns of response between abusers and nonabusers. Whereas marijuana increased cerebellar metabolism in all patients, it increased metabolism in anterior cingulate gyrus and in OFC only in the abusers but not in the controls (reviewed in Volkow et al., 2003).

Frequent marijuana users at baseline show substantially lower brain blood flow (as measured with O-15 water) than controls in a large region of posterior cerebellum (which is linked to an internal timing system), indicating altered brain function may underlie alterations of time sense, which is common following marijuana smoking (Block et al., 2000). Expanding on this, the effects of marijuana on brain perfusion and internal timing were assessed in occasional and chronic marijuana users who performed a paced counting task during the PET study (Ponto et al., 2004). The study showed that smoking marijuana increased rCBF in the ventral forebrain and cerebellar cortex and appears to accelerate a cerebellar clock altering self-paced behaviors.

Recent PET studies also show that smokers who were abstinent with marijuana (25 days) have persistent deficits in blood flow in prefrontal brain regions that are the regions responsible for executive cognitive functioning even though they do not differ from controls in the performance of a modified version of the Stroop task (Eldreth et al., 2004). The authors speculated that users of marijuana recruit an alternative neural network as a compensatory mechanism during performance of this task and that prefrontal deficits may be a common denominator in the evolution of maladaptive behaviors such as substance abuse and other neuropsychiatric disorders. Consistent with this is a recent study in which measurement of brain blood flow in heavy users of marijuana during performance of a gambling task revealed greater activation in the left cerebellum and less activation in the right lateral OFC and the right dorsolateral PFC (DLPFC) and impaired decision making compared to the control group (Bolla et al., 2005). Specifically, the heavy users of marijuana may focus on only the immediate reinforcing aspects of a situation (that is, getting high) while ignoring the negative consequences. Poor decision making could make an individual more prone to addictive behavior and more resistant to treatment.

VULNERABILITY

The question of why some people who experiment with drugs become addicted whereas others do not is important in the context of understanding mechanisms underlying addictive behavior. The finding of low DA D_2 receptors in individuals who are addicted raise important mechanistic questions: (*1*) In the absence of drug addiction, does an individual's baseline level of DA D_2 receptors influence the behavioral response to a stimulant drug? (*2*) Does short-term exposure to a stimulant drug change DA D2 receptor levels and, if so, do these changes persist after protracted withdrawal? (*3*) Can environmental changes affect DA D2 receptor levels? and (*4*) Are high DA D_2 receptors protective in individuals at risk? These questions have been addressed through imaging studies in normal individuals who were not abusing drugs in whom the confounds of neurobiological changes due to prolonged drug exposure are eliminated and in laboratory animals.

Although individuals addicted to cocaine, METH, heroin, or alcohol as a group have significant decrements in DA D_2 receptors, there is considerable overlap in receptor values with those from individuals who are not addicted (reviewed in Volkow et al., 2003). This large variability among individuals formed the basis for a study that showed that healthy individuals who did not abuse drugs with low DA D_2 receptors found an intravenous dose of the stimulant drug methylphendiate pleasant, but those with high DA D2 receptor levels found it aversive (Volkow et al., 1999). This supports the notion that individuals with low DA receptors may have an understimulated reward system and, as a result, they perceive a pleasurable sensation when subjected to a drug-induced elevation in DA. It follows that an individual who takes a drug and finds it pleasant is more likely to repeat the behavior. This finding was recently reinforced in a preclinical PET study with [^{11}C]raclopride that demonstrated that nucleus accumbens D_2/D_3 receptor availability predicts trait impulsivity and cocaine reinforcement in rats (Dalley et al., 2007).

Reduced DA D_2 receptors in abusers of cocaine raise an important question as to the extent to which these reductions preceded the use of cocaine. Although it is not possible to obtain this information in humans, studies in monkeys have addressed this question by imaging DA D2 receptors at baseline and through a 1-year course of cocaine administration followed by a 1-year abstinence period, tracking receptor levels throughout with PET (Nader et al., 2006). This study showed that D_2 receptor availability decreased by 15%–20% within 1 week of initiating self-administration and remained reduced by approximately 20% during 1 year of exposure. Decreases persisted for up to 1 year of abstinence in some monkeys. Monkeys with higher baseline DA D_2 receptor levels self-administered less cocaine, providing evidence for a predisposition to self-administer cocaine based on D_2 receptor availability, and demonstrated a rapid decrease in DA D_2 receptor level following cocaine. This supports the notion that biological vulnerability (that is, low DA D_2 receptors at the outset) as well as cocaine-induced vulnerability (cocaine-induced reductions in DA D_2 receptors) could predispose an individual to cocaine administration.

Highlighting the impact of environmental factors on DA D_2 receptor availability, this same group assessed the effect of changing the social environment of monkeys on DA D_2 receptor availability and on cocaine self-administration using PET (Morgan et al., 2002). Individually housed monkeys had a baseline PET scan to assess DA D_2 receptor levels and were given access to cocaine. Whereas DA D_2 receptor level did not differ among individually housed animals, social housing increased the DA D_2 receptors in the dominant, but not the subordinate, monkeys. In parallel, cocaine use decreased in the dominant animals and increased in the subordinate animals. This study, which occurred over a 3-month time frame, puts forth the notion that DA D_2 receptor level can change within the time frame of normal social activities (Nader and Czoty, 2005).

In animals, repeated exposure to stimulant drugs leads to an enhanced drug-induced psychomotor response and increased DA release that has been postulated to confer vulnerability to drug addiction or drug-induced psychosis in humans. A recent PET study with [^{11}C]raclopride determined whether brief exposure to amphetamine (three oral doses—0.3 mg/kg—on days 1, 3, and 5) in normal healthy individuals in a laboratory setting would alter DA release, producing behavioral and neurochemical sensitization (Boileau et al., 2006). Dopamine release in response to amphetamine was measured on the first exposure (day 1) and at 14 days and 1 year after the third exposure with [^{11}C]raclopride binding. Consistent with a sensitization-like phenomenon, 14 and 365 days after the third dose of amphetamine, there was a greater psychomotor response and increased DA release relative to the initial dose. Moreover, high novelty-seeking and impulsivity personality traits predicted proneness to sensitization. This study with only limited amphetamine exposure demonstrated that sensitization to stimulants achieved in healthy men in the laboratory, that it is associated with enhanced DA release, and that the phenomenon persists for at least 1 year.

Predisposition to alcoholism is likely an interaction between genetic and environmental factors that confer vulnerability and protection. Individuals with an alcohol addiction have low levels of DA D_2 receptors in striatum, and increasing D_2 receptor levels in laboratory animals reduces alcohol consumption (Thanos et al., 2001). A recent study with [^{11}C]raclopride to measure dopamine D_2 receptors and ^{18}FDG to measure brain glucose metabolism compared individuals without an alcohol addiction with a positive family history of alcoholism with individuals without an alcohol addiction with a negative family history (Volkow, Wang, Begleiter, et al., 2006). Dopamine D_2 receptor levels were significantly higher for the family positive group. In addition, significant associations between D_2 receptors and metabolism in frontal regions involved with emotional reactivity and executive control suggest that high levels of D_2 receptors could protect against alcoholism by regulating circuits involved in inhibiting behavioral responses and in controlling emotions. On the other hand, a PET study that measured changes in DA in striatum induced by amphetamine found no differences as a function of family history of alcoholism (Munro et al., 2006).

OUTLOOK

In spite of the increasing reliance of the biomedical sciences, including substance abuse research, on molecular imaging, the development of new radiotracers remains a slow and even rate-limiting process. For example, we still need good radiotracers for many neurotransmitters and neurotransmitter subtypes (including the cannabinoid receptor, the opioid receptor subtypes [kappa and delta], the glutamate and GABA systems, and others, including cellular signaling processes). However, even the familiar radiopharmaceuticals that are the backbone of imaging sciences are the product of enormous effort and even serendipity. Yet the value of radiopharmaceuticals in almost every area of clinical research is of such enormous importance that it justifies a more focused effort in identifying the impediments and in setting scientific and medical priorities. There are a number of urgent requirements to be able to develop radiotracers that can visualize and quantify a single biochemical process in the human body where all of the chemical reactions of life are occurring. These include research in chemistry, training of chemists, advances in molecular design, and the targeting and streamlining of translation of new developments to humans. In addition, as nuclear imaging is combined with other modalities and with measures of genetics and behavior, the need for advanced postprocessing, and quantification and statistical analysis of large datasets, becomes imperative in order to extract meaningful relationships between brain chemistry and behavior.

ACKNOWLEDGMENT

This work was performed in part at Brookhaven National Laboratory under contract DE-AC02-98CH10886 with the U.S. Department of Energy and was supported by its Office of Biological and Environmental Research and by the National Institutes of Health.

REFERENCES

Abi-Dargham, A., Krystal, J.H., Anjilvel, S., Scanley, B.E., Zoghbi, S., Baldwin, R.M., Rajeevan, N., Ellis, S., Petrakis, I.L., Seibyl, J.P., Charney, D.S., Laruelle, M., and Innis, R.B. (1998) Alterations of benzodiazepine receptors in type II alcoholic subjects measured with SPECT and [^{123}I]iomazenil. *Am. J. Psychiatry* 155(11):1550–1555.

Ahlenius, S., Carlsson, A., Engel, J., Svensson, T., and Sodersten, P. (1973) Antagonism by alpha methyltyrosine of the ethanol-induced stimulation and euphoria in man. *Clin. Pharmacol. Ther.* 14:586–591.

Balster, R.L., and Schuster, C.R. (1973) Fixed-interval schedule of cocaine reinforcement: effect of dose and infusion duration. *J. Exp. Anal. Behav.* 20(1):119–129.

Barr, A.M., Panenka, W.J., MacEwan, G.W., Thornton, A.E., Lang, D.J., Honer, W.G., and Lecomte, T. (2006) The need for speed: an update on MAMP addiction. *J. Psychiatry Neurosci.* 31: 301–313.

Bencherif, B., Wand, G.S., McCaul, M.E., Kim, Y.K., Ilgin, N., Dannals, R.F., and Frost, J.J. (2004) Mu-opioid receptor binding measured by [^{11}C]carfentanil positron emission tomography is related to craving and mood in alcohol dependence. *Biol. Psychiatry* 55(3): 255–262.

Berding, G., Schneider, U., Gielow, P., Buchert, R., Donnerstag, F., Brandau, W., Knapp, W.H., Emrich, H.M., and Müller-Vahl, K. (2006) Feasibility of central cannabinoid CB1 receptor imaging with [124I]AM281 PET demonstrated in a schizophrenic patient. *Psychiatry Res.* 147(2/3):249–256.

Block, R.I., O'Leary, D.S., Hichwa, R.D., Augustinack, J.C., Ponto, L.L., Ghoneim, M.M., Arndt, S., Ehrhardt, J.C., Hurtig, R.R., Watkins, G.L., Hall, J.A., Nathan, P.E., and Andreasen, N.C. (2000) Cerebellar hypoactivity in frequent marijuana users. *Neuroreport* 11:749–753.

Boileau, I., Dagher, A., Leyton, M., Gunn, R.N., Baker, G.B., Diksic, M., and Benkelfat, C. (2006) Modeling sensitization to stimulants in humans: an [^{11}C]raclopride/positron emission tomography study in healthy men. *Arch. Gen. Psychiatry* 63(12):1386–1395.

Bolla, K.I., Eldreth, D.A., Matochik, J.A., and Cadet, J.L. (2005) Neural substrates of faulty decision-making in abstinent marijuana users. *NeuroImage* 26(2):480–492.

Brody, A.L., Mandelkern, M.A., London, E.D., Childress, A.R., Lee, G.S., Bota, R.G., Ho, M.L., Saxena, S., Baxter, L.R., Jr., Madsen, D., and Jarvik, M.E. (2002) Brain metabolic changes during cigarette craving. *Arch. Gen. Psychiatry* 59(12):1162–1172.

Brody, A.L., Mandelkern, M.A., London, E.D., Olmstead, R.E., Farahi, J., Scheibal, D., Jou, J., Allen, V., Tiongson, E., Chefer, S.I., Koren, A.O., and Mukhin, A.G. (2006) Cigarette smoking saturates brain alpha 4 beta 2 nicotinic acetylcholine receptors. *Arch. Gen. Psychiatry* 63(8):907–915.

Brody, A.L., Olmstead, R.E., London, E.D., Farahi, J., Meyer, J.H., Grossman, P., Lee, G.S., Huang, J., Hahn, E.L., and Mandelkern, M.A. (2004) Smoking-induced ventral striatum dopamine release. *Am. J. Psychiatry* 161(7):1211–1218.

Brown, A.K., George, D.T., Fujita, M., Liow, J.S., Ichise, M., Hibbeln, J., Ghose, S., Sangare, J., Hommer, D., and Innis, R.B. (2007) PET [^{11}C]DASB imaging of serotonin transporters in patients with alcoholism. *Alcohol Clin. Exp. Res.* 31(1):28–32.

Buchert, R., Thiele, F., Thomasius, R., Wilke, F., Petersen, K., Brenner, W., Mester, J., Spies, L., and Clausen, M. (2006) Ecstasy-induced reduction of the availability of the brain serotonin transporter as revealed by [^{11}C](+)McN5652-PET and the multi-linear reference tissue model: loss of transporters or artifact of tracer kinetic modelling? *J. Psychopharmacol.* November 8 [Epub ahead of print].

Buchert, R., Thomasius, R., Wilke, F., Petersen, K., Nebeling, B., Obrocki, J., Schulze, O., Schmidt, U., and Clausen, M. (2004) A voxel-based PET investigation of the long-term effects of "Ecstasy" consumption on brain serotonin transporters. *Am. J. Psychiatry* 161(7):1181–1189.

Burns, H.D., Van Laere, K., Sanabria-Bohórquez, S., Hamill, T.G., Bormans, G., Eng, W.S., Gibson, R., Ryan, C., Connolly, B., Patel, S., Krause, S., Vanko, A., Van Hecken, A., Dupont, P., De Lepeleire, I., Rothenberg, P., Stoch, S.A., Cote, J., Hagmann, W.K., Jewell, J.P., Lin, L.S., Liu, P., Goulet, M.T., Gottesdiener, K., Wagner, J.A., de Hoon, J., Mortelmans, L., Fong, T.M.,and Hargreaves, R.J. (2007) [^{18}F]MK-9470, a positron emission tomography (PET) tracer for in vivo human PET brain imaging of the cannabinoid-1 receptor. *Proc. Natl. Acad. Sci. USA* 104(23):9800–9805.

Castagnoli, K., Petzer, J.B., Steyn, S.J., van der Schyf, C.J., and Castagnoli, N., Jr. (2003) Inhibition of human MAO-A and MAO-B by a compound isolated from flue-cured tobacco leaves and its neuroprotective properties in the MPTP mouse model of neurodegeneration. *Inflammopharmacology* 11(2):183–188.

Chang, L., and Haning, W. (2006) Insights from recent positron emission tomographic studies of drug abuse and dependence. *Curr. Opin. Psychiatry* 19(3):246–252.

Childress, A.R., Mozley, P.D., McElgin, W., Fitzgerald, J., Reivich, M., and O'Brien, C.P. (1999) Limbic activation during cue-induced cocaine craving. *Am. J. Psychiatry* 156(1):11–18.

Cowan, R.L. (2007) Neuroimaging research in human MDMA users: a review. *Psychopharmacology (Berl)* 189(4):539–556.

Dalley, J.W., Fryer, T.D., Brichard, L., Robinson, E.S., Theobald, D.E., Laane, K., Pena, Y., Murphy, E.R., Shah, Y., Probst, K., Abakumova, I., Aigbirhio, F.I., Richards, H.K., Hong, Y., Baron, J.C., Everitt, B.J., and Robbins, T.W. (2007) Nucleus accumbens D2/3 receptors predict trait impulsivity and cocaine reinforcement. *Science* 315(5816):1267–1270.

Ding, Y.S., and Fowler, J.S. (2005) New-generation radiotracers for nAChR and NET. *Nucl. Med. Biol.* 32(7):707–718.

Eldreth, D.A., Matochik, J.A., Cadet, J.L., and Bolla, K.I. (2004) Abnormal brain activity in prefrontal brain regions in abstinent marijuana users. *NeuroImage* 23(3):914–920.

Fallon, J.H., Keator, D.B., Mbogori, J., Taylor, D., and Potkin, S.G. (2005) Gender: a major determinant of brain response to nicotine. *Int. J. Neuropsychopharmacol.* 8(1):17–26.

Fowler, J.S., Ding, Y.S., and Volkow, N.D. (2003) Radiotracers for positron emission tomography imaging. *Semin. Nucl. Med.* 33(1): 14–27.

Fowler, J.S., and Ido, T. (2002) Initial and subsequent approach for the synthesis of ^{18}FDG. *Semin. Nucl. Med.* 32(1):6–12.

Fowler, J.S., Logan, J., Volkow, N.D., and Wang, G.J. (2005) Translational neuroimaging: positron emission tomography studies of monoamine oxidase. *Mol. Imaging Biol.* 7(6):377–387.

Fowler, J.S., and Volkow, N.D. (2004) Neuroimaging in substance abuse research. In: Charney, D.S., and Nestler, E.J., eds. *Neurobiology of Mental Illness*, 2nd ed. New York: Oxford University Press, pp. 740–752.

Fowler, J.S., Volkow, N.D., Wang, G.J., Ding, Y.S., and Dewey, S.L. (1999) PET and drug research and development. *J. Nucl. Med.* 40(7): 1154–1163.

Gatley, S.J., Lan, R., Volkow, N.D., King, P., Wong, C.T., Gifford, A.N., Pyatt, B., and Makriyannis, A. (1998) Imaging the brain marijuana receptor: development of a radioligand that binds to cannabinoid CB1 receptors in vivo. *J. Neurochem.* 70:417–423.

Gatley, S.J., Volkow, N.D., Wang, G.J., Fowler, J.S., Logan, J., Ding, Y.S., and Gerasimov, M. (2005) PET imaging in clinical drug abuse research. *Curr. Pharm. Des.* 11(25):3203–3219.

George, T.P., Vessichio, J.C., and Termine, A. (2003) A preliminary, placebo controlled trial of selegiline hydrochloride for smoking cessation. *Biol. Psychiatry* 53:136–143.

Gilman, S., Koeppe, R.A., Adams, K., Johnson-Greene, D., Junck, L., Kluin, K.J., Brunberg, J.B., Martorello, S., and Lohman, M. (1996) Positron emission tomographic studies of cerebral benzodiazepine-receptor binding in chronic alcoholics. *Ann. Neurol.* 40:163–171.

Gilman, S., Koeppe, R.A., Adams, K.M., Junck, L., Kluin, K.J., Johnson-Greene, D., Martorello, S., Heumann, M., and Bandekar, R. (1998) Decreased striatal monoaminergic terminals in severe chronic alcoholism demonstrated with (+)[^{11}C]dihydrotetrabenazine and positron emission tomography. *Ann. Neurol.* 44(3): 326–333.

Gorelick, D.A., Kim, Y.K., Bencherif, B., Boyd, S.J., Nelson, R., Copersino, M., Endres, C.J., Dannals, R.F., and Frost, J.J. (2005) Imaging brain mu-opioid receptors in abstinent cocaine users: time course and relation to cocaine craving. *Biol. Psychiatry* 57(12): 1573–1582.

Grant, S., London, E.D., Newlin, D.B., Villemagne, V.L., Liu, X., Contoreggi, C., Phillips, R.L., Kimes, A.S., and Margolin, A. (1996) Activation of memory circuits during cue-elicited cocaine craving. *Proc. Natl. Acad. Sci. USA* 93(21):12040–12045.

Greenwald, M.K., Johanson, C.E., Moody, D.E., Woods, J.H., Kilbourn, M.R., Koeppe, R.A., Schuster, C.R., and Zubieta, J.-K. (2003) Effects of buprenorphine maintenance dose on mu-opioid receptor availability, plasma concentrations, and antagonist blockade in heroin-dependent volunteers. *Neuropsychopharmacology* 28:2000–2009.

Guardia, J. Catafau, A.M., Batlle, F., Martin, J.C., Segura, L. Gonzalvo, B., Prat, G., Carrio, I., and Casas, M. (2000) Striatal dopaminergic D(2) receptor density measured by [(^{123})I]iodobenzamide SPECT in the prediction of treatment outcome of alcohol-dependent patients. *Am. J. Psychiatry* 157:127–129.

Heinz, A., Ragan, P., Jones, D.W., Hommer, D., Williams, W., Knable, M.B., Gorey, J.G., Doty, L., Geyer, C., Lee, K.S., Coppola, R., Weinberger, D.R., and Linnoila, M. (1998) Reduced central serotonin transporters in alcoholism. *Am. J. Psychiatry* 155:1544–1549.

Heinz, A., Reimold, M., Wrase, J., Hermann, D., Croissant, B., Mundle, G., Dohmen, B.M., Braus, D.F., Schumann, G., Machulla, H.J., Bares, R., and Mann, K. (2005) Correlation of stable elevations in striatal mu-opioid receptor availability in detoxified alcoholic patients with alcohol craving: a positron emission tomography study using carbon 11-labeled carfentanil. *Arch. Gen. Psychiatry* 62(1):57–64.

Heinz, A., Siessmeier, T., Wrase, J., Buchholz, H.G., Grunder, G., Kumakura, Y., Cumming, P., Schreckenberger, M., Smolka, M. N., Rosch, F., Mann, K., and Bartenstein, P. (2005) Correlation of alcohol craving with striatal dopamine synthesis capacity and D2/3 receptor availability: a combined [^{18}F]DOPA and [^{18}F]DMFP PET study in detoxified alcoholic patients. *Am. J. Psychiatry* 162(8): 1515–1520.

Heinz, A., Siessmeier, T., Wrase, J., Hermann, D., Klein, S., Grusser, S.M., Flor, H., Braus, D.F., Buchholz, H.G., Grunder, G., Schreckenberger, M., Smolka, M.N., Rosch, F., Mann, K., and Bartenstein, P. (2004) Correlation between dopamine D(2) receptors in the ventral striatum and central processing of alcohol cues and craving. *Am. J. Psychiatry* 161:1783–1789.

Herkenham, M., Lynn, A.B., Little, M.D., Johnson, M.R., Melvin, L.S., de Costa, B.R., and Rice, K.C. (1990) Cannabinoid receptor localization in brain. *Proc. Natl. Acad. Sci. USA* 87:1932–1936.

Hietala, J., West, C., Syvalahti, E., Nagren, K., Lehikoinen, P., Sonninen, P., and Ruotsalainen, U. (1994) Striatal D2 dopamine receptor binding characteristics in vivo in patients with alcohol dependence. *Psychopharmacology (Berl)* 116:285–290.

Horti, A.G., and Villemagne, V.L. (2006) The quest for Eldorado: development of radioligands for in vivo imaging of nicotinic acetylcholine receptors in human brain. *Curr. Pharm. Des.* 12(30): 3877–3900.

Huether, G., Zhou, D., and Rüther, E. (1997) Causes and consequences of the loss of serotonergic presynapses elicited by the consumption of 3,4-methylenedioxy methamphetamine (MDMA, "ecstasy") and its congeners. *J. Neural Transm.* 104:771–794.

Ingman, K., Hagelberg, N., Aalto, S., Nagren, K., Juhakoski, A., Karhuvaara, S., Kallio, A., Oikonen, V., Hietala, J., and Scheinin, H. (2005) Prolonged central mu-opioid receptor occupancy after single and repeated nalmefene dosing. *Neuropsychopharmacology* 30(12):2245–2253.

Jacobsen, L.K., Staley, J.K., Malison, R.T., Zoghbi, S.S., Seibyl, J.P., Kosten, T.R., and Innis, R.B. (2000) Elevated central serotonin transporter binding availability in acutely abstinent cocaine-dependent patients. *Am. J. Psychiatry* 157:1134–1140.

Kalman, D., Morissette, S.B., and George, T.P. (2005) Co-morbidity of smoking in patients with psychiatric and substance use disorders. *Am. J. Addict.* 14(2):106–123.

Khalil, A.A., Steyn, S., and Castagnoli, N. (2000) Isolation and characterization of monoamine oxidase inhibitor from tobacco leaves. *Chem. Res. Toxicology* 13:31–35.

Kim, S.J., Lyoo, I.K., Hwang, J., Sung, Y.H., Lee, H.Y., Lee, D.S., Jeong, D.U., and Renshaw, P.F. (2005) Frontal glucose hypometabolism in abstinent methamphetamine users. *Neuropsychopharmacology* 30(7):1383–1391.

Kling, M.A., Carson, R.E., Borg, L., Zametkin, A., Matochik, J.A., Schluger, J., Herscovitch, P., Rice, K.C., Ho, A., Eckelman, W.C., and Kreek, M.J. (2000) Opioid receptor imaging with positron emission tomography and [(18)F]cyclofoxy in long-term, methadone-treated former heroin addicts. *J. Pharmacol. Exp. Ther.* 295(3):1070–1076.

Koob, G.F., Roberts, A.J., Schulteis, G., Parsons, L.H., Heyser, C.J., Hyytia, P., Merlo-Pich, E., and Weiss, F. (1998) Neurocircuitry targets in ethanol reward and dependence. *Alcohol Clin. Exp. Res.* 22(1):3–9.

Kuikka, J.T.Y., Repo, E., Bergstrom, K.A., Tupala, E., and Tiihonen, J. (2000) Specific binding and laterality of human extrastriatal dopamine D2/D3 receptors in late onset type 1 alcoholic patients. *Neurosci. Lett.* 292:57–59.

Kung, H.F., Kung, M.P., and Choi, S.R. (2003) Radiopharmaceuticals for single-photon emission computed tomography brain imaging. *Semin. Nucl. Med.* 33(1):2–13.

Laine, T.P., Ahonen, A., Torniainen, P., Heikkila, J., Pyhtinen, J., Rasanen, P., Niemela, O., and Hillbom, M. (1999) Dopamine transporters increase in human brain after alcohol withdrawal. *Mol. Psychiatry* 4(2):104–105, 189–191.

Lecchi, M., Ottobrini, L., Martelli, C., Del Sole, A., and Lucignani, G. (2007) Instrumentation and probes for molecular and cellular imaging. *Q. J. Nucl. Med. Mol. Imaging* 51(2):111–126.

Lever, J.R. (2007) PET and SPECT imaging of the opioid system: receptors, radioligands and avenues for drug discovery and development. *Curr. Pharm. Des.* 13(1):33–49.

Lindsey, K.P., Gatley, S.J., and Volkow, N.D. (2003) Neuroimaging in drug abuse. *Curr. Psychiatry Rep.* 5(5):355–361.

Lingford-Hughes, A. (2005) Human brain imaging and substance abuse. *Curr. Opin. Pharmacol.* 5(1):42–46.

Lingford-Hughes, A.R., Acton, P.D., Gacinovic, S., Boddington, S.J., Costa, D.C., Pilowsky, L.S., Ell, P.J., Marshall, E.J., and Kerwin, R.W. (2000) Levels of gamma-aminobutyric acid-benzodiazepine receptors in abstinent, alcohol-dependent women: preliminary findings from an ^{123}I-iomazenil single photon emission tomography study. *Alcohol Clin. Exp. Res.* 24(9):1449–1455.

Lingford-Hughes, A.R., Wilson, S.J., Cunningham, V.J., Feeney, A., Stevenson, B., Brooks, D.J., and Nutt, D.J. (2005) GABA-benzodiazepine receptor function in alcohol dependence: a combined ^{11}C-flumazenil PET and pharmacodynamic study. *Psychopharmacology (Berl)* 180(4):595–606.

London, E.D., Berman, S.M., Voytek, B., Simon, S.L., Mandelkern, M.A., Monterosso, J., Thompson, P.M., Brody, A.L., Geaga, J. A., Hong, M.S., Hayashi, K.M., Rawson, R.A., and Ling, W. (2005) Cerebral metabolic dysfunction and impaired vigilance in recently abstinent methamphetamine abusers. *Biol. Psychiatry* 58(10):770–778.

London, E.D., Simon, S.L., Berman, S.M., Mandelkern, M.A., Lichtman, A.M., Bramen, J., Shinn, A.K., Miotto, K., Learn, J., Dong, Y., Matochik, J.A., Kurian, V., Newton, T., Woods, R., Rawson, R., and Ling, W. (2004) Mood disturbances and regional cerebral metabolic abnormalities in recently abstinent methamphetamine abusers. *Arch. Gen. Psychiatry* 61(1):73–84.

Lyvers, M. (2006) Recreational ecstasy use and the neurotoxic potential of MDMA: current status of the controversy and methodological issues. *Drug Alcohol Rev.* 25(3):269–276.

Mann, K., Agartz, I., Harper, C., Shoaf, S., Rawlings, R.R., Momenan, R., Hommer, D.W., Pfefferbaum, A., Sullivan, E.V., Anton, R.F., Drobes, D.J., George, M.S., Bares, R., Machulla, H.J., Mundle, G., Reimold, M., and Heinz, A. (2001) Neuroimaging in alcoholism: ethanol and brain damage. *Alcohol Clin. Exp. Res.* 25(5 Suppl ISBRA):104S–109S.

Martinez, D., Broft, A., Foltin, R.W., Slifstein, M., Hwang, D-R., Huang, Y., Perez, A., Frankel, W.G., Cooper, T., Kleber, H.D., Fischman, M.W., and Laruelle, M. (2004) Cocaine dependence and d2 receptor availability in the functional subdivisions of the striatum: relationship with cocaine-seeking behavior. *Neuropsychopharmacology* 29:1190–1202.

Martinez, D., Gil, R., Slifstein, M., Hwang, D.R., Huang, Y., Perez, A., Kegeles, L., Talbot, P., Evans, S., Krystal, J., Laruelle, M., and Abi-Dargham, A. (2005) Alcohol dependence is associated with blunted dopamine transmission in the ventral striatum. *Biol. Psychiatry* 58(10):779–786.

Mason, B.J., Salvato, F.R., Williams, L.D., Ritvo, E.C., and Cutler, R.B. (1999) A double-blind, placebo-controlled study of oral nalmefene for alcohol dependence. *Arch. Gen. Psychiatry* 56(8):719–724.

McBride, W.J., Chernet, E., Dyr, W., Lumeng, L., and Li, T.K. (1993) Densities of dopamine D2 receptors are reduced in CNS regions of alcohol-preferring P rats. *Alcohol* 10:387–390.

McCann, U.D., Ricaurte, G.A., and Molliver, M.E. (2001) "Ecstasy" and serotonin neurotoxicity: new findings raise more questions. *Arch. Gen. Psychiatry* 58:907–908.

McCann, U.D., Szabo, Z., Seckin, E., Rosenblatt, P., Mathews, W.B., Ravert, H.T., Dannals, R.F., and Ricaurte, G.A. (2005) Quantitative PET studies of the serotonin transporter in MDMA users and controls using [^{11}C]McN5652 and [^{11}C]DASB. *Neuropsychopharmacology* 30(9):1741–1750.

McClernon, F.J., and Gilbert, D.G. (2004) Human functional neuroimaging in nicotine and tobacco research: basics, background, and beyond. *Nicotine Tob. Res.* 6(6):941–959.

Melichar, J.K., Hume, S.P., Williams, T.M., Daglish, M.R., Taylor, L.G., Ahmad, R., Malizia, A.L., Brooks, D.J., Myles, J.S., Lingford-Hughes, A., and Nutt, D.J. (2005) Using [^{11}C]diprenorphine to image opioid receptor occupancy by methadone in opioid addiction: clinical and preclinical studies. *J. Pharmacol. Exp. Ther.* 312(1):309–315.

Morgan, D., Grant, K.A., Gage, H.D., Mach, R.H., Kaplan, J.R., Prioleau, O., Nader, S.H., Buchheimer, N., Ehrenkaufer, R.L., and Nader, M.A. (2002) Social dominance in monkeys: dopamine D2 receptors and cocaine self-administration. *Nat. Neurosci.* 5(2):169–174.

Munro, C.A., McCaul, M.E., Oswald, L.M., Wong, D.F., Zhou, Y., Brasic, J., Kuwabara, H., Kumar, A., Alexander, M., Ye, W., and Wand, G.S. (2006) Striatal dopamine release and family history of alcoholism. *Alcohol Clin. Exp. Res.* 30(7):1143–1151.

Nader, M.A,. and Czoty, P.W. (2005) PET imaging of dopamine D2 receptors in monkey models of cocaine abuse: genetic predisposition versus environmental modulation. *Am. J. Psychiatry* 162(8):1473–1482.

Nader, M.A., Morgan, D., Gage, H.D., Nader, S.H., Calhoun, T.L., Buchheimer, N., Ehrenkaufer, R., and Mach, R.H. (2006) PET imaging of dopamine D2 receptors during chronic cocaine self-administration in monkeys. *Nat. Neurosci.* 9(8):1050–1056.

Nowak, K.L., McBride, W.J., Lumeng, L., Li, T.K., and Murphy, J. M. (2000) Involvement of dopamine D2 autoreceptors in the ventral tegmental area on alcohol and saccharin intake of the alcohol-preferring P rat. *Alcohol Clin. Exp. Res.* 24:476–483.

Obrocki, J., Schmoldt, A., Buchert, R., Andresen, B., Petersen, K., and Thomasius, R. (2002) Specific neurotoxicity of chronic use of ecstasy. *Toxicol. Lett.* 127(1-3):285–297.

O'Leary, D.S., Block, R.I., Flaum, M., Schultz, S.K., Boles, Ponto, L.L., Watkins, G.L., Hurtig, R.R., Andreasen, N.C., and Hichwa, R.D. (2000) Acute marijuana effects on rCBF and cognition: a PET study. *Neuroreport* 11:3835–3841.

Perry, D.C., Davila-Garcia, M.I., Stockmeier, C.A., and Kellar, K.J. (1999) Increased nicotinic receptors in brains from smokers: membrane binding and autoradiography studies. *J. Pharmacol. Exp. Ther.* 289(3):1545–1552.

Pfeffer, A.O., and Samson, H.H. (1986) Effect of pimozide on home cage ethanol drinking in the rat: dependence on drinking session length. *Drug Alcohol Depend.* 17:47–55.

Phillips, P.E., Stuber, G.D., Heien, M.L., Wightman, R.M., and Carelli, R.M. (2003) Subsecond dopamine release promotes cocaine seeking. *Nature* 422:614–618.

Phillips, T.J., Brown, K.J., Burkhart-Kasch, S., Wenger, C.D., Kelly, M.A., Rubinstein, M., Grandy, D.K., and Low, M.J. (1998) Alcohol preference and sensitivity are markedly reduced in mice lacking dopamine D2 receptors. *Nat. Neurosci.* 1:610–615.

Ponto, L.L., O'Leary, D.S., Koeppel, J., Block, R.I., Watkins, G.L., Richmond, J.C., Ward, C.A., Clermont, D.A., Schmitt, B.A., and Hichwa, R.D. (2004) Effect of acute marijuana on cardiovascular function and central nervous system pharmacokinetics of [(15)O]water: effect in occasional and chronic users. *J. Clin. Pharmacol.* 44(7):751–766.

Quickfall, J., and Crockford, D. (2006) Brain neuroimaging in cannabis use: a review. *J. Neuropsychiatry Clin. Neurosci.* 18(3): 318–332.

Quinton, M.S., and Yamamoto, B.K. (2006) Causes and consequences of methamphetamine and MDMA toxicity. *AAPS J.* 8(2):E337–E347.

Reneman, L., Booij, J., de Bruin, K., Reitsma, J.B., de Wolff, F.A., Gunning, W.B., den Heeten, G.J., and van den Brink, W. (2001) Effects of dose, sex, and long-term abstention from use on toxic effects of MDMA (ecstasy) on brain serotonin neurons. *Lancet* 358(9296):1864–1869.

Reneman, L., de Win, M.M., van den Brink, W., Booij, J., and den Heeten, G.J. (2006) Neuroimaging findings with MDMA/ecstasy: technical aspects, conceptual issues and future prospects. *J. Psychopharmacol.* 20(2):164–175.

Repo, E., Kuikka, J.T., Bergstrom, K.A., Karhu, J., Hiltunen, J., and Tiihonen, J. (1999) Dopamine transporter and D2-receptor density in late-onset alcoholism. *Psychopharmacology (Berl)* 147: 314–318.

Ricaurte, G.A., Forno, L.S., Wilson, M.A., DeLanney, L.E., Irwin, I., Molliver, M.E., and Langston, J.W. (1988) (+/–)3,4-Methylenedioxymethamphetamine selectively damages central serotonergic neurons in nonhuman primates. *JAMA* 260:51–55.

Ritz, M.C., Lamb, R.J., Goldberg, S.R., and Kuhar, M.J. (1987) Cocaine receptors on dopamine transporters are related to self-administration of cocaine. *Science* 237(4819):1219–1223.

Rolls, E.T. (2000) The orbitofrontal cortex and reward. *Cereb. Cortex* 10(3):284–294.

Rose, J.E. (2006) Nicotine and nonnicotine factors in cigarette addiction. *Psychopharmacology (Berl)* 184(3-4):274–285.

Rose, J.E., Behm, F.M., Salley, A.N., Bates, J.E., Coleman, R.E., Hawk, T.C., and Turkington, T.G. (2007) Regional brain activity correlates of nicotine dependence. *Neuropsychopharmacology* 32(12):2441–2452.

Scott, D.J., Domino, E.F., Heitzeg, M.M., Koeppe, R.A., Ni, L., Guthrie, S., and Zubieta, J.K. (2007) Smoking modulation of mu-opioid and dopamine D2 receptor-mediated neurotransmission in humans. *Neuropsychopharmacology* 32(2):450–457.

Scott, W.K., Zhang, F., Stajich, J.M., Scott, B.L., Stacy, M.A., and Vance, J.M. (2005) Family-based case-control study of cigarette smoking and Parkinson disease. *Neurology* 64(3):442–447.

Sekine, Y., Iyo, M., Ouchi, Y., Matsunaga, T., Tsukada, H., Okada, H., Yoshikawa, E., Futatsubashi, M., Takei, N., and Mori, N. (2001) Methamphetamine-related psychiatric symptoms and reduced brain dopamine transporters studied with PET. *Am. J. Psychiatry* 158:1206–1214.

Sekine, Y., Minabe, Y., Ouchi, Y., Takei, N., Iyo, M., Nakamura, K., Suzuki, K., Tsukada, H., Okada, H., Yoshikawa, E., Futatsubashi, M. and Mori, N. (2003) Association of dopamine transporter loss in the orbitofrontal and dorsolateral prefrontal cortices with methamphetamine-related psychiatric symptoms. *Am. J. Psychiatry* 160(9):1699–1701.

Sekine, Y., Ouchi, Y., Takei, N., Yoshikawa, E., Nakamura, K., Futatsubashi, M., Okada, H., Minabe, Y., Suzuki, K., Iwata, Y., Tsuchiya, K.J., Tsukada, H., Iyo, M., and Mori, N. (2006) Brain serotonin transporter density and aggression in abstinent methamphetamine abusers. *Arch. Gen. Psychiatry* 63(1):90–100.

Soyka, M., and Roesner, S. (2006) New pharmacological approaches for the treatment of alcoholism. *Expert Opin. Pharmacother.* 7(17):2341–2353.

Sprenger, T., Berthele, A., Platzer, S., Boecker, H., and Tolle, T.R. (2005) What to learn from in vivo opioidergic brain imaging? *Eur. J. Pain* 9(2):117–121.

Staley, J.K., Krishnan-Sarin, S., Cosgrove, K.P., Krantzler, E., Frohlich, E., Perry, E., Dubin, J.A., Estok, K., Brenner, E., Baldwin, R.M., Tamagnan, G.D., Seibyl, J.P., Jatlow, P., Picciotto, M.R., London, E.D., O'Malley, S., and van Dyck, C.H. (2006) Human tobacco smokers in early abstinence have higher levels of beta2* nicotinic acetylcholine receptors than nonsmokers. *J. Neurosci.* 26(34): 8707–8714.

Stefanini, E., Frau, M., Garau, M.G., Garau, B., Fadda, F., and Gessa, G.L. (1992) Alcohol-preferring rats have fewer dopamine D2 receptors in the limbic system. *Alcohol Alcohol.* 27:127–130.

Thanos, P.K., Taintor, N.B., Rivera, S.N., Umegaki, H., Ikari, H., Roth, G., Ingram, D.K., Hitzemann, R., Fowler, J.S., Gatley, S.J., Wang, G.J., and Volkow, N.D. (2004) DRD2 gene transfer into the nucleus accumbens core of the alcohol preferring and nonpreferring rats attenuates alcohol drinking. *Alcohol Clin. Exp. Res.* 28:720–728.

Thanos, P.K., Volkow, N.D., Freimuth, P., Umegaki, H., Ikari, H., Roth, G., Ingram, D.K., and Hitzemann, R. (2001) Overexpression of dopamine D2 receptors reduces alcohol self-administration. *J. Neurochem.* 78:1094–1103.

Thomasius, R., Zapletalova, P., Petersen, K., Buchert, R., Andresen, B., Wartberg, L., Nebeling, B., and Schmoldt, A. (2006) Mood, cognition and serotonin transporter availability in current and former ecstasy (MDMA) users: the longitudinal perspective. *J. Psychopharmacol.* 20(2):211–225.

Tupala, E., Hall, H., Bergstrom, K., Mantere, T., Rasanen, P., Sarkioja, T., and Tiihonen, J. (2003) Dopamine D2 receptors and transporters in type 1 and 2 alcoholics measured with human whole hemisphere autoradiography. *Hum. Brain Mapp.* 20:91–102.

Tupala, E., Hall, H., Bergstrom, K., Sarkioja, T., Rasanen, P., Mantere, T., Callaway, J., Hiltunen, J., and Tiihonen, J. (2001) Dopamine D(2)/D(3)-receptor and transporter densities in nucleus accumbens and amygdala of type 1 and 2 alcoholics. *Mol. Psychiatry* 6:261–267.

Vander Borght, T., Kilbourn, M., Desmond, T., Kuhl, D., and Frey, K. (1995) The vesicular monoamine transporter is not regulated by dopaminergic drug treatments. *Eur. J. Pharmacol.* 294(2/3): 577–583.

Volkow, N.D., Chang, L., Wang, G.-J., Fowler, J.S., Franceschi, D., Sedler, M.J., Gatley, S.J., Hitzemann, R., Ding, Y.S., Wong, C., and Logan J. (2001) Higher cortical and lower subcortical metabolism in detoxified methamphetamine abusers. *Am. J. Psychiatry* 158:383–389.

Volkow, N.D., Chang, L., Wang, G-J., Fowler, J.S., Franceschi, D., Sedler, M., Gatley, S.J., Miller, E., Hitzemann, R., Ding, Y.S., and Logan, J. (2001) Loss of dopamine transporters in methamphetamine abusers recovers with protracted abstinence. *J. Neurosci.* 21(23):9414–9418.

Volkow, N.D., Wang, G.J., Fowler, J.S., Logan, J., Gatley, S.J., Gifford, A., Hitzemann, R.,Ding, Y.S., and Pappas, N. (1999) Prediction of reinforcing responses to psychostimulants in humans by brain dopamine D2 receptor levels. *Am. J. Psychiatry* 156(9):1440–1443.

Volkow, N.D., and Fowler, J.S. (2000) Addiction, a disease of compulsion and drive: involvement of the orbitofrontal cortex. *Cereb. Cortex* 10:318–325.

Volkow, N.D., Fowler, J.S., Ding, Y.S., Wang, G-J., and Gatley, S.J. (1999) Imaging the neurochemistry of nicotine actions: studies with positron emission tomography. *Nicotine Tob. Res.* 1(Suppl 2):S127–S132; discussion S139–S140.

Volkow, N.D., Fowler, J.S., and Wang, G-J. (2003) Positron emission tomography and single-photon emission computed tomography in substance abuse research. *Semin. Nucl. Med.* 33(2): 114–128.

Volkow, N.D., Fowler, J.S., and Wang, G-J. (2004) The addicted human brain viewed in the light of imaging studies: brain circuits and treatment strategies. *Neuropharmacology* 47(Suppl 1):3–13.

Volkow, N.D., Fowler, J.S., Wolf, A.P., Hitzemann, R., Dewey, S., Bendriem, B., Alpert, R., and Hoff, A. (1991) Changes in brain glucose metabolism in cocaine dependence and withdrawal. *Am. J. Psychiatry* 148(5):621–626.

Volkow, N.D., Wang, G-J., Begleiter, H., Porjesz, B., Fowler, J.S., Telang, F., Wong, C., Ma, Y., Logan, J., Goldstein, R., Alexoff, D., and Thanos, P.K. (2006) High levels of dopamine D2 receptors in unaffected members of alcoholic families: possible protective factors. *Arch. Gen. Psychiatry* 63(9):999–1008.

Volkow, N.D., Wang, G-J., Fischman, M.W., Foltin, R., Fowler, J.S., Franceschi, D., Franceschi, M., Logan, J., Gatley, S.J., Wong, C., Ding, Y.S., Hitzemann, R., and Pappas, N. (2000) Effects of route of administration on cocaine induced dopamine transporter blockade in the human brain. *Life Sci.* 67(12):1507–1515.

Volkow, N.D., Wang, G-J, Fowler, J.S., Hitzemann, R., Angrist, B., Gatley, S.J., Logan, J., Ding, Y.S., and Pappas, N. (1999) Association of methylphenidate-induced craving with changes in right striato-orbitofrontal metabolism in cocaine abusers: implications in addiction. *Am. J. Psychiatry* 156:19–26.

Volkow, N.D., Wang, G-J., Fowler, J.S., Logan, J., Gatley, S.J., Hitzemann, R., Chen, A.D., Dewey, S.L., and Pappas, N. (1997) Decreased striatal dopaminergic responsiveness in detoxified cocaine-dependent subjects. *Nature* 386(6627):830–833.

Volkow, N.D., Wang, G-J., Fowler, J.S., Logan, J., Hitzemann, R., Ding, Y.S., Pappas, N., Shea, C., and Piscani, K. (1996) Decreases in dopamine receptors but not in dopamine transporters in alcoholics. *Alcohol Clin. Exp. Res.* 20:1594–1598.

Volkow, N.D., Wang, G-J., Fowler, J.S., Logan, J., Jayne, M., Franceschi, D., Wong, C., Gatley, S.J., Gifford, A.N., Ding, Y.S., and Pappas, N. (2002) "Nonhedonic" food motivation in humans involves dopamine in the dorsal striatum and methylphenidate amplifies this effect. *Synapse* 44(3):175–180.

Volkow, N.D., Wang, G-J., Franceschi, D., Fowler, J.S., Thanos, P.P., Maynard, L., Gatley, S.J., Wong, C., Veech, R.L., Kunos, G., and Li, T.K. (2006) Low doses of alcohol substantially decrease glucose metabolism in the human brain. *Neuroimage* 29(1):295–301.

Volkow, N.D., Wang, G-J., Hitzemann, R., Fowler, J.S., Overall, J.E., Burr, G., and Wolf, A.P. (1994) Recovery of brain glucose metabolism in detoxified alcoholics. *Am. J. Psychiatry* 151(2): 178–183.

Volkow, N.D., Wang, G-J., Ma, Y., Fowler, J.S., Wong, C., Ding, Y.S., Hitzemann, R., Swanson, J.M., and Kalivas, P. (2005) Activation of orbital and medial prefrontal cortex by methylphenidate in cocaine-addicted subjects but not in controls: relevance to addiction. *J. Neurosci.* 25(15):3932–3939.

Volkow, N.D., Wang, G-J., Maynard, L., Fowler, J.S., Jayne, B., Telang, F., Logan, J., Ding, Y.S., Gatley, S.J., Hitzemann, R., Wong, C., and Pappas, N. (2002) Effects of alcohol detoxification on dopamine D2 receptors in alcoholics: a preliminary study. *Psychiatry Res.* 116(3):163–172.

Volkow, N.D., Wang, G-J., Overall, J.E., Hitzemann, R., Fowler, J.S., Pappas, N., Frecska, E., and Piscani, K. (1997) Regional brain metabolic response to lorazepam in alcoholics during early and late alcohol detoxification. *Alcohol Clin. Exp. Res.* 21(7): 1278–1284.

Volkow, N.D., Wang, G-J., Fischman, M., Foltin, R., Fowler, J.S., Abumrad, N.N., Vitkun, S., Logan, J., Gatley, S.J., Pappas, N., Hitzemann, R., and Shea, C.E. (1997) Relationship between subjective effects of cocaine and dopamine transporter occupancy. *Nature* 386(6627):827–830.

Volkow, N.D., Wang, G-J., Telang, F., Fowler, J.S., Logan, J., Childress, A.R., Jayne, M., Ma, Y., and Wong, C. (2006) Cocaine cues and dopamine in dorsal striatum: mechanism of craving in cocaine addiction. *J. Neurosci.* 26(24):6583–6588.

Wang, G-J., Volkow, N.D., Chang, L., Miller, E., Sedler, M., Hitzemann, R., Zhu, W., Logan, J., Ma, Y., and Fowler, J.S. (2004) Partial recovery of brain metabolism in methamphetamine abusers after protracted abstinence *Am. J. Psychiatry* 161(2):242–248.

Wang, G-J., Volkow, N.D., Fowler, J.S., Cervany, P., Hitzemann, R.J., Pappas, N.R., Wong, C.T., and Felder, C. (1999) Regional brain metabolic activation during craving elicited by recall of previous drug experiences. *Life Sci.* 64(9):775–784.

Wang, G-J., Volkow, N.D., Fowler, J.S., Franceschi, D., Wong, C.T., Pappas, N.R., Netusil, N., Zhu, W., Felder, C., and Ma, Y. (2003) Alcohol intoxication induces greater reductions in brain metabolism in male than in female subjects. *Alcohol Clin. Exp. Res.* 27(6):909–917.

Wang, G-J., Volkow, N.D., Fowler, J.S., Pappas, N.R., Wong, C.T., Pascani, K., Felder, C.A., and Hitzemann, R.J. (1998) Regional cerebral metabolism in female alcoholics of moderate severity does not differ from that of controls. *Alcohol Clin. Exp. Res.* 22(8):1850–1854.

Waniewski, R.A., and Martin, D.L. (1998) Preferential utilization of acetate by astrocytes is attributable to transport, *J. Neurosci.* 18:5225–5233.

Wilson, J.M., Kalasinsky, K.S., Levey, A.I., Bergeron, C., Reiber, G., Anthony, R.M., Schmunk, G.A., Shannak, K., Haycock, J.W., and Kish, S.J. (1996) Striatal dopamine nerve terminal markers in human, chronic methamphetamine users. *Nat. Med.* 2:699–703.

Wong, D.F., Kuwabara, H., Schretlen, D.J., Bonson, K.R., Zhou, Y., Nandi, A., Brasic, J.R., Kimes, A.S., Maris, M.A., Kumar, A., Contoreggi, C., Links, J., Ernst, M., Rousset, O., Zukin, S., Grace, A.A., Lee, J.S., Rohde, C., Jasinski, D.R., Gjedde, A., and London, E.D. (2006) Increased occupancy of dopamine receptors in human striatum during cue-elicited cocaine craving. *Neuropsychopharmacology* 31(12):2716–2727.

Yang, Y.K., Yao, W.J., McEvoy, J.P., Chu, C.L., Lee, I.H., Chen, P.S., Yeh, T.L., and Chiu, N.T. (2006) Striatal dopamine D2/D3 receptor availability in male smokers. *Psychiatry Res.* 146(1): 87–90.

Yoder, K.K., Kareken, D.A., Seyoum, R.A., O'Connor, S.J., Wang, C., Zheng, Q.H., Mock, B., and Morris, E.D. (2005) Dopamine D(2) receptor availability is associated with subjective responses to alcohol. *Alcohol Clin. Exp. Res.* 29:965–970.

Zahniser, N.R., and Doolen, S. (2001) Chronic and acute regulation of Na+/Cl- -dependent neurotransmitter transporters: drugs, substrates, presynaptic receptors, and signaling systems. *Pharmacol. Ther.* 92(1):21–55.

Zhu, J.P.Q., Xu, W., and Angulo, J.A. (2006) MAMP-induced cell death: selective vulnerability in neuronal subpopulations of the striatum in mice. *Neuroscience* 140:607–622.

Zubieta, J.K., Gorelick, D.A., Stauffer, R., Ravert, H.T., Dannals, R.F., and Frost, J.J. (1996) Increased mu opioid receptor binding detected by PET in cocaine-dependent men is associated with cocaine craving. *Nat. Med.* 2(11):1225–1229.

Zubieta, J., Greenwald, M.K., Lombardi, U., Woods, J.H., Kilbourn, M.R., Jewett, D.M., Koeppe, R.A., Schuster, C.R., and Johanson, C.E. (2000) Buprenorphine-induced changes in mu-opioid receptor availability in male heroin-dependent volunteers: a preliminary study. *Neuropsychopharmacology* 23:326–334.

Zubieta, J.K., Heitzeg, M.M., Xu, Y., Koeppe, R.A., Ni, L., Guthrie, S., and Domino, E.F. (2005) Regional cerebral blood flow responses to smoking in tobacco smokers after overnight abstinence. *Am. J. Psychiatry* 162(3):567–577.

50 Brain Reward and fMRI

P. READ MONTAGUE AND PEARL H. CHIU

Questions about brain reward representations and neurobiological substrates of reward and reward processing form one of the broadest areas of neuroscience. The reason for this breadth derives from the fact that reward pursuit is one of the primary functions of a mobile creature, and so it is not surprising that the neural machinery devoted to reward processing is vast, multileveled, and related to every aspect of human cognition. Three decades ago, experiments on reward representation and processing focused almost exclusively on animal studies, and since that time, this work has evolved dramatically up and down. It has extended down to networks of identified molecular interactions (e.g., Hyman et al., 2006) and up to circuits underlying reward-guided choice and decision making in nonuman primates (e.g., Montague, Hyman, et al., 2004; Morris et al., 2004; Morris et al., 2006; Schultz, 2007). In this chapter, we focus on brain reward systems in humans using functional magnetic resonance imaging (fMRI) as the neural probe of choice and restrict our focus further to approaches in this area that lean on either computational modeling of brain reward systems or neuroeconomic probes during decision making. This chapter is taken almost verbatim from Montague (2007) in *Functional Neurology*.

Any discussion of reward processing in humans must first clarify the very broad use of the term *reward* and the kinds of stimuli, behavioral acts, internal mental states, and so on that can act as rewards for humans. More specifically, one must first specify what qualifies as a reward and why, and identify the quantitative settings in which rewards are defined and pursued. It is our general perspective here that by examining the way that rewards guide valuation and decision making, we can clarify and differentiate the uses of the term.

NEUROECONOMIC APPROACHES TO REWARD PROCESSING

Webster's *New Millennium™ Dictionary of English* defines *neuroeconomics* as "the study of the brain in making economic decisions, esp. to build a biological model of decision-making in economic environments." This same dictionary account of the word lists its birth date as the year 2002. The question on many scientists' minds, especially those interested in how any nervous system makes a decision, is just how different is neuroeconomics from behavioral and neuroscience research that has been going on for the last 50 years? Well, in terms of the issues raised, it is not, but in terms of its focus and future outlook, it is indeed opening new areas of inquiry. From the neuroscience side, neuroeconomics stands on the shoulders of a lot of behavioral and neural evidence derived from creatures ranging from fruit flies to humans. However, many issues in decision making and its neural and computational underpinnings, though not uniquely human, take a certain form in humans that is not always directly comparable in model systems such as rodents and fruit flies. Also, as alluded to, much of the work taking place in neuroeconomics has natural connections to computational neuroscience and, through that connection, to practical applications in psychiatry, neurology, and beyond. Last, it is altogether possible that the term *neuroeconomics* is unnecessarily limiting, and for neuroscientists should be thought of as "decision neuroscience" in the same manner that we naturally accept the term *molecular neuroscience*.

Efficiency and the Reward-Harvesting Problem

There are two natural neuroeconomics. The first, let's call it *neuroeconomics I*, addresses the way that neural tissue is built, sustains itself through time, and processes information efficiently. *Neuroeconomics II* concerns itself with the behavioral algorithms running on such neural tissue. This review focuses on neuroeconomics II but begins by highlighting important unanswered issues that arise in neuroeconomics I, and the most important issue is the efficient use of energy.

Modern-day computing devices generate an enormous amount of wasted heat, devoting only a small fraction of their thermal degrees of freedom to the computing itself. The wasted heat derives from many sources, but mainly from a design luxury not available to any evolved biological computers—a wall socket, that is, an ongoing and seemingly inexhaustible source of energy. Modern computers do not have to consider how to obtain their next volt or whether the program they are running is more efficient than some other equivalent way to solve the problem at hand. Without these worries troubling their design, modern computers compute with extremely high speed and accuracy, and they communicate information internally at high rates. All these features contribute to the generation of entropy (Montague, 2006). But most important, a modern computer's life has never depended on making choices about differentially allocating power to computing speed, energy usage, precision, or algorithm efficiency. This example provides a dramatic contrast to the computing economics of evolved biological systems.

In contrast to the example above, biological computers run on batteries that they must recharge using the behavioral strategies at their disposal; consequently, neural hardware and neural software of real creatures never had the option to be grossly inefficient (e.g., Bialek, 1987; Laughlin, 1994). This latter observation is beguiling because it seems so obvious, but it has crafted remarkable efficiency into the nervous system wherever we have been able to look closely, including visual processing (Barlow, 1961; Atick, 1992; Barlow, 2001; Simoncelli and Olshausen, 2001). The human brain runs on about 20–25 watts, representing 20%–25% of an 80- to 100-watt basal power consumption. All the processes that the brain controls—vision, audition, olfaction, standing, running, digestion, and so on—must share this extremely small energy consumption rate. No matter how one divides this energy consumption among ongoing neural computations, an unavoidable conclusion arises: evolved nervous systems compute with an almost freakish efficiency (e.g., Levy and Baxter, 1996; Laughlin et al., 1998; Laughlin, 2001; Attwell and Laughlin, 2001; Laughlin, 2004).

To be this efficient, biological computing devices must take account of investments—efficiencies in the operation of their parts and the algorithms running on those parts—and returns (expected increases in fitness). Collectively, these issues constitute what we call *neuroeconomics I*, the efficient operation of neural tissue. In the visual system, this kind of question has blossomed into a rich area of investigation that falls under the heading "natural visual statistics" approach to vision (or some congener of this name). The central idea is that the neural representations (processing strategies and organizational principles) in the visual system represent a "matching" of the encoding strategy in vision to the natural statistical structure present in the input "signals" (Ruderman, 1994; for review, see Simoncelli and Olshausen, 2001).

This efficiency perspective is important because it has not been applied systematically to the problem of harvesting rewards (Fig. 50.1A). Figure 50.1 does not do justice to the complexities of a creature wandering about and deciding where it should search for prey or whether such searches are worth it. It is a deeply economic problem, but it depends on the statistics of likely reward distributions in the world, and it depends on the internal states and goals of the creature: a creature's internal state changes the way it processes and values external stimuli. The idea of quantifying the statistics of external reward and variables related to internal state is implicit to work on optimal foraging—how an animal should choose to search to maximize its net return on some food or prey (Smith, 1982; Kamil et al., 1987; see Krebs et al., 1978, for a classic example). In summary, the "natural statistics of reward-harvesting" depends on (*1*) the internal "signals" of the organism type, (*2*) the possible redundancies latent in these signals, and (*3*) the way that both "match" the statistics of external stimuli and behavioral options. It is just a harder problem.

Why Should Heat Measures Correlate with Cognitive Variables?

The above efficiency perspective also invites and answers broadly an important question that arises in the context of modern neuroimaging experiments: Why should "heat measures" (fMRI measures) taken from small volumes of neural tissue encode information about the computations being carried out nearby? (Fig. 50.1B) The broad answer is efficiency. One should expect an extremely efficient device to couple the dynamics of ongoing power demands directly to the computations it is performing. In the most efficient scenario (generally impossible to achieve), the dynamics of metabolic demand in a small volume of neural tissue would be exactly equivalent to the computations carried out by that volume. These demand measures would exist across a range of time and space scales; therefore, one should not expect a measurement as crude as fMRI to detect all of them. Nevertheless, efficiency hypotheses provide some insight into why "heat measures" should relate in any sensible way to cognition. If neuroeconomics (as defined above) is to produce a truly biological account of decision making, then it must descend further into the efficient mechanisms that compose the nervous system. In short, it must reconnect deeply with neuroscience and take more seriously the styles of computation required to implement efficient behavioral algorithms in real neural tissue. The incipient steps of neuroeconomics have in large part tested decision making in humans and nonhuman primates with fMRI, positron emission tomography (PET), or single-unit electrophysiology as the neural probes of choice. But the really important connections will come when detailed mechanisms can be reconnected with the interesting behavioral and imaging work.

The second neuroeconomics, neuroeconomics II, chooses as its starting point behavioral algorithms and neural responses associated broadly with decision making and the kinds of valuations that underlie it. And it is explicitly here where portions of economics and neuroscience are beginning to find fruitful common ground. In particular, they find much common ground in computa-

A

+ Internal variables
Infer efficient decisions using statistics and value of rewards within natural scenes
Natural scenes equipped with 'rewards'

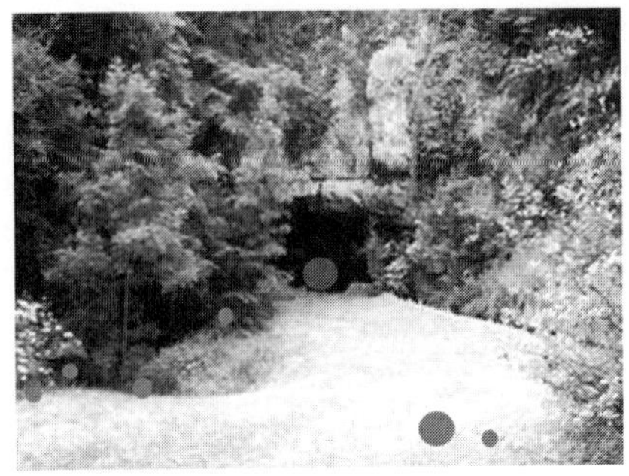

B

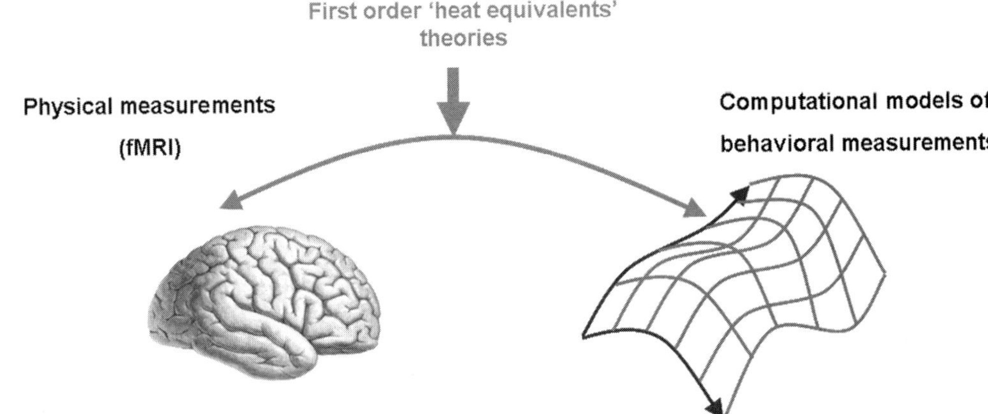

FIGURE 50.1 Efficient representations and their coupling to brain responses. (*A*) Reward harvesting is a complex problem that depends on processing cues from the world efficiently to "harvest prey" (circles) that may be difficult to find or catch. External sensory cues are only part of the problem. As indicated, the other source of signal originates within the creature seeking the rewards—the collection of "internal" signals that define its needs and goals. These variables can change dramatically the value of external stimuli. An efficient nervous system should contain representations that match the internal needs of the creature to the external signals that meet those needs. This is clearly a complex and dynamic problem. (*B*) Because of their dependence on local changes in blood flow and other proxies for metabolic demand, current non-invasive imaging approaches to human brain function (PET and fMRI) implicitly draw a relationship (not an equivalence) between cognitive variables and something akin to a "heat" measure. PET: positron emission tomography; fMRI: functional magnetic resonance imaging.

tional models or explanations grounded in an area called reinforcement learning (RL) (Sutton and Barto, 1998).

Reward-Harvesting, Reinforcement Learning (RL) Models, and Dopamine

As outlined above, the problem of efficiently harvesting rewards from the real world is a complex task that depends on signals inside and outside the organism. In short, a creature needs efficient internal representations that match its collection of internal needs to the external signals that meet those needs. One approach to these problems is called *reinforcement learning* (RL), a modeling approach that casts the reward-harvesting problem explicitly as an interaction between the internal needs of the creature, the external signals from the environment, and an internal teaching signal that depends on both (Sutton and Barto, 1998). Biologically, RL models have provided insight into the computations distributed by midbrain dopamine (DA) neurons, an important neuromodulatory system involved in reward processing and decision making related to reward harvesting (see Daw and Doya, 2006, for a recent review). We review the essence of these models here before showing their application to imaging experiments in humans.

Modeling work on midbrain DA neurons has progressed dramatically over the last decade, and the research community is now equipped with a collection of computational models that depict very explicitly the kinds of information thought to be constructed and broadcast by this system (Montague et al., 1993; Montague and Sejnowski, 1994; Montague et al., 1996; Schultz et al.,

1997; Dayan and Balleine, 2002; Daw and Doya, 2006; for overall review, see Montague, McClure, et al., 2004; for application to addiction, see Redish, 2004). These models arose initially to account for detailed single-unit electrophysiology in midbrain DA neurons recorded while primates carry out simple learning and decision-making tasks (Ljungberg et al., 1992; Quartz et al., 1992; Montague et al., 1994, 1996) or to account for decision making in honeybees equipped with similar neurons (Montague et al., 1995). A large subset of the midbrain DA neurons participate in circuits that learn to value and to predict future rewarding events, especially the delivery of primary rewards such as food, water, and sex (Montague et al., 1996; Schultz et al., 1997; Schultz, 1998; Schultz and Dickinson, 2000; Waelti et al., 2001; Dayan and Abbott, 2001; Montague and Berns, 2002; Bayer and Glimcher, 2005; also see Delgado et al., 2000).

Collectively, these findings have motivated a specific computational hypothesis suggesting that DA neurons emit reward prediction errors encoded in modulations in their spike output (Montague and Sejnowski, 1994; Montague et al., 1996; Schultz et al., 1997). This hypothesis is strongly supported by the timing and amplitude of burst and pause responses in the spike trains of these neurons (Quartz et al., 1992; Montague and Sejnowski, 1994; Montague et al., 1996; Schultz et al., 1997; Waelti et al., 2001; Montague, McClure, et al., 2004; Bayer and Glimcher, 2005). In recent years, this work has evolved significantly, and this model is correct for a subset of transient responses, but clearly not all transient responses (Ikemoto and Panksepp, 1999; Redgrave et al., 1999; theory to explain anomalies: Kakade and Dayan, 2002; also see: Morris et al., 2006; Redgrave and Gurney, 2006). Also, the model does not account at all for slow changes in DA levels that would be detectable with methods such as microdialysis. The complaints about the theory ride on top of the reward prediction error hypothesis, that is, they posit extra information being carried by DA transients. The most coherent theoretical account is that by Kakade and Dayan (2002) and posits an extra "bonus" signal for exploration encoded in dopaminergic transients, an idea followed up on by Redgrave and Gurney (2006).

Despite these open issues, the reward prediction error hypothesis for rapid changes in dopaminergic spike activity continues to explain an important part of the repertoire of responses available to these neurons (Fig. 50.2). In words, *increases* in spike activity (from background rates) mean "things are better than expected," *decreases* mean "things are worse than expected," and *no change* means "things are just as expected." In this interpretation, this system is always emitting information to downstream neural structures because even no change in firing rate carries meaning. The reward prediction error (RPE) takes the following form:

RP error = **current** reward + γ (**next** reward prediction) – (**current** reward prediction),

where γ is a scaling factor between 0 and 1 and represents a way to weight the near-term future more heavily than the distant future. For our purposes, two aspects of this equation are critical: (*1*) The system uses "forward models" to produce an online estimate of the next reward prediction, which is constantly combined with the current experienced reward and current reward prediction. (*2*) The predictions and their comparison across time represent an underlying value function stored in the animal's brain. To see this, we write the model as:

RP error = **current** reward + γV (**next** internal state) – V (**current** internal state).

Here, the function V, called a *value function*, is written as a function of the internal state of the animal. In this expression, valuation takes the form of a value function that associates with each internal state a number, its "value," which represents the total reward that can be expected (on average) from that state into the distant future (reviewed in Montague, McClure, et al., 2004; Daw and Doya, 2006). This kind of stored value is like a long-term judgment; it "values" each state. And it is these values that can be updated through experience and under the guidance of reinforcement signals like the DA reward prediction error. Notice one important fact implicit here—the values are silent, stored numbers. There is no natural way to read out values directly; therefore, experiments on valuation must tease out the underlying value functions indirectly (Fig. 50.3).

The RPE signal highlighted above is exactly the learning signal used in the temporal difference (TD) algorithm familiar to the machine learning field (Kaelbling et al., 1996; Sutton and Barto, 1998). In this computer science context, the learning signal is called the *TD error* and is used in dual modes (*1*) to learn better predictions of future rewards and (*2*) to choose actions that lead to rewarding outcomes. This dual use of the TD error signal is called an *actor-critic system* (Fig. 50.3). We use the terms *TD error* and *reward prediction error* interchangeably.

When used as a learning signal, the RPE can be used to improve predictions of the value of the states of the organisms using simple Hebbian (correlational) learning rules (Montague et al., 1995; Montague et al., 1996; Schultz et al., 1997). A collection of adaptive weights (w) used to represent these predicted values are updated directly in proportion to this TD error—that is, the weights change (Δw) in proportion to the (signed) reward prediction error:

$\Delta w \, \alpha$ TD error (learning rule).

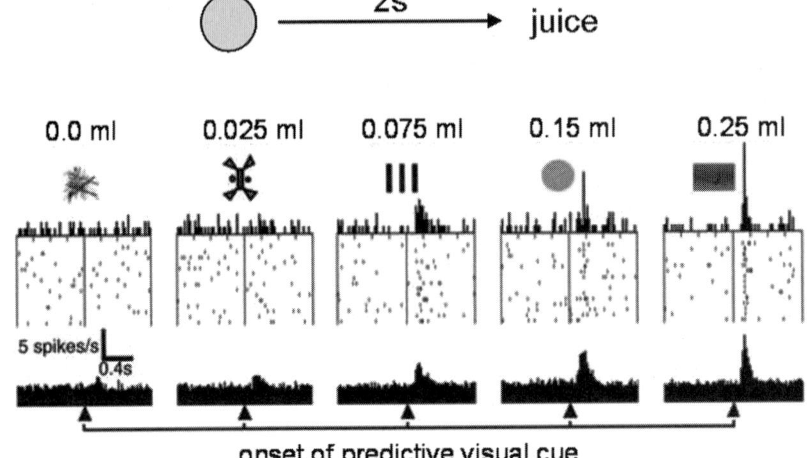

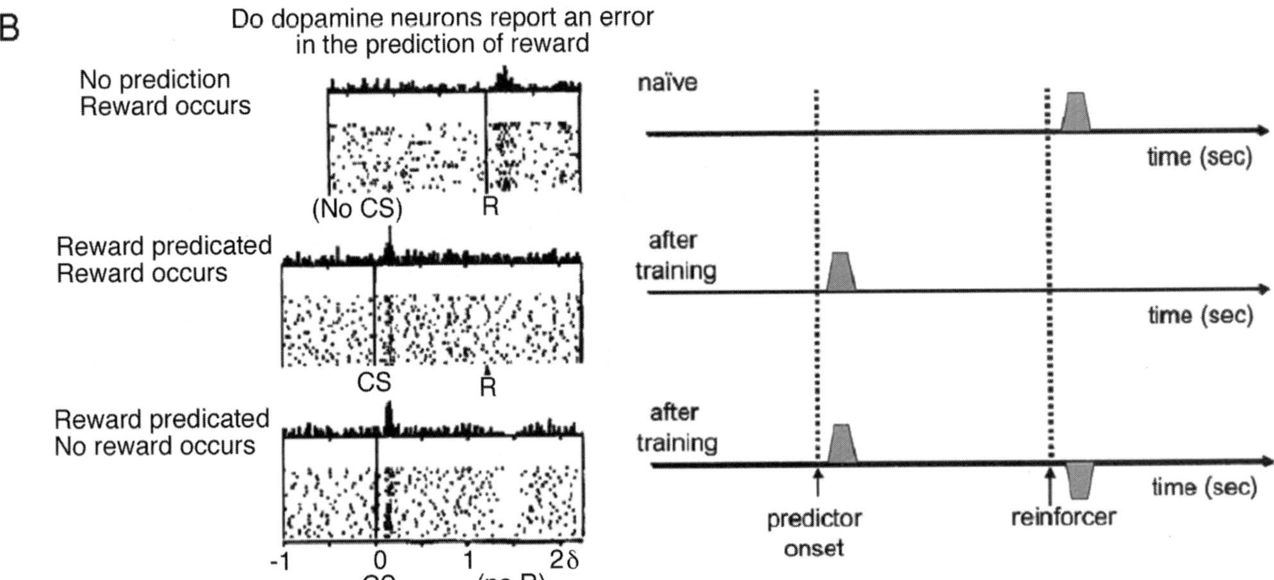

FIGURE 50.2 Dopamine transients encode prediction errors in expected value of future reward. (*A*) Dopamine spike activity and expected value of future reward. During training, each visual cue predicted reward 2 seconds later (recordings from alert monkey), but with differing expected values. The expected value of the future reward (probability p of reward × magnitude m of reward) was (left to right) 0 ml ($p = 1 \times m = 0$ ml), 0.025 ml ($p = 0.5 \times m = 0.05$ ml), 0.075 ml ($p = 0.5 \times m = 0.15$ ml), 0.15 ml ($p = 1.0 \times m = 0.15$ ml), and 0.25 ml ($p = 0.5 \times m = 0.50$ ml). Bin width is 10 ms. Single dopamine neurons spike activity is shown at top with their overlying spike histograms. Spike histograms over 57 neurons are shown at bottom (adapted from Tobler et al., 2005). The TD error signal $r_t + \gamma V(S_{t+1}) - V(S_t)$ accounts for exactly this pattern of change with learning, where S_t is the state of the animal at time t. It also accounts for changes in firing when the timing of reward is changed because this changes dramatically the expected value of reward at the trained time. (*B*) Spike modulation in dopamine neurons carries reward prediction error. (*Top panel*) Dopamine neuron increases its spiking rate at the unexpected delivery of a rewarding fluid (spike histogram on top, individual spike trains beneath). (*Middle panel*) After repeated pairings of visual cue (CS) with fluid reward delivery 1 second later, the transient modulation to reward delivery (R) drops back into baseline and transfers to the time of the predictive cue (CS). (*Bottom panel*) On catch trials, omission of reward delivery causes pause response in dopamine neuron at the time that reward delivery should have occurred based on previous training. (Traces recorded from alert monkey; adapted from Schultz et al., 1997; Montague and Berns, 2002.) The TD error signal $r_t + \gamma V(S_{t+1}) - V(S_t)$ accounts for exactly this pattern of change with learning, where S_t is the state of the animal at time t.

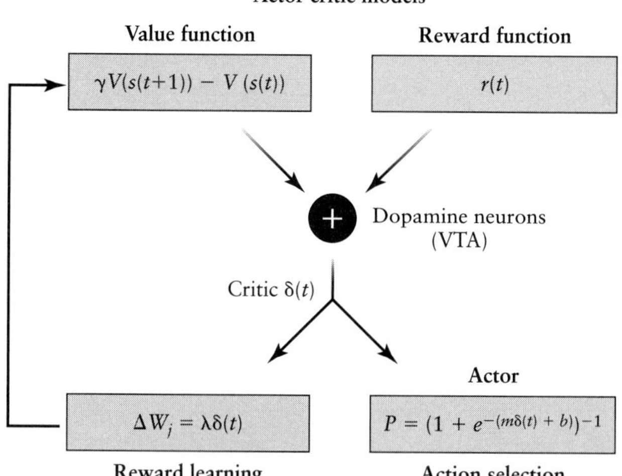

FIGURE 50.3 Hypothesized relationships of actor–critic models to dopamine neuron spike output. Value function information (across states and through time) and reward information combine linearly at the level of dopamine neurons. This combination, if encoded in spike modulations, means that changes in activity encode RPEs $\delta(t)$. This signal is a signed quantity and can be used in target neural structures for learning and action choice. (Adapted from Montague et al., 1996; Montague, Hyman, and Cohen, 2004; also see McClure et al., 2003.)

The congruence of the TD error signal to measured dopaminergic spike activity is quite remarkable. The TD model predicts that the expected value (probability of reward × magnitude of reward) of the delivered reward will be encoded in the transient modulation of DA spike activity. This feature can be seen in Figure 50.2A for conditioned cues that predict different expected values for future rewards. In this figure, each cue predicted fluid delivery 2 seconds into the future, and the amounts listed above each cue are the expected value of that delivery, that is, the probability of delivery × magnitude. The results reproduced here show dopaminergic neuron activity after overtraining on the displayed visual cues (Tobler et al., 2005).

As shown in Figure 50.2B, the model also predicts important temporal features of spike activity changes during conditioning tasks. For example, the unexpected delivery of food and fluid rewards causes burst responses in these neurons (R in Fig. 50.2B). If a preceding sensory cue, such as a light or sound, consistently predicts the time and expected value of the future reward, two dramatic changes occur as learning proceeds: (*1*) the transient response to reward delivery drops back to baseline firing levels and (*2*) a transient response occurs at the time of the earliest predictive sensory cue (CS in middle panel, Fig. 50.2B). However, the system keeps track of the expected time of reward delivery; if reward is not delivered at the expected time after the predictive cue, the firing rate decreases dramatically at the expected time of reward. Recent experiments by Bayer and Glimcher (2005) quantified precisely dopaminergic spiking behavior during reward-dependent saccade experiments in alert monkeys and concluded that these neurons indeed encode a quantitative RPE signal.

To be clear about the scope of this model, it applies strictly to rapid transients in spike rates in the 50–250 millisecond range and does not apply to other timescales of dopaminergic modulation that may well carry other information important for cognitive processing and behavioral control. For example, the model is agnostic with regard to baseline DA levels or even fluctuations on slightly slower timescales such as minutes to hours. Consequently, the model would not account for microdialysis results whose measurements lie in these temporal regimes.

Reward Prediction Error Model Guides fMRI Experiments in Humans

Passive and active conditioning tasks

The RPE model has now been extended to fMRI experiments in humans. Numerous reward expectancy experiments have now been carried out that probe human blood oxygen level dependent (BOLD) responses that correlate with RPEs (Knutson et al., 2000; Berns et al., 2001; Knutson et al., 2001; McClure, Berns, and Montague, 2003; O'Doherty et al., 2003; O'Doherty et al., 2004; for reviews, see O'Doherty, 2004; Montague et al., 2006). This work consistently demonstrates a BOLD response in the ventral striatum and ventral parts of the dorsal striatum that correlate with a TD error expected throughout the task in question (Fig. 50.4A).

One extremely important finding by O'Doherty et al. (2004) is that the BOLD-encoded RPE signals can be dissociated in the dorsal and ventral striatum according to whether an action is required for the acquisition of the reward. This finding is depicted in Figure 50.4B. For passive tasks, the RPE is evident not only in ventral striatum and in active tasks; it is evident in both, but with a strong component in the dorsal striatum (Fig. 50.4B). These findings and the model-based analysis that uncovered them suggest that stimulus–response learning typical of actor–critic circuits in humans may be associated with activation in the dorsal striatum.

Reward Prediction Error Signals Tracked During Sequential Decision Making

The decision task shown in Figure 50.5 (see also COLOR FIGURE 50.5 in separate insert) is a modification of a task meant to test a theory of decision making under uncertainty called *melioration* (Herrnstein and Prelec, 1991; Egelman et al., 1998). This task can be envis-

A

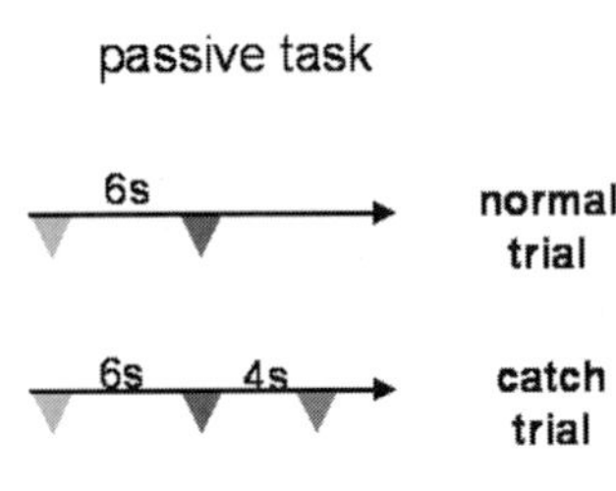

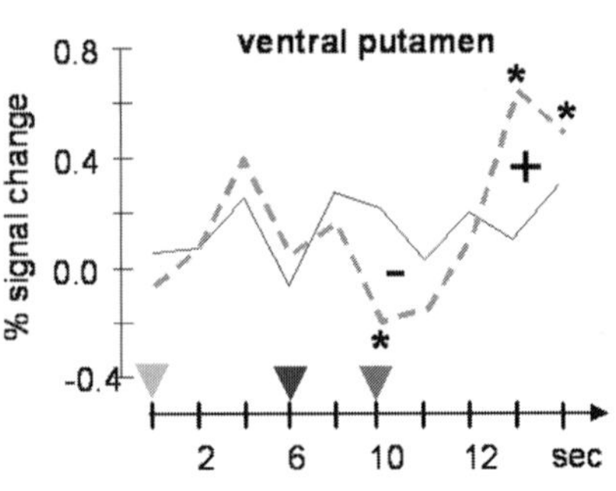

B

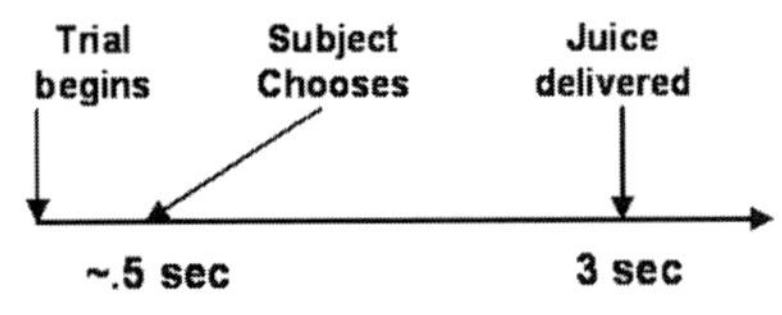

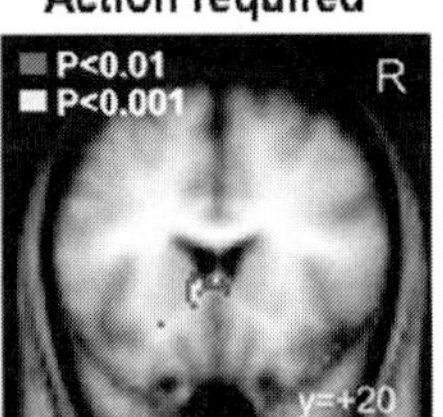

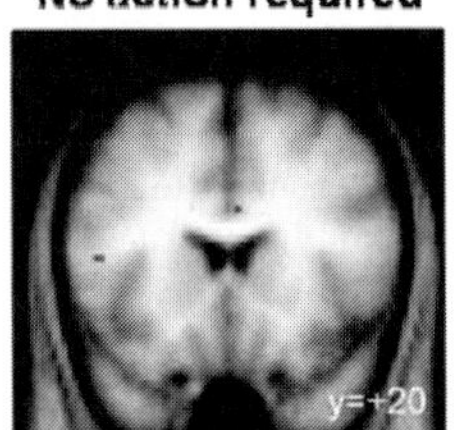

FIGURE 50.4 Actor and critic signals in humans detected by fMRI. (*A*) A simple conditioning task reveals a TD-like prediction-error signal (critic signal; see Fig. 50.3) encoded in hemodynamic responses in the human brain. On a normal training trial, a cue (light gray arrowhead) is followed by the passive delivery of pleasant-tasting juice (dark gray arrowhead) while subjects are scanned (TR = 2 seconds). After training on these contingencies, catch trials were randomly interleaved, and the reward delivery was delayed. Reward reliability continued at 100%, only the time of delivery was changed. The TD model predicts a negative prediction error at the time juice was expected but not delivered and a positive prediction error at the (unexpected) delayed time. At these moments, the expected value of reward deviates positively and negatively from that learned during training. Taking hemodynamic delays into account (~4 seconds), a prediction error of each polarity (positive and negative) can be seen in the ventral putamen during a surprising catch trial. The thin line is the average hemodynamic response during a normal trial, and the dashed line is the average hemodynamic response during a catch trial (original data from McClure, Berns, and Montague, 2003). (*B*) Identification of potential actor response in dorsal striatum (see Fig. 50.3). A conditioning task is carried out in two modes requiring (*1*) a button press (an action) and (*2*) no action at all. The dorsal striatum—a region involved in action selection—responds only during the mode where action is required and shows no response when an action is not required. This is the first demonstration of an actor response detected in the human brain. (Legend adapted from Montague, Hyman, and Cohen, 2004, Fig. 4; original data from O'Doherty et al., 2004). fMRI: functional magnetic resonance imaging.

aged as a simple way to model real-world choices, where the rewards from a choice change as that choice is sampled. In Figure 50.5, the payoff functions for each choice (A or B) change as a function of the fraction of choices allocated to button A in the last 20 choices (Li et al., 2006; also see Daw and Doya, 2006, for review). As choice A is selected, the individual is moved to the right on the *x* axis (fraction allocated to A increases), and so choosing A (red) near the crossing point in the curves causes the returns from subsequent choices to A to decrease, whereas the returns from B increase (magnified in inset). The reward functions model a common scenario encountered by creatures in the real world.

Imagine a bee sampling one flower type repeatedly while ignoring a second flower that it might also sample. All things being equal, as the flower is sampled, its nectar returns decrease (analogue to A, red) whereas the other unsampled flower (analogue to B, blue) type refills, thereby increasing its nectar return the next time it is sampled. A decision model like an actor–critic architecture (Fig. 50.3) that uses a TD error signal as its input gets stuck sampling near such crossing points because this is a stable point for the dynamics of the model (explained in the appendix of Montague and Berns, 2002). Behaviorally, humans do indeed get stuck near the crossing point; however, these data show that a "TD regressor" for the entire 250-choice experiment identifies a strong neural correlate of TD error in the putamen (right panel of Fig. 50.5). Figure 50.5B shows that the model also captures the choice behavior exhib-

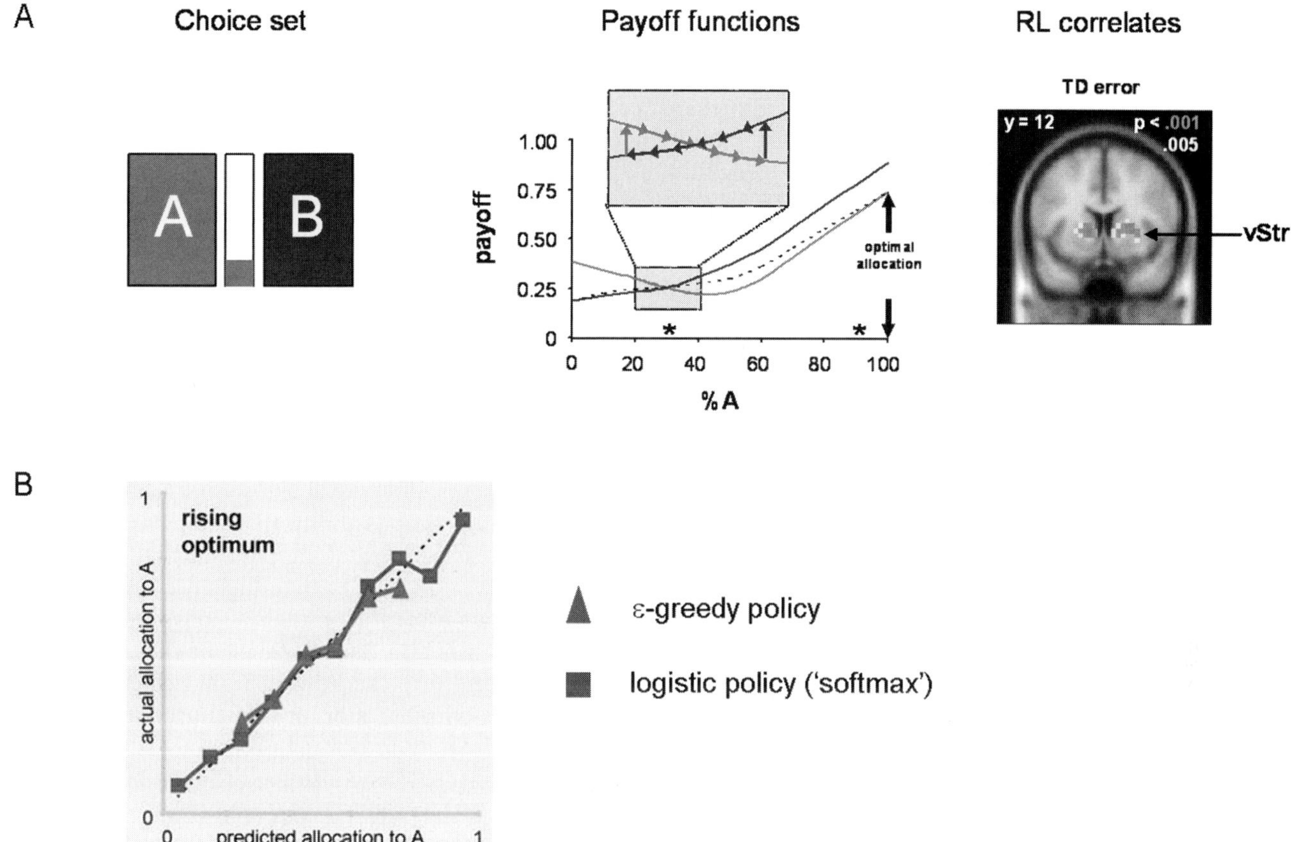

FIGURE 50.5 Actor–critic signals during sequential two-choice decision task. (*A*) Neural correlate of reward prediction error during sequential choice task. (Left) Two-choice task with returns encoded by centrally placed slider bar. (Middle) Inset shows the average behavior of a temporal difference (TD)-error-driven actor–critic model near the crossing point in the reward function. The colored arrows (see COLOR FIGURE 50.5 in separate insert) show what happens when red (A) or blue (B) is chosen, and they indicate the direction that the participants move along the x axis. The inset shows how these functions model one typical real-world occurrence for simple choices—choosing to sample A (red) tends to decrease returns from A while the unsampled returns from B increase, like flowers refilling with nectar while they are not being sampled. An actor–critic model will tend to stick near crossing points (explained in Montague and Berns, 2002). (Right) The hemodynamic correlate of a TD error signal throughout the entire 250 choices in this task is shown at two levels of significance (.001 and .005 [random effect]; $N = 46$; y = 12 mm). The payoff functions for this task are modified from a task originally proposed by Herrnstein and Prelec (1991) to test a theory of choice called *melioration* (adapted almost verbatim from Li et al., 2006). (*B*) Actor–critic model captures choice behavior. Participant decisions were predicted using a reinforcement learning model with two different methods to determine the probability to choose an action (ε-greedy method and sigmoid method). For both methods, we assume that participants maintained independent estimates of the reward expected for each choice, A and B, and updated these values based on experienced rewards using a choice-dependent TD-error (that is, the Rescorla-Wagner learning algorithm). Choices were assumed to be (*1*) probabilistically related to choice values according to a sigmoid function (softmax method, green curve) or (*2*) have a fixed probability of $1\text{-}\varepsilon/2$ for choice associated with bigger weight (ε-greedy method, pink curve). Decisions were binned (x axis) based on predicted likelihood that subjects would choose A. Y values indicate the actual average allocation to A for all choices within each bin. Linear regression shows there is a strong correlation between predicted and actual choices. (MS: $r = 0.97$, RO: $r = 0.99$, FR: $r = 0.97$, PR: $r = 0.97$ for softmax method; MS: $r = 0.97$, RO: $r = 0.99$, FR: $r = 0.95$, PR: $r = 0.99$ for ε-greedy method). (Adapted almost verbatim from Li et al., 2006.) MS: Matching Shoulder; RO: Rising Optimum; FR: Flat Return; PR: Pseudorandom.

ited by humans on this task. Here, the model is the simple actor–critic architecture illustrated in Figure 50.3 and using a sigmoid decision function ("softmax" function) that takes the TD error as input. In Figure 50.13, we illustrate how neural correlates of components of computational models (here the "TD regressor") can be identified during reward-guided decision tasks (see Montague, McClure, et al., 2004; Daw and Doya, 2006; Montague et al., 2006; Lohrenz et al., 2007; Chiu et al., 2008).

On this simple two-choice decision task, the computational model is a central component in the identification of hemodynamic responses that correlate with the TD error signal (see "RL correlates" in Fig. 50.5). The procedure for identifying these RL correlates is straightforward. For each individual, we model the TD error signal throughout the entire task, use this model to generate a sequence of choices using the actor–critic choice model shown in Figure 50.3, and extract three parameters (learning rate and two initial weights for each button) that minimize the difference between the predicted sequence of choices and the individual's measured sequence of choices. This is done separately for each individual. The fitted parameters that produce the best behavioral match are used to compute the TD error signal throughout the entire experiment (250 choices). This best-fit TD error is idiosyncratic for each individual because individuals generate different sequences of choices on the task. The best-fit TD error signal is then convolved with the hemodynamic response function to produce the predicted hemodynamic response for the TD error (see Fig. 50.13 for illustration). The predicted hemodynamic response is then entered into a standard general linear model regression with the measured MR data (Friston et al., 1994; Ashburner and Friston, 1999), and regions of the brain that show the same hemodynamic profile are identified using *t* tests. This is the "RL correlate" shown in Figure 50.5 in the putamen. In contrast to this method, the TD correlate shown in Figure 50.4A is a fluctuation measured directly in the average hemodynamic response (McClure, Berns, and Montague, 2003; O'Doherty et al., 2003; O'Doherty et al., 2004). All details of the fitting procedures can be found clearly in Li et al. (2006).

Anticipation of Secondary Reward (Money) Also Activates Striatum

In this chapter, we are focusing on model-based approaches to reward processing as detected by fMRI; however, human reward responses generate very consistent activations across a common set of subcortical and cortical areas. Some of the earliest work in this area using fMRI was carried out by Breiter and colleagues and others (Breiter et al., 1997; Thut et al., 1997; Breiter et al., 2001). This group recorded responses to cocaine injections and found pronounced activation in the orbitofrontal cortex and the nucleus accumbens among a collection of reward-related regions. Early work by Knutson and colleagues also showed pronounced activation of the nucleus accumbens, but this group showed accumbal activations anticipating the receipt of reward (money) (Knutson et al., 2000; Knutson et al., 2001; see Figure 50.6). In addition, they found that the peak accumbal responses correlated with the amount of money received. Delgado et al. (2000) and Elliott et al. (2003) also identified, early on, large striatal responses to monetary rewards and punishments. Collectively, this work was important in establishing the possibility that more sophisticated reward processing was taking place at the level of the striatum. It is now almost paradigmatic that one can make such an assertion, but these reward-processing experiments using a noninvasive probe that could look "deep enough" into the human brain helped motivate more serious consideration of the striatum as a region involved intimately in reward processing. Prior to this time, the striatum was considered to be a brain region primarily (but not exclusively) involved in the selection and sequencing of motor behaviors (for review, see Wickens, 1993).

HARVESTING REWARDS FROM OTHER AGENTS

We have now seen consistent fMRI-detectable responses to reward delivery, anticipation of reward delivery, and the sequential delivery of rewards predicated on a se-

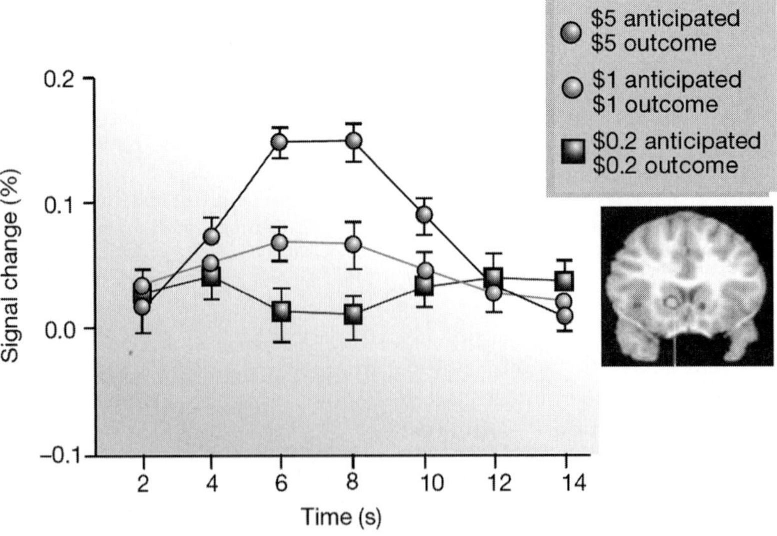

FIGURE 50.6 Anticipation of reward activates striatum. Hemodynamic response to reward delivery grows with time from a cue until reward is delivered. The peak response scales with the amplitude of the monetary reward. (Adapted from Knutson et al., 2001.)

quence of actions. Many of these results were guided, either in their design or interpretation, by reinforcement learning models of reward processing and decision making, or at least were motivated in part by these models. As with any model-based approach, the model is always too simple an account of the reality exposed by the experiments, but it is not a stretch to claim that the reinforcement learning models have significantly structured our arguments and approaches to the vast array of problems associated with adaptively defining procuring rewards. We turn now to a class of behavior most important for humans—harvesting rewards through interaction with other humans. It is in this domain that the idea of a reward signal becomes most abstract, and in the case of empathy and norm enforcement (see Figs. 50.15, 50.16), rewards (both signs) can pass from one individual to another without any exchange of material between the two individuals. This is the sense in which fairness norms and deviations from them form a true common currency within and across individual humans. Although we cannot yet compute the exchange rates of such currencies across individuals, we can indeed see their impact. We start with fairness games derived from the behavioral and experimental economic fields.

It is a rather intuitive claim that fairness between two humans is equivalent in some currency to a trade where both parties feel satisfied with the outcome without being coerced to feel this way. Almost by construction, the idea of fairness implies some understood norm of what is expected from another human when an exchange is carried out. In addition, we all recognize that the idea of a fair exchange between individuals extends well beyond the exchange of material goods (Camerer, 2003). Despite these expansive possibilities, fairness, like many other social sentiments, can be operationalized and probed with mathematically portrayed games (or staged interactions) played with other humans (Camerer, 2003; Camerer and Fehr, 2006).

Economic Games Expose Fairness Norms and Abstract Prediction Error Responses

In exchanges with other humans, efficient reward harvesting—in the form of immediate rewards, favors, or future promises of either—requires an agent to be able to model his or her partner and future interactions with that partner. An individual lacking this modeling capacity is literally incapable of protecting his or her own interests in interactions with others (Camerer and Fehr, 2006). It is well known that mental illness in many forms debilitates one's capacity to interact and exchange fruitfully with other humans, and such incapacities are one important part of human cognition that psychiatry seeks to repair. Consequently, it is particularly important to be able to probe brain responses during active social exchanges among humans and place the results into some quantitative framework. Currently, neuroimaging work in this area has been focused on two-person interactions (Rilling et al., 2002; de Quervain et al., 2004; Rilling et al., 2004a, 2004b; King-Casas et al., 2005; Singer et al., 2006; Tomlin et al., 2006), with one notable exception: using a social conformity experiment in the style of Asch (Asch, 1951; Berns et al., 2005).

One particularly fruitful approach has been the use of economic exchange games. Figure 50.7 illustrates the Ultimatum Game, probably better termed "take-it-or-leave-it." Player X is endowed with an amount of money (or some other valuable resource) and offers a split of this endowment to player Y, who can either accept or reject the offer. If player Y accepts, both players walk away with money; however, if player Y rejects, then no one gets anything. A "rational agent" account of this game would predict that player Y should accept all nonzero offers (Guth et al., 1982; also see Camerer, 2003; Fig. 50.7). Humans reject at a rate of about 50% at roughly a 70:30 to 80:20 split. The data in figure 50.7B (right panel) show a 50% rejection rate at around 70:30 (adapted from Camerer and Fehr, 2006). The reader might stop to "simulate" what they might accept or reject. Notice that the rejection rate changes when the number of responders increases—the presence of second responder causes both responders to accept a poorer split from the proposer. This game and others like it (Rilling et al., 2002) probe fairness norms and in the context of fMRI show that deviations from fairness norms act like rewards and punishments and even change behaviors and brain responses quite significantly (Rilling et al., 2002; Sanfey et al., 2003; Rilling et al., 2004a; King-Casas et al., 2005).

Figure 50.8 shows a bilateral insula response to unfair offers from other humans (deviation from fairness norm shown in Fig. 50.7B), a finding consistent with its responses to negative emotional outcomes (Phillips et al., 1997; Damasio et al., 2000; Sanfey et al., 2003). This response was found to be diminished for a given level of unfairness if individuals played on a computer (Sanfey et al., 2003). Of course, negative emotions may follow the neural signal flagging a deviation from the fairness norm, but the important point here is that in the economic game, it is easy to quantify the norm. Damage to the insula is consistent with its role in computing deviations from norms if we allow that norms are continually being updated by experience (Dani and Montague, 2007). In chronic smokers, damage to the insula appears to create a state where smokers do not generate feelings that they need to smoke—they find it subjectively easier to avoid relapse after quitting (Naqvi et al., 2007). They may have lost their ability to compare their norms to their internal state or to link such comparison to negative emotional states, which becomes the proximate motivating mechanism to smoke again. The Ultimatum Game is particularly clarifying in suggest-

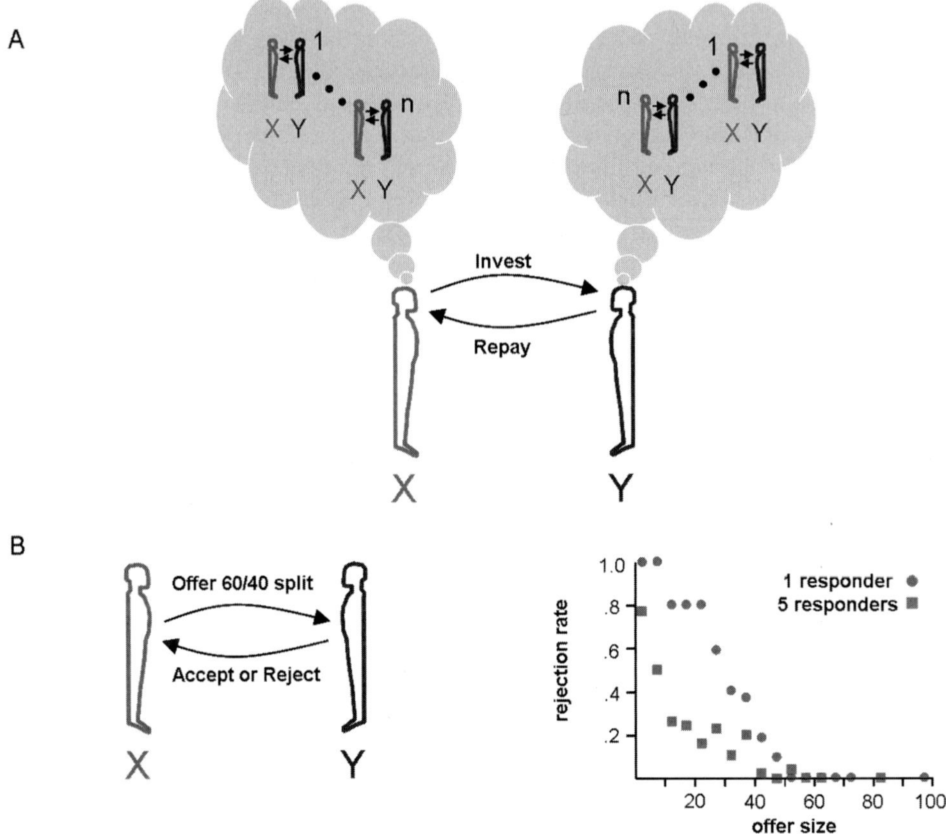

FIGURE 50.7 Two-person economic games expose fairness norms. (*A*) Exchange games between humans engage internal models of others, which may simulate interactions forward for a variable number of exchanges. These interactions evolved in the context of social exchange where multiple encounters were not only likely but were the norm. On these grounds, it is not unreasonable to expect such games to engender models of others that simulate multiple iterations with a partner. (*B*) Ultimatum game (take-it-or-leave-it). On-shot game where a player starts with a fixed amount of money and offers some split (here, 60:40) to the partner. If the partner accepts, both players walk away with money (take it). If the player rejects the offer, neither player gets anything (leave it). A rational agent should accept any nonzero offers (Guth et al., 1982; also see Camerer, 2003), but, in fact, the human rejection rate is 50% at 80:20 split, and, as illustrated here, will change as the number of responders increases. One interpretation of these results is that humans possess well-established fairness norms (Fehr and Schmidt, 1999).

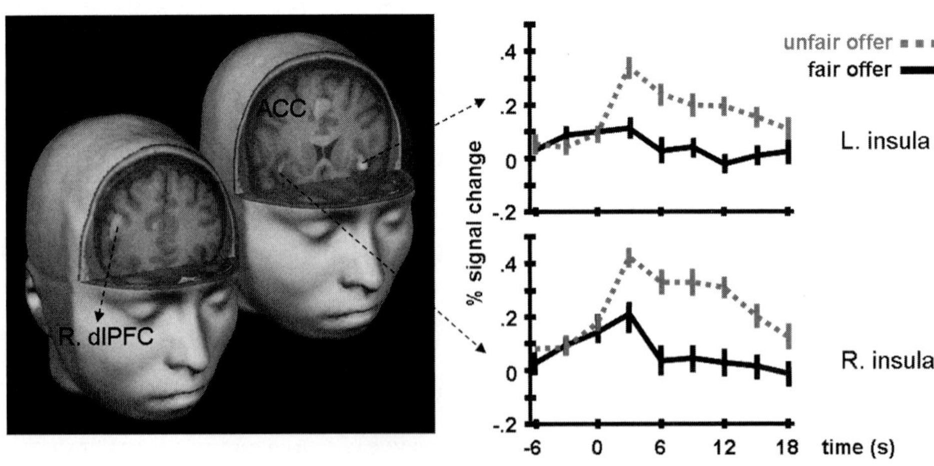

FIGURE 50.8 Insula responds to norm violation in a fairness game. Average hemodynamic responses of the right (R.) and left (L.) insula to the revelation of the proposer's offer in an ultimatum game. Traces are separated by the fairness of the proposer's offer. On this particular version, $10 was split between the players in integral dollar amounts. The behavior showed that offers less than or equal to $2 from a human partner were treated as unfair, that is, rejected at a rate of ~50%. dlPFC = dorso-lateral prefrontal cortex; ACC = anterior cingulate cortex. (Adapted from Sanfey et al., 2003, and data kindly provided by the authors.)

ing these possibilities and useful because the possibilities are easily put into a quantitative model. The exact answer awaits future work.

The Ultimatum Game gives a one-shot probe of norms and norm violation, but without any reputations forming between the interacting humans. In normal life, reputations built with another human form the basis of relationships with others—another area where mental illness can have devastating consequences. However, reputation formation, like one-shot fairness norms, can also be operationalized and turned into a quantitative probe for social interactions. Figures 50.9 (see also COLOR FIGURE 50.9 in separate insert) and 50.10 show fMRI data from a trust game carried out in a large cohort ($N = 100$) of interacting humans. This particular game is a multiround version of a game first suggested by Camerer and Weigelt (1988) but given its name and current form by Berg et al. (1995). Here, we show a multiround adaptation of this game, where two players play 10 rounds of pay–repay cycles (Fig. 50.9). One important difference with the one-shot Ultimatum Game is that reputations form between the players (see King-Casas et al., 2005, for details on reputation formation in this game). They develop a model of their partner's likely response to giving too little or too much money—in short, they form a shared norm of what is expected of one another and respond briskly (good or bad) when that norm is violated.

A number of new results have been discovered using this game while scanning both interacting brains (Montague et al., 2002); however, here, we emphasize just one: a RPE-like signal in the caudate nucleus that occurs on the "intention" to change the level of trust on the next round of play (Fig. 50.10). In early rounds (rounds 3–4), this signal appears in the trustee's caudate nucleus at the revelation of the investor's decision, but in later rounds (rounds 7–8), it occurs before the investor's decision is revealed. So the signal trans-

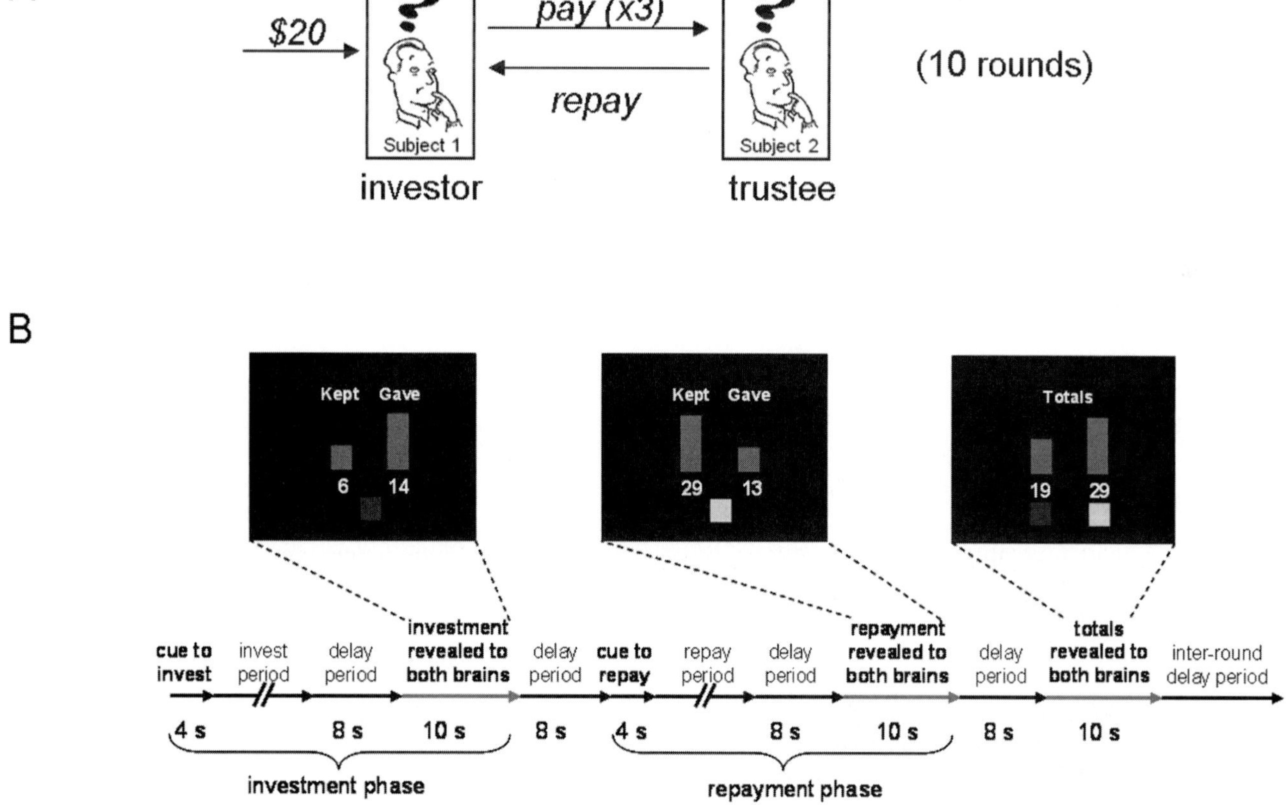

FIGURE 50.9 Multiround trust game: harvesting rewards from other humans. (*A*) On each round, one player called the *investor* is endowed with $20 and can send ("trust") the other player (called the *trustee*) any fraction of this amount. The amount sent is tripled en route to the trustee, who then decides what fraction of the tripled amount to repay. Players execute 10 rounds of this pay–repay cycle. Players maintain their respective roles throughout the entire task, permitting the development of reputations with one another. (*B*) Timeline for events in the multiround trust game. Outcome screens are revealed simultaneously to both players; both interacting brains were scanned simultaneously (see King-Casas et al., 2005; multiround trust game is a variation on the game proposed by Camerer and Weigelt, 1988; Berg et al., 1995).

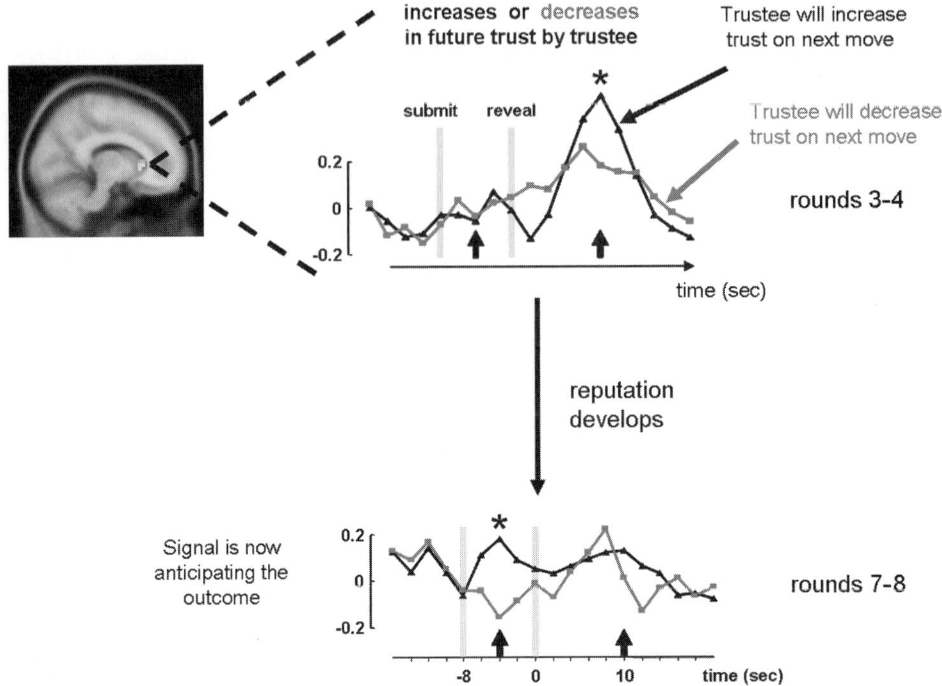

FIGURE 50.10 Correlates of reciprocity and future intentions (trustee brain). (Left brain inset) Bilateral ventral caudate nucleus activation identified by contrasting the brain response to positive reciprocity and negative reciprocity (see King-Casas et al., 2005). *Reciprocity* is defined as relative differences in across-round payment between the players. For example, neutral reciprocity means that one player's fractional change in available money sent was followed by the same fractional change in available money sent by the partner. *Positive reciprocity* means that the partner responded with a greater fractional change in money sent, and *negative reciprocity* means that the partner responded with a lesser fractional change in money sent. Contrasting brain responses to positive and negative reciprocity identified the ventral caudate nucleus. (medium gray and black traces) Average time series in the identified caudate region in early rounds (top; rounds 3–4) and later rounds (bottom; rounds 7–8). The traces have been separated according to the trustee's next move but are shown here at the time that the investor's decision is revealed to both players. The trustee's next move does not happen for ~22 seconds, so this response correlates with the trustee's intention to increase (black trace) or decrease (medium gray trace) their repayment in the near future. Notice the difference between the intention to increase (black trace) and decrease (medium gray trace) repayment shifts 14 seconds earlier as trials progress and reputations build. This shift means that in later rounds (7–8), this signal difference is occurring before the investor's decision is revealed. This is a shift analogous to that seen in simpler conditioning experiments (see Fig. 50.2). (Adapted from King-Casas et al., 2005; Tomlin et al. 2006.)

fers from reacting to the investor's choice to anticipating the investor's choice. The response shows up in a strongly dopaminoceptive structure (caudate) and exhibits exactly the temporal transfer expected for a RPE signal (Fig. 50.2 and Supplementary Online Materials [SOM]; King-Casas et al., 2005). A very clever use of a single-shot version of the trust game by Delgado and colleagues shows that the caudate signals can be dramatically modulated by information about the moral character ("moral priors") of one's partner (Delgado et al., 2005; Fig. 50.11). Once again, we see that reward-processing systems can flexibly and rapidly adapt their function to the problem at hand and can integrate a wide array of information that shows up as measurable changes in BOLD responses. The flexibility of the reward-harvesting systems can also be illustrated by experiments using information about "what might have happened" to generate measurable dynamic responses in the same reward-processing structures (caudate and putamen).

Lohrenz and colleagues have used a market investment game to track fictive error signals, a type of signal related to the ongoing difference between what one "might have earned" and what one "actually earned" (Lohrenz et al., 2007; Figs. 50.12–50.14) (see also COLOR FIGURE 50.14 in separate insert). These investigators show that the brain tracks fictive outcomes using the same reward pathways that generate and distribute reward prediction error signals—ongoing differences between what was expected and what was experienced. So real experience and fictive experience can generate reward error signals, both of which appear to influence an individual's next choice in the investment game (Lohrenz et al., 2007). This game is particularly useful because it might be used to explore brain responses in drug addicts, where the capacity to allow negative out-

A

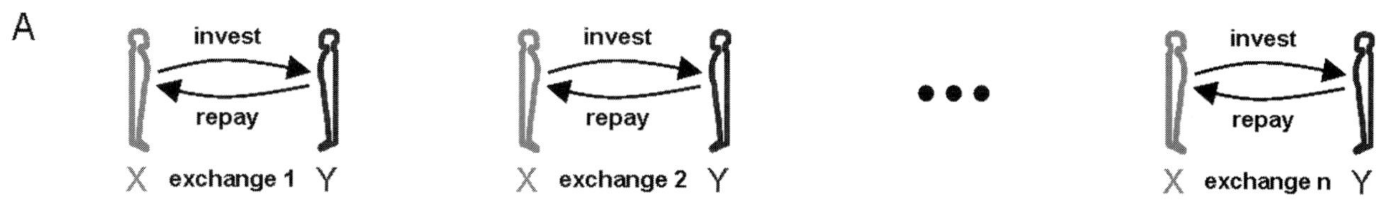

B

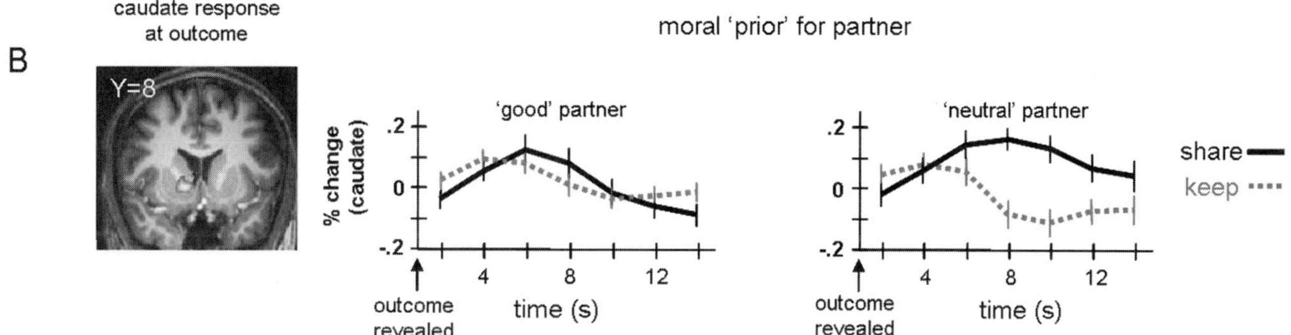

FIGURE 50.11 The influence of moral priors on striatal reward responses to revealed trust. (*A*) Single-shot trust task was played multiple times, but brain responses and behavior were altered by "moral priors" about one's partner. Three partners were used: good, neutral, and bad ("suspect moral character," according to the authors of the study). Players were shown a picture and read a "cover story" about the moral character of their opponent. Players consistently chose to trust the "good" partner more. (*B*) The authors of the study describe the outcome best: "As expected from previous studies, activation of the caudate nucleus differentiated between positive and negative feedback, but only for the 'neutral' partner. Notably, it did not do so for the 'good' partner and did so only weakly for the 'bad' partner, suggesting that prior social and moral perceptions can diminish reliance on feedback mechanisms in the neural circuitry of trial-and-error reward learning." Here, we show the average time series in the caudate at the time the outcome is revealed. The responses illustrate clearly the influence of the "moral prior" on measured responses. (Adapted from Delgado et al., 2005.)

comes that "might happen" to influence drug-taking habits appears to be severely diminished or lost altogether. While chronic smokers generate neural error signals associated with what "might" happen to them, these signals appear to be ignored in a way consonant with addicts' drug use in the clear presence of negative outcomes that might occur or positive outcomes that may be foregone (Chiu et al., 2008).

Common currencies: From fairness to pain

We have now reviewed evidence that reward processing in the human brain can be tracked using fMRI across a wide spectrum of stimuli or internal states that qualify as rewarding. In Figure 50.4, a passive and active conditioning experiment using fruit juice as the "reward" generated hemodynamic responses in the striatum (caudate and putamen) that correlated with a prediction error in the expected value of juice delivery. From primary rewards such as sugar water, we extended to sequential decision making, social exchange with other humans, and the influence of "moral biases" in these exchanges, and we even illustrated fMRI-detectable signals that correlated with fictive reward error signals (Lohrenz et al., 2007; Figs. 50.12–50.14).

This remarkable range of "rewarding" dimensions illustrates a very basic point that we made much earlier—that is, the signal source that controls the reward input to striatum/midbrain system defines implicitly the current goal of the creature and thus the external stimulus or internal state that the creature values at the moment. It is reasonable to hypothesize that in humans, reward-harvesting machinery has the capacity to be redeployed in pursuit of literally any representation that can control the reward function r(t) as depicted in Figure 50.3. This is a powerful way to flexibly control a creature's behavior and to induce cognitive innovation. A new idea or concept gains control of the reward function r(t), and the reward-harvesting machinery that we share with every other vertebrate on the planet takes over, computes RPEs and other quantities (Kakade and Dayan, 2002), and directs learning and decision making for some time. It is now clear why the brain must have a way to gate and filter the kinds of representations (probably intimately dependent on prefrontal cortex) allowed to govern reward-harvesting

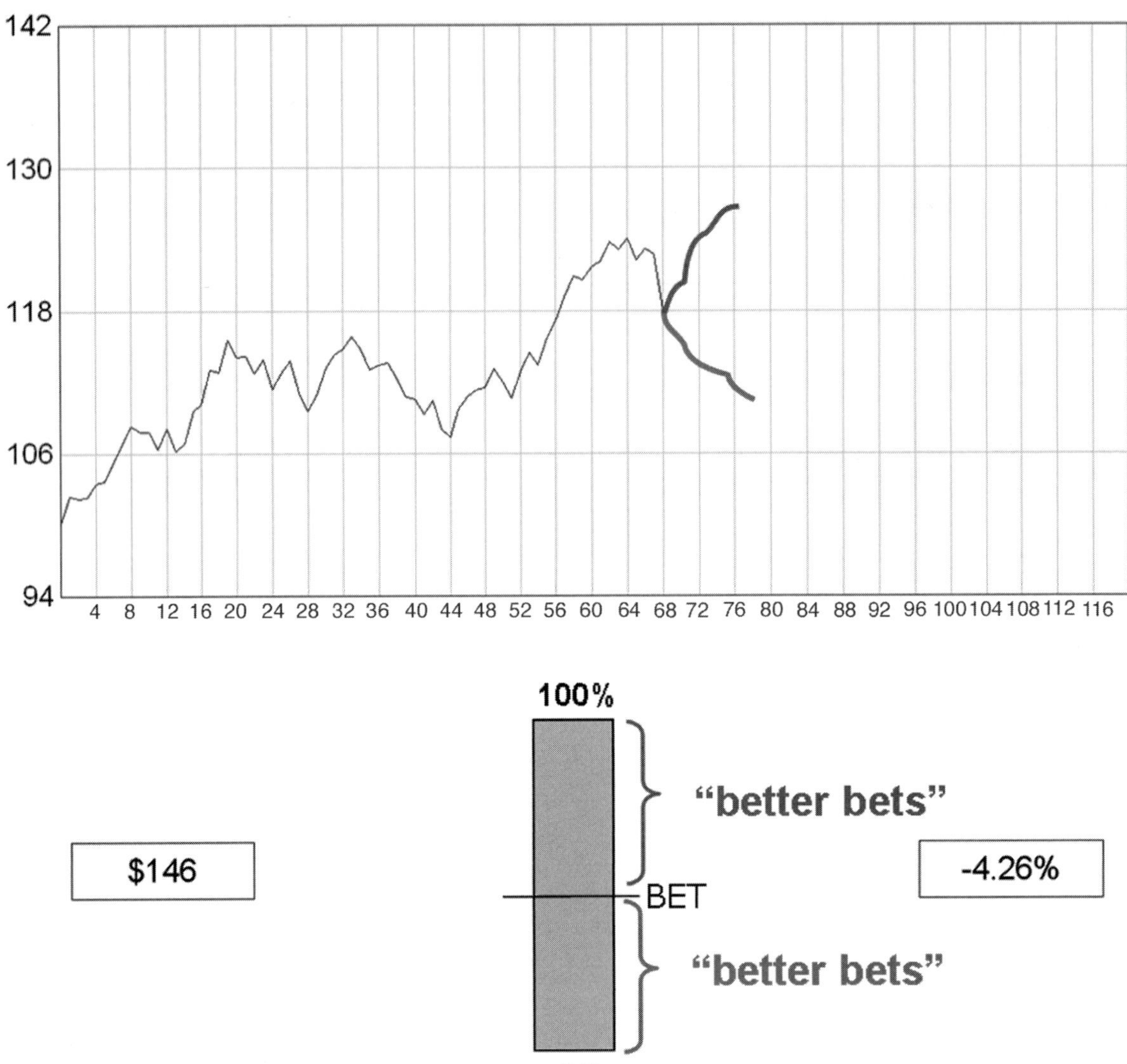

FIGURE 50.12 Fictive errors and the neural substrates of "what might have been." A market investment task where market history is shown as decisions are made. Participants are shown their total available (lower left box) and the fractional percentage change from the last choice (lower right box). Participants move a centrally placed slider bar at each decision point (vertical gray lines) to indicate the fraction of their total to commit into the market (ranging from 0% to 100% in 10% increments). The "riskless" choice in this game is to "cash out" (0% invested). After the bet is placed, the market fluctuates to the next decision point—at that moment, if the market goes up, then all higher bets were better (higher gains); if it goes down, then all lower bets were better (smaller losses). This task was used to track the behavioral and neural influence of "what might have been" (fictive error signal over gains)—that is, the ongoing temporal difference between the best that "might have been" gained and the actual gain. Figure 50.13 shows how such a signal was tracked during this experiment. Twenty equally spaced decisions were made per market, and 20 markets were played (adapted from Lohrenz et al., 2007; Chiu et al., 2008). In behavioral regressions, other than the last bet and the market fluctuation, this "fictive error over gains" was the best predictor of changes in the participants' next bet, showing that it had measurable neural and behavioral influence.

machinery (Miller and Cohen, 2001), and why ideas about RPEs and gating in the prefrontal cortex should be taken seriously and be mathematically extended (O'Reilly et al., 1999; O'Reilly et al., 2002—DA gating hypothesis).

We close our chapter on brain reward and fMRI by touching lightly upon very recent work exploring another rewarding dimension—punishment, that is, why humans are motivated to punish and the proximate brain responses and behavioral contexts that surround the desire to punish. This is an important area, in part because the "valuation function issue" surrounding punishment of other humans relates directly to the nature of social norms, their enforcement, and the way that they would encourage or discourage particular kinds of social structures. This is an area where brain reward processing intersects with the way that humans organize themselves and others into institutions.

Two of the more interesting experiments in this area are illustrated in Figures 50.15 and 50.16. Figure 50.15

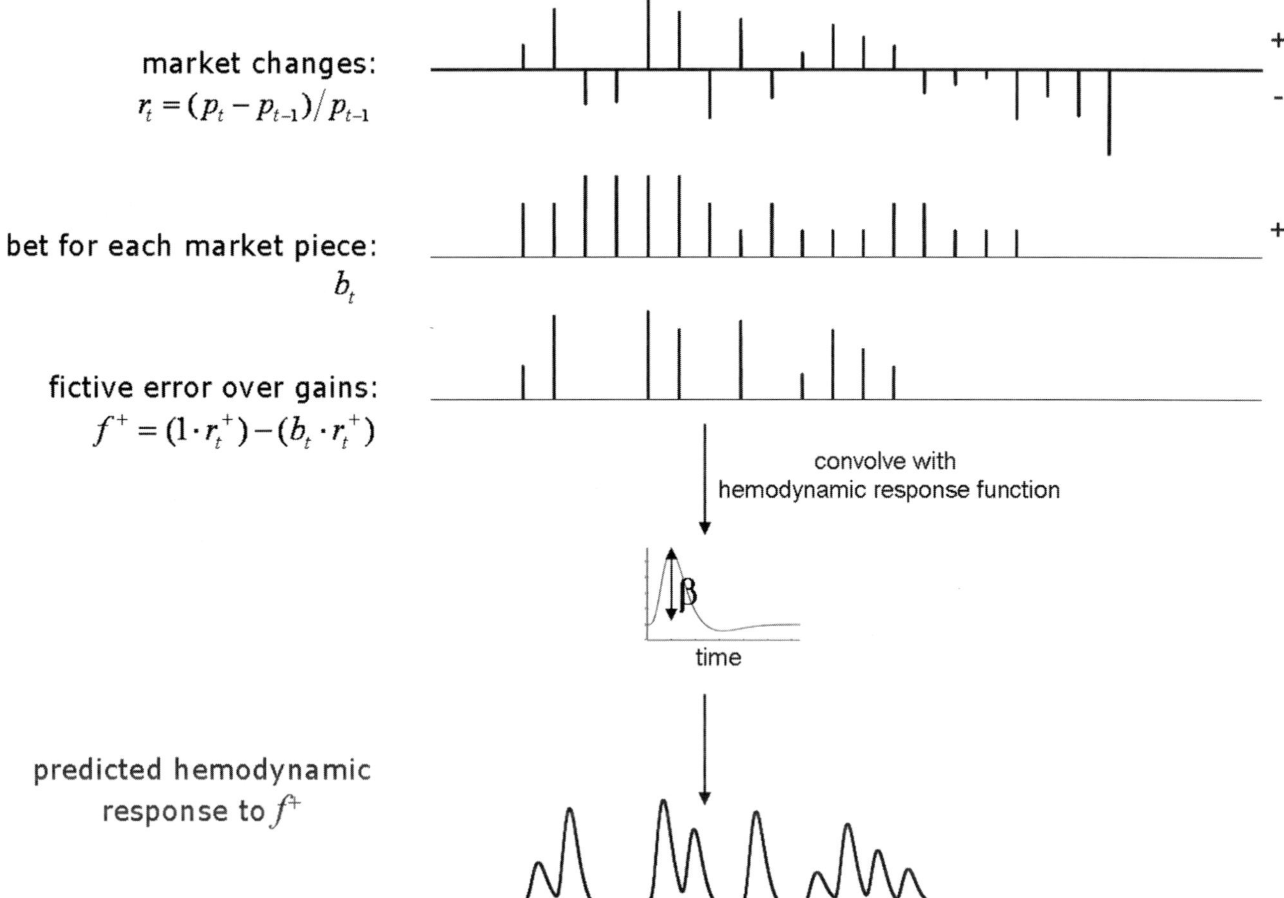

FIGURE 50.13 Building a regressor for fictive errors. To track the "fictive error over gains," we computed the fictive error over gains at each decision point where a gain was earned. The time between decisions is a free variable, and so normally the time of decision occurs at irregular time intervals. For display purposes, we have shown decisions on regular time intervals, but otherwise, these data were taken from a participant in the experiment. The fictive error over gains is then convolved with a hemodynamic response function (impulse response) to produce the hemodynamic response dynamic predicted for the fictive error signal. This trace is best fit to the hemodynamic response in each measured voxel, where the free parameter at hand is the height of the response function *b*. Using standard statistical methods, we identified the voxels whose measured signal correlates best with this expected response dynamic throughout the entire decision-making task. This method amounted to seeking a temporal pattern of blood flow changes that matched the fictive error signal.

is a two-part experiment that addresses the way that norm violations in one domain (fairness in an exchange with another human) translates into brain responses related to another domain (empathic responses to pain in others). Following the theme of this chapter, it is not surprising that reward circuitry is again engaged. In Figure 50.15, an individual witnesses two other individuals playing a game of cooperation/defection (sequential prisoner's dilemma game; Singer et al., 2006). As illustrated, one of the players is a confederate who has been told to play fairly or unfairly. The individual, after watching the game transpire, is then put in a scanner and allowed to watch the confederate receive a painful stimulus. In earlier work (Singer et al., 2004), these same investigators had helped to identify brain responses (using fMRI) that correlate with empathizing with observed pain in others. In this experiment, males and females showed empathy-related fMRI responses when observing pain being delivered to a "fair" confederate. However, for "unfair" confederates, the male brains diverged significantly from the female brains. Male brains showed dramatically reduced responses in empathy-related regions and showed activation in reward-related areas (nucleus accumbens). Even more remarkably, the nucleus accumbens response correlated with the male individuals' reported desire for revenge as subjectively reported (see Singer et al., 2006, for details and Fig. 50.16B). These are revealing findings in that the neural signatures correspond quite well with a behavioral account that casts males as norm enforcers (Singer et al., 2006). Figure 50.16A agrees with these general findings, but it shows an experiment that directly tested brain responses correlating with the act of punishment and not merely the desire to punish. These investigators (de Quervain et al., 2004) used PET imaging and an ultimatum game to probe directly neural responses associ-

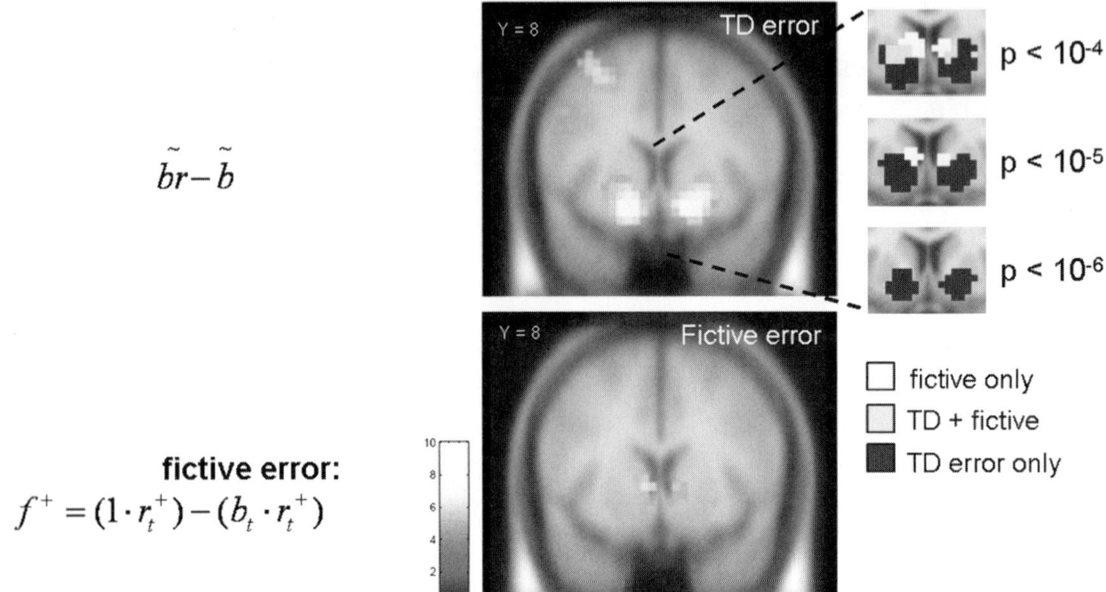

FIGURE 50.14 Separable neural responses for reward prediction error and fictive error. The fictive error signal (Figs. 50.12, 50.13) and the experiential error signal (version of a temporal difference [TD] error signal) are sometimes colinear and must be mathematically separated. This figure shows those activations (at the prescribed statistical threshold) associated with the TD error alone, the fictive error alone, and both. The fictive error is computed as explained in Figure 50.13. At each decision, the experiential error is taken as the difference between the *z*-scored bet $\tilde{b}$ (proxy for expected value of return) and the actual return $\tilde{b}r_t$. Here, r_t is the market as defined in Figure 50.13 (relative fractional change in the price; adapted from Lohrenz et al., 2007; also see Montague et al., 2006; Chiu et al., 2008).

ated with monetary punishment of an unfair player. The results showed a clear activation in dorsal striatum of male brains to punishment of another human who is perceived as "bad," a defector that has abused trust in an exchange with another human.

Valuation Diseases

The reinforcement learning models of reward processing in the brain are clearly incomplete and oversimplified. Two things are clear from single unit recordings in DA neurons in the midbrain: (*1*) they are capable of

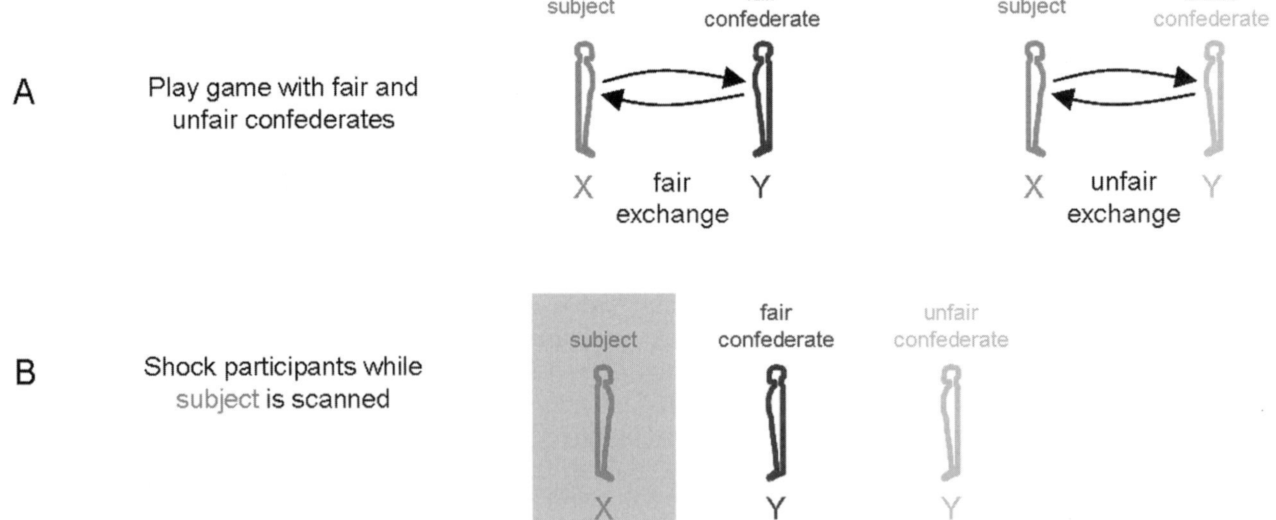

FIGURE 50.15 Common currencies crossing domain boundaries: from fairness to pain. A two-part experiment showing how norm violation in one domain (deviation from fairness in a sequential prisoner's dilemma game) is "credited" and paid for in another domain (experience of pain) (Singer et al., 2006). (*A, B*) After playing the economic game (a sequential prisoner's dilemma game fairly or unfairly), the participants observed the confederates receiving a painful stimulus. *(cont. on next page)*

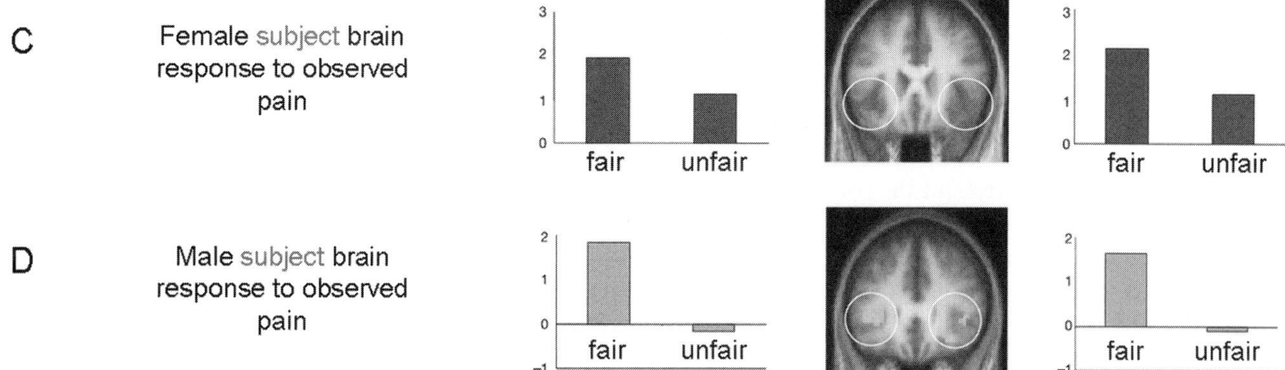

FIGURE 50.15 *(continued)* (*C*) Males and females exhibited brain responses in empathy-related areas like the anterior cingulate cortex and frontal-insular cortex, both shown here (see Singer et al., 2006, for details). (*D*) Male brains demonstrated dramatically reduced empathy-related responses when they viewed unfair players receiving pain but showed increased activation during this time in reward-related areas. These reward responses correlated with the males subjectively reported desire for revenge toward the players perceived as unfair (Fig. 50.16B).

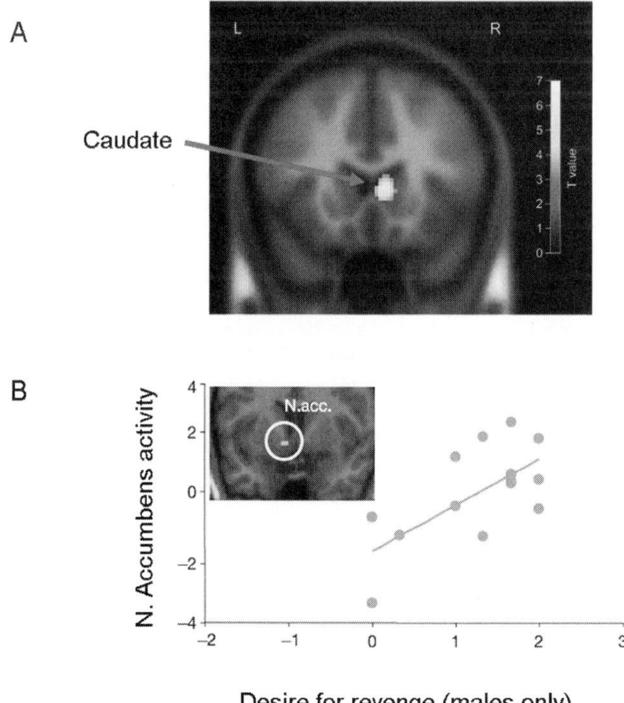

FIGURE 50.16 Reward responses and the punishment of norm violators. (*A*) In an ultimatum game where punishment is possible, the desire to punish activates caudate nucleus (PET experiment using O15 water; de Quervain et al., 2004). Activation in dorsal striatum of male brains to punishment of another human who is perceived as "bad"; a defector that has abused trust in an exchange with another human. This activation scaled with the participants' desire to punish a perceived offender. These responses are consistent with these brains treating the punishment of a defector like a reward. (*B*) Correlation between the subjective desire for revenge (in male brains) toward an unfair player (in Fig. 50.15) and the nucleus accumbens (N. acc.) activation. PET: positron emission tomography.

encoding in their spike rate a reward prediction error signal for summed future reward (Montague et al., 1996; Schultz et al., 1997; reviewed in Schultz, 1998), and (2) they also communicate a host of other responses not related to this class of error signal (Schultz, 1998). We reviewed previously some of the evidence showing that the model was incomplete. Nevertheless, it has provided a way to understand error signals recorded in the striatum using fMRI across a wide array of task demands. In fact, a temporal difference reinforcement learning model has been applied by Redish (2004) to explain a number of features of drug addiction. The essence of that model is that drugs of abuse generate an unpredicted increase in DA that causes overvaluation of cues associated with drug taking. Cast this way, addiction becomes a valuation disease caused by drug-induced DA increases that cannot be learned by the underlying value function. The underlying value function grows without bound (Redish, 2004), which means that the value of drug-predicting cues grows without bound. Ironically, this RL perspective links drug addiction to movement disorders (for example, Parkinson's disease) and might suggest novel treatment strategies or research approaches.

In Parkinson's disease, DA neurons are reduced to ~10% of their normal number by some unknown set of pathological processes. The reward prediction errors generated by such a small number of DA neurons run into a serious signal-to-noise problem. Fluctuations in dopaminergic activity in these few remaining neurons produce an extremely noisy prediction error signal, which would be difficult for downstream neural targets to interpret—they would have difficulty inferring "real" fluctuations from the increased noise level in the few remaining cells.

Consequently, it is difficult to read out differences in the values of the underlying state space—what this means practically is that all behavioral options or internal mental states would appear to have the same value as the current state. In this case, downstream decision-making mechanisms "see" that no other state is any more valuable than the current state, and they would naturally want to remain in that state. The most efficient choice to make is to freeze in the current state in the face of a flat value function. In this depiction, Parkinson's disease becomes a kind of "rational freezing disease" under the influence of a very noisy DA-encoded prediction error system. So the RL framework, which gave us a way to understand the wide range of reward tasks in humans, also provides a new way to connect addiction and movement disorders under a common computational framework.

We expect efforts along these lines to progress in neurology and psychiatry and would expect computational psychiatry and computational neurology to be reasonable subfields emerging in the coming years.

REFERENCES

Asch, S.E. (1951) Effects of group pressure upon the modification and distortion of judgment. In: Guetzkow, H., ed. *Groups, Leadership and Men.* Pittsburgh, PA: Carnegie Press, pp. 177–190.

Ashburner, J., and Friston, K.J. (1999) Nonlinear spatial normalization using basis functions. *Hum. Brain Mapp.* 7:254–266.

Atick, J.J. (1992) Could information-theory provide an ecological theory of sensory processing? *Network* 3:213–251.

Attwell, D., and Laughlin, S.B. (2001) An energy budget for signalling in the grey matter of the brain. *J. Cereb. Blood Flow Metab.* 21:1133–1145.

Barlow, H.B. (1961) Possible principles underlying the transformation of sensory messages. In: Rosenblith, W., ed. *Sensory Communication.* Cambridge, MA: MIT Press, pp. 217–234.

Barlow, H.B. (2001) Redundancy reduction revisited. *Network: Computation in Neural Systems* 12:241–253.

Bayer, H.M., and Glimcher, P.W. (2005) Midbrain dopamine neurons encode a quantitative reward prediction error signal. *Neuron* 47(1):129–141.

Berg, J., Dickhaut, J., and McCabe, K. (1995) Trust, reciprocity, and social history. *Games Econ. Behav.* 10:122–142.

Berns, G.S., Chappelow, J., Zink, C.F., Pagnoni, G., Martin-Skurski, M.E., and Richards, J. (2005) Neurobiological correlates of social conformity and independence during mental rotation. *Biol. Psychiatry* 58:245–253.

Berns, G.S., McClure, S.M., Pagnoni, G., and Montague, P.R. (2001) Predictability modulates human brain response to reward. *J. Neurosci.* 21:2793–2798.

Bialek, W. (1987) Physical limits to sensation and perception. *Ann. Rev. Biophys. Biophys. Chem.* 16:455–478.

Breiter, H.C., Aharon, I., Kahneman, D., Dale, A., and Shizgal, P. (2001) Functional imaging of neural responses to expectancy and experience of monetary gains and losses. *Neuron* 30:619–630.

Breiter, H.C., Gollub, R.L., Weisskoff, R.M., Kennedy, D.N., Makris, N., Berke, J.D., et al. (1997) Acute effects of cocaine on human brain activity and emotion. *Neuron* 19:591–611.

Camerer, C.F. (2003) *Behavioral Game Theory.* Princeton, NJ: Princeton University Press.

Camerer, C.F., and Fehr, E. (2006) When does "economic" man dominate social behavior? *Science* 311:47–52.

Camerer, C.F., and Weigelt, K. (1988) Reputation and corporate strategy: a review of recent theory and applications. *Strategic Management Journal* 9:443–454.

Chiu, P.H., Lohrenz, T.M., and Montague, P.R. (2008) Smokers' brains compute but ignore a fictive error signal in a sequential investment game. *Nat. Neurosci.* 11:514–520.

Damasio, A.R., Grabowski, T.J., Bechara, A., Damasio, H., Ponto, L.L., Parvizi, J., and Hichwa, R.D. (2000) Subcortical and cortical brain activity during the feeling of self-generated emotions. *Nat. Neurosci.* 3:2978–2986.

Dani, J.A., and Montague, P.R. (2007) Disrupting addiction through the loss of drug-associated internal states. *Nat. Neurosci.* 10: 403–404.

Daw, N.D., and Doya, K. (2006) The computational neurobiology of learning and reward. *Curr. Opin. Neurobiol.* 16(2):199–204.

Dayan, P. (1992) The convergence of TD (lambda) for general lambda. *Machine Learn.* 8:341–362.

Dayan, P., and Abbott, L.F. (2001) *Theoretical Neuroscience.* Cambridge, MA: MIT Press.

Dayan, P., and Balleine, B.W. (2002) Reward, motivation and reinforcement learning. *Neuron* 36:285–298.

de Quervain, D.J., Fischbacher, U., Treyer, V., Schellhammer, M., Schnyder, U., et al. (2004) The neural basis of altruistic punishment. *Science* 305:1254–1258.

Delgado, M.R., Frank, R.H., and Phelps, E.A. (2005) Perceptions of moral character modulate the neural systems of reward during the trust game. *Nat. Neurosci.* 8:1611–1618.

Delgado, M.R., Nystrom, L.E., Fissell, C., Noll, D.C., and Fiez, J.A. (2000) Tracking the hemodynamic responses to reward and punishment in the striatum. *J. Neurophysiol.* 84:3072–3077.

Egelman, D.M., Person, C., and Montague, P.R. (1998) A computational role for dopamine delivery in human decision-making. *J. Cogn. Neurosci.* 10:623–630.

Elliott, R., Newman, J.L., Longe, O.A., and Deakin, J.F. (2003) Differential response patterns in the striatum and orbitofrontal cortex to financial reward in humans: a parametric functional magnetic resonance imaging study. *J. Neurosci.* 23(1):303–307.

Fehr, E., and Schmidt, K.M. (1999) A theory of fairness, competition, and cooperation. *Quarterly J. Econ.* 114:817–868.

Friston, K.J., Jezzard, P., and Turner, R. (1994) The analysis of functional MRI time-series. *Hum. Brain Mapp.* 1, 153–171.

Guth, W., Schmittberger, R., and Schwarze, B. (1982) An experimental analysis of ultimatum bargaining. *J. Econ. Behav. Organ.* 3:367–388.

Herrnstein, R.J., and Prelec, D. (1991) Melioration: a theory of distributed choice. *J. Econ. Perspect.* 5:137–156.

Hyman, S.E., Malenka, R.C., and Nestler, E.J. (2006) Neural mechanisms of addiction: the role of reward-related learning and memory. *Annu. Rev. Neurosci.* 29:565–598.

Ikemoto, S., and Panksepp, J. (1999) The role of nucleus accumbens dopamine in motivated behavior: a unifying interpretation with special reference to reward-seeking. *Brain Res. Rev.* 31:6–41.

Kaelbling, L.P., Littman, M.L., and Moore, AW. (1996) Reinforcement learning: a survey. *J. Artif. Intellig. Res.* 4:237–285.

Kakade, S., and Dayan, P. (2002) Dopamine: generalization and bonuses. *Neural Networks* 15: 549–559.

Kamil, A.C., Krebs, J.R., and Pulliam, H.R. (1987) *Foraging Behavior.* New York: Plenum Press.

King-Casas, B., Tomlin, D., Anen, C., Camerer, C.F., Quartz, S.R., and Montague, P.R. (2005) Getting to know you: reputation and trust in a two-person economic exchange. *Science* 308:78–83.

Knutson, B., Fong, G.W., Adams, C.M., Varner, J.L., and Hommer, D. (2001) Dissociation of reward anticipation and outcome with event-related fMRI. *Neuroreport* 12:3683–3687.

Knutson, B., Westdorp, A., Kaiser, E., and Hommer, D. (2000) FMRI visualization of brain activity during a monetary incentive delay task. *NeuroImage* 12:20–27.

Krebs, J.R., Kacelnik, A., and Taylor, P. (1978) Tests of optimal sampling by foraging great tits. *Nature* 275:27–31.

Lau, B., and Glimcher, P.W. (2005) Dynamic response-by-response models of matching behavior in rhesus monkeys. *J. Exp. Anal. Behav.* 84(3):555–579.

Laughlin, S.B. (1994) Matching coding, circuits, cells, and molecules to signals. General principles of retinal design in the fly's eye *Prog. Retinal Eye Res.* 13:165–196.

Laughlin, S.B. (2001) Energy as a constract on the coding and processing of sensory information. *Curr. Opin. Neurobiol.* 11(4):475–480.

Laughlin, S.B. (2004) The implications of metabolic energy requirements in the representation of information in neurons. In: Gazzaniga, M.S., ed. *The Cognitive Neurosciences III*. Cambridge MA: MIT Press, pp. 187–196.

Laughlin, S.B., de Ruyter van Stevenick, R.R., and Anderson, J.C. (1998) The metabolic cost of neural information. *Nat. Neurosci.* 1(1):36–41.

Levy, W.B., and Baxter, R.A. (1996) Energy efficient neural codes. *Neural Comp.* 8(3):531–543.

Li, J., McClure, S.M., King-Casas, B., and Montague, P.R. (2006) Policy adjustment in a dynamic economic game. *PloS One*, 1:e103.

Ljungberg, T., Apicella, P., and Schultz, W. (1992) Responses of monkey dopamine neurons during learning of behavioral reactions. *J. Neurophysiol.* 67(1):145–163.

Lohrenz, T., McCabe, K., Camerer, C.F., and Montague, P.R. (2007) Neural signature of fictive learning signals in a sequential investment task. *Proc. Natl. Acad. Sci. USA* 104:9493–9498.

McClure, S.M., Berns, G.S., and Montague, P.R. (2003) Temporal prediction activates human striatum. *Neuron* 38:339–346.

McClure, S.M., Daw, N., and Montague, P.R. (2003) A computational substrate for incentive salience. *Trends Neurosci.* 26(8): 423–428.

Miller, E.K., and Cohen, J.D. (2001) An integrative theory of prefrontal cortex function. *Annu. Rev. Neurosci.* 24:167–202.

Montague, P.R. (2006) *Why Choose This Book?* New York: Penguin Group.

Montague, P.R. (2007) Neuroeconomics: A view from neuroscience. *Functional Neurology* 22(4):219–234.

Montague, P.R., and Berns, G.S. (2002) Neural economics and the biological substrates of valuation. *Neuron* 36:265–284.

Montague, P.R., Berns, G.S., Cohen, J.D., McClure, S.M., Pagnoni, G., et al. (2002) Hyperscanning: simultaneous fMRI during linked social interactions. *NeuroImage* 16(4):1159–1164.

Montague, P.R., Dayan, P., Nowlan, S.J., Pouget, A., and Sejnowski, T.J. (1993) Using aperiodic reinforcement for directed self-organization. *Adv. Neural Info. Proc. Systems* 5:969–976.

Montague, P.R., Dayan, P., Person, C., and Sejnowski, T.J. (1995) Bee foraging in uncertain environments using predictive Hebbian learning. *Nature* 377:725–728.

Montague, P.R., Dayan, P., and Sejnowski, T.J. (1996) A framework for mesencephalic dopamine systems based on predictive Hebbian learning. *J. Neurosci.* 16(5):1936–1947.

Montague, P.R., Dayan, P., and Sejnowski, T.J. (1994) Foraging in an uncertain environment using predictive Hebbian learning. *Adv. Neural Info. Proc. Systems* 6:598–605.

Montague, P.R., Hyman, S.E., and Cohen, J.D. (2004) Computational roles for dopamine in behavioural control. *Nature* 431: 760–767.

Montague, P.R., King-Casas, B., and Cohen, J.D. (2006) Imaging valuation models in human choice. *Annu. Rev. Neurosci.* 29:417–448.

Montague, P.R., McClure, S.M., Baldwin, P.R., Phillips, P.E.M., Budygin, E.A., et al. (2004) Dynamic gain control of dopamine delivery in freely moving animals. *J. Neurosci.* 24(7):1754–1759.

Montague, P.R., and Sejnowksi, T.J. (1994) The predictive brain: temporal coincidence and temporal order in synaptic learning mechanims. *Learn. Memory* 1(1):1–33.

Morris, G., Arkadir, D., Nevet, A., Vaadia, E., and Bergman, H. (2004) Coincident but distinct messages of midbrain dopamine and striatal tonically active neurons. *Neuron* 43(1):133–143.

Morris, G., Nevet, A., Arkadir, D., Vaadia, E., and Bergman, H. (2006) Midbrain dopamine neurons encode decisions for future action. *Nat. Neurosci.* 9(8):1057–1063.

Naqvi, N.H., Rudrauf, D., Damasio, H., and Bechara, A. (2007) Damage to the insula disrupts addiction to cigarette smoking. *Science* 315:531–534.

O'Doherty, J.P. (2004) Reward representations and reward-related learning in the human brain: insights from neuroimaging. *Curr. Opin. Neurobiol.* 14(6):769–776.

O'Doherty, J.P., Dayan, P., Friston, K., Critchley, H., and Dolan, R.J. (2003) Temporal difference models and reward related learning in the human brain. *Neuron* 38:329–337.

O'Doherty, J.P., Dayan, P., Schultz, J., Deichmann, R., Friston, K., and Dolan, R.J. (2004) Dissociable roles of ventral and dorsal striatum in instrumental conditioning. *Science* 304:452–454.

O'Doherty, J.P., Deichmann, R., Critchley, H.D., and Dolan, R.J. (2002) Neural responses during anticipation of a primary taste reward. *Neuron* 33(5):815–826.

O'Reilly, R.C., Braver, T.S., and Cohen, J.D. (1999) A biologically-based neural network model of working memory. In: Miyake, A., and Shah, P., eds., *Models of Working Memory: Mechanisms of Active Maintenance and Executive Control*. New York: Cambridge University Press, pp. 375–411.

O'Reilly, R.C., Noelle, D.C., Braver, T.S., and Cohen, J.D. (2002) Prefrontal cortex and dynamic categorization tasks: representational organization and neuromodulatory control. *Cereb. Cortex* 12:246–257.

Phillips, M.L., Young, A.W., Senior, C., Brammer, M., Andrew, C., Calder, A.J., et al. (1997) A specific neural substrate for perceiving facial expressions of disgust. *Nature* 389:495–498.

Quartz, S., Dayan, P., Montague, P.R., and Sejnowski, T. (1992) Expectation learning in the brain using diffuse ascending connections. *Soc. Neurosci. Abst.* 18:1210.

Redgrave, P., and Gurney, K. (2006) The short-latency dopamine signal: a role in discovering novel actions? *Nat. Rev. Neurosci.* 7: 967–975.

Redgrave, P., Prescott, T.J., and Gurney, K. (1999) Is the short-latency dopamine response too short to signal reward error? *Trends Neurosci.* 22:146–151.

Redish, A.D. (2004) Addiction as a computational process gone awry. *Science* 306:1944–1947.

Rilling, J.K., Gutman, D.A., Zeh, T.R., Pagnoni, G., Berns, G.S., and Kilts, C.D. (2002) A neural basis for social cooperation. *Neuron* 35:395–405.

Rilling, J.K., Sanfey, A.G., Aronson, J.A., Nystrom, L.E., and Cohen, J.D. (2004a) The neural correlates of theory of mind within interpersonal interactions. *NeuroImage* 22:1694–1703.

Rilling, J.K., Sanfey, A.G., Aronson, J.A., Nystrom, L.E., and Cohen, J.D. (2004b) Opposing BOLD responses to reciprocated and unreciprocated altruism in putative reward pathways. *Neuroreport* 15:2539–2543.

Ruderman, D.L. (1994) The statistics of natural images. *Network* 5:517–548.

Sanfey, A.G., Loewenstein, G., McClure, S.M., and Cohen, J.D. (2006) Neuroeconomics: cross-currents in research on decision-making. *Trends Cog. Sci.* 10(3):108–116.

Sanfey, A.G., Rilling, J.K., Aronson, J.A., Nystrom, L.E., and Cohen, J.D. (2003) The neural basis of economic decision-making in the Ultimatum Game. *Science* 300:1755–1758.

Schultz, W., and Dickinson, A. (2000) Neuronal coding of prediction errors. *Annu. Rev. Neurosci.* 23:473–500.

Schultz, W. (1998) Predictive reward signal of dopamine neurons. *J. Neurophysiol.*, 80:1–27.

Schultz, W. (2007) Multiple dopamine functions at different time courses. *Annu. Rev. Neurosci.* 30:259–288.

Schultz, W., Dayan, P., and Montague, P.R. (1997) A neural substrate of prediction and reward. *Science* 275:1593–1599.

Simoncelli, E., and Olshausen, B.A. (2001) Natural image statistics and neural representation *Annu. Rev. Neurosci.* 24:1193–1215.

Singer, R., Seymour, B., O'Doherty, J., Kaube, H., Dolan, R.J., and Frith, C.D. (2004) Empathy for pain involves the affective but not sensory components of pain. *Science* 303:1157–1162.

Singer, T., Seymour, B., O'Doherty, J.P., Stephan, K.E., Dolan, R.J., and Frith, C.D. (2006) Empathic neural responses are modulated by the perceived fairness of others. *Nature* 439:466–469.

Smith, J.M. (1982) *Evolution and the Theory of Games*. Cambridge, UK: Cambridge University Press.

Sutton, R.S., and Barto, A.G. (1998) *Reinforcement Learning*. Cambridge, MA: MIT Press.

Thut, G., Schultz, W., Roelcke, U., Nienhusmeier, M., Missimer, J., Maguire, R.P., and Leenders, K.L. (1997) Activation of the human brain by monetary reward. *Neuroreport* 8:1225–1228.

Tobler, P.N., Fiorillo, C.D., and Schultz, W. (2005) Adaptive coding of reward value by dopamine neurons. *Science* 307:1642–1645.

Tomlin, D., Kayali, M.A., King-Casas, B., Anen, C., Camerer, C.F., Quartz, S.R., and Montague, P.R. (2006) Agent-specific responses in the cingulate cortex during economic exchanges. *Science* 312: 1047–1050.

Waelti, P., Dickinson, A., and Schultz, W. (2001) Dopamine responses comply with basic assumptions of formal learning theory. *Nature* 412:43–48.

Wickens, J. (1993) *A Theory of the Striatum*. Oxford, UK: Pergamon Press.

51 Principles of the Pharmacotherapy of Addictive Disorders

CHARLES P. O'BRIEN AND CHARLES DACKIS

The modern definition of *addiction* emphasizes uncontrolled drug use rather than tolerance and physical dependence as essential features of the disorder. It is generally recognized that addiction has strong hereditary influences and, once established, behaves as a chronic brain disorder with relapses and remissions over the long term (McLellan et al., 2000). *Tolerance*, a finding commonly present in addiction, is produced by homeostatic neuroadaptations to repeated drug exposure that diminish the pharmacological response (American Psychiatric Association [APA], 1994). *Physical dependence* is a state manifested by withdrawal symptoms that occur when drug taking is terminated or significantly reduced and reflects a "rebound" in unopposed neuroadaptations to repeated drug exposure. Thus, withdrawal symptoms are generally opposite in direction to initial drug effects (O'Brien, 2005b). It is important to note that tolerance and withdrawal symptoms occur commonly among patients who are not addicted, especially those treated for chronic pain, and who are treated with any of the common medications to which the body adapts. These include medications for high blood pressure, anxiety, depression, and pain. Indeed, the fear of producing addiction leads to the undertreatment of pain (Stalnikowicz et al., 2005) and needless suffering despite the availability of effective pain medication (Foley, 1997). Neuroimaging studies in human patients and findings from animal models of addiction suggest that more persistent neuroadaptations contribute other features of addiction, including craving, loss of control, and even denial.

Addictive agents produce euphoria by acutely activating brain reward pathways that have evolved to ensure survival, which largely explains the compelling nature of drug reward. Repeated exposure to addictive agents disrupts neurotransmitter systems (Dackis and O'Brien, 2005b), alters gene expression (Nestler, 2004), and even distorts neuronal morphology in reward-related brain regions (Robinson and Kolb, 2004), suggesting that these agents chronically dysregulate reward pathways. With active drug use, euphoria alternates with craving to establish a cycle of addiction that becomes increasingly entrenched and uncontrollable, despite medical and psychosocial hazards. Craving can be precipitated by environmental cues, stress, and exposure to a small dose of the addictive agent. Cue-induced craving has been associated with limbic activation in a large number of human neuroimaging studies utilizing positron emission tomography (PET) and functional magnetic resonance imaging (fMRI) (Dackis and O'Brien, 2005b), and this pernicious and persistent phenomenon might be reversed by agents that dampen limbic activation. Human neuroimaging studies also demonstrate reductions in frontal metabolism with stimulant, opioid, and alcohol dependence, whereas animal studies indicate that chronic exposure to several addictive agents (for example, opioids, stimulants, nicotine) dysregulates reward function (Koob et al., 2004). These findings support a biological basis for addiction and are guiding neuronal strategies that target specific clinical components of addiction.

The clinical data fit best when addiction is considered to be a syndrome characterized by compulsive drug-seeking behavior that impairs psychosocial functioning or damages health. Whereas initial drug use is voluntary, once addicted, the individual is beset by strong urges to continue or to resume drug taking. Even after detoxification and long periods of abstinence, relapse frequently occurs despite sincere efforts to avoid further drug use. People or situations previously associated with drug use elicit involuntary reactions and may provoke relapse (Wikler, 1973; O'Brien, 1975). The biological mechanisms for these apparently reflex patterns are suggested by data from animal models at the neurochemical level (Chapter 45) and the molecular level (Chapter 38). At the clinical level, conditioned cues (people, places, and things) produce intense craving through involuntary limbic activation, leading to self-destructive drug use even after long periods of abstinence. A key point for the clinician to realize is that the proneness to relapse is based on changes in brain function that continue for months or years after the last use of the drug. Of course, these changes in brain function interact with environmental factors such as social stress and situational triggers.

If tolerance and withdrawal symptoms were the only elements of addictive illness, treatment would simply consist of *detoxification,* a process that allows the body to cleanse itself while receiving descending doses of a medication that reduces withdrawal symptoms (O'Brien, 2006). If drug taking does not resume, homeostatic mechanisms will gradually readapt to the absence of the drug (LeBlanc et al., 1969), and tolerance will be diminished or lost. We now know that detoxification is, at best, a first step in treatment and that simply achieving a drug-free state is not the most significant accomplishment. The more difficult aspect is prevention of relapse to drug-taking behavior.

PRINCIPLES OF RELAPSE PREVENTION

As our understanding of the chronic nature of addictive disorders improved, it became apparent that treatment should be based on a chronic disease model such as diabetes or asthma rather than an acute disease model such as pneumonia. Although the shift from an acute or short-term treatment model to a chronic model is still in progress, there is considerable resistance to this change (McLellan et al., 2000). There are two steps in addiction treatment: detoxification and prevention of relapse. In the United States, the health care system has traditionally paid for detoxification but not for long-term relapse prevention (Dackis and O'Brien, 2005b) that is essential to attaining a favorable clinical outcome.

As a chronic disorder, addiction requires long-term treatment that is usually measured in months and years. The strategies for preventing relapse have traditionally involved counseling or psychotherapy, and more recently included pharmacotherapies that target clinical components of addictive illness. When psychiatric disorders co-occur with addiction, they must be treated concomitantly and preferably by the same treatment team. In this chapter, we focus on medication for the primary addictive disorder, but counseling and medication of comorbid disorders are equally important. This chapter focuses on the principles involved in pharmacotherapy, but the reader is referred to the extensive scientific literature on the evidence-based counseling procedures that should be employed along with medication (Volpicelli et al., 2001).

By the time a person with an addiction presents for treatment, there are usually numerous complicating interpersonal, occupational, legal, and medical problems that affect the prognosis and clinical presentation. The typical patient evolves from drug user to abuser to dependent or addicted person over a period of years. During this time, it is common for social, occupational, family, medical, and legal problems to develop. The Addiction Severity Index (McLellan et al., 1980; Cacciola et al., 2007) contains seven classes of variables that are assessed in a structured interview to obtain a severity rating. Those patients who rank at the severe level only on quantity of drugs used and not on other dimensions have a reasonably good prognosis. In contrast, those with severe psychosocial complications scoring high in the non-drug areas have a poor prognosis and are likely to relapse regardless of their level of drug use severity (Woody et al., 1984).

MANAGEMENT OF COEXISTING MENTAL DISORDERS

Psychiatric disorders commonly coexist with addictive disorders. These include anxiety disorders, psychotic disorders, and affective disorders such as depression. Although some of these dual diagnosis cases are simply a coincidental occurrence of common disorders, the overlap is greater than would be expected by chance based on population prevalence (Kessler et al., 1996). There are three kinds of possible relationships, and each probably occurs in different groups of drug users. A preexisting psychiatric disorder could increase the likelihood of initiating drug use as an attempt at self-medicating the psychiatric symptoms (Woody et al., 1974; Khantzian, 1985). Second, chronic drug taking could produce changes in the brain and in social interactions that predispose to the development of psychiatric disorders. This latter hypothesis is supported by the observation that many of the psychiatric symptoms associated with addictive disorders begin after the addictive process and resolve spontaneously after several weeks of abstinence from drugs of abuse (Schuckit et al., 1997). Finally, addictive and psychiatric illness may present together as independent disorders. Although substance-induced psychiatric disorders may resolve spontaneously with abstinence, independent psychiatric disorders must be stabilized with appropriate medications.

DETOXIFICATION

It is unfortunate that the majority of persons who are drug dependent are merely treated with detoxification and little or no long-term follow-up care. This is not logical, but it is a fact of the current health care system in the United States (McLellan et al., 2005). Detoxification is actually performed by the patient's own metabolic processes. Thus, it can be accomplished voluntarily (although not necessarily safely) through sheer willpower by ceasing drug use or involuntarily when a person with an addiction is incarcerated or placed in a treatment program where access to drugs is denied. The withdrawal syndrome from opiate addiction can be very uncomfortable, but it is not life threatening unless the patient has preexisting medical problems. The symptoms consist of sweating, muscle aches, cramps, nausea, diarrhea, vomiting, tearing of the eyes, rhinorrhea, tremors, tachycardia, and other signs of autonomic nervous system hyperactivity. The discomfort has been compared to a bad case of the flu. Several sorts of treatment of these symptoms are available. Withdrawal from sedatives, alcohol, and stimulants is considered below.

Replacing the drug of dependence or using another drug in the same category in gradually decreasing doses is a direct way to block withdrawal symptoms. As in all forms of detoxification, transfer from a short-acting drug such as heroin to a longer-acting drug such as methadone provides a smooth transition to the drug-free state. By appropriate dosing, detoxification can be achieved with minimal discomfort. A recent innovation for opiate dependence involves using the partial agonist *buprenorphine* as a transition to the drug-free state. The patient can be switched from dependence on heroin or methadone to buprenorphine, which is then stopped with few or no withdrawal symptoms. Buprenorphine was approved by the Food and Drug Administration (FDA) in 2002 as a treatment for opiate dependence.

The same principles apply in the detoxification from nicotine dependence and from sedative (alcohol) dependence, except the untreated sedative withdrawal syndrome is much more dangerous than that of opiates or nicotine. Stimulant withdrawal has not traditionally been treated by detoxification regimens, even though it is associated with poor clinical outcome.

In the treatment of patients dependent on alcohol or other sedatives, appropriate detoxification is critical because the sedative withdrawal syndrome is potentially life threatening. Whereas the acute administration of alcohol and sedatives increases γ-aminobutyric acid (GABA) and decreases glutamate pathways, the reverse occurs with chronic exposure, producing a GABA-deficiency state and glutamate hyperactivity that increases the risk of seizures during withdrawal (Dackis and O'Brien, 2003). There is evidence that sensitization to alcohol withdrawal symptoms occurs, so repeated withdrawals become progressively more severe while the treatment of withdrawal symptoms may retard the sensitization process (Brown et al., 1988). Benzodiazepines effectively suppress the withdrawal syndrome, and with proper attention to electrolytes and vitamins, the vast majority of patients can be safely eased into the alcohol-abstinent state in preparation for a long-term rehabilitation program.

Symptoms of nicotine withdrawal can be diminished by nicotine replacement therapy including chewing gum, patch, or nasal spray. Nicotine gum and nicotine patch do not achieve the peak plasma levels seen with cigarettes, and thus they do not produce the same magnitude of nicotine's subjective effects. Comparisons with placebo treatment show large benefits for nicotine replacement at 6 weeks, but the effect diminishes with time.

The withdrawal syndrome from stimulants such as cocaine and amphetamine consists of hypersomnia, hyperphagia, bradycardia, and a number of depressive symptoms that usually resolve over several days. Interestingly, cocaine withdrawal symptoms appear to be predictive of treatment outcome. Kampman and colleagues (2002) measured cocaine withdrawal symptoms in several trials using the Cocaine Selective Severity Assessment. They found that more withdrawal symptoms in patients at the start of treatment accurately predicted their poorer outcome following treatment. Given these findings, the pharmacological reversal of cocaine withdrawal symptoms with agents like modafinil may improve clinical outcome (Dackis, 2005).

Patients with heavy marijuana use also develop a physical dependence and may present for treatment when they are unable to stop daily use on their own (Haney, 2005). The symptoms consist of irritability, anxiety, marijuana craving, decreased quality and quantity of sleep, and decreased food intake. Various medications have been tried to alleviate these symptoms, and some clinicians have reported success with dronabinol, the oral form of delta 9 tetra hydro cannabinol, but clinical trials are absent (Haney et al., 2004).

Detoxification by Suppression of Autonomic Hyperactivity

For opiate detoxification, methadone is not always available due to legal limitations, and buprenorphine may be undesirable because it is an opiate partial agonist. Clonidine, a nonopiate that reverses opiate withdrawal, is an alternative option in these instances. Lofexidine, a similar medication, is currently in clinical trials as an aid to opiate detoxification. These α_2 agonists act as autoreceptors and produce presynaptic inhibition of locus coeruleus activity, effectively reducing the large adrenergic component of opioid withdrawal (Gerra et al., 2001). Thus, clonidine and lofexidine have found a place in the clinic for treating the symptoms of opioid withdrawal.

Rapid Detoxification for Opiate Addiction

Because persons who are opiate addicts are often afraid to detoxify, there have been efforts to make the process more rapid and less frightening so as to improve the transition to the protection of an opiate antagonist. These efforts began in the 1980s and progressed to the present fad of rapid detoxification while under general anesthesia. A mixture of medications that is typically kept confidential as a "trade secret" is used, but the known commonalities are as follows: After induction of general anesthesia, detoxification is precipitated by an opiate antagonist such as naloxone or naltrexone or a combination of the two; opiates are displaced from their receptors and metabolized, but the patient is not aware of withdrawal symptoms while anesthetized; in some cases, naltrexone may be implanted subcutaneously (L. Gooberman, personal communication, Seminar at University of Pennsylvania, 4/12/97) to prevent relapse to opiate use for varying periods of time after the procedure. The patient is awakened after 6–8 hours and is considered detoxified. This procedure is expensive and carries the risks of general anesthesia. A randomized controlled comparison of rapid detoxification under anesthesia versus buprenorphine detoxification was conducted, and there was no apparent advantage for the procedure under anesthesia (Collins et al., 2005). At this time, there is no evidence that speed of detoxification has any long-term advantage over the usual procedure over several days. Whatever the method, relapse after detoxification is very common.

MEDICATIONS FOR PREVENTION OF RELAPSE

The treatment of patients with an addiction must always be individualized. This requires a complete evaluation so that coexisting medical, psychiatric, and social problems can be addressed as needed. There are, however, common elements to treatment programs. Treatments for addictive disorders may begin with detoxification, but the key to successful treatment is long-term prevention of relapse by behavioral and pharmacological means. Usually these approaches should be combined, but the insistence on behavioral treatment alone and the avoidance of medication remain a significant weakness in many treatment programs. The types of medication that have shown efficacy in combination with behavioral therapy in the prevention of relapse can be classified as agonists (including partial agonists), antagonists, and anticraving medications that work through a variety of mechanisms. Vaccines are an experimental approach that is currently being evaluated in clinical trials (Sofuoglu and Kosten, 2006).

Agonists and Partial Agonists

The first use of an agonist for the treatment of addiction was reported by Vincent Dole (Dole and Nyswander, 1965), who demonstrated that daily methadone treatment could transform the behavior of patients with an opiate addiction. Opiates, which are derivates of the opium poppy, and opioids, which may be peptides or synthetic compounds, activate opiate receptors that are located throughout the nervous system as well as in the endocrine, cardiovascular, gastrointestinal, and other systems of the body. The behavioral effects of opiates include intense euphoria and calming. The user becomes satisfied and relaxed, a state quite different from the euphoric excitement produced by stimulants. Among the other effects of opiates is the activation of an endogenous pain control system, so a person in severe pain experiences relaxation and relief of severe pain.

Although opiates produce prompt physical dependence with repeated use, addiction seldom occurs in patients receiving opiates and opioids for relief of pain (Adams et al., 2006). Of course, prescription opiates and opioids can be abused, and it is the responsibility of the physician to provide humane pain relief to patients in need while exercising caution to reduce the likelihood that the prescribed medication will be obtained by deliberate abusers. The use of heroin or other opiates purchased on the street for the purpose of obtaining a "high" has a significant risk of producing addiction. Currently, it is estimated that there are over one million heroin and other opiate addicts in the United States, and the purity of heroin sold on the street is at an historic high. Much is known about the mechanisms involved in opiate dependence, resulting in a wider variety of effective medications than are found for other types of addiction.

Detoxification is not applicable for those patients who are opioid dependent who prefer maintenance using methadone or buprenorphine (Kreek, 1992). In the mid-1960s, Dole and Nyswander (1965) found that methadone given in a level dose could be used to stabilize patients who were addicted to opiates, block withdrawal symptoms, and reduce or eliminate the craving for heroin. This discovery opened the way for the medical treatment of addictive disorders (Dole and Nyswander, 1965). Methadone has a slow onset by the oral route. It is a long-acting mu-opiate receptor agonist that largely prevents reward or euphoria if the patient "slips" and takes a dose of an opiate. The mechanism for preventing euphoria is based on cross-tolerance in which tolerance (insensitivity) acquired by the use of one drug in a category conveys tolerance to all drugs in that category. Of course, the maintenance dose of methadone must be adjusted to the purity of heroin on the street. A dose of heroin significantly higher in opioid equivalents than the maintenance dose of methadone would override the cross-tolerance effect. Patients can be maintained for many years on a properly adjusted dose of methadone. Craving for opioids is diminished or absent, and patients are able to engage in constructive activities. Cognition and alertness are not impaired, and complex tasks including higher education can be accomplished (Kreek, 1992). Currently, about 200,000 people formerly addicted to illegal opioids are being maintained on methadone in the United States. Those with significant psychosocial problems require counseling or psychotherapy in addition to the medication.

A major change in the treatment of opiate addiction in the United States came in 2000, when legislation was enacted that made it possible to treat persons with an addiction to opiates in a doctor's office rather than requiring a specialized methadone clinic. The medication that was intended for this treatment is buprenorphine. This medication is a partial agonist at the mu receptor and an antagonist at kappa receptors (Bickel and Amass, 1995). As a partial agonist, buprenorphine produces limited opiate effects, and thus overdose is rare. Because of its affinity for the mu receptor, buprenorphine effectively prevents the effects of other opiates and opioids, thus reducing the likelihood that heroin will be used. Patients treated with buprenorphine become dependent on it, as with methadone and levo-alpha-acetylmethadyl (LAAM), but the withdrawal symptoms from buprenorphine are quite mild. A limitation of buprenorphine is the ceiling on opiate agonist effects giving a maximal efficacy of about 40–50 mg of methadone. Persons with an addiction using large doses of street heroin may find that buprenorphine is not sufficiently potent to block withdrawal or drug craving.

After 2 years of debate over how many restrictions to place on the prescribing of this medication, buprenorphine was approved in 2002 as a Schedule III opioid. Prescribing is limited to physicians who take extra training and obtain certification. The rules initially limited doctors to no more than 30 patients per physician. Recently, the limit was raised to 100 because experience and monitoring over the past 4 years has found very little abuse. An important reason may be the fact that buprenorphine is marketed in combination with the opiate antagonist naloxone in a 4:1 ratio of buprenorphine to naloxone. When the medication is taken sublingually, the naloxone is poorly absorbed, and the agonist effects of buprenorphine are not blocked. If a person who wishes to obtain euphoria injects the combination either intravenously or intramuscularly, the naloxone acts as a powerful antagonist, blocking the mu-opioid effects and producing minimal desirable effects, possibly even mild withdrawal, depending on the prior state of the patient (Mendelson et al., 1999).

Another approved opiate agonist that can be used for maintenance is LAAM. This drug has long-acting metabolites that block withdrawal and craving for over 72 hours, and it need be taken only 2 to 3 times per week. Use of LAAM is now a second-line therapy due to the finding of prolonged QT interval corrected (QTc) on cardiograms and the risk of serious cardiac rhythm abnormalities (Marsch et al., 2005).

A similar agonist principle is the use of nicotine replacement therapy in the treatment of tobacco use disorder. The administration of nicotine as a patch, gum, or nasal spray can replace the nicotine received through smoking, thus blocking withdrawal symptoms. The nicotine can be stopped after 1 to 2 weeks without discomfort, although craving may return. The nicotine can be continued as a maintenance for extended periods, as is the case with methadone. The levels obtained via a nicotine patch usually do not produce the pleasant responses achieved through smoking, and there are usually no withdrawal symptoms on stopping the patch. Theoretically, smokers should be able to switch their nicotine dependence from administration via smoking to nicotine delivered by patch, chewing gum, or nasal spray. Although some smokers continue to chew nicotine gum for many months after giving up cigarettes, most stop nicotine replacement after a few weeks. The tendency to relapse may be strong, and thus it is important to teach patients behavioral techniques to resist the urge to smoke. An interesting combination that showed some efficacy in clinical trials is the combination of nicotine and mecamylamine to prevent relapse to smoking. It was hypothesized that stimulation of receptors by an agonist and an antagonist would be more effective, and the side effects of the two drugs would tend to cancel each other out (Rose et al., 2001). The clinical data on this combination have been mixed, and more studies are needed.

A very recent medication that applies the partial agonist principle in the treatment of tobacco use disorder is varenicline (Foulds, 2006). This is an $\alpha_4 \beta_2$ nicotinic receptor partial agonist that has been reported to relieve cigarette craving and to result in a significantly higher rate of abstinence at 52 weeks (23%) than placebo (10.3%) or bupropion (14.6%) in company-sponsored double-blind trials (Jorenby et al., 2006).

Although agonist treatment is effective in opioid and nicotine addiction, agonists have not been found effective in patients addicted to stimulants. Experiments using methylphenidate or dextro-amphetamine as agonists for cocaine and methamphetamine addiction have not been successful (Gorelick et al., 2004). Similarly, benzodiazepine treatment for alcohol or sedative dependence is ineffective. It is unclear why agonist treatment does not work in patients addicted to these substances.

The pharmacological reversal of clinically significant neuroadaptations has long been employed with detoxification regimens, and the normalization of more persistent neuroadaptations might identify agents with anti-craving action (O'Brien, 2005a). In addition to chronic neuroadaptations in reward-related pathways, prefrontal cortical dysregulation has been demonstrated in stimulant, opioid, and alcohol dependence (Dackis and O'Brien, 2005a) and is now viewed as a core component of addiction that contributes to poor impulse control, reduced motivation, and denial in individuals with an addiction (Dackis and O'Brien, 2005a). Consequently, agents that enhance prefrontal cortical metabolism hold promise in the treatment of addiction.

Antagonist Treatment

Advances in understanding how opioids interact with opiate receptors to produce their pharmacological effects led to the development of specific antagonists that have high affinity for these receptors but do not activate the chain of cellular events producing opioid drug effects. Naltrexone is an antagonist that has great affinity for mu-opiate receptors and significant but less affinity for delta and kappa opiate receptors. Unlike methadone, it has no agonist effects, so there are no opioid calming or other subjective effects. When first introduced, naltrexone was thought to be an ideal medication for heroin addiction because it occupied opiate receptors and blocked the effects of subsequent heroin injections. Experience has shown that most persons addicted to heroin prefer methadone because it provides mild opioid-reinforcing effects that are absent in naltrexone. Thus, naltrexone has been used very little except for white-collar individuals with an addiction to opiates such as physicians, nurses, and individuals with a history of opioid addiction recently released from prison on probation (Cornish et al., 1997). The effects of blocking opiate receptors probably depend on the degree of tonic activation of the endogenous opioid system. Some normal volunteers given naltrexone experience nausea and dysphoria, while others experience no reaction. Although long-term blockade of opiate receptors might be expected to produce impairment of neuroendocrine function, remarkably few effects have been noted even in patients who have taken naltrexone daily for several years.

In 2006, a slow-release (depot) injectable preparation of naltrexone was given FDA approval and made available for prescription. Paradoxically, it was approved only for alcoholism because it was discovered in animal models that alcohol activated endogenous opioids (Altshuler et al., 1980), and blocking opiate receptors with naltrexone was found to improve treatment for alcoholism (Volpicelli et al., 1990; Volpicelli et al., 1992). Of course, the depot form of naltrexone is also effective for the treatment of opioid addiction (Comer et al., 2006), and clinical trials are under way that will eventually lead to FDA approval for that indication in addition to alcoholism. Thus, opiate receptor antagonists have been found to be effective in the treatment of opiate addiction and alcoholism. The availability of a depot form is expected to significantly improve the adherence to medication for this treatment method.

Response to naltrexone is similar across all patients with an addiction to opiates because the medication blocks the site of major drug effect. For patients with an alcohol addiction, however, there is great variability. Some patients with an alcohol addiction report that alcohol stimulation is blocked and rehabilitation is greatly aided by the medication. Others report little or no effect. A recent development is the discovery of a functional variant in the mu-opiate receptor gene that is a main target of naltrexone. The variant is an A to G substitution at position 118 of Exon 1 and results in a receptor with reported greater affinity for beta endorphin (Bond et al., 1998). Individuals with this allele have been found to perceive greater stimulation from a given dose of alcohol (Ray and Hutchison, 2004), and the stimulation was found to be blocked by naltrexone pretreatment (Ray, personal communication). A retrospective analysis of patients with an alcohol addiction in a naltrexone clinical trial found that those with the G allele did poorly when randomized to placebo but had a significantly better outcome when randomized to naltrexone (Oslin et al., 2003). This finding was replicated in another clinical trial (Anton et al., 2008) but not in a third (Gelernter et al., 2007).

Blockade of Euphoria

There are different mechanisms whereby medications can block or diminish the euphoria produced by drugs of abuse. Antagonist treatment prevents the addictive agent from effectively binding to brain receptors that mediate the euphoric response. This is best illustrated by naltrexone treatment in opiate dependence because the mechanism of opiate euphoria results from the stimulation of mu-opiate receptors. The mechanism of stimulant euphoria is not well understood, so it has been more difficult to develop medications to block this essential clinical phenomenon. An alternative means of diminishing drug euphoria involves the agonist approach. Opiate agonists block euphoria by cross tolerance. Thus, a steady dose of methadone not only satisfies the drive to obtain opiates but also produces cross tolerance to all other opiates and opioids. If a patient on methadone decides to try to get high anyway, an injection of heroin will result in little or no euphoria (Kreek, 1992). Levo-alpha-acetylmethadyl works in a similar fashion. Buprenorphine, as a partial agonist with very strong affinity for mu receptors, has both the cross-tolerance effect and a blocking effect as it deprives the injected opiate of access to mu receptors (Comer et al., 2005). Nicotine replacement therapy for smokers can reduce the pleasure of smoking by a cross-tolerance mechanism similar to that of methadone for heroin euphoria.

Modafinil, a medication that retards sleep onset, has been shown to block cocaine-induced euphoria in three human laboratory studies of predominately male cocaine users (Dackis et al., 2003; Malcolm et al., 2006; Hart et al., 2008). The mechanism of this blockade is unknown. Other medications block cocaine reward in animal (but not yet reliably demonstrated in human) studies by increasing GABA inhibitory effects on reward pathways such as ventral tegmental–ventral striatal dopamine (DA) pathways. These include medications such as topiramate (Johnson et al., 2004; Kampman et al., 2004), vigabatrin (Brodie et al., 2005), and baclofen (Weerts et al., 2007). Animal models suggest that this GABA-enhancing mechanism may block the rewarding effects of other drugs as well as cocaine.

Medications That Produce an Aversive Response

Until 1995, disulfiram was the only medication available to prevent relapse to uncontrolled drinking in detoxified persons with an alcohol addiction. This medication blocks the metabolism of alcohol, causing the accumulation of acetaldehyde, a noxious by-product. The resulting acetaldehyde reaction is so unpleasant that it effectively prevents patients from consuming any alcohol. Disulfiram has a place in the pharmacopeia of medications for alcoholism, but its usefulness is limited. Despite treatment contracts and even legal coercion, most persons with an alcohol addiction will not take disulfiram regularly, and randomized clinical trials have not shown disulfiram to be efficacious (Fuller et al., 1986). Aversive conditioning has also been tried by timing an injection of emetine to produce vomiting while presenting the smell and taste of alcohol (Childress et al., 1985). Short-term success has been reported, but the technique has never become widespread.

Anticraving Medications

Acamprosate, a completely different medication that appears to decrease the desire for alcohol, was developed in Europe and has been available in the United States since 2004. Acamprosate appears to reduce the long-lasting neuronal hyperexcitability that follows chronic alcohol use (Anton, O'Malley, et al., 2006). The mechanisms are unclear but may include alterations in glutamate receptor gene expression. This medication suppresses the intake of alcohol in rats and, as with naltrexone, activity in the animal model predicts clinical efficacy. In double-blind studies, acamprosate has been shown to increase the likelihood of continuous abstinence in patients with an alcohol addiction and to shorten the period of drinking if the patient "slips" and consumes some alcohol.

The opiate receptor antagonist naltrexone has been reported in several clinical trials to reduce alcohol craving (O'Brien, 2005b) as well as alcohol reward. Human laboratory studies of alcohol priming in nontreatment seeking patients with an alcohol addiction demonstrated a reduction in alcohol craving and alcohol drinking in spite of the alcohol priming drink in participants who were not seeking treatment (O'Malley et al., 2002).

Preclinical data have also shown an effect of alcohol on serotonergic systems. This has motivated trials using medications affecting that system. Ritanserin, a 5-hydroxytryptamine-2 (5-HT_2) receptor antagonist, was found to be no more effective than placebo in the treatment of alcoholism (Johnson et al., 1996). Ondansetron, a 5-HT_3 antagonist, was found to reduce drinking in early-onset patients with an alcohol addiction alone (Johnson et al., 2000) and in combination with naltrexone (Ait-Daoud et al., 2001). Specific craving studies have not been addressed with the serotonergic medications.

STIMULANT ADDICTION

Stimulant use tends to occur in epidemics. In the United States, cocaine use peaked during 1985 with 8.6 million occasional users and 5.8 million regular users. More than 23 million Americans are estimated to have used cocaine at some time, but the number of current users declined steadily to 2.9 million in 1988 and further to 1.5 million in 1995. Lifetime prevalence rates peaked at 2.7% in 2002 (Volkow, 2004). Unfortunately, the number of frequent users (at least weekly) has remained steady since 1991 at about 600,000.

The pharmacological effects of this drug in humans have been observed in the laboratory. Cocaine produces a dose-related increase in wakefulness, improved performance on tasks of vigilance and alertness, sexual arousal, and a sense of self-confidence and well-being. This is accompanied by increased heart rate and blood pressure. Higher doses produce a brief euphoria followed by a desire for more drug. Involuntary motor activity, stereotyped behavior, and paranoia may occur. Irritability, personality change, and increased risk of violence are found among heavy chronic users. The half-life of cocaine in plasma is about 50 minutes, but inhalant (crack) users typically desire more cocaine after 10 to 30 minutes. Intranasal and intravenous use also results in briefer euphoria than would be predicted by plasma cocaine levels, suggesting that a declining plasma concentration is associated with termination of the high and increased craving for cocaine. This theory is supported by PET imaging studies using ^{11}C-labeled cocaine that show that the time course of subjective euphoria parallels the uptake and displacement of the drug in the corpus striatum (Chapter 49).

Addiction is the most common complication of cocaine use although some users, especially those using intranasally, can continue intermittent use for years. Others become compulsive users despite elaborate methods to maintain control. Stimulants tend to be used much more irregularly than opiates, nicotine, and alcohol. Binge use is very common, and a binge may last for hours to days, terminating only when supplies of the drug are exhausted or when use is interrupted by behavioral toxicity such as hallucinations.

Cocaine Sensitization

Sensitization, a consistent finding in animal studies of cocaine and other stimulants, has not been clearly demonstrated in humans with an addiction to cocaine. Sensitization is typically measured by increased behavioral hyperactivity when the same dose is given daily to an animal. In human cocaine users, sensitization for euphoric effects of cocaine is not typically seen. To the contrary, some experienced users report requiring more cocaine over time to obtain euphoria, that is, tolerance. In the laboratory, tachyphylaxis (rapid tolerance) has been observed with reduced effects when the same dose was given repeatedly in one session. Because not all animals show behavioral sensitization to cocaine, and not all human cocaine users become addicted, it is possible that the failure to sensitize predisposes one to cocaine addiction.

Sensitization in humans has been linked to paranoid, psychotic manifestations of cocaine use. This idea is based on the fact that binge-limited paranoia begins after long-term cocaine use (mean interval, 35 months) in vulnerable users (Satel and Edell, 1991). Thus, repeated administration may be required to sensitize the patient to experience paranoia. The phenomenon of kindling has also been invoked to explain cocaine sensitization. Subconvulsive doses of cocaine given repeatedly will eventually produce seizures in rats (Post et al., 1987). This observation has been compared to electrical kindling of seizures and may underlie the gradual development of paranoia.

Cocaine users experience intense craving when exposed to cocaine-related cues, which typically include the neighborhood where they have used cocaine, the sight of cocaine, cocaine paraphernalia, and cash. This response has been measured in the laboratory when abstinent users of cocaine are shown video scenes associated with cocaine use (Ehrman et al., 1992). The conditioned response consists of physiological arousal and increased drug craving. Cue-induced craving is a pernicious phenomenon that leads directly to relapse in patients with an addiction, even after long periods of abstinence. Medications that block limbic activation in response to cocaine cues may prove effective against this pernicious phenomenon.

Relapse prevention is usually the major challenge encountered by clinicians who treat patients with an addiction to cocaine. Effective rehabilitation programs use individual and group psychotherapy based on the principles of Alcoholics Anonymous and/or behavioral treatments such as those based on reinforcing cocaine-free urine tests using vouchers that can be exchanged for goods and services (Alterman and McLellan, 1993; Higgins et al., 1994). These programs produce improvement and varying periods of abstinence, but the risk of relapse remains after months or years of abstinence.

Numerous studies have been conducted on medications that might aid in the rehabilitation of individuals with an addiction to cocaine. A detailed review would not be useful because most are no longer used. Among those medications still under study for possible approval by the FDA as a treatment for stimulant addiction are modafinil (Dackis et al., 2005) and disulfiram (Carroll et al., 1998).

Buprenorphine, a partial opioid agonist, has been found to reduce cocaine self-administration in monkeys (Mello et al., 1989), but studies in patients who were dependent upon cocaine have yielded mixed results. A recent controlled study of buprenorphine in a population of combined patients who were dependent on both opiates and cocaine showed a positive effect in reducing the use of cocaine and opiates (Montoya et al., 2004). The results were consistent with the hypothesis that buprenorphine is effect for cocaine only in higher doses, 16 mg or greater.

Studies in animals have consistently shown that enhancement of GABA activity reduces cocaine self-administration (Roberts et al., 1996). Preliminary results from clinical trials using baclofen, a GABA-B agonist, and topiramate, which activates GABA-A receptors, suggest that this approach may reduce cocaine use in humans as well (Shoptaw et al., 2003). Studies in patients with cocaine and methamphetamine addictions using vigabatrin, an inhibitor of GABA transaminase, are just beginning (Brodie et al., 2005).

Another recent novel approach uses modafinil, a drug that produces alerting via a complex mechanism involving enhanced glutamate activity. A controlled study reported that modafinil-treated patients significantly reduced their use of cocaine when compared to placebo-treated patients (Dackis et al., 2005). Modafinil is currently under intense investigation as a first-line treatment for cocaine dependence.

Other Stimulants

Amphetamine, dextroamphetamine, methamphetamine, phenmetrazine, methylphenidate, and diethylpropion all produce behavioral activation similar to that of cocaine. Amphetamines increase synaptic DA levels primarily by stimulating presynaptic DA release rather than by blockade of reuptake at the DA transporter, as is the case with cocaine. Intravenous or smoked methamphetamine is an important drug of abuse in the western half of the United States, and it produces an abuse/dependence syndrome similar to that of cocaine. Paranoid psychosis is more common with amphetamine abuse. In some sections, methamphetamine abuse has reached epidemic proportions, and there are intensive efforts to develop behavioral and medication treatments for this serious addiction (Rawson et al., 2000).

A different picture arises when oral stimulants are prescribed in a weight reduction program. These drugs do reduce appetite and weight on a short-term basis, but the effects diminish over time as tolerance develops. In rodents, there is a rebound of appetite and weight gain when amphetamine use is stopped. In humans who are obese, weight loss after amphetamine treatment is usually temporary. Anorectic medications, therefore, are not considered to be a treatment for obesity by themselves, but rather a short-term adjunct to behavioral treatment programs. It is noteworthy that drug abuse manifested by drug-seeking behavior occurs in only a small proportion of patients given stimulants to facilitate weight reduction.

Cannabinoids (Marijuana)

Cannabis is a plant that has been cultivated for the production of hemp fiber and for presumed medicinal and psychoactive properties of the plant's products. The smoke from burning cannabis contains 61 different cannabinoids, but virtually all of the psychoactive effects of smoked marijuana can be produced by one of them, Δ-9-tetrahydrocannabinol. In the United States, marijuana is the most commonly used illicit drug. Usage peaked during the late 1970s, when about 60% of high school seniors reported having used marijuana and about 10% reported daily use. Lifetime use declined to 40% and daily use to 2% in the mid-1990s, but 2005 data for 12th graders was 45% lifetime prevalence and for 29- to 30-year-olds, 60% lifetime prevalence (Johnston, 2006).

The actions of cannabis in the brain are becoming better understood. A cannabinoid receptor has been identified (Devane et al., 1988) and cloned (Matsuda et al., 1990), and two subtypes have been identified. These receptors are widely dispersed throughout the brain and in certain other organs. High densities occur in the cerebral cortex, hippocampus, striatum, and cerebellum (Herkenham, 1993). An arachadonic acid derivative has been identified as an endogenous ligand and named anandamide (Devane et al., 1992).

The effects of marijuana depend on the route of administration, the dose, the experience of the user, and the setting in which it is used. Changes in mood, perception, and motivation are reported by most users. The giddiness and relaxed feeling called a "high" lasts about 2 hours. During this time, there is impairment of cognitive functions, perception, reaction time, learning, and memory. Impairment of coordination and eye-tracking behavior has been reported to persist for several hours beyond the perception of a high. Anxiety reactions may occur, especially with higher doses and with oral rather than smoked marijuana.

Although there is no convincing evidence that marijuana can produce a schizophrenic-like syndrome, there are numerous clinical reports that marijuana use can precipitate a relapse in patients recovering from a schizophrenic episode. Marijuana has also been reported to produce an amotivational syndrome. This is not an official diagnosis, but it has been used to describe individuals who withdraw from social activities and show little interest in school, work, or other goal-directed activity. When heavy marijuana use accompanies these symptoms, the drug is often cited as the cause. There are no data that demonstrate a causal relationship, although most authorities recommend that treatment of such patients include cessation of marijuana use. There is no evidence that marijuana damages brain cells or produces any permanent functional changes, and heavy marijuana users show gradual improvement in mental state after stopping its use. This is consistent with animal data indicating impairment of maze learning that persists for weeks after the last dose of the drug.

Tolerance to the effects of marijuana has been demonstrated in humans and animals (Jones et al., 1981). Withdrawal symptoms and signs are not typically seen in clinical populations, but some patients report compulsive frequent marijuana use. In 2002, over 280,000 people entered treatment for cannabis dependence (National Institute on Drug Abuse, 2007). There is no specific treatment for marijuana dependence at this time, but cannabinoids receptor antagonists are logical candidates for investigation. The withdrawal syndrome does not require medication unless persistent signs of depression are present. Prevention of relapse is accomplished by behavioral treatments such as those used in the treatment of alcoholism or cocaine addiction (Stephens et al., 2002).

Several beneficial effects of marijuana have been described. These include reduction of nausea, muscle-relaxing effects, anticonvulsant effects, and reduction of intraocular tension for the treatment of glaucoma. There are also clinical reports asserting that marijuana stimulates appetite and reverses the muscle wasting seen in acquired immune deficiency syndrome and other conditions. When it is taken as a medication rather than as a recreational drug, the psychoactive effects are also present and may impair normal occupational functions. At present, there are insufficient data to claim that cannabinoids are superior to standard treatments, but some controlled studies are in progress. A major problem in assessing the medicinal use of smoked marijuana is the uncertain delivery of multiple substances and variable doses. With the cloning of cannabinoid receptors and the discovery of an endogenous ligand, it is hoped that derivatives of cannabinoids with medicinal uses will be developed.

Hallucinogenic Drugs

Drugs that primarily produce perceptual, thought, or mood disturbances at low doses, with minimal effects on memory and orientation, are classed as hallucinogenic drugs. Examples are lysergic acid diethylamide (LSD), phencyclidine (PCP), methylenedioxymethamphetamine (MMDA, "ecstasy"), and a variety of anticholinergic drugs (atropine, benztropine). Lysergic acid diethylamide was discovered in 1945, but experimental and recreational use peaked in the 1960s and 1970s and then declined. During the 1990s, use again increased. In 1993, 11.8% of college students reported some use of these drugs during their lifetime, and the increase was most striking in younger cohorts beginning in the eighth grade.

Lysergic acid diethylamide is the most potent hallucinogenic drug, producing significant psychedelic effects with a total dose of as little as 25–50 mg. Thus, it is over 3,000 times more potent than mescaline. In humans, the effects of hallucinogenic drugs are variable even in the same individual at different times. In addition to the dose of the drug, individual variables and the setting in which the drug is given are important. At doses of 100 micrograms, LSD produces perceptual distortions and hallucinations; mood changes, including elation, paranoia, or depression; intense arousal; and sometimes a feeling of panic. Signs of LSD ingestion include pupillary dilation, increased blood pressure and pulse, flushing, salivation, lacrimation, and hyperreflexia. The user typically reports prominent visual effects. Colors seem more intense; shapes may appear altered, and the user may focus attention on unusual items such as the pattern of hairs on the back of his or her hand. Claims have been made about the potential of these drugs for enhancing psychotherapy and for treating addictions and other mental disorders. These claims have not been supported by controlled treatment outcome studies; thus, there is no current indication for these drugs as medications.

Medical attention may be sought when an unpleasant reaction occurs. A "bad trip" usually consists of severe anxiety, although at times it is marked by intense depression and suicidal thoughts. The bad trip from LSD may be difficult to distinguish from reactions to anticholinergic drugs and PCP. There are no documented toxic fatalities from LSD use, but fatal accidents and suicides have occurred during or shortly after the trip.

Prolonged psychotic reactions lasting 2 days or more may occur after the ingestion of a hallucinogen. Schizophrenic episodes may be precipitated in susceptible individuals, and there is some evidence that chronic use of these drugs is associated with the development of persistent psychotic disorders (McLellan et al., 1979).

When a user is brought to the emergency room after a bad trip, the severe agitation can be ameliorated with benzodiazepines (that is, diazepam 20 mg orally) or simply "talked down" by reassurance. Neuroleptic medications (DA receptor antagonists) should be avoided as they may intensify the experience. A particularly troubling aftereffect of the use of LSD and other similar drugs is the occurrence of episodic visual disturbances in a small proportion of former users. These are called *flashbacks*, and they resemble the experiences of prior LSD trips. There is now an official diagnostic category called the hallucinogen persisting perception disorder (HPPD) (APA, 1994). The symptoms include false fleeting perceptions in the peripheral fields, flashes of color, geometric pseudohallucinations, and positive afterimages (Abraham and Aldridge, 1993). The visual disorder appears stable in half of the cases and thus represents an apparently permanent alteration of the visual system. These symptoms may be precipitated by stress, fatigue, emergence into a dark environment, marijuana use, neuroleptic use, and anxiety states.

Methylenedioxymethamphetamine

Methylenedioxymethamphetamine (MDMA) and methylenedioxyamphetamine (MDA) are phenylethylamines that have stimulant as well as psychedelic effects. Known as "ecstasy," MDMA in the past was recommended by some psychotherapists as an aid to gaining insight, although no data exist to support this contention. The drug became popular during the 1980s on some college campuses because of testimonials that it enhances self-knowledge. The acute effects are dose-dependent and include tachycardia, dry mouth, jaw clenching, muscle aches, and, at higher doses, visual hallucinations, agitation, hyperthermia, and panic attacks.

Animal data showing degeneration of serotonergic nerve cells and axons have been reported (Ricaurte et al., 1985). In humans, cerebrospinal fluid of individuals with chronic MDMA use has been found to have low levels of serotonin metabolites, but brain studies similar to those reported in animals have not been done. Some residual effects have been reported (Bolla et al., 1998), and there is no evidence that the claimed benefits of MDMA actually occur.

Phencyclidine

Phencyclidine (PCP) is available throughout the United States through illicit channels. It was originally developed as an anesthetic in the 1950s but was abandoned because of a high frequency of postoperative delirium with hallucinations. It was classed as a dissociative anesthetic because, in the anesthetized state, the patients remain conscious, with staring gaze, flat facies, and rigid muscles. As little as 0.05 mg/kg produces emotional withdrawal, concrete thinking, and bizarre responses to projective psychological testing. The symptoms produced by PCP include catatonic posturing and resemble the symptoms of schizophrenia. Abusers taking higher doses may exhibit hostile or assaultive behavior. Anesthetic effects increase with the dosage, and stupor or coma may occur with muscular rigidity, rhabdomyolysis, and hyperthermia. Patients who are intoxicated and in the emergency room may change quickly from aggressive behavior to coma, with elevated blood pressure and enlarged, nonreactive pupils.

Phencyclidine binds with high affinity to sites located in the cortex and limbic structures, resulting in blocking of *N*-methyl-D-aspartic acid (NMDA)-type glutamate receptors. Lysergic acid diethylamide and other psychedelics do not bind to these receptors. There is evidence that NMDA receptors are involved in ischemic neuronal death caused by high levels of excitatory amino acids. Thus, there is interest in potentially therapeutic analogues of PCP that also block NMDA channels but with fewer psychotic effects.

There are no specific treatments for hallucinogenic drug abuse. Patients frequently have to be admitted to the hospital because of brief psychotic episodes, but the most difficult aspect of treatment is the long-term prevention of relapse.

Inhalants

Anesthetic gases such as nitrous oxide or halothane are sometimes taken by medical personnel to produce a "high." Nitrous oxide used in whipping cream canisters may be abused by food service employees. Nitrous oxide produces euphoria and analgesia followed by loss of consciousness. Compulsive use and chronic toxicity are rarely reported, but there are obvious risks of overdosage associated with the abuse of this anesthetic.

Chemicals that are volatile at room temperature and produce abrupt changes in mental state when inhaled are abused by some groups in specific parts of the United States. Examples include toluene (from airplane glue), kerosene, gasoline, carbon tetrachloride, amyl nitrate, and nitrous oxide. Each substance has a characteristic pattern. Solvents such as toluene are typically used by children beginning at age 12. The child places the material in a plastic bag and inhales the vapors. After several minutes of inhalation, dizziness and intoxication occur. Aerosol sprays containing fluorocarbon propellants are used in a similar fashion. Prolonged exposure or daily use may result in damage to several organ systems. Clinical problems include cardiac arrhythmias, bone marrow depression, cerebral degeneration, and damage to liver, kidney, and peripheral nerves. Cardiac arrhythmias and death have occasionally been attributed to inhalant abuse.

Amyl nitrate was used in the past for the treatment of angina because it produces dilation of smooth muscle and relieves coronary artery constriction. In recent years, amyl nitrate and butyl nitrate have been used to relax smooth muscle and enhance orgasm, particularly by male homosexuals. Sold as room deodorizers, these nitrates can produce the feeling of a "rush," flushing, and dizziness. Adverse effects include palpitations, postural hypotension, and headache progressing to loss of consciousness.

DEVELOPMENTAL THERAPEUTICS

The Vaccine Approach

Immunization against the effects of an abused drug was first tested using morphine. Monkeys were immunized with morphine-6-hemisuccinate-BSA (bovine serum albumin), and the resultant morphine antibodies were found to reduce self-administration of heroin but not cocaine (Killian et al., 1978). Recently, active immunization with a new, stable cocaine conjugate has been found to suppress cocaine- but not amphetamine-induced locomotor activity and stereotyped behavior in rats (Rocio et al., 1995). Brain levels of cocaine were also lowered by the antibodies, and rats and mice were found to reduce intravenous cocaine self-administration after passive transfer of cocaine antibodies (Fox et al., 1996; Kantak et al., 2000). A clinical trial involving 34 patients showed that the vaccine caused few side effects and produced dose-related levels of antibodies (Kosten et al., 2002). Recent studies have shown further improvement in the vaccine, but additional studies involving dose-response relationships to clinical response are necessary (Martell et al., 2005). In spite of cocaine antibodies, relapse may still be possible by using a high dose of the drug or by taking a different stimulant.

CLOSING COMMENTS

Medications that target discrete clinical phenomena of addiction, such as euphoria, withdrawal, and craving, are being developed as adjunctive treatments that may significantly improve clinical outcome. The development of these agents has been greatly facilitated by research revealing the underlying neuronal mechanisms of these phenomena. Although the many types of drug use disorders have common aspects, there are also many differences that must be specifically addressed with different pharmacological strategies. In addition, all patients require a full evaluation and tailored treatment plans that take their unique set of problems into account. It is especially important to identify and stabilize co-occurring medical and psychiatric disorders in the addicted population. Approved medications that target cardinal features of addiction are now available for some addictive disorders, and more will certainly be developed through continued research. When viewed in the context of chronic disease, the current treatments for addiction are quite successful (O'Brien and McLellan, 1996; McLellan et al., 2000). Long-term treatment is accompanied by improvements in physical status as well as in mental, social, and occupational functions.

REFERENCES

Abraham, H.D., and Aldridge, A. (1993) Adverse consequences of lysergic acid diethylamide. *Addiction* 88:1327.

Adams, E.H., Breiner, S., Cicero, T.J., Geller, A., Inciardi, J.A., Schnoll, S.H., et al. (2006) A comparison of the abuse liability of tramadol, NSAIDs, and hydrocodone in patients with chronic pain. *J. Pain Symptom Manage.* 31:465–476.

Ait-Daoud, N., Johnson, B.A., Javors, M., Roache, J.D., and Zanca, N.A. (2001) Combining ondansetron and naltrexone treats biological alcoholics: corroboration of self-reported drinking by serum carbohydrate deficient transferrin, a biomarker. *Alcohol Clin. Exp. Res.* 25:847–849.

Alterman, A.I., and McLellan, A.T. (1993) Inpatient and day hospital treatment services for cocaine and alcohol dependence. *J. Subst. Abuse Treat.* 10:269–275.

Altshuler, H.L., Phillips, P.A., and Feinhandler, D.A. (1980) Alteration of ethanol self-administration by naltrexone. *Life Sci.* 26: 679–688.

American Psychiatric Association. (1994) *Diagnostic and Statistical Manual of Mental Disorders*, 4th ed. Washington, DC: Author.

Anton, R., Couper, D., Swift, R., Pettinati, H., Goldman, D., and Oraczi, G. (2008) An evaluation of the mu opiate receptor gene as a predictor of response to naltrexone in the treatment of alcoholism? Results from the COMBINE study. *Arch. Gen. Psychiatry* 65:135–144.

Anton, R., O'Malley, S., Ciraulo, D., Cisler, R., Couper, D., Donovan, D., et al. (2006) Combined pharmacotherapies and behavioral interventions for alcohol dependence—The COMBINE Study: a randomized controlled trial. *JAMA* 295(17):2003–2007.

Bickel, W.K., and Amass, L. (1995) Buprenorphine treatment of opioid dependence: a review. *Exper. Clin. Psychopharmacol.* 3(4): 477–489.

Bolla, K., McCann, U., and Ricaurte, G. (1998): Memory impairment in abstinent MDMA ("ecstasy") users. *Neurology* 51(6): 1532–1537.

Bond, C., LaForge, K., Tian, M., Melia, D., Shengwen, Z., Borg, L., et al. (1998) Single-nucleotide polymorphism in the human mu opioid receptor gene alters b-endorphin binding and activity: Possible implications for opiate addiction. *Proc. Natl. Acad. Sci.* 95:9608–9613.

Brodie, J.D., Figueroa, E., Laska, E.M., and Dewey, S.L. (2005) Safety and efficacy of gamma-vinyl GABA (GVG) for the treatment of methamphetamine and/or cocaine addiction. *Synapse* 55: 122–125.

Brown, M.E., Anton, R.F., Malcolm, R., and Ballenger, J.C. (1988) Alcohol detoxification and withdrawal seizures: clinical support for a kindling hypothesis. *Biol. Psychiatry* 23:507–514.

Cacciola, J.S., Alterman, A.I., McLellan, A.T., Lin, Y.T., Lynch, K.G. (2007) Initial evidence for the reliability and validity of a "Lite" version of the Addiction Severity Index. *Drug Alcohol Depend.* 87:297–302.

Carroll, K.M., Nich, C., Ball, S.A., McCance, E., and Rounsavile, B.J. (1998) Treatment of cocaine and alcohol dependence with psychotherapy and disulfiram. *Addiction* 93:713–727.

Childress, A.R., McLellan, A.T., and O'Brien, C.P. (1985) Behavioral therapies for substance abuse. *Intl. J. Addictions* 20(6&7): 947–969.

Collins, E.D., Kleber, H.D., Whittington, R.A., and Heitler, N.E. (2005) Anesthesia-assisted vs buprenorphine- or clonidine-assisted heroin detoxification and naltrexone induction: a randomized trial. *JAMA* 294:903–913.

Comer, S.D., Sullivan, M.A., Yu, E., Rothenberg, J.L., Kleber, H.D., Kampman, K., et al. (2006) Injectable, sustained-release naltrexone for the treatment of opioid dependence: a randomized, placebo-controlled trial. *Arch. Gen. Psychiatry* 63:210–218.

Comer, S.D., Walker, E.A., and Collins, E.D. (2005) Buprenorphine/naloxone reduces the reinforcing and subjective effects of heroin in heroin-dependent volunteers. *Psychopharmacology* 181(4):664–675.

Cornish, J.W., Metzger, D., Woody, G.E., Wilson, D., McLellan, A.T., Vandergrift, B., and O'Brien, C.P. (1997) Naltrexone pharmacotherapy for opioid dependent federal probationers. *J. Subst. Abuse Treat.* 14:529–534.

Dackis, C.A. (2005) New treatments for cocaine abuse. *Drug Discovery Today* 2:79–86.

Dackis, C.A., and O'Brien, C.P. (2003) The neurobiology of alcoholism. In: Gershon, S., and Soires, R., eds. *Handbook of Psychiatric Disorders*. New York: Marcel Dekker, pp. 563–580.

Dackis, C., and O'Brien, C. (2005a) Neurobiology of addiction: treatment and public policy ramifications. *Nat. Neurosci.* 8:1431–1436.

Dackis, C., and O'Brien, C. (2005b) Neurobiology of addiction: treatment and public policy ramifications (commentary). *Nat. Neurosci.* 8(11):1431–1436.

Dackis, C.A., Kampman, K.M., Lynch, K.G., Pettinati, H.M., and O'Brien, C.P. (2005) A double-blind, placebo-controlled trial of modafinil for cocaine dependence. *Neuropsychopharmacology* 30:205–211.

Dackis, C.A., Lynch, K.G., Yu, E., Samaha, F.F., Kampman, K.M., Cornish, J.W., et al. (2003) Modafinil and cocaine: a double-blind, placebo-controlled drug interaction study. *Drug Alcohol Depend.* 70:29–37.

Devane, W.A., Dysarz, F.A., Johnson, M.R., Melvin, L.S., and Howlett, A.C. (1988) Determination and characterization of a cannabinoid receptor in rat brain. *Mol. Pharm.* 34:605–613.

Devane, W.A., Hanus, L., Breuer, A., Pertwee, R.G., Stevenson, L.A., Griffin, G., et al. (1992) Isolation and structure of a brain constituent that binds to the cannabinoid receptor. *Science* 258: 1946–1949.

Dole, V.P., and Nyswander, M. (1965) A medical treatment for diacetylmorphine (heroin) addiction: a clinical trial with methadone hydrochloride. *JAMA* 193:80–84.

Ehrman, R., Robbins, S., Childress, A.R., and O'Brien, C.P. (1992) Conditioned responses to cocaine-related stimuli in cocaine abuse patients. *Psychopharmacology* 107:523–529.

Foley, K. (1997) Competent care for the dying instead of physician-assisted suicide. *New Engl. J. Med.* 336(1):54–58.

Foulds, J. (2006) The neurobiological basis for partial agonist treatment of nicotine dependence: varenicline. *Int. J. Clin. Pract.* 60: 571–576.

Fox, B.S., Kantak, K.M., Edwards, M.A., Black, K.M., Bollinger, B.K., Botka, A.J., et al. (1996) Efficacy of a therapeutic cocaine vaccine in rodent models [see comments]. *Nat. Med.* 2:1129–1132.

Fuller, R.K., Branchey, L., Brightwell, D.R., Derman, R.M., Emrick, C.D., Iber, F.L., et al. (1986) Disulfiram treatment of alcoholism. A Veterans Administration cooperative study. *JAMA* 256: 1449–1455.

Gelernter, J., Gueorguieva, R., Kranzler, H.R., Zhang, H., Cramer, J., Rosenheck, R., and Krystal, J.H. (2007) Opioid receptor gene (OPRM1, OPRK1, and OPRD1) variants and response to naltrexone treatment for alcohol dependence: results from the VA Cooperative Study. *Alcohol Clin. Exp. Res.* 31:555–563.

Gerra, G., Zaimovic, A., Giusti, F., Di Gennaro, C., Zambelli, U., Gardini, S., and Delsignore, R. (2001) Lofexidine versus clonidine in rapid opiate detoxification. *J. Subst. Abuse Treat.* 21:11–17.

Gorelick, D.A., Gardner, E.L., and Xi, Z.X. (2004) Agents in development for the management of cocaine abuse. *Drugs* 64: 1547–1573.

Haney, M. (2005) The marijuana withdrawal syndrome: diagnosis and treatment. *Curr. Psychiatry Rep.* 7:360–366.

Haney, M., Hart, C.L., Vosburg, S.K., Nasser, J., Bennett, A., Zubaran, C., and Foltin, R.W. (2004) Marijuana withdrawal in humans: effects of oral THC or divalproex. *Neuropsychopharmacology* 29:158–170.

Hart, C.L., Haney, M., Vosburg, S.K., Rubin, E., and Foltin, R.W. (2008) Smoked cocaine self-administration is decreased by modafinil. *Neuropsychopharmacology* 33:761–768.

Herkenham, M.A. (1993) Localization of cannabinoid receptors in brain; relationship to motor and reward systems. *Biological Basis of Substance Abuse* 3:187–200.

Higgins, S.T., Budney, A.J., Bickel, W.K., Badger, G.J., Foerg, F.E., and Ogden, D. (1994) Outpatient behavioral treatment for cocaine dependence: one-year outcome. *Exp. Clin. Psychopharmacol.* 3(2):205–212.

Johnson, B.A., Ait-Daoud, N., Akhtar, F.Z., and Ma, J.Z. (2004) Oral topiramate reduces the consequences of drinking and improves the quality of life of alcohol-dependent individuals: a randomized controlled trial. *Arch. Gen. Psychiatry* 61:905–912.

Johnson, B.A., Jasinski, D.R., Galloway, G.P., Kranzler, H., Weinrieb, R., Anton, R.F., et al. (1996) Ritanserin in the treatment of alcohol dependence—a multi-center clinical trial. *Psychopharmacology* 128:206–215.

Johnson, B.A., Roache, J.D., Javors, M.A., DiClemente, C.C., Cloninger, C.R., Prihoda, T.J., et al. (2000) Ondansetron for reduction of drinking among biologically predisposed alcoholic patients: A randomized controlled trial [see comments]. *JAMA* 284: 963–971.

Johnston, L. (2006). Monitoring the future 2005. In: Johnston, L., O'Malley, P., Bachman, J., and Schulenberg, J., eds. *Monitoring The Future, National Survey Results on Drug Use, 1975–2005*, Vol I, Secondary School Students. Bethesda, MD: National Institute on Drug Abuse, pp. 139–262.

Jones, R.T., Benowitz, N.L., and Herning, R.I. (1981) Clinical review of cannabis tolerance and dependence. *J. Clin. Pharmacol.* 21:143S–152S.

Jorenby, D.E., Hays, J.T., Rigotti, N.A., Azoulay, S., Watsky, E.J., Williams, K.E., et al. (2006) Efficacy of varenicline, an alpha-4beta2 nicotinic acetylcholine receptor partial agonist, vs placebo or sustained-release bupropion for smoking cessation: a randomized controlled trial. *JAMA* 296:56–63.

Kampman, K.M., Pettinati, H., Lynch, K.G., Dackis, C., Sparkman, T., Weigley, C., and O'Brien, C.P. (2004) A pilot trial of topiramate for the treatment of cocaine dependence. *Drug Alcohol Depend.* 75:233–240.

Kampman, K.M., Volpicelli, J.R., Mulvaney, F., Rukstalis, M., Alterman, A.I., Pettinati, H., et al. (2002) Cocaine withdrawal severity and urine toxicology results from treatment entry predict outcome in medication trials for cocaine dependence. *Addict. Behav.* 27:251–260.

Kantak, K., Collins, S., Lipman, E., Bond, J., Giovanoni, K., and Fox, B. (2000) Evaluation of anti-cocaine antibodies and a cocaine vaccine in a rat self-administration model. *Psychopharmacology* 148:251–262.

Kessler, R.C., Nelson, C.B., McGonagle, K.A., Edlund, M.J., Frank, R.G., and Leaf, P.J. (1996) The epidemiology of co-occurring addictive and mental disorders: implications for prevention and service utilization. *Am. J. Orthopsychiatry* 66:17–31.

Khantzian, E.J. (1985) the self-medication hypothesis of addictive disorders: focus on heroin and cocaine dependence. *Am. J. Psychiatry* 142:1259–1264.

Killian, A., Bonese, K., Rothberg, R., Wainer, B., and Schuster, C. (1978) Effects of passive immunization against morphine on heroin self-administration. *Pharmacol. Biochem. Behav.* 9(3):347–352.

Koob, G.F., Ahmed, S.H., Boutrel, B., Chen, S.A., Kenny, P.J., Markou, A., et al. (2004) Neurobiological mechanisms in the transition from drug use to drug dependence. *Neurosci. Biobehav. Rev.* 27:739–749.

Kosten, T., Rosen, M., Bond, J., Settles, M., Roberts, J., Shields, J., et al. (2002) Human therapeutic cocaine vaccine: safety and immogenicity. *Vaccine* 29(8):1196–1204.

Kreek, M.J. (1992). Rationale for maintenance pharmacotherapy of opiate dependence. In: O'Brien, C.P., and Jaffe, J., eds. *Addictive States*. New York: Raven Press, pp. 205–230.

LeBlanc, A., Kalant, H., Gibbins, R., and Berman, N. (1969) Acquisition and loss of tolerance to ethanol by the rat. *J. Pharmacol. Exp. Ther.* 168:244.

Malcolm, R., Swayngim, K., Donovan, J.L., DeVane, C.L., Elkashef, A., Chiang, N., et al. (2006) Modafinil and cocaine interactions. *Am. J. Drug Alcohol Abuse* 32:577–587.

Marsch, L.A., Stephens, M.A., Mudric, T., Strain, E.C., Bigelow, G.E., and Johnson, R.E. (2005) Predictors of outcome in LAAM, buprenorphine, and methadone treatment for opioid dependence. *Exp. Clin. Psychopharmacol.* 13:293–302.

Martell, B.A., Mitchell, E., Poling, J., Gonsai, K., and Kosten, T.R. (2005) Vaccine pharmacotherapy for the treatment of cocaine dependence. *Biol. Psychiatry* 58:158–164.

Matsuda, L.A., Lolait, S.J., Brownstein, M.J., Young, A.C., Bonner, T.I. (1990) Structure of a cannabinoid receptor and functional expression of the cloned cDNA. *Nature* 346:561–564.

McLellan, A., Luborsky, L., O'Brien, C., and Woody, G. (1980) An improved diagnostic instrument for substance abuse patients: The Addiction Severity Index. *J. Nerv. Ment. Dis.* 168:26–33.

McLellan, A.T., Lewis, D.C., O'Brien, C.P., and Kleber, H.D. (2000) Drug dependence, a chronic medical illness: implications for treatment, insurance, and outcomes evaluation. *JAMA* 284:1689–1695.

McLellan, A.T., Weinstein, R.L., Shen, Q., Kendig, C., and Levine, M. (2005) Improving continuity of care in a public addiction treatment system with clinical case management. *Am. J. Addict.* 14:426–440.

McLellan, A.T., Woody, G.E., and O'Brien, C.P. (1979) Development of psychiatric illness in drug abusers. *N. Eng. J. Med.* 301: 1310–1314.

Mello, N.K., Mendelson, J.H., Bree, M.P., and Lukas, S.E. (1989) Buprenorphine suppresses cocaine self-administration by rhesus monkeys. *Science* 245:859–862.

Mendelson, J., Jones, R.T., Welm, S., Baggott, M., Fernandez, I., Melby, A.K., and Nath, R.P. (1999) Buprenorphine and naloxone combinations: the effects of three dose ratios in morphine-stabilized, opiate-dependent volunteers. *Psychopharmacology* 141:37–46.

Montoya, I.D., Gorelick, D.A., Preston, K.L., Schroeder, J.R., Umbricht, A., Cheskin, L.J., et al. (2004) Randomized trial of buprenorphine for treatment of concurrent opiate and cocaine dependence. *Clin. Pharmacol. Ther.* 75:34–48.

National Institute on Drug Abuse. (2007) *Marijuana Facts*. http://www.nida.nih.gov/MarijBroch/parentpg17-18N.html#Addicted.

Nestler, E.J. (2004) Molecular mechanisms of drug addiction. *Neuropharmacology* 47(Suppl 1):24–32.

O'Brien, C.P. (1975) Experimental analysis of conditioning factors in human narcotic addiction. *Pharmacological Rev.* 27:535–543.

O'Brien, C.P. (2005a) Anti-craving (relapse prevention) medications: possibly a new class of psychoactive medication. *Am. J. Psychiatry* 162:1423–1431.

O'Brien, C.P. (2005b) Drug addiction and drug abuse. In: Brunton, L., ed. *Goodman & Gilman's The Pharmacological Basis of Therapeutics*, 11th ed. New York: McGraw-Hill, pp. 607–627.

O'Brien, C.P. (2006). Drug addiction and drug abuse. In: Brunton, L., Lazo, J., and Parker, K., eds., *Goodman & Gilman's The Pharmacological Basis of Therapeutics*, 11th ed. New York: McGraw- Hill, pp. 607–627.

O'Brien, C.P., and McLellan, A.T. (1996) Myths about the treatment of addiction. *Lancet* 347:237–240.

O'Malley, S.S., Krishnan-Sarin, S., Farren, C., Sinha, R., and Kreek, M.J. (2002) Naltrexone decreases craving and alcohol self-administration in alcohol-dependent subjects and activates the hypothalamo-pituitary-adrenocortical axis. *Psychopharmacology (Berl)* 160:19–29.

Oslin, D.W., Berrettini, W., Kranzler, H.R., Pettinati, H., Gelernter, J., Volpicelli, J.R., and O'Brien, C.P. (2003) A functional polymorphism of the mu-opioid receptor gene is associated with naltrexone response in alcohol-dependent patients. *Neuropsychopharmacology* 28:1546–1552.

Post, R.M., Weiss, S.R.B., Pert, A., and Uhde, T.W. (1987). Chronic cocaine administration: sensitization and kindling effects. In: Fisher, S., and Uhlenhuth, E. H., eds. *Cocaine: Clinical and Biobehavioral Aspects*. New York: Oxford University Press, pp. 109–173.

Rawson, R., Huber, A., Brethen, P., Obert, J., Gulati, V., Shoptaw, S., and Ling, W. (2000) Methamphetamine and cocaine users: differences in characteristics and treatment retention. *J. Psychoactive Drugs* 32:233–238.

Ray, L.A., and Hutchison, K.E. (2004) A polymorphism of the mu-opioid receptor gene (OPRM1) and sensitivity to the effects of alcohol in humans. *Alcohol Clin. Exp. Res.* 28:1789–1795.

Ricaurte, G., Bryan, G., Strauss, L., Seiden, L., and Schuster, C. (1985) Hallucinogenic amphetamine selectively destroys brain serotonin nerve terminals. *Science* 229:986–988.

Roberts, D.C., Andrews, M.M., and Vickers, G.J. (1996) Baclofen attenuates the reinforcing effects of cocaine in rats. *Neuropsychopharmacology* 15:417–423.

Robinson, T.E., and Kolb, B. (2004) Structural plasticity associated with exposure to drugs of abuse. *Neuropharmacology* 47(Suppl 1): 33–46.

Rocio, M., Carrera, A., Ashley, J.A., Parsons, L.H., Wirsching, P., Koob, G.F., and Janda, K.D. (1995) Suppression of psychoactive effects of cocaine by active immunization. *Nature* 378:727–730.

Rose, J.E., Behm, F.M., and Westman, E.C. (2001) Acute effects of nicotine and mecamylamine on tobacco withdrawal symptoms, cigarette reward and ad lib smoking. *Pharmacol. Biochem. Behav.* 68:187–197.

Satel, S.L., and Edell, W.S. (1991) Cocaine-induced paranoia and psychosis proneness. *Am. J. Psychiatry* 148(12):1708–1711.

Schuckit, M., Tipp, J., Bergman, M., Reich, W., Hesselbrock, V., and Smith, T. (1997) Comparison of induced and independent major depressive disorders in 2,945 alcoholics. *Am. J. Psychiatry* 154:948–957.

Shoptaw, S., Yang, X., Rotheram-Fuller, E.J., Hsieh, Y.C., Kintaudi, P.C., Charuvastra, V.C., and Ling, W. (2003) Randomized placebo-controlled trial of baclofen for cocaine dependence: preliminary effects for individuals with chronic patterns of cocaine use. *J. Clin. Psychiatry* 64:1440–1448.

Sofuoglu, M., and Kosten, T.R. (2006) Emerging pharmacological strategies in the fight against cocaine addiction. *Expert Opin. Emerg. Drugs* 11:91–98.

Stalnikowicz, R., Mahamid, R., Kaspi, S., and Brezis, M. (2005) Undertreatment of acute pain in the emergency department: a challenge. *Int. J. Qual. Health Care* 17:173–176.

Stephens, R.S., Babor, T.F., Kadden, R., and Miller, M. (2002) The Marijuana Treatment Project: rationale, design and participant characteristics. *Addiction* 97(Suppl 1):109–124.

Volkow, N. (2004) *Cocaine abuse and addiction (from the director)*. National Institute on Drug Abuse Research Report Series. http://www.nida.nih.gov/ResearchReports/Cocaine/Cocaine.html

Volpicelli, J., Pettinati, H., McLellan, A., and O'Brien, C. (2001) *Combining medication and psychosocial treatment for addiction—The BRENDA approach*. New York: Guilford Press.

Volpicelli, J.R., Alterman, A.I., Hayashida, M., and O'Brien, C.P. (1992) Naltrexone in the treatment of alcohol dependence. *Arch. Gen. Psychiatry* 49:876–880.

Volpicelli, J.R., O'Brien, C.P., Alterman, A.I., and Hayashida, M. (1990). Naltrexone and the treatment of alcohol dependence: initial observations. In: Reid, L.B., ed. *Opioids, Bulimia, Alcohol Abuse and Alcoholism*. New York: Springer-Verlag, pp. 195–214.

Weerts, E.M., Froestl, W., Kaminski, B.J., and Griffiths, R.R. (2007) Attenuation of cocaine-seeking by GABA B receptor agonists baclofen and CGP44532 but not the GABA reuptake inhibitor tiagabine in baboons. *Drug Alcohol Depend.* 89:206–213.

Wikler, A. (1973) Dynamics of drug dependence: implications of a conditioning theory for research and treatment. *Arch. Gen. Psychiatry* 28:611–616.

Woody, G.E., McLellan, A.T., Luborsky, L., O'Brien, C.P., Blaine, J., Fox, S., et al. (1984) Severity of psychiatric symptoms as a predictor of benefits from psychotherapy: the Veterans Administration-Penn study. *Am. J. Psychiatry* 141:1172–1177.

Woody, G., O'Brien, C.P., and Rickels, K. (1974) *Depression and anxiety in heroin addicts: a placebo-controlled study of doxepin in combination with methadone*. Presented at the National Academy of Sciences/National Research Council Committee on Problems of Drug Dependence. Washington, DC: National Academy of Sciences, pp. 1160–1167.

VII DEMENTIA

MARY SANO

OVER the past decade major advances have taken place at virtually every level of understanding Alzheimer's disease (AD) and other dementias. New genetic abnormalities have been identified, pathophysiological mechanisms have been elucidated with therapeutic agents targeting these mechanisms in clinical development, and both diagnostic tests and prognostic indicators are present with new ones on the horizon. While these extraordinary advances are apparent in the research questions we ask and they way we address this disease clinically, fundamental questions remain unanswered.

Any discussion of the pathophysiology and treatment of dementias must consider the function and anatomy of the normal brain. In Chapter 55, Wenk reviews the functional neuroanatomy of the different systems involved in learning and memory and the consequences of these pathways' disruption. Complementing this discussion is Berger-Sweeney and colleagues' review of the neurotransmitter systems involved in learning and memory in Chapter 56. In Chapter 53, Kaufer and DeKosky review the current diagnostic classifications of dementia and how they relate to the neurobiology of AD, Parkinson's disease, dementia with Lewy bodies, and other cognitive disorders. In Chapter 57, Bobinski and colleagues discuss the neuropathological and neuroimaging findings associated with normal aging and AD. The central role of the hippocampus in early disease is reviewed. To date, neuroimaging studies provide the most likely candidates as predictors of cognitive decline and dementia in nonsymptomatic aging cohorts. Clinicopathological examination of autopsied patients who had neuropsychological testing and neuroimaging studies at different stages of cognitive impairment prior to death is invaluable for gaining a better understanding of the distinction between normal aging and AD, and of the transitional state just prior to the development of frank dementia. Perl's review of the abnormalities in brain structures in dementia is a natural extension of the earlier chapters in this section. In Chapter 58, Perl discusses advances that have been made in determining the distinction between normal aging and dementia, and delineates the pathological lesions that are emblematic of AD and other dementias.

In Chapter 52, Hardy and colleagues describe mutations in chromosomes 21, 1, and 14 which have all been implicated in familial forms of AD. These mutations affect three different proteins: amyloid precursor protein (APP), presenilin I, and presenilin II. It has been argued that since all these mutations increase the level of AB1-42 in plasma or in cell culture systems, amyloid deposition must be the final common pathway in AD. As compelling as this analysis may be, it is still not definitive. Much of the literature has focused on the role of AB1-42 in the pathophysiology of AD. The neurotoxicity of AB is concentration-dependent and best demonstrated in cell culture systems. Assays permitting examination of human cerebrospinal fluid (CSF) measures of these components provide further support to the story of amyloid toxicity. In addition, recent attention has been paid to soluble abeta and oligomers which currently dominate the thinking in the field as toxic entities. However, the precise mechanism by which cells are killed remain to be identified. Other credible candidates for a central role in cell death include microglial activation with complement expression. It would be a mistake to dismiss the role of the neurofibrillary tangle in the pathophysiology of AD. Perl underlines the importance of tangles in the pathology of AD and implicitly raises the question of how this molecule could not have a critical role in the cognitive deficits observed in AD patients. Although this pathological element of the affected brain has received somewhat less attention than amyloid, it may still be a critical component. This possibility is strengthened when consideration is given to the fact that relatively large depositions of amyloid can occur in aged individuals who have no cognitive impairment. In contrast, large-scale deposition of tangles is almost inevitably associated with cognitive impairment. Some of the earliest pathological changes in AD include tangle formation in entorhinal cortex. Lastly, there is a certain parsimony to attributing disturbed neuronal function to the deposition of intercellular pathology, such as the tangle, rather than to extracellular pathology, such as the plaque. The development of transgenic animal models further clarifies the pathophysiology of AD and establishes a platform for testing potential therapeutic agents. In Chapter 54, Elder reviews this field, retracing the history of the early attempts to overexpress APP without generating plaque or other AD type pathology. Barely a decade ago, mouse models began to appear that reliably mimicked human AD pathology. A concerted effort has been made to gain insight into the etiology of AD by attempting to re-create some the gene-related and/or pathophysiology-related abnormalities in animal models. Genetic manipulations have produced mice that express, overexpress, or underexpress particular genes (APP, presenilin, apolipoprotein E4) and their proteins that are implicated in the pathophysiology of AD. The most recent advances include transgenic animals with new phenotypes that include additional aspects of Alzheimer pathology. Recent *presenilin-1* (PS1) and familial Alzheimer's disease (FAD) mutants can now model age-related neurodegenerative changes, neuronal loss, and recently age-related neurofibrillary tangles (NFTs) like inclusions. Broadening the ability to model these typical pathological features will further our understanding of AD and widen the net of targets for drug development beyond those involved exclusively in amyloid.

The areas where we most urgently need advances are diagnostics and therapeutics. One of the most intriguing possibilities is that imaging techniques may yield a specific diagnostic test for AD, particularly when the illness is in its earliest stages. The chapters by Bobinski and colleagues (57) and Buchsbaum and colleagues (59) raise the possibility that the very early changes in AD may be detectable with magnetic resonance imaging (MRI) and positron emission tomography (PET), respectively. The increasing availability and accuracy of MRI give this technology a potentially broad application. The hippocampal formation may well prove to be a brain region that will provide the earliest window into the process of AD. The ability to detect abnormalities in the hippocampal formation in individuals at risk for AD and to monitor this area's changes with illness progression may suggest that the MRI study of the hippocampus will provide a biological surrogate for the testing and development of drugs designed to alter the progression of the disease. Perhaps such a marker would provide a vehicle to conduct more expeditious clinical trials.

Chapter 60 by Bergmann and Sano reviews progress underlying the therapeutics of AD. Compared to the clinical nihilism that surrounded this disease only 2 decades ago, the availability of approved drugs in two classes (cholinesterase inhibitors and *N*-methyl-D-aspartate [NMDA] receptor antagonist) that have beneficial effects in Alzheimer's patients is a triumph. As Chapter 60 reports, newer treatments targeting amyloid accumulation by various mechanisms including vaccines and secretase modulation are in clinical trials at this very moment which will test the amyloid hypothesis and may provide new hope for patients and practitioners. Development of many of these agents began with the early transgenic models described above and led to full fledged clinical trials. The availability of newer models is already providing leads for new treatment concepts targeting tau and gene.

Chapters 61–63 highlight the importance of subcortical structures in dementia. Using multiple sclerosis as a paradigm, Hyde reviews in Chapter 61 the neuropsychological profile associated with neuropathological lesions observed in these patients. While deficits in working memory and executive function are not uncommon in multiple sclerosis, the more classical neuropsychological deficits in cortical syndromes such as aphasia, agnosia, and apraxia are rarely observed in these patients. Chapters 62 and 63 review two other causes of dementia, dementia with Lewy bodies and Parkinson's disease, respectively. A chapter (65) has been added on frontotemporal dementia (FTD) in which Miller makes the compelling argument that this condition may be more common than previously recognized. FTD is the most common of early onset dementias yet a quarter of the cases occur after the 6th decade. Themes from earlier chapters describing anatomy and imaging resonate as the role of frontal lobe and executive function in clinical phenomenology so characteristic of this disease is described in this chapter. These chapters describe the phenomenology, neuroimaging findings, cognitive profiles, clinical course, genetics, pharmacological management, neurochemical deficits, and neuropathological findings associated with these dementias. While AD, dementia with Lewy bodies, and Parkinson's disease have some common characteristics, it appears that they do represent distinct, yet possibly related, illnesses. It is hoped that further investigation into the interface between these three dementias will achieve a better understanding of their pathophysiology and optimize their treatments.

Two new chapters have been added describing mild cognitive impairment by Peterson (64), and vascular dementia by Chui (66). Both highlight the growing awareness of even subtle cognitive compromise in memory as well as other domains. These chapters describe the clinical presentation of these conditions, demonstrate how cognitive and clinical profiles predict further compromise and incapacity, and address the need to develop treatment algorithms that can address even mild impairment.

Taken together the work summarized in these chapters highlights the importance of cognition in mental health; provides a road map for defining conditions and understanding their phenomenology and pathology; and even provides proof that this dissection of mechanisms of impairment can enlighten our treatment of these conditions.

52 The Genetics and Pathogenesis of Alzheimer's Disease and Related Dementias

JOHN A. HARDY

The role that genetic analysis has played in dissecting the aetiology and pathogenesis of Alzheimer's disease (AD) is the primary focus of this review. The impact of this analysis in terms of animal modeling and clinical investigations is also covered. Other dementing illnesses, including Lewy body disease, prion diseases, Worster Drought syndrome, and frontotemporal dementia, are discussed to the extent that they shed light on the pathogenesis of AD. Progress toward mechanistic therapy is outlined.

INTRODUCTION

In our aging societies, dementias, especially AD but also frontal temporal dementias and Lewy body disease, are increasing societal problems, afflicting perhaps 5% of those older than age 65 years and 20% of those older than 80 years. Treatment for these diseases, as in all neurodegenerative diseases, remains palliative. However, based largely on genetic analysis, we now have an outline of the pathogenic mechanisms involved in these diseases, and we also have a clearer view of the progression of the disease. This increased understanding has led to the identification of several plausible drug targets for these diseases and a general sense of optimism that mechanistic therapy may soon be available. The purpose of this review is to discuss this progress. I focus on AD and discuss other dementias to the extent to which they contribute to our understanding of AD.

ALZHEIMER'S DISEASE

AD is the major cause of dementia in the elderly and afflicts ~4 million Americans (U.S. population ~300 million). Although most cases are late onset and show familial clustering, a small proportion has onset ages younger than age 60 years and shows autosomal dominant inheritance. It seems that all cases with early-onset, autosomal dominant AD have mutations in either the amyloid precursor protein (*APP*) gene or in the presenilin 1 (*PSEN1*) or presenilin 2 (*PSEN2*) genes (Rogaeva, 2002). The only currently accepted genetic risk factor for late-onset AD is the apolipoprotein E (*ApoE*) gene, in which the ε4 allele is risk factor and the ε2 allele is protective (Farrer et al., 1997). Although it is widely believed that there must be other genetic risk factors for late-onset disease, a recent genome screen suggested that there were unlikely to be any other alleles that had as large an effect as *ApoE* (Coon et al., 2007).

APP and Alzheimer's Disease

The occurrence of Alzheimer pathology in Down syndrome (trisomy 21) has long been recognized, and when Glenner and Wong identified the Aβ peptide in the meninges of, first, typical Alzheimer cases (Glenner and Wong, 1984b) and then the same peptide sequence in Down syndrome (Glenner and Wong, 1984a), they commented that it was likely that the gene was on chromosome 21 and was mutated in AD. These remarkable predictions were shown to be correct with the cloning of *APP* and the identification of *APP* mutations in a few AD cases (Goate et al., 1991). Examination of cases of Down syndrome with translocations distal of the *APP* gene showed that these individuals, although they had the obvious features of Down syndrome, did not develop AD (Prasher et al., 1998): this made it clear that the relationship between AD and Down syndrome specifically relates to overexpression of the *APP* gene rather than a nonspecific relationship with the full trisomy.

In general, families with *APP* missense mutations have typical AD with onset ages in the 50s with little variance. However, some cases, particularly those with mutations within the Aβ sequence, have a phenotype that resembles hereditary cerebral hemorrhage with amyloidosis (Dutch type) (HCHWA-D) (Levy et al., 1990). The reason for the variability in the phenotype is not clear. More recently, several families with duplications of the *APP* gene have been identified. Individuals with these duplications also have a variable phenotype with approximately half the duplication carriers developing hemorrhagic strokes and half developing typical AD (Rovelet-Lecrux et al., 2006). These data, of course, fit very well with the observations in Down syndrome, yet hemorrhagic stroke is rare in Down syndrome. The reason for this slight discrepancy is unclear.

ApoE genotype affects the age of onset in families with *APP* mutations and dementia but does not affect the age of onset of hemorrhagic stroke. In dementia, essentially single copies of the ε4 allele reduce the age of onset 5 years relative to ε3 homozygotes, and ε4 homozygotes have an onset age 10 years earlier. Single copies of the ε2 allele increase the age of onset by 5 years, and ε2 homozygotes have an onset age 10 years later (Houlden et al., 1993). These general rules of thumb appear also to be true for AD in Down syndrome (Royston et al., 1994).

One large gap in our current knowledge is that we have little idea about the function of *APP*. When it was first cloned, it was suggested to be a receptor (Kang et al., 1987), and that seems likely to be the case. But its ligand and downstream targets are not known. This means we do not know whether, in some way, Alzheimer pathogenesis relates to the normal function of *APP* (see below).

The Presenilins

A minority of families (~10%) had mutations in the *APP* gene. Genetic linkage analysis showed that the majority of families showed linkage to chromosome 14 (Schellenberg et al., 1992), whereas a minority, largely of Russo-German origin, showed linkage to chromosome 1 (Levy-Lahad et al., 1995). Position cloning identified the genes for the former, which are the majority (~80%), as mutations in the *PSEN1* gene (Sherrington et al., 1995), whereas the others (~10%), including the Russo-German families, had mutations in their homologue, *PSEN2* (Rogaev et al., 1995). Most of the mutations are simple missense variants, but some in frame deletions, most notably *PSEN1* Δex9, have also been described. No nonsense or frameshift mutations have been identified suggesting that the mutations are not simple loss of function variants but not eliminating the possibility that the mutations lead to a partial loss of function.

A very large number of families with *PSEN1* and *PSEN2* mutations have now been described (http://www.molgen.ua.ac.be/ADMutations/) (see Fig. 52.1). In general, families with *PSEN1* mutations have typical AD with ages of onset from 35 to 50, with some of the variability in onset age being accounted for by *ApoE* genotype as with *APP* families (Pastor et al., 2003). Families with *PSEN2* mutations have a very variable onset age, and though a proportion of the variance is accounted for by *ApoE* genotype, much of the variance remains unexplained (Wijsman et al., 2005). Some families with *PSEN1* mutations have an unusual phenotype of initial spastic paraparesis, and these families are generally characterized by have large "cotton wool" plaques rather than neuritic plaques (Crook et al., 1998). Although the reason for the difference in pathogenesis is not clear, it seems that the mutations involved are those that have the largest effect on *APP* processing (Houlden et al., 2000).

In contrast to *APP*, the function of the presenilins are now well understood in outline. They are the central subunit of intramembranous proteases which are responsible for the regulated cleavage of Notch, *APP*, and many other type-1 membrane proteins (see Fig. 52.1).

The effects of pathogenic mutations: The amyloid hypothesis of Alzheimer's disease. In general terms, we have a clear understanding of the effects of the *APP* and presenilin mutations: most *APP* mutations and all presenilin mutations alter *APP* processing such that Aβ deposition is a more likely event (Scheuner et al., 1996) (see Fig. 52.2). Slightly less certain and less well studied is the possibility that some of the intra-Aβ mutations' primary effect is on reducing the solubility of Aβ without altering the position of cleavage (Wisniewski et al., 1991).

Although the general framework of the effects of the pathogenic mutations is clear, the details are not, and the precise mechanisms of the effects of the mutations on *APP* cleavage are not understood. γ-secretase's action is complex and seems to involve an initial cleavage between codons 721 and 722 (Aβ49 and Aβ50) before trimming back the sequence to final cleavage after codon 711 (Aβ40) or 713 (Aβ42) (Weidemann et al., 2002).

Despite this uncertainty over the molecular detail of the effects of the mutations, most researchers have reached a consensus that, in general, the effects of the mutations are directly related to their effects on *APP* processing, and this has been the basis for the amyloid hypothesis of the disorder (Hardy and Selkoe, 2002). Recently, two groups have independently suggested an alternative: that the crucial effect is that all the mutations cause a partial inhibition of presenilin function (Sambamurti et al., 2006; Shen and Kelleher, 2007). They point out that γ-secretase has many vital functions and is involved in the processing of many type-1 membrane proteins beyond *APP* including Notch cleav-

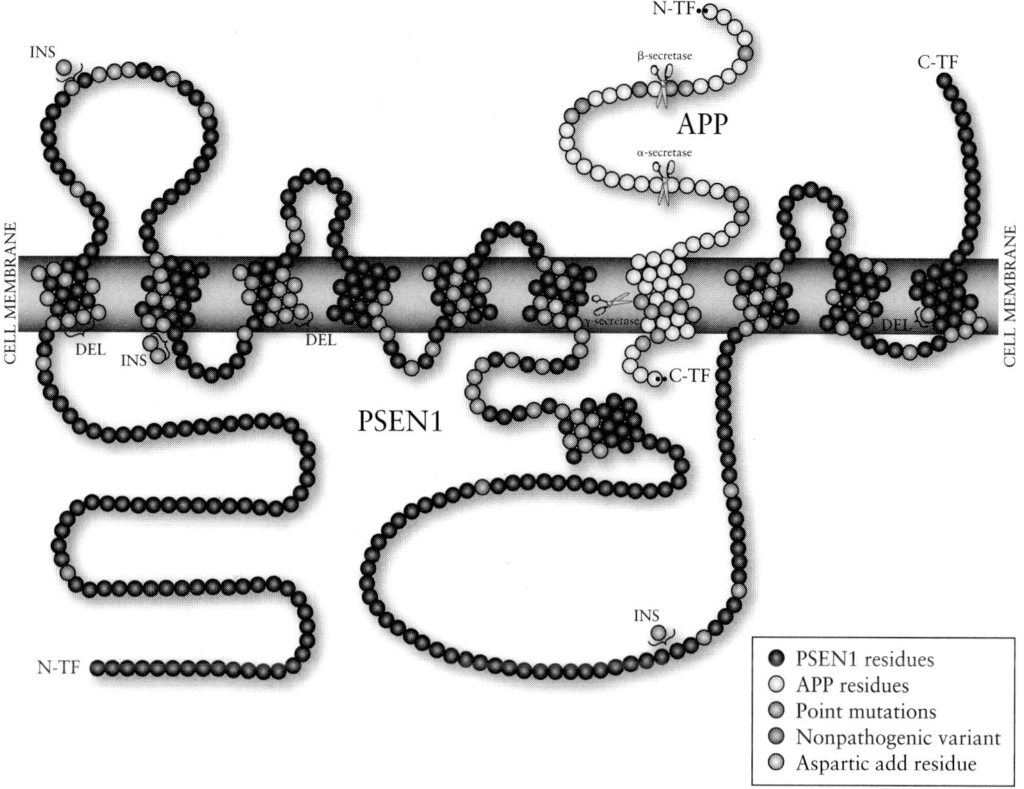

FIGURE 52.1 A diagram of the central structure of γ-secretase with *APP* in the active site of *Presenilin 1 (PSEN1)*. The central role of presenilins in γ-secretase action was shown by the creation of presenilin knock out mice, which fail to metabolize the C-terminal stub of *APP* (De Strooper et al., 1998). The critical aspartate residues at the active site were identified by mutagenesis experiments (Wolfe et al., 1999). The whole active γ-secretase complex containing presenilin and other accessory proteins has been reconstituted in yeast (Edbauer et al., 2003). The structure of *PSEN1* is derived from Laudon et al. (2005). This diagram was drawn by Richard Crook with advice from Wim Annaert.

age but that *APP* is the major substrate in terms of expression. They argue that all the pathogenic mutations may act to inhibit γ-secretase either directly in the case of presenilin mutations, or indirectly through the effects of mutations in, or increased dose of, its major substrate. This argument fits equally well with the genetic data as the amyloid hypothesis, but it seems less likely when one considers the admittedly inconclusive evidence suggesting a neurotoxicity of Aβ and also when one considers the analogy with the other plaque and tangle diseases, Worster Drought syndrome, and some prion dementias. In these latter diseases there are amyloid deposits, tangles, and cell death; and in these the pathogenic mutations are, as in AD, in the extracellular deposited amyloid protein. This analogy suggests that the route to cell death directly involves the deposited protein. Neither of these arguments against the presenilin inhibition hypothesis of AD is conclusive, and this hypothesis remains a credible alternative.

As detailed above, most, but not all, researchers would acknowledge that the most likely mechanism leading to AD in the early-onset kindreds and in Down syndrome is the amyloid hypothesis. However, the applicability of the amyloid hypothesis to late-onset AD is much more widely debated (see below).

Late-Onset Alzheimer's Disease

Apolipoprotein ε. The only established risk factor for late onset disease is the *ApoE* ε4 (Corder et al., 1993). A single copy of the ε4 allele appears to shift the risk curve for developing AD forward by 5 years, in general, in Down syndrome (Royston et al., 1994), in families with *APP* mutations (Houlden et al., 1993), and in families with presenilin mutations (Pastor et al., 2003; Wijsman et al., 2005). Being the homozygote for the ε4 allele shifts the risk curves forward by 10 years, and it seems likely that a single copy of the ε2 allele shifts the curve back by 5 years and two copies, back by 10 years (Corder et al., 1993; Farrer et al., 1997). However, the increase in familial clustering encoded at the *ApoE* ε locus is widely believed not to be sufficient to account for more than a modest proportion of the total famil-

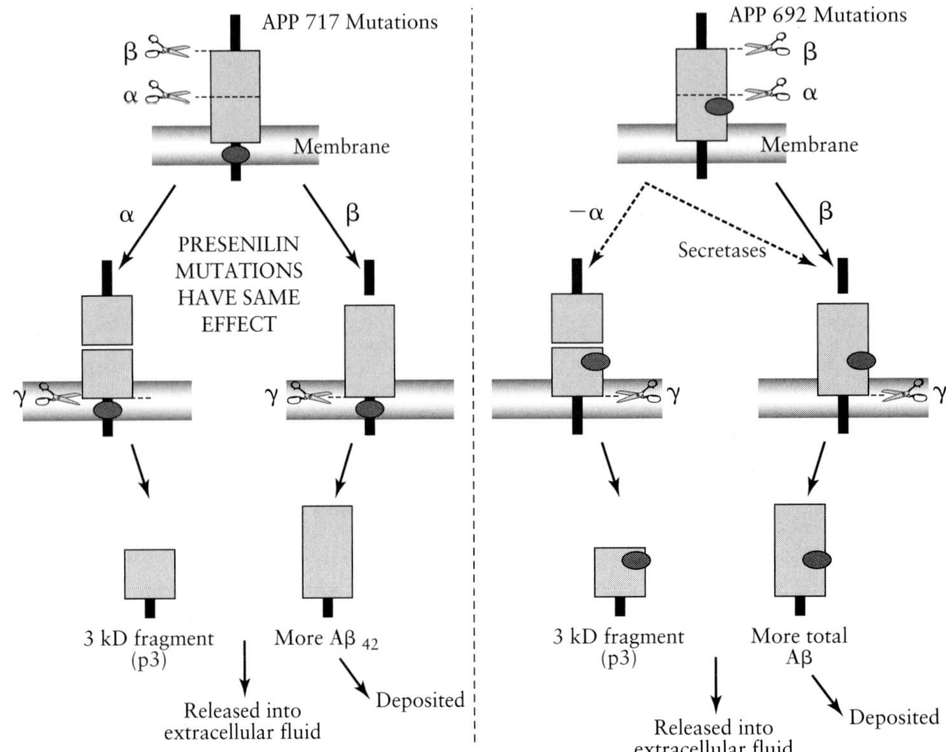

FIGURE 52.2 A simplistic diagram showing *APP* processing. *APP* processing occurs through two alternative pathways (Haass et al., 1992). In the first pathway, *APP* is cleaved at codon 671 by the enzyme β-secretase (BACE; Vassar et al., 1999) and then by γ-secretase. This pathway releases Aβ. In the second pathway, α-secretase cleavage occurs within the Aβ sequence, predominantly at residue 682 by a mixture of ADAM 10 and ADAM 17 (Asai et al., 2003) followed by γ-secretase cleavage. This yields a fragment designated p3 (Haass et al., 1992). The *APP670/1* mutation potentiates BACE cleavage yielding more total Aβ (Cai et al., 1993; Citron et al., 1995; Vassar et al, 1999). Some of the mutations in the *APP* sequence, particularly the *APP692* mutation, inhibit the α-secretase cleavage, indirectly causing more flux through a β cleavage pathway (De Jonghe et al., 1998). *APP* mutations close to the C-terminal of the Aβ sequence marginally alter the final length of a proportion ofAβ causing an increase in the proportion of Aβ42 (Suzuki et al., 1994). Presenilin mutations have essentially the same effect (Scheuner et al., 1996).

The approximate positions of mutations are indicated by the ovals and strength and number of the arrows illustrates the amount of flux through the pathway. The γ-secretase cleavage is a more complex event than conveyed in the diagram (see text and Weidemann et al., 2002).

ial clustering, leading to the belief that there is likely to be on the order of ~5 other genetic risk loci (Daw et al., 2000).

Are there other Alzheimer risk genes? Extensive study using linkage approaches and candidate gene association studies has so far failed to give consistent proof that any of the other candidates are involved in the aetiology of the disease. The Alzgene website (http://www.alzforum.org/res/com/gen/alzgene/default.asp) keeps a continually updated meta-analysis of genes that have been extensively tested for involvement (Bertram et al., 2007). Only two genes, *ACE* and *IL1B,* presently (July 2007) pass the criteria of 95% confidence intervals not including unity when the initial report is excluded and the analysis is confined to a single ethnic group (the standard practice in meta-analysis). Both of these have reported odds ratios of between 1.1 and 1.2: far lower than the odds ratios > 3.5 reported for the *ApoE* ε4 locus.

This finding is consistent with the first reports of a whole genome study in AD, which clearly identified the *ApoE* ε4 locus (Coon et al., 2007), but found nothing else before the sample was fractionated by *ApoE* ε genotype (Reiman et al., 2007). There are many possible explanations for this—the coverage of the whole genome chip arrays is not complete, and this methodology would not pick up genes that had many different risk alleles—but the simplest explanation is that there are no other alleles of major effect. This would suggest that the rest of the risk of disease is predisposed to by common alleles with low risk ratios (> 1.5) or by rare variants with large effect size but low population attributable risk, as well, of course, by environmental influences and chance. The recent success of the dissection of type II diabetes by whole-genome association studies suggests that that the best initial approach to this problem is through the pooling of the data from several large studies to achieve very large sample sizes.

One particularly plausible risk gene is the *APP* gene because we know from the example of Down syndrome and the *APP* duplication families that increases of expression of 50% (three copies of the gene) give disease with ages of onset in the 50s. This means that if there are alleles in the general population with a relative expression level increased by 25%, when homozygote, these, too, would be associated with disease onset at the same age, and presumably, slightly lower expression alleles would be associated with a higher-onset age. In addition, in the other protein deposition disorders where autosomal dominant genes have been found, genetic variability in the expression of the same protein has shown a robust association with the sporadic disease (Singleton et al., 2004). Recently two studies have reported such an association (Brouwers et al., 2006; Guyant-Maréchal et al., 2007), and genetic linkage analysis has also suggested that chromosome 21 may be involved (Wavrant-De Vrieze et al., 1999): however, a recent and thorough analysis failed to confirm this association (Nowotny et al., 2007); so even with this plausible candidate, strict genetic evidence for involvement is lacking.

Does the amyloid hypothesis apply to late-onset Alzheimer's disease? Parsimony would suggest that the overall mechanism of disease in late-onset disease would be generally similar to the mechanism in the autosomal dominant kindreds. However, this point has rightly been much more extensively debated than the mechanism of pathogenesis of the autosomal dominant kindreds. A major gap in our knowledge is a precise understanding of the functions of *APP*. From the perspective of the amyloid hypothesis, one worrying suggestion is that amyloid deposition is a damage-response mechanism. One known function of *APP* is in the blood clotting cascade (Smith et al., 1990), and one intriguing suggestion is that amyloid deposition is a physiological response to microhemorrhaging (Cullen et al., 2006): certainly, there is extensive, though not incontrovertible, evidence that plaque formation occurs centered on blood vessel walls (Miyakawa et al., 1982; Kumar-Singh et al., 2005). In such a scheme, the amyloid deposition may initially, at least, have a damage-response role (Atwood et al., 2002), though such an idea is difficult to reconcile with the development of the disease in the autosomal dominant kindreds. Some have suggested that this damage response role underlies the side-effect profile of the amyloid vaccine (see below).

This debate will be helped as we develop an understanding of the role of *APP* and as we identify and understand more risk factor genes. Most important, however, it will be resolved when/if we develop treatments for the disorder.

INSIGHTS FROM OTHER DEMENTING DISEASES

Although AD is easily the most prevalent dementing disease, other rarer dementias offer useful comparators. These include dementia with Lewy bodies, prion disease, Worster Drought syndrome (British dementia), and frontal temporal dementia with tangles (FTDP-17T).

Dementia with Lewy Bodies

The nosological separations of dementia with Lewy bodies from AD and from Parkinson's disease have proved extremely difficult (McKeith et al., 1996). In some cases of AD, including those with *APP* mutations (Lantos et al., 1994), Down syndrome (Lippa et al., 1999), and presenilin (Lippa et al., 1998) mutations, there are a variable number of Lewy bodies whose presence has become much more clear with the advent of first ubiquitin, and later α-synuclein staining. This observation suggests that Lewy formation, like tangle formation, can be a downstream pathology to *APP* mismetabolism (Hardy, 2003). Individuals with large numbers of cortical Lewy bodies have a dementing phenotype that, on a group though not on an individual level, is distinguishable from typical AD in having a fluctuating course and some parkinsonian features. This latter phenotype, unsurprisingly, overlaps with that in individuals who present with Parkinson's disease and later develop dementia (Lippa et al., 2007). Parkinson's disease and Parkinson's dementia can occasionally be caused by α-synuclein mutations (Polymeropoulos et al., 1997), including gene duplications (Singleton et al., 2003), and the sporadic diseases show a genetic association with the α-synuclein haplotype (Farrer et al., 2001).

Insights into Alzheimer's disease. The nosological confusion between AD and dementia with Lewy Bodies is likely to obscure a rather simple and revealing underlying biology. As is true for prion (see below), tau (see below), and *APP* (see above), α-synuclein deposition is influenced by the α-synuclein haplotype (Singleton et al., 2004). In addition, as is true for tau, α-synuclein deposition is also increased by *APP* mismetabolism (Masliah et al., 2000; Masliah et al., 2001). These data suggest that α-synuclein can be downstream of *APP* mismetabolism in an analogous way to tau (see Fig. 52.3). Experimental support for this notion has come from transgenic experiments which show that α-synuclein deposition in transgenic mice is hastened by an *APP* transgene in an analogous manner to tau deposition (Masliah et al., 2001) (see Fig. 52.3 and below). From

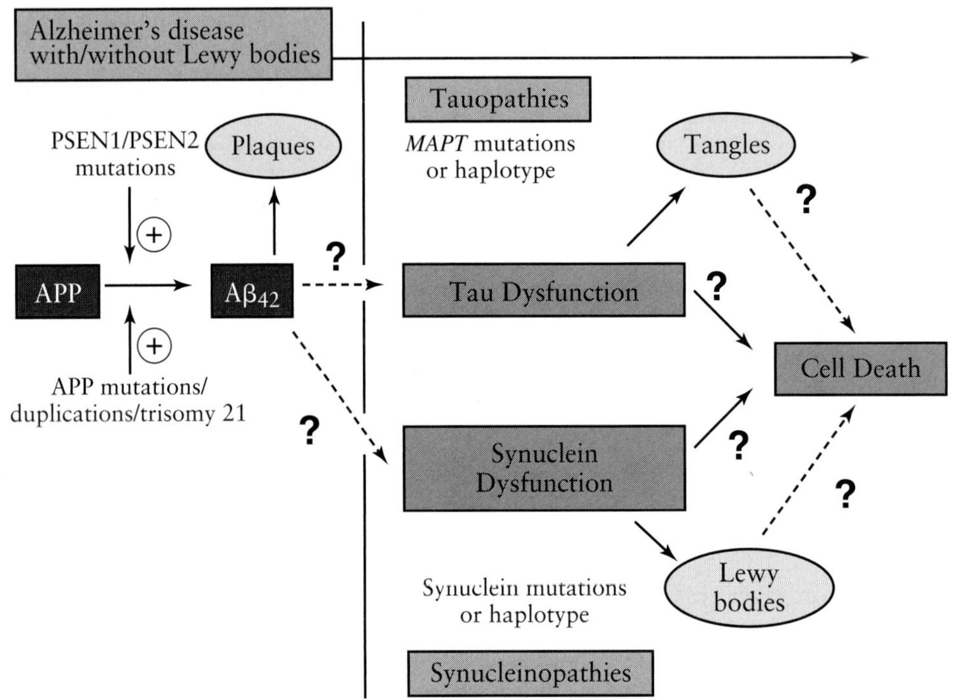

FIGURE 52.3 The proposed relationship between $A\beta$ and tau and α-synuclein and between Alzheimer's disease and dementia with Lewy bodies (Hardy et al., 1998; Hardy, 2003). The genetic data on British dementia and the prion diseases suggest that the cognate proteins (ABri and prion) can behave in a similar way to $A\beta42$.

a treatment perspective, the implication of overlap between AD and dementia with Lewy bodies is that one might expect both syndromes to respond to anti-$A\beta$ therapies but differently to antitau and antisynuclein therapies.

Prion Disease

A full description of prion diseases is beyond the scope of this chapter (see Prusiner, 2001). Prion diseases fall into three classes: hereditary, acquired (infectious, iatrogenic, cannibalistic), and sporadic. At the center of these aetiologies is the prion protein: mutations in the prion gene cause the hereditary disorder. A pathologic conformation of the protein is the infectious agent in the human- and animal-acquired forms of the disease, and genetic variability in the prion gene contributes to the risk of the sporadic disease.

Insights into Alzheimer's disease. There are a number of interesting parallels between prion diseases and AD. First, the obvious similarity that both disorders involve abnormal aggregates of the cognate protein. Some forms of prion diseases involve extracellular depositions of the prion protein as plaques that have a superficial resemblance to the amyloid plaques of AD. However, there are other, perhaps deeper, parallels. Some of the hereditary prion diseases have secondary tangle and Lewy body pathology (Hsiao et al., 1992) indicating that these pathologies can also be secondary to a prion aetiology as they are to an $A\beta$ aetiology. Also, genetic variability in prion expression contributes to the risk of the sporadic disease, with high expressors being at higher risk for disease in a broadly analogous way to the way in which *APP* expression can cause AD (Mead et al., 2001). Perhaps most interesting has been the recent demonstration that extracts of Alzheimer brain amyloid (but not synthetic $A\beta$) can precipitate plaque pathology in *APP* transgenic mice (Meyer-Luehmann et al., 2006), suggesting that the difference between the prion diseases' infectivity and the spread of Alzheimer pathology in AD is, at its basis, a quantitative difference and not a qualitative difference. Perhaps all these diseases of β-sheet protein deposition are diseases of pathologic templating (Hardy, 2005).

Worster Drought Syndrome (British Dementia)

Worster Drought syndrome (Worster-Drought et al., 1933) (now unfortunately redesignated as British dementia) refers to a large English family that has a plaque and tangle disease that, before immunostaining, was considered to be a form of either early-onset AD or hereditary prion disease. The disease is caused by a stop codon mutation at the C-terminus of a type 2 membrane protein (ABri). This frameshift mutation adds

23 nonsense amino acids to the protein (Vidal et al., 1999). Furin cleavage of the 34 terminal amino acids yields an amyloidogenic peptide that is deposited as a congophilic angiopathy and neuritic plaque (Kim et al., 1999).

Insights into Alzheimer's disease. Tangles are the secondary pathology in this disease as it is in AD. The importance of this disease for AD is that it shows that the deposition of a completely unphysiological amyloidogenic peptide can lead to plaque and tangle disease. Through the manipulation of the ABri sequence in mouse transgenics and a replacement of the pathological ABr sequence with either Aβ42 or Aβ40, McGowan and colleagues (McGowan et al., 2005) showed that Aβ42 was essential for deposition to occur.

Frontal Temporal Dementia (FTD) with Parkinsonism Linked to Chromosome 17 with Tangles (*FTDP-17T:* Pick's Disease) and Other "Tangle-Only" Diseases

Hereditary FTD has long been recognized as a comparatively rare cause of morbidity and mortality, but its nosology has been extremely difficult. In the last 10 years, genetic analysis has considerably clarified this difficult issue. So far, three genes have been found, though it is likely that there are others. A nonsense mutation in *CHMP2b* probably explains the disease in a single Danish family (Skibinski et al., 2005), but the majority of families showed genetic linkage to chromosome 17 markers (Foster et al., 1997). About half of these families had tau pathology (Spillantini et al., 1998)—either tangles, Pick bodies, or wispy tau filaments—and about half of them had ubiquitin positive inclusions (Mackenzie and Feldman, 2005). Initially these were grouped together as a single entity, *FTDP-17* (Foster et al., 1997), but we now know they are unrelated diseases despite their clinical and genetic linkage similarities. Those with tau pathology have mutations in the tau (*MAPT*) (Hutton et al., 1998; Poorkaj et al., 1998) gene whereas those with ubiquitin inclusions have mutations in the progranulin (*PGRN*) gene (Baker et al., 2006; Cruts et al., 2006), and have the ribonucleic acid (RNA) binding protein, TDP-43 (Neumann et al., 2006) as the central protein in their inclusions. In this chapter, only the pathogenesis of those dementias with *MAPT* mutations will be discussed because these offer insight into AD.

Two types of *MAPT* mutations have been discovered: missense changes that decrease the binding of tau to microtubules and increase tau's propensity to aggregate (Hong et al., 1998) and splicing mutations that increase the inclusion of exon 10 in the protein (Hutton et al., 1998). Exon 10 encodes one of the four microtubule binding domains, so this form of the protein is commonly described as 4-repeat tau.

Interestingly, the sporadic tangle diseases (including progressive supranuclear palsy; Baker et al., 1999), corticobasal degeneration (Houlden et al., 2001), and Parkinson's dementia complex of Guam (Poorkaj et al., 2001) show a genetic association with the *MAPT* gene. The *MAPT* haplotype that shows association with progressive supranuclear palsy and corticobasal degeneration (CBD) (designated H1c in Europeans; Pittman et al., 2005) is that which shows greatest expression of 4-repeat tau (Myers et al., 2007). The simplest way of thinking of this is to consider these diseases as the same disorder as *FTDP-17T*, but separated from it by an accident of nosology, because both their pathological and clinical features also overlap with this latter disorder.

Mice with *MAPT* transgenes containing *FTDP-17T* mutations develop tangles and cell loss clearly implicating tau dysfunction in neuronal cell death (Lewis et al., 2000).

Insights into Alzheimer's disease. The importance of *FTDP-17* in our understanding of the pathogenesis of cell death in AD is clear. The fact that tau mutations cause tangles and cell death suggests that this is likely the same cell death pathway as the predominant pathway in AD. This suggestion is strengthened by the observation that crossing mutant *APP* transgenic mice with such *MAPT* mice leads to an augmentation of the tangle pathology without altering the amyloid pathology (Lewis et al., 2001). This observation is consistent with the view that Aβ is upstream of *MAPT* in AD (see Fig. 52.3) and is thus also consistent with the amyloid hypothesis of the disorder (Hardy and Selkoe, 2002). Also consistent with this view are observations that reducing tau levels reduces Aβ toxicity on cells (Rapoport et al., 2002) and decreases the behavioral decrements induced by Aβ overexpression in transgenic mice (Roberson et al., 2007).

In addition, some (Myers et al., 2005), though not all, studies (Mukherjee et al., 2007) have reported that the same H1c *MAPT* haplotype that shows an association with progressive supranuclear palsy and corticobasal degeneration shows a weaker association with AD suggesting that increased expression of 4-repeat tau increases the likelihood of developing AD (Myers et al., 2007).

Genetics Based Clinical Progress in Alzheimer's Disease

If we are to develop mechanism-based therapies for AD, then we will want to be able to diagnose the disease accurately and early, and we will want to be able to monitor whether therapies are having beneficial effects. In both of these areas, use of the families with autosomal dominant disease has proven extremely useful because of the predictable nature of the disease.

Such families have been used extensively to determine the earliest clinical symptoms of the disease (Fox et al., 1998). However, possibly the most promising techniques for assessing preclinical change and the rate of progression of disease are imaging techniques: two different and complementary approaches are being used: magnetic resonance imaging (MRI) registration (Freeborough et al., 1996) and positron emission tomography (PET) amyloid imaging (Klunk et al., 2004).

MRI registration is a technique for measuring atrophy as a change in volume in a single person over time (Freeborough et al., 1996), and its use has shown that detectable hippocampal atrophy begins about 6 years before clinical symptoms of disease are apparent and that a more generalized atrophy is detectable about 3 years before the onset of clinical symptoms (Ridha et al., 2006). The analysis also showed that the global rate was relatively similar between persons at the same stage of the development of disease but that the rate of atrophy increased as the disease spread to affect different brain regions (Chan et al., 2003). The clinical utility of the approach was shown when it was used to assess the effects of Aβ immunization when it showed the unexpected outcome that brain volume was decreased by the immunization (Fox et al., 2005) although it remains unclear as to whether this reflected a reduction in brain mass or was caused by loss of amyloid or a change in brain water balance (Fox et al., 2005; Gilman et al., 2005).

PET amyloid imaging has recently been developed using radiolabeled, Pittsburgh Compound B (PIB), an analogue of thioflavin S (Klunk et al., 2004). This compound allows imaging of amyloid deposition in vivo and has shown that this deposition process begins many years (~10) before clinical symptoms appear in presenilin mutation carriers (Klunk et al., 2007) and, when combined with MR registration, that the rate of atrophy correlates with the amyloid load (Edison et al., 2007).

Animal Models and Experimental Therapeutics

The genetic findings outlined above have enabled the creation of transgenic mice that model parts of the disease process. Mice with mutant *APP* transgenes develop plaques (Games et al., 1995) but no tangles, little cell loss (Takeuchi et al., 2000), and only subtle behavioral changes (Hsiao et al., 1996): crossing in presenilin mice increased this pathology but did not change its basic pattern (Duff et al., 1996; Borchelt et al., 1997). These mice have, therefore, been extremely useful in developing anti-amyloid therapies (Duff and Suleman, 2004). As one example among many, the amyloid immunization therapy came directly from such mouse experiments (Schenk et al., 1999; Bard et al., 2000). Mice with mutant *MAPT* genes develop tangles and extensive cell loss (Lewis et al., 2000), and have been useful in developing antitangle therapies (Noble et al., 2005). Mice with mutant *APP* and mutant *MAPT* genes have increased tangle formation, and such mice could be used to explore the relationship between the pathologies (Lewis et al., 2000; Oddo et al., 2003) although this important relationship has not yet been extensively explored.

These mice and the mechanistic understanding we have developed offer a plethora of molecular targets for intervention (see Golde, 2006). The amyloid therapeutic approach that has attracted the most attention has been the amyloid vaccine approach. This approach was borne out of the surprising observation that immunization of *APP* transgenic mice led to the partial clearance of plaque deposits and almost immediate improvement of the *APP* transgenic mice on behavioral testing (Schenk et al., 1999; Morgan et al., 2000; Golde, 2006). Clinical trials of amyloid immunization were stopped after a small proportion of patients who received the test, but not the control immunization, developed meningioencephalitis for reasons that are unclear (Nicoll et al., 2003; Gilman et al., 2005). Although this trial could be seen as hopeful in that it clearly showed that amyloid plaques could be cleared (Nicoll et al., 2003) from the Alzheimer brain, because the trial was aborted, it has remained unclear whether this has beneficial behavioral consequences. It is also unclear whether the meningioencephalitis was merely an unfortunate side effect or whether it reflected an unanticipated role for Aβ in the pathological brain. Thus, this trial has been seen by amyloid optimists as useful proof of principle (Schenk, 2004) and by amyloid pessimists as a harbinger of other likely unsuccessful trials (Atwood et al., 2003).

Many potential therapies have passed the test of working in the transgenic mice: in most cases, human trials are either under way or in the planning stage. If they work, they will be a powerful validation of the pathologic gene through transgenic animals to test therapies as a route to treat all neurologic diseases. If none of them work, then it should cause us to reevaluate all of our assumptions, not just about the amyloid hypothesis, but also about this whole approach to disease.

CONCLUSION

Genetic analysis of AD has led to a widespread belief that we have a basic understanding of the pathogenesis of the disease. It has also led to the development of animal models that appear to replicate aspects of this pathogenesis as well as to the identification of credible molecular targets for therapy. Finally, it has helped in the accurate characterization of the prodrome and clinical course of the disease. However, though there have been many successful therapies in the mouse models of the disease, none has yet shown utility in clinical trials. Although patients with AD are undoubtedly better treated then they were 15 years ago, the only direct benefit to patients from this gene-based approach to research to date has been the availability of genetic testing in the kindreds with *APP* and presenilin mutations.

ACKNOWLEDGMENTS

The author's laboratory is supported by the Medical Research Council. Thanks to Richard Crook for Figure 1.

REFERENCES

Asai, M., Hattori, C., Szabo, B., et al. (2003) Putative function of ADAM9, ADAM10, and ADAM17 as APP alpha-secretase. *Biochem. Biophys. Res. Commun.* 301(1):231–235.

Atwood, C.S., Bishop, G.M., Perry, G., and Smith, M.A. (2002) Amyloid-beta: a vascular sealant that protects against hemorrhage? *J. Neurosci. Res.* 70(3):356.

Atwood, C.S., Perry, G., and Smith, M.A. (2003) Cerebral hemorrhage and amyloid-beta. *Science* 299:1014.

Baker, M., Litvan, I., Houlden, H., et al. (1999) Association of an extended haplotype in the tau gene with progressive supranuclear palsy. *Hum. Mol. Genet.* 8(4):711–715.

Baker, M., Mackenzie, I.R., Pickering-Brown, S.M., Gass, J., et al. (2006) Mutations in progranulin cause tau-negative frontotemporal dementia linked to chromosome 17. *Nature* 442(7105): 916–919.

Bales, K.R., Verina, T., Cummins, D.J., Du, Y., et al. (1999) Apolipoprotein E is essential for amyloid deposition in the APP(V717F) transgenic mouse model of Alzheimer's disease. *Proc. Natl. Acad. Sci. USA* 96(26):15233–15238.

Bard, F., Cannon, C., Barbour, R., et al. (2000) Peripherally administered antibodies against amyloid beta-peptide enter the central nervous system and reduce pathology in a mouse model of Alzheimer disease. *Nat. Med.* 6(8):916–919.

Bertram, L., McQueen, M.B., Mullin, K., Blacker, D., and Tanzi, R.E. (2007) Systematic meta-analyses of Alzheimer disease genetic association studies: the AlzGene database. *Nat. Genet.* 39(1):17–23.

Borchelt, D.R., Ratovitski, T., van Lare, J., et al. (1997) Accelerated amyloid deposition in the brains of transgenic mice coexpressing mutant presenilin 1 and amyloid precursor proteins. *Neuron* 19(4): 939–945.

Brouwers, N., Sleegers, K., Engelborghs, S., et al. (2006) Genetic risk and transcriptional variability of amyloid precursor protein in Alzheimer's disease. *Brain* 129(Pt 11):2984–2991.

Cai, X.D., Golde, T.E., and Younkin, S.G. (1993) Release of excess amyloid beta protein from a mutant amyloid beta protein precursor. *Science* 259(5094):514–516.

Chan, D., Janssen, J.C., Whitwell, J.L., et al. (2003) Change in rates of cerebral atrophy over time in early-onset Alzheimer's disease: longitudinal MRI study. *Lancet* 362(9390):1121–1122.

Citron, M., Teplow, D.B., and Selkoe, D.J. (1995) Generation of amyloid beta protein from its precursor is sequence specific. *Neuron* 14(3):661–670.

Coon, K.D., Myers, A.J., Craig, D.W., et al. (2007) A high-density whole-genome association study reveals that APOE is the major susceptibility gene for sporadic late-onset Alzheimer's disease. *J. Clin. Psychiatry* 68(4):613–618.

Corder, E.H., Saunders, A.M., Strittmatter, W.J., et al. (1993) Gene dose of apolipoprotein E type 4 allele and the risk of Alzheimer's disease in late onset families. *Science* 261(5123):921–923.

Crook, R., Verkkoniemi, A., Perez-Tur, J., et al. (1998) A variant of Alzheimer's disease with spastic paraparesis and unusual plaques due to deletion of exon 9 of presenilin 1. *Nat. Med.* 4(4):452–455.

Cruts, M., Gijselinck, I., van der Zee, J., et al. (2006) Null mutations in progranulin cause ubiquitin-positive frontotemporal dementia linked to chromosome 17q21. *Nature* 442(7105):920–924.

Cullen, K.M., Kocsi, Z., and Stone, J. (2006) Microvascular pathology in the aging human brain: evidence that senile plaques are sites of microhaemorrhages. *Neurobiol. Aging* 27(12):1786–1796.

Daw, E.W., Payami, H., Nemens, E.J., et al. (2000) The number of trait loci in late-onset Alzheimer disease. *Am. J. Hum. Genet.* 66(1):196–204.

De Jonghe, C., Zehr, C., Yager, D., et al. (1998) Flemish and Dutch mutations in amyloid beta precursor protein have different effects on amyloid beta secretion. *Neurobiol. Dis.* 5(4):281–286.

De Strooper, B., Saftig, P., Craessaerts, K., et al. (1998) Deficiency of presenilin-1 inhibits the normal cleavage of amyloid precursor protein. *Nature* 391(6665):387–390.

Duff, K., Eckman, C., Zehr, C., et al. (1996) Increased amyloid-beta42(43) in brains of mice expressing mutant presenilin 1. *Nature* 383(6602):710–713.

Duff, K., and Suleman, F. (2004) Transgenic mouse models of Alzheimer's disease: how useful have they been for therapeutic development? *Brief Funct. Genomic Proteomic.* 3(1):47–55.

Edbauer, D., Winkler, E., Regula, J.T., Pesold, B., Steiner, H., and Haass, C. (2003) Reconstitution of gamma-secretase activity. *Nat. Cell Biol.* 5(5):486–488.

Edison, P., Archer, H.A., Hinz, R., et al. (2007) Amyloid, hypometabolism, and cognition in Alzheimer disease: an [11C]PIB and [18F]FDG PET study. *Neurology* 68(7):501–508.

Farrer, L.A., Cupples, L.A., Haines, J.L., et al. (1997) Effects of age, sex, and ethnicity on the association between apolipoprotein E genotype and Alzheimer disease. A meta-analysis. APOE and Alzheimer Disease Meta Analysis Consortium. *JAMA* 278(16): 1349–1356.

Farrer, M., Maraganore, D.M., Lockhart, P., et al. (2001) alpha-synuclein gene haplotypes are associated with Parkinson's disease. *Hum. Mol. Genet.* 10(17):1847–1851.

Foster, N.L., Wilhelmsen, K., Sima, A.A., Jones, M.Z., D'Amato, C.J., and Gilman, S. (1997) Frontotemporal dementia and parkinsonism linked to chromosome 17: a consensus conference. *Ann. Neurol.* 41(6):706–715.

Fox, N.C., Black, R.S., Gilman, S., Rossor, M.N., et al. (2005) Effects of Abeta immunization (AN1792) on MRI measures of cerebral volume in Alzheimer disease. *Neurology* 64(9):1563–1572.

Fox, N.C., Warrington, E.K., Seiffer, A.L., Agnew, S.K., and Rossor, M.N. (1998) Presymptomatic cognitive deficits in individuals at risk of familial Alzheimer's disease. A longitudinal prospective study. *Brain* 121(Pt 9):1631–1639.

Freeborough, P.A., Woods, R.P., and Fox, N.C. (1996) Accurate registration of serial 3D MR brain images and its application to visualizing change in neurodegenerative disorders. *J. Comput. Assist. Tomogr.* 20(6):1012–1022.

Games, D., Adams, D., Alessandrini, R., et al. (1995) Alzheimer-type neuropathology in transgenic mice overexpressing V717F beta-amyloid precursor protein. *Nature* 373(6514):523–527.

Gilman, S., Koller, M., Black, R.S., et al. (2005) Clinical effects of Abeta immunization (AN1792) in patients with AD in an interrupted trial. *Neurology* 64(9):1553–1562.

Glenner, G.G., and Wong, C.W. (1984a) Alzheimer's disease and Down's syndrome: sharing of a unique cerebrovascular amyloid fibril protein. *Biochem. Biophys. Res. Commun.* 122(3):1131–1135.

Glenner, G.G., and Wong, C.W. (1984b) Alzheimer's disease: initial report of the purification and characterization of a novel cerebrovascular amyloid protein. *Biochem. Biophys. Res. Commun.* 120(3):885–890.

Goate, A., Chartier-Harlin, M.C., Mullan, M., et al. (1991) Segregation of a missense mutation in the amyloid precursor protein gene with familial Alzheimer's disease. *Nature* 349(6311): 704–706.

Golde, T.E. (2006) Disease modifying therapy for AD? *J. Neurochem.* 99(3):689–707.

Guyant-Maréchal, L., Rovelet-Lecrux, A., Goumidi, L., et al. (2007) Variations in the APP gene promoter region and risk of Alzheimer disease. *Neurology* 68:684–687.

Haass, C., Schlossmacher, M.G., Hung, A.Y., et al. (1992) Amyloid beta-peptide is produced by cultured cells during normal metabolism. *Nature* 359(6393):322–324.

Hardy, J. (2003) The relationship between Lewy body disease, Parkinson's disease, and Alzheimer's disease. *Ann. N. Y. Acad. Sci.* 991:167–170.

Hardy, J. (2005) Expression of normal sequence pathogenic proteins for neurodegenerative disease contributes to disease risk: "permissive templating" as a general mechanism underlying neurodegeneration. *Biochem. Soc. Trans.* 33(Pt 4):578–581.

Hardy, J., Duff, K., Gwinn-Hardy, K., Perez-Tur, J., and Hutton, M. (1998) Genetic dissection of Alzheimer's disease and related dementias: amyloid and its relationship to tau. *Nat. Neurosci.* 1(5): 355–358.

Hardy, J., and Selkoe, D.J. (2002) The amyloid hypothesis of Alzheimer's disease: progress and problems on the road to therapeutics. *Science* 297(5580):353–356.

Hong, M., Zhukareva, V., Vogelsberg-Ragaglia, V., et al. (1998) Mutation-specific functional impairments in distinct tau isoforms of hereditary FTDP-17. *Science* 282(5395):1914–1917.

Houlden, H., Baker, M., McGowan, E., et al. (2000) Variant Alzheimer's disease with spastic paraparesis and cotton wool plaques is caused by PS-1 mutations that lead to exceptionally high amyloid-beta concentrations. *Ann. Neurol.* 48(5):806–808.

Houlden, H., Baker, M., Morris, H.R., et al. (2001) Corticobasal degeneration and progressive supranuclear palsy share a common tau haplotype. *Neurology* 56(12):1702–1706.

Houlden, H., Collinge, J., Kennedy, A., et al. (1993) Apolipoprotein E genotype and Alzheimer's disease. Alzheimer's Disease Collaborative Group. *Lancet* 342(8873):737–738.

Hsiao, K., Chapman, P., Nilsen, S., et al. (1996) Correlative memory deficits, Abeta elevation, and amyloid plaques in transgenic mice. *Science* 274(5284):99–102.

Hsiao, K., Dlouhy, S.R., Farlow, M.R., et al. (1992) Mutant prion proteins in Gerstmann-Straussler-Scheinker disease with neurofibrillary tangles. *Nat. Genet.* 1(1):68–71.

Hutton, M., Lendon, C.L., Rizzu, P., et al. (1998) Association of missense and 5'-splice-site mutations in tau with the inherited dementia FTDP-17. *Nature* 393(6686):702–705.

Janus, C., Pearson, J., McLaurin, J., et al. (2000) A beta peptide immunization reduces behavioural impairment and plaques in a model of Alzheimer's disease. *Nature* 408(6815):979–982.

Kang, J., Lemaire, H.G., Unterbeck, A., et al. (1987) The precursor of Alzheimer's disease amyloid A4 protein resembles a cell-surface receptor. *Nature* 325(6106):733–736.

Kim, S.H., Wang, R., Gordon, D.J., et al. (1999) Furin mediates enhanced production of fibrillogenic ABri peptides in familial British dementia. *Nat. Neurosci.* 2(11):984–988.

Klunk, W.E., Engler, H., Nordberg, A., et al. (2004) Imaging brain amyloid in Alzheimer's disease with Pittsburgh Compound-B. *Ann. Neurol.* 55(3):306–319.

Klunk, W.E., Price, J.C., Mathis, C.A., et al. (2007) Amyloid deposition begins in the striatum of presenilin-1 mutation carriers from two unrelated pedigrees. *J. Neurosci.* 27(23):6174–6184.

Kumar-Singh, S., Pirici, D., McGowan, E., et al. (2005) Dense-core plaques in Tg2576 and PSAPP mouse models of Alzheimer's disease are centered on vessel walls. *Am. J. Pathol.* 167(2):527–543.

Lantos, P.L., Ovenstone, I.M., Johnson, J., Clelland, C.A., Roques, P., and Rossoor, M.N. (1994) Lewy bodies in the brain of two members of a family with the 717 (Val to Ile) mutation of the amyloid precursor protein gene. *Neurosci. Lett.* 172(1/2): 77–79.

Laudon, H., Hansson, E.M., Melen, K., et al. (2005) A nine-transmembrane domain topology for presenilin 1. *J. Biol. Chem.* 280(42):35352–35360.

Levy, E., Carman, M.D., Fernandez-Madrid, I.J., Power, M.D., et al. (1990) Mutation of the Alzheimer's disease amyloid gene in hereditary cerebral hemorrhage, Dutch type. *Science* 248(4959): 1124–1126.

Levy-Lahad, E., Wijsman, E.M., Nemens, E., et al. (1995) A familial Alzheimer's disease locus on chromosome 1. *Science* 269(5226): 970–973.

Lewis, J., Dickson, D.W., Lin, W.L., et al. (2001) Enhanced neurofibrillary degeneration in transgenic mice expressing mutant tau and APP. *Science* 293(5534):1487–1491.

Lewis, J., McGowan, E., Rockwood, J., et al. (2000) Neurofibrillary tangles, amyotrophy and progressive motor disturbance in mice expressing mutant (P301L) tau protein. *Nat. Genet.* 25(4):402–405.

Lippa, C.F., Duda, J.E., Grossman, M., et al. (2007) DLB and PDD boundary issues: diagnosis, treatment, molecular pathology, and biomarkers. *Neurology* 68(11):812–819.

Lippa, C.F., Fujiwara, H., Mann, D.M., et al. (1998) Lewy bodies contain altered alpha-synuclein in brains of many familial Alzheimer's disease patients with mutations in presenilin and amyloid precursor protein genes. *Am. J. Pathol.* 153(5):1365–1370.

Lippa, C.F., Schmidt, M.L., Lee, V.M., and Trojanowski, J.Q. (1999) Antibodies to alpha-synuclein detect Lewy bodies in many Down's syndrome brains with Alzheimer's disease. *Ann. Neurol.* 45(3):353–357.

Mackenzie, I.R., and Feldman, H.H. (2005) Ubiquitin immunohistochemistry suggests classic motor neuron disease, motor neuron disease with dementia, and frontotemporal dementia of the motor neuron disease type represent a clinicopathologic spectrum. *J. Neuropathol. Exp. Neurol.* 64(8):730–739.

Masliah, E., Rockenstein, E., Veinbergs, I., et al. (2000) Dopaminergic loss and inclusion body formation in alpha-synuclein mice: implications for neurodegenerative disorders. *Science* 287(5456): 1265–1269.

Masliah, E., Rockenstein, E., Veinbergs, I., et al. (2001) Beta-amyloid peptides enhance alpha-synuclein accumulation and neuronal deficits in a transgenic mouse model linking Alzheimer's disease and Parkinson's disease. *Proc. Natl. Acad. Sci. USA* 98(21): 12245–12250.

McGowan, E., Pickford, F., Kim, J., et al. (2005) Abeta42 is essential for parenchymal and vascular amyloid deposition in mice. *Neuron* 47(2):191–199.

McKeith, I.G., Galasko, D., Kosaka, K., et al. (1996) Consensus guidelines for the clinical and pathologic diagnosis of dementia with Lewy bodies (DLB): report of the consortium on DLB international workshop. *Neurology* 47(5):1113–1124.

Mead, S., Mahal, S.P., Beck, J., Campbell, T., Farrall, M., Fisher, E., and Collinge, J. (2001) Sporadic—but not variant—Creutzfeldt-Jakob disease is associated with polymorphisms upstream of PRNP exon 1. *Am. J. Hum. Genet.* 69(6):1225–1235.

Meyer-Luehmann, M., Coomaraswamy, J., Bolmont, T., et al. (2006) Exogenous induction of cerebral beta-amyloidogenesis is governed by agent and host. *Science* 313(5794):1781–1784.

Miyakawa, T., Shimoji, A., Kuramoto, R., and Higuchi, Y. (1982) The relationship between senile plaques and cerebral blood vessels in Alzheimer's disease and senile dementia. Morphological mechanism of senile plaque production. *Virchows Arch. B Cell Pathol. Incl. Mol. Pathol.* 40:121–129.

Morgan, D., Diamond, D.M., Gottschall, P.E., et al. (2000) A beta peptide vaccination prevents memory loss in an animal model of Alzheimer's disease. *Nature* 408(6815):982–985.

Mukherjee, O., Kauwe, J.S., Mayo, K., Morris, J.C., and Goate, A.M. (2007) Haplotype-based association analysis of the MAPT locus in late onset Alzheimer's disease. *BMC Genet.* 8:3.

Myers, A.J., Kaleem, M., Marlowe, L., et al. (2005) The H1c haplotype at the MAPT locus is associated with Alzheimer's disease. *Hum. Mol. Genet.* 14(16):2399–2404.

Myers, A.J., Pittman, A.M., Zhao, A.S., et al. (2007) The MAPT H1c risk haplotype is associated with increased expression of tau and especially of 4 repeat containing transcripts. *Neurobiol. Dis.* 25(3):561–570.

Neumann, M., Sampathu, D.M., Kwong, L.K., et al. (2006) Ubiquitinated TDP-43 in frontotemporal lobar degeneration and amyotrophic lateral sclerosis. *Science* 314(5796):130–133.

Nicoll, J.A., Wilkinson, D., Holmes, C., Steart, P., Markham, H., and Weller, R.O. (2003) Neuropathology of human Alzheimer disease after immunization with amyloid-beta peptide: a case report. *Nat. Med.* 9(4):448–485.

Noble, W., Planel, E., Zehr, C., et al. (2005) Inhibition of glycogen synthase kinase-3 by lithium correlates with reduced tauopathy and degeneration in vivo. *Proc. Natl. Acad. Sci. USA* 102(19): 6990–6995.

Nowotny, P., Simcock, X., Bertelsen, S., et al. (2007) Association studies testing for risk for late-onset Alzheimer's disease with common variants in the beta-amyloid precursor protein (APP). *Am. J. Med. Genet. B Neuropsychiatr. Genet.* 144(4):469–474.

Oddo, S., Caccamo, A., Shepherd, J.D., et al. (2003) Triple-transgenic model of Alzheimer's disease with plaques and tangles: intracellular Abeta and synaptic dysfunction. *Neuron* 39(3): 409–421.

Pastor, P., Roe, C.M., Villegas, A., et al. (2003) Apolipoprotein epsilon4 modifies Alzheimer's disease onset in an E280A PS1 kindred. *Ann. Neurol.* 54(2):163–169.

Pittman, A.M., Myers, A.J., Abou-Sleiman, P., et al. (2005) Linkage disequilibrium fine mapping and haplotype association analysis of the tau gene in progressive supranuclear palsy and corticobasal degeneration. *J. Med. Genet.* 42(11):837–846.

Polymeropoulos, M.H., Lavedan, C., Leroy, E., et al. (1997) Mutation in the alpha-synuclein gene identified in families with Parkinson's disease. *Science* 276(5321):2045–2047.

Poorkaj, P., Bird, T.D., Wijsman, E., et al. (1998) Tau is a candidate gene for chromosome 17 frontotemporal dementia. *Ann. Neurol.* 43(6):815–825.

Poorkaj, P., Tsuang, D., Wijsman, E., et al. (2001) TAU as a susceptibility gene for amyotropic lateral sclerosis–parkinsonism dementia complex of Guam. *Arch. Neurol.* 58(11):1871–1878.

Prasher, V.P., Farrer, M.J., Kessling, A.M., et al. (1998) Molecular mapping of Alzheimer-type dementia in Down's syndrome. *Ann. Neurol.* 43(3):380–383.

Prusiner, S.B. (2001) Shattuck lecture—neurodegenerative diseases and prions. *N. Engl. J. Med.* 344(20):1516–1526.

Rapoport, M., Dawson, H.N., Binder, L.I., Vitek, M.P., and Ferreira, A. (2002) Tau is essential to beta-amyloid-induced neurotoxicity. *Proc. Natl. Acad. Sci. USA* 99(9):6364–6369.

Reiman, E.M., Webster, J.A., Myers, A.J., et al. (2007) GAB2 alleles modify Alzheimer's risk in APOE epsilon4 carriers. *Neuron* 54(5): 713–720.

Ridha, B.H., Barnes, J., Bartlett, J.W., et al. (2006) Tracking atrophy progression in familial Alzheimer's disease: a serial MRI study. *Lancet Neurol.* 5(10):828–834.

Roberson, E.D., Scearce-Levie, K., Palop, J.J., et al. (2007) Reducing endogenous tau ameliorates amyloid beta-induced deficits in an Alzheimer's disease mouse model. *Science* 316(5825):750–754.

Rogaev, E.I., Sherrington, R., Rogaeva, E.A., et al. (1995) Familial Alzheimer's disease in kindreds with missense mutations in a gene on chromosome 1 related to the Alzheimer's disease type 3 gene. *Nature* 376(6543):775–778.

Rogaeva, E. (2002) The solved and unsolved mysteries of the genetics of early-onset Alzheimer's disease. *Neuromolecular Med.* 2(1): 1–10.

Rovelet-Lecrux, A., Hannequin, D., Raux, G., et al. (2006) APP locus duplication causes autosomal dominant early-onset Alzheimer disease with cerebral amyloid angiopathy. *Nat. Genet.* 38(1): 24–26.

Royston, M.C., Mann, D., Pickering-Brown, S., et al. (1994) Apolipoprotein E epsilon 2 allele promotes longevity and protects patients with Down's syndrome from dementia. *Neuroreport* 5(18): 2583–2585.

Sambamurti, K., Suram, A., Venugopal, C., Prakasam, A., Zhou, Y., Lahiri, D.K., and Greig, N.H. (2006) A partial failure of membrane protein turnover may cause Alzheimer's disease: a new hypothesis. *Curr. Alzheimer Res.* 3(1):81–90.

Schellenberg, G.D., Bird, T.D., Wijsman, E.M., et al. (1992) Genetic linkage evidence for a familial Alzheimer's disease locus on chromosome 14. *Science* 258(5082):668–671.

Schenk, D. (2004) Hopes remain for an Alzheimer's vaccine. *Nature* 431(7007):398.

Schenk, D., Barbour, R., Dunn, W., et al. (1999) Immunization with amyloid-beta attenuates Alzheimer-disease-like pathology in the PDAPP mouse. *Nature* 400(6740):173–177.

Scheuner, D., Eckman, C., Jensen, M., et al. (1996) Secreted amyloid beta-protein similar to that in the senile plaques of Alzheimer's disease is increased in vivo by the presenilin 1 and 2 and APP mutations linked to familial Alzheimer's disease. *Nat. Med.* 2(8): 864–870.

Shen, J., and Kelleher, R.J., III. (2007) The presenilin hypothesis of Alzheimer's disease: evidence for a loss-of-function pathogenic mechanism. *Proc. Natl. Acad. Sci. USA* 104(2):403–409.

Sherrington, R., Rogaev, E.I., Liang, Y., et al. (1995) Cloning of a gene bearing missense mutations in early-onset familial Alzheimer's disease. *Nature* 375(6534):754–760.

Singleton, A., Myers, A., and Hardy, J. (2004) The law of mass action applied to neurodegenerative disease: a hypothesis concerning the etiology and pathogenesis of complex diseases. *Hum. Mol. Genet.*13(Spec No 1):R123–R126.

Singleton, A.B., Farrer, M., Johnson, J., et al. (2003) alpha-Synuclein locus triplication causes Parkinson's disease. *Science* 302(5646): 841.

Skibinski, G., Parkinson, N.J., Brown, J.M., et al. (2005) Mutations in the endosomal ESCRTIII-complex subunit CHMP2B in frontotemporal dementia. *Nat. Genet.* 37(8):806–808.

Smith, R.P., Higuchi, D.A., Broze, G.J., Jr. (1990) Platelet coagulation factor XIa-inhibitor, a form of Alzheimer amyloid precursor protein. *Science* 248(4959):1126–1128.

Spillantini, M.G., Bird, T.D., and Ghetti, B. (1998) Frontotemporal dementia and Parkinsonism linked to chromosome 17: a new group of tauopathies. *Brain Pathol.* 8(2):387–402.

Suzuki, N., Cheung, T.T., Cai, X.D., et al. (1994) An increased percentage of long amyloid beta protein secreted by familial amyloid beta protein precursor (beta APP717) mutants. *Science* 264(5163): 1336–1340.

Takeuchi, A., Irizarry, M.C., Duff, K., et al. (2000) Age-related amyloid beta deposition in transgenic mice overexpressing both Alzheimer mutant presenilin 1 and amyloid beta precursor protein Swedish mutant is not associated with global neuronal loss. *Am. J. Pathol.* 157(1):331–339.

Vassar, R., Bennett, B.D., Babu-Khan, S., et al. (1999) Beta-secretase cleavage of Alzheimer's amyloid precursor protein by the transmembrane aspartic protease BACE. *Science* 286(5440):735–741.

Vidal, R., Frangione, B., Rostagno, A., et al. (1999) A stop-codon mutation in the BRI gene associated with familial British dementia. *Nature* 399(6738):776–781.

Wavrant-De Vrieze, F., Crook, R., Holmans, P., et al. (1999) Genetic variability at the amyloid-beta precursor protein locus may contribute to the risk of late-onset Alzheimer's disease. *Neurosci. Lett.* 269:67–70.

Weidemann, A., Eggert, S., Reinhard, F.B.M., et al. (2002) A novel ε-cleavage within the transmembrane domain of the Alzheimer amyloid precursor protein demonstrates homology with Notch processing. *Biochem.* 41:2825–2835.

Wijsman, E.M., Daw, E.W., Yu, X., et al. (2005) APOE and other loci affect age-at-onset in Alzheimer's disease families with PS2 mutation. *Am. J. Med. Genet. B Neuropsychiatr. Genet.* 132(1): 14–20.

Wisniewski, T., Ghiso, J., and Frangione, B. (1991) Peptides homologous to the amyloid protein of Alzheimer's disease containing a glutamine for glutamic acid substitution have accelerated amyloid fibril formation. *Biochem. Biophys. Res. Commun.* 180(3): 1528.

Wolfe, M.S., Xia, W., Ostaszewski, B.L., Diehl, T.S., Kimberly, W.T., and Selkoe, D.J. (1999) Two transmembrane aspartates in presenilin-1 required for presenilin endoproteolysis and gamma-secretase activity. *Nature* 398(6727):513–517.

Worster-Drought, C., Hill, T.R., and McMenemey, W.H. (1933) Familial presenile dementia with spastic paralysis. *J. Neurol. Psychopath.* 14:27–34.

53 Diagnostic Classifications: Relationship to the Neurobiology of Dementia

DANIEL I. KAUFER AND STEVEN T. DEKOSKY

The diagnostic classification of dementia bridges two levels of analysis. Clinically defined syndromes based on typical signs and symptoms occupy one level, and neuropathologically based criteria derived from retrospective correlations between characteristic structural brain alterations and clinical features form the other. A common approach to classifying degenerative dementias entails identifying associations between specific clinical and pathological features to define probabilistic categories (probable and possible) of clinical diagnostic certainty. Although a neuropathologically based classification of dementia is more objective, such information is usually not available in a clinical setting. Moreover, neuropathological hallmarks of neurodegenerative dementias are usually present before overt clinical signs and symptoms become manifest. These points highlight the need for systematic longitudinal clinical assessment and for prospective clinical validation of neuropathological diagnostic criteria. Accurate clinical characterization and differentiation of dementia syndromes is essential to guiding laboratory diagnostic evaluation and identifying genetic and other biological diagnostic markers and, ultimately, disease-specific interventions.

DEMENTIA: CLINICAL OVERVIEW

Definition of Dementia

Dementia refers to an acquired and persistent syndrome of intellectual impairment, reflecting a variety of disease processes (Cummings and Benson, 1992). As defined in *Diagnostic and Statistical Manual of Mental Disorders*, 4th ed. (*DSM-IV*), the two essential diagnostic features of dementia are (*1*) memory and other cognitive deficits and (*2*) an impairment in social and occupational functioning (American Psychiatric Association [APA], 2000). Delirium and any primary psychiatric disorder that could account for the symptoms must be excluded.

Neuropsychiatric symptoms often accompany dementia and are incorporated into the specific diagnostic criteria for some dementing illnesses, such as Lewy body dementia (LBD) and frontotemporal dementia (FTD). Although memory impairment is the sine qua non of Alzheimer's disease (AD; the most common cause of dementia in middle and late life), other intellectual or neuropsychiatric disturbances may be the initial or predominant clinical manifestation of a dementia syndrome.

DSM-IV requires compromise in social and occupational roles, and this imparts a measure of ecological validity to the diagnosis of dementia. Discrepancies between this criterion and population-based cutoff scores on neuropsychological tests between normal and dementia may reflect individual differences in real-world competence related to age, educational level, cultural background, or medical and psychiatric comorbidity. With emerging biomarkers heralding the era of preclinical diagnosis, the distinction between a pathological disease state and clinical syndrome that jointly define a specific dementia will need to become more explicit.

Dementia Versus Delirium

Delirium (acute confusional state or encephalopathy) is a common syndrome of acquired cognitive dysfunction. Key clinical features distinguishing delirium from dementia are the primary attentional deficits associated with the former and the chronic nature of the latter. The defining characteristics of delirium are a disturbance in consciousness, attentional deficits, brief duration of symptoms, and fluctuation in symptoms over time (APA, 2000). Initial diagnosis of a dementia cannot be made reliably in the presence of delirium. In general, dementia syndromes involve functionally, metabolically, or neurochemically mediated impairment of cognitive functioning associated with structural brain alterations. By contrast, delirium states typically reflect functional brain deficits that can occur in the absence of structural lesions.

This distinction is more relative than absolute, reflecting a dynamic balance between cerebral, functional, and structural perturbations. Individuals with dementia are more susceptible to delirium-producing insults and metabolic derangements that, if unattended, may exacerbate the underlying dementia or ultimately result in death. Potential reversibility is not an inherent feature of dementia as it is for delirium. Reversibility is determined principally by the nature, severity, and duration of the pathophysiologic insult or agent, as well as age of the patient.

PATHOLOGICAL CLASSIFICATION

Etiologies

Etiologies of dementia may be divided into two broad categories: degenerative and nondegenerative (Table 53.1). The first category primarily reflects pathophysiologic processes that are intrinsic to the central nervous system (CNS). Whether a dementia involves degenerative or nondegenerative processes or a combination of the two, individual factors (such as education, gender, age-related changes, preexisting brain disease, environmental exposures, and medical and psychiatric comorbidity) may influence the clinical expression of the dementing process.

Nondegenerative dementias, sometimes referred to as acquired or secondary dementias, are a heterogeneous group of disorders reflecting diverse etiologies: vascular, endocrine, traumatic, demyelinating, neoplastic, infectious, inflammatory, hydrocephalic, systemic, nutritional deficiency, and toxic conditions. Well-defined derangements of cerebral metabolism that result in highly specific cellular degeneration, as exemplified by inherited leukodystrophies and genetically determined heavy metal accumulation disorders (for example, Wilson's disease), occupy a transitional category of metabolic dementias.

TABLE 53.1 *Degenerative and Nondegenerative Dementias*

Degenerative	*Nondegenerative*
Amyloid/tau pathology	*Vascular dementias*
Alzheimer's disease	Multiple cortical infarcts
α-synuclein pathology	Binswanger's disease
Parkinson's disease (dementia)	Lacunar state
Dementia with Lewy bodies	*Infectious dementia*
Multisystem atrophy	HIV dementia
Tau pathology	Whipple's disease
Frontotemporal dementia	Neurosyphilis
Progressive supranuclear palsy	*Demyelinating dementia*
Corticobasal degeneration	Multiple sclerosis
Trinucleotide repeat	*Miscellaneous dementias*
Huntington's disease	Symptomatic hydrocephalus
Spinocerebellar ataxias	*Heavy metal (storage) disorders*
Toxic/metabolic disorders	Dementia syndrome of depression
Wilson's disease (copper)	Deficiencies (vitamin B12, niacin)
Hallevorden–Spatz syndrome (iron)	Endocrinopathies (thyroid, etc.)
Leukodystrophy	Chronic alcohol/drug abuse
Metachromatic leukodystrophy	Wernicke–Korsakoff syndrome
Prion-related dementias[a]	Marchiafava–Bignami disease
Creutzfeldt–Jakob disease	Industrial/environmental toxins
Gerstmann–Straussler–Scheinker syndrome	*Vasculitides (systemic and CNS)*
Fatal familial insomnia (thalamic dementia)	Lupus erythematosus
Variant Creutzfeldt–Jakob disease (BSE)	Sjogren's disease

[a]Inherited, sporadic, and directly transmissable forms. BSE: bovine spongiform encephalopathy; CNS: central nervous system; HIV: human immunodeficiency virus.

Degenerative Dementias: Overview

Neurodegenerative disorders account for the vast majority of adult-onset dementias. Most occur in late life and involve aberrant protein processing that is under variable genetic control (Table 53.2) (Martin, 1999; Pruisner, 2001). Four major classes of pathological protein-related neurodegenerative dementias are (*1*) amyloidopathies, (*2*) α-synucleinopathies, (*3*) tauopathies, and (*4*) trinucleotide repeat disorders. In many cases, familial and sporadic forms of a specific disorder have been described, representing the existence of disease-causing genetic mutations and other genetic factors that modify the risk. Exemplifying our expanding knowledge of such protein-misfolding or mismetabolizing disorders, a new class of disorders referred to as trans-activation-response (TAR) deoxyribonucleic acid (DNA)-binding protein 43 (TDP-43) proteinopathies have been described in association with ubiquitin-positive, tau-negative inclusions that are present in FTD and motor neuron disease (Neumann et al., 2006; Neumann et al., 2007) (see Fig. 53.1).

Amyloidopathies

In AD, autosomal dominant mutations in three distinct genes (presenilin 1 and 2 and the amyloid precursor protein) account for less than 5% of all cases. Genetic polymorphism of the apolipoprotein E gene modulates the risk of developing AD. The E4 allelic variant (one of 3 ApoE alleles: E2, E3, or E4) is associated with higher risk, and the E2 allele may be associated with lower risk.

TABLE 53.2 *Prevalence and Pathological Features of Selected Degenerative Dementias*

Disease	*Prevalence*[a]	*Genetic Factors (chrom. #) (F = familial, S = sporadic)*	*Abnormal Proteins*	*Pathological Features*
Alzheimer's disease	4,000,000	F: APP (21), PS1 (14), PS2 (1) S: apolipoprotein E (19)	β-Amyloid Tau (phosphorylated)	Amyloid (neuritic) plaques, Neurofibrillary tangles
Parkinson's disease	500,000	F: α-synuclein (4) Parkin (recessive) S: CYP2D6	α-Synuclein	Lewy bodies (brain stem), loss of pigmented neurons
Dementia with Lewy bodies Parkinson's disease with dementia	100,000 (est.)	F: SNCA (α-Synuclein) S: apolipoprotein E (19)	α-Synuclein $\pm$ β-Amyloid, $\pm$ Tau	Lewy bodies (diffuse), Lewy neurites, $\pm$ neuritic plaques, $\pm$ neurofibrillary tangles
Frontotemporal dementia	45,000	F: tau (17); progranulin (17) S: ?	Tau, TDP-43	Frontotemporal atrophy $\pm$ tau or TDP-43 inclusions
Huntington's disease	30,000	F: Huntingtin (4) S: ?	Huntingtin	Striatal and cortical atrophy, intraneuronal inclusions
Progressive supranuclear palsy	15,000	F: ? S: ?	Tau	Midbrain atrophy, globose neurofibrillary tangles
Multisystem atrophy	10,000	F: ? S: ?	α-Synuclein	Glial and neuronal inclusions
Creutzfeldt–Jakob disease	400	F: Prion protein gene S: ?	Prion protein (β-pleated sheet)	Amyloid plaques (prion protein)

[a]Estimated prevalence in the United States (2000). *Sources:* Martin (1999), Pruisner (2001), Baker et al. (2006).

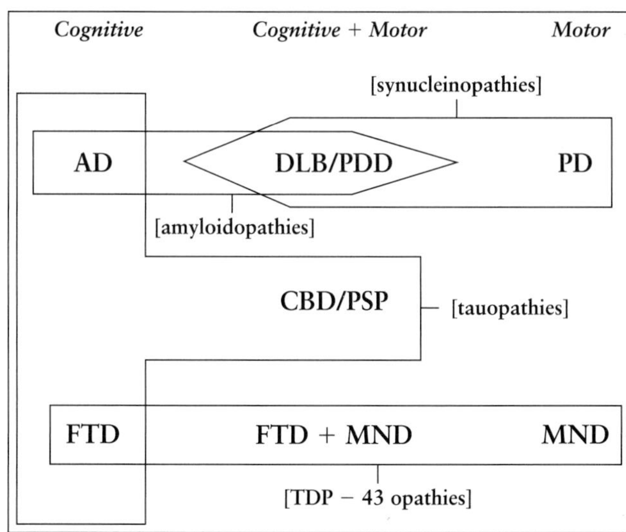

FIGURE 53.1 Clinical syndromes in relation to protein pathology. The spectral relationship between cognitive and motor syndromes in selected neurodegenerative disorders is schematically illustrated. Most cases of DLB and PDD have concomitant amyloid pathology. FTD clinical syndromes are associated primarily with either tau or TDP-43 protein pathology. TDP-43 pathology is associated with "pure" FTD, "pure" MND, and the combination of FTD and MND. AD: Alzheimer's disease; CBD: corticobasal degeneration; DLB: dementia with Lewy bodies; FTD: frontotemporal dementia; MND: motor neuron disease; PDD: Parkinson's disease with dementia; PSP: progressive supranuclear palsy.

Routine clinical testing for genotype, however, is not recommended (Plassman and Breitner, 1996; Mayeux et al., 1999; Knopman et al., 2001).

Despite the genetic diversity of AD, the pathological features are similar. These include the extracellular accumulation of β-amyloid (Aβ) plaques and the intracellular accumulation of neurofibrillary tangles in selected brain regions (The National Institute on Aging and the Reagan Institute Working Group, 1997). The former derive from alternative proteolytic processing of the amyloid-precursor protein (APP), whereas the latter accrue from hyperphosphorylation and extensive cross linking of the microtubule-associated protein tau, which normally stabilizes the neuronal cytoskeleton. Reduced levels of the synthetic enzyme for acetylcholine (choline acetyltransferase) and severe cell loss in basal forebrain cholinergic nuclei are pathological concomitants of AD; but recent evidence suggests that though functional alterations in cholinergic neurotransmission occur early in the course, structural cholinergic deficits do not become prominent until later stages of the disease process (Davis et al., 1999; DeKosky et al., 2002). The topographic distribution and spread of neurofibrillary tangles is the basis for pathologically staging AD (Braak and Braak, 1991; Delacourte et al., 1999). All known genetic mutations underlying familial forms of AD cause aberrant processing of Aβ, and other evidence suggests that amyloid pathology may have a preeminent etiological role (Selkoe, 2000). Although the primary etiology of sporadic AD remains controversial and may well be multifactorial, amyloid mismetabolism remains central to the pathological cascade.

Prion-related diseases are unique in that they may arise as either a genetically determined, infectiously transmitted, or sporadic disorder (Pruisner, 2001). Creutzfeldt–Jakob disease (CJD), the most common prion disorder, occurs by all these mechanisms, whereas fatal familial insomnia (thalamic dementia) and Gerstmann–Straussler–Scheinker syndrome are only associated with a dominantly inherited mutation in the prion protein gene. Infectious transmission represents less than 1% of all cases of prion diseases, typically resulting from direct contact with contaminated instruments or tissue. There is, however, the potential for widespread transmission, as suggested by the 100 or so cases of human variant CJD (bovine spongiform encephalopathy) that have occurred in the United Kingdom. Pathological alteration of the normal prion protein results in a conformational shift from a primarily α-helical to a mostly β-pleated-sheet structure that tends to form amyloid deposits. The altered form of the prion protein is rendered infectious by inducing a similar conformational change in other normal prion proteins. This process underlies the protean and rapidly progressive clinical manifestations of CJD. The previous designation of cerebrospinal fluid (CSF) protein 14–3-3 as a "gold standard" diagnostic marker for CJD (Knopman et al., 2001) has been questioned, with current efforts focusing on diffusion-weighted magnetic resonance imaging (MRI) and serum biomarkers in addition to 14–4-3 (Shiga et al., 2004).

α-Synucleinopathies

Parkinson's disease (PD) is defined by the presence of α-synuclein-containing intracytoplasmic inclusions (Lewy bodies) that accumulate in the substantia nigra and other pigmented nuclei of the brain stem. Dementia with Lewy bodies (DLB), a recently defined class of degenerative dementia, is characterized by brain stem and cortical Lewy bodies and abnormal neurofilaments (Lewy-related neurites) in the CA2–3 region of the hippocampus (McKeith et al., 1996; Perry et al., 1996). Lewy body pathology is seen in 15%—25% of all dementia cases, most commonly in conjunction with pathological features of AD (that is, amyloid plaques), referred to as the Lewy body variant of AD by some authors (Hansen et al., 1990) and as mixed AD/DLB by others. Three pathological subtypes of DLB based on the topographical distribution of Lewy bodies are recognized: (*1*) brain-stem predominant, (*2*) limbic (transitional), and (*3*) neocortical. Neurotransmitter deficits in DLB include the loss of dopaminergic neurons from the substantia nigra, as in PD, and more severe reductions in neocortical cholinergic markers compared to AD (Tiraboschi et al., 2000; Bohnen et al., 2003).

Multisystem atrophy (MSA) refers to a degenerative parkinsonian disorder with variable associated features, including autonomic, cerebellar, and pyramidal tract dysfunction. Three clinical variants of MSA are recognized: (*1*) striatonigral degeneration (SND), (*2*) Shy–Drager syndrome (SDS), and (*3*) olivopontocerebellar atrophy (OPCA; Wenning et al., 1994). All have a common pathological substrate of α-synuclein-containing glial cytoplasmic inclusions that are variably distributed in the cortex and subcortical regions, cerebellum, spinal cord, and dorsal root ganglia (Penney, 1995; Tu et al., 1998). Consensus diagnostic criteria for MSA have suggested two main forms, based on the predominant clinical feature: (*1*) MSA—Parkinson (MSA-P) or (*2*) MSA—cerebellar (MSA-C) (Gilman et al., 1999). Previously described cases of SND and SDS are classified as MSA-P, and sporadic OPCA is referred to as MSA-C.

Tauopathies

Frontotemporal dementia (FTD) is a spectrum of clinicopathological disorders and is divided into three main types: (*1*) Pick's disease, (*2*) non-Pick's FTD, and (*3*) FTD with motor neuron disease (The Lund and Manchester Groups, 1994; McKhann et al., 2001). These FTD variants are virtually indistinguishable with respect to dementia symptoms and gross pathological changes. Microscopic alterations (ballooned neurons and tau-positive Pick bodies) define Pick's disease and are associated with other pathological features common to all three variants: selective frontal-temporal cortical atrophy and neuronal loss, widespread astrocytic gliosis, and a variable degree of spongiform changes. An autosomal dominant mutation on chromosome 17 has been identified as one cause of familial FTD that is typically associated with extrapyramidal motor signs (Wilhelmsen et al., 1994; Yamaoka et al., 1996). Mutations in a gene coding for microtubule associated tau (MAPT) protein on chromosome 17 have been associated with familial cases of FTD, usually with parkinsonian features (Hong et al., 1998). Abnormal structure or altered splicing of the MAPT gene results in impaired binding of tau protein to microtubules and its subsequent polymerization into neurofibrillary tangles. The most common form of familial FTD is associated with mutations in the progranulin gene that, like the MAPT gene, is also located on chromosome 17 (Baker et al., 2006).

Two other degenerative dementias classified as tauopathies are progressive supranuclear palsy (PSP) and corticobasal degeneration (CBD), which exhibit pathological features that overlap with those of FTD (Feany et al., 1996; Litvan et al., 1996; Sergeant et al., 1999). Progressive supranuclear palsy is distinguished by the presence of globose neurofibrillary tangles (distinct from those of AD) composed of aggregated tau protein and accompanied by neuronal loss and gliosis in the subthalamic nucleus, globus pallidus, substantia nigra, and other subcortical nuclei. The pathological hallmarks of CBD are large, achromatic neurons and astrocytic plaques; these tend to be asymmetrically distributed in posterior cortical areas and subcortical regions affected in PSP. A specific tau polymorphism is common to PSP and CBD (Houlden et al., 2001).

TDP-43 Proteinopathies

Although a number of familial cases of FTD were associated with MAPT mutations on chromosome 17, it has been known that other familial cases of FTD were not associated with tau pathology. Recent work has identified TDP-43 as the major component of pathologic inclusions associated with FTD cases that are tau-negative, including sporadic and familial forms of the disease (Neumann et al., 2006, 2007). TDP-43 is also a pathologic hallmark of amyotrophic lateral sclerosis (ALS), a form of motor neuron disease, providing a common link between FTD and ALS. The prominent role of TDP-43 in different forms of FTD, including non-tau-sporadic and familial forms, and FTD associated with motor neuron disease, has led to a recent revision to the classification of FTD-associated disorders (Cairns et al., 2007).

Trinucleotide repeats. Huntington's disease (HD) is somewhat unique in that all cases are inherited in an autosomal dominant pattern. In HD, a disease-causing mutation in the huntingtin gene located on chromosome 4 results in an abnormally long cytosine-adenosine-guanine (CAG) trinucleotide repeat sequence (Huntington's Disease Research Collaborative Group, 1993). An abnormal form of huntingtin protein is deposited in neurons in vulnerable areas of the brain. A higher number of trinucleotide repeats is associated with younger age of onset. Spinocerebellar ataxias are another class of neurodegenerative disorders characterized by inherited trinucleotide repeat sequences; dementia is a variable feature.

PATHOPHYSIOLOGY

Neurotransmitter Systems

There are two general types of central neurotransmitter systems: (*1*) local or interneuron neurotransmitters, such as γ-aminobutyric acid (GABA) and neuropeptides, and (*2*) projection neurotransmitters, including acetylcholine, dopamine, serotonin, and norepinephrine (Cummings and Coffey, 1994). The principal excitatory (glutamate) and inhibitory (GABA) neurotransmitters of the CNS mediate neuronal information transfer in local cortical-cortical and cortical-subcortical circuits. Aberrant or dysregulated activation of excitatory amino acid transmitter receptors for glutamate and *N*-methyl-D-aspartate (NMDA) can trigger a pathological cascade resulting in toxic levels of intracellular calcium. Excitotoxic mechanisms have been hypothesized to play a role in a wide range of neurological disorders by precipitating neurotoxic neuronal death in specific systems (Lipton and Rosenberg, 1994).

Classic neurotransmitters have been associated most closely with cognitive and neuropsychiatric symptoms in dementia. Collectively, cholinergic and monoaminergic projection systems regulate the excitatory and inhibitory tone of multiple cortical and subcortical neural circuits, exerting a modulatory influence on cognitive processes, mood, emotional states, and goal-directed behavior (Mesulam, 1990; Cooper et al., 1991; Cummings and Coffey, 1994). Disruption of these projection systems contributes to cognitive dysfunction (for example, of attention, memory, language) and neuropsychiatric symptoms (for example, depression, apathy, psychosis) in AD and other dementing illnesses. Efforts to relieve symptoms in AD by augmenting cholinergic function may have beneficial neuropsychiatric as well as cognitive effects (Cummings and Kaufer, 1996), but they are limited by neuronal death, synapse loss, and metabolic dysfunction induced by neurofibrillary tangles (DeKosky and Scheff, 1990; DeKosky, 1995).

Neuroimaging

Structural imaging techniques (computed tomography [CT]) and MRI are useful in the evaluation and differential diagnosis of dementing disorders (Knopman et al., 2001). Mass lesions, cerebrovascular disease, demyelination, and focal or regionally selective atrophy are associated with some degenerative dementias. Quantitative MRI methods also show promise in the differential diagnosis of dementia and in preclinical detection of early AD (Kaufer et al., 1997; Jack et al., 1999). In addition to gross structural alterations, underlying metabolic or cerebral perfusion derangements may be detectable by MRI spectroscopy or with functional neuroimaging techniques (Pritchard and Brass, 1992). Functional imaging based on quantitative radioactive tracer measurements of cerebral blood perfusion with single photon emission computed tomography (SPECT) or brain glucose metabolism with positron emission tomography (PET) may identify regional cerebral functional abnormalities that parallel the distribution of pathology in selected diseases. Alzheimer's disease is typically associated with functional deficits in temporal and parietal lobe areas, whereas FTD is characterized by decreased metabolism or perfusion in frontal and anterior temporal lobe regions (Miller et al., 1991). Functional imaging techniques with radioactive tracers to assess the functional integrity of striatal dopamine and cardiac sympathetic (norepinephrine) terminals have also been recognized as having diagnostic utility in DLB (McKeith et al., 2005). Hypoperfusion on SPECT scan or glucose hypometabolism on PET scan in the occipital lobes in conjunction with abnormalities in temporal and parietal patterns shows promise for distinguishing DLB from AD (Lobotesis et al., 2000; Minoshima et al., 2001). Although functional imaging is not recommended for routine use in the diagnosis of dementia (Knopman et al., 2001), PET imaging for diagnosing or confirming dementia highlights has potential utility as an ancillary clinical diagnostic tool (Silverman et al., 2001). Burgeoning research applications of PET include the advent of in vivo amyloid imaging with Pittsburgh Compound B (Klunk et al., 2004) and other putative tracers for preclinical AD (Small et al., 2006), as well as distinguishing AD and FTD (Foster et al., 2007). In particular, neuroimaging for detection of disease-specific proteins (DeKosky and Marek, 2003) will be utilized in specific diagnosis, assessing pharmacologic interventions, and in preclinical detection (Mintun et al., 2006).

CLINICAL SYNDROMES

Functional Classification: Cortical and Subcortical

Neurodegenerative processes selectively involve topographically or functionally related neural systems. For example, pathological involvement in AD is concentrated in medial temporal, limbic, and temporal-parietal association cortices, whereas FTD primarily affects frontal and anterior temporal neocortical and limbic-related regions. By contrast, HD, PD, and PSP are degenerative disorders in which subcortical brain regions, particularly the striatum, are the principal loci of pathological alterations. Although the anatomical regions and functional systems affected by various degenerative dementias are relatively well characterized, the determinants of selective vulnerability underlying specific disease processes are poorly understood.

A systematic approach to the differential diagnosis of dementia is aided by recognition of two distinctive patterns of clinical features: cortical and subcortical (Cummings and Benson, 1992). Cerebral cortical areas represent functional domains that are interconnected in modular serial and parallel networks subserving specific information processing functions (Mesulam, 1990). Structural or functional disturbances in these cortically based networks may produce deficits in instrumental intellectual skills including memory, language, or visuospatial functions. Anatomically, the striatum (caudate and putamen), globus pallidus, anterior and medial thalamus, and substantia nigra are interconnected with frontal cortical regions in a series of circuits with motor and neurobehavioral affiliations (Alexander et al., 1986; Cummings, 1993).

In contrast to the specific nature of intellectual disturbances in a cortical dementia, a subcortical dementia entails more diffuse impairment of mental functioning, including dilapidated thinking, cognitive slowing, memory retrieval deficits, and executive dysfunction (for example, impaired judgment and planning). Subcortical dementia is frequently associated with extrapyramidal dysfunction. Parkinson's disease, HD, and PSP, as well as subcortical vascular disease, white matter diseases, and hydrocephalus, all exhibit clinical symptoms that reflect involvement of the basal ganglia and interconnected structures (Albert et al., 1974; Cummings and Benson, 1984). Although the cortical-subcortical functional classification of dementia does not strictly correlate with regions affected by pathology, it provides a useful heuristic differential diagnostic framework.

Differential Diagnosis

The differential diagnosis of dementia outlined below derives from the cortical-subcortical dichotomy but emphasizes elementary clinical features as the organizing principle (Fig. 53.2; Table 53.3). The first major branch point of this classification is based on attention versus memory deficits. If memory deficit is a primary feature, further distinction is based on the type of memory disturbance (learning vs. retrieval). The nonspecific initial manifestations of some dementias are addressed by inclusion under multiple headings. The American Academy of Neurology practice parameter details guidelines for the clinical evaluation of dementia (Knopman et al., 2001).

Isolated Cognitive or Psychiatric Symptoms

The initial manifestations of a dementia may include only neuropsychiatric symptoms or an isolated cognitive impairment (for example, memory, language, or visuospatial disturbance) in the absence of significant attentional or memory disturbances. Depending on the clinical circumstances, a CT or MRI brain scan may be indicated to rule out a primary CNS process (for example, neoplasm, stroke, subdural hematoma). Frontotemporal dementia may present with primarily neuropsychiatric manifestations, often beginning with disinhibited personality changes or depressive symptoms (Miller et al., 1991). Two clinical subtypes of FTD may also present as isolated language disturbances involving either expressive (primary progressive aphasia) or receptive (semantic dementia) linguistic functions (Neary et al., 1999). Initial manifestations of DLB may include prominent visual hallucinations and fluctuating attentional disturbances in the absence of a frank dementia (McKeith et al., 1996; McKeith et al., 2005).

TABLE 53.3 *Clinico-anatomical Features of Selected Degenerative Dementias*

Etiology	*Clinical Features*	*Anatomical Correlates*	*Neuroimaging Findings MRI (M)/PET (P)*
Alzheimer's	Memory deficit (L)	Medial temporal, nucleus basalis	Hippocampal atrophy (M)
disease	Aphasia, apraxia, agnosia	Temporal and parietal neocortex	↓ Temporal-parietal (P)
Frontotemporal	Memory deficit (R)	Dorsolateral prefrontal cortex	Frontal-temporal atrophy (M)
dementia	Speech/language disorders	Frontal/temporal neocortex (left)	↓ Frontal-temporal (P)
	Disinhibition	Orbitofrontal cortex (right)	
	Hyperorality (Kluver–Bucy)	Amygdala/anterior temporal cortex	
Dementia with	Memory deficit (L or R)	Medial temporal, prefrontal cortex	↓ Temporal-parietal-occipital
Lewy bodies	Fluctuating attention	Reticular activating system (?)	(P)
	Extrapyramidal signs	Substantia nigra	↓ striataldopamine binding
	Psychosis (hallucinations)	Temporal cortex, striatum (?)	(P)
Progressive	Supranuclear gaze palsy	Midbrain	Midbrain atrophy (M)
supranuclear	Dysarthria/dysphagia	Bulbar cranial nerves	↓ Frontal-thalamic (P)
palsy	Gait/balance disturbances, axial rigidity	Globus pallidus, subthalamic nucleus, substantia nigra	
Corticobasal	Unilateral limb signs (dystonia, myoclonus)	Subthalamic nucleus, thalamus, globus pallidus	Focal or asymmetric cortical atrophy (M)
degeneration			↓ Cortical (focal or asymmetric) (P)
	Cortical sensory loss, apraxia, alien hand	Parietal/frontal neocortex (focal and asymmetric)	
	Rigidity, gaze palsy (late)	Midbrain	
Huntington's	Memory deficit (R)	Frontal-striatal (caudate)	Caudate atrophy (M)
disease	Executive dysfunction	Frontal-striatal (caudate)	↓ Striatal-frontal (P)
	Choreiform movements	Putamen, subthalamic nucleus, globus pallidum	
Creutzfeldt–	Memory deficit (L or R)	Medial temporal/frontal-striatal	Diffusion-weighted hyperintensities (M)
Jakob disease	Ataxia, myoclonus	Cerebellar, basal ganglia	↓ Multifocal/diffuse (P)
	Language disturbances	Frontal-temporal	

L: learning deficit; R: retrieval deficit; MRI: magnetic resonance imaging; PET: positron emission tomography (glucose metabolism).

The fluctuating level of consciousness in DLB may mimic a delirium, but it is distinguished by its persistent nature and the absence of metabolic disturbances. Focal, asymmetric degenerative syndromes can produce isolated language or visuospatial disturbances, as in the initial stages of CBD (Mesulam, 1982; Rinne et al., 1994; Caselli, 1995). Mild cognitive impairment (MCI) is characterized by short-term memory deficits (amnestic form) in the absence of other cognitive deficits or functional impairment (Petersen et al., 1999). Up to 50% of individuals classified as having MCI will develop AD within 5 years, underscoring the importance of MCI as a risk factor or potential diagnostic marker for AD and as an entry point for therapeutic intervention (Petersen et al., 2001). Clinico-pathological data suggest that neurofibrillary tangle pathology is commonly present in amnestic MCI (Markesbery et al., 2006). Cerebrospinal fluid studies in MCI indicate that an "AD-like" pattern of lower-than-normal Aβ and elevated tau or phospho-tau predicts conversion to AD in 90% of such cases (Hansson et al., 2006). Importantly, absence of these CSF changes was associated with less than 10% of these cases not converting to AD, indicating that amnestic MCI is not invariably AD, and careful evaluation and longitudinal follow-up are necessary.

Memory Deficit: Learning versus Retrieval

The ability to learn new information is strongly dependent on the integrity of the hippocampus and related medial temporal lobe limbic circuits; a deficit in the ability to form new memory traces is referred to as anterograde amnesia. The inability to recall previously learned information, referred to as retrograde amnesia, is dependent in part on frontal lobe and related subcortical circuits. In learning and retrieval types of memory disorders, spontaneous recall is impaired. Clinically, a retrieval memory deficit is distinguished from a deficit in learning by the ability to recognize target stimuli from a learning trial (for example, a word list) after a delay, either with the aid of cues (cued recall) or from among choices that include target and nontarget stimuli (Cummings and Benson, 1992).

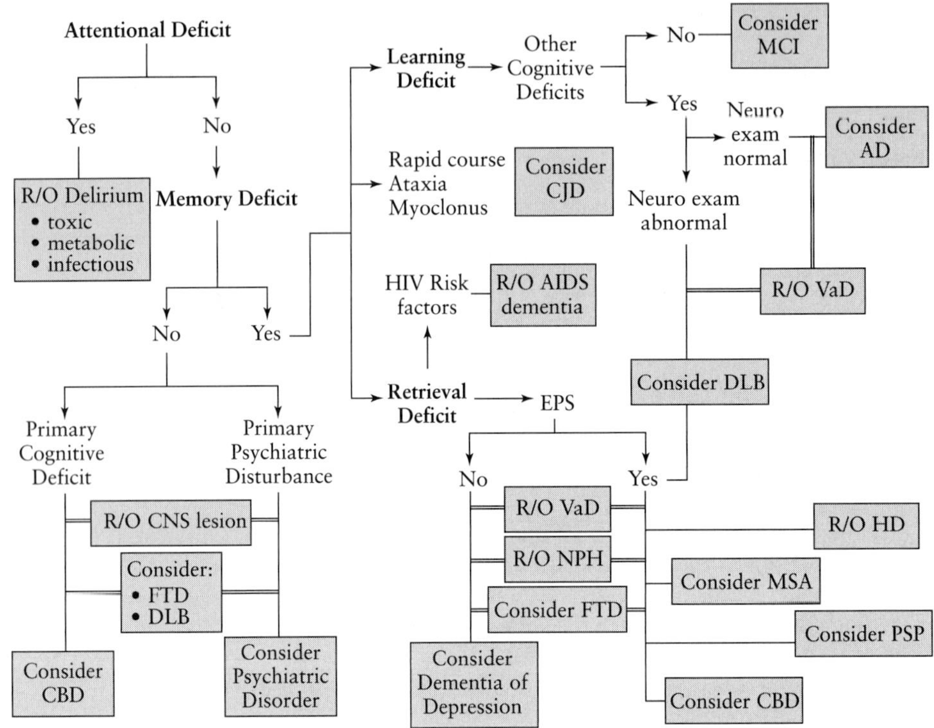

FIGURE 53.2 Differential diagnosis of dementia. R/O: "Rule out"; AIDS: acquired immunodeficiency syndrome; AD: Alzheimer's disease; CBD: corticobasal degeneration; CJD: Creutzfeldt–Jakob disease; CNS: central nervous system; DLB: dementia with Lewy bodies; EPS: extrapyramidal signs; FTD: frontotemporal dementia; HIV: human immunodeficiency virus; HD: Huntington's disease; MCI: mild cognitive impairment; MSA: multisystem atrophy; NPH: normal-pressure hydrocephalus; PSP: progressive supranuclear palsy; VaD: vascular dementia.

Learning Deficit: Differential Diagnosis

Impaired learning (anterograde amnesia) is also referred to as an *amnestic syndrome*; head trauma, Korsakoff's syndrome, herpes encephalitis, and hypoxia are among the most common causes. Alzheimer's disease may present with memory impairment only (that is, MCI) and should be considered as a provisional diagnosis in the absence of other identifiable aetiologies. If AD is the cause, memory functions will continue to decline and other cortically based cognitive disturbances, such as executive, language, and visuospatial disturbances, will emerge. Laboratory screening for aberrant metabolic factors (that is, thyroid function and vitamin B-12 level) and a CT or MRI brain scan to evaluate possible CNS lesions should be pursued to rule out alternative etiologies, particularly those that may be reversible. Vascular dementia (VaD) syndromes usually manifest focal or lateralized neurologic signs. Dementia with Lewy bodies may involve either a learning or retrieval type of memory impairment; concomitant delirium-like features and extrapyramidal signs may help distinguish DLB from AD (Mega et al., 1996), although AD is frequently a concomitant diagnosis.

Alzheimer's disease is the prototypic cortical dementia, principally involving neocortical association areas and related medial temporal lobe structures, with relative preservation of primary motor and sensory areas. In addition to progressive short-term memory loss, core symptoms are "cortical" deficits: aphasia, apraxia, and agnosia (McKhann et al., 1984). Visuospatial dysfunction and word-finding difficulties are common early manifestations. Apathetic indifference, diminished insight or lack of awareness of deficits, and impaired abstract thinking frequently accompany the core neuropsychological deficits. Focal neurological signs are usually absent early on; extrapyramidal motor dysfunction, myoclonus, or seizures may develop late in the course. If extrapyramidal symptoms emerge concurrently with cognitive problems, the diagnosis of DLB must be considered.

National Institute for Neurological and Communication Disorders and Stroke–Alzheimer's Disease and Related Disorders Association (NINCDS-ADRDA) criteria for probable AD include age of onset between 40 and 90 years, deficits in two or more cognitive domains, progression of deficits for at least 6 months, undisturbed consciousness, and the absence of another reasonable diagnosis (McKhann et al., 1984). Possible AD is reserved for cases that, in addition to meeting the above criteria, have an atypical clinical presentation or have another brain-based disorder that is not thought to contribute significantly to the clinical manifestations. Increasing knowledge of biomarkers as early indicators of incipient disease has led to the proposal of research criteria for AD that include only amnestic disorder and the presence of a biomarker of AD (Dubois et al., 2007).

Retrieval Deficit: Differential Diagnosis

Some clinical syndromes of dementia with retrieval memory deficits are accompanied by extrapyramidal signs, reflecting dysfunction in one or more frontal-subcortical circuits. A retrieval type of memory deficit in association with other features of a "subcortical" dementia characterizes acquired immune deficiency syndrome (AIDS)-related cognitive impairment. Two types of dementia-related syndromes, based on severity, have been proposed and clinically validated: (*1*) human immunodeficiency virus (HIV)-1-associated dementia complex (ADC) and (*2*) HIV-1-associated minor cognitive/motor disorder (The Dana Consortium on Therapy for HIV Dementia and Related Cognitive Disorders, 1996). Testing for HIV should be pursued if appropriate risk factors are present in conjunction with relevant signs and symptoms.

Frontotemporal dementia is associated with extrapyramidal signs (for example, familial FTD-17) or features of motor neuron disease in 10%–20% of cases (The Lund and Manchester Groups, 1994; Cairns et al., 2007). In cases where depression is prominent, a history of depression is present, and signs of other neurological disorders are lacking, the possibility of dementia associated with depression (pseudodementia or dementia syndrome of depression) may warrant a diagnostic "challenge" with antidepressants (Caine, 1981). In cases where depression is accompanied by significant cognitive deficits, antidepressant therapy may relieve the mood disturbance and reveal an underlying dementia, most commonly AD.

Extrapyramidal features may also be present in VaD syndromes, particularly those due to multiple lacunar infarcts or diffuse and severe periventricular white matter ischemia (Binswanger's disease). Normal-pressure hydrocephalus (NPH) produces a rapidly progressive and potentially reversible subcortical dementia accompanied by incontinence and gait disturbance. Computed tomography or MRI typically shows ventricular enlargement out of proportion to the degree of cortical gyral atrophy, but clinical correlation is essential. Clinical symptoms, particularly the gait disturbance, may resolve with a ventriculo-peritoneal shunt; shorter duration and an identifiable etiology (for example, meningitis, subdural hematoma) may predict a better response to shunting; Graff-Radford et al., 1989).

Vascular dementia is a heterogeneous syndrome with multiple clinical presentations, depending on lesion type and location (Roman et al., 1993). Infarctions in the territory of large cerebral vessels produce characteristic syndromes of higher intellectual dysfunction, such as aphasias, neglect, or visuospatial difficulties, with or without motor signs, depending on the regions and the extent of brain damage. The occurrence of a single stroke may predict subsequent cognitive decline that is not accompanied by further clinically apparent strokes (Moroney et al., 1996). The pathological mechanism of progressive dementia in this context remains unclear. Diffuse or multifocal small vessel ischemic disease can result in dementia arising from multiple lacunar infarcts. This form of VaD is associated with a preponderance of lesion sites in the frontal lobe white matter or basal ganglia, implicating disruption of frontal-subcortical circuit pathways as the relevant pathological mechanism (Ishii et al., 1986). More diffuse involvement of subcortical white matter secondary to small vessel ischemia (so-called Binswanger's disease) also functionally disconnects cortical and subcortical regions. Vascular dementia occurs more commonly as a mixed dementia syndrome in conjunction with AD than in isolation (Bennett et al., 2005, 2006).

National Institute for Neurological Disorders and Stroke-Association Internationale pour la Recherche et l'Enseignement en Neurosciences (NINDS-AIRENS) diagnostic criteria for probable VaD (Roman et al., 1993) include the presence of dementia, focal neurological signs, relevant cerebrovascular lesions on brain imaging, and an imputed relationship between the dementia syndrome and the cerebrovascular lesions. This relationship must either reflect onset of dementia within 3 months of a stroke, abrupt cognitive deterioration, or fluctuating stepwise progression. Possible VaD is used when the 3-month time requirement is not met. Validation studies for the NINDS-AIRENS and other criteria for VaD have generally shown low sensitivity (Knopman et al., 2001).

A genetically determined VaD syndrome, cerebral autosomal dominant arteriopathy with subcortical infarctions and leukoencephalopathy (CADASIL), has been described and linked to Notch3 mutations on chromosome 19 (Tournier-Lasserve et al., 1993; Joutel et al., 1996). Typically, CADASIL presents in early to middle adulthood and is associated with multiple subcortical infarcts and confluent subcortical white matter ischemic changes of the Binswanger's type and (in contrast to other VaD syndromes) is independent of vascular risk factors.

Extrapyramidal signs in conjunction with retrieval memory deficits are central features of many degenerative dementing illnesses. Huntington's disease typically presents in early to middle adulthood with choreiform movements and behavior and personality changes, including irritability, depression, and impulsivity (Folstein, 1989; Shoulson, 1990). Early-onset cases are more commonly associated with paternal inheritance, seizures, and parkinsonian features. Parkinson's disease is the prototypical extrapyramidal syndrome characterized by resting tremor, bradykinesia, limb rigidity, and postural imbalance. Frank depression and dementia occur in 30%–40% of individuals who are affected (Cummings and

Benson, 1992); with longer duration of the PD, dementia may be over 50%.

Consensus diagnostic criteria for DLB (McKeith et al., 1996) require dementia, one or more core features (fluctuating attention, extrapyramidal signs, visual hallucinations), and supportive clinical features (for example, sensitivity to neuroleptics, frequent falls). These provide a probabilistic clinical diagnosis of DLB. Probable DLB is used when two or more of the core features are present with dementia, and *possible DLB* refers to a dementia syndrome with one of the core features. A prospective validation study by Lopez and colleagues (2002) suggested that consensus diagnostic criteria for DLB have high specificity but low sensitivity, particularly when concomitant AD pathological features are present. Recently revised criteria for DLB (McKeith et al., 2005) identify two other clinical features as "suggestive": rapid-eye-movement (REM) sleep behavior disorder and neuroleptic sensitivity. Either of these two features counts as a core feature if at least one other core feature is present. The revised DLB criteria also include provisions for a probabilistic basis for the pathological diagnosis of DLB based on the predominance of cortical and limbic Lewy bodies relative to the density of neurofibrillary tangles. This addition to the criteria explicitly addresses the problem of overlapping etiologies. Although the consensus criteria view DLB and PD dementia (PDD) as separate disorders, another recent study (Apaydin et al., 2002) observed limbic and neocortical Lewy bodies to be the best predictor of dementia in PDD. The similarities between DLB and PDD are evident in diagnostic criteria for PDD (Emre et al., 2007) and have been suggested to form a spectrum of "Lewy body disorders" distinguished primarily by the predominant initial clinical features (Lippa et al., 2007).

Progressive supranuclear palsy is distinguished from PD by the absence of a resting tremor, the presence of axial (neck and trunk) rigidity, more severe speech and swallowing difficulties, a greater degree of gait and balance impairment, and limitation in voluntary downward gaze (supranuclear gaze palsy) (Collins et al., 1995). Midbrain atrophy on MRI may be a helpful diagnostic sign (Oba et al., 2005; Reich, 2006). Corticobasal degeneration is a rare disorder that may present with unilateral or asymmetric signs of rigidity, myoclonus, apraxia (manifested as "alien hand" phenomena, which refers to a limb that feels "foreign" and may act in an autonomous manner; Riley et al., 1990; Rinne et al., 1994). Other features include visuospatial (nondominant hemisphere) or language (dominant hemisphere) dysfunction and extrapyramidal motor signs akin to those of PSP.

Multisystem atrophy is a group of parkinsonian dementia syndromes that respond poorly to dopaminergic therapy. Compared to PD, striatonigral degeneration (SND) is distinguished by the absence of a resting tremor, symmetrical motor signs, more severe autonomic dysfunction, and more rapid functional decline. The presence of laryngeal stridor and pyramidal tract signs (for example, Babinski sign) may also help distinguish SND from PD. Cognitive function in SND is relatively preserved, although executive deficits are characteristically observed on formal neuropsychological testing (Robbins et al., 1992). Patients with SND may initially respond to levodopa to a limited degree, but the duration of benefit is typically short lived, and treatment is not well tolerated in many cases. Shy–Drager syndrome is distinguished by early, severe dysautonomia, including orthostatic hypotension, urinary problems, constipation, impotence, and sweating. Orthostatic hypotension may be particularly disabling and can be exacerbated by levodopa and other dopaminergic drugs. Sporadic OPCA is distinguished primarily by dysarthria and ataxia in association with marked cerebellopontine atrophy on structural brain imaging. Parkinsonian motor signs and dysautonomia are variably present. Impaired saccadic eye movements and vertical gaze palsy may also occur. Sporadic OPCA, viewed as a form of MSA, is typically distinguished from hereditary forms of OPCA, which are a subtype of spinocerebellar ataxia.

Sporadic CJD occurs in approximately 4 out of 1,000,000 adults aged 60 years or older (Pruisner, 2001). The initial clinical presentation is often nonspecific and may include ataxia or other elementary neurological signs. Disease progression is relentless, with the average duration from symptom onset to death being approximately 9 months. In addition to dementia, language disturbances and myoclonic jerking of the limbs are common features. A CSF test result of 14–3-3 protein may aid the diagnosis, but the specificity of this test is controversial (Knopman et al., 2001; Pruisner, 2001). A periodic spike discharge pattern on electroencephalogram (EEG) often develops later in the course, and recent studies have called attention to the presence of multifocal subcortical signal hyperintensities on diffusion-weighted MRI imaging (Mittal et al., 2002).

SUMMARY AND FUTURE DIRECTIONS

Current classifications of dementia involve mapping the intersection of clinical and neuropathological features. Although the NINCDS-ADRDA diagnostic criteria for AD have been well validated, probabilistic diagnostic classifications for VaD and DLB have not (Knopman et al., 2001). There is significant clinical and pathological overlap among disorders (Langa et al., 2004), where the boundaries between syndromes may be more accurately represented along a spectrum of clinical-pathological features, as depicted in Figure 53.1. Clinical diagnostic heterogeneity within such overlap zones reflects the variable clinical expression of underlying pathological substrates. Increased information about genetic and environmental contributions to dementia risk and etiology should yield a more precise, neurobiologically based differential diagnosis. Eventually, preclinical detection of AD and other degenerative dementias should be possible, along with prophylactic therapies that slow or stop the emergence of dementia symptoms. As fundamental mechanisms of aberrant protein processing in neurodegenerative disorders become elucidated, more definitive diagnostic and therapeutic approaches to dementing disorders will converge.

REFERENCES

Albert, M.L., Feldman, R.G., and Willis, A.L. (1974) The "subcortical dementia" of progressive supranuclear palsy. *J. Neurol. Neurosurg. Psychiatry* 37:121–130.

Alexander, G.E., Delong, M.R., and Strick, P.L. (1986) Parallel organization of functional circuits linking basal ganglia and cortex. *Annu. Rev. Neurosci.* 9:357–381.

American Psychiatric Association. (2000) *Diagnostic and Statistical Manual of Mental Disorders*, 4th ed., text rev. Washington, DC: Author.

Apaydin, H., Ahlskog, E.A., Parisi, J.E., Boeve, B.F., and Dickson, D.W. (2002) Parkinson disease neuropathology: Later-developing dementia and loss of the levodopa response. *Arch. Neurol.* 59: 102–112.

Baker, M., Mackenzie, I.R., Pickering-Brown, S.M., et al. (2006) Mutations in progranulin cause tau-negative frontotemporal dementia linked to chromosome 17. *Nature* 442:916–919.

Bennett, D.A., Schneider, J.A., Arvanitakis, Z., et al. (2006) Neuropathology of older persons without cognitive impairment from two community-based studies. *Neurology* 66:1837–1844.

Bennett, D.A., Schneider, J.A., Bienias, J.L., Evans, D.A., and Wilson, R.S. (2005) Mild cognitive impairment is related to Alzheimer disease pathology and cerebral infarctions. *Neurology* 64:834–841.

Bohnen, N.I., Kaufer, D.I., Hendrickson, R., et al (2003) Cortical cholinergic function is more severely affected in parkinsonian dementia than Alzheimer's disease: an in vivo positron emission tomography study. *Arch. Neurol.* 60:1745–1748.

Braak, H., and Braak, E. (1991) Neuropathological staging of Alzheimer-related staging. *Acta Neuropathol.* 82:239–259.

Caine, E. (1981) Pseudodementia. Current concepts and future directions. *Arch. Gen. Psychiatry* 38:1359–1364.

Cairns, N.J., Bigio, E.H., Mackenzie, I.R., et al. (2007) Neuropathologic diagnostic and nosologic criteria for frontotemporal lobar degeneration: consensus of the Consortium for Frontotemporal Lobar Degeneration. *Acta Neuropathol. (Berl)* 114:5–22.

Caselli, R.J. (1995) Focal and asymmetric cortical degeneration syndromes. *Neurologist* 1:1–19.

Collins, S.J., Ahlskog, E., Parisi, J.E., and Maraganore, D.M. (1995) Progressive supranuclear palsy: neuropathologically based diagnostic clinical criteria. *J. Neurol. Neurosurg. Psychiatry* 58:167–173.

Cooper, J.R, Roth, R.H., and Bloom, F.E. (1991) *The Biochemical Basis of Neuropharmacology*, 6th ed. New York: Oxford University Press.

Cummings, J.L. (1993) Frontal-subcortical circuits and human behavior. *Arch. Neurol.* 50:873–880.

Cummings, J.L. (2000) Cholinesterase-inhibitors: a new class of psychotropic compounds. *Am. J. Psychiatry* 157:4–15.

Cummings, J.L., and Benson, D.F. (1984) Subcortical dementia. *Arch. Neurol.* 41:874–879.

Cummings, J.L., and Benson, D.F. (1992) *Dementia: A Clinical Approach*, 2nd ed. Boston: Heinemann-Butterworths.

Cummings, J.L., and Coffey, C.E. (1994) Neurobiological basis of behavior. In Coffey, C.E., and Cummings, J.L., eds. *Textbook of Geriatric Neuropsychiatry*. Washington, DC: American Psychiatric Press, pp. 72–96.

Cummings, J.L., and Kaufer, D.I. (1996) Neuropsychiatric aspects of Alzheimer's disease: the cholinergic hypothesis revisited. *Neurology* 46:876–883.

The Dana Consortium on Therapy for HIV Dementia and Related Cognitive Disorders. (1996) Clinical confirmation of the American Academy of Neurology algorithm for HIV-1-associated cognitive/motor disorder. *Neurology* 47:1247–1253.

Davis, K.L., Mohs, R.C., Marin, D., et al. (1999) Cholinergic changes and synaptic alterations in Alzheimer's disease. *JAMA* 281: 1401–1406.

DeKosky, S.T. (1995) Searching for the holy grail: what is the structural correlate of cognition? *Neurobiol. Aging* 16:298–300.

DeKosky, S.T., Ikonomovic, M.D., Styren, S.D., et al. (2002) Upregulation of choline acetylcholinestrase activity in hippocampus and frontal cortex of elderly subjects with mild cognitive impairment. *Ann. Neurol.* 51:145–155.

DeKosky, S.T., and Marek, K. (2003) Looking backward to move forward: Early detection of neurodegenerative disorders. *Science* 302:830–834.

DeKosky, S.T., and Scheff, S.W. (1990) Synapse loss in frontal cortex biopsies in Alzheimer's disease: correlation with cognitive severity. *Ann. Neurol.* 27:457–464.

Delacourte, A., David, J.P., Sergeant, N., et al. (1999) The biochemical pathway of neurofibrillary degeneration in aging and Alzheimer's disease. *Neurology* 52:1158–1165.

Dubois, B., Feldman, H.H., Jacova, C., et al. (2007) Research criteria for the diagnosis of Alzheimer's disease: revising the NINCDS-ADRDA criteria. *Lancet Neurol.* 6:734–746.

Emre, M., Aarsland, D., Brown, R., et al. (2007) Clinical diagnostic criteria for dementia associated with Parkinson's disease. *Mov. Disord.* 22:1689–1707.

Feany, M.B., Mattiace, L.A., and Dickson, D.W. (1996) Neuropathologic overlap of progressive supranuclear palsy, Pick's disease, and corticobasal degeneration. *J. Neuropathol. Exp. Neurol.* 55:53–67.

Folstein, S. (1989) *Huntington's Disease*. Baltimore: Johns Hopkins University Press.

Foster, N.L., Heidebrink, J.L., Clark, C.M., et al. (2007) FDG-PET improves accuracy in distinguishing frontotemporal dementia and Alzheimer's disease. *Brain* 130:2616–2635.

Gilman, S., Low, P.A., Quinn, N, et al. (1999) Consensus statement on the diagnosis of multiple system atrophy. *J. Neurol. Sci.* 163: 94–98.

Graff-Radford, N.R., Godersky, J.C., and Jones, M.P. (1989) Variables predicting surgical outcome in symptomatic hydrocephalus in the elderly. *Neurology* 39:1601–1604.

Hansen, L., Salmon, D., Galasko, D., et al. (1990) The Lewy body variant of Alzheimer's disease: a clinical and pathological entity. *Neurology* 40:1–8.

Hansson, O., Zetterberg, H., Buchhave, P., Londos, E., Blennow, K., and Minthon, L. (2006) Association between CSF biomarkers and incipient Alzheimer's disease in patients with mild cognitive impairment: a follow-up study. *Lancet Neurol.* 5:228–234.

Hong, M., Zhukareva, V., Vogelsberg-Ragalia, V., et al. (1998) Mutation-specific functional impairments in distinct isoforms of hereditary FTDP-17. *Science* 282:1914–1917.

Houlden, H., Baker, M., Morris, H.R., et al. (2001) Corticobasal degeneration and progressive supranuclear palsy share a common tau haplotype. *Neurology* 56:1702–1706.

Huntington's Disease Research Collaborative Group. (1993) A novel gene containing a trinucleotide repeat that is expanded and unstable on Huntington's disease chromosomes. *Cell* 72:971–983.

Ishii, N., Nishihara, Y., and Imamura, T. (1986) Why do frontal lobe symptoms predominate in vascular dementia with lacunes? *Neurology* 36:340–345.

Jack, C.R., Petersen, R.C., Xu, Y.C., et al. (1999) Prediction of AD with MRI-based hippocampal volume in mild cognitive impairment. *Neurology* 52:1397–1403.

Joutel, A., Corpechot, C., Ducros, A., et al. (1996) Notch3 mutations in CADASIL, a hereditary adult-onset condition causing stroke and dementia. *Nature* 383:707–710.

Kaufer, D.I., and Cummings J.L. (1996) Delirium and dementia: an overview. In: Feinberg, T., and Farah, M., eds. *Behavioral Neurology and Neuropsychology*. New York: McGraw-Hill, pp. 499–520.

Kaufer, D.I., Itti, L., Miller, B.L., Fairbanks, L., Li, J., Kushi, J, Fishman, J., and Cummings, J.L. (1997) Midline cerebral morphometry distinguishes frontotemporal dementia and Alzheimer's disease. *Neurology* 48:978–985.

Klunk, W.E., Engler, H., Nordberg, A., et al. (2004) Imaging brain amyloid in Alzheimer's disease with Pittsburgh Compound-B. *Ann. Neurol.* 55:306–319.

Knopman, D.S., DeKosky, S.T., Cummings, J.L., et al. (2001) Practice parameter: diagnosis of dementia (an evidence-based review). *Neurology* 56:1143–1153.

Langa, K.M., Foster, N.L., and Larson, E.B. (2004) Mixed dementia: emerging concepts and therapeutic implications. *JAMA* 292: 2901–2908.

Lippa, C.F., Duda, J.E., Grossman, M., et al. (2007) DLB and PDD boundary issues: diagnosis, treatment, molecular pathology, and biomarkers. *Neurology* 68:812–819.

Lipton, S.A., and Rosenberg, P.A. (1994) Excitatory amino acids as a final common pathway for neurological disorders. *N. Engl. J. Med.* 330:613–622.

Litvan, I., Agid, Y., Calne, D., et al. (1996) Clinical research criteria for the diagnosis of progressive supranuclear palsy (Steele-Richardson-Olszewski syndrome): report of the NINDS-SPSP international workshop. *Neurology* 47:1–9.

Lobotesis, K., Fenwick, J.D., Phipps, A., et al. (2000) Occipital hypoperfusion on SPECT in dementia with Lewy bodies but not AD. *Neurology* 56:643–649.

Lopez, O.L., Becker, J.T., Kaufer, D.I., Hamilton, R.L., Sweet, R.A., Klunk, W., and DeKosky, S.T. (2002) Research evaluation and diagnosis of dementia with Lewy bodies. *Arch. Neurol.* 59:43–47.

The Lund and Manchester Groups. (1994) Clinical and neuropathological criteria for frontotemporal dementia: the Lund and Manchester Groups. *J. Neurol. Neurosurg. Psychiatry* 57:416–418.

Markesbery, W.R., Schmitt, F.A., Kryscio, R.J., Davis, D.G., Smith, C.D., and Wekstein, D.R. (2006) Neuropathologic substrate of mild cognitive impairment. *Arch. Neurol.* 63:38–46.

Martin, J.B. (1999) Molecular basis of the neurodegenerative disorders. *N. Engl. J. Med.* 340:1970–1980.

Mayeux, R., Saunders, A.M., Shea, S., et al. (1999) Utility of the apolipoprotein E genotype in the diagnosis of Alzheimer's disease. Alzheimer's Disease Centers Consortium on Apolipoprotein E and Alzheimer's disease. *N. Engl. J. Med.* 338:506–511.

McKeith, I.G., Dickson, D.W., Lowe, J., et al. (2005) Diagnosis and management of dementia with Lewy bodies: third report of the DLB Consortium. *Neurology* 65:1863–1872.

McKeith, I.G., Galasko, D., Kosaka, K., et al. (1996) Consensus guidelines for the clinical and pathologic diagnosis of dementia with Lewy bodies (DLB): report of the consortium on DLB international workshop. *Neurology* 47:1113–1124.

McKhann, G., Drachman, D., Folstein, M., Katzman, R., Price, D., and Stadlan, E.M. (1984) Clinical diagnosis of Alzheimer's disease: report of the NINCDS-ADRDA Work Group under the auspices of the Department of Health and Human Services Task Force on Alzheimer's disease. *Neurology* 34:939–944.

McKhann, G. M., Albert, M. S., Grossman, M., et al. (2001) Clinical and pathological diagnosis of frontotemporal dementia: Report of the Work Group on Frontotemporal Dementia and Pick's Disease. *Arch. Neurol.* 58:1803–1809.

Mega, M.S., Masterman, D.L., Benson, D.F., et al. (1996) Dementia with Lewy bodies: reliability and validity of clinical and pathologic criteria. *Neurology* 47:1403–1409.

Mesulam, M.-M. (1982) Slowly progressive aphasia without generalized dementia. *Ann. Neurol.* 11:592–598.

Mesulam, M.-M. (1990) Large scale neurocognitive networks and distributed processing for attention, language, and memory. *Ann. Neurol.* 28:597–613.

Miller, B.L., Cummings, J.L., Vilanueva-Meyer, J., Boone, K., Mehringer, C.M., Lesser, I.M., and Mena, I. (1991) Frontal lobe degeneration: clinical, neuropsychological, and SPECT characteristics. *Neurology* 41:1374–1382.

Minoshima, S., Foster, N.L., Sima, A.A.F., et al. (2001) Alzheimer's disease versus dementia with Lewy bodies: cerebral metabolic distinction with autopsy confirmation. *Ann. Neurol.* 50:358–365.

Mintun, M.A., Larossa, G.N., Sheline, Y.I., et al. (2006) [11C]PIB in a nondemented population: potential antecedent marker of Alzheimer disease. *Neurology* 67:446–452.

Mittal, S.J., Farmer, P., Kalina, P., Kingsley, P.B., and Halperin, J. (2002) Correlation of diffusion-weighted magnetic resonance imaging with neuropathology in Creutzfeldt-Jakob disease. *Arch. Neurol.* 59:128–134.

Moroney, J.T., Bagiella, E., Desmond, D.W., et al. (1996) Risk factors for incident dementia after stroke. Role of hypoxic and ischemic disorders. *Stroke* 27:1283–1289.

The National Institute on Aging, and the Reagan Institute Working Group on the Diagnostic Criteria for the Neuropathological Assessment of Alzheimer's Disease. (1997) Consensus recommendations for the post-mortem diagnosis of Alzheimer's disease. *Neurobiol. Aging* 18:S1–S2.

Neary, D., Snowden, J.S., Gustafson, L., et al. (1999) Frontotemporal lobar degeneration: a consensus on clinical diagnostic criteria. *Neurology* 51:1546–1554.

Neumann, M., Kwong, L.K., Sampathu, D.M., Trojanowski, J.Q., and Lee, V.M. (2007) TDP-43 proteinopathy in frontotemporal lobar degeneration and amyotrophic lateral sclerosis: protein misfolding diseases without amyloidosis. *Arch. Neurol.* 64:1388–1394.

Neumann, M., Sampathu, D.M., Kwong, L.K., et al. (2006) Ubiquitinated TDP-43 in frontotemporal lobar degeneration and amyotrophic lateral sclerosis. *Science* 314:130–133.

Oba, H., Yagishita, A., Terada, H., et al. (2005) New and reliable MRI diagnosis for progressive supranuclear palsy. *Neurology* 64:2050–2055.

Penney, J.B. (1995) Multiple systems atrophy and nonfamilial olivopontocerebellar atrophy are the same disease. *Ann. Neurol.* 37: 553–554.

Perry, R., McKeith, I.G., and Perry, E. (1996) *Dementia with Lewy Bodies: Clinical, Pathological and Treatment Issues*. Cambridge, UK: Cambridge University Press.

Petersen, R.C., Smith, G.E., Waring, S.C., et al. (1999) Mild cognitive impairment: clinical characteristics and outcome. *Arch. Neurol.* 56:303–308.

Petersen, R.C., Stevens, J.C., Ganguli, M., Tangalos, E., Cummings, J.L., and DeKosky, S.T. (2001) Practice parameter: early detection of dementia: mild cognitive impairment (an evidence-based review). *Neurology* 56:1133–1142.

Plassman, B.L., and Breitner, J.C.S. (1996) Recent advances in the genetics of Alzheimer's disease and vascular dementia with an emphasis on gene-environment interactions. *J. Am. Geriatr. Soc.* 44:1242–1250.

Prichard, J.W., and Brass, L.M. (1992) New anatomical and functional imaging methods. *Ann. Neurol.* 32:395–400.

Pruisner, S.B. (2001) Shattuck lecture—Neurodegenerative diseases and prions. *N. Engl. J. Med.* 344:1516–1526.

Reich, S.G. (2006) Can mid-sagittal MRI be used to diagnose progressive supranuclear palsy? *Nat. Clin. Pract. Neurol.* 2:12–13.

Riley, D.E., Lang, A.E., Lewis, A., Resch, L., Ashby, P., Hornykiewicz, O., and Black, S. (1990) Cortical-basal ganglionic degeneration. *Neurology* 40:1203–1212.

Rinne, J.R., Lee, M.S., Thompson, P.D., and Marsden, C.D. (1994) Corticobasal degeneration. A clinical study of 36 cases. *Brain* 117:1183–1196.

Robbins, T.W., James, M., Lange, K.W., et al. (1992) Cognitive performance in multisystem atrophy. *Brain* 115:271–291.

Roman, G.C., Tatemichi, T.K., Erkinjuntti, T., et al. (1993) Vascular dementia: diagnostic criteria for research studies. Report of the NINDS-AIREN International Workshop. *Neurology* 43:250–260.

Selkoe, D. (2000) Toward a comprehensive theory for Alzheimer's disease. Hypothesis: Alzheimer's disease is caused by the cerebral accumulation and cytotoxicity of amyloid beta-protein. *Ann. N. Y. Acad. Sci.* 924:17–25.

Sergeant, N., Wattez, A., and Delacourte, A. (1999) Neurofibrillary degeneration in progressive supranuclear palsy and corticobasal degeneration: tau pathologies with exclusively "exon 10" isoforms. *J. Neurochem.* 72:1243–1249.

Shiga, Y., Miyazawa, K., Sato, S., et al. (2004) Diffusion-weighted MRI abnormalities as an early diagnostic marker for Creutzfeldt-Jakob disease. *Neurology* 63:443–449.

Shoulson, I. (1990) Huntington's disease: cognitive and psychiatric features. *Neuropsychiatry Neuropsychol. Behav. Neurol.* 3:15–22.

Silverman, D.H.S., Small, G.W., Chang, C.Y., et al. (2001) Positron emission tomography in evaluation of dementia: regional brain metabolism and long-term outcome. *JAMA* 286:2120–2127.

Small, G.W., Kepe, V., Ercoli, L.M., et al. (2006) PET of brain amyloid and tau in mild cognitive impairment. *N. Engl. J. Med.* 355: 2652–2663.

Snowden, J.S., Pickering-Brown, S.M., Mackenzie, I.R., et al. (2006) Progranulin gene mutations associated with frontotemporal dementia and progressive non-fluent aphasia. *Brain* 129:2808–2810.

Tiraboschi, P., Hansen, L.A., Alford, M., et al. (2000) Cholinergic dysfunction in diseases with Lewy bodies. *Neurology* 54:407–411.

Tournier-Lasserve, E., Joutel, A., Melki, J., et al. (1993) Cerebral autosomal dominant arteriopathy with subcortical infarcts and leukoencephalopathy maps to chromosome 19q12. *Nat. Genet.* 3:256–259.

Tu, P.H., Galvin, J.E., Baba, M., et al. (1998) Glial cytoplasmic inclusions in white matter oligodendrocytes of multiple system atrophy brains contain insoluble α-synuclein. *Ann. Neurol.* 44: 415–422.

Wenning, G.K., Ben-Schlomo, Y., Magalhaes, M., et al. (1994) Clinical features and natural history of multiple system atrophy in 100 cases. *Brain* 117:835–845.

Wilhelmsen, K.C., Lynch, T., Pavlou, E., Higgins, M., and Nygaard, T.G. (1994) Localization of disinhibition-dementia-parkinsonism-amyotrophy complex to 17q21–22. *Am. J. Hum. Genet.* 55:1159–1165.

Yamaoka, L.H., Welsh-Bohmer, K.A., Hulette, C.M., et al. (1996) Linkage of frontotemporal dementia to chromosome 17: Clinical and neuropathological characterization of phenotype. *Am. J. Hum. Genet.* 59:1306–1312.

54 | Transgenic Models of Dementias

GREGORY A. ELDER

GENERAL CONSIDERATIONS

Requirements for a Transgenic Model

Animal models offer the opportunity to model human diseases allowing testing of therapeutic strategies as well as investigation of disease course and underlying pathophysiology in a manner that is impractical or unethical in humans. Transgenic technologies introduce genetic modifications into animals. Their use for disease modeling therefore requires that a genetic lesion be associated with a disease or at least that a hypothesis regarding the disorder exists that can be modeled by a genetic modification. Successful modeling also requires that the transgenic organism can exhibit the essential features of the human disease be it pathological, physiological, or behavioral.

Transgenic Organisms

Transgenic technology exists for many organisms, including fish, flies, and worms as well as mammalian species including mice, rats, sheep, and pigs. Modeling in invertebrates such as *Drosophila* or *C. elegans* or in vertebrates such as zebra fish offers advantages including the degree of experimental control and the relatively short life span of the organisms. They suffer the disadvantage though of being far removed phylogenetically from mammals. Although efforts to model human neurodegenerative diseases in these systems continue, they have had less impact than models using mammalian systems and are not discussed further. The interested reader is however referred to several recent reviews that have discussed transgenic modeling of Alzheimer's disease in *Drosophila* and *C. elegans* (Link, 2005; Wu and Luo, 2005) and invertebrate modeling of human tauopathies (Gotz et al., 2007).

Among vertebrates, mice have become by far the species of choice. Transgenic modeling in mice is relatively inexpensive. Mice also have a relatively short life span, and the techniques for performing genetic modifications in them are well developed. Although transgenic rats exist, this technology is not as widely available as for mice.

Methods for Generating Transgenic Organisms

In mice, two general techniques exist for introducing genetic modifications. The first to be developed generates transgenic animals by pronuclear injection. A one-cell embryo at the pronuclear stage is injected with a transgene containing the gene of interest. Transgenes typically consist of plasmid deoxyribonucleic acid (DNA) in which a complementary deoxyribonucleic acid (cDNA) for the protein of interest is linked to a heterologous promoter that drives expression. Natural or artificial introns are often included to allow the primary transcript to be spliced that generally enhances messenger ribonucleic acid (mRNA) stability and a polyadenylation sequence is added to allow proper mRNA processing. Alternatively bacterial, plasmid, or yeast artificial chromosomes may be injected that have the advantage of being able to accommodate even large genes. The injected transgene integrates randomly, typically at a single site and in multiple copies. Because there is no corresponding allele on the homologous chromosome opposite the integration site, these mice are referred to as "hemizygous" rather than "heterozygous." The mouse typically contains its own endogenous version of the gene of interest; therefore, the transgene is in most cases expressed on top of the expression of the endogenous mouse gene leading to an overexpression system.

A second technique, rather than introducing a foreign transgene, modifies an existing gene in the mouse. This approach uses specialized cells termed *embryonic stem (ES) cells* that are cell lines derived from early-stage mouse embryos. These lines can be maintained indefinitely in vitro in an undifferentiated state yet retain the capacity that when injected back into a mouse embryo, they can mix with the endogenous cells of the embryo and contribute to all tissues of the developing mouse including the germ line. The gene of interest is modified in ES cells by introducing a targeting vector that consists of a modified version of the endogenous gene. In ES cells, the targeting vector recombines with the homologous endogenous gene, thereby introducing the modification of interest. Modified ES cells are injected into a blastocyst-stage mouse embryo that generates a chimeric mouse containing endogenous blastocyst cells as well as ES cells. Successful integration of the ES cells into the germ line allows the genetic modification to be propagated as part of the mouse genome, creating stable transgenic lines.

Embryonic stem cell technology has been most commonly used to produce null mutants or gene "knockouts." However it can also be used to modify endogenous mouse genes down to the level of creating single nucleotide changes, producing what are known as "knockin" mice. In contrast to pronuclear injection where multiple copies of a transgene insert randomly in the genome, with ES cell–based methods the native mouse gene is modified in its normal chromosomal location. Thus, though in pronuclear injection a transgene is typically overexpressed and often misexpressed spatially and temporally due to its coupling to a heterologous promoter, with homologous recombination the altered gene is expressed at normal levels with a normal temporal and spatial expression pattern.

ALZHEIMER'S DISEASE

Alzheimer's disease (AD) is the most common cause of senile dementia in the United States and Europe, accounting for some 50%–80% of cases. Alzheimer's disease may in many ways be regarded as the ideal disease for modeling in transgenic systems. It first has a well-recognized pathology, consisting of senile plaques and neurofibrillary tangles (NFTs). The major components of plaques and tangles are well defined, consisting of accumulations of β-amyloid (Aβ) peptide in plaques and hyperphosphorylated forms of tau in NFTs. It has other well-recognized pathological features, including neuronal and synaptic loss, dystrophic neurites, and the presence of reactive astrocytes and activated microglia, all changes that can be modeled in the mouse. Alzheimer's disease also has a well-defined behavioral phenotype, including memory impairments that can be modeled in the mouse as well. Perhaps most important, though, most cases occur sporadically, there are families in which the disease is inherited in an autosomal dominant fashion. These cases of familial Alzheimer's disease (FAD) mimic the sporadic disease clinically and pathologically except for a typically earlier age of onset. Mutations in three genes, the *amyloid precursor protein* (APP), *presenilin-1* (PS1) and *presenilin-2* (PS2) have been identified as causes of FAD (Ertekin-Taner, 2007).

Transgenic Models Based on Overexpression of APP FAD Mutants

In AD, the 39-42 amino acid Aβ peptide deposits in senile plaques. Various in vitro and in vivo studies have demonstrated that Aβ can be neurotoxic. The amyloid cascade hypothesis postulates that Aβ production sets off a chain of events in AD brain that eventually leads to cell death (Selkoe, 2001). The Aβ peptide itself is derived from processing of a larger precursor protein known as APP. The amyloid hypothesis was greatly bolstered by the finding that mutations in APP can cause FAD. Modeling in transgenic mice has been vigorously pursued based on the amyloid hypothesis and has been the subject of several recent reviews (Codita et al., 2006; Games et al., 2006; McGowan et al., 2006).

Early attempts at generating transgenic models in the mouse before the discovery of FAD mutations focused on overexpressing wild-type APP in transgenic mice by pronuclear injection using a variety of promoters. However, none of these efforts produced anything that looked like an amyloid plaque or other recognizable AD-type pathology. It was not until 1995 and 1996 with the reports of PDAPP (Games et al., 1995) and Tg2576 (Hsiao et al., 1996) mice that models mimicking many of the features of human AD began to appear. These mice are described in some detail because they illustrate a general approach that would prove successful in the hands of many investigators and for other neurodegenerative diseases as well.

In the first report, Games et al. (1995) used the platelet derived growth factor-β (PDGF) promoter to drive a splicible human APP minigene capable of expressing all three major APP isoforms and containing an FAD mutation at codon 717 in which a valine was mutated to a phenylalanine (V717F). The PDGF promoter was chosen because, despite its name, it was known to be highly expressed in the central nervous system (CNS) and to drive strong expression of exogenous transgenes in neurons. In the line that was generated (termed *PDAPP* because of the PDGF promoter plus APP), 40 copies of the transgene integrated, resulting in an ≈18-fold elevation of APP RNA and ≈10-fold elevation of human APP protein, both compared to the endogenous mouse APP. Proportionate increases in human Aβ were seen as well. PDAPP mice exhibited age-dependent amyloid deposition in brain parenchyma with the appearance of thioflavin-S positive plaques, including compacted plaques with dense cores that were highly reminiscent of those seen in human AD. Dystrophic neuritis, reactive astrocytes, and activated microglia were all found near plaques. Plaque deposition was minimal at 6 months of age, but readily apparent by 9 months and increased dramatically by 12–15 months (Reilly et al., 2003). PDAPP mice were subsequently shown to develop age-related learning defects (Chen et al., 2000) and synapse loss (Dodart et al., 2000).

Hsiao et al. (1996) independently took a relatively similar approach overexpressing a human APP minigene containing the APP695 form, which is the isoform most highly expressed in neurons. The transgene contained the "Swedish" FAD mutation (K670N/M671L) and was driven by the hamster prion (PrP) promoter that drives expression widely in the nervous system. These mice, termed Tg2576 mice, expressed human APP at levels greater than five-fold above those of the endogenous mouse APP. Aβ40 and 42 levels increased in an age-dependent manner without any change in expression of full-length APP. As in PDAPP mice, Tg2576 mice exhibited an age-dependent deposition of amyloid, resulting in thioflavin-S positive plaques that exhibited the essential features of senile plaques in AD, including gliosis and dystrophic neurites. In Tg2576 mice, plaque amyloid was first clearly seen by 11–13 months, eventually becoming widespread in cortical and limbic structures. Water maze learning was found to be normal in 3-month-old animals but impaired in 9- to 10-month-old mice. The Tg2576 mouse line has been made widely available and is currently the most utilized transgenic model of AD.

Subsequently, many other transgenic lines were developed using relatively similar approaches to those taken for developing PDAPP and Tg2576 mice (reviewed in Codita et al., 2006; Games et al., 2006; McGowan et al., 2006), relying on typically strong promoters to drive expression of APP transgenes containing one or sometimes multiple FAD mutations. Common features of the models were the production of Aβ containing plaques, dystrophic neurites, and gliosis. Cognitive and behavioral deficits were also common (Games et al., 2006). Many other electrophysiological, neurochemical, and neuropathological changes that model aspects of AD in humans have also been reported.

Although the models exhibit many similarities, they differ in certain aspects, one being the time of onset of plaque deposition. TgCRND8 mice that express multiple APP mutations exhibit plaques by 3 months of age (Chishti et al., 2001). The APP23 line, in which a thy1 promoter was used to drive expression of the APP Swedish mutation, is notable for its prominent cerebrovascular amyloid deposition (Calhoun et al., 1999). PDAPP and Tg2576 mice indeed differ in certain aspects—among them, Tg2576 mice increase production of both Aβ40 and Aβ42, whereas in PDAPP mice, Aβ42 is selectively increased (Hsiao et al., 1996; Fryer et al., 2003). In Tg2576 mice most amyloid is found in dense cored plaques with relatively few of the diffuse deposits found in PDAPP mice. Tg2576 mice are also known for their giant plaques (Sasaki et al., 2002) and exhibit more congophilic angiopathy (Fryer et al., 2003), the latter being largely absent in PDAPP mice.

Variations between lines likely reflect the different promoters used to drive expression, the different mutations or combinations of mutations and the genetic backgrounds on which the transgenes have been maintained. PDAPP mice, for example, have been mostly studied on a highly mixed C57BL6/DBA/Swiss-Webster background. By contrast, Tg2576 mice have been typically studied on a mixed C57BL6/SJL background, and the Tg2576 transgene has been difficult to move off this background. Indeed, the Tg2576 transgene leads to early death when present on an FVB/N background (Hsiao et al., 1995).

Transgenic Mice Expressing Presenilin-Associated FAD Mutations

Presenilin-1 (PS1) was discovered in the search for an early-onset FAD gene associated with chromosome 14 (Ertekin-Taner, 2007). More than 160 mutations in PS1 have been linked to FAD, and mutations in PS1 are the most commonly recognized cause of early-onset FAD. Shortly after PS1's discovery, a related gene was identified on chromosome 1 (Ertekin-Taner, 2007). Mutations in this gene, now called *presenilin 2* (PS2), although a less common cause than PS1 also result in FAD. Functionally, presenilins are best known for their role in the γ-secretase cleavage of many transmembrane proteins including APP (Vetrivel et al., 2006). Presenilin FAD mutations in particular shunt APP processing towards the more amyloidogenic Aβ42 species (Vetrivel et al., 2006), an observation that can be been seen as further support for the amyloid hypothesis.

A variety of PS1 FAD mutant lines have been generated using many of the same promoters used to create APP lines, including PDGF (Duff et al., 1996) and PrP (Borchelt et al., 1996; Citron et al., 1997). Some PS2 FAD mutant lines also exist. Several PS1 FAD mutations have also been knocked in to the endogenous mouse PS1 gene (Flood et al., 2002; Guo et al., 1999; Nakano et al., 1999). Presenilin FAD mutant mice have consistently shown selective elevations of Aβ42 with little if any effect on Aβ40. When crossed with plaque-forming APP lines, the PS1 FAD mutants cause earlier and more extensive plaque deposition (Borchelt et al., 1996; Holcomb et al., 1998), although single transgenic PS1 or PS2 mice have never been observed to exhibit plaque formation.

Although PS1/APP bigenic mice have been frequently studied, the parental presenilin lines have been less studied likely due to their lack of a more robust AD pathology. However, PS1 and PS2 FAD mutant lines show exaggerated hippocampal damage following kainite induced excitotoxicity (Guo et al., 1999; Grilli et al., 2000; Schneider et al., 2001), and PS1 FAD mutants render animals more sensitive to trimethyltin-induced hippocampal damage (Kassed et al., 2003). Lesioning of the perforant path also induces excessive neuronal loss in the entorhinal cortex in mice harboring the deltaE9 PS1 FAD mutant (Lazarov et al., 2006). Increased protein oxidation and lipid peroxidation have also been reported in PS1 FAD mutant brain (Mohmmad Abdul et al., 2004; Schuessel et al., 2006), and several studies have documented impaired hippocampal neurogenesis in adult PS1 FAD mutant mice (Wen et al., 2004; Chevallier et al., 2005). One study has reported age-related neurodegenerative changes and neuronal loss in a PS1 FAD mutant line (Chui et al., 1999), and recently age-related NFT-like inclusions were described in a PS1 knockin line (Tanemura et al., 2006). Thus, presenilin FAD mutant mice exhibit a phenotype. What is less apparent is why they fail to exhibit the full range of AD related changes in mice given the potency of the mutations in humans.

Relevance as Models of Alzheimer's Disease

The success of transgenic models such as PDAPP and Tg2576 have depended on the overexpression of APP transgenes containing FAD-associated mutations. In one sense, the models are problematic because of their reliance on overexpressed proteins. One might argue that overexpression of any protein becomes toxic at some level and that it is hardly surprising that overexpression of an amyloidogenic protein at some level causes amyloid deposits. Yet there is no evidence for APP overexpression in sporadic AD.

It is also interesting to compare these overexpression models to APP knockin mice in which the Swedish mutation was introduced into the mouse APP gene (Reaume et al., 1996). These mice should represent the most authentic model of human FAD in the mouse and because the three amino acid differences between mouse and human in the Aβ region were modified as well, they produce human Aβ. In these mice, though Aβ production is increased, no amyloid plaques or any substantial neuropathology develops.

The models have also been troubled by the difficulty of producing the full spectrum of AD pathology including neuronal loss and NFTs. Despite extensive amyloid deposition, PDAPP and Tg2576 exhibit no neuronal loss (Irizarry et al., 1997a, 1997b). APP23 mice show very modest losses of CA1 pyramidal cells (about 15%) (Calhoun et al., 1998) but far below that observed in AD. More substantial neuronal loss has been reported in mice expressing multiple PS1 and APP mutations. In one study (Schmitz et al., 2004), APP transgenic mice expressing APPSwe and V717I-London were crossed with mice harboring the PS1 M146L mutation and a 35% loss of hippocampal neurons was reported. In another study, two APP (APPSwe/APPLondon) mutations expressed from transgenes were crossed onto a mouse line that had two presenilin FAD mutations (M233T/L235P) knocked in to the mouse PS1 gene. Besides amyloid pathology, extensive neuronal loss (> 50%) occurred in the hippocampus. Finally, recently three APP and two PS1 FAD mutations were combined to create a 5X FAD mutant mouse, and neuronal loss was observed (Oakley et al., 2006). Thus, neuronal loss can be induced in the mouse but only, it would seem, by combining multiple mutations that are individually sufficient to cause disease in humans.

A second problem with the models has been the general difficulty of inducing NFT-like pathology. Neurofibrillary tangles are recognized by their propensity to label with certain histological stains, including thioflavin-S and Congo red, and by being ultrastructurally composed of paired helical filaments (PHF). Hyperphosphoryated forms of tau are found in NFTs, and conformationally altered tau epitopes appear that can be recognized by specific antibodies. PDAPP mice accumulate phosphorylated tau epitopes within dystrophic neurites but only in animals older than 14 months of age (Masliah et al., 2001). Within these neurites, 12–15 nm filaments can be found but no PHF and no lesions with the histological staining properties of NFTs. Various hypotheses have been advanced for the difficulty of inducing NFT-like lesions in the mouse including differences between human and mouse tau and the shorter life span of the mouse.

Recently, mice have been produced that exhibit NTF-like lesions and plaques by combining FAD mutations with mutant forms of tau associated with a distinct form of dementia known as frontotemporal dementia with parkinsonian features (FTDP-17). Although clinically distinct from AD (see below), FTDP-17 cases exhibit NFTs like those found in AD, and mutations in tau cause a subset of FTDP-17 cases.

Lewis et al. (2001) first crossed a transgenic line known as JNPL3 that expresses the P301L mutation associated with FTDP-17 with Tg2576 mice. Singly transgenic JPNL3 mice were known to develop NFT-like lesions and the bigenic progeny called TAPP mice exhibited NFTs and amyloid plaques. More recently, Oddo et al. (2003) generated a triple transgenic model (3xTg-AD) by coinjecting independent transgenes harboring APPSwe and the P301L FTDP-17 mutation into fertilized eggs harvested from homozygous PS1M146V knockin mice. The resulting transgenic lines thus express mutations in APP and tau from exogenous transgenes on a background of a PS1 FAD mutation expressed from the endogenous mouse gene. With aging, these mice had increased Aβ40 and Aβ42 levels, accumulated intraneuronal Aβ, and exhibited amyloid plaques and NFT-like lesions that could be immunostained by antibodies that recognize conformationally altered tau epitopes. Amyloid plaques appeared by 6 months of age and preceded tau pathology that was not evident until about 1 year of age. 3xTg-AD mice also developed age-dependent synaptic dysfunction, including altered long-term potentiation and deficits in memory (Oddo et al., 2003; Billings et al., 2005).

These mice thus exhibit a broader spectrum of AD pathology. The question again arises, however: are they models of AD? The mice do exhibit the much-sought-after plaques with tangle pathology. They, however, represent a composite of two distinct diseases that do not naturally occur together. Plaque development is almost certainly driven by the APP and PS1 FAD mutations, with tangle-like pathology driven by the tau mutation. Indeed, in 3xTg-AD mice, the pathologies arise in spatially distinct patterns with Aβ deposition initiating in neocortex and progressing to hippocampus, and tau pathology beginning in hippocampus and progressing to neocortex. It does appear, however, that the mutations do interact, as in TAPP mice, NFTs are found in regions that rarely or never exhibit NFTs in single transgenic JNPL3 animals. In addition, intracerebral injections of anti-Aβ antibodies into the hippocampus of 3xTg-AD mice not only reduced extracellular and intracellular accumulation of Aβ but also resulted in clearance of early tau pathology, although later-stage lesions were resistant (Oddo et al., 2004). These studies thus show that modulating Aβ affects tau pathology and suggest that tau pathology may be induced by Aβ generation. This notion has also been supported by recent studies showing that behavioral deficits in APP FAD mutant mice were reduced when endogenous tau was removed by breeding the APP transgene onto a tau null background (Roberson et al., 2007).

Uses of Transgenic Models to Study AD Pathophysiology: Effects of Different Species of Aβ

In vitro Aβ42 promotes fibril formation more strongly than Aβ40. Recently, the relative plaque forming ability of Aβ40 and Aβ42 was investigated in vivo by generating transgenic mice that selectively express either Aβ40 or Aβ42 (McGowan et al., 2005). These mice were created by fusing Aβ40 and Aβ42 peptide sequences to the C-terminus of the BRI protein. BRI is a transmembrane protein that undergoes a constitutive cleavage near its C-terminal end that releases a soluble 23 amino acid peptide. Aβ40 or Aβ42 selective expression systems were created by replacing the 23 amino acid native BRI peptide with human Aβ40 or Aβ42 sequences. Interestingly, BRI-Aβ42 mice accumulated insoluble Aβ42 and with aging developed amyloid plaques, diffuse deposits, and extensive congophilic angiopathy. By contrast, BRI-Aβ40 mice developed no amyloid pathology at any age. Aβ40 is found in plaque amyloid and is especially common in vascular amyloid. These studies are thus consistent with models suggesting that Aβ42 is required to "seed" parenchymal and vascular deposits of Aβ40.

Transgenic mice have also been used to assess factors that affect patterns of amyloid deposition. Interestingly, though a number of FAD mutations in APP reside near the β and γ-secretase cleavage sites, other mutations lie within the Aβ domain itself. These latter mutations typically do not produce substantial parenchymal deposition in the form of plaques but rather result in extensive vascular deposits. One such mutation is E693Q also known as the Dutch mutation rather than resulting in AD causes a hereditary form of recurrent intracerebral hemorrhage.

Herzig et al. (2004) developed transgenic lines that expressed human wild-type APP, APP-Dutch, or APP-Dutch crossed with a PS1 FAD mutant. These lines exhibited different ratios of Aβ40/42, with APP Dutch being greater than wild-type APP, which was in turn greater than APP-Dutch/PS1. The high ratio of Aβ40/42 in the APP-Dutch mice resulted in extensive congophilic angiopathy with essentially no parenchymal deposition. By contrast, APP-Dutch/PS1 with nearly half the Aβ40/42 ratio of APP-Dutch mice developed parenchymal plaques with little vascular deposition, and wild-type APP mice with intermediate Aβ40/42 ratios had mixed parenchymal and vascular deposition. These results, though not inconsistent with the notion that Aβ42 is necessary as a seed for amyloid deposition in either compartment, suggest that Aβ40 promotes vascular deposition while Aβ42 shifts deposition towards parenchymal amyloid. Other studies (Cheng et al., 2004) have found, however, that transgenic mice harboring a distinct 693 mutation (E693G/Arctic) combined with APP Swedish and Indiana mutations develop prominent parenchymal plaque deposits with little congophilic angiopathy despite high Aβ40/42 ratios. Thus, some other property of mutations at the 693 site besides their effect on Aβ40/42 ratios must also influence parenchymal versus vascular deposition.

The Rise of the Aβ Oligomer

The original amyloid hypothesis regarded Aβ deposited in plaque amyloid as the toxic material. However, subsequently it became clear that plaque counts correlate relatively poorly with the level of cognitive decline and that NFTs, in fact, correlate more strongly than plaques with the degree of dementia. This led to a reevaluation of what form of amyloid might constitute the most toxic species, and recently soluble forms of Aβ have been proposed as the more toxic species.

Soluble Aβ species are toxic in cell culture systems (Walsh and Selkoe, 2007). APP transgenic mice have provided strong circumstantial support for their toxicity in vivo by showing that many pathological and functional changes in these mice occur before plaque pathology. For example, a series of studies in PDAPP mice have shown that volume loss and other anatomic changes in the dentate gyrus are present in 100-day-old mice well before plaque deposition (Redwine et al., 2003; Wu et al., 2004). Tg2576 mice also exhibit electrophysiological and behavioral changes months before plaque deposition (Jacobsen et al., 2006). Behavioral and electrophysiological changes have been described in other lines of APP mice before amyloid deposition as well

(Holcomb et al., 1998; Hsia et al., 1999; Moechars et al., 1999), and in Tg2576 mice, axonal swellings may be present for up to a year before amyloid deposition (Stokin et al., 2005). Indeed, recently a 56-kDa oligomeric Aβ species was identified in Tg2576 mice (Lesne et al., 2006). Levels of this species that has been termed Aβ*56 correlates strongly with the degree of memory impairment in Tg2576 mice; and when injected into rats, Aβ*56 also disrupts cognitive functioning. The finding of pathophysiological changes in PS1 FAD mutant mice (see above) that have elevated Aβ but no plaques is also consistent with a toxic role for soluble forms of Aβ.

Aβ Immunization as a Therapeutic Strategy in Alzheimer's Disease

APP transgenic animals have been widely used to study factors that affect Aβ deposition. For example, the role that apolipoprotein ε4 (ApoE4) and its various isoforms play in the development of plaque pathology has been extensively studied using ApoE4 transgenic and knockout mice (Bales et al., 1997; Holtzman et al., 2000; Fagan et al., 2002). Studies examining how dietary cholesterol affects plaque pathology (Refolo et al., 2001) have formed part of the basis for the interest in statins as a potential AD treatment. Indeed, APP transgenic mice have been used for a range of preclinical studies evaluating factors that influence plaque pathology ranging from inflammatory modulators, metal chelators, and natural products that bind Aβ to lifestyle factors including exercise, environmental enrichment, caloric restriction, and even wine consumption (Adlard et al., 2005; Lazarov et al., 2005; Patel et al., 2005; Games et al., 2006; Wang et al., 2006).

However, nowhere have transgenic mice played a larger role than in the development of immunotherapy as a potential treatment for AD. Indeed, though the initial impetus for immune approaches came from in vitro studies showing that anti-Aβ antibodies could prevent fibril formation as well as disaggregate preformed fibrils (Solomon et al., 1996), without studies in transgenic mice demonstrating their potential effectiveness in vivo, it seems unlikely that these approaches would have ever made their way into human trials. These studies have recently been extensively reviewed by Morgan (2006).

Schenk et al. (1999) first investigated Aβ vaccination in vivo. They initially immunized 6-week-old PDAPP mice (well before the age of plaque deposition in this line) with an Aβ vaccine injected on a monthly basis for 11 months. The mice developed high titers of anti-Aβ antibodies and at 12 months of age showed dramatic reductions in plaque loads. In a second set of studies, 11-month-old mice (after the onset of plaque deposition) were given monthly injections and were examined at 15 and 18 months. At both ages, plaque burdens were dramatically reduced, raising the hope that Aβ vaccination might be beneficial even after parenchymal deposits are present. Subsequent studies confirmed the beneficial effect of Aβ immunotherapy in other transgenic lines, also showing that active immunization could reverse memory deficits in APP and PS/APP mice (Janus et al., 2000; Morgan, 2006).

How active immunization works remains uncertain. Schenk et al. (1999) proposed that anti-Aβ antibodies might coat amyloid deposits and promote phagocytosis by microglia and other immune cells. Later studies found, however, that immunization also induces massive increases in plasma Aβ (DeMattos et al., 2001), suggesting that vaccination might induce movement of Aβ from brain into what has been referred to as a peripheral sink for Aβ. A third possibility is that anti-Aβ antibodies directly impede new fibril formation.

Subsequently, it was found that passive immunization by administering anti-Aβ antibodies peripherally also reduces amyloid deposition (Dodart et al., 2002; Kotilinek et al., 2002). Indeed, multiple studies have shown that even short-term administration of anti-Aβ antibodies improves performance in tests of learning and memory. Interestingly, improvements occur even though no detectible effect is seen on deposits of plaque amyloid, providing further support for the notion that a soluble pool of Aβ may be critical for toxicity.

Whatever its mechanism of action, studies in transgenic mice were sufficiently compelling that Aβ immunization was taken into clinical trials in humans. Although phase 1 studies indicated good immunological responses and tolerability of the vaccine, phase 2 studies in patients with AD were halted due to the appearance of an autoimmune meningoencephalitis in some patients (Orgogozo et al., 2003). Although these initial studies were ultimately disappointing, a retrospective analysis found that those patients with the highest anti-Aβ titers had significantly less cognitive decline than those with low titers (Hock et al., 2003), suggesting that Aβ immunization remains a viable strategy if autoimmune side effects can be overcome. Passive immunization strategies remain attractive, as well, due to the greater control over antibody levels that can be achieved, although some studies in transgenic mice have suggested that adoptive transfer may cause more congophilic angiopathy (Morgan, 2006). Although effective immunomodulatory strategies remain a goal rather than a reality, attempts to develop safer active or passive immunization strategies continue and will without doubt continue to make use of transgenic models.

TAUOPATHY-ASSOCIATED DEMENTIAS

Besides AD, hyperphosphorylated forms of tau accumulate in NFTs in the absence of plaques in a number of neurodegenerative diseases including Pick's disease, progressive supranuclear palsy, corticobasal degeneration, and FTD. Frontotemporal dementia cases present clinically with often prominent behavioral disturbances or isolated language defects and relatively preserved memory, initially. Some cases also exhibit parkinsonian features (FTDP). Pathologically, atrophy—especially frontotemporal—is prominent with neuronal loss, NFTs, and sometimes spongioform change.

Frontotemporal dementia is a less common form of dementia than AD, accounting for 5%–7% of cases in some autopsy series. Like AD, most cases occur sporadically. However, in some families with FTDP, the disease is caused by mutations in the tau gene on chromosome 17 (FTDP-17) (Haugarvoll et al., 2007). Mutations—including exonic point mutations that alter the protein coding sequence as well as intronic mutations that affect splicing or the level of tau expression—have all been identified. In addition to FTDP, tau mutations cause clinical syndromes resembling progressive supranuclear palsy, corticobasal degeneration, Pick's disease, and a disease known as progressive subcortical gliosis.

Tau is a microtubule binding protein that undergoes a complex transcriptional and posttranscriptional regulation producing multiple isoforms (Mandelkow et al., 2007). Tau's only known function is to bind to microtubules, leading to their stabilization. Binding occurs through a microtubule binding domain, and tau isoforms can be broadly divided into those that contain three or four repeats of this domain. Phosphorylation reduces tau binding to microtubules. In AD as well as in human tauopathies, tau becomes hyperphosphoryated, and conformationally altered epitopes appear that can be recognized by specific antibodies. In addition, phosphorylated forms of tau that are normally found in axons become redistributed to the somato-dendritic compartment.

Transgenic Models of Tauopathies

Transgenic modeling of tauopathies has been approached in a manner very similar to that which was successful for AD. Tau transgenes containing FTDP-17 mutations have been typically overexpressed using strong promoters. JPNL3 mice (Lewis et al., 2000) were mentioned briefly above. In these mice, the mouse PrP promoter was used to express the four repeat form of human tau containing the P301L mutation associated with FTDP-17. Hemizygous mice expressed human tau at levels approximately equal to the endogenous mouse tau, leading to about a twofold increase in total tau. JPNL3 mice exhibited marked tangle-like pathology and gliosis in brain as well as spinal cord, with neuronal loss in both regions. In addition to neuronal inclusions, filamentous accumulations of tau occurred in astrocytes and oligodendrocytes (Lin et al., 2003a). These lesions stained with Congo red and thioflavin-S as well as other stains that recognize human NFTs and also, like human NFTs, reacted with anti-tau antibodies that see phosphorylated as well as conformationally altered tau epitopes. Insoluble forms of tau not normally detected in mouse brain accumulated, and a mixture of 10–20 nm diameter straight as well as wavy filaments was visible by electron microscopy, though no true PHFs were found (Lin et al., 2003b). JNPL3 mice developed a progressive motor disorder that became evident as early as 6½ months of age in hemizygous mice and 4½ months in homozygous mice. The motor disorder was associated with a nearly 50% reduction of spinal motor neurons, peripheral nerve degeneration, and neurogenic atrophy. As a control for tau overpression itself, mice were created with the same PrP promoter driving expression of human wild-type tau. These mice exhibited no clinical phenotype, and though neurons in the hippocampus and other regions stained with antibodies that recognize conformationally altered tau epitopes, these neurons did not develop NFTs (Lewis et al., 2000).

Subsequently, many transgenic lines have been made expressing FTDP-17 associated tau mutations under a variety of promoters that drive expression in neurons and glia (reviewed in Gotz et al., 2007). A common feature of these models has been the induction of filamentous tau pathology in neurons and glia that, unlike transgenic AD models, has been readily associated with neuronal loss. Behavioral impairments have been reported, and motor neuron disease has been common, the latter a feature also frequently found in association with human FTD. Differences between models almost certainly reflect variables such as the promoter utilized, the tau isoform expressed, the transgene integration site, and the genetic backgrounds on which the studies were conducted.

As with AD models, questions arise as to whether the disturbances primarily result from the FTDP-17 mutations or could be caused by tau overexpression itself, and indeed a number of studies have shown that overexpression of wild-type human tau can lead to clinical and pathological effects in transgenic mice. Ishihara et al. (1999), for example, used the mouse PrP promoter to overexpress the shortest form of human tau, known as T44, that is most prominently expressed during fetal development. The mice that were created had total tau elevations of 5- to 15-fold in most CNS regions. Young mice exhibited motor weakness, and nonfilamentous tau aggregates could be detected in neurons that stained with phosphorylation and conformation-dependent tau antibodies that recognize NFTs. However, only old mice (18–20 months) developed mature lesions that exhibited the staining properties of NFTs (Ishihara et al., 2001). Similarly, transgenic mice expressing human tau from a P1 artificial chromosome on a mouse tau–/– background accumulated hyperphosphorylated tau at 6 months of age but only developed thioflavin-S positive lesions at 15 months (Andorfer et al., 2003).

Other studies (Spittaels et al., 1999; Probst et al., 2000) have observed that even modest 1.5-fold overexpression of wild-type human tau under the control of the thy-1 promoter induced a redistribution of phosphorylated tau into the cell body and the appearance of conformation-dependent tau epitopes but without the development of lesions having the staining properties of NFTs. Interestingly, though, it is less prone to induce NFT-like lesions, wild-type tau seems more prone to induce axonal spheroids than FDTP-17 mutant tau (Terwel et al., 2005). Expression of human wild-type tau from the mouse Tα1 α-tubulin promoter that is active in glial cells and neurons has also been reported to induce a glial pathology resembling the astrocytic plaques of corticobasal degeneration (Higuchi et al., 2002). Thus, overexpression of wild-type human tau can clearly cause neuropathology, although its propensity to induce NFT-like lesions seems less than FTDP-17 mutant tau. These effects of wild-type tau may, however, be physiologically relevant in that a number of FTDP-17 mutants involve noncoding mutations and, in some cases, missense mutations that result in relative overexpression of certain tau isoforms (Haugarvoll et al., 2007).

Implications for Pathophysiology and Treatment of Human Tauopathies

Although intracellular inclusions like NFTs might intuitively seem to be toxic, recently it has been suggested that the inclusions found, for example, in Huntington's disease may actually be neuroprotective (Ross and Poirier, 2005). In one set of very informative studies, transgenic mice in which tau expression could be regulated were used to examine the relationship between NFT pathology and neuronal dysfunction. In these studies, transgenic mice were created using the tetracycline (tet)-off inducible system (Ramsden et al., 2005; Santacruz et al., 2005). The tetracycline-operon response element (TRE) was used to drive the four repeat form of human tau harboring the P301L FTDP-17 mutation. On a second transgene, the calcium calmodulin kinase II (CaMKII) promoter was used to drive expression of the tet-off transactivator (rTA). Due to the specificity of the CaMKII promoter, these mice expressed high levels of transgenic tau principally in forebrain regions. In the nonrepressed state, transgenic tau levels were increased 7–13-fold relative to endogenous mouse tau, and after treatment with doxycycline that turns transgene expression off, levels fell to approximately 15% of their maximum levels (though still about 2.5-fold above endogenous mouse tau). Without doxycycline suppression, mice in the highest expressing line (rTg4510) developed NFT-like lesions at 4 to 5 months of age in cortex and hippocampus with accumulation of abnormally phosphorylated tau and a 60% loss of CA1 pyramidal neurons. With aging, extensive neurodegeneration occurred in cortical and limbic structures, leading to gross forebrain atrophy and reduced brain weight. Spatial memory deficits were apparent by 2.5 to 4 months of age before NFTs appeared. Interestingly, no motor deficits were detected in rTg4510 mice, likely reflecting the predominately forebrain expression pattern of the transgene.

When 2½-month-old mice were treated with doxycycline and examined at 4 months, the number of NFTs did not change, suggesting that transgene suppression stopped new NFTs from developing without clearing old ones. However, when animals at 4 months of age or older were treated, NFTs continued to accumulate despite transgene suppression, arguing that NFT formation had become transgene independent. Yet despite continued NFT accumulation in the doxycycline-treated animals, brain weight and neuronal numbers stabilized. In addition, both young and old mice treated with doxycycline improved their performance on the Morris water maze, even with relatively short-term treatments.

These findings argue that NFT formation is not necessary for neurodegeneration, and indeed, cognitive impairment in the absence of NFT formation has also been found in other lines of FTDP-17 transgenic mice (Gotz et al., 2007). This dissociation appears to be true for glial pathology as well, as when the P301L mutation was expressed using an oligodendrocyte-specific promoter, myelin disruption and impaired axonal transport preceded the appearance of thioflavin-S stained inclusions in oligodendrocytes (Higuchi et al., 2005). Thus, spatial memory deficits and neuronal loss can be temporally separated from NFT formation, and progressive NFT formation does not necessarily lead to neurodegeneration.

Instead of implicating a direct toxic role for NFTs, such observations suggest the existence of a toxic pre-NFT tau species, offering an interesting parallel to the story of soluble Aβ species. Indeed, recent studies have identified a multimeric species of tau in tau transgenic mice as well as cases of human FTDP-17 and AD (Berger et al., 2007). These tau multimers have been suggested to be responsible for toxicity, although besides a toxic gain of function, it remains possible that imbalances in tau isoforms or altered microtubule binding by tau mutants may lead to a loss of function as well (Ballatore et al., 2007).

Whatever the basis for the effect, studies in rTg4510 transgenic mice argue that neuronal dysfunction can be reversed, suggesting that in human tauopathies—including AD—there may be a phase of the disease that is reversible. Modulation of tau phosphorylation has attracted attention as one therapeutic strategy, and protein kinase inhibitors exist that can be administered orally and penetrate the blood–brain barrier (Gotz et al., 2007). Synthetic analogs of one such inhibitor—K252a, a non-specific protein kinase inhibitor—has been tested in JNPL3 mice and shown to reduce soluble hyperphosphorylated tau as well as delay or prevent development of severe motor impairments (Le Corre et al., 2006), thus offering important preclinical support for this approach to treating human tauopathies.

OTHER DEMENTIAS

Dementia occurs in the context of many other neurodegenerative disorders. One group of disorders that includes Parkinson's disease, diffuse Lewy body disease, and multiple system atrophy is characterized by cytoplasmic inclusions in neurons and glial cells called *Lewy bodies*. Lewy bodies contain high levels of the protein α-synuclein, and missense mutations as well as triplication of the α-synuclein gene have been identified in families with autosomal dominant Parkinson's disease. Transgenic mice that overexpress wild-type or mutant α-synuclein have been made using a variety of neuronal and glial promoters (Fernagut and Chesselet, 2004). Ubiquitin and α-synuclein positive inclusions have been induced by wild-type and mutant α-synuclein, with the extent of pathology generally correlating with transgene expression level. Motor disorders have been common in these mice, although the models have been somewhat disappointing in the lack of dopaminergic cell loss.

British and Danish familial dementias are caused by mutations in a gene on chromosome 13 known as BRI2. Pathologically, the disorders exhibit amyloid plaques composed of BRI protein rather than Aβ. Attempts to model these disorders in transgenic mice have been recently reviewed (Pickford et al., 2006). Prion diseases are also associated with dementia and exhibit amyloid plaques containing prion protein. These diseases, though mostly sporadic, also exist in familial forms, and some transgenic mouse models have been created (Li et al., 2007). Dementia is also associated with Huntington's disease, and a number of transgenic Huntington's models have been developed (Walker, 2007).

CONCLUSIONS

Transgenic models now dominate approaches to animal modeling of human neurodegenerative diseases. The models are in one sense limited by their requirement for a genetic modification. However, the existence of familial forms for most of the common human senile dementias has allowed transgenic models to be created that reproduce the most critical aspects of the disease pathology. These models have improved understanding of disease pathogenesis and have led to new therapeutic approaches. They will, without doubt, continue to play central roles for years to come in preclinical testing and as tools for developing insight into the biological basis of human dementias.

REFERENCES

Adlard, P.A., Perreau, V.M., Pop, V., and Cotman, C.W. (2005) Voluntary exercise decreases amyloid load in a transgenic model of Alzheimer's disease. *J. Neurosci.* 25:4217–4221.

Andorfer, C., Kress, Y., Espinoza, M., de Silva, R., Tucker, K.L., Barde, Y.A., Duff, K., and Davies, P. (2003) Hyperphosphorylation and aggregation of tau in mice expressing normal human tau isoforms. *J. Neurochem.* 86:582–590.

Bales, K.R., Verina, T., Dodel, R.C., Du, Y., Altstiel, L., Bender, M., Hyslop, P., Johnstone, E.M., Little, S.P., Cummins, D.J., Piccardo, P., Ghetti, B., and Paul, S.M. (1997) Lack of apolipoprotein E dramatically reduces amyloid beta-peptide deposition. *Nat. Genet.* 17:263–264.

Ballatore, C., Lee, V.M., and Trojanowski, J.Q. (2007) Tau-mediated neurodegeneration in Alzheimer's disease and related disorders. *Nat. Rev. Neurosci.* 8:663–672.

Berger, Z., Roder, H., Hanna, A., Carlson, A., Rangachari, V., Yue, M., Wszolek, Z., Ashe, K., Knight, J., Dickson, D., Andorfer, C., Rosenberry, T.L., Lewis, J., Hutton, M., and Janus, C. (2007) Accumulation of pathological tau species and memory loss in a conditional model of tauopathy. *J. Neurosci.* 27:3650–3662.

Billings, L.M., Oddo, S., Green, K.N., McGaugh, J.L., and LaFerla, F.M. (2005) Intraneuronal abeta causes the onset of early Alzheimer's disease-related cognitive deficits in transgenic mice. *Neuron* 45:675–688.

Borchelt, D.R., Thinakaran, G., Eckman, C.B., Lee, M.K., Davenport, F., Ratovitsky, T., Prada, C.M., Kim, G., Seekins, S., Yager, D., Slunt, H.H., Wang, R., Seeger, M., Levey, A.I., Gandy, S.E., Copeland, N.G., Jenkins, N.A., Price, D.L., Younkin, S.G., and Sisodia, S.S. (1996) Familial Alzheimer's disease-linked presenilin 1 variants elevate Abeta1-42/1-40 ratio in vitro and in vivo. *Neuron* 17:1005–1013.

Calhoun, M.E., Burgermeister, P., Phinney, A.L., Stalder, M., Tolnay, M., Wiederhold, K.H., Abramowski, D., Sturchler-Pierrat, C., Sommer, B., Staufenbiel, M., and Jucker, M. (1999) Neuronal overexpression of mutant amyloid precursor protein results in prominent deposition of cerebrovascular amyloid. *Proc. Natl. Acad. Sci. USA* 96:14088–14093.

Calhoun, M.E., Wiederhold, K.H., Abramowski, D., Phinney, A.L., Probst, A., Sturchler-Pierrat, C., Staufenbiel, M., Sommer, B., and Jucker, M. (1998) Neuron loss in APP transgenic mice. *Nature* 395:755–756.

Chen, G., Chen, K.S., Knox, J., Inglis, J., Bernard, A., Martin, S.J., Justice, A., McConlogue, L., Games, D., Freedman, S.B., and Morris, R.G. (2000) A learning deficit related to age and beta-amyloid plaques in a mouse model of Alzheimer's disease. *Nature* 408:975–979.

Cheng, I.H., Palop, J.J., Esposito, L.A., Bien-Ly, N., Yan, F., and Mucke, L. (2004) Aggressive amyloidosis in mice expressing human amyloid peptides with the Arctic mutation. *Nat. Med.* 10: 1190–1192.

Chevallier, N.L., Soriano, S., Kang, D.E., Masliah, E., Hu, G., and Koo, E.H. (2005) Perturbed neurogenesis in the adult hippocampus associated with presenilin-1 A246E mutation. *Am. J. Pathol.* 167:151–159.

Chishti, M.A., Yang, D.S., Janus, C., Phinney, A.L., Horne, P., Pearson, J., Strome, R., Zuker, N., Loukides, J., French, J., Turner, S., Lozza, G., Grilli, M., Kunicki, S., Morissette, C., Paquette, J., Gervais, F., Bergeron, C., Fraser, P.E., Carlson, G.A., George-Hyslop, P.S., and Westaway, D. (2001) Early-onset amyloid deposition and cognitive deficits in transgenic mice expressing a double mutant form of amyloid precursor protein 695. *J. Biol. Chem.* 276:21562–21570.

Chui, D.H., Tanahashi, H., Ozawa, K., Ikeda, S., Checler, F., Ueda, O., Suzuki, H., Araki, W., Inoue, H., Shirotani, K., Takahashi, K., Gallyas, F., and Tabira, T. (1999) Transgenic mice with Alzheimer presenilin 1 mutations show accelerated neurodegeneration without amyloid plaque formation. *Nat. Med.* 5:560–564.

Citron, M., Westaway, D., Xia, W., Carlson, G., Diehl, T., Levesque, G., Johnson-Wood, K., Lee, M., Seubert, P., Davis, A., Kholodenko, D., Motter, R., Sherrington, R., Perry, B., Yao, H., Strome, R., Lieberburg, I., Rommens, J., Kim, S., Schenk, D., Fraser, P., St George Hyslop, P., and Selkoe, D.J. (1997) Mutant presenilins of Alzheimer's disease increase production of 42-residue amyloid beta-protein in both transfected cells and transgenic mice. *Nat. Med.* 3:67–72.

Codita, A., Winblad, B., and Mohammed, A.H. (2006) Of mice and men: more neurobiology in dementia. *Curr. Opin. Psychiatry* 19: 555–563.

DeMattos, R.B., Bales, K.R., Cummins, D.J., Dodart, J.C., Paul, S. M., and Holtzman, D.M. (2001) Peripheral anti-A beta antibody alters CNS and plasma A beta clearance and decreases brain A beta burden in a mouse model of Alzheimer's disease. *Proc. Natl. Acad. Sci. USA* 98:8850–8855.

Dodart, J.C., Bales, K.R., Gannon, K.S., Greene, S.J., DeMattos, R.B., Mathis, C., DeLong, C.A., Wu, S., Wu, X., Holtzman, D.M., and Paul, S.M. (2002) Immunization reverses memory deficits without reducing brain Abeta burden in Alzheimer's disease model. *Nat. Neurosci.* 5:452–457.

Dodart, J.C., Mathis, C., Saura, J., Bales, K.R., Paul, S.M., and Ungerer, A. (2000) Neuroanatomical abnormalities in behaviorally characterized APP(V717F) transgenic mice. *Neurobiol. Dis.* 7:71–85.

Duff, K., Eckman, C., Zehr, C., Yu, X., Prada, C.M., Perez-tur, J., Hutton, M., Buee, L., Harigaya, Y., Yager, D., Morgan, D., Gordon, M.N., Holcomb, L., Refolo, L., Zenk, B., Hardy, J., and Younkin, S. (1996) Increased amyloid-beta42(43) in brains of mice expressing mutant presenilin 1. *Nature* 383:710–713.

Ertekin-Taner, N. (2007) Genetics of Alzheimer's disease: a centennial review. *Neurol. Clin.* 25:611–667.

Fagan, A.M., Watson, M., Parsadanian, M., Bales, K.R., Paul, S.M., and Holtzman, D.M. (2002) Human and murine ApoE markedly alters A beta metabolism before and after plaque formation in a mouse model of Alzheimer's disease. *Neurobiol. Dis.* 9:305–318.

Fernagut, P.O., and Chesselet, M.F. (2004) Alpha-synuclein and transgenic mouse models. *Neurobiol. Dis.* 17:123–130.

Flood, D.G., Reaume, A.G., Dorfman, K.S., Lin, Y.G., Lang, D.M., Trusko, S.P., Savage, M.J., Annaert, W.G., De Strooper, B., Siman, R., and Scott, R.W. (2002) FAD mutant PS-1 gene-targeted mice: increased A beta 42 and A beta deposition without APP overproduction. *Neurobiol. Aging* 23:335–348.

Fryer, J.D., Taylor, J.W., DeMattos, R.B., Bales, K.R., Paul, S.M., Parsadanian, M., and Holtzman, D.M. (2003) Apolipoprotein E markedly facilitates age-dependent cerebral amyloid angiopathy and spontaneous hemorrhage in amyloid precursor protein transgenic mice. *J. Neurosci.* 23:7889–7896.

Games, D., Adams, D., Alessandrini, R., Barbour, R., Berthelette, P., Blackwell, C., Carr, T., Clemens, J., Donaldson, T., Gillespie, F., Guido, T., Hagoplan, S., Johnson-Wood, K., Khan, K., Lee, M., Lelbowitz, P., Lieberburg, I., Little, S., Masliah, E., McConlogue, L., Montoya-Zavala, M., Mucke, L., Paganini, L., Pennlman, E., Power, M., Schenk, D., Seubert, P., Snyder, B., Wadsworth, S., Wolozin, B., and Zhao, J. (1995) Alzheimer-type neuropathology in transgenic mice overexpressing V717F beta-amyloid precursor protein. *Nature* 373:523–527.

Games, D., Buttini, M., Kobayashi, D., Schenk, D., and Seubert, P. (2006) Mice as models: transgenic approaches and Alzheimer's disease. *J. Alzheimers Dis.* 9:133–149.

Gotz, J., Deters, N., Doldissen, A., Bokhari, L., Ke, Y., Wiesner, A., Schonrock, N., and Ittner, L.M. (2007) A decade of tau transgenic animal models and beyond. *Brain Pathol.* 17:91–103.

Grilli, M., Diodato, E., Lozza, G., Brusa, R., Casarini, M., Uberti, D., Rozmahel, R., Westaway, D., St George-Hyslop, P., Memo, M., and Ongini, E. (2000) Presenilin-1 regulates the neuronal threshold to excitotoxicity both physiologically and pathologically. *Proc. Natl. Acad. Sci. USA* 97:12822–12827.

Guo, Q., Sebastian, L., Sopher, B.L., Miller, M.W., Ware, C.B., Martin, G.M., and Mattson, M.P. (1999) Increased vulnerability of hippocampal neurons from presenilin-1 mutant knock-in mice to amyloid beta-peptide toxicity: central roles of superoxide production and caspase activation. *J. Neurochem.* 72:1019–1029.

Haugarvoll, K., Wszolek, Z.K., and Hutton, M. (2007) The genetics of frontotemporal dementia. *Neurol. Clin.* 25:697–715.

Herzig, M.C., Winkler, D.T., Burgermeister, P., Pfeifer, M., Kohler, E., Schmidt, S.D., Danner, S., Abramowski, D., Sturchler-Pierrat, C., Burki, K., van Duinen, S.G., Maat-Schieman, M.L., Staufenbiel, M., Mathews, P.M., and Jucker, M. (2004) Abeta is targeted to the vasculature in a mouse model of hereditary cerebral hemorrhage with amyloidosis. *Nat. Neurosci.* 7:954–960.

Higuchi, M., Ishihara, T., Zhang, B., Hong, M., Andreadis, A., Trojanowski, J., and Lee, V.M. (2002) Transgenic mouse model of tauopathies with glial pathology and nervous system degeneration. *Neuron* 35:433–446.

Higuchi, M., Zhang, B., Forman, M.S., Yoshiyama, Y., Trojanowski, J.Q., and Lee, V.M. (2005) Axonal degeneration induced by targeted expression of mutant human tau in oligodendrocytes of transgenic mice that model glial tauopathies. *J. Neurosci.* 25: 9434–9443.

Hock, C., Konietzko, U., Streffer, J.R., Tracy, J., Signorell, A., Muller-Tillmanns, B., Lemke, U., Henke, K., Moritz, E., Garcia, E., Wollmer, M.A., Umbricht, D., de Quervain, D.J., Hofmann, M., Maddalena, A., Papassotiropoulos, A., and Nitsch, R.M. (2003) Antibodies against beta-amyloid slow cognitive decline in Alzheimer's disease. *Neuron* 38:547–554.

Holcomb, L., Gordon, M.N., McGowan, E., Yu, X., Benkovic, S., Jantzen, P., Wright, K., Saad, I., Mueller, R., Morgan, D., Sanders, S., Zehr, C., O'Campo, K., Hardy, J., Prada, C.M., Eckman, C., Younkin, S., Hsiao, K., and Duff, K. (1998) Accelerated Alzheimer-type phenotype in transgenic mice carrying both mutant amyloid precursor protein and presenilin 1 transgenes. *Nat. Med.* 4:97–100.

Holtzman, D.M., Bales, K.R., Tenkova, T., Fagan, A.M., Parsadanian, M., Sartorius, L.J., Mackey, B., Olney, J., McKeel, D., Wozniak, D., and Paul, S.M. (2000) Apolipoprotein E isoform-dependent amyloid deposition and neuritic degeneration in a mouse model of Alzheimer's disease. *Proc. Natl. Acad. Sci. USA* 97:2892–2897.

Hsia, A.Y., Masliah, E., McConlogue, L., Yu, G.Q., Tatsuno, G., Hu, K., Kholodenko, D., Malenka, R.C., Nicoll, R.A., and Mucke, L. (1999) Plaque-independent disruption of neural circuits in Alzheimer's disease mouse models. *Proc. Natl. Acad. Sci. USA* 96: 3228–3233.

Hsiao, K., Chapman, P., Nilsen, S., Eckman, C., Harigaya, Y., Younkin, S., Yang, F., and Cole, G. (1996) Correlative memory deficits, abeta elevation, and amyloid plaques in transgenic mice. *Science* 274:99–102.

Hsiao, K.K., Borchelt, D.R., Olson, K., Johannsdottir, R., Kitt, C., Yunis, W., Xu, S., Eckman, C., Younkin, S., Price, D., Iadecola, C., Clark, B., and Carlson, G. (1995) Age-related CNS disorder and early death in transgenic FVB/N mice overexpressing Alzheimer amyloid precursor proteins. *Neuron* 15:1203–1218.

Irizarry, M.C., McNamara, M., Fedorchak, K., Hsiao, K., and Hyman, B.T. (1997a) APPSw transgenic mice develop age-related A beta deposits and neuropil abnormalities, but no neuronal loss in CA1. *J. Neuropathol. Exp. Neurol.* 56:965–973.

Irizarry, M.C., Soriano, F., McNamara, M., Page, K.J., Schenk, D., Games, D., and Hyman, B.T. (1997b) Abeta deposition is associated with neuropil changes, but not with overt neuronal loss in the human amyloid precursor protein V717F (PDAPP) transgenic mouse. *J. Neurosci.* 17:7053–7059.

Ishihara, T., Hong, M., Zhang, B., Nakagawa, Y., Lee, M.K., Trojanowski, J.Q., and Lee, V.M. (1999) Age-dependent emergence and progression of a tauopathy in transgenic mice overexpressing the shortest human tau isoform. *Neuron* 24:751–762.

Ishihara, T., Zhang, B., Higuchi, M., Yoshiyama, Y., Trojanowski, J.Q., and Lee, V.M. (2001) Age-dependent induction of congophilic neurofibrillary tau inclusions in tau transgenic mice. *Am. J. Pathol.* 158:555–562.

Jacobsen, J.S., Wu, C.C., Redwine, J.M., Comery, T.A., Arias, R., Bowlby, M., Martone, R., Morrison, J.H., Pangalos, M.N., Reinhart, P.H., and Bloom, F.E. (2006) Early-onset behavioral and synaptic deficits in a mouse model of Alzheimer's disease. *Proc. Natl. Acad. Sci. USA* 103:5161–5166.

Janus, C., Pearson, J., McLaurin, J., Mathews, P.M., Jiang, Y., Schmidt, S.D., Chishti, M.A., Horne, P., Heslin, D., French, J., Mount, H.T., Nixon, R.A., Mercken, M., Bergeron, C., Fraser, P.E., St George-Hyslop, P., and Westaway, D. (2000) A beta peptide immunization reduces behavioural impairment and plaques in a model of Alzheimer's disease. *Nature* 408:979–982.

Kassed, C.A., Butler, T.L., Navidomskis, M.T., Gordon, M.N., Morgan, D., and Pennypacker, K.R. (2003) Mice expressing human mutant presenilin-1 exhibit decreased activation of NF-kappaB p50 in hippocampal neurons after injury. *Mol. Brain Res.* 110: 152–157.

Kotilinek, L.A., Bacskai, B., Westerman, M., Kawarabayashi, T., Younkin, L., Hyman, B.T., Younkin, S., and Ashe, K.H. (2002) Reversible memory loss in a mouse transgenic model of Alzheimer's disease. *J. Neurosci.* 22:6331–6335.

Lazarov, O., Peterson, L.D., Peterson, D.A., and Sisodia, S.S. (2006) Expression of a familial Alzheimer's disease-linked presenilin-1 variant enhances perforant pathway lesion-induced neuronal loss in the entorhinal cortex. *J. Neurosci.* 26:429–434.

Lazarov, O., Robinson, J., Tang, Y.P., Hairston, I.S., Korade-Mirnics, Z., Lee, V.M., Hersh, L.B., Sapolsky, R.M., Mirnics, K., and Sisodia, S.S. (2005) Environmental enrichment reduces Abeta levels and amyloid deposition in transgenic mice. *Cell* 120:701–713.

Le Corre, S., Klafki, H.W., Plesnila, N., Hubinger, G., Obermeier, A., Sahagun, H., Monse, B., Seneci, P., Lewis, J., Eriksen, J., Zehr, C., Yue, M., McGowan, E., Dickson, D.W., Hutton, M., and Roder, H.M. (2006) An inhibitor of tau hyperphosphorylation prevents severe motor impairments in tau transgenic mice. *Proc. Natl. Acad. Sci. USA* 103:9673–9678.

Lesne, S., Koh, M.T., Kotilinek, L., Kayed, R., Glabe, C.G., Yang, A., Gallagher, M., and Ashe, K.H. (2006) A specific amyloid-beta protein assembly in the brain impairs memory. *Nature* 440: 352–357.

Lewis, J., Dickson, D.W., Lin, W.L., Chisholm, L., Corral, A., Jones, G., Yen, S.H., Sahara, N., Skipper, L., Yager, D., Eckman, C., Hardy, J., Hutton, M., and McGowan, E. (2001) Enhanced neurofibrillary degeneration in transgenic mice expressing mutant tau and APP. *Science* 293:1487–1491.

Lewis, J., McGowan, E., Rockwood, J., Melrose, H., Nacharaju, P., Van Slegtenhorst, M., Gwinn-Hardy, K., Paul Murphy, M., Baker, M., Yu, X., Duff, K., Hardy, J., Corral, A., Lin, W.L., Yen, S.H., Dickson, D.W., Davies, P., and Hutton, M. (2000) Neurofibrillary tangles, amyotrophy and progressive motor disturbance in mice expressing mutant (P301L) tau protein. *Nat. Genet.* 25: 402–405.

Li, A., Piccardo, P., Barmada, S.J., Ghetti, B., and Harris, D.A. (2007) Prion protein with an octapeptide insertion has impaired neuroprotective activity in transgenic mice. *Embo. J.* 26:2777–2785.

Lin, W.L., Lewis, J., Yen, S.H., Hutton, M., and Dickson, D.W. (2003a) Filamentous tau in oligodendrocytes and astrocytes of transgenic mice expressing the human tau isoform with the P301L mutation. *Am. J. Pathol.* 162:213–218.

Lin, W.L., Lewis, J., Yen, S.H., Hutton, M., and Dickson, D.W. (2003b) Ultrastructural neuronal pathology in transgenic mice expressing mutant (P301L) human tau. *J. Neurocytol.* 32:1091–1105.

Link, C.D. (2005) Invertebrate models of Alzheimer's disease. *Genes Brain Behav.* 4:147–156.

Mandelkow, E., von Bergen, M., Biernat, J., and Mandelkow, E.M. (2007) Structural principles of tau and the paired helical filaments of Alzheimer's disease. *Brain Pathol.* 17:83–90.

Masliah, E., Sisk, A., Mallory, M., and Games, D. (2001) Neurofibrillary pathology in transgenic mice overexpressing V717F beta-amyloid precursor protein. *J. Neuropathol. Exp. Neurol.* 60:357–368.

McGowan, E., Eriksen, J., and Hutton, M. (2006) A decade of modeling Alzheimer's disease in transgenic mice. *Trends Genet.* 22: 281–289.

McGowan, E., Pickford, F., Kim, J., Onstead, L., Eriksen, J., Yu, C., Skipper, L., Murphy, M.P., Beard, J., Das, P., Jansen, K., Delucia, M., Lin, W.L., Dolios, G., Wang, R., Eckman, C.B., Dickson, D.W., Hutton, M., Hardy, J., and Golde, T. (2005) Abeta42 is essential for parenchymal and vascular amyloid deposition in mice. *Neuron* 47:191–199.

Moechars, D., Dewachter, I., Lorent, K., Reverse, D., Baekelandt, V., Naidu, A., Tesseur, I., Spittaels, K., Haute, C.V., Checler, F., Godaux, E., Cordell, B., and Van Leuven, F. (1999) Early phenotypic changes in transgenic mice that overexpress different mutants of amyloid precursor protein in brain. *J. Biol. Chem.* 274: 6483–6492.

Mohmmad Abdul, H., Wenk, G.L., Gramling, M., Hauss-Wegrzyniak, B., and Butterfield, D.A. (2004) APP and PS-1 mutations induce brain oxidative stress independent of dietary cholesterol: implications for Alzheimer's disease. *Neurosci. Lett.* 368:148–150.

Morgan, D. (2006) Immunotherapy for Alzheimer's disease. *J. Alzheimers Dis.* 9:425–432.

Nakano, Y., Kondoh, G., Kudo, T., Imaizumi, K., Kato, M., Miyazaki, J.I., Tohyama, M., Takeda, J., and Takeda, M. (1999) Accumulation of murine amyloidbeta42 in a gene-dosage-dependent manner in PS1 "knock-in" mice. *Eur. J. Neurosci.* 11:2577–2581.

Oakley, H., Cole, S.L., Logan, S., Maus, E., Shao, P., Craft, J., Guillozet-Bongaarts, A., Ohno, M., Disterhoft, J., Van Eldik, L., Berry, R., and Vassar, R. (2006) Intraneuronal beta-amyloid aggregates, neurodegeneration, and neuron loss in transgenic mice with five familial Alzheimer's disease mutations: potential factors in amyloid plaque formation. *J. Neurosci.* 26:10129–10140.

Oddo, S., Billings, L., Kesslak, J.P., Cribbs, D.H., and LaFerla, F.M. (2004) Abeta immunotherapy leads to clearance of early, but not late, hyperphosphorylated tau aggregates via the proteasome. *Neuron* 43:321–332.

Oddo, S., Caccamo, A., Shepherd, J.D., Murphy, M.P., Golde, T.E., Kayed, R., Metherate, R., Mattson, M.P., Akbari, Y., and LaFerla, F.M. (2003) Triple-transgenic model of Alzheimer's disease with plaques and tangles: intracellular Abeta and synaptic dysfunction. *Neuron* 39:409–421.

Orgogozo, J.M., Gilman, S., Dartigues, J.F., Laurent, B., Puel, M., Kirby, L.C., Jouanny, P., Dubois, B., Eisner, L., Flitman, S., Michel, B.F., Boada, M., Frank, A., and Hock, C. (2003) Subacute meningoencephalitis in a subset of patients with AD after Abeta42 immunization. *Neurology* 61:46–54.

Patel, N.V., Gordon, M.N., Connor, K.E., Good, R.A., Engelman, R.W., Mason, J., Morgan, D.G., Morgan, T.E., and Finch, C.E. (2005) Caloric restriction attenuates Abeta-deposition in Alzheimer transgenic models. *Neurobiol. Aging* 26:995–1000.

Pickford, F., Coomaraswamy, J., Jucker, M., and McGowan, E. (2006) Modeling familial British dementia in transgenic mice. *Brain Pathol.* 16:80–85.

Probst, A., Gotz, J., Wiederhold, K.H., Tolnay, M., Mistl, C., Jaton, A.L., Hong, M., Ishihara, T., Lee, V.M., Trojanowski, J.Q., Jakes, R., Crowther, R.A., Spillantini, M.G., Burki, K., and Goedert, M. (2000) Axonopathy and amyotrophy in mice transgenic for human four-repeat tau protein. *Acta. Neuropathol. (Berl)* 99:469–481.

Ramsden, M., Kotilinek, L., Forster, C., Paulson, J., McGowan, E., SantaCruz, K., Guimaraes, A., Yue, M., Lewis, J., Carlson, G., Hutton, M., and Ashe, K.H. (2005) Age-dependent neurofibrillary tangle formation, neuron loss, and memory impairment in a mouse model of human tauopathy (P301L). *J. Neurosci.* 25: 10637–10647.

Reaume, A.G., Howland, D.S., Trusko, S.P., Savage, M.J., Lang, D. M., Greenberg, B.D., Siman, R., and Scott, R.W. (1996) Enhanced amyloidogenic processing of the beta-amyloid precursor protein in gene-targeted mice bearing the Swedish familial Alzheimer's disease mutations and a "humanized" Abeta sequence. *J. Biol. Chem.* 271:23380–23388.

Redwine, J.M., Kosofsky, B., Jacobs, R.E., Games, D., Reilly, J.F., Morrison, J.H., Young, W.G., and Bloom, F.E. (2003) Dentate gyrus volume is reduced before onset of plaque formation in PDAPP mice: a magnetic resonance microscopy and stereologic analysis. *Proc. Natl. Acad. Sci. USA* 100:1381–1386.

Refolo, L.M., Pappolla, M.A., LaFrancois, J., Malester, B., Schmidt, S.D., Thomas-Bryant, T., Tint, G.S., Wang, R., Mercken, M., Petanceska, S.S., and Duff, K.E. (2001) A cholesterol-lowering drug reduces beta-amyloid pathology in a transgenic mouse model of Alzheimer's disease. *Neurobiol. Dis.* 8:890–899.

Reilly, J.F., Games, D., Rydel, R.E., Freedman, S., Schenk, D., Young, W.G., Morrison, J.H., and Bloom, F.E. (2003) Amyloid deposition in the hippocampus and entorhinal cortex: quantitative analysis of a transgenic mouse model. *Proc. Natl. Acad. Sci. USA* 100:4837–4842.

Roberson, E.D., Scearce-Levie, K., Palop, J.J., Yan, F., Cheng, I.H., Wu, T., Gerstein, H., Yu, G.Q., and Mucke, L. (2007) Reducing endogenous tau ameliorates amyloid beta-induced deficits in an Alzheimer's disease mouse model. *Science* 316:750–754.

Ross, C.A., and Poirier, M.A. (2005) Opinion: What is the role of protein aggregation in neurodegeneration? *Nat. Rev. Mol. Cell. Biol.* 6:891–898.

Santacruz, K., Lewis, J., Spires, T., Paulson, J., Kotilinek, L., Ingelsson, M., Guimaraes, A., DeTure, M., Ramsden, M., McGowan, E., Forster, C., Yue, M., Orne, J., Janus, C., Mariash, A., Kuskowski, M., Hyman, B., Hutton, M., and Ashe, K.H. (2005) Tau suppression in a neurodegenerative mouse model improves memory function. *Science* 309:476–481.

Sasaki, A., Shoji, M., Harigaya, Y., Kawarabayashi, T., Ikeda, M., Naito, M., Matsubara, E., Abe, K., and Nakazato, Y. (2002) Amyloid cored plaques in Tg2576 transgenic mice are characterized by giant plaques, slightly activated microglia, and the lack of paired helical filament-typed, dystrophic neurites. *Virchows Arch.* 441:358–367.

Schenk, D., Barbour, R., Dunn, W., Gordon, G., Grajeda, H., Guido, T., Hu, K., Huang, J., Johnson-Wood, K., Khan, K., Kholodenko, D., Lee, M., Liao, Z., Lieberburg, I., Motter, R., Mutter, L., Soriano, F., Shopp, G., Vasquez, N., Vandevert, C., Walker, S., Wogulis, M., Yednock, T., Games, D., and Seubert, P. (1999) Immunization with amyloid-beta attenuates Alzheimer-disease-like pathology in the PDAPP mouse. *Nature* 400:173–177.

Schmitz, C., Rutten, B.P., Pielen, A., Schafer, S., Wirths, O., Tremp, G., Czech, C., Blanchard, V., Multhaup, G., Rezaie, P., Korr, H., Steinbusch, H.W., Pradier, L., and Bayer, T.A. (2004) Hippocampal neuron loss exceeds amyloid plaque load in a transgenic mouse model of Alzheimer's disease. *Am. J. Pathol.* 164:1495–1502.

Schneider, I., Reverse, D., Dewachter, I., Ris, L., Caluwaerts, N., Kuiperi, C., Gilis, M., Geerts, H., Kretzschmar, H., Godaux, E., Moechars, D., Van Leuven, F., and Herms, J. (2001) Mutant presenilins disturb neuronal calcium homeostasis in the brain of transgenic mice, decreasing the threshold for excitotoxicity and facilitating long-term potentiation. *J. Biol. Chem.* 276:11539–11544.

Schuessel, K., Frey, C., Jourdan, C., Keil, U., Weber, C.C., Muller-Spahn, F., Muller, W.E., and Eckert, A. (2006) Aging sensitizes toward ROS formation and lipid peroxidation in PS1M146L transgenic mice. *Free Radic. Biol. Med.* 40:850–862.

Selkoe, D.J. (2001) Alzheimer's disease: genes, proteins, and therapy. *Physiol. Rev.* 81:741–766.

Solomon, B., Koppel, R., Hanan, E., and Katzav, T. (1996) Monoclonal antibodies inhibit in vitro fibrillar aggregation of the Alzheimer beta-amyloid peptide. *Proc. Natl. Acad. Sci. USA* 93: 452–455.

Spittaels, K., Van den Haute, C., Van Dorpe, J., Bruynseels, K., Vandezande, K., Laenen, I., Geerts, H., Mercken, M., Sciot, R., Van Lommel, A., Loos, R., and Van Leuven, F. (1999) Prominent axonopathy in the brain and spinal cord of transgenic mice overexpressing four-repeat human tau protein. *Am. J. Pathol.* 155: 2153–2165.

Stokin, G.B., Lillo, C., Falzone, T.L., Brusch, R.G., Rockenstein, E., Mount, S.L., Raman, R., Davies, P., Masliah, E., Williams, D.S., and Goldstein, L.S. (2005) Axonopathy and transport deficits early in the pathogenesis of Alzheimer's disease. *Science* 307: 1282–1288.

Tanemura, K., Chui, D.H., Fukuda, T., Murayama, M., Park, J.M., Akagi, T., Tatebayashi, Y., Miyasaka, T., Kimura, T., Hashikawa, T., Nakano, Y., Kudo, T., Takeda, M., and Takashima, A. (2006) Formation of tau inclusions in knock-in mice with familial Alzheimer disease (FAD) mutation of presenilin 1 (PS1). *J. Biol. Chem.* 281:5037–5041.

Terwel, D., Lasrado, R., Snauwaert, J., Vandeweert, E., Van Haesendonck, C., Borghgraef, P., and Van Leuven, F. (2005) Changed conformation of mutant tau-P301L underlies the moribund tauopathy, absent in progressive, nonlethal axonopathy of tau-4R/2N transgenic mice. *J. Biol. Chem.* 280:3963–3973.

Vetrivel, K.S., Zhang, Y.W., Xu, H., and Thinakaran, G. (2006) Pathological and physiological functions of presenilins. *Mol. Neurodegener.* 1:4.

Walker, F.O. (2007) Huntington's disease. *Lancet* 369:218–228.

Walsh, D.M., and Selkoe, D.J. (2007) A beta oligomers—a decade of discovery. *J. Neurochem.* 101:1172–1184.

Wang, J., Ho, L., Zhao, Z., Seror, I., Humala, N., Dickstein, D.L., Thiyagarajan, M., Percival, S.S., Talcott, S.T., and Pasinetti, G.M. (2006) Moderate consumption of Cabernet Sauvignon attenuates Abeta neuropathology in a mouse model of Alzheimer's disease. *FASEB J.* 20:2313–2320.

Wen, P.H., Hof, P.R., Chen, X., Gluck, K., Austin, G., Younkin, S. G., Younkin, L.H., DeGasperi, R., Gama Sosa, M.A., Robakis, N.K., Haroutunian, V., and Elder, G.A. (2004) The presenilin-1 familial Alzheimer disease mutant P117L impairs neurogenesis in the hippocampus of adult mice. *Exp. Neurol.* 188:224–237.

Wu, C.C., Chawla, F., Games, D., Rydel, R.E., Freedman, S., Schenk, D., Young, W.G., Morrison, J.H., and Bloom, F.E. (2004) Selective vulnerability of dentate granule cells prior to amyloid deposition in PDAPP mice: digital morphometric analyses. *Proc. Natl. Acad. Sci. USA* 101:7141–7146.

Wu, Y., and Luo, Y. (2005) Transgenic C. elegans as a model in Alzheimer's research. *Curr. Alzheimer Res.* 2:37–45.

55 Functional Neuroanatomy of Learning and Memory

GARY L. WENK

INTRODUCTION TO MULTIPLE MEMORY SYSTEMS

The predominant theme in recent studies of the neuroanatomy of human learning and memory has been that memory does not rely upon a single system of the brain but is composed of many separate systems that can function independent of each other (Mishkin and Appenzeller, 1987; Zola-Morgan and Squire, 1993; Mishkin and Murray, 1994). The dissociations between different types of memory abilities reflect the nature and organization of this distributed system of brain regions. The classic distinctions between long- and short-term memory have evolved into more complicated dichotomies organized around the concepts of declarative (or explicit) and nondeclarative (or implicit) memory systems (Squire, 1992; Schacter and Tulving, 1994). Declarative memories include factual knowledge, such as the multiplication tables and the ability to recognize specific objects, and the events or episodes in one's life. Declarative memories can be acquired quickly within a single learning experience and can be expressed as explicit statements of knowledge. Declarative memories are primarily associated with the medial temporal lobe structures, including the hippocampus and related entorhinal, perirhinal, and parahippocampal cortices.

In contrast, nondeclarative memories are usually acquired more slowly across many learning sessions, with a few notable exceptions, such as taste aversion, and are closely tied to the original learning situation. Nondeclarative memories include a broad range of nonconscious abilities, such as skills or habits controlled by the striatum (Knowlton et al., 1996), and motor responses to classically conditioned stimuli such as the eye-blink reflex organized by the cerebellum (Krupa et al., 1993). Simple reflexes organized by the brain stem and spinal cord that respond to peripheral stimuli are also considered types of nondeclarative memory. Finally, the ability to recall recently acquired information following presentation of some component of the memory, that is, priming, is another type of nondeclarative memory that is thought to require the neocortex (Tulving and Schacter, 1990). These structures are clearly involved in the acquisition of memories. Recent evidence suggests that our long-term memories are ultimately stored in the cortical and subcortical neuronal networks that originally mediated the experience, that is, association cortex and higher-order secondary cortex (Squire, 1992; Roland and Gulyas, 1994) as well as the hippocampus (Rolls, 2000). These distinctions of locus of function have been based upon studies of experimental animals that have been given specific and discrete lesions to the related brain structures mentioned above, as well as upon studies of patients who were amnestic. Finally, it must always be kept in mind that the same brain structure or cortical region may participate in different kinds of learning and memory and that some types of memories require the activation of many different brain regions.

APPROACHES TO THE STUDY OF THE NEUROANATOMY OF MEMORY SYSTEMS: LESION ANALYSES VERSUS STIMULATION VERSUS RECORDING STUDIES

The analysis of the effects of lesions is probably the oldest, and still most widely used, approach to the problem of structure–function analyses and the determination of the neuroanatomy of memory systems in the brain. In humans, the behavioral effects of lesions resulting from head injury, tumors, vascular accidents, or neurosurgery are compared to the behavior of normal patients on a variety of standardized behavioral tasks. Similar research has been completed using nonhuman species such as primates and rodents, with the fundamental difference that the brain lesions are more precisely produced and more discrete in their effects upon behavior. Lesions are typically produced by one of the following methods: aspirating small regions out of the brain; electrolytic lesioning, that is, the passing of electric currents into the specific brain region; heating or cooling of the tissue to produce transient inactivation of the region; or the injection of selective neurotoxins into specific brain regions that may be selectively vulnerable to the action of these toxins. Although brain lesions are relatively easy to produce, the interpretation of their effects can be quite difficult and requires that the experimenter have a thorough understanding of the consequences of each type of manipulation: nonspecific effects of the lesion, transynaptic degeneration of nearby brain regions, effects of the subsequent cell loss upon neuroinflammatory processes, and so on.

Lesions can produce a variety of effects upon behavior that make interpretation difficult. For example, lesions can alter performance in tasks that are sensitive to learning and memory because the critical brain region for that function has been damaged or destroyed, or because that brain region was initially responsible for inhibiting a specific behavior that has now been released from inhibition. Lesions can also cause the expression of the expected behavior to be disorganized so that the patient cannot reliably perform the task in an appropriate manner.

Stimulation of the brain nonspecifically by electrical current, or specifically by the application of pharmacological agents, can produce one of the following responses: (*1*) a relatively specific and discrete effect, such as the activation of a small muscle group, a change in body temperature, or activation of a specific neural system or (*2*) an overall activating effect, such as the aggression response following stimulation of the amygdala or feeding behavior following stimulation of the lateral hypothalamus. Determining which of the above effects of the stimulation might underlie a particular behavior is often quite difficult. The advantage of stimulation studies using recently designed minimal stimulation techniques, over the lesion analyses, however, is that one is working with an intact, functioning, and relatively normal neural system. Recording the brain's neural activity, either electrical or chemical, and interpreting these studies presents a unique series of challenges. Electrophysiological recordings using in-dwelling electrodes can provide instantaneous information on the relationship between the activity of individual neurons, or groups of neurons, within a specific brain region and selected behaviors. The simultaneous recording of the activity of hundreds of neurons can provide information on how neurons interact with each other to produce specific behaviors. The combination of these techniques can provide valuable insights on brain regions involved in specific types of memory. Neuroimaging studies have been used to confirm the results obtained using these methods and extend them by monitoring multiple regions in the healthy or injured brain.

Electrophysiological methods, however, do not allow the determination of the neurotransmitter identity of the neural system being recorded, that is, whether the neurons are acetylcholinergic, dopaminergic, serotonergic, and so on. The determination of the release of specific neurotransmitter substances, for example by microdialysis or by using a push–pull cannula, provides important information on the specificity of the neurotransmitter changes within a particular neural system, but it cannot provide information on instantaneous changes in neuronal activity. Neuroimaging methods can be used to monitor selected aspects of the behavior of specific neurotransmitter systems, such as receptor density and metabolite levels that can then be related to specific mnemonic abilities.

Taken together, these approaches have provided considerable insights into the ways in which memory systems are distributed and organized within the human brain. The following sections present information on the specific brain systems involved in our ability to learn and remember.

MIDLINE DIENCEPHALON STRUCTURES

Medial Dorsal Thalamus

A role for the medial dorsal thalamic nucleus in memory has been based upon the finding that this region is consistently injured in alcoholic Korsakoff's syndrome. This syndrome is associated with a severe anterograde and retrograde amnesia. Patients typically have normal nondeclarative or implicit memory but impaired declarative memory. Patients with medial dorsal thalamic damage following cerebrovascular infarctions also demonstrate significant memory impairments (Winocur et al., 1984; Graff-Radford et al., 1990). Well-circumscribed lesions of this thalamic region can impair performance in a delayed nonmatching to sample task in monkeys (Aggleton and Mishkin, 1983) and rats (Mumby and Pinel, 1994). In addition, when the medial dorsal nucleus (and mammillary bodies) are damaged following administration of the antithiamine drug *pryithiamine*, rats demonstrate significant impairments on a variety of tasks that require learning and memory (Mair et al., 1991). A recent positron emission tomography (PET) study was conducted (Andreasen et al., 1999) to investigate the activity of the medial dorsal thalamus when patients intentionally recalled a specific past personal experience. The silent recall of a consciously retrieved episodic memory produces activation of the left medial dorsal thalamus. This region may therefore assist in the initiation and monitoring of the conscious retrieval of episodic memories. The prefrontal cortex efferents of the medial dorsal thalamus are so extensive that they have been used to define the region (Fuster, 1997). Functional magnetic resonance imaging (fMRI) studies have demonstrated that the human thalamus is involved in verbal memory (Crespo-Facorro et al., 1999) and sequence learning (Rauch et al., 1998).

Mammillary Nucleus

Damage to the mammillothalamic tracts that connect the anterior nucleus of the thalamus with the mammillary bodies located in the posterior hypothalamus also produces a memory impairment (Malamut et al., 1992). The mammillary bodies are a component of the extended hippocampal system; anterograde and retrograde memories are affected following injury to this system (Gilboa et al., 2006). Degeneration of the mammillary bodies is also sometimes reported in patients with Korsakoff's syndrome (Victor et al., 1989). In monkeys, bilateral lesions of the mammillary bodies impair memory (Aggleton and Mishkin, 1985). Two famous clinical cases demonstrate the difficulty in interpreting the consequences of thalamic nucleus versus mammillary nucleus injury in humans. Patient N.A. was a U.S. Air Force radar technician when his barracks roommate accidentally thrust a miniature fencing foil through his right nostril. The foil pierced the cribriform plate and passed into the left medial dorsal nucleus. Computed tomography (CT) scans confirmed that N.A. also has bilateral injury to the mammillothalamic tracts (Squire et al., 1989). N.A. has a slight retrograde amnesia and profound anterograde amnesia. As might be predicted from the above discussion, N.A. has difficulty with declarative but not nondeclarative memories; that is, he can learn motor skills but cannot remember recent events. In contrast, patient B.J. presented with a nearly identical memory disorder (Dusoir et al., 1990) following injury to only the mammillary bodies produced by having a snooker cue thrust through his left nostril. Rats with lesions of the mammillary bodies show similar impairments. Rats show a spatial learning deficit following damage of this structure that may be specific to remembering one or more places over a given time (Sziklas and Petrides, 2000).

THE BASAL FOREBRAIN REGION

The basal forebrain region contains a population of large cholinergic (Ch) neurons within the medial septal area (MSA) that send an efferent projection to the hippocampus, and within the nucleus basalis of Meynert (NBM) that innervates the entire cortical mantle, olfactory bulbs, and amygdala (Wenk and Olton, 1987). Interest in this brain region followed the suggestion that a decline in the number of Ch cells may be responsible for some of the cognitive impairments associated with aging and Alzheimer's disease (AD) (Coyle et al., 1983).

Behavioral deficits associated with lesions of the NBM were initially interpreted as being the result of impairments in learning and memory abilities (for a review, see Olton and Wenk, 1987). The possibility that forebrain Ch systems might not always play a role in the neural processes that underlie memory was initially demonstrated in an elegant study by Dunnett and colleagues (1987) that found that the degree of destruction of NBM Ch neurons did not correlate with the degree of impairment in a spatial memory task. Subsequent studies concluded that NBM Ch neurons may be important for specific aspects of attention (Olton et al., 1988; Robbins et al., 1989; Muir et al., 1992; Wenk, 1993, 1997). More recent studies have confirmed that the Ch projection to neocortex is involved in the control of attention (Everitt and Robbins, 1997; Sarter et al., 2005).

Electrophysiological evidence has also implicated NBM Ch cells in attentional processes. Attention to biologically relevant stimuli was associated with an increase in the activity of basal forebrain neurons in primates (Richardson and DeLong, 1991; Wilson and Rolls, 1990). Single units within the NBM and the nucleus of the diagonal band of Broca were selectively responsive to visual or auditory stimuli that were associated with the expectation of food reward (Wilson and Rolls, 1990). Overall, then, the corticopetal NBM Ch system may be involved in the control of shifting attention to potentially relevant, and brief, sensory stimuli that predict a biologically relevant event, such as the availability of a food reward.

In contrast, MSA Ch efferents to the hippocampus may play a more direct role in the neural processes that underlie learning and memory. However, the influence of MSA Ch cells may be task dependent. For example, selective Ch lesions impaired performance in a delayed nonmatching to position operant task (M.P. McDonald et al., 1997) but did not impair performance in the Morris water maze (Berger-Sweeney et al., 1994).

MEDIAL TEMPORAL LOBE

Overall, the medial temporal region is critical for the development of declarative memories that are required for the long-term storage and conscious recall of specific events or episodes and factual knowledge. Recent lesion analysis studies have confirmed that the severity and nature of declarative memory impairments depend upon the location and extent of injury to specific regions within the temporal lobe. Although injury to the hippocampus can impair declarative memory abilities, the combined destruction of the hippocampus, entorhinal cortices, and parahippocampal gyrus produces far more severe and long-lasting impairments. Lesion analyses have demonstrated that these various regions are involved in controlling different aspects of mnemonic ability (Murray, 1996).

Hippocampus

The hippocampus may mediate the representation of spatial and temporal memories by association of stimuli from all sensory modalities. The kinds of memories that the hippocampus stores have also been referred to as relational, that is, information on how specific objects or events, existing in some spatial or temporal arrangement, are related to each other (Eichenbaum et al., 1994). The key aspect of these kinds of memories is that they are relational, flexible, and permit creative behavior (Nadel, 1996). The hippocampus is critical for encoding information about an animal's environment and the episodes that occur within those environments. In so doing, it forms and stores representations of spaces and spatial contexts; these are called cognitive maps (O'Keefe and Nadel, 1978). Experimental support for these ideas has come from many different approaches to the study of hippocampal function (Eichenbaum et al., 1992). For example, in rats and monkeys, hippocampal neurons increase their firing rate when the animal moves into a specific location in its immediate environment (O'Keefe and Nadel, 1978). These "place field" cells contribute information about the place and time when a memory occurs that becomes part of the context of the memory (Smith and Mizumori, 2006). The cognitive map theory of hippocampal function suggests that discrete and selective lesions of the hippocampus will produce a deficit in place learning or exploration of a novel environment (Nadel, 1996). Functional magnetic resonance imaging studies on humans have confirmed that the hippocampus is active during context-dependent tasks (Nadel et al., 2000) and inferential tasks where the patient integrates previously learned information to perform successfully under novel conditions (Greene et al., 2006). Historically, it has been assumed that the hippocampus also temporarily stores information that has been recently obtained and that is useful for the current task at hand or is destined for long-term storage elsewhere. Recent evidence, however, obtained from patients with temporal lobe injury (for example, H.M.) suggests that the hippocampus may also store information for many years.

Entorhinal and Parahippocampal Cortices

Combined lesions of the entorhinal and parahippocampal cortices impair performance on tasks that require learning and memory almost as seriously as large temporal lobe lesions that include these structures and the hippocampus as well (Zola-Morgan, Squire, Amaral, and Suzuki, 1989b; Suzuki et al., 1993; Zola-Morgan et al., 1994). This fact is better appreciated when one considers that these structures are a critical route for cortical sensory information entering the hippocampus (Insausti et al., 1987). Surprisingly, the bilateral destruction of the entorhinal cortex alone produced only a transient impairment in a delay-dependent form of memory, that is, the delayed nonmatch to sample task (Leonard et al., 1995). Impaired performance in this task was longer lasting when the parahippocampal gyrus was also included with the entorhinal lesion (Zola-Morgan, Squire, Amaral, and Suzuki, 1989b; Suzuki et al., 1993). This delayed nonmatch to sample task is the most sensitive task that is used to demonstrate memory impairments related to the function of the entorhinal cortex. It is a recognition task that requires the animal to distinguish between a novel object and an object seen prior to a delay period. New pairs of objects are used on each trial.

Overall, the perirhinal and entorhinal cortical areas are important for stimulus recognition memory and stimulus-stimulus associations across sensory modalities (Murray, 1996). These ventral temporal cortical areas are probably more important for the consolidation of long-term memories for facts and events, that is, semantic knowledge, than are the amygdala and hippocampus (Squire, 1992; Murray, 1996). Recent studies using fMRI techniques also implicate an interaction between activity within the parahippocampal cortex and hippocampus during the retrieval of autobiographical events (Maguire et al., 2001) and remote memories (Squire and Bayey, 2007).

Amygdala

The amygdala mediates the memory of affective or emotional information and may encode memories for the emotional significance of events (LeDoux, 1993). This type of memory has been given the name valence memory (Nadel, 1996). Support for this concept comes from electrophysiological studies of the activity of amygdala neurons and from studies of the effects of discrete lesions. Amygdala neurons respond most vigorously to stimuli that have affective salience; that is, they predict whether a stimulus will be positively or negatively rewarding (Nishijo et al., 1988). Recent investigations of the primate amygdala are consistent with this hypothesis; amygdala neurons transmit information about a large array of complex sensory, particularly visual in primates, stimuli. This information is processed to allow facial recognition (Gothard et al., 2007). Animals with lesions of the amygdala are impaired in tasks that require a distinction between responses to stimuli that are, or are not, associated with a food reward (R.J. McDonald and White, 1993). However, amygdala lesions do not impair performance in tasks that only require delay-dependent forms of memory, such as in a delayed nonmatch to sample task (Zola-Morgan, Squire, and Amaral, 1989a). The amygdala also seems to code the relative magnitude of the reward (Kesner and Williams, 1995; Rolls et al., 1999). Therefore, the amygdala probably is important for remembering information that is associated with a particular affect. It most likely contributes this information to the adjacent hippocampal system to enhance the consolidation and remembrance of information that is of particular importance to the animal—for example, that certain sensory cues predict significant reward or danger (Aggleton, 2001).

CEREBELLUM

The cerebellum has traditionally been considered to be dedicated to motor functions and is required for the acquisition and expression of the conditioned response (Christian and Thompson, 2005). Its connectivity and phylogenetic development patterns suggest that it also plays a role in higher cognitive processes (Lee and Thompson, 2006). The cerebellum is responsible for implicit memories of sensorimotor learning. The classic example of learning that is controlled by the cerebellum is the eye-blink response (Desimone, 1992; Krupa et al., 1993). Rabbits will blink their eyes in response to an air puff directed to the cornea. When this air puff is repeatedly paired with a tone, the rabbit will learn to blink in response to the tone. Rabbits with cerebellar lesions do not acquire this association. Damage to the cerebellum can impair other learned sensorimotor responses, such as the ability to perform complex motor skills that have been well rehearsed—for example, skiing, golfing, playing musical instruments, speech, or the control of eye movements (Glickstein and Yeo, 1990).

BASAL GANGLIA

The basal ganglia are thought to play a critical role in motor planning and movement sequencing. Studies using fMRI have shown that the basal ganglia may modulate activity in the thalamus during working memory–guided movement sequencing. The globus pallidus may contribute to the planning and temporal organization of motor sequencing (Menon et al., 2000). The caudate nucleus may be responsible for memories of motor responses (for example, estimates of the distance that one moved a lever) as well as habit learning (for example, patterns of specific movements). This type of learning is more gradual than that established by the hippocampus and requires repeated associations of the stimuli to be learned (Knowlton et al., 1996). In addition to habit learning, the caudate may be critical for remembering the spatial relationship of objects with regard to oneself, that is, egocentric memory (Kesner et al., 1993). This is in contrast to the type of memory that may be organized by the hippocampus, that is, memory for the spatial relation of objects in relation to each other (Kesner et al., 1993). In support of this concept, recent studies have shown that neurons in the caudate are active when a monkey is picking up a piece of food or manipulating objects within its environment (Rolls et al., 1983). Connections between the striatum and prefrontal cortex may enable behavioral flexibility that involves extradimensional shifts, particularly for learning and memory of visual cue and response information (Ragozzino et al., 2002; Eschenko and Mizumori, 2007).

PREFRONTAL CORTEX

The prefrontal cortex influences our memory for the temporal order of events rather than the actual memory of those events. Operationally, the neurons within this brain region may control neuronal activity in premotor and motor cortex to inhibit temporally inappropriate behaviors (Narayanan and Laubach, 2006). Therefore, monkeys with lesions of the prefrontal cortex are impaired in a delayed nonmatching to sample task when the sample objects recur again and again across each trial. To perform this task, the monkey must remember which object was seen most recently, inhibit the same response, and therefore choose the other object. In contrast, prefrontal lesions do not impair performance of this task when novel objects are used on each trial. In this instance, the monkey need only recall that an object is novel (never been seen before) and choose that object. Studies using PET suggest that the prefrontal cortex is active during word encoding and that it coordinates its function with the dorsal hippocampus (Leube et al., 2001). Finally, it has become clear that a neural circuit comprising the prefrontal cortex and various limbic structures, in particular the amygdala, normally implements the self-regulation of emotions.

ANTERIOR CINGULATE

Multiple functions that underlie memory have been associated with the anterior cingulate gyrus, perhaps the most important being attention (Posner and Rothbart, 1998). Not surprisingly, healthy elderly adults who demonstrate a dysfunction in attention have decreased activation of this brain region (Milham et al., 2002; Pardo et al., 2007). Single neuron activity recorded during training suggests that the rabbit anterior cingulate cortex cAC is part of an attentional mechanism detecting coincidence between temporally related environmental stimuli (Weible et al., 2003).

ACKNOWLEDGMENT

Preparation of this chapter was supported in part by the National Institute of Aging, RO1 AG030331.

REFERENCES

Aggleton, J.P. (2001) *The Amygdala*. Oxford, UK: Oxford University Press.

Aggleton, J.P., and Mishkin, M. (1983) Memory impairments following restricted medial thalamic lesions. *Exp. Brain Res.* 52: 199–209.

Aggleton, J.P., and Mishkin, M. (1985) Mammillary body lesions and visual recognition in monkeys. *Exp. Brain Res.* 58:190–197.

Andreasen, N.C., O'Leary, D.S., Paradiso, S., Cizadla, T., Arndt, S., Watkins, G.L., Ponto, L.L., and Hichwa, R.D. (1999) The cerebellum plays a role in conscious episodic memory retrieval. *Hum. Brain Mapp.* 8:226–234.

Berger-Sweeney, J., Heckers, S., Mesulam, M.M., Wiley, R.G., Lappi, D.A., and Sharma, M. (1994) Differential effects on spatial navigation of immunotoxin-induced cholinergic lesions of the medial septal area and nucleus basalis magnocellularis. *J. Neurosci.* 14: 4507–4519.

Christian, K.M., and Thompson R.F. (2005) Long-term storage of an associative memory trace in the cerebellum. *Behav. Neurosci.* 119:526–537.

Coyle, J.T., Price, D.L., and DeLong, M.R. (1983) Alzheimer's disease: a disorder of cortical cholinergic innervation. *Science* 219: 1184–1190.

Crespo-Facorro, B., Paradiso, S., Andreasen, N.C., O'Leary, D.S., Watkins, G.L., Boles Ponto, L.L., and Hichwa, R.D. (1999) Recalling word lists reveals cognitive dysmetria in schizophrenia: a positron emission tomography study. *Am. J. Psychiatry* 156:386–392.

Desimone, R. (1992) The physiology of memory: recordings of things past. *Science* 258:245–246.

Dunnett, S.B., Whishaw, I.Q., Jones, G.H., and Bunch, S.T. (1987) Behavioral, biochemical and histochemical effects of different neurotoxic amino acids injected into nucleus basalis magnocellularis of rats. *Neuroscience* 20:653–669.

Dusoir, H., Kapur, N., Byrnes, D.P., McKinstry, S., and Hoare, R.D. (1990) The role of diencephalic pathology in human memory disorder. *Brain* 113:1695–1706.

Eichenbaum, H., Otto, T., and Cohen, N.J. (1992) Review: the hippocampus—what does it do? *Behav. Neural Biol.* 57:2–36.

Eichenbaum, H., Otto, T., and Cohen, N.J. (1994) Two functional components of the hippocampal memory system. *Behav. Brain Sci.* 17:449–518.

Eschenko, O., and Mizumori, S.J.Y. (2007) Memory influences on hippocampal and striatal neural codes: effects of a shift between task rules. *Neurobiol. Learn. Memory* 87:495–509.

Everitt B.J., and Robbins T.W. (1997) Central cholinergic systems and cognition. *Annu. Rev. Psychol.* 48:649–684.

Fuster, J. M. (1997) *The Prefrontal Cortex: Anatomy, Physiology, and Neuropsychology of the Frontal Lobe*, 3rd ed. Philadelphia: Lippincott–Raven.

Gilboa, A., Winocur, G., Rosenbaum, R.S., Poreh, A., Gao, F.Q., Black, S.E., Westmacott, R., and Moscovitch, M. (2006) Hippocampal contributions to recollection in retrograde and anterograde amnesia. *Hippocampus* 16:966–980.

Glickstein, M., and Yeo, C. (1990) The cerebellum and motor learning. *J. Cogn. Neurosci.* 2:69–80.

Gothard, K.M., Battaglia, F.P., Erickson, C.A., Spitler, K.M., and Amaral, D.G. (2007) Neural responses to facial expression and face identity in the monkey amygdala. *J. Neurophysiol.* 97:1671–1683.

Graff-Radford, N.R., Tranel, D., Van Hoesen, G.W., and Brandt, J. (1990) Diencephalic amnesia. *Brain* 113:1–25.

Greene, A.J., Gross, W.L., Elsinger, C.L., and Rao, S.M. (2006) An fMRI analysis of the human hippocampus: inference, context, and task awareness *J. Cogn. Neurosci.* 18:1156–1173.

Insausti, R., Amaral, D.G., and Cowan, W.M. (1987) The entorhinal cortex of the monkey: II. cortical afferents. *J. Comp. Neurol.* 264:356–395.

Kesner, R.P., Bolland, B.L., and Dakis, M. (1993) Memory for spatial locations, motor responses, and objects: triple dissociation among the hippocampus, caudate nucleus, and extrastriate visual cortex. *Exp. Brain Res.* 93:462–470.

Kesner, R.P., and Williams, J.M. (1995) Memory for magnitude of reinforcement: dissociation between the amygdala and hippocampus. *Neurobiol. Learn. Mem.* 64:237–244.

Knowlton, B.J., Mangels, J.A., and Squire, L.R. (1996) A neostriatal habit learning system in humans. *Science* 273:1399–1402.

Krupa, D.J., Thompson, J.K., and Thompson, R.F. (1993) Localization of a memory trace in the mammalian brain. *Science* 260: 989–991.

LeDoux, J.E. (1993) Emotional memory systems in the brain. *Behav. Brain Res.* 58:69–79.

Lee, K.H., and Thompson, R.F. (2006) Multiple memory mechanisms in the cerebellum? *Neuron* 51:680–682.

Leonard, B.W., Amaral, D.G., Squire, L.R., and Zola-Morgan, S. (1995) Transient memory impairment in monkeys with bilateral lesions of the entorhinal cortex. *J. Neurosci.* 15:5637–5659.

Leube, D.T., Erb, M., Grodd, W., Bartels, M., and Kircher, T.T. (2001) Differential activation in parahippocampal and prefrontal cortex during word and face encoding tasks. *Neuroreport* 12: 2773–2777.

Maguire, E.A., Vargha-Khadem, F., and Mishkin M. (2001) The effects of bilateral hippocampal damage on fMRI regional activations and interactions during memory retrieval. *Brain* 124:1156–1170.

Mair, R.G., Knoth, R.L., Rabehenuk, S.A., and Langlais, P.J. (1991) Impairment of olfactory, auditory, and spatial serial reversal learning in rats recovered from pyrithiamine induced thiamine deficiency. *Behav. Neurosci.* 105:360–374.

Malamut, B.L., Graff-Radford, N., Chawluk, J., Grossman, R.I., and Guy, R.C. (1992) Memory in a case of bilateral thalamic infarction. *Neurology* 42:163–169.

McDonald, M.P., Wenk, G.L., and Crawley, J.N. (1997) Analysis of galanin and galanin antagonist, M40, on delayed non-matching to position performance in rats lesioned with the cholinergic immunotoxin 192 IgG-saporin. *Behav. Neurosci.* 111:552–563.

McDonald, R.J., and White, N.M. (1993) A triple dissociation of memory systems: hippocampus, amygdala, and dorsal striatum. *Behav. Neurosci.* 107:3–22.

Menon, V., Anagnoson, R.T., Glover, G.H., and Pfefferbaum, A. (2000) Basal ganglia involvement in memory-guided movement sequencing. *Neuroreport* 11:3641–3645.

Milham, M.P., Erickson, K.I., Banich, M.T., Kramer, A.F., Webb, A., Wszalek, T., and Cohen, N.J. (2002) Attentional control in the aging brain: insights from an fMRI study of the Stroop task. *Brain Cogn.* 49:277–296.

Mishkin, M., and Appenzeller, T. (1987) The anatomy of memory. *Sci. Am.* 256:80–89.

Mishkin, M., and Murray, E.A. (1994) Stimulus recognition. *Curr. Opin. Neurobiol.* 4:200–206.

Muir, J.L., Dunnett, S.B., Robbins, T.W., and Everitt, B.J. (1992) Attentional functions of the forebrain cholinergic systems: effects of intraventricular hemicholinium, physostigmine, basal forebrain lesions and intracortical grafts on a multiple-choice serial reaction time task. *Exp. Brain Res.* 89:611–622.

Mumby, D.G., and Pinel, J.P.J. (1994) Rhinal cortex lesions and object recognition in rats. *Behav. Neurosci.* 108:11–18.

Murray, E.A. (1996) What have ablation studies told us about the neural substrates of stimulus memory? *Semin. Neurosci.* 8:13–22.

Nadel, L. (1996) The hippocampus: selective functions in memory. In: Ono, T., McNaughton, B.L., Molotchnikoff, S., Rolls, E.T., and Nishijo, H., eds. *Perception, Memory, Emotion: Frontiers in Neuroscience*. Oxford, UK: Elsevier, pp. 305–317.

Nadel, L., Samsonovich, A., Ryan, L., and Moscovitch, M. (2000) Multiple trace theory of human memory: Computational, neuroimaging, and neuropsychological results. *Hippocampus* 10:352–368.

Narayanan, N.S., and Laubach, M. (2006) Top-down control of motor cortex ensembles by dorsomedial prefrontal cortex. *Neuron* 52:921–931.

Nishijo, H., Ono, T., and Nishino, H. (1988) Single neuron responses in amygdala of alert monkey during complex sensory stimulation with affective significance. *J. Neurosci.* 8:3570–3583.

O'Keefe, J., and Nadel, L. (1978) *The Hippocampus as a Cognitive Map*. Oxford, UK: Clarendon Press.

Olton, D.S., and Wenk, G.L. (1987) Dementia: Animal models of the cognitive impairments produced by degeneration of the basal forebrain cholinergic system. In: Meltzer, H.Y., ed. *Psychopharmacology: The Third Generation of Progress*. New York: Raven Press, pp. 941–953.

Olton, D.S., Wenk, G.L., Church, R.M., and Meck, W.H. (1988) Attention and the frontal cortical cortex as examined by simultaneous temporal processing. *Neuropsychology* 26:307–318.

Pardo, J.V., Lee, J.T., Sheikh, S.A., Surerus-Johnson, C., Shah, H., et al. (2007) Where the brain grows old: Decline in anterior cingulate and medial prefrontal function with normal aging. *Neuroimage* 35:1231–1237.

Posner, M.I., and Rothbart, M.K. (1998) Attention, self-regulation and consciousness. *Philos. Trans. R. Soc. Lond. B. Biol. Sci.* 353: 1915–1927.

Ragozzino, M.E., Ragozzino, K.E., Mizumori, S.J.Y., and Kesner, R.P. (2002) Role of the dorsomedial striatum in behavioral flexibility for response and visual cue discrimination learning. *Behav. Neurosci.* 116:105–115.

Rauch, S. L., Whalen, P. J., Curran, T., McInerney, S., Heckers, S., and Savage, C. R. (1998) Thalamic deactivation during early implicit sequence learning: a functional MRI study. *Neuroreport* 9:865–870.

Richardson, R.T., and DeLong, M.R. (1991) Functional implications of tonic and phasic activity changes in nucleus basalis neurons. In: Richardson, R.T., ed. *Activation to Acquisition: Functional Aspects of the Basal Forebrain Cholinergic System*. Boston: Birkhauser, pp. 135–166.

Robbins, T.W., Everitt, B.J., Marston, H.M., Wilkinson, J., Jones, G.H., and Page, K.J. (1989) Comparative effects of ibotenic acid- and quisqualic acid-induced lesions of the substantia innominata on attentional function in the rat: further implications for the role of the cholinergic neurons in the nucleus basalis in cognitive processes. *Behav. Brain Res.* 35:221–224.

Roland, P.E., and Gulyas, B. (1994) Visual imagery and visual representation. *Trends Neurosci.* 17:281–297.

Rolls, E.T. (2000) Memory systems in the brain. *Annu. Rev. Psychol.* 51:599–630.

Rolls, E.T., Critchley, H.D., Browning, A.S., Hernadi, A., and Lenard, L. (1999) Responses to the sensory properties of fat of neurons in the primate orbitofrontal cortex. *J. Neurosci.* 19: 1532–1540.

Rolls, E.T., Thorpe, S.J., and Maddison, S.P. (1983) Responses of striatal neurons in the behaving monkey. 1. Head of the caudate nucleus. *Behav. Brain Res.* 7:179–210.

Sarter, M., Hasselmo, M.E., Bruno, J.P. and Givens, B. (2005) Unraveling the attentional functions of cortical cholinergic inputs: interactions between signal-driven and cognitive modulation of signal detection. *Brain Res. Rev.* 48:98–111.

Schacter, D.L., and Tulving, E. (1994) *Memory Systems*. Cambridge, MA: MIT Press.

Smith, D.M., and Mizumori, S.J.Y. (2006) Hippocampal place cells, context and episodic memory. *Hippocampus* 16:716–729.

Squire, L.R. (1992) Declarative and nondeclarative memory: multiple brain systems supporting learning and memory. *J. Cogn. Neurosci.* 4:232–243.

Squire, L.R., Amaral, D.G., Zola-Morgan, S., Kritchevsky, M., and Press, G. (1989) Description of brain injury in the amnesic patient N.A. based on magnetic resonance imaging. *Exp. Neurol.* 105:23–35.

Squire, L.R., and Bayey, P.J. (2007) The neuroscience of remote memory. *Curr. Opin. Neurobiol.* 17:185–196.

Suzuki, W., Zola-Morgan, S., Squire, L.R., and Amaral, D.G. (1993) Lesions of the perirhinal and parahippocampal cortices in the monkey produce long-lasting memory impairment in the visual and tactual modalities. *J. Neurosci.* 13:2430–2451.

Sziklas, V., and Petrides, M. (2000) Selectivity of the spatial learning deficit after lesions of the mammillary region in rats. *Hippocampus* 10:325–328.

Tulving, E., and Schacter, D.L. (1990) Priming and human memory systems. *Science* 247:301–306.

Victor, M., Adams, R.D., and Collins, G.H. (1989) *The Wernicke-Korsakoff Syndrome and Related Neurological Disorders Due to Alcoholism and Malnutrition*, 2nd ed. Philadelphia: F.A. Davis.

Weible, A.P., Weiss, C., and Disterhoft, J.F. (2003) Activity profiles of single neurons in caudal anterior cingulate cortex during trace eyeblink conditioning in the rabbit. *J. Neurophysiol.* 90:599–612.

Wenk, G.L. (1993) A primate model of Alzheimer's disease. *Behav. Brain Res.* 57:117–122.

Wenk, G.L. (1997) The nucleus basalis magnocellularis cholinergic system: 100 years of progress. *Neurobiol. Learn. Mem.* 67:85–95.

Wenk, G.L., and Olton, D.S. (1987) Basal forebrain cholinergic neurons and Alzheimer's disease. In: Coyle, J.T., ed. *Animal Models of Dementia: A Synaptic Neurochemical Perspective*. New York: Alan R. Liss, pp. 81–101.

Wilson, F.A.W., and Rolls, E.T. (1990) Neuronal responses related to the novelty and familiarity of visual stimuli in the substantia innominata, diagonal band of Broca and periventricular region of the primate basal forebrain. *Exp. Brain Res.* 80:104–120.

Winocur, G., Oxbury, S., Roberts, R., Agnetti, V., and Davis, D. (1984) Amnesia in a patient with bilateral lesions to the thalamus. *Neuropsychology* 22:123–143.

Zola-Morgan, S., and Squire, L.R. (1993) Neuroanatomy of memory. *Annu. Rev. Neurosci.* 16:547–563.

Zola-Morgan, S., Squire, L.R., and Amaral, D.G. (1989a) Lesions of the amygdala that spare adjacent cortical regions do not impair memory or exacerbate the impairment following lesions of the hippocampal formation. *J. Neurosci.* 9:1922–1936.

Zola-Morgan, S., Squire, L.R., Amaral, D.G., and Suzuki, W. (1989b) Lesions of perirhinal and parahippocampal cortex that spare the amygdala and the hippocampal formation produce severe memory impairment. *J. Neurosci.* 9:4355–4370.

Zola-Morgan, S., Squire, L.R., and Ramus, S.J. (1994) Severity of memory impairment in monkeys as a function of locus and extent of damage within the medial temporal lobe memory system. *Hippocampus* 4:483–495.

56 Neurochemical Systems Involved in Learning and Memory

JOANNE BERGER-SWEENEY, LAURA R. SCHAEVITZ, AND KARYN M. FRICK

During the past decades, considerable experimental evidence has linked specific neurotransmitter systems to learning and memory processes. Although acetylcholine (ACh) and glutamate have been most extensively studied in relation to memory, considerable evidence also links γ-aminobutyric acid (GABA), dopamine (DA), norepinephrine (NE), and serotonin (5-HT) to memory. Recently, it has become clear that studying the individual contribution of classical neurotransmitters to memory processes is not a feasible approach to studying the neurochemistry of memory because of numerous interactions among transmitters and of modulation by neuroactive peptides, steroid hormones, and trophic factors.

The insights gained from studying neurotransmitters related to learning and memory are particularly relevant to the study of dementia. Dementia is characterized by a progressive, irreversible deterioration of higher cognitive functions, including learning and memory (Coyle et al., 1984). Failure of neurotransmission, particularly in regions of the brain such as the hippocampus and neocortex, is likely to be a fundamental defect responsible for cognitive impairments in dementia. Additionally, it has become increasingly clear that cognitive impairments, including alterations in learning and memory, are prominent features of numerous neurological and psychiatric disorders, such as Parkinson's and Huntington's diseases and schizophrenia. Pharmacological treatments that improve motor deficits in Parkinson's and Huntington's and positive psychiatric symptoms in schizophrenia still leave some higher cognitive functions impaired, such as learning and memory. Understanding the neurochemistry of learning and memory, therefore, is a first step toward relating the symptoms of dementia to underlying biochemical processes.

CONSIDERABLE EVIDENCE SUGGESTS THAT CHOLINERGIC NEURONS PLAY A CRITICAL ROLE IN ACQUISITION AND ATTENTIONAL PROCESSES

Pharmacological studies in numerous species, using a variety of experimental paradigms, have linked ACh to learning and memory processes. In general, cholinergic agonists (for example, physostigmine) improve memory, whereas cholinergic antagonists (for example, scopolamine) impair memory (Bartus et al., 1985) (Table 56.1). Centrally-acting cholinergic agonists improve memory; however, peripherally administered agonists, which do not cross into the central nervous system (CNS), do not improve memory, suggesting that the effects of cholinergic compounds on memory are likely mediated through central mechanisms. Moreover, the dose of a given drug administered to an animal is critical in determining the magnitude and direction of the mnemonic effect; the same compound can either improve or impair memory, depending on the dose administered. Muscarinic and nicotinic receptors are thought to mediate cholinergic effects on learning and memory (Jones et al., 1999; Dani and Bertrand 2007).

Classic lesion studies have identified populations of cholinergic neurons and projections that are critical for learning and memory. These neurons are located in the basal forebrain and project to the hippocampus and neocortex. The basal forebrain region includes the medial septal area (MSA) and the vertical limb of the diagonal band of Broca (dbB), which project primarily to the hippocampus, and the horizontal limb of the dbB and nucleus basalis magnocellularis (nBM), which project to the neocortex. Lesions of the MSA and nBM in rodents impair performance on a variety of mnemonic tasks, including spatial reference and working memory

TABLE 56.1 *Life Cycles and Pharmacological Characteristics of Six Classical Neurotransmitters*

Neurotransmitter	*Synthetic Pathway*	*Degradative Pathway*	*Primary CNS Receptor Subtypes*	*Common Agonists*	*Common Antagonists*
Acetylcholine (ACh)	Choline and acetyl CoA → ACh ↑ ChAT	ACh → Choline and acetic acid ↑ AChE	Muscarinic: M1, M2, M3, M4, M5 Nicotinic: α(2–10) β(2–4)	Muscarine Oxotremorine Carbachol Physostigmine Nicotine	Scopolamine Atropine Pirenzepine mecamylamine Bungarotoxin
Glutamate	Glutamine → Glutamate ↑ Glutaminase Aspartate → Glutamate Glucose → Glutamate	Glutamate → Glutamine Glutamate → GABA ↑ GAD	Ionotrophic: NMDA (1, 2A–D) AMPA (GluR1–3) Kainate Metabotropic: mGluR1–8	Kainic, ibotenic, and quisqualic acids NMDA AMPA DHPG L-AP4	D-AP5 Ketamine MK-801 PCP AIDA
GABA	Glutamate → GABA ↑ GAD	GABA → succinic semialdehyde ↑ GABA transaminase	GABA–A: α(1–6), β(1–3), γ(1–3), δ, ε, θ, ρ(1–3) GABA–B (1–2)	Muscimol Baclofen Benzodiazepines Barbiturates	Bicuculline Picrotoxin Phaclofen Flumazenil
Dopamine	L-tyrosine → L-DOPA ↑ tyrosine hydroxylase L-DOPA → DA ↑ DOPA decarboxlase	Reuptake Dopamine → Norepinephrine ↑ DA β-hydroxylase Dopamine → DOPAC ↑ MAO Dopamine → HVA ↑ COMT and MAO	D_1, D_2, D_3, D_4, D_5	Amphetamine Cocaine SKF38393 Quinpirole Apomorphine Deprenyl	Reserpine Neuroleptics SCH23390 SCH39166 Raclopride Haloperidol
Norepinephrine	Dopamine → NE ↑ Dopamine β-hydroxylase	Reuptake NE → Epinephrine ↑ PNMT NE → MHPG and VMA ↑ COMT and MAO	α1(A,B,D), α2(A–C) β1, β2, β3	Amphetamine Epinephrine Tricyclic antidepressants Clonidine Guanfacine	Reserpine Phentolamine Propranolol Yohimbine
Serotonin	Tryptophan → 5-HTP ↑ tryptophan hydroxylase 5-HTP → 5-HT ↑ amino acid decarboxylase	Reuptake 5-HT → 5-HIAA ↑ MAO and aldehyde dehydrogenase 5-HT → Melatonin (pineal)	5-HT_1(A–F) 5-HT_2(A–C) 5-HT_3, 5-HT_4, 5-HT_{5A}, 5-HT_{5B} 5-HT_6, 5-HT_7	LSD Anxiolytics Sumatriptan Imipramine Fluoxetine (Prozac)	Reserpine Clozapine Clomipramine Antidepressants Methiothepin

Source: Largely from Cooper et al., 1996; Siegel et al., 1999; Nestler et al., 2001.

Note: ↑ denotes the action of an enzyme on the substrate to the upper left of the arrow. For further information on the above or on the anatomical projections of the above listed systems, see Nestler et al. (2001).

5-HT: serotonin; 5-HIAA: 5-hydroxyindoleacetic acid; 5-HTP: 5-hydroxytryptophan; ACh: acetylcholine; AChE: acetylcholinesterase; ACPD: aminocyclopentyl dicarboxylic acid; AIDA: 1-aminoindan-1,5 dicarboxylic acid; AMPA: α-amino-3-hydroxy-5-methyl-4-isoxazole-propionic acid; ChAT: choline acetyltransferase; CNS: central nervous system; CoA: coenzyme A; COMT: catechol-O-methyltransferase; D-AP5: D-2-amino-5 phosphonopentanoate; DA: dopamine; DHPG: 3,5-dihydroxyphenylglycine; DOPAC: dihydroxyphenylacetic acid; GABA: γ-aminobutyric acid; GAD: glutamic acid decarboxylase; HVA: homovanillic acid; L-AP4: L-2-amino-4-phosphonopropionic acid; LSD: lysergic acid diethylamide; MAO: monoamine oxidase; MHPG: 3-methoxy-4-hydroxyphenlglycol; NE: norepinephrine; NMDA: *N*-methyl-D-aspartate; PCP: phencyclidine; PNMT: phenylethanolamine *N*-methyltransferase; VMA: vanillylmandelic acid.

tasks such as the Morris water maze and T-maze alternation. Reference memory and working memory, a dichotomy used extensively in the rodent literature, refer to information to be remembered across trials (reference memory) or for a single trial (working memory) (Olton et al., 1979).

The critical flaw in the early lesion studies was the use of nonspecific lesion techniques. Many studies used electrolytic lesions (which destroy neurons as well as fibers of passage) or excitotoxins such as ibotenic acid (which spare fibers of passage but kill cholinergic and noncholinergic neurons). More specific lesion techniques, such as the immunotoxin 192 IgG saporin, produce selective cholinergic lesions of the basal forebrain. In general, the deficits seen on spatial memory tasks following 192 IgG saporin lesions are considerably less robust than those observed after nonspecific toxin lesions (Baxter and Chiba, 1999). This finding has led many investigators to question the link between the cholinergic system and memory. Recent studies document impairments following either developmental or adult 192 IgG saporin lesions in tasks designed to measure attention, suggesting that basal forebrain cholinergic neurons may be involved in attentional processes. Furthermore, basal forebrain cholinergic neurons appear critical in reorganizing cortical representations of behaviorally important sensory stimuli and may regulate the cortical plasticity necessary for laying down a memory trace (Rasmusson, 2000). Thus, ACh may contribute more to the acquisition and processing of sensory information than to the retention of this information. It is noteworthy that acetylcholinerase inhibitors, which prevent the enzymatic breakdown of acetylcholine, are the most widely prescribed pharmacological treatments for Alzheimer's disease (Musial et al., 2007). These drugs improve, albeit temporarily and only moderately, cognitive impairments in a significant number of patients with Alzheimer's disease.

GLUTAMATE IS INVOLVED IN LONG-TERM POTENTIATION, A PUTATIVE MECHANISM OF LEARNING AND MEMORY

The excitatory amino acid *glutamate* is the most abundant amino acid in the CNS. However, glutamate was not identified as a neurotransmitter until the early 1980s because of its multiple roles in the CNS, including involvement in fatty acid synthesis, ammonia regulation, and as a precursor for GABA. Glutamate receptors are widespread throughout the CNS but are particularly concentrated in the hippocampus and neocortex.

The most obvious connection between glutamate and memory is glutamate's involvement in long-term potentiation (LTP), an artificially induced form of lasting neuronal plasticity originally observed in the hippocampus (Bliss and Lømo, 1973). Long-term potentiation is a putative mechanism of associative learning because its three main characteristics—cooperativity, associativity, and input specificity—closely resemble D.O. Hebb's postulation that a synapse linking two cells will be strengthened if the two cells are active simultaneously (Hebb, 1949). *N*-methyl-D-aspartate (NMDA)-dependent LTP involves induction (in which the initial increase in synaptic potentiation occurs) and maintenance (in which the increase persists for a prolonged period). To induce LTP, a postsynaptic membrane must first be depolarized by the binding of glutamate to postsynaptic α-amino-3-hydroxy-5 methylisoxazole-4-proprionic acid (AMPA) receptors. This depolarization releases a Mg^{2+} blockade of postsynaptic NMDA channels that occurs normally at the resting potential. Glycine and serine act as coagonists at NMDA receptors. Removal of the Mg^{2+} blockade allows an influx of Ca^{2+} into the postsynaptic terminal, which activates a cascade of Ca^{2+}-dependent kinases that leads eventually to potentiation of the postsynaptic neuron. To maintain this potentiation, increased presynaptic glutamate release is required, which involves an unidentified retrograde messenger (MacDonald et al., 2006).

In one of the first links between NMDA receptors and memory it was shown that D-AP5, an NMDA channel blocker, impairs spatial reference memory in rats tested in the Morris water maze (Morris, 1986). Doses sufficient to impair memory also block LTP, suggesting that intact LTP is required for performance of the task. Recent attention has focused on drugs that facilitate AMPA receptor-mediated transmission in the hippocampus (Bannerman et al., 2006). Drugs that facilitate the induction of LTP in vivo improve the retention of several types of memory in rats as well as in aged humans. Together, these studies suggest that pharmacological blockade of LTP results in memory impairment, whereas facilitation of LTP results in memory enhancement.

Knockout studies in mice have offered further insight into the function of the Ca^{2+} ionophore in dendrites, related AMPA and NMDA receptors, and control of intraneuronal kinases important in the initiation of LTP. Mice with a deletion of a portion of the NMDA gene restricted to the CA1 region of the hippocampus exhibit impaired LTP and impaired spatial reference memory in the Morris water maze. Kinases important for LTP initiation, such as α-calcium calmodulin-dependent kinase II (CaMKII), may be under activity-dependent local translational control (L. Wu et al., 1998). Mutations of CaMKII or the fyn tyrosine kinase impair LTP initiation and spatial water-maze learning. Also, the maintenance of LTP putatively involves kinases that are different from those involved in LTP initiation. Cyclic adenosine monophosphate (cAMP)-dependent protein kinase A (PKA) and mitogen-activated protein kinases (MAPKs) are involved in LTP maintenance and can activate transcriptional factors, such as cAMP response element binding (CREB) proteins that activate immediate- and late-response genes. These genes then putatively regulate structural and functional alterations in the neuron that can serve as a substrate for long-term storage of information and may serve as a physical substrate for neuronal plasticity. However, spatial learning can occur even if LTP is completely blocked pharmacologically, a result that highlights the fact that the connection between LTP and memory has yet to be firmly established. Nevertheless, much recent research has been devoted to developing glutamatergic-based drugs to enhance cognition in normal aging and Alzheimer's disease (Knopman, 2006).

GABAERGIC INHIBITION IN THE SEPTOHIPPOCAMPAL SYSTEM CAN PROFOUNDLY INFLUENCE MEMORY

GABA is the primary inhibitory neurotransmitter in the CNS. Its distribution is ubiquitous in the brain, and cell bodies are prominent in several regions involved in learning and memory including the neocortex, nBM, medial septum, hippocampus, striatum, and amygdala. In the medial septum, GABAergic neurons interact extensively with cholinergic neurons, and both of these cell populations send projections to and receive them from the hippocampus. Because the $GABA_A$ receptor complex has multiple binding sites, there are several ways to modulate the GABAergic system pharmacologically. This chloride channel complex includes five major binding sites: GABA (opens the channel), barbiturates (decrease the frequency of channel opening and increase opening duration), benzodiazepines (BDZs; increase the frequency of channel opening), picrotoxin (blocks the channel), and steroids (Sieghart, 2006). The $GABA_B$ receptor is a simple ion channel (K^+ or Ca^{2+}) and is not modulated by the aforementioned compounds.

Breen and McGaugh (1961) first demonstrated GABAergic modulation of memory by showing that posttraining peripheral administration of picrotoxin enhanced maze learning in rats. Posttraining peripheral injection of the $GABA_A$ antagonist *bicuculline* also produces a dose-dependent improvement of passive avoidance retention. Conversely, peripheral injection of the $GABA_A$ agonist *muscimol* impairs passive avoidance retention.

The effects of direct intraseptal modulation of the $GABA_A$ receptor are consistent with those of peripheral injections (Walsh and Stackman, 1992). In general, pre- and posttraining facilitation of $GABA_A$ activation with muscimol or the BDZ agonist chlordiazepoxide impairs memory on a wide variety of tasks including T-maze alternation, the radial arm maze, and the Morris water maze. These infusions also disrupt cholinergic function in the septum and hippocampus. This detrimental effect on memory is particularly interesting in light of the amnesic side effects observed in humans treated with BDZs to relieve anxiety. Conversely, antagonizing the BDZ site can reverse the amnesic effects of several BDZs in humans and rats. Several neuroactive steroids also modulate the $GABA_A$ receptor and affect memory via GABAergic mechanisms. Facilitation of $GABA_B$ activity with the agonist *baclofen* impairs spatial memory and decreases hippocampal cholinergic function, suggesting similar mnemonic and neurochemical consequences of modulating the two GABA receptors. Interestingly, recent work suggests that the cognitive effects of intraseptal cholinergic agonist treatment are not due to increased ACh release but to increased septohippocampal GABA signaling (M. Wu et al., 2000). Such an increase would reduce GABAergic neurotransmission in the hippocampus, thereby disinhibiting hippocampal pyramidal neurons and allowing for increased excitatory plasticity.

The amygdala is also important for the retention of some aversively motivated tasks, and GABAergic mechanisms in this structure may modulate aversive learning. Similar to peripheral injections, intra-amygdala infusion of bicuculline or picrotoxin enhances passive avoidance retention, whereas infusion of muscimol or baclofen impairs retention. It is possible that the amygdala and septohippocampal GABAergic systems interact to affect anxiety and fear and their relationship to memory formation and storage.

DOPAMINERGIC FUNCTION IN THE PREFRONTAL CORTEX IS CRITICAL FOR WORKING MEMORY

Most catecholaminergic neurons originate in discrete nuclei in the brain stem that project widely to the neocortex, limbic system, and striatum. In addition to the striatum, dopaminergic neurons in the ventral tegmental area and substantia nigra project to the prefrontal cortex, anterior cingulate cortex, perirhinal and entorhinal cortices, basal forebrain, hippocampus, and amygdala.

Many studies have examined the effects of peripheral injection of dopaminergic compounds on learning and memory. However, the results are inconsistent, depending on the drug and the task used, as well as on whether the injection is given pre- or posttraining. Peripheral treatments generally disrupt non-mnemonic parameters such as motor function (for example, increased latency to respond) and appetitive behavior, making it difficult to dissociate the effects of dopaminergic compounds on memory from performance effects.

Injections of dopaminergic compounds directly into the CNS suggest that DA modulates memory in part through an interaction with ACh in the septohippocampal system (Decker and McGaugh, 1991). Intraseptal injection of the DA antagonist *haloperidol* increases hippocampal ACh turnover; similar increases in ACh turnover can be produced by intraseptal or ventral tegmental injections of the DA toxin 6-hydroxydopamine

(6-OHDA). These results suggest that the dopaminergic input to the septum inhibits septohippocampal cholinergic activity. Thus, decreasing septal dopaminergic function may improve memory. Indeed, septal 6-OHDA lesions (with desmethylimipramine [DMI] to protect noradrenergic neurons) enhance spatial memory in several tasks, and this improvement is correlated with increased septohippocampal cholinergic activity.

Even more compelling is the role of dopaminergic projections to the prefrontal cortex (PFC) in working memory. Monkeys with bilateral lesions of the PFC are severely impaired on spatial working memory tasks, whereas they are unimpaired on object recognition tasks. Humans with PFC damage show similar memory deficits. Specific dopaminergic lesions of the dorsolateral PFC made by injections of 6-OHDA and DMI result in mnemonic deficits in monkeys similar to those in monkeys with cortical ablations (Brozoski et al., 1979), suggesting a specific role of prefrontal DA in working memory. Peripheral administration of the DA precursor *L-DOPA* or the DA agonist *apomorphine* improves the mnemonic performance of the monkeys whose DA is depleted. Prefrontal cortex injections of D_1 receptor antagonists in monkeys impair memory in an oculomotor delayed-response task without affecting sensory or motor functions (Sawaguchi and Goldman-Rakic, 1991), further implicating the dopaminergic system in working memory function. Recent pharmacological, cellular, and electrophysiological studies in rodents provide evidence that DA can not only mediate plasticity and improve working memory, but can also enhance spatial, reversal, and incentive learning (El-Ghundi et al., 2007).

Some evidence implicates reduced DA function in the cognitive impairments common in several neurodegenerative diseases. Dopaminergic drugs may improve aspects of working memory in individuals with these diseases, as well as in normal individuals (Chamberlain et al., 2006). Patients with Parkinson's disease and schizophrenia commonly exhibit working memory deficits, which is interesting given that reduced DA function in the PFC has been observed in both disorders. Increasing DA levels in patients with schizophrenia using amphetamine or in patients with Parkinson's disease using L-DOPA improves their performance on tests of working memory. The PFC may also be particularly vulnerable to deterioration with increasing age. Aged rats and aged monkeys exhibit a significant loss of DA from the PFC, a finding that is correlated with spatial working memory deficits.

NOREPINEPHRINE AFFECTS MEMORY THROUGH AROUSAL STATES AND MODULATION OF ACETYLCHOLINE AND DOPAMINE

The widespread noradrenergic projections from locus coeruleus (LC) to the neocortex have been implicated in general arousal and attentional states. Noradrenergic fibers originating in the brain stem are divided into two pathways: dorsal and ventral. The ventrally located cell bodies innervate the brain stem and hypothalamus. Dorsally located cell bodies are contained in the LC and innervate the spinal cord, cerebellum, amygdala, septum, hippocampus, and the entire cerebral cortex. Reciprocal connections also project from LC to the PFC. Norepinephrine (NE) has the highest affinity for α_2 andrenergic receptors in the neocortex, which are coupled to G-proteins that inhibit cAMP pathways.

Several studies have failed to observe a direct effect of noradrenergic modulation on memory. For instance, in rodents, NE depletion has little effect on a variety of memory tasks including the radial arm maze and passive avoidance tasks. Other studies in rats and monkeys suggest that α_2 agonists can improve working memory in aged animals and catecholamine-depleted animals. These improvements appear to be restricted to cognitive functions related to the PFC, such as working memory, given that these agonists do not affect spatial reference memory or recognition memory (Ramos and Arnste, 2007). Although most work relating NE to memory focuses on PFC, a recent study suggests that noradrenergic projections to hippocampus may influence LTP (Schimanski et al., 2007). In addition, because most types of memory storage involve arousal and focused attention, the LC's involvement in these processes points towards NE as a modulator of memory function.

The LC can modify septohippocampal cholinergic function and, therefore, NE can modulate memory function indirectly (Decker and McGaugh, 1991). Intraseptal injection of NE increases hippocampal ACh turnover and alters the hippocampal theta rhythm. This relationship between NE and ACh appears to be reciprocal; muscarinic stimulation of the hippocampus inhibits NE synthesis and release, whereas cholinergic depletion increases NE synthesis and release. In addition, nicotine can increase the turnover of NE in the hippocampus and ACh can activate the LC. Behaviorally, neither an LC lesion nor administration of the cholinergic antagonist *scopolamine* affects retention of active avoidance training alone; however, when the two treatments are combined, they produce a severe deficit. Thus, NE and ACh appear to act synergistically to affect some types of memory. Recent evidence suggests that reductions in NE levels are correlated with deficits in hippocampal LTP.

The LC's projections to the PFC also may be indirectly involved in memory. In monkeys and humans, PFC lesions lead to increased distractibility and increased susceptibility to interference by irrelevant stimuli, effects that likely contribute to the observed working memory impairments. The PFCs of patients with attention-deficit/hyperactivity disorder are smaller and less active than those of age-matched controls, and these patients exhibit working memory and attentional impairments, further supporting a role for the PFC in attention. The α_2 agonist *clonidine* significantly ameliorates mnemonic and attentional deficits in young NE-depleted monkeys, suggesting that NE in the PFC may affect memory by reducing interference by distracting or irrelevant stimuli. Because DA is also involved in PFC-dependent tasks, it is likely that NE and DA interact in this area to affect working memory (Ramos and Arnste, 2007).

SEROTONIN INFLUENCES MEMORY AND LONG-TERM POTENTIATION

Almost all serotonergic cell bodies are located in the medial brain-stem region as discrete nuclei termed the *dorsal and medial raphé nuclei*. Projections from these cell bodies extend to virtually all areas of the CNS including the amygdala, thalamus, hypothalamus, olfactory bulb, striatum, basal forebrain, hippocampus, and all regions of the cortex. Its ubiquitous nature and multifaceted functions have made discrete cause-and-effect relationships concerning serontonin's (5-HT's) role in learning and memory difficult to determine (Meneses, 1999). However, characterization of new 5-HT receptor subtypes, as well as new chemical probes that can act with relative specificity toward these receptors, have assisted in this endeavor. Studies in knockout mice and antisense tools also have opened new areas of investigation.

Depletion of 5-HT in certain brain regions, in particular the hippocampus, can impair memory (Buhot et al., 2000). Furthermore, depletion of tryptophan (the amino acid precursor to 5-HT) in the diet of otherwise healthy individuals is correlated with an acute and reversible loss of learning and memory functions. Conversely, 5-HT depletion in PFC in rats is associated with increased plasticity in pyramidal neurons, which in turn potentiates short-term memory.

Of the many 5-HT receptors, 5-HT_{1A}, 5-HT_4, and 5-HT_5 receptors have been associated most consistently with learning and memory (e.g., Malleret et al., 1999). Pharmacological studies, as well as studies in receptor knockout mice, suggest that the 5-HT_{1A} receptors play a role in passive avoidance retention. The 5-HT_4 receptors modulate LTP and long-term depression (LTD). Pharmacological studies, as well as those using receptor antisense oligonucleotides, point to a critical role of 5-HT_6 receptors in enhancing spatial memory in the Morris water maze. 5-HT_7 may also play a role in learning and memory, but this role remains unclear, as 5-HT_7 knockout mice are impaired in contextual fear conditioning but not spatial reference memory in a Barnes maze (Roberts et al., 2004). Some of these changes may take place not via LTP/LTD mechanisms, but by synaptic plasticity and sensory input reorganization, as has been noted in the cholinergic system (Cassel and Jeltsch, 1995).

In addition, 5-HT may influence memory via interactions with the gaseous neurotransmitter nitric oxide (NO). eNOS knockout mice exhibit improved Morris water maze performance and decreased 5-HT turnover in hippocampus and neocortex, suggesting a link between NO and 5-HT. Some behavioral changes might be related to extraneuronal processes, such as blood flow, which NO and 5-HT regulate. Evidence for this 5-HT/NO interaction is bolstered by experiments involving 5-HT_{1B} receptor knockout mice that also show enhanced spatial memory similar to that seen in eNOS knockout mice. It remains to be seen whether this improvement is due specifically to enhanced spatial learning or is a by-product of eNOS alterations of other brain functions that contribute to performance of this task.

VARIOUS NEUROACTIVE PEPTIDES CAN ALSO MODULATE MEMORY

A growing number of peptides have been shown to modulate synaptic plasticity and learning and memory. Many peptides coexist with a variety of classical neurotransmitters and modulate their release in brain regions associated with learning and memory. Examples include ACh and galanin in the septum, GABA and somatostatin in the cortex and hippocampus, and NE and neurotensin in the LC. Several peptides modulate memory including opioids, galanin, oxytocin, vasopressin, neuropeptide Y, cholecystokinin, somatostatin, insulin, neurokinin, and substance P.

Administration of opiate agonists impairs memory, whereas administration of opiate antagonists enhances memory (Decker and McGaugh, 1991). This appears to be true for peripheral administration as well as for intracranial injections. However, intracranial infusions reveal a dissociation between the septohippocampal and amygdalar systems, which are both innervated by opiate peptides. Appetitively motivated tasks testing working memory are affected by intraseptal opiate infusions but not by intra-amygdala infusions, whereas aversively motivated avoidance tasks testing reference memory are affected only by intra-amygdala infusions. In the septum, infusion of the opioid receptor agonist β-endorphin decreases hippocampal ACh turnover, and this effect is blocked by the opioid receptor antagonist *naltrexone*. This result may be due to activation of septal GABAergic interneurons, which inhibit cholinergic neurons that project to the hippocampus. In the amygdala, NE depletion blocks the facilatory effects of naloxone on a passive avoidance task, suggesting an interaction between NE and opioids. Moreover, the naloxone-induced improvements in avoidance and Y-maze discrimination tasks are blocked by injection of noradrenergic β-receptor antagonists injected directly into the amygdala, but not into the striatum or cortex, indicating that NE receptors in the amygdala interact with opiate peptides to affect these types of memory.

The neuromodulatory peptide *galanin* (along with neuropeptide Y) modulates hippocampal function and plays a key role in memory. Galanin impairs a variety of learning and memory tasks including those testing spatial learning, retention, and consolidation (Givens et al., 1992; Wrenn and Crawley, 2001). The inhibitory effects may result from alterations in functional synapses and/or neurotransmitter release in the hippocampus. They may also be mediated through interactions with monoamines. Galanin is colocalized with 5-HT in the dorsal raphé, as well as with NE in the LC, and ACh in the septum. Hence, galanin may modulate the effects of the monoamines and influence cognitive processes via these interactions.

The neurohypophyseal hormones *oxytocin* and *vasopressin* affect memory antagonistically. Vasopressin facilitates memory consolidation and retrieval in rats tested in a variety of avoidance tasks, whereas oxytocin impairs memory in these tasks. The septohippocampal system and raphé nuclei appear to be important for the memory-consolidating effects of these peptides, whereas the amygdala is involved in effects on retrieval (de Wied, 1984). In addition, basal forebrain cholinergic neurons are also innervated by substance P, which enhances retention of passive avoidance if injected into the septum or nBM. The potential importance of substance P to hippocampal-dependent learning and memory is suggested by the fact that knockout mice missing the substance P receptor *neurokinin 3* exhibit cognitive deficits in passive avoidance as well as spatial water maze.

NEUROTROPHIC FACTORS AFFECT LEARNING AND MEMORY VIA MODULATION OF THE CHOLINERGIC AND GLUTAMATERGIC SYSTEMS

Learning and memory are processes that likely include chemical and morphological changes in neurons (Kandel, 2001). It is therefore not surprising that neurotrophic factors, which regulate synaptic modeling and influence neuronal survival, are implicated in learning and memory processes. The first neurotrophic factor was discovered in the peripheral nervous system in the early 1950s (Levi-Montalcini, 1987). This growth-promoting substance was termed *nerve growth factor* (NGF). Since then, other closely related neurotrophins have been discovered, including brain-derived neurotrophic factor (BDNF) and neurotrophins-3 and -4/5 (NT-3, NT-4/5). Three high-affinity receptors appear to be the principal receptors involved in signal transduction. These high-affinity receptors are all transmembrane tyrosine kinases (Trks): TrkA (binds NGF), TrkB (binds BDNF), and TrkC (binds NT-3). NT-4/5 binds to either TrkA or TrkB. All four neurotrophins can also bind a low-affinity receptor termed *p75* or *NGFR*. The hippocampus and neocortex, the main targets of cholinergic innervation from the basal forebrain, contain the highest levels of NGF, BDNF, and NT-3 messenger ribonucleic acids (mRNA) in the mammalian brain. These four trophic factors are target derived and are retrogradely transported to cholinergic projection neuron cell bodies where they appear to interact with receptors on the neurons. Behavioral studies examining animals missing a single neurotrophin or its receptor, as well as animals in which a single neurotrophin has been reintroduced, indicate that all neurotrophic factors play important roles in learning and memory.

Early studies indicated that NGF modulates learning and memory by promoting the survival of basal forebrain cholinergic neurons. Nerve growth factor infusion directly into the brain of rats with transections of the fimbria-fornix, a lesion that results in extensive degeneration of septohippocampal cholinergic neurons and severe spatial memory deficits, significantly reduces septohippocampal cholinergic deterioration and spatial memory deficits induced by the lesion. Similar effects have been demonstrated throughout the basal forebrain. More recent studies indicate that intracranial NGF infusions reduce deficits in memory tasks associated with the age-related loss of basal forebrain cholinergic neurons. The improvement to memory in aging animals has been mirrored in recent clinical trials in which patients with Alzheimer's disease showed some cognitive improvement following treatment with NGF (Williams et al., 2006).

Brain-derived neurotrophic factor, the most abundant neurotrophin in the brain, NT-3, and NT-4/5 all appear to affect learning and memory by modulating LTP (Yamada et al., 2002). Brain-derived neurotrophic factor and TrkB are localized to glutamatergic synapses and may affect synaptic consolidation through immediate early gene signalling cascades. Expression of BDNF and TrkB mRNA increase after spatial and contextual learning. Further, BDNF mRNA levels are up-regulated following exercise, and this increase is correlated with improved cognitive function in several species. Interestingly, heterozygous BDNF knockout mice exhibit impaired LTP and spatial learning, and both of these deficits can be rescued by BDNF. Similarly, a conditional knockout of NT-3 and a knockout of NT-4/5 exhibit impaired LTP, as well as deficits in several hippocampal and amygdala-dependent learning and memory tasks. Despite the tremendous potential of neurotrophins to improve cognitive function in normal patients and patients with dementia, technical problems with drug delivery continue to be a limiting factor in their clinical use (Arancio and Chao, 2007).

STEROID RECEPTORS IN HIPPOCAMPUS AND NEOCORTEX LIKELY MEDIATE STEROID EFFECTS ON MEMORY THROUGH A VARIETY OF MECHANISMS

Steroid hormones, such as estrogens, progestins, and androgens, profoundly affect the function of the hippocampus and neocortex. Receptors for all three of these hormones are found throughout both brain regions, and evidence exists to suggest that all three can modulate hippocampal and cortical function. For example, in female rodents, progesterone modulates hippocampal synaptogenesis, and acute, but not chronic, treatment with progesterone improves spatial and object-recognition memory. Testosterone deprivation impairs spatial working memory in male rats, and testosterone replacement can reverse these deficits (Sandstrom, Kim, and Wasserman, 2006). However, the vast majority of research has focused on estrogens. Estradiol, the most potent form of estrogen, regulates hippocampal dendritic branching and synaptogenesis, enhances membrane excitability and LTP, promotes neurogenesis, and stimulates the activation of numerous intracellular signaling cascades (Woolley, 2007). Estrogens can bind to nuclear (ERα and ERβ) and nonnuclear receptors (identities unknown, possibly associated with the plasma membrane) to influence long- and short-term neural plasticity. Through receptor binding and interactions with modulators such as growth factors, estrogens promote gene transcription, thereby influencing neuronal structure and function. However, directly linking these alterations to memory modulation has proven to be a challenge.

Estrogens released around the time of birth organize female and male hippocampi differently and lead to sex-dependent differences in spatial learning in adulthood. In adulthood, estrogens continue to influence spatial memory: for example, some studies in rodents show subtle variations in spatial memory across the estrous cycle. Other studies find that estradiol treatment improves various types of memory in young and aged female rodents. Estradiol may exert its effects on memory through a variety of mechanisms, including interactions with neurotransmitter systems. For example, estradiol can influence hippocampal excitability by altering cholinergic function in the basal forebrain (Gibbs & Gabor, 2003). Within the hippocampus, estradiol decreases BDNF expression and GABAergic neurotransmission in inhibitory interneurons, leading to disinhibition of pyramidal neurons and formation of new dendritic spines (Segal & Murphy, 2001). Although these alterations are likely the result of estradiol binding to nuclear estrogen receptors, the rapidity of some of estradiol's effects on neural function suggest a critical role for nonnuclear receptors in modulating memory. Data indicating that estradiol is produced locally in the hippocampus present an intriguing new method for rapid estradiol action. For example, estradiol rapidly activates intracellular signal transduction cascades such as the mitogen activated protein kinase (MAP kinase) cascade, and recent data indicate that an estradiol-induced increase in MAPK signaling is necessary for estradiol to improve hippocampal-dependent object memory. Further, this effect can be mediated exclusively by estradiol binding to the plasma membrane, suggesting that memory can be modulated by membrane-associated mechanisms separate from binding to traditional estrogen receptors.

CONCLUSIONS

It should be clear from this brief review that several neurochemical systems are intricately involved in learning and memory processes. Pharmacological studies have provided information about the mnemonic consequences of augmentation or reduction of specific systems, as well as about receptors and secondary and tertiary messenger systems involved in these effects. Lesion studies have provided detailed information about the anatomical distribution of these neurochemical systems and about the alterations in mnemonic processes that result from the absence of a particular transmitter or transmitters. Recent studies have highlighted interactions among transmitters and neuromodulators, making it clear that no neurochemical system influences memory in isolation. In the hippocampus, for example, ACh, glutamate, GABA, NE, 5-HT, peptides, NGF, and hormones all play a role in determining the nature of spatial memories that will be formed and subsequently retrieved. Future investigations will likely continue to focus on the elaborate interplay among transmitters and modulators in learning and memory processes and the specific plastic mechanisms that underlie these effects. Because disturbances of multiple transmitter systems may produce the complex cognitive dysfunction associated with dementia, understanding the intricate interactions among neurochemicals in the brain will be essential for designing effective treatments for dementia.

REFERENCES

Arancio, O., and Chao, M.V. (2007) Neurotrophins, synaptic plasticity and dementia. *Curr. Opin. Neurobio.* 17:325–330.

Bartus, R.T., Dean, R.L., Pontecorvo, M.J., and Flicker, C. (1985) The cholinergic hypothesis: a historical overview, current perspective, and future directions. *Ann. N.Y. Acad. Sci.* 444:332–358.

Baxter, M.G., and Chiba, A.A. (1999) Cognitive functions of the basal forebrain. *Curr. Opin. Neurobiol.* 9:178–183.

Bannerman, D.M., Rawlins, J.N., and Good, M.A. (2006) The drugs don't work—or do they? Pharmacological and transgenic studies of the contribution of NMDA and GluR-A-containing AMPA receptors to hippocampal-dependent memory. *Psychophamacology* 188:552–566.

Bliss, T.V.P., and Lømo, T. (1973) Long-lasting potentiation of synaptic transmission in the dentate area of the anaesthetized rabbit following stimulation of the perforant path. *J. Physiol.* 232: 331–356.

Breen, R.A., and McGaugh, J.L. (1961) Facilitation of maze learning with posttrial injections of picrotoxin. *J. Comp. Physiol. Psychol.* 54:495–501.

Brozoski, T.J., Brown, R.M., Rosvold, H.E., and Goldman, P.S. (1979) Cognitive deficit caused by regional depletion of dopamine in prefrontal cortex of rhesus monkey. *Science* 205:929–932.

Buhot, M.C., Martin, S., and Segu, L. (2000) Role of serotonin in memory impairment. *Ann. Med.* 32:210–221.

Cassel, J.C., and Jeltsch, H. (1995) Serotonergic modulation of cholinergic function in the central nervous system: cognitive implications. *Neuroscience* 69:1–41.

Chamberlain, S.R., Muller, U., Robbins, T.W., and Sahakian B.J. (2006) Neuropharmacological modulation of cogntition. *Curr. Opin. Neurol.* 19:607–612.

Cooper, J.R., Bloom, F.E., and Roth, R.H. (1996) *The Biochemical Basis of Neuropharmacology*, 7th ed. New York: Oxford University Press.

Coyle, J.T., Singer, H., McKinney, M., and Price, D. (1984) Neurotransmitter specific alterations in dementing disorders: insights from animal models. *J. Psychiatr. Res.* 18:501–512.

Dani, J.A., and Bertrand, D. (2007) Nicotinic acetylcholine receptors and nicotinic cholinergic mechanisms of the central nervous system. *Ann. Rev. Pharmacol. Toxicol.* 47:699–729.

Decker, M.W., and McGaugh, J.L. (1991) Role of interactions between the cholinergic system and other neuromodulatory systems in learning and memory. *Synapse* 7:151–168.

de Wied, D. (1984) Neurohypophyseal hormone influences on learning and memory processes. In: Lynch, G., McGaugh, J.L., and Weinberger, N.M., eds. *Neurobiology of Learning and Memory*. New York: Guilford Press, pp. 289–312.

El-Ghundi, M., O'Dowd, B.F., and George, S.R. (2007) Insights into the role of dopamine receptor systems in learning and memory. *Rev. Neurosci.* 18:37-66.

Ellis, K.A., and Nathan, P.J. (2001) The pharmacology of human working memory. *Int. J. Neuropsychopharmacol.* 4:299–313.

Feng, R., Rampon, C., et al. (2001) Deficient neurogenesis in forebrain-specific presenilin-1 knockout mice is associated with reduced clearance of hipppocampal memory traces. *Neuron* 32: 911–926.

Gibbs, R.B., and Gabor, R. (2003) Estrogen and cognition: Applying preclinical findings to clinical perspectives. *J. Neurosci. Res.* 74: 637–643.

Givens, B.S., Olton, D.S., and Crawley, J.N. (1992) Galanin in the medial septal area impairs working memory. *Brain Res.* 582:71–77.

Hebb, D.O. (1949) *The Organization of Behavior.* New York: John Wiley & Sons.

Henderson, V.W., Paganini-Hill, A., Emanuel, C.K., Dunn, M.E., and Buckwalter, J.G. (1994) Estrogen replacement therapy in older women. Comparisons between Alzheimer's disease cases and nondemented control subjects. *Arch. Neurol.* 51:896–900.

Jones, S., Sudweeks, S., and Yakel, J.L. (1999) Nicotinic receptors in the brain: correlating physiology with function. *Trends Neurosci.* 22:555–561.

Kandel, E.R. (2001) The molecular biology of memory storage: a dialogue between genes and synapses. *Science* 294:1030–1038.

Knopman, D.S. (2006) Current treatment of mild cognitive impairment and Alzheimer's disease. *Curr. Neurol. Neurosci. Rep.* 6: 365–371.

Levi-Montalcini, R. (1987) The nerve growth factor 35 years later. *Science* 237:1154–1162.

MacDonald, J.F., Jackson, M.F., and Beazely, M.A. (2006) Hippocampal long-term synaptic plasticity and signal amplification of NMDA receptors *Crit. Rev. Neurobiol.* 18:71–84.

Malleret, G., Hen, R., Guillou, J.L., Segu, L., and Buhot, M.C. (1999) 5-HT1B receptor knock-out mice exhibit increased exploratory activity and enhanced spatial memory performance in the Morris water maze. *J. Neurosci.* 19(14):6157–6168.

McEwen, B.S. (2001) Tracking the estrogen receptor in neurons: implications for estrogen-induced synapse formation. *Proc. Natl. Acad. Sci. USA* 98:7093–7100.

Meneses, A. (1999) 5-HT system and cognition. *Neurosci. Biobehav. Rev.* 23:1111–1125.

Morris, R.G.M. (1986) Selective impairment of learning and blockade of long-term potentiation by an N-methyl-D-aspartate receptor antagonist, AP5. *Nature* 319:774–776.

Musial, A., Bajda, M., and Malawska, B. (2007) Recent developments in cholinesterase inhibitors for Alzheimer's disease treatment. *Curr. Med. Chem.* 14:2654–2679.

Nestler, E.J., Hymam, S.E., and Malenka, R.C. (2001) *Molecular Neuropharmacology*. New York: McGraw-Hill Medical Publishing.

Olton, D.S., Becker, J.T., and Handelmann, G.E. (1979) Hippocampus, space, and memory. *Behav. Brain Sci.* 2:313–365.

Ramos, B.P., and Arnste, A.F. (2007) Adrenergic pharmacology and cognition: focus on the prefrontal cortex. *Pharmacol. Ther.* 113: 523–536.

Rasmusson, D.D. (2000) The role of acetylcholine in cortical synaptic plasticity. *Behav. Brain Res.* 115:205–218.

Roberts, A.J., Krucker, T., Levy, C.L., Slanina, K.A., Sutcliffe, J.F., and Hedlund, P.B. (2004) Mice lacking 5-HT receptors show specific impairments in contextual learning. *Eur. J. Neurosci.* 19:1913–1922.

Sandstrom, N.J., Kim, J. H., and Wasserman, M.A. (2006) Testosterone modulates performance on a spatial working memory task in male rats. *Horm. Behav.* 50:18–26.

Sawaguchi, T., and Goldman-Rakic, P.S. (1991) D1 dopamine receptors in prefrontal cortex: involvement in working memory. *Science* 251:947–950.

Schimanski, L.A., Ali, D.W., Baker, G.B., and Nquyen, P.V. (2007) Impaired hippocampal LTP in inbred mouse strains can be rescued by beta-adrenergic receptor activation. *Eur. J. Neurosci.* 25: 1589–1598.

Segal, M., and Murphy, D. (2001) Estradiol induces formation of dendritic spines in hippocampal neurons: functional correlates. *Horm. Behav.* 40, 156–159.

Siegel, G.W., Agranof, B.W., Albers, R.W., Fisher, S.K., and Uhler, M.D., eds. (1999) *Basic Neurochemistry: Molecular, Cellular, and Medical Aspects*, 6th ed. New York: Lippincott-Raven.

Sieghart, W. (2006) Structure, pharmacology, and function of $GABA_A$ recptor subtypes. *Adv. Pharmacol.* 54:231–63.

Walsh, T.J., and Stackman, R.W. (1992) Modulation of memory by benzodiazepine-acetylcholine interactions. In: Levin, E.D., Decker, M.W., and Butcher, L.L., eds. *Neurotransmitter Interactions and Cognitive Function*. Boston: Birkhauser, pp. 312–328.

Williams, B.J., Eriksdotter-Jonhagen, M., and Granholm, A.C. (2006) Nerve growth factor in treatment and pathogenesis of Alzheimer's disease. *Prog. Neurobiol.* 80:114–128.

Woolley, C.S. (2007) Acute effects of estrogen on neuronal physiology. *Annu. Rev. Pharmacol. Toxicol.* 47:657–680.

Wrenn, C.C., and Crawley, J.N. (2001) Pharmacological evidence supporting a role for galanin in cognition and affect. *Prog. Neuropsychopharmacol. Biol. Psychiatry* 25:283–299.

Wu, L., Wells, D., Tay, J., Mendis, D., Abbott, M.A., Barnitt, A., Quinlan, E., Heynen, A., Fallon, J.R., and Ritchter, J.D. (1998) CPEB-mediated cytoplasmic polyadenylation and the regulation of experience-dependent translation of alpha-CaMKII and mRNA at synapses. *Neuron* 21:1129–1139.

Wu, M., Shanabrough, M., Leranth, C., and Alreja, M. (2000) Cholinergic excitation of septohippocampal GABA but not cholinergic neurons: implications for learning and memory. *J. Neurosci.* 20:3900–3908.

Yamada, K., Mizuno, M., and Nabeshima, T. (2002) Role for brain-derived neurotrophic factor in learning and memory. *Life Sci.* 70:735–744.

57 Neuropathological and Neuroimaging Studies of the Hippocampus in Normal Aging and in Alzheimer's Disease

EFFIE M. MITSIS, MATTHEW BOBINSKI, MIROSLAW BRYS, LIDIA GLODZIK-SOBANSKA, SUSAN DeSANTI, YI LI, BYEONG-CHAE KIM, LISA MOSCONI, AND MONY J. DE LEON

This chapter was revised by Effie M. Mitsis, PhD, from an earlier version written and published in this textbook by the NYU group.

Recent estimates suggest that Alzheimer's disease (AD), the most common type of dementia seen after age 60 years, affects an estimated 15 million people worldwide. In the year 2000, there were 4.5 million people with AD in the U.S. population, and prevalence projections estimate that this number will increase by threefold to 13.2 million people by the year 2050 (Hebert et al., 2003). Other data show that for every patient with dementia, there are approximately eight individuals with no dementia with cognitive deterioration adversely affecting their quality of life (Larrabee and Crook, 1994). Prevalence rates for individuals older than age 65 years with mild cognitive impairment (MCI), considered a prodromal stage of AD, range between 3% for a neuropsychologically defined amnestic subtype (Ganguli et al., 2004; Manly et al., 2005) to as high as 25% when all cognitive subtypes of MCI are considered (Manly et al., 2005). Therefore, with respect to the above estimates, a staggering number of elderly persons with mild to severe cognitive impairments, perhaps 10–20 million, can be expected in the next 35 years, representing a great human and economic toll. Cross-sectional and longitudinal studies commonly observe subtle declines in cognitive functioning associated with aging, and the underlying brain anatomy and physiological mechanisms responsible for these age-related declines in cognition are becoming better understood. Neuropathology and structural neuroimaging studies consistently point to the hippocampal formation as a key structure in understanding age-related cognitive changes, particularly memory impairments.

Neuropathology studies identify the neurons of the hippocampal formation, which includes the entorhinal cortex (EC), hippocampus, and subiculum, as the most vulnerable to the age-related deposition of neurofibrillary tangles (NFT; Braak and Braak, 1991), a diagnostic feature of AD, with synaptic dysfunction (Braak and Braak, 1991), synaptic loss (Scheff et al., 2007), and neuronal loss leading to gross atrophy (Hyman et al., 1984; Gomez-Isla et al., 1996; Bobinski et al., 1997). Moreover, for many elderly patients with MCI, NFT deposition in the hippocampal formation is a relatively focal phenomenon (Giannakopoulos et al., 1994). With the progression of clinical symptoms, there is a correlated progression of the neuropathology with increasing involvement of the neocortex (Braak and Braak, 1991). Similarly, in-vivo neuroimaging studies have demonstrated anatomically specific volume reductions in the hippocampus of patients with MCI (Convit et al., 1997; Jack et al., 1999; De Santi et al., 2001; Jack et al., 2005; van de Pol et al., 2007). As a group, patients with MCI are at increased risk to develop symptoms of AD within a few years. Longitudinal neuroimaging studies show that hippocampal volume and measures of delayed verbal recall are accurate predictors of future dementia in patients with MCI. In neuropathology and neuroimaging studies, the dementia symptoms of AD are associated with hippocampal formation and neocortical pathology. Magnetic resonance imaging (MRI) studies in patients with AD have shown that cortical atrophy occurs in defined sequences as the disease progresses, which is comparable to the pattern of NFT accumulation seen in cross-section at autopsy (Thompson, 2003). Severe EC and hippocampal atrophy is consistently found in patients with mild AD (Jack et al, 1992; Convit et al., 1997), whereas volume reductions in cortical regions are apparent in the more advanced stages of disease (Convit et al., 1997). As our ability to detect the anatomic changes in the hippocampal formation improves, so does our ability to detect patients at increased risk for AD. Improved early detection of AD-related brain changes will be of value in future therapeutic studies examining patients with MCI and possibly even patients at earlier preclinical stages.

The purpose of this chapter is threefold: (*1*) to describe the normal anatomy of the hippocampal formation and the sites vulnerable to neuropathological changes in normal aging and AD; particular emphasis will be placed on the hippocampus proper, with descriptions using histological criteria and the gross landmarks visible with in-vivo structural neuroimaging; (*2*) to briefly review relationships between hippocampal formation damage and neuropsychological performances; and (*3*) to present data that support the hypothesis that hippocampal formation atrophy occurs early in the natural history of AD and actually precedes neocortical involvement.

HIPPOCAMPAL FORMATION NEUROANATOMY

The hippocampal formation is one of the major parts of the allocortex (a phylogenetically older cortex that is part of the rhinencephalon). It consists of the hippocampus proper (hippocampus), dentate gyrus, subicular complex, and EC (Rosene and Van Hoesen, 1987; Amaral and Insausti, 1990).

General Boundaries of the Hippocampus

In the human brain, the hippocampus proper is particularly well developed, occupying the temporal lobe in the floor of the temporal (inferior) horn of the lateral ventricle. The hippocampus is known for its seahorse-like appearance, and much of its gross anatomy can be viewed in vivo with MRI. The length of the hippocampus is about 4 to 5 cm, with a maximal width of about 2 cm and a maximal height of about 1.5 cm (Duvernoy, 1988).

The boundaries of the hippocampus vary along its rostrocaudal length. To illustrate these boundaries at four levels along the hippocampal length, we will use in-vivo T1-weighted MRI scans and postmortem sections stained with cresyl violet (Fig. 57.1A–H). Note that the numbers in brackets in the text correspond to those indicated in the figures. Figures 57.1A and 57.1B represent the anterior hippocampus at the level of the amygdaloid body. At this level the hippocampus ⟨1⟩ is bounded dorsally by the amygdala ⟨2⟩, laterally by the temporal horn ⟨3⟩, inferiorly by the subiculum ⟨4⟩ and the white matter of the parahippocampal gyrus (PG) ⟨5⟩, and medially by the ambient cistern ⟨6⟩. The PG ⟨5⟩ is bounded laterally by the collateral sulcus ⟨7⟩ and inferiorly by the entorhinal ⟨8⟩ and transentorhinal cortices. At this level, the EC extends medially to cover the ambiens ⟨9⟩ and semilunar gyri ⟨10⟩. The boundary between the hippocampus and the amygdala is somewhat indistinct. However, using sagittal views, which are readily obtained with MRI, the visual separation between amygdala and hippocampus can be facilitated (Convit et al., 1999). More posteriorly, at the level of the hippocampal head (also referred to as the pes hippocampus or uncus) (Fig. 57.1C, D), the hippocampus ⟨11⟩ is more complex in shape. Posterior levels of the hippocampus have the shape of a figure eight lying on its side with the temporal horn ⟨3⟩ laterally; the uncal sulcus ⟨11⟩, the white matter of the PG, and the subiculum ⟨4⟩ inferiorly; the choroid plexus of the temporal horn ⟨3a⟩ superiorly; and the ambient cistern ⟨6⟩ medially. The PG is bounded inferiorly and medially by the tentorium cerebelli ⟨12⟩ and laterally by the collateral sulcus. The entorhinal cortex at this level is bounded mainly between the collateral sulcus and the medial aspect (uncus) of the PG. Figures 57.1E and 57.1F represent the level of the body of the hippocampus. At this level the lateral and superior hippocampus boundaries are the temporal horn ⟨3⟩ and choroid plexus of the lateral ventricle. The inferior boundary is the subiculum ⟨4⟩ and the white matter of the PG ⟨5⟩. On the dorsal and medial border of the hippocampus is the fimbria (Fi) ⟨13⟩, which is made up of white matter fibers that extend posteriorly to form the fornix. The cerebrospinal fluid space medial to the body of the hippocampus is the transverse fissure of Bichat ⟨14⟩, which bounds the dentate gyrus medially and separates the subiculum ⟨4⟩ from the thalamus (lateral geniculate level) ⟨15⟩ over the length of the body and tail of the hippocampus. Figures 57.1G and 57.1H represent the tail of the hippocampus at the level of the splenium of the corpus callosum ⟨17⟩. At this level, the hippocampus ⟨1⟩ is inferior and lateral to the fornix ⟨16⟩ and the splenium of the corpus callosum.

The Hippocampus

The individual fields of the hippocampus can be pictured as a stacked bundle of tissue strips running rostrocaudally in the temporal lobe. The distinctive C shape of the hippocampus is present when the bundled strips fold over each other mediolaterally, as seen in the midportion or body of the hippocampus (Fig. 57.1F). On

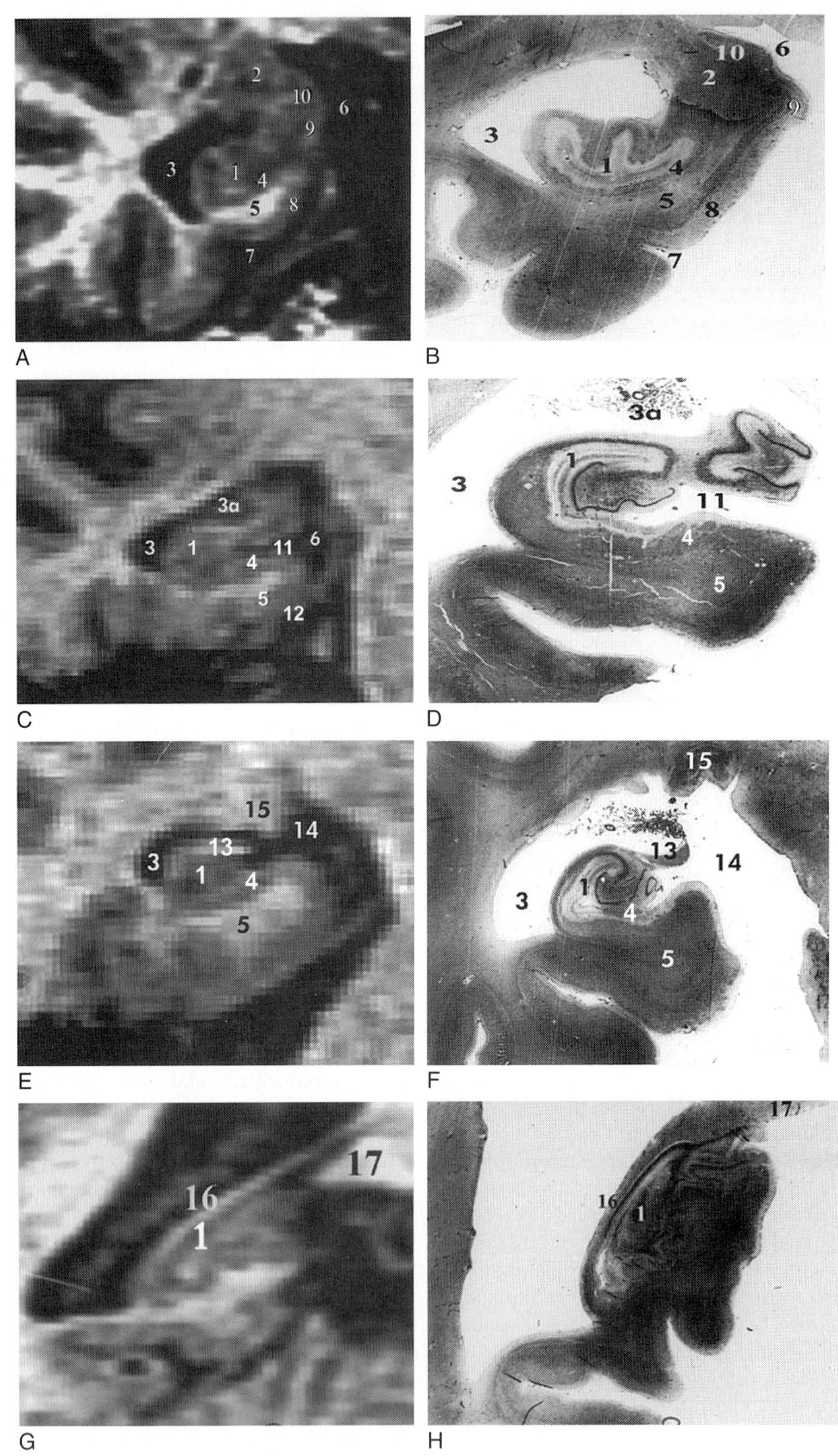

FIGURE 57.1 (*A–H*) Postmortem histological sections stained with cresyl violet and T1-weighted in vivo magnetic resonance imaging coronal images depicting the normal anatomy of the hippocampal region.

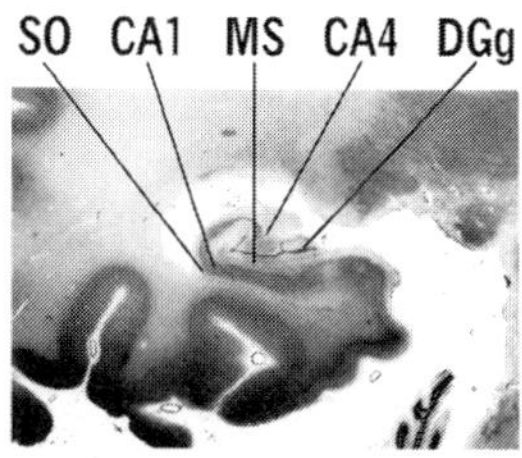

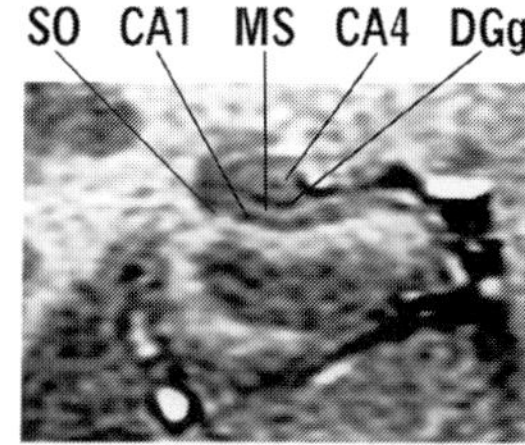

FIGURE 57.2 Postmortem histological slice and corresponding high-resolution coronal magnetic resonance image through the hippocampal body depicting the alveus and the stratum oriens (SO); stratum pyramidale of the CA1 (CA1); a multistrata layer composed of the stratum radiatum, lacunosum, and moleculare of the cornu Ammonis and the molecular layer of the dentate gyrus (MS); sector CA4 (CA4); and the granule layer of the dentate gyrus (DGg).

more rostral sections, the hippocampus bends sharply in a medial and then in a caudal direction. The more rostral levels of the hippocampal structure are more complex, mostly due to a varied number of rostrocaudal flexures. At caudal levels (hippocampal tail), the hippocampus bends dorsally and ascends toward the splenium. As part of allocortex, the cornu Ammonis (hippocampus proper) has three major layers: (*1*) the stratum oriens, (*2*) the stratum pyramidale, and (*3*) a layer that blends the strata radiatum, lacunosum, and moleculare. Aspects of these layers can be appreciated using MRI (Fig. 57.2). On the basis of types of the pyramidal neurons, the cornu Ammonis can be divided into four sectors: CA1 to CA4.

Subicular Complex

The subicular complex is divided into three parts: the subiculum proper, presubiculum, and parasubiculum. Subicular complex subdivisions consist of two layers: (*1*) the molecular layer and (*2*) the pyramidal layer. In the presubiculum, a layer interposed between the molecular and the pyramidal layers, the parvopyramidal layer, is distinguished.

Entorhinal Cortex

The EC and the transentorhinal cortex form a major part of the anterior PG. Phylogenetically, they are relatively old structures. Based on histology and connectivity, the EC is transitional between the hippocampus and the neocortex. The term *entorhinal cortex* was introduced by Brodmann (1909) as a synonym for his area 28. Subsequent studies divided the entorhinal cortex into many fields (Vogt and Vogt, 1919; Braak, 1972) and increased the number to as many as 23 different fields (Rose, 1927). Recent cytoarchitectonic studies showed that parcellation of the entorhinal cortex in humans is largely parallel to that in the monkey and distinguishes only eight different fields (Amaral et al., 1987; Insausti et al., 1995). However, to date, little is known about the physiological function and the consequences of pathology in these fields.

The EC is made up of six layers (Amaral and Insausti, 1990; Insausti et al., 1995). Layer II is one of the most outstanding and distinguishing areas of the EC and is made up of islands of large, modified pyramidal and stellate cells. Compared with the neocortex, one of the most characteristic features of the EC in all species is the absence of an internal granular layer. In its place is an acellular layer of dense fibers called the lamina dissecans.

The EC is adjacent to the more lateral perirhinal cortex (areas 35 and 36 of Brodmann). There is no clear-cut border between area 35 and the EC, and these two fields appear to have an obliquely oriented boundary, where the deep layers of the EC extend somewhat more laterally than the superficial layers. This distinctly angled border between area 35 and the EC has been emphasized by Braak (1980), who has labeled the region of overlap the transentorhinal cortex. With serial coronal MRI sections, one may reliably identify gyral landmarks that are approximate boundaries for the EC region. These landmarks include, on the medial surface, the semilunar gyrus and the gyrus semianularis. The lateral boundary is approximated at anterior levels by the rhinal sulcus and posteriorly by the collateral sulcus.

Hippocampal Formation Connections

The EC, the gateway to the hippocampus, receives massive synaptic input from neocortical association areas and less pronounced input from primary sensory areas (Van Hoesen, 1982; Suzuki and Amaral, 1994). In addition, it receives input from many subcortical regions, including the midbrain raphé nuclei, the ventral tegmental area, the locus coeruleus, the septum, the thalamus and hypothalamus, the amygdala, the magnocellular basal forebrain nuclei, and the claustrum (Insausti et al., 1987). The EC provides the major source of afferent information to the hippocampus via the perforant path (Witter and Amaral, 1991). The predominant component of the perforant path has been regarded as the projection from the stellate layer II neurons of the EC that synapses in the molecular layer on the dendrites of the granular cells of the dentate gyrus. In the classical model of the trisynaptic circuit, this is the first link, followed by the mossy fiber connections to CA3 pyramidal cells and completed by the Schaffer collateral input to CA1. This simplified circuit diagram has been modified recently as it has been shown that there is actually a second distinct projection from the entorhinal cortex, the alternative perforant pathway, that contributes fibers to all the hippocampal fields and to the subiculum (Witter and Amaral, 1991). The alternative

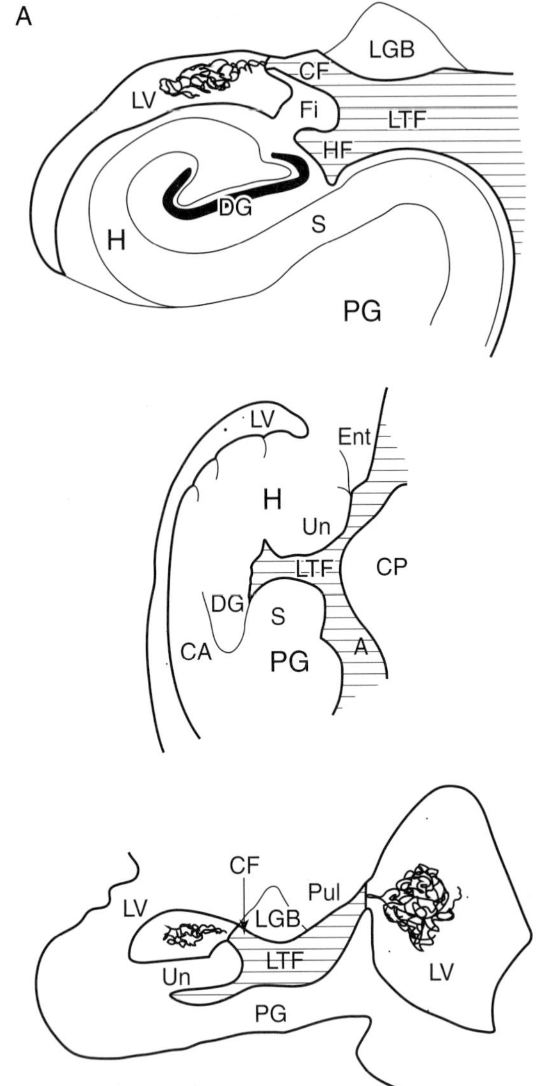

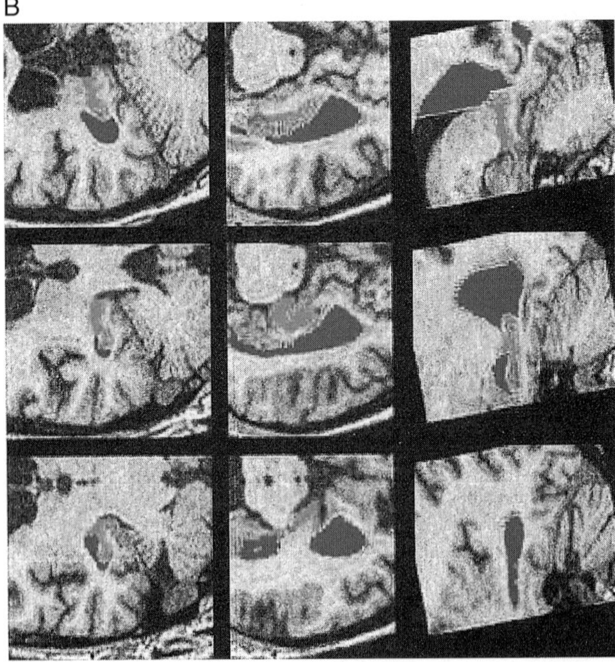

perforant pathway is formed by projection from neurons of layers II and III of the EC to the subiculum, CA1, CA2, and CA3. Much hippocampal output is also directed back to the EC and neocortex directly from CA1 and via relays in the subiculum. Thus, the EC occupies the key position with respect to gating the interactions, output as well as input, between the hippocampus and the rest of the brain.

Cerebrospinal Fluid Anatomy of the Hippocampus

Cerebrospinal fluid (CSF) marks the boundary of the hippocampus over a large surface area. This includes the temporal horn and a complex of CSF containing fissures and cisterns. Figures 57.3A and 57.3B (see also COLOR FIGURE 57.3B in separate insert) depict the orientation of the transverse fissure relative to the hippocampus, PG, thalamic structures, and ventricular CSF in three orthogonal planes. These CSF landmarks are of particular interest for in-vivo imaging, as they provide high-contrast boundaries between the hippocampus and surrounding structures such as the thalamus. In addition, increases in these CSF spaces reflect regional tissue atrophy, and they are therefore of interest in the clinical evaluation. In the coronal view (see Fig. 57.3A, top panel), the lateral boundaries of the transverse fissure of Bichat (also known as the lateral transverse fissure [LTF]) is the medial aspect of the dentate gyrus (DG) and the Fi. The coronal view best permits separation of the choroidal fissure (CF) and hippocampal fissure (HF) extensions of the LTF. In the horizontal or axial view, the LTF begins at the posterior border of the pes hippocampus or uncus (Un) (Fig. 57.3A, middle panel). Medially, the LTF communicates with the

FIGURE 57.3 (*A*) Schematic representations of coronal (top panel), axial (middle panel), and sagittal (bottom panel) views of the hippocampal region. A: ambient cistern; CA: cornu Ammonis; CF: choroids fissure recess; CP: cerebral peduncle; DG: dentate gyrus; Ent: entorhinal cortex; Fi: fimbria; H: hippocampus; HF: hippocampal fissure; LGB: lateral geniculate body; LTF: lateral tranverse fissure; LV: lateral ventricle; PG: parahippocampal gyrus; Pul: pulvinar; S: subiculum; and Un: uncus. (*B*) The magnetic resonance imaging scans were obtained on a General Electric Advantage 1.5T imager using a spoiled gradient echo sequence of 35/9/1 (TR/TE/excitations), a 60 degree flip angle, an 18 cm field of view, and a 256 × 128 acquisition matrix. We obtained 124 contiguous coronal images with a slice thickness of 1.3 mm. On 56 of these images, using a twofold image magnification to aid in region drawing (pixel size = 0.35 mm), we outlined and coded in yellow (see Figure 57.3B in color insert) the hippocampal fissures. Also, the cerebrospinal fluid (CSF) of the lateral ventricle was outlined and coded in red. The top panel shows 3 of the 56 slices coded. All 56 coronal images and the coded regions were reformatted and displayed as 5 mm contiguous slices in a negative angulation axial plane (middle panel) and in a sagittal plane (bottom panel). The reformatted axial images and sagittal images depict the anatomical relationship of the two CSF compartments.

ambient cistern kAl, which borders the cerebral peduncles kCPl. The coronal and sagittal planes (Fig. 57.3A, bottom panel) of section permit identification of the structures bounding the ventral surface of the transverse fissure, namely, the subiculum of the PG, as well as the identification of those thalamic structures bounding the dorsal margin, the lateral geniculate body (LGB), and the pulvinar (Pul).

NEUROPATHOLOGY

Hippocampal Atrophy in Alzheimer's Disease

Impairment of memory is one of the earliest features of AD. Clinical symptoms slowly increase in severity and are accompanied by personality changes, deterioration of language functions, and involvement of the extrapyramidal motor system (Reisberg et al., 1982). Disease severity is associated with a hierarchy of pathological changes progressing from the EC and hippocampus to involvement of the neocortex (Braak and Braak, 1991). Hippocampal atrophy rates, detectable on MRI up to 5 years prior to clinical expression of the disease (Fox et al., 1999; Schott et al., 2003), may be considered a surrogate marker for disease progression and predict progressive cognitive decline (Jack et al., 2000; Barnes et al., 2004; Jack et al., 2005; Mungas et al., 2005) even in aging individuals without subjective memory complaint and with normal baseline scores on cognitive tasks (den Heijer et al., 2006). After disease onset, the spreading sequence of neocortical atrophy mirrors the progressive spread of amyloid plaques and NFT in the brain (Braak and Braak, 1997).

Postmortem histopathological studies show that the hippocampal formation, especially the entorhinal and transentorhinal cortices, is one of the earliest and most severely affected structures in AD (Hyman et al., 1984; Braak and Braak, 1991). Morphological studies of the hippocampal formation reveal neurofibrillary changes and granulovacuolar degeneration of neurons, synaptic and neuronal loss, and amyloid β deposition in plaques and vascular walls (Ball et al., 1985; Braak and Braak, 1991). Neurofibrillary degeneration and the loss of projection neurons responsible for the majority of afferent and efferent connections of the hippocampal formation cause the disruption of intrahippocampal connections and functional isolation of the hippocampal formation from other parts of the memory system (Hyman et al., 1984). Neuronal loss in the hippocampal formation appears to be a major component of the memory impairment seen in AD (Hyman et al., 1984; Bobinski et al., 1997). Neurofibrillary degeneration has been put forth as a cause of neuronal loss and atrophy of the hippocampal formation (Hyman et al., 1984; Davies et al., 1992; Bobinski et al., 1996; Bobinski et al., 1997). The later onset of amyloid deposits in the hippocampal formation subdivisions and the topographical differences in distribution and number suggest that amyloid and neurofibrillary changes develop independently (Bouras et al., 1994). The impact of amyloid deposits on hippocampal formation atrophy is not known.

The severe atrophy of the hippocampal formation in AD is found, to a similar extent, in cellular and fiber layers (Bobinski et al., 1995; Bobinski et al., 1996). Our detailed volumetric study of the hippocampal formation showed marked volume losses in the pyramidal layer of the cornu Ammonis (61%), in the stratum radiatum (74%), and in the lacunosum/moleculare (66%) in patients severely affected by AD compared to normal controls (Bobinski et al., 1995). The volumetric loss of the pyramidal layer reflects the loss of pyramidal cells, whereas the decrease in the volume of the stratum radiatum and lacunosum/moleculare encompasses the loss of (*1*) apical dendrites of the pyramidal cells and (*2*) the perforant fibers and Schaffer collaterals. In the subicular complex, patients severely affected by AD also showed a 68% volumetric loss of the pyramidal layer. This volume loss is a direct effect of loss of cell bodies and perineuronal processes. The atrophy of the apical dendrites of pyramidal cells, and of the dense network of fibers running through the molecular layer of the subicular complex, probably accounts for the 54% decrement in the volume of this layer. The DG is the only hippocampal subdivision that does not manifest a significant volumetric decrement relative to controls. The granular layer is mostly spared in the course of AD and is affected by neurofibrillary pathology only in late-stage AD (Braak and Braak, 1991). In this study, neuronal counts were not made in the EC.

In another pathological study (Bobinski et al., 1995), the volume of the hippocampal formation subdivisions was examined for their relationship to the stage (as determined by the Functional Assessment Staging [FAST] procedure scale) and the duration of AD. Using the FAST scale, the following significant relationships were observed with regional volume measures: CA1 (r52.79), subiculum (r52.75), and EC (r52.62) (Fig. 57.4; see also COLOR FIGURE 57.4 in separate insert).

Over the estimated duration of clinically manifest AD, calculations projected an overall decrease of 60% in the volume of the hippocampal formation. These volumetric decreases in the cornu Ammonis, subicular complex, and EC were 64%, 70%, and 51%, respectively. These cross-sectionally derived results suggest that changes occur in the hippocampal formation and most of its structural components throughout the course of AD (Fig. 57.5).

Determination of the subvolumes of the whole hippocampal formation and estimation of the total number of neurons, NFT, and amyloid deposits in these volumes enabled analysis of the relationships between pathological lesions, neuronal number, and volume of

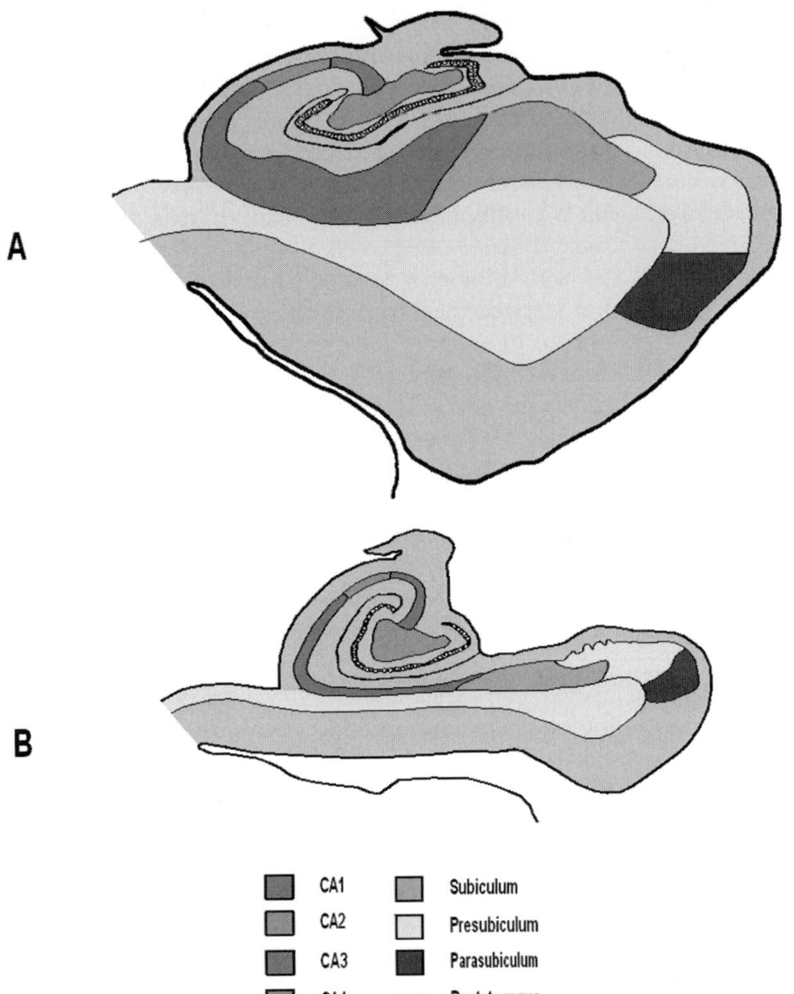

FIGURE 57.4 Schematic drawings of histologically derived volumes of the hippocampus and subicular complex. (*A*) is the average normal control and (*B*) is the average Alzheimer's disease (AD) patient.

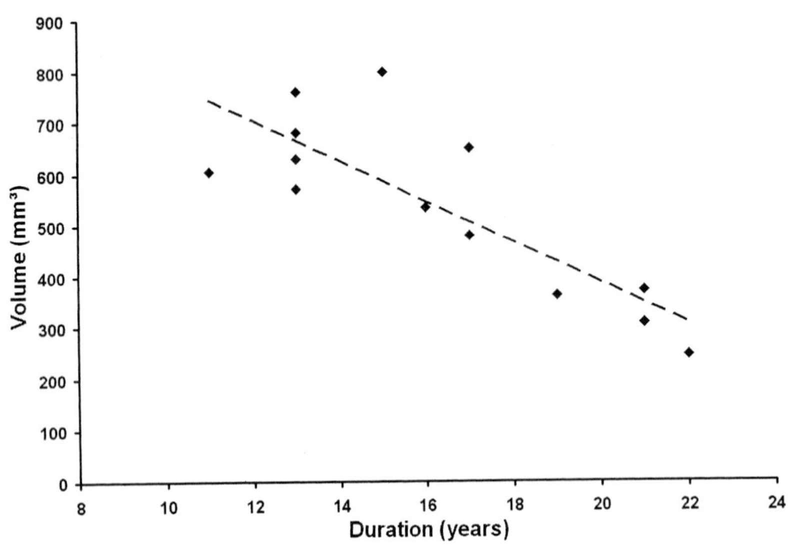

FIGURE 57.5 Scattergram plotting volume of CA1 with disease duration.

the hippocampal subdivisions (Bobinski et al., 1996). Specifically, the volume in the hippocampus proper, as determined by either histological criteria or postmortem MRI studies, correlated linearly with number of neurons (r5.91; Fig. 57.6). This finding, as well as the observation that the volume of the hippocampus as determined by MRI reflects the actual size of the structure (Bobinski et al., 2000), is of particular relevance to in-vivo neuroimaging. These data support the contention that in-vivo neuroimaging measures of atrophy reflect actual histological damage and neuronal loss (see below).

Alzheimer's Disease–Related Neuronal Loss

Neuronal loss in the hippocampal formation in AD has been described by many authors. However, NFT lesions account for only a small proportion of hippocampal neuronal loss (Kril et al., 2002). The EC, CA1, and subiculum are consistently affected severely, whereas the granular layer of the DG is generally spared (Davies et al., 1992; West et al., 1994; Gomez-Isla et al., 1996). Studies of the hippocampus proper show that the number of subdivisions showing neuronal loss depends to a great extent on the duration of the illness and/or the clinical stage of AD in the patients investigated (Bobinski et al., 1997). For those individuals clinically least affected, significant neuronal loss was observed in the CA1 and subiculum. For the patients with more severe AD, significant neuronal loss was observed in CA1, CA2, CA3, CA4, and the subiculum. Recent studies of the EC add to our understanding by demonstrating clear evidence for early neuronal loss (Gomez-Isla et al., 1996). Moreover, neuronal loss correlates with the percentage of neurons with neurofibrillary changes among all neurons (r5.73) (Bobinski et al., 1996). This suggests that neurofibrillary pathology is a possible etiological factor in neuronal and volumetric loss in the hippocampal formation of patients with AD. On the other hand, no significant relationships were found between either neuronal counts or volumes of the hippocampal formation subdivisions and the numerical density of plaques, or the total number of plaques, or the area occupied by amyloid, or the density of vessels with amyloid angiopathy. Therefore, the data indicate that unlike tangle pathology, plaque pathology may not be associated with neuronal loss.

Despite the complex connectivity in the hippocampal formation, neurofibrillary pathology and neuronal loss appear to develop in a structure-specific fashion. Braak and Braak (1991) described a staging scheme of neurofibrillary changes in the brain based on the temporal and topographical distribution of these lesions. According to these authors, neurofibrillary changes develop first in the transentorhinal cortex and then in the EC (*transentorhinal stages*). Further progression involves CA1, the subiculum, and CA4, then sectors CA2 and CA3 of the cornu Ammonis and the parvopyramidal layer of the presubiculum. This was referred to as the *limbic stage* of pathology. The changes in the dentate gyrus and all isocortical association areas (neocortex) appear in the last stage of this classification, the *isocortical stages*.

These observations have been extended to include specific layers in the hippocampal formation (Thal et al., 2000). The first abnormally phosphorylated tau is located in perikarya and dendrites of layer II neurons of the entorhinal and transentorhinal cortices. Next, it appears in the pyramidal layer of CA1 and subiculum, then in the stratum radiatum and oriens, and finally in the outer molecular layer of the DG, which is the perforant pathway target zone. The involvement of the

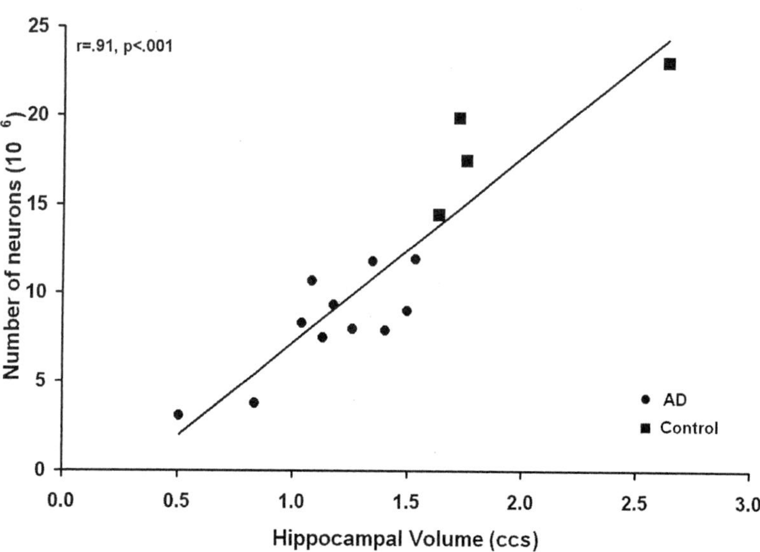

FIGURE 57.6 Scattergram depicting the relationship between hippocampal volume and hippocampal neuronal counts in Alzheimer's disease (AD) patients and controls.

stratum oriens, together with the stratum radiatum and the outer molecular layer of the DG, is seen almost exclusively in individuals with dementia (Thal et al., 2000).

West et al. (1994), who, using unbiased stereological techniques, estimated the total number of neurons in several hippocampal formation subdivisions, also reported structure-specific neuronal loss in AD. Among normal controls they found neuronal losses in two subdivisions, the hilus (CA4) and the subiculum. In the AD group they also observed additional loss of neurons in CA1. Therefore, the pathology of AD does not simply reflect an acceleration of normal aging. The regional pattern of neuronal loss in AD is qualitatively and quantitatively different from that observed in normal aging.

Selective vulnerability of the CA1 sector is supported by observation of marked neuronal loss in the limbic stages (Braak's stage III and IV) (Rossler et al., 2002). Compared to stage I, the number of pyramidal neurons in CA1 was reduced by 33% in stage IV and by 51% in stage V. In the subiculum, significant neuronal loss was found only in stage V (22%).

In a detailed stereology study performed on brains of patients with moderate to severe AD and normal controls, we examined the number of neurons and NFT in the hippocampus (Bobinski et al., 1997). The CA1 sector was severely affected by neurofibrillary pathology and neuronal loss. In this sector there was a profound loss of neurons (86%), and 71% of the surviving neurons were affected by neurofibrillary changes. The subiculum showed somewhat less pathology: the neuronal loss was 68%, and 52% of surviving neurons were affected by neurofibrillary pathology. Other structures, such as CA2, CA3, and CA4, are much less affected by neuronal loss (75%, 53%, and 55%, respectively) and neurofibrillary pathology (33%, 26%, and 28% of surviving neurons, respectively). Finally, the granular layer of the DG was the only hippocampal subdivision without significant neuronal loss over the course of AD. This surprising finding may reflect a unique lack of vulnerability of these cells or may be related to increased cellular plasticity in this region. In the AD group, only 4% of the neurons in the granular layer of the DG showed neurofibrillary changes. Overall, these results support the hypothesis that there is a selective pattern of neuronal vulnerability in AD.

Postmortem studies have documented the presence of NFT in the EC and transentorhinal cortex of elderly individuals with no dementia (Hof et al., 1992). In the brains of patients with early-stage AD, neurofibrillary changes are always detectable in the EC and transentorhinal cortex. Consequently, pathology limited to the EC and transentorhinal cortex may represent a clinically silent phase of the disease (Hof et al., 1992). Neurons of layers II and IV are particularly susceptible to degeneration. Eventually during the course of AD, virtually all neurons in layer II contain NFT (Hirano and Zimmerman, 1962; Kemper, 1978; Hyman et al., 1984; Mann and Esiri, 1989; Braak and Braak, 1991). Layer II is also the first cortical layer showing ghost tangles (clusters of extracellular filaments that are remnants of a degenerated neuron) (Braak and Braak, 1991). Layer IV is affected after layer II. Only a comparatively few NFT are found in layers III and V, and these usually develop late in the course of AD (Braak and Braak, 1991).

It has been suggested that the degeneration of much of the neuronal architecture of the EC destroys a large functional part of hippocampal input and output, and that this destruction results in the memory and cognitive deficits associated with the early stages of AD (Hyman et al., 1984). In a detailed stereological study, Gomez-Isla et al. (1997) found that patients with very mild cognitive impairment (Clinical Dementia Rating [CDR] = 0.5) had 32% fewer neurons in the EC than controls. In layer II, neuronal loss reached 60%. In severe dementia cases (CDR53), the total number of neurons in layer II decreased by 90% and in layer IV by 70%. Moreover, neuronal numbers were negatively correlated with tangle and plaque densities. This study showed that significant neuronal loss in layer II of the EC distinguished even very mild AD from nondemented aging (Gomez-Isla et al., 1996).

In summary, modern stereological techniques have recently shown that CA1 of the hippocampus and layers II and IV of the EC are the most vulnerable to AD pathology and are potentially specific for AD (West et al., 1994; Gomez-Isla et al., 1996).

There is growing evidence suggesting that more than one mechanism of neuronal loss occurs in AD (Gomez-Isla et al., 1997; Broe et al., 2001; Rossler et al., 2002). Apoptosis has been suggested to play a role in AD (de la Monte et al., 1998; Broe et al., 2001). Almost one fourth of the remaining neurons in AD show abnormal nuclear morphology and deoxyribonucleic acid (DNA) fragmentation (Broe et al., 2001). In addition, there is no correlation between apoptotic morphology and tau deposition, suggesting that non-NFT-related neuronal degeneration plays a significant role in AD.

Hippocampal Formation Pathology in Normal Aging

Studies of normal elderly persons typically show that NFT accumulation in the EC and/or hippocampus dramatically increases with increasing age (Price et al., 1991; Arriagada et al., 1992; Giannakopoulos et al., 1994; Langui et al., 1995; Price et al., 2001). Specifically, a pattern of early hippocampal formation NFT deposition (Hubbard et al., 1990; Giannakopoulos et al., 1994; Giannakopoulos et al., 2003), with relative sparing of the neocortex (Price et al., 1991; Arriagada et al., 1992; Ulrich, 1985), is found in studies of elderly individuals with no dementia (normal and MCI). It is informative that strong age relationships remain despite methodological differences in patient recruitment, cognitive evaluation, staining procedures, and anatomical sampling. These differences across studies appear more likely to affect the relative numbers of patients affected rather than the pattern of brain region change. For example, Giannakopoulos et al. (1994) examined 1131 brains of elderly person who were normal and mildly affected but with no dementia derived from a hospital-based medical and surgical service. They observed NFT in the CA1 of the hippocampus in 25% of the sample. By comparison, NFT was uncommon in these patients in the superior frontal (4%) and occipital cortices (3%). Langui et al. (1995) examined the EC and hippocampus from 167 brains of normal patients. The diagnosis of normal was based on clinical notes; no cognitive testing was performed. They observed that AD changes (NFT or senile plaques) were found in less than 20% of patients younger than age 60 years, in over 80% of those between 60 and 80 years, and in nearly 100% of the 56 patients older than age 80 years. The predominant form of pathology was the NFT, either alone or frequently in combination with senile plaques. Only 2% of normal brains showed senile plaques in the absence of NFT. A recent longitudinal study that followed a small cohort of elderly individuals (age range 74–95 years, median age 85 years) who were cognitively intact at time of death found relatively low burdens of AD neuropathology, with 87% of the sample (34 out of 39 patients) having a Braak stage < IV (Knopman et al., 2003).

Summarizing several other studies that examined the hippocampal formation along with neocortical sites, patients with no dementia appear to show a strong age-related tendency toward NFT accumulation that is concentrated in the hippocampal formation (Morris et al., 1991; Price et al., 1991; Arriagada et al., 1992). Although senile plaques also tend to accumulate with age, typically they accumulate at later ages and have a preference for the neocortex rather than the hippocampal formation (Arriagada et al., 1992; Giannakopoulos et al., 1994).

In a recently proposed model, neurofibrillary changes occur in all persons during aging but affect relatively few neurons before 85 to 90 years and are insufficient to cause significant neuronal loss or cognitive impairment (Price et al., 2001). With a substantial amyloid burden, the amount of neurofibrillary change increases during the preclinical stage of AD. There is still insufficient neuronal degeneration to produce detectable cognitive impairment, but autopsied cases in this stage generally meet pathological criteria for AD. Further amyloid deposition and accelerated neurofibrillary change result in significant neuronal dysfunction and death and associated MCI (Price et al., 2001).

These data, which support the Braak model, suggest that age-associated hippocampal formation lesions are the earliest lesions associated with AD. Moreover, it appears that in association with these early lesions, there is a reduction in the volume of the affected tissue, thus making this observation a target for early diagnosis using in-vivo neuroimaging. It was reported that normal elderly individuals with NFT lesions in the hippocampus showed hippocampal volume reductions compared with normal age-matched elderly persons without NFTs (de la Monte, 1989). It therefore appears that the inverse relationship between NFT deposition and hippocampal volume extends throughout the range of normal to severely demented AD. Such neuropathology findings have encouraged the more comprehensive in-vivo examination of the hippocampal formation in aging and AD. To date, longitudinal in-vivo imaging studies are becoming an important bridge between clinical and neuropathology based staging models (Mosconi, Tsui, et al., 2007).

NEUROPSYCHOLOGY

Systematic research with monkeys and rats and related research with humans has identified structures and connections important for memory in the medial temporal lobe and the midline diencephalon. These important structures within the medial temporal lobe are the hippocampus, the subicular complex, and the adjacent and anatomically related entorhinal, perirhinal, and parahippocampal cortices (Mishkin, 1978; Moss et al., 1981; Zola-Morgan et al., 1994). The amygdaloid contribution to memory is modest (Zola-Morgan et al., 1989). Studies of the medial temporal lobe in monkeys showed that the severity of memory impairment depended on the locus and the extent of medial temporal lobe damage (Zola-Morgan et al., 1994). Damage limited to the hippocampus produced mild memory impairment (Zola-Morgan and Squire, 1986). When the damage was increased to include the adjacent entorhinal and parahippocampal cortices, more severe memory impairment was produced. Finally, when the above lesion was extended rostrally to include the more anterior aspects of the EC and the perirhinal cortex, the memory impairment was even greater (Zola-Morgan et al., 1989; Zola-Morgan et al., 1993; Zola-Morgan et al., 1994). These findings suggest that whereas damage to the hippocampus proper produces measurable memory impairment, a substantial part of the severe memory impairment produced by large medial temporal lobe lesions in humans and monkeys can be attributed to damage to the entorhinal, perirhinal, and parahippocampal cortices adjacent to the hippocampus.

Selective hippocampal lesions produce memory storage deficits while preserving immediate recall, remote recall (historical memories), and intelligence (Squire,

1992). Some evidence exists that the measures most sensitive to hippocampal integrity, such as secondary memory tasks emphasizing delayed recall, are somewhat resistant to longitudinal decline over short study intervals in normal aging (Colsher and Wallace, 1991). These observations have led to the successful use of delayed recall tasks in the clinical differentiation of persons with normal aging from patients with no dementia but with MCI who are considered at risk for AD (Welsh et al., 1991; Blacker et al., 2007; for a detailed review, see Twamley et al., 2006). There is a general consensus among the numerous studies that have used delayed recall tasks to investigate neuropsychological function in AD that episodic memory decline is an early and prominent feature of AD, with declines occurring years before significant cognitive and behavioral changes required for a diagnosis of AD. Neuroimaging studies investigating the relationship between neuropathology and cognitive changes have demonstrated that atrophy primarily of the hippocampus correlates with episodic memory impairment in AD (de Leon et al., 1997), with subsequent decline in other cognitive domains consistent with the spread to neocortical regions of the underlying neuropathology.

In summary, the pathological and neuropsychological data offer excellent justification for examining the integrity of the hippocampal formation as a potentially informative anatomy for evaluation of the transition between normal aging, MCI, and AD-related memory decline. However, efficient memory functioning is not simply based on the integrity of the hippocampal formation. Many different locations of brain damage have been associated with memory dysfunctions (Mesulam, 1990), and generalized atrophic changes that are known to occur in normal-aged individuals may also contribute to memory changes (de Leon et al., 1984). Consequently, the determination of meaningful brain–memory relationships in aging humans requires qualitative and quantitative characterization of the cognitive deficits, as well as examination of the anatomical specificity of any statistically significant brain-memory relationship.

NEUROIMAGING STUDIES

In the late 1980s and early 1990s, several laboratories reported that the hippocampal region could be reliably studied with structural neuroimaging (de Leon et al., 1988; Seab et al., 1988; de Leon et al., 1989; Press et al., 1989; Kesslak et al., 1991; de Leon et al., 1993). This advance was partly facilitated by the availability of MRI. Thus, numerous research efforts were directed away from more general markers of brain atrophy (ventricular size and cortical atrophy) to anatomically better-defined regional assessments. In the AD literature, a growing consensus exists among in-vivo neuroimaging studies regarding the involvement of the hippocampus. All studies report hippocampal atrophy relative to age-matched controls.

These results initially were reflected in indirect measures including qualitative ratings of the amount of CSF accumulating in the hippocampal fissures (de Leon et al., 1988; de Leon et al., 1989; de Leon et al., 1993; de Leon et al., 1997); linear two-dimensional estimates of hippocampal width (Scheltens et al., 1992; Jobst et al., 1994); measures of medial temporal lobe gray matter volume (Stout et al., 1996); the size of the suprasellar cistern (Aylward et al., 1996); and the distance between the right and left Un (see de Leon et al., 1994, for review). Subsequently, direct measures of hippocampal volume loss were employed with the advent of new and more sophisticated MRI sequences, as well as the use of precise and validated volumetric methods (Seab et al., 1988; Jack et al., 1992; Convit et al., 1993; Ikeda et al., 1994; Lehericy et al., 1994; Convit, de Leon, Hoptman, et al., 1995; Convit et al., 1997; Jack et al., 1997; Insausti et al., 1998; Laakso et al., 1998; Bobinski et al., 1999; Goncharova et al., 2001).

However, before hippocampal atrophy can be considered a diagnostic marker for early (preclinical) AD, several lines of investigation need to be developed further. Specifically, we need to improve our understanding of the prevalence and severity of hippocampal atrophy over the stages of AD and as a function of age, gender, and genetic factors. The diagnostic specificity of hippocampal atrophy for AD needs to be established, and the relationship between the imaging-determined atrophy and neuropathological features of the disease needs to be validated. Results from more recent longitudinal studies of normal aging show that MCI and AD has begun to demonstrate that structural imaging has potential to predict outcome and that hippocampal and medial temporal lobe changes appear to be the most important predictors of future decline (Glodzik-Sobanska et al., 2005).

CROSS-SECTIONAL HIPPOCAMPAL STUDIES OF NORMAL AGING AND ALZHEIMER'S DISEASE

The decline from normal to MCI and AD has been investigated mainly by MRI studies. These studies have shown, overall, that the rate of medial temporal lobe (MTL) volume reduction correlates with the decline from normal to MCI (Rusinek et al., 2003; Jack et al., 2004). Cross-sectional and longitudinal studies show that imaging the hippocampal formation alterations is of use in the evaluation of age-related memory changes, and in the prediction of future dementia and a diagnosis of AD. Moreover, these in-vivo data support the Braak model. In this model, the earliest stages of AD are marked by selective involvement of the EC followed by hippocampal changes, and finally by progressive neocortical pathology. Recent studies using in-vivo MRI imaging techniques demonstrate the pattern and rate of regional atrophy, with tissue losses of 20%–50% in regions of the hippocampal formation corresponding to the CA1 and subiculum in patients with AD (Frisoni et al., 2006). Importantly, these CA1 and subicular involvements were associated with an increased risk for conversion from MCI to AD (Apostolova et al., 2006). In another study (Apostolova et al., 2006), comparing patients with amnestic MCI and patients with mild AD demonstrated that patients with mild AD have significantly greater bilateral atrophy of the lateral hippocampus an area corresponding to the CA1 region and in the right hippocampus in areas corresponding to the CA2 and CA3 subfields. These findings are in agreement with pathological observations of damage to the hippocampus proper in AD (Bobinski et al., 1995; Bobinski et al., 1997; Schonheit et al., 2004).

Memory decline with aging is closely associated with hippocampal formation integrity. One published MRI study followed a large cohort of normal individuals until the onset of dementia including AD and showed an association between hippocampal and amygdala volumes during normal aging and shorter times until onset of dementia on average 6 years later (den Heijer et al., 2006). The risk for dementia was threefold increased per 1 standard deviation (*SD*) decrease in hippocampal volumes, and twofold increased per 1 *SD* decrease in amygdala volumes (den Heijer et al., 2006).

The distinction between whether memory loss is part of normal aging or a pathological state was explored in a cross-sectional study of younger and older adults using a functional MRI protocol that was specifically developed to perform regional analysis of the hippocampal formation (Small et al., 2002). To determine the frequency of age-related hippocampal decline in the elderly group, the hippocampal circuit of each older patient was compared to the youngest age group using a multivariate linear regression, where the independent variables were the four hippocampal subregions and the dependent variable was group. Patients were then dichotomized into those in which the hippocampal signal did not significantly differ from the younger age group and those who had at least one hippocampal subregion showing significant decline in signal. The findings from this study showed that function in two hippocampal subregions—the subiculum and the DG—declines normally with age, whereas function in the EC was found to decline pathologically (Small et al., 2002). Similarly, entorhinal glucose utilization reductions were found to predict the decline from normal aging to MCI (de Leon et al., 2001). Moreover, this study showed that reduced hippocampal metabolism followed the EC changes among subjects that showed cognitive decline.

An early computed tomography (CT)-based study of a large cohort (405 patients) showed that hippocampal atrophy was significantly more prevalent in all clinical groups compared with controls (de Leon et al., 1997). Seventy-eight percent of the MCI group, 84% of the mild AD group, and 96% of the moderate to severe AD groups showed hippocampal atrophy. Hippocampal atrophy was shown in 29% of controls. Normal controls showed striking age dependence for hippocampal atrophy, whereas the cognitively impaired groups showed prevalence rates independent of age.

Numerous studies have demonstrated the ability of MRI-based volumetric measurements of the hippocampal formation to differentiate between patients with AD and normal controls (Fig. 57.7). Hippocampal formation atrophy has been shown to be one of the most robust and consistently documented findings (Jack et al., 1992; Convit et al., 1997; de Leon et al., 1997; Jack et al., 1997; Laakso et al., 1998).Recently, there has been increased interest in identifying patients at the earliest stages of AD so that effective treatment, when available, can be initiated. Therefore, neuroimaging studies have been performed on patients with no dementia who are at increased risk for AD, including those with family history of AD or the apolipoprotein (ApoE) genotype, and patients with no dementia with mild MCI. The hippocampus size is significantly reduced in patients with MCI compared with normal controls (Convit, de Leon, Tarshish, et al., 1995; Convit et al., 1997; de Leon et al., 1997; Laakso et al., 1998). The volume of the hippocampus is decreased by 11% to 15% in patients with MCI and by 12% to 35% in patients with AD compared to normal controls (Juottonen et al., 1998; Bobinski et al., 1999; De Santi et al., 2001; Du et al., 2001; Glodzik-Sobanska et al., 2005).

With the observation that transentorhinal/EC rather than hippocampus is the site of the earliest pathological changes, several studies demonstrated significant volume loss of this region in patients with MCI compared with normal controls (Killiany et al., 2000; Xu et al., 2000; Du et al., 2001; Pennanen et al., 2004; Devanand et al., 2007). Entorhinal cortex was found to be smaller than normal by 13% in MCI and by 27% to 40% in AD (Juottonen et al., 1998; Bobinski et al., 1999; Du et al., 2001).

These considerable differences in the degree of hippocampal and entorhinal atrophy probably result from different measuring methods and different subjects (severity of impairment). In our recent validation study, we showed that very accurate volumetric measurements of the whole hippocampal formation can be obtained by using an MRI protocol (Bobinski et al., 2000). Strong correlations were found between MRI and histological measurements for the hippocampus (r5.97), hippocampus/subiculum (r5.95), and hippocampus/PG (r5.89). Moreover, strong correlations between MRI subvolumes and neuronal counts were found for the hip-

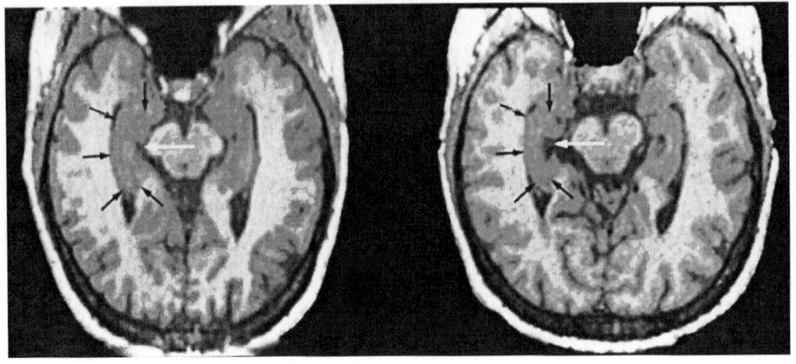

FIGURE 57.7 Axial magnetic resonance imaging scan depicting the hippocampal area from a normal control subject (left) and an age-matched Alzheimer's disease (AD) patient (right). Black arrows mark the boundary of the hippocampus; white arrows point to the region of the hippocampal fissure.

pocampus (r5.90) and the hippocampus/subiculum subvolume (r5.84), suggesting the anatomical validity of MRI volume measurements.

LONGITUDINAL STUDIES PREDICTING THE DEVELOPMENT OF DEMENTIA

The results of many cross-sectional studies of hippocampal atrophy showed that hippocampal changes frequently occur in patients with MCI and thereby may predict the development of symptoms consistent with the course of AD. In our pioneering CT-based studies, 72% of patients with MCI and 4% of controls deteriorated to receive the diagnosis of AD (de Leon et al., 1989; de Leon et al., 1993). The results of this study pointed to the need for longitudinal study of the temporal relation between hippocampal atrophy, neocortical atrophy, and the development of intellectual dysfunction. As only 4% of our normal elderly sample deteriorated to dementia, while 15% had baseline hippocampal atrophy, this study also suggested that to carefully evaluate the predictive risk of hippocampal atrophy, we must also (*1*) extend the period of observation beyond 4 years, (*2*) use more sensitive indices of hippocampal integrity, and (*3*) use more fine-grained assessments of neuropsychological performance.

Subsequent longitudinal studies confirmed and extended our results (Jack et al., 1999; Jack et al., 2000; Dickerson et al., 2001; Killiany et al., 2002). The annual rate of hippocampal atrophy was reported to be 3% in MCI and 3.5% in AD group (Jack et al., 2000). Our studies show that the medial temporal lobe atrophy rate measured with the regional boundary shift method over a 2-year interval was the most significant predictor of decline, in a group of initially healthy individuals who converted to MCI or AD at the 6-year follow-up. Overall prediction accuracy was 89% (Rusinek et al., 2003).

Not all patients with MCI decline to clinical AD. It is estimated that 50%–70% will convert to AD (Kluger et al., 1999). Heterogeneity among patients with MCI may be related to several factors, APoE status being one of them. Polymorphism of the APOE gene is a significant risk factor for developing late-onset AD (Corder et al., 1993). The ε4 allele confers an increased risk of developing AD and lowers the age at onset in a dose-dependent fashion, whereas the ε2 allele is protective. Annual hippocampal atrophy is significantly different in AD patients with (9.8%) and without the APoE ε4 allele (7%) (Mori et al., 2002).

Many studies demonstrated that hippocampal and entorhinal volumes accurately predict future conversion of MCI to AD (Jack et al., 1999; Jack et al., 2000; Killiany et al., 2000; Dickerson et al., 2001; Killiany et al., 2002; Jack et al., 2004). We reported the first evidence that EC glucose use reductions in normal elderly persons, as measured by positron emission tomography (PET), uniquely predict conversion to MCI (Fig. 57.8) (de Leon et al., 2001), and that in MCI and AD metabolism reductions exceed volume losses (De Santi et al., 2001). Using a newly developed automated hippocampal sampling procedure, we demonstrated that hippocampal glucose metabolic rate is a sensitive preclinical predictor of future cognitive impairment, as well as a longitudinal correlate of the decline from normal aging (Mosconi, 2005). More recently, fluorodeoxyglucose (FDG) PET imaging was used longitudinally to predict and monitor cognitive decline from normal aging (Mosconi, Tsui, et al., 2007). Baseline hippocampal glucose metabolic rates predicted decline from normal to AD with 81% accuracy, from normal to other dementias with 77% accuracy, and from normal to MCI with 71% accuracy. Greater rates of hippocampal and cortical glucose metabolic rates were found in the declining as compared to the nondeclining normal patients. Reduced hippocampal glucose metabolic rate was associated with a shorter duration of survival time as normal (Mosconi, Brys, et al., 2007).

Numerous cross-sectional and longitudinal neuroimaging AD studies confirm the involvement of the MTL structures previously described in the neuropathologic literature. Furthermore, structural imaging has demonstrated potential to predict future decline in normal

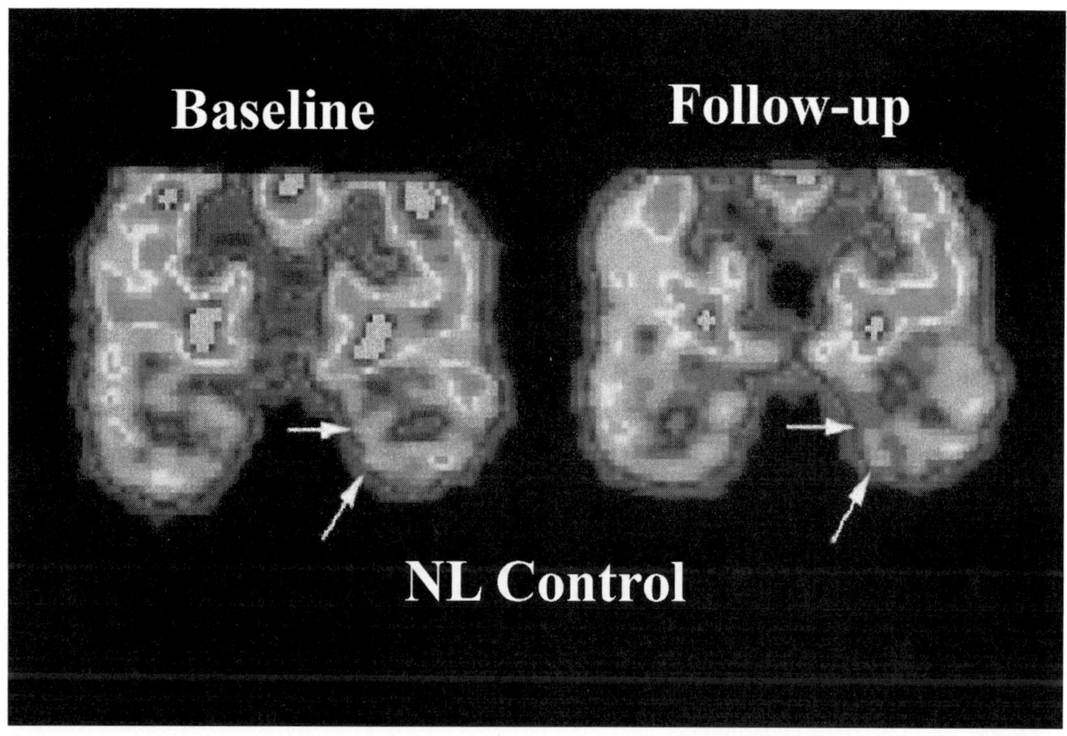

A

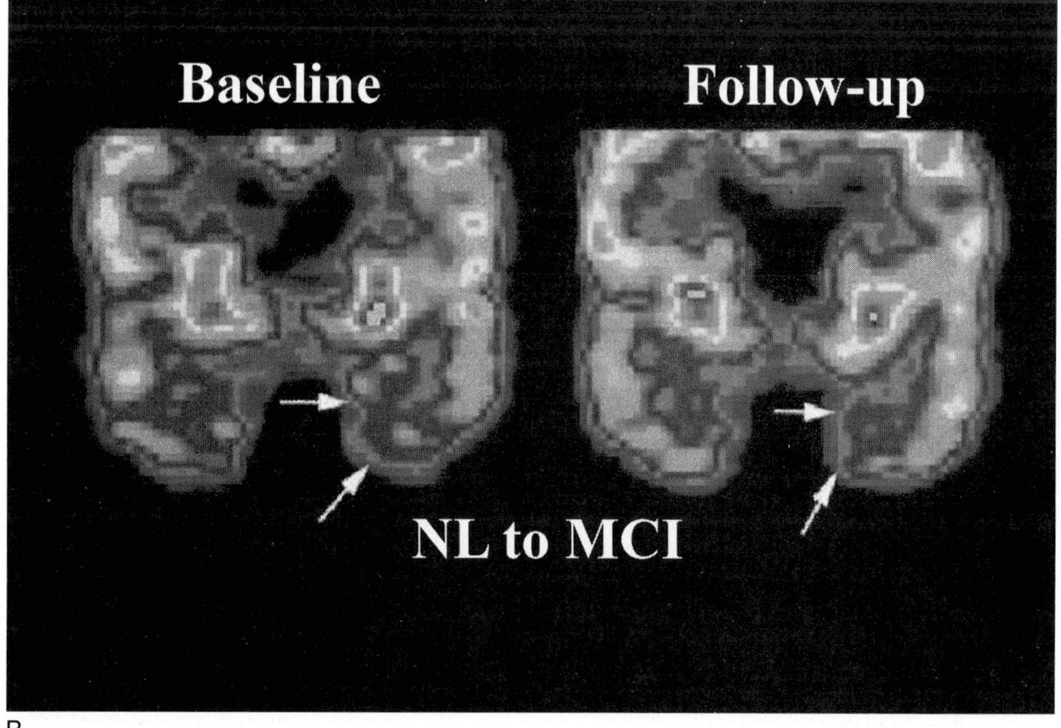

B

FIGURE 57.8 Fluorodeoxyglucose-positron emission tomography (FDG-PET) images in a longitudinal study (baseline and follow-up) demonstrating the region of the entorhinal cortex (arrows) in two normal elderly subjects, one of whom remained normal at the 3-year follow-up (*A*) and the other who declined to mild cognitive impairment (MCI) (*B*). Note the decrease in FDG uptake in the entorhinal cortex of the patient who declined at MCI.

individuals and in individuals with MCI, and hippocampal and MTL changes appear to be the most important regional predictors. In the first published prediction study (de Leon et al., 1989), the hippocampal atrophy qualitatively assessed at baseline was present in more than 90% of 48 patients who had MCI who developed dementia over a 3-year period. Only 19% of patients with MCI whose condition did not worsen had atrophy. Our replication study that applied the same axial image acquisition protocol and the same visual rating scale confirmed the ability of qualitative hippocampal atrophy assessment to predict further evolution to AD at the 4-year follow-up. The baseline assessment of hippocampal atrophy predicted decline with 91% accuracy (de Leon et al., 1993). The results showed that MTL atrophy was sufficient to predict conversion to AD 3 to 4 years in advance.

In summary, consistent with pathological findings, MR studies point to the hippocampus and EC as the first sites for atrophic changes in AD. Entorhinal cortex glucose metabolism reductions predict the transition between normal aging and MCI, and hippocampal volume is a useful predictor of future dementia from MCI. Positron emission tomography MCI studies have identified patterns of hypometabolism in the parietotemporal and posterior cingulate cortex that are also associated with the MCI transition to AD. The temporal relationships between EC, hippocampus, and neocortical hypometabolism are under investigation (see Mosconi et al., 2004, for review).

RELATIONSHIP BETWEEN HIPPOCAMPAL ATROPHY AND MEMORY IN NORMAL AGING

Memory tests that involve medial temporal lobe structures for execution are the best indices of early cognitive impairment. Among normal controls, hippocampal volume correlates with delayed memory performance but not with primary or immediate memory performance (Golomb et al., 1994). Moreover, after a follow-up interval of 4 years, we observed in this same elderly cohort that smaller baseline hippocampal volumes were predictive of disproportionately greater reductions in delayed recall performance (Golomb et al., 1996). These results suggest that hippocampal atrophy may play an important independent role in contributing to the memory loss experienced by many aging adults. Several longitudinal studies showed that the volume of hippocampal formation decreases with age, with annual rates of volume loss ranging from 1.55% to 2.1% (Kaye et al., 1997; Jack et al., 2000). A very strong inverse correlation was found between hippocampal volume and age among normal patients older than age 60 (r52.93) but not among individuals aged 40–60 (Mu et al., 1999). On the other hand, the volume of the EC does not correlate with age (Insausti et al., 1998).

THE ANATOMIC SPECIFICITY OF HIPPOCAMPAL VOLUME LOSS IN PATIENTS AT RISK FOR ALZHEIMER'S DISEASE

The early diagnosis of AD continues to be difficult and requires experience and skill (McKhann et al., 1984). Therefore, many studies have explored the role of noninvasive imaging as a potential aid in the early diagnosis of AD, such as MRI measures of the hippocampus and EC. Research shows that measures of the hippocampus or the EC are significantly different in patients with mild AD versus controls. However, there is less agreement about which of these structures is more useful in differentiating patients with AD in the preclinical stage of disease (Juottonen et al., 1998; Bobinski et al., 1999; Xu et al., 2000; Killiany et al., 2002).

Our early study on anatomical specificity demonstrated that the hippocampal volume separated normal controls from patients with MCI, correctly classifying 74% (Convit, de Leon, Tarshish, et al., 1995). In addition, measurement of the fusiform gyrus volume uniquely improved the ability of hippocampal volume measurement to separate patients with MCI from patients with AD from 74% to 80%. Our cross-sectional data showed that, within the temporal lobe, specific hippocampal volume reductions separated the group at risk for AD from the normal group. By the time impairments are sufficient to allow a diagnosis of AD to be made, in addition to the medial temporal lobe volume reductions, the lateral temporal lobe is showing volume reductions, most saliently involving the fusiform gyrus. Using a longitudinal approach, Jack et al. (2004) measured annualized rates of change in the volume of hippocampus, EC, whole brain, and ventricles with serial MRI measurements in a relatively large sample ($N = 160$) of normal elderly individuals with MCI and patients with probable AD. They found that atrophy rates in the four structures were greater among normal elderly patients who converted to MCI or AD than among those who remained stable, greater among patients with MCI who converted to AD than among those who remained stable, and greater among individuals with fast-progressing AD as compared to those with slow-progressing AD. The MRI changes were related to disease progression rather than to disease stage at baseline.

To address the issue of early involvement of the EC, we measured the hippocampal and superior temporal gyrus volumes as well as the validated landmark method for the EC (Bobinski et al., 1999). In a series of univariate logistic regression models, measurement of the EC correctly classified 100% of the control and 87.5% of the AD group. Measurement of the hippocampus classified 87.5% of the control group and 75% of the AD group. In addition, regression models showed superiority of the entorhinal measures over the hippocampal measures in overall classification accuracy. Other studies confirmed our early observations regarding the superiority of entorhinal measurement over hippocampus measurement in differentiating persons with mild AD from normal controls (Juottonen et al., 1998; Killiany et al., 2002). Subsequently, studies showed that EC accurately differentiates normal controls from those destined to develop dementia and those destined to develop MCI, as well as differentiating patients with MCI and patients with AD (Dickerson et al., 2001; Du et al., 2001; Killiany et al., 2002; Devanand et al., 2007).

Hippocampal volumes may be valuable not only in distinguishing individuals with AD from normal controls but also in identifying individuals with AD neuropathology who have yet to demonstrate dementia or even clinically evident memory impairment. Based on data from the Nun Study, Gosche et al. (2002) showed that hippocampal volumes from postmortem MRI studies distinguished Braak stages III and IV from Braak stages II and below among patients with no dementia. Moreover, among patients who were cognitively intact, the hippocampus distinguished those in Braak stage II from those in stage I or below. The strong correlation between antemortem hippocampal volume and Braak stage (r52.63) was confirmed by another group (Jack et al., 2002).

DIFFERENTIAL DIAGNOSIS

Magnetic resonance imaging techniques have been used to examine diagnostic specificity of different dementing illnesses. Alzheimer's disease is the most common cause of late-life dementia, accounting for 70%–80% of cases. Vascular dementia is the second most common cause of dementia, often occurring together with AD and therefore making accurate differential diagnosis between the two difficult. Other causes of dementia include frontotemporal dementia (FTD) and dementia with Lewy bodies (DLB). Although MTL atrophy is found in patients with AD who have FTD, regional patterns differentiate these two disorders. Frisoni and colleagues (1996) demonstrated that frontal atrophy, enlargement of the left temporal horn, and sparing of the MTL region characterized FTD, whereas more severe MTL loss was typical for AD. Comparison of hippocampal and EC volume loss between patients with AD and those with FTD revealed greater extent of hippocampal atrophy in the AD group. Comparison of patients with AD and patients with vascular dementia has shown a consistent pattern of more severe hippocampal atrophy in AD (Barber et al., 2000). No specific pattern of atrophy has been observed in AD as compared to vascular dementia (Barber et al., 2000; O'Brien et al., 2001; Varma et al., 2002). However, hippocampus and EC correctly discriminate between patients with AD and those with subcortical ischemic vascular dementia (SIVD). Volume losses of the hippocampus and entorhinal complex are less severe in SIVD than in AD (Du et al., 2002). Hippocampal volume distinguishes 82% of patients with SIVD from normal controls and 63% of patients with SIVD from patients with AD. Adding global cerebral changes to hippocampus substantially improves the classification to 96% between patients with SIVD and normal controls and to 83% between patients with SIVD and those with AD. Entorhinal cortex does not improve the discrimination when added to hippocampus (Du et al., 2002). Larger volumes of the whole temporal lobe, the hippocampus, and amygdala (Barber et al., 2000) and smaller putamen volumes (Cousins et al., 2003) distinguish patients who have DLB from patients with AD. There are no studies comparing MCI with other degenerative diseases; therefore, the ability of MRI to discriminate between AD at the MCI stage and other dementing illnesses remains unanswered.

AUTOMATED IMAGE ANALYSIS METHODS

Improved MRI resolution has allowed for precise volumetry of individual MTL structures and new techniques, such as voxel-based morphometry (VBM), have facilitated more rapid image analysis (Glodzik-Sobanska et al., 2005). Voxel-based morphometry is an automated method of measuring atrophy of the entire brain. Whereas volumetric studies use the region of interest (ROI) method, which depends upon the expertise of an imaging technician outlining preselected structures in a series of sections on a computer screen, VBM objectively maps gray matter density changes, on a voxel-by-voxel basis, in the entire brain. Automated techniques such as VBM have been developed to enable automatic analyses of whole-brain structural MRI scans to avoid shortcomings associated with the ROI method (that is, preselected regions and the inherent difficulties associated with reliance upon inter- and intra-individual variability in placement of ROIs).

Voxel-based morphometry has been applied in numerous studies in AD and has been recently applied in individuals with MCI (Rombouts et al., 2000; Baron et al., 2001; Chetelat et al., 2002; Busatto et al., 2003; Pennanen et al., 2005). In addition to "classic" MTL pathology, the VBM method of whole-brain analysis has captured different foci of interest such as posterior cingulate and generally diffuse cerebral atrophy between patients with AD and healthy controls. In what may be the first study to use VBM in individuals with MCI (Chetelat et al., 2002), extensive gray matter loss involving hippocampal and infero-lateral temporal regions was found in MCI relative to age-matched controls with greater gray matter loss found in patients with AD than in patients with MCI in superior and posterior brain, primarily involving the posterior polymodal association cortex.

Other automated procedures such as brain boundary shift integral (BSI), developed for the assessment of global cerebral atrophy rate was also designed to overcome the problems of intra- and interobserver reliability with manual measurement. This method involves computation of change in whole brain volume using a registration and subtraction of two scans. Summary data with this method, comparing 11 patients with AD and 11 matched healthy controls, demonstrated a median volume reduction of 12.3 mL compared to 0.3 mL for controls. Although the annualized rate of atrophy with this method (< 1%) is less than that for hippocampal volume, it has yielded excellent discrimination between patients with AD and controls. Serial annual MRI scans over a 5- to 8-year period, with subsequent analysis of atrophy rate with BSI, demonstrated that patients who are symptom free and at risk for dementia (from families with early-onset AD) have significantly greater rate of global brain atrophy than controls (1% per year vs. 0.24%) (Fox et al., 2001). The semiautomated method has been shown to be superior to volumetric measurement. A 1% increase in atrophy rate, as measured with hippocampal BSI, was associated with an 11-fold increase in the odds of AD diagnosis, whereas for the same manually measured rate, the odds increased only threefold (Barnes et al., 2004).

We recently published longitudinal findings using regional brain boundary shift analysis and spatial coregistration to determine whether rate of medial temporal lobe atrophy over the initial time interval of a 6-year, three time-point longitudinal study is predictive of future memory decline in 45 healthy, elderly patients (Rusinek et al., 2003). After 6 years of observations, 32 patients remained healthy and 13 showed cognitive decline and received a diagnosis of MCI ($n = 9$) or mild to severe AD ($n = 4$). MTL atrophy rate, through its interactions with sex and age, was the most significant predictor of decline. The overall accuracy of prediction was 89% (in 40 of 45 patients), with 91% specificity (in 29 of 32 patients) and 85% sensitivity (in 11 of 13 patients). An annual MTL atrophy rate of 0.7% best enabled the separation of patients who were declining from patients who were nondeclining. As per our knowledge, we demonstrated for the first time that increased MTL atrophy rate is predictive of future memory decline in healthy, elderly volunteer patients (Rusinek et al., 2003). Longitudinal studies such as these reveal the importance and time course of increased rates of global and regional atrophy.

With longitudinal assessment, the issue of atrophy rate stability arises. In a healthy elderly population, the atrophy rate is low and relatively constant over time, whereas in patients with AD, cerebral atrophy rate is greater and accelerates with disease progression (see Glodzik-Sobanska et al., 2005). As estimated with BSI, change in whole-brain atrophy rate was 0.31% per year (Chan et al., 2003). New imaging techniques that allow assessment of tissue integrity on a microstructural level (MTI-facilitating indirect assessment of proteins and membranes; diffusion-weighted imaging—reflecting direction and magnitude of water diffusion) may shed light on early, global, and regional changes. These newer approaches have not yet provided enough data to offer diagnostic conclusions, but they have already shown promise in revealing new anatomic damage and better characterization of tissue volume loss.

CONCLUSIONS

In-vivo techniques not only have shed a new light on the pathogenesis of AD, but they also appear to be of descriptive value over the clinical course of AD and stand ready to contribute to an increased understanding of MCI. The data indicate that visually detected hippocampal changes appear early in the natural history of AD and are progressive. Such changes are relatively uncommon in normal elderly persons. However, when such atrophic changes are present, they are associated with mild memory deficits. The data suggest that in individuals who are mildly impaired, clinically recognizable hippocampal atrophy appears to be related to the AD process, as it predicts with high sensitivity and specificity the decline to AD levels of cognitive performance (de Leon et al., 1989; de Leon et al., 1993). This conclusion is supported in part by postmortem studies that show AD-related pathology in the hippocampal formation of patients with MCI (Price et al., 1991). Moreover, it is universally observed at postmortem examination that hippocampal atrophy occurs in AD. We now extend these observations in vivo by showing a remarkably high frequency of hippocampal atrophy among individuals with probable AD and MCI. The imaging data also show the consistent and necessary involvement of the lateral temporal lobe in the statistical classification of patients with AD relative to patients with MCI. Overall, in patients with no dementia, these findings now permit the identification of brain changes that indicate increased risk for AD. It is anticipated that future therapeutic studies will probably use brain imaging measures as a surrogate markers of cognitive decline, which are relatively free of educational and cultural bias, for selection purposes and as outcome measures.

REFERENCES

Amaral, D.G., and Insausti, R. (1990) Hippocampal formation. In: Paxinos, G., ed. *The Human Nervous System*. San Diego, CA: Academic Press, pp. 711–755.

Amaral, D.G., Insausti, R., and Cowan, W.M. (1987) The entorhinal cortex of the monkey: I. Cytoarchitectonic organization. *J. Comp. Neurol.* 264:326–355.

Apostolova, L.G., Dinov, I.D., Dutton, R.A., Hayashi, K.M., Toga, A.W., Cummings, J.L., and Thompson, P.M. (2006) 3D comparison of hippocampal atrophy in amnestic mild cognitive impairment and Alzheimer's disease. *Brain* 129:2867–2873.

Apostolova, L.G., Dutton, R.A., Dinov, I.D., Hayashi, K.M., Toga, A.W., Cummings, J.L., and Thompson, P.M. (2006) Conversion of mild cognitive impairment to Alzheimer disease predicted by hippocampal atrophy maps. *Arch. Neurol.* 63:693–699.

Arriagada, P.V., Marzloff, K., and Hyman, B.T. (1992) Distribution of Alzheimer-type pathologic changes in nondemented elderly individuals matches the pattern in Alzheimer's disease. *Neurology* 42:1681–1688.

Aylward, E.H., Rasmusson, D.X., Brandt, J., Raimundo, L., Folstein, M., and Pearlson, G.D. (1996) CT measurement of suprasellar cistern predicts rate of cognitive decline in Alzheimer's disease. *J. Int. Neuropsychol. Soc.* 2:89–95.

Ball, M.J., Hachinski, V., Fox, A., Kirshen, A.J., Fisman, M., Blume, W., Kral, V.A., and Fox, H. (1985) A new definition of Alzheimer's disease: a hippocampal dementia. *Lancet* 5:14–16.

Barber, R., Ballard, C., McKeith, I.G., Gholkar, A., and O'Brien, J.T. (2000) MRI volumetric study of dementia with Lewy bodies: a comparison with AD and vascular dementia. *Neurology* 54: 1304–1309.

Barnes, J., Scahill, R.I., Boyes, R.G., Frost, C., Lewis, E.B., Rossor, C.L., Rossor, M.N., and Fox, N.C. (2004) Differentiating AD from aging using semiautomated measurement of hippocampal atrophy rates. *Neuroimage* 23:574–581.

Baron, J.C., Chetelat, G., Desgranges, B., Perchey, G., Landeau, B., de la Sayette, V., and Eustache, F. (2001) In vivo mapping of gray matter loss with voxel-based morphometry in mild Alzheimer's disease. *Neuroimage* 14:298–309.

Blacker, D., Lee, H., Muzikansky, A., Martin, E.C., Tanzi, R., McArdle, J.J., Moss, M., and Albert, M. (2007) Neuropsychological measures in normal individuals that predict subsequent cognitive decline. *Arch. Neurol.* 64:862–871.

Bobinski, M., de Leon, M.J., Convit, A., De Santi, S., Wegiel, J., Tarshish, C.Y., Saint-Louis, L.A., and Wisniewski, H.H. (1999) MRI of entorhinal cortex in mild Alzheimer's disease. *Lancet* 353:38–40.

Bobinski, M., de Leon, M.J., Wegiel, J., De Santi, S., Convit, A., Saint Louis, L.A., Rusinek, H., and Wisniewski, H.M. (2000) The histological validation of postmortem magnetic resonance imaging-determined hippocampal volume in Alzheimer's disease. *Neuroscience* 95:721–725.

Bobinski, M., Wegiel, J., Tarnawski, M., Reisberg, B., de Leon, M.J., Miller, D.C., and Wisniewski, H.M. (1997) Relationships between regional neuronal loss and neurofibrillary changes in the hippocampal formation and duration and severity of Alzheimer's disease. *J. Neuropathol. Exp. Neurol.* 56:414–420.

Bobinski, M.J., Wegiel, J., Wisniewski, H.M., Tarnawski, B., Bobinski, M., Reisberg, B., de Leon, M.J., and Miller, D.C. (1996) Neurofibrillary pathology—correlation with hippocampal formation atrophy in Alzheimer disease. *Neurobiol. Aging* 17: 909–919.

Bobinski, M., Wegiel, J., Wisniewski, H.M., Tarnawski, M., Reisberg, B., Mlodzik, B., de Leon, M.J., and Miller, D.C. (1995) Atrophy of hippocampal formation subdivisions correlates with stage and duration of Alzheimer disease. *Dementia* 6:205–210.

Bouras, C., Hof, P.R., Giannakopoulos, P., Michel, J.P., and Morrison, J.H. (1994) Regional distribution of neurofibrillary tangles and senile plaques in the cerebral cortex of elderly patients: a quantitative evaluation of a one-year autopsy population from a geriatric hospital. *Cereb. Cortex* 4:138–150.

Braak, H. (1972) Zur pigmentoarchitektonic der Grosshirnrinde des Menschen [ ]. *I. Regio entorhinalis. Z. Zellforsch.* 127:407–438.

Braak, H. (1980) *Architectonics of the Human Telencephalic Cortex*. Berlin: Springer-Verlag.

Braak, H., and Braak, E. (1991) Neuropathological staging of Alzheimer-related changes. *Acta Neuropathol.* 82:239–259.

Braak, H., and Braak, E. (1997) Diagnostic criteria for neuropathologic assessment of Alzheimer's disease. *Neurobiol. Aging* 18: S85–S88.

Brodmann, K. (1909) *Vergleichende lokalisationslehre der grosshirnrinde in ihren prinzipien dargestellt auf grund des zellenbaues* [ ]. Leipzig, Germany: Barth.

Broe, M., Shepherd, C.E., Milward, E.A., and Halliday, G.M. (2001) Relationship between DNA fragmentation, morphological changes and neuronal loss in Alzheimer's disease and dementia with Lewy bodies. *Acta Neuropathol.* 101:616–624.

Busatto, G.F., Garrido, G.E., Almeida, O.P., Castro, C.C., Camargo, C.H., Cid, C.G., Buchpiguel, C.A., Furuie, S., and Bottino, C.M. (2003) A voxel-based morphometry study of temporal lobe gray matter reductions in Alzheimer's disease. *Neurobiol. Aging* 24: 221–231.

Chan, D., Janssen, J.C., Whitwell, J.L., Watt, H.C., Jenkins, R., Frost, C., Rossor, M.N., and Fox, N.C. (2003) Change in rates of cerebral atrophy over time in early-onset Alzheimer's disease: longitudinal MRI study. *Lancet* 362:1121–1122.

Chetelat, G., Desgranges, B., De La Sayette, V., Viader, F., Eustache, F., and Baron, J.C. (2002) Mapping gray matter loss with voxel-based morphometry in mild cognitive impairment. *Neuroreport* 13:1939–1943.

Clark, R.F., and Goate, A.M. (1993) Molecular genetics of Alzheimer's disease. *Arch. Neurol.* 50:1164–1172.

Colsher, P.L., and Wallace, R.B. (1991) Longitudinal application of cognitive function measures in a defined population of community-dwelling elders. *Ann. Epidemiol.* 1:215–230.

Convit, A., de Leon, M.J., Golomb, J., George, A.E., Tarshish, C.Y., Bobinski, M., Tsui, W., De Santi, S., Wegiel, J., and Wisniewski, H.M. (1993) Hippocampal atrophy in early Alzheimer's disease: anatomic specificity and validation. *Psychiatr. Q.* 64:371–387.

Convit, A., de Leon, M.J., Hoptman, M.J., Tarshish, C., De Santi, S., and Rusinek, H. (1995) Age-related changes in brain. I. Magnetic resonance imaging measure of temporal lobe volumes in normal subjects. *Psychiatr. Q.* 66:343–355.

Convit, A., de Leon, M.J., Tarshish, C., De Santi, S., Kluger, A., Rusinek, H., and George, A. (1995) Hippocampal volume losses in minimally impaired elderly. *Lancet* 345:266.

Convit, A., de Leon, M.J., Tarshish, C., De Santi, S., Tsui, W., Rusinek, H., and George, A.E. (1997) Specific hippocampal volume reductions in individuals at risk for Alzheimer's disease. *Neurobiol. Aging* 18:131–138.

Convit, A., McHugh, P.R., Wolf, O.T., de Leon, M.J., Bobinski, M., De Santi, S., Roche, A., and Tsui, W. (1999) MRI volume of the amygdala: a reliable method allowing separation from the hippocampal formation. *Psychiatry Res. Neuroimag.* 90:113–123.

Corder, E.H., Saunders, A.M., Strittmatter, W.J., Schmechel, D.E., Gaskell, P.C., Small, G.W., Roses, A.D., Haines, J.L., and Pericak-Vance, M.A. (1993) Gene dose of apolipoprotein E type 4 allele and the risk of Alzheimer's disease in late onset families. *Science* 261:921–923.

Cousins, D.A., Burton, E.J., Burn, D., Gholkar, A., McKeith, I.G., and O'Brien, J.T. (2003) Atrophy of the putamen in dementia with Lewy bodies but not Alzheimer's disease: an MRI study. *Neurology* 61:1191–1195.

Davies, D.V., Horwood, N., Isaacs, S.L., and Mann, D.M.A. (1992) The effect of age and Alzheimer's disease on pyramidal neuron density in the individual fields of the hippocampal formation. *Acta Neuropathol.* 83:510–517.

de la Monte, S.M. (1989) Quantitation of cerebral atrophy in preclinical and end-stage Alzheimer's disease. *Ann. Neurol.* 25:450–459.

de la Monte, S.M., Sohn, Y.K., Ganju, N., and Wands, J.R. (1998) P53- and CD95-associated apoptosis in neurodegenerative diseases. *Lab. Invest.* 78:401–411.

de Leon, M.J., Convit, A., Wolf, O.T., Tarshish, C.Y., De Santi, S., Rusinek, H., Tsui, W., Kandil, E., Scherer, A.J., Roche, A., Imossi, A., Thorn, E., Bobinski, M., Caraos, C., Lesbre, P., Schlyer, D., Poirier, J., Reisberg, B., and Fowler, J. (2001) Prediction of cognitive decline in normal elderly subjects with 2-(^{18}F)fluoro-2-deoxy-D-glucose/positron-emission tomography (FDG/PET). *Proc. Natl. Acad. Sci. USA* 98:10966–10971.

de Leon, M., deSanti, S., Zinkowski, R., Mehta, P., Pratico, D., Segal, S., Clark, C., Kerkman, D. D., Debernardi, J., Li, J., Lair, L., Reisber, B., and Tsui, W. (2004) MRI and CSF studies in the early diagnosis of Alzheimer's disease. *J. Inter. Med.* 256:205–223.

de Leon, M.J., George, A.E., Convit, A., De Santi, S., Golomb, J., Tarshish, C., Rusinek, H., Ferris, S.H., Bobinski, M., and Arena, L. (1994) MR measurement of the medial temporal lobe changes in Alzheimer disease: The case for the interuncal distance. *Am. J. Neuroradiol.* 15:1286–1290.

de Leon, M.J., George, A.E., Ferris, S.H., Christman, D.R., Fowler, J.S., Gentes, C., Brodie, J., Resiberg, B., and Wolf, A.P. (1984) Positron emission tomography and computed tomography assessments of the aging human brain. *J. Comput. Assist. Tomogr.* 8:88–94.

de Leon, M.J., George, A.E., Golomb, J., Tarshish, C., Convit, A., Kluger, A., De Santi, S., McRae, T., Ferris, S.H., Reisberg, B., Ince, C., Rusinek, H., Bobinski, M., Quinn, B., Miller, D.C., and Wisniewski, H.M. (1997) Frequency of hippocampal formation atrophy in normal aging and Alzheimer's disease. *Neurobiol. Aging* 18:1–11.

de Leon, M., Mosconi, L., Blennow, S., DeSanti, S., Zinkowski, R., Mehta, P., Pratico, D., Tsui, W., Saint Louis, L., Sobanska, L., Brys, M., Li, Y., Rich, K., Rinne, J., and Rusinek, H. (2007) Imaging and CSF studies in the preclinical diagnosis of Alzheimer's disease. *Ann. N. Y. Acad. Sci.* 1097:114–145.

de Leon, M.J., George, A.E., Stylopoulos, L.A., Smith, G., and Miller, D.C. (1989) Early marker for Alzheimer's disease: the atrophic hippocampus. *Lancet* 2:672–673.

de Leon, M.J., Golomb, J., George, A.E., Convit, A., Tarshish, C.Y., McRae, T., De Santi, S., Smith, G., Ferris, S.H., Noz, M., and Rusinek, H. (1993) The radiologic prediction of Alzheimer's disease: the atrophic hippocampal formation. *Am. J. Neuroradiol.* 14:897–906.

de Leon, M.J., McRae, T., Tsai, J.R., George, A.E., Marcus, D.L., Freedman, M., Wolf, A.P., and McEwen, B. (1988) Abnormal cortisol response in Alzheimer's disease linked to hippocampal atrophy. *Lancet* 2:391–392.

den Heijer, T., Geerlings, M.I., Hoebeek, F.E., Hofman, A., Koudstaal, P.J., and Breteler, M.M. (2006) Use of hippocampal and amygdalar volumes on magnetic resonance imaging to predict dementia in cognitively intact elderly people. *Arch. Gen. Psychiatry* 63: 57–62.

De Santi, S., de Leon, M.J., Rusinek, H., Convit, A., Tarshish, C.Y., Boppana, M., Tsui, W.H., Daisley, K., Wang, G.J., and Schlyer, D. (2001) Hippocampal formation glucose metabolism and volume losses in MCI and AD. *Neurobiol. Aging* 22:529–539.

Devanand, D.P., Pradhaban, G., Liu, X., Khandji, A., De Santi, S., Segal, S., Rusinek, H., Pelton, G.H., Honig, L.S., Mayeux, R., Stern, Y., Tabert, M.H., and de Leon, M.J. (2007) Hippocampal and entorhinal atrophy in mild cognitive impairment: prediction of Alzheimer disease. *Neurology* 68:828–836.

Dickerson, B.C., Goncharova, I., Sullivan, M.P., Forchetti, C., Wilson, R.S., Bennett, D.A., Beckett, L.A., and Detoledo-Morrell, L. (2001) MRI-derived entorhinal and hippocampal atrophy in incipient and very mild Alzheimer's disease. *Neurobiol. Aging* 22: 747–754.

Du, A.T., Schuff, N., Amend, D., Laaskso, M.P., Hsu, Y.Y., Jagust, W.J., Yaffe, K., Kramer, J.H., Reed, B., Norman, D., Chui, H.C., and Weiner, M.W. (2001) Magnetic resonance imaging of the entorhinal cortex and hippocampus in mild cognitive impairment and Alzheimer's disease. *J. Neurol. Neurosurg. Psychiatry* 71: 441–447.

Du, A.T., Schuff, N., Laakso, M.P., Zhu, X.P., Jagust, W.J., Yaffe, K., Kramer, J.H., Miller, B.L., Reed, B.R., Norman, D., Chui, H.C., and Weiner, M.W. (2002) Effects of subcortical ischemic vascular dementia and AD on entorhinal cortex and hippocampus. *Neurology* 58:1635–1641.

Duvernoy, H.M. (1988) *The Human Hippocampus: An Atlas of Applied Anatomy*. Munich, Germany: J.F. Bergmann Verlag.

Fox, N.C., Crum, W.R., Scahill, R.I., Stevens, J.M., Janssen, J.C., and Rossor, M.N. (2001) Imaging of onset and progression of Alzheimer's disease with voxel-compression mapping of serial magnetic resonance images. *Lancet* 358:201–205.

Fox, N.C., Scahill, R.I., Crum, W.R., and Rossor, M.N. (1999) Correlation between rates of brain atrophy and cognitive decline in AD. *Neurology* 52:1687–1689.

Frisoni, G.B., Beltramello, A., Geroldi, C., Weiss, C., Bianchetti, A., and Trabucchi, M. (1996) Brain atrophy in frontotemporal dementia. *J. Neurol. Neurosurg. Psychiatry* 61:157–165.

Frisoni, G.B., Sabattoli, F., Lee, A.D., Dutton, R.A., Toga, A.W., and Thompson, P.M. (2006) In vivo neuropathology of the hippocampal formation in AD: a radial mapping MR-based study. *Neuroimage* 32:104–110.

Ganguli, M., Dodge, H.H., Shen, C., and DeKosky, S.T. (2004) Mild cognitive impairment, amnestic type: an epidemiologic study. *Neurology* 63:115–121.

Giannakopoulos, P., Herrmann, F.R., Bussiere, T., Bouras, C., Kovari, E., Perl, D.P., Morrison, J.H., Gold, G., and Hof, P.R. (2003) Tangle and neuron numbers, but not amyloid load, predict cognitive status in Alzheimer's disease. *Neurology* 60:1495–1500.

Giannakopoulos, P., Hof, P.R., Mottier, S., Michel, J.P., and Bouras, C. (1994) Neuropathological changes in the cerebral cortex of 1258 cases from a geriatric hospital: retrospective clinicopathological evaluation of a 10-year autopsy population. *Acta Neuropathol.* 87:456–468.

Glodzik-Sobanska, L., Rusinek, H., Mosconi, L., Li, Y., Zhan, J., De Santi, S., Convit, A., Rich, K.E., Brys, M., and de Leon, M.J. (2005) The role of quantitative structural imaging in the early diagnosis of Alzheimer's disease. *Neuroimaging Clin. N. Am.* 15: 803–826.

Golomb, J., Kluger, A., de Leon, M.J., Ferris, S.H., Convit, A., Mittelman, M.S., Cohen, J., Rusinek, H., De Santi, S., and George, A. (1994) Hippocampal formation size in normal human aging: a correlate of delayed secondary memory performance. *Learn. Mem.* 1:45–54.

Golomb, J., Kluger, A., de Leon, M.J., Ferris, S.H., Mittelman, M.S., Cohen, J., and George, A.E. (1996) Hippocampal formation size predicts declining memory performance in normal aging. *Neurology* 47:810–813.

Gomez-Isla, T., Hollister, R., West, H., Mui, S., Growdon, J.H., Petersen, R.C., Parisi, J.E., and Hyman, B.T. (1997) Neuronal loss correlates with but exceeds neurofibrillary tangles in Alzheimer's disease. *Ann. Neurol.* 41:17–24.

Gomez-Isla, T., Price, J.L., McKeel, D.W., Jr., Morris, J.C., Growdon, J.H., and Hyman, B.T. (1996) Profound loss of layer II entorhinal cortex neurons occurs in very mild Alzheimer's disease. *J. Neurosci.* 16:4491–4500.

Goncharova, I.I., Dickerson, B.C., Stoub, T.R., and Detoledo-Morrell, L. (2001) MRI of human entorhinal cortex: a reliable protocol for volumetric measurement. *Neurobiol. Aging* 22:737–745.

Gosche, K.M., Mortimer, J.A., Smith, C.D., Markesbery, W.R., and Snowdon, D.A. (2002) Hippocampal volume as an index of

Alzheimer neuropathology: findings from the Nun Study. *Neurology* 58:1476–1482.

Hebert, L.E., Scherr, P.A., Bienias, J.L., Bennett, D.A., and Evans, D.A. (2003) Alzheimer disease in the US population: prevalence estimates using the 2000 census. *Arch. Neurol.* 60:11119–11122.

Hirano, A., and Zimmerman, H.M. (1962) Alzheimer's neurofibrillary changes. *Arch. Neurol.* 7:227–242.

Hof, P.R., Bierer, L.M., Perl, D.P., Delacourte, A., Buee, L., Bouras, C., and Morrison, J.H. (1992) Evidence for early vulnerability of the medial and inferior aspects of the temporal lobe in an 82-year-old patient with preclinical signs of dementia: regional and laminar distribution of neurofibrillary tangles and senile plaques. *Arch. Neurol.* 49:946–953.

Hubbard, B.M., Fenton, G.W., and Anderson, J.M. (1990) A quantitative histological study of early clinical and preclinical Alzheimer's disease. *Neuropathol. Appl. Neurobiol.* 16:111–121.

Hyman, B.T., Van Hoesen, G.W., Damasio, A.R., and Barnes, C.L. (1984) Alzheimer's disease: cell-specific pathology isolates the hippocampal formation. *Science* 225:1168–1170.

Ikeda, M., Tanabe, H., Nakagawa, Y., Kazui, H., Oi, H., Yamazaki, H., Harada, K., and Nishimura, T. (1994) MRI-based quantitative assessment of the hippocampal region in very mild to moderate Alzheimer's disease. *Neuroradiology* 36:7–10.

Insausti, R., Amaral, D.G., and Cowan, W.M. (1987) The entorhinal cortex of the monkey: III. Subcortical afferents. *J. Comp. Neurol.* 264:396–408.

Insausti, R., Juottonen, K., Soininen, H., Insausti, A.M., Partanen, K., Vainio, P., Laakso, M.P., and Pitkanen, A. (1998) MR volumetric analysis of the human entorhinal, perirhinal, and temporopolar cortices. *Am. J. Neuroradiol.* 19:659–671.

Insausti, R., Tunon, T., Sobreviela, T., Insausti, A.M., and Gonzalo, L.M. (1995) The human entorhinal cortex: a cytoarchitectonic analysis. *J. Comp. Neurol.* 355:171–198.

Jack, C.R., Dickson, D.W., Parisi, J.E., Xu, Y.C., Cha, R.H., O'Brien, P.C., Edland, S.D., Smith, G.E., Boeve, B.F., et al. (2002) Antemortem MRI findings correlate with hippocampal neuropathology in typical aging and dementia. *Neurology* 58:750–757.

Jack, C.R., Petersen, R.C., O'Brien, P.C., and Tangalos, E.G. (1992) MR-based hippocampal volumetry in the diagnosis of Alzheimer's disease. *Neurology* 42:183–188.

Jack, C.R., Petersen, R.C., Xu, Y., O'Brien, P.C., Smith, G.E., and Ivnik, R.J. (2000) Rates of hippocampal atrophy correlate with change in clinical status in aging and AD. *Neurology* 55: 484–489.

Jack, C.R., Jr., Petersen, R.C., Xu, Y., O'Brien, P.C., Smith, G.E., Ivnik, R.J., Boeve, B.F., Tangalos, E.G., and Kokmen, E. (2000) Rates of hippocampal atrophy correlate with change in clinical status in aging and AD. *Neurology* 55:484–489.

Jack, C.R., Petersen, R.C., Xu, Y.C., O'Brien, P.C., Smith, G.E., Ivnik, R.J., Boeve, B.F., Waring, S.C., Tangalos, E.G., and Kokmen, E. (1999) Prediction of AD with MRI-based hippocampal volume in mild cognitive impairment. *Neurology* 52:1397–1403.

Jack, C.R., Petersen, R.C., Xu, Y.C., Waring, S.C., O'Brien, P.C., Tangalos, E.G., Smith, G.E., Ivnik, R.J., and Kokmen, E. (1997) Medial temporal atrophy on MRI in normal aging and very mild Alzheimer's disease. *Neurology* 49:786–794.

Jack, C. R., Jr., Shiung, M.M., Gunter, J.L., O'Brien, P.C., Weigand, S.D., Knopman, D.S., Boeve, B.F., Ivnik, R.J., Smith, G.E., Cha, R.H., Tangalos, E.G., and Petersen, R.C. (2004) Comparison of different MRI brain atrophy rate measures with clinical disease progression in AD. *Neurology* 62:591–600.

Jack, C.R., Jr., Shiung, M.M., Weigand, S.D., O'Brien, P.C., Gunter, J.L., Boeve, B.F., Knopman, D.S., Smith, G.E., Ivnik, R.J., Tangalos, E.G., and Petersen, R.C. (2005) Brain atrophy rates predict subsequent clinical conversion in normal elderly and amnestic MCI. *Neurology* 65:1227–1231.

Jobst, K.A., Smith, A.D., Szatmari, M., Esiri, M.M., Jaskowski, A., Hindley, N., McDonald, B., and Molyneux, A.J. (1994) Rapidly progressing atrophy of medial temporal lobe in Alzheimer's disease. *Lancet* 343:829–830.

Juottonen, K., Laakso, M.P., Insausti, R., Lehtovirta, M., Pitkanen, A., Partanen, K., and Soininen, H. (1998) Volumes of the entorhinal and perirhinal cortices in Alzheimer's disease. *Neurobiol. Aging* 19:15–22.

Kaye, J.A., Swihart, T., Howieson, D., Dame, A., Moore, M.M., Karnos, T., Camicioli, R., Ball, M., Oken, B., and Sexton, G. (1997) Volume loss of the hippocampus and temporal lobe in healthy elderly persons destined to develop dementia. *Neurology* 48:1297–1304.

Kemper, T.L. (1978) Senile dementia: a focal disease in the temporal lobe. In: Nandy, E., ed. *Senile Dementia: A Biomedical Approach*. New York: Elsevier, pp. 105–113.

Kesslak, J.P., Nalcioglu, O., and Cotman, C.W. (1991) Quantification of magnetic resonance scans for hippocampal and parahippocampal atrophy in Alzheimer's disease. *Neurology* 41:51–54.

Killiany, R.J., Gomez-Isla, T., Moss, M., Kikinis, R., Sandor, T., Jolesz, F., Tanzi, R., Jones, K., Hyman, B., and Albert, M.S. (2000) Use of structural magnetic resonance imaging to predict who will get Alzheimer's disease. *Ann. Neurol.* 47:430–439.

Killiany, R.J., Hyman, B.T., Gomez-Isla, T., Moss, M.B., Kikinis, R., Jolesz, F., Tanzi, R., Jones, K., and Albert, M.S. (2002) MRI measures of entorhinal cortex vs. hippocampus in preclinical AD. *Neurology* 58:1188–1196.

Kluger, A., Ferris, S.H., Golomb, J., Mittelman, M.S., and Reisberg, B. (1999) Neuropsychological prediction of decline to dementia in nondemented elderly. *J. Geriatr. Psychiatr. Neurol.* 12:168–179.

Knopman, D.S., Parisi, Salviati, A., Floriach-Robert, M., Boeve, B.F., Ivnik, R.J., Smith, G.E., Dickson, D.W., Johnson, K.A., Petersen, L.E., McDonald, W.C., Braak, H., and Petersen, R.C. (2003) Neuropathology of cognitively normal elderly. *J. Neuropathol. Exp. Neurol.* 62:1087–1095.

Kril, J.J., Patel, S., Harding, A.J., and Halliday, G.M. (2002) Neuron loss from the hippocampus of Alzheimer's disease exceeds extracellular neurofibrillary tangle formation. *Acta Neuropathol.* 103:370–376.

Laakso, M.P., Soininen, H., Partanen, K., Lehtovirta, M., Hallikainen, M., Hanninen, T., Helkala, E.-L., Vainio, P., and Riekkinen, P.J., Sr. (1998) MRI of the hippocampus in Alzheimer's disease: sensitivity, specificity, and analysis of the incorrectly classified subjects. *Neurobiol. Aging* 19:23–31.

Langui, D., Probst, A., and Ulrich, J. (1995) Alzheimer's changes in non-demented and demented patients: a statistical approach to their relationships. *Acta Neuropathol.* 89:57–62.

Larrabee, G.J., and Crook, T.H. (1994) Estimated prevalence of age-associated memory impairment derived from standardized tests of memory function. *Int. Psychogeriat.* 6:95–104.

Lehericy, S., Baulac, M., Chiras, J., Pierot, L., Martin, N., Pillon, B., Deweer, B., Dubois, B., and Marsault, C. (1994) Amygdalohippocampal MR volume measurements in the early stages of Alzheimer disease. *Am. J. Neuroradiol.* 15:929–937.

Manly, J.J., Bell-McGinty, S., Tang, M.X., Schupf, N., Stern, Y., and Mayeux, R. (2005) Implementing diagnostic criteria and estimating frequency of mild cognitive impairment in an urban community. *Arch. Neurol.* 62:1739–1746.

Mann, D.M.A., and Esiri, M.M. (1989) The pattern of acquisition of plaques and tangles in the brains of patients under 50 years of age with Down syndrome. *J. Neurol. Sci.* 89:169–179.

McKhann, G., Drachman, D., Folstein, M., Katzman, R., Price, D., and Stadlan, E.M. (1984) Clinical diagnosis of Alzheimer's disease: report of the NINCDS-ADRDA work group under the auspices of Department of Health and Human Services Task Force on Alzheimer's disease. *Neurology* 34:939–944.

Mesulam, M.M. (1990) Large-scale neurocognitive networks and distributed processing for attention, language, and memory. *Neurol. Prog.* 28(5):597–613.

Mishkin, M. (1978) Memory in monkeys severely impaired by combined but not by separate removal of amygdala and hippocampus. *Nature* 273:297–298.

Mori, E., Lee, K., Yasuda, M., Hashimoto, M., Kazui, H., Hirono, N., and Matsui, M. (2002) Accelerated hippocampal atrophy in Alzheimer's disease with apolipoprotein E epsilon4 allele. *Ann. Neurol.* 51:209–214.

Morris, J.C., McKeel, D.W., Storandt, M., Rubin, E.H., Price, J.L., Grant, E.A., Ball, M.J., and Berg, L. (1991) Very mild Alzheimer's disease: informant-based clinical, psychometric, and pathological distinction from normal aging. *Neurology* 41:469–478.

Mosconi, L. (2005) Brain glucose metabolism in the early and specific diagnosis of Alzheimer's disease. FDG-PET studies in MCI and AD. *Eur. J. Nucl. Med. Mol. Imaging* 32:486–510.

Mosconi, L., Brys, M., Glodzik-Sobanska, L., De Santi, S., Rusinek, H., and de Leon, M.J. (2007) Early detection of Alzheimer's disease using neuroimaging. *Exp. Gerontol.* 42:129–138.

Mosconi, L., De Santi, S., Rusinek, H., Convit, A., and de Leon, M.J. (2004) Magnetic resonance and PET studies in the early diagnosis of Alzheimer's disease. *Expert Rev. Neurother.* 4:831–849.

Mosconi, L., Tsui, W.H., Pupi, A., De Santi, S., Drzezga, A., Minoshima, S., and de Leon, M.J. (2007) (18)F-FDG PET database of longitudinally confirmed healthy elderly individuals improves detection of mild cognitive impairment and Alzheimer's disease. *J. Nucl. Med.* 48:1129–1134.

Moss, M., Mahut, H., and Zola-Morgan, S. (1981) Concurrent discrimination learning of monkeys after hippocampal, entorhinal, or fornix lesions. *J. Neurosci.* 3:227–240.

Mu, Q., Xie, J., Wen, Z., Weng, Y., and Shuyun, Z. (1999) A quantitative MR study of the hippocampal formation, the amygdala, and the temporal horn of the lateral ventricle in healthy subjects 40 to 90 years of age. *Am. J. Neuroradiol.* 20:207–211.

Mungas, D., Harvey, D., Reed, B.R., Jagust, W.J., DeCarli, C., Beckett, L., Mack, W.J., Kramer, J.H., Weiner, M.W., Schuff, N., and Chui, H.C. (2005) Longitudinal volumetric MRI change and rate of cognitive decline. *Neurology* 65:565–571.

O'Brien, J.T., Paling, S., Barber, R., Williams, E.D., Ballard, C., McKeith, I.G., Gholkar, A., Crum, W.R., Rossor, M.N., and Fox, N.C. (2001) Progressive brain atrophy on serial MRI in dementia with Lewy bodies, AD, and vascular dementia. *Neurology* 56:1386–1388.

Paykel, E.S., Brayne, C., Huppert, F.A., Gill, C., Barkley, C., Gehlhaar, E., Beardsall, L., Girling, D.M., Pollitt, P., and O'Connor, D. (1994) Incidence of dementia in a population older than 75 years in the United Kingdom. *Arch. Gen. Psychiatry* 51:325–332.

Pennanen, C., Kivipelto, M., Tuomainen, S., Hartikainen, P., Hanninen, T., Laakso, M.P., Hallikainen, M., Vanhanen, M., Nissinen, A., Helkala, E.L., Vainio, P., Vanninen, R., Partanen, K., and Soininen, H. (2004) Hippocampus and entorhinal cortex in mild cognitive impairment and early AD. *Neurobiol. Aging* 25:303–310.

Pennanen, C., Testa, C., Laakso, M.P., Hallikainen, M., Helkala, E. L., Hanninen, T., Kivipelto, M., Kononen, M., Nissinen, A., Tervo, S., Vanhanen, M., Vanninen, R., Frisoni, G.B., and Soininen, H. (2005) A voxel based morphometry study on mild cognitive impairment. *J. Neurol. Neurosurg. Psychiatry* 76:11–14.

Petrella, J.R., Coleman, R.E., and Doraiswamy, P.M. (2003) Neuroimaging and early diagnosis of Alzheimer disease: a look to the future. *Radiology* 226:315–336.

Press, G.A., Amaral, D.G., and Squire, L.R. (1989) Hippocampal abnormalities in amnesic patients revealed by high-resolution magnetic resonance imaging. *Nature* 341:54–57.

Price, J.L., Davis, P.B., Morris, J.C., and White, D.L. (1991) The distribution of tangles, plaques and related immunohistochemical markers in healthy aging and Alzheimer's disease. *Neurobiol. Aging* 12:295–312.

Price, J.L., Ko, A.I., Wade, M.J., Tsou, S.K., McKeel, D.W., and Morris, J.C. (2001) Neuron number in the entorhinal cortex and CA1 in preclinical Alzheimer disease. *Arch. Neurol.* 58:1395–1402.

Reisberg, B., Ferris, S.H., de Leon, M.J., and Crook, T. (1982) The global deterioration scale for assessment of primary degenerative dementia. *Am. J. Psychiatry* 139:1136–1139.

Rombouts, S.A., Barkhof, F., Witter, M.P., and Scheltens, P. (2000) Unbiased whole-brain analysis of gray matter loss in Alzheimer's disease. *Neurosci. Lett.* 285:231–233.

Rose, M. (1927) Die sog, Riechrinde beim Menschen und beim Affem. II. Teil des "Allocortex bei Tier und Mensch" [ ]. *J. Psychol. Neurol.* 34:261–401.

Rosene, D.L., and Van Hoesen, G.W. (1987) The hippocampal formation of the primate brain: a review of some comparative aspects of cytoarchitecture and connections. In: Jones, E.G. and Peters, A., eds. *Cerebral Cortex*. New York: Plenum Press, pp. 345–456.

Rossler, M., Zarski, R., Bohl, J., and Ohm, T.G. (2002) Stage-dependent and sector-specific neuronal loss in hippocampus during Alzheimer's disease. *Acta Neuropathol.* 103:363–369.

Rusinek, H., De Santi, S., Frid, D., Tsui, W., Tarshish, C., Convit, A., et al. (2003) Regional brain atrophy rate predicts future cognitive decline: 6-year longitudinal MR imaging study of normal aging. *Radiology* 229:691–696.

Rusinek, H., Endo, Y., De Santi, S., Frid, D., Tsui, W.H., Segal, S., Convit, A., and de Leon, M.J. (2004) Atrophy rate in medial temporal lobe during progression of Alzheimer disease. *Neurology* 63:2354–2359.

Scheff, S.W., Price, D.A., Schmitt, F.A., DeKosky, S.T., and Mufson, E.J. (2007) Synaptic alterations in CA1 in mild Alzheimer disease and mild cognitive impairment. *Neurology* 68:1501–1508.

Scheltens, P., Leys, D., Barkhof, F., Huglo, D., Weinstein, H.C., Vermersch, P., Kuiper, M., Steinling, M., Wolters, E.C., and Valk, J. (1992) Atrophy of medial temporal lobes on MRI in "probable" Alzheimer's disease and normal aging: diagnostic value and neuropsychological correlates. *J. Neurol. Neurosurg. Psychiatry* 55:967–972.

Schoenberg, B.S. (1986) Epidemiology of Alzheimer's disease and other dementing disorders. *J. Chronic Dis.* 39:1095–1104.

Schonheit, B., Zarski, R., and Ohm, T. G. (2004) Spatial and temporal relationships between plaques and tangles in Alzheimer-pathology. *Neurobiol. Aging* 25:697–711.

Schott, J.M., Fox, N.C., Frost, C., Scahill, R.I., Janssen, J.C., Chan, D., Jenkins, R., and Rossor, M.N. (2003) Assessing the onset of structural change in familial Alzheimer's disease. *Ann. Neurol.* 53:181–188.

Seab, J.P., Jagust, W.S., Wang, S.F.S., Roos, M.S., Reed, B.R., and Budinger, T.F. (1988) Quantitative NMR measurements of hippocampal atrophy in Alzheimer's disease. *Magn. Reson. Med.* 8:200–208.

Small, S.A., Tsai, W.Y., DeLaPaz, R., Mayeux, R., and Stern, Y. (2002) Imaging hippocampal function across the human life span: is memory decline normal or not? *Ann. Neurol.* 51:290–295.

Squire, L.R. (1992) Memory and the hippocampus: a synthesis from findings with rats, monkeys, and humans. *Psychol. Rev.* 99: 195–231.

Stout, J.C., Jernigan, T.L., Archibald, S.L., and Salmon, D.P. (1996) Association of dementia severity with cortical gray matter and abnormal white matter volume in dementia of Alzheimer type. *Arch. Neurol.* 53:742–749.

Suzuki, W.A., and Amaral, D.G. (1994) Perirhinal and parahippocampal cortices of the macaque monkey: cortical afferents. *J. Comp. Neurol.* 350:497–533.

Thal, D.R., Holzer, M., Rub, U., Waldmann, G., Gunzel, S., Zedlick, D., and Schober, R. (2000) Alzheimer-related tau-pathology in the perforant path target zone and in the hippocampal stratum oriens and radiatum correlates with onset and degree of dementia. *Exp. Neurol.* 163:98–110.

Thompson, L.K. (2003) Unraveling the secrets of Alzheimer's beta-amyloid fibrils. *Proc. Natl. Acad. Sci. USA*, 100:383–385.

Twamley, E.W., Ropacki, S.A., and Bondi, M.W. (2006) Neuropsychological and neuroimaging changes in preclinical Alzheimer's disease. *J. Int. Neuropsychol. Soc.* 12:707–735.

Ulrich, J. (1985) Alzheimer changes in nondemented patients younger than sixty-five: possible early stages of Alzheimer's disease and senile dementia of Alzheimer type. *Ann. Neurol.* 17:273–277.

van de Pol, L.A., van der Flier, W.M., Korf, E.S., Fox, N.C., Barkhof, F., and Scheltens, P. (2007) Baseline predictors of rates of hippocampal atrophy in mild cognitive impairment. *Neurology* 69: 1491–1497.

Van Hoesen, G.W. (1982) The parahippocampal gyrus: new observations regarding its cortical connections in the monkey. *Trends Neurosci.* 5:345–350.

Varma, A.R., Adams, W., Lloyd, J.J., Carson, K.J., Snowden, J.S., Testa, H.J., Jackson, A., and Neary, D. (2002) Diagnostic patterns of regional atrophy on MRI and regional cerebral blood flow change on SPECT in young onset patients with Alzheimer's disease, frontotemporal dementia and vascular dementia. *Acta Neurol. Scand.* 105:261–269.

Vogt, C., and Vogt, O. (1919) Allgemeinere Ergebnisse unserer Hirnforschung [ ]. *J. Psychol. Neurol.* 25:279–462.

Welsh, K., Butters, N., Hughes, J., Mohs, R., and Heyman, A. (1991) Detection of abnormal memory decline in mild cases of Alzheimer's disease using CERAD neuropsychological measures. *Arch. Neurol.* 48:278–281.

West, M.J., Coleman, P.D., Flood, D.G., and Troncoso, J.C. (1994) Differences in the pattern of hippocampal neuronal loss in normal ageing and Alzheimer's disease. *Lancet* 344:769–772.

Witter, M.P., and Amaral, D.G. (1991) Entorhinal cortex of the monkey: V. Projections to the dentate gyrus, hippocampus, and subicular complex. *J. Comp. Neurol.* 307:437–459.

Xu, Y., Jack, C.R., O'Brien, P.C., Kokmen, E., Smith, G.E., Ivnik, R.J., Boeve, B.F., Tangalos, R.G., and Petersen, R.C. (2000) Usefulness of MRI measures of entorhinal cortex versus hippocampus in AD. *Neurology* 54:1760–1767.

Zola-Morgan, S., and Squire, L.R. (1986) Memory impairment in monkeys following lesions limited to the hippocampus. *Behav. Neurosci.* 2:155–160.

Zola-Morgan, S., Squire, L.R., and Amaral, D.G. (1989) Lesions of the amygdala that spare adjacent cortical regions do not impair memory or exacerbate the impairment following lesions of the hippocampal formation. *J. Neurosci.* 9:1922–1936.

Zola-Morgan, S., Squire, L.R., Clower, R.P., and Rempel, N.L. (1993) Damage to the perirhinal cortex exacerbates memory impairment following lesions to the hippocampal formation. *J. Neurosci.* 13:251–265.

Zola-Morgan, S., Squire, L.R., and Ramus, S.J. (1994) Severity of memory impairment in monkeys as a function of locus and extent of damage within the medial temporal lobe memory system. *Hippocampus* 4:483–495.

58 Abnormalities in Brain Structure on Postmortem Analysis of Dementia

DANIEL P. PERL

In the absence of reliable biological markers for the clinical evaluation of any of the major dementing disorders, the autopsy continues to play a critical role in establishing the definitive diagnosis for patients who suffer from dementia. Furthermore, in the absence of a truly valid animal model for the major disorder associated with dementia, Alzheimer's disease (AD), postmortem tissues derived from patients with this disease continue to play an invaluable role for researchers investigating a wide variety of aspects of this condition. Over the past two decades, major advances have been made in identifying relevant changes in brain structure related to the presence of various dementing disorders as well as recognizing those changes that occur in the course of the normal aging process.

NORMAL AGING

Traditionally, it has been taught that normal aging is accompanied by a modest degree of loss of neurons in several regions of the brain. However, the extent of that loss is currently being reassessed using the techniques of systematic nonbiased sampling (stereology). Preliminary data using these nonbiased sampling techniques indicate that such neuronal losses in normal aging are difficult to verify in most regions studied (for review see Peters et al., 1998). Additional studies of this kind will be required to confirm if this impression is correct. Neurofibrillary tangles and senile plaques, lesions to be discussed in detail in "Alzheimer's Disease," are frequently seen in relatively small numbers in the entorhinal cortex, hippocampus, and even neocortex of brains obtained from individuals of advanced age with normal cognitive function. In general, the extent of these lesions in the normal elderly, though variable, is considerably less than that found in patients with clinically apparent AD. However, the distinction between normal-aged individuals and those with mild cognitive impairment can involve subtle distinctions.

ALZHEIMER'S DISEASE

Any of the grossly visible alterations in brain structure that can be seen in patients with AD are entirely nonspecific in nature and overlap extensively with those encountered in brain specimens derived from elderly individuals who had shown normal cognitive function during life. In general, the brain of any individual older than age 60 years shows some increase in fibrous tissue within the leptomeninges, particularly involving the parasaggital regions over the vertex of the cerebral hemispheres. This age-related fibrosis produces a variable degree of whitening and opacification of the membranes. The degree of this change in patients with AD is indistinguishable from that seen in elderly patients with no dementia.

Most brain specimens derived from patients with AD show some degree of cerebral cortical atrophy. This atrophy is most notable in the frontotemporal association cortex and tends to spare primary motor, sensory, and visual areas. Once again, in elderly patients, particularly those of advanced age, there is extensive overlap between brain weight and measures of cortical atrophy between age-matched individuals with normal cognitive function and those with AD. Indeed, the overlap is so extensive that brain weight or cortical thickness measured on the brain specimen of any individual cannot be reliably employed to predict the presence of dementia (Terry, 1986). When taken as a group, such differences were difficult to establish on a statistical basis. However, it should be noted that in cases of AD of presenile onset (that is, arbitrarily set at an onset younger than 65 years), comparisons of brain weight or degree of cortical atrophy with age-matched controls reveal a clear and obvious difference upon gross inspection of the brain.

The loss of brain tissue associated with AD generally leads to a symmetrical dilatation of the lateral ventricles (hydrocephalus ex vacuo). Again, based on this finding, one cannot accurately distinguish between age-matched normals and persons with AD. However, grossly visible atrophy of the hippocampus, with selective dilatation of the temporal horn, does represent a reasonably reliable clue, upon dissection of the brain, that the specimen will ultimately show microscopic evidence of AD. Similarly, the absence of this finding indicates that other explanations for the underlying cause of dementia will likely need to be sought.

Microscopic Changes

The histopathological evaluation of the brain tissues of victims of AD reveals a series of morphological alterations upon which the neuropathological diagnosis is based. Once again, virtually all of these alterations may also be encountered, to some degree, in the brains of elderly patients who during life had demonstrated normal cognitive function. Some of these changes do not correlate with the extent of cognitive loss, whereas for others, the distinction between AD and normal aging involves complex evaluation regarding the extent and distribution of the particular abnormality. Indeed, correlations between the extent and distribution of such lesions are currently undergoing detailed scientific study using brain specimens derived from individuals in large cohorts of elderly patients who have undergone rigorous longitudinal neuropsychological studies.

Neurofibrillary Tangles

In his initial description of the disease that would eventually bear his name, Alois Alzheimer (1907) identified the presence of abnormal fibrous inclusions within the neuronal perikaryal cytoplasm. These inclusions are referred to as *Alzheimer neurofibrillary tangles,* and they are one of the cardinal microscopic lesions associated with the disease. It is difficult to specifically visualize the neurofibrillary tangle using hematoxylin and eosin, the traditional morphological histological stain of pathology. In general, a variety of silver impregnation stains, such as the modified Bielschowski or Gallyas techniques, or the fluorochrome dye *thioflavin S*, are typically employed to better visualize and quantify these changes. With better characterization of the protein constituents of the neurofibrillary tangle, immunohistochemical approaches have also been widely used for this purpose. These have mostly employed antibodies to abnormally phosphorylated tau (see below) (Yen et al., 1987; Dickson et al., 1988; Iwatsubo et al., 1994). Because these techniques require either specialized equipment (in the case of the thioflavin S stain) or experienced histotechnologists (in the case of silver impregnation stains), many anatomical pathologists in general practice are usually unable to evaluate properly brain specimens submitted for the diagnosis of AD. Such specimens are best referred to specialized neuropathology laboratories with the experience and facilities needed to evaluate various neurodegenerative disorders.

Using these special stains, within neurons with a pyramidal perikaryal shape, such as the large neurons of the CA1 sector of the hippocampus and the layer V neurons of the association cortex, the neurofibrillary tangle appears as parallel aggregates of thickened fibrils that frequently surround the nucleus and extend toward the apical dendrite (Fig. 58.1). When neurons with a more rounded configuration are involved by a neurofibrillary tangle, such as neurons of the substantia nigra and locus coeruleus, the inclusion appears as interweaving swirls of fibers and here they are referred to as *globoid tangles*. The vast majority of neurons that contain a neurofibrillary tangle, based on light microscopic and ultrastructural examination, appear to be morphologically intact. However, particularly in areas of the brain with severe neurofibrillary tangle formation, one will encounter examples of tangles lying free in the neuropil and without any associated host neurons. Such structures are referred to as *extracellular* or *ghost tangles* and are thought to represent tangle-bearing neurons that have died, leaving the tangle as a remnant that the brain cannot effectively remove.

The nature of the neurofibrillary tangle has been the subject of considerable research over the past several decades, and much has been learned about its structural components. Ultrastructurally, the neurofibrillary tangle is composed of parallel skeins of abnormal fibrils that measure 10 nm in diameter. The fibrils are paired and wound in a helical fashion having a regular periodicity of 80 nm (Kidd, 1963; Wisniewski et al., 1976). Based on these observations, such structures are generally referred to as *paired helical filaments* (PHF). It took many years to decipher the biochemical nature of these abnormal fibrils because they are extremely resistant to solubilization. The primary constituent of the

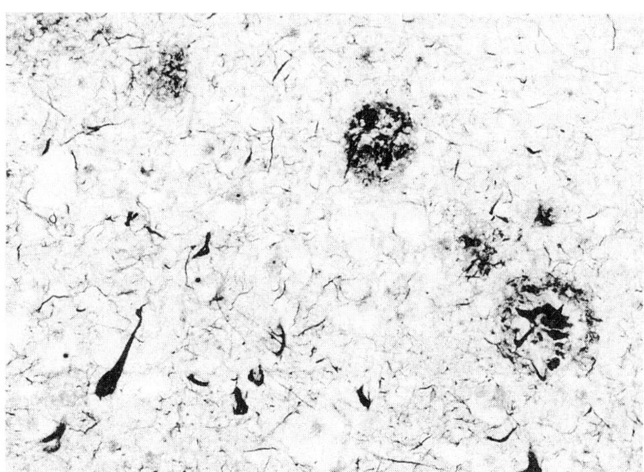

FIGURE 58.1 Alzheimer's disease in the hippocampus (CA1). Modified Bielschowski stain shows neurofibrillary tangles and senile plaques.

neurofibrillary tangle is a microtubule-associated protein called *tau*. The tau within neurofibrillary tangles is abnormally phosphorylated, with phosphate groups attached to specific sites on the molecule (Lee et al., 1991). The neurofibrillary tangle also contains a number of other protein constituents such as ubiquitin (Perry et al., 1987; Love et al., 1988), cholinesterases (Mesulam and Moran, 1987), and β-amyloid (Aβ; see below) (Hyman et al., 1989), the major constituent of the amyloid accumulations seen in senile plaques and leptomeningeal and cerebral cortical blood vessels (see below).

The pattern of distribution of neurofibrillary tangles present in cases of AD is, for the most part, rather distinct and predictable. Severe involvement is seen in the layer II neurons of the entorhinal cortex, the CA1 and subicular regions of the hippocampus, the amygdala, and the deep layers (layers V and superficial VI) of the neocortex (Morrison and Hof, 1997). Studies have shown that the extent and distribution of neurofibrillary tangles in cases of AD do correlate with the degree of dementia and the duration of illness (Arriagada et al., 1992; Hof et al., 1995). This suggests that this neuronal alteration does have some direct impact on the functioning capacity of the individual who is affected. However, it is clear that other factors contribute to the clinical features of the disease.

It is important to recognize that though the neurofibrillary tangle is one of the cardinal histopathological features of AD, this neuropathological alteration may also be encountered in association with a large variety of other disease states (Wisniewski et al., 1979). These include disorders such as postencephalitic parkinsonism, post-traumatic dementia or dementia pugalistica, type C Niemann–Pick disease, and amyotrophic lateral sclerosis/parkinsonism dementia complex of Guam. It remains unclear why diseases with such a wide range of underlying etiological mechanisms should all show this one particular neuronal abnormality.

Senile Plaque

The other major histopathological alteration encountered in patients suffering from AD is the senile or neuritic plaque. Senile plaques are relatively complex lesions but are defined by the presence of a central core accumulation of a 4 kD protein with a β-pleated sheet configuration referred to as Aβ or β–amyloid (Masters et al., 1985; Kang et al., 1987; Beyreuther and Masters, 1990). The β-pleated sheet configuration of the protein confers on the molecule the ability to bind the planar dye Congo Red and produce birefringence when illuminated by polarized light, the physical definition of an amyloid.

Several different forms of plaque are associated with brain aging and AD, and at times the nomenclature employed in the literature can be confusing. The neuritic plaque has a central core of Aβ protein arranged in a radial fashion and is surrounded by a corona of abnormally formed neurites or neuronal processes (either dendrites or axons). The abnormal or dystrophic neurites stain strongly with the same silver impregnation stains (Fig. 58.2) used to identify the neurofibrillary tangles, and ultrastructurally these structures contain dense bodies, membranous profiles, and packets of paired helical filaments. In the periphery of the neuritic plaque, one may also commonly encounter one or two microglial cells and, less frequently, reactive astrocytes.

With the availability of immunohistochemical techniques using antibodies raised against portions of the Aβ protein, it has been recognized that focal diffuse deposits of this amyloid protein may occur in the cerebral cortex in the absence of accompanying dystrophic neurites (Yamaguchi et al., 1989). Such diffuse deposits of Aβ are now referred to as *diffuse plaques*. Diffuse plaques are commonly encountered in the brains of elderly individuals and can be seen in relatively large numbers in the absence of any associated evidence of cognitive impairment (Gentleman et al., 1989; Morris et al., 1996; Wolf et al., 1999).

A third form of plaque has also been identified, consisting of a dense core of Aβ that may or may not be accompanied by a small number of surrounding dystrophic neurites. Such plaques are generally referred to as *burned-out* or *end-stage plaques* and are considered to be the remnants of what was once a neuritic plaque (Wisniewski et al., 1982). Because all neuropathological observations of such lesions are, by their very nature, cross-sectional with respect to time, these interpretations are best thought of as speculation.

The Aβ protein is derived from a larger amyloid precursor protein (APP), which is a highly conserved transmembrane glycoprotein (Kang et al., 1987). The Aβ portion of the precursor protein is formed through the

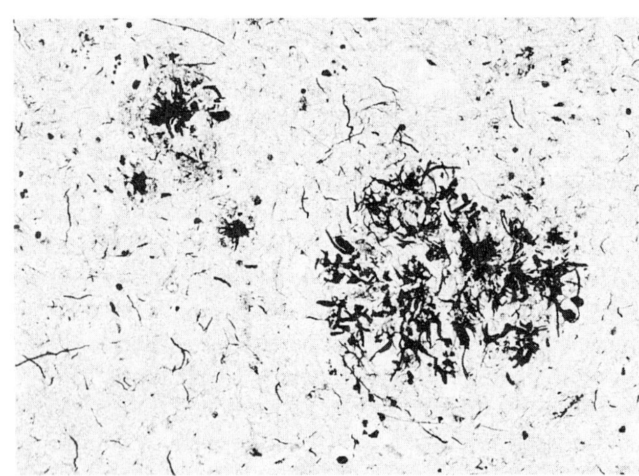

FIGURE 58.2 Alzheimer's disease in the neocortex. Modified Bielschowski stain shows senile or neuritic plaques.

action of two secretases, which split the amino and carboxyl terminals of the 4 kD segment that then accumulates in the tissues (Selkoe et al., 1996; Selkoe, 1998, 2001). The carboxyl end cleavage is ragged, with longer forms (having a total of 42 or 43 amino acids) tending to be deposited within the senile plaques and a shorter form (containing 40 amino acids) tending to accumulate within the leptomeningeal and cerebral cortical blood vessels in the form of congophilic angiopathy (see below) (Prelli et al., 1988). Senile plaques have been shown to accumulate a number of other proteins, for example, heparan sulfate glycoproteins (Maresh et al., 1996; Snow et al., 1996; Castillo et al., 1997), apolipoprotein ε4 (Namba et al., 1991; Dickson et al., 1997; Nishiyama et al., 1997), complement proteins (Dickson and Rogers, 1992; Rogers et al., 1992; McGeer et al., 1994), and alpha-1-antichymotrypsin (Abraham et al., 1990).

Congophilic Angiopathy

Not only does Aβ accumulate in the form of senile plaque cores, there is also a tendency for this molecule to accumulate in the walls of the cerebral blood vessels. This phenomenon is referred to as *congophilic angiopathy*. The vessels that become involved by this process are the small arteries and arterioles of the leptomeninges and those of the gray matter of the cerebral cortex. It has been found that the shorter forms of the Aβ polypeptide, that is, the 1–40 form, predominates in these deposits (Prelli et al., 1988). These accumulations do not appear to exert any deleterious effect on the function of these vessels, although with a severe degree of involvement the vessel becomes prone to spontaneous intraparenchymal rupture, with focal accumulation of blood in the brain tissues. Such hemorrhages are not generally encountered in and around the lenticular nuclei and thalamus, such as that seen as a consequence of uncontrolled systemic hypertension. The hemorrhages associated with congophilic angiopathy tend to occur in the frontal and occipital white matter and may also be multiple. Due to their more isolated location, such lesions are commonly referred to as *lobar hemorrhages*.

Granulovacuolar Degeneration/Eosinophilic Rod-Like Inclusions (Hirano Bodies)

Granulovacuolar degeneration was first identified by Simchowitz in 1911. This poorly understood lesion consists of small vacuoles measuring 2–4 mm in diameter, each containing a small, dense basophilic granule, which typically measures approximately 1 mm in diameter. These granule-containing vacuoles are encountered almost exclusively within the perikaryal cytoplasm of pyramidal neurons of the hippocampus, most typically at the junction between the CA2 and CA1 sectors. They also are seen in lesser numbers in the neurons of the remainder of the CA1 hippocampal region. Ultrastructurally, they are described as a membrane-bound structure with a clear vacuolar matrix containing an electron-dense central granule (Hirano et al., 1968). These central granules stain darkly with silver impregnation stains and are decorated with antibodies directed against phosphorylated neurofilaments *tubulin*, *tau*, and *ubiquitin* (Kahn et al., 1985; Dickson et al., 1987; Ikegami et al., 1996). Little is known about the nature of these lesions or their significance. They may clearly be seen in brain specimens derived from elderly individuals with normal cognitive function. However, two studies have shown that the presence of large numbers of such lesions in the boundary zone between the CA1 and CA2 regions of the caudal aspect of the hippocampus correlates well with a diagnosis of AD (Tomlinson and Kitchener, 1972; Ball and Lo, 1977).

Eosinophilic rod-like inclusions, or Hirano bodies, are encountered within the CA1 region of the hippocampus. These intensely eosinophilic lesions were first identified by Asao Hirano in his pioneering clinico-neuropathological studies of amyotrophic lateral sclerosis/parkinsonism–dementia complex of Guam and are now commonly referred to as *Hirano bodies* (Hirano, 1994). In this disease, confined to the native population of Guam, large numbers of such lesions are commonly encountered. Subsequently, similar inclusions in lesser numbers were noted in some but not all cases of AD. Finally, such lesions may also be identified in the brains of normal-aged individuals with intact cognition, but typically there are very few of these lesions in such specimens. Hirano bodies have a distinct ultrastructural appearance consisting of parallel fibers that interweave in a regular crossing pattern that is strongly reminiscent of the appearance of a tweed fabric. Immunohistochemical studies have revealed the presence of epitopes of actin, tropomyosin, and vinculin in these bodies (Goldman, 1983; Galloway, Perry, and Gambetti, 1987; Galloway, Perry, Kosik, and Gambetti, 1987). At the present time, the Hirano body appears to be a nonspecific alteration, and its significance is unknown.

Synaptic Loss

Studies by Masliah and Terry (Masliah et al., 1989; Terry et al., 1991; Masliah and Terry, 1993; Masliah et al., 1993) and by Scheff and coworkers (Scheff and Price, 1993; Scheff et al., 1993; DeKosky et al., 1996; Scheff and Price, 1998; Scheff et al., 2001) have shown that a substantial loss of synaptic profiles occurs in the brains of patients with AD. This has been investigated using quantification of immunohistochemical markers against synaptic proteins such as synaptophysin and by quantitative electron microscopy. Masliah and coworkers have shown a mean decrease of 45% in the amount of staining of presynaptic boutons in cases of AD, representing a dramatic loss in these critical elements that support cell-to-cell communication (Masliah et al., 1989). These coauthors have argued that this loss constitutes the major morphological counterpart to cognitive loss in AD and that it correlates highly with the degree of functional impairment (Terry et al., 1991).

Diagnostic Criteria for Alzheimer's Disease

In the absence of a specific clinical and/or laboratory diagnostic test for AD, it is correctly stated that one cannot make a definitive clinical diagnosis of this disorder, and confirmation at autopsy is ultimately required. This places the burden of establishing the definitive diagnosis on the neuropathologist. In the majority of cases, particularly those with severe impairment at the end stage of the disease, that task is relatively straightforward, and the brain specimen typically demonstrates extensive and widespread involvement by virtually all of the lesions described above. However, in a significant number of cases, either the extent of involvement by these lesions or the presence of other superimposed pathological processes makes the establishment of a clear-cut diagnosis problematic. Panels of neuropathologists with expertise in the evaluation of such cases have been convened over the years with the task of articulating usable criteria for establishing a neuropathological diagnosis of AD.

Over the years, three major criteria have been proposed by groups of pathologists with expertise in AD, and each has been employed with variable success. The first such criterion was articulated by a group of neuropathologists organized by the National Institute on Aging (NIA) and the American Association of Retired Persons (AARP). The results of their deliberations became known in the literature as the *NIA/AARP* or *Khachaturian Criteria* after the organizer of the group, Dr. Zaven Khachaturian (Khachaturian, 1985). The Khachaturian Criteria sought to establish an approach to the diagnosis of AD based on the use of an age-related senile plaque score that was determined by the density of senile plaques in the neocortex. For example, in individuals dying between the ages of 66 and 75 years, more than 10 neocortical plaques per microscopic field with a total area of 1 mm^2 were required for the diagnosis of AD. However, for individuals dying at an age older than 75 years, 15 plaques per microscopic field were required to establish the diagnosis. This approach attempted to deal with the reality that some elderly individuals could have overtly intact cognitive function yet still show a moderate degree of senile plaque formation in the cerebral cortex.

The second major effort to introduce criteria for the diagnosis of AD was carried out by the Consortium to Establish a Registry for Alzheimer's Disease (CERAD) (Mirra et al., 1991). This group developed a protocol aimed at standardizing the approach for assessing the density of senile plaques in a semiquantitative fashion. They also sought a method to standardize the collection of other measures of the extent of AD-related lesions. For establishing a neuropathological diagnosis, the CERAD group also employed an age-related senile plaque score (plaque density), expressed as being possible, probable, or definite AD. Whether a case is considered possible, probable, or definite relates to the extent of plaque formation in regard to the age of the patient plus information on whether dementia was present on clinical evaluation.

Most recently, consensus recommendations have emerged from the National Institute on Aging/Reagan Institute Working Group on Diagnostic Criteria for the Neuropathological Assessment of Alzheimer's Diseases (Hyman and Trojanowski, 1997). The so-called NIA/Reagan Institute recommendations endorse the use of the CERAD approach for standardized semiquantitative assessments of senile plaque densities and also suggest that the extent and distribution of neurofibrillary tangles present (using the Braak and Braak [1991] stages; see below) be added to the diagnostic assessment. The overall assessment is expressed in terms of a low, medium, or high probability that the dementia present was related to AD.

EARLY-STAGE VERSUS LATE-STAGE ALZHEIMER'S DISEASE

Until relatively recently, the vast majority of the neuropathological literature related to clinico-pathological correlation tended to involve descriptions of the end stages of AD. Because patients with AD do not typically die as a direct consequence of the disease itself, most patients tend to survive to its advanced stages. They tend to linger on in a severely impaired condition for a variable amount of time until a superimposed infection or another disorder emerges to serve as the cause of death. Accordingly, the brain specimen from such a patient will typically demonstrate a severe, widely distributed burden of neurodegenerative lesions. Typically, in the final years of their illness, such patients will have deteriorated so severely that they are completely noncommunicative and are virtually unable to be tested using standard neuropsychological batteries. The brain specimens of such terminal patients will typically show a heavy burden of neurofibrillary tangles and senile plaques. This situation is particularly prevalent among relatively young patients with AD, the patients likely to be diagnosed and followed longitudinally by research groups interested in AD. Accordingly, such patients are likely to be involved in a variety of research studies and eventually undergo autopsy and donation of the brain for use in postmortem studies. Indeed, over the years, the overwhelming proportion of published studies that use postmortem tissues have involved end-stage patients.

However, it must be recognized that AD is a slowly progressive condition that takes many years, perhaps a decade or more, to progress to clinical stages where a diagnosis can first be made. This is generally followed by many years of further progression from early to middle stages of the disorder. Because AD is a distinctly age-related disorder, it is anticipated that a proportion of elderly patients would actually die in the early stages of AD related to the presence of other disease states, frequently before the diagnosis was formally suggested.

It is clear that the incidence and prevalence of AD are strongly correlated with advanced age and that the vast majority of cases are encountered after the age of 80. Recognizing that advanced age, with its inherent frailties and multiple medical comorbidities, leads to a high death rate, it would therefore be anticipated that many elderly individuals would die of unrelated causes while also passing through the early clinical stages of AD. Additionally, it would be anticipated that some elderly individuals would die during the period when the disease was just starting but had not had enough time to produce a sufficient number of lesions to attract clinical attention, neuropsychological workup, and eventual diagnosis. What happens when such a patient comes to a neuropathologist for diagnostic evaluation? It is clear that in many of these cases, the neuropathological changes found would be considered to be part of normal aging. Over the years, many such cases were described, and a literature emerged in which partial expression of the neuropathology of AD was considered a normal counterpart of the aging process and was thought to be separable from AD.

More recently, a number of laboratories have begun to look in a disciplined fashion at the progressive development of the lesions of AD. One of the major objectives of such work has been to clarify the nature of the earliest morphological features of the disease. What appears to be a reproducible pattern for the sequential development of the disease has begun to emerge. This work has come predominantly from the laboratories of several cortical neuroanatomists who have recognized the importance of specific underlying cortical pathways in defining the spread of the lesions as the disease progresses. The work, among others, of Pearson and colleagues (1985), Van Hoesen and Hyman (1990), Morrison and Hof (1997), and Braak and Braak (1991) has made major contributions. This has culminated in a proposed sequence by Eva and Heiko Braak of the progression of AD in six stages of increasing involvement of the brain. Stages 1 and 2 show relatively selective involvement by neurofibrillary tangles in the transentrohinal cortex. This is followed by stages 3 and 4, with increasing limbic lobe involvement, followed by two final stages (5 and 6) with a more typical widespread pattern of involvement in the neocortex. The Braak and Braak stages were developed by evaluating the pattern of neurodegenerative changes present in a series of 83 brain specimens derived from elderly individuals. The stages were constructed by looking at the comparative extent and distribution of lesion development in the brains used in the study, but no associated clinical data were available from the patients from whom these specimens were obtained. Despite this obvious weakness, the Braak and Braak stages have been quite useful and, for the most part, have provided a format for the morphologist to use in evaluating the relative stage of development of the disease.

A small number of research groups have now begun to enroll relatively large cohorts of elderly individuals who demonstrate intact cognitive function and follow them longitudinally over a period of years. In advanced age, some individuals will retain undiminished cognitive capacities, while others will begin to show deterioration, presumably related in some cases to the development of AD. If the cohort is sufficiently large and of advanced age, a significant proportion of deaths will occur each year due to a number of common age-related medical conditions. With an active autopsy procurement program, after several years a number of brain specimens derived from such normal or individuals who were mildly impaired can be collected and made available for study. This has been the design of several ongoing studies, such as the Religious Order Study at Rush-Presbyterian–St. Luke's (Mufson et al., 2000; Kordower et al., 2001; Mitchell et al., 2002), the Nun Study at the University of Kentucky (Snowdon et al., 2000; Gosche et al., 2002; Riley et al., 2002), the Memory and Aging Study at Washington University, St. Louis (Price and Morris, 1999; Morris and Price, 2001; Morris et al., 2001; Price et al., 2001), and the Jewish Home for the Aged Study at the Mount Sinai School of Medicine (Haroutunian et al., 1998; Davis et al., 1999; Bussiere et al., 2002). Such study groups have begun to publish reports on aspects of early AD and have provided important clinico-pathological correlational data. These studies have shown that neurofibrillary tangles and senile plaques correlate with the degree of dementia in patients with mild AD.

DEMENTIA WITH LEWY BODIES (DIFFUSE CORTICAL LEWY BODY DISEASE)

In 1817, James Parkinson, in his classic essay on shaking palsy, noted that the disease that now bears his name left the intellect unimpaired (Parkinson, 1955). Despite the validity of his otherwise remarkably precise clinical description of the disease, it is now known that dementia is a common consequence of this disorder, particularly when it affects elderly individuals. Some studies have shown that more than 50% of patients with Parkinson's disease will eventually develop significant cognitive impairment (Pirozzolo et al., 1993). Extrapyramidal clinical features are also commonly encountered in patients with AD (Molsa et al., 1984).

Some neuropathological studies have shown that approximately one-fourth of patients with a progressive dementia considered consistent with a clinical diagnosis of AD show at autopsy significant numbers of neurofibrillary tangles and senile plaques but also demonstrate degeneration of the dopaminergic neurons of the substantia nigra, pars compacta in association with Lewy bodies in remaining pigmented neurons (Ditter and Mirra, 1987). In such cases, a varying number of weakly eosinophilic spherical cytoplasmic inclusions are also noted in cerebral cortical neurons. Such inclusions stain prominently with antibodies raised against ubiquitin and α-synuclein and are referred to as *cortical Lewy bodies*. The use of such immunohistochemical approaches has allowed the ready identification of large numbers of cases of dementia associated with both nigral and cortical Lewy bodies (Dickson, 1999). To further confuse matters, it is now recognized that at autopsy, virtually all cases of Parkinson's disease show some degree of cortical Lewy body formation (Hughes et al., 1992). This has led to considerable disagreement and controversy regarding how such cases should be categorized diagnostically.

Some have claimed that dementia with Lewy bodies is a distinct and separable clinical and neuropathological entity that is actually quite common, and a consensus conference has proposed specific clinical and neuropathological diagnostic criteria for this condition (McKieth et al., 1996; Lowe and Dickson, 1997). We have pointed out that cases that begin with extrapyramidal features and subsequently develop dementia are virtually indistinguishable neuropathologically from those cases that present with dementia and then show neuropsychiatric and extrapyramidal features (Perl et al., 1998). Indeed, of 76 pathologically established Parkinson's disease cases examined at the United Kingdom Brain Bank, four met the proposed neuropathological diagnostic criteria for dementia with Lewy bodies (Hughes et al., 1992). For these and other reasons, we have raised concerns about considering dementia with Lewy bodies as a distinct clinical entity and have noted that the extensive overlap between AD and Parkinson's disease is far greater than one would anticipate by chance alone (Perl et al., 1998). This has led to the suggestion that such overlap may represent common pathogenetic mechanisms affecting a variety of specific vulnerable neuronal populations. These disagreements remain unresolved and continue to be the subject of active investigation and discussion.

OTHER CAUSES OF DEMENTIA

Multi-Infarct Dementia

Stroke, in the form of brain infarction, is a relatively common disorder in elderly individuals. Indeed, studies have shown that the incidence of clinically apparent brain infarction is about 3 times greater among individuals 75 years of age or older than among individuals younger than 65 years of age. A neuropathological study performed many years ago indicated that over 30% of brain specimens from individuals dying at older than 90 years of age evaluated neuropathologically showed evidence of either acute or healed infarcts in the cerebral hemispheres (Peress et al., 1972). Of the patients in this series who had been noted to be diabetic, the incidence was approximately 50%. In cases in which there is cumulative destruction of vital cerebral structures, such as occurs as a result of multiple cerebral infarctions, clinical evidence of cognitive impairment may be noted. In such cases, the term *multi-infarct dementia* is commonly employed.

Traditionally, this term is reserved for cases in which the cerebrovascular lesions alone are thought to be responsible for the cognitive failure. In our experience, such cases are relatively rare. In the Mount Sinai/Bronx Veterans Administration Alzheimer's Disease Research Center brain bank repository, only 7% of dementia cases coming to neuropathological evaluation were diagnosed as multi-infarct dementia. Of course, patients with AD, particularly those of advanced age, may commonly suffer from superimposed cerebral infarction. In such cases, it may be difficult for the neuropathologist to determine the relative importance of the infarctive lesion or lesions in producing the relative extent of cognitive failure shown in any patient of this type. Such cases are generally referred to as *mixed dementia* and should not be considered examples of true multi-infarct dementia.

In multi-infarct dementia, the extent and distribution of the infarcts present show considerable case-to-case variability. As a general rule, the lesions are multiple, bilateral, and of varying age, typically involving the cerebral cortex, basal ganglia, and/or subcortical white matter. In most cases, one of these general areas will be predominantly involved. In our experience, multiple cerebral cortical areas of infarction represent the most commonly encountered pattern. As a general rule, the total combined volume of cerebral cortical tissue destruction is almost invariably in excess of 50 ml.

Infarctions involving the basal ganglia leading to dementia tend to be smaller than their cerebral cortical counterparts, frequently representing multiple lacunar infarcts, each less than 1 cm in greatest dimension. Such lesions are virtually always bilateral, and involvement of the thalamus is very common (Fig. 58.3). These lesions

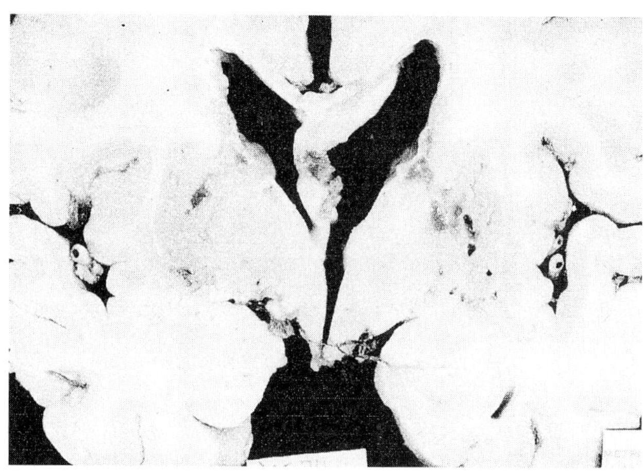

FIGURE 58.3 Gross appearance of a brain with multi-infarct dementia showing several bilateral lacunar infarcts.

represent a consequence of arteriosclerotic disease of the proximal middle cerebral artery and its lenticulostriate perforating branches. Multi-infarct dementia with lacunar and cerebral cortical involvement is also a common pattern of distribution.

In a very small number of cases of multi-infarct dementia, the infarctive process selectively involves the subcortical white matter. Such lesions produce widespread demyelinization, with relative sparing of the overlying cerebral cortex. The ensuing dementia is thought to represent a cortical disconnection syndrome. Such cases are usually referred to as *subacute arteriosclerotic encephalopathy* or *Binswanger's disease*, and this is apparently the rarest form of multi-infarct dementia (Caplan and Schoene, 1978; Caplan, 1995).

Frontotemporal Lobar Degeneration (FTLD)

In patients with presenile onset of dementia (that is, prior to age 65 years), there is a significant proportion of cases that show a clearly demonstrable pattern of cerebral degeneration that selectively involves the frontal and temporal lobes. Such cases are categorized, in general, as examples of frontotemporal lobar degeneration (FTLD). Within this group, there has emerged a rather complex subclassification based on associated clinical features (such as motor neuron disease, parkinsonism, etc.), molecular pathology, and the presence or absence of specific accompanying neuropathologic features (for example, Pick bodies, ubiquitinated intraneuronal inclusions, etc.). This is a rapidly expanding area as new cases are reported and analyzed.

Cases of FTLD in all forms tend to share clinical features that are referred to as *frontotemporal dementia* that includes a nonfluent aphasia with notable deficits in speech production and semantic dementia (preservation of episodic memory—that is, recollections of day-to-day events), and profoundly impaired semantic memory—that is, the understanding of the meaning of verbal and visual stimuli. Poor judgment, disinhibition, and other problems with executive function are also noted in such patients.

Neuropathologists have begun to classify cases of FTLD into those with tau-immunopositive inclusions and those with ubiquitin immunopositive inclusions (FTLD-U). The classic FTLD tau-positive disorder is Pick's disease. Pick's disease is characterized neuropathologically by striking frontotemporal atrophy, with relative sparing of the remainder of the cerebral cortex and the presence of Pick bodies, characteristic inclusions in affected neurons. In its classic presentation, Pick's disease is characterized by emotional and behavioral changes indicative of temporal lobe and amygdala pathology. These patients may show many characteristics of the Kluver–Bucy syndrome, with apathy, hyperorality, and changes in sexual and eating habits. Dementia may be profound. Some cases of Pick's disease may be clinically indistinguishable from AD.

Grossly, the brain with Pick's disease typically shows strikingly severe "knife-edge" atrophy of the frontotemporal cortex (lobar atrophy). The parietal and occipital cortices typically have a normal appearance, with a sharp boundary between the affected and unaffected regions. Symmetrical dilatation of the lateral ventricles is obvious in fully evolved cases, with particularly striking enlargement of the temporal horns. This reflects extensive loss of tissue through severe involvement of the hippocampus and amygdala. Brain weights of these patients are commonly below 1,000 g.

In the affected cortex, one usually finds severe neuronal loss with accompanying reactive gliosis. The few remaining neurons are somewhat swollen and contain a large, spherical inclusion body within the perikaryal cytoplasm. Such inclusions stain prominently with silver impregnation stains (Fig. 58.4). They are best seen in the hippocampus but, to a variable extent, may also be seen in other areas of involved cortex. In regions with severe neuronal loss, it may be difficult to identify any characteristic inclusions, although swollen ("ballooned") neurons with clear chromatolytic cytoplasm (so-called Pick cells) may be encountered. The cytoplasm of such cells generally does not stain with silver stains, although faint argyrophilia may be seen. When neocortical Pick bodies are more extensive, they tend to involve layers II and VI, a pattern of distribution that is strikingly different from the laminar distribution pattern observed in the neurofibrillary tangles of AD (Hof et al., 1994).

Pick bodies in the neocortex may be superficially confused with cortical Lewy bodies, as both lesions are spherical and may be argyrophilic (cortical Lewy bodies tend to be more weakly argyrophilic). Although both inclusions show immunoreactivity to ubiquitin, Pick bodies stain strongly with antitau antibodies, while cor-

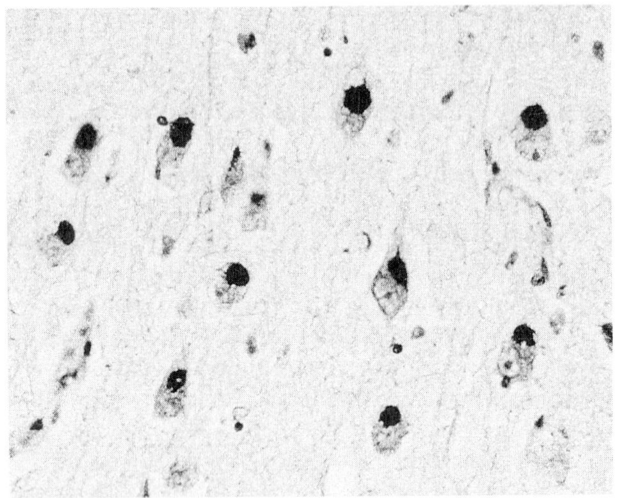

FIGURE 58.4 Pick's disease in the hippocampus. Modified Bielschowski stain shows numerous Pick bodies in pyramidal cells.

tical Lewy bodies do not (Love et al., 1988; Lowe et al., 1988).

Finally, anti-α-synuclein immunostaining marks cortical Lewy bodies prominently but fails to delineate Pick bodies. Ultrastructural studies have shown the Pick body to be a non-membrane-bound inclusion consisting of a randomly arranged accumulation of straight filaments measuring 14–16 nm in diameter and of variable length (Murayama et al., 1990). These filaments are admixed with a variable amount of twisted filaments having a periodicity and diameter distinctly different from those of the paired helical filaments of AD neurofibrillary tangles.

In the hippocampus there may be dramatic involvement of the large pyramidal neurons of the CA1 region by Pick bodies. Smaller similar lesions are also typically encountered in the small neurons of the dentate fasciculus. Most recently, immunohistochemical preparations using antitau antibodies have shown the presence of glial cytoplasmic inclusions in Pick's disease (Iwatsubo et al., 1994). It should be noted that some cases of Pick's disease show, in addition to Pick bodies, neurofibrillary tangles and even senile plaques. In such Pick's disease cases with superimposed AD-related pathology, the clinical presentation and other neuropathological features appear to be no different than those seen in more typical Pick's disease. Finally, the molecular nature of the tau accumulation seen in Pick's disease is distinctly different from that of AD (Delacourte et al., 1996). The tau encountered in AD migrates on a Western blot to reveal three major bands (at 55, 66, and 69 kD), whereas the tau associated with Pick's disease shows only two major bands (at 55 and 66 kD). It has been suggested that this observation may serve as a molecular means for differentiating the two diseases. Finally, recent investigations into other forms of FTLD (see below) have led to the suggestion that this entity be called *frontotemporal lobar degeneration with Pick bodies* (FTLD with Pick bodies) (Cairns et al., 2007).

Those FTLD-U cases are characterized by the presence of ubiquitin immunopositive intraneuronal inclusions that are tau negative and α-synuclein negative (Josephs, 2007). Such frontotemporal lobar degeneration with ubiquitin positive inclusions (FTLD-U) may be seen with or without associated motor neuron disease. Recently, the protein that is ubiquitinated in these inclusions has been identified as TAR-DNA binding protein 43 (TDP-43) (Neumann, et al., 2006). Of interest is that TDP-43 immunoreactive inclusions have also been identified in motor neurons of sporadic cases of amyotrophic lateral sclerosis. Frontotemporal lobar degeneration with ubiquitin positive inclusions may also be linked to mutations to several other proteins, such as progranulin and valsolin-containing protein. This has led to a rather complex approach to classification for which, as further cases are identified and studied, additional modifications will be needed (Cairns et al., 2007).

Frontotemporal Dementia and Parkinsonism Linked to Chromosome 17 (FTDP-17)

An additional form of frontotemporal dementia has been identified that is associated with clinical parkinsonism. Approximately 60% of such cases show evidence of familial clustering, typically with an autosomal dominant inheritance pattern. Studies of such families have demonstrated linkage to chromosome 17q21–22. Because these cases show evidence of accompanying parkinsonism, the nosologic term *frontotemporal dementia and parkinsonism linked to chromosome 17* (FTDP-17) has been introduced (Spillantini et al., 1998).

Clinically, such cases may demonstrate a wide variety of manifestations. Many show the clinical features typical of frontotemporal dementia with a loss of frontal lobe executive functions, hyperorality, stereotyped and perseverative behaviors, a progressive paucity of speech but preserved spatial orientation. The disease typically begins in the 50s, although cases have been reported with onset in the 30s to the 70s. Inappropriate behavior and impulsivity are also common. Prominent psychiatric symptoms similar to those of schizophrenia have also been reported, including auditory hallucinations, delusions, and paranoia. Judgment is impaired, as well as planning and reasoning capabilities. In the later phases of the disease, a more profound global dementia occurs that may often be difficult to separate from that of AD. Signs of parkinsonism, including bradykinesia, limb rigidity, and postural instability, are evident in most cases. Typically, these features do not respond to 3,4-dihydroxyphenylalanine (L-DOPA) therapy. Motor weakness accompanied by muscular wasting in the limbs, and fasciculations has also been reported in some cases.

A relatively small number of morphological descriptions have been reported in documented cases of FTDP-17 (Hulette et al., 1999). Such cases typically show evidence of cerebral cortical atrophy of the frontal and temporal lobes as well as of the amygdala and basal ganglia. In the involved areas, there is evidence of rather severe neuronal loss with accompanying gliosis. In most cases, there is relative sparing of the hippocampus and substantia nigra. In those areas of involvement, tau-immunoreactive intraneuronal inclusions are seen with the appearance of neurofibrillary tangles, as well as tau-positive inclusions in glial cells. Typically, stains for $A\beta$ accumulation are negative. To make the situation even more confusing, some cases of FTDP-17 have been reported with Pick bodies. At present, it remains unclear to what extent such FTDP-17 cases represent a substrate of progressive dementia and/or parkinsonism, particularly when encountered in a familial setting. This also appears to be a situation where the more one looks, the more one finds.

Prion-Related Diseases (Creutzfeldt–Jakob Disease, Gerstmann–Straussler–Scheinker Syndrome, Fatal Familial Insomnia)

Creutzfeldt–Jakob disease (CJD) is an extremely rare form of rapidly progressive dementia. It is seen sporadically and in familial clusters throughout the world. Patients show evidence of a rapidly advancing dementia typically associated with motor disturbances, a characteristic electroencephalographic pattern (so-called triphasic waves), and myoclonic jerks. The disease is invariably fatal, with patients typically dying within a year of onset. Although AD may be confused with CJD at its initial presentation, this characteristically rapid course readily distinguishes CJD from the much more slowly progressive AD. Creutzfeldt–Jakob disease is characterized neuropathologically by neuronal loss, intense reactive gliosis, and spongiform changes. The extent of neuronal loss and the accompanying gliosis correlate well with the length of the illness, generally reflecting the attentiveness of supporting nursing care provided to the patient. Intracerebral inoculation of homogenates of the brain tissue of patients with CJD into nonhuman primates has produced a similar syndrome following a prolonged incubation period and serves as the basis for considering this condition to be transmissible (Gibbs et al., 1968). The nature of the transmissible agent is an abnormally folded protein (PrP protein) that is capable of initiating replication in the host and is referred to generically as a *prion* (Prusiner, 1991). Owing to the potentially infectious nature of affected tissues, organs from suspected patients with CJD (cornea, kidney, etc.) should not be employed for transplantation since they are capable of transmitting disease iatrogenically (Gajdusek et al., 1977).

Gerstmann–Strausler–Scheinker syndrome is an extremely rare disorder (approximately 2–5 cases/100 million population) that is also a prion-related condition. Clinically, it is characterized by cerebellar ataxia, dysmetria, hyporeflexia, and a positive Babinski sign. Neuropathological examination shows prominent plaque-like amyloid deposits in the molecular layer of the cerebellum. The amyloid protein that accumulates is composed of PrP protein and not $A\beta$, as is seen in AD. Gerstmann–Strausler–Scheinker syndrome is inherited in an autosomal dominant fashion, and in most cases a proline to leucine substitution is found at the 102 codon of the PrP molecule (Hsiao et al., 1989).

Fatal familial insomnia (FFI) is also an extremely rare prion-related disorder and in most cases is related to mutations of the 129 codon of the PrP molecule (Gambetti et al., 1995). Patients with FFI show prominent disturbances in sleep–wake cycles, hallucinations, ataxia, myoclonus, dysarthria, and pyramidal signs. This disorder is also invariably fatal, typically with a course of less than 1 year. Neuropathological features include prominent neuronal loss with astrocytosis and spongiform changes localized particularly to the thalamus.

Posttraumatic Dementia (Dementia Pugalistica)

The clinical studies of Critchley (1957) and the clinico-neuropathological findings of Corselis (Corsellis and Brierly, 1959; Corsellis et al., 1973) have helped to characterize a progressive dementing disorder that develops as a consequence of the delayed effects of severe repeated head trauma. This disorder, referred to as *posttraumatic dementia*, *punch drunk syndrome*, or *dementia pugalistica*, is classically encountered in retired boxers, although additional cases are reported following other forms of severe trauma to the head. In a study of 250 randomly selected retired boxers in Great Britain, 26 showed clinical evidence of a posttraumatic encephalopathic condition characterized by extrapyramidal signs, frequently accompanied by a variable extent of dementia (Roberts et al., 1990). Typically, the progression of the dementia was rather slow. However, in some cases, there was such marked functional impairment that institutional placement was required.

Neuropathological examination of patients with dementia pugalistica typically shows thinning and perforation of the septum pellucidum, depigmentation of the substantia nigra, and rather extensive neurofibrillary tangle formation in the frontotemporal cerebral cortex. The distribution of tangles in the cortex predominates in layers II and III, compared to layer V, a pattern that is the reverse of that seen in AD (Hof et al., 1992). Although this condition was classically described by Corselis as being free of senile plaque formation, the sensitive immunohistochemical procedures developed subsequently showed rather dramatic Aβ accumulation (Roberts et al., 1991). Parkinsonian symptoms are related to profound loss of the pigmented neurons in the substantia nigra; however, Lewy bodies are not encountered. Dementia pugalistica is a poorly understood entity, and the pathogenetic mechanisms responsible for progressive neurodegeneration following repeated blows to the head remain entirely obscure.

REFERENCES

Abraham, C.R., Shirahama, T., and Potter, H. (1990) Alpha 1-antichymotrypsin is associated solely with amyloid deposits containing the beta-protein. Amyloid and cell localization of alpha 1-antichymotrypsin. *Neurobiol. Aging* 11:123–129.

Alzheimer, A. (1907) Ueber eine eigenartige erkrankung der hirnrinde [About a peculiar disease of the cerebral cortex]. *Z. Gesamte Neurol. Psychiat.* 18:177–179.

Arriagada, P.V., Growdon, J.H., Hedley-White, T., and Hyman, B.T. (1992) Neurofibrillary tangles and not senile plaques parallel duration and severity of Alzheimer's disease. *Neurology* 42:1681–1688.

Ball, M.J., and Lo, L. (1977) Granulovacuolar degeneration in the ageing brain and in dementia. J. *Neuropathol. Exp. Neurol.* 36: 474–487.

Beyreuther, K., and Masters, C.L. (1990) Nomenclature of amyloid A4 proteins and their precursors in Alzheimer's disease and Down's syndrome. *Neurobiol. Aging* 11:66–68.

Braak, H., and Braak, E. (1991) Neuropathological stageing of Alzheimer-related changes. *Acta Neuropathol. (Berl)* 82:239–259.

Bussiere, T., Friend, P.D., Sadeghi, N., Wicinski, B., Lin, G.I., Bouras, C., Giannakopoulos, P., Robakis, N.K., Morrison, J.H., Perl, D.P., and Hof, P.R. (2002) Stereologic assessment of the total cortical volume occupied by amyloid deposits and its relationship with cognitive status in aging and Alzheimer's disease. *Neuroscience* 112:75–91.

Cairns, N.J., Bigio, E.H., Mackenzie, I.R.A., Neumann, M., Lee, V.M.Y., Hatanpaa, K.J., et al. (2007) Neuropathologic diagnostic and nosologic criteria for frontotemporal lobar degeneration: consensus of the consortium for frontotemporal lobar degeneration. *Acta Neuropathol.* 114:5–22.

Caplan, L.R. (1995) Binswanger's disease–revisited. *Neurology* 45: 626–633.

Caplan, L.R., and Schoene, W.C. (1978) Clinical features of subcortical arteriosclerotic encephalopathy (Binswanger disease). *Neurology* 28:1206–1215.

Castillo, G.M., Ngo, C., Cummings, J., Wight, T.N., and Snow, A.D. (1997) Perlecan binds to the beta-amyloid proteins (A beta) of Alzheimer's disease, accelerates A beta fibril formation, and maintains A beta fibril stability. *J. Neurochem.* 69:2452–2465.

Corsellis, J.A.N., and Brierly, J.B. (1959) Observations on the pathology of insidious dementia following head injury. *J. Mental. Sci.* 105:715–720.

Corsellis, J.A.N., Bruton, C.J., and Freeman-Browne, D. (1973) The aftermath of boxing. *Psychol. Med.* 3:270–303.

Critchley, M. (1957) Medical aspects of boxing particularly from a neurological standpoint. *Br. Med. J.* 1:357.

Davis, K.L., Mohs, R.C., Marin, D., Purohit, D.P., Perl, D.P., Lantz, M., Austin, G., and Haroutunian, V. (1999) Cholinergic markers in elderly patients with early signs of Alzheimer disease. *JAMA* 281:1401–1406.

DeKosky, S.T., Scheff, S.W., and Styren, S.D. (1996) Structural correlates of cognition in dementia: quantification and assessment of synapse change. *Neurodegeneration* 5:417–421.

Delacourte, A., Robitaille, Y., Sergeant, N., Buee, L., Hof, P.R., Wattez, A., Laroche Cholette, A., Mathieu, J., Chagnon, P., and Gauvreau, D. (1996) Specific pathological Tau protein variants characterize Pick's disease. *J. Neuropathol. Exp. Neurol.* 55:159–168.

Dickson, D.W. (1999) Tau and synuclein and their role in neuropathology. *Brain Pathol.* 9:657–661.

Dickson, D.W., Farlo, J., Davies, P., Crystal, H., Fuld, P., and Yen, S.H. (1988) Alzheimer's disease. A double-labeling immunohistochemical study of senile plaques. *Am. J. Pathol.* 132:86–101.

Dickson, D.W., Ksiezak-Reding, H., Davies, P., and Yen, S.H. (1987) A monoclonal antibody that recognizes a phosphorylated epitope in Alzheimer neurofibrillary tangles, neurofilaments and tau proteins immunostains granulovacuolar degeneration. *Acta Neuropathol. (Berl)* 73:254–258.

Dickson, D.W., and Rogers, J. (1992) Neuroimmunology of Alzheimer's disease: a conference report. *Neurobiol. Aging* 13:793–798.

Dickson, T.C., Saunders, H.L., and Vickers, J.C. (1997) Relationship between apolipoprotein E and the amyloid deposits and dystrophic neurites of Alzheimer's disease. *Neuropathol. Appl. Neurobiol.* 23:483–491.

Ditter, S.M., and Mirra, S.S. (1987) Neuropathologic and clinical features of Parkinson's disease in Alzheimer's disease patients. *Neurology* 37:754–760.

Gajdusek, D.C., Gibbs, C.J., Jr., Asher, D.M., Brown, P., Diwan, A., Hoffman, P., Nemo, G., Rohwer, R., and White, L. (1977) Precautions in medical care of, and in handling materials from, patients with transmissible virus dementia (Creutzfeldt-Jakob disease). *N. Engl. J. Med.* 297:1253–1258.

Galloway, P.G., Perry, G., and Gambetti, P. (1987) Hirano bodies contain actin and actin-associated proteins. *J. Neuropathol. Exp. Neurol.* 46:185–199.

Galloway, P.G., Perry, G., Kosik, K., and Gambetti, P. (1987) Hirano bodies contain tau protein. *Brain Res.* 403:337–340.

Gambetti, P., Parchi, P., Petersen, R.B., Chen, S.G., and Lugaresi, E. (1995) Fatal familial insomnia and familial Creutzfeldt-Jakob disease: clinical, pathological and molecular features. *Brain Pathol.* 5:43–51.

Gentleman, S.M., Bruton, C., Allsop, D., Lewis, S.J., Polak, J.M., and Roberts, G.W. (1989) A demonstration of the advantages of immunostaining in the quantification of amyloid plaque deposits. *Histochemistry* 92:355–358.

Gibbs, C.J., Jr., Gajdusek, D.C., Asher, D.M., Alpers, M.P., Beck, E., Daniel, P.M., and Matthews, W.B. (1968) Creutzfeldt-Jakob disease (spongiform encephalopathy): transmission to the chimpanzee. *Science* 161:388–389.

Goldman, J.E. (1983) The association of actin with Hirano bodies. *J. Neuropathol. Exp. Neurol.* 42:146–152.

Gosche, K.M., Mortimer, J.A., Smith, C.D., Markesbery, W.R., and Snowdon, D.A. (2002) Hippocampal volume as an index of Alzheimer neuropathology: findings from the Nun Study. *Neurology* 58:1476–1482.

Haroutunian, V., Perl, D.P., Purohit, D.P., Marin, D., Khan, K., Lantz, M., Davis, K.L., and Mohs, R.C. (1998) Regional distribution of neuritic plaques in the nondemented elderly and subjects with very mild Alzheimer disease. *Arch. Neurol.* 55:1185–1191.

Hirano, A. (1994) Hirano bodies and related neuronal inclusions. *Neuropathol. Appl. Neurobiol.* 20:3–11.

Hirano, A., Dembitzer, H.M., Kurland, L.T., and Zimmerman, H.M. (1968) The fine structure of some intraganglionic alterations. Neurofibrillary tangles, granulovacuolar bodies and "rod-like" structures as seen in Guam amyotrophic lateral sclerosis and parkinsonism-dementia complex. *J. Neuropathol. Exp. Neurol.* 27:167–182.

Hof, P.R., Bierer, L.M., Purohit, D.P., Carlin, L., Schmeidler, J.M., Davis, K.L., and Perl, D.P. (1995) Neurofibrillary tangles correlate with dementia severity in Alzheimer's disease. *Arch. Neurol.* 52:81–88.

Hof, P.R., Bouras, C., Buee, L., Delacourte, A., Perl, D.P., and Morrison, J.H. (1992) Differential distribution of neurofibrillary tangles in the cerebral cortex of dementia pugilistica and Alzheimer's disease cases. *Acta Neuropathol. (Berl)* 85:23–30.

Hof, P.R., Bouras, C., Perl, D.P., and Morrison, J.H. (1994) Quantitative neuropathologic analysis of Pick's disease cases: cortical distribution of Pick bodies and coexistence with Alzheimer's disease. *Acta Neuropathol. (Berl)* 87:115–124.

Hsiao, K., Baker, H.F., Crow, T.J., Poulter, M., Owen, F., Terwilliger, J.D., Westaway, D., Ott, J., and Prusiner, S.B. (1989) Linkage of a prion protein missense variant to Gerstmann-Straussler syndrome. *Nature* 338:342–346.

Hughes, A.J., Daniel, S.E., Kilford, L., and Lees, A.J. (1992) Accuracy of clinical diagnosis of idiopathic Parkinson's disease: a clinico-pathological study of 100 cases. *J. Neurol. Neurosurg. Psychiatry* 55:181–184.

Hulette, C.M., Pericak-Vance, M.A., Roses, A.D., Schmechel, D.E., Yamaoka, L.H., Gaskell, P.C., Welsh-Bohmer, K.A., Crowther, R.A., and Spillantini, M.G. (1999) Neuropathological features of frontotemporal dementia and parkinsonism linked to chromosome 17q21–22 (FTDP-17): Duke Family 1684. *J. Neuropathol. Exp. Neurol.* 58:859–866.

Hyman, B.T., and Trojanowski, J.Q. (1997) Consensus recommendations for the postmortem diagnosis of Alzheimer's disease from the National Institute on Aging and the Reagan Institute working group on diagnostic criteria for the neuropathological assessment of Alheimer's disease. *J. Neuropathol. Exp. Neurol.* 56: 1095–1097.

Hyman, B.T., Van Hoesen, G.W., Beyreuther, K., and Masters, C.L. (1989) A4 amyloid protein immunoreactivity is present in Alzheimer's disease neurofibrillary tangles. *Neurosci. Lett.* 101:352–355.

Ikegami, K., Kimura, T., Katsuragi, S., Ono, T., Yamamoto, H., Miyamoto, E., and Miyakawa, T. (1996) Immunohistochemical examination of phosphorylated tau in granulovacuolar degeneration granules. *Psychiatry Clin. Neurosci.* 50:137–140.

Iwatsubo, T., Hasegawa, M., and Ihara, Y. (1994) Neuronal and glial tau-positive inclusions in diverse neurologic diseases share common phosphorylation characteristics. *Acta Neuropathol. (Berl)* 88:129–136.

Josephs, K. (2007) Frontotemporal lobar degeneration. *Neurologic Clinics* 25:683–696.

Kahn, J., Anderton, B.H., Probst, A., Ulrich, J., and Esiri, M.M. (1985) Immunohistological study of granulovacuolar degeneration using monoclonal antibodies to neurofilaments. *J. Neurol. Neurosurg. Psychol.* 48:924–926.

Kang, J., Lemaire, H.G., Unterbeck, A., Salbaum, J.M., Masters, C.L., Grzeschik, K.H., Multhaup, G., Beyreuther, K., and Muller Hill, B. (1987) The precursor of Alzheimer's disease amyloid A4 protein resembles a cell-surface receptor. *Nature* 325:733–736.

Khachaturian, Z.S. (1985) Diagnosis of Alzheimer's disease. *Arch. Neurol.* 42:1097–1105.

Kidd, M. (1963) Paired helical filaments in electron microscopy of Alzheimer's disease. *Nature* 197:192–193.

Knopman, D.S., Mastri, A.R., Frey, W.H., Sung, J.H., and Rustan, T. (1990) Dementia lacking distinctive histologic features: a common non-Alzheimer degenerative dementia. *Neurology* 40:251–256.

Kordower, J.H., Chu, Y., Stebbins, G.T., DeKosky, S.T., Cochran, E.J., Bennett, D., and Mufson, E.J. (2001) Loss and atrophy of layer II entorhinal cortex neurons in elderly people with mild cognitive impairment. *Ann. Neurol.* 49:202–213.

Lee, V.M.Y., Balin, B.J., Otvos, L., Jr., and Trojanowski, J.Q. (1991) A major subunit of paired helical filaments and derivatized forms of normal tau. *Science* 251:675–678.

Love, S., Saitoh, T., Quijada, S., Cole, G.M., and Terry, R.D. (1988) Alz-50, ubiquitin and tau immunoreactivity of neurofibrillary tangles, Pick bodies and Lewy bodies. *J. Neuropathol. Exp. Neurol.* 47:393–405.

Lowe, J., Blanchard, A., Morrell, K., Lennox, G., Reynolds, L., Billett, M., Landon, M., and Mayer, R.J. (1988) Ubiquitin is a common factor in intermediate filament inclusion bodies of diverse type in man, including those of Parkinson's disease, Pick's disease, and Alzheimer's disease, as well as Rosenthal fibres in cerebellar astrocytomas, cytoplasmic bodies in muscle, and mallory bodies in alcoholic liver disease. *J. Pathol.* 155:9–15.

Lowe, J., and Dickson, D. (1997) Pathological diagnostic criteria for dementia associated with cortical Lewy bodies: review and proposal for a descriptive approach. *J. Neural Transm Suppl.* 51:111–120.

Maresh, G.A., Erezyilmaz, D., Murry, C.E., Nochlin, D., and Snow, A.D. (1996) Detection and quantitation of perlecan mRNA levels in Alzheimer's disease and normal aged hippocampus by competitive reverse transcription-polymerase chain reaction. *J. Neurochem.* 67:1132–1144.

Masliah, E., Mallory, M., Hansen, L., DeTeresa, R., and Terry, R.D. (1993) Quantitative synaptic alterations in the human neocortex during normal aging. *Neurology* 43:192–197.

Masliah, E., and Terry, R. (1993) The role of synaptic proteins in the pathogenesis of disorders of the central nervous system. *Brain Pathol.* 3:77–85.

Masliah, E., Terry, R.D., DeTeresa, R.M., and Hansen, L.A. (1989) Immunohistochemical quantification of the synapse-related protein synaptophysin in Alzheimer disease. *Neurosci. Lett.* 103: 234–239.

Masters, C.L., Multhaup, G., Simms, G., Pottgiesser, J., Martins, R.N., and Beyreuther, K. (1985) Neuronal origin of a cerebral amyloid: neurofibrillary tangles of Alzheimer's disease contain the same protein as the amyloid of plaque cores and blood vessels. *EMBO J.* 4:2757–2763.

McGeer, P.L., Rogers, J., and McGeer, E.G. (1994) Neuroimmune mechanisms in Alzheimer disease pathogenesis. *Alzheimer Dis. Assoc. Disord.* 8:149–158.

McKieth, I.G., Galasko, D., Kosaka, K., Perry, E.K., Dickson, D.W., Hansen, L.A., Salmon, D.P., Lowe, J., Mirra, S.S., and Byrne, E.J. (1996) Consensus guidelines for the clinical and pathologic diagnosis of dementia with Lewy bodies (DLB): report of the consortium on DLB international workshop. *Neurology* 47:1113–1124.

Mesulam, M.M., and Moran, M.A. (1987) Cholinesterases within neurofibrillary tangles related to age and Alzheimer's disease. *Ann. Neurol.* 22:223–228.

Mirra, S.S., Heyman, A., McKeel, D., et al. (1991) The consortium to establish a registry for Alzheimer's disease (CERAD). Part II. Standardization of the neuropathologic assessment of Alzheimer's disease. *Neurology* 41:479–486.

Mitchell, T.W., Mufson, E.J., Schneider, J.A., Cochran, E.J., Nissanov, J., Han, L.Y., Bienias, J.L., Lee, V.M., Trojanowski, J.Q., Bennett, D.A., and Arnold, S.E. (2002) Parahippocampal tau pathology in healthy aging, mild cognitive impairment, and early Alzheimer's disease. *Ann. Neurol.* 51:182–189.

Molsa, P.K., Marttila, R.J., and Rinne, U.K. (1984) Extrapyramidal signs in Alzheimer's disease. *Neurology* 34:1114–1116.

Morris, J.C., and Price, A.L. (2001) Pathologic correlates of nondemented aging, mild cognitive impairment, and early-stage Alzheimer's disease. *J. Mol. Neurosci.* 17:101–118.

Morris, J.C., Storandt, M., McKeel, D.W., Jr., Rubin, E.H., Price, J.L., Grant, E.A., and Berg, L. (1996) Cerebral amyloid deposition and diffuse plaques in "normal" aging: evidence for presymptomatic and very mild Alzheimer's disease. *Neurology* 46: 707–719.

Morris, J.C., Storandt, M., Miller, J.P., McKeel, D.W., Price, J.L., Rubin, E.H., and Berg, L. (2001) Mild cognitive impairment represents early-stage Alzheimer disease. *Arch. Neurol.* 58:397–405.

Morrison, J.H., and Hof, P.R. (1997) Life and death of neurons in the aging brain. *Science* 278:412–419.

Mufson, E.J., Ma, S.Y., Cochran, E.J., Bennett, D.A., Beckett, L.A., Jaffar, S., Saragovi, H.U., and Kordower, J.H. (2000) Loss of nucleus basalis neurons containing trkA immunoreactivity in individuals with mild cognitive impairment and early Alzheimer's disease. *J. Comp. Neurol.* 427:19–30.

Murayama, S., Mori, H., Ihara, Y., and Tomonaga, M. (1990) Immunocytochemical and ultrastructural studies of Pick's disease. *Ann. Neurol.* 27:394–405.

Namba, Y., Tomonaga, M., Kawasaki, H., Otomo, E., and Ikeda, K. (1991) Apolipoprotein E immunoreactivity in cerebral amyloid deposits and neurofibrillary tangles in Alzheimer's disease and kuru plaque amyloid in Creutzfeldt-Jakob disease. *Brain Res.* 541: 163–166.

Neumann, M., Sampathu, D.M., Kwong, L.K., Truax, A.C., Micsenyi, M.C., Chou, T.T., et al. (2006) Ubiquitinated TDP-43 in frontotemporal lobar degeneration and amyotrophic lateral sclerosis. *Science* 314: 130–133.

Nishiyama, E., Iwamoto, N., Ohwada, J., and Arai, H. (1997) Distribution of apolipoprotein E in senile plaques in brains with Alzheimer's disease: investigation with the confocal laser scan microscope. *Brain Res.* 750:20–24.

Parkinson, J. (1955) An essay on the shaking palsy. London, 1817. In: Critchley, M., ed. *James Parkinson (1755–1824)*. London: Macmillan, pp. 145–218.

Pearson, R.C.A., Esiri, M.M., Hiorns, R.W., Wilcock, R.W., and Powell, T.P.S. (1985) Anatomical correlates of the distribution of the pathological changes in the neocortex in Alzheimer's disease. *Proc. Natl. Acad. Sci. USA* 82:4531–4534.

Peress, N.S., Kane, W.C., and Aronson, S.M. (1972) Central nervous system findings in a tenth decade autopsy population. *Prog. Brain Res.* 40:473–483.

Perl, D.P., Olanow, C.W., and Calne, D. (1998) Alzheimer's disease and Parkinson's disease: distinct entities or extremes of a spectrum of neurodegeneration? *Ann. Neurol.* 44:S19–S31.

Perry, G., Friedman, R., Shaw, G., and Chau, C. (1987) Ubiquitin is detected in neurofibrillary tangles and senile plaque neurites of Azheimer's disease brains. *Proc. Natl. Acad. Sci. USA* 84:3033–3036.

Peters, A., Morrison, J.H., Rosene, D.L., and Hyman, B.T. (1998) Are neurons lost from the primate cerebral cortex during normal aging? *Cereb. Cortex* 8:295–300.

Pirozzolo, F.J., Swihart, A.A., Rey, G.J., Mahurin, R., and Jankovic, J. (1993) Cognitive impairments associated with Parkinson's disease and other movement disorders. In: Jankovic, J., and Tolosa, E., eds. *Parkinson's Disease and Other Movement Disorders*. Baltimore: Williams & Wilkins, pp. 493–510.

Prelli, F., Castano, E., Glenner, G.G., and Frangione, B. (1988) Differences between vascular and plaque core amyloid in Alzheimer's disease. *J. Neurochem.* 51:648–651.

Price, J.L., Ko, A.I., Wade, M.J., Tsou, S.K., McKeel, D.W., and Morris, J.C. (2001) Neuron number in the entorhinal cortex and CA1 in preclinical Alzheimer disease. *Arch. Neurol.* 58:1395–1402.

Price, J.L., and Morris, J.C. (1999) Tangles and plaques in nondemented aging and "preclinical" Alzheimer's disease. *Ann. Neurol.* 45:358–368.

Prusiner, S.B. (1991) Molecular biology of prion diseases. *Science* 252:1515–1522.

Riley, K.P., Snowdon, D.A., and Markesbery, W.R. (2002) Alzheimer's neurofibrillary pathology and the spectrum of cognitive function: findings from the Nun Study. *Ann. Neurol.* 51:567–577.

Roberts, G.W., Allsop, D., and Bruton, C. (1990) The occult aftermath of boxing. *J. Neurol. Neurosurg. Psychiatry* 53:373–378.

Roberts, G.W., Gentleman, S.W., Lynch, A., and Draham, D.I. (1991) Beta A4 amyloid protein deposition in brain after head trauma. *Lancet* 338:1422–1423.

Rogers, J., Cooper, N.R., Webster, S., Schultz, J., McGeer, P.L., Styren, S.D., Civin, W.H., Brachova, L., Bradt, B., Ward, P., et al. (1992) Complement activation by beta-amyloid in Alzheimer disease. *Proc. Natl. Acad. Sci. USA* 89:10016–10020.

Scheff, S.W., and Price, D.A. (1993) Synapse loss in the temporal lobe in Alzheimer's disease. *Ann. Neurol.* 33:190–199.

Scheff, S.W., and Price, D.A. (1998) Synaptic density in the inner molecular layer of the hippocampal dentate gyrus in Alzheimer disease. *J. Neuropathol. Exp. Neurol.* 57:1146–1153.

Scheff, S.W., Price, D.A., and Sparks, D.L. (2001) Quantitative assessment of possible age-related change in synaptic numbers in the human frontal cortex. *Neurobiol. Aging* 22:355–365.

Scheff, S.W., Sparks, L., and Price, D.A. (1993) Quantitative assessment of synaptic density in the entorhinal cortex in Alzheimer's disease. *Ann. Neurol.* 34:356–361.

Selkoe, D.J. (1998) The cell biology of beta-amyloid precursor protein and presenilin in Alzheimer's disease. *Trends Cell. Biol.* 8:447–453.

Selkoe, D.J. (2001) Alzheimer's disease: genes, proteins, and therapy. *Physiol. Rev.* 81:741–766.

Selkoe, D.J., Yamazaki, T., Citron, M., Podlisny, M.B., Koo, E.H., Teplow, D.B., and Haass, C. (1996) The role of APP processing and trafficking pathways in the formation of amyloid beta-protein. *Ann. N.Y. Acad. Sci.* 777:57–64.

Simchowicz, T. (1911) Histologische studien über die senile dementz [Histologic studies of senile dementia]. *Histol. und Histopathol Arbeiten Åber die Grosshirnrinde* 4:267–444.

Snow, A.D., Nochlin, D., Sekiguichi, R., and Carlson, S.S. (1996) Identification in immunolocalization of a new class of proteoglycan (keratan sulfate) to the neuritic plaques of Alzheimer's disease. *Exp. Neurol.* 138:305–317.

Snowdon, D.A., Greiner, L.H., and Markesbery, W.R. (2000) Linguistic ability in early life and the neuropathology of Alzheimer's disease and cerebrovascular disease. Findings from the Nun Study. *Ann. N.Y. Acad. Sci.* 903:34–38.

Spillantini, M.G., Bird, T.D., and Ghetti, B. (1998) Frontotemporal dementia and Parkinsonism linked to chromosome 17: a new group of tauopathies. *Brain Pathol.* 8:387–402.

Terry, R.D. (1986) Interrelations among the lesions of normal and abnormal aging of the brain. *Prog. Brain Res.* 70:41–48.

Terry, R.D., Masliah, E., Salmon, D.P., Butters, N., Deteresa, R., Hill, R., Hansen, L.A., and Katzman, R. (1991) Physical basis of cognitive alterations in Alzheimer's disease: synapse loss is the major correlate of cognitive impairment. *Ann. Neurol.* 30:572–580.

Tomlinson, B.E., and Kitchener, D. (1972) Granulovacuolar degeneration of hippocampal pyramidal cells. *J. Pathol.* 106:165–185.

Van Hoesen, G.W., and Hyman, B.T. (1990) Hippocampal formation: anatomy and the patterns of pathology in Alzheimer's disease. *Prog. Brain Res.* 83:445–457.

Wisniewski, H.M., Narang, H.K., and Terry, R.D. (1976) Neurofibrillary tangles of paired helical filaments. *J. Neurol. Sci.* 27:173–181.

Wisniewski, H.M., Vorbrodt, A.W., Moretz, R.C., Lossinsky, A.S., and Grundke-Iqbal, I. (1982) Pathogenesis of neuritic (senile) and amyloid plaque formation. *Exp. Brain Res. Suppl.* 5: 3–9.

Wisniewski, K., Jervis, G.A., Moretz, R.C., and Wisniewski, H.M. (1979) Alzheimer neurofibrillary tangles in diseases other than senile and presenile dementia. *Ann. Neurol.* 5:288–294.

Wolf, D.S., Gearing, M., Snowdon, D.A., Mori, H., Markesbery, W.R., and Mirra, S.S. (1999) Progression of regional neuropathology in Alzheimer disease and normal elderly: findings from the Nun study. *Alzheimer Dis. Assoc. Disord.* 13:226–231.

Yamaguchi, H., Hirai, S., Morimatsu, M., Shoji, M., and Nakazato, Y. (1989) Diffuse type of senile plaques in the cerebellum of Alzheimer-type dementia demonstrated by beta protein immunostain. *Acta. Neuropathol.* 77:314–319.

Yen, S.H., Dickson, D.W., Crowe, A., Butler, M., and Shelanski, M.L. (1987) Alzheimer's neurofibrillary tangles contain unique epitopes and epitopes in common with the heat-stable microtubule associated proteins tau and MAP2. *Am. J. Pathol.* 126:81–91.

59 Functional Brain Imaging Studies in Dementia

MONTE S. BUCHSBAUM, ADAM BRICKMAN, JING ZHANG, AND ERIN A. HAZLETT

The underlying pathophysiological mechanisms resulting in dementia may result from a variety of causes ranging from the relatively well-understood interruptions of blood flow of vascular dementia to the less well-characterized alterations of Alzheimer's disease (AD), Pick's disease, and alcoholic dementia. The clinical diagnosis of dementia in ICD-10 requires a decline in memory and thinking sufficient to impair personal activities of daily living. Similarly, the *Diagnostic and Statistical Manual of Mental Disorders*, 4th ed. (*DSM-IV*; American Psychiatric Association, 1994) requires memory impairment and one or more other cognitive disturbances including aphasia, apraxia, agnosia, and disturbance of executive functioning sufficient to cause impairment in social or occupational function. The criteria of dual cognitive impairment, always including memory deficit, tend to suggest that (*1*) dementia is associated with two brain sites of involvement (for example, temporal lobe memory operations and frontal lobe executive dysfunction) or that (*2*) good memory function depends on the coordination of more than one brain area, leading to the frequent association of memory loss with other cognitive dysfunctions in diseases with general cerebral effects. This coordination of multiple brain regions involved in the strategy of memory may draw especially on frontal lobe resources.

The heterogeneous manifestations of cognitive loss, the confounding effects of executive dysfunction on all cognitive ability, and the widely prevalent comorbidity of central nervous system (CNS) diseases in the elderly make the diagnosis of dementia and its subtypes problematic. As increasingly specific and effective drugs to treat AD, Parkinson's disease, the pseudodementia of depression, and other dementing illnesses are developed, the differential diagnosis of these varieties of dementia will be increasingly critical for good psychiatric care and scientific pharmacotherapy. Functional brain imaging is providing a key tool for mapping the compromised brain areas, assessing regional effects of medication treatment, and even selecting behavioral therapies to exploit undamaged brain resources. This review focuses on the important advances made in positron emission tomography (PET) studies of brain metabolism in dementing illnesses over the past 10 years. There are other useful reviews that cover the earlier literature (Arnold and Kumar, 1993; Herholz, 1995; Messa et al., 1995).

THE ^{18}F-FLUORODEOXYGLUCOSE METHOD AND POSITRON EMISSION TOMOGRAPHY STUDIES IN DEMENTIA

The final common path for the bioenergetics of all neurochemical processes in the brain is glucose use. Fluorodeoxyglucose (FDG) uptake parallels energy consumption (Sokoloff et al., 1977; Hertz and Peng, 1992) that can be quantitatively determined with PET (typically presented as a relative glucose metabolic rate) and is sensitive to the effects of pharmacological treatments in dementia (for example, donepezil) (Teipel et al., 2006) and individual differences in pharmacological response (Buchsbaum, Potkin, Marshall, et al., 1992; Buchsbaum, Potkin, Siegel, et al., 1992). Studies with nuclear magnetic resonance imaging (MRI) phosphorous spectroscopy and PET have suggested that "glucose metabolism is reduced early in AD (reflecting decreased basal synaptic functioning) and is unrelated to a rate limitation in glucose delivery [or] abnormal glucose metabolism" (Murphy et al., 1993, p. 341). Fluorodeoxyglucose metabolic rates are stable over time (Bartlett et al., 1988; Maquet et al., 1990; Bartlett et al., 1991; Wang et al., 1994) with most subjects showing whole brain metabolic variability below 10%. Because individuals differ widely in whole brain metabolic rate, regional differences are often best assessed when data are converted to a relative metabolic rate by dividing by a standard brain area (most commonly the average whole brain glucose metabolic rate). Relative rates are usually more statistically powerful in demonstrating the effects of cognitive and perceptual tasks or patterns of regional decrease (for example, temporal but not occipital decreases in AD compared to the regional pattern in normal subjects).

However, relative measures may be less reliable in following patients over time than the absolute metabolic rate in two situations: (*1*) a patient who loses metabolic rate uniformly across the brain would show no relative change on a follow-up scan and (*2*) large metabolic rate decreases across the cortex (lowering the whole brain metabolic rate) would create large apparent subcortical increases even if subcortical structures remained entirely unchanged over time. The ability to calculate absolute metabolic rates is a significant advantage of PET with FDG over such alternative approaches as functional MRI (fMRI) or cerebral blood flow studies, which do not yield absolute units. However, the latter two approaches offer advantages in the ease with which many behavioral tasks can be administered for the detailed examination of cognitive change; fMRI yields values in individuals being evaluated for dementia that are modestly correlated with the relative metabolic rate (34% of variance shared; $r = 0.58$) (Gonzalez et al., 1995).

NORMAL AGING AND AGE-RELATED MEMORY IMPAIRMENT

Frontal Lobe Deficits in Aging and Memory

The cortical atrophy of age may be more pronounced in the frontal lobe (Coffey et al., 1992), and cognitive decline has been related to the gradual loss of cortical neurons. Because the frontal lobe is important in executive functioning—the sequencing and controlling of tasks—and has the most pronounced reciprocal connections to other cortical areas of any cortical area (Stuss and Benson, 1986), its decline could lead to changes in the cortical areas where cognitive tasks are carried out and the efficiency with which tasks are executed. Functional imaging studies have tended to demonstrate the activation of frontal (Tulving et al., 1994; Kapur et al., 1995) or frontal and temporal areas (Grady et al., 1995). These findings suggest that combined frontal/temporal deficits may be a common feature of dementia.

Metabolic Changes With Age And Dementia

Because there are systematic changes with age, it is important to differentiate age-related change and dementia-related change. Most studies using PET have demonstrated a significant age-associated decrease in cerebral glucose metabolism (A. Martin et al., 1991; Loessner et al., 1995; Moeller et al., 1996; Buchsbaum and Hazlett, 1997; Hazlett et al., 1998). Although a few other studies found age-related functional change to be more marked in the temporal lobe (Takada et al., 1992) or unchanged with age (Tempel and Perlmutter, 1992).

Although many regions have been implicated, age-associated metabolic decreases in the frontal lobe have been consistently reported (Loessner et al., 1995; Buchsbaum and Hazlett, 1997; Hazlett et al., 1998), during task (Hazlett et al., 1998; Reuter-Lorenz et al., 2000) and resting states (De Santi et al., 1995; Kuhl et al., 1982; Loessner et al., 1995). Consistent with a frontal aging hypothesis, we have previously shown an age-associated shift from anterior regions to more posterior regions of the frontal lobe in normal individuals performing a verbal learning task (Hazlett et al., 1998; Brickman et al., 2003). Moreover, in a review of functional neuroimaging studies of normal aging, Cabeza (2001) described consistent findings of either lower activation or absent activation in older normal adults compared to younger adults during tasks of episodic encoding or semantic retrieval. Areas of the frontal lobe were particularly involved, including anterior cingulate/medial frontal lobe (Brodmann areas 24 and 32), dorsolateral prefrontal cortex (Brodmann areas 44, 45, and 46), orbital frontal lobe (Brodmann area 47), and lateral frontal lobe (Brodmann areas 6, 8, and 10).

Our own studies have shown similar findings (Hazlett et al., 1998). Specifically, we used coregistered FDG-PET and MRI to characterize brain function in 70 healthy volunteers aged 20–87. All volunteers performed a verbal memory task (Serial Verbal Learning Task) during the PET scan. Frontal activity showed an age-related decline that remained significant after statistical control for atrophy measured on coregistered MRI. Analyses of young and old subgroups matched on memory performance revealed that young good performers activated frontal regions, whereas old good performers relied on occipital regions. Although activating different cortical regions, good performers of all ages used the same cognitive strategy—semantic clustering. Hazlett et al. (1998) concluded that age-related functional change may reflect dynamic reallocation in a network of brain areas, not merely anatomically fixed neuronal loss or diminished capacity to perform. The eventual diagnostic fate of these memory-impaired volunteers with no dementia will be of interest in understanding cognitive decline with age. The cognitive impairments of elderly monkeys also seem to be mediated by the prefrontal cortex (Gallagher and Rapp, 1997). The pattern of relative frontal decline that appears to be a common characteristic of normal aging may provide a background that interacts with the imaging characteristics and behavioral expression of each of the dementing illnesses described below.

ALZHEIMER'S DISEASE

Regional Neuropathology in Alzheimer's Disease

Neuropathological confirmation is necessary to ultimately confirm the diagnosis of AD; changes in association areas are more severe than those in the primary sensory and motor cortices and may be more severe in temporal regions (Pearson et al., 1985; Rogers and Morrison, 1985; Lewis et al., 1987; Van Hoesen and Damasio, 1987; Hof et al., 1990; Hof and Morrison, 1990; Arnold et al., 1991; Hof and Morrison, 1994).

Regional Metabolic Changes in Alzheimer's Disease

In probable AD, single photon emission tomography (SPECT) and PET studies have revealed decreases in glucose metabolic rate that are relatively greater in temporal and parietal than frontal lobes and may precede full development of AD behaviorally (Fig. 59.1) or structurally (Fig. 59.2). Moreover, the finding in imaging studies that AD tends not to affect primary sensory areas provides a striking parallel to the findings of neuropathological studies (Jagust et al., 1988; McGeer et al., 1990; Buchsbaum et al., 1991; Kumar et al., 1991; Nyback et al., 1991; DeCarli et al., 1992; Jobst et al., 1992; Pearlson et al., 1992; Jagust et al., 1993; Minoshima et al., 1995; Valladares-Neto et al., 1995; Sakamoto et al., 2002). Ratios between metabolic rates in major brain areas have proved more effective than the absolute metabolic rate in a single area for discriminating patients and controls (Heiss et al., 1991; Azari et al., 1993; Jagust et al., 1993; Mielke et al., 1993, 1994).

In difficult diagnostic cases where cerebral infarction versus AD needs to be discriminated, FDG-PET and SPECT may be valuable (Fig. 59.3). Even if the clinical onset is progressive, suggesting AD, FDG-PET, and other forms of neuroimaging can demonstrate unambiguous infarction (Sarangi et al., 2000). It has been found that FDG-PET is more sensitive than SPECT in separating normal elderly individuals from patients when areas in the temporoparietal and posterior cingulate were used (Herholz et al., 2002). Single photon emission tomography visually inspected was also found superior to anatomical MRI for AD and multi-infarct dementia (Honda et al., 2002). In the hippocampus, FDG was also found to separate normal elderly persons, those with mild cognitive impairment, and patients with AD more accurately than MRI-assessed volumetric loss (De Santi et al., 2001).

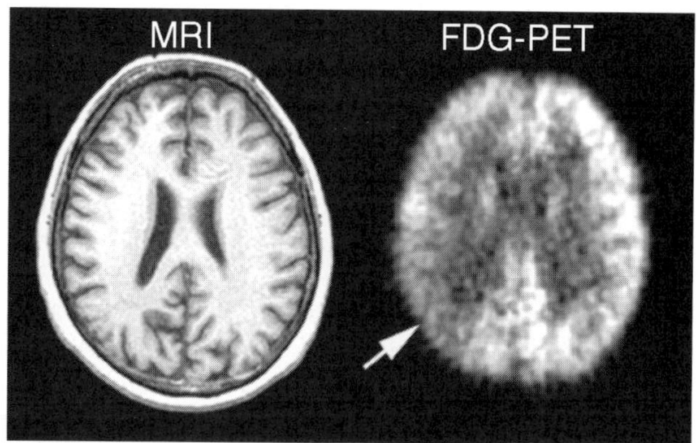

FIGURE 59.2 A PET scan and a MRI scan from a 66-year-old woman with gradual onset of difficulty remembering recent events such as wrapping presents and placing an ironed shirt on a hanger. Neuropsychological tests indicate a parietal lobe deficit and memory impairment. The MRI scan is normal for age, but the PET scan shows an asymmetrical parietal deficit consistent with a cognitive deficit. PET: positron emission tomography; MRI: magnetic resonance imaging.

Changes on FDG-PET scans appear closely related to histopathological change observed in subsequent postmortem exam and indicate the validity of PET in the differential diagnosis of dementias. Negative correlations were observed between postmortem regional neurofibrillary tangle density and a prospectively obtained relative metabolic rate with PET (DeCarli et al., 1992; Mielke et al., 1996). In a large study, 22 individuals with difficult-to-characterize memory loss or dementia using clinical criteria received PET, and ultimate pathological confirmation of AD was achieved in 12. The sensitivity of the clinical diagnosis was 63%, while that

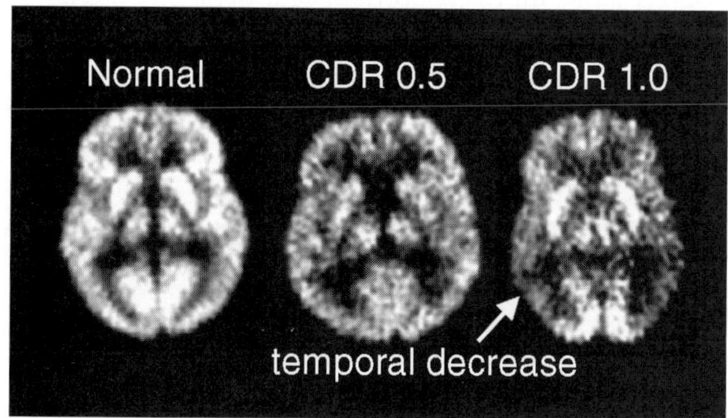

FIGURE 59.1 Positron emission tomography scans from a normal elderly patient, a patient with no dementia with memory impairment, and a patient with probable Alzheimer's disease (AD). Bilateral temporal lobe metabolic decrease is clearly visible in the patient with AD.

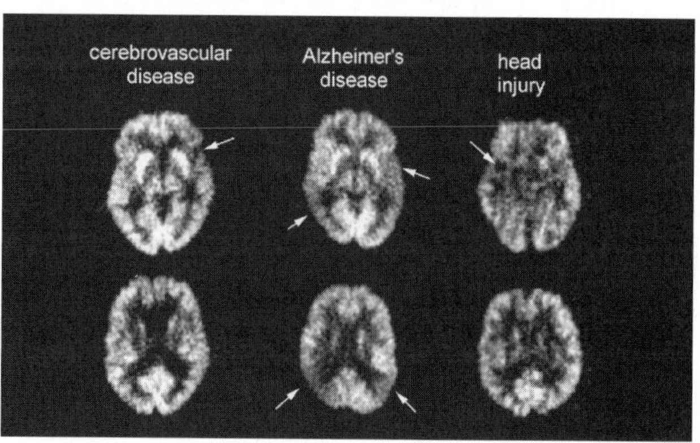

FIGURE 59.3 Differential diagnosis in dementia. Cerebrovascular disease shows a single very low metabolic area; Alzheimer's disease shows a typical bitemporal soft-edged metabolic decrease; head injury shows a single discrete, limited hypometabolic area.

of the PET criteria of bitemporal decrease visually assessed was 93%, indicating the value of PET as a diagnostic tool in memory loss (Hoffman et al., 2000). Visual ratings of FDG-PET showed superior sensitivity to clinical evaluation (0.84 vs. 0.76) and superior specificity (0.74) when compared to the clinical initial evaluation and final evaluation 4 years later (0.58 and 0.63) when evaluated against postmortem findings (Jagust et al., 2007). Statistical mapping techniques have also been confirmed as effective in diagnosing AD and in the differential diagnosis of Alzheimer's (n = 34) and frontotemporal dementia (n = 14) (Higdon et al., 2004) in a sample of patients with imaging and postmortem confirmation. Further, though FDG-PET was slightly better, when voxel-by-voxel statistical mapping was used diagnostic sensitivity and specificity of PET and SPECT were similar (Nihashi et al., 2007). Although this literature suggests that as a diagnostic tool PET is superior to an initial clinical evaluation and more specific than clinical evaluation at a follow-up several years later, its clinical utility (as opposed to scientific validity) must be judged against a standard of selecting treatments. Although the differential treatment of AD with cholinesterase inhibitors and cerebrovascular disease with anticoagulants is established, the measurable cognitive improvement in AD is not large. In a useful review of neurotransmitter deficits in dementia, Huey et al. (2006) concluded that patients with frontotemporal dementia show deficiencies in the serotonin (e.g., Lanctot et al., 2007) and dopamine neurotransmitter systems while the acetylcholine system appears relatively intact. Thus, patient trials of antidementia drugs would appear to profit from functional neuroimaging because of its greater specificity than clinical diagnosis and good agreement with postmortem diagnosis. The lack of specificity in drug trials could lead to a diminution of effect size with underestimation of efficacy. Further, because many inpatients with dementia are treated with low-dose risperidone, a dopamine and serotonin blocker, separating vascular, Alzheimer, and frontotemporal dementia with FDG imaging might have a larger clinical impact than currently appreciated.

Prediction of Development of Alzheimer's Disease

Progression from mild cognitive impairment to AD has been observed longitudinally with FDG-PET (see reviews in Pakrasi and O'Brien, 2005; Prvulovic et al., 2005; Uttner et al., 2006). Hippocampal hypometabolism predicted decline from normal to AD with 81% accuracy, which was confirmed in two cases by postmortem examination (Mosconi et al., 2005; de Leon et al., 2007). For cortical areas, patients with frontotemporal, thalamic, and cingulate changes were more likely to progress to having AD (Hunt et al., 2007). FDG-PET was superior to cerebrospinal fluid (CSF)-phospho-tau in predicting conversion to dementia in patients with mild cognitive impairment (Fellgiebel et al., 2007).

REGIONAL fMRI AND 015 CHANGES IN ALZHEIMER'S DISEASE

Functional MRI studies in AD have consistently demonstrated altered patterns of activation in the medial temporal lobe (hippocampus) and neocortex during memory encoding compared with healthy controls (S.A. Small et al., 1999; Rombouts et al., 2000; Machulda et al., 2003; Sperling et al., 2003). Greater medial temporal lobe activation during a memory encoding task was present in a subgroup of individuals with mild cognitive impairment who demonstrated cognitive decline 2½ years after scanning, compared with a subgroup that remained clinically stable (Dickerson et al., 2004). Greater hippocampal activation predicted greater degree and rate of subsequent cognitive decline over 5.9 years of follow-up after scanning (S.L. Miller et al., 2007). Greater task-related increase in the fusiform and inferior frontal region in patients with AD than normals has also been found (Anderson et al., 2007). These findings suggest that increased activation of medial temporal lobe regions including the hippocampus and frontal lobes may reflect a compensatory response to AD pathology.

AMALOID AND PLAQUE IMAGING IN ALZHEIMER'S DISEASE

Amyloid deposits can be visualized in patients using Pittsburgh Compound B (Klunk et al., 2004) and other compounds (for a review, see Nordberg, 2007). Although this is primarily a structural imaging technique, its greater inclusion of frontal abnormalities, similarities in pattern to FDG uptake, and potential responsiveness to blood flow suggest its mention here.

Frontotemporal Dementia

Primary progressive aphasia, a progressive loss of language with sparing of other cognitive domains, is considered a variant of frontotemporal dementia (FTD). A longitudinal study found a markedly asymmetrical left superior and middle temporal lobe circumscribed area of hypometabolism expanding in a 1-year follow-up (Uttner et al., 2006). In patients with FDG with incontinence, right-hemispheric hypometabolic clusters were found in the premotor/anterior cingulate cortex and the putamen/claustrum/insula (Perneczky et al., 2008).

Subtypes of Alzheimer's Disease

In AD, large individual differences, especially in cortical brain areas affected, as well as in neuropsychological deficit and rate of clinical progression, are characteristic. In a novel analysis, the coefficient of variation of the global metabolic pattern was found to be higher in patients with AD than normal controls (Volkow et al.,

2002). Three major explanations may be proposed for this heterogeneity: (*1*) the existence of subtypes due to differing genetic and/or environmental interactions with predilections for varying anatomical areas and resulting symptom patterns; (*2*) parietal, frontal, and temporal metabolic decreases, often surprisingly asymmetrical, merely reflect variable regional expressions of a common underlying diffuse pathological process; (*3*) cross-sectional studies reveal different stages of progression from a pathological process initiated in the medial temporal lobe that spreads transynaptically through the corticocortical projections to the lateral temporal, frontal, and parietal lobes (e.g., Morrison, 1993).

Most patients with AD show sparing of the visual regions on PET imaging; however, a subgroup with prominent visual symptoms including simultagnosia, visual agnosia, and Balint's syndrome (visual inattention, oculomotor apraxia, and optic ataxia) showed marked metabolic decreases in the parietal and occipital cortex including the primary visual area (Pietrini et al., 1996; Nestor et al., 2003). A subsample of these patients had the diagnosis of AD confirmed at autopsy, suggesting that concurrent cerebrovascular disease was not important in these symptoms. Another behavioral subgroup of patients with AD with delusional misidentification syndrome (Mentis et al., 1995) shared the delusion that their husbands, wives, or physicians were impostors or that similar events had happened in the past. False beliefs in doubles and duplicates have been termed *reduplicative paramnesias* and include the Capgras syndrome. These patients showed lower metabolic rates in the orbitofrontal and neighboring cingulate gyrus regions than a comparison group of patients with AD without these symptoms. Reduplicative paramnesia has been seen after closed head injury, cerebral infarcts, and a variety of other neurological conditions (for a review, see Mentis et al., 1995), with a preponderance of focal lesions in frontal and temporal regions. The role of the frontal lobe in mnemonic organization and time sequencing would appear to be important in this disorder, as the reduplicated person is not typically an unrecognized stranger (as may appear in advanced AD) but rather an intimate companion as a quite accurate copy. Patients with AD and with apathy also have reduced medial frontal and anterior cingulate activity (Benoit et al., 2002).

Information about the Apolipoprotein ε4 (ApoE4) allele may be a valuable way of subtyping patients with AD. Relatives with no dementia at risk for AD (G.W. Small et al., 1995) and patients with AD (Mosconi et al., 2008) with the E4 allele showed lower FDG-PET metabolic rates than individuals without the E4 allele.

Somewhat random variation in the cortical area that is affected first in a progressive global brain illness could be related to the specific symptoms of a particular patient with AD. For example, the finding that patients with lower left-sided metabolism tend to show greater verbal intellectual impairment, whereas those with right hypometabolism show visuospatial impairments (Foster et al., 1983; Haxby et al., 1985; Koss et al., 1985; Grady et al., 1986; Haxby et al., 1986), would be consistent with this hypothesis (although Ober et al., 1991, did not show left–right hemisphere differentiation in visuoconstructive performance). The finding that right–left asymmetries of baseline and follow-up PET scans remain highly correlated over time (Mielke et al., 1994) suggests, however, that a regional predilection of the disease may occur with symptomatic subtypes. The presence of a stable factor structure would also tend to refute the random cortical area decrease hypothesis and support functional and etiological subgroups. Because factor analysis of metabolic rate in multiple brain areas requires large samples, there are only two such reports; one found parieto-temporal, paralimbic, left hemisphere, and frontoparietal factors (Grady et al., 1990), and the other found frontostriatal, central-occipital, fronto-striatal-temporal-occipital, striato-temporoparietal, and mesial temporal-mesial frontal factors (Ichimiya et al., 1994). Although the factor structures are not entirely similar, they provide some data supporting the idea that AD does not strike random patches of cortex. Anatomically limited factors (frontostriatal, centro-occipital, and mesial temporal) showed no correlation with the Mini-Mental State Examination (MMSE) or clinical global dementia ratings, whereas the factors with wide weighting in the frontal, temporal, and parietal regions showed significant correlations (Ichimiya et al., 1994). This supports the important role of frontal connections with many other areas in the development of dementia; there appears to be no single anatomical lesion that alone yields high dementia rating scores. A potentially important subgrouping variable for AD is age of onset. Earlier age of onset has been associated with less subcortical and more widespread cortical metabolic loss (Ichimiya et al., 1994; Sakamoto et al., 2002).

Progression of the illness may also account for variation in the PET metabolic decreases (Fig. 59.1). Metabolic rates in posterior cingulate, hippocampus, and temporal association areas (Schroder et al., 2001; Desgranges et al., 2002) and parietal regions (Santens et al., 2001) are significantly correlated with MMSE scores. Memory function in AD assessed by the selective reminding test was significantly correlated with hippocampal perfusion (Rodriguez et al., 2000). A longitudinal study indicated that decreases in the frontal lobe were most marked (Alexander et al., 2002), perhaps consistent with AD first striking the temporal lobe and then, once patients are identified, progressively affecting the frontal lobe.

Cognitive Tasks in Alzheimer's Disease

Given that the defining behavioral characteristic of dementia is memory deficit, and given that activation with memory tasks has been well demonstrated with functional imaging, memory paradigms seem particularly useful in functional imaging in AD and other dementias. However, most investigators have used a resting condition. Higher test–retest reliability over a short interval for an activation task than in a resting condition was found in normal patients and patients with dementia (Duara et al., 1987). Six studies compared patients and normals and used a task salient for the hallmark behavioral memory deficit of AD during the uptake period (Miller et al., 1987; Buchsbaum et al., 1991; Kessler et al., 1991; Duara et al., 1992; Kessler et al., 1996; Valladares-Neto et al., 1995). These studies found the same temporo/parietal and frontal metabolic decreases during activation that were found in the resting studies. Duara et al. (1992) made a rigorous test of the differential power of resting versus activation conditions to identify patients and found them to be similar. Grady et al. (1993) used a face-matching task that did not have a memory component and observed the usual middle tempora/parietal decreases in AD across the face task and a control sensorimotor task. Surprisingly, at the occipital pole and in frontal premotor cortex, there was significantly greater activation in patients with mild to moderate AD. The authors interpreted this to suggest that patients with AD may have an increased attentional load during the face-matching task and are apparently still able to activate frontal regions. These results could indicate that early in the disease the initial temporal lobe decrease is relatively well fixed across resting, nonmemory, and memory tasks, but that frontal and sensory areas that are less completely affected can still be brought into play by the patient. Task studies in patients with more severe dementia might show the frontal deficits becoming more fixed. Although it could be argued that imaging under resting conditions makes comparability across studies more feasible, an activation task condition may be no more or less problematic than the resting state. In a recent article, Andreasen termed the so-called resting state random episodic silent thinking (REST) (Andreasen et al., 1995). They reviewed which cognitive activities may be activated in rest and presented data on which brain areas may be associated with memory activities at rest. Such strategic shifts in memory access involving the frontal lobe would clearly confound the interpretation of rest activities, especially early in the course of AD, when compensatory frontal activity (Grady et al., 1993) may occur.

Memory tasks that stress a vulnerable system may be especially useful in high-risk studies that attempt to predict which patients with mild memory disturbance or which unaffected relatives of patients with AD will ultimately receive a diagnosis of AD. An analogy with high-risk studies of offspring of patients with schizophrenia could prove instructive. In such studies, more difficult versions of attentional tasks such as the continuous performance task were required to identify patients who would go on to develop schizophrenia, whereas easier versions of the task, which show marked abnormalities in patients with manifest schizophrenia, did not elicit abnormal performance in the patients with preschizophrenia (Cornblatt and Erlenmeyer-Kimling, 1985).

Course of Illness in Alzheimer's Disease

Serial scans of patients with AD from first memory impairment to end-stage illness could demonstrate an atrophic region restricted to the hippocampus that spreads to involve sequentially the lateral temporal lobe, the parietal lobe, and finally frontal cortex (Morrison, 1993). Alternatively, either lateral temporal, frontal, or parietal atrophy directly following hippocampal atrophy might appear, indicating global cortical change or random patchy cortical atrophy unrelated to rate of progression. To differentiate these possibilities, a data set would need methodologically consistent images and a sufficient sample size to allow testing of subgroup hypotheses. Although longitudinal studies in large samples of patients are lacking, PET studies have tended to find a wider range of cortical areas involved. Metabolic changes preceded neuropsychological changes in some patients with early-onset AD (Haxby et al., 1986). Restudy of a small sample of six patients 15 months apart demonstrated that progression in the parietal lobe was greater than in the frontal lobe (Jagust et al., 1988); this finding could reflect progression in a largely parietal-deficit subgroup, but the sample size and follow-up duration are small. Two studies have suggested that low frontal activity may predict more rapid decline. Decreased flow on SPECT predicted rapid decline in a longitudinal study (Hanyu et al., 1995), and frontal reduction in FDG-PET studies was associated with a more rapid clinical course (Mann et al., 1992). In addition, left prefrontal metabolic rate was the best predictor of premorbid function (Alexander et al., 1997). Although not a predictor of decline, changes in frontal and left temporal, but not whole hemisphere, measures of regional cerebral blood flow were correlated with changes in scores on the MMSE (Sachdev et al., 1997). Thus, a decline in frontal activity seems more closely linked to change in the clinical course early in the illness than a decline in activity in occipital cortical areas, a finding not inconsistent with the temporal to frontal to generalized cortical decrease pattern hypothesized by Morrison (1993), but longer-term follow-up is clearly necessary. Generalized decreases in cortical glucose metabolism in late-onset AD and more focal frontal and temporoparietal deficits in early-onset cases have been found (Mielke et al., 1991). Almost all of these studies suggest a more severe metabolic impairment in patients with early-onset disease, which may suggest a more virulent course. The lack of follow-up in these studies leaves unresolved the issue of regional progression, although they do support the view of a heterogeneous disorder.

PICK'S DISEASE

Pick's disease is a rare dementing disorder with greater metabolic decrease and atrophy of the frontal lobe (Fig. 59.4) than other brain regions and correspondingly greater personality change in its early stages than in AD. Stereotypic behavior is common in Pick's disease and frontotemporal degeneration (Shigenobu et al., 2002). Pathological changes (Dickson, 1998) consist of intraneuonal inclusions (Pick bodies). In a study of an autopsy-confirmed case of dementia with Pick's disease (Friedland et al., 1993), the patient was scanned 4 years after the onset of illness, which was characterized by problems in understanding spoken language and agitation; the appearance of visual hallucinations was noted in the year of the PET scan. The greatest relative decrease (13%) was in the right frontal lobe in comparison with control values (0.90 vs. 1.03), whereas right temporal cortex was actually relatively greater than in controls (1.04 vs. 1.01). Specific reduction of frontal metabolic activity has been seen in other recent studies (Lieberman et al., 1998). Decreased frontal function, usually bilateral and combined with temporal lobe decreases, is seen in frontotemporal lobar degeneration (Schumann et al., 2000).

In studies of Fahr's disease, a frontal lobe/hyperkinetic-hypotonic syndrome, reductions in metabolic rate in the frontal lobe and in the putamen, globus pallidus, and temporal regions have been observed (Hempel et al., 2001). Differentiation of AD and frontotemporal dementia demonstrated greater parietal loss in AD but similar temporal findings (Santens et al., 2001).

VASCULAR DEMENTIA

Quite similar localization in PET and anatomical MRI may be seen with large, complete cerebral infarcts, whereas smaller infarcts may show up less clearly on MRI. Scanning with FDG-PET may be valuable in the differential diagnosis (Figs. 59.3 and 59.5). In an important study, patients who had vascular dementia on clinical diagnosis and no cortical infarcts on MRI scans were studied (Sultzer et al., 1995). Frontal metabolic rates were lower in patients with infarcts in the basal ganglia and thalamus or anterior periventricular white matter abnormalities, whereas temporal metabolic rates were lower in individuals with posterior white matter change. This suggests that a disruption of frontostriatal and frontothalamic connections may be important in these remote cortical metabolic change patterns. Sultzer et al. (1995) noted that the PET images in their patients were similar to those seen in AD. With different treatments for vascular and Alzheimer's dementia, this differentiation is important. In a population of vascular, AD, mixed, and frontotemporal dementia, PET showed greater sensitivity and specificity in identifying the different types of early dementia, especially in detecting AD (sensitivity 44%, specificity 83%), than SPECT (Dobert et al., 2005).

SUBCORTICAL DEMENTIA

Parkinson's Disease

Patients with Parkinson's disease and dementia may show temporoparietal PET changes similar to those seen in AD in comparison to patients with no dementia (Peppard et al., 1992). Patients with Parkinson's disease without dementia showed the greatest differences from normals in posterior regions—primary visual, visual association, and parietal cortex—with no significant frontal lobe decrease (Eberling et al., 1994). In a rare study in which a PET scan was available for a patient initially diagnosed

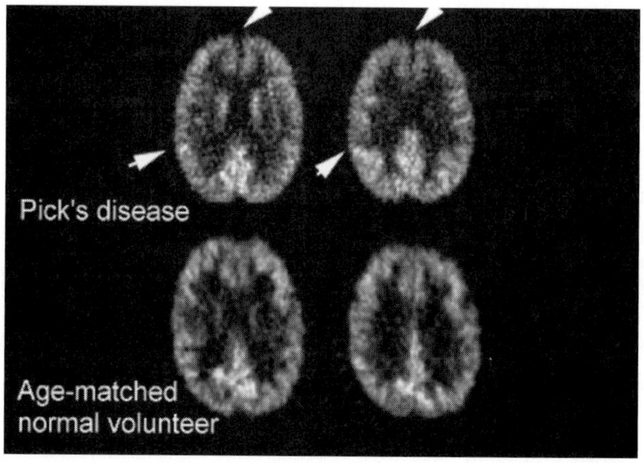

FIGURE 59.4 Pick's disease. Marked frontal decrease extends from the lower arrow to the upper arrow, with a relatively sharp margin bilaterally. The interhemispheric fissure is prominent.

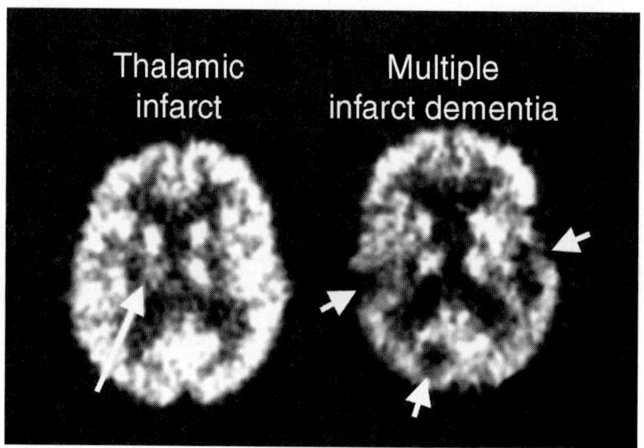

FIGURE 59.5 Cerebrovascular disease. Left: isolated thalamic lacunar infarct associated with deja vue. Right: Multiple areas of marked decrease in metabolic rate associated with severe dementia.

as having AD but found to have only Parkinson's disease at autopsy, a temporoparietal decrease in metabolic rate was found, but frontal decreases were more marked than in a comparison group of patients with AD alone (Schapiro et al., 1993). Patients with diffuse Lewy body disease and AD had a temporoparietal-frontal pattern of metabolic decrease similar to that found in AD (Yong et al., 2007) but with decreases in primary visual areas as well (Albin et al., 1996). These patterns suggest that the dementia of Parkinson's disease, like other dementias, usually is characterized by a widespread reduction in cortical metabolic rate, often involving frontal and temporal regions.

Huntington's Disease

Huntington's disease occurs in adulthood, sometimes first appearing as a psychiatric illness, a dementia, or a motor disorder. It is an autosomal dominant condition possibly associated with CAG repeats on chromosome 4 (Berrios et al., 2001) and affects the basal ganglia, causing a dramatic disappearance of the caudate and putamen on FDG-PET images (Dierks et al., 1999) (Figure 59.6). Presymptomatic gene carriers have significant decreases in caudate and putamen FDG metabolic rates as well as increases in occipital cortex (Feigin et al., 2001; Ciarmiello et al., 2006).

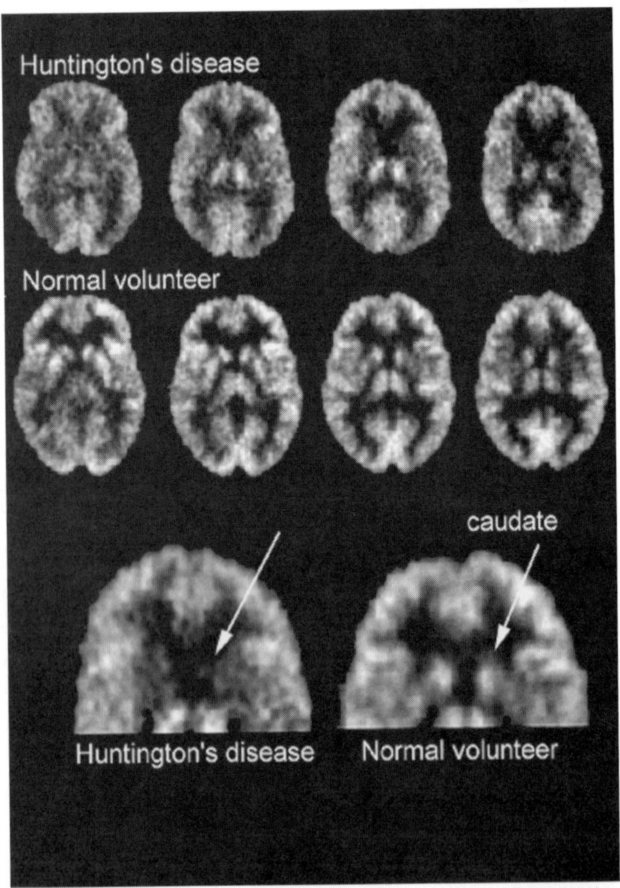

FIGURE 59.6 Huntington's disease. Top row: A patient's metabolic rate in the caudate and putamen is close to white matter values. Middle row: A normal volunteer shows the caudate and putamen clearly. Bottom row: Enlarged view of the striatal region with the caudate nucleus marked. Note near absence of uptake in caudate in Huntington's disease.

ALCOHOLIC KORSAKOFF'S DEMENTIA

Patients with Korsakoff's syndrome showed FDG-PET decreases in the cingulate and precuneate areas (Joyce et al., 1994), and these differences were maintained even after correction for (CSF volume as measured on computed tomography (CT). Acute effects of alcohol appear primarily in the cortex (Volkow et al., 1990), but long-term effects after 6–8 weeks of abstinence were seen in the cingulate and orbitofrontal cortex (Volkow et al., 1997). Anterior temporal and frontal decreases have also been observed in detoxified patients with alcoholic organic mental disorders (P.R. Martin et al., 1992).

OTHER DEMENTIAS

Patients with myotonic dystrophy, a disease with autosomal dominant inheritance, show characteristic changes in muscle, heart, and the endocrine system as well as cerebral involvement. They often have associated organic personality disorders but tend not to show memory deficits as prominently as patients with AD do. Fluorodeoxyglucose-PET has shown significant metabolic decreases in the frontal cortex and lentiform nucleus of patients with myotonic dystrophy rather than in temporal areas, as frequently seen in AD (Mielke et al., 1993). In Creutzfeldt–Jakob disease, widespread metabolic decreases are noted that may appear in occipital, cerebellar, frontal, and perisylvian regions, unlike AD or Pick's disease (Matochik et al., 1995; Henkel et al., 2002).

IS CHRONIC SCHIZOPHRENIA A DEMENTING ILLNESS?

Dementia praecox, an early name for schizophrenia and the gradual appearance of deficits in executive function and memory with progressive impairment in social or occupational function, certainly characterizes many patients with schizophrenia. Schizophrenia shares the pattern of temporal and frontal decreases in metabolic rate seen in AD and other dementias (for reviews of the more than 40 PET and regional cerebral blood flow studies, see Williamson, 1987; Buchsbaum, 1990; Andreasen et al., 1992; Chua and McKenna, 1995; Buchsbaum and Hazlett, 1998). Occipital metabolism, typically spared from decrease in AD, is often similarly spared or even elevated in patients with schizophrenia. Schultz et al. (2002) examined the relationship between age and cerebral blood flow (015-PET) in 49 unmedicated patients with schizophrenia during a resting condition and found negative correlations in anterior cingulate, frontal and parietal cortex bilaterally. The finding of reduced function in the anterior cingulate and frontal lobe with aging is consistent with previous findings in healthy individuals. However, the reduced regional cerebral blood flow (rCBF) observed in the parietal regions may be unique to schizophrenia.

A study of elderly patients with schizophrenia with chronic illness and extended hospital stays indicates that a substantial number of them met clinical criteria for dementia, with global cognitive impairment (Davidson et al., 1995). Patients with AD and patients with schizophrenia who had the same level of overall cognitive impairment based on the MMSE showed different patterns of disabilities (Davidson et al., 1996). The patients with schizophrenia performed more poorly than the patients with AD on the naming and constructional praxis tests but were less impaired on the delayed recall measure. Thus, rapid forgetting of new information distinguishes AD from normal aging and also from the cognitive impairments of chronic schizophrenia (Welsh et al., 1991; Welsh et al., 1992). The evidence from this line of research suggests that the neural mechanisms underlying dementia in late-life schizophrenia and AD are dissimilar. Neurodegeneration (neuron loss, neurofibrillary tangles, astrocytosis, microgliosis) has generally not been found in elderly patients with schizophrenia (Falke et al., 2000). However, aspects of dementia, including disorganization, negative symptoms, and psychoticism, all correlated with blood flow in the cerebellum, suggesting a communality with the dementia of schizophrenia conceptualized as cognitive dysmetria (Kim et al., 2000). And like patients with AD, patients with schizophrenia showed frontal decrease (Carter et al., 1998), and frontal and hippocampal activation was seen on PET scans during memory tasks (Carter et al., 1998; Crespo-Facorro et al., 2001).

COMPUTER METHODS IN DEMENTIA IMAGE ANALYSIS

Significance Probability Mapping and Dementia Subtyping

Voxel-by-voxel mapping of brain imaging, first described as significance probability mapping by Bartels and Subach (1976) and later as statistical parametric mapping (Friston et al., 1991), is a useful adjunct to visual inspection of the scans (Fig. 59.7) (Minoshima et al., 1995; Burdette et al., 1996; Schroder et al., 2001; Alexander et al., 2002; Herholz et al., 2002; Sakamoto et al., 2002; Shigenobu et al., 2002). The technique has the advantage of being able to explore the entire brain systematically in the search for specific areas of metabolic change, but its successful application requires that the region of change be in a similar pixel location in most patients. This requires the assumption that the same anatomical brain area is affected in most patients and the methodology to allow individual brains to be aligned so that the same anatomical areas in each patient appear at the same Cartesian coordinates. The first assumption, reviewed above, is met for AD, although clinical subtypes and individual variation cause slightly different areas in temporal and parietal lobes to be affected, sometimes asymmetrically (Ishii et al., 2001); if the centers of areas with the lowest FDG uptake fail to line up, t test comparisons may not be significant for the group. The second methodological requirement can be met through stable head positioning (Ruttimann et al., 1995) and image warping to align brains to the same coordinates (Fig. 59.8). The results of pixel-by-pixel analyses in AD demonstrate bilateral temporal and parietal change and, to a much lesser extent, medial temporal metabolic decreases with no frontal lobe change, perhaps suggesting that changes outside the lateral temporal cortex may be too variable in position to appear in aligned images. Images can be computed for each individual showing how far each voxel value is from the mean of a control group (typically

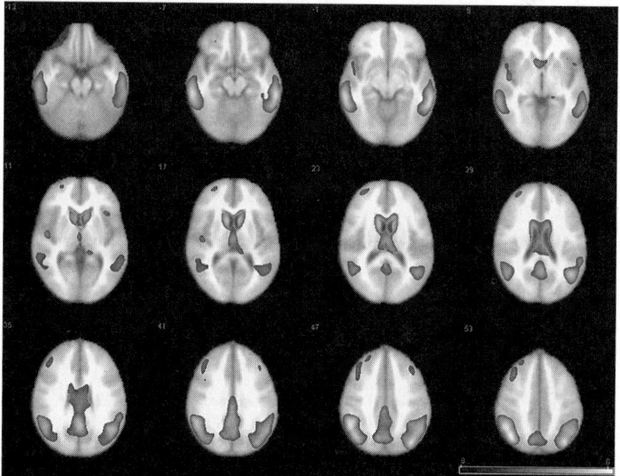

FIGURE 59.7 Statistical comparison of normal (n = 47) and AD (n = 37) positron emission tomography scans after coregistration with MRI, brain extraction from skull and scalp, and 12-parameter standardizing to the shape of the normal brain. The image background is the Montreal Neurological Institute average anatomical MRI brain. Superimposed are patches which indicate areas where t tests reach or exceed $p < .05$, two-tailed (1.99) for a decrease. Note the lower relative metabolic rate in the temporal and parietal lobes in AD. AD: Alzheimer's disease; MRI: magnetic resonance imaging.

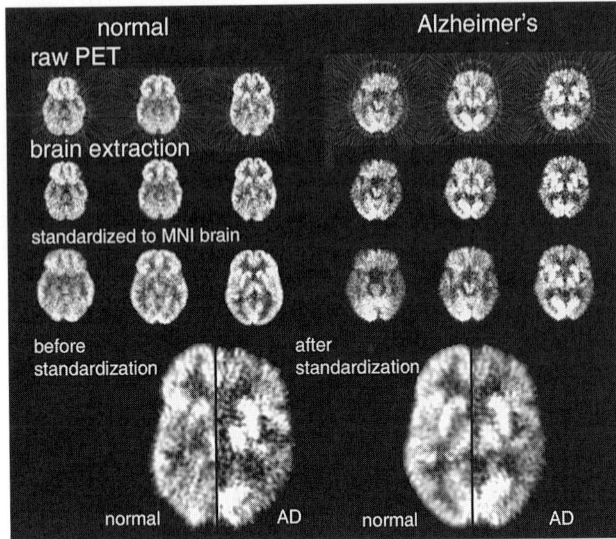

FIGURE 59.8 MRI scan in a normal elderly patient and a patient with AD. Top row: Unaltered FDG-PET scan. Second row: Brain extracted to remove FDG uptake in scalp and scatter. Third row: Images warped to adjust width (x), length (y) and height (z), x, y, and z position and x, y, and z tilt to standard Montreal Neurological Institute anatomical MRI brain created by averaging patients together. Bottom left: Normal patient image (left) and AD patient image (right) placed together before standardization. Bottom right: Normal patient image (left) and AD patient image (right) placed together after standardization. Note the low metabolism in the temporal lobe. Images are now sufficiently similar in shape so that they can be used in statistical analysis. MRI: Magnetic resonance imaging; AD: Alzheimer's disease; FDG: fluorodeoxyglucose; PET: positron emission tomography.

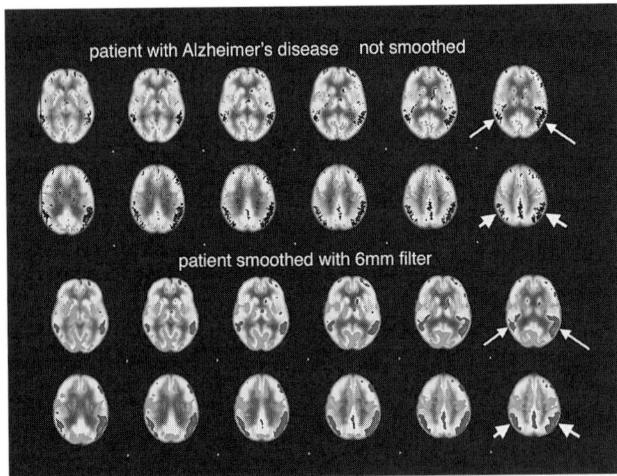

FIGURE 59.9 Individual patient with AD showing comparison with 70 normal volunteers. Black patches mark areas where patient is more than two standard deviations below the group normal. The bitemporal (long arrows) and biparietal (short arrows) decreases indicate the characteristic AD pattern. Light gray patches are areas where relative metabolic rate is above normal and show preservation of parts of the primary occipital cortex striatum and thalamus. Unsmoothed data shows maximum scanner resolution and 6-mm smoothing preserves areas of abnormality and eliminates many small regions which may have appeared due to noise and cortical folding patterns. AD: Alzheimer's disease.

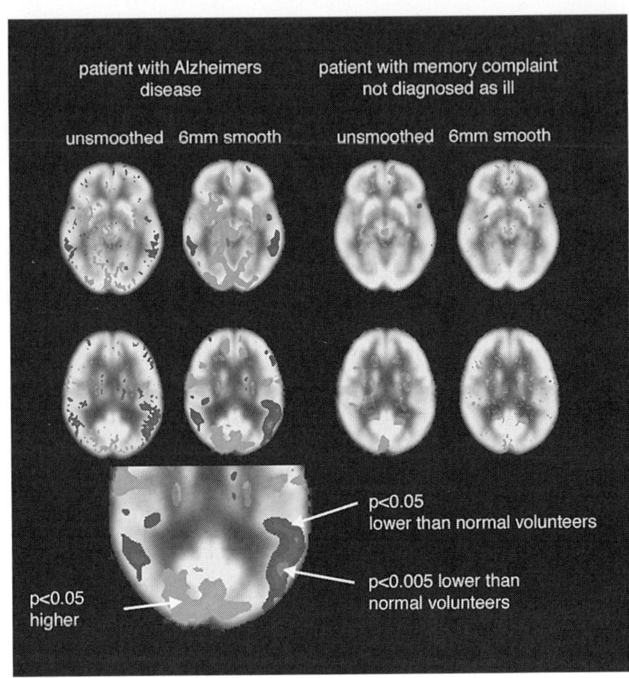

FIGURE 59.10 Significance probability mapping of individual patient with AD and age-matched patient. Patient has extensive areas of temporal lobe decrease not found in typical patient not meeting criteria for AD or MCI. Insert box: Patient with schizophrenia shows frontal decrease in contrast to AD and normal. AD: Alzheimer's disease; MCI: mild cognitive impairment.

expressed as Z scores and indicating the number of standard deviations the patient is from the control group). Human viewers tend to have better performance in diagnostic experiments when viewing these statistical images (Shidahara et al., 2006), and this is illustrated in Figures 59.9 and 59.10.

Regional Area Measurements

Although whole slice significance probability maps can survey the entire brain, smaller areas such as the superior temporal gyrus or the hippocampus may have variable positions with respect to the outer brain margin and may be more accurately analyzed by tracing them on the MRI and assessing these values on PET. Tracing the hippocampus (Fig. 59.11) on each patient's coregistered MRI scan may minimize this variation, allow medial temporal change to be visualized, and greatly improve patient/normal difference determination, as wisely done by some investigators (De Santi et al., 2001). This time-consuming process may be speeded up by the point-counting method, which yields the anatomical volume accurately (MacFall et al., 1994; Keshavan et al., 1995); with coregistered PET, a volumetric metabolic rate method may also be obtained. In our experience, the point-counting method is approximately six- to eightfold faster than outlining methods, but it has been little employed in quantification.

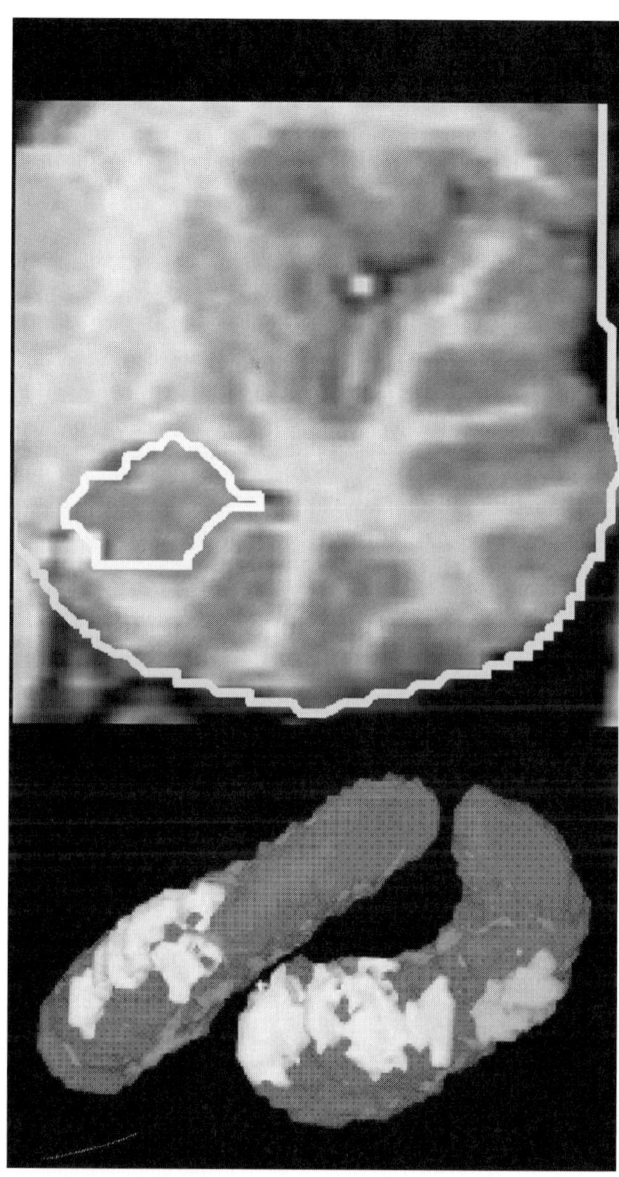

FIGURE 59.11 Top: Coronal section of the temporal lobe with the hippocampus traced. Bottom: Three-dimensional visualization of the hippocampus based on 50–70 coronal sections in the same patients shown in Figure 57.6. Light gray areas are *t* tests where patients with AD have lower values than normal controls. AD: Alzheimer's disease.

Sulcal Enlargement, Structural Shrinkage, and Metabolic Rate

The characteristic sulcal widening associated with cortical shrinkage seen in dementias opens areas of the cerebral cortex to CSF, which is inactive metabolically. With the 4–6 mm resolution of PET, these sulcal areas are not fully resolved, and the cortical mantle could thus reflect an apparent reduction in metabolic rate per unit area of the slice image whereas the actual cortical metabolic rate per unit area of gray matter was unchanged. This would be possible if the cortical shrinkage was due exclusively or largely to loss of histological contents with very low metabolic rates, hypermetabolic compensation by remaining neurons, or to merely closer packing of neurons, a supposition not clearly supported by most microscopic tissue examination. Further, two forms of analysis suggest that this anatomical change is not the sole reason for metabolic decrease. Cortical atrophy on MRI scans was used in analysis of covariance with regional CSF estimates as covariates to demonstrate that the degree of metabolic decrease in AD was much greater than expected on the basis of brain atrophy alone (Smith et al., 1992). An MRI-based partial volume correction procedure did not remove differences between patients and controls and enhanced rather than diminished correlations between regional glucose metabolic rate and neuropsychological test performance (Meltzer et al., 1996). The significance of relative metabolic rate decreases with age in the frontal lobes of men were preserved in eight of nine brain areas after partial volume correction (Yanase et al., 2005). These studies suggest the value of coregistered MRI templates with functional imaging and indicate that metabolic data offer additional information rather than merely duplicating the information provided by structural imaging.

SUMMARY

In the dementia literature, general parallels are observed between data provided by functional imaging and by neuropathological studies. The two approaches converge in suggesting that processes involving the temporal and frontal lobes together are often associated with dementia. Findings in the primary sensory cortex or the occipital and parietal lobes without temporal or frontal involvement are less likely to be associated with dementia. Although neuropathology supplies microscopic detail and quantitative cell counts, quite obviously it cannot in itself be useful as a prognostic measure. Structural resolution with MRI provides gross anatomical resolution but does not reveal regional cortical deficits or correlations with behavioral dysfunction. Combined functional/structural brain imaging strategies are clearly necessary for precise assessment of the functional neuroanatomy. Techniques that examine relationships between metabolic rates in brain regions through correlation coefficients or path analysis may be especially promising for understanding the network of cortical communication that is diminished in dementia (Mentis et al., 1994; Horwitz et al., 1995). Older studies, which lacked high-resolution coregistered anatomical templates and were performed with PET instruments of lower resolution than are currently available, may have been unable to discern the function of key regions for the illness or assess the contribution of sulcal enlargement in the cortex to measures of metabolic rate. New prospective studies are needed to take advantage of the dramatically better resolution imaging now available and to accumulate samples of adequate size to facilitate an understanding of the biological heterogeneity of AD and other dementias. Longitudinal observation of the progression of dementia will allow us to determine whether these diffuse brain deficits follow a specific neuroanatomical program (for example, medial temporal, lateral temporal, frontal in AD) or attack cortical regions in a random and diffuse manner, with symptoms resulting from the particular neuroanatomical deficit but not being etiologically informative.

ACKNOWLEDGMENTS

The authors thank the Charles A. Dana Foundation for supporting their study of normal aging and acknowledge support of NIH Anatomy and function of the thalamus in schizophrenia MH60023.

REFERENCES

Albin, R.L., Minoshima, S., D'Amato, C.J., Frey, K.A., Kuhl, D.A., and Sima, A.A. (1996) Fluoro-deoxyglucose positron emission tomography in diffuse Lewy body disease. *Neurology* 47:462–466.

Alexander, G.E., Chen, K., Pietrini, P., Rapoport, S.I., and Reiman, E.M. (2002) Longitudinal PET evaluation of cerebral metabolic decline in dementia: a potential outcome measure in Alzheimer's disease treatment studies. *Am. J. Psychiatry* 159:738–745.

Alexander, G.E., Furey, M.L., Grady, C.L., et al. (1997) Association of premorbid intellectual function with cerebral metabolism in Alzheimer's disease: implications for the cognitive reserve hypothesis. *Am. J. Psychiatry* 154:165–172.

American Psychiatric Association. (1994) *Diagnostic and Statistical Manual of Mental Disorders*, 4th ed. Washington, DC: Author.

Anderson, K.E., Brickman, A.M., Flynn, J., Scarmeas, N., Van Heertum, R., Sackeim, H., et al. (2007) Impairment of nonverbal recognition in Alzheimer disease: a PET O-15 study. *Neurology* 69:32–41.

Andreasen, N., O'Leary, D.S., Cizadlo, T., et al. (1995) Remembering the past: two facets of episodic memory explored with positron emission tomography. *Am. J. Psychiatry* 152:1576–1585.

Andreasen, N.C., Rezai, K., Alliger, R., et al. (1992) Hypofrontality in neuroleptic-naive patients and in patients with chronic schizophrenia. Assessment with xenon 133 single-photon emission computed tomography and the Tower of London. *Arch. Gen. Psychiatry* 49:943–958.

Arndt, S., Rajarethinam, R., Cizadlo, T., O'Leary, D., Downhill, J., and Andreasen, N.C. (1996) Landmark-based registration and measurement of magnetic resonance images: a reliability study. *Psychiatry Res.* 67:145–154.

Arnold, S.E., Hyman, B.T., Flory, J., Damasio, A.R., and Van Hoesen, G.W. (1991) The topographical and neuroanatomical distribution of neurofibrillary tangles and neuritic plaques in the cerebral cortex of patients with Alzheimer's disease. *Cereb. Cortex* 1: 103–116.

Arnold, S.E., and Kumar, A. (1993) Reversible dementias. *Med. Clin. North Am.* 77:215–230.

Azari, N.P., Pettigrew, K.D., Schapiro, M.B., et al. (1993) Early detection of Alzheimer's disease: a statistical approach using positron emission tomographic data. *J. Cereb. Blood Flow Metab.* 13:438–447.

Bartels, P., and Subach, J. (1976) Significance probability mappings and automated interpretation of complex pictorial scenes. In: Preston, E., and Onoe, M., eds. *Digital Processing of Biomedical Imagery*. New York: Academic Press, pp. 101–114.

Bartlett, E., Brodie, J., Wolf, A., Christman, D., Laska, E., and Meissner, M. (1988) Reproducibility of cerebral glucose metabolic measurements in resting human subjects. *J. Cereb. Blood Flow Metab.* 8:502–512.

Bartlett, E.J., Barouche, F., Brodie, J.D., et al. (1991) Stability of resting deoxyglucose metabolic values in PET studies of schizophrenia. *Psychiatry Res.* 40:11–20.

Benoit, M., Koulibaly, P.M., Migneco, O., Darcourt, J., Pringuey, D.J., and Robert, P.H. (2002) Brain perfusion in Alzheimer's disease with and without apathy: a SPECT study with statistical parametric mapping analysis. *Psychiatry Res.* 114:103–111.

Berrios, G.E., Wagle, A.C., Markova, I.S., et al. (2001) Psychiatric symptoms and CAG repeats in neurologically asymptomatic Huntington's disease gene carriers. *Psychiatry Res.* 102:217–225.

Brickman, A.M., Buchsbaum, M.S., Shihabuddin, L., Hazlett, E.A., Borod, J.C., and Mohs, R.C. (2003) Striatal size, glucose metabolic rate, and verbal learning in normal aging. *Brain Res. Cogn. Brain Res.* 17:106–116.

Buchsbaum, M., and Hazlett, E. (1998) Positron emission tomography studies of abnormal glucose metabolism in schizophrenia. *Schizophr. Bull.* 24:343–364.

Buchsbaum, M.S. (1990) Frontal lobes, basal ganglia, temporal lobes—three sites for schizophrenia? *Schizophr. Bull.* 16:377–378.

Buchsbaum, M.S., and Hazlett, E.A. (1997) Functional brain imaging and aging in schizophrenia. *Schizophr. Res.* 27:129–141.

Buchsbaum, M.S., Kesslak, J.P., Lynch, G., et al. (1991) Temporal and hippocampal metabolic rate during an olfactory memory task assessed by positron emission tomography in patients with dementia of the Alzheimer type and controls. preliminary studies. *Arch. Gen. Psychiatry* 48:840–847.

Buchsbaum, M.S., Potkin, S., Marshall, J., et al. (1992) Effects of clozapine and thiothixene on glucose metabolic rate in schizophrenia. *Neuropsychopharmacology* 6:155–163.

Buchsbaum, M.S., Potkin, S.G., Siegel, B.V. Jr., et al. (1992) Striatal metabolic rate and clinical response to neuroleptics in schizophrenia. *Arch. Gen. Psychiatry* 49:966–974.

Burdette, J.H., Minoshima, S., Vander Borght, T., Tran, D.D., and Kuhl, D.E. (1996) Alzheimer disease: improved visual interpretation of PET images by using three-dimensional stereotaxic surface projections. *Radiology* 198:837–843.

Cabeza, R. (2001) Cognitive neuroscience of aging: contributions of functional neuroimaging. *Scand. J. Psychol.* 42:277–286.

Carter, C.S., Perlstein, W., Ganguli, R., Brar, J., Mintun, M., and Cohen, J.D. (1998) Functional hypofrontality and working memory dysfunction in schizophrenia. *Am. J. Psychiatry* 155:1285–1287.

Chua, S.E., and McKenna, P.J. (1995) Schizophrenia—a brain disease? A critical review of structural and functional cerebral abnormality in the disorder. *Br. J. Psychiatry* 166:563–582.

Ciarmiello, A., Cannella, M., Lastoria, S., Simonelli, M., Frati, L., Rubinsztein, D.C., et al. (2006) Brain white-matter volume loss and glucose hypometabolism precede the clinical symptoms of Huntington's disease. *J. Nucl. Med.* 47:215–222.

Coffey, C.E., Wilkinson, W.E., Parashos, I.A., et al. (1992) Quantitative cerebral anatomy of the aging human brain: a cross-sectional study using magnetic resonance imaging. *Neurology* 42: 527–536.

Cornblatt, B.A., and Erlenmeyer-Kimling, L. (1985) Global attentional deviance as a marker of risk for schizophrenia: specificity and predictive validity. *J. Abnorm. Psychol.* 94:470–486.

Crespo-Facorro, B., Wiser, A.K., Andreasen, N.C., et al. (2001) Neural basis of novel and well-learned recognition memory in schizophrenia: a positron emission tomography study. *Hum. Brain. Mapp.* 12:219–231.

Davidson, M., Harvey, P.D., Powchik, P., et al. (1995) Severity of symptoms in chronically institutionalized geriatric schizophrenic patients. *Am. J. Psychiatry* 152:197–207.

Davidson, M., Harvey, P., Welsh, K.A., Powchik, P., Putnam, K.M., and Mohs, R.C. (1996) Cognitive functioning in late-life schizophrenia: a comparison of elderly schizophrenic patients and patients with Alzheimer's disease. *Am. J. Psychiatry* 153:1274–1279.

DeCarli, C., Atack, J., Ball, M., et al. (1992) Post-mortem regional neurofibrillary tangle densities but not senile plaque densities are related to regional cerebral metabolic rates for glucose during life in Alzheimer's disease patient. *Neurodegeneration* 1:113–121.

de Leon, M.J., Mosconi, L., Blennow, K., DeSanti, S., Zinkowski, R., Mehta, P.D., et al. (2007) Imaging and CSF studies in the preclinical diagnosis of Alzheimer's disease. *Ann. N.Y. Acad. Sci.* 1097:114–145.

DeQuardo, J.R., Bookstein, F.L., Green, W.D., Brunberg, J.A., and Tandon, R. (1996) Spatial relationships of neuroanatomic landmarks in schizophrenia. *Psychiatry Res.* 67:81–95.

De Santi, S., de Leon, M., Convit, A., et al. (1995) Age-related changes in brain: II. Positron emission tomography of frontal and temporal lobe glucose metabolism in normal subjects. *Psychiatry Q.* 66:357–370.

De Santi, S., de Leon, M.J., Rusinek, H., et al. (2001) Hippocampal formation glucose metabolism and volume losses in MCI and AD. *Neurobiol. Aging* 22:529–539.

Desgranges, B., Baron, J.C., Lalevee, C., et al. (2002) The neural substrates of episodic memory impairment in Alzheimer's disease as revealed by FDG-PET: relationship to degree of deterioration. *Brain* 125:1116–1124.

Dickerson, B.C., Salat, D.H., Bates, J.F., Atiya, M., Killiany, R.J., Greve, D.N., et al. (2004) Medial temporal lobe function and structure in mild cognitive impairment. *Ann. Neurology* 56:27–35.

Dickson, D.W. (1998) Pick's disease: a modern approach. *Brain Pathol.* 8:339–354.

Dierks, T., Linden, D.E., Hertel, A., et al. (1999) Multimodal imaging of residual function and compensatory resource allocation in cortical atrophy: a case study of parietal lobe function in a patient with Huntington's disease. *Psychiatry Res.* 90:67–75.

Dobert, N., Pantel, J., Frolich, L., Hamscho, N., Menzel, C., and Grunwald, F. (2005) Diagnostic value of FDG-PET and HMPAO-SPET in patients with mild dementia and mild cognitive impairment: metabolic index and perfusion index. *Dement. Geriatr. Cogn. Disord.* 20:63–70.

Duara, R., Barker, W.W., Chang, J., Yoshii, F., Loewenstein, D.A., and Pascal, S. (1992) Viability of neocortical function shown in behavioral activation state PET studies in Alzheimer disease. *J. Cereb. Blood Flow Metab.* 12:927–934.

Duara, R., Gross-Glenn, K., Barker, W.W., et al. (1987) Behavioral activation and the variability of cerebral glucose metabolic measurements. *J. Cereb. Blood Flow Metab.* 7:266–271.

Eberling, J.L., Richardson, B.C., Reed, B.R., Wolfe, N., and Jagust, W.J. (1994) Cortical glucose metabolism in Parkinson's disease without dementia. *Neurobiol. Aging* 15:329–335.

Falke, E., Han, L.Y., and Arnold, S.E. (2000) Absence of neurodegeneration in the thalamus and caudate of elderly patients with schizophrenia. *Psychiatry Res.* 93:103–110.

Feigin, A., Leenders, K.L., Moeller, J.R., et al. (2001) Metabolic network abnormalities in early Huntington's disease: an [(18)F]FDG PET study. *J. Nucl. Med.* 42:1591–1595.

Fellgiebel, A., Scheurich, A., Bartenstein, P., and Muller, M.J. (2007) FDG-PET and CSF phospho-tau for prediction of cognitive decline in mild cognitive impairment. *Psychiatry Res.* 155:167–171.

Foster, N.L., Chase, T.N., Fedio, P., Patronas, N.J., Brooks, R.A., and Di Chiro, G. (1983) Alzheimer's disease: focal cortical changes shown by positron emission tomography. *Neurology* 33:961–965.

Friedland, R.P., Koss, E., Lerner, A., et al. (1993) Functional imaging, the frontal lobes, and dementia. *Dementia* 4:192–203.

Friston, K.J., Frith, C., Liddle, P., and Frackowiak, R. (1991) Plastic transformation of PET images. *J. Comput. Assist. Tomogr.* 15:634–659.

Gallagher, M., and Rapp, P.R. (1997) The use of animal models to study the effects of aging on cognition. *Annu. Rev. Psychol.* 48:339–370.

Gonzalez, R.G., Fischman, A.J., Guimaraes, A.R., et al. (1995) Functional MR in the evaluation of dementia: correlation of abnormal dynamic cerebral blood volume measurements with changes in cerebral metabolism on positron emission tomography with fludeoxyglucose F 18. *Am. J. Neuroradiol.* 16:1763–1770.

Grady, C.L., Haxby, J.V., Horwitz, B., et al. (1993) Activation of cerebral blood flow during a visuoperceptual task in patients with Alzheimer-type dementia. *Neurobiol. Aging* 14:35–44.

Grady, C.L., Haxby, J.V., Schapiro, M.B., et al. (1990) Subgroups in dementia of the Alzheimer type identified using positron emission tomography. *J. Neuropsychiatry Clin. Neurosci.* 2:373–384.

Grady, C.L., Haxby, J.V., Schlageter, N.L., Berg, G., and Rapoport, S.I. (1986) Stability of metabolic and neuropsychological asymmetries in dementia of the Alzheimer type. *Neurology* 36:1390–1392.

Grady, C.L., McIntosh, A.R., Horwitz, B., et al. (1995) Age-related reductions in human recognition memory due to impaired encoding. *Science* 269:218–221.

Hanyu, H., Nakano, S., Abe, S., Arai, H., Iwamoto, T., and Takasaki, M. (1995) [Longitudinal study of neuropsychological and cerebral blood flow changes in Alzheimer-type dementia]. *Nippon Ronen Igakkai Zasshi* 32:728–735.

Haxby, J.V., Duara, R., Grady, C.L., Cutler, N.R., and Rapoport, S.I. (1985) Relations between neuropsychological and cerebral metabolic asymmetries in early Alzheimer's disease. *J. Cereb. Blood Flow Metab.* 5:193–200.

Haxby, J.V., Grady, C.L., Duara, R., Schlageter, N., Berg, G., and Rapoport, S.I. (1986) Neocortical metabolic abnormalities precede nonmemory cognitive defects in early Alzheimer's-type dementia. *Arch. Neurol.* 43:882–885.

Hazlett, E., Buchsbaum, M., Mohs, R., et al. (1998) Age-related shift in brain region allocation during successful memory performance. *Neurobiol. Aging* 19:437–445.

Heiss, W.D., Szelies, B., Kessler, J., and Herholz, K. (1991) Abnormalities of energy metabolism in Alzheimer's disease studied with PET. *Ann. N.Y. Acad. Sci.* 640:65–71.

Hempel, A., Henze, M., Berghoff, C., Garcia, N., Ody, R., and Schroder, J. (2001) PET findings and neuropsychological deficits in a case of Fahr's disease. *Psychiatry Res.* 108:133–140.

Henkel, K., Zerr, I., Hertel, A., et al. (2002) Positron emission tomography with [(18)F]FDG in the diagnosis of Creutzfeldt-Jakob disease (CJD). *J. Neurol.* 249:699–705.

Herholz, K. (1995) FDG PET and differential diagnosis of dementia. *Alzheimer Dis. Assoc. Disord.* 9:6–16.

Herholz, K., Schopphoff, H., Schmidt, M., et al. (2002) Direct comparison of spatially normalized PET and SPECT scans in Alzheimer's disease. *J. Nucl. Med.* 43:21–26.

Hertz, L., and Peng, L. (1992) Energy metabolism at the cellular level of the CNS. *Can. J. Physiol. Pharmacol.* 70:S145–S157.

Higdon, R., Foster, N.L., Koeppe, R.A., DeCarli, C.S., Jagust, W.J., Clark, C.M., et al. (2004) A comparison of classification methods for differentiating fronto-temporal dementia from Alzheimer's disease using FDG-PET imaging. *Stat. Med.* 23:315–326.

Hof, P.R., Cox, K., and Morrison, J.H. (1990) Quantitative analysis of a vulnerable subset of pyramidal neurons in Alzheimer's disease: I. Superior frontal and inferior temporal cortex. *J. Comp. Neurol.* 301:44–54.

Hof, P.R., and Morrison, J.H. (1990) Quantitative analysis of a vulnerable subset of pyramidal neurons in Alzheimer's disease: II. Primary and secondary visual cortex. *J. Comp. Neurol.* 301:55–64.

Hof, P., and Morrison, J. (1994) The cellular basis of cortical disconnection in Alzheimer's disease and related dementing conditions. In: Terry, R., Katzman, R., and Bick, K., eds. *Alzheimer Disease*. New York: Raven Press, pp. 197–229.

Hoffman, J.M., Welsh-Bohmer, K.A., and Hanson, M., et al. (2000) FDG PET imaging in patients with pathologically verified dementia. *J. Nucl. Med.* 41:1920–1928.

Honda, N., Machida, K., Hosono, M., Matsumoto, T., Matsuda, H., Oshima, M., et al. (2002) Interobserver variation in diagnosis of dementia by brain perfusion SPECT. *Radiat. Med.* 20: 281–289.

Horwitz, B., McIntosh, A.R., Haxby, J.V., et al. (1995) Network analysis of PET-mapped visual pathways in Alzheimer type dementia. *Neuroreport* 6:2287–2292.

Huey, E.D., Putnam, K.T., and Grafman, J. (2006) A systematic review of neurotransmitter deficits and treatments in frontotemporal dementia. *Neurology* 66:17–22.

Hunt, A., Schonknecht, P., Henze, M., Seidl, U., Haberkorn, U., and Schroder, J. (2007) Reduced cerebral glucose metabolism in patients at risk for Alzheimer's disease. *Psychiatry Res.* 155: 147–154.

Ichimiya, A., Herholz, K., Mielke, R., Kessler, J., Slansky, I., and Heiss, W.D. (1994) Difference of regional cerebral metabolic pattern between presenile and senile dementia of the Alzheimer type: a factor analytic study. *J. Neurol. Sci.* 123:11–17.

Ishii, K., Willoch, F., Minoshima, S., et al. (2001) Statistical brain mapping of 18F-FDG PET in Alzheimer's disease: validation of anatomic standardization for atrophied brains. *J. Nucl. Med.* 42:548–557.

Jagust, W.J., Eberling, J.L., Richardson, B.C., et al. (1993) The cortical topography of temporal lobe hypometabolism in early Alzheimer's disease. *Brain Res.* 629:189–198.

Jagust, W.J., Friedland, R.P., Budinger, T.F., Koss, E., and Ober, B. (1988) Longitudinal studies of regional cerebral metabolism in Alzheimer's disease. *Neurology* 38:909–912.

Jagust, W., Reed, B., Mungas, D., Ellis, W., and Decarli, C. (2007) What does fluorodeoxyglucose PET imaging add to a clinical diagnosis of dementia? *Neurology* 69:871–877.

Jobst, K.A., Smith, A.D., Barker, C.S., et al. (1992) Association of atrophy of the medial temporal lobe with reduced blood flow in the posterior parietotemporal cortex in patients with a clinical and pathological diagnosis of Alzheimer's disease. *J. Neurol. Neurosurg. Psychiatry* 55:190–194.

Joyce, E.M., Rio, D.E., Ruttimann, U.E., et al. (1994) Decreased cingulate and precuneate glucose utilization in alcoholic Korsakoff's syndrome. *Psychiatry Res.* 54:225–239.

Kapur, S., Craik, F.I., Jones, C., Brown, G.M., Houle, S., and Tulving, E. (1995) Functional role of the prefrontal cortex in retrieval of memories: a PET study. *Neuroreport* 6:1880–1884.

Keshavan, M.S., Anderson, S., Beckwith, C., Nash, K., Pettegrew, J.W., and Krishnan, K.R. (1995) A comparison of stereology and segmentation techniques for volumetric measurements of lateral ventricles in magnetic resonance imaging. *Psychiatry Res.* 61: 53–60

Kessler, J., Ghaemi, M., Mielke, R., Herholz, K., and Heiss, W.D. (1996) Visual versus auditory memory stimulation in patients with probable Alzheimer's disease. A PET study with 18 FDG. *Ann. N.Y. Acad. Sci.* 777:233–238.

Kessler, J., Herholz, K., Grond, M., and Heiss, W.D. (1991) Impaired metabolic activation in Alzheimer's disease: a PET study during continuous visual recognition. *Neuropsychologia* 29:229–243.

Kim, J.J., Mohamed, S., Andreasen, N.C., et al. (2000) Regional neural dysfunctions in chronic schizophrenia studied with positron emission tomography. *Am. J. Psychiatry* 157:542–548.

Klunk, W.E., Engler, H., Nordberg, A., Wang, Y., Blomqvist, G., Holt, D.P., et al. (2004) Imaging brain amyloid in Alzheimer's disease with Pittsburgh Compound-B. *Ann. Neurology* 55:306–319.

Koss, E., Friedland, R.P., Ober, B.A., and Jagust, W.J. (1985) Differences in lateral hemispheric asymmetries of glucose utilization between early- and late onset Alzheimer-type dementia. *Am. J. Psychiatry* 142:638–640.

Kuhl, D.E., Metter, E.J., Riege, W.H., and Phelps, M.E. (1982) Effects of human aging on patterns of local cerebral glucose utilization determined by the [18F]fluorodeoxyglucose method. *J. Cereb. Blood Flow Metab.* 2:163–171.

Kumar, A., Schapiro, M.B., Grady, C., et al. (1991) High-resolution PET studies in Alzheimer's disease. *Neuropsychopharmacology* 4:35–46.

Lanctot, K., Herrmann, N., Ganjavi, H., Black, S., Rusjan, P., Houle, S., et al. (2007) Serotonin-1A receptors in frontotemporal dementia compared to controls. *Psychiatry Res.* 156(3):247–250.

Leenders, K.L., Perani, D., Lammertsma, A.A., et al. (1990) Cerebral blood flow, blood volume and oxygen utilization. Normal values and effect of age. *Brain* 113:27–47.

Lewis, D.A., Campbell, M.J., Terry, R.D., and Morrison, J.H. (1987) Laminar and regional distributions of neurofibrillary tangles and neuritic plaques in Alzheimer's disease: a quantitative study of visual and auditory cortices. *J. Neurosci.* 7:1799–1808.

Lieberman, A.P., Trojanowski, J.Q., Lee, V.M., et al. (1998) Cognitive, neuroimaging, and pathological studies in a patient with Pick's disease. *Ann. Neurol.* 43:259–265.

Loessner, A., Alavi, A., Lewandrowski, K.U., Mozley, D., Souder, E., and Gur, R.E. (1995) Regional cerebral function determined by FDG-PET in healthy volunteers: normal patterns and changes with age. *J. Nucl. Med.* 36:1141–1149.

MacFall, J.R., Byrum, C.E., Parashos, I., et al. (1994) Relative accuracy and reproducibility of regional MRI brain volumes for point-counting methods. *Psychiatry Res.* 55:167–177.

Machulda, M.M., Ward, H.A., Borowski, B., Gunter, J.L., Cha, R.H., O'Brien, P.C., et al. (2003) Comparison of memory fMRI response among normal, MCI, and Alzheimer's patients. *Neurology* 61:500–506.

Mann, U.M., Mohr, E., Gearing, M., and Chase, T.N. (1992) Heterogeneity in Alzheimer's disease: progression rate segregated by distinct neuropsychological and cerebral metabolic profiles. *J. Neurol. Neurosurg. Psychiatry* 55:956–959.

Maquet, P., Dive, D., Salmon, E., von Frenckel, R., and Franck, G. (1990) Reproducibility of cerebral glucose utilization measured by PET and the [18F]-2-fluoro-2-deoxy-d-glucose method in resting, healthy human subjects. *Eur. J. Nucl. Med.* 16:267–273.

Martin, A., Friston, K., Colebatch, J., and Frackowiak, R. (1991) Decreases in regional cerebral blood flow with normal aging. *J. Cereb. Blood Flow Metab.* 11:684–689.

Martin, P.R., Rio, D., Adinoff, B., et al. (1992) Regional cerebral glucose utilization in chronic organic mental disorders associated with alcoholism. *J. Neuropsychiatry Clin. Neurosci.* 4:159–167.

Matochik, J.A., Molchan, S.E., Zametkin, A.J., Warden, D.L., Sunderland, T., and Cohen, R.M. (1995) Regional cerebral glucose metabolism in autopsy-confirmed Creutzfeldt-Jakob disease. *Acta Neurol. Scand.* 91:153–157.

McGeer, E.G., Peppard, R.P., McGeer, P.L., et al. (1990) 18Fluorodeoxyglucose positron emission tomography studies in presumed Alzheimer cases, including 13 serial scans. *Can. J. Neurol. Sci.* 17:1–11.

Meguro, K., Yamaguchi, S., Yamazaki, H., et al. (1996) Cortical glucose metabolism in psychiatric wandering patients with vascular dementia. *Psychiatry Res.* 67:71–80.

Meltzer, C.C., Zubieta, J.K., Brandt, J., Tune, L.E., Mayberg, H.S., and Frost, J.J. (1996) Regional hypometabolism in Alzheimer's disease as measured by positron emission tomography after correction for effects of partial volume averaging. *Neurology* 47: 454–461.

Mentis, M.J., Salerno, J., Horwitz, B., et al. (1994) Reduction of functional neuronal connectivity in long-term treated hypertension. *Stroke* 25:601–607.

Mentis, M.J., Weinstein, E.A., Horwitz, B., et al. (1995) Abnormal brain glucose metabolism in the delusional misidentification syndromes: a positron emission tomography study in Alzheimer disease. *Biol. Psychiatry* 38:438–449.

Messa, C., Fazio, F., Costa, D.C., and Ell, P.J. (1995) Clinical brain radionuclide imaging studies. *Semin. Nucl. Med.* 25:111–143.

Mielke, R., Herholz, K., Fink, G., Ritter, D., and Heiss, W.D. (1993) Positron emission tomography in myotonic dystrophy. *Psychiatry Res.* 50:93–99.

Mielke, R., Herholz, J., Grond, M., Kessler, J., and Heiss, W. (1991) Differences in regional cerebral glucose metabolism between presenile and senile dementia of Alzheimer type. *Neurobiol. Aging* 13:93–98.

Mielke, R., Herholz, K., Grond, M., Kessler, J., and Heiss, W.D. (1992) Severity of vascular dementia is related to volume of metabolically impaired tissue. *Arch. Neurol.* 49:909–913.

Mielke, R., Herholz, K., Grond, M., Kessler, J., and Heiss, W.D. (1994) Clinical deterioration in probable Alzheimer's disease correlates with progressive metabolic impairment of association areas. *Dementia* 5:36–41.

Mielke, R., Schroder, R., Fink, G.R., Kessler, J., Herholz, K., and Heiss, W.D. (1996) Regional cerebral glucose metabolism and postmortem pathology in Alzheimer's disease. *Acta Neuropathol.* 91:174–179.

Miller, J.D., de Leon, M.J., Ferris, S.H., et al. (1987) Abnormal temporal lobe response in Alzheimer's disease during cognitive processing as measured by 11C-2-deoxy-d-glucose and PET. *J. Cereb. Blood Flow Metab.* 7:248–251.

Miller, S.L., Fenstermacher, E., Bates, J., Blacker, D., Sperling, R.A., and Dickerson, B.C. (2007) Hippocampal activation in adults with mild cognitive impairment predicts subsequent cognitive decline. *J. Neurol. Neurosurg. Psychiatry*. Sept 10 [Epub ahead of print]

Minoshima, S., Frey, K.A., Koeppe, R.A., Foster, N.L., and Kuhl, D.E. (1995) A diagnostic approach in Alzheimer's disease using three-dimensional stereotactic surface projections of fluorine-18-FDG PET. *J. Nucl. Med.* 36:1238–1248.

Moeller, J., Ishikawa, T., Dhawan, V., et al. (1996) The metabolic topography of normal aging. *J. Cereb. Blood Flow Metab.* 16: 385–398.

Morrison, J.H. (1993) Differential vulnerability, connectivity, and cell typology. *Neurobiol. Aging* 14:51–54; discussion 55–56.

Mosconi, L., De Santi, S., Brys, M., Tsui, W.H., Pirraglia, E., Glodzik-Sobanska, L., et al. (2008) Hypometabolism and altered cerebrospinal fluid markers in normal apolipoprotein E E4 carriers with subjective memory complaints. *Biol. Psychiatry* 63(6): 609–618.

Mosconi, L., Tsui, W.H., De Santi, S., Li, J., Rusinek, H., Convit, A., et al. (2005) Reduced hippocampal metabolism in MCI and AD: automated FDG-PET image analysis. *Neurology* 64:1860–1867.

Murphy, D.G., Bottomley, P.A., Salerno, J.A., et al. (1993) An in vivo study of phosphorus and glucose metabolism in Alzheimer's disease using magnetic resonance spectroscopy and PET. *Arch. Gen. Psychiatry* 50:341–349.

Murphy, D.G., DeCarli, C., McIntosh, A.R., et al. (1996) Sex differences in human brain morphometry and metabolism: an in vivo quantitative magnetic resonance imaging and positron emission tomography study on the effect of aging. *Arch. Gen. Psychiatry* 53:585–594.

Nestor, P.J., Caine, D., Fryer, T.D., Clarke, J., and Hodges, J.R. (2003) The topography of metabolic deficits in posterior cortical atrophy (the visual variant of Alzheimer's disease) with FDG-PET. *J. Neurol. Neurosurg. Psychiatry* 74:1521–1529.

Nihashi, T., Yatsuya, H., Hayasaka, K., Kato, R., Kawatsu, S., Arahata, Y., et al. (2007) Direct comparison study between FDG-PET and IMP-SPECT for diagnosing Alzheimer's disease using 3D-SSP analysis in the same patients. *Radiat. Med.* 25:255–262.

Nordberg, A. (2007) Amyloid imaging in Alzheimer's disease. *Curr. Opin. Neurol.* 20:398–402.

Nordberg, A., Lilja, A., Lundqvist, H., et al. (1992) Tacrine restores cholinergic nicotinic receptors and glucose metabolism in Alzheimer patients as visualized by positron emission tomography. *Neurobiol. Aging* 13:747–758.

Nyback, H., Nyman, H., Blomqvist, G., Sjogren, I., and Stone-Elander, S. (1991) Brain metabolism in Alzheimer's dementia: studies of 11C-deoxyglucose accumulation, CSF monoamine metabolites and neuropsychological test performance in patients and healthy subjects. *J. Neurol. Neurosurg. Psychiatry* 54:672–678.

Ober, B.A., Jagust, W.J., Koss, E., Delis, D.C., and Friedland, R.P. (1991) Visuoconstructive performance and regional cerebral glucose metabolism in Alzheimer's disease. *J. Clin. Exp. Neuropsychol.* 13:752–772.

Pakrasi, S., and O'Brien, J.T. (2005) Emission tomography in dementia. *Nucl. Med. Comm.* 26:189–196.

Pearlson, G.D., Harris, G.J., Powers, R.E., et al. (1992) Quantitative changes in mesial temporal volume, regional cerebral blood flow, and cognition in Alzheimer's disease. *Arch. Gen. Psychiatry* 49: 402–408.

Pearson, R.C., Esiri, M.M., Hiorns, R.W., Wilcock, G.K., and Powell, T.P. (1985) Anatomical correlates of the distribution of the pathological changes in the neocortex in Alzheimer disease. *Proc. Natl. Acad. Sci. USA* 82:4531–4534.

Peppard, R.F., Martin, W.R., Carr, G.D., et al. (1992) Cerebral glucose metabolism in Parkinson's disease with and without dementia. *Arch. Neurol.* 49:1262–1268.

Perneczky, R., Diehl-Schmid, J., Forstl, H., Drzezga, A., May, F., and Kurz, A. (2008) Urinary incontinence and its functional anatomy in frontotemporal lobar degenerations. *Eur. J. Nucl. Med. Mol. Imaging* 35(3):605–610.

Pietrini, P., Furey, M.L., Graff-Radford, N., et al. (1996) Preferential metabolic involvement of visual cortical areas in a subtype of Alzheimer's disease: clinical implications. *Am. J. Psychiatry* 153: 1261–1268.

Poon, L. (1985) Differences in human memory with aging: nature, causes, and clinical implications. In: Birren, J., and Schaie, K., eds. *Handbook of the Psychology of Aging*. New York: Van Nostrand Reinhold, pp. 427–462.

Prvulovic, D., Van de Ven, V., Sack, A.T., Maurer, K., and Linden, D.E. (2005) Functional activation imaging in aging and dementia. *Psychiatry Res.* 140:97–113.

Reuter-Lorenz, P., Jonides, J., Smith, E., Hartley, A., Miller, A., Marshuetz, C., et al. (2000) Age differences in frontal lateralization of verbal and spatial working memory revealed by PET. *J. Cogn. Neurosci.* 12:174–187.

Rodriguez, G., Vitali, P., Calvini, P., et al. (2000) Hippocampal perfusion in mild Alzheimer's disease. *Psychiatry Res.* 100:65–74.

Rogers, J., and Morrison, J.H. (1985) Quantitative morphology and regional and laminar distributions of senile plaques in Alzheimer's disease. *J. Neurosci.* 5:2801–2808.

Rombouts, S.A., Barkhof, F., Veltman, D.J., Machielsen, W.C., Witter, M.P., Bierlaagh, M.A., et al. (2000) Functional MR imaging in Alzheimer's disease during memory encoding. *Am. J. Neuroradiol.* 21:1869–1875.

Ruttimann, U.E., Andreason, P.J., and Rio, D. (1995) Head motion during positron emission tomography: is it significant? *Psychiatry Res.* 61:43–51.

Sachdev, P., Gaur, R., Brodaty, H., et al. (1997) Longitudinal study of cerebral blood flow in Alzheimer's disease using single photon emission tomography. *Psychiatry Res.* 68:133–141.

Sakamoto, S., Ishii, K., Sasaki, M., et al. (2002) Differences in cerebral metabolic impairment between early and late onset types of Alzheimer's disease. *J. Neurol. Sci.* 200:27–32.

Salmon, E., Maquet, P., Sadzot, B., Degueldre, C., Lemaire, C., and Franck, G. (1991) Decrease of frontal metabolism demonstrated by positron emission tomography in a population of healthy elderly volunteers. *Acta Neurol. Belg.* 91:288–295.

Santens, P., De Bleecker, J., Goethals, P., et al. (2001) Differential regional cerebral uptake of (18)F-fluoro-2-deoxy-d-glucose in Alzheimer's disease and frontotemporal dementia at initial diagnosis. *Eur. Neurol.* 45:19–27.

Sarangi, S., San Pedro, E.C., and Mountz, J.M. (2000) Anterior choroidal artery infarction presenting as a progressive cognitive deficit. *Clin. Nucl. Med.* 25:187–190.

Schapiro, M.B., Pietrini, P., Grady, C.L., et al. (1993) Reductions in parietal and temporal cerebral metabolic rates for glucose are not specific for Alzheimer's disease. *J. Neurol. Neurosurg. Psychiatry* 56:859–864.

Schroder, J., Buchsbaum, M.S., Shihabuddin, L., et al. (2001) Patterns of cortical activity and memory performance in Alzheimer's disease. *Biol. Psychiatry* 49:426–436.

Schultz, S.K., O'Leary, D.S., Boles Ponto, L.L., Arndt, S., Magnotta, V., Watkins, G.L., et al. (2002) Age and regional cerebral blood flow in schizophrenia: age effects in anterior cingulate, frontal, and parietal cortex. *J. Neuropsychiatry Clin. Neurosci.* 14:19–24.

Schumann, G., Halsband, U., Kassubek, J., et al. (2000) Combined semantic dementia and apraxia in a patient with frontotemporal lobar degeneration. *Psychiatry Res.* 100:21–29.

Shidahara, M., Inoue, K., Maruyama, M., Watabe, H., Taki, Y., Goto, R., et al. (2006) Predicting human performance by channelized Hotelling observer in discriminating between Alzheimer's dementia and controls using statistically processed brain perfusion SPECT. *Ann. Nucl. Med.* 20:605–613.

Shigenobu, K., Ikeda, M., Fukuhara, R., et al. (2002) The Stereotypy Rating Inventory for frontotemporal lobar degeneration. *Psychiatry Res.* 110:175–187.

Small, G.W., Mazziotta, J.C., Collins, M.T., et al. (1995) Apolipoprotein E type 4 allele and cerebral glucose metabolism in relatives at risk for familial Alzheimer disease. *JAMA* 273:942–947.

Small, G.W., Okonek, A., Mandelkern, M.A., et al. (1994) Age-associated memory loss: initial neuropsychological and cerebral metabolic findings of a longitudinal study. *Int. Psychogeriatr.* 6:23–44; discussion 60–62.

Small, S.A., Perera, G.M., DeLaPaz, R., Mayeux, R., and Stern, Y. (1999) Differential regional dysfunction of the hippocampal formation among elderly with memory decline and Alzheimer's disease. *Ann. Neurol.* 45:466–472.

Smith, G.S., de Leon, M.J., George, A.E., et al. (1992) Topography of cross-sectional and longitudinal glucose metabolic deficits in Alzheimer's disease. pathophysiologic implications. *Arch. Neurol.* 49:1142–1150.

Sokoloff, L., Reivich, M., Kennedy, C., et al. (1977) The [14C]deoxyglucose method for the measurement of local cerebral glucose utilization: theory, procedure, and normal values in the conscious and anesthetized albino rat. *J. Neurochem.* 28: 897–916.

Sperling, R.A., Bates, J.F., Chua, E.F., Cocchiarella, A.J., Rentz, D.M., Rosen, B.R., et al. (2003) fMRI studies of associative encoding in young and elderly controls and mild Alzheimer's disease. *J. Neurol. Neurosurg. Psychiatry* 74:44–50.

Stuss, D., and Benson, D. (1986) *The Frontal Lobes.* New York: Raven Press.

Sultzer, D.L., Mahler, M.E., Cummings, J.L., Van Gorp, W.G., Hinkin, C.H., and Brown, C. (1995) Cortical abnormalities associated with subcortical lesions in vascular dementia. Clinical and position emission tomographic findings. *Arch. Neurol.* 52: 773–780.

Takada, H., Nagata, K., Hirata, Y., et al. (1992) Age-related decline of cerebral oxygen metabolism in normal population detected with positron emission tomography. *Neurol. Res.* 14:128–131.

Teipel, S.J., Drzezga, A., Bartenstein, P., Moller, H.J., Schwaiger, M., and Hampel, H. (2006) Effects of donepezil on cortical metabolic response to activation during (18)FDG-PET in Alzheimer's disease: a double-blind cross-over trial. *Psychopharmacology* 187: 86–94.

Tempel, L.W., and Perlmutter, J.S. (1992) Vibration-induced regional cerebral blood flow responses in normal aging. *J. Cereb. Blood Flow Metab.* 12:554–561.

Tulving, E., Kapur, S., Craik, F., Moscovitch, M., and Houle, S. (1994) Hemispheric encoding/retrieval asymmetry in episodic memory: positron emission tomography findings. *Proc. Natl. Acad. Sci. USA* 91:2016–2020.

Uttner, I., Mottaghy, F.M., Schreiber, H., Riecker, A., Ludolph, A.C., and Kassubek, J. (2006) Primary progressive aphasia accompanied by environmental sound agnosia: a neuropsychological, MRI and PET study. *Psychiatry Res.* 146:191–197.

Valladares-Neto, D.C., Buchsbaum, M.S., Evans, W.J., et al. (1995) EEG delta, positron emission tomography, and memory deficit in Alzheimer's disease. *Neuropsychobiology* 31:173–181.

Van Hoesen, G., and Damasio, A. (1987) Neural correlates of cognitive impairment in Alzheimer's disease. In: Mountcastle, V., Plum, F., and Geiger, S., eds. *Handbook of Physiology: The Nervous System, Vol. V, Higher Functions of the Brain.* Bethesda, MD: American Physiological Society, pp. 871–898.

Volkow, N.D., Hitzemann, R., Wolf, A.P., et al. (1990) Acute effects of ethanol on regional brain glucose metabolism and transport. *Psychiatry Res.* 35:39–48.

Volkow, N.D., Wang, G.J., Overall, J.E., et al. (1997) Regional brain metabolic response to lorazepam in alcoholics during early and late alcohol detoxification. *Alcohol Clin. Exp. Res.* 21:1278–1284.

Volkow, N.D., Zhu, W., Felder, C.A., et al. (2002) Changes in brain functional homogeneity in subjects with Alzheimer's disease. *Psychiatry Res.* 114:39–50.

Wang, G.J., Volkow, N.D., Wolf, A.P., Brodie, J.D., and Hitzemann, R.J. (1994) Intersubject variability of brain glucose metabolic measurements in young normal males. *J. Nucl. Med.* 35:1457–1466.

Welsh, K., Butters, N., Hughes, J., Mohs, R., and Heyman, A. (1991) Detection of abnormal memory decline in mild cases of Alzheimer's disease using CERAD neuropsychological measures. *Arch. Neurol.* 48:278–281.

Welsh, K.A., Butters, N., Hughes, J.P., Mohs, R.C., and Heyman, A. (1992) Detection and staging of dementia in Alzheimer's disease. Use of the neuropsychological measures developed for the Consortium to Establish a Registry for Alzheimer's disease. *Arch. Neurol.* 49:448–452.

Williamson, P. (1987) Hypofrontality in schizophrenia: a review of the evidence. *Can. J. Psychiatry* 32:399–404.

Yanase, D., Matsunari, I., Yajima, K., Chen, W., Fujikawa, A., Nishimura, S., et al. (2005) Brain FDG PET study of normal aging in Japanese: effect of atrophy correction. *Eur. J. Nucl. Med. Mol. Imaging* 32:794–805.

Yong, S.W., Yoon, J.K., An, Y.S., and Lee, P.H. (2007) A comparison of cerebral glucose metabolism in Parkinson's disease, Parkinson's disease dementia and dementia with Lewy bodies. *Eur. J. Neurol.* 14(12):1357–1362.

60 Principles of the Pharmacotherapy of Dementia

CHRISTINE BERGMANN AND MARY SANO

The awareness of cognitive loss and dementia has grown dramatically in the past 10 years, leading to routine diagnosis of many of these diseases, including the most common, Alzheimer's disease (AD). Alzheimer's disease is a neurodegenerative condition characterized by progressive cognitive and functional deterioration with an estimated prevalence of over 4 million in the United States. Treatments for AD have been the focus of considerable research. In the past decade, five treatments, representing two classes of drugs, have been approved. Currently, over 160 registered trials in the United States are recruiting patients for the treatment of AD, and many others have been completed and reported. This chapter reviews the pharmacology underlying the currently approved treatments; describes completed trials representing mechanisms and hypotheses identified by clinical observations, epidemiological findings, and basic science; and surveys ongoing clinical trials evaluating new possible mechanisms.

We begin by reviewing currently approved medications for the treatment of dementia. Next, we describe strategies that target amyloid, the current most likely mechanism for intervention. Many different mechanisms of action have been proposed based on laboratory data, animal models, and clinical observation; we present the results of clinical trials testing these mechanisms.

CHOLINESTERASE INHIBITORS

After its release into the synaptic cleft, the neurotransmitter *acetylcholine* is degraded rapidly by the hydrolytic activity of cholinesterases. In the human brain, the most prominent enzyme involved in acetylcholine hydrolysis in acetylcholinesterase. Additional evidence suggests that butyrylcholinesterase can also hydrolyze acetylcholine in the human brain and may be involved in cholinergic transmission (Mesulam et al., 2002). Reductions in the activities of acetylcholinesterase and choline acetyltransferase, enzymes involved in the synthesis and degradation of acetylcholine, were found in brain tissues from patients with AD (Davies and Maloney, 1976). Butyrylcholinesterase constitutes only a small percentage of brain cholinesterase activity in normal aging but has been shown to be increased to 30% in the brains of patients with AD (Mesulam and Geula, 1994). These findings led to the cholinergic hypothesis of AD. According to this hypothesis, the destruction of cholinergic neurons in the basal forebrain and the resulting deficit in central cholinergic transmission contribute substantially to the cognitive deficits and behavioral symptoms observed in patients suffering from AD (Bartus et al., 1982). Inhibition of cholinesterases leads to an increase of acetylcholine concentration in the synaptic cleft and is thought to enhance cholinergic transmission and ameliorate cholinergic deficit. Four cholinesterase inhibitors are available: tacrine, donepezil, rivastigmine, and galantamine. Of these, the first commercially available cholinesterase inhibitor, *tacrine*, is now rarely used because of its hepatotoxic side effects in 40% of all patients (Watkins et al., 1994). The three second-generation cholinesterase inhibitors, *donepezil*, *rivastigmine*, and *galantamine*, are approved for the treatment of AD and are considered the standard of care by the American Academy of Neurology (Doody et al., 2001). Donepezil and galantamine are selective inhibitors of acetylcholinesterase, whereas rivastigmine also inhibits butyrylcholinesterase (Cutler et al, 1998). This class of medications was originally approved for the treatment of patients with mild to moderate disease, and in 2007 the indication for donepezil was expanded to severe AD.

Systematic reviews of all available randomized, double-blind, multicenter, placebo-controlled studies by the Cochrane Collaboration showed moderate benefits of cholinesterase inhibitors on cognitive, behavioral, and functional symptoms for donepezil (Birks and Harvey, 2003), rivastigmine (Birks et al., 2000), and galantamine (Loy and Schneider, 2004). Clinical benefits from the cholinesterase inhibitors were also reported by several other meta-analyses (Ritchie et al., 2004; Whitehead et al., 2004; Takeda et al., 2006), whereas another systematic review questioned the scientific basis for recommendations of cholinesterase inhibitors for treatment of AD, raising issues of methodology and clinical relevance of outcome measures (Kaduszkiewicz et al., 2005). Despite this controversy, the ability to affect cognitive outcome has been robust. Most recently, a trial of donepezil for patients with severe AD and agitation found that there was a modest cognitive benefit, even though no behavioral benefit was observed (Howard et al., 2007).

Memantine

Glutamate represents the main excitatory neurotransmitter in the central nervous system, and a physiological level of glutamate-receptor activity is essential for normal brain function (Kornhuber and Weller, 1997). Glutamate excitotoxicity mediated through excessive activation of *N*-methyl-D-aspartate (NMDA) receptors is believed to play a role in the neuronal cell death observed in AD and other neurodegenerative diseases by causing increases in intracellular calcium that then triggers downstream events that cause cell death (Hynd et al., 2004). Thus, NMDA-receptor antagonists may have a therapeutic potential for neuronal protection from glutamate-mediated neurotoxicity.

Memantine is a low-to-moderate affinity, voltage-dependent, noncompetitive NMDA receptor antagonist with rapid gating kinetics (Danysz et al., 2000). Its fast on/off kinetics and low-to-moderate affinity are key to memantine's action because it ameliorates the effects of excessive glutamate while preserving the physiologic activation of NMDA receptors required for learning and memory. Like other NMDA receptor antagonists, memantine at high concentrations can inhibit mechanisms of synaptic plasticity that are believed to underlie learning and memory, but studies have shown that at lower, clinically relevant concentrations memantine actually promotes synaptic plasticity and preserves or enhances memory in animal models of AD (Johnson and Kotermanski, 2006). However, it is not a cholinesterase inhibitor and therefore offers a different target from the cholinesterase inhibitors that previously were the only approved treatment for AD. Memantine was approved in the United States for treatment of moderate to severe AD in 2003. Systematic reviews of all available randomized, double-blind, multicenter, placebo-controlled studies by the Cochrane Collaboration showed that memantine treatment resulted in significant benefits compared with placebo in cognitive, functional, and behavioral assessments in the treatment group compared to placebo in patients with moderate to severe AD (Areosa-Sastre et al., 2005).

Memantine does not affect the inhibition of acetylcholinesterase by cholinesterase inhibitors, and an open-label European trial indicated that tolerability was not affected when donepezil or other cholinesterase inhibitors were administered to patients already receiving memantine or vice versa (Hartmann and Moebius, 2003; Tariot et al., 2004). Memantine is usually well tolerated, although adverse effects, including confusion, insomnia, and headache, occurred in a small percentage of the study participants (Tariot et al., 2004).

Modulation of Aβ Production

β-amyloid (Aβ) peptides are proteolytic fragments of a larger protein termed *amyloid precursor protein* (APP) which consists of a large extramembranous region, a transmembrane region, and a small cytosolic C-terminal tail (Kang et al., 1987). β-amyloid is generated from APP by sequential cleavages by two proteases termed *β-* and *γ-secretase*. β-amyloid is secreted constitutively by normal cells (Haass et al., 1992) and can be detected in plasma and cerebrospinal fluid (CSF) of normal individuals (Seubert et al., 1992). Amyloid precursor protein is also cleaved by another protease termed *α-secretase* that precludes Aβ generation because the cleavage site within the Aβ sequence produces a small nonamyloidogenic peptide termed *p3* (Esch et al., 1990). Nonneuronal cells preferentially use α-secretase at the expense of β-secretase cleavage whereas neurons predominately use β-secretase cleavage and thus generate mostly Aβ (Simons et al., 1996). β-secretase (BACE-I) was cloned in 1999 (Vassar et al., 1999). BACE-I knockout mice were found to have a normal phenotype, while they abolished Aβ generation (Luo et al., 2001), making BACE-I a major focus of drug discovery efforts ever since. γ-secretase was found to be a protein complex composed of presenilin, nicastrin, PEN2, and APH-1, with presenilin providing the active core of the secretase complex (review in De Strooper, 2003). A major concern regarding potential side effects of γ-secretase inhibitors comes from the identification of several γ-secretase substrates other than APP, including Notch-1 (De Strooper et al., 1999). Safety and tolerability of a γ-secretase inhibiting compound (LY450139) not affecting Notch-1 by Eli Lilly was recently tested in healthy volunteers (Siemers et al., 2005) and patients with AD (Siemers et al., 2006). The compound was well tolerated and reduced plasma Aβ levels but failed to reduce CSF Aβ. A larger study testing the effect of LY450139 on cognition is currently under way.

Aβ Immunotherapy

Active immunization with Aβ attenuates AD-like pathology in a transgenic mouse model of AD (Schenk et al., 1999). Passive immunization with antibodies against Aβ also reduces amyloid deposition (Bard et al., 2000), and both forms of immunization against Aβ reduce learning deficits of APP transgenic mice (Janus et al., 2000; Morgan et al., 2000). The exact underlying mechanism to explain how antibodies reduce Aβ deposition in the brain is unclear. Multiple injections of an Aβ1–42 synthetic peptide (AN1792 by Elan Pharmaceuticals) demonstrated safety and tolerability in a phase I trial (Gilman et al., 2005). In the phase II trial of AN1792, 372 patients with mild to moderate AD were randomized to receive either intramuscular injections of AN1792 or placebo. Among those receiving AN1792, 19.7% developed the predetermined concentration of the Aβ-specific antibody (Bayer et al., 2005). Unfortunately, 18 (6%) patients treated with AN1792 (and none of the placebo group) developed meningoencephalitis, a result that led to prompt discontinuation of the trial. Of the 18 patients with meningoencephalitis, 12 recovered to baseline within several weeks whereas 6 developed long-term neurological or cognitive sequelae (Orgogozo et al., 2003). All study participants were followed longitudinally after cessation of the trial. No significant differences were found between treatment and placebo groups on performance in cognitive testing, although a small subset of the antibody-responder patients had a significantly slower cognitive decline than the antibody nonresponders (Hock et al., 2003). These patients were found to have greater brain volume decreases on neuroimaging analysis than nonresponders, and this decrease in brain volume was associated with better cognitive performance (Fox et al., 2005). In brain autopsies of a subset of patients from this clinical trial, both with and without meningoencephalitis, areas of apparent clearing of amyloid plaques in the cerebral cortex were observed, with an abundance of Aβ-immunoreactive microglia cells (Nicoll et al., 2003; Ferrer et al., 2004; Masliah et al., 2005). The cases of meningoencephalitis did not correlate with the presence or concentration of Aβ antibody titers, and this concentration is now believed to be caused by a T-cell response against Aβ (Monsonego et al., 2003). Currently, there are two phase I clinical trials of active immunization under way using either Aβ derivatives or an Aβ fragment coupled to a carrier (Schenk et al., 2004).

Passive administration of an Aβ-specific humanized monoclonal antibody is currently undergoing a phase II clinical trial in patients with AD. A potential caveat to this form of therapy might be the finding of a study with APP transgenic mice with high levels of cerebral amyloid angiopathy in which passive Aβ immunization caused local microhemorrhages associated with amyloid-bearing vessels (Pfeifer et al., 2002).

Another approach to vaccination, which avoids the use of anti-Aβ antibodies and thus circumvents the risk of meningoencephalitis, was demonstrated in APP transgenic mice by immunizing them with the random amino-acid copolymer *glatiramer acetate* (Frenkel et al., 2005). Glatiramer acetate, which has been successfully used to treat patients with multiple sclerosis, was shown to activate microglial cells, which lead to Aβ clearance without causing encephalitis. Studies in humans are under way.

ANTI-INFLAMMATORY DRUGS

Although inflammation is not considered a hallmark of AD, deposition of Aβ in form of plaques causes a potentially pathological immune response. Senile plaques are often surrounded by activated astrocytes and microglial cells and can also induce activation of the complement cascade (McGeer and McGeer, 2001). Cyclooxygenase (COX) enzymes mediate the conversion of arachidonic acid to prostaglandins, which are crucial components of the proinflammatory process. The main target of nonsteroidal anti-inflammatory drugs (NSAIDs) is COX enzymes. The inducible COX isoform, COX2, is up-regulated in brains of patients with AD (Yasojima et al., 1999), indicating that NSAIDs might be beneficial in AD by reducing neurotoxic inflammation. A subset of NSAIDs have been found to lower Aβ levels independently of COX enzyme activity, apparently by directly modeling γ-secretase activity that enzymatically cleaves Aβ from its larger precursor protein (Weggen et al., 2001). One agent that is particularly effective in modulating γ-secretase activity and ultimately in selective Aβ–42 lowering in animal models is flurizan (Tarenflurbil). In a phase II study, the agent had no effect on cognitive outcomes in mild to moderate AD. Secondary analyses including only patients with mild AD identified a trend toward benefit at the highest dose (800 mg) (Wilcock et al., 2007). This prompted modulation of a phase III study to determine efficacy in this selected population.

Epidemiological studies show a reduced prevalence of AD among chronic users of NSAIDS (McGeer and McGeer, 2007). Transgenic animal studies are clearly providing the rational support for the data derived from the epidemiological studies (Cole et al., 2004). Unfortunately many of the recent long-term, prospective, randomized, double-blind, placebo-controlled clinical trials of NSAIDS in patients with AD have produced negative results and had high drop-out rates because of gastrointestinal side effects (Ho et al., 2006). Because selective COX2 inhibitors have a reduced rate of gastrointestinal side effects, they have been used in clinical trials of patients with AD. Early clinical trials of COX2 inhibitors have not succeeded in reducing cognitive or behavioral deficits in patients either with AD (Aisen et al., 2003) or with mild cognitive impairment (Thal et al., 2005). Selective COX2 inhibitors have recently been shown to increase the risk of cardiovascular events (Mukherjee et al., 2001), which resulted in the withdrawal of some of these drugs from the market and the early termination of several clinical trials, including a trial of dementia prevention with naproxen and celecoxib in AD. At the time the trial was halted, both naproxen and celecoxib were associated with trends toward increased risk of dementia (ADAPT Research Group et al., 2007).

COMPLEMENTARY AND ALTERNATIVE MEDICINES IN THE TREATMENT OF DEMENTIA

Alternative medicines may have potential beneficial results in treating dementia and related symptoms as well as slowing disease progression. Primary mechanisms of action include modifications in neurotransmitter synthesis, inhibition of neurotransmitter reuptake, enzyme-induced neurotransmitter breakdown, and antioxidant activity. Unfortunately, many studies of alternative medicines in dementia are inconclusive and characterized by methodological deficiencies such as small sample sizes and inadequate controls. Extracts of the leaves of the maidenhair tree, Ginkgo biloba, have long been used in China, and more recently in several European countries, as a traditional medicine for various disorders of health. Although some recent trials of Ginkgo biloba showed inconsistent results (Kanowski et al., 1996; Le Bars et al., 1997; van Dongen et al., 2000), a published meta-analysis of clinical studies of Ginkgo biloba showed inconsistent and unconvincing evidence of improvement in cognition and functional activities (Birks et al., 2007). A natural cholinesterase inhibitor, huperzine A, has been isolated from a Chinese herb. Huperzine has been found to improve memory in a small study of short duration (Zhang et al., 2002); other trials are under way. Several small studies using extracts of the herbs *melissa officinalis* or *salvia lavandulaefolia* found slight improvement in cognitive function or behavioral symptoms in the treatment groups (Ballard et al., 2002; Akhondzadeh et al., 2003a; Akhondzadeh et al., 2003b; Perry et al., 2003). Several epidemiologic studies showed a protective effect of increased fish consumption and ω-3 fatty acid intake for the development of AD (Barberger-Gateau et al., 2002; Morris et al., 2003). Meta-analysis of all available biological, epidemiological and observational data suggested a protective effect of ω-3 fatty acids (Lim et al., 2006), but so far only one randomized clinical trial of ω-3 fatty acids showed a positive effect, and only in patients with very mild AD (Freund-Levi et al., 2006). Further trials are in progress.

Levacecarnine is the most common natural short-chain acetyl carnitine ester of L-carnitine and functions physiologically as a shuttle between the cytoplasm and mitochondria for long-chain fatty acids. In animal studies, it has been reported to protect central and peripheral nervous system synapses in neurodegenerative and ageing models and to improve cognitive deficits in aged rats (Barnes et al., 1990). In a meta-analysis, levacecarnine showed some evidence of effect on clinical global impression; however, the authors concluded that the evidence is currently inadequate to recommend its routine use in clinical practice (Hudson and Tabet, 2003).

Another therapeutical strategy is to reduce Aβ neurotoxcitity by attenuation of Aβ–metal ion interactions. β-amyloid accumulation and toxicity are influenced by zinc and copper ions (Bush et al., 1994). These metals are enriched in Aβ deposits, and their removal results in the solubilization of Aβ. The antibiotic *clioquinol*, which is a copper-zinc chelator, increases the solubilization of Aβ in the AD plaque from postmortem human brain tissue, reduces hydrogen peroxide generation from Aβ, and results in a significant decrease in brain Aβ deposition in a transgenic mouse model of AD (Cherny et al., 2001). In a short-term clinical trial, Ritchie et al. (2003) reported that clioquinol therapy significantly slowed the rate of cognitive decline in a subset of patients with AD, as compared with that in controls. The slowing of cognitive decline in patients treated with clioquinol was seen only in those who were more severely affected. A meta-analysis of the use of clioquinol for AD, however, came to the conclusion that trials of longer duration are needed before any recommendations about the use of clioquinol can be given (Jenagaratnam and McShane, 2006).

Clinical trials using the antioxidant *idebenone* had mixed results (Senin et al., 1992; Weyer et al., 1997; Thal et al., 2003). Two other antioxidants, the curry spice *curcumin* and coenzyme Q10, have been shown to destabilize Aβ fibrils in vitro (Ono et al., 2004; Ono et al., 2005). A population-based cohort study found better cognition in elderly Asian patients with high curcumin consumption (Ng et al., 2006); a clinical trial is currently under way (Ringman et al., 2005). As of yet, there are no clinical trials using coenzyme Q10 in patients with AD.

Several observational studies have shown that moderate consumption of wine is associated with a lower incidence of AD (Truelsen et al., 2002; Luchsinger and Mayeux, 2004). Wine is enriched in antioxidant compounds with potential neuroprotective activities. Resveratrol, a polyphenol that occurs in abundance in grapes and red wine, is used by the plant to defend itself against fungal and other attacks. In the early 1990s, the presence of resveratrol was detected in red wine. It is hypothesized to afford antioxidant and neuroprotective properties (Miller and Rice-Evans, 1995) and therefore to contribute to the beneficial effects of red wine consumption on neurodegeneration (Savaskan et al., 2003; Han et al. 2004). Additionally, resveratrol is thought to facilitate the utilization of electrons in the nonmitochondrial portions of the cell (Fauconneau et al., 1997). In a recent study, it was shown that resveratrol promotes intracellular degradation of Aβ via a mechanism that involves the proteasome (Marambaud et al., 2005). Resveratrol does not influence the Aβ producing enzymes and therefore does not inhibit Aβ generation. A small clinical trial of resveratrol in patients with AD has shown encouraging results (Blass and Gibson, 2006); a larger clinical trial is currently under way.

However, clinical trials to evaluate treatment of AD with antioxidant supplements or with food containing large amounts of antioxidants have so far failed to show clinically significant benefits.

Modification of Cardiovascular Risk Factors as a Treatment of Dementia

Traditionally, AD has been thought to be a primary neurodegenerative disorder and not of vascular origin. However, in recent years, epidemiologic studies have identified risk factors for vascular disease that are also associated with cognitive impairment and AD (Breteler, 2000). Cardiovascular risk factors are highly prevalent in the elderly population and rarely exist in isolation. Diabetes mellitus, hypertension, hyperlipidemia, and coronary artery disease often coexist, and this constellation of cardiovascular risk factors has been found to increase the risk for cognitive decline, vascular dementia, and AD (Luchsinger and Mayeux, 2004). The risk of AD has been found to increase with the number of vascular risk factors present in an individual (Luchsinger et al., 2005).

Cell culture and transgenic animal experiments have shown that an increased cholesterol concentration causes an increased generation of AD plaques (Refolo et al., 2000) whereas cholesterol depletion inhibits Aβ formation in vitro and in vivo (Fassbender et al., 2001). Elevated cholesterol is associated with a higher plaque load in patients with AD (Kivipelto et al., 2002), and patients with AD with hypercholesterolemia suffer from more rapid cognitive decline (Evans et al., 2004). Some early epidemiological studies have suggested that statins reduce the risk of AD by as much as 60%–70% (Jick et al., 2000; Wolozin et al., 2000). However, a meta-analysis of recent studies showed statins do not exert a beneficial effect on the risk of dementia and AD (Zhou et al., 2007). A post hoc analysis of pooled data from three clinical trials of patients with AD randomized to galantamine or placebo and also taking a statin or not showed no association between the use of statins and cognitive function; there was also no interaction between statins and galantamine in their effect on cognition (Winblad et al., 2007).

Preliminary results from a double-blind, placebo-controlled, randomized clinical trial of atorvastatin in patients with mild to moderate AD demonstrated a significant benefit on a cognitive measure compared to placebo (Sparks et al., 2005). This benefit was more prominent among individuals with elevated cholesterol levels and higher scores on memory testing at study entry time (Sparks et al., 2006). However, patients in this study were selected regardless of lipid levels, and some may have had cardiovascular risk-reduction benefit; the observed benefit may have derived from this etiology rather than by affecting AD pathology. Two other multicenter trials to examine the effect of statins on slowing the clinical progression of AD are ongoing, and both are recruiting only patients with normal lipid levels. Thus, if a benefit is seen it may be distinct from a cardiovascular risk reduction. Recruitment is complete in both, and these 18-month trials may have results in 2008.

Hypertension is a well-known risk factor for cardiovascular disease and stroke, and thus for vascular dementia. Recent evidence demonstrated that there is a vascular contribution to AD (De La Torre, 2004), although it is not clear if the contribution is simply an added deficit within the clinical profile or if it contributes to the pathophysiology of AD. Observational studies provide support for the association between hypertension and cognitive deficit, including AD; however, they are confounded by many variables, including interventions with various mechanisms of action and changing treatment guidelines.

In fact, a systematic review found the relation of blood pressure to cognitive function and dementia is both complex and inconsistent, differing by the age at which blood pressure was ascertained (middle age or old age), whether having treated or untreated hypertension, and in cross-sectional verses longitudinal studies (Qiu et al., 2005). It is worth noting that these observational studies often include few or no very old subjects (age ≥85), making extrapolation to this population difficult. The successful effect of antihypertensive medication in containing stroke rates provides hope for similar effects on the prevention of cognitive decline and dementia. Observational studies addressing the relationship of the treatment of hypertension and cognitive decline had mixed results. In several longitudinal cohort studies, individuals treated with antihypertensive drugs showed a decreased risk for cognitive decline (Tzourio et al., 1999) or less evident increased risk of cognitive decline and dementia due to hypertension (Elias et al., 1993; Launer et al., 2000). Several trials in which the primary outcome was a measure of cardiovascular risk reduction added a cognitive assessment. In several trials, there were either only benefits in a subset of trial participants (Skoog et al., 2005) or only with long-term use of antihypertensive medication (Cervilla et al., 2000). In one large trial, active therapy with antihypertensive medication decreased the incidence of dementia by 50% over two years (Forette et al., 1998), and another trial in elderly patients with probable AD showed that the mean decline on the Mini Mental State Examination (MMSE) score was much lower in the group on brain-penetrating angiotensin converting enzyme (ACE) inhibitors than in the control group (Ohrui et al., 2004).

Diabetes mellitus has been shown to be associated with changes in cognition; however, the finding of an association between diabetes and AD has been inconsistent (Biessels et al., 2006). In type 1 diabetes, cognitive deficits include mild slowing of mental speed and a diminished mental flexibility (Brands et al., 2005). In type 2 diabetes, cognitive impairment mainly affects learning and memory, mental speed, and flexibility (Allen et al., 2004). The association between diabetes mellitus and AD is particularly strong among carriers of the apolipoprotein ε4 (ApoE4) allele (Peila et al., 2002) and in patients treated with insulin (Ott et al., 1999; Mogi et al., 2004). Brain atrophy in elderly patients with diabetes mellitus is more severe in patients treated with insulin (Ushida et al., 2001). A likely explanation is that only severe cases of diabetes mellitus require insulin treatment. One observational study demonstrated that women with diabetes mellitus had a fourfold increased risk of a major cognitive decline on a verbal fluency test after 4 years compared to women without diabetes mellitus (Kanaya et al., 2004), and improved glucose control as measured by glycohemoglobin could ameliorate this decline. There was no significant difference in cognitive test performance at baseline or follow-up in men regardless of glucose tolerance status or glycohemoglobin level.

A study of a cohort of elderly Mexican Americans showed that one third of the study participants were identified as having type 2 diabetes at baseline, and 58.3% of these diabetics were using either oral antidiabetic medications or insulin or a combination of both. During a 2-year period, there was significantly less physical and cognitive decline among patients receiving treatment with antidiabetic medications compared to those without treatment (Wu et al., 2003). Combination therapy of antidiabetic agents appeared to be more effective than monotherapy in preventing the decline in physical and cognitive functioning for patients. No randomized, double-blind, placebo-controlled clinical trials of tighter blood glucose control and cognitive decline or incident dementia have been reported, but one large clinical trial addressing these questions is currently under way.

There is substantial epidemiologic evidence that cardiovascular risk factors such as hypertension, hyperlipidemia, and diabetes mellitus are associated with cognitive decline, vascular dementia, and perhaps AD. However, at present the exact mechanisms by which these cardiovascular risk factors may increase the risk of cognitive decline and dementia and their relative importance in the pathogenesis of AD are unknown. In this context, further studies to elucidate these mechanisms are needed. Additionally, the incidence of cognitive decline, vascular dementia, and AD should constitute a major outcome measure of future trials comparing different antihypertensive, cholesterol-lowering, and antidiabetic drugs to determine the best clinical strategy for prevention of dementia.

HORMONAL TREATMENT OF DEMENTIA

Systematic meta-analyses of cohort and case-control studies have reported estrogen use to be associated with a reduction in the risk of developing AD of approximately 30% (LeBlanc et al., 2001). However, randomized clinical trials have failed to find any clinically meaningful evidence of benefit in treating patients with preexisting mild-to-moderate AD with estrogen, and the Cochrane review concluded that hormone replacement therapy is not indicated in patients with AD (Hogervorst et al., 2002). The Women's Health Initiative Memory Study, a primary prevention trial, examined the possible benefit of hormone replacement therapy in reducing the incidence or delaying the time of onset of dementia (Shumaker et al., 2004). Adverse outcomes led to the study being terminated early. Treatment was linked to an increased risk of stroke and coronary artery disease and actually increased the risk of dementia (Hazard ratio: 1.76; 95% confidence interval [CI]: 1.19–2.60).

ANTIOXIDANTS AND VITAMINS

The free radical hypothesis of aging proposes that free radical reaction that damages cells are the primary mechanism by which aging occurs (Harman, 1956). Surrogate markers of injury attributable to free radicals are present in patients with AD, particularly near plaque and tangle sites (Grünblatt et al., 2005). Vitamins C and E have been found to protect from oxidative deoxyribonucleic acid (DNA) damage (Huang et al., 2000), and vitamin E protects nerve cells from Aβ peptide toxicity (Behl et al., 1992).

Several population-based prospective observational studies that have used questionnaires to monitor the intake of vitamins C and E on the risk of developing dementia had mixed results (Boothby and Doering, 2005). A placebo-controlled, clinical trial of vitamin E and selegiline in patients with moderately advanced AD was conducted by the Alzheimer's Disease Cooperative Study (Sano et al., 1997). Patients in the vitamin E group were treated with 2000 IU (1342 alpha-tocopherol equivalents) vitamin E per day. The results indicated that vitamin E may slow functional deterioration, leading to nursing home placement. Another clinical trial with vitamin E was conducted in patients with mild cognitive impairment with the primary endpoint being the time to development of possible or probable AD (Petersen et al., 2005). There were no significant differences in the rate of progression to AD between the vitamin E and placebo groups. Despite the lack of high-level evidence to support an association between cognitive benefits or decreased incidence of AD with vitamin C and E use, the use of these vitamins has become commonplace in clinical practice. Unfortunately, there are also safety concerns with the use of vitamin E. A clinical trial of long-term vitamin E supplementation studying the effects on cardiovascular events and cancer not only showed that vitamin E does not prevent cancer or major cardiovascular events, but that it also increases the risk of heart failure (Lonn et al., 2005). A meta-analysis of randomized controlled trials examining the potential dose–response relationship between vitamin E supplementation and total mortality showed dose-dependent and significantly increased all-cause mortality with the use of vitamin E (Miller et al., 2005). Recent recommendations are therefore not to advocate the use of vitamin E in individuals at risk of or affected by AD (Ames and Ritchie, 2007).

Elevated plasma homocysteine levels are a risk factor for cardiovascular disease and stroke and may be related to an increased risk of AD (Seshadri et al., 2002). Deficiencies of folic acid and vitamins B12 and B6 intake increase homocysteine plasma levels. Folic acid and vitamins B12 are needed for the conversion of homocysteine to methionine, and vitamin B6 is needed for the conversion of homocysteine to cysteine. High dietary intake of folic acid and vitamin B12 and B6 decreased homocysteine levels in adults (Homocysteine Lowering Trialists' Collaboration, 2005). A recent longitudinal cohort study reported higher folate intake to decrease the risk of incident AD independent of levels of vitamin B6 and B12 (Luchsinger et al., 2007). However, meta-analyses of clinical trials addressing the influence of folic acid, vitamin B6, and vitamin B12 intake failed to show any beneficial effect on cognitive function (Malouf and Areosa Sastre, 2003; Malouf and Grimley Evans, 2003; Malouf et al., 2003). Furthermore, two recent clinical trials on folic acid and vitamins B6 and B12 failed to show any reduction of the risk of major cardiovascular events and stroke (Bonaa et al., 2006; Lonn et al., 2006). One study of supplementation over a 3-year period in older individuals with no dementia selected for their relatively high homocysteine levels indicated a favorable influence on cognitive function (Durga et al., 2007), whereas a 2-year study in older individuals not selected on homocysteine levels did not (McMahon et al., 2006). Recently reported results of a U.S. multicenter clinical trial of B vitamins and folic acid in the treatment of AD over a 10-month period failed to demonstrate a benefit and was associated with an increase in depressive symptoms (Aisen et al., 2007). In this study, patients had relatively normal homocysteine levels, suggesting that benefits of supplementation may only be observed in those with high homocysteine and low folate intake.

DOPAMINERGIC ENHANCEMENT OF COGNITIVE FUNCTION

The ascending dopamine (DA) system of the mammalian brain has been associated with regulation of motor output, reward-related behavior, executive functions, and short-term memory (Thierry et al., 1998). Dopaminergic projections to the prefrontal cortex and striatum are involved in spatial working memory functions, and striatal and amygdala ascending DA tracts are important for learning and conditioning (Goldman-Rakic, 1998). Research in experimental animals suggests that damage to the lateral prefrontal cortex in monkeys impairs spatial working memory (Brozoski et al., 1979), stimulation of DA D1 receptors by DA D1 receptor agonists can ameliorate these deficits (Cai and Arnsten, 1997).

Studies in healthy humans have suggested that spatial working memory and other executive functions might be improved by administration of low doses of DA, D1, and D2 receptor agonists (Luciana et al., 1992; Mueller et al., 1998; Schuck et al., 2002). Patients with cognitive deficits caused by traumatic brain injury displayed improved performance of executive function and attention but not spatial memory (Lal et al., 1988; McDowell et al., 1998). *Aphasia* describes linguistic difficulties following brain lesions, most often caused by a stroke. The cortical localization of brain damage resulting in aphasia is varied. A review for the Cochrane Database failed to show any positive effects of DA receptor agonists or stimulants on treatment of aphasia poststroke (Greener et al., 2001).

Stimulant drugs such as amphetamine, methamphetamine, and methylphenidate can influence DA neurotransmission by blocking reuptake at the transporter site, thereby increasing extracellular levels of DA. However stimulants also have effects at the noradrenaline and serotonin transporter sites, making attribution of possible cognitive-enhancing properties specifically to DA neurotransmission problematic (Kuczenski and Segal, 1997). Psychomotor stimulants are widely used for the treatment of attention-deficit/hyperactivity disorder (ADHD), as they have an established ability to improve attention and spatial working memory in these patients (Mehta et al., 2004) and even in young healthy volunteers (Camp-Bruno and Herting, 1994; Elliott et al., 1997). Interestingly, these findings do not apply for elderly volunteers (Turner et al., 2003). So far, there has been only one study that attempted to separate dopaminergic and noradrenergic effects on cognitive function by comparing the effects of methylphenidate; 3,4-dihydroxyphenylalanine (L-DOPA); and desipramine (noradrenaline reuptake inhibitor) on attention and inhibition in children with ADHD. The study showed that neither a pure dopaminergic nor noradrenergic explanation is sufficient for an explanation (Overtoom et al., 2003).

Dopaminergic enhancement via monoamine oxidase inhibition has also been examined. The type B monoamine oxidase inhibitor *selegiline* was shown to delay nursing home placement and to mildly improve subsets of neuropsychological testing (Burke et al., 1993; Sano et al., 1997; Filip and Kolibas, 1999) in patients with AD. Yet a meta-analysis came to the conclusion that there was no evidence of any meaningful clinical benefits and thus no justification to use selegiline in the treatment of AD (Birks and Flicker, 2003).

Clinical trials with rasagiline, an irreversible type B monoamine oxidase inhibitor, are currently under way. Oxidative stress occurs when the cellular production of reactive oxygen species overwhelms the natural defense of antioxidants leading to cell death through apoptosis and necrosis and may be important in the development of dementia.

Noradrenergic Modulation of Memory

Ascending noradrenergic projections from the locus coeruleus to higher cortical regions are implicated in arousal and modulate cognitive functions dependent upon prefrontal cortex and associated circuitry. *Working memory* refers to short-term storage, and manipulation of items in memory is dependent upon prefrontal cortex activity (Baddeley, 1986). Animal studies have shown that moderate levels of noradrenaline enhance working memory, whereas higher concentrations impair this function. These findings appear attributable to dissociable effects of noradrenaline at α_1- and α_{2a} adrenoreceptors (Arnsten and Li, 2005). Long-term (emotional) memory appears to be mediated by the amygdalae, with mediotemporal structures being crucial for conditioned fear learning and fearful responses in animals (McGaugh, 2004). Augmentation of noradrenaline transmission has been shown to enhance long-term memory, whereas such effects are reversed by β blockade (van Steegeren et al., 2002; Cahill and Alkire, 2003). The lipophilic β blocker *propranolol* impaired working memory in multiple studies, whereas less lipophilic β blockers such as atenolol had no effect on memory, suggesting that central blockade might be necessary for modulatory effects on memory (Mueller et al., 2005). The α_2 adrenoreceptor agonist *clonidine* was found to impair working memory in most studies (Jakala et al., 1999), whereas findings for other α agonists and selective noradrenaline reuptake inhibitors were inconsistent (Mueller et al., 2005).

SEROTONERGIC MODULATION OF COGNITIVE FUNCTION

Serotonin has long been implicated in a wide range of behavioral functions, especially in mood regulation, aggression, and impulsivity. In recent years, experimental studies with animals and humans have shown that serotonin may also play an important role in normal and impaired cognitive function as well as in specific human memory processes. Lowering of serotonergic activity in healthy volunteers is associated with impairment of long-term memory performance, specifically delayed recall and delayed recognition of pictures (Rowley et al., 1998; Rubinsztein et al., 2001). Studies of the effect of serotonin stimulation on memory function in healthy volunteers have yielded inconsistent results (Schmitt et al., 2001; Harmer et al., 2002).

A depressive episode is often accompanied by extensive cognitive impairment across a wide range of cognitive domains, including impairment of long-term memory functioning, executive function, attention, and concentration. Central serotonergic dysfunction is considered to be one of the neuronal substrates of depression; however, central catecholaminergic activity, the neuroendocrine system, and the immune system are also impaired. Clinical improvement of memory function in patients who were depressed was observed after treatment with selective serotonin reuptake inhibitors (SSRIs) (Richardson et al., 1994; La Pia et al., 2001).

There is increasing evidence for alterations in the function of the serotonin system in AD that may be responsible for many of the behavioral aspects of the disease, including the frequent coexistence of depression. Serotonin receptor binding decreases dramatically with aging in a variety of brain regions (Sheline et al., 2002). Low serotonin has been related to cognitive deficits seen in AD (Lai et al., 2002), and serotonin dysregulation can occur separately or in conjunction with that of the cholinergic system (Buhot et al., 2000). Acute serotonin depletion caused impaired performance on memory testing in patients with AD compared to healthy elderly controls (Porter et al., 2000). There are no randomized controlled trials as of yet of the use SSRIs in patients with AD with the purpose of enhancing cognition.

In frontotemporal dementia, SSRIs have been shown to mildly ameliorate behavioral symptoms such as impulsivity, carbohydrate craving, and compulsion (Swartz et al., 1997); however, they have been found to mildly impair cognitive function (Deakin et al., 2004).

Recently the serotonin 5-HT$_4$ receptor, which has been shown to increase cyclic adenosine monophosphate (cAMP) production, has also been implicated in APP processing. Specifically, it appears to stimulate α-secretase. The therapeutic potential of activation of this receptor has been advanced by the identification of receptor agonists that have been used in transgenic models to demonstrate regulation of the nonamyloidagenic precursor protein (Lezoualc'h, 2007). The development of agonists for this receptor provides a mechanism for therapeutic interventions for AD. In fact, one compound, PRX-03140, a small-molecule agonist of 5-HT$_4$, has been described in the lay literature as having benefit in patients with AD, although the details of the trial and the true effect size has been less clear (http://www.epixpharma.com/products/prx-03140.asp). Registered trials are ongoing (NCT00384423).

SUMMARY

The availability of treatments for AD is now a reality, although the search continues for more effective treatments for dementia and its prodromal conditions. Some leads from epidemiologic data and early laboratory studies have proven ineffective, allowing for a more precise understanding of how to approach treatment. Further, the impact of treatments affecting common comorbidities, such as cerebrovascular and cardiovascular conditions, may have direct and indirect effects on cognition, and these benefits are being sorted out. Methodologies now exist to design and implement clinical trials to assess treatments with extended efficacy, in subjects with milder conditions, and that target potential disease etiologies. New drug classes are currently being evaluated, and any reasonable assessment of the state of the field leads to the conclusion that important results and expanding treatment options are imminent.

REFERENCES

ADAPT Research Group, Lyketsos, C.G., Breitner, J.C., Green, R.C., Martin, B.K., Meinert, C., Piantadosi, S., and Sabbagh, M. (2007) Naproxen and celecoxib do not prevent AD in early results from a randomized controlled trial. *Neurology* 68(21): 1800–1808.

Aisen, P.S., Jin, S., Thomas, R.G., Sano, M., Diaz-Arrastia, R., and Thal, L. for the Alzheimer's Disease Cooperative Study. (2007) The effect of high dose supplements to reduce homocysteine in Alzheimer's disease: The ADCS Homocysteine Trial. International Conference on the Prevention of Dementia, Washington, DC, June 2007.

Aisen, P.S., Schafer, K.A., Grundman, M., Pfeiffer, E., Sano, M., Davis, K.L., Farlow, M.R., Jin, S., Thomas. R.G., and Thal, L.J. (2003) Alzheimer's Disease Cooperative Study. Effects of rofecoxib or naproxen vs placebo on Alzheimer's disease progression: a randomized controlled trial. *JAMA* 289:2819–2826.

Akhondzadeh, S., Noroozian, M., Mohammadi, M., Ohadinia, S., Jamshidi, A.H., and Khani, M. (2003a) Melissa officinalis extract in the treatment of patients with mild to moderate Alzheimer's disease: a double-blind, randomized, placebo controlled trial. *J. Neurol. Neurosurg. Psychiatry* 74:863–866.

Akhondzadeh, S., Noroozian, M., Mohammadi, M., Ohadinia, S., Jamshidi, A.H., and Khani, M. (2003b) Salvia officinalis extract in the treatment of patients with mild to moderate Alzheimer's disease: a double-blind, randomized and placebo controlled trial. *J. Clin. Pharm. Ther.* 28:53–59.

Allen, K.V., Frier, B.M., and Strachan, M.W.J. (2004) The relationship between type 2 diabetes and cognitive dysfunction: longitudinal studies and their methodological limitations. *Eur. J. Pharmacol.* 490:169–175.

Ames, D., and Ritchie, C. (2007) Antioxidants and Alzheimer's disease: time to stop feeding vitamin E to dementia patients? *Int. Psychogeriatr.* 19:1–8.

Areosa-Sastre, A., McShane, R., and Sherriff, F. (2005) Memantine for dementia. *Cochrane Database Syst. Rev.* (2):CD003154.

Arnsten, A.F., and Li, B.M. (2005) Neurobiology of executive functions: catecholamine influences on prefrontal cortical functions. *Biol. Psychiatry* 57:1377–1384.

Baddeley, A. (1986) *Working Memory*. Clarendon: Oxford Science Publications.

Ballard, C.G., O'Brien, J.T., Reichelt, K., and Perry, E.K. (2002) Aromatherapy as a safe and effective treatment of the management of agitation in severe dementia: the results of a double-blind, placebo-controlled trial with Melissa. *J. Clin. Psychiatry* 63:553–558.

Barberger-Gateau, P., Letenneur, L., Deschamps, V., Peres, K., Dartigues, J.F., and Renaud, S. (2002) Fish, meat and risk of dementia: cohort study. *Br. Med. J.* 325:932–933.

Bard, F., Cannon, C., Barbour, R., Burke, R.L., Games, D., Grajeda, H., Guido, T., Hu, K., Huang, J., Johnson-Wood, K., Khan, K., Kholodenko, D., Lee, M., Lieberburg, I., Motter, R., Nguyen, M., Soriano, F., Vasquez, N., Weiss, K., Welch, B., Seubert, P., Schenk, D., and Yednock, T. (2000) Peripherally administered antibodies against amyloid-β enter the central nervous system and reduce pathology in a mouse model of Alzheimer's disease. *Nature Med.* 6:916–919.

Barnes, C.A., Markowska, A.L., Ingram, D.K., Kametani, H., Spangler, E.L., Lemken, V.J., and Olton, D.S. (1990) Acetyl-L-carnitine 2: effects on learning and memory performance of aged rats in simple and complex mazes. *Neurobiol. Aging* 11:499–506.

Bartus, R.T., Dean, R.L. III, Beer, B., and Lippa, A.S. (1982) The cholinergic hypothesis of geriatric memory dysfunction. *Science* 217:408–414.

Bayer, A.J., Bullock, R., Jones, R.W., Wilkinson, D., Paterson, K.R., Jenkins, L., Millais, S.B., and Donoghue, S. (2005) Evaluation of the safety and immunogenicity of synthetic Aβ 42 (AN 1792) in patients with AD. *Neurology* 64:94–101.

Behl, C., Davis, J., Cole, G.M., and Schubert, D. (1992) Vitamin E protects nerve cells from amyloid-beta toxicity. *Biochem. Biophys. Res. Commun.* 186:944–950.

Biessels, G.J., Staekenborg, S., Brunner, E., Brayne, C., and Scheltens, P. (2006) Risk of dementia in diabetes mellitus: a systematic review. *Lancet Neurol.* 5(1):64–74.

Birks, J., Grimley, and Evans, J. (2007) Ginkgo biloba for cognitive impairment and dementia (Cochrane Review). *Cochrane Database Syst Rev.* (2):CD003120.

Birks, J.S., and Harvey, R. (2003) Donepezil for dementia due to Alzheimer's disease. *Cochrane Database Syst. Rev.*:CD001190.

Birks, J., and Flicker, L. (2003) Selegiline for Alzheimer's disease. *Cochrane Database Syst. Rev.*:CD000442.

Birks, J.S., Iakovidou, V., and Tsolaki, M. (2000) Rivastigmine for Alzheimer's disease. *Cochrane Database Syst. Rev.*:CD001191.

Blass, J.P., and Gibson, G.E. (2006) Correlations of disability and biologic alterations in Alzheimer brain and test of significance by a therapeutic trial in humans. *J. Alzheimers Dis.* 9:207–218.

Bonaa, K.H., Njolstad, I., Ueland, P.M., Schirmer, H., Tverdal, A., Steigen, T., Wang, H., Nordrehaug, J.E., Arnesen, E., Rasmussen, K., NORVIT Trial Investigators. (2006) Homocysteine lowering and cardiovascular events after acute myocardial infarction. *N. Eng. J. Med.* 354(15):1578–1588.

Boothby, L.A., and Doering, P.L. (2005) Vitamin C and vitamin E for Alzheimer's disease. *Ann. Pharmacother.* 39:2073–2030.

Brands, A.M., Biessels, G.J., De Haan, E.H., Kappelle, L.J., and Kessels, R.P. (2005) The effects of type 1 diabetes on cognitive performance: a meta-analysis. *Diabetes Care* 28:726–735.

Breteler, M.M.B. (2000) Vascular risk factors for Alzheimer's disease: an epidemiologic perspective. *Neurobiol. Aging* 21:153–160.

Brozoski, T.J., Brown, R.M., Rosvold, H.E., and Goldman, P.S. (1979) Cognitive deficit caused by regional depletion of dopamine in prefrontal cortex of the rhesus monkey. *Science* 205: 929–932.

Buhot, M.C., Martin, S., and Segu, L. (2000) Role of serotonin in memory impairment. *Ann. Med.* 32:210–221.

Burke, W.J., Roccaforte, W.H., Wengel, S.P., Bayer, B.L., Ranno, A.E., and Willcockson, N.K. (1993) L-deprenyl in the treatment of mild dementia of the Alzheimer type: results of a 15-month trial. *J. Am. Geriatr. Soc.* 41:1219–1225.

Bush, A.I., Pettingell, W.H., Multhaup, G., Paradis, M.,Vonsattel, J.P., Gusella, J.F., Beyreuther, K., Masters, C.L., and Tanzi, R.E. (1994) Rapid induction of Alzheimer Aβ amyloid formation by zinc. *Science* 265:1464–1467.

Cahill, L., and Alkire, M.T. (2003) Epinephrine enhancement of human memory consolidation: interaction with arousal at encoding. *Neurobiol. Learn. Mem.* 79:194–198.

Cai, J.X., and Arnsten, A.F. (1997) Dose-dependent effects of the dopamine D1 receptor agonists A77636 or SKF81297 on spatial working memory in aged monkeys. *J. Pharmacol. Exp. Ther.* 283:183–189.

Camp-Bruno, J.A., and Herting, R.L. (1994) Cognitive effects of milacemide and methylphenidate in healthy young adults. *Psychopharmacology* 115:46–52.

Cervilla, J.A., Prince, M., Joels, S., Lovestone, S., and Mann, A. (2000) Long-term predictors of cognitive outcome in a cohort of older people with hypertension. *Br. J. Psychiatry* 177:66–71.

Cherny, R.A., Atwood, C.S., and Xilinas, M.E. (2001) Treatment with a copper-zinc chelator markedly and rapidly inhibits β-amyloid accumulation in Alzheimer's disease transgenic mice. *Neuron* 30: 665–676.

Cole, G.M., Morihara, T., Lim, G.P., Yang, F., Begum, A., and Frautschy, S.A. (2004) NSAID and antioxidant prevention of Alzheimer's disease: lessons from in vitro and animal models. *Ann. N.Y. Acad. Sci.* 1035:68–84.

Cutler, N.R., Polinsky, R.J., Sramke, J.J., Enz, A., Jhee, S.S., Mancione, L., Hourani, J., and Zolnouni, P. (1998) Dose-dependent CSF acetylcholinesterase inhibition by SDZ ENA 713 in Alzheimer's disease. *Acta Neurol. Scand.* 97:244–250.

Danysz, W., Parsons, C.G., Moebius, H.J., Stoeffler, A., and Quack, G. (2000) Neuroprotective and symptomatological action of memantine relevant for Alzheimer's disease-a unified glutamatergic hypothesis on the mechanism of action. *Neurotoxicity Res.* 2:85–98.

Davies, P., and Maloney, A.J. (1976) Selective loss of central cholinergic neurons in Alzheimer's disease. *Lancet.* 2(8000):1403.

Deakin, J.B., Nestor, P.J., Hodges, J.R., and Sahakian, B.J. (2004) Paroxetin does improve symptoms and impairs cognition in frontotemporal dementia: a double-blind randomized controlled trial. *Psychopharmacology* 172:400–408.

De La Torre, J.C. (2004) Is Alzheimer's disease a neurodegenerative or vascular disorder? Data, dogma and dialectics. *Lancet Neurol.* 3:184–190.

De Strooper, B. (2003) APH-1, PEN2, nicastrin with presenilin generate an active γ-secretase complex. *Neuron* 38:9–12.

De Strooper, B., Annaert, W., Cupers, P., Saftig, P., Craessaerts, K., Mumm, J.S., Schroeter, E.H., Schrijvers, V., Wolfe, M.S., Ray, W.J., Goate, A., and Kopan, R. (1999) A presenilin-1-dependent gamma-secretase-like protease mediates release of Notch intracellular domain. *Nature* 398(6727):518–522.

Doody, R.S., Stevens, J.C., Beck, C., Dubinsky, R.M., Kaye, J.A., Gwyther, L., et al. (2001) Practice parameter: management of dementia (an evidence-based review). Report of the Quality Standards Subcommittee of the American Academy of Neurology. *Neurology* 56:1154–1156.

Durga, J., van Boxtel, M.P., Schouten, E.G., Kok, F.J., Jolles, J., Katan, M.B., et al. (2007) Effect of 3-year folic acid supplementation on cognitive function in older adults in the FACIT trial: a randomised, double blind, controlled trial. *Lancet* 369(9557): 208–216.

Elias, M.F., Wolf, P.A., D'Agostino, R.B., Cobb, J., and White, L.R. (1993) Untreated blood pressure level is inversely related to cognitive functioning: The Framingham Study. *Am. J. Epidemiol.* 6:353–364.

Elliott, R., Sahakian, B.J., Matthews, K., Bannerjea, A., Rimmer, J., and Robbins, T.W. (1997) Effects of methylphenidate on spatial working memory and planning in healthy young adults. *Psychopharmacology* 131:196–206.

Esch, F.S., Keim, P.S., Beattie, E.C., Blacher, R.W., Culwell, A.R., Oltersdorf, T., McClure, D., and Ward, P.J. (1990) Cleavage of amyloid beta peptide during constitutive processing of its precursor. *Science* 248:1122–1124.

Evans, R.M., Hui, S., Perkins, A., Lahiri, D.K., Poirier, J., and Farlow, M.R. (2004) Cholesterol and APOE genotype interact to influence Alzheimer disease progression. *Neurology* 62: 1869–1871.

Fassbender, K., Simons, M., Bergmann, C., Stroick, M., Lutjohann, D., Keller, P., Runz, H., Kuhl, S., Bertsch, T., von Bergmann, K., Hennerici, M., Beyreuther, K., and Hartmann, T. (2001) Simvastatin strongly reduces levels of Alzheimer's disease beta-amyloid petides Abeta 42 and Abeta 40 in vitro and in vivo. *Proc. Natl. Acad. Sci. USA* 98:5856–5861.

Fauconneau, B., Waffo-Teguo, P., Huguet, F., Barrier, L., Decendit, A., and Merillon, J.M. (1997) Comparative study of radical scavenger and antioxidant properties of phenolic compounds from Vitis vinifera cell cultures using in vitro tests. *Life Sci.* 61:2103–2110.

Ferrer, I., Boada Rovira, M., Sanchez Guerra, M.L., Rey, M.J., and Costa-Jussa, F. (2004) Neuropathology and pathogenesis of encephalitis following amyloid-β immunization in Alzheimer's disease. *Brain Pathol.* 14:11–20.

Filip, V., and Kolibas, E. (1999) Selegiline in the treatment of Alzheimer's disease: a long-term randomized placebo-controlled trial. Czech and Slovak Senile Dementia of Alzheimer Type Study Group. *J. Psychiatry Neurosci.* 24:234–243.

Forette, F., Seux, M.L., Staessen, J.A., Thijs, L., Birkenhager, W.H., Babarskiene, M.R., Babeanu, S., Bossini, A., Gil-Extremera, B., Girerd, X., Laks, T., Lilov, E., Moisseyev, V., Tuomilehto, J., Vanhanen, H., Webster, J., Yodfat, Y., and Fagard, R. (1998) Prevention of dementia in randomized double-blind placebo-controlled systolic hypertension in Europe (SYST-EUR) trial. *Lancet* 352:1347–1351.

Fox, N.C., Black, R.S., Gilman, S., Rossor, M.N., Griffith, S.G., Jenkins, L., and Koller, M. (2005) AN1792(QS-21)-201 Study. Effects of Aβ-immunization (AN 1792) on MRI measures of cerebral volume in Alzheimer disease. *Neurology* 64:1563–1572.

Frenkel, D., Maron, R., Burt, D.S., and Weiner, H.L. (2005) Nasal vaccination with a proteosome-based adjuvant and glatiramer acetate clears β-amyloid in a mouse model of Alzheimer's disease. *J. Clin. Invest.* 115:2423–2433.

Freund-Levi, Y., Eriksdotter-Jonhagen, M., Cederholm, T., Basun, H., Faxen-Irving, G., Garlind, A., Vedin, I., Vessby, B., Wahlund, L.O., and Palmblad, J. (2006) Omega-3 fatty acid treatment in 174 patients with mild to moderate Alzheimer disease: OmegAD study: a randomized double-blind trial. *Arch. Neurol.* 63: 1402–1408.

Gilman, S., Koller, M., Black, R.S., Jenkins, L., Griffith, S.G., Fox, N.C., Eisner, L., Kirby, L., Rovira, M.B., Forette, F., and Orgogozo, J.M. (2005) AN1792(QS-21)-201 Study Team. Clinical effects of Aβ immunization (AN 1792) in patients with AD in an interrupted trial. *Neurology* 64:1553–1562.

Goldman-Rakic, P.S. (1998) The cortical dopamine system: role in memory and cognition. *Adv. Pharmacol.* 42:707–711.

Greener, J., Enderby, P., and Whurr, R. (2001) Pharmacological treatment for aphasia following stroke. *Cochrane Database Syst. Rev.*:CD000424.

Grünblatt, E., Schlösser, R., Fischer, P., Fischer, M.O., Li, J., Koutsilieri, E., Wichart, I., Sterba, N., Rujescu, D., Möller, H.J., Adamcyk, W., Dittrich, B., Müller, F., Oberegger, K., Gatterer, G., Jellinger, K.J., Mostafaie, N., Jungwirth, S., Huber, K., Tragl, K.H., Danielczyk, W., and Riederer, P. (2005) Oxidative stress related markers in the "VITA" and the centenarian projects. *Neurobiol. Aging* 26(4):429–438.

Haass, C., Schlossmacher, M.G., Hung, A.Y., Vigo-Pelfrey, C., Mellon, A., Ostaszewski, B.L., Lieberburg, I., Koo, E.H., Schenk, D., Teplow, D.B., and Selkoe, D. (1992) Amyloid beta-peptide is produced by cultured cells during normal metabolism. *Nature* 359:322–325.

Han, Y.S., Zheng, W.H., Bastianetto, S., Chabot, J.G., and Quirion, R. (2004) Neuroprotective effects of Resveratrol against beta-amyloid induced neurotoxicity in rat hippocampal neurons: involvement of protein kinase C. *Br. J. Pharmacol.* 141:997–1005.

Harman, D. (1956) Aging: a theory based on free radical and radiation chemistry. *J. Gerontol.* 11:298–300.

Harmer, C.J., Bhagwagar, Z., Cowen, P.J., and Goodwin, G.M. (2002) Acute administration of citalopram facilitates memory consolidation in healthy volunteers. *Psychopharmacol.* 163:106–110.

Hartmann, S., and Moebius, H.J. (2003) Tolerability of memantine in combination with cholinesterase inhibitors in dementia therapy. *Int. Clin. Psychopharmacol.* 18:81–85.

Ho, L., Qin, W., Stetka, B.S., and Pasinetti, G.M. (2006) Is there a future for cyclo-oxygenase inhibitors in Alzheimer's disease? *CNS Drugs* 20:85–98.

Hock, C., Konietzko, U., Streffer, J.R., Tracy, J., Signorell, A., Muller-Tillmanns, B., Lemke, U., Henke, K., Moritz, E., Garcia, E., Wollmer, M.A., Umbricht, D., de Quervain, D.J., Hofmann, M., Maddalena, A., Papassotiropoulos, A., and Nitsch, R.M. (2003) Antibodies against β-amyloid slow cognitive decline in Alzheimer's disease. *Neuron* 38:547–554.

Hogervorst, E., Yaffe, K., Richards, M., and Huppert, F. (2002) Hormone replacement therapy to maintain cognitive function in women with dementia. *Cochrane Database Syst. Rev.* (3):CD003799.

Homocysteine Lowering Trialists' Collaboration. (2005) Dose-dependent effects of folic acid on blood concentrations of homocysteine: a meta-analysis of the randomized trials. *Am. J. Clin. Nutr.* 82:806–812.

Howard, R.J., Juszczak, E., Ballard, C.G., et al. (2007) Donepezil for the treatment of agitation in Alzheimer's disease. *N. Engl. J. Med.* 57:182–192.

Huang, H.Y., Helzlsouer, K.J., and Appel, L.J. (2000) The effects of vitamin C and vitamin E on oxidative DNA damage: results from a randomized controlled trial. *Cancer Epidemiol. Biomarkers Prev.* 9:647–652.

Hudson, S., and Tabet, N. (2003) Acetyl-L-carnitine for dementia. *Cochrane Database for Dementia*:CD003158.

Hynd, M.R., Scott, H.L., and Dodd, P.R. (2004) Glutamate-mediated excitotoxicity and neurodegeneration in Alzheimer's disease. *Neurochem. Int.* 45:583–595.

Jakala, P., Riekkinen, M., Sirvio, J., Koivisto, E., Kejonen, K., Vanhanen, M., and Riekkinen, P., Jr. (1999) Guanfacine, but not clonidine, improves planning and working memory performance in humans. *Neuropsychopharmacology* 20:460–470.

Janus, C., Pearson, J., McLaurin, J., Mathews, P.M., Jiang, Y., Schmidt, S.D., Chishti, M.A., Horne, P., Heslin, D., French, J., Mount, H.T., Nixon, R.A., Mercken, M., Bergeron, C., Fraser, P.E., St George-Hyslop, P., and Westaway, D. (2000) A beta peptide immunization reduces behavioural impairment and plaques in a model of Alzheimer's disease. *Nature* 408(6815):979–982.

Jenagaratnam, L., and McShane, R. (2006) Clioquinol for the treatment of Alzheimer's disease. *Cochrane Database Syst. Rev.*:CD005380.

Jick, H., Zornberg, G.L., Jick, S.S., et al. (2000) Statins and the risk of dementia. *Lancet* 356: 627–1631.

Johnson, J.W., and Kotermanski, S.E. (2006) Mechanism of action of memantine. *Curr. Opin. Pharmacol.* 6:61–67.

Kaduszkiewicz, H., Zimmermann, T., Beck-Bornholdt, H.P., and van den Bussche, H. (2005) Cholinesterase inhibitors for patients with Alzheimer's disease: systematic review of randomized clinical trials. *Br. Med. J.* 331:321–327.

Kanaya, A.M., Barrett-Connor, E., Gildengorin, G., and Yaffe, K. (2004) Change in cognitive function by glucose tolerance status in older adults. *Arch. Intern. Med.* 164:1327–1333.

Kang, J., Lemaire, H.G., Unterbeck, A., Salbaum, J.M., Masters, C.L., Grzeschik, K.H., Multhaup, G., Beyreuther, K., and Muller-Hill, B. (1987) The precursor of Alzheimer's disease amyloid A4 protein resembles a cell-surface receptor. *Nature* 325:733–736.

Kanowski, S., Herrmann, W.M., Stephan, K., Wierich, W., and Hörr, R. (1996) Proof of efficacy of the ginkgo biloba special extract EGb 761 in outpatients suffering from mild to moderate primary degenerative dementia of the Alzheimer type or multi-infarct dementia. *Pharmacopsychiatry* 29(2):47–56.

Kivipelto, M., Helkala, E.L., Laakso, M., et al. (2002) Apolipoprotein E e4 allele, elevated midlife total cholesterol level and high midlife systolic blood pressure are independent risk factors for late-life Alzheimer disease. *Ann. Intern. Med.* 137:149–155.

Kornhuber, J., and Weller, M. (1997) Psychotogenicity and *N*-methyl-D-aspartate receptor antagonism: implications for neuroprotective pharmacotherapy. *Biol. Psychiatry* 41:135–144.

Kuczenski, R., and Segal, D.S. (1997) Effects of methylphenidate on extracellular dopamine, serotonin and norepinephrine: comparison with amphetamine. *J. Neurochem.* 68:2032–2037.

Lal, S., Merbtiz, C.P., and Grip, J.C. (1988) Modification of function in head-injured patients with Sinemet. *Brain Inj.* 2(3):225–233.

Lai, M.K.P., Tsang, S.W.Y., Francis, P.T., Keene, J., Hope, T., and Esiri, M.M. (2002) Postmortem serotonergic correlated of cognitive decline in Alzheimer's disease. *Neuroreport* 13:1175–1178.

La Pia, S., Fuschillo, C., Giorgio, D., Ciriello, R., Pinto, A., and Rivellini, M. (2001) Serotonin (5-HT)-related symptoms and fluoxetine in geriatric depression. *Arch. Gerontol. Geriatr.* 33(Suppl. 1): 213–225.

Launer, L.J., Ross, G.W., Petrovitch, H., Masaki, K., Foley, D., White, L.R., and Havlik, R.J. (2000) Midlife blood pressure and dementia: the Honolulu-Asia aging study. *Neurobiol. Aging* 21: 49–55.

Le Bars, P.L., Katz, M.M., Berman, N., Itil, T.M., Freedman, A.M., and Schatzberg, A.F. (1997) A placebo-controlled, double-blind, randomized trial of an extract of Ginkgo biloba for dementia. North American EGb Study Group. *JAMA* 278(16):1327–1332.

LeBlanc, E.S., Janowsky, J., Chan, B.K., and Nelson, H.D. (2001) Hormone replacement therapy and cognition: systematic review and meta-analysis. *JAMA* 285:1489–1499.

Lezoualc'h, F. (2007) 5-HT4 receptor and Alzheimer's disease: the amyloid connection. *Exp. Neurol.* 205:325–329.

Lim, W.S., Gammack, J.K., Van Niekerk, J., and Dangour, A.D. (2006) Omega 3 fatty acid for the prevention of dementia. *Cochrane Database Syst. Rev.*:CD005379.

Lonn, E., Bosch, J., Yusuf, S., Sheridan, P., Pogue, J., Arnold, J.M., Ross, C., Arnold, A., Sleight, P., Probstfield, J., Dagenais, G.R., HOPE and HOPE-TOO Trial Investigators. (2005) Effects of long-term vitamin E supplementation on cardiovascular events and cancer: a randomized controlled trial. *JAMA* 293:1338–1347.

Lonn, E., Yusuf, S., Arnold, M.J., Sheridan, P., Pogue, J., Micks, M., McQueen, M.J., Probstfield, J., Fodor, G., Held, C., Genest, J., Jr., Heart Outcomes Prevention Evaluation (HOPE) 2 Investigators. (2006) Homocysteine lowering with folic acid and B vitamins in vascular disease. *N. Eng. J. Med.* 354:1567–1577.

Loy, C., and Schneider, L. (2004) Galantamine for Alzheimer's disease. *Cochrane Database Syst. Rev.*:CD001747.

Luchsinger, J.A., and Mayeux, R. (2004) Cardiovascular risk factors and Alzheimer's disease. *Curr. Atheroscl. Rep.* 6:261–266.

Luchsinger, J.A., Reitz, C., Honig, L.S., and Mayeux, R. (2005) Aggregation of vascular risk factors and risk of incident Alzheimer disease. *Neurology* 65:545–551.

Luchsinger, J.A., Tang, M.X., Miller, J., Green, R., and Mayeux, R. (2007) Relation of higher folate intake to lower risk of Alzheimer disease in the elderly. *Arch. Neurol.* 64:86–92.

Luchsinger, J.A., Tang, M.X., Siddiqui, M., Shea, S., and Mayeux, R. (2004) Alcohol intake and risk of dementia. *J. Am. Geriatr. Soc.* 52:540–546.

Luciana, M., Depue, R.A., Arbisi, P., and Leon, A. (1992) Facilitation of working memory in humans by a D2 dopamine receptor agonist. *J. Cogn. Neurosci.* 4:330–347.

Luo, Y., Bolon, B., Kahn, S., Bennett, B.D., Babu-Khan, S., Denis, P., Fan, W., Kha, H., Zhang, J., Gong, Y., Martin, L., Louis, J.C., Yan, Q., Richards, W.G., Citron, M., and Vassar, R. (2001) Mice deficient in BACE-I, the Alzheimer's β-secretase, have normal phenotype and abolished β-amyloid generation. *Nat. Neurosci.* 4:231–232.

Maki, P., and Hogervorst, E. (2003) The menopause and HRT. HRT and cognitive decline. *Best Pract. Res. Clin. Endocrinol. Metab.* (1):105–122.

Malouf, M., Grimley, E.J., and Areosa, S.A. (2003) Folic acid with or without vitamin B12 for cognition and dementia. *Cochrane Database Syst. Rev.*:CD004514.

Malouf, M., and Grimley Evans, J. (2003) The effect of vitamin B6 on cognition. *Cochrane Database Syst. Rev.*:CD004393.

Malouf, M., and Areosa Sastre, A. (2003) Vitamin B12 for cognition. *Cochrane Database Syst. Rev.*:CD004326.

Marambaud, P., Zhao, H., and Davies, P. (2005) Resveratrol promotes clearance of Alzheimer's disease amyloid peptides. *J. Biol. Chem.* 280:37377–37382.

Masliah, E., Hansen, L., Adame, A., Crews, L., Bard, F., Lee, C., Seubert, P., Games, D., Kirby, L., and Schenk, D. (2005) Aβ vaccination effects on plaque pathology in the absence of encephalitis in Alzheimer's disease. *Neurology* 64:129–131.

McDowell, S., Whyte, J., and D'Esposito, M. (1998) Differential effect of a dopaminergic agonist on prefrontal function in traumatic brain injury patients. *Brain* 121:1155–1164.

McGaugh, J.L. (2004) The amygdale modulates the consolidation of memories of emotionally arousing experiences. *Ann. Rev. Neurosci.* 27:1–28.

McGeer, P.L., and McGeer, E.G. (2001) Inflammation, autotoxicity and Alzheimer's disease. *Neurobiol. Aging* 22:799–809.

McGeer, P.L., and McGeer, E.G. (2007) NSAIDs and Alzheimer's disease: epidemiological, animal model and clinical studies. *Neurobiol. Aging* 28:639–647.

McGuiness, B., Todd, S., Passmore, P., and Bullock, R. (2006) The effects of blood pressure lowering on development of cognitive impairment and dementia in patients without apparent prior cerebrovascular disease. *Cochrane Database Syst. Rev.*:CD004034.

McMahon, J.A., Green, T.J., Skeaff, C.M., Knight, R.G., Mann, J.I., and Williams, S.M. (2006) A controlled trial of homocysteine lowering and cognitive performance. *N. Engl. J. Med.* 354(26): 2764–2472.

Mehta, M.A., Goodyer, I.M., and Sahakian, B.J. (2004) Methylphenidate improves working memory and set-shifting in AD/HD: relationships to baseline memory capacity. *J. Child Psychol. Psychiatry* 45:293–305.

Mesulam, M.M., and Geula, C. (1994) Butyrylcholinesterase reactivity differentiates the amyloid plaques of aging from those of dementia. *Ann. Neurol.* 36:722–727.

Mesulam, M., Guillotzet, A., Shaw, P., and Quinn, B. (2002) Widely spread butyrylcholinesterase can hydrolyze acetylcholine in normal and Alzheimer brain. *Neurbiol. Dis.* 9:88–93.

Miller, E.R. 3rd, Pastor-Barriuso, R., Dalal, D., Riemersma, R.A., Appel, L.J., and Guallar, E. (2005) Meta-analysis: high-dosage vitamin E supplementation may increase all-cause mortality. *Ann. Intern. Med.* 142:37–46.

Miller, N.J., and Rice-Evans, C.A.(1995) Antioxidant activity of resveratrol in red wine. *Clin. Chem.* 41(12 Pt 1):1789.

Mogi, N., Umegaki, H., Hattori, A., Maeda, N., Miura, H., Kuzuya, M., Shimokata, H., Ando, F., Ito, H., and Iguchi, A. (2004) Cognitive function in Japanese elderly with type 2 diabetes mellitus. *J. Diabet. Comp.* 18:42–46.

Monsonego, A., Zota, V., Karni, A., Krieger, J.I., Bar-Or, A., Bitan, G., Budson, A.E., Sperling, R., Selkoe, D.J., and Weiner, H.L. (2003) Increased T-cell reactivity to amyloid β protein in older humans and patients with Alzheimer's disease. *J. Clin. Inves.* 112:415–422.

Morgan, D., Diamond, D.M., Gottschall, P.E., Ugen, K.E., Dickey, C., Hardy, J., Duff, K., Jantzen, P., DiCarlo, G., Wilcock, D., Connor, K., Hatcher, J., Hope, C., Gordon, M., and Arendash, G.W. (2000) A beta peptide vaccination prevents memory loss in an animal model of Alzheimer's disease. *Nature* 408(6815): 982–985.

Morris, M.C., Evans, D.A., Bienias, J.L., Tangney, C.C., Bennett, D.A., Wilson, R.S., Aggarwal, N., and Schneider, J. (2003) Consumption of fish and n-3 fatty acids and risk of incident Alzheimer disease. *Arch. Neurol.* 60:940–946.

Mueller, U., von Cramon, D.Y., and Pollmann, S. (1998) D1- versus D2-receptor modulation of visuospatial working memory in humans. *J. Neurosci.* 18:2720–2728.

Mueller, U., Mottweiler, E., and Bublak, P. (2005) Noradrenergic blockade and numeric working memory in humans. *J. Psychopharmacol.* 19:21–28.

Mukherjee, D., Nissen, S.E., and Topol, E.J. (2001) Risk of cardiovascular events associated with selective COX-2 inhibitors. *JAMA* 286:954–959.

Ng, T.P., Chiam, P.C., Lee, T., Chua, H.C., Lim, L., and Kua, E.H. (2006) Curry consumption and cognitive function in the elderly. *Am. J. Epidemiol.* 164:898–906.

Nicoll, J.A., Wilkinson, D., Holmes, C., Steart, P., Markham, H., and Weller, R.O. (2003) Neuropathology of human Alzheimer disease after immunization with amyloid-β pepetide: a case report. *Nature Med.* 9:448–452.

Ohrui, T., Tomita, N., Sato-Nakagawa, T., Matsui, T., Maruyama, M., Niwa, K., Arai, H., and Sasaki, H. (2004) Effects of brain-penetrating ACE inhibitors on Alzheimer disease progression. *Neurology* 63:1324–1325.

Ono, K., Hasegawa, K., Haiki, H., and Yamada, M. (2004) Curcumin has potent anti-amyloidogenic effects for Alzheimer's beta-amyloid fibrils in vitro. *J. Neurosci. Res.* 75:742–750.

Ono, K., Hasegawa, K., Haiki, H., and Yamada, M. (2005) Preformed beta-amyloid fibrils are destabilized by coenzyme Q10 in vitro. *Biochem. Biophys. Res. Commun.* 330:111–116.

Orgogozo, J.M., Gilman, S., Dartigues, J.F., Laurent, B., Puel, M., Kirby, L.C., Jouanny, P., Dubois, B., Eisner, L., Flitman, S., Michel, B.F., Boada, M., Frank, A., and Hock, C. (2003) Subacute meningoencephalitis in a subset of patients with AD after Aβ42 immunization. *Neurology* 61:46–54.

Ott, A., Stolk, R.P., van Harskamp, F., Pols, H.A., Hofman, A., and Breteler, M.M. (1999) Diabetes mellitus and the risk of dementia: The Rotterdam Study. *Neurology* 53:1937–1942.

Overtoom, C.C., Verbaten, M.N., Kemner, C., Kenemans, J.L., van Engeland, H., Buitelaar, J.K., van der Molen, M.W., van der Gugten, J., Westenberg, H., Maes, R.A., and Koelega, H.S. (2003) Effects of methylphenidate, desipramine, and L-dopa on attention and inhibition in children with attention deficit hyperactivity disorder. *Behav. Brain Res.* 145:7–15.

Peila, R., Rodriguez, B.L., and Launer, L.J. (2002) Type 2 diabetes, ApoE gene and the risk for dementia and related pathologies. The Honolulu-Asia Aging Study. *Diabetes* 51:1256–1262.

Perry, N.S.L., Bollen, C., Perry, E.K., and Ballard, C. (2003) Salvia for dementia therapy: review of pharmacological activity and pilot tolerability clinical trial. *Pharmacol. Biochem. Behav.* 75:651–659.

Petersen, R.C., Thomas, R.G., Grundman, M., Bennett, D., Doody, R., Ferris, S., Galasko, D., Jin, S., Kaye, J., Levey, A., Pfeiffer, E., Sano, M., van Dyck, C.H., Thal, L.J., Alzheimer's Disease Cooperative Study Group. (2005) Vitamin E and donepezil for the treatment of mild cognitive impairment. *N. Engl. J. Med.* 352: 2379–2388.

Pfeifer, M., Boncristiano, S., Bondolfi, L., Stalder, A., Deller, T., Staufenbiel, M., Mathews, P.M., and Jucker, M. (2002) Cerebral hemorrhage after passive anti-Aβ immunotherapy. *Science* 298: 1379.

Porter, R.J., Lunn, B.S., Walker, L.L., Gray, J.M., Ballard, C.G., and O'Brien, J.T. (2000) Cognitive deficit induced by acute tryptophan depletion in patients with Alzheimer's disease. *Am. J. Psychiatry* 157:638–640.

Qiu, C., Winblad, B., and Fratiglioni, L. (2005) The age-dependent relation of blood pressure to cognitive function and dementia. *Lancet Neurol.* 4:487–499.

Refolo, L.M., Malester, B., LaFrancois, J., Bryant-Thomas, T., Wang, R., Tint, G.S., Sambamurti, K., Duff, K., and Pappolla, M.A. (2000) Hypercholesterolemia accelerates the Alzheimer's amyloid pathology in a transgenic mouse model. *Neurobiol. Dis.* 7:321–331.

Richardson, J.S., Keegan, D.L., Bowen, R.C., Blackshaw, S.L., Cebrian Perez, S., and Dayal, N. (1994) Verbal learning by major depressive disorder patients during treatment with fluoxetine or amitriptyline. *Int. Clin. Psychopharmacol.* 9:35–40.

Ringman, J.M., Frautschy, S.A., Cole, G.M., Masterman, D.L., and Cummings, J.L. (2005) A potential role of the curry spice curcumin in Alzheimer's disease. *Curr. Alzheimer Res.* 2:131–136.

Ritchie, C.W., Ames, D., Clayton, T., and Lai, R. (2004) Metaanalysis of randomized trials of the efficacy and safety of donepezil, galantamine and rivastigmine for the treatment of Alzheimer's disease. *Am. J. Geriatr. Psychiatry* 12:358–369.

Ritchie, C.W., Bush, A.I., Mackinnon, A., Macfarlane, S., Mastwyk, M., MacGregor, L., Kiers, L., Cherny, R., Li, Q.X., Tammer, A., Carrington, D., Mayros, C., Volitakis, I., Xilinas, M., Ames, D., Davis, S., Beyreuther, K., Tanzi, R.E., and Masters, C.L. (2003) Metal-protein attenuation with iodochlorhydroxyquin (clioquinol) targeting Aβ amyloid depostion and toxicity in Alzheimer disease: a pilot phase 2 clinical trial. *Arch Neurol.* 60:1685–1691.

Rowley, B., Van, F., Mortimore, C., and Connell, J. (1998) Effects of acute tryptophan depletion on tests of frontal and temporal lobe function. *J. Psychopharmacol.* 12:A60.

Rubinsztein, J., Rogers, R.D., Riedel, W.J., Mehta, M.A., Robbins, T.W., and Sahakian, B.J. (2001) Acute dietary tryptophan depletion impairs affective shifting and delayed visual recognition in healthy volunteers. *Psychopharmacol.* 154:319–326.

Sano, M., Ernesto, C., Thomas, R.G., Klauber, M.R., Schafer, K., Grundman, M., Woodbury, P., Growdon, J., Cotman, C.W., Pfeiffer, E., Schneider, L.S., and Thal, L.J. (1997) A controlled trial of selegiline, alpha-tocopherol, or both as treatment for Alzheimer's disease. The Alzheimer's Disease Cooperative Study. *N. Engl. J. Med.* 336:1216–1222.

Savaskan, E., Olivieri, G., Meier, F., Seifritz, E., Wirz-Justice, A., and Müller-Spahn, F. (2003) Red wine ingredient resveratrol protects from beta-amyloid neurotoxicity. *Gerontology* 49(6): 380–383.

Schenk, D., Barbour, R., Dunn, W., Gordon, G., Grajeda, H., Guido, T., Hu, K., Huang, J., Johnson-Wood, K., Khan, K., Kholodenko, D., Lee, M., Liao, Z., Lieberburg, I., Motter, R., Mutter, L., Soriano, F., Shopp, G., Vasquez, N., Vandevert, C., Walker, S., Wogulis, M., Yednock, T., Games, D., and Seubert, P. (1999) Immunization with amyloid-β attenuates Alzheimer-disease-like pathology in the PDAPP mouse. *Nature* 400:173–177.

Schenk, D., Hagen, M., and Seubert, P. (2004) Current progress in β-amyloid immunotherapy. *Curr. Opin. Immunol.* 16:599–606.

Schmitt, J.A.J., Kruizinga, M., and Riedel, W.J. (2001) Non-serotonergic pharmacological profiles and associated cognitive effects of serotonin reuptake inhibitors. *J. Psychopharmacol.* 15: 173–179.

Schuck, S., Bentue-Ferrer, D., Kleinermans, D., Reymann, J.M., Polard, E., Gandon, J.M., and Allain, H. (2002) Psychomotor and cognitive effects of piribedil, a dopamine agonist, in young healthy volunteers. *Fundam. Clin. Pharmacol.* 16:57–65.

Senin, U., Parnetti, L., Barbagallo-Sangiorgi, G., Bartorelli, L., Bocola, V., Capurso, A., Cuzzupoli, M., Denaro, M., Marigliano, V., Tammaro, A.E., and Fioravanti, M. (1992) Idebenone in senile dementia of Alzheimer type: a multicentre study. *Arch. Gerontol. Geriatr.* 15:249–260.

Seshadri, S., Beiser, A., Selhub, J., Jacques, P.F., Rosenberg, I.H., D'Agostino, R.B., Wilson, P.W., and Wolf, P.A. (2002) Plasma homocysteine as a risk factor for dementia and Alzheimer's disease. *N. Eng. J. Med.* 346:476–483.

Seubert, P., Vigo-Pelfrey, C., Esch, F., Lee, M., Dovey, H., Davis, D., Sinha, S., Schlossmacher, M., Whaley, J., and Swindlehurst, C. (1992) Isolation and quantification of soluble Alzheimer's beta-peptide from biological fluids. *Nature* 359:325–327.

Sheline, Y.I., Mintun, M.A., Moerlein, S.M., and Snyder, A.Z. (2002) Greater loss of 5-HT(2A) receptors in midlife than in late life. *Am. J. Psychiatry* 159:430–435.

Shumaker, S.A., Legault, C., Kuller, L., Rapp, S.R., Thal, L., Lane, D.S., Fillit, H., Stefanick, M.L., Hendrix, S.L., Lewis, C.E., Masaki, K., Coker, L.H., Women's Health Initiative Memory Study. (2004) Conjugated equine estrogens and incidence of probable dementia and mild cognitive impairment in postmenopausal women: Women's Health Initiative Memory Study. *JAMA* 291:2947–2958.

Siemers, E.R., Quinn, J.F., Kaye, J., Farlow, M.R., Porsteinsson, A., Tariot, P., Zoulnouni, P., Galvin, J.E., Holtsman, D.M., Knopman, D.S., Satterwhite, J., Gonzales, C., Dean, R.A., and May, P.C. (2006) Effects of a γ-secretase inhibitor in a randomized study of patients with Alzheimer's disease. *Neurology* 66:602–604.

Siemers, E.R., Skinner, M., Dean, R.A., Gonzales, C., Satterwhite, J., Farlow, M., Ness, D., and May, P.C. (2005) Safety, tolerability and changes in amyloid-β concentrations after administration of a γ-secretase inhibitor in volunteers. *Clin. Neuropharmacol.* 28: 126–132.

Simons, M., De Strooper, B., Multhaupt, G., Tienari, P.J., Dotti, C. G., and Beyreuther, K. (1996) Amyloidogenic processing of the human amyloid precursor protein in primary cultures of rat hippocampal neurons. *J. Neurosci.* 16:899–908.

Skoog, I., Lithell, H., Hansson, L., Elmfeldt, D., Hofman, A., Olofsson, B., Trenkwalder, P., Zanchetti, A., SCOPE Study Group. (2005) Effect of baseline cognitive function and antihypertensive treatment on cognitive and cardiovascular outcomes: study on cognition and prognosis in the elderly (SCOPE). *Am. J. Hypertension* 18:1052–1059.

Sparks, D.L., Connor, D.J., Sabbagh, M.N., Petersen, R.B., Lopez, J., and Browne, P. (2006) Circulating cholesterol levels, apolipoprotein E genotype and dementia severity influence the benefit of atorvastatin treatment in Alzheimer's disease: results of the Alzheimer's Disease Cholesterol-Lowering Treatment (ADCLT) trial. *Acta Neurol. Scand.* 185(Suppl):3–7.

Sparks, D.L., Sabbagh, M., Connor, D.J., Lopez, J., Launer, L.J., Browne, P., Wasser, D., Johnson-Traver, S., Lochhead, J., and Ziolwolski, C. (2005) Atorvastatin for the treatment of mild to moderate Alzheimer's disease. *Arch. Neurol.* 62:753–757.

Swartz, J.R., Miller, B.L., Lesser, I.M., and Darby, A.L. (1997) Frontotemporal dementia: Treatment response to serotonin selective reuptake inhibitors. *J. Clin. Psychiatry* 58:212–216.

Takeda, A., Loveman, E., Clegg, A., Kirby, J., Picot, J., Payne, E., and Green, C. (2006) A systematic review of the clinical effectiveness of donepezil, rivastigmine and galantamine on cognition, quality of life and adverse effects in Alzheimer's disease. *Int. J. Geriatr. Psychiatry* 21:17–28.

Tariot, P.N., Farlow, M.R., Grossberg, G.T., Graham, S.M., McDonald, S., Gergel, I., for the Memantine Study Group. (2004) Memantine treatment in patients with moderate to severe Alzheimer disease already receiving treatment. *JAMA* 291:317–324.

Thal, L.J., Ferris, S.H., Kirby, L., Block, G.A., Lines, C.R., Yuen, E., Assaid, C., Nessly, M.L., Norman, B.A., Baranak, C.C., Reines, S.A., Rofecoxib Protocol 078 Study Group. (2005) A randomized, double-blind study of rofecoxib in patients with mild cognitive impairment. *Neuropsychopharmacology* 30:1204–1215.

Thal, L.J., Grundman, M., Berg, J., Ernstrom, K., Margolin, R., Pfeiffer, E., Weiner, M.F., Zamrini, E., and Thomas, R.G. (2003) Idebenone treatment fails to slow cognitive decline in Alzheimer's disease. *Neurology* 61:1498–1502.

Thierry, A.M., Pirot, S., Gioanni, Y., and Glowinski, J. (1998) Dopamine function in the prefrontal cortex. *Adv. Pharmacol.* 42:717–720.

Truelsen, T., Thudium, D., and Gronbaek, M. (2002) Amount and type of alcohol and risk of dementia. *Neurology* 59:1313–1319.

Turner, D.C., Robbins, T.W., Clark, L., Aron, A.R., Dowson, J., and Sahakian, B.J. (2003) Relative lack of cognitive effects of methylphenidate in elderly male volunteers. *Psychopharmacology* 168(4): 455–464.

Tzourio, C., Dufouil, C., Ducimetiere, P., and Alperovitch, A. (1999) Cognitive decline in individuals with high blood pressure: a longitudinal study in the elderly-EVA study group. Epidemiology of vascular aging. *Neurology* 53:1948–1952.

Ushida, C., Umegaki, H., and Hattori, A. (2001) Assessment of brain atrophy in elderly subjects with diabetes mellitus by computed tomography. *Geriatr. Gerontol. Int.* 1:33–37.

Vassar, R., Bennett, B.D., Babu-Khan, S., Kahn, S., Mendiaz, E.A., Denis, P., Teplow, D.B., Ross, S., Amarante, P., Loeloff, R., Luo, Y., Fisher, S., Fuller, J., Edenson, S., Lile, J., Jarosinski, M.A., Biere, A.L., Curran, E., Burgess, T., Louis, J.C., Collins, F., Treanor, J., Rogers, G., and Citron, M. (1999) Beta-secretase cleavage of Alzheimer's amyloid precursor protein by the transmembrane aspartic protease BACE. *Science* 286:735–741.

van Dongen, M.C., van Rossum, E., Kessels, A.G., Sielhorst, H.J., and Knipschild, P.G. (2000) The efficacy of ginkgo for elderly people with dementia and age-associated memory impairment: new results of a randomized clinical trial. *J. Am. Geriatr. Soc.* 48(10):1183–1194.

Van Steegeren, A.H., Everaerd,W., and Gooren, L.J. (2002) The effect of beta-adrenergic blockade after encoding on memory of an emotional event. *Psychopharmacol.* 163:202–212.

Watkins, P.B., Zimmermann, H.J., Knapp, M.J., Gracon, S.I., and Lewis, K.W. (1994) Hepatotoxic effects of tacrine administration in patients with Alzheimer's disease. *JAMA* 271:992–998.

Weggen, S., Eriksen, J.L., Das, P., Sagi, S.A., Wang, R., Pietrzik, C.U., Findlay, K.A., Smith, T.E., Murphy, M.P., Bulter, T., Kang, D.E., Marquez-Sterling, N., Golde, T.E., and Koo, E.H. (2001) A subset of NSAIDs lower amyloidogenic Aβ42 independently of cyclooxygenase activity. *Nature* 414:212–216.

Weyer, G., Babej-Dolle, R.M., Hadler, D., Hofmann, S., and Herrmann, W.M. (1997) A controlled study of 2 doses of idebenone in the treatment of Alzheimer's disease. *Neuropsychobiology* 36:73–82.

Whitehead, A., Perdomo, C., Pratt, R.D., Birks, J., Wilcock, G.K., and Evans, J.G. (2004) Donepezil for the symptomatic treatment of patients with mild to moderate Alzheimer's disease: a meta-analysis of individual patient data from randomized controlled trials. *Int. J. Geriatr. Psychiatry* 19:624–633.

Winblad, B., Jelic, V., Kershaw, P., and Amatniek, J. (2007) Effects of statins on cognitive function in patients with Alzheimer's disease in galantamine clinical trials. *Drugs Aging* 24:57–61.

Wilcock, G., Black, S., Hendrix, S., Zavitz, K., Laughlin, M., and Swabb, E. (2007, Aug. 25–28) *Flurizan in AD: Efficacy and Safety in a 24 month Study*. Paper presented at the European Federation of Neurological Societies (EFNS), Brussels, Belgium.

Wolozin, B., Kellman, W., Ruosseau, P., Celesia, G.G., and Siegel, G. (2000) Decreased prevalence of Alzheimer's disease associated with 3-hydroxy-3-methylglutaryl Coenzyme A reductase inhibitors. *Arch. Neurol.* 57:1439–1443.

Wu, J.H., Haan, M.N., Liang, J., Ghosh, D., Gonzalez, H.M., and Herman, W.H. (2003) Impact of antidiabetic medications on physical and cognitive functioning of older Mexican Americans with diabetes mellitus: a population-based cohort study. *Ann. Epidemiol.* 13:369–376.

Yasojima, K., Schwab, C., McGeer, E.G., and McGeer, P.L. (1999) Distribution of cyclooxygenase-1 and cyclooxygenase-2 mRNAs and proteins in human brain and peripheral organs. *Brain Res.* 830:226–236.

Zhang, Z., Wang, X., Chen, Q., Shu, L., Wang, J., and Shan, G. (2002) Clinical efficacy and safety of huperzine alpha in treatment of mild to moderate Alzheimer disease, a placebo-controlled, double-blind, randomized trial. *Chin. Med. J.* 82:2231–2252.

Zhou, B., Teramukai, S., and Fukushima, M. (2007) Prevention and treatment of dementia or Alzheimer's disease by statins: a meta-analysis. *Dement. Geriatr. Cogn. Disord.* 23:194–201.

61 Cognitive Impairment in Demyelinating Disease

THOMAS M. HYDE

Multiple sclerosis (MS) is a chronic yet episodic demyelinating disorder of the central nervous system (CNS), often involving the brain, spinal cord, and/or cranial nerves. The traditional definition includes the criteria of events "separated by time and space." Practically speaking, this means that signs and symptoms occur, remit, and recur over a period of many years (time) in different locations in the CNS (space). The neurological manifestations are as varied as the functions of the CNS. The exact manifestations in a given case depend upon the location of the inflammatory destructive lesion(s). Common clinical features include weakness, paralysis, loss of vision, double vision, dysarthria, intention tremor, incoordination, imbalance, sensory changes, and bladder problems. Cognitive impairment can also occur and is frequently overlooked. The pattern of relapse and remission is common in the early phases of the illness. Later on, many patients convert to a chronic progressive disorder.

The diagnosis of MS is made based on the clinical history and laboratory findings. The hallmark of MS is a relapsing and remitting pattern of multiple focal neurological deficits occurring over several years. Laboratory and neuroimaging studies are useful for confirmation. Traditionally, examination of the cerebrospinal fluid (CSF) is particularly helpful. During an acute flare, the CSF often shows a mild mononuclear pleocytosis and/or elevated protein level. The gamma globulins in the CSF are synthesized within the nervous system, and in MS on gel electrophoresis form an abnormal pattern termed *oligoclonal bands*. Oligoclonal bands are present in the CSF of the overwhelming majority of patients with MS. Bands have also been reported in neurosyphilis and subacute sclerosing panencephalitis. The presence of bands in the CSF but not in the blood is helpful in confirming the diagnosis of MS, but often they are not present following the first episode.

Modern neuroimaging and electrophysiology have increased the accuracy of diagnosis in MS. Neuroimaging studies, particularly magnetic resonance imaging (MRI), are exceedingly helpful in confirming the diagnosis of MS. In fact, MRI can reveal clinically silent plaques throughout the nervous system. Multifocal lesions, often in the white matter and frequently with a periventricular distribution pattern, are the classic MRI finding in MS. Acute lesions can enhance on occasion with the injection of gadolinium. In addition, atrophy of white matter structures, such as the corpus callosum or medullary pyramids, often occurs later in the course of the disease. Evoked potentials, an electrophysiological measure, can also be useful in MS. Because MS is an inflammatory condition with a preference for myelinated fiber pathways, conductance along known fiber pathways is often slowed in patients with MS. Typically, visual, auditory, and somatosensory evoked potentials are measured to test the competence of signal transmission along their respective pathways in the nervous system. Taken together, laboratory studies can be a useful adjunct to the clinical history and examination in suspected cases of MS.

The differential diagnosis of MS includes CNS manifestations of many systemic illnesses, including autoimmune diseases. These include systemic lupus erythematosus, Sjögren syndrome, polyarteritis nodosa, sarcoidosis, Behçet's disease, Lyme disease, neurosyphilis, progressive multifocal leukoencephalopathy, vitamin B12 deficiency, metachromatic leukodystrophy, Fabry's disease, adrenoleukodystrophy, lymphoma, arteriovenous malformations, and recurrent small embolic or thrombotic infarcts of the CNS (Trojano and Paolicelli, 2001). Careful histories, examinations, and laboratory studies help differentiate between these entities and MS.

The epidemiology of MS has spawned a number of theories about the etiology of this disorder. The prevalence ranges from 1 to 100 per 100,000, increasing with increasing distance from the equator (Weinshenker, 1996; Kurtzke, 2000). The gradient is less prominent but present in the Southern Hemisphere. Individuals of northern European ancestry are at highest risk (Weinshenker, 1996). Individuals who migrate from a high-risk to a low-risk latitude retain some of the risk of their place of birth, especially if they migrate after 15 years of age (Dean, 1967). In addition, there have been reports of "epidemics" of MS theoretically ascribed to the immigration of individuals from high-risk areas (Kurtzke and Hyllested, 1985). Taken together, these findings support a transmissible environmental factor in the etiology of MS. Many environmental factors have been proposed for MS, yet none has been clearly and reproducibly established.

Genetic factors also play a role in the genesis of MS. The disease occurs in relatives of patients with MS with a frequency 10–50 times greater than that in the general population, with the highest risk occurring in siblings (Sadovnick et al., 1988). Twin studies also support a heritable factor in the etiology of MS. There is an eightfold greater risk in monozygotic twins compared to dizygotic twins (Ebers et al., 1986; Sadovnick et al., 1993). The pattern of genetic transmission does not follow that of strict Mendelian inheritance. Additionally, an increased risk in family members of index cases is not strict evidence of a genetic factor because family members share environmental risk factors in addition to genes. However, the discrepancy between dizygotic and monozygotic twins is the strongest evidence for a genetic predisposition toward the development of MS. In all likelihood, MS is caused by the effects of environmental factor(s) acting upon individuals with a genetic susceptibility towards this illness.

Recently, two separate groups have reported that variations in the interleukin 7 receptor alpha chain gene influence the risk of multiple sclerosis (Gregory et al., 2007; Lundmark et al., 2007). The first citation relied upon data from four independent family-based or case-control data sets. Moreover, the latter group also found altered expression of the genes encoding for the interleukin 7 receptor alpha chain and its ligand (interleukin 7) in the CSF of individuals with MS. As more sophisticated techniques become widely employed, the precise nature of the genetic factors influencing risk for MS should be forthcoming in the near future.

Women are more at risk of developing MS than men, in some studies up to 3 times more so (Baum and Rothschild, 1981). The risk of disease is highest between 20 and 40 years of age and then declines. Many late-life cases might represent reactivation of dormant or clinically silent disease that began decades before clinical presentation. Neuropathology studies suggest that clinically silent MS may be more common than was previously believed (Gilbert and Sadler, 1983). Understanding the role of gender and age may ultimately help unravel the environmental and genetic factors that underlie MS.

COGNITIVE IMPAIRMENT IN MULTIPLE SCLEROSIS

Cognitive impairment can appear anytime during the clinical course of MS, although it most often appears later in the illness. Cognitive impairment is often overlooked, especially in its early stages, because of the dramatic and more obvious elemental neurological deficits of most patients with MS. Between 40% and 65% of all patients with MS develop significant levels of cognitive disability (Rao, Leo, Bernardin, et al., 1991; DeSousa et al., 2002). Several large studies have placed the incidence in community-based patients with MS at around 50% (LaRocca, 1984). In nursing home populations of patients with MS, which might be expected to have a greater frequency of cognitive impairment, only about 50% were thought to be impaired although the scale employed was not very sophisticated or detailed (Buchanan et al., 2001). Ascertainment bias is a significant issue when assessing the frequency of cognitive impairment in the MS patient population. The frequency varies, depending upon the source of the patients, the age of the patients, the duration of illness, the type of MS, and the instruments used to perform the cognitive assessment. For example, patients with the relapsing-remitting form of MS tend to have fewer cognitive deficits than those with the chronic progressive form (Heaton et al., 1985; Wishart and Sharpe, 1997).

Testing for cognitive processing deficits can be extremely difficult in MS. The motor and sensory deficits make neuropsychological testing difficult and may confound the results. For example, in a patient with severe diplopia, tests relying upon the visual system may appear to reveal severe impairment. One might mistakenly interpret this as a deficit in cortical processing of visually based information, when in fact it may be due to a deficit in the more elemental aspects of the visual system. Careful neuropsychological studies must take these issues into consideration in patient selection and data interpretation. Heterogeneity of disease severity must also be considered when comparing studies. Patients who are more severely affected by MS, not surprisingly, are predisposed toward cognitive deficits. However, even in the early stages of illness, patients with MS have shown deficits in verbal memory and abstract reasoning (Amato et al., 1995). The course of illness—relapsing-remitting, primary progressive, and secondary progressive—may also play a role in the type of cognitive impairment observed. Patient populations should be carefully characterized and classified into subtypes before inclusion in a study (Peyser et al., 1990). There is no uniform pattern of cognitive impairment in patients with MS. Most commonly, deficits occur in recent memory, attention span, abstract and conceptual reasoning, and rate of information processing. Language is affected less frequently. In general, cognitive deficits in MS appear to follow a profile usually associated with so-called subcortical dementias.

Memory is the most commonly impaired cognitive domain in patients with MS. Defining the nature of this memory deficit has been a work in progress. Different groups use different memory tests. Pure replications have been infrequent. In addition, definitions of the aspects of memory vary from group to group. In general, patients with MS show deficits both in working memory, a "prefrontal cortical task," and episodic recall, a "mesial temporal task."

Working memory, the aspect of memory that permits the manipulation and application of information to problem solving, is also impaired in patients with MS. The frontal lobes seem to be preferentially vulnerable to the development of lesions in MS (Sperling et al., 2001; Lazeron et al., 2005). Heaton et al. (1985) found that patients with MS make more perseveration errors than controls. Using a different paradigm, Rao and Hammeke (1984) also found that patients with chronic progressive MS tend to perseverate and do not modify their problem-solving strategy even with verbal cueing. Working memory dysfunction may be more common in secondary progressive rather than primary progressive MS (Comi et al., 1995). Rovaris et al. (2000) found that a significant proportion of patients with MS perform poorly on a battery of tests of executive function and working memory. Using a wide variety of tests of executive function combined with careful exclusion criteria, Foong et al. (1997) showed that the deficits in executive function were not attributable to primary visual system abnormalities. Patients with frontal white matter lesions tend to have more working memory deficits than other MS patient groups (Arnett et al., 1994). Even early in the course of illness, patients with MS may suffer from working memory deficits (Schulz et al., 2006). As with many other aspects of the illness, only a subset of patients with MS have difficulty with concept formation, set shifting, and modification of responses and problem-solving strategies even with environmental feedback.

Working memory deficits seem to be a feature primarily of the progressive rather than the relapsing-remitting form of the illness (Archibald and Fisk, 2000). In general, working memory deficits usually implicate dysfunction of the dorsolateral prefrontal cortex (Berman et al., 1995; D'Esposito and Postle, 1999). However, most studies that have associated prefrontal cortical function with working memory emphasize the role of prefrontal gray matter rather than white matter. In MS, the lesions either interrupt input to or output from the prefrontal cortex, suggesting that any working memory deficits in MS are related to disconnection of the neural network subserving working memory.

Short-term memory is usually unaffected, but spontaneous and free recall is often deficient (Beatty and Monson, 1996). Fisher (1988) found impairment in general memory, verbal memory, visual memory, and delayed recall. Camp et al. (1999) also found deficits in verbal memory, whereas Rendell et al. (2007) found impairments in prospective memory. Rao et al. (1984; Rao et al., 1993) found deficiencies in immediate and delayed recall. Episodic memory, which is used for day-to-day functions such as the retrieval of appointment times, recall of lists, and recall of places (Rao et al., 1984; Rao, Leo, and St. Aubin-Faubert, 1989; Minden et al., 1990), is more affected than semantic memory, which is used for the retrieval of overlearned names and facts (Beatty et al., 1989; Filley et al., 1989). Automatic memory, which is involved in the most simple coding and categorization of a stimulus, is preserved, in contrast to the more effortful free and cued-recall measures in patients with MS (Grafman et al., 1991; Rao et al., 1993).

Thornton and Raz (1997) conducted a meta-analysis of 36 studies investigating memory function in patients with MS. They concluded that there is significant impairment in all memory domains, not just in retrieval in long-term memory. Another group found abnormalities in reaction time, nonverbal memory, and planning (Schulz et al., 2006). Other groups have found that the primary memory deficit in patients with MS is in the learning of new information (Rao et al., 1984; Gaudino et al., 2001). Verbal memory deficits were associated with the progressive forms of MS. Retrieval failure was noted only in the progressive form of MS. Patients with MS perform normally on tests of motor learning (Rao et al., 1993). Part of the difficulty in interpreting these data is due to the variability in memory deficits in patients with MS. Rao et al. (1984) found that one third of patients with chronic progressive MS performed normally on memory testing, and only 21% were severely affected. In general, learning, recall, and effortful memory measures are abnormal in patients with MS, whereas short-term memory capacity is unimpaired.

Attention span may be abnormal in patients with MS, particularly those with progressive forms of the illness (Fisher, 1988; Filley et al., 1989; Rao, Leo, Bernardin, et al., 1991; Ron et al., 1991; Feinstein, Kartsounis, et al., 1992; Feinstein, Youl, et al., 1992; Camp et al., 1999; Sperling et al., 2001; Schulz et al., 2006). The tasks used to measure attention span vary across these studies, and some do not actually address attention as much as short-term or working memory. Visual and auditory attention are often impaired (Ron et al., 1991). In one study, attention deficits were found relatively early in the course of MS (Feinstein, Kartsounis, et al., 1992; Feinstein, Youl, et al., 1992). However, another group reported that attention deficits appeared only with an extended duration of illness (Amato et al., 2001). A more detailed investigation of attention span in different clinical subtypes of MS might help resolve these discrepancies. Attention involves a widely distributed cortical and subcortical network of interconnected structures (Mesulam, 1981). It is not surprising that at least in some patients with MS, the function of this network is disrupted.

Visuospatial perception and memory also are impaired in some patients with MS (Rao, Leo, Bernardin, et al., 1991; Comi et al., 1995). It is not clear if this is due to abnormalities within the primary visual system (that are common in MS) or to second- and third-order deficits in complex visuospatial processing in association cortex. Parietal white matter is often the site of lesions in patients with MS (Sperling et al., 2001). Lesions in visual association cortex, particularly in the occipito-temporo-parietal junction, are often implicated in visuospatial perception impairment (Cogan, 1979). Additional investigation would be useful.

Cognitive processing speed is slowed in many patients with MS (Kail, 1998; Demaree et al., 1999; Archibald and Fisk, 2000; Sperling et al., 2001). Auditory and visual information processing speed are diminished in patients with MS; however, when these patients are given sufficient time, their performance rises to that of controls (Demaree et al., 1999). This is not an unexpected finding because a delay in conductance along well-recognized primary visual and auditory pathways has long been recognized as a feature of MS as a consequence of demyelination. In fact, it is the basis of the use of evoked potential measurements for the diagnosis of this disease. The use of reaction time as a measure of cognitive processing speed must be interpreted cautiously. Incoordination, weakness, and tremor may impede the speed of the motor response, whereas the speed of the conceptual formulation of the response may be within normal limits.

More classic neurological syndromes of cognitive impairment, such as aphasia, agnosia, and apraxia, are rarely observed in patients with MS. This may be related to the nature of the pathology in MS. In general, MS lesions tend to be relatively small. To produce aphasia or any of the classic cortical lesion syndromes, extensive damage must occur to a precise region of cortex or to fiber pathways arising from the region. The lesions in MS rarely are that extensive, in contrast to strokes, where such syndromes are common. Cognitive functions that are subserved by a more extensive network of structures, such as memory, learning, and attention span, may be more vulnerable to the accumulated effects of small but widely distributed lesions. There has been some systematic investigation of language function in patients with MS. In general, though abnormalities in language function have been reported, they tend to be relatively mild compared to other aspects of cognitive dysfunction in patients with MS (Jambor, 1969; Heaton et al., 1985). Classic aphasia syndromes are quite rare (Olmos-Lau et al., 1977). There are very few reports of classic agnosia or apraxia.

Cognitive impairment markedly alters the quality of life for patients with MS. Their activities of daily living may be severely affected in social and vocational spheres. Their ability to function independently may also be diminished. Those with cognitive deficits are less likely to be employed, are more socially withdrawn, and have greater difficulty performing routine household tasks (Rao, Leo, Ellington, et al., 1991). However, at least in one longitudinal study of 1 year's duration, most patients with MS, regardless of subtype, did not show significant cognitive decline (Hohol et al., 1997).

MAGNETIC RESONANCE IMAGING ABNORMALITIES AND COGNITIVE IMPAIRMENT IN MULTIPLE SCLEROSIS

Prior to the advent of MRI, it was difficult to perform lesion assessment with available neuroimaging techniques. With the exception of active lesions that enhance with contrast injections, MS lesions are difficult to delineate by computed tomography (CT) scan. Therefore, initial neuroimaging studies using this modality focused on ventricular size. Two groups reported that ventricular enlargement correlated with cognitive impairment in MS by CT scan (Rao et al., 1985; Rabins et al., 1986). Because ventricular enlargement is often a correlate of cerebral atrophy, such a correlation is not surprising. In a refined approach to the same issue using MRI measures, Edwards et al. (2001) found that a lower volume of cerebral white matter correlated with poorer performance on a battery of neuropsychological tests, though this group was not able to correlate ventricular enlargement as measured on MRI with poor test performance. Performance on a comprehensive measure of cognitive ability inversely correlated with global gray matter volume in patients with relapsing-remitting MS (Morgen et al., 2006).

Neuroimaging studies with MRI have been invaluable in improving diagnostic accuracy in MS. Several groups have tried to correlate lesion location and number/density with cognitive deficits in patients with MS. For example, several groups have found that patients with MS who were impaired on a neuropsychological screening battery had more brain lesions on MRI than unimpaired patients (Franklin et al., 1988; Ron et al., 1991; Comi et al., 1995; Hohol et al., 1997; Rovaris et al., 1998; Camp et al., 1999; Rovaris et al., 2000). There is disagreement as to the relationship between the clinical subtype of MS, the extent of lesion load, and the degree of neuropsychological impairment (Comi et al., 1995; Hohol et al., 1997; Camp et al., 1999; Fulton et al., 1999). There appears to be a preferential involvement of frontoparietal white matter in MS by MRI analysis (Sperling et al., 2001). Cognitive dysfunction generally correlates with lesions located at the gray-white junction in the prefrontal, limbic, and association cortical regions (Charil et al., 2003).

It should be noted that lesion load as measured with conventional MRI may underestimate the extent of the pathology in MS (Davie et al., 1994). Moreover, MRI measures as presently constituted do not differentiate between active inflammation and gliotic scarring. Finally, lesion expansion and regression may be more common in MS than clinical measures of disease activity might suggest (Isaac et al., 1988; Harris et al., 1991). So-called asymptomatic lesions may actually be symptomatic, depending upon the sensitivity and breadth of the clinical instruments employed. Nevertheless, at least in a small longitudinal study, patients with active disease as measured by lesion load on MRI scan had a fall-off in performance on neuropsychological testing, especially in tests of attention and information-processing speed. This functional deterioration was not present in patients with MS with static MRI measures (Feinstein et al., 1993).

Working memory and executive function impairment may be closely correlated with lesion load in the frontal lobes. Three groups have reported that poor performance on the Wisconsin Card Sort Test is directly correlated with the severity of frontal involvement as measured on MRI scan (Swirsky-Sacchetti et al., 1992; Arnett et al., 1994; Nocentini et al., 2001). Abstraction and conceptual reasoning are most often impaired in patients with MS with a high lesion load (Rao, Leo, Haughton, et al., 1989). Working memory performance inversely correlated with prefrontal and global grey matter volume in patients who were mildly disabled with relapsing-remitting MS (Morgen et al., 2006). In a study that used multiple measures of working memory and executive function in MS, Foong et al. (1997) found that poorer performance on spatial working memory and planning tasks was correlated with the frontal lesion load in MS. However, this correlation disappeared when the result was normalized by total lesion load (Foong et al., 1997). The authors interpreted this to mean that a widespread pathology may underlie executive dysfunction in MS, not just a frontal lesion load. A similar finding was noted by two other groups (Rovaris et al., 1998; Rovaris et al., 2000; Nocentini et al., 2001). One interpretation holds that neuropsychological tests purporting to assess frontal lobe function actually depend upon a more widely distributed neural network. Alternatively, patients with a higher lesion load in the frontal cortex might be expected to have an overall increase in brain lesion load. Correcting for total brain lesion load may obscure the role of frontal lobe lesions in executive function and working memory in MS. The only way to address this issue definitively is to study that probably rare group of patients with MS with predominantly frontal lobe lesions or those with relative sparing of the frontal lobes.

Verbal and visual memory deficits are correlated with lesion load in MS (Ron et al., 1991). The greater the total lesion area, the worse patients with MS perform on measures of recent memory (Rao, Leo, Haughton, et al., 1989). In addition, long-term memory deficits in patients with relapsing-remitting MS also correlate with lesion load. However, short-term memory deficits may not correlate with lesion load in this patient subset (Fulton et al., 1999). Volume loss in cerebral white matter has been correlated with poor performance on a test of visuospatial memory (Edwards et al., 2001).

As noted previously, attention deficits are common in patients with MS. Even in patients early in their clinical course, attention deficits may already be present (Feinstein, Kartsounis, et al., 1992; Feinstein, Youl, et al., 1992; Schulz et al., 2006). Moreover, attention deficits are often associated with clinically silent and unsuspected cerebral lesions on MRI scan. Worsening attention deficits correlate closely with increasing lesion load on MRI (Hohol et al., 1997; Sperling et al., 2001). Auditory attention is impaired in individuals with a high lesion load in MS (Ron et al., 1991). However, lesion load does not correlate with attention measures by all groups (Rao, Leo, Haughton, et al., 1989). Sperling et al. (2001) found that total, frontal, and parietal lesion load all correlated with attentional performance.

Other aspects of neuropsychological function have been examined in the context of lesion load on MRI scan. Abnormalities in information processing speed correlate directly with progressive increases in lesion load on MRI (Hohol et al., 1997; Fulton et al., 1999). The functional substrate of this finding might benefit from more refined anatomical distribution studies of lesion load.

The corpus callosum is an easily measured white matter structure. Atrophy of the corpus callosum has been associated with poor performance on a dichotic listening task in patients with MS (Rao, Bernardin, et al., 1989). Cross-callosal pathways are essential to proper performance of this task. The degradation of fiber pathways contributing to reduced interhemispheric communication produced by MS probably underlies this finding. In addition, atrophy of the corpus callosum has been correlated with poor performance on tests of sustained attention, rapid problem solving, and mental arithmetic (Rao, Leo, Haughton, et al., 1989) and on two tests of verbal fluency, a frontal task (Nocentini et al., 2001). In a more recent study, Edwards et al. (2001) found that corpus callosum atrophy correlated with overall performance on a battery encompassing a wide variety of neuropsychological measures. Therefore, the secondary effects of MS lesions on the integrity of fiber pathways distant from the actual lesion site cannot be underestimated. This limits the value, in part, of focal lesion quantification and cognitive correlates in MS, as well as in other disorders produced by disruption of fiber pathways.

TREATMENT OPTIONS FOR COGNITIVE IMPAIRMENT IN MULTIPLE SCLEROSIS

There are two approaches to the treatment of cognitive impairment in MS. The first is to prevent cognitive impairment or, once it occurs, to prevent its progression. The second is to ameliorate or reverse preexisiting cognitive impairment with agents that enhance cognitive performance. To prevent progression in relapsing-remitting MS, regular injections of interferon β-1b (Betaseron), interferon β-1a (Avonex), and glatiramer acetate (Copaxone) have proven to be highly effective. The administration of such agents should help to slow the development of cognitive impairment or, once it occurs, slow its progression, in patients with relapsing-remitting MS. A recent study suggests that over a 1-year interval, treatment with interferon β-1b actually improved complex attention, concentration, visual learning, and recall, while other neuropsychological dimensions were unchanged. In the untreated MS control group, complex attention, verbal fluency, visual learning, and recall deteriorated, while other dimensions of cognition did not progress (Barak and Achiron, 2002). This finding suggests that prevention of disease progression not only prevents cognitive deterioration, but might also allow compensatory changes that result in cognitive enhancement. Furthermore, Rudick et al. (1999) found that interferon β-1a reduced brain atrophy by 55% during the 2nd year of a 2-year trial in patients with relapsing-remitting MS. In another study, treatment of patients with relapsing-remitting MS with glatiramer acetate had no effect on sustained attention, perceptual processing, verbal and visuospatial memory, and semantic retrieval after 1 and 2 years of treatment. By contrast, in the control untreated group, mean neuropsychological test scores actually rose at 1 and 2 years. The lack of measurable decline in the control group limits the possibility of detecting a therapeutic effect of this agent at least in this patient sample (Weinstein et al., 1999). The study of the effects of these immunomodulatory therapies on cognitive dysfunction in MS clearly deserves more attention.

A variety of other medications have been used to enhance cognitive function in patients with MS. Geisler et al. (1996) studied the effects of amantidine and pemoline on cognitive function in MS. Both medications are used widely to treat the fatigue that frequently occurs in patients with MS. Unfortunately, neither one improved cognitive performance over a 6-week treatment period. However, another group found that amantadine signficiantly reduced fatigue whereas pemoline did not (Krupp et al., 1995). In a more recent study, amantidine was found to improve reaction time (Sailer et al., 2000). This is not unexpected because amantidine enhances dopamine-mediated motor function. Other aspects of cognitive function were not examined in this limited study. Donepezil HCl (Aricept), an acetylcholinesterase inhibitor widely used in Alzheimer's disease to improve cognition, improved attention, memory, and executive function in a short open trial in patients with MS tested at 4 and 12 weeks (Greene et al., 2000). Another group found similar results (Christodoulou et al., 2006). Additional study should be devoted to the use of cognition-enhancing medications in MS, especially as new agents become available. For example, modafinil, a novel nonamphetamine stimulant, has cognition-enhancing qualities that might be beneficial to patients with MS (Baranski and Pigeau, 1997). Disappointingly, modafinil did not improve fatigue in patients with MS in a large randomized double-blind trial (Stankoff et al., 2005). Stimulated by the observation that males are less likely to develop MS than females, a trial of testosterone supplementation was undertaken in male patients with MS. Daily testosterone treatment for 12 months improved cognitive performance and slowed brain atrophy in a small pilot study (Sicotte, et al., 2007). Clearly, much more attention needs to be devoted to interventions designed to slow or reverse the cognitive deficits associated with MS.

SUMMARY

Cognitive impairment is much more frequently associated with MS than is widely appreciated. The cognitive domains most often affected are working memory and executive function, recall, attention, and cognitive processing speed. Although neuropsychological deficits can appear early in the course of the illness, they tend to be more common as the disease progresses. Increasing lesion load as measured on MRI scans is correlated with many measures of neuropsychological dysfunction. Cognitive processes that rely most heavily on distributed and interconnected neural networks, such as executive function, episodic memory, and encoding, may be most vulnerable to the accumulated effects of widely distributed white matter lesions. Deficits in processing speed may be the signature of the central demyelinating lesions that are the hallmark of MS. Corpus callosum atrophy, which probably reflects accumulated axonal damage and regression, is another MRI measure frequently associated with impaired cognitive processing. Primary prevention of disease progression with immunomodulatory therapy may prevent neuropsychological deterioration, at least in patients with the relapsing-remitting form of illness. Cognition-enhancing agents such as acetylcholinesterase inhibitors hold the promise of ameliorating some of the deficits incurred by patients with MS.

ACKNOWLEDGMENTS

The author would like to thank Dr. Terry Goldberg for his advice and guidance in the preparation of this work, and Jamie Rosenthal for assistance in updating and revising this chapter.

REFERENCES

Amato, M.P., Ponziani, G., Pracucci, G., Bracco, L., Siracusa, G., and Amaducci, L. (1995) Cognitive impairment in early-onset multiple sclerosis: pattern, predictors, and impact on everyday life in a 4 year follow-up. *Arch. Neurol.* 52:168–172.

Amato, M.P., Ponziani, G., Siracusa, G., and Sorbi, S. (2001) Cognitive dysfunction in early-onset multiple sclerosis: a reappraisal after 10 years. *Arch. Neurol.* 58:1602–1606.

Archibald, C.J., and Fisk, J.D. (2000) Information processing efficiency in patients with multiple sclerosis. *J. Clin. Exp. Neuropsychol.* 22:686–701.

Arnett, P.A., Rao, S.M., Bernardin, L., Grafman, J., Yetkin, F.Z., and Lobeck, L. (1994) Relationship between frontal lobe lesions and Wisconsin Card Sorting Test performance in patients with multiple sclerosis. *Neurology* 44:420–425.

Barak, Y., and Achiron, A. (2002) Effect of interferon-beta-1b on cognitive functions in multiple sclerosis. *Eur. Neurol.* 47:11–14.

Baranski, J.V., and Pigeau, R.A. (1997) Self-monitoring cognitive performance during sleep deprivation: effects of modafinil, d-amphetamine and placebo. *J. Sleep Res.* 6:84–91.

Baum, H.M., and Rothschild, B.B. (1981) The incidence and prevalence of reported multiple sclerosis. *Ann. Neurol.* 10:420–428.

Beatty, W.W., Goodkin, D.E., Monson, N., and Beatty, P.A. (1989) Cognitive disturbances in patients with relapsing-remitting multiple sclerosis. *Arch. Neurol.* 46:1113–1119.

Beatty, W.W., and Monson, N. (1996) Problems solving by patients with multiple sclerosis: comparison of performance on the Wisconsin and California Card Sorting Tests. *J. Int. Neuropsychol. Soc.* 2:134–140.

Berman, K.F., Ostrem, J.L., Randolph, C., Gold, J., Goldberg, T.E., Coppola, R., Carson, R.E., Hersovitch, P., and Weinberger, D.R. (1995) Physiological activation of a cortical network during performance of the Wisconsin Card Sorting Test: a positron emission tomography study. *Neuropsychologia* 33:1027–1046.

Buchanan, R.J., Wang, S., Huang, C., and Graber, D. (2001) Profiles of nursing home residents with multiple sclerosis using the minimum data set. *Multiple Sclerosis* 7:189–200.

Camp, S.J., Stevenson, V.L., Thomapson, A.J., Miller, D.H., Borras, C., Auriacombe, S., Brochet, B., Falautano, M., Fillipi, M., Hérissé-Dulo, L., Montalban, X., Parrcira, E., Polman, C.H., De Sa, J., and Langdon, D.W. (1999) Cognitive function in primary progressive and transitional progressive multiple sclerosis. A controlled study with MRI correlates. *Brain* 122:1341–1348.

Charil, A., Zijdenbos, A.P., Taylor, J., Boelman, C., Worsley, K.J., Evans, A.C., and Dagher, A. (2003) Statistical mapping analysis of lesion location and neurological disability in multiple sclerosis: application to 452 data sets. *NeuroImage* 19:532–544.

Christodoulou, C., Melville, P., Scherl, W.F., MacAllister, W.S., Elkins, L.E., and Krupp, L.B. (2006) Effects of donepezil on memory and cognition in multiple sclerosis. *J. Neurol. Sci.* 245:127–136.

Cogan, D.G. (1979) Visuospatial dysgnosia. *Am. J. Ophthalmol.* 88: 361–368.

Comi, G., Filippi, M., Martinelli, V., Campi, A., Rodegher, M., Alberoni, M., Siribian, G., and Canal, N. (1995) Brain MRI correlates of cognitive impairment in primary and secondary progressive multiple sclerosis. *J. Neurol. Sci.* 132:222–227.

Davie, C.A., Hawkins, C.P., Barker, G.J., Brennan, A., Tofts, P.S., Miller, D.H., and McDonald, W.I. (1994) Serial proton magnetic resonance spectroscopy in acute multiple sclerosis lesions. *Brain* 117:49–58.

Dean, G. (1967) Annual incidence, prevalence and mortality of multiple sclerosis in white South African-born and in white immigrants to South Africa. *Br. Med. J.* 2:724–730.

Demaree, H.A., DeLuca, J., Gaudino, E.A., and Diamond, B.J. (1999) Speed of information processing as a key deficit in multiple sclerosis: implications for rehabilitation. *J. Neurol. Neurosurg. Psychiatry* 67:661–663.

DeSousa, E.A., Albert, R.H., and Kalman, B. (2002) Cognitive impairments in multiple sclerosis: a review. *Am. J. Alzheimers Dis. Other Demen.* 17:23–29.

D'Esposito, M., and Postle, B.R. (1999) The dependence of span and delayed-response performance on prefrontal cortex. *Neuropsychologia* 37:1303–1315.

Ebers, G.C., Bulman, D.E., Sadovnick, A.D., Paty, D.W., Warren, S., Hader, W., Murray, T.J., Seland, T.P., Duquette, P., Grey, T., et al. (1986) A population-based study of multiple sclerosis in twins. *N. Engl. J. Med.* 315:1638–1642.

Edwards, S.G.M., Liu, C., and Blumhardt, L.D. (2001) Cognitive correlates of supratentorial atrophy on MRI in multiple sclerosis. *Acta Neurol. Scand.* 104:214–223.

Feinstein, A., Kartsounis, L.D., Miller, D.H., Youl, B.D., and Ron, M.A. (1992) Clinically isolated lesions of the type seen in multiple sclerosis: a cognitive, psychiatric, and MRI follow up study. *J. Neurol. Neurosurg. Psychiatry* 55:869–879.

Feinstein, A., Ron, M., and Thompson, A. (1993) A serial study of psychometric and magnetic resonance imaging changes in multiple sclerosis. *Brain* 116:569–602.

Feinstein, A., Youl, B., and Ron, M. (1992) Acute optic neuritis: a cognitive and magnetic resonance imaging study. *Brain* 115:1403–1415.

Filley, C.M., Heaton, R.K., Nelson, L.M., Burks, J.S., and Franklin, G.M. (1989) A comparison of dementia in Alzheimer's disease and multiple sclerosis. *Arch. Neurol.* 46:157–161.

Fisher, J.S. (1988) Using the Wechsler memory scale-revised to detect and characterize memory deficits in multiple sclerosis. *Clin. Neuropsychol.* 2:149–172.

Foong, J., Rozewicz, L., Quaghebeur, G., Davie, C.A., Kartsounis, L.D., Thompson, A.J., Miller, D.H., and Ron, M.A. (1997) Executive function in multiple sclerosis. The role of frontal lobe pathology. *Brain* 120:15–26.

Franklin, G.M., Heaton, R.K., Nelson, L.M., Filley, C.M., and Seibert, C. (1988) Correlation of neuropsychological and MRI findings in chronic/progressive multiple sclerosis. *Neurology* 38:1826–1829.

Fulton, J.C., Grossman, R.I., Udupa, J., Mannon, L.J., Grossman, M., Wei, L., Polansky, M., and Kolson, D.L. (1999) MR lesion load and cognitive function in patients with relapsing-remitting multiple sclerosis. *Am. J. Neuroradiol.* 20:1951–1955.

Gaudino, E.A., Chiaravalloti, N.D., DeLuca, J., and Diamond, B.J. (2001) A comparison of memory performance in relapsing-remitting, primary progressive and secondary progressive multiple sclerosis. *Neuropsychiatr. Neuropsychol. Behav. Neurol.* 14:32–44.

Geisler, M.W., Sliwinski, M., Coyle, P.K., Masur, D.M., Doscher, C., and Krupp, L.B. (1996) The effects of amantadine and pemoline on cognitive functioning in multiple sclerosis. *Arch. Neurol.* 53:185–188.

Gilbert, J.J., and Sadler, M. (1983) Unsuspected multiple sclerosis. *Arch. Neurol.* 40:533–536.

Grafman, J., Rao, S., Bernardin, L., and Leo, G.J. (1991) Automatic memory processes in patients with multiple sclerosis. *Arch. Neurol.* 48:1072–1075.

Greene, Y.M., Tariot, P.N., Wishart, H., Cox, C., Holt, C.J., Schwid, S., and Noviasky, J. (2000) A 12-week open trial of donepezil hydrochloride in patients with multiple sclerosis and associated cognitive impairments. *J. Clin. Psychopharmacol.* 20:350–356.

Gregory, S.G., Schmidt, S., Seth, P., Oksenberg, J.R., Hart, J., Prokop, A., Caillier, S.J., Ban, M., Goris, A., Barcellos, L.F., Lincoln, R., McCauley, J.L., Sawcer, S.J., Compston, D.A., Dubois, B., Hauser, S.L., Garcia-Blanco, M.A., Pericak-Vance, M.A., Haines, J.L., for the Multiple Sclerosis Genetics Group. (2007) Interleukin 7 receptor alpha chain (IL7R) shows allelic and functional association with multiple sclerosis. *Nat. Genet.* 39:1083–1091.

Harris, J.O., Frnak, J.A., Patronas, N., Mcarlin, D.E., and McFarland, H.F. (1991) Serial gadolinium-enhanced magnetic resonance imaging scans in patients with early, relapsing-remitting multiple sclerosis: implications for clinical trials and natural history. *Ann. Neurol.* 29:548–555.

Heaton, R.K., Nelson, L.M., Thompson, D.S., Burks, J.S., and Franklin, G.M. (1985) Neuropsychological findings in relapsing-remitting and chronic progressive MS. *J. Consult. Clin. Psychol.* 53:103–110.

Hohol, M.J., Guttman, C.R.G., Orav, J., Mackin, G.A., Kikinis, R., Khoury, S.J., Lolesz, F.A., and Weiner, H.L. (1997) Serial neuropsychological assessment and magnetic resonance imaging analysis in multiple sclerosis. *Arch. Neurol.* 54:1018–1025.

Isaac, C., Li, D.K.B., Genton, M., Jardine, C., Grochowski, E., Palmer, M., Kastrukoff, L.F., Oger, J., and Paty, D.W. (1988) Multiple sclerosis: a serial study using MRI in relapsing patients. *Neurology* 38:1511–1515.

Jambor, K.L. (1969) Cognitive functioning in multiple sclerosis. *Br. J. Psychiatry* 115:765–775.

Kail, R. (1998) Speed of information processing in patients with multiple sclerosis. *J. Clin. Exp. Neuropsychol.* 20:98–106.

Krupp, L.B., Coyle, P.K., Doscher, C., Miller, A., Cross, A.H., Jandorf, L., Halper, J., Johnson, B., Morgante, L., and Grimson, R (1995) Fatigue therapy in multiple sclerosis: results of a double-blind, randomized, parallel trial of amantidine, pemoline, and placebo. *Neurol.* 45:1956–1961.

Kurtzke, J.F. (2000) Epidemiology of multiple sclerosis. Does this really point toward an etiology? *Neurol. Sci.* 21:383–403.

Kurtzke, J.F., and Hyllested, K. (1985) Multiple sclerosis in the Faroe Islands II. Clinical update, transmission, and the nature of MS. *Neurology* 36:307–328.

LaRocca, N.G. (1984) Psychosocial factors in multiple sclerosis and the role of stress. *Ann. N.Y. Acad. Sci.* 436:435–442.

Lazeron, R.H.C., Boringa, J.B., Schouten, M., Uitedehaag, B.M.J., Bergers, E. Lindeboom, J. Eikelenboom, M.J., Scheltens, P.H., Barkhof, F. and Polman, C.H. (2005) Brain atrophy and lesion load as explaining parameters for cognitive impairment in multiple sclerosis. *Multiple Sclerosis* 11:524–531.

Lundmark, F., Duvefelt, K., Iacobaeus, E., Kockum, I., Wallstrom, E., Khademi, M., Oturai, A., Ryder, L.P., Saarela, J., Harbo, H.F., Celius, E.G., Salter, H., Ollson, T. and Hillert, J. (2007) Variations in interleukin 7 receptor alpha chain (IL7R) influences risk of multiple sclerosis. *Nat. Genet.* 39: 1108–1113.

Mesulam, M.M. (1981) A cortical network for directed attention and unilateral neglect. *Ann. Neurol.* 10:309–325.

Minden, S.L., Moes, E.J., Orav, J., Kaplan, E., and Reich, P. (1990) Memory impairment in multiple sclerosis. *J. Clin. Exp. Neuropsychol.* 12:566–586.

Morgen, J., Sammer, G., Courtney, S.M., Wolters, T., Melchior, H., Blecker, C.R., Oschmann, P., Kaps, M., and Vaitl, D. (2006) Evidence for a direct association between cortical atrophy and cognitive impairment in relapsing-remitting MS. *NeuroImage* 30:891–898.

Nocentini, U., Rossini, P.M., Carlesimo, G.A., Graceffa, A., Grasso, M.G., Lupoi, D., Oliveri, M., Orlacchio, A., Pozzilli, C., Rizzato, B., and Caltagirone, C. (2001) Patterns of cognitive impairment in secondary progressive stable phase of multiple sclerosis: correlations with MRI findings. *Eur. Neurol.* 45:11–18.

Olmos-Lau, N., Ginsberg, M.D., and Geller, J.B. (1977) Aphasia in multiple sclerosis. *Neurology* 27:623–626.

Peyser, J.M., Rao, S.M., LaRocca, N.G., and Kaplan, E. (1990) Guidelines for neuropsychological research in multiple sclerosis. *Arch. Neurol.* 47:94–97.

Rabins, P.V., Brooks, B.F., O'Donnell, P., Pearlson, G.D., Moberg, P., Jubelt, B., Coyle, P., Dalos, N., and Folstein, M.F. (1986) Structural brain correlates of emotional disorder in multiple sclerosis. *Brain* 109:585–597.

Rao, S.M., Bernardin, L., Leo, G.J., Ellington, L., Ryan, S.B., and Burg, L.S. (1989) Cerebral disconnection in multiple sclerosis. *Arch. Neurol.* 46:918–920.

Rao, S.M., Glatt, S., Hammeke, T.A., McQuillen, M.P., Khatri, B.O., Rhodes, A.M., and Pollard, S. (1985) Chronic/progressive multiple sclerosis: relationship between cerebral ventricular size and neuropsychological impairment. *Arch. Neurol.* 42:678–682.

Rao, S.M., Grafman, J., DiGiulio, D., Mittenberg, W., Bernardin, L., Leo, G.J., Luchetta, T., and Unverzagt, F. (1993) Memory dysfunction in multiple sclerosis: its relation to working memory, semantic encoding, and implicit learning. *Neuropsychology* 7: 364–374.

Rao, S.M., and Hammeke, T.A. (1984) Hypothesis testing in patients with chronic progressive multiple sclerosis. *Brain Cogn.* 3:94–104.

Rao, S.M., Hammeke, T.A., McQuillen, M.P., Khatri, B.O. and Lloyd, D. (1984) Memory disturbance in chronic progressive multiple sclerosis. *Arch. Neurol.* 41:625–631.

Rao, S.M., Leo, G.J., Bernardin, L., and Unverzagt, F. (1991) Cognitive dysfunction in multiple sclerosis. I. Frequency, patterns, and prediction. *Neurology* 41:685–691.

Rao, S.M., Leo, G.J., Ellington, L., Nauertz, T., Bernardin, L., and Unverzagt, F. (1991) Cognitive dysfunction in multiple sclerosis. II. Impact on employment and social functioning. *Neurology* 41: 692–696.

Rao, S.M., Leo, G.J., Haughton, V.M., St. Aubin-Faubert, P., and Bernardin, L. (1989) Correlation of magnetic resonance imaging with neuropsychological testing in multiple sclerosis. *Neurology* 39:161–166.

Rao, S.M., Leo, G.J., and St. Aubin-Faubert, P. (1989) On the nature of memory disturbance in multiple sclerosis. *J. Clin. Exp. Neuropsychol.* 11:699–712.

Rendell, P.G., Jensen, and Henry, J.D. (2007) Prospective memory in multiple sclerosis. *J. Internat. Neurophys. Soc.* 13:410–416.

Ron, M.A., Callanan, M.M., and Warrington, E.K. (1991) Cognitive abnormalities in multiple sclerosis: a psychometric and MRI study. *Psychol. Med.* 21:59–68.

Rovaris, M., Filippi, M., Falautano, M., Minicucci, L., Rocca, M. A., Martinelli, V., and Comi, G. (1998) Relations between MR abnormalities and patterns of cognitive impairment in multiple sclerosis. *Neurology* 50:1601–1608.

Rovaris, M., Filippi, M., Minicucci, L., Iannucci, G., Santuccio, G., Possa, F., and Comi, G. (2000) Cortical/subcortical disease burden and cognitive impairment in patients with multiple sclerosis. *Am. J. Neuroradiol.* 21:402–408.

Rudick, R.A., Fisher, E., Lee, J.-C., Simon, J., Jacobs, L., and the Multiple Sclerosis Collaborative Research Group. (1999) Use of the brain parenchymal fraction to measure whole brain atrophy in relapsing-remitting MS. *Neurol.* 53:1698–1704.

Sadovnick, A.D. Armstrong, H., Rice, G.P.A., Bulman, D., Hashimoto, L., Paty. D.W., Hashimoto, S.A., Warren, S., Hader, W., Murray, T.J., et al. (1993) A population-based study of multiple sclerosis in twins: update. *Ann. Neurol.* 33:281–285.

Sadovnick, A.D., Baird, P.A., and Ward, R.H. (1988) Multiple sclerosis: updated risks for relatives. *Am. J. Med. Genet.* 29:533–541.

Sadovnick, A.D., Ebers, G.C., Dyment, D.A., and Risch, N.J. (1996) Evidence for a genetic basis for multiple sclerosis. The Canadian Collaborative Study Group. *Lancet* 347:1728–1730.

Sailer, M., Heinze, H.-J., Schoenfeld, M.A., Hauser, U., and Smid, H.G.O.M. (2000) Amantadine influences cognitive processing in patients with multiple sclerosis. *Pharmacopsychiatry* 33:28–37.

Schulz, D., Kopp, B., Kunkel, A., and Faiss, J.H. (2006) Cognition in the early stage of multiple sclerosis. *J. Neurol.* 253:1002–1010.

Sicotte, N.L., Glesser, B.S., Tandon, V., Klutch, R., Steiner, B., Drain, A.E., Shattuck, D.W., Hull, L., Wang, H.-J., Elashoff, R.M., Swerdloff, R.S., and Voskuhl, R.R. (2007) Testosterone treatment in multiple sclerosis. *Arch. Neurol.* 64:683–688.

Sperling, R.A., Guttman, C.R., Hohol, M.J., Warfield, S.K., Jakab, M., Parente, M. Diamond, E.L., Daffner, K.R., Olek, M.J., Orav, E.J., Kikinis, R., Jolesz, F.A., and Weiner, H.L. (2001) Regional magnetic resonance imaging lesion burden and cognitive function in multiple sclerosis. *Arch. Neurol.* 58:115–121.

Stankoff, B., Waubant, E., Confavreux, C., Edan, G., Debouverie, M., Rumbach, L., Moreau, T., Pelletier, J., Lubetzki, C., Clanet, M., and the French Modafinil Study Group. (2005) Modafinial for fatigue in MS: a randomized placebo-controlled double-blind study. *Neurol.* 64:1139–1143.

Swirsky-Sacchetti, T., Mitchell, D.R., Seward, J., Gonzales, C., Lublin, F., Knobler, R., and Field, H.L. (1992) Neuropsychological and structural brain lesions in multiple sclerosis: a regional analysis. *Neurology* 42:1291–1295.

Thornton, A.E., and Raz, N. (1997) Memory impairment in multiple sclerosis: a quantitative review. *Neuropsychology* 11:357–366.

Trojano, M., and Paolicelli, D. (2001) The differential diagnosis of multiple sclerosis: classification and clinical features of relapsing and progressive neurological syndromes. *Neurol. Sci.* 22:S98–S102.

Weinshenker, B.G. (1996) Epidemiology of multiple sclerosis. *Neurol. Clin.* 14:291–308.

Weinstein, A., Schwid, S.I., Schiffer, R.B., McDermott, M.P., Giang, D.W., and Goodman, A.D. (1999) Neuropsychologic status in multiple sclerosis after treatment with glatiramer. *Arch. Neurol.* 56:319–324.

Wishart, H., and Sharpe, D. (1997) Neuropsychological aspects of multiple sclerosis: a quantitative review. *J. Clin. Exp. Neuropsychol.* 19:810–824.

62 Dementia with Lewy Bodies

DAVID J. BURN, ELAINE K. PERRY, JOHN T. O'BRIEN, NEIL ARCHIBALD, ELIZABETA B. MUKAETOVA-LADINSKA, JOAQUIM CEREJEIRA, DANIEL COLLERTON, EVELYN JAROS, ROBERT PERRY, MARGARET A. PIGGOTT, CHRIS M. MORRIS, ANDREW MCLAREN, CLIVE G. BALLARD, AND IAN G. MCKEITH

Dementia with Lewy bodies (DLB) is a primary neurodegenerative dementia sharing several clinical and pathological characteristics with Parkinson's disease (PD). The first case reports of DLB appeared in 1961, when Okazaki published a report of two patients, aged 69 and 70 years, presenting with dementia who died shortly afterward with severe extrapyramidal rigidity. Autopsy showed Lewy body (LB) pathology in the cerebral cortex (Okazaki et al., 1961). The advent of anti-ubiquitin immunocytochemical staining methods allowed the frequency and distribution of cortical LBs to be defined more easily, and the clinico-pathological boundaries of DLB began to emerge. More recently, α-synuclein antibodies have revealed even more extensive pathological changes in DLB and have demonstrated a neurobiological link with other synucleinopathies, PD, and multiple system atrophy (MSA).

Between 15% and 20% of all cases of the elderly with dementia reaching autopsy have DLB, making it the second most common cause of degenerative dementia after Alzheimer's disease (AD). Patients with DLB have a poorer quality of life and consume more resources than patients with AD (Boström et al., 2007a, 2007b) making the impact of this dementia syndrome even more striking. Exquisite, not infrequently fatal, sensitivity to neuroleptic drugs and encouraging trial results for the use of cholinesterase inhibitors mean that an accurate diagnosis of DLB is more than merely of academic interest. This chapter reviews the clinical features, diagnosis, and investigation of DLB, together with its neuropathology, neurochemistry, and genetics. Finally, the chapter considers the management of this progressive and disabling disorder.

CLINICAL FEATURES AND NATURAL HISTORY

Dementia with Lewy bodies is characterized by a variable combination of fluctuating cognition, neuropsychiatric disturbance, and parkinsonism. Autonomic dysfunction and sleep disorders may also be prominent features, the former contributing to falls.

Fluctuating Cognition

Variation in cognitive performance is commonly observed in many late-onset dementias. It is frustrating to carers and has a major impact upon the patient's ability to perform everyday activities reliably. Fluctuating cognition (FC) may present in several ways, depending upon the severity and diurnal pattern. Carers of patients with DLB describe spontaneous, periodic, and transient episodes of fluctuation, affecting functional abilities (Bradshaw et al., 2004) quite different from the more prolonged, situation-dependent variability seen in AD. Fluctuation occurs in 80% or more of people suffering from DLB, 30%–60% of individuals with vascular dementia (VaD), and 20% of people with AD. Evaluation of fluctuating cognition can be difficult and requires detailed questioning of patients and carers. Several clinical scales have been validated to quantify FC in DLB such as The Clinician Assessment of Fluctuation Scale (Walker et al., 2000a) and The Mayo Fluctuations Composite Scale (Ferman et al., 2004). In the latter study, informant endorsement of three of four questions (Does the patient experience excessive daytime sleepiness? Do they sleep more than 2 hours during the day? Do their words occasionally come out jumbled? Are there times when they stare into space for long periods?) had a positive predictive value of 83% for a diagnosis of DLB versus AD.

Computer-based testing systems offer an alternative method of assessing FC with measures of attention demonstrating marked variation in the DLB population (Walker et al., 2000b). This variation can be detected over very short periods of time (on a second-to-second basis), suggesting that FC arises from dysregulation of continuously active arousal systems. Fluctuating cognition may also be an important determinant of poor prognosis, according to a retrospective analysis of 243 autopsy-confirmed cases of DLB and Parkinson's disease with dementia (PDD) (Jellinger et al., 2007).

Psychiatric Symptoms

At least 80% of patients with DLB experience some neuropsychiatric symptoms, such as visual hallucinations, auditory hallucinations, delusions, delusional misidentification, and depression (Campbell et al., 2001). Visual hallucinations are the most common symptom, with a mean frequency of 50% (range, 13%–80%) in prospective studies, compared with 20%–30% in patients with AD from a meta-analysis of standardized reports. The person with DLB typically sees adults, children, or animals of normal size, sometimes with accompanying auditory hallucinations, which are far less frequent in AD. Visual hallucinations are not only more frequent in patients with DLB compared to AD but also more persistent. Hallucinations can be quantified to monitor change using the North East Visual Hallucinations Inventory (Mosimann et al., 2008).

Extrapyramidal Features

Estimates of the frequency of parkinsonian features at presentation in DLB range between 10% and 78%, whereas 40%–100% of patients display extrapyramidal signs (EPS) at some stage of the illness (McKeith, Perry, et al., 1992; Gnanalingham et al., 1997; Louis et al., 1997; Del Ser et al., 2000). Differences between series are most likely to represent ascertainment bias and the variable definition of clinical phenomenology. There is no consensus on whether the parkinsonism associated with DLB differs phenotypically from that associated with PD. Interpretation of the literature is hindered by a dearth of prospective clinico-pathological data. In a review of 75 case reports of DLB published between 1961 and 1991, Lennox (1992) determined the frequency of parkinsonism to be 90%, with 50% of the patients having three or more of the following symptoms: rigidity, tremor, bradykinesia, gait disorder, and flexed posture. Reduced rest tremor, greater symmetry of signs, myoclonic jerks, and a reduced response to levodopa have all been reported in DLB, although these have not been confirmed by others (Gnanalingham et al., 1997; Louis et al., 1997).

In a large international multicenter study, parkinsonism was reported in 92.4% of 120 patients with DLB (Del Ser et al., 2000). There was a small but statistically significant difference between male and female patients on the five-item Unified Parkinson's Disease Rating Scale (UPDRS) subscore (Ballard et al., 1997), with male patients being more severely affected. Older patients with DLB tended to have higher UPDRS scores, but the difference was not statistically significant. Patients with more severe cognitive impairment (defined as a Mini-Mental State Examination [MMSE] score, 18) had significantly more severe EPS than those with less cognitive decline using the full UPDRS part III, but when this relationship was reexamined using the five-item UPDRS subscore, no difference was found between the groups. This apparent disparity may be interpreted as meaning that patients with more severe dementia have difficulty understanding and executing some of the instructions.

Aarsland and colleagues (2001) described more severe action tremor, rigidity, bradykinesia, difficulty arising from a chair, greater facial impassivity, and gait disturbance in 98 patients with DLB compared with 130 patients with PD. Overall, 68% of the patients with DLB had EPS. Burn and colleagues (2003) describe postural instability and gait difficulty as being significantly more common in DLB compared to PD. Significant parkinsonism was more frequent in patients with DLB (71%) than in those with AD (7%) or VaD (10%) (Ballard, O'Brien, Swann, et al., 2000). The degree of cognitive impairment had no influence on the occurrence of EPS. Patients with DLB with established parkinsonism had an annual increase in severity, assessed using the UPDRS, of 9%, a figure comparable with that seen in PD. In common with PD, progression was more rapid (49% increase in the motor UPDRS score in 1 year) in patients with DLB with early parkinsonism. A postural instability-gait difficulty (PIGD) motor phenotype is overrepresented in DLB (and dementia associated with PD) compared with PD patients with no dementia. In one cross-sectional study, 69% of 26 patients with DLB were classified as PIGD phenotype, compared with only 30% of 38 patients with PD (Burn et al., 2003). The involvement of brain-stem cholinergic nuclei, notably the pedunculopontine nucleus, may be responsible for the expression of this phenotype.

A supranuclear gaze paresis has been described in DLB (Fearnley et al., 1991; de Bruin et al., 1992). In combination with cognitive impairment and falls, this may cause diagnostic confusion with progressive supranuclear palsy. It may sometimes be difficult to ascertain, however, whether the patient with DLB has a true gaze paresis, oculomotor apraxia, or is simply inattentive to the examiner's command.

Sleep disorders

Rapid-eye-movement (REM) sleep behavior disorder (RBD) is a common sleep disturbance in neurodegenerative disorders (Schenck et al., 1993; Sforza et al., 1997; Olson et al., 2000). It is characterized by loss of normal skeletal muscle atonia during REM sleep with resultant motor activity and "acting out of dreams." Patients demonstrate a variety of movements ranging from verbal outbursts to pugilistic movements and even more dramatic motor activity. Injuries to patients and bed partners are common.

REM sleep behavior disorder can present in isolation, that is, not in association with concurrent medical diagnoses, or in the context of medical, and often neurological, disorders. The former is termed "idiopathic" and the latter "secondary." There is a marked sex difference in reported cases of RBD. Over 85% of patients in several large case series were male (Olson et al., 2000; Schenck and Mahowald, 2002), and this male preponderance is also seen in the "secondary" neurodegenerative cases (Iranzo et al., 2006; Boeve, Silber, Parisi, et al., 2003). The reason for this difference is not clear but may reflect a less "aggressive" clinical phenotype in females, leading to fewer medical consultations (Schenck and Mahowald, 2002).

The diagnosis is made on clinical grounds and careful questioning of bed partners is therefore vital. Clinical suspicion may then be backed up by video polysomnography (PSG), utilizing audiovisual footage to confirm the physical features of RBD in addition to electromyography, electro-oculography, electroencephalogram (EEG), and oxygen saturation recordings during sleep. The diagnostic criteria are summarized in Table 62.1.

Estimates from prospective studies in specialist centers place the frequency of RBD at 50%–80% in DLB (Boeve et al., 2004). Prospective population-based studies are needed to assess the true incidence and prevalence of RBD in neurodegenerative disorders in general, and DLB, PD, and MSA in particular. Several studies (Wetter et al., 2000; Boeve et al., 2001; Gagnon et al., 2002; Iranzo et al., 2005) have demonstrated that RBD is common in conditions associated with the intraneuronal deposition of α-synuclein (synucleinopathies such as PD, MSA, and DLB), and this is in contrast to the nonsynucleinopathies such as Progressive Supranuclear Palsy (PSP) and AD (Boeve et al., 2001). This finding has been backed up by several studies in AD (Gagnon et al., 2006) that found clinically evident RBD to be uncommon in patients with AD. In their autopsy study of 15 patients with RBD and a neurodegenerative disorder (Boeve, Silber, and Ferman, 2003), 10 (66.7%) had a diagnosis of RBD predating the development of dementia or parkinsonism by a median of 10 years (range 2 to 29). The neuropathologic diagnoses were LB disease in 12 and MSA in 3. Iranzo et al. (2006) retrospectively assessed 44 consecutive patients diagnosed with idiopathic RBD for the subsequent development of neurodegenerative disorders. Twenty (45%) patients developed a neurological disorder, predominantly PD (9) and DLB (6) and mild cognitive impairment with prominent visuospatial dysfunction (4), after a mean of over 11 years from reported onset of RBD symptoms (range 5–23).

The suggestion that RBD may provide an early clue to the development of "synucleinopathy" in patients who are otherwise asymptomatic may allow insight into the early pathophysiology of these conditions as well as provide better diagnostic accuracy and the potential for earlier treatment when this becomes available. For these reasons, the presence of RBD has now been included in the new consensus criteria for the diagnosis to DLB as a "suggestive" feature (McKeith et al., 2005).

TABLE 62.1 *The Recently Published Second Edition of the International Classification of Sleep Disorders Requires the Following for the Clinical Diagnosis of RBD*

Presence of RSWA on PSG
At least one of the following:
sleep-related, injurious, potentially injurious, or disruptive behaviors by history (that is, dream enactment behavior) and/or
abnormal REM sleep behavior documented during polysomnographic monitoring.
Absence of EEG epileptiform activity during REM sleep unless RBD can be clearly distinguished from any concurrent REM sleep-related seizure disorder.
The sleep disorder is not better explained by another sleep disorder, medical or neurological disorder, mental disorder, medication use, or substance use disorder.

Source: Taken from: American Academy of Sleep Medicine, 2005.

EEG: electroencephalogram; PSG: polysomongram; REM: rapid eye movement; RSWA: REM sleep without atonia.

Autonomic Features

Falls are an important feature of DLB, with over one third of patients suffering more than 20 per year (Ballard et al., 1999). One of the most common causes of falls is abnormal cardiovascular autonomic function, which may predate the onset of parkinsonism and dementia by several years or develop with other clinical features (Kaufmann et al., 2004). Orthostatic hypotension and carotid sinus hypersensitivity are common in DLB (Ballard et al., 1998) and associated with burden of hyperintense lesions on magnetic resonance imaging (MRI) brain scanning (Ballard, O'Brien, Barber, et al., 2000). Patients with DLB demonstrate impairment of sympathetic and parasympathetic function on autonomic testing (Allan et al., 2007), and these changes are associated with reduced cardiac uptake of ^{123}I-meta-iodobenzylguanidine (MIBG), a marker of postganglionic myocardial sympathetic innervation (Oka et al., 2007). Yoshita and colleagues (2006) examined cardiac MIBG scans in 37 patients with DLB and 42 with AD compared to controls. Uptake was significantly reduced in the DLB group compared to AD and control groups. In contrast, no significant differences were found between patients with AD and controls. This suggests a possible use for cardiac MIBG scanning in differentiating DLB from AD, although further work is required. Other autonomic symptoms include urinary incontinence, constipation, erectile dysfunction, and eating and swallowing difficulties (Horimoto et al., 2003, Thaisetthawatkul et al., 2004).

CLINICAL DIAGNOSIS

Consensus clinical diagnostic criteria were first published in 1996 and were updated in 1999 and, most recently, in 2005 (Table 62.2). The criteria characterize the central feature of DLB as a progressive disorder in which episodic memory impairment is often minimal in the early stages, whereas attentional, executive, and visuospatial deficits may be disproportionately prominent (McKeith et al., 1996). The presence of two or more of three core clinical features (fluctuating attention and alertness, recurrent visual hallucinations, parkinsonism), together with the variable presence of suggestive or supportive features, indicates probable DLB. Suggestive features now included in the criteria are RBD, severe neuroleptic sensitivity, and abnormal dopamine (DA) uptake on single photon emission computed tomography (SPECT) or positron emission tomography (PET) imaging. These have a similar diagnostic weighting as the core features but require further validation before being considered sufficient for a diagnosis of probable DLB without the presence of core features. Features considered as supportive of a diagnosis of DLB (listed in Table 62.2) and discussed in this chapter lack specificity because they may also occur in a variety of other disorders (McKeith et al., 1999).

When DLB presents as a primary dementia syndrome, the key differential diagnoses are AD, VaD, delirium secondary to systemic or pharmacological toxicity, prion disease, or other neurodegenerative syndromes. In these circumstances, consensus guidelines for the clinical diagnosis of DLB have been shown to have prospective diagnostic accuracy at least as good as those for AD. Their discriminating value is greatest at an early stage, suggesting that DLB should be considered in any new dementia presentation (McKeith, Ballard, et al., 2000). Inability of patients with DLB who are moderately impaired to copy pentagons accurately has been reported with a sensitivity of 88% and a specificity of 59% compared with AD, suggesting this as a useful screening test (Ala et al., 2001). As described above, EPS are strong diagnostic indicators because parkinsonism is uncommon in early AD or VaD (Ballard, O'Brien, Swann, et al., 2000).

The DLB Consortium recommended that if a patient has had motor symptoms of PD for more than 1 year prior to the diagnosis of dementia, then a diagnosis of PDD is most appropriate. If mental symptoms occur within 12 months of onset of motor disability, then a primary diagnosis of DLB may be more appropriate. This approach is entirely consistent with guidelines for the clinical diagnosis of PD (Gelb et al., 1999) and, more recently, PDD (Emre et al., 2007). It should be remembered, however, that these different patterns of clinical presentation share similar underlying neurodegenerative pathologies, including abnormal α-synuclein deposition and formation of Lewy neurites/bodies. LB parkinsonism and DLB may thus represent a spectrum of LB syndromes. Attempts to draw absolute boundaries between them, such as the 12-month rule, are only arbitrary conventions designed to help in clinical practice because there is strong evidence that the clinical end points of DLB and PDD are similar (Mosimann et al., 2004; Mosimann et al., 2006)

INVESTIGATIONS

Clinical examination and investigations should establish the presence of cognitive, psychiatric, and neurological signs and exclude hematological, biochemical, or pharmacological causes. The EEG is usually abnormal in DLB, with a greater degree of background slowing compared with AD, but this is too nonspecific to be of use in an individual case. Transient slow wave (delta) activity is seen in the temporal lobes of 50% of DLB cases (18% AD) and is associated with a clinical history of loss of consciousness (Briel et al., 1999). No clinically useful laboratory tests have yet been established for the diagnosis of DLB based on plasma or cerebrospinal fluid (CSF) analysis, although CSF Ab42 levels were decreased and tau levels were normal in 11 patients with clinically diagnosed DLB, compatible with the neuropathological findings of high-plaque but low-tangle counts in the DLB brain (Kanemaru et al., 2000).

Neuroimaging

Structural imaging changes in dementia with lewy bodies

Relatively few studies to date have investigated computed tomography (CT) or MRI changes in DLB. An initial report of eight patients diagnosed as having AD during life but with LB pathology at postmortem found more pronounced frontal lobe atrophy on CT than in pure AD cases (Förstl et al., 1993). Larger studies using MRI have failed to replicate this finding.

Instead, the main structural imaging change emerging as characteristic of DLB is relative preservation of the hippocampus and medial temporal lobe compared to the reduction seen in AD (Barber et al., 2000; Whitwell et al., 2007), possibly helping to explain the preservation of mnemonic function in such cases. Although hippocampal volume is slightly reduced, by about 15% compared to controls, the reduction is considerably less than that seen in AD, with some 40% of cases having no evidence of atrophy. Patients with DLB show relatively little cortical gray matter loss when compared to patients

TABLE 62.2 *Revised Criteria for the Clinical Diagnosis of Dementia with Lewy Bodies (DLB)*

1. *Central feature (essential for a diagnosis of possible or probable DLB)*

   Dementia defined as progressive cognitive decline of sufficient magnitude to interfere with normal social or occupational function. Prominent or persistent memory impairment may not necessarily occur in the early stages but is usually evident with progression. Deficits on tests of attention, executive function, and visuospatial ability may be especially prominent.

2. *Core features (two core features are sufficient for a diagnosis of probable DLB, one for possible DLB)*

   Fluctuating cognition with pronounced variations in attention and alertness

   Recurrent visual hallucinations that are typically well formed and detailed

   Spontaneous features of parkinsonism

3. *Suggestive features (If one or more of these is present in the presence of one or more core features, a diagnosis of probable DLB can be made. In the absence of any core features, one or more suggestive features is sufficient for possible DLB. Probable DLB should not be diagnosed on the basis of suggestive features alone.)*

   REM sleep behavior disorder

   Severe neuroleptic sensitivity

   Low dopamine transporter uptake in basal ganglia demonstrated by SPECT or PET imaging

4. *Supportive features (commonly present but not proven to have diagnostic specificity)*

   Repeated falls and syncope

   Transient, unexplained loss of consciousness

   Severe autonomic dysfunction, for example, orthostatic hypotension, urinary incontinence

   Hallucinations in other modalities

   Systematized delusions

   Depression

   Relative preservation of medial temporal lobe structures on CT/MRI scan

   Generalized low uptake on SPECT/PET perfusion scan with reduced occipital activity

   Abnormal (low uptake) MIBG myocardial scintigraphy

   Prominent slow wave activity on EEG with temporal lobe transient sharp waves

5. *A diagnosis of DLB is less likely*

   In the presence of cerebrovascular disease evident as focal neurologic signs or on brain imaging

   In the presence of any other physical illness or brain disorder sufficient to account in part or in total for the clinical picture

   If parkinsonism only appears for the first time at a stage of severe dementia

6. *Temporal sequence of symptoms*

   DLB should be diagnosed when dementia occurs before or concurrently with parkinsonism (if it is present). The term *Parkinson's disease with dementia* (PDD) should be used to describe dementia that occurs in the context of well-established Parkinson's disease. In a practice setting, the term that is most appropriate to the clinical situation should be used, and generic terms such as LB disease are often helpful. In research studies in which distinction needs to be made between DLB and PDD, the existing 1-year rule between the onset of dementia and parkinsonism DLB continues to be recommended. Adoption of other time periods will simply confound data pooling or comparison between studies. In other research settings that may include clinicopathologic studies and clinical trials, both clinical phenotypes may be considered collectively under categories such as LB disease or α-synucleinopathy.

From: McKeith et al., 2005.

REM: rapid-eye-movement; SPECT: single photon emission computed tomography; PET: positron emission tomography; CT: computed tomography; MRI: magnetic resonance imaging; MIBG: ^{123}I-meta-iodobenzylguanidine; EEG: electroencephalogram.

with AD (Whitwell et al., 2007). Rather, when 72 patients with DLB were compared to similar numbers with AD and age-matched controls, the most striking findings on volumetric analysis were focal atrophy of the midbrain, hypothalamus, and substantia inominata in DLB compared to a more generalized atrophy of the temporo-parietal cortex and medial temporal lobes in AD. It has been suggested that temporal lobe atrophy on MRI might be a marker of concurrent tangle pathology in DLB, although larger studies are needed to examine this issue further.

More general measures of atrophy have also been examined in DLB, with patients having a degree of ventricular enlargement similar to that seen in AD (Barber et al., 2000). The rate of volume loss over time using serial MRI has been studied, but no consistent pattern has emerged. O'Brien and colleagues (2001) found similar rates in DLB (1.4%) and AD (2.0%), though Whitwell et al. (2007) found "pure" DLB cases to have similar rates of progression to controls, with increased rates only seen in those with mixed DLB and AD pathology. White matter lesions (WML) are increased in AD and may contribute, together with degenerative pathology, to the severity of cognitive impairment. A similar increase has been described in DLB cases (Barber et al., 1999), although the effects on cognitive function have not yet been determined, though rates of WML progression over time are similar in DLB to AD (Burton et al., 2006).

Functional imaging changes in dementia with Lewy bodies

There have been several studies investigating PET and SPECT changes in DLB. Positron emission tomography studies of glucose metabolism and SPECT investigations using blood flow markers such as Tc-HMPAO have demonstrated many similarities to the patterns seen in AD (Donnemiller et al., 1997; Defebvre et al., 1999; Ishii et al., 1999; Lobotesis et al., 2001). Pronounced biparietal hypoperfusion is seen together with variable deficits in frontal and temporal lobes, which again are usually symmetric. Biparietal hypoperfusion in DLB is even more extensive than in patients with AD matched for age and dementia severity, particularly in Brodmann area 7, an area that mediates important aspects of visuospatial function. Similar patterns of hypoperfusion in the parieto-occipital cortex are seen in patients with DLB and PDD and differ from those in AD (Firbank et al., 2003). Pronounced hypoperfusion in this area may underpin the pronounced visuospatial impairments characteristic of DLB.

Occipital hypometabolism on PET and hypoperfusion on PET and SPECT have been strongly associated with DLB and appear to affect primary visual cortex as well as visual association areas (Brodmann areas 17–19). In contrast, temporal lobe perfusion is relatively preserved, paralleling the findings from structural imaging studies described above. Minoshima and colleagues (2001) reported a sensitivity of 90% and a specificity of 80% for occipital hypometabolism in separating DLB from AD, although only 11 DLB cases were studied. In a larger SPECT study, occipital hypoperfusion had reasonable specificity (86%) in distinguishing DLB from AD and controls, although sensitivity was lower at 64% (Lobotesis et al., 2001).

Labeling of muscarinic acetylcholine receptors using ^{123}I-iodo-quinuclidinyl-benzilate (QNB) has shown an increase in ^{123}I-QNB binding in the right occipital lobe in DLB and right and left occipital lobes in PDD using SPECT imaging (Colloby et al., 2006). It is uncertain whether such occipital changes are related to the occurrence of visual hallucinations.

Studies using PET and SPECT have also investigated changes in the dopaminergic and cholinergic systems. Donnemiller and colleagues (1997) found significant reductions in DLB but not AD in striatal binding of β-carbomethoxy-iodophenyl-tropane (CIT), a ligand with high affinity for the dopamine transporter (DAT), using PET. One disadvantage of CIT is that imaging has to be delayed until 24 hours postinjection. A ligand with faster imaging kinetics, FP (fluoropropyl)-CIT, is now commercially available in many countries and demonstrates DAT reductions even in patients with early PD.

The results of several trials have demonstrated the clinical utility of FP-CIT SPECT in the diagnosis of DLB (Z. Walker et al., 2002; O'Brien et al., 2004). A large, multicenter phase III trial of the technique has been completed (McKeith et al., 2007). Comparing DLB and non-DLB dementia (predominantly AD), abnormal scans had a sensitivity of 77.7% for detecting clinically probable DLB, with a specificity of 90.4% for excluding non-DLB dementia and an overall diagnostic accuracy of 85.7%. Evidence of abnormal DAT activity in the basal ganglia on FP-CIT SPECT scanning has now been incorporated into the Consensus Criteria for DLB as a suggestive feature.

In addition, O'Brien et al. (2004) and Z. Walker et al. (2004) have shown that the pattern of abnormality on FP-CIT SPECT is different in PD and DLB, with more marked reduction of dopaminergic uptake in the caudate head in DLB and PDD compared to PD. In contrast, patients with PD demonstrate greater asymmetry of uptake in the posterior putamina. The lack of asymmetry on FP-CIT SPECT imaging in DLB may help to explain the symmetrical motor features often seen in DLB as well as the association between symmetrical parkinsonism and dementia. Reduced DA D_2 receptor density in basal ganglia using ^{123}I iodobenzamide has also been reported in DLB (Z. Walker et al., 1997).

Neuropsychological Assessment

Increased variability

Dementia with Lewy bodies is characterized by increased variability in performance on cognitive tasks, within and between patients and when compared to age-matched controls and patients with AD (Ballard, O'Brien, Gray, et al., 2001; Ballard, O'Brien, Morris, et al., 2001; Collerton et al., 2005). This variability is particularly evident in executive and attentional tasks. Too few studies have compared DLB with PD or VaD to allow a clear pattern to emerge. This may partly reflect the more variable pathology of DLB, but it is also a feature of the fluctuations that characterize the disease process itself. The effects of these fluctuations are reflected not only in an increase in the variance of scores in DLB groups, but also in the conflicting findings reported on the same tasks.

Differences in performances on specific tasks

In terms of group differences, patients with DLB always do worse than age-matched controls on neuropsychological tasks, with particularly poor performance on visual perceptual and learning tasks, visual semantic tasks, and praxis tasks. Simple global measures of performance (for example, the MMSE) are usually equivalent to those of patients with AD of comparable severity, perhaps reflecting the insensitivity of these measures to attentional impairments. Patients with DLB tend to perform better than patients with AD on verbal memory and orientation tasks. Performance on visual tasks, particularly recognition tasks, is consistently more impaired than in AD (for detailed reviews, see Simard et al., 2000; Lambon et al., 2001; Collerton et al., 2005). The pattern is reversed in comparisons with PD, with patients with DLB generally performing worse in all areas except visual and motor tasks.

Effects of progression on the disease process

Neuropsychological changes as DLB progresses are not well characterized, though differences from AD appear to be particularly pronounced in the early stages and lessen as the disease progresses. Rate of progression, as evidenced by change in global cognitive measures such as the MMSE or Cambridge Cognitive Examination (CAMCOG), is equivalent to or faster than that seen in AD and VaD, with a decline of 4–5 MMSE points per year (Simard et al., 2000; Ballard, O'Brien, Morris, et al., 2001; Johnson et al., 2005).

Clinical utility of neuropsychological assessment

Given that similar tasks have produced different results in different studies, and that effect sizes in comparison with patient groups are generally below 1, single test performances cannot be used in isolation to distinguish between DLB and other dementing illnesses. Patterns of performance on verbal and visuospatial tasks can be used to reliably classify prediagnosed groups of patients with DLB, AD, and VaD. Although the predictive value of test results in the general dementia population is not established, preliminary results are encouraging (Tiraboschi et al., 2006).

At present, the major utility of the neuropsychological assessment of DLB is in defining the effects of this variable disease on the individual patient, to allow the development of evidence-based rehabilitative or compensatory strategies and to monitor progression in that patient.

NEUROPATHOLOGY

Described as the neuropathological hallmark of PD by Friedrich Lewy in 1912, Lewy bodies were first associated with dementia in 1961 by Okazaki et al. Lewy bodies are spherical, intracytoplasmic, eosinophilic, neuronal inclusions with a dense hyaline core and a clear halo. On electron microscopy (EM), they are composed of a core of filamentous and granular material surrounded by radially oriented filaments 10–20 nm in diameter. Subcortical LBs are easily seen using conventional hematoxylin and eosin staining. The presence of LBs in pigmented brain stem nuclei, and in the substantia nigra (SN) in particular, coupled with neuronal loss and gliosis, constitute the characteristic pathological findings in the prototypic LB disease, PD.

Cortical LBs lack the characteristic core and halo appearance of their brain-stem counterparts and were difficult to detect until the late 1980s, when anti-ubiquitin immunocytochemical staining methods allowed their frequency to be determined (Lennox and Lowe, 1997). Ubiquitin antibodies also identified Lewy neurites (LNs) in the hippocampal CA2/3 region of DLB, which were absent in AD. More recently, the presynaptic protein α-synuclein was shown to be a major component of cortical and subcortical LBs and neurites (Spillantini et al., 1997). α-synuclein antibodies label greater numbers of cortical and hippocampal CA2/3 LNs and intraneuronal inclusions than ubiquitin, including fine granular and diffuse deposits and LBs, indicating that accumulation of α-synuclein precedes its ubiquitination (Spillantini et al., 1998; Gómez-Tortosa, Newell, et al., 2000). α-Synuclein antibodies have also identified novel non-ubiquitinated inclusions in hippocampal pyramidal cells of patients with DLB.

Purified LBs contain full-length as well as partially truncated forms and high molecular aggregates of α-synuclein (Baba et al., 1998). Using EM, immunoreactivity to α-synuclein is associated with filaments 5–10 nm wide and 50–700 nm long (Baba et al., 1998). α-synuclein is a widespread neuronal presynaptic protein found in the central nervous system, Schwann cells, cultured oligodendrocytes, platelets, and CSF. Monomeric α-synuclein exists in equilibrium between free and plasma membrane- or vesicle-bound states (McLean et al., 2000). One of α-synuclein protein's crucial functions in vivo is the protection of the nerve terminals against injury via cooperation with cystein string protein (CSPα and soluble *N*-Ethylmaleimide-sensitive factor (NSF) (Bonini and Giasson, 2005). This may play a role in the prevention of neuronal neurodegeneration because α-synuclein abolishes the lethality and neurodegeneration caused by deletion of CSPα and maintains soluble NSF attachment receptor (SNARE) complex assembly (Chandra et al., 2005).

Over-expression of α-synuclein in neuronal cell lines results in changes in membrane fluidity and changes cellular fatty acid uptake and metabolism (Sharon et al., 2003; Castagnet et al., 2005; Golovko et al., 2005), with the earliest defects being inhibition of endoplasmic reticulum-associated degeneration (Cooper et al., 2006). Its self-aggregation and filament formation is extensively modulated by environmental factors (Uversky, 2007).

Prior to assembly into filaments, α-synuclein protein may undergo a transition from a random coil to a β-pleated sheet conformation (Serpell et al., 2000). In vitro studies show that α-synuclein is more likely to self-aggregate when it is overexpressed (Stefanova et al., 2002) or in the presence of some coadjuvant factors (for example, amyloid protein, metal ions, trifluorethanol, septons, heparin, agrin, oxidative stress, low pH, proteosomal inhibition, constituents of chromatin, etc.). The overexpression of α-synuclein also results in selective nigral DA neuronal loss, restricted to the embryogenesis (Wakamatsu et al., 2007).

Post-translational modifications of α-synuclein (for example, phosphorylation, nitration, lipoxidation) also promote fibril formation (Fujiwara et al., 2002; Dalfó and Ferrer, 2008). Phosphorylation of this protein is present in 26% of the elderly human brains and is found in LBs, LNs, white matter axons, and dot-like structures similar to argyrophilic grains. Nitrated α-synuclein is found in cortical LBs and dystrophic neurites in SN and hippocampal neurons that show diffuse cytoplasmic staining (Gómez-Tortosa et al., 2002), suggesting that nitration may be a prerequisite for α-synuclein aggregation. Diffuse presence of nitrated α-synuclein has now been described in the frontal lobe in Pick's disease in the absence of LB formation (Dalfó et al., 2006).

The presence of a large number of other neuronal proteins within LBs may provide further clues to their formation. Cytoskeletal proteins, such as neurofilaments, and microtubules are thought to become trapped within the α-synuclein fibrillary aggregates. The presence of ubiquitin, a cofactor in the ubiquitin-proteasome system of intracellular proteolysis, and catalytic enzymes are considered part of a cell stress response to eliminate abnormal and damaged proteins from cells. Most recently, chaperone proteins, like parkin (a ubiquitin-protein ligase), torsin A, and heat shock proteins (for example, HSP70) known to participate in refolding misfolded proteins and/or directing proteins towards degradation have been also localized in brain stem and cortical LBs and neurites (McNaught and Jenner, 2001; Uryu et al., 2006; Leverenz et al., 2007). These findings, together with the evidence that in the SN of patients with PD, the ubiquitin-proteasome pathway is impaired, have been interpreted to indicate that altered protein handling leads to accumulation of damaged α-synuclein within LBs and to neuronal degeneration (McNaught and Jenner, 2001).

In the hippocampus of patients with DLB and patients with PD, axon pathology involves not only α- but also β- and γ-synuclein (Galvin et al., 1999). Antibodies to β-synuclein reveal accumulations of vesicles in presynaptic mossy fiber terminals of the hippocampal hilus, and antibodies to γ-synuclein detect axonal spheroid-like structures in the dentate molecular layer. Animal and tissue culture studies suggest that β-synuclein may be neuroprotective. Thus, the formation of LBs and motor function deficits are significantly ameliorated in α- and β-synuclein bigenic mice compared to single α-synuclein transgenic mice (Hashimoto et al., 2001; Fan et al., 2006). In tissue culture, the overexpression of β-synuclein directly inhibits α-synuclein aggregation and protofibrillar formation of α-synuclein (Hashimoto et al., 2001; Uversky et al., 2002; Park and Lansbury, 2003). This has been further confirmed in vitro, with β-synuclein dimmers blocking the aggregation of α-synuclein into ring-like oligomers, and also disrupting the already formed α-synuclein aggregates (Tsigelny et al., 2007). In contrast, the overexpression of β-synuclein mutants (P123H and V70M) enhances lysosomal pathology (Wei et al., 2007), and this may play a role in stimulating neurodegeneration. Although γ-synuclein inhibits α-synuclein aggregation (Uversky et al., 2002), its role in neuroprotection is not well understood.

Neuropathological Criteria for DLB

High cortical senile plaque counts are found in the majority of patients with DLB, but their composition differs from those found in pure AD. When present, the dystrophic neurites decorating plaques in DLB are α-synuclein immunoreactive and seldom tau immunoreactive. In 80%–90% of DLB cases, there is no evidence of significant neocortical tau pathology, paired helical filaments, or neurofibrillary tangles (Harrington et al., 1994). Whether or not DLB is considered to be a variant of AD depends upon the pathological definition of AD being used. When using the 1996 DLB criteria (which required only the presence of LB for the pathologic diagnosis) and the Consortium to Establish a Registry for Alzheimer's Disease (CERAD) criteria for AD (a definition of AD that is heavily dependent upon plaque density), 77% of the cases would fulfill both diagnoses. By contrast, 80%–90% of cases would fail to fulfill definitions of AD requiring supra-threshold numbers of neocortical neurofibrillary tangles (E.K. Perry, Smith, et al., 1990).

These findings, alongside with clinical studies showing clinical diagnostic accuracy for DLB to be higher in patients with low-burden AD pathology (Del Ser et al., 2001; Lopez et al., 2002; Merdes et al., 2003), have resulted in a recent revision of the neuropathological criteria for diagnosing DLB (McKeith et al., 2005). This combines the National Institute on Aging (NIA)/Reagan criteria and the modified Consensus DLB guidelines, based on semiquantitative assessment of α-synuclein pathology. Thus, these revised criteria acknowledge that a pathological diagnosis of both diseases should be made on a probabilistic basis, taking into account the extent and the contribution of the different pathological findings (Table 62.3).

Neuropathological assessment of clinical cases of DLB should evaluate Lewy and AD-type pathology to pro-

TABLE 62.3 *Assessment of Likelihood of LB and Alzheimer Pathologies to Be Associated with DLB Clinical Syndrome*

Lewy Body Pathology	*Alzheimer-Type Pathology*		
	NIA-Reagan Low (BST 0-II)	*NIA-Reagan Intermediate (BST III-IV)*	*NIA-Reagan High (BST V-VI)*
Brain-stem predominant	Low	Low	Low
Limbic (transitional)	High	Intermediate	Low
Diffuse neocortical	High	High	Intermediate

From: Mckeith et al., 2005.
DLB: dementia with Lewy bodies; BST: Braak stage; NIA: National Institute on Aging.

vide a degree of likelihood (high, intermediate, or low) that α-synuclein pathology is underlying the clinical syndrome. A diagnosis of DLB becomes less likely as AD-related pathology, staged by NIA/Reagan criteria, increases. According to the new revised criteria, DLB and pure AD will be pathologically distinct in the majority of cases. The validity of the newly proposed criteria still needs to be tested in clinico-neuropathological studies.

Clinico-pathological Correlations

Cognitive and neuropsychiatric correlations

The relationship between cognitive impairment and neuropathological features characteristic for DLB is not clear. In DLB and PDD, severity of cognitive impairment is positively correlated with the density of cortical LBs in frontal and temporal lobes and with the density of LNs in the hippocampal CA2 field, though not with LB density in anterior cingulate cortex (Gómez-Tortosa et al., 1999; Hurtig et al., 2000). However, the contribution of AD pathology (when analyzed according to Braak stages) seems, in some instances, to prevail over the LB staging (Welsman et al., 2007). Fluctuating cognition, in contrast, shows no correlation with LB density in either neocortical, paralimbic, or nigral areas (Gómez-Tortosa et al., 1999). The nucleus basalis of Meynert shows more profound neuron loss in DLB than in AD, as well as extensive LB/α-synuclein pathology, and is therefore likely to contribute significantly to the cognitive decline in DLB (Lippa et al., 1999).

Noncognitive changes in DLB appear to be independent of the presence of LBs. No significant regional differences in LB densities have been reported between cases with and without cognitive fluctuation, hallucinations, delusions, recurrent falls (Gómez-Tortosa, Irizarry et al., 2000), and delusional misidentification (Förstl et al., 1994). Neuropathological studies in patients with DLB and well-formed visual hallucinations (VH) have demonstrated high LB densities in the amygdala and parahippocampus, with early hallucinations relating to higher densities in parahippocampal and inferior temporal cortices (Harding et al., 2002). A higher burden of LBs in the amygdala and in frontal, temporal, and parietal neocortex is also present in patients with PD with VH (Papapetropoulos et al., 2006). However, these findings have not been replicated in a recent DLB study (Yamamoto et al., 2007). Depression, frequently reported in DLB, appears not to be associated with cortical and subcortical LBs (Samuels et al., 2004). However, late-onset major depression appears to be related to the frequent presence of LB pathology (Sweet et al., 2004), whereas presence of LBs in the amygdala in AD increases significantly the risk of developing major depression (odds ratio [OR] = 8.56) (Lopez et al., 2006).

Neurological correlations

The density of LB in the SN does not differ significantly between cases starting with parkinsonism and those evolving initially with dementia (Gómez-Tortosa et al., 1999). Mild or moderate neuron loss in SN has been found to be restricted to DLB cases without parkinsonism, whereas DLB cases with parkinsonism have shown neuron loss in the ventrolateral tier of SN of similar severity to that seen in PD. Brain-stem LBs seem to underlie the presence of essential tremor in some patients with DLB and PD (Louis et al., 2006).

Other features

Although the increased falls reported in DLB may be multifactorial, it is likely that more widespread brain-stem involvement of nondopaminergic nuclei is a contributing factor. Degeneration of the predominantly cholinergic pedunculopontine nucleus and minimal involvement of the SN and locus coeruleus (LC), harboring LBs and LNs but no overt neuronal loss, is a likely candidate because neuronal loss in this structure has been associated with postural instability (Zweig et al., 1989).

Pathologic studies in RBD have suggested dysfunction of one or several brain-stem neuronal pathways. Candidate sites include the SN, LC-subcoeruleus complex, pedunculopontine, dorsal vagus and dorsal raphé nucleus, and the gigantocellular reticular nucleus (Uchiyama et al., 1995; Turner et al., 2000). These nuclei utilize a number of neurotransmitters including dopminergic, noradrenergic, cholinergic, and serotoninergic connections, all of which may play a role in the development of RBD. Eisensehr and colleagues (2003) demonstrated abnormalities in DAT SPECT in patients with subclinical and clinically evident RBD, with increasing severity of abnormality in those patients with overt RBD. These changes are similar to those seen in idiopathic PD. Unfortunately, the numbers of cases in which pathological information is available is small, and more work is necessary to elucidate these complex interactions further.

The pathological correlates for autonomic dysfunction in DLB are likely to be similar to those in cases with pure autonomic failure, where pathology includes neuronal loss, LB, and LN in autonomic nuclei of the brain stem, intermediolateral cell columns of the spinal cord, and sympathetic and parasympathetic ganglia. Indeed, a recent pathological study suggests that the common presence of α-synuclein aggregates in peripheral autonomic neurons and adrenal glands may represent an early presymptomatic phase in the development of LB disorders (Minguez-Castellanos et al., 2007; Fumimura et al., 2007). Carotid sinus hypersensitivity, consisting of falls and dizziness, is highly prevalent in DLB and other neurodegenerative disorders, including AD and PD. The neuropathological correlate of this is hyperphosphorylated tau in tyrosine hydroxylase-containing neurons (catecholaminergic neurons), in the absence of neuronal loss (Miller et al., 2007).

NEUROCHEMISTRY

Dementia with Lewy bodies has more severe and widespread cholinergic deficits than AD, but postsynaptic receptor coupling is intact; and though DA loss is not as great in DLB as in PD, the "compensatory" changes in the DA system that occur in PD are absent in DLB. Clinical differences between AD and DLB/PDD reflect distinct neurochemical profiles underlying specific symptoms and having treatment implications such as response to cholinesterase inhibitors and levodopa, and neuroleptic sensitivity.

The Dopaminergic System

Presynaptic dopaminergic measures

Reduced SN neuron density and low DA concentration in the caudate nucleus were early reports in DLB (E.K. Perry, Marshall, Perry, et al., 1990; R.H. Perry, Irving, et al., 1990; Marshall et al., 1994). Subsequently, DA concentration and DATs have been shown to be reduced in posterior striatum even in DLB cases with no EPS (Piggott et al., 1999; Piggott et al., in press) (Fig. 62.1). Dopamine loss in DLB is less selectively focused on the posterior putamen than in PD, and the caudate is more affected (Piggott et al., 1999). This reflects the pattern of SN neuron loss, with relative sparing of the medial SN in PD. Substantia nigra and DAT loss in DLB are also more symmetric between hemispheres than in PD (Ransmayr et al., 2001; O'Brien et al., 2004; Z. Walker et al., 2004). Dopamine transporter loss affecting caudate and putamen rostrocaudally in DLB has been shown in vivo (Z. Walker et al., 2004; Colloby et al., 2005), and imaging DAT by SPECT and PET can assist differentiation of DLB from AD (Hu et al., 2000; O'Brien et al., 2004; Z. Walker et al., 2007), and such an abnormal scan is now part of the Consensus Criteria as a suggestive feature (McKeith et al., 2007).

Reduced nigrostriatal DA is the most likely substrate for the parkinsonism of DLB. It may be that moderate reduction in dopaminergic input results in more severe EPS in DLB than it would in PD because there is a lack of compensatory changes such as increased turn-

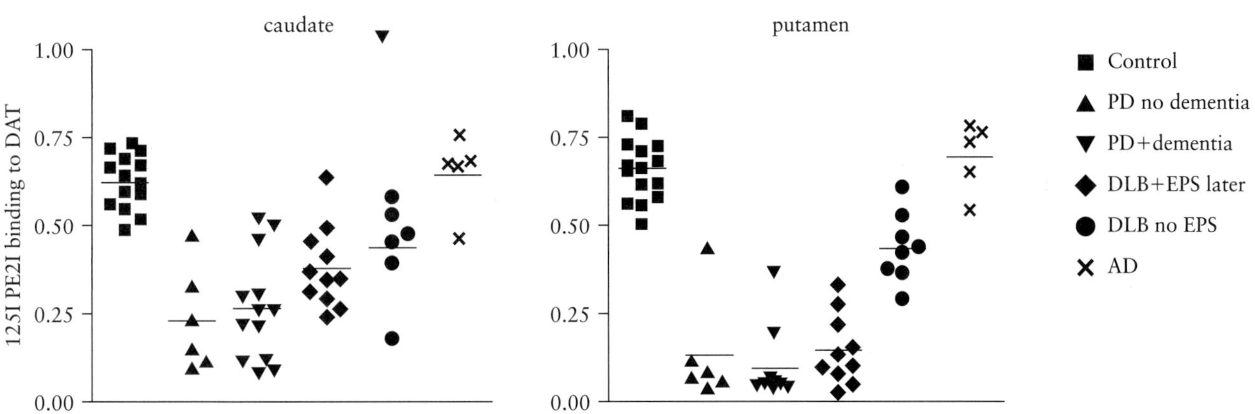

FIGURE 62.1 Dopamine transporter density (fmol 125I PE 2I/mg tissue) in striatum from cases of PD without dementia, PDD, DLB with EPS later, DLB without EPS, AD, and normal elderly control tissue.
Source: Piggot et al., in press.

over of DA and up-regulation of D_2 receptors, which occur in PD (Piggott et al., 1999). Nigrothalamic DA is also likely to be reduced in DLB. The thalamus receives DA via nigro-caudate collaterals, which show depleted DAT immunoreactivity in the 1-methyl-4-phenyl-1,2,3,6-tetrahydropyridine (MPTP)-treated monkey model of PD (Freeman et al., 2001). Other neurotransmitter system changes probably contribute to the movement disorder of DLB, as evidenced by the axial predominance and relative levodopa resistance (Bonelli et al., 2004).

Postsynaptic dopaminergic measures

Striatal DA D_2 receptor density is up-regulated in PD without dementia by > 70% (Piggott et al., 1999) and is doubled in thalamus (Piggott, Ballard, Dickinson, et al., 2007). In DLB there is a slight reduction (↓17%) in D_2 density in the striatum (Piggott et al., 1999), with D_2 density lowest in cases that had severe neuroleptic sensitivity and slightly higher in cases tolerant of neuroleptics (Piggott et al., 1998); it may be that cases with lower D_2 density are more at risk of sudden catastrophic receptor blockade by the D_2 antagonist action of neuroleptics. Failure to up-regulate D_2 receptors in DLB could be due to intrinsic striatal pathology, with β-amyloid (Aβ) and synuclein pathology reported (Duda et al., 2002), or perhaps to deficits in other systems, for example in thalamo-striatal afferents or the cholinergic system.

In the thalamus there is lower D_2 binding in all regions in DLB without EPS; in DLB with EPS there is limited, slight but significant up-regulation in two nuclei only; whereas in PDD cases moderate, significant up-regulation occurs in the motor ventrointermedius nucleus alone (Piggott, Ballard, Dickinson, et al., 2007). Thalamic D_2 receptor binding in DLB and PDD does not vary with cognitive decline or visual hallucinations but is significantly higher with increased EPS (Piggott, Ballard, Dickinson, et al., 2007). In DLB and PDD there is higher thalamic D_2 binding in cases with FC, particularly in the reticular nucleus (Piggott, Ballard, Dickinson, et al., 2007). Inhibitory D_2 receptors located on reticular nucleus γ-aminobutyric acid (GABA)ergic neurons (also inhibitory) will therefore help maintain thalamic and cortical activity, thus enabling fluctuations. In an environment of reduced transmitter concentration, higher D_2 receptors can amplify small transmitter changes leading to variations in consciousness and attention. Similarly, nicotinic receptors were higher in some thalamic nuclei in cases with FC (Pimlott et al., 2006) (see below), possibly suggesting that combined cholinergic and dopaminergic therapy is required to treat FC in DLB.

In temporal cortex in DLB and PDD, D_2 receptors are significantly reduced (> 40%) and are also reduced in DLB cases with concomitant Alzheimer pathology, but are not reduced in pure AD (Piggott, Ballard, Rowan, et al., 2007). Reduced temporal cortical D_2 density correlated with cognitive decline but not with hallucinations or delusions, suggesting neuroleptic use would have a deleterious effect on cognition.

Dopamine D_1 and D_3 receptors in the striatum were not altered in DLB in a postmortem study mainly involving cases with little or no parkinsonism (Piggott et al., 1999).

The Cholinergic System

Presynaptic changes

Presynaptic cholinergic cortical activities are generally more reduced than in AD, and there are also losses in the striatum and in the projection from the pedunculopontine nucleus to the thalamus. As in AD, there is consistent involvement of the nucleus basalis of Meynert, but with LB pathology and more extensive cell loss (Tiraboschi et al., 2000). In the cortex, choline acetyltransferase (ChAT) and acetyl cholinesterase (AChE) (the synthesizing and degrading enzymes of acetylcholine) losses determined postmortem exceed those in AD (in which they are particularly pronounced in the hippocampus) and are apparent early in the disease course (E.K. Perry, Kerwin, et al., 1990; E.K. Perry, Marshall, Kerwin, et al., 1990; Tiraboschi et al., 2002). Cholinergic losses are correlated with cognitive decline in DLB (E.K. Perry, Marshall, Perry, et al., 1990; Samuel et al., 1997; Tiraboschi et al., 2002), and in PD (E.K. Perry et al., 1985; Mattila et al., 2001; Bohnen et al., 2006). Choline acetyltransferase deficits are greater in some visual cortical areas in DLB cases with visual hallucinations compared to those without (E.K. Perry, Kerwin, et al., 1990; Ballard, Piggott, et al., 2000).

Neocortical binding to nicotinic acetylcholine receptors (nAChRs) containing $\alpha4$ and $\beta2$ subunits ($\alpha4^*$ and $\beta2^*$) is reduced in DLB and AD (E.K. Perry, Smith, et al., 1990; Gotti et al., 2006), but unlike AD, in DLB there is an apparent correlation between this nAChR deficit and cortical ChAT reduction (Reid et al., 2000). Somewhat surprisingly, nAChR binding is relatively preserved in the temporal cortex (and in thalamus) in cases of DLB with FC (Ballard, Court, et al., 2002; Pimlott et al., 2006). Because patients with FC are able to be more alert some of the time, the neurotransmitter systems must be capable of reaching the higher level of awareness. When cholinergic losses are severe, a higher density of nicotinic receptors may enable small transmitter fluctuations to lead to variations in consciousness and attention. Whether cortical $\alpha7^*$ receptors are reduced generally in DLB is equivocal (Reid et al., 2000; Gotti et al., 2006), but it is most likely to occur in DLB cases with hallucinations (Court et al., 2001).

In the striatum nAChRs are more reduced in DLB and PD than in AD, notably $\alpha6^*$, $\alpha4^*$, $\beta2^*$, and $\beta3^*$ subtypes (Gotti et al., 2006). Reduced nAChR binding in striatum (partly on dopaminergic terminals) is as severe in DLB as in PD (E.K. Perry et al., 1995; Gotti et al., 2006), perhaps indicating that loss of these receptors occur at an early stage of nigrostriatal degeneration (E.K. Perry et al., 1995). In contrast, $\alpha 4^{*}\beta 2^{*}$ nAChRs were not generally reduced in the thalamus in DLB (although there were reductions in PD), significant deficits only being observed in cases without FC (Pimlott et al., 2006). Reduced $\alpha 7$ receptor binding has been noted in the thalamic reticular nucleus in DLB (and in AD), a region innervated by cholinergic neurons from the basal forebrain (Court et al., 1999).

Loss of nAChRs in DLB is likely to reflect reduced cholinergic innervation (cortex and thalamus), dopaminergic innervation (striatum), and also attenuation of pre- and postsynaptic receptors on glutamatergic, GABAergic, and serotonergic neurons.

Muscarinic receptor changes

Postsynaptically, there is less neuronal damage in DLB than in AD (Tiraboschi et al., 2000; O'Brien et al., 2001). Type 1 cortical muscarinic receptors (M1), unchanged or slightly reduced in severe AD and with defective coupling, have been reported to be up-regulated in temporal and parietal cortex in DLB (E.K. Perry, Smith, et al., 1990; Ballard, Piggott, Johnson, et al., 2000) and higher in frontal cortex in PDD and DLB compared to AD (Warren et al., 2008). M1 up-regulation in temporal cortex in DLB is associated with delusions (Ballard, Piggott, Johnson, et al., 2000). Coupling to G protein–second-messenger systems is preserved in DLB compared to AD in temporal cortex (E.K. Perry et al., 1998) and in frontal cortex (Warren et al., 2008). In contrast, immunohistochemical M1 expression is reduced in selected subfields of hippocampus (Shiozaki et al., 2001). Unlike in cortex, striatal M1 receptor binding is reduced, in parallel with D_2 receptors, in DLB (M1 and D_2 are distributed mainly on the same population of striatal projection neurons) (Piggott et al., 2003).

M2 receptor binding was higher in cingulate cortex compared to controls, and higher M2 and M4 cingulate binding was associated with visual hallucinations (Teaktong et al., 2005). M4 receptors are raised in cingulate in DLB with FC (Teaktong et al., 2005), and in the insular cortex with the symptom of delusions, whereas in thalamus M4 receptors are reduced in DLB (Warren et al., 2007).

Cholinesterase inhibitor therapy may be particularly successful in DLB for a constellation of reasons, including up-regulated, efficiently coupled cortical M1 receptors, severely reduced acetylcholine, little or no cortical atrophy or tangle burden, the potential for higher function to be stabilized in patients with FC, and low M1 receptors in striatum avoiding worsening EPS.

Serotonin

LB pathology and neuron loss have been reported in the raphé nucleus in DLB (Langlais et al., 1993), but not always (Benarroch et al., 2005), and reduced serotonin (5-HT) has been reported in striatum and cortex in DLB (Langlais et al., 1993; E.K. Perry et al., 1993; Ohara et al., 1998). Serotonin transporter binding is reduced (70%) in temporal and parietal cortex in DLB, and 5-HT_{2A} receptors are reduced by 50% in putamen in PD (Piggott et al., 2000), with 5-HT_{2A} receptors also reduced in temporal cortex in DLB and PDD (Cheng et al., 1991). Depression is a frequent symptom in PD and DLB, but a link between serotonin loss and depression remains to be clarified. There is no evidence that selective serotonin reuptake inhibitors are effective in depression in PD (Ghazi-Noori et al., 2003), and patients with untreated PD with depression showed no differences in CSF serotonin metabolites compared to patients without depression (Kuhn et al., 1996). Patients with DLB with a history of major depression actually had relatively higher serotonin transporter binding in parietal cortex than cases without (Ballard, Johnson, et al., 2002). There is however an increase in the numbers of 5-HT_{1A} receptors in temporal cortex in DLB and PDD with depression (Sharp et al., in preparation), and in PD 5-HT_{1A} receptors are increased in frontal and temporal cortex compared to controls (although any relationship to depression was not assessed in this study) (Chen et al., 1998). Treatment of depression in DLB may be more efficacious with a 5-HT_{1A} antagonist.

Greater preservation of serotonergic function may be related to behavioral and psychological symptoms in DLB. Patients with visual hallucinations show a relative preservation of 5HT markers and also have markedly reduced cholinergic parameters (Cheng et al., 1991; E.K. Perry, Marshall, Kerwin, et al., 1990; E.K. Perry et al., 1993).

Glutamate

Excitatory amino acid transmission occurs between several components of the basal ganglia circuit, which are likely to be affected in DLB, and excitotoxic mechanisms are implicated in the progress of neurodegenerative diseases. In PD there is increased excitatory output from the subthalamic nucleus, and glutamate antagonists have been used therapeutically. However, investigations of glutamate markers have been few, with no change in glutamate transporter protein in cortex in two DLB cases (H.L. Scott et al., 2002), no change in *N*-methyl-D-aspartate (NMDA) receptor immunoreactivity in entorhinal cortex and hippocampus (Thorns et al., 1997), and no reduction in glutamate in CSF (Molina et al., 2005). Glutamate receptor (GluR)2/3 α-amino-3-hydroxy-5-methyl-4-isoxasolepropionic acid (AMPA) receptor immunoreactivity was decreased in entorhinal cortex and hippocampus (Thorns et al., 1997), and group I metabotropic GluRs (mGluRs) were reduced in DLB (Albasanz et al., 2005), but these reductions were in cases with Alzheimer pathology. Further studies are needed to determine the extent of GLuR changes in DLB.

GABA

Although anxiety and insomnia are common complaints in DLB, and GABAergic systems are likely affected, there are few published reports of GABAergic changes. Selective dendritic derangement of GABAergic medium spiny neurons in the caudate have been reported and suggested to be linked to disrupted executive function (Zaja-Milatovic et al., 2005; Zaja-Milatovic et al., 2006). However, there was no change in benzodiazepine binding (GABA-A receptor) in the striatum in DLB (Suzuki et al., 2002), and no difference in GABA CSF concentration between controls and DLB (Molina et al., 2005).

Noradrenaline

Degeneration of the LC has been reported in PD and suggested to be linked to symptoms of mood disorder and subtle cognitive change (Cash et al., 1987), and this loss is more extensive in PDD (Cash et al., 1987; Zweig et al., 1993) and DLB (Leverenz et al., 2001; Szot et al. 2006). Locus coeruleus neuron loss correlates with cognitive decline, and there was evidence of compensation in the remaining LC neurons (Szot et al., 2006). α_2 adrenergic receptor density was increased slightly in DLB in frontal cortex (Leverenz et al., 2001). In DLB and AD, there was reduced α_{1D} and α_{2C} adrenergic receptor messenger ribonucleic acid (mRNA) in hippocampus (Szot et al., 2006). Noradrenaline system changes in limbic areas may contribute to depression and to behavioral symptoms such as aggression and pacing, in cortex to cognitive decline, and in basal ganglia to movement disorder; but in the main, these relationships are still to be investigated.

GENETICS

Owing to the similarities between the clinical and pathological manifestations of DLB with AD and PD, it is not surprising that the search for genes that are associated with AD and PD has been used to identify genetic associations with DLB. One report of presumed autosomal dominant DLB (though not according to consensus criteria) in a 67-year-old woman who developed parkinsonism and then dementia, together with her two sons, may indicate a strong genetic basis (Wakabayashi et al., 1998). The relatively late onset of DLB and a poor family history may be one reason why so few DLB families have been identified to date.

Alzheimer's Disease Genes in Dementia with Lewy Bodies

Because of the association of the e4 allele of the apolipoprotein ε4 (ApoE4) gene on chromosome 19 and AD, and the presence of Aβ in DLB, several groups have reported genotyping studies. In DLB, the e4 allele frequency is elevated in a manner analogous to that found in AD. In PD, no association is observed with ApoE4. There are, however, subtle differences in the ApoE4 allele frequencies between AD and DLB, with a higher e2 allele frequency and a reduced frequency of the e4/4 genotype in DLB. Differences in the ApoE4 frequencies may account for some of the differences between the two diseases in terms of clinical presentation and pathology, but it is unlikely that one single genetic determinant accounts for the differences between DLB and AD.

Apolipoprotein ε4 is associated with both senile plaques (SPs) and neurofibrillary tangles (NFTs), and a biochemical effect of the ApoE4 genotype in AD has been proposed (Strittmatter et al., 1993). However, DLB appears not to show a dose-dependant correlation of SP or NFT counts with ApoE4 allele dose, and given the markedly reduced NFT counts seen in DLB compared with AD, this may suggest that ApoE4 does not play a major role in NFT formation.

Recent work indicates potentially four other major loci for AD alone, with regions on chromosomes 4, 6, 12, and 20 being of interest. A recent series of whole-genome scans identified loci on chromosomes 1, 5, 6, 9, 10, 12, 19, 21, and X that appear to associate with AD. One locus on chromosome 12 has been suggested to be due to the α_2-macroglobulin gene. In DLB, our studies have not shown an association with this locus. Others have, however, suggested that the chromosome 12 locus involved in AD is actually in the immediate pericentromeric region of chromosome 12 and may associate with the low-density lipoprotein receptor-like protein or the transcription factor LBP-1c (Taylor et al., 2001). Several studies have eliminated the low-density receptor-like protein in AD and also in DLB. The strongest association with the chromosome 12 locus may be in late-onset dementia families with pathological evidence of DLB rather than AD (W.K. Scott et al., 2000).

The butyrylcholinesterase gene K variant (*BCHE K*) is also a risk factor for AD in conjunction with ApoE4, increasing the risk of AD 18-fold compared to the ApoE4 allele alone. Current studies do not, however, indicate a role for *BCHE* in specifying the risk of DLB. Variation at BCHE may have a bearing on the suggestion that patients with DLB are more likely to respond to cholinergic therapy than patients with AD (see next page). Patients with DLB who are homozygous for the K allele are significantly better at performing an attentional task than wild-type or heterozygous individuals. Cholinesterase inhibitors are, however, ineffective in *BCHE-K* homozygotes, probably because these individuals are at ceiling performance, though wild-type and heterozygous individuals benefit from this treatment since the inhibition of butyrylcholinesterase (and acetylcholinesterase) brings acetylcholine levels to those of *BCHE-K* homozygotes. Screening at the *BCHE* locus for mutations with reduced activity could therefore be used to identify individuals who are likely to have a good response to cholinergic therapy.

No associations have been found with DLB with polymorphisms in the genes for *presenilin 1*, *presenilin 2*, and *α-1 antichymotrypsin*. These genes are therefore unlikely to have a major influence on the pathogenesis of DLB.

Parkinson's Disease Genes in Dementia with Lewy Bodies

Much of the genetics of PD has focused on a candidate gene approach in disease association studies, perhaps because of the assumption that the majority of PD is sporadic. Mutations in the cytochrome P450 gene *CYP2D6* (debrisoquine 4-hydroxylase) and related enzymes have been extensively studied because of the suggestion that PD may be due to an environmental toxin interacting with a specific gene. Elevated frequencies of the common *CYP2D6* mutant allele, *CYP2D6B*, have been inconsistently found among patients compared with controls. Study of the *CYP2D6* gene in DLB has been equally controversial, with one report suggesting findings similar to those in PD, with an increased frequency of the B allele (Saitoh et al., 1995) and one study showing no association (Bordet et al., 1994).

A candidate gene approach to the study of genetic influences in PD has focused upon the dopaminergic system. It would be of interest to ascertain the status of these genes in DLB, given the dopaminergic dysfunction and pathology seen in DLB. An association of the N-acetyltransferase (*NAT*) 2 gene locus with familial PD is also of interest given its role in xenobiotic metabolism and the suggested role of these enzymes in detoxifying DA metabolites (Bandmann et al., 1997). Our own studies, however, do not suggest any association with the *NAT2* locus and DLB.

Mitochondrial mutations are found in DLB at similar levels to those found in AD and PD, arguing that they may be an acquired function of neurodegeneration, though still potentially capable of accelerating the disease process. There is a higher frequency of allele 2 of the DA receptor D_3 gene (*DRD3*) in patients with PD with hallucinations compared to those without hallucinations (Goetz et al., 2001). Unlike AD, there is no significant difference between the frequencies of allele 2 homozygotes and heterozygotes and no association with ApoE4. The *DRD3* receptor may thus be a factor involved in hallucinations and may merit study in DLB.

α-Synuclein has previously been identified as a major component of SP in AD, and this prompted study of the role of the gene in AD. To date, no mutations or associated polymorphisms have been linked to AD. The identification of mutations in *α*-synuclein (Polymeropoulos et al., 1996) and of the protein in LB will no doubt provide an impetus to search for other mutations in PD and also to search for associations with DLB. No simple association has been found with the synuclein gene in PD and DLB. More sophisticated investigations of the *α*-synuclein gene in PD have revealed a possible haplotype linked to the disease, and studies are currently under way in DLB to determine if this is also the case. Other proteins that are implicated in the genetic aetiology of PD could potentially be associated with the pathogenesis of DLB. Synphilin, an *α*-synuclein interacting protein, is present in the PD brain in LBs (Engelender et al., 1999) but does not appear to associate with disease risk in either PD (Bandopadhyay et al., 2001) or DLB (C.M. Morris, unpublished observations).

MANAGEMENT

Establishing an accurate and timely diagnosis is fundamental to planning management and treatment interventions in DLB. This, in turn, relies on acquiring a detailed clinical history supplemented by relevant examinations and investigations (see above). It is then necessary to identify key symptoms and evaluate their significance. A problem list of cognitive, psychiatric, and motor disabilities needs to be established in addition to the usual assessments of functioning, risk, and carer burden.

Until safe and effective medications become available, the mainstay of clinical management is to educate patients and carers about the nature of the symptoms of DLB and suggest strategies to cope with them. Interventions can be targeted for each of the three core symptoms. Strategies for cognitive symptoms include orientation and memory prompts and attentional cues. For psychiatric symptoms, options include explanation, education, reassurance, and targeted behavioral interventions (Collerton and Dudley, 2004). Motor impairments may benefit from physiotherapy and mobility aids.

There are no disease-modifying pharmacological therapies for DLB. Better understanding of the neurobiology of synuclein may lead to the development of novel therapeutic interventions applicable to a diverse group of neurodegenerative disorders including DLB, PD, and MSA, but until then, only symptomatic treatments are available. Alleviation of psychosis, cognitive deficits, and affective and motor symptoms may be required but can be extremely difficult because treatment introduced for one set of symptoms may lead to deterioration in others. In particular, patients treated with antipsychotic medication, especially those with high D_2 receptor antagonism, can experience an exacerbation of parkinsonian symptoms. Further, approximately 50% of all patients who receive neuroleptics experience life-threatening adverse effects, termed *neuroleptic sensitivity* (McKeith, Fairbairn, et al., 1992). This is characterized by sedation, immobility, rigidity, postural instability, falls, and increased confusion. Deterioration can be rapid, and patients are unable to maintain adequate fluid and food intake. The reaction is associated with a poor outcome and a two- to threefold increase in mortality.

Because of these concerns, managing patients with DLB with psychotic symptoms is often complex (McKeith, Galasko, et al., 1995). Factors exacerbating psychosis should be identified and excluded. For patients being treated with antiparkinsonian drugs, dose reduction or even withdrawal should be considered, at least on a trial basis. Empirically, drugs for PD could be reduced or withdrawn in the following order: anticholinergics, amantadine, l-deprenyl (selegiline), DA agonists, and levodopa preparations. If there is no improvement, then a cautious trial of an antipsychotic agent may be considered. Functional impairment in DLB is related to the degree of parkinsonism (McKeith et al., 2006), suggesting that antiparkinsonian therapy has an important role in the management of DLB. 3,4-dihydroxyphenylalanine (L-DOPA) is generally well tolerated in DLB and can still produce worthwhile benefit, although motor responsiveness is generally less than that observed in PD (Bonelli et al., 2004; Molloy et al., 2005). Younger DLB cases may be likely to respond to dopaminergic treatment. The use of levodopa was not associated with any adverse cognitive or neuropsychiatric effects after 3 months of treatment in one study (Molloy et al., 2006).

Treatment of RBD lacks a double-blind, placebo-controlled evidence base. Clonazepam has been reported as effective and well tolerated (Olson et al., 2000) in suppressing the motor features but does not restore REM-sleep atonia (Lapierre and Montplaisir, 1992). Melatonin has also proved beneficial, with control of symptoms or significant improvement being noted in 10 of 14 patients who had failed to respond to clonazepam or were unable to tolerate therapeutic doses (Boeve, Silber, Ferman, et al., 2003). Further work is needed to investigate the potential role of cholinesterase inhibitors and dopaminergic therapies as treatment strategies for RBD.

Following initial positive case reports of the use of newer atypical antipsychotics in DLB, further case studies indicate that neuroleptic sensitivity does occur, especially as the dose is increased (McKeith, Ballard, et al., 1995; Burke et al., 1998; Z. Walker, Grace, et al., 1999). Quetiapine does not appear to significantly worsen motor symptoms in a recent, small placebo-controlled trial of 36 patients with DLB (Kurlan et al., 2007) but was not associated with significant improvement in psychiatric or cognitive outcome measures. Until more robust clinical trials are completed, specific recommendations are limited, but overall, atypical antipsychotics are probably safer than traditional agents in DLB. Low dosing may be more important than the use of any specific drug.

A rational, effective, and safer alternative to treating DLB may be to compensate for the cholinergic deficits previously described by the use of cholinesterase inhibitors. Open studies have shown improvements in cognitive and noncognitive symptoms with donepezil and rivastigmine, without significant deterioration in motor function (Shea et al., 1998). Apathy, anxiety, impaired attention, hallucinations, delusions, sleep disturbance, and cognitive test performance are the most frequently cited treatment-responsive symptoms. Improvements are generally reported as greater than those achieved with similar doses of these drugs in AD, and a recent open-label study found evidence of sustained efficacy after 2 years of treatment (Grace et al., 2001). A multicenter, randomized, placebo-controlled trial of rivastigmine in DLB confirmed these observational studies (McKeith, Spano, et al., 2000). A total of 120 patients with DLB were treated with daily doses of rivastigmine of up to 12 mg or placebo for 20 weeks. Patients had a clinical diagnosis of probable and possible DLB and an MMSE score of greater than 10. Approximately twice as many patients on rivastigmine (63.4%) as on placebo (30.0%) showed at least a 30% improvement from baseline in DLB-typical psychiatric symptoms. Patients also showed improvements on computer-based tests of attention. Adverse effects were similar to those observed with the drug in AD and to those reported for other cholinesterase inhibitors. Parkinsonian symptoms did not worsen on treatment, although emergent tremor was noted in a small number of treated patients.

Similar findings have been noted in two trials of cholinesterase inhibitors in patients with PDD. The largest (Emre et al., 2004) was a randomized multicenter placebo-controlled trial of rivastigmine, at doses of 3 mg–12 mg, in over 500 patients, using dementia rating scales (Alzheimer's Disease Assessment Scale – Cognitive subscale [ADAS-cog] and Clinician's Global Impression of Change subscale [ADAS-CGIC]), cognitive function, and behavioral symptoms (neuropsychiatric inventory, MMSE, Cognitive Drug Research power of attention tests, clock drawing and verbal fluency) as primary and secondary outcome measures, respectively. There was a moderate but significant benefit in the treatment group compared to placebo but at the expense of adverse side effects such as nausea, vomiting, and worsening tremor (10%). Smaller studies, also in PDD (Aarsland et al., 2002; Ravina et al., 2005), have demonstrated similar benefits with donepezil. Head-to-head studies between cholinesterase inhibitors have not been performed to permit advice on which drug should be used first line in the management of DLB and PDD.

Cholinesterase inhibitors should therefore probably be the first choice for symptomatic treatment of the core symptoms of DLB, particularly because they do not carry the adverse risks associated with neuroleptic agents. Further large-scale trials in patients with DLB and PDD are required to support this proposal.

CONCLUSION

DLB is now established as a commonly occurring clinical syndrome accounting for up to 1 in 6 cases of dementia in older people. Recognition of cases with the characteristic clinical symptoms of attentional deficits, visuoperceptual abnormalities, visual hallucinations, fluctuating arousal, and parkinsonism is associated with a high probability of LB pathology and diagnostic accuracy. Unfortunately, a substantial number of cases do not present with such clearly recognizable clinical features and this appears often to be due to the co-existence of significant cortical Alzheimer pathology. The clinician must therefore adopt a high index of suspicion for cases with less florid presentations (possible DLB) and pursue these further by specific inquiry about suggestive clinical features and use of appropriate neuroimaging techniques. Lack of hippocampal atrophy, reduced perfusion of occipital cortex, and reduced striatal dopamine re-uptake are all supportive of a DLB diagnosis compared with AD, which is the usual differential. No other biomarkers have yet been established as useful in the diagnosis of DLB.

When the term DLB was adopted in 1996, it was done so "as a generic term for such cases, because it acknowledges the presence of LB without specifying their relative importance in symptom formation." Although this remark was made predominantly with respect to other degenerative and vascular pathologies, it also holds true in relation to LB themselves. Clinico-pathological correlations between LB and LN density and severity of clinical features are infrequent, consistent with recent opinion that these are end-stage and possibly cytoprotective lesions. Neurotoxic species of α-synuclein have not yet been identified but may well comprise small oligomeric aggregates at the synaptic level. This has major implications for targeting drug development, and further work in this area must be a research priority. The symptomatic and possibly even neuroprotective value of cholinesterase inhibition in the treatment of DLB also needs to be further explored further in large multicenter trials. Levodopa responsiveness of the parkinsonism associated with DLB is poorly documented, and controlled studies are also clearly needed.

REFERENCES

Aarsland, D., Ballard, C., McKeith, I., Perry, R.H., and Larsen, J.P. (2001) Comparison of extrapyramidal signs in dementia with Lewy bodies and Parkinson's disease. *J. Neuropsychiatry Clin. Neurosci.* 13:374–379.

Aarsland, D., Laake, K., Larsen, J.P., and Janvin, C. (2002) Donepezil for cognitive impairment in Parkinson's disease: a randomised controlled study. *J. Neurol. Neurosurg. Psychiatry* 72:708–712.

Ala, T.A., Hughes, L.F., Kyrouac, G.A., Ghobrial, M.W., and Elble, R.J. (2001) Pentagon copying is more impaired in dementia with Lewy bodies than in Alzheimer's disease. *J. Neurol. Neurosurg. Psychiatry* 70:483–488.

Albasanz, J.L., Dalfó, E., Ferrer, I., and Martin, M. (2005) Impaired metabotropic glutamate receptor/phospholipase C signaling pathway in the cerebral cortex in Alzheimer's disease and dementia with Lewy bodies correlates with stage of Alzheimer's-disease-related changes. *Neurobiol. Dis.* 20:685–693.

Allan, L.M., Ballard, C.G., Allen, J., Murray, A., Davidson, A.W., McKeith, I.G., and Kenny, R.A. (2007) Autonomic dysfunction in dementia. *J. Neurol. Neurosurg. Psychiatry* 78(7):671–677.

American Academy of Sleep Medicine. (2005) *The International Classification of Sleep Disorders: Diagnostic and Coding Manual*, 2nd ed. Westchester, IL.

Baba, M., Nakajo, S., Tu, P.H., Tomita, T., Nakaya, K., Lee, V.M., Trojanowski, J.Q., and Iwatsubo, T. (1998) Aggregation of alpha-synuclein in Lewy bodies of sporadic Parkinson's disease and dementia with Lewy bodies. *Am. J. Pathol.* 152:879–884.

Ballard, C., Johnson, M., Piggott, M., et al. (2002) A positive association between 5HT re-uptake binding sites and depression in dementia with Lewy bodies. *J. Affect. Dis.* 69:219–223.

Ballard, C.G., Court, J.A., Piggott, M., et al. (2002) Disturbances of consciousness in dementia with Lewy bodies associated with alteration in nicotinic receptor binding in the temporal cortex. *Conscious. Cogn.* 11:461–474.

Ballard, C.G., McKeith, I., Burn, D., Harrison, R., O'Brien, J., Lowery, K., Campbell, M., Perry, R., and Ince, P. (1997) The UPDRS scale as a means of identifying extrapyramidal signs in patients suffering from dementia with Lewy bodies. *Acta Neurol. Scand.* 96:366–371.

Ballard, C.G., O'Brien, J., Barber, B., et al. (2000) Neurocardiovascular instability, hypotensive episodes and MRI lesions in neurodegenerative dementia. *Ann. N.Y. Acad. Sci.* 903:442–445.

Ballard, C.G., O'Brien, J., Gray, A., Cormack, F., Ayre, G., Rowan, E., Thompson, P., Bucks, R., McKeith, I., Walker, M., and Tovee, M. (2001) Attention and fluctuating attention in patients with dementia with Lewy bodies and Alzheimer's disease. *Arch. Neurol.* 58:977–982.

Ballard, C.G., O'Brien, J., Morris, C.M., Barber, R., Swann, A., Neill, D., and McKeith, I. (2001) The progression of cognitive impairment in dementia with Lewy bodies, vascular dementia and Alzheimer's disease. *Int. J. Geriatr. Psychiatry* 16:499–503.

Ballard, C.G., O'Brien, J., Swann, A., Neill, D., Lantos, P., Holmes, C., Burn, D., Ince, P., Perry, R., and McKeith, I. (2000) One year follow-up of parkinsonism in dementia with Lewy bodies. *Dement. Geriatr. Cogn. Disord.* 11:219–222.

Ballard, C.G., Piggott, M., Johnson, M., Cairns, N.J., Perry, R., McKeith, I., Jaros, E., O'Brien, J., Holmes, C., and Perry, E. (2000) Delusions associated with elevated muscarinic binding in dementia with Lewy bodies. *Ann. Neurol.* 48:868–876.

Ballard, C.G., Shaw, F., Lowery, K., McKeith, I., and Kenny, R. (1999) The prevalence, assessment and associations of falls in dementia with Lewy bodies and Alzheimer's disease. *Dement. Geriatr. Cogn. Disord.* 10:97–103.

Ballard, C.G., Shaw, F., McKeith, I., and Kenny, R. (1998) High prevalence of neurovascular instability in neurodegenerative dementias. *Neurology* 51:1760–1762.

Bandmann, O., Vaughan, J., Holmans, P., Marsden, C.D., and Wood, N.W. (1997) Association of slow acetylator genotype for *N*-acetyl transferase 2 with familial Parkinson's disease. *Lancet* 350:1136–1139.

Bandopadhyay, R., de Silva, R., Khan, N., Graham, E., Vaughan, J., Engelender, S., Ross, C., Morris, H., Morris, C., Wood, N.W.,

Daniel, S., and Lees, A. (2001) No pathogenic mutations in the synphilin-1 gene in Parkinson's disease. *Neurosci. Lett.* 307: 125–127.

Barber, R., Ballard, C.G., McKeith, I.G., Gholkar, A., and O'Brien, J.T. (2000) MRI volumetric study of dementia with Lewy bodies: a comparison with AD and vascular dementia. *Neurology* 54: 1304–1309.

Barber, R., Gholkar, A., Scheltens, P., Ballard, C.G., McKeith, I.G., and O'Brien, J.T. (1999) Medial temporal lobe atrophy on MRI in dementia with Lewy bodies. *Neurology* 52:1153–1158.

Benarroch, E.E., Schmeichel, A.M., Low, P.A., Boeve, B.F., Sandroni, P., and Parisi, J.E. (2005) Involvement of medullary regions controlling sympathetic output in Lewy body disease. *Brain* 128:338–344.

Boeve, B., Silber, M., and Ferman, T. (2004) REM sleep behavior disorder in Parkinson's disease and dementia with Lewy bodies. *J. Ger. Psychiatry Neurol.* 17:146–157.

Boeve, B.F., Dickson, D.W., Olson, E.J., Shepard, J.W., Silber, M.H., Ferman, T.J., Ahlskog, J.E., and Benarroch, E.F. (2006) Insights into REM sleep behavior disorder pathophysiology in brainstem-predominant Lewy body disease. *Sleep Med.* 8:60–64.

Boeve, B.F., Silber, M.H., and Ferman, T.J. (2003) Melatonin for treatment of REM sleep behavior disorder in neurologic disorders: results in 14 patients. *Sleep Med.* 4: 281–284.

Boeve, B.F., Silber, M.H., Ferman, T.J., Kokmen, E., Smith, G.E., Ivnik, R.J., Parisi, J.E., Olson, E.J., and Petersen, R.C. (1998) REM sleep behavior disorder and degenerative dementia: an association likely reflecting Lewy body disease. *Neurology* 51:363–370.

Boeve, B.F., Silber, M.H., Ferman, T.J., Lucas, J.A., and Parisi, J.E. (2001) Association of REM sleep behavior disorder and neurodegenerative disease may reflect an underlying synucleinopathy. *Mov. Disord.* 16:622–630.

Boeve, B.F., Silber, M.H., Parisi, J.E., Dickson, D.W., Ferman, T.J., Benarroch, E.E., Schmeichel, A.M., Smith, G.E., Petersen, R.C., Ahlskog, J.E., Matsumoto, J.Y., Knopman, D.S., Schenck, C.H., and Mahowald, M.W. (2003) Synucleinopathy pathology and REM sleep behavior disorder plus dementia or parkinsonism. *Neurology* 61(1):40–45.

Bohnen, N.I., Kaufer, D.I., Hendrickson, R., et al. (2006) Cognitive correlates of cortical cholinergic denervation in Parkinson's disease and parkinsonian dementia. *J. Neurology* 253:242–247.

Bonelli, S.B., Ransmayr, G., Steffelbauer, M., Lukas, T., Lampl, C., and Deibl, M. (2004) L-dopa responsiveness in dementia with Lewy bodies, Parkinson's disease with and without dementia. *Neurology* 63:376–378.

Bonini, N.M., and Giasson, B.I. (2005) Snaring the function of alpha-synuclein. *Cell* 123(3):359–361.

Bordet, R., Broly, F., Destee, A., and Libersa, C. (1994) Genetic polymorphism of cytochrome P450 2D6 in idiopathic Parkinson's disease and diffuse Lewy body disease. *Clin. Neuropharmacol.* 17:484–488.

Boström, F., Jonsson, L., Minthon, L., and Londos, E. (2007a) Patients with Lewy body dementia have more impaired quality of life than patients with Alzheimer's disease. *Alzheimers Dis. Assoc. Disord.* 21:150–154.

Boström, F., Jonsson, L., Minthon, L., and Londos, E. (2007b) Patients with Lewy body dementia use more resources than those with Alzheimer's disease. *Int. J. Ger. Psychiat.* 22:713–719.

Bradshaw, J., Slaing, M., Hopwood, M., Anderson, V., and Brodtmann, A. (2004) Fluctuating cognition in dementia with Lewy bodies and Alzheimer's disease is qualitatively distinct. *J. Neurol. Neurosurg. Psychiatry* 75(3):382–387.

Briel, R.C., McKeith, I.G., Barker, W.A., Hewitt, Y., Perry, R.H., Ince, P.G., and Fairbairn, A.F. (1999) EEG findings in dementia with Lewy bodies and Alzheimer's disease. *J. Neurol. Neurosurg. Psychiatry* 66:401–403.

Burke, W.J., Pfeiffer, R.F., and McComb, R.D. (1998) Neuroleptic sensitivity to clozapine in dementia with Lewy bodies. *J. Neuropsychiatry Clin. Neurosci.* 10:227–229.

Burn, D.J., Rowan, E.N., Minett, T., et al. (2003) Extrapyramidal features in Parkinson's disease with and without dementia and dementia with Lewy bodies: a cross-sectional comparative study. *Mov. Disord.* 18: 884–889.

Burton, E.J., McKeith, I.G., Burn, D.J., Firbank, M.J., O'Brien, J.T. (2006) Progression of white matter hyperintensities in Alzheimer disease, dementia with Lewy bodies, and Parkinson disease dementia: a comparison with normal ageing. *Am. J. Geriatr. Psychiatry* 14(10):842–849.

Campbell, S., Stephens, S., and Ballard, C. (2001) Dementia with Lewy bodies: clinical features and treatment. *Drugs Ageing* 18: 397–407.

Cash, R., Dennis, T., L'Heureux, R., Raisman, R., Javoy-Agid, F., and Scatton, B. (1987) Parkinson's disease and dementia: norepinephrine and dopamine in locus ceruleus. *Neurology* 37:42–46.

Castagnet, P.I., Golovko, M.Y., Barceló-Coblijn, G.C., et al. (2005) Fatty acid incorporation is decreased in astrocytes cultured from alpha-synuclein gene-ablated mice. *J. Neurochem.* 94(3):839–849.

Chandra, S., Gallardo, G., Fernández-Chacón, R., et al. (2005) Alpha-synuclein cooperates with CSP alpha in preventing neurodegeneration. *Cell* 123(3):383–396.

Chen, C.P., Alder, J.T., Bray, L., Kingsbury, A.E., Francis, P.T., and Foster, O.J. (1998) Post-synaptic 5-HT1A and 5-HT2A receptors are increased in Parkinson's disease neocortex. *Ann. N.Y. Acad. Sci.* 861:288–289.

Cheng, A.V., Ferrier, I.N., Morris, C.M., et al. (1991) Cortical serotonin-S2 receptor binding in Lewy body dementia, Alzheimer's and Parkinson's diseases. *J. Neurol. Sci.* 106:50–55.

Collerton, D., Burn, D., McKeith, I., and O'Brien, J. (2003) Systematic review and meta-analysis show that dementia with Lewy bodies is a visual-perceptual and attentional-executive dementia [erratum appears in *Dement. Geriatr. Cogn. Disord.* 2005;19(1):56]. *Dement. Geriatr. Cogn. Disord.* 16: 229–237.

Collerton, D., and Dudley, R. (2004) A cognitive behavioural framework for the treatment of distressing visual hallucinations in older people. *Behav. Cogn. Psychother.* 32:443–455.

Collerton, D., Perry, E., and McKeith, I. (2005) Why people see things that are not there. A novel perception and attention deficit model for recurrent complex visual hallucinations. *Behav. Brain Sci.* 28:737–794.

Colloby, S.J., Pakrasi, S., Firbank, M.J., Perry, E.K., Piggott, M.A., et al. (2006) In vivo SPECT imaging of muscarinic acetylcholine receptors using (R,R) 123I-QNB in dementia with Lewy bodies and Parkinson's disease dementia. *NeuroImage* 33(2):423–429.

Colloby, S.J., Williams, E.D., Burn, D.J., Lloyd, J.J., McKeith, I.G., and O'Brien, J.T. (2005) Progression of dopaminergic degeneration in dementia with Lewy bodies and Parkinson's disease with and without dementia assessed using 123I-FP-CIT SPECT. *Eur. J. Nucl. Med. Mol. Imag.*32:1176–1185.

Cooper, A.A., Gitler, A.D., Cashikar, A., et al. (2006) Alpha-synuclein blocks ER-Golgi traffic and Rab1 rescues neuron loss in Parkinson's models. *Science* 313(5785):324–328.

Court, J., Spurden, D., Lloyd, S., et al. (1999) Neuronal nicotinic receptors in dementia with Lewy bodies and schizophrenia: a-bungarotoxin and nicotine binding in the thalamus. *J. Neurochem.* 73:1590–1597.

Court, J.A., Ballard, C.G., Piggott, M.A., Johnson, M., O'Brien, J. T., Holmes, C., Cairns, N., Lantos, P., Perry, R.H., Jaros, E., and Perry, E.K. (2001) Visual hallucinations are associated with lower a-bungarotoxin binding in dementia with Lewy bodies. *Pharmacol. Biochem. Behav.* 70:571–579.

Del Ser, T., Hachinski, V., Merskey, H., and Munoz, D.G. (2001) Clinical and pathologic features of two groups of patients with dementia with Lewy bodies: Effect of coexisting Alzheimer-type lesion load. *Alzheimer Dis. Assoc. Disord.* 15:31–44.

Dalfó, E., and Ferrer, I. (2008) Early a-synuclein lipoxidation in neocortex in Lewy bodies diseases. *Neurobiol. Aging* 29(3):408–417.

Dalfó, E., Martinez, A., Muntane, G., and Ferrer, I. (2006) Abnormal a-synuclein solubility, aggregation and nitration in the frontal cortex in Pick's disease. *Neurosci. Lett.* 400:125–129.

de Bruin, V.M., Lees, A.J., and Daniel, S.E. (1992) Diffuse Lewy body disease presenting with supranuclear gaze palsy, parkinsonism, and dementia: a case report. *Mov. Disord.* 7:355–358.

Defebvre, L.J., Leduc, V., Duhamel, A., et al. (1999) Technetium HMPAO SPECT study in dementia with Lewy bodies. *J. Nucl. Med.* 40:956–962.

Del Ser, T., McKeith, I., Anand, R., Cicin-Sain, A., Ferrara, R., and Spiegel, R. (2000) Dementia with Lewy bodies: findings from an international multicentre study. *Int. J. Geriatr. Psychiatry* 15:1034–1045.

Donnemiller, E., Heilmann, J., Wenning, G.K., et al. (1997) Brain perfusion scintigraphy with ^{99m}Tc-HMPAO or ^{99m}Tc-ECD and ^{123}I-beta-CIT single-photon emission tomography in dementia of the Alzheimer-type and diffuse Lewy body disease. *Eur. J. Nucl. Med.* 24:320–325.

Duda, J.E., Giasson, B.I., Mabon, M.E., Lee, V.M., and Trojanowski, J.Q. (2002) Novel antibodies to synuclein show abundant striatal pathology in Lewy body diseases. *Ann. Neurol.* 52:205–210.

Eisensehr, I., Linke, R., Tatsch, K., et al. (2003) Increased muscle activity during rapid eye movement sleep correlates with decrease of striatal presynaptic dopamine transporters. IPT and IBZM SPECT imaging in subclinical and clinically manifest idiopathic REM sleep behavior disorder, Parkinson's disease, and controls. *Sleep* 26:507–512.

Emre, M., Aarsland, D., Albanese, A., et al. (2004) Rivastigmine for dementia associated with Parkinson's disease. *N. Engl. J. Med.* 351:2509–2518.

Emre, M., Aarsland, D., Brown, R., et al. (2007) Clinical diagnostic criteria for dementia associated with Parkinson's disease. *Mov. Disorder* 22(12):1689–1707.

Engelender, S., Kaminsky, Z., Guo, X., et al. (1999) Synphilin-1 associates with α-Synuclein and promotes the formation of cytosolic inclusions. *Nat. Genet.* 22:110–114.

Fan, Y., Limprasert, P., Murray, I.V., Smith, A.C., Lee, V.M., Trojanowski, J.Q., Sopher, B.L., La and Spada, A.R. (2006) Beta-synuclein modulates α-synuclein neurotoxicity by reducing alpha-synuclein protein expression. *Hum. Mol. Genet.* 15:3002–3010.

Farde, L., Suhara, T., Nyberg, S., Karlsson, P., Nakashima, Y., Hietala, J., and Halldin, C. (1997) A PET study of [11C]FLB 457 binding to extrastriatal D2-dopamine receptors in healthy subjects and antipsychotic drug-treated patients. *Psychopharmacology* 133:396–404.

Fearnley, J.M., Revesz, T., Brooks, D.J., Frackowiak, R.S., and Lees, A.J. (1991) Diffuse Lewy body disease presenting with a supranuclear gaze palsy. *J. Neurol. Neurosurg. Psychiatry* 54:159–161.

Ferman, T.J., Boeve, B.F., Smith, G.E., Silber, M.H., Kokmen, E., Petersen, R.C., and Ivnik, R.J. (1999) REM sleep behaviour disorder and dementia: Cognitive differences when compared with AD. *Neurology* 52:951–957.

Ferman, T.J., Smith, G.E., Boeve, B.F., Ivnik, R.J., Petersen, R.C., Knopman, D., Graff-Radford, N., Parisi, J., and Dickson, D.W. (2004) DLB fluctuations: specific features that reliably differentiate from AD and normal ageing. *Neurology* 62:181–187.

Firbank, M.J., Colloby, S.J., Burn, D.J., McKeith, I.G., and O'Brien, J.T. (2003) Regional cerebral blood flow in Parkinson's disease with and without dementia. *NeuroImage* 20:1309–1319.

Förstl, H., Burns, A., Levy, R., and Cairns, N. (1994) Neuropathological correlates of psychotic phenomena in confirmed Alzheimer's disease. *Br. J. Psychiatry* 165:53–59.

Förstl, H., Burns, A., Luthert, P., et al. (1993) The Lewy-body variant of Alzheimer's disease. Clinical and pathological findings. *Br. J. Psychiatry* 162:385–392.

Freeman, A., Ciliax, B., Bakay, R., et al. (2001) Nigrostriatal collaterals to thalamus degenerate in parkinsonian animal models. *Ann. Neurol.*, 50:321–329.

Fujiwara, H., Hasegawa, M., Dohmae, N., et al. (2002) α-Synuclein is phosphorylated in synucleinopathies. *Nat. Cell Biol.* 4:160–164.

Fumimura, Y., Ikemura, M., Saito, Y., Sengoku, R., Kanemura, K., et al. (2007) Analysis of the adrenal gland is useful for evaluating pathology of the peripheral autonomic nervous system in Lewy body disease. *J. Neuropathol. Exp. Neurol.* 66:354–362.

Gagnon, J.F., Bedard, M.A., Fantini, M.L., Petit, D., Panisset, M., Rompre, S., Carrier, J., and Montplaisir, J. (2002) REM sleep behaviour disorder and REM sleep without atonia in Parkinson's disease. *Neurology* 59:585–589.

Gagnon, J.F., Petit, D., Fantini, M.L., Pompre, S., Gauthier, S., Panisset, M., Robillard, A., and Montplaisir, J. (2006) REM sleep behaviour disorder and REM sleep without atonia in probable Alzheimer's disease. *Sleep* 29(10):1321–1325.

Galvin, J.E., Uryu, K., Lee, V.M., and Trojanowski, J.Q. (1999) Axon pathology in Parkinson's disease and Lewy body dementia hippocampus contains alpha-, beta-, and gamma-synuclein. *Proc. Natl. Acad. Sci. USA* 96:13450–13455.

Gelb, D.J., Oliver, E., and Gilman, S. (1999) Diagnostic criteria for Parkinson's disease. *Arch. Neurol.* 56:33–39.

Ghazi-Noori, S., Chung, T.H., Deane, K., Rickards, H., and Clarke, C.E. (2003) Therapies for depression in Parkinson's disease. *Cochrane Database Sys. Rev.*:CD003465.

Gnanalingham, K.K., Byrne, E.J., Thornton, A., Sambrook, M.A., and Bannister, P. (1997) Motor and cognitive function in Lewy body dementia: comparison with Alzheimer's and Parkinson's disease. *J. Neurol. Neurosurg. Psychiatry* 62:243–252.

Gnanalingham, K.K., Smith, L.A., Hunter, A.J., Jenner, P., and Marsden, C.D. (1993) Alterations in striatal and extrastriatal D-1 and D-2 dopamine receptors in the MPTP-treated common marmoset: an autoradiographic study. *Synapse* 14:184–194.

Goetz, C.G., Burke, P.F., Leurgans, S., Berry-Kravis, E., Blasucci, L.M., Raman, R., and Zhou, L. (2001) Genetic variation analysis in Parkinson disease patients with and without hallucinations: case-control study. *Arch. Neurol.* 58:209–213.

Golovko, M.Y., Faergeman, N.J., Cole, N.B., et al. (2005) Alpha-synuclein gene deletion decreases brain palmitate uptake and alters the palmitate metabolism in the absence of alpha-synuclein palmitate binding. *Biochemistry* 44(23):8251–8259.

Gómez-Tortosa, E., Gonzalo, I., Newell, K., et al. (2002) Patterns of protein nitration in dementia with Lewy bodies and striatonigral degeneration. *Acta Neuropathol.* 103(5):495–500.

Gómez-Tortosa, E., Irizarry, M.C., Gomez-Isla, T., and Hyman, B.T. (2000) Clinical and neuropathological correlates of dementia with Lewy bodies. *Ann. N.Y. Acad. Sci.* 920:9–15.

Gómez-Tortosa, E., Newell, K., Irizarry, M.C., Albert, M., Growdon, J.H., and Hyman, B.T. (1999) Clinical and quantitative pathologic correlates of dementia with Lewy bodies. *Neurology* 53:1284–1291.

Gómez-Tortosa, E., Newell, K., Irizarry, M.C., Sanders, J.L., and Hyman, B.T. (2000) Alpha-synuclein immunoreactivity in dementia with Lewy bodies: morphological staging and comparison with ubiquitin immunostaining. *Acta Neuropathol. (Berl)* 99:352–357.

Gotti, C., Moretti, M., Bohr, I., et al. (2006) Selective nicotinic acetylcholine receptor subunit deficits identified in Alzheimer's disease, Parkinson's disease and dementia with Lewy bodies by immunoprecipitation. *Neurobiol. Dis.* 23:481–489.

Grace, J., Daniel, S., Stevens, T., Shankar, K.K., Walker, Z., Byrne, E.J., Butler, S., Wilkinson, D., Woolford, J., Waite, J., and McKeith, I.G. (2001) Long-term use of rivastigmine in patients with dementia with Lewy bodies: An open label trial. *Int. Psychogeriatr.* 13:199–205.

Harding, A.J., Broe, G.A., and Halliday, G.M. (2002) Visual hallucinations in Lewy body disease relate to Lewy bodies in the temporal lobe. *Brain* 125:391–403.

Harrington, C.R., Perry, R.H., Perry, E.K., Hurt, J., McKeith, I.G., Roth, M., and Wischik, C.M. (1994) Senile dementia of Lewy body type and Alzheimer type are biochemically distinct in terms of paired helical filaments and hyperphosphorylated tau protein. *Dementia* 5:215–228.

Hashimoto, M., Rockenstein, E., Mante, M., Mallory, M., and Masliah, E. (2001) Beta-synuclein inhibits alpha-synuclein aggregation: a possible role as an anti-parkinsonian factor. *Neuron* 32:213–223.

Horimoto, Y., Matsumoto, M., Akatsu, H., Ikari, H., Kojima, K., Yamamoto, T., Otsuka, Y., Ojika, K., Ueda, R., and Kosaka, K. (2003) Autonomic dysfunctions in dementia with Lewy bodies. *J. Neurol.* 250(5):530–533.

Hu, X.S., Okamura, N., Arai, H., et al. (2000) 18F-fluorodopa PET study of striatal dopamine uptake in the diagnosis of dementia with Lewy bodies. *Neurology* 55:1575–1577.

Hurtig, H.I., Trojanowski, J.Q., Galvin, J., Ewbank, D., Schmidt, M.L., Lee, V.M., Clark, C.M., Glosser, G., Stern, M.B., Gollomp, S.M., and Arnold, S.E. (2000) Alpha-synuclein cortical Lewy bodies correlate with dementia in Parkinson's disease. *Neurology* 54:1916–1921.

Iranzo, A., Molinuevo, J.L., Santmaria, J., Serradell, M., Marti, M.J., Valldeoriola, F., and Tolosa, E. (2006) Rapid-eye-movement sleep behaviour disorder as an early marker for a neurodegenerative disorder: a descriptive study. *Lancet Neurol.* 5:572–577.

Iranzo, A., Santamaria, J., Rye, D.B., Valldeoriola, F., Marti, M.J., Munoz, E., Vilaseca, I., and Tolosa, E. (2005) Characteristics of idiopathic REM sleep behaviour disorder and that associated with MSA and PD. *Neurology* 65:247–252.

Ishii, K., Yamaji, S., Kitagaki, H., Imamura, T., Hirono, N., and Mori, E. (1999) Regional cerebral blood flow difference between dementia with Lewy bodies and AD. *Neurology* 53:413–416.

Jellinger, K.A., Wenning, G.K., and Seppi, K. (2007) Predictors of survival in dementia with Lewy bodies and Parkinson dementia. *Neurodegener. Dis.* 4:428–430.

Johnson, D.K., Morris, J.C., and Galvin, J.E. (2005) Verbal and visuospatial deficits in dementia with Lewy bodies. *Neurology* 65: 1232–1238.

Kaasinen, V., Nagren, K., Hietala, J., Oikonen, V., Vilkman, H., Farde, L., Halldin, C., and Rinne, J.O. (2000) Extrastriatal dopamine D2 and D3 receptors in early and advanced Parkinson's disease. *Neurology* 54:1482–1487.

Kanemaru, K., Kameda, K., and Yamanouchi, H. (2000) Decreased CSF amyloid b42 and normal tau levels in dementia with Lewy bodies. *Neurology* 54:1875–1876.

Kaufmann, H., Nahm, K., Purohit, D., and Wolfe, D. (2004) Autonomic failure as the initial presentation of Parkinson disease and dementia with Lewy bodies. *Neurology* 63:1093–1095.

Kenny, R.A., Shaw, F.E., O'Brien, J.T., Scheltens, P.H., Kalaria, R., and Ballard, C. (2004) Carotid sinus syndrome is common in dementia with Lewy bodies and correlates with deep white matter lesions. *J. Neurol. Neurosurg. Psychiatry* 75(7):966–971.

Kuhn, W., Muller, T., Gerlach, M., et al. (1996) Depression in Parkinson's disease: biogenic amines in CSF of "de novo" patients. *J. Neural Trans.* 103:1441–1445.

Kurlan, R., Cummings, J., Raman, R., and Thal, L. (2007) Quetiapine for agitation or psychosis in patients with dementia and parkinsonism. For the Alzheimer's Disease Cooperative Study Group *Neurology* 68(17):1356–1363.

Lambon, R.M.A., Powell, J., Howard, D., Whitworth, A.B., Garrard, P., and Hodges, J.R. (2001) Semantic memory is impaired in both dementia with Lewy bodies and Alzheimer's disease: a comparative neuropsychological study and literature review. *J. Neurol. Neurosurg. Psychiatry* 70:149–156.

Langlais, P.J., Thal, L., Hansen, L., Galasko, D., Alford, M., and Masliah, E. (1993) Neurotransmitters in basal ganglia and cortex of Alzheimer's disease with and without Lewy bodies. *Neurology* 43:1927–1934.

Lapierre, O., and Montplaisir, J. (1992) Polysomnographic features of REM sleep behavior disorder: development of a scoring method. *Neurology* 42:1371–1374.

Lennox, G.G. (1992) Lewy body dementia. *Baillieres Clin. Neurol.* 1:653–676.

Lennox, G.G., and Lowe, J.S. (1997) Dementia with Lewy bodies. *Baillieres Clin. Neurol.* 6:147–166.

Leverenz, J., Umar, I., Wang, Q., et al. (2007) Proteomic identification of novel proteins in cortical Lewy bodies. *Brain Pathol.* 17: 139–145.

Leverenz, J.B., Miller, M.A., Dobie, D.J., Peskind, E.R., and Raskind, M.A. (2001) Increased alpha 2-adrenergic receptor binding in locus coeruleus projection areas in dementia with Lewy bodies. *Neurobiol. Aging* 22:555–561.

Lippa, C.F., Smith, T.W., and Perry, E. (1999) Dementia with Lewy bodies: choline acetyltransferase parallels nucleus basalis pathology. *J. Neural Transm.* 106:525–535.

Lobotesis, K., Fenwick, J., Phipps, A., Ryman, A., Swann, A., Ballard, C., McKeith, I.G., and O'Brien, J.T. (2001) Occipital hypoperfusion on SPECT in dementia with Lewy bodies but not AD. *Neurology* 56:643–649.

Lopez, O.L., Becker, J.T., Kaufer, D.I., et al. (2002) Research evaluation and prospective diagnosis of dementia with Lewy bodies. *Arch. Neurol.* 59:43–46.

Lopez, O.L., Becker, J.T., Sweet, R.A., et al. (2006) Lewy bodies in the amygdala increase risk for major depression in subjects with Alzheimer disease. *Neurology* 67(4):660–665.

Louis, E.D., Klatka, L.A., Liu, Y., and Fahn, S. (1997) Comparison of extrapyramidal features in 31 pathologically confirmed cases of diffuse Lewy body disease and 34 pathologically confirmed cases of Parkinson's disease. *Neurology* 48:376–380.

Louis, E.D., Vonsattel, J.P., and Honig, L.S. (2006) Neuropathologic findings in essential tremor. *Neurology* 66(11):1756–1759.

Marshall, E.F., Perry, E.K., Perry, R.H., McKeith, I.G., Fairbairn, A.F., and Thompson, P. (1994) Dopamine metabolism in postmortem caudate nucleus in neurodegenerative disorders. *Neurosci. Res. Commun.* 14:17–25.

Mattila, P.M., Roytta, M., Lonnberg, P., Marjamaki, P., Helenius, H., and Rinne, J.O. (2001) Choline acetytransferase activity and striatal dopamine receptors in Parkinson's disease in relation to cognitive impairment. *Acta Neuropath.* 102:160–166.

McKeith, I., O'Brien, J., Walker, Z., Tatsch, K., Booji, J., et al. (2007) Sensitivity and specificity of dopamine transporter imaging with 123I-FP-CIT SPECT in dementia with Lewy bodies: a phase III, multicentre study *Lancet Neurol.* 6(4):305–313.

McKeith, I.G., Ballard, C.G., and Harrison, R.W. (1995) Neuroleptic sensitivity to risperidone in Lewy body dementia. *Lancet* 346: 699.

McKeith, I.G., Ballard, C.G., Perry, R.H., et al. (2000) Prospective validation of consensus criteria for the diagnosis of dementia with Lewy bodies. *Neurology* 54:1050–1058.

McKeith, I.G., Burn, D., O'Brien, J., Perry, R., and Perry, E.K. (2002) Dementia with Lewy bodies. In: Davis, K.L., Charney, D., Coyle, J.T., and Nemeroff, C., eds. *Neuropsychopharmacology: The 5th Generation of Progress*. Philadelphia: Lippincott, Williams & Wilkins, pp. 1301–1315.

McKeith, I.G., Dickson, D.W., Lowe, J., et al. (2005) Diagnosis and management of dementia with Lewy bodies: third report of the DLB Consortium. *Neurology* 65(12):1863–1872.

McKeith, I.G., Fairbairn, A., Perry, R., Thompson, P., and Perry, E. (1992) Neuroleptic sensitivity in patients with senile dementia of Lewy body type. *Br. Med. J.* 305:673–678.

McKeith, I.G., Galasko, D., Kosaka, K., et al. (1996) Consensus guidelines for the clinical and pathological diagnosis of dementia with Lewy bodies (DLB): report of the consortium on DLB international workshop. *Neurology* 47:1113–1124.

McKeith, I.G., Galasko, D., Wilcock, G.K., and Byrne, E.J. (1995) Lewy body dementia—diagnosis and treatment. *Br. J. Psychiatry* 167:709–717.

McKeith, I.G., Perry, E.K., and Perry, R. (1999) Report of the second dementia with Lewy body international workshop. *Neurology* 53:902–905.

McKeith, I.G., Perry, R.H., Fairbairn, A.F., Jabeen, S., and Perry, E.K. (1992) Operational criteria for senile dementia of Lewy body type (SDLT). *Psychol. Med.* 22:911–922.

McKeith, I.G., Rowan, E., Askew, K., Naidu, A., Allen, L., Barnett, N., Lett, D., Mosimann, U.P., Burn, D., and O'Brien, J.T. (2006) More severe functional impairment in dementia with Lewy bodies than Alzheimer disease is related to extrapyramidal motor dysfunction. *Am. J. Ger. Psychiat.* 14(7):582–588.

McKeith, I.G., Spano, P.F., Del Ser, T., Emre, M., Wesnes, K., Anand, R., Cicin-Sain, A., Ferrara, R., and Spiegel, R. (2000) Efficacy of rivastigmine in dementia with Lewy bodies: a randomised, double-blind, placebo-controlled international study. *Lancet* 356:2031–2036.

McLean, P.J., Kawamata, H., Ribich, S., and Hyman, B.T. (2000) Membrane association and protein conformation of alpha-synuclein in intact neurons. Effect of Parkinson's disease-linked mutations. *J. Biol. Chem.* 275(12):8812–8816.

McNaught, K.S., and Jenner, P. (2001) Proteasomal function is impaired in substantia nigra in Parkinson's disease. *Neurosci. Lett.* 297:191–194.

Merdes, A.R., Hansen, L.A., Jeste, D.V., et al. (2003) Influence of Alzheimer pathology on clinical diagnosis accuracy in dementia with Lewy bodies. *Neurology* 60:1586–1690.

Miller, V.M., Kenny, R.A., Slade, J.Y., Oakley, A.E., and Kalaria, R.N. (2007) Medullary autonomic pathology of carotid sinus hypersensitivity. *Neuropathol. Appl. Neurobiol.* [Epub ahead of print].

Minguez-Castellanos, A., Chamorro, C.E., Escamilla-Sevilla, F., et al. (2007) Do alpha-synuclein aggregates in autonomic plexuses predate Lewy body disorders?: A cohort study. *Neurology* 68:2012–2018.

Minoshima, S., Foster, N.L., Sima, A.A., Frey, K.A., Albin, R.L., and Kuhl, D.E. (2001) Alzheimer's disease versus dementia with Lewy bodies: cerebral metabolism distinction with autopsy confirmation. *Ann. Neurol.* 50:358–365.

Molina, J.A., Gomez, P., Vargas, C., et al. (2005) Neurotransmitter amino acid in cerebrospinal fluid of patients with dementia with Lewy bodies. *J. Neural Transm.* 112:557–563.

Molloy, S., McKeith, I.G., O'Brien, J.T., and Burn, D.J. (2005) The role of levodopa in the management of dementia with Lewy bodies. *J. Neurol. Neurosurg. Psychiatry* 76:1200–1203.

Molloy, S., Rowan, E.N., McKeith, I.G., O'Brien, J.T., and Burn, D.J. (2006) The effect of levodopa on cognitive function in Parkinson's disease with and without dementia and dementia with Lewy bodies. *J. Neurol. Neurosurg. Psychiatry* 77:1323–1328.

Mosimann, U., Rowan, E., Partington, C., Collerton, D., et al. (2006) Characteristics of visual hallucinations in Parkinson's disease dementia and dementia with Lewy bodies. *Am. J. Geriatr. Psychiatry* 14:154–160.

Mosimann, U.P., Collerton, D., Dudley, R., Meyer, T.D., Graham, G., Dean, J.L., Bearn, D., Killen, A., Dickinson, L., Clarke, M.P., and McKeith, I.G. (2008) A semi-structured interview to assess visual hallucinations in older people. *Int. J. Geriatr. Psychiatry* [Epub ahead of print].

Mosimann, U.P., Mather, G., Wesnes, K.A., O'Brien, J.T., Burn, D.J., and McKeith, I.G. (2004) Visual perception in Parkinson disease dementia and dementia with Lewy bodies. *Neurology* 63:2091–2096.

O'Brien, J.T., Colloby, S., Fenwick, J., Williams, E.D., Firbank, M., Burn, D., et al. (2004) Dopamine transporter loss visualized with FP-CIT SPECT in the differential diagnosis of dementia with Lewy bodies. *Arch. Neurol.* 61:919–925.

O'Brien, J.T., Paling, S., Barber, R., et al. (2001) Progressive brain atrophy on serial MRI in dementia with Lewy bodies, AD, and vascular dementia. *Neurology* 56:1386–1388.

O'Brien, J.T., Paling, S., Barber, R., Williams, E.D., Ballard, C., McKeith, I.G., Gholkar, A., Crum, W.R., Rossor, M.N., and Fox, N.C. (2001) Progressive brain atrophy on serial MRI in dementia with Lewy bodies, AD and vascular dementia. *Neurology* 56: 1386–1388.

Ohara, K., Kondo, N., and Ohara, K. (1998) Changes of monoamines in post-mortem brains from patients with diffuse Lewy body disease. *Pro. Neuro-Psychopharm. Biol. Psychiatry* 22: 311–317.

Oka, H., Yoshioka, M., Morita, M., Onouchi, K., Suzuki, M., Ito, Y., Hirai, T., Mochio, S., and Inoue, K. (2007) Reduced cardiac 123I-MIBG uptake reflects cardiac sympathetic dysfunction in Lewy body disease. *Neurology* 69(14):1460–1465.

Okazaki, H., Lipton, L.S., and Aronson, S.M. (1961) Diffuse intracytoplasmic ganglionic inclusions (Lewy type) associated with progressive dementia and quadraparesis in flexion. *J. Neurol. Neurosurg. Psychiatry* 20:237–244.

Olson, E.J., Boeve, B.F., and Silber, M.H. (2000) Rapid eye movement sleep behaviour disorder: demographic, clinical and laboratory findings in 93 cases. *Brain* 123:331–339

Papapetropoulos, S., McCorquodale, D.S., Gonzalez, J., Jean-Gilles, L., and Mash, D.C. (2006) Cortical and amygdalar Lewy body burden in Parkinson's disease patients with visual hallucinations. *Parkinsonism Rel. Disord.* 12:253–256.

Park, J.Y., and Lansbury, P.T., Jr. (2003) Beta-synuclein inhibits formation of alpha-synuclein protofibrils: a possible therapeutic strategy against Parkinson's disease. *Biochemistry* 42: 3696–3700.

Perry, E.K., Court, J., Goodchild, R., Griffiths, M., Jaros, E., Johnson, M., Lloyd, S., Piggott, M., Spurden, D., Ballard, C., McKeith, I., and Perry, R. (1998) Clinical neurochemistry: developments in dementia research based on brain bank material. *Journal of Neural Transmission (Budapest)* 105:915–933.

Perry, E.K., Curtis, M., Dick, D.J., et al. (1985) Cholinergic correlates of cognitive impairment in Parkinson's disease: comparisons with Alzheimer's disease. *J. Neurol. Neurosurg. Psychiatry* 48:413–421.

Perry, E.K., Kerwin, J., Perry, R.H., Irving, D., Blessed, G., and Fairbairn, A. (1990) Cerebral cholinergic activity is related to the incidence of visual hallucinations in senile dementia of Lewy body type. *Dementia* 1:2–4.

Perry, E.K., Marshall, E., Kerwin, J., et al. (1990) Evidence of a monoaminergic-cholinergic imbalance related to visual hallucinations in Lewy body dementia. *J. Neurochem.* 55:1454–1456.

Perry, E.K., Marshall, E., Perry, R.H., et al. (1990) Cholinergic and dopaminergic activities in senile dementia of Lewy body type. *Alzheimer Dis. Assoc. Disord.* 4:87–95.

Perry, E.K., Marshall, E., Thompson, P., et al. (1993) Monoaminergic activities in Lewy body dementia: relation to hallucinosis and extrapyramidal features. *J. Neural Transm. – Parkinson's Dis. Dement. Sect.* 6:167–177.

Perry, E.K., Morris, C.M., Court, J.A., et al. (1995) Alteration in nicotine binding sites in Parkinson's disease, Lewy body dementia and Alzheimer's disease: possible index of early neuropathology. *Neuroscience* 64:385–395.

Perry, E.K., Smith, C.J., Court, J.A., and Perry, R.H. (1990) Cholinergic nicotinic and muscarinic receptors in dementia of Alzheimer, Parkinson and Lewy body types. *J. Neural Transm. – Parkinson's Dis. Dement. Sect.* 2:149–158.

Perry, R.H., Irving, D., Blessed, G., Fairbairn, A., and Perry, E.K. (1990) Senile dementia of Lewy body type. A clinically and neuropathologically distinct form of Lewy body dementia in the elderly. *J. Neurol. Sci.* 95:119–139.

Piggott, M.A., Ballard, C.G., Burn, D.J., Rowan, E., McKeith, I.G., Perry, R.H., Jaros, E., Perry, E.K. (in press) Dopamine transporter loss in Dementia with Lewy bodies and Parkinson's Disease Dementia.

Piggott, M.A., Ballard, C.G., Dickinson, H.O., McKeith, I.G., Perry, R.H., and Perry, E.K. (2007) Thalamic D2 receptors in dementia with Lewy bodies, Parkinson's disease, and Parkinson's disease dementia. *Int. J. Neuropsychopharm.* 10(2):231–244.

Piggott, M.A., Ballard, C.G., Rowan, E., Holmes, C., McKeith, I.G., Jaros, E., Perry, R.H., and Perry, E.K. (2007) Selective loss of dopamine D2 receptors in temporal cortex in dementia with Lewy bodies, association with cognitive decline. *Synapse* 61(11):903–911.

Piggott, M., Goodchild, R., Johnson, M., Ballard, C., and Perry, E. (2000, April) Serotonin receptor changes in dementing diseases of the elderly. Paper presented at the International Psychogeriatrics Association, Newcastle.

Piggott, M.A., Marshall, E.F., Thomas, N., et al. (1999) Striatal dopaminergic markers in dementia with Lewy bodies, Alzheimer's and Parkinson's diseases: rostrocaudal distribution. *Brain* 122: 1449–1468.

Piggott, M.A., Owens, J., O'Brien, J., et al. (2003) Muscarinic receptors in basal ganglia in dementia with Lewy bodies, Parkinson's disease and Alzheimer's disease. *J. Chem. Neuroanat.* 25:161–173.

Piggott, M.A., Perry, E.K., Marshall, E.F., et al. (1998) Nigrostriatal dopaminergic activities in dementia with Lewy bodies in relation to neuroleptic sensitivity: comparisons with Parkinson's disease. *Biol. Psychiatry* 44:765–774.

Pimlott, S.L., Piggott, M., Ballard, C., McKeith, I., Perry, R., Kometa, S., Owens, J., Wyper, D., and Perry, E. (2006) Thalamic nicotinic receptors implicated in disturbed consciousness in dementia with Lewy bodies. *Neurobiol. Dis.* 21(1):50–56.

Polymeropoulos, M.H., Higgins, J.J., Golbe, L.I., and Nussbaum, R.L. (1996) Mapping of a gene for Parkinson's disease to chromosome 4q21-q23. *Science* 274:1197–1198.

Ransmayr, G., Seppi, K., Donnemiller, E., et al. (2001) Striatal dopamine transporter function in dementia with Lewy bodies and Parkinson's disease. *Eur. J. Nucl. Med.* 28:1523–1528.

Ravina, B., Putt, M., Siderowf, A., et al. (2005) Donepezil for dementia in Parkinson's disease: a randomised, double blind, placebo controlled, crossover study. *J. Neurol. Neurosurg. Psychiatry* 76:934–939.

Reid, R.T., Sabbagh, M.N., Corey-Bloom, J., Tiraboschi, P., and Thal, L.J. (2000) Nicotinic receptor losses in dementia with Lewy bodies: comparisons with Alzheimer's disease. *Neurobio. Aging* 21: 741–746.

Saitoh, T., Xia, Y., Chen, X., Masliah, E., Galasko, D., Shults, C., Thal, L.J., Hansen, L.A., and Katzman, R. (1995) The CYP2D6B mutant allele is overrepresented in the Lewy body variant of Alzheimer's disease. *Ann. Neurol.* 37:110–112.

Samuel, W., Alford, M., Hofstetter, C.R., and Hansen, L. (1997) Dementia with Lewy bodies versus pure Alzheimer disease: differences in cognition, neuropathology, cholinergic dysfunction, and synapse density. *J. Neuropath. Exp. Neurol.* 56:499–508.

Samuels, S.C., Brickman, A.M., Burd, J.A., Purohit, A.C., Quereshi, P.Q., and Serby, M. (2004) Depression in autopsy-confirmed dementia with Lewy bodies and Alzheimer's disease. *Mt. Sinai J. Med.* 71:55–62.

Schenck, C.H., Hurwitz, T.D., and Mahowlad, M.W. (1993) Normal and abnormal REM sleep regulation: REM sleep behaviour disorder: an update on a series of 96 patients and a review of the world literature. *J. Sleep Res.* 2:224–231.

Schenck, C.H., and Mahowald, M.W. (2002) REM sleep behaviour disorder: clinical, developmental and neuroscience perspectives 16 years after its formal identification in sleep. *Sleep* 25:120–138.

Scott, H.L., Pow, D.V., Tannenberg, A.E., and Dodd, P.R. (2002) Aberrant expression of the glutamate transporter excitatory amino acid transporter 1 (EAAT1) in Alzheimer's disease. *J. Neurosci.* 22:RC206.

Scott, W.K., Grubber, J.M., Conneally, P.M., Small, G.W., Hulette, C.M., Rosenberg, C.K., Saunders, A.M., Roses, A.D., Haines, J.L., and Pericak-Vance, M.A. (2000) Fine mapping of the chromosome 12 late-onset Alzheimer disease locus: potential genetic and phenotypic heterogeneity. *Am. J. Hum.Genet.* 66:922–932.

Serpell, L.C., Berriman, J., Jakes, R., Goedert, M., and Crowther, R.A. (2000) Fiber diffraction of synthetic alpha-synuclein filaments shows amyloid-like cross-beta conformation. *Proc. Natl. Acad. Sci. USA* 97:4897–4902.

Sforza, E., Krieger, J., and Petiau, C. (1997) REM sleep behaviour disorder: clinical and physiopathological findings. *Sleep Med. Rev.* 1:57–69.

Sharon, R., Bar-Joseph, I., Frosch, M.P., et al. (2003) The formation of highly soluble oligomers of alpha-synuclein is regulated by fatty acids and enhanced in Parkinson's disease. *Neuron* 37(4): 583–595.

Sharp, S.I., Ballard, C.G., Ziabreva, I., Piggott, M.A., Perry, R.H., Perry, E.K., McKeith, I.G., Aarsland, D., Ehrt, U., Larsen, J.-P., and Paul T. Francis. Serotonin 1A receptor levels associated with depression in patients with Dementia with Lewy bodies and Parkinson's disease dementia. Manuscript submitted for publication.

Shea, C., MacKnight, C., and Rockwood, K. (1998) Donepezil for treatment of dementia with Lewy bodies: a case series of nine patients. *Int. Psychogeriatr.* 10:229–238.

Shinotoh, H., Aotsuka, A., Ota, T., Tanaka, N., Fukushi, K., Nagatsuka, S., Tanada, S., and Ivie, T. (2001) Brain cholinergic function in dementia with Lewy bodies and Alzheimer's disease measured by PET. *Abstracts, Proc 5th Int Conference on Progress in PD and AD*:74.

Shiozaki, K., Iseki, E., Hino, H., and Kosaka, K. (2001) Distribution of M1 muscarinic acetylcholine receptors in the hippocampus of patients with Alzheimer's disease and dementia with Lewy bodies-an immunohistochemical study. *J. Neurol. Sci.* 193:23–28.

Shiozaki, K., Iseki, E., Uchiyama, H., et al. (1999) Alterations of muscarinic acetylcholine receptor subtypes in diffuse Lewy body disease: relation to Alzheimer's disease. *J. Neurol. Neurosurg. Psychiatry* 67:209–213.

Simard, M., van Reekum, R., and Cohen, T. (2000) A review of the cognitive and behavioural symptoms in dementia with Lewy bodies. *J. Neuropsychiatry Clin. Neurosci.* 12:425–450.

Spillantini, M.G., Crowther, R.A., Jakes, R., Hasegawa, M., and Goedert, M. (1998) Alpha-synuclein in filamentous inclusions of Lewy bodies from Parkinson's disease and dementia with Lewy bodies. *Proc. Natl. Acad. Sci. USA* 95:6469–6473.

Spillantini, M.G., Schmidt, M.L., Lee, V.M., Trojanowski, J.Q., Jakes, R., and Goedert, M. (1997) Alpha-synuclein in Lewy bodies. *Nature* 388:839–840.

Stefanova, N., Emgård, M., Klimaschewski, L., et al. (2002) Ultrastructure of alpha-synuclein-positive aggregations in U373 astrocytoma and rat primary glial cells. *Neurosci Lett.* 323(1):37–40.

Strittmatter, W.J., Saunders, A.M., Schmechel, D., Pericak-Vance, A.M., Enghild, J., Salvesen, G.S., and Roses, A.D. (1993) Apolipoprotein E: high avidity binding to b-amyloid and increased frequency of type 4 allele in late-onset familial Alzheimer's disease. *Proc. Natl. Acad. Sci. USA* 90:1977–1981.

Suzuki, M., Desmond, T.J., Albin, R.L., and Frey, K.A. (2002) Striatal monoaminergic terminals in Lewy body and Alzheimer's dementias. *Ann. Neurol.* 51:767–771.

Sweet, R.A., Hamilton, R.I., Butters, M.A., Mulsant, B.H., Pollock, B.G., Lewis, D.A., Lopez, O.I., DeKosky, S.T., and Reynolds, C.F. (2004) Neuropathologic correlates of late-onset major depression. *Neuropsychopharmacology* 29:2242–2250.

Szot, P., White, S.S., Greenup, J.L., Leverenz, J.B., Peskind, E.R., and Raskind, M.A. (2006) Compensatory changes in the noradrenergic nervous system in the locus ceruleus and hippocampus of postmortem subjects with Alzheimer's disease and dementia with Lewy bodies. *J. Neurosci.* 26:467–478.

Taylor, A.E., Yip, A., Brayne, C., Easton, D., Evans, J.G., Xuereb, J., Cairns, N., Esiri, M.M., and Rubinsztein, D.C. (2001) Genetic association of an LBP-1c/CP2/LSF gene polymorphism with late onset Alzheimer's disease. *J. Med. Genet.* 38:232–233.

Teaktong, T., Piggott, M.A., McKeith, I.G., Perry, R.H., Ballard, C., and Perry, E. (2005) Muscarinic M2 and M4 receptors in anterior cingulate cortex: relation to neuropsychiatric symptoms in dementia with Lewy bodies. *Behav. Brain Res.* 161:299–305.

Thaisetthawatkul, P., Boeve, B.F., Benarroch, E.E., Sandroni, P., Ferman, T.J., Petersen, R., and Low, P.A. (2004) Autonomic dysfunction in dementia with Lewy bodies. *Neurology* 62:1804–1809.

Thorns, V., Mallory, M., Hansen, L., and Masliah, E. (1997) Alterations in glutamate receptor 2/3 subunits and amyloid precursor protein expression during the course of Alzheimer's disease and Lewy body variant. *Acta Neuropathol.* 94:539–548.

Tiraboschi, P., Hansen, L.A., Alford, M., et al. (2000) Cholinergic dysfunction in diseases with Lewy bodies. *Neurology* 54:407–411.

Tiraboschi, P., Hansen, L.A., Alford, M., et al. (2002) Early and widespread cholinergic losses differentiate dementia with Lewy bodies from Alzheimer disease. *Arch. Gen. Psychiatry* 59:946–951.

Tiraboschi, P., Salmon, D.P., Hansen, L.A., Hofstetter, R.C., Thal, L.J., and Corey-Bloom, J. (2006) What best differentiates Lewy body from Alzheimer's disease in early stage dementia. *Neurology* 129:729–735.

Tsigelny, I.F., Bar-On, P., Sharikov, Y., Crews, L., Hashimoto, M., Miller, M., Keller, S.H., Platoshyn, O., Yuan, J.X.-Y., and Masliah, E. (2007) Dynamics of a-synuclein aggregation and inhibition of pore-like oligomer development by b-synuclein. *FEBS J.* 274: 1862–1877.

Turner, R.S., D'Amato, C.J., Chervin, R.D., and Blaivas, M. (2000) The pathology of REM sleep behavior disorder with comorbid Lewy body dementia. *Neurology* 55:1730–1732.

Uchiyama, M., Isse, K., Tanaka, K., et al. (1995) Incidental Lewy body disease in a patient with REM sleep behavior disorder. *Neurology* 45:709–712.

Uryu, K., Richter-Landsberg, C., and Welsh, W. (2006) Convergence of heat shock protein 90 with ubiquitin in filamentous alpha-synuclein inclusions of alpha-synucleinopathies. *Am. J. Pathol.* 168:947–961.

Uversky, V. (2007) Neuropathology, biochemistry and biophysics of a-synuclein aggregation. *J. Neurochem.* 103:17–37.

Uversky, V.N., Li, J., Souillac, P., Millett, I.S., Doniach, S., Jakes, R., Goedert, M., and Fink, A. (2002) Biophysical properties of the synucleins and their propensities to fibrillate: inhibition of alpha-synuclein assembly by beta and gamma-synucleins. *J. Biol. Chem.* 277:11970–11978.

Wakabayashi, K., Hayashi, S., Ishikawa, A., Hayashi, T., Okuizumi, K., Tanaka, H., Tsuji, S., and Takahashi, H. (1998) Autosomal dominant diffuse Lewy body disease. *Acta Neuropathol. (Berl)* 96:207–210.

Wakamatsu, M., Ashii, A., Iwata, S., Sakagami, J., Ukai, Y., Ono, M., Kanbe, D., Muramatsu, S., Kobayashi, K., Iwatsubo, T., and Yoshimoto, M. (2007) Selective nigral dopamine neurons induced by overexpression of truncated human a-synuclein in mice. *Neurobiol Aging* 29(4):574–585.

Walker, M.P., Ayre, G.A., Cummings, J.L., Wesnes, K., McKeith, I.G., O'Brien, J.T., and Ballard, C.G. (2000a) The Clinician Assessment of Fluctuation and the One Day Fluctuation Assessment Scale. Two methods to assess fluctuating confusion in dementia. *Br. J. Psychiatry* 177:252–256.

Walker, M.P., Ayre, G.A., Cummings, J.L., Wesnes, K., McKeith, I.G., O'Brien, J.T., and Ballard, C.G. (2000b) Quantifying fluctuation in dementia with Lewy bodies, Alzheimer's disease, and vascular dementia. *Neurology* 54:1616–1624.

Walker, Z., Grace, J., Overshot, R., Satarasinghe, S., Swan, A., Katona, C.L., and McKeith, I.G. (1999) Olanzapine in dementia with Lewy bodies: a clinical study. *Int. J. Geriatr. Psychiatry* 14: 459–466.

Walker, Z., Costa, D.C., Ince, P., McKeith, I.G., and Katona, C.L. (1999) In-vivo demonstration of dopaminergic degeneration in dementia with Lewy bodies. *Lancet* 354:646–647.

Walker, Z., Costa, D.C., Janssen, A.G., Walker, R.W., Livingstone, G., and Katona, C.L. (1997) Dementia with Lewy bodies: a study of post-synaptic dopaminergic receptors with iodine-123 iodobenzamide single-photon emission tomography. *Eur. J. Nucl. Med.* 24:609–614.

Walker, Z., Costa, D.C., Walker, R.W., Lee, L., Livingston, G., Jaros, E., Perry, R., McKeith, I.G., and Katona, C.L. (2004) Striatal dopamine transporter in dementia with Lewy bodies and Parkinson disease A comparison. *Neurology* 62:1568–1572.

Walker, Z., Costa, D.C., Walker, R.W.H., et al. (2002) Differentiation of dementia with Lewy bodies from Alzheimer's disease using a dopaminergic presynaptic ligand. *J. Neurol. Neurosurg. Psychiatry* 73:134–140.

Walker, Z., Jaros, E., Walker, R.W.H., Lee, L., Costa, D.C., Livingston, G., Ince, P.G., Perry, R., McKeith, I., and Katona, C.L.E. (2007) Dementia with Lewy bodies: a comparison of clinical diagnosis, FP-CIT single photon emission computed tomography imaging and autopsy. *J. Neurol. Neurosurg. Psychiatry* 78(11):1176–1181.

Warren, N.M., Piggott, M.A., Lees, A.J., and Burn, D.J. (2007) Muscarinic receptors in the thalamus in progressive supranuclear palsy and other neurodegenerative disorders. *J. Neuropathol. Exp. Neurol.* 66(5):399–404.

Warren, N.M., Piggott, M.A., Lees, A.J., Perry, E.K., and Burn, D.J. (2008) Intact coupling of M1 receptors and preserved M2 and M4 receptors in the cortex in progressive supranuclear palsy: contrast with other dementia. *J. Chem. Neuroanat.* 35(3):268–274.

Wei, J., Fujita, M., Nakai, M., Waragai, M., Watabe, K., Akatsu, H., Rockenstein, E., Masliah, E., and Hashimoto, M. (2007) Enhanced lysosomal pathology caused by b-synuclein mutants linked to dementia with Lewy bodies. *J. Biol. Chem.* 282:28904–28914.

Welsman, D., Cho, M., Taylor, C., Adams, A., Thal, L.J., and Hansan, L.A. (2007) In dementia with Lewy bodes, Braak stage determines phenotype, not Lewy body distribution. *Neurology* 69:356–359.

Wetter, T.C., Collado-Seidel, V., Pollmacher, T., Yassouridis, A., and Trenkwalder, C. (2000) Sleep and periodic leg movement patterns in drug-free patients with Parkinson's disease and multiple system atrophy. *Sleep* 23:361–367.

Whitwell, J.L., Weigand, S.D., Shiung, M.M., Boeve, B.F., Ferman, T.J., et al. (2007) Focal atrophy in dementia with Lewy bodies on MRI: a distinct pattern from Alzheimer's disease. *Brain* 130: 708–719.

Yamamoto, R., Iseki, E., Murayama, N., Minegishi, M., Marui, W., Togo, T., Katsuse, O., Kosaka, K., Kato, M., Iwatsubo, T., and Arai, H. (2007) Correlation in Lewy pathology between the claustrum and visual areas in brains of dementia with Lewy bodies. *Neurosci Lett.* 415:219–224.

Yoshita, M., Taki, J., Yokoyama, K., Noguchi-Shinohara, M., Matsumoto, Y., Nakajima, K., and Yamada, M. (2006) Value of 123I-MIBG radioactivity in the differential diagnosis of DLB from AD. *Neurology* 66:1850–1854.

Zaja-Milatovic, S., Keene, C.D., Montine, K.S., Leverenz, J.B., Tsuang, D., and Montine, T.J. (2006) Selective dendritic degeneration of medium spiny neurons in dementia with Lewy bodies. *Neurology* 66:1591–1593.

Zaja-Milatovic, S., Milatovic, D., Schantz, A.M., et al. (2005) Dendritic degeneration in neostriatal medium spiny neurons in Parkinson disease. *Neurology* 64:545–547.

Zweig, R.M., Cardillo, J.E., Cohen, M., Giere, S., and Hedreen, J.C. (1993) The locus ceruleus and dementia in Parkinson's disease. *Neurology* 43:986–991.

Zweig, R.M., Jankel, W.R., Hedreen, J.C., Mayeux, R., and Price, D.L. (1989) The pedunculopontine nucleus in Parkinson's disease. *Ann. Neurol.* 26:41–46.

63 Dementia in Parkinson's Disease

MARTIN GOLDSTEIN AND C. WARREN OLANOW

Parkinson's disease (PD) is an age-related neurodegenerative disorder that is clinically characterized primarily by motor dysfunction. The cardinal features are resting tremor, rigidity, bradykinesia, and gait dysfunction with postural disturbances. Pathologically, the hallmark of PD is degeneration of dopaminergic (DA-ergic) neurons in the substantia nigra pars compacta (SNc), intracellular protein aggregates in affected neurons known as Lewy bodies (LBs), and a consequent loss of DA-ergic input to the striatum as well as other basal ganglia, thalamic, and cerebral regions (Olanow et al., 2001). Although interest has traditionally focused on motor dysfunction, nonmotor features are increasingly recognized as intrinsic components of PD phenomenology (Poewe, 2007). Among the most important of these nonmotor features is cognitive dysfunction, which is common (Caballol et al., 2007) and can progress to meet clinical criteria of dementia (Goldmann Gross et al., 2008). Indeed, PD-related cognitive disturbances can profoundly affect occupational and social adaptation (Alpert et al., 1990; Dubinsky et al., 1991; Goetz et al., 1995), comprise a major source of disability (Ahlskojg, 2007; Green and Camicioli, 2007), worsen prognosis (Goetz et al., 1995; Aarsland et al., 1996; Litvan, 1998; Aarsland et al., 2000), and shorten survival (Ebmeir et al., 1990a; Louis et al., 1997; Fernandez and Lapane, 2002; Levy, Tang, Louis, et al., 2002). To enhance awareness and clarify terminology, the Movement Disorder Society recently introduced standardized diagnostic criteria (Emre et al., 2007) and assessment strategies (Dubois et al., 2007) that hopefully will be incorporated into the *Diagnostic and Statistical Manual of Mental Disorders*, 5th ed. (*DSM-V*). This review focuses on PD-related cognitive dysfunction and contrasts the clinical, neuropsychological, and pathological features of the dementia that occurs in PD with those associated with other major neurodegenerative disease states.

NOSOLOGY

Although *Parkinson's disease with dementia* (PDD) is a common clinical term, its emergence as a well-defined syndrome remains incomplete, and clinicopathologic definitions remain poorly operationalized (McKeith, 2007). Even nosologic characterization of cognitive dysfunction in PD represents a layered challenge. First, cognitive dysfunction in PD can be multifactorial, as detailed in Figure 63.1. Second, standard treatments for PD can negatively affect cognitive function. Third, comorbidity with other age-associated dementias (for example, cerebrovascular disease, Alzheimer's disease, etc.) is common and can be significant (Leibson et al., 2006). Fourth, the distinction between PDD and dementia with Lewy bodies (DLB) can be difficult (Boeve, 2007); indeed, the distinction between PDD and DLB is somewhat arbitrary, and it remains unclear if they are different disorders or merely variations of a single disease spectrum (Lippa et al., 2007).

EPIDEMIOLOGY

Parkinson's disease is the second most common neurodegenerative disorder after Alzheimer's disease (AD), affecting up to 1% of individuals older than the age of 60 years (Tanner and Goldman, 1996; Khandhar and Marks, 2007). In his original monograph, James Parkinson noted that cognition and behavior were unaffected (Parkinson, 1817). The presence of cognitive disturbances in PD was recognized by Charcot (1877) (who was also the first to apply the term *Parkinson's disease*), and it is now known that cognitive dysfunction commonly occurs in PD (Caballol et al., 2007; Goldmann Gross et al., 2008). Indeed, up to 90% of patients with PD eventually develop cognitive deficits, and a large percentage of these patients progress to frank dementia (Aarsland et al., 2003). Epidemiologic recognition that cognitive dysfunction, including dementia, is widely prevalent in PD has been a principal driving force for the increasing attention that has focused on the nonmotor aspects of PD (McKeith, 2007). Indeed, long-term follow-up studies of patients with PD indicate that dementia and other non-DA features are the primary source of disability (Hely et al., 2005).

The reported incidence and prevalence of cognitive dysfunction in PD vary considerably. This is likely at least in part due to heterogeneities of the patient populations studied, the methodology used to assess cognitive function, and the criteria for diagnosing dementia that

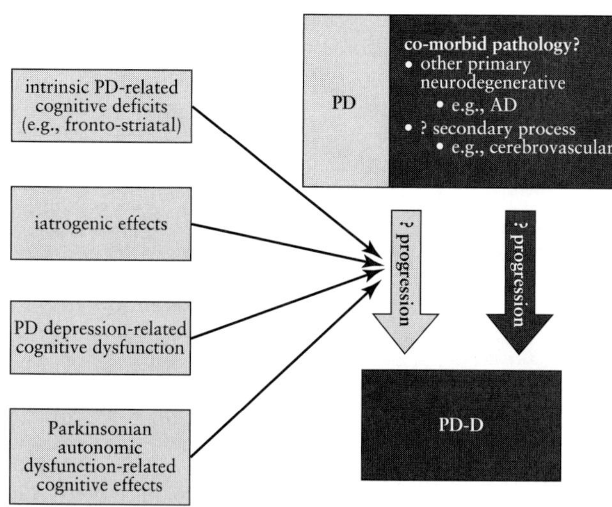

FIGURE 63.1 Multi-factorial conversion of Parkinson's disease to Parkinson's disease with dementia.

were employed (Brown and Marsden, 1984; Boyd et al., 1991; Ebmeier et al., 1991; Pillon et al., 1991; Emre et al., 2007). For example, PDD prevalence has conventionally been studied in hospital clinic–based populations, which consequently limits the generalizability of the data (Emre et al., 2007). Prevalence of dementia among patients with PD was long thought to be about 25% (McKeith, 2007), an estimate influenced by the predominance of movement disorder clinic settings of many studies. However, patients with PD with cognitive impairment may be cared for at a memory clinic or in an institutional care setting and are thus excluded from movement disorder clinic–based prevalence estimates (McKeith, 2007), yielding an artifactually low estimate of PDD. Also, early studies often did not distinguish patients with PDD from patients with DLB (Cummings et al., 1988; Emre et al., 2007), perhaps correctly. Further, PD-related dementia has historically been defined using criteria developed for AD, which may be insensitive to the dementia that occurs in PD and again yielding artificially low prevalence estimates. These types of confounds should be reduced by the establishment of PDD-specific diagnostic criteria (Emre et al., 2007).

Nonetheless, despite epidemiologic challenges, data indicate that intellectual impairment meeting standardized criteria for dementia is common in PD, particularly in the later stages of the disease (Elizan et al., 1986; Ebmeier et al., 1991; Biggins et al., 1992; Lieberman, 1998; Caballol et al., 2007; Goldmann Gross et al., 2008). In a seminal review, Cummings (1988) analyzed 27 studies representing over 4,000 patients with PD and found a mean dementia prevalence of 40%. Mayeux et al. (1992) performed a community-based population study and found that 41.3% of patients with PD had dementia (Mayeux et al., 1992). In a meta-analysis, Aarsland et al. (2005) noted that there was a dementia prevalence of 31.5% among patient populations with PD. They further determined that up to 4% of dementia cases in the general population were due to PDD (Aarsland et al., 2005). They estimated the prevalence of PDD in the general population aged 65 and older to be 0.2%–0.5% (Aarsland et al., 2005). Other studies have reported prevalence rates for dementia among patients with PD of 48% (Hobson and Meara, 2004), 23% (Athey et al., 2005), and 22% (de Lau et al., 2005). Interestingly, even among patients with newly diagnosed PD, the dementia prevalence has been reported as being up to 17% (Foltynie et al., 2004; Kang et al., 2005). Overall, estimates place the prevalence of dementia in PD at 6 times that of age-matched controls (Mayeux et al., 1992; Poewe, 2006; Emre et al., 2007; McKeith, 2007).

Due to the higher mortality rate of PDD relative to patients with PD (Levy, Tang, Louis, et al., 2002), the extent of dementia may be underestimated by prevalence surveys (Mayeux et al., 1990; Marder et al., 1991). More informative data is therefore derived from longitudinal studies affording incidence estimates (Emre et al., 2007). Community-based studies have reported yearly dementia incidence rates of approximately 10% among patients with PD, and relative risks of developing dementia up to 5.9% in comparison to patients with no PD (Aarsland et al., 2001; Hobson et al., 2005; Rippon and Marder, 2005). In a controlled longitudinal study of the incidence of dementia among patients with PD, Biggins et al. (1992) found that 19% of patients with PD developed dementia over a 4½-year period. Patients with PD who developed dementia tended to be older at time of disease onset and to have a longer duration of PD than those who did not develop dementia. Similar results have been reported in a longitudinal cohort study (Williams-Gray et al., 2007), a case-control study (Rajput et al., 1984), and a hospital-based study (Mayeux et al., 1990). Cumulative incidence rates for dementia among patients with PD in carefully performed studies have been reported to be as high as 80% (Aarsland et al., 2003; Burton et al., 2004).

Reid et al. (1996) prospectively followed patients with newly diagnosed PD to assess dementia incidence. They observed that 28% of patients developed dementia after 5 years (Reid et al. 1996). Aarsland et al. (2003) found a 78% cumulative prevalence of dementia in PD after 8 years. In this study, a prominent age effect was observed, with dementia prevalence increasing from 12.4% in the 50- to 59-year age group, to 68.7% in those older than 80 years of age. The mean time course from the onset of PD to development of dementia varies in different studies, ranging between 3 years (Williams-Gray et al., 2007) and 10 years from diagnosis (Hughes et al., 2000; Aarsland et al., 2003). This corresponded to an annual dementia incidence of 30.0 per 1,000 person-years (Williams-Gray et al., 2007).

Although more contemporary prevalence rates of PDD are high in comparison to older studies, they may still underestimate the extent of cognitive impairment in PD. Potential confounds include sampling problems, lack of appropriate controls, use of variable diagnostic criteria, and failure to consider premorbid intelligence. Also, patients with PD are traditionally managed by neurologists who focus on motor dysfunction and place less emphasis on the detection and reporting of behavioral phenomenology.

NEUROPATHOLOGY AND PATHOPHYSIOLOGY OF PDD

Although the precise pathophysiology of cognitive dysfunction in PD remains incompletely understood, scientific advances are yielding increasing insights (Calabresi et al., 2006). It was long thought that much, if not all, dementia in PD was coincidental with brain aging or concomitant AD. However, the realization that patients with PD have a much higher risk of developing dementia than age-matched controls made this theory inadequate (McKeith, 2007). That PDD can incorporate a dysexecutive syndrome, an amnestic "Alzheimer-like" profile (less common), and/or a DLB-like pattern further suggests multifactorial contributors to the development of PDD.

The characteristic neuropathologic feature of PD is degeneration of nigro-striatal DA-ergic neurons coupled with intracellular proteinaceous inclusions known as LBs (Agid et al., 1987; Jellinger, 1987). Within the SNc there is specific involvement of ventro-lateral neurons with relative sparing of DA neurons in the more medial ventral tegmental area (Fearnley and Lees, 1991). With the advent of ubiquitin and α-synuclein staining, it is now appreciated that pathology in PD is extensive (Uversky, 2007). Neuronal loss, frequently associated with LBs, can be found in epinephrine neurons of the locus coeruleus (LC), cholinergic (ACh-ergic) neurons of the nucleus basalis of Meynert (NBM), serotonin neurons of the midline raphé, in the olfactory areas, and in multiple regions of the cerebral hemisphere, brain stem, spinal cord, and peripheral autonomic system (Braak et al., 2006a; Braak et al., 2006b). Indeed, recent studies by Braak and colleagues (Braak et al., 2003; Braak, et al., 2006a) suggest that degeneration in non-DA-ergic regions of the lower brain stem (dorsal motor nucleus of the vagus) and olfactory system precede DA-ergic pathology.

Lewy body pathology in cortical and mesocortical regions is thought to represent the principal pathological correlate of dementia in PD (Hurtig et al., 2000; Emre et al., 2007). Parkinson's disease with dementia can also be associated with AD-type pathology (that is, senile plaques [SPs] and neurofibrillary tangles [NFTs]) that occurs more frequently than in the general populations; McKeith (2007) has suggested a pathologic probability matrix, depicted in Figure 63.2, to help conceptualize these different pathologic processes.

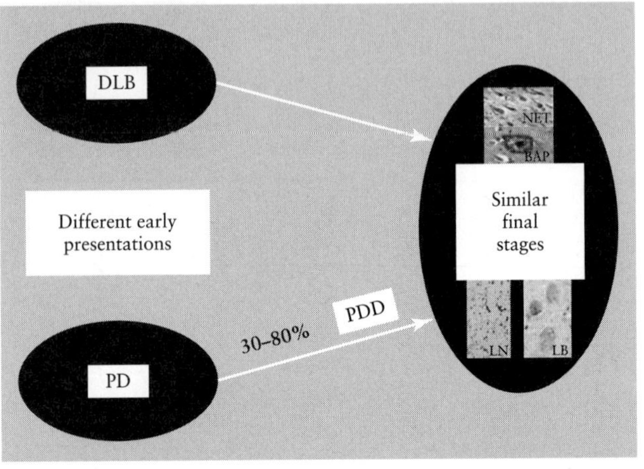

FIGURE 63.2 Converging neuropathologic relationship of Parkinson's disease with dementia (PDD) and dementia with Lewy bodies (DLB).

Cognitive Impairment Secondary to Nigro-Striatal-Frontal Dysfunction

The primary pathologic defect of PD, nigro-striatal DA neuron loss, can lead to dysfunction in striato-frontal loops yielding a variety of cognitive defects (Zgaljardic et al., 2003; Owen, 2007). Although detailed understanding of how nigro-striatal-frontal pathophysiology produces PD-related cognitive impairment remains elusive, broad categories of executive dysfunction represent the core cognitive feature of PD (Alexander et al., 1986; Cummings, 1995; Tinaz et al., 2008). Parkinson's disease–related cognitive dysfunction suggests involvement of each of the major prefrontal cortico-subcortical circuit domains. For example, PDD phenomenology includes semantic, working memory, and task control deficiencies (implicating dorsolateral prefrontal dysfunction), inhibitory dyscontrol (implicating orbitofrontal dysfunction), and initiative/agency failure (implicating medial frontal dysfunction), among other defects (Cummings, 1995; Mesulam, 2000; Frank et al., 2007). Functional neuroimaging offers significant potential for elucidating the specific frontostriatal substrates that underlie the individual PDD clinical features (Monchi et al., 2007).

Neurotransmitter Systems Implicated in PD-Related Neuropsychiatric Dysfunction

Extensive efforts have been made to characterize neurotransmitter profiles associated with cognitive impairment in PD (Francis and Perry, 2007). Dopamine and non-DA systems are affected in PD, including serotonergic (Ser-ergic) neurons in the median raphé, noradrenergic (norepinephrine [NE]-ergic) neurons in the LC, and ACh-ergic neurons in the NBM (Agid et al., 1987; Braak et al., 2006a: Braak et al., 2006b). Speculations as to the basis of such multitransmitter system pathology include excitotoxic damage in targets of the subthalamic nucleus whose glutamatergic neurons are overactive in PD (Rodriguez et al., 1998).

Dopamine system

The reduction in striatal DA secondary to degeneration of SNc DA neurons correlates with, and to a large extent is responsible for, the motor abnormalities that characterize PD. It should be appreciated that the SNc also provides DA-ergic innervation to the entire basal ganglia complex, and portions of the thalamus and cerebral cortex, particularly frontal areas (Parent et al., 2000; Smith and Kieval, 2000). Increasing attention is being devoted to the role of DA depletion in nonmotor aspects of PD, including sleep disturbance, affective dysregulation, and cognitive impairment (Bédard et al., 1998; Brooks and Piccini, 2006; Calabresi et al., 2006; Chaudhuri et al., 2006; Cropley et al., 2006). Extensive animal model, neuropathologic, neurophysiologic, and functional neuroimaging data indicate that DA systems are involved in a myriad of neuropsychological functions, and that DA depletion as occurs in PD can lead to a variety of behavioral disorders (El-Ghundi et al., 2007). The negative symptomatology of schizophrenia (for example, apathy, affective blunting, cognitive slowing) that is thought to be related to DA inhibition offers potential insights into the pathophysiology of dementia in PD (Fournet et al., 2000). Dopamine excess can also be associated with multiple cognitive and behavioral derangements (for example, schizophrenia, amphetamine-induced psychosis, etc.) (Taylor et al., 1990; Zahrt et al., 1997; Goldman-Rakic, 1998, 1999). In PD, DA depletion and iatrogenic DA excess represent potential contributors to the neuropsychiatric dysfunction that can be seen in this disorder (Burn and Troster, 2004).

Norepinephrine (NE) system

The NE system is involved in multiple cognitive and affective functions (Ramos and Amsten, 2007). Many psychotropic agents function via noradrenergic mechanisms, and abnormal increases and decreases in NE activity can adversely affect cognitive function (Ordway and Klimek, 2001). Norepinephrine activity changes in the prefrontal cortex can especially affect prefrontally mediated executive processes (Arnsten et al., 1999; Birnbaum et al., 1999). Extensive data implicate noradrenergic alterations in PD as a contributing factor that leads to neurobehavioral and cognitive dysfunction in PD (Agid et al., 1987; Brooks, 1998; Emre, 2003; Bosboom et al., 2004).

Serotonin (5-HT) system

Considerable data implicate 5-HT systems in affective regulation, impulse control, and aggression (Wrase et al., 2006). Derangements of 5-HT system function have been detected in PD (Kish, 2003; Kish et al., 2008), with the potential to significantly contribute to neuropsychological dysfunction in these domains (Chamberlain et al., 2006; Alex and Pehek, 2007). Further, decarboxylase activity in 5-HT neurons may facilitate conversion of exogenously administered levodopa (LD) to DA (Yamada et al., 2007) and thereby perhaps contribute to cognitive dysfunction associated with changes in DA availability. For all of these reasons, there has been increasing interest in the role of 5-HT in the neurobehavioral features of PD.

Cholinergic (ACh) system

Cholinergic systems play a crucial role in cognitive function, especially memory processes (Cooper et al., 1992). Cholinergic system involvement in the pathogenesis of cognitive dysfunction in AD has directed attention to these systems in patients with PDD (Contestabile et al., 2007), where prominent degeneration is detected in the NBM, the primary source of cholinergic input to the cerebral cortex. The dynamic relationship between DA and ACh has long been a focus of pathophysiologic attention in PD (Calabresi et al., 2006; Schliebs and Arendt, 2006), prompting the early introduction of anticholinergic agents as a treatment for PD. Indeed, such therapies have long been known to adversely affect cognitive function, and these drugs are contraindicated in patients with PD with cognitive dysfunction (Olanow et al., 2001). Interest in the ACh–DA balance has been renewed, with the increasing focus on cognitive dysfunction in PD and the identification of numerous cholinergic neuronal subtypes that might have different functional effects (Calabresi et al., 2006). In fact, cholinergic deficits may be more pronounced in PD than in AD and may occur at an earlier stage of the disease (Bohnen and Frey, 2007). Recent data have demonstrated the clinical utility of cholinesterase inhibitors for PDD (Emre et al., 2004; Cummings and Winblad, 2007).

Cognitive Dysfunction Secondary to Iatrogenic Complications of PD

Medications used to treat PD have complex cognitive effects that remain incompletely understood. Antiparkinsonian drugs can improve and adversely influence cognitive function.

Anti-ACh agents

Anticholinergic activity can impair cognitive function and even cause delirium, especially in the elderly (Koller, 1984; Van Spaendonck et al., 1993; Bédard et al., 1999). Anti-ACh agents (for example, benztropine, trihexyphenidyl) have been long known to be associated with cognitive impairment in PD. For example, in a controlled study of patients with PD, 2 weeks of treatment with the anti-ACh agent trihexyphenidyl caused executive deficits (Bédard et al., 1999), and 4 months of treatment resulted in impaired short-term memory (Cooper et al., 1992). As these drugs typically have minimal antiparkinsonian effects (mostly acting only on tremor), they are rarely employed in the modern era and contraindicated in patients with impaired cognitive functions and the elderly (Olanow et al., 2001).

Dopamine agents

Dopaminergic anti-PD agents have complicated effects on cognitive performance (Molloy et al., 2006; Schultz, 2007a, 2007b). In the early stages of PD, LD can potentially improve select cognitive functions, with variable reports of improvement in wakefulness, verbal fluency, working memory, conditional learning, and cognitive sequencing, as well as reductions in perseveration and global bradyphrenia (Gotham et al., 1988; Cooper et al., 1992; Owen, Roberts, et al., 1993; Cools, 2006; McNamara and Durso, 2006). It has been suggested that one of the ways that LD might ameliorate some high-level cognitive deficits in PD is by inducing increased perfusion to the dorsolateral prefrontal cortex (Cools et al., 2001b; Cools et al., 2002). However, DA-ergic agents also have the potential to cause a wide range of neurobehavioral abnormalities especially when used in more advanced stages of the illness, at higher dosages, and/or in the elderly (Cools et al., 2001b; Olanow et al., 2001; Cools, 2006).

Anti-PD surgery

Surgical treatments are now widely employed in the management of patients with advanced PD (Olanow and Brin, 2001). Striking clinical benefits have been observed in patients who have failed medical therapy, particularly with disability related to motor complications. Ablative lesions for PD (for example, pallidotomy and thalamotomy) have been largely replaced by deep brain stimulation (DBS) because of the increased safety of the latter and a reduced risk of inducing side effects associated with brain lesions (particularly bilateral brain lesions). However, DBS typically involves multiple needle passes through the brain to precisely identify the desired brain target and can induce cognitive impairment, especially in those with preexisting dysfunction (Appleby et al., 2007). Neuropsychological screening to exclude patients with cognitive impairment is now recommended.

Ablative procedures

Cognitive dysfunction following surgical lesions relate to the site and size of the lesion, and whether procedures are performed bilaterally or unilaterally (Lombardi et al., 2000; Trépanier et al., 2000). Nonlateralizing attentional and hemisphere-specific impairments of frontostriatal cognitive function can follow unilateral ablative procedures (Trépanier et al., 2000). A dysexecutive syndrome coupled with behavioral changes of a "frontal nature" has been reported in up to 30% of patients with PD following unilateral pallidotomy (Trépanier et al., 1998). Left-sided pallidotomy is associated with impaired verbal learning and verbal fluency, whereas right-sided pallidotomy causes a loss of visuospatial constructional abilities, which frequently persist (Trépanier et al., 2000). Reports of adverse effects are even more common after bilateral pallidotomy (Parkin et al., 2002), which can include a wide range of neuro-behavioral dysfunctions including affective (depression), comportmental (for example, abulia), impulse control (for example, obsessive–compulsive disorder [OCD]), and assorted cognitive disturbances (for example, apraxias) as well as dysphagia, and dysphonia. Accordingly, physicians have been reluctant to recommend bilateral pallidotomies even to patients who are cognitively intact and with bilateral PD symptoms (Ghika et al., 1999; Olanow and Brin, 2001).

Deep brain stimulation (DBS). Deep brain stimulation has become the surgical procedure of choice for PD (Olanow et al., 2001). High-frequency stimulation simulates the effect of a lesion without necessitating the production of a destructive lesion (Obeso et al., 2001). Deep brain stimulation also permits the performance of bilateral procedures with relative safety, and the targeting of relevant brain structures such as the subthalamic nucleus (STN) that physicians have been reluctant to lesion because of the risk of a potentially fatal hemiballismus (Obeso et al., 2001). This procedure also permits periodic readjustment of stimulator settings to maximize benefits and minimize adversity, and stimulation can be stopped in the case of undesired adverse events.

Cognitive aspects of DBS represent an area of intense study for a variety of reasons. First, DBS has become an important therapy for PD. Second, DBS carries the potential for multifactorial cognitive complications (Voon et al., 2006). For example, immediate cognitive sequelae can result from the multiple needle passes through the frontal lobes required to precisely identify the target site and to place the permanent electrode. More important, however, are the ongoing neuro-behavioral effects associated with continued stimulation, which, though widely commented upon, remain poorly defined (Appleby et al., 2007). For example, stimulation in the region of the STN can lead to profound depression with increased suicide rates, transient periods of uproarious laughter, and impulse control dysfunction (see below). Finally, the evolving application of DBS for the treatment of a range of neuropsychiatric disorders such as depression and OCD (Wichamann and DeLong, 2006) has further prompted curiosity about the neurobehavioral effects of stimulating a variety of brain targets. Immediate and evolving long-term cognitive effects of PD can be complicated by any preexisting neurobehavioral dysfunction; this has prompted recommendations that neuropsychological assessment be an essential component of evaluation for a DBS procedure (Okun et al., 2007).

Unilateral thalamic stimulation is relatively well tolerated (Woods et al., 2001), but this procedure is now rarely employed because superior results are obtained with DBS-STN or globus pallidus pars interna (GPi). The cognitive effects of unilateral or bilateral DBS-GPi remain somewhat controversial (Ardouin et al., 1999; Fields et al., 1999; Saint-Cyr et al., 2000). One group found no evidence of impairment following bilateral DBS-GPi on a full battery of neuropsychological tests (Fields et al., 1999). In fact, they reported significant improvement in delayed recall, as well as subjective anxiolysis. In contrast, another study observed deterioration in lexical fluency following DBS-GPi (Ardouin et al., 1999). Relative to DBS-STN, patients who have DBS-GPi have been noted to have a higher suicide rate (Appleby et al., 2007). Nonetheless, in a study of patients with DBS-GPi, Rodrigues et al. (2007) found improved quality of life measures, including cognition.

Deep brain stimulation-STN has emerged as the predominant surgical treatment modality, and there is increasing focus on the cognitive sequelae for this procedure (Aybek et al., 2007). An early study investigating cognitive aspects of DBS-STN found improved performance on the random number generation test, Wisconsin Card Sorting Test, and on paced serial addition and missing digit tests, but that performance worsened conditional associative learning (Jahanshahi et al., 2000). Morrison et al. (2000) designed a neuropsychological program to try to distinguish the cognitive effects of surgical implantation from stimulation in patients undergoing bilateral DBS-STN. In a study of 17 patients, they demonstrated that the surgical procedure itself adversely affected attention and concentration and tended to adversely affect verbal learning, naming, and verbal fluency (Morrison et al., 2004). No detectable adverse effects on cognition or depression were associated with stimulation (Morrison et al., 2004). Pillon et al. (2000) also tried to discriminate the acute effects on cognition of surgical implantation from those of chronic STN stimulation. They reported no impairment of memory or executive functions for up to 6 months after DBS surgery but did find mild impairment in lexical fluency at 12 months (Pillon et al., 2000). They also noted small but significant improvements in psychomotor speed and working memory when the stimulator was turned on compared to when it was turned off. Saint-Cyr and colleagues (2000) reported significant declines in multiple cognitive processes (working memory, speed of mental processing, bimanual motor speed and coordination, set switching, phonemic fluency, long-term consolidation of verbal material, and encoding of visuospatial material) in the first year after surgery, particularly in older patients with bilateral DBS-STN. In trying to interpret these studies, it is important to realize that (a) there are variations in surgical technique and in the number of needle passes required to identify the target, (b) the precise location of the electrode is not known with precision, (c) stimulation of different sites within the same brain target can lead to opposite effects (that is, though stimulation in the ventral pallidum improves parkinsonian features, stimulation in the dorsal GPi can worsen them), and (d) stimulation has the potential to affect distant as well as near brain regions.

Parsons et al. (2006) performed a quantitative meta-analysis to better ascertain the cognitive consequences of DBS-STN. Analyzing studies published between 1990 and 2006, the investigators found small declines in executive functions, verbal learning, and memory; moderate declines were only reported in semantic and phonemic verbal fluency. Changes in verbal fluency were not related to patient age, disease duration, stimulation parameters, or change in DA-ergic therapy after surgery. York et al. (2007) investigated cognitive and other neuropsychiatric outcomes at 6 months in patients who had bilateral DBS-STN compared to those who received best medical treatment. Compared to controls, patients who had DBS-STN demonstrated significant declines in verbal memory and inhibition of a dominant response, with trends for declines in verbal fluency, verbal long-term recall, and set-shifting. Patients who had DBS-STN demonstrated no significant changes in depression or anxiety scores, but one patient who had DBS developed dementia over 6 months compared to none of the PD controls. This data prompted the study authors to recommend counseling candidates for DBS-STN about the risk of mild linguistic and executive cognitive declines associated with the procedure.

Conflicting results obviously may reflect differences in patient population, neural target for stimulation, laterality, and status of the stimulator at the time of neurobehavioral evaluation. Of particular interest are case reports of patients who experienced profound depression with suicidal ideations following STN stimulation (Burkhard et al., 2004; Appleby et al., 2007) and a possible role of STN in impulse control disorders (Wichamann and DeLong, 2006; Hardesty and Sackeim, 2007).

Further studies are required to better inform us about the neurophysiologic and neurobehavioral consequences of DBS.

RELATIONSHIP OF PDD TO OTHER NEURODEGENERATIVE COGNITIVE DISORDERS

Nosologic classification of the neurodegenerative dementias represents an evolving construct, as progressively improving clinical, pathologic, and mechanistic understanding emerges. Diagnostic classification has historically been influenced by what type of patients a physician is likely to see. For example, a patient with dementia and parkinsonism might be diagnosed as having "Alzheimer disease with parkinsonism" in a memory disorder clinic but with "PD-dementia" in a movement disorder clinic. The neuropathologist who finds pathological evidence consistent with PD and AD may also struggle to provide an exact diagnosis and may be understandably prejudiced by the clinical history in providing a final diagnosis. In these instances, the pathology report may represent less of a diagnostic "gold standard" than simply a reflection of the clinical orientation of the physicians, who in turn were hoping to be informed by pathologic findings (Perl et al., 1998).

Multidisciplinary neuroscientific insights have generated increasing interest in the commonalities between PDD and other neurodegenerative cognitive disorders, and the question as to whether they are separate diseases or merely part of a spectrum of neurodegeneration (Love, 2005; Metzler-Baddeley, 2007). Clinical and neuropathologic overlap of PDD, AD with parkinsonism, and DLB have especially driven hypotheses regarding their respective relationships and the possibility of a common underlying neurodegenerative process (Perl et al., 1998; Galvin, 2006). For example, many patients diagnosed during life with PDD demonstrate classic degenerative changes in the SNc postmortem but also show NFTs and SPs sufficient to make a diagnosis of AD and/or diffuse cortical LBs consistent with DLB-related pathology (Byrne et al., 1987; Perl et al., 1998; Noe et al., 2004; Burn, 2006a, 2006b). These pathologic admixtures, along with their corresponding clinical overlap, have prompted consideration of the possibility that these disorders comprise various cognitive-motor permutations of a neurodegenerative spectrum, with consequent implications for nosologic classification. Although such theorizing, and their empiric bases, remain an evolving process, it is useful to briefly review currently known pathologic relationships among PD and other major neurodegenerative cognitive disorders to clinico-pathologically contextualize PD-related cognitive dysfunction. Table 63.1 provides a summary of the pathologic findings among the major neurodegenerative cognitive disorders (Boeve, 2007).

TABLE 63.1 *Neurodegenerative Cognitive Disorders and Associated Dysfunctional Proteins*

Dysfunctional Protein	*Neurodegenerative Syndrome*
Amyloid	AD
(amyloidopathies)	Down syndrome
Tau	AD
(tauopathies)	Pick's disease
	CBGD
	PSP
	FTDP-17 with mutation in the microtubule-associated protein tau (FTDP-17 MAPT)
α-synuclein	PDD
(synucleinopathies)	DLB
	MSA
TAR DNA-binding protein 43 (TDP-43)	FTLD ubiquitin-positive inclusions (FTLD-U)
huntingtin	HD

Adapted from Boeve (2003).
AD: Alzheimer's disease; CBGD: cortico basal ganglionic degeneration; PSP: progressive supranuclear palsy; PDD: Parkinson's disease with dementia; DLB: dementia with Lewy bodies; MSA: multiple system atrophy; FTLD: frontotemporal lobar dementia; HD: Huntington's disease.

PD and AD

Although AD and PD are relatively common disorders of the elderly, the overlap of clinical and pathological features between the two conditions exceeds that which would be expected to occur by chance alone (Perl et al., 1998), further driving interest in potentially unifying their pathogenic mechanisms. That said, there exist fundamental differences in the patterns of evolution of AD and PD dementias that support their clinicopathologic individualization (Stern et al., 1998).

Patients with PD have increased risk of developing dementia, and there is increased frequency of parkinsonian motor features in patients with AD. There is increased risk of AD in siblings of patients with PDD compared with siblings of matched normal patients (Marder et al., 1999). Traumatic brain injury, hypertension, and diabetes are risk factors for the development of AD (Schofield et al., 1997), but not for PDD (Levy, Tang, Cote, et al., 2002).

Spectrum conceptualizations of neurodegenerative cognitive disorders have driven increasing interest in the relationship between the cognitive profiles of PDD and AD (Bronnick et al., 2007).

Parkinsonism in AD

Numerous clinical studies have reported on the presence of parkinsonian features in patients with AD (Chui et al., 1985; Mayeux et al., 1985; Kurlan et al., 2000). In these cases, AD-related parkinsonian motor abnormalities are usually characterized by rigidity and bradykinesia rather than resting tremor (Mitchell, 1999; Kurlan et al., 2000). As with cognitive dysfunction in PD, the prevalence of AD-related parkinsonian features is likely to be underestimated because most reports come from AD clinics focusing primarily on cognitive function and without expertise in movement disorders. Reports of the prevalence of parkinsonism in patient populations with AD vary considerably, with some extending to 90%, particularly in studies performed by movement disorder specialists (Molsa et al., 1984; Lippa et al., 1998; Mitchell, 1999). For example, in one study conducted by investigators with PD expertise, 92% (n = 143) of patients with AD were found to have extrapyramidal signs (Molsa et al., 1984). In a 66-month prospective longitudinal study, extrapyramidal features developed in 36% of patients with mild AD (n = 44) who were preselected on the basis of not having motor dysfunction at baseline; this compared to 5% (n = 58) in age-matched controls (Morris et al., 1989). Parkinsonian motor features can be detected at any stage of the AD-related dementia process (Morris et al., 1989).

Neuropsychological overlap and distinctions between AD and PD

In general, cognitive impairment is more extensive in AD than in PDD. Although executive dysfunction is the core feature of PDD, anterograde amnesia is the hallmark of AD (McKeith, 2007). However, despite their respective relative cortical versus subcortical bases, there is significant overlap in the cognitive profiles of PDD and AD (Bronnick et al., 2007; McKeith, 2007), as depicted in Figure 63.3. Investigators have attempted to determine if there exists a meaningful distinction in the cognitive profile of patients with AD complicated by parkinsonism (ADP) versus AD without parkinsonism. In a study comparing these groups matched for age, education, and disease duration, patients with ADP, relative to their AD counterparts, were more impaired on tests of short-term learning and memory, orientation, naming, verbal fluency, and construction, but not on tests of long-term memory, abstract reasoning, or verbal comprehension (Richards, Bell, et al., 1993). Such data suggest that parkinsonism within the context of AD may be a useful marker for a cognitive deficit profile distinct from that characterizing AD uncomplicated by parkinsonism, representing in part a mixture of PDD and AD pathology.

Pathological overlap and distinctions: evidence of PD changes in AD, and AD changes in PD

Postmortem studies provide evidence of pathologic overlap between PD and AD, with numerous reports documenting a high prevalence of neuropathological features of PD in patients diagnosed antemortem with AD (Byrne et al., 1987; Perl et al., 1998; Noe et al., 2004; Burn, 2006a, 2006b). In the Morris et al. (1989) study of patients with AD with extrapyramidal motor signs described above, postmortem nigral changes consistent with PD-related pathology were identified in addition to expected AD changes. In another study, 18 of 40 consecutively presenting patients with "autopsy-confirmed" AD also had neurodegenerative changes in the SN consistent

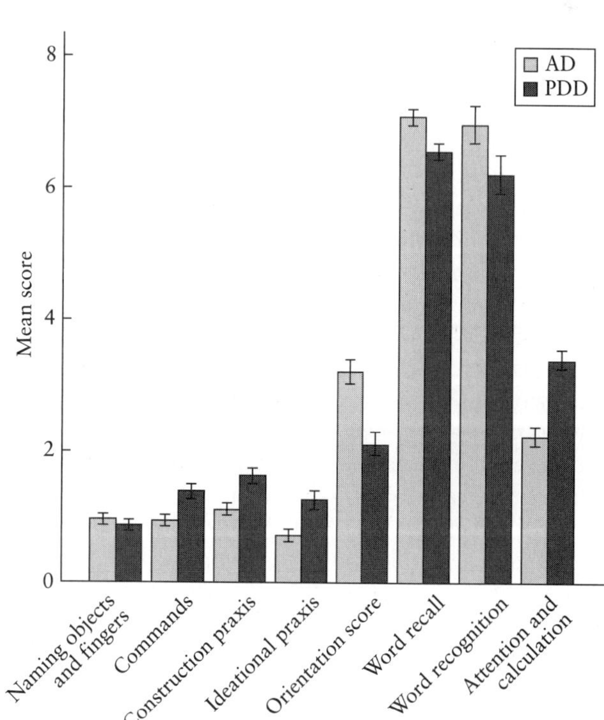

Higher scores indicate worse performance. Values are mean (95% CI).

FIGURE 63.3 Cognitive profile of Parkinson's disease with dementia (PDD) compared with Alzheimer's disease (AD).

with a diagnosis of PD (Leverenz and Sumi, 1986). Ditter and Mira (1987) studying 20 consecutively presenting patients with "pathologically confirmed" AD observed that 55% also had nigral degeneration with LBs in the SNc consistent with a pathological diagnosis of PD. In another study, 23% of patients with AD specifically selected because they met the Consortium to Establish a Registry for Alzheimer's Disease (CERAD) clinical and neuropathological criteria for "definite AD" had PD-consistent changes in the SN at postmortem (Hulette et al., 1995).

Studies in patients clinically diagnosed with PD show parallel evidence of AD-related pathology. For example, an autopsy study of 36 patients with "autopsy-proven" PD noted SPs and NFTs consistent with a pathological diagnosis of AD in 42% of patients (Boller et al., 1980). Alzheimer's disease-related pathologic changes were more severe in patients with PD with dementia than in patients with PD with no dementia, and the frequency of AD pathology was 6 times higher than that expected in an age-matched control population (Boller et al., 1980). Another study compared the prevalence of AD pathology in patients with dementia and patients with no dementia with "pathologically proven" PD and in age-matched controls. Senile plaques and NFTs sufficient to make a diagnosis of AD were present in 75% of the PD group and in 94% of those patients with PDD (Gaspar and Gray, 1984).

In sum, there exists significant clinical and pathological overlap between PD and AD, but the overall etiologic significance of this remains unknown.

Parkinsonian Spectrum Processes

A group of disorders termed "Parkinson's plus" or "atypical Parkinsonism" comprise syndromes marked by more widespread degeneration than is seen with PD (usually striatum and pallidum in addition to SNc) combined with a variety of additional motor and nonmotor features (cerebellar degeneration, eye movement disorders, autonomic dysfunction). In general, atypical parkinsonian syndromes are characterized by early-onset speech and gait disturbance, axial greater than appendicular rigidity, relative absence of tremor, and a poor response to LD (Olanow et al., 2001). They include multiple system atrophy (MSA), progressive supranuclear palsy (PSP), and cortico basal ganglionic degeneration (CBGD). Each of these include variable parkinsonian and cognitive features (Litvan, Agid, Calne, et al., 1996; Schneider et al., 1997; Kertesz et al., 2000; Wenning et al., 2000). The cognitive profiles associated with each of these syndromes tend to manifest distinctive neuropsychological patterns (Lauterbach, 2004; Robbins et al., 1994).

Dementia with Lewy bodies (DLB) has become the preferred term used to describe the dementia that occurs in association with parkinsonian features and diffusely distributed cortical LBs (McKeith et al, 1996; McKeith, 2007). Dementia with Lewy bodies is now thought to be the second most frequent neuropathologically diagnosed degenerative dementia (Aarsland, 2002; Ransmayr, 2002). Dementia with Lewy bodies is a clinically defined syndrome consisting of a predominantly dysexecutive dementia, prominent visual hallucinations, and fluctuating sensorium in addition to parkinsonian motor features (McKeith, 2007). The presence of cognitive dysfunction characterized by at least two of three core features qualifies for a diagnosis of probable DLB, which in turn is 90% predictive of LB pathology at autopsy (McKeith et al., 2005; McKeith, 2007). Other common features include depression, rapid-eye-movement (REM) behavior sleep disorder (RBD), prominent gait instability, and syncope (McKeith et al., 1996; Aarsland, 2002; Ransmayr, 2002).

Dementia with Lewy bodies is pathologically characterized by widely distributed cortical and subcortical (SNc, LC, dorsal vagal nucleus, NBM) LBs, in association with nigral degeneration and AD-type lesions (McKeith et al., 1996; Verny and Duyckaerts, 1998). Neurochemical findings include marked reductions of cortical acetylcholine and nigro-striatal DA (McKeith et al., 1996; McKeith et al., 2004). Mean age at disease onset ranges between 60 and 68 years; mean disease duration averages 6 to 7 years (McKeith et al., 2004). Males are more frequently affected than females (McKeith et al., 2004).

A key, though somewhat arbitrary, differential diagnostic feature distinguishing PDD and DLB is the temporal sequence of the onset of motor and cognitive dysfunction: dementia occurring prior to, or within 1 year after the onset of PD features is diagnosed as DLB, whereas dementia developing more than 1 year after the onset of PD is diagnosed as PDD (McKeith et al., 2005). This is known as the "one year rule." Many question the legitimacy of the "one year rule" as a principal nosologic distinction between DLB and PDD (Lippa et al., 2007). The absence of empiric foundation for a diagnostic rule that categorizes a dementia beginning 11 months after PD diagnosis as DLB but one beginning 13 months later as PDD seems somewhat contrived and raises the question of whether they are not in fact a part of the same neurodegenerative disorder.

The cognitive dysfunction of DLB is usually more severe than the dementia of PDD, particularly for prefrontally mediated (Downes et al., 1998) and visual processing tasks (McKeith, 2007). For example, a recent study by Mondon et al. (2007) attempted to compare cognitive profiles of PDD and DLB. Despite global similarities in cognitive performances, patients with DLB consistently had worse performance on tasks requiring higher-order visuospatial processing.

In contrast to the general trend in PDD, psychosis can occur in DLB regardless of DA-ergic treatment (McKeith et al., 2005). Approximately 75% of patients with DLB experience hallucinations, and more than 50% suffer from delusions (Aarsland et al., 2001). In a study by Aarsland and colleagues (2000) comparing DLB, PDD, and PD without dementia, delusions and hallucinations were most common in the DLB group (57% and 76%, respectively), followed by the PDD group (29% and 54%, respectively), and finally the PD without dementia group (7% and 14%, respectively). Patients with DLB are reported to be exquisitely sensitive to neuroleptics, though historically this issue may have been exaggerated (Aarsland et al., 2005).

In sum, there is striking clinical, pathological, and biochemical overlap among DLB, PDD, and AD with parkinsonism. It remains to be determined whether DLB represents a discrete nosological entity or merely an anticipated intermediary on the neurodegenerative spectrum between PD and AD. Boeve (2007) published an exhaustive review of parkinsonian spectrum neurodegenerative processes; see Table 63.2 for an inventory of characteristic features.

RISK FACTORS FOR DEVELOPMENT OF COGNITIVE DYSFUNCTION IN PD

Genetic

Genetic factors have been implicated in the aetiology of PD. Several different genetic mutations have been identified in small numbers of patients with autosomal dominant and recessive forms of familial PD (De Marco et al., 2008; Kahle, 2008). Of particular note are mutations in *LRRK2* gene that are found not only in early-onset familial cases, but also in older patients with no family history and with clinical and pathologic fea-

TABLE 63.2 *Features of Other Neurodegenerative Cognitive Disorders Presenting with Parkinsonism*

Disorder	*Parkinsonian Findings*	*Principal Cognitive Features*
DLB	Masked facies, stooped posture, reduced arm swing similar to PD and PDD, but tremor less asymmetric and more postural than resting. Features tend to develop after cognitive features.	• severe progression of mixed subcortical and cortical features • visual hallucinations • fluctuating sensorium • neuroleptic sensitivity
CBGD	Markedly asymmetric rigidity (dystonia), often with coexisting jerky tremor, myoclonus; parkinsonism is minimally levodopa responsive.	Cortical dysfunction as reflected by at least one of the following: • focal or asymmetric ideomotor apraxia • alien limb phenomenon • cortical sensory loss • visual or sensory hemineglect • constructional apraxia • apraxia of speech or nonfluent aphasia
PSP	Parkinsonism with early gait impairment and postural instability, impaired vertical eye movements, wide-eyed stare, reduced eye-blink frequency, axial greater than appendicular rigidity.	Early onset of cognitive impairment including at least two of the following: apathy, impairment in abstract thought, decreased verbal fluency, utilization or imitation behavior, or frontal release signs.
MSA	Parkinsonism with early speech and balance impairment, axial rigidity, minimal asymmetry; minimal LD responsivity in the striatonigral variant (MSA-P); ataxia and spasticity prominent in the olivopontocerebellar atrophy variant (MSA-C); orthostatic hypotension and autonomic dysfunction prominent in the Shy–Drager syndrome variant.	• variable • overall milder / more subtle / more gradual progression
FTLD-P17	Variable parkinsonism, sometimes LD responsive, often similar findings to those in CBGD.	mixed dysexecutive
AD+p	Parkinsonism tends to be later in course; rigidity, bradykinesia, tremor (resting or postural) most obvious.	• anterograde amnesia • dysnomia

Source: Adapted from Boeve, 2007.

DLB: dementia with Lewy bodies; CBGD: cortico basal ganglionic degeneration; PSP: progressive supranuclear palsy; MSA: multisystem atrophy; FTLD-P17: frontotemporal lobar dementia with parkinsonism associated with chromosome 17 mutation; AD+p: Alzheimer's Disease with parkinsonism; PDD: Parkinson's disease with dementia; LD: levodopa.

tures typical of sporadic PD. First-degree relatives of patients with sporadic PD also have an increased risk of developing PD (Warner and Schapira, 2003).

As for PDD specifically, genetic data is sparse. A positive family history of parkinsonism or dementia imposes a modest increase in the chance that a patient with PD will convert to PDD (Marder et al., 1990; Schrag et al., 1998). Genetic predisposition for PDD has only been systematically studied for apolipoprotein ε4 (ApoE4) genotypes, with conflicting results (Emre et al., 2007). A positive correlation of E2 or E4 alleles with PDD was reported in some studies (Harhangi et al., 2000; Parsian et al., 2002; de Lau et al., 2005) whereas a negative association with E4 was found in others (Koller et al., 1995; Inzelberg et al., 1998; Camicioli et al., 2005). Dementia has been reported in familial forms of PD characterized by *PARK1* (Zarranz et al., 2004) and *PARK8* (Wszolek et al., 1997) genes, whereas PDD is rare in those familial PD forms characterized by *PARK2, PARK6,* and *PARK7* genes (Emre et al., 2007).

Age

Significant interactions exist between age, age at time of PD onset, and PD-associated cognitive deterioration (Richards, Stern, et al., 1993; Marder et al., 1995; Glatt et al., 1996; Schrag et al., 1998; Graham and Sagar, 1999; Emre et al., 2007). Several studies have demonstrated that in PD, advancing age is associated with a faster rate of development of extrapyramidal motor dysfunction, more severe gait and postural instability, decreased LD responsivity, and more profound cognitive impairment including dementia (Levy, 2007). In general, it appears that age and overall disease severity are synergistic risk factors for developing dementia in PD (Levy, Schupf, et al., 2002; Levy, 2007). It was previously inferred that the apparently low incidence of cognitive deficits in patients with young-onset PD may relate to their ability to compensate for PD-related degenerative changes (Dubois et al., 1990). However, a study by Aarsland, Kvaloy, et al. (2007) found that, after adjusting for age, age at PD onset does not influence the risk for later dementia development.

Education Level

As in AD, education level correlates inversely with cognitive decline in PD (Glatt et al., 1996; Cohen et al., 2007; Verbaan et al., 2007). Although the association between high educational attainment and lower risk of developing cognitive dysfunction suggests the potential for education to modulate cognitive performance in PD, interpretation of such findings is complicated by multiple potential confounds (Ngandu et al., 2007). For example, a potential association of greater academic achievement with higher premorbid cognitive performance would imply greater cognitive reserve capacity, with consequent resilience to the neurodegenerative dementia processes (Ngandu et al., 2007).

Environmental Exposure

Epidemiological studies have noted an inverse correlation between smoking and PD, with epidemiologic studies consistently demonstrating that smokers have a seemingly reduced risk of developing PD (Morens et al., 1995). By contrast, Levy, Tang, Cote, et al. (2002) noted a positive association between smoking and dementia in patients with PD; in particular, current smoking was more strongly associated with incident dementia than past smoking.

Type, Severity, and Levodopa Responsivity of Motor Symptoms

There is a strong correlation between the severity of parkinsonian motor signs and the severity of cognitive deficits (Ebmeier et al., 1990b; Richards, Stern, et al., 1993; Marder et al., 1995; Glatt et al., 1996; Levy, Schupf, et al., 2002). Motor deficit and advanced age have a particularly synergistic effect on the risk of developing cognitive impairment: Levy, Schupf, et al. (2002) found that patients with older age and high severity of motor symptoms had a relative risk of incident dementia of 9.7% compared with a younger age/lower severity group.

In general, akinetic-rigid forms of PD are associated with a higher risk of dementia (Ebmeier et al., 1991; Emre et al., 2007; Williams-Gray et al., 2007). Akinetic-rigid forms of PD are characterized by features that classically do not respond to LD including axial, gait, posture, balance, facial reactivity, and speech disturbances (Elizan et al., 1986; Emre et al., 2007). Aarsland et al. (2004) further found that LD-unresponsive features are associated with accelerated cognitive decline. Levy and colleagues (2000) found that speech impairment, bradykinesia, and axial instability had the strongest associations with incident dementia in PD. A cross-sectional study by Burn et al. (2003) found an overrepresentation of the postural instability gait difficulty (PIGD) motor subtype to be present in 88% of patients with PDD compared with 38% of patients with PD without dementia. In the PD group, tremor dominant (TD) and PIGD subtypes were evenly represented compared to the predominant PIGD pattern in PDD (Burn et al., 2003). This observation was further supported by a prospective follow-up study of 40 patients with PD where 25% of those with the PIGD subtype developed dementia, compared with none who had TD or indeterminate phenotypes (Burn et al., 2006). Williams-Gray et al. (2007) also observed that in a cohort of patients with PD, those who did not have a TD PD phenotype at baseline had a greater risk of developing dementia. It should be appreciated that patients with the PIGD subtype are also more likely to have an atypical parkinsonism and to have a more aggressive rate of decline in motor features as well (Emre et al., 2007). In contrast, tremor dominance at presentation has been associated with relative cognitive resilience and a reduced risk of developing dementia (Elizan et al., 1986). In fact, Alves and colleagues (2006) found that dementia did not occur among patients with persistent TD subtype, and patients with TD subtype at baseline did not develop dementia unless they transitioned to PIGD subtype. Patients who suffer from dystonic dyskinesias have been variably associated with increased risk for PDD (Emre et al., 2007).

Perceptual Disturbance (Hallucinations)

Visual hallucinations (VH) are a marker for increased risk of the subsequent development of dementia in patients with PD (Mayeux et al., 1992; Stern et al., 1993; Marder et al., 1995; Aarsland et al., 2003). Ramirez-Ruiz et al. (2007) found that 45% of patients with PD and no dementia who experienced hallucinations developed dementia over the course of a 1-year period. In the same study, more than 80% of patients with PD with no dementia who had hallucinations had mild cognitive impairment (MCI) compared to only 30% of patients with PD with no dementia who did not have hallucinations (Ramirez-Ruiz et al., 2007). Cognitive functions involving higher visual processing, including visual memory, were especially affected in those with hallucinations.

Sleep Disturbance

Sleep disturbances with excessive daytime sleepiness (EDS) are common in PD (Brodsky et al., 2003), with multiple potential complicating influences on cognitive and affective function. Excessive daytime sleepiness has been reported to be a risk factor for the development of dementia in a patient with PD (Gjerstad et al., 2007). REM behavior disorder (RBD), a parasomnia frequently reported in PD, may also be a risk factor for dementia (Sinforiani et al., 2006). For example, patients with PD with concomitant RBD show significantly worse performance on neuropsychological tests measuring episodic verbal memory, executive functions, and visuoperceptual processing compared to patients with PD without RBD (Vendette et al., 2007). In a consecutive series of RBD patients, 10 of 25 with PD had dementia (Olson et al., 2000). Although there have been longitudinal studies demonstrating that RBD is a risk factor for PD (Schenck et al., 1996), there have not been similar studies with respect to PDD. It should be appreciated that RBD is also commonly seen in other synucleinopathies that are associated with dementia such as DLB and MSA.

CLINICAL FEATURES OF PDD

Cognitive Profile

Cognitive dysfunction in PD can range from exquisitely subtle changes requiring sensitive neuropsychological instruments to detect, to frank dementia where the patient requires continuous supervision to ensure safety. When slight, the patient, caregivers, and even experienced clinicians may not recognize the presence of any cognitive problem (Marjama-Lyons and Koller, 2001). Although onset is typically insidious, progression to dementia is usually inexorable, with mean annual rate of decline in Mini-Mental State Examination (MMSE) score ranging from 1 to 4.5 points (Aarsland et al., 2004; Burn et al., 2006). Recognition that dementia becomes increasingly prevalent in PD populations over time prompted the need to develop standardized criteria for diagnosing PDD (McKeith, 2007). A Movement Disorder Society Task Force (MDSTF) charged with this responsibility recently reported its findings (Emre et al., 2007). Based on an extensive literature review, this group recently published a definitive compilation of the neuropsychiatric profile characterizing PDD. We here briefly review the characteristic features of PDD, which are inventoried in Table 63.3.

Early stages: Sentinel neuropsychological deficits

Although Graham and Sagar (1999) suggested the existence of a "motor-only" stage of PD characterized by progressive motor dysfunction in the absence of cognitive impairment, neuropsychological deficits can be noted in the vast majority of patients even in the early stages of the disease (Pirozzolo et al., 1982; Taylor et al., 1990; Cooper et al., 1991; Janvin et al., 2005; Lewis et al., 2005; Williams-Gray et al., 2007). Cognitive deficits in early PD are marked by significant heterogeneity among a variety of different cognitive domains, including executive, linguistic, memory, and complex visual (Taylor et al., 1990; Cooper et al., 1991; Dubois and Pillon, 1997; Cools et al., 2001a; Janvin et al., 2005; Lewis et al., 2005; Williams-Gray et al., 2007). Although the relationship between the initial deficit pattern and the subsequent dementia remains to be clarified (Emre et al., 2007), data derived from prospective studies suggest that certain deficit patterns may herald later cognitive decline (Mahieux et al., 1998; Janvin et al., 2005). For example, a longitudinal community-based epidemiological study of patients with PD showed that baseline performance on verbal fluency tasks was significantly associated with subsequent incident dementia (Jacobs et al., 1995). Results of several other studies also suggest that poor performance on tests of verbal fluency may be a distinct characteristic of the "preclinical" phase of dementia in PD (Emre et al., 2007). As mentioned

TABLE 63.3 *Clinical Features of PDD*

Core features	• insidious onset • slow progression • impairment in more than one cognitive domain • deficits severe enough to impair daily life (social, occupational, or personal care) • impairment independent of that attributable to motor or autonomic symptoms
Associated clinical features	• cognitive features: ○ impaired attention ▪ may fluctuate during the day and from day to day ○ impaired executive functions ▪ especially initiation, planning, concept formation, rule finding, set shifting ▪ deficient set maintenance ▪ reduced mental speed (bradyphrenia) ○ impaired visuo-spatial functions ▪ deficient performance on tasks requiring visual-spatial orientation, perception, or construction ○ impaired memory function ▪ reduced recent memory ▪ poor performance on free recall tasks ▪ recognition usually better than free recall ○ linguistic dysfunction ▪ dysnomia ▪ impaired complex comprehension • perceptual disturbances ○ hallucinations: mostly visual, usually complex, formed objects • thought content disturbance ○ delusions • mood dysregulation ○ depression ○ anxiety • comportmental features: ○ apathy: decreased spontaneity; reduced motivation, interest, and effortful behavior ○ changes in personality • excessive daytime sleepiness

Source: Adapted from Emre et al. (2007).

(under Epidemiology), Williams-Gray et al. (2007) longitudinally followed a community-based cohort of patients with newly diagnosed idiopathic PD. Although 10% developed dementia at a mean of 3.5 years from diagnosis, 57% showed some evidence of cognitive impairment. Deficits attributable to frontostriatal dysfunction was the predominant deficit among the group with no dementia; however, the most important clinical predictors of subsequent global cognitive decline (following correction for age) were impaired performance on neuropsychological tasks thought to be mediated by posterior cortical substrates, including semantic fluency and visuospatial functions (especially visuomotor construction) (Williams-Gray et al., 2007).

Neuropsychological studies of PD emphasize the early prominence of dysexecutive features (Mahieux et al., 1998). For example, patients with early PD demonstrate impaired learning of novel tasks requiring internally driven processing (that is, set acquisition) (Taylor and Saint-Cyr, 1995). Reduced working memory in early PD can manifest as nonspecific bradyphrenia (Wilson et al., 1980; Cooper and Sagar, 1993a; Cooper et al., 1994) and prolonged decision making in tasks with high cognitive load (Zimmermann, et al., 1992). Retrieval deficits and impaired abstraction have also been observed in the early stages of PD (Dubois and Pillon, 1998), although in contrast to PD, these patients are frequently improved by cuing, suggesting a more fundamental problem with retrieval rather than encoding of memory.

The presence of MCI in a patient with PD (Foltynie et al., 2002) has prompted research to determine if a sentinel dementia profile can be defined that represents a sentinel pattern for PDD as has been considered in AD. For example, Janvin et al. (2006) investigated whether certain MCI patterns are harbingers for subsequent dementia development in PD. Janvin et al. (2006) longitudinally tracked patients with PD with intact cognition and with various MCI subtypes and found 62% of patients with PD with MCI, compared to 20% of patients with PD who were cognitively intact, developed dementia. Single-domain nonamnesic MCI and multidomain slightly impaired MCI were associated with PDD development, while amnesic MCI subtype was not (Janvin et al., 2006). This pattern is distinct from the natural history of AD, where amnesic MCI has been identified as a principal sentinel for AD conversion (Mariani et al., 2007). These findings may have important therapeutic implications for treatment of dementia in PD where MCI may turn out to be a more reliable index of future disability than it has in AD.

PDD cognitive profile

Executive dysfunction. Extensive evidence indicates that executive dysfunction constitutes a central characteristic of PDD (Emre et al., 2007). Neuropsychological assays sensitive to frontal lobe dysfunction (for example, tests of planning, working memory, set maintenance, set shifting, impulse control, conflict detection, etc.) reveal progressive executive failure in PD (Van Spaendonck et al., 1993). Further, the executive dysfunction of PD gives rise to secondary impairments in multiple other cognitive domains (for example, memory retrieval impairment due to failure of ancillary executive processes) (Pillon et al., 1993). Importantly, the presence of dominant executive dysfunction constitutes a key clinical feature distinguishing PDD from AD dementia (Cahn-Weiner et al., 2002).

Attention is a core executive function that is disrupted in PD (Ballard et al., 2002). Because many attentional assessment instruments confound attention with other executive processes and motor speed, methodologic issues complicate interpretation of attentional studies in PD (Emre et al., 2007). Nonetheless, based on reports from several studies (e.g., Ballard et al., 2002), it seems clear that attentional impairment represents a core attribute of PDD, with prominent tendency for fluctuation in concentration that is distinct from other cortical neurodegenerative disorders such as AD (Cahn-Weiner et al., 2002; Emre et al., 2007).

Patients with PD also demonstrate excessive dependence on external cues for task initiation, struggling to perform motor and cognitive tasks that require utilization of an internal strategy (Hsieh et al., 1995; Berger et al., 1999). Consequently, patients with PD require increased processing time to formulate task goals (set acquisition) (Owen et al., 1992; Dubois and Pillon, 1998). Dependence on external cues to execute a serial learning strategy appears to also correlate with motor dysfunction, primarily bradykinesia (Berger et al., 1999).

Patients with PD develop progressive deficiency implementing efficient and accurate task control operations (Owen et al., 1992; Dubois and Pillon, 1998). Impaired attentional set-shifting ability (Cools et al., 2001a; Woodward et al., 2002) becomes prominent with PD progression. Impaired set shifting has been suggested to underlie the difficulty patients with PD manifest in performing bimanual simultaneous motor tasks (Horstink et al., 1990). It appears that the difficulty is more in initiating a response set for a new relevant dimension rather than in disengaging from a previously reinforced category (Brown and Marsden, 1988; Owen, Roberts, et al., 1993; Partiot et al., 1996). Set-shifting impairment in particular is associated with motor severity (particularly rigidity) as inventoried by the Unified Parkinson's Disease Rating Scale (UPDRS) (Van Spaendonck et al., 1996). Because of diminished set acquisition and set-shifting proficiency, patients with PDD frequently experience a progressive diminution in multitasking capacity (Brown et al., 1993).

Concept formation (that is, abstract inductive reasoning) can be tested using a variety of neuropsychological instruments (for example, Conceptualization subscale of the Mattis Dementia Rating Scale [DRS], Similarities subtest of the Wechsler Adult Intelligence Scale [WAIS], Raven's Progressive Matrices [RPM], and Wisconsin Card Sorting Test [WCST]) (Dubois et al., 2007; Emre et al., 2007). Patients with PDD show consistently impaired performance on such measures compared to patients with PD with no dementia (Paolo et al., 1996; Van Spaendonck et al., 1996; Marié et al., 1999; Emre et al., 2007).

Several studies have contrasted the executive functions in PDD and AD (e.g., Cahn-Weiner et al., 2002). Although select data indicate that patients with PDD are no more perseverative than patients with AD on WCST performance (Paolo et al., 1996), it is likely that set shifting and other dysexecutive features yield increased vulnerability to perseveration in PD (Cools et al., 1984; Owen et al., 1992; Downes et al., 1993). Compared to patients with AD, patients with PDD commit more total errors on the WCST, but not on any other index of performance (Paolo et al., 1996). Patients with PDD have also been noted to perform worse than patients with AD on the RPM (Starkstein et al., 1996). Although performing better on memory subscores, patients with PDD are noted to perform worse than patients with AD on select executive function DRS subscales (Aarsland et al., 2003).

Linguistic dysfunction. Several studies have documented verbal fluency deficits in PDD (Emre et al., 2007), especially those employing the DRS, where verbal fluency assessment constitutes a large portion of the Initiation and Perseveration subscale (Aarsland et al., 2003; Paolo et al., 1995). However, data are heterogeneous regarding phonemic or semantic vulnerability predominance (Piatt et al., 1999; Noe et al., 2004). With the exception of prosody, overall linguistic function is less impaired in PDD than in AD (Cummings et al., 1988), where dysnomia in particular is a fundamental hallmark.

Learning and memory impairment. Memory impairment is the presenting problem in approximately two thirds or fewer of patients with PDD (compared to 94% with DLB and 100% with AD) (Noe et al., 2004). Several types of learning and memory impairment plague patients with PD, evolving with disease stage progression (Owen, Beksinska, et al., 1993), with neuropsychological studies of memory function in PDD yielding variable and sometimes inconsistent results (Emre et al., 2007). Phenomenologic and methodologic complexities contribute to this variability. Phenomenologically, many memory functions are dependent on executive processes and are consequently directly vulnerable to PD-related frontostriatal dysfunction (Pillon et al., 1993). Methodologically, neuropsychological assays of memory functions often involve executive processes intrinsic to those memory processes being measured and are therefore not solitary probes of memory function.

Reports suggest that anterograde memory function, mediating short-term and recent memory capacities, progressively dwindles with PD progression (Sullivan et al., 1989). Encoding and storage abilities per se are relatively spared in PD (Sullivan and Sagar, 1991; Pillon et al., 1996). However, PD-related attentional reduction, with secondarily deleterious effects on storage, especially contributes to impaired new memory formation when conducted within the context of interfering stimuli (Sullivan and Sagar, 1991; Cooper and Sagar, 1993a; Marié et al., 1999). Retrograde memory performance is especially vulnerable to the effects of progressive failure of ancillary executive processes essential to long-term memory performance. Memory-affecting executive processes vulnerable to PD-related degeneration include internally driven search strategies (Buytenhuijs et al., 1994), information retrieval (Dubois and Pillon, 1998), and dating capacity (Sagar, Cohen, et al., 1988). It is important to note, however, that evidence for dysexecutive-related mechanisms of memory dysfunction in PD primarily derives from studies of patients with PD with no dementia who demonstrate preserved recognition memory and performance enhancement when given retrieval cues (Emre et al., 2007), thereby suggesting preservation of memory function per se. However, patients with PD who meet criteria for a formal diagnosis of dementia are in fact impaired on cued recall tasks (Pillon et al., 1993; Higginson et al., 2005), including recognition deficits for verbal (Noe et al., 2004; Higginson et al., 2005) and nonverbal stimuli (Noe et al., 2004), suggesting primary memory failure (Whittington et al., 2000) at least at the later stages of the dementia process.

Working memory, which consists of the ability to scan, manipulate, and/or process newly registered information, becomes increasingly impaired in PD (Owen, Iddon, et al., 1997; Fournet et al., 2000; Hoppe et al., 2000). Because working memory relies on a complex interdependence of multiple executive (attention, set maintenance, task control operations, etc.) and memory functions, coordinated by a complex frontally based neural network, it is not surprising that working memory would decompensate under the weight of the PD-related frontostriatal pathology. Patients with PD are capable of schema learning but require more practice than controls to achieve comparable levels of performance (Soliveri et al., 1992). Learning of conditional associations by trial and error also becomes impaired (Sprengelmeyer et al., 1995). Over time, procedural learning deficits become increasingly prominent as well (Saint-Cyr et al., 1988; Ferraro et al., 1993; Pascual-Leone et al., 1993; Haaland et al., 1997; Sarazin et al., 2001).

Several studies have attempted to identify those memory features which distinguish PDD and AD. Although results have been frequently inconsistent, data overall indicate that verbal and visual memory are overall less impaired in PDD than in AD (Kuzis et al., 1999; Cahn-Weiner et al., 2002; Higginson et al., 2005).

Visuospatial dysfunction. Visuospatial deficits have long been noted to complicate PD (Bowen et al., 1972). The mechanism underlying visuospatial impairment has not been well-delineated (Bradley et al., 1989), and it is not clear if these deficits are independent of attentional (M.J. Wright et al., 1990; Filoteo and Maddox, 1999) and/or other executive impairments (Brown and Marsden, 1986; Brown and Marsden, 1988; Growdon et al., 1990; Raskin et al., 1992; Bondi et al., 1993; Berry et al., 1999; Blanchet et al., 2000). Overall, patients with PDD have more impaired visuo-perceptual function than patients with PD with no dementia (Mosimann et al., 2004), and patients with PDD tend to perform worse than patients with AD in many visuo-perceptual domains (Mosimann et al., 2004).

Dyspraxia. Praxis assessment necessarily involves assaying multiple cognitive and even motor domains (for example, executive, visuospatial, visuomotor control, fine motor, etc.). Consequently, it is not surprising that patients with PDD typically perform poorly on praxis assessments, especially those involving drawing/construction (Emre et al., 2007). For example, patients with PDD show significantly impaired performance on the Clock Drawing Test and other design construction tasks, with layered deficits of planning, organization, and visuomotor control (Cahn-Weiner et al., 2003; Cormack et al., 2004). Overall, data suggest that visuomotor praxis is more impaired in PDD than AD (Cormack et al., 2004; Emre et al., 2007).

Neuropsychiatric Dysregulation

Psychiatric disturbances developing within the context of PD can be multifactorial in their genesis and complex in their consequences. The same, or closely related, mechanisms generating cognitive impairment in PD can also yield affective dysregulation, thought content derangement, perceptual disturbance, impulse dyscontrol, and comportmental dysregulation (Taylor et al., 1990; Weintraub and Hurtig, 2007; Weintraub and Potenza, 2006). In turn, psychiatric phenomenology can (*1*) aetiologically contribute to, (2) exacerbate, and/or (*3*) complicate the management of PD-related cognitive dysfunction. Psychiatric disturbances complicating PD even without dementia can be extensive. For example, Pacchetti et al. (2005), studying 289 consecutive outpatients with PD, found 18% had hallucinations, 7% had hallucinations plus "confusion," and 4% had hallucinations plus delusions. Another investigation by Aarsland, Brønnick, and Her (2007) exhaustively explored the profile of neuropsychiatric symptoms in PDD. In this study of over 500 patients with PDD using the Neuropsychiatric Inventory (NPI), they found that 89% of patients had least one neuropsychiatric symptom. The most common symptoms were depression (58%), apathy (54%), anxiety (49%), and hallucinations (44%). Patients with PD with psychosis and agitation symptom clusters had the lowest MMSE, highest UPDRS, and highest caregiver distress scores (Aarsland, Brønnick, and Her, 2007). Psychotic symptoms can be aggravated by DA-ergic medications and accordingly limit the ability to use these medications to better control PD motor features. The prominence of psychotic symptoms complicating PD has prompted formulation of standardized diagnostic criteria for these features (Ravina et al., 2007). We briefly review core neurospychiatric dysregulation complicating the neurobehavioral profile of PDD.

Mood dysregulation: Depression and anxiety

Depressed mood is common in PD, with prevalence rates approximating 50% (Dooneief et al., 1992). Major depression has been reported to occur in 13% of patients with PDD (Aarsland et al., 2001). Depression within the context of PD may represent the most complexly layered affective dysregulation. As depicted in Figure 63.4, depression in PD can be a consequence of multiple possible aetiologic mechanisms. It has long been debated if depression in PD is related to endogenous or exogenous mechanisms. It is not surprising that patients who have a chronic, progressive, neurodegenerative condition might become depressed. Alternatively, neurodegeneration with involvement of multiple monoamine neurotransmitter systems might cause depression as an inherent component of the PD process. New concepts are also emerging. Although it has long been appreciated that the masked facies of PD can mimic depression, data suggest a more insidious effect than mere mimicry. If facial expression is constrained by an impaired capacity to recruit facial mimetic muscles, brain regions involved in affective responsivity may be similarly restrained. Another hypothetical mechanism by which masked facies can reflect or be causative of depression invokes the evolving concept of mirror neurons. This concept hypothesizes that an inability to "mirror" the socioemotional facial expressions of others can have an impact on the activation of socioemotionally relevant mirror neuron functioning.

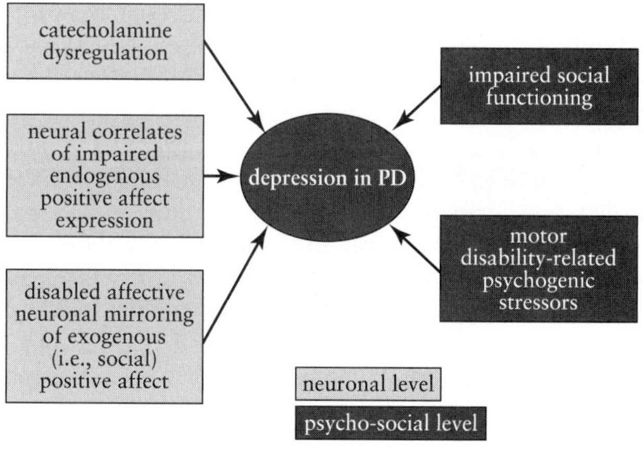

FIGURE 63.4 Depressogenic mechanisms in Parkinson's disease.

As in other clinical contexts, depression can itself cause secondary cognitive dysfunction (for example, pseudodementia). Patients who are depressed can appear to have dementia but remain cognitively intact, which can be readily recognized after treatment of the depression. On the other hand, patients with PD with depression tend to be more cognitively impaired on tests of memory function and language fluency than patients with PD without comorbid depression matched for age, education, gender, age at disease onset, disease duration, and disease severity (Tröster, Paolo, et al., 1995; Tröster, Stalp, et al., 1995). Thus, depression might also occur as a consequence of the dementia process.

Parkinsonian motor and cognitive features include many that phenomenologically suggest depression, including affective blunting, bradyphrenia, and apathy (Koller, 1984). Further, typical neurovegetative indices of depression (for example, sleep disturbance, appetite) can be deranged by PD, and so their reliability as markers of affective dysregulation is compromised. Therefore, an essential component of PD clinical evaluation is a comprehensive affective assessment that includes probing the patient's subjective experience to confirm whether or not a dysthymic state exists. Although PD-associated depression typically appears as a psychomotor retardation due to PD-related masking and bradykinesia, the subjective experience can include significant agitated depression-type features. In general, the pattern and severity of depression appear to be significantly influenced by the severity of motor dysfunction and degree of overall functional disability (Gotham et al., 1986a; Brown et al., 1988).

Mood swings frequently accompany the motor fluctuations associated with LD treatment, with depression being more pronounced during off periods. Depression has been reported to occur in approximately two thirds of patients with PD with motor fluctuations, with consequent impact on patient quality of life (Nissenbaum et al., 1987). Therefore interventions designed to reduce motor fluctuations may be helpful in ameliorating PD-related depression (Olanow et al., 2001) and consequent depression-related cognitive complications.

Subjective anxiety appears to occur at similar rates as dysphoria, and the two disturbances are often comorbid (Menza et al., 1993; Emre et al., 2007). Anxiety can also be more prominent in off periods. Indeed, some patients with PD suffer severe panic episodes confined to off episodes that can be dramatically relieved by manipulation of pharmacotherapy for PD. Anxiety tends to be more pronounced in patients with PDD; however, objective irritability appears to be less prevalent than in other neurodegenerative dementias (Engelborghs et al., 2005).

Apathy is another common mood disturbance in PD. Prevalence rates in PDD have been reported to be as high as 54% (Aarsland, Brønnick, and Her, 2007), compared to frequencies of 17% in patient populations with PDD with no dementia (Aarsland et al., 2001).

Hallucinations

Perceptual disturbances or hallucinations commonly complicate PD (Fénelon et al., 2000, 2006), and occur in up to 65% of patients with PDD (Aarsland, Brønnick, and Her, 2007; Williams et al., 2007). Visual hallucinations occur at least twice as frequently as auditory hallucinations (Emre et al., 2007). They are predominantly composed of visual images that are typically complex, formed, and represent real (animals, people) but nonthreatening objects (Fénelon et al., 2000; Mosimann et al., 2006). Patients with PDD generally retain insight regarding the hallucinatory nature of the perceptual derangement until more advanced stages (Aarsland, Brønnick, and Her, 2007). In many instances the hallucinations are more disturbing to family members than to patients. In more advanced cases, patients may develop hallucinations in association with paranoid ideations, particularly involving marital infidelity.

PD-associated hallucinations can be multifactorial in origin (Holroyd et al., 2001). They may occur spontaneously or be induced by LD and other DA-ergic medications. Dopamine agonists in particular can induce hallucinations, even in the early stages of the disease (Rascol et al., 2000; Olanow et al., 2001). Cortical LBs and prominent cholinergic deficits are frequent postmortem findings in patients with PD who experience hallucinations with or without dementia (Aarsland et al., 2001; Assal and Cummings, 2002). Parkinsonism associated with prominent hallucinations should prompt consideration of underlying DLB pathology (Williams et al., 2007).

Visual hallucinations tend to be associated with multiple cognitive deficits, including frontal dysfunction and memory deterioration (Ozer et al., 2007). Santangelo et al. (2007) studied cognitive function in patients with PD in a 2-year study, comparing those with hallucinations at baseline, those who developed hallucinations during the course of follow-up, and those who remained hallucination free throughout the study. Cognitive performance significantly declined in all three groups, but at end point, patients with PD who had hallucinations scored significantly lower than those who did have hallucinations on phonological and semantic fluency tasks, immediate free recall, and go/no-go tasks (Santangelo et al., 2007). Hallucinations and poor phonological fluency independently predicted the later development of diffuse cognitive impairment (Santangelo et al., 2007). Visual hallucinations are reported to occur with similar frequency and severity in PDD and DLB (Emre et al., 2007), contrasting with significantly lower prevalence rates in AD (Hirono et al., 1999).

The development of hallucinations can restrict the ability to adequately treat patients with PD, as higher doses of DA-ergic medications can induce/aggravate hallucinatory behavior and cognitive impairment. Treatment with atypical neuroleptics such as quetiapine or clozapine, even in very low doses (for example, 12.5–50 mg) can provide dramatic benefit for patients with PD and permit higher doses of LD to be employed to treat parkinsonian motor features. Most studies have shown that clozapine is more effective than quetiapine, but typically the latter is tried first to avoid the risk of agranulocytosis and the need for periodic monitoring required with clozapine. Atypical neuroleptics are frequently associated with sedation and may cause worsening parkinsonism.

Thought content disturbance

Disturbances of thought content, sometimes rising to the level of delusionality, can complicate PD (Aarsland et al., 1999; Aarsland et al., 2001; Holroyd et al., 2001). In general, delusions are less common than hallucinations in PDD, although the two are often comorbid (Emre et al., 2007). Although occurring in up to 17% of patients with PD in general (Aarsland et al., 1999; Marsh et al., 2004), the frequency of delusions in PDD is reported to be up to 30% (Aarsland, Brønnick, and Her, 2007), generally lower than prevalence rates reported in DLB (Aarsland et al., 2001). However, Mosimann et al. (2006) observed that there was a similar frequency, content, and severity of delusions over time in PDD and DLB; paranoid and "phantom boarder" type are among the most common in PDD and DLB (Aarsland et al., 2001).

Impulse dyscontrol

Impulse control disorders (ICDs) including pathological gambling, hypersexuality, and varied compulsions (for example, eating, shopping) have recently been described in patients with PD (Weintraub and Potenza, 2006; Voon and Fox, 2007). Intrinsic PD pathology and iatrogenic effects (especially treatment with DA-ergic agents) are thought to contribute to impulse control impairment (Pontone et al., 2006; Pagonabarraga et al., 2007; Mamikonyan et al., 2008). Risk factors include young age, dopamine agonists particularly in high doses, and preexisting depression or an ICD (Dodd et al., 2005; Voon and Fox, 2007). Impulse control disorders have now been described in association with multiple DA agonists (pramipexole, ropinirole, pergolide) and appear to be a class effect (Mamikonyan et al., 2008). How DA agonists lead to ICDs is not known, but it is fascinating that DA is known to be closely linked to reward (Schultz, 1998). It has been speculated that DA agonists might induce ICDs through activation of specific DA receptor subtypes, but it is possible that DA agonists act by restoring DA-ergic tone that permits expression of their baseline personality. In that context, however, it is noteworthy that these problems are not typically seen with LD. In contrast, LD has been associated with a DA dysregulation syndrome and a condition known as "punding" where patients repeatedly perform meaningless activities such as gathering and assembling and disassembling objects (Evans et al., 2004). These in turn have not been described with DA agonists. Further studies are required to determine the precise frequency of ICDs in PD in comparison to the general public; such studies must take into account that there is now more ready access to gambling (for example, Internet, more widely accessible casinos) and that the risk of pathologic gabling (PG) is greater in individuals who are retired or have a disabling illness (Weintraub and Potenza, 2006). Impulse control disorders can represent an especially delicate management challenge when they occur within the context of PDD.

CLINICAL ASSESSMENT

Traditional clinical inventories including the MMSE and UPDRS remain the staples of routine cognitive assessment in PD and have a reasonably adequate capacity to identify major cognitive and affective dysfunction (Starkstein and Merello, 2007). However, there has been evolving need to formulate more sensitive and detailed assessment strategies that are more specifically focused on the problems that occur in PD. Consequently, the MDSTF has recently published a practice guideline of methodologies for diagnosing dementia in PD (Dubois et al., 2007); we review these below.

Routine Examination

The MMSE has long been used as a screening instrument for dementia in community-based samples (Folstein et al., 1975; Wells et al., 1992). However, the MMSE is not a particularly sensitive instrument for PD, where deficits primarily affect executive domains, particularly in the early stages of the illness. Thus, for instance, a patient with PD with an MMSE score of 27 may have considerably more cognitive impairment than would be expected for an individual in the general population. The MDSTF has developed guidelines for routine office-based assessment that augment the MMSE by adding domain-specific screening tasks (Dubois et al., 2007); see Table 63.4 for a summary inventory of these assessments.

Neuropsychological Assessment

Neuropsychologic testing provides a standardized method for gauging cognitive dysfunction that can be used as a baseline for future evaluations, aid in differential diagnosis, and inform treatment planning (Litvan, Agid, Goetz, et al., 1996; Litvan, Mega, et al., 1996). Unlike an office-based clinical screen, standardized neuropsychological testing establishes precise, objective measurements. Patient scores on cognitive tests are compared to a standardized, "expectable" reference value derived from normative data sets that control for such factors as gender, age, and education. With population-based and patient-specific reference points in mind, the typical neuropsychological evaluation measures a wide array of skills. Overlearned skills and novel problem-solving abilities are assessed. Because most neuropsychological instruments de facto test more than one cognitive skill (for example, attentional capacity impacts other directed measures of cognitive functions), assessment batteries typically rely on a combination of measures within and across cognitive domains to systematically eliminate confounds. Pattern analysis serves to highlight salient findings in building a cognitive profile while providing context for excluding erroneous scores or discrepancies. Qualitative behavioral observations throughout the assessment offer valuable additional data regarding factors such as

TABLE 63.4 *MDSTF Guidelines for Office-based Screening of PD-related Cognitive Deficits*

Cognitive Domain	*Method of Evaluation*	*Pass/Fail Criteria*
General intellectual functioning	MMSE	Cut-off score for impairment: <26
Mental tracking	Months of the year in reverse order	Omission of two or more months, incorrect sequencing of months, or failure to carry out task within 90 seconds
Lexical verbal fluency	Number of words beginning with "s" generated within 60 seconds	Fewer than 10 items
Planning/organization	Clock Drawing Test ("set hands to 'ten past two'")	Inability to insert the correct clock-face numbers or hands pointing to an incorrect time
Constructional praxis	MMSE intersecting pentagons	Copy should include two pentagons which overlap
Memory	MMSE 3-word recall	Failure to recall all three words suggests the existence of a memory storage or memory retrieval problem

Source: Adapted from Dubois et al. (2007).
MDSTF: Movement Disorder Society Task Force; PD: Parkinson's disease; MMSE: Mini-Mental State Examination.

anxiety and compensatory strategies, which can negatively affect test validity.

Neuropsychological test inventory

See Table 63.5 for a summary inventory of MDSTF-recommended neurospsychological assays applicable to characterizing PDD.

Test interpretation

A formal diagnosis of PDD is generally conferred when the following criteria are met: (*1*) impaired cognitive function representing a decline from premorbid ability, (*2*) memory impairment in addition to impairment of at least one other cognitive domain, (*3*) deficit severity sufficient to impair functioning in daily life, and (*4*) presence of at least one associated behavioral feature (for example, apathy, hallucinations, excessive daytime sleepiness) (Dubois et al., 2007). Deficits in only one cognitive domain (for example, memory or executive dysfunction) may justify a diagnosis of MCI but do not satisfy criteria for a formal dementia diagnosis. Likewise, cognitive decline that has yet to cause functional disability does not fall into the category of dementia per se.

Neuroimaging

Structural and functional neuroimaging modalities can be helpful in clarifying the aetiology, and possibly informing the management, of cognitive dysfunction in PD (Sawle et al., 1994; Brooks, 2000). Although practice guidelines continue to evolve regarding its utilization, neuroimaging has become a valuable diagnostic tool in evaluating cognitive dysfunction in general. The ability of neuroimaging to aid in the differential diagnosis of cognitive dysfunction arising within the context of parkinsonism is manifold. In addition to detecting imaging-specific features of parkinsonism, patients presenting with a combination of cognitive dysfunction and parkinsonian motor signs often possess layered comborbid neuropathology. In addition to the age-related multiple syndromes that are capable of producing admixtures of cognitive and motor dysfunction, patients need to be screened for the presence, and relative contributions, of neurodegenerative, cerebrovascular, neoplastic, hemorrhagic, and other pathologies that might cause or contribute to the cognitive dysfunction.

Structural imaging

Computed tomography (CT). Computed tomography has diagnostic utility for the urgent evaluation of acute mental status changes that arise within the context of parkinsonism and/or dementia. However, magnetic resonance imaging (MRI) has supplanted CT as the structural imaging modality of choice, as it provides superior ability to visualize brain structures and pathology, particularly in the posterior fossa. An exception is Fahr's disease, an idiopathic syndrome manifest by calcification in the basal ganglia, which can present with parkinsonism and can best be detected on CT. Computed tomography is also valuable for the identification of disorders associated with calcium deposits and hemorrhage.

Magnetic resonance imaging (MRI). Many pathologic problems that contribute to the development of cognitive/extrapyramidal motor syndromes can be detected on MRI. Magnetic resonance imaging is also especially valuable for evaluating the distribution and severity of cerebrovascular disease, neoplasia, subdural hematomas, hydrocephalus, prion diseases, and so on, which could contribute to parkinsonism and dementia. Magnetic resonance imaging can be useful in the differential diagnosis of the atypical parkinsonisms (Hauser and Olanow, 1994). Magnetic resonance imaging studies demonstrate pronounced low-signal abnormalities in the striatum on T2-weighted MRI images in patients with atypical parkinsonism (Olanow, 1992) that can help distinguish these conditions from PD. These changes are due to iron accumulation and reflect neurodegeneration in the striatum that is not typically found in idiopathic PD. Cerebellar and brain-stem atrophy are features of olivoponto cerebellar atrophy (OPCA) or MSA-cerebellar type (MSA-C) (Bhattacharya et al., 2002). Bilateral symmetric high-signal abnormalities in the globus pallidus and SN pars reticulate on T1-weighted MRI are indicative of exposure to manganese, which in high concentration has the potential to cause a form of parkinsonism (Olanow, 2004).

Serial volumetric T1-weighted MRI images in patients with PD demonstrate a significant loss of brain volume compared to age-matched controls (Hu et al., 2001). Atrophy of the substantia innominata, measured on coronal thin-section T2-weighted MR images, can reflect degeneration of the NBM that is pronounced in patients with AD and PDD (Hanyu et al., 2002). Burton et al. (2004) performed a cross-sectional study to determine if a specific pattern of cerebral atrophy is associated with PDD. Using voxel-based morphometry (VBM), the investigators found reduced gray matter volume in patients with PDD relative to controls in bilateral temporal and occipital lobes as well as in right frontal, left parietal, and some subcortical regions. In contrast, patients with PD without dementia showed only reduced gray matter volume primarily in the frontal lobe compared with controls. In another VBM MRI study, Beyer, Janvin, et al. (2007) found gray matter reductions in frontal, parietal, limbic, and temporal lobes in patients with PDD compared with PD patients with no dementia. In patients with PD with MCI and no dementia, reduced

TABLE 63.5 *Neuropsychological Tests Commonly Used to Evaluate Cognitive Functioning in PD*

Cognitive Domain		*Neuropsychological Test*
Global intellectual functioning		Mattis DRS
Estimated level of premorbid cognitive ability		North American Adult Reading Test (NART-R)
		Shipley Institute of Living Skills
		Vocabulary (WAIS-III)
Executive functions	Working memory	Digit Span
		Spatial Span (CANTAB, WMS-III)
		Letter-Number Sequencing (WMS-III)
	Conceptualization	Similarities, Matrix Reasoning (WAIS-III)
		Wisconsin Card Sort Test
		Tower of London
	Set activation	Verbal Fluency (FAS, Animal Naming)
	Set shifting	TMT
	Set maintenance	Stroop Test
		Odd Man Out Test
Motor function	Speed	Finger-tapping test
	Dexterity	Grooved Pegboard
	Strength	Hand Dynamometer
Memory	Verbal memory	California Verbal Learning Test
		Logical Memory (WMS-III)
	Visual memory	Family Pictures (WMS-III)
		Visual Reproduction (WMS-R)
Language		Boston Naming Test
		North American Reading Test (NART-R)
Visual and spatial skills	Visuoconstructive	Copy of the Clock
		Visual-Motor Integration
	Visuospatial	Judgment of Line Orientation
		Cube Analysis (VOSP)
		Hooper Visual Organization Test
	Visuoperceptual	Benton Facial Recognition
		Fragmented Letters (VOSP)
Neuropsychiatric	Apathy	Marin Apathy Scale
		Frontal Systems Behavior Scale
	Depression	MADRS
		Hamilton Depression Inventory
		Geriatric Depression Scale
	Anxiety	Beck Anxiety Inventory
		YBOCS
	Visual hallucination	PPQ
	Psychosis	SCID
		NPI
Caregiver rating scales		ABAS-II
		Frontal Systems Behavior Scale, caregiver survey

Source: Adapted from Dubois et al. (2007).

gray matter was detected in left frontal and both temporal lobes (Beyer, Janvin, et al., 2007). Finally, Matsui and colleagues (2007) used diffusion tensor imaging (DTI) to compare fractional anisotropy (FA) values between patients with PD with and without dementia. The PDD group showed significant FA reduction in the bilateral posterior cingulate bundles compared with PD patients with no dementia, and FA values in the left posterior cingulate bundle correlated with several cognitive parameters (Matsui et al., 2007). While no significant volumetric differences were observed in one study of PDD in comparison with DLB (Burton et al., 2004), a more recent study detected more pronounced cortical atrophy in temporal, parietal, and occipital cortical regions in patients with DLB than in patients with PDD despite similarities in the severity of the dementia (Beyer, Larsen, et al., 2007). In sum, MRI is useful in evaluating the patient with PDD but does not permit specific diagnosis of PDD versus other neurodegenerative dementias.

Functional imaging

Nuclear: Single Photon Emission Computed Tomography (SPECT) and Positron Emission Tomography (PET). As with structural neuroimaging, functional imaging can also provide useful information in patients with cognitive and motor dysfunction. Single photon emission computed tomography (SPECT) and positron emission tomography (PET) each offers the potential to image blood flow and perfusion (for example, $H_2{}^{15}O$), metabolic activity (for example, flouro-deoxyglucose [FDG]), and measures of nigro-striatal function including markers of presynaptic DA transporter (carbomethoxy-iodophenyltropane [CIT]), postsynaptic DA receptors, and decarboxylase activity (F-dopa uptake) (Brooks, 1999; Hu et al., 2000). Striatal β-CIT SPECT and FD-PET provide a quantitative measure of nigro-striatal function and can be used for diagnosis of PD and for monitoring disease progression (Sawle et al., 1994; Brooks, 1998; Marek et al., 1998; Ito et al., 1999; Rakshi et al., 1999; Brooks and Samuel, 2000). Positron emission tomography studies have a greater signal-to-noise ratio than SPECT and are generally thought to be more accurate but are less widely available. FD-PET and β-CIT SPECT reveal reduced striatal uptake in patients with PD (Brooks, 1998; Marek et al., 1998). Changes are most pronounced in the posterolateral striatum, the primary projection target of affected nigral neurons, and tend to be asymmetric. FD-PET studies have been used to investigate differences in global DA-ergic function in patients with PD with and without dementia, as well as in normal controls (Ito et al., 2002). No changes in imaging markers of nigrostriatal function were detected between patients with PDD and PD patients without dementia with equivalent parkinsonian motor disability in one study (Ito et al., 2002). In another, patients with PDD demonstrated a greater reduction in 18F-dopa uptake in the ventral striatum and midbrain, as well as reduced uptake in anterior cingulate regions in comparison to patients with PD with no dementia (Rakshi et al., 1999). These results suggested that dementia in PD is associated with impaired mesolimbic and ventrostriatal DA-ergic function (Ito et al., 2002). Positron emission tomography studies have also been reported to show reduced uptake of 5-HT and noradrenergic markers in patients with PDD compared to patients with PD with no dementia (Brooks, 1998).

In patients with PD, ^{18}FDG-PET studies demonstrate hypometabolism in posterior parietal and temporal cortical regions (Hu et al., 2000). In addition, $H_2{}^{15}O$-PET studies reveal reduced blood flow in prefrontal areas during performance on tasks that recruit frontostriatal circuits in comparison with age-matched healthy controls (Cools et al., 2002). However, in patients with early-stage PD with no dementia who performed as well as normal controls on a planning task, perfusion studies showed normal frontal lobe activation during the planning phase despite abnormal processing within the basal ganglia (Dagher et al., 2001). By contrast, patients demonstrated enhanced hippocampal activity; the investigators speculated this could represent a shift to the declarative memory system as a compensation for insufficient working memory capacity within the frontostriatal system (Dagher et al., 2001). Parkinson's disease–associated derangement of basal ganglia outflow might thus partially underlie the dysexecutive features that are frequently observed in this group of patients (Owen et al., 1998).

In general, a variety of frontal, temporal, and parietal metabolic changes have been reported in PDD (Kuhl et al., 1984; Peppard et al., 1992; Vander-Borght et al., 1997), similar to changes reported in AD (Foster et al., 1984) and DLB (Hu et al., 2000), even when LB pathology is restricted to the brain stem (Turjanski and Brooks, 1997). Finally, in comparison to patients with PD, patients with PDD and patients with DLB show decreased metabolism in the inferior and medial frontal lobes bilaterally, and in the right parietal lobe. In contrast, in comparison with patients with PDD, patients with DLB had a greater decrease in metabolic activity in the anterior cingulate region (Yong et al., 2007).

Magnetic Resonance Spectroscopy (MRS). The diagnostic utility of magnetic resonance spectroscopy (MRS) derives from its capacity to provide a "chemical biopsy" of a focal region of brain parenchyma. Magnetic resonance spectroscopy can be used to assay neuronal integrity and determine abnormal levels of various markers associated with particular pathogenic processes. Proton MRS (1H MRS) in particular has been used to detect cortical dysfunction in PD and has been correlated with neuropsychological measures (Hu et al., 1999). Early studies in patients with PD found increased cerebral lactate levels, a nonspecific MRS marker of metabolic alterations and neuropathology, and even greater increases in those with PDD (Bowen et al., 1995; Brooks, 1999; Hu et al., 2000). A significant reduction in *N*-acetyl aspartate (NAA), an MRS marker of neuronal integrity, has been found in temporo-parietal regions of patients with PD (Taylor-Robinson et al., 1999). These changes correlate with measures of global cognitive decline independent of motor impairment (Hu et al., 1999). Summerfield et al. (2002) found decreased NAA in the occipital lobes in PDD as compared to PD. Bowen et al. (1995) found that in comparison to healthy controls, there was increased lactate/NAA ratio in the occipital lobes in PD, and even more so in patients with PDD, suggesting impaired oxidative metabolism, particularly in PDD (Bowen et al., 1995).

Another potential marker for assessing cognitive decline in PD is 31P-MRS, which is useful for assaying the neuronal bioenergetic state. Significant changes in the inorganic phosphate (Pi)/adenosine triphosphate (ATP) ratio, signifying impaired cellular energy and metabolism, have been found in temporo-parietal cortex of patients with PD compared with controls (Hu et al., 2000). These changes were found to correlate with estimated reductions in cognitive functions. Magnetic resonance spectroscopy studies of patients with PD may thus provide markers of current and possibly future cognitive impairment (Hu et al., 1999, 2000).

Functional MRI (fMRI). Functional MRI has become the principal methodology for functional brain mapping and is finding increasing application as a tool for investigating cognitive function in PD. Novel neuropsychological activation paradigms and integrated cognitive-motor-autonomic measurement techniques are being developed to more thoroughly study differences in neuronal activity and metabolism in patients with PD and patients with PDD (Dagher and Nagano-Saito, 2007). A full discussion of this area is beyond the scope of this chapter, but it is anticipated that fMRI will provide insight into cognitive and other neuropsychiatric disorders in patients with PD.

Electroenecephalography

No specific electroencephalogram (EEG) pattern identifies patients with PD or PDD. However, patients with PDD have been reported to have slower baseline EEG background activity than patients with PD with no dementia (Neufeld et al., 1994). Significant decreases in relative alpha power have also been reported in PDD compared to PD (Sinanovic et al., 2005). A positive correlation between EEG frequency and MMSE scores has also been reported (Sinanovic et al., 2005). Abnormal EEG patterns of spike bursts and suppression raises the possibility of dementia due to prion disease or advanced AD.

Nuclear cardiac scanning

A number of investigators have applied cardiac nuclear scanning to investigate markers that might potentially distinguish PDD from other neurodegenerative dementias (Emre et al., 2007). Cardiac uptake of metaiodobenzylguanidine (MIBG), a marker for noradrenergic transporters, is reduced in patients with PD and patients with DLB (Orimo et al., 1999; Satoh et al., 1999) due to degeneration of postganglionic sympathetic fibers (Orimo et al., 1999). Future studies are needed to determine if there are different patterns in patients with PD and patients with PDD. Cardiac MIBG has been shown to be useful for the differentiation of PD from MSA (Braune et al., 1999) and PSP (Yoshita, 1998) because cardiac MIBG uptake usually remains normal in these conditions.

MANAGEMENT

We summarize below a step-wise algorithm for managing patients with PDD (Cooper et al., 1992; Saint-Cyr et al., 1993; Goetz and Stebbins, 1995; Tröster, Paolo, et al., 1995; Graham et al., 1997; Bédard et al., 1999; Rascol et al., 2000; Marjama-Lyons and Koller, 2001; Olanow et al., 2001; Wilson et al., 2002; Alexopoulos et al., 2005; Cummings and Winblad, 2007; Liepelt et al., 2007):

1. Screen for and treat reversible comorbid conditions, for example:
    a. metabolic
    b. endocrine
    c. nutritional
    d. infectious
    e. toxic

2. Eliminate or minimize iatrogenic etiologic and/or exacerbating agents—These agents can potentiate confusion and other DA-ergic side effects, including hallucinations, particularly in patients with advanced PD with preexisting cognitive vulnerabilities:
    a. non-PD agents
        i. sedatives, hypnotics
        ii. other central nervous system active agents
    b. PD agents—remove in the following order
        i. anticholinergics
        ii. amantadine
        iii. monoamine oxidase-B inhibitors (for example, selegiline)
        iv. dopamine agonists

3. Optimize LD— If the patient still has impaired cognitive function despite the above measures, it is appropriate to gradually lower the LD dose to see if this provides any improvement in cognitive function. It may be preferable to compromise motor control to find an LD dose that does not worsen mental function.

4. Treat sleep dysregulation.
5. Treat mood dysregulation.
6. Low-dose atypical neuroleptic medications if mental picture is confounded by psychotic signs (hallucinations, delusions, comportmental dysregulation) (see Weintraub and Hurtig, 2007, for a detailed review). Note that these drugs are good for the treatment of hallucinations but typically are not helpful for the treatment of confusion or cognitive impairment.
7. Acetylcholinesterase-inhibitor (AChase-I) trial
   a. As in AD, acetylcholinesterase inhibitors may provide benefits for patients with PD, primarily by temporarily slowing cognitive degeneration. Rivastigmine and Aricept have been shown to improve cognitive dysfunction and to reduce the rate of decline, but benefits have been modest. Rivastigmine is now available in a transdermal patch formulation for the treatment of PDD. (see Table 63.6 for a summary of relevant clinical trials of acetylcholinesterase-inhibitors [AChaseI] use in PDD.)
8. assess for and implement environmental/behavioral interventions to ensure adequate
   a. safety and supervision
   b. daily structured activities
   c. caregiver support

There is considerable interest in testing the value of acetylcholinesterase inhibitors in patients with PD with MCI. Although results have been inconclusive in patients with AD, there are reasons to suspect that results are more likely to be positive in patients with PD. First, it is not clear that patients in the general population with MCI have or will develop a neurodegenerative process. In contrast, patients with PD already have a neurodegenerative process in which the large majority will go on to develop cognitive dysfunction in the later stages of the disease. In addition, the cholinergic deficit in PD is more severe than it is in AD and develops at an earlier stage of the disease. For these reasons, there is some optimism that treatment of MCI in PD will prevent or delay the development of PDD.

PROGNOSIS

If there are reversible or exacerbating influences that are amenable to some of the above interventions, then select patients with PDD can improve and/or stabilize for sustained time periods. For most, the dementia inexorably advances, eventually contributing to significantly increased morbidity and mortality (Marder et al., 1991; Louis et al., 1997). An analysis by Jellinger et al. (2007) summarized many important prognostic features. In a retrospective analysis of 243 autopsy-confirmed cases of PDD and DLB, the average age at symptom onset was 67, and median survival was 5 years from symptom onset. Older age at symptom onset, fluctuating cognition, early-onset hallucinations, and comorbid AD pathology predicted shorter survival (Jellinger et al., 2007). In contrast, initial parkinsonism without or with delayed onset of dementia is associated with improved survival. When adjusted for age, gender, and AD comorbidity, early dementia onset was identified as the best predictor of poor outcome (Jellinger et al., 2007).

Although great progress has been made in recent years in treating the motor features of PD, this review reveals the extensive interest in the nonmotor and non-DA-ergic features of PD, and enhanced awareness of their frequency and potential to cause disability for patients with PD and their caregivers (Olanow et al., in press). As stated, the majority of patients with PD develop cognitive dysfunction and more than one half of patients

TABLE 63.6 *Placebo-controlled Trials of Cholinesterase Inhibitors in PDD*

Study	*N started/ N completed*	*Duration (weeks)*	*AChase-I*	*Diagnosis*	*Outcome*
Aarsland, 2002	14/12	20	donepezil	PDD	no change in mean UPDRS score
Leroi et al., 2004	16/10	18	donepezil	PDD	no treatment effect for change in NPI score
Emre et al., 2004	541/410	24	rivastigmine	PDD	positive treatment effect for change in NPI score; positive treatment effect for fewer hallucinations as adverse event
Ravina et al., 2005	22/19	10	donepezil	PDD	no treatment effect for change in BPRS total score or BPRS psychosis subscale score

Source: Adapted from Weintraub and Hurtig, 2007.

AChase-I: Cholinesterase-inhibitor; PDD: Parkinson's disease with dementia; UPDRS: Unified Parkinson's Disease Rating Scale; NPI: Neuropsychiatric Inventory; BPRS: Brief Psychiatric Rating Scale.

will ultimately develop dementia. Indeed, it is now appreciated that dementia is the most important cause of disability for patients with advanced PD and is the most common cause of nursing home placement (Goetz and Stebbins, 1993; Aarsland et al., 2000; Weintraub et al., 2004). It is hoped that with the advent of new insights into the nature of the cognitive dysfunction and neuropsychiatric problems that occur in PD, soon there will be innovative neuroprotective and restorative therapies that will minimize and even prevent the development of these problems.

REFERENCES

Aarsland, D. (2002) Dementia with Lewy bodies. *Tidsskr. Nor Laegeforen.* 122(5):525–529.

Aarsland, D., Andersen, K., Larsen, J.P., et al. (2001) Risk of dementia in Parkinson's disease: a community-based, prospective study. *Neurology* 56:730–736.

Aarsland, D., Andersen, K., Larsen, J.P., et al. (2004) The rate of cognitive decline in Parkinson's disease. *Arch. Neurol.* 61: 1906–1911.

Aarsland, D., Andersen, K., Larsen, J.P., Lolk, A.L., and Kragh-Sorensen, P. (2003) Prevalence and characteristics of dementia in Parkinson disease: an 8-year prospective study. *Arch. Neurol.* 60:387–392.

Aarsland, D., Ballard, C., Larsen, J.P., and McKeith, I. (2001) A comparative study of psychiatric symptoms in dementia with Lewy bodies and Parkinson's disease with and without dementia. *Int. J. Geriatr. Psychiatry* 16(5):528–536.

Aarsland, D., Brønnick, K., and Her, U. (2007) Neuropsychiatric symptoms in patients with Parkinson's disease and dementia: frequency, profile and associated care giver stress. *J. Neurol. Neurosurg. Psychiat.* 78(1):36–42.

Aarsland, D., Kvaloy, J.T., Andersen, K., et al. (2007) The effect of age of onset of PD on risk of dementia. *J. Neurol.* 254(1): 38–45.

Aarsland, D., Larsen, J.P., Lim, N.G., Janvin, C., Karlsen, K., Tandberg, E., and Cummings, J.L. (1999) Range of neuropsychiatric disturbances in patients with Parkinson's disease. *J. Neurol. Neurosurg. Psychiatry* 67(4):492–496.

Aarsland, D., Larsen, J.P., Tandberg, E., and Laake, K. (2000) Predictors of nursing home placement in Parkinson's disease: a population-based, prospective study. *J. Am. Geriatr. Soc.* 48(8): 938–942.

Aarsland, D., Perry, R., Larsen, J.P., McKeith, I.G., O'Brien, J.T., Perry, E.K., Burn, D., and Ballard, C.G. (2005) Neuroleptic sensitivity in Parkinson's disease and parkinsonian dementias. *J. Clin. Psychiatry* 66(5):633–637.

Aarsland, D., Tandberg, E., Larsen, J.P., and Cummings, J.L. (1996) Frequency of dementia in Parkinson's disease. *Arch. Neurol.* 53(6):538–542.

Aarsland, D., Zaccai, J., and Brayne, C. (2005) A systematic review of prevalence studies of dementia in Parkinson's disease. *Mov. Disord.* 20:1255–1263.

Agid, Y., Javoy-Agid, F., and Ruberg, M. (1987) Biochemistry of neurotransmitters in Parkinson's disease. In: Marsden, C.D., and Fahn, S., eds. *Movement Disorders 2: Neurology, Vol. 7.* London: Butterworths, pp. 166–230.

Ahlskojg, J.E. (2007) Beating a dead horse: dopamine and Parkinson disease. *Neurology* 69(17):1701–1711.

Albert, M.L., Feldman, R.G., and Willis, A.L. (1974) The "subcortical dementia" of progressive supranuclear palsy. *J. Neurol. Neurosurg. Psychiatry* 37(2):121–130.

Alex, K.D., and Pehek, E.A. (2007) Pharmacologic mechanisms of serotonergic regulation of dopamine neurotransmission. *Pharmacol. Ther.* 113(2):296–320.

Alexander, G.E., DeLong, M.R., and Strick, P.L. (1986) Parallel organization of functionally segregated circuits linking basal ganglia and cortex. *Annu. Rev. Neurosci.* 9:357–381.

Alexopoulos, G.S., Jeste, D.V., Chung, H., et al. (2005) The expert consensus guideline series. Treatment of dementia and its behavioral disturbances. Introduction: methods, commentary, and summary. *Postgrad. Med.* Jan (Spec No): 6–22

Alpert, M., Rosen, A., Welkowitz, J., and Lieberman, A. (1990) Interpersonal communication in the context of dementia. *J. Commun. Disord.* 23(4/5):337–346.

Alves, G., Larsen, J.P., Emre, M., Wentzel-Larsen, T., and Aarsland, D. (2006) Changes in motor subtype and risk for incident dementia in Parkinson's disease. *Mov. Disord.* 21:1123–1130.

Anthony, J.C., LeResche, L., Niaz, U., von Korff, M.R., and Folstein, M.F. (1982) Limits of the "Mini-Mental State" as a screening test for dementia and delirium among hospital patients. *Psychol. Med.* 12(2):397–408.

Appleby, B.S., Duggan, D.S., Regenberg, A., and Rabins, P.V. (2007) Psychiatric and neuropsychiatric adverse events associated with deep brain stimulation: A meta-analysis of ten years' experience. *Mov. Disord.* 22(12):1722–1728.

Ardouin, C., Pillon, B., Peiffer, E., Bejjani, P., Limousin, P., Damier, P., Arnulf, I., Benabid, A.L., Agid, Y., and Pollak, P. (1999) Bilateral subthalamic or pallidal stimulation for Parkinson's disease affects neither memory nor executive functions: a consecutive series of 62 patients. *Ann. Neurol.* 46(2):217–223.

Arnsten, A.F., Mathew, R., Ubriani, R., Taylor, J.R., and Li, B.M. (1999) Alpha-1 noradrenergic receptor stimulation impairs prefrontal cortical cognitive function. *Biol. Psychiatry* 45(1):26–31.

Assal, F., and Cummings, J.L. (2002) Neuropsychiatric symptoms in the dementias. *Curr. Opin. Neurol.* 15(4):445–450.

Athey, R.J., Porter, R.W., and Walker, R.W. (2005) Cognitive assessment of a representative community population with Parkinson's disease (PD) using the Cambridge Cognitive Assessment-Revised (CAMCOG-R). *Age Ageing* 34:268–273.

Aybek, S., Gronchi-Perrin, A., Berney, A., et al. (2007) Long-term cognitive profile and incidence of dementia after STN-DBS in Parkinson's disease. *Mov. Disord.* 22(7):974–981.

Ballard, C.G., Aarsland, D., McKeith, I., et al. (2002) Fluctuations in attention: PD dementia vs DLB with parkinsonism. *Neurology* 59:1714–1720.

Baronti, F. (2002) [Psychological and cognitive problems in Parkinson disease—therapeutic possibilities] [German]. *Schweiz. Rundsch. Med. Prax.* 91(10):411–417.

Bédard, M.A., el Massioui, F., Malapani, C., Dubois, B., Pillon, B., Renault, B., and Agid, Y. (1998) Attentional deficits in Parkinson's disease: partial reversibility with naphtoxazine (SDZ NVI-085), a selective noradrenergic alpha 1 agonist. *Clin. Neuropharmacol.* 21(2):108–117.

Bédard, M.A., Pillon, B., Dubois, B., Duchesne, N., Masson, H., and Agid, Y. (1999) Acute and long-term administration of anticholinergics in Parkinson's disease: specific effects on the subcortico-frontal syndrome. *Brain Cogn.* 40(2):289–313.

Bejjani, B.P., Damier, P., Arnulf, I., et al. (1999) Transient acute depression induced by high-frequency deep brain stimulation. *N. Engl. J. Med.* 340:1476–1480.

Berding, G., Odin, P., Brooks, D.J., Nikkhah, G., Matthies, C., Peschel, T., Shing, M., Kolbe, H., van Den Hoff, J., Fricke, H., Dengler, R., Samii, M., and Knapp, W.H. (2001) Resting regional cerebral glucose metabolism in advanced Parkinson's disease studied in the off and on conditions with [(18)F]FDG-PET. *Mov. Disord.* 16(6):1014–1022.

Berger, H.J., van Es, N.J., van Spaendonck, K.P., Teunisse, J.P., Horstink, M.W., van't Hof, M.A., and Cools, A.R. (1999) Relationship between memory strategies and motor symptoms in Parkinson's disease. *J. Clin. Exp. Neuropsychol.* 21(5):677–684.

Bergman, J., and Lerner, V. (2002) Successful use of donepezil for the treatment of psychotic symptoms in patients with Parkinson's disease. *Clin. Neuropharmacol.* 25(2):107–110.

Berry, E.L., Nicolson, R.I., Foster, J.K., Behrmann, M., and Sagar, H.J. (1999) Slowing of reaction time in Parkinson's disease: the involvement of the frontal lobes. *Neuropsychologia* 37(7):787–795.

Beyer, M.K., Janvin, C.C., Jan, P., Larsen, J.P., and Dag Aarsland, D. (2007) A magnetic resonance imaging study of patients with Parkinson's disease with mild cognitive impairment and dementia using voxel-based morphometry. *J. Neurol. Neurosurg. Psychiatry* 78:254–259.

Beyer, M.K., Larsen, J.P., and Aarsland, D. (2007) Gray matter atrophy in Parkinson disease with dementia and dementia with Lewy bodies. *Neurology* 69:747–754.

Bhattacharya, K., Saadia, D., Eisenkraft, B., Yahr, M.D., Olanow, W., Drayer, B., and Kaufmann, H. (2002) Brain magnetic resonance imaging in multiple system atrophy and Parkinson's disease. A diagnostic algorithm. *Arch. Neurol.* 59:835–842.

Biggins, C.A., Boyd, J.L., Harrop, F.M., Madeley, P., Mindham, R.H., Randall, J.I., and Spokes, E.G. (1992) A controlled, longitudinal study of dementia in Parkinson's disease. *J. Neurol. Neurosurg. Psychiatry* 55(7):566–571.

Birnbaum, S., Gobeske, K.T., Auerbach, J., Taylor, J.R., and Arnsten, A.F. (1999) A role for norepinephrine in stress-induced cognitive deficits: alpha-1-adrenoceptor mediation in the prefrontal cortex. *Biol. Psychiatry* 46(9):1266–1274.

Blanchet, S., Marie, R.M., Dauvillier, F., Landeau, B., Benali, K., Eustache, F., and Chavoix, C. (2000) Cognitive processes involved in delayed non-matching-to-sample performance in Parkinson's disease. *Eur. J. Neurol.* 7(5):473–483.

Boeve, B. (2003) Diagnosis and management of the non-Alzheimer dementias. In: Noseworth, J.W., ed. *Neurological Therapeutics*. London: Martin Dunitz, pp. 2826–2854.

Boeve, B.F. (2007) Parkinson-related dementias. *Neurol. Clin.* 25(3): 761–781.

Bohnen, N.I., and Frey, K.A. (2007) Imaging of cholinergic and monoaminergic neurochemical changes in neurodegenerative disorders. *Mol. Imaging Biol.* 9(4):243–257.

Boller, F., Mizutani, T., Roessmann, U., and Gambetti, P. (1980) Parkinson disease, dementia and Alzheimer disease: clinicopathological correlations. *Ann. Neurol.* 7:329–335.

Boller, F., Passafiume, D., Keefe, N.C., Rogers, K., Morrow, L., and Kim, Y. (1984) Visuospatial impairment in Parkinson's disease. Role of perceptual and motor factors. *Arch. Neurol.* 41(5): 485–490.

Bondi, M.W., Kaszniak, A.W., Bayles, K.A., and Vance, K.T. (1993) Contribution of frontal system dysfunction to memory and perceptual ability in Parkinson's disease. *Neuropsychology* 7:89–102.

Bosboom, J.L., Stoffers, D., and Wolters, E. Ch. (2004) Cognitive dysfunction and dementia in Parkinson's disease. *J. Neural Transm.* 111(10/11):1303–1315.

Bowen, B.C., Block, R.E., Sanchez-Ramos, J., Pattany, P.M., Lampman, D.A., Murdoch, J.B., and Quencer, R.M. (1995) Proton MR spectroscopy of the brain in 14 patients with Parkinson disease. *Am. J. Neuroradiol.* 16(1):61–68.

Bowen, F.P., Hoehn, M.M., and Yahr, M.D. (1972) Parkinsonism: alterations in spatial orientation as determined by a route-walking test. *Neuropsychologia* 10(3):355–361.

Bowen, F.P., Kamienny, R.S., Burns, M.M., and Yahr, M. (1975) Parkinsonism: effects of levodopa treatment on concept formation. *Neurology* 25(8):701–704.

Boyd, J.L., Cruickshank, C.A., Kenn, C.W., Madeley, P., Mindham, R.H., Oswald, A.G., Smith, R.J., and Spokes, E.G. (1991) Cognitive impairment and dementia in Parkinson's disease: a controlled study. *Psychol. Med.* 21(4):911–921.

Braak, H., Del Tredici, K., Rub, U., et al. (2003) Staging of brain pathology related to sporadic Parkinson's disease. *Neurobiol. Aging* 24(2):197–211.

Braak, H., Muller, C.M., Rub, U., et al. (2006a) Pathology associated with sporadic Parkinson's disease--where does it end? *J. Neural Transm. Suppl.* (70):89–97.

Braak, H., Rub, U., and Del Tredici, K. (2006b) Cognitive decline correlates with neuropathological stage in Parkinson's disease. *J. Neurol. Sci.* 248(1/2):255–258.

Bradley, V.A., Welch, J.L., and Dick, D.J. (1989) Visuospatial working memory in Parkinson's disease. *J. Neurol. Neurosurg. Psychiatry* 52(11):1228–1235.

Braune, S., Reinhardt, M., Schnitzer, R., Riedel, A., and Lucking, C.H. (1999) Cardiac uptake of [123I]MIBG separates Parkinson's disease from multiple system atrophy. *Neurology* 53:1020–1025.

Brodsky, M.A., Godbold, J., Roth, T., and Olanow, C.W. (2003) Sleepiness in Parkinson's disease: a controlled study. *Mov. Disord.* 18:668–672.

Bronnick, K., Emre, M., Lane, R., Tekin, S., and Aarsland, D. (2007) Profile of cognitive impairment in dementia associated with Parkinson's disease compared with Alzheimer's disease. *J. Neurol. Neurosurg. Psychiatry.* 78(10):1064–1068.

Brooks, D.J. (1998) The early diagnosis of Parkinson's disease. *Ann. Neurol.* 44(3 Suppl 1):S10–S18.

Brooks, D.J. (1999) Functional imaging of Parkinson's disease: is it possible to detect brain areas for specific symptoms? *J. Neural. Transm. Suppl.* 56:139–153.

Brooks, D.J. (2000) Morphological and functional imaging studies on the diagnosis and progression of Parkinson's disease. *J. Neurol.* 247(Suppl 2):II11–II18.

Brooks, D.J., and Piccini, P. (2006) Imaging in Parkinson's disease: the role of monoamines in behavior. *Biol. Psychiatry* 59(10): 908–918.

Brooks, D.J., and Samuel, M. (2000) The effects of surgical treatment of Parkinson's disease on brain function: PET findings. *Neurology* 55(12 Suppl 6):S52–S59.

Brown, R.G., and Marsden, C.D. (1984) How common is dementia in Parkinson's disease? *Lancet* 2(8414):1262–1265.

Brown, R.G., and Marsden, C.D. (1986) Visuospatial function in Parkinson's disease. *Brain* 109(Pt 5):987–1002.

Brown, R.G., and Marsden, C.D. (1988) Internal versus external cues and the control of attention in Parkinson's disease. *Brain* 111(Pt 2):323–345.

Brown, R.G., and Marsden, C.D. (1990) Cognitive function in Parkinson's disease: from description to theory. *Trends Neurosci.* 13(1):21–29.

Brown, R.G., Jahanshahi, M., and Marsden, C.D. (1993) The execution of bimanual movements in patients with Parkinson's, Huntington's and cerebellar disease. *J. Neurol. Neurosurg. Psychiatry* 56(3):295–297 [comment in: *J. Neurol. Neurosurg. Psychiatry* (1994) 57(1):126].

Brown, R.G., MacCarthy, B., Gotham, A.M., Der, G.J., and Marsden, C.D. (1988) Depression and disability in Parkinson's disease: a follow-up of 132 cases. *Psychol. Med.* 18(1):49–55.

Brown, R.G., Marsden, C.D., Quinn, N., and Wyke, M.A. (1984) Alterations in cognitive performance and affect-arousal state during fluctuations in motor function in Parkinson's disease. *J. Neurol. Neurosurg. Psychiatry* 47(5):454–465.

Burkhard, P.R., Vingerhoets, F.J., Berney, A., Bogousslavsky, J., Villemure, J.G., and Ghika, J. (2004) Suicide after successful deep brain stimulation for movement disorders. *Neurology* 63(11):2170–2172.

Burn, D.J. (2006a) Cortical Lewy body disease and Parkinson's disease dementia. *Curr. Opin. Neurol.* 19:572–579.

Burn, D.J. (2006b) Parkinson's disease dementia: what's in a Lewy body? *J. Neural Transm. Suppl.* 70:361–365.

Burn, D.J., Rowan, E.N., Allan, L.M., Molloy, S., O'Brien, J.T., and McKeith, I.G. (2006) Motor subtype and cognitive decline in Parkinson's disease, Parkinson's disease with dementia, and dementia with Lewy bodies *J. Neurol. Neurosurg. Psychiatry* 77: 585–589.

Burn, D.J., Rowan, E.N., Minnett, T., et al. (2003) Extrapyramidal features in Parkinson's disease with and without dementia and dementia with Lewy bodies: a cross-sectional comparative study. *Mov. Disord.* 18:884–889.

Burn, D.J., and Troster, A.I. (2004) Neuropsychiatric complications of medical and surgical therapies for Parkinson's disease. *J. Geriatr. Psychiatry Neurol.* 17(3):172–180.

Burton, E.J., McKeith, I.G., Burn, D.J., Williams, E.D., and O'Brien, J.T. (2004) Cerebral atrophy in Parkinson's disease with and without dementia: a comparison with Alzheimer's disease, dementia with Lewy bodies and controls. *Brain* 127(4):791–800.

Buytenhuijs, E.L., Berger, H.J., Van Spaendonck, K.P., Horstink, M.W., Borm, G.F., and Cools, A.R. (1994) Memory and learning strategies in patients with Parkinson's disease. *Neuropsychologia* 32(3):335–342.

Byrne, E.J., Lowe, J., Godwin-Austen, R.B., Arie, T., and Jones, R. (1987) Dementia of Parkinson's disease associated with diffuse cortical Lewy bodies. *Lancet* 1:501.

Caballol, N., Picconi, M.J., and Tolosa, E. (2007) Cognitive dysfunction and dementia in Parkinson disease. *Mov. Disord.* (Suppl 17):S358–S366.

Cahn-Weiner, D.A., Grace, J., Ott, B.R., Fernandez, H.H., Friedman, J.H. (2002) Cognitive and behavioral features discriminate between Alzheimer's and Parkinson's disease. *Neuropsychiatry Neuropsychol. Behav. Neurol.* 15:79–87.

Cahn-Weiner, D.A., Williams, K., Grace, J., Tremont, G., Westervelt, H., and Stern, R.A. (2003) Discrimination of dementia with Lewy bodies from Alzheimer disease and Parkinson disease using the clock drawing test. *Cogn. Behav. Neurol.* 16:85–92.

Calabresi, P., Picconi, B., Parnetti, L., and DiFilippo, M. (2006) A convergent model for cognitive dysfunctions in Parkinson's disease: the critical dopamine-acetylcholine synaptic balance. *Lancet Neurol.* 5(11):974–983.

Camicioli, R., Rajput, A., Rajput, M., et al. (2005) Apolipoprotein E-ε4 and catechol-O-methyltransferase alleles in autopsy-proven Parkinson's disease: relationship to dementia and hallucinations. *Mov. Disord.* 20:989–994.

Chamberlain, S.R., Muller, U., Robbins, T.W., and Sahakian, B.J. (2006) Neuropharmacological modulation of cognition. *Curr. Opin. Neurol.* 19(6):607–612.

Charcot, J.M. (1877) *Leçons sur les Maladies du Système Nerveux Faites à la Salpêtrière. Recueillies par Bourneville.* Tome I, 3rd ed. Paris: pp. 155–188.

Chaudhuri, K.R., Healy, D.G., and Schapira, A.H. (2006) Non-motor symptoms of Parkinson's disease: diagnosis and management. *Lancet Neurol.* 5(3):235–245.

Chow, T.W., Miller, B.L., Hayashi, V.N., and Geschwind, D.H. (1999) Inheritance of frontotemporal dementia. *Arch. Neurol.* 56(7):817–822.

Chui, H.C., Teng, E.L., Henderson, V.W., and Moy, A.C. (1985) Clinical subtypes of dementia of the Alzheimer type. *Neurology* 35:1544–1550.

Cohen, O.S., Vakil, E., Tanne, D., Nitsan, Z., Schwartz, R., and Hassin-Baer, S. (2007) Educational level as a modulator of cognitive performance and neuropsychiatric features in Parkinson disease. *Cogn. Behav. Neurol.* 20(1):68–72.

Contestabile, A., Ciani, E, and Contestabile, A (2007) The place of choline acetyltransferase activity measurement in the "cholinergic hypothesis" of neurodegenerative diseases. *Neurochem. Res.* 33(2): 318–327.

Cools, A.R., van den Bercken, J.H., Horstink, M.W., van Spaendonck, K.P., and Berger, H.J. (1984) Cognitive and motor shifting aptitude disorder in Parkinson's disease. *J. Neurol. Neurosurg. Psychiatry* 47(5):443–453.

Cools, R. (2006) Dopaminergic modulation of cognitive function-implications for L-DOPA treatment in Parkinson's disease. *Neurosci. Biobehav. Rev.* 30(1):1–23.

Cools, R., Barker, R.A., Sahakian, B.J., and Robbins, T.W. (2001a) Enhanced or impaired cognitive function in Parkinson's disease as a function of dopaminergic medication and task demands. *Cereb. Cortex* 11(12):1136–1143.

Cools, R., Barker, R.A., Sahakian, B.J., and Robbins, T.W. (2001b) Mechanisms of cognitive set flexibility in Parkinson's disease. *Brain* 124(Pt 12):2503–2512.

Cools, R., Stefanova, E., Barker, R.A., Robbinson, T.W., and Owen, A.M. (2002) Dopaminergic modulation of high-level cognition in Parkinson's disease: the role of the prefrontal cortex revealed by PET. *Brain* 125(Pt 3):584–594.

Cooper, J.A., and Sagar, H.J. (1993a) Encoding deficits in untreated Parkinson's disease. *Cortex* 29(2):251–265.

Cooper, J.A., and Sagar, H.J. (1993b) Incidental and intentional recall in Parkinson's disease: an account based on diminished attentional resources. *J. Clin. Exp. Neuropsychol.* 15(5):713–731.

Cooper, J.A., Sagar, H.J., Doherty, S.M., Jordan, N., Tidswell, P., and Sullivan, E.V. (1992) Different effects of dopaminergic and anticholinergic therapies on cognitive and motor function in Parkinson's disease. A follow-up study of untreated patients. *Brain* 115(Pt 6):1701–1725.

Cooper, J.A., Sagar, H.J., Jordan, N., Harvey, N.S., and Sullivan, E.V. (1991) Cognitive impairment in early, untreated Parkinson's disease and its relationship to motor disability. *Brain* 114(Pt 5): 2095–2122.

Cooper, J.A., Sagar, H.J., Tidswell, P., and Jordan, N. (1994) Slowed central processing in simple and go/no-go reaction time tasks in Parkinson's disease. *Brain* 117(Pt 3):517–529.

Cormack, F., Aarsland, D., Ballard, C., and Tovee, M.J. (2004) Pentagon drawing and neuropsychological performance in Dementia with Lewy bodies, Alzheimer's disease, Parkinson's disease and Parkinson's disease with dementia. *Int. J. Geriatr. Psychiatry* 19:371–377.

Critchley, H. (2005) Neural mechanisms of autonomic, affective, and cognitive integration. *J. Comparative Neurol.* 493(1):154–166.

Cropley, V.L., Fujita, M., Innis, R.B., and Nathan, P.J. (2006) Molecular imaging of the dopaminergic system and its association with human cognitive function. *Biol. Psych.* 59(10):898–907.

Cummings, J., and Winblad, B. (2007) A rivastigmine patch for the treatment of Alzheimer's disease and Parkinson's disease dementia. *Expert Rev. Neurother.* 7(11):1457–1463.

Cummings, J.L. (1988) Intellectual impairment in Parkinson's disease: clinical, pathologic, and biochemical correlates. *J. Geriatr. Psychiatry Neurol.* 1:24–36.

Cummings, J.L. (1995) Anatomic and behavioral aspects of frontal-subcortical circuits. *Ann. N.Y. Acad. Sci.* 15(769):1–13.

Cummings, J.L., Darkins, A., Mendez, M., Hill, M.A., and Benson, D.F. (1988) Alzheimer's disease and Parkinson's disease: comparison of speech and language alterations. *Neurology* 38:680–684.

Dagher, A., and Nagano-Saito, A. (2007) Functional and anatomical magnetic resonance imaging in Parkinson's disease. *Mol. Imaging Biol.* 9(4):234–242.

Dagher, A., Owen, A.M., Boecker, H., and Brooks, D.J. (2001) The role of the striatum and hippocampus in planning: a PET activation study in Parkinson's disease. *Brain* 124(Pt 5):1020–1032.

de Lau, L.M., Schipper, C.M., Hofman, A., Koudstaal, P.J., and Breteler, M.M. (2005) Prognosis of Parkinson disease: risk of dementia and mortality: the Rotterdam Study. *Arch. Neurol.* 62: 1265–1269.

De Marco, E.V., Tarantino, P., Rocca, F.E., et al. (2008) Alpha-synuclein promoter haplotypes and dementia in Parkinson's disease. *Am. J. Med. Genet. B Neuropsychiatr. Genet.* 147(3):403–407.

Ditter, S.M., and Mirra, S.S. (1987) Neuropathologic and clinical features of Parkinson's disease in Alzheimer's disease patients. *Neurology* 37:754–760.

Dodd, M.L., Klos, K.J., Bower, J.H., Geda, Y.E., Josephs, K.A., and Ahlskog, J.E. (2005) Pathological gambling caused by drugs used to treat Parkinson disease. *Arch. Neurol.* 62(9):1377–1381.

Dooneief, G., Mirabello, E., Bell, K., Marder, K., Stern, Y., and Mayeux, R. (1992) An estimate of the incidence of depression in idiopathic Parkinson's disease. *Arch. Neurol.* 49(3):305–307.

Downes, J.J., Priestley, N.M., Doran, M., Ferran, J., Ghadiali, E., and Cooper, P. (1998) Intellectual, mnemonic, and frontal functions in dementia with Lewy bodies: a comparison with early and advanced Parkinson's disease. *Behav. Neurol.* 11(3):173–183.

Downes, J.J., Sharp, H.M., Costall, B.M., Sagar, H.J., and Howe, J. (1993) Alternating fluency in Parkinson's disease. An evaluation of the attentional control therapy of cognitive impairment. *Brain* 116(Pt 4):887–902.

Dubinsky, R.M., Gray, C., Husted, D., Busenbark, K., Vetere-Overfield, B., Wiltfong, D., Parrish, D., and Koller, W.C. (1991) Driving in Parkinson's disease. *Neurology* 41(4):517–520.

Dubois, B., Burn, D., Goetz, C., et al. (2007) Movement Disorder Society Task Force practical strategies for the diagnosis of Parkinson's disease dementia. *Mov. Disord.* 22:2314–2324.

Dubois, B., and Pillon, B. (1997) Cognitive deficits in Parkinson's disease. *J. Neurol.* 244(1):2–8.

Dubois, B., and Pillon, B. (1998) Cognitive and behavioral aspects of movement disorders. In: Jankovic, J., and Tolosa, E., eds. *Parkinson's Disease and Movement Disorders*. Baltimore: Williams & Wilkins, pp. 837–858.

Dubois, B., Pillon, B., Sternic, N., Lhermitte, F., and Agid, Y. (1990) Age-induced cognitive disturbances in Parkinson's disease. *Neurology* 40(1):38–41.

Ebmeier, K.P., Calder, S.A., Crawford, J.R., Stewart, L., Besson, J.A., and Mutch, W.J. (1990a) Clinical features predicting dementia in idiopathic Parkinson's disease: a follow-up study. *Neurology* 40(8):1222–1224.

Ebmeier, K.P., Calder, S.A., Crawford, J.R., Stewart, L., Besson, J.A., and Mutch, W.J. (1990b) Mortality and causes of death in idiopathic Parkinson's disease: results from the Aberdeen whole population study. *Scott. Med. J.* 35(6):173–175.

Ebmeier, K.P., Calder, S.A., Crawford, J.R., Stewart, L., Cochrane, R.H., and Besson, J.A. (1991) Dementia in idiopathic Parkinson's disease: prevalence and relationship with symptoms and signs of parkinsonism. *Psychol. Med.* 21(1):69–76.

Ebmeier, K.P., Potter, D.D., Cochrane, R.H., Crawford, J.R., Stewart, L., Calder, S.A., Besson, J.A., and Salzen, E.A. (1992) Event related potentials, reaction time, and cognitive performance in idiopathic Parkinson's disease. *Biol. Psychol.* 33(1):73–89.

El-Ghundi, M., O'Dowd, B.F., and George, S.R. (2007) Insights into the role of dopamine receptor systems in learning and memory. *Rev. Neurosci.* 18(1):37–66.

Elizan, T.S., Sroka, H., Maker, H., Smith, H., and Yahr, M.D. (1986) Dementia in idiopathic Parkinson's disease. Variables associated with its occurrence in 203 patients. *J. Neural. Transm.* 65(3/4):285–302.

Emre, M. (2003) What causes mental dysfunction in Parkinson's disease? *Mov. Disord.* 18(Suppl 6):S63–S71.

Emre, M., Aarsland, D., Albanese, A., et al. (2004) Rivastigmine for dementia associated with Parkinson's disease. *N. Engl. J. Med.* 351(24):2509–2518.

Emre, M., Aarsland, D., Brown, R., et al. (2007) Clinical diagnostic criteria for dementia associated with Parkinson's disease. *Mov. Disord.* 22:1689–1707.

Engelborghs, S., Maertens, K., Nagels, G., et al. (2005) Neuropsychiatric symptoms of dementia: cross-sectional analysis from a prospective, longitudinal Belgian study. *Int. J. Geriatr. Psychiatry* 20:1028–1037.

Evans, A.H., Katzenschlager, R., Paviour, D., et al. (2004) Punding in Parkinson's disease: its relation to the dopamine dysregulation syndrome. *Mov. Disord.* 19:397–405.

Factor, S.A., Feustel, P.J., Friedman, J.H., Comella, C.L., Goetz, C.G., Kurlan, R., Parsa, M., Pfeiffer, R., and the Parkinson Study Group. (2003) Longitudinal outcome of Parkinson's disease patients with psychosis. *Neurology* 60:1756–1761.

Fearnley, J.M., and Lees, A.J. (1991) Ageing and Parkinson's disease: substantia nigra regional selectivity. *Brain* 114:2283–2301.

Fénelon, G., Goetz, C.G., and Karenberg, A. (2006) Hallucinations in Parkinson disease in the prelevodopa era. *Neurology* 66:93–98.

Fénelon, G., Mahieux, F., Huon, R., and Ziegler, M. (2000) Hallucinations in Parkinson's disease: prevalence, phenomenology, and risk factors. *Brain* 123:733–745.

Fernandez, H.H., and Lapane, K.L. (2002) Predictors of mortality among nursing home residents with a diagnosis of Parkinson's disease. *Med. Sci. Monit.* 8(4):CR241–CR246.

Ferraro, F.R., Balota, D.A., and Connor, L.T. (1993) Implicit memory and the formation of new associations in nondemented Parkinson's disease individuals and individuals with senile dementia of the Alzheimer type: a serial reaction time (SRT) investigation. *Brain Cogn.* 21(2):163–180.

Fields, J.A., Troster, A.I., Wilkinson, S.B., Pahwa, R., and Koller, W.C. (1999) Cognitive outcome following staged bilateral pallidal stimulation for the treatment of Parkinson's disease. *Clin. Neurol. Neurosurg.* 101(3):182–188.

Filoteo, J.V., and Maddox, W.T. (1999) Quantitative modeling of visual attention processes in patients with Parkinson's disease: effects of stimulus integrality on selective attention and dimensional integration. *Neuropsychology* 13(2):206–222.

Folstein, M.F., Folstein, S.E., and McHugh, P.R. (1975) "Mini-mental state." A practical method for grading the cognitive state of patients for the clinician. *J. Psychiatr. Res.* 12(3):189–198.

Foltynie, T., Brayne, C., and Barker, R.A. (2002) The heterogeneity of idiopathic Parkinson's disease. *J. Neurol.* 249:138–145.

Foltynie, T., Brayne, C.E., Robbins, T.W., and Barker, R.A. (2004) The cognitive ability of an incident cohort of Parkinson's patients in the UK. The CamPaIGN study. *Brain* 127:550–560.

Foster, N.L., Chase, T.N., Mansi, L., et al. (1984) Cortical abnormalities in Alzheimer's disease. *Ann. Neurol.* 16:649–654.

Fournet, N., Moreaud, O., Roulin, J.L., Naegele, B., and Pellat, J. (2000) Working memory functioning in medicated Parkinson's disease patients and the effect of withdrawal of dopaminergic medication. *Neuropsychology* 14(2):247–253.

Francis, P.T., and Perry, E.K. (2007) Cholinergic and other neurotransmitter mechanisms in Parkinson's disease, Parkinson's disease dementia, and dementia with Lewy bodies. *Mov. Disor.* Suppl 17:S351–S357.

Frank, M.J., Scheres, A., and Sherman, S.J. (2007) Understanding decision-making deficits in neurological conditions: insights from models of natural action selection. *Philos. Trans. R Soc. Lond. B Biol. Sci.* 362(1485):1641–1654.

Galvin, J.E. (2006) Cognitive change in Parkinson disease. *Alzheimer Dis. Assoc. Disord.* 20(4):302–310.

Gaspar, P., and Gray, F. (1984) Dementia in idiopathic Parkinson's disease: a neuropathological study of 32 cases. *Acta Neuropathol.* 64:43–52.

Gelb, D.J., Oliver, E., and Gilman, S. (1999) Diagnostic criteria for Parkinson disease. *Arch. Neurol.* 56:33–39.

Gemmell, H.G., Sharp, P.F., Smith, F.W., Besson, J.A., Ebmeier, K.P., Davidson, J., Evans, N.T., Roeda, D., Newton, R., and Mallard, J.R. (1989) Cerebral blood flow measured by SPECT as a diagnostic tool in the study of dementia. *Psychiatry Res.* 29(3):327–329.

Ghika, J., Ghika-Schmid, F., Fankhauser, H., Assal, G., Vingerhoets, F., Albanese, A., Bogousslavsky, J., and Favre, J. (1999) Bilateral contemporaneous posteroventral pallidotomy for the treatment of Parkinson's disease: neuropsychological and neurological side effects. Report of four cases and review of the literature. *J. Neurosurg.* 91(2):313–321; comment in: *J. Neurosurg.* 2000 92(3):509.

Giladi, N., Treves, T.A., Paleacu, D., Shabtai, H., Orlov, Y., Kandinov, B., Simon, E.S., and Korczyn, A.D. (2000) Risk factors for dementia, depression, and psychosis in long-standing Parkinson's disease. *J. Neural Transm.* 10:759–771.

Gjerstad, M.D., Boeve, B., Wentzel-Larsen, T., et al. (2007) Occurrence and clinical correlates of REM sleep behavior disorder in patients with Parkinson's disease over time. *J. Neurol. Neurosurg. Psychiatry* 79(4):387–391.

Glatt, S.L., Hubble, J.P., Lyons, K., Paolo, A., Troster, A.I., Hassanein, R.E., and Koller, W.C. (1996) Risk factors for dementia in Parkinson's disease: effect of education. *Neuroepidemiology* 15(1):20–25.

Goetz, C.G., and Stebbins, G.T. (1993) Risk factors for nursing home placement in advanced Parkinson's disease. *Neurology* 43(11): 2227–2229.

Goetz, C.G., and Stebbins, G.T. (1995) Mortality and hallucinations in nursing home patients with advanced Parkinson's disease. *Neurology* 45(4):669–671.

Goldmann Gross, R., Siderowf, A., and Hurtig, H.I. (2008) Cognitive impairment in Parkinson's disease and dementia with Lewy bodies: a spectrum of disease. *Neurosignals* 16(1):24–34.

Goldman-Rakic, P.S. (1998) The cortical dopamine system: role in memory and cognition. *Adv. Pharmacol.* 42:707–711.

Goldman-Rakic, P.S. (1999) The physiological approach: functional architecture of working memory and disordered cognition in schizophrenia. *Biol. Psychiatry*46(5):650–661.

Gotham, A.M., Brown, R.G., and Marsden, C.D. (1986a) Depression in Parkinson's disease: a quantitative and qualitative analysis. *J. Neurol. Neurosurg. Psychiatry* 49(4):381–389.

Gotham, A.M., Brown, R.G., and Marsden, C.D. (1986b) Levodopa treatment may benefit or impair "frontal" function in Parkinson's disease. *Lancet* 2(8513):970–971.

Gotham, A.M., Brown, R.G., and Marsden, C.D. (1988) "Frontal" cognitive function in patients with Parkinson's disease "on" and "off" levodopa. *Brain* 111(Pt 2):299–321.

Graham, J.M., Grunewald, R.A., and Sagar, H.J. (1997) Hallucinosis in idiopathic Parkinson's disease. *J. Neurol. Neurosurg. Psychiatry* 63(4):434–440.

Graham, J.M., and Sagar, H.J. (1999) A data-driven approach to the study of heterogeneity in idiopathic Parkinson's disease: identification of three distinct subtypes. *Mov. Disord.* 14(1):10–20.

Green, T., and Camicioli, R. (2007) Depressive symptoms and cognitive status affect health-related quality of life in older patients with Parkinson's disease. *J. Am. Geriatr. Soc.* 55(11):1888–1890.

Growdon, J.H., Corkin, S., and Rosen, T.J. (1990) Distinctive aspects of cognitive dysfunction in Parkinson's disease. *Adv. Neurol.* 53:365–376.

Haaland, K.Y., Harrington, D.L., O'Brien, S., and Hermanowicz, N. (1997) Cognitive-motor learning in Parkinson's disease. *Neuropsychology* 11(2):180–186.

Hanyu, H., Asano, T., Sakurai, H., Tanaka, Y., Takasaki, M., and Abe, K. (2002) MR analysis of the substantia innominata in normal aging, Alzheimer disease, and other types of dementia. *Am. J. Neuroradiol.* 23(1):27–32; comment in: *Am. J. Neuroradiol.* 23(1):33–34.

Hardesty, D.E., and Sackeim, H.A. (2007) Deep brain stimulation in movement and psychiatric disorders. *Biol. Psychiatry* 61(7):831–835.

Harhangi, B.S., de Rijk, M.C., van Duijin, C.M., Van Vroeckhoven, C., Hofman, A., and Breteler, M.M.B. (2000) APOE and the risk of PD with or without dementia in a population-based study. *Neurology* 54:1272–1276.

Harrington, D.L., Haaland, K.Y., Yeo, R.A., and Marder, E. (1990) Procedural in memory in Parkinson's disease: impaired motor but not visuoperceptual learning. *J. Clin. Exp. Neuropsychol.* 12(2):323–339.

Hauser, R.A., and Olanow, C.W. (1994) MRI of neurodegenerative diseases. *J. Neuroimaging* 4:146–158.

Hay, J.F., Moscovitch, M., and Levine, B. (2002) Dissociating habit and recollection: evidence from Parkinson's disease, amnesia and focal lesion patients. *Neuropsychologia* 40(8):1324–1334.

Hely, M.A., Morris, J.G., Reid, W.G., and Trafficante, R. (2005) Sydney Multicenter Study of Parkinson's Disease: non-L-dopa-responsive problems dominate at 15 years. *Mov. Disord.* 20: 190–199.

Henderson, J.M., Gai, W.P., Hely, M.A., Reid, W.G., Walker G.L., and Halliday, G.M. (2001) Parkinson's disease with late Pick's dementia. *Mov. Disord.* 16(2):311–319.

Higginson, C.I., Wheelock, V.L., Carroll, K.E., and Sigvardt, K.A. (2005) Recognition memory in Parkinson's disease with and without dementia: evidence inconsistent with the retrieval deficit hypothesis. *J. Clin. Exp. Neuropsychol.* 27:516–528.

Hirono, N., Mori, E., Tanimukai, S., et al. (1999) Distinctive neurobehavioral features among neurodegenerative dementias. *J. Neuropsychiatry Clin. Neurosci.* 11:498–503.

Hobson, P., Gallacher, J., and Meara, J. (2005) Cross-sectional survey of Parkinson's disease and parkinsonism in a rural area of the United Kingdom. *Mov. Disord.* 20:995–998.

Hobson, P., and Meara, J. (2004) Risk and incidence of dementia in a cohort of older subjects with Parkinson's disease in the United Kingdom. *Mov. Disord.* 19:1043–1049.

Holroyd, S., Currie, L., and Wooten, G.F. (2001) Prospective study of hallucinations and delusions in Parkinson's disease. *J. Neurol. Neurosurg. Psychiatry* 70(6):734–738.

Hoppe, C.D., Muller, U.D., Werheid, K.D., Thone, A.D., and von Cramon, Y.D. (2000) Digit Ordering Test: clinical, psychometric, and experimental evaluation of a verbal working memory test. *Clin. Neuropsychol.* 14(1):38–55.

Horstink, M.W., Berger, H.J., van Spaendonck, K.P., van den Bercken, J.H., and Cools, A.R. (1990) Bimanual simultaneous motor performance and impaired ability to shift attention in Parkinson's disease. *J. Neurol. Neurosurg. Psychiatry* 53(8):685–690.

Hovestadt, A., de Jong, G.J., and Meerwaldt, J.D. (1987) Spatial disorientation as an early symptom of Parkinson's disease. *Neurology* 37(3):485–487.

Hsieh, S., Lee, C.Y., and Tai, C.T. (1995) Set-shifting aptitude in Parkinson's disease: external versus internal cues. *Psychol. Rep.* 77(1):339–349.

Hu, M.T., Taylor-Robinson, S.D., Chaudhuri, K.R., Bell, J.D., Labbe, C., Cunningham, V.J., Koepp, M.J., Hammers, A., Morris, R.G., Turjanski, N., and Brooks, D.J. (2000) Cortical dysfunction in non-demented Parkinson's disease patients: a combined (31)P-MRS and (18)FDG-PET study. *Brain* 123(Pt 2):340–352.

Hu, M.T., Taylor-Robinson, S.D., Chaudhuri, K.R., Bell, J.D., Morris, R.G., Clough, C., Brooks, D.J., and Turjanski, N. (1999) Evidence for cortical dysfunction in clinically non-demented patients with Parkinson's disease: a proton MR spectroscopy study. *J. Neurol. Neurosurg. Psychiatry* 67(1):20–26.

Hu, M.T., White, S.J., Chaudhuri, K.R., Morris, R.G., Bydder, G.M., and Brooks, D.J. (2001) Correlating rates of cerebral atrophy in Parkinson's disease with measures of cognitive decline. *J. Neurol. Transm.* 108(5):571–580.

Hughes, T.A., Ross, H.F., Musa, S., et al. (2000) A 10-year study of the incidence of and factors predicting dementia in Parkinson's disease. *Neurology* 54:1596–1602.

Hulette, C., Mirra, S., Wilkinson, W., et al. (1995) The Consortium to Establish a Registry for Alzheimer's Disease (CERAD). Part IX. A prospective cliniconeuropathologic study of Parkinson's features in Alzheimer's disease. *Neurology* 45:1991–1995.

Hulette, C.M., Pericak-Vance, M.A., Roses, A.D., Schmechel, D.E., Yamaoka, L.H., Gaskell, P.C., Welsh-Bohmer, K.A., Crowther,

R.A., and Spillantini, M.G. (1999) Neuropathological features of frontotemporal dementia and parkinsonism linked to chromosome 17q21-22 (FTDP-17): Duke Family 1684. *J. Neuropathol. Exp. Neurol.* 58(8):859–866.

Hurtig, H.I., Trojanowski, J.Q., Galvin, J., et al. (2000) Alphasynuclein cortical Lewy bodies correlate with dementia in Parkinson's disease. *Neurology* 54:1916–1921.

Inzelberg, R., Chapman, J., Treves, T.A., et al. (1998) Apolipoprotein E4 in Parkinson disease and dementia: new data and meta-analysis of published studies. *Alzheimer Dis. Assoc. Disord.* 12:45–48.

Ito, K., Morrish, P.K., Rakshi, J.S., Uema, T., Ashburner, J., Bailey, D.L., Friston, K.J., and Brooks, D.J. (1999) Statistical parametric mapping with 18F-dopa PET shows bilaterally reduced striatal and nigral dopaminergic function in early Parkinson's disease. *J. Neurol. Neurosurg. Psychiatry* 66(6):754–758.

Ito, K., Nagano-Saito, A., Kato, T., Arahata, Y., Nakamura, A., Kawasumi, Y., Hatano, K., Abe, Y., Yamada, T., Kachi, T., and Brooks, D.J. (2002) Striatal and extrastriatal dysfunction in Parkinson's disease with dementia: a 6-[18F]fluoro-L-dopa PET study. *Brain* 125(Pt 6):1358–1365.

Jacobs, D.M., Marder, K., Cote, L.J., Sano, M., Stern, Y., and Mayeux, R. (1995) Neuropsychological characteristics of preclinical dementia in Parkinson's disease. *Neurology* 45(9):1691–1696; comment in: *Neurology* 1997 48(2):546–547.

Jahanshahi, M., Ardouin, C.M., Brown, R.G., Rothwell, J.C., Obeso, J., Albanese, A., Rodriguez-Oroz, M.C., Moro, E., Benabid, A.L., Pollak, P., and Limousin-Dowsey, P. (2000) The impact of deep brain stimulation on executive function in Parkinson's disease. *Brain* 123(Pt 6):1142–1154.

Jahanshahi, M., Brown, R.G., and Marsden, C.D. (1993) A comparative study of simple and choice reaction time in Parkinson's, Huntington's and cerebellar disease. *J. Neurol. Neurosurg. Psychiatry* 56(11):1169–1177.

Janvin, C.C., Aarsland, D., and Larsen, J.P. (2005) Cognitive predictors of dementia in Parkinson's disease: a community-based, 4-year longitudinal study. *J. Geriatr. Psychiatry Neurol.* 18:149–154.

Janvin, C.C., Larsen, J.P., Aarsland, D., and Hugdahl, K. (2006) Subtypes of mild cognitive impairment in Parkinson's disease: progression to dementia. *Mov. Disord.* 21(9):1343–1349.

Jellinger, K. (1987) The pathology of parkinsonism. In: Marsden, C.D., and Fahn, S., eds. *Movement Disorders 2*. London: Butterworths, pp. 124–165.

Jellinger, K.A. (2007) Morphological substrates of parkinsonism with and without dementia: a retrospective clinico-pathological study. *J. Neural Transm. Suppl.*(72):91–104.

Jellinger, K.A., Wenning, G.K., and Seppi, K. (2007) Predictors of survival in dementia with Lewy bodies and Parkinson dementia. *Neurodegen. Dis.* 4(6):428–430.

Kahle, P.J. (2008) α-Synucleinopathy models and human neuropathology: similarities and differences *Acta Neuropathol (Berl)* 115(1):87–95.

Kang, G.A., Bronstein, J.M., Masterman, D.L., Redelings, M., Crum, J.A., and Ritz, B. (2005) Clinical characteristics in early Parkinson's disease in a central California population-based study. *Mov. Disord.* 20:1133–1142.

Kertesz, A., Martinez-Lage, P., Davidson, W., and Munoz, D.G. (2000) The corticobasal degeneration syndrome overlaps progressive aphasia and frontotemporal dementia. *Neurology* 55:1368–1375.

Khandhar, S.M., and Marks, W.J. (2007) Epidemiology of Parkinson's disease. *Dis. Mon.* 53(4):200–205.

Kish, S.J. (2003) Biochemistry of Parkinson's disease: is a brain serotonergic deficiency a characteristic of idiopathic Parkinson's disease? *Adv. Neurol.* 91:39–49.

Kish, S.J., Tong, J., Hornykiewicz, O., Rajput, A., Chang, L.J., Guttman, M., and Furukawa, Y. (2008) Preferential loss of serotonin markers in caudate versus putamen in Parkinson's disease. *Brain* 131(Pt 1):120–131.

Koller, W.C. (1984) Disturbance of recent memory function in parkinsonian patients on anticholinergic therapy. *Cortex* 20(2):307–311.

Koller, W.C., Glatt, S.L., Hubble, J.P., et al. (1995) Apolipoprotein E genotypes in Parkinson's disease with and without dementia. *Ann. Neurol.* 37:242–245.

Korczyn, A.D. (2001) Dementia in Parkinson's disease. *J. Neurol.* 248(Suppl 3):III1–III4.

Kuhl, D.E., Metter, E.J., and Riege, W.H. (1984) Patterns of local cerebral glucose utilisation determined in Parkinson's disease by the 18F-fluorodeoxyglucose method. *Ann. Neurol.* 15:419–424.

Kurlan, R., Richard, I.H., Papka, M., and Marshall, F. (2000) Movement disorders in Alzheimer's disease: more rigidity of definitions is needed. *Mov. Disord.* 15(1):24–29.

Kuzis, G., Sabe, L., Tiberti, C., Merello, M., Leiguarda, R., and Starkstein, S.E. (1999) Explicit and implicit learning in patients with Alzheimer disease and Parkinson disease with dementia. *Neuropsychiatry Neuropsychol. Behav. Neurol.* 12:265–269.

Lauterbach, E.C. (2004) The neuropsychiatry of Parkinson's disease and related disorders. *Psychiatr. Clin. North Am.* 27(4):801–825.

Lavernhe, G., Pollak, P., Brenier, F., Gaio, J.M., Hommel, M., Pellat, J., and Perret, J. (1989) Alzheimer's disease and Parkinson's disease: neuropsychological differentiation [French]. *Rev. Neurol. (Paris)* 145(1):24–30.

Lees, A.J., and Smith, E. (1983) Cognitive deficits in the early stages of Parkinson's disease. *Brain* 106:257–270.

Leibson, C.L., Maraganore, D.M., Bower, J.H., et al. (2006) Comorbid conditions associated with Parkinson's disease: a population-based study. *Mov. Disord.* 22(7):1054–1055.

Leverenz, J., and Sumi, S.M. (1986) Parkinson's disease in patients with Alzheimer's disease. *Arch. Neurol.* 43:662–664.

Levin, B.E., Llabre, M.M., and Weiner, W.J. (1989) Cognitive impairments associated with early Parkinson's disease. *Neurology* 39:557–561.

Levy, G. (2007) The relationship of Parkinson disease with aging. *Arch. Neurol.* 64(9):1242–1246.

Levy, G., Schupf, N., Tang, M.X., Cote, L.J., Louis, E.D., Mejia, H., Stern, Y., and Marder, K. (2002) Combined effect of age and severity on the risk of dementia in Parkinson's disease. *Ann. Neurol.* 51(6):722–729.

Levy, G., Tang, M.X., Cote, L.J., Louis, E.D., Alfaro, B., Mejia, H., Stern, Y., and Marder, K. (2000) Motor impairment in PD: relationship to incident dementia and age. *Neurology* 55(4):539–544.

Levy, G., Tang, M.X., Cote, L.J., Louis, E.D., Alfaro, B., Mejia, H., Stern, Y., and Marder, K. (2002) Do risk factors for Alzheimer's disease predict dementia in Parkinson's disease? An exploratory study. *Mov. Disord.* 17(2):250–257.

Levy, G., Tang, M.X., Louis, E.D., et al. (2002) The association of incident dementia with mortality in PD. *Neurology* 59:1708–1713.

Lewis, S.J.G., Foltynie, T., Blackwell, A.D., Robbins, T.W., Owen, A.M., and Barker, R.A. (2005) Heterogeneity of Parkinson's disease in the early clinical stages using a data driven approach. *J. Neurol. Neurosurg. Psychiatry* 76:343–348.

Lieberman, A. (1998) Managing the neuropsychiatric symptoms of Parkinson's disease. *Neurology* 50(Suppl 6):S33–S38; discussion S44–S48.

Liepelt, I., Maetzler, W., Blaicher, H.P., Gasser, T., and Berg, D. (2007) Treatment of dementia in parkinsonian syndromes with cholinesterase inhibitors. *Dement. Geriatr. Cogn. Disord.* 23(6):351–367.

Lippa, C.F., Dud, J.E., Grossman, M., et al. (2007) DLB and PDD boundary issues: diagnosis, treatment, molecular pathology, and biomarkers. *Neurology* 68(11):812–819.

Lippa, C.F., Smith, T.W., and Swearer, J. (1998) Dementia with parkinsonism: Alzheimer's disease is more common than dementia with Lewy bodies. *Am. J. Alzheimer's Dis. Demen.* 13(5):229–235.

Litvan, I. (1998) Parkinsonism-dementia syndromes. In: Jankovic, J., and Tolosa, E., Eds. *Parkinson's Disease and Movement Disorders*. Baltimore: Williams & Wilkins, pp. 819–836.

Litvan, I., Agid, Y., Calne, D., et al. (1996) Clinical research criteria for the diagnosis of progressive supranuclear palsy (Steele-Richardson-Olszewski syndrome): report of the NINDS-SPSP international workshop. *Neurology* 47:1–9.

Litvan, I., Agid, Y., Goetz, C., Jankovic, J., Wenning, G.K., Brandel, J.P., Lai, E.C., Verny, M., Mangone, C.A., and Pearce, R.K. (1996) Accuracy of clinical criteria for the diagnosis of progressive supranuclear palsy (Steele-Richardson-Olszewski syndrome). *Neurology* 46(4):922–930.

Litvan, I., Mega, M.S., Cummings, J.L., and Fairbanks, L. (1996) Neuropsychiatric aspects of progressive supranuclear palsy. *Neurology* 47(5):1184–1189.

Lombardi, W.J., Gross, R.E., Trepanier, L.L., Lang, A.E., Lozano, A.M., and Saint-Cyr, J.A. (2000) Relationship of lesion location to cognitive outcome following microelectrode-guided pallidotomy for Parkinson's disease: support for the existence of cognitive circuits in the human pallidum. *Brain* 123(Pt 4):746–758.

Louis, E.D., Marder, K., Cote, L., Tang, M., and Mayeux, R. (1997) Mortality from Parkinson disease. *Arch. Neurol.* 54(3):260–264.

Love, S. (2005) Neuropathological investigation of dementia: a guide for neurologists. *J. Neurol. Neurosurg. Psychiatry* 76(Suppl 5): v8–v14.

Mahieux, F., Fenelon, G., Flahault, A., Manifacier, M.J., Michelet, D., and Boller, F. (1998) Neuropsychological prediction of dementia in Parkinson's disease. *J. Neurol. Neurosurg. Psychiatry* 64:178–183.

Mamikonyan, E., Siderowf, A.D., Duda, J.E., Potenza, M.N., Horn, S., Stern, M.B., and Weintraub, D. (2008) Long-term follow-up of impulse control disorders in Parkinson's disease. *Mov. Disord.* 23(1):75–80.

Marder, K. (2002) Donepezil for cognitive impairment in Parkinson's disease: a randomized controlled trial. *Curr. Neurol. Neurosci. Rep.* 2(5):390–391.

Marder, K., Flood, P., Cote, L., and Mayeux, R. (1990) A pilot study of risk factors for dementia in Parkinson's disease. *Mov. Disord.* 5(2):156–161.

Marder, K., Leung, D., Tang, M., Bell, K., Dooneief, G., Cote, L., Stern, Y., and Mayeux, R. (1991) Are demented patients with Parkinson's disease accurately reflected in prevalence surveys? a survival analysis. *Neurology* 41(8):1240–1243.

Marder, K., Tang, M.X., Alfaro, B., Mejia, H., Cote, L., Jacobs, D., Stern, Y., Sano, M., and Mayeux, R. (1998) Postmenopausal estrogen use and Parkinson's disease with and without dementia. *Neurology* 50(4):1141–1143.

Marder, K., Tang M.X., Alfaro, B., Mejia, H., Cote, L., Lovis, E., Stern, T., and Mayeux, R. (1999) Risk of Alzheimer's disease in relatives of a Parkinson's disease patient with and without dementia. *Neurology* 52(4):719–724.

Marder, K., Tang, M.X., Cote, L., Stern, Y., and Mayeux, R. (1995) The frequency and associated risk factors for dementia in patients with Parkinson's disease. *Arch. Neurol.* 52(7):695–701.

Marek, K.L., Innis, R.B., and Seibyl, J. (1998) Assessment of Parkinson's disease progression with b-CIT and SPECT imaging. *Mov. Disord.* 13(Suppl 2):238–230.

Mariani, E., Monastero, R., and Mecocci, P. (2007) Mild cognitive impairment: a systematic review. *J. Alzheimers Dis.* 12(1):23–35.

Marié, R.M., Barre, L., Dupuy, B., Viader, F., Defer, G., and Baron, J.C. (1999) Relationships between striatal dopamine denervation and frontal executive tests in Parkinson's disease. *Neurosci. Lett.* 260(2):77–80.

Marié, R.M., Barre, L., Rioux, P., Allain, P., Lechevalier, B., and Baron, J.C. (1995) PET imaging of neocortical monoaminergic terminals in Parkinson's disease. *J. Neural. Transm. Park. Dis. Dement. Sect.* 9(1):55–71.

Marjama-Lyons, J.M., and Koller, W.C. (2001) Parkinson's disease. Update in diagnosis and symptom management. *Geriatrics* 56(8): 24–25, 29–30, 33–35.

Marsh, L., Williams, J.R., Rocco, M., Grill, S., Munro, C., and Dawson, T.M. (2004) Psychiatric comorbidities in patients with Parkinson disease and psychosis. *Neurology* 63:293–300.

Matsui, H., Nishinaka, K., Oda, M., et al. (2007) Dementia in Parkinson's disease: diffusion tensor imaging. *Acta Neurol. Scand.* 116(3):177–181.

Mayeux, R., Chen, J., Mirabello, E., Marder, K., Bell, K., Dooneief, G., Cote, L., and Stern, Y. (1990) An estimate of the incidence of dementia in idiopathic Parkinson's disease. *Neurology* 40(10): 1513–1517.

Mayeux, R., Denaro, J., Hemenegildo, N., Marder, K., Tang, M.X., Cote, L.J., and Stern, Y. (1992) A population-based investigation of Parkinson's disease with and without dementia. Relationship to age and gender. *Arch. Neurol.* 49(5):492–497.

Mayeux, R., Stern, Y., Rosenstein, R., Marder, K., Hauser, A., Cote, L., and Fahn, S. (1998) An estimate of the prevalence of dementia in idiopathic Parkinson's disease. *Arch. Neurol.* 45(3):260–262.

Mayeux, R., Stern, Y., and Spanton, S. (1985) Heterogeneity in dementia of the Alzheimer type: evidence of subgroups. *Neurology* 35:453–461.

McGeer, P.L., Itagaki, S., Boyes, B.E., and McGeer, E.G. (1988) Reactive microglia are positive for HLA-DR in the substantia nigra of Parkinson's and Alzheimer's disease brains. *Neurology* 38: 1285–1291.

McKeith, I. (2007) Dementia with Lewy bodies and Parkinson's disease with dementia: where two worlds collide. *Practical Neurology* 7:374–382.

McKeith, I., Mintzer, J., Aarsland, D., et al. (2004) Dementia with Lewy bodies. *Lancet Neurol.* 3:19–28.

McKeith, I.G., Dickson, D.W., Lowe, J., et al. (2005) Consortium on DLB: Diagnosis and management of dementia with Lewy bodies: third report of the DLB consortium. *Neurology* 65:1863–1872.

McKeith, I.G., Galasko, D., Kosaka, K., et al. (1996) Consensus guidelines for the clinical and pathological diagnosis of dementia with Lewy bodies: report of the consortium on DLB international workshop. *Neurology* 47:1113–1124.

McKeith, I.G., Grace, J.B., Walker, Z., Byrne, E.J., Wilkinson, D., Stevens, T., and Pery, E.K. (2000) Rivastigmine in the treatment of dementia with Lewy bodies: preliminary findings from an open trial. *Int. J. Geriatr. Psychiatry* 15(5):387–392.

McNamara, P., and Durso, R. (2006) Neuropharmacological treatment of mental dysfunction in Parkinson's disease. *Behav. Neurol.* 17(1):43–51.

Menza, M.A., Robertson, H.D., and Bonapace, A.S. (1993) Parkinson's disease and anxiety: comorbidity with depression. *Biol. Psychiatry* 34:465–470.

Mesulam, M.M. (2000) Behavioral neuroanatomy. In: M.M. Mesulam, ed. *Principles of Behavioral and Cognitive Neurology*. New York: Oxford University Press, pp. 1–120.

Metzler-Baddeley, C. (2007) A review of cognitive impairments in dementia with Lewy bodies relative to Alzheimer's Disease and Parkinson's Disease with Dementia. *Cortex* 43(5):583–600.

Mitchell, S.L. (1999) Extrapyramidal features in Alzheimer's disease. *Age Ageing* 28(4):401–409.

Molloy, S.A., Rowan, E.N., O'Brien, J.T., McKeith, I.G., Wesnes, K., and Burn, D.J. (2006) Effect of levodopa on cognitive function in Parkinson's disease with and without dementia and dementia with Lewy bodies. *J. Neurol. Neurosurg. Psychiatry* 77(12): 1323–1328.

Molsa, P.K., Marttila, R.J., and Rinne, U.K. (1984) Extrapyramidal signs in Alzheimer's disease. *Neurology* 34:1114–1116.

Monchi, O., Petrides, M., Mejia-Constain, B., et al. (2007) Cortical activity in Parkinson's disease during executive processing depends on striatal involvement. *Brain* 130(Pt 1):233–244.

Mondon, K., Gochard, A., Marqué, A., et al. (2007) Visual recognition memory differentiates dementia with Lewy bodies and Parkinson's disease dementia. *J. Neurol. Neurosurg. Psychiatry* 78: 738–741.

Morens, D.M., Grandinetti, A., Reed, D., et al. (1995) Cigarette smoking and protection from Parkinson's disease: false association or etiologic clue? *Neurology* 45:1041–1051.

Morris, J.C., Drazner, M., Fulling, K., et al. (1989) Clinical and pathological aspects of parkinsonism in Alzheimer's disease. *Arch. Neurol.* 46:651–657.

Morrison, C.E., Borod, J.C., Brin, M.F., Raskin, S.A., Germano, I.M., Weisz, D.J., and Olanow, C.W. (2000) A program for neuropsychological investigation of deep brain stimulation (PNIDBS) in movement disorder patients: program development and preliminary data. *Neuropsychiatry Neuropsychol. Behav. Neurol.* 13: 204–219.

Morrison, C.E., Borod, J., Perrine, K., et al. (2004) Neuropsychological functioning following bilateral subthalamic nucleus stimulation in Parkinson's disease. *Arch. Clin. Neuropsychology* 19(2): 165–181.

Mosimann, U.P., Mather, G., Wesnes, K.A., O'Brien, J.T., Burn, D.J., and McKeith, I.G. (2004) Visual perception in Parkinson disease dementia and dementia with Lewy bodies. *Neurology* 63: 2091–2096.

Mosimann, U.P., Rowan, E.N., Partington, C.E., et al. (2006) Characteristics of visual hallucinations in Parkinson disease dementia and dementia with lewy bodies. *Am. J. Geriatr. Psychiatry* 14:153–160.

Nasreddine, Z.S., Loginov, M., Clark, L.N., Lamarche, J., Miller, B.L., Lamontagne, A., Zhukareva, V., Lee, V.M., Wilhelmsen, K.C., and Geschwind, D.H. (1999) From genotype to phenotype: a clinical pathological, and biochemical investigation of frontotemporal dementia and parkinsonism (FTDP-17) caused by the P301L tau mutation. *Ann. Neurol.* 45(6):704–715.

Neufeld, M.Y., Blumen, S., Aitkin, I., Parmet, Y., and Korczyn, A.D. (1994) EEG frequency analysis in demented and nondemented parkinsonian patients. *Dementia* 5:23–28.

Ngandu, T., von Strauss, E., Helkala, E.L., et al. (2007) Education and dementia: What lies behind the association? *Neurology* 69:1442–1450.

Nissenbaum, H., Quinn, N.P., Brown, R.G., Toone, B., Gotham, A.M., and Marsden, C.D. (1987) Mood swings associated with the "on-off" phenomenon in Parkinson's disease. *Psychol. Med.* 17(4):899–904.

Noe, E., Marder, K., Bell, K.L., Jacobs, D.M., Manly, J.J., and Stern, Y. (2004) Comparison of dementia with Lewy bodies to Alzheimer's disease and Parkinson's disease with dementia. *Mov. Disord.* 19:60–67.

Obeso, J.A., Olanow, C.W., Rodriguez-Oroz, M.C., et al. (2001) Deep-brain stimulation of the subthalamic nucleus or the pars interna of the globus pallidus in Parkinson's disease. The Deep-Brain Stimulation for Parkinson's Disease Study Group. *N. Eng. J. Med.* 345(13):956–963.

Okun, M.S., Rodriguez, R.L., Mikos, A., Miller, K., Kellison, I., Kirsch-Darrow, L., Wint, D.P., Springer, U., Fernandez, H.H., Foote, K.D., Crucian, G., and Bowers, D. (2007) Deep brain stimulation and the role of the neuropsychologist. *Clin. Neuropsychol.* 21(1):162–189.

Olanow, C.W., Lang, A.E., and Stocchi, F. (in press) *The non-motor and non-dopamine features of Parkinson's disease*. London: Wiley-Blackwell Press.

Olanow, C.W. (1992) Magnetic resonance imaging in parkinsonism. *Neurol. Clin. North Am.* 10(2):405–420.

Olanow, C.W. (2004) Manganese-induced parkinsonism and Parkinson's disease. *Ann. N.Y. Acad. Sci.* 1012:209–223.

Olanow, C.W., and Brin, M.F. (2001) Surgery for Parkinson's disease: a physician's perspective. *Adv. Neurol.* 86:421–433.

Olanow, C.W., Brin, M., and Obeso, J.A. (2000) The role of deep brain stimulation as a surgical treatment for Parkinson's disease. *Neurology* 55(Suppl 6):60–66.

Olanow, C.W., Good, P.F., and Perl, D.P. (1999) Evidence of damage to the globus pallidus pars interna and pedunculopontine nucleus in Parkinson's disease: implications for neuroprotection. *Soc. Neurosci. Abstr.* 25:1342.

Olanow, C.W., and Tatton, W.G. (1999) Etiology and pathogenesis of Parkinson's disease. *Annu. Rev. Neurosci.* 22:123–144.

Olanow, C.W., Watts, R.L., and Koller, W.C. (2001) An algorithm (decision tree) for the management of Parkinson's disease: treatment guidelines. *Neurology* 56(11 Suppl 5):S1–S88.

Olson, E.J., Boeve, B.F., and Silber, M.H. (2000) Rapid eye movement sleep behaviour disorder: demographic, clinical and laboratory findings in 93 cases. *Brain* 123:331–339.

Ordway, G.A., and Klimek, V. (2001) Noradrenergic pathology in psychiatric disorders: postmortem studies. *CNS Spectr.* 6(8):697–703.

Orimo, S., Ozawa, E., Nakade, S., Sugimoto, T., and Mizusawa, H. (1999) (123)I-metaiodobenzylguanidine myocardial scintigraphy in Parkinson's disease. *J. Neurol. Neurosurg. Psychiatry* 67:189–194.

Owen, A.D., Schapira, A.H., Jenner, P., and Marsden, C.D. (1997) Indices of oxidative stress in Parkinson's disease, Alzheimer's disease and dementia with Lewy bodies. *J. Neural. Transm. Suppl.* 51:167–173.

Owen, A.M. (2007) Cognitive dysfunction in Parkinson's disease: the role of frontostriatal circuitry. *Neuroscientist* 10(6):525–537.

Owen, A.M., Beksinska, M., James, M., Leigh, P.N., Summers, B.A., Marsden, C.D., Quinn, N.P., Sahakian, B.J., and Robbins, T.W. (1993) Visuospatial memory deficits at different stages of Parkinson's disease. *Neuropsychologia* 31(7):627–644.

Owen, A.M., Doyon, J., Dagher, A., Sadikot, A., and Evans, A.C. (1998) Abnormal basal ganglia outflow in Parkinson's disease identified with PET. Implications for higher cortical functions. *Brain* 121(Pt 5):949–965.

Owen, A.M., Iddon, J.L., Hodges, J.R., Summers, B.A., and Robbins, T.W. (1997) Spatial and non-spatial working memory at different stages of Parkinson's disease. *Neuropsychologia* 35(4): 519–532.

Owen, A.M., James, M., Leigh, P.N., Summers, B.A., Marsden, C.D., Quinn, N.P., Lange, K.W., and Robbins, T.W. (1992) Fronto-striatal cognitive deficits at different stages of Parkinson's disease. *Brain* 115(Pt 6):1727–1751.

Owen, A.M., Roberts, A.C., Hodges, J.R., Summers, B.A., Polkey, C.E., and Robbins, T.W. (1993) Contrasting mechanisms of impaired attentional set-shifting in patients with frontal lobe damage or Parkinson's disease. *Brain* 116(Pt 5):1159–1175.

Ozer, F., Meral, H., Lutfu, H., et al. (2007) Cognitive impairment patterns in Parkinson's disease with visual hallucinations. *J. Clin. Neurosci.* 14(8):742–746.

Pacchetti, C., Manni, R., Zangaglia, R., Mancini, F., Marchioni, E., Tassorelli, C., Terzaghi, M., Ossola, M., Martignoni, E., Moglia, A., and Nappi, G. (2005) Relationship between hallucinations, delusions, and rapid eye movement sleep behavior disorder in Parkinson's disease. *Mov. Disord.* 20:1439–1448.

Pagonabarraga, J., Garcia-Sanchez, C., Llebaria, G., Pascual-Sedano, B., Gironell, A., and Kulisevsky, J. (2007) Controlled study of decision-making and cognitive impairment in Parkinson's disease. *Mov. Disord.* 22(10):1430–1435.

Paolo, A.M., Axelrod, B.N., Troster, A.I., Blackwell, K.T., and Koller, W.C. (1996) Utility of a Wisconsin card sorting test short form in persons with Alzheimer's and Parkinson's disease. *J. Clin. Exp. Neuropsychol.* 18:892–897.

Paolo, A.M., Troster, A.I., Glatt, S.L., Hubble, J.P., and Koller, W.C. (1995) Differentiation of the dementias of Alzheimer's and Parkinson's disease with the dementia rating scale. *J. Geriatr. Psychiatry Neurol.* 8(3):184–188.

Parent, A., Sato, F., Wu, Y., et al. (2000) Axonal collateralization as a general principle of organization in the basal ganglia. *Trends Neurosci.* 23:20–27.

Parkin, S.G., Gregory, R.P., Scott, R., Bain, P., Silburn, P., Hall, B., Boyle, R., Joint, C., and Aziz, T.Z. (2002) Unilateral and bilateral pallidotomy for idiopathic Parkinson's disease: a case series of 115 patients. *Mov. Disord.* 17(4):682–692.

Parkinson, J. (1817) *An Essay on the Shaking Palsy*. London: Whitingham and Rowland.

Parsian, A., Racette, B., Goldsmith, L.J., and Perlmutter, J.S. (2002) Parkinson's disease and apolipoprotein E: possible association with dementia but not age at onset. *Genomics* 79:458–461.

Parsons, T., Rogers, S., Braaten, A., Woods, S., and Tröster, A. (2006) Cognitive sequelae of subthalamic nucleus deep brain stimulation in Parkinson's disease: a meta-analysis. *Lancet Neurol.* 5(7):578–588.

Partiot, A., Verin, M., Pillon, B., Teixeira-Ferreira, C., Agid, Y., and Dubois, B. (1996) Delayed response tasks in basal ganglia lesions in man: further evidence for a striato-frontal cooperation in behavioural adaptation. *Neuropsychologia* 34(7):709–721.

Pascual-Leone, A., Grafman, J., Clark, K., Stewart, M., Massaquoi, S., Lou, J.S., and Hallett, M. (1993) Procedural learning in Parkinson's disease and cerebellar degeneration. *Ann. Neurol.* 34(4): 594–602.

Peppard, R.F., Martin, W.R.W., Carr, G.D., et al. (1992) Cerebral glucose metabolism in Parkinson's disease with and without dementia. *Arch. Neurol.* 49:1262–1268.

Perl, D.P., Olanow, C.W., and Calne, D. (1998) Alzheimer's disease and Parkinson's disease: distinct entities or extremes of a spectrum of neurodegeneration? *Ann. Neurol.* 44(3):19–31.

Piatt, A.L., Fields, J.A., Paolo, A.M., Koller, W.C., and Tröster, A.I. (1999) Lexical, semantic, and action verbal fluency in Parkinson's disease with and without dementia. *J. Clin. Exp. Neuropsychol.* 21(4):435–443.

Pillon, B., Deweer, B., Agid, Y., and Dubois, B. (1993) Explicit memory in Alzheimer's disease, Huntington's disease, and Parkinson's disease. *Arch. Neurol.* 50:374–379.

Pillon, B., Ardouin, C., Damier, P., Krack, P., Houeto, J.L., Klinger, H., Bonnet, A.M., Pollak, P., Benabid, A.L., and Agid, Y. (2000) Neuropsychological changes between "off" and "on" STN or GPi stimulation in Parkinson's disease. *Neurology* 55(3):411–418.

Pillon, B., Dubois, B., and Agid, Y. (1991) Severity and specificity of cognitive impairment in Alzheimer's, Huntington's, and Parkinson's diseases and progressive supranuclear palsy. *Ann. N.Y. Acad. Sci.* 640:224–227.

Pillon, B., Ertle, S., Deweer, B., Sarazin, M., Agid, Y., and Dubois, B. (1996) Memory for spatial location is affected in Parkinson's disease. *Neuropsychologia* 34(1):77–85.

Pirozzolo, F.J., Hansch, E.C., Mortimer, J.A., Webster, D.D., and Kuskowski, M.A. (1982) Dementia in Parkinson disease: a neuropsychological analysis. *Brain Cogn.* 1(1):71–83.

Poewe, W. (2006) The natural history of Parkinson's disease. *J. Neurol.* 253(Suppl 7):VII2–VII6.

Poewe, W. (2007) Dysautonomia and cognitive dysfunction in Parkinson's disease. *Mov. Disord.* 22(Suppl 17):S374–S378.

Pontone, G., Williams, J.R., Bassett, S.S., and Marsh, L. (2006) Clinical features associated with impulse control disorders in Parkinson disease. *Neurology* 67(7):1258–1261.

Rabins, P.V., and Folstein, M.F. (1983) The dementia patient: evaluation and care. *Geriatrics* 38(8):99–103, 106.

Rajput, A.H., Offord, K.P., Beard, C.M., and Kurland, L.T. (1984) Epidemiology of parkinsonism: incidence, classification and mortality. *Ann. Neurol.* 16:278–283.

Rakshi, J.S., Uema, T., Ito, K., Bailey, D.L., Morrish, P.K., Ashburner, J., Dagher, A., Jenkins, I.H., Friston, K.J., and Brooks, D.J. (1999) Frontal, midbrain and striatal dopaminergic function in early and advanced Parkinson's disease. A 3D [(18)F]dopa-PET study. *Brain* 122(Pt 9):1637–1650.

Ramirez-Ruiz, B., Junque, C., Marti, M.J., Valldeoriola, F., and Tolosa, E. (2007) Cognitive changes in Parkinson's disease patients with visual hallucinations. *Dement. Geriatr. Cogn. Disord.* 23(5): 281–288.

Ramos, B.P., and Amsten, A.F. (2007) Adrenergic pharmacology and cognition: focus on the prefrontal cortex. *Pharmacol. Ther.* 113(3): 523–536.

Ransmayr, G. (2002) [Dementia with Lewy bodies] [German]. *Wien Med. Wochenschr.* 152(3/4):81–84.

Rascol, O., Brooks, D.J., Korczyn, A.D., et al. (2000) A five year study of the incidence of dyskinesia in patients with early Parkinson's disease who were treated with ropinirole or levodopa. *N. Engl. J. Med.* 342:1484–1491.

Raskin, S.A., Borod, J.C., and Tweedy, J.R. (1992) Set-shifting and spatial orientation in patients with Parkinson's disease. *J. Clin. Exp. Neuropsychol.* 14(5):801–821.

Ravina, B., Marder, K., Fernandez, H.H., et al. (2007) Diagnostic criteria for psychosis in Parkinson's disease: report of an NINDS, NIMH work group. *Mov. Disord.* 22(8):1061–1068.

Reid, W.G.J., Hely, M.A., Morris, J.G.L., et al. (1996) A longitudinal study of Parkinson's disease: clinical and neuropsychological correlates of dementia. *J. Clin. Neurosci.* 3:327–333.

Richards, M., Bell, K., Dooneief, G., Marder, K., Sano, M., Mayeux, R., and Stern, Y. (1993) Patterns of neuropsychological performance in Alzheimer's disease patients with and without extrapyramidal signs. *Neurology* 43(9):1708–1711.

Richards, M., Stern, Y., Marder, K., Cote, L., and Mayeux, R. (1993) Relationships between extrapyramidal signs and cognitive function in a community-dwelling cohort of patients with Parkinson's disease and normal elderly individuals. *Ann. Neurol.* 33(3):267–274.

Ring, H.A., Bench, C.J., Trimble, M.R., Brooks, D.J., Frackowiak, R.S., and Dolan, R.J. (1994) Depression in Parkinson's disease. A positron emission study. *Br. J. Psychiatry* 165(3):333–339.

Rinne, J.O., Laine, M., Kaasinen, V., Norvasuo-Heila, M.K., Nagren, K., and Helenius, H. (2002) Striatal dopamine transporter and extrapyramidal symptoms in frontotemporal dementia. *Neurology* 58(10):1489–1493.

Rippon GA, and Marder KS (2005) Dementia in Parkinson's disease. *Adv. Neurol.* 96:95–113.

Robbins, T.W., James, M., Owen, A.M., Lange, K.W., Lees, A.J., Leigh, P.N., Marsden, C.D., Quinn, N.P., and Summers, B.A. (1994) Cognitive deficits in progressive supranuclear palsy, Parkinson's disease, and multiple system atrophy in tests sensitive to frontal lobe dysfunction. *J. Neurol. Neurosurg. Psychiatry* 57(1):79–88.

Rodrigues, J.P., Walters, S.E., Watson, P., Stell, R., and Mastaglia, F.L. (2007) Globus pallidus stimulation improves both motor and nonmotor aspects of quality of life in advanced Parkinson's disease. *Mov. Disord.* 22(13):1866–1870.

Rodriguez, M.C., Obeso, J.A., and Olanow, C.W. (1998) Subthalamic nucleus-mediated excitotoxicity in Parkinson's disease: a target for neuroprotection. *Ann. Neurol.* 44(3):175–188.

Rosler, M. (2002) The efficacy of cholinesterase inhibitors in treating the behavioural symptoms of dementia. *Int. J. Clin. Pract. Suppl.* 127:20–36.

Sagar, H.J. (1987) Clinical similarities and differences between Alzheimer's disease and Parkinson's disease. *J. Neural. Transm. Suppl.* 24:87–99.

Sagar, H.J., Cohen, N.J., Sullivan, E.V., Corkin, S., and Growdon, J.H. (1988) Remote memory function in Alzheimer's disease and Parkinson's disease. *Brain* 111(Pt 1):185–206.

Sagar, H.J., Sullivan, E.V., Gabrieli, J.D., Corkin, S., and Growdon, J.H. (1988) Temporal ordering and short-term memory deficits in Parkinson's disease. *Brain* 111(Pt 3):525–539.

Saint-Cyr, J.A., Taylor, A.E., and Lang, A.E. (1988) Procedural learning and neostriatal dysfunction in man. *Brain* 111(Pt 4): 941–959.

Saint-Cyr, J.A., Taylor, A.E., and Lang, A.E. (1993) Neuropsychological and psychiatric side effects in the treatment of Parkinson's disease. *Neurology* 43(12 Suppl 6):S47–S52.

Saint-Cyr, J.A., Trépanier, L.L., Kumar, R., Lozano, A.M., and Lang, A.E. (2000) Neuropsychological consequences of chronic bilateral stimulation of the subthalamic nucleus in Parkinson's disease. *Brain* 123(Pt 10):2091–2108.

Santangelo, G., Trojano, L., Vitale, C., et al. (2007) A neuropsychological longitudinal study in Parkinson's patients with and without hallucinations. *Mov. Disord.* 22(16):2418–2425.

Sarazin, M., Deweer, B., Merkl, A., Von Poser, N., Pillon, B., and Dubois, B. (2002) Procedural learning and striatofrontal dysfunction in Parkinson's disease. *Mov. Disord.* 17(2):265–273.

Sarazin, M., Deweer, B., Pillon, B., Merkl, A., and Dubois, B. (2001) [Procedural learning and Parkinson disease: implication of striatofrontal loops] [French]. *Rev. Neurol. (Paris)* 157(12):1513–1518.

Satoh, A., Serita, T., Seto, M., et al. (1999) Loss of 123I-MIBG uptake by the heart in Parkinson's disease: assessment of cardiac sympathetic denervation and diagnostic value. *J. Nucl. Med.* 40:371–375.

Sawle, G.V., Playford, E.D., Burn, D.J., Cunningham, V.J., and Brooks, D.J. (1994) Separating Parkinson's disease from normality. Discriminant function analysis of fluorodopa F 18 positron emission tomography data. *Arch. Neurol.* 51(3):237–243.

Schenck, C.H., Bundlie, S.R., and Mahowald, M.W. (1996) Delayed emergence of a parkinsonian disorder in 38% of 29 older men initially diagnosed with idiopathic rapid eye movement sleep behaviour disorder. *Neurology* 46:388–393.

Schliebs, R., and Arendt, T. (2006) The significance of the cholinergic system in the brain during aging and in Alzheimer's disease. *J. Neural Transm.* 113(11):1625–1644.

Schneider, J.A., Watts, R.L., Gearing, M., et al. (1997) Corticobasal degeneration: neuropathologic and clinical heterogeneity. *Neurology* 48:959–969.

Schofield, P.W., Tang, M., Marder, K., Bell, K., Dooneief, G., Chun, M., Sano, M., Stern, Y., and Mayeux, R. (1997) Alzheimer's disease after remote head injury: an incidence study. *J. Neurol. Neurosurg. Psychiatry* 62(2):119–124.

Schrag, A., Ben-Shlomo, Y., Brown, R., Marsden, C.D., and Quinn, N. (1998) Young-onset Parkinson's disease revisited—clinical features, natural history, and mortality. *Mov. Disord.* 13(6):885–894.

Schultz, W. (1998) Predictive reward signal of dopamine neurons. *J. Neurophysiol.* 80:1–27.

Schultz, W. (2007a) Behavioral dopamine signals. *Trends Neurosci.* 30(5):203–210.

Schultz, W. (2007b) Multiple dopamine functions at different time courses. *Annu. Rev. Neurosci.* 30:259–288.

Sinanovic, O., Kapidzic, A., Kovacevic, L., Hudic, J., and Smajlovic, D. (2005) EEG frequency and cognitive dysfunction in patients with Parkinson's disease. *Med. Arch.* 59:286–287.

Sinforiani, E., Zangaglia, R., Manni, R., et al. (2006) REM sleep behavior disorder, hallucinations, and cognitive impairment in Parkinson's disease. *Mov. Disord.* 21:462–466.

Smith, Y., and Kieval, J.Z. (2000) Anatomy of the dopamine system in the basal ganglia. *Trends Neurosci.* 23:28–33.

Snowden, M.B., Bowen, J.D., Hughes, J., and Larson, E.B. (1995) Study of Alzheimer's dementia patients with parkinsonian features. *J. Geriatr. Psychiatry Neurol.* 8(3):154–158.

Soliveri, P., Brown, R.G., Jahanshahi, M., and Marsden, C.D. (1992) Effect of practice on performance of a skilled motor task in patients with Parkinson's disease. *J. Neurol. Neurosurg. Psychiatry* 55(6):454–460.

Sprengelmeyer, R., Canavan, A.G., Lange, H.W., and Homberg, V. (1995) Associative learning in degenerative neostriatal disorders: contrasts in explicit and implicit remembering between Parkinson's and Huntington's diseases. *Mov. Disord.* 10(1):51–65.

Sroka, H., Elizan, T.S., Yahr, M.D., Burger, A., and Mendoza, M.R. (1981) Organic mental syndrome and confusional states in Parkinson's disease. Relationship to computerized tomographic signs of cerebral atrophy. *Arch. Neurol.* 38(6):339–342.

Starkstein, S., and Merello, M. (2007) The Unified Parkinson's Disease Rating Scale: Validation study of the mentation, behavior, and mood section. *Mov. Disord.* 22(15):2156–2161.

Starkstein, S.E., Sabe, L., Petracca, G., et al. (1996) Neuropsychological and psychiatric differences between Alzheimer's disease and Parkinson's disease with dementia. *J. Neurol. Neurosurg. Psychiatry* 61:381–387.

Stern, Y., Marder, K., Tang, M.X., and Mayeux, R. (1993) Antecedent clinical features associated with dementia in Parkinson's disease. *Neurology* 43(9):1690–1692; comment in: *Neurology* 1994 44(8):1553.

Stern, Y., Tang, M.X., Jacobs, D.M., Sano, M., Marder, K., Bell, K., Dooneief, G., Schofield, P., and Cote, L. (1998) Prospective comparative study of the evolution of probable Alzheimer's disease and Parkinson's disease dementia. *J. Int. Neuropsychol. Soc.* 4(3): 279–284.

Stuss, D.T., and Benson, D.F. (1986) *The Frontal Lobes*. New York: Raven Press.

Sullivan, E.V., and Sagar, H.J. (1989) Nonverbal recognition and recency discrimination deficits in Parkinson's disease and Alzheimer's disease. *Brain* 112(Pt 6):1503–1517.

Sullivan, E.V., and Sagar, H.J. (1991) Double dissociation of short-term and long-term memory for nonverbal material in Parkinson's disease and global amnesia. A further analysis. *Brain* 114(Pt 2): 893–906.

Sullivan, E.V., Sagar, H.J., Gabrieli, J.D., Corkin, S., and Growdon, J.H. (1989) Different cognitive profiles on standard behavioral tests in Parkinson's disease and Alzheimer's disease. *J. Clin. Exp. Neuropsychol.* 11(6):799–820.

Summerfield, C., Gomez-Anson, B., Tolosa, E., et al. (2002) Dementia in Parkinson disease: a proton magnetic resonance spectroscopy study. *Arch. Neurol.* 59:1415–1420.

Tang, M.X., Jacobs, D., Stern, Y., Marder, K., Schofield, P., Gurland, B., Andrews, H., and Mayeux, R. (1996) Effect of oestrogen during menopause on risk and age at onset of Alzheimer's disease. *Lancet* 348(9025):429–432; comment in: *A.C.P. J Club.* 1997 126(1):21; *Lancet* 1996 348(9025):420–421; *Lancet* 1996 348(9033):1027–1028; discussion 1029–1030.

Tanner, C.M., and Goldman, S.M. (1996) Epidemiology of Parkinson's disease. *Neurol. Clin.* 14:317–335.

Taylor, A.E., and Saint-Cyr, J.A. (1990) Depression in Parkinson's disease: reconciling physiological and psychological perspectives. *J. Neuropsychiatry Clin. Neurosci.* 2(1):92–98.

Taylor, A.E., and Saint-Cyr, J.A. (1995) The neuropsychology of Parkinson's disease. *Brain Cogn.* 28(3):281–296.

Taylor, A.E., Saint-Cyr, J.A., and Lang, A.E. (1990) Memory and learning in early Parkinson's disease: evidence for a "frontal lobe syndrome." *Brain Cogn.* 13(2):211–232.

Taylor-Robinson, S.D., Turjanski, N., Bhattacharya, S., Seery, J.P., Sargentoni, J., Brooks, D.J., Bryant, D.J., and Cox, I.J. (1999) A proton magnetic resonance spectroscopy study of the striatum and cerebral cortex in Parkinson's disease. *Metab. Brain Dis.* 14(1): 45–55.

Tinaz, S., Schendan, H.E., and Stern, C.E. (2008) Fronto-striatal deficit in Parkinson's disease during semantic event sequencing. *Neurobiol. Aging* 29(3):397–407.

Trépanier, L.L., Kumar, R., Lozano, A.M., Lang, A.E., and Saint-Cyr, J.A. (2000) Neuropsychological outcome of GPi pallidotomy and GPi or STN deep brain stimulation in Parkinson's disease. *Brain Cogn.* 42(3):324–347.

Trépanier, L.L., Saint-Cyr, J.A., Lozano, A.M., and Lang, A.E. (1998) Neuropsychological consequences of posteroventral pallidotomy for the treatment of Parkinson's disease. *Neurology* 51(1):207–215.

Tröster, A.I., Paolo, A.M., Lyons, K.E., Glatt, S.L., Hubble, J.P., and Koller, W.C. (1995) The influence of depression on cognition in

Parkinson's disease: a pattern of impairment distinguishable from Alzheimer's disease. *Neurology* 45(4):672–676.

Tröster, A.I., Stalp, L.D., Paolo, A.M., Fields, J.A., and Koller, W.C. (1995) Neuropsychological impairment in Parkinson's disease with and without depression. *Arch. Neurol.* 52(12):1164–1169.

Turjanski, N., and Brooks, D.J. (1997) PET and the investigation of dementia in the parkinsonian patient. *J. Neurol. Transm. Suppl.* 51:37–48.

Uversky, V.N. (2007) Neuropathology, biochemistry, and biophysics of alpha-synuclein aggregation. *J. Neurochem.* 103(1):17–37.

Van Spaendonck, K.P., Berger, H.J., Horstink, M.W., Buytenhuijs, E.L., and Cools, A.R. (1993) Impaired cognitive shifting in parkinsonian patients on anticholinergic therapy. *Neuropsychologia* 31(4):407–411.

Van Spaendonck, K.P., Berger, H.J., Horstink, M.W., Buytenhuijs, E.L., and Cools, A.R. (1996) Executive functions and disease characteristics in Parkinson's disease. *Neuropsychologia* 34(7):617–626.

Vander-Borght, T., Minoshima, S., Giordani, B., et al. (1997) Cerebral metabolic differences in Parkinson's and Alzheimer's disease matched for dementia severity. *J. Nucl. Med.* 38:797–802.

Vendette, M., Gagnon, J.F., Decary, A., et al. (2007) REM sleep behavior disorder predicts cognitive impairment in Parkinson disease without dementia. *Neurology* 69(19):1843–1849.

Verbaan, D., Marinus, J., Visser, M., van Rooden, S.M., Stiggelbout, A.M., Middelkoop, H.A., and van Hilten, J.J. (2007) Cognitive impairment in Parkinson's disease. *J. Neurol. Neurosurg. Psychiatry* 78(11):1182–1187.

Verny, M., and Duyckaerts, C. (1998) Dementia with Lewy bodies. *Ann. Med. Interne (Paris)* 149(4):209–215.

Voon, V., and Fox, S.H. (2007) Medication-related impulse control and repetitive behaviors in Parkinson disease. *Arch. Neurol.* 64(8): 1089–1096.

Voon, V., Kubu, C., Krack, P., Houeto, J.L., and Tröster, A.I. (2006) Deep brain stimulation: neuropsychological and neuropsychiatric issues. *Mov. Disord.* 21(Suppl 14):S305–S327.

Warner, T.T., and Schapira, A.H.V. (2003) Genetic and environmental factors in the aetiology of Parkinson's disease. *Ann. Neurol.* 53:516–523.

Weintraub, D., and Hurtig, H.I. (2007) Presentation and management of psychosis in Parkinson's disease and dementia with Lewy bodies. *Am. J. Psychiatry* 164:1491–1498.

Weintraub, D., Moberg, P.J., Duda, J.E., Katz, I.R., and Stern, M.B. (2004) Effect of psychiatric and other nonmotor symptoms on disability in Parkinson's disease. *J. Am. Geriatr. Soc.* 52(5):784–788.

Weintraub, D., and Potenza, M.N. (2006) Impulse control disorders in Parkinson's disease. *Curr. Neurol. Neurosci. Rep.* 6(4):302–306.

Wells, J.C., Keyl, P.M., Chase, G.A., Aboraya, A., Folstein, M.F., and Anthony, J.C. (1992) Discriminant validity of a reduced set of Mini-Mental State Examination items for dementia and Alzheimer's disease. *Acta Psychiatr. Scand.* 86(1):23–31.

Wenning, G.K., Ben-Shlomo, Y., Hughes, A., et al. (2000) What clinical features are most useful to distinguish definite multiple system atrophy from Parkinson's disease? *J. Neurol. Neurosurg. Psychiatry* 68:434–440.

Werber, E.A., and Rabey, J.M. (2001) The beneficial effect of cholinesterase inhibitors on patients suffering from Parkinson's disease and dementia. *J. Neural. Transm.* 108(11):1319–1325.

Whittington, C.J., Podd, J., and Kan, M.M. (2000) Recognition memory impairment in Parkinson's disease: power and meta-analyses. *Neuropsychology* 14: 233–246.

Wichamann, T., and DeLong, M.R. (2006) Deep brain stimulation for neurologic and neuropsychiatric disorders. *Neuron* 52(1):197–204.

Williams, D.R., Warren, J.D., and Lees, A.J. (2007) Using the presence of visual hallucinations to differentiate Parkinson's disease from atypical Parkinsonism. *J. Neurol. Neurosurg. Psychiatry* http://jnnp.bmj.com/cgi/rapidpdf/jnnp.2007.124677v1.

Williams-Gray, C.H., Foltynie, T., Brayne, C.E., et al. (2007) Evolution of cognitive dysfunction in an incident Parkinson's disease cohort. *Brain* 130(Pt 7):1787–1798.

Wilson, R.S., Kaszniak, A.W., Klawans, H.L., and Garron, D.C. (1980) High speed memory scanning in parkinsonism. *Cortex* 16(1):67–72.

Wilson, R.S., Mendes De Leon, C.F., Barnes, L.L., Schneider, J.A., Bienias, J.L., Evans, D.A., and Bennett, D.A. (2002) Participation in cognitively stimulating activities and risk of incident Alzheimer disease. *JAMA* 287(6):742–748.

Woods, S.P., Fields, J.A., Lyons, K.E., Koller, W.C., Wilkinson, S.B., Pahwa, R., and Troster, A.I. (2001) Neuropsychological and quality of life changes following unilateral thalamic deep brain stimulation in Parkinson's disease: a one-year follow-up. *Acta Neurochir. (Wien)* 143(12):1273–1277; discussion 1278.

Woodward, T., Bub, D., and Hunter, M. (2002) Task switching deficits associated with Parkinson's disease reflect depleted attentional resources. *Neuropsychologia* 40(12):1948.

Wrase, J., Reimold, M., Puls, I., Kienast, T., and Heinz, A. (2006) Serotonergic dysfunction: brain imaging and behavioral correlates. *Cogn. Affect Behav. Neurosci.* 6(1):53–61.

Wright, M.J., Burns, R.J., Geffen, G.M., and Geffen, L.B. (1990) Covert orientation of visual attention in Parkinson's disease: an impairment in the maintenance of attention. *Neuropsychologia* 28(2):151–159.

Wright, S.L., and Persad, C. (2007) Distinguishing between depression and dementia in older persons: neuropsychological and neuropathological correlates. *J. Geriatr. Psychiatry Neurol.* 20(4):189–198.

Wszolek, Z.K., Vieregge, P., Uittis, R.J., et al. (1997) German-Canadian Family (Family A) with parkinsonism, amyotrophy, and dementia: longitudinal observation. *Parkinsonism Rel. Disord.* 3:125–136.

Yamada, H., Aimi, Y., Nagatsu, I., et al. (2007) Immunohistochemical detection of L-DOPA-derived dopamine within serotonergic fibers in the striatum and the substantia nigra pars reticulata in Parkinsonian model rats. *Neurosci. Res.* 59(1):1–7.

Yong, S.W., Yoon, J.K., An, Y.S., and Lee, P.H. (2007) A comparison of cerebral glucose metabolism in Parkinson's disease, Parkinson's disease dementia and dementia with Lewy bodies. *Eur. J. Neurology* 14(12):1357–1362.

York, M.K., Dulay, M., Macias, A., et al. (2007) Cognitive declines following bilateral subthalamic nucleus deep brain stimulation for the treatment of Parkinson's disease. *J. Neurol. Neurosurg. Psychiatry* http://jnnp.bmj.com/cgi/rapidpdf/jnnp.2007.118786v1.

Yoshita, M. (1998) Differentiation of idiopathic Parkinson's disease from striatonigral degeneration and progressive supranuclear palsy using iodine-123 meta-iodobenzylguanidine myocardial scintigraphy. *J. Neurol. Sci.* 155:60–67.

Zahrt, J., Taylor, J.R., Mathew, R.G., and Arnsten, A.F. (1997) Supranormal stimulation of D1 dopamine receptors in the rodent prefrontal cortex impairs spatial working memory performance. *J. Neurosci.* 17(21):8528–8535.

Zareparsi, S., Wirdefeldt, K., Burgess, C.E., Nutt, J., Kramer, P., Schalling, M., and Payami, H. (1999) Exclusion of dominant mutations within the FTDP-17 locus on chromosome 17 for Parkinson's disease. *Neurosci. Lett.* 272(2):140–142.

Zarranz, J.J., Alegre, J., Gémez-Esteban, J., et al. (2004) The new mutation, E46K, of α-synuclein causes Parkinson and Lewy body dementia. *Ann. Neurol.* 55:164–173.

Zgaljardic, D.J., Borod, J.C., Foldi, N.S., and Mattis, P. (2003) A review of the cognitive and behavioral sequelae of Parkinson's disease: relationship to frontostriatal circuitry. *Cogn. Behav. Neurol.* 16(4):193–210.

Zimmermann, P., Sprengelmeyer, R., Fimm, B., and Wallesch, C.W. (1992) Cognitive slowing in decision tasks in early and advanced Parkinson's disease. *Brain Cogn.* 18(1):60–69.

64 Mild Cognitive Impairment

BRENDAN J. KELLEY AND RONALD C. PETERSEN

Mild cognitive impairment (MCI) defines a population experiencing cognitive decline in excess of that associated with normal cognitive changes of aging, but which does not reach the threshold of the earliest clinical features of dementia. In general, there is minimal if any impact on the individual's daily activities. *Mild cognitive impairment* initially referred to memory impairment with preserved nonmemory cognitive performance, but more recently the term has been expanded to include other (nonmemory) cognitive domains. Most research has focused on the amnestic (memory predominant) form of MCI, a likely precursor of Alzheimer's disease (AD). Over the past decade, research has demonstrated the MCI criteria to be reliable, and some data regarding patient outcomes has been established. Investigation of factors that may predict progression from MCI to AD remains an active area of research. Neuropathological studies have confirmed findings intermediate between those of AD and normal aging. Brain structural and functional neuroimaging documents a transitional state (between normal and AD) in MCI. One clinical trial suggested that donepezil may provide symptomatic benefit for a limited period of time in MCI, although most randomized clinical trials have been essentially negative. We discuss the implications of MCI for clinical practice and future research.

INTRODUCTION AND CONCEPTUAL FRAMEWORK

Clinicians are frequently asked to evaluate the importance of a patient's forgetfulness. Elderly individuals who feel that their memory has changed are frequently (and understandably) concerned about developing AD. Neurodegenerative conditions such as AD are characterized by insidious onset and gradually progressive decline. The proposal of a "latent" stage of disease during which neuropathological changes occur but with subclinical or mild functional manifestations would seem reasonable. Mild cognitive impairment attempts to identify these "partially symptomatic" individuals who may be slightly forgetful but with preservation of other cognitive and functional abilities (Petersen et al., 1999; Petersen, Doody, et al., 2001; Petersen, 2003a).

Although superficially simple, the construct and clinical relevance of MCI has several important implications.

Cognitive Changes of Normal Aging

Discussion of MCI implies knowledge about the cognitive changes associated with normal aging. Characterization of these cognitive changes has remained an area of active research, without general agreement on the nature or degree of impairment or the neuropathological substrate of those impairments. Consequently, characterization of the early changes of MCI remains difficult (Ivnik et al., 1999). Normative data for the performance of elderly individuals on a variety of neuropsychological tests exist (Sliwinski et al., 1996; Petersen, 2003a). However, some argue that these normative values are contaminated by the inclusion of persons who would meet current definitions of MCI, and consequently they reflect more impairment than should be expected as a consequence of normal aging (Sliwinski et al., 1996). It is unclear how large an effect this may have on the normative values, or precisely how one would exclude such patients without prior knowledge of where the cutoff should exist. Although research efforts continue to more precisely delineate the cognitive changes associated with normal aging, clinical judgment remains the most reliable means to assess MCI at present.

Dementia

Also implicit to this discussion is a general agreement upon the definition of *dementia*. The general features that define dementia in the *Diagnostic and Statistical Manual* 3rd ed., rev. (*DSM-III-R*) remain a useful reference point (American Psychiatric Association [APA], 1987). These require memory impairment beyond that associated with normal aging and impairment of at least one other cognitive domain such as attention, language, visuospatial skills, or problem solving. These cognitive deficits are of sufficient severity to compromise daily functional activities and do not occur in the setting of altered sensorium such as delirium or an acute confusional state.

In the *DSM-III-R* definition, memory impairment is an essential feature of dementia. Although this is true of many dementias, it is conceivable that patients with frontotemporal dementia or Lewy body dementia might present with significant impairment of nonmemory cognitive domains (and relatively spared memory functioning) early in the disorder. A more general definition of *dementia* as cognitive decline of sufficient severity to compromise a person's daily function might be more inclusive of non-Alzheimer's dementia subtypes.

Proposed Benefit for Early Detection of Dementia

Clinical and research efforts to define and to detect MCI presume a benefit to the earlier diagnosis of degenerative disease. In the context of the aging of the world's population (Sloane et al., 2002), degenerative dementias represent an issue of growing global concern and hold a looming burden on healthcare resources. One major strategy for addressing this potential crisis involves delaying the onset and/or progression of these diseases. Early diagnosis then becomes paramount in trying to prevent subsequent disability. In a clinical context, detection of MCI may identify individuals at a greater risk of subsequent transition to AD and provide clinicians the opportunity to counsel these patients more effectively.

Along these lines, the American Academy of Neurology (AAN) practice parameter addressing MCI concluded that persons with memory impairment who meet criteria for MCI are at increased risk of progressing to clinically probable AD and should be counseled and followed accordingly (Petersen, Stevens, et al., 2001). Ideally, identification of these individuals would allow for intervention to reduce the risk of progression to dementia at a stage where cognitive impairment has remained mild. At present, no such treatment exists. Candidate treatments include cholinesterase inhibitors, antioxidants, anti-inflammatory agents, and nootropics among others (Geda and Petersen, 2001).

HISTORICAL CONTEXT

Earlier cognitive investigations of older individuals had focused on those cognitive changes associated with normal aging. Terms such as *aging-associated cognitive decline* (AACD), *age-associated memory impairment* (AAMI), *benign senescent forgetfulness*, and *late-life forgetfulness* have been variably applied to these changes (Gauthier et al., 2006). By contrast, the MCI construct refers to an abnormal process, with the intent of identifying individuals in the prodromal stages of a dementing condition. By definition, it is fundamentally different from normal aging.

Early MCI criteria focused on individuals having memory impairment (amnestic MCI) with the aim of identifying the prodromal state of AD. As our understanding of the importance of the early diagnosis of dementia has grown, a more general construct of MCI and of specific subtypes of MCI has emerged. The general framework of MCI as the prodromal phase of a degenerative disease has remained a core concept to this evolving construct.

DIAGNOSTIC CRITERIA

The original criteria for MCI, designed to characterize the early stages of an AD-like process, were thus centered on memory impairment (Petersen et al., 1999). As discussed above, the construct of MCI has expanded to include many other types of intermediate cognitive impairment that may be precursors to a variety of dementing disorders. Figure 64.1 shows the diagnostic algorithm currently being used by the National Institute on Aging (NIA)–sponsored Alzheimer's Disease Centers Program and the Alzheimer's Disease Neuroimaging Initiative (ADNI) to diagnose MCI (Mueller et al., 2005). It should be emphasized that these criteria for MCI are clinical. Although neuropsychological testing may be helpful in characterizing the cognitive deficits in individuals having MCI, attempts to define arbitrary cutoffs on neuropsychological measures to retrospectively identify individuals with MCI have demonstrated that application of these cutoff values in the absence of clinical judgment results in an unstable diagnostic paradigm and eliminates the predictive value of the MCI diagnosis (Ritchie et al., 2001).

An international conference on diagnostic criteria helped to translate these findings into a clinical construct useful for primary care practitioners because these are the individuals most likely to first encounter persons in this mild range of cognitive impairment (Petersen, 2004; Winblad et al., 2004).

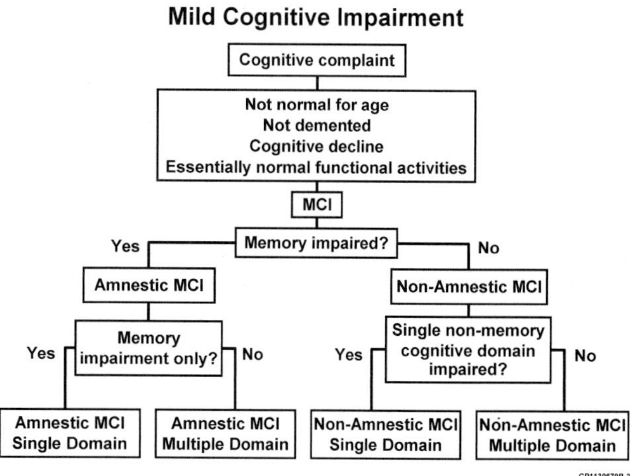

FIGURE 64.1 Algorithm for diagnosing and subtyping mild cognitive impairment. From Petersen, 2004. Reprinted by permission.

CLINICAL DIAGNOSIS AND MCI SUBTYPES

Clinical Diagnosis of MCI

The importance of an accurate clinical history, preferably corroborated by an informant who knows the patient well, has remained paramount to the diagnosis of MCI. The first criterion for the diagnosis of MCI involves a cognitive concern on the part of the patient or an informant (Daly et al., 2000). Although these individuals are typically mildly affected and are aware of their deficits, corroboration by an informant is quite useful (Daly et al., 2000). The second criterion requires objective demonstration of cognitive impairment relative to age- and education-adjusted expectations (Ivnik et al., 1992; Smith et al., 1996). Some high-functioning patients who fall within the normal range of memory function may in fact have experienced a decline from their baseline level of function, and in these individuals, it may be appropriate to diagnose MCI.

The combination of history, mental status exam, neuropsychological testing, and any additional information available is then used to determine whether the patient's cognitive function is normal or compatible with dementia. If the patient has no dementia but has experienced a decline in cognitive function, and if most daily activities have been preserved, the patient can be designated as having MCI.

Once an individual has been diagnosed as having MCI, the clinician evaluates whether a memory impairment is present. Screening memory tests such as a word list with a delayed recall component or more detailed neuropsychological testing can be useful to document memory functioning. As discussed above, though no particular reference point for normal aging is entirely accurate, normative data based upon patients of similar demographic characteristics may be useful. Patients with MCI tend to fall 1.5 standard deviations below their age- and education-matched expectations on measures of learning and recall, but it must again be emphasized that these are only guidelines and not cutoff scores for MCI.

A screening mental status examination, such as the Mini-Mental State Examination (MMSE), Modified Mini-Mental State (3MS) Examination, and Kokmen Short Test of Mental Status (Folstein et al., 1975; Teng and Chui, 1987; Kokmen et al., 1991), should be administered in addition to the general neurological examination. However, these screening examinations are often insensitive in the MCI range of cognitive function. Patients with MCI may score in the 26 to 28 range on the MMSE, which is typically reported as normal. A mental status exam instrument without a significant memory component will not accurately differentiate patients with relatively isolated memory impairment from those experiencing normal aging. Consequently, the clinician may consider augmenting the screening cognitive instrument with an additional memory test (Knopman and Ryberg, 1989; Petersen, 1991).

Subtypes of MCI

If a memory impairment is present, then the subtype of MCI is amnestic MCI (aMCI). Neuropsychological testing can further aid in determining whether other cognitive domains such as language, executive function, or visuospatial skills are also impaired. If the individual has an isolated memory difficulty, the MCI subtype would be aMCI-single domain. If another cognitive domain is impaired in addition to memory, then the MCI subtype is aMCI-multiple domain.

Analogously, if the patient is determined to have cognitive impairment in the MCI range (not normal, no dementia) but without a significant memory impairment, the clinician then determines which cognitive domains are impaired (Fig. 64.1). Nonamnestic MCI (naMCI) is subtyped similarly to aMCI, with single domain (naMCI-single domain) or multiple domain (naMCI-multiple domain) designations. The goal of such subtyping in clinical practice is to accurately describe the individual's clinical syndrome.

Evaluation

Physical examination and medical laboratory tests similar to those used in the evaluation of dementia may identify medical issues that could affect cognitive function. Although depression can often be differentiated from AD, it may present with subtle memory impairment in its early stages, and clinicians should remain attuned to possible psychiatric etiologies as well.

Mild cognitive impairment is a clinical diagnosis, and although neuropsychological testing alone does not establish the diagnosis of MCI, it can be suggestive in the appropriate clinical context (Petersen, 2000). The neuropsychological testing battery must include sufficiently difficult learning and recall tasks to help to differentiate patients with MCI from those experiencing normal aging. Figure 64.2 illustrates typical neuropsychological testing profiles of individuals with MCI, normal aging, and very mild clinically probable Alzheimer's disease (Clinical Dementia Rating Scale [CDR] 0.5). On measures of general cognitive function such as the MMSE and full scale IQ, the individual with MCI performs more similar to a normal elderly patient, whereas memory function on delayed verbal recall (Logical Memory II) and nonverbal delayed recall (Visual Reproductions II) more closely resembles mild AD (Petersen et al., 1999).

After describing the patient's symptom complex, the clinician attempts to determine the etiology of these symptoms. Similar to evaluation of the etiology of

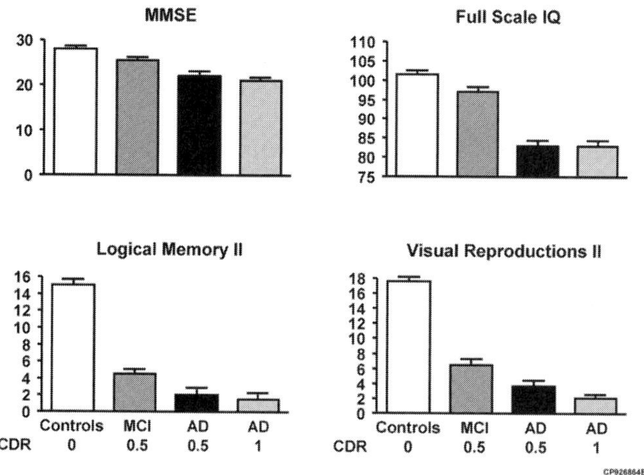

FIGURE 64.2 Cognitive profiles comparing individuals having mild cognitive impairment with performance of normal patients and patients with AD. The Mini-Mental State Exam (MMSE) and Full Scale IQ represent measures of general intellectual function (top two panels). Measures of verbal memory function (Logical Memory II) and nonverbal memory function (Visual Reproductions II) are shown in the bottom two panels. From Petersen et al., 1999. Reprinted by permission.

dementia, historical, neuroimaging, or laboratory data may suggest the cause of MCI is of a degenerative, vascular, psychiatric, or traumatic etiology or secondary to a medical illness. The clinician then uses this available data to classify the MCI syndrome by likely etiology: degenerative (gradual onset, insidious progression), vascular (abrupt onset, stepwise decline, vascular risk factors, history of strokes, transient ischemic attack [TIAs]), psychiatric (depressed mood or anxiety), or secondary to concomitant medical disorders (for example, congestive heart failure, diabetes mellitus, systemic cancer).

OUTCOMES

Combining the clinical MCI subtype with the presumed etiology, the clinician can make a reliable prediction about the outcome of the MCI syndrome as illustrated in Figure 64.3. It should be acknowledged that part of the construct illustrated in Figure 64.3 is theoretical and not yet validated at this time. Amnestic MCI of a degenerative etiology is very likely to progress to AD, and the AAN has endorsed this construct in its practice parameter (Petersen, Stevens, et al., 2001). The corresponding outcomes of patients having naMCI subtypes are currently under investigation.

Patients diagnosed with aMCI using the criteria outlined in Figure 64.1 and having a presumed degenerative etiology will progress to dementia (usually AD) at a rate of 10%–15% per year (Petersen et al., 1999; Petersen et al., 2005). Some variability in the reported rate of progression exists within the literature, due in part to variation in the definition and operationalization of the MCI criteria.

Epidemiologic studies, particularly those that retrofitted neuropsychological criteria to existing databases, have reported variable rates of progression, with some studies reporting lower progression rates (Daly et al., 2000; Aggarwal et al., 2005; Gauthier et al., 2006; Fischer et al., 2007). In the large clinical trials studying MCI, progression rates have varied from 5%–16% per year (Petersen et al., 2005). Despite the variability in the precise rate of progression reported, all of these studies have reported progression rates far higher than the population incidence figures for AD of 1%–2% per year.

The data from longitudinal studies suggests that individuals meeting criteria for MCI, particularly aMCI of a degenerative etiology, progress to dementia at a rate of 10% per year. The majority of individuals having aMCI of a degenerative etiology progress to AD. A large prospectively designed trial conducted in Germany reported that patients with MCI diagnosed using the criteria in Figure 64.1 progressed to dementia at rates of 7.2%–10.2% per year (Busse et al., 2006). In this study, some patients improved from MCI to normal (approximately 5% per year), but a subset who initially improved subsequently declined, implying instability of the clinical course during progression to dementia. The vast majority of dementia cases were believed to represent AD.

For patients presenting for evaluation of a cognitive concern in a typical neurology practice, the progression rate is likely to be in the 10%–15% per year range for those meeting the criteria for aMCI. Community studies enrolling more heterogeneous patient populations suggest that in those populations the rates to be lower, perhaps in the 8%–10% per year range. It is important to

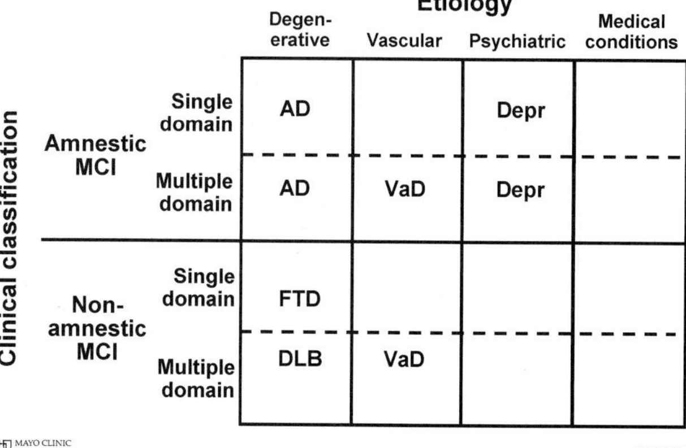

FIGURE 64.3 Predicted outcome of mild cognitive impairment subtypes according to presumed etiology. Adapted from Petersen, 2003a. Reprinted by permission.

inform patients that a small fraction of individuals with MCI will improve and that others may remain clinically stable for many years. Thus, though MCI (and particularly aMCI) of a presumed degenerative etiology identifies individuals at increased risk of developing dementia, the diagnosis of MCI is not deterministic of progression to dementia. A progression rate of 10%–12% per year is probably a reasonably accurate estimate to use in counseling patients.

PREDICTORS OF PROGRESSION

Identification of clinical, genetic, and surrogate biomarker factors that may aid in identifying patients with MCI likely to progress to dementia or AD more rapidly than others remains a major area of research interest. In addition to the obvious benefit in counseling patients and family members, those designing clinical trials of potential therapeutics would like to stratify patients to enroll those at increased risk of progressing to AD within the time frame of the study. Several potential predictors of progression have emerged: (*1*) clinical severity, (*2*) Apolipoprotein ε4 (ApoE4) carrier status, (*3*) MRI hippocampal volumes, (*4*) cerebrospinal fluid (CSF) and plasma biomarkers, (*5*) fluorodeoxyglucose (FDG)-positron emission tomography (FDG-PET), and (*6*) ligand-bound PET imaging. Although very preliminary, the predictive value of several plasma signaling proteins recently reported to be dysregulated in AD (Ray et al., 2007) will likely be investigated in the near future.

Clinical Severity

Individuals with more severe memory impairment progress to AD more rapidly than those having less severe memory impairment. This may account for some of the variability observed in the clinical trials to be discussed later and for some of the variability in the epidemiologic data. Individuals having the aMCI-multiple domain subtype will probably progress more rapidly than those having aMCI-single domain. A recent study reported that individuals with aMCI-multiple domain subtype actually had poorer overall survival than individuals with aMCI-single domain subtype (Hunderfund et al., 2006).

Apolipoprotein ε Genotype

The genetic features of MCI are similar to those of clinically probable AD. Apolipoprotein ε4 carrier status is a recognized risk factor for the development of AD (Corder et al., 1993). Apolipoprotein ε4 carrier status has been demonstrated to have predictive value for progression from MCI to AD in several studies, including the Alzheimer's Disease Cooperative Study (ADCS) MCI Treatment Trial and the Religious Order Study (Petersen et al., 1995; Tierney et al., 1996; Aggarwal et al., 2005). Apolipoprotein ε4 carrier status correlates with more rapid progression of hippocampal atrophy on magnetic resonance imaging (MRI) in adults who are cognitively normal as well (Jak et al., 2007). Although ApoE4 carrier status may predict a higher rate of progression to AD among those diagnosed with aMCI, it is not currently recommended for routine clinical use (Farrer et al., 1997).

MRI Volumetric Studies

A great deal of data exist regarding volumetric analyses of structural MRI as a predictor of progression from MCI to AD. Hippocampal atrophy was shown to be a prominent and important predictor of subsequent progression from MCI to dementia and AD (Jack et al., 1999) (Fig. 64.4). Volumetric measurements of entorhinal cortex volume, whole-brain volume, and ventricular volume have also shown utility (Jack et al., 2005). An analysis employing a combined measurement of entorhinal and hippocampal volume reported a small but detectable predictive utility for this combined measurement independent of age and cognitive variables (Devanand et al., 2007). Another study suggests that subjective visual assessments of the hippocampal formation may provide predictive utility as well (DeCarli et al., 2007). An investigation of the longitudinal rate of hippocampal atrophy identified several baseline characteristics (age, worse baseline cognitive performance, ApoE4 carrier status, and baseline hippocampal volumes) predicted a higher rate of hippocampal atrophy over the subsequent 2 years (van de Pol et al., 2007).

Evaluating the usefulness of volumetric assessments has been complicated by the variable algorithms used to segment MRI volumes as well as variability in the

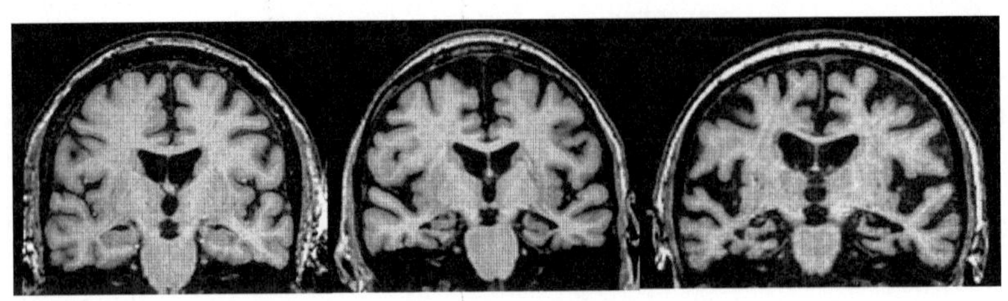

FIGURE 64.4 Coronal magnetic resonance imaging showing degrees of hippocampal atrophy in normal (left), mild cognitive impairment (middle), and Alzheimer's disease (right) patients.

populations studied. Although some studies have demonstrated a small added predictive value, the magnitude of this among patients having less readily detectable cognitive impairment has yet to be determined. The ADNI is intended, in part, to address these issue (Mueller et al., 2005).

CSF and Plasma Biomarkers

Cerebrospinal fluid and plasma biomarkers are in the early stages of development. Some studies have suggested that CSF measures of beta-amyloid ($A\beta$) and tau may aid in differentiating patients with MCI from those experiencing normal aging (Galasko et al., 1997; Galasko et al., 1998; Growdon, 1999), and others have suggested that these markers may have utility in predicting progression from MCI to AD (Sunderland et al., 1999; Stefani et al., 2006). A multinational study found that baseline CSF levels of tau phosphorylated at threonine 231, but not total tau protein levels, correlated with cognitive decline and conversion from MCI to AD (Buerger et al., 2002). This was confirmed by another study investigating several biomarkers longitudinally (Brys et al., 2007). Pathological studies in AD reported a correlation between neocortical neurofibrillary pathology and tau phosphorylated at threonine 231 (p-tau_{231}) but not tau phosphorylated at threonine 181 (p-tau_{181}) (Buerger et al., 2006). A study investigating the utility of CSF concentrations of $A\beta$ 1–42, total tau (T-tau), and p-tau_{181} in predicting progression from MCI to AD over a 4-year observation window reported a sensitivity of 95% and specificity of 83% using the combination of elevated T-tau and lowered $A\beta$ 1–42 (Hansson et al., 2006). A similarly designed study that used a 2-year observation window reported sensitivity and specificity of 70%–80% for p-tau_{231} and for the ratios of T-tau/$A\beta_{42/40}$ and T-tau/$A\beta_{42/40}$, suggesting that these biomarkers may have predictive value even when investigated in a 2-year trial (Brys et al., 2007).

The obvious hope is that biochemical markers associated with AD pathology may augment clinical insights to provide improved prediction of the likelihood of progression from MCI to AD at the earliest possible stage. Although CSF biomarkers continue to be explored in large clinical trials (such as ADNI; Mueller et al., 2005), the currently available data are insufficient to recommend the use of CSF biomarkers in evaluation of MCI.

A recent report on the dependence of CSF $A\beta$ levels upon time of day and activity may imply that careful design of the conditions under which CSF is collected may make predictions based upon the measurements of these biomarkers more robust (Bateman et al., 2007). Study of plasma $A\beta$ levels is less well developed, but this or another plasma biomarker may prove useful in the future (van Oijen et al., 2006; Graff-Radford et al., 2007).

FDG-PET Imaging

Some evidence suggests that metabolic changes in the brain may precede structural changes in AD and, therefore, metabolic functional imaging might detect pathological changes at an earlier point than structural neuroimaging. Clearly, this would provide valuable prognostic information directly relevant to individuals having MCI. Investigations of FDG-PET have reported FDG-PET changes suggestive of evolving AD among patients who were cognitively normal genetically predisposed to develop AD (Small et al., 1995; Reiman et al., 1996). Further, several studies indicate that AD patterns of PET at the MCI stage predict progression to AD (Anchisi et al., 2005; Drzezga et al., 2005). Although intuitive, this technique requires further validation before it could be recommended for routine clinical use.

Ligand-bound FDG-PET

Recently, imaging techniques that attempt in vivo identification of proteins implicated in AD pathology have been developed. Such imaging techniques could potentially have prognostic value in predicting progression of MCI.

The Pittsburgh compound B (PiB) (Klunk et al., 2004) employs FDG bound to a ligand that binds to amyloid in an attempt to image amyloid deposition in the brain. Initial studies have suggested utility in distinguishing between patients who are normal, patients with MCI, and patients with AD. The limited data available investigating this compound in MCI indicate three patterns: PiB retention similar to that of patients who are normal, PiB retention mimicking patients with AD, and intermediate patterns. The clinical meaning of the three subgroups that these patterns of uptake define has not yet been defined, and only very limited longitudinal data are available regarding the outcome of these patients with MCI. It must also be acknowledged that PiB retention is not specific to amyloid deposition related to AD and that increased PiB retention has also been reported in cerebral amyloid angiopathy (Johnson et al., 2007; Lockhart et al., 2007).

2-(1-[6-[(2-[^{18}F]fluoroethyl)(methyl)amino]amino]-2-naphthyl]ethylidene)malononitrile (FDDNP), developed at University of California at Los Angeles (UCLA), is a ligand-bound FDG tracer that labels amyloid and tau proteins. This agent theoretically labels neuritic elements in the brain, including neuritic plaques and neurofibrillary tangles (NFTs) (Small et al., 2006). By labeling amyloid and tau, FDDNP may be less specific for amyloid pathology but may prove more sensitive at imaging the total pathological burden. Again, these data are very preliminary, and longitudinal studies of FDDNP, PiB, and other ligand-bound agents will be needed to quantify and validate their performance (Ryu and Chen, 2008).

NEUROPATHOLOGICAL CORRELATES

The neuropathological substrate of MCI, particularly aMCI of presumed degenerative etiology, continues to be a topic of active research and debate. Some investigators contend that in patients with aMCI the neuropathological substrate of AD is already in place and, therefore, we should diagnose these patients as having AD (Markesbery et al., 2006). In support of this, a Washington University study asserted that AD exists neuropathologically in MCI (Morris et al., 2001). However, investigators at Washington University did not use MCI as a clinical designation and, therefore, likely see only patients at a more clinically advanced stage than MCI. Further, this study did not include autopsy data from patients at the MCI stage or even the CDR 0.5 stage. Most patients had progressed clinically to CDR 1 by the time of autopsy. Thus, these data are perhaps more correctly viewed as an outcome study, rather than a cross-sectional study of patients with mild degrees of cognitive impairment. As such, it would be reasonably expected that their neuropathological data demonstrate AD.

Several studies have reported on the neuropathology of patients who died with the clinical classification of MCI (Bennett et al., 2005; Petersen et al., 2006). Pathological data in the Religious Order Study demonstrated an intermediate pathology between the neuropathological changes of normal aging and those of very early AD (Bennett et al., 2005). These investigators reported that a combination of neuropathological findings, including neurodegeneration and vascular pathology, contributed to the clinical picture of MCI.

A recent Mayo Clinic study found neuropathologic features intermediate between changes of normal aging and AD in patients who died though their clinical classification was aMCI (Petersen et al., 2006). Most of these patients had some degree of medial temporal lobe pathology, usually NFTs, but only sparse diffuse plaques in the neocortex. They had mostly low NIA-Reagan scores for the probability of meeting neuropathology criteria for AD.

A study from the University of Kentucky reported pathological findings similar to those of early AD among patients with aMCI (Markesbery et al., 2006). These investigators acknowledged that the patients with MCI may have been more clinically advanced than in other studies, and that the patients with AD used for comparison were in the early clinical stages of AD.

A second study from Mayo investigated the pathological outcomes of patients with aMCI. As predicted, the majority of patients had progressed to AD. However, as many as 20% had other types of dementing disorders such as frontotemporal dementia, dementia with Lewy bodies, progressive supranuclear palsy, and vascular dementia, although taken singly, each of these disorders was uncommon (Fig. 64.5) (Jicha et al., 2006).

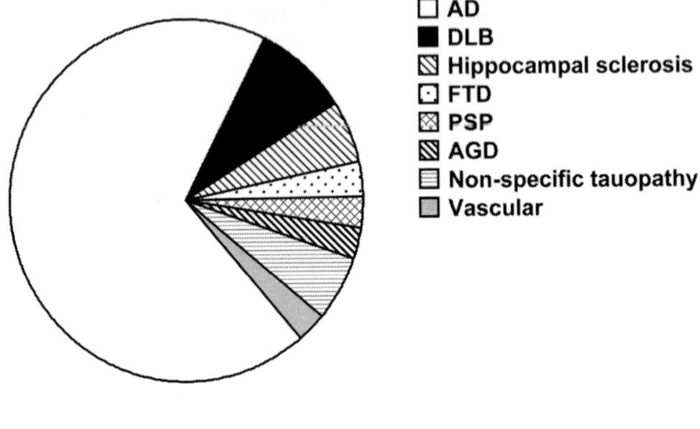

FIGURE 64.5 Neuropathological outcome of subjects with history of mild cognitive impairment. From Petersen, 2007b. Reprinted by permission.

Therefore, although most aMCI cases progress to AD, some develop other clinical syndromes.

In summary, the actual pathologic substrate of most patients with aMCI appears to be one of evolving AD. That is, the full AD neuropathologic spectrum is not present at the MCI stage, but many incipient features are evolving.

EPIDEMIOLOGICAL DATA REGARDING MCI

There are a number of cohort studies that have investigated MCI prospectively (Lopez et al., 2003). However, due to MCI being a relatively recently defined construct, several epidemiological studies were already under way without having been designed to incorporate MCI criteria. Various attempts have been made to "retrofit" MCI criteria into these already designed studies, with variable success. These considerations likely account for the substantial variability in reported prevalence figures. Table 64.1 shows the reported prevalence rates for MCI and other related constructs (such as AACD) among studies that retrofitted MCI criteria to ongoing longitudinal studies, as well as newer studies employing MCI criteria prospectively.

Among studies using current MCI criteria prospectively, the reported prevalence rates have generally been about 12%–18% among patients with no dementia older than age 65 years. As would be expected, lower rates are reported when the entire population, including patients with dementia, serves as the denominator (Unverzagt et al., 2001; Bennett et al., 2002). These figures depend somewhat on the specific subtype of MCI studied and the methods used to operationalize the MCI criteria. For example, using a neuropsychological algorithm to define MCI, prevalence figures are quite variable (Ritchie et al., 2001), likely reflecting the arbitrary selection of the neuropsychological instruments and the

TABLE 64.1 *Selected MCI Epidemiology/Cohort Studies*

Reference	Population	Number of Participants	Retrospective/ Prospective	Diagnosis Clinical/Algorithmic	Prevalence %		
					CIND	AACD	MCI
Busse et al., 2006	Germany	980	P	A		9	3-5
Graham et al., 1997	Canada	2,914	R	C	17		5
Unverzagt et al., 2001	African American, Indianapolis, IN	351	P	C	23		12
Bennett et al., 2002	Catholic clergy	798	P	C			26
Ritchie et al., 2001	France	833	R	A		21	3
Lopez et al., 2003	Multicenter	927	P	C			18
Hanninen et al., 2002	Finland	806	P	A			5
Boeve et al., 2003	Rochester, MN	111	P	C			12
Petersen et al., 2007	Rochester, MN	1,704	P	C			16
Jungwirth et al., 2005	Austria	592	P	A			24
Di Carlo et al., 2007	Italy	2,768	R	A	9.5		16
Das et al., 2007	India	745	P	C			14
Luck et al., 2007	Germany	3,327	P	C			15

CIND: cognitive impairment not demented; AACD: aging-associated cognitive decline; MCI: mild cognitive impairment.

arbitrary definition of cutoff scores. Some studies have implied longitudinal instability of the MCI construct, although this instability may simply have reflected the test–retest variability of the neuropsychological instruments that had been used to define MCI (Ritchie et al., 2001; Larrieu et al., 2002), rather than instability of the clinically defined MCI construct described here.

Clearly, the numerous methodological considerations of these various studies complicate the interpretation of the available epidemiologic data on MCI. Overall, the data in Table 64.1 indicate that the prevalence of MCI is probably in the 12%–15% range among individuals 65 years and older, with an incidence in the range of 1% per year. These figures are similar to those reported for AD.

TREATMENT

There is no Food and Drug Administration (FDA)-approved treatment intervention for MCI. Given the discussion above, one would not expect an overall treatment indication of MCI any more than one would expect an overall indication for dementia. Analogous to the subtyping of dementia into diseases such as AD, vascular dementia, frontotemporal dementia, and so on, subtyping of MCI may identify populations at risk of progressing to specific dementia subtypes, thereby identifying individuals in whom specific targeted therapies could be investigated. For the reasons discussed above, aMCI may provide a potential target for interventions directed towards the prodromal stage of AD.

Symptomatic Treatment in AD

Five drugs have been approved by the FDA for the treatment of clinically probable AD, although only four are commonly used. Three of these four are acetylcholinesterase inhibitors, used in response to research indicating a cholinergic deficit in AD (Bowen et al., 1976; Davies and Maloney, 1976; Petersen, 1977; Whitehouse et al. 1981). In the past decade, acetylcholinesterase inhibitors have been shown to be effective at modulating the symptoms of AD and currently form the mainstay of treatment in clinically probable AD.

Disease Modifying Treatment in AD

Considerable research supports a role of oxidative damage in the pathophysiology of AD, and some epidemiologic data suggest that antioxidants may be associated with a lower incidence of AD (Goodwin et al., 1983; Gale et al., 1996; La Rue et al., 1997; Perrig et al., 1997; Morris et al., 1998). A clinical trial of patients with moderate AD reported a benefit for vitamin E and selegiline in slowing the progression of moderate AD

(Sano et al., 1997). Following that study, an AAN practice parameter recommended that vitamin E at 1000 IU twice daily be considered as a treatment to slow the progression of AD (Doody et al., 2001). Recent meta-analyses that raised concerns of an increased risk of death among those taking greater than 400 IU per day of supplemental vitamin E (Miller et al., 2005) have cooled enthusiasm for recommending this treatment, although the applicability of those meta-analysis findings to typical AD patients is unclear.

CLINICAL TRIAL DATA IN MCI

Five major drug trials investigating compounds used for the symptomatic treatment of AD in MCI populations have taken place. These are summarized in Table 64.2. Taken together, these trials enrolled 4,000–5,000 patients in numerous centers around the world. Unfortunately, none has been notably positive, with one possible exception (Petersen, 2003b). The numerous possible reasons for this outcome are discussed later.

Donepezil and Vitamin E Trials

The ADCS enrolled 769 patients with aMCI among 69 centers in the United States and Canada and (Petersen et al., 2005). Patients were randomized to three treatment groups: donepezil (10 mg per day), vitamin E (2,000 IU per day), or placebo. All participants received a multivitamin. Each patient was followed with clinical evaluations every 6 months for up to 3 years. The entry criteria included those outlined in Figure 64.1 for aMCI, a score on the MMSE of 24 or greater, and performance 1.5 to 2 standard deviations below education-adjusted normative values on a modified version of the Wechsler Memory Scale–Revised Logical Memory II subtest. These criteria ensured that the patients were sufficiently memory impaired to be close to transitioning to AD, yet did not meet criteria for dementia. The primary outcome measure was clinical progression to AD. The study planners projected a progression rate of 10%–15% per year for the patients with aMCI and powered the study to detect a reduction in that rate of 33%.

The patients with aMCI progressed to AD at a rate of 16% per year in this study, similar to the design projection. Neither of the two active treatment arms reduced the risk of progression to AD over the entire 3 years of the study. However, donepezil did reduce the risk of progression to AD for the first 12 months of the study in all patients, and this effect persisted up to 24 months among ApoE4 carriers. In analyzing this data, it should be noted that of the 214 conversions from aMCI to AD encountered in the trial, 76% were ApoE4 carriers. There was no treatment effect for vitamin E. The secondary outcome measures generally corroborated these primary outcome findings regarding the risk and rate of progression from aMCI to AD. Of the 214 conversions to dementia, 212 were diagnosed with possible or probable AD, indicating that the aMCI criteria were quite specific in identifying individuals at higher risk for developing AD.

The authors of this study concluded that although donepezil could not be generally recommended for the treatment of aMCI, clinicians should discuss the potential role of this medication with patients on an individual basis. Although there is no FDA-approved treatment for MCI, the off-label use of donepezil could be considered for treatment of aMCI on an individualized basis. On the basis of this study, the authors did not advocate using ApoE4 genotyping with the aim of identifying individuals having a higher likelihood of a clinical progression to AD at an earlier stage in the disease process, in accord with the many consensus panels that have argued against this type of testing. As the first clinical trial to show the ability of an intervention to delay the onset of clinical AD, this was an important study that provides evidence for the conceptual framework and feasibility of attempts to intervene at the MCI stage.

TABLE 64.2 *MCI Clinical Trials*

Sponsor	*Compound*	*Number Enrolled*	*Duration (years)*	*Primary Outcome*	*Progression Rate*	*Result*	*Reference*
ADCS	Donepezil Vitamin E	769	3	AD	16%	Partially Positive	Petersen et al., 2005
Johnson and Johnson[a]	Galantamine	2048	2	CDR 1	5%	Negative	Gold et al., 2004
Novartis	Rivastigmine	1018	4	AD	5%	Negative	Feldman et al., 2007
Merck	Rofecoxib	1457	3-4	AD	5%	Negative	Thal et al., 2005

[a]Two trials.
AD: Alzheimer's disease; ADCS: Alzheimer's Disease Cooperative Study; CDR: Clinical Dementia Rating Scale.

Galantamine

Johnson and Johnson sponsored two studies investigating the impact of galantamine on the progression from aMCI to AD (Gold et al., 2004). These multinational studies assessed the rate of progression from aMCI to AD using progression on the CDR from 0.5 to 1 as their primary end point. This important distinction, using progression on the CDR rather than clinical criteria for AD, renders the results of the study more difficult to interpret. For example, a patient may progress from aMCI to AD while remaining at the CDR level of 0.5, which could result in decreased sensitivity due to the study design. These two trials enrolled 2,048 patients in total, among whom 43% were ApoE4 carriers. Overall, 13% on galantamine progressed from aMCI to AD (vs. 18% in the placebo group) in one trial and 17% of the galantamine group progressed (vs. 21% of the placebo group) in the second trial. Although this trend in favor of galantamine was present, neither trial reached statistical significance. Magnetic resonance imaging was performed on many of the participants, with a suggestion that galantamine may have reduced the rate of whole-brain atrophy over the 2-year study period. Thus, although there were no significant treatment effects in these trials, there was some suggestion of a drug effect, possibly corroborated with MRI volumetric measures. Both studies showed a greater number of deaths in the galantamine treated groups relative to placebo, necessitating a warning about this possibility. It is possible that fewer than expected deaths occurred in the placebo groups, but this is uncertain.

Rivastigmine

Novartis investigated its acetylcholinesterase inhibitor rivastigmine (Feldman et al., 2007) in a 3-year study that enrolled 1,018 patients with aMCI and assessed progression from aMCI to AD. This multinational study had many of the same features as the ADCS but encountered difficulties with the operationalizing diagnostic criteria and neuropsychological measures. The study was conducted across 14 countries and required multiple translations of the neuropsychological instruments employed. Further, this study enrolled patients at a milder stage than that in the ADCS trial of donepezil (Petersen, 2007a). Likely as a consequence of these operational difficulties, the conversion rate was much lower than expected, necessitating extension of the study to 4 years to achieve an adequate number of events. Over the 4-year time period, 17.3% of patients taking rivastigmine progressed to AD compared to 21.4% of patients on placebos. Although the difference was in the predicted direction, it did not reach statistical significance. Similarly, there was no significant difference between treatment arms in the various neuropsychological measures used as secondary end points. Another criticism of the study design was that ApoE4 genotyping was performed in only a subset of patients, which did not allow this important stratifying variable to be included in the data analysis. The investigators speculated that the inclusion criteria (which were different from those used in the donepezil trial) as well as the exclusion of patients having symptoms of depression at baseline may have contributed to the lower-than-anticipated observed conversion rate of 5% per year. It should be noted that despite the low conversion rate, nearly all patients who progressed to dementia were diagnosed with AD.

Rofecoxib

Merck sponsored a large trial of the Cyclooxygenase-2 (COX 2) inhibitor rofecoxib in patients with aMCI (Thal et al., 2005). This 2-year trial enrolled 1,457 patients and used progression from aMCI to AD as the primary outcome measure. The observed progression rate was lower than anticipated, necessitating extension of the study to 3–4 years. This study reported annual conversion rates to AD of 6.4% in the rofecoxib group and 4.5% for the placebo group, achieving statistical significance (p = .011) in favor of the placebo group. The cognitive measures used as secondary outcomes did not corroborate the finding of the primary outcome, and consequently the authors tended to dismiss the significance of the finding in favor of placebo. The authors identified several factors that correlated with an increased risk of progression to AD, including lower MMSE score, ApoE4 carrier status, age, gender, and prior use of ginkgo biloba. Including these measures in a multivariate prediction model, the statistical significance of the primary outcome was no longer present. The investigators in this trial had modified the memory inclusion criteria, accepting a lesser degree of impairment than in other MCI studies. It is unclear if this design resulted in a more mildly affected study population overall, but it may have contributed to the low observed conversion rate. It is uncertain whether the findings of this study suggest that use of rofecoxib increased the rate of progression to AD, or whether this finding was simply spurious. In either case, it did not demonstrate the predicted benefit.

Discussion of Available Clinical Trial Data

Considered together, these trials allow some important conclusions. Many factors likely contributed to the variability in rate of progression from aMCI to AD among these clinical trials, including differences in the patient populations recruited and, importantly, the operationalization of the aMCI criteria and the primary outcome measures (Petersen, 2007a). Pertinent to the multinational trials, translation of the evaluative instruments and cultural variability as to what constitutes dementia or AD or aMCI may have had a significant impact on the trial outcomes. Due to differing normative expectations of daily functioning, the clinical threshold for a diagnosis of dementia or AD varies widely among cultures. Extending this reasoning, one would expect these cultural differences to be magnified in making the more subtle clinical determination of aMCI. Although multinational clinical trials present opportunities to investigate an intervention in a wider population, logistical difficulties relevant to studies in aMCI and AD may have hampered the ability to produce reliable results.

These studies varied in the implementation procedures used to satisfy the memory criteria of the aMCI diagnosis. These seemingly harmless differences in cutoff scores, when used as inclusion criteria, may significantly affect the composition of the study groups. For example, defining milder degrees as inclusion criteria for patients with aMCI may result in very mild aMCI and possibly patients who were normal (which would have been in the control group of another trial) being included in the treatment groups, resulting in a lower than expected conversion rate.

Because ApoE4 carrier status is a strong predictor of progression to AD among aMCI populations, the variable ApoE4 carrier rates among these studies are another important factor that likely influenced the outcomes.

All of these trials used conversion to AD as a primary outcome measure, but they differed in the method by which this end point was determined. In addition to cultural differences in the clinical diagnosis of AD, these studies also varied as to how the primary outcome measure was operationalized. One study used a change in the CDR to determine conversion to AD, whereas others used clinical diagnosis of AD by the investigators to determine this end point. Because these studies rely upon identification and definition of subtle phenomenon of the incipient stages of AD, seemingly innocuous differences in implementation criteria may lead to significant impacts on outcome measures.

A few important points relevant to the construct of aMCI emerge from these studies. First, although the overall progression rate ranged from 5% to 16%, all of these rates are much higher than the population incidence rate for AD of 1%–2%. The rate of 16% per year in the ADCS donepezil trial far exceeds this general population rate by severalfold. Even the "least successful" trial employing aMCI criteria identified a population that was at 2 or 3 times the risk of developing AD when compared to the general population. Therefore, although the treatments studied were essentially ineffective, the trials themselves documented the success and utility of using aMCI criteria to enroll a population enriched for individuals at higher risk of developing AD during the time frame of a clinical trial. As disease-modifying treatments for AD move into clinical trials, the ability to identify a group of patients likely to progress at an accelerated rate would provide an excellent clinical substrate for testing compounds targeting the underlying disease process. These clinical trials confirm that the aMCI construct does identify such individuals.

MCI IN CLINICAL PRACTICE

Ultimately, the clinical utility of MCI as a diagnostic entity will be determined by its usefulness for clinicians in caring for and counseling patients. Most literature to date has investigated the aMCI subtype of a degenerative etiology, a likely prodrome of AD. Therefore, this discussion primarily pertains to that clinical subtype.

In 2001, the AAN endorsed the construct of MCI (Petersen, Stevens, et al., 2001). This evidence-based practice parameter found sufficient evidence to encourage clinicians to identify and evaluate patients in their practices for the diagnosis of MCI. Based on many of the data discussed above, these individuals are at increased risk of developing dementia in the future and should be counseled appropriately. Although no disease-modifying treatment currently exists, therapeutic interventions may become available for these patients in the future. In the years since the publication of this practice parameter, a tremendous increase in the available data regarding MCI has occurred and consequently, the practice parameter will likely be updated in the near future.

As older individuals represent a continually increasing segment of U.S. society, the number of patients presenting with subtle cognitive concerns will increase, as will the demands, desires, and concerns of these individuals. Clinicians will require a diagnostic framework in which to evaluate, classify, and ultimately treat these individuals. If one accepts the premise that individuals pass through a stage of "partial symptoms" en route to developing a degenerative dementia such as AD, then the construct of MCI provides such a framework.

It must be noted that diagnostic classifications such as MCI are arbitrary. The distinctions between categories such as MCI and clinically probable AD are artificial when considered in the context of the gradual evolution of AD. Nevertheless, this terminology addresses the need to communicate clearly and effectively with our patients and with each other. The clinical designation of aMCI can be quite useful in characterizing people who do not meet diagnostic criteria for AD or dementia and avoids the stigma that labels such as dementia or AD may carry.

HOW SHOULD I COUNSEL PATIENTS HAVING MCI?

It would be appropriate to place the evolving nature of the construct of MCI into context. That is, there certainly remains discussion in the literature regarding the precise characterization of the diagnostic criteria for MCI within the research literature. With that said, a patient who meets the criteria outlined in Figure 64.1 and whose symptoms are felt to be due to a degenerative process is likely at a 10%–15% per year risk of progressing to clinically probable AD. To the extent a patient deviates from these criteria, this prediction could be adjusted upward or downward. For example, an ApoE4 carrier (keeping in mind that ApoE4 testing is not recommended in this clinical situation) having hippocampal atrophy evident on MRI would presumably be at a higher risk of progressing more rapidly. Alternatively, an individual not carrying the ApoE4 genotype with no family history of dementia and having normal appearing hippocampal structures would presumably progress less rapidly. Of course, regular clinical reevaluation remains the best adjunct for making this determination.

Discussion of the implications of the MCI diagnosis is perhaps the most important aspect of counseling at this time. Although a patient is cognitively competent, they may wish to begin planning for the future and addressing financial issues, retirement, living arrangements, and so on.

As discussed above, there is no medication with an FDA-approved indication for MCI. The results from the ADCS trial provide an excellent framework for discussion of the possible use of a cholinesterase inhibitor. A 63-year-old high-functioning professional may regard the modest symptomatic benefit demonstrated in that trial as important to his or her ability to continue to function in the work environment and may be inclined towards early treatment with donepezil. Alternatively, a 75-year-old retiree primarily engaged in leisure activities may choose to defer treatment until a stage of greater impairment. As these simple caricatures illustrate, the choice of whether and when to initiate treatment with a cholinesterase inhibitor is ultimately a personal decision that must be made following a frank discussion between the clinician and patient of realistic aims and expectations.

Many physicians recommend a variety of lifestyle modifications in an attempt to minimize the rate of progression, although definitive data here are limited. Frequently, physicians recommend that patients remain physically active, intellectually engaged, socially active, and that they follow a heart-healthy diet (Fratiglioni et al., 2004; Rovio et al., 2005). Although insufficient data exist to support a direct impact on progression from aMCI to AD, these lifestyle modifications may improve an older individual's overall quality of life, irrespective of an impact on progression to AD. Some preliminary evidence suggests possible benefit for cognitive rehabilitation in patients with MCI, although large studies with meaningful long-term follow-up are lacking (Belleville, 2008).

Lasty, patients may derive substantial encouragement and reassurance from the recognition that MCI is a rapidly evolving topic of investigation and that they should remain in touch with their physician regarding future advancements that will likely be made in this area.

FUTURE RESEARCH PROSPECTS

The MCI construct has become useful in research and clinical practice and is being considered for inclusion in the next revision of the *Diagnostic and Statistical Manual of Mental Disorders–V* (Petersen and O'Brien, 2006). As stated earlier, the clinical value of the MCI construct ultimately will be determined by practicing clinicians.

Many research efforts aim to improve the accuracy of outcome prediction for patients with aMCI. It has been demonstrated that patients carrying ApoE4 genotypes and having atrophic hippocampi on MRI will likely progress more rapidly. Cerebral metabolic patterns seen on FDG-PET and CSF biomarkers, such as phosphorylated tau and Aβ 1–42, may also provide useful prognostic data. Newer molecular imaging techniques employing PiB and FDDNP may provide valuable antemortem detection of underlying pathology associated with aMCI in the future. Studies investigating these agents in aMCI are already under way.

Currently, clinical criteria (Fig. 64.1) can be used to identify patients having MCI. Consideration of the suspected etiology will then allow discussion of likely outcomes with the patient (Fig. 64.2). In the research setting, a combination of these clinical considerations, augmented with some combination of the technological measures mentioned above, will be evaluated to identify combinations that improve prognostication. Although these techniques will initially be restricted to research settings, if they are proven useful, they may be adopted into practice at tertiary care centers for the adjudication of difficult cases.

A large number of agents proposed to have a disease-modifying effect in AD are at various stages of investigation. These include nonsteroidal anti-inflammatory medications proposed to modulate the biochemical processing of amyloid, active, and passive immunization strategies and monoclonal antibodies, among others. The construct of aMCI may identify individuals more likely to benefit from these agents due to intervention occurring at a time when symptoms are minimal, and as such may play an important role in structuring the enrollment and end points of future clinical trials of such disease-modifying agents (Cummings et al., 2007).

CONCLUSION

Intervention for individuals likely to develop AD during an asymptomatic or minimally symptomatic state holds the greatest promise, as well as poses the greatest challenges, for disease-modifying therapies. Most existing research supports the finding that aMCI identifies individuals likely to develop AD in the future. When disease-modifying therapies directed at AD emerge, the MCI construct may prove useful to identify individuals at an early stage in the course of the disease who stand to benefit significantly from an intervention that halts or slows the disease process prior to the development of significant functional disability. In the ultimate extension of this line of reasoning, individuals at risk for developing these diseases may be identified while still clinically normal, and intervention may allow for disease prevention in the future. Further, the construct of MCI aids in sensitizing clinicians to earlier presenting features of dementing disorders. Having been expanded to include nonmemory cognitive deficits, MCI can be viewed as a precursor stage to many dementias, and subtypes of MCI may ultimately be demonstrated to predict specific dementia subtypes.

REFERENCES

Aggarwal, N.T., Wilson, R.S., Beck, T.L., Bienias, J.L., and Bennett, D.A. (2005) Mild cognitive impairment in different functional domains and incident Alzheimer's disease. *J. Neurol. Neurosurg. Psychiatry* 76(11):1479–1484.

Aggarwal, N.T., Wilson, R.S., Beck, T.L., Bienias, J.L., Berry-Kravis, E., and Bennett, D.A. (2005) The apolipoprotein E epsilon4 allele and incident Alzheimer's disease in persons with mild cognitive impairment. *Neurocase* 11(1):3–7.

American Psychiatric Association. (1987) *Diagnostic and Statistical Manual of Mental Disorders*, 3rd ed., rev. Washington, DC: Author.

Anchisi, D., Borroni, B., Franceschi, M., Kerrouche, N., Kalbe, E., Beuthien-Beumann, B., Cappa, S., Lenz, O., Ludecke, S., Marcone, A., Mielke, R., Ortelli, P., Padovani, A., Pelati, O., Pupi, A., Scarpini, E., Weisenbach, S., Herholz, K., Salmon, E., Holthoff, V., Sorbi, S., Fazio, F., and Perani, D. (2005) Heterogeneity of brain glucose metabolism in mild cognitive impairment and clinical progression to Alzheimer disease. *Arch. Neurol.* 62(11):1728–1733.

Bateman, R.J., Wen, G., Morris, J.C., and Holtzman, D.M. (2007) Fluctuations of CSF amyloid-beta levels: implications for a diagnostic and therapeutic biomarker. *Neurology* 68(9):666–669.

Belleville, S. (2008) Cognitive training for persons with mild cognitive impairment. *Int. Psychogeriatr.* 20(1):57–66.

Bennett, D.A., Schneider, J.A., Bienias, J.L., Evans, D.A., and Wilson, R.S. (2005) Mild cognitive impairment is related to Alzheimer disease pathology and cerebral infarctions. *Neurology* 64(5):834–841.

Bennett, D.A., Wilson, R.S., Schneider, J.A., Evans, D.A., Beckett, L.A., Aggarwal, N.T., Barnes, L.L., Fox, J.H., and Bach, J. (2002) Natural history of mild cognitive impairment in older persons. *Neurology* 59(2):198–205.

Boeve, B., McCormick, J., Smith, G., Ferman, T., Rummans, T., Carpenter, T., Ivnik, R., Kokmen, E., Tangalos, E., Edland, S., Knopman, D., and Petersen, R. (2003) Mild cognitive impairment in the oldest old. *Neurology* 60(3):477–480.

Bowen, D.M., Smith, C.B., White, P., and Davison, A.N. (1976) Neurotransmitter-related enzymes and indices of hypoxia in senile dementia and other abiotrophies. *Brain* 99(3):459–496.

Brys, M., Pirraglia, E., Rich, K., Rolstad, S., Mosconi, L., Switalski, R., Glodzik-Sobanska, L., De Santi, S., Zinkowski, R., Mehta, P., Pratico, D., Saint Louis, L.A., Wallin, A., Blennow, K., and de Leon, M.J. (2007) Prediction and longitudinal study of CSF biomarkers in mild cognitive impairment. *Neurobiol. Aging* 24 doi:10.1016/j.neurobiolaging.2007.08.010.

Buerger, K., Ewers, M., Pirttila, T., Zinkowski, R., Alafuzoff, I., Teipel, S.J., DeBernardis, J., Kerkman, D., McCulloch, C., Soininen, H., and Hampel, H. (2006) CSF phosphorylated tau protein correlates with neocortical neurofibrillary pathology in Alzheimer's disease. *Brain* 129(Pt 11):3035–3041.

Buerger, K., Teipel, S.J., Zinkowski, R., Blennow, K., Arai, H., Engel, R., Hofmann-Kiefer, K., McCulloch, C., Ptok, U., Heun, R., Andreasen, N., DeBernardis, J., Kerkman, D., Moeller, H., Davies, P., and Hampel, H. (2002) CSF tau protein phosphorylated at threonine 231 correlates with cognitive decline in MCI subjects. *Neurology* 59(4):627–629.

Busse, A., Hensel, A., Guhne, U., Angermeyer, M.C., and Riedel-Heller, S.G. (2006) Mild cognitive impairment: long-term course of four clinical subtypes. *Neurology* 67(12):2176–2185.

Corder, E.H., Saunders, A.M., Strittmatter, W.J., Schmechel, D.E., Gaskell, P.C., Small, G.W., Roses, A.D., Haines, J.L., and Pericak-Vance, M.A. (1993) Gene dose of apolipoprotein E type 4 allele and the risk of Alzheimer's disease in late onset families. *Science* 261(5123):921–923.

Cummings, J.L., Doody, R., and Clark, C. (2007) Disease-modifying therapies for Alzheimer disease: challenges to early intervention. *Neurology* 69(16):1622–1634.

Daly, E., Zaitchik, D., Copeland, M., Schmahmann, J., Gunther, J., and Albert, M. (2000) Predicting conversion to Alzheimer disease using standardized clinical information. *Arch. Neurol.* 57(5):675–680.

Das, S.K., Bose, P., Biswas, A., Dutt, A., Banerjee, T.K., Hazra, A.M., Raut, D.K., Chaudhuri, A., and Roy, T. (2007) An epidemiologic study of mild cognitive impairment in Kolkata, India. *Neurology* 68(23):2019–2026.

Davies, P., and Maloney, A.J. (1976) Selective loss of central cholinergic neurons in Alzheimer's disease. *Lancet* 2(8000):1403.

DeCarli, C., Frisoni, G.B., Clark, C.M., Harvey, D., Grundman, M., Petersen, R.C., Thal, L.J., Jin, S., Jack, C.R., Jr., and Scheltens, P. (2007) Qualitative estimates of medial temporal atrophy as a predictor of progression from mild cognitive impairment to dementia. *Arch. Neurol.* 64(1):108–115.

Devanand, D.P., Pradhaban, G., Liu, X., Khandji, A., De Santi, S., Segal, S., Rusinek, H., Pelton, G.H., Honig, L.S., Mayeux, R., Stern, Y., Tabert, M.H., and de Leon, M.J. (2007) Hippocampal and entorhinal atrophy in mild cognitive impairment: prediction of Alzheimer disease. *Neurology* 68(11):828–836.

Di Carlo, A., Lamassa, M., Baldereschi, M., Inzitari, M., Scafato, E., Farchi, G., and Inzitari, D. (2007) CIND and MCI in the Italian elderly: frequency, vascular risk factors, progression to dementia. *Neurology* 68(22):1909–1916.

Doody, R.S., Stevens, J.C., Beck, C., Dubinsky, R.M., Kaye, J.A., Gwyther, L., Mohs, R.C., Thal, L.J., Whitehouse, P.J., DeKosky, S.T., and Cummings, J.L. (2001) Practice parameter: management of dementia (an evidence-based review). Report of the Quality Standards Subcommittee of the American Academy of Neurology. *Neurology* 56(9):1154–1166.

Drzezga, A., Grimmer, T., Riemenschneider, M., Lautenschlager, N., Siebner, H., Alexopoulus, P., Minoshima, S., Schwaiger, M., and Kurz, A. (2005) Prediction of individual clinical outcome in MCI by means of genetic assessment and (18)F-FDG PET. *J. Nucl. Med.* 46(10):1625–1632.

Farrer, L.A., Cupples, L.A., Haines, J.L., Hyman, B., Kukull, W.A., Mayeux, R., Myers, R.H., Pericak-Vance, M.A., Risch, N., and van Duijn, C.M. (1997) Effects of age, sex, and ethnicity on the association between apolipoprotein E genotype and Alzheimer disease. A meta-analysis. APOE and Alzheimer Disease Meta Analysis Consortium. *JAMA* 278(16):1349–1356.

Feldman, H.H., Ferris, S., Winblad, B., Sfikas, N., Mancione, L., He, Y., Tekin, S., Burns, A., Cummings, J., Del Ser, T., Inzitari, D., Orgogozo, J.M., Sauer, H., Scheltens, P., Scarpini, E., Herrmann, N., Farlow, M., Potkin, S., Charles, H.C., Fox, N.C., and Lane, R. (2007) Effect of rivastigmine on delay to diagnosis of Alzheimer's disease from mild cognitive impairment: the InDDEx Study. *Lancet Neurol.* 6(6):501–512.

Fischer, P., Jungwirth, S., Zehetmayer, S., Weissgram, S., Hoenigschnabl, S., Gelpi, E., Krampla, W., and Tragl, K.H. (2007) Conversion from subtypes of mild cognitive impairment to Alzheimer dementia. *Neurology* 68(4):288–291.

Folstein, M., Folstein, S., and McHugh, P. (1975) "Mini-mental state." A practical method for grading the cognitive state of patients for the clinician. *J. Psychiatry Res.* 12:189–198.

Fratiglioni, L., Paillard-Borg, S., and Winblad, B. (2004) An active and socially integrated lifestyle in late life might protect against dementia. *Lancet Neurol.* 3(6):343–353.

Galasko, D., Chang, L., Motter, R., Clark, C.M., Kaye, J., Knopman, D., Thomas, R., Kholodenko, D., Schenk, D., Lieberburg, I., Miller, B., Green, R., Basherad, R., Kertiles, L., Boss, M.A., and Seubert, P. (1998) High cerebrospinal fluid tau and low amyloid beta42 levels in the clinical diagnosis of Alzheimer disease and relation to apolipoprotein E genotype. *Arch. Neurol.* 55(7):937–945.

Galasko, D., Clark, C., Chang, L., Miller, B., Green, R.C., Motter, R., and Seubert, P. (1997) Assessment of CSF levels of tau protein in mildly demented patients with Alzheimer's disease. *Neurology* 48(3):632–635.

Gale, C.R., Martyn, C.N., and Cooper, C. (1996) Cognitive impairment and mortality in a cohort of elderly people. *Br. Med. J.* 312(7031):608–611.

Gauthier, S., Reisberg, B., Zaudig, M., Petersen, R.C., Ritchie, K., Broich, K., Belleville, S., Brodaty, H., Bennett, D., Chertkow, H., Cummings, J.L., de Leon, M., Feldman, H., Ganguli, M., Hampel, H., Scheltens, P., Tierney, M.C., Whitehouse, P., and Winblad, B. (2006) Mild cognitive impairment. *Lancet* 367(9518):1262–1270.

Geda, Y.E., and Petersen, R.C. (2001) Clinical trials in mild cognitive impairment. In: Gauthier, S. and Cummings, J.L., eds. *Alzheimer's Disease and Related Disorders Annual 2001*. London: Martin Dunitz, pp. 69–83.

Gold, M., Francke, S., Nye, J.S., Goldstein, H.R., Fijal, B., Truyen, L., and Cohen, N. (2004) Impact of APOE genotype on the efficacy of galantamine for the treatment of mild cognitive impairment. *Neurobiol. Aging* 25(Suppl 2):S521.

Goodwin, J.S., Goodwin, J.M., and Garry, P.J. (1983) Association between nutritional status and cognitive functioning in a healthy elderly population. *JAMA* 249(21):2917–2921.

Graff-Radford, N.R., Crook, J.E., Lucas, J., Boeve, B.F., Knopman, D.S., Ivnik, R.J., Smith, G.E., Younkin, L.H., Petersen, R.C., and Younkin, S.G. (2007) Association of low plasma Abeta42/Abeta40 ratios with increased imminent risk for mild cognitive impairment and Alzheimer disease. *Arch. Neurol.* 64(3):354–362.

Graham, J.E., Rockwood, K., Beattie, B.L., Eastwood, R., Gauthier, S., Tuokko, H., and McDowell, I. (1997) Prevalence and severity of cognitive impairment with and without dementia in an elderly population. *Lancet* 349(9068):1793–1796.

Growdon, J.H. (1999) Biomarkers of Alzheimer disease. *Arch. Neurol.* 56(3):281–283.

Hanninen, T., Hallikainen, M., Tuomainen, S., Vanhanen, M., and Soininen, H. (2002) Prevalence of mild cognitive impairment: a population-based study in elderly subjects. *Acta Neurol. Scand.* 106(3):148–154.

Hansson, O., Zetterberg, H., Buchhave, P., Londos, E., Blennow, K., and Minthon, L. (2006) Association between CSF biomarkers and incipient Alzheimer's disease in patients with mild cognitive impairment: a follow-up study. *Lancet Neurol.* 5(3):228–234.

Hunderfund, A.L., Roberts, R.O., Slusser, T.C., Leibson, C.L., Geda, Y.E., Ivnik, R.J., Tangalos, E.G., and Petersen, R.C. (2006) Mortality in amnestic mild cognitive impairment: a prospective community study. *Neurology* 67(10):1764–1768.

Ivnik, R.J., Malec, J.F., Smith, G.E., Tangalos, E.G., Petersen, R.C., Kokmen, E., and Kurland, L.T. (1992) Mayo's Older Americans Normative Studies: WAIS-R, WMS-R and AVLT norms for ages 56 to 97. *Clin. Neuropsychol.* 6(Suppl):1–104.

Ivnik, R.J., Smith, G.E., Lucas, J.A., Petersen, R.C., Boeve, B.F., Kokmen, E., and Tangalos, E.G. (1999) Testing normal older people three or four times at 1- to 2-year intervals: defining normal variance. *Neuropsychology* 13(1):121–127.

Jack, C.R., Jr., Petersen, R.C., Xu, Y.C., O'Brien, P.C., Smith, G.E., Ivnik, R.J., Boeve, B.F., Waring, S.C., Tangalos, E.G., and Kokmen, E. (1999) Prediction of AD with MRI-based hippocampal volume in mild cognitive impairment. *Neurology* 52(7):1397–1403.

Jack, C.R., Jr., Shiung, M.M., Weigand, S.D., O'Brien, P.C., Gunter, J.L., Boeve, B.F., Knopman, D.S., Smith, G.E., Ivnik, R.J., Tangalos, E.G., and Petersen, R.C. (2005) Brain atrophy rates predict subsequent clinical conversion in normal elderly and amnestic MCI. *Neurology* 65(8):1227–1231.

Jak, A.J., Houston, W.S., Nagel, B.J., Corey-Bloom, J., and Bondi, M.W. (2007) Differential cross-sectional and longitudinal impact of APOE genotype on hippocampal volumes in nondemented older adults. *Dement. Geriatr. Cogn. Disord.* 23(6):282–289.

Jicha, G.A., Parisi, J.E., Dickson, D.W., Johnson, K., Cha, R., Ivnik, R.J., Tangalos, E.G., Boeve, B.F., Knopman, D.S., Braak, H., and Petersen, R.C. (2006) Neuropathologic outcome of mild cognitive impairment following progression to clinical dementia. *Arch. Neurol.* 63(5):674–681.

Johnson, K.A., Gregas, M., Becker, J.A., Kinnecom, C., Salat, D.H., Moran, E.K., Smith, E.E., Rosand, J., Rentz, D.M., Klunk, W.E., Mathis, C.A., Price, J.C., Dekosky, S.T., Fischman, A.J., and Greenberg, S.M. (2007) Imaging of amyloid burden and distribution in cerebral amyloid angiopathy. *Ann. Neurol.* 62(3):229–234.

Jungwirth, S., Weissgram, S., Zehetmayer, S., Tragl, K.H., and Fischer, P. (2005) VITA: subtypes of mild cognitive impairment in a community-based cohort at the age of 75 years. *Int. J. Geriatr. Psychiatry* 20(5):452–458.

Klunk, W.E., Engler, H., Nordberg, A., Wang, Y., Blomqvist, G., Holt, D.P., Bergstrom, M., Savitcheva, I., Huang, G.F., Estrada, S., Ausen, B., Debnath, M.L., Barletta, J., Price, J.C., Sandell, J., Lopresti, B.J., Wall, A., Koivisto, P., Antoni, G., Mathis, C.A., and Langstrom, B. (2004) Imaging brain amyloid in Alzheimer's disease with Pittsburgh Compound-B. *Ann. Neurol.* 55(3):306–319.

Knopman, D.S., and Ryberg, S. (1989) A verbal memory test with high predictive accuracy for dementia of the Alzheimer type. *Arch. Neurol.* 46(2):141–145.

Kokmen, E., Smith, G.E., Petersen, R.C., Tangalos, E., and Ivnik, R.C. (1991) The short test of mental status. Correlations with standardized psychometric testing. *Arch. Neurol.* 48(7):725–728.

La Rue, A., Koehler, K.M., Wayne, S.J., Chiulli, S.J., Haaland, K.Y., and Garry, P.J. (1997) Nutritional status and cognitive functioning in a normally aging sample: a 6-y reassessment. *Am. J. Clin. Nutr.* 65(1):20–29.

Larrieu, S., Letenneur, L., Orgogozo, J.M., Fabrigoule, C., Amieva, H., Le Carret, N., Barberger-Gateau, P., and Dartigues, J.F. (2002) Incidence and outcome of mild cognitive impairment in a population-based prospective cohort. *Neurology* 59(10):1594–1599.

Lockhart, A., Lamb, J.R., Osredkar, T., Sue, L.I., Joyce, J.N., Ye, L., Libri, V., Leppert, D., and Beach, T.G. (2007) PIB is a non-specific imaging marker of amyloid-beta (Abeta) peptide-related cerebral amyloidosis. *Brain* 130(Pt 10):2607–2615.

Lopez, O.L., Jagust, W.J., DeKosky, S.T., Becker, J.T., Fitzpatrick, A., Dulberg, C., Breitner, J., Lyketsos, C., Jones, B., Kawas, C., Carlson, M., and Kuller, L.H. (2003) Prevalence and classification of mild cognitive impairment in the Cardiovascular Health Study Cognition Study: part 1. *Arch. Neurol.* 60(10):1385–1389.

Luck, T., Riedel-Heller, S.G., Kaduszkiewicz, H., Bickel, H., Jessen, F., Pentzek, M., Wiese, B., Koelsch, H., van den Bussche, H., Abholz, H.H., Moesch, E., Gorfer, S., Angermeyer, M.C., Maier, W., and Weyerer, S. (2007) Mild cognitive impairment in general practice: age-specific prevalence and correlate results from the German study on aging, cognition and dementia in primary care patients (AgeCoDe). *Dement. Geriatr. Cogn. Disord.* 24(4):307–316.

Markesbery, W.R., Schmitt, F.A., Kryscio, R.J., Davis, D.G., Smith, C.D. and Wekstein, D.R. (2006) Neuropathologic substrate of mild cognitive impairment. *Arch. Neurol.* 63(1):38–46.

Miller, E.R. 3rd, Pastor-Barriuso, R., Dalal, D., Riemersma, R.A., Appel, L.J., and Guallar, E. (2005) Meta-analysis: high-dosage vitamin E supplementation may increase all-cause mortality. *Ann. Intern. Med.* 142(1):37–46.

Morris, J.C., Storandt, M., Miller, J.P., McKeel, D.W., Price, J.L., Rubin, E.H., and Berg, L. (2001) Mild cognitive impairment represents early-stage Alzheimer disease. *Arch. Neurol.* 58(3):397–405.

Morris, M.C., Beckett, L.A., Scherr, P.A., Hebert, L.E., Bennett, D.A., Field, T.S., and Evans, D.A. (1998) Vitamin E and vitamin C supplement use and risk of incident Alzheimer disease. *Alzheimer Dis. Assoc. Disord.* 12(3):121–126.

Mueller, S.G., Weiner, M.W., Thal, L.J., Petersen, R.C., Jack, C., Jagust, W., Trojanowski, J.Q., Toga, A.W., and Beckett, L. (2005) The Alzheimer's disease neuroimaging initiative. *Neuroimaging Clin. N. Am.* 15(4):869–877, xi-xii.

Perrig, W.J., Perrig, P., and Stahelin, H.B. (1997) The relation between antioxidants and memory performance in the old and very old. *J. Am. Geriatr. Soc.* 45(6):718–724.

Petersen, R., Roberts, R., Knopman, D., Ivnik, R., Pankratz, V.S., Boeve, B., and Rocca, W. (2007) Prevalence of mild cognitive impairment in a population-based study. *Neurology* 68(12 Suppl 1): A237.

Petersen, R.C. (1977) Scopolamine induced learning failures in man. *Psychopharmacol. (Berl)* 52(3):283–289.

Petersen, R.C. (1991) Memory assessment at the bedside. In: Yanagihara, T. and Petersen, R.C., eds. *Memory Disorders*. New York, Dekker, pp. 137–152.

Petersen, R.C. (2000) Mild cognitive impairment: transition between aging and Alzheimer's disease. *Neurologia* 15(3):93–101.

Petersen, R.C. (2003a) *Mild Cognitive Impairment: Aging to Alzheimer's Disease*. Oxford, UK, and New York: Oxford University Press.

Petersen, R.C. (2003b) Mild cognitive impairment clinical trials. *Nat. Rev. Drug Discov.* 2(8):646–653.

Petersen, R.C. (2004) Mild cognitive impairment as a diagnostic entity. *J. Intern. Med.* 256(3):183–194.

Petersen, R.C. (2007a) MCI treatment trials: failure or not? *Lancet Neurol.* 6(6):473–475.

Petersen, R.C. (2007b) Mild cognitive impairment. *Continuum: Lifelong Learning in Neurology* 13(2):15–38.

Petersen, R.C., Doody, R., Kurz, A., Mohs, R.C., Morris, J.C., Rabins, P.V., Ritchie, K., Rossor, M., Thal, L., and Winblad, B. (2001) Current concepts in mild cognitive impairment. *Arch. Neurol.* 58(12):1985–1992.

Petersen, R.C., and O'Brien, J. (2006) Mild cognitive impairment should be considered for DSM-V. *J. Geriatr. Psychiatry Neurol.* 19(3):147–154.

Petersen, R.C., Parisi, J.E., Dickson, D.W., Johnson, K.A., Knopman, D.S., Boeve, B.F., Jicha, G.A., Ivnik, R.J., Smith, G.E., Tangalos, E.G., Braak, H., and Kokmen, E. (2006) Neuropathologic features of amnestic mild cognitive impairment. *Arch. Neurol.* 63(5):665–672.

Petersen, R.C., Smith, G.E., Ivnik, R.J., Tangalos, E.G., Schaid, D.J., Thibodeau, S.N., Kokmen, E., Waring, S.C., and Kurland, L.T. (1995) Apolipoprotein E status as a predictor of the development of Alzheimer's disease in memory-impaired individuals. *JAMA* 273(16):1274–1278.

Petersen, R.C., Smith, G.E., Waring, S.C., Ivnik, R.J., Tangalos, E.G., and Kokmen, E. (1999) Mild cognitive impairment: clinical characterization and outcome. *Arch. Neurol.* 56(3):303–308.

Petersen, R.C., Stevens, J.C., Ganguli, M., Tangalos, E.G., Cummings, J.L., and DeKosky, S.T. (2001) Practice parameter: early detection of dementia: mild cognitive impairment (an evidence-based review). Report of the Quality Standards Subcommittee of the American Academy of Neurology. *Neurology* 56(9):1133–1142.

Petersen, R.C., Thomas, R.G., Grundman, M., Bennett, D., Doody, R., Ferris, S., Galasko, D., Jin, S., Kaye, J., Levey, A., Pfeiffer, E., Sano, M., van Dyck, C.H., and Thal, L.J. (2005) Vitamin E and donepezil for the treatment of mild cognitive impairment. *N. Engl. J. Med.* 352(23):2379–2388.

Ray, S., Britschgi, M., Herbert, C., Takeda-Uchimura, Y., Boxer, A., Blennow, K., Friedman, L.F., Galasko, D.R., Jutel, M., Karydas, A., Kaye, J.A., Leszek, J., Miller, B.L., Minthon, L., Quinn, J.F., Rabinovici, G.D., Robinson, W.H., Sabbagh, M.N., So, Y.T., Sparks, D.L., Tabaton, M., Tinklenberg, J., Yesavage, J.A., Tibshirani, R., and Wyss-Coray, T. (2007) Classification and prediction of clinical Alzheimer's diagnosis based on plasma signaling proteins. *Nat. Med.* 13(11):1359–1362.

Reiman, E.M., Caselli, R.J., Yun, L.S., Chen, K., Bandy, D., Minoshima, S., Thibodeau, S.N., and Osborne, D. (1996) Preclinical evidence of Alzheimer's disease in persons homozygous for the epsilon 4 allele for apolipoprotein E. *N. Engl. J. Med.* 334(12):752–758.

Ritchie, K., Artero, S., and Touchon, J. (2001) Classification criteria for mild cognitive impairment: a population-based validation study. *Neurology* 56(1):37–42.

Rovio, S., Kareholt, I., Helkala, E.L., Viitanen, M., Winblad, B., Tuomilehto, J., Soininen, H., Nissinen, A., and Kivipelto, M. (2005) Leisure-time physical activity at midlife and the risk of dementia and Alzheimer's disease. *Lancet Neurol* 4(11):705–711.

Ryu, E.K., and Chen, X. (2008) Development of Alzheimer's disease imaging agents for clinical studies. *Front. Biosci.* 13:777–789.

Sano, M., Ernesto, C., Thomas, R.G., Klauber, M.R., Schafer, K., Grundman, M., Woodbury, P., Growdon, J., Cotman, C.W., Pfeiffer, E., Schneider, L.S., and Thal, L.J. (1997) A controlled trial of selegiline, alpha-tocopherol, or both as treatment for Alzheimer's disease. The Alzheimer's Disease Cooperative Study. *N. Engl. J. Med.* 336(17):1216–1222.

Sliwinski, M., Lipton, R.B., Buschke, H. and Stewart, W. (1996) The effects of preclinical dementia on estimates of normal cognitive functioning in aging. *J. Gerontol. B Psychol. Sci. Soc. Sci.* 51(4): P217–P225.

Sloane, P.D., Zimmerman, S., Suchindran, C., Reed, P., Wang, L., Boustani, M., and Sudha, S. (2002) The public health impact of Alzheimer's disease, 2000–2050: potential implication of treatment advances. *Annu. Rev. Public Health* 23:213–231.

Small, G.W., Kepe, V., Ercoli, L.M., Siddarth, P., Bookheimer, S.Y., Miller, K.J., Lavretsky, H., Burggren, A.C., Cole, G.M., Vinters, H.V., Thompson, P.M., Huang, S.C., Satyamurthy, N., Phelps, M.E., and Barrio, J.R. (2006) PET of brain amyloid and tau in mild cognitive impairment. *N. Engl. J. Med.* 355(25):2652–2663.

Small, G.W., Mazziotta, J.C., Collins, M.T., Baxter, L.R., Phelps, M.E., Mandelkern, M.A., Kaplan, A., La Rue, A., Adamson, C. F., Chang, L., et al. (1995) Apolipoprotein E type 4 allele and cerebral glucose metabolism in relatives at risk for familial Alzheimer disease. *JAMA* 273(12):942–947.

Smith, G.E., Petersen, R.C., Parisi, J.E., Ivnik, R.J., Tangalos, E., and Waring, S. (1996) Definition, course, and outcome of mild cognitive impairment. *Aging Neuropsychol. Cogn.* 3(2):141–147.

Stefani, A., Martorana, A., Bernardini, S., Panella, M., Mercati, F., Orlacchio, A., and Pierantozzi, M. (2006) CSF markers in Alzheimer disease patients are not related to the different degree of cognitive impairment. *J. Neurol. Sci.* 251(1/2):124–128.

Sunderland, T., Wolozin, B., Galasko, D., Levy, J., Dukoff, R., Bahro, M., Lasser, R., Motter, R., Lehtimaki, T., and Seubert, P. (1999) Longitudinal stability of CSF tau levels in Alzheimer patients. *Biol. Psychiatry* 46(6):750–755.

Teng, E.L., and Chui, H.C. (1987) The Modified Mini-Mental State (3MS) examination. *J. Clin. Psychiatry* 48(8):314–318.

Thal, L.J., Ferris, S.H., Kirby, L., Block, G.A., Lines, C.R., Yuen, E., Assaid, C., Nessly, M.L., Norman, B.A., Baranak, C.C., and Reines, S.A. (2005) A randomized, double-blind, study of rofecoxib in patients with mild cognitive impairment. *Neuropsychopharm.* 30(6):1204–1215.

Tierney, M.C., Szalai, J.P., Snow, W.G., Fisher, R.H., Tsuda, T., Chi, H., McLachlan, D.R., and St. George-Hyslop, P.H. (1996) A prospective study of the clinical utility of ApoE genotype in the prediction of outcome in patients with memory impairment. *Neurology* 46(1):149–154.

Unverzagt, F.W., Gao, S., Baiyewu, O., Ogunniyi, A.O., Gureje, O., Perkins, A., Emsley, C.L., Dickens, J., Evans, R., Musick, B., Hall, K.S., Hui, S.L., and Hendrie, H.C. (2001) Prevalence of cognitive impairment: data from the Indianapolis Study of Health and Aging. *Neurology* 57(9):1655–1662.

van de Pol, L.A., van der Flier, W.M., Korf, E.S., Fox, N.C., Barkhof, F., and Scheltens, P. (2007) Baseline predictors of rates of hippocampal atrophy in mild cognitive impairment. *Neurology* 69(15): 1491–1497.

van Oijen, M., Hofman, A., Soares, H.D., Koudstaal, P.J., and Breteler, M.M. (2006) Plasma Abeta(1–40) and Abeta(1–42) and the risk of dementia: a prospective case-cohort study. *Lancet Neurol.* 5(8):655–660.

Whitehouse, P.J., Price, D.L., Clark, A.W., Coyle, J.T., and DeLong, M.R. (1981) Alzheimer disease: evidence for selective loss of cholinergic neurons in the nucleus basalis. *Ann. Neurol.* 10(2): 122–126.

Winblad, B., Palmer, K., Kivipelto, M., Jelic, V., Fratiglioni, L., Wahlund, L.O., Nordberg, A., Backman, L., Albert, M., Almkvist, O., Arai, H., Basun, H., Blennow, K., de Leon, M., DeCarli, C., Erkinjuntti, T., Giacobini, E., Graff, C., Hardy, J., Jack, C., Jorm, A., Ritchie, K., van Duijn, C., Visser, P., and Petersen, R.C. (2004) Mild cognitive impairment—beyond controversies, towards a consensus: report of the International Working Group on Mild Cognitive Impairment. *J. Intern. Med.* 256(3):240–246.

65 | Frontotemporal Dementia

STEVEN Z. CHAO, INDRE VISKONTAS, AND BRUCE L. MILLER

Over a century ago, Prague neuropsychiatrist Arnold Pick (1851–1924) noted that some cases of dementia were caused by focal atrophy to the anterior portions of the brain and were not associated with a distributed neurodegeneration (Pick, 1892). In his paper "On the Relationship between Senile Cerebral Atrophy and Aphasia" (translated title), Pick reported a case of 71-year-old-man with progressive cognitive impairments, including deficits in language and aggressive behavior. Upon pathology, Pick found focal left temporal lobe atrophy. He was fascinated by the presence of a regional rather than diffuse neurodegeneration and the aphasia that followed. Twelve years later, Pick published descriptions of several more cases with combined behavioral and language disturbances with "circumscribed atrophies" (Pick, 1904). In the following decade, Alois Alzheimer observed swollen neurons and argyrophylic inclusions in a patient who showed a degenerative frontal cortical syndrome (Alzheimer, 1911). These inclusions later were called "Pick bodies." The clinical presentation and pathology continued to be characterized into the 1920s, when the first comprehensive description of what is now called "Pick's disease" was published (Gans, 1922; Onari and Spatz, 1926).

From the late 1920s until the 1980s, Pick's disease was largely ignored, as Alzheimer's disease (AD) usurped the vast majority of scientific resources devoted to the study of dementia. A resurgence of research into the non-Alzheimer's dementias began with a description by Marcel Mesulam of a series of patients with language deficits in the face of asymmetric degeneration of the left hemisphere: he named this disorder "primary progressive aphasia" (PPA) (Mesulam, 1982). Shortly thereafter, patients with progressive symmetric frontal atrophy were described, and eventually the term *frontotemporal dementia* (FTD) was applied to this disorder (Neary et al., 1986; Gustafson, 1987).

The clinical criteria for FTD were refined in the 1990s, first by the Lund-Manchester groups and later by an international consortium led by David Neary (The Lund and Manchester Groups, 1994; Neary et al., 1998). The Neary criteria renamed the disorder *frontotemporal lobar degeneration* (FTLD) and divided FTLD into three distinct subtypes: (*1*) *progressive nonfluent aphasia* (PNFA), in which patients show primarily deficits in verbal expression and predominantly left-frontal atrophy; (*2*) *frontotemporal dementia* (FTD), in which first symptoms are generally behavioral disturbances and atrophy is symmetrical and predominantly frontal; and (*3*) *semantic dementia* (SD), in which patients gradually loss access to semantic concepts (that is, meanings of words) and temporal atrophy.

EPIDEMIOLOGY

Previously considered a rare disease, in fact, FTLD is a relatively common condition and is the most common cause of early-onset (< 65 years of age) dementia (Ratnavalli et al., 2002; Knopman et al., 2004). The variability in clinical presentation, often psychiatric, and the lack of distinctive pathological markers contributed to the misdiagnosis and underdiagnosis of FTLD. Despite the recent improvements in antemortem diagnostic tools, the gold standard for diagnosis remains pathology.

In a study by Knopman and colleagues in Rochester, Minnesota, the incidence rates (new cases per 100,000 people) were 2.2 for people aged 40 to 49 years, 3.3 for people aged 50 to 59 years, and 8.9 for people aged 60 to 69 years. In comparison, the corresponding rates for AD were found to be 0.0, 3.3, and 8.9, respectively (Knopman et al., 2004). Similarly, researchers in the Netherlands found the prevalence of FTD (cases per 100,000 people) to be 3.6 in the 50 to 59 years age group, 9.4 for the 60 to 69 years age group, and 3.8 for the 70 to 79 years age group (Rosso et al., 2003). If the overlapping atypical parkinsonian syndromes such as progressive supranuclear palsy (PSP), cortical basal degeneration (CBD), and amyotrophic lateral sclerosis (ALS) are considered part of the spectrum of FTLD, the prevalence of the disorder greatly exceeds these conservative estimates.

Although FTLD most commonly presents in the sixties, up to one fourth of cases are patients older than the age of 65 (Rosso et al., 2003; Johnson et al., 2005). Progressive nonfluent aphasia typically presents slightly later than the other subtypes of FTLD, often in the seventies (Johnson et al., 2005). Frontotemporal lobar degeneration cases presenting anywhere from the thirties to nineties have been reported (Knopman et al.,

1990; Barker et al., 2002; Ratnavalli et al., 2002; Rosso et al., 2003; Johnson et al., 2005).

GENETICS

Frontotemporal lobar degeneration is strongly genetic, and in up to 40% of cases there is a family history of dementia; in approximately 10% of cases, an autosomal dominant inheritance pattern is suggested (Stevens et al., 1998; Chow et al., 1999; Goldman et al., 2005). The first association of FTLD with mutations on chromosome 17 was reported in 1994 (Lynch et al., 1994; Wilhelmsen et al., 1994), although the actual mutation was not found until 1998, when four groups reported that FTLD with parkinsonism was caused by mutations in the microtubule associated protein tau (MAPT) (Clark et al., 1998; Hutton et al., 1998; Spillantini et al., 1998; Poorkaj et al., 1998). Tau is a neuron-specific microtubule-associated protein that interacts with tubulin to stabilize and assemble microtubules. Mutated tau can cause disease by aggregating into various species of insoluble tau protein including the Pick body and the neurofibrillary tangle (Hasegawa et al., 1998; Neumann et al., 2001; Hayashi et al., 2002; Pickering-Brown et al., 2004). Alternatively, mutations can also cause impaired microtubule binding, assembly, or axonal transport (Hasegawa et al., 1998; Hong et al., 1998). Carriers of tau mutations generally show frontal/executive deficits on neuropsychological tests decades before the onset of dementia, raising the possible association of neurodevelopmental deficits with abnormal tau (Geschwind et al., 2001).

Recently mutations in the progranulin (*PGRN*) gene were found to account for many other genetic FTLD cases (Baker et al., 2006; Cruts et al., 2006; Gass et al., 2006). *PGRN* is widely expressed and is thought to be a secreted growth factor that plays a role in development and tumorogenesis. It is metabolized to granulin, a protein that is involved in wound repair and inflammation (He et al., 2003). So far, all pathogenic mutations have been found to be nonsense, splice-site, or frameshift mutations leading to premature coding termination and null alleles. The exact pathogenic mechanism remains unknown, but putative mechanisms include inadequate growth factor activity or an impairment in the inflammatory response (Baker et al., 2006). Although intraneuronal and cytoplasmic inclusions composed of the deoxyribonucleic acid (DNA)-binding protein TDP-43 are seen with PGRN mutations, a direct link between TDP-43 and progranulin has yet to be established (Baker et al., 2006; Neumann et al., 2006).

More than 40 mutations in MAPT and 44 mutations in *PGRN* have been described to date (Gass et al., 2006). Familial FTLD has also been associated with mutations of genes other than tau and *PGRN*. For example, mutations in the valosin protein have been linked to the FTD syndrome associated with Paget's disease and inclusion body myositis (Schroder et al., 2005). In addition, mutations in the ESCRTIII-complex subunit on chromosome 3 have been identified in one Dutch family with an FTD-like phenotype (Gydesen et al., 2002; Skibinski et al., 2005).

These mutations do not account for all of the familial cases of FTLD, as families with autosomal dominant patterns of inheritance linked to chromosome 17 (Wilhelmsen et al., 2004) and chromosome 9 (Hosler et al., 2000), but without MAPT or *PGRN* mutations, have been reported. The apolipoprotein ε4 (ApoE4) allele, strongly associated with AD, does not appear to be a strong risk factor for FTLD (Geschwind et al., 1998; Pickering-Brown et al., 2000).

CLINICAL SYNDROMES

As mentioned above, diagnostic criteria were first defined in 1994 by the Lund and Manchester groups and refined by an international consortium on FTD led by David Neary in 1998 (The Lund and Manchester Groups, 1994; Neary et al., 1998). The Neary criteria divided these syndromes into three clinical subtypes under the term *frontotemporal lobar degeneration* (FTLD). The three syndromes are frontotemporal dementia (FTD), in which early symptoms are primarily behavioral, and atrophy is generally focused bilaterally in the frontal lobes; semantic dementia (SD), which is characterized by a progressive loss of word meaning or the ability to recognize emotions and empathize with others, and either right or left asymmetrical anterior temporal lobe atrophy; and progressive nonfluent aphasia (PNFA), first symptoms of which include a progressive impairment in verbal fluency and word-finding, with early atrophy in the left-perisylvian region and in the left frontal and insular areas (Neary et al., 1998) (see Figure 65.1).

Although the classification of FTLD into three subtypes was initially undertaken to capture syndromes

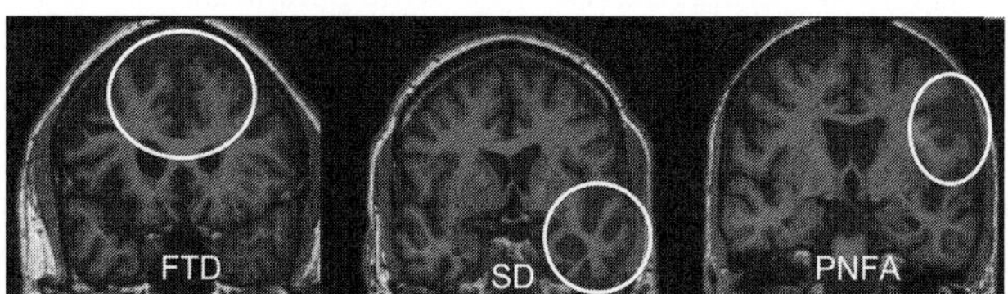

FIGURE 65.1 Heterogeneity of atrophy in FTLD subtypes. T1-weighted MRI scans (coronal slices) of three patients, each with a unique FTLD subtype. FTD patients shown primarily bilateral frontal atrophy, SD patients show asymmetric temporal lobe atrophy and PNFA patients show primarily left frontal atrophy. FTLD: frontotemporal lobar degeneration; MRI: magnetic resonance imaging; FTD: frontotemporal dementia; SD: semantic dementia; PNFA: progressive nonfluent aphasia.

that were presumed to have the same underlying neuropathology, differences at the molecular level between the subtypes are now emerging. For example, though patients with FTD are generally equally likely to have tau or ubiquitin-TDP-43 inclusions, patients with SD generally show ubiquitin inclusions whereas patients with PNFA are more likely to show tau inclusions, not ubiquitin, postmortem and usually present with symptoms that lead to a diagnosis of either CBD or PSP (Gorno-Tempini, Murray, et al., 2004; Roberson et al., 2005; Josephs et al., 2006).

FRONTOTEMPORAL DEMENTIA (FTD; FRONTAL-VARIANT FTLD)

Frontotemporal dementia is characterized by frontal lobe atrophy, resulting in prominent behavioral and personality changes. Cognitive impairments are typically less pronounced than behavioral changes in the early stages of the disease. Deficits in executive function are usually present by the time patients seek medical care, and patients are disorganized, inattentive, exhibit poor judgment, and have difficulty with planning, multitasking, and problem solving. When FTD affects dorsomedial prefrontal structures, patients become apathetic and passive and lose interest in personal affairs. Conversely, when the disease affects orbitofrontal and ventromedial frontal cortex, patients become disinhibited with an inappropriately euphoric affect (Miller et al., 1991; Neary et al., 1998; Rosen et al., 2002). In many patients, features of apathy and disinhibition are intermixed.

Many patients exhibit stereotyped and repetitive motor behaviors that are in many ways similar to those seen in patients with autism and schizophrenia, that is, rubbing, picking, clapping, and rocking (Mendez et al., 2005). Overeating and weight gain are common and characteristic features of FTD (Woolley et al., 2007). Patients may also have an uncontrollable urge to "use" objects in view. This use behavior may include grasping items within reach, repeatedly opening and closing doors, and switching lights on and off.

Given the dramatic behavioral and personality changes, patients frequently present to psychiatric clinics. Apathetic behavior is easily misjudged as a symptom of depression, and disinhibited behavior can be mistaken for mania (Gustafson, 1987). Delusions can be present, but hallucinations are rare. Suicidal ideations and guilt are uncommon in FTD (Perry and Miller, 2001).

Memory complaints can occur but are not typically presenting symptoms. In many cases, patients score normally on bedside screening tests such as the Mini-Mental State Examination (MMSE; Gregory et al., 1999) but show deficits on frontal/executive tasks upon comprehensive neuropsychological evaluations. These deficits include impairments in working memory, attention, verbal fluency, mental flexibility, response inhibition, and abstract reasoning. Verbal memory, spatial memory, and orientation are relatively spared in FTD (Kramer et al., 2003; Rosen et al., 2004; Neary et al., 2005). Therefore, impairment on frontal/executive tasks with relative preservation of memory or visuospatial function usually helps to differentiate FTD from AD.

Loss of empathy, coldness, emotional blunting, and abnormal nonverbal communication (for example, loss of facial expression and prosody) are early deficits in social behavior (Edwards-Lee et al., 1997; Rosen et al., 2002). In contrast, patients with AD usually show sparing of social skills until late into the course of the disease. Lack of insight is characteristic of most patients with FTD and some with patients with AD.

SEMANTIC DEMENTIA (SD; TEMPORAL-VARIANT FTLD)

Anatomically, SD is associated with progressive atrophy in anterior temporal asymmetrically either left or right. Clinically, patients with predominantly-left temporal atrophy show a profound anomia, progressively losing conceptual knowledge of words, whereas patients with right temporal atrophy lose the ability to recognize emotions in faces and empathize with others (Neary et al., 1998). The ratio of left to right temporal patients is around 3:1 (Thompson et al., 2003; Seeley et al., 2005).

Patients with predominantly left-sided atrophy present with a fluent, anomic aphasia, marked by word-finding difficulties and trouble naming objects, places, and people. Word meanings are lost, but the ability to read, write, and spell these words is retained. This word-meaning deficit follows a hierarchical pattern. First, patients lose specific exemplars of a category, such as poodle, beagle, and greyhound in the category "dogs"; next, the category name itself is lost, with "dogs" being referred to simply as animals; and finally, all categories are lost, and patients refer to all objects as "things." This anomic pattern in SD can be differentiated from anomia in AD, such that though patients with AD can generally describe some aspects of the object in question such as its function or features, patients with SD can no longer access any information about the item.

In most cases, recent episodic memory is preserved in the early stages of the disease, whereas memory for remote autobiographical events occurring in childhood or early adulthood may be lost. Upon neuropsychological evaluation, impairments in object naming, word-to-picture matching, surface dyslexia, and category fluency are observed. Episodic memory, spatial memory, executive functions, and orientation to time and place are relatively preserved early in the disease.

Like FTD, behavioral disturbances commonly develop with SD, probably reflecting the common orbitofrontal involvement of both syndromes (Rosen et al., 2006). Patients may develop visually oriented compulsions, such as collecting bright objects, and new artistic talents may emerge (Miller et al., 1998).

Patients with predominantly right-sided atrophy present with a behavioral syndrome characterized by flat affect, emotional blunting, and changes in social interactions. This pattern of symptoms is thought to result from deficits in emotion recognition (Rosen et al., 2002). Patients usually show a lack of insight. Many patients develop prosopagnosia (an inability to recognize faces) or associative agnosia (difficulty assigning meaning to an object; Neary et al., 1998). Patients may develop compulsions involving symbolic stimuli (for example, working on word puzzles or playing solitaire; Seeley et al., 2005). Loss of empathy is an early feature of the right temporal variant (Rankin et al., 2006).

Although patients initially show asymmetrical atrophy, regional degeneration becomes bilateral with disease progression. As atrophy spreads to the contralateral temporal lobe, patients show symptoms of right and left-sided SD (Seeley et al., 2005). Very late in the disease course, as degeneration encroaches upon frontal cortex, patients develop additional behavioral symptoms reminiscent of FTD (Liu et al., 2004).

PROGRESSIVE NONFLUENT APHASIA

Progressive nonfluent aphasia is characterized by deficits in verbal fluency. Anatomically, PNFA is characterized by left fronto-insular and perisylvian atrophy. Patients show decreased word output and shortened sentences. Commonly, agrammatism is observed, characterized by telegraphic speech. Reading is nonfluent and effortful, and writing is agrammatic and often riddled with phonemic errors. Many patients have trouble repeating multisyllabic, consonant-rich words, particularly those requiring an alternation between labial or coronal consonants, and dorsal, radical, or laryngeal consonants (for example, *artillery* or *Methodist Episcopal*). Patients retain the ability to produce single-syllable sounds. This apparent motor deficit speech production primary motor weakness is also known as *speech apraxia*.

In contrast to FTD, personal and interpersonal conduct, behavior, and insight are preserved early in PNFA. Spatial skills and short-term memory are also preserved until late in the course (Gorno-Tempini et al., 2004). Despite the dramatic change in the ability to communicate, many patients with PNFA continue to live and work independently, even late into the disease. Neuropsychological test performance in these patients is usually compromised by the aphasia. There may be a large discrepancy between cognitive test results and daily life function.

As the disease progresses, neurological examination may reveal rigidity, limb apraxia, up gaze palsies, or gait disturbance, all symptoms of PSP or CBD. Most patients with PNFA develop these syndromes, and all three are linked by tau pathology.

Frontotemporal Lobar Degeneration with Motor Neuron Disease

The relationship between dementia and motor neuron disease was first recognized more than a century ago, but only recently has the link between FTLD and ALS been studied comprehensively. Fueled by the discovery of overlapping genetics linking familial cases to chromosome 9 (Hosler et al., 2000), and common neuropathology (Cooper et al., 1995; Jackson et al., 1996) showing tau-negative, ubiquitin-positive inclusions, neurologists have defined an FTD-ALS syndrome. In a prospective study, up to 15% of patients with FTD had possible or probable ALS, and 50% of patients with ALS had measurable cognitive or behavioral symptoms of FTD, many of whom met criteria for an FTLD syndrome (Lomen-Hoerth et al., 2002; Lomen-Hoerth et al., 2003).

Patients with FTD-ALS may present with either cognitive or motor symptoms. Patients with bulbar-onset ALS may be at increased risk of developing dementia compared to patients with limb-onset ALS (Lomen-Hoerth et al., 2003). The presence of motor neuron disease significantly worsens the prognosis of FTLD (Hodges et al., 2003; Roberson et al., 2005).

DIAGNOSIS

As described above, diagnosis of FTLD is largely based on clinical presentation and careful neuropsychological evaluations, but definitive diagnosis requires pathology. Although several centers are in the process of developing effective antemortem diagnostic tools, the current criteria remain insufficient. There are ancillary tests that can help in making or excluding the diagnosis.

NEUROIMAGING

Structural neuroimaging with magnetic resonance imaging (MRI) has become an essential part of the evaluation of suspected FTLD. Unfortunately, very early in the disease MRI may fail to capture abnormalities, although with higher resolution scanners, normal MRI scans are rare (Miller et al., 1991). As the disease progresses, atrophy of frontal and anterior temporal structures is nearly universal (Miller and Gearhart, 1999).

As mentioned above, patients with FTD show predominantly bilateral frontal atrophy, throughout dorsolateral prefrontal cortex and medial premotor regions (Rosen et al., 2002). In SD, temporal lobe atrophy is usually asymmetric but can be either right or left sided. Patients with PNFA show selective atrophy in left frontoinsular cortex and the left perisylvian region. Patients with FTD/ALS usually present with atrophy in motor and premotor cortex, and sometimes in the anterior temporal lobes (Chang et al., 2005).

Functional imaging using Tc99-hexamethyl-propyleneamine (HMPAO)-spect and 2-deoxy-2-[18F] luorodeoxyglucose (18FDG) typically shows bifrontal hypoperfusion or hypometabolism (Miller et al., 1991; Hoffman et al., 2000), consistent with structural imaging findings. Functional imaging may be more sensitive than MRI early in the disease and is also helpful in differentiating FTLD from AD and other dementias.

Molecular imaging of amyloid with Pittsburgh compound B has shown significant promise in differentiating FTLD from AD, due to the fact that patients with FTLD normally do not have significant amyloid deposits.

CEREBROSPINAL FLUID

The basic cerebrospinal fluid (CSF) profile in FTLD is normal. Using levels of CSF beta-amyloid (Aβ) and unphosphorylated and phosphorylated tau, some investigators have found reasonable separations from AD and healthy controls. Although promising, these approaches will require better sensitivity and specificity (Grossman et al., 2007). Lumbar puncture should be pursued only to exclude infectious, inflammatory, or other conditions.

TREATMENT

Until recently, research into the diagnosis of FTLD was stymied by a paucity of treatment options. At this time, there is no proven pharmacotherapy available for FTLD or any of its associated diseases; however, animal models of FTLD have been recently developed, paving the way towards an effective treatment. At this time, treatment is focused on alleviating specific symptoms.

Symptomatic treatment for behavioral symptoms, including altered mood, impulsive behavior, and agitation, involves the administration of selective serotonin reuptake inhibitors (SSRIs), shown to be effective by improving behavior in small non-placebo-controlled studies (Swartz et al., 1997; Moretti et al., 2003). These findings were not replicated in one small placebo-controlled study (Deakin et al., 2004). Low-dose atypical neuroleptics (for example, quetiapine) are sometimes necessary to control aggressive behaviors, but these drugs should be used with caution as the Food and Drug Administration (FDA) has reported increased mortality in elderly patients. The co-association of extrapyramidal and motor neuron degeneration in FTD makes the atypical neuroleptics particularly worrisome. Memantine, a partial *N*-methyl-D-aspartate (NMDA)–antagonist used to treat AD, is under active investigation, and a therapeutic clinical trial is under way.

Besides the traditional pharmacotherapy, education and support for caregivers and families of patients with FTLD is monumental. Understanding the biological basis of inappropriate behaviors helps families come to terms with the disease. In FTD, impaired social interaction can result in the loss of independent living early in the disease. Anticipating the progression of illness can help families make difficult decisions (for example, transition to long-term-care facility living and end-of-life care) in a more gradual and controlled manner. In most cases, the patient relies heavily on others to survive and to minimize damage to his or her self or others. This causes significant physical and psychological stress to his or her caregivers. Participation in support groups can be very helpful. Caregivers of patients with dementia are at risk for depression and medical illness (Schulz et al., 1995), and regular help for the caregiver is essential. Patients with language deficits, such as those with SD or PNFA, should be referred to speech therapy and seek alternative communication devices. Caregiver and family education about aphasia helps to facilitate communication.

In protecting patients' socioeconomic integrity, the patient and family should be warned about the importance of avoiding situations in which a patient's poor judgment or impulsivity can have dire consequences (for example, driving, financial or political decision making; Perry and Miller, 2001). In the end stages of disease, the physician should guide families towards setting goals of care and making decisions according to the patient's wishes premorbidly.

REFERENCES

Alzheimer, A. (1911) Über eigenartige Krankheitsfälle des späteren Alters [On certain peculiar diseases of old age]. *Zeitschrift für die gesamte Neurologie und Psychiatrie* 4:356–385.

Baker, M., Mackenzie, I.R., Pickering-Brown, S.M., Gass, J., Rademakers, R., Lindholm, C., Snowden, J., Adamson, J., Sadovnick, A.D., Rollinson, S., Cannon, A., Dwosh, E., Neary, D., Melquist, S., Richardson, A., Dickson, D., Berger, Z., Eriksen, J., Robinson, T., Zehr, C., Dickey, C.A., Crook, R., McGowan, E., Mann, D., Boeve, B., Feldman, H., and Hutton, M. (2006) Mutations in progranulin cause tau-negative frontotemporal dementia linked to chromosome 17. *Nature* 442(7105):916–919.

Barker, W.W., Luis, C.A., Kashuba, A., Luis, M., Harwood, D.G., Loewenstein, D., Waters, C., Jimison, P., Shepherd, E., Sevush, S., Graff-Radford, N., Newland, D., Todd, M., Miller, B., Gold, M., Heilman, K., Doty, L., Goodman, I., Robinson, B., Pearl, G., Dickson, D., and Duara, R. (2002) Relative frequencies of Alzheimer disease, Lewy body, vascular and frontotemporal dementia, and hippocampal sclerosis in the State of Florida Brain Bank. *Alzheimer Dis. Assoc. Disord.* 16(4):203–212.

Benussi, L., Binetti, G., Sina, E., Gigola, L., Bettecken, T., Meitinger, T., and Ghidoni, R. (2008) A novel deletion in progranulin gene is associated with FTDP-17 and CBS. *Neurobiol. Aging* 29(3): 427–435.

Chan, D., Walters, R.J., Sampson, E.L., Schott, J.M., Smith, S.J., and Rossor, M.N. (2004) EEG abnormalities in frontotemporal lobar degeneration. *Neurology* 62(9):1628–1630.

Chang, J.L., Lomen-Hoerth, C., Murphy, J., Henry, R.G., Kramer, J.H., Miller, B.L., and Gorno-Tempini, M.L. (2005) A voxel-based morphometry study of patterns of brain atrophy in ALS and ALS/FTLD. *Neurology* 65(1):75–80.

Chow, T.W., Miller, B.L., Hayashi, V.N., and Geschwind, D.H. (1999) Inheritance of frontotemporal dementia. *Arch. Neurol.* 56(7):817–822.

Clark, L.N., Poorkaj, P., and Wszolek, Z. et al. (1998) Pathogenic implications of mutations in the tau gene in pallido-ponto-nigral degeneration and related neurodegenerative disorders linked to chromosome 17. *Proc. Natl. Acad. Sci. USA* 95(22):13103–13107.

Cooper, P.N., Jackson, M., Lennox, G., Lowe, J., and Mann, D.M. (1995) Tau, ubiquitin, and alpha B-crystallin immunohistochemistry define the principal causes of degenerative frontotemporal dementia. *Arch. Neurol.* 52(10):1011–1015.

Cruts, M., Kumar-Singh, S., and Van Broeckhoven, C. (2006) Progranulin mutations in ubiquitin-positive frontotemporal dementia linked to chromosome 17q21. *Curr. Alzheimer Res.* 3(5):485–491.

Deakin, J.B., Rahman, S., Nestor, P.J., Hodges, J.R., and Sahakian, B.J. (2004) Paroxetine does not improve symptoms and impairs cognition in frontotemporal dementia: a double-blind randomized controlled trial. *Psychopharmacol. (Berl)* 172(4):400–408.

Edwards-Lee, T., Miller, B.L., Benson, D.F., Cummings, J.L., Russell, G.L., Boone, K., and Mena, I. (1997) The temporal variant of frontotemporal dementia. *Brain* 120(6):1027–1040.

Gans, A. (1922) Betrachtungen über Art und Ausbreitung des krankhaften Prozesses in einem Fall von Pickscher Atrophie des Stirnhirns [Reflections on the nature and spread of diseased processes in the decline of Pick's atrophy of the frontal lobe]. *Zeitschrift für die gesamte Neurologie und Psychiatrie* 80:10–28.

Gass, J., Cannon, A., Mackenzie, I.R., Boeve, B., Baker, M., Adamson, J., Crook, R., Melquist, S., Kuntz, K., Petersen, R., Josephs, K., Pickering-Brown, S.M., Graff-Radford, N., Uitti, R., Dickson, D., Wszolek, Z., Gonzalez, J., Beach, T.G., Bigio, E., Johnson, N., Weintraub, S., Mesulam, M., White, C.L. III, Woodruff, B., Caselli, R., Hsiung, G.Y., Feldman, H., Knopman, D., Hutton, M., and Rademakers, R. (2006) Mutations in progranulin are a major cause of ubiquitin-positive frontotemporal lobar degeneration. *Hum. Mol. Genet.* 15(20):2988–3001.

Geschwind, D., Karrim, J., Nelson, S.F., and Miller, B. (1998) The apolipoprotein E epsilon4 allele is not a significant risk factor for frontotemporal dementia. *Ann. Neurol.* 44(1):134–138.

Geschwind, M., Rosen, H., Kramer, J., et al. (2001) Dementia in PSP—Subcortical or frontal? In: *53rd Meeting of the American Academy of Neurology, Abstract #1592*. Philadelphia, PA.

Goldman, J.S., Farmer, J.M., Van Deerlin, V.M., Wilhelmsen, K.C., Miller, B.L., and Grossman, M. (2004) Frontotemporal dementia: genetics and genetic counseling dilemmas. *Neurologist* 10(5): 227–234.

Goldman, J.S., Farmer, J.M., Wood, E.M., Johnson, J.K., Boxer, A., Neuhaus, J., Lomen-Hoerth, C., Wilhelmsen, K.C., Lee, V.M., Grossman, M., and Miller, B.L. (2005) Comparison of family histories in FTLD subtypes and related tauopathies. *Neurology* 65(11):1817–1819.

Gorno-Tempini, M.L., Dronkers, N.F., Rankin, K.P., Ogar, J.M., Phengrasamy, L., Rosen, H.J., Johnson, J.K., Weiner, M.W., and Miller, B.L. (2004) Cognition and anatomy in three variants of primary progressive aphasia. *Ann. Neurol.* 55(3):335–346.

Gorno-Tempini, M.L., Murray, R.C., Rankin, K.P., Weiner, M.W., and Miller, B.L. (2004) Clinical, cognitive and anatomical evolution from nonfluent progressive aphasia to corticobasal syndrome: a case report. *Neurocase* 10(6):426–436.

Gregory, C.A., Serra-Mestres, J., and Hodges, J.R. (1999) Early diagnosis of the frontal variant of frontotemporal dementia: how sensitive are standard neuroimaging and neuropsychologic tests? *Neuropsychiatry. Neuropsychol. Behav. Neurol.* 12(2):128–135.

Grossman, M., Wood, E.M., Moore, P., Neumann, M., Kwong, L., Forman, M.S., Clark, C.M., McCluskey, L.F., Miller, B.L., Lee, V.M., and Trojanowski, J.Q. (2007) TDP-43 pathologic lesions and clinical phenotype in frontotemporal lobar degeneration with ubiquitin-positive inclusions. *Arch. Neurol.* 64(10):1449–1454.

Gustafson, L. (1987) Frontal lobe degeneration of non-Alzheimer type. II. Clinical picture and differential diagnosis. *Arch. Gerontol. Geriatr.* 6(3):209–223.

Gydesen, S., Brown, J.M., Brun, A., Chakrabarti, L., Gade, A., Johannsen, P., Rossor, M., Thusgaard, T., Grove, A., Yancopoulou, D., Spillantini, M.G., Fisher, E.M., Collinge, J., and Sorensen, S. A. (2002) Chromosome 3 linked frontotemporal dementia (FTD-3). *Neurology* 59(10):1585–1594.

Hasegawa, M., Smith, M.J., and Goedert, M. (1998) Tau proteins with FTDP-17 mutations have a reduced ability to promote microtubule assembly. *FEBS Lett.* 437(3):207–210.

Hayashi, S., Toyoshima, Y., Hasegawa, M., Umeda, Y., Wakabayashi, K., Tokiguchi, S., Iwatsubo, T., and Takahashi, H. (2002) Late-onset frontotemporal dementia with a novel exon 1 (Arg5His) tau gene mutation. *Ann. Neurol.* 51(4):525–530.

He, Z., Ong, C.H., Halper, J., and Bateman, A. (2003) Progranulin is a mediator of the wound response. *Nat. Med.* 9(2):225–229.

Hodges, J.R., Davies, R., Xuereb, J., Kril, J., and Halliday, G. (2003) Survival in frontotemporal dementia. *Neurology* 61(3):349–354.

Hoffman, J.M., Welsh-Bohmer, K.A., Hanson, M., Crain, B., Hulette, C., Earl, N., and Coleman, R.E. (2000) FDG PET imaging in patients with pathologically verified dementia. *J. Nucl. Med.* 41(11): 1920–1928.

Hong, M., Zhukareva, V., Vogelsberg-Ragaglia, V., et al. (1998) Mutation-specific functional impairments in distinct tau isoforms of hereditary FTDP-17. *Science* 282(5395):1914–1917.

Hosler, B.A., Siddique, T., Sapp, P.C., Sailor, W., Huang, M.C., Hossain, A., Daube, J.R., Nance, M., Fan, C., Kaplan, J., Hung, W.Y., McKenna-Yasek, D., Haines, J.L., Pericak-Vance, M.A., Horvitz, H.R., and Brown, R.H., Jr. (2000) Linkage of familial amyotrophic lateral sclerosis with frontotemporal dementia to chromosome 9q21-q22. *JAMA* 284(13):1664–1669.

Hutton, M., Lendon, C.L., Rizzu, P., Baker, M., Froelich, S., Houlden, H., Pickering-Brown, S., Chakraverty, S., Isaacs, A., Grover, A., Hackett, J., Adamson, J., Lincoln, S., Dickson, D., Davies, P., Petersen, R.C., Stevens, M., de Graaff, E., Wauters, E., van Baren, J., Hillebrand, M., Joosse, M., Kwon, J.M., Nowotny, P., Heutink, P., et al. (1998) Association of missense and 5'-splice-site mutations in tau with the inherited dementia FTDP-17. *Nature* 393(6686):702–705.

Jackson, M., Lennox, G., and Lowe, J. (1996) Motor neuron disease-inclusion dementia. *Neurodegeneration* 5(4):339–350.

Johnson, J.K., Diehl, J., Mendez, M.F., Neuhaus, J., Shapira, J.S., Forman, M., Chute, D.J., Roberson, E.D., Pace-Savitsky, C., Neumann, M., Chow, T.W., Rosen, H.J., Forstl, H., Kurz, A., and Miller, B.L. (2005) Frontotemporal lobar degeneration: demographic characteristics of 353 patients. *Arch. Neurol.* 62(6): 925–930.

Josephs, K.A., Duffy, J.R., Strand, E.A., et al. (2006) Clinicopathological and imaging correlates of progressive aphasia and apraxia of speech. *Brain* 129(6):1385–1398.

Knopman, D.S., Mastri, A.R., Frey, W.H.D., Sung, J.H., and Rustan, T. (1990) Dementia lacking distinctive histologic features: a common non-Alzheimer degenerative dementia. *Neurology* 40(2): 251–256.

Knopman, D.S., Petersen, R.C., Edland, S.D., Cha, R.H., and Rocca, W.A. (2004) The incidence of frontotemporal lobar degeneration in Rochester, Minnesota, 1990 through 1994. *Neurology* 62:506–508.

Kramer, J.H., Jurik, J., Sha, S.J., Rankin, K.P., Rosen, H.J., Johnson, J.K., and Miller, B.L. (2003) Distinctive neuropsychological patterns in frontotemporal dementia, semantic dementia, and Alzheimer disease. *Cogn. Behav. Neurol.* 16(4):211–218.

Lebert, F., Stekke, W., Hasenbroekx, C., and Pasquier, F. (2004) Frontotemporal dementia: a randomised, controlled trial with trazodone. *Dement. Geriatr. Cogn. Disord.* 17(4):355–359.

Lee, V.M., Wilhelmsen, K.C., and Geschwind, D.H. (1999) From genotype to phenotype: a clinical pathological, and biochemical investigation of frontotemporal dementia and parkinsonism (FTDP-17) caused by the P301L tau mutation. *Ann. Neurol.* 45(6): 704–715.

Liu, W., Miller, B.L., Kramer, J.H., Rankin, K., Wyss-Coray, C., Gearhart, R., Phengrasamy, L., Weiner, M., and Rosen, H.J. (2004) Behavioral disorders in the frontal and temporal variants of frontotemporal dementia. *Neurology* 62(5):742–748.

Lomen-Hoerth, C., Anderson, T., and Miller, B. (2002) The overlap of amyotrophic lateral sclerosis and frontotemporal dementia. *Neurology* 59(7):1077–1079.

Lomen-Hoerth, C., Murphy, J., Langmore, S., Kramer, J.H., Olney, R.K., and Miller, B. (2003) Are amyotrophic lateral sclerosis patients cognitively normal? *Neurology* 60(7):1094–1097.

The Lund and Manchester Groups. (1994) Clinical and neuropathological criteria for frontotemporal dementia. *J. Neurol. Neurosurg. Psychiatry* 57(4):416–418.

Lynch, T., Sano, M., Marder, K.S., Bell, K.L., Foster, N.L., Defendini, R.F., Sima, A.A., Keohane, C., Nygaard, T.G., Fahn, S., et al. (1994) Clinical characteristics of a family with chromosome 17-linked disinhibition-dementia-parkinsonism-amyotrophy complex. *Neurology* 44(10):1878–1884.

Masellis, M., Momeni, P., Meschino, W., Heffner, R., Jr., Elder, J., Sato, C., Liang, Y., St. George-Hyslop, P., Hardy, J., Bilbao, J., Black, S., and Rogaeva, E. (2006) Novel splicing mutation in the progranulin gene causing familial corticobasal syndrome. *Brain* 129(Pt 11):3115–3123.

Mendez, M.F., Shapira, J.S., and Miller, B.L. (2005) Stereotypical movements and frontotemporal dementia. *Mov. Disord.* 20(6): 742–745.

Mesulam, M.M. (1982) Slowly progressive aphasia without generalized dementia. *Ann. Neurol.* 11(6):592–598.

Mesulam, M., Johnson, N., Krefft, T.A., Gass, J.M., Cannon, A.D., Adamson, J.L., Bigio, E.H., Weintraub, S., Dickson, D.W., Hutton, M.L., and Graff-Radford, N.R. (2007) Progranulin mutations in primary progressive aphasia: the PPA1 and PPA3 families. *Arch. Neurol.* 64(1):43–47.

Miller, B.L., Lesser, I.M., Boone, K.B., Hill, E., Mehringer, C.M., and Wong, K. (1991) Brain lesions and cognitive function in late-life psychosis. *Br. J. Psychiatry* 158:76–82.

Miller, B.L., Cummings, J., Mishkin, F., Boone, K., Prince, F., Ponton, M., and Cotman, C. (1998) Emergence of artistic talent in frontotemporal dementia. *Neurology* 51(4):978–982.

Miller, B.L., and Gearhart, R. (1999) Neuroimaging in the diagnosis of frontotemporal dementia. *Dement. Geriatr. Cogn. Disord.* 10(Suppl 1):71–74.

Moretti, R., Torre, P., Antonello, R.M., Cazzato, G., and Bava, A. (2003) Frontotemporal dementia: paroxetine as a possible treatment of behavior symptoms. A randomized, controlled, open 14-month study. *Eur. Neurol.* 49(1):13–19.

Neary, D., Snowden, J.S., Bowen, D.M., Sims, N.R., Mann, D.M., Benton, J.S., Northen, B., Yates, P.O., and Davison, A.N. (1986) Neuropsychological syndromes in presenile dementia due to cerebral atrophy. *J. Neurol. Neurosurg. Psychiatry* 49(2):163–174.

Neary, D., Snowden, J.S., Gustafson, L., Passant, U., Stuss, D., Black, S., Freedman, M., Kertesz, A., Robert, P.H., Albert, M., Boone, K., Miller, B.L., Cummings, J., and Benson, D.F. (1998) Frontotemporal lobar degeneration: a consensus on clinical diagnostic criteria. *Neurology* 51(6):1546–1554.

Neary, D., Snowden, J., and Mann, D. (2005) Frontotemporal dementia. *Lancet Neurol.* 4(11):771–780.

Neumann, M., Schulz-Schaeffer, W., Crowther, R.A., Smith, M.J., Spillantini, M.G., Goedert, M., and Kretzschmar, H.A. (2001) Pick's disease associated with the novel Tau gene mutation K369I. *Ann. Neurol.* 50(4):503–513.

Neumann, M., Sampathu, D.M., Kwong, L.K., Truax, A.C., Micsenyi, M.C., Chou, T.T., Bruce, J., Schuck, T., Grossman, M., Clark, C.M., McCluskey, L.F., Miller, B.L., Masliah, E., Mackenzie, I.R., Feldman, H., Feiden, W., Kretzschmar, H.A., Trojanowski, J.Q., and Lee, V.M. (2006) Ubiquitinated TDP-43 in frontotemporal lobar degeneration and amyotrophic lateral sclerosis. *Science* 314(5796):130–133.

Onari, K., and Spatz, H. (1926) Anatomische Beiträge zur Lehre von der Pickschen umschriebenen Grobhirnrinden-Atrophie ("Picksche Krankheit") [Anatomical contributions to the study of Pick's described brain degeneration ("Pick's Disease")]. *Zeitschrift für die gesamte Neurologie und Psychiatrie* 101:470–511.

Perry, R.J., and Miller, B.L. (2001) Behavior and treatment in frontotemporal dementia. *Neurology* 56(11 Suppl 4):S46–S51.

Pick, A. (1892) Über die Beziehungen der senilen Atrophie zur Aphasie [On the relationship between senile cerebral atrophy and aphasia]. *Prager Medizinische Wochenschrift* 17:165–167.

Pick, A. (1904) Zur Symptomatologie der linksseitigen Schläfenlappenatrophie [On the symptamatology of left temporal lobe atrophy]. *Monatsschrift für Psychiatrieund Neurologie* 16:378–388.

Pickering-Brown, S.M., Owen, F., Isaacs, A., Snowden, J., Varma, A., Neary, D., Furlong, R., Daniel, S.E., Cairns, N.J., Mann, and D.M. (2000) Apolipoprotein E epsilon4 allele has no effect on age at onset or duration of disease in cases of frontotemporal dementia with pick- or microvacuolar-type histology. *Exp. Neurol.* 163(2):452–456.

Pickering-Brown, S.M., Baker, M., Nonaka, T., Ikeda, K., Sharma, S., Mackenzie, J., Simpson, S.A., Moore, J.W., Snowden, J.S., de Silva, R., Revesz, T., Hasegawa, M., Hutton, M., and Mann, D.M. (2004) Frontotemporal dementia with Pick-type histology associated with Q336R mutation in the tau gene. *Brain* 127(Pt 6): 1415–1426.

Poorkaj, P., T.D. Bird, E. Wijsman, et al. (1998) Tau is a candidate gene for chromosome 17 frontotemporal dementia. *Ann. Neurol.* 43(6):815–825.

Rankin, K.P., Gorno-Tempini, M.L., Allison, S.C., Stanley, C.M., Glenn, S., Weiner, M.W., and Miller, B.L. (2006) Structural anatomy of empathy in neurodegenerative disease. *Brain* 129(11): 2945–2956.

Ratnavalli, E., Brayne, C., Dawson, K., and Hodges, J.R. (2002) The prevalence of frontotemporal dementia. *Neurology* 58(11): 1615–1621.

Roberson, E.D., Hesse, J.H., Rose, K.D., Slama, H., Johnson, J.K., Yaffe, K., Forman, M.S., Miller, C.A., Trojanowski, J.Q., Kramer, J.H., and Miller, B.L. (2005) Frontotemporal dementia progresses to death faster than Alzheimer disease. *Neurology* 65(5):719–725.

Rosen, H.J., Allison, S.C., Ogar, J.M., Amici, S., Rose, K., Dronkers, N., Miller, B.L., and Gorno-Tempini, M.L. (2006) Behavioral features in semantic dementia vs other forms of progressive aphasias. *Neurology* 67(10):1752–1756.

Rosen, H.J., Perry, R.J., Murphy, J., Kramer, J.H., Mychack, P., Schuff, N., Weiner, M., Levenson, R.L., and Miller, B.L. (2002) Emotion comprehension in the temporal variant of frontotemporal dementia. *Brain* 125:2286–2295.

Rosen, H.J., Narvaez, J.M., Hallam, B., Kramer, J.H., Wyss-Coray, C., Gearhart, R., Johnson, J.K., and Miller, B.L. (2004) Neuropsychological and functional measures of severity in Alzheimer disease, frontotemporal dementia, and semantic dementia. *Alzheimer Dis. Assoc. Disord.* 18(4):202–207.

Rosso, S.M., Donker Kaat, L., Baks, T., Joosse, M., de Koning, I., Pijnenburg, Y., de Jong, D., Dooijes, D., Kamphorst, W., Ravid, R., Niermeijer, M.F., Verheij, F., Kremer, H.P., Scheltens, P., van Duijn, C.M., Heutink, P., and van Swieten, J.C. (2003) Frontotemporal dementia in the Netherlands: patient characteristics and prevalence estimates from a population-based study. *Brain* 126(Pt 9):2016–2022.

Schroder, R., Watts, G.D., Mehta, S.G., Evert, B.O., Broich, P., Fliessbach, K., Pauls, K., Hans, V.H., Kimonis, V., and Thal, D.R. (2005) Mutant valosin-containing protein causes a novel type of frontotemporal dementia. *Ann. Neurol.* 57(3):457–461.

Schulz, R., O'Brien, A.T., Bookwala, J., and Fleissner, K. (1995) Psychiatric and physical morbidity effects of dementia caregiving: prevalence, correlates, and causes. *Gerontologist* 35(6):771–791.

Seeley, W.W., Bauer, A.M., Miller, B.L., Gorno-Tempini, M.L., Kramer, J.H., Weiner, M., and Rosen, H.J. (2005) The natural history of temporal variant frontotemporal dementia. *Neurology* 64(8):1384–1390.

Skibinski, G., Parkinson, N.J., Brown, J.M., Chakrabarti, L., Lloyd, S.L., Hummerich, H., Nielsen, J.E., Hodges, J.R., Spillantini, M. G., Thusgaard, T., Brandner, S., Brun, A., Rossor, M.N., Gade, A., Johannsen, P., Sorensen, S.A., Gydesen, S., Fisher, E.M., and Collinge, J. (2005) Mutations in the endosomal ESCRTIII-complex subunit CHMP2B in frontotemporal dementia. *Nat. Genet.* 37(8): 806–808.

Sparks, D., and Markesbery, W.R. (1991) Altered serotonergic and cholinergic synaptic markers in Pick's disease. *Arch. Neurol.* 48:796–799.

Spillantini, M.G., Murrell, J.R., Goedert, M., Farlow, M.R., Klug, A., and Ghetti, B. (1998) Mutation in the tau gene in familial multiple system tauopathy with presenile dementia. *Proc. Natl. Acad. Sci. USA* 95(13):7737–7741.

Stevens, M., van Duijn, C.M., Kamphorst, W., de Knijff, P., Heutink, P., van Gool, W.A., Scheltens, P., Ravid, R., Oostra, B.A., Niermeijer, M.F., and van Swieten, J.C. (1998) Familial aggregation in frontotemporal dementia. *Neurology* 50(6):1541–1545.

Swartz, J.R., Miller, B.L., Lesser, I.M., Booth, R., Darby, A., Wohl, M., and Benson, D.F. (1997) Behavioural phenomenology in Alzheimer's disease, frontotemporal dementia, and late-life depression: A retrospective analysis. *J. Geriatr. Psychiatry Neurol.* 10:67–74.

Thompson, S.A., Patterson, K., and Hodges, J.R. (2003) Left/right asymmetry of atrophy in semantic dementia: behavioral-cognitive implications. *Neurology* 61(9):1196–1203.

Valdmanis, P.N., Dupre, N., Bouchard, J.P., Camu, W., Salachas, F., Meininger, V., Strong, M., and Rouleau, G.A. (2007) Three families with amyotrophic lateral sclerosis and frontotemporal dementia with evidence of linkage to chromosome 9p. *Arch. Neurol.* 64(2):240–245.

Wilhelmsen, K., Lynch, T., Pavlou, E., et al. (1994) Localization of disinhibition-dementia-parkinsonism-amyotrophy complex to 17q21–22. *Am. J. Hum. Genet.* 6:1159–1165.

Wilhelmsen, K.C. (1997) Frontotemporal dementia is on the MAP-tau. *Ann. Neurol.* 41(2):139–140.

Wilhelmsen, K.C., Forman, M.S., Rosen, H.J., et al. (2004) 17q-linked frontotemporal dementia-amyotrophic lateral sclerosis without tau mutations with tau and alpha-synuclein inclusions. *Arch. Neurol.* 61(3):398–406.

Woolley, J.D., Gorno-Tempini, M.L., Seeley, W.W., Rankin, K., Lee, S.S., Matthews, B.R., and Miller, B.L. (2007) Binge eating is associated with right orbitofrontal-insular-striatal atrophy in frontotemporal dementia. *Neurology* 69(14):1424–1433.

66 | Vascular Dementia

NANCY NIELSEN-BROWN AND HELENA C. CHUI

Cerebrovascular disease (CBVD) accounts for the second largest group of dementias, either alone or in combination with Alzheimer's disease (AD). Unlike AD, vascular cognitive impairment/vascular dementia is not itself a disease. Vascular cognitive impairment is a syndrome or phenotype that results when vascular risk factors lead to CBVD, then to vascular brain injury that disrupts brain networks for memory and thinking. Vascular cognitive impairment encompasses all instances where cognitive impairment is attributed to CBVD and is greater than expected for normal aging. Vascular dementia is a subset of vascular cognitive impairment where the cognitive impairment is sufficiently severe to interfere with everyday social and occupational function. There is tremendous heterogeneity in the spectrum of vascular dementia: a host of risk factors, types of CBVD, types of brain injury, profiles of cognitive impairment (for example, dysexecutive syndrome, aphasia, neglect), behavioral symptoms (for example, depression, apathy), and clinical subtypes of vascular cognitive impairment.

It is a heterogeneous phenotype that may result from a variety of risk factors, blood vessel pathologies, types of vascular brain injury, and regional distribution of infarcts and hemorrhages. The spectrum of cognitive impairment due to vascular causes includes the following subtypes:

- *Mild vascular cognitive impairment:* Most frequent in elderly persons, this subtype comprises those with memory or other cognitive deficits who are within normal limits in activities of daily functioning. They may demonstrate evidence of silent or white matter changes on computed tomography (CT) or magnetic resonance imaging (MRI) scans.
- *Subcortical ischemic vascular dementia:* includes lacunar state, strategic infarct dementia, and Binswanger's syndrome. This group of dementias results from structural changes in the walls of small penetrating vessels, subsequent complete or incomplete infarction, and/or gliosis of the surrounding neuropil. A rare autosomal dominant subtype (cerebral autosomal dominant arteriopathy with subcortical infarcts and leukoencephalopathy, or CADASIL) develops multiple small infarcts in the thalamus, pons, basal ganglia, and white matter.
- *Lacunar infarct dementia:* a result of multiple small-vessel occlusions with resultant parenchymal cavitary lesions. These bilateral occlusions occur most frequently in the deep gray matter, internal capsule, and white matter. The ongoing progression of vascular damage leads to a progressive dementia.
- *Strategic infarct dementia:* occurs due to a single infarct in a strategic location such as the parietal lobe, thalamus, or the anterior cerebral artery circulation. Onset is usually abrupt.
- *Binswanger's syndrome:* is also termed *subcortical leukoencephalopathy*. Arterial degeneration and stenosis lead to widespread incomplete infarction of deep white matter. This is associated with chronic hypertension; therefore, small and larger vessels are affected, resulting in chronic hypoperfusion of the white matter. Due to the gradual increase in small vessel wall injury, cognitive decline in subcortical vascular dementias (SVDs) is slowly progressive. Thus, this type can often be mistaken for AD.
- *Cortical "multi-infarct" dementia:* occurs with infarcts of the cortex in more than one area, with associated neurological deficits on physical examination. These infarcts occur in large arteries and are therefore clinically characteristic of the hemisphere and the particular lobes affected. Signs include aphasia, apraxia, and motor deficits in addition to the memory deficit. The abrupt onset and "step-wise" pattern of deficits were characteristics identified early in dementia research to distinguish cortical dementia from AD, although a gradual, fluctuating course also occurs. Atherosclerosis and embolic sources from the heart or carotid arteries are major risk factors.
- *Poststroke dementia:* A single stroke may lead to dementia, or double the risk of developing subsequent dementia (Ivan et al., 2004). Preexisting cognitive impairment and risk factors for embolic stroke, such as atrial fibrillation or cardiac valvular disease, are frequent findings. The frequency of dementia is similar for hemorrhagic stroke as for ischemic stroke.

A glossary of terms related to vascular cognitive impairment is provided (Table 66.1).

PREVALENCE AND INCIDENCE

Estimates of prevalence and incidence of vascular dementia vary depending on the choice of criteria and

TABLE 66.1 *Glossary of Vascular Dementia Terminology*

AD	Alzheimer's disease: accelerated β-amyloidosis and tauopathy associated with progressive amnesia and cortical dementia
Arteriosclerosis	Pathologic term encompassing atherosclerosis and arteriolosclerosis
Atherosclerosis	Pathologic term referring to inflammatory, cholesterol lesion involving the intimal layer of large arteries with internal elastic lamina
Arteriolosclerosis	Pathologic term referring to hyaline degeneration of the smooth muscle of small arterioles (600–900 microns in diameter)
CAA	Cerebral amyloid angiopathy
CADASIL	Cerebral autosomal dominant arteriopathy with subcortical infarcts and leukoencephalopathy
CBVD	Cerebrovascular disease
	Disorders affecting blood circulation to the brain and transport of substrates across the blood brain barrier
Infarct	Pathologic term referring to loss of brain tissue due to ischemia
Lacune	French word for "hole." Used pathologically to include lacunar infarcts and dilated perivascular spaces
Leukoaraiosis	Rarefaction of the white matter noted on CT
MID	Multi-infarct dementia: Subtype of vascular dementia defined by multiple infarcts large and small
Silent infarct	Infarct (pathologically confirmed) or presumed infarct (on MRI) without history of corresponding neurological event
	Note: Silent stroke is oxymoron because stroke refers to a clinical event
Stroke	Clinical term for sudden loss of neurologic function due to cerebrovascular dysfunction
Stroke dementia	Subtype of vascular dementia which follows a symptomatic stroke
SVD	Subcortical vascular dementia: associated with vascular lesions apparently confined to white matter and subcortical gray matter
Symptomatic infarct	Infarct (pathologically confirmed) or presumed infarct (by characteristics on structural imaging) with corresponding history of sudden loss of neurological function
VaD	Vascular dementia
VCI	Vascular cognitive impairment: Cognitive impairment or dementia resulting from vascular brain injury
WMH	White matter hyperintensity
WML	White matter lesion
	Hyperintensities are the cerebral white matter visualized on T-2 weighted, proton density, or FLAIR MRI sequences

CT: computed tomography; MRI: magnetic resonance imaging; FLAIR: fluid-attenuated inversion recovery.

the use of neuroimaging. Currently, several consensus clinical criteria are in use for the diagnosis of vascular dementia, but there is no agreed-upon criteria for the diagnosis of mild vascular cognitive impairment. Modified versions of the dementia criteria have been proposed but are not yet widely in use, and prevalence and prognosis are under study (Frisoni et al., 2002). Magnetic resonance imaging often reveals unsuspected, subclinical evidence of vascular brain injury (for example, silent infarcts and deep white matter changes) in this group. Although the lifetime risk of stroke is greater than AD (Seshadri et al., 2006), incidence rates for vascular dementia following stroke are generally five- to tenfold less; about 25%–32% of persons meet criteria for dementia 3 months poststroke (Pohjasvaara et al., 1998; Desmond et al., 2000).

In epidemiological surveys, vascular dementia is identified as the second most common contributor to dementia after AD. Incidence rates for vascular dementia of 11 per 1,000 person years among persons older than 65 years have been reported in two recent epidemiological surveys (Fitzpatrick et al., 2004; Ravaglia et al., 2005). No differences in rates of incident dementia were noted for patients with small- versus large-vessel stroke (Desmond et al., 2002). Ethnic comparisons in the Cardiovascular Health Study showed nearly twofold higher incidence rates among African Americans compared to Whites (Fitzpatrick et al., 2004). On the other hand, five-fold lower rates were reported in a retrospective study of Whites living in Rochester, Minnesota (Knopman et al., 2002). The wide ranges in incidence rates of vascular dementia may reflect differences in ethnicity, socioeconomic status, and study methodology.

Cross sectional studies have observed that 26%–32% of patients hospitalized for stroke meet *Diagnostic and Statistical Manual of Mental Disorders*, 3rd ed., rev.

(*DSM-III*: American Psychiatric Association [APA], 1987) criteria for dementia (Pohjasvaara et al., 1998; Desmond et al., 2000). Incidence of stroke dementia can be determined by selecting stroke patients who are dementia free at baseline, matching them to a stroke-free control group, and following them prospectively. In the Framingham study, 20% of stroke cases dementia free at baseline compared to 11% of the controls developed dementia during 10 years of follow-up (hazard ratio [HR]: 2.0, 95% confidence interval [CI]: 1.4–2.9) (Ivan et al., 2004). Even higher incident rates were reported in the Columbia Stroke Study (Desmond et al., 2002): crude incident rate of dementia was 8.49 per 100 person years in the stroke group versus 1.37 cases in a stroke-free control group (relative risk [RR]: 3.83, 95% CI: 2.14–6.84).

DIAGNOSIS

The diagnosis of vascular cognitive impairment is developed sequentially by considering clinical, neuropsychological, imaging, and pathologic findings. A history of vascular risk factors, the presence of focal neurological signs, and the presence of vascular lesions on neuroimaging are key elements in the diagnosis. Currently, the clinical diagnosis of vascular dementia is based on first- or second-generation consensus criteria. As a first step toward developing a third-generation approach to the diagnosis of vascular cognitive impairment, guidelines to improve harmonization of data collection were published (Hachinski et al., 2006).

Clinical Diagnosis of Mild Vascular Cognitive Impairment (VCI)

As mild cognitive impairment may be a prodrome to vascular dementia (Meyer et al., 2002; Laukka et al., 2004; Ingles et al., 2007), patients with vascular mild cognitive impairment need to be identified and risk factors modified early. There is an increased risk of dementia following stroke in these patients not present in matched patients suffering stroke without mild vascular cognitive impairment (Gamaldo et al., 2006). Unlike the mild cognitive impairment (MCI) with predominant amnesia that precedes AD, there are no agreed upon criteria for mild vascular cognitive impairment (VCI). Severity of memory impairment is generally not as severe in mild VCI as in AD, and responds better to cueing or recognition. Otherwise, the pattern of cognitive domains affected in mild VCI may vary greatly, depending upon the location of vascular brain injury. Criteria for mild VCI include objective evidence of memory, executive, language, visual-spatial impairment, or slowing in psychomotor speed without impairment in work or activities of daily living. Patients with mild VCI are typically aware of the deficit and seek evaluation.

Clinical Diagnosis of Subcortical Ischemic Vascular Dementia

Lacunar infarcts represent approximately 25% of symptomatic ischemic strokes. The accumulation of small infarcts in the deep white and gray matter may lead to SVD, also referred to as *lacunar state*, *strategic infarct dementia*, or *Binswanger's syndrome*. A single strategically placed symptomatic infarct (for example, in the anterior or dorsomedial thalamus, genu of the internal capsule) can lead to the dementia syndrome, by disrupting frontal-subcortical loops. Criteria have also been proposed for the SVD subtype of VCI (Erkinjuntti et al., 2000); these criteria emphasize slowing of cognition, executive dysfunction, depression, extrapyramidal signs, and gait disturbance. The *dysexecutive syndrome* refers to impairment of selective attention, abstract reasoning, and mental flexibility. In SVD, memory impairment is variable, less severe, and more likely to respond to cueing than is noted in Alzheimer's dementia.

Subcortical lacunar infarct dementia is characterized by impaired memory and executive functions, slowing of information processing, and alterations in personality and affect. The apathy, depression, and behavioral changes may be more prominent than the cognitive deficits. Physical examination findings include parkinsonian gait disturbances, sudden hemiparesis, dysarthria, pseudobulbar palsy, and incontinence. Prefrontal lobe lesions lead to behavioral signs including a lack of volition and akinetic mutism.

Strategic infarct dementia

Bilateral infarction in the distribution of the paramedian thalamic artery is associated with a dementia syndrome. At times, a single paramedian branch arising from the basilar artery often supplies anteromedial thalamic regions. The dementia syndrome associated with such strategic infarcts is characterized by marked apathy, impaired attention and mental control, and anterograde and retrograde amnesia (Bogouslavsky et al., 1988), a picture characteristic of executive dysfunction.

Binswanger's syndrome

Binswanger's syndrome refers to the combination of severe, confluent, deep white matter changes, together with a slowly progressive decline in cognition and gait. The white matter changes are postulated to result from chronic hypoperfusion, incomplete infarction, and demyelination in periventricular and deep white border zones.

The clinical features of Binswanger's syndrome include insidiously progressive dementia, persistent hypertension or systemic vascular disease, lengthy clinical course with long plateaus, and accumulation of focal neurologic signs, including asymmetric weakness, pyramidal signs, pseudobulbar palsy, and gait disturbance. The neurobehavioral features of Binswanger's syndrome include apathy, lack of drive, mild depression, and alterations of mood (Bennett et al., 1990). The periods of slowly progressive dementia may be mistaken for AD. The presence of gait disturbance, urinary incontinence, and ventriculomegaly may be mistaken for normal pressure hydrocephalus, although on neuroimaging, cerebral atrophy and widening of the cortical sulci distinguish Binswanger's syndrome.

Clinical Diagnosis of Cortical Vascular "Multi-infarct" Dementia

For several decades, the Hachinski ischemic score (HIS) (Hachinski et al., 1975) and later the *DSM* served as the mainstays for the diagnosis of multi-infarct dementia. Early guidelines did not distinguish cortical from subcortical subtypes. Guidelines for interpreting neuroimaging findings were incorporated into at least four new sets of criteria for vascular dementia, published from 1990 to 1995. These second-generation criteria require three basic elements for a diagnosis of vascular dementia: (*1*) evidence of dementia or cognitive impairment, (*2*) evidence of vascular brain injury, and (*3*) presumptive evidence of a causal relationship between cognitive impairment and vascular brain injury.

The criteria differ in the way they operationalize each of these three diagnostic elements (Table 66.2). The traditional and, later, modified HIS relies on a characteristic phenotype (for example, the presence of an abrupt onset, focal neurological symptoms and signs, and hypertension) (Hachinski et al., 1975), rather than explicitly assessing causal relationship. The National Institute of Neurological Disorders and Stroke and Association Internationale pour la Recherché et l'Enseignement en Neurosciences (NINDS-AIREN) criteria (Román et al., 1993) are conservative at each level, requiring (*1*) evidence of impairment in memory plus two other cognitive domains, (*2*) evidence of CBVD (that is, focal neurological signs and infarcts/white matter changes on neuroimaging), and (*3*) onset of dementia within 3 months of stroke. The Alzheimer's Disease Diagnostic and Treatment Centers (ADDTC) criteria (Chui et al., 1992) are more liberal, as they (*1*) do not require prominent memory disturbance, (*2*) do not require focal neurological signs, and (*3*) allow either one infarct with a temporal relationship to onset of cognitive impairment or evidence of two infarcts outside of the cerebellum as sufficient evidence for a diagnosis of probable ischemic vascular dementia. The *DSM-IV* (APA, 1994) and *International Classification of Diseases*, 10th rev. (*ICD-10*; World Health Organization, 1993) criteria do not operationalize criteria for causality, leaving the individual clinician to decide whether there is "significant cerebrovascular disease that is judged to be etiologically related to the disturbance."

Although the criteria follow a common motif, they lead to different patient classifications and are not interchangeable. A patient meeting ADDTC criteria for probable ischemic vascular dementia often will not meet NINDS-AIREN criteria for probable vascular dementia. Among 480 cases of incident dementia in the Cardiovascular Health Study Cognition Study, the number of cases classified as probable vascular dementia by ADDTC, *DSM-IV*, and NINDS-AIREN criteria were 117, 62, and 42, respectively (Lopez et al., 2005). The NINDS-AIREN criteria have been most widely adopted in pharmacological drug trials.

Mixed Alzheimer's disease/vascular dementia

The possibility of concomitant AD often clouds the relationship between vascular brain ischemia and cognitive impairment. The likelihood of CBVD and AD increases with age, and in autopsy studies, mixed pathology is frequently found in older individuals.

At the present time, there is little consensus on how to identify and classify mixed AD/vascular dementia cases in a clinical setting. The National Institute of Neurological and Communicative Disorders and Stroke–Alzheimer Disease and Related Disorders Association (NINDS-ARDRA)(McKhann et al., 1984) criteria for AD downgrade the diagnosis from probable to possible AD in the presence of an alternate etiology, which might contribute to the dementia. The NINDS-AIREN criteria for vascular dementia were developed for epidemiologic surveys and expressly discourage a diagnosis of mixed AD/vascular dementia. In contrast, the ADDTC criteria support a mixed diagnosis by allowing the clinician to make a diagnosis of probable/possible AD and/or vascular cognitive impairment on their own independent merits. A neurobehavioral approach to diagnosis may also be taken:

1. Consider the pattern and severity of cognitive impairment (memory, executive, or other disturbance of higher cognitive function).
2. Consider the size and location of vascular ischemia (symptomatic infarcts, silent infarcts, white matter changes).
3. Consider the severity and pattern of atrophy (hippocampus, frontal, temporal, parietal).

TABLE 66.2 *Clinical Criteria for Vascular Dementia (VaD)*

Diagnostic Criteria		*Dementia*	*VBI*		*Evidence of causal relationship*
Hachinski ischemic score (HIS; Hachinski et al., 1975) (Total: 0–18 points) HIS ≥ 7 suggests MID HIS 5–6 suggests MIX HIS ≤ 4 suggests AD		No specific criteria.	2 points: Abrupt onset, fluctuating course, history of stroke, focal neurologic symptoms, focal neurologic signs 1 point: Stepwise progression, nocturnal confusion, relative preservation of personality, depression, somatic complaints, emotional incontinence, hypertension, atherosclerosis		Not required
DSM-IV (APA, 1994)		Memory loss sufficient to interfere with everyday function. No clouding of consciousness.	Stepwise deteriorating course and "patchy" distribution of deficits Focal neurologic signs and symptoms		Evidence from the history, physical examination, or laboratory tests of significant cerebrovascular disease that is judged to be etiologically related to the disturbance
ICD-10 (WHO, 1993)		Unequal distribution of deficits in higher cognitive functions, with some affected and others relatively spared.	There is evidence of focal brain damage, manifest as at least one of the following: Unilateral spastic weakness of the limbs, unilaterally increased tendon reflexes, an extensor plantar response, pseudobulbar palsy		From the history, examination, or test, there is evidence of significant cerebrovascular disease, which may reasonably be judged to be etiologically related to the dementia (history of stroke, evidence of cerebral infarction)
ADDTC (Chui et al., 1992)	Probable	Multifaceted cognitive impairment sufficient to interfere with customary affairs of life.	Two or more strokes or infarct outside cerebellum by imaging		Or 1 infarct with temporal relationship to onset of cognitive impairment
	Possible		1 infarct outside cerebellum by imaging or confluent white matter change CHS ≥ 7		Not required
NINDS-AIREN (Román et al., 1993)	Probable	Memory loss plus impairment in two other cognitive domains.	Focal signs on neurologic exam	Imaging findings of VBI	And onset of dementia within 3 months following a recognized stroke or abrupt deterioration in cognitive function or fluctuating, stepwise progression of cognitive deficits
	Possible			Either imaging findings or temporal relationship or abrupt onset or stepwise. Fluctuating course.	

VBI: vascular brain injury; HIS: Hachinski ischemic score; MID: Multi-infarct dementia; MIX: Mixed Alzheimer/vascular dementia; AD: Alzheimer's disease; *DSM-IV*: *Diagnostic and Statistical Manual of Mental Disorders*, 4th ed.; *ICD*: *International Classification of Diseases*, 10th rev.; ADDTC: Alzheimer's Disease Diagnostic and Treatment Centers; NINDS-AIREN: National Institute of Neurological Disorders and Stroke Association International pour la Recherché et l'Enseignement en Neurosciences; CHS: Cardiovascular Health Study.

4. Assess the extent to which vascular brain ischemia can explain the severity and pattern of cognitive impairment.

5. If vascular brain ischemia cannot adequately explain the cognitive impairment, consider the likelihood that AD is also present.

Clinical Diagnosis of Poststroke Dementia

The clinical findings in poststroke dementia are often overshadowed by the motor and sensory neurologic deficits of the stroke. The type (hemorrhagic or ischemic) or location of the stroke were not found to be determinants of poststroke dementia (Barba et al., 2000). A history of preexisting cognitive impairment should be sought with all patients admitted for stroke, as it is a risk factor for subsequent dementia.

Neuropsychological Evaluation of Vascular Cognitive Impairment/Vascular Dementia

There is no single cognitive impairment profile that characterizes VCI. Attention and executive function, language and visuospatial abilities, memory, and learning may be affected in various degrees and combinations, related to the size and location of vascular injury. The domains most often impaired include abstraction, mental flexibility, information processing speed, and working memory (Desmond et al., 2000), with verbal memory, especially retention, being somewhat less affected (Sachdev et al., 2004a). Sachdev et al. (2004b) concluded that the picture of VCI in stroke/transient ischemic attack (TIA) patients shows subcortical deficits embellished by cognitive deficits from cortical infarctions.

• Middle cerebral artery strokes are associated with aphasia (dominant hemisphere) and neglect (nondominant hemisphere).
• Anterior cerebral artery syndromes produce apathy, abulia, and akinetic mutism.
• Posterior cerebral artery syndromes are characterized by amnesia, anomia, and agnosia.
• Subcortical infarcts and deep white matter changes tend to disrupt frontal-subcortical networks and are associated with a subcortical dementia or dysexecutive syndrome.

In keeping with such heterogeneity, neuropsychological protocols must be sensitive to a wide range of cognitive impairments. The Folstein Mini-Mental State Examination (MMSE), though a fairly good screening instrument for AD, does not assess speed or executive function and is relatively insensitive to SVD. The Modified MMSE (3MS) redresses some of these issues by adding verbal fluency, similarities, and cued-recall items. The Neuropsychological Working Group for Vascular Cognitive Impairment Harmonization Standards (Hachinski et al., 2006) has recommended long-, intermediate-, and short-assessment protocols, which take 60, 30, or 5 minutes, respectively, to administer (Table 66.3). Instruments to assess neurobehavioral change and mood, which often accompany VCI, are also suggested.

Neuroimaging of Vascular Cognitive Impairment/ Vascular Dementia

Magnetic resonance imaging or CT confirm the size and location of symptomatic strokes and detect many forms of silent ischemic and hemorrhagic vascular brain injury. Microinfarcts fall below the threshold of detection, even for MRI, and are discovered primarily at autopsy. Anoxic brain injury manifests as diffuse atrophy without discrete areas of hyperintensity or encephalomalacia. Thus, though MRI is essential for the state-of-the-art clinical evaluation of vascular cognitive impairment, it does not disclose all forms of vascular injury.

TABLE 66.3 *Proposed 60-Minute, 30-Minute, and 5-Minute Neuropsychological Protocols*

Domain	*60 Minute*	*30 Minute*	*5 Minute*
Screening Test	MMSE	(Supplemental: MMSE)	
Semantic Fluency	Animal Naming	Animal Naming	
Phonemic Fluency	Controlled Oral Word Association	Controlled Oral Word Association	1-letter phonemic fluency
Association Test	Digit Symbol Substitution (WAIS-III)	Digit Symbol Substitution (WAIS-III)	
Association Test	Trail Making	(Supplemental: Trail Making)	
Memory and Learning	Hopkins Verbal Learning Test–Revised (Alternate: California Verbal Learning Test–2)	Hopkins Verbal Learning Test–Revised	5-word memory task (registration, recall, recognition) 6-item orientation
Language/Lexical Retrieval	Boston Naming Test – second ed., short form (Supplemental: BNT Recognition)		
Visual-Spatial	Rey Osterrieth Complex Figure copy (Supplemental: Memory) (Supplemental: Digit Symbol Coding Incidental Learning) Future Use: Simple and Choice Reaction Time		
Mood		Depression Scale Center for Epidemiologic Studies	
Behavior		Neuropsychiatric Inventory (NPI-Q)	
Activities of Daily Living	IQ-CODE		

Source: Hachinski et al., 2006.
MMSE: Mini-Mental State Examination; WAIS: Wechsler Adult Intelligence Scale; BNT: Boston Naming Test; IQ-CODE: Informant Questionnaire on Cognitive Decline in the Elderly; NPI-Q: Neuropsychiatric Inventory Brief Questionnaire Form.

TABLE 66.4 *Key MRI Measures and Their Clinical Significance*

MRI Lesion	*MRI Measure*	*Clinical Significance*
Silent infarcts	The location of discrete infarcts and SI in areas strategically important for cognition should be sought.	Strategic locations include: head of caudate Anterior and dorsomedial thalamus Genu and anterior limb of the internal capsule. Multimodal association cortex.
White matter hyperintensities	Quantitative volumes or semiquantitative rating scales are recommended for grading WMH, and the likely contribution of WMH grade to cognitive impairment should be assessed.	Changes in bedside mental status scores do not usually become apparent until there is severe, confluent WMH (CHS grade ≥ 7).
Microhemorrhages		Numerous microhemorrhages on T-2* weighted MRI suggest small vessel angiopathy (e.g., due to hypertension, CAA, or CADASIL).
Hippocampal atrophy/volume	Quantitative volumes or semiquantitative rating scales are recommended for grading hippocampal atrophy.	Hippocampal atrophy is characteristic of AD but is also associated with hippocampal sclerosis.
Cerebral cortical atrophy/ volume	Quantitative volumes or semiquantitative rating scales are recommended for grading cerebral cortical atrophy.	Cerebral atrophy correlates with global cognition and predicts regardless of the etiological subtype, and can be associated with pure VBI without AD.

MRI: magnetic resonance imaging; SI: silent infarcts; WMH: white matter hyperintensities; CHS: Cardiovascular Health Study; CAA: cerebral amyloid angiopathy; CADASIL: cerebral autosomal dominant arteriopathy with subcortical infarcts and leukoencephalopathy; AD: Alzheimer's disease; VBI: vascular brain injury.

Key MRI measures and their clinical significance are summarized in Table 66.4.

Symptomatic infarcts

Among patients with symptomatic stroke, a corresponding cortical or subcortical lesion can usually be found on CT or MRI. Cortical infarcts typically appear as wedge-shaped lesions that conform either to the distribution of a single occluded artery or to the border zone between two arteries. Subcortical or lacunar infarcts are round lesions, ranging in size from 3 to 15 mm in diameter, in the distribution of small penetrating arterioles. Acute infarcts are bright on diffusion weighted images. Over time, macrophages clear necrotic brain tissue, and the infarct becomes cystic.

Silent infarcts

Among elderly persons without a clinical history of stroke, small discrete lesions > 3 mm in diameter may be seen in the subcortical gray and white matter. On MRI, they are hyperintense on T-2, proton density, and fluid-attenuated inversion recovery (FLAIR) sequences and variably hypointense on T-1 weighted images. Although there have been few pathologic studies to confirm their underlying histology, these lesions are generally labeled *silent infarcts*. The prevalence of silent infarcts increases with age and hypertension (Longstreth et al., 2002; Vermeer et al., 2002). Silent infarcts are associated with increased risk of stroke and cognitive impairment (Vermeer, Den Heijer, et al., 2003; Vermeer, Prins, et al., 2003).

Dilated perivascular spaces

Dilated perivascular spaces or Virchow–Robin spaces should be distinguished from silent infarcts. In general, perivascular spaces appear isointense relative to cerebrospinal fluid (CSF), whereas silent infarcts appear hyperintense to CSF on proton density or FLAIR MRI. Two exceptions should be noted: (*1*) cystic infarcts, which are usually > 1 cm in size, may have isointense centers and (*2*) giant perivascular spaces (up to 1 cm) may be found below the putamen, adjacent to lateral portion of the anterior commissure (Pullicino et al., 1995).

White matter hyperintensities

Diffuse hyperintensities on proton density, T-2 weighted, or FLAIR MRI are observed frequently in the periventricular and deep white matter of asymptomatic as well as symptomatic elderly persons. On CT, corresponding areas of decreased attenuation or rarefaction are labeled "leukoaraiosis." The deep cerebral white matter is susceptible to hypoperfusion, as these regions depend for their blood supply upon long, high resistance, end-arterioles. Widespread stenosis of these arterioles, most commonly due to arteriolosclerosis, places the deep white matter at ischemic risk (O'Sullivan et al., 2002). Severe white matter hyperintensities are associated pathologically with progressive loss of myelin and later axons (Yamanouchi, 1991). Associations between white matter hyperintensities and hypertension, stroke, and executive processing speed are now well-established by cross-sectional and longitudinal data (Longstreth et al., 2005; Prins et al., 2005). For clinical practice, semiquantitative rating scales, such as Age-Related White Matter Change (ARWMC) (Wahlund et al., 2001) or Cardiovascular Health Study (CHS) (Yue et al., 1997) white matter hyperintensity scales, can be used, but with a caveat. The semiquantitative rating scales show ceiling effects, and the highest score is assigned well before white matter hyperintensities, volumes have plateaued (van Straaten et al., 2006).

Microhemorrhages

Gradient-echo (GE) or T-2 weighted MRI are capable of detecting millimeter-sized paramagnetic blood products, including hemosiderin stored in macrophages, associated with leakage of small blood vessels in the basal ganglia or subcortical white matter. Microbleeds appear as rounded hypointense foci < 5 mm that are located in the brain parenchyma. They should be distinguished from vascular flow voids, leptomeningeal hemosiderosis, and subcortical mineralization. Because of "blooming" of magnetic susceptibility effects, microhemorrhages are magnified on GE sequences and appear larger than their actual tissue size. Microhemorrhages are associated with hypertension and CADASIL (Viswanathan and Chabirat, 2006).

Hippocampal atrophy

The most common cause of medial temporal lobe or hippocampal atrophy in late life is AD-type neurofibrillary degeneration. However, hippocampal atrophy may also result from hippocampal sclerosis. In the setting of late-life dementia, as opposed to early- or mid-life medial temporal lobe epilepsy, atrophy-related to hippocampal sclerosis is not accompanied by hyperintensity on T-2 or FLAIR sequences. Because AD and hippocampal sclerosis are characterized by amnesia and hippocampal atrophy, the clinical differentiation remains challenging. In patients with clinical diagnosis of AD, subcortical ischemic vascular dementia (SIVD), and normal aging, hippocampal volume is correlated with learning and memory, explaining 44% of the variance (Mungas et al., 2001). In the absence of concomitant hippocampal sclerosis, hippocampal volume is generally preserved in cases with VCI (Zarow et al., 2005). Hippocampal volume is best quantified using computerized algorithms. However, for clinical practice, semiquantitative rating scales (for example, Scheltens' rating of medial temporal lobe atrophy; Korf et al., 2004) may be used.

Cortical atrophy

Diffuse cerebral cortical atrophy is a typical hallmark of AD but is associated with other causes of dementia, including CBVD. Cortical gray matter atrophy is correlated with the overall severity of cognitive impairment (Mungas et al., 2001) and predicts longitudinal rate of cognitive decline (Mungas et al., 2005). Cortical gray matter volume is best quantified by computerized segmentation algorithms. Several semiquantitative rating scales have also been adopted (Manolio et al., 1994) but have not been widely adopted in clinical practice.

Pathologic Diagnosis of Vascular Cognitive Impairment

At the present time, there are no agreed-upon criteria for the pathologic diagnosis of VCI/vascular dementia. Variability and heterogeneity in the type, distribution, and severity of vascular brain ischemia has impeded the development of a staging instrument for VCI/vascular dementia, akin to the Braak and Braak staging for neurofibrillary degeneration or the Consortium to Establish a Registry for Alzheimer's Disease (CERAD) neuritic plaque score used for the neuropathologic diagnosis of AD. As for clinical and imaging data, efforts are now being made to standardize the collection of pathology data (Hachinski et al., 2006). Recent studies including the Nun Study, Oxford Project to Investigate Memory and Aging (OPTIMA), Honolulu Asia Aging Study, and the Religious Orders Study indicate that brain infarction and AD contribute additively to cognitive impairment. So far, the data do not show that these effects are multiplicative or synergistic; however, given the vast heterogeneity of vascular brain injury, it is plausible to predict variability and range in the strength of interactions between CBVD and AD.

Neuropathologic examination provides a sensitive and independent measure of vascular brain injury and

- confirms or newly detects vascular brain injury, especially for lesions that fall below the threshold of detection by neuroimaging (for example, incomplete infarction, selective neuronal loss, microinfarcts).
- confirms or identifies the type of underlying CBVD (for example, atherosclerosis, arteriolosclerosis, CADASIL).
- ascertains the presence and extent of AD pathology.

A meta-analysis of the HIS for 312 autopsied cases with dementia showed the best cutoff scores to distinguish multi-infarct dementia from AD was as originally proposed (HIS ≥ 7 for multi-infarct dementia; HIS ≤ 4 for Alzheimer's dementia); the diagnosis of the mixed dementia remained difficult (Moroney et al., 1997). Gold et al. (2002) compared the four new clinical criteria against a pathologic diagnosis of vascular dementia for 89 autopsy cases. In this study, vascular dementia was defined pathologically by the presence of cortical infarcts in at least three areas, exclusive of primary and secondary visual cortices. (Note: In this study, vascular lesions confined to subcortical structures were not considered sufficient for a diagnosis of vascular dementia.) In general, the clinical criteria proved to be highly specific but relatively insensitive, suggesting that current clinical criteria underestimate the extent of actual ischemic brain injury.

PROGNOSIS

The two types of outcomes considered in this chapter are mortality and rate of cognitive decline. The discussion below includes population studies, longitudinal cohort studies, and pharmacological trials for vascular dementia rather than milder forms of VCI. In general, mortality is greater in vascular dementia than AD, though rate of cognitive decline is slower. Magnetic resonance imaging findings hold promise for individualizing prognosis and incorporating the combined effects of AD and CBVD.

Mortality

In the 1990s, mortality associated with vascular dementia and AD was reported in several large, Scandinavian, community-based studies. In a study of incident dementia among persons older than 75 years, mortality was higher for persons with vascular dementia compared to persons with AD, with mean survival times of 2.8 years (95% CI: 2.2–3.4) and 3.1 years (95% CI: 2.8–3.5), respectively (Agüero-Torres et al., 1999). Within the vascular dementia group, excess mortality was higher for men and for cases with more severe dementia and functional disability. These differences most likely reflect the effects of more severe cardiovascular comorbidity and physical disability in vascular dementia compared to the AD group. Similarly, in a retrospective study in Rochester, Minnesota, cases with vascular dementia showed 50% survival rates of 3–4 years and a twofold higher mortality risk than AD (Knopman et al., 2003). Within the vascular dementia group, there was a relative protective effect associated with antiplatelet/anticoagulant medication and higher diastolic blood pressure. Treatment of vascular risk factors may narrow the differential mortality rates between AD and vascular dementia.

Cognitive decline

Community vascular dementia studies. Cognitive decline was assessed in a 7-year follow-up of a representative sample of elderly persons with dementia living in Kungsholmen, Sweden (Agüero-Torres et al., 1998). In the initial prevalence survey, 225 cases of dementia were identified, including 121 AD, 52 vascular dementia, and 80 other dementias. During the first 3-year follow-up period, the average annual rate of change on the MMSE was greater for AD (–2.75, 95% CI: –3.32–2.18, $n = 51$) than vascular dementia (–1.75, 95% CI: –2.67–0.85, $n = 19$). A diagnosis of AD, greater functional disability, and greater cognitive impairment predicted greater cognitive decline.

Hospital-based stroke cohort studies. In a 1-year follow-up study of the first 151 patients in the Columbia-Presbyterian Stroke Cohort, neuropsychological performance improved for some individuals (Desmond et al., 1996). Probability of improvement was 54% for a patient with left hemisphere stroke or major hemispheral syndrome but only 12% for patients with diabetes mellitus. The reason for poorer prognosis in the latter group is not clear but may be related to more widespread and progressive small-vessel CBVD associated with diabetes.

In an African American stroke cohort followed with annual neuropsychological testing for up to 7 years, slower rate of cognitive decline was reported for vascular dementia or stroke without dementia (SWD) compared to AD (Nyenhuis et al., 2002). On the MMSE, the mean annual decline was –0.87 points for the vascular dementia ($n = 79$) and –0.20 for SWD ($n = 56$), compared to –1.86 for AD ($n = 113$). In the Sidney Stroke Study (Sachdev et al., 2004b), patients with stroke had a mean decline of –0.83 points on the MMSE, compared to an increase of +0.76 for controls. The occurrence of an interval stroke significantly increased the mean decline in MMSE to –2.0 points. Thus, among patients with stroke, baseline dementia and intercurrent stroke are associated with greater rate of cognitive decline.

TREATMENT

At the present time, there is no specific tool to assess risk for VCI or risk of recurrent stroke. Careful attention to vascular risk factors, such as hypertension or cardiac disease, is essential. The Framingham Stroke Risk Profile is a useful tool to estimate the 10-year risk for stroke for men and women aged 55–80 years old, based on age, systolic blood pressure, diabetes, smoking, cardiovascular disease, atrial fibrillation, and left ventricular hypertrophy (Wolf et al., 1991; D'Agostino et al., 1994). The Stroke Profile Score is based on a good history, blood pressure, and electrocardiogram. The score can be recalculated after the patient embarks on a risk-reduction treatment plan and differentiates the risk associated with untreated and treated hypertension. The literature suggests that diabetes mellitus (Desmond et al., 2000) may be particularly salient to cognitive impairment associated with CBVD. Principles of supportive care to optimize quality of life are similar and equally important for families with vascular dementia as for families with AD.

Tertiary Amelioration (Symptomatic and Supportive Care)

Tertiary amelioration refers to symptomatic improvement of cognition, behavior, or mood. Several agents have shown modest efficacy on cognitive function in randomized controlled clinical trials of vascular dementia. These agents include piracetam, oxiracetam, nicergoline, citicoline, pentoxyfylline, propentofylline, nimodipine, triflusal, and gingko biloba (for review, see Kaye, 2002). The efficacy and safety of the calcium antagonist nimodipine versus placebo was studied in 230 patients with SVD (Pantoni et al., 2005). At 52 weeks, no significant differences were noted in the Sandoz Clinical Assessment Geriatric, but there were fewer dropouts and adverse events in the nimodipine group, suggesting a possible beneficial effect on cardiovascular comorbidity. In a study of mild to moderate vascular dementia (N = 321), 20 mg/day of memantine, a noncompetitive *N*-methyl-D-aspartate (NMDA) receptor antagonist, was associated with improved cognition, stabilization of global function and behavior, and good tolerance and safety (Orgogozo et al., 2002).

Cholinesterase inhibitors have been studied in vascular dementia as well as in AD. Erkinjuntti et al. (2002) reported a 2.7 point difference in the Alzheimer Disease Assessment Scale (ADAS-cog) in the galantamine ($n = 396$) versus placebo ($n = 196$) in patients with probable vascular dementia or AD/CBVD. Auchus et al. (2007) reported that VaD patients treated with galantamine ($n = 396$) showed greater improvement in ADAS-cog than in placebo group ($n = 390$) (–1.8 vs. –0.3). Similarly, Pratt et al. (2002; $N = 893$) and Wilkinson et al. (2003; $N = 616$) reported approximately a 2-point benefit in a randomized, double-blind, placebo-controlled, 24-week study of donepezil among patients with probable vascular dementia (for review, see Román et al., 2005). By way of caveat, a meta-analysis undertaken by Kavirajan and Schneider (2007) showed increased mortality associated with donepezil (odds ratio [OR]: 1.44, 95% CI: 0.68–3.02; $p = .04$) in two of three vascular dementia trials.

Attention should be paid to affective and behavioral symptoms in vascular dementia. Depression and apathy are common affective symptoms associated with vascular dementia. Selective serotonin reuptake inhibitors (SSRIs) are generally well tolerated and effective. The older tricyclic antidepressants can also be effective but are less well tolerated; those with significant anticholinergic side effects (for example, amitriptyline) should be avoided. Agitation, psychotic symptoms, and disruptive behavior occur less commonly in vascular dementia than in AD. Because vascular dementia may be accompanied by extrapyramidal signs, antipsychotic medications may increase imbalance and risk of falls. Atypical antipsychotic medications with fewer extrapyramidal side effects (for example, respiridone, olanzepinem, quetiapine) may be considered but should be monitored carefully. A proactive, interdisciplinary, and holistic approach should be taken to address risk reduction, patient safety, advanced directives, palliative care, and quality of life.

REFERENCES

Agüero-Torres, H., Fratiglioni, L., Guo, Z., Viitanen, M., and Winblad, B. (1998) Prognostic factors in very old demented adults: A seven-year follow-up from a population-based survey in Stockholm. *J. Am. Geriatr. Soc.* 46:444–452.

Agüero-Torres, H., Fratiglioni, L., Guo, Z., Viitanen, M., and Winblad, B. (1999) Mortality from dementia in advanced age: A 5-year follow-up study of incident dementia cases. *Clin. Epidmiol.* 52: 737–743.

American Psychiatric Association. (1987) *Diagnostic and Statistical Manual of Mental Disorders*, 3rd ed., rev. Washington, DC: Author.

American Psychiatric Association. (1994) *Diagnostic and Statistical Manual of Mental Disorders*, 4th ed. Washington, DC: Author.

Auchus, A.P., Brashear, H.R., Salloway, S., Korczyn, A.D., De Deyn, P.P., and Gassmann-Mayer, C., for the GAL-INT-26 Study Group. (2007) Galantamine treatment of vascular dementia. A randomized trial. *Neurology* 69:448–458.

Barba, R., Martínez-Espinosa, S., Rodríguez-García, E., Pondal, M., Vivancos, J., and Del Ser, T. (2000) Poststroke dementia: clinical features and risk factors. *Stroke* 31:1494–1501.

Bennett, D.A., Wilson, R.S., Gilley, D.W., and Fox, J.H. (1990) Clinical diagnosis of Binswanger's disease. *J. Neurol. Neurosurg. Psychiatry* 53:961–965.

Bogouslavsky, J., Regli, F., and Uske, A. (1988) Thalamic infarcts: clinical syndrome, etiology and prognosis. *Neurology* 38:837–848.

Chui, H.C., Victoroff, J.I., Margolin, D., Jagust, W., Shankle, R., and Katzman, R. (1992) Criteria for the diagnosis of ischemic vascular dementia proposed by the State of California Alzheimer Disease Diagnostic and Treatment Centers (ADDTC). *Neurology* 42:473–480.

D'Agostino, R.B., Wolf, P.A., Belanger, A.J., and Kannel, W.B. (1994) Stroke risk profile: Adjustment for anti-hypertensive medication: The Framingham Study. *Stroke* 25:40–43.

Desmond, D.W., Moroney, J.T., Paik, M.C., et al. (2000) Frequency and clinical determinants of dementia after stroke. *Neurology* 54:1124–1131.

Desmond, D.W., Moroney, J.T., Sano, M., and Stern, Y. (2002) Incidence of dementia after ischemic stroke: Results of a longitudinal study. *Stroke* 33:2254–2262.

Desmond, D.W., Moroney, J.T., Sano, M., and Stern, Y. (1996) Recovery of cognitive function after stroke. *Stroke* 27:1798.

Erkinjuntti, T., Inzitari, D., Pantoni, L., Wallin, A., Scheltens, P., Rockwood, K., Roman, G.C., Chui, H., and Desmond, D.W. (2000) Research criteria for subcortical vascular dementia in clinical trials. *J. Neural Transm.* 59:23–30.

Erkinjuntti, T., Kurz, A., Gauthier, S., Bullock, R., Lilienfeld, S., Damaraju, C.V. (2002) Efficacy of galantamine in probable vascular dementia and Alzheimer's disease combined with cerebrovascular disease: a randomized trial. *Lancet* 359:1283–1290.

Fitzpatrick, A.L., Kuller, L.H., Ives, D.G., et al. (2004) Incidence and prevalence of dementia in the Cardiovascular Health Study. *Am. Geriatr. Soc.* 52:195–204.

Frisoni, G.B., Galluzzi, S., Bresciani, L., Zanetti, O., and Geroldi, C. (2002) Mild cognitive impairment with subcortical vascular features—Clinical characteristics and outcome. *J. Neurol.* 249: 1423–1432.

Gamaldo, A., Moghekar, A., Kilada, S., Resnick, S.M., Zonderman, A.B., and O'Brien, R. (2006) Effect of a clinical stroke on the risk of dementia in a prospective cohort. *Neurology* 67:1363–1369.

Gold, G., Bouras, C., Canuto, A., Bergallo, M.F., Herrmann, F.R., Hof, P.R., Mayor, P.-A., Michel, J.-P., and Giannakopoulos, P. (2002) Clinicopathological validation study of four sets of clinical criteria for vascular dementia. *Am. J. Psychiatry* 159:82–87.

Hachinski, V., Iadecola, C., Petersen, R.C., et al. (2006) National Institute of Neurological Disorders and Stroke—Canadian Stroke Network Vascular Cognitive Impairment Harmonization Standards. *Stroke* 37:2220–2241.

Hachinski, V.C., Iliff, L.D., Zilkha, E., et al. (1975) Cerebral blood flow in dementia. *Arch. Neurol.* 32:632–637.

Ingles, J.L., Boulton, D.C., Fisk, J.D., and Rockwood, K., (2007) Preclinical vascular cognitive impairment and Alzheimer disease. *Stroke* 38:1148–1153.

Ivan, C.S., Seshadri, S., Beiser, A., et al. (2004) Dementia after stroke: The Framingham Study. *Stroke* 35:1264–1269.

Kavirajan, H., and Schneider, L.S. (2007) The efficacy and adverse effects of cholinesterase inhibitors and memantine in vascular dementia: a systematic review and meta-analysis of controlled trials. *The Lancet Neurology*, 6:782–792.

Kaye, J. (2002) Treatment of vascular dementia. In: Qizilbash, N., Schneider, L.S., Chui, H., Tariot, P., Brodaty, H., Kaye, J., and Erkinjuntti, T., eds. (2002) *Evidence-Based Dementia Practice.* Oxford, UK: Blackwell Science, pp. 589–607.

Knopman, D., Rocca, W.A., Cha, R.H., et al. (2003) Survival study of vascular dementia in Rochester, Minnesota. *Arch. Neurol.* 60:85–90.

Knopman, D.S., Rocca, W.A., Cha, R.H., Edland, S.D., and Kokmen, E. (2002) Incidence of vascular dementia in Rochester, MN, 1985–1989. *Arch. Neurol.* 59:1605–1610.

Korf, E.S.C., Wahlund, L.-O., Visser, P.J., and Scheltens, P. (2004) Medial temporal lobe atrophy on MRI predicts dementia in patients with mild cognitive impairment. *Neurology* 63:94–100.

Laukka, E.J., Jones, S., Fratiglioni, L., and Bäckman, L. (2004) Cognitive functioning in preclinical vascular dementia: a 6-year follow-up. *Stroke* 35:1805–1809.

Longstreth, W.T., Jr., Dulberg, C., Manolio, T.A., Lewis, M.R., Beauchamp, N.J., Jr., O'Leary, D., Carr, J., and Furberg, C.D. (2002) Incidence, manifestations, and predictors of brain infarcts by serial cranial magnetic resonance imaging in the elderly: the Cardiovascular Health Study. *Stroke* 33:2376–2382.

Longstreth, W.T., Arnold, A., Beauchamp, N.J., et al. (2005) Incidence, manifestations, and predictors of worsening white matter on serial cranial magnetic resonance imaging in the elderly: the Cardiovascular Health Study. *Stroke* 36:56–61.

Lopez, O.L., Kuller, L.H., Becker, J.T., Jagust, W.J., DeKosky, S.T., Fitzpatrick, A., Breitner, J., Lyketsos, C., Kawas, C., and Carlson, M. (2005) Classification of vascular dementia in the Cardiovascular Health Study Cognition Study. *Neurology* 64:1539–1547

McKhann, G., Drachman, D., Folstein, M., Katzman, R., Price, D., Stadlan, E. (1984) Clinical diagnosis of Alzheimer's disease: Report of the NINCDS-ADRDA Work Group under the auspices of Department of Health and Human Services Task Force on Alzheimer's Disease. *Neurology* 34:939–944.

Manolio, T.A., Kronmal, R.A., Burke, G.L., Poirer, V., O'Leary, D. H., Gardin, J.M., Fried, L.P., Steinberg, E.P., and Bryan, R.N. (1994) Magnetic resonance abnormalities and cardiovascular disease in older adults. The Cardiovascular Health Study. *Stroke* 25:318–327.

Meyer, J.S., Xu, G., Thornby, J., Chowdhury, M.H., and Quach, M. (2002) Is mild cognitive impairment prodromal for vascular dementia like Alzheimer's disease? *Stroke* 33:1981–1985.

Moroney, J.T., Bagiella, E., Desmond, D.W., et al. (1997) Meta-analysis of the Hachinski Ischemic Store in pathologically verified dementias. *Neurology* 49:1096–1105.

Mungas, D., Harvey, D., Reed, B.R., Jagust, W.J., DeCarli, C., Beckett, L., Mack, W.J., Kramer, J.H., Weiner, M.W., Schuff, N., and Chui, H.C. (2005) Longitudinal volumetric MRI change and rate of cognitive decline. *Neurology* 65:565–571.

Mungas, D., Jagust, W.J., Reed, B.R., Kramer, J.H., Weiner, M.W., Schuff, N., Norman, D., Mack, W.J., Willis, L., and Chui, H.C. (2001) MRI predictors of cognition in subcortical ischemic vascular disease and Alzheimer disease. *Neurology* 57:2229–2235.

Nyenhuis, D.L., Gorelick, P.B., Freels, S., and Garron, D.C. (2002) Cognitive and functional decline in African Americans with vascular dementia, AD, and stroke without dementia. *Neurology* 58:56–61.

O'Sullivan, M., Jarosz, J.M., Martin, R.J., Deasy, N., Powell, J.F., and Markus, H.S. (2001) MRI hyperintensities of the temporal lobe and external capsule in patients with CADASIL. *Neurology* 56:628–634.

O'Sullivan, M., Lythgoe, D.J., Pereira, A.C., Summers, P.E., Jarosz, J.M., Williams, S.C.R., and Markus, H.S. (2002) Patterns of cerebral blood flow reduction in patients with ischemic leukoaraiosis. *Neurology* 59:321–326.

Orgogozo, J.M., Rigaud, A.-S., Stoffler, A., Mobius, H.J., and Forette, F. (2002) Efficacy and safety of memantine patients with mild to moderate vascular dementia: a randomized placebo controlled trial (MMM 300). *Stroke* 33:1834–1839.

Pantoni, L., del Ser, T., Soglian, A.G., Amigoni, S., Spadari, G., Binelli, D., and Inzitari, D. (2005) Efficacy and safety of nimodipine in subcortical vascular dementia: a randomized placebo-controlled trial. *Stroke* 36:619–624.

Pohjasvaara, T., Erkinjuntti, T., Ylikoski, R., Hietanen, M., Vataja, R., and Kaste, M. (1998) Clinical determinants of post-stroke dementia. *Stroke* 29:75–81.

Pratt, R.D., Perdomo, C.A., and the Donepezil VaD 307 and 308 Study Groups. (2002) Donepezil-treated patients with probable vascular dementia demonstrate cognitive benefits. *Ann. NY Acad. Sci.* 977:513–522.

Prins, N.D., van Dijk, E.J., den Heijer, T., Vermeer, S.E., Jolles, J., Koudstaal, P.J., Hofman, A., and Breteler, M.M. (2005) Cerebral small-vessel disease and decline in information processing speed, executive function and memory. *Brain* 128:2034–2041.

Pullicino, P.M., Miller, L.L., Alexandrov, A., and Ostrow, P.T. (1995) Infraputaminal "lacunes." Clinical and pathological correlations. *Stroke* 26:1598–1602.

Ravaglia, G., Forti, P., Maioli, F., et al. (2005) Incidence and etiology of dementia in a large elderly Italian population. *Neurology* 64:1525–1530.

Román, G.C., Tatemichi, T.K., Erkinjuntti, T., et al. (1993) Vascular dementia: diagnostic criteria for research studies. Report of the NINDS-AIREN International Workshop. *Neurology* 43: 250–260.

Román, G.C., Wilkinson, D.G., Doody, R.S., Black, S.E., Salloway, S.P., Schindler, R.J. (2005) Donepezil in vascular dementia: combined analysis of two-large scale clinical trials. *Dement. Geriatr. Cogn. Disord.* 20:338–344.

Sachdev, P.S., Brodaty, H., Valenzuela, M.J., Lorentz, L., Looi, J.C.L., Wen, W., and Zagami, A.S. (2004a) The neuropsychological profile of vascular cognitive impairment in stroke and TIA patients. *Neurology* 62:912–919.

Sachdev, P.S., Brodaty, H., Valenzuela, M.J., Lorentz, L., Koschera, A. (2004b) Progression of cognitive impairment in stroke patients. *Neurology* 63:1618–1623.

Seshadri, S., Beiser, A., Kelly-Hayes, M., Kase, C.S., Au, R., Kannel, W.B., and Wolf, P.A. (2006) The lifetime risk of stroke: estimates from the Framingham Study. *Stroke* 37:345–350.

Van Straaten, E.C., Fazekas, F., Rostrup, E., Scheltens, P., Schmidt, R., Pantoni, L., Inzitari, D., Waldemar, G., Erkinjuntti, T., Mantyla, R., Wahlund, L.O., LADIS Group, and Barkhof, F. (2006) Impact of white matter hyperintensities scoring method on correlations with clinical data: the LADIS study. *Stroke* 37:836–840.

Vermeer, S.E., Den Heijer, T., Koudstaal, P.J., Oudkerk, M., Hofman, A., and Breteler, M.M. (2003) Incidence and risk factors of silent brain infarcts in the population-based Rotterdam Scan Study. *Stroke* 34:392–396.

Vermeer, S.E., Koudstaal, P.J., Oudkerk, M., Hofman, A., and Breteler, M.M. (2002) Prevalence and risk factors of silent brain infarcts in the population-based Rotterdam Scan Study. *Stroke* 33:21–25.

Vermeer, S.E., Prins, N.D., den Heijer, T., Hofman, A., Koudstaal, P.J., and Breteler, M.M. (2003) Silent brain infarcts and the risk of dementia and cognitive decline. *N. Engl. J. Med.* 348:1215–1222.

Viswanathan, A., and Chabirat, H. (2006) Cerebral microhemorrhages. *Stroke* 37:550–555.

Wahlund, L.O., Barkhof, F., Fazekas, F., Bronge, L., Augustin, M., Sjogren, M., Wallin, A., Ader, H., Leys, D., Pantoni, L., Pasquier, F., Erkinjuntti, T., Scheltens, P. (2001) A new rating scale for age-related white matter changes applicable to MRI and CT. *Stroke* 32:1318–1322.

Wilkinson, D., Doody, R., Helme, R., Taubman, K., Mintzer, J., Kertesz, A., Pratt, R.D., and the Donepezil 308 Study Group. (2003) Donepezil in vascular dementia: A randomized, placebo-controlled study. *Neurology* 61:479–486.

Wolf, P.A., D'Agostino, R.B., Belanger, A.J., and Kannel, W.B. (1991) Probability of stroke: a risk profile from the Framingham study. *Stroke* 22:312–318.

World Health Organization. (1993) *International Classification of Diseases, Tenth Revision.* Geneva, Switzerland: Author.

Yamanouchi, H. (1991) Loss of white matter oligodendrocytes and astrocytes in progressive subcortical vascular encephalopathy of Binswanger type. *Acta Neurol. Scand.* 83:301–305.

Yue, N.C., Arnold, A.M., Longstreth, W.T., Jr., Elster, A.D., Jungreis, C.A., O'Leary, D.H., Poirier, V.C., and Byran, R.N. (1997) Sulcal, ventricular, and white matter changes at the MR imaging of the brain. *Radiology* 202:33–39.

Zarow, C., Vinters, H.V., Ellis, W.G., Weiner, M.W., Mungas, D., White, L., and Chui, H.C. (2005) Correlates of hippocampal neuron number in Alzheimer's disease and ischemic vascular dementia. *Ann. Neurol.* 57:896–903.

VIII PSYCHIATRIC DISORDERS OF CHILDHOOD ONSET

DANIEL S. PINE

Current conceptualizations of mental illness have been shaped heavily by two major research themes manifest during the past three decades. First, as perhaps best exemplified by the three editions of this volume, advances in neuroscience make it increasingly clear that mental illnesses reflect individual differences in neural processes. Thus, one major research theme examines the manner in which individual differences in one or another neural process relate to individual differences in risk for or expressions of psychopathology. Second, most mental illnesses are now conceptualized as developmental conditions where the pathophysiologic process that ultimately manifest as one or another illness begin during childhood. Thus, the second major research theme examines the manner in which events and individual characteristics during childhood relate to risk for or expressions of psychopathology throughout life. This second major theme has emerged following a few consistent observations. These include the observation that mental illnesses manifest during childhood predict a high risk for mental illness in adulthood among children and adolescents who were previously affected. Perhaps equally important are observations from family studies noting strong aggregation between mental illnesses in parents and their children, coupled with observations from research demonstrating robust developmental influences in rodents and nonhuman primates on neural systems implicated in mental illnesses. In the current section, these two major themes coalesce in a series of chapters examining one or another aspect of neurobiology as it relates to expressions of mental illness during childhood. These chapters can be arranged loosely into three broad sections, reflecting three interrelated research themes.

Four of the 12 chapters in this section focus on recent methodological advances and associated theoretical implications that exert broad effects on conceptualizations of many if not all pediatric mental illnesses. Thus, the material presented in Chapter 77 from Michael Rutter provides an amazingly broad context through which to view all of the other chapters in the section. This chapter concisely summarizes data on which the current developmental conceptualization rests for many mental illnesses. Three other chapters delineate the manner in which one or another modern research technique might allow precise specification of developmental processes that culminate in mental illness, manifest in adulthood. Thus, in Chapter 68, B.J. Casey and Sarah Durston describe how research in cognitive neuroscience holds the hope of implicating specific information processing functions and their associated neural circuitry in specific developmental psychopathologies. Similarly, in Chapter 74, Jay N. Giedd and colleagues describe manifestations of a changing neural template, as assessed through measures of brain structure visualized with structural magnetic resonance imaging (MRI), from which the functions noted by Casey and Durston emerge. Finally, Jeremy Veenstra-VanderWeele, Randy D. Blakely, and Edwin H. Cook review the manner in which genetic factors contribute to developmental psychopathology.

In addition to these four chapters, focused on processes applicable to many psychiatric disorders, five chapters focus on specific sets of psychiatric conditions that can loosely be grouped together. Many of these conditions fit within the family of syndromes described by Rutter as "neurodevelopmental syndromes," disorders characterized by a relatively persistent course, early onset, male predominance, and overt signs of perturbed brain function. Thus, Hardan and Reiss review in Chapter 67 recent findings on disorders associated with marked intellectual disability, typically in association with frank neuro-developmental delay; Swedo and colleagues review in Chapter 78 data on autism and pervasive developmental disorders; Gogtay and Rapoport review data on pediatric psychotic disorders; Lombroso, Bloch, and Leckman review data on tic-related disorders; Plessen and Peterson review data on attention-deficit/hyperactivity disorder. For each of these syndromes, advances in brain imaging have been particularly helpful in shaping current developmental conceptualizations and increasingly strong focus on neurobiology. Observations of shared clinical features may eventually lead to findings linking this family of syndromes based on the role of one or another biological process.

Finally, in three other chapters, data are reviewed pertinent to families of disorders primarily characterized by profound disturbances in emotional processes. For these disorders, advances in affective neuroscience and developmental applications thereof have stimulated an increasingly strong focus on neural processes in children that have been implicated previously in emotional processes in rodents and nonhuman primates. For the disorders considered in these three chapters, relative to neurodevelopmental disorders considered in the other chapters, onset tends to be relatively late, with less evidence of male preponderance and even perhaps a female preponderance; moreover, the course in these emotion-related conditions tends to be more episodic, and research on pathophysiology delineates strong influences of environmental factors. These findings suggest that the core underlying pathophysiology in families of syndromes, such as "neurodevelopmental" or "emotion-related" conditions, may eventually be differentiated on developmental grounds. Thus, Leibenluft reviews recent data on manifestations of bipolar-spectrum illnesses; Monk and Pine review data on anxiety; whereas Kaufman, Martin, and Blumberg view data on trauma-related syndromes, with a particular focus on depressive syndromes.

In some ways, the 12 chapters in this section represent a culmination. Following many years of research, two streams of research can coalesce, one focusing on neurobiology and the other focusing on development. In other respects, these chapters represent a beginning. Now that development and neurobiology can be more integrally connected in research on mental illnesses, the next decade holds the hope of ushering in major conceptual changes, shaped by the mutually influential insights that a melding of developmental and neurobiological focuses might bring to research in many aspects of mental illness.

67 The Neurobiology of Intellectual Disabilities

ANTONIO Y. HARDAN AND ALLAN L. REISS

Intellectual disabilities (ID), previously known as mental retardation, are conditions of heterogeneous etiologies defined by cognitive impairment coupled with deficits in adaptive functioning arising during the course of development, occurring prior to 18 years of age. According to *Diagnostic and Statistical Manual of Mental Disorders*, text rev. (*DSM-IV-TR*) criteria, the diagnosis of an intellectual disability is made when an individual displays substantial deficits in intellectual functioning by scoring lower than 2 standard deviations below the population mean on IQ measures, and when these intellectual deficits are accompanied by impairment in several areas of adaptive functioning, such as in self-care, school functioning, or interpersonal skills (American Psychiatric Association [APA], 2000). Based upon these parameters, the prevalence of ID is estimated at 1% of the general population, with most individuals (approximately 85%) functioning in the mild range of disability with IQ score ranging between 50/55 and 69. However, this rate varies by age, sex, and socioeconomic classification. Rates are thought to increase with age until early adulthood, at which point there is a decrease. The increase through childhood is attributed in part to the fact that children are assessed and diagnosed during the school years, when they begin to demonstrate difficulty mastering academic skills at the expected level.

Comorbid psychiatric conditions have been recognized to occur in individuals with ID at rates exceeding those in the general population with estimates ranging from 27% to 71% (Bregman, 1991). Psychiatric evaluation of individuals with an ID is complicated by the patients' cognitive levels and communication skills, as well as the tendency of individuals unfamiliar with cognitive disabilities to dismiss symptoms as merely manifestations of the ID, resulting in widespread underdiagnosis of psychiatric illnesses in this population. Symptoms may be expressed somewhat differently from those commonly observed in the specific conditions, and the tendency of individuals with ID is to communicate dysphoria, anxiety, anger, and frustration in nonverbal forms, such as self-injurious behavior, stereotyped rocking, aggression, and self-stimulation (APA, 2000; Feinstein and Reiss, 1996). Additionally, associated deficits, particularly communication and cognitive impairments, may make it difficult to obtain reliable information about symptoms from the individual; therefore, diagnosis is often made using objectively observable symptoms that can be reported by collateral sources. Conditions found to be occurring at a higher rate in individuals with ID include pervasive developmental disorders, attention-deficit/hyperactivity disorder, conduct disorders, mood disorders, anxiety disorders, and stereotypic movement disorders.

Estimates of prevalence fail to characterize adequately the diversity of neurocognitive, behavioral, and psychiatric presentations of individuals with ID. This chapter discusses the neurobiology of several diverse causes of ID. Each condition has been selected to represent a specific etiologic risk factor for the development of an ID. Fragile X syndrome (FXS) serves as an example of a single-gene disorder caused by a mutation on the X chromosome. In spite of the seemingly simple etiology, the absence of one protein in this condition has been shown to have widespread ramifications in the development and functioning of the brain. The condition is also notable for bringing to the forefront of psychiatric research the genetic phenomenon of triplet repeat expansion. Tuberous sclerosis complex (TSC) is an autosomal dominant multisystem disorder characterized by the development of multiple hamartomas in different organ systems including the brain. This condition illustrates how a mutation in one of two different genes, either *TSC1* or *TSC2*, can result in the same phenotype. Williams syndrome is an oligogenic disorder, typically resulting from the loss of 17–20 contiguous genes on chromosome 7. Research is ongoing in the exploration of the relationship between deleted genes and the characteristic physical and neurocognitive profile of individuals with Williams syndrome. Down syndrome results from genetic aberrations on a chromosomal level. Disorders of aneuploidy require the consideration of at least scores of genes in the understanding of the resulting neurobiology. Finally, fetal alcohol syndrome is the most common example of the widespread and deleterious effects of an exogenous agent on central nervous system development.

FRAGILE X SYNDROME

Fragile X (FXS) is the most common inherited cause of neurodevelopmental disability, occurring at a frequency of approximately 1 in every 4,000 to 8,000 live births. Fragile X is prototype of a single-gene disorder resulting in brain dysfunction and intellectual disability. The syndrome arises from the disruption in expression of the FXS mental retardation 1 (*FMR1*) gene, which is most commonly caused by expansion of a cytosine-guanine-guanine (CGG) repeat stretch in the *FMR1* gene with resultant hypermethylation and silencing of expression. The extent of expansion of CGG repeats corresponds with two different clinical stages of the syndrome. The premutation state of the gene is associated with approximately 50–200 CGG repeats, is typically not hypermethylated, and is not associated with significant clinical symptoms. The full mutation consists of about 200 CGG repeats or more and is associated with hypermethylation of the gene and the consequent syndrome. The phenotype of FXS is modified by sex of the person with FXS as *FMR1* is an X-linked gene. As such, males (with one X chromosome only) are more affected than females (who have two X chromosomes, one with the mutation). The phenotype can be further influenced by the presence of a gradation of severity that is dependent on the degree of expression of *FMR1* protein. Even partial expression of *FMR1* in some males may result in partial sparing of cognition (Hagerman et al., 1994). Because the syndrome is caused by the deficiency in expression of a single gene, FXS serves as an important model of inquiry in the effort to understand the pathway between genotype and phenotype in intellectual disability.

Cellular and Molecular Aspects

The syndrome acquired its name through the means of its first genetic diagnostic test. A fragile site was found to be induced at site Xq27.3 in metaphase spreads of peripheral lymphocytes in folate-deficient media (Krawczun et al., 1985). The specific gene responsible, *FMR1*, was then identified in 1991 (Fu et al., 1991), along with the mechanism by which the condition is transmitted—trinucleotide repeat expansion. Deoxyribonucleic acid (DNA) analysis of individuals with FXS revealed a hypermethylated CpG site and overlong CGG repeat proximal to the coding region of *FMR1*. Furthermore, in contrast to the normal *FMR1* gene, the number of trinucleotide repeats in either the premutation and full mutation allele could significantly increase in subsequent generations—a phenomenon known as "genetic anticipation." The means of transmission has been shown to be affected by the parent of origin, with the expansion occurring in FXS almost exclusively through maternal transmission, another non-Mendelian feature of FXS known as genetic "imprinting." The expansion leads to excessive methylation of the CpG island and consequent silencing of the gene.

The FXS mental retardation protein (FMRP), the gene product of *FMR1*, has been shown to be expressed throughout embryonic development and has also been found to be expressed broadly throughout the body in adult tissues. It is particularly abundant in neurons, localized in the perikaryon and in the proximal part of axons and dendrites (Feng et al., 1997). Fragile X mental retardation protein has been shown to be a ribonucleic acid (RNA) binding protein associated with polyribosomes and is thought to play a role in the control of messenger ribonucleic acid (mRNA) translation. Moreover, *FMR1* mRNA has been found in high concentration in synaptosomal fractions, suggesting a specific role in modulation of protein synthesis at synapses (Weiler et al., 1997). Characterizations of regions of FMRP and analysis of the presence of specific portions of FMRP in different cellular regions also have led to the premise that the protein is involved in the shuttling of mRNA between the nucleus and cytoplasm (Feng et al., 1997).

More recently, there is growing evidence that FMRP acts as a regulator of translation. For example, FMRP has been shown to inhibit translation of various mRNAs (Laggerbauer et al., 2001; Li et al., 2001). Abnormal regulation of protein synthesis as caused by reduction in FMRP could then in turn potentially affect synaptic maturation and plasticity. As protein synthesis following synaptic input has been found to be critical in the conversion of such input into learning and memory, the accumulation of evidence suggests that FMRP plays a crucial role in behavior as conceptualized at a cellular level.

The absence or reduction of FMRP in FXS has been shown to result in neuronal morphologic changes, particularly in dendritic spines. Neurons in FXS knockout mice have increased spine density and spine length in pyramidal cells of the visual cortex (Comery et al., 1997). Fragile X mice have longer, more immature dendritic spines than control mice. Histologic examination in humans with FXS has shown increased numbers of dendritic spines and significantly more dendritic spines with an immature morphology in temporal and visual cortices (Irwin et al., 2001). These findings strongly suggest FMRP involvement in the development and pruning of synaptic structures.

The relationship of FMRP and several receptors and neurotransmitter pathways have recently been examined. First, studies of the *FMR1* knockout mouse indicate that α-amino-3-hydroxy-5-methylisoxazile-4-propionic acid (AMPA) receptors are reduced significantly in number and activity (Arai et al., 1996). These receptors play an important role in synaptic transmission, and a recent study was conducted to examine the efficacy of an

AMPA receptor modulator in individuals with FXS. Unfortunately, initial findings did not show clear benefit for individuals who were affected (Berry-Kravis et al., 2006). Second, the link between FXS and the cholinergic system has also received some attention. Findings from the animal knock out model and humans indicate that the cyclic adenosine monophosphate (cAMP) cascade is significantly altered (Berry-Kravis and Huttenlocher, 1992; Berry-Kravis and Sklena, 1993; Berry-Kravis et al., 1995; Bielarczyk et al., 2003). Given that cAMP mediates cholinergic neurotransmission (Lauder, 1993; Felder, 1995), it follows that alterations to cAMP cascade function in FXS would impact cholinergic neurotransmission. A strong association in non-FXS neural tissue between FMRP overexpression and increased cAMP production upon stimulation of adenylate cyclase has been shown (Berry-Kravis and Ciurlionis, 1998). Further, more recent studies of fly and mouse FXS neural models and human neural tissue from individuals with FXS also show lower than expected levels of cAMP in response to stimulation of adenylate cyclase (Kelley et al., 2007). In light of this association between cAMP and cholinergic neurotransmission, the examination of the efficacy of acetylcholinesterase inhibitors in FXS appears to be warranted. Finally, deficit in the γ-aminobutyric acid (GABA)ergic inhibitory system have been associated with epilepsy, autistic-like syndromes, and sensory-motor gating observed in FXS. These observations are supported by a recent study providing evidence of alterations in GABA-releasing interneurons in the mouse model of FXS warranting the examination of GABAergic agents in this disorder (Selby et al., 2007).

Physical and Neuropsychiatric Characteristics

Physical and behavioral features are typically more prominent in males, given the X chromosome linked nature of the disorder (males with the syndrome have only one X chromosome that carries the mutation). However, in comparison to other genetic and chromosomal syndromes such as Down syndrome, males with FXS may not be easily recognized as having the syndrome based on physical characteristics alone. Associated physical features include long and narrow face, prominent ears, narrow intereye distance, macro-orchidism in males, various musculoskeletal problems, and mitral valve prolapse. Nearly all males with the full mutation have mild to severe ID (Rousseau et al., 1994) with about 15%–20 % developing seizures (Hagerman and Hagerman, 2002). Approximately 50% of females with the full mutation have moderate ID to borderline IQ levels. Although individuals with the premutation form of *FMR1* were at first thought to be completely spared the cognitive and behavioral symptoms of FXS, recent evidence has suggested that the presence of premutation state might result in milder clinical symptoms, particularly when the repeat size is closer to the full mutation range (that is, >100 repeats).

Additional behavioral and psychiatric features of the FXS full mutation include hyperactivity, marked gaze aversion, and motor stereotypies. Social anxiety as well as schizotypal and avoidant personality disorders are frequently observed in females (Franke et al., 1998). The frequency of autistic-like symptoms is higher than expected in a general developmentally delayed population and has been variously estimated between 5% and 40% of males with FXS (Hagerman, 1996). Individuals with FXS may also present a unique profile of autistic symptoms, including more stereotypies and unusual nonverbal interactions and more difficulty with peer interactions compared to adult interactions. Finally, males with FXS demonstrate a distinctive greeting in which they may show interest in engaging socially but then withdraw by avoiding eye contact and turning their body away from the person (Tsiouris and Brown, 2004). These anxiety-related behaviors appear to be associated with abnormal cortisol reactivity and are consistent with a number of documented hypothalamic-pituitary abnormalities including precocious puberty and elevated gonadotrophins levels (Hessl et al., 2004; Hessl et al., 2006).

Individuals with FXS also demonstrate a particular profile of intellectual strengths and weaknesses. This profile is similar in quality for both genders, though females typically function at a much higher overall intellectual level and manifest less severe deficits than do males. The characteristic cognitive profile includes weaknesses in attentional/executive function, visual memory and perception, mental manipulation of visual–spatial relationships among objects, visual–motor coordination, processing of arithmetical stimuli, and theory of mind (Grigsby et al., 1990; Hagerman et al., 1992; Mazzocco et al., 1993; Sobesky et al., 1994; Hinton et al., 1995; Reiss et al., 1995; Riddle et al., 1998; Munir et al., 2000; Bennetto et al., 2001). In contrast, studies assessing verbal-based skills show females with FXS to have relative strengths or spared abilities in this area (Kemper et al., 1986; Freund and Reiss, 1991; Mazzocco et al., 1993). Further, an *FMR1* knockout mouse model demonstrated impaired inhibitory control and sustained and selective attention compared to wild-type littermates (Moon et al., 2006). Working memory deficits are also frequently demonstrated in individuals with FXS (Kemper et al., 1986; Grigsby et al., 1990; Mazzocco et al., 1993). Kirk et al. (2005) demonstrated that girls with FXS made more errors on a test of working memory than did IQ-matched controls, indicating that difficulties with working memory were not solely attributable to a lower IQ.

Neuroanatomy

Magnetic resonance imaging (MRI) studies have begun to examine the effects of the *FMR1* full mutation on brain development and have thus begun to establish a neuroanatomical phenotype. Like autism, mild macrocephaly can be observed in this condition and may be more prominent in females with FXS compared to normal controls. Males and females with FXS have been shown to have decreased size of posterior cerebellar vermis and increased size of the fourth ventricle (Reiss et al., 1991; Mostofsky et al., 1998). Caudate nucleus, thalamic nucleus, and lateral ventricular volumes are increased in FXS as well (Mostofsky et al., 1998; Reiss et al., 1995; Lee et al., 2007) (Fig. 67.1; see also COLOR FIGURE 67.1 in separate insert). The volumetric differences in posterior cerebellar vermis, caudate nucleus, and lateral ventricles correlate with performance on IQ and other neurocognitive measures in individuals with FXS (Mostofsky et al., 1998; Reiss et al., 1995). Differences in volume of temporal lobe structures include increase in amygdalar volumes, age-related increase in hippocampal volume, and age-related decrease in the volume of the superior temporal gyrus (Reiss et al., 1995). Analysis of developmental changes in brain anatomy in children and adolescents with FXS show typical age-related decrease in gray matter and increase in white matter (Eliez et al., 2001). However, in contrast to controls, patients with FXS showed no significant correlations between IQ scores and volumes of cortical or subcortical gray matter.

While most studies have focused on gray matter regions, some investigations have examined white matter anatomy. A diffusion tensor imaging study found that females with FXS had aberrant white matter structure in frontostriatal pathways and parietal sensory-motor tracts (Barnea-Goraly et al., 2003). More recently, increased white matter volumes were observed in parietal and temporal regions in a sample of males and females with FXS through the use of an automated morphometric procedure called *tensor-based morphometry* (Lee et al., 2007). Although FMRP is primarily expressed in the cell body and postsynaptic region, it is probable that abnormalities in dendrites and synapse formation could affect the development of axons linking brain regions and consequently affecting white matter structures. In fact, several lines of evidence support these observations, including a recent investigation of a mosaic mouse model of FXS reporting that presynaptic *FMR1* genotype influences the degree of synaptic connectivity (Hanson and Madison, 2007).

A growing number of imaging studies have focused on the functional neuroanatomy of FXS. Differences in brain activation patterns have been observed in females with FXS when performing several cognitive tasks, including a visuospatial working memory task (Kwon et al., 2001), an arithmetic task (Rivera et al., 2002), and a cognitive interference task (Tamm et al., 2002). More recently, activation patterns were examined during an episodic memory task and revealed significantly reduced levels of brain activation localized to the basal forebrain and hippocampus in females with FXS (Greicius et al., 2003) (Fig. 67.2).

These findings suggest the existence of deficits in frontostriatal connections and in parietal and hippocampal regions. More importantly, these investigations have provided direct evidence that decreased FMRP expression underlies cognitive deficits with higher level being associated with more typical/healthy patterns of brain activation (Hessl et al., 2004).

Conclusion

Fragile X syndrome serves as a potent reminder to the difficulties involved in the elucidation of the pathogenesis of neurogenetic and neurodevelopmental disorders. In spite of the clearly identified genetic cause and increasingly well-characterized neuropsychological, molecular, cellular, and neuroanatomic features, FXS is far from being clearly understood. It is evident that even with a single-gene disorder, the final behavioral and cognitive outcomes of individuals with FXS also reflect the regulatory effects of FMRP on other genes and the complex interaction between genetic and environmental factors (Dyer-Friedman et al., 2002).

TUBEROUS SCLEROSIS

The tuberous sclerosis complex (TSC) is a typical autosomal dominant disorder of which abnormal cellular differentiation and proliferation are key features. The prevalence rate is estimated to be 1:6000 (Osborne et al., 1991) with a neurocognitive profile that includes individuals with severe levels of cognitive abilities to normal intelligence. It is characterized by the development of hamartomas in virtually every organ system,

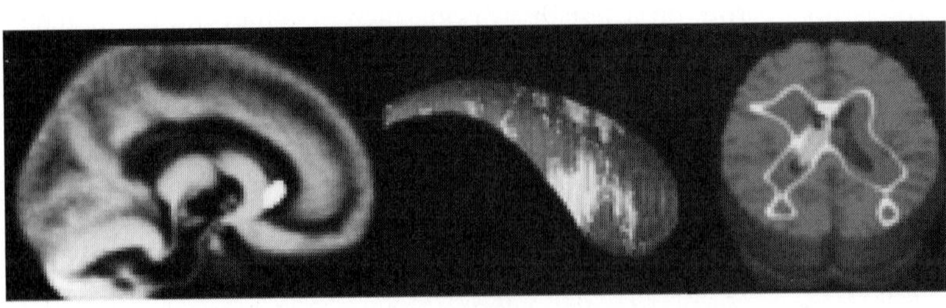

FIGURE 67.1 Increased caudate size as measured by voxel-based morphometry (left), surface-based mapping (middle), and tensor-based morphometry (right) (Lee et al., 2007).

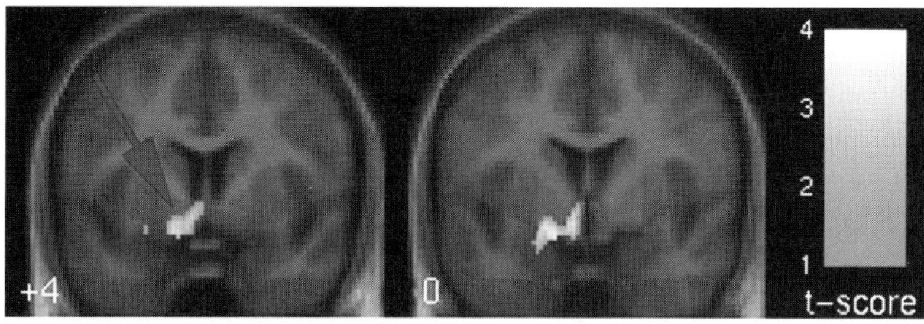

FIGURE 67.2 Coronal images showing deficient basal forebrain activation in individuals with Fragile X syndrome when compared to controls while performing a recognition task (Greicius et al., 2003).

including the heart and kidneys. In the brain, hamartomas appear as cerebral cortical and subcortical tubers, subependymal nodules (SENs), and subependymal giant cell astrocytomas (SEGAs). Multiple distinctive dermatologic manifestations such as shagreen patches, hypopigmented macules, periungual fibromas, and facial angiofibromas have led to this condition being termed a neurocutaneous disorder.

Genetics

The two genes associated with TSC are *TSC1* and *TSC2* and are located on chromosome 9q34 and l6p13.3, respectively (Van Slegtenhorst et al., 1997; DiMario, 2004). *TSC1* and *TSC2* encode two proteins: *hamartin* and *tuberin*, respectively (Van Slegtenhorst et al., 1997). In familial cases of TSC, half are due to mutations in *TSC1*, and the other half are due to mutations in *TSC2*. Despite the autosomal dominant inheritance pattern, there are a significant number of spontaneous cases resulting from new mutations of these genes.

Mutations of *TSC1* and *TSC2* lead to tuber formation resulting in the same phenotype (Van Slegtenhorst et al., 1998). However, the precise mechanisms involved in the pathogenesis of this phenotype are not clear. The function of hamartin is unknown, although some studies have suggested that it may play a role in cellular growth regulation (Van Slegtenhorst et al., 1997). Tuberin, which in animal models has been shown to function as a guanosine-5' triphosphate (GTP)ase-activating protein (GAP), is thought to play a role in neuronal migration, differentiation, and/or development. These two proteins appear to be interrelated because hamartin and tuberin have been shown to interact in vivo (Van Slegtenhorst et al., 1998), and studies of rat fibroblasts with *TSC1* and *TSC2* mutations demonstrated that hamartin is a growth inhibitory protein whose biologic effects are probably dependent on its interaction with tuberin (Benvenuto et al., 2000).

Neuropsychiatric Characteristics

Epilepsy is a common occurrence in TSC, estimated to occur in 70%–90% of individuals who are affected who come to medical attention (Gomez, 1988). The seizure type most commonly described in infancy is infantile spasms. Although these seizures typically disappear spontaneously over a period of weeks to months, they may evolve into other seizure types, such as symptomatic generalized epilepsy, partial epilepsy, and mixtures of seizure types (Webb et al., 1996). A very high incidence of autism has been found in individuals with TSC. Estimates of the occurrence of autism in TSC range from 17% to 68% by the age of 5 years (Gillberg et al., 1994; Gutierrez et al., 1998). The wide range in reporting is most likely due to differing methods used in the diagnosis of TSC and autism. Learning disorders have also been described, including in those with normal intelligence. Memory impairments, speech delay, dyscalculia, visuospatial disturbances, and dyspraxia have all been reported in individuals with TSC (Jambaque et al., 1991). Finally, several behavioral difficulties have been described, with hyperactivity (59%–86%) and aggressive behavior (13%) being the most common (Gillberg et al., 1994).

The relationship between tuber location and neuropsychiatric manifestations has also been examined. Overall, a greater number of identified tubers and subependymal nodules are correlated with higher seizure frequency, greater cognitive impairment, and fewer self help skills (Yorns et al., 2001). Tubers in the temporal lobe and cerebellum have also been associated with autism. Although tubers in the temporal region have been linked to symptoms of autism, this association has been questioned in light of the extensive temporal lobe involvement in some individuals with TSC but without any autistic symptomatology. High number, of tubers in the cerebellum have also been linked to symptoms of autism (Weber et al., 2000); this association appears to be more robust with recent evidence of association between specific social deficits, such as social isolation, and lesions in the right cerebellum (Eluvathingal et al., 2006).

Neuropathology and Neuroanatomy

In the brain, TSC lesions consist of tubers, subependymal nodules, SEGAs, white matter abnormalities, and microscopic anomalies such as microdysgenesis, heterotopic gray matter, and lamination defects. Tubers are pervasive, occurring in a large percentage of patients with TSC, and they most commonly occur in the frontal, temporal, and parietal cortex. Subependymal nodules are well-circumscribed lesions that are usually found along the surface of the lateral ventricles and less commonly within the aqueduct and the fourth ventricle. These nodules can extend into the surrounding brain structures and can undergo malignant transformation. Subependymal giant cell astrocytomas share similar cellular characteristics with SENs, including giant cells, and also are found frequently along the surface of lateral ventricles. These tumors can also become malignant and cause acute obstruction in the ventricular system, resulting in signs of increased intracranial pressure, seizures, or mental status changes.

Structural MRI has become the primary imaging tool to examine the existence and the localizations of brain lesions in TSC such as tubers and nodules (Luat et al., 2007). In addition, there is evidence of more widespread and subtle abnormalities in normal-appearing regions of the brain. Magnetic resonance imaging studies analyzing gray and white matter volumes comparing individuals with TSC and controls have shown gray matter volume reduction in selected regions of the brain, including the medial temporal lobe, posterior cingulate gyrus, basal ganglia, and thalamus (Ridler et al., 2001). White matter volumes were also reduced in the major intrahemispheric tracts, such as the right inferior longitudinal fasiculi and the bilateral occipito-frontal fasiculi (Ridler et al., 2001). Diffusion tensor imaging studies are also consistent with these observations, reporting the presence of widespread white matter ultrastructural changes (Garaci et al., 2004).

Conclusion

Tuberous sclerosis complex is a neuronal migration disorder with focal and widespread anatomic and histologic abnormalities. Elucidating the neurobiologic underpinnings of TSC and its brain lesions will likely contribute to our understanding of its different neurobehavioral phenotypes.

Consequently, the study of TSC may be useful as a genetic model for neurodevelopmental disorders and behaviors of unclear etiologies such as autism, attention-deficit/hyperactivity disorder, aggression, and cognitive impairment.

WILLIAMS SYNDROME

Williams syndrome (WS) is a rare neurogenetic disorder occurring in up to 1 in 10,000 births (Meyer-Lindenberg et al., 2006). Williams syndrome is caused by the deletion of more than 20 contiguous genes on chromosome 7 (Ewart et al., 1993). The syndrome results in a characteristic pattern of physical manifestations. Facial features include a flat nasal bridge, prominent lips and wide mouth, malar flattening, full cheeks, long philtrum, small mandible, epicanthal folds, and periorbital fullness. Abnormal reaction to sound is quite common in WS and is one of the most common early behavioral features (Morris, 2006). Also known as "auditory hyperacusis," it is observed in the absence of increased ability to detect low amplitude sounds (Levitin et al., 2005). The deletion of elastin in WS is responsible for common cardiac manifestations, including supravalvular aortic stenosis, and other connective tissue symptoms such as joint and skin laxity.

Individuals with WS usually fall within the mild to moderately mentally retarded range, with IQ scores ranging from 40 to 90 with a mean of approximately 55. In comparison to other cognitive domains, some linguistic skills appear to be preserved or even enhanced in individuals with WS, but this contention has been questioned recently (Brock, 2007). Interesting aspects of language in WS include a proclivity for the use of unusual words and great facility with affectively laden language (Bellugi et al., 2000). Visuomotor and visuospatial aspects of WS include impairment in the copying of geometric patterns and shapes and difficulty in processing of global, as opposed to local, features of visual representation. A notable exception to the generalized impairments in visuospatial processing is the remarkable ability of individuals with WS to recognize, discriminate, and remember familiar and unfamiliar faces (Rossen et al., 1995), a feature of particular interest in the context of their exceptionally strong appetitive social drive.

Genetics

Williams syndrome is caused by a contiguous microdeletion on band 7q11.23 of chromosome 7 that involves the gene encoding elastin and more than 20 other genes (Ewart et al., 1993). The vast majority (> 95%) of cases of WS are caused by the deletion of the typical region on chromosome 7. However, a smaller percentage of cases of WS involve atypical patterns of genetic deletion. If these cases of atypical deletion can be correlated with partial expression of the phenotype of WS, the hope is that greater specificity can be achieved in identifying the individual genes that are responsible for or contribute to the different aspects of the phenotype of WS.

Neurophysiology

Electrophysiological studies have examined the timing and organization of neural systems in two areas of cognition thought to be different in WS. First, individuals with WS appear to have significantly different sensory processing. A series of studies have found that brainstem auditory processing is normal in WS, suggesting a cortical source to the auditory hyperexcitability seen in this condition (Mills et al., 2000). Event-related potential (ERP) studies examining auditory semantic processing and illusionary contour perception found unusual patterns of brain organization and activation in individuals with WS (Mills et al., 2000; Grice et al., 2003). Second, face processing was shown to produce abnormal patterns of ERP response in WS, possibly due to structural abnormalities in the temporo-occipital regions including the fusiform gyrus (Mills et al., 2000). Results also suggested a dissociation between face perception, which is abnormal in WS, and face recognition, which shows normally organized, but delayed, development.

Neuroanatomy and Functional Abnormalities

Gross anatomical analysis of four brains of individuals with WS revealed small brains with parietal and occipital hypoplasia, with a characteristic curtailment of the dorsal-ventral axis (Galaburda and Bellugi, 2000).

Dorsomedial gyral patterns were noted to be abnormal on gross anatomic examination and MRI analysis (Galaburda et al., 2001). No abnormalities were seen in the laminar and columnar arrangement of neurons, glia, myelin content, and vascularization. However, there is evidence for atypical neuron size and cell packing density (Galaburda et al., 2002).

Magnetic resonance imaging studies have shown that compared to age-matched controls, patients with WS have a 13% decrease in cerebral volume, relatively preserved cerebellar volume, relative sparing of cerebral gray matter volume, and disproportionate reduction in cerebral white matter (Jernigan and Bellugi, 1990; Reiss et al., 2000). There also appears to be an atypical pattern of proportionally greater anterior to posterior cerebral tissue, as defined by frontal compared to parietal plus occipital volumes. Superior temporal gyrus volume also is proportionately larger in individuals with WS, a finding which is of interest given the function of this region in auditory and language processing.

Regional and morphological differences in brain structures have been reported while applying different methods of MRI analysis. Cerebral shape, as measured by the curvature of the corpus callosum and cerebral hemispheres, has been shown to be abnormally flattened in WS (Fig. 67.3; see also COLOR FIGURE 67.3 in separate insert) (Schmitt et al., 2001a). Direct cross-sectional area measurements of corpus callosum showed decreased tissue in posterior portions of the this structure (Schmitt et al., 2001b). Consistent with these observations, a recent investigation applying mesh-based geometrical modeling methods found the corpus callosum in individuals with WS to be shorter, less curved, and with thinner posterior regions (Luders et al., 2007). Analysis of cerebral gyral patterns have revealed abnormalities in the dorsal, but not ventral, portions of the central sulcus (Galaburda et al., 2001) with increased gyrification bilaterally in occipital regions (Gaser et al., 2006).

Functional studies have also been conducted in individuals with WS to investigate visuospatial deficits, hippocampal function, and social/emotional processing. Studies of visuospatial construction suggest neural processing abnormalities in the dorsal stream (spatial processing), with relatively intact ventral stream function (visual processing) (Paul et al., 2002). Investigation of hippocampal function suggests impairment of this region as evidenced by a reduction in blood flow, decreased *N*-acetylaspartate (NAA) levels, and diminished functional responsivity in the absence of gross structural abnormalities (Meyer-Lindenberg et al., 2005). The social domain in WS has received a lot of interest in light of the excessive-appetitive social behavior in the presence of deficits in the social-perceptual and social-cognitive components of theory of mind. These investigations suggest that orbitofrontal cortex dysfunction may be contributing to social disinhibition and reduced reactivity to social cues (Meyer-Lindenberg et al., 2005).

Taken together, these anatomical and functional findings suggest the existence of hippocampal abnormalities, functional and structural abnormalities of dorsal cortical regions, and dysregulation of amygdalar and orbitofrontal function in WS. The precise behavioral and cognitive correlates of these neural findings remain to be elucidated.

Conclusion

Williams syndrome provides a distinct opportunity to understand the development of cognition and its neuronal pathways in light of the co-existence of areas of deficits and strengths in various cognitive abilities. This profile can be examined in humans by focusing on cases of atypical deletions (Korenberg et al., 2000). However, as atypical deletion cases are rare, progress

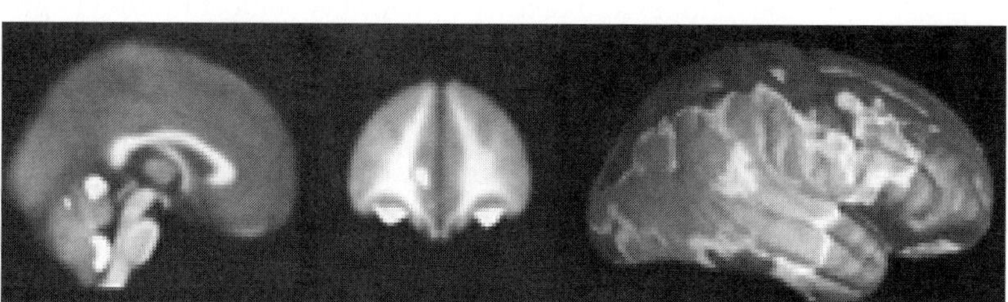

FIGURE 67.3 Structural abnormalities in individuals with Williams syndrome: increased cerebellar vermis and orbito-frontal region as measured by voxel-based morphometry (left); and increased cortical thickness including superior temporal gyrus (STG) (Gaser et al., 2006).

in understanding gene-brain-behavior relations in WS is probably best served using knockout mouse models. This strategy has started yielding some results with the development of models for candidate genes for neurobehavioral abnormalities. Preliminary findings are promising such as the potential correlation of LIM-Kinase 1 (LIM refers to the three gene products Lin-11, Isl-1 and Mec-3) with visuospatial constructive deficit (Frangiskakis et al., 1996). This research will ultimately allow a better understanding of the underlying neurobiologic abnormalities of WS and consequently the cognitive and behavioral abnormalities observed in this disorder.

DOWN SYNDROME

Down syndrome (DS) is the most common genetic cause of intellectual disability, with an average prevalence of 14 per 10,000 (Centers for Disease Control and Prevention [CDC], 2006). Physical characteristics include short stature, midfacial hypoplasia, low nasal bridge, epicanthal folds, protrusion of tongue, hyperflexibility of joints, and hypotonia. The neurocognitive profile includes IQ scores of approximately 45–50, relative strengths in visuospatial skills, and a particular weakness in face recognition. Language development is generally delayed. Over time, expressive language remains impoverished, whereas receptive language eventually becomes a relative strength (Wang and Bellugi, 1993). Individuals with DS are at significant risk for neuropsychiatric disorders with estimates of comobidity ranging from 18% to 38% (Dykens et al., 2002; Capone et al., 2006). The most common comorbid conditions in childhood and adolescence include attention-deficit/hyperactivity disorder (ADHD), oppositional defiant disorder, and conduct disorder, although females with DS tend to have fewer problems than males (Lund, 1988). Autistic symptoms also can occur in individuals with DS (Rasmussen et al., 2001). Later in life, individuals with DS have a markedly higher incidence of Alzheimer's disease (AD), likely related to the presence of genetic loci that are established risk factors for AD on chromosome 21 (Isacson, 2002). The prevalence of dementia by age 65 is estimated to be between 30% and 75% (Zigman et al., 1997), with an average age of onset between 50 and 55 (Lai and Williams, 1989).

Molecular Genetics

The most common etiology of DS is trisomy 21, which occurs as a result of nondisjunction during gamete formation. The vast majority of cases result from full trisomy 21 of maternal origin (Antonarakis, 1991). More uncommon forms are due to mosaicism, in which nondisjunction occurs following fertilization with resultant trisomic and euploid cell lines, and to partial or full translocation of chromosome 21 to another chromosome (Capone, 2001).

Chromosome 21 is the smallest human autosome and, as such, potentially represents the most comprehensible opportunity for analysis of chromosomal aneuploidy. The entire sequence of 21q, which contains approximately 225 genes, was published in 2000 (Hattori et al., 2000). The shorter arm, 21p, is not associated with the DS phenotype and is not considered important in the pathophysiology of the clinical phenotype. In spite of the relatively small size of the chromosome, the elucidation of the pathophysiology of DS is daunting as it requires the consideration of the proximal and downstream effects of genes on 21q. The study of cases of partial trisomy 21 resulting from partial translocations suggests the presence of a 4 Mb region on 21q, termed the *DS critical region* (DSCR) (Antonarakis, 1998), which is most important for the development of the syndrome. The triplication of this region has been associated with numerous features of DS, including flat nasal bridge, protruding tongue, palatal abnormalities, short and broad hands, and intellectual disability. However, the DSCR is not the only region critical to the development of DS, as several cases of phenotypic DS have been found with triplications not including the DSCR (Korenberg et al., 1994). Nevertheless, the study of the DSCR may serve as a model for attempts to link multigenic sites to specific phenotypic features of DS.

Despite the increase in our understanding of DS, a considerable number of questions remain to be answered including how an extra copy of chromosome 21 genes is linked to the phenotype of DS. For a number of genes, a dosage effect has been observed in DS, with higher levels of protein product resulting from the presence of a third copy of the gene. Increased levels of protein product may then lead to different aspects of the phenotype of DS. Alternatively, increased protein products may affect the expression of other genes or gene products, with potentially deleterious effects on various aspects of neural development and function. Many other genes present in triplicate in individuals with DS have been found to have normal levels of protein product expression, possibly as a result of regulatory feedback mechanisms (Chrast et al., 2000).

Neuropathological Findings

Postmortem investigations have revealed reduction in the number and density of neurons in most brain regions. Specifically, interneurons and pyramidal neurons in the cerebral cortex are reduced in number (Ross et al., 1984; Wisniewski et al., 1986). Reduced synaptic density and complexity of synaptic connections have been observed postnatally, suggesting an abnormal pattern of synaptic pruning (Huttenlocher, 1984). These observations were recently highlighted with the discovery of morphological abnormalities of the dendritic spines in the brains of Ts65Dn, one of the existing mouse models for DS (Belichenko et al., 2004). Delays in myelination have also been noted in children who were affected, though less consistently.

Neuroanatomic Findings

Autopsy examination of the brain has revealed decreased size and weight, decreased anterior-posterior diameter, decreased gyral complexity, and narrow superior temporal gyrus (Coyle et al., 1986; Wisniewski, 1990). Magnetic resonance imaging studies in children and adults have found decreased size of the brain, decreased anterior-posterior diameter, disproportionately smaller cerebellum and brainstem, and relatively preserved subcortical structures (Aylward, Habbak, et al., 1997; Aylward, Li, et al., 1997; Weis et al., 1991). Magnetic resonance imaging studies also have shown decreased hippocampal size and relative preservation of parietal gray matter, findings that may shed light on the neurobiological substrate for relative weaknesses in memory and relative strengths in visuospatial skills (Aylward et al., 1999; Pinter et al., 2001). In older adults with DS, decreasing volume of the hippocampus, amygdala, and posterior parahippocampal gyrus have been correlated with increasing age and onset of dementia (Krasuski et al., 2002). Finally, two recent voxel-based morphometry studies reported findings consistent with the region-of-interest investigations of decreased gray matter in the hippocampus (White et al., 2003) and the parahippocampus (Teiple et al., 2004).

Conclusion

Similar to other genetic disorders, DS provides another opportunity to learn about the relationship of specific genes and the development of cognitive and neuropsychiatric disorders. At least two genes in the DSCR are known to be overexpressed in DS: the minibrain gene (MNB) and the gene encoding amyloid precursor protein (APP). Mutations in the gene for APP have been associated with rare forms of familial AD as well as one form of cerebroarterial amyloidosis, which results in amyloid deposition in the brain (Goate et al., 1991). These observations have led to an increased interest in DS because elucidating its neurobiology will contribute to a better understanding of AD and other disorders, such as leukemia, which are commonly observed in individuals with DS.

FETAL ALCOHOL SPECTRUM DISORDERS

Fetal alcohol spectrum disorders (FASD) is a nondiagnostic, umbrella term used to describe the entire range of effects resulting from gestational alcohol exposure. In light of the challenges of accurate ascertainment, the exact prevalence rate is somewhat difficult to determine. In contrast, the rate of fetal alcohol syndrome (FAS), the most clearly defined condition, ranges from 0.5 per 1,000 births in the United States (May and Gossage, 2001) to 46.4 per 1,000 births in South Africa (May et al., 2000). The condition was first described systematically in 1973 when diagnostic criteria were formulated and the defects were specifically attributed to maternal alcohol use and abuse during pregnancy. These criteria included pre- and postnatal growth retardation, as evidenced by height, weight, and head circumference below the 10th percentile; distinctive pattern of facial anomalies, including a thin upper lip, epicanthal folds, and an indistinct philtrum; and central nervous system dysfunction, as evidenced by low IQ scores and behavioral problems. However, it has become clear more recently that the effects of prenatal alcohol exposure fall on a continuum that is roughly correlated with the extent of exposure, with FAS merely representing one end. These observations led to the development of the FASD and the recommendations of a careful specialized evaluation when a history of in utero alcohol exposure exists (Manning and Hoyme, 2007).

Fetal alcohol syndrome is the leading cause of intellectual disability in the general population. Intellectual functioning is generally impaired in children with FAS with an average IQ of 70, although the range can be between 20 and 100 (Streissguth et al., 1991). Lower IQ also is observed in children with prenatal alcohol exposure not meeting criteria for FAS (Mattson, 1997). In children of either normal or below-average IQ who are prenatally exposed, symptoms of hyperactivity and inattention have been observed. Studies suggest the presence of impairments in learning and memory encoding, and less consistently, in language function, motor abilities, and visuospatial skills (Mattson and Riley, 1998). These behavioral and cognitive symptoms are far more sensitive indicators of prenatal alcohol exposure than the physical anomalies typically associated with FAS.

Alcohol Exposure and Neural Development

Investigations in laboratory animals have been conducted to examine the effects of alcohol on neural development. Rodent studies have identified phases of prenatal brain development particularly affected by alcohol exposure, and these phases in turn have been correlated with specific periods of human gestation (Guerri, 1998). Alcohol exposure during the first trimester has been correlated with increased incidence of major craniofacial and neural tube abnormalities (Ernhart et al., 1987). The second gestational trimester marks the period of neuronal generation and migration, as well as differentiation of most areas of the nervous system. Impairment in neuronal proliferation and migration throughout the brain have been associated with alcohol exposure during this period (Miller and Robertson, 1993). The last trimester marks a period of substantial brain growth, development and proliferation of glial cells, and development of synapses and dendrites. Exposure during this time leads to severe neuronal loss, changes in synaptogenesis and myelination, reactive gliosis, microcephaly, and particular susceptibility to cerebellar and hippocampal damage (Guerri, 1998).

Cellular Physiology

A variety of mechanisms have been identified through which alcohol is known to affect neurons and glia. Damage to embryonic radial glia cells, which are important in directing neuronal migration, likely contributes to abnormalities in neuronal migration and neuroglial heterotopies (Miller, 1992). Alcohol has been shown to interfere with the proliferation and differentiation of astrocytes, resulting in dysfunction in their supportive role in brain development and homeostasis (Kennedy and Mukerji, 1986). For example, neurotrophic factors produced by astrocytes have been shown to be depleted by alcohol. Alcohol-induced neuronal apoptosis has been documented, including through effects on *N*-methyl-D-aspartate (NMDA) and GABA receptors (Ikonomidou et al., 2000) and through modulation of expression of cytotoxic receptors in the brain (Cheema et al., 2000). The effect of alcohol on oligodendrocytes was strongly suggested through the observation of delayed myelination and aberrant morphology of myelin sheaths (Guerri et al., 2001). In a more generalized way, alcohol may induce other types of damage such as hypoxia and ischemia, leading to impaired development and structural damage.

Neuroanatomy

Autopsy reports have indicated a wide variety of structural problems resulting from alcohol exposure, but with no specific pattern of brain malformations being described consistently. However, it should be noted that postmortem examinations of cases of FAS have generally been performed on the individuals who were most severely affected. Microcephaly, hydrocephalus, cerebral dysgenesis, and anteriorly fused frontal lobes have all been reported in many cases of FAS. Dysgenesis or agenesis of the corpus callosum, cerebellum, and brain stem have also been reported. Other miscellaneous findings include abnormalities in the olfactory bulb, hippocampus, and basal ganglia.

Magnetic resonance imaging studies have been consistent with observations reported in postmortem studies with evidence supporting a direct relationship between imaging findings and the degree of prenatal alcohol exposure. Several studies have reported a decrease in total brain volume involving gray and white matte structures (Roebuck et al., 1998; McGee and Riley, 2006). However, a recent study examining individuals with a history of prenatal alcohol exposure, either with or without facial dysmorphology, found that cerebral white matter volumes were more affected than gray matter volumes (Archibald et al., 2001). The corpus callosum shows a variety of defects ranging from subtle size and shape differences to frank agenesis (Sowell et al., 2001; Bookstein et al., 2002), occurring at a significantly higher incidence in individuals with a history of prenatal alcohol exposure compared to other individuals who are developmentally disabled. In patients with FAS, these callosal changes have been correlated with symptoms of inattention, hyperactivity, and impaired verbal intellectual functioning. Basal ganglia, including the caudate nucleus, have been found to be disproportionately reduced in more severe cases of prenatal alcohol exposure (Mattson et al., 1996). Cerebellar gray and white matter volumes are decreased in individuals diagnosed with FAS (Archibald et al., 2001), and cerebellar vermal lobules I–V are observed to be disproportionately reduced in size in human and animal studies (Sowell et al., 1996). Magnetic resonance imaging examination of the hippocampus is of interest due to neurobehavioral impairments associated with FAS, including poor spatial learning and memory. However, imaging studies of the hippocampus in FAS have found only differences in left–right symmetry (Riikonen et al., 1999) or no disproportionate reduction in overall volume (Archibald et al., 2001).

Conclusion

Prenatal alcohol exposure has been shown to have effects on cognitive, emotional, and behavioral functioning that could occur independently of the physical characteristics. The examination of these deficits allows the investigation of the effects of an external toxic agent at different times of brain development. Information provided will increase our understanding not only of the pathophysiology of FASD but numerous other disorders where an external insult is suspected to be a contributing or causal factor.

SUMMARY

Attempts to understand the biological basis of ID must begin by considering the process of normal brain development. This enormously complex process involves the temporal and spatial coordination of numerous genetic, neurochemical, and neuromorphological factors. None of these factors exists in isolation of other processes, thereby making it difficult to trace the direct pathway between an etiological risk factor and its numerous

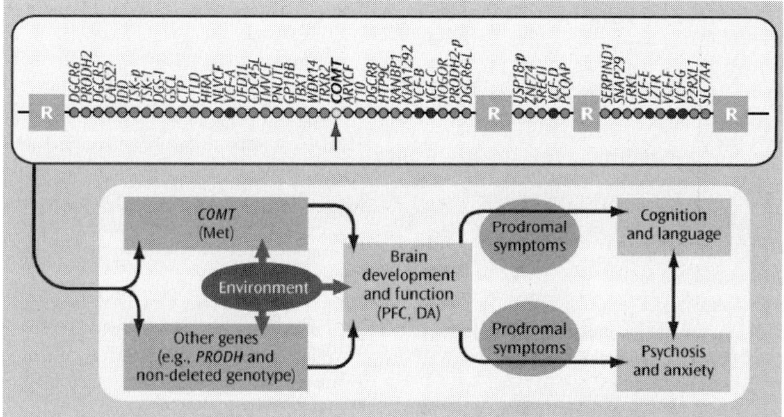

FIGURE 67.4 Velocardiofacial syndrome is due to a microdeletion located in the long arm of chromosome 22. This disorder illustrates the complexity of intellectual disabilities with the involvement of numerous genetic, neurochemical, and neuromorphological factors. It is the most common microdeletion genetic disorder, occurring in at least 1:5000 live births (Botto et al., 2003). This syndrome is also an attractive model for the study of psychotic disorders, since about 30% of all individuals who are affected develop schizophrenia-like symptoms (Gothelf et al., 2007). Individuals with 22q11.2 deletions have only one copy of the catechol-O-methyltransferase (*COMT*) gene because this gene resides in the region that is deleted. A variant of the *COMT* genes is the polymorphism resulting from a substitution of the amino acid *methionine* (Met) for that of valime (Val). The presence of Met has been associated with slower breakdown and greater availability of dopamine. The existence of Met allele and symptoms of psychosis and anxiety or depression was associated with increase risk of psychosis (Gothelf, Eliez, et al., 2005). Reprinted with permission from Kates (2007).

consequences. However, new research methods, such as the study of more homogeneous model disorders, provides real promise for beginning to unravel the complex interplay among genetic risk (and protective) factors, neurobiological processes and environmental influences (for example, see Fig. 67.4).

The genetic contributions to behavior and cognition include the correct encoding, transcription, and translation of genes necessary for brain development and function. The absence, lack, or overproduction of proteins encoded by these genes will obviously have a widespread impact on different aspects of development. At an ultrastructural level, distinct cellular morphology has been noted in several conditions associated with ID. Most prominently, dendritic anomalies have been associated with conditions such as FXS, DS, and Rett syndrome. At a cellular level, abnormalities in specific types of cells in the central nervous system (that is, neurons and glia) will result in neural dysfunction. Cytoarchitectonic organization may result from abnormalities in neural cell differentiation, migration, proliferation, and programmed death. Finally, environment and experience will have direct effects on the biological outcome of neural development. The increased understanding of the neurobiologic underpinnings of ID will not only contribute to the field of developmental disorders but also to the evolving understanding of human brain function and organization.

REFERENCES

American Psychiatric Association. (2000) *Diagnostic and Statistical Manual of Mental Disorders*, 4th ed. Washington, DC: Author.

Antonarakis, S.E. (1998) 10 years of genomics, chromosome 21, and Down syndrome. *Genomics* 51:1–16.

Antonarakis, S.E. (1991) Parental origin of the extra chromosome in trisomy 21 as indicated by analysis of DNA polymorphisms. Down Syndrome Collaborative Group. *N. Engl. J. Med.* 324:872–876.

Arai, A., Kessler, M., Rogers, G., and Lynch, G. (1996) Effects of a memory-enhancing drug on DL-alpha-amino-3-hydroxy-5-methyl-4-isoxazolepropionic acid receptor currents and synaptic transmission in hippocampus. *J. Pharmacol. Exp. Ther.* 278:627–638.

Archibald, S.L., Fennema-Notestine, C., Gamst, A., Riley, E.P., Mattson, S.N., and Jernigan, T.L. (2001) Brain dysmorphology in individuals with severe prenatal alcohol exposure. *Dev. Med. Child. Neurol.* 43:148–154.

Aylward, E.H., Habbak, R., Warren, A.C., Pulsifer, M.B., Barta, P.E., Jerram, M., et al. (1997) Cerebellar volume in adults with Down syndrome. *Arch. Neurol.* 54:209–212.

Aylward, E.H., Li, Q., Habbak, Q.R., Warren, A., Pulsifer, M.B., Barta, P.E., et al. (1997) Basal ganglia volume in adults with Down syndrome. *Psychiatry Res.* 74:73–82.

Aylward, E.H., Li, Q., Honeycutt, N.A., Warren, A.C., Pulsifer, M.B., Barta, P.E., et al. (1999) MRI volumes of the hippocampus and amygdala in adults with Down's syndrome with and without dementia. *Am. J. Psychiatry* 156: 564–568.

Barnea-Goraly, N., Eliez, S., Hedeus, M., Menon, V., White, C.D., Moseley, M., et al. (2003) White matter tract alterations in fragile X syndrome: preliminary evidence from diffusion tensor imaging. *Am. J. Med. Genet. B Neuropsychiatr. Genet.* 118:81–88.

Belichenko, P.V., Masliah, E., Kleschevnikov, A.M., Villar, A.J., Epstein, C.J., Salehi, A., et al. (2004) Synaptic structural abnormalities in the Ts65Dn mouse model of Down syndrome. *J. Comp. Neurol.* 480:281–298.

Bellugi, U., Lichtenberger, L., Jones, W., Lai, Z., and St. George, M.I. (2000) The neurocognitive profile of Williams syndrome: a complex pattern of strengths and weaknesses. *J. Cogn. Neurosci.* 12:7–29.

Bennetto, L., Pennington, B.F., Porter, D., Taylor, A.K., and Hagerman, R.J. (2001) Profile of cognitive functioning in women with the fragile X mutation. *Neuropsychology* 15:290–299.

Benvenuto, G., Li, S., Brown, S.J., Braverman, R., Vass, W.C., Cheadle, J.P., et al. (2000) The tuberous sclerosis-1 (TSC1) gene product harmartin suppresses cell growth and augments the expression of the TSC2 product tuberin by inhibiting its ubiquitination. *Oncogene* 19:6303–6316.

Berry-Kravis, E., and Ciurlionis, R. (1998) Overexpression of fragile X gene (FMR-1) transcripts increases cAMP production in neural cells. *J. Neurosci. Res.* 51:41–48.

Berry-Kravis, E., Hicar, M., and Ciurlionis, R. (1995) Reduced cyclic AMP production in fragile X syndrome: cytogenetic and molecular correlations. *Pediatr. Res.* 38:638–643.

Berry-Kravis, E., and Huttenlocher, P.R. (1992) Cyclic AMP metabolism in fragile X syndrome. *Ann. Neurol.* 31:22–26.

Berry-Kravis, E., Krause, S.E., Block, S.S., Guter, S., Wuu, J., Leurgans, S., et al. (2006) Effect of CX516, an AMPA-modulating compound, on cognition and behavior in fragile X syndrome: a controlled trial. *J. Child Adolesc. Psychopharmacol.* 16:525–540.

Berry-Kravis, E., and Sklena, P. (1993) Demonstration of abnormal cyclic AMP production in platelets from patients with fragile X syndrome. *Am. J. Med. Genet.* 45:81–87.

Bielarczyk, H., Tomaszewicz, M., Madziar, B., Cwikowska, J., Pawelczyk, T., and Szutowicz, A. (2003) Relationships between cholinergic phenotype and acetyl-CoA level in hybrid murine neuroblastoma cells of septal origin. *J. Neurosci. Res.* 73:717–721.

Bookstein, F.L., Streissguth, A.P., Sampson, P.D., Connor, P.D., and Barr, H.M. (2002) Corpus callosum shape and neuropsychological deficits in adult males with heavy fetal alcohol exposure. *NeuroImage* 15:233–251.

Botto, L.D., May, K., Fernhoff, P.M., Correa, A., Coleman, K., Rasmussen, S.A., et al. (2003) A population-based study of the 22q11.2 deletion: phenotype, incidence, and contribution to major birth defects in the population. *Pediatrics* 112:101–107.

Bregman, J.D. (1991) Current developments in the understanding of mental retardation. Part II: Psychopathology. *J. Am. Acad. Child Adolesc. Psychiatry* 30:861–872.

Brock, J. (2007) Language abilities in Williams syndrome: a critical review. *Dev. Psychopathol.* 19:97–127.

Capone, G., Goyal, P., Ares, W., and Lannigan, E. (2006) Neurobehavioral disorders in children, adolescents, and young adults with Down syndrome. *Am. J. Med. Genet. C Semin. Med. Genet.* 142:158–172.

Capone, G.T. (2001) Down syndrome: advances in molecular biology and the neurosciences. *J. Dev. Behav. Pediatr.* 22:40–59.

Centers for Disease Control and Prevention. (2006) CDC Wonder: Population Information. http://wonder.cdc.gov/population.html.

Cheema, Z.F., West, J.R., and Miranda, R.C. (2000) Ethanol induces Fas/Apo [apoptosis]-1 mRNA and cell suicide in the developing cerebral cortex. *Alcohol Clin. Exp. Res.* 24:535–543.

Chrast, R., Scott, H.S., Papasavvas, M.P., Rossier, C., Antonarakis, E.S., Barras, C., et al. (2000) The mouse brain transcriptome by SAGE: differences in gene expression between P30 brains of the partial trisomy 16 mouse model of Down syndrome (Ts65Dn) and normals. *Genome Res.* 10:2006–2021.

Comery, T.A., Harris, J.B., Willems, P.J., Oostra, B.A., Irwin, S.A., Weiler, I.J., et al. (1997) Abnormal dendritic spines in fragile X knockout mice: maturation and pruning deficits. *Proc. Natl. Acad. Sci. USA* 94:5401–5404.

Coyle, J.T., Oster-Granite, M.L., and Gearhart, J.D. (1986) The neurobiologic consequences of Down syndrome. *Brain Res. Bull.* 16: 773–787.

DiMario, F.J., Jr. (2004) Brain abnormalities in tuberous sclerosis complex. *J. Child Neurol.*19:650–657.

Dyer-Friedman, J., Glaser, B., Hessl, D., Johnston, C., Huffman, L.C., Taylor, A., et al. (2002) Genetic and environmental influences on the cognitive outcomes of children with fragile X syndrome. *J. Am. Acad. Child Adolesc. Psychiatry* 41:237–244.

Dykens, E.M., Shah, B., Sagun, J., Beck, T., and King, B.H. (2002) Maladaptive behaviour in children and adolescents with Down's syndrome. *J. Intellect. Disabil. Res.* 46:484–492.

Eliez, S., Blasey, C.M., Freund, L.S., Hastie, T., and Reiss, A.L. (2001) Brain anatomy, gender and IQ in children and adolescents with fragile X syndrome. *Brain* 124: 1610–1618.

Eluvathingal, T.J., Behen, M.E., Chugani, H.T., Janisse, J., Bernardi, B., Chakraborty, P., et al. (2006) Cerebellar lesions in tuberous sclerosis complex: neurobehavioral and neuroimaging correlates. *J. Child Neurol.* 21:846–851.

Ernhart, C.B., Sokol, R.J., Martier, S., Moron, P., Nadler, D., Ager, J.W., et al. (1987) Alcohol teratogenicity in the human: a detailed assessment of specificity, critical period, and threshold. *Am. J. Obstet. Gynecol.* 156:33–39.

Ewart, A.K., Morris, C.A., Atkinson, D., Jin, W., Sternes, K., Spallone, P., et al. (1993) Hemizygosity at the elastin locus in a developmental disorder, Williams syndrome. *Nat. Genet.* 5:11–16.

Feinstein, C., and Reiss, A.L. (1996) Psychiatric disorder in mentally retarded children and adolescents: The challenges of meaningful diagnosis. *Ment. Retard.* 5:827–852.

Felder, C.C. (1995) Muscarinic acetylcholine receptors: signal transduction through multiple effectors. *FASEB J.* 9:619–625.

Feng, Y., Gutekunst, C.A., Eberhart, D.E., Yi, H., Warren, S.T., Hersch, S.M. (1997) Fragile X mental retardation protein: nucleocytoplasmic shuttling and association with somatodendritic ribosomes. *J. Neurosci.* 17:1539–1547.

Frangiskakis, J.M., Ewart, A.K., Morris, C.A., Mervis, C.B., Bertrand, J., Robinson, B.F., et al. (1996) LIM-kinase1 hemizygosity implicated in impaired visuospatial constructive cognition. *Cell* 86:59–69.

Franke, P., Leboyer, M., Gansicke, M., Weiffenbach, O., Biancalana, V., Cornillet-Lefebre, P., et al. (1998) Genotype-phenotype relationship in female carriers of the premutation and full mutation of FMR-1. *Psychiatry Res.* 80:113–127.

Freund, L.S., and Reiss, A.L. (1991) Cognitive profiles associated with the fra(X) syndrome in males and females. *Am. J. Med. Genet.* 38:542–547.

Fu, Y.H., Kuhl, D.P., Pizzuti, A. (1991) Variation of the CGG repeat at the fragile X site results in genetic instability: resolution of the Sherman paradox. *Cell* 67:1047–1058.

Galaburda, A.M., and Bellugi, U.V. (2000) Multi-level analysis of cortical neuroanatomy in Williams syndrome. *J. Cogn. Neurosci.* 12:74–88.

Galaburda, A.M., Holinger, D.P., Bellugi, U., and Sherman, G.F. (2002) Williams syndrome: neuronal size and neuronal-packing density in primary visual cortex. *Arch. Neurol.* 59:1461–1467.

Galaburda, A.M., Schmitt, J.E., Atlas, S.W., Eliez, S., Bellugi, U., and Reiss, A.L. (2001) Dorsal forebrain anomaly in Williams syndrome. *Arch. Neurol.* 58:1865–1869.

Garaci, F.G., Floris, R., Bozzao, A., Manenti, G., Simonetti, A., Lupattelli, T., et al. (2004) Increased brain apparent diffusion coefficient in tuberous sclerosis. *Radiology* 232(2):461–465.

Gaser, C., Luders, E., Thompson, P.M., Lee, A.D., Dutton, R.A., Geaga, J.A., et al. (2006) Increased local gyrification mapped in Williams syndrome. *NeuroImage* 33:46–54.

Gillberg, I.C., Gillberg, C., and Ahlsen, G. (1994) Autistic behavior and attention deficits in tuberous sclerosis. A population-based study. *Dev. Med. Child Neurol.* 36:50–56.

Goate, A., Chartier-Harlin, M.C., Mullan, M., Brown, J., Crawford, F., Fidani, L., et al. (1991) Segregation of a missense mutation in the amyloid precursor protein gene with familial Alzheimer's disease. *Nature* 349:704–706.

Gomez, M.R. (1988) Neurologic and psychiatric features. In: Gomez, M.R., ed. *Tuberous sclerosis*. New York: Raven Press, pp. 21–36.

Gothelf, D., Eliez, S., Thompson, T., Hinard, C., Penniman, L., Feinstein, C., et al. (2005) COMT genotype predicts longitudinal cognitive decline and psychosis in 22q11.2 deletion syndrome. *Nat. Neurosci.* 8:1500–1502.

Gothelf, D., Penniman, L., Gu, E., Eliez, S., Reiss, A.L.(2007) Developmental trajectories of brain structure in adolescents with 22q11.2 deletion syndrome: a longitudinal study. *Schizophr. Res.* 96:72–81.

Greicius, M.D., Krasnow, B., Boyett-Anderson, J.M., Eliez, S., Schatzberg, A.F., Reiss, A.L., et al. (2003) Regional analysis of hippocampal activation during memory encoding and retrieval: fMRI study. *Hippocampus* 13:164–174.

Grice, S.J., Haan, M.D., Halit, H., Johnson, M.H., Csibra, G., Grant, J., et al. (2003) ERP abnormalities of illusory contour perception in Williams syndrome. *Neuroreport* 6(14):1773–1777.

Grigsby, J.P., Kemper, M.B., Hagerman, R.J., and Myers, C.S. (1990) Neuropsychological dysfunction among affected heterozygous fragile X females. *Am. J. Med. Genet.* 35:28–35.

Guerri, C., Pascual, M., and Renau-Piqueras, J. (2001) Glia and fetal alcohol syndrome. *Neurotoxicology* 22:593–599.

Guerri, C. (1998) Neuroanatomical and neurophysiological mechanisms involved in central nervous system dysfunctions induced by prenatal alcohol exposure. *Alcohol Clin. Exp. Res.* 22:304–312.

Gutierrez, G.C., Smalley, S.L., and Tanguay, P.E. (1998) Autism in tuberous sclerosis complex. *J. Autism Dev. Disord.* 28:97–103.

Hagerman, R.J., and Hagerman, P.J. (2002) The fragile X premutation: into the phenotypic fold. *Curr. Opin. Genet. Dev.* 12:278–283.

Hagerman, R.J., Hull, C.E., Safanda, J.F., Carpenter, I., Staley, L.W., O'Connor, R.A., et al. (1994) High functioning fragile X males: demonstration of an unmethylated fully expanded FMR-1 mutation associated with protein expression. *Am. J. Med. Genet.* 51: 298–308.

Hagerman, R.J., Jackson, C., Amiri, K., Silverman, A.C., O'Connor, R., and Sobesky, W. (1992) Girls with fragile X syndrome: physical and neurocognitive status and outcome. *Pediatrics* 89:395–400.

Hagerman, R.J. (1996) Physical and behavioral phenotype. In: Hagerman, R.J., and Cronister, A., eds. *Fragile X syndrome: diagnosis, treatment, and research.* Baltimore and London: Johns Hopkins University Press, pp. 46–47.

Hanson, J.E., and Madison, D.V. (2007) Presynaptic FMR1 genotype influences the degree of synaptic connectivity in a mosaic mouse model of fragile X syndrome. *J. Neurosci.* 27:4014–4018.

Hattori, M., Fujiyama, A., Taylor, T.D., Watanabe, H., Yada, T., Park, H.S., et al. (2000) The DNA sequence of human chromosome 21. *Nature* 405:311–319.

Hessl, D., Glaser, B., Dyer-Friedman, J., and Reiss, A.L. (2006) Social behavior and cortisol reactivity in children with fragile X syndrome. *J. Child Psychol. Psychiatry* 47:602–610.

Hessl, D., Rivera, S.M., and Reiss, A.L. (2004) The neuroanatomy and neuroendocrinology of fragile X syndrome. *Ment. Retard. Dev. Disabil. Res. Rev.* 10:17–24.

Hinton, V.J., Halperin, J.M., Dobkin, C.S., Ding, X.H., Brown, W.T., and Miezejeski, C.M. (1995) Cognitive and molecular aspects of fragile X. *J. Clin. Exp. Neuropsychol.* 17:518–528.

Huttenlocher, P.R. (1984) Synapse elimination and plasticity in developing human cerebral cortex. *Am. J. Ment. Defic.* 88:488–496.

Ikonomidou, C., Bittigau, P., Ishimaru, M.J., Wozniak, D.F., Koch, C., Genz, K., et al. (2000) Ethanol-induced apoptotic neurodegeneration and fetal alcohol syndrome. *Science* 287:1056–1060.

Irwin, S.A., Patel, B., Idupulapati, M., Harris, J.B., Crisostomo, R.A., Larsen, B.P., et al. (2001) Abnormal dendritic spine characteristics in the temporal and visual cortices of patients with fragile-X syndrome: a quantitative examination. *Am. J. Med. Genet.* 98: 161–167.

Isacson, O., Seo, H., Lin, L., Albeck, D., and Granholm, A.C. (2002) Alzheimer's disease and Down's syndrome: roles of APP, trophic factors and ACh. *Trends Neurosci.* 25:79–84.

Jambaque, I., Cusmai, R., Curatolo, P., et al. (1991) Neuropsychological aspects of tuberous sclerosis in relation to epilepsy and MRI findings. *Dev. Med. Child Neurology* 33:698–705.

Jernigan, T.L., and Bellugi, U. (1990) Anomalous brain morphology on magnetic resonance images in Williams syndrome and Down syndrome. *Arch. Neurol.* 47:529–533.

Kates, W.R. (2007) Inroads to mechanisms of disease in child psychiatric disorders. *Am. J. Psychiatry* 164:547–551.

Kelley, D.J., Davidson, R.J., Elliott, J.L., Lahvis, G.P., Yin, J.C., and Bhattacharyya, A. (2007) The cyclic AMP cascade is altered in the fragile X nervous system. *PLoS ONE.* 2(9):e931.

Kemper, M.B., Hagerman, R.J., Ahmad, R.S., and Mariner, R. (1986) Cognitive profiles and the spectrum of clinical manifestations in heterozygous fra (X) females. *Am. J. Med. Genet.* 23:139–156.

Kennedy, L.A., and Mukerji, S. (1986) Ethanol neurotoxicity. 2. Direct effects on differentiating astrocytes. *Neurobehav. Toxicol. Teratol.* 8:17–21.

Kirk, J.W., Mazzocco, M.M., and Kover, S.T. (2005) Assessing executive dysfunction in girls with fragile X or Turner syndrome using the Contingency Naming Test (CNT). *Dev. Neuropsychol.* 28:755–777.

Korenberg, J.R., Chen, X.N., Hirota, H., Lai, Z., Bellugi, U., Burian, D., et al. (2000) VI. Genome structure and cognitive map of Williams syndrome. *J. Cogn. Neurosci.* 12:89–107.

Korenberg, J.R., Chen, X.N., Schipper, R., Sun, Z., Gonsky, R., Gerwehr, S., et al. (1994) Down syndrome phenotypes: the consequences of chromosomal imbalance. *Proc. Natl. Acad. Sci. USA* 91:4997–5001.

Krasuski, J.S., Alexander, G.E., Horwitz, B., Rapoport, S.I., and Schapiro, M.B. (2002) Relation of medial temporal lobe volumes to age and memory function in nondemented adults with Down's syndrome: implications for the prodromal phase of Alzheimer's disease. *Am. J. Psychiatry* 159:74–81.

Krawczun, M.S., Jenkins, E.C., and Brown, W.T. (1985) Analysis of the fragile-X chromosome: localization and detection of the fragile site in high resolution preparations. *Hum. Genet.* 69:209–211.

Kwon, H., Menon, V., Eliez, S., Warsofsky, I.S., White, C.D., Dyer-Friedman, J., et al. (2001) Functional neuroanatomy of visuospatial working memory in fragile X syndrome: relation to behavioral and molecular measures. *Am. J. Psychiatry* 158:1040–1051.

Laggerbauer, B., Ostareck, D., Keidel, E.M., Ostareck-Lederer, A., and Fischer, U. (2001) Evidence that fragile X mental retardation protein is a negative regulator of translation. *Hum. Mol. Genet.* 10:329–338.

Lai, F., and Williams, R.S. (1989) A prospective study of Alzheimer disease in Down syndrome. *Arch. Neurol.* 46:849–853.

Lauder, J.M. (1993) Neurotransmitters as growth regulatory signals: role of receptors and second messengers. *Trends Neurosci.* 16: 233–240.

Lee, A.D., Leow, A.D., Lu, A., Reiss, A.L., Hall, S., Chiang, M.C., et al. (2007) 3D pattern of brain abnormalities in fragile X syndrome visualized using tensor-based morphometry. *NeuroImage* 34:924–938.

Levitin, D.J., Cole, K., Lincoln, A., and Bellugi, U. (2005) Aversion, awareness, and attraction: investigating claims of hyperacusis in the Williams syndrome phenotype. J. *Child Psychol. Psychiatry* 46:514–523.

Li, Z., Zhang, Y., Ku, L., Wilkinson, K.D., Warren, S.T., and Feng, Y. (2001) The fragile X mental retardation protein inhibits translation via interacting with mRNA. *Nucleic Acids Res.* 29:227.

Luat, A.F., Makki, M., and Chugani, H.T. (2007) Neuroimaging in tuberous sclerosis complex. *Curr. Opin. Neurol.* 20:142–150.

Luders, E., Di Paola, M., Tomaiuolo, F., Thompson, P.M., Toga, A.W., Vicari, S., et al. (2007) Callosal morphology in Williams syndrome: a new evaluation of shape and thickness. *Neuroreport* 18:203–207.

Lund, J. (1988) Psychiatric aspects of Down's syndrome. *Acta Psychiatr. Scand.* 78:369–374.

Manning, M.A., and Hoyme, H.E. (2007) Fetal alcohol spectrum disorders: a practical clinical approach to diagnosis. *Neurosci. Biobehav. Rev.* 31:230.

Mattson, M.P. (1997) Cellular actions of beta-amyloid precursor protein and its soluble and fibrillogenic derivatives. *Physiol. Rev.* 77:1081–1132.

Mattson, S.N., Riley, E.P., Sowell, E.R., Jernigan, T.L., Sobel, D.F., and Jones, K.L. (1996) A decrease in the size of the basal ganglia in children with fetal alcohol syndrome. *Alcohol Clin. Exp. Res.* 20:1088–1093.

Mattson, S.N., and Riley, E.P. (1998) A review of the neurobehavioral deficits in children with fetal alcohol syndrome or prenatal exposure to alcohol. *Alcohol Clin. Exp. Res.* 22:279–294.

May, P.A., Brooke, L., Gossage, J.P., Croxford, J., Adams, C., Jones, K.L, et al. (2000) Epidemiology of fetal alcohol syndrome in a South African community in the Western Cape Province. *Am. J. Pub. Health* 90:1905–1912.

May, P.A., and Gossage, J.P. (2001) Estimating the prevalence of fetal alcohol syndrome. A summary. *Alcohol Res. Health* 25:159–167.

Mazzocco, M.M., Pennington, B.F., and Hagerman, R.J. (1993) The neurocognitive phenotype of female carriers of fragile X: additional evidence for specificity. *J. Dev. Behav. Pediatr.* 14:328–335.

McGee, C.L., and Riley, E.P. (2006) Brain imaging and fetal alcohol spectrum disorders. *Ann. Ist. Super. Sanita* 42:46–52.

Meyer-Lindenberg, A., Hariri, A.R., Munoz, K.E., Mervis, C.B., Mattay, V.S., Morris, C.A., et al. (2005) Neural correlates of genetically abnormal social cognition in Williams syndrome. *Nat. Neurosci.* 8:991–1003.

Meyer-Lindenberg, A., Mervis, C.B., and Berman, K.F. (2006) Neural mechanisms in Williams syndrome: a unique window to genetic influences on cognition and behaviour. *Nat. Rev. Neurosci.* 7:380–393.

Miller, M.W., and Robertson, S. (1993) Prenatal exposure to ethanol alters the postnatal development and transformation of radial glia to astrocytes in the cortex. *J. Comp. Neurol.* 337:253–266.

Miller, M.W. (1992) The effects of prenatal exposure to ethanol on cell proliferation and neuronal migration. In: Miller, M.W., ed. *Development of the Central Nervous System: Effects of Alcohol and Opiates*. New York: Alan R. Liss, pp. 47–69.

Mills, D.L., Alvarez, T.D., St. George, M., Appelbaum, L.G., Bellugi, U., and Neville, H., III. (2000) Electrophysiological studies of face processing in Williams syndrome. *J. Cogn. Neurosci.* 12:47–64.

Moon, J., Beaudin, A.E., Verosky, S., Driscoll, L.L., Weiskopf, M., Levitsky, D.A., Crnic, L.S., and Strupp, B.J. (2006) Attentional dysfunction, impulsivity, and resistance to change in a mouse model of fragile X syndrome. *Behav. Neurosci.* 120:1367–1379.

Morris, C.A. (2006) *The Dysmorphology, Genetics, and Natural History of Williams-Beauren Syndrome*. Baltimore: John Hopkins University Press, pp. 3–17.

Mostofsky, S.H., Mazzocco, M.M., Aakalu, G., Warsofsky, I.S., Denckla, M.B., and Reiss, A.L. (1998) Decreased cerebellar posterior vermis size in fragile X syndrome: correlation with neurocognitive performance. *Neurology* 50:121–130.

Munir, F., Cornish, K.M., and Wilding, J. (2000) A neuropsychological profile of attention deficits in young males with fragile X syndrome. *Neuropsychologia* 38:1261–1270.

Osborne, J.P., Fryer, A., and Webb, D. (1991) Epidemiology of tuberous sclerosis. *Ann. N.Y. Acad. Sci.* 615:125–127.

Paul, B.M., Stiles, J., Passarotti, A., Bavar, N., and Bellugi, U. (2002) Face and place processing in Williams syndrome: evidence for a dorsal-ventral dissociation. *Neuroreport* 13:1115–1119.

Pinter, J.D., Brown, W.E., Eliez, S., Schmitt, J.E., Capone, G.T., and Reiss, A.L. (2001) Amygdala and hippocampal volumes in children with Down syndrome: a high-resolution MRI study. *Neurology* 56: 972–974.

Rasmussen, P., Borjesson, O., Wentz, E., and Gillberg, C. (2001) Autistic disorders in Down syndrome: background factors and clinical correlates. *Dev. Med. Child Neurol.* 43:750–754.

Reiss, A.L., Abrams, M.T., Greenlaw, R., Freund, L., and Denckla, M.B. (1995) Neurodevelopmental effects of the FMR-1 full mutation in humans. *Nat. Med.* 1:159–167.

Reiss, A.L., Eliez, S., Schmitt, J.E., Straus, E., Lai, Z., Jones, W., et al. (2000) Neuroanatomy of Williams syndrome: a high-resolution MRI study. *J. Cogn. Neurosci.* 12:65–73.

Reiss, A.L., Freund, L., Tseng, J.E., and Joshi, P.K. (1991) Neuroanatomy in fragile X females: the posterior fossa. *Am. J. Hum. Genet.* 49:279–288.

Riddle, J.E., Cheema, A., Sobesky, W.E., Gardner, S.C., Taylor, A.K., Pennington, B.F., et al. (1998) Phenotypic involvement in females with the FMR1 gene mutation. *Am. J. Ment. Retard.* 102:590–601.

Ridler, K., Bullmore, E.T., DeVries, P.J., Suckling, J., et al. (2001) Widespread anatomical abnormalities of gray and white matter structure in tuberous sclerosis. *Psychol. Med.* 31:1437–1446.

Riikonen, R., Salonen, I., Partanen, K., and Verho, S. (1999) Brain perfusion SPECT and MRI in fetal alcohol syndrome. *Dev. Med. Child Neurol.* 41:652–659.

Rivera, S.M., Menon, V., White, C.D., Glaser, B., and Reiss, A.L. (2002) Functional brain activation during arithmetic processing in females with fragile X syndrome is related to FMR1 protein expression. *Hum. Brain Mapp.* 16:206–218.

Roebuck, T.M., Mattson, S.N., and Riley, E.P. (1998) A review of the neuroanatomical findings in children with fetal alcohol syndrome or prenatal exposure to alcohol. *Alcohol Clin. Exp. Res.* 22: 339–344.

Ross, M.H., Galaburda, A.M., and Kemper, T.L. (1984) Down's syndrome: is there a decreased population of neurons? *Neurology* 34:909–916.

Rossen, M.L., Jones, W., Wang, P.P., and Klima, E.S. (1995) Face processing: remarkable sparing in Williams syndrome. *Genet. Counsel.* 6:138–140.

Rousseau, F., Heitz, D., Tarleton, J., MacPherson, J., Malmgren, H., Dahl, N., et al. (1994) A multicenter study on genotype-phenotype correlations in the fragile X syndrome, using direct diagnosis with probe StB12.3: the first 2,253 cases. *Am. J. Hum. Genet.* 55: 225–237.

Schmitt, J.E., Eliez, S., Bellugi, U., and Reiss, A.L. (2001a) Analysis of cerebral shape in Williams syndrome. *Arch. Neurol.* 58:283–287.

Schmitt, J.E., Eliez. S., Warsofsky. I.S., Bellugi, U., Reiss, A.L. (2001b) Corpus callosum morphology of Williams syndrome: relation to genetics and behavior. *Dev. Med. Child Neurol.* 43:155–159.

Selby, L., Zhang, C., and Sun, Q.Q. (2007) Major defects in neocortical GABAergic inhibitory circuits in mice lacking the fragile X mental retardation protein. *Neurosci. Lett.* 412:227–232.

Sobesky, W.E., Hull, C.E., and Hagerman, R.J. (1994) Symptoms of schizotypal personality disorder in fragile X women. *J. Am. Acad. Child Adolesc. Psychiatry* 33:247–255.

Sowell, E.R., Jernigan, T.L., Mattson, S.N., Riley, E.P., Sobel, D.F., and Jones, K.L. (1996) Abnormal development of the cerebellar vermis in children prenatally exposed to alcohol: size reduction in lobules I-V. *Alcohol Clin. Exp. Res.* 20:31–34.

Sowell, E.R., Mattson, S.N., Thompson, P.M., Jernigan, T.L., Riley, E.P., and Toga, A.W. (2001) Mapping callosal morphology and cognitive correlates: effects of heavy prenatal alcohol exposure. *Neurology* 57:235–244.

Streissguth, A.P., Aase, J.M., Clarren, S.K., Randels, S.P., LaDue, R.A., and Smith, D.F. (1991) Fetal alcohol syndrome in adolescents and adults. *JAMA* 265:1961–1967.

Tamm, L., Menon, V., Johnston, C.K., Hessl, D.R., and Reiss, A.L. (2002) fMRI study of cognitive interference processing in females with fragile X syndrome. *J. Cogn. Neurosci.* 14:160–171.

Teiple, S.J., Alexander, G.E., Schapiro, M.B., Moller, H.J., Rapoport, S.I., and Hampel, H. (2004) Age-related cortical gray matter reductions in non-demented Down's syndrome adults determined by MRI with voxel-based morphometry. *Brain* 127:811–824.

Tsiouris, J.A., and Brown, W.T. (2004) Neuropsychiatric symptoms of fragile X syndrome: pathophysiology and pharmacotherapy. *CNS Drugs* 18:687–703.

Van Slegtenhorst, M., de Hoogt, R., Hermans, C., et al. (1997) Identification of the tuberous sclerosis gene TSC1 on chromosome 9q34. *Science* 277:805–808.

Van Slegtenhorst, M., Nellist, M., Negelkerken, B., et al. (1998) Interaction between hamartin and tuberin, the TSC1 and TSC2 gene products. *Hum. Mol. Genetics* 7:1053–1057.

Wang, P.P., and Bellugi, U. (1993) Williams syndrome, Down syndrome, and cognitive neuroscience. *Am. J. Dis. Child.* 147:1246–1251.

Webb, D.W., Fryer, A.E., and Osbourne, J.P. (1996) Morbidity associated with tuberous sclerosis: A population study. *Dev. Med. Child Neurol.* 38:146–155.

Weber, A.M., Egelhoff, J.C., McKellop, J.M., and Franz, D.N. (2000) Autism and the cerebellum: evidence from tuberous sclerosis. *J. Autism Dev. Disord.* 30:511–517.

Weiler, I.J., Irwin, S.A., Klintsova, A.Y., Spencer, C.M., Brazelton, A.D., Miyashiro, K., et al. (1997) Fragile X mental retardation protein is translated near synapses in response to neurotransmitter activation. *Proc. Natl. Acad. Sci. USA* 94:5395–5400.

Weis, S., Weber, G., Neuhold, A., and Rett, A. (1991) Down syndrome: MR quantification of brain structures and comparison with normal control subjects. *Am. J. Neuroradiol.* 12:1207–1211.

White, N.S., Alkire, M.T., and Haier, R.J. (2003) A voxel-based morphometric study of nondemented adults with Down syndrome. *NeuroImage* 20:393–403.

Wisniewski, K.E., Laure-Kamionowska, M., and Connell, F. (1986) Neuronal density and synaptogenesis in the postnatal stage of brain maturation in Down syndrome. In: Epstein, C.J., ed. *The Neurobiology of Down Syndrome.* New York: Raven Press, pp. 29–45.

Wisniewski, K.E. (1990) Down syndrome children often have brain with maturation delay, retardation of growth, and cortical dysgenesis. *Am. J. Med. Genet. Suppl.* 7:274–281.

Yorns, W., Burleson, J.A., and DiMario, F.J. (2001) Brain morphometry in tuberous sclerosis complex. *J. Invest. Med.* 49:221A.

Zigman, W., Schupf, N., Haveman, M., and Silverman, W. (1997) The epidemiology of Alzheimer disease in intellectual disability: results and recommendations from an international conference. *J. Intellect. Disabil. Res.* 41:76–80.

68 Cognitive Neuroscience Approaches to Typical and Atypical Development

B.J. CASEY AND SARAH DURSTON

Only recently have we begun to understand and appreciate the complexities of human brain development with the emergence of noninvasive imaging techniques. At the forefront of these methodological advances has been the development of functional capabilities of magnetic resonance imaging (MRI). This work hinges on the precision of behavioral measures in capturing the psychological constructs and behavioral phenomenon that change with development and/or are disrupted in child and adolescent psychiatric disorders. Although structural changes in the brain are important, functional brain changes are critical in more directly linking the behavior to the underlying neural circuitry. Normal developmental changes are the focus of this chapter, but examples of abnormal development are provided, focusing predominantly on the prevalent childhood disorder of attention-deficit/hyperactivity disorder (ADHD). A general discussion of molecular genetics of childhood psychiatric disorder is presented in Chapter 71, but it is useful to consider these factors and their impact on human development typical and atypical here.

This introduction to a cognitive neuroscience approach highlights some of the key methodological advances important in the assessment of human brain development. Assessment of behavioral and brain development requires methods that provide the opportunity to assess changes that occur as the child moves into and out of stages of development or pathological progressions. The chapter is divided into three general sections: First, we consider methodologies for examining neurodevelopment in humans, then provide an overview of major developmental findings from these methods, and finally highlight new approaches that provide further insight to mechanisms related to childhood psychiatric disorders.

METHODS FOR EXAMINING HUMAN BRAIN AND COGNITIVE DEVELOPMENT

Magnetic resonance technologies have introduced a new set of tools for capturing features of brain development in living, developing humans. The most common MR methods used in the study of human brain development are illustrated below. These methods have provided scientists with the opportunity to safely track cognitive and neural processes underlying human development. These imaging methods became especially important to cognitive and developmental scientists when functional imaging techniques were developed. Whereas MRI is used to produce structural images of the brain useful for anatomical and morphometric studies, the functional component of functional MRI (fMRI) allows an in vivo measure of brain activity. The functional methodology measures changes in blood oxygenation in the brain that are assumed to reflect changes in neural activity (Logothettis et al., 2001) and eliminates the need for exogenous contrast agents, including radioactive isotopes (Kwong et al., 1992; Ogawa et al., 1990). Diffusion tensor imaging (DTI), a relatively new MR technique, can detect changes in white matter microstructure based on properties of diffusion (Pierpaoli et al., 1996). Diffusion of water in white matter tracts is affected by myelin and the orientation and regularity of fibers and provides an index of brain connectivity. Because all three of these MR techniques are noninvasive, development and learning can be tracked more precisely within individuals with repeat scans over short or long intervals of time (that is, days to years) (Fig. 68.1; see also COLOR FIGURE 68.1 in separate insert).

Human imaging methods have advanced the field of developmental neuroscience by providing evidence of changes in structural architecture and functional organization in the developing brain in vivo. However, these measures provide only an indirect measure of brain structure and function. Changes in the volume of a structure or amount of activity as measured by fMRI methods lack the resolution to definitely characterize the mechanism of change. Histological evidence suggests that brain development is a dynamic process of regressive and progressive changes. As such, MRI-based cortical changes observed with development may be a combination of myelination, dendritic pruning, and changes in the vascular, neuronal, and glial density. These methodologies provide information about regional development that in conjunc-

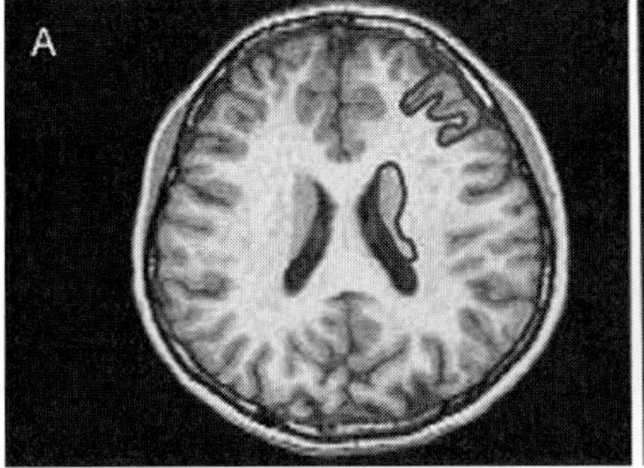

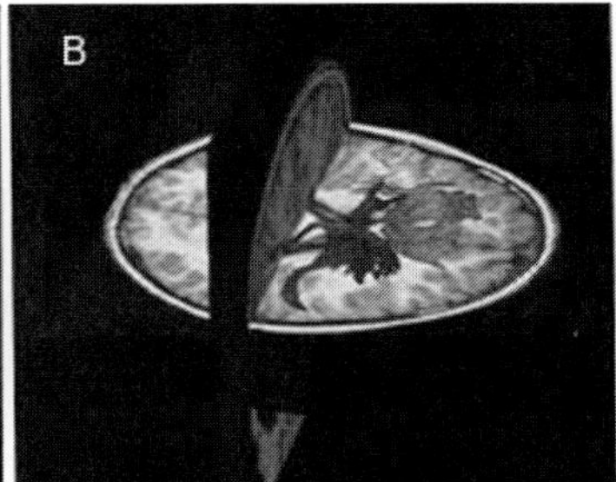

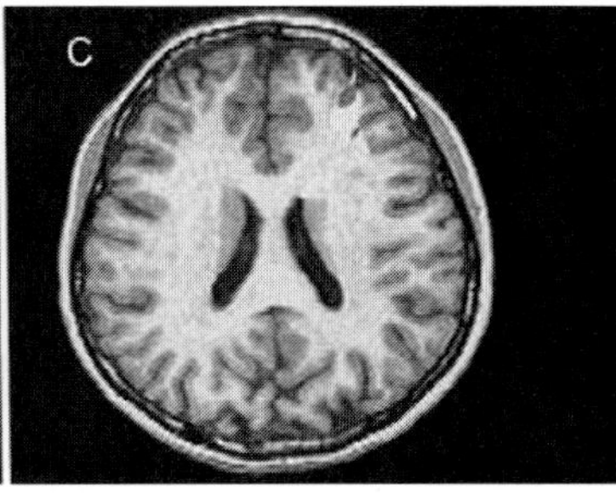

FIGURE 68.1 Structural magnetic resonance imaging (MRI) is used to produce structural images of the brain useful for anatomical and morphometric studies (Panel A), diffusion tensor imaging (DTI) measures fiber tracts between anatomical structures (Panel B), and functional MRI (fMRI) measures patterns of brain activity within those structures (Panel C). From Casey et al. (2002).

tion with postmortem and animal histological studies have the potential to tease these processes apart. Further, because these tools permit not only scanning of children but repeated scanning of the same individual over time, they can provide measurement of general neuroanatomical changes with learning and development. This chapter highlights MR-based measures of change in neuroanatomy, cortical connectivity, and cortical function with learning and development.

NEUROANATOMICAL DEVELOPMENT OF THE HUMAN BRAIN

A number of structural imaging studies have mapped the neuroanatomical course of human brain development. The findings parallel many of the postmortem histologic findings providing validity for in vivo imaging measures and also parallel behavioral and cognitive development. Investigators could inappropriately view as causal, coincidental changes in brain and behavioral development by simply assuming linear changes across systems and direct associations between these changes. Nonetheless, the synchrony in time course of the changes reported in MRI-based anatomical studies and cognitive development have driven more direct tests of these associations in functional imaging studies. For this reason, MRI-morphometric studies of change in structural architecture are highlighted.

The most compelling reports of structural changes with development over the period of childhood and adolescence have come from longitudinal MRI studies (e.g., Gogtay et al., 2004; Sowell et al., 2004). In general, the sequence in which the cortex matures parallels cognitive milestones in human development. Regions subserving primary functions, such as motor and sensory systems, mature first, with temporal and parietal association cortices associated with basic language skills and spatial attention maturing next. Higher-order association areas, such as the prefrontal and lateral temporal cortices, which integrate primary sensorimotor processes and modulate basic attention and language processes, appear to mature last. Specifically, MRI-based measures showed that cortical gray matter loss occurred earliest in the primary sensorimotor areas and latest in the dorsolateral prefrontal cortex. These findings are consistent with nonhuman and human primate postmortem studies showing that the prefrontal cortex matures at a more protracted rate than sensorimotor cortex in synaptic density (Huttenlocher, 1979; Bourgeois et al., 1994). Cross-sectional studies of normative brain maturation during childhood and adolescence have shown somewhat similar patterns, concluding that gray matter loss during this period reflects a sculpting process of the immature brain into the fully functioning mature one (Sowell et al., 2003). As such, the pattern of development observed is suggested to reflect the ongoing neuronal regressive events, such as pruning and the elimination of connections.

Developmental changes in subcortical regions occur over this period of development as well. One of the more reliable patterns reported is in subcortical regions to which association cortex projects. For example, cross-sectional (Sowell et al., 1999) and longitudinal studies (Gogtay et al., 2004) show patterns of development in portions of the basal ganglia to which the prefrontal cortex directly projects. Again, this pattern may reflect the gradual elimination of connections, with strengthening of others.

What is the corresponding pattern of change in white matter volume over this period? In contrast to an inverted *U*-shape pattern of development in most gray matter areas with age, white matter volume increases in a roughly linear pattern, increasing throughout development until approximately young adulthood, paralleling changes in volume and density. These changes presumably reflect ongoing myelination of axons by oligodendrocytes enhancing neuronal conduction and communication. Connections are being fine-tuned with the elimination of an overabundance of synapses and strengthening of relevant connections with development and experience.

How do these structural changes relate to cognitive changes? Developmental changes in cortical development have been found to correlate with behavioral performance measures. Sowell and colleagues (2001) showed an association between prefrontal lobe structural maturation and memory function using neuropsychological measures. Similar associations have been reported between MRI-based prefrontal volume and specific measures of cognitive control ability to override an inappropriate response in favor of another (Casey et al., 1997). Together these studies suggest that, perhaps not surprisingly, functional changes in brain development are reflected in structural changes.

ATYPICAL DEVELOPMENT OF THE HUMAN BRAIN

Magnetic resonance imaging has been used to study a host of developmental disorders. The majority of these studies have focused on the common childhood disorder of ADHD, with a prevalence rate of approximately 5% to 8%. This disorder is used as an example throughout this chapter. Over two decades of structural MRI, studies of abnormalities in ADHD have reliably shown smaller-than-normal brain volumes. In addition to an overall reduction in total brain volume, four major findings about regional differences are notable. Relative to controls, individuals with ADHD show (*1*) smaller MRI-based volumes of the caudate nucleus, (*2*) smaller prefrontal volumes, (*3*) smaller cerebellum vermis, and (*4*) smaller white matter tracts. However, of note, some debate persists on the degree to which these regionally specific changes are independent of the overall reductions in brain volume. Longitudinal MRI-based anatomical studies of individuals with ADHD (Castellanos et al., 2002; Shaw et al., 2006) suggest that these neuranatomical abnormalities are present early in childhood. As such, these differences appear to be due to early environmental and/or genetic effects.

REGIONAL DEVELOPMENT OF WHITE MATTER

Magnetic resonance imaging–based morphometry studies suggest that cortical connections are being fine-tuned with the elimination of an overabundance of synapses and strengthening of relevant connections with development and experience. Recent advances in MR technology, such as DTI, provide a potential tool for examining the role of white matter tracts in the development of cognitive and brain development with greater detail. This method provides information on directionality and regularity of myelinated fiber tracts.

Until recently, few studies have linked brain connectivity measures with cognitive development (Klingberg et al., 1999), although indirect measures of white matter suggest regional development in prefrontal cortex and presumably function. Of these studies, one showed that development of working memory capacity was positively correlated with prefrontal-parietal connectivity (Klingberg et al., 2002) consistent with imaging studies showing differential recruitment of these regions in children relative to adults. Using a similar approach, Liston and colleagues (2005) showed that DTI-based connectivity in frontostriatal and posterior fiber tracts correlated with age, but only frontostriatal connectivity correlated with efficient (fast and accurate) performance on a go/no-go task. The prefrontal fiber tracts examined were defined by regions of interest identified in an fMRI study using the same task (Durston et al., 2002). Similar combined DTI and fMRI analytical approaches have shown the importance of the maturation of prefrontal-parietal connectivity in performance of a working memory task. As such, DTI and fMRI-based measures with these regions correlated across age. Across these studies, measures of brain connectivity were correlated with development, but specificity of the involvement of particular fiber tracts in cognitive performance was shown by dissociating the particular tract or cognitive ability. These dissociations are important when distinguishing between performance and age-related differences in imaging measures.

ATYPICAL DEVELOPMENT OF WHITE MATTER

Many studies have linked prefrontal structure to cognitive deficits in ADHD. Few studies have examined the role of white matter tracts between the prefrontal cortex and other structures implicated in the disorder, or the extent to which white matter tract myelination or regularity correlate in family members with the disorder. Functional imaging maps from a go/no-go task were used to identify portions of the ventral prefrontal cortex and striatum, involved in suppressing an inappropriate action (that is, cognitive control), in parent–child dyads (Casey et al., 2007). Specifically, structural connectivity in right prefrontal fiber tracts correlated with functional activity in the frontostriatal regions and with performance of a go/no-go task in parent–child dyads with ADHD. A role of prefrontal connectivity in disruption of cognitive control in ADHD was supported further by an association between white matter integrity in this region in ADHD children and their parents. Connectivity in the ADHD parent and child in prefrontal regions was tightly associated. Together, these findings suggest that heritability in myelination and regularity of frontostriatal fibers may contribute to individual differences in the efficient recruitment of cognitive control that may underlie deficits in this ability in ADHD. Such evidence highlights the need to consider genetic and environmental factors that may alter myelin and synapse formation (for example, neurotrophin factors and white matter injury).

FUNCTIONAL ORGANIZATION OF THE DEVELOPING HUMAN BRAIN

What do the previously described changes in brain structure, such as prolonged development of the prefrontal gray and white matter, mean in terms of function? The development of the prefrontal cortex is believed to play an important role in the maturation of higher cognitive abilities. Mature cognition is characterized by the ability to filter and suppress irrelevant information and actions (sensorimotor processes) in favor of relevant ones (Casey et al., 2002). A child's capacity to filter information and suppress inappropriate actions in favor of appropriate ones continues to develop across the first two decades of life, with susceptibility to interference from competing sources lessening with maturity. Many paradigms used to study cognitive development require cognitive control such as the Stroop and go/no-go tasks. Collectively, imaging studies using these tasks show a shift from diffuse to focal prefrontal activations with development as these brain regions become fine-tuned with experience (Casey et al., 2005). Based on cross-sectional and longitudinal studies (Durston et al., 2006) the pattern of activity within brain regions central to task performance (that correlate with reaction time and accuracy) appear to become more focal or fine-tuned with increased activity, whereas regions not correlated with task performance decrease in activity with age. This pattern of activity, observed across a variety of paradigms, might reflect development within, and refinement of, projections to and from these regions (consistent with the DTI findings presented in the previous section).

The region-specific differences in activation with age that have been reported may reflect maturation but may also reflect simple performance differences. For this reason, the collection of behavioral responses is critical across these studies. Children almost always perform worse on higher cognitive tasks. Therefore, it is difficult to specify whether the activation differences are age related or simply reflect an overall difference in performance, without equating performance between age groups or controlling for performance differences. To address this issue, investigators have adopted different approaches for teasing apart age versus performance-driven differences. One key strategy is to use performance matching to equate behavioral performance (Schlaggar et al., 2002). Post hoc, patients are divided into subgroups based on behavioral performance that is either matched across groups or not matched to assess age differences that are independent of performance and performance differences that are independent of age. These patterns help identify the basis of the observed activation and/or regional differences and how they relate to the task demands. As such, this approach provides a better understanding of how maturation relates to increased cognitive abilities. For instance, in a study of cognitive control that showed performance-related neural recruitment (Bunge et al., 2002) children were divided into "better and worse performers." Children with effective response inhibition did not recruit the same prefrontal regions as those activated by adults, suggesting an age-related recruitment in this region. However, they did recruit a subset of the same posterior association areas (parietal regions) consistently activated in adults. Children with poor behavioral regulation did not recruit these posterior regions, suggesting that improved ability to withhold an inappropriate response may first require mature activation of posterior parietal regions that is task specific.

As not all tasks yield comparable performance across age groups, a second approach that has been used to equate performance across groups is to parametrically manipulate task difficulty (Durston et al., 2002). In a parametric design, task difficulty is titrated with increases in task demands (for example, increased response competition, memory load, or stimulus degradation) allowing comparisons between children and adults on trials equated for accuracy. Durston and colleagues (2002) used a version of a go/no-go task that parametrically manipulated the number go trials (responses) preceding a no-go trial (withhold response). Behaviorally, children and adults had more errors as the number of responses preceding a no-go trial increased. Children, however, had as many errors for no-go trials following a single go trial as adults had when a no-go trial followed as many as five go trials. The imaging data from adults showed a monotonic increase in association areas of the ventral prefrontal and posterior parietal cortices as the number of go trials preceding a no-go trial increased, but children maximally activated these regions regardless of whether they had to withhold a response following one, three, or five go trials (responses). These data are consistent with other reports showing that immature cognition is characterized by an enhanced sensitivity to interference from competing sources (for example, response competition) that coincides with immature association cortex, specifically in prefrontal and posterior parietal related circuitry.

The majority of developmental observations described above have relied on cross-sectional samples or even comparisons across studies. However, cross-sectional analyses may falsely suggest changes over time or fail to detect the specificity or magnitude of these changes given the large individual variability in brain structure among individuals, especially during development. Recent longitudinal work tracking cognitive and brain development from late childhood into early adolescence during performance of go/no-go tasks with fMRI showed a developmental shift in patterns of cortical activation from diffuse to focal activity similar to those reported in large cross-sectional studies (Durston et al., 2006).

Regions uncorrelated with task performance were recruited less with age, whereas a region in ventral prefrontal cortex that correlated with performance (speed and accuracy) showed enhanced recruitment. This change in pattern of activity was associated with enhanced performance of the cognitive control task. Activation in earlier developing regions such as the primary motor cortex remained unchanged. A parallel cross-sectional analysis based on a second group of children (the same ages as the longitudinal group) showed less specific results, supporting the importance of longitudinal studies in evaluating cortical changes with age.

Although most pediatric imaging studies have focused on cortical changes, there are significant subcortical changes with development as well. Galvan and colleagues (2006) tested the hypothesis that differential development of subcortical regions relative to cortical control regions may explain suboptimal decision making in adolescence. Development of both of these regions (cortical and subcortical) is immature in childhood and mature in adulthood, but during adolescence limbic regions appear to be similar in functional development to that of adults, whereas cortical regions remain immature. Accordingly, protracted development of the prefrontal cortex relative to functionally mature limbic subcortical regions during this period may result in less efficient regulation of behavior during emotionally charged contexts. Individual differences in recruitment of these subcortical regions have been shown to be related to suboptimal decisions. These studies together with the longitudinal MRI-based morphometry studies suggest differential developmental trajectories for sensorimotor and subcortical regions relative to association areas like the prefrontal cortex. Both the imaging-based neuroanatomical and functional studies highlight the importance of examining changes in ability within individuals over time. As such, this work can begin to delineate processes specific to learning or development and their disruption in developmental disorders.

COGNITIVE NEUROSCIENCE APPROACH TO UNDERSTANDING ATYPICAL DEVELOPMENT

As noted throughout this chapter, a cornerstone of human behavioral development is the ability to regulate inappropriate thoughts and actions in favor of appropriate ones (that is, cognitive control). Recently, theories of cognitive ability and its disruption in a number of developmental disorders have begun to emphasize learning mechanisms, based largely (Casey, Durston, et al., 2006) on computational and animal studies of operant conditioning, of executive functions. The basic assumption of these theories is that learning when, what, or in which contexts to expect an event is critical for adjusting behavior appropriately in different contexts over time. Control of behavior should be implemented when something unexpected or motivationally relevant (for example, signal of safety or danger) occurs to adjust behavior to that situation. Implicit in this notion is that the child must be able to learn to predict future events to detect unpredicted ones. This ability is essential in planning and maintaining appropriate thoughts and actions in different social contexts over time.

Deficits in learning to detect regularities or irregularities in the environment could lead to less signaling of control systems to help alter or adjust behavior accordingly. Such deficits could mimic those observed when top-down control systems themselves are impaired. Put another way, the control systems may function adequately when "on line" but may not be brought on line when needed, due to failures in these bottom-up signaling mechanisms. Likewise, intact signaling but inefficient top-down control could result in poor regulation of behavior but, presumably, in a more general way. The variability in cognitive performance reported in the clinical literature may be partly due to such differences. Targeting top-down and bottom-up contributions to cognitive control may help to isolate the etiology of developmental disorders and to target biologically relevant interventions.

Let us consider functional imaging studies of ADHD from this perspective. Like the structural imaging studies, fMRI studies show multiple neural systems are involved in this disorder, including the prefrontal cortex, caudate nucleus, cerebellum, and parietal cortex. Most of these studies show hypoactivation of these regions that appears to normalize with stimulant medication. Figure 68.2 depicts a cartoon of the many different brain regions activated across recent imaging studies of ADHD. At first glance, these regions may seem to suggest disparate findings within the literature. However, each of these regions (basal ganglia, cerebellum, and parietal cortex) is part of unique circuits that project to and from prefrontal cortex, thus providing a means for signaling prefrontal regions when top-down control needs to be imposed. Ineffective signaling of control systems by any one of these regions could lead to poor regulation of behavior, but with subtle differences, depending on the system involved or the behavior task used. For example, the basal ganglia and cerebellum have been implicated in learning about the frequency and the timing of events (that is, learning what to expect and when). These regions may signal the prefrontal cortex when an unexpected or competing event occurs at an unpredicted time, to adjust behavior appropriately. The posterior parietal region has been implicated in signaling prefrontal cortex when competing stimuli require top-down biasing of attention in favor of one stimulus attribute or location over another.

Consistent with this view, Durston and colleagues (2007) showed that children with ADHD benefit less

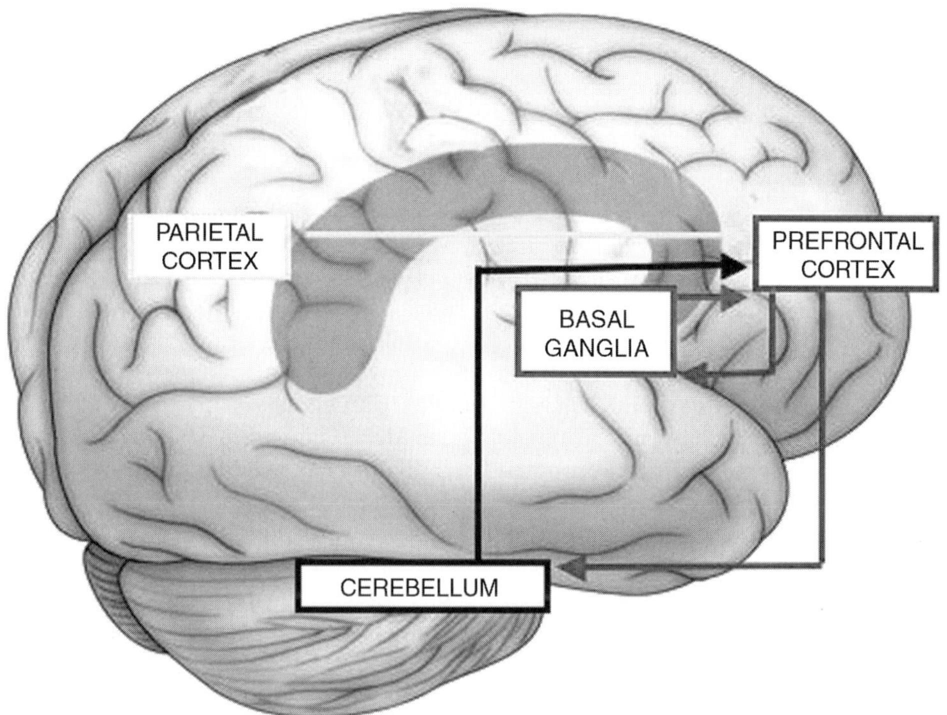

FIGURE 68.2 Brain circuitry implicated in attention-deficit/hyperactivity disorder. Each circuit has projections both to and from the prefrontal cortex. The basal ganglia, cerebellum, and posterior systems signal the prefrontal cortex when new or competing sensory information is encountered so that the prefrontal cortex can immediately determine whether it provides new and important information or whether it can safely be ignored (Casey and Durston, 2006).

from events being predictable in terms of their reaction time than control children and are less accurate when events occur at unpredictable times. Furthermore, they had decreased activity in cerebellum when events were temporally unpredictable. These findings are consistent with the view that some forms of ADHD may be related to an impaired ability to learn from temporal and contextual cues in the environment, thus hindering the ability to alter behavior when contexts change.

In sum, development of cognitive control and its disruption in developmental disorders involves a number of prefrontal circuits. Because brain regions within this circuitry mature at different rates, development must be considered in delineating the contributions of different brain regions (for example, cortical and subcortical) to cognitive control and its disruption in ADHD. Identification of which of these systems is altered within individuals could help individualize and target interventions and treatments (Casey et al., 2007).

IMPACT OF METHODOLOGICAL ADVANCES ON THE FIELD

Developments in the Human Genome Project and in MRI methods provide us with the opportunity to more directly examine the effects of early experience on gene expression and plasticity in the developing human brain. These methods also offer new directions in biological psychiatry. We are in an explosive era of methodological development that has opened new doors for examining the developing human brain in vivo. Functional neuroimaging is providing new insights into the dynamics of neural circuits involved in cognitive and emotional development, and genomic research is producing an abundance of new target molecules for the treatment of developmental disorders. With this progress, new efforts are under way to unify the understanding of functional brain anatomy with physiological, cellular, and molecular processes that influence behavior. Cognitive neuroscientists have begun to show how genetic variants can affect the activity of brain regions implicated in well-defined behaviors with combined imaging and genetic studies (Egan et al., 2001). Such approaches are only beginning to be used with developmental and clinical populations and are most informative when grounded in parallel transgenic mouse models. A unified understanding of mechanisms involved in cognitive and emotional development may open up new avenues for therapeutic intervention for clinical populations at the pharmacological, genetic, and behavioral levels.

Although the major psychiatric disorders display a substantial heritable component, very few genetic associations to these phenotypes have proven to be reliable.

The majority of allelic associations with neurobehavioral phenotypes are not consistently replicated. For instance, a recent meta-analysis of 24 studies (comprising more than 3,000 participants) of the association between the serotonin transporter-linked polymorphic region and anxiety-related personality traits found "that the effect, if present, is small" (Munafo et al., 2005). Genetic risk is likely distributed across many allelic variants in psychiatric illness. Thus the effect size of any single risk factor for disorders will be small and difficult to reliably identify.

Endophenotypes are heritable, distinct endpoints in biology such as anatomy, biochemistry, and behavior that reflect discrete components of pathophysiologic processes. These refined phenotypes have been proposed as attractive targets for human genetic studies because they are less biologically complex than disease phenotypes and can be more objectively and reliably ascertained than categorical disorders. These attributes suggest that genetic correlation with a specific endophenotype should prove more reliable than associations with disease phenotype, but to date, this is often not the case. To ensure the utility of endophenotypes, candidate gene studies must be focused on validated endophenotypes that are biologically more simple, relate more closely to the biology of the candidate gene, and can be more precisely measured than categorical disorder phenotypes. Specifically, endophenotypes must fulfill several criteria: (*1*) reflect a biological process that is a component of the more complex disorder phenotype, (*2*) be more biologically simple than the disorder phenotype to ensure that the effect size of any particular risk factor is relatively large, and (*3*) the biology of the endophenotype must be understood well enough that it can be related to specific candidate risk factors including genetic, environmental, and developmental ones. Endophenotypes that fail to meet these criteria may yield similar findings as diagnostic-based phenotypes (Flint and Munafo, 2007).

In this context, cognitive neuroscientists have begun to combine imaging and genetic studies in examining these endophenotypes in psychiatric disorders. One example is illustrated in recent research on biological substrates of ADHD that has been characterized by impulsivity and inattention for which a dopamine-deficit hypothesis has been posited (Swanson et al., 2007). Dopamine genes have been a target of inquiry in understanding risk factors for the disorder. Specifically, the dopamine-transporter (*DAT1*) gene has been implicated repeatedly in ADHD (Cook et al., 1995), although the mechanism by which it exerts its effects remains unknown. The polymorphism associated with ADHD has been shown to affect expression of the transporter. Dopamine transporters are predominantly expressed in the striatum, and stimulant medication that is often effective in treating impulse control in ADHD is believed to exert its therapeutic effects by blocking dopamine transporters in this region. Genetic imaging studies have begun to examine *DAT1* gene effects on brain activation patterns in individuals with ADHD. In one study, a sample of sibling-pairs discordant for ADHD and individuals matched on age and gender were tested using a version of go/no-go task with fMRI (Durston et al., 2007). Dopamine-transporter genotype affected activation in striatum in individuals with familial risk for ADHD (affected and unaffected siblings) but not controls. These results suggest that DAT gene effects in the striatum may be involved in translating genetic risk for ADHD into a neurobiological substrate, as only those individuals at risk for the disorder showed gene effects on striatal activation. This and similar findings may point towards long-term possibilities for tailoring individual therapies by *DAT1*-genotype: If this genotype has differential effects on striatal activation, it may become possible to use this polymorphism as a surrogate end point in individualized treatments targeting genotype/fMRI-activation profiles.

SUMMARY

Clearly, imaging and genetic techniques will continue to inform us about progressions in typically developing and atypically developing populations. This chapter suggests that biological and child psychiatry is in a new era, moving from solely behavioral and psychopharmacological investigations of biological substrates of disorders. The field is now moving toward a more unified understanding of neural mechanisms involved in childhood psychiatric disorders with the use of imaging and genetic methods from a cognitive neuroscience approach. Such an approach may open up new avenues for therapeutic intervention for clinical populations at the pharmacological, genetic, and behavioral levels and identify windows of development that may be most optimal to treatment.

REFERENCES

Bourgeois, J.P., Goldman-Rakic, P.S., and Rakic, P. (1994) Synaptogenesis in the prefrontal cortex of rhesus monkeys. *Cereb. Cortex* 4:78–96.

Bunge, S.A., Dudukovic, N.M., Thomason, M.E., Vaidya, C.J., and Gabrieli, J.D. (2002) Immature frontal lobe contributions to cognitive control in children: evidence from fMRI. *Neuron.* 33:301–311.

Casey, B. J. (2002) Windows into the developing human brain. *Science* 296:1408–1409.

Casey, B.J., Amso, D., and Davidson, M.C. (2007) Learning about learning and development with neuroimaging. In: Johnsons, M., and Munakata, Y., eds. *Attention and Performance XXI: Processes of Change in Brain and Cognitive Development.* Cambridge, MA: MIT.

Casey, B.J., and de Haan, M. (2002) Imaging methods in developmental science. *Dev. Sci.* 5(3):265–267.

Casey, B.J. and Durston S. (2006) From behavior to cognition to the brain and back: What have we learned from functional imaging studies of ADHD. *Am. J. Psychiatry* 163(6):957–960.

Casey, B.J., Epstein, J., Buhle, J. et al. (2007) Frontostriatal connectivity and its role in cognitive control in parent-child dyads with ADHD. *Am. J. Psychiatry* 164:1–7.

Casey, B.J., and Munakata, Y. (2002) Converging methods in developmental science: an introduction. *Dev. Psychobiol.* 40(3):197–199.

Casey, B.J., Thomas, K.M., Davidson, M.C., Kunz, K., and Franzen P.L. (2002) Dissociating striatal and hippocampal function developmentally with a stimulus-response compatibility task. *J. Neurosci.* 22:8647–8652.

Casey, B.J., Tottenham, N., Liston, C., and Durston, S. (2005) Imaging the developing brain: what have we learned about cognitive development? *Trends Cogn. Sci.* 9:104–110.

Casey, B.J., Trainor, R.J., Orendi, J.L., Schubert, A.B., Nystrom, L.E., Giedd, J.N., et al. (1997) A developmental functional MRI study of prefrontal activation during performance of a go-no-go task. *J. Cogn. Neurosci.* 9:835–847.

Castellanos, X., Lee, P.P., Sharp, W., Jeffries, N.O., Greenstein, D.K., Clasen, L.S., Blumenthal, J.D., James, R.S., Ebens, C.L., Walter, J.M., Zijdenbos, A., Evans, A.C., Giedd, J.N., and Rapoport, J.L. (2002) Developmental trajectories of brain volume abnormalities in children and adolescents with attention-deficit/hyperactivity disorder. *JAMA.* 288(14):1740–1748.

Cook, E.H., Jr., Stein, M.A., Krasowski, M.D., Cox, N.J., Olkon, D.M., Kieffer, J.E., and Leventhal, B.L. (1995) Association of attention-deficit disorder and the dopamine transporter gene. *Am. J. Hum. Genet.* 56(4):993–998.

DeCasper, A.J., and Fifer, W.P. (1980) Of human bonding: newborns prefer their mothers' voices. *Science* 208:1174–1176.

Durston, S., Davidson, M.C., Mulder, M.J., Spicer, J.A., Galvan, A., Tottenham, N., Scheres, A., Castellanos, F.X., van Engeland, H., and Casey, B.J. (2007) Neural and behavioral correlates of expectancy violations in attention-deficit hyperactivity disorder. *J. Child Psychol. Psychiatry* 48(9):881–889.

Durston, S., Davidson, M.C., Tottenham, N., et al. (2006) A shift from diffuse to focal cortical activity with development. *Dev. Sci.* 9:1–8.

Durston, S., Thomas, K., Yang, Y., et al. (2002) A neural basis for the development of inhibitory control. *Dev. Sci.* 5(4):F9–F16.

Durston, D., Fossella, J.A., Mulder, M.J., Casey, B.J., Ziermans, T.B. Vessaz, M.N., and van Engeland, H. (2008) Dopamine-transporter genotype conveys familial risk for attention-deficit/hyperactivity disorder through striatal activation. *J. Am. Acad. Child Adolesc. Psychiatry* 47(1):61–67.

Egan, M.F., Goldberg, T.E., Kolachana, B.S., Callicott, J.H., Mazzanti, C.M., Straub, R.E., Goldman, D., and Weinberger, D.R. (2001) Effect of COMT Val108/158 Met genotype on frontal lobe function and risk for schizophrenia. *Proc. Natl. Acad. Sci. USA* 98(12): 6917–6922.

Ellis, A.W., and Lambon Ralph, M.A. (2000) Age of acquisition effects in adult lexical processing reflect loss of plasticity in maturing systems: insights from connectionist networks. *J. Exp. Psychol. Learn. Mem. Cogn.* 26(5):1103–1123.

Fan, J., Fossella, J., Sommer, T., Wu, Y., and Posner, M.I. (2003) Mapping the genetic variation of executive attention onto brain activity. *Proc. Natl. Acad. Sci. USA* 100(12):7406–7411.

Flint, J., and Munafo, M. (2007) The endophenotype concept in psychiatric genetics. *Psychol. Med.* 37:163–180.

Fifer, W.P., and Moon, C.M. (1995) The effects of fetal experience with sound. In: Lecanuet, J.-P., Fifer, W.P., Krasnegor, N. A., and Smotherman, W.P., eds. *Fetal Development—A Psychobiological Perspective*. Hillsdale, NJ: Lawrence Erlbaum, pp. 351–368.

Galvan, A., Hare, T.A., and Parra, C.E. (2006) Earlier development of the accumbens relative to orbitofrontal cortex might underlie risk-taking behavior in adolescents. *Neuroscience* 26(25):6885–6892.

Gogtay, N., Giedd, J.N., Lusk, L., Hayashi, K.M., Greenstein, D., Vaituzis, A.C., Nugent, T.F., III, Herman, D.H., Clasen, L.S., Toga, A.W., Rapoport, J.L., and Thompson, P.M. (2004) Dynamic mapping of human cortical development during childhood through early adulthood. *Proc. Natl. Acad. Sci. USA* 101:8174–8179

Hepper, P.G. (1987) The amniotic fluid: an important priming role in kin recognition. *Anim. Behav.* 35(5):1343–1346.

Hertz-Pannier, L., Gaillard, W.D., Mott, S.H., Cuenod, C.A., Bookheimer, S.Y., Weinstein, S., Conroy, J., Papero, P.H., Schiff, S.J., Le Bihan, D., and Theodore, W.H. (1997) Noninvasive assessment of language dominance in children and adolescents with functional MRI: a preliminary study. *Neurology* 48(4):1003–1012.

Huttenlocher, P.R. (1979) Synaptic density in human frontal cortex-developmental changes and effects of aging. *Brain Reseach* 163: 195–205.

Johnson, M.H. (2001) Functional brain development in humans. *Nat. Rev. Neurosci.* 2:475–483.

Karni, A., Meyer, G., Jezzard, P., Adams, M.M., Turner, R., and Ungerleider, L.G. (1995) Functional MRI evidence for adult motor cortex plasticity during motor skill learning. *Nature* 377(6545): 155–158.

Klingberg, T., Forssberg, H., and Westerberg, H. (2001) Increased brain activity in frontal and parietal cortex underlies the development of visuospatial working memory capacity during childhood. *J. Cogn. Neurosci.* 14:1–10.

Klingberg, T., Forssberg, H., and Westerberg, H. (2002) Increased brain activity in frontal and parietal cortex underlies the development of visuospatial working memory capacity during childhood. *J. Cogn. Neurosci.* 14(1):1–10.

Klingberg, T., Vaidya, C.J., Gabrieli, J.D., Moseley, M.E., and Hedehus, M. (1999) Myelination and organization of the frontal white matter in children: a diffusion tensor MRI study. *Neuroreport* 10(13):2817–2821.

Kwong, K.K., Belliveau, J.W., Chesler, D.A., Goldberg, I.E., Weisskoff, R.M., Poncelet, B.P., Kennedy, D.N., Hoppel, B.E., Cohen, M.S., and Turner, R. (1992) Dynamic magnetic resonance imaging of human brain activity during primary sensory stimulation. *Proc. Natl. Acad. Sci. USA* 89:5675–5679.

Liston, C., Watts, R., Tottenham, N., Davidson, M.C., Niogi, S., Ulug, A.M., et al. (2005) Frontostriatal microstructure modulates efficient recruitment of cognitive control. *Cerebral Cortex* 16:553–560.

Logothetis, N.K., Pauls, J., Augath, M., Trinath, T., and Oeltermann, A. (2001) Neurophysiological investigation of the basis of the fMRI signal. *Nature* 412:150–157.

McClelland, J.L., Thomas, A.G., McCandliss, B.D., and Fiez, J.A. (1999) Understanding failures of learning: Hebbian learning, competition for representational space, and some preliminary experimental data. *Prog. Brain Res.* 121:75–80.

McEwen, B. (2003) Early life influence on life-long patterns of behavior and health. *Ment. Retard. Dev. Disabil. Res. Rev.* 9(3):149–154.

Munafo, M.R., Clark, T., and Flint, J. (2005) Does measurement instrument moderate the association between the serotonin transporter gene and anxiety-related personality traits? A meta-analysis. *Mol. Psychiatry* 10(4):415–419.

Ogawa, S., Lee, T.M., Snyder, A.Z., and Raichle, A.Z. (1990) Oxygenation-sensitive contrast in magnetic resonance image of rodent brain at high magnetic fields. *Mag. Reson. Med.* 14:68–78.

Pierpaoli, C., Jezzard, P., Basser, P.J., Barnett, A., and DiChiro, G. (1996) Diffusion tensor MR imaging of the human brain. *Radiology* 201:637–648.

Posner, M.I., Rothbart, M., Farah, M., and Bruer, J. (2001) The developing human brain. *Dev. Sci.* 4(3):253–387.

Schlaggar, B.L., Brown, T.T., Lugar, H.M., Visscher, K.M., Miezin, F.M., and Peterson, S.E. (2002) Functional neuroanatomical differences between adults and school-age children in the processing of single words. *Science* 296:1476–1479.

Shaw, P., Lerch, J., Greenstein, D., Sharp, W., Clasen, L., Evans, A., Giedd, J., Castellanos, F.X., and Rapoport, J. (2006) Longitudinal mapping of cortical thickness and clinical outcome in children and adolescents with attention-deficit/hyperactivity disorder. *Arch. Gen. Psychiatry* 63(5):540–549.

Sowell, E.R., Delis, D., Stiles, J., and Jernigan, T.L. (2001) Improved memory functioning and frontal lobe maturation between childhood and adolescence: a structural MRI study. *J. Int. Neuropsychol. Soc.* 7(3):312–322.

Sowell, E.R., Peterson, B.S., Thompson, P.M., Welcome, S.E., Henkenius, A.L., and Toga, A.W. (2003) Mapping cortical change across the human life span. *Nat. Neurosci.* 6:309–315.

Sowell, E.R., Thompson, P.M., Leonard, C.M., Welcome, S.E., Kan, E., and Toga, A.W. (2004) Longitudinal mapping of cortical thickness and brain growth in normal children. *J. Neurosci.* 24: 8223–8231.

Sowell, E.R., Thompson, P.M., Holmes, C.J., Jernigan, T.L., and Toga, A.W. (1999) In vivo evidence for post-adolescent brain maturation in frontal and striatal regions. *Nat. Neurosci.* 2(10):859–861.

Sullivan, R. M., Hofer, M. A., and Brake, S. C. (1986) Olfactory-guided orientation in neonatal rats is enhanced by a conditioned change in behavioral state. *Dev. Psychobio.* 19(6):615–623.

Swanson, J.M., Kinsbourne, M., Nigg, J., Lanphear, B., Stefanatos, G.A., Volkow, N., Taylor, E., Casey, B.J., Castellanos, F.X., and Wadhwa, P.D. (2007) Etiologic subtypes of attention-deficit/hyperactivity disorder: brain imaging, molecular genetic and environmental factors and the dopamine hypothesis. *Neuropsychol. Rev.* 17(1):39–59.

Swedo, S.E., Leonard, H.L., Garvey, M., Mittleman, B., Allen, A.J., Perlmutter, S., Louge, L., Dow, S., Zamkoff, J., and Dubbert, B.K. (1998) Pediatric autoimmune neuropsychiatric disorders associated with streptococcal infections: clinical description of the first 50 cases. *Am. J. Psychiatry* 155(2):264–271.

Wolf, S.S., Jones, D.W., Knable, M.B., Gorey, J.G., Lee, K.S., Hyde, T.M., Coppola, R., and Weinberger, D.R. (1996) Tourette syndrome: prediction of phenotypic variation in monozgotic twins by caudate nucleus D2 receptor binding. *Science* 273(5279): 1225–1227.

Zevin, J., and Seidenberg, M. (2002) Age of acquisition effects in reading and other tasks. *J. Mem. Lang.* 47:1–29.

69 The Neurobiology of Impulsivity and Self-Regulatory Control in Children with Attention-Deficit/Hyperactivity Disorder

KERSTIN J. PLESSEN AND BRADLEY S. PETERSON

Attention-deficit/hyperactivity disorder (ADHD) is the most frequently diagnosed psychiatric disorder in children, with a worldwide prevalence of 5.3% (Polanczyk et al., 2007). It is defined by the presence of inattention, hyperactivity, and impulsivity (American Psychiatric Association [APA], 1994). This triad of symptom domains is thought to reflect an inability to control, or self-regulate, thought and behavior (Barkley, 1997, 2006). Thus, understanding the neural basis and ontogeny of impulsivity and self-regulatory control is crucially important for understanding the pathophysiology of ADHD and for developing improved, rationally based treatments for the disorder.

The clinical presentation of ADHD is heterogeneous in terms of its profile of symptoms, the intensities of those symptoms across diagnostic subtypes, and their longitudinal course. The current diagnostic system (*Diagnostic and Statistical Manual of Mental Disorders*, 4th ed. [*DSM-IV*]; APA, 1994) distinguishes three subtypes of ADHD: predominantly hyperactive/impulsive, inattentive, and combined. The symptoms of ADHD usually attenuate during adolescence, with approximately half of children remaining substantially affected into adulthood (Mannuzza et al., 1991; Biederman et al., 1993; Willoughby, 2003; Kessler et al., 2006). Some have argued, however, that symptoms often do not necessarily improve but rather change in presentation, with inattention either persisting or worsening but hyperactivity declining across time (Biederman et al., 2000).

The clinical evolution of ADHD symptoms is often complicated further by the presence of comorbid conditions, such as anxiety disorders, tic disorders, obsessive–compulsive disorder (OCD), or depression (Milberger et al., 1995; Jensen et al., 1997; Graetz et al., 2001; Peterson et al., 2001; Sukhodolsky et al., 2003; Blackman et al., 2005). A substantial subgroup of children with ADHD are at risk of developing oppositional defiant disorder (ODD) and conduct disorder (CD), both of which benefit from early clinical identification and treatment (Coté et al., 2002; Cunningham, 2002; Gillberg et al., 2004). In addition, children diagnosed with the combined or hyperactive/impulsive subtype of ADHD are at higher risk for the development not only of CD but also drug abuse, criminality, and other risk-taking behaviors (Biederman et al., 1997; Pratt et al., 2002; Barkley, 2004; Thapar et al., 2006). Finally, ADHD often co-occurs with bipolar disorder, perhaps in part because these conditions overlap in several of their diagnostic criteria, but likely beyond what would be expected given these shared criteria (Biederman et al., 1996; Leibenluft et al., 2003). These conditions may represent impairment in the self-regulatory control of affect, motoric behavior, aggressive drives, and social interactions, extending beyond the dysregulation that presumably produces the core symptomatic triad that constitutes ADHD.

IMPULSIVITY AND SELF-REGULATORY CONTROL

Impulsivity and impaired self-regulatory control are closely related constructs (Ainslie, 1975; Logue, 1988; Evenden and Ryan, 1996). *Impulsivity* has been defined as "a predisposition toward rapid, unplanned reactions to internal or external stimuli without regard to the negative consequences of these reactions to themselves or others" (Moeller et al., 2001, p. 1784). Impulsivity comprises a broad range of behaviors, from simple motor responses to more complex, goal-directed action sequences that, when exhibited with sufficient frequency for long durations, constitute a behavioral trait. Thus, children with ADHD often have trouble delaying or inhibiting behavioral responses on neuropsychological tasks, a trait captured in current *DSM-IV* diagnostic criteria as having difficulty waiting in line, blurting out answers before questions are completed, or interrupting others in conversation. Impulsivity is manifest independent of the child's emotional state (N. Eisenberg et al., 2006).

Impaired self-regulatory control is a related, but broader, construct that describes a difficulty in filtering, coordinating, and temporally organizing perceptions, affective experience, memories, thoughts, and stress responses during the planning, execution, and monitoring of goal-directed behaviors (Tucker et al., 1995; M.I. Posner and Rothbart, 2000). Thus, the construct of *impulsivity* refers more specifically to the behavioral consequences of impaired self-regulatory control, particularly when they occur in the context of difficulty in inhibiting a prepotent (a "primed" or "automatic") response. Impaired self-regulatory control, in contrast, includes difficulty in inhibiting or regulating emotions and thought processes even in the absence of overt behavioral response, and in that sense captures the symptoms of inattention and hyperactivity within the diagnostic criteria for ADHD, not only the symptoms of impulsivity.

The capacity to self-regulate thought, emotion, and behavior may be regarded as one of the defining ontological features of human development, and children with ADHD are often regarded by adults and even friends as relatively immature compared with same-age peers. Current diagnostic criteria for ADHD, in fact, stipulate that inattention, hyperactivity, and impulsive symptoms are present "to a degree that is maladaptive and inconsistent with developmental level" (APA, 1994), and they may not necessarily have been classified as deviant had they been present earlier in development. Most children do in fact begin developing a capacity to regulate thought, emotion, and behavior, including the ability to postpone gratification and to inhibit prepotent responses, during the first years of life, and consequently ADHD can be diagnosed reliably even in preschool-aged children (Kollins et al., 2006).

The emergence of self-regulatory control during development is influenced by several genetically and environmentally determined features and abilities of the child, such as temperament, personality, and intelligence (Zuckerman et al., 1991; Rothbart and Bates, 1998; M.I. Posner and Rothbart, 2000). We review these features and abilities in turn, along with their neurobiologic underpinnings, that are thought to contribute to the normal ontogeny of self-regulatory control, and we consider deviance of this development that is thought to lead to the emergence of ADHD symptoms. Approaching a review of the neurobiology and pathophysiology of ADHD from the perspective of impaired self-regulatory control will therefore not represent an exhaustive review of all literature pertaining to ADHD but will rather focus on one of the more unifying constructs through which this condition can be understood (Barkley, 1997; Evenden, 1999).

THE GENETICS OF IMPULSIVITY AND ITS RELEVANCE TO ADHD

The strongest and most replicated findings from family-based and molecular genetic studies of ADHD are reviewed elsewhere in this volume (refer to Chapter 71). We discuss here briefly some of the larger conceptual issues concerning study of the genetic and neurobiological basis of impulsivity and self-regulatory control as they may relate to understanding the pathophysiology of ADHD.

Dimensional Phenotypes

Genetic studies of ADHD are complicated by the heterogeneity of the disorder's clinical symptoms and the pathophysiological subtypes of ADHD (Swanson et al., 2007). In addition, the core symptoms of ADHD are distributed on a spectrum that is continuous with normal behavior, complicating the dichotomous classification of inattention, hyperactivity, and impulsivity as either deviant or not (Stevenson et al., 2005). The use of dimensional measures, in addition to categorical diagnostic criteria, is therefore likely to be crucially important in genetic studies of ADHD that aim to associate genetic variation with the quantitative variation in ADHD symptoms across individuals (refer to Chapter 71). In addition to considering the core symptoms of ADHD as dimensional variables, some investigators have tried to reduce these symptoms to even simpler, more precisely measured, and more behaviorally distinct constructs (Alessi and Petry, 2003; Congdon and Canli, 2005). *Impulsivity* has been variously fractionated, for example, into a disturbance in inhibitory control, an aversion to the delay of rewards, excessively rapid decision making due to a deficit in reflective capacity, and impaired attentional control (Evenden, 1999; Winstanley et al., 2004). These more basic dimensional constructs, also termed *endophenotypes* or *intermediate phenotypes*, may aid the search for genetic contributions to impulsivity (Gottesman and Gould, 2003; Meyer-Lindenberg and Weinberger, 2006). One such construct for measuring impulsivity in humans and animals, for example, is *delay discounting*, a task that assesses the preference of a smaller, immediate reward over a larger delayed one (Logue, 1988). Impulsivity measured with this task has been associated with the interaction of polymorphisms on genes encoding two different dopamine receptor subtypes, DRD2 and DRD4, suggesting that the functional interaction of these two dopaminergic systems may determine individual variability in impulsive decision making (D.T. Eisenberg et al., 2007).

Genetic Influences on Neurotransmitter Systems

Genetic studies support the validity of conceptualizing impulse control or self-regulation as lying on a single continuum (Kalenscher et al., 2006). Individual variations on this continuum have been associated with sequencing variants of genes associated with serotonergic (Soubrie, 1986; Evenden, 1999) or dopaminergic neurotransmission (Congdon and Canli, 2005). Although the role of the serotonergic system in ADHD has been relatively underexplored, probably because effective medications for the treatment of ADHD do not obviously act via serotonergic receptors or transporters and do not prominently alter serotonin metabolism (Zametkin and Rapoport, 1987; Spencer et al., 2000; Volkow et al., 2005), recent genetic and other neurobiological findings have suggested that the serotonergic system may be important in the modulation of impulse control and the symptoms of ADHD (Manor et al., 2001; Kent et al., 2002; Flory et al., 2007). In a recent prospective follow-up study of children with ADHD aged 7–11 years, a lower serotonergic responsivity, as measured in a provocation test with fenfluramine, was predictive of developing antisocial personality disorder later in life (Flory et al., 2007).

Genes linked to dopamine (DA) receptors and the DA transporter (DAT) may also help to determine the capacity for impulse control, perhaps through the crucial role they play in the development and functional integrity of frontostriatal circuits (Kreek et al., 2005). Polymorphisms in various genes related to the DA system, for example, seem to influence inhibitory control in the prefrontal cortex (PFC) and striatum, and they have been implicated strongly in the pathophysiology of ADHD (Bilder et al., 2004; Cools, 2006; refer to Chapter 71). This genetic evidence for the importance of the dopaminergic system in the pathophysiology of ADHD is consistent with the well-documented effectiveness of stimulant medications that target dopaminergic neurotransmission in the treatment of ADHD (Volkow et al., 2005).

An X-linked gene, monoamine oxidase A (MAO-A), is an important determinant of the catabolism of serotonin and DA, and it also influences impulsivity. Polymorphisms in this gene in healthy individuals influence the reactivity and volume of limbic and other brain regions during the performance of inhibitory tasks (Meyer-Lindenberg et al., 2006; Passamonti et al., 2006). Moreover, the effects of this genotype on the risk for developing conduct disorder in childhood and violent behaviors in adult life is moderated by the degree of exposure to adverse life events. Children who carry the functional polymorphism of this gene that is associated with low levels of MAO-A expression (MAO-A-L) exhibit more problem behaviors if they experienced maltreatment (Caspi et al., 2002). This finding represents an example of a Gene × Environment (G × E) interaction, in which the effects of a genotype varies with the degree of exposure to a particular environmental influence (Caspi and Moffitt, 2006). Other genes implicated in the regulation of impulsivity are those of the catechol-O-methyltransferase (COMT) and noradrenergic systems that have also been implicated in ADHD (Kreek et al., 2005). Thus, the polygenic basis of ADHD is mirrored in the polygenic basis of impulse control.

ENVIRONMENTAL RISK FACTORS

Despite the current emphasis on the study of genetic influences in ADHD, knowing the weight of specific epigenetic influences in the interaction between genetic and environmental influences is indispensable for estimating the predisposition of a child to develop ADHD and other psychiatric disorders (Rutter et al., 1997; Insel and Collins, 2003). Environmental factors conventionally are assumed to have a direct and often dose-related biological influence on specific symptoms (Needleman et al., 1990). The study of environmental influences, however, is hindered by assessment methods that are often of questionable validity and reliability, such as subjective reports of smoking and alcohol use during pregnancy or of parenting strategies and styles experienced during early childhood (Rutter, 2005a). In addition, understanding the complex interplay and interactions of environmental influences with genetic vulnerabilities requires increasingly sophisticated, nonlinear models that are either rudimentary in their development or insufficiently understood and used by investigators (Caspi and Moffitt, 2006). Moreover, many environmental influences may be mediated through various epigenetic mechanisms, such as methylation, histone modification, or genomic imprinting, that may permanently induce complex, nonlinear modifications of gene expression (Kraemer et al., 2001; Weaver et al., 2004; Rutter, 2005b; Goos et al., 2007).

Early Childhood Adversity

Indicators of childhood adversity increase the risk for developing ADHD and other psychiatric impairments (Biederman, Milberger, et al., 1995). Findings from the Isle of Wight Study confirmed that the accumulation of several risk factors (severe marital discord, low social class, large family size, paternal criminality, maternal mental disorder, and foster care placement) rather than one single risk factor predicted mental health problems in children (Rutter et al., 1976). The same factors were found to increase the risk for developing ADHD, although males were more vulnerable to these influences than were females (Biederman et al., 2002). Exposure to numerous childhood adversities is thought to impair development of self-regulatory control, which likely predisposes to ADHD and other psychiatric disorders (Cicchetti et al., 1997). The observational nature of these studies, however, does not allow a definitive distinction between environmental and genetic influences on the development of ADHD (Rutter, 1989).

Parenting Styles

Parenting style may mediate the effects of childhood adversity on developing ADHD (Kazdin et al., 1997; Masten et al., 1999). Indeed, children who are impulsive often challenge the skills of even the best caregivers, provoking parenting styles that include use of aggressive disciplinary methods, controlling and authoritarian directives, frequent displays of disapproval, and fewer rewards than parents of age-matched peers (Bell, 1968; Barkley et al., 1991; C. Johnston, 1996; Woodward et al., 1998).

Many parents of children with ADHD themselves suffer from impairments in impulse control, contributing to a disorganized parenting style that can influence the development of ADHD in their children (Biederman et al., 1990; Biederman, Faraone, et al., 1995). These influences differ across developmental stages of the child, with their effects being most pivotal early in development, even in the preschool years, in determining a child's self-regulatory capacity, which in turn is of paramount importance in determining the quality of a child's interpersonal relationships (Bowlby, 1988; Fonagy, 2002; Sugarman, 2006). The neurobiological mechanisms through which parenting styles contribute to the development of ADHD, however, remain largely unknown and should be mapped through longitudinal studies that assess the interactions of parenting style and genotypes on the development of self-regulatory control and ADHD symptoms (Nigg, 2005).

Low Birth Weight

Children who are born prematurely or at low birth weight are at considerably elevated risk for developing ADHD and other cognitive impairments (Bhutta et al., 2002). The degree of maternal warmth that these children experience, however, modifies expression of these difficulties (Tully et al., 2004). Anatomical imaging studies have shown that many brain regions in children who are born prematurely are comparatively smaller in infancy relative to controls who are born at term, disturbances that seem to persist into later childhood. The magnitudes of these abnormalities predict the degree of cognitive impairment that these preterm children exhibit (Peterson et al., 2000; Peterson et al., 2003).

Maternal Smoking

Maternal smoking during pregnancy has been shown repeatedly in longitudinal studies of large populations to increase by more than twofold the risk of developing ADHD and other externalizing behaviors, including aggression and delinquency (Weitzman et al., 1992; Milberger et al., 1996; G.M. Williams et al., 1998; Brennan et al., 1999; Linnet et al., 2005; Braun et al., 2006; Romano et al., 2006). These risks may be independent of genetic contributions, as they have been detected in a population-based sample of twins (N = 1,452 twin-pairs aged 5–16 years) that controlled for genetic influences (Thapar et al., 2003). The effects are also independent of those carried by low birth weight, which increases with smoking, and of the effects of maternal alcohol use during pregnancy, with which smoking often co-occurs (G.M. Williams et al., 1998; Mick et al., 2002). Moreover, smoking has been shown to produce hyperactive offspring in animal studies (Johns et al., 1982). Chronic exposure to nicotine is thought to increase impulsivity in part through an up-regulation of nicotine receptors (Hagino, 1985; Ernst et al., 2001).

Lead Exposure

Although the association of lead blood levels with reduced IQ and impaired visuomotor integration is best documented, other studies have reported an association of lead levels with aggressive behavior and impulsivity (Needleman et al., 1990). Recently, one large epidemiological survey demonstrated associations of more severe symptoms of ADHD with lead levels under 10 μg/dl, the threshold level for safety recommended by the Centers for Disease Control and Prevention (Centers for Disease Control and Prevention [CDC], 2005; Braun et al., 2006). Indeed, inattention has been reported even with extremely low serum levels of lead (≤ 3 μg/dl)—an alarming finding, given that approximately 5% of Mexican American children had serum lead levels of 10 μg/dl (Pirkle et al., 1994; Chiodo et al., 2004).

Television

Much of the research that has associated the amount of television exposure to mental health outcomes in children is descriptive, cross-sectional, and based on small, selected populations with short-term follow-up (Christakis and Zimmerman, 2006). Nevertheless, meta-analyses (Bushman and Anderson, 2001) and long-term follow-up studies (Johnson and Johnson, 2002) have shown that the amount of TV watching in childhood correlates with the frequency of violent behaviors exhibited later in life, which some investigators attribute to the violent content of TV programs and video games (Uhlmann and Swanson, 2004). The relevance of TV watching and the playing of video games for the development of symptoms and behavior more specific to ADHD, rather than those related to violent behaviors in general, is largely unknown. Some have speculated that some of the more complex neuropsychological deficits associated with ADHD may derive from certain characteristics of TV watching, such as the frequent attentional shifts and interruptions that occur during most TV programs (Nigg, 2006).

Parents often report that children with impulsive behavior and inattention spend large amounts of time watching TV or playing video games (Obel et al., 2004). Some have interpreted these findings in light of evidence that video games and TV watching activate circuitry involved in reward processing, and that this reward is particularly gratifying to children with ADHD (Barkley, 2006). In addition, the frequency of TV viewing at ages 1 and 3 years has predicted attentional problems at age 7, suggesting that perhaps excessive TV watching may play a causal role in the development of ADHD symptoms (Christakis et al., 2004). In this study, ADHD symptoms, however, were loosely defined, and other studies have had difficulty replicating its findings using more stringent behavioral criteria (Bertholf and Goodison, 2004; Obel et al., 2004).

The associations of TV watching with ADHD symptoms do not prove causality, however, and studies have not adequately disentangled the effects of excessive TV watching from other characteristics of the home environment, parenting style, and genetic endowment with which it is likely correlated, including the presence of parental ADHD. Children with ADHD, for example, are more likely than children without ADHD to have parents who also have ADHD. The children and their parents with ADHD, moreover, are likely to share genes that confer a vulnerability to developing ADHD. Parents who have either ADHD or these vulnerability genes may be more likely to allow or encourage their children to watch television or to play video games, for example, in that children who are difficult to manage may be placed in front of the TV to keep them calm (Nigg, 2006), and parents with ADHD conceivably may be more likely to avail themselves of this coping strategy. This sort of circumstance would then give rise to a correlation of a specific genetic vulnerability (for ADHD) with a feature of the environment (TV watching) that could easily produce, and therefore be confused with, the correlation of environmental exposure (TV watching) with the child's disorder (ADHD).

GENE–ENVIRONMENT CORRELATIONS AND INTERACTIONS

Although a relatively new area of study, the exploration of interactions between genetic and environmental factors has yielded important new leads in the understanding of childhood psychiatric disorders, and it has helped to bridge our understanding of the roles of "nature" and "nurture" in the genesis of childhood psychopathologies (Ridley, 2003; Gottesman and Hanson, 2005; Caspi and Moffitt, 2006). Gene × Environment interactions may help explain the discrepancy between the high heritability of ADHD (estimated in family genetic studies to be approximately 0.8) with the difficulty in robustly and reproducibly identifying vulnerability genes for ADHD (Faraone et al., 2005; refer to Chapter 71).

Gene × Environment interactions likely determine who develops ADHD, when in the course of development it begins, what its degree of severity will be, whether symptoms will attenuate with age, and what its response to treatment will be (Thapar et al., 2007). A genetic marker associated with ADHD (a haplotype in a gene encoding the DAT), for example, interacts with maternal use of alcohol during pregnancy to increase the risk for developing ADHD (Brookes et al., 2006). Identification of these G × E interactions is also likely to be important in understanding why certain children with ADHD develop CD (Wilens et al., 2002). Children with ADHD who carry a particular allele of the COMT gene, for example, are more susceptible to the effects of low birth weight that contribute to the development of antisocial behavior (Thapar et al., 2005). In addition, even though the DAT gene has been implicated in the pathophysiology of ADHD (refer to Chapter 71), a recent large prospective study of adolescents at risk for developing ADHD has reported that adverse childhood experiences moderate the influence of the DAT gene on ADHD symptoms, in that the genetic effect was observed only in adolescents exposed previously to high levels of psychosocial adversity (Laucht et al., 2007).

Gene–environment correlations, in contrast, are defined as the genetic liability to be exposed to specific environmental circumstances (Rutter and Silberg, 2002). A genetically determined behavioral trait can produce a systematic variation in the environment that confuses the direction of causality attributed to the associations of either genetic or environmental factors with the behavioral traits under investigation. Children with the impulsive symptoms of ADHD, for example, have an increased probability of exposing themselves to risk-taking and sensation-seeking situations; thus, risk taking and the experiences in their environment to which it exposes them is not independent of their underlying genetic vulnerability to ADHD, producing a gene–environment correlation that can therefore hinder the measurement of G × E interactions (Hur and Bouchard, 1997; Ryb et al., 2006). The example already provided for TV watching and ADHD is another example of a possible gene–environment correlation that can confound, or at least complicate, the assessment of a G × E interaction.

ANIMAL MODELS

Animal models are invaluable in many fields of biomedical research for testing models of pathophysiology and for developing novel therapeutics. The development of valid animal models of developmentally based psychopathologies, however, remains challenging because of the polygenic nature of these disorders, the uncertainty and nonspecificity of animal behaviors in their relevance to human psychiatric disease, and our poor knowledge of the underlying disease mechanisms when constructing the animal model (Overall, 2000). Appropriate animal models should have good face validity, so that they produce behavioral traits that correspond to symptoms typical in individuals with the disorder. They should also have good construct validity, being constructed from clearly stated models of pathophysiology for the disorder. Finally, they should have good predictive validity, predicting characteristics of the disorder that were previously unknown, such as associated neurobiological abnormalities or the effects of novel therapeutic agents (Davids et al., 2003).

Genetic knockout (KO) mouse mutants offer particularly good construct validity in animal models because they target specific genes associated with an illness. Further, a number of inbred rat strains are commonly used in the study of ADHD, including the spontaneous hypertensive rat (SHR), the Wistar–Kyoto hyperactive rat, and the Naples high-excitability rat, all of which share good face validity for hyperactive behavior. Several genetic mouse models have also been developed, such as the hyperactive wheel-running mouse, the coloboma mutant mouse, the acallosal mouse, and the thyroid receptor β mutant mouse. Models for ADHD have also been induced by neurotoxins or lesions that target certain brain structures to produce symptoms mimicking those of ADHD. These include, for example, intracisternally administered 6-hydroxydopamine (6-OHDA) lesions in neonatal rats, or the induction of neonatal hypoxia (van der Kooij and Glennon, 2007).

Several animal models thus far seem to be especially promising or popular in the study of ADHD. One of the more promising models is the DAT KO mouse, which in addition to having good construct validity offers excellent face validity in terms of producing hyperactive and impulsive behavior, which most animal models do not (Gainetdinov et al., 1999). Moreover, the DAT KO mouse offers good predictive validity for modelling the therapeutic effects of stimulant medication (van der Kooij and Glennon, 2007). One of the most widely used animal models is the SHR, which offers a high degree of face validity for hyperactivity (Sagvolden et al., 2005). This model, however, also includes traits not found in children with ADHD, such as arterial hypertension (Okamoto and Aoki, 1963), and stimulants have been found by some (Hynes et al., 1985; Amini et al., 2004) but not by others (Sagvolden et al., 2005) to increase hyperactive symptoms in the SHR model, thus reflecting poorly on its predictive validity.

THE ONTOGENY OF NEUROPSYCHOLOGICAL DEFICITS

Mapping the neuropsychological deficits in children with ADHD is important for several reasons. First, identifying these deficits helps in identifying and acquiring needed services (Luria, 1973). Second, knowing the neuropsychological deficits associated with ADHD should provide clues to its underlying pathophysiology (Nigg et al., 2005). Third, neuropsychological measures, when combined with other information, such as symptom scores, genetic information, or neuroimaging data, may identify joint biomarkers that can be used to advance diagnostic tools (Niculescu et al., 2006).

Executive functions (those abilities that facilitate plan for future contingencies, the inhibition of automatic responses, and the pursuit of long-term goals) and self-regulatory control depend largely on neural activity within cortico-subcortical circuits. These circuits execute their regulatory functions through distinct but parallel neural pathways that connect the cortex with various parts of the striatum and limbic system, then with the thalamus, and subsequently with the cortex (Alexander et al., 1986). The PFC plays a particularly important role in self-regulatory control and executive functioning via its projections to the striatum, and in reward behavior and motivation via its connections within mesocorticolimbic circuits (see Fig. 69.1). The neurotransmitters involved in these circuits are predominantly do-

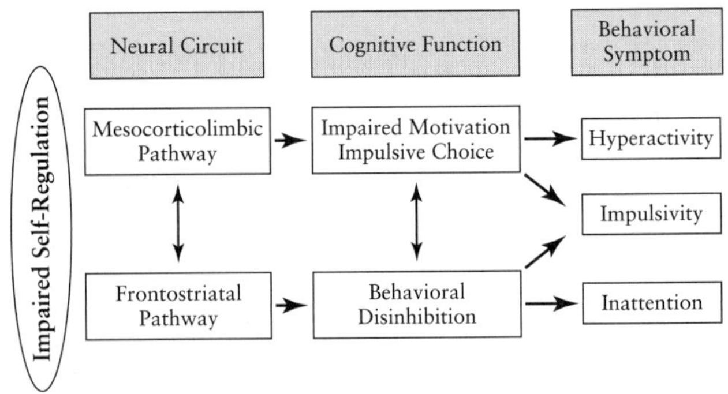

FIGURE 69.1 Elements of impaired self-regulation in attention-deficit/hyperactivity disorder (ADHD). Impaired self-regulation is thought to arise from dysfunction in frontostriatal and mesocorticolimbic circuits. This dysfunction may underlie the neuropsychological disturbances most commonly reported in ADHD, particularly in the executive functions and inhibitory control that are based primarily within frontostriatal circuits, and in decision making and reward that are thought to be based primarily within mesocorticolimbic circuits. Together these dysfunctions support one or more of the typical triad of symptoms in ADHD.

paminergic and glutamatergic, although serotonin and noradrenalin play important neuromodulatory roles as well (Siegel et al., 2006).

Deficits in the self-regulatory functions that cortico-subcortical circuits subserve, however, are not unique to ADHD, as they cut across multiple diagnostic domains, including schizophrenia, bipolar disorder, depression, Tourette syndrome, OCD, borderline personality disorder, and substance abuse (Robbins, 1990; Elliott et al., 1996; Brodsky et al., 1997; Rosenberg et al., 1997; Peterson et al., 1998; Jentsch and Taylor, 1999; Willcutt et al., 2005; Leibenluft et al., 2007). Future studies will need to identify which portions of these circuits contribute to specific aspects of self-regulatory control and their involvement in each of these various diagnostic syndromes (Banaschewski et al., 2005). This presumably will require including more diagnostic groups within individual studies and comparing self-regulatory functions across them, rather than simply comparing children with ADHD and healthy controls (Sukhodolsky et al., 2003). The deficits in the neural circuits that subserve self-regulatory control, however, could represent a common biological vulnerability to a number of neuropsychiatric disorders that manifests as a distinct behavioral phenotype when superimposed on the additional background of genetic, environmental, and developmental influences that are unique to that phenotype (Nigg and Casey, 2005; Jensen et al., 2007).

Impulsive behavior generally can be conceptualized as either the impairment of behavioral inhibition or the aversion to a delay of reward (Evenden, 1999). Likewise, the neuropsychological impairments of children with ADHD are generally conceptualized as either predominantly cognitive and inhibitory—and therefore relating to executive functioning (EF)—or as motivational and reward related (Castellanos et al., 2006). These two hypothesized domains of impairment presumably map to differing portions of cortico-subcortical circuits, suggesting that dysfunction in one or both of these "dual pathways" produces two primary subtypes of ADHD, one characterized by deficits primarily in cognitive inhibitory control, and the other by disturbances in primarily motivational, reward-related behavior (Sonuga-Barke, 2003). This distinction between cognitive and emotional domains is increasingly difficult to maintain, however, given that integration of these two conceptual poles is increasingly gaining conceptual favor (Ochsner, 2004; J. Posner et al., 2005; Zelazo and Cunningham, 2006; Blair et al., 2007) (Fig. 69.2).

Development of Frontostriatal Circuits

Inhibitory executive functions are based primarily in frontostriatal portions of cortico-subcortical circuits, those connecting the dorsolateral PFC (DLPFC) and anterior cingulate cortex (ACC) to the dorsal striatum. Functions of these frontostriatal loops include, but are not limited to, inhibition of prepotent responses, working memory, and planning of goal-directed behaviors. These functional capacities develop rapidly and progressively during childhood and adolescence (Davidson et al., 2006). Recent functional magnetic resonance imaging (fMRI) studies have reported that brain activation during inhibitory tasks becomes more focused within PFCs during adolescence (Durston, Davidson, et al., 2006; Marsh et al., 2006; Rubia et al., 2006), likely reflecting the progressive pruning of exuberant synapses (Huttenlocher, 1979) and the myelination of white matter tracts in the frontal lobe, both of which occur contemporaneously with the emergence of im-

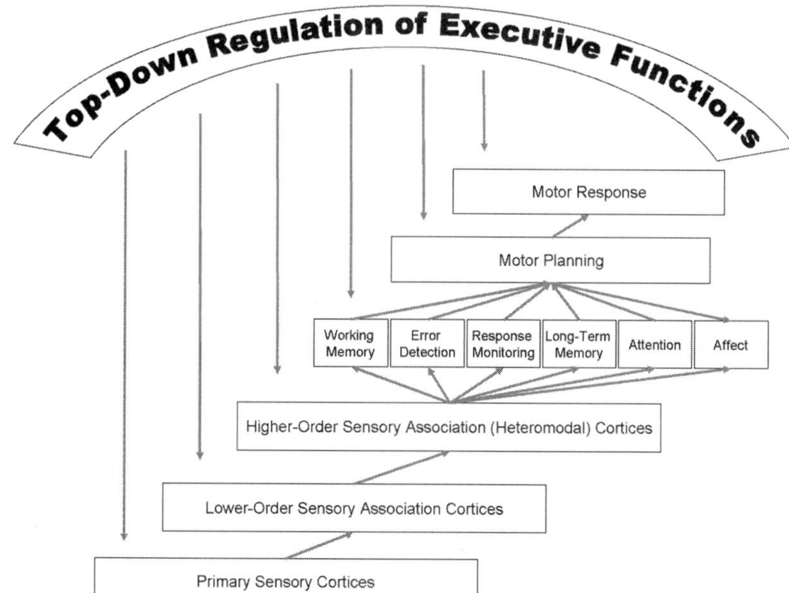

FIGURE 69.2 Top-down regulation of sensory input, information processing, and motoric output executive functions strongly influence all stages of sensorimotor processing, from perception to specific cognitive processes and motor output (Gilbert and Sigman, 2007; Saalmann et al., 2007).

pulse control during adolescence (Giedd et al., 1999; Sowell, Peterson, et al., 2003).

Development of Mesocorticolimbic Circuits

Although the anatomical and functional maturation of mesocorticolimbic circuits is not mapped as robustly as that of frontostriatal circuits, their importance for the proper development of self-regulation is increasingly recognized (Kerr and Zelazo, 2004; Levy, 2004). The development of mesocorticolimbic pathways parallels the development during adolescence of the reduction in risk-taking behaviors and the improved capacity to work toward goals in the distant future (N. Eisenberg et al., 2006; Scheres et al., 2006). The capacity to regulate emotions and impulses is typically attributed to the portions of these circuits that connect ventromedial and orbitofrontal cortices with the amygdala, hippocampus, ACC, and ventral striatum (Hariri et al., 2002; Meyer-Lindenberg et al., 2006). The orbital frontal cortex (OFC) plays a central role in reward circuitry, in that lesions in macaque monkeys impair performance on tasks that involve learning the salience of reward and nonreward cues and the appropriate change of behavior with changes in reinforcement cues (Jones and Mishkin, 1972; G.V. Williams et al., 1993; Rolls, 1994, 2000). In addition, many lesion, animal, and neuropsychological studies have demonstrated the salience of reciprocal connections between the amygdala and OFC in decision-making behaviors (Damasio et al., 1994; Schoenbaum et al., 1998; Bechara et al., 2000). Thus, orbitofrontal-limbic projections, together with the ACC and ventral striatum, seem to mediate decision making, motivational control, and nonimpulsive responding.

Executive Functioning

Broadly defined, EFs are flexible, top-down processes that enable individuals to follow rules and to pursue goals over time (Goldman-Rakic, 1996; Miyake et al., 2000; K. Johnston et al., 2007). For the purposes of categorizing and measuring deficits, EF has been subdivided into the inhibition of prepotent responses, initiating and discontinuing of actions, ignoring of task-irrelevant information, monitoring of performance, and above all, pursuing long-term goals at the expense of the immediate satisfaction of drives (Davidson et al., 2006). In that EFs help to inhibit impulses and to ignore distracting stimuli, they may be considered as a prerequisite to, and an inherent part of, self-regulatory control (Pennington and Ozonoff, 1996). The impulsivity, hyperactivity, and distractibility of ADHD reflects a broad class of EF impairment that likely comprises smaller and more precisely specified units of executive dysfunction, such as decreased inhibitory control, aversion to delay of rewards, overrapid decision making, poor self-reflective capacities, and an impaired ability to sustain attention (Evenden, 1999; Winstanley et al., 2004). When mapping deficits in inhibitory and self-regulatory control in children with ADHD, these various component processes of executive functioning will need to be parsed from one another and from potential disturbances in arousal and motivation (Nigg, 2006).

Mapping Inhibitory Deficits

Neuropsychological tests that assess the executive functions of suppressing prepotent responses include the widely used "go/no-go" and "stop" tests (Spreen and Strauss, 1998). Both require making rapid responses to a number of sequential stimuli while withholding responses to a minority of stimuli. When such tests are used in fMRI studies, the inhibition of a prepotent response usually produces right lateralized activation of the inferior frontal gyrus (Garavan et al., 1999). Moreover, lesions of this region increase Stop Signal Reaction Times (SSRT; that is, the ability to inhibit a response that has already been initiated) (Aron et al., 2003). Meta-analyses have shown that children with ADHD exhibit a fairly robust deficit in performance on the stop task compared with healthy controls (Oosterlaan et al., 1998; Willcutt et al., 2005); difficulties in withholding prepotent impulses and inhibitory control thus have been hypothesized to constitute the core deficit in neuropsychological functioning that subsequently disrupts other EFs (Barkley, 1997, 2006).

Impairment of Interference

The Stroop, Simon, and Flanker tasks all measure somewhat more complex cognitive abilities (Stroop, 1935; Simon, 1969; Eriksen and Eriksen, 1974). The Stroop task, for example, requires probands to inhibit a prepotent behavior (the highly automated task of word reading) in favor of a less automatic behavior (the naming of colors in which the words are written). Thus, the test measures the ability to overcome the cognitive interference generated when using a rule to overcome automated behavior, considered a prototypical requirement of self-regulatory control (Peterson et al., 2002). Brain activation during performance of such tasks involves a widely distributed network that includes the anterior cingulate, prefrontal, motor, temporal, parietal, and peristriate cortices as well as the basal ganglia (Peterson et al., 1999; Bush et al., 2000). A meta-analysis has shown that children with ADHD typically perform less well than controls on the Stroop task, although the effect size is quite low (van Mourik et al., 2005).

Complex Tests of EF

Other neuropsychological tests used to study ADHD measure even more complex cognitive capabilities, such as the identification of current and changing rules in the

Wisconsin Card Sorting Test (WCST), constructs closely related to set-shifting. Given difficulties that children with ADHD have when performing simpler inhibitory tests of only a single cognitive function, the difficulty that they have with these demanding tasks, which has been confirmed in several meta-analyses, is perhaps not surprising (Frazier et al., 2004; Romine et al., 2004; Willcutt et al., 2005). Although more complex tasks are more difficult to interpret, they also are closer to real-life experiences than are some of the simpler neuropsychological tests, and therefore they may have greater ecological validity.

Clinical and experimental neuropsychological testing takes place in settings that differ strikingly from real-life situations. Children with ADHD are exposed in their daily lives not only to sensory distractions but also to emotional influences that accompany the distractions. Together, these emotional disruptions contribute to greater difficulties with attentional regulation and impulse control, perhaps explaining the modest effect sizes (0.5 to 0.8 for most tasks) reported in meta-analyses of studies of executive functioning in children with ADHD compared with healthy controls (Martinussen et al., 2005; Nigg, 2005). These modest effect sizes have provoked criticism of the thesis that inhibitory deficits are of central importance in ADHD, and they have led some investigators to suggest either that findings from neuropsychological testing should be related to measures of regulation of emotional state or that cognitive tests should be combined with assessment of motivational factors (Kerr and Zelazo, 2004; Nigg, 2005; Castellanos et al., 2006).

Deficits of Attention

Although difficulties in sustaining attention are commonly regarded as the core problem in ADHD, attentional problems arguably could be a consequence of more central problems with inhibitory control, in that an inability to suppress the perception of task-irrelevant information could produce difficulties in sustaining attention and goal-directed activity (Evenden, 1999). Findings from experimental studies of attention in children with ADHD, in fact, have in general been highly variable, and the few existing studies have tended to demonstrate the sparing of sustained attention in children with ADHD (Nigg, 2006). Meta-analyses suggest instead that a substantial proportion of children with ADHD experience problems when performing the Continuous Performance Test, most specifically in the differentiation of a target from a nontarget, a problem that has been most closely related to disturbances in arousal (Losier et al., 1996; Willcutt et al., 2005). Similar findings in other psychiatric populations, however, suggest that these deficits in attention and arousal may be relatively nonspecific (Corkum and Siegel, 1993; Halperin et al., 1993; Hall et al., 1997).

Working Memory

Recent meta-analyses suggest that problems in spatial working memory, a construct that likely depends on and contributes to selective attention, interference control, and short-term memory, thus far is one of the most replicable neuropsychological deficits detected in children with ADHD (Martinussen et al., 2005; Willcutt et al., 2005). Meta-analyses of studies that have assessed verbal working memory have also found replicable deficits that seem to be less robust than those reported for spatial working memory (Martinussen et al., 2005; Willcutt et al., 2005).

Delay Aversion and Impaired Time Perception

Difficulty with waiting one's turn in line or in conversation are two of the current diagnostic criteria for ADHD that may represent a more general aversion of delay in children with ADHD (Sonuga-Barke et al., 1992). Delay aversion may also account for the documented preference of these children for smaller immediate rewards compared with larger delayed ones, a trade-off that may be a consequence of an altered sensitivity to reinforcers or to underlying problems with the accurate perception of time and with temporal sequencing (Toplak et al., 2006). Problems with tolerating delay and perceiving time may be a consequence of cortical hypoarousal, which could also account for the presence of increased stimulus-seeking behavior as a compensatory phenomenon in children with ADHD (G. Shaw and Brown, 1999; Antrop et al., 2000). Similarly, deficits in the perception of time may account for problems with motor timing and the characteristic problems with gross motor control, clumsiness, and more variable reaction times in children with ADHD, problems that have been attributed to the cerebellum and the basal ganglia (Rasmussen and Gillberg, 2000; Castellanos and Tannock, 2002; Salman, 2002; Castellanos et al., 2005). The variability in reaction times has in fact been hypothesized to be one of the core problems in children with ADHD, particularly as it relates to spontaneous fluctuations in neural activity and sustained attention that can compete with goal-directed activities. These fluctuations are present in healthy children and may be exaggerated in children with ADHD (Castellanos and Tannock, 2002; Castellanos et al., 2005; Sonuga-Barke and Castellanos, 2007).

NEUROIMAGING STUDIES OF IMPULSIVITY AND ADHD

Functional and anatomical neuroimaging are powerful methods for improving our understanding of the pathophysiology of ADHD. Functional neuroimaging, which includes fMRI, single photon emission computed tomography (SPECT), and positron emission tomography (PET), can map differences in functional activation across groups of patients and controls even when neuropsychological testing reveals that the performance of a given task across diagnostic groups is similar. Such differences in functional activation can indicate, for example, the presence of adaptive strategies associated with a particular disorder that do not manifest in actual differences in performance, or they can depict the primary functional deficit. Functional MRI has an advantage over PET and SPECT for the study of children with ADHD in that it measures brain activity noninvasively and without the use of radioactive substances, thereby facilitating the study of larger samples of children at younger ages, and across multiple time points, to visualize longitudinally the maturation of cognitive functions and their anatomical substrates in developing children. Anatomical brain imaging, in contrast, reveals deviations in brain structure that may represent either a vulnerability to developing ADHD, a compensatory response to the presence of dysfunction elsewhere in the brain, or simply downstream, epiphenomenal effects of more central pathophysiological disturbances located elsewhere in the brain (Peterson, 2003; Viding et al., 2006).

Despite publication of a growing number of imaging studies, the influence of imaging technologies on the understanding and treatment of ADHD thus far has been limited. The relative paucity of robust, reproducible findings may be a consequence of small sample sizes, disease heterogeneity in the patient groups, varying degrees of psychiatric comorbidity, and differing technical and methodological approaches across studies, including differences in acquisition and processing of the images (Peterson, 2003; Bush et al., 2005; Mitterschiffthaler et al., 2006; Plessen et al., 2007). Nevertheless, a number of imaging findings in ADHD do seem to be reproducible. These findings can be grouped into those that implicate either the frontostriatal circuits thought to subserve self-regulation, inhibitory control, and executive functions, or the mesocorticolimbic circuits that are thought to subserve tolerance of delay, the processing of rewards, and decision making (Fig. 69.3A and Fig. 69.3B).

Frontostriatal Systems Subserving Self-Regulation and Inhibitory Control

Functional imaging studies have helped to link the impaired performance of children with ADHD on tasks of inhibitory control with disturbances in frontostriatal circuits. Most fMRI paradigms have relied on widely used tests of inhibition, such as the "go/no-go" and the "stop" tasks. Inhibitory tasks activate networks in healthy individuals throughout the cortex, but predominantly in the right hemisphere, and particularly in the right inferior cortex (Aron and Poldrack, 2005). A recent meta-analysis of findings from 16 fMRI studies of individuals with ADHD reported widespread hypoactivation in children and adults with ADHD when performing a task of response inhibition, particularly in the PFCs bilaterally, the cingulate cortex, the left parietal lobe, and the right caudate nucleus (Dickstein et al., 2006). Individuals with ADHD, however, exhib-

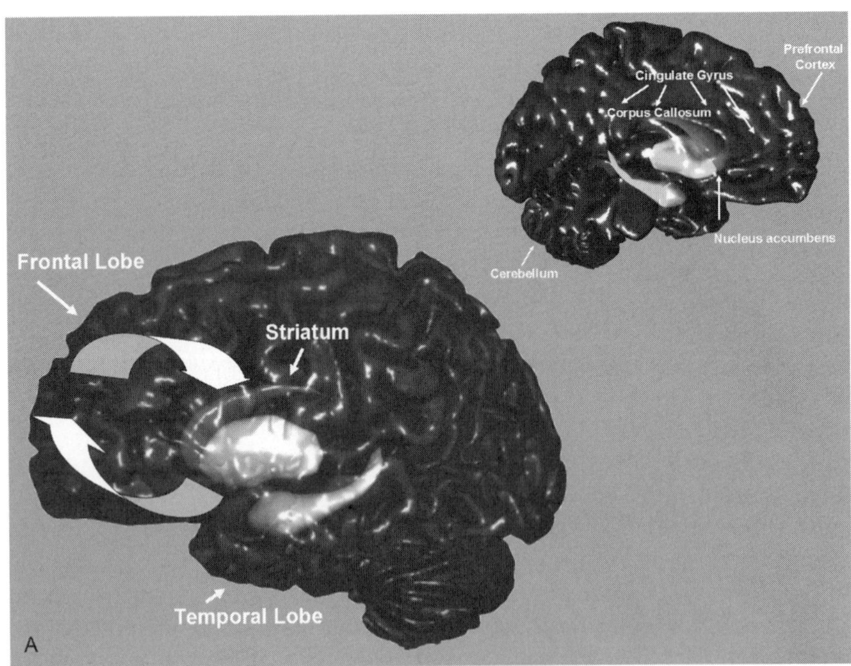

FIGURE 69.3(*A*): Neural circuits most commonly implicated in the pathogenesis of attention-deficit/hyperactivity disorder (ADHD) Views of frontostriatal circuits, in lateral and midsagittal views (upper thumbnail) and the anatomical regions most commonly implicated in the pathogenesis of ADHD.

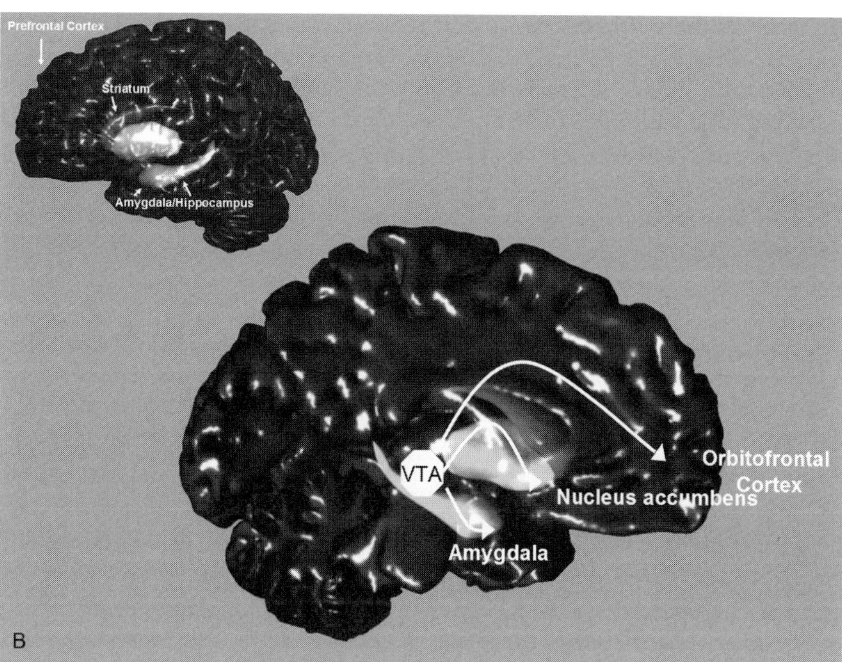

FIGURE 69.3 (*B*): Views of mesocorticolimbic circuits in midsagittal and lateral views (upper thumbnail).

ited greater activation than controls in medial frontal and right paracentral regions. Findings of the meta-analysis were not altered by exclusion of five studies that included adults with ADHD (Bush et al., 1999; Schweitzer et al., 2000; Ernst et al., 2003; Schweitzer et al., 2004; Valera et al., 2005) or when including only studies of individuals who are medication naïve (Rubia et al., 2005; Silk et al., 2005; Pliszka et al., 2006; Smith et al., 2006). In a separate study, affected individuals with ADHD and their unaffected siblings showed reduced ventral frontal activation during an inhibitory task, suggesting that activation during successful inhibition is determined by a familial vulnerability for developing ADHD (Durston, Mulder, et al., 2006).

Reduced striatal activity was first identified in a series of SPECT studies of persons with ADHD (Lou et al., 1984; Lou et al., 1989; Lou et al., 1998). Positron emission tomography studies subsequently revealed a diffuse reduction in frontostriatal metabolism in ADHD that was particularly prominent in females (Zametkin et al., 1990; Zametkin et al., 1993; Ernst et al., 1994; Ernst et al., 1998). Reduced striatal activity was then supported by several fMRI studies in which patients with ADHD performed tasks requiring inhibitory control (Vaidya et al., 1998; Durston et al., 2003; Tamm et al., 2004). The typically poor performance of children with ADHD on inhibitory tasks, however, makes difficult the determination of whether reduced neural activation originates with impaired task performance or is a trait disturbance independent of performance level. Indeed, one study suggested that caudate activation may depend only on the performance level and cognitive load of a task (Vaidya et al., 1998).

Functional MRI studies have consistently reported reduced activity of the ACC, positioned within the medial PFC, in children and adults with ADHD during the performance of inhibitory tasks (Bush et al., 1999; Rubia et al., 1999; Durston et al., 2003; Tamm et al., 2004). The ACC is involved in the monitoring of conflict and reward and in detecting errors, and it is thought to be a central determinant of self-regulatory control (Devinsky et al., 1995; Peterson et al., 1999). The ACC activates strongly during self-regulatory tasks such as the Stroop (Stroop, 1935), Simon (Simon, 1969), and Flanker (Eriksen and Eriksen, 1974) tasks (Peterson et al., 1999; Bunge et al., 2002; Peterson et al., 2002). Some investigators suggest that the cingulum should be divided into functionally distinct regions, including its anterior (executive functioning), posterior (emotional valence), dorsal (cognitive), and ventral (emotional) components (Bush et al., 2000). Based on this diversity of functions and its pattern of anatomical connectivity, the ACC is thought to operate as a cross-road between, and an integrator of activity in, the frontostriatal and mesocorticolimbic systems.

Morphology of Frontal and Striatal Regions

Abnormalities in brain activity in persons with ADHD have been paralleled by findings of similar regional abnormalities in brain structure. Which of these abnormalities is primary, however, and which is secondary remains unknown. The most reproducible morphological abnormalities reported in ADHD thus far have been reduced volumes of the frontal lobes, basal ganglia, and cerebellum (Valera et al., 2007). Reduced volumes of prefrontal regions (especially the right frontal cortex) may produce difficulties with inhibiting prepotent responses and decreased brain activity during inhibitory tasks in children with ADHD (Casey et al., 1997). Reduced activity and smaller volumes of the basal ganglia, particularly in the caudate nucleus, have been reported frequently in individuals with ADHD (Castellanos et al., 1994; Castellanos et al., 1996; Filipek et al., 1997; Semrud-Clikeman et al., 2000; Castellanos et al., 2001; Castellanos et al., 2002). Moreover, the integrity of white matter fibers connecting the frontal cortices with the basal ganglia has been reported in a preliminary diffusion tensor imaging (DTI) study of children with ADHD (Ashtari et al., 2005). Finally, the cerebellum participates in the motor planning and attentional control that frontostriatal circuits subserve (Allen et al., 1997; Thach, 1998), and the cerebellar vermis has been reported smaller in numerous studies of ADHD (Berquin et al., 1998; Mostofsky et al., 1998; Castellanos et al., 2001; Castellanos et al., 2002; Mackie et al., 2007). Together these findings suggest that hypoplasia is widespread in self-regulatory control systems in children with ADHD.

A reduced overall brain size in patients with ADHD that is not simply attributable to reductions in volume of the frontal cortex has also been reported in several studies (Castellanos et al., 1996; Filipek et al., 1997; Castellanos et al., 2001; Rapoport et al., 2001; Castellanos et al., 2002; Sowell, Thompson, et al., 2003). The detection of a statistically significant reduction in overall brain size, however, may be a consequence of including anatomically heterogeneous clinical and genetic subtypes of ADHD, each of which may affect a specific brain region or set of regions, but which as a statistical aggregate appear as reductions across all brain regions, a seemingly generalized effect across the brain (Mill et al., 2006; Valera et al., 2007). The largest anatomical study thus far, consisting of scans from 152 children with ADHD and 139 controls, reported a reduction in overall brain volume in the ADHD group (Castellanos et al., 2002). After controlling for overall brain volume, the only regional volume that remained statistically significant was the cerebellum, likely because its volume did not correlate substantially with overall brain volume and head size, whereas volumes of cortical regions did. Nevertheless, the region with the largest percent difference in volume between groups (22%) was in the temporal lobe, compared with considerably smaller percent differences in other cortical regions and cerebellum (5%–12%), suggesting that anatomical disturbances may be most prominent in the temporal lobe. This finding and its interpretation would be consistent with a finer-grained analysis of the morphological features of the cortical surface, which reported prominent volume reductions in the temporal and frontal cortices in children with ADHD compared with matched controls (Sowell, Thompson, et al., 2003).

The corpus callosum (CC) connects the frontal and prefrontal cortices across the midline and is therefore of interest in understanding frontal connectivity in ADHD (Roessner et al., 2004; Plessen et al., 2007). Numerous studies have reported smaller rostral portions of the CC, the subregion containing axons that connect PFCs in particular (Hynd et al., 1990, 1991; Giedd et al., 1994; Semrud-Clikeman et al., 1994; Baumgardner et al., 1996; Lyoo et al., 1996). A recent meta-study, however, revealed that a reduced size of the splenium (connecting parietal and occipital cortices across the midline) is actually the most reliable finding in the CC (Valera et al., 2007).

Longitudinal findings in children with ADHD are beginning to emerge. The earlier mentioned, large anatomical MRI study combined a cross-sectional and longitudinal design. Analyses of the changes in volume across time revealed that overall brain volume, which was smaller in the ADHD group, was evident early in life and persisted until at least adolescence (Castellanos et al., 2002). The change in cerebral volumes with age paralleled those of the healthy controls, with volumes in the ADHD group being smaller than control volumes at all ages. One exception was the volume of the caudate nucleus, the trajectory of which tended to flatten with increasing age, whereas volumes of the controls continued to decline, thereby "normalizing" caudate volumes in the ADHD group during adolescence. Furthermore, additional analyses localized reductions in cortical size to the medial and superior prefrontal and precentral cortices (P. Shaw et al., 2006). Children with more severe symptoms exhibited more prominent thinning of the left medial PFC compared with children with less severe symptoms and with healthy controls.

Furthermore, throughout childhood and adolescence the ADHD group had nonprogressive reductions in volume of the superior cerebellar vermis, a structure subserving the processing and estimation of time as well as functions of regulation (Schmahmann, 1996; Ackermann et al., 1999; Mackie et al., 2007). Volumes of the right and left inferior-posterior cerebellar lobes decreased in children with ADHD with worse clinical outcomes compared with those who had more favorable outcomes and the controls. The high rate of comorbidity with anxiety and ODD in children with smaller cerebellar volumes suggested that the cerebellum may subserve a neuromodulatory function, and that this function is disrupted in children with ADHD whose symptoms persist throughout adolescence (Mackie et al., 2007).

Imaging Studies of the Mesocorticolimbic System

The presence of delay aversion, altered reward values, and impulsive decision making suggest involvement of the mesocorticolimbic reward system in the pathophysiology of ADHD. Neuroimaging studies in individuals with ADHD, however, have not yet adequately assessed the functional integrity of this system. A recent study did report decreased striatal activation in adolescents with ADHD during a reward anticipation task, with reduced activity accompanying greater severity of hyperactivity and impulsivity, but not inattention (Knutson et al., 2001; Scheres et al., 2007). The striatal hyporesponsiveness during reward anticipation was hypothesized to increase stimulus-seeking behavior, which if confirmed would link striatal hyporesponsiveness with impulsive behavior in humans (Robbins and Everitt, 1999; Scheres et al., 2007).

Few structural MRI studies have assessed brain anatomy in regions involved in reward processing. Although two studies reported normal hippocampus volumes in children and adolescents with ADHD (Filipek et al., 1997; Castellanos et al., 2001), a more recent study reported larger hippocampi bilaterally, especially in more anterior portions of the hippocampus, in children and adolescents with ADHD (Plessen et al., 2006). Further, increased hippocampus size correlated inversely with the severity of symptoms of ADHD, suggesting that the findings were compensatory in nature. The hypertrophy was hypothesized to improve deficits of temporal perception and temporal sequencing, which may originate elsewhere, possibly in prefrontal cortex and cerebellum. Although overall volumes of the amygdala did not differ between patients with ADHD and controls, surface analyses showed that several amygdala subregions were smaller in children with ADHD than in controls, and these same regions generally correlated significantly and positively with the severity of ADHD symptoms. Finally, interregional correlations suggested that connectivity between the amygdala and the orbitofrontal cortex was disrupted in the ADHD group. The altered connectivity between amygdala and orbitofrontal cortex presumably could contribute to impulsive behavior and impulsive decision making through reduced self-regulatory influences of the orbitofrontal cortex on emotional processing in the amygdala.

TREATMENT

Medication

Stimulants (methylphenidate [MPH], dextroamphetamine, and related preparations) produce a clear therapeutic effect on the symptoms of ADHD in over 70% of children who take them (The MTA Cooperative Group, 1999b; Greenhill et al., 2002). The number of randomized, double-blind clinical trials of stimulant medications exceeds those for all other psychotropic medications in children, and their efficacy in treating the symptoms of ADHD is beyond dispute (Schachter et al., 2001; Solanto et al., 2001). Although the mechanisms of action of medications for ADHD are not yet completely identified, they include increasing extracellular DA in the striatum and frontal cortex—MPH does so by blocking presynaptic DATs (and norepinephrine), whereas amphetamine releases DA from the presynaptic terminal through the DAT (Volkow et al., 2005). Although the medication is generally well tolerated, side effects of stimulant medications can include suppression of appetite, weight loss, modest reductions in height, and insomnia. Rare side effects include motor stereotypies, nervousness, and, extremely rarely, psychosis (Greenhill et al., 1999; Rapport and Moffitt, 2002). All are reversible upon reduction or discontinuation of the medication. Although dextroamphetamine has similar therapeutic and adverse effects as MPH, amphetamine may cause less suppression of appetite and a greater increase in tics (Castellanos et al., 1997; Efron et al., 1997).

Several additional concerns about stimulant use have arisen recently. First, sudden cardiac death has been reported in several children on stimulant medications. Although a clear causal relationship of medication use with cardiac death has not been established, the reports spurred the recommendation to assess cardiovascular status before medication is started and close monitoring following its initiation (Biederman et al., 2006; Vitiello, 2007). Second, one study reported an increase in the number of white blood cells and chromosomal aberrations after three months of MPH treatment in children, raising concern about its potential mutagenic effects (El-Zein et al., 2005). The methodology of this small study has been questioned (Preston et al., 2005), and a subsequent laboratory study did not detect any clastogenic effect of MPH in vitro (Suter et al., 2006). Nevertheless, the report highlights the absence of rigorous, long-term follow-up studies in children taking stimulants (Andersen, 2005; Martin, 2006). Third, several developmental animal studies of repeated low-dose exposure to stimulants have reported changes in brain DA metabolism, behavioral alterations, and aberrant responses to the reinforcing properties of cocaine in adulthood (Bolanos et al., 2003; Brandon et al., 2003; Carlezon et al., 2003). These findings cannot be extrapolated directly to humans, however, and in contrast to what these animal data might predict, the preponderance of available evidence suggests that stimulants do not increase the liability to substance abuse but instead may actually reduce the risk for later substance abuse (Biederman et al., 1999; Wilens et al., 2003). The animal studies do suggest, however, that more study of the long-term effects of stimulant medications in children may be warranted (Volkow and Insel, 2003).

Nonstimulant medications include atomoxetine, a noradrenalin reuptake blocker that has good clinical efficacy and tolerability, including a seemingly safe cardiovascular profile (Michelson et al., 2001; Spencer et al., 2001). Rare events of hepatotoxity that resolve after discontinuation of the medication have been described (Lim et al., 2006). Similar to other antidepressant medications, infrequent suicidal ideation has been described following its use, and this therefore needs to be monitored (Food and Drug Administration [FDA], 2005; Himpel et al., 2005). The recent introduction of atomoxetine to the marketplace is responsible for the relatively more limited clinical experience with this medication and the relatively low number of efficacy studies compared with the stimulant medications.

Adolescents with ADHD who have never taken stimulant medications are at a higher risk of developing drug abuse than are adolescents without ADHD. Several preliminary studies suggest that treatment with stimulants reduces the risk of drug abuse later in life (Biederman et al., 1997; Biederman et al., 1999; Sullivan and Rudnik-Levin, 2001; Barkley et al., 2003; Wilens et al., 2003). Preclinical studies are more equivocal, however, which suggest that the dopaminergic effects of MPH and amphetamine reproduce the reinforcing effects of drugs of abuse (Andersen et al., 2002; Carlezon et al., 2003; Volkow, 2006). Nevertheless, MPH when administered orally has a low abuse potential, probably because its slow rate of delivery does not elicit euphoria, probably the best predictor of a drug's abuse potential (Volkow et al., 2001; Volkow et al., 2002; Volkow et al., 2005; Hyman et al., 2006).

Behavioral Treatments

A number of behavioral therapies that specifically address the importance of parenting strategies in children with ADHD have been developed and validated (Anastopoulos et al., 1993; Kazdin, 1997; Pelham et al., 1998; Sonuga-Barke et al., 2001; Webster-Stratton et al., 2001). Such approaches generally aim to strengthen the external supports that parents can provide to enhance self-regulatory functions in their children. A comprehensive review of behavioral treatments is beyond the scope of this chapter (Chronis et al., 2004). Nevertheless, it warrants mention here that the efficacy of well-designed and carefully administered behavioral therapy as a stand-alone treatment for ADHD was shown in a rigorous and randomized, multicenter clinical trial to be no better than the treatment that children with ADHD receive in the community (which included medication administration in some), and that it was substantially inferior to the efficacy of optimally managed treatment with stimulant medications (The MTA Cooperative Group, 1999b). The design and findings of this study are discussed in more detail below.

A number of alternative treatment approaches have been developed as behavioral therapies for ADHD and related problems. These include cognitive retraining strategies and self-regulatory control training using neurofeedback (Holtmann and Stadler, 2006). Although these therapies remain of considerable research interest, only one has been shown in a randomized controlled trial to improve ADHD symptoms significantly when compared with a reasonable control treatment. That study reported improved response inhibition and reasoning, as well as reduced parent-rated symptoms of inattention, following the systematic training of working memory over a 5-week period (Klingberg et al., 2005). If these findings are confirmed in other controlled studies, they would support the hypothesized central role of frontostriatal circuits in the pathogenesis of ADHD and related problems in self-regulatory control.

The Multimodal Treatment of ADHD (MTA) Study

The Multimodal Treatment Study of Children with ADHD (MTA study) study is the largest systematic study undertaken thus far for the treatment of ADHD (The MTA Cooperative Group, 1999b). It randomized 579 children (ages 7–9.9 years) to four different treatment arms: (*1*) intensive medication treatment only, (*2*) behavioral treatment only, (*3*) a combination of medication and behavioral treatments, and (*4*) community-treated comparison group (The MTA Cooperative Group, 1999b). Medication management consisted of four different doses of MPH over the titration period, ending with an individually determined "best dose." Behavioral treatment consisted of 27 parenting group sessions, 8 individual sessions, 8 weeks of full-time summer treatment program, 10 sessions of teacher consultation, and 60 half-days of a teacher's aide at school.

Primary end-point analyses after 14 months of treatment showed that medication accounted for the largest clinical improvement, with children in the medication-only and the combined groups improving to comparable degrees in their symptoms of inattention and impulsivity-hyperactivity (The MTA Cooperative Group, 1999b). Children in the behavioral treatment alone and in the community-treated comparison group did not improve to this extent, even though their symptoms improved relative to baseline. Thus, the MTA study confirmed the efficacy of treatment with MPH up to 14 months in duration. The primary planned analyses also suggested that the best behavioral therapy that the field had to offer at that time did not afford a greater improvement in ADHD symptoms beyond the improvement that optimal medication management alone could provide.

Nevertheless, secondary outcome analyses did show that combined therapy provided modestly greater improvements in non-ADHD symptom domains, including social skills, and in overall parent satisfaction with treatment (The MTA Cooperative Group, 1999b; Hinshaw et al., 2000; Wells et al., 2000). Children in the combined treatment group also required lower dosages of MPH (31.2 mg) than did children in the medication-only group (37.7 mg) (The MTA Cooperative Group,

1999b). Furthermore, constructive parenting strategies in the combined group were significantly improved compared with either medication or behavioral treatments alone (Wells et al., 2006). Other significant moderators of the response of ADHD symptoms to treatment detected in exploratory analyses included the presence of comorbid anxiety disorders (March et al., 2000; Jensen et al., 2001), comorbid ODD/CD (Jensen et al., 2001), single parent status (The MTA Cooperative Group, 1999a), parental depression (Owens et al., 2003), childhood IQ (Owens et al., 2003), race (Arnold et al., 2003), and socioeconomic status (The MTA Cooperative Group, 1999a; Rieppi et al., 2002). Of these effects, the moderating effects of comorbid anxiety disorder seem especially strong (March et al., 2000; Jensen et al., 2001; Swanson et al., 2001). Behavioral therapy reduced ADHD symptoms in those with comorbid anxiety (33.5% of the sample) significantly more (the effect size—as measured by parental perceived inattention in the group with comorbid anxiety—was .70 versus .03 in children who were not anxious). Moreover, combined treatment yielded a greater improvement in ADHD symptoms (effect size = 1.02 in children with comorbid anxiety, compared to .78 in medication treatment alone) (March et al., 2000). These findings suggest that children with ADHD and comorbid anxiety do benefit particularly and specifically from behavioral treatment, and that this may be a subgroup with a unique underlying neurobiology, developmental trajectory, and treatment responsiveness (Jensen et al., 2001).

For ethical reasons, the study did not include a non-treated placebo control group of children with ADHD. Consequently, 67% of children in the community-treated comparison group received some form of medication treatment, turning this into an active treatment group with ill-defined treatment options, and setting a high goal for documenting beneficial effects in the remaining three arms of active treatment (Swanson et al., 2002). Moreover, the medication group received their medication for the entire 14-month treatment period, whereas the intensive behavioral therapy was tapered during the last months of the study, a design that may have favored the medication intervention at the 14-month end-point assessment (Pelham, 1999). The first follow-up at 24 months (10 months after concluding active treatment) revealed a persistent effect in the medication-only and combined treatment groups, albeit with a marked reduction in effect size (The MTA Cooperative Group, 2004).

CONCLUSION

The development of adequate impulse control and a more general capacity for self-regulation is an intricate interplay of genetic and environmental determinants that, when disturbed in a myriad of ways, can produce the symptoms of impulsivity, hyperactivity, and distractibility that are diagnosed as ADHD. The highly variable profiles of symptoms, neuropsychological deficits, and measures of brain structure and function in children with ADHD suggest that a diversity of underlying causal pathways can produce this general behavioral phenotype. Family-genetic, twin, and adoption studies, along with molecular genetic studies, all support the contention that ADHD is a neurobehavioral syndrome that has a multiplicity of causes and etiological subtypes. Neuropsychological and brain imaging studies suggest that these various etiologies likely affect adversely the anatomical and functional development of circuits that subserve self-regulatory control generally, disturbing in particular the frontostriatal circuits that subserve inhibitory control and executive functions and mesocorticolimbic circuits that subserve motivation and reward-based learning. Frontostriatal circuits have received far greater attention thus far in neuropsychological and imaging studies of ADHD than have mesocorticolimbic circuits.

Although the mechanisms of action of medications for ADHD are not yet completely known, the action of stimulant medications involves at least in part an increase in striatal DA via the blocking of DA and norepinephrine transporters. The neural pathways through which behavioral therapies exert their effects are even less well known, although the most effective treatments seem often to support the development of an improved capacity for self-regulation. Improvement of these capacities during adolescence in most children with ADHD suggest either that the neural systems subserving self-regulatory control catch up following a maturational lag, or that compensatory neural systems develop sufficiently to help to bolster these capacities with time. Neurobiological studies of normal development and children with ADHD thus far suggest that both mechanisms contribute to the improvement of symptoms with age. Identifying the neural bases for these developmental effects and for the efficacies of known treatments is vitally important for the development of rationally based improvements in the safety and effectiveness of the therapies available for children suffering from ADHD.

ACKNOWLEDGMENTS

This work was supported by the Center for Child and Adolescent Mental Health, University of Bergen, Norway, and in part by National Institute of Mental Health grants MH01232, MH59139, MH068318, and K02-74677, and the Suzanne Crosby Murphy Endowment at Columbia University College of Physicians and Surgeons. We thank Dr. Xuejun Hao for his technical help and Dr. Jason Royal for his editorial assistance.

REFERENCES

Ackermann, H., Graber, S., Hertrich, I., and Daum, I. (1999) Cerebellar contributions to the perception of temporal cues within the speech and nonspeech domain. *Brain Lang.* 67(3):228–241.

Ainslie, G. (1975) Specious reward: a behavioral theory of impulsiveness and impulse control. *Psychol. Bull.* 82(4):463–496.

Alessi, S.M., and Petry, N.M. (2003) Pathological gambling severity is associated with impulsivity in a delay discounting procedure. *Behav. Processes* 64(3):345–354.

Alexander, G.E., DeLong, M.R., and Strick, P.L. (1986) Parallel organization of functionally segregated circuits linking basal ganglia and cortex. *Annu. Rev. Neurosc.* 9:357–381.

Allen, G., Buxton, R.B., Wong, E.C., and Courchesne, E. (1997) Attentional activation of the cerebellum independent of motor involvement. *Science* 275(5308):1940–1943.

American Psychiatric Association. (1994) *Diagnostic and Statistical Manual of Mental Disorders*, 4th ed. Washington, DC: Author.

Amini, B., Yang, P. B., Swann, A. C., and Dafny, N. (2004) Differential locomotor responses in male rats from three strains to acute methylphenidate. *Int. J. Neurosci.* 114(9):1063–1084.

Anastopoulos, A.D., Shelton, T.L., DuPaul, G.J., and Guevremont, D.C. (1993) Parent training for attention-deficit hyperactivity disorder: its impact on parent functioning. *J. Abnorm. Child Psychol.* 21(5):581–596.

Andersen, S.L. (2005) Stimulants and the developing brain. *Trends Pharmacol. Sci.* 26(5):237–243.

Andersen, S.L., Arvanitogiannis, A., Pliakas, A.M., LeBlanc, C., and Carlezon, W.A. (2002) Altered responsiveness to cocaine in rats exposed to methylphenidate during development. *Nat. Neurosci.* 5(1):13–14.

Antrop, I., Roeyers, H., Van Oost, P., and Buysse, A. (2000) Stimulation seeking and hyperactivity in children with ADHD. *J. Child Psychol. Psychiatry* 41(2):225–231.

Arnold, L.E., Elliot, M., Sachs, L., Bird, H., Kraemer, H.C., Wells, K.C., Abikoff, H.B., Comarda, A., Conners, C.K., Elliott, G.R., Greenhill, L.L., Hechtman, L., Hindshaw, S.P., Hoza, B., Jensen, P.S., March, J.S., Newcorn, J.H., Pelham, W.E., Severe, J.B., Swanson, J.M., Vitiello, B., and Wigal, T. (2003) Effects of ethnicity on treatment attendance, stimulant response/dose, and 14-month outcome in ADHD. *J. Consult. Clin. Psychol.* 71(4):713–727.

Aron, A.R., Fletcher, P.C., Bullmore, E.T., Sahakian, B.J., and Robbins, T.W. (2003) Stop-signal inhibition disrupted by damage to right inferior frontal gyrus in humans. *Nat. Neurosci.* 6(2):115–116.

Aron, A.R., and Poldrack, R.A. (2005) The cognitive neuroscience of response inhibition: relevance for genetic research in attention-deficit/hyperactivity disorder. *Biol. Psychiatry* 57(11):1285–1292.

Ashtari, M., Kumra, S., Bhaskar, S. L., Clarke, T., Thaden, E., Cervellione, K.L., Rhinewine, J., Kane, J.M., Adesman, A., Milanaik, R., Maytal, J., Diamond, A., Szeszko, P., and Ardekani, B. A. (2005) Attention-deficit/hyperactivity disorder: A preliminary diffusion tensor imaging study. *Biol. Psychiatry* 57(5):448–455.

Banaschewski, T., Hollis, C., Oosterlaan, J., Roeyers, H., Rubia, K., Willcutt, E. and Taylor, E. (2005) Towards an understanding of unique and shared pathways in the psychopathophysiology of ADHD. *Dev. Sci.* 8(2):132–140.

Barkley, R.A. (1997) Behavioral inhibition, sustained attention, and executive functions: constructing a unifying theory of ADHD. *Psychol. Bull.* 121(1):65–94.

Barkley, R.A. (2004) Driving impairments in teens and adults with attention-deficit/hyperactivity disorder. *Psychiat. Clin. N. Am.* 27(2): 233–260.

Barkley, R.A. (2006) *Attention Deficit Hyperactivity Disorder: A Handbook for Diagnosis and Treatment.* New York, London: Guilford Press.

Barkley, R.A., Fischer, M., Edelbrock, C., and Smallish, L. (1991) The adolescent outcome of hyperactive children diagnosed by research criteria–III. Mother-child interactions, family conflicts and maternal psychopathology. *J. Child Psychol. Psychiatry* 32(2):233–255.

Barkley, R.A., Fischer, M., Smallish, L., and Fletcher, K. (2003) Does the treatment of attention-deficit/hyperactivity disorder with stimulants contribute to drug use/abuse? A 13-year prospective study. *Pediatrics* 111(1):97–109.

Baumgardner, T.L., Singer, H.S., Denckla, M.B., Rubin, M.A., Abrams, M.T., Colli, M.J., and Reiss, A.L. (1996) Corpus callosum morphology in children with Tourette syndrome and attention deficit hyperactivity disorder. *Neurology* 47(2):477–482.

Bechara, A., Damasio, H., and Damasio, A. R. (2000) Emotion, decision making and the orbitofrontal cortex. *Cereb. Cortex* 10(3): 295–307.

Bell, R.Q. (1968) A reinterpretation of the direction of effects in studies of socialization. *Psychol. Rev.* 75(2):81–95.

Berquin, P.C., Giedd, J.N., Jacobsen, L.K., Hamburger, S.D., Krain, A.L., Rapoport, J.L., and Castellanos, F.X. (1998) Cerebellum in attention-deficit hyperactivity disorder: a morphometric MRI study. *Neurology* 50(4):1087–1093.

Bertholf, R.L., and Goodison, S. (2004) Television viewing and attention deficits in children. *Pediatrics* 114(2):511–512; au. reply: 511–512.

Bhutta, A.T., Cleves, M.A., Casey, P.H., Cradock, M.M., and Anand, K.J. (2002) Cognitive and behavioral outcomes of school-aged children who were born preterm: a meta-analysis. *JAMA* 288(6): 728–737.

Biederman, J., Faraone, S.V., Keenan, K., Knee, D., and Tsuang, M.T. (1990) Family-genetic and psychosocial risk factors in *DSM-III* attention deficit disorder. *J. Am. Acad. Child Adolesc. Psychiatry* 29(4):526–533.

Biederman, J., Faraone, S.V., Mick, E., Spencer, T., Wilens, T., Kiely, K., Guite, J., Ablon, J.S., Reed, E., and Warburton, R. (1995) High risk for attention deficit hyperactivity disorder among children of parents with childhood onset of the disorder: a pilot study. *Am. J. Psychiatry* 152(3):431–435.

Biederman, J., Faraone, S., Mick, E., Wozniak, J., Chen, L., Ouellette, C., Marrs, A., Moore, P., Garcia, J., Mennin, D., and Lelon, E. (1996) Attention-deficit hyperactivity disorder and juvenile mania: an overlooked comorbidity? *J. Am. Acad. Child Adolesc. Psychiatry* 35(8):997–1008.

Biederman, J., Faraone, S.V., and Monuteaux, M.C. (2002) Differential effect of environmental adversity by gender: Rutter's index of adversity in a group of boys and girls with and without ADHD. *Am. J. Psychiatry* 159(9):1556–1562.

Biederman, J., Faraone, S.V., Spencer, T., Wilens, T., Norman, D., Lapey, K.A., Mick, E., Lehman, B.K., and Doyle, A. (1993) Patterns of psychiatric comorbidity, cognition, and psychosocial functioning in adults with attention deficit hyperactivity disorder. *Am. J. Psychiatry* 150(12):1792–1798.

Biederman, J., Mick, E., and Faraone, S.V. (2000) Age-dependent decline of symptoms of attention deficit hyperactivity disorder: impact of remission definition and symptom type. *Am. J. Psychiatry* 157(5):816–818.

Biederman, J., Milberger, S., Faraone, S.V., Kiely, K., Guite, J., Mick, E., Ablon, S., Warburton, R., and Reed, E. (1995) Family-environment risk factors for attention-deficit hyperactivity disorder. A test of Rutter's indicators of adversity. *Arch. Gen. Psychiatry* 52(6): 464–470.

Biederman, J., Spencer, T.J., Wilens, T.E., Prince, J.B., and Faraone, S.V. (2006) Treatment of ADHD with stimulant medications: response to Nissen perspective in the New England Journal of Medicine. *J. Am. Acad. Child Adolesc. Psychiatry* 45(10):1147–1150.

Biederman, J., Wilens, T., Mick, E., Faraone, S.V., Weber, W., Curtis, S., Thornell, A., Pfister, K., Jetton, J.G., and Soriano, J. (1997) Is ADHD a risk factor for psychoactive substance use disorders? Findings from a four-year prospective follow-up study. *J. Am. Acad. Child Adolesc. Psychiatry* 36(1):21–29.

Biederman, J., Wilens, T., Mick, E., Spencer, T., and Faraone, S.V. (1999) Pharmacotherapy of attention-deficit/hyperactivity disorder reduces risk for substance use disorder. *Pediatrics* 104(2): e20.

Bilder, R. M., Volavka, J., Lachman, H.M., and Grace, A.A. (2004) The catechol-O-methyltransferase polymorphism: relations to the tonic-phasic dopamine hypothesis and neuropsychiatric phenotypes. *Neuropsychopharmac.* 29(11):1943–1961.

Blackman, G.L., Ostrander, R., and Herman, K.C. (2005) Children with ADHD and depression: a multisource, multimethod assessment of clinical, social, and academic functioning. *J. Atten. Disord.* 8(4):195–207.

Blair, K.S., Smith, B.W., Mitchell, D.G., Morton, J., Vythilingam, M., Pessoa, L., Fridberg, D., Zametkin, A., Sturman, D., Nelson, E.E., Drevets, W.C., Pine, D.S., Martin, A., and Blair, R.J. (2007) Modulation of emotion by cognition and cognition by emotion. *NeuroImage* 35(1):430–440.

Bolanos, C.A., Barrot, M., Berton, O., Wallace-Black, D., and Nestler, E.J. (2003) Methylphenidate treatment during pre- and periadolescence alters behavioral responses to emotional stimuli at adulthood. *Biol. Psychiatry* 54(12):1317–1329.

Bowlby, J. (1988) *A Secure Base: Parent-Child Attachment and Healthy Human Development*. New York: Basic Books.

Brandon, C.L., Marinelli, M., and White, F.J. (2003) Adolescent exposure to methylphenidate alters the activity of rat midbrain dopamine neurons. *Biol. Psychiatry* 54(12):1338–1344.

Braun, J.M., Kahn, R.S., Froehlich, T., Auinger, P., and Lanphear, B.P. (2006) Exposures to environmental toxicants and attention deficit hyperactivity disorder in U.S. children. *Environ. Health Perspect.* 114(12):1904–1909.

Brennan, P.A., Grekin, E.R. and Mednick, S.A. (1999) Maternal smoking during pregnancy and adult male criminal outcomes. *Arch. Gen. Psychiatry* 56(3):215–219.

Brodsky, B.S., Malone, K.M., Ellis, S.P., Dulit, R.A., and Mann, J.J. (1997) Characteristics of borderline personality disorder associated with suicidal behavior. *Am. J. Psychiatry* 154(12):1715–1719.

Brookes, K.J., Mill, J., Guindalini, C., Curran, S., Xu, X., Knight, J., Chen, C.K., Huang, Y.S., Sethna, V., Taylor, E., Chen, W., Breen, G., and Asherson, P. (2006) A common haplotype of the dopamine transporter gene associated with attention-deficit/hyperactivity disorder and interacting with maternal use of alcohol during pregnancy. *Arch. Gen. Psychiatry* 63(1):74-81.

Bunge, S.A., Dudukovic, N.M., Thomason, M.E., Vaidya, C.J., and Gabrieli, J.D. (2002) Immature frontal lobe contributions to cognitive control in children: evidence from fMRI. *Neuron* 33(2): 301–311.

Bush, G., Frazier, J.A., Rauch, S.L., Seidman, L.J., Whalen, P.J., Jenike, M.A., Rosen, B.R., and Biederman, J. (1999) Anterior cingulate cortex dysfunction in attention-deficit/hyperactivity disorder revealed by fMRI and the counting Stroop. *Biol. Psychiatry* 45(12):1542–1552.

Bush, G., Luu, P., and Posner, M.I. (2000) Cognitive and emotional influences in anterior cingulate cortex. *Trends Neurosci.* 4(6): 215–222.

Bush, G., Valera, E.M., and Seidman, L.J. (2005) Functional neuroimaging of attention-deficit/hyperactivity disorder: a review and suggested future directions. *Biol. Psychiatry* 57(11):1273–1284.

Bushman, B.J., and Anderson, C.A. (2001) Media violence and the American public. Scientific facts versus media misinformation. *Am. Psychol.* 56(6/7):477–489.

Carlezon, W.A., Mague, S.D., and Andersen, S.L. (2003) Enduring behavioral effects of early exposure to methylphenidate in rats. *Biol. Psychiatry* 54(12):1330–1337.

Casey, B.J., Castellanos, F.X., Giedd, J.N., Marsh, W.L., Hamburger, S.D., Schubert, A.B., Vauss, Y.C., Vaituzis, A.C., Dickstein, D.P., Sarfatti, S.E., and Rapoport, J.L. (1997) Implication of right frontostriatal circuitry in response inhibition and attention-deficit/ hyperactivity disorder. *J. Am. Acad. Child Adolesc. Psychiatry* 36(3):374–383.

Caspi, A., McClay, J., Moffitt, T.E., Mill, J., Martin, J., Craig, I. W., Taylor, A., and Poulton, R. (2002) Role of genotype in the cycle of violence in maltreated children. *Science* 297(5582):851–854.

Caspi, A., and Moffitt, T.E. (2006) Gene-environment interactions in psychiatry: joining forces with neuroscience. *Nat. Rev. Neurosci.* 7(7):583–590.

Castellanos, F.X., Giedd, J.N., Berquin, P.C., Walter, J.M., Sharp, W., Tran, T., Vaituzis, A.C., Blumenthal, J.D., Nelson, J., Bastain, T.M., Zijdenbos, A., Evans, A.C., and Rapoport, J.L. (2001) Quantitative brain magnetic resonance imaging in girls with attention-deficit/hyperactivity disorder. *Arch. Gen. Psychiatry* 58(3):289–295.

Castellanos, F.X., Giedd, J.N., Eckburg, P., Marsh, W.L., Vaituzis, A. C., Kaysen, D., Hamburger, S.D., and Rapoport, J.L. (1994) Quantitative morphology of the caudate nucleus in attention deficit hyperactivity disorder. *Am. J. Psychiatry* 151(12):1791–1796.

Castellanos, F.X., Giedd, J.N., Elia, J., Marsh, W.L., Ritchie, G.F., Hamburger, S.D., and Rapoport, J.L. (1997) Controlled stimulant treatment of ADHD and comorbid Tourette's syndrome: effects of stimulant and dose. *J. Am. Acad. Child Adolesc. Psychiatry* 36(5): 589–596.

Castellanos, F.X., Giedd, J.N., Marsh, W.L., Hamburger, S.D., Vaituzis, A.C., Dickstein, D.P., Sarfatti, S.E., Vauss, Y.C., Snell, J.W., Lange, N., Kaysen, D., Krain, A.L., Ritchie, G.F., Rajapakse, J.C., and Rapoport, J.L. (1996) Quantitative brain magnetic resonance imaging in attention-deficit hyperactivity disorder. *Arch. Gen. Psychiatry* 53(7):607–616.

Castellanos, F.X., Lee, P.P., Sharp, W., Jeffries, N.O., Greenstein, D.K., Clasen, L.S., Blumenthal, J.D., James, R.S., Ebens, C.L., Walter, J.M., Zijdenbos, A., Evans, A. C., Giedd, J.N., and Rapoport, J. L. (2002) Developmental trajectories of brain volume abnormalities in children and adolescents with attention-deficit/hyperactivity disorder. *JAMA* 288(14):1740–1748.

Castellanos, F.X., Sonuga-Barke, E.J., Milham, M.P., and Tannock, R. (2006) Characterizing cognition in ADHD: beyond executive dysfunction. *Trends Cogn. Sci.* 10(3):117–123.

Castellanos, F.X., Sonuga-Barke, E.J.S., Scheres, A., Di Martino, A., Hyde, C., and Walters, J.R. (2005) Varieties of attention-deficit/ hyperactivity disorder-related intra-individual variability. *Biol. Psychiatry* 57(11):1416–1423.

Castellanos, F.X., and Tannock, R. (2002) Neuroscience of attention-deficit/hyperactivity disorder: the search for endophenotypes. *Nat. Rev. Neurosci.* 3(8):617–628.

Centers for Disease Control and Prevention. (2005) *Preventing Lead Poisoning in Young Children*. Atlanta, GA: Author.

Chiodo, L.M., Jacobson, S.W., and Jacobson, J.L. (2004) Neurodevelopmental effects of postnatal lead exposure at very low levels. *Neurotoxicol. Teratol.* 26(3):359–371.

Christakis, D.A., and Zimmerman, F.J. (2006) Media as a public health issue. *Arch. Pediatr. Adolesc. Med.* 160(4):445–446.

Christakis, D.A., Zimmerman, F.J., DiGiuseppe, D.L., and McCarty, C.A. (2004) Early television exposure and subsequent attentional problems in children. *Pediatrics* 113(4):708–713.

Chronis, A.M., Chacko, A., Fabiano, G.A., Wymbs, B.T., and Pelham, W.E. (2004) Enhancements to the behavioral parent training paradigm for families of children with ADHD: review and future directions. *Clin. Child Fam. Psychol. Rev.* 7(1):1–27.

Cicchetti, D., Rogosch, F.A., Toth, S.L., and Spagnola, M. (1997) Affect, cognition, and the emergence of self-knowledge in the toddler offspring of depressed mothers. *J. Exp. Child Psychol.* 67(3):338–362.

Congdon, E., and Canli, T. (2005) The endophenotype of impulsivity: reaching consilience through behavioral, genetic, and neuroimaging approaches. *Behav. Cogn. Neurosci. Rev.* 4(4):262–281.

Cools, R. (2006) Dopaminergic modulation of cognitive function-implications for L-DOPA treatment in Parkinson's disease. *Neurosci. Biobehav. Rev.* 30(1):1–23.

Corkum, P.V., and Siegel, L.S. (1993) Is the continuous performance task a valuable research tool for use with children with attention-deficit-hyperactivity disorder? *J. Child Psychol. Psychiatry* 34(7):1217–1239.

Coté, S., Tremblay, R.E., Nagin, D.S., Zoccolillo, M., and Vitaro, F. (2002) Childhood behavioral profiles leading to adolescent conduct disorder: risk trajectories for boys and girls. *J. Am. Acad. Child Adolesc. Psychiatry* 41(9):1086–1094.

Cunningham, C.E. (2002) Preschoolers at risk for attention-deficit hyperactivity disorder and oppositional defiant disorder: family, parenting, and behavioral correlates. *J. Abnorm. Child Psychol.* 30(6):555.

Damasio, H., Grabowski, T., Frank, R., Galaburda, A.M., and Damasio, A.R. (1994) The return of Phineas Gage: clues about the brain from the skull of a famous patient. *Science* 264(5162):1102–1105.

Davids, E., Zhang, K., Tarazi, F.I., and Baldessarini, R.J. (2003) Animal models of attention-deficit hyperactivity disorder. *Brain Res. Brain Res. Rev.* 42(1):1–21.

Davidson, M.C., Amso, D., Anderson, L.C., and Diamond, A. (2006) Development of cognitive control and executive functions from 4 to 13 years: evidence from manipulations of memory, inhibition, and task switching. *Neuropsychologia* 44(11):2037–2078.

Devinsky, O., Morrell, M.J., and Vogt, B.A. (1995) Contributions of anterior cingulate cortex to behaviour. *Brain* 118(Pt 1):279–306.

Dickstein, S.G., Bannon, K., Castellanos, F.X., and Milham, M.P. (2006) The neural correlates of attention deficit hyperactivity disorder: an ALE meta-analysis. *J. Child. Psychol. Psychiatry* 47(10): 1051–1062.

Durston, S., Davidson, M.C., Tottenham, N., Galvan, A., Spicer, J., Fossella, J.A., and Casey, B.J. (2006) A shift from diffuse to focal cortical activity with development. *Dev. Science* 9(1):1–8.

Durston, S., Mulder, M., Casey, B.J., Ziermans, T., and van Engeland, H. (2006) Activation in ventral prefrontal cortex is sensitive to genetic vulnerability for attention-deficit hyperactivity disorder. *Biol. Psychiatry* 60(10):1062–1070.

Durston, S., Tottenham, N.T., Thomas, K.M., Davidson, M.C., Eigsti, I.M., Yang, Y., Ulug, A.M., and Casey, B.J. (2003) Differential patterns of striatal activation in young children with and without ADHD. *Biol. Psychiatry* 53(10):871–878.

Efron, D., Jarman, F., and Barker, M. (1997) Side effects of methylphenidate and dexamphetamine in children with attention deficit hyperactivity disorder: a double-blind, crossover trial. *Pediatrics* 100(4):662–666.

Eisenberg, D.T., Mackillop, J., Modi, M., Beauchemin, J., Dang, D., Lisman, S.A., Lum, J. K., and Wilson, D.S. (2007) Examining impulsivity as an endophenotype using a behavioral approach: a DRD2 TaqI A and DRD4 48-bp VNTR association study. *Behav. Brain Funct.* 3:2.

Eisenberg, N., Hofer, C., and Vaughan, J. (2006) Effortful control and its socioemotional consequences. *In*: Gross, J.J., ed. *Handbook of Emotion Regulation*. New York, London: Guilford Press, pp. 287–306.

El-Zein, R.A., Abdel-Rahman, S.Z., Hay, M.J., Lopez, M.S., Bondy, M.L., Morris, D.L., and Legator, M.S. (2005) Cytogenetic effects in children treated with methylphenidate. *Cancer Lett.* 230(2): 284–291.

Elliott, R., Sahakian, B.J., McKay, A.P., Herrod, J.J., Robbins, T.W., and Paykel, E.S. (1996) Neuropsychological impairments in unipolar depression: the influence of perceived failure on subsequent performance. *Psychol. Med.* 26(5):975–989.

Eriksen, B.A., and Eriksen, C.W. (1974) Effects of noise letters upon the identification of a target letter in a nonsearch task. *Percept. Psychophys.* 16:143–149.

Ernst, M., Kimes, A.S., London, E.D., Matochik, J.A., Eldreth, D., Tata, S., Contoreggi, C., Leff, M., and Bolla, K. (2003) Neural substrates of decision making in adults with attention deficit hyperactivity disorder. *Am. J. Psychiatry* 160(6):1061–1070.

Ernst, M., Liebenauer, L.L., King, A.C., Fitzgerald, G.A., Cohen, R.M., and Zametkin, A.J. (1994) Reduced brain metabolism in hyperactive girls. *J. Am. Acad. Child Adolesc. Psychiatry* 33(6): 858–868.

Ernst, M., Moolchan, E.T., and Robinson, M.L. (2001) Behavioral and neural consequences of prenatal exposure to nicotine. *J. Am. Acad. Child Adolesc. Psychiatry* 40(6):630–641.

Ernst, M., Zametkin, A.J., Matochik, J.A., Jons, P.H., and Cohen, R.M. (1998) DOPA decarboxylase activity in attention deficit hyperactivity disorder adults. A [fluorine-18]fluorodopa positron emission tomographic study. *J Neurosci.* 18(15):5901–5907.

Evenden, J.L. (1999) Varieties of impulsivity. *Psychopharmacol. (Berl)* 146(4):348–361.

Evenden, J.L., and Ryan, C.N. (1996) The pharmacology of impulsive behaviour in rats: the effects of drugs on response choice with varying delays of reinforcement. *Psychopharmacol. (Berl)* 128(2):161–170.

Faraone, S.V., Perlis, R.H., Doyle, A.E., Smoller, J.W., Goralnick, J. J., Holmgren, M.A., and Sklar, P. (2005) Molecular genetics of attention-deficit/hyperactivity disorder. *Biol. Psychiatry* 57(11): 1313–1323.

Food and Drug Administration. (2005) http://www.fda.gov/medwatch /safety/2005/nov05.htm.

Filipek, P.A., Semrud-Clikeman, M., Steingard, R.J., Renshaw, P.F., Kennedy, D.N., and Biederman, J. (1997) Volumetric MRI analysis comparing subjects having attention-deficit hyperactivity disorder with normal controls. *Neurology* 48(3):589–601.

Flory, J.D., Newcorn, J.H., Miller, C., Hart, Y.S., and Halperin, J.M. (2007) Serotonergic function in children with attention-deficit hyperactivity disorder: relationship to later antisocial personality disorder. *Br. J. Psychiatry* 190(5):410–414.

Fonagy, P. (2002) *Affect Regulation, Mentalization, and the Development of the Self*. New York: Other Press.

Frazier, T.W., Demaree, H.A., and Youngstrom, E.A. (2004) Meta-analysis of intellectual and neuropsychological test performance in attention-deficit/hyperactivity disorder. *Neuropsychology* 18(3): 543–555.

Gainetdinov, R.R., Wetsel, W.C., Jones, S.R., Levin, E.D., Jaber, M., and Caron, M.G. (1999) Role of serotonin in the paradoxical calming effect of psychostimulants on hyperactivity. *Science* 283(5400):397–401.

Garavan, H., Ross, T.J., and Stein, E.A. (1999) Right hemispheric dominance of inhibitory control: an event-related functional MRI study. *Proc. Natl. Acad. Sci. USA* 96(14):8301–8306.

Giedd, J.N., Blumenthal, J., Jeffries, N., Castellanos, F., Liu, H., Zijdenbos, A., Paus, T., Evans, A., and Rapoport, J. (1999) Brain development during childhood and adolescence: a longitudinal MRI study. *Nat. Neurosci.* 2:861–863.

Giedd, J.N., Castellanos, F.X., Casey, B.J., Kozuch, P., King, A.C., Hamburger, S.D., and Rapoport, J.L. (1994) Quantitative morphology of the corpus callosum in attention deficit hyperactivity disorder. *Am. J. Psychiatry* 151(5):665–669.

Gilbert, C.D., and Sigman, M. (2007) Brain states: top-down influences in sensory processing. *Neuron* 54(5):677–696.

Gillberg, C., Gillberg, I.C., Rasmussen, P., Kadesjö, B., Söderström, H., Råstam, M., Johnson, M., Rothenberger, A., and Niklasson, L. (2004) Co-existing disorders in ADHD—implications for diagnosis and intervention. *Eur. Child Adol. Psychiatry* 13(Suppl 1): 80–92.

Goldman-Rakic, P.S. (1996) The prefrontal landscape: implications of functional architecture for understanding human mentation and the central executive. *Phil. Trans. Royal Soc. London. Series B, Biol. Sci.* 351(1346):1445–1453.

Goos, L.M., Ezzatian, P., and Schachar, R. (2007) Parent-of-origin effects in attention-deficit hyperactivity disorder. *Psychiatry Res.* 149(1/3):1–9.

Gottesman, I.I., and Gould, T.D. (2003) The endophenotype concept in psychiatry: etymology and strategic intentions. *Am. J. Psychiatry* 160(4):636–645.

Gottesman, I.I., and Hanson, D.R. (2005) Human development: biological and genetic processes. *Annu. Rev. Psychol.* 56:263–286.

Graetz, B.W., Sawyer, M.G., Hazell, P.L., Arney, F., and Baghurst, P. (2001) Validity of DSM-IVADHD subtypes in a nationally representative sample of Australian children and adolescents. *J. Am. Acad. Child Adolesc. Psychiatry* 40(12):1410–1417.

Greenhill, L.L., Halperin, J.M., and Abikoff, H. (1999) Stimulant medications. *J. Am. Acad. Child Adolesc. Psychiatry* 38(5):503–512.

Greenhill, L.L., Pliszka, S., Dulcan, M.K., Bernet, W., Arnold, V., Beitchman, J., Benson, R.S., Bukstein, O., Kinlan, J., McClellan, J., Rue, D., Shaw, J.A., and Stock, S. (2002) Practice parameter for the use of stimulant medications in the treatment of children, adolescents, and adults. *J. Am. Acad. Child Adolesc. Psychiatry* 41(2 Suppl):26S–49S.

Hagino, N. (1985) Effect of maternal nicotine on the development of sites for [3H] nicotine binding in the fetal brain. *Int. J. Dev. Neurosci.* 3(5):567.

Hall, S.J., Halperin, J.M., Schwartz, S.T., and Newcorn, J.H. (1997) Behavioral and executive functions in children with attention-deficit hyperactivity disorder and reading disability. *J. Atten. Disord.* 1(4):235–243.

Halperin, J.M., Newcorn, J.H., Matier, K., Sharma, V., McKay, K.E., and Schwartz, S. (1993) Discriminant validity of attention-deficit hyperactivity disorder. *J. Am. Acad. Child Adolesc. Psychiatry* 32(5):1038–1043.

Hariri, A.R., Mattay, V.S., Tessitore, A., Kolachana, B., Fera, F., Goldman, D., Egan, M.F., and Weinberger, D.R. (2002) Serotonin transporter genetic variation and the response of the human amygdala. *Science* 297(5580):400–403.

Himpel, S., Banaschewski, T., Heise, C.A., and Rothenberger, A. (2005) The safety of non-stimulant agents for the treatment of attention-deficit hyperactivity disorder. *Expert Opin. Drug Saf.* 4(2):311–321.

Hinshaw, S.P., Owens, E.B., Wells, K.C., Kraemer, H.C., Abikoff, H.B., Arnold, L.E., Conners, C.K., Elliott, G., Greenhill, L.L., Hechtman, L., Hoza, B., Jensen, P.S., March, J.S., Newcorn, J.H., Pelham, W.E., Swanson, J.M., Vitiello, B., and Wigal, T. (2000) Family processes and treatment outcome in the MTA: negative/ineffective parenting practices in relation to multimodal treatment. *J. Abnorm. Child Psychol.* 28(6):555–568.

Holtmann, M., and Stadler, C. (2006) Electroencephalographic biofeedback for the treatment of attention-deficit hyperactivity disorder in childhood and adolescence. *Expert Rev. Neurother.* 6(4):533–540.

Hur, Y.M., and Bouchard, T.J., Jr. (1997) The genetic correlation between impulsivity and sensation seeking traits. *Behav. Genet.* 27(5):455–463.

Huttenlocher, P.R. (1979) Synaptic density in human frontal cortex—developmental changes and effects of aging. *Brain Res.* 163(2):195–205.

Hyman, S.E., Malenka, R.C., and Nestler, E.J. (2006) Neural mechanisms of addiction: the role of reward-related learning and memory. *Ann. Rev. Neurosci.* 29:565–598.

Hynd, G.W., Semrud-Clikeman, M., Lorys, A.R., Novey, E.S., and Eliopulos, D. (1990) Brain morphology in developmental dyslexia and attention deficit disorder/hyperactivity. *Arch. Neurol.* 47(8):919–926.

Hynd, G.W., Semrud-Clikeman, M., Lorys, A.R., Novey, E.S., Eliopulos, D., and Lyytinen, H. (1991) Corpus callosum morphology in attention deficit-hyperactivity disorder: morphometric analysis of MRI. *J. Learn. Disabil.* 24(3):141–146.

Hynes, M.D., Langer, D.H., Hymson, D.L., Pearson, D.V., and Fuller, R.W. (1985) Differential effects of selected dopaminergic agents on locomotor activity in normotensive and spontaneously hypertensive rats. *Pharmacol. Biochem. Behav.* 23(3):445–448.

Insel, T.R., and Collins, F.S. (2003) Psychiatry in the genomics era. *Am. J. Psychiatry* 160(4):616–620.

Jensen, P.S., Hinshaw, S.P., Kraemer, H.C., Lenora, N., Newcorn, J.H., Abikoff, H.B., March, J.S., Arnold, L.E., Cantwell, D.P., Conners, C.K., Elliott, G.R., Greenhill, L.L., Hechtman, L., Hoza, B., Pelham, W.E., Severe, J.B., Swanson, J.M., Wells, K.C., Wigal, T., and Vitiello, B. (2001) ADHD comorbidity findings from the MTA study: comparing comorbid subgroups. *J. Am. Acad. Child Adolesc. Psychiatry* 40(2):147–158.

Jensen, P.S., Martin, D., and Cantwell, D.P. (1997) Comorbidity in ADHD: implications for research, practice, and *DSM-V. J. Am. Acad. Child Adolesc. Psychiatry* 36(8):1065–1079.

Jensen, P.S., Youngstrom, E.A., Steiner, H., Findling, R.L., Meyer, R.E., Malone, R.P., Carlson, G.A., Coccaro, E.F., Aman, M.G., Blair, J., Dougherty, D., Ferris, C., Flynn, L., Green, E., Hoagwood, K., Hutchinson, J., Laughren, T., Leve, L.D., Novins, D.K., and Vitiello, B. (2007) Consensus report on impulsive aggression as a symptom across diagnostic categories in child psychiatry: implications for medication studies. *J. Am. Acad. Child Adolesc. Psychiatry* 46(3):309–322.

Jentsch, J.D., and Taylor, J.R. (1999) Impulsivity resulting from frontostriatal dysfunction in drug abuse: implications for the control of behavior by reward-related stimuli. *Psychopharmacol.* 146(4):373–390.

Johns, J.M., Louis, T.M., Becker, R.F., and Means, L.W. (1982) Behavioral effects of prenatal exposure to nicotine in guinea pigs. *Neurobehav. Toxicol. Teratol.* 4(3):365–369.

Johnson, J.G., and Johnson, J.G. (2002) Television viewing and aggressive behavior during adolescence and adulthood. *Science* 295(5564):2468.

Johnston, C. (1996) Parent characteristics and parent-child interactions in families of nonproblem children and ADHD children with higher and lower levels of oppositional-defiant behavior. *J. Abnorm. Child Psychol.* 24(1):85–104.

Johnston, K., Levin, H.M., Koval, M.J., and Everling, S. (2007) Top-down control-signal dynamics in anterior cingulate and prefrontal cortex neurons following task switching. *Neuron* 53(3):453–462.

Jones, B., and Mishkin, M. (1972) Limbic lesions and the problem of stimulus—reinforcement associations. *Exp. Neurol.* 36(2):362–377.

Kalenscher, T., Ohmann, T., and Gunturkun, O. (2006) The neuroscience of impulsive and self-controlled decisions. *Int. J. Psychophysiol.* 62(2):203–211.

Kazdin, A.E. (1997) Parent management training: evidence, outcomes, and issues. *J. Am. Acad. Child Adolesc. Psychiatry* 36(10):1349–1356.

Kazdin, A.E., Kraemer, H.C., Kessler, R.C., Kupfer, D.J., and Offord, D.R. (1997) Contributions of risk-factor research to developmental psychopathology. *Clin. Psychol. Rev.* 17(4):375–406.

Kent, L., Doerry, U., Hardy, E., Parmar, R., Gingell, K., Hawi, Z., Kirley, A., Lowe, N., Fitzgerald, M., Gill, M., and Craddock, N. (2002) Evidence that variation at the serotonin transporter gene influences susceptibility to attention deficit hyperactivity disorder (ADHD): analysis and pooled analysis. *Mol. Psychiatry* 7(8):908–912.

Kerr, A., and Zelazo, P.D. (2004) Development of "hot" executive function: The children's gambling task. *Brain Cogn.* 55(1):148–157.

Kessler, R.C., Adler, L., Barkley, R., Biederman, J., Conners, C.K., Demler, O., Faraone, S. V., Greenhill, L.L., Howes, M.J., Secnik, K., Spencer, T., Ustun, T.B., Walters, E. E., and Zaslavsky, A.M. (2006) The prevalence and correlates of adult ADHD in the United States: results from the National Comorbidity Survey Replication. *Am. J. Psychiatry* 163(4):716–723.

Klingberg, T., Fernell, E., Olesen, P.J., Johnson, M., Gustafsson, P., Dahlstrom, K., Gillberg, C.G., Forssberg, H., and Westerberg, H. (2005) Computerized training of working memory in children with ADHD—a randomized, controlled trial. *J. Am. Acad. Child Adolesc. Psychiatry* 44(2):177–186.

Knutson, B., Adams, C.M., Fong, G.W., and Hommer, D. (2001) Anticipation of increasing monetary reward selectively recruits nucleus accumbens. *J. Neurosci.* 21(16):RC159.

Kollins, S.G., Greenhill, L., Swanson, J., Wigal, S., Abikoff, H., McCracken, J., Riddle, M., McGough, J., Vitiello, B., Wigal, T., Skrobala, A., Posner, K., Ghuman, J., Davies, M., Cunningham, C., and Bauzo, A. (2006) Rationale, design, and methods of the Preschool ADHD Treatment Study (PATS). *J. Am. Acad. Child Adolesc. Psychiatry* 45(11):1275–1283.

Kraemer, H.C., Stice, E., Kazdin, A., Offord, D., and Kupfer, D. (2001) How do risk factors work together? Mediators, moderators, and independent, overlapping, and proxy risk factors. *Am. J. Psychiatry* 158(6):848–856.

Kreek, M.J., Nielsen, D.A., Butelman, E.R., and LaForge, K.S. (2005) Genetic influences on impulsivity, risk taking, stress responsivity and vulnerability to drug abuse and addiction. *Nat. Neurosci.* 8(11):1450–1457.

Laucht, M., Skowronek, M.H., Becker, K., Schmidt, M.H., Esser, G., Schulze, T.G., and Rietschel, M. (2007) Interacting effects of the dopamine transporter gene and psychosocial adversity on attention-deficit/hyperactivity disorder symptoms among 15-year-olds from a high-risk community sample. *Arch. Gen. Psychiatry* 64(5):585–590.

Leibenluft, E., Charney, D.S., and Pine, D.S. (2003) Researching the pathophysiology of pediatric bipolar disorder. *Biol. Psychiatry* 53(11):1009–1020.

Leibenluft, E., Rich, B.A., Vinton, D.T., Nelson, E.E., Fromm, S.J., Berghorst, L.H., Joshi, P., Robb, A., Schachar, R.J., Dickstein, D.P., McClure, E.B., and Pine, D.S. (2007) Neural circuitry engaged during unsuccessful motor inhibition in pediatric bipolar disorder. *Am. J. Psychiatry* 164(1):52–60.

Levy, F. (2004) Synaptic gating and ADHD: a biological theory of comorbidity of ADHD and anxiety. *Neuropsychopharmacol.* 29(9): 1589–1596.

Lim, J.R., Faught, P.R., Chalasani, N.P., and Molleston, J.P. (2006) Severe liver injury after initiating therapy with atomoxetine in two children. *J. Pediatr.* 148(6):831–834.

Linnet, K.M., Wisborg, K., Obel, C., Secher, N.J., Thomsen, P.H., Agerbo, E., and Henriksen, T.B. (2005) Smoking during pregnancy and the risk for hyperkinetic disorder in offspring. *Pediatrics* 116(2):462–467.

Logue, A.W. (1988) Research on self-control: an integrated framework. *Behav. Brain Res.* 11:665–709.

Losier, B.J., McGrath, P.J., and Klein, R.M. (1996) Error patterns on the continuous performance test in non-medicated and medicated samples of children with and without ADHD: a meta-analytic review. *J. Child Psychol. Psychiatry* 37(8):971–987.

Lou, H.C., Andresen, J., Steinberg, B., McLaughlin, T., and Friberg, L. (1998) The striatum in a putative cerebral network activated by verbal awareness in normals and in ADHD children. *Eur. J. Neurol.* 5(1):67–74.

Lou, H.C., Henriksen, L., and Bruhn, P. (1984) Focal cerebral hypoperfusion in children with dysphasia and/or attention deficit disorder. *Arch. Neurol.* 41(8):825–829.

Lou, H.C., Henriksen, H., Bruhn, P., Borner, H., and Nielsen, J.B. (1989) Striatal dysfunction in attention deficit and hyperkinetic disorder. *Arch. Neurol.* 46:48–52.

Luria, A.R. (1973) *The Working Brain: an Introduction to Neuropsychology*. New York: Basic Books.

Lyoo, I.K., Noam, G.G., Lee, C.K., Lee, H.K., Kennedy, B.P., and Renshaw, P.F. (1996) The corpus callosum and lateral ventricles in children with attention-deficit hyperactivity disorder: a brain magnetic resonance imaging study. *Biol. Psychiatry* 40(10):1060–1063.

Mackie, S., Shaw, P., Lenroot, R., Pierson, R., Greenstein, D.K., Nugent, T.F. 3rd, Sharp, W.S., Giedd, J.N., and Rapoport, J.L. (2007) Cerebellar development and clinical outcome in attention deficit hyperactivity disorder. *Am. J. Psychiatry* 164(4):647–655.

Mannuzza, S., Klein, R.G., Bonagura, N., Malloy, P., Giampino, T.L. and Addalli, K.A. (1991) Hyperactive boys almost grown up. V. Replication of psychiatric status. *Arch. Gen. Psychiatry* 48(1):77–83.

Manor, I., Eisenberg, J., Tyano, S., Sever, Y., Cohen, H., Ebstein, R. P., and Kotler, M. (2001) Family-based association study of the serotonin transporter promoter region polymorphism (5-HTTLPR) in attention deficit hyperactivity disorder. *Am. J. Med. Genet.* 105(1): 91–95.

March, J.S., Swanson, J.M., Arnold, L.E., Hoza, B., Conners, C.K., Hinshaw, S.P., Hechtman, L., Kraemer, H.C., Greenhill, L.L., Abikoff, H.B., Elliott, L.G., Jensen, P.S., Newcorn, J.H., Vitiello, B., Severe, J., Wells, K.C., and Pelham, W.E. (2000) Anxiety as a predictor and outcome variable in the multimodal treatment study of children with ADHD (MTA). *J. Abnorm. Child Psychol.* 28(6):527–541.

Marsh, R., Zhu, H., Schultz, R.T., Quackenbush, G., Royal, J., Skudlarski, P., and Peterson, B.S. (2006) A developmental fMRI study of self-regulatory control. *Hum. Brain Mapp.* 27(11):848–863.

Martin, A. (2006) Stimulating: prescribing amidst controversy. *Am. J. Psychiatry* 163(4):574–577.

Martinussen, R., Hayden, J., Hogg-Johnson, S., and Tannock, R. (2005) A meta-analysis of working memory impairments in children with attention-deficit/hyperactivity disorder. *J. Am. Acad. Child Adolesc. Psychiatry* 44(4):377–384.

Masten, A.S., Hubbard, J.J., Gest, S.D., Tellegen, A., Garmezy, N., and Ramirez, M. (1999) Competence in the context of adversity: pathways to resilience and maladaptation from childhood to late adolescence. *Dev. Psychopathol.* 11(1):143–169.

Meyer-Lindenberg, A., Buckholtz, J.W., Kolachana, B., Hariri, A.R., Pezawas, L., Blasi, G., Wabnitz, A., Honea, R., Verchinski, B., Callicott, J.H., Egan, M., Mattay, V., and Weinberger, D.R. (2006) Neural mechanisms of genetic risk for impulsivity and violence in humans. *Proc. Natl. Acad. Sci. USA* 103(16):6269–6274.

Meyer-Lindenberg, A., and Weinberger, D.R. (2006) Intermediate phenotypes and genetic mechanisms of psychiatric disorders. *Nat. Rev. Neurosci.*7(10):818–827.

Michelson, D., Faries, D., Wernicke, J., Kelsey, D., Kendrick, K., Sallee, F.R., and Spencer, T. (2001) Atomoxetine in the treatment of children and adolescents with attention-deficit/hyperactivity disorder: a randomized, placebo-controlled, dose-response study. *Pediatrics* 108(5):e83.

Mick, E., Biederman, J., Faraone, S.V., Sayer, J., and Kleinman, S. (2002) Case-control study of attention-deficit hyperactivity disorder and maternal smoking, alcohol use, and drug use during pregnancy. *J. Am. Acad. Child Adolesc. Psychiatry* 41(4):378–385.

Milberger, S., Biederman, J., Faraone, S.V., Chen, L., and Jones, J. (1996) Is maternal smoking during pregnancy a risk factor for attention deficit hyperactivity disorder in children? *Am. J. Psychiatry* 153(9):1138–1142.

Milberger, S., Biederman, J., Faraone, S.V., Murphy, J., and Tsuang, M.T. (1995) Attention deficit hyperactivity disorder and comorbid disorders: issues of overlapping symptoms. *Am. J. Psychiatry* 152(12):1793–1799.

Mill, J., Caspi, A., Williams, B.S., Craig, I., Taylor, A., Polo-Tomas, M., Berridge, C.W., Poulton, R., and Moffitt, T.E. (2006) Prediction of heterogeneity in intelligence and adult prognosis by genetic polymorphisms in the dopamine system among children with attention-deficit/hyperactivity disorder: evidence from 2 birth cohorts. *Arch. Gen. Psychiatry* 63(4):462–469.

Mitterschiffthaler, M.T., Ettinger, U., Mehta, M.A., Mataix-Cols, D., and Williams, S.C. (2006) Applications of functional magnetic resonance imaging in psychiatry. *J. Magn. Res. Imag.* 23(6):851–861.

Miyake, A., Friedman, N.P., Emerson, M.J., Witzki, A.H., and Wager, T.D. (2000) The unity and diversity of executive functions and their contributions to complex "frontal lobe" tasks: A latent variable analysis. *Cogn. Psychol.* 41(1):49–100.

Moeller, F.G., Barratt, E.S., Dougherty, D.M., Schmitz, J.M., and Swann, A.C. (2001) Psychiatric aspects of impulsivity. *Am. J. Psychiatry* 158(11):1783–1793.

Mostofsky, S.H., Reiss, A.L., Lockhart, P., and Denckla, M.B. (1998) Evaluation of cerebellar size in attention-deficit hyperactivity disorder. *J. Child Neurol.* 13(9):434–439.

The MTA Cooperative Group. (1999a) A 14-month randomized clinical trial of treatment strategies for attention-deficit/hyperactivity disorder. *Arch. Gen. Psychiatry* 56(12):1073–1086.

The MTA Cooperative Group. (1999b) Moderators and mediators of treatment response for children with attention-deficit/hyperactivity disorder: the Multimodal Treatment Study of children with attention-deficit/hyperactivity disorder. *Arch. Gen. Psychiatry* 56(12):1088–1096.

The MTA Cooperative Group. (2004) National Institute of Mental Health Multimodal Treatment Study of ADHD Follow-up: changes in effectiveness and growth after the end of treatment. *Pediatrics* 113(4):762–769.

Needleman, H.L., Schell, A., Bellinger, D., Leviton, A., and Allred, E. N. (1990) The long-term effects of exposure to low doses of lead in childhood. An 11-year follow-up report. *N. Engl. J. Med.* 322(2):83–88.

Niculescu, A.B., Lulow, L.L., Ogden, C.A., Le-Niculescu, H., Salomon, D.R., Schork, N.J., Caligiuri, M.P., and Lohr, J.B. (2006) Phenochipping of psychotic disorders: a novel approach for deconstructing and quantitating psychiatric phenotypes. *Am. J. Med. Gen. Part B, Neuropsych. Genet.* 141(6):653–662.

Nigg, J.T. (2005) Neuropsychologic theory and findings in attention-deficit/hyperactivity disorder: the state of the field and salient challenges for the coming decade. *Biol. Psychiatry* 57(11):1424–1435.

Nigg, J.T. (2006) *What Causes ADHD?* New York, London: Guilford Press.

Nigg, J.T., and Casey, B.J. (2005) An integrative theory of attention-deficit/ hyperactivity disorder based on the cognitive and affective neurosciences. *Dev. Psychopathol.* 17(3):785–806.

Nigg, J.T., Willcutt, E.G., Doyle, A.E., and Sonuga-Barke, E.J. (2005) Causal heterogeneity in attention-deficit/hyperactivity disorder: do we need neuropsychologically impaired subtypes? *Biol. Psychiatry* 57(11):1224–1230.

Obel, C., Henriksen, T.B., Dalsgaard, S., Linnet, K.M., Skajaa, E., Thomsen, P.H., and Olsen, J. (2004) Does children's watching of television cause attention problems? Retesting the hypothesis in a Danish cohort. *Pediatrics* 114(5):1372–1373; au. reply: 1373–1374.

Ochsner, K.N. (2004) Current directions in social cognitive neuroscience. *Curr. Opin. Neurobiol.* 14(2):254–258.

Okamoto, K., and Aoki, K. (1963) Development of a strain of spontaneously hypertensive rats. *Jpn. Circ. J.* 27:282–293.

Oosterlaan, J., Logan, G.D., and Sergeant, J.A. (1998) Response inhibition in AD/HD, CD, comorbid AD/HD + CD, anxious, and control children: a meta-analysis of studies with the stop task. *J. Child Psychol. Psychiatry* 39(3):411–425.

Overall, K.L. (2000) Natural animal models of human psychiatric conditions: assessment of mechanism and validity. *Prog. Neuropsychopharmacol. Biol. Psychiatry* 24(5):727–776.

Owens, E.B., Hinshaw, S.P., Kraemer, H.C., Arnold, L.E., Abikoff, H.B., Cantwell, D.P., Conners, C.K., Elliott, G., Greenhill, L.L., Hechtman, L., Hoza, B., Jensen, P.S., March, J.S., Newcorn, J.H., Pelham, W.E., Severe, J.B., Swanson, J.M., Vitiello, B., Wells, K.C., and Wigal, T. (2003) Which treatment for whom for ADHD? Moderators of treatment response in the MTA. *J. Consult. Clin. Psychol.* 71(3):540–552.

Passamonti, L., Fera, F., Magariello, A., Cerasa, A., Gioia, M.C., Muglia, M., Nicoletti, G., Gallo, O., Provinciali, L., and Quattrone, A. (2006) Monoamine oxidase-a genetic variations influence brain activity associated with inhibitory control: new insight into the neural correlates of impulsivity. *Biol. Psychiatry* 59(4):334–340.

Pelham, W.E., Jr. (1999) The NIMH multimodal treatment study for attention-deficit hyperactivity disorder: just say yes to drugs alone? *Can. J. Psychiatry* 44(10):981–990.

Pelham, W.E., Jr., Wheeler, T., and Chronis, A. (1998) Empirically supported psychosocial treatments for attention deficit hyperactivity disorder. *J. Clin. Child Psychol.* 27(2):190–205.

Pennington, B.F., and Ozonoff, S. (1996) Executive functions and developmental psychopathology. *J. Child Psychol. Psychiatry* 37(1):51–87.

Peterson, B.S. (2003) Conceptual, methodological, and statistical challenges in brain imaging studies of developmentally based psychopathologies. *Dev. Psychopathol.* 15(3):811–832.

Peterson, B.S., Anderson, A.W., Ehrenkranz, R., Staib, L.H., Tageldin, M., Colson, E., Gore, J.C., Duncan, C.C., Makuch, R.W., and Ment, L.R. (2003) Regional brain volumes and their later neurodevelopmental correlates in term and preterm infants. *Pediatrics* 111(5 Pt 1):939–948.

Peterson, B.S., Kane, M.J., Alexander, G.M., Lacadie, C., Skudlarski, P., Leung, H.C., May, J., and Gore, J.C. (2002) An event-related functional MRI study comparing interference effects in the Simon and Stroop tasks. *Brain Res. Cogn. Brain Res.* 13(3):427–440.

Peterson, B.S., Pine, D.S., Cohen, P., and Brook, J.S. (2001) Prospective, longitudinal study of tic, obsessive-compulsive, and attention-deficit/hyperactivity disorders in an epidemiological sample. *J. Am. Acad. Child Adolesc. Psychiatry* 40(6):685–695.

Peterson, B.S., Skudlarski, P., Anderson, A.W., Zhang, H., Gatenby, J.C., Lacadie, C.M., Leckman, J.F., and Gore, J.C. (1998) A functional magnetic resonance imaging study of tic suppression in Tourette syndrome. *Arch. Gen. Psychiatry* 55(4):326–333.

Peterson, B.S., Skudlarski, P., Gatenby, J.C., Zhang, H., Anderson, A.W., and Gore, J.C. (1999) An fMRI study of Stroop word-color interference: evidence for cingulate subregions subserving multiple distributed attentional systems. *Biol. Psychiatry* 45(10):1237–1258.

Peterson, B.S., Vohr, B., Staib, L.H., Cannistraci, C.J., Dolberg, A., Schneider, K.C., Katz, K.H., Westerveld, M., Sparrow, S., Anderson, A.W., Duncan, C.C., Makuch, R.W., Gore, J.C., and Ment, L.R. (2000) Regional brain volume abnormalities and long-term cognitive outcome in preterm infants. *JAMA* 284(15):1939–1947.

Pirkle, J.L., Brody, D.J., Gunter, E.W., Kramer, R.A., Paschal, D.C., Flegal, K.M., and Matte, T.D. (1994) The decline in blood lead levels in the United States. The National Health and Nutrition Examination Surveys (NHANES). *JAMA* 272(4):284–291.

Plessen, K.J., Bansal, R., Zhu, H., Whiteman, R., Amat, J., Quackenbush, G.A., Martin, L., Durkin, K., Blair, C., Royal, J., Hugdahl, K., and Peterson, B.S. (2006) Hippocampus and amygdala morphology in attention-deficit/hyperactivity disorder. *Arch. Gen. Psychiatry* 63(7):795–807.

Plessen, K.J., Royal, J., and Peterson, B.S. (2007) Neuroimaging of tic disorders with coexisting attention-deficit/hyperactivity disorder. *Eur. Child Adolesc. Psychiatry* 16(Suppl. I):60–70.

Pliszka, S.R., Glahn, D.C., Semrud-Clikeman, M., Franklin, C., Perez, R., III, Xiong, J., and Liotti, M. (2006) Neuroimaging of inhibitory control areas in children with attention deficit hyperactivity disorder who were treatment naive or in long-term treatment. *Am. J. Psychiatry* 163(6):1052–1060.

Polanczyk, G., de Lima, M.S., Horta, B.L., Biederman, J., and Rohde, L.A. (2007) The worldwide prevalence of ADHD: a systematic review and metaregression analysis. *Am. J. Psychiatry* 164(6):942–948.

Posner, J., Russell, J.A., and Peterson, B.S. (2005) The circumplex model of affect: an integrative approach to affective neuroscience, cognitive development, and psychopathology. *Dev. Psychopathol.* 17(3):715–734.

Posner, M.I., and Rothbart, M.K. (2000) Developing mechanisms of self-regulation. *Dev. Psychopathol.* 12(3):427–441.

Pratt, T.C., Cullen, F.T., Blevins, K.R., Daigle, L., and Unnever, J.D. (2002) The relationship of attention deficit hyperactivity disorder to crime and delinquency: a meta-analysis. *Int. J. Police Sci. Mgmt.* 4(4):344–360.

Preston, R.J., Kollins, S.H., Swanson, J.M., Greenhill, L.L., Wigal, T., Elliott, G.R., and Vitiello, B. (2005) Comments on "Cytogenetic effects in children treated with methylphenidate" by El-Zein et al. *Cancer Lett.* 230(2):292–294.

Rapoport, J.L., Castellanos, F.X., Gogate, N., Janson, K., Kohler, S., and Nelson, P. (2001) Imaging normal and abnormal brain development: new perspectives for child psychiatry. *Aust. N. Z. J. Psychiatry* 35(3):272–281.

Rapport, M.D., and Moffitt, C. (2002) Attention deficit/hyperactivity disorder and methylphenidate. A review of height/weight, cardiovascular, and somatic complaint side effects. *Clin. Psychol. Rev.* 22(8):1107–1131.

Rasmussen, P., and Gillberg, C. (2000) Natural outcome of ADHD with developmental coordination disorder at age 22 years: a controlled, longitudinal, community-based study. *J. Am. Acad. Child Adolesc.* 39(11):1424–1431.

Ridley, M. (2003) *Nature versus Nuture*. New York: Harper Collins.

Rieppi, R., Greenhill, L.L., Ford, R.E., Chuang, S., Wu, M., Davies, M., Abikoff, H.B., Arnold, L.E., Conners, C.K., Elliott, G.R., Hechtman, L., Hinshaw, S.P., Hoza, B., Jensen, P.S., Kraemer, H.C., March, J.S., Newcorn, J.H., Pelham, W.E., Severe, J.B., Swanson, J.M., Vitiello, B., Wells, K.C., and Wigal, T. (2002) Socioeconomic status as a moderator of ADHD treatment outcomes. *J. Am. Acad. Child Adolesc. Psychiatry* 41(3):269–277.

Robbins, T.W. (1990) The case of frontostriatal dysfunction in schizophrenia. *Schizophr. Bull.* 16(3):391–402.

Robbins, T.W., and Everitt, B.J. (1999) Drug addiction: bad habits add up. *Nature* 398(6728):567–570.

Roessner, V., Banaschewski, T., Uebel, H., Becker, A., and Rothenberger, A. (2004) Neuronal network models of ADHD —lateralization with respect to interhemispheric connectivity reconsidered. *Eur. Child Adolesc. Psychiatry* 13(Suppl 1): I71–I79.

Rolls, E.T. (1994) Neurophysiology and cognitive functions of the striatum. *Revue Neurolog.* 150(8/9):648–660.

Rolls, E.T. (2000) The orbitofrontal cortex and reward. *Cereb. Cortex* 10(3):284–294.

Romano, E., Tremblay, R.E., Farhat, A., and Cote, S. (2006) Development and prediction of hyperactive symptoms from 2 to 7 years in a population-based sample. *Pediatrics* 117(6):2101–2110.

Romine, C.B., Lee, D., Wolfe, M.E., Homack, S., George, C., and Riccio, C.A. (2004) Wisconsin Card Sorting Test with children: a meta-analytic study of sensitivity and specificity. *Arch. Clin. Neuropsychol.* 19(8):1027–1041.

Rosenberg, D.R., Dick, E.L., O'Hearn, K.M., and Sweeney, J.A. (1997) Response-inhibition deficits in obsessive-compulsive disorder: an indicator of dysfunction in frontostriatal circuits. *J. Psychiatry Neurosci.* 22(1):29–38.

Rothbart, M.K., and Bates, J.E. (1998) Temperament. *In*: Damon, W., and Eisenberg, N, eds. *Handbook of child psychology. Vol. 3. Social, emotional, and personality development*, 5th ed. New York: Wiley, pp. 105–176.

Rubia, K., Overmeyer, S., Taylor, E., Brammer, M., Williams, S.C., Simmons, A., and Bullmore, E.T. (1999) Hypofrontality in attention deficit hyperactivity disorder during higher-order motor control: a study with functional MRI. *Am. J. Psychiatry* 156(6):891–896.

Rubia, K., Smith, A.B., Brammer, M.J., Toone, B., and Taylor, E. (2005) Abnormal brain activation during inhibition and error detection in medication-naive adolescents with ADHD. *Am. J. Psychiatry* 162(6):1067–1075.

Rubia, K., Smith, A.B., Woolley, J., Nosarti, C., Heyman, I., Taylor, E., and Brammer, M. (2006) Progressive increase of frontostriatal brain activation from childhood to adulthood during event-related tasks of cognitive control. *Hum. Brain Mapp.* 27(12):973–993.

Rutter, M. (1989) Isle of Wight revisited: twenty-five years of child psychiatric epidemiology. *J. Am. Acad. Child Adolesc. Psychiatry* 28(5):633–653.

Rutter, M. (2005a) Environmentally mediated risks for psychopathology: research strategies and findings. *J. Am. Acad. Child Adolesc. Psychiatry* 44(1):3–18.

Rutter, M. (2005b) How the environment affects mental health. *Br. J. Psychiatry* 186:4–6.

Rutter, M., Dunn, J., Plomin, R., Simonoff, E., Pickles, A., Maughan, B., Ormel, J., Meyer, J., and Eaves, L. (1997) Integrating nature and nurture: implications of person-environment correlations and interactions for developmental psychopathology. *Dev. Psychopathol.* 9(2):335–364.

Rutter, M., and Silberg, J. (2002) Gene-environment interplay in relation to emotional and behavioral disturbance. *Annu. Rev. Psychol.* 53:463–490.

Rutter, M., Tizard, J., Yule, W., Graham, P., and Whitmore, K. (1976) Research report: Isle of Wight Studies, 1964-1974. *Psychol. Med.* 6(2):313–332.

Ryb, G.E., Dischinger, P.C., Kufera, J.A., and Read, K.M. (2006) Risk perception and impulsivity: association with risky behaviors and substance abuse disorders. *Accid. Anal. Prev.* 38(3):567–573.

Saalmann, Y.B., Pigarev, I.N., and Vidyasagar, T.R. (2007) Neural mechanisms of visual attention: how top-down feedback highlights relevant locations. *Science* 316(5831):1612–1615.

Sagvolden, T., Russell, V.A., Aase, H., Johansen, E.B., and Farshbaf, M. (2005) Rodent models of attention-deficit/hyperactivity disorder. *Biol. Psychiatry* 57(11):1239–1247.

Salman, M.S. (2002) The cerebellum: it's about time! But timing is not everything—new insights into the role of the cerebellum in timing motor and cognitive tasks. *J. Child Neurol.* 17(1):1–9.

Schachter, H.M., Pham, B., King, J., Langford, S., and Moher, D. (2001) How efficacious and safe is short-acting methylphenidate for the treatment of attention-deficit disorder in children and adolescents? A meta-analysis. *CMAJ* 165(11):1475–1488.

Scheres, A., Dijkstra, M., Ainslie, E., Balkan, J., Reynolds, B., Sonuga-Barke, E., and Castellanos, F.X. (2006) Temporal and probabilistic discounting of rewards in children and adolescents: effects of age and ADHD symptoms. *Neuropsychologia* 44(11):2092–2103.

Scheres, A., Milham, M.P., Knutson, B., and Castellanos, F.X. (2007) Ventral striatal hyporesponsiveness during reward anticipation in attention-deficit/hyperactivity disorder. *Biol. Psychiatry* 61(5): 720–724.

Schmahmann, J.D. (1996) From movement to thought: Anatomic substrates of the cerebellar contribution to cognitive processing. *Hum. Brain Mapp.* 4(3):174–198.

Schoenbaum, G., Chiba, A.A., and Gallagher, M. (1998) Orbitofrontal cortex and basolateral amygdala encode expected outcomes during learning. *Nat. Neurosci.* 1(2):155–159.

Schweitzer, J.B., Faber, T.L., Grafton, S.T., Tune, L.E., Hoffman, J.M., and Kilts, C.D. (2000) Alterations in the functional anatomy of working memory in adult attention deficit hyperactivity disorder. *Am. J. Psychiatry* 157(2):278–280.

Schweitzer, J.B., Lee, D.O., Hanford, R.B., Zink, C.F., Ely, T.D., Tagamets, M.A., Hoffman, J.M., Grafton, S.T., and Kilts, C.D. (2004) Effect of methylphenidate on executive functioning in adults with attention-deficit/hyperactivity disorder: Normalization of behavior but not related brain activity. *Biol. Psychiatry* 56(8):597–606.

Semrud-Clikeman, M., Filipek, P.A., Biederman, J., Steingard, R., Kennedy, D., Renshaw, P., and Bekken, K. (1994) Attention-deficit hyperactivity disorder: magnetic resonance imaging morphometric analysis of the corpus callosum. *J. Am. Acad. Child Adolesc. Psychiatry* 33(6):875–881.

Semrud-Clikeman, M., Steingard, R.J., Filipek, P., Biederman, J., Bekken, K., and Renshaw, P.F. (2000) Using MRI to examine brain-behavior relationships in males with attention deficit disorder with hyperactivity. *J. Am. Acad. Child Adolesc. Psychiatry* 39(4):477–484.

Shaw, G., and Brown, G. (1999) Arousal, time estimation, and time use in attention-disordered children. *Dev. Neuropsychol.* 16(2): 227–242.

Shaw, P., Lerch, J., Greenstein, D., Sharp, W., Clasen, L., Evans, A., Giedd, J., Castellanos, F.X., and Rapoport, J. (2006) Longitudinal mapping of cortical thickness and clinical outcome in children and adolescents with attention-deficit/hyperactivity disorder. *Arch. Gen. Psychiatry* 63(5):540–549.

Siegel, G.J., Albers, R.W., Brady, S.T., and Price, D.L. (2006) *Basic Neurochemistry: Molecular, Cellular, and Medical Aspects.* Boston: Elsevier Academic Press.

Silk, T., Vance, A., Rinehart, N., Egan, G., O'Boyle, M., Bradshaw, J.L., and Cunnington, R. (2005) Fronto-parietal activation in attention-deficit hyperactivity disorder, combined type: functional magnetic resonance imaging study. *Br. J. Psychiatry* 187(3):282–283.

Simon, J.R. (1969) Reactions toward the source of stimulation. *J. Exp. Psychol.* 81:174–176.

Smith, A.B., Taylor, E., Brammer, M., Toone, B., and Rubia, K. (2006) Task-specific hypoactivation in prefrontal and temporoparietal brain regions during motor inhibition and task switching in medication-naive children and adolescents with attention deficit hyperactivity disorder. *Am. J. Psychiatry* 163(6):1044–1051.

Solanto, M., Arnstein, A., and Castellanos, F.X. (2001) *Stimulant Drugs and ADHD. Basic and Clinical Neuroscience.* London: Oxford University Press.

Sonuga-Barke, E.J. (2003) The dual pathway model of AD/HD: an elaboration of neuro-developmental characteristics. *Neurosci. Biobehav. Rev.* 27(7):593–604.

Sonuga-Barke, E.J., and Castellanos, F.X. (2007) Spontaneous attentional fluctuations in impaired states and pathological conditions: A neurobiological hypothesis. *Neurosci. Biobehav. Rev.* 31(7): 977–986.

Sonuga-Barke, E.J., Daley, D., Thompson, M., Laver-Bradbury, C., and Weeks, A. (2001) Parent-based therapies for preschool attention-deficit/hyperactivity disorder: a randomized, controlled trial with a community sample. *J. Am. Acad. Child Adolesc. Psychiatry* 40(4):402–408.

Sonuga-Barke, E.J., Taylor, E., Sembi, S., and Smith, J. (1992) Hyperactivity and delay aversion—I. The effect of delay on choice. *J. Child Psychol. Psychiatry* 33(2):387–398.

Soubrie, P. (1986) Reconciling the role of central serotonin neurons in human and animal behavior. *Behav. Brain Res.* 9(2):319–364.

Sowell, E.R., Peterson, B.S., Thompson, P.M., Welcome, S.E., Henkenius, A.L., and Toga, A.W. (2003) Mapping cortical change across the human life span. *Nat. Neurosci.* 6(3):309–315.

Sowell, E.R., Thompson, P.M., Welcome, S.E., Henkenius, A.L., Toga, A.W., and Peterson, B.S. (2003) Cortical abnormalities in children and adolescents with attention-deficit hyperactivity disorder. *Lancet* 362(9397):1699–1707.

Spencer, T., Biederman, J., Heiligenstein, J., Wilens, T., Faries, D., Prince, J., Faraone, S.V., Rea, J., Witcher, J., and Zervas, S. (2001) An open-label, dose-ranging study of atomoxetine in children with attention deficit hyperactivity disorder. *J. Child Adolesc. Psychopharmacol.* 11(3):251–265.

Spencer, T., Biederman, J., and Wilens, T. (2000) Pharmacotherapy of attention deficit hyperactivity disorder. *Child Adolesc. Psychiatr. Clin. N. Am.* 9(1):77–97.

Spreen, O., and Strauss, E. (1998) *A Compendium of Neuropsychological Tests: Administration, Norms, and Commentary.* New York: Oxford University Press.

Stevenson, J., Asherson, P., Hay, D., Levy, F., Swanson, J., Thapar, A., and Willcutt, E. (2005) Characterizing the ADHD phenotype for genetic studies. *Dev. Sci.* 8(2):115–121.

Stroop, J.R. (1935) Studies of interference in serial verbal reactions. *J. Exp. Psychol.* 18:643–662.

Sugarman, A. (2006) Attention deficit hyperactivity disorder and trauma. *Int. J. Psychoanal.* 87(Pt 1):238–241.

Sukhodolsky, D.G., Scahill, L., Zhang, H., Peterson, B.S., King, R.A., Lombroso, P.J., Katsovich, L., Findley, D., and Leckman, J.F. (2003) Disruptive behavior in children with Tourette's syndrome: association with ADHD comorbidity, tic severity, and functional impairment. *J. Am. Acad. Child Adolesc. Psychiatry* 42(1):98–105.

Sullivan, M.A., and Rudnik-Levin, F. (2001) Attention deficit/hyperactivity disorder and substance abuse. Diagnostic and therapeutic considerations. *Ann. N. Y. Acad. Sci.* 931:251–270.

Suter, W., Martus, H.J., and Elhajouji, A. (2006) Methylphenidate is not clastogenic in cultured human lymphocytes and in the mouse bone-marrow micronucleus test. *Mutat. Res.* 607(2):153–159.

Swanson, J.M., Arnold, L.E., Vitiello, B., Abikoff, H.B., Wells, K.C., Pelham, W.E., March, J.S., Hinshaw, S.P., Hoza, B., Epstein, J.N., Elliott, G.R., Greenhill, L.L., Hechtman, L., Jensen, P.S., Kraemer, H.C., Kotkin, R., Molina, B., Newcorn, J.H., Owens, E.B., Severe, J., Hoagwood, K., Simpson, S., Wigal, T., and Hanley, T. (2002) Response to commentary on the multimodal treatment study of ADHD (MTA): mining the meaning of the MTA. *J. Abnorm. Child Psychol.* 30(4):327–332.

Swanson, J.M., Kinsbourne, M., Nigg, J., Lanphear, B., Stefanatos, G.A., Volkow, N., Taylor, E., Casey, B.J., Castellanos, F.X., and Wadhwa, P.D. (2007) Etiologic subtypes of attention-deficit/hyperactivity disorder: brain imaging, molecular genetic and environmental factors and the dopamine hypothesis. *Neuropsychol. Rev.* 17(1):39–59.

Swanson, J.M., Kraemer, H.C., Hinshaw, S.P., Arnold, L.E., Conners, C.K., Abikoff, H.B., Clevenger, W., Davies, M., Elliott, G.R., Greenhill, L.L., Hechtman, L., Hoza, B., Jensen, P.S., March, J.S., Newcorn, J.H., Owens, E.B., Pelham, W.E., Schiller, E., Severe, J.B., Simpson, S., Vitiello, B., Wells, K., Wigal, T., and Wu, M. (2001) Clinical relevance of the primary findings of the MTA: success rates based on severity of ADHD and ODD symptoms at the end of treatment. *J. Am. Acad. Child Adolesc. Psychiatry* 40(2): 168–179.

Tamm, L., Menon, V., Ringel, J., and Reiss, A.L. (2004) Event-related fMRI evidence of frontotemporal involvement in aberrant response inhibition and task switching in attention-deficit/hyperactivity disorder. *J. Am. Acad. Child Adolesc. Psychiatry* 43(11): 1430–1440.

Thach, W.T. (1998) What is the role of the cerebellum in motor learning and cognition? *Trends Cogn. Sci.* 2(9):331–337.

Thapar, A., Fowler, T., Rice, F., Scourfield, J., van den Bree, M., Thomas, H., Harold, G., and Hay, D. (2003) Maternal smoking during pregnancy and attention deficit hyperactivity disorder symptoms in offspring. *Am. J. Psychiatry* 160(11):1985–1989.

Thapar, A., Langley, K., Asherson, P., and Gill, M. (2007) Gene-environment interplay in attention-deficit hyperactivity disorder and the importance of a developmental perspective. *Br. J. Psychiatry* 190:1–3.

Thapar, A., Langley, K., Fowler, T., Rice, F., Turic, D., Whittinger, N., Aggleton, J., Van den Bree, M., Owen, M., and O'Donovan, M. (2005) Catechol-O-methyltransferase gene variant and birth weight predict early-onset antisocial behavior in children with attention-deficit/hyperactivity disorder. *Arch. Gen. Psychiatry* 62(11):1275–1278.

Thapar, A., van den Bree, M., Fowler, T., Langley, K., and Whittinger, N. (2006) Predictors of antisocial behaviour in children with attention deficit hyperactivity disorder. *Eur. Child Adolesc. Psychiatry* 15(2):118–125.

Toplak, M.E., Dockstader, C., and Tannock, R. (2006) Temporal information processing in ADHD: findings to date and new methods. *J. Neurosci. Meth.* 151(1):15–29.

Tucker, D.M., Luu, P., and Pribram, K.H. (1995) Social and emotional self-regulation. *Ann. N.Y. Acad. Sci.* 769(1):213–239.

Tully, L.A., Arseneault, L., Caspi, A., Moffitt, T.E., and Morgan, J. (2004) Does maternal warmth moderate the effects of birth weight on twins' attention-deficit/hyperactivity disorder (ADHD) symptoms and low IQ? *J. Consult. Clin. Psychol.* 72(2):218–226.

Uhlmann, E., and Swanson, J. (2004) Exposure to violent video games increases automatic aggressiveness. *J. Adolesc.* 27(1):41–52.

Vaidya, C.J., Austin, G., Kirkorian, G., Ridlehuber, H.W., Desmond, J.E., Glover, G.H., and Gabrieli, J.D.E. (1998) Selective effects of methylphenidate in attention deficit hyperactivity disorder: A functional magnetic resonance study. *Proc. Natl. Acad. Sci. USA* 95(24):14494–14499.

Valera, E.M., Faraone, S.V., Biederman, J., Poldrack, R.A., and Seidman, L.J. (2005) Functional neuroanatomy of working memory in adults with attention-deficit/hyperactivity disorder. *Biol. Psychiatry* 57(5):439–447.

Valera, E.M., Faraone, S.V., Murray, K.E., and Seidman, L.J. (2007) Meta-analysis of structural imaging findings in attention-deficit/hyperactivity disorder. *Biol. Psychiatry* 61(12):1361–1369.

van der Kooij, M.A., and Glennon, J.C. (2007) Animal models concerning the role of dopamine in attention-deficit hyperactivity disorder. *Neurosci. Biobehav. Rev.* 31(4):597–618.

van Mourik, R., Oosterlaan, J., and Sergeant, J.A. (2005) The Stroop revisited: a meta-analysis of interference control in AD/HD. *J. Child Psychol. Psychiatry* 46(2):150–165.

Viding, E., Williamson, D.E., and Hariri, A.R. (2006) Developmental imaging genetics: challenges and promises for translational research. *Dev. Psychopathol.* 18(3):877–892.

Vitiello, B. (2007) Research in child and adolescent psychopharmacology: recent accomplishments and new challenges *Psychopharmacol.* 191:5–13.

Volkow, N.D. (2006) Stimulant medications: how to minimize their reinforcing effects? *Am. J. Psychiatry* 163(3):359–361.

Volkow, N.D., Fowler, J.S., Wang, G., Ding, Y., and Gatley, S.J. (2002) Mechanism of action of methylphenidate: insights from PET imaging studies. *J. Atten. Disord.* 6(Suppl 1):43.

Volkow, N.D., and Insel, T.R. (2003) What are the long-term effects of methylphenidate treatment? *Biol. Psychiatry* 54(12):1307–1309.

Volkow, N.D., Wang, G.J., Fowler, J.S., and Ding, Y.S. (2005) Imaging the effects of methylphenidate on brain dopamine: new model on its therapeutic actions for attention-deficit/hyperactivity disorder. *Biol. Psychiatry* 57(11):1410–1415.

Volkow, N.D., Wang, G.-J., Fowler, J.S., Logan, J., Gerasimov, M., Maynard, L., Ding, Y.-S., Gatley, S.J., Gifford, A., and Franceschi, D. (2001) Therapeutic doses of oral methylphenidate significantly increase extracellular dopamine in the human brain. *J. Neurosci.* 21(2):121RC-125RC.

Weaver, I.C., Cervoni, N., Champagne, F.A., D'Alessio, A.C., Sharma, S., Seckl, J.R., Dymov, S., Szyf, M., and Meaney, M.J. (2004) Epigenetic programming by maternal behavior. *Nat. Neurosci.* 7(8):847–854.

Webster-Stratton, C., Reid, J., and Hammond, M. (2001) Social skills and problem-solving training for children with early-onset conduct problems: who benefits? *J. Child Psychol. Psychiatry* 42(7):943–952.

Weitzman, M., Gortmaker, S., and Sobol, A. (1992) Maternal smoking and behavior problems of children. *Pediatrics* 90(3):342–349.

Wells, K.C., Epstein, J.N., Hinshaw, S.P., Conners, C.K., Klaric, J., Abikoff, H.B., Abramowitz, A., Arnold, L.E., Elliott, G., Greenhill, L.L., Hechtman, L., Hoza, B., Jensen, P.S., March, J.S., Pelham, W., Pfiffner, L., Severe, J., Swanson, J.M., Vitiello, B., and Wigal, T. (2000) Parenting and family stress treatment outcomes in attention deficit hyperactivity disorder (ADHD): an empirical analysis in the MTA study. *J. Abnorm. Child Psychol.* 28(6):543–553.

Wells, K.C., Chi, T.C., Hinshaw, S.P., Epstein, J.N., Pfiffner, L., Nebel-Schwalm, M., Owens, E.B., Arnold, L.E., Abikoff, H.B., Conners, C.K., Elliott, G.R., Greenhill, L.L., Hechtman, L., Hoza, B., Jensen, P.S., March, J., Newcorn, J.H., Pelham, W.E., Severe, J.B., Swanson, J., Vitiello, B., and Wigal, T. (2006) Treatment-related changes in objectively measured parenting behaviors in the multimodal treatment study of children with attention-deficit/hyperactivity disorder. *J. Consult. Clin. Psychol.* 74(4):649–657.

Wilens, T.E., Biederman, J., and Spencer, T.J. (2002) Attention deficit/hyperactivity disorder across the lifespan. *Annu. Rev. Med.* 53: 113–131.

Wilens, T.E., Faraone, S.V., Biederman, J., and Gunawardene, S. (2003) Does stimulant therapy of attention-deficit/hyperactivity disorder beget later substance abuse? a meta-analytic review of the literature. *Pediatrics* 111(1):179–185.

Willcutt, E.G., Doyle, A.E., Nigg, J.T., Faraone, S.V., and Pennington, B.F. (2005) Validity of the executive function theory of attention-deficit/hyperactivity disorder: a meta-analytic review. *Biol. Psychiatry* 57(11):1336–1346.

Williams, G.M., O'Callaghan, M., Najman, J.M., Bor, W., Andersen, M.J., Richards, D.D., and Chinlyn, U. (1998) Maternal cigarette smoking and child psychiatric morbidity: a longitudinal study. *Pediatrics* 102(1):e11.

Williams, G.V., Rolls, E.T., Leonard, C.M., and Stern, C. (1993) Neuronal responses in the ventral striatum of the behaving macaque. *Behav. Brain Res.* 55(2):243–252.

Willoughby, M.T. (2003) Developmental course of ADHD symptomatology during the transition from childhood to adolescence: a review with recommendations. *J. Child Psychol. Psychiatry* 44(1): 88–106.

Winstanley, C.A., Dalley, J.W., Theobald, D.E., and Robbins, T.W. (2004) Fractionating impulsivity: contrasting effects of central 5-HT depletion on different measures of impulsive behavior. *Neuropsychopharmacol.* 29(7):1331–1343.

Woodward, L., Taylor, E., and Dowdney, L. (1998) The parenting and family functioning of children with hyperactivity. *J. Child Psychol. Psychiatry* 39(2):161–169.

Zametkin, A.J., Liebenauer, L.L., Fitzgerald, G.A., King, A.C., Minkunas, D.V., Herscovitch, P., Yamada, E.M., and Cohen, R.M. (1993) Brain metabolism in teenagers with attention-deficit hyperactivity disorder. *Arch. Gen. Psychiatry* 50(5):333–340.

Zametkin, A.J., Nordahl, T.E., Gross, M., King, A.C., Semple, W.E., Rumsey, J., Hamburger, S., and Cohen, R.M. (1990) Cerebral glucose metabolism in adults with hyperactivity of childhood onset. *N. Eng. J. Med.* 323(20):1361–1366.

Zametkin, A.J., and Rapoport, J. (1987) Noradrenergic hypothesis of attention deficit disorder with hyperactivity: a critical review. *In*: Meltzer, H. Y., ed. *Psychopharmacology: The Third Generation of Progress*. New York: Raven Press, pp. 837–842.

Zelazo, P.D., and Cunningham, W.A. (2006) Executive function: Mechanisms underlying emotion regulation. In: Gross, J.J., ed. *Handbook of Emotion Regulation*. New York, London: Guilford Press, pp. 135–158.

Zuckerman, M., Kuhlman, D.M., Thornquist, M., and Kiers, H. (1991) Five (or three) robust questionnaire scale factors of personality without culture. *Person. Indiv. Diff.* 12(9):929–941.

70 Childhood Anxiety Disorders: A Cognitive Neurobiological Perspective

CHRISTOPHER S. MONK AND DANIEL S. PINE

Major insights on the neurobiology of pediatric anxiety disorders have emerged from two research approaches: (*1*) epidemiological studies on relationship between anxiety disorders and other forms of psychopathology across development and generations and (*2*) psychobiological studies conducted in patients with disorders. In this chapter, findings from both approaches are integrated with research on preclinical aspects of fear to generate insights on pathophysiology. Together, this integration engenders interest in the role of cognitive processing in patients with anxiety disorders. In this setting, the term *cognitive* is used broadly to refer to a suite of information processing functions that facilitate decision making. From this perspective, cognitive processes define the manner in which new information is processed by the brain and integrated within existing information stores to effectively influence behavior. Thus, affective processes can be conceptualized as the subset of cognitive processes where stimuli and associated decisions concern motivationally significant events, those with potential impact on fitness. For anxiety, these events concern the assessment of and response to danger.

Available cognitive findings effectively bridge prior findings from epidemiological, clinical/biological, and preclinical/biological perspectives, permitting a more complete portrait of anxiety disorders. Three specific aspects of research on cognition facilitate this bridging.

1. The neural bases of information processing are more finely delineated than the neural bases of psychopathology. Therefore, by including cognitive processes as part of emotional tasks, more precise hypotheses on pathophysiology can be developed.
2. Cognitive tasks are amenable to neuroimaging techniques suitable for studies in children, including functional magnetic resonance imaging (fMRI). These imaging procedures are particularly informative when participants are engaged in tasks that involve discrete events in time, as provided by many cognitive tasks.
3. Tasks that involve precise cognitive components that are directly related to core symptoms can be used to examine neurobiological markers with neuroimaging as they relate to trait or state effects of anxiety.

The current chapter considers data on five specific anxiety disorders: generalized anxiety disorder (GAD) or *overanxious disorder* (the term used in the *Diagnostic and Statistical Manual of Mental Disorders*, 3rd ed. revised [*DSM-III-R*]; American Psychiatric Association, 1987, for children presenting with symptoms of GAD), social phobia, specific phobia, panic disorder with and without agoraphobia, and posttraumatic stress disorder (PTSD). Obsessive–compulsive disorder (OCD) is minimally discussed as it is considered a unique anxiety disorder with a distinct etiology and course, covered in other chapters. The initial section of the chapter reviews preclinical research to provide novel insights on perturbed brain function in clinical anxiety. This review is followed by an overview of research on epidemiology and clinical correlates of anxiety disorders in children. The third section provides a cognitive integrative approach to the study of anxiety disorders in children.

PRECLINICAL RESEARCH

Fear and anxiety-related behaviors are well conserved across species. This conservation is reflected in the fact that dangerous stimuli and situations precipitate similar changes in behavior, autonomic physiology, cognitive function, and brain engagement across a range of mammalian species. Given these cross-species similarities, research on anxiety provides an unusually strong opportunity for efforts to link animal-model investigations into the neurobiology of behavior to databases from clinical studies. Moreover, the strong role of developmental factors in shaping anxiety across species further attests to the relevance of integrative perspectives on anxiety. From such integrative work, a neurophysiological and molecular understanding of fear-related behaviors in animals has developed, with potential key applicability to clinical anxiety disorders, conceptualized through the lens of development.

Fear Circuitry

Research in the basic sciences has stimulated considerable interest in brain systems engaged by dangerous stimuli or events, stimuli that an organism will extend efforts to avoid. Much of this interest derives from research on fear conditioning, a learning-based phenomenon whereupon a neutral conditioned stimulus (CS+) is repeatedly paired with an intrinsically aversive unconditioned stimulus, such as an electric shock or aversive air puff (unconditioned stimulus or UCS). Following CS/UCS pairings, the CS comes to elicit responses formerly associated with only the UCS. Interest in fear conditioning derives at least partially from the precise delineation of brain circuits engaged by the process. In particular, changes in response to the CS involve changes within an amygdala-based circuit. Figure 70.1 illustrates a framework that depicts the broad outlines of this circuit while also delineating the manner in which functioning in this circuit can be linked to clinical constructs. This includes measures of information processing and clinical phenotype.

Enhanced understanding of neural processes engaged by fear conditioning has stimulated interest in various related areas. With respect to research that may inform developmental theories of clinical anxiety, four topics appear particularly relevant: (*1*) research that differentiates responses to innately aversive (UCS) stimuli as opposed to conditioned (CS+) stimuli; (*2*) research relating functioning within neural structures engaged by fear conditioning experiments to cognitive or neurohormonal systems that exhibit dysfunction in clinical disorders; (*3*) research examining the effects of environmental adversity during development on fear conditioning circuitry; and (*4*) research on the interactions among genes, brain lesions, development, and fear.

Fear versus anxiety

Clinical studies consistently find that patients with anxiety disorders exhibit abnormal responses to circumstances that provoke fear in the absence of previous exposures to such circumstances (Pine, 2007). For example, even in the absence of previous direct experience, various mildly noxious stimuli produce greater fear responses in patients than healthy patients. These stimuli include a range of agents or experiences, such as carbon dioxide

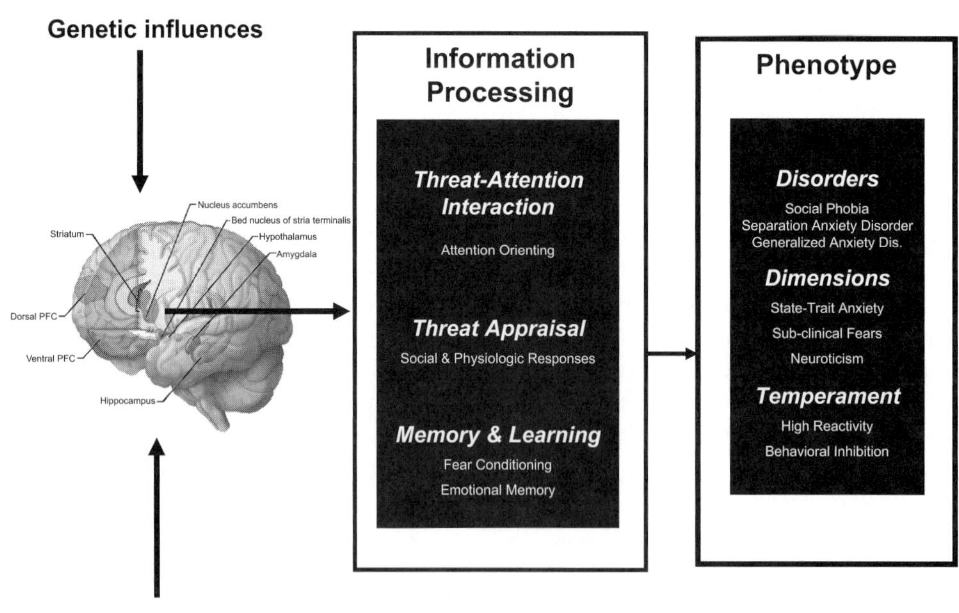

FIGURE 70.1 A framework for integrating neuroscience and clinical work on pediatric anxiety disorders. This figure displays a framework for psychobiological influences on anxiety disorders and associated clinical phenotypes, as displayed in the box on the right. Genes and the environment contribute to risk for clinical phenotypes by influencing functioning in a distributed neural circuit. Key components of this circuit are illustrated in the figure on the left. These genetic and environmental influences do not directly map onto currently conceptualized phenotypes. Rather, they shape information processing functions depicted in the box adjacent to the illustrated neural circuit. These functions include attention, appraisal, and learning as well as other processes not reviewed in the current chapter.

inhalation, threat of a painful experience, or presentation of mildly upsetting photographs. Clearly, anticipation plays a role in these differences, as physiological perturbations in patients prior to stimulus presentation represent strong predictors of anxiety responses during stimulus presentation. These heightened responses in patients with anxiety disorder to innately dangerous stimuli appear more consistently abnormal than responses in learning paradigms, such as during classic fear conditioning paradigms (Lissek et al., 2005). These findings in humans parallel preclinical investigations that have attempted to separate the neurobiology of two key constructs, anxiety versus fear.

In recent preclinical studies, the term *fear* has been used to describe neural responses to briefly presented explicit fear cues that acquire fear-evoking properties through learning, as in the classic fear conditioning experiment. Behavioral and physiologic responses to these situations rapidly remit once the feared stimulus is removed. In contrast, the term *anxiety* has been used to describe neural responses to sustained threats that possess innately fear-provoking capabilities. Such responses are tonically maintained, as modeled in rodents by exposure to an innately dangerous scenario, such as a well-lit room or an open field (Davis, 1998). Work by Davis and colleagues implicates the central nucleus of the amygdala in the "fear" response, as opposed to the bed nucleus of the stria terminalis, a structure closely related to the amygdala, which is implicated in "anxiety-like" behaviors (Davis, 1998). The anatomical locations of these structures appear in Figure 70.1.

These findings relate to a basic question of anxiety research: when is fear and anxiety normal and when do they become pathological? The above results separate in animal models "anxiety-like" behaviors from "fear-like" behaviors, with the former bearing closer relationships with behaviors and physiological perturbations seen in clinical disorders. Other work, however, suggests other possible distinctions between normal and abnormal anxiety behaviors, beyond the "fear–anxiety" distinction. For example, Grillon and Bouton each suggested that the ability categorize ambiguous stimuli differs among healthy patients and patients with anxiety, with Grillon emphasizing the role of categorization based on stimulus type or the context of an aversive exposure and Bouton emphasizing the role of categorization based on temporal factors (Bouton, 2002; Grillon, 2002). These differences invoke anatomy distinct from that emphasized by Davis. Thus, for Grillon, circuitry encompassing the hippocampus has been implicated in categorization of threat based on context, whereas for Bouton, the prefrontal cortex (PFC) has been implicated in categorization based on temporal factors. Anatomical locations of these structures also appear in Figure 70.1.

Despite differences in some particulars, for Grillon (2002), Bouton (2002), and Davis (1998), each perspective suggests that efforts to more definitively link preclinical findings with findings from clinical studies benefit from precise definitions of behavioral responses to varying classes of threat stimuli. As such, future attempts at basic clinical integration might benefit from research linking functioning in fear circuits in lower mammals with precisely defined behaviors and regulatory systems implicated in clinical disorders.

Fear circuitry and systems perturbed in clinical anxiety

From the clinical perspective, hypervigilance, exaggerated attention to threat, and other aspects of perturbed threat–attention interaction represent one cardinal feature of many anxiety disorders (see below). These cognitive processes allow stimuli with fear-provoking qualities, such as angry faces, to become more efficiently processed. Preclinical research on attention regulation suggests that such hypervigilance may reflect the influence of fear-relevant circuitry on brain systems devoted to attention allocation. Preexisting dysregulation during a fear response or alterations in regulation following a fear-provoking event may relate to the neurobiological profile that is seen in patients with various anxiety disorders. Preclinical work has begun to delineate the neural circuitry involved in perceiving and responding to threat cues. The amygdala translates the perception of threat and initiates the biochemical reaction (LeDoux, 1990). As one part of this fear response, neural systems engaged in perception may become attuned to selectively process potential threat stimuli.

Beyond perturbations in attention to threat cues, dysfunction in the hypothalamic-pituitary-adrenal (HPA) axis represents a second area where patients with various psychiatric disorders demonstrate consistent abnormalities. Such dysfunction is not unexpected, given anatomical connections illustrated in Figure 70.1 among the amygdala, bed nucleus of the stria terminalis, and the hypothalamus. The data appear most consistent in certain forms of major depression among adults, though data in various adult anxiety disorders, particularly those associated with acute stress or trauma, also implicate HPA axis dysfunction. Of note, findings in these areas appear decidedly stronger among adult mood and anxiety disorders, relative to pediatric mood and anxiety disorders. Considerable work shows that neuroendocrine cascades lead to inhibition of corticotrophin-releasing hormone (CRH) release from the hypothalamus along the HPA axis. In tandem with this negative feedback, CRH appears to also produce positive feedback on stress-sensitive behaviors regulated by the amygdala (Schulkin et al., 1998). This counterregulatory phenomenon has been documented using a psychological stressor (Makino et al., 1999) and following the administration of stress-levels of glucocorticoids (Makino et al., 1994). Moreover, the infusion of CRH into the amygdala potentiates the fear response (Takahashi et al., 1989). These results combined with the work of Davis (1998) noted above suggest that the CRH infusion may affect the stria terminalis and lead to increased fear-related behavior. Given the consistency of findings implicating HPA axis disturbance in adult patients with clinical disorders, these results may clarify neural pathways associated with the amygdala that contribute to such abnormalities.

Adversity and the developing brain

A wealth of research in rodents delineates the degree to which environmental adversity can alter brain systems engaged by fear conditioning experiments. One of the most fascinating results from research in this area reveals a long-standing developmental change in the sensitivity of these brain systems to environmental perturbation. Among young rodent pups, increased pup licking, grooming, and arched-back nursing (LG-ABN) leads to alterations in the long-term functioning of the HPA axis and medial temporal lobe (MTL) (Francis et al., 1999). Relative to manipulations in mature organisms, these environmental perturbations lead to much longer-term changes in regulation of the HPA axis, consistent with a resetting in the regulatory capacity of this system.

These changes have been clearly linked to specific changes within the environment and within brain systems involved in fear-related behaviors. These effects are depicted in Figure 70.1 as an arrow running directly from environmental influences to the fear circuit. For example, in a cross-fostering study, pups that received low levels of LG-ABN evidenced reduced glucocorticoid receptor messenger ribonucleic acid (mRNA) expression in the hippocampus, increased CRH mRNA in the periventricular nucleus, and decreased numbers of amygdalar benzodiazepine receptors (Francis et al., 1999). In addition, a reduction in LG-ABN levels is associated with lower α_2 adrenoreceptor and γ-aminobutyric acid (GABA-A) receptor density in the locus coeruleus, and these animals also present increases in fear-related behaviors in novel situations (Caldji et al., 1998). Moreover, rat pups that experienced reduced LG-ABN revealed a host of neuroanatomical and neurochemical alterations in the hippocampus, a structure known to be involved in memory in many species. Interestingly, these animals were also impaired in a test of spatial memory. The HPA axis, amygdala, hippocampus, and locus coeruleus constitute a neural circuit that permits organisms to respond to threat, and this system may be modified in development.

Similar findings have been documented in nonhuman primates. Adult nonhuman primates who were mistreated in early development displayed a suppressed cortisol response to a CRH challenge compared to nonabused controls (E.O. Johnson et al., 1996). In another investigation, adult macaques reared when their mothers were exposed to a variable foraging demand condition show alterations in CRH and cortisol concentrations relative to animals experiencing either the high or low foraging demands (Coplan et al., 1996). In the same set of animals, the noradrenergic probe, yohimbine, increases behavioral inhibition in monkeys from the variable foraging condition (Rosenblum et al., 1994). These studies indicate that adversity in early development leads to long-term alterations in the HPA axis, norepinephrine, MTL structures, and also memory.

Developmental perturbations and fear

Studies of environmental adversity clearly document the plasticity of the immature fear circuit. Given the robustness of these findings, considerable work in areas beyond environmental adversity further explores the degree to which development shapes long-term trajectories of fear-related behaviors. Two sets of findings appear most robust, one related to genetics and the other related to anatomical changes.

Genetic research further confirms the plastic nature of the rodent fear circuit, as alluded to in Figure 70.1 by the arrow running directly from genes to the fear circuit. Perhaps the strongest data emerge for studies of serotonin (5HT) manipulations. Perturbation of 5HT consistently produces alterations in fear-related behaviors among mice. At least for some 5HT manipulations, these effects occur in a developmental context, such that 5HT alterations in juveniles, even when they are transiently induced, produce long-lasting alterations in anxiety. Conversely, the same alterations made during adulthood and actively present in mature mice produce no such concurrently expressed alterations in anxiety. These findings have been demonstrated for manipulations of the 5HT1a receptor and of the 5HT transporter (Ansorge et al., 2004; Gross and Hen, 2004). They suggest that 5HT gene effects on anxiety arise through organizational rather than acute effects on fear-circuit function. These findings generate considerable interest for extensions to humans, given recent findings in humans documenting relationships among environmental adversity, a 5HT transporter polymorphism, amygdala function, and various psychiatric outcomes (Caspi and Moffitt, 2006).

Findings from lesions studies further suggest that alterations in amygdala-based circuitry influence fear behaviors in a developmental context. The most convincing findings show that the effects of amygdala lesions on fear in monkeys vary based on the age at which the injury is sustained and the nature of the threat. Thus, lesions in immature and mature monkeys produce reduced fear of snakes but markedly different responses to social threats. Here, lesions in immature monkeys lead to increases in social fear, whereas lesions in mature monkeys produce the opposite effect (Prather et al., 2001). Given that the intrinsic connectivity of the amygdala is established early in life, these developmental effects are likely to reflect changes in amygdala connections with frontal or temporal aspects of association cortex (Pine, 2003).

In summary, considerable enthusiasm has emerged for efforts to integrate preclinical and clinical research in anxiety, as this might inform research among children. This enthusiasm derives from a confluence of findings. First, neural circuits involved in anxiety-related behaviors, as depicted in Figure 70.1, have been precisely delineated through research on fear conditioning. Second, these initial advances have stimulated efforts to distinguish fear-related behaviors that represent normal adaptive responses to danger from behaviors that represent signs of pathology. Finally, recent studies delineate developmentally sensitive periods during which fear circuits can be selectively altered, either through direct effects on the environment, direct effects on genes, or direct effects on the neural circuitry. When coupled with research reviewed below on the prevalence of clinical anxiety disorders in children, these findings raise hopes that such integrative so-called translational research might impact a sizable proportion of individuals.

EPIDEMIOLOGICAL INVESTIGATIONS

From the clinical perspective, much of the most influential developmental research examining anxiety disorders adopts an epidemiological perspective. This work focuses on a range of clinical phenotypes depicted in the right-hand margin of Figure 70.1. This includes clinically defined anxiety disorders, dimensional measures of anxiety, or anxiety disorder precursors, as measured by personality scales (for example, neuroticism) or in measures of early childhood temperament (for example, high reactivity, behavioral inhibition). Studies in this area, as reviewed below, delineate three major questions concerning heterogeneity. First, studies on the prevalence of childhood anxiety disorders raise questions on differences between developmental fluctuations in anxiety disorders as opposed to developmentally appropriate anxieties. Second, longitudinal studies document moderately strong associations between child and adult anxiety disorders, but questions arise on factors that distinguish children with transient as opposed to persistent problems. Finally, family studies note consistent associations between parental mood or anxiety disorders and childhood anxiety, but questions emerge on factors that distinguish at-risk children who ultimately manifest chronic problems with anxiety as opposed to transient or no problems.

Prevalence and Onset of Anxiety Disorders

Anxiety disorders represent the most common group of psychiatric disorder affecting children and adolescents. Conservative estimates suggest that approximately 5%–15% of children will exhibit symptoms of an impairing anxiety disorder at some point during development (Pine and Klein, in press). However, reported rates vary widely, from a minimum of 1.8% (Anderson et al., 1987) to a maximum of 23.5% (Verhulst et al., 1997). Such marked cross-study variation could support recent views emphasizing a focus on anxiety dimensions and viewing psychiatric conditions as tail ends of normally distributed traits, with prevalence variations reflecting variation in cut-points. Data examining the marked effect of cut-point variation on prevalence support this view (Shaffer et al., 1996). Hence, variation in prevalence would reflect the inclusion of "cases" in some studies considered "noncases" in other studies. These findings emphasize the continued need for refinements in assessment as well as the need to refine understandings of pathological processes that underlie anxiety disorders.

Risk for specific anxiety disorders exhibits important fluctuations across development, raising further questions on factors that distinguish unique subgroups of children with pathological as opposed to slightly excessive "normal" levels of anxiety. For example, peak onset of separation anxiety disorder and specific phobia occur relatively early in childhood. Similarly, the prevalence of social phobia in adolescence ranges from 1.6% to 4%, but prevalence appears considerably lower during childhood (Essau et al., 1999; Wittchen et al., 1999). These adolescent changes in risk for a pathological condition parallel broader changes in social concerns or anxiety, as a normal developmental phenomenon (Pine et al., 1998). Meanwhile, panic disorder exhibits prevalence in the 1%–2% ranges between late adolescence and early adulthood (Reed and Wittchen,1998). This condition is extremely rare before puberty and exhibits a steady increase as adolescents mature. Such changes parallel increases in rates of isolated reports of spontaneous panic (Pine et al., 1998).

Longitudinal Associations

At least seven studies have followed children with anxiety symptoms or disorders as they mature through adolescence and into adulthood (Pine and Klein, in press). As a group, these studies suggest that anxiety disorders present during childhood confer an approximate two- to fivefold increase in risk for various later-life psychopathologies. Most prominently, this risk applies to major depression and specific adolescent or adult anxiety disorders. Viewed from another perspective, these associations between childhood anxiety and later disorders reflect two trends. First, most pediatric anxiety disorders resolve, but most adults with either major depression or an anxiety disorder exhibit signs of an anxiety disorder during childhood (Pine et al., 1998). Thus, a crucial issue is to identify the anxious pediatric subgroup that goes on to retain anxiety or develop other forms of psychopathology.

Research comparing outcomes for specific anxiety disorders provides little clarification on this issue (Pine and Klein, in press). Limited specificity in longitudinal outcome emerges. Although childhood anxiety disorders are not associated with behavioral disorders at long-term follow-up, individual anxiety disorders show associations with a broad range of adult mood and anxiety disorders. Thus, though specific phobia does relate selectively to specific phobia, subclinical specific fears also exhibit robust associations with major depression (Weissman et al., 1997; Wickramaratne and Weissman, 1998; Pine et al., 2001). Similarly, adolescent panic attacks and separation anxiety disorder may relate to panic disorder in later life (R.G. Klein, 1995). Obsessive–compulsive disorder during childhood also predicts risk for a range of various other conditions, including tic disorders and attention-deficit/hyperactivity disorder (ADHD) (Peterson et al., 2001). Similarly, GAD or overanxious disorder in childhood predicts a wide range of later adult disorders, including GAD as well as major depression (Pine et al., 1998; Gregory et al., 2007).

Familial Risk

As with research on longitudinal course, studies on the familial aggregation generate a set of relatively clear conclusions. However, a parallel set of questions emerges in data from familial and longitudinal studies.

Some of the most consistent associations emerge in research relating parent panic disorder to increased risk for child anxiety disorders, particularly separation anxiety disorder (Pine and Klein, in press). As with longitudinal studies, however, this association is not unique to either adult panic disorder or child separation anxiety disorder. Namely, parental depression also predicts a high risk of separation anxiety disorder in children (Biederman, Faraone, et al., 2001), whereas parental panic disorder may also exhibit an association with childhood overanxious disorder (Last et al., 1991). For other anxiety disorders, studies document some evidence of specificity in the link between social anxiety disorder in parents and their children (Fyer, 1993; Lieb et al., 2000). On the other hand, studies examining children of parents who are depressed provide perhaps the strongest evidence of nonspecificity in associations between parental disorders and childhood anxiety disorders. Children of parents who are depressed exhibit increased risk for a range of anxiety disorders. Interestingly, paralleling some findings in longitudinal studies, the strongest and most consistent associations emerge between parental depression and either specific fears or overanxious disorder among children (Weissman et al., 1997). Nevertheless, as noted above, children of parents who are depressed also exhibit an increased risk for separation anxiety disorder (Biederman, Faraone, et al., 2001).

These results, documenting strong cross-generational transmission of anxiety, raise questions on the specific role of environmental and genetic factors in broad conferral of risk as well as in the nonspecific transmission of risk across a range of disorder subtypes. The most consistent effort to address these questions relies on twin studies. Although much of this research examines adults, findings from a series of large, rigorously conducted studies in children and adolescents are also emerging (Pine and Klein, in press). Research remains in early stages, but twin studies in children and adults already are beginning to yield potentially crucial insights. For example, consistent with results from longitudinal and family studies, twin studies demonstrate a strong association among the genetic factors related to GAD and major depressive disorder (MDD) (Kendler et al., 1995). This suggests that a common set of genes may confer risk for various forms of mood and anxiety and manifest as pervasive worry in some individuals or at some points in life as opposed to pervasive depression in other individuals or at other points in life.

Clinical Correlates of Anxiety

Dissatisfied with the heterogeneity of epidemiological studies, recent investigations have sought to identify meaningful subgroups of children who are anxious. Such meaningful subgroups would be expected to ultimately differ in terms of familial risk or longitudinal course. As of this writing, most research in this area has documented relatively simple associations between anxiety and one or another correlate, manifest in a demographic, family-based, temperamental, or biological variable. However, this research has stimulated efforts to use such correlates to subdivide subgroups of children in terms of longitudinal course or family risk.

Virtually all large-scale epidemiological studies of anxiety disorders note a consistent association with female gender. This association appears strongest and most consistent for specific phobia, GAD, agoraphobia, or panic, with less consistent evidence in social anxiety and obsessive–compulsive disorders (Kessler et al., 1994). Interestingly, unlike in depression, where female preponderance arises at puberty, a female preponderance for anxiety disorders may appear as early as 6 years of age (Lewinsohn et al., 1998).

As suggested in Figure 70.1, variations in infant temperament are also associated with anxiety. Interest in this association follows from research on high reactivity in infancy and its association with behavioral inhibition, which refers to the tendency for toddlers to react with hesitancy in the face of novelty, particularly social novelty (Kagan et al., 1999; Perez-Edgar and Fox, 2005). Inhibited, relative to noninhibited, children face an elevated risk for anxiety disorders, in general, and social anxiety disorder in particular (Perez-Edgar and Fox, 2005). Familial associations also emerge in this area, such that parental panic disorder confers a high risk for childhood behavioral inhibition. However, as with work on clinical anxiety disorders, behavioral inhibition shows only moderate specificity with adolescent or adult outcomes. Longitudinal and family-based studies also demonstrate relationships with adult major depression.

Some research indicates that parental style is associated with the development of anxiety. However, associations appear neither strong nor specific with anxiety but may rather reflect associations with various psychopathologies (Wood et al., 2003). Similarly, prospective research finds a strong association between parental rejection or overprotection and adolescent social anxiety disorder (Lieb et al., 2000). These findings raise questions on the degree to which risk or protective factors in the family environment, respectively, might facilitate or inhibit the transmission of disorders from parents to children. For example, family adversity may facilitate parental rejection, which in turn may facilitate transmission. Similarly, these environmental factors may interact with genetic risks (Caspi and Moffitt, 2006). Such findings on family adversity raise broader questions on the degree to which environmental factors relate to onset, persistence, and resistant anxiety in children. Children with persistent anxiety disorders may differ systematically in terms of their exposure to adverse environments from children with transient disorders. As shown in Figure 70.1, such effects are likely to be manifested through influences of genes and the environment on underlying brain circuitry.

Considerable research delineates associations between environmental adversity and anxiety symptoms. Specifically, adverse events in adulthood are a major predictor of psychopathology (Brown et al., 1994; Brown et al., 1996; Post et al., 1996). Moreover, recent evidence suggests that adverse life events are also risk factors for children and adolescents as well (Mirza et al., 1998; Pine and Cohen, 2002). Importantly, this includes findings from prospective research noting a specific increase in the risk for panic attacks and GAD associated with earlier environmental adversity (Pine and Cohen, 2002). Similarly, using another approach, motor vehicle accidents led to a 75% rate of PTSD 6 weeks and 6 months after the incident in children and adolescents (Mirza et al., 1998). Following a natural disaster, adolescents exhibited high levels of post-traumatic stress and symptom severity correlated with the mortality and destruction in the given region (Goenjian et al., 2001). Nevertheless, though many children experience trauma and other adverse events, not all go on to develop an anxiety or mood disorder. Further, how and what neurobiological mechanisms are altered by adverse events are far from clear (Pine, 2003). Clarifying the neurobiological pathways that mediate experience and pathology may help to identify why some individuals may be at higher risk for developing a disorder following trauma.

These findings relating environmental adversity to anxiety symptoms raise questions on the degree to which these associations are mediated through effects of environmental adversity on brain systems associated with anxiety. As noted above, preclinical research documents developmentally sensitive effects of stress on brain systems involved in anxiety. Neurobiological studies in humans reveal findings that are consistent with this preclinical evidence. For example, traumatized adults with PTSD show high levels of cerebral spinal fluid CRH and normal or low levels of cortisol (Yehuda et al., 1990; Yehuda et al., 1991; Yehuda et al., 1995; Yehuda et al., 1996; Bremner, Licino, et al., 1997; Baker et al., 1999; Rasmusson et al., 2001). Adults who were traumatized as children also evidence HPA axis dysregulation. In particular, women who suffered early sexual abuse showed enhanced dexamethasone suppression of cortisol (Stein et al., 1997). Anatomically, adults who were victims of early abuse evidence reduced hippocampal volume (Bremner, Randall, et al., 1997; Bremner et al., 2003). Recently, findings from rodents demonstrated that an early-life CRH infusion was associated with a reduced number of hippocampal CA3 neurons and up-regulation of CRH expression in adults (Brunson et al., 2001). This effect does not require glucocorticoids (Brunson et al., 2001). These results indicate that the elevated CRH levels early in life may be involved in the reduced hippocampal volume found in early trauma-related PTSD.

Turning to children, studies on the neurobiological aspects of trauma and PTSD have yielded discrepant results. In an examination of children who were maltreated and with PTSD, urinary-free cortisol was higher relative to controls (De Bellis, Baum, et al., 1999). However, in another study, children who were abused and depressed presented higher adrenocorticotropic hormone (ACTH) secretion following a CRH pharmacological challenge, but no differences in cortisol were revealed (Kaufman et al., 1997). With regard to anatomical effects of abuse history in children, De Bellis and colleagues (De Bellis, Keshavan, et al., 1999) found that though patients with PTSD presented relatively small intracranial volumes, cerebral structures, and corpus callosum, no differences were found in the hippocampus or amygdala. These results suggest that the anatomical aberrations in the adult hippocampus might not occur until later in development.

Summary

Evidence from preclinical and clinical investigations converge to indicate that alterations in a broad circuit involving the amygdala, stria terminalis, and the HPA axis are implicated in fear response as well as anxiety symptoms. Findings from developmental epidemiology indicate that familial or prior anxiety confers risk of subsequent anxiety. However, the specificity for risk for anxiety type and the markers to identify subgroups that retain the disorder have not been delineated. In the following section, results from cognitive investigations of anxiety are reviewed. Cognitive tasks that tap anxiety-related symptoms permit a more precise understanding of how behavior varies from normal in clinical populations. Moreover, the use of a cognitive framework in the study of anxiety would facilitate links to the field of cognitive neuroscience. Developing tasks that tap anxiety-related symptoms and are derived from cognitive neuroscience procedures would permit the brain bases for this disorder to be better understood.

A COGNITIVE APPROACH TO THE STUDY OF ANXIETY DISORDERS IN CHILDREN

Clinical studies suggest that anxiety during childhood represents a risk for later psychopathology as well as a possible observable manifestation of increased familial risk for various conditions, including panic disorder and major depression. Preclinical studies delineate a distributed circuit encompassing the amygdala that is engaged by fear-provoking circumstances. Researchers remain quite interested in delineating the degree to which this circuit participates in normal and pathological expressions of anxiety, in the hopes of clarifying the nature of associations between child and adult anxiety. Given the sophisticated understanding of fear response in preclinical research, extrapolations to clinical research might provide valuable insights on key clinical questions, including questions on the heterogeneity of anxiety in development and across generations. Existing efforts to forge ties between preclinical and clinical domains have raised as many questions as answers. Future efforts might benefit from an integration of methods in cognitive neuroscience with methods in clinical research on pediatric anxiety. As shown in Figure 70.1, future investigations integrate research on fear-circuit function, and clinical phenotypes might benefit from a focus on information processing functions (depicted in the center of Figure 70.1) that can be tied to brain circuit function and to clinical phenotypes.

A wealth of clinical research recognizes the salience of perturbed information processing in the expression of anxiety disorders among adults and children. Theories in this area suggest that individual variability in information processing may be crucial to the origins, maintenance, and treatment of anxiety disorders (Beck et al., 1985; Eysenck, 1992; Beck and Clark, 1997). In particular, as is described below, variations in cognitive regulatory processes, such as attention, appraisal, and memory, may play a role in the course of the anxiety disorder. Major questions remain concerning the degree to which these processes play a role in the causes of anxiety, as opposed to simply reflecting the effects of anxiety. Although anxiety can directly influence cognitive functions, treatment studies provide compelling evidence that cognitive factors represent more than epiphenomena or complications of the anxious state. Rather, such factors are likely to play some role in the initiation and/or maintenance of anxiety disorders, given that manipulations in the form of cognitive-behavioral therapies produce robust changes in cognitive correlates and symptoms of anxiety. These treatments invoke the therapist to assist patients in learning to alter maladaptive patterns of thought, presuming that these patterns play a role in pathogenesis (Beck et al., 1985; Barrett et al., 2001; Barrowclough et al., 2001).

This rich tradition of clinical research has become increasingly relevant for preclinical studies, in light of recent advances in cognitive neuroscience. Established tasks in cognitive neuroscience delineate neural circuits engaged by many of the cognitive constructs targeted in clinical studies of cognition as it relates to anxiety. As shown in Figure 70.1, this allows research on cognition to bridge actively between clinical and preclinical research on anxiety-related behaviors. This linking ties findings from anxiety-related epidemiological findings to the larger corpus of neuroscience research. Specifically, via fMRI and electroencephalogram (EEG) methods, neuroscience findings and theory could eventually be brought to bear on clinical questions, given the strong understanding in preclinical studies of brain mechanisms involved in anxiety.

In the examination of cognition in anxiety, our focus is on the processes involved in perception and response to threat cues, changes in organisms following exposure to threatening situations, and also variations in cognitive styles (for example, dwelling on potentially adverse events) that might increase the likelihood of anxiety. Specifically, four cognitive processes are enumerated that relate to anxiety disorders: (*1*) attention, (*2*) subjective reactions to fear provocation as occurs during threat appraisal, (*3*) memory, and (*4*) rumination.

Attention

Subjective states of fear elicit changes in information processing. Humans and lower mammals selectively monitor potential signs of danger, a process that involves changes in attention focus. Beyond changes in attention induced by acute fear states, susceptibility to and maintenance of anxiety disorders may be associated with biases in attention to threat. Interestingly, this association is unique to anxiety, whereas depression is often related to alterations in memory processing. This dissociation between attention and memory biases in anxiety and depression may provide insight into relation between anxiety disorders and depression across generations as well as development.

Experimental tasks were developed to better understand how anxiety symptoms relate to attention. Attention reflects a complex suite of discrete functions; these include the maintenance of an aroused state, the detection of, orientation towards, and response to salient environmental events, as well as the focusing of cognitive resources towards isolated pieces of information selected from a complex stimulus array. Discrete anatomical regions have been implicated in each of these attention processes (Posner, 1986; Desimone, 1998; Miller and Cohen, 2001).

As reviewed in recent meta-analyses, considerable data implicate perturbed attention in anxiety (Bar-Haim et al., 2007). One type of attention task is based on the suggestion that individuals who are anxious may attend to threat more rapidly or have difficulty disengaging from a threatening stimulus. In one paradigm (the modified Stroop) designed to study this attentional bias, words are presented to patients in different colors. Patients are instructed to identify the color. When presented with a threatening word (for example, *kill*), reaction time to color identification is increased relative to when the word is nonthreatening. Such results indicate that threatening words interfere with the processes involved in declaring the color. In psychopathology, multiple studies report that patients with anxiety disorders show exaggerated increases in reaction time for color identification with threat stimuli in GAD (MacLeod et al., 1986; Mogg et al., 1995), panic disorder (McNally et al., 1990), social phobia (Mattia et al., 1993), specific phobia but only when the threat word is related to the phobia (Watts et al., 1986), and PTSD (Foa et al., 1991). Meanwhile, patients who are depressed typically do not show attentional bias to negative stimuli (MacLeod et al., 1986; Mogg et al., 1993; Bradley, Mogg, Millar, and White, 1995). Moreover, this effect is reliably found in children and adults. However, though alterations in performance on the Stroop task may be due to early attention processes, this task is also sensitive to differences in motoric output (that is, color naming). Consequently, though these data are consistent with the hypothesis that individuals who are anxious show an attentional bias to threat stimuli, variations of reaction time in mounting a motoric response may explain the results (Mogg et al., 2000).

The probe detection task provides results that more precisely target the location of the cognitive disturbance. Figure 70.2 depicts one example of this task. Following the presentation of a fixation cross, neutral and threat

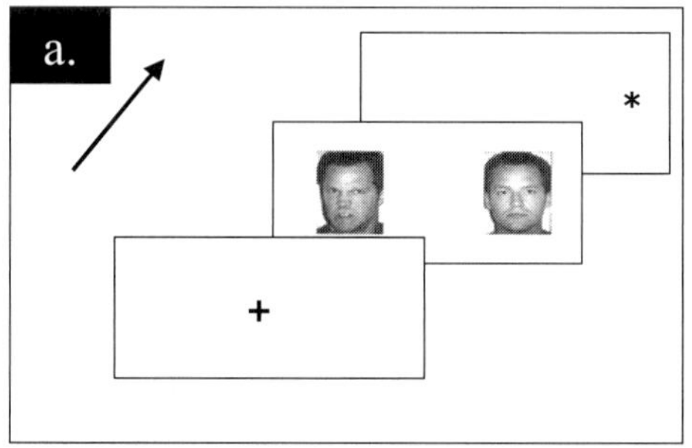

Attention Orienting Task

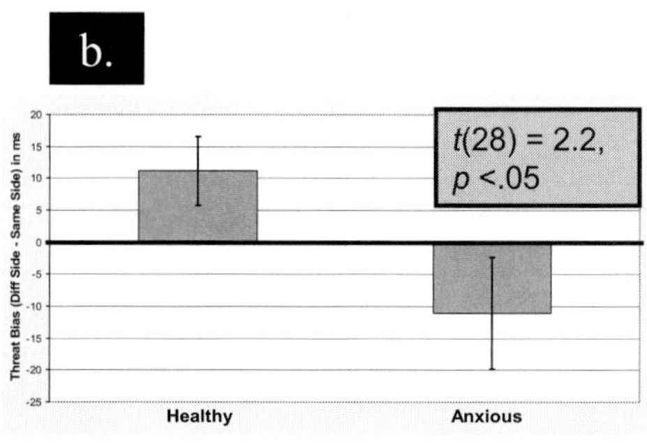

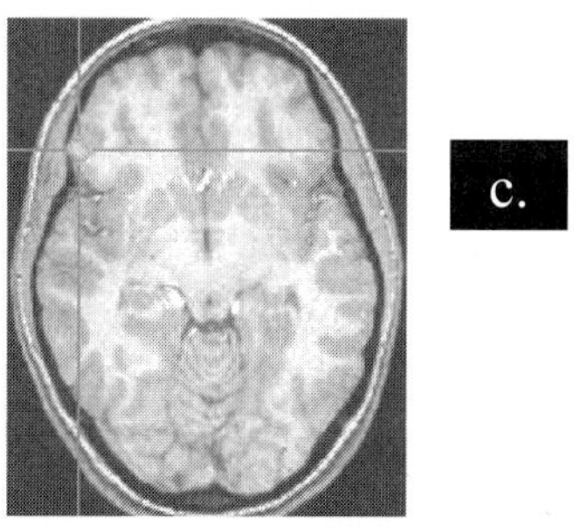

FIGURE 70.2 The dot-probe threat attention task. Figure 70.2a depicts a single trial in a dot-probe task. The trial begins with a "warning," signaled by the presence of the fixation-cross, presented in the middle of the visual field. This is followed by presentation of two stimuli depicted in opposite hemi-fields, one threat-related stimulus and a second neutral stimulus. Finally, the orienting of attention is monitored based on reaction time to the dot-probe, as indicated by the asterisk that replaces the neutral face. Figure 70.2b shows behavioral data on this paradigm, as reported elsewhere (Monk et al., 2006). As shown, adolescent patients with generalized anxiety disorder (GAD) exhibit a bias away from the threat stimulus, as indicated by a negative threat bias, whereas healthy adolescents show a bias towards threat, as indicated by a positive bias. Figure 70.2c maps brain regions differentially engaged across all threat trials in GAD relative to healthy adolescents. The figure reveals greater right ventro-lateral prefrontal cortical engagement in GAD relative to healthy adolescents.

stimuli are briefly presented on two spatial locations of a computer screen, as depicted in Figure 70.2a, where an angry and neutral face are presented side-by-side. Immediately following this presentation, a probe is presented in the location of one of the stimuli. Patients are instructed to press the button that corresponds to the location of the probe. If a patient attends more to the location where a threat stimulus is presented, that patient will exhibit a faster reaction time to the probes that follow the location of the threat stimuli than the probes that follow the neutral stimuli. Therefore, this task indexes the spatial location of patients' attention at the offset of threat and nonthreat stimuli. At least among adults, patients with anxiety disorders or with subclinical anxiety, but not with depression, consistently exhibit faster reaction times to probes that follow threat words relative to controls (MacLeod et al., 1986; Mogg et al., 1995; Mogg et al., 1997).

Although findings in children and adolescents also reveal perturbed attention bias, these findings tend to vary based on the nature of the paradigm. When words are used as threat stimuli, children and adolescents with PTSD show an attentional bias to socially threatening stimuli and away from depression-related stimuli (Dalgleish et al., 2001). In GAD, children showed a bias to threat stimuli relative to controls, whereas pediatric patients with mixed anxiety-depression did not evidence attentional bias to threat- or depression-related stimuli (Taghavi et al., 1999). Similarly, children with a range of anxiety disorders and children with high-test anxiety demonstrated an attentional bias to threat words (Vasey et al., 1995; Vasey et al., 1996). However, when pictures are used as stimuli, children with PTSD or GAD have exhibited a bias away from threat stimuli whereas healthy juveniles exhibit a bias towards threat (Monk et al., 2006; Pine, Mogg, et al., 2005). Figure 70.2b also shows data from one of these studies. In this figure, the negative bar in the patients with GAD depicts a faster reaction time to the probe trial shown in Figure 70.2a where a probe replaces a neutral face, relative to a trial where a probe would replace the neutral face. The opposite trend occurs in the healthy patients, showing a facilitation of responding to the probe behind the threat. These findings suggest that threats exert nonlinear influences on attention among healthy patients and patients with disorders, with initial monitoring during low-level threat, followed by avoidance during extreme threat (Pine, 2007).

Recent research has begun to determine whether this attentional bias is due to attracting attention or to inability to disengage attention. Results to this question have implications for different core features of the cognitive profile in anxiety. One study attempted to disentangle these effects of attention drawing versus attention holding using an attention cuing paradigm (Fox et al., 2001). The results indicate that anxiety is related to difficulty in disengaging from threat stimuli and not the initial orienting of attention. Individuals with this cognitive propensity would dedicate resources to the processing of threatening information: a behavior that could maintain and possibly induce anxiety symptoms.

This tendency to dwell on threat involves a rapidly responding neural network that requires minimal levels of awareness. Paradigms that involve masking the stimulus impede patients' ability to be aware of the stimulus. In a masking design, a stimulus is presented for a very brief duration (< 30 ms) followed by another stimulus (the mask) in the same location. Although this makes it difficult to consciously detect the stimulus, the stimulus may influence behavior, as in the probe detection and the Stroop tasks (MacLeod and Rutherford, 1992; Mogg et al., 1993; Bradley, Mogg, Millar, and White, 1995; Bradley et al., 1997). Therefore, combined with the evidence from Fox and colleagues (2001), these data indicate that awareness does not mediate the impaired ability to disengage from threat stimuli; rather, anxiety may lead patients to automatically dwell on threat stimuli. However, further work is needed to disentangle the roles of variability in attention-drawing versus attention-holding processes.

The neural basis for this automatic process is becoming clearer. In animals and humans, the neural processing of threat stimuli involves two pathways: a slow and a fast pathway (Morris et al., 1999). The fast pathway bypasses the cortex and directly engages the amygdala, allowing the organism to respond more quickly to threat. The amygdala is a structure that is activated in response to perceived threat (LeDoux, 2000), and patients with anxiety disorders show amygdala hyperresponsivity to threat stimuli (Rauch et al., 2000; Thomas, Drevets, Dahl, et al., 2001).

Furthermore, tasks where stimuli can be consciously processed may also activate the amygdala in adults and children (Breiter et al., 1996; Thomas, Drevets, Whalen, et al., 2001). In one study, adults exhibited amygdala activation to fearful relative to neutral faces, but this pattern was not found in children (Thomas, Drevets, Whalen, et al., 2001). Children did show activation to fearful and neutral faces relative to fixation (Thomas, Drevets, Whalen, et al., 2001). This is consistent with earlier work that revealed amygdala activation in children in response to fearful relative to nonsense stimuli (Baird et al., 1999). Thus, children's amygdala activation does not appear to discriminate between fearful and neutral facial expressions. Turning to patients, patients with combat PTSD showed activation in the amygdala in response to combat sounds, while the combat controls and the normal controls did not exhibit this activation (Liberzon et al., 1999). Similarly, in patients with social phobias, amygdala activation correlated with self-reported fear in a public and private speaking task (Tillfors et al., 2001). In addition, children and adolescents with GAD or panic disorder showed more amygdala activation to fearful faces than controls, while children who were depressed showed less amygdala activation to these faces (Thomas, Drevets, Dahl, et al., 2001).

Neuroimaging tasks focusing specifically on the interactions between attention and threat may further shed light on factors contributing to developmental variation in threat circuitry engagement. Although work in this area is only beginning, such research is starting to clarify the manner in which development, brain circuitry, and information processing interact to shape clinical phenotypes. For example, this work shows that other brain structures implicated in the fear circuit depicted in Figure 70.1 may influence amygdala activation, contributing to developmental and between-person variation in anxiety.

Figure 70.2c displays data consistent with this possibility. Here, brain regions are mapped where pediatric patients with GAD and healthy adolescents differ in terms of activation during the attention-threat task shown in Figure 70.2a. Patients with GAD exhibit enhanced activation in the ventrolateral PFC (vlPFC) (Monk et al., 2006), encompassing regions that exhibit strong anatomical and functional connectivity with the amygdala. Moreover, the magnitude of this vlPFC activation predicted lower levels of anxiety in GAD, suggesting that vlPFC serves to regulate underlying perturbations in the amygdala, consistent with a wealth of other data (Bouton, 2002; Pezawas et al., 2005).

Eliciting Fear in the Laboratory

The tendency to feel frightened by objects or situations experienced by most individuals as nonthreatening represents a cardinal feature of most clinical anxiety disorders. This increased tendency to experience the subjective state of fear is associated with a variety of cognitive correlates, including the tendency to think about feared objects or situations when they are not present, to scan the environment for signs of danger, and to neglect other nonfrightening aspects of the environment. This tendency is also associated with signs of physiological hypersensitivity to cues of potentially frightening objects or situations. This tendency has been termed an abnormal *appraisal bias* in clinical anxiety (Pine, 2007).

From the clinical perspective, this heightened tendency to subjectively experience fear in situations that most individuals do not fear can be reliably probed in the laboratory. Patients with anxiety disorders, when exposed to cues of various dangers, have been reliably shown to exhibit greater increases in fear than either healthy individuals or individuals who were psychiatrically impaired without anxiety. This represents one of the most reproducible results in clinical psychiatry, found across diagnoses as well as age groups.

On the surface, this may appear to be a relatively trivial finding because anxiety disorders, by definition, are characterized by subjectively reported hypersensitivity to fear-provoking stimuli or situations. Nevertheless, the consistency with which symptoms of anxiety disorders can be reproduced in the laboratory provides clinical investigators with a unique tool. Researchers can reliably elicit states of fear in various gradations, while monitoring the degree to which changes in fear herald changes in physiology and cognition. Moreover, researchers can invoke cognitive or pharmacological manipulations in the laboratory, to consider the degree to which these manipulations alter fear susceptibility and associated cognitive or physiological correlates. This may carry significant implications for understanding therapeutic mechanisms. Finally, with refinements in EEG and fMRI technologies, this aspect of anxiety disorders also allows investigators to examine the degree to which changes in subjective state, physiology, and cognition are associated with the engagement of particular neural circuits. Figure 70.3a presents data that illustrate the potential utility of this approach. Interestingly, some distinctions emerge across the various anxiety disorders, with respect to responses to a range of potentially fearful objects or situations.

A reliable method for inducing a stress response in humans is to ask them to speak or perform a task in public. Given the prominence of concerns about such situations in social anxiety disorder, one might expect particularly high levels of fear among these patients. However, heightened anxiety occurs in a range of patient groups. For example, using a regimented form of the social stress test, adolescents with anxiety disorders (GAD and GAD with separation anxiety disorder) have been shown to exhibit greater increases in ACTH levels (Gerra et al., 2000). Following the test, the same group exhibited enhanced norepinephrine levels. These results resemble findings in behavioral inhibition, where children who were inhibited exhibit elevated cortisol in novel, mildly stressful social situations. Kagan and colleagues developed paradigms to evaluate young children's reactivity to novel situations, particularly social novelty. Children classified as reactive in response to novelty in infancy were more likely to develop anxious symptoms (Kagan et al., 1999) particularly social phobia (Biederman, Hirshfeld-Becker, et al., 2001). Similarly, children at risk for anxiety disorders evidence behavioral inhibition (Rosenbaum et al., 1988). This tendency has been linked to perturbations in the amygdale among children who were formerly inhibited and studied with fMRI as adults (Schwartz et al., 2003).

Among adults acutely affected with social anxiety disorder, Davidson and colleagues (2000) demonstrated distinct subjective as well as EEG profiles during a similar form of social provocation. However, some inconsistencies emerge in this area. For example, with respect to HPA axis findings, adolescent girls with social phobia did not show a difference from healthy controls

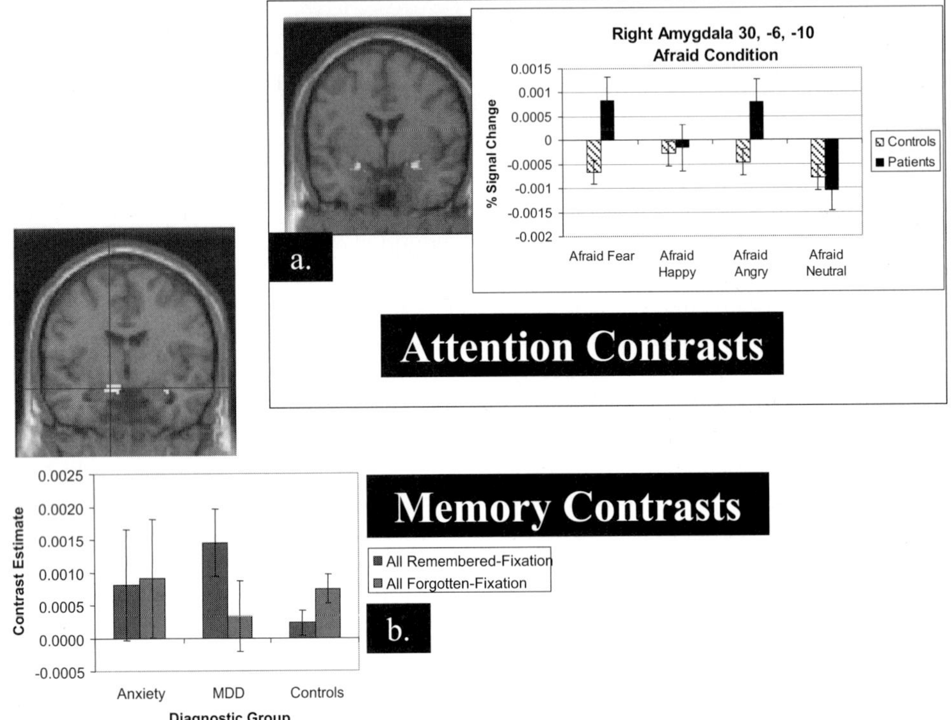

FIGURE 70.3 Using cognitive neuroscience to dissociate amygdala correlates of pediatric anxiety and pediatric depression. Figure 70.3a presents data from a recent study implicating amygdala dysfunction in pediatric generalized anxiety disorder (GAD) (McClure et al., 2007). The coronal brain picture depicts the location of bilateral amygdala activation differences in 15 patients with GAD, relative to 20 healthy adolescents. The graph shows that these differences in the right amgydala occur for fear faces and angry faces, relative to happy and neutral faces, specifically when patients attend to their experienced state of fear. Figure 70.3b presents data from a recent study implicating amygdala dysfunction in pediatric MDD but not anxiety (Roberson-Nay et al., 2006). The coronal brain picture depicts the location of bilateral amygdala activation differences in 11 adolescents with depression, relative to 10 adolescents who were anxious, and 23 healthy adolescents. The graph displays the manner in which the difference in the left amygdala reflects enhanced activation in major depressive disorder (MDD), relative to adolescents who are anxious and healthy adolescents, specifically for correctly remembered faces.

during social challenge (Martel et al., 1999). Similarly, Heim et al. (2000) found HPA axis abnormalities in response to laboratory-induced social stress among adults with major depression as opposed to those with anxiety disorders, though some HPA axis abnormalities in this group resulted from the effects of early trauma and associated PTSD symptoms.

Finally, other tasks narrow this focus on social threat to core aspects of social experience by asking patients to monitor their internally experienced fear level while they view social stimuli, such as faces of varying emotions. This manipulation allows investigators to actively monitor in the laboratory or the neuroimaging environment neural and cognitive processes engaged during appraisal of social threat. Work in this area shows that adolescents with social phobia show an abnormal behavioral or attention response to face-emotion displays, as do adolescents who are not anxious at high familial risk for anxiety (Pine et al., 2005b). Moreover, this abnormality in information processing is reflected in abnormal engagement of underlying neural circuitry (McClure et al., 2007). As shown in Figure 70.3a, adolescents with GAD or social phobia show enhanced engagement of the amygdala when viewing negative-valence face-emotion photographs and rating experienced level of fear. This enhancement also occurs in medial and ventral expanses of the PFC, but it only occurs when attention is directed towards experienced level of fear. Finally, consistent with behavioral data in adolescents who are at risk, brain imaging research among adolescents who were formerly inhibited without anxiety disorders also shows that amygdale perturbation only occurs in this same attention state (Perez-Edgar et al., 2007). Thus, during exposure to social threat, abnormal attention and amygdala activation is associated with the expression of overt anxiety and risk for anxiety in adolescence.

Another frequently used method for manipulating fear states in humans extends findings implicating monoamine abnormalities in the regulation of fear states among animals. In primates, manipulations of the noradrenergic system reliably alter levels of fear. Consistent with these findings, adults with panic disorder as well as children with separation anxiety disorder display alterations in adrenergic functioning. Physiological challenges that target the adrenergic system reveal aberrations in the subjective reaction and physiological response among children with anxiety. In response to a yohimbine challenge, children with separation anxiety disorder showed increases in self-rated anxiety and blunting in growth hormone (GH) relative to controls, indicating dysfunction in the noradrenergic system (Sallee et al., 2000). Using another noradrenergic probe, clonidine, anxious children again showed increased ratings for anxiety, but GH was increased relative to controls (Sallee et al., 1998). Other signs of neuroendocrinological dyregulation in GH systems emerge in studies of children with major depression as well as children without depression and at risk for depression (Birmaher et al., 2000). In line with this evidence that anxiety is associated with a disturbance in GH regulation, childhood separation anxiety and overanxious disorder may predict shorter stature among females in early adulthood (Pine et al., 1996).

Some data suggest that patients with anxiety may be particularly sensitive to subjective somatic experiences, especially changes in respiratory regulation. Moreover, these data also suggest that such hypersensitivity relates to specific subclasses of pediatric anxiety disorders, when contrasted with data on the response to social threat in other pediatric anxiety disorders. Perhaps the most extensive evidence in this realm documents subjective hypersensitivity to various respiratory manipulations among adults with panic disorder but not a select group of other anxiety disorders, such as OCD (D.F. Klein, 1993). Interestingly, such abnormalities are paralleled by dysfunction in physiological systems and genetics. Finally, abnormal response to respiratory manipulations is found among asymptomatic adults at high risk for panic disorder.

These data suggest that hypersensitivity to respiratory change represents a risk marker for a relatively narrow family of anxiety disorders each related to spontaneous panic. Consistent with this view, children with anxiety disorders, particularly separation anxiety disorder, exhibit subjective and physiological abnormalities during carbon dioxide inhalation (Pine et al., 2000). Moreover, unlike the heightened response to social threat, which occurs in pediatric social phobia but not separation anxiety disorder, the heightened response to respiratory threat occurs in separation anxiety disorder but not social anxiety disorder. Of note, this unique, relatively specific response to direct respiratory challenge differs from the response to the threat of respiratory challenge. Specifically, though response to respiratory challenge relates to specific disorders, abnormal response to anticipation of a carbon dioxide challenge is independent of specific pediatric anxiety disorder diagnosis (Pine et al., 2005a; Terleph et al., 2006).

These findings indicate that dysregulation of respiration may be a risk factor for a specific set of anxiety disorders. In support of this, investigations have found a link between anxiety and smoking, a behavior that creates a respiratory challenge. In particular, prospective longitudinal studies indicate that smoking predicts anxiety disorder, but anxiety in nonsmokers did not predict later smoking (Breslau and Klein, 1999; J.G. Johnson et al., 2000). However, data in children who were asymptomatic born to parents with panic disorder do not support this view. Here, respiratory dysregulation does show a consistent relationship with childhood separation anxiety disorder. Nevertheless, respiratory profiles appear similar among unaffected offspring of parents with panic disorder, major depression, or no psychopathology (Pine et al., 2005a).

Each of these studies documents subjective and physiological abnormalities in laboratory conditions, where patients are explicitly told that they may be exposed to fear-provoking situations. Independent of the particular stimulus that is feared, individuals with anxiety disorders may exhibit signs of hypersensitivity to threats, such as the experience of entering laboratory environments knowing that fear may be provoked. As noted above, abnormalities when anticipating threats appear to be nonspecific correlates of various anxiety disorders. Similarly, in a series of studies, Grillon et al. (1997, 1998, 2005) have examined the degree to which startle magnitude reflects hypersensitivity to potentially dangerous contexts, as modeled by many laboratory-based studies of anxiety. Individuals with anxiety disorders or even at risk for anxiety are hypothesized to exhibit enhanced fear in these contexts. Consistent with this possibility, Grillon et al. (1997) found enhanced baseline startle, an index of reactivity related to anxiety-like behaviors in animals (Davis et al., 1993) and in adolescents at risk for anxiety disorders (Grillon et al., 1997). However, in another study by the same group, only female patients at risk for anxiety displayed this same pattern, while males who were at risk showed enhanced fear-potentiated startle and a normal response at baseline (Grillon and Ameli, 1998). Moreover, consistent with heterogeneity in associations, such abnormalities also relate to risk for depression (Grillon et al., 2005). Further work in this area will reveal how anxiety, fear, and gender influence the startle response.

Memory

As in attention, memory functioning has been extensively studied in individuals with anxiety disorders. One set of studies in this area relies on iterations of the fear-conditioning paradigm, one specific form of memory. Studies in this area generally find weak associations between anxiety disorders and fear conditioning (Lissek et al., 2005). Another set of studies relies on memory tests designed to evaluate predictions posited by Beck and colleagues (Beck et al., 1985; Beck and Clark, 1997) that patients with mood or anxiety disorders would show mood congruent memory. That is, a patient with GAD, for instance, would evidence enhanced memory for threat-related stimuli whereas patients who were depressed would show better memory for sad or depressing information. In addition, like attention, the brain–behavior associations for memory have been intensively investigated; and, therefore, disturbances in aspects of memory function in anxiety disorders provide clues to the neural bases of the disorder.

Two types of memory are explicit and implicit (Schacter and Tulving, 1994). Explicit memory involves the recollection of facts as well as events (Richardson-Klavehn and Bjork, 1988). Implicit memory subsumes several different types of memory that do not require awareness. In particular, implicit includes priming (facilitated performance due to prior exposure) and procedural learning (motor skills, conditioning, and associative learning). In seminal work by Milner, resections of the medial temporal lobe that included the hippocampus led to profound memory impairments (Scoville and Milner, 1957). Later evidence arose that these structures are not necessary for priming and skill learning (Milner, 1962; Gabrieli et al., 1990). Current literature provides support for a double dissociation of explicit and implicit memory whereby patients with damage to the MTL are impaired in explicit memory and individuals with damage to structures including the visual cortex (Fleischman et al., 1995; Gabrieli et al., 1995), basal ganglia (Gabrieli et al., 1997), or cerebellum (Sanes et al., 1990) are impaired in implicit tasks. Recent imaging work also indicates that the MTL subserves explicit memory, whereas the basal ganglia is involved in implicit memory (Poldrack et al., 2001). Furthermore, the neural bases for types of working memory, the ability to hold and manipulate information for a brief interval of time, are also becoming clearer. Although it is not possible to give a full account of the literature of cognitive neuroscience for memory in this chapter, work with nonhuman primates and neuroimaging has revealed many processes and subprocesses of memory systems. Thus, a clinical population that has a disturbance in a particular memory function suggests where the neural basis for the disorder might arise.

Although consistent support has emerged for mood congruent memory in depression (Bradley, Mogg, and Williams, 1995), the data are much less clear for anxiety (MacLeod and Matthews, 2004). Multiple studies using a range of tasks document that panic disorder in adults is related to enhanced explicit memory for threat or anxiety-related words (McNally et al., 1989; Cloitre and Liebowitz, 1991; Becker et al., 1994; Cloitre et al., 1994; Lundh et al., 1997; Becker et al., 1999; but see Otto et al., 1994; Banos et al., 2001). Meanwhile, the effects of social phobia on memory are mixed. Two studies using positive and negative facial expressions found an explicit memory bias for negative or critical faces (Lundh and Ost, 1996; Foa et al., 2000). In another study using socially relevant positive and negative words, patients with social phobia needed less practice to learn the negative words and experienced less mnemonic interference from competing information (Amir et al., 2001). However, other similar investigations with patients with social phobias did not find a memory bias (Rapee et al., 1994; Cloitre et al., 1995) whereas one study found a memory bias for reassuring faces and overall impaired explicit memory that was possibly due to heightened state anxiety (Perez-Lopez and Woody, 2001). One study documented an implicit memory bias in patients with social phobias for socially threatening sentences (Amir et al., 2000). For GAD, findings are similarly inconsistent (Mathews et al., 1989; Mogg and Marden, 1990; MacLeod and McLaughlin, 1995). Thus, though attentional biases to threat are consistently found in anxiety disorders, memory biases to threat stimuli are only consistently documented in panic disorders. Typically, attention to a stimulus is thought to lead to enhanced memory (Norman, 1969). Further research is necessary to investigate why attention bias does not translate into memory bias. For example, some anxiety disorders may be associated with a degree of cognitive interference that dampens the mnemonic effects of attention.

Turning to PTSD, intrusive memory is a cardinal symptom. Although this symptom clearly reflects memory system impairment, researchers are only beginning to elucidate the precise nature of memory involvement in PTSD. For explicit memory, consistent abnormalities emerge in two processes. The first concerns a form of emotional memory. Healthy adults consistently exhibit a mnemonic bias for emotionally arousing stimuli (Christianson and Loftus, 1991; Christianson and Hübinette, 1993; Christianson and Engelberg, 1999) and individuals with PTSD exhibit an exaggeration of this bias, manifest as a greater tendency to recall emotionally negative information than comparison patients (Zeitlin and McNally, 1991; Vrana et al., 1995). Importantly, this enhanced bias is found relative to healthy, psychiatric, and trauma comparisons. Moreover, this bias emerges early in development (Moradi et al., 2000). In particular, children and adolescents with PTSD showed overall explicit memory impairment for words and also evidence a bias for negative words.

The second explicit memory process concerns aspects of source monitoring and autobiographical memory, which involves source memory in the coding of event times and locations. In one set of studies, patients with PTSD exhibit a reduced ability to recall specific personal memories that previously had been experimentally paired with neutral and affectively laden words (McNally et al., 1995). Similarly, adolescents who were traumatized show impairments in autobiographical memories (Meesters et al., 2000). Another set of studies relies on a standard false memory paradigm, which presents a series of word lists that each relate to unpresented, thematic words, the so-called critical lures (Deese, 1959; Roediger and McDermott, 1995). In two studies, patients with PTSD exhibited a greater tendency to recognize such critical lures (Bremner, Shobee, et al., 2000; Zoellner et al., 2000) indicating a deficiency in source monitoring. Deficient source memory may act in concert with a mnemonic bias for negative information to facilitate the creation of intrusive memories.

Although implicit memory has been less intensively studied, recent studies also implicate implicit memory bias in PTSD. The most consistent findings emerge in studies that rely upon conceptually rich stimuli, such as complex trauma-related sentences (McNally and Amir, 1996) suggesting that the detection of implicit memory bias requires the engagement of complex elaborative processes.

Although current theory views memory abnormalities as precursors for PTSD or other anxiety disorders, studies have only just begun to consider the role of trait versus state-anxiety effects on memory abnormalities. Moreover, the weight of the evidence from studies in adults and in adolescents implicates abnormal emotional memory in depression but not in anxiety, where some abnormalities in nonemotional memory have been documented (Hertel, 2004; Vasa et al., 2007). Of note, these data in adolescents and adults document a dissociation between depression, characterized by emotion-related bias in memory but not attention, and anxiety, characterized by emotion-related bias in attention but not memory. Finally, this behavioral dissociation also may provide insights on specificity in the neural correlates of anxiety and depression. Figure 70.3b shows brain-imaging data from an emotional memory paradigm on which adolescents with depression but not adolescents with anxiety disorders show deficits (Pine et al., 2004; Roberson-Nay et al., 2006). As shown in Figure 70.3b, amygdala dysfunction manifests on a memory paradigm in adolescent depression but not anxiety, a disorder that involves amygdala dysfunction on the attention paradigm, as shown in Figure 70.3a. Thus, not only does research on information processing provide clues on cognitive specificity for associations with anxiety relative to depression, but such research also provides clues on specificity in associated neural architecture.

Fears, Worry, and Rumination

Fears, worrying, and ruminating are normal and certainly serve adaptive functions, but excessive levels of these cognitive processes are related to psychopathology and, in particular, GAD. Relative to controls and patients with social phobias, patients with GAD evidence a greater number of worries, have more topics that they worry about, experience more distress during worrying, feel lower subjective controllability, and experience more bodily sensations related to the worry (Hoyer et al., 2001). Similarly, worrying and anxiety are related in childhood (Silverman et al., 1995; Weems et al., 2000), and children at risk for anxiety disorders have a higher number of fears (Turner et al., 1987). In addition, those with enhanced startle in the dark reported excessive fear of the dark in childhood, indicating that this neurophysiological marker for anxiety may relate to childhood fears (Grillon et al., 1997).

Typically, fears and worries decrease with development (Gullone et al., 2001), perhaps partly due to the maturation of cognitive capacities such as inhibition and the ability to generate reassuring memories for past events. However, with these increased cognitive capacities comes the ability to create more flexible mental representations, permitting an increased capacity to formulate more vivid, realistic worries or fears. Indeed, with development in adolescents, the content of worries becomes more complex and less reliant on perceptually salient characteristics (Stattin, 1984). Thus, though most children experience a reduction of fears with development, there may be a subgroup whose fears become more salient and impairing.

FUTURE RESEARCH IN CHILDHOOD ANXIETY DISORDERS

Psychiatric diagnoses are rough approximations of dysfunctional neurobiological systems. Given the high degree of comorbidity, low level of predictive power, and heterogeneity of outcome in particular disorders, it is unlikely that current diagnoses cleanly map onto particular neurobiological disturbances. By more precisely relating symptoms to neurobiology, it may be possible to develop more refined diagnoses. Furthermore, considerable data suggest that research on cognition bridges clinical and biological research on anxiety. As such, cognitive tasks can be constructed to isolate key components of anxiety symptoms. The normal and abnormal development of performance on these tasks can be documented and related to risk for the disorder. In addition, fMRI can map abnormal engagement of neural systems probed by these tasks across development. Given the extensive knowledge base linking cognition to brain function, work in this area allows delineation of precise integrative hypotheses.

In devising studies to examine the development of anxiety disorders, it is useful to consider four separate lines of research. First, epidemiological investigations provide the basis for the generation of hypotheses linking particular anxiety disorders to the onset of cognitive abilities, the maturation of neural systems, and the possible neurobiological relationship between disorders that frequently co-occur. Second, key clinical symptoms can be documented and used as starting points for developing tasks that tap these symptoms. Third, task development should also draw from patients with brain lesions, animal models, and neuroimaging procedures that involve relevant neural systems. Moreover, though the examination of humans and animals with brain lesions indicates how the brain functions without a particular structure, brain activation in neuroimaging only reveals structures that are responsive to the task and not whether they are necessary for successful performance of that task (Gabrieli, 1998). Thus, the development of hypotheses relating symptoms to brain systems would benefit from considering research from lesion and neuroimaging approaches.

REFERENCES

American Psychiatric Association (1987) *Diagnostic and Statistical Manual of Mental Disorders*, 3rd ed. rev. Washington, DC: Author.

Amir, N., Coles, M.E., Brigidi, B., and Foa, E.B. (2001) The effect of practice on recall of emotional information in individuals with generalized social phobia. *J. Abnorm. Psychol.* 110:76–82.

Amir, N., Foa, E.B., and Coles, M.E. (2000) Implicit memory bias for threat-relevant information in individuals with generalized social phobia. *J. Abnorm. Psychol.* 109:713–720.

Anderson, J., Williams, S., McGee, R., and Silva, P.A. (1987) *DSM-III* disorders in preadolescent children: prevalence in a large sample from the general population. *Arch. Gen. Psychiatry* 44:69–76.

Ansorge, M.S., Zhou, M., Lira, A., Hen, R., and Gingrich, J.A. (2004) Early-life blockade of the 5-HT transporter alters emotional behavior in adult mice. *Science* 306:879–881.

Baird, A.A., Gruber, S.A., Fein, D.A., Maas, L.C., Steingard, R.J., Renshaw, P.F., Cohen, B.M., and Yurgelun-Todd, D.A. (1999) Functional magnetic resonance imaging of facial affect recognition in children and adolescents. *J. Am. Acad. Child Adol. Psychiatry* 38:195–199.

Baker, D.G., West, S.A., Nicholson, W.E., Ekhator, N.N., Kasckow, J.W., Hill, K.K., Bruce, A.B., Orth, D.N., and Geracioti, T.D., Jr. (1999) Serial CSF corticotropin-releasing hormone levels and adrenocortical activity in combat veterans with posttraumatic stress disorder. *Am. J. Psychiatry* 156:585–588.

Banos, R.M., Medina, P.M., and Pascual, J (2001) Explicit and implicit memory biases in depression and panic disorder. *Behav. Res. Ther.* 39:61–74.

Bar-Haim, Y., Lamy, D., Pergamin, L., Bakermans-Kranenburg, M.J., and van IJzendoorn, M.H. (2007) Threat-related attentional bias in anxious and non-anxious individuals: a meta-analytic study. *Psych. Bull.* 133:1–24.

Barrett, P., Duffy, A., Dadds, M., and Rapee, R. (2001) Cognitive-behavioral treatment of anxiety disorders in children: long-term (6-year) follow-up. *J. Consult. Clin. Psychol.* 69:135–149.

Barrowclough, C., King, P., Colville, J., Russell, E., Burns, A., and Tarrier, N. (2001) A randomized trial of the effectiveness of cognitive-behavioral therapy and supportive counseling for anxiety symptoms in older adults. *J. Consult. Clin. Psychol.* 69:756–762.

Beck, A., Emery, G., and Greenberg, R.L. (1985) *Anxiety Disorders and Phobias: A Cognitive Perspective*. New York: Basic Books.

Beck, A.T., and Clark, D.A. (1997) An information processing model of anxiety: automatic and strategic processes. *Behaviour Research and Therapy* 35:49–58.

Becker, E., Rinck, M., and Margraf, J. (1994) Memory bias in panic disorder. *J. Abnorm. Psychol.* 103:396–399.

Becker, E.S., Roth, W.T., Andrich, M., and Margraf, J. (1999) Explicit memory in anxiety disorders. *J. Abnorm. Psychol.* 108: 153–163.

Biederman, J., Faraone, S.V., Hirshfeld-Becker, D.R., Friedman, D., Robin, J.A., and Rosenbaum, J.F. (2001) Patterns of psychopathology and dysfunction in high-risk children of parents with panic disorder and major depression. *Am. J. Psychiatry* 158:49–57.

Biederman, J., Hirshfeld-Becker, D.R., Rosenbaum, J.F., Herot, C., Friedman, D., Snidman, N., Kagan, J., and Faraone, S.V. (2001) Further evidence of association between behavioral inhibition and social anxiety in children. *Am. J. Psychiatry* 158:1673–1679.

Birmaher, B., Dahl, R.E., Williamson, D.E., Perel, J.M., Brent, D.A., Axelson, D.A., Kaufman, J., Dorn, L.D., Stull, S., Rao, U., and Ryan, N.D. (2000) Growth hormone secretion in children and adolescents at high risk for major depressive disorder. *Arch. Gen. Psychiatry* 57:867–872.

Bouton, M.E. (2002) Context, ambiguity, and unlearning: sources of relapse after behavioral extinction. *Biol. Psychiatry* 52:976–986.

Bradley, B.P., Mogg, K., and Lee, S.C. (1997) Attentional biases for negative information in induced and naturally occurring dysphoria. *Behav. Res. Ther.* 35:911–927.

Bradley, B.P., Mogg, K., Millar, N., and White, J. (1995) Selective processing of negative information: effects of clinical anxiety, concurrent depression, and awareness. *J. Abnorm. Psychol.* 104: 532–536.

Bradley, B.P., Mogg, K., and Williams, R. (1995) Implicit and explicit memory for emotion-congruent information in clinical depression and anxiety. *Behav. Res. Ther.* 33:755–770.

Breiter, H.C., Etcoff, N.L., Whalen, P.J., Kennedy, W.A., Rauch, S.L., Buckner, R.L., Strauss, M.M., Hyman, S.E., and Rosen, B.R. (1996) Response and habituation of the human amygdala during visual processing of facial expression. *Neuron* 17:875–887.

Bremner, J.D., Licino, J., Darnell, A., Krystal, J.H., Owens, M.J., Southwick, S.M., Nemeroff, C.B., and Charney, D.S. (1997) Elevated CSF corticotropin-releasing factor concentrations in PTSD. *Am. J. Psychiatry* 154:624–629.

Bremner, J. D., Vythilingam, M., Vermetten, E., Southwick, S. M., McGlashan, T., Nazeer, A., et al. (2003) MRI and PET study of deficits in hippocampal structure and function in women with childhood sexual abuse and posttraumatic stress disorder. *Am. J. Psychiatry* 160:924–932.

Bremner, J.D., Randall, P., Vermetten, E., Staib, L., Bronen, R.A., Mazure, C., Capelli, S., McCarthy, G., Innis, R.B., and Charney, D.S. (1997) Magnetic resonance imaging-based measurement of hippocampal volume in posttraumatic stress disorder related to childhood physical and sexual abuse—a preliminary report. *Biol. Psychiatry* 41:23–32.

Bremner, J.D., Shobe, K.K., and Kihlstrom, J.F. (2000) False memories in women with self-reported childhood sexual abuse: an empirical study. *Psychol. Sci.* 11:333–337.

Breslau, N., and Klein, D.F. (1999) Smoking and panic attacks: an epidemiologic investigation. *Arch. Gen. Psychiatry* 56:1141–1147.

Brown, G.W., Harris, T.O., and Eales, M.J. (1996) Social factors and comorbidity of depressive and anxiety disorders. *Br. J. Psychiatry Suppl.* 30:50–57.

Brown, G.W., Harris, T.O., and Hepworth, C. (1994) Life events and endogenous depression. A puzzle reexamined. *Arch. Gen. Psychiatry* 51:525–534.

Brunson, K.L., Eghbal-Ahmadi, M., Bender, R., Chen, Y., and Baram, T.Z. (2001) Long-term, progressive hippocampal cell loss and dysfunction induced by early-life administration of corticotropin-releasing hormone reproduce the effects of early-life stress. *Proc. Natl. Acad. Sci. USA* 98:8856–8861.

Caldji, C., Tannenbaum, B., Sharma, S., Francis, D., Plotsky, P.M., and Meaney, M.J. (1998) Maternal care during infancy regulates the development of neural systems mediating the expression of fearfulness in the rat. *Proc. Natl. Acad. Sci. USA* 95:5335–5340.

Caspi, A., and Moffitt, T.E. (2006) Gene-environment interactions in psychiatry: joining forces with neuroscience. *Nat. Rev. Neurosci.* 7:583–590.

Christianson, A.-S., and Engelberg, E. (1999) Memory and emotional consistency: the MS Estonia ferry disaster. *Memory* 7:471–482.

Christianson, S.A., and Hübinette, B. (1993) Hands up! A study of witnesses' emotional reactions and memories associated with bank robberies. *Appl. Cogn. Psychol.* 7:365–379.

Christianson, S.A., and Loftus, E.F. (1991) Remembering emotional events: the fate of detailed information. *Cogn. Emot.* 5:81–108.

Cloitre, M., Cancienne, J., Heimberg, R.G., Holt, C.S., and Liebowitz, M. (1995) Memory bias does not generalize across anxiety disorders. *Behav. Res. Ther.* 33:305–307.

Cloitre, M., and Liebowitz, M.R. (1991) Memory bias in panic disorder: An investigation of the cognitive avoidance hypothesis. *Cogn. Ther. Res.* 15:371–386.

Cloitre, M., Shear, M.K., Cancienne, J., and Zeitlin, S.B. (1994) Implicit and explicit memory for catastrophic associations to bodily sensation words in panic disorder. *Cogn. Ther. Res.* 18:225–240.

Coplan, J.D., Andrews, M.W., Rosenblum, L.A., Owens, M.J., Friedman, S., Gorman, J.M., and Nemeroff, C.B. (1996) Persistent elevations of cerebrospinal fluid concentrations of corticotropin-releasing factor in adult nonhuman primates exposed to early-life stressors: implications for the pathophysiology of mood and anxiety disorders. *Proc. Natl. Acad. Sci. USA* 93:1619–1623.

Dalgleish, T., Moradi, A.R., Taghavi, M.R., Neshat-Doost, H.T., and Yule, W. (2001) An experimental investigation of hypervigilance for threat in children and adolescents with post-traumatic stress disorder. *Psychol. Med.* 31:541–547.

Davidson, R., Marshall, J., Tomarken, A., and Henriques, J. (2000) While a phobic waits: regional brain electrical and autonomic activity in social phobics during anticipation of public speaking. *Biol. Psychiatry* 15:85–95.

Davis, M. (1998) Are different parts of the extended amygdala involved in fear versus anxiety? *Biol. Psychiatry* 44:1239–1247.

Davis, M., Falls, W.A., Campeau, S., and Kim, M. (1993) Fear-potentiated startle: a neural and pharmacological analysis. *Behav. Brain Res.* 58:175–198.

De Bellis, M.D., Baum, A.S., Birmaher, B., Keshavan, M.S., Eccard, C.H., Boring, A.M., Jenkins, F.J., and Ryan, N.D. (1999) Developmental traumatology part I: biological stress systems. *Biol. Psychiatry* 45:1259–1270.

De Bellis, M.D., Keshavan, M.S., Clark, D.B., Casey, B.J., Giedd, J.N., Boring, A.M., Frustaci, K., and Ryan, N.D. (1999) A.E. Bennett Research Award. Developmental traumatology. Part II: Brain development. *Biol. Psychiatry* 45:1271–1284.

Deese, J. (1959) On the prediction of occurrence of particular verbal intrusions in immediate recall. *J. Exp. Psychol.* 58:17–22.

Desimone, R. (1998) Visual attention mediated by biased competition in extrastriate visual cortex. *Philos. Trans. R Soc. Lond. B Biol. Sci.* 353:1245–1255.

Essau, C., Conradt, J., and Petermann, F. (1999) Frequency and comorbidity of social phobia and social fears in adolescents. *Behav. Res. Ther.* 37:831–843.

Eysenck, M.W. (1992) *Anxiety: The Cognitive Perspective*. Hillsdale, NJ: Lawrence Erlbaum.

Fleischman, D., Gabrieli, J., Reminger, S., Rinaldi, J., Morrell, F., and Wilson, R. (1995) Conceptual priming in perceptual identification for patients with Alzheimer's disease and a patient with a right occipital lobectomy. *Neuropsychology* 9:187–197.

Foa, E.B., Gilboa-Schechtman, E., Amir, N., and Freshman, M. (2000) Memory bias in generalized social phobia: remembering negative emotional expressions. *J. Anxiety Disord.* 14:501–519.

Foa, E.B., Rothbaum, B.O., Riggs, D.S., and Murdock, T.B. (1991) Treatment of posttraumatic stress disorder in rape victims: a comparison between cognitive-behavioral procedures and counseling. *J. Consult. Clin. Psychol.* 59:715–723.

Fox, E., Russo, R., Bowles, R., and Dutton, K. (2001) Do threatening stimuli draw or hold visual attention in subclinical anxiety? *J. Exp. Psychol.: Gen.* 130:681–700.

Francis, D., Diorio, J., Liu, D., and Meaney, M.J. (1999) Nongenomic transmission across generations of maternal behavior and stress responses in the rat. *Science* 286:1155–1158.

Fyer, A.J. (1993) Heritability of social anxiety: a brief review. *J. Clin. Psychiatry* 54(Suppl):10–12.

Gabrieli, J., Fleischman, D., Keane, M., Reminger, S., and Morrell, F. (1995) Double dissociation between memory systems underlying explicit and implicit memory in the human brain. *Psychol. Sci.* 6:76–82.

Gabrieli, J., Stebbins, G., Singh, J., Willingham, D., and Goetz, C. (1997) Intact mirror-tracing and impaired rotary-pursuit skill learning in patients with Huntington's disease: evidence for dissociable memory systems in skill learning. *Neuropsychol.* 11:272–281.

Gabrieli, J.D., Milberg, W., Keane, M.M., and Corkin, S. (1990) Intact priming of patterns despite impaired memory. *Neuropsychologia* 28:417–427.

Gabrieli, J.D.E. (1998) Cognitive neuroscience of human memory. *Annu. Rev. Psychol.* 49:87–115.

Gerra, G., Zaimovic, A., Zambelli, U., Timpano, M., Reali, N., Bernasconi, S., and Brambilla, F. (2000) Neuroendocrine responses to psychological stress in adolescents with anxiety disorder. *Neuropsychobiol.* 42:82–92.

Goenjian, A.K., Molina, L., Steinberg, A.M., Fairbanks, L.A., Alvarez, M.L., Goenjian, H.A., and Pynoos, R.S. (2001) Posttraumatic stress and depressive reactions among Nicaraguan adolescents after hurricane Mitch. *Am. J. Psychiatry* 158:788–794.

Gregory, A.M., Caspi, A., Moffitt, T.E., Koenen, K., Eley, T.C., and Poulton, R. (2007) Juvenile mental health histories of adults with anxiety disorders. *Am. J. Psychiatry* 164:301–308.

Grillon, C. (2002) Associative learning deficits increase symptoms of anxiety in humans. *Biol. Psychiatry* 51:851–858.

Grillon, C., and Ameli, R. (1998) Effects of threat and safety signals on startle during anticipation of aversive shocks, sounds, or airblasts. *J. Psychophysiol.* 12:329–337.

Grillon, C., Dierker, L., and Merikangas, K.R. (1997) Startle modulation in children at risk for anxiety disorders and/or alcoholism. *J. Am. Acad. Child Adolesc. Psychiatry* 36:925–932.

Grillon, C., Warner, V., Hille, J., Merikangas, K.R., Bruder, G.E., Tenke, C.E., Nomura, Y., Leite, P., and Weissman, M.M. (2005) Families at high and low risk for depression: a three-generation startle study. *Biol. Psychiatry* 57:953–960.

Gross, C., and Hen, R. (2004) The developmental origins of anxiety. *Nat. Rev. Neurosci.* 5:545–552.

Gullone, E., King, N.J., and Ollendick, T.H. (2001) Self-reported anxiety in children and adolescents: a three-year follow-up study. *J. Genet. Psychol.* 162:5–19.

Heim, C., Newport, D.J., Heit, S., Graham, Y.P., Wilcox, M., Bonsall, R., Miller, A.H., and Nemeroff, C.B. (2000) Pituitary-adrenal and autonomic responses to stress in women after sexual and physical abuse in childhood. *JAMA* 284:592–597.

Hertel, P. (2004) Memory for emotional and nonemotional events in depression: a question of habit? *In*: Reisberg, D.H.P., ed. *Memory and Emotion*. New York: Oxford University Press, pp. 186–216.

Hoyer, J., Becker, E.S., and Roth, W.T. (2001) Characteristics of worry in GAD patients, social phobics, and controls. *Depress. Anxiety* 13:89–96.

Johnson, E.O., Kamilaris, T.C., Calogero, A.E., Gold, P.W., and Chrousos, G.P. (1996) Effects of early parenting on growth and development in a small primate. *Ped. Res.* 39:999–1005.

Johnson, J.G., Cohen, P., and Brook, J.S. (2000) Associations between bipolar disorder and other psychiatric disorders during adolescence and early adulthood: a community-based longitudinal investigation. *Am. J. Psychiatry* 157:1679–1681.

Kagan, J., Snidman, N., Zentner, M., and Peterson, E. (1999) Infant temperament and anxious symptoms in school age children. *Dev. Psychopathol.* 11:209–224.

Kaufman, J., Birmaher, B., Perel, J., Dahl, R.E., Moreci, P., Nelson, B., Wells, W., and Ryan, N.D. (1997) The corticotropin-releasing hormone challenge in depressed abused, depressed nonabused, and normal control children. *Biol. Psychiatry* 42:669–679.

Kendler, K.S., Walters, E.E., Neale, M.C., Kessler, R.C., Heath, A.C., and Eaves, L.J. (1995) The structure of the genetic and environmental risk factors for six major psychiatric disorders in women. Phobia, generalized anxiety disorder, panic disorder, bulimia, major depression, and alcoholism. *Arch. Gen. Psychiatry* 52:374–383.

Kessler, R.C., McGonagle, K.A., Zhao, S., Nelson, C.B., Hughes, M., Eshleman, S., Wittchen, H.U., and Kendler, K.S. (1994) Lifetime and 12-month prevalence of *DSM-III-R* psychiatric disorders in the United States. Results from the National Comorbidity Survey. *Arch. Gen. Psychiatry* 51:8–19.

Klein, D.F. (1993) False suffocation alarms, spontaneous panics, and related conditions. An integrative hypothesis. *Arch. Gen. Psychiatry* 50:306–317.

Klein, R.G. (1995) Is panic disorder associated with childhood separation anxiety disorder? *Clin. Neuropharmacol.* 18:S7–S14.

Last, C.G., Hersen, M., Kazdin, A., Orvaschel, H., and Perrin, S. (1991) Anxiety disorders in children and their families. *Arch. Gen. Psychiatry* 48:928–934.

LeDoux, J.E. (1990) Information flow from sensation to emotion: Plasticity in the neural computation of stimulus value. *In*: Moore, G.M., ed. *Learning and Computational Neuroscience: Foundations of Adaptive Networks*. Cambridge, MA: MIT Press, pp. 2–51.

LeDoux, J.E. (2000) Emotion circuits in the brain. *Annu. Rev. Neurosci.* 23:155–184.

Lewinsohn, P.M., Gotlib, I.H., Lewinsohn, M., Seeley, J.R., and Allen, N.B. (1998) Gender differences in anxiety disorders and anxiety symptoms in adolescents. *J. Abnorm. Psychol.* 107:109–117.

Liberzon, I., Taylor, S.F., Amdur, R., Jung, T.D., Chamberlain, K.R., Minoshima, S., Koeppe, R.A., and Fig, L.M. (1999) Brain activation in PTSD in response to trauma-related stimuli. *Biol. Psychiatry* 45:817–826.

Lieb, R., Wittchen, H.U., Hofler, M., Fuetsch, M., Stein, M.B., and Merikangas, K.R. (2000) Parental psychopathology, parenting styles, and the risk of social phobia in offspring: a prospective-longitudinal community study. *Arch. Gen. Psychiatry* 57:859–866.

Lissek, S., Powers, A.S., McClure, E.B., Phelps, E.A., Woldehawariat, G., Grillon C., and Pine, D.S. (2005) Classical fear conditioning in the anxiety disorders: a meta-analysis. *Behav. Res. Ther.* 43:1391–1424.

Lundh, L.G., Czyzykow, S., and Ost, L.G. (1997) Explicit and implicit memory bias in panic disorder with agoraphobia. *Behav. Res. Ther.* 35:1003–1014.

Lundh, L.G., and Ost, L.G. (1996) Recognition bias for critical faces in social phobics. *Behav. Res. Ther.* 34:787–794.

MacLeod, C., and Mathews, A. (2004) Selective memory effects in anxiety disorders: an overview of research findings and their implications. *In*: Reisberg, D.H.P., ed. *Memory and Emotion*. New York: Oxford University Press, pp. 155–185.

MacLeod, C., Mathews, A., and Tata, P. (1986) Attentional bias in emotional disorders. *J. Abnorm. Psychol.* 95:15–20.

MacLeod, C., and McLaughlin, K. (1995) Implicit and explicit memory bias in anxiety: a conceptual replication. *Behav. Res. Ther.* 33:1–14.

MacLeod, C., and Rutherford, E.M. (1992) Anxiety and the selective processing of emotional information: mediating roles of awareness, trait and state variables, and personal relevance of stimulus materials. *Behav. Res. Ther.* 30:479–491.

Makino, S., Gold, P.W., and Schulkin, J. (1994) Corticosterone effects on corticotropin-releasing hormone mRNA in the central nucleus of the amygdala and the parvocellular region of the paraventricular nucleus of the hypothalamus. *Brain Res.* 640:105–112.

Makino, S., Shibasaki, T., Yamauchi, N., Nishioka, T., Mimoto, T., Wakabayashi, I., Gold, P.W., and Hashimoto, K. (1999) Psychological stress increased corticotropin-releasing hormone mRNA and content in the central nucleus of the amygdala but not in the hypothalamic paraventricular nucleus in the rat. *Brain Res.* 850:136–143.

Martel, F.L., Hayward, C., Lyons, D.M., Sanborn, K., Varady, S., and Schatzberg, A.F. (1999) Salivary cortisol levels in socially phobic adolescent girls. *Depress. Anxiety* 10:25–27.

Mathews, A., Mogg, K., May, J., and Eysenck, M. (1989) Implicit and explicit memory bias in anxiety. *J. Abnorm. Psychol.* 98:236–240.

Mattia, J.I., Heimberg, R.G., and Hope, D.A. (1993) The revised Stroop color-naming task in social phobics. *Behav. Res. Ther.* 31:305–313.

McClure, E.B., Monk, C.S., Nelson, E.E., Parrish, J.M., Adler, A., Blair, R.J., Fromm, S., Charney, D.S., Leibenluft, E., Ernst, M., and Pine, D.S. (2007) Abnormal attention modulation of fear circuit function in pediatric generalized anxiety disorder. *Arch. Gen. Psychiatry* 64:97–106.

McNally, R.J., and Amir, N. (1996) Perceptual implicit memory for trauma-related information in post-traumatic stress disorder. *Cogn. Emot.* 10:551–556.

McNally, R.J., Foa, E.B., and Donnell, C.D. (1989) Memory bias for anxiety information in patients with panic disorder. *Cogn. Emot.* 3:27–44.

McNally, R.J., Kaspi, S.P., Riemann, B.C., and Zeitlin, S.B. (1990) Selective processing of threat cues in posttraumatic stress disorder. *J. Abnorm. Psychol.* 99:398–402.

McNally, R.J., Lasko, N.B., Macklin, M.L., and Pitman, R.K. (1995) Autobiographical memory disturbance in combat-related posttraumatic stress disorder. *Behav. Res. Ther.* 33:619–630.

Meesters, C., Merckelbach, H., Muris, P., and Wessel, I. (2000) Autobiographical memory and trauma in adolescents. *J. Behav. Ther. Exp. Psychiatry* 31:29–39.

Miller, E.K., and Cohen, J.D. (2001) An integrative theory of prefrontal cortex function. *Annu. Rev. Neurosci.* 24:167–202.

Milner, B. (1962) Les troubles de la memoire accompagnant des lesions hippocampiques bilaterales [Memory impairment accompanying bilateral hippocampal lesions]. *In*: Passouant, P., ed. *Physiologie de l'hippocampe*. Paris: Centre National de la Recherche Scientifique, pp. 257–272.

Mirza, K.A., Bhadrinath, B.R., Goodyer, I.M., and Gilmour, C. (1998) Post-traumatic stress disorder in children and adolescents following road traffic accidents. *Br. J. Psychiatry* 172:443–447.

Mogg, K., Bradley, B.P., de Bono, J., and Painter, M. (1997) Time course of attentional bias for threat information in non-clinical anxiety. *Behav. Res. Ther.* 35:297–303.

Mogg, K., Bradley, B.P., Millar, N., and White, J. (1995) A follow-up study of cognitive bias in generalized anxiety disorder. *Behav. Res. Ther.* 33:927–935.

Mogg, K., Bradley, B.P., Williams, R., and Mathews, A. (1993) Subliminal processing of emotional information in anxiety and depression. *J. Abnorm. Psychol.* 102:304–311.

Mogg, K., and Marden, B. (1990) Processing of emotional information in anxious subjects. *Br. J. Clin. Psychol.* 29:227–229.

Mogg, K., Millar, N., and Bradley, B.P. (2000) Biases in eye movements to threatening facial expressions in generalized anxiety disorder and depressive disorder. *J. Abnorm. Psychol.* 109:695–704.

Monk, C.S., Nelson, E.E., McClure, E.B., Mogg, K., Bradley, B.P., Leibenluft, E., Blair, R.J., Chen, G., Charney, D.S., Ernst, M., and Pine, D.S. (2006) Ventrolateral prefrontal cortex activation and attentional bias in response to angry faces in adolescents with generalized anxiety disorder. *Am. J. Psychiatry* 163:1091–1097.

Moradi, A.R., Taghavi, R., Neshat-Doost, H.T., Yule, W., and Dalgleish, T. (2000) Memory bias for emotional information in children and adolescents with posttraumatic stress disorder: a preliminary study. *J. Anxiety Disord.* 14:521–534.

Morris, J.S., Ohman, A., and Dolan, R.J. (1999) A subcortical pathway to the right amygdala mediating "unseen" fear. *Proc. Natl. Acad. Sci. USA* 96:1680–1685.

Norman, D.A. (1969) Memory while shadowing. *Q. J. Exp. Psychol.* 21:85–93.

Otto, M.W., McNally, R.J., Pollack, M.H., Chen, E., and Rosenbaum, J.F. (1994) Hemispheric laterality and memory bias for threat in anxiety disorders. *J. Abnorm. Psychol.* 103:828–831.

Perez-Edgar, K., and Fox, N.A. (2005) Temperament and anxiety disorders. *Child Adolesc. Psychiatry Clin. N. Am.* 14:681–706, viii.

Perez-Edgar, K., Roberson-Nay, R., Hardin, M.G., Poeth, K., Guyer, A.E., Nelson, E.E., McClure, E.B., Henderson, H.A., Fox, N.A., Pine, D.S., and Ernst, M. (2007) Attention alters neural responses to evocative faces in behaviorally inhibited adolescents. *Neuroimage* 35:1538–1546.

Perez-Lopez, J.R., and Woody, S.R. (2001) Memory for facial expressions in social phobia. *Behav. Res. Ther.* 39:967–975.

Peterson, B.S., Pine, D.S., Cohen, P., and Brook, J.S. (2001) Prospective, longitudinal study of tic, obsessive-compulsive, and attention-deficit/hyperactivity disorders in an epidemiological sample. *J. Am. Acad. Child Adolesc. Psychiatry* 40:685–695.

Pezawas, L., Meyer-Lindenberg, A., Drabant, E.M., Verchinski, B.A., Munoz, K.E., Kolachana, B.S., Egan, M.F., Mattay, V.S., Hariri, A.R., and Weinberger, D.R. (2005) 5-HTTLPR polymorphism impacts human cingulate-amygdala interactions: a genetic susceptibility mechanism for depression. *Nat. Neurosci.* 8:828–834.

Pine, D. S. (2007) A neuroscience perspective on pediatric anxiety disorders. *J. Child Psychol. Psychiatry* 48:631–648.

Pine, D.S. (2003) Developmental psychobiology and response to threats: relevance to trauma in children and adolescents. *Biol. Psychiatry* 53:796–808.

Pine, D.S., and Cohen, J.A. (2002) Trauma in children and adolescents: risk and treatment of psychiatric sequelae. *Biol. Psychiatry* 51:519–531.

Pine, D.S., Cohen, P., and Brook, J. (1996) Emotional problems during youth as predictors of stature during early adulthood: results from a prospective epidemiologic study. *Pediatrics* 97:856–863.

Pine, D.S., Cohen, P., and Brook, J. (2001) Adolescent fears as predictors of depression. *Biol. Psychiatry* 50:721–724.

Pine, D.S., Cohen, P., Gurley, D., Brook, J., and Ma, Y. (1998) The risk for early-adulthood anxiety and depressive disorders in adolescents with anxiety and depressive disorders. *Arch. Gen. Psychiatry* 55:56–64.

Pine, D.S., and Klein, R.G. (in press) Anxiety disorders. *In*: Rutter, M., Bishop, D., Pine, D.S., Scott, S., Stevenson, J., Taylor, E., Thapar, A., eds. *Rutter's Child and Adolescent Psychiatry*, 5th ed. Oxford, UK: Blackwell Publishing.

Pine, D.S., Klein, R.G., Coplan, J.D., Papp, L.A., Hoven, C.W., Martinez, J., Kovalenko, P., Mandell, D.J., Moreau, D., Klein, D.F., and Gorman, J.M. (2000) Differential carbon dioxide sensitivity in childhood anxiety disorders and nonill comparison group. *Arch. Gen. Psychiatry* 57:960–967.

Pine, D.S., Klein, R.G., Roberson-Nay, R., Mannuzza, S., Moulton, J.L. III, Woldehawariat, G., and Guardino, M. (2005a) Response to 5% carbon dioxide in children and adolescents: relationship to panic disorder in parents and anxiety disorders in subjects. *Arch. Gen. Psychiatry* 62:73–80.

Pine, D.S., Klein, R.G., Roberson-Nay, R., Mannuzza, S., Moulton, J.L., Woldehawariat, G., and Guardino, M. (2005b) Face emotion processing and risk for panic disorder in youth. *J. Am. Acad. Child Adolesc. Psychiatry* 44:664–672.

Pine, D.S., Lissek, S., Klein, R.G., Mannuzza, S., Moulton, J.L. 3rd, Guardino, M., and Woldehawariat, G. (2004) Face-memory and emotion: associations with major depression in children and adolescents. *J. Child Psychol. Psychiatry* 45:1199–1208.

Pine, D.S., Mogg, K., Bradley, B.P., Montgomery, L., Monk, C.S., McClure, E., Guyer, A.E., Ernst, M., Charney, D.S., and Kaufman, J. (2005) Attention bias to threat in maltreated children: implications for vulnerability to stress-related psychopathology. *Am. J. Psychiatry* 162:291–296.

Poldrack, R.A., Clark, J., Pare-Blagoev, E.J., Shohamy, D., Creso Moyano, J., Myers, C., and Gluck, M.A. (2001) Interactive memory systems in the human brain. *Nature* 414:546–550.

Posner, M.I. (1986) A framework for relating cognitive to neural systems. *Electroencephalogr. Clin. Neurophysiol Suppl.* 38:155–166.

Post, R.M., Weiss, S.R.B., Leverich, G.S., George, M.S., Frye, M., and Ketter, T.A. (1996) Developmental psychobiology of cyclic affective illness: implications for early therapeutic intervention. *Dev. Psychopathol.* 8:273–305.

Prather, M.D., Lavenex, P., Mauldin-Jourdain, M.L., Mason, W.A., Capitanio, J.P., Mendoza, S.P., and Amaral, D.G. (2001) Increased social fear and decreased fear of objects in monkeys with neonatal amygdala lesions. *Neurosci.* 106:653–658.

Rapee, R.M., McCallum, S.L., Melville, L.F., Ravenscroft, H., and Rodney, J.M. (1994) Memory bias in social phobia. *Behav. Res. Ther.* 32:89–99.

Rasmusson, A.M., Lipschitz, D.S., Wang, S., Hu, S., Vojvoda, D., Bremner, J.D., Southwick, S.M., and Charney, D.S. (2001) Increased pituitary and adrenal reactivity in premenopausal women with posttraumatic stress disorder. *Biol. Psychiatry* 50:965–977.

Rauch, S.L., Whalen, P.J., Shin, L.M., McInerney, S.C., Macklin, M.L., Lasko, N.B., Orr, S.P., and Pitman, R.K. (2000) Exaggerated amygdala response to masked facial stimuli in posttraumatic stress disorder: a functional MRI study. *Biol. Psychiatry* 47:769–776.

Reed, V., and Wittchen, H.U. (1998) DSM-IV panic attacks and panic disorder in a community sample of adolescents and young adults: How specific are panic attacks. *Psychiatric Res.* 32:335–345.

Richardson-Klavehn, A., and Bjork, R.A. (1988) Measures of memory. *Annu. Rev. Psychol.* 36:475–543.

Roberson-Nay, R., McClure, E.B., Monk, C.S., Nelson, E.E., Guyer, A.E., Fromm, S.J., Charney, D.S., Leibenluft, E., Blair, J., Ernst, M., and Pine, D.S. (2006) Increased amygdala activity during successful memory encoding in adolescent major depressive disorder: an fMRI study. *Biol. Psychiatry* 60:966–973.

Roediger, H.L., and McDermott, K.B. (1995) Creating false memories: remembering words not presented in lists. *J. Exp. Psychol.: Learn. Mem. Cogn.* 21:803–814.

Rosenbaum, J.F., Biederman, J., Gersten, M., Hirshfeld, D.R., Meminger, S.R., Herman, J.B., Kagan, J., Reznick, J.S., and Snidman, N. (1988) Behavioral inhibition in children of parents with panic disorder and agoraphobia. A controlled study. *Arch. Gen. Psychiatry* 45:463–470.

Rosenblum, L.A., Coplan, J.D., Friedman, S., Bassoff, T., Gorman, J.M., and Andrews, M.W. (1994) Adverse early experiences affect noradrenergic and serotonergic functioning in adult primates. *Biol. Psychiatry* 35:221–227.

Sallee, F.R., Richman, H., Sethuraman, G., Dougherty, D., Sine, L., and Altman-Hamamdzic, S. (1998) Clonidine challenge in childhood anxiety disorder. *J. Am. Acad. Child Adolesc. Psychiatry* 37:655–662.

Sallee, F.R., Sethuraman, G., Sine, L., and Liu, H. (2000) Yohimbine challenge in children with anxiety disorders. *Am. J. Psychiatry* 157:1236–1242.

Sanes, J.N., Dimitrov, B., and Hallett, M. (1990) Motor learning in patients with cerebellar dysfunction. *Brain* 113:103–120.

Schacter, D.L., and Tulving, E. (1994) What are the memory systems of 1994? *In*: Schacter, D.L., and Tulving, E., eds. *Memory Systems 1994*. Cambridge, MA: MIT Press, pp 1–38.

Schulkin, J., Gold, P.W., and McEwen, B.S. (1998) Induction of corticotropin-releasing hormone gene expression by glucocorticoids: implications for understanding the states of fear and anxiety and allostatic load. *Psychoneuroendocrinol.* 23:219–243.

Schwartz, C.E., Wright, C.I., Shin, L.M., Kagan, J., and Rauch, S.L. (2003) Inhibited and uninhibited infants "grown up": adult amygdalar response to novelty. *Science* 300:1952–1953.

Scoville, W.B., and Milner, B. (1957) Loss of recent memory after bilateral hippocampal lesions. *J. Neurol. Neurosurg. Psychiatry* 20: 11–21.

Shaffer, D., Gould, M.S., Fisher, P., Trautman, P., Moreau, D., Kleinman, M., and Flory, M. (1996) Psychiatric diagnosis in child and adolescent suicide. *Arch. Gen. Psychiatry* 53:339–348.

Silverman, W.K., La Greca, A.M., and Wasserstein, S. (1995) What do children worry about? Worries and their relation to anxiety. *Child Dev.* 66:671–686.

Stattin, H. (1984) Developmental trends in the appraisal of anxiety-provoking situations. *J. Pers.* 52:46–57.

Stein, M.B., Yehuda, R., Koverola, C., and Hanna, C. (1997) Enhanced dexamethasone suppression of plasma cortisol in adult women traumatized by childhood sexual abuse. *Biol. Psychiatry* 42:680–686.

Taghavi, M.R., Neshat-Doost, H.T., Moradi, A.R., Yule, W., and Dalgleish, T. (1999) Biases in visual attention in children and adolescents with clinical anxiety and mixed anxiety-depression. *J. Abnorm. Child Psychol.* 27:215–223.

Takahashi, L.K., Kalin, N.H., Vanden Burgt, J.A., and Sherman, J.E. (1989) Corticotropin-releasing factor modulates defensive-withdrawal and exploratory behavior in rats. *Behav. Neurosci.* 103: 648–654.

Terleph, T.A., Klein, R.G., Roberson-Nay, R., Mannuzza, S., Moulton, J.L., Woldehawariat, G., Guardino, M., and Pine, D.S. (2006) Stress-responsivity and HPA-axis activity in juveniles: results from a home-based CO_2-inhalation study. *Am. J. Psychiatry* 163: 738–740.

Thomas, K.M., Drevets, W.C., Dahl, R.E., Ryan, N.D., Birmaher, B., Eccard, C.H., Axelson, D., Whalen, P.J., Casey, B.J. (2001) Amygdala response to fearful faces in anxious and depressed children. *Arch. Gen. Psychiatry* 58:1057–1063.

Thomas, K.M., Drevets, W.C., Whalen, P.J., Eccard, C.H., Dahl, R.E., Ryan, N.D., and Casey, B.J. (2001) Amygdala response to facial expressions in children and adults. *Biol. Psychiatry* 49:309–316.

Tillfors, M., Furmark, T., Marteinsdottir, I., Fischer, H., Pissiota, A., Langstrom, B., and Fredrikson, M. (2001) Cerebral blood flow in subjects with social phobia during stressful speaking tasks: a PET study. *Am. J. Psychiatry* 158:1220–1226.

Turner, S.M., Beidel, D.C., and Costello, A. (1987) Psychopathology in the offspring of anxiety disorders patients. *J. Consult. Clin. Psychol.* 55:229–235.

Vasa, R.A., Roberson-Nay, R., Klein, R.G., Mannuzza, S., Moulton, J.L. 3rd, Guardino, M., Merikangas, A., Carlino, A.R., and Pine, D.S. (2007) Memory deficits in children with and at risk for anxiety disorders. *Depress. Anxiety* 24:85–94.

Vasey, M.W., Daleiden, E.L., Williams, L.L., and Brown, L.M. (1995) Biased attention in childhood anxiety disorders: a preliminary study. *J. Abnorm. Child Psychol.* 23:267–279.

Vasey, M.W., el-Hag, N., and Daleiden, E.L. (1996) Anxiety and the processing of emotionally threatening stimuli: distinctive patterns of selective attention among high- and low-test- anxious children. *Child Dev.* 67:1173–1185.

Verhulst, F.C., van der Ende, J., Ferdinand, R.F., and Kasius, M.C. (1997) The prevalence of *DSM-III-R* diagnoses in a national sample of Dutch adolescents. *Arch. Gen. Psychiatry* 54:329–336.

Vrana, S.R., Roodman, A., and Beckham, J.C. (1995) Selective processing of trauma-relevant words in posttraumatic stress disorder. *J. Anxiety Disord.* 9:515–530.

Watts, F.N., Trezise, L., and Sharrock, R. (1986) Processing of phobic stimuli. *Br. J. Clin. Psychol.* 25:253–259.

Weems, C.F., Silverman, W.K., and La Greca, A.M. (2000) What do youth referred for anxiety problems worry about? Worry and its relation to anxiety and anxiety disorders in children and adolescents. *J. Abnorm. Child Psychol.* 28:63–72.

Weissman, M.M., Warner, V., Wickramaratne, P., Moreau, D., Olfson, M. (1997) Offspring of depressed parents. 10 Years later. *Arch. Gen. Psychiatry* 54:932–940.

Wickramaratne, P.J., and Weissman, M.M. (1998) Onset of psychopathology in offspring by developmental phase and parental depression. *J. Am. Acad. Child Adol. Psychiatry* 37:933–942.

Wittchen, H.-U., Stein, M.B., and Kessler, R.C. (1999) Social fears and social phobia in a community sample of adolescents and young adults: Prevalence, risk factors and co-morbidity. *Psychol. Med.* 29:309–323.

Wood, J.J., McLeod, B.D., Sigman, M., Hwang, W.C., and Chu, B.C. (2003) Parenting and childhood anxiety: theory, empirical findings, and future directions. *J. Child Psychol. Psychiatry* 44: 134–151.

Yehuda, R., Kahana, B., Binder-Brynes, K., Southwick, S., Mason, J.W., and Giller, E.L. (1995) Low urinary cortisol excretion in Holocaust survivors with posttraumatic stress disorder. *Am. J. Psychiatry* 152:982–-986.

Yehuda, R., Southwick, S., Giller, E.L., Ma, X., and Mason, J.W. (1991) Low urinary cortisol excretion and severity of PTSD symptoms in Vietnam combat veterans. *J. Nerv. Ment. Disord.* 180:321–325.

Yehuda, R., Southwick, S.M., Nussbaum, G., Wahby, V., Giller, E.L., Jr., and Mason, J.W. (1990) Low urinary cortisol excretion in patients with posttraumatic stress disorder. *J. Nerv. Ment. Dis.* 178:366–369.

Yehuda, R., Teicher, M.H., Trestman, R.L., Levengood, R.A., and Siever, L.J. (1996) Cortisol regulation in posttraumatic stress disorder and major depression: a chronobiological analysis. *Biol. Psychiatry* 40:79–88.

Zeitlin, S.B., and McNally, R.J. (1991) Implicit and explicit memory bias for threat in post-traumatic stress disorder. *Behav. Res. Ther.* 29:451–457.

Zoellner, L.A., Foa, E.B., Brigidi, B.D., and Przeworski, A. (2000) Are trauma victims susceptible to "false memories." *J. Abnorm. Psychol.* 109:517–524.

71 Molecular Genetics of Childhood and Adolescent Onset Psychiatric Disorders

JEREMY M. VEENSTRA-VANDERWEELE, RANDY D. BLAKELY, AND EDWIN H. COOK, JR.

Much more is unknown than known in the molecular genetics of child and adolescent onset psychiatric disorders. Useful genetic information is just beginning to emerge, primarily in disorders associated with chromosomal abnormalities and disorders that feature simple inheritance patterns involving only one gene. A few genes have been implicated in disorders with more complex patterns of inheritance. These appear to be genes of small effect that increase risk of a disorder but cannot be thought of as causing the disorder. Although child psychiatric genetics remains in its infancy, the long-term goals are to increase understanding of pathophysiology with the goal of improved treatments and a better understanding of genetic, environmental, and gene–environment interactions.

Child and adolescent psychiatry presents a specific set of possibilities and obstacles to the geneticist. A general discussion of epidemiological and molecular genetic methodology is presented elsewhere, but it is useful to consider the application of these methods to the special situation of childhood disorders. The flow of human development complicates any study that assigns phenotype definitions to children, but the study of childhood disorders also offers some luxuries that are missing in adult psychiatry genetics, such as the easier availability of parents, siblings, and extended families.

The introduction highlights some of the key genetic concepts important in the study of childhood psychiatric disorders. The chapter then is divided into four sections covering chromosomal disorders, relatively simple genetic disorders, complex genetic disorders, and finally disorders that are frequently comorbid in child psychiatry. Most psychiatric disorders with variable age of onset, such as mood disorders and anxiety disorders, are covered in their corresponding chapters (26 and 38) elsewhere in the text. One exception is obsessive–compulsive disorder (OCD), which is covered here because a substantial proportion of cases have onset before adulthood, particularly in familial OCD (Samuels et al., 2006).

SIMPLE OR COMPLEX GENETICS

A number of contrasts affect the study of child psychiatry genetics. First among these is the distinction between relatively simple and complex genetic disorders. Genetic defects in a single gene cause relatively simple genetic disorders such as autosomal dominant susceptibility to breast cancer (*BRCA1*). Even here, it is important to note that within each of these relatively simple genetic disorders, penetrance and expression may vary. Variable expression can be seen in women with mutations in *BRCA1* because some women develop ovarian cancer or other types of cancer instead of breast cancer (Friedman et al., 1995). Variable penetrance is also evident because there are those with *BRCA1* mutations who never develop breast cancer. Penetrance is a particularly relevant concept in child psychiatry, where penetrance rates may depend on age and environment.

A few disorders with onset in childhood, such as Rett syndrome (RTT), Fragile X syndrome (FXS), and maternally inherited chromosome 15q11-q13 duplications and triplications are relatively simple genetic disorders. More single-gene or chromosomal disorders will likely be identified as coherent entities within heterogeneous syndromes such as autism; however, simple genetic disorders are unlikely to account for the majority of children and adolescents with genetic susceptibility to mental illness.

Most psychiatric disorders are best described as arising from complex genetics, where multiple gene variants converge to increase susceptibility to a given disorder. Because multiple gene variants must occur together to produce disease in an individual, each variant is typically frequent in the overall population. Instead of describing these common variants as "mutations" or "defects," they are more appropriately called "variants" to reflect the notion that they do not cause disease except in interaction with other gene variants or environmental factors. No complex genetic disorders have as yet been parsed to identify all susceptibility genes, but some potential patterns of gene interactions have been proposed, including additive and multiplicative effects. The pattern of genetic risk in psychiatric disorders is likely to include interactions between an array of gene variants that may individually make small or large contributions to the overall pattern of risk. Other gene variants may actually serve a protective role, whether decreasing risk, modifying severity, or altering expression of the phenotype.

LOCUS OR ALLELIC HETEROGENEITY

Locus heterogeneity means that defects in different loci, or genes, may cause the same phenotype. The concept arose in relatively simple genetics, where, for example, defects in one of a few different genes can cause hereditary nonpolyposis colorectal cancer (HNPCC) (Nystrom-Lahti et al., 1994). This idea becomes much more complicated in more complex genetic disorders, where different (likely overlapping) groups of genetic variants may cause susceptibility to disease. Locus heterogeneity will likely be very common in psychiatric syndromes because within a single disorder, symptoms can be quite different from patient to patient.

Allelic heterogeneity means that different defects in the same gene may lead to different patterns of genetic disease. This concept also arose in simple genetic disorders, where different mutations in the same gene can lead to different phenotype patterns. For example, many different mutations in a single gene (*CFTR*) have been described in cystic fibrosis, some of which are associated with particularly mild forms of the disorder or may lead to more pancreatic than lung findings (The Cystic Fibrosis Genotype-Phenotype Consortium, 1993). As rare and common variants in relevant genes (for example, the serotonin transporter [SERT] *SLC6A4*; Devlin et al., 2005; Sutcliffe et al., 2005) are better understood, allelic heterogeneity may also become relevant in complex genetic disorders in psychiatry.

ASSOCIATION OR LINKAGE MAPPING

With a few notable exceptions, tests of genetic association have been used to study candidate genes in disease. Tests of association are considerably more powerful than tests of linkage at a given locus, allowing genes of weaker effect to be detected (Elston and Spence, 2006). These tests compare the observed alleles in individuals with a disease to those expected by chance. The candidate gene approach has proven more fruitful in child than in adult psychiatry, particularly in attention-deficit/hyperactivity disorder (ADHD). This approach is dependent on some understanding of the biology of a given disorder. This understanding can be based on response to medication, such as stimulants in ADHD, or on a biochemical finding, such as hyperserotonemia in autism. Each of these approaches has proven fruitful. Seven different candidate genes within the dopamine (DA), norepinephrine, and serotonin systems have led to replicated association findings in ADHD and have yielded five identified functional variants. The serotonin transporter was the first candidate gene in autism because of its role in platelet serotonin uptake, and it has been found to harbor rare and common functional variants associated with autism. Unfortunately, however, we have only a very limited understanding of the pathophysiology of any psychiatric disorder, so the number of potential candidate genes in a given disorder is large, given the large number of genes expressed during brain development.

For these reasons, genome-wide approaches have been favored for identifying areas of linkage within families. Based on experience in the study of other complex genetic disorders ranging from diabetes to bipolar mood disorder, investigators currently favor nonparametric approaches that make no assumptions about disease transmission. These approaches typically use affected sibling pairs to identify increased sharing of alleles at particular points in the genome, but similar approaches may be applied to larger families, when available.

CHROMOSOMAL DISORDERS RELEVANT TO CHILD PSYCHIATRY

Although they cannot explain the origin of most disorders, chromosomal abnormalities may provide important clues to genes and protein systems relevant in child psychiatry. A few of the more common chromosomal disorders are discussed below. The core clinical features of these disorders are given in Table 71.1. Uncommon chromosomal anomalies associated with specific psychiatric disorders are discussed in the Complex Genetic Disorders section.

22q11 Deletion Syndrome

Deletion of chromosome 22q11, sometimes called *velocardiofacial syndrome*, is associated with an elevated incidence of schizophrenia and bipolar disorder in adults (Carlson et al., 1997). Recent research suggests a complex phenotype in children with 22q11 deletions, including autism spectrum disorders, attention problems, and early-onset psychosis (Vorstman et al., 2006). Although

TABLE 71.1 *Summary of Chromosomal Disorders with a High Rate of Childhood Psychiatric Comorbidity*

Disorder	*Core Features*	*Chromosomal Anomaly or Gene*	*Psychiatric Comorbidity*
22q11 deletion / Velocardiofacial syndrome	Characteristic facial features, intellectual disability, cardiac defects, and multiple midline defects including cleft palate and brain malformations	Chromosome 22q11 deletion	Hyperactivity, autism spectrum disorder (ASD), mood instability, psychosis
Prader–Willi syndrome	Hypotonia, mild intellectual disability, short stature, hypogonadism, and compulsive eating behavior with obesity	Paternally inherited deletion of chromosome 15q11-q13 or maternal uniparental disomy	Compulsive behavior
Angelman syndrome	Characteristic facial features, intellectual disability, ataxia, hypotonia, epilepsy, absence of speech, and predominant smiling and laughter	Maternally inherited deletion of chromosome 15q11-q13, paternal uniparental disomy, or mutation of *UBE3A*	ASD
Maternal chromosome 15q11-q13 duplication syndrome	Hypotonia, intellectual disability, epilepsy, autism spectrum disorder	Maternally inherited duplication of chromosome 15q11-q13	ASD, hyperactivity, mood instability
Turner syndrome	Short stature, webbing of the posterior neck, sternal deformities, streak ovaries, and mild cognitive impairment	Monosomy of the X chromosome	Hyperactivity, social impairment
Williams syndrome	Characteristic facial features, intellectual disability, supravalvular aortic stenosis, infantile hypercalcemia, short stature	Microdeletion of chromosome 7q11.23	Social disinhibition, specific phobias, generalized anxiety (Dykens, 2003)

it is not yet entirely clear what gene or genes are responsible for the psychiatric symptoms in chromosome 22q11 deletion syndrome, a few strong candidate genes have emerged, including the T-Box transcription factor gene *TBX1* (Paylor et al., 2006), the proline dehydrogenase gene *PRODH* (Raux et al., 2007), and the catechol-O-methyltransferase gene *COMT* (Gothelf et al., 2007).

Prader–Willi and Angelman Syndromes

Prader–Willi and Angelman syndromes reflect genetic imprinting of a region of chromosome 15. Prader–Willi syndrome (PWS) most commonly results from deletion of the paternal chromosome 15q11-q13 region. No single gene has been identified as responsible for the PWS phenotype, and the disorder is thought to result from the imprinting of multiple genes that are only expressed from the paternal chromosome. Absence of a paternally expressed small nucleolar ribonucleic acid (RNA) (snoRNA), HBII-52, may account for some of the features of PWS (Kishore and Stamm, 2006). HBII-52 is a noncoding RNA transcript that binds to the exon Vb sequence of the serotonin 5-HT_{2C} receptor gene, thereby facilitating inclusion of a nonedited form of this exon. In PWS, where HBII-52 is absent, the nonedited form of the 5-HT_{2C} gene transcript is decreased, which would lead to decreased sensitivity to serotonin at this receptor (Wang et al., 2000). Altered serotonin signaling in PWS could relate to the obesity or compulsive behavior seen in PWS and make this relatively simple disorder a potential model for more complex neurobehavioral syndromes such as eating disorders or OCD.

Angelman syndrome (AS) results from the absence or mutation of the *UBE3A* gene in the maternal chromosome 15q11-q13 region. Patients with deletions or uniparental disomy, where both chromosomes have been inherited from the father, have more severe phenotypes, suggesting that other genes nearby, such as the γ-aminobutyric acid (GABA) receptor subunit genes (*GABRB3*, *GABRA5*, *GABRG3*) may contribute to the more severe phenotype in deletion cases (Moncla et al., 1999). Interestingly, disruption of *UBE3A* function in mice leads to an inhibition of α-calcium/calmodulin-dependent kinase type 2 (CaMKII), and preventing this CaMKII inhibition corrected the seizures, poor coordination, and learning problems typically seen in these mice (van Woerden et al., 2007).

Turner Syndrome

Turner syndrome affects females who have only one copy of the X chromosome (45, X) and is associated with social and cognitive impairments, including an elevated risk of autism and ADHD. Girls with an X chromosome from their mother (45, X^m) (that is, in whom the X chromosome from the father was absent) have significantly worse social cognition, behavioral inhibition, and verbal and visuospatial memory than those who received their X chromosome from their father (45, X^p) (Skuse et al., 1997). The parent-of-origin effect suggests an imprinted locus (a gene on the X chromosome expressed only when inherited from the father) that could have an effect on differences between male and female psychosocial development because males do not receive an X chromosome from their father. Ongoing work to understand this altered social function has identified association between the novel gene *EFHC2* and recognition of fearful facial expressions in girls with Turner syndrome (Weiss et al., 2007).

SIMPLE GENETIC DISORDERS WITH CHILDHOOD PSYCHIATRIC PHENOTYPES

Simple genetic disorders are rare and often include psychiatric problems and other clinical features. The core clinical features and associated psychiatric comorbidities of some important simple genetic disorders are given in Table 71.2. A number of relatively simple genetic syndromes primarily affect other systems but also have prominent child psychiatry phenotypes. For example, Smith–Lemli–Opitz syndrome (SLOS), which results from a defect in cholesterol biosynthesis, prominently includes self-injurious behavior and symptoms of autism in a majority of children (Tierney et al., 2001). Smith–Lemli–Opitz syndrome is an important disorder to detect because cholesterol supplementation may correct portions of the phenotype (Starck et al., 2002). Unlike simple genetic syndromes that include child psychiatric manifestations as a smaller part of their overall phenotype, RTT and FXS manifest predominantly as neuropsychiatric disorders.

Rett Syndrome

Rett syndrome (RTT) is an uncommon X-linked disorder with almost all cases being sporadic. Girls with RTT develop normally until approximately 6–18 months of age, when they lose speech and purposeful hand movements and then progress to develop autistic behavior, microcephaly, seizures, and eventually abnormal breathing patterns that typically lead to death before adulthood. Mutations in *MECP2*, the gene encoding methyl-CpG binding protein 2 (MeCP2), cause RTT (Amir et al., 1999). Remarkably, other forms of variation at *MECP2*, including missense mutations and gene region duplications, have now also been associated with intellectual disability and progressive neurological symptoms in males (Van Esch et al., 2005). (Please note that here and throughout the chapter, the term *intellectual disability* is used to replace the diagnostic category historically termed as *mental retardation*, as suggested by leading clinical and advocacy organizations; Schalock et al., 2007.) The MeCP2 protein normally binds methylated CpG dinucleotides and forms part of the complex that deacetylates histones to repress gene expression. Therefore, RTT is thought to be a result of inappropriate gene overexpression. Mice that lack *MECP2* develop a neurological dysfunction that parallels RTT, but restoring *MECP2* gene function in mature animals

TABLE 71.2 *Summary of Relatively Simple Genetic Disorders with a High rate of Childhood Psychiatric Comorbidity*

Disorder	*Core Features*	*Gene*	*Psychiatric Comorbidity*
Rett syndrome	Loss of speech and purposeful hand movements at 6–18 months and progression to microcephaly, seizures, ataxia, stereotypic hand movements, and abnormal breathing patterns	*MECP2*	ASD
Fragile X syndrome	Macroorchidism, large ears, prominent jaw, intellectual disability and high-pitched speech	*FMR1*	Hyperactivity, ASD
Smith–Lemli–Opitz syndrome (SLOS)	Characteristic facial features, microcephaly, hypotonia, syndactyly, and hypogenitalism	*DHCR7*	ASD, self-injurious behavior
Tuberous sclerosis	Facial angiofibromas, ashleaf spots, shagreen patches, multiple hamartomatous lesions including brain, skin, heart, and kidney, risk of cancer, risk of seizures, intellectual disability	*TSC1, TSC2*	ASD, ADHD (de Vries et al., 2005)
Lesch–Nyhan syndrome	Choreoathetosis, dystonia, compulsive self-injury and intellectual disability	*HPRT*	Self-injurious behavior (Nyhan, 1997)
PTEN hamartoma tumor syndrome	Multiple hamartomatous lesions including skin, mucous membranes, or intestines, risk of cancer, macrocephaly, and cognitive impairment	*PTEN*	ASD (Buxbaum et al., 2007)

PTEN: protein tyrosine phosphatase; ASD: autism spectrum disorders; ADHD: attention-deficit/hyperactivity disorder.

reverses this phenotype (Guy et al., 2007), suggesting that the deficit may relate to neuronal or synaptic stability rather than irreversible neuropathology.

Fragile X Syndrome

Fragile X syndrome (FXS) is the prototypical genetic syndrome caused by a trinucleotide repeat expansion. Increased rates of autism spectrum disorders and ADHD are observed in FXS (Hessl et al., 2001). Although interest is appropriately focused on the relatively high rate of autistic features in patients with FXS, the rate of FXS in the population of referred psychiatric patients with autism is low. The responsible gene variant is a cytosine-guanine-guanine (CGG) triplet repeat that can increase in number when passed down from parent to child. When the repeat sequence increases past 200 copies, the *FMR1* gene on chromosome Xq27 is hypermethylated and the protein is no longer expressed. As an X-linked disorder, FXS typically affects boys, but it may also affect girls to a milder degree, and the level of familial mental retardation protein (FMRP) expression in girls may correlate with the degree of behavior problems (Hessl et al., 2001). The exact role of the *FMR1* protein (FMRP) in neurons is not entirely clear, but FMRP interacts with messenger ribonucleic acids (mRNAs) and ribosomes, suggesting a role in protein synthesis. Familial mental retardation protein is synthesized in dendritic spines in response to stimulation of group 1 metabotropic glutamate receptors including mGluR5 (Bear et al., 2004). Immature dendritic spine size and shape have been noted in FXS patients and *FMR1* knockout mice (Grossman et al., 2006). Study of the pathophysiology of FXS has led to development of mGluR5 antagonists that have at least partially reversed FXS genetic models in fruit flies and mice (McBride et al., 2005; Yan et al., 2005). This is an example of a disorder in which targeted clinical trials are being planned based on the pathophysiological information provided from the identification of the genetic cause of the syndrome (Dolen and Bear, 2005).

COMPLEX GENETIC DISORDERS WITH CHILDHOOD OR ADOLESCENT PSYCHIATRIC PHENOTYPES

Complex genetic disorders constitute the bulk of child psychiatric disease. For each disorder, evidence for genetic susceptibility to the disease is briefly reviewed. Chromosomal abnormalities, candidate gene studies, and genomic linkage and association results are then detailed to demonstrate the current state of molecular genetics of the disorder. Disorders that by definition have onset in childhood are discussed first. Disorders with variable-onset, including onset in childhood or adolescence, are discussed second and in less detail. Finally, disorders that are frequently relevant in child psychiatry, such as communication disorders, reading disability, and nocturnal enuresis, are discussed briefly.

Autistic Disorder

Evidence suggests that autism is a genetic disorder with complex inheritance. The current prevalence of autism is approximately 0.2% (Chakrabarti and Fombonne, 2001). Approximately 4 times as many boys are affected than girls. The broader definition of autism spectrum disorder may include as many as 0.7% of children (Kuehn, 2007). Twin studies show a 60%–91% concordance rate in monozygotic twins, depending on whether a narrow or broad phenotype is considered, in contrast to 0%–10% concordance in dizygotic twins (Bailey et al., 1995). Sibling recurrence rate has been estimated to be 4.5%–10% (Jorde et al., 1991). The pattern of relative risk in autism is consistent with multiplicative inheritance, with multiple gene variants converging to lead to risk of the disorder.

Molecular genetic research in autism is further along than any of the other childhood onset neuropsychiatric disorders discussed here. This progress has resulted largely from a mobilization of family advocacy and federal funding that has engaged clinical and basic science researchers. The emerging picture reveals a disorder with multiple chromosomal anomalies, a few rare variants or mutations of large effect in synaptic development genes, and functional common variants of smaller effect in multiple brain development genes. Additional genes show evidence of association in more than one study but without a clearly identified functional variant that could account for autism risk. This pattern probably results as much from the technology available for finding genes and demonstrating that gene variants are functional as from the true underlying pattern of genetic risk alleles.

Chromosomal anomalies have increased rates in autism, but no single anomaly is found in more than 4% of autism samples. The most frequent chromosomal disorder in nonsyndromal autism is maternally inherited duplication or triplication of 15q11-q13 (either interstitial duplications of 15q11-q13 or supernumerary inverted duplications) (Schroer et al., 1998). Expression changes of genes in this region have been reported in autism, including both the AS gene *UBE3A* and the GABA receptor *GABRB3* gene (Baron et al., 2006; Hogart et al., 2007). Quite a number of smaller, primarily de novo, deletions, duplications, or rearrangements scattered throughout the genome have been reported in autism and may account for as many as 10% of cases (Sebat et al., 2007; Szatmari et al., 2007). Although most of these chromosomal anomalies likely disrupt multiple genes, making it difficult to narrow down the gene responsible, balanced translocations may disrupt only one gene. In one patient with autism and intellectual disability, a balanced translocation has been found to disrupt the potassium channel subunit gene *KCNMA1* on chromosome 10q22.

Paralleling the association of rare de novo chromosomal anomalies with autism, rare mutations in a few genes have been found to confer a greatly heightened risk of autism. Four genes with rare mutations or deletions implicated in one or two families with autism all encode proteins that are involved in synapse formation. Disruption of the postsynaptic neuroligin-4 gene (*NLGN4* on chromosome Xp22) is associated with X-linked intellectual disability and autism, although with variable penetrance for each disorder (Jamain et al., 2003; Laumonnier et al., 2004). A rare amino acid variant that causes retention of neuroligin-3 (*NLGN3* on chromosome Xq13) in the endoplasmic reticulum has also been described in two brothers with autism (Jamain et al., 2003; Comoletti et al., 2004). Consistent with a role of altered neuroligin signaling in autism, missense variants and a de novo deletion in the gene encoding the presynaptic neuroligin binding partner, neurexin 1β (*NRXN1* on 2p16), have also been detected in autism (Feng et al., 2006; Szatmari et al., 2007). Finally, a de novo autism mutation was detected that leads to truncation of *SHANK3* (on 22q13), which encodes an intracellular postsynaptic scaffolding protein that binds to neuroligins (Durand et al., 2007). The 22q13 microdeletion syndrome that includes *SHANK3* also sometimes includes autistic symptoms (Durand et al., 2007). Taken together, these uncommon mutation events point to disruption of the genes responsible for synaptic regulation in a very small group of patients with autism, most of whom also have severe cognitive or speech deficits.

Elevated platelet serotonin levels in about one-fourth of patients with autism led to investigation of the SERT (*SLC6A4* on 17q11) as a primary candidate gene. Association at the common functional variant 5-HTTLPR has been reported and replicated in many studies including the largest study (Devlin et al., 2005). However, the variability across studies may reflect the presence of multiple functional variants throughout the gene or a complex relationship between different SERT gene variants or alleles and particular symptoms of autism (Brune et al., 2006). Several different uncommon amino acid variants in the SERT gene *SLC6A4* have now been reported in several families with autism spectrum disorder and compulsive behavior (Ozaki et al., 2003; Sutcliffe et al., 2005). The association with autism spectrum disorder appears limited to males in these families, in agreement with the linkage peak in this region that is limited to families containing males but not females affected with autism (Sutcliffe et al., 2005). Remarkably, each of the six reported *SLC6A4* variants associated with autism or OCD leads to increased SERT (Prasad et al., 2006). Future work may clarify whether other variants outside of the coding region contribute to autism susceptibility in the larger group of patients with autism.

Association at a common functional promoter variant in the hepatocyte growth factor receptor gene (*MET* on 7q31) was found in two populations within a single study (Campbell et al., 2006). The allele that leads to lower gene transcription is associated with an increased risk of autism. Interestingly, *MET* is important not only in cortical and cerebellar development, but also in immune and gastrointestinal function, which is sometimes reported to be altered in autism.

The remaining linkage and association studies in autism have identified several regions and genes of interest but without pointing to a clear functional gene variant that contributes to risk. The strongest and most consistent linkage signals have been reported on chromosomes 2q, 7q, 11p, and 17q, but several other linkage peaks have been reported (International Molecular Genetic Study of Autism Consortium, 1998, 2001; Yonan et al., 2003; Szatmari et al., 2007). Many single studies have reported association of a particular gene with autism. Association has been reported in multiple samples at a possibly functional promoter polymorphism in *RELN* (Persico et al., 2001); although replication attempts have been inconsistent. Replication studies have also confirmed association at *GABRB3*, *SLC25A12*, and *EN2*, although no functional variants have been identified (Cook et al., 1998; Buxbaum et al., 2001; Gharani et al., 2004).

Multiple studies have now considered subgroups, intermediate phenotypes, or endophenotypes in attempts to identify genes for autism. The most common approach has been subgrouping probands based upon language development in linkage studies (Alarcón et al., 2002). An example of the endophenotype approach is a genome-wide association study that identified *ITGB3* as a quantitative trait locus for platelet serotonin in an inbred population (Weiss et al., 2004). Other candidate traits for gene mapping include macrocephaly, language level, general level of intellectual functioning, degree of social and communication impairment, presence of seizure disorder, gender of proband, dysmorphology, and severity or specific nature of restricted and repetitive behaviors (Fig. 71.3).

Tourette Syndrome and Tic Disorders

Gilles de la Tourette Syndrome (GTS) has prevalence rates of around 0.05% and significant evidence for a genetic component. Twin studies have found a monozygotic concordance rate of 53%–56% and a dizygotic concordance rate of 8% (Price et al., 1985; Hyde et al., 1992). This is consistent with a reported first-degree relative recurrence rate of around 9%. The recurrence rate is higher among male relatives. When affection status is broadened to include chronic tics or OCD, a much higher recurrence rate is observed.

A number of chromosomal anomalies have been reported in GTS, a de novo inversion event on chromosome 13q in one patient led State and colleagues to

TABLE 71.3 *Summary of Genetic Findings in Autism Spectrum Disorder*

Replicated Cytogenetic Findings	*Chromosomes with Most Significant Evidence for Linkage*	*Genes with Rare Functional Variants or Mutations*	*Genes with Associated Common Functional Variants*	*Genes with Replicated Association but no Known Functional Variant*
Maternally inherited chromosome 15q11-q13 duplications	2q	*NLGN3*	*SLC6A4*	*GABRB3*
	7q	*NLGN4*	*MET*	*SLC25A12*
Numerous other chromosomal abnormalities and copy number variants	11p	*SHANK3*	*RELN*	*EN2*
	17q	*SLC6A4*		
		NRXN1		

screen the Slit and trk-like 1 gene (*SLITRK1*), where they identified a truncation mutation in one family that cosegregated with GTS or trichotillomania. This truncation mutation disrupted the ability of *SLITRK1* expression to induce dendritic outgrowth (Abelson et al., 2005). They also identified a rare variant in two patients in the distal untranslated region of the gene that altered micro-RNA binding; although this variant may be enriched in Ashkenazi Jewish populations independent of GTS (Keen-Kim et al., 2006).

Other chromosomal anomalies have been found in GTS that disrupt a gene, but no other mutations or functional variants have been detected. Inverted duplication of chromosome 7q22.1-q31.1 disrupted *IMMP2L*, the inner mitochondrial membrane peptidase subunit 2-like gene (Petek et al., 2001). An inversion on chromosome 18q21-q22 alters replication timing but does not clearly disrupt a single gene.

Linkage analysis in GTS has been less fruitful than was initially expected. Despite a number of focused linkage studies, no evidence has been found for linkage to the regions implicated by chromosomal findings. Regions with some evidence for linkage include chromosomes 2p, 3q, 4q, 8p and 11q (The Tourette Syndrome Association International Consortium for Genetics [TSAICG], 1999; Merette et al., 2000; Verkerk et al., 2006; TSAICG, 2007). A few gene association findings have been reported, but none have been consistent across studies.

Attention-Deficit/Hyperactivity Disorder

Attention-deficit/hyperactivity disorder (ADHD) is the most common childhood psychiatric disorder, with prevalence rates of 7%–11% in school-age children and much higher prevalence in males than in females. Twin studies have found a monozygotic concordance rate of 51%–58% and a dizygotic concordance rate of 31%–33% (Goodman and Stevenson, 1989; Sherman et al., 1997). The recurrence rate in first-degree relatives is approximately 25%, with higher rates in males (Biederman et al., 1992). Higher recurrence rates are identified when subgroups of ADHD are considered (Faraone et al., 2000).

The candidate gene approach in ADHD has generated some encouraging results within the monoamine systems. The overall picture of association at multiple genes suggests that many common alleles with small effects lead to risk for ADHD. Cook and colleagues (1995) originally reported association at a variable number tandem repeat (VNTR) in the 3' untranslated region (UTR) of the DA transporter (DAT) gene *SLC6A3*. This 3' UTR VNTR acts as a transcriptional enhancer in transfection DA neurons (Michelhaugh et al., 2001). Caution in considering the 3' UTR VNTR as more than a marker is suggested by subsequent studies finding considerable variability in association signals across samples, and stronger evidence for association when other polymorphisms are also included in analyses (Asherson et al., 2007). Recent studies suggest that *SLC6A3* genotype may interact with prenatal exposure to alcohol or nicotine to confer risk of ADHD (Kahn et al., 2003; Brookes et al., 2006). Patients who were homozygous for the less active form of the *SLC6A3* 3' VNTR have a poorer response to methylphenidate (Stein et al., 2005). Further subgroup or quantitative trait analyses will be needed to clarify the role of DAT variants in ADHD susceptibility (Mazei-Robinson and Blakely, 2006).

Multiple studies in ADHD have also found significant association at a VNTR polymorphism in exon 3 of the DA receptor D_4 gene (*DRD4*) (Ebstein et al., 1996). The seven-copy repeat leads to a less responsive version of the receptor and is associated with ADHD across multiple samples (Li et al., 2006). Despite the functional nature of the exon 3 polymorphism, other polymorphisms could also be involved, and evidence for association has also been found at a promoter repeat element (McCracken et al., 2000).

Associations have also been reported in ADHD at common functional variants in the SERT gene *SLC6A4* (Kent et al., 2002), the norepinephrine transporter gene *SLC6A2* (Kim et al., 2006), and the DA β-hydroxylase gene (*DBH*) (Daly et al., 1999; Tang et al., 2006). Multiple other gene associations have been reported in ADHD without clear identification of a functional polymorphism. Replicated family-based associations have also been reported for the synaptic vesicle docking protein gene *SNAP25* and the serotonin receptor 5-HT_{1B} gene (*HTR1B*) (Barr et al., 2000; Hawi et al., 2002).

Despite multiple candidate gene variants with evidence for association, initial linkage studies appear to

TABLE 71.4 *Summary of Genetic Findings in Attention-Deficit/Hyperactivity Disorder*

Chromosomes with Most Significant Evidence for Linkage	*Candidate Genes with Associated Common Functional Variants*	*Candidate Genes with Replicated Association but no Known Functional Variant*
5p	*SLC6A3*	*SNAP25*
17p	*DRD4*	*HTR1B*
	SLC6A4	
	SLC6A3	
	DBH	

point to other gene variants that may contribute a larger risk of ADHD. Multiple linkage studies have pointed to regions on chromosomes 5p (Hebebrand et al., 2006) and 17p (Ogdie et al., 2004), with significant peaks also reported for 4q, 11q, and 16p (Smalley et al., 2002; Arcos-Burgos et al., 2004). Quantitative trait approaches may be quite helpful in ADHD but will likely need to use more extensive behavior rating scales than simply the *Diagnostic and Statistical Manual of Mental Disorders*, 4th ed. (*DSM-IV*; American Psychiatric Association, 1994) criteria. More sophisticated quantitative trait analyses have already been explored in association studies (Waldman et al., 1998; Curran et al., 2001). (Fig. 71.4)

Eating Disorders

Anorexia nervosa (AN) and bulimia nervosa (BN) typically have onset in adolescence and appear to have some overlapping genetic susceptibility. Anorexia nervosa has an incidence of about 0.5%, and BN has an incidence of about 1.5% among women. The largest twin study in AN found a monozygotic concordance rate of 56% in comparison to 5% among dizygotic twins (Holland et al., 1988). Twin studies in BN report monozygotic concordance rates ranging from 8% to 23% compared to 0%–9% in dizygotic twins (Bulik et al., 2000). A recent large family study used anorexia and bulimia probands to demonstrate a significant overlap in genetic susceptibility. The rate of AN was 3.4% in first-degree relatives of AN probands. The rate of BN was 4% in first-degree relatives of BN probands. The rates of each disorder in the relatives of probands with the other disorder were almost identical (Strober et al., 2000).

The first eating disorders linkage study identified a region on chromosome 1p in families with two or more relatives with restricting AN (Grice et al., 2002). Subsequent studies with an expanded group of families have identified additional linkage peaks with quantitative traits thought to underlie the AN and BN phenotypes (Devlin et al., 2002; Bacanu et al., 2005). Two association studies have now separately reported association findings within the serotonin receptor 1D gene (*HTR1D*) and the opioid receptor delta 1 gene (*OPRD1*) under the chromosome 1p linkage peak (Bergen et al., 2003; Brown et al., 2007). Numerous other candidate genes have been considered without replication across studies.

Obsessive–Compulsive Disorder

Obsessive–compulsive disorder has a variable onset that includes children and adolescents. Family studies using adult probands have found that an early age at onset of obsessive–compulsive symptoms is strongly related to a more familial form of the disorder (Nestadt et al., 2000). Family studies using child and adolescent probands have also consistently indicated that OCD is familial with a recurrence risk of 17%–23% in first-degree relatives (Chabane et al., 2005; do Rosario-Campos et al., 2005). Recurrence risk clusters in families, with a minority of early-onset OCD probands having an affected first-degree relative, and most of those having multiple relatives who are affected within a single family, suggest a subgroup with higher genetic risk (do Rosario-Campos et al., 2005).

The first small genome screen in extended families ascertained through early-onset OCD probands found suggestive linkage on chromosome 9p24 (Hanna et al., 2002). A replication study on 9p24 found a nearly identical linkage signal using the same analysis parameters in families ascertained through adult OCD probands (Willour et al., 2004). Two studies have now detected association at the glutamate transporter gene *SLC1A1* on 9p24, with both studies finding stronger association in male probands (Arnold et al., 2006; Dickel et al., 2006); although no functional allele has been identified.

Other linkage studies in OCD have also been promising but have not generated significant evidence for linkage. A second small genome screen in early-onset OCD identified a suggestive linkage signal on chromosome 10p. Fine mapping in this region revealed an association signal at three adjacent polymorphisms including an amino acid change at a conserved residue in *ADAR3*, which encodes an adenosine deaminase enzyme involved in RNA editing (Hanna et al., 2007). The ADAR enzyme family is responsible for editing the mRNA transcripts of multiple neurotransmitter receptors, including the serotonin 5-HT_{2C} receptor (see PWS section above) and glutamate receptors (Nishikura, 2006). Fruit flies lacking the single ADAR gene present in *Drosophila* show uncoordinated movements and markedly increased grooming behavior (Palladino et al., 2000), although multiple steps are necessary before this should be viewed as a genetic model for OCD. The largest linkage study using adult probands with OCD found one region on chromosome 3q that nearly met criteria for significance (Shugart et al., 2006). Linkage studies of hoarding behavior within OCD or GTS pedigrees have identified significant evidence for linkage on chromosomes 4q, 5q, 14q, and 17q (Zhang et al., 2002; Samuels et al., 2007).

The candidate gene approach in OCD has focused on the serotonin system. Pooled analysis supports association of the long allele of the SERT gene 5-HTTLPR promoter polymorphism across published studies in OCD (Dickel et al., 2007). Functional studies show that the 5-HTTLPR long allele has increased transcription in comparison to the short allele (Heils et al., 1996), but a single nucleotide polymorphism (SNP) also alters transcription (Hu et al., 2006). Inclusion of this SNP in the analyses strengthened evidence for association to OCD in one sample (Hu et al., 2006). Adding further support for SERT gain-of-function alleles in OCD, an uncommon SERT amino acid variant has been detected in several families with a complex pattern of psychiatric disorders, including OCD, autism spectrum disorders, and anorexia (Ozaki et al., 2003). This isoleucine to valine change (Ile425Val) results in increased cell surface expression of SERT and increased 5-HT transport (Prasad et al., 2005).

COMPLEX GENETIC DISORDERS THAT ARE FREQUENTLY COMORBID IN CHILD PSYCHIATRY

Reading Disability

Susceptibility to specific reading disability (RD), also called *developmental dyslexia*, has a substantial genetic component. Reading disability is a common disorder with a prevalence of 5%–10%, with a male–female ratio as high as 4:1. The largest twin study finds a concordance rate of 68% in monozygotic twins, in comparison to 38% in dizygotic twins (DeFries and Alarcon, 1996). Family studies have found a recurrence rate of around 35%–45% in first-degree relatives (Pennington et al., 1991).

A number of genetic findings have been consistently replicated in RD. Chromosome 15q contains the *DYX1C1* gene first identified through translocation mapping and subsequently associated with RD (Taipale et al., 2003). Two adjacent genes, *KIAA0319* and *DCDC2*, within a linkage region on chromosome 6p, are strongly associated with RD (Cope et al., 2005; Meng et al., 2005). Finally, single studies have implicated the *ROBO1* gene on chromosome 3p and the *MRPL19* and *C2ORF3* genes on chromosome 2p (Hannula-Jouppi et al., 2005; Anthoni et al., 2007). Remarkably, each of these genes appears to play a role in neuronal migration, which is the most common abnormality in brain imaging studies in RD (McGrath et al., 2006). Regions of linkage on chromosomes 1p, 18p, and Xq suggest that additional genes may also be implicated (McGrath et al., 2006).

Communication Disorders

Communication disorders can be divided into two types: speech disorders and language disorders. Stuttering is a disorder of speech fluency. Twin and family studies have shown that stuttering has a significant genetic component. A significant linkage signal has been reported on chromosome 12q (Riaz et al., 2005), and a significant linkage signal confined to females has been reported on chromosome 21 (Suresh et al., 2006).

Specific language impairment (SLI) refers to a developmental disorder leading to language deficits in children with otherwise intact cognition. Twin studies suggest that SLI has a significant genetic component as well; however, most families with language disorders show complex patterns of inheritance. One four-generation extended family with autosomal dominant orofacial dyspraxia and deficits in language processing allowed identification of the first speech and language disorder susceptibility gene on chromosome 7q31, *FOXP2*, which encodes a putative transcription factor (Lai et al., 2001). Linkage studies have identified significant evidence on other chromosomes including 13q, 16q, and 19q (Bartlett et al., 2002; Specific Language Impairment Consortium, 2004).

SUMMARY

The dominant theme in child psychiatry genetics is complexity. Even relatively simple genetic disorders such as RTT have allelic heterogeneity leading to different phenotypes depending on the mutation. Syndromes such as autism are likely to show locus heterogeneity, with variants in many different gene combinations producing clinically indistinguishable phenotypes, at least at this point. Within most of the childhood psychiatric disorders, investigators will find oligogenic inheritance, with multiple genetic variants required to produce susceptibility to disease. Some disorders, like attention deficit disorder, may be the summation of multiple quantitative trait loci that produce a spectrum with maladaptive behavior at its extreme.

As we learn to sort out the complex relationships between genetic variants and disease, we must also start considering the relationship between genetic and environmental influences. With advancing molecular genetic methods, we will be able to identify all of the susceptibility variants for a given child psychiatric disease; however, our mission does not stop there. Although it is possible to identify environmental factors in multifactorial diseases without any genetic knowledge, this task will become much easier when the genetic susceptibility of each individual can be calculated. For example, Caspi and colleagues (2003) identified the short allele of the *SLC6A4* 5-HTTLPR polymorphism as a risk factor for depression in the context of stressful life events. The intersection of genetic and environmental studies may yield unsuspected maternal, placental, and childhood environmental factors that increase susceptibility to disease.

It is important to note that susceptibility genes are often protective genes in other genetic and environmental contexts. The classic example is the protection against malaria conferred by heterozygosity for the sickle cell trait, which leads to sickle cell anemia in homozygous individuals (Aidoo et al., 2002). A hypothetical example in child psychiatry would be a genetic variant that would increase susceptibility to autism in one context but increase concentration and focus in another context (for example, in patients who have other risk factors for ADHD). It is also important to remember that the advantage of susceptibility genes in other contexts may not be related to brain development, but instead to resistance to infectious or cardiac disease.

Despite the caution that must be exercised in using limited genetic knowledge (as well as other knowledge that is incomplete) to make decisions with far-reaching consequences, the potential rewards of molecular genetic studies in child psychiatry are great. Genetic studies will enable identification of novel protein systems that lead to disease. New drugs will be developed that relieve symptoms. It is important to note that the insulin locus is a weak susceptibility gene in Type I diabetes, but a powerful treatment. When six or more genes act in concert to cause disease (for example, most complex genetic disorders), it may be possible to prevent or treat disease by correcting only one of their RNA or protein products.

REFERENCES

Abelson, J.F., Kwan, K.Y., O'Roak, B.J., Baek, D.Y., Stillman, A.A., Morgan, T.M., Mathews, C.A., Pauls, D.L., Rasin, M.R., Gunel, M., Davis, N.R., Ercan-Sencicek, A.G., Guez, D.H., Spertus, J.A., Leckman, J.F., Dure, L.St., Kurlan, R., Singer, H.S., Gilbert, D.L., Farhi, A., Louvi, A., Lifton, R.P., Sestan, N., and State, M.W. (2005) Sequence variants in SLITRK1 are associated with Tourette's syndrome. *Science* 310:317–320.

Aidoo, M., Terlouw, D.J., Kolczak, M.S., McElroy, P.D., ter Kuile, F.O., Kariuki, S., Nahlen, B.L., Lal, A.A., and Udhayakumar, V. (2002) Protective effects of the sickle cell gene against malaria morbidity and mortality. *Lancet* 359:1311–1312.

Alarcón, M., Cantor, R., Liu, J., Gilliam, T., Autism Genetic Resource Exchange Consortium, and Geschwind, D. (2002) Evidence for a language quantitative trait locus on chromosome 7q in multiplex autism families. *Am. J. Hum. Genet.* 70:60–71.

American Psychiatric Association. (1994) *Diagnostic and Statistical Manual of Mental Disorders*, 4th ed. Washington, DC: Author.

Amir, R.E., Van den Veyver, I.B., Wan, M., Tran, C.Q., Francke, U., and Zoghbi, H.Y. (1999) Rett syndrome is caused by mutations in X-linked MECP2, encoding methyl-CpG-binding protein 2. *Nat. Genet.* 23:185–188.

Anthoni, H., Zucchelli, M., Matsson, H., Muller-Myhsok, B., Fransson, I., Schumacher, J., Massinen, S., Onkamo, P., Warnke, A., Griesemann, H., Hoffmann, P., Nopola-Hemmi, J., Lyytinen, H., Schulte-Korne, G., Kere, J., Nothen, M.M., and Peyrard-Janvid, M. (2007) A locus on 2p12 containing the co-regulated MRPL19 and C2ORF3 genes is associated to dyslexia. *Hum. Mol. Genet.* 16:667–677.

Arcos-Burgos, M., Castellanos, F.X., Pineda, D., Lopera, F., Palacio, J.D., Palacio, L.G., Rapoport, J.L., Berg, K., Bailey-Wilson, J.E., and Muenke, M. (2004) Attention-deficit/hyperactivity disorder in a population isolate: linkage to loci at 4q13.2, 5q33.3, 11q22, and 17p11. *Am. J. Hum. Genet.* 75:998–1014.

Arnold, P.D., Sicard, T., Burroughs, E., Richter, M.A., and Kennedy, J.L. (2006) Glutamate transporter gene SLC1A1 associated with obsessive-compulsive disorder. *Arch. Gen. Psychiatry* 63:769–776.

Asherson, P., Brookes, K., Franke, B., Chen, W., Gill, M., Ebstein, R.P., Buitelaar, J., Banaschewski, T., Sonuga-Barke, E., Eisenberg, J., Manor, I., Miranda, A., Oades, R.D., Roeyers, H., Rothenberger, A., Sergeant, J., Steinhausen, H.C., and Faraone, S.V. (2007) Confirmation that a specific haplotype of the dopamine transporter gene is associated with combined-type ADHD. *Am. J. Psychiatry* 164:674–677.

Bacanu, S.A., Bulik, C.M., Klump, K.L., Fichter, M.M., Halmi, K.A., Keel, P., Kaplan, A.S., Mitchell, J.E., Rotondo, A., Strober, M., Treasure, J., Woodside, D.B., Sonpar, V.A., Xie, W., Bergen, A.W., Berrettini, W.H., Kaye, W.H., and Devlin, B. (2005) Linkage analysis of anorexia and bulimia nervosa cohorts using selected behavioral phenotypes as quantitative traits or covariates. *Am. J. Med. Genet. B Neuropsychiatr. Genet.* 139:61–68.

Bailey, A., Le Couteur, A., Gottesman, I., Bolton, P., Simonoff, E., Yuzda, E., and Rutter, M. (1995) Autism as a strongly genetic disorder: Evidence from a British twin study. *Psychol. Med.* 25: 63–78.

Baron, C.A., Tepper, C.G., Liu, S.Y., Davis, R.R., Wang, N.J., Schanen, N.C., and Gregg, J.P. (2006) Genomic and functional profiling of duplicated chromosome 15 cell lines reveal regulatory alterations in UBE3A-associated ubiquitin-proteasome pathway processes. *Hum. Mol. Genet.* 15:853–869.

Barr, C.L., Feng, Y., Wigg, K., Bloom, S., Roberts, W., Malone, M., Schachar, R., Tannock, R., and Kennedy, J.L. (2000) Identification of DNA variants in the SNAP-25 gene and linkage study of these polymorphisms and attention-deficit hyperactivity disorder. *Mol. Psychiatry* 5:405–409.

Bartlett, C.W., Flax, J.F., Logue, M.W., Vieland, V.J., Bassett, A.S., Tallal, P., and Brzustowicz, L.M. (2002) A major susceptibility locus for specific language impairment is located on 13q21. *Am. J. Hum. Genet.* 71:45–55.

Bear, M.F., Huber, K.M., and Warren, S.T. (2004) The mGluR theory of fragile X mental retardation. *Trends Neurosci.* 27:370–377.

Bergen, A.W., van den Bree, M.B., Yeager, M., Welch, R., Ganjei, J.K., Haque, K., Bacanu, S., Berrettini, W.H., Grice, D.E., Goldman, D., Bulik, C.M., Klump, K., Fichter, M., Halmi, K., Kaplan, A., Strober, M., Treasure, J., Woodside, B., and Kaye, W.H. (2003) Candidate genes for anorexia nervosa in the 1p33-36 linkage region: serotonin 1D and delta opioid receptor loci exhibit significant association to anorexia nervosa. *Mol. Psychiatry* 8:397–406.

Biederman, J., Faraone, S., Keenan, K., Benjamin, J., Krifcher, B., Moore, C., Sprich-Buckminster, S., Ugaglia, K., Jellinek, M., Steingard, R., Spencer, T., Norman, D., Kolodny, R., Kraus, I., Perrin, J., Keller, M., and Tsuang, M. (1992) Further evidence for family-genetic risk factors in attention deficit hyperactivity disorder: Patterns of comorbidity in probands and relatives in psychiatrically and pediatrically referred samples. *Arch. Gen. Psychiatry* 49:728–738.

Brookes, K.J., Mill, J., Guindalini, C., Curran, S., Xu, X., Knight, J., Chen, C.K., Huang, Y.S., Sethna, V., Taylor, E., Chen, W., Breen, G., and Asherson, P. (2006) A common haplotype of the dopamine transporter gene associated with attention-deficit/hyperactivity disorder and interacting with maternal use of alcohol during pregnancy. *Arch. Gen. Psychiatry* 63:74–81.

Brown, K.M., Bujac, S.R., Mann, E.T., Campbell, D.A., Stubbins, M.J., and Blundell, J.E. (2007) Further evidence of association of OPRD1 & HTR1D polymorphisms with susceptibility to anorexia nervosa. *Biol. Psychiatry* 61:367–373.

Brune, C.W., Kim, S.J., Salt, J., Leventhal, B.L., Lord, C., Cook, E.H. Jr. (2006) 5-HTTLPR genotype-specific phenotype in children and adolescents with autism. *Am. J. Psychiatry* 163:2148–2156.

Bulik, C.M., Sullivan, P.F., Wade, T.D., and Kendler, K.S. (2000) Twin studies of eating disorders: a review. *Int. J. Eat. Disord.* 27:1–20.

Buxbaum, J.D., Cai, G., Chaste, P., Nygren, G., Goldsmith, J., Reichert, J., Anckarsater, H., Rastam, M., Smith, C.J., Silverman, J.M., Hollander, E., Leboyer, M., Gillberg, C., Verloes, A., and Betancur, C. (2007) Mutation screening of the PTEN gene in patients with autism spectrum disorders and macrocephaly. *Am. J. Med. Genet. B Neuropsychiatr. Genet.* 144:484–491.

Buxbaum, J.D., Silverman, J.M., Smith, C.J., Kilifarski, M., Reichert, J., Hollander, E., Lawlor, B.A., Fitzgerald, M., Greenberg, D.A., and Davis, K.L. (2001) Evidence for a susceptibility gene for autism on chromosome 2 and for genetic heterogeneity. *Am. J. Hum. Genet.* 68:1514–1520.

Campbell, D.B., Sutcliffe, J.S., Ebert, P.J., Militerni, R., Bravaccio, C., Trillo, S., Elia, M., Schneider, C., Melmed, R., Sacco, R., Persico, A.M., and Levitt, P. (2006) A genetic variant that disrupts MET transcription is associated with autism. *Proc. Natl. Acad. Sci. USA* 103:16834–16839.

Carlson, C., Papolos, D., Pandita, R.K., Faedda, G.L., Veit, S., Goldberg, R., Shprintzen, R., Kucherlapati, R., and Morrow, B. (1997) Molecular analysis of velo-cardio-facial syndrome patients with psychiatric disorders. *Am. J. Hum. Genet.* 60:851–859.

Caspi, A., Sugden, K., Moffitt, T.E., Taylor, A., Craig, I.W., Harrington, H., McClay, J., Mill, J., Martin, J., Braithwaite, A., and Poulton, R. (2003) Influence of life stress on depression: moderation by a polymorphism in the 5-HTT gene. *Science* 301: 386–389.

Chabane, N., Delorme, R., Millet, B., Mouren, M.C., Leboyer, M., and Pauls, D. (2005) Early-onset obsessive-compulsive disorder: a subgroup with a specific clinical and familial pattern? *J. Child Psychol. Psychiatry* 46:881–887.

Chakrabarti, S., and Fombonne, E. (2001) Pervasive developmental disorders in preschool children. *JAMA* 285:3093–3099.

Comoletti, D., De Jaco, A., Jennings, L.L., Flynn, R.E., Gaietta, G., Tsigelny, I., Ellisman, M.H., and Taylor, P. (2004) The Arg451Cys-neuroligin-3 mutation associated with autism reveals a defect in protein processing. *J. Neurosci.* 24:4889–4893.

Cook, E., Stein, M., Krasowski, M., Cox, N., Olkon, D., Kieffer, J., and Leventhal, B. (1995) Association of attention deficit disorder and the dopamine transporter gene. *Am. J. Hum. Genet.* 56:993–998.

Cook, E.H., Jr., Courchesne, R.Y., Cox, N.J., Lord, C., Gonen, D., Guter, S.J., Lincoln, A., Nix, K., Haas, R., Leventhal, B.L., and Courchesne, E. (1998) Linkage-disequilibrium mapping of autistic disorder, with 15q11-13 markers. *Am. J. Hum. Genet.* 62: 1077–1083.

Cope, N., Harold, D., Hill, G., Moskvina, V., Stevenson, J., Holmans, P., Owen, M.J., O'Donovan, M.C., and Williams, J. (2005) Strong evidence that KIAA0319 on chromosome 6p is a susceptibility gene for developmental dyslexia. *Am. J. Hum. Genet.* 76:581–591.

Curran, S., Mill, J., Sham, P., Rijsdijk, F., Marusic, K., Taylor, E., and Asherson, P. (2001) QTL association analysis of the DRD4 exon 3 VNTR polymorphism in a population sample of children screened with a parent rating scale for ADHD symptoms. *Am. J. Med. Genet.* 105:387–393.

The Cystic Fibrosis Genotype-Phenotype Consortium. (1993) Correlation between genotype and phenotype in patients with cystic fibrosis. *N. Engl. J. Med.* 329:1308–1313.

Daly, G., Hawi, Z., Fitzgerald, M., and Gill, M. (1999) Mapping susceptibility loci in attention deficit hyperactivity disorder: preferential transmission of parental alleles at DAT1, DBH and DRD5 to affected children. *Mol. Psychiatry* 4:192–196.

de Vries, P., Humphrey, A., McCartney, D., Prather, P., Bolton, P., and Hunt, A. (2005) Consensus clinical guidelines for the assessment of cognitive and behavioural problems in tuberous sclerosis. *Eur. Child Adolesc. Psychiatry* 14:183–190.

DeFries, J.C., and Alarcon, M. (1996) Genetics of specific reading disability. *Ment. Retard. Dev. Disabil. Res. Rev.* 2:39–47.

Devlin, B., Bacanu, S.A., Klump, K.L., Bulik, C.M., Fichter, M.M., Halmi, K.A., Kaplan, A.S., Strober, M., Treasure, J., Woodside, D.B., Berrettini, W.H., and Kaye, W.H. (2002) Linkage analysis of anorexia nervosa incorporating behavioral covariates. *Hum. Mol. Genet.* 11:689–696.

Devlin, B., Cook, E.H., Coon, H., Dawson, G., Grigorenko, E.L., McMahon, W., Minshew, N., Pauls, D., Smith, M., Spence, M. A., Rodier, P.M., Stodgell, C., and Schellenberg, G.D. (2005) Autism and the serotonin transporter: the long and short of it. *Mol. Psychiatry* 10:1110–1116.

Dickel, D., Veenstra-VanderWeele, J., Bivens, N., Wu, X., Fischer, D., Van Etten-Lee, M., Himle, J., Leventhal, B., Cook, E., and Hanna, G. (2007) Association studies of serotonin system candidate genes in early-onset obsessive-compulsive disorder. *Biol. Psychiatry* 61:322–329.

Dickel, D.E., Veenstra-VanderWeele, J., Cox, N.J., Wu, X., Fischer, D.J., Van Etten-Lee, M., Himle, J.A., Leventhal, B.L., Coo, E.H., Jr., and Hanna, G.L. (2006) Association testing of the positional and functional candidate gene SLC1A1/EAAC1 in early-onset obsessive-compulsive disorder. *Arch. Gen. Psychiatry* 63:778–785.

do Rosario-Campos, M.C., Leckman, J.F., Curi, M., Quatrano, S., Katsovitch, L., Miguel, E.C., and Pauls, D.L. (2005) A family study of early-onset obsessive-compulsive disorder. *Am. J. Med. Genet. B Neuropsychiatr. Genet.* 136:92–97.

Dolen, G., and Bear, M.F. (2005) Courting a cure for fragile X. *Neuron* 45:642–644.

Durand, C.M., Betancur, C., Boeckers, T.M., Bockmann, J., Chaste, P., Fauchereau, F., Nygren, G., Rastam, M., Gillberg, I.C., Anckarsater, H., Sponheim, E., Goubran-Botros, H., Delorme, R., Chabane, N., Mouren-Simeoni, M.C., de Mas, P., Bieth, E., Roge, B., Heron, D., Burglen, L., Gillberg, C., Leboyer, M., and Bourgeron, T. (2007) Mutations in the gene encoding the synaptic scaffolding protein SHANK3 are associated with autism spectrum disorders. *Nat. Genet.* 39:25–27.

Dykens, E.M. (2003) Anxiety, fears, and phobias in persons with Williams syndrome. *Dev. Neuropsychol.* 23:291–316.

Ebstein, R.P., Novick, O., Umansky, R., Priel, B., Osher, Y., Blaine, D., Bennett, E.R., Nemanov, L., Katz, M., and Belmaker, R.H. (1996) Dopamine D4 receptor (D4DR) exon III polymorphism associated with the human personality trait of novelty seeking. *Nat. Genet.* 12:78–80.

Elston, R.C., and Spence, A.M. (2006) Advances in statistical human genetics over the last 25 years. *Stat. Med.* 25:3049–3080.

Faraone, S.V., Biederman, J., and Monuteaux, M.C. (2000) Toward guidelines for pedigree selection in genetic studies of attention deficit hyperactivity disorder. *Genet. Epidemiol.* 18:1–16.

Feng, J., Schroer, R., Yan, J., Song, W., Yang, C., Bockholt, A., Cook, E.H., Jr., Skinner, C., Schwartz, C.E., and Sommer, S.S. (2006) High frequency of neurexin 1beta signal peptide structural variants in patients with autism. *Neurosci. Lett.* 409:10–13.

Friedman, L., Szabo, C., Ostermeyer, E., Dowd, P., Butler, L., Park, T., Lee, M., Goode, E., Rowell, S., and King, M. (1995) Novel inherited mutations and variable expressivity of BRCA1 alleles, including the founder mutation 185delAG in Ashkenazi Jewish families. *Am. J. Hum. Genet.* 57:1284–1297.

Gharani, N., Benayed, R., Mancuso, V., Brustowicz, L.M., and Millonig, J.H. (2004) Association of the homeobox transcription factor, ENGRAILED 2 with autism spectrum disorder. *Mol. Psychiatry* 9:474–484.

Goodman, R., and Stevenson, J. (1989) A twin study of hyperactivity—II. The aetiological role of genes, family relationships and perinatal adversity. *J. Child Psychol. Psychiatry* 30:691–709.

Gothelf, D., Feinstein, C., Thompson, T., Gu, E., Penniman, L., Van Stone, E., Kwon, H., Eliez, S., and Reiss, A.L. (2007) Risk factors for the emergence of psychotic disorders in adolescents with 22q11.2 deletion syndrome. *Am. J. Psychiatry* 164:663–669.

Grice, D.E., Halmi, K.A., Fichter, M.M., Strober, M., Woodside, D.B., Treasure, J.T., Kaplan, A.S., Magistretti, P.J., Goldman, D., Bulik, C.M., Kaye, W.H., and Berrettini, W.H. (2002) Evidence for a susceptibility gene for anorexia nervosa on chromosome 1. *Am. J. Hum. Genet.* 70:787–792.

Grossman, A.W., Aldridge, G.M., Weiler, I.J., and Greenough, W.T. (2006) Local protein synthesis and spine morphogenesis: Fragile X syndrome and beyond. *J. Neurosci.* 26:7151–7155.

Guy, J., Gan, J., Selfridge, J., Cobb, S., and Bird, A. (2007) Reversal of neurological defects in a mouse model of Rett syndrome. *Science* 315:1143–1147.

Hanna, G., Veenstra-Vander Weele, J., Cox, N., Boehnke, M., Himle, J., Curtis, G., Leventhal, B., and Cook, E. (2002) Genome-wide linkage analysis of families with obsessive-compulsive disorder ascertained through pediatric probands. *Am. J. Med. Genet. (Neuropsychiat. Genet.)* 114:541–552.

Hanna, G., Veenstra-VanderWeele, J., Cox, N., Van Etten, M., Fischer, D., Himle, J., Bivens, N., Wu, X., Roe, C., Hennessy, K., Dickel, D., Leventhal, B., and Cook, E. (2007) Evidence for a susceptibility locus on chromosome 10p15 in early-onset obsessive-compulsive disorder. *Biol. Psychiatry* 62:856–862.

Hannula-Jouppi, K., Kaminen-Ahola, N., Taipale, M., Eklund, R., Nopola-Hemmi, J., Kaariainen, H., and Kere, J. (2005) The axon guidance receptor gene ROBO1 is a candidate gene for developmental dyslexia. *PLoS Genet.* 1:e50.

Hawi, Z., Dring, M., Kirley, A., Foley, D., Kent, L., Craddock, N., Asherson, P., Curran, S., Gould, A., Richards, S., Lawson, D., Pay, H., Turic, D., Langley, K., Owen, M., O'Donovan, M., Thapar, A., Fitzgerald, M., and Gill, M. (2002) Serotonergic system and attention deficit hyperactivity disorder (ADHD): a potential susceptibility locus at the 5-HT(1B) receptor gene in 273 nuclear families from a multi-centre sample. *Mol. Psychiatry* 7:718–725.

Hebebrand, J., Dempfle, A., Saar, K., Thiele, H., Herpertz-Dahlmann, B., Linder, M., Kiefl, H., Remschmidt, H., Hemminger, U., Warnke, A., Knolker, U., Heiser, P., Friedel, S., Hinney, A., Schafer, H., Nurnberg, P., and Konrad, K. (2006) A genome-wide scan for attention-deficit/hyperactivity disorder in 155 German sib-pairs. *Mol. Psychiatry* 11:196–205.

Heils, A., Teufel, A., Petri, S., Stoeber, G., Riederer, P., Bengel, D., and Lesch, K.P. (1996) Allelic variation of human serotonin transporter gene expression. *J. Neurochem.* 66:2621–2624.

Hessl, D., Dyer-Friedman, J., Glaser, B., Wisbeck, J., Barajas, R.G., Taylor, A., and Reiss, A.L. (2001) The influence of environmental and genetic factors on behavior problems and autistic symptoms in boys and girls with fragile x syndrome. *Pediatrics* 108:88.

Hogart, A., Nagarajan, R.P., Patzel, K.A., Yasui, D.H., and Lasalle, J.M. (2007) 15q11-13 GABAA receptor genes are normally biallelically expressed in brain yet are subject to epigenetic dysregulation in autism-spectrum disorders. *Hum. Mol. Genet.* 16:691–703.

Holland, A.J., Sicotte, N., and Treasure, J. (1988) Anorexia nervosa: evidence for a genetic basis. *J. Psychosom. Res.* 32:561–571.

Hu, X.Z., Lipsky, R.H., Zhu, G., Akhtar, L.A., Taubman, J., Greenberg, B.D., Xu, K., Arnold, P.D., Richter, M.A., Kennedy, J.L., Murphy, D.L., and Goldman, D. (2006) Serotonin transporter promoter gain-of-function genotypes are linked to obsessive-compulsive disorder. *Am. J. Hum. Genet.* 78:815–826.

Hyde, T.M., Aaronson, B.A., Randolph, C., Rickler, K.C., and Weinberger, D.R. (1992) Relationship of birth weight to the phenotypic expression of Gilles de la Tourette's syndrome in monozygotic twins. *Neurology* 42:652–658.

International Molecular Genetic Study of Autism Consortium. (1998) A full genome screen for autism with evidence for linkage to a region on chromosome 7q. *Hum. Mol. Genet.* 7:571–578.

International Molecular Genetic Study of Autism Consortium. (2001) A genome wide screen for autism: Strong evidence for linkage to chromosomes 2q, 7q and 16p. *Am. J. Hum. Genet.* 69:570–581.

Jamain, S., Quach, H., Betancur, C., Rastam, M., Colineaux, C., Gillberg, I.C., Soderstrom, H., Giros, B., Leboyer, M., Gillberg, C., Bourgeron, T., Paris Autism Research International Sibpair Study. (2003) Mutations of the X-linked genes encoding neuroligins NLGN3 and NLGN4 are associated with autism. *Nat. Genet.* 34:27–29.

Jorde, L., Hasstedt, S., Ritvo, E., Mason-Brothers, A., Freeman, B., Pingree, C., McMahon, W., Peterson, B., Jenson, W., and Moll, A. (1991) Complex segregation analysis of autism. *Am. J. Hum. Genet.* 49:932–938.

Kahn, R.S., Khoury, J., Nichols, W.C., and Lanphear, B.P. (2003) Role of dopamine transporter genotype and maternal prenatal smoking in childhood hyperactive-impulsive, inattentive, and oppositional behaviors. *J. Pediatr.* 143:104–110.

Keen-Kim, D., Mathews, C.A., Reus, V.I., Lowe, T.L., Herrera, L.D., Budman, C.L., Gross-Tsur, V., Pulver, A.E., Bruun, R.D., Erenberg, G., Naarden, A., Sabatti, C., and Freimer, N.B. (2006) Overrepresentation of rare variants in a specific ethnic group may confuse interpretation of association analyses. *Hum. Mol. Genet.* 15:3324–3328.

Kent, L., Doerry, U., Hardy, E., Parmar, R., Gingell, K., Hawi, Z., Kirley, A., Lowe, N., Fitzgerald, M., Gill, M., and Craddock, N. (2002) Evidence that variation at the serotonin transporter gene influences susceptibility to attention deficit hyperactivity disorder (ADHD): analysis and pooled analysis. *Mol. Psychiatry* 7:908–912.

Kim, C.H., Hahn, M.K., Joung, Y., Anderson, S.L., Steele, A.H., Mazei-Robinson, M.S., Gizer, I., Teicher, M.H., Cohen, B.M., Robertson, D., Waldman, I.D., Blakely, R.D., and Kim, K.S. (2006) A polymorphism in the norepinephrine transporter gene alters promoter activity and is associated with attention-deficit hyperactivity disorder. *Proc. Natl. Acad. Sci. USA* 103:19164–19169.

Kishore, S., and Stamm, S. (2006) The snoRNA HBII-52 regulates alternative splicing of the serotonin receptor 2C. *Science* 311: 230–232.

Kuehn, B.M. (2007) CDC: autism spectrum disorders common. *JAMA* 297:940.

Lai, C.S., Fisher, S.E., Hurst, J.A., Vargha-Khadem, F., and Monaco, A.P. (2001) A forkhead-domain gene is mutated in a severe speech and language disorder. *Nature* 413:519–523.

Laumonnier, F., Bonnet-Brilhault, F., Gomot, M., Blanc, R., David, A., Moizard, M.P., Raynaud, M., Ronce, N., Lemonnier, E., Calvas, P., Laudier, B., Chelly, J., Fryns, J.P., Ropers, H.H., Hamel, B.C., Andres, C., Barthelemy, C., Moraine, C., and Briault, S. (2004) X-linked mental retardation and autism are associated with a mutation in the NLGN4 gene, a member of the neuroligin family. *Am. J. Hum. Genet.* 74:552–557.

Li, D., Sham, P.C., Owen, M.J., and He, L. (2006) Meta-analysis shows significant association between dopamine system genes and attention deficit hyperactivity disorder (ADHD). *Hum. Mol. Genet.* 15:2276–2284.

Mazei-Robinson, M.S., and Blakely, R.D. (2006) ADHD and the dopamine transporter: are there reasons to pay attention? *Handb. Exp. Pharmacol.* 175:373–415.

McBride, S.M., Choi, C.H., Wang, Y., Liebelt, D., Braunstein, E., Ferreiro, D., Sehgal, A., Siwicki, K.K., Dockendorff, T.C., Nguyen, H.T., McDonald, T.V., and Jongens, T.A. (2005) Pharmacological rescue of synaptic plasticity, courtship behavior, and mushroom body defects in a Drosophila model of fragile X syndrome. *Neuron* 45:753–764.

McCracken, J.T., Smalley, S.L., McGough, J.J., Crawford, L., Del'Homme, M., Cantor, R.M., Liu, A., and Nelson, S.F. (2000) Evidence for linkage of a tandem duplication polymorphism upstream of the dopamine D4 receptor gene (DRD4) with attention deficit hyperactivity disorder (ADHD). *Mol. Psychiatry* 5:531–536.

McGrath, L.M., Smith, S.D., and Pennington, B.F. (2006) Breakthroughs in the search for dyslexia candidate genes. *Trends Mol. Med.* 12:333–341.

Meng, H., Smith, S.D., Hager, K., Held, M., Liu, J., Olson, R.K., Pennington, B.F., DeFries, J.C., Gelernter, J., O'Reilly-Pol, T., Somlo, S., Skudlarski, P., Shaywitz, S.E., Shaywitz, B.A., Marchione, K., Wang, Y., Paramasivam, M., LoTurco, J.J., Page, G.P., and Gruen, J.R. (2005) DCDC2 is associated with reading disability and modulates neuronal development in the brain. *Proc. Natl. Acad. Sci. USA* 102:17053–17058.

Merette, C., Brassard, A., Potvin, A., Bouvier, H., Rousseau, F., Emond, C., Bissonnette, L., Roy, M.A., Maziade, M., Ott, J., and Caron, C. (2000) Significant linkage for Tourette syndrome in a large French Canadian family. *Am. J. Hum. Genet.* 67: 1008–1013.

Michelhaugh, S., Fiskerstrand, C., Lovejoy, E., Bannon, M., and Quinn, J.P. (2001) The dopamine transporter gene (SLC6A3) variable number of tandem repeats domain enhances transcription in dopamine neurons. *J. Neurochem.* 79:1033–1038.

Moncla, A., Malzac, P., Voelckel, M.A., Auquier, P., Girardot, L., Mattei, M.G., Philip, N., Mattei, J.F., Lalande, M., and Livet, M.O. (1999) Phenotype-genotype correlation in 20 deletion and 20 non-deletion Angelman syndrome patients. *Eur. J. Hum. Genet.* 7:131–139.

Nestadt, G., Samuels, J., Riddle, M., Bienvenu, O.J. 3rd, Liang, K.Y., LaBuda, M., Walkup, J., Grados, M., and Hoehn-Saric, R. (2000) A family study of obsessive-compulsive disorder. *Arch. Gen. Psychiatry* 57:358–363.

Nishikura, K. (2006) Editor meets silencer: crosstalk between RNA editing and RNA interference. *Nat. Rev. Mol. Cell. Biol.* 7: 919–931.

Nyhan, W. (1997) The recognition of Lesch-Nyhan syndrome as an inborn error of purine metabolism. *J. Inherit. Metab. Dis.* 20: 171–178.

Nystrom-Lahti, M., Parsons, R., Sistonen, P., Pylkkanen, L., Aaltonen, L.A., Leach, F.S., Hamilton, S.R., Watson, P., Bronson, E., Fusaro, R., et al. (1994) Mismatch repair genes on chromosomes 2p and 3p account for a major share of hereditary nonpolyposis colorectal cancer families evaluable by linkage. *Am. J. Hum. Genet.* 55:659–665.

Ogdie, M.N., Fisher, S.E., Yang, M., Ishii, J., Francks, C., Loo, S.K., Cantor, R.M., McCracken, J.T., McGough, J.J., Smalley, S.L., and Nelson, S.F. (2004) Attention deficit hyperactivity disorder: fine mapping supports linkage to 5p13, 6q12, 16p13, and 17p11. *Am. J. Hum. Genet.* 75:661–668.

Ozaki, N., Goldman, D., Kaye, W., Plotnikov, K., Greenberg, B., Rudnick, G., and Murphy, D. (2003) A missense mutation in the serotonin transporter is associated with a complex neuropsychiatric phenotype. *Mol. Psychiatry* 8:933–936.

Palladino, M.J., Keegan, L.P., O'Connell, M.A., and Reenan, R.A. (2000) A-to-I pre-mRNA editing in Drosophila is primarily involved in adult nervous system function and integrity. Cell 102: 437–449.

Paylor, R., Glaser, B., Mupo, A., Ataliotis, P., Spencer, C., Sobotka, A., Sparks, C., Choi, C.H., Oghalai, J., Curran, S., Murphy, K.C., Monks, S., Williams, N., O'Donovan, M.C., Owen, M.J., Scambler, P.J., and Lindsay, E. (2006) Tbx1 haploinsufficiency is linked to behavioral disorders in mice and humans: implications for 22q11 deletion syndrome. *Proc. Natl. Acad. Sci. USA* 103: 7729–7734.

Pennington, B.F., Gilger, J.W., Pauls, D., Smith, S.A., Smith, S.D., and DeFries, J.C. (1991) Evidence for major gene transmission of developmental dyslexia. *JAMA* 266:1527–1534.

Persico, A., D'Agruma, L., Maiorano, N., Totaro, A., Militerni, R., Bravaccio, C., Wassink, T., Schneider, C., Melmed, R., Trillo, S., Montecchi, F., Palermo, M., Pascucci, T., Puglisi-Allegra, S., Reichelt, K.-L., Conciatori, M., Marino, R., Quattrocchi, C., Baldi, A., Zelante, L., Gasparini, P., and Keller, F. (2001) Reelin gene alleles and haplotypes as a factor predisposing to autistic disorder. *Mol. Psychiatry* 6:150–159.

Petek, E., Windpassinger, C., Vincent, J.B., Cheung, J., Boright, A.P., Scherer, S.W., Kroisel, P.M., and Wagner, K. (2001) Disruption of a novel gene (IMMP2L) by a breakpoint in 7q31 associated with Tourette syndrome. *Am. J. Hum. Genet.* 68:848–858.

Prasad, H.C., Sutcliffe, J.S., and Blakely, R.D. (2006, October) *Serotonin transporter variants identified in subjects with autism confer a gain-of-function phenotype arising from distinct mechanisms.* Paper presented at Society for Neuroscience Annual Meeting, Atlanta, GA.

Prasad, H.C., Zhu, C.B., McCauley, J.L., Samuvel, D.J., Ramamoorthy, S., Shelton, R.C., Hewlett, W.A., Sutcliffe, J.S., and Blakely, R.D. (2005) Human serotonin transporter variants display altered sensitivity to protein kinase G and p38 mitogen-activated protein kinase. *Proc. Natl. Acad. Sci. USA* 102:11545–11550.

Price, R.A., Kidd, K.K., Cohen, D.J., Pauls, D.L., and Leckman, J.F. (1985) A twin study of Tourette syndrome. *Arch. Gen. Psychiatry* 42:815–820.

Raux, G., Bumsel, E., Hecketsweiler, B., van Amelsvoort, T., Zinkstok, J., Manouvrier-Hanu, S., Fantini, C., et al. (2007) Involvement of hyperprolinemia in cognitive and psychiatric features of the 22q11 deletion syndrome. *Hum. Mol. Genet.* 16:83–91.

Riaz, N., Steinberg, S., Ahmad, J., Pluzhnikov, A., Riazuddin, S., Cox, N.J., and Drayna, D. (2005) Genomewide significant linkage to stuttering on chromosome 12. *Am. J. Hum. Genet.* 76: 647–651.

Samuels, J., Shugart, Y.Y., Grados, M.A., Willour, V.L., Bienvenu, O.J., Greenberg, B.D., Knowles, J.A., McCracken, J.T., Rauch, S.L., Murphy, D.L., Wang, Y., Pinto, A., Fyer, A.J., Piacentini, J., Pauls, D.L., Cullen, B., Rasmussen, S.A., Hoehn-Saric, R., Valle, D., Liang, K.Y., Riddle, M.A., and Nestadt, G. (2007) Significant linkage to compulsive hoarding on chromosome 14 in families with obsessive-compulsive disorder: results from the OCD Collaborative Genetics Study. *Am. J. Psychiatry* 164:493–499.

Samuels, J.F., Riddle, M.A., Greenberg, B.D., Fyer, A.J., McCracken, J.T., Rauch, S.L., Murphy, D.L., Grados, M.A., Pinto, A., Knowles, J.A., Piacentini, J., Cannistraro, P.A., Cullen, B., Bienvenu, O.J. 3rd, Rasmussen, S.A., Pauls, D.L., Willour, V.L., Shugart, Y.Y., Liang, K.Y., Hoehn-Saric, R., and Nestadt, G. (2006) The OCD collaborative genetics study: methods and sample description. *Am. J. Med. Genet. B Neuropsychiatr. Genet.* 141:201–207.

Schalock, R.L., Luckasson, R.A., Shogren, K.A., Borthwick-Duffy, S., Bradley, V., Buntinx, W.H., Coulter, D.L., Craig, E.M., Gomez, S.C., Lachapelle, Y., Reeve, A., Snell, M.E., Spreat, S., Tasse, M.J., Thompson, J.R., Verdugo, M.A., Wehmeyer, M.L., and Yeager, M.H. (2007) The renaming of mental retardation: understanding the change to the term intellectual disability. *Intellect. Dev. Disabil.* 45:116–124.

Schroer, R.J., Phelan, M.C., Michaelis, R.C., Crawford, E.C., Skinner, S.A., Cuccaro, M., Simensen, R.J., Bishop, J., Skinner, C., Fender, D., Stevenson, R.E. (1998) Autism and maternally derived aberrations of chromosome 15q. *Am. J. Med. Genet.* 76: 327–336.

Sebat, J., Lakshmi, B., Malhotra, D., Troge, J., Lese-Martin, C., Walsh, T., Yamrom, B., et al. (2007) Strong association of de novo copy number mutations with autism. *Science* 316:445–449.

Sherman, D.K., McGue, M.K., and Iacono, W.G. (1997) Twin concordance for attention deficit hyperactivity disorder: a comparison of teachers' and mothers' reports. *Am. J. Psychiatry* 154:532–535.

Shugart, Y.Y., Samuels, J., Willour, V.L., Grados, M.A., Greenberg, B.D., Knowles, J.A., McCracken, J.T., Rauch, S.L., Murphy, D.L., Wang, Y., Pinto, A., Fyer, A.J., Piacentini, J., Pauls, D.L., Cullen, B., Page, J., Rasmussen, S.A., Bienvenu, O.J., Hoehn-Saric, R., Valle, D., Liang, K.Y., Riddle, M.A., and Nestadt, G. (2006) Genomewide linkage scan for obsessive-compulsive disorder: evidence for susceptibility loci on chromosomes 3q, 7p, 1q, 15q, and 6q. *Mol. Psychiatry* 11:763–770.

Skuse, D., James, R., Bishop, D., Coppin, B., Dalton, P., Aamodt-Leeper, G., Bacarese-Hamilton, M., Creswell, C., McGurk, R., and Jacobs, P. (1997) Evidence from Turner's syndrome of an imprinted X-linked locus affecting cognitive function. *Nature* 387:705–708.

Specific Language Impairment Consortium. (2004) Highly significant linkage to the SLI1 locus in an expanded sample of individuals affected by specific language impairment. *Am. J. Hum. Genet.* 74:1225–1238.

Smalley, S.L., Kustanovich, V., Minassian, S.L., Stone, J.L., Ogdie, M.N., McGough, J.J., McCracken, J.T., MacPhie, I.L., Francks, C., Fisher, S.E., Cantor, R.M., Monaco, A.P., and Nelson, S.F. (2002) Genetic linkage of attention-deficit/hyperactivity disorder on chromosome 16p13, in a region implicated in autism. *Am. J. Hum. Genet.* 71:959–963.

Starck, L., Lovgren-Sandblom, A., and Bjorkhem, I. (2002) Cholesterol treatment forever? The first Scandinavian trial of cholesterol supplementation in the cholesterol-synthesis defect Smith-Lemli-Opitz syndrome. *J. Intern. Med.* 252:314–321.

Stein, M.A., Waldman, I.D., Sarampote, C.S., Seymour, K.E., Robb, A.S., Conlon, C., Kim, S.J., and Cook, E.H. (2005) Dopamine transporter genotype and methylphenidate dose response in children with ADHD. *Neuropsychopharmacol.* 30:1374–1382.

Strober, M., Freeman, R., Lampert, C., Diamond, J., and Kaye, W. (2000) Controlled family study of anorexia nervosa and bulimia nervosa: evidence of shared liability and transmission of partial syndromes. *Am. J. Psychiatry* 157:393–401.

Suresh, R., Ambrose, N., Roe, C., Pluzhnikov, A., Wittke-Thompson, J.K., Ng, M.C., Wu, X., Cook, E.H., Lundstrom, C., Garsten, M., Ezrati, R., Yairi, E., and Cox, N.J. (2006) New complexities in the genetics of stuttering: significant sex-specific linkage signals. *Am. J. Hum. Genet.* 78:554–563.

Sutcliffe, J.S., Delahanty, R.J., Prasad, H.C., McCauley, J.L., Han, Q., Jiang, L., Li, C., Folstein, S.E., and Blakely, R.D. (2005) Allelic heterogeneity at the serotonin transporter locus (SLC6A4) confers susceptibility to autism and rigid-compulsive behaviors. *Am. J. Hum. Genet.* 77:265–279.

Szatmari, P., Paterson, A.D., Zwaigenbaum, L., Roberts, W., Brian, J., Liu, X.Q., Vincent, J.B., et al. (2007) Mapping autism risk loci using genetic linkage and chromosomal rearrangements. *Nat. Genet.* 39:319–328.

Taipale, M., Kaminen, N., Nopola-Hemmi, J., Haltia, T., Myllyluoma, B., Lyytinen, H., Muller, K., Kaaranen, M., Lindsberg, P.J., Hannula-Jouppi, K., and Kere, J. (2003) A candidate gene for developmental dyslexia encodes a nuclear tetratricopeptide repeat domain protein dynamically regulated in brain. *Proc. Natl. Acad. Sci. USA* 100:11553–11558.

Tang, Y., Buxbaum, S.G., Waldman, I., Anderson, G.M., Zabetian, C.P., Kohnke, M.D., and Cubells, J.F. (2006) A single nucleotide polymorphism at DBH, possibly associated with attention-deficit/hyperactivity disorder, associates with lower plasma dopamine beta-hydroxylase activity and is in linkage disequilibrium with two putative functional single nucleotide polymorphisms. *Biol. Psychiatry* 60:1034–1038.

Tierney, E., Nwokoro, N.A., Porter, F.D., Freund, L.S., Ghuman, J. K., Kelley, R.I. (2001) Behavior phenotype in the RSH/Smith-Lemli-Opitz syndrome. *Am. J. Med. Genet.* 98:191–200.

The Tourette Syndrome Association International Consortium for Genetics. (1999) A complete genome screen in sib pairs affected by Gilles de la Tourette syndrome. *Am. J. Hum. Genet.* 65:1428–1436.

The Tourette Syndrome Association International Consortium for Genetics. (2007) Genome scan for Tourette disorder in affected-sibling-pair and multigenerational families. *Am. J. Hum. Genet.* 80:265–272.

Van Esch, H., Bauters, M., Ignatius, J., Jansen, M., Raynaud, M., Hollanders, K., Lugtenberg, D., Bienvenu, T., Jensen, L.R., Gecz, J., Moraine, C., Marynen, P., Fryns, J.P., and Froyen, G. (2005) Duplication of the MECP2 region is a frequent cause of severe mental retardation and progressive neurological symptoms in males. *Am. J. Hum. Genet.* 77:442–453.

van Woerden, G.M., Harris, K.D., Hojjati, M.R., Gustin, R.M., Qiu, S., de Avila Freire, R., Jiang, Y.H., Elgersma, Y., and Weeber, E.J. (2007) Rescue of neurological deficits in a mouse model for Angelman syndrome by reduction of alphaCaMKII inhibitory phosphorylation. *Nat. Neurosci.* 10:280–282.

Verkerk, A.J., Cath, D.C., van der Linde, H.C., Both, J., Heutink, P., Breedveld, G., Aulchenko, Y.S., and Oostra, B.A. (2006) Genetic and clinical analysis of a large Dutch Gilles de la Tourette family. *Mol. Psychiatry* 11:954–964.

Vorstman, J.A., Morcus, M.E., Duijff, S.N., Klaassen, P.W., Heineman-de Boer, J.A., Beemer, F.A., Swaab, H., Kahn, R.S., and van Engeland, H. (2006) The 22q11.2 deletion in children: high rate of autistic disorders and early onset of psychotic symptoms. *J. Am. Acad. Child Adolesc. Psychiatry* 45:1104–1113.

Waldman, I., Rowe, D., Abramowitz, A., Kozel, S., Mohr, J., Sherman, S., Cleveland, H., Sanders, M., Gard, J., and Stever, C. (1998) Association and linkage of the dopamine transporter gene and attention-deficit hyperactivity disorder in children: Heterogeneity owing to diagnostic subtype and severity. *Am. J. Hum. Genet.* 63:1767–1776.

Wang, Q., O'Brien, P.J., Chen, C.X., Cho, D.S., Murray, J.M., and Nishikura, K. (2000) Altered G protein-coupling functions of RNA editing isoform and splicing variant serotonin2C receptors. *J. Neurochem.* 74:1290–1300.

Weiss, L.A., Purcell, S., Waggoner, S., Lawrence, K., Spektor, D., Daly, M.J., Sklar, P., and Skuse, D. (2007) Identification of EFHC2 as a quantitative trait locus for fear recognition in Turner syndrome. *Hum. Mol. Genet.* 16:107–113.

Weiss, L.A., Veenstra-Vanderweele, J., Newman, D.L., Kim, S.J., Dytch, H., McPeek, M.S., Cheng, S., Ober, C., and Cook, E.H., Jr., Abney M (2004) Genome-wide association study identifies ITGB3 as a QTL for whole blood serotonin. *Eur. J. Hum. Genet.* 12:949–954.

Willour, V.L., Yao Shugart, Y., Samuels, J., Grados, M., Cullen, B., Bienvenu, O.J. 3rd, Wang, Y., Liang, K.Y., Valle, D., Hoehn-Saric, R., Riddle, M., and Nestadt, G. (2004) Replication study supports evidence for linkage to 9p24 in obsessive-compulsive disorder. *Am. J. Hum. Genet.* 75:508–513.

Yan, Q.J., Rammal, M., Tranfaglia, M., and Bauchwitz, R.P. (2005) Suppression of two major Fragile X Syndrome mouse model phenotypes by the mGluR5 antagonist MPEP. *Neuropharmacol.* 49:1053–1066.

Yonan, A.L., Alarcon, M., Cheng, R., Magnusson, P.K., Spence, S.J., Palmer, A.A., Grunn, A., Juo, S.H., Terwilliger, J.D., Liu, J., Cantor, R.M., Geschwind, D.H., and Gilliam, T.C. (2003) A genome-wide screen of 345 families for autism-susceptibility loci. *Am. J. Hum. Genet.* 73:886–897.

Zhang, H., Leckman, J.F., Pauls, D.L., Tsai, C.P., Kidd, K.K., and Campos, M.R. (2002) Genomewide scan of hoarding in sib pairs in which both sibs have Gilles de la Tourette syndrome. *Am. J. Hum. Genet.* 70:896–904.

72 Pediatric Bipolar Disorder

ELLEN LEIBENLUFT

Bipolar disorder (BD) in adults has received considerably more research attention than BD in youth, and more readers will have had the opportunity to observe the illness in adults than in children or adolescents. Therefore, this chapter begins with a brief discussion of how the clinical presentation, research opportunities, and methodological challenges differ between adult and pediatric BD.

A number of claims have been made about how the clinical presentation of BD in youth differs from that in adults. For example, articles frequently state that (*1*) BD in youth is characterized by a chronic, nonepisodic course; (*2*) pediatric mania is characterized by irritability, whereas euphoria is prominent in adult mania; and (*3*) comorbid attention-deficit/hyperactivity disorder (ADHD) is more common in youth with BD than in adults with BD, complicating the diagnostic process in children (Biederman, 2006).

However, not all of these claims are consistent with recent data. For example, studies of youth using assessment techniques similar to those used in adults identify samples of children and adolescents with clear-cut manic episodes meeting *Diagnostic and Statistical Manual of Mental Disorders* (*DSM-IV*; American Psychiatric Association, 1994) criteria (Kowatch et al., 2005; Axelson et al., 2006; Birmaher et al., 2006). Furthermore, 86% of these young patients with BD report euphoria during mania (Axelson et al., 2006), indicating that elated mood is the rule, rather than the exception, in pediatric mania. These same studies also show, however, that youth with BD cycle more rapidly than do adults with the illness, with a mean of 15.7 ± 17.5 changes in mood polarity per year versus 3.5 ± 7.4 in adults (Birmaher et al., 2006).

Data do support the claim that comorbid ADHD is more common in youth with BD than in adults with BD (for example, over 50% in youth vs. approximately 10% in adults) (Kowatch et al., 2005; Nierenberg et al., 2005; Birmaher et al., 2006). These rates apply when ADHD is diagnosed based on symptoms during euthymia, thus diminishing the confounding effect of symptom overlap between ADHD and mania. Important research questions include whether, and how, ADHD in a youth with BD differs pathophysiologically from ADHD in a youth without BD, and dissociating the impact of comorbid ADHD from that of BD on brain function in patients meeting criteria for both illnesses.

Given the contention that the clinical presentation of pediatric BD differs markedly from its adult presentation, some suggest that assessment techniques and diagnostic criteria used in adults should not be applied to children (Tillman and Geller, 2003; Mick et al., 2005). Different groups have proposed different modifications, complicating efforts to synthesize findings across research groups. Thus, readers of the literature should pay close attention to diagnostic criteria and assessment methods in studies of pediatric BD. It is particularly important to determine whether, and how, full-duration manic or hypomanic episodes were identified, to ensure that patients meet *DSM-IV* criteria for BD. Although the study of children with nonepisodic, impairing irritability and ADHD-like symptoms is an important area of research, such children do not meet *DSM-IV* criteria for BD, and it should not be assumed that the neurobiology of their illness is identical to that of youth meeting *DSM-IV* criteria for BD (Davanzo et al., 2003; Volk and Todd, 2006; Rich et al., 2007).

Thus, questions about the clinical presentation of pediatric BD have complicated neurobiological research. In addition, there are differences inherent in research with pediatric, rather than adult, patients. Some research techniques that are acceptable in adults are not so in children (for example, positron emission tomography [PET]), and some research methodologies are more feasible in youth than adults (for example, obtaining genetic trios). Also, youth with BD have not had lengthy exposure to either illness or psychotropic medication and are more likely than adults to have "affectively loaded" pedigrees (see below).

Finally, research on pediatric psychopathology is complex, in that it involves studying brain function that is being shaped by the trajectories of both normal development and an unfolding pathological process. Although this presents challenges to investigators, it also provides the opportunity to study pathology as it develops in young patients and in those at risk for highly heritable illnesses such as BD.

The literature on the neurobiology of pediatric BD is considerably more limited than the corresponding adult literature. Although most published research is phenomenological and descriptive, more investigators are now performing neurobiological studies. The chapter begins with a discussion of studies of cognitive and emotional information processing. This is followed by a review of the neuroimaging literature and of genetic studies. As will be seen, research indicates that youth with BD have specific deficits processing cognitive and emotional information. Structural and functional neuroimaging studies implicate prefrontal-amygdala-striatal circuitry in the pathophysiology of pediatric BD, consistent with studies in BD adults. Genetic studies in pediatric BD are so preliminary as to preclude conclusions at this time.

LABORATORY-BASED STUDIES OF COGNITIVE AND AFFECTIVE PROCESSES

In pediatric and adult BD, considerably more data have been collected on cognitive than affective processing. Because the core deficit of BD is mood dysregulation, more data regarding affective processing would be welcome. The cognitive domains most studied in pediatric BD are memory, sustained attention, response flexibility/set-shifting/motor inhibition, and responses to emotional stimuli. Deficits in verbal memory and sustained attention have been identified in youth with BD, as in adults, although the contribution of comorbid ADHD to such deficits is unclear. Studies also suggest that youth with BD perform poorly on set-shifting and/or response reversal tasks, as well as in labeling facial emotion.

Memory

Verbal memory and attentional deficits are the most commonly reported cognitive dysfunction in adults with BD (Glahn et al., 2004). Six studies (Doyle et al., 2005; Glahn et al., 2005; McClure, Treland, Snow, Dickstein, et al., 2005; Olvera et al., 2005; Pavuluri, Schenkel, et al., 2006; Rucklidge, 2006) document verbal memory deficits in youth with BD. Three of these find deficits only in youth with BD and comorbid ADHD (McClure, Treland, Snow, Dickstein, et al., 2005; Olvera et al., 2005; Rucklidge, 2006) whereas two find deficits in BD youth without comorbid ADHD (Doyle et al., 2005; Pavuluri, Schenkel, et al., 2006). In addition, three studies report diminished working memory for objects in patients versus controls (Dickstein et al., 2004; McClure, Treland, Snow, Dickstein, et al., 2005; Pavuluri, Schenkel, et al., 2006).

Sustained Attention

In adults with BD, variants of the continuous performance test (CPT) have been used to document sustained attention deficits, including trait-related target detection deficits and increased commission errors in mania (Clark and Goodwin, 2004). In pediatric BD, the literature is mixed. Three studies (Doyle et al., 2005; McClure, Treland, Snow, Schmajuk, et al., 2005; Pavuluri, Schenkel, et al., 2006) report deficient sustained attention in youth with BD, whereas two others (Robertson et al., 2003; DelBello et al., 2004) do not. One positive study (Pavuluri, Schenkel, et al., 2006) found that comorbid ADHD exacerbated the attentional deficit. Two studies (McClure, Treland, Snow, Schmajuk, et al., 2005; Pavuluri, Schenkel, et al., 2006) report that attentional deficits are present in patients with euthymia.

Response Flexibility/Set-Shifting/Motor Inhibition

Parents frequently observe that youth with BD have emotional outbursts when asked to shift from one activity to another. Such response inflexibility can result from perseveration, deficits in attentional set-shifting, motor disinhibition, or other pathology. A number of tasks assess these related domains, including the Wisconsin Card Sort Test (WCST), the Intradimensional/Extradimensional Shift (ID/ED), response reversal (RR) tasks, and stop signal or stop-change tasks.

Six studies using set-shifting or RR tasks demonstrate deficits in youth with BD (Dickstein et al., 2004; Doyle et al., 2005; Gorrindo et al., 2005; McClure, Treland, Snow, Schmajuk, et al., 2005; Olvera et al., 2005; Pavuluri, Schenkel, et al., 2006), with only one negative study (Robertson et al., 2003) (Table 72.1). Thus, the evidence for response inflexibility in youth with BD is rather strong. Such deficits may be independent of ADHD (Dickstein et al., 2004; Doyle et al., 2005; Gorrindo et al., 2005; although also see Olvera et al., 2005; Pavuluri, Schenkel, et al., 2006) and present in patients with euthymia (Dickstein et al., 2004; Gorrindo et al., 2005; Pavuluri, Schenkel, et al., 2006). Meyer et al. (2004) also reported increased perseveration on the WCST in youth at risk for BD who later develop the illness (Meyer et al., 2004).

Remarkably, given the high comorbidity with ADHD, relatively little attention has focused on motor inhibition in pediatric BD. One study (McClure, Treland, Snow, Schmajuk, et al., 2005) in pediatric BD used the stop signal task and reported a trend ($p < .07$) toward delayed inhibition in youth with BD versus controls. In the same study, youth with BD but without comorbid ADHD were significantly slower than controls on the stop-change task, which requires inhibiting one response and substituting an alternate one (McClure, Treland, Snow, Schmajuk, et al., 2005). In a related series of findings, investigators have reported slow processing speed in youth with BD (Doyle et al., 2005; Rucklidge, 2006).

TABLE 72.1 *Studies of Response Flexibility in Youth with Bipolar Disorder (BD)*

Citation	*Sample*	*Mean Age ± SD (y)*	*% ADHD (current) in BD*	*Task*	*Significant Findings in BD*
Robertson et al., 2003	44 BD 30 MDD 45 C	19.4 ± 2.9 18.5 ± 2.8 18.2 ± 1.6	7	Wisconsin Card Sort	None
Dickstein et al., 2004	21 BD 21 C	12.47 ± 2.37 12.68 ± 2.36	57	Intra/Extradimensional Shift	deficits on simple reversal
Doyle et al., 2005	57 BD 46 C	13.3 ± 2.4 13.6 ± 2.2	74[a]	Wisconsin Card Sort	↑ nonperseverative errors
Gorrindo et al., 2005	24 BD 25 C	13.6 ± 2.6 14.5 ± 1.8	67	Probabilistic Response Reversal	reversal learning deficit
McClure, Treland, Snow, Schmajuk, et al., 2005	40 BD 22 C	12.9 ± 2.7 13.5 ± 2.0	58	Stop-Change	slower to execute alternate response
Olvera et al., 2005	36 BD 16 C	15.3 ± 1.04 14.9 ± 1.44	67[b]	Wisconsin Card Sort	↑ perseverative and non-perseverative errors
Pavuluri, Schenkel, et al., 2006	56 BD[c] 28 C	12.01 ± 3.21 11.19 ± 2.57	52	Cogtest Set Shifting	↑ total error

ADHD: attention-deficit/hyperactivity disorder; BD: bipolar disorder; MDD: major depressive disorder; C: controls
[a]17% of C also had ADHD.
[b]25% of C also had ADHD; figures are for lifetime.
[c]50% unmedicated.

Responses to Emotional Stimuli

Three laboratory-based studies (McClure et al., 2003; McClure, Treland, Snow, Schmajuk, et al., 2005; Rich et al., in press), and behavioral data from one functional magnetic resonance imaging (fMRI) study described below (Rich et al., 2006), indicate that youth with BD have deficits labeling facial emotion. The deficit is not specific to a particular facial emotion (Rich et al., in press), is unrelated to mood state or comorbidity (McClure, Treland, Snow, Schmajuk, et al., 2005; Rich et al., in press), and distinguishes youth with BD from those with anxiety disorders and/or major depression, and from those with ADHD and/or conduct disorder (Guyer et al., 2007). Because pragmatic language deficits and face-labeling deficits are present in youth with autism spectrum disorders, it is interesting to note that pragmatic language deficits have also been reported in youth with BD (McClure, Treland, Snow, Schmajuk, et al., 2005; Towbin et al., 2005; Goldstein et al., 2006).

Two studies find that emotion impacts more adversely on attention in patients with BD than controls. In one, controls, but not youth with BD, devoted extra attentional resources, as indicated by increased P3 parietal amplitude, to a task as it became more frustrating. In another study, children with BD and comorbid anxiety disorders (ANX) showed an attentional bias toward threat faces; this bias differentiated them from controls, BD without ANX, and youth with ANX alone (Brotman et al., 2007). As more research focuses on affective processing, ANX comorbidity will require as much attention as ADHD comorbidity in studies of youth with BD.

Summary

In just a few years, a body of literature has developed documenting deficits in verbal memory, response flexibility, and face emotion labeling, although the latter findings are from one laboratory and require independent replication. Object memory and sustained attention require more study, as do emotion–attention interactions. Larger studies will clarify the effects of mood state, medication, and comorbid illnesses (ANX as well as ADHD). Future research should elucidate genetic influences on cognitive and affective information processing and include children at risk for BD.

These behavioral data are an important complement to structural MRI (sMRI) and fMRI studies (reviewed below). Response flexibility deficits are consistent with fMRI and lesion studies implicating ventral prefrontal cortex (PFC) in the pathophysiology of BD (Starkstein and Robinson, 1997; Blumberg, Leung, et al., 2003; Chang et al., 2004; Pavuluri, Schenkel, et al., 2006; Rich et al., 2006; Leibenluft et al., 2007). Deficits in emotional face processing are consistent with reports of decreased amygdala volume in pediatric BD, and with fMRI studies showing amygdala hyperactivation (vs. controls) in response to facial stimuli (Rich et al., 2006; Pavuluri, Schenkel, et al., 2006). Children and adults with BD have verbal memory deficits, and an fMRI study of verbal memory in adults with BD implicates the left dorsolateral PFC (DLPFC) (BA 46/9) (Deckersbach et al., 2006). The latter results, along with behavioral data suggesting adverse attention–emotion interactions in pediatric BD and sMRI and fMRI studies reviewed below, highlight the need for more research on cortical structure and function in pediatric BD.

NEUROIMAGING

Structural MRI

Of all the modalities used to study the neurobiology of pediatric BD, sMRI has been the most widely employed. Approximately 20 studies have been published, although only three (Lyoo et al., 2002; Frazier, Breeze, et al., 2005; Frazier, Chiu, et al., 2005) have a sample size greater than 25 patients. These small samples, combined with significant differences in methodology, preclude drawing firm conclusions; in particular, negative findings must be interpreted cautiously.

Nonetheless, several preliminary conclusions can be drawn. As detailed below, amygdala volume appears to be decreased in pediatric BD versus controls. Evidence also suggests decreased cortical gray matter in BD, although its precise location and extent bears further study. Finally, white matter hyperintensities (WMH) may be more common in BD than controls, but not in BD versus other childhood psychopathology.

Subcortical Structures

The most consistent finding in sMRI studies of pediatric BD is decreased amygdala volume relative to controls. In contrast, amygdala volume in adult BD has been reported to be increased, decreased, or unchanged (Lyoo et al., 2006). Six studies report amygdala volume in BD youth (Table 72.2). Four found significantly smaller volumes in patients versus controls (Blumberg, Kaufman, et al., 2003; DelBello, Zimmerman, et al., 2004; Chang, Karchemskiy, et al., 2005; Dickstein et al., 2005), one reported a trend (Chen et al., 2004), and the sixth and largest ($N = 43$ patients; Frazier, Chiu, et al., 2005) found no difference. One study rescanned 10 patients after 2 years and found persistently decreased amygdala volume (Blumberg et al., 2005). Another (Chang, Karchemskiy, et al., 2005) found that patients exposed to lithium or valproate tended to have larger amygdala volume than patients without such exposure, consistent with adult data (Bowley et al., 2002). Given evidence, reviewed below, suggesting that youth with BD have amygdala hyperactivity in certain emotional contexts, it is possible that decreased amygdala volume in this population may be due to glutamatergic neurotoxicity.

Data on hippocampal volume are mixed: two studies found decreased hippocampal volume in patients (Blumberg, Kaufman, et al., 2003; Frazier, Chiu, et al., 2005), but others have not (Chen et al., 2004; Chang, Karchemskiy, et al., 2005; Dickstein et al., 2005). As noted above, negative findings should be interpreted cautiously. Striatal data are limited, with three positive findings reported (DelBello, Zimmerman, et al., 2004; Wilke et al., 2004; Dickstein et al., 2005). Other studies (DelBello, Zimmerman, et al., 2004; Chang, Barnea-Goraly, et al., 2005; Frazier, Chiu, et al., 2005; Sanches, Roberts, et al., 2005) have not found between-group differences in striatal or thalamic volume. Morphometric studies in adults with BD have yielded similarly

TABLE 72.2 *Amygdala Volume in Pediatric Bipolar Disorder*

Citation	*Sample*	*Mean Age ± SD (y)*	*MR Methods*	*Analytic Method*	*Finding in BD vs. C*
Blumberg, Kaufman, et al., 2003	14 BD 23 C	Not provided[b]	1.5 T 1.2 mm slices	manual tracing	↓total AMYG, $p = .001$
DelBello, Zimmerman, et al., 2004	23 BD 20 C	16.3 ± 2.4 17.2 ± 1.9	1.5 T 1.5 mm slices	manual tracing	↓ total AMYG, $p = .02$
Chen et al., 2004	16 BD 21 C	16 ± 3.0 16 ± 4.0	1.5 T 1.5 mm slices	manual tracing	↓ L AMYG, $p = .06$
Chang, Karchemskiy, et al., 2005	20 BD[a] 20 C	14.6 ± 2.8 14.1 ± 2.8	3 T 1.5 mm slices	manual tracing	↓ L AMYG, $p = .046$ ↓ R AMYG, $p = .009$
Dickstein et al., 2005	20 BD 20 C	13.4 ± 2.5 13.3 ± 2.3	1.5 T 1.2 mm slices	voxel-based morphometry	↓ L AMYG, $p < .01$
Frazier, Chiu, et al., 2005	43 BD 20 C	11.3 ± 2.7 11.0 ± 2.6	1.5 T 1.5 mm slices	manual tracing	No difference

BD: bipolar disorder; C: controls; AMYG: amygdala; MR: magnetic resonance.
[a]all BD had familial illness.
[b]Range 10–22 years.

mixed results with regard to hippocampal, striatal, and thalamic abnormalities (Lyoo et al., 2006).

Cortical Volume

The most detailed study of cortical gray matter in pediatric BD found diffuse decreases in patients' cortical gray (Frazier, Breeze, et al., 2005), including the fusiform and parahippocampal gyri, consistent with literature suggesting deficits in face processing and memory. Diffuse cortical deficits were also found in a much smaller study that used voxel-based morphometry (Wilke et al., 2004). Another study reported decreased gray matter in the DLPFC (BA 9) (Dickstein et al., 2005), whereas others found no between-group differences in subgenual frontal volume (Sanches, Sassi, et al., 2005) or total cerebral volume (Chang, Barnea-Goraly, et al., 2005). Chen et al. (2004) found that patients had smaller superior temporal gyri than controls due to deficits in white, not gray, matter.

White Matter Hyperintensities (WMH)

White matter hyperintensities are among the most consistent sMRI findings in adults with BD (Lyoo et al., 2006). The prevalence of WMH increases with age, and risk factors for WMH include hypertension, alcohol abuse, and other confounding variables more common in adults than children. Therefore, the question of whether youth with BD have WMH is of interest. The largest study (Lyoo et al., 2002) examined 408 youth who were psychiatrically hospitalized, of whom 56 had BD. White matter intensities were more common in youth with BD rather than schizophrenia or controls (17.9%, 2.4%, and 1.2%, respectively), but WMH were as common in unipolar depression (13.8%) or conduct disorder/ADHD (13.6%) as BD. Thus, in children with BD as in adults (Breeze et al., 2003), WMH are more common in patients than in controls, but WMH are not specific to BD.

Functional MRI

Although the number of fMRI studies in pediatric BD remains small, there are many ongoing studies. The current literature, like that in adult BD, implicates a circuit including the amygdala, anterior cingulate cortex (ACC), striatum, and ventral and dorsal PFC.

Three fMRI studies in pediatric BD involve processing of emotional faces. In one event-related study (Rich et al., 2006), children with BD, compared to controls (*1*) saw neutral faces as more hostile; (*2*) were more afraid of neutral faces; and (*3*) had increased amygdala, striatal, and ventral PFC activation when assessing the hostility of the neutral face or their response to it (Figures 72.1a and 72.1b). A second, block design study found increased amygdala and decreased ventral and dorsal PFC activation in patients versus controls when viewing happy faces, suggesting diminished top-down control (Pavuluri, O'Connor, et al., 2006); similar findings have been reported in some, but not all, studies in adults with BD (for a review, see Yurgelun-Todd and Ross, 2006). A third study (Dickstein et al., 2007) found that, compared to controls, patients with BD had increased striatal and ACC activation when encoding happy faces and increased ventral PFC activation when encoding angry faces.

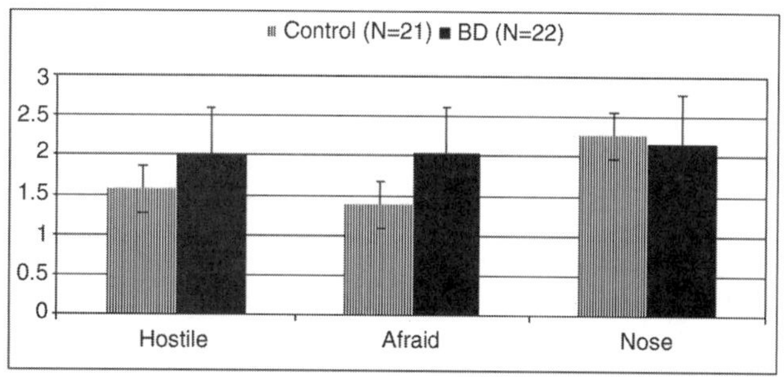

FIGURE 72.1a Patients view neutral faces and rate, on a 1–5 scale, the hostility on the face, how afraid they are of the face, and the width of the nose on the face. Patients with bipolar disorder (BD) view neutral faces as more hostile than do controls and are more afraid of them than are controls, but rate there are no between-group differences in nose width ratings. Thus, patients' ratings differ from controls when there attention is drawn to an emotional, but not to a nonemotional, facial feature (see Rich et al., 2006, for details).

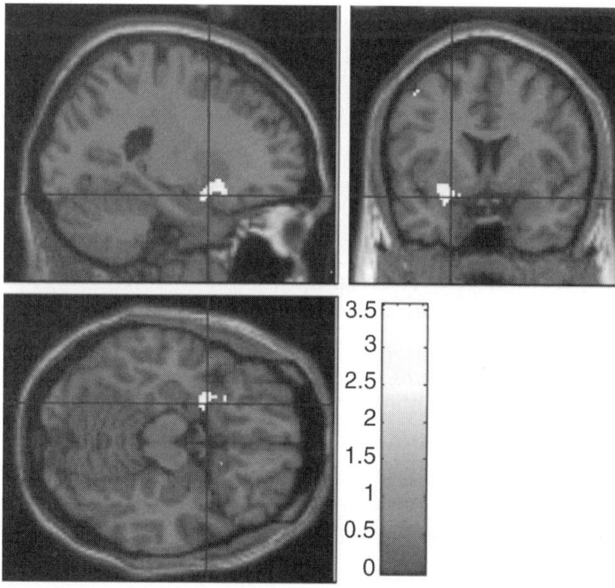

FIGURE 72.1b Neural activation when patients ($N = 22$ bipolar disorder, 21 controls) view neutral faces and rate the hostility on the face, versus rating nose width. Map shows regions activated more by patients than controls. Threshold $p < .005$, uncorrected. Area of increased activation in patients vs. controls includes left amygdala, $x = -22$, $y = 6$, $z = -16$, $t = 3.56$, $p < .001$ (see Rich et al., 2006, for details).

Thus, studies of face processing implicate the amygdala, striatum, and PFC, whereas studies using other behavioral paradigms further implicate the striatum and PFC. One found decreased striatal and ventral PFC activation in BD, versus controls, during failed motor inhibition, suggesting that patients may have a deficient striatal "error signal" (Leibenluft et al., 2007); similar findings were reported in a study of adults with euthymia with BD performing a Stroop task (Strakowski et al., 2005). In contrast, however, Blumberg, Martin, et al. (2003) found striatal hyperactivity in youth with BD performing a Stroop task (Blumberg, Martin, et al., 2003). These inconsistent results may be due to methodological and/or sample differences among studies. On a response flexibility task, Nelson et al. (2007) reported increased DLPFC activation in patients versus controls when successfully executing the flexible response (Nelson et al., 2007). Finally, Chang et al. (2004) found widespread between-group differences in striatal and limbic activation on a visuospatial working memory task and while rating responses to emotional pictures.

In sum, the fMRI literature in pediatric BD is just emerging. A major challenge for researchers will be to design tasks that probe psychological processes central to the disorder. Out-of-scanner studies, such as those reviewed above, can guide researchers in this regard. It is important to specify not only which circuits are dysfunctional in pediatric BD, but also the manner in which such dysfunction relates to particular behaviors as occurring in precise psychological contexts. Future studies will also address associations between neuroimaging results and clinical presentation, course, and genotype. Finally, no published fMRI studies compare adults and children performing the same task; such studies would be useful to identify the developmental trajectory of neural dysfunction in patients with BD.

Magnetic Resonance Spectroscopy

Magnetic resonance spectroscopy (MRS) studies in pediatric BD have focused on *N*-acetylaspartate (NAA), myoinostol (mI), and the glutamate/glutamine peak (Glx). Sample sizes are quite small, with the largest BD sample being 17 (Cecil et al., 2002).

For mI, one study found that youth with BD had higher ACC mI concentrations than controls or youth with intermittent explosive disorder (Davanzo et al., 2003), whereas another found that lithium treatment reduced ACC mI concentrations in youth with BD (Davanzo et al., 2001). These results replicate a finding in adult BD and are consistent with the hypothesis that lithium's effectiveness in BD results from its ability to decrease inositol (Moore et al., 1999). Given protein kinase C's (PKC) involvement in the phosphoinositide pathway, these results are also consistent with data indicating significantly lower PKC activity in youth with BD than controls (Pandey et al., 2007). Also, youth with mood disorders and a parent with BD had a 16% increase in frontal mI compared to controls, further implicating increased frontal mI in pediatric BD (Cecil et al., 2003).

Two studies comparing patients on medication to controls found that patients had decreased frontal NAA (Cecil et al., 2002). Regarding Glx, an early report suggested that youth with BD who were medication free had increased Glx compared to controls (Castillo et al., 2000), but more recent work suggests that ACC Glx elevation may be associated with comorbid ADHD in BD, rather than BD itself (Moore et al., 2006; Moore et al., 2007).

Thus, preliminary evidence suggests that pediatric BD may be associated with decreased NAA, increased mI, and/or increased Glx in frontal regions, with a particular emphasis on the ACC. Stork and Renshaw (2005) suggested that similar findings in adults implicate mitochondrial dysfunction in BD (Stork and Renshaw, 2005). Future MRS studies will require larger samples, preferably in patients who are medication free.

FAMILY AND GENETIC STUDIES

For several reasons, the genetics of pediatric BD are of particular interest. In a number of illnesses, early-onset cases are more "genetically loaded" than later-onset ones, and genetic research in the early-onset cases has been fruitful (Bishop, 1999; Imbimbo et al., 2005). Studies suggest that first-degree relatives (FDR) of early-onset BD probands have a higher prevalence of BD than do FDR of later-onset probands (Rice et al., 1987; Strober et al., 1988; Pauls et al., 1992; Todd et al., 1993; Neuman et al., 1997; Grigoroiu-Serbanescu et al., 2001; Somanath et al., 2002). Although the definition of early-onset ranges from prepubertal (Strober et al., 1988) to before age 25 (Grigoroiu-Serbanescu et al., 2001) in these studies, several give remarkably consistent prevalence estimates, that is, 8.9%–11.9% BD in FDR of early-onset probands, compared to 3.1%–5.5% BD in FDR of adult onset (Neuman et al., 1997; Grigoroiu-Serbanescu et al., 2001; Somanath et al., 2002). Geller et al. (2006) obtained a higher rate of BP-I disorder, 28.2%, in the parents of youth with BD, a difference that may stem from methodological differences in the assessment techniques used in youth and their parents. Finally, one study suggests that the mode of transmission may differ between early- and late-onset BD, with the early-onset form being more likely to involve a major gene of effect, albeit with polygenic components (Grigoroiu-Serbanescu et al., 2001).

Data also indicate that the age of onset of BD is familial (Leboyer et al., 1998; Lin et al., 2006) and heritable, with heritability estimates of 0.4–0.5 (Faraone et al., 2004; Visscher et al., 2001). This, along with research suggesting that familial early-onset BD may be relatively homogeneous clinically (that is, characterized by rapid switching) (MacKinnon et al., 2003) and/or associated with ADHD (Faraone et al., 2003), has encouraged researchers to conduct association studies in pediatric BD. Many of these studies use trio designs, which control for population stratification and are particularly feasible in samples with young probands. Five such association studies have been conducted in BD youth. All are small, and four (Geller and Cook, Jr., 1999; Geller and Cook, 2000; Geller et al., 2005; Baumer et al., 2006) are negative. The fifth, positive study found that the Val66 brain-derived neurotrophic factor (BDNF) polymorphism was preferentially transmitted in 53 trios with a prepubertal-onset BD proband, compared to control trios (Geller et al., 2004).

A related line of research consists of association and linkage studies attempting to identify genetic mechanisms determining age of onset in BD. Participants in these studies are adult patients with BD, and age of onset is determined retrospectively. Benedetti et al. (Benedetti et al., 2004) identified an association between the wild variant (T/T) of the glycogen synthase kinase 3-B promoter gene and earlier age of onset in two independent samples of adults with BD (Benedetti et al., 2004), whereas Bellivier et al. (2002) found evidence of an association between serotonin transporter gene polymorphism and age of onset (Bellivier et al., 2002). Using linkage techniques, Faraone et al. (2004) found suggestive, but not significant, evidence that loci on chromosomes 12, 14, and 15 influence the age of onset of BD (Faraone et al., 2004). The same group (Faraone et al., 2006) also found linkage between a locus on 9q34 and mania onset before age 20 in 58 families with BD.

Finally, attention has focused on early onset BD because of the suggestion that the genetic mechanism of anticipation may be involved in the pathophysiology of BD (McInnis et al., 1993). Anticipation is characterized clinically by earlier age of onset in successive generations, and genetically by unstable trinucleotide repeats. A number of studies suggest earlier age of onset of BD in successive generations, although interpretation of the data are complicated by a possible cohort effect (Visscher et al., 2001; Lange and McInnis, 2002). Also, data implicating trinucleotide repeats in BD are very preliminary (Lindblad et al., 1998; Verheyen et al., 1999; O'Donovan et al., 2003).

In sum, genetic research on pediatric BD is only beginning. Future directions will include pharmacogenomic and genetic imaging studies. Multisite studies, which have proven to be important in adult BD genetic research, will be essential in pediatric BD genetic research, given the relatively low prevalence of the latter.

CONCLUSIONS AND FUTURE DIRECTIONS

Both out-of-scanner and neuroimaging studies implicate prefrontal-striatal-amygdala circuitry in the pathophysiology of pediatric BD. Specifically, out-of-scanner studies document deficits in response inflexibility and face emotion processing, both of which are mediated by prefrontal-striatal-amygdala circuitry. Data also suggest that youth with BD may have sustained attention and verbal memory deficits, congruent with literature indicating decreased cortical volume and/or cortical dysfunction in pediatric BD. And, finally, there is evidence for decreased frontal mI in children with BD. None of these neurobiological findings in pediatric BD are strikingly different from those reported in adult BD although, as noted above, there have been no published neuroimaging studies directly comparing adults and youth with BD.

As noted above, comorbidity with ADHD and anxiety disorders complicates data interpretation in studies of pediatric BD. Other important confounding variables include mood state and medication. Indeed, because youth with BD tend to have relatively severe illness (Birmaher et al., 2006), it is difficult to study patients who are unmedicated. To address these potential confounds, studies must have sample sizes large enough to allow adequately powered subgroup analyses. In a relatively uncommon illness such as pediatric BD, multisite studies may be needed to ensure large samples for pathophysiological and genetic studies; for this to be possible, investigators will need to agree on diagnostic criteria and assessment techniques.

Important emerging research approaches in pediatric BD, as with other populations, include imaging genetics and pharmacogenetics (Hariri et al., 2006; McMahon et al., 2006). In addition, a number of research groups are studying unaffected youth at risk for BD. Such studies allow investigators to dissociate neurobiological dysfunction causing BD from dysfunction secondary to BD; in addition, unaffected at-risk youth are medication naïve. Whereas researchers studying schizophrenia have made considerable progress identifying potential endophenotypes for the illness (Braff et al., 2007), similar research in BD is in its infancy. Studies of youth at risk for BD should facilitate the identification of BD endophenotypes while, eventually, helping to provide information that will allow not only more effective treatment of BD, but perhaps even its prevention.

REFERENCES

American Psychiatric Association. (1994) *Diagnostic and Statistical Manual of Mental Disorders,* 4th ed. Washington, DC: Author.

Axelson, D., Birmaher, B., Strober, M., Gill, M.K., Valeri, S., Chiappetta, L., Ryan, N., Leonard, H., Hunt, J., Iyengar, S., Bridge, J., and Keller, M. (2006) Phenomenology of children and adolescents with bipolar spectrum disorders. *Arch. Gen. Psychiatry* 63:1139–1148.

Baumer, F.M., Howe, M., Gallelli, K., Simeonova, D.I., Hallmayer, J., and Chang, K.D. (2006) A pilot study of antidepressant-induced mania in pediatric bipolar disorder: Characteristics, risk factors, and the serotonin transporter gene. *Biol. Psychiatry* 60: 1005–1012.

Bellivier, F., Leroux, M., Henry, C., Rayah, F., Rouillon, F., Laplanche, J.L., and Leboyer, M. (2002) Serotonin transporter gene polymorphism influences age at onset in patients with bipolar affective disorder. *Neurosci. Lett.* 334:17–20.

Benedetti, F., Bernasconi, A., Lorenzi, C., Pontiggia, A., Serretti, A., Colombo, C., and Smeraldi, E. (2004) A single nucleotide polymorphism in glycogen synthase kinase 3-beta promoter gene influences onset of illness in patients affected by bipolar disorder. *Neurosci. Lett.* 355:37–40.

Biederman, J. (2006) The evolving face of pediatric mania. *Biol. Psychiatry* 60:901–902.

Birmaher, B., Axelson, D., Strober, M., Gill, M.K., Valeri, S., Chiappetta, L., Ryan, N., Leonard, H., Hunt, J., Iyengar, S., and Keller, M. (2006) Clinical course of children and adolescents with bipolar spectrum disorders. *Arch. Gen. Psychiatry* 63:175–183.

Bishop, D.T. (1999) BRCA1 and BRCA2 and breast cancer incidence: a review. *Ann. Oncol.* 10(Suppl 6):113–119.

Blumberg, H.P., Fredericks, C.A., Wang, F., Kalmar, J.H., Spencer, L., Papademetris, X., Pittman, B., Martin, A., Peterson, B.S., Fulbright, R.K., and Krystal, J.H. (2005) Preliminary evidence for persistent abnormalities in amygdala volumes in adolescents and young adults with bipolar disorder. *Bipolar Disord.* 7:570–576.

Blumberg, H.P., Kaufman, J., Martin, A., Whiteman, R., Zhang, J.H., Gore, J.C., Charney, D.S., Krystal, J.H., and Peterson, B.S. (2003) Amygdala and hippocampal volumes in adolescents and adults with bipolar disorder. *Arch. Gen. Psychiatry* 60:1201–1208.

Blumberg, H.P., Leung, H.C., Skudlarski, P., Lacadie, C.M., Fredericks, C.A., Harris, B.C., Charney, D.S., Gore, J.C., Krystal, J.H., and Peterson, B.S. (2003) A functional magnetic resonance imaging study of bipolar disorder: state- and trait-related dysfunction in ventral prefrontal cortices. *Arch. Gen. Psychiatry* 60:601–609.

Blumberg, H.P., Martin, A., Kaufman, J., Leung, H.C., Skudlarski, P., Lacadie, C., Fulbright, R.K., Gore, J.C., Charney, D.S., Krystal, J.H., and Peterson, B.S. (2003) Frontostriatal abnormalities in adolescents with bipolar disorder: preliminary observations from functional MRI. *Am. J. Psychiatry* 160:1345–1347.

Bowley, M.P., Drevets, W.C., Ongur, D., and Price, J.L. (2002) Low glial numbers in the amygdala in major depressive disorder. *Biol. Psychiatry* 52:404–412.

Braff, D.L., Freedman, R., Schork, N.J., and Gottesman, I.I. (2007) Deconstructing schizophrenia: an overview of the use of endophenotypes in order to understand a complex disorder. *Schizophr. Bull.* 33:21–32.

Breeze, J.L., Hesdorffer, D.C., Hong, X., Frazier, J.A., and Renshaw, P.F. (2003) Clinical significance of brain white matter hyperintensities in young adults with psychiatric illness. *Harvard Rev. Psychiatry* 11:269–283.

Brotman, M.A., Rich, B.A., Schmajuk, M., Reising, M., Monk, C., Dickstein, D.P., Mogg, K., Bradley, B.P., Pine, D., and Leibenluft, E. (2007) Attention bias to threat faces in children with bipolar disorder and comorbid lifetime anxiety disorders. *Biol. Psychiatry* 61:819–821.

Castillo, M., Kwock, L., Courvoisie, H., and Hooper, S.R. (2000) Proton MR spectroscopy in children with bipolar affective disorder: preliminary observations. *Am. J. Neuroradiol.* 21:832–838.

Cecil, K.M., DelBello, M.P., Morey, R., and Strakowski, S.M. (2002) Frontal lobe differences in bipolar disorder as determined by proton MR spectroscopy. *Bipolar Disord.* 4:357–365.

Cecil, K.M., DelBello, M.P., Sellars, M.C., and Strakowski, S.M. (2003) Proton magnetic resonance spectroscopy of the frontal lobe and cerebellar vermis in children with a mood disorder and a familial risk for bipolar disorders. *J. Child Adolesc. Psychopharmacol.* 13:545–555.

Chang, K., Adleman, N.E., Dienes, K., Simeonova, D.I., Menon, V., and Reiss, A. (2004) Anomalous prefrontal-subcortical activation in familial pediatric bipolar disorder: a functional magnetic resonance imaging investigation. *Arch. Gen. Psychiatry* 61:781–792.

Chang, K., Barnea-Goraly, N., Karchemskiy, A., Simeonova, D.I., Barnes, P., Ketter, T., and Reiss, A.L. (2005) Cortical magnetic resonance imaging findings in familial pediatric bipolar disorder. *Biol. Psychiatry* 58:197–203.

Chang, K., Karchemskiy, A., Barnea-Goraly, N., Garrett, A., Simeonova, D.I., and Reiss, A. (2005) Reduced amygdalar gray matter volume in familial pediatric bipolar disorder. *J. Am. Acad. Child Adolesc. Psychiatry* 44:565–573.

Chen, B.K., Sassi, R., Axelson, D., Hatch, J.P., Sanches, M., Nicoletti, M., Brambilla, P., Keshavan, M.S., Ryan, N.D., Birmaher, B., and Soares, J.C. (2004) Cross-sectional study of abnormal amygdala development in adolescents and young adults with bipolar disorder. *Biol. Psychiatry* 56:399–405.

Clark, L., and Goodwin, G.M. (2004) State- and trait-related deficits in sustained attention in bipolar disorder. *Eur. Arch. Psychiatry Clin. Neurosci.* 254:61–68.

Davanzo, P., Thomas, M.A., Yue, K., Oshiro, T., Belin, T., Strober, M., and McCracken, J. (2001) Decreased anterior cingulate myo-inositol/creatine spectroscopy resonance with lithium treatment in children with bipolar disorder. *Neuropsychopharmacol.* 24: 359–369.

Davanzo, P., Yue, K., Thomas, M.A., Belin, T., Mintz, J., Venkatraman, T.N., Santoro, E., Barnett, S., and McCracken, J. (2003) Proton magnetic resonance spectroscopy of bipolar disorder versus intermittent explosive disorder in children and adolescents. *Am. J. Psychiatry* 160:1442–1452.

Deckersbach, T., Dougherty, D.D., Savage, C., McMurrich, S., Fischman, A.J., Nierenberg, A., Sachs, G., and Rauch, S.L. (2006) Impaired recruitment of the dorsolateral prefrontal cortex and hippocampus during encoding in bipolar disorder. *Biol. Psychiatry* 59:138–146.

DelBello, M.P., Adler, C.M., Amicone, J., Mills, N.P., Shear, P.K., Warner, J., and Strakowski, S.M. (2004) Parametric neurocognitive task design: a pilot study of sustained attention in adolescents with bipolar disorder. *J. Affect. Disord.* 82(Suppl 1):S79–S88.

DelBello, M.P., Zimmerman, M.E., Mills, N.P., Getz, G.E., and Strakowski, S.M. (2004) Magnetic resonance imaging analysis of amygdala and other subcortical brain regions in adolescents with bipolar disorder. *Bipolar Disord.* 6:43–52.

Dickstein, D.P., Milham, M.P., Nugent, A.C., Drevets, W.C., Charney, D.S., Pine, D.S., and Leibenluft, E. (2005) Frontotemporal alterations in pediatric bipolar disorder: results of a voxel-based morphometry study. *Arch. Gen. Psychiatry* 62:734–741.

Dickstein, D.P., Rich, B.A., Roberson-Nay, R., Vinton, D.T., Berghorst, L.H., Pine, D. S., and Leibenluft, E. (2007) Neural activation during encoding of emotional faces in pediatric bipolar disorder. *Bipolar Disorder.* 9:679–692

Dickstein, D.P., Treland, J.E., Snow, J., McClure, E.B., Mehta, M.S., Towbin, K.E., Pine, D.S., and Leibenluft, E. (2004) Neuropsychological performance in pediatric bipolar disorder. *Biol. Psychiatry* 55:32–39.

Doyle, A.E., Wilens, T.E., Kwon, A., Seidman, L.J., Faraone, S.V., Fried, R., Swezey, A., Snyder, L., and Biederman, J. (2005) Neuropsychological functioning in youth with bipolar disorder. *Biol. Psychiatry* 58:540–548.

Faraone, S.V., Glatt, S.J., Su, J., and Tsuang, M.T. (2004) Three potential susceptibility loci shown by a genome-wide scan for regions influencing the age at onset of mania. *Am. J. Psychiatry* 161:625–630.

Faraone, S.V., Glatt, S.J., and Tsuang, M.T. (2003) The genetics of pediatric-onset bipolar disorder. *Biol. Psychiatry* 53:970–977.

Faraone, S.V., Lasky-Su, J., Glatt, S.J., Van Eerdewegh, P., and Tsuang, M.T. (2006) Early onset bipolar disorder: possible linkage to chromosome 9q34. *Bipolar Disord.* 8:144–151.

Frazier, J.A., Breeze, J.L., Makris, N., Giuliano, A.S., Herbert, M.R., Seidman, L., Biederman, J., Hodge, S.M., Dieterich, M.E., Gerstein,

E.D., Kennedy, D.N., Rauch, S.L., Cohen, B.M., and Caviness, V.S. (2005) Cortical gray matter differences identified by structural magnetic resonance imaging in pediatric bipolar disorder. *Bipolar Disord.* 7:555–569.

Frazier, J.A., Chiu, S., Breeze, J.L., Makris, N., Lange, N., Kennedy, D.N., Herbert, M.R., Bent, E.K., Koneru, V.K., Dieterich, M.E., Hodge, S.M., Rauch, S.L., Grant, P.E., Cohen, B.M., Seidman, L.J., Caviness, V.S., and Biederman, J. (2005) Structural brain magnetic resonance imaging of limbic and thalamic volumes in pediatric bipolar disorder. *Am. J. Psychiatry* 162:1256–1265.

Geller, B., Badner, J.A., Tillman, R., Christian, S.L., Bolhofner, K., and Cook, E.H. Jr. (2004) Linkage disequilibrium of the brain-derived neurotrophic factor Val66Met polymorphism in children with a prepubertal and early adolescent bipolar disorder phenotype. *Am. J. Psychiatry* 161:1698–1700.

Geller, B., and Cook, E.H. Jr. (1999) Serotonin transporter gene (HTTLPR) is not in linkage disequilibrium with prepubertal and early adolescent bipolarity. *Biol. Psychiatry* 45:1230–1233.

Geller, B., and Cook, E.H. Jr. (2000) Ultradian rapid cycling in prepubertal and early adolescent bipolarity is not in transmission disequilibrium with val/met COMT alleles. *Biol. Psychiatry* 47: 605–609.

Geller, B., Tillman, R., Badner, J.A., and Cook, E.H. Jr. (2005) Are the arginine vasopressin V1a receptor microsatellites related to hypersexuality in children with a prepubertal and early adolescent bipolar disorder phenotype? *Bipolar Disord.* 7:610–616.

Geller, B., Tillman, R., Bolhofner K., Zimmerman, B., Strauss, N.A., and Kaufmann, P. (2006) Controlled, blindly rated, direct-interview family study of a prepubertal and early-adolescent bipolar I disorder phenotype: Morbid risk, age of onset, and comorbidity. *Arch. Gen. Psychiatry* 63:1130–1138.

Glahn, D.C., Bearden, C.E., Caetano, S., Fonseca, M., Najt, P., Hunter, K., Pliszka, S.R., Olvera, R.L., and Soares, J.C. (2005) Declarative memory impairment in pediatric bipolar disorder. *Bipolar Disord.* 7:546–554.

Glahn, D.C., Bearden, C.E., Niendam, T.A., and Escamilla, M.A. (2004) The feasibility of neuropsychological endophenotypes in the search for genes associated with bipolar affective disorder. *Bipolar Disord.* 6:171–182.

Goldstein, T.R., Miklowitz, D.J., and Mullen, K.L. (2006) Social skills knowledge and performance among adolescents with bipolar disorder. *Bipolar Disord.* 8:350–361.

Gorrindo, T., Blair, R.J., Budhani, S., Dickstein, D.P., Pine, D.S., and Leibenluft, E. (2005) Deficits on a probabilistic response-reversal task in patients with pediatric bipolar disorder. *Am. J. Psychiatry* 162:1975–1977.

Grigoroiu-Serbanescu, M., Martinez, M., Nothen, M.M., Grinberg, M., Sima, D., Propping, P., Marinescu, E., and Hrestic, M. (2001) Different familial transmission patterns in bipolar I disorder with onset before and after age 25. *Am. J. Med. Genet.* 105:765–773.

Guyer, A.E., McClure, E.B., Adler, A., Brotman, M.A., Rich, B.A., Kimes, A.S., Pine, D., Ernst, M., and Leibenluft, E. (2007) Specificity of facial expression labeling deficits in childhood psychopathology. *J. Child Psychol. Psychiatry* 48:863–871.

Hariri, A.R., Drabant, E.M., and Weinberger, D.R. (2006) Imaging genetics: perspectives from studies of genetically driven variation in serotonin function and corticolimbic affective processing. *Biol. Psychiatry* 59:888–897.

Imbimbo, B.P., Lombard, J., and Pomara, N. (2005) Pathophysiology of Alzheimer's disease. *Neuroimaging Clin. N. Am.* 15:727–753, ix.

Kowatch, R.A., Youngstrom, E.A., Danielyan, A., and Findling, R.L. (2005) Review and meta-analysis of the phenomenology and clinical characteristics of mania in children and adolescents. *Bipolar Disord.* 7:483–496.

Lange, K.J., and McInnis, M.G. (2002) Studies of anticipation in bipolar affective disorder. *CNS Spectr.* 7:196–202.

Leboyer, M., Bellivier, F., McKeon, P., Albus, M., Borrman, M., Perez-Diaz, F., Mynett-Johnson, L., Feingold, J., and Maier, W. (1998) Age at onset and gender resemblance in bipolar siblings. *Psychiatry Res.* 81:125–131.

Leibenluft, E., Rich, B.A., Vinton, D.T., Nelson, E.E., Fromm, S.J., Berghorst, L.H., Joshi, P., Robb, A., Schachar, R.J., Dickstein, D.P., McClure, E.B., and Pine, D.S. (2007) Neural circuitry engaged during unsuccessful motor inhibition in pediatric bipolar disorder. *Am. J. Psychiatry* 164:52–60.

Lin, P.I., McInnis, M.G., Potash, J.B., Willour, V., MacKinnon, D.F., DePaulo, J.R., and Zandi, P.P. (2006) Clinical correlates and familial aggregation of age at onset in bipolar disorder. *Am. J. Psychiatry* 163:240–246.

Lindblad, K., Nylander, P.O., Zander, C., Yuan, Q.P., Stahle, L., Engstrom, C., Balciuniene, J., Pettersson, U., Breschel, T., McInnis, M., Ross, C.A., Adolfsson, R., and Schalling, M. (1998) Two commonly expanded CAG/CTG repeat loci: involvement in affective disorders? *Mol. Psychiatry* 3:405–410.

Lyoo, I.K., Hwang, J., Sim, M., Dunn, B.J., and Renshaw, P.F. (2006) Advances in magnetic resonance imaging methods for the evaluation of bipolar disorder. *CNS Spectr.* 11:269–280.

Lyoo, I.K., Lee, H.K., Jung, J.H., Noam, G.G., and Renshaw, P.F. (2002) White matter hyperintensities on magnetic resonance imaging of the brain in children with psychiatric disorders. *Compr. Psychiatry* 43:361–368.

MacKinnon, D.F., Zandi, P.P., Gershon, E., Nurnberger, J.I., Jr., Reich, T., and DePaulo, J.R. (2003) Rapid switching of mood in families with multiple cases of bipolar disorder. *Arch. Gen. Psychiatry* 60:921–928.

McClure, E.B., Pope, K., Hoberman, A.J., Pine, D.S., and Leibenluft, E. (2003) Facial expression recognition in adolescents with mood and anxiety disorders. *Am. J. Psychiatry* 160:1172–1174.

McClure, E.B., Treland, J.E., Snow, J., Dickstein, D.P., Towbin, K.E., Charney, D.S., Pine, D.S., and Leibenluft, E. (2005) Memory and learning in pediatric bipolar disorder. *J. Am. Acad. Child Adolesc. Psychiatry* 44:461–469.

McClure, E.B., Treland, J.E., Snow, J., Schmajuk, M., Dickstein, D.P., Towbin, K.E., Charney, D.S., Pine, D.S., and Leibenluft, E. (2005) Deficits in social cognition and response flexibility in pediatric bipolar disorder. *Am. J. Psychiatry* 162:1644–1651.

McInnis, M.G., McMahon, F.J., Chase, G.A., Simpson, S.G., Ross, C.A., and DePaulo, J.R. Jr. (1993) Anticipation in bipolar affective disorder. *Am. J. Hum. Genet.* 53:385–390.

McMahon, F.J., Buervenich, S., Charney, D., Lipsky, R., Rush, A.J., Wilson, A.F., Sorant, A.J., Papanicolaou, G.J., Laje, G., Fava, M., Trivedi, M.H., Wisniewski, S.R., and Manji, H. (2006) Variation in the gene encoding the serotonin 2A receptor is associated with outcome of antidepressant treatment. *Am. J. Hum. Genet.* 78:804–814.

Meyer, S.E., Carlson, G.A., Wiggs, E.A., Martinez, P.E., Ronsaville, D.S., Klimes-Dougan, B., Gold, P.W., and Radke-Yarrow, M. (2004) A prospective study of the association among impaired executive functioning, childhood attentional problems, and the development of bipolar disorder. *Dev. Psychopathol.* 16:461–476.

Mick, E., Spencer, T., Wozniak, J., and Biederman, J. (2005) Heterogeneity of irritability in attention-deficit/hyperactivity disorder subjects with and without mood disorders. *Biol. Psychiatry* 58: 576–582.

Moore, C.M., Biederman, J., Wozniak, J., Mick, E., Aleardi, M., Wardrop, M., Dougherty, M., Harpold, T., Hammerness, P., Randall, E., Lyoo, I.K., and Renshaw, P.F. (2007) Mania, glutamate/glutamine and risperidone in pediatric bipolar disorder: A proton magnetic resonance spectroscopy study of the anterior cingulate cortex. *J. Affect. Disord* 99:19–25.

Moore, C.M., Biederman, J., Wozniak, J., Mick, E., Aleardi, M., Wardrop, M., Dougherty, M., Harpold, T., Hammerness, P., Randall, E., and Renshaw, P.F. (2006) Differences in brain chemistry in children and adolescents with attention deficit hyperactivity disorder with and without comorbid bipolar disorder: a proton magnetic resonance spectroscopy study. *Am. J. Psychiatry* 163:316–318.

Moore, G.J., Bebchuk, J.M., Parrish, J.K., Faulk, M.W., Arfken, C.L., Strahl-Bevacqua, J., and Manji, H.K. (1999) Temporal dissociation between lithium-induced changes in frontal lobe myo-inositol and clinical response in manic-depressive illness. *Am. J. Psychiatry* 156:1902–1908.

Nelson, E.E., Vinton, D.T., Berghorst, L., Towbin, K.E., Hommer, R.A., Dickstein, D.P., Rich, B.A., Brotman, M.A., Pine, D.S., and Leibenluft, E. (2007) Brain systems underlying response flexibility in healthy and bipolar adolescents: an event-related fMRI study. *Bipolar Disord.* 9:810–819.

Neuman, R.J., Geller, B., Rice, J.P., and Todd, R.D. (1997) Increased prevalence and earlier onset of mood disorders among relatives of prepubertal versus adult probands. *J. Am. Acad. Child Adolesc. Psychiatry* 36:466–473.

Nierenberg, A.A., Miyahara, S., Spencer, T., Wisniewski, S.R., Otto, M.W., Simon, N., Pollack, M.H., Ostacher, M.J., Yan, L., Siegel, R., and Sachs, G.S. (2005) Clinical and diagnostic implications of lifetime attention-deficit/hyperactivity disorder comorbidity in adults with bipolar disorder: data from the first 1000 STEP-BD participants. *Biol. Psychiatry* 57:1467–1473.

O'Donovan, M., Jones, I., and Craddock, N. (2003) Anticipation and repeat expansion in bipolar disorder. *Am. J. Med. Genet. C Semin. Med. Genet.* 123:10–17.

Olvera, R.L., Semrud-Clikeman, M., Pliszka, S.R., and O'Donnell, L. (2005) Neuropsychological deficits in adolescents with conduct disorder and comorbid bipolar disorder: a pilot study. *Bipolar Disord.* 7:57–67.

Pandey, G.N., Ren, X., Dwivedi, Y., and Pavuluri, M.N. (2008) Decreased protein kinase C (PKC) in platelets of pediatric bipolar patients: Effect of treatment with mood stabilizing drugs. *J. Psychiatry Res.* 21:101–116.

Pauls, D.L., Morton, L.A., and Egeland, J.A. (1992) Risks of affective illness among first-degree relatives of bipolar I old-order Amish probands. *Arch. Gen. Psychiatry* 49:703–708.

Pavuluri, M.N., O'Connor, M.M., Harral, E., and Sweeney, J.A. (2006) Affective neural circuitry during facial emotion processing in pediatric bipolar disorder. *Biol. Psychiatry* 62:158–167.

Pavuluri, M.N., Schenkel, L.S., Aryal, S., Harral, E.M., Hill, S.K., Herbener, E.S., and Sweeney, J.A. (2006) Neurocognitive function in unmedicated manic and medicated euthymic pediatric bipolar patients. *Am. J. Psychiatry* 163:286–293.

Rice, J., Reich, T., Andreasen, N.C., Endicott, J., Van Eerdewegh, M., Fishman, R., Hirschfeld, R.M., and Klerman, G.L. (1987) The familial transmission of bipolar illness. *Arch. Gen. Psychiatry* 44:441–447.

Rich, B.A., Grimley, M.E., Schmajuk, M., Blair, K.S., Blair, R.J.R., Leibenluft, E. (in press) Face emotion labeling deficits in children with bipolar disorder and severe mood dysregulation. *Dev. Psychopathol.*

Rich, B.A., Schmajuk, M., Perez-Edgar, K.E., Fox, N.A., Pine, D.S., and Leibenluft, E. (2007) Different psychophysiological and behavioral responses elicited by frustration in pediatric bipolar disorder and severe mood dysregulation. *Am. J. Psychiatry* 164: 309–317.

Rich, B.A., Vinton, D.T., Roberson-Nay, R., Hommer, R.E., Berghorst, L.H., McClure, E.B., Fromm, S.J., Pine, D.S., and Leibenluft, E. (2006) Limbic hyperactivation during processing of neutral facial expressions in children with bipolar disorder. *Proc. Natl. Acad. Sci. USA* 103:8900–8905.

Robertson, H.A., Kutcher, S.P., and Lagace, D.C. (2003) No evidence of attentional deficits in stabilized bipolar youth relative to unipolar and control comparators. *Bipolar Disord.* 5:330–339.

Rucklidge, J.J. (2006) Impact of ADHD on the neurocognitive functioning of adolescents with bipolar disorder. *Biol. Psychiatry* 60:921–928.

Sanches, M., Roberts, R.L., Sassi, R.B., Axelson, D., Nicoletti, M., Brambilla, P., Hatch, J.P., Keshavan, M.S., Ryan, N.D., Birmaher, B., and Soares, J.C. (2005) Developmental abnormalities in striatum in young bipolar patients: a preliminary study. *Bipolar Disord.* 7:153–158.

Sanches, M., Sassi, R.B., Axelson, D., Nicoletti, M., Brambilla, P., Hatch, J.P., Keshavan, M.S., Ryan, N.D., Birmaher, B., and Soares, J.C. (2005) Subgenual prefrontal cortex of child and adolescent bipolar patients: a morphometric magnetic resonance imaging study. *Psychiatry Res.* 138:43–49.

Somanath, C.P., Jain, S., and Reddy, Y.C. (2002) A family study of early-onset bipolar I disorder. *J. Affect. Disord.* 70:91–94.

Starkstein, S.E., and Robinson, R.G. (1997) Mechanism of disinhibition after brain lesions. *J. Nerv. Ment. Disord.* 185:108–114.

Stork, C., and Renshaw, P.F. (2005) Mitochondrial dysfunction in bipolar disorder: evidence from magnetic resonance spectroscopy research. *Mol. Psychiatry* 10:900–919.

Strakowski, S.M., Adler, C.M., Holland, S.K., Mills, N.P., DelBello M.P., and Eliassen, J.C. (2005) Abnormal FMRI brain activation in euthymic bipolar disorder patients during a counting Stroop interference task. *Am. J. Psychiatry* 162:1697–1705.

Strober, M., Morrell, W., Burroughs, J., Lampert, C., Danforth, H., and Freeman, R. (1988) A family study of bipolar I disorder in adolescence. Early onset of symptoms linked to increased familial loading and lithium resistance. *J. Affect. Disord.* 15:255–268.

Tillman, R., and Geller, B. (2003) Definitions of rapid, ultrarapid, and ultradian cycling and of episode duration in pediatric and adult bipolar disorders: a proposal to distinguish episodes from cycles. *J. Child Adolesc. Psychopharmacol.* 13:267–271.

Todd, R.D., Neuman, R., Geller, B., Fox, L.W., and Hickok, J. (1993) Genetic studies of affective disorders: should we be starting with childhood onset probands? *J. Am. Acad. Child Adolesc. Psychiatry* 32:1164–1171.

Towbin, K.E., Pradella, A., Gorrindo, T., Pine, D.S., and Leibenluft, E. (2005) Autism spectrum traits in children with mood and anxiety disorders. *J. Child Adolesc. Psychopharmacol.* 15:452–464.

Verheyen, G.R., Del Favero, J., Mendlewicz, J., Lindblad, K., Van Zand, K., Aalbregtse, M., Schalling, M., Souery, D., and Van Broeckhoven, C. (1999) Molecular interpretation of expanded RED products in bipolar disorder by CAG/CTG repeats located at chromosomes 17q and 18q. *Neurobiol. Dis.* 6:424–432.

Visscher, P.M., Yazdi, M.H., Jackson, A.D., Schalling, M., Lindblad, K., Yuan, Q.P., Porteous, D., Muir, W.J., and Blackwood, D.H. (2001) Genetic survival analysis of age-at-onset of bipolar disorder: evidence for anticipation or cohort effect in families. *Psychiatric Genet.* 11:129–137.

Volk, H.E., and Todd, R.D. (2006) Does the child behavior checklist juvenile bipolar disorder phenotype identify bipolar disorder? *Biol. Psychiatry* 62:115–120.

Wilke, M., Kowatch, R.A., DelBello, M.P., Mills, N.P., and Holland, S.K. (2004) Voxel-based morphometry in adolescents with bipolar disorder: first results. *Psychiatry Res.* 131:57–69.

Yurgelun-Todd, D.A., and Ross, A.J. (2006) Functional magnetic resonance imaging studies in bipolar disorder. *CNS Spectr.* 11: 287–297.

73 Neurobiology of Child and Adolescent Depression

JOAN KAUFMAN, ANDRÉS MARTIN, AND HILARY BLUMBERG

Major depression disorder (MDD) in children and adolescents is common, recurrent, and associated with significant morbidity and mortality (Birmaher, Ryan, Williamson, et al., 1996; Costello et al., 2002; Brent and Weersing, 2007). The point prevalence of MDD is 2% in children and 5%–8% in adolescents (Lewinsohn et al., 1999; Costello et al., 2002). Within 5 years of the onset of MDD, 70% of clinically referred children and adolescents with depression experience a recurrence (Kovacs, 1996; Brent and Weersing, 2007). High rates of recurrence, with continuity between adolescent and adult MDD, are also reported in epidemiological studies (Pine et al., 1998; Lewinsohn et al., 1999). In addition, longitudinal follow-up studies suggest that children with depression have persistent functional impairment after recovery (Ryan, 2005), and in some (Rao et al., 1995; Geller et al., 2001) but not all studies (Weissman et al., 1999), children with MDD have been found to be at elevated risk for the onset of bipolar disorders. Most sobering, however, is the finding that more than 5% of adolescents with depression will complete suicide within 15 years of their initial episode of MDD (Rao et al., 1993; Weissman et al., 1999).

In 1999, at the time of the first publication of this text, sleep and neuroendocrine parameters were the primary focus of most investigations of the neurobiology of child- and adolescent-onset depression (Kaufman and Ryan, 1999). These studies revealed continuities and discontinuities in the psychobiological correlates of MDD across the life cycle. Specifically, though electroencephalographic (EEG) sleep and basal hypothalamic-pituitary-adrenal (HPA) axis abnormalities were frequently reported in adults with depression, they were rarely observed in children. In contrast, studies using the Dexamethasone Suppression Test (DST) and various growth hormone probes showed greater continuity across the life cycle. At the time of the first publication of this text, only two neuroimaging studies had been completed in juvenile cohorts. One reported reduced frontal lobe volume in children with depression when compared to psychiatric controls (Steingard et al., 1996), and the other reported reduced regional cerebral blood flow (rCBF) in this region (Tutus et al., 1998). Given the paucity of work in this area at the time of the first publication of this text, it was impossible to draw conclusions regarding the neuroanatomical correlates of MDD in children.

Over the next 5 years, additional imaging studies suggested that early-onset depression, like adult depression, might be associated with structural and functional changes in frontal and subcortical structures (Kaufman, Blumberg, and Young, 2004). This conclusion, however, was based on a limited number of studies, with no independent replication of pediatric neuroimaging findings. At the time of the publication of the second edition of this text, developmental differences in children, adolescents, and adults with MDD became most evident in pharmacological treatment studies. Although questions about the efficacy of tricyclic antidepressants (TCAs) in children were raised previously (Hazell et al., 1995; Martin et al., 2000), conclusions from the early TCA studies were limited due to small sample size (Birmaher, Ryan, Williamson, Brent, and Kaufman, 1996). A definitive study published in 2001 unequivocally demonstrated that TCAs are comparable to placebo in children and suggested that selective serotonin reuptake inhibitors (SSRIs) were effective in pediatric populations (Keller et al., 2001).

Since the publication of the second edition of this text, there has been a black box warning added to the label of SSRI medications; new evidence for frontotemporal brain circuitry involvement in pediatric depression from multiple neuroimaging studies; a burgeoning literature on the role, and interaction of, genetic and environmental (G × E) factors in the etiology of depression (Caspi et al., 2003); and the emergence of the field of imaging genomics (Hariri and Weinberger, 2003; Hariri et al., 2005). This latter development has yet to be incorporated into the design of studies examining the neurobiology of child- and adolescent-onset depression. Consequently, this chapter is organized into three sections: (*1*) a brief review and discussion of pharmacological treatment studies of MDD in children and adolescents and the role of SSRI administration in youth; (*2*) an update and synthesis of extant imaging studies in pediatric MDD; and (*3*) a review of emerging G × E and imaging genomics findings with a discussion of the role of this work in guiding future studies on the neurobiology of child- and adolescent-onset depression. Currently, methods to diagnose and treat pediatric MDD are largely extrapolated from those in adults. However, available research suggests that there are some important developmental differences in MDD across the life cycle. Unfortunately, the nature and extent of these differences remains to be fully elucidated.

PHARMACOLOGICAL TREATMENT STUDIES OF CHILDREN AND ADOLESCENTS WITH DEPRESSION

In 1997, Emslie and colleagues published the first double-blind, randomized, placebo-controlled trial of an SSRI antidepressant in children and adolescents with MDD, showing clear superiority for fluoxetine over placebo (Emslie et al., 1997). At the time of the publication of this study, the efficacy of TCAs in children was still debated. In 2001, however, a multisite, double-blind, placebo-controlled trial of 275 outpatients with depression who were 12–19 years of age randomized to paroxetine, imipramine, or placebo provided conclusive evidence for the inefficacy of TCA medications in juvenile cohorts (Keller et al., 2001). Patients randomized to imipramine received ratings comparable to those of patients receiving placebo on all of the clinical outcome measures. In contrast, in this first study paroxetine preliminarily proved superior to placebo on measures of affect, global improvement, and remission of depressive symptoms.

In subsequent years, additional investigations further demonstrated the efficacy of SSRI medications in the treatment of child and adolescent depression, such that in 2002, U.S. physicians wrote nearly 11 million prescriptions for youth for SSRIs and other non-TCA antidepressants (Vasa et al., 2006). The following year, however, the Food and Drug Administration (FDA) began issuing warnings against the use of SSRI medications in children due to concerns about medication-induced suicidality. These warnings culminated with the issuing of a black box label against SSRIs on October 15, 2004. Specifically, the FDA warned that "Antidepressants increased the risk of suicidal thinking and behavior (suicidality) in short-term studies in children and adolescents with major depressive disorder and other psychiatric disorders." The FDA decision was based on an analysis of pediatric suicidality data from 4,582 children and adolescents treated in 24 randomized clinical trials, showing that 4% of SSRI-treated youths developed new-onset suicidal ideation (as opposed to gestures, or completed suicides), compared to 2% of those treated with placebo (Hammad et al., 2006), yielding a relative risk for SSRIs of 1.66 (95% confidence interval [CI], 1.28–2.98).

The ongoing prescription of SSRI medications for youth with depression has been argued based on the following findings (Vasa et al., 2006): (*1*) As discussed at the onset of this chapter, pediatric MDD is associated with significant morbidity and mortality; (*2*) the majority of adolescents who commit suicide suffer from an untreated mood disorder; (*3*) SSRIs are effective for the treatment of anxiety disorders that frequently predate and complicate the course of MDD in children and adolescents; and (*4*) in the only study to directly compare cognitive-behavioral therapy (CBT) to SSRI (fluoxetine) treatment for adolescent depression (March et al., 2006), SSRI treatment was superior to CBT, with the latter treatment not statistically different than placebo. (See Brent, 2006, for discussion of other more effective CBT treatment studies in adolescents with depression.)

A more recent meta-analysis of randomized controlled trials of SSRI and other non-TCA antidepressants included three additional studies and 700 more children and adolescents with depression than the analysis conducted by the FDA (Bridge et al., 2007). The authors of this latter meta-analysis concluded the benefits of SSRI antidepressant treatment far outweigh the potential risks for suicidality in this age group. The meta-analysis included 15 pediatric MDD trials, 6 pediatric obsessive–compulsive disorder (OCD) trials, and 6 non-OCD anxiety disorder pediatric trials. Relative to placebo, antidepressants were found to be efficacious for pediatric MDD, OCD, and non-OCD anxiety disorders, with the effects strongest for non-OCD anxiety disorders and most modest for MDD. In addition, the rate of suicidal ideation or suicide attempt associated with drug therapy, though greater than with placebo, was not statistically greater with drug therapy for any diagnostic group, and there were no completed suicides in any of the clinical trials included in the meta-analysis.

Studies have shown that in the wake of the black box and related advisories, there has been a marked reduction in the prescription of antidepressants for children and adolescents, a prescribing shift away from pediatricians and family practitioners onto psychiatrists, and growing concerns that the resulting undertreatment of MDD in this age group has led to increased deaths by suicide (Kurian et al., 2007; Nemeroff et al., 2007). Indeed, in 2004 the youth suicide rate increased for the first time after a decade of gradual and steady decline (Hamilton et al., 2007). A recent study indicates SSRI prescriptions for youth decreased 22% in the United States between 2003 and 2005, and youth suicide rates increased 14% between 2003 and 2004, which is the largest year-to-date change in suicide rates in the United States since the Centers for Disease Control and Prevention began systematically collecting suicide data in

1979 (Gibbons et al., 2007). A similar drop in SSRI prescriptions in the Netherlands was associated with a 49% increase in youth suicide (Gibbons et al., 2007).

The SSRI medications appear less potent in juvenile cohorts than in adults with depression, with fluoxetine the only demonstrated effective SSRI for children 12 years of age or younger (Bridge et al., 2007). To date, they are the most effective agents available, with only modest and nonsignificant benefits on most outcome measures documented in studies of the efficacy of venlafaxine, nefazadone, and mirtazapine in adolescents. Differences in the mechanism of action of TCA and SSRI antidepressants may provide insights into the pathophysiology of early-onset MDD and suggest alternative targets for pharmacological treatment interventions (Kaufman et al., 2001). For example, though TCAs and SSRIs enhance serotonergic transmission and reduce *N*-methyl-D-aspartate (NMDA) glutamate receptor function (Kilts, 1994), amelioration of depressive symptoms with SSRI treatment is uniquely correlated with increases in the neurosteroid *3-alpha, 5-alpha, tetrahydroprogesterone* (ALLO) (Guidotti and Costa, 1998). *3-alpha, 5-alpha, tetrahydroprogesterone* binds with high affinity to γ-aminobutyric acid (GABA-A) receptors and potently facilitates GABA transmission at these sites. It is the hope that better understanding of the brain systems and regulatory pathways involved in early-onset MDD will lead to the identification of novel and potentially more efficacious treatments for child and adolescent depression. More research, however, is needed in this area.

NEUROIMAGING STUDIES OF CHILDREN AND ADOLESCENTS WITH DEPRESSION

Emerging studies suggest that MDD is characterized by deficits in two overlapping neural circuits: *(1)* a "fear" circuit that is involved in regulation of the threat response and emotion processing and that encompasses amygdala, hippocampus, and associated prefrontal cortex (PFC) regions (for example, subgenual PFC, anterior cingulate) and *(2)* a "reward" circuit that is involved in the regulation of reward-related behaviors and that encompasses the striatum, orbitofrontal cortex (OFC), and amygdala as well (Vasa et al., 2006). In this section we review neuroimaging studies in children and adolescents with depression that have examined the role of these frontotemporal corticolimbic neural systems. Structural neuroimaging studies are reviewed first, then functional neuroimaging studies, followed by a discussion of magnetic resonance spectroscopy (MRS) studies that point to molecular mechanisms that might underlie the structural and functional abnormalities in children and adolescents with depression. Throughout, we focus on the studies that directly assess children and adolescents with MDD as well as discuss the findings from the studies in youths within the context of the literature in adults with MDD. Continuities and discontinuities will again be evident across the life cycle, with too few studies to draw definitive conclusions regarding developmental differences in the neural underpinnings of MDD in children, adolescents, and adults.

STRUCTURAL NEUROIMAGING

The structural neuroimaging literature is the largest neuroimaging literature in pediatric MDD to date; thus, only this section is subdivided by brain region. The key findings of the structural neuroimaging research studies discussed below are summarized in Table 73.1.

Frontal Lobe

Steingard and colleagues (1996) conducted the first published structural magnetic resonance imaging (MRI) report of differences in frontal lobe morphology in pediatric depressive disorders. They compared a group of 65 children and adolescents with depressive disorders to 18 children and adolescents in a psychiatric control group without depressive disorders. In their study, *frontal lobe volume* was defined as a comprehensive region that included all tissue anterior to a plane between the left and right prefrontal sulci. Children with depressive disorders were found to have reduced frontal lobe/cerebral volume ratios, compared to the psychiatric controls. Additionally, the investigators noted a significant inverse association between frontal lobe volume and age. These findings were consistent with findings of PFC volume reductions in adults with MDD, providing some of the first evidence to suggest that PFC abnormalities might be early abnormalities in MDD associated with vulnerability to MDD. However, ability to draw conclusions about MDD in youth from this important initial study is limited by the lack of a comparison group without psychiatric illness. The findings of decreases in frontal lobe volume with age raised interesting questions about whether PFC abnormalities in MDD might represent an acceleration of normal decreases in PFC volume with age, as has been suggested to contribute to PFC abnormalities in other mood disorders (Blumberg et al., 2006).

In 2002, three new structural MRI studies of frontal morphology in pediatric MDD emerged that provided direct comparisons between children and adolescents with MDD and age-matched normal controls (NC). Nolan and colleagues (2002) extended earlier studies (Steingard et al., 1996) with a structural MRI study of PFC volume in 22 children and adolescents with MDD, and 22 age and gender-matched NCs. No differences were initially observed between the patients with depression and controls on volumetric measurements. Secondary anal-

TABLE 73.1 *Structural Neuroimaging Studies of Children and Adolescents with Major Depression*

Reference	*Sample*	*Ages*	*Method*	*Results*
Steingard et al., 1996	65 DD 18 PC	6–17	1.5 Tesla, 5 mm slice thickness	DD < PC frontal lobe volume
Nolan et al., 2002	22 MDD 22 NC	9–17	1.5 Tesla 1.5 mm slice thickness	familial MDD ≤ NC < nonfamilial MDD left PFC volume (12 familial MDD, 10 non-familial)
Botteron et al., 2002	30 MDD 8 NC	17–23	1.5 Tesla, 1 mm slice thickness	MDD < NC left subgenual PFC volume
Steingard et al., 2002	19 MDD 38 NC	13–17	1.5 Tesla, 1.5 mm slice thickness	MDD < NC whole brain volume, frontal white matter volume MDD > NC frontal gray matter volume
Rosso et al., 2005	20 MDD 24 NC	11–17	1.5 Tesla, 1.5 mm slice thickness	MDD < NC amygdala volumes MDD = NC hippocampal volumes
MacMillan et al., 2003	23 MDD 23 NC	8–17	1.5 Tesla, 1.5 mm slice thickness	MDD = NC amygdala and hippocampal volumes
MacMaster et al., 2008	32 MDD 35 NC	8–21	1.5 Tesla, 1.5 mm slice thickness	MDD = NC amygdala volume MDD < NC hippocampal volume
Munn et al., 2007	26 MDD twins 24 HR twins 18 LR twins	15–23	1.5 Tesla, 1 mm slice thickness	MDD = HR = LR amygdala volumes $r = 0.75$, $p < .01$, correlation LR co-twin amygdala volume correlation MDD-HR twin pairs not reported
MacMaster and Kusumakar, 2004a	17 MDD 17 NC	13–18	1.5 Tesla, 1.5 mm slice thickness	MDD < NC hippocampal volume
MacMaster and Kusumakar, 2004b	17 MDD 17 NC	7–20	1.5 Tesla, 1.5 mm slice thickness	MDD > NC pituitary volume
MacMaster et al., 2006	35 MDD 35 NC	8–17	1.5 Tesla, 1.5 mm slice thickness	MDD > NC pituitary volume

DD: depressive disorders (major depression and/or dysthymia); HR: high risk, co-twin has history of major depression disorder (MDD) diagnosis with at least 4 weeks duration and positive family history for MDD; LR: no lifetime history of MDD for either co-twin, and no first-degree relatives with a lifetime history of any mood disorder; NC: normal controls; PC: psychiatric controls; PFC: prefrontal cortex.

yses detected significant group differences when the depressed cohort was stratified according to family loading for depression. Children without a family history of depression were found to have greater PFC volume than NCs and patients with a family loading of affective illness. Children in the latter group had smaller PFC volume than the NCs, although this difference failed to reach statistical significance. The importance of family loading of affective illness in explaining variability in neuroimaging findings has been demonstrated in adult studies of patients with depression as well (Drevets et al., 1997), with adults with depression who have family loading for pure depressive illness found to have reduction in subgenual PFC volume, and adults with family loading for depressive spectrum disorders such as substance use and antisocial personality disorder not found to have reduced subgenual PFC volume (Drevets et al., 1997). Although the methods used to characterize family loading for psychiatric illness were different in this child and the other adult study, the results highlight the importance of obtaining family loading for psychiatric illness data in neuroimaging studies (Kaufman et al., 2001).

In addition to differing in definitions of family loading, the previously described studies used different parameters to assess PFC volume. The PFC definition used by Nolan and colleagues (Nolan et al., 2002) included all gray and white matter tissue anterior to the genu of the corpus callosum, whereas Drevets and colleagues (1997) studied a much more focal region of left subgenual PFC gray matter. In an investigation of this specific PFC subregion, Botteron and colleagues (2002) studied 30 young women with adolescent-onset MDD compared to 8 age-matched controls and also found a 19% reduction in left subgenual PFC volumes (Botteron et al., 2002). A recent study by Tang and colleagues (2007) similarly demonstrated ventral anterior cingulate cortex (vACC) volume decreases in women who were psychotropic medication naïve with MDD experiencing their first depressive episode, suggesting that this volume reduction is present at illness onset and may represent a vulnerability factor that is not related to medication exposure or duration of depressive disorder.

In 2002, Steingard and colleagues compared 19 adolescents with MDD (73% with a family loading for affective illness) and 38 NCs and used a similar definition of PFC as Nolan and colleagues (2002). Steingard and colleagues (2002) further subdivided PFC into white matter and gray matter and found a dissociation between the type of matter and the direction of the group differences. Adolescents with MDD, as compared to NC, had significant reductions in PFC white matter but increases in PFC gray matter. The inconsistency between this finding of increases in PFC gray matter and previous reports of PFC gray matter decreases could have resulted from differences in sample characteristics and methods used to define PFC subregions. Replication of the gray–white matter finding is warranted.

Mesial Temporal Lobe

Amygdala

More recently, investigators have examined mesial temporal lobe structures that share substantial connectivity with the PFC in children and adolescents with MDD. Rosso and colleagues (2005) compared a group of 20 adolescents who were unmedicated with MDD to a group of 24 NC adolescents and found that amygdala volumes were on average 12% smaller in the adolescents with MDD. Three other somewhat larger investigations, however, failed to replicate this finding (MacMillan et al., 2003; Munn et al., 2007; Macmaster et al., 2008).

Hippocampus

MacMaster and Kusumakar (2004a) found hippocampus volume decreases in a study of 17 adolescents with MDD as compared to 17 age- and sex-matched NC adolescents, and in an expanded sample of 32 children and adolescents (ages 8–21) with MDD (Macmaster et al., 2008). In the study discussed above, however, Rosso and colleagues (2005) did not detect decreases in hippocampus volumes in adolescents with MDD. It is possible that the differences in the findings reflect sex differences in hippocampus involvement in MDD. The MacMaster and Kusumakar study found a more prominent decrease in hippocampal volume in males than in females, and the Rosso MDD sample was predominantly female. Frodl and colleagues (2002), in a study of female and male adults experiencing their first MDD episode, found decreased hippocampus volumes only in males with MDD. However, reductions in hippocampal volumes have been reported in studies of adults with MDD that included females and males with MDD (Sheline et al., 1996; Bremner et al., 2000; Mervaala et al., 2000; MacQueen et al., 2003). It is possible that hippocampus volume abnormalities are more prominent in males early in the course of MDD but that the magnitude of hippocampal abnormalities converges between the sexes later in the course of the disorder. Sexually dimorphic features of hippocampus development have been reported (Giedd et al., 1997), theorized to result from differences in sex hormones, especially at puberty. Further study of the effects of sex hormones on the neural circuitry of MDD may help to elucidate the mechanisms that underlie the shift from the equivalent rate of MDD in girls and boys prior to puberty, to the higher rate in females after puberty.

Sex difference, however, is just one of the many factors that have been suggested to influence the expression of hippocampus abnormalities in MDD. Sample differences in family loading for affective illnesses (MacMaster et al., 2008), number of prior episodes of MDD (Sheline et al., 1996; MacQueen et al., 2003; Caetano et al., 2004), and exposure to antidepressant medications (Sheline et al., 2003) are three additional factors that may account for discrepancies across prior studies.

Environmental factors may also influence hippocampus abnormalities in MDD. In a recent study of adult twins (de Geus et al., 2007)—7 pairs concordant for lifetime anxiety and depression symptomatology, 15 pairs concordant for an absence of significant lifetime anxiety and depression symptomatology, and 10 pairs discordant on anxiety and depression symptom history—comparison of concordant symptomatic and concordant asymptomatic twins yielded no significant group differences in brain morphometry. Hippocampal volume differences were only evident in individuals with a lifetime history of anxiety and depression symptoms when compared to discordant co-twins, with co-twins with a lifetime history of anxiety and depression apt to report a history of chronic stress from major life events and lower social supports. These latter factors have also been shown to be relevant in moderating genetic risk for depression (Kaufman, Yang, et al., 2004; Kaufman et al., 2006).

In contrast to the results of the twin study discussed above, there has been some suggestion that reduced hippocampal volume represents a preexisting, inherent vulnerability factor rather than a consequence of trauma exposure, given one study found combat exposed twins with post-traumatic stress disorder (PTSD) and their unexposed co-twins had smaller hippocampal volumes than twins who were combat exposed without PTSD and their co-twins who were unexposed (Gilbertson et al., 2002). This interpretation has to be accepted with caution, however, as the veterans who were combat exposed who developed PTSD and their unexposed co-twins were more likely to have had a history of childhood physical and/or sexual abuse, highlighting the potential importance of early developmental insults on hippocampal structure. As is discussed later in this chapter, the emerging picture in the field is that the simultaneous examination of genetic and environmental factors is critical to explain heterogeneity in studies of brain morphology and psychiatric illness.

Other Implicated Brain Regions

Given the relationship between stress and MDD, and the observation of HPA axis abnormalities during depressive episodes, the pituitary is another structure that has been examined in adult and child neuroimaging studies. Consistent with a previous report in adults with MDD of increased pituitary volume (Krishnan et al., 1991), increased pituitary volume has been detected in two independent juvenile cohorts of patients with MDD (MacMaster and Kusumakar, 2004b; MacMaster et al., 2006). Increases in pituitary volume in psychiatric patients have also been found to be associated with elevated cortisol postdexamethasone (Axelson et al., 1992), one of the few HPA axis abnormalities frequently reported in child and adolescent cohorts with depression (Kaufman and Ryan, 1999). Future neuroimaging studies of HPA structures may provide important insights into endocrinological contributions to the pathophysiology of MDD.

FUNCTIONAL NEUROIMAGING

The functional neuroimaging studies reviewed in this section are summarized in Table 73.2. Early studies of regional brain function in adolescents with MDD were conducted using single photon emission computed tomography (SPECT) measures of rCBF of participants at rest during scanning. Tutus and colleagues (1998) included 14 adolescents with depression and 11 NCs in their SPECT study and, consistent with findings in adults (Baxter et al., 1989; Bench et al., 1993), found reductions in left anterolateral rCBF in the adolescents with depression. They also noted decreases in temporal lobe rCBF. However, in a study of seven adolescents with depression and seven matched NCs, Kowatch and colleagues (1999) found increased rCBF in the temporal lobe. Thus, early functional neuroimaging studies in pediatric MDD were consistent with the adult literature in finding frontotemporal abnormalities, although the direction of the temporal abnormalities was inconsistent across available studies.

More recent functional neuroimaging studies of pediatric MDD have consisted of functional MRI (fMRI) investigations. In addition to providing improvements in spatial and temporal resolution as compared to SPECT, fMRI has the advantage that it does not require the use of radioisotopes for study. Moreover, it provides the opportunity to investigate dynamic changes in regional brain response while research participants perform tasks that target the behavior and the neural circuitry that subserves them. A growing neuropsychological literature on pediatric MDD implicates early abnormalities in the processing of stimuli of emotional and motivational relevance. Adults with depression have shown deficits in

TABLE 73.2 *Functional Neuroimaging Studies of Children and Adolescents with Major Depression*

Reference	*Sample*	*Ages*	*Method*	*Results*
Tutus et al., 1998	14 MDD 11 NC	11–15	^{99}Tc HMPAO brain SPECT	MDD < NC rCBF left anterolateral and temporal lobes
Kowatch et al., 1999	7 MDD 7 NC	13–18	^{99}Tc HMPAO brain SPECT	MDD > NC rCBF temporal lobe subregions
Forbes et al., 2006	14 MDD 17 NC	9–17	1.5 Tesla; reward task	Decision phase of task MDD < NC ACC, caudate, inferior OFC MDD > NC middle/superior OFC Outcome phase of task MDD < NC ACC, caudate, OFC (during loss or low reward) MDD > NC amygdala, OFC (high reward condition)
Roberson-Nay et al., 2006	10 MDD 23 NC	9–17	3.0 Tesla; View angry, fearful, happy, and neutral faces plus postscanner recognition memory task	MDD < NC memory for faces Successful vs. unsuccessful face encoding MDD > NC left amygdala activation
Thomas et al., 2001	5 MDD 5 NC	8–16	1.5 Tesla; Passive viewing of fearful and neutral faces	Fearful expressions vs. fixation MDD < NC left amygdala activation

ACC: anterior cingulate cortex; MDD: major depression disorder; NC: normal controls; OFC: orbitofrontal cortex; SPECT: single photon emission computed tomography; ^{99}Tc HMPAO: Technetium-99m hexamethylpropylene amine oxime; rCBF: regional cerebral blood flow.

processing facial affect (Rubinow and Post, 1992) and mood-congruent biases toward negative emotional stimuli such as increased likelihood of interpreting facial affect as sadness, and to selectively attend to negative facial expressions (Suslow et al., 2001). Pediatric MDD studies suggest that these behavioral abnormalities may have their origins early in the disorder as evidence is accumulating in children and adolescents with MDD of perturbations in the processing of fearful facial stimuli, a response bias towards sad stimuli, as well as diminished sensitivity to rewarding stimuli (Pine et al., 2004; Ladouceur et al., 2006; Forbes et al., 2007).

Paradigms based on these implicated behavioral systems have begun to be implemented in fMRI studies of pediatric MDD. For example, Forbes and colleagues (2006) studied 14 children and adolescents with MDD and 17 NCs with fMRI performed during a reward-related decision-making task. Youth with depression exhibited disrupted responding in the reward decision/anticipation and reward outcome phase of the task. In the decision phase, children with depression exhibited blunted responses in the ACC, bilateral caudate, and inferior OFC, especially during high-magnitude reward conditions. This pattern is consistent with decreased emotional reactivity to reward. In addition, children with depression had increased activation in the middle and superior OFC bilaterally, especially during the low-magnitude reward condition, which is consistent with overregulation of emotional responses. In the outcome phase of the task, children with depression had a blunted response in the ACC, caudate, and OFC, particularly during loss and low-magnitude rewards. After low- and high-magnitude rewards, children with depression exhibited increased amygdala activation, with increased OFC activation also observed in response to high rewards. These findings are consistent with findings in the adult MDD literature that reports blunted response of ventral striatum and excessive ventromedial PFC response to positive emotional and rewarding stimuli (Keedwell et al., 2005; Epstein et al., 2006). In adults, this pattern was associated with *adhedonia*, a decreased interest and ability to derive pleasure from activities, suggesting that it may also contribute to anhedonic symptoms in children with MDD.

Excesses in amygdala response to motivationally and emotionally relevant stimuli have been further observed in adults and adolescents with MDD. In adults with MDD, Sheline and colleagues (2001) observed elevated response to emotional faces, especially faces depicting fear. In a preliminary small study comparing five girls with MDD (ages 8–16 years) to five girls with anxiety disorders and five NCs, Thomas and colleagues (2001) reported the opposite finding—decreased amygdala activation in association with MDD. However, in a subsequent study, as depicted in Figure 73.1, Roberson-Nay and colleagues (2006) found increases in amygdala activation in a face-processing task. This study included a larger sample of 10 adolescents with MDD, as compared to 11 with anxiety and 23 NCs. Another distinction of this study was the behavioral paradigm employed, in which the successful and unsuccessful encoding of emotional facial stimuli were measured. Increases in amygdala activation were detected in the adolescents with MDD when successful face encoding was assessed (Roberson-Nay et al., 2006). Increased activation in amygdala activation when processing emotional stimuli may be a trait marker for MDD, as it has recently also been observed in nondepressed child and adolescent offspring of adults with MDD (Monk et al., 2008).

The similar regional distribution of the findings between the structural and the functional neuroimaging studies suggests that the structural abnormalities may underlie the regional dysfunction. In the study of structure–function relationships in adults with MDD, an association was found between decreased core amygdala volumes and increases in amygdala response to words with negative valence (Siegle et al., 2003). Future studies of structure–function relationship in pediatric MDD may provide important insights into the pathophysiology of the disorder.

Adult studies provide promising evidence that antidepressant treatments have the potential to reverse the functional abnormalities of MDD. For example, Sheline and colleagues (2001) found that pretreatment elevations in amygdala response to emotional faces were reduced following antidepressant treatment. Mayberg and colleagues (2000) also found that pretreatment hyperactivity of the vACC was associated with response to antidepressant treatment. Moreover, posttreatment reductions in vACC occurred in a time course coincident

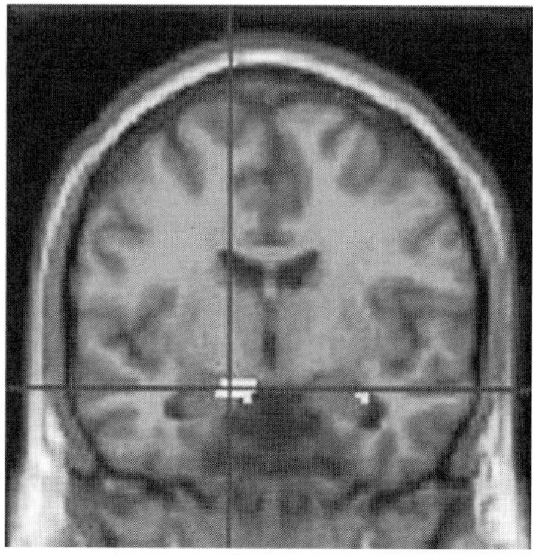

FIGURE 73.1 Amygdala activation in response to facial stimuli in adolescents with depression. Adolescents with major depression disorder (MDD), when compared to healthy controls, show greater activation in the amygdala when contrasting activations were obtained for successfully remembered minus unsuccessfully remembered faces. Reprinted from Roberson-Nay et al., 2006.

with the time course for depression recovery (Mayberg et al., 2000). This finding has been replicated by other groups, and the finding has been extended to show that nonpharmcological treatments may also have a salutary effect on the circuitry. Cognitive-behavioral therapy treatments, for example, may provide top-down effects on the circuitry by strengthening PFC functioning, which in turn may better regulate vACC activity (Brody et al., 2001; Goldapple et al., 2004).

MAGNETIC RESONANCE SPECTROSCOPY

The magnetic resonance spectroscopy studies reviewed in this section are summarized in Table 73.3. Steingard and colleagues (2000) examined proton MRS in the OFC of 22 adolescents with depression (ages 13–17 years), compared to 43 NC adolescents, and found adolescents with depression to have increases in choline to creatinine (Cho/Cr) and Cho/*N*-acetylaspartate (Cho/NAA) ratios in the OFC. This suggests that alterations in cell membrane stability might contribute to abnormalities in structure in ventral regions of PFC in pediatric MDD. Differences in Cho have also been detected in the dorsolateral PFC (DLPFC) in pediatric MDD, although reports are inconclusive regarding the direction of differences reported in association with pediatric MDD. Farchione and colleagues (2002) found increases in DLPFC Cho in 11 adolescents who were treatment naïve with depression, compared to 11 NCs. More recently, however, Caetano and colleagues (2005) found lower levels of DLPFC Cho in 14 children and adolescents with depression (ages 9–17 years), compared to 22 matched NCs. Kusumakar and colleagues (2001) also found reductions in Cho/Cr ratios in left amygdala in 11 adolescents with MDD. This latter finding is in contrast to studies in adults, in which patients with depression were found to have increased mesial temporal lobe Cho/Cr ratios (Mervaala et al., 2001). The reasons for the discrepancy between the direction of the findings in these frontotemporal regions are not clear. Future study of Cho in adolescents with MDD may help to elucidate abnormalities in cellular integrity that may contribute to the early changes in cortico-limbic structure.

The Caetano study (Caetano et al., 2005) is also intriguing in reporting higher levels of myoinositol (mI) in the left DLPFC in adolescents with MDD. Elevations in mI may be reflective of abnormalities in the phosphatidyl-inositol signaling pathway. This pathway has been especially implicated in bipolar disorder (BD) and indeed increases in mI were reported in adolescents with BD, compared to NCs as well as a comparison group with intermittent explosive disorder (Davanzo et al., 2003). Moreover, the mood-stabilizing treatment lithium is associated with reductions in pretreatment mI elevations (Davanzo et al., 2003). This suggests the potential for mI as a marker not only for mood disorders but also for response to mood disorder treatments and raises questions about what affects lithium might have in a pediatric MDD group.

Rosenberg and colleagues (2004) and Mirza et al. (2004) found decreases in the anterior cingulate in the glutamatergic Glx peak, which includes glutamate and glutamine measures, in 13 adolescents who were psychotropic medication naïve with depression compared to NC adolescents. Their group subsequently used MRS methods to quantify the contributions of glutamate and glutamine in an independent sample of 28 additional adolescents

TABLE 73.3 *Magnetic Resonance Spectroscopy Studies of Children and Adolescents with Major Depression*

Reference	*Sample*	*Ages*	*Method*	*Results*
Steingard et al., 2000	22 MDD	13–17	1.5 Tesla	MDD > NC orbitofrontal cytostolic Cho/Cr ratios
	43 NC			MDD > NC orbitofrontal cytostolic Cho/NAA ratios
Farchione et al., 2002	11 MDD	10–16	1.5 Tesla	MDD > NC left dorsolateral PFC Cho
	11 NC			MDD = NC dorsolateral PFC NAA and Cr
Caetano et al., 2005	14 MDD	9–17	1.5 Tesla	MDD < NC dorsolateral PFC Cho
	22 NC			MDD > NC left dorsolateral PFC mI
Mirza et al., 2004	13 MDD	10–19	1.5 Tesla	MDD < NC anterior cingulate Glx
	13 NC			
Rosenberg et al., 2004	14 MDD	11–17	1.5 Tesla	MDD < NC anterior cingulate glutamate
	14 NC			MDD = NC anterior cingulate glutamine
Kusumakar et al., 2001	11 MDD	14–18	1.5 Tesla	MDD < NC left amygdala Cho/Cr ratios
	11 NC			MDD = NC right amygdala Cho/Cr ratios; and right and left NAA/Cr ratios

Cho: choline compounds; Cr: creatine-phosphocreatine; Glx: glutamate + glutamine; MDD: major depression disorder; mI: myoinositol; NAA: *N*-acetylaspartate; NC: normal control; PFC: prefrontal cortex.

(Rosenberg et al., 2004). Consistent with a finding in adults with MDD (Auer et al., 2000), decreases in glutamate, but not glutamine, were demonstrated in the adolescents with MDD (Rosenberg et al., 2004). In the Caetano study described above (Caetano et al., 2005), glutamate levels in the DLPFC were inversely related to the duration of illness and number of depressive episodes. In adolescents with BD, frontal increases in Glx have been reported (Castillo et al., 2000). This raises the question of whether differences in the direction of frontal abnormalities in glutamate might differentiate MDD and BD. Direct comparisons between these disorders are warranted.

Taken together, the data suggest that MRS studies provide intriguing potential for the detection of early abnormalities in cell membrane integrity, as well as abnormalities in glutamate and phosphatidyl-inositol signaling pathways, that may underlie abnormalities in cortico-limbic structure and function in MDD. These may point to specific pathophysiological mechanisms in child and adolescent MDD that could be targeted in treatments.

FUTURE DIRECTIONS

Genes and environment have long been hypothesized to be relevant to the etiology of mood disorders. Since the original publication by Caspi and colleagues (2003) documenting an interaction between the serotonin transporter (5-HTTLPR) gene and stressful life events in the etiology of MDD, more than 20 studies have replicated this finding (Moffit, personal communication, May 21, 2007). Although child-onset depression has been associated with various candidate genes in single investigations (Strauss et al., 2004; Adams et al., 2005), interactions between 5-HTTLPR and adverse life events have been reported in three studies with children and adolescents (Eley et al., 2004; Kaufman, Yang, et al., 2004; Kaufman et al., 2006), and a fourth study has documented an association between 5-HTTLPR, stress, and behavioral inhibition in children, a related phenotype (Fox et al., 2005).

There is emerging consensus on the importance of considering G × E factors in mood disorders research—not only in studies examining MDD onset but also in studies examining the neural underpinnings of MDD. In 2002, Hariri and colleagues published one of the first papers demonstrating that variation in the 5-HTTLPR could modulate amygdala activation in response to emotionally arousing stimuli. Since the seminal paper by Hariri and colleagues (2002), which documented that the presence of the short ("s"), as opposed to the long ("l), allele of 5-HTTLPR is associated with increased amygdala activation to aversive stimuli, this finding has been replicated in eight independent reports: seven studies with healthy volunteers (Bertolino et al., 2005; Canli et al., 2005; Hariri et al., 2005; Heinz et al., 2005; Pezawas et al., 2005; Canli et al., 2006; Smolka et al., 2007) and one study with adults with depression (Dannlowski et al., 2007). Effects have been demonstrated with paradigms using diverse stimuli, including fearful faces (Hariri et al., 2002; Bertolino et al., 2005; Hariri et al., 2005; Pezawas et al., 2005; Canli et al., 2006; Dannlowski et al., 2007), unpleasant pictures (Heinz et al., 2005; Smolka et al., 2007), and negative words (Canli et al., 2005). There is one report suggesting that the increased activation in response to aversive compared to neutral stimuli is due to tonic activation and decreased activation in response to neutral stimuli (Canli et al., 2005). There are also preliminary data suggesting that amygdala activation is susceptible to the effects of genes and environment in interaction (Canli et al., 2006), and is under control of multiple genes (Smolka et al., 2007).

We conducted one small pilot study in this area (Herrington et al., 2007). These preliminary data highlight the value of incorporating imaging genomics strategies into future studies of the pathophysiology of child and adolescent MDD. Participants ($N = 11$) were stratified according to environmental stress (for example, maltreatment vs. no significant lifetime stressors) and genetic risk (for example, s/s vs. l/l, s/l excluded) and were administered a slightly modified version of the fMRI dichotic listening task developed by Vuilleumier and colleagues (Grandjean et al., 2005). This task includes two nonsense words recorded by male and female speakers in angry and neutral tones. Two stimuli were presented simultaneously, one to each ear on each trial. Participants selectively attended to either left or right ear and performed a gender decision of voice heard on the target side. Because children who were maltreated have been found to have atrophy of the corpus callosum in multiple independent studies (De Bellis et al., 1999; Teicher et al., 2000; De Bellis et al., 2002), and reduction in corpus collosal fractional anisotropy, a measure of axonal integrity (Jackowski et al., 2008), this prosody task was chosen because it requires interhemispheric transfer through the region of the corpus showing deficits in children who were maltreated. It also involves affective processing circuits, with key anatomical structures involved in these circuits sensitive to variation in 5-HTTLPR and environmental stress. This task also avoids racial biasing effects inherent in face-processing tasks that can be problematic to employ in ethnically diverse samples. In our preliminary analysis of the data, main effects were found for genetic risk. When comparing angry to neutral words, participants who were high risk (s/s) showed significantly decreased right superior temporal sulcus (STS) activity and increased right amygdala activation. In the attended/nonattended ear contrast, participants who were high risk (s/s) also showed decreased left OFC activation when compared to participants who were low risk (l/l). A similar pattern of results was found for environmental risk, and G × E interactions will be examined when the sample is expanded. These preliminary results and other emerging work in the area demonstrate the power of using candidate gene and G × E approaches together with fMRI to understand the pathophysiology of stress-related psychiatric disorders such as child-onset depression.

CONCLUDING REMARKS

The field of neuroimaging research in pediatric mood disorders is still in its infancy. The convergence of findings across the structural, functional, and spectroscopy studies is beginning to implicate frontotemporal abnormalities in child and adolescent MDD, as reported in adults with MDD. The utilization of imaging genomic approaches promises to help further elucidate the neural underpinnings of this disorder and will likely help to explain inconsistencies in results across studies. MDD in children and adolescents is a serious disorder, and more research is needed in this area to optimize clinical interventions for this vulnerable population.

REFERENCES

Adams, J.H., Wigg, K.G., King, N., et al. (2005) Association study of neurotrophic tyrosine kinase receptor type 2 (NTRK2) and childhood-onset mood disorders. *Am. J. Med. Genet. B Neuropsychiatr. Genet.* 132:90–95.

Auer, D.P., Putz, B., Kraft, E., Lipinski, B., Schill, J., and Holsboer, F. (2000) Reduced glutamate in the anterior cingulate cortex in depression: an in vivo proton magnetic resonance spectroscopy study. *Biol. Psychiatry* 47:305–313.

Axelson, D.A., Doraiswamy, P.M., Boyko, O.B., et al. (1992) In vivo assessment of pituitary volume with magnetic resonance imaging and systematic stereology: relationship to dexamethasone suppression test results in patients. *Psychiatry Res.* 44:63–70.

Baxter, L.R., Schwartz, J.M., Phelps, M.E., et al. (1989) Reduction of prefrontal cortex glucose metabolism common to three types of depression. *Arch. Gen. Psychiatry* 46:243–250.

Bench, C.J., Friston, K.J., Brown, R.G., Frackowiak, R.S., and Dolan, R.J. (1993) Regional cerebral blood flow in depression measured by positron emission tomography: the relationship with clinical dimensions. *Psychol. Med.* 23:579–590.

Bertolino, A., Arciero, G., Rubino, V., et al. (2005) Variation of human amygdala response during threatening stimuli as a function of 5-HTTLPR genotype and personality style. *Biol. Psychiatry* 57:1517–1525.

Birmaher, B., Ryan, N.D., Williamson, D.E., Brent, D.A., and Kaufman, J. (1996) Childhood and adolescent depression: a review of the past 10 years. Part II. *J. Am. Acad. Child Adolesc. Psychiatry* 35:1575–1583.

Birmaher, B., Ryan, N.D., Williamson, D.E., et al. (1996) Childhood and adolescent depression: a review of the past 10 years. Part I. *J. Am. Acad. Child Adolesc. Psychiatry* 35:1427–1439.

Blumberg, H.P., Krystal, J.H., Bansal, R., et al. (2006) Age, rapid-cycling, and pharmacotherapy effects on ventral prefrontal cortex in bipolar disorder: a cross-sectional study. *Biol. Psychiatry* 59:611–618.

Botteron, K.N., Raichle, M.E., Drevets, W.C., Heath, A.C., and Todd, R.D. (2002) Volumetric reduction in left subgenual prefrontal cortex in early onset depression. *Biol. Psychiatry* 51:342–344.

Bremner, J.D., Narayan, M., Anderson, E.R., Staib, L.H., Miller, H.L., and Charney, D.S. (2000) Hippocampal volume reduction in major depression. *Am. J. Psychiatry* 157:115–118.

Brent, D.A. (2006) Glad for what TADS adds, but many TADS grads still sad. *J. Am. Acad. Child Adolesc. Psychiatry* 45:1461–1464.

Brent, D.A., and Weersing, R. (2007) Depressive disorders. In: A. Martin and F. Volkmar, eds. *Lewis's Child and Adolescent Psychiatry: A Comprehensive Textbook*, 4th ed. Philadelphia: Wolters Kluwer/Lippincott Wiliams & Wilkins, pp. 503–513.

Bridge, J.A., Iyengar, S., Salary, C.B., et al. (2007) Clinical response and risk for reported suicidal ideation and suicide attempts in pediatric antidepressant treatment: a meta-analysis of randomized controlled trials. *JAMA* 297:1683–1696.

Brody, A.L., Saxena, S., Mandelkern, M.A., Fairbanks, L.A., Ho, M.L., and Baxter, L.R. (2001) Brain metabolic changes associated with symptom factor improvement in major depressive disorder. *Biol. Psychiatry* 50:171–178.

Caetano, S.C., Fonseca, M., Olvera, R.L., et al. (2005) Proton spectroscopy study of the left dorsolateral prefrontal cortex in pediatric depressed patients. *Neurosci. Lett.* 384:321–326.

Caetano, S.C., Hatch, J.P., Brambilla, P., et al. (2004) Anatomical MRI study of hippocampus and amygdala in patients with current and remitted major depression. *Psychiatry Res.* 132:141–147.

Canli, T., Omura, K., Haas, B.W., Fallgatter, A., Constable, R.T., and Lesch, K.P. (2005) Beyond affect: a role for genetic variation of the serotonin transporter in neural activation during a cognitive attention task. *Proc. Natl. Acad. Sci. USA* 102:12224–12229.

Canli, T., Qiu, M., Omura, K., et al. (2006) Neural correlates of epigenesis. *Proc. Natl. Acad. Sci. USA* 103:16033–16038.

Caspi, A., Sugden, K., Moffitt, T.E., et al. (2003) Influence of life stress on depression: moderation by a polymorphism in the 5-HTT gene. *Science* 301:386–389.

Castillo, M., Kwock, L., Courvoisie, H., and Hooper, S.R. (2000) Proton MR spectroscopy in children with bipolar affective disorder: preliminary observations. *Am. J. Neuroradiol.* 21:832–838.

Costello, E.J., Pine, D.S., Hammen, C., et al. (2002) Development and natural history of mood disorders. *Biol. Psychiatry* 52:529–542.

Dannlowski, U., Ohrmann, P., Bauer, J., et al. (2007) Serotonergic genes modulate amygdala activity in major depression. *Genes Brain Behav.* 6(7):672–676.

Davanzo, P., Yue, K., Thomas, M.A., et al. (2003) Proton magnetic resonance spectroscopy of bipolar disorder versus intermittent explosive disorder in children and adolescents. *Am. J. Psychiatry* 160:1442–1452.

De Bellis, M.D., Keshavan, M.S., Clark, D.B., et al. (1999) Developmental traumatology. Part II: Brain development. *Biol. Psychiatry* 45:1271–1284.

De Bellis, M.D., Keshavan, M.S., Shifflett, H., et al. (2002) Brain structures in pediatric maltreatment-related posttraumatic stress disorder: a sociodemographically matched study. *Biol. Psychiatry* 52:1066–1078.

de Geus, E.J., van't Ent, D., Wolfensberger, S.P., et al. (2007) Intrapair differences in hippocampal volume in monozygotic twins discordant for the risk for anxiety and depression. *Biol. Psychiatry* 61:1062–1071.

Drevets, W.C., Price, J.L., Simpson, J.R., Jr., et al. (1997) Subgenual prefrontal cortex abnormalities in mood disorders. *Nature* 386: 824–827.

Eley, T.C., Sugden, K., Corsico, A., et al. (2004) Gene-environment interaction analysis of serotonin system markers with adolescent depression. *Mol. Psychiatry* 9:908–915.

Emslie, G.J., Rush, A.J., Weinberg, W.A., et al. (1997) A double-blind, randomized, placebo-controlled trial of fluoxetine in children and adolescents with depression. *Arch. Gen. Psychiatry* 54: 1031–1037.

Epstein, J., Pan, H., Kocsis, J.H., et al. (2006) Lack of ventral striatal response to positive stimuli in depressed versus normal subjects. *Am. J. Psychiatry* 163:1784–1790.

Farchione, T.R., Moore, G.J., and Rosenberg, D.R. (2002) Proton magnetic resonance spectroscopic imaging in pediatric major depression. *Biol. Psychiatry* 52:86–92.

Forbes, E.E., Christopher May, J., Siegle, G.J., et al. (2006) Reward-related decision-making in pediatric major depressive disorder: an fMRI study. *J. Child Psychol. Psychiatry* 47:1031–1040.

Forbes, E.E., Shaw, D.S., and Dahl, R.E. (2007) Alterations in reward-related decision making in boys with recent and future depression. *Biol. Psychiatry* 61:633–639.

Fox, N.A., Nichols, K.E., Henderson, H.A., et al. (2005) Evidence for a gene-environment interaction in predicting behavioral inhibition in middle childhood. *Psychol. Sci.* 16:921–926.

Frodl, T., Meisenzahl, E.M., Zetzsche, T., et al. (2002) Hippocampal changes in patients with a first episode of major depression. *Am. J. Psychiatry* 159:1112–1118.

Geller, B., Zimerman, B., Williams, M., Bolhofner, K., and Craney, J.L. (2001) Bipolar disorder at prospective follow-up of adults who had prepubertal major depressive disorder. *Am. J. Psychiatry* 158:125–127.

Gibbons, R.D., Brown, C.H., Hur, K., et al. (2007) Early evidence on the effects of regulators' suicidality warnings on SSRI prescriptions and suicide in children and adolescents. *Am. J. Psychiatry* 164:1356–1363.

Giedd, J.N., Castellanos, F.X., Rajapakse, J.C., Vaituzis, A.C., and Rapoport, J.L. (1997) Sexual dimorphism of the developing human brain. *Prog. Neuropsychopharmacol. Biol. Psychiatry* 21: 1185–118201.

Gilbertson, M., Shenton, M.E., Ciszewski, A., et al. (2002) Smaller hippocampal volume predicts pathologic vulnerability to psychological trauma. *Nat. Neurosci.* 5:1242–1247.

Goldapple, K., Segal, Z., Garson, C., et al. (2004) Modulation of cortical-limbic pathways in major depression: treatment-specific effects of cognitive behavior therapy. *Arch. Gen. Psychiatry* 61:34–41.

Grandjean, D., Sander, D., Pourtois, G., et al. (2005) The voices of wrath: brain responses to angry prosody in meaningless speech. *Nat. Neurosci.* 8:145–146.

Guidotti, A., and Costa, E. (1998) Can the antidysphoric and anxiolytic profiles of selective serotonin reuptake inhibitors be related to their ability to increase brain 3 alpha, 5 alpha-tetrahydroprogesterone (allopregnanolone) availability? *Biol. Psychiatry* 44:865–873.

Hamilton, B.E., Minino, A.M., Martin, J.A., Kochanek, K.D., Strobino, D.M., and Guyer, B. (2007) Annual summary of vital statistics: 2005. *Pediatrics* 119:345–360.

Hammad, T.A., Laughren, T., and Racoosin, J. (2006) Suicidality in pediatric patients treated with antidepressant drugs. *Arch. Gen. Psychiatry* 63:332–339.

Hariri, A.R., Drabant, E.M., Munoz, K.E., et al. (2005) A susceptibility gene for affective disorders and the response of the human amygdala. *Arch. Gen. Psychiatry* 62:146–152.

Hariri, A.R., Mattay, V.S., Tessitore, A., et al. (2002) Serotonin transporter genetic variation and the response of the human amygdala. *Science* 297:400–403.

Hariri, A.R., and Weinberger, D.R. (2003) Imaging genomics. *Br. Med. Bull.* 65:259–270.

Hazell, P., O'Connell, D., Heathcote, D., Robertson, J., and Henry, D. (1995) Efficacy of tricyclic drugs in treating child and adolescent depression: a meta-analysis. *BMJ* 310:897–901.

Heinz, A., Braus, D.F., Smolka, M.N., et al. (2005) Amygdala-prefrontal coupling depends on a genetic variation of the serotonin transporter. *Nat. Neurosci.* 8:20–21.

Herrington, J., Douglas-Palumberi, H., Meadows, A., et al. (2007, May) *fMRI study of prosody processing in maltreated children.* Paper presented at the Annual Meeting of the Society of Biological Psychiatry, San Diego, CA.

Jackowski, A.P., Douglas-Palumberi, H., Jackowski, M., et al. (2008) Corpus callosum in maltreated children with PTSD: A diffusion tensor imaging study. *Psychiatric Res.: Neuroimaging,* 162(3):256–261.

Kaufman, J., Blumberg, H.P., and Young, C.M. (2004) Neurobiology of early onset mood disorders. In: Charney, D.S., Nestler, E.J., eds. *Neurobiology of Mental Illness*, 2nd ed. New York: Oxford University Press, pp. 1007–1021.

Kaufman, J., Martin, A., King, R., and Charney, D. (2001) Are child-, adolescent-, and adult-onset depression one and the same disorder? *Biol. Psychiatry* 49:1012–1033.

Kaufman, J., and Ryan, N. (1999) The neurobiology of child and adolescent depression. In: Charney, D., Nestler, E., and Bunny, B., eds. *The Neurobiological Foundation of Mental Illness.* New York: Oxford University Press, pp. 810–821.

Kaufman, J., Yang, B.Z., Douglas-Palumberi, H., et al. (2004) Social supports and serotonin transporter gene moderate depression in maltreated children. *Proc. Natl. Acad. Sci. USA* 101:17316–17321.

Kaufman, J., Yang, B.Z., Douglas-Palumberi, H., et al. (2006) Brain-derived neurotrophic factor-5-HTTLPR gene interactions and environmental modifiers of depression in children. *Biol. Psychiatry* 59:673–680.

Keedwell, P.A., Andrew, C., Williams, S.C., Brammer, M.J., and Phillips, M.L. (2005) A double dissociation of ventromedial prefrontal cortical responses to sad and happy stimuli in depressed and healthy individuals. *Biol. Psychiatry* 58:495–503.

Keller, M.B., Ryan, N., Birmaher, B., et al. (2001) Multi-center trial of paroxetine and imipramine in the treatment of adolescent depression. *J. Am. Acad. Child Adolesc. Psychiatry* 40(7):762–772.

Kilts, C.D. (1994) Recent pharmacologic advances in antidepressant therapy. *Am. J. Med.* 97:3S–12S.

Kovacs, M. (1996) Presentation and course of major depressive disorder during childhood and later years of the life span. *J. Am. Acad. Child Adolesc. Psychiatry* 35:705–715.

Kowatch, R.A., Devous, M.D. Sr., Harvey, D.C., et al. (1999) A SPECT HMPAO study of regional cerebral blood flow in depressed adolescents and normal controls. *Prog. Neuropsychopharmacol. Biol. Psychiatry* 23:643–656.

Krishnan, K.R., Doraiswamy, P.M., Lurie, S.N., et al. (1991) Pituitary size in depression. *J. Clin. Endocrinol. Metab.* 72:256–259.

Kurian, B.T., Ray, W.A., Arbogast, P.G., Fuchs, D.C., Dudley, J.A., and Cooper, W.O. (2007) Effect of regulatory warnings on antidepressant prescribing for children and adolescents. *Arch. Pediatr. Adolesc. Med.* 161:690–696.

Kusumakar, V., MacMaster, F.P., Gates, L., Sparkes, S.J., and Khan, S.C. (2001) Left medial temporal cytosolic choline in early onset depression. *Can. J. Psychiatry* 46:959–964.

Ladouceur, C.D., Dahl, R.E., Williamson, D.E., et al. (2006) Processing emotional facial expressions influences performance on a go/nogo task in pediatric anxiety and depression. *J. Child Psychol. Psychiatry* 47:1107–1115.

Lewinsohn, P.M., Rohde, P., Klein, D.N., and Seeley, J.R. (1999) Natural course of adolescent major depressive disorder: I. Continuity into young adulthood. *J. Am. Acad. Child Adolesc. Psychiatry* 38:56–63.

MacMaster, F.P., and Kusumakar, V. (2004a) Hippocampal volume in early onset depression. *BMC Med.* 2:2.

MacMaster, F.P., and Kusumakar, V. (2004b) MRI study of the pituitary gland in adolescent depression. *J. Psychiatry Res.* 38:231–236.

MacMaster, F.P., Mirza, Y., Szeszko, P.R., et al. (2008) Amygdala and hippocampal volumes in familial early onset major depressive disorder. *Biological Psychiatry.* 63(4):385–390.

MacMaster, F.P., Russell, A., Mirza, Y., et al. (2006) Pituitary volume in treatment-naive pediatric major depressive disorder. *Biol. Psychiatry* 60:862–866.

MacMillan, S., Szeszko, P.R., Moore, G.J., et al. (2003) Increased amygdala: hippocampal volume ratios associated with severity of anxiety in pediatric major depression. *J. Child Adolesc. Psychopharmacol.* 13:65–73.

MacQueen, G.M., Campbell, S., McEwen, B.S., et al. (2003) Course of illness, hippocampal function, and hippocampal volume in major depression. *Proc. Natl. Acad. Sci. USA* 100:1387–1392.

March, J., Silva, S., and Vitiello, B. (2006) The Treatment for Adolescents with Depression Study (TADS): methods and message at 12 weeks. *J. Am. Acad. Child Adolesc. Psychiatry* 45:1393–1403.

Martin, A., Kaufman, J., and Charney, D. (2000) Pharmacotherapy of early-onset depression. Update and new directions. *Child Adolesc. Psychiatry Clin. N. Am.* 9:135–157.

Mayberg, H.S., Brannan, S.K., Tekell, J.L., et al. (2000) Regional metabolic effects of fluoxetine in major depression: serial changes and relationship to clinical response. *Biol. Psychiatry* 48:830–843.

Mervaala, E., Fohr, J., Kononen, M., et al. (2000) Quantitative MRI of the hippocampus and amygdala in severe depression. *Psychol. Med.* 30:117–25.

Mervaala, E., Kononen, M., Fohr, J., et al. (2001) SPECT and neuropsychological performance in severe depression treated with ECT. *J. Affect. Disord.* 66:47–58.

Mirza, Y., Tang, J., Russell, A., et al. (2004) Reduced anterior cingulate cortex glutamatergic concentrations in childhood major depression. *J. Am. Acad. Child Adolesc. Psychiatry* 43:341–348.

Monk, C.S., Klein, R., Telzer, B., et al. (2008) Amygdala and nucleus accumbens activation to emotional facial expressions in children and adolescents at risk for major depression. *Am. J. Psychiatry* 165(1):90–98.

Munn, M.A., Alexopoulos, J., Nishino, T., et al. (2007) Amygdala volume analysis in female twins with major depression. *Biol. Psychiatry* 62:415–422.

Nemeroff, C.B., Kalali, A., Keller, M.B., et al. (2007) Impact of publicity concerning pediatric suicidality data on physician practice patterns in the United States. *Arch. Gen. Psychiatry* 64:466–472.

Nolan, C.L., Moore, G.J., Madden, R., et al. (2002) Prefrontal cortical volume in childhood-onset major depression: preliminary findings. *Arch. Gen. Psychiatry* 59:173–179.

Pezawas, L., Meyer-Lindenberg, A., Drabant, E.M., et al. (2005) 5-HTTLPR polymorphism impacts human cingulate-amygdala interactions: a genetic susceptibility mechanism for depression. *Nat. Neurosci.* 8:828–834.

Pine, D.S., Cohen, P., Gurley, D., Brook, J., and Ma, Y. (1998) The risk for early-adulthood anxiety and depressive disorders in adolescents with anxiety and depressive disorders. *Arch. Gen. Psychiatry* 55:56–64.

Pine, D.S., Lissek, S., Klein, R.G., et al. (2004) Face-memory and emotion: associations with major depression in children and adolescents. *J. Child Psychol. Psychiatry* 45:1199–1208.

Rao, U., Ryan, N.D., Birmaher, B., et al. (1995) Unipolar depression in adolescents: clinical outcome in adulthood. *J. Am. Acad. Child Adolesc. Psychiatry* 34:566–578.

Rao, U., Weissman, M.M., Martin, J.A., and Hammond, R.W. (1993) Childhood depression and risk of suicide: a preliminary report of a longitudinal study. *J. Am. Acad. Child Adolesc. Psychiatry* 32:21–27.

Roberson-Nay, R., McClure, E.B., Monk, C.S., et al. (2006) Increased amygdala activity during successful memory encoding in adolescent major depressive disorder: An FMRI study. *Biol. Psychiatry* 60:966–973.

Rosenberg, D.R., Mirza, Y., Russell, A., et al. (2004) Reduced anterior cingulate glutamatergic concentrations in childhood OCD and major depression versus healthy controls. *J. Am. Acad. Child Adolesc. Psychiatry* 43:1146–1153.

Rosso, I.M., Cintron, C.M., Steingard, R.J., Renshaw, P.F., Young, A.D., and Yurgelun-Todd, D.A. (2005) Amygdala and hippocampus volumes in pediatric major depression. *Biol. Psychiatry* 57:21–26.

Rubinow, D.R., and Post, R.M. (1992) Impaired recognition of affect in facial expression in depressed patients. *Biol. Psychiatry* 31:947–953.

Ryan, N.D. (2005) Treatment of depression in children and adolescents. *Lancet* 366:933–940.

Sheline, Y.I., Barch, D.M., Donnelly, J.M., Ollinger, J.M., Snyder, A.Z., and Mintun, M.A. (2001) Increased amygdala response to masked emotional faces in depressed subjects resolves with antidepressant treatment: an fMRI study. *Biol. Psychiatry* 50:651–658.

Sheline, Y.I., Gado, M.H., and Kraemer, H.C. (2003) Untreated depression and hippocampal volume loss. *Am. J. Psychiatry* 160: 1516–1518.

Sheline, Y.I., Wang, P.W., Gado, M.H., Csernansky, J.G., and Vannier, M.W. (1996) Hippocampal atrophy in recurrent major depression. *Proc. Natl. Acad. Sci. USA* 93:3908–3913.

Siegle, G. J., Konecky, R. O., Thase, M. E., and Carter, C. S. (2003) Relationships between amygdala volume and activity during emotional information processing tasks in depressed and never-depressed individuals: an fMRI investigation. *Ann. NY Acad. Sci.* 985:481–484.

Smolka, M.N., Buhler, M., Schumann, G., et al. (2007) Gene-gene effects on central processing of aversive stimuli. *Mol. Psychiatry* 12:307–317.

Steingard, R.J., Renshaw, P.F., Hennen, J., et al. (2002) Smaller frontal lobe white matter volumes in depressed adolescents. *Biol. Psychiatry* 52:413–417.

Steingard, R.J., Renshaw, P.F., Yurgelun-Todd, D., et al. (1996) Structural abnormalities in brain magnetic resonance images of depressed children. *J. Am. Acad. Child Adolesc. Psychiatry* 35: 307–311.

Steingard, R.J., Yurgelun-Todd, D.A., Hennen, J., et al. (2000) Increased orbitofrontal cortex levels of choline in depressed adolescents as detected by in vivo proton magnetic resonance spectroscopy. *Biol. Psychiatry* 48:1053–1061.

Strauss, J., Barr, C.L., George, C.J., et al. (2004) Association study of brain-derived neurotrophic factor in adults with a history of childhood onset mood disorder. *Am. J. Med. Genet. B Neuropsychiatr. Genet.* 131:16–19.

Suslow, T., Junghanns, K., and Arolt, V. (2001) Detection of facial expressions of emotions in depression. *Percept. Mot. Skills* 92: 857–868.

Tang, Y., Wang, F., Xie, G., Liu, J., Li, L., Su, L., et al. (2007) Reduced ventral anterior cingulate and amygdala volumes in medication-naive females with major depressive disorder: A voxel-based morphometric magnetic resonance imaging study. *Psychiatry Res.* 156(1):83–86.

Teicher, M.H., Anderson, S.L., Dumont, Y., et al. (2000) Childhood neglect attenuates development of the corpus callosum. *Soc. Neurosci. Abstr.* 26(2000):549.

Thomas, K.M., Drevets, W.C., Dahl, R.E., et al. (2001) Amygdala response to fearful faces in anxious and depressed children. *Arch. Gen. Psychiatry* 58:1057–1063.

Tutus, A., Kibar, M., Sofuoglu, S., Basturk, M., and Gonul, A.S. (1998) A technetium-99m hexamethylpropylene amine oxime brain single-photon emission tomography study in adolescent patients with major depressive disorder. *Eur. J. Nucl. Med.* 25: 601–606.

Vasa, R.A., Carlino, A.R., and Pine, D.S. (2006) Pharmacotherapy of depressed children and adolescents: current issues and potential directions. *Biol. Psychiatry* 59:1021–1028.

Weissman, M.M., Wolk, S., Goldstein, R.B., et al. (1999) Depressed adolescents grown up. *JAMA* 281:1707–1713.

74 Structural Magnetic Resonance Imaging of Typical Pediatric Brain Development

JAY N. GIEDD, SAMANTHA L. WHITE, AND MARK CELANO

Many psychiatric disorders, even those with adult onset such as schizophrenia, are increasingly being viewed from a neurodevelopmental perspective. Advances in imaging technology, such as magnetic resonance imaging (MRI), allow exploration of the biological substrates that may underlie differences in healthy and unhealthy brain development. Magnetic resonance imaging is particularly well-suited for pediatric studies because unlike other imaging modalities such as computerized tomography (CT) or positron emission tomography (PET), MRI does not use ionizing radiation. The safety and tolerability of MRI allows not only the scanning of children but also repeated scans of the same individuals throughout development. This capability to accurately characterize in vivo cerebral anatomy and physiology throughout development has launched a new era of pediatric neuroscience.

Studies of typical maturation are important to provide a "yardstick" from which to assess deviations in clinical populations and also to elucidate fundamental features of brain development that may serve as heuristics to guide future interventions or research initiatives. In this chapter, the focus is on structural (or anatomic) MRI.

METHODOLOGIC CONSIDERATIONS

The smallest units of MRI pictures are called *pixels* (picture elements) or their three dimensional counterparts, *voxels* (volume elements). Each voxel is assigned a single value based on the average magnetic properties of the tissue in that box. The size of the voxel can vary depending on magnet strength, and reductions in voxel size can be purchased with the currency of time. Most of the literature is from scans producing voxels of 1 to 3 ml in volume. It is worth noting that even a 1 ml voxel may contain millions of neurons and trillions of synaptic connections that confer substantial, but often unheeded, implications for interpretation.

A general goal of structural image analysis is to classify each voxel according to tissue type (for example, gray matter [GM], white matter [WM], cerebrospinal fluid [CSF], vasculature), as well as to assign it to the structure or region in which it belongs. The classification usually employs computer algorithms that combine information about the intensity of the voxel with atlases that inform the probability of tissue type based on the voxel's location in the brain (Collins et al., 1995).

Once the voxels have been classified, their number in a specific region can be counted to provide volume estimates. To the extent that one can create a one-to-one correspondence between the same parts in different brain images, "average" brains for groups can be created. Averaged brains lend themselves to powerful statistical analyses, but high individual variation in brain morphometry makes achieving meaningful one-to-one correspondence challenging. Anchoring each individual image on the least variable sulci has enhanced the utility of this approach (Thompson et al., 2004).

DEVELOPMENTAL ANATOMIC TRAJECTORIES DURING TYPICAL CHILDHOOD AND ADOLESCENCE

Magnetic resonance imaging studies of typical child and adolescent brain development began to be reported in the 1990s (Jernigan and Tallal, 1990; Jernigan et al., 1991; Pfefferbaum et al., 1994; Caviness et al., 1996; Giedd, Snell, et al., 1996; Reiss et al., 1996; Sowell and Jernigan, 1998; Caviness et al., 1999; Sowell, Thompson, Holmes, Batth, et al., 1999; Sowell, Thompson, Holmes, Jernigan, and Toga, 1999). Although early studies were cross-sectional and data for the typical populations were often from scans acquired for clinical indications that were subsequently read as normal, the results indicating moderate changes in total brain size but substantial changes in GM, WM, and CSF volumes were in general agreement.

In 1989, Markus Krusei, MD, began an ongoing longitudinal imaging project at the Child Psychiatry Branch (CPB) of the National Institute of Mental Health (NIMH). The study design is for typical and atypically developing participants to return for scans and neuropsychological testing at approximately 2-year intervals. Unless otherwise indicated the results in the following sections are from the most recent analyses of the CPB data consisting of 829 scans from 387 subjects, ages 3 to 27 years.

Total Cerebral Volume

In the CPB cohort total cerebral volume peaks at 10.5 years in females and 14.5 years in males (Lenroot et al., 2007). By age 6 years the brain is at approximately 95% of this peak (see Fig. 74.1a). That total cerebral volume decreases during adolescence was not previously detected

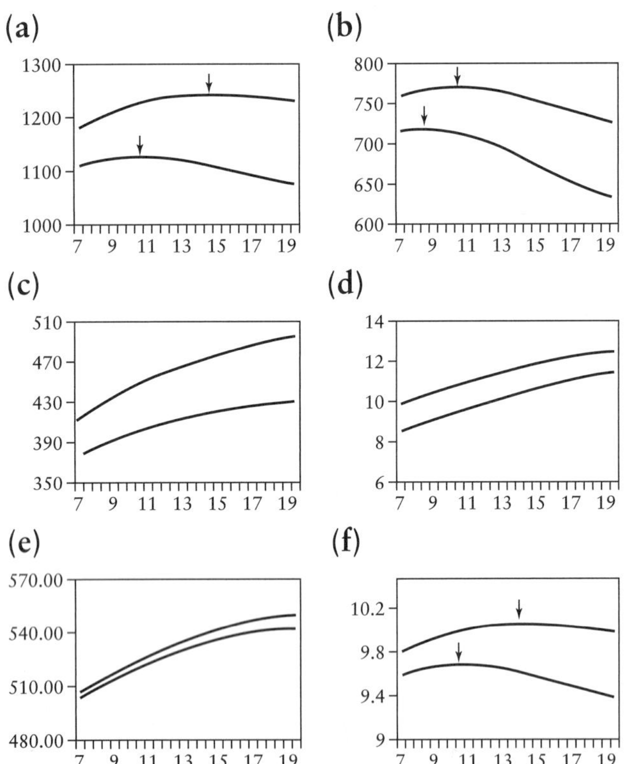

FIGURE 74.1 Mean volume by age in years for males (N = 475 scans) and females (N = 354 scans). Middle lines in each set of three lines represent mean values, and upper and lower lines represent upper and lower 95% confidence intervals. All curves differed significantly in height and shape with the exception of lateral ventricles, in which only height was different, and mid-sagittal area of the corpus callosum, in which neither height nor shape was different. (*a*) Total brain volume, (*b*) gray matter volume, (*c*) white matter volume, (*d*) lateral ventricle volume, (*e*) mid-sagittal area of the corpus callosum, and (*f*) caudate volume.

with postmortem data (Dekaban, 1977; Dekaban and Sadowsky, 1978) or cross-sectional MRI studies (Jernigan and Tallal, 1990; Giedd, Snell, et al., 1996). Consistent with previous reports (Goldstein et al., 2001), mean total cerebral volume is approximately 10% larger in males. Total brain size differences should not be interpreted as imparting any sort of functional advantage or disadvantage. Gross structural measures may not reflect sexually dimorphic differences in functionally relevant factors such as neuronal connectivity and receptor density. Of note is the high variability of brain size, even in this group of rigorously screened children and adolescents who were healthy. Children who were healthy and normally functioning at the same age may have as much as a 50% difference in total brain volume, further highlighting the need to be cautious regarding functional implications of absolute brain sizes.

Ventricles

Consistent with previous reports of greater ventricular volume in adults versus children (Jernigan and Tallal, 1990), lateral ventricular volume increased robustly with age in the CPB sample of children and adolescents who were healthy (see Fig. 74.1d). This is noteworthy because increased ventricular volumes are associated with a broad range of neuropsychiatric conditions. That ventricular volume is highly variable, and increases in healthy pediatric development complicates interpretation of ventricular volume changes in patient populations.

White Matter

Magnetic resonance imaging voxels containing a sufficient amount of myelinated axons are classified as WM. Myelination is the wrapping of oligodendrocytes around axons that increases the speed of neuronal signal transmission and modulates the timing and synchrony of neuronal firing patterns that convey meaning in the brain (Fields and Stevens-Graham, 2002).

Consistent with previous reports (Pfefferbaum et al., 1994; Giedd et al., 1995; Reiss et al., 1996; Giedd, Blumenthal, Jeffries, Castellanos, et al., 1999; Giedd, Blumenthal, Jeffries, Rajapakse, et al., 1999; Sowell et al., 2001; Sowell et al., 2003; Lenroot et al., 2007), WM volumes increase throughout childhood and adolescence (see Fig. 74.1c). The rate of increase is age dependent (Giedd, Blumenthal, Jeffries, Castellanos, et al., 1999) and can increase as much as 50% in small regions of interest (Thompson et al., 2000), but at the lobar level (frontal, temporal, and parietal lobes) developmental WM trajectories are similar.

The most prominent WM structure is the corpus callosum (CC), consisting of approximately 200 million axons connecting homologous areas of the left and right cortex. The organization of the CC is roughly topographic, with anterior, middle, and posterior segments containing fibers from their corresponding cortical regions. The functions of the CC can generally be thought of as integrating the activities of the left and right cerebral hemispheres, including functions related to the unification of sensory fields (Shanks et al., 1975; Berlucchi, 1981), memory storage and retrieval (Zaidel and Sperry, 1974), attention and arousal (Levy, 1985), and enhancement of language and auditory functions (Cook, 1986). The relationship between improved capacities for these functions during childhood and adolescence and the noted morphologic changes is intriguing. Several studies have indicated that CC development continues to progress throughout adolescence (Allen et al., 1991; Cowell et al., 1992; Pujol et al., 1993; Rauch and Jinkins, 1994; Thompson et al., 2000), raising the question of whether this may be related to the improvement in these cognitive capacities seen during childhood and adolescence. In the CPB sample, total midsagittal CC area increased robustly from ages 4 to 20 years (see Fig. 74.1e).

The growing interest in exploring neural circuitry has encouraged the development of newer MR techniques, such as magnetization transfer (MT) imaging and diffusion tensor imaging (DTI), which allow characterization of the microstructure of WM and the direction of axons. These techniques have begun to be applied to pediatric populations.

Diffusion tensor imaging studies of typical child and adolescent development have consistently shown decreases of overall diffusion and increases in anisotropy (a measure of the directionality or nonrandomness of the diffusion; see Cascio et al., 2007, for review). High anisotropy measures are thought to reflect coherently bundled myelinated axons and axonal pruning (Suzuki et al., 2003) that allow greater efficiency of neuronal communication.

A growing body of literature documents a relationship between anisotropy measures and cognitive abilities. In a study, of 23 healthy subjects aged 7 to 18 years, high anisotropy in the temporal lobe correlated with memory capacity and high anisotropy in the frontal lobe correlated with language ability (Nagy et al., 2004). High anisotropy in frontal and occipitoparietal association areas correlated with IQ in a DTI study of 47 healthy subjects ages 5 to 18 years (Schmithorst et al., 2005). A positive correlation between anisotropy in temporal and parietal areas and reading ability has been reported in three pediatric DTI studies (Beaulieu et al., 2005; Deutsch et al., 2005; Niogi and McCandliss, 2006). A DTI study, of 21 subjects aged 7 to 31 years, demonstrated decreased diffusion of WM fibers connecting the ventral prefrontal cortex to the caudate nucleus that was paralleled by improvements in reaction time and cognitive performance (Liston et al., 2006).

Magnetization transfer imaging relates the number of protons bound to macromolecules to the number of unbound (free) protons, reflected as the magnetization transfer ratio (MTR) (Rovaris et al., 2003). Magnetization transfer ratio values are decreased with demyelination or axonal loss (Brochet and Dousset, 1999) and increase with myelination. Studies of children and adolescents who are healthy have reported MTR values increasing with maturation (Engelbrecht et al., 1998; van Buchem et al., 2001; Mukherjee and McKinstry, 2006), although only an adult study has linked MTR values to cognitive performance (Lee et al., 2004).

Gray Matter

The composition of MRI voxels classified as GM may vary by region but by default are voxels with not enough myelin to be classified as WM or enough fluid to be classified as CSF. Unlike WM during childhood and adolescence, GM trajectories follow an inverted *U*-shaped path with total GM peaking at age 8.5 years in females and 10.5 years in males (see Fig. 74.1b). This decoupling of developmental curves for GM and WM belies the inseparable connection among neurons, glial cells, and myelin, which are fellow components in neural circuits and are bound by lifelong reciprocal relationships (Fields and Stevens-Graham, 2002).

Cortical Gray Matter

At the lobar level peak volumes of cortical GM vary by region and occur earlier in girls. Gray matter volumes peak in the frontal lobes at 9.5 years in girls and 10.5 years in boys, in the temporal lobes at 10.0 years in girls and 11.0 years in boys, and in the parietal lobes at 7.5 years in girls and 9 years in boys (see Fig. 74.2).

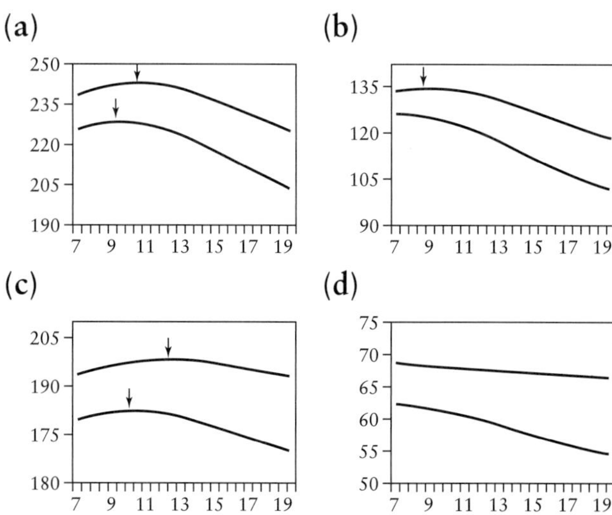

FIGURE 74.2 Gray matter subdivisions: (*a*) frontal lobe, (*b*) parietal lobe, (*c*) temporal lobe, and (*d*) occipital lobe.

To assess cortical GM at greater spatial resolution we examined change in GM from ages 4 to 20 years on a voxel-by-voxel basis in a group of 13 subjects who had each been scanned 4 times at approximately 2-year intervals (Gogtay et al., 2004). An animation of these changes is available at http://www.loni.ucla.edu/~thompson/DEVEL/dyanamic.html. As with the lobar measurements, childhood GM increase is followed by loss beginning at different ages in different regions. Cortical GM loss occurs earliest in the primary sensorimotor areas and latest in the dorsolateral prefrontal cortex (DLPFC), inferior parietal, and superior temporal gyrus. Areas subserving primary functions, such as motor and sensory systems, mature earliest. Higher order association areas that integrate those primary functions mature later. For example, the late-maturing superior temporal gyrus (along with prefrontal and inferior parietal cortices) serves as a heteromodal association site integrating memory, audio-visual input, and object recognition functions (Mesulam, 1998; Calvert, 2001; Martin and Chao, 2001).

Elucidating the cellular events underlying the GM volume changes is an area of active inquiry in neuroimaging research. Postmortem studies suggest that part of the GM changes may be related to synaptic proliferation and pruning (Huttenlocher, 1994). A study acquiring MRI and quantified electroencephalogram (EEG) in 138 healthy subjects from ages 10 to 30 years found that curvilinear reductions in frontal and parietal GM were matched by similar curvilinear reductions in EEG power of the corresponding regions, supporting the connection between GM volume reductions, EEG changes, and synaptic pruning (Whitford et al., 2007). Myelination may change classification of voxels along the interior cortical border from GM to WM resulting in cortical thinning as assessed by MR volumetrics but would not necessarily entail changes in synaptic density (Sowell et al., 2001). Knowledge of the degree to which these and other phenomena may be driving the MR changes has profound implications for interpreting the imaging results. Imaging of nonhuman primates with postmortem validation may help in this regard.

Subcortical Gray Matter

Basal Ganglia

The basal ganglia are a collection of subcortical nuclei that are involved in circuits mediating movement, higher cognitive functions, attention, and affective states. Anomalous volumes of basal ganglia structures have been reported for almost all neuropsychiatric disorders that have been investigated by neuroimaging (Giedd et al., 2006). The basal ganglia comprise the caudate, putamen, globus pallidus, subthalamic nucleus, and substantia nigra. Because of the small size and ambiguity of MR signal contrast of the borders defining the structures, only the first three are readily quantifiable by MRI, and automated techniques have only been established as reliable for measurement of the caudate. Like the cortical GM structures, the caudate nucleus follows an inverted *U*-shape developmental trajectory. Caudate size peaks at age 10.5 years in girls and 14.0 years in boys (see Fig. 74.1f). The shape of the caudate developmental trajectory is more similar to that of frontal and parietal GM than temporal. This supports the notion that brain regions that share extensive connections also share similar developmental courses.

Amygdala and Hippocampus

The temporal lobes, amygdala, and hippocampus are integral players in the arenas of emotion, language, and memory (Nolte, 1993). Human capacity for these functions changes markedly between the ages of 4 and 18 years (Jerslid, 1963; Wechsler, 1974; Diener et al., 1985), although the relationship between the development of these capacities and morphological changes in the structures subserving these functions is poorly understood.

The amygdala and hippocampus have not been quantified for the longitudinal sample. In a previous report from a cross-sectional sample subset of the NIMH sample, amygdala volume increased significantly only in males, and hippocampal volume increased significantly with age only in females (Giedd, Vaituzis, et al., 1996). This pattern of gender-specific maturational volumetric changes is consistent with nonhuman primate studies indicating a relatively high number of androgen receptors in the amygdala (Clark et al., 1988) and a relatively higher number of estrogen receptors in the hippocampus (Morse et al., 1986), although direct links between receptor density and growth patterns have not been established.

INFLUENCES ON DEVELOPMENTAL TRAJECTORIES OF BRAIN ANATOMY DURING CHILDHOOD AND ADOLESCENCE

Nature/Nurture

One of the fundamental challenges for understanding what factors affect the trajectories is to discern genetic from nongenetic influences. Twin studies are best suited to address these types of questions, and in 2001 we began collaborating with a team of experts in twin research at the Virginia Institute for Psychiatric and Behavioral Genetics and Department of Psychiatry, Virginia Commonwealth University. To date, the sample from the longitudinal study consists of approximately 600 scans from 90 monozygotic (MZ) and dizygotic (60) DZ twin pairs.

Structural equation modeling (SEM), which typically uses numeric optimization of a likelihood function to produce parameter values that provide the best fit to the data, is applied to correlation differences between MZ and DZ twins to determine the relative contributions to phenotypic variance of (A) additive genetic, (C) shared environmental, or (E) unique environmental factors (Neale and Cardon, 1992). Additive genetic effects (that is, "heritability") are high, and shared environmental effects are low for most brain morphometric measures (Wallace et al., 2006). Additive genetic effects for total cerebrum and lobar volumes (including GM and WM subcompartments) ranged from 0.77 to 0.88, for the caudate nucleus were 0.80, and for the CC 0.85.

The cerebellum has a distinctive heritability profile with an additive genetic effect of only 0.49 (although wide confidence intervals merit cautious interpretation). Pediatric cerebellar development is also noteworthy as being the most sexually dimorphic and among the latest to reach peak volume. These features make the cerebellum a prime target for pediatric neuroimaging studies. Prominent environmental influences on cerebellar development are consistent with its preferential susceptibility to insults such as alcohol, lead, or anoxia. Postnatal neurogenesis of cerebellar Purkinje cells may also be related to environmental susceptibility (Welsh et al., 2002), although the relationship between this process and volumetric changes remains to be elucidated. Also unclear is whether the unique development and heritability characteristics of the cerebellum are related to its divergence from the other regions soon after neural tube formation; whereas cerebrum, CC, and subcortical structures all are derived from the embryonic prosencephalon, cerebellar tissue is primarily derived from the rombencephalon (Kandel et al., 2000).

Highly heritable brain morphometric measures provide biological markers for inherited traits and may serve as targets for genetic linkage and association studies. These intermediate phenotypes may increase the power to detect quantitative trait loci (QTLs) influencing critical behavioral functions and liability to psychopathology (Gottesman and Gould, 2003). A greater understanding of the forces that guide brain development will help provide a heuristic for developing and implementing more effective interventions in the treatment of brain-based disorders.

Multivariate analyses allow assessment of the degree to which the same genetic or environmental factors contribute to multiple neuroanatomic structures. Like the univariate variables, these interstructure correlations can be parceled into relationships of either genetic or environmental origin. This knowledge is vitally important for interpretation of most of the twin data, including understanding the impact of genes that may affect distributed neural networks and interventions that may have global brain impacts.

Multivariate analyses indicate that shared genetic effects account for more of the variance than structure-specific effects, with a single factor accounting for 60% of genetic variability in cortical thickness (Schmitt et al., 2007). Six factors account for 58% of the remaining variance, with five groups of structures strongly influenced by the same underlying genetic factors. That most of the genetic variance is determined by genes that are shared between the major gross neural subdivisions is consistent with evolutionary genetic models of brain development that hypothesize global, genetically mediated differences in cell division as the driving force behind interspecies differences in total brain volume (Finlay and Darlington, 1995) as well as with the radial unit hypothesis of neocortical expansion proposed by Rakic (1995).

Comparative neuroanatomic analyses of multiple mammalian species have shown that total brain volume is highly correlated with regional volumes, irrespective of region (including neocortex, striatum, thalamus, and cerebellum), and accounts for the vast majority (> 96%) of the observed volumetric variance in all regions measured except for the olfactory bulb (Fishell, 1997; Darlington et al., 1999). Such strong correlations are thought to reflect a generalized adaptation to specific selective pressures; although it is more expensive, in terms of energy, to expand the computational resources of the entire brain when only specific functions are needed, the molecular adjustments required are far fewer than those required to completely repattern gross neural architecture.

An important aspect of developmental twin studies is assessment of age by heritability interactions. Vulnerabilities of highly heritable neuropsychiatric illnesses such as anxiety, bipolar disorder, depression, eating disorder, psychosis, and substance abuse are presumably present at birth. However, the peak age for emergence of symptoms in all of these disorders is during adolescence. Age-related changes in heritability may be linked to the timing of gene expression and related to the age of onset of disorders. Knowledge of when certain brain structures are particularly sensitive to genetic or environmental influences during development could also have important educational and/or therapeutic implications. For lobar volumes, WM additive genetic effects account for a greater proportion of the variance with increasing age whereas for GM unique environment effects account for a greater proportion of the variance with increasing age.

Sex

Given that nearly all neuropsychiatric disorders have different prevalence, age of onset, and symptomatology between males and females, sex differences in typical developmental trajectories are highly relevant for studies of pathology. Robust sex differences in developmental trajectories were noted for nearly all structures with peak volumes generally occurring 1 to 3 years earlier for females. Differences in trajectory shapes indicate that male/female differences are not only due to later onset of puberty in boys. The sex differences are also not due solely to body size. Male/female brain size difference remains highly significant when covaried for height and/or weight.

To assess the relative contributions of sex chromosomes and hormones, our group is studying patients with anomalous sex chromosome variations (for example, XXY, XXX, XXXY, XYY) and patients with anomalous hormone levels (for example, congenital adrenal hyperplasia, familial male precocious puberty, Cushing's syndrome).

Specific Genes

As with any quantifiable neuropsychological, clinical, or behavioral feature, people can be categorized into groups based on genotype and the averaged brains of the different genotype groups can be compared statistically. One of the most frequently studied genes in adult populations has been apolipoprotein 4 (*ApoE4*). Alleles of the *ApoE4* gene modulate risk for Alzheimer's disease with carriers of the 4 allele being at increased risk and carriers of 2 possibly at decreased risk compared with noncarriers. To explore the question of whether *ApoE4* alleles have distinct neuroanatomic signatures identifiable in childhood and adolescence, we examined 529 scans from 239 healthy subjects aged 4 to 20 years (Shaw et al., 2007). Although there were no significant IQ by genotype interactions, there was a stepwise effect on cortical thickness in the entorhinal and right hippocampal regions with the 4 group the thinnest, the 3 homozygotes in the middle, and the 2 group the thickest. These data suggest that pediatric assessments might one day be informative for adult onset disorders.

Brain–Behavior Correlations

As behaviors emanate from the integrated activity of distributed networks, demonstrating straightforward relationships between the size of a given brain structure and a particular behavior or ability has been elusive. Nonetheless, correlations have been identified between some aspects of brain structure and functional capacity. Several studies have shown that there are correlations of brain structural measures with IQ on whole-brain and regional levels (Thompson et al., 2001; Posthuma et al., 2002; Haier et al., 2004; Toga and Thompson, 2005). Relationships between memory function and hippocampal size have also been noted in several species. Food-storing species of birds have larger hippocampi than related nonfood-storing species (Krebs et al., 1989; Sherry et al., 1989), whereas in mammals a similar example can be found in voles. Male voles of the polygamous species travel far and wide in search of mates. They perform better than their female counterparts on laboratory measures of spatial ability and have significantly larger hippocampi (Sherry et al., 1992). Conversely, in the monogamous vole species, which do not show male–female differences in spatial ability, no sexual dimorphism of hippocampal size is seen (Jacobs et al., 1990). In humans also, correlations between memory for stories and left hippocampal volume have also been noted (Lencz et al., 1992; Goldberg et al., 1994). A study of taxi drivers in London found that they had larger hippocampi than controls, thought to be related to their extensive amount of navigational memory required for their work (Maguire et al., 2000).

An important consideration in linking form and function in the brain is that differences in the trajectories of development may in some cases be more informative than the final adult differences. For instance, in our longitudinal study looking at the relationship between cortical thickness and IQ differences in age by cortical thickness developmental curves were more predictive of IQ than differences in cortical thickness at age 20 years (Shaw et al., 2006).

CONCLUSION

Group differences in anatomical MRI have been reported for nearly all neuropsychiatric disorders. However, because of the large overlap in structure sizes or developmental trajectories, MRI is currently not of diagnostic utility for psychiatric disorders (except to rule out possible central nervous system insults such as tumors, intracranial bleeds, or congenital anomalies as etiologies for the symptoms). There is no identified "lesion" common to all, or even most, children with the most frequently studied disorders of autism, attention-deficit/hyperactivity disorder, childhood-onset schizophrenia, dyslexia, Fragile X, juvenile-onset bipolar disorder, posttraumatic stress disorder, Sydenham's chorea, or Tourette's syndrome.

A more immediately useful aspect of anatomical imaging may be to provide endophenotypes in typical or atypical populations. Endophenotypes are biological markers that may serve as intermediaries between genes and behavior or diagnostic syndromes. Endophenotypes related to a disease may be found in milder forms in family members without the full-blown syndrome. Current nonimaging examples in schizophrenia research include eye-tracking abnormalities (Holzman et al., 1974; Calkins and Iacono, 2000) and deficits in P50 suppression (Braff et al., 2001; Braff and Freedman, 2002).

Using brain morphometry as an endophenotype has the potential to create more biologically driven subtypes (to address the important issue of heterogeneity in current polythetic diagnostic schemes such as the *Diagnostic and Statistical Manual of Mental Disorders*, 4th ed., that combines historical tradition, compatibility with International Classification of Diseases [ICD]-10, clinical and research data, and consensus of the field) and may be more directly related to specific gene effects.

Remarkable advances in the field of pediatric neuroimaging have opened new windows into our understanding of the living, growing human brain. The mapping of developmental trajectories in typical development lays the groundwork for the next stages of exploring the influences on those trajectories and ultimately using this knowledge to optimize brain development in healthy and clinical populations.

REFERENCES

Allen, L.S., Richey, M.F., Chai, Y.M., and Gorski, R.A. (1991) Sex differences in the corpus callosum of the living human being. *J. Neurosci.* 11:933–942.

American Psychiatric Association. (1994) *Diagnostic and Statistical Manual of Mental Disorders,* 4th ed. Washington, DC: Author.

Beaulieu, C., Plewes, C., Paulson, L.A., Roy, D., Snook, L., Concha, L., et al. (2005) Imaging brain connectivity in children with diverse reading ability. *NeuroImage* 25(4):1266–1271.

Berlucchi, G. (1981) Interhemispheric asymmetries in visual discrimination: a neurophysiological hypothesis. *Doc. Opthal. Proc. Ser.* 30:87–93.

Braff, D.L., and Freedman, R. (2002) Endophenotypes in studies of the genetics of schizophrenia. In Davis, K.L., Charney, D.S., Coyle, J.T., and Nemeroff, C.B., eds. *Neuropsychopharmacology: The Fifth Generation of Progress*. Philadelphia: Lippincott Williams & Wilkins, pp. 703–716.

Braff, D.L., Geyer, M.A., and Swerdlow, N.R. (2001) Human studies of prepulse inhibition of startle: normal subjects, patient groups, and pharmacological studies. *Psychopharmacology (Berl)* 156(2/3):234–258.

Brochet, B., and Dousset, V. (1999) Pathological correlates of magnetization transfer imaging abnormalities in animal models and humans with multiple sclerosis. *Neurology* 53(5 Suppl 3):7.

Calkins, M.E., and Iacono, W.G. (2000) Eye movement dysfunction in schizophrenia: a heritable characteristic for enhancing phenotype definition. *Am. J. Med. Genet.* 97(1):72–76.

Calvert, G.A. (2001) Crossmodal processing in the human brain: insights from functional neuroimaging studies. *Cereb. Cortex* 11(12): 1110–1123.

Cascio, C.J., Gerig, G., and Piven, J. (2007) Diffusion tensor imaging: Application to the study of the developing brain. *J. Am. Acad. Child Adolesc. Psychiatry* 46(2):213–223.

Caviness, V.S.J., Kennedy, D.N., Richelme, C., Rademacher, J., and Filipek, P.A. (1996) The human brain age 7–11 years: a volumetric analysis based on magnetic resonance images. *Cereb. Cortex* 6(5):726–736.

Caviness, V.S.J., Lange, N.T., Makris, N., Herbert, M.R., and Kennedy, D.N. (1999) MRI-based brain volumetrics: emergence of a developmental brain science. *Brain Dev.* 21(5):289–295.

Clark, A.S., MacLusky, N.J., and Goldman-Rakic, P.S. (1988) Androgen binding and metabolism in the cerebral cortex of the developing rhesus monkey. *Endocrinology* 123:932–940.

Collins, D.L., Holmes, C.J., Peters, T.M., and Evans, A.C. (1995) Automatic 3-D model-based neuroanatomical segmentation. *Hum. Brain Mapp.* 3:190–208.

Cook, N.D. (1986) *The Brain Code. Mechanisms of Information Transfer and the Role of the Corpus Callosum*. London: Methuen.

Cowell, P.E., Allen, L.S., Zalatimo, N.S., and Denenberg, V.H. (1992) A developmental study of sex and age interactions in the human corpus callosum. *Dev. Brain Res.* 66:187–192.

Darlington, R.B., Dunlop, S.A., and Finlay, B.L. (1999) Neural development in metatherian and eutherian mammals: variation and constraint. *J. Comp. Neurol.* 411(3):359–368.

Dekaban, A.S. (1977) Tables of cranial and orbital measurements, cranial volume, and derived indexes in males and females from 7 days to 20 years of age. *Ann. Neurol.* 2:485–491.

Dekaban, A.S., and Sadowsky, D. (1978) Changes in brain weight during the span of human life: relation of brain weights to body heights and body weights. *Ann. Neurol.* 4:345–356.

Deutsch, G.K., Dougherty, R.F., Bammer, R., Siok, W.T., Gabrieli, J. D., and Wandell, B. (2005) Children's reading performance is correlated with white matter structure measured by diffusion tensor imaging. *Cortex* 41(3):354–363.

Diener, E., Sandvik, E., and Larsen, R.F. (1985) Age and sex effects for affect intensity. *Dev. Psychology* 21:542–546.

Engelbrecht, V., Rassek, M., Preiss, S., Wald, C., and Modder, U. (1998) Age-dependent changes in magnetization transfer contrast of white matter in the pediatric brain. *Am. J. Neuroradiol.* 19(10): 1923–1929.

Fields, R.D., and Stevens-Graham, B. (2002) New insights into neuron-glia communication. *Science* 298(5593):556–562.

Finlay, B.L., and Darlington, R.B. (1995) Linked regularities in the development and evolution of mammalian brains. *Science* 268: 1578–1584.

Fishell, G. (1997) Regionalization in the mammalian telencephalon. *Curr. Opin. Neurobiol.* 7(1):62–69.

Giedd, J.N., Blumenthal, J., Jeffries, N.O., Castellanos, F.X., Liu, H., Zijdenbos, A., et al. (1999) Brain development during childhood and adolescence: a longitudinal MRI study. *Nat. Neurosci.* 2(10):861–863.

Giedd, J.N., Blumenthal, J., Jeffries, N.O., Rajapakse, J.C., Vaituzis, A.C., Liu, H., et al. (1999) Development of the human corpus callosum during childhood and adolescence: A longitudinal MRI study. *Prog. Neuro-Psychopharmacol. Biol. Psychiatry* 23(4):571–588.

Giedd, J.N., Castellanos, F.X., Rajapakse, J.C., Kaysen, D., Vaituzis, A.C., Vauss, Y.C., et al. (1995) Cerebral MRI of human brain development—ages 4–18. *Biol. Psychiatry* 37(9):657.

Giedd, J.N., Shaw, P., Wallace, G.L., Gogtay, N., and Lenroot, R. (2006) Anatomic brain imaging studies of normal and abnormal brain development in children and adolescents. In: Cicchetti, D., ed. *Developmental Psychopathology*, 2nd ed., Vol. 2. Hoboken, NJ: Wiley, pp. 127–196.

Giedd, J.N., Snell, J.W., Lange, N., Rajapakse, J.C., Casey, B.J., Kozuch, P.L., et al. (1996) Quantitative magnetic resonance imaging of human brain development: ages 4-18. *Cereb. Cortex* 6(4):551–560.

Giedd, J.N., Vaituzis, A.C., Hamburger, S.D., Lange, N., Rajapakse, J.C., Kaysen, D., et al. (1996) Quantitative MRI of the temporal lobe, amygdala, and hippocampus in normal human development: ages 4-18 years. *J. Comp. Neurol.* 366(2):223–230.

Gogtay, N., Giedd, J.N., Lusk, L., Hayashi, B.S., Greenstein, D., Vaituzis, A.C., et al. (2004) Dynamic mapping of human cortical development during childhood through early adulthood. *Proc. Natl. Acad. Sci. USA* 101(21):8174–8179.

Goldberg, T.E., Torrey, E.F., Berman, K.F., and Weinberger, D.R. (1994) Relations between neuropsychological performance and brain morphological and physiological measures in monozygotic twins discordant for schizophrenia. *Psychiatry Res.* 55:51–61.

Goldstein, J.M., Seidman, L.J., Horton, N.J., Makris, N.K., Kennedy, D.N., Caviness, V.S. Jr., et al. (2001) Normal sexual dimorphism of the adult human brain assessed by in vivo magnetic resonance imaging. *Cereb. Cortex* 11(6):490–497.

Gottesman, I., and Gould, T.D. (2003) The endophenotype concept in psychiatry: etymology and strategic intentions. *Am. J. Psychiatry* 160(4):636–645.

Haier, R.J., Jung, R.E., Yeo, R.A., Head, K., and Alkire, M.T. (2004) Structural brain variation and general intelligence. *NeuroImage* 23(1):425–433.

Holzman, P.S., Proctor, L.R., Levy, D.L., Yasillo, N.J., Meltzer, H.Y., and Hurt, S.W. (1974) Eye-tracking dysfunctions in schizophrenic patients and their relatives. *Arch. Gen. Psychiatry* 31(2):143–151.

Huttenlocher, P.R. (1994). Synaptogenesis in human cerebral cortex. In: Dawson, G., and Fischer, K., eds. *Human Behavior and the Developing Brain*. New York: Guilford Press, pp. 137–152.

Jacobs, L.F., Gaulin, S.J., Sherry, D.F., and Hoffman, G.E. (1990) Evolution of spatial cognition: sex-specific patterns of spatial behavior predict hippocampal size. *Proc. Natl. Acad. Sci. USA* 87:6349–6352.

Jernigan, T.L., and Tallal, P. (1990) Late childhood changes in brain morphology observable with MRI. *Dev. Med Child Neurol.* 32: 379–385.

Jernigan, T.L., Trauner, D.A., Hesselink, J.R., and Tallal, P.A. (1991) Maturation of human cerebrum observed in vivo during adolescence. *Brain* 114:2037–2049.

Jerslid, A.T. (1963) *The Psychology of Adolescence*, 2nd ed. New York: Macmillan.

Kandel, E.R., Schwartz, J.H., and Jessell, T.M. (2000) *Principles of Neural Science*, 4th ed. New York: McGraw-Hill, Health Professions Division.

Krebs, J.R., Sherry, D.F., Healy, S.D., Perry, V.H., and Vaccarino, A.L. (1989) Hippocampal specialization of food-storing birds. *Proc. Natl. Acad. Sci. USA* 86:1388–1392.

Lee, K.Y., Kim, T.K., Park, M., Ko, S., Song, I.C., and Cho, I.H. (2004) Age-related changes in conventional and magnetization transfer MR imaging in elderly people: comparison with neurocognitive performance. *Kor. J. Radiol.* 5(2):96–101.

Lencz, T., McCarthy, G., Bronen, R.A., Scott, T.M., Inserni, J.A., Sass, K.J., et al. (1992) Quantitative magnetic resonance imaging in temporal lobe epilepsy: relationship to neuropathology and neuropsychological function. *Ann. Neurol.* 31:629–637.

Lenroot, R.K., Gogtay, N., Greenstein, D.K., Wells, E.M., Wallace, G.L., Clasen, L.S., et al. (2007) Sexual dimorphism of brain developmental trajectories during childhood and adolescence. *NeuroImage* 36(4):1065–1073.

Levy, J. (1985) Interhemispheric collaboration: single mindedness in the asymmetric brain. In: Best, C. T., ed. *Hemisphere Function and Collaboration in the Child*. New York: Academic Press, pp. 11–32.

Liston, C., Watts, R., Tottenham, N., Davidson, M.C., Niogi, S., Ulug, A.M., et al. (2006) Frontostriatal microstructure modulates efficient recruitment of cognitive control. *Cereb Cortex* 16(4):553–560.

Maguire, E.A., Gadian, D.G., Johnsrude, I.S., Good, C.D., Ashburner, J., Frackowiak, R.S., et al. (2000) Navigation-related structural change in the hippocampi of taxi drivers. *Proc. Natl. Acad. Sci. USA* 97(8):4398–4403.

Martin, A., and Chao, L.L. (2001) Semantic memory and the brain: structure and processes. *Curr. Opin. Neurobiol.* 11(2):194–201.

Mesulam, M.M. (1998) From sensation to cognition. *Brain* 121(Pt 6):1013–1052.

Morse, J.K., Scheff, S.W., and DeKosky, S.T. (1986) Gonadal steroids influence axonal sprouting in the hippocampal dentate gyrus: a sexually dimorphic response. *Exp. Neurol.* 94:649–658.

Mukherjee, P., and McKinstry, R.C. (2006) Diffusion tensor imaging and tractography of human brain development. *Neuroimaging Clin. N. Am.* 16(1):19–43, vii.

Nagy, Z., Westerberg, H., and Klingberg, T. (2004) Maturation of white matter is associated with the development of cognitive functions during childhood. *J. Cogn. Neurosci.* 16(7):1227–1233.

Neale, M.C., and Cardon, L.R. (1992) *Methodology for Genetic Studies of Twins and Families*. Dordrecht, the Netherlands: Kluwer Academic.

Niogi, S.N., and McCandliss, B.D. (2006) Left lateralized white matter microstructure accounts for individual differences in reading ability and disability. *Neuropsychologia* 44(11):2178–2188.

Nolte, J. (1993) Olfactory and limbic systems. In: Farrell, R., ed. *The Human Brain. An Introduction to its Functional Anatomy*, 3rd ed. St. Louis: Mosby-Year Book, Inc., pp. 397–413.

Pfefferbaum, A., Mathalon, D.H., Sullivan, E.V., Rawles, J.M., Zipursky, R.B., and Lim, K.O. (1994) A quantitative magnetic resonance imaging study of changes in brain morphology from infancy to late adulthood. *Arch. Neurol.* 51(9):874–887.

Posthuma, D., De Geus, E.J., Baare, W.F., Hulshoff Pol, H.E., Kahn, R.S., and Boomsma, D.I. (2002) The association between brain volume and intelligence is of genetic origin. *Nat. Neurosci.* 5(2): 83–84.

Pujol, J., Vendrell, P., Junque, C., Marti-Vilalta, J.L., and Capdevila, A. (1993) When does human brain development end? Evidence of corpus callosum growth up to adulthood. *Ann. Neurol.* 34: 71–75.

Rakic, P. (1995) A small step for the cell, a giant leap for mankind: a hypothesis of neocortical expansion during evolution. *Trends Neurosci.* 18(9):383–388.

Rauch, R.A., and Jinkins, J.R. (1994) Analysis of cross-sectional area measurements of the corpus callosum adjusted for brain size in male and female subjects from childhood to adulthood. *Behav. Brain Res.* 64:65–78.

Reiss, A.L., Abrams, M.T., Singer, H.S., Ross, J.L., and Denckla, M.B. (1996) Brain development, gender and IQ in children. A volumetric imaging study. *Brain* 119(Pt 5):1763–1774.

Rovaris, M., Iannucci, G., Cercignani, M., Sormani, M.P., De Stefano, N., Gerevini, S., et al. (2003) Age-related changes in conventional, magnetization transfer, and diffusion-tensor MR imaging findings: study with whole-brain tissue histogram analysis. *Radiology* 227(3):731–738.

Schmithorst, V.J., Wilke, M., Dardzinski, B.J., and Holland, S.K. (2005) Cognitive functions correlate with white matter architecture in a normal pediatric population: a diffusion tensor MRI study. *Hum. Brain Mapp.* 26(2):139–147.

Schmitt, J.E., Wallace, G.L., Rosenthal, M.A., Molloy, E.A., Ordaz, S., Lenroot, R., et al. (2007) A multivariate analysis of neuroanatomic relationships in a genetically informative pediatric sample. *NeuroImage* 35(1):70–82.

Shanks, M.F., Rockel, A.J., and Powel, T.P.S. (1975) The commissural fiber connections of the primary somatic sensory cortex. *Brain Res.* 98:166–171.

Shaw, P., Greenstein, D., Lerch, J., Clasen, L., Lenroot, R., Gogtay, N., et al. (2006) Intellectual ability and cortical development in children and adolescents. *Nature* 440(7084):676–679.

Shaw, P., Lerch, J.P., Pruessner, J.C., Taylor, K.N., Rose, A.B., Greenstein, D., et al. (2007) Cortical morphology in children and adolescents with different apolipoprotein E gene polymorphisms: an observational study. *Lancet Neurol.* 6(6):494–500.

Sherry, D.F., Jacobs, L.F., and Gaulin, S.J. (1992) Spatial memory and adaptive specialization of the hippocampus [see comments]. *Trends Neurosci.* 15:298–303.

Sherry, D.F., Vaccarino, A.L., Buckenham, K., and Herz, R.S. (1989) The hippocampal complex of food-storing birds. *Brain Behav. Evol.* 34:308–317.

Sowell, E.R., and Jernigan, T.L. (1998) Further MRI evidence of late brain maturation: Limbic volume increases and changing asymmetries during childhood and adolescence. *Dev. Neuropsychol.* 14(4):599–617.

Sowell, E.R., Peterson, B.S., Thompson, P.M., Welcome, S.E., Henkenius, A.L., and Toga, A.W. (2003) Mapping cortical change across the human life span. Nat. *Neurosci.* 6(3):309–315.

Sowell, E.R., Thompson, P.M., Holmes, C.J., Batth, R., Jernigan, T.L., and Toga, A.W. (1999) Localizing age-related changes in brain structure between childhood and adolescence using statistical parametric mapping. *NeuroImage* 9(6 Pt 1):587–597.

Sowell, E.R., Thompson, P.M., Holmes, C.J., Jernigan, T.L., and Toga, A.W. (1999) In vivo evidence for post-adolescent brain maturation in frontal and striatal regions. *Nat. Neurosci.* 2(10):859–861.

Sowell, E.R., Thompson, P.M., Tessner, K.D., and Toga, A.W. (2001) Mapping continued brain growth and gray matter density reduction in dorsal frontal cortex: Inverse relationships during postadolescent brain maturation. *J. Neurosci.* 21(22):8819–8829.

Suzuki, Y., Matsuzawa, H., Kwee, I.L., and Nakada, T. (2003) Absolute eigenvalue diffusion tensor analysis for human brain maturation. *NMR Biomed.* 16(5):257–260.

Thompson, P.M., Cannon, T.D., Narr, K.L., van Erp, T., Poutanen, V.P., Huttunen, M., et al. (2001) Genetic influences on brain structure. *Nat. Neurosci.* 4(12):1253–1258.

Thompson, P.M., Giedd, J.N., Woods, R.P., MacDonald, D., Evans, A.C., and Toga, A.W. (2000) Growth patterns in the developing brain detected by using continuum mechanical tensor maps. *Nature* 404(6774):190–193.

Thompson, P.M., Hayashi, K.M., Sowell, E.R., Gogtay, N., Giedd, J.N., Rapoport, J.L., et al. (2004) Mapping cortical change in Alzheimer's disease, brain development, and schizophrenia. *NeuroImage* 23(Suppl 1):S2–S18.

Toga, A.W., and Thompson, P.M. (2005) Genetics of brain structure and intelligence. *Annu. Rev. Neurosci.* 28:1–23.

van Buchem, M.A., Steens, S.C., Vrooman, H.A., Zwinderman, A. H., McGowan, J.C., Rassek, M., et al. (2001) Global estimation of myelination in the developing brain on the basis of magnetization transfer imaging: a preliminary study. *Am. J. Neuroradiol.* 22(4):762–766.

Wallace, G.L., Schmitt, J.E., Lenroot, R.K., Viding, E., Ordaz, S., Rosenthal, M.A., et al. (2006) A pediatric twin study of brain morphometry. *J. Child Psychol. Psychiatry* 47(10):987–993.

Wechsler, D. (1974) *Wechsler Intelligence Scale for Children—Revised*. New York: The Psychological Corporation.

Welsh, J.P., Yuen, G., Placantonakis, D.G., Vu, T.Q., Haiss, F., O'Hearn, E., et al. (2002) Why do Purkinje cells die so easily after global brain ischemia? Aldolase C, EAAT4, and the cerebellar contribution to posthypoxic myoclonus. *Adv. Neurol.* 89:331–359.

Whitford, T.J, Rennie, C.J., Grieve, S.M, Clark, C.R., Gordon, E. E., and Williams, L. M. (2007) Brain maturation in adolescence: concurrent changes in neuroanatomy and neurophysiology. *Hum Brain Mapp.* 28(3):228–237.

Zaidel, D., and Sperry, R. W. (1974) Memory impairment after commissurotomy in man. *Brain* 97:263–272.

75 Tourette's Syndrome and Tic-Related Disorders in Children

PAUL J. LOMBROSO, MICHAEL H. BLOCH, AND
JAMES F. LECKMAN

A decade ago, Tourette's syndrome (TS) was a promising territory for psychiatrically oriented geneticists. It was considered a model neuropsychiatric disorder with a complex phenotype believed to be associated with mutations at a single autosomal locus. Characterization of the TS gene would be a major advance and would lead to clarification of how nongenetic factors might modulate the expression of the phenotype. Although TS remains a promising territory for geneticists, particularly those interested in oligogenetic disorders, it has become a focus of research for a remarkable diversity of disciplines, ranging from psychometricians and prenatal epidemiologists to experts in the neural circuits that link the cortex with the basal ganglia and neuroimmunologists interested in brain-based autoimmune phenomena. Even mathematical types have tried to sort out the temporal sequence of bouts of tics using tools associated with nonlinear, chaotic, dynamical systems. In this chapter, we present a brief summary of current research on TS and elaborate a provisional model of pathogenesis.

PHENOMENOLOGY

Tics are sudden, repetitive movements, gestures, or vocalizations that frequently mimic some aspect of normal behavior. Tic disorders are classified in the *Diagnostic and Statistical Manual of Mental Disorders*, 4th ed. (*DSM-IV*; American Psychiatric Association [APA], 1994) according to type, being either motor or phonic, and duration, being either transient or chronic (Table 75.1). The criterion that stipulates marked distress or significant impairment in important areas of functioning is no longer considered necessary for diagnosis, as many individuals have obvious tic symptomatology without impaired functioning, and this criterion has been removed from *DSM-IV-TR* (APA, 2000). Transient tic disorder is a condition of childhood characterized by the time-limited expression of one or more simple motor or phonic tics. The tics generally vary in severity over weeks or months, and a conservative approach to treatment is usually indicated. The distribution of the tics is for the most part limited to the head, neck, or upper extremities. Although transient tics may be purely phonic, these are less frequent seen. Typically, the disorder has an onset between 3 and 10 years of age, and boys are at greater risk to develop symptoms. As currently defined, the symptoms can be present for only up to 1 year.

Chronic motor tic disorder is a condition that has a broad range of severity and is observed in children and adults. In most cases, the tics involve the face, head, neck, or shoulders. Like other tic disorders, chronic motor tic disorder has a waxing and waning course that often appears in bouts and is typically aggravated by stress and fatigue. Chronic motor tic disorder may be characterized by vocal tics only. However, like transient tics, this condition is rarely seen clinically.

When motor and phonic tics are present, the disorder is known by the eponym *Tourette's syndrome*. The disorder typically begins in early childhood (mean age of 7) with simple eye blinking or facial tics. The range of tic symptoms varies tremendously from one individual to the next and within the same individual over time. Most frequently seen are tics that involve the muscles of the eyes, face, neck, and shoulders. Vocalizations typically begin 1 to 2 years after motor tics and most often consist of repetitive throat clearing, sniffling, or grunting. More complex phonic tics such as barking, echolalia, nonsense syllables, abrupt changes in speech, or coprolalia occur in less than one fourth of cases. There has been a recent increase in appreciation for sensory phenomena that may immediately precede the tic symptomatology. These sensations are variously described as a feeling of pressure, an urge, or an itch that impels the person to perform the tic to relieve the sensation (Leckman et al., 1993; Leckman et al., 1994; Scahill et al., 1995).

Most individuals with TS report that their symptoms occur in bouts usually lasting a few minutes at most and wax and wane over longer intervals of time (weeks to months). The temporal occurrence of tics has led to

TABLE 75.1 *Diagnostic Criteria for Tourette's Syndrome and Various Tic Disorders*

Diagnostic criteria for Tourette's syndrome (307.23)

A. Both multiple motor and one or more vocal tics have been present at some time during the illness, although not necessarily concurrently.

B. The tics occur many times a day (usually in bouts), nearly every day or intermittently throughout a period of more than a year; and during this period, there is never a tic-free period of more than 3 consecutive months.

C. Onset before age 18.

D. Not due to the direct physiological effects of a substance (for example, stimulants) or a general medical condition (for example, Huntington's chorea or postviral encephalitis).

Diagnostic criteria for chronic motor disorder (307.22)

A. Single or multiple motor or vocal tics, but not both, have been present at some time during the illness.

B. The tics occur many times a day, nearly every day, or intermittently throughout a period of more than a year; and during this period, there is never a tic-free interval of more than 3 months.

C. Onset before age 18.

D. Not due to the direct physiological effects of a substance (for example, stimulants) or a general medical condition (for example, Huntington's chorea or postviral encephalitis).

E. Has never met the criteria for Tourette's disorder.

Diagnostic criteria for transient tic disorder (307.21)

A. Single or multiple motor and/or vocal tics.

B. The tics occur many times a day, nearly every day for at least 4 weeks, but for no longer than 12 consecutive months.

C. Onset before age 18.

D. Not due to the direct physiological effects of a substance (for example, stimulants) or a general medical condition (for example, Huntington's chorea or postviral encephalitis).

E. Has never met the criteria for Tourette's disorder or chronic motor or vocal disorder.

Diagnostic criteria for tic disorder not otherwise specified (307.20)

This category is for a tic disorder that does not meet criteria for a specific tic disorder. Examples include tics lasting less than 4 weeks or tics with an onset after age 18.

Source: American Psychiatric Association, 2000.

efforts to apply nonlinear dynamic models to TS, and to determine if the bout-like occurrence of tics over seconds to minutes and the waxing and waning of tics over weeks to months is a product of the same underlying fractal process (Peterson and Leckman, 1998).

The worst period for many patients is from 8 to 12 years of age, with the majority of individuals experiencing a significant reduction of their tics during their late adolescence (Leckman et al., 1998; Bloch et al., 2006). Nonetheless, a substantial minority (25%) of patients who are clinically identified become chronically disabled in adulthood by constant paroxysms of tics, including coprolalia and self-injurious tics (A.K. Shapiro et al., 1988). Population-based studies also support the conclusion that the frequency and intensity of tics diminish with age (Peterson et al., 2001).

EPIDEMIOLOGY

Estimates for the prevalence for transient tics, chronic motor tic disorder, and TS have varied over the years. Transient tics appear to be a relatively common disorder, with between 4% and 10% of school-age children affected (Rutter and Hemming, 1970; Zahner et al., 1988; Costello et al., 1996; Khalifa and von Knorring, 2006). The prevalence of chronic tic disorder is between 1% and 10%, depending on the population under study (Burd et al., 1986a, 1986b; Apter et al., 1993; Khalifa and von Knorring, 2006). Combining these two estimates, childhood tic disorders are the most common form of movement disorders, with a population prevalence of approximately 4%–10%.

The differences that have been found between studies can be attributed to a large extent to variations in the methodologies used for each survey. For example, significant differences in prevalence rates will be obtained, depending on the ascertainment of the population (clinic vs. community-based surveys), as well as the ages of the sample (children vs. adolescent populations), or the instruments being used (self-reports vs. direct interviews). As might be expected, the highest prevalence rates were obtained in those studies that used clinic samples and among children between the ages of 7 and 11.

In one of the more methodologically sophisticated studies, Apter and colleagues (1993) conducted a survey of all adolescents being inducted into the Israeli army and observed a point prevalence of 4.3 per 10,000 for TS. Although the study did not directly estimate the prevalence for all tic disorders among this sample, it can be estimated from the available data to be approximately an order of magnitude higher, or 4.7 per 1000. The expression of tic disorders has been consistently found to be higher among boys than girls (3–8:1), and TS appears in all social, racial, and ethnic groups (Burd et al., 1986a, 1986b; Costello et al., 1996).

COMORBID DISORDERS

In his original descriptions of the syndrome, Gilles de la Tourette (1885) described nine cases in which he hinted at the genetics of the disorder, as well as the presence in his patients of several comorbid illnesses. Today, it is generally agreed that TS is associated with a spectrum of psychopathology. Several reports of clinical samples have documented unexpectedly high rates of inattention and hyperactivity, aggressiveness, obsessive–compulsive disorder (OCD), depression, and anxiety in individuals with TS. Other commonly noted difficulties include sleep disturbance, learning disabilities, and speech problems. However, it is still not clear what the underlying relationship is between these various behavioral and emotional problems and TS. The central issue is whether there is a single genetic factor that contributes to some, or all, of the associated syndromes or whether they are disorders with independent etiologies. About 50% of patients with TS referred to clinics have sufficient attentional, impulsive, and hyperactive symptoms to warrant the diagnosis of attention-deficit/hyperactivity disorder (ADHD) (Comings and Comings, 1987; Bruun and Budman, 1992; Cohen et al., 1992). In many children, the attentional and disruptive behaviors produce greater impairment than the tics themselves. Some have questioned whether these clinically referred cases reflect a bias of ascertainment whereby children with more than one disorder are more likely to be referred to clinicians than are children with only one disorder (Berkson, 1946). However, data from epidemiological studies among schoolchildren with TS have suggested that referral bias does not account for the association of ADHD with TS. Khalifa and von Knorring (2006) studied 25 identified probands who met diagnostic criteria for TS in their epidemiological sample, and 17 (68%) of these were also diagnosed with ADHD. This was more than an eightfold increase in the frequency of ADHD compared to that found in the general population (8%).

Over 60% of patients with TS also report OC symptoms during the course of their illness (Pauls et al., 1986; Pauls et al., 1991). Typically, these symptoms begin in prepuberty (Jagger et al., 1982). The obsessional thoughts and compulsive behaviors often become more prominent during later adolescence, and in some cases, the full-blown OCD symptom picture becomes even more burdensome then the original tic symptomatology. The OCD symptoms are more likely to have aggressive or sexual content than those of patients with OCD without tics (George et al., 1993; Leckman et al., 1997). Another interesting difference that is emerging is that tic-related forms of OCD are frequently associated with a need to "even things up" or to repeat actions until they feel "just right" (Leckman et al., 1993; Leckman et al., 1994; Leckman et al., 1997). Data from genetic and epidemiological studies also indicate that childhood-onset OCD and TS are closely related conditions. Khalifa and von Knorring (2006) studied 25 identified probands who met diagnostic criteria for TS in their epidemiological sample, and four (16%) of these were also diagnosed with OCD. Pauls et al. (1986) reported that 10%–15% of the first-degree relatives of individuals with TS were diagnosed with OCD, whether or not the index case had OCD. Also, OC symptoms, when present, in children with TS, appear more likely to persist into adulthood than the tics themselves (Bloch et al., 2006).

The co-occurrence of depression and anxiety symptoms with TS are commonplace and may reflect the cumulative psychosocial burden of having tics or shared biological diatheses or both (Robertson and Orth, 2006; Robertson et al., 2006). Antecedent depressive symptoms do predict modest increases in tic severity (Lin et al., 2007). However, this study also documented that future depression severity is more closely associated with antecedent worsening of psychosocial stress and OC symptoms than it is with future measures of tic severity.

Children with a range of other neurodevelopmental disorders are also at increased risk for tic disorders. Kurlan and colleagues (1994) reported a fourfold increase in the prevalence of tic disorders among children in special educational settings in a single school district in upstate New York. These children were not mentally challenged but did have significant learning disabilities or other speech or physical impairments. Children with autism and other pervasive developmental disorders are also at higher risk for developing TS (Baron-Cohen et al., 1999).

MODELS OF PATHOGENESIS

The basal ganglia are a group of nuclei that have been described as a critical way station in a somatotopically organized pathway that runs from the cerebral cortex to the basal ganglia and then passes to the thalamus before returning to the cortex (Alexander et al., 1990; Goldman-Rakic and Selemon, 1990; Mink, 2001). These circuits run parallel to each other, are minimally overlapping, and interconnect the cortex, striatum, globus pallidus, substantia nigra, and thalamus. They are believed to carry information concerning a variety of motor, somatosensory, cognitive, and emotional ideations. As reviewed below, neuroimaging studies have pointed to volumetric changes within the basal ganglia and cerebral cortices among patients with TS. A current hypothesis is that TS is caused by inhibitory failure in one or more of these pathways, and considerable effort is currently concentrated on investigating whether disruptions of these pathways exist in patients with TS (Singer, 1997; Leckman and Riddle, 2000; Leckman, 2002).

A possible model of the pathogenesis of TS is shown in Figure 75.1. It is likely that one or more genes are active early during central nervous system (CNS) development and, either directly or through their interrelationship with environmental factors, set the stage for vulnerability to tic disorders. One of the hallmarks of TS is that tic symptoms are often exacerbated by stress or periods of heightened excitement. The vast majority of patients commonly report that anxiety, fatigue, or emotional trauma increases their tics (Bornstein et al., 1990). This has recently been confirmed in longitudinal studies (Lin et al., 2007).

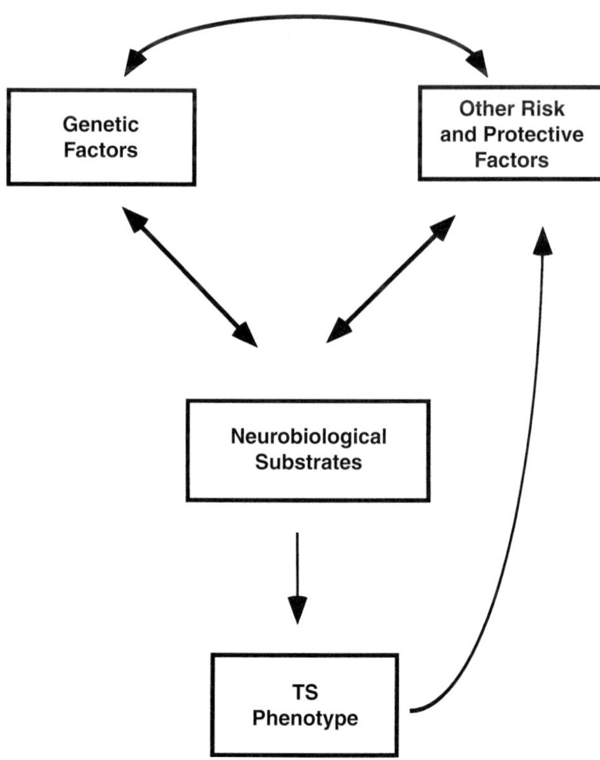

FIGURE 75.1 Model of pathogenesis of Tourette's syndrome (TS). This model predicts the existence of one or more susceptibility genes acting in concert with epigenetic risk factors during the course of brain development. These interactions constrain later brain development and/or leave it vulnerable to injury. The net result is altered or functionally imbalanced neural circuits that link the basal ganglia with specific regions in the cortex and thalamus. This imbalance leads to a disinhibition of thalamocortical projections and the symptoms of the disease, see Leckman and Riddle (2000) and Leckman et al. (2006) for reviews.

Tic severity may be influenced by prenatal environment factors, especially ones that affect weight and neurodevelopment (Pasamanick and Kawi, 1956; Leckman et al., 1990; Hyde et al., 1992; Whitaker et al., 1997), by postnatal factors such as gender-specific hormonal surges (Peterson et al., 1994), and by recurrent streptococcal infections (Kiessling et al., 1993; Swedo et al., 1994; Swedo et al., 1998). Some patients with TS are also vulnerable to specific stressors such as exposure to psychostimulants (Golden, 1974; Riddle et al., 1995) and thermal stress (Lombroso et al., 1991; Scahill et al., 2001). Such observations point to a stress-diathesis model for TS in which the severity of the syndrome is the product of an interaction between inherited vulnerability factors and cumulative environmental stresses occurring at critical periods of brain development (Leckman et al., 1991).

GENETIC FACTORS

Gilles de la Tourette was the first to suggest a familial pattern of expression among his patients with TS. Modern twin and family studies provide evidence that genetic factors are involved in the vulnerability to TS and related disorders (Pauls and Leckman, 1986). The concordance rate for TS among monozygotic twin pairs is greater than 50%, whereas the concordance of dizygotic twin pairs is about 10% (Price et al., 1985). If cotwins with chronic motor tic disorder are included, these concordance figures increase to 77% for monozygotic and 30% for dizygotic twin pairs. These differences in the concordance of monozygotic and dizygotic twin pairs indicate that genetic factors play an important role in the etiology, but the fact that concordance for monozygotic twins is less than 100% also indicates that nongenetic factors are critical in determining the nature and severity of the clinical syndrome.

Other studies indicate that first-degree family members of probands with TS are at substantially higher risk for developing TS, chronic motor tic disorder, and OCD than unrelated individuals (Pauls et al., 1991). The rates are substantially higher than might be expected by chance in the general population and greatly exceed the rates for these disorders among the relatives of individuals with other psychiatric disorders except OCD.

The pattern of vertical transmission among family members has led several groups of investigators to test specific genetic hypotheses. Although not definitive, segregation analyses could not rule out autosomal transmission (Pauls and Leckman, 1986). However, subsequent efforts to identify susceptibility genes within large multigenerational families or using affected sibling pair designs have met with limited success (The Tourette Syndrome Association International Consortium for Genetics, 1999, 2007).

Identity-by-descent (IBD) approaches have also been used in population isolates in Canada, South Africa, and Costa Rica. The South African study implicated regions near the centromere of chromosome 2, as well as on markers 6p, 8q, 11q, 14q, 20q, and 21q. Of interest, the 11q marker in the French Canadian family that was associated with the highest log of odds ratio (LOD) score was the same marker for which significant linkage disequilibrium with TS was recently detected in the Afrikaner population of South Africa (Simonic et al., 1998; Merette et al., 2000; Simonic et al., 2001).

In addition, a number of cytogenetic abnormalities have been reported in TS families (Cuker et al., 2004). Among the more recent findings, Verkerk and colleagues (2003) reported the disruption of the contactin-associated protein 2 gene on chromosome 7. This gene encodes a membrane protein located at nodes of Ranvier of axons that may be important for the distribution of the K(+) channels, which would affect signal conduction along myelinated neurons. In addition, using a candidate gene approach identified by chromosomal anomalies, Abelson et al. (2005) identified and mapped a de novo chromosome 13 inversion in a patient with TS. The gene *SLITRK1* was identified as a brain-expressed candidate gene mapping approximately 350 kilobases from the 13q31 breakpoint. Mutation screening of 174 patients was undertaken with the resulting identification of a truncating frame-shift mutation in a second family affected with TS. In addition, two examples of a rare variant were identified in a highly conserved region of the 3' untranslated region of the gene corresponding to a brain expressed micro-ribonucleic acid (miRNA) binding domain. None of these anomalies were demonstrated in 3600 controls. In vitro studies showed that the frame-shift and the miRNA binding site variant had functional potential and were consistent with a loss-of-function mechanism. Studies of *SLITRK1* and the miRNA predicted to bind in the variant-containing 3' region showed expression in multiple neuroanatomical areas implicated in TS neuropathology including the cortical plate, striatum, globus pallidus, thalamus, and subthalamic nucleus.

NEUROBIOLOGY

Although neuropathological studies of postmortem TS brains are few in number, a recent stereological study indicates that there is a marked alteration in the number and density of γ-aminobutyric acid (GABA)ergic parvalbumin-positive cells in basal ganglia structures (Kalanithi et al., 2005). In the caudate there was a greater than 50% reduction in the GABAergic fast-spiking interneurons and a 30%–40% reduction of these same cells in the putamen. This same study found a reduction of the GABAergic parvalbumin-positive projection neurons in the external segment globus pallidus (GPe) as well as a dramatic increase (>120%) in the number and proportion of GABAergic projection neurons of the internal segment of the GPe. These alterations are consistent with a developmental defect in tangential migration of some GABAergic neurons. Further studies are needed to confirm and extend these findings, such as toward a more complete understanding of how the different striatal interneurons are affected, and determine how alterations in GABAergic interneurons and GPe projection neurons could lead to a form of thalamocortical dysrhythmia (Llinas et al., 2005; Leckman et al., 2006).

AUTOIMMUNE HYPOTHESIS

Recent reports have suggested that autoimmune mechanisms may play a role in certain individuals with tic disorders (Kiessling et al., 1993; Murphy et al., 1997; Singer et al., 1998; Swedo et al., 1998; Peterson et al., 2000; Morshed et al., 2001). In such patients, the presence of tics or OC symptoms has been linked to an earlier infection with group A beta-hemolytic streptococci (GABHS; Swedo et al., 1997; Singer et al., 1998), although other infectious agents have also been suggested (Allen, 1997). The most compelling evidence of an etiological link between these disorders and GABHS infection comes from a study that found an increased proportion of GABHS infections (odds ratio = 13.6) within the preceding 12 months in children newly diagnosed with TS compared to well-matched controls (Mell et al., 2005).

The role of T-cell immunity has been clearly demonstrated in rheumatic heart disease (Cunningham et al., 1997; Guilherme and Kalil, 2004), but much less is understood about T-cell immunity in pediatric autoimmune neuropsychiatric disorders associated with streptococcal infections (PANDAS). Molecular mimicry between streptococcus pyogenes and cardiac proteins likely contributes to the autoimmune reactions in rheumatic heart disease. In assessing the examination of investigators, cardiac myosin has been shown as a putative autoantigen recognized by auto-antibodies of patients with rheumatic fever. Isolating T cells from cardiac tissue revealed that a significant portion of the clones showed cross-reactivity with myosin, valve-derived proteins, and specific streptococcal M proteins.

In relation to prevention of autoimmunity and maintenance of immune tolerance, the suppressive function regulatory T cells (Tregs) was shown in experimental animal models (Sakaguchi et al., 1995). This small population of $CD4^+CD25^+$ T cells is a potent inhibitor of $CD4^+$, $CD8^+$ T lymphocytes, as well as B lymphocytes (Piccirillo and Shevach, 2004). Recently, reduced frequencies of $CD4^+CD25^+$ Treg cells were demonstrated in patients with a variety of autoimmune diseases, including multiple sclerosis, systemic lupus erythematosus, type 1 diabetes, and rheumatoid arthritis, as well as TS (Kawikova et al., 2007). Immune responses are also associated with release of multiple cytokines. There have been relatively few studies that have examined the possible role of cytokines in PANDAS, but there are some data that suggest that interleukin-12 and tumor necrosis factor alpha concentrations are elevated in some patients with TS at baseline and during periods of symptom exacerbation (Leckman et al., 2005).

B cells are also likely to be involved. The hypothesis predicts that individuals who are susceptible produce antibodies against streptococci in a normal fashion. However, the antibodies then recognize self-proteins within the CNS (Kansy et al., 2006). As a consequence of this cross-reactivity, the CNS is compromised and neurological symptoms emerge. Repeated infections in individuals who are vulnerable are thought to exacerbate clinical symptoms. Based on this hypothesis, several groups have attempted to develop animal models of the disorder by infusing putative auto-antibodies bilaterally into the striatum in an effort to reproduce symptoms of the disorder. Results of these efforts have been mixed, with some groups recording significant increases in the production of stereotypies in rats infused with sera from patients with TS compared to those infused with sera from normal controls (Hallett et al., 2000; Taylor et al., 2002). However, others have been unable to replicate these findings (Singer et al., 2005).

A line of research has shown that antineural antibodies from Sydenham's chorea and PANDAS cases react with the neuronal cell surface to induce high levels of calcium/calmodulin-dependent protein (CaM) kinase II activity in human neuroblastoma cells (Kirvan et al., 2003; Kirvan et al., 2006) and that this activation can lead to an increased dopaminergic innervation of the striatum (Kirvan et al., 2006).

NEUROIMAGING

The pathophysiology of TS and other tic disorders has long been thought to involve anatomical and functional disturbances of the basal ganglia, a belief based primarily on circumstantial evidence compiled from clinical observations of TS and preclinical studies of basal ganglia function. Despite strong circumstantial evidence that the pathophysiology of TS involves structural and functional disturbances of the basal ganglia, inconsistent findings in relatively small in vivo TS imaging studies have yielded contradictory results concerning the role of abnormal basal ganglia morphology in the pathophysiology of TS (Peterson et al., 1993; Singer et al., 1993; Castellanos, Giedd, Hamburger, et al., 1996; Castellanos, Giedd, Marsh, et al., 1996; Moriarty et al., 1997). Recently, basal ganglia volumes were measured on high-resolution magnetic resonance images acquired in 154 patients with TS and 130 healthy children and adults (Peterson et al., 2003). Repeated-measures analyses tested hypotheses concerning regional specificity, age effects, and abnormal asymmetries in the TS basal ganglia. In contrast to earlier reports, the only significant finding was that caudate nucleus volumes were significantly smaller in children and adults with TS. Lenticular nucleus volumes also were smaller in adults and children with TS, but this was true only of those individuals with a diagnosis of comorbid OCD. In addition, regional volumes did not correlate significantly with the severity of tic, OCD, or ADHD symptoms. Furthermore, a recent study associated decreased childhood caudate volume in children with TS with increased adulthood tic severity (Bloch et al., 2005).

In contrast, a recent magnetic resonance imaging (MRI) study using the same sample of patients found support for a disturbance in the cortical components of the cortico-striato-thalamo-cortical circuitry. High-resolution images were acquired in 155 patients with TS and 131 healthy controls. The patients with TS were found to have larger volumes in prefrontal and parieto-occipital cortical regions, and smaller inferior occipital volumes (Peterson et al., 2001). In this study, the orbitofrontal and parieto-occipital cerebral volumes were significantly associated with tic severity in adults, but they were negligible in children. The authors concluded that the pathophysiology of TS includes a broadly distributed disturbance in cortical systems.

Functional in vivo neuroimaging studies are consistent with this result. Several studies have attempted to dissociate the neural patterns specific to tics from those associated with other aspects of TS. Tic severity has been reported to be related to decreased activity in the cingulate and striatum (Chase et al., 1986; Moriarty et al., 1995) as well as in frontal cortex (Chase et al., 1986) and left medial temporal cortex (Moriarty et al., 1995). Stern and colleagues (2000) utilized an $[^{15}0]$ H_20 positron emission tomography (PET) and identified activations in the supplementary motor area (SMA), premotor, and primary motor cortices, anterior cingulate, prefrontal cortex, the insula and claustrum, and portions of putamen and caudate nucleus as being synchronous with tics. A recent event-related functional MRI (fMRI) study observed a similar pattern of activity prior to and during tics in 10 patients (Bohlhalter et al., 2006). Activations were found in several areas prior to tics including the SMA and premotor cortex, insula, putamen, thalamus, cerebellum, parietal operculum, and anterior cingulate. During tics, activity progressed into dorsolateral prefrontal cortex, sensorimotor regions (including primary motor cortex), and the superior parietal lobule. These findings provide our first view of the temporal pattern of brain activity associated with tics, but they fail to address whether this sequence differs from that involved in intentional movements. The central role of the SMA activation prior to tic onset has been confirmed by a functional neuroimaging study that included normal controls imitating specific tics (Hampson et al., 2008). The region showing the most robust difference in time course across groups was the SMA. It is interesting to note that Bohlhalter et al. (2006) reported the SMA to be more active prior to tics than during tics in their patients with TS. Although our results do not suggest that the region has a peak in hemodynamic response prior to motor cortex, it does show a broader temporal profile in the patients with tics than in the controls. This suggests that the region may have abnormally elevated activity in the seconds preceding and following tic execution. Cortical areas have also been implicated in studies of tic suppression. For example, in a study of tic suppression in TS, significant changes in signal intensity were seen in the basal ganglia and thalamus and in anatomically connected cortical regions (Peterson et al., 1998). In addition, the magnitudes of regional signal change in the basal ganglia and thalamus correlated inversely with the severity of tic symptoms. These findings again suggest that the pathogenesis of tics involves an impaired modulation of neuronal activity in cortical as well as subcortical neural circuits.

Disturbances in dopamine (DA) neurotransmission have been put forward on the basis of several lines of evidence. Clinically, the majority of patients (80%) report significant reduction of tic symptoms when placed on haloperidol or other neuroleptics that selectively block dopaminergic D_2 receptors (A.K. Shapiro and Shapiro, 1988; E.S. Shapiro et al., 1989). In contrast, tic symptoms are often aggravated following withdrawal from neuroleptic treatment or after exposure to medications that increase central DAergic activity, such as CNS stimulants. Studies of cerebrospinal fluid (CSF) have reported altered levels of homovanillic acid (HVA), the major metabolite of DA, in TS populations compared to control groups (Butler et al., 1979; Cohen et al., 1979; Leckman et al., 1988). This led to a DA receptor hypersensitivity hypothesis that proposed that TS was due to the supersensitivity of postsynaptic DA receptors through increases in their number or affinity for DA. Thus far, PET studies examining striatal DA metabolism in adults with TS have found a higher density of DA D_2 receptor density in the more severely affected member of disconcordant monozygotic twin pairs (Wolf et al., 1996), increased right ventral striatal DA receptor density (Albin et al., 2003) and increased amphetamine-induced DA release in the putamen compared to normal controls (Singer et al., 2002). Single photon emission computed tomography (SPECT) studies have demonstrated increased striatal DA transporter (DAT) density in children and adults with TS compared to normal controls (Cheon et al., 2004; Serra-Mestres et al., 2004). Results from a recent postmortem study have identified consistent increases of DAT and DA D_2 receptor density in many areas of the frontal cortex (Yoon et al., 2007).

NEUROPHYSIOLOGY

Two studies using transcranial magnetic stimulation (TMS) have documented defective paired-pulse inhibition and reduced motor thresholds in TS and early-onset, tic-related OCD and suggest possible primary motor cortex abnormalities in these disorders (Zieman et al., 1997; Greenberg et al., 2000). That defective intracortical inhibition is found in early-onset OCD and TS is consistent with the view that the similar and frequently overlapping symptoms and heritability of these two illnesses may reflect common pathophysiology in cortico-striatal-thalamic-cortical circuits. Pharmacological studies have shown that intracortical inhibition measured by TMS procedures depends to a large degree on a balance between inhibitory GABAergic and excitatory glutaminergic mechanisms, so that the observed reduced intracortical inhibition could result from activity in thalamocortical inputs producing relatively less GABAergic inhibition or relatively more glutamate-mediated excitation of the cortical output neurons.

More recently, investigators have focused on the crucial role that neural oscillations play in maintaining normal CNS function. Neurons form behavior-dependent oscillating networks of various sizes and frequencies that bias input selection and facilitate synaptic plasticity, mechanisms that cooperatively support temporal representation as well as the transfer and long-term consolidation of information. Coherent network activity is likely to modulate sensorimotor gating as well as focused motor actions. Disruption of these normal oscillatory circuits and the emergence of aberrant oscillatory activity has been postulated to play a role in the moment-to-moment pathophysiology of TS (Leckman et al., 2006). Briefly, there is clear evidence of sensorimotor deficits in TS (Swerdlow et al., 2006) and emerging evidence that thalamocortical dysrhythmias are present in individuals with TS (Moran et al., 2005). In addition, the known electrophysiological effects of medications (Leckman et al., 2006; Swerdlow et al., 2006), the beneficial effects of low-frequency repetitive TMS targeting the SMA (Mantovani et al., 2006), and surgical interventions used to treat TS likely have an ameliorative effect on these aberrant oscillations (Bajwa et al., 2007). Similarly, a strong case can be made that successful behavioral treatments involve the willful training regions of the prefrontal cortex to engage in tic suppression and the performance of competing motor responses to unwanted sensory urges such that these prefrontal regions become effective modulators of aberrant thalamocortical rhythms. The SMA has also been found to show an increase in alpha coherence (linked with prefrontal and somatosensory sites) during periods of tic suppression (Serrien et al., 2005), suggesting its potential role in tic control as well as tic onset. In conclusion, a deeper understanding of neural oscillations may illuminate the complex, challenging, enigmatic, internal world that is TS (Leckman et al., 2006).

TOWARD AN INTEGRATED DEVELOPMENTAL THEORY OF PATHOGENESIS

If tics, like stereotypies, vary according to the balance of activity of medium spiny neurons in the striosome and matrix compartments of the striatum, then it should be possible to examine the clinical impact of genetic and/or developmental insults that affect the relative number and sensitivity of medium spiny neurons in the two striatal compartments (Leckman, 2002). For example, perinatal ischemic and hypoxic insults involving parenchymal lesions increase the risk of tic disorders eightfold (Whitaker et al., 1997). Further, this model may provide a meaningful integration of knowledge about tics drawn from a number of clinical observations. These include the stress responsiveness of tics (limbic activation), the presence of premonitory sensory urges (as sensory motor and primary motor cortical inputs converge on the fewer than normal medium spiny neurons in the matrix), the reduction of tics when an individual is engaged in acts that require selective attention and guided motor action (heightened activity within the matrix compartment), and the need to "even up" sensory and motor stimuli in a bilaterally symmetrical fashion (convergence of information from both ipsi- and contralateral primary motor neurons on medium spiny neurons within the matrix). The timing of tics and the course of tic disorders may be reflected in the collective burst firing of dopaminergic neurons (Peterson and Leckman, 1998) and there is clear evidence to support the presence of a hyperdopaminergic state in many patients with severe TS (Wolf et al., 1996; Singer et al., 2002; Albin et al., 2003; Cheon et al., 2004; Serra-Mestres et al., 2004; Yoon et al., 2007).

From a developmental perspective, it is clear that many of the GABAergic interneurons of the cerebral cortex migrate tangentially from the same embryonic regions in the ganglionic eminence that also give rise to the GABAergic medium spiny neurons of the striatum (Anderson et al., 2001). Could adverse events occurring at a specific point in development account for the striatal imbalance and the intracortical deficits seen in some patients with TS? The recent postmortem finding of Kalanthi et al. (2005) provides empirical support for this speculation. These anatomical changes might well lead to the aberrant oscillatory rhythms seen in TS (Moran et al., 2005; Leckman et al., 2006).

Finally, it is tempting to speculate that in Sydenham's chorea and in postinfectious forms of TS, the functional activity of the medium spiny neurons of the matrix is differentially impaired as a result of the autoimmune response (Leckman and Riddle, 2000). Indeed, one plausible hypothesis is that the antineural antibodies found in a subset of patients with TS may modulate synaptic transmission and alter the balance of activity within neurons of the striosomal and matrisomal compartments of the striatum (Kirvan et al., 2006).

FUTURE DIRECTIONS

The next decade of research on TS and related disorders will build on some of the recent findings presented in this chapter. Although immunological, neuroimaging, neurochemical, and family genetic studies, as well as the clinical investigations of the phenomenology and natural history of the disorder, will doubtless provide useful clues to the biological processes involved in this disorder, the field needs to continue to develop animal models that will permit a more complete exploration of the neurobiological mechanisms involved in TS.

ACKNOWLEDGMENTS

This work was supported in part by the Tourette Syndrome Association, National Association for Research in Schizophrenia and Affective Disorders, the Donaghue Foundation, and National Institutes of Health and National Institute of Mental Health Grants MH52711, MH01527, MH44843, MH49351, MH00508, NS16648, HD03008, RR00125, and RR06022.

REFERENCES

Abelson, J.F., Kwan, K.Y., O'Roak, B.J., Baek, D.Y., Stillman, A.A., Morgan, T.M., Mathews, C.A., Pauls, D.L., Rasin, M.R., Gunel, M., Davis, N.R., Ercan-Sencicek, A.G., Guez, D.H., Spertus, J.A., Leckman, J.F., Dure, L.S. IV, Kurlan, R., Singer, H.S., Gilbert, D.L., Farhi, A., Louvi, A., Lifton, R.P., Sestan, N., and State, M.W. (2005) Sequence variants in SLITRK1 are associated with Tourette's syndrome. *Science* 310:317–320.

Albin, R.L., Koeppe, R.A., Bohnen, N.I., Nichols, T.E., Meyer, P., Wernette, K., Minoshima, S., Kilbourn, M.R., and Frey, K.A. (2003) Increased ventral striatal monoaminergic innervation in Tourette syndrome. *Neurology* 61:310–315.

Alexander, G.E., Crutcher, M.D., and DeLong, M.R. (1990) Functional architecture of basal ganglia circuits: neural substrates of parallel processing. *Trends Neurosci.* 13:266–271.

Allen, A. (1997) Group A streptococcal infections and childhood neuropsychiatric disorders. *CNS Drugs* 8:267–275.

American Psychiatric Association. (1994) *Diagnostic and Statistical Manual of Mental Disorders*, 4th ed. Washington, DC: Author.

American Psychiatric Association. (2000) *Diagnostic and Statistical Manual of Mental Disorders*, 4th ed., text rev. Washington, DC: Author.

Anderson, S.A., Marin, O., Horn, C., Jennings, K., and Rubenstein, J.L. (2001) Distinct cortical migrations from the medial and lateral ganglionic eminences. *Development* 128:353–363.

Apter, A., Pauls, D.L., Bleich, A., Zohar, A.H., Kron, S., Ratzoni, G., Dycian, A., Kotler, M., Weizman, A., Gadot, N., and Cohen, D.J. (1993) An epidemiological study of Gilles de la Tourette's syndrome in Israel. *Arch. Gen. Psychiatry* 50:734–738.

Bajwa, R.J., de Lotbinière, A.J., King, R.A., Jabbari, B., Kunze, K., Quatrano, S., Scahill, L., and Leckman, J.F. (2007) Deep brain stimulation in Tourette's syndrome. *Mov Disord.* 22(9):1346–1350.

Balthazar, K. (1957) Über das anatomische substrat der generalisierten tic-krankeit (maladie des tics, Gilles de la Tourette): Entwicklungshemmung des corpus striatum [The anatomical substratum of the generalized tic disease (maladie des tics, Gilles de la Tourette); arrest of development of the corpus striatum]. Archiv für Psychiatrie und Zeitschrift f.d.ges. *Neurologie* 195: 531–549.

Baron-Cohen, S., Mortimore, C., Moriarty, J., Izaguirre, J., and Robertson, M. (1999) The prevalence of Gilles de la Tourette's syndrome in children and adolescents with autism. *J. Child Psychol. Psychiatry* 40:213–218.

Berkson, J.B. (1946) Limitations of the application of fourfold table analysis to hospital data. *Biometrics* 2:47–51.

Bloch, M.H., Leckman, J.F., and Peterson, B.S. (2005) Basal ganglia volumes and future tic severity in children with Tourette syndrome. *Neurology* 65:1253–1258.

Bloch, M.H., Peterson, B.S., Scahill, L., Otka, J., Katsovich, L., Zhang, H., and Leckman, J.F. (2006) Adulthood outcome of tic and obsessive-compulsive symptom severity in children with Tourette syndrome. *Arch. Pediatr. Adolesc. Med.* 160:65–69.

Bohlhalter, S., Goldfine, A., Matteson, S., Garraux, G., Hanakawa, T., Kansaku, K., Wurzman, R. and Hallett, M., et al. (2006) Neural correlates of tic generation in Tourette syndrome: an event-related functional MRI study. *Brain* 129:2029–2037.

Bornstein, R.A., Stefl, M.E., and Hammond, L. (1990) A survey of Tourette syndrome patients and their families: The 1987 Ohio Tourette Survey. *Neuropsychiatry Clin. Neurosci.* 2:275–281.

Brett, P., Robertson, M.M., Gurling, H., and Curtis, D. (1993) Failure to find linkage and increased homozygosity for the dopamine D3 receptor. *Lancet* 341:1225.

Brooks, D.J., Turjanski, N., Sawle, G.V., Playford, E.D., and Lees, A.J. (1992) PET studies on the integrity of the pre and postsynaptic dopaminergic system in Tourette syndrome. *Adv. Neurol.* 58:227–231.

Bruun, R.D., and Budman, C.L. (1992) The natural history of Tourette syndrome. *Adv. Neurol.* 58:1–6.

Burd, L., Kerbeshian, L., Wikenheiser, M., and Fisher, W. (1986a) Prevalence of Gilles de la Tourette's syndrome in North Dakota adults. *Am. J. Psychiatry* 143:787.

Burd, L., Kerbeshian, L., Wikenheiser, M., and Fisher, W. (1986b) A prevalence study of Gilles de la Tourette's syndrome in North Dakota in school-age children. *J. Am. Acad. Child Adolesc. Psychiatry* 25:552–553.

Butler, I.J., Koslow, S.H., Seifert, W.E., Jr., Caprioli, R.M., and Singer, H.S. (1979) Biogenic amine metabolism in Tourette syndrome. *Ann. Neurol.* 6:37–39.

Castellanos, F.X., Giedd, J.N., Hamburger, S.D., Marsh, W.L., and Rapoport, J.L. (1996) Brain morphometry in Tourette's syndrome: the influence of comorbid attention-deficit/hyperactivity disorder. *Neurology* 47:1581–1583.

Castellanos, F.X., Giedd, J.N., Marsh, W.L., Hamburger, S.D., Vaituzis, A.C., Dickstein, D.P., Sarfatti, S.E., Vauss, Y.C., Snell, J.W., Lange, N., Kaysen, D., Krain, A.L., Ritchie, G.F., Rajapakse, J.C., and Rapoport, J.L. (1996) Quantitative brain magnetic resonance imaging in attention-deficit hyperactivity disorder. *Arch. Gen. Psychiatry* 53:607–616.

Chappell, P.B., Leckman, J.F., Riddle, M.A., Anderson, G.M., Listwak, S.J., Ort, S.I., Hardin, M.T., Scahill, L.D., and Cohen, D.J. (1992) Neuroendocrine and behavioral responses to naloxone in Tourette's syndrome. *Adv. Neurol.* 58:253–262.

Chase, T.N., Geoffrey, V., Gillespie, M., and Burrows, G.H. (1986) Structural and functional studies of Gilles de la Tourette syndrome. *Rev. Neurol.* 142:851–855.

Cheon, K.A., Ryu, Y.H., Namkoong, K., Kim, C.H., Kim, J.J., and Lee, J.D. (2004) Dopamine transporter density of the basal ganglia assessed with [123] IPT SPECT in drug-naive children with Tourette's disorder. *Psychiatry Res.* 130:85–95.

Cohen, D.J., Friedhoff, A.J., Leckman, J.F., and Chase, T.N. (1992) Tourette syndrome: extending basic research to clinical care, the clinical phenotype, and natural history. *Adv. Neurol.* 58:341–362.

Cohen, D.J., Shaywitz, B.A., Caparulo, B.K., Young, J.G., and Bowers, M.B. (1979) Chronic multiple tics of Gilles de la Tourette's disease: CSF acid monoamine metabolites after probenecid administration. *Arch. Gen. Psychiatry* 35:245–250.

Comings, D.E., and Comings, B.G. (1987) Tourette's syndrome and attention deficit disorder with hyperactivity. *Arch. Gen. Psychiatry* 44(11):1023–1026.

Comings, D.E., Wu, S., Chiu, C., Ring, R.H., Gade, R., Ahn, C., MacMurray, J.P., Dietz, G., and Muhleman, D. (1996) Polygenic inheritance of Tourette syndrome, stuttering, attention deficit hyperactivity, conduct, and oppositional defiant disorder. *Am. J. Med. Genet. Neuropsychiatry Genet.* 67:264–288.

Costello, E.J. Angold, A., Burns, B.J., Stangl, D.K., Tweed, D.L., Erkanli, A., and Worthman, C.M. (1996) The Great Smoky Mountains study of youth. *Arch. Gen. Psychiatry* 53:1129–1136.

Cuker, A., State, M. W., King, R. A., Davis, N., and Ward, D. C. (2004) Candidate locus for Gilles de la Tourette syndrome/obsessive compulsive disorder/chronic tic disorder at 18q22. *Am. J. Med. Genetics, sec. A* 130:37–39.

Cunningham, M.W., Antone, S.M., Smart, M., Liu, R., and Kosanke, S. (1997) Molecular analysis of human cardiac myosin-cross-reactive B- and T-cell epitopes of the group A streptococcal M5 protein. *Infect. Immun.* 65:3913–3923.

Curtis, D., Robertson, M.M., and Gurling, H.M. (1992) Autosomal dominant gene transmission in a large kindred with Gilles de la Tourette syndrome. *Br. J. Psychiatry* 160:845–849.

de la Tourette, G. (1885) Etude sur une affection nerveuse caracterisee par de l'incoordination motrice accompagnee d'echolalie et de copralalie [Study of a neurological condition characterized by motor in-coordination accompanied by echolalia and coprolalia]. *Arch. Neurol.* 9:19–42.

Devor, E.J., Grandy, D.K., and Civelli, O. (1990) Genetic linkage is excluded for the D2-dopamine receptor lambda HD2G1 and flanking loci on chromosome 11q22-q23 in Tourette syndrome. *Hum. Hered.* 40:105–108.

Dewulf, A., and van Bogaert, L. (1940) Etudes anatomo-cliniques de sydromes hypercinetiques complexes [Studies of the clinical-anatomy of complex hyperkinetic syndromes]. *J. Psychiatry Neurol.* 104:53–61.

Donnai, D. (1987) Gene location in Tourette syndrome. *Lancet* 1:627.

George, M.S., Trimble, M.R., Ring, H.A., Sallee, F.R., and Robertson, M.M. (1993) Obsessions in obsessive-compulsive disorder with and without Gilles de la Tourette's syndrome. *Am. J. Psychiatry* 150:93–97.

Golden, G.S. (1974) Gilles de la Tourette syndrome following methylphenidate administration. *Dev. Med. Child Neurol.* 16:76–78.

Goldman-Rakic, P.S., and Selemon, L.D. (1990) New frontiers in basal ganglia research. *Trends Neurosci.* 13:241–244.

Greenberg, B.D., Ziemann, U., Cora-Locatelli, G., Harmon, A., Murphy, D.L., Keel, J.C., and Wassermann, E.M. (2000) Altered cortical excitability in obsessive-compulsive disorder. *Neurology* 54:142–147.

Grice, D.E., Leckman, J.F., Pauls, D.L., Kurlan, R., Kidd, K.K., Pakstis, A.J., Chang, F.M., Buxbaum, J.D., Cohen, D.J., and Glernter, J. (1996) Linkage disequilibium between an allele at the dopamine D4 receptor locus and Tourette syndrome, by the transmission-disequilibrium test. *Am. J. Hum. Genet.* 59:644–652.

Guilherme, L., and Kalil, J. (2004) Rheumatic fever: From sore throat to autoimmune heart lesions. *Int. Arch. Allergy Immunol.* 134:56–64.

Haber, S.N., Kowall, N.W., Vonsattel, J.P., Bird, E.D., and Richardson, E.P. Jr. (1986) A postmortem neuropathological and immunohistochemical study. *J. Neurol. Sci.* 75:225–241.

Hallett, J.J., Harling-Berg, C.J., Knopf, P.M., Stopa, E.G., and Kiessling, L.S. (2000) Anti-telencephalic antibodies in Tourette syndrome cause neuronal dysfunction. *J. Neuroimmunol.* 111: 195–202.

Hampson, M., Tokoglu, F., King, R.A., and Constable, T.R. (2008) *Differential brain activity during chronic motor tics and intentional movements of healthy controls.* Manuscript submitted for publication.

Hyde, T.M., Aaronson, B.A., Randolph, C., Rickler, K.C., and Weinberger, D.R. (1992) Relationship of birth weight to the phenotypic expression of Gilles de la Tourette's syndrome in monozygotic twins. *Neurology* 42:652–658.

Jagger, J., Prusoff, B.A., Cohen, D.J., Kidd, K.K., Carbonari, C.M., and John, K. (1982) The epidemiology of Tourette syndrome: a pilot study. *Schizophr. Bull.* 8:267–278.

Kalanithi, P.S., Zheng, W., Kataoka, Y., DiFiglia, M., Grantz, H., Saper, C. B., Schwartz, M.L., Leckman, J.F., and Vaccarino, F.M. (2005) Altered parvalbumin-positive neuron distribution in basal ganglia of individuals with Tourette syndrome. *Proc. Nat. Acad. Sci. USA* 102:13307–13312.

Kansy, J.W., Leckman, J.F., McIver, K., Katsovich, L., Lombroso, P. J., Zabriskie, J.B., and Bibb, J.A. (2006) Identification of pyruvate kinase as an antigen associated with Tourette syndrome. *J. Neuroimmunol.* 181:165–176.

Kawikova, I., Leckman, J.F., Kronig, H., Katsovich, L., Bessen, D., Ghebremichael, M., and Bothwell, A.L.M. (2007) Decreased number of regulatory T cells suggests impaired immune tolerance in children with Tourette's syndrome. *Biol. Psychiatry* 61:273–278.

Khalifa, N., and von Knorring, A.L. (2006) Psychopathology in a Swedish population of school children with tic disorders. *J. Am. Acad. Child Adolesc. Psychiatry* 45:1346–1353.

Kiessling, L.S., Marcotte, A.C., and Culpepper, L. (1993) Antineuronal antibodies in movement disorders. *Pediatrics* 92:39–43.

Kirvan, C.A., Swedo, S.E., Heuser, J.S., and Cunningham, M.W. (2003) Mimicry and autoantibody-mediated neuronal cell signaling in Sydenham chorea. *Nat. Med.* 9(7):914–920.

Kirvan, C.A., Swedo, S.E., Kurahara, D., and Cunningham, M.W. (2006) Streptococcal mimicry and antibody-mediated cell signaling in the pathogenesis of Sydenham's chorea. *Autoimmunity* 39: 21–29.

Kurlan, R., Behr, J., Medved, L., Shoulson, I., Pauls, D., Kidd, J.R., and Kidd, K.K. (1986) Familial Tourette's syndrome: report of a large pedigree and potential for linkage analysis. *Neurology* 36: 772–776.

Kurlan, R., Whitmore, D., Irvine, C., McDermott, M. P., and Como, P. G. (1994) Tourette's syndrome in a special education population: a pilot study involving a single school district. *Neurology* 44:699–702.

Leckman, J.F. (2002) Tourette's syndrome. *Lancet* 360:1577–1586.

Leckman, J.F., Dolnansky, E.S., Hardin, M.T., Clubb, M., Walkup, J.T., Stevenson, J., and Pauls, D.L. (1990) Perinatal factors in the expression of Tourette's syndrome: an exploratory study. *J. Am. Acad. Child Adolesc. Psychiatry* 2:220–226.

Leckman, J.F., Grice, D.E., Boardman, J., Zhang, H., Vitale, A., Bondi, C., Alsobrook, J., Peterson, B.S., Cohen, D.J., Rasmussen, S.A., Goodman, W.K., McDougle, C.J., and Pauls, D.L. (1997) Symptoms of obsessive compulsive disorder. *Am. J. Psychiatry* 154:911–917.

Leckman, J.F., Katsovich, L., Kawikova, I., Lin, H., Zhang, H., Krönig, H., Morshed, S., Parveen, S., Grantz, H., Findley, D.B., Lombroso, P.J., and King, R.A. (2005) Increased serum levels of Tumour Necrosis Factor-alpha and IL-12 in Tourette's syndrome. *Biol. Psychiatry* 57(6):667–673.

Leckman, J.F., Knorr, A., Rasmusson, A.M., and Cohen, D.J. (1991) Another frontier for basal ganglia research: Tourette's syndrome and related disorders. *Trends Neurosci.* 3:207–211.

Leckman, J.F., Pauls, D.L., Peterson, B.S., Riddle, M.A., Anderson, G.M., and Cohen, D.J. (1992) Pathogenesis of Tourette's syndrome: clues from the clinical phenotype and natural history. *Adv. Neurol.* 58:15–23.

Leckman, J.F., Price, R.A., Walkup, J.T., Ort, S.I., Pauls, D.L., and Cohen, D.J. (1987) Birthweights of monozygotic twins discordant for Tourette's syndrome. *Arch. Gen. Psychiatry* 44:100.

Leckman, J.F., and Riddle, M.A. (2000) Tourette's syndrome: when habit forming units form habits of their own? *Neuron* 28:349–354.

Leckman, J.F., Riddle, M.A., Berrettini, W.H., Anderson, G.M., Hardin, M.T., Chappell, P.B., Bissette, G., Nemeroff, C.B., Goodman, W.K., and Cohen, D.J. (1988) Elevated CSF dynorphin A[1-8] in Tourette's syndrome. *Life Sci.* 43:2015–2023.

Leckman, J.F., Vaccarino, F.M., Kalanithi, P.S., and Rothenberger, A. (2006) Tourette syndrome: A relentless drumbeat. *J. Child Psychol. Psychiatry* 47:537–550.

Leckman, J.F., Walker, D.E., and Cohen, D.J. (1993) Premonitory urges in Tourette's syndrome. *Am. J. Psychiatry* 150:98–102.

Leckman, J.F., Walker, D.E., Goodman, W.K., Pauls, D.L., and Cohen, D.J. (1994) "Just right" perceptions associated with compulsive behaviors in Tourette's syndrome. *Am. J. Psychiatry* 151:675–680.

Leckman, J.F., Zhang, H., Vitale, A., Lahnin, F., Lynch, K., Bondi, C., Kim, Y.-S., and Peterson, B.S. (1998) Course of tic severity in Tourette's syndrome: the first two decades. *Pediatrics* 102:14–19.

Lin, H., Katsovich, L., Ghebremichael, M., Findley, D.B., Grantz, H., Lombroso, P.J., King, R.A., Zhang, H., and Leckman, J.F (2007) Psychosocial stress predicts future symptom severities in children and adolescents with Tourette syndrome and/or obsessive-compulsive disorder. *J. Child Psychol. Psychiatry* 48:157–166.

Llinas, R., Urbano, F. J., Leznik, E., Ramirez, R. R., and van Marle, H. J. (2005) Rhythmic and dysrhythmic thalamocortical dynamics: GABA systems and the edge effect. *Trends Neurosci.* 28:325–333.

Lombroso, P.J., Mack, G., Scahill, L., King, R., and Leckman, J.F. (1991) Exacerbation of Tourette's syndrome associated with thermal stress: a family study. *Neurology* 41:1984–1987.

Malison, R.T., McDougle, C.J., van Dyck, C.H., Scahill, L., Baldwin, R.M., Seibyl, J.P., Price, L.H., Leckman, J.F., and Innis, R.B. (1995) [^{123}I]beta-CIT SPECT imaging of striatal dopamine transporter binding in Tourette's disorder. *Am. J. Psychiatry* 152: 1359–1361.

Mantovani, A., Lisanby, S.H., Pieraccini, F., Ulivelli, M., Castrogiovanni, P., and Rossi. S. (2006) Repetitive transcranial magnetic stimulation (rTMS) in the treatment of obsessive-compulsive disorder (OCD) and Tourette's syndrome (TS). *Int. J. Neuropsychopharmacol.* 9: 95–100.

Mell, L.K., Davis, R.L., and Owens, D. (2005) Association between streptococcal infection and obsessive-compulsive disorder, Tourette's syndrome, and tic disorder. *Pediatrics* 116:56–60.

Merette, C., Brassard, A., Potvin, A., Bouvier, H., Rousseau, F., Emond, C., Bissonnette, L., Roy, M.A., Maziade, M., Ott, J., and Caron, C. (2000) Significant linkage for Tourette syndrome in a large French Canadian family. *Am. J. Hum. Genet.* 67:1008–1013.

Mink, J. (2001) Neurobiology of basal ganglia circuits. In: Cohen, D.J., Jankovic, J., and Goetz, C.G., eds. *Tourette Syndrome.* Philadelphia: Lippincott, Williams & Wilkins, pp. 113–122.

Moran, K.A., Leckman, J.F., Vaccarino, F.M., Walton, K.D., and Llinas, R.R. (2005) *Neuromagnetic correlates of Gilles de la Tourette syndrome.* Paper presented at the 35th Annual Meeting of the Society for Neuroscience, November 2005, Washington, DC.

Moriarty, J., Costa, D.C., Schmitz, B., Trimble, M.R., Ell, P.J., and Robertson, M.M. (1995) Brain perfusion abnormalities in Gilles de la Tourette's syndrome. *Br. J. Psychiatry* 167(2):249–254.

Moriarty, J., Varma, A.R., Stevens, J., Fish, M., Trimble, M.R., and Robertson, M.M. (1997) A volumetric MRI study of Gilles de la Tourette's syndrome. *Neurology* 49:410–415.

Morshed, S.A., Parveen, S., Leckman, J.F., Mercadante, M.T., Bittencourt-Kiss, M.H., Miguel, E.C., Arman, A., Yazgan, Y., Fujii, T., Paul, S., Peterson, B.S., Zhang, H., King, R., Scahill, L., and Lombroso, P.J. (2001) Antibodies against neural, nuclear, cytoskeletal and streptococcal epitopes in children and adults with Tourette's syndrome. Sydenham's chorea, and autoimmune disorders. *Biol. Psychiatry* 50:566–577.

Murphy, T.K., Goodman, W.K., Fudge, M.W., Williams, R.C., Ayoub, E.M., Dalal, M., Lewis, M.H., and Zabriskie, J.B. (1997) B-lymphocyte antigen D8/17: a peripheral marker for childhood-onset obsessive-compulsive disorder and Tourette's syndrome? *Am. J. Psychiatry* 154:402–407.

Pasamanick, B., and Kawi, A. (1956) A study of the association of prenatal and perinatal factors in the development of tics in children. *J. Pediatr.* 48:596.

Pauls, D.L., Cohen, D.J., and Heimbuch, R., Detlor, J., and Kidd, K.K. (1981) Familial pattern and transmission of Gilles de la Tourette syndrome and multiple tics. *Arch. Gen. Psychiatry* 38: 1091–1093.

Pauls, D.L., and Leckman, J.F. (1986) The inheritance of Gilles de la Tourette's syndrome and associated behaviors: evidence for autosomal dominant transmission. *N. Engl. J. Med.* 315:993–997.

Pauls, D.L., Pakstis, A., Kurlan, R., Kidd, K.K., Leckman, J.F., Cohen, D.J., Kidd. J.R., Como, P., and Sparkes, R. (1990) Segregation and linkage analyses of Tourette's syndrome and related disorders. *J. Am. Acad. Child Adolesc. Psychiatry* 29:195–203.

Pauls, D.L., Raymond, C., Stevenson, J., and Leckman, J.F. (1991) A family study of Gilles de la Tourette syndrome. *Am. J. Hum. Genet.* 48:154–163.

Pauls, D.L., Towbin, K.E., Leckman, J.F., Zahner, G., and Cohen, D.J. (1986) Gilles de la Tourette's syndrome and obsessive-compulsive disorder: evidence supporting a genetic relationship. *Arch. Gen. Psychiatry* 43:1180–1182.

Peterson, B.S., and Leckman, J.F. (1998) The temporal dynamics of tics in Gilles de la Tourette syndrome. *Biol. Psychiatry* 44:1337–1348.

Peterson, B.S., Leckman, J.F., Scahill, L., Naftolin, F., Keefe, D., Charest, N.J., King, R.A., Hardin, M.T., and Cohen, D.J. (1994) Steroid hormones and Tourette's syndrome: early experience with antiandrogen therapy. *J. Clin. Psychopharmacol.* 14:131–135.

Peterson, B.S., Leckman, J.F., Tucker, D., Scahill, L., Staob, L., Zhang, H., King, R., Cohen, D., Gore, J.C., and Lombroso, P.J. (2000) Preliminary findings of antistreptococcal antibody titers and basal ganglia volumes in tic, obsessive-compulsive, and attention-deficit/hyperactivity disorders. *Arch. Gen. Psychiatry* 57:364–372.

Peterson, B.S., Riddle, M.A., Cohen, D.J., Katz, L.D., Smith, J.C., Hardin, M.T., and Leckman, J.F. (1993) Reduced basal ganglia volumes in Tourette's syndrome using 3-dimensional reconstruction techniques from magnetic resonance images. *Neurology* 43: 941–949.

Peterson, B.S., Skudlarski, P., Anderson, A.W., Zhang, H., Gatenby, J.C., Lacadie, C.M., Leckman, J.F., and Gore, J.C. (1998) A functional magnetic resonance imaging study of tic suppression in Tourette syndrome. *Arch. Gen. Psychiatry* 55:326–333.

Peterson, B.S., Staib, L., Scahill, L., Zhang, H., Anderson, C., Leckman, J.F., Cohen, D.J., Gore, J.C., Albert, J., and Webster, R. (2001) Regional brain and ventricular volumes in Tourette syndrome. *Arch. Gen. Psychiatry* 58:427–440.

Peterson, B.S., Thomas, P., Kane, M.J., Scahill, L., Zhang, H., Bronen, R., King, R.A., Leckman, J.F., and Staib, L. (2003) Basal ganglia volumes in Tourette syndrome. *Arch. Gen. Psychiatry* 60:415–424.

Piccirillo, C.A., and Shevach, E.M. (2004) Naturally-occurring CD4+CD25+ immunoregulatory T cells: Central players in the arena of peripheral tolerance. *Semin. Immunol.* 16:81–88.

Price, R.A., Kidd, K.K., Cohen, D.J., Pauls, D.L., and Leckman, J.F. (1985) A twin study of Tourette syndrome. *Arch. Gen. Psychiatry* 42:815–820.

Riddle, M., Lynch, K., Scahill, L., DeVries, A., Cohen, D., and Leckman, J. (1995) Methylphenidate discontinuation and reinitiation during long-term treatment of children with Tourette's disorder and attention-deficit hyperactivity disorder: a pilot study. *J. Child Adolesc. Psychopharmacol.* 5:205–214.

Robertson, M.M. (2006) Mood disorders and Gilles de la Tourette's syndrome: An update on prevalence, etiology, comorbidity, clinical associations, and implications. *J. Psychosom. Res.* 61(3):349–358.

Robertson, M.M., and Orth, M. (2006) Behavioral and affective disorders in Tourette syndrome. *Adv. Neurol.* 99:39–60.

Robertson, M.M., Banerjee, S., Kurlan, R., Cohen, D.J., Leckman, J.F., McMahon, W., Pauls, D.L., Sandor, P., and van de Wetering, B.J. (1999) The Tourette syndrome diagnostic confidence index: development and clinical associations. *Neurology* 53:2108–2112.

Rutter, M., and Hemming, M. (1970) Individual items of deviant behavior: their prevalence and clinical significance. In: Rutter, M., Tizard, J., and Whitmore, K., eds. *Education, Health, and Behavior.* London: Longman, pp. 202–232.

Sakaguchi, S., Sakaguchi, N., Asano, M., Itoh. M., and Toda, M. (1995) Immunologic self-tolerance maintained by activated T cells expressing IL-2 receptor alpha-chains (CD25). Breakdown of a single mechanism of self-tolerance causes various autoimmune diseases. *J. Immunol.* 155:1151–1164.

Scahill, L., Leckman, J., and Marek, K. (1995) Sensory phenomena in Tourette's syndrome. *Adv. Neurol.* 65:273–280.

Scahill, L., Lombroso, P.J., Mack, G., Van Wattum, P.J., Zhang, H., Vitale, A., and Leckman, J.F. (2001) Thermal sensitivity in Tourette syndrome. *Percep. Mot. Skills* 92:419–432.

Serra-Mestres, J., Ring, H.A., Costa, D.C., Gacinovic, S., Walker, Z., Lees, A.J., Robertson, M.M., and Trimble, M.R. (2004) Dopamine transporter binding in Gilles de la Tourette syndrome: a [123I]FP-CIT/SPECT study. *Acta Psychiatrica Scand.* 109:140–146.

Serrien, D.J., Orth, M., Evans, A.H., Lees, A.J., and Brown, P. (2005) Motor inhibition in patients with Gilles de la Tourette syndrome: functional activation as revealed by EEG coherence. *Brain* 128:116–125.

Shapiro, A.K., and Shapiro, E.S. (1988) Treatment of tic disorders with haloperidol. In: Cohen, D.J., Bruun, R.D., and Leckman J.F., eds. *Tourette's Syndrome and Tic Disorders.* New York: Wiley, pp. 267–289.

Shapiro, A.K., Shapiro, E.S., and Bruun, R.D. (1978) *Gilles de la Tourette Syndrome.* New York: Raven Press.

Shapiro, A.K., Shapiro, E.S., Young, J.G., and Feinberg, T.E. (1988) History of Tourette and tic disorders. In: Shapiro, A.K., Shapiro, E.S., Young, J.G., and Feinberg, T.E., eds. *Gilles de la Tourette Syndrome.* New York: Raven Press, pp. 1–27.

Shapiro, E.S., Shapiro, A.K., Fulop, G., Hubbard, M., Mandeli, J., Nordlie, J., and Phillips, R.A. (1989) Controlled study of haloperidol, pimozide, and placebo for the treatment of Gilles de la Tourette's syndrome. *Arch. Gen. Psychiatry* 46:722–730.

Simonic, I., Gericke, G.S., Ott, J., and Weber, J.L. (1998) Identification of genetic markers associated with Gilles de la Tourette syndrome in an Afrikaner population. *Am. J. Hum. Genet.* 63:839–846.

Simonic, I., Nyholt, D.R., Gericke, G.S., Gordon, D., Matsumoto, N., Ledbetter, D.H., Ott, J., and Weber, J.L. (2001) Further evidence for linkage of Gilles de la Tourette syndrome (GTS) susceptibility loci on chromosomes 2p11, 8q22 and 11q23-24 in South African Afrikaners. *Am. J. Med. Genet.* 105:163–167.

Singer, H.S. (1997) Neurobiology of Tourette syndrome. *Neurol. Clin.* 15:357–379.

Singer, H.S., Giuliano, J.D., Hansen, B.H., Hallett, J.J., Laurino, J. P., Benson, M., and Kiessling, L.S. (1998) Antibodies against human putamen in children with Tourette syndrome. *Neurology* 50:1618–1624.

Singer, H.S., Hahn, I.-H., and Moran, T.H. (1991) Abnormal dopamine uptake sites in postmortem striatum from patients with Tourette's syndrome. *Ann. Neurol.* 30:558–562.

Singer, H.S., Mink, J.W., Loiselle, C.R., Burke, K.A., Ruchkina, I., Morshed, S., Parveen, S., Leckman, J.F., Hallett, J.J., and Lombroso, P.J. (2005) Microinfusion of antineuronal antibodies into rodent striatum: failure to differentiate between elevated and low titers. *J. Neuroimmunol.* 163:8–14.

Singer, H.S., Reiss, A.L., Brown, J., Aylward, E.H., Shih, B., Chee, E., Harris, E.L., Reader, M.J., Chase, G.A., Bryan, N., and Denckla, M.B. (1993) Volumetric MRI changes in basal ganglia of children with Tourette's syndrome. *Neurology* 43:950–956.

Singer, H.S., Wong, D.F., Brown, J.E., Brandt, J., Krafft, L., Shaya, E., Dannals, R.F., and Wagner, H.N. (1992) Positron emission tomography evaluation of dopamine D-2 receptors in adults with Tourette syndrome. *Adv. Neurol.* 58:233–239.

Singer, H,S., Szymanski, S., Giuliano, J., Yokoi, F., Dogan, A.S., Brasic, J.R., Zhou, Y., Grace, A.A., and Wong, D.F. (2002) Elevated intrasynaptic dopamine release in Tourette's syndrome measured by PET. *Am. J. Psychiatry* 159:1329–1336.

Stern, E., Silbersweig, DA., Cheem, K.-Y., Holmes, A., Robertson, M.M., Trimble, M., Frith, C.D., Frackowiak, R.S., and Dolan, R.J. (2000) A functional neuroanatomy of tics in Tourette syndrome. *Arch. Gen. Psychiatry* 57:741–748.

Swedo, S.E., Leonard, H.L., Garvey, M., Mittleman, B., Allen, A.J., Perlmutter, S., Lougee, L., Dow, S., Zamkoff, J., and Dubbert, B.K. (1998) Pediatric autoimmune neuropsychiatric disorders associated with streptococcal infections: clinical description of the first 50 cases. *Am. J. Psychiatry* 155:264–271.

Swedo, S.E., Leonard, H.L., and Kiessling, L.S. (1994) Speculations on antineuronal antibody-mediated neuropsychiatric disorders of childhood. *Pediatrics* 93:323–326.

Swedo, S.E., Leonard, H.L., Mittleman, B.B., Allen, A.J., Rapoport, J.L., Dow, S.P., Kanter, M.E., Chapman, F., and Zabriskie, J. (1997) Identification of children with pediatric autoimmune neuropsychiatric disorders associated with streptococcal infections by a marker associated with rheumatic fever. *Am. J. Psychiatry* 154:110–112.

Swerdlow, N.R., Bongiovanni, M.J., Tochen, L., and Shoemaker, J.M. (2006) Separable noradrenergic and dopaminergic regulation of prepulse inhibition in rats: implications for predictive validity and Tourette Syndrome. *Psychopharmacol. (Berl)* 186(2): 246–254.

Taylor, J.R., Morshed, S., Parveen, S., Leckman, J., and Lombroso, P.J. (2002) An animal model of Tourette's syndrome. *Am. J. Psychiatry* 159:657–690.

The Tourette Syndrome Association International Consortium for Genetics. (1999) A complete genome screen in sib-pairs affected with Gilles de la Tourette syndrome. *Arch. Gen. Psychiatry* 65: 1428–1436.

Tourette Syndrome Association International Consortium for Genetics. (2007) Genome scan for Tourette disorder in affected-sibling-pair and multigenerational families. *Am. J. Hum. Genet.* 80(2): 265–272.

Verkerk, A.J., Mathews, C.A., Joosse, M., Eussen, B.H., Heutink, P., Oostra, B.A., and Tourette Syndrome Association International Consortium for Genetics. (2003) CNTNAP2 is disrupted in a family with Gilles de la Tourette syndrome and obsessive compulsive disorder. *Genomics* 82:1–9.

Whitaker, A.H., Van Rossem, R., Feldman, J.F., Schonfeld, I.S., Pinto-Martin, J.A., Tore, C., et al. (1997) Psychiatric outcomes in low-birth-weight children at age 6 years: relation to neonatal cranial ultrasound abnormalities. *Arch. Gen. Psychiatry* 54:847–856.

Wolf, S.S., Jones, D.W., Knable, M.B., Gorey, J.G., Lee, K.S., Hyde, T.M., Coppola, R., and Weinberger, D. (1996) Tourette syndrome: prediction of phenotypic variation in monozygotic twins by caudate nucleus D2 receptor binding. *Science* 273:1225–1227.

Yoon, D.Y., Gause, C.D., Leckman, J.F., and Singer, H.S. (2007) Frontal dopaminergic abnormality in Tourette syndrome: A postmortem analysis. *J. Neurol. Sci.* 255:50–56.

Zahner, G.E.P., Clubb, M.M., Leckman, J.F., and Pauls, D.L. (1988) The epidemiology of Tourette's syndrome. In: Cohen, D.J., Bruun, RD., and Leckman, J.F., eds. *Tourette's Syndrome and Tic Disorders*. New York: Wiley, pp. 79–89.

Ziemann, U., Paulus, W., and Rothenberger, A. (1997) Decreased motor inhibition in Tourette's disorder: evidence from transcranial magnetic stimulation. *Am. J. Psychiatry* 154:1277–1284.

76 The Neurobiology of Childhood Psychotic Disorders

NITIN GOGTAY AND JUDITH RAPOPORT

Psychotic disorders are rare in children, but as is often the case with very early-onset illnesses (Childs and Scriver, 1986), they tend to be more severe than their adult counterparts. Transient psychotic symptoms, however, are more common in healthy children than generally recognized (Caplan, 1994; Schreier, 1999; McGee et al., 2000). Although the existence of childhood schizophrenia was acknowledged early in the 20th century (Kraepelin, 1919), systematic research has been limited by diagnostic uncertainty and the general lack of knowledge about the psychotic processes at any age (Nicolson and Rapoport, 1999). Initially, the term *childhood psychosis* was used broadly to include the spectrum of severe behavioral disorders and autism, which were equated with schizophrenia (Volkmar, 1996).

In 1971, Kolvin established a clinical distinction between autism and other psychotic disorders of childhood. However, even today, high rates of over diagnosis of childhood schizophrenia remain due to symptom overlap and the presence of relatively fleeting hallucinations in pediatric patients who are not psychotic (Lukianowicz, 1969; McKenna et al., 1994). Although anxiety and stress are probably the most common causes of hallucinations in preschool children, and the prognosis of these symptoms is usually benign (Rothstein, 1981), in school-age children, psychotic phenomena generally tend to be more persistent and are more likely to be associated with drug toxicity or significant mental illness (Davison, 1983; Abramowicz, 1993; Schreier, 1999; McGee et al., 2000). However, recent epidemiologic data show self-reported psychotic symptoms at age 11 to have predictive power (odds ratio [OR] = 16.4, confidence interval [CI]: 3.9–67.8) for schizophreniform diagnosis at age 26, suggesting that psychotic symptoms probably exist as a continuous phenotype rather than an all-or-none phenomenon (Poulton et al., 2000).

CLINICAL PHENOMENOLOGY AND TREATMENT

Differential Diagnosis

Hallucinations are more common than generally recognized in normal preschool as well as school-age children (Caplan, 1994; Schreier, 1999; McGee et al., 2000). Children with conduct disorder and various other behavioral disturbances can show hallucinations (Garralda, 1984a, 1984b). Childhood-onset schizophrenia is very rare (estimated to be about 1/300th the rate of the adult disorder) and must be distinguished from various other childhood conditions that manifest psychotic symptoms and/or deterioration in function. The disorders most commonly misdiagnosed as childhood onset schizophrenia (COS) are

1. Affective disorders: Hallucinations are relatively common in pediatric bipolar disorder and major depression (Chambers et al., 1982; Varanka et al., 1988). However, the psychotic symptoms in these conditions tend to be mood congruent, and follow-up studies on this population generally suggest a stable clinical outcome (Garralda, 1984b; McClellan and McCurry, 1999; Ulloa et al., 2000)
2. Organic psychosis and substance abuse disorders may mimic withdrawal states or negative symptoms (Garralda, 1984a; Caplan et al., 1991).
3. Pervasive developmental disorders and childhood disintegrative disorder may cause thought disorder and social withdrawal.
4. Conduct disorder and various other behavioral disturbances can also be associated with hallucinations (Garralda, 1984a, 1984b)
5. Finally, a sizeable, heterogeneous group of children with transient psychotic symptoms and multiple developmental abnormalities are not adequately characterized by existing *Diagnostic and Statistical Manual of Mental Disorders*, 4th ed. (*DSM-IV*; American Psychiatric Association [APA], 1994) categories (McKenna et al., 1994; Kumra et al., 1998). In *DSM*, these patients might be coded as psychosis not otherwise specified (NOS). Many meet criteria for attention-deficit/hyperactivity disorder (ADHD) but also have striking affective dysregulation. Similarities in neuropsychological test profiles, brain morphologic and eye movement abnormalities, and of familial risk factors suggested that some of these children would fall within schizophrenia spectrum (Kumra et al., 1998; Kumra, 2000). However, these atypical cases can be distinguished from schizophrenia by the transient

nature of the psychotic symptoms and relatively intact social interest. Most important, this group, provisionally labeled *multidimensionally impaired* (MDI), appears to have a different course as a recent 2- to 8-year prospective follow-up study showed that none progressed to schizophrenia (Nicolson et al., 2001) while about 38% progressed to become bipolar I (Gogtay et al., 2007).

The psychosis of COS can usually be distinguished by its severe and pervasive nature and its nonepisodic, unremitting course. Poor premorbid functioning in the areas of speech and language development, and social interactions (isolation and withdrawal) seen in childhood schizophrenia may also differentiate these patients.

Although psychotic symptoms may occur in otherwise healthy populations as noted above, recent epidemiological data from a 15-year prospective study based in Dunedin, New Zealand, suggest that clear psychotic phenomena at age 12 predict psychotic disorders at age 25. Thus, even transient psychotic phenomena in childhood may in fact be a prodrome for later manifestation of psychotic illness (Poulton et al., 2000).

Treatment

The cornerstone of treatment is antipsychotic drugs, but these patients also require an array of services, including education about their illness, special social and educational training, and family and individual counseling. Because of its rarity, few controlled trials of antipsychotic medications have been conducted in children or adolescents with schizophrenia. Two such trials with typical antipsychotics showed partial response and high incidence of side effects (Pool et al., 1976; Green et al., 1992; Spencer and Campbell, 1994).

The atypical antipsychotics *risperidone, olanzapine,* and *quetiapine* are now first-line agents for child and adolescent schizophrenia, based primarily on studies of adult-onset schizophrenia (AOS). The first controlled trial of an atypical antipsychotic was in a group of 21 children and adolescents with treatment-refractory schizophrenia (Kumra et al., 1996). In this double-blind comparison of haloperidol and clozapine, clozapine (mean dose 176 ± 149 mg/day) was more effective for positive and negative symptoms of schizophrenia than was haloperidol (mean dose 16 ± 8 mg/day). As expected for this refractory group, little benefit was seen from haloperidol; however, as there was no placebo arm in the study, it is hard to assess the true effect size for clozapine, and relatively high rates of neutropenia and seizures were seen in the clozapine group. A more recent double-blind randomized control trial of comparing clozapine ($n = 12$) with olanzapine ($n = 13$) showed a significant advantage for clozapine in the alleviation of negative symptoms of schizophrenia, which was not correlated with improvement in mood or extrapyramidal side effects. As anticipated, clozapine was associated with more overall side effects, including enuresis, tachycardia, hypertension, and significant weight gain at 2 years (Shaw et al., 2006).

Due to the ethical constraints, none of the ongoing pediatric trials were placebo controlled, and all were limited to comparisons with other atypical agents. The results of our prior study and studies in patients with AOS (Davis et al., 2003; Moncrieff, 2003) show that clozapine has the greatest antipsychotic efficacy, although its toxicity limits its use to patients with the most severe treatment-refractory schizophrenia.

Children and adolescents may be more susceptible to adverse effects of atypical antipsychotics. The lack of risk for tardive dyskinesia associated with clozapine represents an important advance but presents a complex tradeoff with physically and socially disabling problems of drowsiness, drooling, hyperglycemia, hypertension, and weight gain. Additionally, children and adolescents treated with clozapine have increased susceptibility to neutropenia and akathisia. Akathisia can frequently manifest as worsening of psychotic symptoms or agitation in children, which frequently results in dosage increment. This side effect is responsive to adjunctive propranolol (Gogtay et al., 2002) treatment.

Clinical Outcome

Childhood-onset schizophrenia is usually chronic (Gordon et al., 1994). The diagnosis is stable, with at least one half of the cases remaining severely impaired (Werry et al., 1991; J. R. Asarnow et al., 1994; R. F. Asarnow et al., 1994) and a substantial minority showing continued deterioration (J. R. Asarnow et al., 1994; Hollis, 2000). As with adults, premorbid function is a good predictor of outcome (Werry et al., 1991). In a recent analysis, rates of remission in COS were determined using the recently proposed standardized remission criteria (Andreasen et al., 2005). At 2-year follow-up, 7 of 62 patients with COS (11.3%) met criteria for sustained remission that was also associated with improved global assessment scores, higher full-scale IQ at admission, and also thicker mean cortical thickness at initial scan (Dr. Deanna Greenstein, unpublished data).

NEUROPSYCHOLOGY AND NEUROBIOLOGY

The continuity between COS and AOS is supported by overlapping abnormalities in neurocognitive functioning (Gochman et al., 2005), smooth pursuit eye movement (Sporn et al., 2005), genetic studies (Addington et al., 2004; Addington et al., 2005), family studies (Nicolson et al., 2003), and structural neuroimaging studies (Rapoport et al., 2005). Because COS is thought to reflect more profound early disturbance in brain development, one would expect the very early onset cases to be more severely impaired.

National Institute of Mental Health Sample

Most of the neurobiological studies of COS have been carried out at the National Institute of Mental Health (NIMH). These cases are between the ages of 6 and 18, with premorbid IQ of 70 or above, meet *DSM-IV* criteria for schizophrenia, and have onset of psychotic symptoms by age 12. Because trials of new agents are part of this study, all patients were required to be refractory or intolerant to several antipsychotics. Patients were diagnosed using structured and unstructured interviews (Gordon et al., 1994). To date, 95 patients have participated in the study, including 55 boys and 41 girls with a mean age of 13.58 ± 2.62 years and mean age of onset of psychosis at 10.18 ± 2.01 years.

Neuropsychological Studies

Neuropsychological function in COS has been studied in depth by Robert Asarnow and colleagues (R. F. Asarnow et al., 1994; R. F. Asarnow et al., 1995; R. F. Asarnow, 1999). Although rote language skills and simple perceptual processing are not impaired, these children perform poorly on tasks involving fine motor coordination, attention, and short-term and working memory (Karatekin and Asarnow, 1998). Evoked-potential studies show diminished amplitude of brain electrical activity during these tasks, suggesting that allocation of necessary attentional resources is deficient. Similar deficits were observed in adults with schizophrenia (R.F. Asarnow et al., 1995). The overall pattern of deficits appears similar to that observed in adult patients who were severely ill with a first episode with significant generalized deficit and a relative deficit of executive functioning in adolescents (Rhinewine et al., 2005). In a recent analyses on 67 parents and 24 siblings with COS, siblings with COS performed significantly more poorly than controls on Trails Making Test B; whereas parents with COS performed more poorly than controls on Trails Making Test A, suggesting that healthy first-degree relatives of COS probands have subtle deficits in tests involving oculomotor/psychomotor speed, working memory, and executive function as has been shown in relatives of AOS probands (Gochman et al., 2004). The long-term (13+ years) trajectory of IQ measures in COS, in spite of chronic illness and concomitant, progressive loss of cortical gray matter (GM), appears stable, similar to that reported for patients with adult onset (Gochman et al., 2005).

Neurobiological Studies

Eye tracking

Eye-tracking abnormalities, as reflected in the poor ability to follow a moving target, have been well described in adult patients with schizophrenia (Levy et al., 1994). These abnormalities are of interest as indirect indicators of frontal lobe function and are also considered genetic markers in schizophrenia. A study of adolescents with schizophrenia found greater catch-up saccade amplitude and a trend for lower gain in this population (Friedman et al., 1992).

The NIMH cohort of children with COS exhibits a pattern of eye-tracking dysfunction similar to that reported for adult patients. Relative to healthy age mates, this pattern is characterized by qualitatively poor eye tracking, higher root mean square error (RMSE), lower gain, and a greater frequency of catch-up saccades (Jacobsen, Hong, et al., 1996; Kumra et al., 2001). In our studies with juveniles, similar abnormalities were seen in patients with COS and in patients with psychotic disorder NOS, although this latter group did not exhibit a higher rate of catch-up saccades. As seen in adult patients, children with schizophrenia exhibit significantly greater eye-tracking impairments than patients who are healthy and patients with ADHD, as reflected by lower gain, greater RMSE, lower percentage of total task time engaged in tracking the target, and greater frequency of "catch-up" saccades.

A recent analysis comparing eye-tracking abnormalities between COS and AOS first-degree relatives showed that both COS and AOS parents had poorer eye-tracking performance than community controls. However, continuous qualitative score and RMSE differed significantly only between COS parents and controls whereas AOS parents did not differ significantly from their control group. Effect sizes for all the eye-tracking measures were higher for COS than AOS groups: (0.50 vs. 0.30 for continuous qualitative score; 0.59 vs. 0.28 for RMSE; 0.10 vs. 0.01 for leading saccades; all p values > .05). These findings suggest that the genetic factors underlying eye-tracking dysfunction appear more salient for COS (Sporn et al., 2005).

Family Studies

Very early onset illnesses tend to have more salient genetic causes (Childs and Scriver, 1986). Because COS is continuous with adult-onset illness (Rapoport et al., 2005; Greenstein et al., 2006), then as with other disorders of presumed multifactorial origin, early-onset cases of schizophrenia should be associated with a greater familial loading. Several studies with AOS suggest that earlier onset is associated with higher familial rates for the disorder (Pulver et al., 1990).

There are very few systematic family studies of childhood schizophrenia. NIMH and University of California, Los Angeles (UCLA) have used structured interviews to obtain diagnostic information for first-degree relatives of children with schizophrenia. Studies so far indicate an increased rate of schizophrenia spectrum disorders in the first-degree relatives of patients. The UCLA family study found a 13.86% rate of narrow spectrum disorder in the relatives of children with schizophrenia compared with 5.4% for ADHD and 0.82% for community controls (R.F. Asarnow et al., 2001) that was higher than that found in relatives of adult-onset cases. Most recently, Nicolson et al. (2003) also found increased incidence of schizophrenia spectrum disorders in parents of children with schizophrenia relative to community controls and the parents of adult cases. Thus, these studies suggest greater salience for some genetic factors in early cases.

There is no clinical evidence of unusual early or current social stress, and a single study of parental expressed emotion (EE) did not find high EE for the early-onset group (R.F. Asarnow and Asarnow, 1994), and other risk factors do not appear to be increased in the NIMH sample. For example, no evidence was found for precocious puberty (Frazier et al., 1997) or pregnancy/birth complications (Nicolson et al., 1999) that was also substantiated recently on a larger sample comparing 60 children with COS and their 48 healthy siblings (Ordonez et al., 2005).

Genetic Studies

Recent advances in molecular genetics and the recent work to sequence the entire human genome offer hope to identify susceptibility genes to a range of simple and complex diseases such as schizophrenia.

Cytogenetic Studies

Cytogenetic abnormalities appear more pronounced for COS. High-resolution banding karyotype and fluorescent in situ hybridization (FISH) analyses are done routinely on all patients with COS and MDI to look for Fragile X, 22q11 deletions, Smith–Magenis (17p11.2del), and 15q11-q13 deletions/duplications. Our cohorts show a rate of almost 10% for 95 COS probands with chromosomal abnormalities. The 22q11 deletion syndrome (22q11DS), manifest as velocardio-facial syndrome (VCFS), is estimated to occur in 1 in 4000 live births (Papolos et al., 1996) and is a known risk factor for schizophrenia (Pulver et al., 1994; Murphy et al., 1999). Four of 90 (4.4%) of our unselected patients with COS have VCFS with spontaneous 22q11 deletion, a rate significantly higher than 0.46% found for the available reports on a total of 870 adult onset cases ($p = .002$). Similarly, 2 of 38 (5.2%) females have mosaic Turner's syndrome, a rate about 500 times higher than expected for this particular subtype of Turner's syndrome.

Candidate genes

With an initial hypothesis that there may be more detrimental/penetrant mutations in known schizophrenia susceptibility genes in COS, to date we have examined a total of 15 genes previously reported positive for AOS and also nine putative autism genes given the higher rates of comorbid pervasive developmental disorder (PDD) with our sample (Sporn et al., 2004; Rapoport et al., 2005). Polymorphisms in seven genes previously implicated in AOS samples show significant association with COS, using a family-based design (Rapoport et al., 2005). In contrast, none of the nine putative autism risk genes showed evidence of association with COS.

BRAIN IMAGING

Brain Morphology

Recent advances in brain magnetic resonance imaging (MRI) allow reliable, automated quantitative measurement of multiple brain regions (Collins et al., 1999). Reports on brain morphologic abnormalities are also scarce, and most come from the NIMH sample, with more recent contributions from other groups (Sowell et al., 2000; Sowell, Levitt, Toga, and Asarrow, 2000; Matsumoto, Simmons, Williams, Hadjulis, et al., 2001; Matsumoto, Simmons, Williams, Pipe, et al., 2001). There is general agreement that children with schizophrenia show increased lateral ventricular volume, decreased GM volume, and increased basal ganglia volume (probably secondary to medication effect) (Rapoport et al., 1997; Rapoport et al., 1999; Sowell, Levitt, et al., 2000) but less agreement with respect to reduced volume of temporal lobe structures (Jacobsen, Giedd, et al., 1996; Matsumoto, Simmons, Williams, Hadjulis, et al., 2001; Matsumoto, Simmons, Williams, Pipe, et al., 2001).

Prospective longitudinal brain MRI studies of the NIMH childhood schizophrenia population have been uniquely informative. Early analyses using whole lobe volume measures showed increasing ventricular volume and decreasing total cortical, frontal, medial temporal, and parietal GM volumes at 2, 4, and 6 years after initial scan (Rapoport et al., 1999; Rapoport et al., 2001), and effect size comparison with adult studies suggested that such changes are more striking during adolescence (Gogate et al., 2001).

Earlier studies were limited to whole lobe GM measurements. Recent advances in computational image analysis permit regional GM density or cortical thickness measurements that provide unprecedented anatomic details of cortical GM detail across the entire brain and can be applied to large samples when automated (Thompson et al., 2000; 2001; Luders et al., 2005).

Using cross-sectional and longitudinal data, and with these state-of-the-art cortical brain mapping methods, we have been able to address some important questions about brain development in COS. Our analyses show that the pattern of cortical brain development in COS progresses in a unique "back to front" (parieto-frontal-temporal) direction (Thompson et al., 2001) and appears to be an exaggerated pattern of normal GM development (Gogtay, Giedd, et al., 2004), suggesting that GM loss in COS may reflect an exaggeration of normal maturational process of synaptic/dendritic pruning during adolescence (Huttenlocher, 1979; Huttenlocher and Dabholkar, 1997). This pattern is illustrated in Figure 76.1 (see also COLOR FIGURE 76.1 in separate insert).

The diagnostic specificity of these findings was established by mapping a subgroup of children with MDI (n = 12, 38%) that has converted to bipolar I diagnosis that showed a left lateralized gain in GM density and GM reduction on the right lateral and bilateral anterior cingulate cortices and a left lateralized gain in GM density and GM reduction on the right lateral and bilateral anterior cingulate cortices (Gogtay et al., 2007) The GM findings in COS appeared to be not due to medications, as quantitative analysis of matched COS (n = 23), MDI (n = 19), and healthy community control (n = 38) groups showed the GM loss to be limited only to the COS group (Gogtay, Sporn, et al., 2004).

Cortical thickness analyses have been completed on 70 patients with COS (age 6–26 years, 330 scans), comparing them to 72 matched healthy controls. This comparison showed that as patients with COS mature, the robust and global GM loss during the adolescent years becomes limited to prefrontal and superior temporal cortices by age 24, thus mimicking a pattern seen in adult patients and further establishing the continuity between the two phenotypes (Greenstein et al., 2006). (Fig. 76.2; see also COLOR FIGURE 76.2 in sepearate insert.)

Finally, our recent studies have addressed the question of whether the cortical GM loss in schizophrenia could be a trait marker. Cortical thickness analyses comparing 56 healthy siblings with COS with 56 matched controls using mixed-effect regression models that included a total of 100 scans for each group showed the healthy siblings with COS to have smaller prefrontal and superior temporal GM thickness in early ages, which appeared to normalize by age 20 (Gogtay, Greenstein, et al., 2007). Given that none of the siblings had schizophrenia spectrum diagnoses and had no medication exposure, these results show that the GM changes in COS are a trait marker. (Fig. 76.3.)

Other Imaging Studies

Thomas and colleagues (1998) conducted a proton magnetic resonance spectroscopy study of 10 children with schizophrenia and 12 healthy children. They found that the ratio of N-acetylaspartate (NAA) to creatine was significantly lower in the frontal lobes of children with schizophrenia than in healthy children. Similarly, lower NAA signals were also seen in hippocampal and dorsolateral prefrontal cortical regions of the NIMH childhood schizophrenia population (Bertolino et al., 1998). Although the role of NAA in brain function has not been

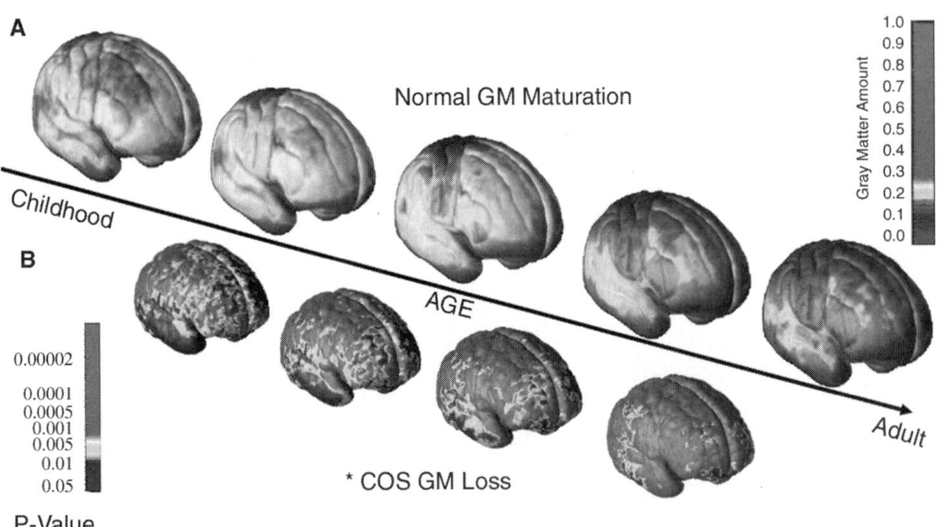

FIGURE 76.1 Comparison of the patterns of cortical gray matter (GM) loss in childhood-onset schizophrenia (COS) (between ages 12 and 16) to that seen in normal cortical maturation (between ages 4 to 22). (*A*) Right lateral view of the dynamic sequences of cortical GM maturation in healthy children between ages 4 and 22 (n = 13; 54 scans; upper panel) rescanned every 2 years. Scale bar shows GM amount at each of the 65,536 cortical points across the entire cortex represented using a color scale (see Figure 76.1 in color insert). Cortical GM maturation appears to progress in a "back to front" (parietotemporal) manner. (*B*) Right lateral view of the dynamic sequence of cortical GM maturation in COS between ages 12 and 16 compared with age- and sex-matched healthy controls (n = 12, 36 scans in each group), where children are rescanned every 2 years. Dynamic maps represent p values for the difference in GM amount between COS and controls at each of the 65,536 cortical points, and p values are represented using a color scale. Cortical GM loss in COS also appears to follow in a "back to front" direction on the lateral surface, thus suggesting that the COS pattern is an exaggeration of the normal GM maturation.

*Data on childhood schizophrenia only age 12 to 16.

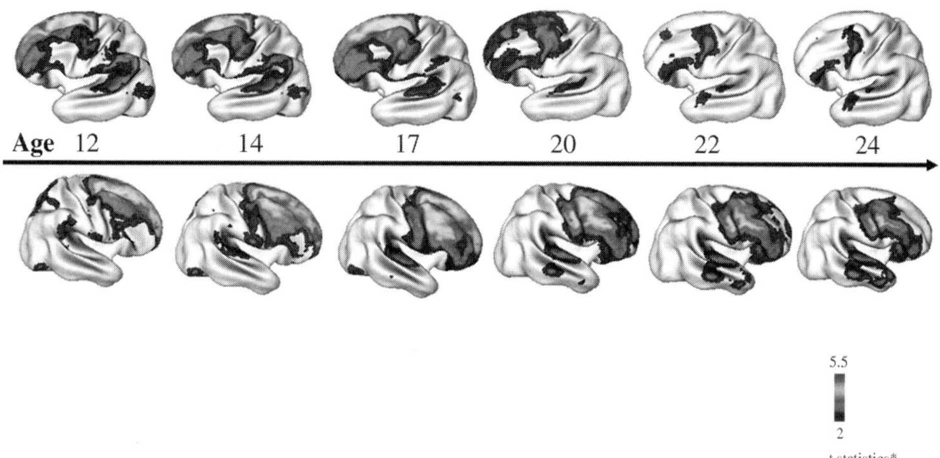

FIGURE 76.2 Progression of cortical gray matter (GM) loss in childhood-onset schizophrenia (COS) (n = 70; 162 scans) relative to age-, sex-, and scan interval–matched healthy controls (n = 72; 168 scans) from adolescence to young adulthood (age 12 to 24). Analyses were done using mixed model regression statistics and covaried for mean cortical thickness. Side bar shows t statistic with threshold to control for multiple comparisons using the false discovery rate (FDR) procedure with q = .05. Differences are from mixed model regression with age centered at approximate 3-year intervals for middle 80% of the age range, and colors (see Figure 76.2 in color insert) represent areas of statistically significant thinning in COS.

firmly established, it is thought to be a marker of neuronal density or neuronal volume (Renshaw et al., 1995).

Few functional imaging studies have been conducted in COS, quite possibly because functional imaging modalities demand that patients be immobile for a fixed period of time and/or that they carry out a cognitive task. Also, positron emission tomography (PET) studies involve exposure to radiation, thus limiting the use of pediatric controls.

Cerebral glucose metabolism was examined in 16 adolescent patients from the NIMH COS sample and 26 healthy adolescents matched for age, sex, and handedness (but not task performance) using PET and ^{18}F-fluorodeoxyglucose (FDG). Positron emission tomography findings indicated mild hypofrontality and abnormal neural circuitry that involved cerebellum in COS (Jacobsen and Rapoport, 1998).

White matter (WM) abnormalities in COS remain largely unexplored. A recent voxel-based diffusion tensor imaging (DTI) study on a small sample of patients with adolescent-onset schizophrenia suggested disrupted structural integrity of WM tracts in the anterior cingulate region (Kumra et al., 2005). Our recent analysis using whole lobe WM volumes on 70 children with COS (ages 7 to 26) with prospective rescans (n = 162 scans) showed that the slope for WM growth was significantly lower in children with COS compared to matched healthy controls in all lobes (p < .05), indicating that the GM reduction in COS is not secondary to WM encroachment (Gogtay et al., 2008). We are currently applying

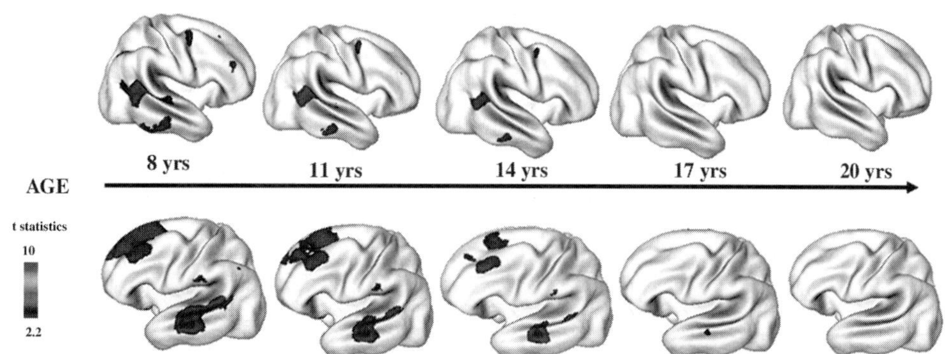

FIGURE 76.3 Cortical gray matter (GM) thickness in healthy childhood-onset schizophrenia (COS) siblings (n = 52; 110 scans) compared to age-, sex-, and scan interval–matched healthy controls (n = 52; 108 scans) between ages 8 through 28. Healthy siblings with COS show significant GM deficits in left prefrontal and bilateral temporal cortices and smaller deficits in right prefrontal and inferior parietal cortices. These deficits in healthy siblings normalize with age, with no abnormalities remaining by age 20. Side bar shows t statistic with threshold to control for multiple comparisons using the false discovery rate (FDR) procedure with q = 0.05. Differences are from mixed model regression with age centered at approximate 3-year intervals for middle 80% of the age range, and shading represent areas of statistically significant thinning in siblings with COS.

the novel tensor-based mapping technique to create dynamic maps of WM growth for these patients.

SUMMARY AND FUTURE DIRECTIONS

Converging evidence implicates abnormal neurodevelopment in schizophrenia that appears more striking in COS. In contrast to later-onset illness, longitudinal studies of the NIMH COS sample suggest more consistent (but nonprogressive) deterioration in intellectual function, and a more severe and progressive loss of cortical brain tissue in adolescence. This, together with the insidious onset of illness in this disorder, suggests that the pathologic processes underlying COS are more pronounced than those for adults and reflect a progressive neurodevelopmental disorder.

The increased rate of cytogenetic abnormalities and candidate risk gene associations in COS suggest that there will be other chromosomal instabilities (duplications or deletions) that are etiologic. This is currently being explored using high-density whole-genome scans in this cohort. Clinically, the COS endophenotypes suggest novel susceptibility genes for speech/language development, and PDDs.

With respect to anatomic brain imaging, advances in neuroimaging and genetic methodology, combined with the availability of longitudinal data, now allow further insights into the disease onset, course, and etiopathologic mechanisms in COS that can be extended to the understanding of schizophrenia pathology in general. Prospective brain-imaging studies of children who are at high risk suggest that at least some of the brain abnormalities are trait markers, and studies linking risk alleles and abnormal brain development will provide further insights.

While new atypical agents have more benign adverse effect profiles, clozapine remains the best alternative for treatment-refractory cases. A safer version of clozapine is needed for this severely ill and vulnerable population.

REFERENCES

Abramowicz, M. (1993) Drugs that cause psychiatric symptoms. *Med. Lett. Drugs Ther.* 35:65–70.

Addington, A.M., Gornick, M., Duckworth, J., Sporn, A., Gogtay, N., Bobb, A., et al. (2005) GAD1 (2q31.1), which encodes glutamic acid decarboxylase (GAD(67)), is associated with childhood-onset schizophrenia and cortical gray matter volume loss. *Mol. Psychiatry* 10(6):581–588.

Addington, A.M., Gornick, M., Sporn, A.L., Gogtay, N., Greenstein, D., Lenane, M., et al. (2004) Polymorphisms in the 13q33.2 gene G72/G30 are associated with childhood-onset schizophrenia and psychosis not otherwise specified. *Biol. Psychiatry* 55(10):976–980.

American Psychiatric Association. (1994) *Diagnostic and Statistical Manual of Mental Disorders*, 4th ed. Washington, DC: Author.

Andreasen, N.C., Carpenter, W.T., Jr., Kane, J.M., Lasser, R.A., Marder, S.R., and Weinberger, D.R. (2005) Remission in schizophrenia: proposed criteria and rationale for consensus. *Am. J. Psychiatry* 162(3):441–449.

Asarnow, J.R., Tompson, M.C., and Goldstein, M.J. (1994) Childhood-onset schizophrenia: a followup study. *Schizophr. Bull.* 20(4):599–617.

Asarnow, R.F. (1999) Neurocognitive impairments in schizophrenia: a piece of the epigenetic puzzle. *Eur. Child Adolesc. Psychiatry* 8(Suppl 1):I5–I8.

Asarnow, R.F., Asamen, J., Granholm, E., Sherman, T., Watkins, J.M., and Williams, M. E. (1994) Cognitive/neuropsychological studies of children with a schizophrenic disorder. *Schizophr. Bull.* 20(4):647–669.

Asarnow, R.F., and Asarnow, J.R. (1994) Childhood-onset schizophrenia: editors' introduction. *Schizophr. Bull.* 20(4):591–597.

Asarnow, R.F., Brown, W., and Strandburg, R. (1995) Children with a schizophrenic disorder: neurobehavioral studies. *Eur. Arch. Psychiatry Clin. Neurosci.* 245(2):70–79.

Asarnow, R.F., Nuechterlein, K.H., Fogelson, D., Subotnik, K.L., Payne, D.A., Russell, A.T., et al. (2001) Schizophrenia and schizophrenia-spectrum personality disorders in the first-degree relatives of children with schizophrenia: the UCLA family study. *Arch. Gen. Psychiatry* 58(6):581–588.

Bertolino, A., Callicott, J.H., Elman, I., Mattay, V.S., Tedeschi, G., Frank, J.A., et al. (1998) Regionally specific neuronal pathology in untreated patients with schizophrenia: a proton magnetic resonance spectroscopic imaging study. *Biol. Psychiatry* 43(9):641–648.

Caplan, R. (1994) Thought disorder in childhood. *J. Am. Acad. Child Adolesc. Psychiatry* 33(5):605–615.

Caplan, R., Shields, W.D., Mori, L., and Yudovin, S. (1991) Middle childhood onset of interictal psychosis. *J. Am. Acad. Child Adolesc. Psychiatry* 30(6):893–896.

Chambers, W.J., Puig-Antich, J., Tabrizi, M.A., and Davies, M. (1982) Psychotic symptoms in prepubertal major depressive disorder. *Arch. Gen. Psychiatry* 39(8):921–927.

Childs, B., and Scriver, C.R. (1986) Age at onset and causes of disease. *Perspect. Biol. Med.* 29(3 Pt 1):437–460.

Collins, D.L., Zijdenbos, A.P., Baare, W.F.C., and Evans, A.C. (1999) ANIMAL+INSECT: Improved cortical structure segmentation. In: *Proceedings of the Annual Conference on Information Processing in Medical Imaging (IPMI)*. Visegrad, Hungary: Springer, pp. 210–223.

Davis, J.M., Chen, N., and Glick, I.D. (2003) A meta-analysis of the efficacy of second-generation antipsychotics. *Arch. Gen. Psychiatry* 60(6):553–564.

Davison, K. (1983) Schizophrenia-like psychoses associated with organic cerebral disorders: a review. *Psychiatr. Dev.* 1(1):1–33.

Frazier, J.A., Alaghband-Rad, J., Jacobsen, L., Lenane, M.C., Hamburger, S., Albus, K., et al. (1997) Pubertal development and onset of psychosis in childhood onset schizophrenia. *Psychiatry Res.* 70(1):1–7.

Friedman, L., Abel, L.A., Jesberger, J.A., Malki, A., and Meltzer, H.Y. (1992) Saccadic intrusions into smooth pursuit in patients with schizophrenia or affective disorder and normal controls. *Biol. Psychiatry* 31(11):1110–1118.

Garralda, M.E. (1984a) Hallucinations in children with conduct and emotional disorders: I. The clinical phenomena. *Psychol. Med.* 14(3):589–596.

Garralda, M.E. (1984b) Hallucinations in children with conduct and emotional disorders: II. The follow-up study. *Psychol. Med.* 14(3):597–604.

Gochman, P.A., Greenstein, D., Sporn, A., Gogtay, N., Keller, B., Shaw, P., et al. (2005) IQ stabilization in childhood-onset schizophrenia. *Schizophr. Res.* 77(2–3):271–277.

Gochman, P.A., Greenstein, D., Sporn, A., Gogtay, N., Nicolson, R., Keller, A., et al. (2004) Childhood onset schizophrenia: familial neurocognitive measures. *Schizophr. Res.* 71(1):43–47.

Gogate, N., Giedd, J., Janson, K., and Rapoport, J.L. (2001) Brain imaging in normal and abnormal brain development: new perspectives for child psychiatry. *Clin. Neurosci. Res.* 1:283–290.

Gogtay, N., Chavez, A., Klunder, A., Lu, A., Leow, A.D., Lee, A.D., Toga, A.W., Rapoport, J.L., and Thompson, P.M. (2008) *3-D brain growth abnormalities in childhood-onset schizophrenia visualized using tensor based morphometry*. Unpublished manuscript.

Gogtay, N., Giedd, J.N., Lusk, L., Hayashi, K.M., Greenstein, D., Vaituzis, A.C., et al. (2004) Dynamic mapping of human cortical development during childhood through early adulthood. *Proc. Natl. Acad. Sci. USA* 101(21):8174–8179.

Gogtay, N., Greenstein, D., Lenane, M., Clasen, L., Sharp, W., Gochman, P., et al. (2007) Cortical brain development in nonpsychotic siblings of patients with childhood onset schizophrenia. *Arch. Gen. Psychiatry* 64(7):772–780.

Gogtay, N., Ordonez, A., Herman, D., Hayashi, K.M., Greenstein, D., Vaituzis, A.C., et al. (2007) Dynamic mapping of cortical development before and after the onset of pediatric bipolar illness. *J. Child Psychol. Psychiatry* 48(9):852–862.

Gogtay, N., Sporn, A., Alfaro, C.L., Mulqueen, A., and Rapoport, J.L. (2002) Clozapine-induced akathisia in children with schizophrenia. *J. Child Adolesc. Psychopharmacol.* 12(4):347–349.

Gogtay, N., Sporn, A., Clasen, L.S., Nugent, T.F. III., Greenstein, D., Nicolson, R., et al. (2004) Comparison of progressive cortical gray matter loss in childhood-onset schizophrenia with that in childhood-onset atypical psychoses. *Arch. Gen. Psychiatry* 61(1):17–22.

Gordon, C.T., Frazier, J.A., McKenna, K., Giedd, J., Zametkin, A., Zahn, T., et al. (1994) Childhood-onset schizophrenia: an NIMH study in progress. *Schizophr. Bull.* 20(4):697–712.

Green, W.H., Padron-Gayol, M., Hardesty, A.S., and Bassiri, M. (1992) Schizophrenia with childhood onset: a phenomenological study of 38 cases. *J. Am. Acad. Child Adolesc. Psychiatry* 31(5):968–976.

Greenstein, D., Lerch, J., Shaw, P., Clasen, L., Giedd, J., Gochman, P., et al. (2006) Childhood onset schizophrenia: cortical brain abnormalities as young adults. *J. Child Psychol. Psychiatry* 47(10): 1003–1012.

Hollis, C. (2000) Adult outcomes of child- and adolescent-onset schizophrenia: diagnostic stability and predictive validity. *Am. J. Psychiatry* 157(10):1652–1659.

Huttenlocher, P.R. (1979) Synaptic density in human frontal cortex–developmental changes and effects of aging. *Brain Res.* 163(2): 195–205.

Huttenlocher, P.R., and Dabholkar, A.S. (1997) Regional differences in synaptogenesis in human cerebral cortex. *J. Comp. Neurol.* 387(2):167–178.

Jacobsen, L.K., Giedd, J.N., Vaituzis, A.C., Hamburger, S.D., Rajapakse, J.C., Frazier, J.A., et al. (1996) Temporal lobe morphology in childhood-onset schizophrenia. *Am. J. Psychiatry* 153(3):355–361.

Jacobsen, L.K., Hong, W.L., Hommer, D.W., Hamburger, S.D., Castellanos, F.X., Frazier, J.A., et al. (1996) Smooth pursuit eye movements in childhood-onset schizophrenia: comparison with attention-deficit hyperactivity disorder and normal controls. *Biol. Psychiatry* 40(11):1144–1154.

Jacobsen, L.K., and Rapoport, J.L. (1998) Research update: childhood-onset schizophrenia: implications of clinical and neurobiological research. *J. Child Psychol. Psychiatry* 39(1):101–113.

Karatekin, C., and Asarnow, R. F. (1998) Working memory in childhood-onset schizophrenia and attention-deficit/hyperactivity disorder. *Psychiatry Res.* 80(2):165–176.

Kolvin, I. (1971) Studies in the childhood psychoses. I. Diagnostic criteria and classification. *Br. J. Psychiatry* 118(545):381–384.

Kraepelin, E. (1919). *Dementia Praecox and Paraphrenia*. Huntington, NY: Robert E Krieger.

Kumra, S. (2000) The diagnosis and treatment of children and adolescents with schizophrenia. "My mind is playing tricks on me." *Child Adolesc. Psychiatry Clin. N. Am.* 9(1):183–199, x.

Kumra, S., Ashtari, M., Cervellione, K.L., Henderson, I., Kester, H., Roofeh, D., et al. (2005) White matter abnormalities in early-onset schizophrenia: a voxel-based diffusion tensor imaging study. *J. Am. Acad. Child Adolesc. Psychiatry* 44(9):934–941.

Kumra, S., Frazier, J.A., Jacobsen, L.K., McKenna, K., Gordon, C.T., Lenane, M.C., et al. (1996) Childhood-onset schizophrenia. A double-blind clozapine-haloperidol comparison. *Arch. Gen. Psychiatry* 53(12):1090–1097.

Kumra, S., Jacobsen, L.K., Lenane, M., Zahn, T.P., Wiggs, E., Alaghband-Rad, J., et al. (1998) "Multidimensionally impaired disorder": is it a variant of very early-onset schizophrenia? *J. Am. Acad. Child Adolesc. Psychiatry* 37(1):91–99.

Kumra, S., Sporn, A., Hommer, D.W., Nicolson, R., Thaker, G., Israel, E., et al. (2001) Smooth pursuit eye-tracking impairment in childhood-onset psychotic disorders. *Am. J. Psychiatry* 158(8): 1291–1298.

Levy, D.L., Holzman, P.S., Matthysse, S., and Mendell, N.R. (1994) Eye tracking and schizophrenia: a selective review. *Schizophr. Bull.* 20(1):47–62.

Luders, E., Narr, K.L., Thompson, P.M., Woods, R.P., Rex, D.E., Jancke, L., et al. (2005) Mapping cortical gray matter in the young adult brain: effects of gender. *NeuroImage* 26(2):493–501.

Lukianowicz, N. (1969) Hallucinations in non-psychotic children. *Psychiatr. Clin. (Basel)* 2(6):321–337.

Matsumoto, H., Simmons, A., Williams, S., Hadjulis, M., Pipe, R., Murray, R., et al. (2001) Superior temporal gyrus abnormalities in early-onset schizophrenia: similarities and differences with adult-onset schizophrenia. *Am. J. Psychiatry* 158(8):1299–1304.

Matsumoto, H., Simmons, A., Williams, S., Pipe, R., Murray, R., and Frangou, S. (2001) Structural magnetic imaging of the hippocampus in early onset schizophrenia. *Biol. Psychiatry* 49(10): 824–831.

McClellan, J., and McCurry, C. (1999) Early onset psychotic disorders: diagnostic stability and clinical characteristics. *Eur. Child Adolesc. Psychiatry* 8(Suppl 1):I13–I19.

McGee, R., Williams, S., and Poulton, R. (2000) Hallucinations in nonpsychotic children. *J. Am. Acad. Child Adolesc. Psychiatry* 39(1):12–13.

McKenna, K., Gordon, C.T., Lenane, M., Kaysen, D., Fahey, K., and Rapoport, J.L. (1994) Looking for childhood-onset schizophrenia: the first 71 cases screened. *J. Am. Acad. Child Adolesc. Psychiatry* 33(5):636–644.

McKenna, K., Gordon, C.T., and Rapoport, J. L. (1994) Childhood-onset schizophrenia: timely neurobiological research. *J. Am. Acad. Child Adolesc. Psychiatry* 33(6):771–781.

Moncrieff, J. (2003) Clozapine v. conventional antipsychotic drugs for treatment-resistant schizophrenia: a re-examination. [see comment]. *Br. J. Psychiatry* 183:161–166.

Murphy, K.C., Jones, L.A., and Owen, M.J. (1999) High rates of schizophrenia in adults with velo-cardio-facial syndrome. *Arch. Gen. Psychiatry* 56(10):940–945.

Nicolson, R., Brookner, F.B., Lenane, M., Gochman, P., Ingraham, L.J., Egan, M.F., et al. (2003) Parental schizophrenia spectrum disorders in childhood-onset and adult-onset schizophrenia. *Am. J. Psychiatry* 160(3):490–495.

Nicolson, R., Lenane, M., Brookner, F., Gochman, P., Kumra, S., Spechler, L., et al. (2001) Children and adolescents with psychotic disorder not otherwise specified: a 2- to 8-year follow-up study. *Compr. Psychiatry* 42(4):319–325.

Nicolson, R., Malaspina, D., Giedd, J.N., Hamburger, S., Lenane, M., Bedwell, J., et al. (1999) Obstetrical complications and childhood-onset schizophrenia. *Am. J. Psychiatry* 156(10):1650–1652.

Nicolson, R., and Rapoport, J.L. (1999) Childhood-onset schizophrenia: rare but worth studying. *Biol. Psychiatry* 46(10):1418–1428.

Ordonez, A.E., Bobb, A., Greenstein, D., Baker, N., Sporn, A., Lenane, M., et al. (2005) Lack of evidence for elevated obstetric complications in childhood onset schizophrenia. *Biol. Psychiatry* 58(1):10–15.

Papolos, D.F., Faedda, G.L., Veit, S., Goldberg, R., Morrow, B., Kucherlapati, R., et al. (1996) Bipolar spectrum disorders in patients diagnosed with velo-cardio-facial syndrome: does a hemizygous deletion of chromosome 22q11 result in bipolar affective disorder? *Am. J. Psychiatry* 153(12):1541–1547.

Pool, D., Bloom, W., Mielke, D.H., Roniger, J.J.J., and Gallant, D.M. (1976) A controlled evaluation of loxitane in seventy-five adolescent schizophrenic patients. *Curr. Ther. Res. Clin. Exp.* 19(1):99–104.

Poulton, R., Caspi, A., Moffitt, T.E., Cannon, M., Murray, R., and Harrington, H. (2000) Children's self-reported psychotic symptoms and adult schizophreniform disorder: a 15-year longitudinal study. *Arch. Gen. Psychiatry* 57(11):1053–1058.

Pulver, A.E., Brown, C.H., Wolyniec, P., McGrath, J., Tam, D., Adler, L., et al. (1990) Schizophrenia: age at onset, gender and familial risk. *Acta Psychiatr. Scand.* 82(5):344–351.

Pulver, A.E., Nestadt, G., Goldberg, R., Shprintzen, R.J., Lamacz, M., Wolyniec, P.S., et al. (1994) Psychotic illness in patients diagnosed with velo-cardio-facial syndrome and their relatives. *J. Nerv. Ment. Dis.* 182(8):476–478.

Rapoport, J.L., Addington, A.M., Frangou, S., and Psych, M.R. (2005) The neurodevelopmental model of schizophrenia: update 2005. *Mol. Psychiatry* 10(5):434–449.

Rapoport, J.L., Castellanos, F.X., Gogate, N., Janson, K., Kohler, S., and Nelson, P. (2001) Imaging normal and abnormal brain development: new perspectives for child psychiatry. *Aust. N. Z. J. Psychiatry* 35(3):272–281.

Rapoport, J.L., Giedd, J., Kumra, S., Jacobsen, L., Smith, A., Lee, P., et al. (1997) Childhood-onset schizophrenia. Progressive ventricular change during adolescence. *Arch. Gen. Psychiatry* 54(10):897–903.

Rapoport, J.L., Giedd, J.N., Blumenthal, J., Hamburger, S., Jeffries, N., Fernandez, T., et al. (1999) Progressive cortical change during adolescence in childhood-onset schizophrenia. A longitudinal magnetic resonance imaging study. *Arch. Gen. Psychiatry* 56(7):649–654.

Renshaw, P.F., Yurgelun-Todd, D.A., Tohen, M., Gruber, S., and Cohen, B.M. (1995) Temporal lobe proton magnetic resonance spectroscopy of patients with first-episode psychosis. *Am. J. Psychiatry* 152(3):444–446.

Rhinewine, J.P., Lencz, T., Thaden, E.P., Cervellione, K.L., Burdick, K.E., Henderson, I., et al. (2005) Neurocognitive profile in adolescents with early-onset schizophrenia: clinical correlates. *Biol. Psychiatry* 58(9):705–712.

Rothstein, A. (1981) Hallucinatory phenomena in childhood. A critique of the literature. *J. Am. Acad. Child Psychiatry* 20(3):623–635.

Schreier, H.A. (1999) Hallucinations in nonpsychotic children: more common than we think? *J. Am. Acad. Child Adolesc. Psychiatry* 38(5):623–625.

Shaw, P., Sporn, A., Gogtay, N., Overman, G. P., Greenstein, D., Gochman, P., et al. (2006) Childhood-onset schizophrenia: A double-blind, randomized clozapine-olanzapine comparison. *Arch. Gen. Psychiatry* 63(7):721–730.

Sowell, E.R., Levitt, J., Thompson, P.M., Holmes, C.J., Blanton, R.E., Kornsand, D.S., et al. (2000) Brain abnormalities in early-onset schizophrenia spectrum disorder observed with statistical parametric mapping of structural magnetic resonance images. *Am. J. Psychiatry* 157(9):1475–1484.

Sowell, E.R., Toga, A.W., and Asarnow, R. (2000) Brain abnormalities observed in childhood-onset schizophrenia: a review of the structural magnetic resonance imaging literature. *Ment. Retard. Dev. Disabil. Res. Rev.* 6(3):180–185.

Spencer, E.K., and Campbell, M. (1994) Children with schizophrenia: diagnosis, phenomenology, and pharmacotherapy. *Schizophr. Bull.* 20(4):713–725.

Sporn, A., Greenstein, D., Gogtay, N., Sailer, F., Hommer, D.W., Rawlings, R., et al. (2005) Childhood-onset schizophrenia: smooth pursuit eye-tracking dysfunction in family members. *Schizophr. Res.* 73(2/3):243–252.

Sporn, A.L., Addington, A.M., Gogtay, N., Ordonez, A.E., Gornick, M., Clasen, L., et al. (2004) Pervasive developmental disorder and childhood-onset schizophrenia: comorbid disorder or a phenotypic variant of a very early onset illness? *Biol. Psychiatry* 55(10):989–994.

Thomas, M.A., Ke, Y., Levitt, J., Caplan, R., Curran, J., Asarnow, R., et al. (1998) Preliminary study of frontal lobe 1H MR spectroscopy in childhood-onset schizophrenia. *J. Magn. Reson. Imaging* 8(4):841–846.

Thompson, P.M., Giedd, J.N., Woods, R.P., MacDonald, D., Evans, A.C., and Toga, A.W. (2000) Growth patterns in the developing brain detected by using continuum mechanical tensor maps. *Nature* 404(6774):190–193.

Thompson, P.M., Vidal, C., Giedd, J.N., Gochman, P., Blumenthal, J., Nicolson, R., et al. (2001) Mapping adolescent brain change reveals dynamic wave of accelerated gray matter loss in very early-onset schizophrenia. *Proc. Natl. Acad. Sci. USA* 98(20): 11650–11655.

Ulloa, R.E., Birmaher, B., Axelson, D., Williamson, D.E., Brent, D.A., Ryan, N.D., et al. (2000) Psychosis in a pediatric mood and anxiety disorders clinic: phenomenology and correlates. *J. Am. Acad. Child Adolesc. Psychiatry* 39(3):337–345.

Varanka, T.M., Weller, R.A., Weller, E.B., and Fristad, M.A. (1988) Lithium treatment of manic episodes with psychotic features in prepubertal children. *Am. J. Psychiatry* 145(12):1557–1559.

Volkmar, F.R. (1996) Childhood and adolescent psychosis: a review of the past 10 years. *J. Am. Acad. Child Adolesc. Psychiatry* 35(7):843–851.

Werry, J.S., McClellan, J.M., and Chard, L. (1991) Childhood and adolescent schizophrenic, bipolar, and schizoaffective disorders: a clinical and outcome study. *J. Am. Acad. Child Adolesc. Psychiatry* 30(3):457–465.

77 Developmental Perspectives on Psychopathology

MICHAEL RUTTER

Over the last couple of decades, there has been a virtual revolution in the ways in which developmental perspectives on psychopathology have been conceptualized (Rutter, 2008). This chapter seeks to outline the most important of these changes in concept—their detailed application being considered in greater detail in other chapters in this volume. Six may be singled out: (*1*) childhood origins of schizophrenia, (*2*) the adult sequelae of childhood neurodevelopmental disorders, (*3*) age differences in effects and neuroplasticity, (*4*) genetic influences and gene-environment interdependence, (*5*) biology of environmental effects, and (*6*) the steps needed to move from observational associations/correlations to causal inference.

CHILDHOOD ORIGINS OF SCHIZOPHRENIA

A generation ago, most psychiatrists viewed schizophrenia as an adult-onset psychosis. By sharp contrast, it is now generally viewed as a neurodevelopmental disorder (Murray and Lewis, 1987; Weinberger, 1987; Keshavan et al., 2004; Rapoport et al., 2005). Three sets of findings have been most influential in this change of concept (Rutter, Maughan, and Kim-Cohen, 2006). First, well-conducted prospective longitudinal studies have shown that, at a group level, individuals who later develop a schizophrenia spectrum disorder tend to show developmental impairments in very early motor and language functions (Cannon et al., 2002; Isohanni et al., 2004). There is nothing very specific about the pattern, but the presence of such impairments does differentiate schizophrenia from bipolar disorder and other psychiatric conditions (Murray et al., 2004). Uncertainty remains on whether these childhood precursors reflect early manifestations of a genetically influenced liability or, rather, some separate environmental risk factor. Second, in late childhood/early adolescence, many children show psychotic-like features (Poulton et al., 2000; Cannon et al., 2002). At first, doubts were expressed on the meaning of these features, but follow-up studies have shown significant associations with the later development of schizophrenia spectrum disorders. Finally, prospective studies of individuals in genetically high-risk families (because of the presence of at least two relatives with a schizophrenia spectrum disorder) have shown that they exhibit prodromal features that tend to lead to the onset of an overt schizophrenia spectrum disorder (Owens and Johnstone, 2006).

Since the pioneering structural imaging study by Crow and Johnstone in 1977 that first demonstrated brain abnormalities in schizophrenia, numerous other investigations (using improved technologies) have confirmed the reality of brain changes in schizophrenia. Yet a surprising number of puzzles remain. The early childhood developmental impairments (usually described as precursors) may be presumed to reflect some form of atypical neural functioning, but what is happening at this early stage, and is it driven by the genetic liability or some yet to be identified environmental risk factor? The Dutch famine findings (Stein et al., 1975; Susser et al., 1996), replicated in the Chinese famine findings (St. Clair et al., 2005), point to the likely involvement of prenatal famine in a causal chain that can lead to schizophrenia, but which brain effects carry the psychopathological risk, and what relevance do these have for schizophrenia as it occurs in more ordinary circumstances? Could the explanation lie in the role of folate deficiency in causing de novo genomic mutations (McClellan et al., 2006)?

Somewhat similar queries arise with respect to the psychotic-like features arising in late childhood. What are the neural changes that are associated, and why does only a minority of these childhood abnormalities lead on to schizophrenia in adult life? Are those that do predispose to schizophrenia different in their qualities from those that do not? Or, is there some type of "two-hit" mechanism by which some second set of risk factors is involved in the transition from precursors to overt schizophrenia?

Another risk factor that is evident a year or two later is the heavy early use of cannabis. The risk does not seem to apply to occasional recreational use of cannabis, and it does not apply to cannabis that is first used only in adult life (Zammit et al., 2002; Arseneault et al., 2004). Animal models have confirmed that the effects of cannabis in adolescence differ from those in adult life (Schneider and Koch, 2003; Pistis et al., 2004). The findings differ, however, from other precursors in seeming to apply only to individuals with a predisposition to schizophrenia. Most strikingly, a significant interaction has been found between heavy early cannabis use and possession of the val/val variant of the catechol-O-methyltransferase (*COMT*) gene (Caspi et al., 2005). The interaction implies (but does not prove) that the genetic variant and the cannabis are operating on the same causal pathway.

Moving up the age span to late adolescence/early adult life, the important high-risk studies from Johnstone's Edinburgh group (Owens and Johnstone, 2006) have confirmed the reality (in individuals with a strong family history of schizophrenia) of prodromal features preceding, but leading on to, an overt schizophrenic psychosis. Schizotypal features and cognitive functions best differentiated those individuals who did and who did not go on to show a schizophrenia spectrum disorder. Brain imaging findings differentiated high-risk subjects from controls; somewhat similar differences were associated with the transition into overt schizophrenia, but the latter were weaker effects. Pantelis et al. (2003) also reported longitudinal magnetic resonance imaging (MRI) data showing brain changes associated with the onset of psychosis. This has also been found more strikingly in the progressive changes during the 5 years after the onset of schizophrenia beginning in childhood (Thompson et al., 2001).

The term *prodromata* implies that they represent the beginnings of schizophrenia, but follow-up studies have shown that about one half do not go on to show schizophrenia (Drake and Lewis, 2005). Why not? Also, what role is played by the brain developments that normally take place during adolescence as shown by postmortem (Huttenlocher, 2002) and brain imaging findings (Giedd et al., 1999; Gogtay et al., 2004; Shaw et al., 2006; Toga et al., 2006).

One further query concerns the additional brain changes that appear to take place following the onset of overt schizophrenia (see above). Of course, it is difficult entirely to rule out the possibility that these reflect the effects of medication rather than disease progression, but the latter seems probable. If confirmed, we will have to conclude that schizophrenia truly reflects neurodevelopmental abnormalities in early childhood, but this does not mean that there is a static pathology; further changes seem likely in late adolescence when there is the transition to overt illness, and yet more changes may follow illness onset. Here I use schizophrenia only as an exemplar of some of the key developmental considerations that apply to the neurobiology of mental illness.

NEURODEVELOPMENTAL DISORDERS OF CHILDHOOD

The focus needs to shift now to the early onset childhood disorders that involve some form of neurodevelopmental impairment—such as autism spectrum disorders (ASDs), attention-deficit/hyperactivity disorder (ADHD), dyslexia, and specific language impairment (SLI). The findings raise a somewhat different set of issues. To begin with, in each case, although the initial diagnoses are not usually made until after infancy, there is substantial evidence of neuropsychological abnormalities in infancy.

Autism Spectrum Disorders

Differences are most obvious by 18 to 24 months, but more subtle features may be seen by 12 months in some cases. Two considerations stand out. First, they highlight the need to conceptualize the neuropsychological abnormalities in terms of ones that are both evident and operating in early life. The best-demonstrated cognitive features associated with ASD are those described as an impairment in theory of mind (ToM) (U. Frith, 2003). Their association with autism is indisputable, but the early manifestations of ASD force attention onto features such as joint attention that are evident before ToM is detectable (Sigman and Ruskin, 1999). Whether or not these constitute a precursor of ToM or something different remains uncertain, but there is the imperative to focus neural investigations on early- rather than late-appearing neurodevelopmental features. Second, home movies have served to confirm earlier clinical observations that a substantial proportion (perhaps one fourth) of children with an ASD shows a transient (sometimes prolonged) loss of language skills—usually about the age of 18 to 24 months (Werner et al., 2005). The meaning of this developmental regression remains quite uncertain, and clearly it warrants systematic study. Clinical observations (and one well-conducted study comparing children with ASD and those with SLI) suggest that this pattern of regression is much more characteristic of ASD than SLI or normal language development (Pickles et al., 2008). If confirmed, it would constitute a useful diagnostic pointer that might provide clues to pathogenesis.

In considering the ways in which the evidence of early manifestations of autism has implications for neural research, three points may be made. First, eye-tracking methods may be useful in studying joint attention skills that ordinarily become manifest at about 12 to 14 months of age (Klin et al., 2002; Klin et al., 2003). Second, functional MRI (fMRI) may be informative on the brain systems involved in early social perception (see Schultz and Robins, 2005). Third, the important discovery of mirror neurons (see Rizzolatti and Craighero, 2004) provides a focus on a neural component that may be of particular relevance to autism (Williams et al., 2001; Dapretto et al., 2005).

A further feature of ASD is the finding (first observed nearly four decades ago; Rutter, 1970) that about one fourth of individuals with ASD develop epilepsy, and that in about two thirds of cases, the onset is in late adolescence/early adult life (Hutton et al., in press). This characteristic age of onset is markedly different from the early childhood onset that is much more typical in the general population and individuals with an intellectual disability. It would seem clear that this late adolescent change is likely to have some important neuropathological significance, but it is not yet known quite what this is.

Another feature of ASD is that although there is a general modest tendency for social functioning to improve somewhat with increasing age, the majority of individuals with a nonverbal IQ in the normal range (that is, the subgroup with the best prognosis) remain quite impaired in adult life (Howlin et al., 2004). It is by no means self-evident why this is so. Is it a function of the basic neural deficit, in which case what is it that is causing the disability when overall cognitive functioning is relatively spared? Or is it a consequence of inadequate services in childhood or adult life?

Two other puzzles warrant mention. First, since Kanner's (1943) initial clinical report, it has been evident that a substantial minority of individuals with ASD show an increased head size (Woodhouse et al., 1996; Fombonne et al., 1999). Imaging studies (Courchesne et al., 2003) have confirmed that this indexes increased brain size. Prospective studies have been informative in showing that head circumference is approximately normal at birth but then increases significantly during the preschool years (DiCicco-Bloom et al., 2006) and possibly plateaus somewhat after that. What neural change does this reflect, and why does it occur in this age period? Second, although ASD is quite strongly associated with late-onset epilepsy and with overall cognitive impairment, neither appear to be features of the broader phenotype as seen in first-degree relatives (Bailey et al., 1998). Why not? Is some additional (genetic or nongenetic) risk process needed to transform the broader phenotype to ASD "proper"?

Dyslexia

Broadly comparable issues arise with other neurodevelopmental disorders. Thus, although dyslexia cannot be diagnosed until school age when typically developing children ordinarily learn to read, prospective high-risk studies (Lyytinen et al., 2004) show evoked response potential (ERP) differences in infancy—differences that are associated with later language skills. The neurobiological basis must be sought in relation to very early developing functions that are relevant for later reading skills but that are evident well before reading develops. Over the years, some reviewers have postulated that dyslexia represents some kind of "maturational lag"—that is, the acquisition of reading follows a basically normal course, but it just takes longer. The high persistence of reading/spelling difficulties into adult life (see Rutter, Maughan, and Kim-Cohen, 2006) raises queries regarding this suggestion, but the brain imaging findings similarly point to a difference rather than a lag (Francis et al., 1996). On the other hand, comparisons of familial high-risk and control groups also suggest that the liability to dyslexia extends much more broadly than the categorical diagnosis would seem to imply (Snowling et al., 2003). The implication is that the neurobiology is likely to apply to individuals with the liability to dyslexia but whose reading falls within normal limits. On the other hand, it is probable that it does not represent just the end of a normal continuum.

Specific Language Impairment

Similar considerations apply to SLI. There are very large individual differences in the age at which children first learn to speak, and such variations do not imply pathology. They are no different in principle from the comparable large individual differences in the age of the eruption of primary or secondary dentition, or the age of reaching puberty. On the other hand, there is a substantial proportion of children who are not only late in speaking, but also who go on to show language impairments that continue into adolescence and adult life. There are three main reasons why this needs to be viewed as separate from normal variation. First, their age of language acquisition extends far beyond the normal curve. Second, their impairment includes some degree of nonverbal functioning and major social impairment—at least in the case of those with a severe disability in receptive language (Clegg et al., 2005). Third, although there is a plateau in the growth of language skills that is evident during adolescence, this occurs at much the same age in children who develop typically and in those with SLI (Francis et al., 1996). Neurobiological studies need to focus on a valid disorder; but, equally, they need to appreciate that the disorder does not constitute a highly modular language disability; rather, it extends much more broadly, even though it does not represent the end of a normal distribution (Bishop et al., 1995).

Commonalities Among Neurodevelopmental Disorders

Two last points need to be made with respect to neurodevelopmental disorders. First, numerous studies have shown a quite substantial degree of co-occurrence among neurodevelopmental disorders (see Bishop and Rutter, 2008). It has sometimes been hoped that these might reflect artefactual diagnostic/behavioral differences and that attention to cognitive functioning would show much more unity. In the event, the one study to test this possibility systematically found as much heterogeneity at the cognitive level as at the behavioral level (Pennington, 2006). Neurobiological studies must take that on board. "Pure" disorders are the exception rather than the rule, and neurobiological studies must accept, and determine the reasons for, the co-occurrence. Second, the commonality among neurodevelopmental disorders points to the desirability of capitalizing on this as part of overall research strategies. For example, it is striking that all of these early-onset neurodevelopmental disorders show a marked male preponderance, which contrasts sharply with the female preponderance found with adolescent-onset disorders (Rutter et al., 2003). Why? What are the biological underpinnings? Theories have been put forward to explain the excess of males with ASD, but the fact that the excess applies to most of the neurodevelopmental disorders (apart from dyscalculia) raises the possibility that although there may be diagnostic-specific specificities, it is quite likely that there is some common feature that accounts for the male preponderance across this group of disorders. Clearly, it cannot be a function of organic brain dysfunction as such because it does not apply to either cerebral palsy or epilepsy. So what is involved?

AGE DIFFERENCES

A massively neglected area in neurobiological studies concerns the basis of age differences in response to external agents of all kinds. The findings would have hugely important theoretical and practical implications. For example, some three decades ago, Rapoport (1980) noted that whereas stimulant medications tended to have a euphoric effect in adults (associated with the use of stimulants as a recreational drug), it tended to have a dysphoric effect in children (so that stimulants did not have a street value as a drug of addiction). It cannot be said that this observation has been well validated by systematic research; but, probably, it is correct. What constitutes its biological basis?

Similar issues arise with respect to apparent age differences in response to cannabis (as shown by both human [Arsenault et al., 2004] and animal studies [Schneider and Koch, 2003; Pistis et al., 2004]), and to the effects of an *N*-methyl-D-aspartate (NMDA) antagonist, as studied in rats (Farber et al., 1995). Both have potential relevance to the question of why overt schizophrenia does not usually develop until late adolescence or early adult life, despite precursors and prodromata being evident at a much earlier age.

There is rather more evidence on alcohol effects (Monti et al., 2005). In brief, the available evidence suggests that adolescents, as compared with adults, are less susceptible to the side effects of alcohol (such as hangovers) and thus are better able to engage in heavy binge drinking without the deterrent of the unpleasant side effects. On the other hand, they may be more susceptible to the negative effects on cognition and attention. The combination of these two contrasting age-related effects is that adolescents may be more likely to engage in dangerous heavy binge drinking and be more vulnerable to the damage from doing so. The biological studies are less solid than desirable, but the evidence is certainly sufficient to highlight the theoretical and practical importance of age differences.

The research literature on drug responses is similarly provocative yet inconclusive. Despite the strong continuities between major depressive disorders in young people and apparently comparable disorders in adults, children and adolescents appear to have much less favorable responses to tricyclics (Hazell et al., 1995). It is possible that this is a consequence of a high placebo response rate in most studies, combined with inadequate attention to pharmacokinetic issues (see Volkow and Swanson, 2008), but it seems unlikely that these fully account for the age differences. If the age difference in response is real, what is its biological meaning? The evidence on selective serotonin reuptake inhibitors (SSRIs) suggests possibly greater benefits in young people, but the evidence is not strong (Brent and Weersing, 2008) and is accompanied by a possible (but disputed) greater effect on suicidal ideation in young people. Once more, what are needed are not just more, and better, randomized controlled trials (RCTs), but also relevant, appropriately focused, biological studies.

One more age difference warrants mention because it raises somewhat different theoretical (and practical) issues. Moffitt (1993) was responsible for identifying the crucially important distinction between "lifecourse-persistent" (LCP) and "adolescence-limited" (AL) antisocial behavior. Her distinction provided the first really useful understanding of the heterogeneity of antisocial behavior; and, with some modifications, it has stood the test of time (meaning multiple research evaluations). It was especially provocative in its implication that an exceptionally early age of onset was associated with a much increased tendency to persist into adult life (that is, the opposite of what is usually found with age differences). The key biological question, however, is what this might mean in terms of mediating mechanisms. Three key findings have begun to shed light on the matter. First, Silberg et al. (1996) found that the genetic component of population variance was much stronger in the case of antisocial behavior associated with hyperactivity. The implication was that the persistence into adult life might be driven not by the age of onset, but rather by the presence of ADHD features (which virtually always manifest themselves in early life). A further twist to this possibility has been provided by the evidence that heritability is highest with antisocial behavior associated with psychopathic features (Viding et al., 2005). Again, however, the implication is that what may matter is the form of the behavior and not its age of onset. Second, longitudinal trajectory analyses by Odgers, Caspi, et al. (2007) showed that, in addition to the LCP and AL varieties of antisocial behavior, there was a large subgroup showing childhood-onset antisocial behavior that did not persist into adult life. Again, the implication was that childhood onset might not constitute the main driving force. A further extension of the work (Odgers, Milne, et al., 2007) showed that a strong predictor of persistence was provided by a family history of antisocial behavior/alcohol problems. Of course, this could reflect either genetic or environmental influences (probably both); but, once more, attention is shifted from age of onset as such to the overall pattern. The implication, in this case, is that the biological studies need to focus on those pattern differences instead of (or in addition to) the age differences in onset.

Neuroplasticity

Neuroplasticity is a term applied to the ability of the nervous system to adapt its structural and functional organization to altered circumstances arising from developmental or environmental (including traumatic) changes (Sheedlo and Turner, 1992). A crucial issue throughout all considerations of plasticity has been the degree to which it applies only or mainly during periods of major brain organization. In animals, it has been investigated using a variety of experimental strategies that include exclusion of particular forms of sensory input (as by the suturing together of the eyelids of one eye), or the creation of specific brain lesions at different ages, or the transplantation of cells from one part of the brain to another part that ordinarily deals with quite different sensory functions. In humans, natural experiments on sensory input have provided parallels—as, for example, through the restoration of vision by the removal of congenital cataracts or the provision of hearing through cochlear implants. The range of natural experiments, however, extends much more broadly in its incorporation of studies comparing congenitally blind and blindfolded sighted participants or the studies of unusual levels of experience (for example, in professional musicians or London taxi drivers' learning of many thousands of routes) or comparisons of language features in children reared in different language environments (including hearing children reared by deaf parents and vice versa), or comparisons of first- and second-language learning at different ages (see Roder and Neville, 2003). The advent of the various forms of structural and functional brain imaging have greatly increased the potential of what can be learned from these human studies. With respect to brain lesions, human studies have included examination of variations according to age of the effects on language development of unilateral lesions affecting the speech areas of the brain (see Stiles, 2000, for a review).

Neuroplasticity incorporates a range of phenomena, but here attention is drawn to just a few with important psychopathological implications. First, with respect to the role of sensory input in driving and shaping normal brain development in key sensitive periods during which the relevant brain structure is being established, a distinction needs to be drawn between experience-expectant and experience-adaptive biological developmental programming (see Rutter, 2006b). The former refers to the circumstances in which normal brain development requires particular sensory input if normal brain development is to take place. It is called *experience-expectant* because in all ordinary circumstances of rearing such input will always be available (Greenough et al., 1987). The best-known example is provided by the Hubel and Weisel (2005) studies showing that this applied to binocular visual input. The next obvious clinical application is the need for early surgical correction of strabismus to ensure later normal binocular vision. Various clinical reviewers have sought to extend the phenomenon to most forms of early rearing experiences, but clearly that is unwarranted, and major questions remain on there being possible parallels with nonvisual experiential input.

Experience-adaptive programming concerns a rather different phenomenon—namely, the particular ways in which brain development (as with other forms of somatic development) is shaped to be adaptive to the environmental circumstances prevailing during the key sensitive period during which the relevant aspect of biological development is taking place. The reality of this variety is supported by much evidence (Bateson et al., 2004), and the best-known psychological example is provided by the extent to which, after about the first 6 months of life, children's ability to make particular phonological discriminations is shaped by their language of rearing (Kuhl, 1994; Kuhl et al., 1997; Maye et al., 2002; Werker, 2003).

Third, there are experience-dependent brain effects—meaning that there are effects of experience on brain structure and function that can occur at any age and that do not involve effects on ordinary brain growth. Thus, animal studies have shown that environmental enrichment/deprivation has brain effects in adult, as well as juvenile, animals. Human brain imaging studies have shown the effects of psychological, as well as pharmacological, interventions (Goldapple et al., 2004). Other brain imaging studies, too, have shown variations in brain structure associated with intensive experiences in adult life (see, e.g., Elbert et al., 1995; Sluming et al., 2007, with respect to musical performance). In the absence of extensive longitudinal data, it is impossible to be sure that the brain changes resulted from (rather than preceded) the musical training, but circumstantial evidence favors the former inference. Also, an intervention study of training in juggling showed that the training had brain effects (Draganski et al., 2004).

The findings on neuroplasticity already have some important psychopathological implications, but major challenges remain. The evidence on the effects of unilateral brain lesions on language have clearly demonstrated that in early and middle childhood, such lesions do not result in aphasic symptomatology and do not lead to a specific impairment of verbal cognitive skills, both of which are typical of comparable lesions in later childhood, adolescence, and adult life (Vargha-Khadem et al., 1992; Vargha-Khadem and Mishkin, 1997; Bates and Roe, 2001). This finding alone always made the search for a unilateral brain lesion that might be responsible for autism or for SLI of developmental origin, or dyslexia, misguided. Accordingly, biological studies have shifted focus to more broadly based brain systems and to the interconnectivity among them. The findings also emphasize that the biology underpinning developmental disorders cannot be inferred from the effects of brain lesions in adult life.

The neural effects of severe experiential deprivation in humans has been most strikingly evident in the sequelae of profound institutional deprivation in children reared in institutions, who have been adopted into generally well-functioning adoptive families (Rutter, Beckett, et al., 2007). Although no sequelae have been detected in children who left institutional care younger than age 6 months, deficits have been found in some two fifths of children adopted after that age (Beckett et al., 2006; Kreppner et al., 2007). Most strikingly, the rate of deficits showed a marked step-wise increase in the second half of the first year with no further increase thereafter. The implication seems to be that profound institutional deprivation takes some months to bring about lasting effects, but thereafter the effects have proved to be remarkably persistent—at least up to age 11 years. The effects of the early deprivation at age 11 were as marked then, at least 7 years after adoption, as they had been 5 years earlier at age 6, or 7 years earlier at age 4. Some form of biological change seems possible, although whether it takes the form of developmental programming (and if so, which variety) or neural damage remains unclear. The lasting effects cannot be attributed to associated subnutrition (present in over one half the children) because the sequelae were evident in children whose weight was within normal limits. Even in the absence of subnutrition, profound deprivation lasting longer than 6 months was associated with a marked impairment in head growth (Sonuga-Barke et al., 2008). Curiously, however, despite the centrality of reduced head circumference, this reduction did not mediate the psychological sequelae. The findings provide a striking example of lasting effects of profound psychological deprivation, but it is necessary to note that the sequelae mainly concerned unusual patterns such as disinhibited attachment (Rutter, Beckett, et al., 2007) or quasi-autistic features (Rutter, Kreppner, et al., 2007), rather than the more ordinary forms of emotional disturbance or disruptive behavior.

Numerous questions remain on the brain mechanisms involved in neuroplasticity, and on the nature and effects of sensitive periods. What is clear, however, is that there are marked variations among psychological functions in the role of sensitive periods. Thus, with respect to language, there is an early sensitive period for phonological discrimination and grammar, but not for semantics. The sensitive period for phonological discrimination operates in the first year, but the period for establishment of language in the nondominant hemisphere if the dominant hemisphere is damaged lasts for 4 to 5 years. With respect to visual and auditory recovery after early sensory deprivation, recovery seems less likely for complex perceptual functions than more elementary ones. With respect to neuroplasticity itself, knowledge is still limited on the degree to which intramodal changes are responsible (so that intact modalities may reorganize, thereby increasing their efficiency); or sensory areas may modify their responsiveness to different forms of sensory input; or functional reallocation is responsible. With respect to the broader implications for psychopathology, perhaps the main implication is to be wary of any assumption that neurodevelopmental disorders necessarily involve a deficit in a whole system. Also, it is necessary to recognize that aberrant neuroplasticity may be implicated in some mental disorders. For example, does the increased head size in early childhood associated with autism reflect impaired neuronal pruning? Might the transition in late adolescence from prodromal symptoms to overt psychosis in schizophrenia be related to brain changes that normally take place in that age period?

GENETIC INFLUENCES AND GENE-ENVIRONMENT INTERDEPENDENCE

Understanding of the role of genetic influences on development and on psychopathology has undergone a virtual revolution in the last two decades or so. First, although a very small proportion of cases of mental disorders may be due to pathogenic Mendelian mutant genes (early-onset dominant Alzheimer's disease and Rett syndrome, to take two examples from opposite ends of the age span, are cases in point), the great majority constitute multifactorial disorders in which the relevant genes constitute common polymorphic variations (Rutter, 2006a). Moreover, each of these genetic variations account for a tiny proportion of the overall population variance to the liability to the disorder in question. Thus, Kendler (2005) calculated that the average odds ratio for replicated susceptibility genes was just 1.3 despite the fact that the cumulative genetic effect (from all relevant genes) was strong.

Second, an important portion of genetic effects are indirect—operating "outside the skin" via gene-environment correlations (rGE) and interactions (G × E)–to use Kendler's terminology (Kendler and Baker, 2007; Rutter, 2007). That is to say, the genetic effects influence exposure and sensitivity to the environment rather than having a direct effect on liability to mental disorder. With respect to rGE, a systematic review of adequate quality published studies showed heritabilities in the range of 15%–35% for parental behaviors and family interactions. The neurobiological challenge lies in the need to determine the mechanism involved. rGE and G × E present different challenges in this connection. With rGE, the effect on exposure comes via the influence of genes on either parental or child behaviors that serve to shape or select environments (Rutter, 2006a). Thus, the genes themselves do not shape or select; rather, it is the behaviors they influence that do that. In the case of parental behaviors, the first need is to identify the specific behaviors that shape rearing experiences that create psychological risk. The degree of heritability of those parental behaviors is very much a subsidiary question of limited importance (other than in respect to the finding that heritability is not zero). Once the most influential parental behaviors have been identified, the prime need shifts to the question of what the key rearing experiences do to the organism. In other words, the question now changes from how genes operate outside the skin to how the environment gets under the skin. By what mechanism does the environment have effects beyond the duration of the experience (see section on next page)?

The needs and challenges in the case of G × E are somewhat different. For many years, behavioral geneticists argued that G × E was of so little importance that it could be ignored without loss. There were always sound theoretical reasons for doubting that claim (see Rutter and Pickles, 1991; Rutter and Silberg, 2002; Rutter, Moffitt, and Caspi, 2006), and there is now a growing number of replicated G × E findings in the field of psychopathology. The research leaders were Caspi and Moffitt with their demonstrations of G × E with respect to a variant of a gene influencing monoamine oxidase A (MAO-A) activity that interacted with child maltreatment in relation to the outcome of antisocial behavior (Caspi et al., 2002); with respect to a 5HTT gene allelic variation that interacted with early child maltreatment and later life stresses in relation to the outcome of depression (Caspi et al., 2003); and with respect to the role of a val/val allelic variation of the *COMT* gene predisposing to schizophrenia spectrum disorders only through an interaction with heavy early use of cannabis (Caspi et al., 2005). The reality of the G × E has been shown by the rigorous methodological checks to investigate validity; by the numerous human replications (with only a few nonreplications); by the confirmatory studies in rhesus monkeys, which also showed that the G × E was associated with neurochemical and neurocognitive effects (Bennett et al., 2002; Champoux et al., 2002; Barr et al., 2004); and by the human imaging studies that showed the effects of the G × E on neural structure and function (Hariri et al., 2002; Hariri et al., 2005; Heinz et al., 2005; Pezawas et al., 2005; Meyer-Lindenberg et al., 2006).

The findings carry several messages. First, with all three of these examples of G × E, there was no main effect of G. The importance of the genetic variant was evident only through the demonstrated interaction with a measured environmental feature. Second, the genetic affect associated with G × E operated in individuals without mental disorder—underlining the inferences that the effect probably operated dimensionally and that it concerned environmental sensitivity and not any direct psychopathological effect. It remains an open question as to whether the sensitivity applies to environmental circumstances generally (as suggested by Boyce, 2007) or only to adverse environments. However, it does appear that the specific G × E found in each case applies only to a relatively narrow range of psychopathological outcomes and not to mental disorder generally. Thus, the MAO-A interaction with maltreatment applied to antisocial behavior but not depression, whereas the 5HTT interaction with maltreatment applied to depression but not antisocial behavior. Developmentally, it is also relevant that the G × E with 5HTT applies to maltreatment in childhood, but its mental disorder consequences applied to depression is only evident some years later. The neurobiological course in the intervening years is yet unknown.

Third, despite the apparent psychopathological specificity of each G × E example, the neural correlates between the 5HTT G and the MAO-A G × E seem to involve the same brain systems in somewhat similar ways (see Pezawas et al., 2005; Meyer-Lindenberg et al., 2006). Of course, it has been known for a long time that many genes tend to have pleiotropic effects (see Rutter, 2006a), but the overlap raises challenges for understanding the neural underpinning of the roots of psychopathology. The same set of findings has also shown that some neural effects apply only to males, and not females. Why?

A fourth message from modern molecular genetic research is that genetic effects on psychopathology may not apply to syndromes as currently conceptualized in contemporary classification systems. Thus, Thapar et al. (2005) found that the val variant of the *COMT* gene was associated with the development of antisocial behavior in children with ADHD—a finding now replicated in two other samples (Caspi et al., 2008). It is notable that the genetic variant was not associated with ADHD as such, or with antisocial behavior in the absence of ADHD. It is also noteworthy that this is the same val variant associated through G × E with the cannabis effect on schizophrenia spectrum disorder. The genetic findings emphasize the need to link the genetics with a much broader range of neurobiological studies and to focus on neurochemical and neural connectivity effects that may not be diagnosis-specific.

There is one other quite different type of gene-environment interdependence of particular developmental importance that must be noted—namely, environmental effects on gene expression and thereby on psychological functioning (Champagne et al., 2004; Weaver et al., 2004; Cameron et al., 2005; Meaney and Szyf, 2005). The studies of Meaney and his colleagues have shown that a particular form of arched back nursing in rats during the first week of life (but not later) is associated with lasting individual differences in the offspring's behavior and response to later stress. Cross-fostering showed that the intergenerational effect was environmentally, and not genetically, mediated. Neurochemical research went on to demonstrate that the effect was mediated by deoxyribonucleic acid (DNA) methylation of a specific glucocorticoid receptor gene promoter in the hippocampus. Clinicians have been tempted to speculate on possible human equivalents of arched back nursing and to argue that the findings mean that environmental effects on gene expression underlie the long-term effects of early child rearing. Neither follows. The rat findings applied only to a particular form of maternal behavior and not to maternal–infant contact as a whole; also, they applied only to the first week of life. The findings are hugely important with respect to environmental effects on gene expression, and hence to a mechanism by which environments "get under the skin." It is quite likely that they are implicated in developmental biological programming (Rutter, 2006b) and may well be involved in prenatal stress effects (Coe and Lubach, 2000). It will be surprising, too, if they did not have an even wider applicability, but it remains still to be determined which environmental effects operate through this mechanism.

BIOLOGY OF ENVIRONMENTAL EFFECTS

Legitimate queries have been raised on whether some of the long-term psychopathological risks associated with an adverse environment may be genetically mediated, and on whether some supposed socialization effects may represent the effects of children on their families, rather than the reverse. Nevertheless, the use of research designs that can take account of genetic influences and that can test for the direction of causal influences has shown that there are long-term environmental effects on the liability to mental disorder that stem from experiences such as physical and sexual abuse, and institutional deprivation (Rutter, 2005a). A key question that arises is what these experiences do to the organism to bring about long-term consequences; how, as it were, they "get under the skin." Numerous possibilities need to be considered. Thus, the evidence of G × E interaction (see previous section on genetics) suggests that the genes and the environment may be operating on the same causal pathway. Insofar as that is the case, effects on neurotransmitters may be implicated. The demonstration of environmentally influenced epigenetic changes affecting gene expression (see previous section on genetics) provides another mechanism. It is not yet known which environmental effects, in what circumstances, involve gene expression, but it is likely that some will do so—perhaps especially prenatal and postnatal stress effects, and also some forms of developmental programming. Animal and human studies have clearly documented long-term effects on neuroendocrine patterning following serious chronic stress and deprivation experiences (Gunnar and Vázquez, 2006). What is less clear at the moment is what are the functional consequences of the changed patterns and whether neuroendocrine alterations mediate the psychopathological sequelae. As noted above, profound institutional deprivation seems to bring about neural programming changes, including effects on head size (and, by extrapolation, brain size). Perhaps, surprisingly, impaired brain growth did not mediate the psychological sequelae indicating the challenges that remain on biological mediating mechanisms. A further possibility is that the early adverse experiences bring about changed patterns of behavior and of interpersonal interactions, which in turn give rise to ongoing stress experiences that predispose to mental disorder (Robins, 1966; Champion et al., 1995). Insofar as that is the case, it may be that early adverse experiences have long-term effects in part because they give rise to later adverse experiences. Yet another possibility is that the mediator of long-term effects of early experiences lies in part in the mental sets or internal working models to which they give rise. Of course, these thought processes will involve neural changes, but it may be that it is the content of the thoughts, rather than the neurochemical changes with which they are associated, that are influential. Over the last couple of decades, much experimental and naturalistic research has demonstrated a range of biological consequences of environmental experiences, but much less is known on the biological mechanisms that mediate the psychopathological risks. This constitutes a relatively neglected area of research and one that should be given high priority.

PROCEEDING FROM CORRELATION TO CAUSAL INFERENCE

A key issue that has come into increasing prominence in recent years is how to proceed from correlational findings based on observational data to inferences about causal mechanisms or processes. Sometimes it has been assumed that this is a problem that applies only to epidemiological case-control investigations, but that is far from the case (Rutter, 2007b). It needs to be appreciated that brain imaging findings and molecular genetic findings are essentially correlational and, hence, open to the same problem. To begin with, both have proved particularly difficult to replicate. But assuming that some finding has been extensively replicated, the dilemma on causal inference needs to be considered (see Schultz et al., 2003; C. Frith and Frith, 2008). If well replicated, it can be concluded that the association between neural structure/functioning and psychopathology is real, but does it reflect causation? The alternative is that it constitutes a response to psychopathology or experience (that is, reverse causation). We know that pharmacological and psychological treatments have effects on imaging findings (see, e.g., Goldapple et al., 2004), and we know that deprivation and enrichment in animals has measurable effects on brain structure/function (Nelson and Jeste, 2008). Reverse causation is a real possibility. A second possibility is that the imaging studies must involve an experimental component if causal inferences are to be made. With respect to causal inferences more generally, there is much to be said for the use of "natural experiments" to pull apart variables that ordinarily go together and, thereby, to provide greater leverage on testing causal hypotheses (Rutter et al., 2001; Rutter, 2007b).

Much the same applies to genetic findings. The finding of a replicated association between a susceptibility gene and some mental disorder outcome provides a good indication that the gene is involved in some way in the causal processes. The question is: "in what way?" The association might mean that the gene has a neurochemical effect that is directly involved in the liability to the disorder being investigated, or it might mean that it has an effect only on some subcomponent of the disorder. Alternatively, it might be influencing neuroendocrine function or immune responses that connect up with the causal pathway to the gene, but only indirectly. Yet another possibility is that the genetic effect is not on any component of the mental disorder as such but, rather, on environmental responsivity that is implicated in causation only insofar as it involves substantial risk or protective processes. The lesson is that imaging and molecular genetic studies can be hugely informative on the underlying neurobiology of mental disorders, but careful attention needs to be paid to what can, and what cannot, be inferred or concluded.

CONCLUSIONS

Developmental psychopathology has become the mainstream perspective on psychopathology in childhood and adult life (see Rutter, 2008). With respect to neurobiology, the main implications are that the research focus needs to be on biologically dynamic developmental processes, and that the mediating mechanisms may involve normal, as well as abnormal, functioning. The key challenge is to elucidate the nature and extent of those continuities and discontinuities over time and over the normality/pathology divide.

REFERENCES

Arseneault, L., Cannon, M., Witton, J., and Murray, R. (2004) Causal association between cannabis and psychosis: examination of the evidence. *Br. J. Psychiatry* 184:110–117.

Bailey, A., Palferman, S., Heavey, L., and Le Couteur, A. (1998) Autism: The phenotype in relatives. *J. Autism Dev. Disord.* 28:381–404.

Barr, C.S., Newman, T.K., Shannon, C., Parker, C., Dvoskin, R.L. Becker, M.L., et al. (2004) Rearing condition and 5-HTTLPR interact to influence limbic-hypothalamic-pituitary-adrenal axis response to stress in infant macaques. *Biol. Psychiatry* 55:733–738.

Bates, E., and Roe, K. (2001) Language development in children with unilateral brain injury. In: Nelson, C.A., and Luciana, M., eds. *Handbook of Developmental Cognitive Neuroscience.* Cambridge, MA: MIT Press, pp. 281–307.

Bateson, P., Barker, D., Clutton-Brock, T., Deb, D., D'Udine, B., Foley, R.A., et al. (2004) Developmental plasticity and human health. *Nature* 430:419–421.

Beckett, C., Maughan, B., Rutter, M., Castle, J., Colvert, E., Groothues, C., et al. (2006) Do the effects of early severe deprivation on cognition persist into early adolescence? Findings from the English and Romanian Adoptees study. *Child Dev.* 77:696–711.

Bennett, A.J., Lesch, K.P., Heils, A., Long, J.D., Lorenz, J.G., Shoaf, S.E., et al. (2002) Early experience and serotonin transporter gene variation interact to influence primate CNS function. *Mol. Psychiatry* 7:118–122.

Bishop, D.V.M., North, T., and Donlan, C. (1995) Genetic basis of specific language impairment: Evidence from a twin study. *Dev. Med. Child Neurol.* 37:56–71.

Bishop, D.V.M., and Rutter, M. (2008) Neurodevelopmental disorders. In: Rutter, M., Bishop, D., Pine, D., Scott, S., Stevenson, J., Taylor, E., and Thapar, A., eds. *Rutter's Child and Adolescent Psychiatry,* 5th ed. Oxford, UK: Blackwell, pp. 32–41.

Boyce, W.T. (2007) A biology of misfortune: Stress, reactivity, social context and the ontogeny of psychopathology in early life. In: Masten, A.F., ed. *Multilevel Dynamics in Developmental Psychopathology: Pathways to the Future. The Minnesota Symposia on Child Psychology, vol 34.* London and Mahwah, NJ: Lawrence Erlbaum, pp. 45–82.

Brent, D., and Weersing, V.R. (2008) Depressive disorders in childhood and adolescence. In: Rutter, M., Bishop, D., Pine, D., Scott, S., Stevenson, J., Taylor, E., and Thapar, A., eds. *Rutter's Child and Adolescent Psychiatry,* 5th ed. Oxford, UK: Blackwell, pp. 589–613.

Cameron, N.M., Parent, C., Champagne, F.A., Fish, E.W., Ozaki-Kuroda, K., and Meaney, M.J. (2005) The programming of individual differences in defensive responses and reproductive strategies in the rat through variations in maternal care. *Neurosci. Biobehav. Rev.* 29:843–865.

Cannon, M., Caspi, A., Moffitt, T., Harrington, H., Taylor, A., et al. (2002) Evidence for early-childhood, pan-developmental impairment specific to schizophrenic disorder. *Arch. Gen. Psychiatry* 59:449–456.

Caspi, A., Langley, K., Milne, B., Moffitt, T.E., O'Donovan, M., Owen, M.J., et al. (2008) A replicated molecular-genetic basis for subtyping antisocial behavior in ADHD. *Arch. Gen. Psychiatry* 65:203–210.

Caspi, A., McClay, J., Moffitt, T.E., Mill, J., Martin, J., Craig, I.W., et al. (2002) Role of genotype in the cycle of violence in maltreated children. *Science* 297:851–854.

Caspi, A., Moffitt, T.E., Cannon, M., McClay, J., Murray, R., Harrington, H., et al. (2005) Moderation of the effect of adolescent-onset cannabis use on adult psychosis by a functional polymorphism in the COMT gene: Longitudinal evidence of a gene-environment interaction. *Biol. Psychiatry* 57:1117–1127.

Caspi, A., Sugden, K., Moffitt, T.E., et al. (2003) Influence of life stress on depression: Moderation by a polymorphism in the 5-HTT gene. *Science* 301:386–389.

Champagne, F., Chretien, P., Stevenson, C.W., Zhang, T.Y., Gratton, A., and Meaney, M.J. (2004) Variations in nucleus accumbens dopamine associated with individual differences in maternal behaviour in the rat. *J. Neurosci.* 24:4113–4123.

Champion, L.A., Goodall, G.M., and Rutter, M. (1995) Behaviour problems in childhood and stressors in early adult life. I. A 20 year follow-up of London school children. *Psychol. Med*, 25:231–246.

Champoux, M., Bennett, A., Shannon, C., Higley, J.D., Lesch, K.P., and Suomi, S.J. (2002) Serotonin transporter gene polymorphism, differential early rearing and behavior in rhesus monkey neonates. *Mol. Psychiatry* 7:1058–1063.

Clegg, J., Hollis, C., Mawhood, L., and Rutter, M. (2005) Developmental language disorders: A follow-up in later adult life. *J. Child Psychol. Psychiatry* 46:128–149.

Coe, S.L., and Lubach, G.R. (2000) Prenatal influences on neuroimmune set points in infancy. *Ann. N. Y. Acad. Sci.* 917:468–477.

Courchesne, E., Carper, R., and Akshoomoff, N. (2003) Evidence of brain overgrowth in the first year of life in autism. *JAMA* 290:337–344.

Crow, T.J., and Johnstone, E.C. (1977) Cerebral atrophy and cognitive impairment in chronic schizophrenia. *Lancet* 1(8007):357.

Dapretto, M., Davies, M.S., Pfeifer, J.H., Scott, A.A., Sigman, M., Bookheimer, S.Y., and Lacoboni, M. (2005) Understanding emotions in others: mirror-neuron dysfunction in children with autism spectrum disorders. *Nat. Neurocsci.* 9:28–30.

DiCicco-Bloom, E., Lord, C., Zwaigenbaum, L., Courchesne, E., Dager, S.R., Schmitz, C., Schultz, R.T., Crawley, J., and Young L.J. (2006) The developmental neurobiology of autism spectrum disorders. *J. Neurosci.* 26:6897–6906.

Draganski, B., Gaser, C., Busch, V., Schuierer, G., Bogdahn, U., and May, A. (2004) Changes in grey matter induced by training. *Nature* 427:311–312.

Drake, R.J., and Lewis, S.W. (2005) Early detection of schizophrenia. *Curr. Opin. Psychiatry* 18:147–150.

Elbert, O.T., Pantev, C., Wienbruch, C., Rockstroh, B., and Taub, E. (1995) Increased cortical representation of the fingers of the left hand in string players. *Science* 270:305–307.

Farber, N.B., Wozniak, D.F., Price, M.T., Labruyere, J., Huss, J., St. Peter, H., and Olney, J.W. (1995) Age-specific neurotoxicity in the rat associated with NMDA receptor blockade: Potential relevance to schizophrenia? *Biol. Psychiatry* 38:788–796.

Fombonne, E., Rogé, B., Claverie, J., Courty, S., and Frémolle, J. (1999) Microcephaly and macrocephaly in autism. *J. Autism Dev. Disord.* 29:113–119.

Francis, D.J., Shaywitz, S.E., Stuebing, K.K., Shaywitz, B.A., and Fletcher, J.M. (1996) Developmental lag versus deficit models of reading disability: A longitudinal, individual growth curves analysis. *J. Educ. Psychology* 88:3–17.

Frith, C. and Frith, U. (2008) What can we learn from structural and functional brain imaging? In: Rutter, M., Bishop, D., Pine, D., Scott, S., Stevenson, J., Taylor, E., and Thapar, A., eds. *Rutter's Child and Adolescent Psychiatry*, 5th ed. Oxford, UK: Blackwell, pp. 134–144.

Frith, U. (2003) *Autism: Explaining the Enigma*, 2nd ed. Oxford, UK: Blackwell.

Giedd, J.N., Blumenthal, J., Jeffries, N., Catellanos, F., Liu, H., Zijdenbos, A., et al. (1999) Brain development during childhood and adolescence: a longitudinal MRI study. *Nat. Neurosci.* 2: 861–863.

Gogtay, N., Giedd, J.N., Lusk, L., Hayashi, K.M., Greenstein, D., Vaituzis, A.C., et al. (2004) Dynamic mapping of human cortical development during childhood through early adulthood. *Proc. Natl. Acad. Sci. USA* 101:8174–8179.

Goldapple, K., Segal, Z., Garson, C., Lau, M., Bieling, P., Kennedy, S., and Mayberg, H. (2004) Modulation of cortical-limbic pathways in major depression: Treatment-specific effects of cognitive behavior therapy. *Arch. Gen. Psychiatry* 61:34–41.

Greenough, W.T., Black, J.E., and Wallace, C.S. (1987) Experience and brain development. *Child Dev.* 58:539–559.

Gunnar, M., and Vázquez, D. M. (2006) Stress, neurobiology and developmental psychopathology. In: Cicchetti, D., and Cohen, D., eds. *Developmental Psychopathology*, Vol. 2. New York: Wiley, pp. 533–577.

Hariri, A.R., Drabant, E.M., Munoz, K.E., Kolachana, B.S., Mattay, V.S., Egan, M.F., et al. (2005) A susceptibility gene for affective disorders and the response of the human amygdale. *Arch. Gen. Psychiatry* 62:146–152.

Hariri, A.R., Mattay, V.S., Tessitore, A., Kolachana, B., Fera, F., Goldman, D., et al. (2002) Serotonin transporter genetic variation and the response of the human amygdale. *Science* 297:400–403.

Hazell, P., Heathcote, D.O.C., Robertson, J., and Henry, D. (1995) Efficacy of tricyclic drugs in treating child and adolescent depression: a meta-analysis. *Br. Med. J.* 310:897–901.

Heinz, A., Braus, D.F., Smolka, M.N., Wrase, J., Puls, I., Hermann, D., et al. (2005) Amygdala-prefrontal coupling depends on a genetic variation of the serotonin transporter. *Nat. Neurosci.* 8:20–21.

Howlin, P., Goode, S., Hutton, J., and Rutter, M. (2004) Adult outcome for children with autism. *J. Child Psychol. Psychiatry* 45:212–229.

Hubel, D.H., and Weisel, T.N. (2005) *Brain and Visual Perception.* Oxford, UK: Oxford University Press.

Huttenlocher, P.R. (2002) *Neural Plasticity: The Effects of Environment on the Development of the Cerebral Cortex.* Cambridge, MA: Harvard University Press.

Hutton, J., Goode, S., Murphy, M., Le Couteur, A., and Rutter, M. (in press) New-onset psychiatric disorders in individuals with autism. *Autism.*

Isohanni, M., Murray, G., Jokelainen, J., Croudave, T., and Jones, P. (2004) The persistence of developmental markers in childhood and adolescence and risk for schizophrenic psychoses in adult life. A 34 year follow-up of the northern Finland 1966 birth cohort. *Schizophr. Res.* 71:213–225.

Kanner L. (1943) Autistic disturbances of affective contact. *Nervous Child* 2:217–250.

Kendler, K.S. (2005) "A gene for ..." The nature of gene action in psychiatric disorders. *Am. J. Psychiatry* 162:1243–1252.

Kendler, K.S., and Baker, J.H. (2007) Genetic influences on measures of the environment: A systematic review. *Psychol. Med.* 37: 615–626.

Keshavan, M.S., Kennedy, J.L., and Murray, R.M., eds. (2004) *Neurodevelopment and Schizophrenia.* London and New York: Cambridge University Press.

Klin, A., Jones, W., Schultz, R., and Volkmar, F.R. (2003) The enactive mind, or from actions to cognition: Lessons from autism. *Philos. Tran. R. Soc. Lond. B Biol. Sci.* 358:345–360.

Klin, A., Jones, W., Schultz, R., Volkmar, F.R., and Cohen D.J. (2002) Defining and quantifying the social phenotype in autism. *Am. J. Psychiatry* 159:895–908.

Kreppner, J., Rutter, M., Beckett, C., Castle, J., Colvert, E., Groothues, C., et al. (2007) Normality and impairment following profound early institutional deprivation? A longitudinal follow-up into early adolescence. *Dev. Psychology* 43:931–946.

Kuhl, P.K. (1994) Learning and representation in speech and language. *Curr. Opin. Neurobio.* 4:812–822.

Kuhl, P.K., Andruski, J.E., Chistovich, I.A., Chistovich, L.A., Kozhevnikova, E.V., Ryskina, V.L., et al. (1997) Cross-language analysis of phonetic units in language addressed to infants. *Science* 277:684–686.

Landa, R., and Garrett-Meyer, E. (2006) Development in infants with autism spectrum disorders: A prospective study. *J. Child Psychol. Psychiatry* 47:629–638.

Lyytinen, H., Ahonen, T., Eklund, K., Guttorm, T., Kulju, P., Laakso, M.-L., Leiwo, M., Lyytinen, P., Poikkeus, A.-M., Richardson, U., Torppa, M., and Viholainen, H. (2004) Early development of children at familial risk for Dyslexia: follow-up from birth to school age. *Dyslexia* 10:146–178.

Maye, J., Werker, J.F., and Gerken, L. (2002) Infant sensitivity to distributional information can affect phonetic discrimination. *Cognition* 82:B101–B111.

McClellan, J.M., Susser, E., and King, M.C. (2006) Maternal famine, de novo mutations and schizophrenia. *JAMA* 296:582–584.

Meaney, M.J., and Szyf, M. (2005) Environmental programming of stress responses through DNA methylation: life at the interface between a dynamic environment and a fixed genome. *Dialog. Clin Neurosci.* 7:103–23.

Meyer-Lindenberg, A., Buckholtz, J.W., Kolachana, B., Hariri, A.R., Pezawas, L., Blasi, G., et al. (2006) Neural mechanisms of genetic risk for impulsivity and violence in humans. *Proc. Natl. Acad. Sci. USA* 103:6269–6274.

Moffitt, T.E. (1993) Adolescence-limited and life-course persistent antisocial behavior: A developmental taxonomy. *Psychol. Rev.* 100:674–701.

Monti, P.M., Miranda, R., Nixon, K., Sher, K.J., Swartzwelder, H.S., Tapert, S.F., et al. (2005) Adolescence: Booze, brains and behavior. *Alcohol.: Clin. Exp. Res.* 29:207–220.

Murray, R.M., and Lewis, S.W. (1987) Is schizophrenia a neurodevelopmental disorder? *Br. Med. J. (Clin. Res. Ed.)* 295:681–682.

Murray, R., Sham, P., Van Os, J., Zanelli, J., Cannon, M., and McDonald, C. (2004) A developmental model for similarities and dissimilarities between schizophrenia and bipolar disorder. *Schizophr. Res.* 71:405–416.

Nelson, C.A., and Jeste, S. (2008) Neurobiological perspectives on developmental psychopathology. In: Rutter, M., Bishop, D., Pine, D., Scott, S., Stevenson, J., Taylor, E., and Thapar, A., eds. *Rutter's Child and Adolescent Psychiatry,* 5th ed. Oxford, UK: Blackwell, pp. 145–159.

Odgers, C.L., Caspi, A., Broadbent, J.M., Dickson, N., Hancox, R.J., Harrington, H-L., Poulton, R., Sears, M.R., Thomson, W.M., and Moffitt, T.E. (2007) Prediction of differential adult health burden by conduct problem subtypes in males. *Arch. Gen. Psychiatry* 64:476–484.

Odgers, C.L., Milne, B., Caspi, A, Crump, R., Poulton, R., and Moffitt, T.E. (2007) Predicting prognosis for the conduct-problem boy: Can family history help? *J. Am. Acad. Child Adol. Psychiatry* 46:1240–1249.

Owens, D.G.C., and Johnstone, E.C. (2006) Precursors and prodromata of schizophrenia: findings from the Edinburgh High Risk Study and their literature context. *Psychol. Med.* 36:1501–1514.

Pantelis, C., Velakoulis, D., McGorry, P.D., Wood, S.J., Suckling, J., Phillips, L.J., et al. (2003) Neuroanatomical abnormalities before and after onset of psychosis: A cross-sectional and longitudinal MRI comparison. *Lancet* 361:281–288.

Pennington, B. (2006) From single to multiple deficit models of developmental disorders. *Cognition* 101:385–413.

Pezawas, O.L., Meyer-Lindenberg, A., Drabant, E.M., Verchinski, B.A., Munoz, K., Kolachana, B., et al. (2005) 5-HTTLPR polymorphism impacts human cingulate-amygdala interactions: a genetic susceptibility mechanism for depression. *Nat. Neurosci.* 8:828–834.

Pickles, A., Simonoff, E., Conti-Ramsden, G., Falcaro, M., Simkin, Z., Charman, T., et al. (2008) *Loss of language in early development of autism and specific language impairment.* Manuscript submitted for publication.

Pistis, M., Perra, S., Pillolla, G., Melis, M., Muntoni, A.L., et al. (2004) Adolescent exposure to cannabinoids induces long-lasting changes in the response to drugs of abuse of rat midbrain dopamine neurons. *Biol. Psychiatry* 15:86–94.

Poulton, R., Caspi, A., Moffitt, T., Cannon, M., Murray, R., and Harrington, H. (2000) Children's self-reported psychotic symptoms and adult schizophrenia disorder. *Arch. Gen. Psychiatry* 57:1053–1058.

Rapoport, J. (1980) Diagnostic significance of drug response in child psychiatry. In: Purcell, E.F., ed. *Psychopathology of Children and Youth.* New York: Josiah Macy Jr. Foundation, pp. 154–170.

Rapoport, J.L., Addington, A.M., and Frangou, S. (2005) The neurodevelopmental model of schizophrenia: update 2005. *Mol. Psychiatry* 10:434–449.

Rizzolatti, G., and Craighero, L. (2004) The mirror-neuron system. *Annu. Rev. Neurosci.* 27:169–192.

Robins, L. (1966) *Deviant Children Grown Up: A Sociological and Psychiatric Study of Sociopathic Personality.* Baltimore: Williams & Wilkins.

Roder, B., and Neville, H. (2003) Developmental functional plasticity. In: Grafman, J., and Robertson, I.H., eds. *Handbook of Neuropsychology*, 2nd ed., Vol 9. St Louis, MO and Oxford, UK: Elsevier Science, pp. 231–270.

Rutter, M. (1970) Autistic children: infancy to adulthood. *Sem. Psychiatry* 2:435–450.

Rutter, M. (2005a) Environmentally mediated risks for psychopathology: Research strategies and findings. *J. Am. Acad. Child Adoles. Psychiatry* 44:3–18.

Rutter, M. (2005b) Incidence of autism spectrum disorders: changes over time and their meaning. *Acta Paediatrica* 94:2–15.

Rutter, M. (2006a) *Genes and Behavior: Nature-Nurture Interplay Explained.* Oxford, UK: Blackwell.

Rutter, M. (2006b) The psychological effects of early institutional rearing. In: Marshall, P.J., and Fox, N.A., eds. *The Development of Social Engagement: Neurobiological Perspectives.* Oxford, UK: Oxford University Press, pp. 355–391.

Rutter, M. (2007a) Gene-environment interdependence. *Dev. Sci.* 10:12–18.

Rutter, M. (2007b) Proceeding from observed correlation to causal inference: The use of natural experiments. *Perspect. Psychol. Sci.* 2:377–395.

Rutter, M. (2008) Developing concepts in developmental psychopathology. In: Hudziak, J.J., ed. *Genetic and Environmental Influences on Developmental Psychopathology and Wellness.* Arlington, VA: American Psychiatric Publishing, pp. 3–22.

Rutter, M., Beckett, C., Castle, J., Colvert, E., Kreppner, J., Mehta, M., et al. (2007) Effects of profound early institutional deprivation: An overview of findings from a UK longitudinal study of Romanian adoptees. *Eur. J. Dev. Psychol* 4:332–350.

Rutter, M., Caspi, A., and Moffitt, T. E. (2003) Using sex differences in psychopathology to study causal mechanisms: unifying issues and research strategies. *J. Child Psychol. Psychiatry* 44:1092–1115.

Rutter, M., Colvert, E., Kreppner, J., Beckett, C., Castle, J., Groothues, C., et al. (2007) Early adolescent outcomes for institutionally-deprived and non-deprived adoptees. I. Disinhibited attachment. *J. Child Psychol. Psychiatry* 48:17–30.

Rutter, M., Kreppner, J., Croft, C., Murin, M., Colvert, E., Beckett, C., et al. (2007) Early adolescent outcomes of institutionally deprived and non-deprived adoptees. III. Quasi-autism. *J. Child Psychol. Psychiatry* 48:1200–1207.

Rutter, M., Maughan, B. and Kim-Cohen, J. (2006) Continuities and discontinuities in psychopathology between childhood and adult life. *J. Child Psychol. Psychiatry* 47:276–295.

Rutter, M., Moffitt, T.E., and Caspi, A. (2006) Gene-environment interplay and psychopathology: Multiple varieties but real effects. *J. Child Psychol. Psychiatry* 47:226–261.

Rutter, M., and Pickles, A. (1991) Person-environment interactions; concepts, mechanisms and implications for data analysis. In: Wachs, T.D., and Plomin, R., eds. *Conceptualization and Measurement of Organism-Environment Interaction.* Washington, DC: American Psychological Association, pp. 105–141.

Rutter, M., Pickles, A., Murray, R., and Eaves, L. (2001) Testing hypotheses on specific environmental causal effects on behavior. *Psychol. Bull.* 127:291–324.

Rutter, M., and Silberg, J. (2002) Gene-environment interplay in relation to emotional and behavioral disturbance. *Annu. Rev. Psychol.* 53:463–490.

Schneider, M., and Koch, M. (2003) Chronic pubertal, but no adult chronic cannabinoid treatment impairs sensorimotor gating, recognition memory, and the performance in a progressive ratio task in adult rats. *Neuropsychopharmacol.* 28:1760–1769.

Schultz, R.T., and Robins, D.L. (2005) Functional neuroimaging studies of autism spectrum disorders. In: Volkmar, F.R., Paul, R., Klin, A., Cohen, D., eds. *Handbook of Autism and Pervasive Developmental Disorders*, Vol. 1. Hoboken, NJ: Wiley and Sons, pp. 515–533.

Schultz, T., Grelotti, D.J., Klin, A., Kleinman, J., Van der Gaag, C., Marois, R., and Skudlarski, P. (2003) The role of the fusiform face area in social cognition: implications for the pathobiology of autism. *Philos. Trans. R. Soc. Lond. B Biol. Sci.* 358:415–427.

Shaw, P., Greenstein, D., Lerch, J., Clasen, L., Lenroot, R., Gogtay, N., Evans, A. Rapoport, J., and Giedd, J. (2006) Intellectual ability and cortical development in children and adolescents. *Nature* 440:676–679.

Sheedlo, H.J., Li, L., and Turner, J.E. (1992) Effects of RPE-cell factors secreted from permselective fibers on retinal cells in vitro. *Brain Res.* 7:327–337.

Sigman, M., and Ruskin, E. (1999) Continuity and change in the social competence of children with autism, Down syndrome, and developmental delays. *Monographs of the Society for Research in Child Development*, 256(64, Serial No. 1).

Silberg, J., Meyer, J., Pickles, A., et al. (1996) Heterogeneity among juvenile antisocial behaviours: findings from the Virginia Twin Study of Adolescent Behavioural Development. In: Bock, G.R., and Goode, J.A., *Genetics of Criminal and Antisocial Behaviour. Ciba Foundation Symposium 194.* Chichester, UK: Wiley, pp. 76–86.

Sluming, V., Brooks, J., Howard, M., Downes, J.J., and Roberts, N. (2007) Broca's area supports enhanced visuospatial cognition in orchestral musicians. *J. Neurosci.* 4:3799–3806.

Snowling, M.J., Gallagher, A., and Frith, U. (2003) Family risk of dyslexia is continuous: Individual differences in the precursors of reading skill. *Child Dev* 74:358–373.

Sonuga-Barke, E.J.S., Beckett, C., Kreppner, J., Castle, J., Colvert, E., Stevens, S., et al. (2008) *Is sub-nutrition necessary for a poor outcome following severe and pervasive early deprivation? Brain growth, cognition and mental health.* Manuscript submitted for publication.

St. Clair, D., Xu, M., Wang, P., Yu, Y., Fang, Y., Zhang, F., Sheng, X., Gu, N., Feng, G., Sham, P., and He, L. (2005) Rates of adult schizophrenia following prenatal exposure to the Chinese famine of 1959-1961. *JAMA* 294:557–562.

Stein, Z.A., Susser, M., Saenger, G., and Marolla, F. (1975) *Famine and Human Development: The Dutch Hunger Winter of 1944-1945.* New York: Oxford University Press.

Stiles, J. (2000) Neural plasticity and cognitive development. *Dev. Neuropsychol.* 18:237–272.

Susser, E., Neugebauer, R., Hoek, H.W., Brown, A.S., Lin, S., Labovitz, D., and Gorman, J.M. (1996) Schizophrenia after prenatal famine: Further evidence. *Arch. Gen. Psychiatry* 53:25–31.

Thapar, A., Langley, K., Fowler, T., Rice, F., Turic, D., Whittinger, N., et al. (2005) Catechol-O-methyltransferase gene variant and birth weight predict early-onset antisocial behavior in children with attention-deficit/hyperactivity disorder. *Arch. Gen. Psychiatry* 62:1275–1278.

Thompson, P.M., Vidal, C., Giedd, J.N., Gochman, P., Blumenthal, J., Nicolson, R., et al. (2001) Mapping adolescent brain changes reveals dynamic wave of accelerated gray matter loss in very early-onset schizophrenia. *Proc. Natl. Acad. Sci. USA* 98:11650–11655.

Toga, A.W., Thompson, P.M., and Sowell, E.R. (2006) Mapping brain maturation. *Trends Neurosc.* 29:148–159.

Vargha-Khadem, F., Isaacs, E., van der Werf, S., Robb, S., and Wilson, J. (1992) Development of intelligence and memory in children with hemiplegic cerebral palsy: The deleterious consequences of early seizures. *Brain* 115:315–329.

Vargha-Khadem, F., and Mishkin, M. (1997) Speech and language outcome after hemispherectomy in childhood. In: Tuxhorn, I., Holthausen, H., and Boenigk, H.E., eds. *Paediatric Epilepsy Syndromes and Their Surgical Treatment.* Sydney, Australia: Libbey, pp. 774–784.

Viding, E., Blair, R.J.R., Moffitt, T.E., and Plomin, R. (2005) Evidence for substantial genetic risk for psychopathy in 7-year-olds. *J. Child Psychol. Psychiatry* 46:592–597.

Volkow, N., and Swanson, J. (2008) Neurochemistry and basic psychopharmacology. In: Rutter, M., Bishop, D., Pine, D., Scott, S., Stevenson, J., Taylor, E., and Thapar, A., eds. *Rutter's Child and Adolescent Psychiatry,* 5th ed. Oxford, UK: Blackwell, pp. 212–231.

Weaver, I.C., Diorio, J., Seckl, J.R., Szyf, M., and Meaney, M.J. (2004) Early environmental regulation of hippocampal glucocorticoid receptor gene expression: characterization of intracellular mediators and potential genomic target. *Ann. N. Y. Acad. Sci.* 1024:182–212.

Weinberger, D.R. (1987) Implications of normal brain development for the pathogenesis of schizophrenia. *Arch. Gen. Psychiatry* 44:660–669.

Werker, J.F. (2003) Baby steps to learning language. *J. Pediatrics* 143:S62–S69.

Werner, E., Dawson, G., Munson, J., and Osterling, J. (2005) Variation in early developmental course in autism and its relation with behavioral outcome at 3-4 years of age. *J. Autism Dev. Disord.* 35:337–350.

Williams, J., Whiten, A., Suddendorf, T., and Perrett, D. (2001) Imitation, mirror neurons and autism. *Neurosci. Biobehav. Rev.* 25:287–295.

Woodhouse, W., Bailey, A., Rutter, M., Bolton, P., Baird, G. and Le Couteur, A. (1996) Head circumference in autism and other pervasive developmental disorders. *J. Child Psychol. Psychiatry* 37:665–671.

Zammit, S., Allebeck, P., Andreasson, S., Lundberg, I., and Lewis, G. (2002) Self reported use as a risk factor for schizophrenia in Swedish conscripts of 1969: historical cohort study. *Br. Med. J.* 325:1199–1203.

78 Neurobiology of Autism and the Pervasive Developmental Disorders

SARAH SPENCE, PAUL GRANT, AUDREY THURM, AND SUSAN E. SWEDO

Autism is a neurodevelopmental disorder that affects individuals across the life span and includes impairments in three domains of functioning: social reciprocity, communication, and repetitive and restrictive behaviors (American Psychiatric Association [APA], 2000). Autistic disorder (autism) is currently classified in the *Diagnostic and Statistical Manual of Mental Disorders,* 4th ed. (*DSM-IV*; APA, 1994) as one of the pervasive developmental disorders (PDD), which also include Asperger's disorder, PDD–not otherwise specified (PDD-NOS), Rett disorder, and childhood disintegrative disorder (CDD) (APA, 2000). Asperger's disorder was newly defined in *DSM-IV* (APA, 1994) and includes the same qualitative impairments in social interaction and restricted, repetitive, and stereotyped interests as autistic disorder, but individuals who are affected do not have significantly impairing communication or cognitive deficits. The diagnosis of PDD-NOS is made when full criteria for autism are not met, but impairing symptoms in social interaction and communication are present. The focus of this chapter will be on autistic disorder and, to a lesser extent, the broader phenotype that includes Asperger's disorder and PDD-NOS.

Autism, Asperger's disorder, and PDD-NOS are usually merged into a single group and referred to as the autism spectrum disorders (ASD). The two other diagnostic classifications in the PDD category—Rett disorder and CDD—are usually considered as unique entities, particularly in neurobiological studies. Rett disorder is found almost exclusively in girls and includes at least 5 months of typical development, followed by deceleration of head growth, loss of purposeful hand movements and the appearance of stereotyped hand movements, at least temporary regression in social interaction, gait/trunk dyscoordination, and impaired language and psychomotor retardation (APA, 2000). Childhood disintegrative disorder is defined by normal development for the first 2 years of life, with appropriate language acquisition and social skills exhibited, and then loss of skills in multiple domains, including motor and cognitive domains (APA, 2000). Rett disorder and CDD have some behavioral symptoms related to autism and are characterized by a regressive course, but they are not usually grouped with other PDDs for neurobiologic study because Rett disorder has been found to be almost exclusively associated with a specific mutation (MECP2) on the X chromosome (Amir et al., 1999), and the later onset and unique deteriorating clinical course of CDD suggest a separate etiology. Further, CDD is quite rare, so acquiring sufficient sample sizes is difficult (Fombonne, 2005).

The most recent reports indicate a prevalence of 1 of 150 for ASD (Rice, 2007), with a male-to-female ratio that approximates 4:1 (Fombonne, 2005). Data from several reports indicate that the prevalence of autism is on the rise, but there are no data on the incidence of the disorder, so it is impossible to accurately assess time trends. Further, the available prevalence data are limited by a number of methodological factors, including changes in diagnostic criteria over time, variable sampling techniques, and small sample sizes (Fombonne, 2005).

The phenomenology of autism includes the behaviors described in the current diagnostic criteria (APA, 2000), as well as other associated developmental, medical, and underlying genetic conditions. Impairments in social abnormalities have been considered to be the "core" deficits in autism since the original report by Leo Kanner in 1943, but language delay is often the first symptom noted and brought to professional attention (Chakrabarti and Fombonne, 2001). Although not part of the diagnostic criteria, cognitive deficits are common among individuals with autism: previous reports indicated that up to 70% of individuals with autism also met criteria for mental retardation, but more recent studies have found lower rates (Chakrabarti and Fombonne, 2001). Approximately one third of individuals with autism are reported to undergo a regression of language and/or social skills between 12 and 36 months of life (Kurita, 1985; Luyster et al., 2005). Werner and Dawson (2005), utilizing home videotapes of children who were developing typically and children with autism (with and without regression), were able to validate parental reports of the onset of regression and demonstrated that the children were using words and gestures normally at their first birthday party. Studies that have tracked the natural history of the individuals with regressive autism generally have found poor prognosis, with respect to factors such as ability to live independently or to have meaningful employment (Nordin and Gillberg, 1998; Howlin et al., 2004).

In the present nosology, autism is a highly heterogeneous diagnostic category, diagnosed exclusively on the basis of behavioral abnormalities. Although severity is typically measured by totaling symptoms in the triad of social, communication, and restrictive/repetitive behavior, studies from typical populations indicate these domains often track independently (Happe et al., 2006). Further, these behavioral traits vary widely across the general population, and determining when an individual's symptoms meet criteria for the autism spectrum disorders can be difficult, particularly early in childhood. Extensive research has been devoted to finding cutoff points that accurately identify individuals who will demonstrate impairments (Gotham et al., 2007). Autism is highly heritable (Geschwind and Levitt, 2007), and subsyndromal symptoms have been found in family members and relatives (Piven, Palmer, et al., 1997). Thus, a broader autism phenotype (BAP) has been proposed (Le Couteur et al., 1996), and several groups are now studying a variety of behavioral and biological phenotypes and endophenotypes. Phenotypes and endophenotypes have been postulated based on characteristics of the clinical progression of the disorder (for example, a regressive phenotype), neurocognitive profiles, or demonstrated neuroimaging abnormalities. Narrowing the phenotype to increase homogeneity of the sample under investigation may facilitate the search for etiologies because phenotype–genotype relationships do not appear plausible at the level of the behavioral disorder (Happe et al., 2006; Hus et al., 2007).

Until recently, autism was most often diagnosed after age 3, the cutoff age for symptom onset. Autism is sometimes diagnosed at earlier ages, and studies are now beginning to investigate prodromal symptoms, early disease markers, and predictors of disease severity. Deficits in developmental social-communication skills such as joint attention (Dawson et al., 2002; Dawson et al., 2004), imitation (Rogers, Hepburn, Stackhouse, and Wehner, 2003), and early social-orienting behaviors (Dawson et al., 2004) are common. Even before an official diagnosis is made, early markers are often present by 12 months of age; these include decreased eye contact, abnormal visual tracking, and disengagement of visual attention, along with reduced social interest, imitation, and social smiling (Zwaigenbaum et al., 2005).

There are reports of multiple behavioral and developmental abnormalities associated with autism. These include sensory impairments, oversensitivity, and undersensitivity, as well as sensory integration deficits (Rogers, Hepburn, and Wehner, 2003); restrictive eating habits and preferences (Schreck et al., 2004; Schreck and Williams, 2006); motor abnormalities such as toe walking (Kielinen et al., 2004); and aggressive behavior and self-injury (McClintock et al., 2003). Seizures occur frequently among individuals who are affected, as discussed below. Psychiatric symptoms are also common, especially compulsions, specific phobias, and symptoms of attention-deficit/hyperactivity disorder (ADHD) (Leyfer et al., 2006).

In laying the groundwork for a review of the neurobiological study of autism, it is important to consider the neuropsychological impairments specific to autism (as opposed to those associated with general developmental delay). Early in life, the autism-specific deficits include abnormalities of joint attention and theory of mind deficits. Later in development, specific deficits are found in executive functioning, such as cognitive inflexibility (Ozonoff et al., 1994; Verte et al., 2006). Comprehensive neuropsychological models of the disorder have been proposed and include a complex information processing model, in which underconnectivity of cortical regions in the brain underlies difficulties in higher-order processing of complex information (for example, concepts) across different neural systems (Minshew et al., 1997). A competing model posits that social motivation is deficient in autism, and this deficit early in life prevents opportunities for learning and using other key social communication skills. The deficits may arise from aberrations of key brain circuits or communication among brain regions (Minshew et al., 2006). Given the complexity of the neuropsychiatric symptomatology of autism, it is likely that there is not just one overarching cognitive deficit, but a number of distinct neurocognitive abnormalities that manifest as distinct but overlapping symptom profiles (Happe et al., 2006).

COMORBIDITIES

Although autism remains a disorder that is defined by a constellation of behavioral symptoms, there is increasing interest in the associated medical and neurological signs and symptoms of autism. Probably the best known and perhaps the most important of these is epilepsy. Since the 1960s, there have been reports of an increased incidence of epilepsy among individuals with autism, although the rates have varied substantially (5%–44%) (Tuchman and Rapin, 2002). This may be because of differences in the definitions of *autism* and/or *epilepsy* and differences in the characteristics of the samples such as the inclusion/exclusion of individuals with other neurogenetic disorders such as Fragile X or tuberous sclerosis that also have increased rates of epilepsy (Ballaban-Gil and Tuchman, 2000); an association of epilepsy with lower IQ (Tuchman et al., 1991; Pavone et al., 2004); and inclusion of older individuals, as there is a bimodal age of onset with many having their first seizure in adolescence (Volkmar and Nelson, 1990). The rate of epilepsy in community-based samples is likely to be lower that these rates, which were obtained from clinics and individuals with significant impairments.

Interestingly, there have also been reports of electroencephalogram (EEG) abnormalities (specifically of an epileptiform nature) among individuals with autism without any clinical seizures. These were once thought to be rare (< 10%; Tuchman and Rapin, 1997), but recently there have been reports of much higher rates (> 50%; Chez et al., 2006; H.L. Kim et al., 2006). The presence of these abnormalities is especially intriguing in the context of the complex relationship that exists between epilepsy/EEG abnormalities and deficits of language and behavior among individuals with autism. Investigators are now questioning whether these abnormalities could be causally related to the autism phenotype (Chez et al., 2006). In this case, these discharges could be seen as a cortical biomarker for ASD and might represent a potential treatment target. However, others argue that the epilepsy and the EEG abnormalities are simply an epiphenomenon of an underlying neural deficit that is responsible for the cognitive, linguistic, and behavioral difficulties seen in ASD (Tharp, 2004).

There is some interest in the overlap of ASD with Landau–Kleffner syndrome (LKS) (a rare childhood epilepsy syndrome) (Landau and Kleffner, 1957) because LKS presents with language regression along with the appearance of seizures and abnormal EEGs. However, it should be noted that LKS can be distinguished from ASD by the specificity of the language loss and the later age at onset of symptoms (grade school aged, rather than prior to age 3 years).

Sensory and Motor Abnormalities

Although the symptoms do not constitute those of primary sensory deficits, reports of abnormal sensory behaviors are common among individuals with ASD. Visual, auditory, tactile, and pain sensitivity have all been shown to be increased and/or decreased (Rogers, Hepburn, and Wehner, 2003). Similarly, obvious motor deficits are not common in ASD, but there are reports of subtle abnormalities including delayed motor milestones (Mayes and Calhoun, 2003), gait disturbances (Kielinen et al., 2004), and balance and coordination problems (Ghaziuddin and Butler, 1998; Minshew et al., 2004). The cortical circuitry underlying these deficits is unknown, but investigators are now turning to functional imaging techniques such as functional magnetic resonance imaging (fMRI), event-related potentials (ERP), magnetoencephalography (MEG), and positron emission tomography (PET) to evaluate regional areas of pathology.

Immunological Abnormalities

Investigation into possible neuroimmune abnormalities in ASD is an area of increasing focus as immunological abnormalities may be one way that environmental factors could affect central nervous system (CNS) function. In the 1980s and 1990s, there were a number of studies demonstrating abnormal immune function in ASD, including abnormal T-cell subset profiles and depressed NK-cell function (for review, see Krause et al., 2002; Ashwood and Van de Water, 2004). However, ensuing investigations have yielded inconsistent results. Some data have suggested a general excess in inflammatory reactions among individuals with autism (Jyonouchi et al., 2001), whereas others have suggested a failure of immunoreactivity. Results from examination of specific cytokine profiles in the sera also have shown variability. Most recently, investigators have demonstrated increased levels of tumor necrosis factor-α (TNF-α) (Ashwood and Wakefield, 2006) and interferon-γ (IFN-γ) (Croonenberghs et al., 2002) in the sera of individuals with autism, whereas others have shown decreased levels of transforming growth factor-β1 (TGF-β1) (Okada et al., 2007). Other investigators have documented a more general increased activation of Th2 and Th1 immune responses, which appear to occur in the absence of the compensatory increase in the regulatory cytokine interleukin-10 (IL-10) (Molloy et al., 2006).

Auto immunity has also been implicated in ASD. Family histories reveal increased rates of autoimmune disorders among first-degree relatives of children with autism (Comi et al., 1999; Sweeten et al., 2003). Antibodies to brain tissue have been found in the sera of children with autism (Singh et al., 1993; Singh et al., 1997; Connolly et al., 1999; Connolly et al., 2006), and investigators are now looking for maternal antibodies reacting against fetal brain tissue.

Research into the role of the immune system in autism is hampered by the inability to assess neuroimmune function directly. Peripheral measures are being used as a surrogate to studying CNS dysfunction without adequate documentation of relevance. However, at least one study has provided us with more direct evidence of neuroimmune dysfunction. Vargas and colleagues (2005) documented a proinflammatory cytokine/chemokine response in the cerebrospinal fluid of children with ASD and provided direct confirmation of microglial activation in postmortem brain tissue. If replicated, these data may not only shed light on a potential etiopathogenesis of autism but also may provide a potential treatment target in ASD.

ABNORMALITIES OF BRAIN STRUCTURE AND FUNCTION

The neuropathology of autism has been reviewed extensively by a number of authors, including an excellent summary coauthored by Schultz and Anderson (2004) in the previous edition of this textbook and recent reviews (Bauman and Kemper, 2005; Pickett and London, 2005). An abbreviated review of the neuropathological reports will not be attempted here, as the issues of study interpretation are complex, and the number of primary reports is small. In fact, there are currently fewer original reports than there are summary reviews of the neuropathology of autism. In part, this is due to the fact that neuropathological investigations have been hampered by a lack of autistic brain, and a paucity of brain tissue from healthy children at various developmental stages of interest (for example, toddlers during the period of onset of developmental regression in autism). The recent establishment of a neurodevelopmental brain bank and the institution of the Autism Tissue Program (ATP) promises to correct these deficiencies, providing sufficient tissue for additional investigations of the structural abnormalities associated with ASD. In the interim, evidence suggestive of autistic brain pathology is being provided by clinical observations and neuroimaging studies.

Clinical Observations

Since Kanner's first description of autism (Kanner, 1943), it has been consistently noted that there is an increase in head size among individuals with ASD. Frank macrocephaly (defined as a head circumference [HC] at the 98th percentile or above) has been found in ~20% of individuals with autism (Fombonne et al., 1999). These data have support from two parallel lines of evidence: brain weight data from pathological studies and the total brain volume data from imaging. This phenomenon may shed light on aberrant brain development, especially early in life. However, there is some controversy over exactly when this occurs in development, with some studies showing the presence of macrocephaly early in life with normalization in later childhood/adulthood, and others showing no effect of age (Woodhouse et al., 1996; Lainhart et al., 1997; Courchesne et al., 2001; Aylward et al., 2002). Perhaps most intriguing are two studies showing rapidly accelerating head growth in early infancy. Both had relatively small samples and performed a retrospective analysis of HC records from birth. Courchesne reported that HC in autism was normal or even slightly smaller than average at birth but then showed an abnormal acceleration of head growth during the first year of life (Courchesne et al., 2003).

Defining rapid growth as a change of more then 25 percentile points between 1 and 2 months of age, Dementieva found that 11/15 patients with autism showed this abnormal growth pattern (Dementieva et al., 2005). It has also been demonstrated that macrocephaly is more common among family members of individuals with autism (Fidler et al., 2000; Miles et al., 2000; Lainhart et al., 2006), suggesting that this may be part of the broader phenotype in autism.

Structural Neuroimaging

Given the paucity of brain tissue, many investigators have attempted to study the structural brain abnormalities in autism via imaging modalities. Unfortunately, methodological differences have led to a myriad of inconsistencies in this literature (see Palmen and van Engeland, 2004; Lainhart, 2006, for reviews). Technological differences in acquisition, postacquisition image processing, and morphometric analysis techniques have all contributed to the variability. There have also been vast differences in characteristics of patients with autism and controls, with differing ages, cognitive levels, behavioral functioning, and medical comorbidities within and across studies.

Perhaps the most consistent result has been that of larger overall brain volumes in individuals with autism (Piven et al., 1995; Courchesne et al., 2001; Hazlett et al., 2005). What these larger brains mean for individuals with autism is still being debated. Some posit that there is an early acceleration of brain growth, followed by premature arrest, both abnormal patterns leading to abnormal brain function (Courchesne, 2004). Others argue that larger brains might be associated with increased modularity and decreased functional integration (Schultz et al., 2000). Data from two lines of investigation may shed light on this question. First, is there an effect of development on these differences? Until recently, the developmental trajectory of this brain enlargement had not been examined, largely because of the difficulties in obtaining scans from young children with ASD. Like the story seen in the head circumference data, it appears that there may be an early brain enlargement that becomes less pronounced as the individuals age; this enlargement may or may not persist into adulthood (see Redcay and Courchesne, 2005, for review). The second question is whether the enlargement is driven by a specific tissue type (for example, gray vs. white matter) and/or brain region. The enlargement appears to involve gray and white matter in some samples (Courchesne et al., 2001). But others have reported significant increases only in gray matter and not in white matter (Lotspeich et al., 2004; Hazlett et al., 2006). Conversely, Herbert and colleagues (2004) suggested that the enlargement was the result of white matter immediately adjacent to the cortex since its size remained increased even after correction for total brain volumes. Some report enlargement in posterior but not frontal regions (Piven et al., 1996); others reported the opposite

(Carper et al., 2002). Still others have reported that the regional differences apply to gray and white matter independently (Piven et al., 1996) and may be affected by age (Carper et al., 2002).

The complex interactions between tissue type, region, age, and even IQ of samples makes replication difficult across sites and samples and creates a real challenge for meaningful interpretation. Even when investigators have limited their examinations to very specific brain structures or regions that are hypothesized to be involved in the behavioral deficits seen in ASD (such as limbic regions, frontal cortex, and cerebellum), the results have been inconsistent. The earliest finding of neocerebellar vermian hypoplasia (Courchesne et al., 1988) is one that has been replicated in some (Kaufmann et al., 2003) but not other (Piven, Saliba, et al., 1997) studies.

Studies of amygdala volume are also numerous and just as inconsistent. Compared to typically developing controls, some studies find increases (Sparks et al., 2002; Schumann et al., 2004), some find decreases (Aylward et al., 1999; Pierce et al., 2001), and still another found no differences (Haznedar et al., 2000). Likewise, inconsistent findings are reported in volumes of hippocampus, basal ganglia, thalamus, and corpus callosum (see Palmen and van Engeland, 2004, for a detailed review). The inconsistency of these results may be merely a result of methodological differences, or it may reflect true heterogeneities of the disorder.

Structural imaging studies can tell us only about differences in relatively gross measures of size and shape, and these measurements may not tell us how neuroanatomical structures contribute to the phenomenology of autism. Thus, structural imaging must be combined with other modalities, such as functional neuroimaging, to further our understanding of the neurobiologic basis of ASD.

Functional Neuroimaging

Within the realm of functional neuroanatomy, studies of autism have mainly used the fMRI approach, investigating behavioral domains impaired in autism, including theory of mind (and joint attention), face/emotion recognition and processing, executive functions, language, and motor/attention (Brambilla et al., 2004). Recent advances in the field of social neuroscience have increased understanding of the neural circuitry for more finely parsed-out aspects of those social behaviors impaired in autism. For example, aspects of these behaviors controlled by the medial frontal cortex include reward valuing, monitoring, mentalizing, and self-reflection (Amodio and Frith, 2006). One of the most studied aspects is mentalizing—required for theory of mind, and important because of the young age (that is, 4 years) at which children without autism accurately respond to false-belief tasks (Baron-Cohen et al., 1985). Extensive work has now implicated neural circuitry for this process, in the posterior part of the superior temporal sulcus, the temporo-parietal junction, the temporal poles, and the medial prefrontal cortex (Frith and Frith, 2006).

Within the realm of face perception, several studies have noted abnormalities in the fusiform gyrus in individuals with autism (e.g., Pierce et al., 2001; Ogai et al., 2003). One of the most interesting recent studies revealed that though there may be fusiform area hypoactivation when engaged in face processing (including recognition tasks), individuals with autism also show increased amygdala activation during tasks with faces; and, furthermore, this activation was correlated with time spent looking at the target (Dalton et al., 2005). This ties into recent eye-tracking studies, finding social impairments in autism correlated with time spent visually monitoring mouths instead of eyes (Klin et al., 2002). These findings are critical to our understanding of how facial recognition and facial processing are faulty in autism. They also help link behavioral findings (that individuals with autism perceive faces differently) to our growing knowledge of the neural circuitry of face processing, which appears to involve visual systems (fusiform gyrus) and systems involved in mirroring, mentalizing, and emotion recognition (Haxby and Ida Gobbini, 2007).

Despite these examples, progress in further pinpointing the neurodevelopmental circuitry and systems specific to autism has been slowed by the lack of data on differences in functional activity at different developmental stages, but investigators now are beginning to fill the void. For example, recent studies have found the location of joint attention activity (typically developed by 1 year) in right ventral medial frontal cortex and left anterior frontal cortex, as well as cingulate cortex, bilateral caudate nuclei, and right anterior frontal lobe, indicating consistency with other mentalistic domains (J.H. Williams et al., 2005). Eye gaze vis-à-vis joint attention has also been studied, with posterior superior temporal sulcus hypoactivation (Pelphrey et al., 2005). Use of quantitative measurements of behavior during these imaging tasks is beginning to allow for the parsing out of reasons for functional differences found among individuals with autism (DiCicco-Bloom et al., 2006).

There has been recent attention on the area of mirror neurons, with the hypothesis that social deficits of autism (such as imitation) may be related to failure of the mirror neuron system as part of larger cortical system abnormalities (J.H. Williams et al., 2001). Among other studies that have used event-related fMRI, Dapretto and colleagues (2006) found that individuals with autism had reduced activity in the pars opercularis area of the inferior frontal gyrus when engaged in imitation of facial emotional expressions.

Techniques such as EEG and MEG have also been used recently to measure brain activity among individuals with autism, while subjects engaged in activities such as attending to visual cues (for example, images of faces) or tests of auditory perception. Using an ERP approach, studies investigating typical development of components of face processing have found that individuals with autism have reduced differentiation of familiar versus unfamiliar faces (Dawson, Carver, et al., 2002), reduced response in brain activity for fearful versus neutral faces (Dawson et al., 2004), and slower responses to faces and a larger response to objects (compared to faces), when compared to children with developmental delay and children who are developing typically (Webb et al., 2006).

GENETICS

Autism is one of the most heritable of all complex neuropsychiatric conditions, with heritability estimates of 60%–90% (Folstein and Rutter, 1977; Ritvo et al., 1985). The degree to which genetics contributes to ASD has been studied using twin and family studies, associations with known chromosomal abnormalities, statistical genetics techniques such as linkage and association studies, and specific candidate gene analysis (see Chapter 71 for further discussion of the role of genetics in psychiatric disorders). The current hypothesis is that there are multiple, as yet unidentified, genes that contribute to the etiology of this complex disorder via gene–gene, epigenetic, and gene–environment interactions. To date, the nature of the interrelationship between genetic and environmental factors is unknown. Although a "quasi-autistic pattern" was observed in a small fraction of Romanian orphans who were severely neglected (Rutter, Andersen-Wood, et al., 1999), not all of the orphaned children were impaired, suggesting that genetic susceptibility may have determined which children manifest autistic symptoms in response to the environmental stressors. Further, many but not all of the children who were affected improved following their adoption, suggesting that "resiliency genes" might also have played a role in determining symptom severity.

The study of autism genetics has exploded over the past two decades with the advent of more reliable diagnostic tests (Autism Diagnostic Interview—Revised and Autism Diagnostic Observation Scale), the establishment of large shared databases (Geschwind et al., 2001) and collaborative projects (Szatmari et al., 2007), and improved molecular and statistical genetics techniques. A PubMed Medline search using the search term *autism and genetics* lists more than 1,600 references, more than one half of which were published in the last 5 years. However, despite this intensive effort, there are no known "autism genes" to date. It is widely believed that the presence of significant genotypic and phenotypic heterogeneity has significantly hampered the search for autism susceptibility genes. A full review is beyond the scope of this chapter, but the key elements of current genetic research are reviewed.

Twin studies, the gold standard for determination of heritability, show a higher concordance for autism in monozygotic (36%–96%) than dizygotic twins (0%–23%) and further increased concordance for the broader autism spectrum (Folstein and Rutter, 1977; Ritvo et al., 1985; Steffenburg et al., 1989; Ritvo et al., 1991; Bailey et al., 1995; Le Couteur et al., 1996). Likewise, sibling recurrence rates are reported at 2%–6% from family studies (Rutter, Silberg, et al., 1999), compared to less than 1% risk in the general population. A number of investigators have ongoing studies looking prospectively at the infant siblings of children with ASD, and it is likely that these studies may give us a more accurate estimate.

The presence of the "broader autism phenotype" detected in the family members who do not have autism of an individual with ASD is another clue to heritability (Bailey et al., 1998). Researchers studying siblings and parents have documented less severe manifestations of ASD such as social and communicative impairments or stereotypic behaviors (Kanner, 1943; Piven et al., 1990; Landa et al., 1991; Piven et al., 1991; Landa et al., 1992; Bolton et al., 1994; Piven et al., 1994; Bailey et al., 1995; Smalley et al., 1995), higher rates of social phobia (Smalley et al., 1995; Piven and Palmer, 1999), obsessive–compulsive behaviors (Hollander, King, et al., 2003), and language delay and other language problems (Bartak et al., 1975; Landa et al., 1991; Landa et al., 1992; Bolton et al., 1994; Folstein et al., 1999).

Overall, it is estimated that 5%–9% of all ASD cases have identifiable chromosomal abnormalities (Lewis et al., 1995; Fombonne et al., 1997; Cook, 2001; Wassink et al., 2001). The most frequently associated conditions include Rett syndrome, Fragile X syndrome, tuberous sclerosis complex (TSC), and a maternally inherited duplication on chromosome 15q. It is important to note that though a high percentage of individuals with these disorders present with an autism phenotype, these disorders account for only a small percentage of all ASD cases. However, study of these syndromes and their genetic defects may provide insight into the molecular mechanisms leading to the pathophysiology of ASD. In TSC, the development of CNS lesions is believed to be due to alterations in neurogenesis and neuronal migration (Curatolo et al., 2002).The presence of seizures (especially infantile spasms) and mental retardation have been noted as risk factors for the development of autism in these patients (Gutierrez et al., 1998; Smalley, 1998). For a discussion of Rett syndome, Fragile X syndrome, and the 15q duplication syndrome, see Chapter 71.

Autism has also been reported in association with many other neurogenetic disorders, some with single gene etiology. These are usually case reports or small case series, so prevalence estimates are not available (either for autism within these disorders or for the occurrence of these disorders in autism populations). Some of these documented in the literature include neurofibromatosis (Gillberg and Forsell, 1984; P.G. Williams and Hersh, 1998), hypomelanosis of Ito (Zappella, 1993), Moebius syndrome (Gillberg and Steffenburg, 1989), Prader–Willi and Angelman syndrome (Steffenburg et al., 1996; Veltman et al., 2005), Joubert syndrome (Ozonoff et al., 1999), Down syndrome (Fombonne et al., 1997; Kent et al., 1999), Williams syndrome (Reiss et al., 1985), Sotos syndrome (Morrow et al., 1990), muscular dystrophy (Komoto et al., 1984; Zwaigenbaum and Tarnopolsky, 2003), Cowden syndrome (Goffin et al., 2001), Cohen syndrome (Howlin and Karpf, 2004), velocardiofacial syndrome (Fine et al., 2005), ARX mutations (Sherr, 2003), and Timothy syndrome (Splawski et al., 2004).

There also have been cases reported of autism occurring in some metabolic disorders such as untreated phenylketonuria (PKU) (Baieli et al., 2003) and Smith–Lemli–Opitz syndrome (SLO) (Tierney et al., 2001). These are especially important because they represent conditions where treatment is available. So, though these particular cases may represent "nonidiopathic" autism, many researchers feel that studying these specific defects is one important avenue to discovering autism susceptibility genes.

Other Chromosomal Abnormalities

The literature is full of case reports of patients with autism who have specific chromosomal anomalies (deletions, translocations, duplications) found on routine cytogenetic analysis. These involve almost every autosome and both sex chromosomes (for reviews, see Gillberg, 1998, and Lauritsen et al., 1999). Newer techniques such as those labeling subtelomeric rearrangements have identified these aberrations in autism as well (Borg et al., 2002; Wolff et al., 2002; Oliveira et al., 2003; Font-Montgomery et al., 2004). Finally, reports of mutations in specific genes known to be related to important neurodevelopmental functions are especially intriguing such as the protein tyrosine phosphatase (PTEN) mutations identified in a group of individuals with large head size (Butler et al., 2005). Protein tyrosine phosphatase is a tumor supressor gene that is known to function in the control of cell proliferation. For more discussion of relevant mutations, see Chapter 71.

Microdeletions and Duplications

Previously, studies reporting chromosomal abnormalities were produced with relatively low-resolution cytogenetic techniques, but recent developments in microarray technology have allowed comprehensive analysis of genome-wide copy number variation (CNV) in autism at much higher resolution. Arrays based on typing of polymorphic markers such as single nucleotide polymorphisms (SNPs) also allow one to assess non-Mendelian inheritance, if parents are also typed. An increase or decrease in hybridization signal or a pattern of non-Mendelian inheritance signals a potential CNV (Sebat et al., 2004). Recent reports show that de novo CNVs are detectable in as many as 10% of autism cases (Sebat et al., 2007; Szatmari et al., 2007). The rate in simplex families is higher than families where multiple members are affected (Sebat et al., 2007). These data so far suggest that the genetic architecture of simplex and multiplex autism may differ. Because most of the CNV are rare mutational events and only a few are seen recurrently, their exact etiological significance is still being debated. Some investigators propose that with increasing resolution of the technology for detection, these microdeletions/duplications may be identifiable in a much larger number of patients (Sebat et al., 2007).

The co-occurrence of autism with single gene disorders and other chromosomal anomalies may give us clues to the pathophysiology of ASD. In fact, some of the genes lie in regions that have also been linked to autism in genome scans (see below), and thus they represent promising candidates for autism susceptibility genes. However, it is generally believed that patients with these disorders are relatively rare and represent "secondary" cases or autism mimics. In general, autism is considered a complex neuropsychiatric disorder and as such is assumed to involve complex genetics with multiple genes at play. Past studies have proposed 2–10 (Pickles et al., 1995) or even 15–20 (Risch et al., 1999) interacting genes contributing to autism susceptibility. Jones proposed a risk factor model suggesting that each gene contributes a small amount to the risk for the disorder and that only individuals who cross a certain threshold will show the full phenotype (Jones and Szatmari, 2002). This could explain the broader phenotype in families who might have a cluster of subthreshold risk alleles (Veenstra-Vanderweele et al., 2003).

Disorders with complex genetics present researchers with many challenges. The search for these genes is made more difficult by the large number of genes, the phenotypic heterogeneity of the disorder, the existence of genetic heterogeneity, and the probability of gene–gene and gene–environment interactions. Nonetheless, this is a field with tremendous activity, and researchers are using many different approaches to identify chromosomal regions that may harbor autism susceptibility genes. A few of these techniques (for example, whole-genome scans, candidate gene analysis, endophenotype analysis) are discussed below.

Linkage

Since 1998, there have been 13 published whole-genome scans from eight different research groups (International

Molecular Genetic Study of Autism Consortium [IMGSAC], 1998; Barrett et al., 1999; Philippe et al., 1999; Risch et al., 1999; IMGSAC, 2001; Liu et al., 2001; Auranen et al., 2002; Shao et al., 2002; Yonan et al., 2003; Philippi et al., 2005; Schellenberg et al., 2006; Ylisaukko-Oja et al., 2006; Szatmari et al., 2007). With the exception of chromosome 7q, where the linkage has been supported by a meta-analysis (Badner and Gershon, 2002), the loci identified in many of these studies are neither definitive nor even consistent across studies. In addition to chromosome 7, regions of interest supported by very strong peaks or multiple studies include 2q (Philippe et al., 1999; IMGSAC, 2001; Buxbaum et al., 2002; Shao et al., 2002), 3 (Auranen et al., 2002; Shao et al., 2002; Ylisaukko-Oja et al., 2006), 4 (IMGSAC, 1998; Barrett et al., 1999; Yonan et al., 2003; Ylisaukko-Oja et al., 2006), 13 (Barrett et al., 1999), 16p (IMGSAC, 2001; Liu et al., 2001; Yonan et al., 2003; Philippi et al., 2005), and 17 (Risch et al., 1999; IMGSAC, 2001; Liu et al., 2001; Yonan et al., 2003; Stone et al., 2004; Cantor et al., 2005; Ylisaukko-Oja et al., 2006). Despite the strong male bias in ASD, the evidence for linkage to the X chromosome remains inconsistent, with only some groups showing suggestive linkage (Auranen et al., 2002; Shao et al., 2002; Yonan et al., 2003).

Overall, these results have been disappointing, with only nominal statistical significance and rare replication in independent samples. However, the inconsistencies do not necessarily signal that the identified regions are unimportant. Rather, methodological issues could be at play. The first is sample size. Because of the time and cost of data collection, small samples have been the rule. However, there has been a move towards collaboration in recent years, and larger samples are being made available to the scientific community for study. The first example of this was the creation of the Autism Genetic Resource Exchange (AGRE) a publicly available gene bank (www.agre.org) (Geschwind et al., 2001). Recently, an even larger collaborative effort has been launched with sponsorship by Autism Speaks. The Autism Genome Project (AGP) represents a combination of many of the existing autism genetic research programs in the United States and abroad with over 150 researchers from 50 institutions (Szatmari et al., 2007).

Another issue is the density of the genotype mapping (for example, the marker being studied could be too far from the actual locus). A final issue is that of genetic heterogeneity (that any given locus accounts for only a small fraction of the autism cases; Jones and Szatmari, 2002), and this is a harder issue to resolve. Perhaps the best example of this is in the results from the AGP, the largest genome scan to date (Szatmari et al., 2007). It was expected that increasing the sample size would result in increased power to detect susceptibility loci. But, despite a huge increase in sample size, results still did not reach genome-wide significance. Clearly, increasing sample size alone does not appear to be the answer. Thus, novel statistical techniques to reduce the impact of genetic heterogeneity and other methods, such as narrowing the phenotype to reduce phenotypic heterogeneity (for example, endophenotype analysis; see below), need to be employed.

Reducing Phenotypic Heterogeneity

Investigators have begun to use endophenotypes related to autism in an attempt to reduce heterogeneity and identify factors that may relate more closely to genetic etiologies than the current broad diagnostic categories. Endophenotypes are components of a more complex phenotype, such as behavioral, cognitive, morphologic, or biochemical features that may be more directly related to the underlying genetic etiologies (Gottesman and Gould, 2003). Narrowing a large and varied sample to those families who show only certain features of the phenotype has been shown to strengthen the linkage signal at various loci. The concept is that each of the many genetic risk factors underlying disease susceptibility may actually contribute to different aspects of the disease phenotype. This tool is especially powerful when applied to quantitative or continuous measures related to the disorder (for example, extent of language delay, severity of social deficit, or behavioral aberrations) rather than categorical definitions of disease (for example, autistic or normal) (Geschwind and Alarcon, 2006).

Endophenotypes that have been successfully utilized to strengthen linkage signals so far include the presence or severity of language delay, which has been linked to regions on chromosome 2q (Buxbaum et al., 2001; Shao et al., 2002; Spence et al., 2006), chromosome 7q (Barrett et al., 1999; Bradford et al., 2001; Alarcon et al., 2002), and chromosome 13q (Bradford et al., 2001). The presence of insistence on sameness (Shao et al., 2003) strengthened linkage on chromosome 15q at the region of the γ-aminobutyric acid (GABA) receptor beta 3 subunit (GABRB3) gene. One group also found strengthened linkage in the same region based on the savant skill endophenotype (Nurmi et al., 2003), but a recent attempt at replication in an independent sample failed (Mulder et al., 2005). Subsetting families according to the presence of obsessive–compulsive behaviors strengthened the signal on chromosome 17 (McCauley, Olson, Dowd, et al., 2004) and on chromosomes 6 and 19, as well as producing new evidence for linkage on chromosome 1 (Buxbaum et al., 2004). Finally, a recent study used the presence of regression in both siblings who were affected to stratify families from the AGRE sample and found relatively strong linkage peaks (NPL >3, $p < 10^{-4}$) despite a small sample size (34 families) (Molloy et al., 2005), but this was not replicated in an independent sample (Schellenberg et al., 2006). Even endophenotypes that do not define the syndrome, but are frequently found in association, such as head circumference, electrophysiologic measures, seizures, as well as new kinds of phenotypes such as gene-expression profiles from peripheral lymphoblasts, may be useful.

Candidate Gene Studies

Another approach taken by investigators is to identify candidate genes and test for their association with autism. Candidate genes can be chosen either because their function is believed to be involved in the underlying pathophysiology of autism (functional candidates) or because they are located in regions implicated in linkage studies (positional candidates). The strongest candidates are those that are positionally and functionally relevant. A large number of candidate genes have been examined in autism. But, like the linkage studies, the results remain inconsistent at best and conflicting at worst, with none having yielded evidence that can be interpreted as more than suggestive. And only a few have been replicated in independent samples.

The genes in which there has been special interest include those with functional relevance for the disorder. For instance, association has been reported with multiple genes involved in many different aspects of brain development: HOXA1 (Ingram et al., 2000) and ENGRAILED (Petit et al., 1995; Gharani et al., 2004) are involved in hindbrain development; REELIN is implicated in neuronal migration (Persico et al., 2001; Zhang et al., 2002; Bonora et al., 2003; Skaar et al., 2005); MET is involved with synaptogenesis (as well as in some non-CNS functions that also are implicated in ASD such as immune and gastrointestinal function) (Campbell et al., 2006). Other pathways of interest include axon path-finding and cellular proliferation (Geschwind and Levitt, 2007). Association has also been reported with genes that affect neurotransmitter systems, specifically: a GABA receptor subunit gene *GABRB3* (Cook et al., 1998; Buxbaum et al., 2002; McCauley, Olson, Delahanty, et al., 2004); a serotonin transporter gene *SCL6A* (Cook et al., 1997; Klauck et al., 1997; Tordjman et al., 2001; Yirmiya et al., 2001; S.J. Kim et al., 2002; Conroy et al., 2004); and a glutamate receptor gene *GRIN2A* (Barnby et al., 2005).

Gene Expression Profiling

With the advent of array technology, this is an area that is just beginning to be explored, but a recent study elegantly demonstrates the strength of this methodology. As proof of principle, Nishimura and colleagues (2007) demonstrated that expression profiling from lymphoblastoid cell lines can be used to differentiate between patients with autism secondary to single gene mutations (FRAX and 15q duplication syndrome). But in addition to identifying those genes differentially expressed between the two patient groups, they also identified a group of common genes that were disregulated compared to nonautistic controls. One with some functional relevance is a gene involved in GABA receptor expression and microtubule networks, *JAKMIP1*. By exploring these overlapping genes, they then identified a potential molecular link between FRAX and 15q duplication syndromes, the cytoplasmic FMR-1 interacting protein 1 (CYFIP1). This protein is up-regulated in the 15q duplication patients and is known to antagonize the gene product of the FMR-1 gene. The functional dependence of FMR1 and CYFIP1 was confirmed in neuronal cell culture, and they were able to show the effect of down-regulation of FMR-1 and up-regulation of CYFIP1 in two key downstream genes JAKMIP1 and GPR155. Turning back to the array technology, they went on to explore the association with autisms by demonstrating that these genes are also differentially expressed in idiopathic autism compared to nonautistic controls. Thus, this is a sophisticated multimodal demonstration of the power of gene expression profiling in identification of possible autism susceptibility loci.

PHARMACOTHERAPY OF PERVASIVE DEVELOPMENTAL DISORDERS

No pharmacologic agent has received Food and Drug Administration (FDA) indication for any core symptom of any of the disorders in the autism spectrum. To achieve such indication, a drug would need to be tested in relatively homogeneous and carefully described samples employing the gold standard double-blind placebo-controlled (DBPC) trials. To date, such trials have not been reported. On the other hand, drugs from many pharmacologic classes have been used in attempt to treat the troubling behaviors associated with ASD, and some have been tested in DBPC trials. To the extent that such drug trials may provide insight into the neurobiology of the disorder, the data are presented here. It must be kept in mind that the clinical picture of the autism spectrum may represent the final common pathway of abnormalities in a variety of brain regions or neurotransmitters and that these derangements may arise from a number of different etiologies. Thus, even a clinically homogenous sample may include patients with symptoms of differing etiologies.

It is instructive when reviewing the pharmacologic treatment of autism to note the experience with secretin. There was anecdotal evidence of benefit for behavioral symptoms in children with autism after they had received this hormone in the course of diagnostic studies (Horvath et al., 1998). But multiple subsequent controlled studies failed to corroborate the effectiveness of the treatment, despite great initial enthusiasm (Sturmey, 2005; K.W. Williams et al., 2005).

The most consistent neurochemical finding in autism has been elevation of whole blood serotonin (5-HT) in patients with autism (McDougle et al., 2003). Levels remain higher than in normal controls through adulthood, unaccounted for by race or medications. Parents and siblings of patients with autism have been reported to have elevated serotonin levels as well (Leboyer et al., 1999).On the other hand, cerebrospinal fluid serotonin metabolite (5-hydroxyindoleacetic acid, [HIAA]) has not been found to be elevated in children with autism compared to controls (Gillberg, Svennerholm, and Hamilton-Hellberg, 1983; Gillberg and Svennerholm, 1987; Narayan et al., 1993). Challenge tests have suggested reduced central 5-HT response (Hoshino et al., 1985; McBride et al., 1989) and increased sensitivity of the 5-HT_{1D} receptor in patients with autism (Hollander et al., 2000; Novotny et al., 2000). Acute tryptophan (serotonin precursor) depletion led to worsening of repetitive behaviors in a sample of adults with autism (McDougle et al., 1993; McDougle, Naylor, Cohen, Aghajanian, et al., 1996). In short, the data implicate the serotonin system, but without clarifying a mechanism.

The few controlled trials using selective serotonin reuptake inhibitors (SSRIs) seem to show benefit among adults (McDougle, Naylor, Cohen, Volkmar, et al., 1996; Buchsbaum et al., 2001; Hollander et al., 2005) as well as in reducing repetitive behaviors among children and adolescents with ASD (Hollander et al., 2005). Larger studies are under way that will attempt to corroborate the effectiveness of SSRIs for repetitive behaviors in autism, as well as a longer term study in very young patients attempting to improve core autistic symptoms.

The data implicating the dopamine (DA) system are largely clinical and based on the effectiveness of DA-blocking drugs in treating symptoms frequently troubling to patients with autism. Peripheral measures of DA or its metabolite homovanillic acid (HVA) or of prolactin level (a surrogate for dopamine function) have failed to find significant differences so far between patients with autism and controls (Launay et al., 1987; Minderaa et al., 1994). Measures of HVA in cerebrospinal fluid have largely demonstrated no differences between patients with autism and controls (Narayan et al., 1993).

The Research Units on Pediatric Psychopharmacology (RUPP; 2005), a consortium of five university medical center research facilities, conducted a trial of risperidone because of its anecdotal effectiveness. In a placebo controlled trial of 101 children with autism, irritability, hyperactivity, and aggression were all significantly improved after 8 weeks (McCracken et al., 2002). A further analysis of the data suggests that there also may have been significant improvements in the core symptoms of restricted, repetitive, and stereotyped behaviors of ASD (McDougle et al., 2005). Other investigators, in a randomized DBPC trial of risperidone in 79 children, found there were significant improvements in the frequently associated symptoms of aggression, self-injury, and tantrums (Shea et al., 2004). On the basis of these findings, risperidone was recently granted approval by the FDA for the treatment of irritability and other behavioral symptoms in children with ASD.

The other monoamine neurotransmitter, norepinephrine (NE), has been measured, along with its metabolite *3-methoxy-4-hydroxyphenylglycol* (MHPG) in patients with autism. In one study, peripheral NE was found to be higher in patients with autism than in controls, and the enzyme *DA-β-hydroxylase* (converting dopamine to NE) was lower in patients and in their family members (Lake et al., 1977). However, plasma MHPG was found to be similar in patients with autism and controls in two studies (J.G. Young et al., 1981; Minderaa et al., 1994), and urinary NE and metabolite were similar overnight in one of the studies (Minderaa et al., 1994). Cerebrospinal fluid MHPG was found similar to controls in two studies of patients with autism (J.G. Young et al., 1981; Gillberg et al., 1983).

Pharmacologic trials partially confirm the results of these investigations. Tricyclic antidepressants and the α-adrenergic agonists *clonidine* and *guanfacine* have been used for symptoms of hyperactivity and inattention in open-label trials. Desipramine and clomipramine have been found to be differentially effective in the repetitive behaviors in autism (Gordon et al., 1992; McDougle et al., 1992; Gordon et al., 1993). In two small controlled trials, clonidine was found to be effective for irritability and hyperactivity in some children with autism (Jaselskis et al., 1992) and in improving social relationships in some children and adults with autism (Fankhauser et al., 1992).

The RUPP consortium conducted a controlled crossover trial of methylphenidate among 66 children with autism who were able to tolerate a test dose. Optimal dose was determined in blinded fashion, and that dose was continued in open-label follow-on study. The stimulant was superior to placebo for hyperactivity in these children, but less effective than in children who were developing typically, and there were more adverse effects (RUPP, 2005). Because there were no effects on core autism symptoms, it is not clear what this trial reveals about the neurobiology of ASD.

There has been hypothetical consideration of glutamate dysfunction in autism (Carlsson, 1998). Thus far, peripheral measures of this amino acid, the primary excitatory neurotransmitter in the brain, have been inconsistent. Some investigators have found elevation of glutamate in patients with autism (and family members) (Moreno-Fuenmayor et al., 1996; Aldred et al., 2003). But another study found lower glutamate in patients with autism compared to age-matched controls (Rolf et al., 1993). Other studies support a disorder of glutamate neurotransmission or receptors (Purcell et al., 2001; Fatemi et al., 2002; Shinohe et al., 2006).

A few controlled trials have sustained the interest in use of glutamatergic agents for autism. Amantadine, a glutamate *N*-methyl-D-aspartate (NMDA) receptor antagonist, was found to be effective for some symptoms in young patients with autism in a controlled trial (King et al., 2001). A partial NMDA agonist, D-cycloserine, also produced significantly greater symptom improvements than placebo in a small group of children with autism, including changes in a core symptom, social responsiveness (Posey et al., 2004). However, a drug that reduces glutamate release, lamotrigine, had no significant effect over placebo (Belsito et al., 2001). A study has just commenced at the National Institute of Mental Health in which riluzole, a glutamate antagonist, will be compared with placebo in children and adolescents with ASD and obsessive–compulsive symptoms. Riluzole has not previously been evaluated for treatment of autistic symptoms, but has shown benefits in childhood-onset obsessive–compulsive disorder (OCD) (Grant et al., 2007).

γ-Amino butyric acid is an amino acid that acts as an inhibitory neurotransmitter in the brain. γ-Amino butyric acid-ergic drugs, in particular the benzodiazepines, are known to be disinhibiting even among healthy children and may exacerbate dyscontrol in patients with autism. However, the key role of GABA in neurocircuits postulated to be involved in autistic behaviors suggests that modulation of GABA may be of therapeutic benefit. One reported trial of a GABA antagonist, flumazenil, in a small number of patients with autism was promising enough to suggest testing its benefits in a larger sample (Wray et al., 2000).

The cholinergic neurotransmitter system has not been investigated with DBPC studies, but some open-label trials of cholinesterase inhibitors have been suggestive of benefit in adults and children with ASD (Hardan and Handen, 2002; Hertzman, 2003; Chez et al., 2004).

Because of their evident importance in the affiliative behaviors in rodents (L.J. Young et al., 2001; Winslow and Insel, 2004), the peptides oxytocin (OT) and vasopressin (AVP) have been investigated in ASD (Panksepp, 1993; Insel et al., 1999; L.J. Young et al., 2002). One group of young males with autism has been found to have lower plasma OT levels compared to controls (Modahl et al., 1998). But only a single study has tested therapeutic effect of OT in patients with autism (Hollander, Novotny, et al., 2003), perhaps because the drug must be administered intravenously and has such a short half-life. That study failed to find significant effect. Further studies will certainly be forthcoming as a long-acting agent becomes available.

Any number of other neuroactive chemicals have been investigated in autism, including hormones, opioids, steroids, and others (for example, melatonin). Only negative results have been reported so far in controlled studies. Vitamins and nutritional supplements are also used, but to date, none has been found uniquely efficacious in a controlled trial.

Although studies indicate that up to 75% of individuals with autism take psychotropic medications for problem behaviors associated with autism (Tsakanikos et al., 2007), virtually all individuals with autism receive behavioral/educational treatment of some form or another throughout their lifetime. Although no medication has yet been found to target core features of autism, controlled trials have found efficacy for some behavioral treatments on outcomes such as cognitive and adaptive functioning. Specifically, comprehensive early intervention approaches (often consisting of variants of applied behavior analysis) have been found to be efficacious in young children, with variable effects depending on factors such as age, amount and duration of treatment, and pretreatment level of functioning (Howard et al., 2005; Cohen et al., 2006). In addition, parent training is a frequently used behavioral technique with reports of benefit (Brookman-Frazee et al., 2006), and there are numerous reports of the utility of therapies targeting specific symptoms, such as specific educational programs, speech/language therapy, occupational therapy, physical therapy, and social skills training. Most children receive a combination of therapeutic interventions, as is fitting for such a complex neuropsychiatric disorder. The RUPP consortium is currently testing a combination of interventions including risperidone and parent training, hypothesizing that this combination will boost the effects found in the risperidone-only trial, and thus exemplifying a comprehensive approach to combining pharmacologic and behavioral treatment.

FUTURE DIRECTIONS

Determining the etiopathogenesis of autism and its related disorders will require increased research into the neurobiology of normal human development, as well as additional efforts directed at fully characterizing the social and communication deficits central to ASD. One of the first steps in this effort is to define the biological and behavioral manifestations of the various "autisms"—groups of patients who not only share clinical characteristics in common, but also have commonalities of etiology, pathophysiology, and prognosis. Such phenotyping efforts are ongoing at several centers, including the newly established autism research program at the National Institute of Mental Health. It is hoped that delineating clinically homogeneous subgroups of patients will result in cleaner research populations and increase the chances of finding the underlying pathology. By concentrating on smaller segments of the population of ASD, it is also possible to provide more meaningful recommendations for therapeutic interventions.

Genetic investigations should continue in autism, but they need to be conducted with well-phenotyped populations and to take phenotypic heterogeneity into the analyses. It is expected that genetic research will focus less on single-genetic disorders in the future and focus more on gene–gene and gene–environment interactions. Increased attention should be paid to the role that environmental factors play in the etiology of autism, as all agree that the environment appears intimately involved in the etiopathogenesis of autism. In addition, well-designed epidemiologic studies are needed to determine the true prevalence rates of autism, and to determine changes across time in incidence. Such studies may pinpoint the introduction of an environmental trigger for autism, just as forensic epidemiologic approaches were successful in determining the disease-producing effects of asbestos, cigarette smoking, and other agents.

Although the major thrust of autism research must remain focused on discovering the cause and cure of autism, "until then" research is also essential. Currently, there are no pharmacologic therapies for the core symptoms of autism, and only a few medications available for the associated medical and neuropsychiatric symptoms. New treatments need to be developed, tested, and made available to individuals who are impaired. Existing behavioral interventions need to be subjected to appropriate evaluations of efficacy and effectiveness in "real-world" settings. When the results of such studies are known, they need to be transmitted quickly to clinicians, so that every individual with autism receives the best possible standard of care.

ACKNOWLEDGMENTS

This work was written as part of our official duties as government employees. The article is freely available for publication without a copyright notice, and there are no restrictions on its use, now or subsequently. The views expressed in this chapter do not necessarily represent the views of the National Institute of Mental Health, National Institutes of Health, Department of Health and Human Services, or the United States government.

REFERENCES

Alarcon, M., Cantor, R. M., Liu, J., Gilliam, T. C., and Geschwind, D. H. (2002) Evidence for a language quantitative trait locus on chromosome 7q in multiplex autism families. *Am. J. Hum. Genet.* 70(1):60–71.

Aldred, S., Moore, K. M., Fitzgerald, M., and Waring, R. H. (2003) Plasma amino acid levels in children with autism and their families. *J. Autism Dev. Disord.* 33(1):93–97.

American Psychiatric Association. (1994) *Diagnostic and Statistical Manual of Mental Disorders*, 4th ed. Washington, DC: Author.

American Psychiatric Association. (2000) *Diagnostic and Statistical Manual of Mental Disorders*, text rev. Washington, DC: Author.

Amir, R.E., Van den Veyver, I.B., Wan, M., Tran, C.Q., Francke, U., and Zoghbi, H.Y. (1999) Rett syndrome is caused by mutations in x-linked MECP2, encoding methyl-CPG-binding protein 2. *Nat. Genet.* 23(2):185–188.

Amodio, D.M., and Frith, C.D. (2006) Meeting of minds: The medial frontal cortex and social cognition. *Nat. Rev. Neurosci.* 7(4):268–277.

Ashwood, P., and Van de Water, J. (2004) Is autism an autoimmune disease? *Autoimmun. Rev.* 3(7/8):557–562.

Ashwood, P., and Wakefield, A.J. (2006) Immune activation of peripheral blood and mucosal CD3+ lymphocyte cytokine profiles in children with autism and gastrointestinal symptoms. *J. Neuroimmunol.* 173(1/2):126–134.

Auranen, M., Vanhala, R., Varilo, T., Ayers, K., Kempas, E., Ylisaukko-Oja, T., Sinsheimer, J.S., Peltonen, L., and Jarvela, I. (2002) A genomewide screen for autism-spectrum disorders: Evidence for a major susceptibility locus on chromosome 3q25-27. *Am. J. Hum. Genet.* 71(4):777–790.

Aylward, E.H., Minshew, N.J., Field, K., Sparks, B.F., and Singh, N. (2002) Effects of age on brain volume and head circumference in autism. *Neurology* 59(2):175–183.

Aylward, E.H., Minshew, N.J., Goldstein, G., Honeycutt, N.A., Augustine, A.M., Yates, K.O., Barta, P.E., and Pearlson, G.D. (1999) MRI volumes of amygdala and hippocampus in non-mentally retarded autistic adolescents and adults. *Neurology* 53(9):2145–2150.

Badner, J.A., and Gershon, E.S. (2002) Regional meta-analysis of published data supports linkage of autism with markers on chromosome 7. *Mol. Psychiatry* 7(1):56–66.

Baieli, S., Pavone, L., Meli, C., Fiumara, A., and Coleman, M. (2003) Autism and phenylketonuria. *J. Autism Dev. Disord.* 33(2):201–204.

Bailey, A., Le Couteur, A., Gottesman, I., Bolton, P., Simonoff, E., Yuzda, E., and Rutter, M. (1995) Autism as a strongly genetic disorder: Evidence from a British twin study. *Psychol. Med.* 25(1):63–77.

Bailey, A., Palferman, S., Heavey, L., and Le Couteur, A. (1998) Autism: The phenotype in relatives. *J. Autism Dev. Disord.* 28(5): 369–392.

Ballaban-Gil, K., and Tuchman, R. (2000) Epilepsy and epileptiform EEG: Association with autism and language disorders. *Ment. Retard. Dev. Disabil. Res. Rev.* 6(4):300–308.

Barnby, G., Abbott, A., Sykes, N., Morris, A., Weeks, D.E., Mott, R., Lamb, J., Bailey, A.J., and Monaco, A.P. (2005) Candidate-gene screening and association analysis at the autism-susceptibility locus on chromosome 16p: Evidence of association at GRIN2A and ABAT. *Am. J. Hum. Genet.* 76(6):950–966.

Baron-Cohen, S., Leslie, A.M., and Frith, U. (1985) Does the autistic child have a "theory of mind"? *Cognition* 21(1):37–46.

Barrett, S., Beck, J.C., Bernier, R., Bisson, E., Braun, T.A., Casavant, T.L., Childress, D., Folstein, S.E., Garcia, M., Gardiner, M.B., Gilman, S., Haines, J.L., Hopkins, K., Landa, R., Meyer, N.H., Mullane, J.A., Nishimura, D.Y., Palmer, P., Piven, J., Purdy, J., Santangelo, S.L., Searby, C., Sheffield, V., Singleton, J., Slager, S., et al. (1999) An autosomal genomic screen for autism. Collaborative linkage study of autism. *Am. J. Med. Genet.* 88(6):609–615.

Bartak, L., Rutter, M., and Cox, A. (1975) A comparative study of infantile autism and specific development receptive language disorder. I. The children. *Br. J. Psychiatry* 126:127–145.

Bauman, M.L., and Kemper, T.L. (2005) Neuroanatomic observations of the brain in autism: A review and future directions. *Int. J. Dev. Neurosci.* 23(2/3):183–187.

Belsito, K.M., Law, P.A., Kirk, K.S., Landa, R.J., and Zimmerman, A.W. (2001) Lamotrigine therapy for autistic disorder: A randomized, double-blind, placebo-controlled trial. *J. Autism Dev. Disord.* 31(2):175–181.

Bolton, P., Macdonald, H., Pickles, A., Rios, P., Goode, S., Crowson, M., Bailey, A., and Rutter, M. (1994) A case-control family history study of autism. *J. Child Psychol. Psychiatry* 35(5):877–900.

Bonora, E., Beyer, K.S., Lamb, J.A., Parr, J.R., Klauck, S.M., Benner, A., Paolucci, M., Abbott, A., Ragoussis, I., Poustka, A., Bailey, A.J., and Monaco, A.P. (2003) Analysis of REELIN as a candidate gene for autism. *Mol. Psychiatry* 8(10):885–892.

Borg, I., Squire, M., Menzel, C., Stout, K., Morgan, D., Willatt, L., O'Brien, P.C., Ferguson-Smith, M.A., Ropers, H.H., Tommerup, N., Kalscheuer, V.M., and Sargan, D.R. (2002) A cryptic deletion of 2q35 including part of the PAX3 gene detected by breakpoint mapping in a child with autism and a de novo 2;8 translocation. *J. Med. Genet.* 39(6):391–399.

Bradford, Y., Haines, J., Hutcheson, H., Gardiner, M., Braun, T., Sheffield, V., Cassavant, T., Huang, W., Wang, K., Vieland, V., Folstein, S., Santangelo, S., and Piven, J. (2001) Incorporating language phenotypes strengthens evidence of linkage to autism. *Am. J. Med. Genet.* 105(6):539–547.

Brambilla, P., Hardan, A.Y., di Nemi, S.U., Caverzasi, E., Soares, J.C., Perez, J., and Barale, F. (2004) The functional neuroanatomy of autism. *Funct. Neurol.* 19(1):9–17.

Brookman-Frazee, L., Stahmer, A., Baker-Ericzen, M.J., and Tsai, K. (2006) Parenting interventions for children with autism spectrum and disruptive behavior disorders: Opportunities for cross-fertilization. *Clin. Child Fam. Psychol. Rev.* 9(3/4):181–200.

Buchsbaum, M.S., Hollander, E., Haznedar, M.M., Tang, C., Spiegel-Cohen, J., Wei, T.C., Solimando, A., Buchsbaum, B.R., Robins, D., Bienstock, C., Cartwright, C., and Mosovich, S. (2001) Effect of fluoxetine on regional cerebral metabolism in autistic spectrum disorders: A pilot study. *Int. J. Neuropsychopharmacol.* 4(2):119–125.

Butler, M.G., Dasouki, M.J., Zhou, X.P., Talebizadeh, Z., Brown, M., Takahashi, T.N., Miles, J.H., Wang, C.H., Stratton, R., Pilarski, R., and Eng, C. (2005) Subset of individuals with autism spectrum disorders and extreme macrocephaly associated with germline PTEN tumour suppressor gene mutations. *J. Med. Genet.* 42(4):318–321.

Buxbaum, J.D., Silverman, J., Keddache, M., Smith, C.J., Hollander, E., Ramoz, N., and Reichert, J.G. (2004) Linkage analysis for autism in a subset families with obsessive-compulsive behaviors: Evidence for an autism susceptibility gene on chromosome 1 and further support for susceptibility genes on chromosome 6 and 19. *Mol. Psychiatry* 9(2):144–150.

Buxbaum, J.D., Silverman, J.M., Smith, C.J., Greenberg, D.A., Kilifarski, M., Reichert, J., Cook, E.H., Jr., Fang, Y., Song, C.Y., and Vitale, R. (2002) Association between a GABRB3 polymorphism and autism. *Mol. Psychiatry* 7(3):311–316.

Buxbaum, J.D., Silverman, J.M., Smith, C.J., Kilifarski, M., Reichert, J., Hollander, E., Lawlor, B.A., Fitzgerald, M., Greenberg, D.A., and Davis, K.L. (2001) Evidence for a susceptibility gene for autism on chromosome 2 and for genetic heterogeneity. *Am. J. Hum. Genet.* 68(6):1514–1520.

Campbell, D.B., Sutcliffe, J.S., Ebert, P.J., Militerni, R., Bravaccio, C., Trillo, S., Elia, M., Schneider, C., Melmed, R., Sacco, R., Persico, A.M., and Levitt, P. (2006) A genetic variant that disrupts met transcription is associated with autism. *Proc. Natl. Acad. Sci. USA* 103(45):16834–16839.

Cantor, R.M., Kono, N., Duvall, J.A., Alvarez-Retuerto, A., Stone, J.L., Alarcon, M., Nelson, S.F., and Geschwind, D.H. (2005) Replication of autism linkage: Fine-mapping peak at 17q21. *Am. J. Hum. Genet.* 76(6):1050–1056.

Carlsson, M.L. (1998) Hypothesis: Is infantile autism a hypoglutamatergic disorder? Relevance of glutamate–serotonin interactions for pharmacotherapy. *J. Neural Transm.* 105(4/5):525–535.

Carper, R.A., Moses, P., Tigue, Z.D., and Courchesne, E. (2002) Cerebral lobes in autism: Early hyperplasia and abnormal age effects. *NeuroImage* 16(4):1038–1051.

Chakrabarti, S., and Fombonne, E. (2001) Pervasive developmental disorders in preschool children. *JAMA* 285(24):3093–3099.

Chez, M.G., Aimonovitch, M., Buchanan, T., Mrazek, S., and Tremb, R.J. (2004) Treating autistic spectrum disorders in children: Utility of the cholinesterase inhibitor rivastigmine tartrate. *J. Child Neurol.* 19(3):165–169.

Chez, M.G., Chang, M., Krasne, V., Coughlan, C., Kominsky, M., and Schwartz, A. (2006) Frequency of epileptiform EEG abnormalities in a sequential screening of autistic patients with no known clinical epilepsy from 1996 to 2005. *Epilepsy Behav.* 8(1):267–271.

Cohen, H., Amerine-Dickens, M., and Smith, T. (2006) Early intensive behavioral treatment: Replication of the UCLA model in a community setting. *J. Dev. Behav. Pediatr.* 27(2 Suppl):S145–S155.

Comi, A.M., Zimmerman, A.W., Frye, V.H., Law, P.A., and Peeden, J.N. (1999) Familial clustering of autoimmune disorders and evaluation of medical risk factors in autism. *J. Child Neurol.* 14(6):388–394.

Connolly, A.M., Chez, M.G., Pestronk, A., Arnold, S.T., Mehta, S., and Deuel, R.K. (1999) Serum autoantibodies to brain in Landau-Kleffner variant, autism, and other neurologic disorders. *J. Pediatr.* 134(5):607–613.

Connolly, A.M., Chez, M., Streif, E.M., Keeling, R.M., Golumbek, P.T., Kwon, J.M., Riviello, J.J., Robinson, R.G., Neuman, R.J., and Deuel, R.M. (2006) Brain-derived neurotrophic factor and autoantibodies to neural antigens in sera of children with autistic spectrum disorders, Landau-Kleffner syndrome, and epilepsy. *Biol. Psychiatry* 59(4):354–363.

Conroy, J., Meally, E., Kearney, G., Fitzgerald, M., Gill, M., and Gallagher, L. (2004) Serotonin transporter gene and autism: A haplotype analysis in an Irish autistic population. *Mol. Psychiatry* 9(6):587–593.

Cook, E. H. Jr. (2001) Genetics of autism. *Child Adolesc. Psychiatr. Clin. N. Am.* 10(2):333–350.

Cook, E. H., Jr., Courchesne, R.Y., Cox, N.J., Lord, C., Gonen, D., Guter, S.J., Lincoln, A., Nix, K., Haas, R., Leventhal, B.L., and Courchesne, E. (1998) Linkage-disequilibrium mapping of autistic disorder, with 15q11-13 markers. *Am. J. Hum. Genet.* 62(5): 1077–1083.

Cook, E. H., Jr., Courchesne, R., Lord, C., Cox, N.J., Yan, S., Lincoln, A., Haas, R., Courchesne, E., and Leventhal, B.L. (1997) Evidence of linkage between the serotonin transporter and autistic disorder. *Mol. Psychiatry* 2(3):247–250.

Courchesne, E. (2004) Brain development in autism: Early overgrowth followed by premature arrest of growth. *Ment. Retard. Dev. Disabil. Res. Rev.* 10(2):106–111.

Courchesne, E., Carper, R., and Akshoomoff, N. (2003) Evidence of brain overgrowth in the first year of life in autism. *JAMA* 290(3): 337–344.

Courchesne, E., Karns, C.M., Davis, H.R., Ziccardi, R., Carper, R.A., Tigue, Z.D., Chisum, H.J., Moses, P., Pierce, K., Lord, C., Lincoln, A.J., Pizzo, S., Schreibman, L., Haas, R.H., Akshoomoff, N.A., and Courchesne, R.Y. (2001) Unusual brain growth patterns in early life in patients with autistic disorder: An MRI study. *Neurology* 57(2):245–254.

Courchesne, E., Yeung-Courchesne, R., Press, G.A., Hesselink, J.R., and Jernigan, T.L. (1988) Hypoplasia of cerebellar vermal lobules vi and vii in autism. *N. Engl. J. Med.* 318(21):1349–1354.

Croonenberghs, J., Wauters, A., Devreese, K., Verkerk, R., Scharpe, S., Bosmans, E., Egyed, B., Deboutte, D., and Maes, M. (2002) Increased serum albumin, gamma globulin, immunoglobulin IGG, and IGG2 and IGG4 in autism. *Psychol. Med.* 32(8): 1457–1463.

Curatolo, P., Verdecchia, M., and Bombardieri, R. (2002) Tuberous sclerosis complex: A review of neurological aspects. *Eur. J. Paediatr. Neurol.* 6(1):15–23.

Dalton, K.M., Nacewicz, B.M., Johnstone, T., Schaefer, H.S., Gernsbacher, M.A., Goldsmith, H.H., Alexander, A.L., and

Davidson, R.J. (2005) Gaze fixation and the neural circuitry of face processing in autism. *Nat. Neurosci.* 8(4):519–526.

Dapretto, M., Davies, M.S., Pfeifer, J.H., Scott, A.A., Sigman, M., Bookheimer, S.Y., and Iacoboni, M. (2006) Understanding emotions in others: Mirror neuron dysfunction in children with autism spectrum disorders. *Nat. Neurosci.* 9(1):28–30.

Dawson, G., Carver, L., Meltzoff, A.N., Panagiotides, H., McPartland, J., and Webb, S.J. (2002) Neural correlates of face and object recognition in young children with autism spectrum disorder, developmental delay, and typical development. *Child Dev.* 73(3):700–717.

Dawson, G., Munson, J., Estes, A., Osterling, J., McPartland, J., Toth, K., Carver, L., and Abbott, R. (2002) Neurocognitive function and joint attention ability in young children with autism spectrum disorder versus developmental delay. *Child Dev.* 73(2):345–358.

Dawson, G., Toth, K., Abbott, R., Osterling, J., Munson, J., Estes, A., and Liaw, J. (2004) Early social attention impairments in autism: Social orienting, joint attention, and attention to distress. *Dev. Psychol.* 40(2):271–283.

Dawson, G., Webb, S.J., Carver, L., Panagiotides, H., and McPartland, J. (2004) Young children with autism show atypical brain responses to fearful versus neutral facial expressions of emotion. *Dev. Sci.* 7(3):340–359.

Dementieva, Y.A., Vance, D.D., Donnelly, S.L., Elston, L.A., Wolpert, C.M., Ravan, S.A., DeLong, G.R., Abramson, R.K., Wright, H. H., and Cuccaro, M.L. (2005) Accelerated head growth in early development of individuals with autism. *Pediatr. Neurol.* 32(2): 102–108.

DiCicco-Bloom, E., Lord, C., Zwaigenbaum, L., Courchesne, E., Dager, S.R., Schmitz, C., Schultz, R.T., Crawley, J., and Young, L.J. (2006) The developmental neurobiology of autism spectrum disorder. *J. Neurosci.* 26(26):6897–6906.

Fankhauser, M.P., Karumanchi, V.C., German, M.L., Yates, A., and Karumanchi, S.D. (1992) A double-blind, placebo-controlled study of the efficacy of transdermal clonidine in autism. *J. Clin. Psychiatry* 53(3):77–82.

Fatemi, S.H., Halt, A.R., Stary, J.M., Kanodia, R., Schulz, S.C., and Realmuto, G.R. (2002) Glutamic acid decarboxylase 65 and 67 KDA proteins are reduced in autistic parietal and cerebellar cortices. *Biol. Psychiatry* 52(8):805–810.

Fidler, D.J., Bailey, J.N., and Smalley, S.L. (2000) Macrocephaly in autism and other pervasive developmental disorders. *Dev. Med. Child Neurol.* 42(11):737–740.

Fine, S.E., Weissman, A., Gerdes, M., Pinto-Martin, J., Zackai, E. H., McDonald-McGinn, D.M., and Emanuel, B.S. (2005) Autism spectrum disorders and symptoms in children with molecularly confirmed 22q11.2 deletion syndrome. *J. Autism Dev. Disord.* 35(4):461–470.

Folstein, S., and Rutter, M. (1977) Infantile autism: A genetic study of 21 twin pairs. *J. Child Psychol. Psychiatry* 18(4):297–321.

Folstein, S.E., Santangelo, S.L., Gilman, S.E., Piven, J., Landa, R., Lainhart, J., Hein, J., and Wzorek, M. (1999) Predictors of cognitive test patterns in autism families. *J. Child Psychol. Psychiatry* 40(7):1117–1128.

Fombonne, E. (2005) Epidemiology of autistic disorder and other pervasive developmental disorders. *J. Clin. Psychiatry* 66(Suppl 10):3–8.

Fombonne, E., Du Mazaubrun, C., Cans, C., and Grandjean, H. (1997) Autism and associated medical disorders in a French epidemiological survey. *J. Am. Acad. Child Adolesc. Psychiatry* 36(11):1561–1569.

Fombonne, E., Roge, B., Claverie, J., Courty, S., and Fremolle, J. (1999) Microcephaly and macrocephaly in autism. *J. Autism Dev. Disord.* 29(2):113–119.

Font-Montgomery, E., Weaver, D.D., Walsh, L., Christensen, C., and Thurston, V.C. (2004) Clinical and cytogenetic manifestations of subtelomeric aberrations: Report of six cases. *Birth Defects Res. Part A Clin. Mol. Teratol.* 70(6):408–415.

Frith, C.D., and Frith, U. (2006) The neural basis of mentalizing. *Neuron* 50(4):531–534.

Geschwind, D.H., and Alarcon, M. (2006) Finding genes in spite of genetic heterogeneity: Endopenotypes, QTL mapping, and expression profiling in autism. In: Moldin S.O., and Rubenstein, J.L.R., eds. *Finding Genes in Spite of Genetic Heterogeneity: Endopenotypes, QTL Mapping, and Expression Profiling in Autism.* Boca Raton: CRC Press, 75–93.

Geschwind, D.H., and Levitt, P. (2007) Autism spectrum disorders: Developmental disconnection syndromes. *Curr. Opin. Neurobiol.* 17(1):103–111.

Geschwind, D.H., Sowinski, J., Lord, C., Iversen, P., Shestack, J., Jones, P., Ducat, L., and Spence, S.J. (2001) The autism genetic resource exchange: A resource for the study of autism and related neuropsychiatric conditions. *Am. J. Hum. Genet.* 69(2): 463–466.

Gharani, N., Benayed, R., Mancuso, V., Brzustowicz, L.M., and Millonig, J.H. (2004) Association of the homeobox transcription factor, engrailed 2, with autism spectrum disorder. *Mol. Psychiatry* 9(5):540.

Ghaziuddin, M., and Butler, E. (1998) Clumsiness in autism and Asperger syndrome: A further report. *J. Intellect. Disabil. Res.* 42(Pt 1):43–48.

Gillberg, C. (1998) Chromosomal disorders and autism. *J. Autism Dev. Disord.* 28(5):415–425.

Gillberg, C., and Forsell, C. (1984) Childhood psychosis and neurofibromatosis—more than a coincidence? *J. Autism Dev. Disord.* 14(1):1–8.

Gillberg, C., and Steffenburg, S. (1989) Autistic behaviour in Moebius syndrome. *Acta Paediatr. Scand.* 78(2):314–316.

Gillberg, C., and Svennerholm, L. (1987) CSF monoamines in autistic syndromes and other pervasive developmental disorders of early childhood. *Br. J. Psychiatry* 151:89–94.

Gillberg, C., Svennerholm, L., and Hamilton-Hellberg, C. (1983) Childhood psychosis and monoamine metabolites in spinal fluid. *J. Autism Dev. Disord.* 13(4):383–396.

Goffin, A., Hoefsloot, L.H., Bosgoed, E., Swillen, A., and Fryns, J.P. (2001) PTEN mutation in a family with Cowden syndrome and autism. *Am. J. Med. Genet.* 105(6):521–524.

Gordon, C.T., Rapoport, J.L., Hamburger, S.D., State, R.C., and Mannheim, G.B. (1992) Differential response of seven subjects with autistic disorder to clomipramine and desipramine. *Am. J. Psychiatry* 149(3):363–366.

Gordon, C.T., State, R.C., Nelson, J.E., Hamburger, S.D., and Rapoport, J.L. (1993) A double-blind comparison of clomipramine, desipramine, and placebo in the treatment of autistic disorder. *Arch. Gen. Psychiatry* 50(6):441–447.

Gotham, K., Risi, S., Pickles, A., and Lord, C. (2007) The autism diagnostic observation schedule: Revised algorithms for improved diagnostic validity. *J. Autism Dev. Disord.* 37(4):613–627.

Gottesman, I.I., and Gould, T.D. (2003) The endophenotype concept in psychiatry: Etymology and strategic intentions. *Am. J. Psychiatry* 160(4):636–645.

Grant, P., Lougee, L., Hirschtritt, M. and Swedo, S.E. (2007) An open-label trial of riluzole, a glutamate antagonist, in children with treatment resistant obsessive-compulsive disorder. *J Child Adolesc Psychopharmacol.* 17(6):761–767.

Gutierrez, G.C., Smalley, S.L., and Tanguay, P.E. (1998) Autism in tuberous sclerosis complex. *J. Autism Dev. Disord.* 28(2):97–103.

Happe, F., Ronald, A., and Plomin, R. (2006) Time to give up on a single explanation for autism. *Nat. Neurosci.* 9(10):1218–1220.

Hardan, A.Y., and Handen, B.L. (2002) A retrospective open trial of adjunctive donepezil in children and adolescents with autistic disorder. *J. Child Adolesc. Psychopharmacol.* 12(3):237–241.

Haxby, J.V., and Ida Gobbini, M. (2007) The perception of emotion and social cues in faces. *Neuropsychologia* 45(1):1.

Hazlett, H.C., Poe, M.D., Gerig, G., Smith, R.G., and Piven, J. (2006) Cortical gray and white brain tissue volume in adolescents and adults with autism. *Biol. Psychiatry* 59(1):1–6.

Hazlett, H.C., Poe, M., Gerig, G., Smith, R.G., Provenzale, J., Ross, A., Gilmore, J., and Piven, J. (2005) Magnetic resonance imaging and head circumference study of brain size in autism: Birth through age 2 years. *Arch. Gen. Psychiatry* 62(12):1366–1376.

Haznedar, M.M., Buchsbaum, M.S., Wei, T.C., Hof, P.R., Cartwright, C., Bienstock, C.A., and Hollander, E. (2000) Limbic circuitry in patients with autism spectrum disorders studied with positron emission tomography and magnetic resonance imaging. *Am. J. Psychiatry* 157(12):1994–2001.

Herbert, M.R., Ziegler, D.A., Makris, N., Filipek, P.A., Kemper, T. L., Normandin, J.J., Sanders, H.A., Kennedy, D.N., and Caviness, V.S. Jr. (2004) Localization of white matter volume increase in autism and developmental language disorder. *Ann. Neurol.* 55(4): 530–540.

Hertzman, M. (2003) Galantamine in the treatment of adult autism: A report of three clinical cases. *Int. J. Psychiatry Med.* 33(4): 395–398.

Hollander, E., King, A., Delaney, K., Smith, C.J., and Silverman, J.M. (2003) Obsessive-compulsive behaviors in parents of multiplex autism families. *Psychiatry Res.* 117(1):11–16.

Hollander, E., Novotny, S., Allen, A., Aronowitz, B., Cartwright, C., and DeCaria, C. (2000) The relationship between repetitive behaviors and growth hormone response to sumatriptan challenge in adult autistic disorder. *Neuropsychopharmacol.* 22(2):163–167.

Hollander, E., Novotny, S., Hanratty, M., Yaffe, R., DeCaria, C.M., Aronowitz, B.R., and Mosovich, S. (2003) Oxytocin infusion reduces repetitive behaviors in adults with autistic and Asperger's disorders. *Neuropsychopharmacol.* 28(1):193–198.

Hollander, E., Phillips, A., Chaplin, W., Zagursky, K., Novotny, S., Wasserman, S., and Iyengar, R. (2005) A placebo controlled crossover trial of liquid fluoxetine on repetitive behaviors in childhood and adolescent autism. *Neuropsychopharmacol.* 30(3):582–589.

Horvath, K., Stefanatos, G., Sokolski, K.N., Wachtel, R., Nabors, L., and Tildon, J.T. (1998) Improved social and language skills after secretin administration in patients with autistic spectrum disorders. *J. Assoc. Acad. Minor Phys.* 9(1):9–15.

Hoshino, Y., Watanabe, M., Tachibana, R., Kaneko, M., and Kumashiro, H. (1985) The TRH and Lh-Rh loading test in autistic children. *Fukushima J. Med. Sci.* 31(1):55–61.

Howard, J.S., Sparkman, C.R., Cohen, H.G., Green, G., and Stanislaw, H. (2005) A comparison of intensive behavior analytic and eclectic treatments for young children with autism. *Res. Dev. Disabil.* 26(4):359–383.

Howlin, P., Goode, S., Hutton, J., and Rutter, M. (2004) Adult outcome for children with autism. *J. Child Psychol. Psychiatry* 45(2): 212–229.

Howlin, P., and Karpf, J. (2004) Using the social communication questionnaire to identify "autistic spectrum" disorders associated with other genetic conditions: Findings from a study of individuals with Cohen syndrome. *Autism* 8(2):175–182.

Hus, V., Pickles, A., Cook, E.H., Jr., Risi, S., and Lord, C. (2007) Using the Autism Diagnostic Interview–Revised to increase phenotypic homogeneity in genetic studies of autism. *Biol. Psychiatry* 61(4):438–448.

International Molecular Genetic Study of Autism Consortium. (1998) A full genome screen for autism with evidence for linkage to a region on chromosome 7q. *Hum. Mol. Genet.* 7(3):571–578.

International Molecular Genetic Study of Autism Consortium. (2001) Further characterization of the autism susceptibility locus auts1 on chromosome 7q. *Hum. Mol. Genet.* 10(9):973–982.

Ingram, J.L., Stodgell, C.J., Hyman, S L., Figlewicz, D.A., Weitkamp, L.R., and Rodier, P.M. (2000) Discovery of allelic variants of HOXA1 and HOXB1: Genetic susceptibility to autism spectrum disorders. *Teratology* 62(6):393–405.

Insel, T.R., O'Brien, D.J., and Leckman, J.F. (1999) Oxytocin, vasopressin, and autism: Is there a connection? *Biol. Psychiatry* 45(2): 145–157.

Jaselskis, C.A., Cook, E.H., Jr., Fletcher, K.E., and Leventhal, B.L. (1992) Clonidine treatment of hyperactive and impulsive children with autistic disorder. *J. Clin. Psychopharmacol.* 12(5):322–327.

Jones, M.B., and Szatmari, P. (2002) A risk-factor model of epistatic interaction, focusing on autism. *Am. J. Med. Genet.* 114(5):558–565.

Jyonouchi, H., Sun, S., and Le, H. (2001) Proinflammatory and regulatory cytokine production associated with innate and adaptive immune responses in children with autism spectrum disorders and developmental regression. *J. Neuroimmunol.* 120(1/2): 170–179.

Kanner, L. (1943) Autistic disturbances of affective contact. *Nervous Child* 10:217–250.

Kaufmann, W.E., Cooper, K.L., Mostofsky, S.H., Capone, G.T., Kates, W.R., Newschaffer, C.J., Bukelis, I., Stump, M.H., Jann, A.E., and Lanham, D.C. (2003) Specificity of cerebellar vermian abnormalities in autism: A quantitative magnetic resonance imaging study. *J. Child Neurol.* 18(7):463–470.

Kent, L., Evans, J., Paul, M., and Sharp, M. (1999) Comorbidity of autistic spectrum disorders in children with Down syndrome. *Dev. Med. Child Neurol.* 41(3):153–158.

Kielinen, M., Rantala, H., Timonen, E., Linna, S.L., and Moilanen, I. (2004) Associated medical disorders and disabilities in children with autistic disorder: A population-based study. *Autism* 8(1): 49–60.

Kim, H.L., Donnelly, J.H., Tournay, A.E., Book, T.M., and Filipek, P. (2006) Absence of seizures despite high prevalence of epileptiform EEG abnormalities in children with autism monitored in a tertiary care center. *Epilepsia* 47(2):394–398.

Kim, S.J., Cox, N., Courchesne, R., Lord, C., Corsello, C., Akshoomoff, N., Guter, S., Leventhal, B L., Courchesne, E., and Cook, E.H. Jr. (2002) Transmission disequilibrium mapping at the serotonin transporter gene (SLC6A4) region in autistic disorder. *Mol. Psychiatry* 7(3):278–288.

King, B.H., Wright, D.M., Handen, B.L., Sikich, L., Zimmerman, A.W., McMahon, W., Cantwell, E., Davanzo, P.A., Dourish, C. T., Dykens, E.M., Hooper, S.R., Jaselskis, C.A., Leventhal, B.L., Levitt, J., Lord, C., Lubetsky, M.J., Myers, S.M., Ozonoff, S., Shah, B.G., Snape, M., Shernoff, E.W., Williamson, K., and Cook, E.H. Jr. (2001) Double-blind, placebo-controlled study of amantadine hydrochloride in the treatment of children with autistic disorder. *J. Am. Acad. Child Adolesc. Psychiatry* 40(6):658–665.

Klauck, S.M., Poustka, F., Benner, A., Lesch, K.P., and Poustka, A. (1997) Serotonin transporter (5-HTT) gene variants associated with autism? *Hum. Mol. Genet.* 6(13):2233–2238.

Klin, A., Jones, W., Schultz, R., Volkmar, F., and Cohen, D. (2002) Visual fixation patterns during viewing of naturalistic social situations as predictors of social competence in individuals with autism. *Arch. Gen. Psychiatry* 59(9):809–816.

Komoto, J., Usui, S., Otsuki, S., and Terao, A. (1984) Infantile autism and Duchenne muscular dystrophy. *J. Autism Dev. Disord.* 14(2):191–195.

Krause, I., He, X.S., Gershwin, M.E., and Shoenfeld, Y. (2002) Brief report: Immune factors in autism: A critical review. *J. Autism Dev. Disord.* 32(4):337–345.

Kurita, H. (1985) Infantile autism with speech loss before the age of thirty months. *J. Am. Acad. Child Psychiatry* 24(2):191–196.

Lainhart, J.E. (2006) Advances in autism neuroimaging research for the clinician and geneticist. *Am. J. Med. Genet. C Semin. Med. Genet.* 142(1):33–39.

Lainhart, J.E., Bigler, E.D., Bocian, M., Coon, H., Dinh, E., Dawson, G., Deutsch, C.K., Dunn, M., Estes, A., Tager-Flusberg, H., Folstein, S., Hepburn, S., Hyman, S., McMahon, W., Minshew,

N., Munson, J., Osann, K., Ozonoff, S., Rodier, P., Rogers, S., Sigman, M., Spence, M.A., Stodgell, C.J., and Volkmar, F. (2006) Head circumference and height in autism: A study by the collaborative program of excellence in autism. *Am. J. Med. Genet. A* 140(21):2257–2274.

Lainhart, J.E., Piven, J., Wzorek, M., Landa, R., Santangelo, S.L., Coon, H., and Folstein, S.E. (1997) Macrocephaly in children and adults with autism. *J. Am. Acad. Child Adolesc. Psychiatry* 36(2):282–290.

Lake, C.R., Ziegler, M.G., and Murphy, D.L. (1977) Increased norepinephrine levels and decreased dopamine-beta-hydroxylase activity in primary autism. *Arch. Gen. Psychiatry* 34(5):553–556.

Landa, R., Folstein, S.E., and Isaacs, C. (1991) Spontaneous narrative-discourse performance of parents of autistic individuals. *J. Speech Hear. Res.* 34(6):1339–1345.

Landa, R., Piven, J., Wzorek, M.M., Gayle, J.O., Chase, G.A., and Folstein, S.E. (1992) Social language use in parents of autistic individuals. *Psychol. Med.* 22(1):245–254.

Landau, W.M., and Kleffner, F.R. (1957) Syndrome of acquired aphasia with convulsive disorder in children. *Neurology* 7(8):523–530.

Launay, J.M., Bursztejn, C., Ferrari, P., Dreux, C., Braconnier, A., Zarifian, E., Lancrenon, S., and Fermanian, J. (1987) Catecholamines metabolism in infantile autism: A controlled study of 22 autistic children. *J. Autism Dev. Disord.* 17(3):333–347.

Lauritsen, M., Mors, O., Mortensen, P.B., and Ewald, H. (1999) Infantile autism and associated autosomal chromosome abnormalities: A register-based study and a literature survey. *J. Child Psychol. Psychiatry* 40(3):335–345.

Leboyer, M., Philippe, A., Bouvard, M., Guilloud-Bataille, M., Bondoux, D., Tabuteau, F., Feingold, J., Mouren-Simeoni, M.C., and Launay, J.M. (1999) Whole blood serotonin and plasma beta-endorphin in autistic probands and their first-degree relatives. *Biol. Psychiatry* 45(2):158–163.

Le Couteur, A., Bailey, A., Goode, S., Pickles, A., Robertson, S., Gottesman, I., and Rutter, M. (1996) A broader phenotype of autism: The clinical spectrum in twins. *J. Child Psychol. Psychiatry* 37(7):785–801.

Lewis, K.E., Lubetsky, M.J., Wenger, S.L., and Steele, M.W. (1995) Chromosomal abnormalities in a psychiatric population. *Am. J. Med. Genet.* 60(1):53–54.

Leyfer, O.T., Folstein, S.E., Bacalman, S., Davis, N.O., Dinh, E., Morgan, J., Tager-Flusberg, H., and Lainhart, J.E. (2006) Comorbid psychiatric disorders in children with autism: Interview development and rates of disorders. *J. Autism Dev. Disord.* 36(7):849–861.

Liu, J., Nyholt, D.R., Magnussen, P., Parano, E., Pavone, P., Geschwind, D., Lord, C., Iversen, P., Hoh, J., Ott, J., and Gilliam, T.C. (2001) A genomewide screen for autism susceptibility loci. *Am. J. Hum. Genet.* 69(2):327–340.

Lotspeich, L.J., Kwon, H., Schumann, C.M., Fryer, S.L., Goodlin-Jones, B.L., Buonocore, M.H., Lammers, C.R., Amaral, D.G., and Reiss, A.L. (2004) Investigation of neuroanatomical differences between autism and Asperger syndrome. *Arch. Gen. Psychiatry* 61(3):291–298.

Luyster, R., Richler, J., Risi, S., Hsu, W.L., Dawson, G., Bernier, R., Dunn, M., Hepburn, S., Hyman, S.L., McMahon, W.M., Goudie-Nice, J., Minshew, N., Rogers, S., Sigman, M., Spence, M.A., Goldberg, W.A., Tager-Flusberg, H., Volkmar, F.R., and Lord, C. (2005) Early regression in social communication in autism spectrum disorders: A CPEA study. *Dev. Neuropsychol.* 27(3):311–336.

Mayes, S.D., and Calhoun, S.L. (2003) Ability profiles in children with autism: Influence of age and IQ. *Autism* 7(1):65–80.

McBride, P.A., Anderson, G.M., Hertzig, M.E., Sweeney, J.A., Kream, J., Cohen, D.J., and Mann, J.J. (1989) Serotonergic responsivity in male young adults with autistic disorder. Results of a pilot study. *Arch. Gen. Psychiatry* 46(3):213–221.

McCauley, J.L., Olson, L.M., Delahanty, R., Amin, T., Nurmi, E.L., Organ, E.L., Jacobs, M.M., Folstein, S.E., Haines, J.L. and Sutcliffe, J.S. (2004) A linkage disequilibrium map of the 1-mb 15q12 GABA(A) receptor subunit cluster and association to autism. *Am. J. Med. Genet. B Neuropsychiatr. Genet.* 131(1):51–59.

McCauley, J.L., Olson, L.M., Dowd, M., Amin, T., Steele, A., Blakely, R.D., Folstein, S.E., Haines, J.L., and Sutcliffe, J.S. (2004) Linkage and association analysis at the serotonin transporter (SLC6A4) locus in a rigid-compulsive subset of autism. *Am. J. Med. Genet.* 127B(1):104–112.

McClintock, K., Hall, S., and Oliver, C. (2003) Risk markers associated with challenging behaviours in people with intellectual disabilities: A meta-analytic study. *J. Intellect. Disabil. Res.* 47(Pt 6):405–416.

McCracken, J.T., McGough, J., Shah, B., Cronin, P., Hong, D., Aman, M.G., Arnold, L.E., Lindsay, R., Nash, P., Hollway, J., McDougle, C.J., Posey, D., Swiezy, N., Kohn, A., Scahill, L., Martin, A., Koenig, K., Volkmar, F., Carroll, D., Lancor, A., Tierney, E., Ghuman, J., Gonzalez, N. M., Grados, M., Vitiello, B., Ritz, L., Davies, M., Robinson, J., and McMahon, D. (2002) Risperidone in children with autism and serious behavioral problems. *N. Engl. J. Med.* 347(5):314–321.

McDougle, C.J., Naylor, S.T., Cohen, D.J., Aghajanian, G.K., Heninger, G.R., and Price, L. H. (1996) Effects of tryptophan depletion in drug-free adults with autistic disorder. *Arch. Gen. Psychiatry* 53(11):993–1000.

McDougle, C.J., Naylor, S.T., Cohen, D.J., Volkmar, F.R., Heninger, G.R., and Price, L.H. (1996) A double-blind, placebo-controlled study of fluvoxamine in adults with autistic disorder. *Arch. Gen. Psychiatry* 53(11):1001–1008.

McDougle, C.J., Naylor, S.T., Goodman, W.K., Volkmar, F.R., Cohen, D.J., and Price, L.H. (1993) Acute tryptophan depletion in autistic disorder: A controlled case study. *Biol. Psychiatry* 33(7):547–550.

McDougle, C.J., Posey, D., and Potenza, M.N. (2003) Neurobiology of serotonin function in autism. In: Hollander E., eds. *Neurobiology of Serotonin Function in Autism.* New York: Marcel Dekker, pp. 199–220.

McDougle, C.J., Price, L.H., Volkmar, F.R., Goodman, W.K., Ward-O'Brien, D., Nielsen, J., Bregman, J., and Cohen, D.J. (1992) Clomipramine in autism: Preliminary evidence of efficacy. *J. Am. Acad. Child Adolesc. Psychiatry* 31(4):746–750.

McDougle, C.J., Scahill, L., Aman, M.G., McCracken, J.T., Tierney, E., Davies, M., Arnold, L.E., Posey, D.J., Martin, A., Ghuman, J.K., Shah, B., Chuang, S.Z., Swiezy, N.B., Gonzalez, N.M., Hollway, J., Koenig, K., McGough, J.J., Ritz, L., and Vitiello, B. (2005) Risperidone for the core symptom domains of autism: Results from the study by the autism network of the research units on pediatric psychopharmacology. *Am. J. Psychiatry* 162(6): 1142–1148.

Miles, J.H., Hadden, L.L., Takahashi, T.N., and Hillman, R.E. (2000) Head circumference is an independent clinical finding associated with autism. *Am. J. Med. Genet.* 95(4):339–350.

Minderaa, R.B., Anderson, G.M., Volkmar, F.R., Akkerhuis, G.W., and Cohen, D.J. (1994) Noradrenergic and adrenergic functioning in autism. *Biol. Psychiatry* 36(4):237–241.

Minshew, N.J., Goldstein, G., and Siegel, D.J. (1997) Neuropsychologic functioning in autism: Profile of a complex information processing disorder. *J. Int. Neuropsychol. Soc.* 3(4):303–316.

Minshew, N.J., Sung, K., Jones, B.L., and Furman, J.M. (2004) Underdevelopment of the postural control system in autism. *Neurology* 63(11):2056–2061.

Minshew, N.J., Webb, S.J., Williams, D., and Dawson, G. (2006) Neuropsychology and neurophysiology of autism spectrum disorders. In: Moldin S.O., and Rubenstein, J.L.R., eds. *Understanding Autism: From Basic Neuroscience to Treatment.* Boca Raton, FL: CRC Press, pp. 379–415.

Modahl, C., Green, L., Fein, D., Morris, M., Waterhouse, L., Feinstein, C., and Levin, H. (1998) Plasma oxytocin levels in autistic children. *Biol. Psychiatry* 43(4):270–277.

Molloy, C.A., Keddache, M., and Martin, L.J. (2005) Evidence for linkage on 21q and 7q in a subset of autism characterized by developmental regression. *Mol. Psychiatry* 10(8):741–746.

Molloy, C.A., Morrow, A.L., Meinzen-Derr, J., Schleifer, K., Dienger, K., Manning-Courtney, P., Altaye, M., and Wills-Karp, M. (2006) Elevated cytokine levels in children with autism spectrum disorder. *J. Neuroimmunol.* 172(1/2):198–205.

Moreno-Fuenmayor, H., Borjas, L., Arrieta, A., Valera, V., and Socorro-Candanoza, L. (1996) Plasma excitatory amino acids in autism. *Invest. Clin.* 37(2):113–128.

Morrow, J.D., Whitman, B.Y., and Accardo, P.J. (1990) Autistic disorder in Sotos syndrome: A case report. *Eur. J. Pediatr.* 149(8): 567–569.

Mulder, E.J., Anderson, G.M., Kema, I.P., Brugman, A.M., Ketelaars, C.E., de Bildt, A., van Lang, N.D., den Boer, J.A., and Minderaa, R.B. (2005) Serotonin transporter intron 2 polymorphism associated with rigid-compulsive behaviors in Dutch individuals with pervasive developmental disorder. *Am. J. Med. Genet. B Neuropsychiatr. Genet.* 133(1):93–96.

Narayan, M., Srinath, S., Anderson, G.M., and Meundi, D.B. (1993) Cerebrospinal fluid levels of homovanillic acid and 5-hydroxyindoleacetic acid in autism. *Biol. Psychiatry* 33(8/9):630–635.

Nishimura, Y., Martin, C.L., Lopez, A.V., Spence, S.J., Alvarez-Retuerto, A.I., Sigman, M., Steindler, C., Pelligrini, S., Schanen, N.C., Warren, S.T., and Geschwind, D.H. (2007) Genome-wide expression profiling of lymphoblastoid cell lines distinguishes different forms of autism and reveals shared pathways. *Hum. Mol. Genet.* Jul 15;16(14):1682–1698. Epub May 21, 2007.

Nordin, V., and Gillberg, C. (1998) The long-term course of autistic disorders: Update on follow-up studies. *Acta Psychiatr. Scand.* 97(2):99–108.

Novotny, S., Hollander, E., Allen, A., Mosovich, S., Aronowitz, B., Cartwright, C., DeCaria, C., and Dolgoff-Kaspar, R. (2000) Increased growth hormone response to sumatriptan challenge in adult autistic disorders. *Psychiatry Res.* 94(2):173–177.

Nurmi, E.L., Dowd, M., Tadevosyan-Leyfer, O., Haines, J.L., Folstein, S.E., and Sutcliffe, J.S. (2003) Exploratory subsetting of autism families based on savant skills improves evidence of genetic linkage to 15q11-q13. *J. Am. Acad. Child Adolesc. Psychiatry* 42(7): 856–863.

Ogai, M., Matsumoto, H., Suzuki, K., Ozawa, F., Fukuda, R., Uchiyama, I., Suckling, J., Isoda, H., Mori, N., and Takei, N. (2003) fMRI study of recognition of facial expressions in high-functioning autistic patients. *Neuroreport* 14(4):559–563.

Okada, K., Hashimoto, K., Iwata, Y., Nakamura, K., Tsujii, M., Tsuchiya, K.J., Sekine, Y., Suda, S., Suzuki, K., Sugihara, G., Matsuzaki, H., Sugiyama, T., Kawai, M., Minabe, Y., Takei, N., and Mori, N. (2007) Decreased serum levels of transforming growth factor-beta1 in patients with autism. *Prog. Neuropsychopharmacol. Biol. Psychiatry* 31(1):187–190.

Oliveira, G., Matoso, E., Vicente, A., Ribeiro, P., Marques, C., Ataide, A., Miguel, T., Saraiva, J., and Carreira, I. (2003) Partial tetrasomy of chromosome 3q and mosaicism in a child with autism. *J. Autism Dev. Disord.* 33(2):177–185.

Ozonoff, S., Strayer, D.L., McMahon, W.M., and Filloux, F. (1994) Executive function abilities in autism and Tourette syndrome: An information processing approach. *J. Child Psychol. Psychiatry* 35(6):1015–1032.

Ozonoff, S., Williams, B.J., Gale, S., and Miller, J.N. (1999) Autism and autistic behavior in Joubert syndrome. *J. Child Neurol.* 14(10):636–641.

Palmen, S.J., and van Engeland, H. (2004) Review on structural neuroimaging findings in autism. *J. Neural Transm.* 111(7):903–929.

Panksepp, J. (1993) Commentary on the possible role of oxytocin in autism. *J. Autism Dev. Disord.* 23(3):567–569.

Pavone, P., Incorpora, G., Fiumara, A., Parano, E., Trifiletti, R.R., and Ruggieri, M. (2004) Epilepsy is not a prominent feature of primary autism. *Neuropediatrics* 35(4):207–210.

Pelphrey, K.A., Morris, J.P., and McCarthy, G. (2005) Neural basis of eye gaze processing deficits in autism. *Brain* 128(Pt 5):1038–1048.

Persico, A.M., D'Agruma, L., Maiorano, N., Totaro, A., Militerni, R., Bravaccio, C., Wassink, T.H., Schneider, C., Melmed, R., Trillo, S., Montecchi, F., Palermo, M., Pascucci, T., Puglisi-Allegra, S., Reichelt, K.L., Conciatori, M., Marino, R., Quattrocchi, C.C., Baldi, A., Zelante, L., Gasparini, P., and Keller, F. (2001) REELIN gene alleles and haplotypes as a factor predisposing to autistic disorder. *Mol. Psychiatry* 6(2):150–159.

Petit, E., Herault, J., Martineau, J., Perrot, A., Barthelemy, C., Hameury, L., Sauvage, D., Lelord, G., and Muh, J.P. (1995) Association study with two markers of a human homeogene in infantile autism. *J. Med. Genet.* 32(4):269–274.

Philippe, A., Martinez, M., Guilloud-Bataille, M., Gillberg, C., Rastam, M., Sponheim, E., Coleman, M., Zappella, M., Aschauer, H., Van Maldergem, L., Penet, C., Feingold, J., Brice, A., Leboyer, M., and van Malldergerme, L. (1999) Genome-wide scan for autism susceptibility genes. Paris Autism Research International Sibpair Study. *Hum. Mol. Genet.* 8(5):805–812.

Philippi, A., Roschmann, E., Tores, F., Lindenbaum, P., Benajou, A., Germain-Leclerc, L., Marcaillou, C., Fontaine, K., Vanpeene, M., Roy, S., Maillard, S., Decaulne, V., Saraiva, J.P., Brooks, P., Rousseau, F., and Hager, J. (2005) Haplotypes in the gene encoding protein kinase c-beta (PRKCB1) on chromosome 16 are associated with autism. *Mol. Psychiatry* 10(10):950–960.

Pickett, J., and London, E. (2005) The neuropathology of autism: A review. *J. Neuropathol. Exp. Neurol.* 64(11):925–935.

Pickles, A., Bolton, P., Macdonald, H., Bailey, A., Le Couteur, A., Sim, C.H., and Rutter, M. (1995) Latent-class analysis of recurrence risks for complex phenotypes with selection and measurement error: A twin and family history study of autism. *Am. J. Hum. Genet.* 57(3):717–726.

Pierce, K., and Courchesne, E. (2001) Evidence for a cerebellar role in reduced exploration and stereotyped behavior in autism. *Biol. Psychiatry* 49(8):655–664.

Pierce, K., Muller, R.A., Ambrose, J., Allen, G., and Courchesne, E. (2001) Face processing occurs outside the fusiform "face area" in autism: Evidence from functional MRI. *Brain* 124(Pt 10): 2059–2073.

Piven, J., and Palmer, P. (1999) Psychiatric disorder and the broad autism phenotype: Evidence from a family study of multiple-incidence autism families. *Am. J. Psychiatry* 156(4):557–563.

Piven, J., Arndt, S., Bailey, J., and Andreasen, N. (1996) Regional brain enlargement in autism: A magnetic resonance imaging study. *J. Am. Acad. Child Adolesc. Psychiatry* 35(4):530–536.

Piven, J., Arndt, S., Bailey, J., Havercamp, S., Andreasen, N.C., and Palmer, P. (1995) An MRI study of brain size in autism. *Am. J. Psychiatry* 152(8):1145–1149.

Piven, J., Chase, G.A., Landa, R., Wzorek, M., Gayle, J., Cloud, D., and Folstein, S. (1991) Psychiatric disorders in the parents of autistic individuals [see comments]. *J. Am. Acad. Child Adolesc. Psychiatry* 30(3):471–478.

Piven, J., Gayle, J., Chase, G.A., Fink, B., Landa, R., Wzorek, M. M., and Folstein, S.E. (1990) A family history study of neuropsychiatric disorders in the adult siblings of autistic individuals [see comments]. *J. Am. Acad. Child Adolesc. Psychiatry* 29(2): 177–183.

Piven, J., Palmer, P., Landa, R., Santangelo, S., Jacobi, D., and Childress, D. (1997) Personality and language characteristics in parents from multiple-incidence autism families. *Am. J. Med. Genet.* 74(4):398–411.

Piven, J., Saliba, K., Bailey, J., and Arndt, S. (1997) An MRI study of autism: The cerebellum revisited [see comments]. *Neurology* 49(2):546–551.

Piven, J., Wzorek, M., Landa, R., Lainhart, J., Bolton, P., Chase, G.A., and Folstein, S. (1994) Personality characteristics of the parents of autistic individuals. *Psychol. Med.* 24(3):783–795.

Posey, D.J., Kem, D.L., Swiezy, N.B., Sweeten, T.L., Wiegand, R.E., and McDougle, C.J. (2004) A pilot study of D-cycloserine in subjects with autistic disorder. *Am. J. Psychiatry* 161(11):2115–2117.

Purcell, A.E., Jeon, O.H., Zimmerman, A.W., Blue, M.E., and Pevsner, J. (2001) Postmortem brain abnormalities of the glutamate neurotransmitter system in autism. *Neurology* 57(9):1618–1628.

Redcay, E., and Courchesne, E. (2005) When is the brain enlarged in autism? A meta-analysis of all brain size reports. *Biol. Psychiatry* 58(1):1–9.

Reiss, A.L., Feinstein, C., Rosenbaum, K.N., Borengasser-Caruso, M.A., and Goldsmith, B.M. (1985) Autism associated with Williams syndrome. *J. Pediatr.* 106(2):247–249.

Rice, C. (2007) Prevalence of autism spectrum disorders–autism and developmental disabilities monitoring network, 14 sites, United States, 2002. *MMWR Surveill. Summ.* 56(1):12–28.

Risch, N., Spiker, D., Lotspeich, L., Nouri, N., Hinds, D., Hallmayer, J., Kalaydjieva, L., McCague, P., Dimiceli, S., Pitts, T., Nguyen, L., Yang, J., Harper, C., Thorpe, D., Vermeer, S., Young, H., Hebert, J., Lin, A., Ferguson, J., Chiotti, C., Wiese-Slater, S., Rogers, T., Salmon, B., Nicholas, P., Myers, R.M., et al. (1999) A genomic screen of autism: Evidence for a multilocus etiology. *Am. J. Hum. Genet.* 65(2):493–507.

Ritvo, E.R., Freeman, B.J., Mason-Brothers, A., Mo, A., and Ritvo, A.M. (1985) Concordance for the syndrome of autism in 40 pairs of afflicted twins. *Am. J. Psychiatry* 142(1):74–77.

Ritvo, E.R., Ritvo, R., and Freeman, B.J. (1991) Debate and argument. Concordance for the syndrome of autism [letter; comment]. *J. Child Psychol. Psychiatry* 32(6):1031–1034.

Rogers, S.J., Hepburn, S., and Wehner, E. (2003) Parent reports of sensory symptoms in toddlers with autism and those with other developmental disorders. *J. Autism Dev. Disord.* 33(6):631–642.

Rogers, S.J., Hepburn, S.L., Stackhouse, T., and Wehner, E. (2003) Imitation performance in toddlers with autism and those with other developmental disorders. *J. Child Psychol. Psychiatry* 44(5):763–781.

Rolf, L.H., Haarmann, F.Y., Grotemeyer, K.H., and Kehrer, H. (1993) Serotonin and amino acid content in platelets of autistic children. *Acta Psychiatr. Scand.* 87(5):312–316.

RUPP Investigators (Research Units on Pediatric Psychopharmacology) (2005) Randomized, controlled, crossover trial of methylphenidate in pervasive developmental disorders with hyperactivity. *Arch. Gen. Psychiatry* 62(11):1266–1274.

Rutter, M., Andersen-Wood, L., Beckett, C., Bredenkamp, D., Castle, J., Groothues, C., Kreppner, J., Keaveney, L., Lord, C., and O'Connor, T.G. (1999) Quasi-autistic patterns following severe early global privation. English and Romanian adoptees (ERA) Study Team. *J. Child Psychol. Psychiatry* 40(4):537–549.

Rutter, M., Silberg, J., O'Connor, T., and Simonoff, E. (1999) Genetics and child psychiatry: II. empirical research findings. *J. Child Psychol. Psychiatry* 40(1):19–55.

Schellenberg, G.D., Dawson, G., Sung, Y.J., Estes, A., Munson, J., Rosenthal, E., Rothstein, J., Flodman, P., Smith, M., Coon, H., Leong, L., Yu, C.E., Stodgell, C., Rodier, P.M., Spence, M.A., Minshew, N., McMahon, W.M., and Wijsman, E.M. (2006) Evidence for multiple loci from a genome scan of autism kindreds. *Mol. Psychiatry* 11(11):979, 1049–1060.

Schreck, K.A., and Williams, K. (2006) Food preferences and factors influencing food selectivity for children with autism spectrum disorders. *Res. Dev. Disabil.* 27(4):353–363.

Schreck, K.A., Williams, K., and Smith, A.F. (2004) A comparison of eating behaviors between children with and without autism. *J. Autism Dev. Disord.* 34(4):433–438.

Schultz, R.T., and Anderson, G.M. (2004) The neurobiology of autism and the pervasive developmental disorders. In: Charney D. S., and Nestler, E.J., eds. *The Neurobiology of Autism and the Pervasive Developmental Disorders*. Oxford, UK and New York: Oxford University Press, pp. 954–967.

Schultz, R.T., Romanski, L., and Tsatsanis, K. (2000) Neurofunctional models of autistic disorder and Asperger's syndrome: Clues from neuroimaging. In: Klin, A., Volkmar, F.R., and Sparrow, S. S., eds. *Neurofunctional Models of Autistic Disorder and Asperger's Syndrome: Clues from Neuroimaging*. New York: Plenum Press, pp. 179–209.

Schumann, C.M., Hamstra, J., Goodlin-Jones, B.L., Lotspeich, L.J., Kwon, H., Buonocore, M.H., Lammers, C.R., Reiss, A.L., and Amaral, D.G. (2004) The amygdala is enlarged in children but not adolescents with autism; the hippocampus is enlarged at all ages. *J. Neurosci.* 24(28):6392–6401.

Sebat, J., Lakshmi, B., Malhotra, D., Troge, J., Lese-Martin, C., Walsh, T., Yamrom, B., Yoon, S., Krasnitz, A., Kendall, J., Leotta, A., Pai, D., Zhang, R., Lee, Y.H., Hicks, J., Spence, S.J., Lee, A.T., Puura, K., Lehtimaki, T., Ledbetter, D., Gregersen, P.K., Bregman, J., Sutcliffe, J.S., Jobanputra, V., Chung, W., Warburton, D., King, M.C., Skuse, D., Geschwind, D.H., Gilliam, T.C., Ye, K., and Wigler, M. (2007) Strong association of de novo copy number mutations with autism. *Science* 316(5823): 445–449.

Sebat, J., Lakshmi, B., Troge, J., Alexander, J., Young, J., Lundin, P., Maner, S., Massa, H., Walker, M., Chi, M., Navin, N., Lucito, R., Healy, J., Hicks, J., Ye, K., Reiner, A., Gilliam, T.C., Trask, B., Patterson, N., Zetterberg, A., and Wigler, M. (2004) Large-scale copy number polymorphism in the human genome. *Science* 305(5683):525–528.

Shao, Y., Cuccaro, M.L., Hauser, E.R., Raiford, K.L., Menold, M.M., Wolpert, C.M., Ravan, S.A., Elston, L., Decena, K., Donnelly, S.L., Abramson, R.K., Wright, H.H., DeLong, G.R., Gilbert, J. R., and Pericak-Vance, M.A. (2003) Fine mapping of autistic disorder to chromosome 15q11-q13 by use of phenotypic subtypes. *Am. J. Hum. Genet.* 72(3):539–548.

Shao, Y., Raiford, K.L., Wolpert, C.M., Cope, H.A., Ravan, S.A., Ashley-Koch, A.A., Abramson, R.K., Wright, H.H., DeLong, R.G., Gilbert, J.R., Cuccaro, M.L., and Pericak-Vance, M.A. (2002) Phenotypic homogeneity provides increased support for linkage on chromosome 2 in autistic disorder. *Am. J. Hum. Genet.* 70(4):1058–1061.

Shao, Y., Wolpert, C.M., Raiford, K.L., Menold, M.M., Donnelly, S.L., Ravan, S.A., Bass, M.P., McClain, C., von Wendt, L., Vance, J.M., Abramson, R.H., Wright, H.H., Ashley-Koch, A., Gilbert, J.R., DeLong, R.G., Cuccaro, M.L., and Pericak-Vance, M.A. (2002) Genomic screen and follow-up analysis for autistic disorder. *Am. J. Med. Genet.* 114(1):99–105.

Shea, S., Turgay, A., Carroll, A., Schulz, M., Orlik, H., Smith, I., and Dunbar, F. (2004) Risperidone in the treatment of disruptive behavioral symptoms in children with autistic and other pervasive developmental disorders. *Pediatrics* 114(5):e634–e641.

Sherr, E.H. (2003) The ARX story (epilepsy, mental retardation, autism, and cerebral malformations): one gene leads to many phenotypes. *Curr. Opin. Pediatr.* 15(6):567–571.

Shinohe, A., Hashimoto, K., Nakamura, K., Tsujii, M., Iwata, Y., Tsuchiya, K.J., Sekine, Y., Suda, S., Suzuki, K., Sugihara, G., Matsuzaki, H., Minabe, Y., Sugiyama, T., Kawai, M., Iyo, M., Takei, N., and Mori, N. (2006) Increased serum levels of glutamate in adult patients with autism. *Prog. Neuropsychopharmacol. Biol. Psychiatry* 30(8):1472–1477.

Singh, V.K., Warren, R., Averett, R., and Ghaziuddin, M. (1997) Circulating autoantibodies to neuronal and glial filament proteins in autism. *Pediatr. Neurol.* 17(1):88–90.

Singh, V.K., Warren, R.P., Odell, J.D., Warren, W.L., and Cole, P. (1993) Antibodies to myelin basic protein in children with autistic behavior. *Brain Behav. Immun.* 7(1):97–103.

Skaar, D.A., Shao, Y., Haines, J.L., Stenger, J.E., Jaworski, J., Martin, E.R., DeLong, G.R., Moore, J.H., McCauley, J.L., Sutcliffe, J.S., Ashley-Koch, A.E., Cuccaro, M.L., Folstein, S.E., Gilbert, J.R., and Pericak-Vance, M.A. (2005) Analysis of the RELN gene as a genetic risk factor for autism. *Mol. Psychiatry* 10(6): 563–571.

Smalley, S.L. (1998) Autism and tuberous sclerosis. *J. Autism Dev. Disord.* 28(5):407–414.

Smalley, S.L., McCracken, J., and Tanguay, P. (1995) Autism, affective disorders, and social phobia. *Am. J. Med. Genet.* 60(1): 19–26.

Sparks, B.F., Friedman, S.D., Shaw, D.W., Aylward, E.H., Echelard, D., Artru, A.A., Maravilla, K.R., Giedd, J.N., Munson, J., Dawson, G., and Dager, S.R. (2002) Brain structural abnormalities in young children with autism spectrum disorder. *Neurology* 59(2):184–192.

Spence, S.J., Cantor, R.M., Chung, L., Kim, S., Geschwind, D.H., and Alarcon, M. (2006) Stratification based on language-related endophenotypes in autism: Attempt to replicate reported linkage. *Am. J. Med. Genet. B Neuropsychiatr. Genet.* 141(6):591–598.

Splawski, I., Timothy, K.W., Sharpe, L.M., Decher, N., Kumar, P., Bloise, R., Napolitano, C., Schwartz, P.J., Joseph, R.M., Condouris, K., Tager-Flusberg, H., Priori, S.G., Sanguinetti, M.C., and Keating, M.T. (2004) Ca(v)1.2 calcium channel dysfunction causes a multisystem disorder including arrhythmia and autism. *Cell* 119(1):19–31.

Steffenburg, S., Gillberg, C., Hellgren, L., Andersson, L., Gillberg, I. C., Jakobsson, G., and Bohman, M. (1989) A twin study of autism in Denmark, Finland, Iceland, Norway and Sweden. *J. Child Psychol. Psychiatry* 30(3):405–416.

Steffenburg, S., Gillberg, C.L., Steffenburg, U., and Kyllerman, M. (1996) Autism in Angelman syndrome: A population-based study. *Pediatr. Neurol.* 14(2):131–136.

Stone, J.L., Merriman, B., Cantor, R.M., Yonan, A.L., Gilliam, T.C., Geschwind, D.H., and Nelson, S.F. (2004) Evidence for sex-specific risk alleles in autism spectrum disorder. *Am. J. Hum. Genet.* 75(6):1117–1123.

Sturmey, P. (2005) Secretin is an ineffective treatment for pervasive developmental disabilities: a review of 15 double-blind randomized controlled trials. *Res. Dev. Disabil.* 26(1):87–97.

Sweeten, T.L., Bowyer, S.L., Posey, D.J., Halberstadt, G.M., and McDougle, C.J. (2003) Increased prevalence of familial autoimmunity in probands with pervasive developmental disorders. *Pediatrics* 112(5):e420.

Szatmari, P., Paterson, A.D., Zwaigenbaum, L., Roberts, W., Brian, J., Liu, X.Q., Vincent, J.B., Skaug, J.L., Thompson, A.P., Senman, L., Feuk, L., Qian, C., Bryson, S.E., Jones, M.B., Marshall, C.R., Scherer, S.W., Vieland, V.J., Bartlett, C., Mangin, L.V., Goedken, R., Segre, A., Pericak-Vance, M.A., Cuccaro, M.L., Gilbert, J.R., Wright, H.H., Abramson, R.K., Betancur, C., Bourgeron, T., Gillberg, C., Leboyer, M., Buxbaum, J.D., Davis, K.L., Hollander, E., Silverman, J.M., Hallmayer, J., Lotspeich, L., Sutcliffe, J.S., Haines, J.L., Folstein, S.E., Piven, J., Wassink, T.H., Sheffield, V., Geschwind, D.H., Bucan, M., Brown, W. T., Cantor, R.M., Constantino, J.N., Gilliam, T.C., Herbert, M., Lajonchere, C., Ledbetter, D.H., Lese-Martin, C., Miller, J., Nelson, S., Samango-Sprouse, C.A., Spence, S., State, M., Tanzi, R.E., Coon, H., Dawson, G., Devlin, B., Estes, A., Flodman, P., Klei, L., McMahon, W.M., Minshew, N., Munson, J., Korvatska, E., Rodier, P.M., Schellenberg, G.D., Smith, M., Spence, M.A., Stodgell, C., Tepper, P.G., Wijsman, E.M., Yu, C.E., Roge, B., Mantoulan, C., Wittemeyer, K., Poustka, A., Felder, B., Klauck, S.M., Schuster, C., Poustka, F., Bolte, S., Feineis-Matthews, S., Herbrecht, E., Schmotzer, G., Tsiantis, J., Papanikolaou, K., Maestrini, E., Bacchelli, E., Blasi, F., Carone, S., Toma, C., Van Engeland, H., de Jonge, M., Kemner, C., Koop, F., Langemeijer, M., Hijimans, C., Staal, W.G., Baird, G., Bolton, P.F., Rutter, M.L., Weisblatt, E., Green, J., Aldred, C., Wilkinson, J.A., Pickles, A., Le Couteur, A., Berney, T., McConachie, H., Bailey, A.J., Francis, K., Honeyman, G., Hutchinson, A., Parr, J.R., Wallace, S., Monaco, A.P., Barnby, G., Kobayashi, K., Lamb, J.A., Sousa, I., Sykes, N., Cook, E.H., Guter, S.J., Leventhal, B.L., Salt, J., Lord, C., Corsello, C., Hus, V., Weeks, D.E., Volkmar, F., Tauber, M., Fombonne, E., and Shih, A. (2007) Mapping autism risk loci using genetic linkage and chromosomal rearrangements. *Nat. Genet.* 39(3):319–328.

Tharp, B.R. (2004) Epileptic encephalopathies and their relationship to developmental disorders: Do spikes cause autism? *Ment. Retard. Dev. Disabil. Res. Rev.* 10(2):132–134.

Tierney, E., Nwokoro, N.A., Porter, F.D., Freund, L.S., Ghuman, J.K., and Kelley, R.I. (2001) Behavior phenotype in the RSH/ Smith-Lemli-Opitz syndrome. *Am. J. Med. Genet.* 98(2):191– 200.

Tordjman, S., Gutknecht, L., Carlier, M., Spitz, E., Antoine, C., Slama, F., Carsalade, V., Cohen, D.J., Ferrari, P., Roubertoux, P.L., and Anderson, G.M. (2001) Role of the serotonin transporter gene in the behavioral expression of autism. *Mol. Psychiatry* 6(4):434–439.

Tsakanikos, E., Costello, H., Holt, G., Sturmey, P., and Bouras, N. (2007) Behaviour management problems as predictors of psychotropic medication and use of psychiatric services in adults with autism. *J. Autism Dev. Disord.* 37(6):1080–1085.

Tuchman, R., and Rapin, I. (2002) Epilepsy in autism. *Lancet Neurol.* 1(6):352–358.

Tuchman, R.F., and Rapin, I. (1997) Regression in pervasive developmental disorders: Seizures and epileptiform electroencephalogram correlates. *Pediatrics* 99(4):560–566.

Tuchman, R.F., Rapin, I., and Shinnar, S. (1991) Autistic and dysphasic children. II: epilepsy. *Pediatrics* 88(6):1219–1225.

Vargas, D.L., Nascimbene, C., Krishnan, C., Zimmerman, A.W., and Pardo, C.A. (2005) Neuroglial activation and neuroinflammation in the brain of patients with autism. *Ann. Neurol.* 57(1):67–81.

Veenstra-VanderWeele, J., Cook, E., Jr., and Lombroso, P.J. (2003) Genetics of childhood disorders: XLVI. Autism, part 5: Genetics of autism. *J. Am. Acad. Child Adolesc. Psychiatry* 42(1):116–118.

Veltman, M.W., Craig, E.E., and Bolton, P.F. (2005) Autism spectrum disorders in Prader-Willi and Angelman syndromes: A systematic review. *Psychiatr. Genet.* 15(4):243–254.

Verte, S., Geurts, H.M., Roeyers, H., Oosterlaan, J., and Sergeant, J.A. (2006) Executive functioning in children with an autism spectrum disorder: Can we differentiate within the spectrum? *J. Autism Dev. Disord.* 36(3):351–372.

Volkmar, F.R., and Nelson, D.S. (1990) Seizure disorders in autism. *J. Am. Acad. Child Adolesc. Psychiatry* 29(1):127–129.

Wassink, T.H., Piven, J., and Patil, S.R. (2001) Chromosomal abnormalities in a clinic sample of individuals with autistic disorder. *Psychiatr. Genet.* 11(2):57–63.

Webb, S.J., Dawson, G., Bernier, R., and Panagiotides, H. (2006) ERP evidence of atypical face processing in young children with autism. *J. Autism Dev. Disord.* 36(7):881–890.

Werner, E., and Dawson, G. (2005) Validation of the phenomenon of autistic regression using home videotapes. *Arch. Gen. Psychiatry* 62(8):889– 895.

Williams, J.H., Waiter, G.D., Perra, O., Perrett, D.I., and Whiten, A. (2005) An fMRI study of joint attention experience. *NeuroImage* 25(1):133–140.

Williams, J.H., Whiten, A., Suddendorf, T., and Perrett, D.I. (2001) Imitation, mirror neurons and autism. *Neurosci. Biobehav. Rev.* 25(4):287–295.

Williams, K.W., Wray, J.J., and Wheeler, D.M. (2005) Intravenous secretin for autism spectrum disorder. *Cochrane Database Syst Rev*(3):CD003495.

Williams, P.G., and Hersh, J.H. (1998) Brief report: The association of neurofibromatosis type 1 and autism. *J. Autism Dev. Disord.* 28(6):567–571.

Winslow, J.T., and Insel, T.R. (2004) Neuroendocrine basis of social recognition. *Curr. Opin. Neurobiol.* 14(2):248–253.

Wolff, D.J., Clifton, K., Karr, C., and Charles, J. (2002) Pilot assessment of the subtelomeric regions of children with autism: Detection of a 2q deletion. *Genet. Med.* 4(1):10–14.

Woodhouse, W., Bailey, A., Rutter, M., Bolton, P., Baird, G., and Le Couteur, A. (1996) Head circumference in autism and other pervasive developmental disorders. *J. Child Psychol. Psychiatry* 37(6):665–671.

Wray, J.A., Yoon, J.H., Vollmer, T., and Mauk, J. (2000) Pilot study of the behavioral effects of flumazenil in two children with autism. *J. Autism Dev. Disord.* 30(6):619–620.

Yirmiya, N., Pilowsky, T., Nemanov, L., Arbelle, S., Feinsilver, T., Fried, I., and Ebstein, R.P. (2001) Evidence for an association with the serotonin transporter promoter region polymorphism and autism. *Am. J. Med. Genet.* 105(4):381–386.

Ylisaukko-Oja, T., Alarcon, M., Cantor, R.M., Auranen, M., Vanhala, R., Kempas, E., von Wendt, L., Jarvela, I., Geschwind, D.H., and Peltonen, L. (2006) Search for autism loci by combined analysis of Autism Genetic Resource Exchange and Finnish Families. *Ann. Neurol.* 59(1):145–155.

Yonan, A.L., Alarcon, M., Cheng, R., Magnusson, P.K., Spence, S.J., Palmer, A.A., Grunn, A., Juo, S.H., Terwilliger, J.D., Liu, J., Cantor, R.M., Geschwind, D.H., and Gilliam, T.C. (2003) A genome-wide screen of 345 families for autism-susceptibility loci. *Am. J. Hum. Genet.* 73(4):886–897.

Young, J.G., Cohen, D.J., Kavanagh, M.E., Landis, H.D., Shaywitz, B.A., and Maas, J.W. (1981) Cerebrospinal fluid, plasma, and urinary MHPG in children. *Life Sci.* 28(25):2837–2845.

Young, L.J., Lim, M.M., Gingrich, B., and Insel, T.R. (2001) Cellular mechanisms of social attachment. *Horm. Behav.* 40(2):133–138.

Young, L.J., Pitkow, L.J., and Ferguson, J.N. (2002) Neuropeptides and social behavior: Animal models relevant to autism. *Mol. Psychiatry* 7(Suppl 2):S38–S39.

Zappella, M. (1993) Autism and hypomelanosis of Ito in twins. *Dev. Med. Child Neurol.* 35(9):826–832.

Zhang, H., Liu, X., Zhang, C., Mundo, E., Macciardi, F., Grayson, D.R., Guidotti, A.R., and Holden, J.J. (2002) REELIN gene alleles and susceptibility to autism spectrum disorders. *Mol. Psychiatry* 7(9):1012–1017.

Zwaigenbaum, L., Bryson, S., Rogers, T., Roberts, W., Brian, J., and Szatmari, P. (2005) Behavioral manifestations of autism in the first year of life. *Int. J. Dev. Neurosci.* 23(2–3):143–152.

Zwaigenbaum, L., and Tarnopolsky, M. (2003) Two children with muscular dystrophies ascertained due to referral for diagnosis of autism. *J. Autism Dev. Disord.* 33(2):193–199.

IX SPECIAL TOPIC AREAS

ANTONIA S. NEW

79 Neuropsychiatry: The Border Between Neurology and Psychiatry

WILLIAM M. MCDONALD AND MICHAEL S. OKUN

In 1864, Wilhelm Griesinger established the first neuropsychiatry curriculum in Berlin. Twenty years earlier, in his classic text *Mental Pathology and Therapeutics*, he developed a thesis that mental illness was the result of brain lesions. By the turn of the 20th century, academic researchers were testing hypotheses that emotion and behavior had a neuroanatomical basis. In Griesinger's vision, neuropsychiatry linked principles common to neurology and psychiatry and extended the laboratory of neuroscience research into the complexities of human behavior and emotion. The basis of neuropsychiatry was the understanding that emotional tone may be determined by neuroanatomy and tempered by the environment. The translational loop is complete when the clinical observations of the neuropsychiatrist form the laboratory investigations in the neurosciences.

The developments in the field of neuroscience, psychiatric research, and clinical practice during the 20th century were dramatic. At the same time Kraepelin was searching for a specific lesion to determine the origin of dementia praecox, Pavlov was explaining behavior in terms of a reflex arc, and Freud was proposing that the unconscious was the basis of human emotion. By the middle of the century, with the discovery of the therapeutic effects of chlorpromazine, psychiatric research had shifted and neuroscientists refocused attention on the neurobiological substrates of mental disorders. The monoamine hypothesis of depression and the dopamine model of schizophrenia developed from clinical observations about the efficacy of specific medications and provided a theoretical basis that later led to laboratory models of mental illness.

Over the past 50 years, the explosion in research techniques including neuroimaging, neuropathology, molecular neurobiology, and neurochemistry has advanced the understanding of the neuroscience of mental illness. The development of these techniques and the role of the clinical neuroscientist have led to a "worldwide renaissance" in neuropsychiatry (Cummings and Hegarty, 1994). This chapter traces these developments from the earliest hypotheses of the neuroanatomy of emotion. Clinical observations and research in neurological disorders have shown that certain disease states (that is, Parkinson's disease [PD] and the movement disorders) may serve as a model of the interaction of neuroanatomy and psychiatric symptoms. This chapter also addresses the role of neuropsychiatry in interpreting basic neuroscience findings within a clinical context. These interpretations have provided insights into new areas of neuroscience research.

THE HISTORY OF THE BIOLOGY OF EMOTION

Hippocrates to Bucy

The biology of human emotion has been the subject of medical debate from the time of Hippocrates. In this era, four humors were believed to affect behavior: mania, melancholia, paranoia, and phrenitis (Lewis, 1934). The appreciation of the role of the brain in psychiatric illness would develop slowly and deviate from this principle. Saint Augustine and other scholars in the 17th and 18th centuries believed that the root of insanity was demonic possession. Commonly held beliefs associated mental illness with immortality or weakness in character.

The advances in the treatment of mental illness in the 19th century were focused on the humane treatment of individuals with mental illness championed by Philippe Pinel (1745–1826) in France and Dorothea Dix (1802–1887) in the United States. Other physicians focused on understanding the neuroanatomical basis for psychosis and mental disorders. Benjamin Rush (1745–1813), in his influential book *Medical Inquiries and Observations on the Diseases of the Mind* (Rush, 1812/2007), proposed that insanity was caused by vascular congestion of cerebral blood vessels and advocated bloodletting as a treatment (Fig. 79.1). The German physician Franz Gall (1758–1828) developed the concept of *phrenology*, in which he proposed that there were 37 organs in the brain controlling psychic function that could be mapped on the skull surface. The doctrine of phrenology soon spread throughout Europe and the United States and was an early attempt to equate neuroanatomical structures

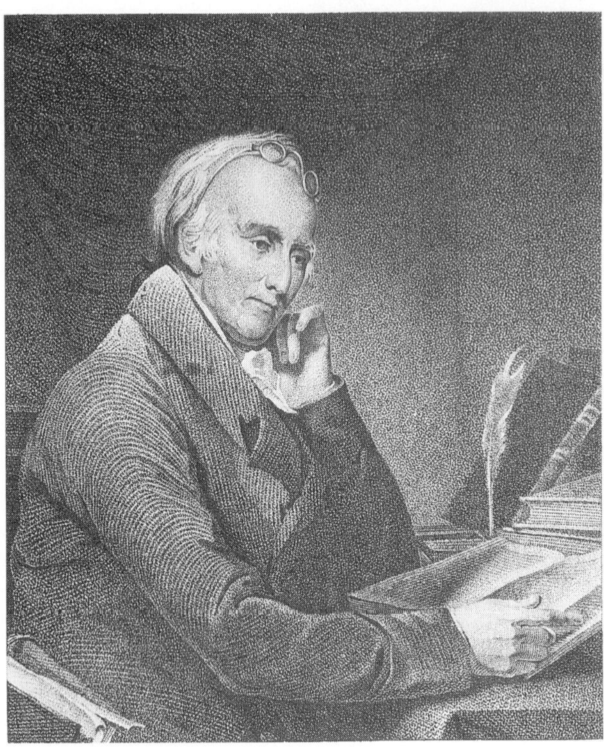

FIGURE 79.1 Benjamin Rush (1745–1813) was one of the early proponents of bloodletting and a strong advocate of its use in a number of medical illnesses including the yellow fever epidemic of 1793. The year before he died, he published *Medical Inquiries and Observations on the Diseases of the Mind*, the first American medical textbook focusing on the treatment of mental illness. Perhaps his greatest contributions were to a number of social and political causes. He was a signer of the Declaration of Independence, a founder of the Philadelphia Dispensary (one of the first hospitals in the United States devoted to the care of the poor), and a strong advocate for education for women and abolition of slavery. His role in the humane treatment of the mentally ill is acknowledged by his portrait on the official seal of the American Psychiatric Association and a bronze plaque placed on his grave with the title, "Father of American Psychiatry."

with mental processes. Kraepelin's (1855–1926) work in defining the course and outcome of mental disorders and distinguishing *dementia praecox* from melancholia and manic-depressive insanity was the beginning of modern psychiatric nosology.

However, neuroanatomists conducted most psychiatric research, and psychiatrists were isolated in large institutions providing care for those with chronic mental illness. Psychiatrists had little academic training or contact with the other medical specialists including neurologists. Diseases of the mind were segregated physically and professionally from diseases of the brain.

Despite these barriers, important advances were being made in understanding organic causes of psychiatric symptoms. In 1890, the Russian psychiatrist S.S. Korsakoff described the association of amnesia with polyneuritis known today as Korsakoff's psychosis. Sixteen years later, Alois Alzheimer presented pathological evidence of a common dementia syndrome. In his original case report, Alzheimer discussed the prominent psychotic features of his patient writing, "at times she believed one intended to murder her . . . and appears to have auditory hallucinations" (Martin, 2002). John Hughlings Jackson (1835–1911) studied epilepsy, and his observation that the clinical features of an epileptic seizure correlated with a specific anatomical focus were important in developing the idea of psychic functions localized to specific areas of the brain. Landmark publications, including Sherrington's *The Integrative Action of the Nervous System* (1906/1948), detailed the reflex arc and served as the foundation for neurology and new areas of research. Klüver and Bucy's experiments demonstrated that bilateral ablation of the temporal lobes caused psychic blindness (that is, visual agnosia) hypersexuality, severe memory loss, and docile behavior in aggressive rhesus monkeys and further stimulated research in understanding brain disease and agitated psychiatric disturbances.

The Treatment of Psychosis

Scientific progress was also being made in the understanding of "lunacy" and therapy for the psychoses. At the turn of the 20th century, syphilis and pellagra were major health problems (Fig. 79.2). Neurosyphilis, or general paresis of the insane, was a significant cause of psychosis. The discovery in 1912 that the spirochete *Treponema pallidum* was the etiological agent in neurosyphilis confirmed that psychosis could be precipitated by organic factors. In 1927, Austrian psychiatrist Julius von Wagner-Jauregg won the Nobel Prize in Medicine for his use of malarial fever to prevent the development of the psychosis associated with tertiary syphilis. His first treatments began in 1917, almost three decades before the discovery of penicillin. In 1937, the discovery that pellagra, a major cause of dementia and psychosis in impoverished areas, was due to a dietary deficiency of nicotinic acid provided a breakthrough in public mental health.

Another public health problem, the epidemic of encephalitis lethargica in 1916 provided evidence of an association between the physical and psychological effects of disease of the subcortical brain structures (Brain, 1958). Patients stricken with the encephalitis had a range of psychiatric symptoms including "shouting fits," psychosis, bizarre behavior, vocal tics, coprolalia, echolalia, echopraxia, palilalia, and parkinsonism. Autopsies of these patients showed significant pathology in many subcortical structures. These findings prompted studies of lesions of the hypothalamus and their effect on behavior (e.g., Bard, 1929) and the endocrine system (e.g., Camus and Roussy, 1922), as well as the effect of lesions in the brain stem on altering the level of consciousness. By the middle of the century, research in neurology

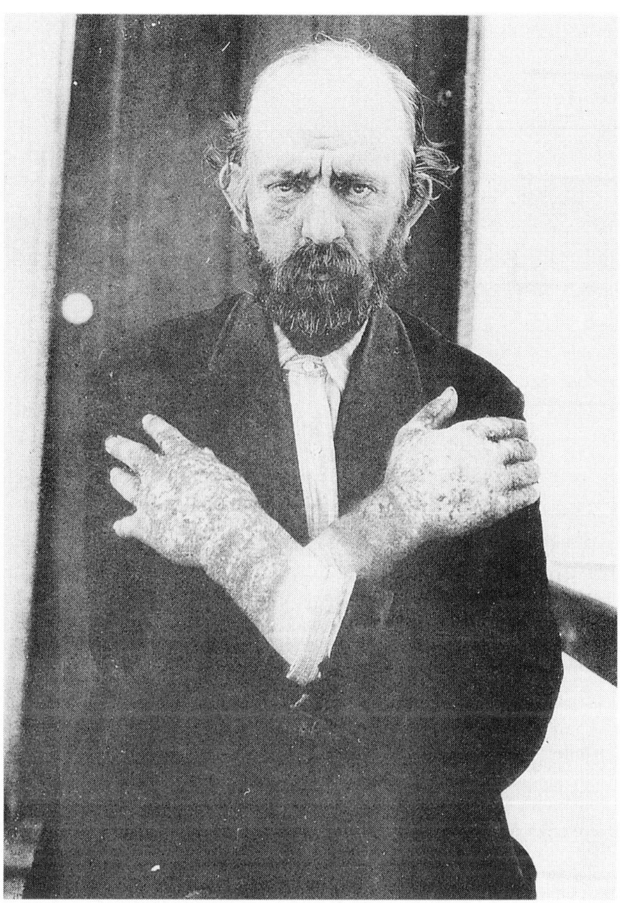

FIGURE 79.2 Man with pellagra, a disease caused by a deficiency of niacin (a B complex vitamin) and manifested by the 4 Ds: diarrhea, dermatitis (scaly skin sores and mucosal changes), dementia (mental changes including dementia and psychosis), and death. Pellagra was first described in Europe in 1762 and was first reported in the United States in 1902 and became epidemic in the American South. In 1912, there were 30,000 cases in South Carolina alone, with a mortality rate of 40%. Dr. Joseph Goldberger of the U.S. Public Health Service linked pellagra to niacin-deficient diets among rural tenant farmers and mill workers. Goldberger's association of dietary deficiency to pellagra is considered one of the landmark public health findings of the twentieth century. Courtesy of the James W. Babcock, M.D., Papers, MSS #294, Waring Historical Library, Medical University of South Carolina, Charleston, SC.

increased the understanding of the relationship of the brain to behavior in three important areas: the association of focal lesions in the brain to clinical symptoms, the relationship of the nervous system to endocrine structures, and the subsequent effects on behavior and understanding of the role of the brain stem in the state of consciousness (Brain, 1958).

Treatments of psychoses were also being advanced. Methods of inducing convulsions in patients with psychoses were developed based on the erroneous assumption that patients with epilepsy could not develop schizophrenia. In 1935, Manfred Sakel used insulin shock therapy and Lazlo Meduna used pentylenetetrazol to induce convulsions and treat psychosis. Three years later, the Italian psychiatrists Ugo Cerletti and Lucio Bini used electroshock treatments, in place of other previous treatments for inducing seizures. A decade later, Egas Moniz and Walter Freeman developed the surgical procedure of prefrontal lobotomy for psychosis. In 1949, Moniz won the Nobel Prize in Medicine for his contributions, which included the development of cerebral angiography. In that same year, over 5,000 lobotomies were performed in the United States.

Freud and Psychodynamic Theory

Hill (1964) argued that two 19th century neurologists, Sigmund Freud (1856–1939) and Carl Wernicke (1848–1905), were responsible for establishing the neuropsychiatric and psychodynamic approaches to psychiatry and, in the process, further separating general psychiatry from neurology and general medicine. Ironically, both men had studied in the lab of Theodor Meynert (1835–1893), who proposed that mental illness resulted from brain dysfunction and cortical circulatory problems. Wernicke related the behavioral symptoms of sensory aphasia and memory problems to specific areas of the brain. Although Wernicke's approach was a model for modern neuropsychiatry, correlating the patient's observable behavior with anatomical brain changes, Freud described the phenomena of aphasia in psychological terms using concepts such as *pathological lesions* that led to "functional retrogression" to an earlier state of development (Stengel, 1954). In parallel with the treatments for psychotic disorders, Freud was developing his method of psychoanalytic treatment. The lay public understood the principles of psychoanalysis and neurosis more easily than the foreign notions of psychosis and treatments such as shock therapy. Psychiatric concepts became more accessible as people became intrigued with dream therapy, slips of the tongue, and other commonly observed manifestations of the unconscious mind.

Although psychodynamic theory has clearly enriched psychiatry, the adoption of psychodynamic principles (and later social and epidemiological psychiatry) by psychiatrists further separated neurology, and the study of the brain, from psychiatry, and the study of the mind (Lishman, 1992). Freud proposed that the mind was a dynamic force. Conscious thought and the mind were not equivalent; preconscious and unconscious thoughts could be understood only by careful observation and interpretation. Neurological and psychiatric symptoms such as conversion hysteria could be understood only by interpreting the experiences of the individual in relation to his or her inner psychic structures (that is, the id, ego, and superego). Data collected by the examiner consisted of the patient's interactions with the examiner and subjective experiences from dreams, fantasies, wishes, and slips of the tongue. Understanding of the psychoses was also proposed to fit into the psychoanalytic model, most notably by Jung in 1906 and Abraham, who in 1908 outlined how the libido theory explained the symptoms of *dementia praecox*. In 1911, Freud expanded the view of the psychoses with the concept of *narcissism* in the Schreber case, in which he compared the psychoses and psychoneuroses as disorders in sexual development and libidinal forces (Hart, 1931).

While Freud developed his theories, highlighting the importance of the individual and subjective experiences, the understanding of the neuroanatomic basis of emotion was progressing in parallel. Mega et al. (1997) outlined the evolution of the limbic system starting with Papez and described the limbic system as "the border between psychiatry and neurology." Papez (1937) defined the evolution of human emotion and integrated basic anatomical studies and clinical observations of patients with specific neurological lesions. The hypothalamus was hypothesized to be important in the expression of emotion because animals could express "sham rage" if the connection between the hypothalamus and brain stem and spinal cord was severed. This reaction would occur even when the connections to the diencephalic and telencephalic structures were severed. This observation, coupled with the evidence that Broca's limbic structures were interconnected with the hypothalamus, led Papez to the conclusion that the hypothalamus was a central structure in emotional expression. The Papez circuit connected the hypothalamus, which was the integral piece in the "expression" of emotion, and the cerebral cortex, which was primarily responsible for the "experience" of emotion (Fig. 79.3).

Fifteen years later, MacLean (1952) defined the limbic system and included the medial circuit of Papez and the lateral cortical structures (orbital frontal cortex, temporal lobe, and insula) and subcortical structures (amygdala and dorsal medial thalamus) described by Yakovlev (1948) (Mega et al., 1997). MacLean defined the limbic system as the "visceral brain that interprets and gives expression to incoming information in terms of feeling." The field of neuropsychiatry has developed in parallel with the evolution of the understanding of structures such as the limbic system as a means of understanding the biology of emotion and behavior.

Advances in Psychiatric Treatment

Advances in the treatment of psychiatric disorders over the past 50 years have changed the nature of the field from investigations based on psychoanalytic theory to investigations of the neuropsychiatric basis of psychiatric illnesses. Additionally, neuropharmacology developed with the discovery of the efficacy of lithium (1949) and iproniazid (1957) for the treatment of mood disorders. The synthesis of the first antipsychotic *chlorpromazine* (1952), the first tricyclic antidepressant *imipramine* (1959), and the first benzodiazepine *chlordiazepoxide* (1960) further expanded neuropharmacology.

The use of medications to treat psychiatric disorders has likely provided the impetus in psychiatry for the acceptance of a more biological view of psychiatric symptoms, especially in disorders such as schizophrenia and melancholia. Neuroscience advances in the understanding of frontal-subcortical loops, including parts of the limbic system that affect motor and nonmotor symptoms in neurological disease, have helped to create models of the etiology of neuropsychiatric symptoms (Alexander et al., 1990). Similarly, research in neurochemistry has provided insights into the role of behavioral symptoms in medical disease. Neuropeptides such as corticotropin-releasing factor, which are processed and transported

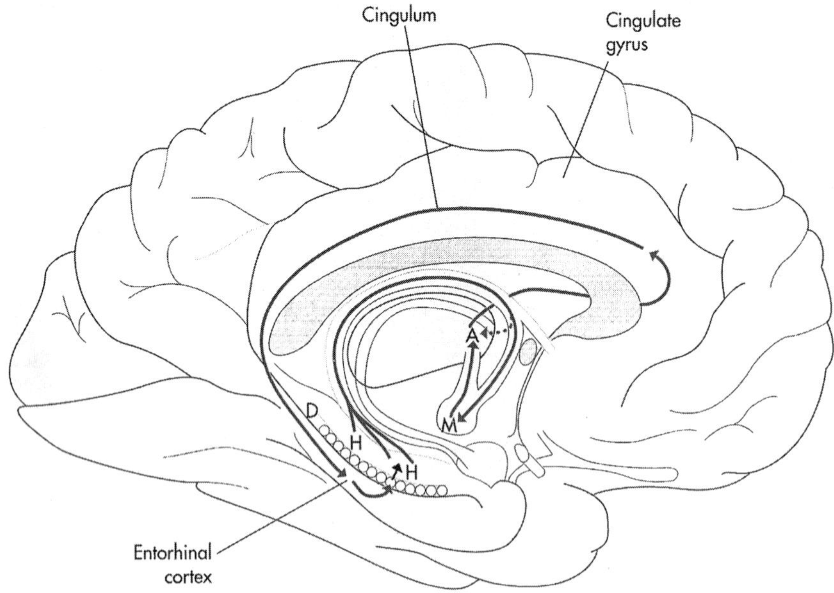

FIGURE 79.3 Schematic view of the Papez circuit hypothesized in the 1930s to integrate basic anatomical studies and understanding of the neuroanatomical basis of emotion. The circuit includes the hippocampus (H) that projects via the fornix to the septal area of the hypothalamus. In turn, the mammillary bodies (M) project via the mammillothalmic tract to the anterior thalamic nuclei (A). The shortcut from the hippocampus directly to the anterior thalamic nucleus is indicated by the dashed line and is not part of the circuit as originally proposed. The anterior thalamic nuclei project via the internal capsule to the cerebral cortex (cingulated gyrus) and via the dentate gyrus (D) back to the hypothalamus.

to nerve terminals, have been associated with a variety of neuropsychiatric symptoms (Nemeroff, 1992). Additionally, neuroendocrine studies have demonstrated the association of hormones to human sexuality (Wood and Naftolin, 1999) and human attachment (Insel and Winslow, 1999).

The study of clinical symptoms in neurological disorders has advanced with improvements in the ability to image the brains of symptomatic patients and understand the neuropathology underlying psychiatric symptoms. Magnetic resonance imaging (MRI) studies have shown a relationship between lesions in the frontal cortex and subcortical structures to depression and mania (Krishnan et al., 1993). The understanding of the neuroanatomical basis of psychiatric symptoms has also been improved with the availability of positron emission tomography (PET) and functional magnetic resonance imaging (fMRI). These techniques measure metabolic activity and functional changes in response to specific tasks and have allowed, for the first time, direct measures of the energy consumption of the brain and are hypothesized to be correlated with neuronal activity.

Advances in the neuroscience of behavior have led to new insights into the etiology of neuropsychiatric symptoms. For example, PET studies of prefrontal-subcortical circuits have confirmed that syndromes associated with obsessive–compulsive disorder (OCD) have the same pattern of metabolic uptake as idiopathic OCD (Cummings, 1993). Clinical neuropsychiatrists have used these research findings to develop models to understand psychiatric symptoms in patients with neurological disease, and also to develop treatment strategies to manage these symptoms. The neurobiology of many of the neuropsychiatric conditions is covered in substance abuse (Part VI), dementia (Part VII), developmental disorders (Part VIII), aggression, personality, and personality disorders (Part IX). In this chapter, the focus is on specific neurological diseases traditionally managed by neurologists (the movement disorders, multiple sclerosis, and stroke) and the occurrence and etiology of psychiatric symptoms. This discussion is not intended to be an exhaustive review, as there are many other neurological conditions with prominent psychiatric symptoms (for example, head injury, infectious diseases such as neurosyphilis and human immunodeficiency virus, to mention only a few). Instead, this chapter is intended as a review of the approach to neuropsychiatric symptoms.

NEUROLOGICAL DISEASE AS A MODEL OF PSYCHIATRIC SYNDROMES

The border between psychiatry and neurology includes comorbid psychiatric conditions that are coincidental with the neurological disorder (for example, substance abuse), a reaction to the neurological disability (for example, adjustment disorder) or an underlying cause of the disorder (for example, conversion reaction). The areas that have received the most attention are the psychiatric symptoms that are hypothesized to be an integral part of the symptom complex of neurological conditions. Many of these syndromes have been shown to be secondary to the underlying neuropathology. The psychiatric symptoms observed in patients with neurological disease may be the most difficult for the physician, caregiver, and patient. These symptoms dramatically increase the caregiver burden as well as the cost of managing the diseases. Movement disorders in particular are associated with significant nonmotor neuropsychiatric symptoms including cognitive dysfunction, psychosis, and profound changes in personality and mood.

Symptom Profile

The diagnosis of depression and anxiety can be particularly difficult in patients with neurological disease. For example, nondepressed patients who suffered a stroke often show a loss of energy, concentration, appetite, and sleep because of the medical complications of the stroke. They may therefore be misdiagnosed as depressed (Rodin and Voshart, 1986). Conversely, depression may be underdiagnosed because the patient who suffered a stroke lacks insight into his or her emotional state because of anosognosia, aprosody, or neglect (Ross et al., 1986). These arguments have been made for many neurological and medical disorders, and they focus on the validity of the *Diagnostic and Statistical Manual of Mental Disorders* (*DSM-IV*) criteria (American Psychiatric Association, 1994) in diagnosing depression in patients with medical problems. By *DSM-IV* criteria, most neurological patients would be classified as having a mood disorder secondary to a medical disorder. This classification may be technically correct, but it is too broad and may include patients with chronic low-grade depression, adjustment disorder with depressed mood, and major depression. A more useful classification scheme would define a group of patients with a course of illness similar to that of major depression and with depressive symptoms that respond to somatic treatments for depression.

A number of variations of the *DSM* criteria for major depression have been compared in patients who were medically ill. Using the inclusive scheme, the rater counts a symptom if it is present. Using the etiologic scheme, the symptom is counted only if the rater determines that it is not due to the underlying medical disorder but is the result of a comorbid mood disorder. For example, the rater would first have to determine if a patient who suffered a stroke met symptom criteria for withdrawal or loss of energy and then make a judgment to determine if those symptoms were physical manifestations of the stroke or were due to depression and not the stroke. Any symptom, if present, would be counted in the inclusive scheme, and only symptoms due to depression would be counted in the etiologic scheme. The etiologic scheme is, of course, subjective, and reliability between observers may be difficult, depending on the experience of the observers, whether caregivers or family are present at the interview, and whether the rater is familiar with the patient. The inclusive scheme is easier to use because the rater need only determine if the symptom is present or absent without making an inference as to the etiology of the symptom.

The inclusive approach has been validated in studies of inpatients who were medically ill (Koenig et al., 1997) and patients who were poststroke (Fedoroff et al., 1991), but not in other neurological disorders. The inclusive strategy would be the most practical for clinicians and would encourage the development of simple checklists to confirm psychiatric diagnoses.

Etiology

Clinical research designed to understand the nature of mood disorders in neurological syndromes has focused on biological research markers for endogenous depression including family history of mood disorders, laboratory tests (for example, the dexamethasone suppression test), course of untreated depression, and response to antidepressant medications. Research has concentrated on three disorders: Alzheimer's disease, stroke, and PD. Few studies have been designed for long-term follow-up of neurological patients with mood disorders, and there are few placebo-controlled clinical trials of psychiatric medications specific to these neurological conditions to determine response and long-term effects. Despite these deficiencies, metabolic imaging studies comparing primary or idiopathic depression with secondary depression from neurological disease have shown a remarkable convergence on the neuropathological basis for these disorders (Robinson et al., 1999), supporting a common pathophysiology and etiology.

The etiology of depression in neurological disease may be one of three, not mutually exclusive, theories: (*1*) depression is a reaction to the disability of the neurological disease, including the psychosocial and individual personality factors; (*2*) depression is the result of medications or treatments for the neurological condition such as dopamine agonists in PD or corticosteroids in multiple sclerosis; and (*3*) depression results from the neuroanatomical or neurophysiological changes that occur as part of the disease.

Cerebrovascular Disease

The association of neuropsychiatric symptoms and neurological disease is most clearly defined in stroke patients, in whom a discrete lesion on neuroimaging studies can be correlated with the onset of symptoms. Studies of patients of acute stroke from several countries have found a mean prevalence of 20% for major depression and 19% for minor depression (Robinson, 1998). In a majority of patients, poststroke depression remitted within a year; however, 25% continued to be depressed for years. Depression was associated with longer times to recovery, cognitive dysfunction, and increased mortality (Robinson, 1998) as well as in treating poststroke depression that was associated with improved recovery in activities of daily living (Chemerinski et al., 2001). Cognitive impairment has also been shown to be associated with depressive symptoms poststroke (Robinson et al., 1984) and some (Kimura et al., 2000), but not all (Robinson et al., 2000), studies have shown an improvement in cognitive function in patients who respond to antidepressant treatment. Finally, poststroke depression has been correlated with premature mortality (Robinson et al., 2000).

Strokes, particularly in the left frontal cortex and left basal ganglia, have been linked to significant depression (Robinson et al., 1984; Starkstein et al., 1987) and patients with depression following a stroke exhibited a pattern of decreased metabolic activity and blood flow in the orbitofrontal cortex and basal ganglia as well as decreased serotonin receptors in the left temporal cortex (Robinson et al., 1999). The phenomenology, response to dexamethasone, cognitive impairment secondary to depression, natural course of untreated depression, and response to antidepressant medication are all similar to those of patients without stroke with major depression (Fedoroff et al., 1991).

Double-blind, placebo-controlled trials of the antidepressants *trazodone* (Reding et al., 1986), *nortriptyline* (Lipsey et al., 1984), *fluoxetine* (Wiart et al., 2000), and *citalopram* (Andersen, 1993) concluded that these medications were more effective than placebo in treating poststroke depression. Lauritzen et al. (1994) compared the combination of treatment with imipramine and mianserin to desipramine and mianserin in poststroke depression and found that imipramine was more effective than desipramine in a melancholia scale, but not on changes in the Hamilton Depression Rating Scale. In an additional study of patients who were depressed after suffering a stroke, comparing two antidepressants, nortriptyline but not fluoxetine, proved more effective than placebo (Robinson et al., 2000). Electroconvulsive therapy (Murray et al., 1986), psychotherapy (Hibbard et al., 1990), and stimulants (Grade et al., 1998; Tharwani et al., 2007) are also effective in treating poststroke depression.

Basal Ganglia Disease

Diseases of the basal ganglia have been strongly associated with high rates of mood and cognitive disorders

(McHugh, 1989) and specific dysfunctions in the nonmotor basal ganglia-thalamo-cortical pathways have been implicated in neuropsychiatric symptoms (Alexander et al., 1986). Using this paradigm, researchers have shown selective involvement of the limbic and prefrontal striatal pathways may lead to neuropsychiatric symptoms. These pathways have a role in modulating emotions (Damasio, 1983). Studies of cerebral blood flow and metabolism in patients with depression without comorbid neurological disease including stroke have shown abnormalities in the striatum and frontal lobes (Baxter et al., 1989; Drevets and Rubin, 1989; Mayberg et al., 1991; Robinson et al., 1999).

Anatomically segregated frontal lobe-subcortical circuits have been described including a motor circuit, an oculomotor circuit, and a prefrontal circuit, each originating in a separate area of cortex (dorsolateral prefrontal cortex, lateral orbital cortex, and anterior cingulate cortex, respectively). These circuits are contiguous and project from the frontal lobes to the striatum then to the output nuclei of the basal ganglia (globus pallidus, substantia nigra, and pars reticulata). The projections then pass to thalamic nuclei and back to the frontal lobes.

Based on studies of patients with specific anatomical lesions, Cummings (1993) outlined three frontal lobe syndromes associated with abnormalities in the frontal-subcortical circuits. The dorsolateral prefrontal syndrome has pronounced executive function deficits (for example, reduced verbal fluency, inability to adapt to changing tasks) and motor programming tasks. The orbitofrontal syndrome is associated with profound personality changes (for example, irritability and disinhibition). Finally, the anterior cingulate syndrome is associated with apathy. Characteristics of each of these syndromes have been described in neurological disorders associated with lesions within the specific frontal-subcortical circuit.

Huntington's disease (HD) is an autosomal dominant movement disorder caused by an increased number of polyglutamine repeats on chromosome 4 that most often results in dementia, as well as progressive chorea. Huntington's disease usually presents in patients who are in their 30s or 40s and often has severe cognitive dysfunction, an orbitofrontal syndrome, and other prominent psychiatric symptoms including depression, psychosis, and suicide rates that are significantly higher than those of the general population. Apathy (Mayeux, 1984), OCD (Cummings, 1992), high rates of antisocial personality disorder, anxiety, irritability, and an explosive disorder (Folstein, 1989) have also been described in patients with HD. Often, personality changes precede the onset of HD (Brothers, 1964) and worsen with the onset of the movement disorder (Mayeux, 1984). Depression, anxiety, and irritability occur in half of the patients (Craufurd et al., 2001) and often precede the onset of motor and cognitive symptoms (Shoulson et al., 1989).

George Huntington (1882) described suicide as one of the major features of HD. In one report, half the patients who committed suicide did so before they were diagnosed, and in older patients, the suicide rate was more than 20 times that of age-matched controls 50–69 years old (Schoenfeld et al., 1984). The impulsivity of the patient with HD makes the prevention of suicide a challenge for the practitioner.

Positron emission tomography has demonstrated a decrease in cerebral glucose metabolism in the para-limbic system (orbito-frontal-inferior prefrontal cortex) of patients with HD who were depressed compared to controls, implicating nonmotor loops of the basal ganglia (Mayberg et al., 1992). This finding was comparable to the para-limbic hypometabolism found in patients with PD with depression (Mayberg et al., 1990) and was supported by the role of this area in emotional tone (Damasio, 1983). The medial caudate is affected first in HD, and these changes are hypothesized to be associated with the personality changes seen early in HD. The ventromedial caudate receives projections from the lateral orbital-frontal cortex and is in the lateral orbital-frontal cortex-ventromedial caudate circuit, where lesions may be associated with marked personality changes (orbitofrontal syndrome) (Cummings, 1993). Degeneration of the dorsomedial caudate has also been hypothesized to be associated with depression in HD (Mayberg et al., 1992). Involvement of the head of the caudate nucleus, which receives projections from the dorsolateral prefrontal cortex, is reflected in the abnormalities on the Wisconsin Card Sort test and other measures of executive function noted in HD patients and correspond to Cummings' (1993) dorsolateral prefrontal syndrome.

James Parkinson (1817) first described the disease that bears his name in *An Essay on the Shaking Palsy*. However, it was not until almost a century later that the degeneration of the corpus striatum (Wilson, 1912) and substantia nigra (Lewy, 1913) was linked to the symptoms of PD. Parkinson noted in his early description of the nonmotor symptoms of PD that "melancholy" was a prominent feature. The diagnosis of depression in PD may be complicated by the fact that the parkinsonian symptoms overlap with symptoms of depression (for example, masked facies and bradykinesia), and there are no reliable and valid diagnostic scales to differentiate depression from PD-related motor symptoms (Leentjens et al., 2000). Parkinson's disease is one of the best-characterized examples of a neuropsychiatric disease with evidence of a neuropathological basis for the cognitive, emotional, and psychotic symptoms associated with the disorder.

The prevalence of major depression in PD is high, with most estimates falling in the range of 20%–30% (Allain et al., 2000; Ranoux, 2000). In a worldwide survey of patients with PD, depression, disease severity, and medication use were the three factors most closely associated with quality of life (Global Parkinson's Disease Survey, 2002). There is evidence that depression in PD is not simply a reaction to the disability. Depression and anxiety syndromes often occur before the onset of motor symptoms (Mayeux et al., 1981; Sano et al., 1989) and patients with PD have higher rates of depression than patients with similar disability from other chronic diseases such as diabetes or arthritis (Mayeux, 1984). There is only a weak correlation between the absolute rate of disability and depression in PD patients (Menza and Mark, 1994; Tandberg et al., 1997).

The medications used to treat PD do not appear to be responsible for depressive symptoms. The dopamine agonists although associated with psychiatric symptoms, including delirium and agitation as well as mood fluctuations secondary to "off" and "on" states (Cummings, 1992), do not cause depression. Depressed mood is associated with an "off" state (Nissenbaum et al., 1987), and patients can have a subjective feeling of panic when going "off." Most patients do not describe depression or anxiety when turning "on" after their medication begins to take effect. Dopamine agonists, instead of causing depression, may be used by the patient as an antidepressant in an effort to prevent the "off" state. Other dopaminergic medications, including the short-lived antidepressant nomifensine and the amphetamines, may be effective antidepressants.

The etiology of depression in PD is associated with the underlying neurodegenerative process (A.J. Hughes et al., 1992). Positron emission tomography studies have demonstrated hypometabolism in the striatum and orbitofrontal cortex that is more pronounced in patients with PD and comorbid depression (Mentis et al., 2002). This pattern was similar to the pattern in patients without PD and major depression (Mayberg et al., 1990; Paulus and Trenkwalder, 1998). The loss of the dopamine neurons in the mesolimbic and mesocortical circuits can also lead to depression. Serotonin cell loss in the median raphé is associated with depressed mood (Mayeux et al., 1984; Mayeux et al., 1986). Additionally, cell loss in cholinergic neurons of the nucleus basalis of Meynert and noradrenergic cell loss in the locus ceruleus were associated with cognitive and behavioral problems (Sagar, 1999). It is hypothesized that because there is a wide range of variability in the cell loss across individuals in each neuroanatomical area, there may be considerable variability in the nonmotor symptoms (Cummings, 1992). Levels of serotonin metabolites are decreased in the cerebrospinal fluid of patients with PD who are depressed (Mayeux et al., 1984). Other biological markers for depression include decreased platelet-imipramine binding (Raisman et al., 1986), a shortened rapid-eye-movement latency (Kostic et al., 1991), and abnormal dexamethasone suppression test (Mayeux et al., 1986). Degeneration of the subcortical loops involving the visual cortex (Middleton and Strick, 2000) may theoretically be associated with visual hallucinations in PD that may be exacerbated by dopamine agonists.

Although there are only a limited number of placebo-controlled trials of somatic therapies in PD and depression, trials using tricyclic antidepressants (Strong and Vaughan, 1965; Laitinen, 1969; Andersen et al., 1980) and bupropion HCL (Goetz et al., 1984) have shown these medications to be effective in treating depressive symptoms without worsening PD symptoms. Open trials of the selective serotonin reuptake inhibitors (SSRIs) have also shown these medications to be effective in treating depression (McCance-Katz et al., 1992; Montastruc et al., 1995; Hauser and Zesiewicz, 1997; Ceravolo et al., 2000; Rampello et al., 2002). However these studies have a number of methodological flaws, including the failure to use standardized scales to diagnose depression and assess depressive symptoms. In addition, acute and maintenance electroconvulsive therapy were found to be effective in the treatment of depression and parkinsonian symptoms in PD (Burke et al., 1988; Kellner et al., 1994; Wengel et al., 1998).

In clinical studies, depression early in the course of PD was associated with an increased rate of dementia over time. Similarly, in a community study, impaired cognitive function and psychosis were significant predictors of depression in PD (Tandberg et al., 1997). Depression at the baseline evaluation was also shown to predict the development of dementia in patients with PD (T.A. Hughes et al., 2000).

In PD, motor symptoms were more likely correlated with degeneration of the putamen, and cognitive function was associated with loss of neurons in the caudate and degeneration of cholinergic and noradrenergic projections to the cerebral cortex (Sagar, 1999). Additionally, PET studies showed that patients with depression have abnormalities in the caudate and orbito-frontal areas that were distinct from the pattern shown in dementia and PD (Mayberg et al., 1990). These early studies are now supported indirectly from the observations of Braak et al., (2004) who have defined a hypothesis for the degenerative process in PD.

Other diseases of the basal ganglia, including progressive supranuclear palsy (PSP) and Wilson's disease (WD), are also associated with high rates of depression. The onset of PSP is in the 60s, and symptoms may include supranuclear gaze palsy, axial rigidity, pseudobulbar palsy, prominent gait disorder, dystonia, and impairment in postural reflexes. The syndrome has a number of psychological symptoms including apathy, depression, irritability, and euphoria. However, the characteristic mood lability associated with the pseudobulbar affect (sudden bursts of laughing or crying) may lead to the misdiagnosis of depression early in the course of the illness and a delay in recognizing the underlying neurological disease (Dalziel and Griffiths, 1977). Progressive supranuclear palsy is unique among the neurological disorders of the basal ganglia in that early in the course of this disease, patients are often misdiagnosed with depression when in fact they are manifesting the early signs of a progressive dementia (Schneider and Chui, 1986). This phenomenon has been designated *pseudodepression* (Morstyn et al., 1982) to distinguish it from the pseudodementia in patients with apparent cognitive disorders who actually have depression (Wells et al., 1979).

Wilson's disease, or hepatolenticular degeneration, is a recessively inherited disorder of copper metabolism with prominent motor symptoms which may include rigidity, tremor, myoclonus, dystonia, and dysarthria. Wilson's disease preferentially affects the liver and brain, and Kayser–Fleisher rings are neurological manifestations that present in nearly all patients with central nervous system involvement. Neuropsychiatric symptoms occur in approximately half the patients, including behavioral changes (incongruous behavior, irritability, and aggression), cognitive impairment, depressed or dysphoric mood and, rarely, psychotic states (Dening and Berrios, 1989). Dening and Berrios' (1989) retrospective analysis of 195 patients with WD found that approximately one fifth of them were evaluated by a psychiatrist prior to their diagnosis of WD. Psychiatric variables (absence of incongruous behavior) were associated with a more favorable outcome, and behavioral changes were associated with some neurological changes (dysarthria, dysphagia, drooling, and rigidity) but not others (tremor). The neuropsychiatric symptoms also were correlated more closely with the degree of central nervous system involvement, suggesting an organic involvement rather than the severity of illness (for example, the result of a reaction to the disability of the disease).

Multiple Sclerosis

Disseminated sclerosis, or multiple sclerosis (MS), was first described by Cruveilhier in 1835, and half a century later, Charcot's classic pathological studies detailed the clinical presentation and neuropathology of the disorder (Murray, 2005). The most common form of MS is the relapsing-remitting form. Neuropsychiatric symptoms include cognitive deficits, depression, and euphoria or an abnormal sense of well-being (Cottrell and Wilson, 1926; Joffe et al., 1987; Rao, 1990; Rao et al., 1991) and have been shown to have a similar relapsing-remitting pattern. They are often the initial presenting symptom of MS (Mendez, 1995). The incidence of depression is more common than in other neurological diseases (Whitlock and Siskind, 1980) and may occur in approximately half of the patients, usually early in the course of the disease (Schubert and Foliart, 1993). Suicide rates are 7½ times those seen in the general population (Sadovnick et al., 1991), and mood disturbances are strongly correlated with a decreased quality of life (Wang et al., 2000; Fruewald et al., 2001). A significant minority of patients have subsyndromal symptoms (for example, 48% of patients in one study complained of emotional dyscontrol) associated with significant psychological distress (Feinstein and Feinstein, 2001). An increased incidence of bipolar disease has also been reported in patients with MS (Sadovnick et al., 1991).

Factors associated with the mood changes in MS patients are demyelination (Pujol et al., 2000), female gender, age younger than 35 years, a family history of depression (Patten et al., 2000), corticosteroid treatment (Franklin et al., 1988), and interferon beta therapy (Walther and Hohlfeld, 1999). Depression in MS has also been shown to occur as a reaction to the disability of the disease (Zorzon et al., 2001). An open label study showed moclobemide to be effective in treating depression in patients with MS (Barak et al., 1999).

Recent studies found a weak but significant correlation between depression and lesions in the right frontal and temporal lobes (Bakshi et al., 2000; Berg et al., 2000; Zorzon et al., 2001). Some studies have found that unlike patients with PD, HD, and idiopathic depression there is no evidence of subcortical disease and depression in patients with MS (Berg et al., 2000). The degree of demyelination and the amount of cognitive dysfunction have been correlated to the severity of depression (Rabins et al., 1986). Many of the neuropsychiatric symptoms in MS are hypothesized to be the result of demyelination of subcortical circuits involving the prefrontal cortex (Mendez, 1995). Interestingly, late in the disease, patients with MS may experience anosodiaphoria or a lack of concern for their neurological deficits. This can be a prominent symptom leading to an abnormal sense of well-being despite significant and increasing neurological deficits (Mendez, 1995).

THE FUTURE OF NEUROPSYCHIATRY

The physicist Erwin Schrödinger, in his book *What Is Life? The Physical Aspects of the Living Cell* (1992), argued that the understanding of the living organism should be evaluated using the scientific disciplines of physics and chemistry. His student, the Nobel laureate Francis Crick, urged that research focus on an understanding of the molecular basis of the mind and called for research that focused on the neurobiological basis of mental activity (Crick, 1994). He described his hypothesis that emotions, memories, aspirations, and a sense of personal identity are all derived from components of the nervous system and associated molecules (Crick, 1994).

In the extreme, the mind can be visualized as an information processing computer with neural circuits that output emotions. The danger of a purely mechanical view of human emotions is that it fails to take into account the richness of the understanding of the human condition that has been described in the psychoanalytic literature (Forrest, 1992). The other extreme is to view the mind as somehow separate from the visceral brain and emotions as epiphenomena. These views of mental processes have polarized psychiatry.

Academic departments of psychiatry are often presented as more "biological" or "psychoanalytic," as though these two viewpoints in psychiatry are mutually exclusive. In his presidential address to the Royal Society of Medicine in 1931, Dr. Bernard Hart acknowledged that it would be difficult to determine whether the psychological or physiological viewpoint is the "right road" to advance psychiatry. He cautioned that although it was reasonable to question whether one approach was more appropriate than the other, "it will be difficult to obtain an answer which is not conditioned by the traditions, habits of thought, and prejudices of the man who gives it" (Hart, 1931, p. 196). Unfortunately, the cautionary note of Dr. Hart about the "intrinsic imperfections" of psychological theories including psychoanalysis remains true today. The "conceptions cannot be so adequately tested by a constant resort to objective observations, and those observations are themselves liable to numerous subjective and distorting factors" (Hart, 1931, pp. 196–197. The challenge to the analytic community is to not only provide a rich descriptive literature on the human condition, but also to base theoretical templates on scientific methodology.

The Nobel laureate, Eric Kandel, wrote that the scientific advances in the neural sciences and psychiatry offer an opportunity for the two disciplines to work together on developing theories that combine insights from both fields (Kandel, 1998). Kandell called for a rapprochement between the disciplines that would enrich the field by allowing psychoanalytic theories to inform the basic neurobiology of behavior. Neuropsychiatry is an understanding of the biological basis of behavior with an appreciation that the behavior occurs in the context of an individual with multiple influences including family, society, and the individual's personal traditions and prejudices. In assessing and treating the patient, the neuropsychiatrist relies heavily on the tools of traditional psychiatry including the diagnostic interview and psychotherapy. The leaders in the field of neuropsychiatry have emphasized the importance of a multidisciplinary approach to understand these complex disorders. Yudofsky and Hales, in editorials in the *Journal of Neuropsychiatry*, have raised the concern that "an increased focus on biology could cause the conceptual pendulum to swing to a reductionist extreme wherein psychosocial aspects of neuropsychiatric disorders are dangerously deemphasized" (Yudofsky and Hales, 1989, p. 4; Yudofsky and Hales, 1999). They described the "delicate balance" that the neuropsychiatrist undertakes in combining an understanding of the brain with an understanding of the interpersonal problems of the patient, as well as social and environmental factors in the expression of symptoms in neurological illness. Clearly, research on the neurobiology of mental illness has brought psychiatry closer to neurology and the scientific understanding of human emotions. However, some argue that the borderland between psychiatry and neurology is really a "no-man's land" and that psychiatrists and neurologists have failed to find common ground for a mutually enriching exchange (Geschwind, 1975).

In the quarter century since that statement was written, the field of neuropsychiatry has developed and added to the understanding of this borderland. Neuropsychiatry is as much a study of the neuroscience data and an interpretation of the expression of psychiatric symptoms in disease as it is the study of the individual and the social and psychological factors that affect the patient. Neuropsychiatrists are in the unique position of understanding the impact of neurological disease on all patients as well as the individual patient. In academic medicine, the neuropsychiatrist can function as a clinician-researcher and/or clinician educator, with the primary goal of understanding the complexity of diagnosing and treating psychiatric symptoms in patients who are neurologically ill. In Griesenger's view of the neuroscientist clinician, the role of the physician is to understand the complexity of human behavior within the context of biology. In this view, we are all individuals and yet have a common genetic basis. This theme was echoed by C.J. Jung in his description of the collective unconscious and by Crick and Watson in the discovery of the double helix of deoxyribonucleic acid (DNA). Neuropsychiatry is the integration of the psychology of the individual and the neurobiology of the human condition.

REFERENCES

Alexander, G.E., Crutcher, M.D., and DeLong, M.R. (1990) Basal ganglia-thalamocortical circuits: parallel substrates for motor, oculomotor, "prefrontal" and "limbic" functions. *Prog. Brain Res.* 85:119–146.

Alexander, G.E., DeLong, M.R., and Strick, P.L. (1986) Parallel organization of functionally segregated circuits linking basal ganglia and cortex. *Ann. Rev. Neurosci.* 9:357–381.

Allain, H., Schuck, S., and Mauduit, N. (2000) Depression in Parkinson's disease. *Br. Med. J.* 320(7245):1287–1288.

American Psychiatric Association. (1994) *Diagnostic and Statistical Manual of Mental Disorders* (4th ed.). Washington, DC: Author.

American Psychiatric Association. (2000) *Diagnostic and Statistical Manual of Mental Disorders* (4th ed., text rev.). Washington, DC: Author.

Andersen, J., Aabro, E., Gulmann, N., et al. (1980) Anti-depressive treatment in Parkinson's disease. A controlled trial of the effect of nortriptyline in patients with Parkinson's disease treated with L-DOPA. *Acta Neurol. Scand.* 62(4):210–219.

Andersen, G., Vestergaard, K., and Riis, J.O. (1993) Citalopram for post-stroke pathological crying. *Lancet* 342(8875):837–839.

Bakshi, R., Czarnecki, D., Shaikh, Z.A., et al. (2000) Brain MRI lesions and atrophy are related to depression in multiple sclerosis. *Neuroreport* 11(6):1153–1158.

Barak, Y., Ur, E., and Achiron, A. (1999) Moclobemide treatment in multiple sclerosis patients with comorbid depression: an open-label safety trial. *J. Neuropsychiatry Clin. Neurosci.* 11(2):271–273.

Bard, P. (1929) The central representation of the sympathetic system. *Arch. Neurol. Psychiatry* 22:230–246.

Baxter, L.R., Schwartz, J.M., Phelps, M.E., et al. (1989) Reduction of prefrontal cortex glucose metabolism common to three types of depression. *Arch. Gen. Psychiatry* 46(3):243–250.

Berg, D., Supprian, T., Thomae, J., et al. (2000) Lesion pattern in patients with multiple sclerosis and depression. *Multiple Sclerosis* 6(3):156–162.

Braak, H., Ghebremedhin, E., Rüb, U., Bratzke, H., and Del Tredici, K. (2004) Stages in the development of Parkinson's disease-related pathology. *Cell Tissue Res.* 318(1):21–134.

Brain, R. (1958) Neurology: past, present, and future. *Br. Med. J.* 1(5067):355–360.

Brothers, C. (1964) Huntington's chorea in Victoria and Tasmania. *J. Neurol. Sci.* 1:405–420.

Burke, W.J., Peterson, J., and Rubin, E.H. (1988) Electroconvulsive therapy in the treatment of combined depression and Parkinson's disease. *Psychosomatics* 29(3):341–346.

Camus, J., and Roussy, G. (1922) Pituitary systems. *Rev. Neurol.* 38:622–642.

Ceravolo, R., Nuti, A., Piccinni, A., et al. (2000) Paroxetine in Parkinson's disease: effects on motor and depressive symptoms. *Neurology* 55:1216–1218.

Chemerinski, E., Robinson, R,G,, Arndt, S., and Kosier, JT. (2001) The effect of remission of poststroke depression on activities of daily living in a double-blind randomized treatment study. *J. Nerv. Ment. Dis.* 189(7):421–425.

Cottrell, S.S., and Wilson, S.A.K. (1926) The affective symptomatology of disseminated sclerosis: a study of 100 cases. *J. Neurol. Psychopath.* 7:1–30.

Craufurd, D., Thompson, J.C., and Snowden, J.S. (2001) Behavioral changes in Huntington disease. *Neuropsychiatry Neuropsychol. Behav. Neurol.* 14(4):219–226.

Crick, F. (1994) *The Astonishing Hypothesis: The Scientific Search for the Soul.* New York: Charles Scribner's Sons.

Cummings, J.L. (1986) Subcortical dementia. Neuropsychology, neuropsychiatry, and pathophysiology. *Br. J. Psychiatry* 149:682–697.

Cummings, J.L. (1992) Depression and Parkinson's disease: a review [see comments]. *Am. J. Psychiatry* 149(4):443–454.

Cummings, J.L. (1993) Frontal-subcortical circuits and human behavior. *Arch. Neurol.* 50(8):873–880.

Cummings, J.L., and Hegarty, A. (1994) Neurology, psychiatry, and neuropsychiatry. *Neurology* 44(2):209–213.

Dalziel, J.A., and Griffiths, R.A. (1977) Progressive supranuclear palsy. *Age Ageing* 6(3):185–191.

Damasio, H. (1983) A computed tomographic guide to the identification of cerebral vascular territories. *Arch. Neurol.* 40(3):138–142.

Dening, T.R., and Berrios, G.E. (1989) Wilson's disease. Psychiatric symptoms in 195 cases. *Arch. Gen. Psychiatry* 46(12):1126–1134.

Drevets, W.C., and Rubin, E.H. (1989) Psychotic symptoms and the longitudinal course of senile dementia of the Alzheimer type. *Biol. Psychiatry* 25(1):39–48.

Fedoroff, J.P., Starkstein, S.E., Parikh, R.M., et al. (1991) Are depressive symptoms nonspecific in patients with acute stroke? *Am. J. Psychiatry* 148(9):1172–1176.

Feinstein, A., and Feinstein, K. (2001) Depression associated with multiple sclerosis. Looking beyond diagnosis to symptom expression. *J. Affect. Disord.* 66(2/3):193–198.

Folstein, M.F. (1989) Heterogeneity in Alzheimer's disease. *Neurobiol. Aging* 10(5):434–435; discussion 446–448.

Forrest, D.V. (1992) A psychiatrist replies to Yudofsky's "Psychoanalysis, psychopharmacology, and the influence of neuropsychiatry." *J. Neuropsychiatry Clin. Neurosci.* 4(1):111–113.

Franklin, G.M., Heaton, R.K., Nelson, L.M., et al. (1988) Correlation of neuropsychological and MRI findings in chronic/progressive multiple sclerosis. *Neurology* 38(12):1826–1829.

Fruewald, S., Loeffler-Stastka, H., Eher, R., et al. (2001) Depression and quality of life in multiple sclerosis. *Acta Neurol. Scand.* 104(5):257–261.

Geschwind, N. (1975) The apraxias: neural mechanisms of disorders of learned movement. *Am. Scientist* 63(2):188–195.

Global Parkinson's Disease Survey Steering Committee. (2002) Factors impacting on quality of life in Parkinson's disease: results from an international survey. *Mov. Disord.* 17:60–67.

Goetz, C.G., Tanner, C.M., and Klawans, H.L. (1984) Bupropion in Parkinson's disease. *Neurology* 34(8):1092–1094.

Grade, C., Redford, B., Chrostowski, J., Toussaint, L., and Blackwell, B. (1998) Methylphenidate in early poststroke recovery: a double-blind, placebo-controlled study. *Arch. Phys. Med. Rehabil.* 79: 1047–1050.

Griesinger, W. (1965) *Mental Pathology and Therapeutics: A Facsimile of the 1987 Edition*, Robertson, C.L., and Rutherford, J., trans. New York: Macmillan.

Hart, B. (1931) Psychology and psychiatry. *Proc. R. Soc. Med.* 25: 187–200.

Hauser, R.A., and Zesiewicz, T.A. (1997) Sertraline for the treatment of depression in Parkinson's disease [see comments]. *Mov. Disord.* 12(5):756–759.

Hibbard, M.R., Grober, S.E., Gordon, W.A., and Aletta, A.G. (1990) Modification of cognitive psychotherapy for the treatment of post-stroke depression. *Behav. Ther.* 13:15–17.

Hill, D. (1964) The bridge between neurology and psychiatry. *Lancet* 1:509–514.

Hughes, A.J., Daniel, S.E., and Kilford, L., et al. (1992) Accuracy of clinical diagnosis of idiopathic Parkinson's disease: a clinico-pathological study of 100 cases. *J. Neurol. Neurosurg. Psychiatry* 55:181–184.

Hughes, T.A., Ross, H.F., Musa, S., et al. (2000) A 10-year study of the incidence of and factors predicting dementia in Parkinson's disease. *Neurology* 54(8):1596–1602.

Huntington, G. (1882) Onchorea. *Med. Surg. Rep.* 26:317–321.

Insel, T.R., and Winslow, J.T. (1999). The neurobiology of social attachment. In: Charney, D.S., Nestler, E.J., and Bunney, B.S., eds. *Neurobiology of Mental Illness.* New York: Oxford University Press, pp. 880–890.

Joffe, R.T., Lippert, G.P., Gray, T.A., Sawa, G., and Horvath, Z. (1987) Mood disorder and multiple sclerosis. *Arch. Neurol.* 44: 376–348.

Kandel, E.R. (1998) A new intellectual framework for psychiatry. *Am. J. Psychiatry* 155:457–469.

Kellner, C.H., Beale, M.D., Pritchett, J.T., et al. (1994) Electroconvulsive therapy and Parkinson's disease: the case for further study. *Psychopharmacol. Bull.* 30(3):495–500.

Kimura, M., Robinson, R.G., and Kosier, J.T. (2000) Treatment of cognitive impairment after poststroke depression: a double-blind treatment trial. *Stroke* 31(7):1482–1486.

Koenig, H.G., George, L.K., Peterson, B.L., and Pieper, C.F. (1997) Depression in medically ill hospitalized older adults: prevalence, characteristics, and course of symptoms according to six diagnostic schemes. *Am. J. Psychiatry* 154(10):1376–1383.

Kostic, V.S., Susic, V., Przedborski, S., et al. (1991) Sleep EEG in depressed and nondepressed patients with Parkinson's disease. *J. Neuropsychiatry Clin. Neurosci.* 3(2):176–179.

Krishnan, K.R., McDonald, W.M., et al. (1993) Neuroanatomical substrates of depression in the elderly. *Eur. Arch. Psychiatry Clin. Neurosci.* 243(1):41–46.

Laitinen, L. (1969) Desipramine in treatment of Parkinson's disease. A placebo-controlled study. *Acta Neurol. Scand.* 45(1):109–113.

Lauritzen, L., Bendsen, B.B., Vilmar, T., et al. (1994) Post-stroke depression: combined treatment with imipramine or desipramine and mianserin: a controlled clinical study. *Psychopharmacology* 114: 119–122.

Leentjens, A.F., Verhey, F.R., Lousberg, R., et al. (2000) The validity of the Hamilton and Montgomery-Asberg depression rating scales as screening and diagnostic tools for depression in Parkinson's disease. *Int. J. Geriatr. Psychiatry* 15(7):644–649.

Lewis, J.L. (1934) Melancholia: a historical review. *J. Ment. Sci.* 80: 1–42.

Lewy, F.H. (1913) Zur pathologischen anatomie der paralysis agitans. *Dtsch. Ztschr. Nervenheilk* 50:50–55.

Lipsey, J.R., Robinson, R.G., et al. (1984) Nortriptyline treatment of poststroke depression: a double-blind study. *Lancet* 1(8372): 297–300.

Lishman, W.A. (1992) What is neuropsychiatry? *J. Neurol. Neurosurg. Psychiatry* 55(11):983–985.

MacLean, P.D. (1952) Some psychiatric implications of physiological studies on frontotemproal portion of limbic system. *EEG Clin. Neurophysiol.* 4:407–418.

Martin, J.B. (2002) The integration of neurology, psychiatry, and neuroscience in the 21st century. *Am. J. Psychiatry* 159:695–704.

Mayberg, H.S., Parikh, R.M., Morris, P.L., et al. (1991) Spontaneous remission of post-stroke depression and temporal changes in cortical S2-serotonin receptors. *J. Neuropsychiatry Clin. Neurosci.* 3(1):80–83.

Mayberg, H.S., Starkstein, S.E., Peyser, C.E., et al. (1992) Paralimbic frontal lobe hypometabolism in depression associated with Huntington's disease. *Neurology* 42(9):1791–1797.

Mayberg, H.S., Starkstein, S.E., Sadzot, B., et al. (1990) Selective hypometabolism in the inferior frontal lobe in depressed patients with Parkinson's disease. *Ann. Neurol.* 28(1):57–64.

Mayeux, R. (1984) Behavioral manifestations of movement disorders. Parkinson's and Huntington's disease. *Neurol. Clin.* 2(3): 527–540.

Mayeux, R., Stern, Y., Cote, L., et al. (1984) Altered serotonin metabolism in depressed patients with Parkinson's disease. *Neurology* 34(5):642–646.

Mayeux, R., Stern, Y., Rosen, J., et al. (1981) Depression, intellectual impairment, and Parkinson disease. *Neurology* 31(6):645–650.

Mayeux, R., Stern, Y., Williams, J.B., et al. (1986) Clinical and biochemical features of depression in Parkinson's disease. *Am. J. Psychiatry* 143(6):756–769.

McCance-Katz, E.F., Marek, K.L., and Price, L.H. (1992) Serotonergic dysfunction in depression associated with Parkinson's disease [see comments]. *Neurology* 42(9):1813–1814.

McHugh, P.R. (1989) The neuropsychiatry of basal ganglia disorders: a triadic syndrome and its explanation. *Neuropsychiatry Neuropsychol. Behav. Neurol.* 2:239–247.

Mega, M.S., Cummings, J.L., Salloway, S., et al. (1997) The limbic system: an anatomic, phylogenetic, and clinical perspective [see comments]. *J. Neuropsychiatry Clin. Neurosci.* 9(3):315–330.

Mender, D. (1996) On neuropsychiatry and society [letter; comment]. *J. Neuropsychiatry Clin. Neurosci.* 8(3):362–363.

Mendez, M.F. (1995) The neuropsychiatry of multiple sclerosis. *Int. J. Psychiatry Med.* 25(2):123–130.

Mentis, M.J., McIntosh, A.R., Perrine, K., et al. (2002) Relationships among the metabolic patterns that correlate with mnemonic, visuospatial, and mood symptoms in Parkinson's disease. *Am. J. Psychiatry* 159:746–754.

Menza, M.A., and Mark, M.H. (1994) Parkinson's disease and depression: the relationship to disability and personality. *J. Neuropsychiatry Clin. Neurosci.* 6(2):165–169.

Middleton, F.A., and Strick, P.L. (2000) Basal ganglia output and cognition: evidence from anatomical, behavioral, and clinical studies. *Brain Cogn.* 42(2):183–200.

Montastruc, J.L., Fabre, N., Blin, O., Senard, J.M., Rascol, O., and Rascol, A. (1995) Does fluoxetine aggravate Parkinson's disease? A pilot prospective study. *Mov. Disord.* 10:355–357.

Morstyn, R., Hochanadel, G., Kaplan, E., et al. (1982) Depression vs. pseudodepression in dementia. *J. Clin. Psychiatry* 43(5):197–199.

Murray, T.J. (2005) *Multiple Sclerosis:The History of a Disease.* New York: Demos Medical Publishing.

Murray, G.B., Shea, V., and Conn, D.K. (1986) Electroconvulsive therapy for poststroke depression. *J. Clin. Psychiatry* 47:258–260.

Nemeroff, C.B. (1992) New vistas in neuropeptide research in neuropsychiatry: focus on corticotropin-releasing factor. *Neuropsychopharmacology* 6(2):69–75.

Nissenbaum, H., Quinn, N.P., Brown, R.G., et al. (1987) Mood swings associated with the "on-off" phenomenon in Parkinson's disease. *Psychol. Med.* 17(4):899–904.

Papez, J.W. (1937) A proposed mechanism of emotion. *Arch. Neurol. Psychiatry* 38:725–743.

Parkinson, J. (1817) *An Essay on the Shaking Palsy.* London: Sherwood, Neely, and Jones.

Patten, S.B., Metz, L.M., and Reimer, M.A. (2000) Biopsychosocial correlates of lifetime major depression in a multiple sclerosis population. *Multiple Sclerosis* 6(2):115–120.

Paulus, W., and Trenkwalder, C. (1998) Imaging of nonmotor symptoms in Parkinson syndromes. *Clin. Neurosci.* 5(2):115–120.

Pujol, J., Bello, J., Deus, J., et al. (2000) Beck Depression Inventory factors related to demyelinating lesions of the left arcuate fasciculus region. *Psychiatry Res.* 99(3):151–159.

Rabins, P.V., Brooks, B.R., O'Donnell, P., et al. (1986) Structural brain correlates of emotional disorder in multiple sclerosis. *Brain* 109:585–597.

Raisman, R., Cash, R., and Agid, Y. (1986) Parkinson's disease: decreased density of 3H-imipramine and 3H-paroxetine binding sites in putamen. *Neurology* 36(4):556–560.

Rampello, L., Chiechio, S., Raffaele, R., Vecchio, I., and Nicoletti, F. (2002) The SSRI, citalopram, improves bradykinesia in patients with Parkinson's disease treated with L-dopa. *Clin. Neuropharmacol.* 25:21–24.

Ranoux, D. (2000) Depression and Parkinson's disease. *Encephale* 26(3):22–26.

Rao, S.M. (1990) Multiple sclerosis in subcortical dementia. In: Cummings, J.L., ed. *Subcortical Dementia.* New York: Oxford University Press, pp. 164–180.

Rao, S.M., Leo, G.J., Bernardin, L., et al. (1991) Cognitive dysfunction in multiple sclerosis. I. Frequency, patterns, and prediction [see comments]. *Neurology* 41(5):685–691.

Reding, M.J., Orto, L.A., Winter, S.W., et al. (1986) Antidepressant therapy after stroke. A double-blind trial. *Arch. Neurol.* 43(8): 763–765.

Richard, I.H., and Kurlan, R. (1997) A survey of antidepressant drug use in Parkinson's disease. Parkinson Study Group. *Neurology* 49(4):1168–1170.

Richard, I.H., Maughn, A., and Kurlan, R. (1999) Do serotonin reuptake inhibitor antidepressants worsen Parkinson's disease? A retrospective case series. *Mov. Disord.* 14(1):155–157.

Robinson, R.G. (1998) Treatment issues in poststroke depression. *Depress. Anxiety* 8(Suppl 1):85–90.

Robinson, R.G., Chemerinski, E., and Jorge, R. (1999) Pathophysiology of secondary depressions in the elderly. *J. Geriatr. Psychiatry Neurol.* 12(3):128–136.

Robinson, R.G., Schultz, S.K., Castillo, C., et al. (2000) Nortriptyline versus fluoxetine in the treatment of depression and in short-term recovery after stroke: a placebo-controlled, double-blind study. *Am. J. Psychiatry* 157(3):351–359.

Robinson, R.G., Starr, L.B., Lipsey, J.R., et al. (1984) A two-year longitudinal study of post-stroke mood disorders: dynamic changes in associated variables over the first six months of follow-up. *Stroke* 15(3):510–517.

Rodin, G., and Voshart, K. (1986) Depression in the medically ill: an overview. *Am. J. Psychiatry* 143(6):696–705.

Ross, E.D., Gordon, W.A., Hibbard, M., et al. (1986) The dexamethasone suppression test, poststroke depression, and the validity of DSM-III-based diagnostic criteria. *Am. J. Psychiatry* 143(9): 1200–1201.

Rush, B. (2007) *Medical Inquiries and Observations on the Diseases of the Mind*. Whitefish, MT: Kessinger Publishing. (Originally published 1812).

Sadovnick, A.D., Bulman, D.E., Hashimoto, L., et al. (1991) The influence of gender on the susceptibility to multiple sclerosis in sibships. *Arch. Neurol.* 48(6):586–568.

Sagar, H.J. (1999) Clinicopathological heterogeneity and non-dopaminergic influences on behavior in Parkinson's disease. *Adv. Neurol.* 80:409–417.

Sano, M., Stern, Y., and Williams, J.E.A. (1989) Coexisting dementia and depression in Parkinson's disease. *Arch. Neurol.* 46(12): 1284–1286.

Schneider, L.S., and Chui, H.C. (1986) Progressive supranuclear palsy manifesting with depressive features. *J. Am. Geriatr. Soc.* 34(9):663–665.

Schoenfeld, M., Myers, R.H., Cupples, L.A., et al. (1984) Increased rate of suicide among patients with Huntington's disease. *J. Neurol. Neurosurg. Psychiatry* 47(12):1283–1287.

Schrödinger, E. (1992) *What is Life? The Physical Aspects of the Living Cell with Mind and Matter and Autobiographical Sketches*. New York: Cambridge University Press.

Schubert, D.S., and Foliart, R.H. (1993) Increased depression in multiple sclerosis patients. A meta-analysis. *Psychosomatics* 34(2):124–130.

Sherrington, C. (1948) *The Integrative Action of the Nervous System*. Cambridge, MA: Yale University Press. (Originally published 1906).

Shoulson, I., Odoroff, C., Oakes, D., et al. (1989) A controlled clinical trial of baclofen as protective therapy in early Huntington's disease. *Ann. Neurol.* 25(3):252–259.

Starkstein, S.E., Parikh, R.M., and Robinson, R.G. (1987) Post-stroke depression and recovery after stroke. *Lancet* 1(8535):743.

Stengel, E.A. (1954) A re-evaluation of Freud's book "On Aphasia": Its significance for psycho-analysis. *Int. J. Psychoanal.* 35:85–89.

Strong, M.S., and Vaughan, C.W. (1965) The test of time. VII. Otolaryngology. *BMQ* 16(3):85–87.

Tandberg, E., Larsen, J.P., Aarsland, D., et al. (1997) Risk factors for depression in Parkinson's disease. *Arch. Neurol.* 54(5):625–630.

Tharwani, H.M., Yerramsetty, P., Mannelli, P., Patkar, A., and Masand, P. (2007) Recent advances in poststroke depression. *Curr. Psychiatry Rep.* 9(3):225–231.

Walther, E.U., and Hohlfeld, R. (1999) Multiple sclerosis: side effects of interferon beta therapy and their management. *Neurology* 53(8):1622–1627.

Wang, J.L., Reimer, M.A., Metz, L.M., et al. (2000) Major depression and quality of life in individuals with multiple sclerosis [see comments]. *Int. J. Psychiatry Med.* 30(4):309–317.

Wells, K.C., Hersen, M., Bellack, A.S., et al. (1979) Social skills training in unipolar nonpsychotic depression. *Am. J. Psychiatry* 136(10):1331–1332.

Wengel, S.P., Burke, W.J., Pfeiffer, R.F., et al. (1998) Maintenance electroconvulsive therapy for intractable Parkinson's disease. *Am. J. Geriatr. Psychiatry* 6(3):263–269.

Whitlock, F.A., and Siskind, M.M. (1980) Depression as a major symptom of multiple sclerosis. J. Neurol. Neurosurg. *Psychiatry* 43(10):861–865.

Wiart, L., Petit, H., Joseph, P.A., Mazaux, J.M., and Barat, M. (2000) Fluoxetine in early poststroke depression: a double-blind placebo-controlled study. *Stroke* 31:1829–1832.

Wichmann, T., and DeLong, M.R. (1996) Functional and pathophysiological models of the basal ganglia. *Curr. Opin. Neurobiol.* 6(6):751–758.

Wilson, S.A.K. (1912) Progressive lenticular degeneration: a familial nervous disease associated with cirrhosis of the liver. *Brain* 34: 295–509.

Wood, R.I., and Natfolin, F. (1999). The neurobiology of human sexuality. In: Charney, D.S., Nestler, E.J., and Bunney, B.S., eds. *Neurobiology of Mental Illness*. New York: Oxford University Press, pp. 872–879.

Yakovlev, P.I. (1948) Motility, behavior and the brain: stereodynamic organization and neural co-ordinates of behavior. *J. Nerv. Ment. Dis.* 107(4):314–335.

Yudofsky, S.C., and Hales, R.E. (1989) The reemergence of neuropsychiatry: definition and direction. *J Neuropsychiatry Clin Neurosci.* 1(1):1–6.

Yudofsky, S.C., and Hales, R.E. (1999) What's new in neuropsychiatry. *J. Neuropsychiatry Clin. Neurosci.* 11(1):1–4.

Zorzon, M., de Masi, R., Nasuelli, D., et al. (2001) Depression and anxiety in multiple sclerosis. A clinical and MRI study in 95 subjects. *J. Neurol.* 248(5):416–421.

80 The Neurobiology of Personality Disorders

ANTONIA S. NEW, JOSEPH TRIEBWASSER, AND MARIANNE GOODMAN

The distinction in the *Diagnostic and Statistical Manual of Mental Disorders* (*DSM*) (American Psychiatric Association [APA], 2000) between Axis I and II disorders initially stemmed from an assumption that the former arise from "biological" predispositions and the latter from "environmental" conditions (Siever and Davis, 1991). This distinction, however, is belied by evidence that personality disorders are highly heritable, with heritability estimates ranging from 0.38 to 0.79 (Torgersen, 2000). Although environmental stress may play a role in the development of personality disorders, this is the case with many illnesses encoded on Axis I as well, including major depressive disorder (MDD), in which environmental factors, in conjunction with vulnerability genes, appear to place individuals at increased risk (Caspi et al., 2003). Although much is yet to be learned about the neuroscience of personality disorders, a number of important advances have been made in delineating the biological underpinnings of a number of them. In this chapter, rather than reviewing all the *DSM* personality disorders, we review findings in the three—borderline, antisocial, and schizotypal personality disorders—that have received the most investigative scrutiny.

BORDERLINE PERSONALITY DISORDER

Borderline personality disorder (BPD) is found in approximately 1%–4% of the general population, making it as prevalent as schizophrenia and bipolar I disorder (Torgersen et al., 2001; Moran et al., 2006). Patients with BPD are heavily represented in clinical populations (Zimmerman et al., 2005) and are disproportionate users of mental health services at all levels of care (Comtois et al., 2003; Bender et al., 2006). Although early factor analyses examining the *DSM* symptoms for BPD suggested that three factors (disturbed relatedness, behavioral dysregulation, and affective dysregulation) underlie the disorder (Sanislow et al., 2000; Sanislow et al., 2002), recent evidence that the three identified factors are very highly correlated with one another lends support to an overarching single construct (Sanislow et al., 2000; Sanislow et al., 2002; Johansen et al., 2004).

Improved diagnostic tools are at the foundation of the recent wave of empirical study of BPD. Semistructured clinical interviews for diagnosing the disorder have achieved a high level of interrater and test–retest reliability. Specifically, good interrater reliability has been demonstrated for the Structured Interview for DSM-IV Personality Disorders (Jane et al., 2006) and the Diagnostic Interview for DSM-IV Personality Disorders (DIPD-IV) (Zanarini et al., 2000), while the Diagnostic Interview for Borderline Personality Disorder–Revised (DIB-R) has demonstrated excellent interrater reliability and good test–retest reliability (Zanarini et al., 2002).

Comorbidity

The Collaborative Longitudinal Personality Disorders Study (CLPS), initiated in the mid-1990s, is a prospective descriptive study of a large clinical sample of patients with schizotypal, borderline, avoidant, and/or obsessive–compulsive personality disorders, or else MDD and no personality disorder (Skodol et al., 1999). The CLPS data showed that the Axis I comorbidities most commonly seen with BPD were post-traumatic stress disorder (PTSD) and substance abuse. While patients with BPD showed a high rate of MDD (79% lifetime), this was not higher than the prevalence across personality disorders (66%–82%). The most common Axis II comorbidities of BPD were antisocial and dependent personality disorders (McGlashan et al., 2000). In patients with MDD, the presence of comorbid BPD seems to complicate the course of the MDD, with an earlier onset of depression, a higher rate of other comorbidity on Axes I and II, a higher likelihood of conduct disorder, and elevated levels of anger/hostility (Sullivan et al., 1994) as well as greater illness burden and less favorable treatment response (Gunderson et al., 2004; Skodol et al., 2005).

Putative Etiologic Factors for Borderline Personality Disorder

The role of trauma

Although it has been assumed that BPD is the result of traumatic experiences, this model has been brought into question by evidence that the disorder is highly heritable (Torgersen, 2000). A further source of doubt about a traumatic etiology for BPD is that much of the research done to assess childhood trauma relies on data obtained retrospectively from adults with BPD, which is subject to the "negative halo" recall bias inevitable with already ill probands (Paris, 2000). This bias may be especially pronounced in patients with BPD, who are prone to caste a negative emotional tone over memories of prior experiences, possibly distorting the accuracy of the memories (Bailey and Shriver, 1999).

Adults with BPD appear to be more likely than those without BPD to give histories of early physical and sexual abuse, witnessed domestic violence, and unfavorable rearing styles (Herman et al., 1989; Paris et al., 1994a, 1994b; Zanarini and Frankenburg, 1997; Bandelow et al., 2005). Data from the CLPS study further suggest that BPD is more strongly correlated with reported childhood abuse and neglect than are MDD or schizotypal, avoidant, or obsessive–compulsive personality disorders (Battle et al., 2004). In addition, a reported history of abuse more strongly predicts adult BPD than a reported history of neglect, and reported exposure to disturbed adult caretakers bestows a greater risk than reported separation from these caretakers (Zanarini et al., 1989). Although childhood abuse or neglect, environmental instability, and parental psychopathology appear to increase the risk of adult BPD, "protective factors" such as artistic talents, superior school performance, and above-average intellectual skills decrease the risk (Helgeland and Torgersen, 2004).

However, even childhood sexual abuse, which has been particularly implicated in BPD, is not an inevitable prerequisite for its development (Goodman and Yehuda, 2002; Soloff et al., 2002). An estimated 20%–45% of patients with BPD have no history of sexual abuse (Goodman and Yehuda, 2002), whereas 80% of those with sexual abuse histories have no personality pathology (Paris, 1998). Longitudinal studies of children who were followed after a report of child abuse show that a substantial number of children with severe abuse remain functionally resilient, with little impairment across social, occupational, and interpersonal domains (McGloin and Widom, 2001). Zanarini and colleagues have concluded that though trauma may be an important etiological factor, it is neither necessary nor sufficient for the development of BPD; rather, childhood abuse may be part of a broader context of family neglect/chaos in the histories of patients with BPD (Zanarini and Frankenburg, 1997).

A meta-analysis of a large number of studies, with over 2,000 participants, looking at BPD and child abuse yielded a pooled effect size of only $r = .28$ (Fossati, Madeddu, and Maffei, 1999). In a sample of participants recruited from newspaper ads, childhood physical and sexual abuse were not predictors for BPD but were for paranoid and antisocial personality disorders (Bierer et al., 2003). A recent study comparing outpatients with BPD to healthy controls showed that familial neurotic spectrum disorders, childhood sexual abuse, separation from parents, and unfavorable parental rearing styles independently predict BPD. These results support a multifactorial model of the etiology of the disorder, with familial psychiatric disorders and sexual abuse as key contributing factors (Bandelow et al., 2005).

Taken together, these studies suggest that patients with BPD appear to have higher rates of child abuse than population averages, but that a number of other factors also play an important role.

Genetic vulnerability

Like many other medical disorders, BPD is likely the result of an interaction of heritable vulnerability with environmental factors that bring out the full phenotype.

Family Studies

Family studies show that first-degree relatives of probands with BPD are 10 times more likely to have been treated for BPD or a "BPD-like personality disorder," and significantly more likely to have been treated for unipolar depression, than the first-degree relatives of probands with schizophrenia (Loranger et al., 1982). A subsequent study examining symptom dimensions in family members of patients with BPD showed that affective instability and impulsivity were significantly more common in first-degree relatives of patients with BPD than of patients with non-BPD personality disorders and than patients with schizophrenia. In addition, unipolar depression was more common in the relatives of patients with BPD than of patients with other personality disorders, regardless of whether the BPD proband had a history of major depression (Silverman et al., 1991). In a large family study of 341 patients with BPD (and 1,580 of their first-degree relatives) and 104 patients with other personality disorders (with 472 of their first-degree relatives), BPD was found to be more common among the relatives of patients with BPD than of Axis II comparison probands. However, five of the criteria for BPD (inappropriate anger, affective instability, paranoia/dissociation, general impulsivity, and intense, unstable relationships) and all four sectors of borderline psychopathology (affect, cognition, impulsivity, and interpersonal relationships) were found to be more common and discriminating than the BPD diagnosis itself (Zanarini et al., 2004). These studies suggest that dimensions of BPD symptoms seem to run in families, more so in fact than the categorical diagnosis.

Genetics and Heritability

Family studies can indirectly reflect genetic heritability; however, only twin studies provide definitive evidence for it. Limited data from twin studies are available for BPD. One study examining 221 twin pairs showed that BPD was substantially heritable, with a heritability score of 0.69 (Torgersen, 2000), although this finding clearly requires replication. A recent study of 324 Chinese twins showed similar heritability rates for cluster B personality disorders of 65%; however, BPD was not independently assessed (Ji et al., 2006). In a study in which parents assessed personality disorder features of their children (ages 4–15 years, 112 twin pairs), 0.76 of the variance in BPD features appeared to be genetic in origin (Coolidge et al., 2001).

Research into specific genes involved in BPD is at an early stage. A recent case-control study showed a significant association between the serotonin transporter (5-HTT) gene and BPD, with higher frequencies of the 10 repeat of the VNTR marker and the S-10 haplotype, and fewer frequencies of the 12 repeat and LA-12 haplotype, in patients with BPD compared with healthy controls (Ni et al., 2006). This result is consistent with findings of a genetic association between the low-expressing S allele and aggressive behavior (Cadoret et al., 2003) as well as NEO Personality Inventory ratings of neuroticism, which is characterized by negative emotionality including anxiety, depression, vulnerability, and hostility (Sen et al., 2004). A simultaneous case-control study of the same gene in BPD, however, failed to replicate the association found by Ni and colleagues (Pascual et al., 2006).

Another gene that has been implicated in impulsive aggression and suicidal behavior, common features of BPD, is that encoding tryptophan hydroxylase (TPH), the rate-limiting enzyme in 5-HT biosynthesis. Two isoforms are known, TPH-1 and TPH-2. Tryptophan hydroxylase-1 has been correlated with various psychiatric and behavioral disorders by gene polymorphism association studies. A recent case-control study of 95 women with BPD and 98 healthy controls showed that one six-single nucleotide polymorphism (SNP) haplotype was absent from the controls but represented about one fourth of all haplotypes in the BPD group (Zaboli et al., 2006). Although these preliminary studies of specific genes implicated in BPD are suggestive and support the presence of a serotonergic abnormality, they all require replication.

Neurocognitive Testing

There is an extensive literature on neurocognitive function in BPD. Early studies focused on global intelligence, employing the Wechsler Adult Intelligence Scale (WAIS), and the Rorschach test. These studies found that intelligence was generally preserved in BPD but that patients showed distortions in projective testing. After the advent of *DSM-III*, some (Burgess, 1991; O'Leary et al., 1991), but not all (Cornelius et al., 1989; Driessen et al., 2000), studies found that patients with BPD manifested neurocognitive impairment. However, no consistent pattern of deficits could be discerned, and studies were often hampered by extensive comorbidity in the samples (Fertuck et al., 2006).

More recently, studies have focused less on broadly defined areas of cognitive functioning and more specifically on tasks related to impulsivity and emotional processing. Studies have shown that patients with BPD demonstrate disinhibited responding and impairment in planning responses (Bazanis et al., 2002). Impaired planning, for example, has been demonstrated with a task assessing the ability to delay monetary reward gratification; patients with BPD were unable to delay reward for longer-term benefit across trials compared to controls (Dougherty et al., 1999).

In a large study, patients with BPD were specifically impaired in the punishment–reward condition of a go/no-go task, reflecting difficulty inhibiting behavior associated with punishment (Leyton et al., 1999); a preliminary report suggested that the subset of patients with BPD with a history of suicide attempts had more commission errors on the punishment–reward component (Leyton et al., 1999). Using a similar go/no-go task, incarcerated women with BPD committed more passive avoidance errors than inmates with no BPD, which was interpreted as reflecting the difficulty of patients with BPD in inhibiting punished responses (Hochhausen et al., 2002). These studies provide consistent support for motoric disinhibition in BPD.

A study employing the Attention Network Task (Fan et al., 2002) showed that patients with BPD were impaired in their ability to engage in cognitive conflict resolution, but that the aspect of attention that included alerting and orienting to the task at hand was intact (Posner et al., 2002). Studies have shown that the Stroop Word Color Interference Task has little relationship to measures of personality and may best be understood as tapping specifically cognitive processes (Golden et al., 1975). Data suggest that this task does not differentiate between patients with BPD and normal controls (Arntz et al., 2000; Mitropoulou et al., 2002). In the Emotional Stroop Task, on the other hand, patients with BPD showed more interference caused by supraliminally presented emotional words with a variety of negative words (including negative views of others, sexual abuse–related words, and negative self-descriptors) compared to healthy controls; however, cluster C patients with personality disorder also demonstrated this effect (Arntz et al., 2000).

Neuropsychological studies of emotional processing show that in the directed forgetting task, patients with BPD compared to controls had enhanced encoding of negatively valenced borderline-salient words and impaired forgetting of these words (Korfine and Hooley, 2000). Although it is well known that patients with BPD show disturbances in interpersonal relationships, few studies have sought to define empirically this population's specific deficits in social cognition. One area that has received some attention is the recognition of facial emotional expression—a crucial domain because the ability to read emotion accurately and appropriately is essential to navigating interpersonal interactions. If patients with BPD have the neuropsychological deficit of overreading and misreading emotional cues, this would go far in explaining the puzzling symptom of exaggerated emotional responses in interpersonal interactions. If, for example, neutral faces appear hostile, this might account for apparently unprovoked anger. The first empirical study to examine facial expression recognition in BPD showed that women patients correctly identified fear and anger and in fact identified them more accurately than controls. The authors interpreted this as reflecting intact emotion recognition in BPD. Interestingly, however, the most significant group difference was that women with BPD misread neutral faces more than controls, specifically overreading anger (Wagner and Linehan, 1999). In a recent study using the Multimorph Facial Affect Recognition Task (Blair et al., 2001), as facial expressions morphed from neutral to maximum intensity, participants with BPD correctly identified facial affect at an earlier stage than did healthy controls, demonstrating that participants with BPD were more sensitive to emotional expressions, regardless of valence. These results lend support to the notion that patients with BPD overread emotional responses.

Neuroendocrine Studies

Biological studies of personality disorder have employed a variety of agents in neuroendocrine challenge studies as well as peripheral markers and have found very widely replicated decreases in serotonergic responsiveness, especially in relation to impulsive-aggressive symptoms and affective instability (Coccaro et al., 1989; Linnoila et al., 1989; O'Keane et al., 1992; Siever and Trestman, 1993; Linnoila et al., 1994; Virkkunen et al., 1994; Dougherty et al., 1999; Goveas et al., 2004). Cerebrospinal fluid (CSF) studies have shown decreased concentrations of the serotonin metabolite 5-HIAA in patients with BPD with suicidal behavior (Brown et al., 1982; Gardner et al., 1990) and with impulsive aggression (Brown et al., 1982), although this is not specific to the BPD diagnosis (Traskman-Bendz et al., 1986; Roy et al., 1988; Linnoila et al., 1989; Linnoila et al., 1994; Virkkunen et al., 1994; Lidberg et al., 2000; Stanley et al., 2000).

Decreased serotonergic responsivity in impulsive aggression in personality disorders has also been supported by studies utilizing hormone responses to pharmacologic stimulation of the serotonergic system, including fenfluramine and meta-chloropiperazine (m-CPP) (Coccaro et al., 1989; O'Keane et al., 1992; Coccaro et al., 1996). Specific studies of peripheral markers in patients with BPD have demonstrated decreased platelet paroxetine binding compared to controls, perhaps reflecting diminished presynaptic serotonergic dysfunction (Ng Ying Kin et al., 2005).

Neuroimaging: Structural findings

Structural brain imaging studies have also supported anatomical differences between patients with BPD and controls in brain areas known to underlie impulsive aggression. Prefrontal cortex (PFC), particularly orbital frontal cortex (OFC) and adjacent ventral medial cortex (including anterior cingulate gyrus [ACG]), plays a central role in the regulation of aggressive behavior (Pribram and Bragshaw, 1953; Singh, 1976; Bear and Fulop, 1987; Damasio et al., 1994; Miller et al., 1997). In addition, injury to OFC early in childhood can result in disinhibited, aggressive behavior later in life (S.W. Anderson et al., 1999).

Anatomical magnetic resonance imaging (MRI) studies comparing patients with BPD to healthy controls show significant volume reduction with manually traced assessment of right ACG (Brodmann area [BA] 24) and left OFC in patients with BPD (Tebartz van Elst et al., 2003), but this was not confirmed in a larger sample using voxel-based morphometry (Rusch et al., 2003). Recent work in a large sample of manually traced MRI scans showed specific reductions in gray matter volume in ACG (BA 24) in patients with BPD compared with controls (Hazlett et al., 2005), replicating in a larger sample the earlier finding of volume reduction in ACG.

Much as prefrontal brain regions play a role in regulating the expression of aggression, amygdala has been viewed as one of the subcortical structures from which emotions may emerge. An early MRI study showed that total amygdala volume tended to be reduced in female patients with BPD compared to controls (Driessen et al., 2000). This was viewed as perhaps reflecting excitotoxicity with volume loss. Two subsequent small studies reported significant decreases in amygdala volume in BPD (Schmahl et al., 2003; Tebartz van Elst et al., 2003), although another study showed no difference in amygdala volume between women with BPD and controls (Brambilla et al., 2004). Two recent studies with much larger samples showed no difference in amygdala volume in BPD compared to controls (Zetzsche et al., 2006; New et al., 2007). Taken together, structural imaging studies lend support to a loss of volume in ACG (BA 24) in BPD but do not converge into a consistent finding of decreased amygdala volume.

Functional Neuroimaging (see Table 80.1)

Resting positron emission tomography

Two resting studies using 18-fluorodeoxyglucose positron emission tomography (^{18}FDG PET), showed decreased metabolism in patients with BPD compared to healthy volunteers in anterior and medial frontal regions (BA 9,10, 32, 46) (De La Fuente et al., 1997; Soloff et al., 2000). Another ^{18}FDG PET study showed that patients with BPD with depression had less relative uptake in ACG (BA 32) at baseline compared to patients who were depressed without BPD (Oquendo et al., 2005). In contrast, one resting PET study showed increased metabolism in female patients with BPD in frontal and anterior cingulate regions (BA 32, 8, 10) (Juengling et al., 2003).

Serotonergic studies

Peripheral evidence for decreased serotonergic responsiveness in BPD led to brain imaging studies to explore central serotonergic responsiveness more directly. A number of studies have demonstrated decreased metabolic activity in OFC and ACG in response to serotonergic challenge in patients who were impulsive and aggressive with BPD compared to healthy controls. One such study,

TABLE 80.1 *Functional Brain Imaging Studies in BPD*

Authors, Year	*Number of Participants*	*Imaging Technique*	*Provocation Condition*	*Regions Underactive in BPD*	*Regions Overactive in BPD*	*Medication*
Resting PET scans						
De la Fuente et al., 1997	10 BPD, 15 HC	^{18}FDG PET	resting	Anterior PFC, ACG	None	None
Soloff et al., 2000	5 BPD, 8 HC	^{18}FDG PET	resting	OFC, right insula	None	None
Oquendo et al., 2005	11 BPD+ MDD, 8 MDD	^{18}FDG PET	resting	ACG	Parieto-temporal cortex	None
Juengling et al., 2003	12 HC, 12 BPD	^{18}FDG PET	resting	Hippocampus, cuneus	ACG	None
Serotonergic stimuli with PET						
Soloff et al., 2000	5 BPD, 8 HC	^{18}FDG PET	d,l-fenfluramine	OFC, right insula	None	None
Oquendo et al., 2005	11 BPD+ MDD, 8 MDD	^{18}FDG PET	d,l-fenfluramine	None	None	None
New et al., 2002	13 HC, 13 BPD-IED	^{18}FDG PET	m-CPP	ACG, OFC	Posterior cingulate	None
New et al., 2004	10 BPD	^{18}FDG PET	fluoxetine 20 mg/ day for 12 weeks	OFC increased after fluoxetine		None except study med
Leyton et al., 2001	13 BPD, 11 HC	alpha-[(11)C] methyl-L-tryptophan trapping PET	resting	Medial frontal gyrus, ACG, STG, striatum	None	None
Frankle et al., 2005	10 IED (mostly BPD), 10 HC	[(11)C]McN 5652 5-HTT PET ligand	resting	ACG binding	None	None
[^{15}O]H_2O PET						
Schmahl et al., 2003	10 BPD, 10 trauma controls	[^{15}O]H_2O PET	abandonment scripts	Right ACG	DLPFC, anterior PFC	On meds

TABLE 80.1 *Functional Brain Imaging Studies in BPD*

Authors, Year	*Number of Participants*	*Imaging Technique*	*Provocation Condition*	*Regions Underactive in BPD*	*Regions Overactive in BPD*	*Medication*
Schmahl et al., 2004	10 BPD, 10 trauma controls	[^{15}O]H_2O PET	Trauma scripts	Right ACG, DLPFC	None	On meds
Functional MRI						
Herpertz et al., 2001	6BPD, 6HC	fMRI BOLD	IAPS pictures, neutral and aversive	Medial temporal gyrus	Amygdala; medial and inferior frontal gyrus	None
Schnell et al., 2007	14 BPD, 14 HC	fMRI BOLD	TAT pictures, aversive pictures	Aversive-neutral: Left ACG, middle temporal gyri, superior medial frontal gyrus	Aversive alone: OFC, insula, left ACG, medial PFC	None
Schnell & Herpertz, 2007	6 BPD, 6 HC	fMRI BOLD	IAPS pictures, neutral and aversive, and after DBT for patients	None	Left dorsomedial, ACG. Group difference less after DBT	None
Beblo et al., 2006	20 BPD, 21 HC	fMRI BOLD	Unresolved vs. resolved life events	Insula, amygdala, ACG, left posterior cingulate	None	None
Schmahl, Bohus et al., 2006	12 BPD, 12 HC	fMRI BOLD	Thermal pain stimulation	Posterior parietal, ACG, amygdala	DLPFC	None
Donegan et al., 2003	15 BPD, 15 HC	fMRI BOLD	Eckman faces	None	Amygdala to neutral and emotional faces	On meds

BOLD: blood oxygen level dependent; ^{18}FDG PET: 18-fluorodeoxyglucose positron emission tomography; fMRI: functional magnetic resonance imaging; BPD: border line personality disorder; HC: healthy controls; MDD: major depressive disorder; IED: intermittent explosive disorder; m-CPP: meta-chloropiperazine; IAPS: International Affective Picture System; TAT: Thematic Apperception Test; DBT: dialectical behavioral therapy; PFC: prefrontal cortex; ACG: anterior cingulate gyrus; OFC: orbital frontal cortex; STG: superior temporal gyrus; DLPFC: dorsolateral prefrontal cortex.

using ^{18}FDG PET, found that though normal patients showed increased metabolism in OFC and ACG following d,l-fenfluramine, patients who were impulsive and aggressive with personality disorders showed significant increases only in inferior parietal lobe (Siever et al., 1999). A larger study in a group of patients with BPD with affective instability but not specifically selected for impulsive aggression also demonstrated hypometabolism in ACG and OFC in response to d,l-fenfluramine compared to healthy controls (Soloff et al., 2000). One study showed baseline lower metabolic activity in patients who were patients with BPD, but this group difference was eliminated after fenfluramine administration (Oquendo et al., 2005). An ^{18}FDG PET study in patients with an impulsive and aggressive personality disorder (all but one of whom had BPD) after m-CPP administration showed reduced metabolic responses in medial OFC and ACG compared to controls (New et al., 2002). Recently, normalization of PFC dysfunction by fluoxetine treatment was shown in patients with impulsive-aggressive BPD (New et al., 2004). In addition, increased metabolic activity was seen in posterior cingulate at rest and in response to m-CPP; posterior cingulate is a brain area that has been specifically implicated in the recognition of facial emotion and therefore is particularly interesting in BPD (Phillips, Bullmore, et al., 1998; Sprengelmeyer et al., 1998).

More recently, the tight coupling of metabolic activity between OFC and amygdala, specifically ventral amygdala, seen in healthy patients was shown to be absent in patients with impulsive-aggressive BPD (New et al., 2007). This raises the possibility that differential connectivity among brain regions may underlie abnormal aggression modulation in BPD, and that brain regions such as ACG (Pietrini et al., 2000) that normally modulate expressions of anger fail to come on line in BPD when needed.

The mechanism of the serotonergic abnormality in BPD has been examined more closely with molecular neuroimaging studies. A PET study of serotonin synthesis showed lower synthesis in men with BPD compared to controls in medial frontal gyrus, ACG, superior temporal gyrus, and corpus striatum; women with BPD had lower serotonin synthesis compared to controls in right ACG and superior temporal gyrus (Leyton et al., 2001). More recently, we employed the 5-HTT PET radiotracer [11C]McN5652 to show reduced availability of 5-HTT in ACG of individuals with impulsive aggression and a personality disorder compared to healthy controls, suggesting reduced serotonergic innervation in this brain region (Frankle et al., 2005). Interestingly, as noted above, evidence shows an association between a particular haplotype of the 5-HTT gene (10 repeat of the VNTR intronic marker and the short form of a promoter polymorphism) and BPD, which lends further support to the notion that genetic differences in the 5-HTT may play a role in the etiology of the disorder (Ni et al., 2006).

Although the strongest case for a deficit in serotonin-mediated activation of OFC and ACG has been made in patients with BPD selected for impulsive aggression, poor emotion regulation is a closely related symptom cluster. Indeed, the same brain regions that modulate the expression of aggression and anger have been implicated in the control of fear and other emotions (Orr et al., 2000; Peri et al., 2000; M.C. Anderson et al., 2004), and affective instability is highly correlated with impulsive aggression in BPD (Fossati, Madeddu, and Maffei, 1999; Sanislow et al., 2000; Johansen et al., 2004). Positron emission tomography studies have suggested underactivity of OFC in response to abandonment scripts in patients with BPD with abuse histories compared to women who were abused and without BPD (Schmahl et al., 2003; Schmahl et al., 2004). Further support for the involvement of impaired OFC function in BPD comes from a study comparing neurological patients with lesions in OFC, patients with lesions in other areas of PFC, patients with BPD, and healthy controls. The patients with OFC lesions and the patients with BPD performed similarly on several measures compared to the other two groups (Berlin et al., 2005).

Use of $[^{15}O]H_2O$ PET permits the measurement of regional brain blood flow under various conditions. This approach has been employed using script-driven imagery of abandonment in BPD and healthy controls during tracer uptake. Memories of abandonment were associated with greater increases in blood flow in dorsolateral prefrontal cortex (DLPFC) and greater decreases in right ACG in women with BPD than in controls (Schmahl et al., 2003). It should be noted, however, that most patients in the BPD group were on psychoactive medications, while most in the control group were not. Using script-driven imagery of child abuse during PET, women with child abuse histories but not BPD showed increased blood flow in right DLPFC, right ACG, and left OFC, but decreased blood flow in left DLPFC, while women with child abuse histories and BPD failed to activate these regions. In this study, too, most patients with BPD were on psychoactive medications, while most in the control group were not (Schmahl et al., 2004).

Functional MRI

Functional MRI (fMRI) provides the opportunity for more finely grained time-resolution of brain activation during specific tasks through event-related designs. Although this approach has been used widely in the study of mental illnesses such as PTSD and depression, such work is still in its early phases in BPD.

A pilot study using exposure to standardized negative emotional images from the International Affective Picture System (IAPS) found increased activity in amygdala in six BPD patients compared to controls, which was interpreted as suggesting a neural substrate for the heightened emotional responsiveness seen in BPD (Herpertz et al., 2001). In a study using affective versus neutral images from the Thematic Apperception Test, patients with BPD failed to show the differential response to emotional versus neutral pictures in amygdala, OFC, and ACG seen in healthy controls; this suggests that individuals with BPD may be equally emotionally responsive to neutral and to emotional stimuli. The authors did not examine group differences in blood oxygen level dependent (BOLD) response to neutral pictures alone. However, in response to emotional pictures, patients with BPD displayed increased BOLD responses in bilateral OFC and insular regions, in left ACG, and in medial PFC compared to controls (Schnell et al., 2007). Interestingly, a small pilot study (BPD, $N = 6$) showed that treatment with dialectical behavior therapy decreased response to negative pictures in right ACG, temporal and posterior cingulate cortices, as well as in left insula, perhaps reflecting treatment-related attenuation of emotional responsiveness to unpleasant stimuli (Schnell and Herpertz, 2007).

In a study exploring individualized autobiographical memories of unresolved and resolved negative life events, when contrasting the former with the latter, patients showed significant bilateral activation of insula, amygdala, ACG, left posterior cingulate cortex, right occipital cortex, bilateral cerebellum, and midbrain not seen in healthy patients (Beblo et al., 2006).

When subjected to painful heat stimuli during fMRI, (Schmahl et al., 2006), patients with BPD showed less activation in posterior parietal cortex, and stronger activation in DLPFC, than controls. In addition, patients but not controls revealed strong deactivation in perigenual ACG.

The recognition of faces appears to involve specific face recognition regions, including fusiform gyrus, areas of right occipital cortex, and right superior temporal lobe (Kesler-West et al., 2001). However, brain regions involved in recognition of facial emotions appear to be left ACG, posterior cingulate gyrus, medial frontal cortex, and OFC (Phillips, Bullmore, et al., 1998; Sprengelmeyer et al., 1998). Specific investigations of regional brain activity in response to emotional faces in BPD have shown overactivation of amygdala to faces, regardless of emotional valence, compared to a fixation point, and postscan debriefing revealed that some patients with BPD had difficulty disambiguating neutral faces or found them threatening (Donegan et al., 2003). This lends further support to the model of an overreading of emotion in patients with BPD and of deficits in activity in brain regions central to "top-down" modulation of emotional responses.

Biologically Informed Treatments

Research findings of decreased 5-HT metabolites and blunted responses to serotonergic challenge led to trials of selective serotonergic reuptake inhibitors (SSRIs) in the treatment of BPD (Rinne et al., 2002) and of impulsive aggression in a mixed group of patients with personality disorders (Coccaro and Kavoussi, 1997). These trials showed mood stabilization and decreased aggressive behavior with SSRIs over placebo. One study also showed an increase in brain metabolic activity, as assessed by ^{18}FDG PET, in OFC in patients with BPD treated with fluoxetine, bringing their pattern of brain metabolic activity to more closely resemble healthy individuals (New et al., 2004). It is important to underscore that though we have argued that this disorder has a fundamental neurobiology, it does not follow that the only effective treatment will be pharmacologic. Like MDD, other neurobiological disorders may well respond to psychotherapy. In fact, the best-proven treatment to date for BPD is dialectical behavior therapy, which specifically employs skills training to improve affect modulation.

ANTISOCIAL PERSONALITY DISORDER

Epidemiology

Antisocial personality disorder (ASPD) affects 5% of the population and is 7 times more common in men than women. It has been associated with negative outcomes including low professional achievement, substance abuse, and legal problems (Moffitt, 2002). The diagnosis is made primarily on the basis of behavioral difficulties, especially criminality, and has been criticized for a lack of affective criteria except for absence of remorse. The resulting characterization of the disorder skews heavily towards individuals with offense histories, and in fact 50%–80% of prisoners meet criteria for ASPD (Ogloff, 2006; Warren and South, 2006), raising questions as to whether it is more a sociological or legal construct than a clinical one. Certainly the focus on behavioral criteria has resulted in a highly heterogeneous population of ASPD "cases," which complicates attempts to define the underlying biological disturbance(s).

A related diagnosis, which is often confused with ASPD, is psychopathy (Table 80.2). However, there are important distinctions between the two, in that psychopathy denotes a more circumscribed and homogenous population. Psychopathy affects 1% of the general community, 3% of psychiatric patients, and 15% of male prisoners (compared to the 50%–80% who meet ASPD criteria). Diagnosed reliably by the Hare Psychopathy Checklist–Revised (PCL-R; Hare, 1991), psychopathy is defined by a combination of interpersonal and affective difficulties and social deviance. Factor analysis of the PCL-R components reveals two factors: (*1*) an emotional component comprising characteristics such as shallowness and lack of guilt and (*2*) antisocial behavioral acts (Hare, 1991). The emotional factor, unlike the behavioral component, does not diminish with age. Moreover, the emotional component is not highly associated with ASPD diagnosis, socioeconomic status, or IQ.

Another important distinction between ASPD and psychopathy is the forms of aggression characteristic of the two disorders. The aggression of ASPD is primarily "reactive," which means it is done impulsively in response to specific circumstances. The aggression of psychopathy includes not only "reactive" but also planned and goal-directed acts, referred to as "instrumental ag-

TABLE 80.2 *Distinguishing Antisocial Personality Disorder from Psychopathy*

	Antisocial Personality Disorder	*Psychopathy*
Epidemiology	• heterogeneous group • 5% population • 50%–80% of prisoners	• homogenous group • 1% population • 15% of prisoners
Phenomenology	• behavioral difficulties • only affective criteria is "absence of remorse"	• behavioral • interpersonal • affective difficulties • social deviance
Type of aggression	• reactive	• reactive and • instrumental
Neuropsychology	• frontal lobe dysfunction	• frontal lobe dysfunction and • poor associative learning • poor status-reinforcement learning
Neuroimaging	• frontal hypoperfusion • frontal-limbic circuitry involved	• frontal hypoperfusion • frontal-limbic circuitry involved and • paralimbic circuitry involved

These diagnoses are often used interchangeably, and yet they are defined quite differently, as is summarized above.

gression." Each form of aggression probably has a distinct pattern of brain region involvement and underlying neurobiology.

Antisocial personality disorder and psychopathy thus probably describe individuals with differing phenomenology, etiological factors, and central nervous system dysfunction; however, the psychiatric literature often does not acknowledge the crucial distinctions between the two conditions, frequently applying findings in one to the other. Moreover, the literature also sometimes conflates antisocial behaviors and symptoms, psychopathic behaviors and symptoms, and criminality, all of which overlap one another but are by no means identical.

Theoretical Models of ASPD and Psychopathy

Reactive aggression, seen in ASPD and BPD, is believed to involve lesions of OFC. When an individual is threatened, a response system mediated by amygdala and OFC offers several options, ranging from a freeze response to a flight response to reactive aggression (Seguin, 2004). Individuals with disordered reactive aggression have impairments in this system, ranging from failure to consider consequences when deciding how to respond to a threat (processes thought to be mediated by OFC and medial frontal cortex; Damasio, 1994), to misjudging response and dominance cues or misreading angry facial expression (Blair et al., 2001). Neurological patients with known OFC lesions show reactive aggression, offering additional support to the OFC model (Damasio, 1994).

Instrumental aggression, seen only in psychopathy, is hypothesized to originate from impaired capacity to form associations between distress cues and social stimuli and from hyporesponsiveness to fear, as described in the violence inhibition mechanism model (Blair et al., 2006), which is based on the notion that empathy is necessary for moral socialization (Blair et al., 2001). The normal mechanism for inhibiting aggression in humans involves the perception of a distress cue: when an individual cries and has sad facial affect, this triggers a submission response in an aggressor, attenuating the aggressive response. This mechanism is thought to be impaired in psychopathy, such that human distress does not inhibit the submissive response (Blair and Cipolotti, 2000). Evidence for this comes from impaired facial emotion recognition in patients with psychopathy (Blair and Cipolotti, 2000; Mitchell et al., 2002), deficits implicating amygdala dysfunction.

Neurocognitive Function in ASPD and Psychopathy

A meta-analysis of 39 studies examining 4,589 patients with antisocial behavior—a heterogeneous sample including patients with ASPD, criminals, patients with conduct disorder, patients with psychopathy, and delinquents—demonstrated that they had impaired performance on executive function measures (by 0.62 standard deviations) (Morgan and Lilienfeld, 2000). However, the findings were less conclusive regarding the relationship between executive function and ASPD.

Neuroimaging in ASPD and Psychopathy

Neuroimaging: Structural findings

Prefrontal abnormalities and deficits have been associated with psychopathic personality traits and antisocial behavior (Lapierre et al., 1995; Davidson et al., 2000), but the data for ASPD itself are far less conclusive (Malloy et al., 1990; Burgess, 1992; Goyer et al., 1994; Kuruoglu et al., 1996; Raine et al., 2000; Crowell et al., 2003). In part, this is due to the heterogeneity of the ASPD diagnosis; also, many studies have not controlled for demographic and psychiatric comorbidities (for an exception, see Crowell et al., 2003). Nonetheless, an anatomical MRI study that did control for the potential confounds of comorbid substance use and other psychiatric disorders found patients with ASPD to have significantly decreased prefrontal gray matter volumes compared to substance dependent and healthy controls (Raine et al., 2000). However, in a sample of patients with psychopathic ASPD with alcoholism, no differences in PFC volumes were found after controlling for duration of alcohol use and years of education, and there was no correlation between prefrontal volumes and degree of psychopathy (Laakso et al., 2002).

Functional neuroimaging

Functional neuroimaging results have been more consistent, with dysfunctional patterns of activation involving prefrontal regions and amygdala for in ASPD and psychopathy. A single photon emission computed tomography (SPECT) study at rest in ASPD revealed marked frontal hypoperfusion (Kuruoglu et al., 1996). Additionally, during the acquisition phase of a differential aversive classical conditioning paradigm, patients with ASPD compared to controls demonstrated differing patterns of activation in amygdala and DLPFC, suggesting that patients required additional effort to form negative emotional associations (Schneider et al., 2000). Similar dysfunction in prefrontal and/or amygdala circuitry has been noted in psychopathy in response to viewing negative pictures (Muller et al., 2003), an affective memory task (Kiehl et al., 2001), script-guided imagery (Li et al., 2006), and processing of emotional words (Intrator et al., 1997). Patients with psychopathy may require recruitment of additional resources when faced with an emotional task because frontal regions, although activated, may function relatively inefficiently and exhibit impaired processing of aversive stimuli in particular.

Development, Childhood Antecedents

Landmark longitudinal studies in the developmental aspects of antisocial behavior distinguished between early- and adolescent-onset cases, with early-onset individuals more likely to become criminals in adulthood and to be characterized by aggression, hyperactivity, and impaired neuropsychological performance (Moffitt, 1990, 1993). Physical anomalies and birth complications, coupled with early psychosocial adversity including poor education, low family income, or being raised by a single parent, increased the risk for violent delinquency (Arseneault et al., 2002). However, alternative developmental trajectories have been proposed for girls (Schaeffer et al., 2006).

Genetics

Although minimal data exist regarding the genetics of ASPD, the literature about antisocial behavior boasts over 100 twin and adoption studies. Meta-analyses suggest that 41%–50% of the variance is due to genetic factors, 16%–20% to shared family experience, and 30%–43% to experiences specific to the individual (Rhee and Waldman, 2002; Moffitt, 2005). However, the heritability of antisocial behavior may be affected by developmental changes, sex differences, and diagnostic subtypes and comorbidities (Slutske, 2001). For example, differing heritability estimates exist for juvenile-onset versus adult-onset antisocial behavior (Lyons et al., 1995), and adolescence-limited versus life course–persistent subtypes (Moffitt, 1993). Although similar heritability estimates exist for females and males, the former require more familial genetic and nongenetic risk factors (Cloninger et al., 1978; Slutske, 2001; Jacobson et al., 2002). Moreover, risk factors for antisocial behavior have considerable overlap with those for other disorders, including alcoholism (Jang et al., 2000; Huang et al., 2006) and attention-deficit/hyperactivity disorder (Silberg et al., 1996), and for higher-order personality traits such as novelty seeking and behavioral disinhibition (Young et al., 2000). The clarification of dispositions and other features that heighten the risk for individuals to commit antisocial acts may help identify susceptibility genes and endophenotypes that underlie the behavioral phenotype. Endophenotypes for antisocial behavior may include descriptive variables such as fearlessness, novelty seeking, and low self-control as well as biological measures including frontal lobe hypoarousal, executive dysfunction, or serotonergic abnormalities (Moffitt, 2005).

More recently, gene–environment (G-E) interactions for antisocial behavior have received widespread attention because of the finding that men with low-activity alleles for a polymorphism for monoamine oxidase A and histories of childhood abuse are at increased risk for antisocial behaviors as adults (Caspi et al., 2002). This synergy between a particular gene and a measured environmental influence has been replicated in some (Foley et al., 2004; Kim-Cohen et al., 2006) but not all (Huizinga et al., 2006; Widom and Brzustowicz, 2006) studies, and the finding may not extend to females (Sjoberg et al., 2007). Subsequent inquiries into G-E interactions have included family dysfunction as an environmental "moderator variable" (Button et al., 2005), socioeconomic status as a shared environmental risk factor (Tuvblad et al., 2006), and adolescent aggression interacting with parental criticism and delinquency (Narusyte et al., 2007).

Summary

The ASPD diagnosis has been criticized for its dependence on behavioral criteria, with a resultant heterogeneous patient population, thereby limiting neurobiological research efforts. Psychopathy, by contrast, defines a relatively homogenous group who demonstrate emotional and behavioral symptoms and is characterized by unique patterns of instrumental aggression. Considerable progress has been made in the understanding of psychopathy, including the roles of OFC, amygdala, and deficits in social learning, empathy, and the processing of fear and emotion.

SCHIZOTYPAL PERSONALITY DISORDER (SPD)

Schizotypal personality disorder (SPD) is defined by *DSM-IV-TR* as a "pervasive pattern of social and interpersonal deficits marked by acute discomfort with, and reduced capacity for, close relationships as well as by cognitive or perceptual distortions and eccentricities of behavior, beginning by early adulthood and present in a variety of contexts" (APA, 2000, p. 697). Although SPD and schizophrenia have numerous clinical and laboratory parameters in common, patients with SPD are spared the psychosis and catastrophic decline in functioning seen in schizophrenia (Siever and Davis, 1991).

The neurobiological exploration of SPD has the potential to reveal much about SPD and the other "odd, eccentric" personality disorders. Perhaps more important, a nuanced understanding of the ways in which the brains of patients with SPD resemble and differ from those of patients with schizophrenia may shed light on the pathophysiology, treatment, and prevention of schizophrenia itself.

Prevalence

Although *DSM-IV-TR* describes the approximate prevalence of SPD as 3%, the best estimate of the frequency in the general population using *DSM-III-R* or *DSM-IV* criteria has been 0.6% (Torgersen et al., 2001) to 0.7% (Maier et al., 1992). Base rates of approximately 2%–6%, in relatives of psychiatric patients and relatives of controls, were found in earlier studies (Baron et al., 1985; Coryell and Zimmerman, 1989; Black et al., 1993) that used *DSM-III*, rather than the more stringent *DSM-III-R* and *DSM-IV*, criteria.

Reliability of the diagnosis

Categorical interrater reliabilities when diagnosing SPD using published instruments have ranged from .55 to .86. In CLPS patients, SPD demonstrated test-retest reliability of .64 using the DIPD-IV, which compared favorably to test-retest reliabilities using the Structured Clinical Interview for *DSM-IV* Axis I Disorders (SCID-I) of .61 for MDD, .60 for obsessive–compulsive disorder (OCD), .59 for social phobia, and .44 for generalized anxiety disorder (Zanarini et al., 2000).

Stability

Very little data exists about the long-term stability of SPD. Retesting at 7–14 months of undergraduate volunteers diagnosed with the disorder using the Schedule for Nonadapative and Adaptive Personality (SNAP) a self-report questionnaire, found a correlation coefficient between the two time points of .59 (Melley et al., 2002). In the CLPS sample, only 34% of individuals with SPD continued to meet the diagnostic threshold 12 months later, though the stability of all personality disorders during the follow-up period was greater than for MDD (Shea et al., 2002). In general, while CLPS data, like Children in the Community Study data, have failed to support the *DSM* concept of categorically defined personality disorders persisting through the lifespan, there appear to be core traits or dimensions within these disorders—perhaps akin to "negative" symptoms of schizophrenia—that do show temporal stability, as opposed to the "positive" symptoms, behaviors, and state-like symptoms that tend to fluctuate with age and clinical status (Pukrop and Krischer, 2005). Also, longitudinal research has demonstrated the strong predictive validity of categorical Axis II diagnoses, in that they are robustly associated with longitudinal functional impairment, especially in the social sphere (Skodol et al., 2005), even in individuals who no longer meet criteria for the personality disorders themselves. Moreover, SPD symptoms in adolescence or early adulthood have been found to be strongly associated with poorer quality of life (Chen, Cohen, Kasen, and Johnson, 2006; Chen, Cohen, Kasen, Johnson, Berenson, and Gordon, 2006) as well as with negative outcomes such as MDD, dysthymic disorder (Johnson et al., 2005), and anxiety disorders (Johnson et al., 2006) a decade or more later.

Comorbidity, illness burden, treatment utilization

Collaborative Longitudinal Personality Disorders Study data suggest that patients with SPD who are treatment seeking or treated have higher rates of Axis I comorbidity than do patients with MDD, and that the rates of most of the major mood, anxiety, substance-related, and eating disorders are higher among patients with SPD than the published frequencies in the general population; the mean number of lifetime Axis I diagnoses in the SPD group was 3.8. The same researchers also found that SPD was associated with a higher rate of Axis II comorbidity than any of the three other personality disorders (avoidant personality disorder, borderline personality disorder, and obsessive-compulsive personality disorder) being studied. Perhaps unsurprisingly, SPD was especially strongly associated with cooccurrence of the other cluster A disorders (paranoid and schizoid personality disorders) (McGlashan et al., 2000). Above and beyond its associations with other psychiatric illnesses, SPD also seems to be correlated with increased severity, worse naturalistic outcomes (Grilo et al., 2005), greater impairment in social and emotional functioning (Skodol et al., 2005), and less robust treatment responses (Catapano et al., 2006) in the comorbid disorders.

Family studies

The modern conceptualization of SPD has its roots, in part, in Danish adoption studies (Kety et al., 1975). Recent analyses of Danish and Copenhagen adoption cohorts have found that the schizophrenia spectrum disorders (SSDs; for example, schizophrenia, schizoaffective disorder, SPD, and paranoid personality disorder), as a group and individually, all show evidence of genetic transmission, and that there is a genetic relationship between schizophrenia and SPD; there was no significant evidence of a genetic relationship between SSDs and psychiatric disorders outside the spectrum (Kendler et al., 1994). The Finnish Adoption Study found that SPD was significantly more common in biological offspring of mothers with SSDs (Tienari et al., 2003), and that the interaction of familial SSDs and childhood environmental dysfunction was strongly predictive of SSDs in adult adoptees (Wynne et al., 2006).

Genetics

The role of catechol-O-methyltransferase valine-158-methionine (COMT val-158-met) polymorphism in schizophrenia has been one of the most intensively studied areas in psychiatric genetics (Williams et al., 2007). No association was found between SPD and COMT val-158-met genotype in a sample of SPD patients with other personality disorders and healthy controls, though a correlation was found between COMT genotype and performance on tests of executive function (Wisconsin Card Sorting Test: WCST) and working memory (Paced Auditory Serial Addition Test; Minzenberg et al., 2006). In randomly selected male conscripts, an association was observed between COMT val-158-met genotype and a dimensional measure of schizotypy, especially in the domains of disorganization and negative symptoms (Stefanis et al., 2004).

Cognitive testing

One of the best-replicated findings in SPD has been a pattern of neuropsychological deficits that appear to be specific to the schizophrenia spectrum. Often, SPD-related impairment is similar to, though less severe than, that seen in schizophrenia. There does, however, appear to be some cognitive dysfunction that is unique to schizophrenia itself.

Cognitive deficits that may be specific to SPD and the other SSDs include those involving verbal learning (Bergman et al., 1998), executive function (Trestman et al., 1995; Raine et al., 2002), sustained attention (Roitman et al., 1997), and working memory (Roitman et al., 2000; Mitropoulou et al., 2002; Mitropoulou et al., 2005), which may represent a "core" spectrum-specific deficit that mediates the others (Mitropoulou et al., 2005; McClure, Romero, et al., 2007). Domains in which SPD has been associated with cognitive scores intermediate between those of patients with schizophrenia and healthy controls include verbal learning (Bergman et al., 1998), attention, overall intellectual functioning (Cadenhead et al., 1999), abstract reasoning (Weiser et al., 2003), working auditory memory, and visuospatial memory (Mitropoulou et al., 2002), whereas patients with SPD have been found to score similarly to patients with schizophrenia on tests of instruction in comprehension and arithmetic, both of which rely primarily on concentration (Weiser et al., 2003). On the Continuous Performance Task (CPT), patients with SPD have evinced the deficits in context representation, but not the deficits in context maintenance, seen in schizophrenia (Barch et al., 2004).

Certain cognitive features of SPD appear to be associated with specific anatomical variables involving caudate: Smaller total relative caudate volumes in female patients with SPD have been found to correlate with worse scores in selected domains of the WCST and California Verbal Learning Test (Koo, Levitt, et al., 2006), and the degree of caudate volume reduction has been found to correlate with severity of perseveration in two separate working memory tasks (Levitt et al., 2004). Also, higher right and left head of the caudate shape index scores (that is, degrees of "edginess") have been found to correlate inversely with visuospatial memory and auditory/verbal working memory performance respectively (Levitt et al., 2004).

In schizophrenia, cognitive impairment has been found to be strongly predictive of overall clinical outcome. Although this relationship has not been firmly established in SPD, inverse correlations have been found between working memory and interpersonal schizotypal symptoms in adults (Mitropoulou et al., 2002) and between Wechsler Intelligence Scale scores and negative and disorganized schizotypal symptoms in adolescents (Trotman et al., 2006) with SPD.

Neuroimaging-Structural

Ventricles and CSF

In an MRI study of ventricular size, patients with schizophrenia were found to have larger left anterior and temporal horns than healthy controls, while patients with SPD showed sizes intermediate between these two groups (Buchsbaum et al., 1997). Men with SPD have been found to have larger CSF volumes than healthy controls, a result consistent with published findings in schizophrenia (Dickey et al., 2000), and women with SPD have been observed to have large sulcal CSF relative volumes compared to controls (Koo, Dickey, et al., 2006).

Cortex

Patients with SPD have been shown to have smaller temporal lobes than healthy comparisons, a finding that is not accounted for by smaller overall brain volumes (Downhill et al., 2001). Patients with SPD have also been found to have a decrease in left superior temporal gyrus gray matter volume similar to that seen in schizophrenia; unlike patients with schizophrenia, however, patients with SPD show relative sparing of the medial temporal lobe (Dickey et al., 1999). A diffusion tensor imaging (DTI) analysis showed bilaterally reduced fractional anisotropy in the uncinate fasciculus of male patients with SPD compared with controls (Nakamura et al., 2005); this suggestion of altered fronto-temporal connectivity in SPD is consistent with white matter tract findings in schizophrenia (Kubicki et al., 2005).

Thalamus

Although a structural MRI study did not find differences in total or relative thalamic volumes between patients with SSD and healthy controls, patients with schizophrenia had shape abnormalities in left anterior thalamus, whereas patients with SPD had shape abnormalities in the right mediodorsal nucleus region (Hazlett et al., 1999). Also, pulvinar volumes—and, correcting for total brain volume, the sums of pulvinar and mediodorsal nucleus volumes—were smaller in patients with schizophrenia and patients with SPD than in healthy controls, with more pronounced findings in left brain (Byne et al., 2001).

Striatum

Patients with SPD have been found to demonstrate size reduction in caudate nucleus (Levitt et al., 2002; Koo, Levitt, et al., 2006), and increased "edginess" of the head of the caudate nucleus (Levitt et al., 2004) compared with healthy controls. In contrast to this finding of decreased size of caudate nucleus, which is consistent with the published literature on schizophrenia, putamen size has been found to be reduced in patients with SPD compared with healthy controls, whereas the same study found putamen size to be increased in patients with schizophrenia (Shihabuddin et al., 2001). Findings involving caudate have been found to be correlated with neuropsychological impairment (see Neurocognitive Testing section).

Midline structures

Posterior corpus callosum in patients with SPD has been found to be intermediate in size between that in patients with schizophrenia and healthy controls. However, the same study found an increase in size of the genu of corpus callosum, and a narrowing of a region of corpus callosum just posterior to the genu, in patients with SPD compared with patients with schizophrenia and controls (Downhill et al., 2000). Females with SPD have been found to have larger cavum septi pellucidi than healthy controls, a finding similar to one in schizophrenia (Dickey et al., 2007).

Functional Neuroimaging

In PET scans performed immediately after a serial verbal learning test, patients with SPD were found to have metabolic rates intermediate between patients with schizophrenia and healthy controls in lateral temporal regions, but higher than normal metabolic rates in medial frontal and medial temporal areas (Buchsbaum et al., 2002). However, only patients with schizophrenia differed from healthy controls in demonstrating lower relative metabolism in an area in the region of the mediodorsal nucleus of thalamus bilaterally (Hazlett et al., 1999). In a further distinction between SPD and schizophrenia, patients with SPD were found to have elevated putamen relative glucose metabolic rates after a verbal learning task compared to patients with schizophrenia and healthy controls (Shihabuddin et al., 2001). Another example of patients with SPD demonstrating activation patterns different from those of healthy controls in response to cognitive demands is provided by fMRI findings of decreased activation among patients with SPD in key frontal regions during the memory retention period of a visuospatial working memory test (Koenigsberg et al., 2005).

Neuroendocrine and ligand studies

Given the implied role of dopaminergic dysfunction in schizophrenia, the dopamine (DA) system has been a focus of research in SPD as well. Patients with SPD have been found to have significantly higher CSF (Siever et al., 1993) and mean plasma (Siever et al., 1991) concentrations of homovanillic acid (HVA), a DA metabolite, than comparison subjects. Furthermore, plasma and CSF HVA concentrations were found to be positively correlated with "psychotic-like" SPD symptoms. A SPECT study of striatal amphetamine-induced DA release found that DA release in patients with SPD was similar to that in patients with remitted schizophrenia but lower than that seen during acute schizophrenia exacerbations (Abi-Dargham et al., 2004).

By contrast, it appears that patients with SPD show responses to hypothalamic-pituitary-adrenal (HPA) activation that are opposite to those seen in schizophrenia: 2-deoxyglucose, an acute glycopyruvic stressor, which induces exaggerated HPA activation in patients with schizophrenia compared to healthy controls, was found to induce lower cortisol elevations in patients with SPD than in controls. This may imply that patients with SPD are better "buffered" against physiological response to stress than healthy individuals (Mitropoulou et al., 2004).

Schizotypal Personality Disorder and Schizophrenia

Schizotypal personality disorder is the prototype of the SSDs, and it is useful to look at SPD's overlap with schizophrenia and at the important differences between them. Put another way, it is worth exploring not only why patients with SPD have SPD, but also why they are spared the frank psychosis and—in the worst cases—inability to live independently seen in schizophrenia.

Possible relationships between SPD and schizophrenia include:

1. A *forme fruste* model, in which the underlying disturbances in SPD are largely the same as in schizophrenia but may be present to a lesser degree. Support for this model comes from variables in which patients with SPD score similarly to patients with schizophrenia and especially from measures in which patients with SPD occupy a middle ground between patients with schizophrenia and healthy controls. The clinical signs and symptoms of SPD as well as most of the published

neurocognitive, neuroimaging, and neuroendocrine data fall into one of these two categories.

2. An added insult model, in which patients with SPD and patients with schizophrenia share certain underlying disturbances, but patients with schizophrenia suffer from some additional disturbance(s) that cause(s) frank psychosis and catastrophic loss of functioning. Support for this model comes from variables in which patients with schizophrenia, but not patients with SPD, show marked abnormalities; such variables include context maintenance on the AX-CPT, medial temporal lobe gray matter volume, shape of left anterior thalamus, and relative metabolism in the mediodorsal nucleus of thalamus after a serial verbal learning task.

3. A buffer or protective factor model, in which patients with SPD and patients with schizophrenia share certain underlying disturbances, but patients with SPD possess some neurobiological features or assets that protect them from full-blown schizophrenia. Support for this model comes from variables in which patients with SPD, but not patients with schizophrenia, show abnormalities; the SPD-specific abnormalities may represent a protective factor. Such variables include shape of the right mediodorsal nucleus region; size of the genu of corpus callosum; width of a region of corpus callosum just posterior to the genu; and medial frontal, medial temporal, and putamen glucose metabolic rates after a serial verbal learning task. Further evidence for this model comes from measures on which patients with SPD and patients with schizophrenia show abnormalities in different directions; again, the SPD-specific abnormalities may represent a protective factor. Such measures include putamen size, which appears to be increased in schizophrenia but reduced in SPD, and HPA axis activation in response to 2-deoxyglucose, which seems to be exaggerated in schizophrenia but blunted in SPD.

Biologically Informed Treatments

The view of SPD as part of the schizophrenia spectrum, and the evidence of psychotic-like symptoms in SPD, led to treatment trials of antipsychotic medications. An early single-blind trial of low-dose haloperidol in SPD found improvements on the Global Assessment Scale overall as well as on scales measuring Ideas of Reference, Odd Communication, and Social Isolation on the Schedule for Interviewing Borderlines (Hymowitz et al., 1986). The second-generation antipsychotics are of particular interest in SPD, given their antipsychotic effects combined with their putative procognitive activity (Harvey and Keefe, 2001; Keefe, Sweeney, et al., 2007), though results of a large, multicenter study failed to show superiority of atypical agents over a conventional antipsychotic (Keefe, Bilder, et al., 2007). An open-label trial of olanzapine in SPD showed improvements in overall functioning and in depression and psychosis scores (Keshavan et al., 2004). In the only placebo-controlled randomized medication trial in SPD alone known to us, low-dose risperidone was associated with improvements in the general, positive, and negative symptom measures of the Positive and Negative Symptom Scale (Koenigsberg et al., 2003). Future pharmacological research in SPD likely will focus on alleviating patients' suspiciousness and perceptual disturbances as well as their cognitive deficits, which may stem from prefrontal dopaminergic hypoactivity and may therefore be aggravated by antidopaminergic agents such as conventional antipsychotics (Goodman et al., 2000). Drugs that enhance D1 and/or noradrenergic activity in prefrontal regions may prove beneficial to patients with SPD by enhancing cognition, perhaps mediated by improvements in working memory. One such agent, the α-2 agonist *guanfacine*, has shown evidence of improving context processing in patients with SPD, as measured by normalization of performance on the AX-CPT (McClure, Barch, et al., 2007).

CONCLUSIONS

Although it is premature to define specific etiologies for even the best-understood personality disorders, it is clear that personality disorders, like other mental illnesses, are grounded in neurobiological vulnerabilities. These vulnerabilities are likely to eventuate in the full-blown disorder in the context of specific developmental and present-day environmental stimuli. Thus personality disorders, like Axis I disorders, are the result of complex G-E interactions. The distinction, encoded in the *DSM* system, between Axes I and II is weakened by the elucidation of the neurobiological underpinnings of personality disorders. As the specific neurobiological mechanisms underlying specific personality disorders are better understood, this distinction may disappear completely.

REFERENCES

Abi-Dargham, A., Kegeles, L.S., Zea-Ponce, Y., Mawlawi, O., Martinez, D., Mitropoulou, V., O'Flynn, K., Koenigsberg, H.W., Van Heertum, R., Cooper, T., Laruelle, M., and Siever, L.J. (2004) Striatal amphetamine-induced dopamine release in patients with schizotypal personality disorder studied with single photon emission computed tomography and [123I]iodobenzamide. *Biol. Psychiatry* 55(10):1001–1006.

American Psychiatric Association. (2000) *Diagnostic and Statistical Manual of Mental Disorders* (4th ed., text rev.). Washington, DC: Author.

Anderson, M.C., Ochsner, K.N., Kuhl, B., Cooper, J., Robertson, E., Gabrieli, S.W., Glover, G.H., and Gabrieli, J.D. (2004) Neural systems underlying the suppression of unwanted memories. *Science* 303(5655):232–235.

Anderson, S.W., Bechara, A., Damasio, H., et al. (1999) Impairment of social and moral behavior related to early damage in human prefrontal cortex. *Nat. Neurosci.* 2:1032–1037.

Arntz, A., Appels, C., and Sieswerda, S. (2000) Hypervigilance in borderline disorder: a test with the emotional Stroop paradigm. *J. Personal Disord.* 14(4):366–373.

Arseneault, L., Tremblay, R.E., Boulerice, B., and Saucier, J.F. (2002) Obstetrical complications and violent delinquency: testing two developmental pathways. *Child Dev.* 73(2):496–508.

Bailey, J.M., and Shriver, A. (1999) Does childhood sexual abuse cause borderline personality disorder? *J. Sex Marital Ther.* 25(1):45–57.

Bandelow, B., Krause, J., Wedekind, D., Broocks, A., Hajak, G., and Ruther, E. (2005) Early traumatic life events, parental attitudes, family history, and birth risk factors in patients with borderline personality disorder and healthy controls. *Psychiatry Res.* 134(2): 169–179.

Barch, D.M., Mitropoulou, V., Harvey, P.D., New, A.S., Silverman, J.M., and Siever, L.J. (2004) Context-processing deficits in schizotypal personality disorder. *J. Abnorm. Psychol.* 113(4):556–568.

Baron, M., Gruen, R., Asnis, L., and Lord, S. (1985) Familial transmission of schizotypal and borderline personality disorders. *Am. J. Psychiatry* 142(8):927–934.

Battle, C.L., Shea, M.T., Johnson, D.M., Yen, S., Zlotnick, C., Zanarini, M.C., Sanislow, C.A., Skodol, A.E., Gunderson, J.G., Grilo, C.M., McGlashan, T.H., and Morey, L.C. (2004) Childhood maltreatment associated with adult personality disorders: findings from the Collaborative Longitudinal Personality Disorders Study. *J. Personal Disord.* 18(2):193–211.

Bazanis, E., Rogers, R.D., Dowson, J.H., Taylor, P., Meux, C., Staley, C., Nevinson-Andrews, D., Taylor, C., Robbins, T.W., and Sahakian, B.J. (2002) Neurocognitive deficits in decision-making and planning of patients with DSM-III-R borderline personality disorder. *Psychol. Med.* 32(8):1395–1405.

Bear, D. M. & Fulop, M. (1987) The neurology of emotion. In: A. Hobson, ed. *Behavioral Biology in Medicine.* South Norwalk CT: Meduration, Inc.

Beblo, T., Driessen, M., Mertens, M., Wingenfeld, K., Piefke, M., Rullkoetter, N., Silva-Saavedra, A., Mensebach, C., Reddemann, L., Rau, H., Markowitsch, H.J., Wulff, H., Lange, W., Berea, C., Ollech, I., and Woermann, F.G. (2006) Functional MRI correlates of the recall of unresolved life events in borderline personality disorder. *Psychol. Med.* 36(6):845–856.

Bender, D.S., Skodol, A.E., Pagano, M.E., Dyck, I.R., Grilo, C.M., Shea, M.T., Sanislow, C.A., Zanarini, M.C., Yen, S., McGlashan, T.H., and Gunderson, J.G. (2006) Prospective assessment of treatment use by patients with personality disorders. *Psychiatr. Serv.* 57(2):254–257.

Bergman, A., Harvey, P., Lees-Roitman, S., Mitropoulou, V., Marder, D., and Siever, L.J. (1998) Verbal learning and memory in schizotypal personality disorder. *Schizophr. Bull.* 24(4):635–641.

Berlin, H.A., Rolls, E.T., and Iversen, S.D. (2005) Borderline personality disorder, impulsivity, and the orbitofrontal cortex. *Am. J. Psychiatry* 162(12):2360–2373.

Bierer, L.M., Yehuda, R., Schmeidler, J., Mitropoulou, V., New, A.S., Silverman, J.M., and Siever, L.J. (2003) Abuse and neglect in childhood: relationship to personality disorder diagnoses. *CNS Spectr.* 8(10):737–754.

Black, D.W., Noyes, R., Jr., Pfohl, B., Goldstein, R.B., and Blum, N. (1993) Personality disorder in obsessive-compulsive volunteers, well comparison subjects, and their first-degree relatives. *Am. J. Psychiatry* 150(8):1226–1232.

Blair, R.J., and Cipolotti, L. (2000) Impaired social response reversal. A case of "acquired sociopathy." *Brain* 123(Pt 6):1122–1141.

Blair, R.J., Colledge, E., Murray, L., and Mitchell, D.G. (2001) A selective impairment in the processing of sad and fearful expressions in children with psychopathic tendencies. *J. Abnorm. Child Psychol.* 29(6):491–498.

Blair, R.J., Peschardt, K.S., Budhani, S., Mitchell, D.G., and Pine, D.S. (2006) The development of psychopathy. *J. Child Psychol. Psychiatry* 47(3/4):262–276.

Brambilla, P., Soloff, P.H., Sala, M., Nicoletti, M.A., Keshavan, M.S., and Soares, J.C. (2004) Anatomical MRI study of borderline personality disorder patients. *Psychiatry Res.* 131(2):125–133.

Brown, G.L., Ebert, M.H., Goyer, P.F., Jimerson, D.C., Klein, W.J., Bunney, W.E., and Goodwin, F.K. (1982) Aggression, suicide, and serotonin relationships to CSF amine metabolites. *Am. J. Psychiatry* 139:741–746.

Buchsbaum, M., Yang, S., Hazlett, E., Siegel, B., Germans, M., Haznedar, M., O'Faithbheartaigh, S., Wei, T., Silverman, J., and Siever, L.J. (1997) Ventricular volume and asymetry in schizotypal personality disorder and schizophrenia assessed with magnetic resonance imaging. *Schizophr. Res.* 27:45–53.

Buchsbaum, M.S., Nenadic, I., Hazlett, E., Spiegel-Cohen, J., Fleischman, M.B., Akhavan, A., Silverman, J.M., and Siever, L.J. (2002) Differential metabolic rates in prefrontal and temporal Brodmann areas in schizophrenia and schizotypal personality disorder. *Schizophr. Res.* 54(1/2):141–150.

Burgess, J.W. (1991) Relationship of depression and cognitive impairment to self-injury in borderline personality disorder, major depression, and schizophrenia. *Psychiatry Res.* 38(1):77–87.

Burgess, J.W. (1992) Neurocognitive impairment in dramatic personalities: histrionic, narcissistic, borderline, and antisocial disorders. *Psychiatry Res.* 42(3):283–290.

Button, T.M., Scourfield, J., Martin, N., Purcell, S., and McGuffin, P. (2005) Family dysfunction interacts with genes in the causation of antisocial symptoms. *Behav. Genet.* 35(2):115–120.

Byne, W., Buchsbaum, M.S., Kemether, E., Hazlett, E., Shinwari, A., and Siever, L.J. (2001) MRI assessment of medial and dorsal pulvinar nuclei of the thalamus in schizophrenia and schizotypal personality disorder. *Arch. Gen. Psychiatry* 58:133–140.

Cadenhead, K.S., Perry, W., Shafer, K.M., and Braff, D.L. (1999) Cognitive functions in schizotypal personality disorder. *Schizophr. Res.* 37(2):123–132.

Cadoret, R.J., Langbehn, D., Caspers, K., Troughton, E.P., Yucuis, R., Sandhu, H.K., and Philibert, R. (2003) Associations of the serotonin transporter promoter polymorphism with aggressivity, attention deficit, and conduct disorder in an adoptee population. *Compr. Psychiatry* 44(2):88–101.

Caspi, A., McClay, J., Moffitt, T.E., Mill, J., Martin, J., Craig, I.W., Taylor, A., and Poulton, R. (2002) Role of genotype in the cycle of violence in maltreated children. *Science* 297(5582):851–854.

Caspi, A., Sugden, K., Moffitt, T.E., Taylor, A., Craig, I.W., Harrington, H., McClay, J., Mill, J., Martin, J., Braithwaite, A., and Poulton, R. (2003) Influence of life stress on depression: moderation by a polymorphism in the 5-HTT gene. *Science* 301(5631): 386–389.

Catapano, F., Perris, F., Masella, M., Rossano, F., Cigliano, M., Magliano, L., and Maj, M. (2006) Obsessive-compulsive disorder: a 3-year prospective follow-up study of patients treated with serotonin reuptake inhibitors OCD follow-up study. *J. Psychiatr. Res.* 40(6):502–510.

Chen, H., Cohen, P., Kasen, S., and Johnson, J.G. (2006) Adolescent axis I and personality disorders predict quality of life during young adulthood. *J. Adolesc. Health* 39(1):14–19.

Chen, H., Cohen, P., Kasen, S., Johnson, J.G., Berenson, K., and Gordon, K. (2006) Impact of adolescent mental disorders and physical illnesses on quality of life 17 years later. *Arch. Pediatr. Adolesc. Med.* 160(1):93–99.

Cloninger, C.R., Christiansen, K.O., Reich, T., and Gottesman, I.I. (1978) Implications of sex differences in the prevalences of antisocial personality, alcoholism, and criminality for familial transmission. *Arch. Gen. Psychiatry* 35(8):941–951.

Coccaro, E., Kavoussi, R., Oakes, M., Cooper, T., and Hauger, R. (1996) 5HT2a/2c receptor blockade by amesergide fully attenuates prolactin response to d-fenfluramine challenge in physically healthy human subjects. *Psychopharmacology (Berl)* 126(1):24–30.

Coccaro, E.F., and Kavoussi, R.J. (1997) Fluoxetine and impulsive aggressive behavior in personality disordered subjects. *Arch. Gen. Psychiatry* 54:1081–1088.

Coccaro, E.F., Siever, L.J., Klar, H.M., Maurer, G., Cochrane, K., Cooper, T., Mohs, R.C., and Davis, K.L. (1989) Serotonergic studies in patients with affective and personality disorders. Correlates with suicidal and impulsive aggressive behavior. *Arch. Gen. Psychiatry* 46:587–599.

Comtois, K.A., Russo, J., Snowden, M., Srebnik, D., Ries, R., and Roy-Byrne, P. (2003) Factors associated with high use of public mental health services by persons with borderline personality disorder. *Psychiatr. Serv.* 54(8):1149–1154.

Coolidge, F.L., Thede, L.L., and Jang, K.L. (2001) Heritability of personality disorders in childhood: a preliminary investigation. *J. Personal Disord.* 15(1):33–40.

Cornelius, J.R., Soloff, P.H., George, A.W.A., Schulz, C., Tarter, R., and Brenner, R.P. (1989) An evaluation of the significant of selected neuropsychiatric abnormalities in the etiology of borderline personality disorder. *J. Personal. Disord.* 3:19–25.

Coryell, W.H., and Zimmerman, M. (1989) Personality disorder in the families of depressed, schizophrenic, and never-ill probands. *Am. J. Psychiatry* 146(4):496–502.

Crowell, T.A., Kieffer, K.M., Kugeares, S., and Vanderploeg, R.D. (2003) Executive and nonexecutive neuropsychological functioning in antisocial personality disorder. *Cogn. Behav. Neurol.* 16(2):100–109.

Damasio, A.R. (1994) *Descartes' Error: Emotion, Rationality and the Human Brain.* New York: Putnam Books.

Damasio, H., Grabowski, T., Frank, R., Galaburda, A., and Damasio, A.R. (1994) The return of Phineas Gage: clues about the brain from the skull of a famous patient. *Science* 264:1102–1105.

Davidson, R.J., Putnam, K.M., and Larson, C.L. (2000) Dysfunction in the neural circuitry of emotion regulation—a possible prelude to violence. *Science* 289:591–594.

De La Fuente, J.M., Goldman, S., Stanus, E., Vizuete, C., Morlan, I., Bobes, J., and Mendlewicz, J. (1997) Brain glucose metabolism in borderline personality disorder. *J. Psychiatr. Res.* 31(5):531–541.

Dickey, C.C., McCarley, R.W., Voglmaier, M.M., Niznikiewicz, M.A., Seidman, L.J., Hirayasu, Y., Fischer, I., Teh, E.K., Van Rhoads, R., Jakab, M., Kikinis, R., Jolescz, F.A., and Shenton, M.E. (1999) Schizotypal personality disorder and MRI abnormalities of temporal lobe gray matter. *Biol. Psychiatry* 45:1393–1402.

Dickey, C.C., McCarley, R.W., Xu, M.L., Seidman, L.J., Voglmaier, M.M., Niznikiewicz, M.A., Connor, E., and Shenton, M.E. (2007) MRI abnormalities of the hippocampus and cavum septi pellucidi in females with schizotypal personality disorder. *Schizophr. Res.* 89(1/3):49–58.

Dickey, C.C., Shenton, M. E., Hirayasu, Y., Fischer, I., Voglmaier, M.M., Niznikiewicz, M.A., Seidman, L.J., Fraone, S., and McCarley, R.W. (2000) Large CSF volumes not attributable to ventricular volume in schizotypal personality disorder. *Am. J. Psychiatry* 157(1):48–54.

Donegan, N.H., Sanislow, C.A., Blumberg, H.P., Fulbright, R.K., Lacadie, C., Skudlarski, P., Gore, J.C., Olson, I.R., McGlashan, T.H., and Wexler, B.E. (2003) Amygdala hyperreactivity in borderline personality disorder: implications for emotional dysregulation. *Biol. Psychiatry* 54(11):1284–1293.

Dougherty, D.M., Bjork, J.M., Huckabee, H., Moeller, F., and Swann, A. (1999) Laboratory measures of aggression and impulsivity in women with borderline personality disorder. *Psychiatry Res.* 85(3):315–326.

Downhill, J.E., Buchsbaum, M.S., Hazlett, E.A., Barth, S., Lees-Roitman, S., Nunn, M., Lekarev, O., Wei, T., and Siever, L.J. (2001) Temporal lobe volume determined by magnetic resonance imaging in schizotypal personality disorder and schizophrenia. *Schizophr. Res.* 48(2/3):187–199.

Downhill, J.E., Buchsbaum, M.S., Wei, T.S., Speigel-Cohen, J., Hazlett, E.A., Haznedar, M.M., Silverman, J., and Siever, L.J. (2000) Shape and size of the corpus callosum in schizophrenia and schizotypal personality disorder. *Schizophr. Res.* 42:193–208.

Driessen, M., Herrmann, J., Stahl, K., Zwaan, M., Meier, S., Hill, A., Osterheider, M., and Petersen, D. (2000) Magnetic resonance imaging volumes of the hippocampus and the amgydala in women with borderline personality disorder and early traumatization. *Arch. Gen. Psychiatry* 57(12):1115–1122.

Driessen, M., Herrmann, J., Stahl, K., Zwaan, M., Meier, S., Hill, A., Osterheider, M., and Petersen, D. (2000) Magnetic resonance imaging volumes of the hippocampus and the amygdala in women with borderline personality disorder and early traumatization. *Arch. Gen. Psychiatry* 57(12):1115–1122.

Fan, J., McCandliss, B.D., Sommer, T., Raz, A., and Posner, M.I. (2002) Testing the efficiency and independence of attentional networks. *J. Cogn. Neurosci.* 14(3):340–347.

Fertuck, E.A., Lenzenweger, M.F., Clarkin, J.F., Hoermann, S., and Stanley, B. (2006) Executive neurocognition, memory systems, and borderline personality disorder. *Clin. Psychol. Rev.* 26(3):346–375.

Foley, D.L., Eaves, L.J., Wormley, B., Silberg, J.L., Maes, H.H., Kuhn, J., and Riley, B. (2004) Childhood adversity, monoamine oxidase a genotype, and risk for conduct disorder. *Arch. Gen. Psychiatry* 61(7):738–744.

Fossati, A., Madeddu, F., and Maffei, C. (1999) Borderline personality disorder and childhood sexual abuse: a meta-analytic study. *J. Personal. Disord.* 13(3):268–280.

Fossati, A., Maffei, C., Bagnato, M., Donati, D., Namia, C., and Novella, L. (1999) Latent structure analysis of DSM-IV borderline personality disorder criteria. *Compr. Psychiatry* 40(1):72–79.

Frankle, W.G., Lombardo, I., New, A.S., Goodman, M., Talbot, P.S., Huang, Y., Hwang, D.R., Slifstein, M., Curry, S., Abi-Dargham, A., Laruelle, M., and Siever, L.J. (2005) Brain serotonin transporter distribution in subjects with impulsive aggressivity: a positron emission study with [11C]McN 5652. *Am. J. Psychiatry* 162(5):915–923.

Fricke, S., Moritz, S., Andresen, B., Jacobsen, D., Kloss, M., Rufer, M., and Hand, I. (2006) Do personality disorders predict negative treatment outcome in obsessive-compulsive disorders? A prospective 6-month follow-up study. *Eur. Psychiatry* 21(5):319–324.

Gardner, D.L., Lucas, P.B., and Cowdry, R.W. (1990) CSF metabolites in borderline personality disorder compared with normal controls. *Biol. Psychiatry* 28:247–254.

Golden, C.J., Marsella, A.J., and Golden, E.E. (1975) Personality correlates of the Stroop Color and Word Test: more negative results. *Percept. Mot. Skills* 41(2):599–602.

Goodman, M., Mitropoulou, V., New, A.S., Koenigsberg, H.W., and Siever, L.J. (2000) Frontal cortex dysfunction and subcortical dopaminergic activity in schizophrenia spectrum. *Biol. Psychiatry* 47:34S.

Goodman, M., and Yehuda, R (2002) The relationship between psychological trauma and borderline personality disorder. *Psychiatric Ann.* 32(6):337–346.

Goveas, J.S., Csernansky, J.G., and Coccaro, E.F. (2004) Platelet serotonin content correlates inversely with life history of aggression in personality-disordered subjects. *Psychiatry Res.* 126(1):23–32.

Goyer, P.F., Andreason, P.J., Semple, W.E., Clayton, A.H., King, A.C., Compton-Toth, B.A., Schulz, S.C., and Cohen, R.M. (1994) Positron-emission-tomography and personality disorders. *Neuropsychopharmacology* 10(1):21–28.

Grilo, C.M., Sanislow, C.A., Shea, M.T., Skodol, A.E., Stout, R.L., Gunderson, J.G., Yen, S., Bender, D.S., Pagano, M.E., Zanarini, M.C., Morey, L.C., and McGlashan, T.H. (2005) Two-year prospective naturalistic study of remission from major depressive disorder as a function of personality disorder comorbidity. *J. Consult. Clin. Psychol.* 73(1):78–85.

Gunderson, J.G., Morey, L.C., Stout, R.L., Skodol, A.E., Shea, M.T., McGlashan, T.H., Zanarini, M.C., Grilo, C.M., Sanislow, C.A., Yen, S., Daversa, M.T., and Bender, D.S. (2004) Major depressive disorder and borderline personality disorder revisited: longitudinal interactions. *J. Clin. Psychiatry* 65(8):1049–1056.

Hare, R. (1991). *The Hare Psychopathology Checklist Revised*. Toronto, Canada: Multi-Health Systems.

Harvey, P.D., and Keefe, R.S. (2001) Studies of cognitive change in patients with schizophrenia following novel antipsychotic treatment. *Am. J. Psychiatry* 158(2):176–184.

Hazlett, E.A., Buchsbaum, M.S., Byne, W., Wei, T.C., Spiegel-Cohen, J., Geneve, C., Kinderlehrer, R., Haznedar, M.M., Shihabuddin, L., and Siever, L.J. (1999) Three-dimensional analysis with MRI and PET of the size, shape and function of the thalamus in the schizophrenia spectrum. *Am. J. Psychiatry* 156:1190–1199.

Hazlett, E.A., New, A.S., Newmark, R., Haznedar, M.M., Lo, J.N., Speiser, L.J., Chen, A.D., Mitropoulou, V., Minzenberg, M., Siever, L.J., and Buchsbaum, M.S. (2005) Reduced anterior and posterior cingulate gray matter in borderline personality disorder. *Biol. Psychiatry* 58(8):614–623.

Helgeland, M.I., and Torgersen, S. (2004) Developmental antecedents of borderline personality disorder. *Compr. Psychiatry* 45(2): 138–147.

Herman, J.L., Perry, J.C., and van der Kolk, B.A. (1989) Childhood trauma in borderline personality disorder. *Am. J. Psychiatry* 146:490–495.

Herpertz, S., Dietrich, T., Wenning, B., Krings, T., Erberich, S., Willmes, K., Thron, A., and Sass, H. (2001) Evidence of abnormal amygdala functioning in borderline personality disorder: a functional MRI study. *Biol. Psychiatry* 50(4):292–298.

Hochhausen, N.M., Lorenz, A.R., and Newman, J.P. (2002) Specifying the impulsivity of female inmates with borderline personality disorder. *J. Abnorm. Psychol.* 111(3):495–501.

Huang, D.B., Kamat, P.P., and Wang, J. (2006) Demographic characteristics and antisocial personality disorder of early and late onset alcoholics identified in a primary care clinic. *Am. J. Addict.* 15(6):478–482.

Huizinga, D., Haberstick, B.C., Smolen, A., Menard, S., Young, S.E., Corley, R.P., Stallings, M.C., Grotpeter, J., and Hewitt, J.K. (2006) Childhood maltreatment, subsequent antisocial behavior, and the role of monoamine oxidase A genotype. *Biol. Psychiatry* 60(7):677–683.

Hymowitz, P., Frances, A., Jacobsberg, L., et al. (1986) Neuroleptic treatment of schizotypal personality disorder. *Compr. Psychiatry* 27:267–271.

Intrator, J., Hare, R., Stritzke, P., Brichtswein, K., Dorfman, D., Harpur, T., Bernstein, D., Handelsman, L., Schaefer, C., Keilp, J., Rosen, J., and Machac, J. (1997) A brain imaging (single photon emission computerized tomography) study of semantic and affective processing in psychopaths. *Biol. Psychiatry* 42(2):96–103.

Jacobson, K.C., Prescott, C.A., and Kendler, K.S. (2002) Sex differences in the genetic and environmental influences on the development of antisocial behavior. *Dev. Psychopathol.* 14(2):395–416.

Jane, J.S., Pagan, J.L., Turkheimer, E., Fiedler, E.R., and Oltmanns, T.F. (2006) The interrater reliability of the Structured Interview for DSM-IV Personality. *Compr. Psychiatry* 47(5):368–375.

Jang, K.L., Vernon, P.A., and Livesley, W.J. (2000) Personality disorder traits, family environment, and alcohol misuse: a multivariate behavioural genetic analysis. *Addiction* 95(6):873–888.

Ji, W.Y., Hu, Y.H., Huang, Y.Q., Cao, W.H., Lv, J., Qin, Y., Pang, Z.C., Wang, S.J., and Li, L.M. (2006) [A twin study of personality disorder heritability]. *Zhonghua Liu Xing Bing Xue Za Zhi* 27(2):137–141.

Johansen, M., Karterud, S., Pedersen, G., Gude, T., and Falkum, E. (2004) An investigation of the prototype validity of the borderline DSM-IV construct. *Acta Psychiatr. Scand.* 109(4):289–298.

Johnson, J.G., Cohen, P., Kasen, S., and Brook, J.S. (2005) Personality disorder traits associated with risk for unipolar depression during middle adulthood. *Psychiatry Res.* 136(2/3):113–121.

Johnson, J.G., Cohen, P., Kasen, S., and Brook, J.S. (2006) Personality disorders evident by early adulthood and risk for anxiety disorders during middle adulthood. *J. Anxiety Disord.* 20(4):408–426.

Juengling, F.D., Schmahl, C., Hesslinger, B., Ebert, D., Bremner, J.D., Gostomzyk, J., Bohus, M., and Lieb, K. (2003) Positron emission tomography in female patients with borderline personality disorder. *J. Psychiatr. Res.* 37(2):109–115.

Keefe, R.S., Bilder, R.M., Davis, S.M., Harvey, P.D., Palmer, B.W., Gold, J.M., Meltzer, H.Y., Green, M.F., Capuano, G., Stroup, T.S., McEvoy, J.P., Swartz, M.S., Rosenheck, R.A., Perkins, D.O., Davis, C.E., Hsiao, J.K., Lieberman, JA; CATIE Investigators; Neurocognitive Working Group. (2007) Neurocognitive effects of antipsychotic medications in patients with chronic schizophrenia in the CATIE Trial. *Arch Gen Psychiatry* 64(6): 633–647.

Keefe, R.S., Sweeney, J.A., Gu, H., Hamer, R.M., Perkins, D.O., McEvoy, J.P., and Lieberman, J.A. (2007) Effects of olanzapine, quetiapine, and risperidone on neurocognitive function in early psychosis: a randomized, double-blind 52-week comparison. *Am. J. Psychiatry* 164(7):1061–1071.

Kendler, K.S. (1985) Diagnostic approaches to schizotypal personality disorder: a historical perspective. *Schizophr. Bull.* 11(4):538–553.

Kendler, K.S., Gruenberg, A.M., and Kinney, D.K. (1994) Independent diagnoses of adoptees and relatives as defined by DSM-III in the provincial and national samples of the Danish Adoption Study of Schizophrenia. *Arch. Gen. Psychiatry* 51(6):456–468.

Keshavan, M., Shad, M., Soloff, P., and Schooler, N. (2004) Efficacy and tolerability of olanzapine in the treatment of schizotypal personality disorder. *Schizophr. Res.* 71(1):97–101.

Kesler-West, M., Andersen, A.H, Smith, C.D., Avison, M.J., Davis, C.E., Kryscio, R.J., and Blonder, L. (2001) Neural substrates of facial emotion processing using fMRI. *Brain Res. Cogn. Brain Res.* 11(2):213–226.

Kety, S.S., Rosenthal, D., Wender, P.H., et al. (1975). Mental illness in the biological and adoptive families of adopted individuals who have become schizophrenic: preliminary report based on psychiatric reviews. In: R. Fieve, D. Rosenthal, and H. Brill, eds. *Genetic Research in Psychiatry*. Baltimore: Johns Hopkins University Press, pp. 147–165.

Kiehl, K.A., Smith, A.M., Hare, R.D., Mendrek, A., Forster, B.B., Brink, J., and Liddle, P.F. (2001) Limbic abnormalities in affective processing by criminal psychopaths as revealed by functional magnetic resonance imaging. *Biol. Psychiatry* 50(9):677–684.

Kim-Cohen, J., Caspi, A., Taylor, A., Williams, B., Newcombe, R., Craig, I.W., and Moffitt, T.E. (2006) MAOA, maltreatment, and gene-environment interaction predicting children's mental health: new evidence and a meta-analysis. *Mol. Psychiatry* 11(10):903–913.

Koenigsberg, H.W., Buchsbaum, M.S., Buchsbaum, B.R., Schneiderman, J.S., Tang, C.Y., New, A., Goodman, M., and Siever, L.J. (2005) Functional MRI of visuospatial working memory in schizotypal personality disorder: a region-of-interest analysis. *Psychol. Med.* 35(7):1019–1030.

Koenigsberg, H.W., Reynolds, D., Goodman, M., New, A.S., Mitropoulou, V., Trestman, R.L., Silverman, J., and Siever, L.J. (2003) Risperidone in the treatment of schizotypal personality disorder. *J. Clin. Psychiatry* 64(6):628–634.

Koo, M.S., Dickey, C.C., Park, H.J., Kubicki, M., Ji, N.Y., Bouix, S., Pohl, K.M., Levitt, J.J., Nakamura, M., Shenton, M.E., and McCarley, R.W. (2006) Smaller neocortical gray matter and larger sulcal cerebrospinal fluid volumes in neuroleptic-naive women with schizotypal personality disorder. *Arch. Gen. Psychiatry* 63(10):1090–1100.

Koo, M.S., Levitt, J.J., McCarley, R.W., Seidman, L.J., Dickey, C.C., Niznikiewicz, M.A., Voglmaier, M.M., Zamani, P., Long, K.R., Kim, S.S., and Shenton, M.E. (2006) Reduction of caudate nucleus volumes in neuroleptic-naive female subjects with schizotypal personality disorder. *Biol. Psychiatry* 60(1):40–48.

Korfine, L., and Hooley, J. (2000) Directed forgetting of emotional stimuli in borderline personality disorder. *J. Abnorm. Psychol.* 109(2):214–221.

Kubicki, M., McCarley, R.W., and Shenton, M.E. (2005) Evidence for white matter abnormalities in schizophrenia. *Curr. Opin. Psychiatry* 18(2):121–134.

Kuruoglu, A.C., Arikan, Z., Vural, G., Karatas, M., Arac, M., and Isik, E. (1996) Single photon emission computerised tomography in chronic alcoholism. Antisocial personality disorder may be associated with decreased frontal perfusion. *Br. J. Psychiatry* 169(3):348–354.

Laakso, M.P., Gunning-Dixon, F., Vaurio, O., Repo-Tiihonen, E., Soininen, H., and Tiihonen, J. (2002) Prefrontal volumes in habitually violent subjects with antisocial personality disorder and type 2 alcoholism. *Psychiatry Res.* 114(2):95–102.

Lapierre, D., Braun, C.M., and Hodgins, S. (1995) Ventral frontal deficits in psychopathy: neuropsychological test findings. *Neuropsychologia* 33(2):139–151.

Levitt, J.J., McCarley, R.W., Dickey, C.C., Voglmaier, M.M., Niznikiewicz, M., Seidman, L.J., Hirayasu, Y., Ciszewski, A.A., Kikinis, R., Jolesz, F.A., and Shenton, M.E. (2002) MRI study of caudate nucleus volume and its cognitive correlates in neuroleptic-naive patients with schizotypal personality disorder. *Am. J. Psychiatry* 159(7):1190–1197.

Levitt, J.J., Westin, C.F., Nestor, P.G., Estepar, R.S., Dickey, C.C., Voglmaier, M.M., Seidman, L.J., Kikinis, R., Jolesz, F.A., McCarley, R.W., and Shenton, M.E. (2004) Shape of caudate nucleus and its cognitive correlates in neuroleptic-naive schizotypal personality disorder. *Biol. Psychiatry* 55(2):177–184.

Leyton, M., Okazawa, H., Diksic, M., Paris, J., Rosa, P., Mzengeza, S., Young, S.N., Blier, P., and Benkelfat, C. (2001) Brain regional alpha-[11C]methyl-L-tryptophan trapping in impulsive subjects with borderline personality disorder. *Am. J. Psychiatry* 158(5): 775–782.

Leyton, M., Young, S., Paris, J., Pihl, R., and Benkelfat, C. (1999) Suicide attempts and impulsivity. *Biol. Psychiatry* 45S(8S):146S.

Li, C.S., Kosten, T.R., and Sinha, R. (2006) Antisocial personality and stress-induced brain activation in cocaine-dependent patients. *Neuroreport* 17(3):243–247.

Lidberg, L., Belfrage, H., Bertilsson, L., Evenden, M.M., and Asberg, M. (2000) Suicide attempts and impulse control disorder are related to low cerebrospinal fluid 5-HIAA in mentally disordered violent offenders. *Acta Psychiatr. Scand.* 101(5):395–402.

Linnoila, M., DeJong, J., and Virkkunen, M. (1989) Family history of alcoholism in violent offenders and impulsive fire setters. *Arch. Gen. Psychiatry* 46:613–616.

Linnoila, M., Virkkunen, M., George, T., Eckardt, M., Higley, J.D., Nielsen, D., and Goldman, D. (1994) Serotonin, behavior and alcohol. In: B. Jansson, H. Jornvall, U. Rydberg, L. Terenius, and L. Vallee, eds. *Toward a Molecular Basis of Alcohol Use and Abuse.* Switzerland: Birkhauser Verlag Base, pp. 155–163.

Loranger, A.W., Oldham, J.M., and Tulis, E.H. (1982) Familial transmission of DSM-III borderline personality disorder. *Arch. Gen. Psychiatry* 39(7):795–799.

Lyons, M.J., True, W.R., Eisen, S.A., Goldberg, J., Meyer, J.M., Faraone, S.V., Eaves, L.J., and Tsuang, M.T. (1995) Differential heritability of adult and juvenile antisocial traits. *Arch. Gen. Psychiatry* 52(11):906–915.

Maier, W., Lichtermann, D., Oehrlein, A., and Fickinger, M. (1992) Depression in the community: a comparison of treated and non-treated cases in two non-referred samples. *Psychopharmacology (Berl)* 106(Suppl):S79–S81.

Malloy, P., Noel, N., Longabaugh, R., and Beattie, M. (1990) Determinants of neuropsychological impairment in antisocial substance abusers. *Addict. Behav.* 15(5):431–438.

McClure, M., Barch, D.M., Romero, M.J., Minzenberg, M.J., Triebwasser, J., Harvey, P.D., and Siever, L.J. (2007) The effects of guanfacine of context processing abnormalities in schizotypal personality disorder. *Biol. Psychiatry* 15(61):1157–1160.

McClure, M.M., Romero, M.J., Bowie, C.R., Reichenberg, A., Harvey, P.D., and Siever, L.J. (2007) Visual-spatial learning and memory in schizotypal personality disorder: continued evidence for the importance of working memory in the schizophrenia spectrum. *Arch. Clin. Neuropsychol.* 22(1):109–116.

McGlashan, T.H., Grilo, C.M., Skodol, A.E., Gunderson, J.G., Shea, M.T., Morey, L.C., Zanarini, M.C., and Stout, R.L. (2000) The Collaborative Longitudinal Personality Disorders Study: baseline Axis I/II and II/II diagnostic co-occurrence. *Acta Psychiatr. Scand.* 102(4):256–264.

McGloin, J.M., and Widom, C.S. (2001) Resilience among abused and neglected children grown up. *Dev. Psychopathol.* 13(4): 1021–1038.

Melley, A.H., Oltmanns, T.F., and Turkheimer, E. (2002) The Schedule for Nonadaptive and Adaptive Personality (SNAP): temporal stability and predictive validity of the diagnostic scales. *Assessment* 9(2):181–187.

Miller, B.L., Darby, A., Benson, D.F., et al (1997) Aggressive, socially disruptive and antisocial behaviour associated with fronto-temporal dementia. *Br. J. Psychiatry* 170:150–154.

Minzenberg, M.J., Xu, K., Mitropoulou, V., Harvey, P.D., Finch, T., Flory, J.D., New, A.S., Goldman, D., and Siever, L.J. (2006) Catechol-O-methyltransferase Val158Met genotype variation is associated with prefrontal-dependent task performance in schizotypal personality disorder patients and comparison groups. *Psychiatr. Genet.* 16(3):117–124.

Mitchell, D.G., Colledge, E., Leonard, A., and Blair, R.J. (2002) Risky decisions and response reversal: is there evidence of orbitofrontal cortex dysfunction in psychopathic individuals? *Neuropsychologia* 40(12):2013–2022.

Mitropoulou, V., Goodman, M., Sevy, S., Elman, I., New, A.S., Iskander, E.G., Silverman, J.M., Breier, A., and Siever, L.J. (2004) Effects of acute metabolic stress on the dopaminergic and pituitary-adrenal axis activity in patients with schizotypal personality disorder. *Schizophr. Res.* 70(1):27–31.

Mitropoulou, V., Harvey, P.D., Maldari, L.A., Moriarty, P.J., New, A.S., Silverman, J.M., and Siever, L.J. (2002) Neuropsychological performance in schizotypal personality disorder: evidence regarding diagnostic specificity. *Biol. Psychiatry* 52(12):1175–1182.

Mitropoulou, V., Harvey, P.D., Zegarelli, G., New, A.S., Silverman, J.M., and Siever, L.J. (2005) Neuropsychological performance in schizotypal personality disorder: importance of working memory. *Am. J. Psychiatry* 162(10):1896–1903.

Moffitt, T.E. (1990) Juvenile delinquency and attention deficit disorder: boys' developmental trajectories from age 3 to age 15. *Child Dev.* 61(3):893–910.

Moffitt, T.E. (1993) Adolescence-limited and life-course-persistent antisocial behavior: a developmental taxonomy. *Psychol. Rev.* 100(4):674–701.

Moffitt, T.E. (2002) Teen-aged mothers in contemporary Britain. *J. Child Psychol. Psychiatry* 43(6):727–742.

Moffitt, T.E. (2005) Genetic and environmental influences on antisocial behaviors: evidence from behavioral-genetic research. *Adv. Genet.* 55:41–104.

Moran, P., Coffey, C., Mann, A., Carlin, J.B., and Patton, G.C. (2006) Dimensional characteristics of DSM-IV personality disorders in a large epidemiological sample. *Acta Psychiatr. Scand.* 113(3):233–236.

Morgan, A.B., and Lilienfeld, S.O. (2000) A meta-analytic review of the relation between antisocial behavior and neuropsychological measures of executive function. *Clin. Psychol. Rev.* 20(1):113–136.

Muller, J.L., Sommer, M., Wagner, V., Lange, K., Taschler, H., Roder, C.H., Schuierer, G., Klein, H.E., and Hajak, G. (2003) Abnormalities in emotion processing within cortical and subcortical regions in criminal psychopaths: evidence from a functional magnetic resonance imaging study using pictures with emotional content. *Biol. Psychiatry* 54(2):152–162.

Nakamura, M., McCarley, R.W., Kubicki, M., Dickey, C.C., Niznikiewicz, M.A., Voglmaier, M.M., Seidman, L.J., Maier, S.E., Westin, C.F., Kikinis, R., and Shenton, M.E. (2005) Frontotemporal disconnectivity in schizotypal personality disorder: a diffusion tensor imaging study. *Biol. Psychiatry* 58(6):468–478.

Narusyte, J., Andershed, A.K., Neiderhiser, J.M., and Lichtenstein, P. (2007) Aggression as a mediator of genetic contributions to the association between negative parent-child relationships and adolescent antisocial behavior. *Eur. Child Adolesc. Psychiatry* 16(2):128–137.

New, A., Hazlett, E., Buchsbaum, M.S., Goodman, M., Reynolds, D., Mitropoulou, V., Sprung, L., Shaw, R.B. Jr., Koenigsberg, H.W., Platholi, J., Silverman, J., and Siever, L. (2002) Blunted prefrontal cortical 18fluorodeoxyglucose positron emission tomography response to meta-chloropiperazine in impulsive aggression. *Arch. Gen. Psychiatry* 59(7):621–629.

New, A.S., Buchsbaum, M.S., Hazlett, E.A., Goodman, M., Koenigsberg, H.W., Lo, J., Iskander, L., Newmark, R., Brand, J., O'Flynn, K., and Siever, L.J. (2004) Fluoxetine increases relative metabolic rate in prefrontal cortex in impulsive aggression. *Psychopharmacology (Berl)* 176(3/4):451–458.

New, A.S., Hazlett, E.A., Buchsbaum, M.S., Goodman, M., Mitelman, S.A., Newmark, R., Trisdorfer, R., Haznedar, M.M., Koenigsberg, H.W., Flory, J., and Siever, L.J. (2007) Amygdala-prefrontal disconnection in borderline personality disorder. *Neuropsychopharmacology* 32:1629–1640.

Ng Ying Kin, N. M., Paris, J., Schwartz, G., Zweig-Frank, H., Steiger, H., and Nair, N.P. (2005) Impaired platelet [3H]paroxetine binding in female patients with borderline personality disorder. *Psychopharmacology (Berl)* 182(3):447–451.

Ni, X., Chan, K., Bulgin, N., Sicard, T., Bismil, R., McMain, S., and Kennedy, J.L. (2006) Association between serotonin transporter gene and borderline personality disorder. *J. Psychiatr. Res.* 40(5): 448–453.

O'Keane, V., Maloney, E., O'Neil, H., O'Connor, A., Smith, C., and Dinan, T.G. (1992) Blunted prolactin response to d-fenfluramine in sociopathy: Evidence for subsensitivity of central serotonergic function. *Br. J. Psychiatry* 160:643–646.

O'Leary, K.M., Brouwers, P., Gardner, D.L., and Cowdry, R.W. (1991) Neuropsychological testing of patients with borderline personality disorder. *Am. J. Psychiatry* 148(1):106–111.

Ogloff, J.R. (2006) Psychopathy/antisocial personality disorder conundrum. *Aust. N. Z. J. Psychiatry* 40(6/7):519–528.

Oquendo, M.A., Krunic, A., Parsey, R.V., Milak, M., Malone, K.M., Anderson, A., van Heertum, R.L., and John Mann, J. (2005) Positron emission tomography of regional brain metabolic responses to a serotonergic challenge in major depressive disorder with and without borderline personality disorder. *Neuropsychopharmacology* 30(6):1163–1172.

Orr, S.P., Metzger, L.J., Lasko, N.B., Macklin, M.L., Peri, T., and Pitman, R.K. (2000) De novo conditioning in trauma-exposed individuals with and without posttraumatic stress disorder. *J. Abnorm. Psychol.* 109(2):290–298.

Paris, J. (1998) Does childhood trauma cause personality disorders in adults? *Can. J. Psychiatry* 43(2):148–153.

Paris, J. (2000) Childhood precursors of borderline personality disorder. *Psychiatr. Clin. North Am.* 23(1):77–88, vii.

Paris, J., Zweig-Frank, H., and Guzder, J. (1994a) Psychological risk factors for borderline personality disorder in female patients. *Compr. Psychiatry* 35(4):301–305.

Paris, J., Zweig-Frank, H., and Guzder, J. (1994b) Risk factors for borderline personality in male outpatients. *J. Nerv. Ment. Dis.* 182(7):375–380.

Pascual, J.C., Soler, J., Barrachina, J., Campins, M.J., Alvarez, E., Perez, V., Cortes, A., and Baiget, M. (2006) Failure to detect an association between the serotonin transporter gene and borderline personality disorder. *J. Psychiatr. Res.* 40(5):448–453.

Peri, T., Ben-Shakhar, G., Orr, S.P., and Shalev, A.Y. (2000) Psychophysiologic assessment of aversive conditioning in posttraumatic stress disorder. *Biol. Psychiatry* 47(6):512–519.

Phillips, M.L., Bullmore, E.T., Howard, R., Woodruff, P.W., Wright, I.C., Williams, S.C., Simmons, A., Andrew, C., Brammer, M., and David, A.S. (1998) Investigation of facial recognition memory and happy and sad facial expression perception: an fMRI study. *Psychiatry Res.* 83(3):127–138.

Phillips, M.L., Young, A.W., Scott, S.K., Calder, A.J., Andrew, C., Giampietro, V., Williams, S.C., Bullmore, E.T., Brammer, M., and Gray, J.A. (1998) Neural responses to facial and vocal expressions of fear and disgust. *Proc. R Soc. Lond. B Biol. Sci.* 265(1408):1809–1817.

Pietrini, P., Guazzelli, M., Vasso, G., Jaffe, K., and Grafman, J. (2000) Neural correlates of imaginal aggressive behavior assessed by positron emission tomography in healthy subjects. *Am. J. Psychiatry* 157(11):1772–1781.

Posner, M.I., Rothbart, M.K., Vizueta, N., Levy, K.N., Evans, D.E., Thomas, K.M., and Clarkin, J.F. (2002) Attentional mechanisms of borderline personality disorder. *Proc. Natl. Acad. Sci. USA* 99(25):16366–16370.

Pribram, K.H., and Bragshaw, M. (1953) Further analysis of the temporal lobe syndrome utilizing frontotemporal ablation. *J. Comp. Neurol.* 99:347–375.

Pukrop, R., and Krischer, M. (2005) Changing views about personality disorders: Comment about the prospective studies CIC, CLPS, and MSAD. *J. Personal. Disord.* 19(5):563–572.

Raine, A., Lencz, T., Bihrle, S., et al. (2000) Reduced prefrontal gray volume and autonomic deficits in antisocial personality disorder. *Arch. Gen. Psychiatry* 57:119–127.

Raine, A., Lencz, T., Yaralian, P., Bihrle, S., LaCasse, L., Ventura, J., and Colletti, P. (2002) Prefrontal structural and functional deficits in schizotypal personality disorder. *Schizophr. Bull.* 28(3):501–513.

Rhee, S.H., and Waldman, I.D. (2002) Genetic and environmental influences on antisocial behavior: a meta-analysis of twin and adoption studies. *Psychol. Bull.* 128(3):490–529.

Rinne, T., van den Brink, W., Wouters, L., and van Dyck, C. (2002) SSRI treatment of borderline personality disorder: a randomized, placebo controlled clinical trial for female patients with borderline personality disorder. *Am. J. Psychiatry* 159(12):2048–2054.

Roitman, S.E., Cornblatt, B.A., Bergman, A., Obuchowski, M., Mitropoulou, V., Keefe, R.S., Silverman, J., and Siever, L.J. (1997) Attentional functioning in schizotypal personality disorder. *Am. J. Psychiatry* 154(5):655–660.

Roitman, S.E., Mitropoulou, V., Keefe, R.S., Silverman, J.M., Serby, M., Harvey, P.D., Reynolds, D.A., Mohs, R.C., and Siever, L.J. (2000) Visuospatial working memory in schizotypal personality disorder patients. *Schizophr. Res.* 41(3):447–455.

Roy, A., Adinoff, B., and Linnoila, M. (1988) Acting out hostility in normal volunteers: negative correlation with levels of 5-HIAA in cerebrospinal fluid. *Psychiatr. Res.* 24:187–194.

Rusch, N., van Elst, L.T., Ludaescher, P., Wilke, M., Huppertz, H.J., Thiel, T., Schmahl, C., Bohus, M., Lieb, K., Hesslinger, B.,

Hennig, J., and Ebert, D. (2003) A voxel-based morphometric MRI study in female patients with borderline personality disorder. *NeuroImage* 20(1):385–392.

Sanislow, C.A., Grilo, C.M., and McGlashan, T.H. (2000) Factor analysis of the DSM-III-R borderline personality disorder criteria in psychiatric inpatients. *Am. J. Psychiatry* 157(10):1629–1633.

Sanislow, C.A., Grilo, C.M., Morey, L.C., Bender, D.S., Skodol, A.E., Gunderson, J.G., Shea, M.T., Stout, R.L., Zanarini, M.C., and McGlashan, T.H. (2002) Confirmatory factor analysis of DSM-IV criteria for borderline personality disorder: findings from the collaborative longitudinal personality disorders study. *Am. J. Psychiatry* 159(2):284–290.

Schaeffer, C.M., Petras, H., Ialongo, N., Masyn, K.E., Hubbard, S., Poduska, J., and Kellam, S. (2006) A comparison of girls' and boys' aggressive-disruptive behavior trajectories across elementary school: prediction to young adult antisocial outcomes. *J. Consult. Clin. Psychol.* 74(3):500–510.

Schmahl, C., Bohus, M., Esposito, F., Treede, R.D., Di Salle, F., Greffrath, W., Ludaescher, P., Jochims, A., Lieb, K., Scheffler, K., Hennig, J., and Seifritz, E. (2006) Neural correlates of antinociception in borderline personality disorder. *Arch. Gen. Psychiatry* 63(6):659–667.

Schmahl, C.G., Elzinga, B.M., Vermetten, E., Sanislow, C., McGlashan, T.H., and Bremner, J.D. (2003) Neural correlates of memories of abandonment in women with and without borderline personality disorder. *Biol. Psychiatry* 54(2):142–151.

Schmahl, C.G., Vermetten, E., Elzinga, B.M., and Bremner, J.D. (2004) A positron emission tomography study of memories of childhood abuse in borderline personality disorder. *Biol. Psychiatry* 55(7):759–765.

Schneider, F., Habel, U., Kessler, C., Posse, S., Grodd, W., and Muller-Gartner, H.W. (2000) Functional imaging of conditioned aversive emotional responses in antisocial personality disorder. *Neuropsychobiology* 42(4):192–201.

Schnell, K., Dietrich, T., Schnitker, R., Daumann, J., and Herpertz, S.C. (2007) Processing of autobiographical memory retrieval cues in borderline personality disorder. *J. Affect. Disord.* 97(1/3): 253–259.

Schnell, K., and Herpertz, S.C. (2007) Effects of dialectic-behavioral-therapy on the neural correlates of affective hyperarousal in borderline personality disorder. *J. Psychiatr. Res.* 41(10):837–847.

Seguin, J.R. (2004) Neurocognitive elements of antisocial behavior: Relevance of an orbitofrontal cortex account. *Brain Cogn.* 55(1): 185–197.

Sen, S., Villafuerte, S., Nesse, R., Stoltenberg, S.F., Hopcian, J., Gleiberman, L., Weder, A., and Burmeister, M. (2004) Serotonin transporter and GABAA alpha 6 receptor variants are associated with neuroticism. *Biol. Psychiatry* 55(3):244–249.

Shea, M., Stout, D.B., Gunderson, J., Morey, L., Grilo, C., McGlashan, T., Skodol, A.E., Dolan-Sewell, R., Dyck, I., and Zanarini, M. (2002) Short-term diagnostic stability of schizotypal, borderline avoidant and obsessive compulsive personality disorders. *Am. J. Psychiatry* 159(12):2036–2041.

Shihabuddin, L., Buchsbaum, M.S., Hazlett, E.A., Silverman, J., New, A., Brickman, A.M., Mitropoulou, V., Nunn, M., Fleishman, M.B., Tang, C., and Siever, L.J. (2001) Striatal size and glucose metabolic rate in schizotypal personality disorder and schizophrenia. *Arch. Gen. Psychiatry* 58:877–884.

Siever, L.J., Amin, F., Coccaro, E.F., Bernstein, D., Kavoussi, R.J., Kalus, O., Horvath, T.B., Warne, P., Davidson, M., and Davis, K. (1991) Plasma homovanillic acid in schizotypal personality disorder patients and controls. *Am. J. Psychiatry* 148:1246–1248.

Siever, L.J., Amin, F., Coccaro, E.F., Trestman, R.L., Silverman, J., Horvath, T.B., Mahon, T.R., Knott, P., Davidson, M., and Davis, K.L. (1993) Cerebrospinal fluid homovanillic acid in schizotypal personality disorder. *Am. J. Psychiatry* 150:149–151.

Siever, L.J., Buchsbaum, M.S., New, A.S., Spiegel-Cohen, J., Wei, T., Hazlett, E.A., Sevin, E., Nunn, M., and Mitropoulou, V. (1999) d,l-fenfluramine response in impulsive personality disorder assessed with [18F]fluorodeoxyglucose positron emission tomography. *Neuropsychopharmacology* 20(5):413–423.

Siever, L.J., and Davis, K.L. (1991) A psychobiologic perspective on the personality disorders. *Am. J. Psychiatry* 148:1647–1658.

Siever, L.J., and Trestman, R.L. (1993) The serotonin system and aggressive personality disorder. *Int. Clin. Psychopharmacology* 8(Suppl 2):33–39.

Silberg, J., Meyer, J., Pickles, A., Simonoff, E., Eaves, L., Hewitt, J., Maes, H., and Rutter, M. (1996) Heterogeneity among juvenile antisocial behaviours: findings from the Virginia Twin Study of Adolescent Behavioural Development. *Ciba Found. Symp.* 194: 76–86; discussion 86–92.

Silverman, J.M., Pinkham, L., Horvath, T.B., Coccaro, E.F., Klar, H., Schear, S., Apter, S., Davidson, M., Mohs, R.C., and Siever, L.J. (1991) Affective and impulsive personality disorder traits in the relatives of patients with borderline personality disorder. *Am. J. Psychiatry* 148(10):1378–1385.

Singh, S.D. (1976) Sociometric analysis of the effects of the bilateral lesion of frontal cortex on the social behavior of rhesus monkeys. *Indian J. Psychol.* 51(2):144–160.

Sjoberg, R.L., Nilsson, K.W., Wargelius, H.L., Leppert, J., Lindstrom, L., and Oreland, L. (2007) Adolescent girls and criminal activity: role of MAOA-LPR genotype and psychosocial factors. *Am. J. Med. Genet. B Neuropsychiatr. Genet.* 144(2):159–164.

Skodol, A.E., Grilo, C.M., Pagano, M.E., Bender, D.S., Gunderson, J.G., Shea, M.T., Yen, S., Zanarini, M.C., and McGlashan, T.H. (2005) Effects of personality disorders on functioning and well-being in major depressive disorder. *J. Psychiatr. Pract.* 11(6): 363–368.

Skodol, A.E., Gunderson, J.G., Shea, M.T., McGlashan, T.H., Morey, L.C., Sanislow, C.A., Bender, D.S., Grilo, C.M., Zanarini, M.C., Yen, S., Pagano, M.E., and Stout, R.L. (2005) The Collaborative Longitudinal Personality Disorders Study (CLPS): overview and implications. *J. Personal Disord.* 19(5):487–504.

Skodol, A.E., Stout, R.L., McGlashan, T.H., Grilo, C.M., Gunderson, J.G., Shea, M.T., Morey, L.C., Zanarini, M.C., Dyck, I.R., and Oldham, J.M. (1999) Co-occurrence of mood and personality disorders: a report from the Collaborative Longitudinal Personality Disorders Study (CLPS). *Depress. Anxiety* 10(4):175–182.

Slutske, W.S. (2001) The genetics of antisocial behavior. *Curr. Psychiatry Rep.* 3(2):158–162.

Soloff, P.H., Lynch, K.G., and Kelly, T.M. (2002) Childhood abuse as a risk factor for suicidal behavior in borderline personality disorder. *J. Personal Disord.* 16(3):201–214.

Soloff, P.H., Meltzer, C.C., Greer, P.J., Constantine, D., and Kelly, T.M. (2000) A fenfluramine-activated FDG-PET study of borderline personality disorder. *Biol. Psychiatry* 47: 540–547.

Sprengelmeyer, R., Rausch, M., Eysel, U.T., and Przuntek, H. (1998) Neural structures associated with recognition of facial expressions of basic emotions. *Proc. Biol. Sci.* 265(1409):1927–1931.

Stanley, B., Molcho, A., Stanley, M., Winchel, R., Gameroff, M.J., Parsons, B., and Mann, J.J. (2000) Association of aggressive behavior with altered serotonergic function in patients who are not suicidal. *Am. J. Psychiatry* 157(4):609–614.

Stefanis, N.C., Van Os, J., Avramopoulos, D., Smyrnis, N., Evdokimidis, I., Hantoumi, I., and Stefanis, C.N. (2004) Variation in catechol-o-methyltransferase val158 met genotype associated with schizotypy but not cognition: a population study in 543 young men. *Biol. Psychiatry* 56(7):510–515.

Sullivan, P.F., Joyce, P.R., and Mulder, R.T. (1994) Borderline personality disorder in major depression. *J. Nerv. Ment. Dis.* 182(9):508–516.

Tebartz van Elst, L., Hesslinger, B., Thiel, T., Geiger, E., Haegele, K., Lemieux, L., Lieb, K., Bohus, M., Hennig, J., and Ebert, D.

(2003) Frontolimbic brain abnormalities in patients with borderline personality disorder: a volumetric magnetic resonance imaging study. *Biol. Psychiatry* 54(2):163–171.

Tienari, P., Wynne, L.C., Laksy, K., Moring, J., Nieminen, P., Sorri, A., Lahti, I., and Wahlberg, K.E. (2003) Genetic boundaries of the schizophrenia spectrum: evidence from the Finnish Adoptive Family Study of Schizophrenia. *Am. J. Psychiatry* 160(9):1587–1594.

Torgersen, S. (2000) Genetics of patients with borderline personality disorder. *Psychiatr. Clin. North Am.* 23(1):1–9.

Torgersen, S., Kringlen, E., and Cramer, V. (2001) The prevalence of personality disorders in a community sample. *Arch. Gen. Psychiatry* 58(6):590–596.

Traskman-Bendz, L., Asberg, M., and Schalling, D. (1986) Serotonergic function and suicidal behavior in personality disorders. *Ann. N. Y. Acad. Sci.* 487:168–174.

Trestman, R.L., Keefe, R.S.E., Harvey, P.D., deVegvar, M.L., Losonczy, M.F., Lees-Roitman, S., Davidson, M., Aronson, A., Silverman, J., and Siever, L.J. (1995) Cognitive function and biological correlates of cognitive performance in schizotypal personality disorder. *Psychiatry Res.* 59:127–136.

Trotman, H., McMillan, A., and Walker, E. (2006) Cognitive function and symptoms in adolescents with schizotypal personality disorder. *Schizophr. Bull.* 32(3):489–497.

Tuvblad, C., Grann, M., and Lichtenstein, P. (2006) Heritability for adolescent antisocial behavior differs with socioeconomic status: gene-environment interaction. *J. Child Psychol. Psychiatry* 47(7):734–743.

Virkkunen, M., Rawlings, R., Tokola, R., Poland, R.E., Guidotti, A., Nemeroff, C., Bisette, G., Kalogera, K., Karonen, S.L., and Linnoila, M. (1994) CSF biochemistries, glucose metabolism, and diurnal activity rhythms in alcoholic violent offenders, fire setters, and healthy volunteers. *Arch. Gen. Psychiatry* 51(1):20–27.

Wagner, A.W., and Linehan, M.M. (1999) Facial expression recognition ability among women with borderline personality disorder: implications for emotion regulation? *J. Personal Disord.* 13(4): 329–344.

Warren, J.I., and South, S.C. (2006) Comparing the constructs of antisocial personality disorder and psychopathy in a sample of incarcerated women. *Behav. Sci. Law* 24(1):1–20.

Weiser, M., Noy, S., Kaplan, Z., Reichenberg, A., Yazvitsky, R., Nahon, D., Grotto, I., and Knobler, H.Y. (2003) Generalized cognitive impairment in male adolescents with schizotypal personality disorder. *Am. J. Med. Genet. B Neuropsychiatr. Genet.* 116(1):36–40.

Widom, C.S., and Brzustowicz, L.M. (2006) MAOA and the "cycle of violence:" childhood abuse and neglect, MAOA genotype, and risk for violent and antisocial behavior. *Biol. Psychiatry* 60(7):684–689.

Williams, H.J., Owen, M.J., and O'Donovan, C. (2007) Is COMT a susceptibility gene for schizophrenia? *Schizophr. Bull.* 33(3): 635–641.

Wynne, L.C., Tienari, P., Nieminen, P., Sorri, A., Lahti, I., Moring, J., Naarala, M., Laksy, K., Wahlberg, K.E., and Miettunen, J. (2006) I. Genotype-environment interaction in the schizophrenia spectrum: genetic liability and global family ratings in the Finnish Adoption Study. *Fam. Process* 45(4):419–434.

Young, S.E., Stallings, M.C., Corley, R.P., Krauter, K.S., and Hewitt, J.K. (2000) Genetic and environmental influences on behavioral disinhibition. *Am. J. Med. Genet.* 96(5):684–695.

Zaboli, G., Gizatullin, R., Nilsonne, A., Wilczek, A., Jonsson, E.G., Ahnemark, E., Asberg, M., and Leopardi, R. (2006) Tryptophan hydroxylase-1 gene variants associate with a group of suicidal borderline women. *Neuropsychopharmacology* 31(9):1982–1990.

Zanarini, M., and Frankenburg, F. (1997) Pathways to the development of borderline personality disorder. *J. Personal. Disord.* 11(1):93–104.

Zanarini, M.C., Frankenburg, F.R., and Vujanovic, A.A. (2002) Inter-rater and test-retest reliability of the Revised Diagnostic Interview for Borderlines. *J. Personal. Disord.* 16(3):270–276.

Zanarini, M.C., Frankenburg, F.R., Yong, L., Raviola, G., Bradford Reich, D., Hennen, J., Hudson, J.I., and Gunderson, J.G. (2004) Borderline psychopathology in the first-degree relatives of borderline and axis II comparison probands. *J. Personal. Disord.* 18(5):439–447.

Zanarini, M.C., Gunderson, J.G., Marino, M.F., Schwartz, E.O., and Frankenburg, F.R. (1989) Childhood experiences of borderline patients. *Compr. Psychiatry* 30(1):18–25.

Zanarini, M.C., Skodol, A.E., Bender, D., Dolan, R., Sanislow, C., Schaefer, E., Morey, L.C., Grilo, C.M., Shea, M.T., McGlashan, T.H., and Gunderson, J.G. (2000) The Collaborative Longitudinal Personality Disorders Study: reliability of axis I and II diagnoses. *J. Personal. Disord.* 14(4):291–299.

Zetzsche, T., Frodl, T., Preuss, U.W., Schmitt, G., Seifert, D., Leinsinger, G., Born, C., Reiser, M., Moller, H.J., and Meisenzahl, E.M. (2006) Amygdala volume and depressive symptoms in patients with borderline personality disorder. *Biol. Psychiatry* 60(3):302–310.

Zimmerman, M., Rothschild, L., and Chelminski, I. (2005) The prevalence of DSM-IV personality disorders in psychiatric outpatients. *Am. J. Psychiatry* 162(10):1911–1918.

81 The Neurobiology of Aggression

R. J. R. BLAIR

Aggression is a serious social concern as well as a considerable economic burden on society. Each year more than 1.5 million people die through violence (Krug et al., 2002), and in the United States alone, more than 3 million violent crimes are committed (Reiss et al., 1994). Patients with a variety of psychiatric disorders including, but not limited to, personality disorders are at increased risk for developing aggression. It is thus important to understand the neurobiology of aggression, particularly maladaptive aggression (Connor et al., 2006).

A TAXONOMY OF HUMAN AGGRESSION: REACTIVE AND PROACTIVE AGGRESSION

Multiple subdivisions of the domain of aggression and antisocial behavior can be made (Hinshaw and Lee, 2003). However, many of these subdivisions have no clear neurobiological basis. One exception to this is the division between reactive (a.k.a. affective, impulsive, or defensive, or RAID; cf. Steiner et al., 2003) and proactive (a.k.a. instrumental or premeditated, or PIP; cf. Steiner et al., 2003) aggression (Linnoila et al., 1983; Berkowitz, 1993; Crick and Dodge, 1996; Barratt et al., 1999).

Numerous investigators have made this distinction between reactive and proactive aggression (Linnoila et al., 1983; Berkowitz, 1993; Crick and Dodge, 1996; Barratt et al., 1999). It has been tied to differential developmental pathways (Vitaro et al., 1998; Connor, 2002). Moreover, considerable data strongly support the existence of two relatively separable populations of individuals who are aggressive: individuals who present with mostly reactive aggression and individuals who present with high levels of mostly proactive and some reactive aggression (Linnoila et al., 1983; Crick and Dodge, 1996; Barratt et al., 1999; Connor, 2002). In addition, the discriminant validity of proactive and reactive aggression has been demonstrated; although reactive and instrumental aggression are substantially correlated, a two-factor model fits the data better than a one-factor model (Poulin and Boivin, 2000).

Reactive Aggression

Reactive aggression is triggered by a frustrating or threatening event and involves unplanned, enraged attacks on the object perceived to be the source of the threat/frustration. The aggression is often accompanied by anger and can be considered "hot." It is initiated without regard for any potential goal.

Reactive aggression appears to be exhibited by all mammalian species (Blanchard et al., 1977; Panksepp, 1998). It is part of the mammalian gradated response to threat. Low levels of danger from distant threats induce freezing. Higher levels of danger from closer threats induce attempts to escape the immediate environment. Higher levels of danger still, when the threat is very close and escape is impossible, initiate reactive aggression (Blanchard et al., 1977).

Animal work indicates that this progressive response to threat is mediated by a basic threat system that runs from medial amygdaloidal areas downward, largely via the stria terminalis to the medial hypothalamus, and from there to the dorsal half of the periaqueductal gray (PAG) (Panksepp, 1998; Gregg and Siegel, 2001). This system is organized in a hierarchical manner such that aggression evoked by stimulation of the amygdala is dependent on the functional integrity of the medial hypothalamus and PAG, but aggression evoked by stimulation of the PAG is not dependent on the functional integrity of the amygdala (Panksepp, 1998; Gregg and Siegel, 2001). This neural system, amygdala-hypothalamus-PAG, is thought to mediate reactive aggression in humans also (Panksepp, 1998; Gregg and Siegel, 2001; R.J.R. Blair, 2004b). This system is regulated by orbital, medial, and ventrolateral frontal cortex (R.J.R. Blair, 2004b). In line with this, recent work reports a gradated response within medial frontal cortex that increases proportionally with the individual's retaliative reactive aggression (Lotze et al., 2007).

There are many social environmental circumstances that increase the risk for reactive aggression. These include physical and sexual abuse (Dodge et al., 1995; Farrington and Loeber, 2000) as well as exposure to a threatening environment (Miller et al., 1999; Schwab-Stone et al., 1999). An increased risk for reactive aggression is found in a variety of psychiatric and neurological conditions. These include post-traumatic stress disorder (PTSD; Silva et al., 2001), childhood bipolar disorder (BD) (Leibenluft et al., 2003), borderline personality disorder (BPD) (Skodol et al., 2002), intermittent explosive disorder (Coccaro, 1998), psychopathy

(Cornell et al., 1996), and "acquired sociopathy" following damage to orbital frontal cortex (Grafman et al., 1996; Damasio, 1998).

Instrumental Aggression

Instrumental aggression is purposeful and goal directed (for example, to obtain the victim's possessions). The aggression need not be accompanied by an emotional state and can be considered "cold" (Steiner et al., 2003). In direct contrast with reactive aggression, it is initiated to achieve a goal.

There have been suggestions that animal work on the neurobiology of predatory aggression might be informative regarding human instrumental aggression (Gregg and Siegel, 2001). Predatory aggression occurs during food seeking in certain omnivorous and carnivorous species. It is mediated by a circuit including dorsolateral hypothalamic sites and the ventral half of the PAG (Gregg and Siegel, 2001). However, there are several reasons to discount an association between human instrumental aggression and predatory aggression (R.J.R. Blair, 2004a). First, predatory aggression in animals is not displayed towards conspecifics (Flynn, 1976). Stimulation of the circuitry mediating predatory aggression in animals will initiate attacks on live prey and the biting of dead prey. It will not, however, initiate attacks on conspecifics (Gregg and Siegel, 2001). In contrast, instrumental aggression in humans is almost always displayed towards conspecifics. Second, instrumental aggression in humans is highly influenced by the individual's learning environment; for example, environmental factors play a large role in determining the choice of weapons from fists to pistols. Such response flexibility is not seen in animal predatory aggression.

As goal-directed motor behavior, instrumental aggression is likely to recruit the same cortical neural systems as any other goal-directed motor program. In brief, these neural systems include temporal cortex, to represent the object, and striatal and premotor cortical neurons, to implement the action behavior (Passingham and Toni, 2001). The amygdala and ventromedial frontal cortex are involved in the associative learning process that allows the selection of the appropriate behavior to achieve the goal (Killcross et al., 1997; Baxter et al., 2000; Passingham et al., 2000). Indeed, recent functional magnetic resonance imaging (fMRI) work examining instrument aggression and prosocial behavior in a virtual environment supports the role of these structures (J.A. King et al., 2006).

Social/individual parameters that increase the risk for instrumental aggression or instrumental antisocial behavior more generally include lowered socioeconomic status and IQ (Frick et al., 1994; Hare, 2003). The only psychiatric condition known to increase the risk for instrumental aggression is psychopathy (Cornell et al., 1996; Frick et al., 2005). This disorder is also associated with an increased risk for reactive aggression (Cornell et al., 1996; Frick et al., 2005).

A Critique of the Reactive–Instrumental Aggression Dichotomy

The distinction between reactive and instrumental aggression was critiqued by Bushman and Anderson (2001). They consider that the distinction faces two main problems (Bushman and Anderson, 2001). First, they argue that it is confounded with the automatic-controlled information processing dichotomy (Shiffrin and Schneider, 1977; Norman and Shallice, 1986). Automatic processing occurs when responses to stimuli are so overlearned that they occur automatically. Controlled processing is typically thought to involve the recruitment of "executive systems" that select the appropriate behavior for the situation. However, this criticism is misplaced. It is possible that some authors have confounded the two dichotomies; but, in principle, reactive and proactive aggression could be either "automatic" or "controlled." The neural systems mediating reactive aggression are under considerable "executive control" (see below): that is, reactive aggression should not be considered simply automatic. Similarly, theoretically at least, instrumental aggression could become a sufficiently overlearned response to an environmental stimulus: that is, instrumental aggression should not be considered necessarily controlled. In short, the reactive–instrumental aggression dichotomy is orthogonal to the automatic-controlled dichotomy.

Their second criticism of the reactive–instrumental aggression dichotomy is that it excludes aggressive acts based on multiple motives. Bushman and Anderson (2001) discussed an example of an insulted individual who either reacts immediately in anger or waits and executes a later revenge. They argue that "the same motive appears operative in both cases" (p. 276) even though the first would be considered reactive and the second instrumental aggression. However, it is important to note that in a reactive episode, the motive is not guiding the behavioral choice: the insult triggers reactive aggression that is not suppressed by regulatory systems. In contrast, in the instrumental case, the motive is one of the factors influencing behavioral selection: the form of the revenge. In short, the criticisms of Bushman and Anderson are valid against some of the vaguer conceptualizations of the distinction. However, they are less applicable to positions based within a neuroscience perspective.

Normative and Maladaptive Aggression

It is important to note that the display of reactive or instrumental aggression does not necessarily imply pathology. Reactive aggression is an appropriate response of the basic threat circuitry to a highly threatening stimulus. Whether or not to use instrumental aggression or antisocial behavior is a result of decision making: Do the benefits of achieving the goal outweigh the costs of harm to others? Stealing another individual's $50 when he or she is not looking and you are starving is clearly not a maladaptive response. Jails contain many individuals who have engaged in instrumental antisocial behavior that has no basis in pathology.

Although the display of reactive or instrumental aggression does not necessarily imply pathology, it may indicate pathology. For example, reactive aggression may imply pathology if it is expressed to stimuli that are not conventionally considered sufficiently threatening, or if it is disproportionate in extent, severity, and persistence and occurs out of a pretext (Connor, 2002). Instrumental aggression may imply pathology if it is used indiscriminately to achieve goals and/or the damage to the victim is clearly disproportionate to the potential gain (for example, clubbing people over the head from behind with an iron bar to take their wallet without threatening them beforehand).

For the remainder of this chapter, the neurobiological bases of maladaptive reactive and instrumental aggression are considered.

Maladaptive Reactive Aggression

Underlying causes: genes and environment

Genetic factors. Twin, adoption, and family studies suggest genetic influences on aggression (Rhee and Waldman, 2002), with heritability estimates for dimensional measures of aggression ranging from 44% to 72% in adults. However, most of these behavioral genetic studies have not attempted to distinguish between reactive and proactive aggression. This is unfortunate, as it is likely that there are independent genetic risk factors that increase the risk that individuals will show reactive aggression alone or reactive and instrumental aggression in conjunction.

Recent molecular genetic work has been very informative however (Meyer-Lindenberg et al., 2006). In particular, genetic variation in monoamine oxidase A (MAO-A, 309850) has been linked to reactive aggression. MAO-A is located on the X chromosome (Xp11.23) and provides the major enzymatic clearing step for serotonin and norepinephrine during brain development. Mouse knockouts for MAO-A have elevated brain levels of serotonin, norepinephrine, and dopamine and exhibited increased aggressive behavior (Cases et al., 1995).

In humans, work in Holland has revealed that homozygous males for a missense mutation in the MAO-A gene (who represent functional gene knockouts) also show increased risk for reactive aggression (Brunner et al., 1993). Moreover, the number of tandem repeats of polymorphism of the MAO-A gene affects transcriptional efficiency: enzyme expression is relatively high for carriers of 3.5 or 4 repeats (MAOA-H) and lower for carriers of 2, 3, or 5 repeats (MAOA-L) (Sabol et al., 1998). In recent work, Meyer-Lindenberg and colleagues (2006) reported that the MAOA-L genotype, relative to the MAOA-H genotype, is associated with (*1*) significant reductions in volume throughout the cingulate gyrus, the amygdala bilaterally, and within the insula and (*2*) increased activity in left amygdala and decreased response of subgenual (BA 25) and supragenual (BA 32) ventral cingulate cortex, left lateral orbital frontal cortex (OFC), and left insular cortex, when engaged in matching judgments for fearful and angry expressions relative to neutral objects (Meyer-Lindenberg et al., 2006). In addition, during the retrieval stage of an emotional memory paradigm, MAOA-L relative to MAOA-H male patients showed increased amygdala and hippocampal activity to negative versus neutral images (the opposite was seen in female patients; MAOA-L relative to MAOA-H female patients showed less amygdala activation) (Fan et al., 2003; Meyer-Lindenberg et al., 2006). Moreover, males who were MAOA-L, relative to MAOA-H, showed deficient activation of dorsomedial frontal cortex during performance of attentional tasks (Fan et al., 2003; Meyer-Lindenberg et al., 2006) and a related area, ventrolateral prefrontal cortex, during performance of a go/no-go task (Passamonti et al., 2006).

In short, data indicate that the association of MAO-A with reactive aggression relates to the role of this gene in determining serotonin/norepinephrine/dopamine levels that in turn are associated with increased responsiveness of the basic threat circuitry (cf. increased amygdala response to emotional expressions; Meyer-Lindenberg et al., 2006) and decreased responsiveness within frontal regulatory systems (Fan et al., 2003; Meyer-Lindenberg et al., 2006; Passamonti et al., 2006). Other genes are also associated with increased responsiveness of the basic threat circuitry and decreased responsiveness within frontal regulatory systems. For example, a relatively common polymorphism (5-HTTLPR) in the promoter region of the human 5-HTT gene (*SLC6A4*) results in two common alleles or variants: the so-called short (S) and long (L), constituting 14 and 16 copies of a 20- to 23-nucleotide repeat cassette, respectively (Heils et al., 1996). Several studies have reported that S allele carriers show greater amygdala responses than L allele homozygotes to emotional expressions (Hariri et al., 2002; Hariri et al., 2005). Moreover, S allele carriers show reduced functional connectivity with potential regulatory regions of frontal cortex such as rostral anterior cingulate cortex (Pezawas et al., 2005). In addition, some studies have reported that S allele carriers are at increased risk for aggression (Hallikainen et al., 1999; Liao et al., 2004; Haberstick et al., 2006), though not all studies have (Sakai et al., 2007), and the form of aggression (reactive only or reactive + instrumental) has not received careful attention. These data are thus suggestive that genetic influences increasing amygdala responsiveness and/or reducing the responsiveness of those regions involved in the regulation of emotional responding will increase the risk for reactive aggression.

Environmental factors. Animal work indicates that environmental threats may elevate the baseline neural responsiveness of the basic threat systems (S.M. King, 1999) and the neurochemical response to threat (Charney, 2003). Moreover, work with humans who have been exposed to extreme threats and developed PTSD supports this. Patients with PTSD show elevated amygdala responses to threatening stimuli (e.g., Rauch et al., 2006). Interestingly, with respect to reactive aggression, there are some suggestions that PTSD is also associated with reduced responsiveness of regions involved in the regulation of emotional responding (e.g., Rauch et al., 2006). There are a variety of social environmental circumstances that increase the risk for reactive aggression: for example, physical and sexual abuse (Dodge et al., 1995; Farrington and Loeber, 2000) and exposure to violence (Miller et al., 1999; Schwab-Stone et al., 1999). These can also lead to PTSD that, as a disorder, is associated with an increased risk for reactive aggression (Silva et al., 2001). Components of the basic threat system, particularly the amygdala, divert attention to environmental threat. If the basic threat system is stressed, the animal shows hypervigilance for threat (S.M. King, 1999). Similarly, reactively aggressive children show "hostile attribution biases" (Crick and Dodge, 1996; Steiner et al., 1997).

Gene–environment interactions. In short, there are genetic and environmental factors that increase the responsiveness of the basic threat circuitry and/or reduce the responsiveness of those regions involved in the regulation of emotional responding. These can interact such that the impact of the genetic predisposition becomes considerably more accentuated following exposure to environmental stressors. Thus, recent research has suggested that the genetic vulnerability to reactive aggression conferred by the low-activity allele of MAOA-L variant is particularly evident (or even only evident) in the presence of an environmental maltreatment (Caspi et al., 2002; though see Sakai et al., 2007).

Neurocognitive Impairments Associated with Maladaptive Reactive Aggression

As noted above, it is thought that reactive aggression is mediated by a basic threat system (amygdala-hypothalamus-PAG) that is cortically regulated by regions of inferior and medial frontal cortex. Whether reactive aggression occurs (as opposed to freezing or flight) is determined by the salience of the threat stimulus—the more salient, the greater the probability that the individual's response will be reactive aggression. The salience of the threat stimulus is determined by exogenous factors (for example, its proximity) as well as endogenous factors (responsiveness of the basic threat circuitry and functional integrity of the frontal regulatory systems). Maladaptive levels of reactive aggression, and the disorders associated with maladaptive levels of reactive aggression, are associated with either overresponsiveness in the basic threat circuitry or underresponsiveness in the regulatory systems or both.

Overresponsiveness of the Basic Threat Circuitry

Of the disorders principally associated with an increased risk for reactive aggression (PTSD, childhood BD, BPD, Intermittent Explosive Disorder [IED], psychopathy, and acquired sociopathy), there have been indications that four might be associated with overresponsiveness of the basic threat circuitry: PTSD, BPD, childhood BD, and IED. Considerable data suggests that PTSD is associated with an elevated amygdala response to a variety of threat-related cues including personalized traumatic narratives (Rauch et al., 1996; Shin et al., 2004), trauma-related cues (Liberzon et al., 1999; Protopopescu et al., 2005), and fearful facial expressions (Rauch et al., 2000; Armony et al., 2005; Shin et al., 2005; Williams et al., 2006; though see Lanius et al., 2001; Shin et al., 1999). Moreover, amygdala-centric models of PTSD are currently dominant (Liberzon and Martis, 2006; Rauch et al., 2006). Data also suggest that patients with BPD show elevated amygdala responses to threat-related cues, including facial expressions (Donegan et al., 2003), particularly fearful expressions (Minzenberg et al., 2007) and aversive images (Herpertz et al., 2001).

The situation is rather less clear with respect to childhood BD and IED. A detailed analysis of both disorders from a cognitive neuroscience perspective is only now beginning. However, recent work with childhood BD and IED has indicated that both might be exaggerated amygdala activity (Rich et al., 2006; Coccaro et al., 2007). However, it is worth noting that in both conditions the exaggerated activity was only seen in specific conditions and, more importantly, not those conditions typically most associated with increased amygdala activity in healthy populations. In considerable work, the amygdala has been shown to be particularly responsive to fearful relative to neutral expressions (e.g., Whalen et al., 2001). However, neither the patients with childhood BD or IED showed an exaggerated response to fearful expressions (Rich et al., 2006; Coccaro et al., 2007), unlike what is seen in patients with PTSD in comparable studies (Rauch et al., 2000; Armony et al., 2005; Shin et al., 2005; Williams et al., 2006). The children with BD showed an exaggerated amygdala response when making threat relevant judgments with respect to neutral expressions (Rich et al., 2006). The exaggerated amygdala response in patients with IED was seen to angry expressions (Coccaro et al., 2007). These preliminary data suggest if the increased risk for reactive aggression seen in childhood BD and IED relates to overresponsiveness of components of the basic threat circuitry it relates to specific stimuli triggers rather than the more general overresponsiveness that does seem to be apparent in PTSD and BPD.

Underresponsiveness in Frontal Systems Involved in the Regulation of Emotional and Reactive Aggressive Responses

All of the disorders associated with an increased risk for reactive aggression have also been associated with dysfunction in frontal systems involved in the regulation of affect. However, it is important to note that though early accounts of the regulation of aggression assumed a single inhibitory system (Davidson et al., 2000), it now appears plausible that there are at least four forms of system that allow the control of emotional responding and consequently reactive aggression:

1. There are regions of frontal cortex that appear to project excitatory connections to potentially inhibitory interneurons within the amygdala, leading to a reduction in amygdala activity (Likhtik et al., 2005). It is possible that such connections are recruited during emotional suppression paradigms where there appears to be direct frontal suppression of the amygdala (Beauregard et al., 2001; Levesque et al., 2003).
2. Considerable data using reappraisal paradigms attest to a role for attentional manipulation of emotional stimuli such that the emotional responses to these stimuli can be suppressed (Ochsner and Gross, 2005). If the individual attends to nonemotional features of a stimulus, the representation of these nonemotional features, following models of attention as representational competition (Desimone and Duncan, 1995), will interfere with the representation of the emotional features of the stimulus and thus reduce consequent emotional responding to these features (Pessoa and Ungerleider, 2004; Mitchell et al., 2006). This form of attentional emotional suppression also occurs when attention to task-relevant features of a stimulus interferes with the representation of the emotional features of the environment (Pessoa et al., 2005; K.S. Blair et al., 2007; Mitchell et al., 2007).
3. Ventromedial prefrontal cortex (vmPFC) appears importantly involved in the detection of reinforcement contingency changes; that is, the detection that an action performed to achieve a goal is no longer achieving that goal (R.J.R. Blair, 2004b). Detection of contingency changes allows reversal learning (that is, response reversal) to occur, and the individual changes his or her behavior so that his or her goal is now achieved. This behavioral change is implemented by dorsomedial and ventrolateral frontal cortex (O'Doherty et al., 2003; Budhani et al., 2007). A failure to achieve successful reversal learning will be associated with frustration; the individual will continue to do the old action that no longer achieves the behavior. Frustration has long been implicated with an increased risk for reactive aggression (Berkowitz, 1993).
4. Ventrolateral and other regions of prefrontal cortex also appear importantly involved in social response reversal: the modulation of behavioral responding according to the social cues of conspecifics (R.J.R. Blair and Cipolotti, 2000; Kringelbach and Rolls, 2003). The regulation of the behavior of others and the maintenance of the social hierarchy is an important part of primate social life. Ventrolateral prefrontal cortex appears to play an important role in regulating threats from conspecifics, in the form of angry expressions, and hierarchy information (R.J.R. Blair et al., 1999). A breakdown in this system is likely to be associated with inappropriate social behavior and reactive confrontations.

A functional analysis with respect to the above systems of the frontal dysfunction seen in the patient groups associated with an increased risk for reactive aggression is only in its infancy. However, it is safe to conclude that frontal lobe damage, if it affects ventromedial and ventrolateral frontal cortex, is associated with an increased risk for reactive aggression in humans (Pennington and Bennetto, 1993; Grafman et al., 1996; Anderson et al., 1999). Moreover, a host of neuroimaging studies have provided evidence of frontal dysfunction in individuals displaying heightened levels of reactive aggression (Volkow and Tancredi, 1987; Goyer et al., 1994; Raine et al., 1998). A study by Raine and colleagues (1998) is worthy of particular note here. In this study, the neural responses of individuals who were reactively as opposed to instrumentally aggressive were contrasted. It was only the individuals who were reactively aggressive who showed indications of reduced activity in right frontal cortex (Raine et al., 1998).

When considering individual conditions related to an increased risk for reactive aggression, a relatively good case can be made for systems involved in the direct suppression of amygdala activity being dysfunctional in PTSD and BPD (Rauch et al., 2006; New et al., 2007). Post-traumatic stress disorder has been associated with decreased responding within regions of middle prefrontal cortex following presentation of traumatic narratives (Lanius et al., 2001; Shin et al., 2004), trauma-related cues (Bremner et al., 1999), fearful facial expressions (Shin et al., 2005; Williams et al., 2006), and during the performance of emotional Stroop interference tasks (Shin et al., 2001; Bremner et al., 2004; though see Shin et al., 1997; Bryant et al., 2005). Patients with BPD have shown impaired rostral anterior cingulate cortex metabolic response to fenfluramine (Siever et al., 1999; Oquendo et al., 2005) and m-chlorophenylpiperazine (New et al., 2002) and more recently a reduced correlated response between amygdala and OFC relative to controls in response to m-chlorophenylpiperazine (New et al., 2007).

With respect to childhood BD, a case can be made that apparent dysfunction in ventrolateral prefrontal cortex might be related to their increased risk for reactive aggression, given the role of this region in reversal learning (and consequently avoiding frustration) and social response reversal. Certainly children with BD show impairment on response reversal paradigms (Gorrindo et al., 2005), generally impaired expression processing, and social cue processing (McClure et al., 2005). Moreover, recent fMRI work using a motor inhibition task paradigm demonstrated reduced ventrolateral prefrontal cortex activity in the children with BD (Leibenluft et al., 2007).

An interesting contrast condition to those above is psychopathy. In this disorder, there is a clear increased risk for reactive aggression (though, in contrast to the other conditions considered above, there is also a clear increased risk for instrumental aggression). However, there is no suggestion of overresponsiveness in the basic threat circuitry. Instead, the majority of studies indicate amygdala responding in individuals with psychopathy to emotional stimuli is reduced (see below; Kiehl et al., 2001; Gordon et al., 2004; Birbaumer et al., 2005).

Reactive aggression in psychopathy appears to be frustration based as opposed to threat based. Consistent with this, individuals with psychopathy show impairment in reversal learning (Budhani and Blair, 2005; Budhani et al., 2006). Continuing with old actions even though they no longer achieve the goal rather than implementing new actions (that is, achieving reversal learning) will increase the risk for frustration. Early work suggested that this might relate to ventrolateral prefrontal cortex dysfunction in psychopathy (Mitchell et al., 2002). However, more recent fMRI work has indicated that the impairment relates to vmPFC dysfunction: individuals with psychopathy fail to show the depression in response within vmPFC following the failure to receive the expected reward. Functionally, this probably relates to an impairment in detecting the contingency change (that is, that the action no longer achieves the goal).

Neuropharmacological factors

A considerable body of work suggests that neuropharmacological factors modulate the risk for aggression. Particularly important contributions appear to be made by:

1. Norepinephrine (NE). Has a considerable role in the innervation of the basic threat systems in animals (Pieribone et al., 1994) and humans (Ferry et al., 1999). Given this, it is unsurprising that increasing NE activity facilitates aggression in several animal species, including reactive aggression in humans (Coccaro, 1996). Moreover, reducing NE activity by agents such as propranolol reduces the incidence of reactive aggression in humans (Volavka et al., 2004).

2. γ-aminobutyric acid (GABA). Alcohol and benzodiazepines have been consistently shown to increase aggression in mammalian species (Fish et al., 2001). In humans, various clinical reports have detailed incidents of aggression following treatment with benzodiazepines varying from 10% in a mixed diagnostic group (Rosenbaum et al., 1984) to 58% in patients with BPD (Gardner and Cowdry, 1985). Controlled laboratory studies have also shown that administration of benzodiazepines is associated with increased behavioral aggression following provocation in patients who were anxious undergoing benzodiazepine treatment (Bond et al., 1995) and in healthy volunteers administered only one dose of a benzodiazepine (Bond and Silveira, 1993).

3. Vasopressin (AVP). Animal work suggests that AVP increases the responsiveness of the basic threat systems: it increases anxiety related behaviors and the neurochemical response to threat (Landgraf et al., 1995). In line with this, animal studies also suggest a positive relationship between central AVP activity and aggression (Ferris, 2005). Work with humans remains in its infancy.

4. Testosterone. Although androgen receptors are widely distributed in the rat brain, their greatest densities are within basic threat system: the amygdala, hypothalamus, and PAG (Hamson et al., 2004). Increased testosterone should facilitate reactive aggression, and work with several animal species confirms this suggestion (Book et al., 2001). The evidence in humans is not compelling. However, the problem here may be methodological. Reactive aggression is a response to environmental threat or frustration; reactive aggression must be provoked—it is not simply spontaneously evoked. Typically, studies using a provocation methodology report that testosterone administration increased aggression (Pope et al., 2000) whereas those not using provocation report testosterone administration did not find increased aggression (O'Connor et al., 2002). Interestingly, recent work has demonstrated that even a single dose of testosterone influences responses to social cues (Hermans et al., 2006), including increasing emotional responses to angry expressions, a provocation cue for reactive aggression (van Honk et al., 2001; Putman et al., 2007).

5. Serotonin. A link between serotonin and the modulation of aggression has long been made. Animal work has shown that serotonin innervates frontal regulatory systems and has a direct inhibitory influence on the PAG (Deakin and Graeff, 1991). In particular, the postsyn-

aptically located 5-HT1B heteroreceptor plays a highly selective role in the modulation of reactive aggression (Olivier, 2004). Consistent with this, considerable animal work, and a growing human literature, indicates an inverse relationship between serotonergic activity and reactive aggression (Coccaro and Kavoussi, 1997; Bjork et al., 2000; New et al., 2002). However, it should be noted that it appears likely that the role of serotonin in regulating aggression is far more complex than a simple inhibitory story allows (Olivier, 2004).

Maladaptive Instrumental Aggression

Instrumental aggression is a form of instrumental behavior—that is, a behavior undertaken to achieve a particular goal. In the case of instrumental aggression, violence is used by the individual in the expectation that this will allow the individual's goal to be met. When faced with a goal ("obtain $50"), the individual has a range of behavioral options (for example, "find a job," "mug someone"). Choosing between these choices will be a function of, first, availability (Can a job/potential victim be found?) and second, action costs (social punishment and the distress of the victims). In short, an individual might choose an antisocial behavior because (*1*) he or she is under social/situational pressure to do so. The antisocial acts are simply the most viable options available. In this case, the instrumental aggression/antisocial behavior, though perhaps socially undesirable, need not be maladaptive—from the individual's perspective, it may be the only way to achieve his or her goals or (*2*) their calculation of the costs related to the actions/empathic responding/use of this information is deficient. In short, instrumental aggression/antisocial behavior can be considered maladaptive if the decision making that leads to the choice of the action is dysfunctional.

Psychopathy appears to represent a disorder where the neural-cognitive systems necessary for socialization are compromised, and there is consequently considerable increased risk for the display of instrumental aggression. Psychopathy is not currently included in *Diagnostic and Statistical Manual of Mental Disorders* (*DSM-IV*; American Psychiatric Association, 1994) and should not be considered synonymous with conduct disorder (CD) or antisocial personality disorder (APD); less than 25% of those meeting diagnosis for CD or APD would meet cut-offs for psychopathy (Hare and Neumann, 2006). Psychopathy has behavioral components (for example, criminal activity and poor behavioral control) but also important affective-interpersonal components (notably a lack of empathy and guilt) (Frick et al., 1994; Harpur and Hare, 1994). It is a developmental disorder (Lynam et al., 2007). Moreover, the relationship between specific forms of positive parenting techniques and reduced antisocial behavior levels does not hold for children who present with the emotional dysfunction associated with psychopathy (Wootton et al., 1997; Oxford et al., 2003).

Underlying causes: Genes and environment

Genetic factors. Recent behavioral genetic work has suggested a genetic contribution to psychopathy (Blonigen et al., 2003; Blonigen et al., 2005; Viding et al., 2005). For example, in a recent large study with around 3,500 twin pairs, callous/unemotional traits were shown to be strongly heritable (67% heritability) at 7 and 9 years (Viding et al., 2005). However, as yet, there has been no molecular genetic work on psychopathy.

Environmental factors. There have been suggestions that psychopathy might be due to early physical/sexual abuse or neglect (Rutter, 2005). However, as noted above, the literature is relatively clear regarding the impact of such stressors on brain development. Animal work indicates that neglect and other stressors increase emotional and amygdala responsiveness to threatening stimuli (Bremner and Vermetten, 2001; Rilling et al., 2001). Similarly, in humans, early physical/sexual abuse is a significant risk factor for the emergence of PTSD that is associated with increased emotional and amygdala responsiveness (Rauch et al., 2006). Increased emotional and amygdala responsiveness is the opposite of the pathopathology observed in psychopathy (see below).

Neurocognitive Impairments Associated with Maladaptive Instrumental Aggression

A crucial process for socialization is the ability to form stimulus-reinforcement associations. To learn that hitting another individual is bad, a representation of this action must be associated with an aversive unconditioned stimulus. A considerable literature implicates the role of the amygdala in the formation and processing of stimulus-reinforcement associations (Baxter and Murray, 2002; Everitt et al., 2003). The aversive unconditioned stimulus that is particularly important for moral socialization is the distress of other individuals, the expressions of fear and sadness (R.J.R. Blair, 2003). The expressions of fear and sadness serve as social reinforcers; as such, they allow caregivers to teach the societal valence of objects and actions to the developing individual (R.J.R. Blair, 2003); actions/objects associated with the sadness/fear of others, in healthy developing children, are to be avoided. A considerable body of work attests to the power of facial expressions to transmit valence information in humans and other primates (Klinnert et al., 1987; Mineka and Cook, 1993; R.J.R. Blair, 2003). The amygdala is crucially involved in the response to fearful and sad expressions (Adolphs, 2002; R.J.R. Blair, 2003).

Moreover, recent fMRI work has shown that the response of the amygdala to fearful expressions is modulated by whether there is an object with which to make the association of the distress of the expression (Hooker et al., 2006). If an object is present, the response of the amygdala to fearful expressions is significantly greater than if it is not present.

Moral socialization by parents and peers helps the developing child appropriately represent the costs of antisocial behavior. An important temperamental variable determining the ease with which a child can be socialized is fearfulness (Kochanska, 1997). This variable can be considered to index the functional integrity of the amygdala. The punishment that best achieves moral socialization is the victim's distress; empathy induction, focusing the transgressor's attention on the victim, particularly fosters moral socialization (Hoffman, 1994; Eisenberg, 2002).

The core deficits seen in psychopathy all relate to the functional role of the amygdala in stimulus-reinforcement learning and in responding to fearful and sad expressions. The impairment of individuals with psychopathy in stimulus-reinforcement association is evidenced by their impairment in aversive conditioning, the augmentation of the startle reflex following the presentation of visual threat primes and passive avoidance learning (Newman and Kosson, 1986; Levenston et al., 2000; Flor et al., 2002). Moreover, recent fMRI work has demonstrated that individuals with psychopathy show reduced amygdala responding during aversive conditioning relative to comparison individuals (Birbaumer et al., 2005). Several studies across groups have now demonstrated impairment in the recognition of fearful and, to a lesser extent, sad expressions in individuals with psychopathy (R.J.R. Blair et al., 2001; Dadds et al., 2006; Dolan and Fullam, 2006; though see Kosson et al., 2002). Moreover, a recent meta-analysis of studies examining expression recognition in instrumentally aggressive populations has more generally demonstrated that these populations are associated with impairment in the recognition of fearful and sad expressions (Marsh and Blair, 2008). In addition, fMRI work has indicated that individuals with psychopathic traits show reduced responding to fearful expressions (Gordon et al., 2004). Other work has shown that individuals with psychopathy show reduced amygdala responding to emotional words in the context of emotional memory paradigms (Kiehl et al., 2001) and less amygdala differentiation in responding when making cooperation relative to defection choices in a prisoner's dilemma paradigm (Rilling et al., 2006).

The amygdala appears to feeds forward reinforcement information associated with stimuli to medial OFC that then represents this outcome information. The function of this representation of reinforcement information within OFC is to allow the normalization of competing outcomes so that the value of differing rewards such as apples and oranges can be compared (Montague and Berns, 2002; Padoa-Schioppa and Assad, 2006; cf. Schoenbaum and Roesch, 2005). This reinforcement expectancy information can then be used in decisions as to whether to approach the object or action or not. Given the suggestion made above that the amygdala's role in stimulus-reinforcement learning is disrupted in psychopathy, it might be expected that individuals with psychopathy will show anomalous medial OFC activity in the context of tasks that activate the amygdala. This is exactly what is seen. In Kiehl's study of emotional memory, the individuals with psychopathy not only showed reduced amygdala responses to the emotional words but also reduced rostral anterior cingulate cortex/medial OFC activation (Kiehl et al., 2001). There was also reduced medial OFC activity in the individuals with psychopathy during aversive conditioning (Birbaumer et al., 2005) as well as less medial OFC differentiation in responding when making cooperation relative to defection choices in the prisoner's dilemma paradigm (Rilling et al., 2006). Moreover, work has demonstrated reduced connectivity between the amygdala and vmPFC in children with psychopathic traits when responding to emotional expressions.

Medial OFC and, to a lesser extent, the amygdala have been consistently identified in neuroimaging studies of harm-based moral reasoning (Greene et al., 2001; Moll et al., 2002; Luo et al., 2006). For example, Greene and colleagues (2001) reported increased medial OFC activity to personal as opposed to impersonal moral choices; the difference between these two situations effectively relates to the salience of the victim. Similarly, Luo et al. (2006) demonstrated increased amygdala and medial OFC activity to more severe relative to less severe moral transgressions. The suggestion has been made that this activity in harm-based moral reasoning paradigms reflects the roles of the amygdala and ventromedial frontal cortex outlined above. The amygdala allows the association of representations of transgressions that harm others (for example, interpersonal violence, property damage/theft) with the emotional response to the victim's fear/sadness (see R.J.R. Blair, 1995; R.J.R. Blair et al., 2005). The individual's "automatic moral attitude" to a moral transgression involves the activation of the amygdala by the conditioned stimulus that is the individual's representation of the moral transgression. The amygdala then provides expected reinforcement (positively and negatively valenced) information that is represented as a valenced outcome within medial OFC. This information is crucial for determining the individual's "attitude" towards the action—his or her tendency to approach or avoid it. Given the nature of the impairment in psychopathy, individuals with psychopathy should and do show notable impairment in the care-based moral reasoning (R.J.R. Blair, 1995; Gray et al., 2003).

SUMMARY

Considerable progress is being made in understanding the neurobiological bases of human adaptive and maladaptive aggression. Importantly, it is clear that reactive and instrumental aggression must be distinguished. Table 81.1 summarizes the main differences between these forms of aggression.

Reactive and instrumental aggression differ not only in their behavioral form but also in the neural architectures that mediate them. Reactive aggression involves a motor response driven by the amygdala, hypothalamus, and PAG and modulated by regions of frontal cortex. Reactive aggression can become maladaptive if either the basic emotional response becomes overly responsive or because the frontal regulatory systems become underresponsive. Disorders associated with an increased risk for reactive aggression include PTSD, BPD, childhood BD, IED, and psychopathy.

Instrumental aggression is mediated by the same neural circuits that mediate other forms of instrumental action. Whether instrumental aggression as opposed to any other form of instrumental action is used by the person to achieve his or her goals is dependent on their prior learning and current decision making. Maladaptive instrumental aggression occurs if the systems necessary for moral socialization or decision making are disrupted. Neural regions particularly implicated include the amygdala and vmPFC. The disorder principally associated with an increased risk for instrumental aggression is psychopathy.

TABLE 81.1 *A Comparison of Reactive and Instrumental Aggression*

	Reactive Aggression	*Instrumental Aggression*
Behavioral form	The aggression involves unplanned, enraged attacks on the object perceived to be the source of the threat/frustration.	The aggression is purposeful, goal directed, and can be described as cold blooded.
Neuroarchitecture involved	Reactive aggression is mediated by a circuit that runs from medial amygdaloid areas to the medial hypothalamus, and then to the dorsal half of the PAG. This circuit is modulation by orbital and medial frontal cortex.	Instrumental aggression is likely to be mediated by the same neural systems that mediate other forms of goal-directed behavior (i.e., temporal and premotor cortex). In healthy individuals, the amygdala and ventromedial frontal cortex are involved in the associative learning process that allows the selection of appropriate behaviors to achieve goals. If these structures, particularly the amygdala, are dysfunctional, then the individual is less likely to learn to avoid antisocial behavior through socialization.
Neurotransmitters involved	Noradrenaline, GABA, vasopression, testosterone, and serotonin have all been implicated in the modulation of reactive aggression.	Largely unknown. However, there may be noradrenergic influences on the associative learning processes mediated by the amygdala that allow appropriate socialization.
Risk factors	An individual may be at higher risk of reactive aggression if either: 1. The neural circuitry mediating reactive aggression has been previously activated through aversive stimulation (e.g., as a consequence of trauma). 2. The modulatory role of frontal cortical regions has been compromised due to neurological insult or neurochemical perturbations.	An individual is at higher risk for instrumental aggression if either: 1. The systems crucial for socialization, in particular the amygdala, are dysfunctional. 2. The individual received inappropriate socialization experiences (e.g., if instrumental aggression is reinforced).
Psychiatric conditions associated with this form of aggression	PTSD, childhood bipolar disorder, borderline personality disorder, IED, psychopathy, and "acquired sociopathy" following damage to orbital frontal cortex.	Psychopathy. Also those individuals with conduct disorder and antisocial personality disorder whose pathology relates to the emotional dysfunction seen in psychopathy.

PAG: periaqueductal gray; GABA: γ-aminobutyric acid; PTSD: post-traumatic stress disorder; IED: intermittent explosive disorder.

REFERENCES

Adolphs, R. (2002) Neural systems for recognizing emotion. *Curr. Opin. Neurobiol.* 12:169–177.

American Psychiatric Association (1994) *Diagnostic and Statistical Manual of Mental Disorders* (4th ed.). Washington, DC: Author.

Anderson, S.W., Bechara, A., Damasio, H., Tranel, D., and Damasio, A.R. (1999) Impairment of social and moral behaviour related to early damage in human prefrontal cortex. *Nat. Neurosci.* 2: 1032–1037.

Armony, J.L., Corbo, V., Clement, M.H., and Brunet, A. (2005) Amygdala response in patients with acute PTSD to masked and unmasked emotional facial expressions. *Am. J. Psychiatry* 162: 1961–1963.

Barratt, E.S., Stanford, M.S., Dowdy, L., Liebman, M.J., and Kent, T.A. (1999) Impulsive and premeditated aggression: a factor analysis of self-reported acts. *Psychiatry Res.* 86:163–173.

Baxter, M.G., and Murray, E.A. (2002) The amygdala and reward. *Nat. Rev. Neurosci.* 3:563–573.

Baxter, M.G., Parker, A., Lindner, C.C., Izquierdo, A.D., and Murray, E.A. (2000) Control of response selection by reinforcer value requires interaction of amygdala and orbital prefrontal cortex. *J. Neurosci.* 20:4311–4319.

Beauregard, M., Levesque, J., and Bourgouin, P. (2001) Neural correlates of conscious self-regulation of emotion. *J. Neurosci.* 21: RC165.

Berkowitz, L. (1993) *Aggression: Its Causes, Consequences, and Control.* Philadelphia: Temple University Press.

Birbaumer, N., Veit, R., Lotze, M., Erb, M., Hermann, C., Grodd, W., et al. (2005) Deficient fear conditioning in psychopathy: a functional magnetic resonance imaging study. *Arch. Gen. Psychiatry* 62:799–805.

Bjork, J.M., Dougherty, D.M., Moeller, F.G., and Swann, A.C. (2000) Differential behavioral effects of plasma tryptophan depletion and loading in aggressive and nonaggressive men. *Neuropsychopharmacology* 22:357–369.

Blair, K.S., Smith, B.W., Mitchell, D.G., Morton, J., Vythilingam, M., Pessoa, L., et al. (2007) Modulation of emotion by cognition and cognition by emotion. *NeuroImage* 35:430–440.

Blair, R.J.R. (1995) A cognitive developmental approach to morality: Investigating the psychopath. *Cognition* 57:1–29.

Blair, R.J.R. (2003) Facial expressions, their communicatory functions and neuro-cognitive substrates. *Philos. Trans. R. Soc. Lond. B Biol. Sci.* 358:561–572.

Blair, R.J.R. (2004a) The neurobiology of aggression. In: Charney, D.S., and Nestler, E.J., ed. *Neurobiology of Mental Illness.* New York: Oxford University Press, pp. 1076–1085.

Blair, R.J.R. (2004b) The roles of orbital frontal cortex in the modulation of antisocial behavior. *Brain Cogn.* 55:198–208.

Blair, R.J.R., and Cipolotti, L. (2000) Impaired social response reversal: A case of "acquired sociopathy." *Brain* 123:1122–1141.

Blair, R.J.R., Colledge, E., Murray, L., and Mitchell, D.G. (2001) A selective impairment in the processing of sad and fearful expressions in children with psychopathic tendencies. *J. Abnorm. Child.*

Blair, R.J.R., Mitchell, D.G.V., and Blair, K.S. (2005) *The Psychopath: Emotion and the Brain.* Oxford, UK: Blackwell.

Blair, R.J.R., Morris, J.S., Frith, C.D., Perrett, D.I., and Dolan, R. (1999) Dissociable neural responses to facial expressions of sadness and anger. *Brain* 122:883–893.

Blanchard, R.J., Blanchard, D.C., and Takahashi, L.K. (1977) Attack and defensive behaviour in the albino rat. *Anim. Behav.* 25:197–224.

Blonigen, D.M., Carlson, S.R., Krueger, R.F., and Patrick, C.J. (2003) A twin study of self-reported psychopathic personality traits. *Personal. Individ. Diff.* 35:179–197.

Blonigen, D.M., Hicks, B.M., Krueger, R.F., Patrick, C.J., and Iacono, W.G. (2005) Psychopathic personality traits: heritability and genetic overlap with internalizing and externalizing psychopathology. *Psychol. Med.* 35:637–648.

Bond, A.J., Curran, H.V., Bruce, M., O'Sullivan, G., and Shine, P. (1995) Behavioural aggression in panic disorder after 8 weeks of treatment with alprazolam. *J. Affect. Disord.* 35:117–123.

Bond, A.J., and Silveira, J.C. (1993) The combination of alprazolam and alcohol on behavioral aggression. *J. Stud. Alcohol Suppl.* 11:30–39.

Book, A.S., Starzyk, K.B., and Quinsey, V.L. (2001) The relationship between testosterone and aggression: a meta-analysis. *Aggress. Viol. Behav.* 6:579–599.

Bremner, J.D., Staib, L.H., Kaloupek, D., Southwick, S.M., Soufer, R., and Charney, D.S. (1999) Neural correlates of exposure to traumatic pictures and sound in Vietnam combat veterans with and without posttraumatic stress disorder: a positron emission tomography study. *Biol. Psychiatry* 45:806–816.

Bremner, J.D., and Vermetten, E. (2001) Stress and development: Behavioral and biological consequences. *Dev. Psychopathol.* 13: 473–489.

Bremner, J.D., Vermetten, E., Vythilingam, M., Afzal, N., Schmahl, C., Elzinga, B., et al. (2004) Neural correlates of the classic color and emotional Stroop in women with abuse-related posttraumatic stress disorder. *Biol. Psychiatry* 55:612–620.

Brunner, H.G., Nelen, M., Breakefield, X.O., Ropers, H.H., van Oost, B.A. (1993) Abnormal behavior associated with a point mutation in the structural gene for monoamine oxidase A. *Science* 262:578–580.

Bryant, R.A., Felmingham, K.L., Kemp, A.H., Barton, M., Peduto, A.S., Rennie, C., et al. (2005) Neural networks of information processing in posttraumatic stress disorder: a functional magnetic resonance imaging study. *Biol. Psychiatry* 58:111–118.

Budhani, S., and Blair, R.J. (2005) Response reversal and children with psychopathic tendencies: success is a function of salience of contingency change. *J. Child Psychol. Psychiatry* 46:972–981.

Budhani, S., Marsh, A.A., Pine, D.S., and Blair, R.J. (2007) Neural correlates of response reversal: Considering acquisition. *NeuroImage* 34:1754–1765.

Budhani, S., Richell, R.A., and Blair, R.J. (2006) Impaired reversal but intact acquisition: probabilistic response reversal deficits in adult individuals with psychopathy. *J. Abnorm. Psychol.* 115: 552–558.

Bushman, B.J., and Anderson, C.A. (2001) Is it time to pull the plug on the hostile versus instrumental aggression dichotomy? *Psychol. Rev.* 108:273–279.

Cases, O., Seif, I., Grimsby, J., Gaspar, P., Chen, K., Pournin, S., et al. (1995) Aggressive behavior and altered amounts of brain serotonin and norepinephrine in mice lacking MAOA. *Science* 268:1763–1766.

Caspi, A., McClay, J., Moffitt, T.E., Mill, J., Martin, J., Craig, I.W., et al. (2002) Role of genotype in the cycle of violence in maltreated children. *Science* 297:851–854.

Charney, D.S. (2003) Neuroanatomical circuits modulating fear and anxiety behaviors. *Acta Psychiatr. Scand. Suppl.* 417:38–50.

Coccaro, E.F. (1996) Neurotransmitter correlates of impulsive aggression in humans. *Ann. N. Y. Acad. Sci.* 794:82–89.

Coccaro, E.F. (1998) Impulsive aggression: a behavior in search of clinical definition. *Harv. Rev. Psychiatry* 5:336–339.

Coccaro, E.F., and Kavoussi, R.J. (1997) Fluoxetine and impulsive aggressive behavior in personality-disordered subjects. *Arch. Gen. Psychiatry* 54:1081–1088.

Coccaro, E.F., McCloskey, M.S., Fitzgerald, D.A., and Phan, K.L. (2007) Amygdala and orbitofrontal reactivity to social threat in individuals with impulsive aggression. *Biol. Psychiatry* 62:168–178.

Connor, D.F. (2002) *Aggression and Anti-Social Behaviour in Children and Adolescents. Research and Treatment.* New York: Guilford Press.

Connor, D.F., Carlson, G.A., Chang, K.D., Daniolos, P.T., Ferziger, R., Findling, R.L., et al. (2006) Juvenile maladaptive aggression: a review of prevention, treatment, and service configuration and a proposed research agenda. *J. Clin. Psychiatry* 67:808–820.

Cornell, D.G., Warren, J., Hawk, G., Stafford, E., Oram, G., and Pine, D. (1996) Psychopathy in instrumental and reactive violent offenders. *J. Consult, Clin. Psychol.* 64:783–790.

Crick, N.R., and Dodge, K.A. (1996) Social information-processing mechanisms on reactive and proactive aggression. *Child Dev.* 67:993–1002.

Dadds, M.R., Perry, Y., Hawes, D.J., Merz, S., Riddell, A.C., Haines, D.J., et al. (2006) Attention to the eyes and fear-recognition deficits in child psychopathy. *Br. J. Psychiatry* 189:280–281.

Damasio, A. (1998) The somatic marker hypothesis and the possible functions of the prefrontal cortex. In: Roberts, A.C., Robbins, T. W., and Weiskrantz, L., eds. *The Prefrontal Cortex*. New York: Oxford University Press, pp. 36–50.

Davidson, R.J., Putnam, K.M., and Larson, C.L. (2000) Dysfunction in the neural circuitry of emotion regulation—a possible prelude to violence. *Science* 289:591–594.

Deakin, J.F.W., and Graeff, F.G. (1991) 5HT and mechanisms of defense. *Psychopharmacology* 5:305–315.

Desimone, R., and Duncan, J. (1995) Neural mechanisms of selective visual attention. *Annu. Rev. Neurosci.* 18:193–222.

Dodge, K.A., Pettit, G.S., Bates, J.E., and Valente, E. (1995) Social information-processing patterns partially mediate the effect of early physical abuse on later conduct problems. *J. Abnorm. Psychol.* 104:632–643.

Dolan, M., and Fullam, R. (2006) Face affect recognition deficits in personality-disordered offenders: association with psychopathy. *Psychol. Med.* 36:1563–1569.

Donegan, N.H., Sanislow, C.A., Blumberg, H.P., Fulbright, R.K., Lacadie, C., Skudlarski, P., et al. (2003) Amygdala hyperreactivity in borderline personality disorder: implications for emotional dysregulation. *Biol. Psychiatry* 54:1284–1293.

Eisenberg, N. (2002) Empathy-related emotional responses, altruism, and their socialization. In: Davidson, R.J., and Harrington, A., eds. *Visions of Compassion: Western Scientists and Tibetan Buddhists Examine Human Nature*. New York: Oxford University Press, pp. 131–164.

Everitt, B.J., Cardinal, R.N., Parkinson, J.A., Robbins, T.W. (2003) Appetitive behavior: impact of amygdala-dependent mechanisms of emotional learning. *Ann. N. Y. Acad. Sci.* 985:233–250.

Fan, J., Fossella, J., Sommer, T., Wu, Y., and Posner, M.I. (2003) Mapping the genetic variation of executive attention onto brain activity. *Proc. Natl. Acad. Sci. USA* 100:7406–7411.

Farrington, D.P., and Loeber, R. (2000) Epidemiology of juvenile violence. *Child Adolesc. Psychiatr. Clin N. Am.* 9:733–748.

Ferris, C.F. (2005) Vasopressin/oxytocin and aggression. *Novartis Found. Symp.* 268:190–198; discussion 198–200, 242–253.

Ferry, B., Roozendaal, B., and McGaugh, J.L. (1999) Involvement of alpha1-adrenoceptors in the basolateral amygdala in modulation of memory storage. *Eur. J. Pharmacol.* 372:9–16.

Fish, E.W., Faccidomo, S., DeBold, J.F., and Miczek, K.A. (2001) Alcohol, allopregnanolone and aggression in mice. *Psychopharmacol. (Berl)* 153:473–483.

Flor, H., Birbaumer, N., Hermann, C., Ziegler, S., and Patrick, C.J. (2002) Aversive Pavlovian conditioning in psychopaths: Peripheral and central correlates. *Psychophysiol.* 39:505–518.

Flynn, J.P. (1976) Neural basis of threat and attack. In: Grenell, R.G., and Abau, S.G., eds. *Biological Foundations of Psychiatry*. New York: Raven Press, pp. 275–295.

Frick, P.J., O'Brien, B.S., Wootton, J.M., and McBurnett, K. (1994) Psychopathy and conduct problems in children. *J. Abnorm. Psychol.* 103:700–707.

Frick, P.J., Stickle, T.R., Dandreaux, D.M., Farell, J.M., and Kimonis, E.R. (2005) Callous-unemotional traits in predicting the severity and stability of conduct problems and delinquency. *J. Abnorm. Child Psychol.* 33:471–487.

Gardner, D.L., and Cowdry, R.W. (1985) Alprazolam-induced dyscontrol in borderline personality disorder. *Am. J. Psychiatry* 146: 98–100.

Gordon, H.L., Baird, A.A., and End, A. (2004) Functional differences among those high and low on a trait measure of psychopathy. *Biol. Psychiatry* 56:516–521.

Gorrindo, T., Blair, R.J., Budhani, S., Dickstein, D.P., Pine, D.S., and Leibenluft, E. (2005) Deficits on a probabilistic response-reversal task in patients with pediatric bipolar disorder. *Am. J. Psychiatry* 162:1975–1977.

Goyer, P.F., Andreason, P.J., Semple, W.E., Clayton, A.H., King, A.C., Compton-Toth, B.A., et al. (1994) Positron-emission tomography and personality disorders. *Neuropsychopharmacol.* 10:21–28.

Grafman, J., Schwab, K., Warden, D., Pridgen, B.S., and Brown, H.R. (1996) Frontal lobe injuries, violence, and aggression: A report of the Vietnam head injury study. *Neurology* 46:1231–1238.

Gray, N.S., MacCulloch, M.J., Smith, J., Morris, M., and Snowden, R.J. (2003) Forensic psychology: Violence viewed by psychopathic murderers. *Nature* 423:497–498.

Greene, J.D., Sommerville, R.B., Nystrom, L.E., Darley, J.M., and Cohen, J.D. (2001) An fMRI investigation of emotional engagement in moral judgment. *Science* 293:1971–1972.

Gregg, T.R., and Siegel, A. (2001) Brain structures and neurotransmitters regulating aggression in cats: implications for human aggression. *Prog. Neuropsychopharmacol. Biol. Psychiatry* 25:91–140.

Haberstick, B.C., Smolen, A., and Hewitt, J.K. (2006) Family-based association test of the 5HTTLPR and aggressive behavior in a general population sample of children. *Biol. Psychiatry* 59:836–843.

Hallikainen, T., Saito, T., Lachman, H.M., Volavka, J., Pohjalainen, T., Ryynanen, O.P., et al. (1999) Association between low activity serotonin transporter promoter genotype and early onset alcoholism with habitual impulsive violent behavior. *Mol. Psychiatry* 4:385–388.

Hamson, D.K., Jones, B.A., and Watson, N.V. (2004) Distribution of androgen receptor immunoreactivity in the brainstem of male rats. *Neuroscience* 127:797–803.

Hare, R.D., and Neumann, C.S. (2006) The PCL-R assessment of psychopathy: Development, structural properties, and new directions. In: Patrick, C.J., ed. *Handbook of Psychopathy*. New York: Guilford Press, pp. 58–90.

Hare, R.D. (2003) *Hare Psychopathy Checklist-Revised* (PCL-R; 2nd ed.). Toronto, Canada: Multi Health Systems.

Hariri, A.R., Drabant, E.M., Munoz, K.E., Kolachana, B.S., Mattay, V.S., Egan, M.F., et al. (2005) A susceptibility gene for affective disorders and the response of the human amygdala. *Arch. Gen. Psychiatry* 62:146–152.

Hariri, A.R., Mattay, V.S., Tessitore, A., Kolachana, B., Fera, F., Goldman, D., et al. (2002) Serotonin transporter genetic variation and the response of the human amygdala. *Science* 297:400–403.

Harpur, T.J., and Hare, R.D. (1994) Assessment of psychopathy as a function of age. *J. Abnorm. Psychol.* 103:604–609.

Heils, A., Teufel, A., Petri, S., Stober, G., Riederer, P., Bengel, D., et al. (1996) Allelic variation of human serotonin transporter gene expression. *J. Neurochem.* 66:2621–2624.

Hermans, E.J., Putman, P., and van Honk, J. (2006) Testosterone administration reduces empathetic behavior: a facial mimicry study. *Psychoneuroendocrinol.* 31:859–866.

Herpertz, S.C., Dietrich, T.M., Wenning, B., Krings, T., Erberich, S.G., Willmes, K., Thron, A., and Sass, H. (2001) Evidence of abnormal amygdala functioning in borderline personality disorder: a functional MRI study. *Biol. Psychiatry* 50:292–298.

Hinshaw, S.P., and Lee, S.S. (2003) Oppositional defiant and conduct disorder. In: Mash, E.J., and Barkley, R.J., eds. *Child Psychopathology*. New York: Guilford Press, pp. 144–198.

Hoffman, M.L. (1994) Discipline and internalisation. *Dev. Psychology* 30:26–28.

Hooker, C.I., Germine, L.T., Knight, R.T., and D'Esposito, M. (2006) Amygdala response to facial expressions reflects emotional learning. *J. Neurosci.* 26:8915–8922.

Kiehl, K.A., Smith, A.M., Hare, R.D., Mendrek, A., Forster, B.B., Brink, J., et al. (2001) Limbic abnormalities in affective processing by criminal psychopaths as revealed by functional magnetic resonance imaging. *Biol. Psychiatry* 50:677–684.

Killcross, S., Robbins, T.W., and Everitt, B.J. (1997) Different types of fear-conditioned behaviour mediated by separate nuclei within amygdala. *Nature* 388:377–380.

King, J.A., Blair, R.J., Mitchell, D.G., Dolan, R.J., and Burgess, N. (2006) Doing the right thing: A common neural circuit for appropriate violent or compassionate behavior. *NeuroImage* 30: 1069–1076.

King, S.M. (1999) Escape-related behaviours in an unstable, elevated and exposed environment. II. Long-term sensitization after repetitive electrical stimulation of the rodent midbrain defence system. *Behav. Brain Res.* 98:127–142.

Klinnert, M.D., Emde, R.N., Butterfield, P., and Campos, J.J. (1987) Social referencing: The infant's use of emotional signals from a friendly adult with mother present. *Annu. Prog. Child Psychiat. Child Dev.* 22:427–432.

Kochanska, G. (1997) Multiple pathways to conscience for children with different temperaments: From toddlerhood to age 5. *Dev. Psychology* 33:228–240.

Kosson, D.S., Suchy, Y., Mayer, A.R., and Libby, J. (2002) Facial affect recognition in criminal psychopaths. *Emotion* 2:398–411.

Kringelbach, M.L., and Rolls, E.T. (2003) Neural correlates of rapid reversal learning in a simple model of human social interaction. *NeuroImage* 20:1371–1383.

Krug, E.G., Dahlberg, L.L., Mercy, J.A., Zwi, A., and Lozano, R. (2002) *World Report on Violence and Health*. Geneva: World Health Organization.

Landgraf, R., Gerstberger, R., Montkowski, A., Probst, J.C., Wotjak, C.T., Holsboer, F., et al. (1995) V1 vasopressin receptor antisense oligodeoxynucleotide into septum reduces vasopressin binding, social discrimination abilities, and anxiety-related behavior in rats. *J. Neurosci.* 15:4250–4258.

Lanius, R.A., Williamson, P.C., Densmore, M., Boksman, K., Gupta, M.A., Neufeld, R.W., et al. (2001) Neural correlates of traumatic memories in posttraumatic stress disorder: a functional MRI investigation. *Am. J. Psychiatry* 158:1920–1922.

Leibenluft, E., Blair, R.J., Charney, D.S., and Pine, D.S. (2003) Irritability in pediatric mania and other childhood psychopathology. *Annu. N. Y. Acad. Sci.* 1008:201–218.

Leibenluft, E., Rich, B.A., Vinton, D.T., Nelson, E.E., Fromm, S.J., Berghorst, L.H., et al. (2007) Neural circuitry engaged during unsuccessful motor inhibition in pediatric bipolar disorder. *Am. J. Psychiatry* 164:52–60.

Levenston, G.K., Patrick, C.J., Bradley, M.M., and Lang, P.J. (2000) The psychopath as observer: Emotion and attention in picture processing. *J. Abnorm. Psychol.* 109:373–386.

Levesque, J., Eugene, F., Joanette, Y., Paquette, V., Mensour, B., Beaudoin, G., et al. (2003) Neural circuitry underlying voluntary suppression of sadness. *Biol. Psychiatry* 53:502–510.

Liao, D.L., Hong, C.J., Shih, H.L., and Tsai, S.J. (2004) Possible association between serotonin transporter promoter region polymorphism and extremely violent crime in Chinese males. *Neuropsychobiol.* 50:284–287.

Liberzon, I., and Martis, B. (2006) Neuroimaging studies of emotional responses in PTSD. *Ann. N. Y. Acad. Sci.* 1071:87–109.

Liberzon, I., Taylor, S.F., Amdur, R., Jung, T.D., Chamberlain, K.R., Minoshima, S., et al. (1999) Brain activation in PTSD in response to trauma-related stimuli. *Biol. Psychiatry* 45:817–826.

Likhtik, E., Pelletier, J.G., Paz, R., and Pare, D. (2005) Prefrontal control of the amygdala. *J. Neurosci.* 25:7429–7437.

Linnoila, M., Virkkunen, M., Scheinin, M., Nuutila, A., Rimon, R., and Goodwin, F.K. (1983) Low cerebrospinal fluid 5-hydroxy indoleacetic acid concentration differentiates impulsive from nonimpulsive violent behavior. *Life Sci.* 33:2609–2614.

Lotze, M., Veit, R., Anders, S., and Birbaumer, N. (2007) Evidence for a different role of the ventral and dorsal medial prefrontal cortex for social reactive aggression: An interactive fMRI study. *NeuroImage* 34:470–478.

Luo, Q., Nakic, M., Wheatley, T., Richell, R., Martin, A., and Blair, R.J. (2006) The neural basis of implicit moral attitude—an IAT study using event-related fMRI. *NeuroImage* 30:1449–1457.

Lynam, D.R., Caspi, A., Moffitt, T.E., Loeber, R., and Stouthamer-Loeber, M. (2007) Longitudinal evidence that psychopathy scores in early adolescence predict adult psychopathy. *J. Abnorm. Psychol.* 116:155–165.

Marsh, A.A., and Blair, R.J.R. (2008) Antisocial behavior is associated with specific deficits in recognition of the fear facial expression: a meta-analysis. *Neurosci. Biobehav. Rev.* 32:454–465.

McClure, E.B., Treland, J.E., Snow, J., Schmajuk, M., Dickstein, D.P., Towbin, K.E., et al. (2005) Deficits in social cognition and response flexibility in pediatric bipolar disorder. *Am. J. Psychiatry* 162:1644–1651.

Meyer-Lindenberg, A., Buckholtz, J.W., Kolachana, B., Hariri, R., Pezawas, L., Blasi, G., et al. (2006) Neural mechanisms of genetic risk for impulsivity and violence in humans. *Proc. Natl. Acad. Sci. USA* 103:6269–6274.

Miller, L.S., Wasserman, G.A., Neugebauer, R., Gorman-Smith, D., and Kamboukos, D. (1999) Witnessed community violence and antisocial behavior in high-risk, urban boys. *J. Clin. Child Psychol.* 28:2–11.

Mineka, S., and Cook, M. (1993) Mechanisms involved in the observational conditioning of fear. J. *Exper. Psychol.: Gen.* 122: 23–38.

Minzenberg, M.J., Fan, J., New, A.S., Tang, C.Y., and Siever, L.J. (2007) Fronto-limbic dysfunction in response to facial emotion in borderline personality disorder: An event-related fMRI study. *Psychiatry Res.* 155:231–243.

Mitchell, D.G., Nakic, M., Fridberg, D., Kamel, N., Pine, D.S., and Blair, R.J. (2007) The impact of processing load on emotion. *NeuroImage* 34:1299–1309.

Mitchell, D.G., Richell, R.A., Leonard, A., and Blair, R.J. (2006) Emotion at the expense of cognition: psychopathic individuals outperform controls on an operant response task. *J. Abnorm. Psychol.* 115:559–566.

Mitchell, D.G.V., Colledge, E., Leonard, A., and Blair, R.J.R. (2002) Risky decisions and response reversal: Is there evidence of orbitofrontal cortex dysfunction in psychopathic individuals? *Neuropsychologia* 40:2013–2022.

Moll, J., De Oliveira-Souza, R., Bramati, I.E., and Grafman, J. (2002) Functional networks in emotional moral and nonmoral social judgments. *NeuroImage* 16:696–703.

Montague, P.R., and Berns, G.S. (2002) Neural economics and the biological substrates of valuation. *Neuron* 36:265–284.

New, A.S., Hazlett, E.A., Buchsbaum, M.S., Goodman, M., Mitelman, S.A., Newmark, R., et al. (2007) Amygdala-prefrontal disconnection in borderline personality disorder. *Neuropsychopharmacol.* 32:1629–1640.

New, A.S., Hazlett, E.A., Buchsbaum, M.S., Goodman, M., Reynolds, D., Mitropoulou, V., et al. (2002) Blunted prefrontal cortical 18fluorodeoxyglucose positron emission tomography response to meta-chlorophenylpiperazine in impulsive aggression. *Arch. Gen. Psychiatry* 59:621–629.

Newman, J.P., and Kosson, D.S. (1986) Passive avoidance learning in psychopathic and nonpsychopathic offenders. *J. Abnorm. Psychol.* 95:252–256.

Norman, D., and Shallice, T. (1986) Attention to action: Willed and automatic control of behaviour. In: Davidson, R.J., Schwartz, G.E., and Shapiro, D., eds. *Consciousness and Self-Regulation.* New York: Plenum Press, pp. 1–18.

Ochsner, K.N., and Gross, J.J. (2005) The cognitive control of emotion. *Trends Cogn. Sci.* 9:242–249.

O'Connor, D.B., Archer, J., Hair, W.M., and Wu, F.C.W. (2002) Exogenous testosterone, aggression and mood in eugonodal and hypogonadal men. *Physiol. Behav.* 75:557–566.

O'Doherty, J., Critchley, H., Deichmann, R., and Dolan, R.J. (2003) Dissociating valence of outcome from behavioral control in human orbital and ventral prefrontal cortices. *J. Neurosci.* 23: 7931–7939.

Olivier, B. (2004) Serotonin and aggression. *Ann. N. Y. Acad. Sci.* 1036:382–392.

Oquendo, M.A., Krunic, A., Parsey, R.V., Milak, M., Malone, K.M., Anderson, A., et al. (2005) Positron emission tomography of regional brain metabolic responses to a serotonergic challenge in major depressive disorder with and without borderline personality disorder. *Neuropsychopharmacol.* 30:1163–1172.

Oxford, M., Cavell, T.A., and Hughes, J.N. (2003) Callous-unemotional traits moderate the relation between ineffective parenting and child externalizing problems: A partial replication and extension. *J. Clin. Child Adoles. Psychol.* 32:577–585.

Padoa-Schioppa, C., and Assad, J.A. (2006) Neurons in the orbitofrontal cortex encode economic value. *Nature* 441:223–226.

Panksepp, J. (1998) *Affective Neuroscience: The Foundations of Human and Animal Emotions.* New York: Oxford University Press.

Passamonti, L., Fera, F., Magariello, A., Cerasa, A., Gioia, M.C., Muglia, M., et al. (2006) Monoamine oxidase-a genetic variations influence brain activity associated with inhibitory control: new insight into the neural correlates of impulsivity. *Biol. Psychiatry* 59:334–340.

Passingham, R.E., Toni, I., and Rushworth, M.F. (2000) Specialisation within the prefrontal cortex: the ventral prefrontal cortex and associative learning. *Exp. Brain Res.* 133:103–113.

Passingham, R.E., and Toni, I. (2001) Contrasting the dorsal and ventral visual systems: guidance of movement versus decision making. *NeuroImage* 14:S125–S131.

Pennington, B.F., and Bennetto, L. (1993) Main effects or transaction in the neuropsychology of conduct disorder? Commentary on "The neuropsychology of conduct disorder." *Dev. Psychopathol.* 5:153–164.

Pessoa, L., Padmala, S., and Morland, T. (2005) Fate of unattended fearful faces in the amygdala is determined by both attentional resources and cognitive modulation. *NeuroImage* 28:249–255.

Pessoa, L., and Ungerleider, L.G. (2004) Neuroimaging studies of attention and the processing of emotion-laden stimuli. *Prog. Brain Res.* 144:171–182.

Pezawas, L., Meyer-Lindenberg, A., Drabant, E.M., Verchinski, B.A., Munoz, K.E., Kolachana, B.S., et al. (2005) 5-HTTLPR polymorphism impacts human cingulate-amygdala interactions: a genetic susceptibility mechanism for depression. *Nat. Neurosci.* 8:828–834.

Pieribone, V.A., Nicholas, A.P., Dagerlind, A., and Hokfelt, T. (1994) Distribution of alpha 1 adrenoceptors in rat brain revealed by in situ hybridization experiments utilizing subtype-specific probes. *J. Neurosci.* 14:4252–4268.

Pope, H.G., Kouri, E.M., and Hudson, J.I. (2000) Effects of supraphysiologic doses of testosterone on mood and aggression in normal men: a randomized controlled trial. *Arch. Gen. Psychiatry* 57:133–140.

Poulin, F., and Boivin, M. (2000) Reactive and proactive aggression: evidence of a two-factor model. *Psychol. Assess.* 12:115–122.

Protopopescu, X., Pan, H., Tuescher, O., Cloitre, M., Goldstein, M., Engelien, W., et al. (2005) Differential time courses and specificity of amygdala activity in posttraumatic stress disorder subjects and normal control subjects. *Biol. Psychiatry* 57:464–473.

Putman, P., Hermans, E.J., and van Honk, J. (2007) Exogenous cortisol shifts a motivated bias from fear to anger in spatial working memory for facial expressions. *Psychoneuroendocrinol.* 32:14–21.

Raine, A., Meloy, J.R., Birhle, S., Stoddard, J., LaCasse, L., and Buchsbaum, M.S. (1998) Reduced prefrontal and increased subcortical brain functioning assessed using positron emission tomography in predatory and affective murderers. *Behav. Sci. Law* 16:319–332.

Rauch, S.L., Shin, L.M., and Phelps, E.A. (2006) Neurocircuitry models of posttraumatic stress disorder and extinction: human neuroimaging research—past, present, and future. *Biol. Psychiatry* 60:376–382.

Rauch, S.L., van der Kolk, B.A., Fisler, R.E., Alpert, N.M., Orr, S.P., Savage, C.R., et al. (1996) A symptom provocation study of posttraumatic stress disorder using positron emission tomography and script-driven imagery. *Arch. Gen. Psychiatry* 53:380–387.

Rauch, S.L., Whalen, P.J., Shin, L.M., McInerney, S.C., Macklin, M.L., Lasko, N.B., et al. (2000) Exaggerated amygdala response to masked facial stimuli in posttraumatic stress disorder: a functional MRI study. *Biol. Psychiatry* 47:769–776.

Reiss, A.J., Miczek, K.A., and Roth, J.A. (1994) *Understanding and Preventing Violence. Vol. 2. Biobehavioral Influences.* Washington, DC: National Academy Press.

Rhee, S.H., and Waldman, I.D. (2002) Genetic and environmental influences on antisocial behavior: a meta-analysis of twin and adoption studies. *Psychol. Bull.* 128:490–529.

Rich, B.A., Vinton, D.T., Roberson-Nay, R., Hommer, R.E., Berghorst, L.H., McClure, E.B., et al. (2006) Limbic hyperactivation during processing of neutral facial expressions in children with bipolar disorder. *Proc. Natl. Acad. Sci. USA* 103:8900–8905.

Rilling, J.K., Glenn, A.L., Jairam, M.R., Pagnoni, G., Goldsmith, D.R., Elfenbein, H.A., et al. (2006) Neural correlates of social cooperation and non-cooperation as a function of psychopathy. *Biol. Psychiatry* 61:1260–1271.

Rilling, J.K., Winslow, J.T., O'Brien, D., Gutman, D.A., Hoffman, J.M., and Kilts, C.D. (2001) Neural correlates of maternal separation in rhesus monkeys. *Biol. Psychiatry* 49:146–157.

Rosenbaum, J.F., Woods, S.W., Groves, J.E., and Klerman, G.L. (1984) Emergence of hostility during alprazolam treatment. *Am. J. Psychiatry* 141:793.

Rutter, M. (2005) Commentary: What is the meaning and utility of the psychopathy concept? *J. Abnorm. Child Psychol.* 33:499–503.

Sabol, S.Z., Hu, S., and Hamer, D. (1998) A functional polymorphism in the monoamine oxidase A gene promoter. *Hum. Genet.* 103:273–279.

Sakai, J.T., Lessem, J.M., Haberstick, B.C., Hopfer, C.J., Smolen, A., Ehringer, M.A., et al. (2007) Case-control and within-family tests for association between 5HTTLPR and conduct problems in a longitudinal adolescent sample. *Psychiatr. Genet.* 17:207–214.

Schoenbaum, G., and Roesch, M. (2005) Orbitofrontal cortex, associative learning, and expectancies. *Neuron* 47:633–636.

Schwab-Stone, M., Chen, C., Greenberger, E., Silver, D., Lichtman, J., and Voyce, C. (1999) No safe haven II: The effects of violence exposure on urban youth. *J. Am. Acad. Child Adoles. Psychiatry* 38:359–367.

Shiffrin, R.M., and Schneider, W. (1977) Controlled and automatic human information processing: II. Perceptual learning, automatic attending, and a general theory. *Psycholog. Rev.* 84:127–190.

Shin, L.M., Kosslyn, S.M., McNally, R.J., Alpert, N.M., Thompson, W.L., Rauch, S.L., et al. (1997) Visual imagery and perception in posttraumatic stress disorder. A positron emission tomographic investigation. *Arch. Gen. Psychiatry* 54:233–241.

Shin, L.M., McNally, R.J., Kosslyn, S.M., Thompson, W.L., Rauch, S.L., Alpert, N.M., et al. (1999) Regional cerebral blood flow during script-driven imagery in childhood sexual abuse-related PTSD: A PET investigation. *Am. J. Psychiatry* 156:575–584.

Shin, L.M., Orr, S.P., Carson, M.A., Rauch, S.L., Macklin, M.L., Lasko, N.B., et al. (2004) Regional cerebral blood flow in the amygdala and medial prefrontal cortex during traumatic imagery in male and female Vietnam veterans with PTSD. *Arch. Gen. Psychiatry* 61:168–176.

Shin, L.M., Whalen, P.J., Pitman, R.K., Bush, G., Macklin, M.L., Lasko, N.B., et al. (2001) An fMRI study of anterior cingulate function in posttraumatic stress disorder. *Biol. Psychiatry* 50: 932–942.

Shin, L.M., Wright, C.I., Cannistraro, P.A., Wedig, M.M., McMullin, K., Martis, B., et al. (2005) A functional magnetic resonance imaging study of amygdala and medial prefrontal cortex responses to overtly presented fearful faces in posttraumatic stress disorder. *Arch. Gen. Psychiatry* 62:273–281.

Siever, L.J., Buchsbaum, M.S., New, A.S., Spiegel-Cohen, J., Wei, T., Hazlett, E.A., et al. (1999) d,l-fenfluramine response in impulsive personality disorder assessed with [18F]fluorodeoxyglucose positron emission tomography. *Neuropsychopharmacol.* 20:413–423.

Silva, J.A., Derecho, D.V., Leong, G.B., Weinstock, R., and Ferrari, M.M. (2001) A classification of psychological factors leading to violent behavior in posttraumatic stress disorder. *J. Forensic Sci.* 46:309–316.

Skodol, A.E., Gunderson, J.G., Pfohl, B., Widiger, T.A., Livesley, W.J., and Siever, L.J. (2002) The borderline diagnosis I: psychopathology, comorbidity, and personality structure. *Biol. Psychiatry* 51:936–950.

Steiner, H., Garcia, I.G., and Matthews, Z. (1997) Posttraumatic stress disorder in incarcerated juvenile delinquents. *J. Am. Acad. Child Adolesc. Psychiatry* 36:357–365.

Steiner, H., Saxena, K., and Chang, K. (2003) Psychopharmacologic strategies for the treatment of aggression in juveniles. *CNS Spectrum* 8:298–308.

van Honk, J., Tuiten, A., Hermans, E., Putman, P., Koppeschaar, H., Thijssen, J., et al. (2001) A single administration of testosterone induces cardiac accelerative responses to angry faces in healthy young women. *Behav. Neurosci.* 115:238–242.

Viding, E., Blair, R.J.R., Moffitt, T.E., and Plomin, R. (2005) Evidence for substantial genetic risk for psychopathy in 7-year-olds. *J. Child Psychol. Psychiatry* 46:592–597.

Vitaro, F., Gendreau, P.L., Tremblay, R.E., and Oligny, P. (1998) Reactive and proactive aggression differentially predict later conduct problems. *J. Child Psychol. Psychiatry* 39:377–385.

Volavka, J., Bilder, R., and Nolan, K. (2004) Catecholamines and aggression: the role of COMT and MAO polymorphisms. *Ann. N. Y. Acad. Sci.* 1036:393–398.

Volkow, N.D., and Tancredi, L. (1987) Neural substrates of violent behaviour. A preliminary study with positron emission tomography. *Br. J. Psychiatry* 151:668–673.

Whalen, P.J., Shin, L.M., McInerney, S.C., Fischer, H., Wright, C.I., and Rauch, S.L. (2001) A functional MRI study of human amygdala responses to facial expressions of fear versus anger. *Emotion* 1:70–83.

Williams, L.M., Kemp, A.H., Felmingham, K., Barton, M., Olivieri, G., Peduto, A., et al. (2006) Trauma modulates amygdala and medial prefrontal responses to consciously attended fear. *NeuroImage* 29:347–357.

Wootton, J.M., Frick, P.J., Shelton, K.K., and Silverthorn, P. (1997) Ineffective parenting and childhood conduct problems: The moderating role of callous-unemotional traits. *J. Consult. Clin. Psychology* 65:292–300.

82 Sexual Dysfunction and Pharmacological Treatments: Biological Interactions

STUART N. SEIDMAN, STEVEN P. ROOSE, AND RAYMOND C. ROSEN

Sexual dysfunctions are common, in general, and are especially prevalent among patients with psychiatric disorders. Sexual disorders are associated with a range of imputed neurobiological, medical, psychological, and interpersonal causes and have a significant impact on interpersonal functioning and quality of life. Moreover, the interaction between comorbid sexual and psychiatric disorders has clinical implications for the diagnosis, course, and treatment of both conditions. In recent years, there has been significant progress in the basic research and clinical therapeutics of sexual medicine, with major advances in our understanding of the mechanisms of sexual response and the effects of pharmacological agents on sexual desire, arousal, and orgasm. Such progress has driven the field of sexual medicine, which had traditionally been dominated by psychodynamic and behavioral paradigms and treatments, toward greater overlap with neurobiological approaches to mental illnesses. In this chapter, we first review the psychobiology of sexual function and dysfunction, then describe diagnostic and therapeutic approaches to sexual dysfunction, and finally consider issues relevant to the interaction between sexual dysfunction and mood disorders. The major emphasis of the chapter is on the introduction of some of the more recent biologically based advances in sexual medicine to the broader arena of clinical neuropsychiatry.

NORMAL SEXUAL FUNCTION

The Psychobiology of Sexual Function

There are four overlapping phases of sexual function: (*1*) drive; (*2*) arousal, marked by erection in men and by vaginal lubrication and engorgement in women; (*3*) climax, marked by orgasm and ejaculation; and (*4*) resolution, which involves some degree of refractoriness.

The neural mechanisms mediating sexual response are virtually identical in both sexes (McKenna, 2001, 2002). Thus, in each phase of sexual response, though characteristic events appear different because of dimorphisms in pelvic anatomy, the underlying neurophysiology is similar. For example, both sexes experience sexual desire characterized by fantasies and imagery, and arousal characterized by genital vasocongestion. This vasocongestion (followed by perineal muscle contractions) can be induced in either sex at the spinal level (via genital stimuli transmitted by the pudendal nerve) or at supraspinal levels (via spinothalamic and spinoreticular pathways to brain stem, midbrain, hypothalamic, and cortical sites). In men and women, orgasm is characterized by nearly identical rhythmic contractions of the striated perineal muscles (that is, approximately 10 contractions at 0.7 second intervals), similar cardiorespiratory changes, and an oxytocin peak (McKenna, 2001, 2002). Finally, in both sexes, specific serotonin reuptake inhibitors (SSRIs) inhibit orgasm (Giuliano and Clement, 2005).

Sexual behavior involves the complex interplay of endocrine, sensory, autonomic, cortical, and limbic neurophysiology. A comprehensive review of the psychobiology of sexual function is beyond the scope of this chapter and has been well reviewed by Meston and Frohlich (2000) and Pfaus (1999). Here, we highlight two components of sexual physiology that are of particular interest to neurobiologists: (*a*) central nervous system modulators of sexual behavior, monoamines and androgens, and (*b*) the neurovascular physiology of genital vasocongestion.

Nervous system

Monoamines and sexual function. In humans, evidence for the primary role of monoamines in sexual function is derived from the side-effect profiles of psychotropic medications, particularly antidepressants (Werneke, Northey, and Bhugra, 2006). We consider this later in this chapter. Here we highlight only the direction of effects supported by the literature. It should be recognized that most neurotransmitters with central effects on sexual function also influence peripheral nervous system control of the genital response. Moreover, there is a balance of interactions—central and peripheral—between neurotransmitters, such as monoamines, and other neuromodulators, such as nitric oxide (NO) and sex steroids. Localizing the sexual effects of neuropharmacological manipulations is therefore difficult.

The catecholamines *dopamine* (DA) and *norepinephrine* (NE) have stimulatory effects on sexual behavior. In the 1970s, it was reported that dopaminergic drugs given for parkinsonism appeared to be prosexual, and clinical consensus has been that DA agonists increase sexual desire and erectile function. In rats, experimental data confirm that DA agonists increase mounting, reduce the latency to ejaculation, and affect lordosis (Hull et al., 1999). Dopamine release in the medial preoptic area (MPOA) stimulates an increased copulatory rate and efficiency. Notably, the presence of testosterone has been shown to be permissive for DA release in the MPOA, probably mediated through NO production (Putnam et al., 2000).

Dopamine antagonists inhibit sexual functioning, particularly orgasm. Norepinephrine levels increase during sexual activity and are positively correlated with arousal in men and women—increasing dramatically at orgasm and then decreasing precipitously in men (for example, to baseline by 2 minutes postorgasm) and gradually in women.

In contrast to the activating effects of catecholamines, serotonin (5-hydroxytryptamine [5-HT]) tends to inhibit sexual behavior. In monkeys, 5-$HT_{1C/1D}$ agonists inhibit sexual behavior. In male rats, activation of the 5-HT_{1A} receptor lowers the threshold for ejaculation, whereas activation of 5-HT_{1B} and 5-HT_{1C} and antagonism of 5-HT_2 all inhibit sexual behavior (Pfaus, 1999). In humans, data suggest that functional polymorphisms in the 5HT_{2A} receptor (and its G-protein second messenger complex) are related to whether or not a patient taking an SSRI will develop sexual dysfunction (Bishop et al. 2006).

Androgens and sexual function. Gonadal steroids are necessary for mating. In all male mammals studied, there is a dramatic reduction in sexual activity following the removal of testosterone by either surgical ablation of the testes or seasonal regression. Castration is typically followed by the loss first of ejaculation, then of intromission, and finally of mounting; androgen replacement (peripherally or via intracerebral implantation to the MPOA) restores these sexual behaviors in reverse order (Michael et al., 1989;Wallen et al., 1991). Although among humans the role of testosterone in the maintenance of male sexual function is more complex, a large body of evidence supports a strong influence. For example, increasing levels of plasma androgens at puberty are correlated with the onset of nocturnal emission, masturbation, dating, and infatuation (Kemper, 1990), and the level of free testosterone is correlated with sexual thoughts (Meston and Frohlich, 2000). Males with an early onset of androgen secretion (that is, precocious puberty) often develop in parallel an early interest in sexuality and erotic fantasies (Feder, 1984). Hypogonadism (that is, reduction in circulating androgens) is characterized by loss of libido and a loss in sleep-associated and spontaneous erections; testosterone replacement leads to a dramatic increase in sexual desire, sexual activity, and frequency of erections (Steidle et al., 2003; McNicholas et al., 2003; Wang et al., 2004). Finally, suppression of testosterone secretion in eugonadal men leads to reduced sexual desire and activity and a decrease in spontaneous and fantasy-driven erections, though no decrease in erectile response to erotic film (that is, externally driven erections) (Davidson and Rosen, 1992; Bagatell et al., 1994; Schmidt et al., 2004).

Testosterone levels in eugonadal men exhibit wide interindividual variability and do not generally correlate with sexual desire or performance. The clinical consensus has been that among men there is a "low testosterone threshold" (which may vary from person to person) below which some aspects of sexual function are impaired, such as internally driven erections and arousal. However, such a threshold is not well established, and some data suggest that testosterone administration to eugonadal men can stimulate arousability and sexual interest (Schiavi et al., 1997).

Data are inconsistent regarding the relation between testosterone and sexual function in women. Following the observation in 1959 that among women who had undergone adrenalectomy and/or ovariectomy (to slow the progression of breast cancer), androgens and not estrogens appeared to be responsible for libido, a large body of conflicting evidence has been accumulated (Basson, 2006b; Basson, 2007a; Wierman et al., 2006), including the following:

1. The reduction in testosterone following oophorectomy and adrenalectomy is associated with a consistent reduction in sexual desire; replacement with exogenous testosterone (with or without estrogen) restores sexual desire (Sherwin, 1988, 2002; Goldstat et al., 2003; Wierman et al., 2006).

2. In premenopausal women, some data from correlational studies support a positive association between androgen level and sexual function, including intercourse frequency (Persky et al., 1982), initiation of coitus (Halpern et al., 1997), masturbation frequency (Bancroft et al., 1983), and vaginal response to erotic stimuli in

the laboratory (Schreiner-Engel et al., 1981). Yet other correlational data provide only limited support: in the Study of Women's Health Across the Nation (SWAN), a multicentered, multiethnic 2-year longitudinal study of 2,961 women aged 42–52 years, all of whom had at least one menses in the past 3 months, there was only a marginal relationship detected between testosterone levels and sexual desire (Santoro et al., 2005). Furthermore, in a community-based, cross-sectional study of 1,021 women aged 18–75 years (Davis et al., 2005), there was no association between testosterone levels and scores on any of the sexual function domains evaluated.

3. In postmenopausal women not receiving hormone replacement therapy (HRT), androgen level is correlated with sexual activity (Leiblum et al., 1983; Bancroft and Cawood, 1996) and sexual desire (Bachmann and Leiblum, 1991).

4. Testosterone levels are not typically lower in women with hypoactive sexual desire disorder.

5. Androgen antagonists do not consistently suppress libido in women (Meston and Frohlich, 2000).

Neurovascular physiology of genital vasocongestion

Male genital vasocongestion (erection). Basic research on neurovascular mechanisms of genital vasocongestion has contributed greatly to our understanding of normal and pathological processes of erection. Smooth muscle contractility is regulated by a delicate balance between neurotransmitter and vasoactive substances mediating erectile tissue contraction (consistent with flaccidity) and relaxation (consistent with erection). Nitric oxide plays a major role in inducing trabecular smooth muscle relaxation. Following release, NO diffuses across smooth muscle cell membranes and binds to soluble guanylate cyclase. The resultant increase in intracellular cyclic guanosine monophosphate (cGMP) leads to binding of cGMP to cGMP-dependent protein kinases and to cGMP-dependent ion channels. The lowered intracellular calcium and activation of myosin light chain phosphatases results in inhibition of smooth muscle contractility and enhancement of erection. Multiple vasoactive agents, including vasoactive intestinal polypeptide, prostaglandin E1, forskolin, phosphodiesterase inhibitors, and α-adrenergic receptor antagonists, affect smooth muscle contractility. Ultimately, all act by affecting intracellular calcium and thereby modulating specific smooth muscle myosin light chain kinases and myosin light chain phosphatases. These enzymes rapidly change the state of myosin phosphorylation and result in either smooth muscle contraction (flaccidity) or relaxation (erection).

Female genital vasocongestion. Genital vasocongestion occurs in women within seconds after erotic stimulation (van Lunsen and Laan, 2004). Nitric oxide and vasointestinal polypeptide (VIP) mediate vasodilatation; and acetylcholine blocks vasoconstrictive mechanisms (via noradrenergic release). Vaginal smooth muscle is relaxed, and arteriolar dilatation increases the transudation of interstitial fluid, leading to lubrication. A striking aspect of female arousal is that subjective arousal is poorly correlated with genital response (Basson, 2006a). For example, increases in genital vasocongestion in response to erotic videos are similar among women who report problems with arousal and women who report no problems with arousal (van Lunsen and Laan, 2004). Furthermore, there is a low correlation between brain activation in areas controlling genital response and simultaneous ratings of subjective arousal (Karama et al., 2002).

SEXUAL DYSFUNCTION

Sexual problems are generally classified according to the four-phase model of sexual response. These phases include (*1*) sexual desire disorders (hypoactive sexual desire disorder [HSDD], sexual aversion disorder); (*2*) sexual arousal disorders (erectile dysfunction [ED], female arousal disorder); (*3*) orgasmic disorders (female orgasmic disorder, premature or delayed ejaculation); and (*4*) sexual pain disorders (dyspareunia, vaginismus) (Table 82.1).

Diagnostic criteria for sexual dysfunctions are operationally defined as follows:

1. Criterion A defines the specific psycho-physiological impairment (for example, lack of orgasm, or erectile dysfunction).
2. Criterion B requires that the disturbance causes marked distress or interpersonal difficulty.
3. Criterion C requires that the dysfunction is not better accounted by another Axis I disorder, general medical condition, or solely due to a substance effect (medication or drug of abuse).

Problems with *Diagnostic and Statistical Manual of Mental Disorders* (*DSM-IV*) (American Psychiatric Association [APA], 2004) definitions of sexual dysfunction include the following:

1. Anchoring the diagnoses of sexual dysfunction to the phases of sexual response does not well capture the reality of these disorders, which frequently overlap (Basson et al., 2004).
2. There is no diagnostic category of "sexual dysfunction due to a psychiatric disorder," though the association of sexual dysfunction with depression, anxiety, schizophrenia, and substance abuse is unequivocal.
3. Validity and reliability of *DSM-IV* criteria for sexual dysfunction have not been well tested.
4. Specific operational criteria for the disorders are not used. Notably, the lack of specific time criteria (for

TABLE 82.1 *Sexual Response Phases, Associated Sexual Dysfunctions, and Relationship to Depression*

Phase	*Characteristics*	*Sexual Dysfunction*	*Treatment with Established Efficacy*	*Depression Correlates*
1. Desire	First phase of sexual response: subjective feelings of sexual interest or appetite, sexual urges, or fantasies. No identifiable physiological correlates.	Hypoactive sexual desire disorder; sexual aversion disorder.	None.	MDD++; DD+; psychotropic medications++
2. Excitement	Second phase of sexual response: subjective and physiological concomitants of sexual arousal. Penile erection in males, vaginal engorgement and lubrication in females.	Female sexual arousal disorder; male ED. Sexual pain disorders: dyspareunia, vaginismus.	Male ED: PDE inhibitors (e.g., sildenafil, vardenafil, tadalafil); penile self-injection therapy; penile prosthesis/vacuum constriction device.	MDD++; psychotropic medications+
3. Orgasm	Third phase of sexual response: climax or peaking of sexual tension, rhythmic contractions of the genital musculature, and intense subjective involvement.	Female orgasmic disorder; male orgasmic disorder; PE.	Male PE: SSRIs, behavior therapy; female orgasmic disorder: behavior therapy, bibliotherapy.	Psychotropic medications++
4. Resolution	Final phase of sexual response: physical release of tension and subjective sense of well-being. Most men have a refractory period for further sexual stimulation.	None.	n/a.	None.

DD: dysthymic disorder; ED: erectile dysfunction; MDD: major depressive disorder; PDE: phosphodiesterase; PE: premature ejaculation; SSRI: serotonin specific reuptake inhibitor.
+: anecdotal; ++: well established

example, ejaculatory latency for PE) or duration criteria (for example, 6 months for ED) makes heterogeneity of diagnoses a large clinical and research problem.

Female Sexual Dysfunction

Sexual dysfunction is more prevalent in women than men overall: large epidemiological studies have found that about 40% of women and 30% of men reported having one or more sexual problems in the past year (Lewis et al., 2004; Laumann et al., 2006; Nicolosi et al., 2006). Two factors that must be considered in the context of female sexual dysfunction are baseline sexual interest and age. Having too little sexual desire is reported by 10%–51% of women surveyed in various countries (Laumann et al., 2006; Nicolosi et al., 2006). Indeed, a notable observation from the SWAN study was that among women in established relationships, sexual desire is an uncommon reason for engaging in sexual activity: 40% of the enrolled women reported that they never or infrequently felt sexual desire (Avis et al., 2005). Even so, most were capable of arousal, and only 13% expressed discontent with their sexual experiences. Such epidemiological data, which are generally consistent across studies, have broad implications for the clinical assessment, treatment, and study of disorders of female sexual function. For example, although diagnostic criteria for HSDD require that this disorder be diagnosed when a woman fails to feel desire at any stage during the sexual experience, sexual thoughts are infrequent in most women (without apparent sexual dissatisfaction), and the frequency of sexual fantasies or sexual thoughts does not generally correlate with sexual satisfaction.

A second factor of great importance is age: the prevalence of female sexual dysfunction increases with age and is associated with the presence of vascular risk factors and menopause (Lewis et al., 2004). Older women experience a reduction in pelvic muscle tension, relaxation of the urethral meatus (with urinary incontinence sometimes associated with orgasm), reduction in orgiastic rectal contractions, vaginal dryness (generally associated with the menopausal decline in estrogen), reduced libido (possibly associated with a decline in testosterone or dehydroepiandrosterone [DHEA] level), reduced engorgement (possibly due to pelvic vascular insufficiency), a decrease in the intensity of orgasm, and an increase in the time needed to achieve orgasm (McKenna, 2002; Basson, 2006b). It has been postulated that, similar to the most common pathophysiological mechanism of male sexual dysfunction, females develop a reduction in pelvic blood flow with age, with a consequent impairment in arousal—specifically, reduced vaginal lubrication and clitoral tumescence. With these caveats in mind, we consider the most commonly diagnosed sexual dysfunctions: hypoactive sexual desire disorder, sexual arousal disorder, anorgasmia, and dyspareunia.

Hypoactive sexual desire disorder (HSDD) is diagnosed when the patient is judged to have persistent or recurrently deficient (or absent) sexual fantasies and desire for sexual activity. It is estimated that about one in three women has HSDD (Lewis et al., 2004; Avis et al., 2005; Laumann et al., 2006; Nicolosi et al., 2006), though lack of desire may be far more common, even normative (Basson, 2006a; Segraves and Segraves, 1991). Important determinants of sexual desire include partner conflicts and the presence of other sexual dysfunctions (for example, anorgasmia).

Diagnostic criteria that have been used in studying HSDD include reported frequency of self-initiated sexual activity once every 2 weeks or less, along with a subjective lack of desire to engage in any sexual behavior and absence or decrease in sexual fantasy. Medical conditions that have been associated with HSDD include endocrine disorders (for example, hypogonadism, hypothyroidism, hyperprolactinemia), temporal lobe lesions, environmental toxins, medications (for example, SSRIs), and substance use (Basson, 2007b; Basson and Schultz, 2007; Bhasin et al., 2007). Major depressive disorder (MDD) is especially important to rule out in women, as the prevalence of MDD is high, and reduced libido is present in the majority of patients who are depressed (West et al., 2004). The degree of personal distress associated with the HSDD varies widely.

Female sexual arousal disorder (FSAD) refers to a persistent lack of subjective or physical arousal during sexual stimulation. Sexual arousal disorder in women is characterized by an inability to achieve an adequate lubrication-swelling response of the vagina and labia for the completion of sexual activity or a lack of subjective arousal during sexual activity; there are no objective criteria (Basson, 2006a). Although women with sexual arousal disorder may have intercourse, the lack of adequate lubrication can cause pain. Large epidemiological surveys have shown that approximately 15%–20% of premenopausal women have difficulty becoming lubricated during sexual stimulation and that such difficulty increases with age (Lewis et al., 2004; Avis et al., 2005; Laumann et al., 2006; Nicolosi et al., 2006;).

Orgasmic disorder is defined by the persistent or recurrent difficulty, delay in, or absence of orgasmic attainment despite adequate sexual stimulation and arousal. It is subclassified into situational, generalized, and mixed situational and depends on the clinician's judgment regarding the patient's sexual experience, age, and adequacy of stimulation (Basson et al., 2004). About 10% of women have never experienced orgasm, and a majority of women have situational orgasmic difficulties (Simons and Carey, 2001; Nicolosi et al., 2006). Important clinical issues include the presence of MDD, the use of antidepressants (particularly serotonergic medications), and relationship conflicts.

Dyspareunia, or pain associated with sexual intercourse, is generally caused by a lack of lubrication or other physical cause. *Vaginismus*, or involuntary spasms of the musculature of the outer third of the vagina, is a significant cause of penetration difficulties in women. These disorders are seen relatively frequently in sex therapy clinics, occurring in approximately 15% of women presenting for treatment. A wide variety of medical and psychological conditions have been associated with these disorders, including hymenal scarring, pelvic inflammatory disease, and vulvar vestibulitis.

Treatment of female sexual dysfunction

Despite its high prevalence, female sexual dysfunction is rarely reported to clinicians and remains mostly untreated. Estrogen replacement and estrogen creams can be effective for postmenopausal vaginal changes, as can the use of water-soluble lubricants (for example, K-Y vaginal jelly). Standard treatment for HSDD consists of individual or couples psychotherapy, with limited demonstrable treatment success (Basson, 2006a). Orgasmic disorder is effectively treated by a combined masturbation and sex therapy approach with individuals, couples, or groups or with bibliotherapy. All of these methods focus on issues of body image, relaxation, self-stimulation, acceptance of sexual feelings, tolerance of higher levels of arousal, loss of control, and partner functioning. Patient and partner education is considered an important component in the management of female sexual dysfunction and should be a continuous element at each phase in the process of care. There has been only limited systematic study of these and other commonly used treatment modalities, such as vaginal lubricants, vaginal dilators, pelvic floor rehabilitation (with biofeedback electromyography), and Kegel exercises.

Other than estrogen therapy for dyspareunia related to genitourinary atrophy, no medications are approved by the Food and Drug Administration (FDA) for the treatment of female sexual dysfunction. Yet many off-label uses of available medications have been considered, including androgens, phosphodiesterase inhibitors (for example, sildenafil, vardenafil, and tadalafil), yohimbine, alcohol, DA agonists, stimulants, and/or antidepressants. Although these agents may stimulate mood changes or other nonspecific (that is, placebo) responses, none have been demonstrated to have specific therapeutic effects on HSDD or other sexual dysfunctions. For example, Segraves et al. (2001) studied bupropion sustained release

(SR) in women with HSDD who were not depressed. Eligible women first received placebo, single-blind, for 4 weeks; nonresponders then received bupropion SR, single-blind, for 8 additional weeks. Of 51 women with placebo-resistant HSDD, 29% responded to open treatment with bupropion SR.

There has been some interest in using phosphodiesterase inhibitors, such as sildenafil, for female sexual dysfunction, based on positive anecdotal reports and open trials. For example, in a small, laboratory-based, randomized trial, a single 50-mg dose of sildenafil increased subjective arousal, genital sensations, and ease of orgasm in some women with arousal disorder (Basson and Brotto, 2003). However, in two 12-week placebo-controlled trials in which 781 women with sexual dysfunction were randomized to receive sildenafil, 25–100 mg, or placebo prior to sexual activity, changes in sexual function were indistinguishable between the groups (Basson et al., 2000; Basson and Brotto, 2003). In a more recent study, 202 postmenopausal women with FSAD were randomized to receive sildenafil (a 50-mg dose adjustable to 100 or 25 mg) or placebo in a 12-week, double-blind, placebo-controlled study. Significant improvements in the Female Intervention Efficacy Index (FIEI) questions 2 (increased genital sensation during intercourse or stimulation, $p = .017$) and 4 (increased satisfaction with intercourse and/or foreplay, $p = .015$) were observed with sildenafil compared to placebo. For women with FSAD without concomitant HSDD, sildenafil was associated with significantly greater improvement than placebo in five of six FIEI items ($p < .02$). No significant improvements were shown for women with concomitant HSDD (Berman et al., 2003). Overall, based on the limited data available, it appears that sildenafil, though well tolerated, offers limited or idiosyncratic benefit to women with sexual dysfunction (Shields and Hrometz, 2006).

Hormonal Treatments

Supraphysiologic androgen therapy has been prescribed for female sexual dysfunction since the 1930s, and more recently, testosterone replacement at physiological doses has been studied in randomized trials. Accumulating evidence suggests that androgen replacement (for example, with testosterone in women who are hormone deficient) has libido and arousal-enhancing effects. Multiple testosterone replacement trials in oophorectomized women have demonstrated improved sexual function, with an increase in sexual fantasy, satisfaction, arousal, libido, energy, and mood; though not consistently in coital frequency and orgasm (Somboonporn et al., 2005). In women who are postmenopausal and who have a loss of libido, testosterone replacement in addition to estrogen HRT is associated with improved sexual function and mood (J.C. Montgomery et al., 1987). For example, in 6-month randomized trials of transdermal testosterone administered to naturally menopausal women with HSDD, testosterone improved sexual function (Shifren et al., 2006). Yet in women who were postmenopausal who did not complain of low libido, testosterone replacement in addition to estrogen HRT has not been shown to be different from estrogen HRT alone (Myers et al., 1990; Sand and Studd, 1995).

A review of randomized controlled trials of testosterone for women who were peri- and postmenopausal taking hormone therapy was published in the Cochrane Library in 2005 (Somboonporn et al., 2005). Study participants included women who had either a natural or surgically induced menopause; the intervention was testosterone plus HRT, versus HRT. There were 1,957 participants included in the meta-analysis, and study duration ranged from 1.5 to 24 months (median 6 months). Adding testosterone to HRT had beneficial effects on sexual function in postmenopausal women for the domains of sexual activity combined with coital frequency, responsiveness, and libido, and for composite sexual function score; and an adverse effect of a significant reduction in high density lipoprotein (HDL) cholesterol. Testosterone did not affect well-being, fatigue, bone health, body composition, menopausal symptoms, cognition, hirsuitism, acne, hostility, plasma viscosity, fibrinogen level, or hematocrit. Long-term effects on breast cancer and coronary heart disease were not known.

In 2006, the European Agency for the Evaluation of Medical Products (EMEA) approved the testosterone patch for female HSDD. The two pivotal clinical trials that demonstrated the effectiveness of testosterone at improving sexual desire and response in women who were surgically postmenopausal were The Intimate Studies SM1 and SM2. Intimate Study SM1 was a 6-month, randomized, double-blind, placebo-controlled clinical trial in which 562 women with bilateral salpingo-oophorectomy and HSDD, ages 26–70 years, all of whom were receiving estrogen HRT, were randomized to testosterone (300 μg/day, $n = 283$) or placebo ($n = 279$) (Simon et al., 2005). After 6 months, the frequency of satisfactory sexual activity (2.10 episodes per 4 weeks) increased only in the testosterone group, and this was clearly superior to the placebo group (0.98 episodes per 4 weeks; $p = .0003$); the testosterone group had a significant improvement in sexual desire and a decrease in distress. The safety profile was similar in both groups. Intimate Study SM2 was a near-identical study ($N = 533$, women with hysterectomy and bilateral oophorectomy, 6-month randomized controlled trial [RCT]) that also demonstrated that those randomized to the testosterone patch had a significant improvement in sexual desire ($p < .001$) and a decrease in distress ($p < .009$). Adverse effects were also similar in the two groups (Buster et al., 2005).

A pooled analysis of these and two other similarly designed RCTs ($N = 1,619$) confirmed the efficacy of a

300-μg testosterone patch applied twice weekly in addition to estrogen (delivered transdermally in one study, orally in another, and by either route in two studies): women receiving testosterone reported 1.9 more sexually satisfying events per month than they had at baseline, as compared with 0.9 more among those receiving placebo; in all four studies, those receiving testosterone had a significant increase in sexual desire and response; and in three of the studies, there were significant reductions in sexual distress (Braunstein et al., 2005; Buster et al., 2005; Davis et al., 2006). Unwanted androgenic effects, including hirsutism, acne, and lowered HDL cholesterol, were uncommon in all studies. Yet, despite such consistent evidence for the short-term efficacy of testosterone in surgically menopausal women, a task force of The Endocrine Society—adhering closely to evidence-based guidelines—published in 2006 a clinical practice guideline recommending against the generalized use of testosterone in women (Wierman et al., 2006).

Finally, *tibolone* is a unique compound that is classified as a selective tissue estrogenic activity regulator (STEAR) and is widely used for the treatment of symptoms of menopause. After oral ingestion, tibolone is converted to three active metabolites: the 3α-OH and 3β-OH-tibolone metabolites have estrogenic effects on the bone, vagina, and menopausal symptoms; the Δ^4 isomer has progestogenic and androgenic properties. Systematic studies have confirmed that tibolone is as effective as estrogenic HRT regimens for menopausal symptoms, such as hot flushes, sweating, insomnia, headache, and fatigue. It has also been shown to reverse vaginal atrophy. Moreover, tibolone leads to improved sexual function, including sexual desire, arousability, sexual fantasies, and vaginal lubrication (Kenemans and Speroff, 2005; Osmanagaoglu et al., 2006). Compared with estrogen HRT regimens, tibolone is associated with significantly greater improvement in coital frequency, enjoyment, and satisfaction. Such prosexual effects may be due to the direct androgenic actions of the Δ^4 isomer or to the increase in free testosterone that occurs because tibolone leads to a decrease in sex hormone binding globulin (SHBG) level.

Male Sexual Dysfunction

Age-associated changes in male sexual response include (*1*) reduced libido, (*2*) reduced number and frequency of morning erections, (*3*) reduced penile sensitivity, (*4*) reduced arousal, including increased latency for and difficulty maintaining erection, (*5*) prolonged plateau phase, (*6*) reduced ejaculatory volume and force of expulsion, and (*7*) a prolonged refractory period (Schiavi et al., 1991). The age-associated decrease in testosterone level may be associated with a reduction in libido and mood, though this is controversial (Feldman et al., 2002; Seidman et al., 2002).

The most common male sexual dysfunctions are HSDD, PE, and ED. These diagnoses require clinical judgment and do not include frequency or duration criteria. As in women, male HSDD is defined by the chronic absence (or deficiency in) sexual fantasies and desire for sexual activity (Segraves and Segraves, 1991). It has been estimated that the 1-year prevalence is 3%, though other estimates are as high as 16% (Lewis et al., 2004; Laumann et al., 2006; Nicolosi et al., 2006). In men, HSDD is especially influenced by the presence of other sexual dysfunctions (for example, ED and PE), psychiatric illness, or medical conditions. It is particularly important to consider comorbid hypogonadism and alcohol abuse, as these conditions are common in men (Basson, 2007b; Basson and Schultz, 2007).

Premature ejaculation (PE) is defined as persistent or recurrent ejaculation with minimal sexual stimulation before, on, or shortly after penetration or before the person wishes it (Rosen, Catania, et al., 2007; Rosen, McMahon, et al., 2007). An important component of the definition of PE is the patient's perception of lack of control over ejaculation. Generally, ejaculation occurs too quickly (less than 1 minute) and before or soon after penetration into the vagina. Ejaculation occurring after vaginal penetration is less easily defined as premature. There are many couples for whom these definitions would be inadequate, and the most useful definition is probably an attitudinal one: ejaculation is premature if either partner perceives it to be. In making the diagnosis, clinicians should consider the circumstances of the problem, including the degree of associated distress in the male and his partner. The current *DSM-IV-TR* definition of PE has a low positive predictive value, and dividing PE into four syndromes has been proposed for *DSM-V* (Waldinger and Schweitzer, 2007).

About one fourth of men in the United States report that in the past year there was a period of several months or more in which they came to a climax too quickly (Lewis et al., 2004; Laumann et al., 2006; Nicolosi et al., 2006). Despite its greater prevalence, PE has attracted less attention among health professionals and the lay public than ED. This may be due, in part, to the fact that men with mild or moderate PE are still able to function sexually (that is, to perform intercourse). In the most severe cases, however, the man ejaculates before penetration is achieved. Far fewer men with PE seek professional help for their problem, including those with the most severe forms of the disorder. This is unfortunate because simple and effective therapies are widely available.

The diagnosis of PE begins with a bio-psycho-social assessment of the patient and partner. Other aspects of sexual functioning should be carefully assessed, particularly because PE can develop as a secondary reaction to ED. Otherwise, little is known about either the pathophysiology or the etiology of the disorder. The known organic factors that can cause PE include trauma to the sympathetic nervous system from abdominal aortic aneurysm surgery, pelvic fractures, and urological pathologies such as prostatic hypertrophy, prostatitis, or urethritis. Spontaneous ejaculation and PE have been described in association with diabetes, arteriosclerosis, cardiovascular disease, venous leakage, polycythemia, polyneuritis, and alcohol withdrawal. Although all of the above have been reported in the literature to be associated with PE, the majority of patients have no detectable organic etiology.

Erectile dysfunction is defined as the inability to obtain and maintain an erection sufficient for satisfactory intercourse or other sexual expression. It is a para-aging phenomenon that affects up to one half of all men between the ages of 40 and 70 years (Feldman et al., 1994; Lue et al., 2004; Nicolosi et al., 2006). Approximately 10% of middle-aged men have *complete ED*, defined as the total inability to achieve or maintain an erection sufficient for sexual performance. An additional 25% of men of this age have intermittent erectile difficulties. The disorder is highly age dependent, as the combined prevalence of moderate to complete ED rises from approximately 22% at age 40 to 49% by age 70 (Feldman et al., 1994; Lue et al., 2004). Erectile dysfunction is associated with, and presumably exacerbated by, poor health: it is more common among men with diabetes, heart disease, hypertension, cigarette smoking, and hyperlipidemia (Feldman et al., 1994; Lue et al., 2004; Nicolosi et al., 2006). There is a strong positive correlation between ED and depressive symptoms, impairment in social and occupational functioning, and reduced quality of life (Feldman et al., 1994; Lue et al., 2004; Nicolosi et al., 2006). Successful treatment of ED appears to ameliorate this morbidity (Rosen et al., 2006; Seidman, Roose, et al., 2001).

Treatment of male sexual dysfunction

Hypoactive sexual desire disorder. Standard treatment for HSDD consists of individual or couples psychotherapy, with limited demonstrable treatment success. Pharmacological treatment with psychotropic agents such as yohimbine, DA agonists, stimulants, and/or antidepressants may stimulate mood changes or nonspecific (that is, placebo) responses but have not been demonstrated to have specific therapeutic effects on HSDD. Testosterone replacement in hypogonadal men stimulates an increase in sexual desire and arousal (Steidle et al., 2003; McNicholas et al., 2003; Wang et al., 2004). In eugonadal men, the sexual effects of exogenous testosterone are indistinguishable from those of placebo (O'Carroll and Bancroft, 1984; Pope et al., 2000).

Premature ejaculation. Premature ejaculation can be treated behaviorally, via the stop, start, or squeeze procedure, or pharmacologically via SSRIs. The current method of choice in treating PE is behavior modification using the procedure described by Masters and Johnson (Haslam, 1975). This method is known as the *pause method* and involves start-and-stop behavior therapy; combined with a frenulum squeeze procedure, it is called the *pause-squeeze technique*. The method involves direct stimulation of the male until premonitory sensations are experienced just prior to orgasm. All stimulation is stopped at this point. After repeated practice over 4–8 weeks, the male becomes more aware of these anticipatory sensations and is able to delay or control his ejaculation to a much greater degree. When practiced regularly by the male and his partner, the conditioning technique is often effective in the short term. However, it demands significant motivation on the part of the couple, and treatment efficacy is not always maintained over time.

Although SSRIs are not approved by the FDA for PE, there is clear evidence in the literature of their effectiveness, and they are in widespread use. Because SSRIs are known to delay ejaculation, the rationale, supported by case reports, was that a medication that delays ejaculation from normal to impaired should also delay ejaculation from premature to normal. The presumed mechanism is via 5-HT_2 receptor activation that is inhibitory to ejaculation—through ascending serotonergic projections to the medial preoptic area and/or descending serotonergic pathways to the lumbosacral motor nuclei. Multiple controlled trials, using a variety of definitions of PE, have supported the efficacy of serotonergic agents in this condition. In double-blind, placebo-controlled trials using patient and partner assessments, clomipramine (CMI) 25–50 mg, paroxetine 20–40 mg, sertraline 50–150 mg, fluoxetine 20–40 mg, and dapoxetine 30–60 mg have been shown to produce significant ejaculatory delay—that is, 2–10 minutes' increased latency to ejaculation, when used 6 hours prior to coitus (Lue et al., 2004; Pryor et al., 2006; Giuliano and Clement, 2006; Waldinger, 2007). A meta-analysis of studies, conducted in accordance with current standards of evidence-based medicine, demonstrated similar efficacies for daily treatment with paroxetine, clomipramine, sertraline, and fluoxetine; paroxetine appeared to have the strongest delaying effect on ejaculation (Giuliano and Clement, 2006).

The SSRI *dapoxetine* has been recently considered as an on-demand medication for men with moderate-to-severe PE. In 12-week randomized, double-blind, placebo-controlled trials done at 121 sites in the United States, men with moderate-to-severe PE in stable, heterosexual relationships took placebo (n = 870), 30 mg dapoxetine (n = 874), or 60 mg dapoxetine (n = 870) as needed, 1–3 hours before anticipated sexual activity. Dapoxetine significantly prolonged intravaginal ejaculatory latency time (IELT), measured by stopwatch ($p < .0001$, all doses vs. placebo). Mean IELT at baseline was 0.90 (SD = .47) minute, 0.92 (.50) minute, and 0.91 (.48) minute, and at study end point (week 12 or final visit) was 1.75 (2.21) minutes for placebo, 2.78 (3.48) minutes for 30 mg dapoxetine, and 3.32 (3.68) minutes for 60 mg dapoxetine. Dapoxetine was effective at the first dose, and adverse events (30 mg and 60 mg dapoxetine, respectively) were nausea (8.7%, 20.1%), diarrhea (3.9%, 6.8%), headache (5.9%, 6.8%), and dizziness (3.0%, 6.2%) (Pryor et al., 2006).

In a study of daily SSRI treatment, men with PE were randomized to receive 60 mg dapoxetine (group 1, n = 115), 20 mg paroxetine (group 2, n = 113), or placebo (group 3, n = 112) daily for 12 weeks. At the end of the treatment, the mean IELT was increased from 38, 31, and 34 seconds to 179, 370, and 55 seconds, in groups 1, 2, and 3, respectively (p = .01 in group 1 and p = .001 in group 2) (Safarinejad, 2006). Most authors currently recommend initial daily use of an SSRI, followed by use as needed. In one study, however, rapid ejaculation resumed shortly after withdrawal of CMI therapy that had been administered for the previous 8 weeks (Waldinger et al., 2006). In many men with PE, daily SSRI administration will be needed.

Ejaculation can also be delayed by on-demand use of topical anaesthetics and tramadol. Phosphodiesterase inhibitors, such as sildenafil, may have some efficacy in PE: in a recent study, 180 men with primary PE (and without ED) were randomized to receive one of three treatments: 50 mg sildenafil as needed, 20 mg paroxetine daily, and squeeze technique daily. After 3 and 6 months, sildenafil was superior to paroxetine, and to squeeze technique in IELT, PE grade, intercourse satisfactory score (ISS) (W.F. Wang et al., 2007). There is no support for treatment of PE with intracavernous injection of vasoactive drugs.

Finally, some animal studies have shown that strong immediate ejaculation delay may be induced by administration of a combination of an SSRI with a 5-HT_{1A} receptor antagonist. The combination of an SSRI and any other compound that immediately and potently raises serotonin neurotransmission and/or use of oxytocin receptor antagonists may form the basis for the development of new on-demand and/or daily drugs for the treatment of PE (Waldinger and Schweitzer, 2005; Waldinger et al., 2006; de Jong et al., 2007; Waldinger, 2007).

Erectile dysfunction. The first-line option for ED is an oral medication such as sildenafil, vardenafil, or tadafil. These medications may be used alone or in combination with sexual counseling or education. Brief sexual or couples counseling is aimed at resolving specific conflicts, such as relationship distress, sexual performance concerns, and dysfunctional communication patterns. Advantages of sexual counseling include its noninvasiveness and relatively broad applicability. The major disadvantages are the lack of acceptability for many patients and uncertain efficacy.

The primary oral medications for the treatment of erectile dysfunction—sildenafil, tadalafil, and vardenafil—are competitive inhibitors of cGMP-specific phosphodiesterase type 5 (PDE-5), the predominant isozyme causing he breakdown of cGMP in the human corpus cavernosum. The mechanism of action is peripheral and involves direct effects on smooth muscle relaxation and vasodilation of the penile arterioles. Efficacy of >50% is generally obtained, depending upon the etiology and severity of ED. The drugs' side effects include headaches, flushing, dyspepsia, and nasal congestion, all of which are generally mild. A small percentage of men (less than 5%) may also experience alterations in color vision (blue hue), visual brightness or sensitivity, or blurred vision. The effects (and side effects) are dose proportional. The absolute contraindication to the administration of PDE-5 inhibitors is the concomitant use of nitrates or NO donors in any form, including oral, sublingual, transdermal, inhalational, or aerosol.

Until the introduction of sildenafil, the primary nonsurgical ED treatment with proven efficacy was penile self-injection therapy. This treatment consists of the injection of vasodilator medications into the penis using a small needle. After the initial test injections in the urologist's office, patients receive instructions in the self-injection technique. Once they have learned the proper technique and reached the satisfactory dose of the medication, patients receive medication and supplies for home injections. Follow-up is conducted through periodic visits to assure compliance and resupply the medication. The most commonly used injectable medication is alprostadil, which is available as a ready-use kit under the brand name Caverject. Injection therapy is effective in most cases of ED, regardless of etiology. It is contraindicated in men with a history of hypersensitivity to the drug employed, in those at risk for priapism (for example, those with sickle cell disease or hypercoagulable states), and in men receiving monoamine oxidase inhibitors. Intracavernosal injections have been shown to be effective in about 70%–80% of men who fail first-line therapy with sildenafil (Shabsigh et al., 2006). However, many men and their partners find this method unacceptable. The current indication for self-injection therapy is as salvage for PDE-5 nonresponders or for those in whom PDE-5s are contraindicated.

Vacuum constriction device (VCD) therapy is a well-established, noninvasive treatment that is approved by the FDA for over-the-counter distribution. It provides a useful treatment alternative for patients for whom pharmacological therapies are contraindicated or who do not desire other interventions. Vacuum constriction devices apply a negative pressure to the flaccid penis, thus drawing venous blood into the penis, which is then retained by the application of an elastic constriction band at the base of the penis. Efficacy rates of 60%–80% have been reported in most studies. Like intracorporal injection therapy, VCD treatment is associated with a high rate of patient discontinuation. The adverse events occasionally associated with VCD therapy include penile pain, numbness, bruising, and delayed ejaculation.

Finally, surgical implantation of a penile prosthesis is appropriate in patients who fail nonsurgical therapy for any reason, such as lack of efficacy, unacceptable side effects, and/or dissatisfaction. Penile prostheses may also be indicated in patients with other conditions in addition to ED, such as Peyronie's disease and other penile deformities. The main advantages of penile prostheses are reliability, permanent availability, and freedom from medications and supplies. Disadvantages include the need for surgery, infection, and malfunction. After long years of development, penile prostheses have become a safe and effective treatment modality.

Psychiatric illness and sexual dysfunction

Psychiatric illnesses can affect sexual function in multiple ways. First, there can be direct neurobiological effects, as with the reversible loss of erectile function in a subset of men with MDD (Seidman and Roose, 2000). Second, there can be indirect effects through the disruption of social and interpersonal relationships. Finally, most of the drugs used in the treatment of psychiatric illnesses are associated with sexual dysfunction. In the setting of comorbid sexual and psychiatric disorders, ascertaining which condition is primary is often difficult.

There are surprisingly few systematic studies detailing the sexual functioning of patients with chronic mental disorders. For example, the effect of schizophrenia on sexual function is unclear, and any neurobiological effects (for example, from medication effects) are likely influenced by the stability of the psychosocial situation, the degree of interpersonal relatedness, the presence of negative symptoms (particularly anhedonia), and the occurrence of positive symptoms (delusions and hallucinations) that can have sexual content (Schiavi, 1994). Sexual functioning in patients with schizophrenia has been variously reported as increased, decreased, and unchanged, and in patients taking traditional antipsychotic medications, impairments in all phases of sexual response have been demonstrated (Üçok et al., 2007). Such effects are likely related to DA antagonism and hyperprolactinemia, both of which are known inhibitors of sexual function.

In a large cross-sectional study of 827 stable outpatients with schizophrenia in Turkey, all of whom were taking antipsychotic medication, patients were interviewed and completed the Arizona Sexual Experience Scale (ASEX). Overall, more than one half (53%) had sexual dysfunction: 54% reported a low sexual desire, and 42% reported problems having an orgasm. Among the men, ED and ejaculation problems were seen in 48% and 64%, respectively; among the women, 25% had amenorrhea. Arizona Sexual Experience Scale score (indicating the severity of sexual dysfunction) was positively correlated with severity of illness ($p = .02$); this remained significant for men only after controlling for other variables ($p = .005$) (Üçok et al., 2007).

Because psychiatric disorders can influence sexual functioning through the consequences of maladaptive developmental experiences, intrapsychic and interpersonal pathology, psychosocial instability, and medication and hormonal effects, the extent to which central neurobiological abnormalities contribute to sexual dysfunction is unknown (Schiavi, 1994). It is likely that the closest neurobiological link exists between mood disorders and sexual dysfunction. In this section, we focus on the relationship between depressive illness, its treatment with medication, and sexual dysfunction.

Depression and Sexual Function

Models of comorbidity

Although sexual dysfunction and depression are highly comorbid, the causal relationship is unclear. There are five models, not mutually exclusive, that may be used to understand the coexistence of both conditions. First, the psychosocial distress that is invariably part of sexual dysfunction might stimulate the development of "secondary" depressive illness in individuals who are vulnerable. Second, sexual dysfunction can be a symptom of depression: MDD is associated with decreased libido, diminished erectile function, and decreased sexual activity. Third, a common factor (for example, alcohol use, cardiovascular disease, or hypogonadism) might be etiologically related to both conditions. Fourth, antidepressant medication might lead to sexual dysfunction. Finally, depression and sexual dysfunction, both relatively common, might be serendipitously comorbid and etiologically unrelated.

Impact of depression on sexual function

Loss of libido is considered a classic vegetative symptom of MDD and has played a prominent role in psychodynamic and other psychological formulations of depressive illness. Systematically collected data confirm that MDD is associated with decreased libido, diminished erectile function in men, and decreased sexual activity, though there are few studies of patients who were unmedicated and depressed (Seidman, 2003). Sexual problems associated with depression and antidepressants in women can be further complicated by neurohormonal status and are not well studied (Rubinow et al., 2002).

The most commonly used instrument for measurement of the male erectile response is a mechanical strain gauge that measures penile tumescence via an increase in penile circumference. The device is simple to use and provides reliable measurement of nocturnal penile tumescence (NPT). Loss of NPT is a hallmark of ED that is presumed to be biologically mediated. Roose and colleagues (1982) first reported that NPT was lost in two men who had MDD, and that this condition improved after remission of the depression. This was then evaluated systematically by Steiger and colleagues (1993) who compared NPT in 25 men with an acute episode of depression to matched controls who were not depressed. Although no statistically significant differences in NPT parameters were found between the depressed and control groups, there was a complete lack of NPT in four (16%) men who were depressed that was reversed after antidepressant therapy. Thase and colleagues (1988) demonstrated a significant reduction in NPT time and decreased penile rigidity in 34 men who were depressed compared with controls who were not depressed. The NPT time was reduced by at least one standard deviation below the control mean in 40% of men who were depressed and was comparable to that in a group of 14 men who were not depressed with a diagnosis of ED due to organic causes. These findings were confirmed in a repeat study with a new group of 51 men with MDD (Thase et al., 1992; Nofzinger et al., 1993). Together, these studies support the conclusion that erectile function is impaired in some men who are depressed, suggesting a neurophysiological link between depression and ED.

The impact of sexual dysfunction on mood

The link between sexual function and mood has not been well characterized. There is, however, suggestive evidence of a strong bidirectional association from a population-based study of middle-aged men, from multiple clinical studies performed at sexual dysfunction clinics, and from ED treatment studies. The Massachusetts Male Aging Study (MMAS) was a cross-sectional, community-based, random-sample survey of health and aging in men aged 40 to 70 years (N = 1,290). Based on the subjects' responses to nine questions that were highly correlated with biological measures of erectile response, levels of ED were graded as nil (48%), minimal (17%), moderate (25%), or complete (10%) (Araujo et al., 1998). Depression and anger were highly correlated with ED. Using the Center for Epidemiologic Studies Depression Scale (CES-D) cutoff of 16 (suggesting clinically significant depressive symptoms), 41% of men with this degree of depressive symptomatology had moderate or complete ED—twice the level of men who were not depressed. Anger also appeared related to higher ED prevalence (Araujo et al., 1998).

In a clinical study, 46 men and women presenting with HSDD were evaluated with structured psychiatric interviews, and those with current Axis I conditions were excluded. Compared to 36 matched controls, the patients (that is, men and women) had an elevated lifetime prevalence of affective disorders (73% of men and 71% of women with HSDD compared to 32% of male and 27% of female controls) (Schreiner-Engel and Schiavi, 1986). Notably, the depressive illness usually preceded the HSDD. In a study from the Netherlands, 111 men and 120 women with HSDD who presented for participation in a study of bibliotherapy were evaluated with a structured diagnostic interview. Among the men with HSDD, the rates of current anxiety disorder (12.6%), lifetime anxiety disorder (17.9%), and lifetime affective disorder (21.6%) were significantly higher than the rates of these conditions in a comparable general Dutch population (6.5%, 13.8%, and 13.6%, respectively). Among the women with HSDD, the rates of current anxiety disorder (18.3%), lifetime anxiety disorder (37.5%), lifetime affective disorder (40.8%), and lifetime eating disorder (3.3%) were significantly higher than the rates of these conditions in a comparable general population (12.9%, 25.0%, 24.5%, and 1.3%, respectively) (van Lankveld and Grotjohann, 2000).

Shabsigh and colleagues (1998) conducted a study of 100 men who presented to a urological clinic with ED, benign prostatic hyperplasia (BPH), or both and were screened for self-reported "depression," defined as above-threshold scores on two questionnaires. Men with ED (n = 66) were 2.6 times more likely to report depression than were men with BPH alone (n = 34). Moreover, among men who received ED treatment (with either penile intracavernosal injection or a vacuum device), all 15 patients in the nondepressed ED group continued treatment and were satisfied with the outcome, whereas only 7/18 (39%) of patients in the depressed ED group continued treatment. Thus, in this sample of men, depression was associated with ED and with treatment discontinuation.

Finally, Seidman, Roose, et al. (2001) and Rosen et al. (2006) conducted placebo-controlled, parallel-group, double-blind clinical trials of the PDE-5 inhibitors sildenafil (50 to 100 mg) and vardenafil (10 to 20 mg) in men with ED and comorbid depression. Patients were older than 18 years, were in stable heterosexual relationships, and had been experiencing ED for over 6 months. Minor depression (sildenafil study) or mild depression (vardenafil study) were diagnosed with a structured clinical interview and severity rated with Hamilton Rating Scale for Depression (HAM-D) scores; enrollment was limited to patients with mild-to-moderate depression. Patients were randomized to the PDE-5 or placebo for 12 weeks. The HAM-D scores were significantly reduced in ED responders compared to ED nonresponders—even among the small number of ED responders treated with placebo. The results of these studies suggest that men who are depressed who respond to ED treatment show robust improvement in depressive symptoms.

Because low testosterone and excess testosterone states can have powerful psychiatric effects, particularly on libido, energy, and mood, it has long been hypothesized that hypogonadism leads to depression, and that exogenous testosterone can help MDD and/or depressive symptoms that evolve with age (that is, andropause). Confirmation that the testosterone level declines significantly with age has given further momentum to the clinical practice of testosterone replacement as an antidepressant strategy for late-life depression. Yet there are few studies in which the efficacy of exogenous testosterone has been assessed using modern psychiatric diagnostic criteria or accepted clinical trials methodology. Indeed, in the more recent methodologically rigorous studies, there has been limited support for efficacy.

Seidman, Spatz, and colleagues (2001) enrolled 30 men with hypogonadal symptoms (defined as having testosterone levels below 350 ng/dl) and comorbid MDD in a double-blind clinical trial of testosterone replacement as an antidepressant treatment. Patients were randomized to receive testosterone, 200 mg/week, or placebo for 6 weeks. Response rates and mean change in Hamilton scores were not distinguishable between the groups. There is some evidence that testosterone replacement is an effective antidepressant in certain subgroups of men who are depressed, such as those with medication resistance (Seidman and Rabkin, 1998; Pope et al., 2003) and/or with human immunodeficiency virus infection (Rabkin et al., 2000), though evidence overall is weak (Seidman et al., 2005).

Psychotropic medication and sexual dysfunction

Many prescription and nonprescription drugs with diverse pharmacological properties have been reported to induce sexual dysfunction, particularly antihypertensives, anti-ulcer drugs, alcohol, sedatives/hypnotics, mood stabilizers, antipsychotics, and antidepressants. Yet most of these reports have been anecdotal, have focused only on men, and have not reliably identified the phase of sexual response that is impaired. More important, none has clearly distinguished the effects of the medication from those of the underlying disease (Basson and Schultz, 2007). This is particularly important in assessing the sexual effects of psychotropic agents because such effects should be considered in the context of behavioral changes in the underlying psychiatric condition associated with therapeutic actions of the drug. In addition, because the prevalence of sexual dysfunction in the nondepressed general population is high, linking sexual dysfunction to specific medications is difficult without population-based controls (S.A. Montgomery et al., 2002).

With the introduction and widespread use of SSRIs, the issue of medication-associated sexual dysfunction assumed greater clinical significance, particularly with respect to treatment compliance and quality-of-life concerns. In addition, in this context, the neurobiological overlap between sexual function, depression, and monoamine physiology is particularly keen.

Antidepressants may cause sexual side effects in the drive phase (for example, decreased libido—though this is difficult to distinguish from the decrease in sexual satisfaction associated with pervasive anhedonia); the arousal phase (for example, ED—though the relation to preexisting organic factors and to MDD complicates this association); and/or the release phase (for example, delayed orgasm or anorgasmia). With serotonergic medications, orgasmic delay appears to be most common, followed by decreased libido and then arousal difficulties. Painful and/or retrograde ejaculation occurs in some men taking tricyclic antidepressants (TCAs) and antipsychotics; it may be related to adrenergic blockade. Estimates of SSRI-associated sexual side effects vary enormously—from less than 1% in postmarketing surveillance studies to greater than 50% in studies using systematic inquiries (Seidman, 2003). The most consistent estimates are that about one third of patients taking SSRIs develop sexual dysfunction. Sexual dysfunction is reported somewhat less frequently with monoamine oxidase inhibitors, even less often with TCAs, and rarely with nefazodone, bupropion, and mirtazepine.

Although low libido and ED are reported during SSRI treatment, the rates are not substantially different from base rates in the general population. In contrast, a significant proportion of patients taking SSRIs report problems occurring during the orgasm phase (that is, delayed ejaculation in men and anorgasmia in women); such problems are uncommon in the general population (Seidman, 2003). The presumed mechanism of orgasmic dysfunction is via 5-HT_2 receptor activation, which is inhibitory to ejaculation—through ascending serotonergic projections to the medial preoptic area and/or descending serotonergic pathways to the lumbosacral motor nuclei. Such activation apparently leads to an increase in genital sensory threshold and the experience of genital anesthesia. Some data suggest that SSRIs may affect sexual function via the reduced production of NO and through noradrenergic actions (Angulo et al., 2001). PDE-5s might have a prosexual effect via an impact on the NO system.

Strategies for treating SSRI-induced sexual dysfunction include (*1*) decreasing the dose, (*2*) waiting for tolerance to develop, (*3*) switching to an antidepressant that does not have sexual side effects (for example, nefazodone, bupropion, or mirtazepine), and/or (*4*) adding an "antidote." In anecdotal case reports, multiple antidotes have been reported, including the α_2-adrenergic receptor antagonist, yohimbine; the 5-HT_2 receptor antagonists, nefazodone and cyproheptadine; the 5-HT_3 receptor antagonist, granisetron; the DA agonist, amantadine; bupropion; buspirone; the PDE-5 inhibitor, sildenafil; psychostimulants and other agents, such as ginkgo biloba (Fava et al., 2006). In uncontrolled trials, "response" rates greater than 50% have been reported for many of these agents. All of these reports varied in dosing, follow-up, gender specificity, sexual dysfunction specificity, and methodology for determining sexual dysfunction remission. None of these strategies has achieved widespread clinical acceptance.

Of the placebo-controlled studies of antidotes for SSRI-associated sexual dysfunction, none has proved promising. Michelson and colleagues (2002) performed two placebo controlled trials in women with SSRI-associated sexual dysfunction: in one, amantadine and buspirone were not distinguishable from placebo (Michelson et al., 2000); in the other, olanzapine, mirtazepine, and yohimbine were not distinguishable from placebo. Similarly, systematic trials have not found bupropion SR, ephedrine, or gingko biloba more effective than placebo for SSRI-associated sexual dysfunction (Kang et al., 2002; Clayton et al., 2004; DeBattista et al., 2005). In one series of sildenafil studies, men who were taking SSRIs and reported treatment-emergent sexual dysfunction were randomized to receive either sildenafil or placebo, and sildenafil administration was associated with improvement in sexual dysfunction (Nurnberg et al., 2002; Nurnberg et al., 2003; Fava et al., 2006). Yet most of the enrolled men had multiple sexual problems at baseline (mean, > three problems). Thus, beyond the established efficacy of sildenafil for ED, specific improvement in ejaculatory delay could not be distinguished from improvement in erectile function in these samples. This is particularly important because for the majority of men with SSRI-induced sexual dysfunction, persistent ejaculatory delay despite improved ED appears to be the norm.

Finally, Seidman and colleagues (2003) treated 21 men with SSRI-related ejaculatory delay with higher than usual doses of sildenafil. Enrolled patients were instructed to use 25 mg of sildenafil 1 hour prior to sexual activity on at least two occasions. If this was not effective for the ejaculatory delay, they were instructed to increase the dose progressively up to a maximum of 200 mg. After the low-dose phase (< 100 mg), 12/14 who had comorbid ED at baseline achieved full ED remission; only 4/21 achieved improvement in ejaculatory delay. Sixteen patients with persistent ejaculatory delay were eligible for the high-dose phase: 5 withdrew from the study, 4 increased to a maximum dose of 150 mg, and 6 increased to a maximum dose of 200 mg. Of the 10 patients who had ejaculatory delay (and no ED) and who chose to take sildenafil (150–200 mg), 9 reported a significant clinical improvement in ejaculatory delay and 7 achieved full remission. These open data suggest that anorgasmia may require a higher sildenafil dose for response than does ED.

CONCLUSION

The association between sexual dysfunction and mental illness is complex and bidirectional, though precise causal relations remain unclear. Sexual dysfunction and the psychosocial distress that frequently accompanies it may precipitate the development of a mood disorder in individuals who are vulnerable, mood dysregulation may cause sexual dysfunction, or both conditions may coexist independently.

Greater attention should be paid to sexual problems in psychiatric patients. First, these patients are at high risk for developing sexual problems, due either to their illness or to medications used in its treatment. Second, sexual problems can seriously reduce the quality of life of these patients. Finally, there are new options available for managing these problems.

REFERENCES

American Psychiatric Association (2004) *Diagnostic and Statistical Manual of Mental Disorders* (4th ed.). Washington, DC: Author.

Angulo, J., Peiro, C., Sanchez-Ferrer, C.F., Gabancho, S., Cuevas, P., Gupta, S., and Saenz de Tejada, I. (2001) Differential effects of serotonin reuptake inhibitors on erectile responses, NO-production, and neuronal NO synthase expression in rat corpus cavernosum tissue. *Br. J. Pharmacol.* 134:1190–1194.

Araujo, A.B., Durante, R., Feldman, H.A., Goldstein, I., and McKinlay, J.B. (1998) The relationship between depressive symptoms and male erectile dysfunction: Cross sectional results from the Massachusetts Male Aging Study. *Psychosom. Med.* 60:458–465.

Avis, N.E., Zhao, X., Johannes, C.B., Ory, M., Brockwell, S., and Greendale, G.A. (2005) Correlates of sexual function among multiethnic middle-aged women: results from the Study of Women's Health Across the Nation (SWAN). *Menopause* 12:385–398.

Bachmann, G., and Leiblum, S.R. (1991) Sexuality in sexagenarian women. *Maturitas* 13:45–50.

Bagatell, C.J., Heiman, J.R., Rivier, J.E., and Bremner, W.J. (1994) Effects of endogenous testosterone and estradiol on sexual behavior in normal young men. *J. Clin. Endocrinol. Metab.* 78:711–716.

Bancroft, J., and Cawood, E.H.H. (1996) Androgens and the menopause: A study of 40–60 year old women. *Clin. Endocrinol.* 45: 577–587.

Bancroft, J., Sanders, D., Davidson, D., and Warner, P. (1983) Mood, sexuality, hormones and the menstrual cycle: III. Sexuality and the role of androgens. *Psychosom. Med.* 45:509.

Basson, R. (2006a) Clinical practice. Sexual desire and arousal disorders in women. *N. Engl. J. Med.* 354:1497–1506.

Basson, R. (2006b) The complexities of women's sexuality and the menopause transition. *Menopause* 13:853–855.

Basson, R. (2007a) Hormones and sexuality: Current complexities and future directions. *Maturitas* 57:66–70.

Basson, R. (2007b) Sexuality in chronic illness: no longer ignored. *Lancet* 369:350–352.

Basson, R., and Brotto, L.A. (2003) Sexual psychophysiology and effects of sildenafil citrate in oestrogenised women with acquired genital arousal disorder and impaired orgasm: a randomised controlled trial. *BJOG* 110:1014–1024.

Basson, R., Leiblum, S., Brotto, L., Derogatis, L., Fourcroy, J., Fugl-Meyer, K., Graziottin, A., Heiman, J.R., Laan, E., Meston, C., Schover, L., van Lankveld, J., and Schultz, W.W. (2004) Revised definitions of women's sexual dysfunction. *J. Sex Med.* 1:40–48.

Basson, R., McInnes, R., Smith, M.D., Hodgson, G., Spain, T., and Koppiker, N. (2000) Efficacy and safety of sildenafil in estrogenized women with sexual dysfunction associated with female sexual arousal disorder. *Obstet. Gynecol.* 95:S54.

Basson, R., and Schultz, W.W. (2007) Sexual sequelae of general medical disorders. *Lancet* 369:409–424.

Berman, J.R., Berman, L.A., Toler, S.M., Gill, J., and Haughie, S. (2003) Safety and efficacy of sildenafil citrate for the treatment of female sexual arousal disorder: a double-blind, placebo controlled study. *J. Urol.* 170:2333–2338.

Bhasin, S., Enzlin, P., Coviello, A., and Basson, R. (2007) Sexual dysfunction in men and women with endocrine disorders. *Lancet* 369:597–611.

Bishop, J.R., Moline, J., Ellingrod, V.L., Schultz, S.K., and Clayton, A.H. (2006) Serotonin 2A-1438 G/A and G-protein Beta3 subunit C825T polymorphisms in patients with depression and SSRI-associated sexual side-effects. *Neuropsychopharmacol.* 31:2281–2288.

Braunstein, G.D., Sundwall, D.A., Katz, M., Shifren, J.L., Buster, J.E., Simon, J.A., Bachman, G., Aguirre, O.A., Lucas, J.D., Rodenberg, C., Buch, A., and Watts, N.B. (2005) Safety and efficacy of a testosterone patch for the treatment of hypoactive sexual desire disorder in surgically menopausal women: a randomized, placebo-controlled trial. *Arch. Intern. Med.* 165:1582–1589.

Buster, J.E., Kingsberg, S.A., Aguirre, O., Brown, C., Breaux, J.G., Buch, A., Rodenberg, C.A., Wekselman, K., and Casson, P. (2005) Testosterone patch for low sexual desire in surgically menopausal women: a randomized trial. *Obstet. Gynecol.* 105:944–952.

Clayton, A.H., Warnock, J.K., Kornstein, S.G., Pinkerton, R., Sheldon-Keller, A., and McGarvey, E.L. (2004) A placebo-controlled trial of bupropion SR as an antidote for selective serotonin reuptake inhibitor-induced sexual dysfunction. *J. Clin. Psychiatry* 65:62–67.

Davidson, J.M., and Rosen, R.C. (1992) Hormonal determinants of erectile function. In: Rosen, R.C., and Leiblum, S.R., eds. *Erectile Disorders: Assessment and Treatment.* New York: Guilford Press, pp. 72–95.

Davis, S.R., Davison, S.L., Donath, S., and Bell, R.J. (2005) Circulating androgen levels and self-reported sexual function in women. *JAMA* 294:91–96.

Davis, S.R., van der Mooren, M.J., van Lunsen, R.H., Lopes, P., Ribot, C., Rees, M., Moufarege, A., Rodenberg, C., Buch, A., and Purdie, D.W. (2006) Efficacy and safety of a testosterone patch for the treatment of hypoactive sexual desire disorder in surgically menopausal women: a randomized, placebo-controlled trial. *Menopause* 13:387–396.

de Jong, T.R., Veening, J.G., Olivier, B., and Waldinger, M.D. (2007) Oxytocin involvement in SSRI-induced delayed ejaculation: a review of animal studies. *J. Sex Med.* 4:14–28.

DeBattista, C., Solvason, B., Poirier, J., Kendrick, E., and Loraas, E. (2005) A placebo-controlled, randomized, double-blind study of adjunctive bupropion sustained release in the treatment of SSRI-induced sexual dysfunction. *J. Clin. Psychiatry* 66:844–848.

Fava, M., Nurnberg, H.G., Seidman, S.N., Holloway, W., Nicholas, S., Tseng, L.J., and Stecher, V.J. (2006) Efficacy and safety of sildenafil in men with serotonergic antidepressant-associated erectile dysfunction: results from a randomized, double-blind, placebo-controlled trial. *J. Clin. Psychiatry* 67:240–246.

Feder, H.H. (1984) Hormones and sexual behavior. *Ann. Rev. Psychol.* 35:165–200.

Feldman, H.A., Goldstein, I., Hatzichristou, D.G., Krane, R.J., and McKinlay, J.B. (1994) Impotence and its medical and psychosocial correlates: results of the Massachusetts Male Aging Study. *J. Urol.* 151:54–61.

Feldman, H.A., Longcope, C., Derby, C.A., Johannes, C.B., Araujo, A.B., Coviello, A.D., Bremner, W.J., and McKinlay, J.B. (2002) Age trends in the level of serum testosterone and other hormones in middle-aged men: longitudinal results from the Massachusetts male aging study. *J. Clin. Endocrinol. Metab.* 87:589–598.

Giuliano, F., and Clement, P. (2005) Physiology of ejaculation: emphasis on serotonergic control. *Eur. Urol.* 48:408–417.

Giuliano, F., and Clement, P. (2006) Serotonin and premature ejaculation: from physiology to patient management. *Eur. Urol.* 50:454–466.

Goldstat, R., Briganti, E., Tran, J., Wolfe, R., and Davis, S.R. (2003) Transdermal testosterone therapy improves well-being, mood, and sexual function in premenopausal women. *Menopause* 10:390–398.

Halpern, C.T., Udry, J.R., and Suchindran, C. (1997) Testosterone predicts initiation of coitus in adolescent females. *Psychosom. Med.* 59:161–171.

Haslam, M.T. (1975) Psycho-sexual disorders and their treatment: Part II. *Curr. Med. Res. Opin.* 3:51–62.

Hull, E.M., Lorrain, D.S., Du, J., Matuszewich, L., Lumley, L.A., Putnam, S.K., and Moses, J. (1999) Hormone-neurotransmitter interactions in the control of sexual behavior. *Behav. Brain Res.* 105:105–116.

Kang, B.J., Lee, S.J., Kim, M.D., and Cho, M.J. (2002) A placebo-controlled, double-blind trial of ginkgo biloba for antidepressant-induced sexual dysfunction. *Hum. Psychopharmacol.* 17:279–284.

Karama, S., Lecours, A.R., Leroux, J.M., Bourgouin, P., Beaudoin, G., Joubert, S., and Beauregard, M. (2002) Areas of brain activation in males and females during viewing of erotic film excerpts. *Hum. Brain Mapp.* 16:1–13.

Kemper, T.D. (1990) *Social Structure and Testosterone.* New Brunswick, NJ: Rutgers University Press.

Kenemans, P., and Speroff, L. (2005) Tibolone: clinical recommendations and practical guidelines. A report of the International Tibolone Consensus Group. *Maturitas* 51:21–28.

Laumann, E.O., Paik, A., Glasser, D.B., Kang, J.H., Wang, T., Levinson, B., Moreira, E.D., Jr., Nicolosi, A., and Gingell, C. (2006) A cross-national study of subjective sexual well-being among older women and men: findings from the Global Study of Sexual Attitudes and Behaviors. *Arch. Sex Behav.* 35:145–161.

Leiblum, S.R., Bachmann, G., Kemmann, E., Colburn, D., and Schwartzman, L. (1983) Vaginal atrophy in the postmenopausal woman: The importance of sexual activity and hormones. *JAMA* 249:2195–2198.

Lewis, R.W., Fugl-Meyer, K.S., Bosch, R., Fugl-Meyer, A.R., Laumann, E.O., Lizza, E., and Martin-Morales, A. (2004) Epidemiology/risk factors of sexual dysfunction. *J. Sex Med.* 1:35–39.

Lue, T.F., Giuliano, F., Montorsi, F., Rosen, R.C., Andersson, K.E., Althof, S., Christ, G., Hatzichristou, D., Hirsch, M., Kimoto, Y., Lewis, R., McKenna, K., MacMahon, C., Morales, A., Mulcahy, J., Padma-Nathan, H., Pryor, J., de Tejada, I.S., Shabsigh, R., and Wagner, G. (2004) Summary of the recommendations on sexual dysfunctions in men. *J. Sex Med.* 1:6–23.

McKenna, K.E. (2001) Neural circuitry involved in sexual function. *J. Spinal Cord. Med.* 24:148–154.

McKenna, K.E. (2002) The neurophysiology of female sexual function. *World J. Urol.* 20:93–100.

McNicholas, T.A., Dean, J.D., Mulder, H., Carnegie, C., and Jones, N.A. (2003) A novel testosterone gel formulation normalizes androgen levels in hypogonadal men, with improvements in body composition and sexual function. *Br. J. Urol.* 91:69–74.

Meston, C.M., and Frohlich, P.F. (2000) The neurobiology of sexual function. *Arch. Gen. Psychiatry* 57:1012–1030.

Michael, R.P., Rees, H.D., and Bonsall, R.W. (1989) Sites in the male primate brain at which testosterone acts as an androgen. *Brain Res.* 502:11–20.

Michelson, D., Bancroft, J., Targum, S., Kim, Y., and Tepner, R. (2000) Female sexual dysfunction associated with antidepressant administration: a randomized, placebo-controlled study of pharmacologic intervention. *Am. J. Psychiatry* 157:239–243.

Michelson, D., Kociban, K., Tamura, R., and Morrison, M.F. (2002) Mirtazapine, yohimbine or olanzapine augmentation therapy for serotonin reuptake-associated female sexual dysfunction: a randomized, placebo controlled trial. *J. Psychiatr. Res.* 36:147–152.

Montgomery, J.C., Appleby, L., Brincat, M., et al. (1987) Effect of oestrogen and testosterone implants on psychological disorders of the climacteric. *Lancet* 339:297–299.

Montgomery, S.A., Baldwin, D.S., and Riley, A. (2002) Antidepressant medications: a review of the evidence for drug-induced sexual dysfunction. *J. Affect. Disord.* 69:119–140.

Myers, L.S., Dixen, J., Morrissette, D., Carmichael, M., and Davidson, J.M. (1990) Effect of oestrogen, androgen, and progestin on sexual psychophysiology and behavior in postmenopausal women: A comparative study. *J. Clin. Endocrinol. Metab.* 70:1124–1131.

Nicolosi, A., Laumann, E.O., Glasser, D.B., Brock, G., King, R., and Gingell, C. (2006) Sexual activity, sexual disorders and associated help-seeking behavior among mature adults in five Anglophone countries from the Global Survey of Sexual Attitudes and Behaviors (GSSAB). *J. Sex Marital Ther.* 32:331–342.

Nofzinger, E.A., Thase, M.E., Reynolds, C.F. III, Frank, E., Jennings, J.R., Garamoni, G.L., Fasiczka, A.L., and Kupfer, D.J. (1993) Sexual function in depressed men. Assessment by self-report, behavioral, and nocturnal penile tumescence measures before and after treatment with cognitive behavior therapy. *Arch. Gen. Psychiatry* 50:24–30.

Nurnberg, H.G., Hensley, P.L., Gelenberg, A.J., Fava, M., Lauriello, J., and Paine, S. (2003) Treatment of antidepressant-associated sexual dysfunction with sildenafil: a randomized controlled trial. *JAMA* 289:56–64.

Nurnberg, H.G., Seidman, S.N., Gelenberg, A.J., Fava, M., Rosen, R., and Shabsigh, R. (2002) Depression, antidepressant therapies, and erectile dysfunction: clinical trials of sildenafil citrate (Viagra®) in treated and untreated patients with depression. *Urology* 60:58–66.

O'Carroll, R., and Bancroft, J. (1984) Testosterone therapy for low sexual interest and erectile dysfunction in men: a controlled study. *Br. J. Psychiatry* 145:146–151.

Osmanagaoglu, M.A., Atasaral, T., Baltaci, D., and Bozkaya, H. (2006) Effect of different preparations of hormone therapy on sexual dysfunction in naturally postmenopausal women. *Climacteric* 9:464–472.

Persky, H., Dreisibach, L., Miller, W.R., et al. (1982) The relation of plasma androgen levels to sexual behaviors and attitudes of women. *Psychosom. Med.* 44:305–319.

Pfaus, J.G. (1999) Neurobiology of sexual behavior. *Curr. Opin. Neurobiol.* 9:751–758.

Pope, H.G.J., Cohane, G.H., Kanayama, G., Siegel, A.J., and Hudson, J.I. (2003) Testosterone gel supplementation for men with refractory depression: a randomized, placebo-controlled trial. *Am. J. Psychiatry* 160:105–111.

Pope, H.G.J., Kouri, E.M., and Hudson, J.I. (2000) Effects of supraphysiologic doses of testosterone on mood and aggression in normal men. A randomized controlled trial. *Arch. Gen. Psychiatry* 57:133–140.

Pryor, J.L., Althof, S.E., Steidle, C., Rosen, R.C., Hellstrom, W.J., Shabsigh, R., Miloslavsky, M., and Kell, S. (2006) Efficacy and tolerability of dapoxetine in treatment of premature ejaculation: an integrated analysis of two double-blind, randomised controlled trials. *Lancet* 368:929–937.

Putnam, S.K., Du, J., Sato, S., and Hull, E.M. (2000) Testosterone restoration of copulatory behavior correlates with medial preoptic dopamine release in castrated male rats. *Horm. Behav.* 39: 216–224.

Rabkin, J.G., Wagner, G., and Rabkin, R. (2000) A double-blind, placebo-controlled trial of testosterone therapy for HIV-positive men with hypogonadal symptoms. *Arch. Gen. Psychiatry* 57: 141–147.

Roose, S.P., Glassman, A.H., Walsh, B.T., and Cullen, K. (1982) Reversible loss of nocturnal penile tumescence during depression: a preliminary report. *Neuropsychobiology* 8:284–288.

Rosen, R., Shabsigh, R., Berber, M., Assalian, P., Menza, M., Rodriguez-Vela, L., Porto, R., Bangerter, K., Seger, M., and Montorsi, F. (2006) Efficacy and tolerability of vardenafil in men with mild depression and erectile dysfunction: the depression-related improvement with vardenafil for erectile response study. *Am. J. Psychiatry* 163:79–87.

Rosen, R.C., Catania, J.A., Althof, S.E., Pollack, L.M., O'Leary, M., Seftel, A.D., and Coon, D.W. (2007) Development and validation of four-item version of Male Sexual Health Questionnaire to assess ejaculatory dysfunction. *Urology* 69:805–809.

Rosen, R.C., McMahon, C.G., Niederberger, C., Broderick, G.A., Jamieson, C., and Gagnon, D.D. (2007) Correlates to the clinical diagnosis of premature ejaculation: results from a large observational study of men and their partners. *J. Urol.* 177:1059–1064.

Rubinow, D.R., Schmidt, P.J., Roca, C.A., and Daly, R.C. (2002) Gonadal hormones and behavior in women: Concentrations versus context. In: Pfaff, D., Arnold, A.P., Etgen, A.M., Fahrbach, S.E., and Rubin, R.T., eds. *Hormones, Brain and Behavior*. New York: Academic Press, pp. 37–73.

Safarinejad, M.R. (2006) Comparison of dapoxetine versus paroxetine in patients with premature ejaculation: a double-blind, placebo-controlled, fixed-dose, randomized study. *Clin. Neuropharmacol.* 29:243–252.

Sand, R., and Studd, J.W.W. (1995) Exogenous androgens in postmenopausal women. *Am. J. Med.* 98:76S–79S.

Santoro, N., Torrens, J., Crawford, S., Allsworth, J.E., Finkelstein, J.S., Gold, E.B., Korenman, S., Lasley, W.L., Luborsky, J.L., McConnell, D., Sowers, M.F., and Weiss, G. (2005) Correlates of circulating androgens in mid-life women: the study of women's health across the nation. *J. Clin. Endocrinol. Metab.* 90:4836–4845.

Schiavi, R.C. (1994) Effect of chronic disease and medication on sexual functioning. In: Rossi, A.S., ed. *Sexuality Across the Life Course*. Chicago: University of Chicago Press, pp. 313–339.

Schiavi, R.C., Mandeli, J., Schreiner-Engel, P., and Chambers, A. (1991) Aging, sleep disorders, and male sexual function. *Biol. Psychiatry* 30:15–24.

Schiavi, R.C., White, D., Mandeli, J., and Levine, A.C. (1997) Effect of testosterone administration on sexual behavior and mood in men with erectile dysfunction. *Arch. Sex. Behav.* 26:231–241.

Schmidt, P.J., Berlin, K.L., Danaceau, M.A., Neeren, A., Haq, N.A., Roca, C.A., and Rubinow, D.R. (2004) The effects of pharmacologically induced hypogonadism on mood in healthy men. *Arch. Gen. Psychiatry* 61:997–1004.

Schreiner-Engel, P., and Schiavi, R.C. (1986) Lifetime psychopathology in individuals with low sexual desire. *J. Nerv. Ment. Dis.* 174:646–651.

Schreiner-Engel, P., Schiavi, R.C., Smith, H., and White, D. (1981) Sexual arousability and the menstrual cycle. *Psychosom. Med.* 43:199–214.

Segraves, K.B., and Segraves, R.T. (1991) Hypoactive sexual desire disorder: prevalence and comorbidity in 906 subjects. *J. Sex Marital Ther.* 17:55–58.

Segraves, R.T., Croft, H., Kavoussi, R., Ascher, J.A., Batey, S.R., Foster, V.J., Bolden-Watson, C., and Metz, A. (2001) Bupropion sustained release (SR) for the treatment of hypoactive sexual desire disorder (HSDD) in nondepressed women. *J. Sex Marital Ther.* 27:303–316.

Seidman, S.N. (2003) The aging male: androgens, erectile dysfunction, and depression. *J. Clin. Psychiatry* 64(Suppl 10):31–37.

Seidman, S.N., Araujo, A.B., Roose, S.P., Devanand, D.P., Xie, S., Cooper, T.B., and McKinlay, J.B. (2002) Low testosterone levels in elderly men with dysthymic disorder. *Am. J. Psychiatry* 159: 456–459.

Seidman, S.N., Miyazaki, M., and Roose, S.P. (2005) Intramuscular testosterone supplementation to selective serotonin reuptake inhibitor in treatment-resistant depressed men: randomized placebo-controlled clinical trial. *J. Clin. Psychopharmacol.* 25:584–588.

Seidman, S.N., Pesce, V.C., and Roose, S.P. (2003) High-dose sildenafil citrate for selective serotonin reuptake inhibitor-associated ejaculatory delay: open clinical trial. *J. Clin. Psychiatry* 64:721–725.

Seidman, S.N., and Rabkin, J.G. (1998) Testosterone replacement therapy for hypogonadal men with SSRI-refractory depression. *J. Affect. Disord.* 48:157–161.

Seidman, S.N., and Roose, S.P. (2000) The relationship between depression and erectile dysfunction. *Curr. Psychiatry Rep.* 2:201–205.

Seidman, S.N., Roose, S.P., Menza, M.A., Shabsigh, R., and Rosen, R.C. (2001) Treatment of erectile dysfunction in men with depressive symptoms: results of a placebo-controlled trial with sildenafil citrate. *Am. J. Psychiatry* 158:1623–1630.

Seidman, S.N., Spatz, E., Rizzo, C., and Roose, S.P. (2001) Testosterone replacement therapy for hypogonadal men with major depressive disorder: a randomized, placebo-controlled clinical trial. *J. Clin. Psychiatry* 62:406–412.

Shabsigh, R., Klein, L.T., Seidman, S.N., Kaplan, S.A., Lehrhoff, B.J., and Ritter, J.S. (1998) Increased incidence of depressive symptoms in men with erectile dysfunction. *Urology* 52:848–852.

Shabsigh, R., Seftel, A.D., Rosen, R.C., Porst, H., Ahuja, S., Deeley, M.C., Garcia, C.S., and Giuliano, F. (2006) Review of time of onset and duration of clinical efficacy of phosphodiesterase type 5 inhibitors in treatment of erectile dysfunction. *Urology* 68:689–696.

Sherwin, B.B. (1988) Affective changes with estrogen and androgen replacement therapy in surgically menopausal women. *J. Affect. Disord.* 14:177–187.

Sherwin, B.B. (2002) Randomized clinical trials of combined estrogen-androgen preparations: effects on sexual functioning. *Fertil. Steril.* 77(Suppl 4):S49–S54.

Shields, K.M., and Hrometz, S.L. (2006) Use of sildenafil for female sexual dysfunction. *Ann. Pharmacother.* 40:931–934.

Shifren, J.L., Davis, S.R., Moreau, M., Waldbaum, A., Bouchard, C., Derogatis, L., Derzko, C., Bearnson, P., Kakos, N., O'Neill, S., Levine, S., Wekselman, K., Buch, A., Rodenberg, C., and Kroll, R. (2006) Testosterone patch for the treatment of hypoactive sexual desire disorder in naturally menopausal women: results from the INTIMATE NM1 Study. *Menopause* 13:770–779.

Simon, J., Braunstein, G., Nachtigall, L., Utian, W., Katz, M., Miller, S., Waldbaum, A., Bouchard, C., Derzko, C., Buch, A., Rodenberg, C., Lucas, J., and Davis, S. (2005) Testosterone patch increases sexual activity and desire in surgically menopausal women with hypoactive sexual desire disorder. *J. Clin. Endocrinol. Metab.* 90:5226–5233.

Simons, J.S., and Carey, M.P. (2001) Prevalence of sexual dysfunctions: results from a decade of research. *Arch. Sex. Behav.* 30: 177–219.

Somboonporn, W., Davis, S., Seif, M.W., and Bell, R. (2005) Testosterone for peri- and postmenopausal women. *Cochrane Database Syst. Rev.* 4:CD004509.

Steidle, C., Schwartz, S., Jacoby, K., Sebree, T., Smith, T., and Bachand, R. (2003) AA2500 testosterone gel normalizes androgen levels in aging males with improvements in body composition and sexual function. *J. Clin. Endocrinol. Metab.* 88:2673–2681.

Steiger, A., Holsboer, F., and Benkert, O. (1993) Studies of nocturnal penile tumescence and sleep electroencephalogram in patients with major depression and in normal controls. *Acta Psychiatr. Scand.* 87:358–363.

Thase, M.E., Reynolds, C.F. III, Jennings, J.R., Frank, E., Garamoni, G.L., Nofzinger, E.A., Fascizka, A.L., and Kupfer, D.J. (1992) Diminished nocturnal penile tumescence in depression: a replication study. *Biol. Psychiatry* 31:1136–1142.

Thase, M.E., Reynolds, C.F. III, Jennings, J.R., Frank, E., Howell, J.R., Houck, P.R., Berman, S., and Kupfer, D.J. (1988) Nocturnal penile tumescence is diminished in depressed men. *Biol. Psychiatry* 24:33–46.

Üçok, A., İncesu, C., Aker, T., and Erkoç, S. (2007) Sexual dysfunction in patients with schizophrenia on antipsychotic medication. *Eur. Psychiatry* 22(5):328–333.

van Lankveld, J.J., and Grotjohann, Y. (2000) Psychiatric comorbidity in heterosexual couples with sexual dysfunction assessed with the composite international diagnostic interview. *Arch. Sex Behav.* 29:479–498.

van Lunsen, R.H., and Laan, E. (2004) Genital vascular responsiveness and sexual feelings in midlife women: psychophysiologic, brain, and genital imaging studies. *Menopause* 11:741–748.

Waldinger, M.D. (2007) Premature ejaculation: definition and drug treatment. *Drugs* 67:547–568.

Waldinger, M.D., and Schweitzer, D.H. (2005) Retarded ejaculation in men: an overview of psychological and neurobiological insights. *World J. Urol.* 23:76–81.

Waldinger, M.D., and Schweitzer, D.H. (2007) The DSM-IV-TR is an inadequate diagnostic tool for premature ejaculation. *J. Sex Med.* 4:822–823.

Waldinger, M.D., Schweitzer, D.H., and Olivier, B. (2006) Dapoxetine treatment of premature ejaculation. *Lancet* 368:1869–1870.

Wallen, K., Eisler, J.A., Tannenbaum, P.L., Nagell, K.M., and Mann, D.R. (1991) Antide (Nal-Lys GnRH antagonist) suppression of pituitary-testicular function and sexual behavior in group-living rhesus monkeys. *Physiol. Behav.* 50:429–435.

Wang, C., Cunningham, G., Dobs, A., Iranmanesh, A., Matsumoto, A.M., Snyder, P.J., Weber, T., Berman, N., Hull, L., and Swerdloff, R.S. (2004) Long-term testosterone gel (AndroGel) treatment maintains beneficial effects on sexual function and mood, lean and fat mass, and bone mineral density in hypogonadal men. *J. Clin. Endocrinol. Metab.* 89:2085–2098.

Wang, W.F., Wang, Y., Minhas, S., and Ralph, D.J. (2007) Can sildenafil treat primary premature ejaculation? A prospective clinical study. *Int. J. Urol.* 14:331–335.

Werneke, U., Northey, S., and Bhugra, D. (2006) Antidepressants and sexual dysfunction. *Acta Psychiatr. Scand.* 114:384–397.

West, S.L., Vinikoor, L.C., and Zolnoun, D. (2004) A systematic review of the literature on female sexual dysfunction prevalence and predictors. *Annu. Rev. Sex Res.* 15:40–172.

Wierman, M.E., Basson, R., Davis, S.R., Khosla, S., Miller, K.K., Rosner, W., and Santoro, N. (2006) Androgen therapy in women: an Endocrine Society Clinical Practice guideline. *J. Clin. Endocrinol. Metab.* 91:3697–3710.

83 The Neurobiology of Social Attachment

THOMAS R. INSEL AND JAMES T. WINSLOW

Beginning with Bowlby's seminal contributions, attachment and separation have become familiar theoretical components of ego psychology, developmental psychology, and psychodynamic theory (Bowlby, 1982). Early descriptions of the devastating consequences of social neglect on development in humans (Spitz, 1946) and nonhuman primates (Harlow and Mears, 1979) provided the impetus for attempts to understand the importance of attachment for normal psychological development. A subsequent generation of studies used a structured interview, the Ainsworth Strange Situation, to define individual differences in patterns of attachment and to investigate the relationship of individual attachment styles to subsequent personality variables (Waters and Sroufe, 1983). In spite of progress in understanding the psychological aspects of attachment, we know relatively little about the neurobiological basis of social attachment. If one considers that abnormal social attachments characterize virtually every form of psychopathology, it seems especially remarkable that the chemistry, the anatomy, and the physiology of social bond formation remain largely unexplored. To be sure, there is a considerable literature on the neurobiology and psychobiology of separation (Kraemer, 1992), but this work may not prove instructive for understanding social bond formation. Attachment is not simply the absence of separation. Accordingly, there is no obvious reason why attachment and separation should be subserved by the same neural pathways.

The behavioral process of attachment is undoubtedly complex, involving such disparate experiences as an infant bonding to his or her mother and two adults falling in love. In spite of their complexity, these diverse behavioral processes should be amenable to neurobiological study because (*1*) attachment (even adult–adult pair bond formation) is not unique to humans and (*2*) each of the forms of attachment can be defined operationally as several discrete, quantifiable behaviors (Table 83.1). These behaviors, like other reproductive behaviors, are critical for species survival; thus, one might expect to find his or her neural substrates highly conserved phylogenetically. Paradoxically, attachment behaviors show profound species differences even between closely related species. Infant attachment, for example, varies between altricial species requiring extensive parental support and precocial species that are relatively independent from the day of birth. Maternal behavior varies from a few minutes of nursing each day (as in rabbits and tree shrews) to nearly continuous contact (as in most primates). And pair bonding (that is, long-term, selective adult–adult attachment) may be restricted to monogamous species, rare in mammals but common among birds. For neurobiologists, these phylogenetic variations provide the opportunity for comparative studies, allowing differences in anatomy and physiology to be correlated with differences in behavior.

This review describes recent neurobiological research on three forms of attachment: infant–mother, mother–infant, and pair bonding (Insel and Young, 2001). In each case, a summary of the neurobiological literature is provided, with attempts to relate these findings to human studies. But first, a comment on the social brain.

IS THERE A SOCIAL BRAIN?

A major debate in systems neuroscience has focused on the existence of modules in the brain, specifically neural systems dedicated to categorical information. Clearly,

TABLE 83.1 *Measures of Mammalian Attachment Behavior*

Dyad	*Operant Measures for Assessment*
Infant–parent	Cling, suckle, separation response
Mother–infant	Nursing, retrieval, nest building, grooming, defense, separation response
Father–infant	Retrieval, nest building, defense, separation grooming, response
Male–female	Shared territory, cohabitation partner preference, mate guarding, separation response
Male–male/ female–female	Reciprocal grooming, proximity, defense

there are systems for sensory processing (for example, visual and auditory pathways) and for motor control, but are there modules for processing higher-order information such as social information? Or, to put the question more succinctly, are we wired for social behavior?

In humans and nonhuman primates, there are brain regions uniquely activated by faces. The fusiform area in the most posterior aspects of the inferior temporal lobe of the human brain is important for face recognition (Kanwisher et al., 1997; Johnson et al., 2005; McKone et al., 2007). Lesions of this area result in prosopagnosia, an inability to recognize faces, and neuroimaging studies demonstrate activation of this region and of the amygdala when people look at faces.

In monkeys, functional magnetic resonance imaging (fMRI) and neurophysiological studies have similarly identified specific regions and select cells within the superior temporal sulcus of the temporal lobe that are activated by faces and social gaze (Pinsk et al., 2005; Afraz et al., 2006; Tsao et al., 2006; see also Emery, 2000). Furthermore, stimulation of cells in this region appears to bias categorization of ambiguous cues as facial cues. Facial expression and other facial information from temporal cortical regions appear to be integrated in nuclei of the amygdala (Gothard et al., 2007).

Although these findings have suggested to some that the brain comes equipped with social domain-specific cells, others have suggested that so-called face cells are not specific for faces. Imaging studies have shown that the fusiform area responds when people look at any category of information that has been organized into many subcategories or individual elements. For instance, most people use this region when looking at pictures of faces, but birders also activate this same region when looking at pictures of birds and realtors when looking at pictures of houses (Gauthier et al., 2000). Indeed, Gauthier has shown that the fusiform region is recruited when subjects are taught to identify many individuals in a collection of greebles, tiny play figures each with unique characteristics (Gauthier et al., 1999; Bukach et al., 2006). The notion, then, is that the brain may have modules that respond to complex categories, of which social information is an important example.

Mindful of this continuing controversy, we can nevertheless be confident that face recognition is likely distinct from object recognition and that the temporal cortex and amygdala are intimately involved in processing social information (Haxby, 2006; Gothard et al., 2007; Hoffman et al., 2007). Certainly in rodents and many other olfactory mammals, there is an entire neural system dedicated to processing pheromones, nonvolatile olfactory signals communicating reproductive and social status (Brennan and Kendrick, 2006). In the primate brain, which is more visual than olfactory, one should not be surprised to find pathways that process complex social information, and one need not be concerned that these same pathways can also process other kinds of information.

Recent studies in nonprimates have taken the social brain concept one step further by looking for genes critical for social behavior. In mice, genes have been identified for social subordination (Long et al., 2004), for social recognition (Ferguson et al., 2000; Bielsky et al., 2005), and even for recognizing the gender of a social companion (Stowers et al., 2002).

The study of social recognition is intriguing in that mice with a knockout of the gene for oxytocin (Ferguson et al., 2000; Choleris et al., 2006) or for the vasopressin V1A receptor (Bielsky et al., 2005) were able to form nonsocial memories but, like people with prosopagnosia, showed a selective deficit in social recognition. This deficit could be completely rescued by injecting oxytocin into the amygdala (Ferguson et al., 2001) or by replacing V1A receptors in the septum (Bielsky et al., 2005; Fig. 83.1).

Although it may seem unlikely that a single gene would code for social memory, an even more remarkable study in the lowly nematode, *Caenorhabditis elegans*, identified a single polymorphism in a neuropeptide receptor gene that separated strains that feed as solitary worms from those that feed socially (de Bono and Bargmann, 1998). That is, a single base change in this species appears responsible for profound differences in social organization. Similarly, the presence or absence of variations in the promoter region of a vasopressin receptor gene may predict monogamy in different species of vole and within the prairie vole: differences in the length of "inserts" in the vasopressin receptor gene appear to account for individual differences in sociality and attachment (Hammock and Young, 2005).

The emerging fields of social neuroscience (Cacioppo, 1994) and sociogenomics (Robinson, 1999) will be identifying genes, proteins, and pathways for social cognition and social behavior. As social behavior has been critical for natural selection, the brain has no doubt evolved to support reproductive and agonistic functions. As a result, we may discover that ostensibly complicated behaviors such as aspects of social organization have relatively simple or at least simply defined molecular and cellular mechanisms.

INFANT ATTACHMENT

The study of attachment in infancy forms the basis of most of what we know about the behavioral process of bonding. Studies of imprinting in birds (Bateson, 1966), early olfactory learning in rabbits (Hudson, 1993), and the development of affectional bonds in nonhuman primates (Harlow and Suomi, 1970) have yielded a rich literature on the process by which the newborn forms a selective attachment to its mother. From a neurobio-

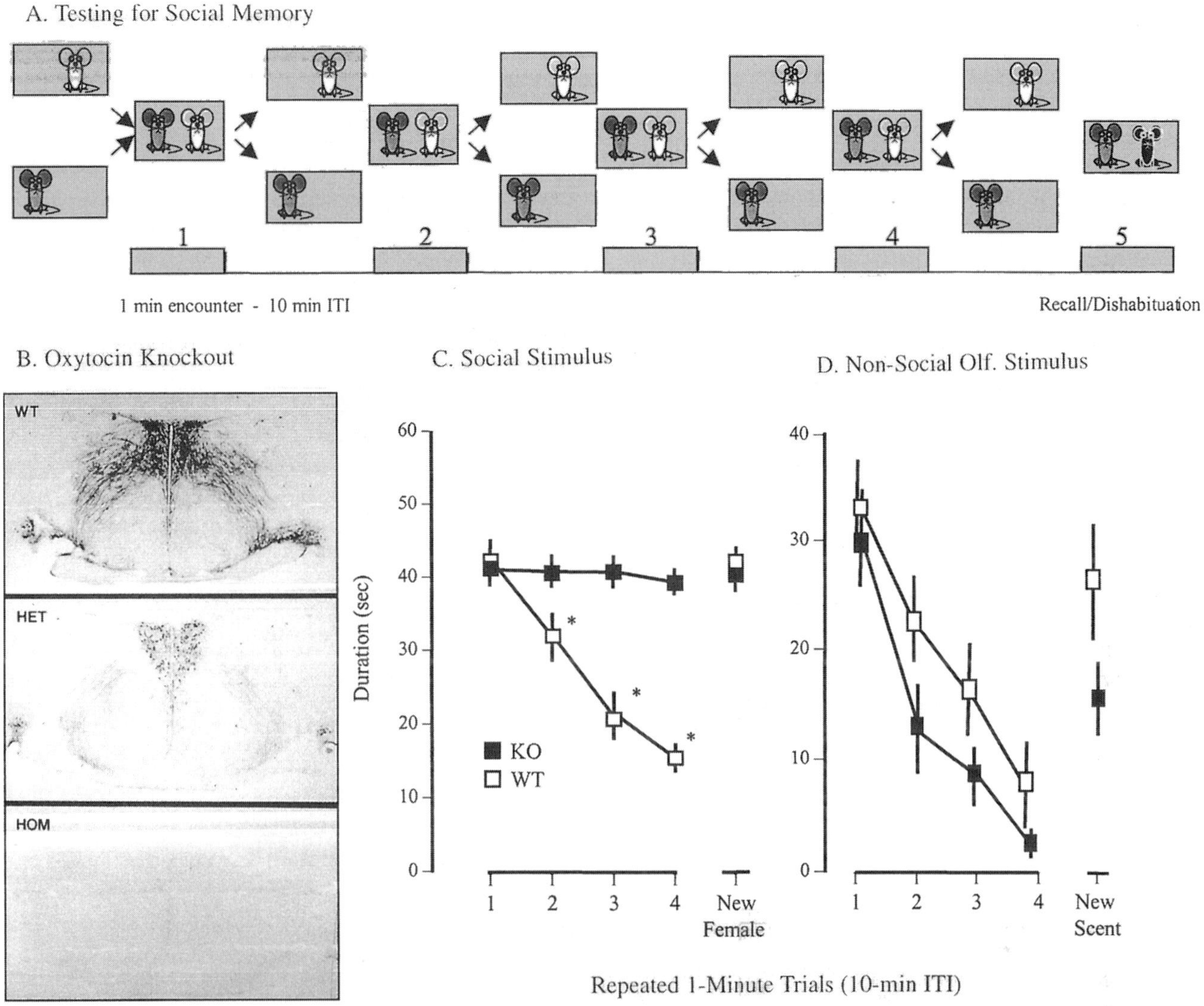

FIGURE 83.1 Social amnesia in an oxytocin knockout (KO) mouse. Social memory in mice can be assessed by repeated tests of social investigation. As shown in *A*, a test mouse is exposed to a novel intruder mouse for 1 minute, then separated for 10 minutes and retested. The time spent investigating the same intruder is compared across four trials. In a fifth trial, a novel intruder mouse is used. In *B*, immunocytochemical staining for oxytocin is shown in the hypothalamus of wild-type (WT), heterozygous (HET), and homozygous (HOM) oxytocin KO mice. In C, using the test for social memory, WT mice show the expected decrease in social investigation over repeated exposures to the same intruder, indicating social recognition. By contrast, oxytocin KO mice show no evidence of recognition, as investigation time does not decrease over repeated trials. WT and KO mice show the expected recognition of a nonsocial stimulus (cotton ball scented with lemon) presented in an identical paradigm. It appears that social memory is distinct from other kinds of memory and that oxytocin is necessary for development of a social memory.

logical perspective, we know more about separation than attachment, but three insights promise to be helpful for future studies of how infants form attachments to their caregivers.

First, we know that learning can occur prenatally. Studies of the rat fetus demonstrate unambiguous evidence of classical conditioning (Smotherman and Robinson, 1994). Of course, the length of gestation and the maturity of the newborn vary greatly across mammals. In the rat, gestation lasts 22 days, and a considerable proportion of brain development occurs postnatally. By contrast, in the development of the human brain, most neurogenesis is complete early in the second trimester of gestation, and much of the elaboration and sculpting of connectivity occurs in the third trimester. Thus, relative to the rat fetus, there may be even more opportunity for prenatal influences on brain and cognitive development in humans. Indeed, this may explain the observation that newborn human infants orient selectively to the sound of their mother's voice (DeCasper and Spence, 1986). It is certainly possible that many of the affectional ties to the mother observed postnatally could be laid down by prenatal experience. Although the human neonate may orient toward maternal cues, most research suggests that if attachment is defined as the selective preference for a single caregiver, then attachment in our species first develops in the second half of the first year.

How infants recognize and develop affiliative preferences for their mothers has been a fruitful area of investigation. For most mammalian infants, the first preference is olfactory. Newborns appear to recognize and preferentially approach sources of maternal scent. The olfactory system matures before the visual and auditory systems, and the process by which early olfactory experience (amniotic fluid, maternal scents, nest odors) leaves lasting imprints on the developing limbic system has been a focus of considerable research (Leon, 1992). These studies have demonstrated the importance of the noradrenergic innervation of the olfactory bulbs, as propranolol reduces and isoproterenol facilitates olfactory learning in the rat pup (Sullivan et al., 1989). Indeed, recent studies suggest that maturation of norepinephrine (NE) connections between the olfactory bulbs, the locus ceruleus, and the amygdala may control the duration of the sensitive period for learning maternal scent (Moriceau and Sullivan, 2005; Moriceau et al., 2006).

In addition, dopaminergic pathways may be recruited, particularly in the consolidation of memories of odor associations, since administration of a dopamine (DA) D_1 antagonist immediately after stimulus pairing blocks the development of odor preference (Leon, 1992). Oxytocin has also been implicated in the formation of maternal-associated olfactory cues (Nelson and Panksepp, 1996). This approach offers an important new perspective on infant–mother attachment focused on recognition and the development of a selective preference, a necessary precondition for the formation of a mother–infant bond.

Finally, Hofer and his colleagues have suggested that the process of mother–infant attachment, which superficially appears relatively simple in a rat, actually involves several independent physiological processes in which the mother serves as a "hidden regulator" for the infant (Hofer, 1984). In a sense, this early postnatal period might be considered extrauterine gestation, with the infant's heart rate, respiratory rate, rate of protein synthesis, and endocrine status under subtle but pervasive maternal control. What is particularly fascinating about this model is the implication that dysregulation between mother and infant could occur in a discrete aspect of function even though no loss or separation is apparent. That is, if a rat mother fails to groom her infant, the pup might show a decreased rate of protein synthesis but a normal heart rate and a normal corticosterone concentration (Schanberg and Field, 1987). Conversely, nongrooming maternal contact appears to be critical for stabilizing the corticosterone level but not for several other physiological indices (Stanton et al., 1987). The way in which maternal behavior and infant physiology interact is no doubt reciprocal and largely dependent on the infant's stage of development.

In a program of elegant studies, Meaney and his colleagues have shown that rat mothers vary naturally in the amount of grooming they provide to their pups and that this difference in grooming has long-term consequences for the behavior of their offspring (for recent review, see Meaney, 2001). The adult offspring of high-grooming mothers are less fearful, less responsive to stress, and have more brain glucocorticoid and benzodiazepine receptors than offspring of low-grooming mothers (Liu et al., 1997). Cross-fostering studies have shown that these differences are due to the rearing condition and not to a genetic difference in high-grooming and low-grooming rats. Indeed, the biological offspring of low-grooming mothers, when raised by a high-grooming mother, not only show the expected decrease in fearfulness, they also show increased grooming of their own pups, providing a nongenomic mechanism for the transmission of behavior across generations (Francis et al., 1999). Recently, these efforts have focused on the molecular mechanisms mediating epigenetic transmission of persistent, intergenerational alterations in the behavioral phenotype of affected animals. Convergent evidence indicates that differing maternal care influences methylation patterns in the chromatin of promoter regions of genes responsible for glucocorticoid receptor expression (Meaney and Szyf, 2005; Weaver et al., 2007). These ingenious studies provide critically important insights about the interaction of gene and experience in the development of neural processes.

Neuroanatomy

The neurobiological data on infant attachment, though scant, focus on the critical stage of olfactory learning, possibly mediated by noradrenergic fibers to the olfactory bulb (Moriceau and Sullivan, 2005). In the primate infant, visual cues no doubt prove important, and the identification of face cells in the inferior temporal cortex early in infancy may be an important substrate for the formation of a selective preference (Rodman et al., 1993). We know considerably more about the neuroanatomical substrates of the infant's separation response. Interestingly, neurophysiological recording and stimulation studies point to the anterior cingulate cortex as a site for the generation of separation calls (Maclean and Newman, 1988). This same area has been shown to be activated by painful stimuli, suggesting that in infancy, and possibly in later life, separation may activate pathways important for pain as well as anxiety, providing a mechanism for the amelioration of the separation distress by opiates (Craig et al., 1996).

Clinical Correlate—Autism

Of particular relevance to the discussion of infant attachment, children with autism frequently fail to develop the recognition and preferential attachment to parental stimuli that is so basic to normal development in primate infants. This deficit in attachment is probably not due to the mental retardation present in 75% of children with autism because infants with other disorders with comparable retardation, such as Down syndrome, exhibit abundant affiliative behavior. The deficits in social attachment in autism may be fundamental to this disorder (Fein et al., 1986). Without a clear picture of the neural substrates of normal infant attachment, the suspects for explaining abnormal attachment remain entirely speculative.

Many of the genes and pathways described above for the social brain have been investigated. Recent findings suggest that hypoactivation of the fusiform area reported when people with autism look at pictures of faces (Schultz et al., 2000; Dalton et al., 2005) may represent deficits in gaze fixation, and these in turn may reflect differences in the way faces are processed by their amygdala (Dalton et al., 2005; Bachevalier and Loveland, 2006). At a neurochemical level, oxytocin (along with NE) appears important for processing social information. Mice with a null deletion of oxytocin cannot process social information (Ferguson et al., 2000), monkeys with autistic features show a reduction in cerebrospinal fluid (CSF) oxytocin (Winslow et al., 2003), and oxytocin concentrations in plasma are reduced in autism (Modahl et al., 1998), but there is still no strong evidence that oxytocin is involved in the pathophysiology of this disorder. Finally, a considerable literature implicates serotonin in autism. Serotonergic lesions reduce separation distress in rat pups (Winslow and Insel, 1990). In several studies of autism, whole blood serotonin is reduced (Cook, 1990), but the relationship of this change to brain serotonergic pathways remains to be demonstrated.

PARENTAL BEHAVIOR

Although research on attachment has focused primarily on the infant's bond to the mother (or other primary caregiver), the parent's bond to the infant is of equal importance. Because in most mammals the female parent provides most if not all of the care, studies of maternal behavior can provide an important perspective on the neurobiology of attachment. The laboratory rat has been an ideal subject for studies of maternal care (Numan, 1994). Unlike many mammals, female rats show little interest in infants of their own species until just before parturition. About a day prior to delivery, they shift from avoiding pups to showing intense interest, with avid nest building, retrieval, grooming, and defense of young. These behaviors persist throughout the period of lactation, then abate with weaning. Rats, therefore, provide an opportunity to study two quite distinct aspects of maternal care: its onset and maintenance. For studies of attachment, the transition from avoidance to intense interest is of particular importance.

Oxytocin

Oxytocin, a nine amino acid neuropeptide important for labor and nursing, has also been implicated in the neural mediation of maternal behavior. The traditional view of oxytocin as an endocrine hormone acting on peripheral organs has recently been revised to consider this peptide as a neurotransmitter with central actions. Not only do hypothalamic cells synthesizing oxytocin project to diverse sites within the brain and brain stem, but receptors have been found throughout the limbic system in the forebrain and autonomic centers in the brain stem (Barberis and Tribollet, 1996). Furthermore, oxytocin is released within the brain following chemical depolarization of the appropriate neurons, and fibers have been demonstrated at the ultrastructural level to make synaptic contacts in the central nervous system (CNS) (Buijs and van Heerikhuize, 1982). Thus, the evidence is quite strong that the brain is a target organ for oxytocin.

Several investigators have reported that oxytocin given centrally to estrogen-primed nulliparous female rats facilitates the onset of maternal behavior. In the first such report, Pedersen and Prange (1979) noted that the effect was specific to oxytocin (the only other neuropeptide with significant albeit weaker effects was vasopressin) and rapid (onset within 30 minutes). Perhaps even more remarkable, blockade of oxytocin neurotransmission with central injection of an antagonist or antiserum, or by lesions of oxytocin-producing cells in the hypothalamus, results in a significant inhibition of maternal behavior (Insel, 1992). These various interventions appear to inhibit the onset but not the maintenance of maternal behavior. An oxytocin antagonist or a lesion has no effect on maternal care once a female begins to show interest in pups (Insel, 1992). These results support the notion that oxytocin is necessary for the transition from maternal avoidance to attachment to pups and that a central increase in oxytocin given under the appropriate gonadal steroid conditions might facilitate the onset of maternal care. In a sense, the role of oxytocin in the uterus and mammary tissue for providing the physiological support of the offspring is matched by a role in the brain for subserving the motivational changes essential for maternal care.

Oxytocin function in the rat brain is regulated at several levels by estrogen. Estrogen (interacting with progesterone) induces oxytocin gene expression in the hypothalamus (Crowley et al., 1995). In addition, estrogen regulates the number of oxytocin receptors, not only in the uterus and mammary myoepithelium but also in a few discrete nuclei in the brain (Insel, 1992). The physiological changes in gonadal steroids that occur during pregnancy appear to be sufficient, as oxytocin receptors increase in two key limbic brain regions—the bed nucleus of the stria terminalis and the ventromedial nucleus of the hypothalamus—at or just before parturition, coincident with the onset of maternal behavior (Winslow and Insel, 1990).

The available data suggest a model in which physiological changes in gonadal steroids increase the synthesis of peptide and the number of receptors. The changes in oxytocin receptors are not ubiquitous. Only those regions rich in estrogen receptors (for example, the bed nucleus of the stria terminalis and the ventromedial nucleus of the hypothalamus) show increased oxytocin receptor binding, but in these regions the changes are rapid and profound (up to 300% increases in hypothalamic binding in 72 hours) (A.E. Johnson et al., 1989). Thus, in select target sites, the sensitivity to endogenous oxytocin increases markedly at parturition. These brain regions appear to be critical for the onset of maternal behavior, as females without this increase in oxytocin neurotransmission may exhibit normal labor but fail to care for their offspring (Insel, 1992).

It is important to recognize that oxytocin is only one link in a very complex neurochemical chain necessary for maternal behavior. It is not yet clear how oxytocin influences other neurotransmitters or even if it functions to increase or decrease neural activity. Some evidence using site-specific injections of an oxytocin antagonist suggests that the peptide may be particularly important for regulating dopaminergic function from the ventral tegmental area (Pedersen et al., 1994). Dopamine has also been implicated in certain aspects of rat maternal behavior (Hansen et al., 1991). Depletion of DA neurons in the ventral tegmentum by chemical lesion produces significant disorganization of established maternal behavior and blocks the development of maternal behavior if administered during pregnancy. Similar disruptions of maternal behavior are obtained after administration of the DA receptor antagonist *haloperidol* and after acute and chronic administration of cocaine. Oxytocin, either via DA or by a direct effect, may also regulate the release of prolactin and opiate peptides, two other neural systems that appear to influence maternal behavior.

Neuroanatomy

The onset of maternal behavior in the rat is associated with increased neuronal activity in the medial preoptic area (MPOA) of the hypothalamus (Numan, 1994). This region of the hypothalamus is still poorly understood, but we know that it receives an important projection from the amygdala via the bed nucleus of the stria terminalis and that it sends projections to the ventral tegmental area, a region involved in incentive reward. The MPOA is rich in estrogen receptors, the onset of maternal behavior is associated with a pronounced increase in local estrogen receptor gene expression, and exogenous administration of estrogen into the MPOA stimulates maternal behavior in nulliparous females (Numan, 1994). Moreover, lesions of the MPOA inhibit maternal behavior and pup stimuli increase the induction of Fos protein in this region, reflecting increased activity. Consequently, projections from the MPOA to the ventral tegmental area may be critical for maternal behavior, possibly allowing pup odors processed via the amygdala and bed nucleus of the stria terminalis to become reinforcing by activation of the ventral tegmental area (Numan, 1994). Febo et al. (2005) recently demonstrated, using fMRI in rats, that suckling and oxytocin administration stimulated activity in the nucleus accumbens consistent with the hypothesis that recruitment of the reward pathways during bonding of a dam to her offspring may be modulated by oxytocin release.

Clinical Correlate—Maternal Neglect

The same neural circuitry—amygdala, bed nucleus of the stria terminalis, MPOA, and ventral tegmental area—is found in the primate brain, but its significance is less evident. The human brain is not only two orders of magnitude larger than the rat brain, it includes a massive cortical mantle with which to govern the amygdala and hypothalamus. Clearly, human maternal behavior does not commence at parturition and does not require either labor or nursing. On the other hand, there are women who appear not to bond to their infants after normal deliveries, demonstrating a syndrome that has been called *maternal neglect*. Preclinical research would suggest two likely mechanisms for the syndrome of maternal neglect. One would be a deficit in estrogen binding in the hypothalamus or bed nucleus of the stria terminalis, resulting from either a defect in estrogen production or an abnormal estrogen receptor. A second hypothetical mechanism would be a deficit in CNS oxytocin neurotransmission, as occurs in animal studies with central oxytocin antagonist administration. In humans, pituitary oxytocin is secreted into the circulation during parturition and nursing. Based on the data from other mammals, one might speculate that the central release of oxytocin during labor or nursing contributes to the affiliative bond formed between mother and infant, and that absence of either the central release of the peptide or a defect in the brain receptor could result in decreased maternal interest. Note that a woman with such a deficit might be able to deliver and nurse normally but would not experience her infant as reinforcing and would not respond normally to signs of her infant's distress.

PAIR BOND FORMATION

The development of adult–adult pair bonds is the least studied form of attachment from a neurobiological perspective. The relative paucity of studies can be attributed to the absence of pair bonds in commonly used laboratory animals, such as rats and mice. By definition, pair bonds occur in monogamous animals, with approximately 3% of mammals currently considered monogamous (Kleiman, 1977). Much of this research has focused on microtine rodents or voles, as this genus includes closely related monogamous and nonmonogamous (that is, polygynous or promiscuous) species.

The prairie vole (*Microtus ochrogaster*) is a mouse-sized rodent that lives in burrows across the American Midwest. Prairie voles are usually found in multigenerational family groups with a single breeding pair (Carter et al., 1995). They manifest the classic features of monogamy: a breeding pair shares the same nest and territory where they are in frequent contact, males participate in parental care, and intruders of either sex are rejected. Following the death of one of the pair, a new mate is accepted only about 20% of the time (the rate is approximately the same whether the male or the female is the survivor). Prairie voles also demonstrate a curious pattern of reproductive development. Offspring remain sexually suppressed as long as they remain within the natal group. For females, puberty occurs not at a specific age but after exposure to a chemosignal in the urine of an unrelated male (Carter et al., 1995). Within 24 hours of exposure to this signal, the female becomes sexually receptive. She mates repeatedly with an unrelated male and, in the process, forms a selective and enduring preference or pair bond.

The closely related montane vole (*Microtus montanus*) looks remarkably similar to the prairie vole and shares many features of its nonsocial behaviors but differs consistently on measures of social behavior. Montane voles are generally found in isolated burrows (in high meadows in the Rockies), show little interest in social contact, and are clearly not monogamous (Jannett, 1980). Males provide little if any parental care, and females frequently abandon their young between 8 and 14 days postpartum (Jannett, 1982). In laboratory studies where prairie voles spend most of their time huddled together, montane voles spend little time in side-by-side contact even within the confines of a mouse cage (Shapiro and Dewsbury, 1990). In contrast to prairie voles, montane pups do not respond to social separation with either isolation calls or corticosterone release, although the pups give both responses to nonsocial stressors (Insel and Shapiro, 1992) (Table 83.2).

Prairie and montane voles thus provide an intriguing natural experiment for studying the neural substrates of pair bonding. Pair bonding in this case can be assessed by the formation of a partner preference that normally follows mating in the monogamous vole. Because of the evidence for oxytocin in the mediation of sexual behavior (Witt, 1995), oxytocin might also influence pair bond formation in the prairie vole. Research with several other species has demonstrated that oxytocin is released with mating (Witt, 1995) and that mating appears important for pair bonding in the prairie vole (Williams et al., 1992). To determine if oxytocin released with mating is necessary or sufficient for pair bonding, prairie voles were treated with either oxytocin (in the absence of mating) or a selective oxytocin antagonist (prior to mating).

TABLE 83.2 *A Comparative Model for the Study of Attachment*

	Prairie Vole	*Montane Vole*
Infant separation calls	High	Low, absent
Maternal behavior	High, enduring	High but transient
Paternal behavior	High, enduring	Absent
Male–female	Monogamous	Promiscuous
Filial (huddle time)	High	Low

Oxytocin (but not vasopressin) given centrally (intracerebroventricularly [ICV]) to females facilitates the development of a partner preference in the absence of mating (Crowley et al., 1995). A selective oxytocin antagonist given ICV prior to mating blocks formation of the partner preference without interfering with mating. This effect appears specific: neither CSF nor a vasopressin antagonist given in an identical fashion blocks partner preference formation. Presumably, the oxytocin antagonist prevents the binding of oxytocin to its receptor and thereby blocks the behavioral consequences of mating. These results suggest that oxytocin released with mating is necessary and sufficient for the formation of a pair bond in the female prairie vole. In the montane vole, central administration of oxytocin increases self-grooming and does not induce a partner preference.

The Neuroanatomy of Pair Bonding

Because oxytocin has such different effects in prairie and montane voles, a map of where oxytocin acts in the prairie vole brain may provide an important clue to the neuroanatomy of pair bond formation. As it turns out, these two vole species differ markedly in the neural distribution of oxytocin receptors, although they appear identical with respect to several other systems (Insel, 1992). Oxytocin receptors show similar binding characteristics (in terms of kinetics and specificity) in the two species, but the receptors are expressed within entirely different pathways (Fig. 83.2a). This species difference in regional receptor distribution indicates that different brain areas are responding to endogenous oxytocin; thus, the central effects of oxytocin should be quite different in prairie and montane voles. For instance, in the prairie vole, oxytocin receptors are found in brain regions associated with reward (nucleus accumbens and prelimbic cortex), suggesting that oxytocin might have reinforcing properties selectively in this species. An oxytocin antagonist injected directly into these areas blocks pair bond formation in female prairie voles (Insel and Young, 2001) (Figs. 83.2b and 2c). Conversely, receptors in the lateral septum, found only in the montane vole, might be responsible for the effect of oxytocin on self-grooming, an effect that is observed in the montane vole but not the prairie vole.

In summary, prairie voles and montane voles show different patterns of oxytocin receptor distribution in brain, and this peptide appears to be important for pair bond formation, a process that occurs in the monogamous prairie vole but not in the promiscuous montane vole. Remarkably, in male prairie voles, oxytocin appears less important than the related neuropeptide *vasopressin* (Winslow et al., 1993) (Fig. 83.3). Apparently, pair bonding in male and female voles involves two different albeit closely related neural systems. Studies with transgenic and viral vector techniques demonstrate that increasing vasopressin receptors in select neural pathways can facilitate social interest and pair bond formation, with the ventral pallidum an important site in male prairie voles (Young et al., 1999; Pitkow et al., 2001).

Molecular studies of both oxytocin and vasopressin receptors suggest that species differences in distribution may result from hypervariable regions found in the promoters of both genes (Hammock and Young, 2005; Wu et al., 2005) (Fig. 83.3c). These differences in gene structure have even suggested a molecular mechanism for monogamy (Hammock and Young, 2005). Whatever the molecular mechanism, monogamous species like prairie voles and marmosets have abundant receptors for either oxytocin or vasopressin in mesolimbic pathways, such as the nucleus accumbens and the ventral pallidum. One current hypothesis is that these receptors link social information to reward circuits in the brain, providing a neurobiological mechanism for pair bonding. In its simplest form, the release of oxytocin or vasopressin with mating would activate these reward pathways in monogamous species, resulting in a conditioned response or preference, just as if the individual had received cocaine or amphetamine. In the nonmonogamous species without receptors in these pathways, the release of the same neuropeptides would not result in a conditioned response, and therefore mating would not lead to a partner preference or pair bond.

Clinical correlate—human bonding

Humans form enduring, selective bonds, but the role of central oxytocin or vasopressin in this process remains largely unexplored. Across human cultures, sexual behavior

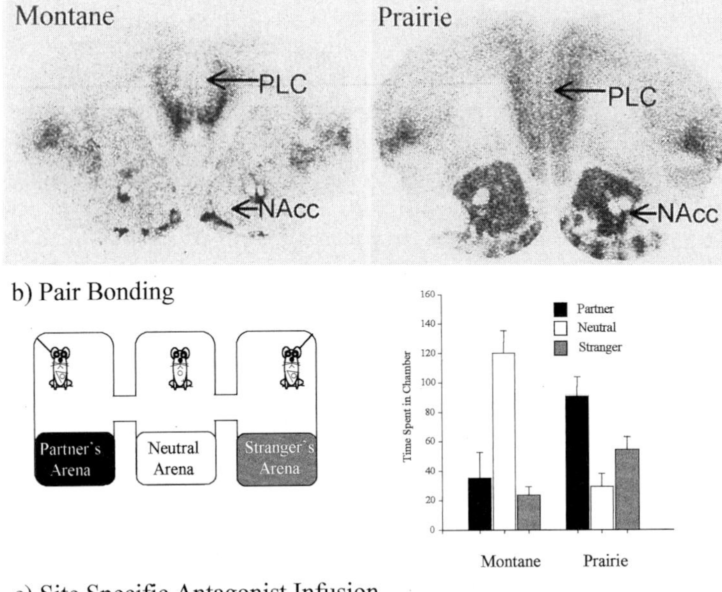

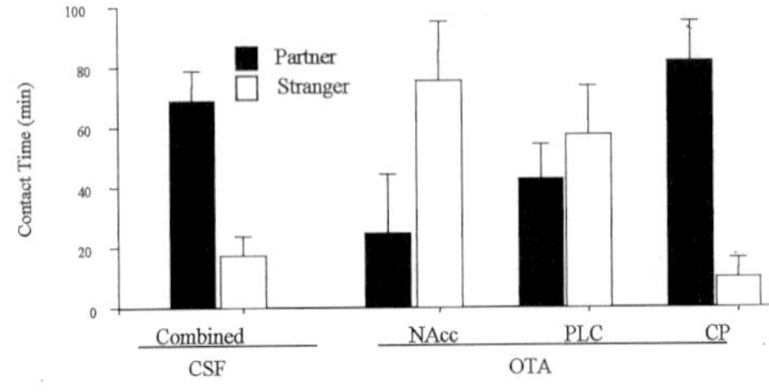

FIGURE 83.2 Oxytocin and social attachment in the monogamous female prairie vole. *A*. Receptor autoradiograms with montane and prairie voles show different distributions of oxytocin receptors in the brain, particularly in the nucleus accumbens (NAcc) and the prelimbic cortex (PLC). *B*. In the laboratory, pair bonding is assessed with a partner preference test. After mating with a "partner," the experimental female vole is placed in a three-chambered arena in which the partner is tethered in one chamber and a novel male or "stranger" (S) is tethered in another chamber. The experimental animal, placed in the neutral (N) chamber, has free access to all three areas. After mating, female prairie voles spend more time in the partner's chamber than in the neutral or stranger's chamber, indicating a partner preference. In contrast, mated montane voles show no preference for either the partner or the stranger, indicating the absence of a mating-induced social attachment. C. Partner preference formation is blocked in the female prairie vole by infusions of an oxytocin receptor antagonist (OTA) into the NAcc as well as into the PLC, while cerebrospinal fluid into either area or OTA infused into the caudate putamen (CP) has no effect on partner preference formation.

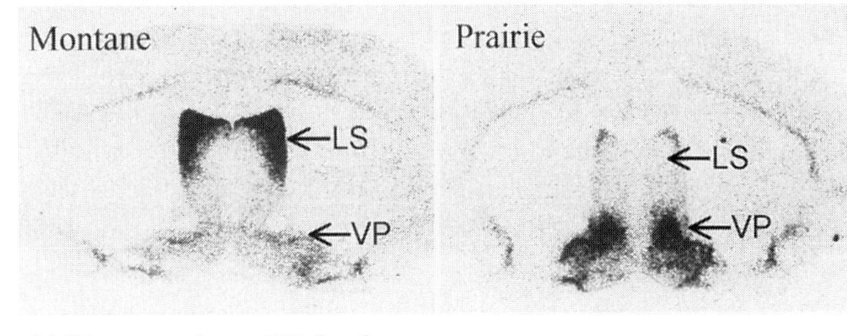

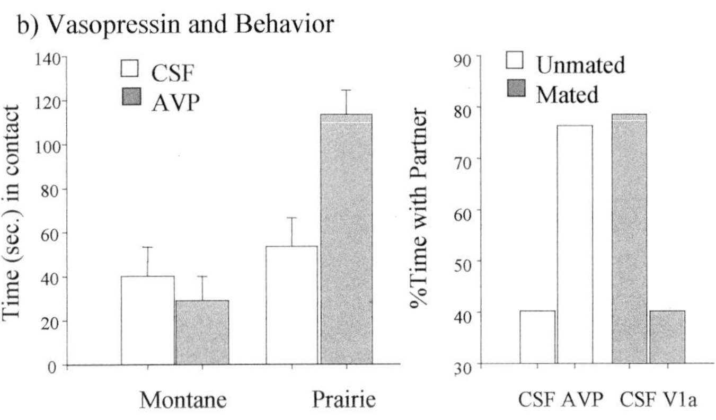

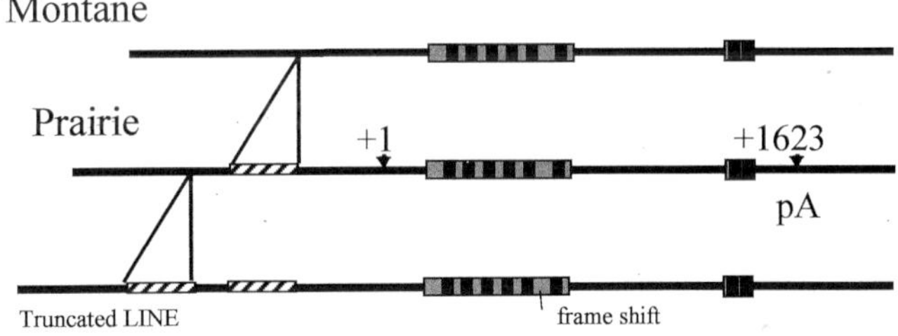

FIGURE 83.3 Vasopressin (V1a) receptor and social attachment in monogamous male voles. *A*. Montane and prairie voles have different distributions of V1a receptor binding, with prairie voles having a high density of receptors in the ventral pallidum (VP) and montane voles having receptors in the lateral septum (LS). *B*. The species differences in receptor distribution are likely responsible for the species differences in the behavioral effects of arginine vasopressin (AVP) and perhaps in the formation of social attachments. In a test of nonspecific affiliative behavior, intracerebroventricular AVP infusions increase social interest in the male prairie vole but not in the montane vole. Furthermore, AVP stimulates the formation of a partner preference in the absence of mating, and V1a receptor antagonists prevent partner preference formation after extensive mating bouts. CSF: cerebrospinal fluid. *C*. These species differences in receptor distribution may be the result of species differences in gene structure. The prairie vole V1a receptor gene has been duplicated, with one copy being downstream of a retrotransposon element (LINE) and also has a frame shift mutation in the coding region. Both copies have a large complex repetitive expansion just over 700 base pairs from the transcription start site. Either the gene duplication or the promoter expansion could contribute to the evolution of the expression pattern. pA: polyadenylation site.

is consistently associated with pair bonding (Fisher, 1992), although sex is neither necessary nor sufficient for human pair bond formation. Oxytocin and vasopressin are released into plasma during human sexual behavior (Murphy et al., 1987), and one might speculate that the simultaneous release into specific neural pathways facilitates the formation of a pair bond, as shown in prairie voles. Of course, to influence pair bond formation in humans, oxytocin receptors would need to be located in sites homologous to those found in monogamous species. In the human brain, the pattern of receptor distribution does not resemble the pattern of either the monogamous prairie vole or the promiscuous montane vole (Loup et al., 1991). Oxytocin receptors are concentrated in the human diagonal band (consistent with a role in memory) and the substantia nigra (consistent with a role in the regulation of dopaminergic neurotransmission). Although there are neither pharmacological nor physiological data from humans with which to support or disprove a role for central oxytocin in pair bonding, Two recent human studies have implicated oxytocin in processes important for the development of trusting relationships (Kosfeld et al., 2005) and reduced fear associated with provocative facial expressions (Kirsch et al., 2005). These findings suggest the possibility that oxytocin in humans may be important in the early stages of social approach critical for the development of new social relationships. In addition, a human neuroimaging study of romantic love also found more activation of mesolimbic DA pathways when people looked at pictures of their romantic partners compared to pictures of familiar but nonromantic friends (Bartels and Zeki, 2000).

SUMMARY

The study of social behavior represents a frontier for neurobiology. Recognizing that processing of simple visual signals involves 20 or 30 cortical domains, the quest for mapping the neural substrates for something as complex as attachment seems especially ambitious. Nevertheless, by attending to discrete aspects of these complex behaviors and by investigating where candidate neurotransmitters act, we are beginning to make progress. Within the various forms of attachment, there may be separate systems for the initiation and maintenance (or the appetitive and consummatory) aspects of the behavior. For instance, oxytocin appears to influence the initiation but not the maintenance of maternal behavior and pair bonding.

It may be useful to consider attachment behavior as a subset of behaviors related to reward. In that sense, the neural substrates of attachment are those pathways that couple social recognition (olfactory, auditory, and visual stimuli) to the neural pathways for reinforcement, such as the mesolimbic projections from the ventral tegmental area to the nucleus accumbens and prefrontal cortex (Insel and Young, 2001). The amygdala nuclei, the bed nucleus of the stria terminalis, and the MPOA are all important in this process. The dense concentration of estrogen receptors in these regions provides a mechanism for linking physiological changes in gonadal hormones at puberty or parturition to the need for enhanced information processing to facilitate reproductive behaviors. Oxytocin receptors, which are exquisitely sensitive to changes in gonadal steroids, are one of the links in this chain.

One of the most important lessons from the study of attachment behavior is the profound variation even among closely related species. Although this variation provides an opportunity for comparative neurobiology—correlating species differences in anatomy with behavior—it also suggests the futility of selecting a single animal model for investigating the neural substrates of normal or abnormal human attachment behavior. The goal of comparative studies is to find underlying principles that guide the evolution of neural systems, not to find a model for pathological behavior. Nevertheless, by demonstrating the importance of a given neural system for a class of behaviors across phylogeny, this approach provides candidates to study in our own species.

Although at the beginning of the chapter we noted that disturbances in attachment behavior characterize virtually every form of psychopathology, the neurobiology of attachment may be most relevant to autism. Autism is characterized by deficits in social interaction as well as abnormalities of language and frequent mental retardation. We know very little about the pathophysiology of autism, but the studies of attachment described above may prove helpful in pointing to candidate genes for this syndrome. For instance, the role of oxytocin in infant, parental, and adult–adult attachment may be instructive. The observation that genetically normal monkeys or humans raised in a socially deprived environment exhibit autistic behaviors (and, in the monkeys, reduced CSF oxytocin) may be instructive. Although most children with genetic autistism are born into nurturing environments, their disorder may effectively impose a form of social deprivation. If early social experience is critical for the development of social pathways, just as early visual experience is critical for the development of ocular dominance columns, then much of what we observe in autism may be the result of the infant's inability to exploit the social world. Intense early interventions might be expected to prevent many of the features we associate with this devastating chronic disorder. Additional research is necessary in this area, but animal studies may prove important in guiding the search for what to look for and where to look in humans with impaired attachment behavior.

REFERENCES

Afraz, S.R., Kiani, R., and Esteky, H. (2006) Microstimulation of inferotemporal cortex influences face categorization. *Nature* 442:692–695.

Bachevalier, J., and Loveland, K.A. (2006) The orbitofrontal-amygdala circuit and self-regulation of social-emotional behavior in autism. *Neurosci. Biobehav. Rev.* 30:97–117.

Barberis, C., and Tribollet, E. (1996) Vasopressin and oxytocin receptors in the central nervous system. *Crit. Rev. Neurobiol.* 10: 119–154.

Bartels, A., and Zeki, S. (2000) The neural basis of romantic love. *Neuroreport* 11:3829–3834.

Bateson, P. (1966) The characteristics and context of imprinting. *Biol. Rev.* 41:177–220.

Bielsky, I.F., Hu, S.B., Ren, X., Terwilliger, E.F., and Young, L.J. (2005) The V1a vasopressin receptor is necessary and sufficient for normal social recognition: a gene replacement study. *Neuron* 47:503–513.

Bowlby, J. (1982) *Attachment and Loss: Attachment*. New York: Basic Books.

Brennan, P.A., and Kendrick, K.M. (2006) Mammalian social odours: attraction and individual recognition. *Philos. Trans. R. Soc. Lond. B Biol. Sci.* 361:2061–2078.

Buijs, R.M., and van Heerikhuize, J.J. (1982) Vasopressin and oxytocin release in the brain—a synaptic event. *Brain Res.* 252:71–76.

Bukach, C.M., Gauthier, I., and Tarr, M.J. (2006) Beyond faces and modularity: the power of an expertise framework. *Trends Cogn. Sci.* 10:159–166.

Cacioppo, J.T. (1994) Social neuroscience: autonomic, neuroendocrine, and immune responses to stress. *Psychophysiology* 31: 113–128.

Carter, C., DeVries, A., and Getz, L. (1995) Physiological substrates of mammalian monogamy: the prairie vole model. *Neurosci. Biobehav. Rev.* 19:303–314.

Choleris, E., Ogawa, S., Kavaliers, M., Gustafsson, J.A., Korach, K.S., Muglia, L.J., et al. (2006) Involvement of estrogen receptor alpha, beta and oxytocin in social discrimination: A detailed behavioral analysis with knockout female mice. *Genes Brain Behav.* 5:528–539.

Cook, E.H. (1990) Autism: review of neurochemical investigation. *Synapse* 6:292–230.

Craig, A.D., Reiman, E.M., Evans, A., and Bushnell, M.C. (1996) Functional imaging of an illusion of pain. *Nature* 384:258–260.

Crowley, R.S., Insel, T.R., O'Keefe, J.A., Kim, N.B., and Amico, J.A. (1995) Increased accumulation of oxytocin messenger ribonucleic acid in the hypothalamus of the female rat: induction by long term estradiol and progesterone administration and subsequent progesterone withdrawal. *Endocrinology* 136:224–231.

Dalton, K.M., Nacewicz, B.M., Johnstone, T., Schaefer, H.S., Gernsbacher, M.A., Goldsmith, H.H., et al. (2005) Gaze fixation and the neural circuitry of face processing in autism. *Nat. Neurosci.* 8:519–526.

de Bono, M., and Bargmann, C. (1998) Natural variation in a neuropeptide Y receptor homolog modifies social behavior and food response in C. elegans. *Cell* 94:679–689.

DeCasper, A.J., and Spence, M.J. (1986) Prenatal maternal speech influences newborns' perception of speech sounds. *Infant Behav. Dev.* 9:133–140.

Emery, N. (2000) The eyes have it: the neuroethology, function and evolution of social gaze. *Neurosci. Biobehav. Rev.* 24:581–604.

Febo, M., Numan, M., and Ferris, C.F. (2005) Functional magnetic resonance imaging shows oxytocin activates brain regions associated with mother-pup bonding during suckling. *J. Neurosci.* 25: 11637–11644.

Fein, D., Pennington, B., Markowitz, P., Braverman, M., and Waterhouse, L. (1986) Toward a neuropsychological model of infantile autism: are the social deficits primary? *J. Am. Acad. Child Psychiatry* 25:198–212.

Ferguson, J.N., Aldag, J.M., Insel, T.R., and Young, L.J. (2001) Oxytocin in the medial amygdala is essential for social recognition in the mouse. *J. Neurosci.* 21:8278–8285.

Ferguson, J.N., Young, L.J., Hearn, E., Insel, T.R., and Winslow, J.T. (2000) Social amnesia in mice lacking the oxytocin gene. *Nature Genet.* 25:284–288.

Fisher, H. (1992) *The Anatomy of Love*. New York: W.W. Norton.

Francis, D., Diorio, J., Liu, D., and Meaney, M.J. (1999) Nongenomic transmission across generations of maternal behavior and stress responses in the rat. *Science* 286:1155–1158.

Gauthier, I., Skudlarski, P., Gore, J., and Anderson, A. (2000) Expertise for cars and birds recruits brain areas involved in face recognition. *Nature Neurosci.* 3:191–197.

Gauthier, I., Tarr, M., Anderson, A., Skudlarski, P., and Gore, J. (1999) Activation of the middle fusiform "face area" increases with expertise in recognizing novel objects. *Nature Neurosci.* 2: 568–573.

Gothard, K.M., Battaglia, F.P., Erickson, C.A., Spitler, K.M., and Amaral, D.G. (2007) Neural responses to facial expression and face identity in the monkey amygdala. *J. Neurophysiol.* 97:1671–1683.

Hammock, E.A., and Young, L.J. (2005) Microsatellite instability generates diversity in brain and sociobehavioral traits. *Science* 308:1630–1634.

Hansen, S., Harthon, C., Wallin, E., Lofberg, I., and Svensson, K. (1991) Mesotelencephalic dopamine system and reproductive behavior in the female rat: effects of ventral tegmental 6-OHDA lesions on maternal and sexual responsiveness. *Behav. Neurosci.* 105:588–598.

Harlow, H.F., and Mears, C. (1979) *The Human Model: Primate Perspectives*. New York: Wiley.

Harlow, H., and Suomi, S. (1970) The nature of love—simplified. *Am. Psychol.* 25:161–168.

Haxby, J.V. (2006) Fine structure in representations of faces and objects. *Nat. Neurosci.* 9:1084–1086.

Hofer, M.A. (1984) Relationships as regulators: a psychobiologic perspective on bereavement. *Psychosom. Med.* 46:183–197.

Hoffman, K.L., Gothard, K.M., Schmid, M.C., and Logothetis, N.K. (2007) Facial-expression and gaze-selective responses in the monkey amygdala. *Curr. Biol.* 17:766–772.

Hudson, R. (1993) Olfactory imprinting. *Curr. Opin. Neurbiol.* 3: 548–552.

Insel, T.R. (1992) Oxytocin: a neuropeptide for affiliation-evidence from behavioral, receptor autoradiographic, and comparative studies. *Psychoneuroendocrinol.* 17:3–33.

Insel, T.R., and Shapiro, L.E. (1992) Oxytocin receptor distribution reflects social organization in monogamous and polygamous voles. *Proc. Natl. Acad. Sci.* 89:5981–5985.

Insel, T.R., and Young, L.J. (2001) The neurobiology of attachment. *Nature Rev. Neurosci.* 3:129–136.

Jannett, F.J. (1980) Social dynamics in the montane vole Microtus montanus as a paradigm. *Biologist* 62:3–19.

Jannett, F.J. (1982) The nesting patterns of adult voles (Microtus montanus) in field populations. *J. Mammol.* 63:495–498.

Johnson, A.E., Ball, G.F., Coirini, H., Harbaugh, C.R., McEwen, B.S., and Insel, T.R. (1989) Time course of the estradiol-dependent induction of oxytocin receptor binding in the ventromedial hypothalamic nucleus of the rat. *Endocrinology* 125:1414–1419.

Johnson, M.H., Griffin, R., Csibra, G., Halit, H., Farroni, T., de Haan, M., et al. (2005) The emergence of the social brain network: evidence from typical and atypical development. *Dev. Psychopathol.* 17:599–619.

Kanwisher, N., McDermott, J., and Chun, M. (1997) The fusiform face area: a module in human extrastriate cortex specialized for face perception. *J. Neurosci.* 17:4302–4311.

Kirsch, P., Esslinger, C., Chen, Q., Mier, D., Lis, S., Siddhanti, S., et al. (2005) Oxytocin modulates neural circuitry for social cognition and fear in humans. *J. Neurosci.* 25:11489–11493.

Kleiman, D.G. (1977) Monogamy in mammals. *Q. Rev. Biol.* 52: 39–69.

Kosfeld, M., Heinrichs, M., Zak, P.J., Fischbacher, U., and Fehr, E. (2005) Oxytocin increases trust in humans. *Nature* 435:673–676.

Kraemer, G. (1992) A psychobiological theory of attachment. *Behav. Brain Sci.* 15:494–551.

Leon, M. (1992) The neurobiology of filial learning. *Annu. Rev. Psychol.* 43:377–398.

Liu, D., Diorio, J., Tannenbaum, B., Caldji, C., Francis, D., Freedman, A., et al. (1997) Maternal care, hippocampal glucocorticoid receptors, and hypothalamic-pituitary-adrenal response to stress. *Science* 277:1659–1662.

Long, J.M., LaPorte, P., Paylor, R., and Wynshaw-Boris, A. (2004) Expanded characterization of the social interaction abnormalities in mice lacking Dvl1. *Genes Brain Behav.* 3:51–62.

Loup, F., Tribollet, E., Dubois-Dauphin, M., and Dreifuss, J.J. (1991) Localization of high-affinity binding sites for oxytocin and vasopressin in the human brain. An autoradiographic study. *Brain Res.* 555:220–232.

Maclean, P.D., and Newman, J.D. (1988) Role of midline frontolimbic cortex in production of isolation calls in squirrel monkeys. *Brain Res.* 450:111–117.

McKone, E., Kanwisher, N., and Duchaine, B.C. (2007) Can generic expertise explain special processing for faces? *Trends Cogn. Sci.* 11:8–15.

Meaney, M.J. (2001) Maternal care, gene expression, and the transmission of individual differences in stress reactivity across generations. *Annu. Rev. Neurosci.* 24:1161–1192.

Meaney, M.J., and Szyf, M. (2005) Maternal care as a model for experience-dependent chromatin plasticity? *Trends Neurosci.* 28: 456–463.

Modahl, C., Green, L., Fein, D., Morris, M., Waterhouse, L., Feinstein, C., et al. (1998) Plasma oxytocin levels in autistic children. *Biol. Psychiatry* 43:270–277.

Moriceau, S., and Sullivan, R.M. (2005) Neurobiology of infant attachment. *Dev. Psychobiol.* 47:230–242.

Moriceau, S., Wilson, D.A., Levine, S., and Sullivan, R.M. (2006) Dual circuitry for odor-shock conditioning during infancy: corticosterone switches between fear and attraction via amygdala. *J. Neurosci.* 26:6737–6748.

Murphy, M.R., Seckl, J.R., Burton, S., Checkley, S.A., and Lightman, S.L. (1987) Changes in oxytocin and vasopressin secretion during sexual activity in men. *J. Clin. Endocrinol. Metab.* 65:738–741.

Nelson, E.E., and Panksepp, J. (1996) Oxytocin and infant-mother bonding in rats. *Behav. Neurosci.* 110:583–592.

Numan, M. (1994) Maternal behavior. In: Knobil, E., and Neill, J., eds. *The Physiology of Reproduction*. New York: Raven Press, pp. 221–302.

Pedersen, C.A., Caldwell, J.O., Walker, C., Ayers, G., and Mason, G.A. (1994) Oxytocin activates the postpartum onset of rat maternal behavior in the ventral tegmental and medial preoptic areas. *Behav. Neurosci.* 108:1163–1171.

Pedersen, C.A., and Prange, A.J., Jr. (1979) Induction of maternal behavior in virgin rats after intracerebroventricular administration of oxytocin. *Proc. Natl. Acad. Sci.* 76:6661–6665

Pinsk, M.A., DeSimone, K., Moore, T., Gross, C.G., and Kastner, S. (2005) Representations of faces and body parts in macaque temporal cortex: a functional MRI study. *Proc. Natl. Acad. Sci. USA* 102:6996–7001.

Pitkow, L., Sharer, C., Ren, X., Insel, T., Terwilliger, E., and Young, L.J. (2001) Facilitation of affiliation and pair-bond formation by vasopressin receptor gene transfer into the ventral forebrain of a monogamous vole. *J. Neurosci.* 21:7392–7396.

Robinson, G.E. (1999) Integrative animal behaviour and sociogenomics. *Trends Ecol. Evol.* 14:202–205.

Rodman, H.R., Scalaidhe, S.P., and Gross, C.G. (1993) Response properties of neurons in temporal cortical visual areas of infant monkeys. *J. Neurophysiol.* 70:1115–1136.

Schanberg, S., and Field, T. (1987) Sensory deprivation stress and supplemental stimulation in the rat pup and preterm human neonate. *Child Dev.* 58:1431–1447.

Schultz, R.T., Gauthier, I., Klin, A., Fulbright, R.K., Anderson, A.W., Volkmar, F., et al. (2000) Abnormal ventral temporal cortical activity during face discrimination among individuals with autism and Asperger syndrome. *Arch. Gen. Psychiatry* 57:331–340.

Shapiro, L.E., and Dewsbury, D.A. (1990) Differences in affiliative behavior, pair bonding, and vaginal cytology in two species of vole. *J. Comp. Psychol.* 104:268–274.

Smotherman, W., and Robinson, S. (1994) Classical conditioning of opioid activity in the fetal rat. *Behav. Neurosci.* 108:951–961.

Spitz, R.A. (1946) Anaclitic depression: an inquiry into the genesis of psychiatric conditions in early childhood, II. *Psychoanal. Study Child.* 2:313–342.

Stanton, M.E., Wallstrom, J., and Levine, S. (1987) Maternal contact inhibits pituitary-adrenal stress responses in preweanling rats. *Dev. Psychobiol.* 20:131–145.

Stowers, L., Holy, T.E., Meister, M., Dulac, C., and Koentges, G. (2002) Loss of sex discrimination and male-male aggression in mice deficient for TRP2. *Science* 295:1493–1500.

Sullivan, R., Wilson, D., and Leon, M. (1989) Norepinephrine and learning-induced plasticity in infant rat olfactory system. *J. Neurosci.* 9:3998–4006.

Tsao, D.Y., Freiwald, W.A., Tootell, R.B., and Livingstone, M.S. (2006) A cortical region consisting entirely of face-selective cells. *Science* 311:670–674.

Waters, E., and Sroufe, L.A. (1983) Social competence as a developmental construct. *Dev. Rev.* 3:79–97.

Weaver, I.C., D'Alessio, A.C., Brown, S.E., Hellstrom, I.C., Dymov, S., Sharma, S., et al. (2007) The transcription factor nerve growth factor-inducible protein a mediates epigenetic programming: altering epigenetic marks by immediate-early genes. *J. Neurosci.* 27:1756–1768.

Williams, J., Catania, K., and Carter, C.S. (1992) Development of partner preferences in female prairie voles (Microtus ochrogaster): the role of social and sexual experience. *Horm. Behav.* 26:339–349.

Winslow, J.T., Hastings, N., Carter, C.S., Harbaugh, C.R., and Insel, T.R. (1993) A role for central vasopressin in pair bonding in monogamous prairie voles. *Nature* 365:545–548.

Winslow, J.T., and Insel, T.R. (1990) Serotonergic modulation of the rat pup's ultrasonic vocal development: studies with MDMA. *J. Pharmacol. Exp. Ther.* 254:212–220.

Winslow, J.T., Noble, P.L., Lyons, C.K., Stark, S.M., and Insel, T.R. (2003) Rearing effects on cerebrospinal fluid oxytocin concentration and social buffering in rhesus monkeys. *Neuropsychopharmacol.* 28(5):910–918.

Witt, D.M. (1995) Oxytocin and rodent sociosexual responses: from behavior to gene expression. *Neurosci. Biobehav. Rev.* 19:315–324.

Wu, S., Jia, M., Ruan, Y., Liu, J., Guo, Y., Shuang, M., et al. (2005) Positive association of the oxytocin receptor gene (OXTR) with autism in the Chinese Han population. *Biol. Psychiatry* 58:74–77.

Young, L.J., Nilsen, R., Waymire, K., MacGregor, G., and Insel, T.R. (1999) Increased affiliative response to vasopressin in mice expressing the V1a receptor from a monogamous vole. *Nature* 400: 766–768.

84 The Neurobiology of Eating Disorders

WALTER KAYE, MICHAEL STROBER, AND DAVID JIMERSON

Anorexia nervosa (AN) and bulimia nervosa (BN) are potentially chronic, disabling conditions, characterized by aberrant patterns of feeding behavior and weight regulation, and deviant attitudes and perceptions toward body weight and shape. In AN, an inexplicable fear of weight gain and unrelenting obsession with fatness, even in the face of increasing cachexia, accounts for its protracted course, extreme medical and psychological morbidity, and mortality rates in prospectively observed cohorts exceeding those of all other psychiatric disorders. Bulimia nervosa, which like AN, is associated with extreme concern with weight and shape, typically emerges after a period of food restriction, which may or may not have been associated with weight loss; binge eating is then followed by either self-induced vomiting or some other means of compensation for the excess of food that has been consumed. The majority of people with BN have highly irregular feeding patterns, and satiety may be impaired. Although abnormally low body weight is an exclusion for the diagnosis of BN, some 25%–30% of patients with BN have a prior history of AN. Moreover, in spite of the broad differences in the topography of their feeding behavior, but reflecting common concerns with weight and shape, the two conditions coaggregate in families (Strober et al., 2000). Likewise, common to individuals with AN or BN are general psychopathological features, in particular low self-esteem, depression, and anxiety.

Each of these diagnostic labels is, perhaps, misleading in several respects. This is because individuals with AN rarely have complete suppression of appetite but rather exhibit a seemingly volitional, and more often than not, ego syntonic resistance to feeding drives, eventually succumbing to near-constant preoccupation with food and eating rituals due to prolonged food deprivation on the one hand, and heightened vigilance to food-related cues due to the psychological drive to avoid mature body weight. Similarly, little evidence exists to suggest that those with BN have a primary, pathological drive to overeat; rather, like individuals with AN, individuals with BN have a seemingly relentless drive to restrain their food intake, an extreme fear of weight gain, and, not infrequently, a distorted view of their actual body shape. Thus, the loss of control of feeding behavior occurs intermittently, sometimes following the onset of dieting behavior, in other cases precipitated by emotional factors. Also, as noted above, there are longitudinal continuities between the two in that episodes of binge eating develop prospectively in a significant proportion of people with AN (Halmi et al., 1991). Thus, given their shared emotional and cognitive features, the frequent diagnostic transitions between syndromes that occur over time (Milos et al., 2005), and their cotransmission in families, it has been argued that AN and BN share at least some risk and liability factors.

Anorexia nervosa and BN are certainly complex phenotypes whose etiology is ascribed to multiple interacting developmental, social, and biological processes; however, knowledge of these causal pathways remains incomplete. Although cultural attitudes toward standards of ideal body shape have obvious relevance to the psychopathology of eating disorders, it is not likely that such influences are paramount insofar as dieting behavior and the drive toward thinness are common in industrialized countries throughout the world, yet AN and BN affect only an estimated 0.3%–0.7%, and 1.7%–2.5%, respectively, of females in the general population. Also significant here is that numerous descriptions of a syndrome reminiscent of AN date from the late 17th century (Treasure and Campbell, 1994), suggesting that factors beyond those deemed culture bound play a central etiologic role. Second, these syndromes, in particular AN, have a relatively stereotypic clinical presentation, sex distribution, and age of onset, underscoring the role played by an intrinsic biological vulnerability, and diagnostic validity of the syndrome itself.

CLINICAL PHENOMENOLOGY

Current diagnostic convention subdivides AN into two subtypes based on variations in feeding behavior that parallels the broader distinction between AN and BN; validity of these subtypes is supported externally by evidence of contrasting patterns of premorbid functioning and psychopathological correlates (Garner et al., 1985). In the restrictor subtype, subnormal body weight and an ongoing malnourished state are maintained by unremitting food avoidance; in the bulimic subtype of AN, there is comparable weight loss and malnutrition, yet the course of illness is marked by supervening episodes of binge eating, usually followed by some type of compensatory action such as self-induced vomiting or laxative abuse. Curiously, individuals with the bulimic subtype of AN are more likely to exhibit a broader pattern of behavioral and affective dysregulation, exemplified in histories of behavioral dyscontrol, substance abuse, and overt family conflict in comparison to those with the restricting subtype (Garfinkel et al., 1980; Casper et al., 1992). Particularly common in individuals with AN are personality traits of marked perfectionism, conformity, obsessionality, constriction of affect and emotional expression, and these traits typically appear in advance of weight loss and persist even after long-term weight recovery, indicating they are not merely epiphenomena of acute malnutrition (Strober, 1980; Casper, 1990; Srinivasagam et al., 1995).

Although individuals with BN remain at normal body weight, they often aspire to ideal weights far below the range of normalcy for their age and height. The core features of BN include repeated episodes of binge eating followed by compensatory self-induced vomiting, laxative abuse, or pathologically extreme exercise, as well as abnormal concern with weight and shape. The *Diagnostic and Statistical Manual of Mental Disorders* (*DSM-IV*; American Psychiatric Association, 1994) has specified a distinction within this group between those individuals with BN who engage in self-induced vomiting or laxative, diuretic, or enema abuse (purging type), and those who exhibit other forms of compensatory action such as fasting or exercise (nonpurging type). Beyond these differences, it has been speculated (Vitousek and Manke, 1994) that there are two clinically divergent subgroups of individuals with BN differing significantly in their core, identifying psychopathological substrate, a so-called multi-impulsive type in whom BN occurs in conjunction with more pervasive difficulties in behavioral self-regulation and affective instability, and a second type whose distinguishing features include self-effacing behaviors, dependence on external rewards, and extreme compliance. Individuals with BN of the multi-impulsive type are far more likely to have histories of substance abuse and display other impulse control problems such as shoplifting and self-injurious behaviors. Considering these differences, it has been postulated that individuals with multi-impulsive bulimia rely on binge eating and purging as a means of regulating intolerable states of tension, anger, and fragmentation, whereas individuals with the latter type of bulimia may have binge episodes precipitated through dietary restraint with compensatory behaviors maintained through reduction of guilty feelings associated with fears of weight gain.

The course of episode recovery in AN is, in most cases, a protracted one; 50%–70% of individuals will eventually have complete, or nearly complete, resolution of the illness, and in some 30% residual features persist long into adulthood. Thus once developed, rarely does AN pursue a chronic, unremitting course late into adult life; an estimated 5% will eventually die from the disease itself, or from suicide (Berkman et al., 2007). For BN, follow-up studies 5 to 10 years after presentation show a 50% rate of recovery, persistence of illness at syndromic levels of intensity in nearly 20%, and subthreshold levels of symptomatic eating disturbance behaviors in a significant proportion of cases (Keel and Mitchell, 1997). Recent studies of long-term course progression (Eddy et al., 2007; Fichter and Quadflieg, 2007) suggest a generally greater morbidity and continuity of disease phenotype in AN compared to BN, and a generally worse outcome among individuals with BN in whom AN was present premorbidly.

FAMILIALITY AND HERITABILITY

Findings from case-control studies (Lilenfeld et al., 1998; Strober et al., 2000) suggest a 7- to 12-fold increase in the prevalence of AN and BN in relatives of eating disordered probands compared to relatives of never ill controls. This significant familial recurrence risk of AN and BN provides impressive evidence of the transmissibility of both phenotypes. However, the relative contribution of genes versus nongenetic familial factors to the observed pattern of familial aggregation remains unknown.

Twin studies can differentiate genetic from environmental effects by comparing concordance for a trait, or disorder, between identical (monozygotic; MZ) and fraternal (dizygotic; DZ) twins. Although few in number, twin studies of AN and BN suggest a significant contribution of genes to liability, with 58%–76% of the variance in AN (Wade et al., 2000; Klump, McGue, and Iacono, 2001) and 54%–83% of the variance in BN (Kendler et al., 1991; Bulik et al., 1998) accounted for by additive genetic factors, in line with estimates of heritability reported for schizophrenia and bipolar disorder.

As already noted, in spite of their differentiating characteristics, AN and BN share at least some underlying familial liability factors. Convergent findings from twin studies indicate an increased coaggregation of AN and BN among identical twins, supporting evidence of a confluence of shared and unique etiopathogenic features characterizing the broader spectrum of eating disorder phenotypes (Lilenfeld et al., 1998).

That the transmitted liability to eating disorders may possibly be mediated by a more diffuse phenotype of continuous behavioral traits is suggested by evidence of

(*1*) significant heritability of disordered eating attitudes, weight preoccupation, dissatisfaction with weight and shape, dietary restraint, binge eating, and self-induced vomiting (Rutherford et al., 1993; Sullivan et al., 1998; Wade et al., 1998; Wade et al., 1999; Klump, McGue, and Iacono, 2000), and (*2*) familiality of subthreshold forms of eating disorders (Strober et al., 2000).

Recent data (Klump, McGue, and Iacono, 2000, 2001) from the Minnesota Twin Family Study (MTFS) illustrate the effects of age and pubertal status on the heritability of eating attitudes and behaviors. In the first of these studies (Klump, McGue, and Iacono, 2000), the differential influence of genetic versus environmental effects was compared between 680 11-year-old twins and 602 17-year-old twins. Whereas genetic influence on weight preoccupation and overall eating pathology was negligible for the younger age cohort, over half of the variance in these attitudes and behaviors could be accounted for by genetic factors in the 17-year-old cohort. The follow-up analysis of the data set (Klump, McGue, and Iacono, 2001), in which the younger cohort was subdivided by pubertal status, revealed a more powerful effect of puberty than age per se, suggesting a potential mediating role of pubertal ovarian steroid activity in activating genes of etiologic significance.

MOLECULAR GENETIC FINDINGS

The first genome-wide search for potential susceptibility genes in AN (see Kaye et al., 2000) was an international collaboration that applied a nonparametric allele sharing linkage analysis to data from 192 kindreds with at least one affected relative pair with AN and related eating disorders, including BN (Grice et al., 2002). Although evidence for linkage in the entire sample was negligible, an analysis using a narrow affection status model comprising relatives with restricting type AN (RAN) only generated a peak multipoint nonparametric linkage score of 3.45 in the 1p33–36 region. Further analysis (B. Devlin et al., 2002) using a covariate-based linkage analysis identified two variables, drive for thinness and obsessionality, incorporated as covariates into the linkage analysis, identified other regions of potential interest, one close to genome-wide significance on chromosome 1q (log of odds ratio: LOD = 3.46). Although considered preliminary, these initial findings suggest genetic heterogeneity in eating disorders and the potential value of applying more refined genomic analyses on large samples of patients with AN.

A growing number of studies using a case-control design have examined the potential association of various candidate genes with AN and BN (see reviews by Klump, Miller, et al., 2001; Tozzi et al., 2002). Evidence linking AN and BN to monoamine functioning have led researchers to target serotonin (5-HT_{2A}, 5-$HT_{1Dß}$, 5-HTT, 5-HT7, tryptophan hydroxylase receptor [TPH]) and dopamine (DA)-related genes ($D_{3,}$ D_4), but findings to date have been inconsistent or negative. The initial report of linkage of RAN to the chromosome 1p region (Grice et al., 2002) was followed up with a report of evidence of significant association with two genes under this linkage peak, the serotonin 1d (HTR1D) and delta opioid (OPRD1) receptor, along with the DA receptor on chromosome 11 (Bergen et al., 2003). A British group has reported a confirmation of the HTR1D and OPRD1 association in a case control study (Brown et al., 2007).

The presumptive role of atypicalities in feeding and energy expenditure in the pathophysiology of AN and BN has lead researchers to examine genes related to these processes. Findings suggest possible associations between the *UCP-2/UCP-3* gene (Campbell et al., 1999), the estrogen receptor ß gene (Rosenkranz et al., 1998), and the gene for agouti-related protein (Vink et al., 2001) and AN, but here, too, no consistently replicated evidence for association with either AN or BN has accrued to date.

Association studies of BN are scant, with one study (Bulik et al., 2003) reporting significant linkage on chromosome 10p, and another (Steiger et al., 2005) suggesting that the short (S) allele in the promoter region of the serotonin transporter gene may confer risk for affective and behavior dysregulation among persons with BN.

In general, the results in this area to date argue convincingly for the importance of characterizing the latent phenotypic structure underlying these conditions and the application of more refined covariate and quantitative trait locus models of genome-wide association and linkage analyses (Bacanu et al., 2005; Bulik et al., 2005) in the search for genes of potential relevance.

BEHAVIORAL SYMPTOMS IN FAMILIES AS POTENTIAL INTERMEDIATE PHENOTYPES

A variety of behavioral symptoms and traits characterize the promorbid state in people with AN or BN, some of which persist following recovery from low body weight or binge eating. That such phenomena may index expression of a genetic diathesis is a notion receiving increasing attention.

Several family and twin studies have examined the covariation between eating disorders and various other psychiatric conditions that co-occur with AN and BN. These studies have been reviewed in detail (Lilenfeld et al., 1998; Strober et al., 2000; Godart et al., 2002). With regard to major affective illness, studies of AN probands have yielded familial risk estimates in the range of 7%–25%, compared to relative risk estimates in normal controls in the range of 2.1–3.4 (Strober et al., 2006). Likewise, studies of BN probands have shown, with rare exception, that their first-degree relatives are several times more likely to develop affective disorders than relatives of control probands. Two recent twin studies are in accord with this conclusion, finding evidence for shared as well as unique genetic influences on major depression and AN and BN (Kendler et al., 1995; Wade et al., 2000), and a recent family study (Strober et al., 2006; Strober et al., 2007) suggests the intriguing possibility that the frequent co-occurrence of AN with affective and anxiety disorders may stem from pleiotropic effects of genes shared by these clinical syndromes.

Family studies investigating rates of substance use disorders suggest relatively low rates among relatives of RAN probands. In contrast, rates are elevated in relatives of probands with BN. However, several studies (Kaye et al., 1996; Schuckit et al., 1996) indicate that there is no evidence of a cross-transmission of BN and substance use disorder in families, and twin data (Kendler et al., 1995) have shown that the genes influencing susceptibility to alcoholism were independent of those underlying risk to BN.

Independent familial transmission of obsessive–compulsive disorder (OCD) and AN and BN was recently found in a controlled family study of eating disorders (Lilenfeld et al., 1998). By contrast, shared transmission was found between broadly defined AN and BN and the childhood anxiety disorders *separation anxiety* and *overanxious disorder* (Miller et al., 1998), and shared genetic transmission was found between BN and phobia and panic disorder (Kendler et al., 1995). Preliminary data suggest common familial transmission of AN and obsessive–compulsive personality disorder (OCPD; Lilenfeld et al., 1998). Findings indicated an increased risk of OCPD in relatives of AN probands compared to controls, even after accounting for the effects of proband comorbidity for these disorders. These results suggest the possible existence of a broad, genetically influenced phenotype with core features of rigid perfectionism and propensity for extreme behavioral constraint.

PERSISTENT SYMPTOMS AFTER RECOVERY

Determining whether behavioral symptoms are a consequence or cause of the eating disorder is problematic. Premorbid studies are not practical, but patients can be studied after long-term recovery from an eating disorder. The assumed absence of confounding nutritional influences in women who recovered from an eating disorder thus raises a possibility that persistent psychobiological abnormalities might be trait related, contributing to the pathogenesis of this disorder. Although no agreed-upon definition of recovery from AN or BN presently exists, investigators tend toward a definition that emphasizes stable and healthy body weight for months or years, the relative absence of pathological eating behavior, and normal cyclical menstruation.

Several reports (Strober, 1980; Casper, 1990; Srinivasagam et al., 1995; Kaye et al., 1998) have found that in many women long-term recovered from AN and BN, there is conspicuous persistence of anxiety, novelty seeking (especially among those with BN), perfectionism, and obsessional behaviors along with feelings of ineffectiveness, a drive for thinness, and unusual habits related to eating behavior. The persistence of these symptoms after recovery thus raises the intriguing question of whether sex-specific disturbances of such behaviors may in fact occur premorbidly and contribute to disease pathogenesis in AN and BN.

NEUROBIOLOGY OF EATING DISORDERS

The role of biology in the etiology of AN has been proposed for many decades (Treasure et al., 1994). New understandings of the neurotransmitter modulation of appetitive behaviors have raised the question of whether such disturbances cause eating disorders (Morley and Blundell, 1988; Fava et al., 1989). Moreover, technologies that permit direct measurements of complex brain function and relationships to behavior are shedding new light on the pathophysiology of these disorders.

Brain Imaging Studies in Eating Disorders

It is well known that patients ill with AN have enlarged ventricles and sulci widening (see review by A.R. Ellison and Fong, 1998). 1H-MRS revealed reduced lipid signals in the frontal white matter and occipital gray matter and was associated with decreased body mass index (Roser et al., 1999). Whether these abnormalities persist to a lesser degree after weight restoration is less certain because some studies show persistent alterations (Katzman et al., 1996) but other studies show normalization of gray and white matter after recovery in AN and BN (Wagner, Greer, et al., 2006).

I. Gordon et al. (1997) found that 13 of 15 patients ill with AN had unilateral temporal lobe hypoperfusion that persisted in the patients studied after weight restoration. A later study (Chowdhury et al., 2001) found adolescent patients with AN had unilateral temporoparietal and frontal lobe hypoperfusion. Kuruoglu et al. (1998) studied 2 patients ill with AN with bilateral hypoperfusion in frontal, temporal, and parietal regions which normalized after 3 months of remission. Takano et al. (2001) found hypoperfusion in the medial prefrontal cortex and anterior cingulate and hyperperfusion in the thalamus and amygdalo-hippocampal complex. Rastam et al. (2001) found temporo-parietal and orbitofrontal hypoperfusion in patients who had recovered from AN. Fewer studies have assessed glucose metabolism using positron emission tomography (PET). Delvenne et al. (1995) studied patients ill with AN who, compared to controls, had frontal and parietal hypometabolism that normalized with weight gain. More recently, resting blood flow in RAN before and after weight restoration suggested reduced blood flow in the anterior cingulate in both state conditions compared to controls using single photon emission computed tomography (SPECT) (Kojima, Nagai, and Nakabeppu, 2005). Taken together, studies in the resting condition most frequently suggest alterations of the temporal, parietal, or cingulate cortex during the ill state. A few older studies suggest persistent alterations in those areas after weight gain. Few brain imaging studies have been done in BN, but several (Wu et al., 1990; Andreason et al., 1992; Nozoe et al., 1995; Delvenne et al., 1999) raise the possibility of frontal or temporal alterations and hemispheric asymmetry.

In summary, these earlier studies show temporal region disturbances in patients with AN when ill and after various degrees of recovery. In addition, other brain areas, such as frontal and cingulate regions, and the parietal cortex are often altered. Although these studies show remarkable consistency, particularly in terms of temporal involvement, it should be noted that numbers of patients in each study tend to be small, and there is often inconsistency in terms of definition of subgroups and states of illness studied. Small sample size and irregular definitions make it difficult to know whether these are lateralizing findings or whether there are differences between subtypes of eating disorders. The meaning of these findings is open to interpretation. At the least, they suggest that regions of the brain involved in the modulation of mood, cognition, impulse control, and decision making may be altered in AN and BN. Still, this is a promising start and should be strong support for further investigations.

BODY IMAGE DISTORTION

A most puzzling symptom of AN is the severe and intense body image distortion in which emaciated individuals perceive themselves as fat. Theoretically, body image distortion might be related to the syndrome of neglect (Mesulam, 1981), which may be coded in parietal, frontal, and cingulate regions that assign motivational relevance to sensory events. It is well known that lesions in the right parietal cortex may not only result in denial of illness or anosognosia, somatoparaphrenia, the numerous misidentification syndromes, but may also produce experiences of disorientation of body parts and body image distortion. It has long been recognized that the parietal cortex mediates perceptions of the body and its activity in physical space (Gerstmann, 1924). Recent work extends this concept to suggest that the parietal lobe contributes to the experience of being an "agent" of one's own actions (Farrar et al., 2003). Wagner and colleagues (2003) confronted patients with AN and age-matched healthy controls with their own digitally distorted body images as well as images of a different person using a computer-based video technique. These studies reported a hyperresponsiveness in brain areas belonging to the frontal visual system and the attention network (BA 9) as well as inferior parietal lobule (BA 40), including the anterior part of the intraparietal (IPL) sulcus. Bailer et al. (2004) reported negative relationships between 5-HT_{2A} receptor activity and the Eating Disorder Inventory Drive for Thinness Scale in the left parietal cortex and other regions. It is intriguing to raise the possibility that left hemisphere disturbances of this pathway may contribute to body image distortion.

APPETITIVE REGULATION

Individuals with AN and those who have had lifetime diagnoses of AN and BN (AN–BN) tend to have negative mood states and dysphoric temperament. There is evidence that there is a dysphoria reducing character to dietary restraint (Vitousek and Manke, 1994; Strober, 1995; Kaye et al., 2003) and binge–purge behaviors (Abraham and Beaumont, 1982; Johnson and Larson, 1982; Kaye et al., 1986). This would suggest some interaction between pathways regulating appetitive behaviors and emotions. In fact, functional magnetic resonance imagining (fMRI) studies support this hypothesis. When emaciated and malnourished AN individuals are shown pictures of food, they display abnormal activity in the insula and orbitofrontal cortex (OFC) as well as in mesial temporal, parietal, and anterior cingulate cortex (Nozoe et al., 1993; Nozoe et al., 1995; Z. Ellison et al., 1998; Naruo et al., 2000; C.M. Gordon et al., 2001; Uher et al., 2004). Studies using SPECT, PET-O15, or fMRI found that when patients ill with AN ate food or were exposed to food, they had activated temporal regions and often increased anxiety (Nozoe et al., 1993; Z. Ellison et al., 1998; Naruo et al., 2000; C.M. Gordon et al., 2001). Those results could be consistent with anxiety provocation and related amygdala activation, and the notion that the emotional value of an experience is stored in the amygdala (LeDoux, 2003). Uher et al. (2003) used pictures of food and nonfood aversive emotional stimuli and fMRI to assess patients who had recovered (REC) from AN. Food stimulated medial prefrontal and anterior cingulate cortex in patients ill with AN and in patients recovered from AN but lateral prefrontal regions only in the REC group. In patients recovered from AN, prefrontal cortex, anterior cingulate cortex (ACC), and cerebellum were more highly activated after food compared to control participants and those chronically ill with AN. This finding suggested that higher ACC and medial prefrontal cortex activity in women ill with AN and women recovered from AN compared to control women (CW) may be a trait marker for AN.

A recent study used fMRI to investigate the effect of administration of nutrients. Compared to controls, patients recovered from AN had a significantly reduced fMRI signal response to the blind administration of sucrose or water in the insula, anterior cingulate, and striatal regions (Fig. 84.1). For CW, self-ratings of pleasantness of the sugar taste were positively correlated to the signal response in the insula, anterior cingulate, and ventral and dorsal putamen. In comparison, individuals recovered from AN failed to show any relationship in these regions to self-ratings of pleasant response to a sucrose taste. A large literature shows that the anterior insula and associated gustatory cortex respond not only to the taste and physical properties of food but also to its rewarding properties (Schultz et al., 2000; O'Doherty et al., 2001; Small et al., 2001). Insular inputs to the ventrolateral striatum are hypothesized to mediate behaviors involving eating, particularly of highly palatable, high-energy foods (Kelley et al., 2002). Patients with AN tend to avoid high-calorie, palatable food. In theory, this is consistent with abnormal responses of insula-striatal circuits that are hypothesized to mediate behavioral responses to the incentive value of food.

THE INSULA AND INTEROCEPTIVE AWARENESS

Do individuals with AN have an insular disturbance specifically related to gustatory modulation, or a more generalized disturbance related to the integration of interoceptive stimuli? The insula is thought to play an important role in processing interoceptive information, which can be defined as the sense of the physiological condition of the entire body (Craig, 2002). Aside from taste, interoceptive information includes sensations such as temperature, touch, muscular and visceral sensations, vasomotor flush, air hunger, and others (Paulus and Stein, 2006). The role of the insula is thus focused on how the value of stimuli might affect the body state. Interoception has long been thought to be critical for self-awareness because it provides the link between cognitive and affective processes and the current body state.

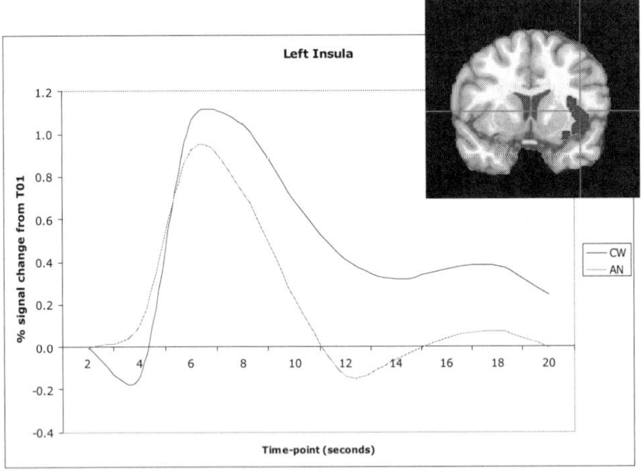

FIGURE 84.1 Coronal view of left insula ROI (x = –41, y = 5, z = 5). Time course of blood oxygen level dependent (BOLD) signal as a mean of all 16 recovered restricting-type anorexia nervosa and 16 control women for taste-related (sucrose and water) response in the left insula. ROI: region of interest.

STUDIES OF NEUROTRANSMITTERS

Neuropeptides

The past decade has witnessed accelerating basic research on the role of neuropeptides in the regulation of feeding behavior. Indirect evidence from clinical studies suggests the possibility that altered regulation of neuropeptides may contribute to abnormal eating patterns in the eating disorders and in obesity. The mechanisms for controlling food intake involve a complicated interplay between peripheral systems (including gustatory stimulation, gastrointestinal peptide secretion, and vagal afferent nerve responses) and central nervous system (CNS) neuropeptides and/or monoamines. Thus, studies in animals show that neuropeptides, such as cholecystokinin, the endogenous opioids (such as β-endorphin), and neuropeptide-Y, regulate the rate, duration, and size of meals, as well as macronutrient selection (Morley and Blundell, 1988; Schwartz et al., 2000; Saper et al., 2002). In addition to regulating eating behavior, a number of CNS neuropeptides participate in the regulation of neuroendocrine pathways. Thus, clinical studies have evaluated the possibility that CNS neuropeptide alterations may contribute to dysregulated secretion of the gonadal hormones, cortisol, thyroid hormones, and growth hormone in the eating disorders (Stoving et al., 1999; Jimerson and Wolfe, 2004).

Although there are relatively few studies to date, most of the neuroendocrine and neuropeptide alterations apparent during symptomatic episodes of AN and BN tend to normalize after recovery. This observation suggests that most of the disturbances are consequences rather than causes of malnutrition, weight loss, and/or altered meal patterns. Still, an understanding of these neuropeptide disturbances may shed light on why many people with AN or BN cannot easily "reverse" their illness. In AN, malnutrition may contribute to a downward spiral sustaining and perpetuating the desire for more weight loss and dieting. Symptoms such as increased satiety, obsessions, and dysphoric mood may be exaggerated by these neuropeptide alterations and thus contribute to this downward spiral. Additionally, mutual interactions between neuropeptide, neuroendocrine, and neurotransmitter pathways may contribute to the constellation of psychiatric comorbidity often observed in these disorders. Even after weight gain and normalized eating patterns, many individuals who have recovered from AN or BN have physiological, behavioral, and psychological symptoms that persist for extended periods of time. Menstrual cycle dysregulation, for example, may persist for some months after weight restoration. The following sections provide a brief overview of studies of neuropeptides in AN and BN.

When underweight, patients with AN have increased plasma cortisol secretion that is thought to be at least in part a consequence of hypersecretion of endogenous CRH (Gold et al., 1986; Kaye, Gwirtsman, et al., 1987; Walsh et al., 1987; Licinio et al., 1996). In that the plasma and cerebrospinal fluid (CSF) measures return toward normal, it appears likely that activation of the hypothalamic–pituitary–adrenal axis (HPA) axis is precipitated by weight loss. The observation of increased CRH activity is of great theoretical interest in AN because intracerebroventricular CRH administration in experimental animals produces many of the physiologic and behavioral changes associated with AN, including markedly decreased eating behavior (Glowa and Gold, 1991).

Opioid Peptides

Studies in laboratory animals raise the possibility that altered endogenous opioid activity might contribute to pathological feeding behavior in eating disorders because opioid agonists generally increase, and opioid antagonists decrease, food intake (Morley et al., 1985). State-related reductions in concentrations of CSF β-endorphin and related opiate concentrations have been found in ill AN patients and in ill BN patients (Kaye, Berrettini, et al., 1987; Lesem et al., 1991; Brewerton et al., 1992). In contrast, using the T-lymphocyte as a model system, Brambilla, Brunetta, Peirone, et al. (1995) found elevated β-endorphin levels in AN, although the levels were normal in BN (Brambilla, Brunetta, Draisci, et al., 1995). If β-endorphin activity is a facilitator of feeding behavior, then reduced CSF concentrations could reflect decreased central activity of this system, which then maintains or facilitates inhibition of feeding behavior in the eating disorders.

Neuropeptide-Y (NPY) and Peptide YY (PYY)

Neuropeptide-Y (NPY) and peptide YY (PYY) are of considerable theoretical interest because they are among the most potent endogenous stimulants of feeding behavior within the CNS (Morley et al., 1985; Kalra et al., 1991; Schwartz et al., 2000). Peptide YY is more potent than NPY in stimulating food intake; both are selective for carbohydrate-rich foods. Underweight individuals with AN have been shown to have elevations of CSF NPY, but normal PYY (Kaye, Berrettini, et al., 1990). Clearly, elevated NPY does not result in increased feeding in underweight patients with anorexia; however, the possibility that increased NPY activity underlies the obsessive and paradoxical interest in dietary intake and food preparation is a hypothesis worth exploring. On the other hand, CSF levels of NPY and PYY have been reported to be normal in women with BN when measured while patients were acutely ill. Although levels of PYY increased above normal when patients were reassessed after 1 month of abstinence from bingeing and vomiting, levels of the peptides were similar to control values in patients who were in long-term recovery (Gendall, 1999).

More recently, it has been reported that the plasma concentration of NPY was lower in patients with anorexia than in controls, whereas patients with bulimia had elevated NPY levels (Baranowska et al., 2001). Other data indicate that basal plasma PYY levels in AN are similar to or elevated in comparison to control values, with variability in postprandial PYY responses also noted across studies (Stock et al., 2005; Misra et al., 2006; Germain et al., 2007; Nakahara et al., 2007; Otto et al., 2007). Initial studies indicate that basal plasma PYY levels in BN are similar to control values, but that the postprandial response is significantly blunted in the patient group (Kojima, Nakahara, et al., 2005; Monteleone et al., 2005). Additional research will be needed to assess the potential behavioral correlates of these findings.

Cholecystokinin

Cholecystokinin (CCK) is a peptide secreted by the gastrointestinal system in response to food intake. Release of CCK is thought to be one means of transmitting satiety signals to the brain by way of vagal afferents (Gibbs et al., 1973). In parallel to its role in satiety in rodents, exogenously administered CCK reduces food intake in humans (Kissileff et al., 1981). The preponderance of data suggests that patients with BN, in comparison to controls, have diminished release of CCK following ingestion of a standardized test meal (Geracioti and Liddle, 1988; Phillipp et al., 1991; Pirke et al., 1994; M.J. Devlin et al., 1997; Keel et al., 2007). Measurements of basal CCK values in blood lymphocytes and in CSF also appear to be decreased in patients with BN (Lydiard et al., 1993; Brambilla, Brunetta, Draisci, et al., 1995). It has been suggested that the diminished CCK response to a meal may play a role in diminished postingestive satiety observed in BN (LaChaussee et al., 1992). The CCK response in patients with bulimia was found to return toward normal following treatment (Geracioti and Liddle, 1988).

Studies of CCK in AN have yielded less consistent findings. Some studies have found elevations in basal levels of plasma CCK (Phillipp et al., 1991; Tamai et al., 1993), as well as increased peptide release following a test meal (Harty et al., 1991; Phillipp et al., 1991). One study found that blunting of CCK response to an oral glucose load normalized in patients with anorexia after partial restoration of body weight (Tamai et al., 1993). Other studies have found that measures of CCK function in AN were similar to or lower than control values (Geracioti et al., 1992; Pirke et al., 1994; Brambilla, Brunetta, Peirone, et al., 1995; Baranowska et al., 2000). Further studies are needed to evaluate the relationship between altered CCK regulation and other indices of abnormal gastric function in patients symptomatic with bulimia and anorexia (Geliebter et al., 1992).

Leptin

Leptin, the protein product of the *ob* gene, is secreted predominantly by adipose tissue cells. In the hypothalamus, leptin interacts with neuropeptide Y, serotonin, and the melanocortins to decrease food intake, thus regulating body fat stores (Zhang et al., 1994; Friedman and Halaas, 1998; Zigman and Elmquist, 2003). In rodent models, defects in the leptin coding sequence resulting in leptin deficiency or defects in leptin receptor function are associated with obesity. In humans, serum and CSF concentrations of leptin are positively correlated with fat mass in individuals across a broad range of body weight, including obesity (Considine et al., 1996; Schwartz et al., 1996). Thus, obesity in humans is not thought to be a result of leptin deficiency per se, although rare genetic deficiencies in leptin production have been associated with familial obesity (Farooqi et al., 2001).

Underweight patients with AN have consistently been found to have significantly reduced serum leptin concentrations in comparison to normal weight controls (Hebebrand et al., 1995; Grinspoon et al., 1996; Mantzoros et al., 1997; Eckert et al., 1998; Baranowska et al., 2001; Monteleone et al., 2004). Based on studies in laboratory animals, it has been suggested that low leptin levels may contribute to amenorrhea and other hormonal changes in the disorder (Mantzoros et al., 1997; Ahima et al., 2000; Holtkamp et al., 2003; Ahima and Osei, 2004). In healthy volunteers, even modest reductions in energy intake result in substantial decreases in circulating leptin levels (Wolfe et al., 2004). Although the reduction in fasting serum leptin levels in AN is correlated with reduction in body mass index, there has been some discussion of the possibility that leptin levels in patients with anorexia may be higher than expected based on the extent of weight loss (Frederich et al., 2002; Jimerson, 2002). Mantzoros et al. (1997) reported an elevated CSF to serum leptin ratio in patients with AN compared to controls, suggesting that the proportional decrease in leptin levels with weight loss is greater in serum than in CSF. A longitudinal investigation during refeeding in AN patients has shown that CSF leptin concentrations reach normal values before full weight restoration, possibly as a consequence of the relatively rapid and disproportionate accumulation of fat during refeeding (Mantzoros et al., 1997). This finding led the authors to suggest that premature normalization of leptin concentration might contribute to difficulty in achieving and sustaining a normal weight in AN. Further research is needed to assess whether serum leptin levels at the time of discharge are predictive of posthospital clinical course (Lob et al., 2003; Holtkamp et al., 2004). Plasma and CSF leptin levels appear to be similar to control values in patients with AN who are long-term recovered (Gendall, 1999).

As recently reviewed (Monteleone et al., 2004), patients with BN, in comparison to carefully matched controls, have significantly decreased leptin concentrations in serum samples obtained after overnight fast (Brewerton et al., 2000; Jimerson et al., 2000; Monteleone et al., 2000; Baranowska et al., 2001; Frederich et al., 2002). Initial findings in individuals who have achieved sustained recovery from BN, when compared to controls with closely matched percent body fat, suggest that serum leptin levels remain decreased. This finding may be related to evidence for a persistent decrease in activity in the HPA axis in patients with BN who are long-term recovered (Wolfe et al., 2000). These alterations could be associated with decreased metabolic rate and a tendency toward weight gain, contributing to the preoccupation with body weight characteristic of BN.

Ghrelin

Intracerebroventricular injections of the gut-related peptide *ghrelin* strongly stimulated feeding in rats and increased body weight gain. When administered to healthy human volunteers, ghrelin results in increased hunger and food intake (Wren et al., 2001). In addition, it has been reported that fasting plasma ghrelin concentrations in humans are negatively correlated with body mass index (BMI) (Shiiya et al., 2002; Tanaka et al., 2002), percentage body fat and fasting leptin and insulin concentrations (Tschop et al., 2001). As recently reviewed, a number of studies have shown elevation in circulating ghrelin levels in AN, with a return to normal levels as patients regain weight (Jimerson and Wolfe, 2006). Further research is needed to explore the possible existence of ghrelin resistance in cachectic states related to the eating disorders.

Studies comparing fasting plasma ghrelin concentrations in patients with BN and healthy controls have yielded variable results (Jimerson and Wolfe, 2006). It is of interest, however, that the postprandial decrease in ghrelin levels appears to be blunted in patients with BN (Kojima, Nagai, and Nakabeppu, 2005; Monteleone et al., 2005), consistent with other evidence for diminished satiety responses in the disorder.

Monoamine Systems

There is an abundance of evidence that individuals with AN and BN have disturbances of monoamine function in the ill state. Although less well studied, monoamine disturbances appear to persist after recovery.

Dopamine

Altered DA activity has been found among patients ill with AN and BN. Homovanillic acid (HVA), the major metabolite of DA in humans, was decreased in CSF of underweight patients with AN (Kaye et al., 1984). While patients ill with BN, as a group, have normal CSF HVA, several studies have shown a significant reduction of CSF HVA in patients with BN with high binge frequency (Kaye, Ballenger, et al., 1990; Jimerson et al., 1992). Individuals with AN have altered frequency of functional polymorphisms of DA D_2 receptor genes that might affect receptor transcription and translation efficiency (Bergen et al., 2005). Central nervous system DA metabolism may explain differences in symptoms between patients with AN, AN–BN, and BN. Our group (Kaye et al., 1999) found that patients recovered from AN had significantly reduced concentrations of CSF HVA, compared to women who recovered from AN–BN or BN (Fig. 84.2). Dopamine neuronal function has been associated with motor activity (Kaye et al., 1999), reward (Blum et al., 1995; Salamone, 1996), and novelty seeking. Individuals with AN have stereotyped and hyperactive motor behavior, anhedonic, restrictive personalities, and reduced novelty seeking.

Serotonin

Serotonin (5-HT) pathways play an important role in postprandial satiety. Treatments that increase intrasynaptic 5-HT, or directly activate 5-HT receptors, tend to reduce food consumption whereas interventions that dampen 5-HT neurotransmission or block receptor activation reportedly increase food consumption and promote weight gain (Blundell, 1984; Leibowitz and Shor-Posner, 1986). Moreover, CNS 5-HT pathways have been implicated in the modulation of mood, impulse regulation and behavioral constraint, and obsessionality, and they affect a variety of neuroendocrine systems.

There has been considerable interest in the role that 5-HT may play in AN and BN (Jimerson et al., 1990; Kaye and Weltzin, 1991; Treasure and Campbell, 1994; Brewerton, 1995; Kaye et al., 1998; Steiger et al., 2005).

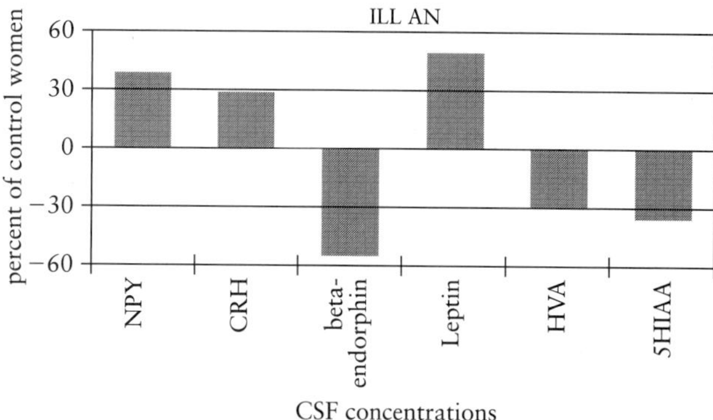

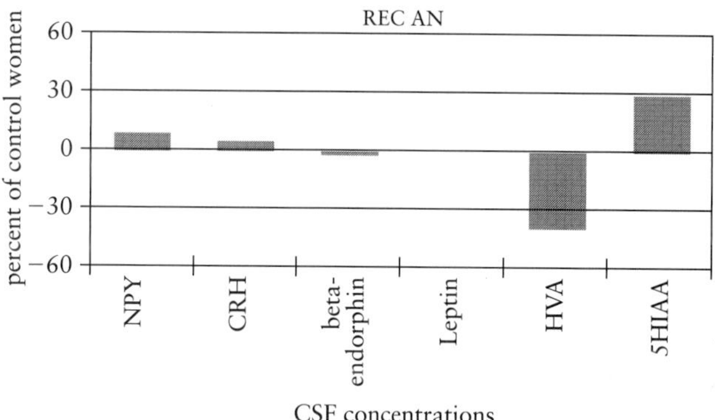

FIGURE 84.2 Comparison of cerebrospinal fluid (CSF) concentrations of neuropeptide and monoamine metabolites in individuals who were ill (underweight) and long-term recovered from anorexia nervosa (AN). CSF values in AN are compared to healthy control women, where control mean values are set to 0.

In part, this is related to the fact that studies have found that AN and BN have alterations in 5-HT metabolism. When underweight, individuals with AN have a significant reduction in basal concentrations of the serotonin metabolite *5-hydroxyindolacetic acid* (5-HIAA) in the CSF compared to healthy controls, as well as blunted plasma prolactin response to drugs with 5-HT activity and reduced ^{3}H-imipramine binding. Together, these findings suggest reduced serotonergic activity, although this may arise secondarily from reductions in dietary supplies of the 5-HT synthesizing amino acid *tryptophan*. By contrast, CSF concentrations of 5-HIAA are reported to be elevated in patients with AN who were long-term weight recovered. These contrasting findings of reduced serotonergic activity in patients acutely ill with AN and heightened serotonergic activity in patients with long-term recovery from AN may seem counterintuitive; however, because dieting lowers plasma tryptophan levels in otherwise healthy women (Anderson et al., 1990), resumption of normal eating in individuals with AN may unmask intrinsic abnormalities in serotonergic systems that mediate certain core behavioral or temperamental underpinnings of risk and vulnerability.

Considerable evidence also exists for a dysregulation of serotonergic processes in BN. Examples include blunted prolactin response to the 5-HT receptor agonists *m-chlorophenylpiperazine* (m-CPP), *5-hydroxytrytophan*, and *dl-fenfluramine*, and enhanced migraine-like headache response to m-CPP challenge. Acute perturbation of serotonergic tone by dietary depletion of tryptophan has also been linked to increased food intake and mood irritability in individuals with BN compared to healthy controls. And, like AN, women with long-term recovery from BN have been shown to have elevated concentrations of 5-HIAA in the CSF as well as increased platelet binding of paroxetine.

There is an extensive literature associating the serotonergic systems and fundamental aspects of behavioral inhibition (Soubrie, 1986; Geyer, 1996). Reduced CSF 5-HIAA levels are associated with increased impulsivity and aggression in humans and nonhuman primates, whereas increased CSF 5-HIAA levels are related to behavioral inhibition (Fairbanks et al., 2001; Westergaard et al., 2003). Thus, it is of interest that women who recovered from AN and BN had elevated CSF 5-HIAA concentrations. Behaviors found after recovery from AN and BN, such as obsessionality with symmetry and exactness, anxiety, and perfectionism, tend to be opposite in character to behaviors displayed by people with low 5-HIAA levels. Together, these studies contribute to a growing literature suggesting that CSF 5-HIAA concentrations may correlate with a spectrum of behavior. Reduced CSF 5-HIAA levels appear to be related to behavioral undercontrol whereas increased CSF 5-HIAA concentrations may be related to behavioral overcontrol.

The possibility of a common vulnerability for BN and AN may seem puzzling given well-recognized differences in behavior in these disorders. However, recent studies suggest that AN and BN have a shared etiologic vulnerability. That is, there is a familial aggregation of a range of eating disorders in relatives of probands with either BN or AN, and these two disorders are highly comorbid in twin studies. Both disorders respond to 5-HT specific medications, and both disorders have high levels of harm avoidance (see Klump, Bulik, et al., 2000), a personality trait hypothesized to be related to increased 5-HT activity. These data raise the possibility that a disturbance of 5-HT activity may create a vulnerability for the expression of a cluster of symptoms that are common to AN and BN. Other factors that are independent of a vulnerability for the development of an eating disorder may contribute to the development of eating disorder subgroups. For example, people with RAN have extraordinary self-restraint and self-control. The risk for OCPD is elevated only in this subgroup and in their families and shows a shared transmission with RAN (Lilenfeld et al., 1998). In other words, an additional vulnerability for behavioral overcontrol and rigid and inflexible mood states, combined with a vulnerability for an eating disorder, may result in RAN.

The contribution of 5-HT to specific human behaviors remains uncertain. Serotonin has been postulated to contribute to temperament or personality traits such as harm avoidance (Cloninger, 1987) or behavioral inhibition (Soubrie, 1986) or to categorical dimensions such as OCD (Barr et al., 1992), anxiety and fear, (Charney et al., 1990) or depression (Grahame-Smith, 1992), as well as satiety for food consumption. It is possible that separate components of 5-HT neuronal systems (that is, different pathways or receptors) are coded for such specific behaviors. However, that may not be consistent with the neurophysiology of 5-HT neuronal function.

Positron emission tomography (PET) studies using 5-HT receptor radioligands

The marriage of PET imaging with selective neurotransmitter radioligands has resulted in a technology permitting new insights into regional binding and specificity of 5-HT and DA neurotransmission in vivo in humans and their relationship to behaviors.

The 5-HT_{1A} autoreceptor is located presynaptically on 5-HT somatodendritic cell bodies in the raphé nucleus, where it functions to decrease 5-HT neurotransmission (Staley et al., 1998). High densities of postsynaptic 5-HT_{1A} exist in the hippocampus, septum, amygdala, and entorhinal and frontal cortex, where they serve to mediate the effects of released 5-HT. Studies in animals and humans implicate the 5-HT_{1A} receptor in anxiety (File et al., 2000) and depression and/or suicide (Mann, 1999). Pharmacological and knockout studies implicate the 5-HT_{1A} receptor in the modulation of anxiety (Gross et al., 2002). Bailer et al. (2007) reported that patients ill with AN had a 50%–70% increase in 5-HT_{1A} receptor binding potential (BP) in subgenual, mesial temporal, orbital frontal, and raphé brain regions, as well as prefrontal, lateral temporal, anterior cingulate, and parietal regions. Increased 5-HT_{1A} postsynaptic activity has been reported in patients ill with BN (Tiihonen et al., 2004). Patients who recovered from AN–BN and BN (Bailer et al., 2005; Kaye, unpublished data) had a significant 20%–40% increase in 5-HT_{1A} receptor BP in these same regions compared to CW (Bailer et al., 2005). In contrast, women who recovered from RAN showed no difference in 5-HT_{1A} receptor BP compared to controls (Bailer et al., 2005).

Anorexia nervosa and BN are frequently comorbid with depression and anxiety disorders. However, reduced 5-HT_{1A} receptor BP has been found in patients ill with depression (Drevets et al., 1999; Sargent et al., 2000) and patients who have recovered from depression (Bhagwagar et al., 2004, as well as in a primate model for depression (Shively et al., 2006). Parsey et al. (2005) found no difference in carbonyl-[^{11}C]WAY100635 BP in major depressive disorder, although a subgroup of patients who were never medicated had elevated carbonyl-[^{11}C]WAY100635 BP. Recent studies have found reduced [^{11}C]WAY100635 BP in social phobia (Lanzenberger et al., 2007) and panic disorder (Neumeister et al., 2004). These findings suggest that AN and BN, mood, and depression share disturbances of common systems but are etiologically different.

Postsynaptic 5-HT_{2A} receptors, which are in high densities in the cerebral cortex and other regions of rodents and humans (Saudou and Hen, 1994; Burnet et al., 1997), are of interest because they have been implicated in the modulation of feeding and mood, as well as serotonin specific reuptake inhibitor (SSRI) response (Simansky, 1996; Stockmeier, 1997; Bonhomme and Esposito, 1998; De Vry and Schreiber, 2000; Bailer et al., 2004). Patients ill with AN have been found to have normal 5-HT_{2A} receptors BP values in one study (Bailer et al., 2007) and reduced BP in another study (Audenaert et al., 2003) in the left frontal, bilateral parietal, and occipital cortex. After recovery, patients with RAN (Frank et al., 2002) had reduced 5-HT_{2A} receptors BP in mesial temporal and parietal cortical areas as well as in subgenual and pregenual cingulate cortex. Similarly, women who recovered from BAN (Bailer et al., 2004) had reduced 5-HT_{2A} receptors BP in left subgenual cingulate, left parietal, and right occipital cortex. And women who recovered from BN only had reduced [^{18}F]altanserin BP relative to controls in the orbital frontal region (Kaye, Frank, et al., 2001).

The PET imaging studies in patients ill with and recovered from AN and BN described above have found significant correlations between harm avoidance and binding for the 5-HT_{1A}, 5-HT_{2A}, and DA D_2/D_3 receptors in mesial temporal and other limbic regions. Bailer et al. (2004) found that patients who recovered from AN–BN showed a positive relationship between [^{18}F]altanserin BP in the left subgenual cingulate and mesial temporal cortex and harm avoidance. For patients ill with AN, [^{18}F]altanserin BP was positively related to harm avoidance in the suprapragenual cingulate, frontal, and parietal regions. 5-HT_{2A} receptor binding and harm avoidance were shown to be negatively correlated in the frontal cortex in healthy participants (Moresco et al., 2002) and in the prefrontal cortex in patients that attempted suicide (van Heeringen et al., 2003). Clinical and epidemiological studies have consistently shown that one or more anxiety disorders occur in the majority of people with AN or BN (Kendler et al., 1995; Walters and Kendler, 1995; Godart et al., 2002; Kaye et al., 2004). Silberg and Bulik (2005), using twins, found a unique genetic effect that influences liability to early anxiety and eating disorder symptoms. When a lifetime anxiety disorder is present, the anxiety most commonly occurs first in childhood, preceding the onset of AN or BN (Deep et al., 1995; Bulik et al., 1997; Godart et al., 2000). Anxiety and harm avoidance remain elevated after recovery from AN, AN–BN, and BN (Wagner, Barbarich, et al., 2006), even if individuals never had a lifetime anxiety disorder diagnosis (Kaye et al., 2004). Finally, anxiety (Spielberger et al., 1970) and harm avoidance from the Cloninger (Cloninger et al., 1994) Temperament and Character Inventory (TCI) have been a robust signal in genetic studies (Bacanu et al., 2005). In summary, the premorbid onset and the persistence of anxiety and harm avoidance symptoms after recovery suggest these are traits that contribute to the pathogenesis of AN and BN. The PET imaging data suggest that such behaviors are related to disturbances of 5-HT and DA neurotransmitter function in limbic and executive pathways.

This technology holds the promise of a new era of understanding the complexity of neuronal systems in human behavior. For example, postsynaptic 5-HT_{1A} receptors (Sibille et al., 2000; Celada et al., 2001; Szabo and Blier, 2001; Richer et al., 2002) have "downstream" effects and interactions with other neuronal systems, such as norepinephrine, glutamate, and γ-aminobutyric acid (GABA). Enhanced 5-HT_{1A} activity in AN and BN may cause or reflect an altered balance between these neuronal systems. Moreover, 5-HT_{1A} receptors interact with other 5-HT receptors such as 5-HT_{2A} (Martin et al., 1997; Szabo and Blier, 2001). 5-HT_{1A} postsynaptic receptors mediate locus coeruleus firing through 5-HT transmission at 5-HT_{2A} receptors (Szabo and Blier, 2001). Theoretically, increased 5-HT_{1A} and reduced 5-HT_{2A} postsynaptic receptor activity in AN might result in an increase in noradrenergic neuròn firing (Szabo and Blier, 2001). Moreover, postsynaptic 5-HT_{1A} receptors hyperpolarize and 5-HT_{2A} receptors depolarize layer V pyramidal neurons (Martin-Ruiz et al., 2001). In AN, synergistic effects of these receptors, which are colocalized on pyramidal neurons, may reduce pyramidal neuronal excitability.

In summary, these PET radioligand studies confirm that altered 5-HT neuronal pathway activity persists after recovery from AN and BN and support the possibility that these psychobiological alterations might contribute to traits, such as increased anxiety, that may contribute to a vulnerability to develop an eating disorder.

TREATMENT

Bulimia Nervosa

Controlled trials have provided convincing evidence for the efficacy of psychological and pharmacological treatments for BN. These studies have been conducted in outpatient settings, given that inpatient treatment for BN is generally limited to patients with acute medical problems (for example, severe hypokalemia) or psychiatric comorbidity (for example, depression with suicidal ideation) (American Psychiatric Association Workgroup on Eating Disorders, 2006). The largest number of controlled trials has focused on manual-based cognitive behavioral treatment (CBT) (Fairburn, Jones, et al., 1993; Arnow, 1997; Shapiro et al., 2007). These studies have shown a decrease in the frequency of binge eating and purging episodes of approximately 60%–70%, with complete abstinence from these behaviors in some 30%–50% of cases. There is also evidence that CBT results in improvements in other psychological symptoms of the disorder, including preoccupation with body shape and weight, and that CBT is more effective than more narrow behavioral approaches in addressing bulimic symptoms. Other data suggest that manual-based interpersonal therapy may achieve reduction in symptoms similar to results achieved with CBT, although the rate of response may be somewhat slower (Fairburn, Marcus, and Wilson, 1993; Agras et al., 2000). Preliminary reports indicate that structured self-help approaches may be of assistance to some individuals (Mitchell et al., 2001; Perkins et al., 2006), consistent with suggestions regarding the potential usefulness of "stepped-care" algorithms in treatment planning.

The efficacy of antidepressant medications in the treatment of BN has been demonstrated in a number of double-blind, placebo-controlled trials (Jimerson et al., 1996; Zhu and Walsh, 2002; Shapiro et al., 2007). Beneficial effects have been seen across a variety of medication classes, including earlier trials with tricyclic agents and monoamine oxidase inhibitors, and more recent studies with SSRIs. Patients participating in these trials typically reported from 8 to 10 episodes of binge eating per week at baseline. The average decrease in binge frequency for patients receiving the antidepressant medication was about 55%, approximately twice the widely variable rate of response for patients randomized to placebo administration. Only a minority of patients in the medication treatment trials actually achieved full abstinence from binge eating and purging behaviors. Although antidepressant administration may contribute to reduction in symptoms of depression, the reduction in bulimic symptoms does not appear to be correlated with the magnitude of the antidepressant response. With similar response rates seen across different classes of antidepressants, initial choice of medication is often based on a range of clinical considerations including typical side-effect profile. Studies have shown that individuals who do not achieve a satisfactory response to an initial trial with one class of medication may respond to a second trial with an alternate agent. In the largest of the antidepressant trials, treatment with the SSRI *fluoxetine* (at a dose of 60 mg/day) resulted in a 67% decrease in the frequency of binge eating and a 56% decrease in self-induced vomiting episodes, significantly greater than the 33% and 5% decreases in binge eating and vomiting, respectively, seen in the placebo-treated group (Fluoxetine Bulimia Nervosa Collaborative Study Group, 1992). Consistent with clinical observations, follow-up data for individuals maintained on fluoxetine over the course of a year indicated a significant benefit for medication in comparison to placebo, although significant rates of clinical relapse occurred and the trial experienced substantial rates of attrition (Romano et al., 2002).

As a follow-up to controlled trials demonstrating efficacy for psychological and pharmacological modalities, a number of investigators have conducted direct comparisons of outcome for patients randomized to psychotherapy, to pharmacotherapy, or to combination treatment (Mitchell et al., 1990; Fichter et al., 1991; Agras et al., 1992; Leitenberg et al., 1994; Goldbloom et al., 1997; Walsh et al., 1997). In general, these trials have demonstrated a greater decrease in frequency of bulimic episodes for psychotherapy (usually CBT) in comparison to pharmacotherapy. Although combined treatment was not notably superior to either treatment alone, this approach may be helpful in decreasing symptoms of depression, anxiety, and eating-related symptoms in some individuals. Currently, there are no established predictors of which patients might respond preferentially to psychotherapy or pharmacotherapy, although it has been suggested that individuals who show little response during the early sessions of CBT or medication treatment may be candidates for alternate treatment interventions (Agras et al., 2000; Walsh, Sysko, and Parides, 2006).

Continued research is needed to develop new treatment approaches for nonresponsive patients, and to decrease relapse in those who do respond. Previous double-blind, placebo-controlled studies have reported mixed results in BN for a range of alternate agents, including naltrexone (Mitchell et al., 1989; Marrazzi et al., 1995), dexfenfluramine (Fahy et al., 1993), lithium (Hsu et al., 1991), and inositol (Gelber et al., 2001). A preliminary trial with the serotonin-3 receptor antagonist *ondansetron* showed a decrease in the frequency of bulimic symptoms in patients who were severely symptomatic (Faris et al., 2000).

Initial controlled trials have also indicated that the antiepileptic drug *topiramate* can reduce the frequency of binge eating and purging episodes in BN, although further studies are needed to assess efficacy and side effects in this patient population (Hoopes et al., 2003; Nickel et al., 2005).

Anorexia Nervosa

Progress in developing new and more effective treatment interventions for patients with AN has been slower than BN (Agras et al., 2004). Psychological approaches to the treatment of the disorder derived from psychoanalytic, family systems, and behaviorally oriented interventions (Arnow, 1997). For patients who are emaciated and hospitalized in psychiatric units experienced in the treatment of eating disorders, interdisciplinary approaches including supportive nursing care and behavioral techniques are frequently helpful in initiating the lengthy process of weight restoration (American Psychiatric Association Workgroup on Eating Disorders, 2006).

More recent controlled trials have demonstrated benefits of family therapy, insight-oriented therapy, and supportive psychotherapy (Russell et al., 1987; Treasure et al., 1995; Eisler et al., 1997; Dare et al., 2001). Family therapy techniques appear to be particularly helpful in younger patients with AN (Lock and le Grange, 2005). Follow-up studies suggest that these interventions may also help prevent relapse in patients who achieve weight restoration. Recent studies have begun more systematic evaluation of the potential benefits of manualized cognitive behavioral and family therapies for this disorder (Kleifield et al., 1996; Fairburn, 2005; Lock and le Grange, 2005).

The role of medication treatment in low-weight patients with AN has been limited (Jimerson et al., 1996; Attia et al., 2005; Bulik et al., 2007). One agent that appeared to accelerate weight gain in an early trial in AN was cyproheptadine (Halmi et al., 1986), although the magnitude of this effect was quite small. In contrast to the effectiveness of antidepressant medications in patients with BN, initial studies showed limited benefit with traditional antidepressant agents. More recently, several studies have failed to demonstrate a beneficial effect for the addition of SSRIs in the treatment of patients who were hospitalized with anorexia (Attia et al., 1998; Ferguson et al., 1999; Strober et al., 1999). Based on the important role of serotonin in the behavioral effects of antidepressant drugs (Blier and de Montigny, 1999), this lack of efficacy may be a result of decreased function in CNS serotonergic pathways which is characteristic of underweight patients with anorexia, and appears to be restored following weight gain (Wolfe et al., 1997; Kaye et al., 2005).

Initial interest in the possible benefit of neuroleptics in the treatment of AN was based on clinical observations of weight gain with these medications. Results from randomized, double-blind controlled trials with pimozide and sulpiride failed to demonstrate accelerated weight gain, however (Vandereycken and Pierloot, 1982; Vandereycken, 1984). Prompted in part by observations of weight gain in other patient groups associated with the use of atypical neuroleptics, promising results have been obtained in pilot studies of olanzapine and other atypical neuroleptic drugs in low-weight patients with anorexia (Barbarich et al., 2004; Bosanac et al., 2005; Mondraty et al., 2005; Steffen et al., 2006).

Patients with anorexia who have achieved weight restoration often have persisting psychological symptomatology accompanied by a significant risk of recurrence of low-weight episodes, leading to interest in studies of relapse prevention. A clinically based, prospective longitudinal follow-up study failed to show significant benefit of fluoxetine treatment in comparison to historical controls (Strober et al., 1997). Subsequently, a double-blind, placebo-controlled trial in patients whose weight was restored demonstrated that fluoxetine treatment was associated with reduced relapse rate and reductions in depression, anxiety, and obsessions and compulsions (Kaye, Nagata, et al., 2001). In contrast, a recent study failed to demonstrate a difference in time to relapse in patients with AN whose weight was restored who were receiving CBT and who were randomly assigned to adjunctive treatment with fluoxetine or placebo (Walsh, Kaplan, et al., 2006).

SUMMARY

There remain daunting challenges to the investigation of neurobiological mediators of risk and clinical pathology in AN and BN. To what extent abnormalities detected are consequences of pathological eating behavior, malnutrition, or their long-term sequelae remains speculative. Data on the functional status of these neurobiological systems are too sparse to allow for definitive conclusions regarding the possible etiological significance of differences reported between patients with an eating disorder and normal controls.

Clearly, many of the alterations in neuropeptide and monoaminergic function in eating disorders are state dependent; however, given the effects of these systems on mood, anxiety, memory organization, and body physiology they may well have significant pathogenic influence, sustaining and exacerbating certain psychological and cognitive elements of these syndromes. Thus, neurobiologically mediated effects may be contributing factors to the frequently long-term, pernicious, and self-sustaining course of illness, at least in many patients. These associations, while remaining speculative, nevertheless underscore the importance of aggressive and sustained treatment of the nutritional and behavioral-psychological elements of the syndromes to allow for stabilization and possible normalization of neuropeptidergic and monoaminergic functions.

Still, several lines of evidence from family, twin, premorbid-retrospective data, and studies after recovery suggest that traits, perhaps related to 5-HT modulation of anxiety and perfectionistic obsessiveness, create a susceptibility for some people to develop an eating disorder.

REFERENCES

Abraham, S., and Beaumont, P. (1982) How patients describe bulimia or binge eating. *Psychol. Med.* 12:625–635.

Agras, W., Brandt, H., Bulik, C., Dolan-Sewell, R., Fairburn, C., Halmi, K., Herzog, D., Jimerson, D., Kaplan, A., Kaye, W., Le Grange, D., Lock, J., Mitchell, J., Rudorfer, M., Street, L., Striegel-Moore, R., Vitousek, K., Walsh, B., and Wilfley, D. (2004) Report of the National Institutes of Health workshop on overcoming barriers to treatment research in anorexia nervosa. *Int. J. Eat. Disord.* 35:509–521.

Agras, W.S., Crow, S.J., Halmi, K.A., Mitchell, J.E., Wilson, G.T., and Kraemer, H.C. (2000) Outcome predictors for the cognitive behavior treatment of bulimia nervosa: Data from a multisite study. *Am. J. Psychiatry* 157:1302–1308.

Agras, W.S., Rossiter, E.M., Arnow, B., Schneider, J.A., Telch, C.F., Raeburn, S.D., Bruce, B., Perl, M., and Koran, L.M. (1992) Pharmacologic and cognitive-behavioral treatment for bulimia nervosa: a controlled comparison. *Am. J. Psychiatry* 149:82–87.

Ahima, R., and Osei, S. (2004) Leptin signaling. *Physiol. Behav.* 81:223–241.

Ahima, R., Saper, C., Flier, J., and Elmquist, J. (2000) Leptin regulation of neuroendocrine systems. *Front. Neuroendocrinol.* 21: 263–307.

American Psychiatric Association. (1994) *Diagnostic and Statistical Manual of Mental Disorders* (4th ed.). Washington, DC: Author.

American Psychiatric Association Workgroup on Eating Disorders. (2006) Practice guideline for the treatment of patients with eating disorders, 3rd edition. *Am. J. Psych.* 163:1–54.

Anderson, I.M., Parry-Billings, M., Newsholme, E.A., Fairburn, C.G., and Cowen, P.J. (1990) Dieting reduces plasma tryptophan and alters brain 5-HT function in women. *Psychol. Med.* 20:785–791.

Andreason, P.J., Altemus, M., Zametkin, A.J., King, A.C., Lucinio, J., and Cohen, R.M. (1992) Regional cerebral glucose metabolism in bulimia nervosa. *Am. J. Psychiatry* 149:1506–1513.

Arnow, B.A. (1997) Psychotherapy of anorexia and bulimia nervosa. In: Jimerson, D.C., and Kaye, W., eds. *Eating Disorders*. London: Balliere Tindall, pp. 235–257.

Attia, E., Haiman, C., Walsh, B.T., and Flater, S.R. (1998) Does fluoxetine augment the inpatient treatment of anorexia nervosa? *Am. J. Psychiatry* 155:548–551.

Attia, E., Wolk, S., Cooper, T., Glasofer, D., and Walsh, B. (2005) Plasma tryptophan during weight restoration in patients with anorexia nervosa. *Biol. Psychiatry* 57:674–678.

Audenaert, K., Van Laere, K., Dumont, F., Vervaet, M., Goethals, I., Slegers, G., Mertens, J., van Heeringen, C., and Dierckx, R. (2003) Decreased 5-HT2a receptor binding in patients with anorexia nervosa. *J. Nucl. Med.* 44:163–169.

Bacanu, S., Bulik, C., Klump, K., Fichter, M., Halmi, K., Keel, P., Kaplan, A., Strober, M., Treasure, J., Woodside, D.B., Berrettini, W., and Kaye, W. (2005) Linkage analysis of anorexia and bulimia nervosa cohorts using selected behavioral phenotypes as quantitative traits or covariates. *Am. J. Med. Genet. B, Neuropsychiatr. Genet.* 139:61–68.

Bailer, U.F., Frank, G., Henry, S., Price, J., Meltzer, C., Mathis, C., Wagner, A., Thornton, L., Hoge, J., Ziolko, S.K., Becker, C., McConaha, C., and Kaye, W.H. (2007) Exaggerated 5-HT_{1A} but normal 5-HT_{2A} receptor activity in individuals ill with anorexia nervosa. *Biol. Psychiatry* 61:1090–1099.

Bailer, U.F., Frank, G.K., Henry, S.E., Price, J.C., Meltzer, C.C., Weissfeld, L., Mathis, C.A., Drevets, W.C., Wagner, A., Hoge, J., Ziolko, S.K., McConana, C.W., and Kaye, W.H. (2005) Altered brain serotonin 5-HT_{1A} receptor binding after recovery from anorexia nervosa measured by positron emission tomography and [^{11}C]WAY100635. *Arch. Gen. Psychiatry* 62:1032.

Bailer, U.F., Price, J.C., Meltzer, C.C., Mathis, C.A., Frank, G.K., Weissfeld, L., McConaha, C.W., Henry, S.E., Brooks-Achenbach, S., Barbarich, N.C., and Kaye, W.H. (2004) Altered 5-HT_{2A} receptor binding after recovery from bulimia-type anorexia nervosa: relationships to harm avoidance and drive for thinness. *Neuropsychopharmacol.* 29:1143–1155.

Baranowska, B., Radzikowska, M., Wasilewska-Dziubinska, E., Roguski, K., and Borowiec, M. (2000) Disturbed release of gastrointestinal peptides in anorexia nervosa and in obesity. *Diabetes Obes. Metab.* 2:99–103.

Baranowska, B., Wolinska-Witort, E., Wasilewska-Dziubinska, E., Roguski, K., and Chmielowska, M. (2001) Plasma leptin, neuropeptide Y (NPY) and galanin concentrations in bulimia nervosa and in anorexia nervosa. *Neuroendocrinol. Letts.* 22:356–358.

Barbarich, N., McConaha, C., Gaskill, J., LaVia, M., Frank, G.K., Brooks, S., Plotnicov, K., and Kaye, W.H. (2004) An open trial of olanzapine in anorexia nervosa. *J. Clin. Psychiatry* 65:1480–1482.

Barr, L.C., Goodman, W.K., Price, L.H., McDougle, C.J., and Charney, D.S. (1992) The serotonin hypothesis of obsessive compulsive disorder: implications of pharmacologic challenge studies. *J. Clin. Psychiatry* 53(Suppl):17–28.

Bergen, A.W., van den Bree, M.B.M., Yeager, M., Welch, R., Ganjei, J.K., Haque, K., Bacanu, S., Berrettini, W.H., Grice, D.E., Bulik, C.M., Klump, K., Fichter, M., Halmi, K., Kaplan, A., Strober, M., Treasure, J., Woodside, D.B., and Kaye, W.H. (2003) Serotonin 1D (HRT1D) and delta opioid (OPRD1) receptor locus sequence variation is significantly associated with anorexia nervosa. *Mol. Psychiatry* 8:397–406.

Bergen, A., Yeager, M., Welch, R., Haque, K., Ganjei, J.K., Mazzanti, C., Nardi, I., van den Bree, M.B.M., Fichter, M., Halmi, K., Kaplan, A., Strober, M., Treasure, J., Woodside, D.B., Bulik, C., Bacanu, A., Devlin, B., Berrettini, W.H., Goldman, D., and Kaye, W. (2005) Association of multiple DRD2-141 polymorphism with anorexia nervosa. *Neuropsychopharm.* 30:1703–1710.

Berkman, N., Lohr, K., and Bulik, C. (2007) Outcomes of eating disorders: A systematic review of the literature. *Int. J. Eat. Disord.* 40:292–309.

Bhagwagar, Z., Rabiner, E., Sargent, P., Grasby, P., and Cowen, P. (2004) Persistent reduction in brain serotonin$_{1A}$ receptor binding in recovered depressed men measured by positron emission tomography with [^{11}C]WAY-100635. *Mol. Psychiatry* 9:386–392.

Blier, P., and de Montigny, C. (1999) Serotonin and drug-induced therapeutic responses in major depression, obsessive-compulsive and panic disorders. *Neuropsychopharmacol.* 21:91S–98S.

Blum, K., Sheridan, P.J., Wood, R.C., Braverman, E.R., Chen, T.J., and Comings, D.E. (1995) Dopamine D2 receptor gene variants: association and linkage studies in impulsive-addictive-compulsive behaviour. *Pharmacogenet.* 5:121–141.

Blundell, J.E. (1984) Serotonin and appetite. *Neuropharmacol.* 23: 1537–1551.

Bonhomme, N., and Esposito, E. (1998) Involvement of serotonin and dopamine in the mechanism of action of novel antidepressant drugs: a review. *J. Clin. Psychopharmacol.* 18:447–454.

Bosanac, P., Norman, T., Burrows, G., and Beaumont, P. (2005) Serotonergic and dopaminergic systems in anorexia nervosa: a role for atypical antipsychotics? *Aust. N. Z. J. Psychiatry* 39:146–153.

Brambilla, F., Brunetta, M., Draisci, A., Peirone, A., Perna, G., Sacerdote, P., Manfredi, B., and Panerai, A.E. (1995) T-lymphocyte cholecystokinin-8 and beta-endorphin in eating disorders: II. Bulimia nervosa. *Psychiatry Res.* 59:51–56.

Brambilla, F., Brunetta, M., Peirone, A., Perna, G., Sacerdote, P., Manfredi, B., and Panerai, A.E. (1995) T-lymphocyte cholecystokinin-8 and beta-endorphin concentrations in eating disorders: I. Anorexia nervosa. *Psychiatry Res.* 59:43–50.

Brewerton, T.D. (1995) Toward a unified theory of serotonin dysregulation in eating and related disorders. *Psychoneuroendocrinol.* 20:561–590.

Brewerton, T.D., Lesem, M.D., Kennedy, A., and Garvey, W.T. (2000) Reduced plasma leptin concentration in bulimia nervosa. *Psychoneuroendocrinol.* 25(7):649–658.

Brewerton, T.D., Lydiard, R.B., Laraia, M.T., Shook, J.E., and Ballenger, J.C. (1992) CSF beta-endorphin and dynorphin in bulimia nervosa. *Am. J. Psychiatry* 149:1086–1090.

Brown, K., Bujac, S., Mann, E., Campbell, D., Stubbins, M., and Blundell, J. (2007) Further evidence of association of OPDR1 & HTR1D polymorphisms with susceptibility to anorexia nervosa. *Biol. Psychiatry* 61:367–373.

Bulik, C., Bacanu, S., Klump, K., Fichter, M., Halmi, K., Keel, P., Kaplan, A., Mitchell, J., Rotondo, A., Strober, M., Treasure, J., Woodside, D.B., Sonpar, V., Xie, W., Bergen, A., Berrettini, W., Kaye, W., and Devlin, B. (2005) Selection of eating-disorder phenotypes for linkage analysis. *Am. J. Med. Genet. B, Neuropsychiatr. Genet.* 139:81–87.

Bulik, C., Berkman, N., Brownley, K., Sedway, J., and Lohr, K. (2007) Anorexia nervosa treatment: a systematic review of randomized controlled trials. *Int. J. Eat. Disord.* 40:310–320.

Bulik, C.M., Devlin, B., Bacanu, S.A., Thornton, L., Klump, K.L., Fichter, M., Halmi, K., Kaplan, A., Strober, M., Woodside, D.B., Bergen, A., Ganjei, J.K., Crow, S., Mitchell, J., Rotondo, A., Mauri, M., Cassano, G., Keel, P.K., Berrettini, W.H., and Kaye, W. (2003) Significant linkage on chromosome 10p in families with bulimia nervosa. *Am. J. Hum. Genet.* 72:200–207.

Bulik, C.M., Sullivan, P.F., Fear, J.L., and Joyce, P.R. (1997) Eating disorders and antecedent anxiety disorders: a controlled study. *Acta Psychiatr. Scand.* 96:101–107.

Bulik, C.M., Sullivan, P.F., and Kendler, K.S. (1998) Heritability of binge-eating and broadly defined bulimia nervosa. *Biol. Psychiatry* 44:1210–1218.

Burnet, P.W., Eastwood, S.L., and Harrison, P.J. (1997) [3H]WAY-100635 for 5-HT1A receptor autoradiography in human brain: a comparison with [3H]8-OH-DPAT and demonstration of increased binding in the frontal cortex in schizophrenia. *Neurochem. Int.* 30:565–574.

Campbell, D.A., Sundaramurthy, D., Gordon, D., Markham, A.F., and Pieri, L.F. (1999) Association between a marker in the UCP-2/UCP-3 gene cluster and genetic susceptibility to anorexia nervosa. *Mol. Psychiatry* 4:68–70.

Casper, R.C. (1990) Personality features of women with good outcome from restricting anorexia nervosa. *Psychosom. Med.* 52:156–170.

Casper, R.C., Hedeker, D., and McClough, J.F. (1992) Personality dimensions in eating disorders and their relevance for subtyping. *J. Am. Acad. Child Adolesc. Psychiatry* 31:830–840.

Celada, P., Puig, M.V., Casanovas, J.M., Guillazo, G., and Artigas, F. (2001) Control of dorsal raphe serotonergic neurons by the medial prefrontal cortex: Involvement of serotonin-1A, $GABA_A$, and glutamate receptors. *J. Neurosci.* 21:9917–9929.

Charney, D.S., Woods, S.W., Krystal, J.H., and Heninger, G.R. (1990) Serotonin function and human anxiety disorders. *Ann. N. Y. Acad. Sci.* 600:558–572.

Chowdhury, U., and Gordon, I., and Lask, B. (2001) Neuroimaging and anorexia nervosa. *J. Am. Acad. Child Adoles. Psychiatry* 40:738.

Cloninger, C.R. (1987) A systematic method for clinical description and classification of personality variants. A proposal. *Arch. Gen. Psychiatry* 44:573–588.

Cloninger, C.R., Przybeck, T.R., Svrakic, D.M., and Wetzel, R.D. (1994) *The Temperament and Character Inventory (TCI): A Guide to Its Development and Use*. St. Louis, MO: Washington University, Center for Psychobiology of Personality.

Considine, R., Sinha, M., Heiman, M., Kriauciunas, A., Stephens, T., Nyce, M., Ohannesian, J., Marco, C., McKee, L., Bauer, T., and Caro, J. (1996) Serum immunoreactive-leptin concentrations in normal-weight and obese humans. *N. Eng. J. Med.* 334:292–295.

Craig, A.D. (2002) How do you feel? Interoception: the sense of the physiological condition of the body. *Nat. Rev. Neurosci.* 3:655–666.

Dare, C., Eisler, I., Russell, G., Treasure, J., and Dodge, L. (2001) Psychological therapies for adults with anorexia nervosa. Randomised controlled trial of out-patient treatments. *Br. J. Psychiatry* 178:216–221.

Deep, A.L., Nagy, L.M., Weltzin, T.E., Rao, R., and Kaye, W.H. (1995) Premorbid onset of psychopathology in long-term recovered anorexia nervosa. *Int. J. Eat. Disord.* 17:291–297.

Delvenne, V., Goldman, S., De Maertelaer, V., and Lotstra, F. (1999) Brain glucose metabolism in eating disorders assessed by positron emission tomography. *Int. J. Eat. Disord.* 25:29–37.

Delvenne, V., Lotstra, F., Goldman, S., Biver, F., De Maertelaer, V., Appelboom-Fondu, J., Schoutens, A., Bidaut, L.M., Luxen, A., and Mendelwicz, J. (1995) Brain hypometabolism of glucose in anorexia nervosa: a PET scan study. *Biol. Psychiatry* 37:161–169.

Devlin, B., Bacanu, S.-A., Klump, K.L., Bulik, C.M., Fichter, M.M,, Halmi, K.A., Kaplan, A.S., Strober, M., Treasure, J., Woodside, D.B., Berrettini, W.H., and Kaye, W.H. (2002) Linkage analysis of anorexia nervosa incorporating behavioral covariates. *Hum. Mol. Genet.* 11:689–696.

Devlin, M.J., Walsh, B.T., Guss, J.L., Kissileff, H.R., Liddle, R.A., and Petkova, E. (1997) Postprandial cholecystokinin release and gastric emptying in patients with bulimia nervosa. *Am. J. Clin. Nutr.* 65:114–120.

De Vry, J., and Schreiber, R. (2000) Effects of selected serotonin 5-HT(1) and 5-HT(2) receptor agonists on feeding behavior: possible mechanisms of action. *Neurosci. Biobehav. Rev.* 24:341–353.

Drevets, W.C., Frank, E., Price, J.C., Kupfer, D.J., Holt, D., Greer, P.J., Huang, Y., Gautier, C., and Mathis, C. (1999) PET imaging of serotonin 1A receptor binding in depression. *Biol. Psychiatry* 46:1375–1387.

Eckert, E.D., Pomeroy, C., Raymond, N., Kohler, P.F., Thuras, P., and Bowers, C.Y. (1998) Leptin in anorexia nervosa. *J. Clin. Endocrinol. Metab.* 83:791–795.

Eddy, K., Dorer, D., Franko, D., Tahilani, K., Thompson-Brenner, H., and Herzog, D. (2007) Should bulimia nervosa be subtyped by history of anorexia nervosa? A longitudinal validation. *Int. J. Eat. Disord.* 40 Suppl:S67–71.

Eisler, I., Dare, C., Russell, G.F., Szmukler, G., Le Grange, D., and Dodge, E. (1997) Family and individual therapy in anorexia nervosa. A 5-year follow-up. *Arch. Gen. Psychiatry* 54:1025–1030.

Ellison, A.R., and Fong, J. (1998) Neuroimaging in eating disorders. In: Hoek, H.W., Treasure, J.L., and Katzman, M.A., eds. *Neurobiology in the Treatment of Eating Disorders*. Chichester, UK: John Wiley & Sons, pp. 255–269.

Ellison, Z., Foong, J., Howard, R., Bullmore, E., Williams, S., and Treasure, J. (1998) Functional anatomy of calorie fear in anorexia nervosa. *Lancet* 352:1192.

Fahy, T.A., Eisler, I., and Russell, G.F. (1993) A placebo-controlled trial of d-fenfluramine in bulimia nervosa. *Br. J. Psychiatry* 162:597–603.

Fairbanks, L., Melega, W., Jorgensen, M., Kaplan, J., and McGuire, M. (2001) Social impulsivity inversely associated with CSF 5-HIAA and fluoxetine exposure in vermet monkeys. *Neuropschopharmacol.* 24:370–378.

Fairburn, C.G. (2005) Evidence-based treatment of anorexia nervosa. *Int. J. Eat. Disord.* 37(Suppl):S26–S30.

Fairburn, C.G., Jones, R., Peveler, R.C., Hope, R.A., and O'Connor, M. (1993) Psychotherapy and bulimia nervosa. Longer-term effects of interpersonal psychotherapy, behavior therapy, and cognitive behavior therapy. *Arch. Gen. Psychiatry* 50:419–428.

Fairburn, C.G., Marcus, M.D., and Wilson, G.T. (1993). Cognitive-behavioral therapy for binge eating and bulimia nervosa: a comprehensive treatment manual. In: Fairburn, C.G., and Wilson, G.T., eds. *Binge Eating: Nature, Assessment, and Treatment*. New York: Guilford Press, pp. 361–404.

Faris, P.L., Kim, S.W., Meller, W.H., Goodale, R.L., Oakman, S.A., Hofbauer, R.D., Marshall, A.M., Daughters, R.S., Banerjee-Stevens, D., Eckert, E.D., and Hartman, B.K. (2000) Effect of decreasing afferent vagal activity with ondansetron on symptoms of bulimia nervosa: a randomised, double-blind trial. *Lancet* 355:792–797.

Farooqi, I.S., Keogh, J.M., Kamath, S., Jones, S., Gibson, W.T., Trussell, R., Jebb, S.A., Li, G.Y., and O'Rahilly, S. (2001) Partial leptin deficiency and human adiposity. *Nature* 414:34–35.

Farrar, C., Franck, N., Georgieff, N., Frith, C., Decety, J., and Jeannerod, M. (2003) Modulating the experience of agency: a positron emission tomography study. *NeuroImage* 18:324–333.

Fava, M., Copeland, P.M., Schweiger, U., and Herzog, D.B. (1989) Neurochemical abnormalities of anorexia nervosa and bulimia nervosa. *Am. J. Psychiatry* 146:963–971.

Ferguson, C.P., La Via, M.C., Crossan, P.J., and Kaye, W.H. (1999) Are serotonin selective reuptake inhibitors effective in underweight anorexia nervosa? *Int. J. Eat. Disord.* 25:11–17.

Fichter, M., and Quadflieg, N. (2007) Long-term stability of eating disorder diagnoses. *Int. J. Eat. Disord.* 40 Suppl:S61–S66.

Fichter, M.M., Leibl, K., Rief, W., Brunner, E., Schmidt-Auberger, S., and Engel, R.R. (1991) Fluoxetine versus placebo: a double-blind study with bulimic inpatients undergoing intensive psychotherapy. *Pharmacopsychiat.* 24:1–7.

File, S.E., Kenny, P.J., and Cheeta, S. (2000) The role of the dorsal hippocampal serotonergic and cholinergic systems in the modulation of anxiety. *Pharmacol. Biochem. Behav.* 66:65.

Fluoxetine Bulimia Nervosa Collaborative Study Group. (1992) Fluoxetine in the treatment of bulimia nervosa. A multicenter, placebo-controlled, double-blind trial. *Arch. Gen. Psychiatry* 49: 139–147.

Frank, G.K., Kaye, W.H., Meltzer, C.C., Price, J.C., Greer, P., McConaha, C., and Skovira, K. (2002) Reduced 5-HT2A receptor binding after recovery from anorexia nervosa. *Biol. Psychiatry* 52:896–906.

Frederich, R., Hu, S., Raymond, N., and Pomeroy, C. (2002) Leptin in anorexia nervosa and bulimia nervosa: importance of assay technique and method of interpretation. *J. Lab. Clin. Med.* 139: 72–79.

Friedman, J., and Halaas, J. (1998) Leptin and the regulation of body weight in mammals. *Nature* 395:763–770.

Garfinkel, D.M.P.E., Moldofsky, H., and Garner, D.M. (1980) The heterogeneity of anorexia nervosa. Bulimia as a distinct subgroup. *Arch. Gen. Psychiatry* 37:1036–1040.

Garner, D.M., Garfinkel, P.E., and O'Shaughnessy, M. (1985) The validity of the distinction between bulimia with and without anorexia nervosa. *Am. J. Psychiatry* 142:581–587.

Gelber, D., Levine, J., and Belmaker, R.H. (2001) Effect of inositol on bulimia nervosa and binge eating. *Int. J. Eat. Disord.* 29: 345–348.

Geliebter, A., Melton, P.M., McCray, R.S., Gallagher, D.R., Gage, D., Hashim, S.A. (1992) Gastric capacity, gastric emptying, and test-meal intake in normal and bulimic women. *Am. J. Clin. Nutr.* 56:656–661.

Gendall, K. (1999) Leptin, neuropeptide Y, and peptide YY in long-term recovered eating disorder patients. *Biol. Psychiatry* 46: 292–299.

Geracioti, T.D., Jr., and Liddle, R.A. (1988) Impaired cholecystokinin secretion in bulimia nervosa. *N. Engl. J. Med.* 319:683–688.

Geracioti, T.D., Jr., Liddle, R.A., Altemus, M., Demitrack, M.A., and Gold, P.W. (1992) Regulation of appetite and cholecystokinin secretion in anorexia nervosa. *Am. J. Psychiatry* 149:958–961.

Germain, N., Galusca, B., Le Roux, C., Bossu, C., Ghatei, M., Lang, F., Bloom, S., and Estour, B. (2007) Constitutional thinness and lean anorexia nervosa display opposite concentrations of peptide YY, glucagon-line peptide 1, ghrelin, and leptin. *Am. J. Clin. Nutr.* 85:957–971.

Gerstmann, J. (1924) Fingeragnosie: eine umschriebene Storung der Orientierung am eigenen Korper [Finger agnosia: a localized body image disturbance]. *Wien Kinische Wochenschr* 37:1010–1013.

Geyer, M.A. (1996) Serotonergic functions in arousal and motor activity. *Behav. Brain Res.* 73:31.

Gibbs, J., Young, R.C., and Smith, G.P. (1973) Cholecystokinin decreases food intake in rats. *J. Comp. Physiol. Psychol.* 84:488–495.

Glowa, J., and Gold, P. (1991) Corticotropin releasing hormone produces profound anorexigenic effects in the rhesus monkey. *Neuropeptides* 18:55–61.

Godart, N.T., Flament, M.F., Lecrubier, Y., and Jeammet, P. (2000) Anxiety disorders in anorexia nervosa and bulimia nervosa: comorbidity and chronology of appearance. *Eur. Psychiatry* 15: 38–45.

Godart, N.T., Flament, M.F., Perdereau, F., and Jeammet, P. (2002) Comorbidity between eating disorders and anxiety disorders: a review. *Int. J. Eat. Disord.* 32:253–270.

Gold, P.W., Gwirtsman, H., Avgerinos, P.C., Nieman, L.K., Gallucci, W.T., Kaye, W., Jimerson, D., Ebert, M., Rittmaster, R., and Loriaux, D.L. (1986) Abnormal hypothalamic-pituitary-adrenal function in anorexia nervosa. Pathophysiologic mechanisms in underweight and weight-corrected patients. *N. Engl. J. Med.* 314:1335–1342.

Goldbloom, D.S., Olmsted, M., Davis, R., Clewes, J., Heinmaa, M., Rockert, W., and Shaw, B. (1997) A randomized controlled trial of fluoxetine and cognitive behavioral therapy for bulimia nervosa: short-term outcome. *Behav. Res. Ther.* 35:803–811.

Gordon, C.M., Dougherty, D.D., Fischman, A.J., Emans, S.J., Grace, E., Lamm, R., Alpert, N.M., Majzoub, J.A., and Rausch, S.L. (2001) Neural substrates of anorexia nervosa: a behavioral challenge study with positron emission tomography. *J. Pediatr.* 139: 51–57.

Gordon, I., Lask, B., Bryant-Waugh, R., Christie, D., and Timimi, S. (1997) Childhood-onset anorexia nervosa: towards identifying a biological substrate. *Int. J. Eat. Disord.* 22:159–165.

Grahame-Smith, D.G. (1992) Serotonin in affective disorders. *Int. Clin. Psychopharmacol.* 6(Suppl 4):5–13.

Grice, D.E., Halmi, K.A., Fichter, M., Strober, M., Woodside, D.B., Treasure, J., Kaplan, A.S., Magistretti, P.J., Goldman, D., Kaye, W.H., Bulik, C.M., and Berrettini, W.H. (2002) Evidence for a susceptibility gene for anorexia nervosa on chromosome 1. *Am. J. Hum. Genet.* 70:787–792.

Grinspoon, S., Gulick, T., Askari, H., Landt, M., Lee, K., Anderson, E., Ma, Z., Vignati, L., Bowsher, R., Herzog, D., and Klibanski, A. (1996) Serum leptin levels in women with anorexia nervosa. *J. Clin. Endocrinol. Metab.* 81:3861–3863.

Gross, C., Zhuang, X., Stark, K., Ramboz, S., Oosting, R., Kirby, L., Santarelli, L., Beck, S., and Hen, R. (2002) Serotonin$_{1A}$ receptor acts during development to establish normal anxiety-like behaviour in the adult. *Nature* 416:396–400.

Halmi, K.A., Eckert, E., LaDu, T.J., and Cohen, J. (1986) Anorexia nervosa. Treatment efficacy of cyproheptadine and amitriptyline. *Arch. Gen. Psychiatry* 43:177–181.

Halmi, K.A., Eckert, E., Marchi, P., Sampugnaro, V., Apple, R., and Cohen, J. (1991) Comorbidity of psychiatric diagnoses in anorexia nervosa. *Arch. Gen. Psychiatry* 48:712–718.

Harty, R.F., Pearson, P.H., Solomon, T.E., and McGuigan, J.E. (1991) Cholecystokinin, vasoactive intestinal peptide and peptide histidine methionine responses to feeding in anorexia nervosa. *Reg. Peptides* 36:141–150.

Hebebrand, J., van der Heyden, J., Devos, R., Kopp, W., Herpertz, S., Remschmidt, H., and Herzog, W. (1995) Plasma concentrations of obese protein in anorexia nervosa. *Lancet* 346:1624–1625.

Holtkamp, K., Hebebrand, J., Mika, C., Heer, M., Heussen, N., and Herpertz-Dahlmann, B. (2004) High serum leptin levels subsequent to weight gain predict renewed weight loss in patients with anorexia nervosa. *Pschoneuroendocrinol.* 29:791–797.

Holtkamp, K., Mika, C., Grzella, I., Heer, M., Pak, H., Hebebrand, J., and Herpertz-Dahlmann, B. (2003) Reproductive function during weight gain in anorexia nervosa. Leptin represents a metabolic gate to gonadotropin secretion. *J. Neural Transm.* 110:427–435.

Hoopes, S., Reimherr, F., and Hedges, D. (2003) Treatment of bulimia nervosa with topiramate in a randomized, double-blind placebo-controlled trial, part 1: improvement in binge and purge measures. *J. Clin. Psychiatry* 64:1335–1341.

Hsu, L.K., Clement, L., Santhouse, R., and Ju, E.S. (1991) Treatment of bulimia nervosa with lithium carbonate. A controlled study. *J. Nerv. Ment. Dis.* 179:351–355.

Jimerson, D.C. (2002) Leptin and the neurobiology of eating disorders. *J. Lab. Clin. Med.* 139:70–71.

Jimerson, D.C., Lesem, M.D., Kaye, W.H., and Brewerton, T.D. (1992) Low serotonin and dopamine metabolite concentrations in cerebrospinal fluid from bulimic patients with frequent binge episodes. *Arch. Gen. Psychiatry* 49:132–138.

Jimerson, D.C., Lesem, M.D., Kaye, W.H., Hegg, A.P., and Brewerton, T.D. (1990) Eating disorders and depression: is there a serotonin connection? *Biol. Psychiatry* 28:443–454.

Jimerson, D.C., Mantzoros, C., Wolfe, B.E., and Metzger, E.D. (2000) Decreased serum leptin in bulimia nervosa. *J. Clin. Endorinol. Metab.* 85:4511–4514.

Jimerson, D.C., and Wolfe, B. (2006). Psychobiology of eating disorders. In: Wonderlich, S.M.J., de Zwaan, M., and Steiger, H., ed. *Annual Review of Eating Disorders: Part 2—2006*. Oxford, UK: Radcliffe Publishing, pp. 1–15.

Jimerson, D.C., Wolfe, B.E., Brotman, A.W., and Metzger, E.D. (1996) Medications in the treatment of eating disorders. *Psychiatr. Clin. North Am.* 19:739–754.

Jimerson, D.C., and Wolfe, B.E. (2004) Neuropeptides in eating disorders. *CNS Spectr.* 9:516–522.

Johnson, C., and Larson, R. (1982) Bulimia: an analysis of mood and behavior. *Psychosom. Med.* 44:341–351.

Kalra, S.P., Dube, M.G., Sahu, A., Phelps, C.P., and Kalra, P.S. (1991) Neuropeptide Y secretion increases in the paraventricular nucleus in association with increased appetite for food. *Proc. Natl. Acad. Sci. USA* 88:10931–10935.

Katzman, D.K., Lambe, E.K., Mikulis, D.J., Ridgley, J.N., Goldbloom, D.S., and Zipursky, R.B. (1996) Cerebral gray matter and white matter volume deficits in adolescent girls with anorexia nervosa. *J. Pediatrics* 129:794–803.

Kaye, W., Bulik, C., Thornton, L., Barbarich, N., Masters, K., Fichter, M., Halmi, K., Kaplan, A., Strober, M., Woodside, D.B., Bergen, A., Crow, S., Mitchell, J., Rotondo, A., Mauri, M., Cassano, G., Keel, P.K., Plotnicov, K., Pollice, C., Klump, K., Lilenfeld, L.R., Devlin, B., Quadflieg, R., and Berrettini, W.H. (2004) Comorbidity of anxiety disorders with anorexia and bulimia nervosa. *Am. J. Psychiatry* 161:2215–2221.

Kaye, W., Frank, G., Bailer, U.F., Henry, S., Meltzer, C.C., Price, J., Mathis, C., and Wagner, A. (2005) Serotonin alterations in anorexia and bulimia nervosa: new insights from imaging studies. *Physiol. Behav.* 85:73–81.

Kaye, W.H., Ballenger, J.C., Lydiard, R.B., Stuart, G.W., Laraia, M.T., O'Neil, P., Fossey, M.D., Stevens, V., Lesser, S., and Hsu, G. (1990) CSF monoamine levels in normal-weight bulimia: evidence for abnormal noradrenergic activity. *Am. J. Psychiatry* 147:225–229.

Kaye, W.H., Barbarich, N.C., Putnam, K., Gendall, K.A., Fernstrom, J., Fernstrom, M., McConaha, C.W., and Kishore, A. (2003) Anxiolytic effects of acute tryptophan depletion in anorexia nervosa. *Int. J. Eat. Disord.* 33:257–267.

Kaye, W.H., Berrettini, W., Gwirtsman, H., and George, D.T. (1990) Altered cerebrospinal fluid neuropeptide Y and peptide YY immunoreactivity in anorexia and bulimia nervosa. *Arch. Gen. Psychiatry* 47:548–556.

Kaye, W.H., Berrettini, W.H., Gwirtsman, H.E., Chretien, M., Gold, P.W., George, D.T., Jimerson, D.C., and Ebert, M.H. (1987) Reduced cerebrospinal fluid levels of immunoreactive proopiomelanocortin related peptides (including beta-endorphin) in anorexia nervosa. *Life Sci.* 41:2147–2155.

Kaye, W.H., Ebert, M.H., Raleigh, M., and Lake, R. (1984) Abnormalities in CNS monoamine metabolism in anorexia nervosa. *Arch. Gen. Psychiatry* 41:350–355.

Kaye, W.H., Frank, G.K., and McConaha, C. (1999) Altered dopamine activity after recovery from restricting-type anorexia nervosa. *Neuropsychopharm.* 21:503–506.

Kaye, W.H., Frank, G.K., Meltzer, C.C., Price, J.C., McConaha, C.W., Crossan, P.J., Klump, K.L., and Rhodes, L. (2001) Altered serotonin 2A receptor activity in women who have recovered from bulimia nervosa. *Am. J. Psychiatry* 158:1152–1155.

Kaye, W.H., Greeno, C.G., Moss, H., Fernstrom, J., Fernstrom, M., Lilenfeld, L.R., Weltzin, T.E., and Mann, J.J. (1998) Alterations in serotonin activity and psychiatric symptomatology after recovery from bulimia nervosa. *Arch. Gen. Psychiatry* 55:927–935.

Kaye, W.H., Gwirtsman, H.E., George, D.T., Ebert, M.H., Jimerson, D.C., Tomai, T.P., Chrousos, G.P., and Gold, P.W. (1987) Elevated cerebrospinal fluid levels of immunoreactive corticotropin-releasing hormone in anorexia nervosa: relation to state of nutrition, adrenal function, and intensity of depression. *J. Clin. Endocrinol. Metab.* 64:203–208.

Kaye, W.H., Gwirtsman, H.E., George, D.T., Weiss, S.R., and Jimerson, D.C. (1986) Relationship of mood alterations to bingeing behaviour in bulimia. *Br. J. Psychiatry* 149:479–485.

Kaye, W.H., Lilenfeld, L.R., Berrettini, W.H., Strober, M., Devlin, B., Klump, K.L., Goldman, D., Bulik, C.M., Halmi, K.A., Fichter, M.M., Kaplan, A., Treasure, J., Plotnicov, K.H., Pollice, C.P., Rao, R., and McConaha, C.W. (2000) A search for susceptibility loci for anorexia nervosa: methods and sample description. *Biol. Psychiatry* 47:794–803.

Kaye, W.H., Lilenfeld, L.R., Plotnicov, K., Merikangas, K.R., Nagy, L., Strober, M., Bulik, C.M., Moss, H., and Greeno, C.G. (1996) Bulimia nervosa and substance dependence: association and family transmission. *Alcohol. Clin. Exp. Res.* 20:878–881.

Kaye, W.H., Nagata, T., Weltzin, T.E., Hsu, L.K., Sokol, M.S., McConaha, C., Plotnicov, K.H., Weise, J., and Deep, D. (2001) Double-blind placebo-controlled administration of fluoxetine in restricting- and restricting-purging-type anorexia nervosa. *Biol. Psychiatry* 49:644–652.

Kaye, W.H., and Weltzin, T.E. (1991) Serotonin activity in anorexia and bulimia nervosa: relationship to the modulation of feeding and mood. *J. Clin. Psychiatry* 52(Suppl):41–48.

Keel, P., Wolfe, B.E., Liddle, R., De Young, K., and Jimerson, D.C. (2007) Clinical features and physiological response to a test meal in purging disorder and bulimia nervosa. *Arch. Gen. Psychiatry* 64:1058–1066.

Keel, P.K., Klump, K.L., Miller, K.B., McGue, M., & Iacono, W.G. (2005) Shared transmission of eating disorders and anxiety disorders. *Int. J. Eat. Disord.* 38(2):99–105.

Keel, P.K., and Mitchell, J.E. (1997) Outcome in bulimia nervosa. *Am. J. Psychiatry* 154:313–321.

Kelley, A.E., Bakshi, V.P., Haber, S., Steininger, T., Will, M., and Zhang, M. (2002) Opioid modulation of taste hedonics within ventral striatum. *Physiol. Behav.* 76:365–377.

Kendler, K.S., MacLean, C., Neale, M., Kessler, R., Heath, A., and Eaves, L. (1991) The genetic epidemiology of bulimia nervosa. *Am. J. Psychiatry* 148:1627–1637.

Kendler, K.S., Walters, E.E., Neale, M.C., Kessler, R.C., Heath, A.C., and Eaves, L.J. (1995) The structure of the genetic and environmental risk factors for six major psychiatric disorders in women. Phobia, generalized anxiety disorder, panic disorder, bulimia, major depression, and alcoholism. *Arch. Gen. Psychiatry* 52:374–383.

Kissileff, H., Pi-Sunyer, F., Thornton, J., and Smith, G. (1981) C-terminal octapeptide of cholecystokinin decreases food intake in man. *Am. J. Clin. Nutr.* 34:154–160.

Kleifield, E.I., Wagner, S., and Halmi, K.A. (1996) Cognitive-behavioral treatment of anorexia nervosa. *Psychiatr. Clin. North Am.* 19: 715–737.

Klump, K.L., Bulik, C.M., Pollice, C., Halmi, K.A., Fichter, M.M., Berrettini, W.H., Devlin, B., Strober, M., Kaplan, A., Woodside, D.B., Treasure, J., Shabbout, M., Lilenfeld, L.R., Plotnicov, K.H., and Kaye, W.H. (2000) Temperament and character in women with anorexia nervosa. *J. Nerv. Ment. Dis.* 188:559–567.

Klump, K.L., McGue, M., and Iacono, W.G. (2000) Age differences in genetic and environmental influences on eating attitudes and behaviors in preadolescent and adolescent female twins. *J. Abnorm. Psychol.* 109:239–251.

Klump, K.L., McGue, M., and Iacono, W.G. (2001) Genetic and environmental influences on anorexia nervosa syndromes in a population-based sample of twins. *Psychol. Med.* 31:737–740.

Klump, K.L., Miller, K.B., Keel, P.K., McGue, M., and Iacono, W.G. (2001) Genetic and environmental influences on anorexia nervosa syndromes in a population-based twin sample. *Psychol. Med.* 31:737–740.

Kojima, S., Nagai, N., and Nakabeppu, Y. (2005) Comparison of regional cerebral blood flow in patients with anorexia nervosa before and after weight gain. *Psychiatry Res.* 140:251–258.

Kojima, S., Nakahara, T., Nagai, N., Muranaga, T., Tanaka, M., Yasuhara, D., Masuda, A., Date, Y., Ueno, H., Nakazato, M., and Naruo, T. (2005) Altered ghrelin and peptide YY responses to meals in bulimia nervosa. *Clin. Endocrinol. (Oxf)* 62:74–78.

Kuruoglu, A.C., Kapucu, O., Atasever, T., Arikan, Z., Isik, E., and Unlu, M. (1998) Technetium-99m-HMPAO brain SPECT in anorexia nervosa. *J. Nucl. Med.* 39:304–306.

LaChaussee, J.L., Kissileff, H., Walsh, B., and Hadigan, C. (1992) The single-item meal as a measure of binge-eating behavior in patients with bulimia nervosa. *Physiol. Behav.* 51:593–600.

Lanzenberger, R., Mitterhauser, M., Spindelegger, C., Wadsak, W., Klein, N., Mien, L., Holik, A., Attarbaschi, T., Mossaheb, N., Sacher, J., Geiss-Granadia, T., Keletter, K., Kasper, S., and Tauscher, J. (2007) Reduced serotonin-1A receptor binding in social anxiety disorder. *Biol. Psychiatry* 61:1081–1089.

LeDoux, J. (2003) The emotional brain, fear, and the amygdala. *Cell. Mol. Neurobiol.* 23:727–738.

Leibowitz, S.F., and Shor-Posner, G. (1986) Brain serotonin and eating behavior. *Appetite* 7:1–14.

Leitenberg, H., Rosen, J.C., Wolf, J., Vara, L.S., Detzer, M.J., Srebnik, D. (1994) Comparison of cognitive-behavior therapy and desipramine in the treatment of bulimia nervosa. *Behav. Res. Ther.* 32:37–45.

Lesem, M.D., Berrettini, W., Kaye, W.H., and Jimerson, D.C. (1991) Measurement of CSF dynorphin A 1-8 immunoreactivity in anorexia nervosa and normal-weight bulimia. *Biol. Psychiatry* 29: 244–252.

Licinio, J., Wong, M.L., and Gold, P.W. (1996) The hypothalamic-pituitary-adrenal axis in anorexia nervosa. *Psychiatry Res.* 62: 75–83.

Lilenfeld, L.R., Kaye, W.H., Greeno, C.G., Merikangas, K.R., Plotnicov, K., Pollice, C., Rao, R., Strober, M., Bulik, C.M., and Nagy, L. (1998) A controlled family study of anorexia nervosa and bulimia nervosa: psychiatric disorders in first-degree relatives and effects of proband comorbidity. *Arch. Gen. Psychiatry* 55:603–610.

Lob, S., Pickel, J., Bidlingmaier, M., Schaaf, L., Backmund, H., Gerlinghoff, M., and Stalla, G. (2003) Serum leptin monitoring in anorectic patients during refeeding therapy. *Exp. Clin. Endocrinol. Diabetes* 111: 278–282.

Lock, J., and le Grange, D. (2005) Family-based treatment of eating disorders. *Int. J. Eat. Disord.* 37(Suppl):S64–S67.

Lydiard, R.B., Brewerton, T.D., Fossey, M.D., Laraia, M.T., Stuart, G., Beinfeld, M.C., and Ballenger, J.C. (1993) CSF cholecystokinin octapeptide in patients with bulimia nervosa and in normal comparison subjects. *Am. J. Psychiatry* 150:1099–1101.

Mann, J.J. (1999) Role of the serotonergic system in the pathogenesis of major depression and suicidal behavior. *Neuropsychopharmacol.* 21:99S–105S.

Mantzoros, C., Flier, J.S., Lesem, M.D., Brewerton, T.D., and Jimerson, D.C. (1997) Cerebrospinal fluid leptin in anorexia nervosa: correlation with nutritional status and potential role in resistance to weight gain. *J. Clin. Endocrinol. Metab.* 82:1845–1851.

Marrazzi, M.S., Bacon, J.P., Kinzie, J., Luby, E.D. (1995) Naltrexone use in the treatment of anorexia nervosa and bulimia nervosa. *Int. Clin. Psychopharmacol.* 10:163–172.

Martin, E.R., Kaplan, N.L., and Weir, B.S. (1997) Tests for linkage and association in nuclear families. *Am. J. Hum. Genet.* 61: 439–448.

Martin-Ruiz, R., Puig, M.V., Celada, P., Shapiro, D.A., Roth, B.L., Mengod, G., and Artigas, F. (2001) Control of serotonergic function in medial prefrontal cortex by serotonin-2A receptors through a glutamate-dependent mechanism. *J. Neurosci.* 21:9856–9866.

Mesulam, M. (1981) A cortical network for directed attention and unilateral neglect. *Ann. Neurol.* 10:309–325.

Miller, K.B., Klump, K.L., Keel, P.K., McGue, M., and Iacono, W.G. (1998) *A population-based twin study of anorexia and bulimia nervosa: Heritability and shared transmission with anxiety disorders.* Paper presented at the Eating Disorders Research Society Meeting, Boston.

Milos, G., Spindler, A., Schnyder, U., and Fairburn, C. (2005) Instability of eating disorder diagnoses: prospective study. *Br. J. Psychiatry* 187:573–578.

Misra, M., Miller, K., Tsai, P., Gallagher, K., Lin, A., Lee, N., Herzog, D., and Klibanski, A. (2006) Elevated peptide YY levels in adolescent girls with anorexia nervosa. *J. Clin. Endocrinol. Metab.* 91:1027–1033.

Mitchell, J.E., Christenson, G., Jennings, J., Huber, M., Thomas, B., Pomeroy, C., and Morley, J. (1989) A placebo-controlled, double-blind crossover study of naltrexone hydrochloride in outpatients with normal weight bulimia. *J. Clin. Psychopharmacol.* 9:94–97.

Mitchell, J.E., Fletcher, L., Hanson, K., Mussell, M.P., Seim, H., Crosby, R., and al Banna, M. (2001) The relative efficacy of fluoxetine and manual-based self-help in the treatment of outpatients with bulimia nervosa. *J. Clin. Psychopharmacol.* 21:298–304.

Mitchell, J.E., Pyle, R.L., Eckert, E.D., Hatsukami, D., Pomeroy, C., and Zimmerman, R. (1990) A comparison study of antidepressants and structured intensive group psychotherapy in the treatment of bulimia nervosa. *Arch. Gen. Psychiatry* 47:149–157.

Mondraty, N., Birmingham, C., Touyz, S.W., Sundakov, V., Chapman, L., and Beaumont, P. (2005) Randomized controlled trial of olanzapine in the treatment of cognitions in anorexia nervosa. *Australas. Psychiatry* 13:72–75.

Monteleone, P., DiLieto, A., Castaldo, E., and Maj, M. (2004) Leptin functioning in eating disorders. *CNS Spectr.* 9:523–529.

Monteleone, P., Di Lieto, A., Tortorella, A., Longobardi, N., and Maj, M. (2000) Circulating leptin in patients with anorexia nervosa, bulimia nervosa or binge-eating disorder: relationship to body weight, eating patterns, psychopathology and endocrine changes. *Psychiatry Res.* 94:121–129.

Monteleone, P., Martiadis, V., Rigamonti, A., Fabrazzo, M., Giordani, C., Muller, E., and Maj, M. (2005) Investigation of peptide YY and ghrelin responses to a test meal in bulimia nervosa. *Biol. Psychiatry* 57:926–931.

Moresco, F.M., Dieci, M., Vita, A., Messa, C., Gobbo, C., Galli, L., Rizzo, G., Panzacchi, A., De Peri, L., Ivernizzi, G., and Fazio, F. (2002) *In vivo* serotonin $5HT_{2A}$ receptor binding and personality traits in healthy subjects: A positron emission tomography study. *NeuroImage* 17:1470–1478.

Morley, J.E., and Blundell, J.E. (1988) The neurobiological basis of eating disorders: some formulations. *Biol. Psychiatry* 23:53–78.

Morley, J.E., Levine, A.S., Gosnell, B.A., Mitchell, J.E., Krahn, D.D., and Nizielski, S.E. (1985) Peptides and feeding. *Peptides* 6:181–192.

Nakahara, T., Kojima, S., Tanaka, M., Yasuhara, D., Harada, T., Sagiyama, K., Muranaga, T., Nagai, N., Nakazato, M., Nozeo, S., Naruo, T., and Inui, A. (2007) Incomplete restoration of the secretion of ghrelin and PYY compared to insulin after food ingestion following weight gain in anorexia nervosa. *J. Psych. Res.* 41:814–820.

Naruo, T., Nakabeppu, Y., Sagiyama, K., Munemoto, T., Homan, N., Deguchi, D., Nakajo, M., and Nozoe, S. (2000) Characteristic regional cerebral blood flow patterns in anorexia nervosa patients with binge/purge behavior. *Am. J. Psychiatry* 157:1520–1522.

Neumeister, A., Brain, E., Nugent, A., Carson, R., Bonne, O., Lucnekbaugh, D., Eckelman, W., Herschovitch, P., Charney, D., and Drevets, W. (2004) Reduced serotonin type 1_A receptor binding in panic disorder. *J. Neurosci.* 24:589–591.

Nickel, C., Tritt, K., Muehlbacher, M., Pedrosa, G., Mitterlehner, F., Kaplan, P., Lahmann, C., Leiberich, P., Krawczyk, J., Kettler, C., Rother, W., Loew, T., and Nickel, M. (2005) Topiramate treatment in bulimia nervosa patients: a randomized, double-blind placebo-controlled trial. *Int. J. Eat. Disord.* 38:295–300.

Nozoe, S., Naruo, T., Nakabeppu, Y., Soejima, Y., Nakajo, M., and Tanaka, H. (1993) Changes in regional cerebral blood flow in patients with anorexia nervosa detected through single photon emission tomography imaging. *Biol. Psychiatry* 34:578–580.

Nozoe, S., Naruo, T., Yonekura, R., Nakabeppu, Y., Soejima, Y., Nagai, N., Nakajo, M., and Tanaka, H. (1995) Comparison of regional cerebral blood flow in patients with eating disorders. *Brain Res. Bull.* 36:251–255.

O'Doherty, J., Rolls, E.T., Francis, S., Bowtell, R., and McGlone, F. (2001) Representation of pleasant and aversive taste in the human brain. *J. Neurophysiol.* 85:1315–1321.

Otto, B., Cuntz, U., Otto, C., Heldwein, W., Reiepi, R., and Tschop, M. (2007) Peptide YY release in anorectic patients after liquid meal. *Appetite* 48:301–304.

Parsey, R.V., Oquendo, M.A., Ogden, R.T., Olvet, D., Simpson, N., Huang, Y., Van Heertum, R., Arango, V., and Mann, J.J. (2005) Altered serotonin 1A binding in major depression: a [carbonyl-C-11]WAY100635 positron emission tomography study. *Biol. Psychiatry* 59:106–113.

Paulus, M., and Stein, M.B. (2006) An insular view of anxiety. *Biol. Psychiatry* 60:383–387.

Perkins, S., Murphy, R., Schmidt, U., and Williams, C. (2006) Self-help and guided self-help for eating disorders. *Cochrane Database of Systematic Reviews* 3.

Phillipp, E., Pirke, K.M., Kellner, M.B., and Krieg, J.C. (1991) Disturbed cholecystokinin secretion in patients with eating disorders. *Life Sci.* 48:2443–2450.

Pirke, K.M., Kellner, M.B., Friess, E., Krieg, J.C., and Fichter, M.M. (1994) Satiety and cholecystokinin. *Int. J. Eat. Disord.* 15:63–69.

Rastam, M., Bjure, J., Vestergren, E., Uvebrant, P., Gillberg, I.C., Wentz, E., and Gillberg, C. (2001) Regional cerebral blood flow in weight-restored anorexia nervosa: a preliminary study. *Dev. Med. Child. Neurol.* 43:239–242.

Richer, M., Hen, R., and Blier, P. (2002) Modification of serotonin neuron properties in mice lacking 5-HT_{1A} receptors. *Eur. J. Pharmacol.* 435:195–203.

Romano, S.J., Halmi, K.A., Sarkar, N.P., Koke, S.C., and Lee, J.S. (2002) A placebo-controlled study of fluoxetine in continued treatment of bulimia nervosa after successful acute fluoxetine treatment. *Am. J. Psychiatry* 159:96–102.

Rosenkranz, K., Hinney, A., Ziegler, A., Hermann, H., Fichter, M., Mayer, H., Siegfried, W., Young, J.K., Remschmidt, H., and Hebebrand, J. (1998) Systematic mutation screening of the estrogen receptor beta gene in probands of different weight extremes: identification of several genetic variants. *J. Clin. Endocrinol. Metab.* 83:4524–4527.

Roser, W., Bubl, R., Buergin, D., Seelig, J., Radue, E.W., and Rost, B. (1999) Metabolic changes in the brain of patients with anorexia and bulimia nervosa as detected by proton magnetic resonance spectroscopy. *Int. J. Eat. Disord.* 26:119–136.

Russell, G.F., Szmukler, G.I., Dare, C., and Eisler, I. (1987) An evaluation of family therapy in anorexia nervosa and bulimia nervosa. *Arch. Gen. Psychiatry* 44:1047–1056.

Rutherford, J., McGuffin, P., Katz, R.J., and Murray, R.M. (1993) Genetic influences on eating attitudes in a normal female twin population. *Psychol. Med.* 23:425–436.

Salamone, J.D. (1996) The behavioral neurochemistry of motivation: methodological and conceptual issues in studies of the dynamic activity of nucleus accumbens dopamine. *J. Neurosci. Meth.* 64:137–149.

Saper, C.B., Chou, T.C., and Elmquist, J.K. (2002) The need to feed: homeostatic and hedonic control of eating. *Neuron* 36:199–211.

Sargent, P.A., Kjaer, K.H., Bench, C.J., Rabiner, E.A., Messa, C., Meyer, J., Gunn, R.N., Grasby, P.M., and Cowen, P.J. (2000) Brain $serotonin_{1A}$ receptor binding measured by positron emission tomography with [^{11}C]WAY-100635: effects of depression and antidepressant treatment. *Arch. Gen. Psychiatry* 57:174–180.

Saudou, F., and Hen, R. (1994) 5-Hydroxytryptamine receptor subtypes in vertebrates and invertebrates. *Neurochem. Int.* 25:503–532.

Schuckit, M.A., Tipp, J.E., Anthenelli, R.M., Bucholz, K.K., Hesselbrock, V.M., and Nurnberger, J.I., Jr. (1996) Anorexia nervosa and bulimia nervosa in alcohol-dependent men and women and their relatives. *Am. J. Psychiatry* 153:74–82.

Schultz, W., Tremblay, L., and Hollerman, J.R. (2000) Reward processing in primate orbitofrontal cortex and basal ganglia. *Cereb. Cortex* 10:272–284.

Schwartz, M.W., Peskind, E., Raskind, M., Boyko, E.J., and Porte, D., Jr. (1996) Cerebrospinal fluid leptin levels: relationship to plasma levels and to adiposity in humans. *Nat. Med.* 2:589–593.

Schwartz, M.W., Woods, S.C., Porte, D., Jr., Seeley, R.J., and Baskin, D.G. (2000) Central nervous system control of food intake. *Nature* 404:661–671.

Shapiro, J., Berkman, N., Brownley, K., Sedway, J., Lohr, K., and Bulik, C. (2007) Bulimia nervosa treatment: a systematic review of randomized controlled trials. *Int. J. Eat. Disord.* 40:321–336.

Shiiya, T., Nakazato, M., Mizuta, M., Date, Y., Mondal, M.S., Tanaka, M., Nozoe, S., Hosoda, H., Kangawa, K., and Matsukura, S. (2002) Plasma ghrelin levels in lean and obese humans and the effect of glucose on ghrelin secretion. *J. Endocrin. Metab.* 87:240–244.

Shively, C., Friedman, D., Gage, H., Bounds, M., Brown-Proctor, C., Blair, J., Henderson, J., Smith, M., and Buchheimer, N. (2006) Behavioral depression and positron emission tomography-determined serotonin 1A receptor binding potential in cynomolgus monkeys. *Arch. Gen. Psychiatry* 63:396–403.

Sibille, E., Pavlides, C., Benke, D., and Toth, M. (2000) Genetic inactivation of the Serotonin(1A) receptor in mice results in downregulation of major GABA(A) receptor alpha subunits, reduction of GABA(A) receptor binding, and benzodiazepine-resistant anxiety. *J. Neuroscience* 20:2758–2765.

Silberg, J., and Bulik, C. (2005) Developmental association between eating disorders symptoms and symptoms of depression and anxiety in juvenile twin girls. *J. Child Psychol. Psychiat.* 46:1317–1326.

Simansky, K.J. (1996) Serotonergic control of the organization of feeding and satiety. *Behav. Brain Res.* 73:37–42.

Small, D., Zatorre, R., Dagher, A., Evans, A., and Jones-Gotman, M. (2001) Changes in brain activity related to eating chocolate: from pleasure to aversion. *Brain* 124:1720–1733.

Soubrie, P. (1986) Reconciling the role of central serotonin neurons in human and animal behavior. *Behav. Brain Sci.* 9:319.

Spielberger, C.D., Gorsuch, R.L., and Lushene, R.E. (1970) *STAI Manual for the State Trait Anxiety Inventory*. Palo Alto, CA: Consulting Psychologists Press.

Srinivasagam, N.M., Kaye, W.H., Plotnicov, K.H., Greeno, C., Weltzin, T.E., and Rao, R. (1995) Persistent perfectionism, symmetry, and exactness after long-term recovery from anorexia nervosa. *Am. J. Psychiatry* 152:1630–1634.

Staley, J., Malison, R., and Innis, R. (1998) Imaging of the serotonergic system: interactions of neuroanatomical and functional abnormalities of depression. *Biol. Psychiatry* 44:534–549.

Steffen, K.L., Roerig, J.L., Mitchell, J., and Uppala, S. (2006) Emerging drugs for eating disorder treatment. *Expert Opin. Emerg. Drugs* 11:315–336.

Steiger, H., Richardson, J., Israel, M., Ng Ying Kin, N., Bruce, K., Mansour, S., and Marie Parent, A. (2005) Reduced density of platelet-binding sites for [3H]paroxetine in remitted bulimic women. *Neuropsychopharmacol.* 30:1028–1032.

Stock, S., Leichner, P., Wong, A., Ghatei, M., Kieffer, T., Bloom, S., and Chanoine, J. (2005) Ghrelin, peptide YY, glucose-dependent insulinotropic polypeptide, and hunger responses to a mixed meal in anorexic, obese, and control female adolescents. *J. Clin. Endocrinol. Metab.* 90:2161–2168.

Stockmeier, C.A. (1997) Neurobiology of serotonin in depression and suicide. *Ann. N. Y. Acad. Sci.* 836:220–232.

Stoving, R.K., Hangaard, J., Hansen-Nord, M., and Hagen, C. (1999) A review of endocrine changes in anorexia nervosa. *J. Psychiatr. Res.* 33:139–152.

Strober, M. (1980) Personality and symptomatological features in young, nonchronic anorexia nervosa patients. *J. Psychosom. Res.* 24:353–359.

Strober, M. (1995) Family-genetic perspectives on anorexia nervosa and bulimia nervosa. In: Brownell, K., and Fairburn, C., eds. *Eating Disorders and Obesity—A Comprehensive Handbook*. New York: Guilford Press, pp. 212–218.

Strober, M., Freeman, R., DeAntonio, M., Lampert, C., and Diamond, J. (1997) Does adjunctive fluoxetine influence the post-hospital course of restrictor-type anorexia nervosa? A 24-month prospective, longitudinal followup and comparison with historical controls. *Psychopharmacol. Bull.* 33:425–431.

Strober, M., Freeman, R., Lampert, C., and Diamond, J. (2007) The association of anxiety disorders and obsessive compulsive personality disorder with anorexia nervosa: Evidence from a family study with discussion of nosological and neurodevelopmental implications. *Int. J. Eat. Disord.* 40 Suppl:S46–S51.

Strober, M., Freeman, R., Lampert, C., Diamond, J., and Kaye, W. (2000) Controlled family study of anorexia nervosa and bulimia nervosa: evidence of shared liability and transmission of partial syndromes. *Am. J. Psychiatry* 157:393–401.

Strober, M., Lilenfeld, L., Kaye, W., and Bulik, C. (2006). Genetics factors in eating disorders. In: Cooper, P., and Stein, A., eds. *Feeding Disorders in Children and Adolescents, 2nd ed.* Chur, Switzerland: Harwood Academic Publishers, pp. 169–189.

Strober, M., Pataki, C., Freeman, R., and DeAntonio, M. (1999) No effect of adjunctive fluoxetine on eating behavior or weight phobia during the inpatient treatment of anorexia nervosa: an historical case-control study. *J. Child Adolesc. Psychopharmacol.* 9:195–201.

Sullivan, P.F., Bulik, C.M., and Kendler, K.S. (1998) The epidemiology and classification of bulimia nervosa. *Psychol. Med.* 28:599–610.

Szabo, S.T., and Blier, P. (2001) Serotonin (1A) receptor ligands act on norepinephrine neuron firing through excitatory amino acid and GABA(A) receptors: a microiontophoretic study in the rat locus coeruleus. *Synapse* 42:203–212.

Takano, A., Shiga, T., Kitagawa, N., Koyama, T., Katoh, C., Tsukamoto, E., and Tamaki, N. (2001) Abnormal neuronal network in anorexia nervosa studied with I-123-IMP SPECT. Psychiatry Research: *NeuroImaging* 107(1):45–50.

Tamai, H., Takemura, J., Kobayashi, N., Matsubayashi, S., Matsukura, S., and Nakagawa, T. (1993) Changes in plasma cholecystokinin concentrations after oral glucose tolerance test in anorexia nervosa before and after therapy. *Metab. Clin. Exp.* 42:581–584.

Tanaka, M., Naruo, T., Muranaga, T., Yasuhara, D., Shiiya, T., Nakazato, M., Matsukura, S., and Nozoe, S. (2002) Increased fasting plasma ghrelin levels in patients with bulimia nervosa. *Eur. J. Endocrin.* 146:R1–R3.

Tiihonen, J., Keski-Rahkonen, A., Lopponen, M., Muhonen, M., Kajander, J., Allonen, T., Nagren, K., Hietala, J., and Rissanen, A. (2004) Brain serotonin 1A receptor binding in bulimia nervosa. *Biol. Psychiatry* 55:871.

Tozzi, F., Bergen, A.W., and Bulik, C.M. (2002) Candidate gene studies in eating disorders. *Psychopharmacol. Bull.* 36:60–90.

Treasure, J., and Campbell, I. (1994) The case for biology in the aetiology of anorexia nervosa. *Psychol. Med.* 24:3–8.

Treasure, J., Todd, G., Brolly, M., Tiller, J., Nehmed, A., and Denman, F. (1995) A pilot study of a randomised trial of cognitive analytical therapy vs. educational behavioral therapy for adult anorexia nervosa. *Behav. Res. Ther.* 33:363–367.

Tschop, M., Wawarta, R., Reiepl, R., Friedrich, S., Bidlingmaier, M., Landgraf, R., and Folwaczny, C. (2001) Post-prandial decrease of circulating human ghrelin levels. *J. Endocrinol. Invest.* 24: RC19–RC21.

Uher, R., Brammer, M., Murphy, T., Campbell, I., Ng, V., Williams, S., and Treasure, J. (2003) Recovery and chronicity in anorexia nervosa: brain activity associated with differential outcomes. *Biol. Psychiatry* 54:934–942.

Uher, R., Murphy, T., Brammer, M., Dalgleish, T., Phillips, M., Ng, V., Andrew, C., Williams, S., Campbell, I., and Treasure, J. (2004) Medial prefrontal cortex activity associated with symptom provocation in eating disorders. *Am. J. Psychiatry* 161:1238–1246.

van Heeringen, C., Audenaert, K., Van Laere, K., Dumont, F., Slegers, G., Mertens, J., Dierckx, R.A. (2003) Prefrontal 5-HT_{2a} receptor binding index, hopelessness and personality characteristics in attempted suicide. *J. Affect. Disord.* 74:149–158.

Vandereycken, W., and Pierloot, R. (1982) Pimozide combined with behavior therapy in the short-term treatment of anorexia nervosa. A double-blind placebo-controlled cross-over study. *Acta Psychiatr. Scand.* 66:445–450.

Vandereycken, W. (1984) Neuroleptics in the short-term treatment of anorexia nervosa. A double-blind placebo-controlled study with sulpiride. *Br. J. Psychiatry* 144:288–292.

Vink, T., Hinney, A., van Elburg, A.A., van Goozen, S.H., Sandkuijl, L.A., Sinke, R.J., Herpertz-Dahlmann, B.M., Hebebrand, J., Remschmidt, H., van Engeland, H., and Adan, R.A. (2001) Association between an agouti-related protein gene polymorphism and anorexia nervosa. *Mol. Psychiatry* 6:325–328.

Vitousek, K., and Manke, F. (1994) Personality variables and disorders in anorexia nervosa and bulimia nervosa. *J. Abnorm. Psychol.* 103:137–147.

Wade, T.D., Bulik, C.M., Neale, M., and Kendler, K.S. (2000) Anorexia nervosa and major depression: Shared genetic and environmental risk factors. *Am. J. Psychiatry* 157:469–471.

Wade, T., Martin, N.G., and Tiggemann, M. (1998) Genetic and environmental risk factors for the weight and shape concerns characteristic of bulimia nervosa. *Psychol. Med.* 28:761–771.

Wade, T., Neale, M.C., Eaves, L.J., Heath, A.C., Kessler, R.C., and Kendler, K.S. (1999) A genetic analysis of the eating and attitudes associated with bulimia nervosa: dealing with the problem of ascertainment. *Behav. Genet.* 29:1–10.

Wagner, A., Aizenstein, H., Frank, G.K., Figurski, J., May, J.C., Putnam, K., Bailer, U.F., Fischer, L., Henry, S.E., McConaha, C., and Kaye, W.H. (2008) Altered insula response to a taste stimulus in individuals recovered from restricting-type anorexia nervosa. *Neuropsychopharmacol.* 33:513–523.

Wagner, A., Barbarich, N., Frank, G., Bailer, U.F., Weissfeld, L., Henry, S., Achenbach, S., Vogel, V., Plotnicov, K., McConaha, C., Kaye, W., and Wonderlich, S. (2006) Personality traits after recovery from eating disorders: do subtypes differ? *Int. J. Eat. Disord.* 39:276–284.

Wagner, A., Greer, P., Bailer, U., Frank, G., Henry, S., Putnam, K., Meltzer, C.C., Ziolko, S.K., Hoge, J., McConaha, C., and Kaye, W.H. (2006) Normal brain tissue volumes after long-term recovery in anorexia and bulimia nervosa. *Biol. Psychiatry* 59:291–293.

Wagner, A., Ruf, M., Braus, D.F., and Schmidt, M.H. (2003) Neuronal activity changes and body image distortion in anorexia nervosa. *Neuroreport* 14:2193–2197.

Walsh, B., Kaplan, A., Attia, E., Olmsted, M., Parides, M., Carter, J., Pike, K., Devlin, M., Woodside, B., Roberto, C., and Rocket, W. (2006) Fluoxetine after weight restoration in anorexia nervosa: a randomized controlled trial. *JAMA* 295:2605–2612.

Walsh, B.T., Roose, S.P., Katz, J.L., Dyrenfurth, I., Wright, L., Vande Wiele, R., and Glassman, A.H. (1987) Hypothalamic-pituitary-adrenal-cortical activity in anorexia nervosa and bulimia. *Psychoneuroendocrinol.* 12:131–140.

Walsh, B.T., Sysko, R., and Parides, M.K. (2006) Early response to desipramine among women with bulimia nervosa. *Int. J. Eat. Disord.* 39:72–75.

Walsh, B.T., Wilson, G.T., Loeb, K.L., Devlin, M.J., Pike, K.M., Roose, S.P., Fleiss, J., and Waternaux, C. (1997) Medication and psychotherapy in the treatment of bulimia nervosa. *Am. J. Psychiatry* 154:523–531.

Walters, E.E., and Kendler, K.S. (1995) Anorexia nervosa and anorexic-like syndromes in a population-based female twin sample. *Am. J. Psychiatry* 152:64–71.

Westergaard, G., Suomi, S., Chavanne, T., Houser, L., Hurley, A., Cleveland, A., Snoy, P., and Higley, J. (2003) Physiological correlates of aggression and impulsivity in free-ranging female primates. *Neuropsychopharmacol.* 28:1045–1055.

Wolfe, B., Jimerson, D., Orlova, C., and Mantzoros, C. (2004) Effect of dieting on plasma leptin, soluble leptin receptor, adiponectin and resistin levels in healthy volunteers. *Clin. Endocrinol. (Oxf)* 61:332–338.

Wolfe, B.E., Metzger, E.D., and Jimerson, D.C. (1997) Research update on serotonin function in bulimia nervosa and anorexia nervosa. *Psychopharmacol. Bull.* 33:345–354.

Wolfe, B., Metzger, E., Levine, J., Finkelstein, D., Cooper, T., and Jimerson, D. (2000) Serotonin function following remission from bulimia nervosa. *Neuropsychopharmacol.* 22:257–263.

Wren, A., Seal, L., Cohen, M., Byrnes, A., Front, G., Murphy, K., Dhillo, W., Ghatei, M., and Bloom, S. (2001) Ghrelin enhances appetite and increases foot intake in humans. *J. Clin. Endocrinol. Metab.* 86:5992–5995.

Wu, J.C., Hagman, J., Buchsbaum, M.S., Blinder, B., Derrfler, M., Tai, W.Y., Hazlett, E., and Sicotte, N. (1990) Greater left cerebral hemisphere metabolism in bulimia assessed by positron emission tomography. *Am. J. Psychiatry* 147:309–312.

Zhang, Y., Proenca, R., Maffei, M., Barone, M., Leopold, L., and Friedman, J. (1994) Positional cloning of the mouse obese gene and its human homologue. *Nat. Genet.* 372:425–432.

Zhu, A., and Walsh, B. (2002) Pharmacologic treatment of eating disorders. *Can. J. Psychiatry* 47:227–234.

Zigman, J., and Elmquist, J. (2003) Minireview: From anorexia to obesity—the yin and yang of body weight control. *Endocrinol.* 144:3749–3756.

85 The Neurobiology of Sleep

GIULIO TONONI AND CHIARA CIRELLI

Sleep is a state of reduced responsiveness to environmental stimuli, usually associated with immobility and stereotyped postures. This reduced responsiveness is rapidly reversible—distinguishing sleep from coma—but is still potentially dangerous. Considering that such a state of reduced responsiveness occupies one third of our life, that it is universal, being present in every animal species studied, and that it is tightly regulated, it is likely to serve some essential function. However, what that function is remains uncertain to this day. What is certain is that if we stay awake much longer than the usual 16 hours a day, we are soon overcome by sleepiness, and we become cognitively impaired. The brain is spontaneously active during sleep, so changes in sleep rhythms can be a sensitive indicator of changes in brain function in neuropsychiatric disorders.

In this chapter, we first examine how sleep is traditionally subdivided into different stages that alternate in the course of the night. We will then consider the brain centers that determine whether we are asleep or awake and examine the negative consequences of sleep deprivation. We then discuss how brain activity changes between sleep and wakefulness and consider how this leads to the characteristic modifications of consciousness experienced during dreaming and dreamless sleep. Finally, we turn to the paramount but still mysterious question of sleep function.

SLEEP STAGES AND CYCLES

The scientific study of sleep and wakefulness came of age in 1928 when Hans Berger developed an amplifier that could record the electrical activity generated by the brain and discovered that the electroencephalogram (EEG) changes dramatically between wakefulness and sleep, mostly because of the appearance of sleep slow waves and spindles (Jung and Berger, 1979). Another key development occurred in 1953, when Aserinsky and Kleitman discovered a stage of sleep during which the EEG was similar to that of wakefulness. Because this stage was associated with bursts of eye movements, it was called *rapid-eye-movement* (REM) sleep. By contrast, all other sleep has come to be called *non-rapid-eye-movement* (NREM) sleep.

Nowadays, sleep is studied for clinical and research purposes by combining behavioral observations with electrophysiological recordings. The EEG records synchronous synaptic activity from millions of neurons underlying electrodes applied to the scalp (Fig. 85.1). The electrooculogram (EOG), which is recorded from electrodes attached to the skin near the eyes, detects small electrical fields generated by eye movements. The electromyogram (EMG), which is generally recorded from electrodes attached to the chin, is used to detect sustained (tonic) and episodic (phasic) changes in muscle activity that correlate with changes in behavioral state. In the course of the night, the EEG, EOG, and EMG patterns undergo coordinated changes that are used to distinguish among different sleep stages.

Wakefulness

During wakefulness, the EEG is characterized by waves of low amplitude and high frequency. This kind of EEG pattern is known as *low-voltage fast-activity* or *activated*. When eyes close in preparation for sleep, EEG alpha activity (8–13 Hz) becomes prominent, particularly in occipital regions. Such alpha activity is thought to correspond to an "idling" rhythm in visual areas.

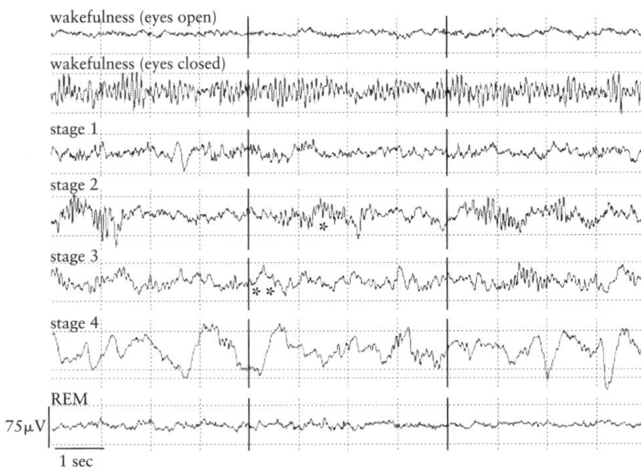

FIGURE 85.1 The human electroencephalogram (EEG) during wakefulness and the different stages of sleep (*: sleep spindles; **: slow wave).

The waking EOG reveals frequent voluntary eye movements and eye blinks. The EMG reveals tonic muscle activity with additional phasic activity related to voluntary movements.

Stage 1

Falling asleep is a gradual phenomenon of progressive disconnection from the environment. Sleep is usually entered through a transitional state, stage 1, characterized by loss of alpha activity and the appearance of a low-voltage mixed-frequency EEG pattern with prominent theta activity (3–7 Hz). Eye movements become slow and rolling, and muscle tone relaxes. Although there is decreased awareness of sensory stimuli, a subject in stage 1 may deny that he was asleep. Motor activity may persist for a number of seconds during stage 1. Occasionally participants experience sudden muscle contractions (hypnic jerks), sometimes accompanied by a sense of falling and dreamlike imagery. Participants deprived of sleep often have "microsleep" episodes that consist of brief (5–10 seconds) bouts of stage 1 sleep; these episodes can have serious consequences in situations that demand constant attention, such as driving a car.

NREM Sleep: Stage 2

After a few minutes in stage 1, people usually progress to stage 2 sleep. Stage 2 is heralded in the EEG by the appearance of K-complexes and sleep spindles, which are especially evident over central regions. K-complexes are made up of a high-amplitude negative sharp wave followed by a positive slow wave and are often triggered by external stimuli. Sleep spindles are waxing and waning oscillations at around 12–15 Hz that last about 1 second and occur 5–10 times a minute. Eye movements and muscle tone are much reduced. Stage 2 qualifies fully as sleep because people are partially disconnected from the environment, meaning that they do not respond to the events around them—their *arousal threshold* is increased. If stimuli are strong enough to wake them up, people in stage 2 will confirm that they were asleep.

NREM Sleep: Stages 3 and 4

Stage 2 is followed, especially at the beginning of the night, by a period comprising stages 3 and 4, during which the EEG shows prominent slow waves in the delta range (≤2 Hz, >75 μV in humans). The distinction between stages 3 and 4 is conventionally based on the proportion of slow waves (respectively less and more than 50% of a 30-second epoch). Eye movements cease during stages 3 and 4, and EMG activity decreases further. Stage 3 and 4 are also referred to as *slow-wave sleep*, *delta sleep*, or *deep sleep* because the threshold for arousal is higher than in stage 2. The process of awakening from slow-wave sleep is drawn out, and participants often remain confused for some time.

REM Sleep

After deepening through stages 2 to 4, NREM sleep lightens and returns to stage 2, after which the sleeper enters REM sleep. As was mentioned, REM sleep derives its name from the frequent bursts of eye movements (Aserinsky and Kleitman, 1953; Carskadon et al., 2002). It is also referred to as *paradoxical sleep* (Jouvet, 1962, 1965, 1998) because the EEG during REM sleep is similar to the activated EEG of waking or of stage 1. Indeed, the EEG of REM sleep is characterized by low-voltage fast-activity, often with increased power in the theta band (3–7 Hz). REM sleep is not subdivided into stages but rather is described in terms of tonic and phasic components. Tonic aspects of REM sleep include the activated EEG and a generalized loss of muscle tone, except for the extraocular muscles that drive the REMs and the diaphragm that keeps us breathing. Rapid-eye-movement sleep is also accompanied by penile erections (their significance is unknown, but their occurrence can rule out neurological causes of impotence). Phasic features of REM include irregular bursts of REMs and muscle twitches. Behaviorally, REM sleep is deep sleep, with an arousal threshold that is as high as in slow-wave sleep.

SLEEP DURING THE LIFE SPAN

Sleep patterns change markedly across the life span (Carskadon et al., 2002; Peirano et al., 2003; Carskadon et al., 2004; Jenni et al., 2004; Jenni and Carskadon, 2004; Ohayon et al., 2004). Newborn infants spend 16–18 hours per day sleeping, with an early version of REM sleep, called *active sleep*, occupying about half of their sleep time. At approximately 3–4 months of age, when sleep starts to become consolidated during the night, the sleep EEG shows more mature waveforms characteristic of NREM and REM sleep. During early childhood, total sleep time decreases, and REM sleep proportion drops to adult levels. The proportion of NREM sleep spent in slow-wave sleep increases during the first year of life, reaches a peak, declines during adolescence and adulthood, and may disappear entirely by age 60.

THE SLEEP CYCLE

The succession of NREM sleep stages followed by an episode of REM sleep is called a *sleep cycle* and lasts approximately 90–110 minutes in humans. As shown in Figure 85.2, there are a total of 4–5 cycles every night. Slow-wave sleep is prominent early in the night, especially during the first sleep cycle, and diminishes as the night progresses. As slow-wave sleep wanes, periods of REM sleep lengthen and show greater phasic activity. The proportion of time spent in each stage and the pattern of stages across the night is fairly consistent in normal adults. A healthy young adult will typically spend about 5% of the sleep period in stage 1 sleep, about 50% in stage 2 sleep, 20%–25% in slow-wave sleep (stages 3 and 4), and 20%–25% in REM sleep.

Brain Centers Regulating Wakefulness and Sleep

Two antagonistic sets of brain structures are responsible for orchestrating the regular alternation between wakefulness and sleep. The neuronal groups that promote wakefulness are located in the basal forebrain, posterior hypothalamus, and in the upper brain stem, whereas those promoting NREM sleep are located in the anterior hypothalamus and basal forebrain (Szymusiak et al., 2001; Jones, 2003; McGinty and Szymusiak, 2003; McGinty et al., 2004; Jones, 2005b; Saper, Scammell, and Lu, 2005). Other cellular groups in the dorsal part of the pons and in the medulla constitute the so-called REM sleep generator (Fig. 85.3) (Jouvet, 1962, 1965; Lai and Siegel, 1988; Chase and Morales, 1990; Jouvet, 1994; McCarley, 2004; Siegel, 2005). The circadian clock, centered on the suprachiasmatic nucleus of the hypothalamus (SCN), exerts an overall control on many of these brain areas, to ensure that sleep occurs at the appropriate time of the 24-hour light–dark cycle (Aston-Jones, 2005; Mistlberger, 2005; Saper, Lu, et al., 2005; Zee and Manthena, 2007).

Maintenance of wakefulness is dependent on several heterogeneous cell groups extending from the upper pons and midbrain (the so-called reticular activating system (RAS) (Lindsley et al., 1949; Moruzzi and Magoun, 1949) to the posterior hypothalamus and basal forebrain. These cell groups are strategically placed so that they can release, over wide regions of the brain, neuromodulators and neurotransmitters that produce EEG activation, such as acetylcholine, hypocretin, histamine, norepinephrine, and glutamate. As we will see, the main mechanism by which these neuromodulators and neurotransmitters produce cortical activation is by closing leakage potassium channels on the cell membrane of cortical and thalamic neurons, thus keeping cells depolarized and ready to fire.

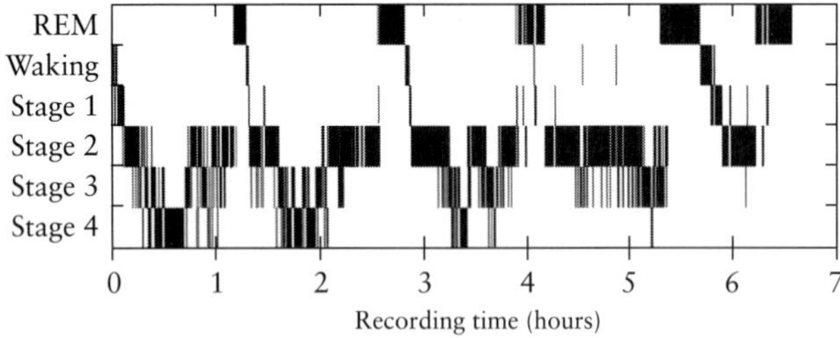

FIGURE 85.2 Hypnogram for an all-night recording in a young man. Note the occurrence of five sleep cycles, the predominance of slow-wave sleep (stages 3 and 4) early in the night, and the increasing length of REM sleep episodes later in the night.

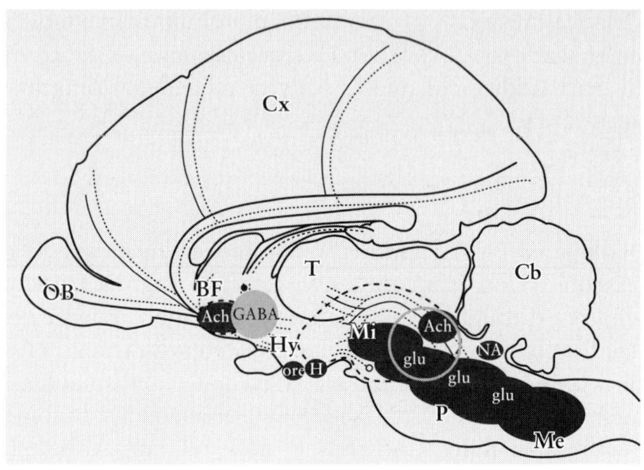

FIGURE 85.3 The major brain areas involved in initiating and maintaining wakefulness (dark gray), NREM sleep (light gray), and REM sleep (light gray circle).

Acetylcholine

Cholinergic cells are located in the basal forebrain and in two small nuclei in the pons: the pedunculopontine tegmental and lateral dorsal tegmental nuclei (PPT/LDT). Basal forebrain and pontine cholinergic cells fire at high rates in wakefulness and REM sleep and decrease or stop firing during NREM sleep (el Mansari et al., 1989; Lee, Hassani, Alonso, and Jones, 2005). Pontine cholinergic cells project to the thalamus, where they help depolarize specific and intralaminar thalamic nuclei. The latter, which are dispersed throughout the thalamus and project diffusely to the cortex, fire at very high frequencies during wakefulness and REM sleep and help to synchronize cortical firing in the gamma (> 28 Hz) range (McCormick, 1989; Steriade, 2004; Jones, 2005a). They also project to other cholinergic and noncholinergic (many of them glutamatergic) cells in the basal forebrain, which in turn provide an excitatory input to the entire cortex (Jones, 2003, 2005b). Indeed, drugs with anticholinergic activity, including tricyclic antidepressants and atropine, can cause sedation and produce slow waves in the EEG (Domino et al., 1968; Itil and Fink, 1968). On the other hand, cholinergic agonists (for example, nicotine) usually enhance arousal (Metherate et al., 1992; Gillin et al., 1994). In patients with Alzheimer's disease, loss of cholinergic cells is associated with slowing of the cortical EEG (Prinz et al., 1982; Soininen et al., 1992; Dierks et al., 1995; Montplaisir et al., 1998).

Histamine

Cholinergic neurons in the pons also project to the posterior hypothalamus, where histaminergic neurons are located in the tuberomammillary nucleus (Brown et al., 2001). Histaminergic neurons, which project throughout the cortex, fire at the highest rates during wakefulness and are inhibited during NREM and REM sleep (Takahashi et al., 2006). They have an important wakefulness-promoting function, as shown by the increased sleep and drowsiness when they are experimentally inactivated (Lin et al., 1989; Lin et al., 1996). Indeed, over-the-counter antihistaminergic drugs are used all over the world to facilitate the induction of sleep (Barbier and Bradbury, 2007).

Glutamate

Probably the largest contingent of the wakefulness-promoting system is made up by cells dispersed throughout the brain-stem reticular formation and the basal forebrain that do not release conventional neuromodulators but rather the ubiquitous neurotransmitter *glutamate*. By binding to metabotropic receptors, glutamate can act as a neuromodulator and influence the excitability of target cells. The firing patterns of these glutamatergic cells are not well characterized (Jones, 2003, 2005a, 2005b).

Norepinephrine

Noradrenergic cells are concentrated in the locus coeruleus in the upper pons, from where they project throughout the brain (Berridge and Waterhouse, 2003; Aston-Jones, 2005). They fire tonically during wakefulness and emit short, phasic bursts of activity during behavioral choices or salient events (Foote et al., 1980; Aston-Jones and Bloom, 1981a, 1981b; Berridge and Abercrombie, 1999; Aston-Jones and Cohen, 2005). The release of norepinephrine increases the response of cortical neurons to incoming stimuli, but it is not necessary for EEG activation (noradrenergic lesions induce mild sedation) (McCormick, 1989; Berridge and Foote, 1991; Cape and Jones, 1998; Berridge and Espana, 2000). However, the release of norepinephrine during wakefulness is essential for the induction of genes such as *P-CREB*, *Arc*, and *BDNF*, which are involved in synaptic potentiation and thereby in learning (Cirelli et al., 1996; Cirelli and Tononi, 2000). By contrast, locus coeruleus neurons decrease their firing during NREM sleep and cease firing altogether during REM sleep: in this way, neural activity during sleep does not translate into long-term synaptic potentiation, so we do not end up learning the wrong things and confuse dreams for reality.

Serotonin

Serotoninergic cells from the dorsal raphé nucleus also project widely throughout the brain. Serotoninergic neurons, like noradrenergic neurons, fire at higher levels in waking, fire at lower levels in NREM sleep, and fall silent during REM sleep. However, in contrast to noradrenergic neurons, serotoninergic neurons are inactivated when animals make behavioral choices or orient to salient stimuli and are activated instead during repetitive motor activity such as locomoting, grooming, or feeding (McGinty and Harper, 1976; Jacobs et al., 2002). As is mentioned later, the inactivity of serotonin cells during sleep may contribute to the sensory disconnection from the environment that occurs during sleep. The role of serotonin in sleep is complicated, however, because it may also be involved in sleep induction, at least in part by inhibiting the cholinergic system (Cape and Jones, 1998; Jouvet, 1999; Jones, 2005a).

Dopamine

Another aminergic neuromodulator is dopamine (DA). Dopamine-containing neurons located in the substantia nigra and ventral tegmental area innervate the frontal cortex, basal forebrain, and limbic structures (Monti and Monti, 2007). Unlike other aminergic cells, dopaminergic neurons do not appear to change their firing rate depending on behavioral state. However, psychostimulants such as amphetamines and cocaine that block reuptake of monoamines, including norepinephrine, DA, and serotonin, promote prolonged wakefulness and increase cortical activation and behavioral arousal (Monti and Monti, 2007).

Hypocretin

The peptide *hypocretin* (also known as *orexin*) is produced by cells in the dorsolateral hypothalamus that provide excitatory input to all components of the waking system (Kilduff and Peyron, 2000; Sakurai, 2007). These cells, too, are most active during waking, especially in relation to motor activity and exploratory behavior, and almost stop firing during NREM and REM sleep (Lee, Hassani, and Jones, 2005; Mileykovskiy et al., 2005). Most patients with *narcolepsy*, a disorder characterized by excessive somnolence and cataplectic attacks, have low or undetectable levels of hypocretin in the cerebrospinal fluid (Dauvilliers et al., 2007).

Hypothalamus, Basal Forebrain, and Sleep

As we seek a quiet, dark, and silent place to fall asleep and close our eyes, the activity of the waking-promoting neuronal groups is decreased due to reduced sensory input. In addition, several of these brain areas are actively inhibited by antagonistic neuronal populations located in the hypothalamic and basal forebrain and become active at sleep onset. When the waking-promoting neuronal groups become nearly silent, the decreasing levels of acetylcholine and other waking-promoting neuromodulators and neurotransmitters lead to the opening of leak potassium channels in cortical and thalamic neurons, which become hyperpolarized and begin oscillating at low frequencies.

The importance of hypothalamic structures for sleep induction was recognized at the beginning of the 20th century during an epidemic of a viral infection of the brain called *encephalitis lethargica*. Von Economo (1931) concluded that if the infection destroyed the posterior hypothalamus, patients indeed became lethargic, but if the anterior hypothalamus was lesioned, patients became severely insomniac. Indeed, subsequent studies confirmed that cell groups within the anterior hypothalamus are involved in the initiation and maintenance of sleep. The ventrolateral preoptic area (VLPO) has been suggested as a possible sleep switch (Sherin et al., 1996; Szymusiak et al., 1998). However, many other neurons scattered through the anterior hypothalamus, for instance in the median preoptic nucleus (Suntsova et al., 2002) and in the basal forebrain, also play a major role in initiating and maintaining sleep. These neurons tend to fire during sleep and stop firing during wakefulness. When they are active, many of them release γ-aminobutyric acid (GABA) and the peptide *galanin*, and inhibit most waking-promoting areas, including cholinergic, noradrenergic, histaminergic, hypocretinergic, and serotonergic cells. In turn, the latter inhibit several sleep-promoting neuronal groups (Szymusiak et al., 2001; McGinty and Szymusiak, 2003; McGinty et al., 2004; Saper, Scammell, and Lu, 2005). This reciprocal inhibition provides state stability, in that each state reinforces itself as well as inhibits the opponent state.

The REM Sleep Generator

The REM sleep generator consists of pontine cholinergic cell groups (LDT and PPT) that we have already encountered as waking-promoting areas, and of nearby cell groups in the medial pontine reticular formation and in the medulla (Jouvet, 1962, 1965; Lai and Siegel, 1988; Chase and Morales, 1990; Jouvet, 1994; McCarley, 2004; Siegel, 2005). Lesions in these areas eliminate REM sleep without significantly disrupting NREM sleep. Rapid eye movement sleep can also be eliminated by certain antidepressants, especially monoamine oxidase inhibitors. As we have seen, pontine cholinergic neurons produce EEG activation by releasing acetylcholine to the thalamus and to cholinergic and glutamatergic basal forebrain neurons that in turn activate the limbic system and cortex. However, though during wakefulness other waking-promoting neuronal groups, such as noradrenergic, histaminergic, hypocretinergic and serotonergic neurons, are also active, they are inhibited during REM sleep. Other REM active neurons in the dorsal pons are responsible for the tonic inhibition of muscle tone during REM sleep. Finally, neurons in the medial pontine reticular formation fire in bursts and produce phasic events of REM sleep, such as REMs and muscle twitches.

The Circadian Clock

In mammals, the primary clock that keeps circadian time is the suprachiasmatic nucleus (SCN) of the hypothalamus. The SCN regulates a number of endocrine and behavioral parameters to coordinate the state of the organism with the 24-hour light–dark cycle, including wakefulness and sleep (Aston-Jones, 2005; Mistlberger, 2005; Saper, Lu, et al., 2005; Deboer et al., 2007; Zee and Manthena, 2007). In diurnal animals, the SCN activates waking-promoting areas and inhibits sleep-promoting areas during the day, maximally at the end of the day, whereas the converse is true at night. This makes it difficult to sleep in the early evening or to be awake in the early morning. In animals in which the SCN has been lesioned, sleep is no longer concentrated in one main episode but is dispersed across the entire 24-hour cycle (Mistlberger et al., 1983; Tobler et al., 1983; Bergmann et al., 1987). Each of the ~20,000 cells of the SCN contain a molecular clock that changes their excitability according to a near-24-hour rhythm and that is reset by light. The SCN produces a coherent output because its cells synchronize among themselves.

Humoral Factors

For a long time, it was assumed that sleep was mediated by the accumulation of some humoral factor during wakefulness—a kind of hypnotoxin. Despite a long search, only a few humoral factors have any well-defined role in sleep physiology. One of the best studied substances is adenosine, not surprising given the well-known antisleep effect of the A1 antagonist *caffeine* (Porkka-Heiskanen et al., 2002; Basheer et al., 2004). Extracellular adenosine accumulates in the basal forebrain area during wakefulness, inhibiting cholinergic neurons and promoting sleep (Porkka-Heiskanen et al., 1997), although the importance of this feedback mechanism has recently been disputed (Blanco-Centurion et al., 2006). Also, in humans, extracellular adenosine does not seem to accumulate in several brain areas as a function of previous wakefulness (Zeitzer et al., 2006). Prostaglandin D_2, another sleep promoting substance, acting on the prostaglandin D (PGD) receptor, indirectly activates adenosine A2A-dependent pathways in the basal forebrain (Huang et al., 2007). However, neither A1 nor PGD receptor knockout mice have abnormal baseline sleep. Similarly, a number of lymphokines, such as interleukin-1 (IL-1) and tumor necrosis factor (TNF) alpha, modulate sleep. These effects are often species specific and could be most relevant in the context of acute inflammation or infection. However, the TNF and IL-1 type I receptor knockouts have abnormal sleep, suggesting also a role in baseline sleep regulation (Krueger et al., 2001).

The pineal hormone *melatonin* is strongly regulated by the circadian clock and peaks at night in diurnal and nocturnal animals (it has been called the "darkness hormone"). Melatonin receptors are highly expressed in the SCN, and melatonin can help reset circadian rhythms and thereby influence sleep (Zee and Manthena, 2007). Light and melatonin can be used to alleviate and correct circadian rhythm disorders and conditions such as jet lag and night-shift work. Melatonin is also effective in regularizing the sleep–wake schedule of light-blind subjects whose sleep–wake periods tend to free-run, as well as in children and in the elderly with brain disorders, for example in the treatment of the "sundowning" often seen in dementia (Arendt, 2005; Richardson, 2005).

SLEEP REGULATION AND SLEEP DEPRIVATION

If we are not allowed to sleep and are forced to stay awake longer than usual, sleep pressure mounts and soon becomes overwhelming. Thus, sleep is homeostatically regulated: the more we stay awake, the longer and more intensely we sleep afterwards: arousal thresholds increase, there are fewer awakenings, and during NREM sleep the amplitude and prevalence of slow waves become much higher (Fig. 85.4; see also COLOR FIGURE 85.4 in separate insert), and there can be a rebound of REM sleep. Sleep pressure only diminishes if one is allowed to sleep, and the number and amplitude of sleep slow waves gradually diminish.

In humans, the most prominent effect of total sleep deprivation, and even of sleep restriction (for several nights), is cognitive impairment, with striking practical consequences (Bonnet and Arand, 2003; Dinges, 2006). For example, each year drowsy driving is responsible for at least 100,000 automobile crashes; 71,000 injuries; and 1,550 fatalities (National Sleep Foundation, 2002; Radun and Summala, 2004). A person who is sleep deprived tends to take longer to respond to stimuli, particularly when tasks are monotonous and low in cognitive demands. However, sleep deprivation produces more than just decreased alertness. Tasks emphasizing higher cognitive functions—such as logical reasoning, encoding, decoding, and parsing complex sentences; complex subtraction tasks; and tasks involving a flexible thinking style and the ability to focus on a large number of goals simultaneously—are all significantly affected even after one single night of sleep deprivation. Tasks requiring sustained attention, such as those including goal-directed activities, can be impaired by even a few hours of sleep loss. For example, a recent study showed that medical interns make more frequent serious diagnostic errors when they worked frequent shifts of 24 hours or more than when they worked shorter shifts (Barger et al., 2006). Unfortunately, subjects who are sleep deprived underestimate the severity of their cognitive impairment, often with tragic consequences. Also, lack of sleep does not completely eliminate the capacity to perform but rather makes the performance inconsistent and unreliable (Doran et al., 2001). Thus, a sleepy driver will either respond normally to an emergency or not at all, due to rapid changes in vigilance state and the sudden intrusion of microsleeps during waking. Similarly, people may still be able to transiently perform at baseline levels in short tests even after 3–4 days of sleep deprivation. However, the same subjects will perform very poorly when engaged in tasks requiring sustained attention. An important issue

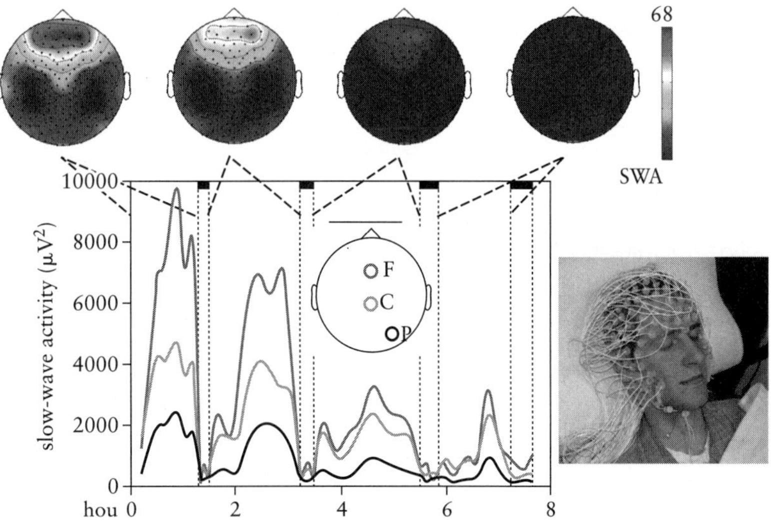

FIGURE 85.4 Sleep slow waves as a marker of sleep pressure. Bottom panel: During early sleep, at the end of a day of wakefulness, sleep pressure is maximal. This is reflected in frequent and large sleep slow waves, measured here as slow-wave activity (power in the 0.5–4 Hz band, in red for a frontal electroencephalogram (EEG) channel, green for a central channel, and blue for an occipital channel). During sleep, slow-wave activity decreases exponentially, reflecting a reduction of sleep pressure. The transitory drops in slow-wave activity correspond to episodes of rapid-eye-movement (REM) sleep. Top panel: Topographic display of slow-wave activity over the scalp for the four sleep cycles. Notice the frontal predominance and the progressive decline in the course of the night. (See Figure 85.4 in color insert.)

that remains unresolved is whether the cognitive impairment seen after sleep deprivation and sleep restriction is exclusively due to sleepiness—the increasing internal pressure to fall asleep presumably mediated by the sleep-promoting areas discussed before—or to progressive cellular dysfunctions in cortical and other circuits that have been awake too long—a veritable form of neuronal tiredness.

It should be mentioned that several well-controlled studies have discredited the once-popular notion that loss of REM sleep might lead to psychosis and suicide. Indeed, REM sleep deprivation as well as total sleep deprivation improves mood in approximately 50% of people who are depressed.

NEURAL CORRELATES OF WAKEFULNESS AND SLEEP

Wakefulness and NREM and REM sleep are accompanied by distinctive molecular changes, changes in spontaneous neural activity and metabolism, and responsiveness to stimuli.

Molecular Changes

It might seem unlikely that the mere change from wakefulness to sleep should lead to changes in the expression of genes in the brain, but this is actually what happens, and on a massive scale. Hundreds of gene transcripts (messenger ribonucleic acids [mRNAs]) are expressed at higher levels in the waking brain, and a different set of transcripts are expressed at higher levels in sleep (Cirelli et al., 2004). Many of these molecular changes are specific to the brain because they do not occur in other tissues such as liver and muscle. Transcripts upregulated during wakefulness code for proteins that help the brain to face high-energy demand, high synaptic excitatory transmission, and high transcriptional activity, as well as the cellular stress that may derive from one or more of these processes. Moreover, wakefulness is associated with the increased expression of several genes that are involved in long-term potentiation of synaptic strength, such as *P-CREB, Arc, NGFI-A,* and *BDNF* (Cirelli et al., 1996; Cirelli and Tononi, 2000) (Fig. 85.5). As we have seen, one reason these genes are expressed in wakefulness and not in sleep has to do with the release of norepinephrine, which is high during wakefulness, when animals make decisions and learn about the environment, but is low during sleep.

By contrast, the genes that increase their expression during sleep include several that may be involved in long-term depression of synaptic strength and possibly in synaptic consolidation (Cirelli et al., 2004). Other sleep-related genes appear to favor the rate of protein synthesis, which is also increased in sleep. Finally, many

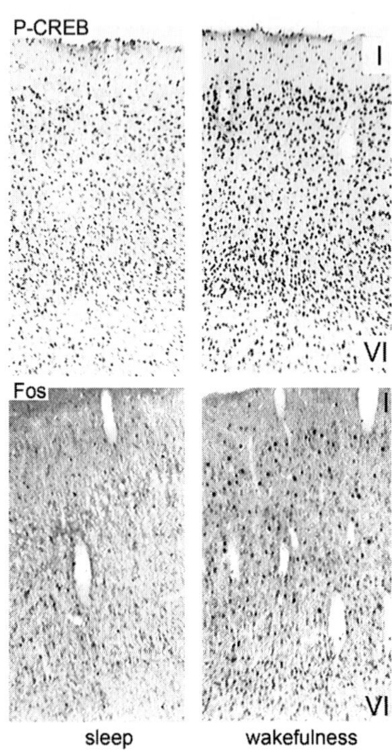

FIGURE 85.5 The expression of the transcription factors P-CREB and Fos is high in wakefulness and low in sleep (rat parietal cortex I and VI, cortical layers I and VI).

sleep-related genes play a significant role in membrane trafficking and maintenance. Thus, these findings suggest that although sleep is a state of behavioral inactivity, it is associated not only with intense neural activity, but also with the increased expression of many genes that may favor specific cellular functions.

Spontaneous Neural Activity

Wakefulness

The waking EEG, characterized by the presence of low-voltage fast-activity, is known as *activated* because most cortical neurons are steadily depolarized close to their firing threshold (Fig. 85.6), and are thus ready to respond to the slightest change in their inputs. The steady depolarization is due to the release of acetylcholine and other neurotransmitters and neuromodulators, which close leakage potassium channels on the membrane of cortical neurons. The readiness to respond of cortical and thalamic neurons enables fast and effective interactions among distributed regions of the thalamocortical system, resulting in a continuously changing sequence of specific firing patterns. Because these firing patterns are not globally synchronous across the cortex, the EEG displays rapid fluctuations of low amplitude rather than high-voltage, low-frequency waves. Nevertheless, superimposed on the low-voltage, fast-activity background of wakefulness one frequently observes rhythmic oscillatory episodes within the alpha (8–13 Hz), beta (14–28 Hz), and gamma (> 28 Hz) range, which are usually localized to specific cortical areas. These waking rhythms are due to the activation of oscillatory mechanisms intrinsic to each cell as well as to the entrainment of oscillatory circuits among excitatory and inhibitory neurons.

NREM sleep

As we have seen, the EEG of NREM sleep is dramatically different from that of wakefulness and is characterized by the occurrence of slow waves (< 2 Hz in humans), K-complexes, and sleep spindles. At the beginning of sleep, the release of acetylcholine and other neuromodulators is much reduced, with the consequence that leakage potassium channels on the membrane of cortical and thalamic cells open, positively charged potassium ions leave the cells, and membrane potentials are drawn towards hyperpolarization. This and other neuromodulatory-mediated changes trigger a series of membrane currents that lead to an oscillation in cellular membrane potential called the *slow oscillation* (Fig. 85.6) (Steriade et al., 2001). As shown by intracellular recordings, the slow oscillation is made up of a hyperpolarization phase, or *down-state*, which lasts a few hundreds of milliseconds, and a slightly longer depolarization phase, or *up-state*. The down-state is associated with the virtual absence of synaptic activity within cortical networks. During the up-state, by contrast, cortical cells fire at rates that are as high as or even higher than those seen in waking and that may even show periods of fast oscillatory activity in the gamma range.

The slow oscillation is found in virtually every cortical neuron and is synchronized across much of the cortical mantle by cortico-cortical connections, which is why the EEG records high-voltage, low-frequency waves. Human EEG recordings using 256 channels have revealed that the slow oscillation behaves as a traveling wave that sweeps across a large portion of the cerebral cortex (Massimini et al., 2004). Most of the time, the sweep starts in the very front of the brain and propagates front to back. These sweeps occur very infrequently during stage 1, around 5 times a minute during stage 2, more than 10 times a minute in stage 3, and 20 times a minute in stage 4. Thus, a wave of depolarization and intense synaptic activity, followed by a wave of hyperpolarization and synaptic silence, sweeps across the brain more and more frequently just as NREM sleep becomes deeper. These waves of activity and inactivity are reminiscent of those of contraction and relaxation that sweep through the cardian tissue triggered by the electrical activity originating in the sinus pacemaker that travels along the conduction system. It is as if, during NREM sleep, the brain were to unveil its own spontaneous "brain beat."

The various EEG waves that characterize NREM sleep are closely associated with the slow oscillation. Slow oscillations can occur every few seconds at a single cortical source or can originate at short intervals at multiple cortical sites, in which case they superimpose or interfere, leading to EEG slow waves that are shorter and more fractured (delta waves, 1–2 Hz in humans). Waves in the delta range are also favored by certain intrinsic currents present in cortical and thalamic neurons. Topographically, slow waves are especially prominent over dorsolateral prefrontal cortex. K-complexes are probably nothing more than slow oscillations, usually triggered by external stimuli, which appear particularly prominent because they are not immediately preceded or followed by other slow waves.

Sleep spindles occur during the depolarized phase of the slow oscillation and are generated in thalamic circuits as a consequence of cortical firing. When the cortex enters an up-state, strong cortical firing excites GABAergic neurons in the reticular nucleus of the thalamus. These in turn strongly inhibit thalamocortical neurons, triggering intrinsic currents that produce a rebound burst of action potentials. These bursts percolate within local thalamoreticular circuits and produce oscillatory firing at around 12–15 Hz. Thalamic spindle sequences reach back to the cortex and are globally synchronized by corticothalamic circuits, where they appear in the EEG as sleep spindles.

REM sleep

During REM sleep, the EEG returns to an activated, low-voltage fast-activity pattern that is similar to that

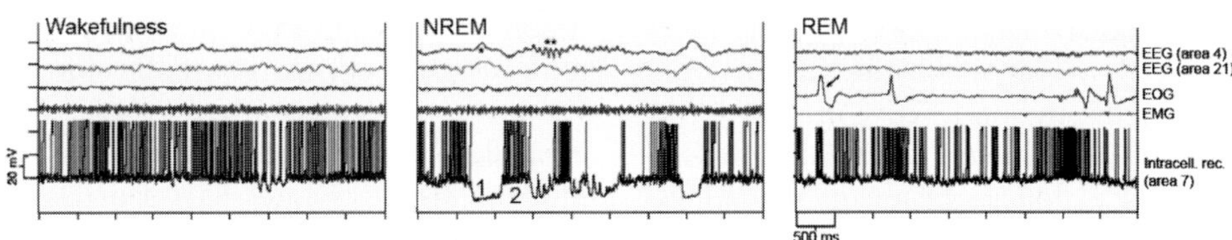

FIGURE 85.6 Simultaneous electroencephalogram (EEG), electrooculogram (EOG), electromyogram (EMG), and intracellular cortical recording in a cat. During non-rapid-eye-movement (NREM) sleep, the EEG trace shows slow waves (*) and sleep spindles (**), while the intracellular trace reveals the occurrence of slow oscillations in membrane potential (1 and 2 indicate down-state and up-state, respectively). During REM sleep, note the absence of muscle tone and the presence of rapid eye movements (arrow).

of quiet wakefulness or stage 1. As in wakefulness, the tonic depolarization of cortical and thalamic neurons is caused by the closure of leakage potassium channels. In fact, during REM sleep acetylcholine and other neuromodulators are released again at high levels, just as in wakefulness, and neuronal firing rates in several brain areas tend to be even higher.

Metabolism and Blood Flow

Recently, the data painstakingly obtained by recording the activity of individual neurons have been complemented by imaging studies that provide a simultaneous picture of synaptic activity over the entire brain, although at much lower resolution (Braun et al., 1997; Maquet et al., 1997).

NREM sleep

Positron emission tomography (PET) studies show that metabolic activity and blood flow are globally reduced in NREM sleep compared to resting wakefulness. During slow-wave sleep, metabolic activity can be reduced by as much as 40%. Metabolic activity is mostly due to the energetic requirements of synaptic transmission, and its reduction during NREM sleep is thus most likely due to the hyperpolarized phase of the slow oscillation, during which synaptic activity is essentially abolished. At a regional level, activation is especially reduced in the thalamus, due to its profound hyperpolarization during NREM sleep. In the cerebral cortex, activation is reduced in dorsolateral prefrontal, orbitofrontal, and anterior cingulate cortex. This deactivation is to be expected given that slow oscillations are especially prominent in these areas. Parietal, precuneus, and posterior cingulate cortex, as well as medial temporal cortex, also show relative deactivations. By contrast, primary sensory cortices are not deactivated compared to resting wakefulness. Basal ganglia and cerebellum are also deactivated, probably because of the reduced inflow from cortical areas.

REM sleep

During REM sleep, absolute levels of blood flow and metabolic activity are high, reaching levels similar to those seen during wakefulness, as would be expected based on the tonic depolarization and high firing rates of neurons. There are, however, interesting regional differences. Some brain areas are more active in REM sleep than in wakefulness. For example, there is a strong activation of limbic areas, including the amygdala and the parahippocampal cortex. Cerebral cortical areas that receive strong inputs from the amygdala, such as the anterior cingulate and the parietal lobule, are also activated, as are extrastriate areas. By contrast, the rest of parietal cortex, precuneus, posterior cingulate, and dorsolateral prefrontal cortex are relatively deactivated. As we will see, these regional activations and inactivations are consistent with the differences in mental state between sleep and wakefulness.

Upon awakening, blood flow is rapidly reestablished in brain stem and thalamus, as well as in the anterior cingulate cortex. However, it can take up to 20 minutes for blood flow to be fully reestablished in other brain areas, notably dorsolateral prefrontal cortex. It is likely that this sluggish reactivation is responsible for the phenomenon of sleep inertia—a postawakening deficit in alertness and performance that can last for tens of minutes.

Responsiveness to Stimuli

The most striking behavioral consequence of falling asleep is a progressive disconnection from the outside world. We stop responding to stimuli and, to the extent that we remain conscious, our experiences become largely independent of the current environment. This disconnection would appear to be important because we make several behavioral adjustments to bring it about: we seek a quiet environment, find a comfortable position, and close our eyes. However, people (especially small children) can fall asleep in a noisy environment and in uncomfortable positions—in the laboratory people can even sleep with their eyes taped open. Everything else being equal, the threshold for responding to peripheral stimuli gradually increases with the succession of NREM sleep stages 1 to 4 and remains high during REM sleep. Because cortical neurons continue to fire actively during sleep, how does this disconnection come about?

NREM sleep

As we have seen, during the transition from wakefulness to NREM sleep, the release of acetylcholine and other neuromodulators is reduced, leading to the progressive hyperpolarization of thalamocortical neurons. As a consequence, sensory stimuli that normally would be relayed to the cortex often fail to do so because they do not manage to fire thalamocortical cells. In addition, the rhythmic hyperpolarization during sleep spindles is especially effective in blocking incoming stimuli because it imposes an intrinsic oscillatory rhythm that effectively decouples inputs from outputs. Thus, the "thalamic gate" to the cerebral cortex is partially closed (Steriade, 2003). However, sensory stimuli in various modalities still elicit evoked potentials from the cerebral cortex, and neuroimaging studies show that primary cortical areas are still being activated (Portas et al., 2000). Recent studies using transcranial magnetic stimulation (TMS) and high-density EEG have employed direct cortical stimulation to bypass the thalamic gate (Massimini et al., 2005). The results show that during wakefulness TMS induces an initial local response followed for about 300 milliseconds by multiple, fast waves of activity associated with rapidly changing configurations of scalp potentials (Fig. 85.7; see also COLOR FIGURE 85.7 in separate insert). With the onset of NREM sleep, however, the brain response to TMS changes markedly. The initial response doubles in amplitude and lasts longer. After this large wave, however, no further TMS-locked activity can be detected, and all TMS-evoked activity ceases by 150 milliseconds. Moreover, this response, which lacks high-frequency components, remains localized and does not propagate to connected brain regions. Apparently, the ability of brain regions to interact causally with each other—their *effective connectivity*—breaks down during NREM sleep.

REM sleep

With the transition from NREM to REM sleep, neurons return to be steadily depolarized much as they are during quiet wakefulness, yet we still ignore sensory stimuli. It is as if we are preoccupied with the brain's intrinsic activity rather than with what goes on in the external world (Llinas and Pare, 1991), similar to what happens during states of intense absorption that can occur even when awake, say when one is engrossed in reading a captivating novel. The underlying mechanisms, however, are not clear. As we have seen, prefrontal and parietal cortical areas are deactivated in REM sleep compared to wakefulness. These regions include brain areas important for directing and sustaining attention to what is going on in sensory cortices. Sensory inputs reaching primary cortices would then find themselves to be systematically unattended. It is likely that the reduced activity in these cortical regions is a direct consequence of changes in the neuromodulatory milieu during REM sleep. The reduction of serotonin release during REM sleep may favor a dissociative-hallucinogenic state, as seen with certain psychoactive compounds.

Nevertheless, in contrast to a person in a coma or a vegetative state, a sleeping person can always be awakened if stimuli are strong enough or especially meaningful. For example, it is well known that the sound of one's name, or the wailing of a baby, are among the most effective signals for awakening.

Consciousness During Sleep

Sleep brings about at once the most common and the most dramatic change in consciousness that we are likely to witness—from the near fading of all experience to the bizarre hallucinations of dreams. Indeed, studying mental activity during sleep offers a unique opportunity to find out how changes in brain activity are associated with changes in consciousness. Typically, subjects are awoken at different times of night and are asked to report whatever was going through their mind (Hobson et al., 2000; Hobson and Pace-Schott, 2002).

Sleep onset

Reports from sleep onset, that is, stage 1, are very frequent (80%–90% of the time), but they are also very short, usually hallucinatory experiences. These are called *hypnagogic hallucinations*, from a Greek word meaning "leading into sleep." In contrast to typical dreams, hypnagogic hallucinations are often static, similar to single snapshots or a short sequence of still frames.

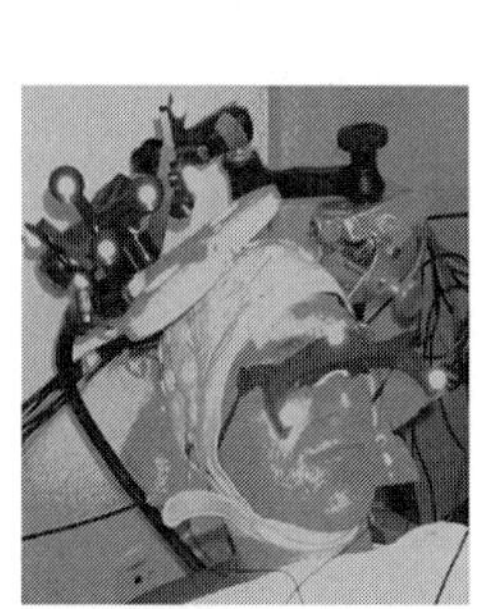

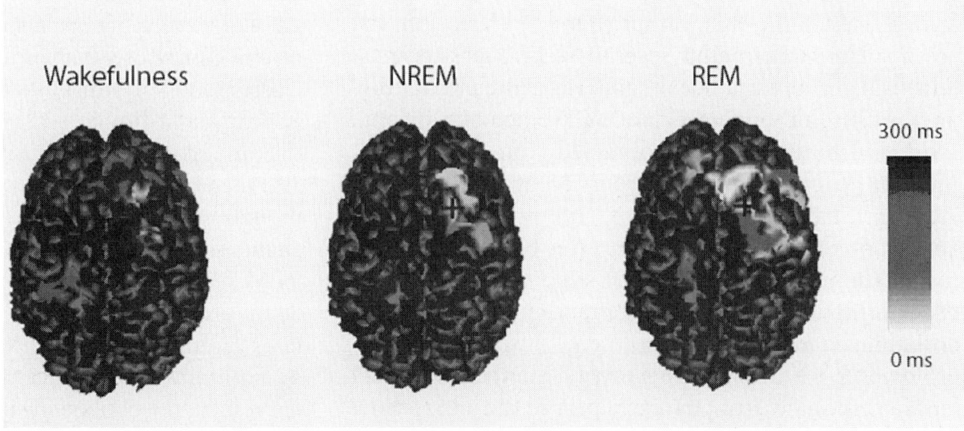

FIGURE 85.7 Spatiotemporal cortical current maps of transcranial magnetic stimulation (TMS)-induced activity during wakefulness, non-rapid-eye-movement (NREM), and REM sleep. On the left is the setup for TMS/EEG. From the electroencephalogram (EEG) data, maximum current sources corresponding to periods of significant activations were plotted and color-coded according to their latency of activation (light blue, 0 ms; red, 300 ms). The yellow cross marks the TMS target on the cortical surface. Note the rapidly changing patterns of activation during wakefulness, lasting up to 300 ms and involving several different areas; the brief activation that remains localized to the area of stimulation during NREM sleep; and an intermediate pattern of activation during REM sleep. (From Massimini, Tononi, et al., 2005; see Figure 85.7 in color insert.)

NREM sleep

Awakenings from NREM sleep yield reports 60%–80% of the time. Thus, there is a substantial number of awakenings from NREM sleep that yield no report whatsoever, especially early in the night when stages 3 and 4 are prevalent. The length of NREM reports is widely distributed. However, there are many very short reports early in the night, and much longer reports later in the night, considerably longer than those typically obtained at sleep onset or even during quiet wakefulness. Reports from NREM sleep, especially early in the night, can be thought like and lack perceptual vividness. However, especially later in the night, they can be much more hallucinatory and, generally speaking, more dream like. Indeed, hallucinatory content increases steeply from waking to sleep onset, and then to NREM sleep and REM sleep, whereas thought-like content behaves in the opposite way.

REM sleep

Awakenings from REM sleep yield reports 80%–90% of the time, a percentage similar to that obtained at sleep onset. Especially in the morning hours, the percentage is close to 100% (the report rate for wakefulness). Remarkably, the median word count of REM sleep reports is even higher than that of wakefulness reports, whether quiet or active. This finding seems to fit with the notion that dreams are single minded and thus less frequently interrupted by extraneous thoughts than waking consciousness. The average length of REM reports increases with the duration of the REM sleep episode. By contrast, there is no such relationship for NREM sleep reports.

These observations lead to several conclusions. Contrary to initial claims, some kind of conscious experience during sleep is the rule, rather than the exception. Especially late in the night, several NREM reports must be considered as bona fide dreams, no matter what criteria one uses, although they are on average not as long, vivid, and bizarre as those obtained from REM sleep. Another general conclusion from recent studies is that the length, hallucinatory content, and overall dream-like quality of reports increase from the beginning to the end of the night, irrespective of sleep stage. Thus, the relationship between sleep stages and dream features is probabilistic rather than absolute.

However, we must not forget that a number of NREM reports, especially from the early part of the night, show little evidence of conscious content. Considering that people awakened from stage 3 and 4 NREM sleep, even when they do report something, often take a long time to wake up and confabulate while still half asleep, it seems reasonable to assume that this may be the only time of our regular existence when we are close to losing consciousness altogether. So why does consciousness fade in NREM sleep early in the night, especially considering that spontaneous activity persists? One possibility is that the down-state of the slow oscillation, which sweeps the cerebral cortex once a second and produces an intermittent, near-global deactivation, results in the effective disconnection of cortical regions. Indeed, as we have seen above, studies of TMS/EEG have shown a breakdown of cortical effective connectivity during early NREM sleep (Massimini et al., 2005). By contrast, at sleep onset, and in stage 2 NREM sleep towards the morning, there are relatively long periods of activation between slow oscillations that may explain why most participants report dream-like experiences, although usually short ones. Finally, the long and vivid dreams of REM sleep can occur because brain activation is not interrupted at all by slow oscillations (Fig. 85.7; see also COLOR FIGURE 85.7 in separate insert).

Finally, though the vivid dreams of REM sleep can at times be hard to distinguish from waking experience, usually they share some features that are remarkably consistent with the changes in brain activation revealed by neuroimaging studies. For example, a key feature of dreaming consciousness is the reduced responsiveness to external stimuli, accompanied by vivid hallucinations, especially visual ones. Accordingly, PET studies of REM sleep show reduced activity in primary visual cortex, accompanied by increased activity in higher visual areas. Another relevant difference between dreaming and waking consciousness concerns the ability to reflect on oneself and one's experience, especially the ability to judge the verisimilitude of dreams. As we have seen, dorsolateral prefrontal cortex, which is involved in volitional control and self-monitoring, is especially deactivated during REM sleep. Reduced activation of dorsolateral prefrontal cortex may also contribute to the disorientation, reduction of directed thinking, and working memory observed in dreams, and contribute to dreaming amnesia. Conversely, dreams are characterized by a high degree of emotional involvement, especially fear and anxiety. Correspondingly, imaging studies have revealed a marked activation of limbic and paralimbic structures such as the amygdala, the anterior cingulate cortex, the insula, and medial orbitofrontal cortex during REM sleep. Although we still do not know what is responsible for the changes in brain regional activation that occur during REM sleep, it is likely that neuromodulatory systems may be involved. For example, because monoaminergic systems are silent during REM sleep, acetylcholine is alone in maintaining brain activation. Consistent with imaging results, the cholinergic innervation is especially strong in limbic and paralimbic areas and much weaker in dorsolateral prefrontal cortex.

THE FUNCTIONS OF SLEEP

Why should we periodically abandon daily activities, relinquish the search for food, forgo our reproductive duties, stop monitoring the environment for dangers or opportunities, and slumber for hours into an altered state of consciousness? An appealing idea is that sleep may have evolved from the circadian rest–activity cycle and may thus represent a default state of inactivity that keeps us out of trouble during the dark hours (or the light hours for nocturnal creatures) when we have nothing better to do. However, it is likely that sleep serves some more fundamental function. First, why should animals engage in prolonged periods of quiescence during which they are dangerously out of touch? Second, sleep seems to be universal. All animal species studied so far sleep, from invertebrates such as fruit flies and bees to birds and mammals. Nor has evolution found an easy way of getting rid of sleep. Some animals who need continuous vigilance while swimming or flying—for example, certain dolphins and migrating birds—have developed alternating unihemispheric sleep rather than eliminating sleep altogether. Third, sleep need is carefully regulated. As we have seen, if sleep is eliminated or restricted for some time, there is a gradual increase in sleep pressure that rapidly becomes irresistible, and the subsequent sleep is longer and more intense. This suggests that ensuring a certain amount of sleep is as important as preserving appropriate levels of temperature, energy, or electrolytes. Many of the hypotheses that have been put forth over the years fall into two main categories: those that propose a role of sleep in memory, and those that envision a role in brain restitution.

Sleep and Memory

A connection between sleep and memory was noted a long time ago. After struggling to learn a new piece of music for much of the day, we often play it better after a night of sleep. Recently, the importance of sleep and even naps occurring after certain types of declarative and nondeclarative learning has been documented in well-controlled experiments (Siegel, 2001; Stickgold and Walker, 2005a, 2005b; Vertes and Siegel, 2005; Born et al., 2006; Walker and Stickgold, 2006). Sleep could indeed offer a favorable context for certain aspects of learning and memory. The sensory disconnection associated with sleep reduces interference between ongoing activities and the consolidation of previously acquired memories. Moreover, sleep permits the repeated reactivation, in an off-line mode, of the neural circuits originally activated during the memorable experience. Studies using multielectrode recordings in animals and PET/functional magnetic resonance imaging (fMRI) in humans have shown that brain areas or cells activated during waking are preferentially reactivated during subsequent sleep. A further advantage of sleep is that the relevant neural circuits can be reactivated in a spaced and interleaved fashion. This would favor the integration of new with old memories and would avoid catastrophic interference. The intense, high-frequency bursts of spontaneous neural activity that occur during sleep may be particularly important for triggering molecular mechanisms of synaptic consolidation and to enlarge the network of associations.

Many unknowns remain, however. Whether sleep may favor the consolidation of newly established memories or the maintenance of older ones is not clear. The molecular correlates of such processes are still unclear. Molecular markers of memory acquisition are turned off during sleep, which may be advantageous given that the intense neural activity of sleep occurs while the animal is disconnected from the environment. Also, much of the early literature connecting sleep and memory was concerned with REM sleep. However, prolonged inhibition of REM sleep in humans through certain antidepressants does not seem to disrupt memory, nor does the complete disappearance of REM sleep after certain brain-stem lesions.

REM Sleep After Certain Brain-Stem Lesions

Sleep and brain restitution

When we have been awake too long we say we are tired, and after sleep we feel refreshed. Not surprisingly, the most intuitively compelling idea about the function of sleep is that sleep may restore some precious fuel or energy charge that was depleted during wakefulness. It is likely that sleep may indeed reduce energy waste by enforcing body rest in animals with high metabolic rates (this is certainly what hibernation does by drastically reducing body and brain metabolism, shutting off brain activity, and reducing temperature). However, in humans the metabolic savings of spending the night asleep rather than quietly awake are no more than a slice of bread (Horne, 1980). Moreover, we also say we are tired after muscle exertions, yet most bodily organs can recover through quiet wakefulness and do not need sleep. The notable exception is the brain: if we do not sleep, even though we may remain immobile, we rapidly suffer cognitive impairment. Therefore, most researchers agree that sleep may be especially important for restoring the brain and provide something not afforded by quiet waking. However, there is great uncertainty when it comes to which chemical or molecular pathway in the brain may be wasted during waking and restored during sleep. For example, it has been suggested that sleep may favor the replenishment of glycogen in glial stores (Benington and Heller, 1995), although recent evidence shows that this may only be true in a few brain regions (Gip et al., 2002; Franken et al., 2003, 2006). The molecular changes that take place between wakefulness and sleep suggest other possibilities as well (Cirelli et al., 2004): sleep could counteract synaptic fatigue by favoring the replenishment of calcium in presynaptic stores, the replenishment of glutamate vesicles, the resting of mitochondria, the synthesis of proteins, or the trafficking and recycling of membranes. Unfortunately, most of these possibilities remain unexplored.

Sleep and Synaptic Homeostasis

Memory consolidation and brain restitution are important perspectives on the function of sleep that are not mutually exclusive. A recent hypothesis reconciles these two perspectives by proposing that the main function of sleep is to control the strength of synapses impinging on neurons in the cortex and elsewhere (Tononi and Cirelli, 2003, 2006). This hypothesis effectively proposes a role for sleep in brain restitution—synaptic strength would increase during wakefulness and return to baseline during sleep. At the same time, the hypothesis claims that sleep is the price we pay because our brains are plastic and is thus related in an important manner to memory.

The hypothesis focuses mostly on NREM sleep, but REM sleep may fulfill a similar role with different mechanisms. The hypothesis says, first, that wakefulness is associated with synaptic potentiation in several cortical circuits (as we have seen, genes involved in synaptic potentiation are indeed unregulated during wakefulness). Although this remarkable plasticity is a good thing, reflecting our ability to learn and adapt, it comes at a cost. Synaptic activity is where the brain spends up to 70% of its energy, and increased synaptic strength means increased energy consumption just to keep the brain running (even if we merely sit and do nothing). Increased synaptic strength also means increased housekeeping and space needs. Neural cells have enormous dendritic trees literally covered with synapses, whose maintenance must burden membrane trafficking mechanisms. Moreover, there is very little room inside the brain for adding new synapses or making them bigger. In short, the brain is prone to synaptic overload, and it should have some homeostatic mechanism to save on energy, space, and supplies, and to prevent the saturation of its plastic abilities.

This is where sleep comes into the picture. As we have seen, the increased amplitude of slow waves after periods of wakefulness is a reliable marker of sleep pressure, although we do not know for sure why. According to the hypothesis, the reason is that, when we fall asleep, the increased strength of cortico-cortical synapses increases synchronization and thus boosts the amplitude of slow waves. More important, the hypothesis says that slow waves may also have a job to do: they cause the proportional reduction in the strength of all synapses impinging on a neuron. This would occur because intense neuronal firing during the up-state, followed by profound hyperpolarization during the down-state, is an ideal stimulus for triggering generalized synaptic depression, also known as *downscaling*. Thus, slow oscillations would progressively bring the total synaptic strength down to a baseline value. This in turn would explain the progressive reduction of slow waves amplitude during sleep. Direct evidence for net synaptic potentiation during waking and net synaptic depression during sleep has recently been obtained in rats (Vyazovskiy et al., 2008).

Given what was said before, it is not difficult to see how such a mechanism for regulating total synaptic strength—that is, for maintaining synaptic homeostasis—would serve an essential function: synaptic downscaling during sleep would make sure synapses strengthened by waking do not burn too much energy, overcrowd the little space that is available, or saturate our ability to learn further. As an added benefit, downscaling could benefit memory processes by cleaning out weaker synapses, and thereby improving performance. A growing body of molecular, electrophysiological, and behavioral evidence supports this hypothesis (Huber et al., 2004; Huber et al., 2006; Huber et al., 2007), but there are alternative explanations, and critical tests still need to be performed.

Sleep and Brain Development

The ideas discussed above are usually framed in terms of adult sleep. However, we have seen that sleep is especially abundant early in development, before birth and during the first year or two. This is a time of intense synaptogenesis as well as remodeling of connections—synaptic density in the cerebral cortex grows exuberantly during the first year of life and then decreases, most prominently during adolescence and then more slowly throughout life. Intriguingly, sleep slow-wave activity exhibits a very similar profile, suggesting once again a tight relationship between synapses and sleep need. Indeed, some experimental evidence supports the notion that sleep early in life is important for brain plasticity. For example, recent experiments have demonstrated a role for NREM sleep for the activity-dependent development of visual system circuits. During a critical period of brain development, occluding the vision of one eye causes a rapid remodeling of the visual cortex and its inputs. It was found that sleep enhances the effects of a preceding period of monocular deprivation on visual cortical responses, but wakefulness in complete darkness does not (Frank et al., 2001). The preponderance of REM sleep early in life, and its strong association with immaturity at birth across and within species, suggests that this sleep stage may be especially important for brain maturation. Indeed, REM sleep deprivation alters lateral geniculate reorganization and recovery after release of monocular occlusion (Marks et al., 1995).

SUMMARY

Sleep is characterized behaviorally by immobility and a reduced responsiveness to environmental stimuli that is rapidly reversible. The EEG, EMG, and EOG reveal distinct stages: a transitional stage 1; stage 2 (EEG spindles), stages 3–4 of NREM sleep (slow waves), and REM sleep (rapid eye movements with wake-like, activated EEG). There are 4–5 NREM–REM cycles every night. The transitions from wakefulness to sleep and between sleep stages are coordinated by a set of subcortical centers that are neurochemically heterogeneous. Broadly speaking, the reticular activating system in the posterior hypothalamus and upper brain-stem sustains brain activation through the release of neuromodulators such as acetylcholine, glutamate, and histamine; the anterior hypothalamus coordinates sleep; the upper pons triggers REM sleep; and the suprachiasmatic nucleus is responsible for the circadian modulation of sleep propensity.

Various aspects of brain activity change during sleep, as shown by molecular, unit recordings, and imaging studies, but the brain by no means shuts off. For example, average firing rates in the cerebral cortex are similar to those of quiet wakefulness. However, during NREM sleep cortical cells undergo a characteristic slow oscillation: up to once a second, their membrane potential becomes hyperpolarized and all synaptic activity ceases for a few hundreds of milliseconds. When depolarization returns, it is often accompanied by sleep spindles—faster oscillations generated by interactions between the reticular thalamic nucleus and the thalamus proper. During NREM sleep, metabolism in prefrontal and associative areas is reduced, and the brain is relatively disconnected from the environment, due in part to a breakdown of effective connectivity among cortical regions. During REM sleep, prefrontal areas are still deactivated, but there is a strong activation of limbic circuits. The interruption of serotonin release during REM sleep may contribute to the persisting disconnection from the environment.

Sleep represents a striking modification of consciousness, which fades early in the night and returns to be vivid later on in the form of dreams. A number of NREM awakenings, especially early in the night, yield little conscious recall. However, more often than not, NREM awakenings result in meaningful reports, and in the later part of the night subjects may report full-fledged dreams. Awakenings from REM sleep almost always produce long and vivid dreams. Dreams are usually highly visual, in full color, but do not lack sound, touch, smell and taste, pleasure and pain. Just as in wakefulness, we experience objects, animals, people, faces, places, and so on. We can also have all sorts of thoughts and emotions, especially fear and anxiety. Thus, the dreaming brain is disconnected from the external world, yet it can generate a virtual, imagined world that is fairly similar to the real one. There are, however, some telltale signs of dreaming, including the fading of voluntary control, attention and reflective thought, and an impairment of working memory and episodic memory. By contrast, dreams rely on a network of associations that is less constrained than in waking life.

The periodic and obligatory alteration of consciousness that is forced upon us by sleep is likely to serve an essential function, but what this function might be remains an open issue. Sleep is potentially dangerous, yet it occupies a large fraction of our lives, it is universal in the animal kingdom, and lack of sleep is followed by increasing sleep pressure and cognitive impairment. Various ideas have been put forth, including a role in memory consolidation, in brain restitution, and in brain development. Finally, an intriguing hypothesis is that sleep may be the price we pay for synaptic plasticity during wakefulness.

REFERENCES

Arendt, J. (2005) Melatonin: characteristics, concerns, and prospects. *J. Biol. Rhythms* 20:291–303.

Aserinsky, E., and Kleitman, N. (1953) Regularly occurring periods of eye motility, and concomitant phenomena, during sleep. *Science* 118:273–274.

Aston-Jones, G. (2005) Brain structures and receptors involved in alertness. *Sleep Med.* 6(Suppl 1):S3–S7.

Aston-Jones, G., and Bloom, F.E. (1981a) Activity of norepinephrine-containing locus coeruleus neurons in behaving rats anticipates fluctuations in the sleep-waking cycle. *J. Neurosci.* 1:876–886.

Aston-Jones, G., and Bloom, F.E. (1981b) Nonrepinephrine-containing locus coeruleus neurons in behaving rats exhibit pronounced responses to non-noxious environmental stimuli. *J. Neurosci.* 1: 887–900.

Aston-Jones, G., and Cohen, J.D. (2005) An integrative theory of locus coeruleus-norepinephrine function: adaptive gain and optimal performance. *Annu. Rev. Neurosci.* 28:403–450.

Barbier, A.J., and Bradbury, M.J. (2007) Histaminergic control of sleep-wake cycles: recent therapeutic advances for sleep and wake disorders. *CNS Neurol. Disord. Drug Targets* 6:31–43.

Barger, L.K., Ayas, N.T., Cade, B.E., Cronin, J.W., Rosner, B., Speizer, F.E., and Czeisler, C.A. (2006) Impact of extended-duration shifts on medical errors, adverse events, and attentional failures. *PLoS Med.* 3:e487.

Basheer, R., Strecker, R.E., Thakkar, M.M., and McCarley, R.W. (2004) Adenosine and sleep-wake regulation. *Prog. Neurobiol.* 73:379–396.

Benington, J.H., and Heller, H.C. (1995) Restoration of brain energy metabolism as the function of sleep. *Prog. Neurobiol.* 45:347–360.

Bergmann, B.M., Mistlberger, R.E., and Rechtschaffen, A. (1987) Period-amplitude analysis of rat electroencephalogram: stage and diurnal variations and effects of suprachiasmatic nuclei lesions. *Sleep* 10:523–536.

Berridge, C.W., and Abercrombie, E.D. (1999) Relationship between locus coeruleus discharge rates and rates of norepinephrine release within neocortex as assessed by in vivo microdialysis. *Neurosci.* 93:1263–1270.

Berridge, C.W., and Espana, R.A. (2000) Synergistic sedative effects of noradrenergic alpha(1)- and beta-receptor blockade on forebrain electroencephalographic and behavioral indices. *Neurosci.* 99:495–505.

Berridge, C.W., and Foote, S.L. (1991) Effects of locus coeruleus activation on electroencephalographic activity in neocortex and hippocampus. *J. Neurosci.* 11:3135–3145.

Berridge, C.W., and Waterhouse, B.D. (2003) The locus coeruleus-noradrenergic system: modulation of behavioral state and state-dependent cognitive processes. *Brain Res. Brain Res. Rev.* 42: 33–84.

Blanco-Centurion, C., Xu, M., Murillo-Rodriguez, E., Gerashchenko, D., Shiromani, A.M., Salin-Pascual, R.J., Hof, P.R., and Shiromani,

P.J. (2006) Adenosine and sleep homeostasis in the basal forebrain. *J. Neurosci.* 26:8092–8100.

Bonnet, M.H., and Arand, D.L. (2003) Clinical effects of sleep fragmentation versus sleep deprivation. *Sleep Med. Rev.* 7:297–310.

Born, J., Rasch, B., and Gais, S. (2006) Sleep to remember. *Neuroscientist* 12:410–424.

Braun, A.R., Balkin, T.J., Wesenten, N.J., Carson, R.E., Varga, M., Baldwin, P., Selbie, S., Belenky, G., and Herscovitch, P. (1997) Regional cerebral blood flow throughout the sleep-wake cycle. An H2(15)O PET study. *Brain* 120(Pt 7):1173–1197.

Brown, R.E., Stevens, D.R., and Haas, H.L. (2001) The physiology of brain histamine. *Prog. Neurobiol.* 63:637–672.

Cape, E.G., and Jones, B.E. (1998) Differential modulation of high-frequency gamma-electroencephalogram activity and sleep-wake state by noradrenaline and serotonin microinjections into the region of cholinergic basalis neurons. *J. Neurosci.* 18:2653–2666.

Carskadon, M.A., Acebo, C., and Jenni, O.G. (2004) Regulation of adolescent sleep: implications for behavior. *Ann. N. Y. Acad. Sci.* 1021:276–291.

Carskadon, M.A., Harvey, K., Duke, P., Anders, T.F., Litt, I.F., and Dement, W.C. (2002) Pubertal changes in daytime sleepiness. 1980. *Sleep* 25:453–460.

Chase, M.H., and Morales, F.R. (1990) The atonia and myoclonia of active (REM) sleep. *Annu. Rev. Psychol.* 41:557–584.

Cirelli, C., Gutierrez, C.M., and Tononi, G. (2004) Extensive and divergent effects of sleep and wakefulness on brain gene expression. *Neuron* 41:35–43.

Cirelli, C., Pompeiano, M., and Tononi, G. (1996) Neuronal gene expression in the waking state: a role for the locus coeruleus. *Science* 274:1211–1215.

Cirelli, C., and Tononi, G. (2000) Differential expression of plasticity-related genes in waking and sleep and their regulation by the noradrenergic system. *J. Neurosci.* 20:9187–9194.

Dauvilliers, Y., Arnulf, I., and Mignot, E. (2007) Narcolepsy with cataplexy. *Lancet* 369:499–511.

Deboer, T., Detari, L., and Meijer, J.H. (2007) Long term effects of sleep deprivation on the mammalian circadian pacemaker. *Sleep* 30:257–262.

Dierks, T., Frolich, L., Ihl, R., and Maurer, K. (1995) Correlation between cognitive brain function and electrical brain activity in dementia of Alzheimer type. *J. Neural Transm. Gen. Sect.* 99: 55–62.

Dinges, D.F. (2006) The state of sleep deprivation: From functional biology to functional consequences. *Sleep Med. Rev.* 10:303–305.

Domino, E.F., Yamamoto, K.I., Dren, A.T. (1968) Role of cholinergic mechanisms in states of wakefulness and sleep. *Progr. Brain Res.* 28:113–133.

Doran, S.M., Van Dongen, H.P., and Dinges, D.F. (2001) Sustained attention performance during sleep deprivation: evidence of state instability. *Arch. Ital. Biol.* 139:253–267.

el Mansari, M., Sakai, K., and Jouvet, M. (1989) Unitary characteristics of presumptive cholinergic tegmental neurons during the sleep-waking cycle in freely moving cats. *Exp. Brain Res.* 76: 519–529.

Foote, S.L., Aston-Jones, G., and Bloom, F.E. (1980) Impulse activity of locus coeruleus neurons in awake rats and monkeys is a function of sensory stimulation and arousal. *Proc. Natl. Acad. Sci. USA* 77:3033–3037.

Frank, M.G., Issa, N.P., and Stryker, M.P. (2001) Sleep enhances plasticity in the developing visual cortex. *Neuron.* 30(1):275–287.

Franken, P., Gip, P., Hagiwara, G., Ruby, N.F., and Heller, H.C. (2003) Changes in brain glycogen after sleep deprivation vary with genotype. *Am. J. Physiol. Regul. Integr. Comp. Physiol.* 285:R413–R419.

Franken, P., Gip, P., Hagiwara, G., Ruby, N.F., and Heller, H.C. (2006) Glycogen content in the cerebral cortex increases with sleep loss in C57BL/6J mice. *Neurosci. Lett.* 402:176–179.

Gillin, J.C., Lardon, M., Ruiz, C., Golshan, S., and Salin-Pascual, R. (1994) Dose-dependent effects of transdermal nicotine on early morning awakening and rapid eye movement sleep time in non-smoking normal volunteers. *J. Clin. Psychopharmacol.* 14:264–267.

Gip, P., Hagiwara, G., Ruby, N.F., and Heller, H.C. (2002) Sleep deprivation decreases glycogen in the cerebellum but not in the cortex of young rats. *Am. J. Physiol. Regul. Integr. Comp. Physiol.* 283:R54–R59.

Hobson, J.A., and Pace-Schott, E.F. (2002) The cognitive neuroscience of sleep: neuronal systems, consciousness and learning. *Nat. Rev. Neurosci.* 3:679–693.

Hobson, J.A., Pace-Schott, E.F., and Stickgold, R. (2000) Dreaming and the brain: toward a cognitive neuroscience of conscious states. *Behav. Brain Sci.* 23:793–842; discussion 904–1121.

Horne, J.A. (1980) Sleep and body restitution. *Experientia* 36:11–13.

Huang, Z.L., Urade, Y., and Hayaishi, O. (2007) Prostaglandins and adenosine in the regulation of sleep and wakefulness. *Curr. Opin. Pharmacol.* 7:33–38.

Huber, R., Ghilardi, M.F., Massimini, M., Ferrarelli, F., Riedner, B.A., Peterson, M.J., and Tononi, G. (2006) Arm immobilization causes cortical plastic changes and locally decreases sleep slow wave activity. *Nat. Neurosci.* 9:1169–1176.

Huber, R., Ghilardi, M.F., Massimini, M., and Tononi, G. (2004) Local sleep and learning. *Nature* 430:78–81.

Huber, R., Tononi, G., and Cirelli, C. (2007) Exploratory behavior, cortical BDNF expression, and sleep homeostasis. *Sleep* 30:129–139.

Itil, T., and Fink, M. (1968) EEG and behavioral aspects of the interaction of anticholinergic hallucinogens with centrally active compounds. *Prog. Brain Res.* 28:149–168.

Jacobs, B.L., Martin-Cora, F.J., and Fornal, C.A. (2002) Activity of medullary serotonergic neurons in freely moving animals. *Brain Res. Brain Res. Rev.* 40:45–52.

Jenni, O.G., Borbely, A.A., and Achermann, P. (2004) Development of the nocturnal sleep electroencephalogram in human infants. *Am. J. Physiol. Regul. Integr. Comp. Physiol.* 286:R528–R538.

Jenni, O.G., and Carskadon, M.A. (2004) Spectral analysis of the sleep electroencephalogram during adolescence. *Sleep* 27:774–783.

Jones, B.E. (2003) Arousal systems. *Front. Biosci.* 8:s438–s451.

Jones, B.E. (2005a) Basic mechanisms of sleep-wake states. In: Kryger, M.H., Roth, T., Dement, W.C., eds. *Principles and Practice of Sleep Medicine*, 4th ed. Philadelphia: Elsevier Saunders, pp. 136–153.

Jones, B.E. (2005b) From waking to sleeping: neuronal and chemical substrates. *Trends Pharmacol. Sci.* 26:578–586.

Jouvet, M. (1962) [Research on the neural structures and responsible mechanisms in different phases of physiological sleep.]. *Arch. Ital. Biol.* 100:125–206.

Jouvet, M. (1965) Paradoxical sleep–a study of its nature and mechanisms. *Prog. Brain Res.* 18:20–62.

Jouvet, M. (1994) Paradoxical sleep mechanisms. *Sleep* 17:S77–S83.

Jouvet, M. (1998) Paradoxical sleep as a programming system. *J. Sleep Res.* 7(Suppl 1):1–5.

Jouvet, M. (1999) Sleep and serotonin: an unfinished story. *Neuropsychopharmacol.* 21:24S–27S.

Jung, R., and Berger, W. (1979) [Fiftieth anniversary of Hans Berger's publication of the electroencephalogram. His first records in 1924–1931 (author's transl)]. *Arch. Psychiatr. Nervenkr.* 227:279–300.

Kilduff, T.S., Peyron, C. (2000) The hypocretin/orexin ligand-receptor system: implications for sleep and sleep disorders. *Trends Neurosci.* 23:359–365.

Krueger, J.M., Obal, F.J., Fang, J., Kubota, T., and Taishi, P. (2001) The role of cytokines in physiological sleep regulation. *Ann. N. Y. Acad. Sci.* 933:211–221.

Lai, Y.Y., and Siegel, J.M. (1988) Medullary regions mediating atonia. *J. Neurosci.* 8:4790–4796.

Lee, M.G., Hassani, O.K., Alonso, A., and Jones, B.E. (2005) Cholinergic basal forebrain neurons burst with theta during waking and paradoxical sleep. *J. Neurosci.* 25:4365–4369.

Lee, M.G., Hassani, O.K., and Jones, B.E. (2005) Discharge of identified orexin/hypocretin neurons across the sleep-waking cycle. *J. Neurosci.* 25:6716–6720.

Lin, J.S., Hou, Y., Sakai, K., and Jouvet, M. (1996) Histaminergic descending inputs to the mesopontine tegmentum and their role in the control of cortical activation and wakefulness in the cat. *J. Neurosci.* 16:1523–1537.

Lin, J.S., Sakai, K., Vanni-Mercier, G., and Jouvet, M. (1989) A critical role of the posterior hypothalamus in the mechanisms of wakefulness determined by microinjection of muscimol in freely moving cats. *Brain Res.* 479:225–240.

Lindsley, D.B., Bowden, J.W., and Magoun, H.W. (1949) Effect upon the EEG of acute injury to the brainstem activating system. *EEG Clin. Neurophysiol.* 1:475–486.

Llinas, R.R., and Pare, D. (1991) Of dreaming and wakefulness. *Neurosci.* 44:521–535.

Maquet, P., Degueldre, C., Delfiore, G., Aerts, J., Péters, J.M., Luxen, A., and Franck, G. (1997) Functional neuroanatomy of human slow wave sleep. *J. Neurosci.* 17:2807–2812.

Marks, G.A., Shaffery, J.P., Oksenberg, A., Speciale, S.G., and Roffwarg, H.P. (1995) A functional role for REM sleep in brain maturation. *Behav. Brain Res.* 69(1/2):1–11.

Massimini, M., Ferrarelli, F., Huber, R., Esser, S.K., Singh, H., and Tononi, G. (2005) Breakdown of cortical effective connectivity during sleep. *Science* 309:2228–2232.

Massimini, M., Huber, R., Ferrarelli, F., Hill, S., and Tononi, G. (2004) The sleep slow oscillation as a traveling wave. *J. Neurosci.* 24:6862–6870.

McCarley, R.W. (2004) Mechanisms and models of REM sleep control. *Arch. Ital. Biol.* 142:429–467.

McCormick, D.A. (1989) Cholinergic and noradrenergic modulation of thalamocortical processing. *Trends Neurosci.* 12:215–221.

McGinty, D., Gong, H., Suntsova, N., Alam, M.N., Methippara, M., Guzman-Marin, R., and Szymusiak, R. (2004) Sleep-promoting functions of the hypothalamic median preoptic nucleus: inhibition of arousal systems. *Arch. Ital. Biol.* 142:501–509.

McGinty, D.J., and Harper, R.M. (1976) Dorsal raphe neurons: depression of firing during sleep in cats. *Brain Res.* 101:569–575.

McGinty, D., and Szymusiak, R. (2003) Hypothalamic regulation of sleep and arousal. *Front. Biosci.* 8:s1074–s1083.

Metherate, R., Cox, C.L., and Ashe, J.H. (1992) Cellular bases of neocortical activation: modulation of neural oscillations by the nucleus basalis and endogenous acetylcholine. *J. Neurosci.* 12: 4701–4711.

Mileykovskiy, B.Y., Kiyashchenko, L.I., and Siegel, J.M. (2005) Behavioral correlates of activity in identified hypocretin/orexin neurons. *Neuron* 46:787–798.

Mistlberger, R.E. (2005) Circadian regulation of sleep in mammals: role of the suprachiasmatic nucleus. *Brain Res. Rev.* 49:429–454.

Mistlberger, R.E., Bergmann, B.M., Waldenar, W., and Rechtschaffen, A. (1983) Recovery sleep following sleep deprivation in intact and suprachiasmatic nuclei-lesioned rats. *Sleep* 6:217–233.

Monti, J.M., and Monti, D. (2007) The involvement of dopamine in the modulation of sleep and waking. *Sleep Med. Rev.* 11:113–133.

Montplaisir, J., Petit, D., Gauthier, S., Gaudreau, H., and Decary, A. (1998) Sleep disturbances and EEG slowing in Alzheimer's disease. *Sleep Res. Online* 1:147–151.

Moruzzi, G., and Magoun, H.W. (1949) Brain stem reticular formation and activation of the EEG. *EEG Clin. Neurophysiol.* 1: 455–473.

National Sleep Foundation. (2002) *Sleep in America Poll.* Available at http://www.sleepfoundation.org.

Ohayon, M.M., Carskadon, M.A., Guilleminault, C., and Vitiello, M.V. (2004) Meta-analysis of quantitative sleep parameters from childhood to old age in healthy individuals: developing normative sleep values across the human lifespan. *Sleep* 27: 1255–1273.

Peirano, P., Algarin, C., and Uauy, R. (2003) Sleep-wake states and their regulatory mechanisms throughout early human development. *J. Pediatr.* 143:S70–S79.

Porkka-Heiskanen, T., Alanko, L., Kalinchuk, A., and Stenberg, D. (2002) Adenosine and sleep. *Sleep Med. Rev.* 6:321–332.

Porkka-Heiskanen, T., Strecker, R.E., Thakkar, M., Bjorkum, A.A., Greene, R.W., and McCarley, R.W. (1997) Adenosine: a mediator of the sleep-inducing effects of prolonged wakefulness. *Science* 276:1265–1268.

Portas, C.M., Krakow, K., Allen, P., Josephs, O., Armony, J.L., and Frith, C.D. (2000) Auditory processing across the sleep-wake cycle: simultaneous EEG and fMRI monitoring in humans. *Neuron* 28:991–999.

Prinz, P.N., Peskind, E.R., Vitaliano, P.P., Raskind, M.A., Eisdorfer, C., Zemcuznikov, N., and Gerber, C.J. (1982) Changes in the sleep and waking EEGs of nondemented and demented elderly subjects. *J. Am. Geriatr. Soc.* 30:86–93.

Radun, I., and Summala, H. (2004) Sleep-related fatal vehicle accidents: characteristics of decisions made by multidisciplinary investigation teams. *Sleep* 27:224–227.

Richardson, G.S. (2005) The human circadian system in normal and disordered sleep. *J. Clin. Psychiatry* 66(Suppl 9):3–9; quiz 42–43.

Sakurai, T. (2007) The neural circuit of orexin (hypocretin): maintaining sleep and wakefulness. *Nat. Rev. Neurosci.* 8:171–181.

Saper, C.B., Lu, J., Chou, T.C., and Gooley, J. (2005) The hypothalamic integrator for circadian rhythms. *Trends Neurosci.* 28:152–157.

Saper, C.B., Scammell, T.E., and Lu, J. (2005) Hypothalamic regulation of sleep and circadian rhythms. *Nature* 437:1257–1263.

Sherin, J.E., Shiromani, P.J., McCarley, R.W., and Saper, C.B. (1996) Activation of ventrolateral preoptic neurons during sleep. *Science* 271:216–219.

Siegel, J.M. (2001) The REM sleep-memory consolidation hypothesis. *Science* 294:1058–1063.

Siegel, J.M. (2005) REM sleep. In: Kryger, M.H., Roth, T., and Dement, W.C., eds. *Principles and Practice of Sleep Medicine*, 4th ed. Philadelphia: Elsevier Saunders, pp. 120–135.

Soininen, H., Reinikainen, K.J., Partanen, J., Helkala, E.L., Paljarvi, L., and Riekkinen, P.J. (1992) Slowing of electroencephalogram and choline acetyltransferase activity in post mortem frontal cortex in definite Alzheimer's disease. *Neurosci.* 49:529–535.

Steriade, M. (2003) The corticothalamic system in sleep. *Front. Biosci.* 8:D878–D899.

Steriade, M. (2004) Acetylcholine systems and rhythmic activities during the waking–sleep cycle. *Prog. Brain Res.* 145:179–196.

Steriade, M., Timofeev, I., and Grenier, F. (2001) Natural waking and sleep states: a view from inside neocortical neurons. *J. Neurophysiol.* 85:1969–1985.

Stickgold, R., and Walker, M.P. (2005a) Memory consolidation and reconsolidation: what is the role of sleep? *Trends Neurosci.* 28: 408–415.

Stickgold, R., and Walker, M.P. (2005b) Sleep and memory: the ongoing debate. *Sleep* 28:1225–1227.

Suntsova, N., Szymusiak, R., Alam, M.N., Guzman-Marin, R., and McGinty, D. (2002) Sleep-waking discharge patterns of median preoptic nucleus neurons in rats. *J. Physiol.* 543:665–677.

Szymusiak, R., Alam, N., Steininger, T.L., and McGinty, D. (1998) Sleep-waking discharge patterns of ventrolateral preoptic/anterior hypothalamic neurons in rats. *Brain Res.* 803:178–188.

Szymusiak, R., Steininger, T., Alam, N., and McGinty, D. (2001) Preoptic area sleep-regulating mechanisms. *Arch. Ital. Biol.* 139: 77–92.

Takahashi, K., Lin, J.S., and Sakai, K. (2006) Neuronal activity of histaminergic tuberomammillary neurons during wake-sleep states in the mouse. *J. Neurosci.* 26:10292–10298.

Tobler, I., Borbely, A.A., and Groos, G. (1983) The effect of sleep deprivation on sleep in rats with suprachiasmatic lesions. *Neurosci. Lett.* 42:49–54.

Tononi, G., and Cirelli, C. (2003) Sleep and synaptic homeostasis: a hypothesis. *Brain Res. Bull.* 62:143–150.

Tononi, G., and Cirelli, C. (2006) Sleep function and synaptic homeostasis. *Sleep Med. Rev.* 10:49–62.

Vertes, R.P., and Siegel, J.M. (2005) Time for the sleep community to take a critical look at the purported role of sleep in memory processing. *Sleep* 28:1228–1229; discussion 1230–1233.

von Economo C. (1931) *Encephalitis lethargica. Its sequelae and treatment.* Transl: Newman, K.O. London: Oxford University Press.

Vyazovskiy, V.V., Cirelli, C., Pfister-Genskow, M., Faraguna, U., and Tononi, G. (2008) Molecular and electrophysiological evidence for net synaptic potentiation in wake and depression in sleep. *Nat. Neurosci.* 11:200–208.

Walker, M.P., and Stickgold, R. (2006) Sleep, memory, and plasticity. *Annu. Rev. Psychol.* 57:139–166.

Zee, P.C., and Manthena, P. (2007) The brain's master circadian clock: implications and opportunities for therapy of sleep disorders. *Sleep Med. Rev.* 11:59–70.

Zeitzer, J.M., Morales-Villagran, A., Maidment, N.T., Behnke, E.J., Ackerson, L.C., Lopez-Rodriguez, F., Fried, I., Engel, J., Jr., and Wilson, C.L. (2006) Extracellular adenosine in the human brain during sleep and sleep deprivation: an in vivo microdialysis study. *Sleep* 29:455–461.

86 The Neurobiology of Resilience

MARGARET HAGLUND, PAUL NESTADT, NICOLE S. COOPER, STEVEN SOUTHWICK, AND DENNIS S. CHARNEY

Resilience is the successful adaptation to severe or chronic stress. Resilient individuals are those who are able to maintain or rapidly regain psychological well-being in the face of extreme stress or trauma exposure. Historically, most research on the effects of severe stress focused on its deleterious effects on well-being. More recently, there has been a great deal of interest in understanding the phenomenon of resilience to stress, and in delineating the neurobiological and psychological profile of resilient individuals. Identifying the factors that set resilient individuals apart from those who are vulnerable to the effects of stress has clinical significance: understanding the neurobiology and psychology of resilience enables researchers and clinicians to develop new therapies for the prevention and treatment of stress-induced psychopathology in nonresilient individuals. Furthermore, motivated individuals can draw from our increasing understanding of the features of resilience to achieve greater personal resilience to stress.

This chapter outlines the current understanding of resilience, from genetic, developmental, psychological, and neurobiological perspectives, and presents promising new therapies for the promotion of resilience to stress.

PREVALENCE OF RESILIENCE

Measuring the prevalence of resilience is inherently difficult because the demonstration of resilience requires surviving severe stress or trauma, which not all individuals experience. Additionally, resilient individuals do not tend to present to physicians. Nevertheless, one can deduce from the low prevalence of posttraumatic stress disorder (PTSD) that resilience is relatively common. The majority of individuals are exposed to trauma during their lifetime: in the United States, lifetime risk of at least one significant traumatic event, such as sudden unexpected death of a loved one, injury in a motor vehicle accident, or experiencing assault, is estimated at 80%–90% (Breslau et al., 1998; Bruce et al., 2001). In contrast, the estimated lifetime prevalence of PTSD is only 8%, and the conditional probability of PTSD after exposure to trauma is only slightly higher, at an estimated 9% (Breslau et al., 1998; Kessler et al., 1995). Certain types of trauma are significantly more likely to cause PTSD, particularly rape (65.0%) and combat exposure (38.8%) for men, and rape (45.9%) and physical abuse (48.5%) for women (Kessler et al., 1995). In general, traumatic events that are severe and unpredictable, intentionally caused by other human beings, and result in loss (of a loved one, property, or physical integrity) are most likely to lead to PTSD (Jordan et al., 1991; Yehuda, 2004). Of note, even in the most severe traumas such as rape and combat, it is estimated that at least 35% of survivors do not go on to develop PTSD. Therefore, it seems likely at least one third of individuals are resilient to the effects of extreme stress.

GENETICS OF RESILIENCE

Scientists are beginning to untangle the genetic contributors of resilience and in some cases have identified specific alleles affecting response to stress. It has long been suspected that anxiety and panic disorders are at least partially heritable. Studies of combat-exposed men enrolled in the Vietnam Twin Registry have found that PTSD, panic disorder, and general anxiety disorder, frequently comorbid conditions, all have significant genetic contributions. It is estimated that up to 40% of the variance in occurrence of these disorders is accounted for by genetic factors, rather than by situation or trauma-related factors (True et al., 1993; Scherrer et al., 2000; Chantarujikapong et al., 2001). At least one chromosomal area that may be involved in the susceptibility to these anxiety and panic disorders has been identified: the q31-34 area of chromosome 4 has been linked to the presence of panic disorders (Kaabi et al., 2006). Interestingly, this same chromosomal area contains the gene for a neuropeptide Y (NPY) receptor. Neuropeptide Y is a peptide released during stress that appears to mitigate the negative effects of the stress response (discussed in more detail later in the chapter). Presumably, variations in NPY receptors affect an individual's ability to adapt to stress; more research is needed to determine which alleles confer resistance to stress, and which are associated with increased susceptibility to stress-induced psychopathology.

The regulation of cortisol, a key hormone involved in adaptation to stress, is affected by genetic factors. Functional polymorphisms of the glucocorticoid receptor (GR) have been identified: at least two of these variants, n363s and bc11, may increase response to cortisol. Certain individuals therefore have a genetic predisposition to be hypersensitive to the effects of stress (DeRijk et al., 2006).

Genetic variations in the serotonergic system also appear to affect susceptibility to stress-induced psychopathology. The short allele of the serotonin (5-HT) transporter promoter gene (*5HTTLPR*), which compared to the long allele results in decreased transporter availability and lower uptake of 5-HT from synaptic clefts, has been implicated in a number of studies in a maladaptive response to stress. Individuals who are carriers for the short allele of *5HTTLPR* appear to have heightened activation of the amygdala and increased coupling between the amygdala and ventro-medial prefrontal cortex (PFC) while viewing fearful or aversive stimuli. Heightened activation of the amygdala and ventro-medial PFC has been previously associated with major depression (Hariri et al., 2002; Heinz et al., 2005). Carriers of the short allele of *5HTTLPR* also appear to be at increased risk for developing PTSD and stress-induced depression (H.J. Lee et al., 2005; Kim et al., 2007).

Genetic polymorphisms affecting resilience to stress have been identified in the noradrenergic system as well as in the serotonergic system. Functional polymorphisms in the gene that produces catechol-O-methyltransferase (*COMT*), an enzyme that degrades dopamine (DA) and norepinephrine (NE), have been identified and found to affect response to stress. Individuals with the low functioning *met* allele for the enzyme, and hence higher circulating levels of DA and NE, tend to exhibit more anxious behaviors and lower resilience against negative moods (Heinz and Smolka, 2006). They also tend to avoid novelty-seeking behaviors, and while viewing aversive images, show heightened activity in the visuospatial attention system as well as increased reactivity and connectivity in cortico-limbic circuits (Drabant et al., 2006), suggesting that they have a heightened awareness for potential threats (Smolka et al., 2005). Another group studying the *COMT* gene found that carriers of the low functioning *met* allele exhibited greater plasma endocrine and subjective stress responses in response to psychologically stressful tasks than did carriers of the high-functioning allele (Jabbi et al., 2007).

Polymorphisms in DA receptors and in the DA transporter gene have also been associated with vulnerability to depression and PTSD (Dunlop and Nemeroff, 2007). In a study of combat veterans for instance, the A1+ allele of the D_2 receptor was associated with more severe PTSD and higher levels of anxiety and depression (Lawford et al., 2006). Finally, a polymorphism in the gene for brain derived neurotrophic factor (BDNF), a widely expressed protein that stimulates neurogenesis and promotes learning and memory, has been linked with an increased likelihood of suffering stress-induced depression (Kim et al., 2007).

Additional genetic polymorphisms involved in resilience to stress are currently being identified; our understanding of the genetics of resilience is likely to increase rapidly in coming years. As more of the genetic factors underlying resilience are uncovered, it may become possible for scientists to design gene or drug therapies specific for individuals with low-resilience genetic profiles.

THE DEVELOPMENT OF RESILIENCE: ROLE OF EARLY LIFE ENVIRONMENT

In addition to genetic make-up, another key contributor to resilience is developmental environment. The study of resilience from a developmental perspective dates back to the early 1970s (Masten and Obradovic, 2006). An important discovery to emerge from this research is that resilience is common, even in children who suffered severe adversity in early life. Studies of adolescents whose development was stunted in childhood due to traumatic experiences such as being orphaned have found that the majority of children rapidly demonstrate "developmental catch-up" when placed in safe and nurturing environments (Masten, 2001). It seems that, under the right circumstances, neural circuits involved in resilience are modifiable for many years after birth, possibly even into adulthood.

Nevertheless, severely traumatic experiences in early life can negatively affect the development of stress response systems, in some cases doing long-lasting damage. Studies of rodents and nonhuman primates indicate that animals abused by their mothers during the first few weeks after birth have delayed independence and a decreased ability to manage stress later in life, demonstrated by high levels of behavioral anxiety, a hyperactive hypothalamic–pituitary–adrenal (HPA) axis, and increased basal levels of the anxiogenic corticotrophin releasing hormone (CRH) in the cerebrospinal fluid (Strome et al., 2002; Claes, 2004; McCormack et al., 2006). Furthermore, nonhuman primates who suffered damage to their stress response systems as a result of abuse in infancy seem more likely to mistreat their own infants, perpetuating the effects of abuse across generations (Maestripieri et al., 2007).

Studies of human survivors of early life stress and abuse have also found long-lasting alterations in central nervous system circuits and structures involved in psychological well-being. Severe prenatal stress and early childhood abuse have been linked to increased HPA axis activity later in life, putting survivors at risk for the adverse effects of chronic hypercortisolemia (Heim et al.,

2000; Vythilingam et al., 2002; Seckl and Meaney, 2006; Janssen et al., 2007). Developmental environment also influences the adult functioning of the locus coeruleus–norepinephrine (LC–NE) system, with severe stress in early life leading to its hyperfunctioning. For instance, one study found that police recruits with a history of childhood trauma had significantly higher levels of a salivary metabolite of NE in response to viewing aversive videos than did healthy controls (Otte, Neylan, Pole, et al., 2005). Other research has found that physical or sexual abuse in childhood can lead to smaller-than-average hippocampal volumes; decreased hippocampal volume is commonly seen in individuals with depression or chronic stress disorders (Janssen et al., 2007). Thus, it appears that early abuse can cause long-standing changes in brain structures and circuits associated with resilience.

There is, then, apparently conflicting evidence: though early life trauma can do lasting damage to stress response systems, survivors of childhood adversity frequently develop into resilient adults. One factor that can partly explain this apparent paradox is the degree to which a traumatic event is manageable by its survivor. Early exposure to unpredictable and uncontrollable traumas commonly leads to later psychopathology. In contrast, exposure to moderately stressful events which can be mastered to an extent (for example, family relocation, illness of a parent, or loss of a friendship) seems to enable children to effectively regulate their stress response systems. Children who have experience successfully coping with difficult situations reap benefits when faced with stressors later in life, experiencing less physiological and psychological distress (Boyce and Chesterman, 1990; Khoshaba and Maddi, 1999). It seems that the experience of mastering stress provides a form of immunity against later challenges. This phenomenon is known as *stress inoculation*, based on the analogy to vaccine-induced inoculation against disease (Rutter, 1993). Just as exposure to a low dose of a pathogen enables the body to mount a long-lasting immune response, exposure to moderate amounts of stress enables organisms to conquer and fight off future stressors.

Research on rodents and primates supports the stress inoculation hypothesis and provides insight into its neurobiological mechanisms. Young monkeys presented with a manageable stressor in the form of periodic short maternal separations experience acute distress during the separation periods, manifested by behavioral agitation and temporarily increased cortisol levels. Later in life, however, the same monkeys demonstrate lower anxiety (for example, increased exploratory behavior in novel environments) and lower basal stress hormone levels than monkeys who never underwent periods of maternal separation (Parker et al., 2004). Furthermore, these stress-inoculated monkeys demonstrate improved performance on tests of prefrontal-dependent cognition compared with their non-stress-inoculated peers (Parker et al., 2005). Poor control of prefrontal cognition has been associated with depression in humans (Murphy et al., 2001; Harvey et al., 2005).

Just as in humans, the degree of control that an animal has over a stressor plays a key role in determining whether the event will lead to subsequent vulnerability or resilience to stress. Animals administered unavoidable and unpredictable shocks tend to develop exaggerated fear responses, heightened anxiety states, and deficits in active coping when faced with subsequent stressors: this condition is known as *learned helplessness* (Overmier and Seligman, 1967). The phenomenon of learned helplessness is a well-known animal model for depression and is thought to lead to dysregulation of the serotonergic neurons in the dorsal raphé nuclei (Greenwood et al., 2003) as well as to reduce hippocampal cell proliferation. Because 5-HT has far-reaching effects in the limbic system, the dysregulations created by learned helplessness likely have serious negative effects on cognition and mood.

In contrast, animals that are administered shocks and given the ability to avoid them by modifying their behavior do not develop learned helplessness. Furthermore, animals that have at one time experienced behavioral control over predictable tail shocks are less likely than naïve animals to develop learned helplessness if they are subsequently exposed to unpredictable and inescapable shocks (Seligman and Maier, 1967). Similarly, human beings that have been "stress inoculated" to one type of stressor by successfully managing the stressor appear to acquire resilience to a broad range of other subsequent stressors (Masten and Obradovic, 2006).

The neural pathways responsible for stress inoculation are currently being elucidated. Rats that have learned behavioral control over a stressor show decreased activity of at least two brain areas normally involved in mediating response to fear, the medial PFC (MPFC) and the serotonergic neurons of the dorsal raphé nucleus (Amat et al., 2006). The pathways involved in mediating stress inoculation in humans have yet to be identified.

It is important to note that even among animals administered unpredictable and unavoidable shocks, not all develop learned helplessness. Similarly, in humans exposed to severe, unpredictable, and uncontrollable traumas, not all go on to develop PTSD or other anxiety or panic disorders. Clearly, genetic factors interact with environmental exposures to affect resilience. In some cases, a resilient genetic profile may be enough to overcome even the most adverse developmental circumstances.

In the following sections, we outline what current research holds to be some of the most important factors, psychological and neurobiological, characterizing resilience to extreme stress in the adult.

PSYCHOBIOLOGICAL FEATURES OF RESILIENCE

Traits and Behaviors

Dispositional optimism

Optimism has been repeatedly correlated with increased psychological well-being and health (Affleck and Tennen, 1996; Goldman et al., 1996) and with greater life satisfaction (Klohnen, 1996). An optimistic disposition is thought to be in large part inherited; however, motivated individuals can increase their optimism with practice. Optimists maintain positive emotions even in the face of adversity because they tend to view problems as temporary and limited in scope. Pessimists, on the other hand, tend to think of their problems as permanent and pervasive and consequently are more prone to depression (Table 86.1).

Positive emotions play an integral role in the capacity to tolerate stress. Positive affect is associated with health-protecting factors including greater social connectedness and adaptive coping mechanisms (Steptoe et al., 2005). Positive emotions also appear to decrease autonomic arousal (Isen et al., 1987; Folkman and Moskowitz, 2000) and as a result lead to better physical health. Positive affect has been associated with reduced use of medical services, fewer stress-related illnesses, decreased neuroendocrine, cardiovascular, and inflammatory reactivity (Scheier et al., 1989; Zeidner

TABLE 86.1 *Selected Psychological Resilience Factors: Attitudes and Behaviors that Can Help Maintain Well-Being During Stress*

1. Positive attitude and optimism
   - Optimism is strongly related to resilience
   - Optimism is in part inherited but can be learned through therapy
   - Putative neurobiological mechanisms: strengthens reward circuits, decreases autonomic activity
2. Cognitive reappraisal/reframing: finding meaning or value in adversity
   - Traumatic experiences can be reevaluated through a more positive lens
   - Trauma can lead to growth: learn to reappraise or reframe adversity, finding its benefits; assimilate the event into personal history; accept its occurrence; and recover
   - Recognize that failure is an essential ingredient for growth
   - Putative neurobiological mechanisms: alters memory reconsolidation, strengthens cognitive control over emotions
3. Active coping: seeking solutions, managing emotions
   - Resilient individuals use active rather than passive coping skills (dealing with problem and with emotions versus withdrawal, resignation, numbing)
   - Can be learned: work on minimizing appraisal of threat, creating positive statements about oneself, focusing on aspects that can be changed
   - Putative neurobiological mechanisms: prevents fear conditioning and learned helplessness, promotes fear extinction
4. Facing fears: learning to move through fear
   - Fear is normal and can be used as a guide for action
   - Facing and overcoming fears can increase self-esteem and sense of self-efficacy
   - Practice undertaking and completing challenging or anxiety-inducing tasks
   - Putative neurobiological mechanisms: promotes fear extinction, stress inoculation
5. Physical exercise: engage in regular physical activity
   - Physical exercise has positive effects on physical and psychological hardiness
   - Effective at increasing mood and self-esteem
   - Putative neurobiological mechanisms: promotes neurogenesis, improves cognition, attenuates HPA activity, aids in regulation of emotion, boost immune system.
6. Social support and role models or mentors
   - Establish and nurture a supportive social network
   - Very few can "go it alone"; resilient individuals derive strength from close relationships
   - Social support is safety net during stress
   - Role models and mentors can help teach resilience: imitation is powerful mode of learning
   - Putative neurobiological mechanisms: oxytocin mediates initial bonding/attachment. "Mirror"/Von Economo neurons involved in neuronal imprinting of human values
7. Moral compass: embrace a set of core beliefs that few things can shatter
   - Live by a set of guiding principles
   - For many, moral compass means religious or spiritual faith
   - Altruism strongly associated with resilience: selfless acts increase our own well being
   - Putative neurobiological mechanisms: spirituality/religiosity associated with strong serotonergic systems. Morality has neural basis, likely evolved because adaptive

and Hammer, 1992; Carver et al., 1993; Danner et al., 2001; Steptoe et al., 2005). Positive emotions have even been correlated with longevity: for example, a study of 180 nuns found that nuns whose diaries from youth reflected optimism lived significantly longer than nuns with more negative diaries (Danner et al., 2001). Optimists are thought to have robust brain reward circuits, which is discussed in further detail later in the chapter.

Positive cognitive reappraisal

Cognitive reappraisal, or the ability to find the silver lining in every cloud, is closely related to optimism and strongly associated with resilience (Gross, 2002; Tugade and Fredrickson, 2004; Southwick et al., 2005). The technique, also known as *cognitive flexibility* or *cognitive reframing*, refers to the purposeful, conscious transformation of emotional experience. Cognitive reframing is the reinterpretation of traumatic events to find their positive meaning, value, or the new opportunity that they provide. It stands in contrast to suppression, which signifies conscious attempts to forget traumatic events. Individuals who use cognitive reappraisal when dealing with trauma have less anger and physiologic arousal than those who use suppression techniques (Gross, 2002).

The ability to find personal meaning in tragedy is extraordinarily helpful in successfully overcoming trauma. Viktor Frankl, psychiatrist and Holocaust survivor, attributes his survival of concentration camps largely to this process of "meaning making"; in fact, meaning making became the basis for the school of psychotherapy that he founded, known as logotherapy. On a long enforced march, weak from hunger and cold, he wrote, "I forced my thoughts to turn to another subject. Suddenly I saw myself standing on the platform of a well-lit, warm and pleasant lecture room. . . . I was giving a lecture on the psychology of the concentration camp!" (Frankl, 1959/2006, p. 73). The conscious construction of this narrative and of the meaning he would derive from his experiences provided Dr. Frankl with the psychological endurance to survive his days in concentration camps.

The importance of synthesizing traumatic events into one's personal life narrative was described over a century ago by Pierre Janet, the French neurologist. Janet noted that his patients with posttraumatic pathology had failed to integrate their traumatic memories into a cohesive story. Janet stressed the necessity of cognitive reappraisal in preventing or overcoming posttraumatic stress; traumatic memories "needed to be modified and transformed, that is, placed in their proper context and reconstructed into neutral or meaningful narratives. Janet saw memory as an act of creation, rather than a static recording of events" (van der Kolk and van der Hart, 1989, p. 1537). Although Janet's theories on the role of cognitive reframing in posttraumatic psychopathology are over 100 years old, they remain apt and useful today in thinking about resilience.

Active Coping Styles

Active coping means deploying productive strategies for solving problems, managing stress, and regulating negative emotions that may arise in the aftermath of adverse events. Active coping behaviors include acknowledging and trying to solve problems, accepting that which cannot be changed, facing fears, using humor and physical exercise to alleviate stress, and seeking out social support and role models. Active coping has repeatedly been associated with hardiness and psychological resilience in various populations (Moos and Schaefer, 1993). In contrast, passive coping, including the blunting of emotions through substance use, denial, disengagement, or resignation, is associated with depression and lower levels of hardiness (Maddi, 1999).

Acceptance

Acceptance is an adaptive coping strategy commonly found among people who are able to tolerate extreme and uncontrollable stress (Siebert, 1996; Manne et al., 2003). Acceptance involves recognizing the uncontrollable aspects of certain stressors, changing expectations about outcome based on reality, and focusing on controllable aspects of the stressor. Acceptance is not to be confused with resignation, which is giving up or coping passively. Acceptance has been linked with better physical and psychological health and lower levels of distress in various populations (Wade et al., 2001). Recent evidence includes the finding that individuals who had an accepting coping style had fewer PTSD symptoms following the terrorist attacks of September 11, 2001 (Silver et al., 2002).

Facing fears

Facing fears is a key component of the active coping paradigm. Fear conditioning, which is discussed in greater detail later in the chapter, plays a major role in the development and maintenance of posttraumatic psychopathology. Individuals with PTSD avoid a wide variety of life's opportunities (people, places, events, etc.) that may serve as reminders of the trauma; thus, conditioned fear is maintained rather than extinguished. In contrast, resilient individuals are more adept at managing fear, using it as a guide to critically appraise threat and to select appropriate action.

Active coping at the time of trauma or when exposed to traumatic reminders appears to attenuate fear conditioning, likely by redirecting activity in the lateral and central nuclei of the amygdala away from the brain stem and toward the motor circuits in the ventral striatum.

This has the effect of reducing brain-stem-mediated responses to fear, such as freezing behavior and autonomic and endocrine responses, and enabling productive action (LeDoux and Gorman, 2002). Resilient individuals have learned to face fears and to actively cope with them; by moving through fear, they avoid fear conditioning and are less likely to develop psychopathology and functional impairments in the aftermath of trauma.

Humor

Humor, frequently used by resilient individuals, has been identified as an adaptive coping style and mature defense mechanism (Vaillant, 1977). It appears that humor decreases the probability of developing stress-induced depression (Deaner and McConatha, 1993; Thorson and Powell, 1994). The use of humor has been studied in resilient Vietnam veterans (Haas and Hendin, 1984), surgical patients (Carver et al., 1993), cancer patients (Culver et al., 2002), and at-risk children (Werner and Smith, 1992; Wolin and Wolin, 1993) and has been shown to be protective against distress. Humor is thought to diminish the threatening nature and negative emotional impact of stressful situations (Folkman, 1997), fostering a more positive perspective on challenging circumstances. The use of humor also relieves tension and discomfort (Vaillant, 1992) and attracts social support. Humor is thought to activate a network of subcortical regions that are critically involved in the dopaminergic reward system (Mobbs et al., 2003).

Physical exercise

Physical exercise has consistently been shown to have positive effects on physical hardiness, mood, and self-esteem. Individuals who exercise regularly report lower depression scores than those who do not exercise (Camacho et al., 1991; Brosse et al., 2002). Physical exercise has effects on a number of neurobiological factors that affect resilience. It attenuates the HPA axis response to stress, increases release of endorphins, and increases levels of plasma monoamines and the 5-HT precursor *tryptophan*. It is also thought to induce the expression of several genes related to neuroplasticity and neurogenesis, such as hippocampal BDNF (Cotman and Berchtold, 2002). A study of high-impact running in humans suggested that the activity has a beneficial impact on cognitive functioning: high-impact running was associated with improved vocabulary learning and retention as well as a lower likelihood of age-related cognitive diminution (Winter et al., 2006).

Social support

The last active coping strategy we discuss is the seeking out of social support. Higher levels of social support have been associated with better mental and physical health outcomes following a wide variety of stressors (Resick, 2001). Social support is thought to decrease appraisals of threat (Fontana et al., 1989), counteract feelings of loneliness (Bisschop et al., 2004), increase sense of self-efficacy, reduce functional impairment (Travis et al., 2004), and increase treatment compliance. Role models and mentors form a valuable part of a strong social support network.

Social isolation and lack of social support are associated with higher rates of mood and anxiety disorders, higher levels of stress, and increased morbidity and mortality from medical illness. Individuals who seek and nurture a supportive social network during times of stress tend to fare better during stress or adversity than inidividuals who are socially isolated.

Moral Compass: A Set of Guiding Ethical Principles

Moral compass, or an internal framework of belief about right and wrong, is another feature common to resilient individuals (Southwick et al., 2005). This construct may but does not have to include adherence to a religious or spiritual system.

Religion and spirituality seem to have a protective effect on physical and psychological well-being. A meta-analysis of 126,000 individuals from 42 independent samples found religious practice or involvement to be associated with lower risk of mortality from all causes (McCullough et al., 2000). In addition, higher levels of religious belief have been correlated with lower incidence of depression and higher rates of remission from depression in a number of populations (Braam et al., 1997; Koenig et al., 1998; Braam et al., 2001). Interestingly, one's particular religious affiliation is not implicated in the overall relationship between religiousness and improved psychological and physical health.

The neurobiology underlying religion and spirituality's positive effects on well-being is not well understood at this time. There is some evidence suggesting that spiritual or self-transcendent experiences are associated with increased density of 5-HT_{1A} receptors in the dorsal raphé nuclei, hippocampus, and neocortex (reviewed by Hasler et al., 2004). The role of the 5-HT system in spiritual experience is further supported by studies showing that drugs known to affect 5-HT (for example, LSD, mescaline, psilocybin) often produce spiritual awareness, a sense of insight, and religious ecstasy (Borg et al., 2003). Chronic stress appears to lead to a down-regulation of 5HT_{1A} receptors; spirituality and religiosity may enhance the functioning of the 5-HT system, fostering resilience and protecting against the development of posttraumatic mental illness.

Religious faith or spirituality is not an essential ingredient in a strong moral compass. In fact, morality appears to have a neural basis and is likely intrinsic to human nature. The idea that morality is inherent to human beings is ancient. Epictetus, a Greek philosopher living in Rome in the first century A.D. wrote: "Every one of us has come into this world with innate conceptions as to good and bad, noble and shameful . . . fitting and inappropriate" (Stockdale, 1991). Moral sense likely developed early in human evolution as our ancestors organized into societies: the successful functioning of society requires cooperation and trust between members. Many studies support the notion that principles of cooperation and reciprocity are ingrained within human nature. Games designed to test participants' morality repeatedly find that human beings act according to the rule that fairness to others should supercede self-interest. For example, in games in which participants are given money to divide between themselves and strangers, most participants choose to divide the money equally among players. Furthermore, participants who play fairly in such games tend to show heightened activation of their dopaminergic reward systems on imaging studies (Fehr and Fischbacher, 2003). These findings provide support for the hypothesis that people know what is right and derive fulfillment from acting accordingly.

The hypothesis that morality has a neural basis is supported by the observation that moral sense can be damaged by injury to the brain. "Acquired sociopathy" can result from trauma to certain areas of the brain, including, for example, the anterior PFC and anterior temporal lobes. Functional brain imaging studies in which participants are asked to make moral judgments show heightened activity in these regions (Moll et al., 2005).

Altruism

Altruism, or putting one's moral compass into action, is a powerful contributor to resilience. For example, research on the behavior of citizens after bombing attacks during World War II showed that those who demonstrated altruism by caring for others suffered fewer trauma-related mood and anxiety symptoms than would be expected. Furthermore, individuals who had been symptomatic preattack experienced a meaningful decrease in psychological distress (Rachman, 1979). It appears that, similar to acting fairly, performing acts of altruism activates brain reward circuits. One study found that participants who gave money to charity, whether voluntarily or through taxation, showed heightened activation of the ventral striatum, an important part in reward pathways (Harbaugh et al., 2007).

Some individuals are able to find meaning in personal tragedy by embracing a survivor mission to help others. Rape survivors who go public with their experience to raise social awareness through events such as Take Back the Night, and the mothers who founded Mothers Against Drunk Driving after their children were injured or killed in drunk driving accidents, are examples of this phenomenon.

We now discuss some of the most important neurobiological factors associated with resilience. Individuals with the psychological features of resilience we have discussed likely have a neurobiological profile characterized by optimal levels of these factors.

NEUROBIOLOGICAL PROFILE OF RESILIENCE

A number of neurotransmitters, neuropeptides, and hormones have been implicated in acute and long-term adaptation to stress. A comprehensive review of the many functions and effects of these factors is beyond the scope of this chapter; we focus specifically on the factors' role in mediating the stress response (Table 86.2, Fig. 86.1; see also COLOR FIGURE 86.1 in separate insert).

Corticotropin Releasing Hormone (CRH)

The hypothalamus releases CRH in conditions of stress, activating the pituitary-adrenal axis and triggering the release of cortisol and dehydroepiandrosterone (DHEA). Corticotropin releasing hormone also has important direct effects in the central nervous system; CRH containing neurons and CRH receptors are distributed widely throughout the brain and gut (Steckler and Holsboer, 1999). Activation of CRH neurons in the amygdala triggers fear-related behaviors, whereas activation of cortical CRH neurons reduces expectation of rewards. It seems that excessive stress in early life can result in abnormally elevated CRH activity in the adult brain (Strome et al., 2002).

Corticotropin releasing hormone acts via two G-coupled receptors, CRH-1 and CRH-2. These receptors appear to have opposite effects in the response to stress (Bale et al., 2002; Grammatopoulos and Chrousos, 2002); the CRH-1 receptor primarily activates the behavioral, endocrine, and visceral responses to stress, whereas CRH-2 generally serves to dampen these effects (Tache and Bonaz, 2007). However, activation of the CRH-2 receptor does produce some anxiogenic effects, for example, enhancing CRH-1 mediated suppression of feeding behavior (Bakshi et al., 2002). More research is necessary to determine the precise role of both receptors.

Abnormally high CRH levels in the cerebrospinal fluid have been linked to major depression and PTSD (Bremner et al., 1997; D.G. Baker et al., 1999; Nemeroff, 2002). Resilient individuals likely have the capacity to effectively regulate CRH levels and/or the relative activity of both receptor subtypes. Corticotropin releasing hormone receptor antagonists are currently under active investigation as potential new pharmacotherapies for anxiety and mood disorders as well as for stress-related

TABLE 86.2 *The Neurochemical Response Patterns to Acute Stress*

Neurochemical	*Acute Effects*	*Brain Region*	*Key Functional Interactions*	*Association with Resilience*	*Association with Psychopathology Potential for treatment?*
CRH	Activated fear behaviors, increased arousal, increased motor activity, inhibited neurovegetative function, reduced reward expectations	Prefrontal cortex, cingulated cortex, amygdala, nucleus accumbens, hippocampus, hypothalamus, bed nucleus of the stria terminalis, periaqueductal gray matter, locus coeruleus, dorsal raphé nuclei	CRH-1 receptor anxiogenic, CRH-2 receptor anxiolytic, increases cortisol and DHEA, activates locus coeruleus–norepinephrine system	Reduced CRH release, adaptive changes in CRH-1 and CRH-2 receptors	Persistently increased CRH concentration may predispose to PTSD and mood disorders as well as stress-related gastrointestinal disorders CRH receptor antagonists under investigation as treatments for mood and stress-related disorders
Cortisol	Mobilized energy, increased arousal, focused attention	Prefrontal cortex, hippocampus, amygdala, hypothalamus	Increases amygdala corticotrophin releasing hormone (CRH), increases hypothalamic CRH	Stress-induced increase rapidly constrained by negative feedback mechanisms	Dysregulated cortisol systems (excessive cortisol release, improperly functioning negative feedback systems) seen in mood disorders and PTSD
Dehydroepi-androsterone (DHEA)	Counteracts deleterious effects of high cortisol Neuroprotective Positive mood effects	Largely unknown; hypothalamus	Antiglucocorticoid actions	High DHEA–cortisol ratios may prevent/ lessen severity of PTSD and depression	Low DHEA response to stress may predispose to PTSD and depression and sensitize to the effects of hypercortisolemia DHEA tested as treatment for depression: should be tested as treatment for PTSD as well
Locus coeruleus–norepinephrine system	General alarm function activated by extrinsic and intrinsic threat; increased arousal, increased attention, fear memory formation, facilitated motor response	Prefrontal cortex, amygdala, hippocampus, hypothalamus	Activates sympathetic axis, inhibits parasympathetic outflow, stimulates hypothalamic CRH	Reduced responsiveness of locus coeruleus–norepinephrine system	Unrestrained functioning of locus coeruleus–norepinephrine system, seen in some patients with PTSD, leads to chronic anxiety, hyper-vigilance, and intrusive memories Beta-receptor blockade may help prevent PTSD

Neuropeptide Y (NPY)	Anxiolytic Improves performance under stress	Amygdala, hippocampus, hypothalamus, septum, periaqueductal gray matter, locus coeruleus	Reduces CRH-related actions at amygdala, reduces rate of firing of locus coeruleus	Adaptive increase in amygdala neuropeptide Y is associated with reduced stress-induced anxiety and depression	Low NPY associated with PTSD Y-1 and Y-2 receptors may be targets for treating mood and anxiety disorders. NPY administration may protect against stress
Galanin	Involved in anxiety and vulnerability to stress; GAL-1 receptor anxiolytic, GAL-3 anxiogenic	Prefrontal cortex, amygdala, hippocampus, locus coeruleus	Reduces the anxiogenic effects of locus coeruleus–norepinephrine system activation	Adaptive increase in amygdala galanin is associated with reduced stress-induced anxiety and depression	Low galanin levels likely related to increased vulnerability to PTSD and depression; yet to be studied
Serotonin (5-HT)	Mixed effects: 5-HT stimulation of 5-HT2 receptors is anxiogenic; 5-HT stimulation of 5-HT_{1A} receptors is anxiolytic	Prefrontal cortex, amygdala, hippocampus, dorsal raphé	High levels of cortisol decrease 5-HT_{1A} receptors	High activity of postsynaptic 5-HT_{1A} receptors may facilitate recovery	Low activity of postsynaptic 5-HT_{1A} receptors may predispose to anxiety and depression
Dopamine	High prefrontal cortex and low nucleus accumbens dopamine levels are associated with anhedonic and helpless behaviors	Prefrontal cortex, nucleus accumbens, amygdala	Reciprocal interactions between cortical and subcortical dopamine systems	Within optimal window of activity, preserves functions involving reward and extinction of fear	Excessive mesocortical dopamine release associated with vulnerability to stress Persistently high levels of prefrontal cortical dopamine associated with chronic anxiety and fear Low levels of circulating dopamine linked to depression

CRH: corticotrophin-releasing hormone; PTSD: post-traumatic stress disorder.

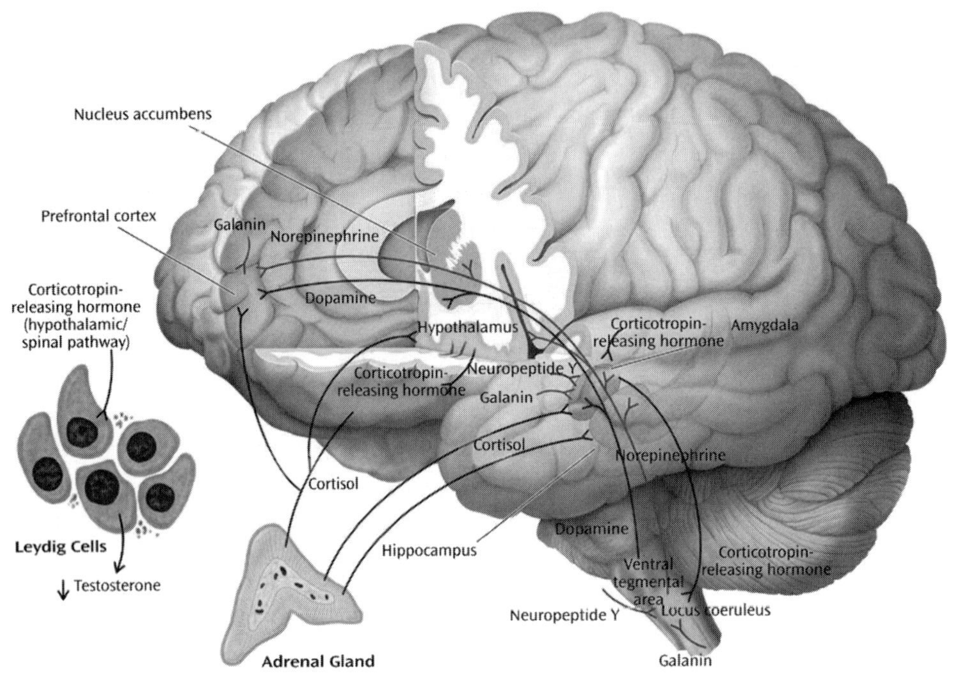

FIGURE 86.1 Neurochemical response patterns to acute stress. This figure illustrates some of the key brain structures involved in the neurochemical response patterns following acute psychological stress. The functional interactions among the different neurotransmitters, neuropeptides, and hormones are emphasized. The functional status of brain regions such as the amygdala (neuropeptide Y, galanin, corticotropin releasing hormone [CRH], cortisol, and norepinephrine), hippocampus (cortisol and norepinephrine), locus coeruleus (neuropeptide Y, galanin, and CRH), and prefrontal cortex (dopamine, norepinephrine, galanin, and cortisol) depends upon the balance among multiple inhibitory and excitatory neurochemical inputs. Functional effects may vary depending on the brain region. For example, cortisol increases CRH concentrations in the amygdala and decreases concentrations in the paraventricular nucleus of the hypothalamus. As described in the text, these neurochemical response patterns may relate to resilience and vulnerability to the effects of extreme psychological stress. (Modified and reprinted with permission from Cambridge University Press, 2007).

gastrointestinal disorders such as irritable bowel syndrome (Zoumakis et al., 2006; Tache and Bonaz, 2007).

Cortisol

Many forms of psychological stress increase the synthesis and release of cortisol, which leads to increased arousal, vigilance, inhibition of growth and reproduction, and containment of the immune response. In resilient individuals, the stress-induced increase in cortisol is effectively constrained via an elaborate negative feedback system involving GR and mineralocorticoid receptors (MR) (de Kloet et al., 2007). Excessive and sustained cortisol secretion can have serious adverse effects, including osteoporosis, immunosuppression, hypertension, metabolic syndrome, depression, and anxiety (Whitworth et al., 2005; Carroll et al., 2007).

Cortisol has important regulatory effects on the hippocampus, amygdala, and PFC. It plays a role in the formation, processing, and retrieval of memories, particularly fearful memories. Cortisol levels appear to be dysregulated in mood and anxiety disorders and in PTSD. Patients with major depressive disorder tend to have higher than normal levels of cortisol and a blunted suppression of cortisol secretion in response to the dexamethasone suppression test (Yehuda, 2001). In contrast, basal circulating cortisol levels are generally lower in individuals with PTSD than in healthy individuals (Griffin et al., 2005; Bierer et al., 2006; Yehuda, Yang, et al., 2006). Correspondingly, individuals with PTSD tend to show higher-than-average cortisol suppression during the dexamethasone suppression test, implying that their HPA-axis GRs are hypersensitive.

That patients with PTSD might have lower-than-average basal cortisol levels suggests that the disorder may develop in the setting of abnormally low cortisol; this hypothesis is supported by a number of studies showing that steroid administration inhibits traumatic memory formation (Bierer et al., 2006). Patients who are pretreated with stress doses of glucocorticoids before surgery and/or hospitalization in the intensive care unit are less likely to have traumatic memories of their hospital stay after discharge than patients treated with placebo (Brunner et al., 2006; Schelling et al., 2006; Weis et al., 2006).

Although there is a great deal of data suggesting that patients with PTSD have lower basal cortisol than healthy controls and that PTSD may develop in the setting of low glucocorticoid levels, there is also conflicting evidence. Some studies have found no difference in cortisol levels between patients with PTSD and healthy controls (Wheler et al., 2006); some have even found that patients with PTSD have higher-than-average basal cortisol levels, and that elevated cortisol at the time of trauma may predict subsequent PTSD development (D.G. Baker et al., 2005; Inslicht et al., 2006). In summary, though it is clear that cortisol is implicated in the encoding of traumatic memories and in the subsequent development of posttraumatic psychopathology, the exact nature of this effect is still under investigation. Undoubtedly though, dysregulation of cortisol secretion has adverse effects on resilience to stress.

Dehydroepiandrosterone (DHEA)

Like cortisol, DHEA is an adrenal steroid released under stress; in contrast to cortisol, DHEA protects against the negative effects of excessive stress. Dehydroepiandrosterone is secreted episodically and synchronously with cortisol (Rosenfeld et al., 1971) and has antiglucocorticoid activity in the brain (Browne et al., 1992). Dehydroepiandrosterone and its metabolites interfere with the normal uptake of GRs in the hippocampus (Kimonides et al., 1998; Bastianetto et al., 1999; Morfin and Starka, 2001) preventing corticosteroid-induced hippocampal neurotoxicity. Dehydroepiandrosterone derivatives also amplify long-term potentiation of hippocampal neurons, likely by modulating transmission at the *N*-methyl-D-aspartate (NMDA) receptor (Chen et al., 2006). The steroid's neuroprotective and potentiating effects in the hippocampus help to facilitate learning and memory.

Dehydroepiandrosterone appears to enhance cognition and performance under stress. In a study of soldiers undergoing rigorous training as part of military survival school, DHEA-S to cortisol ratios were highest in those soldiers who demonstrated the best performance during training. Thus, DHEA-S to cortisol ratios may index the degree to which an individual is buffered against the negative effects of stress (Morgan et al., 2004).

Recovery from severe stress also appears to be facilitated by high levels of DHEA. A study of veterans recovering from PTSD found that symptom improvement and effective coping predicted higher plasma DHEA levels (Yehuda, Brand, Golier, et al., 2006). In another study of women with PTSD, DHEA release in response to adrenocorticotrophic hormone (ACTH) injections was greatest in women with the lowest symptom severity, and the DHEA to cortisol ratios were correlated with better mood. A large capacity for adrenal DHEA release may be associated with strong recovery from PTSD (Rasmusson et al., 2004).

Other studies have also found a negative correlation between plasma DHEA levels and depressive symptoms (Goodyer et al., 1998; Gallagher and Young, 2002; Young et al., 2002). Research is currently being conducted regarding the efficacy of DHEA as an antidepressant. In a recent placebo-controlled trial of DHEA as a treatment for depression in patients with HIV/AIDS, DHEA was significantly more effective than placebo as an antidepressant (Rabkin et al., 2006). More research is needed to determine whether DHEA could also be an effective treatment for other patients with depression and patients with PTSD.

The Locus Coeruleus–Norepinephrine System

Stress activates the locus coeruleus (LC), which results in increased norepinephrine (NE) release in projection sites of the LC, including the amygdala, PFC, and hippocampus. The LC is activated by a variety of stressors, intrinsic (for example, hypoglycemia, hypotension) and extrinsic (environmental threats). Such activation serves as a general alarm function and is adaptive in a life-threatening situation. Activation of the LC contributes to the sympathetic nervous system and HPA axis stimulation and inhibits parasympathetic outflow and neurovegetative function, including eating and sleep. A high level of activation of the LC–NE system inhibits function of the PFC, thereby favoring instinctual responses over more complex cognition (Charney, 1999).

The activation of the HPA and LC–NE systems under acute stress facilitates the encoding and relay of aversively charged emotional memories, beginning at the amygdala. Animal studies have shown that injections of NE into the amygdala enhance memory consolidation; on the other hand, blocking NE activity during stress impedes the encoding of fearful memories. In rats, blocking the lateral nucleus of the amygdala to the effects of NE during reactivation of a fearful memory prevents the process of memory reconsolidation and appears to permanently impair that memory (Debiec and LeDoux, 2006). Based on the evidence from animal studies showing that β-receptor blockade prior to or immediately after learning a task inhibits some aspects of memory consolidation, there have been recent studies in humans investigating whether β-blockers given shortly after trauma might be an effective treatment for PTSD. Results have been mixed. A pilot study found that trauma survivors who received the β-blocker *propanolol* immediately on their presentation to the emergency room exhibited less physiological reactivity when recalling memories of their trauma 3 months later than did patients who received placebo (Pitman et al., 2002). However, subsequent studies in humans have failed to show a consistent effect of propanolol on cued or contextual fear conditioning (Orr et al., 2006). More work is needed to determine whether β-adrenergic blockade has potential as an effective treatment for PTSD.

If unchecked, persistent hyperresponsiveness of the LC–NE system contributes to chronic anxiety, fear, intrusive memories, and an increased risk of cardiovascular disease and hypertension. In some patients with panic disorder, PTSD, and major depression, there is evidence of heightened LC–NE activity (Charney et al., 1987; Charney et al., 1992; Southwick et al., 1997; Geracioti et al., 2001). In addition, in one study of 598 patients with coronary disease, those with depressive symptoms had higher urinary NE excretion than those without (Otte, Neylan, Pipkin, et al., 2005).

Neuropeptide Y (NPY)

Neuropeptide Y is an abundant peptide that is widely distributed throughout the brain and acts via at least five G-protein coupled receptors, Y1–Y5 (Pieribone et al., 1992; R.A. Baker and Herkenham, 1995; Risold and Swanson, 1997; Makino et al., 2000; Karl et al., 2006). Neuropeptide Y produces anxiolytic effects and appears to enhance cognitive functioning under stress. There are important functional interactions between NPY and CRH (Heilig et al., 1994; Britton et al., 2000): NPY counteracts the anxiogenic effects of CRH at various locations within the stress/anxiety circuit, including the amygdala, hippocampus, hypothalamus, and LC (Sajdyk et al., 2006). It may be that the balance between NPY and CRH neurotransmission is critical to maintaining a homeostatic emotional state during stress (Kask et al., 1997; Eva et al., 2006; Sajdyk et al., 2006).

High levels of NPY appear to protect against depression and anxiety, with the Y1 and Y2 receptors playing important roles in the peptide's effects on mood (Heilig et al., 1993; Heilig, 1995). Neuropeptide Y activation of the Y-1 receptor inhibits several metabolic and behavioral stress responses, including gastrointestinal distress, anxious behavior, and decreased sleep (Eva et al., 2006). Antidepressant drugs and electroconvulsive therapy increase NPY in rodent brains as they decrease depression; this effect is likely mediated by the Y-1 receptor (Karl et al., 2006). A variety of antidepressant drugs increase NPY levels in humans as well (Husum and Mathe, 2002). Y-2 knockout mice exhibit fewer anxious and depressed behaviors and are more adventurous (Carvajal et al., 2006). The Y1- and Y2-receptors may therefore be useful targets for treating mood and anxiety disorders in humans.

Low NPY levels are also associated with PTSD. In a study of combat veterans with and without PTSD, plasma NPY levels varied: veterans with a past history of PTSD had higher NPY levels than veterans with current PTSD, and NPY levels were predicted by extent of symptom improvement (Yehuda, Brand, and Yang, 2006). Other patients with PTSD have been shown to have reduced plasma NPY levels and a blunted yohimbine-induced increase in NPY (Rasmusson et al., 2000).

Finally, elevated NPY levels are associated with better performance under stress. Preliminary work with special operations soldiers under extreme training stress indicates that high NPY levels are associated with better performance (Morgan et al., 2000). Neuropeptide Y's protective effects against depression, anxiety, and posttraumatic psychopathology, in addition to its beneficial effects on performance under stress, suggest that the peptide could be an effective pharmacotherapy for enhancing resilience to stress. However, it will first be necessary to design a drug delivery method that enables the peptide to penetrate into the CSF; intranasal administration may be effective in this regard.

Galanin

Galanin, another abundant neuropeptide, has been shown to be involved in a number of physiological and behavioral functions, including anxiety, stress, and alcohol intake (Moller et al., 1999; A. Holmes et al., 2002). Understanding of galanin's mechanisms of action and effects is still at an early stage; however, overall the peptide appears to mitigate the effects of stress.

Three receptors for galanin have been identified, and two of these (GAL-1 and GAL-3) have been found to affect stress and anxiety (Walton et al., 2006). The GAL-1 receptor, expressed in the amygdala, hypothalamus, and bed nucleus of the stria terminalis, acts as an auto-receptor (Sevcik et al., 1993; Gustafson et al., 1996; Xu et al., 2001) and appears to be involved in anxiolysis: knockout mice for the GAL-1 receptor show increased anxiety-like behaviors (F.E. Holmes et al., 2003). The GAL-3 receptor, on the other hand, produces anxiogenic effects when activated (Swanson et al., 2005). In humans, certain polymorphisms of the gene for the GAL-3 receptor have been linked with anxiety and alcoholism (Belfer et al., 2006).

It has been suggested that galanin recruitment during periods of stress may diminish negative emotions caused by hyperactivity of the noradrenergic system (Karlsson and Holmes, 2006). Galanin appears to inhibit NE, serotonin (5-HT), and DA neurons from firing, reducing release of these neurotransmitters in forebrain target regions. Further evidence that galanin mitigates hyperactivity of the noradrenergic system comes from the finding that galanin agonists reduce behavioral signs of opiate withdrawal in mice (A. Holmes and Picciotto, 2006). Additionally, galanin-overexpressing transgenic mice are unresponsive to the anxiogenic effects of the α_2 receptor antagonist yohimbine. Consistent with this observation, galanin injected directly into the central nucleus of rodent amygdalas blocked the anxiogenic effects of stress, which is associated with increased NE release in the central nucleus of the amygdala (Khoshbouei et al., 2002).

Galanin's anxiolytic effects are reflected by its close association with ascending monoamine pathways. A dense galanin immunoreactive fiber system originating in the LC innervates forebrain and midbrain structures, including the hippocampus, hypothalamus, amygdala, and PFC (Perez et al., 2001). However, galanin does not appear to be coreleased from noradrenergic terminals—examinations of rodent brains whose stress system was activated by yohimbine suggest that galanin is released from separate afferent neurons (Barrera et al., 2006). Galanin-releasing neurons are most likely located immediately adjacent to the central amygdala and appear to be activated by nonnoradrenergic afferents that themselves are activated by NE activity; therefore, targeting galanin for antidepressant or anti-anxiety treatment will likely be challenging (Barrera et al., 2005). To our knowledge, galanin function has not been studied in patients exposed to traumatic stress or patients with PTSD or major depression.

Serotonin

Serotonin (5-HT) is well known as one of the neurotransmitters most relevant to mood. As a neuromodulater, 5-HT also regulates other neurotransmitter systems involved in mood and anxiety, and dysregulation of the 5-HT system may cause a cascade of changes in brain chemistry.

Acute stress results in increased 5-HT turnover in the PFC, nucleus accumbens, amygdala, and lateral hypothalamus (Kent et al., 2002). Serotonin release may have anxiogenic and anxiolytic effects, depending on the region of the forebrain involved and the receptor subtype activated. 5-HT_{1A} receptors are anxiolytic and may be responsible for adaptive responses to aversive events, whereas anxiogenic effects appear to be mediated by 5-HT_{2A} receptors (Charney and Drevets, 2002). $5HT_{1A}$ knock-out mice show an increase in anxiety-like behaviors (Heisler et al., 1998; Parks et al., 1998), including behavioral inhibition in ambiguous environments (settings that contain neutral and fear-conditioned cues). This type of behavior represents an inappropriate generalization of fearful behavior, a phenomenon that occurs in some human anxiety disorders, including panic disorder, specific phobias, and PTSD (Klemenhagen et al., 2006). Therefore, lower-than-normal activation of $5HT_{1A}$ receptors may be involved in the pathophysiology of human anxiety disorders.

A scenario has been proposed in which early life stress increases CRH and cortisol levels, which, in turn, downregulate 5-HT_{1A} receptors, resulting in a lower threshold for tolerating stressful life events. Alternatively, 5-HT_{1A} receptor density may be partly genetic. The density of 5-HT_{1A} receptors in patients who are depressed is lower than in patients who are not depressed when they are depressed and when they are in remission (Drevets et al., 1999). It has been recently demonstrated that 5-HT_{1A} receptor density is also lower in patients with panic disorder than in healthy controls (Neumeister et al., 2004). However, data so far do not support the hypothesis that decreased 5-HT_{1A} binding plays a role in PTSD: a positron emission tomography (PET) study scanning receptor status in individuals with PTSD found no differences in $5HT_{1A}$ receptor distribution, binding potential, or tracer delivery (Bonne et al., 2005).

Dopamine

Dopamine is released in some areas of the brain and inhibited in others during extreme stress. Stress activates DA release in the MPFC (Cabib et al., 2002) and inhibits DA release in the nucleus accumbens, one of the regions associated with human experience of pleasure and reward (Cabib and Puglisi-Allegra, 1996). Lesions of the amygdala in a conditioned stress model block stress-induced DA activation in the MPFC, implying amygdalar control over stress-induced DA release (Goldstein et al., 1996; Cabib et al., 2002). The degree to which an individual's DA system is activated by stress is in part genetically determined, and individuals whose genetic profile results in excessive mesocortical DA release after stressful events may have a tendency towards vulnerability to stress (Cabib et al., 2002). As mentioned in the earlier discussion on NE, studies of individuals with low-functioning variants of the *COMT* gene, leading to less DA degradation, display higher anxiety and lower resistance to stress (Heinz and Smolka, 2006).

Although hyperactivity of the dopaminergic system may increase susceptibility to suffering negative effects of stress, it appears that underactivity of dopaminergic neurons in the PFC may be implicated in sustaining posttraumatic stress disorders. Lesions of dopaminergic neurons in the MPFC delay extinction of the conditioned fear response (Morrow et al., 1999), which can sustain PTSD symptoms.

Reduced levels of circulating DA have also been implicated in depression in a number of studies (Dunlop and Nemeroff, 2007). This link is supported by the fact that individuals with Parkinson's disease (and decreased DA production) have high rates of depression. Postmortem studies of patients who were depressed have found reduced DA metabolites in the cerebrospinal fluid and in brain areas regulating mood and motivation.

Dopamine plays an important role in the brain's reward pathways, which we now discuss. The proper functioning of reward pathways is critical to resilience.

NEURAL CIRCUITRY OF REWARD: HOW REWARD PATHWAYS IMPACT RESILIENCE TO STRESS

A stable and well-functioning system of reward pathways and response to pleasant stimuli is a prerequisite for dealing successfully with stress and traumatic life experiences. The ability to respond appropriately to positive events and situations is vital to the preservation of reward expectation, optimism, and positive self-concept following stress or trauma. Resilient individuals likely

TABLE 86.3 *Neural Mechanisms Related to Resilience and Vulnerability to Extreme Stress (modified and reprinted with permission from Cambridge University Press 2007)*

Mechanism	Neurochemical Systems	Brain Regions	Association With Resilience	Association With Psychopathology
Reward	Dopamine, dopamine receptors, glutamate, N-methyl-D-aspartic acid (NMDA) receptors, γ-aminobutyric acid (GABA), opioids, cAMP response element binding protein, ΔFosB	Medial prefrontal cortex, orbital frontal cortex, nucleus accumbens, amygdala, hippocampus, ventral tegmental area, hypothalamus	In resilient individuals, stress does not produce impairment in neurochemical or transcription factor-mediated reward	Stress-induced reduction in dopamine and increases in cAMP response–element binding protein transcription produces a dysfunction in reward circuitry leading to anhedonia and hopelessness
Reconsolidation	Glutamate, NMDA receptors norepinephrine, β-adrenergic receptors, cAMP response-element binding protein	Amygdala, hippocampus	The lability of the memory trace allows a reorganization of original memory that is less traumatic	Repeated reactivation and reconsolidation may further strengthen the memory trace and lead to persistence of trauma-related symptoms
Extinction	Glutamate, NMDA receptors, voltage-gated calcium channels norepinephrine, dopamine, GABA	Medial prefrontal sensory cortex, amygdala	An ability to quickly attenuate learned fear through a powerful extinction process	Failure in neural mechanisms of extinction may relate to persistent traumatic memories, reexperiencing symptoms, hyperarousal, and phobic behaviors

cAMP: cyclic adenosine monophosphate; NMDA: *N*-methyl-D-aspartate.

have a robust reward system, which is hypersensitive to reward and/or resistant to change (Table 86.3, Fig. 86.2; see also COLOR FIGURE 86.2 in separate insert).

The dopaminergic system is involved in mediating elements of the reward system, including motivation, incentive, and hedonic tone (Barrot et al., 2002; Wise, 2002). Dopaminergic neurons increase firing when rewards are unexpected or better than expected (Schultz, 2002) and decrease their rate of firing when rewards are absent or less than predicted. Imaging research suggests that the anticipation of reward involves mesolimbic DA pathways through the ventral striatum (Knutson and Cooper, 2005) and other subcortical limbic structures including the dorsal striatum, amygdala, and midbrain ventral tegmental area.

The roles of the orbital frontal and MPFCs in reward are somewhat more complex. The orbital frontal cortex, taking input from the nucleus accumbens, assists in discriminating the motivational value of rewarding stimuli (Martin-Soelch et al., 2001; Schultz, 2002). The MPFC appears to be involved in assessing the likelihood of receiving a given reward (as opposed to its magnitude) (Knutson and Cooper, 2005) and providing feedback along glutamatergic projections to the nucleus accumbens and the ventral tegmental area. The anterior insula is involved in producing aversion to risks in the pursuit of reward (Kuhnen and Knutson, 2005). In making decisions about behavior, it appears that a stimulus's potential rewards are assessed in subcortical areas before being analyzed in the MPFC (Knutson and Cooper, 2005).

Strength, persistence, and emotional value of reward memory are modulated by circuits formed by the amygdala, subiculum, bed nucleus of the stria terminalis, nucleus accumbens, and MPFC. Specifically, the cyclic adenosine monophosphate (cAMP) pathway and expression of cAMP response-element binding protein in the amygdala strengthen positive as well as negative associations (Hall et al., 2001; Josselyn et al., 2001). Rodents have been shown to develop persistent anhedonia when increased cAMP response element binding is present in the nucleus accumbens (Barrot et al., 2002).

Stresses, chronic and acute, are correlated with decreased sensitivity to rewarding stimuli and increased sensitivity to aversive stimuli (Pliakas et al., 2001; Bogdan and Pizzagalli, 2006). Although exposure to acute stress has the potential to alter reward circuits, decreasing positive response to reward, it seems that resilient individuals are less sensitive to the effects of stress, maintaining highly functional reward systems under adverse conditions. The neurobiology underlying robust reward systems is not well understood; however, there is

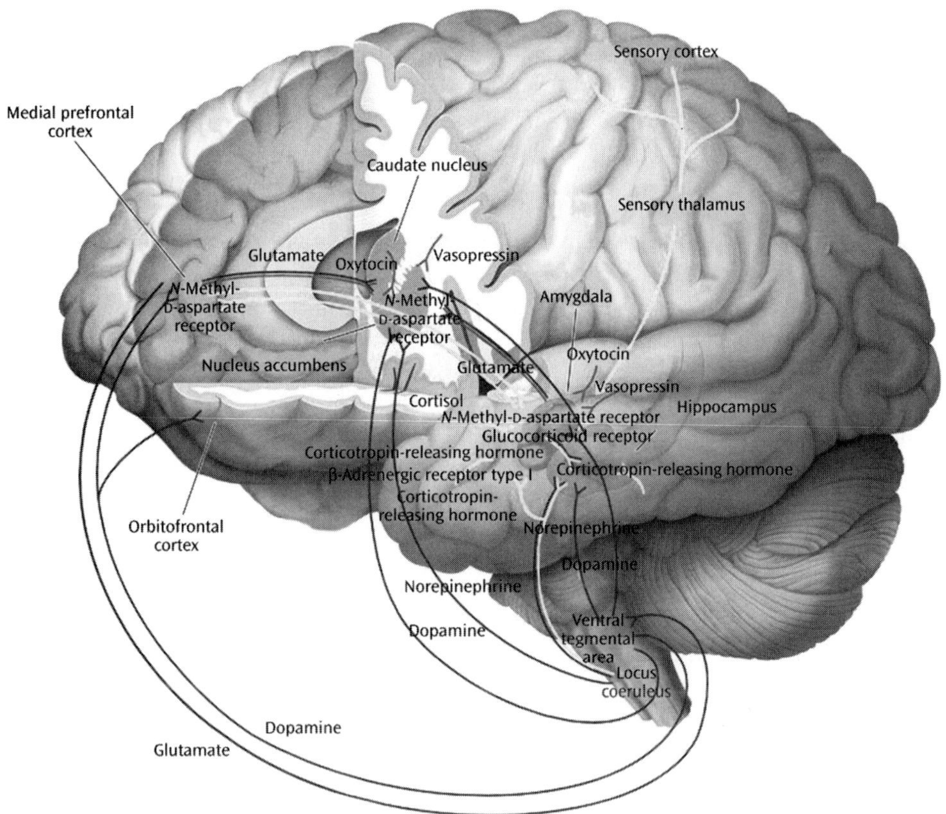

FIGURE 86.2 Neural circuits associated with reward, fear conditioning, and social behavior. The figure depicts a simplified summary of some of the brain structures and relevant neurochemistry mediating the neural mechanisms of reward (purple paths), fear conditioning and extinction (yellow paths), and social behaviors (blue paths). Only a subset of the many known interconnections among these various regions is shown, and relevant interneurons are not illustrated, yet it can be seen there is considerable overlap in the brain structures associated with these neural mechanisms. This suggests that there may be clinically relevant functional interactions among the circuits. For example, a properly functioning reward circuit may be necessary for the reinforcement of positive social behaviors. An overly responsive fear circuit or impaired extinction process may negatively influence functioning of the reward system. The assessment of these neural mechanisms must be considered in the context of their neurochemical regulation. Alterations in one neurotransmitter, neuropeptide, or hormone system will affect more than one circuit. Several receptors that may be targeted by new anti-anxiety and antidepressant drugs are illustrated. The functional status of these circuits has important influences on stress-related psychopathology and the discovery of novel therapeutics (see text). (Modified and reprinted with permission from Cambridge University Press, 2007; see Figure 86.2 in color insert).

some evidence from animal models that is beginning to provide insight into potential mechanisms. In rodent models, chronic exposure to stressful stimuli will lead to an enduring aversion to social contact. Researchers have found that knocking out *BDNF* in the mesolimbic DA system of the rodents seems to produce a reward system that has lost its plasticity, remaining resistant to change when the rats are subsequently presented with stressors. After undergoing this mesolimbic DA pathway-specific knockdown of *BDNF*, mice become inoculated to the effects of repeated social aggression (Berton et al., 2006). These findings highlight the major role of the reward system's plasticity in determining resilience and indicate a possible mechanism through which a resistant reward system plays a part in allowing resilient individuals to endure hardships without developing posttraumatic psychopathology.

THE NEURAL CIRCUITRY OF ANXIETY AND FEAR: THE ROLE OF FEAR LEARNING IN RESILIENCE TO STRESS

Fear Conditioning

Individuals with PTSD suffer distress when they encounter traumatic reminders. Over time, patients suffering from PTSD tend to "overgeneralize" fear cues: they begin to associate more and more features in their environment with their past traumas. Often, fear cues are objectively nonthreatening and unrelated to trauma. The process through which previously neutral stimuli become fear inducing is known as *fear conditioning*. In the terminology of fear conditioning, previously neutral stimuli become "conditioned" stimuli by virtue of their association with aversive ("unconditioned") stimuli (Blair et al., 2001).

Resilience to the effects of severe stress may be characterized in part by the capacity to avoid overgeneralizing fear-inducing triggers. Resilient individuals are also likely adept at extinguishing of fearful memories; in other words, those who are resistant to stress have an easier time letting go of frightening memories and associations.

Cue-specific conditioned stimuli are transmitted to the thalamus by external and visceral pathways. Afferents reach the lateral amygdala by means of two parallel circuits: a rapid subcortical path directly from the dorsal (sensory) thalamus and a slower regulatory cortical pathway encompassing the primary somatosensory cortices, the insula, and the anterior cingulate/PFC. Contextual conditioned stimuli are projected to the lateral amygdala from the hippocampus and the bed nucleus of the stria terminalis. The lateral nucleus of the amygdala is likely a site of fear memory storage as well as fear acquisition (Schafe et al., 2005). The existence of the long loop pathway (passing through cortical regions) indicates that sensory information relayed to the amygdala undergoes substantial higher-level processing, thereby enabling assignment of significance based on prior exposure to stimuli. This potential for higher-level processing of conditioned stimuli is important because it implies that there is potential for modifying the processing of fear-conditioned stimuli with cognitive therapies.

The lateral amygdala, once engaged, projects to the central and medial nuclei of the amygdala, which project indirectly to the acoustic startle pathway in the brain stem (Davis, 2006). The central nucleus of the amygdala appears to be the primary output nucleus involved in initial memory consolidation; infusions of anisomycin, a protein synthesis inhibitor, into the central nucleus during fear training disrupts consolidation of fear memory (Debiec and LeDoux, 2006). The central nucleus projects to the hypothalamus and brain stem, triggering the cascade of autonomic, endocrine, and behavioral responses associated with fear (Schafe et al., 2001).

The molecular processes underlying fear conditioning is an area of active investigation. Consolidation of fear conditioning is thought to occur via long-term potentiation of synapses in the lateral amygdala. A recent study found that fear-conditioned rats show increases in an actin-polymerization protein, profilin, in dendritic spines in the lateral amygdala; this finding could contribute to a greater understanding of the specific changes underlying synaptic plasticity (Schafe et al., 2005). However, our understanding of the cellular mechanisms underlying the process remains far from complete (Sigurdsson et al., 2007). The currently accepted model to explain how long-term potentiation in the lateral amygdala might lead to the consolidation of fear conditioning was proposed by LeDoux and colleagues (LeDoux, 2000). The model proposes that calcium entry through NMDA receptors and voltage-gated calcium channels initiates the molecular processes to consolidate synaptic changes into long-term memory; short-term memory requires only calcium entry through NMDA receptors (Blair et al., 2001).

Because NMDA receptors are critical in fear learning, which is mediated by glutamate acting in the central nucleus of the amygdala (Davis, 2006), we may be able to impair fear learning by blocking NMDA receptors in the amygdala during stress. This has been demonstrated in rodents (Walker and Davis, 2000; Rodrigues et al., 2001) but has yet to be tested in humans. Blockade of voltage-gated calcium channels may also prove useful in preventing PTSD in those who are exposed to stress. Of course, because these are mechanisms of initial fear consolidation, it would be necessary to initiate receptor blockade treatment prior to trauma exposure to prevent posttraumatic stress. This might be feasible and useful in populations that are certain to encounter severe stress, for example, soldiers to be deployed in combat, or disaster relief workers.

Reconsolidation and Extinction

Existing memories, when retrieved or "reactivated" by remembering, become labile and prone to change. Reactivated memories may go down one of two pathways: they may either be strengthened by reconsolidation, or weakened by extinction (Eisenhardt and Menzel, 2007). The processes appear to be mutually exclusive, and may compete for cellular resources (Dudai and Eisenberg, 2004). The processes of memory reactivation, reconsolidation, and extinction involve NMDA and β-adrenergic receptors and require cAMP response element binding protein induction, indicating that nuclear protein synthesis is necessary (Kida et al., 2002). Reconsolidation and extinction are impaired by NMDA and β-adrenergic blockade, and enhanced by the NMDA partial agonist D-cycloserine (Przybyslawski et al., 1999; Royer et al., 2000; Charney and Drevets, 2002; Chhatwal et al., 2006; Debiec and LeDoux, 2006; Sotres-Bayon et al., 2007). Whether the process of reconsolidation or of extinction will be engaged appears to depend on the timing and type of memory retrieval; short memory reactivation sessions tend to lead to reconsolidation, whereas long and intensive extinction training is necessary to achieve extinction (J.L. Lee et al., 2006). In mice, fear reconsolidation is best achieved by repeated exposures to fearful stimuli, spaced over time. In contrast, the most effective way to induce extinction is with "massed exposures" to conditioned stimuli (Chhatwal et al., 2006).

Reconsolidation and extinction of a memory are affected by the age of the memory in question (Fulton, 2006). As would be expected, younger memories are more prone to being altered by either process, although intensifying the memory reactivation process helps enhance the lability of older memories (Suzuki et al., 2004). The time frame during which reconsolidation occurs is still under debate, with some groups finding that the process can be disrupted up to several weeks after initial fear training (Nader et al., 2000; Davis and Myers, 2002; Debiec et al., 2002; Dudai and Eisenberg, 2004; Milekic and Alberini, 2002). At some point, though, it is thought that reconsolidation is complete and it is no longer possible to reactivate the process.

Similarly, the process of extinction changes over time. Extinction induced immediately after fear acquisition (between 10 minutes and 1 hour later) is thought to occur by "erasing" the learned fear (Myers et al., 2006). However, extinction induced 24–72 hours after initial fear training appears to be a new form of learning altogether (Myers and Davis, 2007). The extinction that is achieved during this later time period may be thought of as the formation of a new, safe association with the original fear cue; this new association is placed, "like a blanket," over the older fear association (Chhatwal et al., 2006). That the original fear association still exists underneath the blanket of safety is suggested by observations that extinguished fears can return spontaneously.

Memory consolidation, reconsolidation, and extinction involve different neural circuits. The central nucleus of the amygdala (CeA) and hippocampus are involved in initial memory consolidation, the lateral amygdala (LA) in reconsolidation, and the basal lateral amygdala (BLA) in extinction (Bahar et al., 2004; Debiec and LeDoux, 2006). The MPFC is a critical structure in extinction. Since the 1980s, studies have found that lesions of the MPFC result in an impairment of normal extinction; the resistance to extinction that is produced by lesions to the MPFC has been described as a form of "emotional perseveration," likening the phenomenon to the cognitive perseveration that is observed subsequent to lesions in the dorsolateral PFC (cited in Sotres-Bayon et al., 2006). Failure to achieve an adequate level of activation of the MPFC might lead to persistent fear responses (Herry and Garcia, 2002). Individuals with the capacity to function well after high-stress experiences may have potent MPFC inhibition of amygdala responsiveness. In contrast, patients with PTSD have been shown to exhibit increased left amygdala activation during fear acquisition and decreased activity of the MPFC/anterior cingulate during extinction.

Reconsolidation and extinction of traumatic memories are implicated in vulnerability and resilience to extreme stress. Individuals who are able to attenuate learned fear through extinction are likely highly stress resilient. Due to our growing understanding of the mechanisms of memory processing, there will likely be ever more possibilities for helping trauma survivors manage their traumatic memories. For example, we know that the NMDA partial agonist *D-cycloserine* enhances memory reconsolidation and memory extinction, and that extinction rather than reconsolidation can be selected if a traumatic memory is reactivated in the context of intensive prolonged exposure therapy in a safe environment. Consistent with this understanding, at least two double-blind placebo-controlled trials in humans with anxiety disorders have found that significant symptom reduction is achieved with a combination of D-cycloserine and prolonged exposure based psychotherapy (Ressler et al., 2004; Hofmann et al., 2006).

Another therapy under active investigation is β-receptor blockade. As discussed previously, because antagonizing β receptors disrupts the process of reconsolidation, recent trials have investigated the efficacy of β-blockers at weakening traumatic memories, and some have shown promise (Przybyslawski and Sara, 1997; Przybyslawski et al., 1999; J.L. Lee et al., 2006). Other receptors known to be involved in extinction, including for example the *BDNF* receptor tyrosine kinase b, are being targeted in preclinical trials and show promise as future PTSD treatments (Chhatwal et al., 2006).

IMPLICATIONS FOR PREVENTION AND TREATMENT OF POSTTRAUMATIC PSYCHOPATHOLOGY

Our growing understanding of genetic, developmental, psychological, and neurobiological resilience factors will likely lead to the development of new therapies, psychotherapeutic and pharmacologic, for enhancing resilience to stress. Stress inoculation training, via exposure to manageable stressors including physical and mental challenges, may be useful in building resistance to adversity in children and adults. Given that resilient individuals tend to use social support, optimism, cognitive reframing, spirituality, altruism, and active coping styles in dealing with adversity, it would be beneficial for all individuals to work on using or strengthening these attitudes and behaviors.

It may also be possible to enhance resilience with pharmacologic means; undoubtedly, pharmacologic therapies will be most beneficial in combination with psychotherapy designed to bolster psychological resilience factors. The likelihood and/or severity of stress-induced psychopathology may be reduced with the use of NPY, DHEA, CRH-1 antagonists, and GAL-1 agonists, for example; further trials are necessary to investigate the potential of these molecules to diminish stress and anxiety in humans. It may even be possible to prevent posttraumatic stress disorders by pretreating individuals at risk for trauma with protective pharmacologic agents. To this end, it would be useful to conduct trials evaluating the efficacy of agents that target receptors involved in fear conditioning and fear extinction, that is, voltage-gated calcium channels, β-adrenergic receptors, tyrosine kinase b receptors, and NMDA receptors. By weakening fear-conditioning mechanisms and enhancing fear-extinction pathways, it may be possible to attenuate the encoding of traumatic memories that often occurs upon exposure to trauma.

Continued progress in understanding the genetic, developmental, biological, and psychological underpinnings of resilience and vulnerability to stress, as well as the interactions between these factors, will aid in moving the field towards the identification, prevention, and treatment of those at risk of developing stress-related psychopathology.

REFERENCES

Affleck, G., and Tennen, H. (1996) Constructing benefits from adversity: Adaptational significance and dispositional underpinnings. *J. Personality* 64:899–922.

Amat, J., Paul, E., Zarza, C., et al. (2006) Previous experience with behavioral control over stress blocks the behavioral and dorsal raphe nucleus activating effects of later uncontrollable stress: role of the ventral medial prefrontal cortex. *J. Neurosci.* 26: 13264–13272.

Bahar, A., Dorfman, N., and Dudai, Y. (2004) Amygdalar circuits required for either consolidation or extinction of taste aversion memory are not required for reconsolidation. *Eur. J. Neurosci.* 19:1115–1118.

Baker, D.G., Ekhator, N.N., Kasckow, J.W., et al. (2005) Higher levels of basal serial CSF cortisol in combat veterans with posttraumatic stress disorder. *Am. J. Psychiatry* 162:992–994.

Baker, D.G., West, S.A., Nicholson, W.E., et al. (1999) Serial CSF corticotropin-releasing hormone levels and adrenocortical activity in combat veterans with posttraumatic stress disorder. *Am. J. Psychiatry* 156:585–588.

Baker, R.A., and Herkenham, M. (1995) Arcuate nucleus neurons that project to the hypothalamic paraventricular nucleus: neuropeptidergic identity and consequences of adrenalectomy on mRNA levels in the rat. *J. Comp. Neurol.* 358:518–530.

Bakshi, V.P., Smith-Roe, S., Newman, S.M., et al. (2002) Reduction of stress-induced behavior by antagonism of corticotropin-releasing hormone 2 (CRH2) receptors in lateral septum or CRH1 receptors in amygdala. *J. Neurosci.* 22:2926–2935.

Bale, T.L., Picetti, R., Contarino, A., et al. (2002) Mice deficient for both corticotropin-releasing factor receptor 1 (CRFR1) and CRFR2 have an impaired stress response and display sexually dichotomous anxiety-like behavior. *J. Neurosci.* 22:193–199.

Barrera, G., Echevarria, D.J., Poulin, J.F., et al. (2005) One for all or one for one: does co-transmission unify the concept of a brain galanin "system" or clarify any consistent role in anxiety? *Neuropeptides* 39:289–292.

Barrera, G., Hernandez, A., Poulin, J.F., et al. (2006) Galanin-mediated anxiolytic effect in rat central amygdala is not a result of corelease from noradrenergic terminals. *Synapse* 59:27–40.

Barrot, M., Olivier, J.D., Perrotti, L.I., et al. (2002) CREB activity in the nucleus accumbens shell controls gating of behavioral responses to emotional stimuli. *Proc. Natl. Acad. Sci. USA* 99:11435–11440.

Bastianetto, S., Ramassamy, C., Poirier, J., et al. (1999) Dehydroepiandrosterone (DHEA) protects hippocampal cells from oxidative stress-induced damage. *Brain Res. Mol. Brain Res.* 66:35–41.

Belfer, I., Hipp, H., McKnight, C., et al. (2006) Association of galanin haplotypes with alcoholism and anxiety in two ethnically distinct populations. *Mol. Psychiatry* 11:301–311.

Berton, O., McClung, C.A., Dileone, R.J., et al. (2006) Essential role of BDNF in the mesolimbic dopamine pathway in social defeat stress. *Science* 311:864–868.

Bierer, L.M., Tischler, L., Labinsky, E., et al. (2006) Clinical correlates of 24-h cortisol and norepinephrine excretion among subjects seeking treatment following the World Trade Center attacks on 9/11. *Ann. N. Y. Acad. Sci.* 1071:514–520.

Bisschop, M.I., Knegsman, D.M.W., Beekman, A.T.F., et al. (2004) Chronic diseases and depression: the modifying role of psychosocial resources. *Soc. Sci. Med.* 59:721–733.

Blair, H.T., Schafe, G.E., Bauer, E.P., et al. (2001) Synaptic plasticity in the lateral amygdala: a cellular hypothesis of fear conditioning. *Learn. Mem.* 8:229–242.

Bogdan, R., and Pizzagalli, D.A. (2006) Acute stress reduces reward responsiveness: implications for depression. *Biol. Psychiatry* 60: 1147–1154.

Bonne, O., Bain, E., Neumeister, A., et al. (2005) No change in serotonin type 1A receptor binding in patients with posttraumatic stress disorder. *Am. J. Psychiatry* 162:383–385.

Borg, J., Andree, B., Soderstrom, H., et al. (2003) The serotonin system and spiritual experiences. *Am. J. Psychiatry* 160:1965–1969.

Boyce, W.T., and Chesterman, E. (1990) Life events, social support, and cardiovascular reactivity in adolescence. *J. Dev. Behav. Pediatr.* 11:105–111.

Braam, A.W., Beekman, A.T.F., Deeg, D.J.H., et al. (1997) Religiosity as a protective or prognostic factor of depression in later life; results from a community survey in The Netherlands. *Acta Psychiatr. Scand.* 96:199–205.

Braam, A.W., Van Den Eeden, P., Prince, M.J., et al. (2001) Religion as a cross-cultural determinant of depression in elderly Europeans: results from the EURODEP collaboration. *Psychol. Med.* 31:803–814.

Bremner, J.D., Licinio, J., Darnell, A., et al. (1997) Elevated CSF corticotropin-releasing factor concentrations in posttraumatic stress disorder. *Am. J. Psychiatry* 154:624–629.

Breslau, N., Kessler, R.C., Chilcoat, H.D., et al. (1998) Trauma and posttraumatic stress disorder in the community: the 1996 Detroit Area Survey of Trauma. *Arch. Gen. Psychiatry* 55:626–632.

Britton, K.T., Akwa, Y., Spina, M.G., et al. (2000) Neuropeptide Y blocks anxiogenic-like behavioral action of corticotropin-releasing factor in an operant conflict test and elevated plus maze. *Peptides* 21:37–44.

Brosse, A.L., Sheets, E.S., Lett, H.S., et al. (2002) Exercise and the treatment of clinical depression in adults—Recent findings and future directions. *Sports Med.* 32:741–760.

Browne, E.S., Wright, B.E., Porter, J.R., et al. (1992) Dehydroepiandrosterone: antiglucocorticoid action in mice. *Am. J. Med. Sci.* 303:366–371.

Bruce, S.E., Weisberg, R.B., Dolan, R.T., et al. (2001) Trauma and posttraumatic stress disorder in primary care patients. *Prim. Care Companion J. Clin. Psychiatry* 3:211–217.

Brunner, R., Schaefer, D., Hess, K., et al. (2006) Effect of high-dose cortisol on memory functions. *Ann. N. Y. Acad. Sci.* 1071:434–437.

Cabib, S., and Puglisi-Allegra, S. (1996) Different effects of repeated stressful experiences on mesocortical and mesolimbic dopamine metabolism. *Neurosci.* 73:375–380.

Cabib, S., Ventura, R., and Puglisi-Allegra, S. (2002) Opposite imbalances between mesocortical and mesoaccumbens dopamine responses to stress by the same genotype depending on living conditions. *Behav. Brain Res.* 129:179–185.

Camacho, T.C., Roberts, R.E., Lazarus, N.B., et al. (1991) Physical-activity and depression—Evidence from the Alameda County Study. *Am. J. Epidem.* 134:220–231.

Carroll, B.J., Cassidy, F., Naftolowitz, D., et al. (2007) Pathophysiology of hypercortisolism in depression. *Acta Psychiatr. Scand.* (Suppl):90–103.

Carvajal, C., Dumont, Y., Herzog, H., et al. (2006) Emotional behavior in aged neuropeptide Y (NPY) Y2 knockout mice. *J. Mol. Neurosci.* 28:239–245.

Carver, C., Pozo, C., Harris, S.D., et al. (1993) How coping mediates the effect of optimism on distress: a study of women with early stage breast cancer. *J. Pers. Soc. Psychology* 65:375–390.

Chantarujikapong, S.I., Scherrer, J.F., Xian, H., et al. (2001) A twin study of generalized anxiety disorder symptoms, panic disorder symptoms and post-traumatic stress disorder in men. *Psychiatry Res.* 103:133–145.

Charney, D.S., and Bunney, B.S. (1999) The neurobiology of anxiety disorder. In: D.S. Charney, and E.J. Nestler, eds. *The Neurobiology of Mental Illness*. New York: Oxford University Press, 605–627.

Charney, D.S., and Drevets, W.D. (2002) The neurobiological basis of anxiety disorders. In: K.L. Davis, D.S. Charney, J.T. Coyle, and C. Nemeroff, eds. *Neuropsychopharmacology: The Fifth Generation of Progress*. Philadelphia: Lippincott, Williams & Wilkins pp. 901–930.

Charney, D.S., Woods, S.W., Goodman, W.K., et al. (1987) Neurobiological mechanisms of panic anxiety: biochemical and behavioral correlates of yohimbine-induced panic attacks. *Am. J. Psychiatry* 144:1030–1036.

Charney, D.S., Woods, S.W., Krystal, J.H., et al. (1992) Noradrenergic neuronal dysregulation in panic disorder: the effects of intravenous yohimbine and clonidine in panic disorder patients. *Acta Psychiatr. Scand.* 86:273–282.

Chen, L., Dai, X.N. and Sokabe, M. (2006) Chronic administration of dehydroepiandrosterone sulfate (DHEAS) primes for facilitated induction of long-term potentiation via sigma 1 (sigma1) receptor: optical imaging study in rat hippocampal slices. *Neuropharmacology* 50:380–392.

Chhatwal, J.P., Stanek-Rattiner, L., Davis, M., et al. (2006) Amygdala BDNF signaling is required for consolidation but not encoding of extinction. *Nat. Neurosci.* 9:870–872.

Claes, S.J. (2004) Corticotropin-releasing hormone (CRH) in psychiatry: from stress to psychopathology. *Ann. Med.* 36:50–61.

Cotman, C.W., and Berchtold, N.C. (2002) Exercise: a behavioral intervention to enhance brain health and plasticity. *Trends Neurosci.* 25:295–301.

Culver, J.L., Arena, P.L., Antoni, M.H., et al. (2002) Coping and distress among women under treatment for early stage breast cancer: Comparing African Americans, Hispanics and non-Hispanic whites. *Psycho-Oncology* 11:495–504.

Danner, D.D., Snowdon, D.A., and Friesen, W.V. (2001) Positive emotions in early life and longevity: findings from the nun study. *J. Pers. Soc. Psychol.* 80:804–813.

Davis, M. (2006) Neural systems involved in fear and anxiety measured with fear-potentiated startle. *Am. Psychol.* 61:741–756.

Davis, M., and Myers, K.M. (2002) The role of glutamate and gamma-aminobutyric acid in fear extinction: Clinical implications for exposure therapy. *Biol. Psychiatry* 52:998–1007.

Deaner, S.L., and McConatha, J.T. (1993) The relation of humor to depression and personality. *Psychological Rep.* 72:755–763.

Debiec, J., and LeDoux, J.E. (2006) Noradrenergic signaling in the amygdala contributes to the reconsolidation of fear memory: treatment implications for PTSD. *Ann. N. Y. Acad. Sci.* 1071:521–524.

Debiec, J., LeDoux, J.E., and Nader, K. (2002) Cellular and systems reconsolidation in the hippocampus. *Neuron* 36:527–538.

de Kloet, E.R., Derijk, R.H. and Meijer, O.C. (2007) Therapy insight: is there an imbalanced response of mineralocorticoid and glucocorticoid receptors in depression? *Nat. Clin. Prac.* 3:168–179.

DeRijk, R.H., Wust, S., Meijer, O.C., et al. (2006) A common polymorphism in the mineralocorticoid receptor modulates stress responsiveness. *J. Clin. Endocr. Metab.* 91:5083–5089.

Drabant, E.M., Hariri, A.R., Meyer-Lindenberg, A., et al. (2006) Catechol O-methyltransferase val158met genotype and neural mechanisms related to affective arousal and regulation. *Arch. Gen. Psychiatry* 63:1396–1406.

Drevets, W.C., Frank, E., Price, J.C., et al. (1999) PET imaging of serotonin 1A receptor binding in depression. *Biol. Psychiatry* 46: 1375–1387.

Dudai, Y., and Eisenberg, M. (2004) Rites of passage of the engram: reconsolidation and the lingering consolidation hypothesis. *Neuron* 44:93–100.

Dunlop, B.W., and Nemeroff, C.B. (2007) The role of dopamine in the pathophysiology of depression. *Arch. Gen. Psychiatry* 64:327–337.

Eisenhardt, D., and Menzel, R. (2007) Extinction learning, reconsolidation and the internal reinforcement hypothesis. *Neurobiol. Learn. Mem.* 87:167–173.

Eva, C., Serra, M., Mele, P., et al. (2006) Physiology and gene regulation of the brain NPY Y1 receptor. *Front. Neuroendocrinol.* 27: 308–339.

Fehr, E., and Fischbacher, U. (2003) The nature of human altruism. *Nature* 425:785–791.

Folkman, S. (1997) Positive psychological states and coping with severe stress. *Soc. Sci. Med.* 45:1207–1221.

Folkman, S., and Moskowitz, J.T. (2000) Positive affect and the other side of coping. *Am. Psychol.* 55:647–654.

Fontana, A.F., Kerns, R.D., Rosenberg, R.L., et al. (1989) Support, stress, and recovery from coronary heart disease: a longitudinal causal model. *Health Psychology* 8:175–193.

Frankl, V.E. (2006) *Man's Search for Meaning*. (I. Lasch, Trans). Boston: Beacon Press. (Original work published 1959)

Fulton, D. (2006) Reconsolidation: does the past linger on? *J. Neuroscience* 26:10935–10936; discussion 10936.

Gallagher, P., and Young, A. (2002) Cortisol/DHEA ratios in depression. *Neuropsychopharmacol.* 26:410.

Geracioti, T.D., Jr., Baker, D.G., Ekhator, N.N., et al. (2001) CSF norepinephrine concentrations in posttraumatic stress disorder. *Am. J. Psychiatry* 158:1227–1230.

Goldman, S.L., Kraemer, D.T., and Salovey, P. (1996) Beliefs about mood moderate the relationship of stress to illness and symptom reporting. *J. Psychosom. Res.* 41:115–128.

Goldstein, L.E., Rasmusson, A.M., Bunney, B.S., et al. (1996) Role of the amygdala in the coordination of behavioral, neuroendocrine, and prefrontal cortical monoamine responses to psychological stress in the rat. *J. Neurosci.* 16:4787–4798.

Goodyer, I.M., Herbert, J. and Altham, P.M. (1998) Adrenal steroid secretion and major depression in 8- to 16-year-olds, III. Influence of cortisol/DHEA ratio at presentation on subsequent rates of disappointing life events and persistent major depression. *Psychol. Med.* 28:265–273.

Grammatopoulos, D.K., and Chrousos, G.P. (2002) Functional characteristics of CRH receptors and potential clinical applications of CRH-receptor antagonists. *Trends Endocrin. Metab.* 13:436–444.

Greenwood, B.N., Foley, T.E., Day, H.E.W., et al. (2003) Freewheel running prevents learned helplessness/behavioral depression: Role of dorsal raphe serotonergic neurons. *J. Neurosci.* 23:2889–2898.

Griffin, M.G., Resick, P.A., and Yehuda, R. (2005) Enhanced cortisol suppression following dexamethasone administration in domestic violence survivors. *Am. J. Psychiatry* 162:1192–1199.

Gross, J.J. (2002) Emotion regulation: affective, cognitive, and social consequences. *Psychophysiol.* 39:281–291.

Gustafson, E.L., Smith, K.E., Durkin, M.M., et al. (1996) Distribution of a rat galanin receptor mRNA in rat brain. *Neuroreport* 7:953–957.

Haas, A.P., and Hendin, H. (1984) *Wounds of War: The Psychological Aftermath of Combat in Vietnam*. New York: Basic Books.

Hall, J., Thomas, K.L., and Everitt, B.J. (2001) Fear memory retrieval induces CREB phosphorylation and Fos expression within the amygdala. *Eur. J. Neurosci.* 13:1453–1458.

Harbaugh, W.T., Mayr, U., and Burghart, D.R. (2007) Neural responses to taxation and voluntary giving reveal motives for charitable donations. *Science* 316:1622–1625.

Hariri, A.R., Mattay, V.S., Tessitore, A., et al. (2002) Serotonin transporter genetic variation and the response of the human amygdala. *Science* 297:400–403.

Harvey, P.O., Fossati, P., Pochon, J.B., et al. (2005) Cognitive control and brain resources in major depression: an fMRI study using the n-back task. *NeuroImage* 26:860–869.

Hasler, G., Drevets, W.C., Manji, H.K., et al. (2004) Discovering endophenotypes for major depression. *Neuropsychopharmacol.* 29: 1765–1781.

Heilig, M. (1995) Antisense inhibition of neuropeptide Y (NPY)-Y1 receptor expression blocks the anxiolytic-like action of NPY in amygdala and paradoxically increases feeding. *Regul. Pept.* 59:201–205.

Heilig, M., Koob, G.F., Ekman, R., et al. (1994) Corticotropin-releasing factor and neuropeptide-y—role in emotional integration. *Trends Neurosci.* 17:80–85.

Heilig, M., McLeod, S., Brot, M., et al. (1993) Anxiolytic-like action of neuropeptide Y: mediation by Y1 receptors in amygdala, and dissociation from food intake effects. *Neuropsychopharmacol.* 8:357–363.

Heim, C., Newport, D.J., Heit, S., et al. (2000) Pituitary-adrenal and autonomic responses to stress in women after sexual and physical abuse in childhood. *JAMA* 284:592–597.

Heinz, A., Braus, D.F., Smolka, M.N., et al. (2005) Amygdala-prefrontal coupling depends on a genetic variation of the serotonin transporter. *Nat. Neurosci.* 8:20–21.

Heinz, A., and Smolka, M.N. (2006) The effects of catechol-O-methyltransferase genotype on brain activation elicited by affective stimuli and cognitive tasks. *Rev. Neurosci.* 17:359–367.

Heisler, L.K., Chu, H.M., Brennan, T.J., et al. (1998) Elevated anxiety and antidepressant-like responses in serotonin 5-HT1A receptor mutant mice. *Proc. Natl. Acad. Sci. USA* 95:15049–15054.

Herry, C., and Garcia, R. (2002) Prefrontal cortex long-term potentiation, but not long-term depression, is associated with the maintenance of extinction of learned fear in mice. *J. Neurosci.* 22: 577–583.

Hofmann, S.G., Meuret, A.E., Smits, J.A., et al. (2006) Augmentation of exposure therapy with D-cycloserine for social anxiety disorder. *Arch. Gen. Psychiatry* 63:298–304.

Holmes, A., and Picciotto, M.R. (2006) Galanin: a novel therapeutic target for depression, anxiety disorders and drug addiction? *CNS Neurol. Disord. Drug Targ.* 5:225–232.

Holmes, A., Yang, R.J., and Crawley, J.N. (2002) Evaluation of an anxiety-related phenotype in galanin overexpressing transgenic mice. *J. Mol. Neurosci.* 18:151–165.

Holmes, F.E., Bacon, A., Pope, R.J., et al. (2003) Transgenic overexpression of galanin in the dorsal root ganglia modulates pain-related behavior. *Proc. Natl. Acad. Sci. USA* 100:6180–6185.

Husum, H., and Mathe, A.A. (2002) Early life stress changes concentrations of neuropeptide Y and corticotropin-releasing hormone in adult rat brain. Lithium treatment modifies these changes. *Neuropsychopharmacol.* 27:756–764.

Inslicht, S.S., Marmar, C.R., Neylan, T.C., et al. (2006) Increased cortisol in women with intimate partner violence-related posttraumatic stress disorder. *Ann. N. Y. Acad. Sci.* 1071:428–429.

Isen, A.M., Daubman, K.A., and Nowicki, G.P. (1987) Positive affect facilitates creative problem-solving. *J. Personal. Soc. Psychology* 52:1122–1131.

Jabbi, M., Kema, I.P., van der Pompe, G., et al. (2007) Catechol-O-methyltransferase polymorphism and susceptibility to major depressive disorder modulates psychological stress response. *Psychiatr. Genet.* 17:183–193.

Janssen, J., Hulshoff Pol, H.E., de Leeuw, F.E., et al. (2007) Hippocampal volume and subcortical white matter lesions in late-life depression: comparison of early- and late-onset depression. *J. Neurol. Neurosurg. Psychiatry* 78(6):638–640.

Jordan, B.K., Schlenger, W.E., Hough, R., et al. (1991) Lifetime and current prevalence of specific psychiatric disorders among Vietnam veterans and controls. *Arch. Gen. Psychiatry* 48:207–215.

Josselyn, S.A., Shi, C., Carlezon, W.A., Jr., et al. (2001) Long-term memory is facilitated by cAMP response element-binding protein overexpression in the amygdala. *J. Neurosci.* 21:2404–2412.

Kaabi, B., Gelernter, J., Woods, S.W., et al. (2006) Genome scan for loci predisposing to anxiety disorders using a novel multivariate approach: strong evidence for a chromosome 4 risk locus. *Am. J. Hum. Genet.* 78:543–553.

Karl, T., Burne, T.H. and Herzog, H. (2006) Effect of Y1 receptor deficiency on motor activity, exploration, and anxiety. *Behav. Brain Res.* 167:87–93.

Karlsson, R.M., and Holmes, A. (2006) Galanin as a modulator of anxiety and depression and a therapeutic target for affective disease. *Amino Acids* 31:231–239.

Kask, A., Rago, L., and Harro, J. (1997) Alpha-helical CRF(9-41) prevents anxiogenic-like effect of NPY Y1 receptor antagonist BIBP3226 in rats. *Neuroreport* 8:3645–3647.

Kent, J.M., Mathew, S.J., and Gorman, J.M. (2002) Molecular targets in the treatment of anxiety. *Biol. Psychiatry* 52:1008–1030.

Kessler, R.C., Sonnega, A., Bromet, E., et al. (1995) Posttraumatic stress disorder in the National Comorbidity Survey. *Arch. Gen. Psychiatry* 52:1048–1060.

Khoshaba, D.M., and Maddi, S.R. (1999) Early experiences in hardiness development. *Consul. Psychol. J.* 51:106–116.

Khoshbouei, H., Cecchi, M., Dove, S., et al. (2002) Behavioral reactivity to stress: amplification of stress-induced noradrenergic activation elicits a galanin-mediated anxiolytic effect in central amygdala. *Pharmacol. Biochem. Behav.* 71:407–417.

Kida, S., Josselyn, S.A., de Ortiz, S.P., et al. (2002) CREB required for the stability of new and reactivated fear memories. *Nat. Neurosci.* 5:348–355.

Kim, J.M., Stewart, R., Kim, S.W., et al. (2007) Interactions between life stressors and susceptibility genes (5-HTTLPR and BDNF) on depression in Korean elders. *Biol. Psychiatry* 62:423–428.

Kimonides, V.G., Khatibi, N.H., Svendsen, C.N., et al. (1998) Dehydroepiandrosterone (DHEA) and DHEA-sulfate (DHEAS) protect hippocampal neurons against excitatory amino acid-induced neurotoxicity. *Proc. Natl. Acad. Sci. USA* 95:1852–1857.

Klemenhagen, K.C., Gordon, J.A., David, D.J., et al. (2006) Increased fear response to contextual cues in mice lacking the 5-HT1A receptor. *Neuropsychopharmacol.* 31:101–111.

Klohnen, E.C. (1996) Conceptual analysis and measurement of the construct of ego-resiliency. *J. Personal. Soc. Psychology* 70:1067–1079.

Knutson, B., and Cooper, J.C. (2005) Functional magnetic resonance imaging of reward prediction. *Curr. Opin. Neurol.* 18:411–417.

Koenig, H.G., George, L.K., and Peterson, B.L. (1998) Religiosity and remission of depression in medically ill older patients. *Am. J. Psychiatry* 155:536–542.

Kuhnen, C.M., and Knutson, B. (2005) The neural basis of financial risk taking. *Neuron* 47:763–770.

Lawford, B.R., Young, R., Noble, E.P., et al. (2006) The D2 dopamine receptor (DRD2) gene is associated with co-morbid depression, anxiety and social dysfunction in untreated veterans with post-traumatic stress disorder. *Eur. Psychiatry* 21:180–185.

LeDoux, J.E. (2000) Emotion circuits in the brain. *Annu. Rev. Neurosci.* 23:155–184.

LeDoux, J.E., and Gorman, J.M. (2002) A call to action: Overcoming anxiety through active coping. *Am. J. Psychiatry* 159: 171–171.

Lee, H.J., Lee, M.S., Kang, R.H., et al. (2005) Influence of the serotonin transporter promoter gene polymorphism on susceptibility to posttraumatic stress disorder. *Depress. Anxiety* 21:135–139.

Lee, J.L., Milton, A.L., and Everitt, B.J. (2006) Reconsolidation and extinction of conditioned fear: inhibition and potentiation. *J. Neuroscience* 26:10051–10056.

Maddi, S.R. (1999) Hardiness and optimism as expressed in coping patterns. *Consul. Psychology J.* 51:95–105.

Maestripieri, D., Lindell, S.G., and Higley, J.D. (2007) Intergenerational transmission of maternal behavior in rhesus macaques and its underlying mechanisms. *Dev. Psychobiol.* 49:165–171.

Makino, S., Baker, R.A., Smith, M.A., et al. (2000) Differential regulation of neuropeptide Y mRNA expression in the arcuate nucleus and locus coeruleus by stress and antidepressants. *J. Neuroendocrinol.* 12:387–395.

Manne, S., Duhamel, K., Ostroff, J., et al. (2003) Coping and the course of mother's depressive symptoms during and after pediatric bone marrow transplantation. *J. Am. Acad. Child Adol. Psychiatry* 42:1055–1068.

Martin-Soelch, C., Leenders, K.L., Chevalley, A.F., et al. (2001) Reward mechanisms in the brain and their role in dependence: evidence from neurophysiological and neuroimaging studies. *Brain Res. Brain Res. Rev.* 36:139–149.

Masten, A.S. (2001) Ordinary magic—Resilience processes in development. *Am. Psychologist* 56:227–238.

Masten, A.S., and Obradovic, J. (2006) Competence and resilience in development. *Ann. N. Y. Acad. Sci.* 1094:13–27.

McCormack, K., Sanchez, M.M., Bardi, M., et al. (2006) Maternal care patterns and behavioral development of rhesus macaque abused infants in the first 6 months of life. *Dev. Psychobiol.* 48: 537–550.

McCullough, M.E., Hoyt, W.T., Larson, D.B., et al. (2000) Religious involvement and mortality: a meta-analytic review. *Health Psychology* 19:211–222.

Milekic, M.H., and Alberini, C.M. (2002) Temporally graded requirement for protein synthesis following memory reactivation. *Neuron* 36:521–525.

Mobbs, D., Greicius, M.D., Abdel-Azim, E., et al. (2003) Humor modulates the mesolimbic reward centers. *Neuron* 40:1041–1048.

Moll, J., Zahn, R., de Oliveira-Souza, R., et al. (2005) Opinion: the neural basis of human moral cognition. *Nat. Rev. Neurosci.* 6: 799–809.

Moller, C., Sommer, W., Thorsell, A., et al. (1999) Anxiogenic-like action of galanin after intra-amygdala administration in the rat. *Neuropsychopharmacol.* 21:507–512.

Moos, R.H., and Schaefer, J.A. (1993) Coping resources and processes: current concepts and measures. In: L. Goldberger and S. Breznits, eds. *Handbook of Stress: Theoretical and Clinical Aspects*. New York: Free Press, pp. 234–257.

Morfin, R., and Starka, L. (2001) Neurosteroid 7-hydroxylation products in the brain. *Int. Rev. Neurobiol.* 46:79–95.

Morgan, C.A. III, Southwick, S., Hazlett, G., et al. (2004) Relationships among plasma dehydroepiandrosterone sulfate and cortisol levels, symptoms of dissociation, and objective performance in humans exposed to acute stress. *Arch. Gen. Psychiatry* 61: 819–825.

Morgan, C.A. III, Wang, S., Mason, J., et al. (2000) Hormone profiles in humans experiencing military survival training. *Biol. Psychiatry* 47:891–901.

Morrow, B.A., Elsworth, J.D., Rasmusson, A.M., et al. (1999) The role of mesoprefrontal dopamine neurons in the acquisition and expression of conditioned fear in the rat. *Neurosci.* 92:553–564.

Murphy, F.C., Rubinsztein, J.S., Michael, A., et al. (2001) Decision-making cognition in mania and depression. *Psycholog. Med.* 31: 679–693.

Myers, K.M., and Davis, M. (2007) Mechanisms of fear extinction. *Mol. Psychiatry* 12:120–150.

Myers, K.M., Ressler, K.J., and Davis, M. (2006) Different mechanisms of fear extinction dependent on length of time since fear acquisition. *Learn. Mem.* 13:216–223.

Nader, K., Schafe, G.E., and LeDoux, J.E. (2000) The labile nature of consolidation theory. *Nat. Rev. Neurosci.* 1:216–219.

Nemeroff, C.B. (2002) Recent advances in the neurobiology of depression. *Psychopharmacol. Bull.* 36(Suppl 2):6–23.

Neumeister, A., Bain, E., Nugent, A.C., et al. (2004) Reduced serotonin type 1A receptor binding in panic disorder. *J. Neurosci.* 24:589–591.

Orr, S.P., Milad, M.R., Metzger, L.J., et al. (2006) Effects of beta blockade, PTSD diagnosis, and explicit threat on the extinction and retention of an aversively conditioned response. *Biol. Psychol.* 73:262–271.

Otte, C., Neylan, T.C., Pipkin, S.S., et al. (2005) Depressive symptoms and 24-hour urinary norepinephrine excretion levels in patients with coronary disease: findings from the Heart and Soul Study. *Am. J. Psychiatry* 162:2139–2145.

Otte, C., Neylan, T.C., Pole, N., et al. (2005) Association between childhood trauma and catecholamine response to psychological stress in police academy recruits. *Biol. Psychiatry* 57:27–32.

Overmier, J.B., and Seligman, M.E. (1967) Effects of inescapable shock upon subsequent escape and avoidance responding. *J. Comp. Physiol. Psychol.* 63:28–33.

Parker, K.J., Buckmaster, C.L., Justus, K.R., et al. (2005) Mild early life stress enhances prefrontal-dependent response inhibition in monkeys. *Biol. Psychiatry* 57:848–855.

Parker, K.J., Buckmaster, C.L., Schatzberg, A.F., et al. (2004) Prospective investigation of stress inoculation in young monkeys. *Arch. Gen. Psychiatry* 61:933–941.

Parks, C.L., Robinson, P.S., Sibille, E., et al. (1998) Increased anxiety of mice lacking the serotonin1A receptor. *Proc. Natl. Acad. Sci. USA* 95:10734–10739.

Perez, S.E., Wynick, D., Steiner, R.A., et al. (2001) Distribution of galaninergic immunoreactivity in the brain of the mouse. *J. Comp. Neurol.* 434:158–185.

Pieribone, V.A., Brodin, L., Friberg, K., et al. (1992) Differential expression of mRNAs for neuropeptide Y-related peptides in rat nervous tissues: possible evolutionary conservation. *J. Neurosci.* 12:3361–3371.

Pitman, R.K., Sanders, K.M., Zusman, R.M., et al. (2002) Pilot study of secondary prevention of posttraumatic stress disorder with propranolol. *Biol. Psychiatry* 51:189–192.

Pliakas, A.M., Carlson, R.R., Neve, R.L., et al. (2001) Altered responsiveness to cocaine and increased immobility in the forced swim test associated with elevated cAMP response element-binding protein expression in nucleus accumbens. *J. Neurosci.* 21:7397–7403.

Przybyslawski, J., Roullet, P., and Sara, S.J. (1999) Attenuation of emotional and nonemotional memories after their reactivation: role of beta adrenergic receptors. *J. Neurosci.* 19:6623–6628.

Przybyslawski, J., and Sara, S.J. (1997) Reconsolidation of memory after its reactivation. *Behav. Brain Res.* 84:241–246.

Rabkin, J.G., McElhiney, M.C., Rabkin, R., et al. (2006) Placebo-controlled trial of dehydroepiandrosterone (DHEA) for treatment of nonmajor depression in patients with HIV/AIDS. *Am. J. Psychiatry* 163:59–66.

Rachman, S. (1979) Concept of required helpfulness. *Behav. Res. Ther.* 17:1–6.

Rasmusson, A.M., Hauger, R.L., Morgan, C.A., et al. (2000) Low baseline and yohimbine-stimulated plasma neuropeptide Y (NPY) levels in combat-related PTSD. *Biol. Psychiatry* 47:526–539.

Rasmusson, A.M., Vasek, J., Lipschitz, D.S., et al. (2004) An increased capacity for adrenal DHEA release is associated with decreased avoidance and negative mood symptoms in women with PTSD. *Neuropsychopharmacol.* 29:1546–1557.

Resick, P.A. (2001) *Clinical Psychology: A Modular Course*. Philadelphia: Taylor & Francis Group.

Ressler, K.J., Rothbaum, B.O., Tannenbaum, L., et al. (2004) Cognitive enhancers as adjuncts to psychotherapy—Use of D-cycloserine in phobic individuals to facilitate extinction of fear. *Arch. Gen. Psychiatry* 61:1136–1144.

Risold, P.Y., and Swanson, L.W. (1997) Chemoarchitecture of the rat lateral septal nucleus. *Brain Res. Brain Res. Rev.* 24:91–113.

Rodrigues, S.M., Schafe, G.E., and LeDoux, J.E. (2001) Intra-amygdala blockade of the NR2B subunit of the NMDA receptor disrupts the acquisition but not the expression of fear conditioning. *J. Neurosci.* 21:6889–6896.

Rosenfeld, R.S., Hellman, L., Roffwarg, H., et al. (1971) Dehydroisoandrosterone is secreted episodically and synchronously with cortisol by normal man. *J. Clin. Endocrinol. Metab.* 33:87–92.

Royer, S., Martina, M., and Pare, D. (2000) Bistable behavior of inhibitory neurons controlling impulse traffic through the amygdala: role of a slowly deinactivating K^+ current. *J. Neurosci.* 20: 9034–9039.

Rutter, M. (1993) Resilience: some conceptual considerations. *J. Adolesc. Health* 14:626–631.

Sajdyk, T.J., Fitz, S.D., and Shekhar, A. (2006) The role of neuropeptide Y in the amygdala on corticotropin-releasing factor receptor-mediated behavioral stress responses in the rat. *Stress* 9:21–28.

Schafe, G.E., Doyere, V., and LeDoux, J.E. (2005) Tracking the fear engram: the lateral amygdala is an essential locus of fear memory storage. *J. Neurosci.* 25:10010–10014.

Schafe, G.E., Nader, K., Blair, H.T., et al. (2001) Memory consolidation of Pavlovian fear conditioning: a cellular and molecular perspective. *Trends Neurosci.* 24:540–546.

Scheier, M.F., Matthews, K.A., Owens, J.F., et al. (1989) Dispositional optimism and recovery from coronary artery bypass surgery: the beneficial effects on physical and psychological well-being. *J. Pers. Soc. Psychol.* 57:1024–1040.

Schelling, G., Roozendaal, B., Krauseneck, T., et al. (2006) Efficacy of hydrocortisone in preventing posttraumatic stress disorder following critical illness and major surgery. *Ann. N. Y. Acad. Sci.* 1071:46–53.

Scherrer, J.F., True, W.R., Xian, H., et al. (2000) Evidence for genetic influences common and specific to symptoms of generalized anxiety and panic. *J. Affect. Disord.* 57:25–35.

Schultz, W. (2002) Getting formal with dopamine and reward. *Neuron* 36:241–263.

Seckl, J.R., and Meaney, M.J. (2006) Glucocorticoid "programming" and PTSD risk. *Ann. N. Y. Acad. Sci.* 1071:351–378.

Seligman, M.E., and Maier, S.F. (1967) Failure to escape traumatic shock. *J. Exp. Psychol.* 74:1–9.

Sevcik, J., Finta, E.P., and Illes, P. (1993) Galanin receptors inhibit the spontaneous firing of locus coeruleus neurons and interact with mu-opioid receptors. *Eur. J. Pharmacol.* 230:223–230.

Siebert, A. (1996) *The Survivor Personality: Why Some People are Stronger, Smarter, and More Skillful at Handling Life's Difficulties . . . and How You Can Be, Too.* New York: Berkely Publishing Group.

Sigurdsson, T., Doyere, V., Cain, C.K., et al. (2007) Long-term potentiation in the amygdala: a cellular mechanism of fear learning and memory. *Neuropharmacol.* 52:215–227.

Silver, R.-C., Holman, E.A., McIntosh, D.-N., et al. (2002) Nationwide longitudinal study of psychological responses to September 11. *JAMA* 288:1235–1244.

Smolka, M.N., Schumann, G., Wrase, J., et al. (2005) Catechol-O-methyltransferase val158met genotype affects processing of emotional stimuli in the amygdala and prefrontal cortex. *J. Neurosci.* 25:836–842.

Sotres Bayon, F., Bush, D.E. and Ledoux, J.E. (2007) Acquisition of fear extinction requires activation of NR2B-containing NMDA receptors in the lateral amygdala. *Neuropsychopharmacol.* 32: 1929–1940.

Sotres-Bayon, F., Cain, C.K., and LeDoux, J.E. (2006) Brain mechanisms of fear extinction: historical perspectives on the contribution of prefrontal cortex. *Biol. Psychiatry* 60:329–336.

Southwick, S.M., Krystal, J.H., Bremner, J.D., et al. (1997) Noradrenergic and serotonergic function in posttraumatic stress disorder. *Arch. Gen. Psychiatry* 54:749–758.

Southwick, S.M., Vythilingam, M., and Charney, D.S. (2005) The psychobiology of depression and resilience to stress: implications for prevention and treatment. *Ann. Rev. Clin. Psychol.* 1:255–291.

Steckler, T., and Holsboer, F. (1999) Corticotropin-releasing hormone receptor subtypes and emotion. *Biol. Psychiatry* 46:1480–1508.

Steptoe, A., Wardle, J., and Marmot, M. (2005) Positive affect and health-related neuroendocrine, cardiovascular, and inflammatory processes. *Proc. Natl. Acad. Sci. USA* 102:6508–6512.

Stockdale, J.B. (1991) *Courage Under Fire: Testing Epictetus' Doctrines in a Laboratory of Human Behavior.* Stanford, CA: Hoover Institution Press.

Strome, E.M., Wheler, G.H., Higley, J.D., et al. (2002) Intracerebroventricular corticotropin-releasing factor increases limbic glucose metabolism and has social context-dependent behavioral effects in nonhuman primates. *Proc. Natl. Acad. Sci. USA* 99:15749–15754.

Suzuki, A., Josselyn, S.A., Frankland, P.W., et al. (2004) Memory reconsolidation and extinction have distinct temporal and biochemical signatures. *J. Neurosci.* 24:4787–4795.

Swanson, C.J., Blackburn, T.P., Zhang, X., et al. (2005) Anxiolytic- and antidepressant-like profiles of the galanin-3 receptor (Gal3) antagonists SNAP 37889 and SNAP 398299. *Proc. Natl. Acad. Sci. USA* 102:17489–17494.

Tache, Y., and Bonaz, B. (2007) Corticotropin-releasing factor receptors and stress-related alterations of gut motor function. *J. Clin. Invest.* 117:33–40.

Thorson, J.A., and Powell, F.C. (1994) Depression and sense of humor. *Psychological Rep.* 75:1473–1474.

Travis, L.A., Lyness, J.M., Shields, C.G., et al. (2004) Social support, depression, and functional disability in older adult primary-care patients. *Am. J. Geriatr. Psychiatry* 12:265–271.

True, W.R., Rice, J., Eisen, S.A., et al. (1993) A twin study of genetic and environmental contributions to liability for posttraumatic stress symptoms. *Arch. Gen. Psychiatry* 50:257–264.

Tugade, M.M., and Fredrickson, B.L. (2004) Resilient individuals use positive emotions to bounce back from negative emotional experiences. *J. Pers. Soc. Psychology* 86:320–333.

Vaillant, G. (1977) *Adaptation to Life.* Boston: Little Brown.

Vaillant, G. (1992) The historical origins and future potential of Sigmund Freud's concept of the mechanisms of defence. *Int. Rev. Psycho Analysis* 19:35–50.

van der Kolk, B.A., and van der Hart, O. (1989) Pierre Janet and the breakdown of adaptation in psychological trauma. *Am. J. Psychiatry* 146:1530–1540.

Vythilingam, M., Heim, C., Newport, J., et al. (2002) Childhood trauma associated with smaller hippocampal volume in women with major depression. *Am. J. Psychiatry* 159:2072–2080.

Wade, S.L., Borawski, E.A., Taylor, H.G., et al. (2001) The relationship of caregiver coping to family outcomes during the initial year following pediatric traumatic injury. *J. Consult. Clin. Psychol.* 69:406–415.

Walker, D.L., and Davis, M. (2000) Involvement of NMDA receptors within the amygdala in short- versus long-term memory for fear conditioning as assessed with fear-potentiated startle. *Behav. Neurosci.* 114:1019–1033.

Walton, K.M., Chin, J.E., Duplantier, A.J., et al. (2006) Galanin function in the central nervous system. *Curr. Opin. Drug Discov. Devel.* 9:560–570.

Weis, F., Kilger, E., Roozendaal, B., et al. (2006) Stress doses of hydrocortisone reduce chronic stress symptoms and improve health-related quality of life in high-risk patients after cardiac surgery: A randomized study. *J. Thor. Cardiov. Surg.* 131:277.

Werner, E., and Smith, R. (1992) *Overcoming the Odds: High-risk Children from Birth to Adulthood.* Ithaca, NY: Cornell University Press.

Wheler, G.H., Brandon, D., Clemons, A., et al. (2006) Cortisol production rate in posttraumatic stress disorder. *J. Clin. Endocrinol. Metab.* 91:3486–3489.

Whitworth, J.A., Williamson, P.M., Mangos, G., et al. (2005) Cardiovascular consequences of cortisol excess. *Vasc. Health Risk Manag.* 1:291–299.

Winter, B., Breitenstein, C., Mooren, F.C., et al. (2006) High impact running improves learning. *Neurobiol. Learn. Mem.* 87(4):597–609.

Wise, R.A. (2002) Brain reward circuitry: insights from unsensed incentives. *Neuron* 36:229–240.

Wolin, S.J., and Wolin, S. (1993) *The Resilient Self: How Survivors of Troubled Families Rise above Adversity*. New York: Villard Books.

Xu, Z.Q., Tong, Y.G., and Hokfelt, T. (2001) Galanin enhances noradrenaline-induced outward current on locus coeruleus noradrenergic neurons. *Neuroreport* 12:1779–1782.

Yehuda, R. (2001) Biology of posttraumatic stress disorder. *J. Clin. Psychiatry* 62(Suppl 17):41–46.

Yehuda, R. (2004) Risk and resilience in posttraumatic stress disorder. *J. Clin. Psychiatry* 65(Suppl 1):29–36.

Yehuda, R., Brand, S.R., Golier, J.A., et al. (2006) Clinical correlates of DHEA associated with post-traumatic stress disorder. *Acta Psychiatr. Scand.* 114:187–193.

Yehuda, R., Brand, S., and Yang, R.K. (2006) Plasma neuropeptide Y concentrations in combat exposed veterans: relationship to trauma exposure, recovery from PTSD, and coping. *Biol. Psychiatry* 59:660–663.

Yehuda, R., Yang, R.K., Buchsbaum, M.S., et al. (2006) Alterations in cortisol negative feedback inhibition as examined using the ACTH response to cortisol administration in PTSD. *Psychoneuroendocrinol.* 31:447–451.

Young, A.H., Gallagher, P., and Porter, R.J. (2002) Elevation of the cortisol-dehydroepiandrosterone ratio in drug-free depressed patients. *Am. J. Psychiatry* 159:1237–1239.

Zeidner, M., and Hammer, A.L. (1992) Coping with missile attack—resources, strategies, and outcomes. *J. Personality* 60:709–746.

Zoumakis, E., Grammatopoulos, D.K., and Chrousos, G.P. (2006) Corticotropin-releasing hormone receptor antagonists. *Eur. J. Endocrinol.* 155:S85–S91.

87 A Brief History of Neural Evolution

DANIEL R. WILSON

Billions of years of evolution, millions of synapses, thousands of epigenetic neural pathways, and a new era of genomics . . . all explained in a brief chapter? Well, no, but Dobzhansky's (1964) aphorism holds true: "nothing in life makes sense except in the light of evolution" (p. 449). In the past century, neuropsychiatric research has recently been enriched by and, to a lesser degree, enriched genomic and evolutionary sciences. Still a far greater degree of mutual benefit is possible as genomic neuroscience and evolutionary behavioral sciences merge. Diverse data from neuroethology, evolutionary epidemiology, evolutionary psychiatry, and genomics spur further integration of and insights in these and other disciplines. Thus, it is useful to outline the truly ancient roots and foundational evolutionary facts of brain and behavior because a clearer picture of neural evolution is to be found in the increasingly complex heuristic systems that underlie the neurobiology of normative behavior and mental illness. To that end, let us first trace events leading to life, then on through many pertinent milestones, and the phylogenetics of neural transmission and higher assemblages of heuristic processes.

The narrative history of life takes us into what astro- and geophysicists term "Deep Time" from when the earth formed 4.567 billion years ago (bya) (Rutherford, 1939). Scientific work concerning how life evolved from nonlife, *abiogenesic biopoesis*, is of direct interest but until the past century was largely uninvestigated (Bernal, 1960). Indeed, folkloric and theogenic explanations prevailed in most cultures and little scientific progress had been made since 500 BCE when the Greek philosopher Anaximander proposed that the organic world evolved from a formless condition, with later transformation of species. Modern interest dates only to 1871, when Sir Joseph Hooker wrote to Charles Darwin that the original spark of life may have begun in a "warm little pond, with all sorts of ammonia and phosphoric salts, light, heat, electricity, etc. present, that a protein compound was chemically formed ready to undergo still more complex changes" (Huxley, 1918, p. 526). Yet insight still accumulated quite slowly, and there is not yet a fully "received" model of life origins although the process is known at least in outline. From primitive fossil microorganisms biologists note life on earth had emerged, by means of auto-catalytic chemical reactions, 3.8 bya (John Paul II, 1996). This geobiologic record also indicates subsequent diversity and complexity of life after oxygenic photosynthesis began 3 bya. This yielded an oxygen-rich environment that led to aerobic cellular respiration about 2 bya. A true science of abiogenesis traces to Aleksandr Oparin in 1924, whose experiments demonstrated Hooker's "primeval soup" could form organic molecules in anaerobic environs catalyzed by sunlight (Oparin, 1952). Moreover, these molecules would not only combine in an ever-more complex fashion until they dissolved into coacervate droplets (a colloidal inclusion cohering in spherical aggregations due to hydrophobic forces of lipid molecules) (Pratt and Pohorille, 2002), but also these proto-cellular droplets would fuse to form larger aggregates that eventually would fission into descendant droplets. Such "reproduction" was evidence of primitive metabolic factors that maintained integrity and survival of prebiotic cells (Pohorille et al., 2003). Thus vesicular bilayers with amphiphilic molecules were not only ancestors of early biotic cells but also were intermediaries by which nonliving matter in the universe came to life (John Paul II, 1996; Eigen and Schuster, 1971; Pohorille, 2007). The famous Miller–Urey experiments in 1953 expanded this line of research demonstrating prebiotic creation not only of bilipids membranes but also basic monomeric biomolecules such as amino acids (S.L. Miller, 1953; S.L. Miller and Urey, 1959). Bilayers built of amphiphilic molecules that form vesicles are protobiologically relevant examples (Deamer and Pashley, 1989; Dworkin et al., 2001). Alone, such vesicles are merely envelopes of encased "seawater" awash with molecules needed for primitive, abiologic chemical reactions. However, these had three major sequelae—adduction of biopolymers from monomers, intermediary stochastic metabolic synthesis of small molecules (including most of what are now termed "neurotransmitters"), and receptors embedded in cell membranes that activate a variety of iononotropic or metabotropic effects—notably signal transduction of transport processes (Engelmann,

1882; Jan and Jan, 1992). Even lacking many complex capacities of modern organisms, proto-cellular vesicles could—depending on composition or environs—undergo complex morphological changes such as growth, fusion, fission, budding, and internal vesicle assembly, as well as vesicle-surface interactions. Remarkably, even 3 bya such included mediation by transmembrane peptides and, perhaps, proteins (Rasmussen et al., 2003; Hanczyc and Szostak, 2004). Moreover, stochastic processes within coacervate vesicles led to polymerized nucleotides that eventually gave rise to ribonucleic acid (RNA) and simple ribozymes capable of self-replication by which coacervate cells entered into selective pressure to optimizing catalytic efficiency. This generated more diverse ribozymes, some that catalyzed peptidyl transfer, and as early ribosomes were organized, protein synthesis became common as oligopeptidergic-RNA complexes iterated more efficient protein catalysts (Tam and Saier, 1993; Andersson et al., 1998; Saier, 2003). By this point, life had been ineffably created.

From this basic sketch of processes by which protocells formed and began to include basic elements of metabolism, let us turn to a summary of how these truly ancient origins led to higher neurobehavioral assemblages. In most organisms, more than one fourth of proteins and a third of all genes relate to neural formation and regulation (McGinnis et al., 1984; Wallin and von Heijne, 1998; Aravind et al., 2003; Caveney et al., 2006). Remarkably, these essential adaptations evolved in the prebiotic era despite their essential contribution to virtually all life processes, notably neural systems. An understanding of such major themes in the evolution of neural life put much of neurobiology and mental illness into clearer context.

MAJOR MILESTONES IN THE EVOLUTION OF NEURAL LIFE

Eukaryotes and Metazoa

Until the past generation, discussion had moved little beyond Aristotle and Linnaeus (Dohrn, 1875). Although after Darwin, scientists increasingly emphasized evolution, phylogenetics had been unable to make any sense of the enormous gap between the earliest common ancestor of all life and the rise of eukaryotes (that is, nearly all complex cells and almost all multicellulates) (Knoll, 1992). Thus, 80% of bioevolution lay beyond science, notably nearly all events after prokaryotic life emerged from the prebionts 3.8 bya until eukaryotes arose some 2 bya (Valentine, 1994; Valentine et al., 1996).

This spans the Proterozoic Period, the 2-billion year geological eon before abundant complex life appeared on Earth 542 million years ago (mya) as the "recent" part of the Pre-Cambrian. Recent evidence indicates that signal transduction and membrane receptor activity arose in this remote era (Koshland, 1988; Hirabayashi and Kasai, 1993; Nelson et al., 1999; Anderson and Greenberg, 2001; Hille, 2001; Liu et al., 2002; Meinhardt, 2002; Golden, 2002; Miljkovic-Licina et al., 2004; Kirk, 2005). More precisely, prokaryotic evolution led to Archean eukaryotes in the Ectasian Period of the Mesoprotozoic Era, at least 1200–1600 mya (Knoll, 1992; Kumar and Rzhetsky, 1996; Butterfield, 2000; Lewis and McCourt, 2004), and perhaps even to 2.7 bya (Brocks et al., 1999; Denes et al., 2007; Sakarya et al., 2007). Details of eukaryotic origins are beyond the present scope, but briefly, eukaryotes are much larger than prokaryotes and, via endosymbiosis, they have unique internal membranous structures, organelles, cytoplasm (through which run cytoskeletal microtubules and filaments), as well as deoxyribonucleic acid (DNA) in proper chromosomes (Heckman et al., 2001; Sanderson, 2003; Yoon et al., 2004).

Definitive animals evolved from flagellated protozoa, the eldest living examples of which are choano-flagellates (collared flagellates akin to sponges) (Vaglia and Hall, 1999; Müller and Müller, 2003). Molecular studies place these in a supergroup called the "Opisthokontia" that include animals, fungi, and a few parasitic protists. Despite remote shared common ancestry, numerous plastid genes and ribosomal DNA are homologous in land plants and algae (Karol et al., 2001). Significantly with regard to the rise of neural assemblages, certain flagellate green algae can perceive sites where light is optimal for photosynthesis via a primitive eye—yet one with optics, photoreceptors, and an elementary signal-transduction chain. This visual apparatus, the earliest quasi-neural systems, dates to some 1,200 mya (Hegemann, 1997). Diplozoa, the earliest eukaryotic lineage diverging toward Metazoa, are defined by two linked eukarotic cells bound by intercellular tight junctions, gap junctions, and desmosomes (Cavalier-Smith et al., 1996). Diplozotes engendered Protosomes, for example, arthropods, annelids, mollusks, or flatworms (Aguinaldo et al., 1997), as well as Deuterostomes, for example, Echinodemata (radially symmetric, exclusively marine organisms such as starfish) and Chordata (more familiar vertebrates, including fish, amphibians, reptiles, birds, and mammals). The first distinct animal fossils include the earliest known complex metazoa, or multicellular organisms that arose in the Ediacaran Period of the Neoprotozoic Era, just preceding the Cambrian biota (Knoll et al., 2004). These appear at the dawn of the Phanaerozoic Eon, the current geologic eon. Apart from ediacarians, most known animal phyla appeared in the "Cambrian Explosion" 542 mya when—in a brief geological phase—all extant phyletic "bauplans," or body templates, of modern animals came into being (in addition to many other now long-extinct alternate forms). Yet nearly all living animals are in a monophylum, the Bilateria. Bilaterian bauplans are (with few curious exceptions) bilaterally symmetric and triploblastic with three well-developed germ layers that give rise to tissues forming distinct organs, and a digestive chamber with two openings (mouth and anus). The fossil record indicates animal phyla widely diverged in the Cambrian. Although the earliest unequivocal presence of bilaterians is from 555-mya fossils, recent calculations suggest Deuterosomia have Proterozoic origins (unimaginable until recent discoveries), with major lineages diverged prior to the first global glaciations in the Cryogenian Period amid the second phase of the Protozoic Era well before the Cambrian. The Cryogenian "snowball earth" was defined by the two heaviest ice ages ever on Earth; the Sturtian and Marinoan glaciations so heavily covered the planet between 850 and 630 mya (Kirschvink, 1992) that the Pannotian supercontinent fractured, causing rapid oceanic and atmospheric changes that brought 200 million years of the global ice age to an end, launching the Cambrian Explosion 542 mya. Such dramatic changes in evolutionary environs inevitably entail equally dramatic phenotypic reactions and extinctions as well as eventual phases of rapid adaptive radiation (E.O. Wilson, 1975; D.R. Wilson, 1998). After the glaciations ended, multicellular evolution accelerated dramatically. Triploblasts diverged by the mid-Proterozoic and chordates split from annelids 1.2 bya, from insects 1.1 bya, and from echinoderms (such as starfish) 1 bya (Wray et al., 1996; Kalyani and Rao, 1998; Seilacher et al., 1998; Schlosser, 2005). Still, in either the shorter fossil or older timeline, bilaterian biota were rather static until the cusp of the Cambrian 542 mya when characteristic Ediacaran fossil assemblages vanished. The dramatic radiation of bilaterians appears to have burgeoned after the end of the Cryogenian, perhaps via release of adaptive innovations due to but also constrained by the unimaginably snowbound conditions of that era.

HOMEOBOX, PLACODES, AND TERRESTRIALIZATION LEADING TO HIGHER NEURAL SYSTEMS

The bilaterian radiation was due, in part, to far more rapid selective dynamics powered by the evolution of sexual reproduction (Darwin, 1871, 1872). It was also an expression of the two most profound phylogenetic innovations for more rapid evolution—Hox genes and placodes. These evolutionary innovations allowed rapid terrestrialization, a major advance eliciting ever higher orders of neurobehavioral assemblages (Brugmann and Moody, 2005).

With the Homeobox came a potent means to direct wide-ranging morphogenesis of animal and plant development from a core bauplan expressed by highly conserved DNA. An entire family of Homeobox genes originated and duplicated at least 700 mya and perhaps 1.2 bya (Garber et al., 1983). This includes a special Hox cluster and a more specific Hox complex that patterns body axes by directing segmentation and growth. Profound diversity of organismic body plans across phyla actually spring from deeply canalized and tightly conserved master control genes that express extraordinary pleiomorphy via operations of the Homeobox complex (Gehring, 1998). Moreover, it has only recently been determined this complex drives many critical embryonic developments via embryonic placodes (Nielsen, 2001; Mazet, 2006; Rasmussen et al., 2007).

PLACODES AND NEUROBEHAVIORAL ASSEMBLAGES

Placodes are columnar thickening of embryonic epithelia from which cephalochordate organs develop. Neurogenic placodes develop atop the neural tube to generate paired sensory organs and ganglia (Goodrich, 1930; LeDouarin, 1982; Wada et al., 1998; Baker and Bronner-Fraser, 2001; Begbie and Graham, 2001; Graham et al., 2004; Holzschuh et al., 2005), diverse cell types (Smeets and González, 1992, 2000), and triune segmentation of the brain (Wada et al., 1998; Schlosser, 2005). Placode differentiation and genetic pathways that underlay their development are now fairly well understood. Evolution of the protoplacode arose at least with the earliest central nervous system (CNS) elements if not with the late eumetazoa up to 1 bya (Blair and Hedges, 2005). While Darwin (1859) long ago noted how human embryos seem more like the larvae of extant marine Ascidians (sea squirt), recent analyses of ascidian neural tubes—with fewer than 400 cells and fewer than 100 neurons—indeed reveal that tube induction closely follows patterns of more complex vertebrate brain (Wada et al., 1998). Moreover, ascidian homologues to vertebrate Homeobox genes controlling CNS development (*Pax-2, Pax-5,* and *Pax-8*) indicate ascidian (*HrPax-258*) arises from a single precursor gene with three later vertebrate genes via duplication and modification. Moreover, in a highly conserved manner, this Homeobox specifies three brain regions: anterior (*Hroth* homologous to vertebrate fore- and midbrain), middle (*HrPax-258* homologous to vertebrate anterior hindbrain and perhaps some midbrain), and posterior (*Hox* homologous to vertebrate hindbrain and spinal cord) (Wada et al., 1998). Subsequent vertebrate placodes gave rise to higher CNS elements including adenohypophysis, olfactory, optic, profundal, trigeminal, otic, lateral line, and epibranchial components (Smeets and González, 1992, 2000). An early next step in evolution of complex brain—mediated by placodes and Homeoboxes in chordates and insects—entailed tripartite anatomical regionalization along the anteroposterior axis: forebrain (prosencephalon), midbrain (mesencephalon), and hindbrain (metencephalon-myelencephalon) (Burnstock, 1969). During fetal development, these regions further subdivide as neurons migrate within subassemblages that address ever greater adaptive specialties including secondary dorsoventral differentiation. Thus, over a billion years of neurophylogeny, Homeobox genes and placodes subsumed increasing hierarchical integration, moving from simple poriferian neural nets to primitive bilaterian neurosensory assemblages, then to basic chordate neural tubes, onto cephalocordate parallel ganglial circuits and true sensory organs, leading to a vertebrate tripartite CNS, all well elaborated in the Paleozoic Era that began at the end of the Cryogenian. The specific genomic events that gave rise to these earliest manifestations of neural centrality are known in broad outline. A basic metazoan genome of nearly 20,000 loci suggests that vertebrate genes numbering 70,000 resulted from two early, massive duplications. Thus, bilaterian innovation—notably including brain evolution—was not so dependent on generation of new mutations as on tinkering with an extant genomic array (D.R. Wilson, 1993a; Adoutte et al., 2000). This new, more integrative phylogeny underscores the importance of developmental regulatory epigenetic networks in evolution (Jacob, 1977; Knoll and Carroll, 1999). Table 87.1 is a summary of the evolutionary sequence of key neuromental assemblages.

Although neurons are distinct from general somatic cells, their evolutionary derivation from less specialized cells is obvious. Living cells inevitably induce microelectrical potentials across membranes. This sets the stage in which phylogentic refinements of transmembrane conductivity evolved from random depolarization phenomena. Disturbance of primitive cell membranes alter electrical potentials only locally, yet rather basic refinements in the spatial and chemical aspects of cells gave rise to propagative depolarization that, coupled with synapsis, is the principle means of interneuronal communication. From such beginnings developed dispersed neural systems as evident in Medusa (jellyfish), with coordinated

TABLE 87.1 *Key Neuromental Assemblages*

Taxonomic Level	*Neural Structure*	*Age*
Prebionts	Monoamines and receptors	~3000 mya
Prokaryotes	Membrane proteins and channels	~2000 mya
Porifera	Neural net and prototissue	1100 mya
Chordates	Homeobox, placodes & spinal cord	>800 mya
Classic Reptilians	Midbrain	270 mya
Late Reptiles	Paleolimbus	120 mya
Early Mammalians	Limbocortex	60 mya
Primato-hominoids	Cortex	~40 mya
Hominids	Neo-cortex	1–2 mya

neural action to maintain a swimming sweep, but nothing anatomically identifiable as a nervous system in a "centralized" sense. The helminths are the earliest taxa with an overt central neural apparatus, that is, worms have a brain from and to which a neural cord entrains the rest of the soma. This arrangement is highly canalized in the HOX gene cluster with imago anatomical referents in all subsequent species (Vernier et al., 1995). Although a central brain of sorts is evident in helminths, much somatic "intellect" is retained at this phylogenetic level; decapitated worms can breed, feed, dig, locomote, and inure to mazes. With insects comes a brain compartmentalized into three sections—protocerebrum, deutocerebrum, and tritocerebrum—that coordinate end-organ activity via "giant fiber tracts." Indeed, insects have a larger sensory organ domain than any other taxonomic level including vertebrates (odors, sound, luminescence, texture, pressure, humidity, temperature, and chemognosis). Concentration of so many complex sense organs in the tiny capitum of insects is a feat of bioengineering efficiency that keeps depolarization circuits all the shorter and more alacritous. This accounts for the uncanny "intellect" all too often on display by insects—no doubt, intimately related to their status as the most numerous of earthly multicellulates. Vertebrates further refined and covered neural assemblages in a calcific armor through which ascending and descending tracts govern more advanced activities. With vertebrates, CNS emerges in as three anterior spinal cord enlargements constituting hindbrain, midbrain, and forebrain. Late reptiles and early mammals retained basic vertebrate structures but further accreted at the forebrain a paleocortical "limbic system" and then a range of domain-specific neocortical centers (Sperry, 1964). The efflorescence, plasticity, and self-awareness of these later structures is especially remarkable among social mammals, notably primates (about which more is discussed later in this article).

Although plants and fungi colonized land only 500 mya, arthropods and other early complex animals rapidly evolved, as sexual selection elaborated diversity while Homeobox/placode systems ensured efficiency in adaptation and canalized the classical terrestrial template of limbs extending along a gastric axis. Tetrapods diverged from lobe-finned fish 430 mya, amphibians 392 mya, and then early Amniotia (with embryonic amnion, chorion, and allantois membranes induced from thick stratified epithelium by thyroid hormone without amphibian metamorphosis) (Blair and Hedges, 2005). The amniotic tetrapod led to vertebrates including Sauropsidia (reptiles, dinosaurs, and birds) 325 mya and later Synapsidia (advanced reptiles and mammals) some 200 mya. Primitive mammalians emerged 200 mya, with subsequent elaboration through 140 mya but truly flourishing with primates from 80 mya to the rise of superfamily Hominoidea 25 mya, and especially genus Homo 2.5 mya (National Research Council, 1990).

This long, rather complex tale is important, as there is now a phylogenetically valid taxonomy from before the first to the present forms of life (Walde, Goto, et al., 1994; Walde, Wick, et al., 1994; Szostak et al., 2001; Pohorille, 2007). This lineage leading up and into the origins of the CNS, pertinent neurobiology, and behavior in higher organisms is not only worthy of further consideration, but also too little is known. With such basic phylogeny traced from prebiotic origins across several billion years, there is a better context to summarize several fundamental aspects of neural evolution that engender all the extraordinary capacities delineated in the other chapters of this book.

The Triune Brain in Evolution

The tripartite model of neuroethology even in an era of complex genomic neuroscience is the best available schematic by which genomic neuroscience can be reconciled with a clinically relevant understanding of normative and pathophenotypic aspects of neurobiological epigenesis. Only a prelude is possible for what will be a lengthy path toward a more coherent picture of neuromental evolution. The triune concept of brain, though now principally associated with the work of Paul MacLean (1990), is actually quite a staple of medical history. The Smith Papyrus, ca. 1750 BCE, is the earliest extant written reference to the neuromental apparatus, or "brain" (Garrison, 1917). However, the Egyptians paid so little regard to the neuromental substance that it was routinely disgorged from the skull and discarded even as the body itself was ritualistically embalmed for mummification and all other major organs were venerated in cenoptic jars. Nevertheless, 2,400 years ago Plato posited a tripartite model of brain in relation to behavioral regulation. This Platonic neuroscience is noteworthy in many respects, not the least by its close resemblance to arrangements of Homeoboxes and MacLean: "*Epithimetikon*" as the basic appetitive level over which operated "*Thimoeides*" as an apparatus of affect, and "*Logistikon*," a more rarified level of rationality. St. Augustine of Hippo, too, had a biotheologic tripartite system. Galen of Pergamum, among his many accomplishments, likewise propounded a triunian concept of neuromentality. Not only was he prescient in fixing "the seat of the soul" in the frontal lobes, he also further noted this lay above mere vegetative and animal levels of the brain. Freud, too, offered a highly influential triune schema with id, ego, and superego having obvious correlates in neuroethology (MacLean, 1952, 1990). Thus, via the extended vitality of Platonic, Augustinian, Galenic, and Freudian ideas, triunian concepts secured primacy for well more than two millennia of early neuroscience. Hence, any triune conceptual system has considerable resonance with essential characteristics of Western culture as well as subtle but inescapably religious overtones. So, old though it is, the triune framework entered the 20th century with remarkable vigor and soon came to explicitly influence contemporary neuroscience.

But other crucial discoveries accrued between the waning days of medieval scholasticism and the extraordinary growth of neuroscience in the new millennium. In 1664, Thomas Willis published the first dissection of distinct subcortical structures and assessment of their functional anatomy, namely, basal ganglia, or corpus striatum (Parent, 1986). The central position of distinct cortical and brainstem tracts led Willis to believe it was perhaps the "sensorium commune" of Aristotle, an imagined structure then thought to originate all motor efferents and receive all sensory afferents. However, neurology soon turned to cortical histology, and efforts to localize higher mental functions as cortical research reigned in the 18th and 19th centuries. Some research continued on the basal ganglia until it was discovered that functions long ascribed to it were properties of adjacent corticospinal paths and the striatum "seemed to fall from its high estate and depreciate in physiological significance" (Kinnier Wilson, 1914). Yet striatal research advanced rapidly in the early 20th century via experimentally induced lesion disorders of motor functions (Ramón y Cajal, 1911; Vogt, 1911; Kinnier Wilson, 1914), as the striatum reemerged amid interest about the "extrapyramidal motor system" in which it was grouped with brain-stem nuclei as a complete, independent motor unit (Carpenter et al., 1981; Parent, 1986). *Basal ganglia* generally refers to these major anatomical telencephalic subcortical nuclei at the base of the forebrain: formally the corpus striatum (striatum and globus pallidus) with the substantia nigra and subthalamic nucleus. Meanwhile in 1878, Broca published his crucial idea of *"le grande lobe limbique"* that began to quash a variety of popular quasi- and pseudoscientific accounts. Here it is necessary only to note how Broca was of a piece with the neuroethology soon to follow. In 1921, Loewi identified the *vagusstoff*—the first neurotransmitter, which has been known for less than a century. From this, a plethora of receptor subtypes and variations upon them continue to be identified in structure and function, as again neuroethology was greatly enriched. Then in 1937, Papez extended Broca's hypothesis toward a description of "mechanisms of emotion" of modern behavioral neuroscience generally and genomic neuroethology in particular.

An Overview of the Genomics of Neurotransmission

There has been an explosion of research data in basic and clinical neuroscience as well as genomics (Hyman and Nestler, 1993; Damasio, 1998) via confluent advances in laboratory and clinical research methods ranging from brain imaging to recombinant molecular medicine, as is well-detailed elsewhere throughout this volume. Indeed, a problem is the sheer abundance of neuroscience data that renders unwieldy any ambition to integrate an evolutionary perspective that, in itself, leverages even more data (D.R. Wilson, 1998). How, then, to proceed with evolutionary neuroscience?

We have traced how the brain evolved in a series of three main assemblages above the merely vegetative. Up to 400–300 mya, vertebrate brain-stem and proto-medullary formation mediated fundamentally asocial and purely self-preservative behaviors. Profound advances in brain occurred during the "age of dinosaurs" some 250 mya as over the next 150 million years this anlage evolved into classical reptilian hindbrain, basal ganglia, and midbrain that mediated agonistic social rank hierarchy based on subconscious, autonomic ritualized agonistic behavior (Price et al., 1994; Reiner et al., 1998). This began with the Permian-Triassic great dyings 251 mya, the most severe of earthly extinctions (96% of marine species and 70% of terrestrial vertebrates died) (Erwin, 1993). Thereafter, into the Jurassic and early Cretaceous Periods from 180 to 110 mya, these early theraspid (proto-social reptiles) neural arrangements passed into the elements of mammalian brain—the paleolimbic mediation of emotive social assessments and relative resource potential (MacLean, 1990). The Mammalian Period began as the thalamocingulate gyrus let mothers recognize distress calls of their pups—such enhancement of reproductive success was among the most fundamental of biogenic resource potentiality (MacLean, 1990). This phase also entailed rapid genomic innovation in all manner of mammalian features such as live birth parturition, mother–offspring bonding from lactation and beyond, thermoregulation, body hair, and advanced hormones and neurotransmitter circuitries, as well as social aggregations that induced kinship selection and eusociality (Gilbert, 1989, 1992; Dawkins, 1989; MacLean, 1990; Wilson, 1993b; Price et al., 1994; D.R. Wilson et al., 1999; Gardner and Wilson, 2004). The Cretaceous-Tertiary boundary 65.5 mya was marked by another major extinction in which many species—and all then extant dinosaurs—vanished in as little as a million years. This dramatic clearing of the competitive environment allowed mammals to flourish, especially eusocial orders such as primates and cetaceans (for example, whales and dolphins). From at least 50 mya, roughly when India began to subduct under Asia, primate-hominoid brain refinements occurred with increasing rapidity, including the refinement of what is now deemed the neolimbic system. In the past 15–20 million years, higher hominoid (apes in the human line) and later hominid (human) developments refined domain-specific, neocortical aspects of small-group behavior among conspecifics (MacLean, 1990; Gilbert, 1992; Price et al., 1994; D.R. Wilson, 1998). Thereafter, greater encephalization followed, with progressively increased neuronal and synaptic density, plasticity, and diversity in forebrain. This enhancement of the range of neural operations fostered brain and behavioral self-regulation of experience by which novel perceptuo-motor abilities, memory, and learning emerged. Talents grew in facial recognition, visuospatial and mathematical analysis, musicality, pictorial art, linguistic expression, and even quasi-theosophical or existential considerations (D.R. Wilson, 1994). This set the stage for further hominid encephalization as cortical capacity exploded over the past few million years.

An overarching and enduring theme of neuromental phylogeny is accretion of successively higher and more plastic reaction via complex integration as behavior channels perceptions in relation to environmental cues (Jaspers, 1963). Moreover, though such cues are directed to a wide spectrum of complex proximal biosocial ends, these are ultimately to maximize reproductive success. Such success is contingent upon acute and sustained recognition—via neuromental representation and summated behavior—of environmental referents. In the most reduced sense and apart from predator avoidance, such realizations must negotiate access to nutritional and fecundity resources. Indeed as seen earlier, even bacteria can sense and react to environmental realities, that is, chemotaxis. However, as biosocial environs become more complex in advanced mammals, so do neuromental processes of representation, analysis, and behavioral response. Such a phylogenetic perspective presumes a rather determined neuromentalistic apparatus. However, selectionist explanations only carry the phenotype so far, particularly with respect to complex behavior. It is certainly true that things are often quite tightly "wired up" (Gilbert, 1989). But complexities of advanced neural systems surpass semiotic encoding capacities of their genomes—human neocortex has some one thousand million million (1.0×10^{15}) synapses, while the total human genome has only 3.5 billion (3.5×10^9) nucleotide base pairs. Thus, genes appear insufficient to wholly specify neural circuitry. Normative neural ontogeny depends on phenotypic adjustments fitting genotype to individual environs. Much phenotypic adjustment is mediated by deselection of neurons within individual development. After in utero "blossoming," neurons undergo severe synaptic "pruning" via "expectant" reaction to experience (Edelman, 1988; Gazzaniga, 1992). This helps account for plasticity of behavioral phenotypes in eusocial animals. Because normal neuromental ontogeny is fashioned by selective loss of synaptic connectivity, it not surprising that the adult brain has increased—if incomplete—constraints on learning and behavior as well as "cortical blindness" due to insufficient expectant-experiential cues. Brains of eusocial animals result from elaborate bauplans, but these templates are modified by developmental experience. Moreover, the degree to which an organism's phenotypic reaction increases along the phylogenetic line (D.R. Wilson, 1993b, 1998).

EVOLUTIONARY EPIDEMIOLOGY OF NEUROTRANSMISSION

Great progress has advanced neurotransmitter biology so rapidly in the past generation that it is impossible to review in detail. Thus, our aim at this juncture is to relate key aspects of human neurotransmitter evolutionary epidemiology to related neuroethological research within a tripartite assemblage of brain in advanced vertebrates. To this end, evolution is being harnessed within a more manageable medical scope via an emerging subdiscipline of medical anthropology: evolutionary epidemiology (D.R. Wilson, 1998).

For the present purpose, it is sufficient to note that evolutionary epidemiology is a synthesis of basic population genetic operations merged with medical epidemiology. Evolutionary epidemiology changes epidemiological prevalence rates into population genetic frequency rates (D.R. Wilson, 2006). Among the applicable principles that, when rearranged, derive unique insights into psychopathology are aspects of population genetics, mutation, phenotypy, and evolutionarily stabilized strategies (Maynard Smith, 1974, 1976, 1982; Maynard Smith and Price, 1973; Maynard Smith and Parker, 1976). These can identify gene systems of population prevalence so high as to be best explained via advantageous natural selection (at least in the past environment of evolution). Indeed, evolutionary epidemiology strongly suggests that some epigenetic psychiatric syndromes are human genomic population polymorphisms (Huxley et al., 1964; D.R. Wilson, 1998; D.R. Wilson and Cory, 2007). We have noted that neuroscience and medicine have little considered the extraordinarily ancient nature of neurotransmitters, much less the degree to which the nervous system has evolved via gene duplication or "autologous cloning" within phylogenetically ancient families that can undergo terminal modifications that render advantageous otherwise merely neutral redundancies of cloned sequences (D.R. Wilson, 1993a; Vernier et al., 1995; Spudich and Jung, 2005; Tasmees et al., 2005). Although there is some consensus as to ancient origin of neurotransmitters, there is only dawning realization that subsequent evolutionary diversification of these moieties into a variety of receptor subtypes follows a hierarchical, triune pattern. Compared across species, subcortical subtypes are quite modal, whereas more phyletic divergence is noted in comparison to limbic microanatomy and remarkably more so in cortical tissues of the primate line leading to *Homo sapiens* (Dickinson, 1988; Fryxell, 1995; Vincent et al., 1998; Androutsellis-Theotokis et al., 2003).

For example, with respect to serotonin (Peroutka and Howell, 1994, p. 319), G protein-coupled receptors are a "superfamily" in species from yeast to man. The primordial 5-HT receptor evolved at least 800–1,100 mya, with the chordate line divergent as early as 700–900 mya. Mammalian 5-HT subtypes differentiated more rapidly over the past 90 million years, especially in the hominoid line over the past 20 million years (Hen, 1993). Similar evidence suggests dopamine receptors evolved via autologous cloning, with especially rapid diversification among mammals in the same time frame (Cardinaud et al., 1997; Cardinaud et al., 1998). Although all bioamine receptor subtypes are expressed in the CNS, generally within rather discrete circuits, the extraordinary proliferation in eusocial mammals arose as a genetic driver of encephalization that subserved more flexible neuromental function amid increasingly complex phenotypic challenges. Clearly, duplicate receptor genes can serve exaptation (Chang et al., 1996), and tissue-specific regulatory transaction factors can mediate advantageous adaptations (Previc, 1999; Seaman et al., 1999). Acquisition of novel "redundant" receptor epigenic range was a major feature of evolution in vertebrates, reptiles, and mammals, and a constellation of neurotransmitter subtypes evolved rapidly most notably in primato-hominids (Livak et al., 1995; Chang et al., 1996; Marchese et al., 1999). These subtypes modulate circuits which organize a variety of abstract cortical functions and cognitive skills critical to human life history—language, thought, fine motor praxia, executive planning, enhanced working memory, cognitive flexibility, abstract reasoning, temporal awareness, social generativity, and the emergence of self-awareness. Newer subtypes also enabled increasing (if incomplete) cortical modulation of reptilian and paleomammalian neuromental repertoires compatible with and validating a tripartite neuroethological hierarchy.

Four decades ago, it was proposed that many aspects of phenotypy may be due to temporo-spatial alterations in regulation of structural gene expression rather than functional changes induced by mutation (Zuckerkandl and Pauling, 1965). If so, morphological and molecular need be entirely codependent—that is, "two organisms may be phenotypically more [or less] different than they are on the basis of the amino acid sequences of their polypeptide chains" (Zuckerkandl and Pauling, 1965, p. 361). That organismic evolution may be modulated by gene regulation rather than mutation has been proposed as the explanation for observed discrepancies between rates of phenotypic and molecular evolution (King and Wilson, 1975; Valentine and Campbell, 1975; Bruce and Ayala, 1978). This affords empirical confirmation of important theoretical work in evolutionary biology, notably phenotypes that are "extended" (Dawkins, 1989) and "reactive" (Mayr, 1963). That natural selection would not eliminate the wasted energy and selective burden of frivolous genetic expression makes sense if extant templates for propitious adaptability are available in the form of structural and regulatory exaptations (D.R. Wilson, 1993a). Hence, examination of structure or activity of variant enzymes is necessary to appreciate distinctive features of related species and polymorphisms across and within species. Dopa decarboxylase (*Ddc*) is taxonomically conserved from alga to man, and the neural functions of *Ddc* are ancient as well. All animals have at least rudimentary catecholamine neural apparatus, and even plants have an analogue of *Ddc* (Rodin and Riggs, 2003). Examples of varieties via gene duplication followed by divergence of expression include several globin genes that evolved unique phenotypic effects (D.R. Wilson, 1998). If so, substantial phenotypic variability may be due to divergent lineages of structural gene regulation derived from a duplicated common ancestral gene rather than an entirely random mutation. This may account for what might otherwise appear to be directed evolution as well as the nuanced texture of phenotypic assemblages within and across species, perhaps particularly phylogenetic and ontogenetic orchestration of the complexities of advanced neurotransmission. To this end, studies have been made of factors necessary in sympathetic, parasympathetic, and enteric ganglia phenotypy—the autonomic nervous system, as derived entirely from early neural crest (Patten et al., 1999). Requisites include transcription factor Mash1, glial derived neurotrophic factor (GDNF; with its receptor subunits), and the neuregulin system. Each is necessary for euphenic differentiation and survival of autonomic neurons. Moreover, mice without Homeobox transcription factor Phox2b had phenotypic failure of all autonomic ganglia as well as three cranial sensory ganglia of the autonomic system. Similarly, Phox2b was needed for proper expression of GDNF-receptor subunit Ret as well as maintenance of Mash1 expression in the enteric nervous system and related peripheral sympathetic ganglia. Phox2b mutation also failed to activate genes for dopamine-beta-hydroxylase (DBH) and tyrosine hydroxylase (TH). Hence, two principal enzymes regulating biosynthesis and metabolism of neurotransmitters, their myriad receptor subtypes, and associated peptides are ontogenically regulated by quite specific cellular mechanisms accrued in phylogeny. Indeed, varieties and assemblages of noradrenergic, dopaminergic, and serotonergic (among other) neural phenotypes have been sculpted with extraordinary complexity and efficiency. Similarly, studies of noradrenergic neurotransmitter identity specification in neural crest stem likewise found Phox2a and/or closely related Phox2b crucial for expression of TH and DBH (Lo et al., 1999). Similar studies of protein transport evolution have given rise to phylogenetic trees (Saier, 1999). Also, neuronal restricted precursors can generate multiple neurotransmitter phenotypes during maturation in culture (Kalyani et al., 1998). These precursors are mitotically active, electrically immature, and express only a subset of neuronal markers, whereas mature cells are not only postmitotic but also synthesize and respond to specific subsets of neurotransmitter molecules including glycine, glutamate, γ-aminobutyric acid (GABA), dopamine, and acetylcholine. Individual precursors are clearly pleomorphic and can engender heterogeneous progeny with respect to neurotransmitter response and synthesis. Differentiation is further modulated by sonic hedgehog and bone morphogenetic protein moeities. Hedgehog is mitogenic and inhibits subtypal differentiation, whereas BMP-2 and BMP-4 inhibit mitosis and promote subtypal differentiation. Single-cell neuronal precursors can differentiate into multiple classes of neurons in response to environmental cues. Recent work on specific gene control of functional unit formation in cortex is revealing. Mouse genes *Emx2* and *Pax6* modulate a cascade of other significant ontogenic genes that are retained in humans with analogous structure and function (Bishop et al., 2000). Removal of *Emx2* reduced visual cortex and expanded motor cortex, whereas *Pax6* had opposite effects. From such work, fuller explanations of normative and pathophenotypic epigenesis has begun. Pertinently, cortical pathophenotypies in arousal (anxiety or abulia), affect (depression and mania), and thought (schizophrenia) all appear to be frequently linked to subtle genomic variance, some of which is due to gene duplication. At a minimum, it is clear that genes can formulate neuromental assemblages in quite specific ways and have done so in three modal aggregates—from the evolution of metazoan animals, through reptiles and early mammals, then on to advanced mammals. With this, it is useful to consider serotonin and dopamine in more detail and with reference to possible clinical applications (D.R. Wilson et al., 1999).

Dopamine and serotonin long have been thought to make up elements of a model of neuromentation in humans that begins to encompass normative and pathophenotypy of special relevance to mood and thought disorders. This preliminary model allows correlations between evolutionary factors, genomic neuroscience, and clinical perspectives. Generally, these moieties have reciprocal physiological effects, with dopamine a modally stimulating neurotransmitter and serotonin an inhibitory stimulating neuro-transmitter. Serotonin and dopamine subsystems clearly coevolved in the course of mammaloprimatoid brain and social evolution. Novel molecular analytic techniques have more fully elucidated evolutionary and genomic complexities of these neurotransmitter systems (Owens and Risch, 1995; whose excellent summary follows briefly here). Dopamine receptors were long thought to exist in only two types. More recently, at least five variant loci have been identified, some with considerable point polymorphism (Owens and Risch, 1995). An even more complex picture is obtained with respect to serotonin (Hen, 1993). There are even more detailed racemes in each of these neurotransmitter receptor families, both of which can be further grouped into at least two clusters of similar function and distribution. With respect to dopamine, five receptors have sprouted in the respective lineages of the original D_1 or D_2 typology. These aggregations reflect similarities in anatomy, physiology, and evolution. The D_2 cluster is of special interest, as D_2, D_3, and D_4 subtypes appeared later phylogenetically and were designed to facilitate higher level cognitive-affective expressions that evolved in response to mammalian evolutionary pressures, notably the mediation of conspecific social interaction. The D_1 cluster is manifestly more primitive. It subserves extrapyramidal tract and midbrain adaptations to more primitive selective pressures that shaped classical reptilian neuromental assemblages now deeply canalized in evolution. The distribution of each protein-typical messenger ribonucleic acid (mRNA) identifies diverse neuronal receptor networks in brain (Chio et al., 1990). Densities of the D_2 cluster localize to hypothalamic, limbic, and frontocortical areas far more than those of D_1. Such differential distribution helps explain efficacy with limited toxicity of antipsychotic drugs active in D_2 circuits (Owens and Risch, 1995). Striatal and pallidal subdivision of the basal ganglia are extant in many amniotes, but only with a paucity of cells, modest tegmental dopaminergic input, and little cortical input (Reiner et al., 1998). Amniote basal ganglia have a primary influence on motor functions via efferent links to the tectum. In sauropsids (modern amniotes, that is, birds and reptiles), striatal and pallidal aspects of basal ganglia are neuronally rich with similar neuronal populations evident across species (the striatum, in particular, receives significant tegmental and cortical dopaminergic input). The functional anatomy of basal ganglia is similarly homologous across amniotes, primarily as evident in motor efferents in cerebral cortex and tectum in mammals as well as sauropsids. Basal ganglia efferents to cortex are more elaborate in mammals than in sauropsids. This evolutionary elaboration occurred in the transition from amphibians to reptiles. These advances enabled amniotes to learn and execute more sophisticated repertoire of behavior—important adaptations for a fully terrestrial habitat. Only in the mammalian line, however, did cerebral cortex emerge as the major target of basal ganglia ennervation. Human striatum receives dopaminergic input from substantia nigra and ventral tegmental area (cell groups A8, A9, and A10) with structural and functional subdivisions rostrocaudally and dorsoventrally. These subserve motor and nonmotor origins for cortical dopaminergic projections to nigra and tegmentum. Distribution of dopaminergic elements through caudate, putamen, and nucleus accumbens vary across coronal sections (Piggott et al., 1999). Dopamine D_1 receptor density declines rostrocaudally in putamen but not caudate. There is significantly lower D_1 binding in structures posterior to the anterior commissure, whereas D_2 receptor density also increases rostrocaudally like the putamen/caudate. Density of dopamine uptake sites increases rostrocaudally in caudate, especially ventrally, but not in putamen. Dopamine D_3 receptors concentrate in ventral striatum, particularly nucleus accumbens, though without a rostrocaudal gradient. D_1 and D_3 receptors concentrate in striosomes, but D_2 receptors and uptake sites have higher densities in the matrix. Dopamine levels were equivalent in caudate and putamen but significantly elevated at accumbens and the anterior commissure. Significant elevations were evident of homovanillic acid and homovanillic acid/dopamine ratios in putamen compared to the caudate, especially caudal to the anterior commissure. Distribution of dopamine receptors and related metabolic markers not only evidence unique domains in striatal function but are germane to in vivo clinical imaging of dopamine transporter and receptor biology in neurological and psychiatric disorders. As molecular neuropsychiatry converges with and influences clinical studies of behavioral pathophenotypies, anatomical-functional anomalies at particular points along rostrocaudal, lateromedial, and dorsoventral brain axes are being delineated for specific diseases (Tsankova et al., 2007).

The rise of serotonin is akin to that of dopamine (Owens and Risch, 1995). However, serotonin is even more widely distributed in the brain (and thus may have less specific subdistribution than dopamine), and it clusters within four types with a total of more than a dozen subtypes. The rapid pace of discoveries in serotonergic neurobiology makes a detailed account of current knowledge not only difficult but also ephemeral and is, in any event, well beyond the range of present basic discussion. Assays of serotonin receptor mRNA densities vary considerably across brain regions; but, taken together, these indicate serotonin mediation of widely diverse cognitive and behavioral activities—notably, projections of the dorsal raphé-striatum. These are phylogenetically earlier features largely fixed in the course of reptilian brain evolution in a mode similar to D_1. Serotonin projections of medial raphé-hippocampal system evolved later to address different phylogenetic demands. Given their robust microanatomical links to limbic structures and functions, these later serotonin innovations modulate affective-cognitive demands that are the hallmark of mammalian social evolution (MacLean, 1990; D.R. Wilson, 1998).

These distinctive receptor subtypes derive from a phylogenetically common ancestral form. Each modification of the template branched off as an innovative subtypal resolution of specific selective pressures extant at different times in the environment of phylogenetic adaptation (MacLean, 1990). In mammalo-primatoid brain, such innovations modulated social behavior in increasingly sophisticated ways. Of course, many multigene and supergene families exist in eukaryote genomes (multigene families with uniform copy members like genes for ribosomal RNA, those with variable members like immunoglobulin genes, and supergene families such as those for various growth factor and hormone receptors; Ohta, 1989). Evolutionary epidemiological analyses indicate that natural selection favors those genomes with more useful mutants arising from templates of duplicated genes. Because any gene has a certain probability of mutation, success in acquiring a new gene by duplication may be expressed as the ratio of probabilities of spreading of useful versus detrimental mutations in redundant gene copies. Analyses show that natural selection and random drift are important for the origin of gene families. In addition, interaction between molecular mechanisms such as unequal crossing-over and gene conversion, and selection or drift, is found to have a large effect on evolution by gene duplication.

Such rapidly accruing insights concerning neurotransmission necessitated revised theoretical formulations in which normal thought and mood are contingent on orchestrated actions and diverse modulators, perhaps especially dopamine and serotonin, as well as many other transmitters, quasi-transmitters, and agents such as neurohormones, peptides, and endogenous opioids. Still, dopamine and serotonin are clearly important modulators of euthymia and sensible thought, whereas derangements in dopamine/serotonin physiology express disease such as psychosis, abulia, mood, and extrapyramidal effects. Psychotic and mood symptoms arise when prefrontal cortex and/or mesolimbic systems are hyperdopaminergic (Janssen et al., 1988; Davis et al., 1991; Meltzer, 1992). Serotonin depletion typically aggravates symptoms via initial escalation of mood and activity followed by irritability and thought disorder frequently accentuated by reduction of serotonergic circuits (P. Keck, personal communication, 31 December 1997). Moreover, compounds with high ratios of raphé-hippocampal-limbic circuit serotonin, S_{rhl}, to dopamine of the limbic type, D_2 (S_{rhl}/D_2) may be especially efficacious in the treatment of psychotic and mood disorders, including severe manic depression (Meltzer, 1992).

Serotonin inhibits dopamine striatal efferents, whereas serotonin reuptake inhibitors rouse mood but inhibit dopaminergic limbic structures, notably the nucleus accumbens, and can induce extrapyramidal effects. Moreover, lesions of serotonergic dorsal raphé tracts reduce neuroleptic-induced catalepsy. Serotonin effects on dopamine are modulated by receptors of the 1_A, 2, and 3 serotonin subtypes. The unique profile of clozapine microphysiology, in vitro and in vivo, is revealing in that it has increased affinity for limbic D_4 receptors and antagonizes 5-HT_2 moieties. These moieties elicit dopamine release "downstream" in the striatum and, thereby, limit extrapyramidal symptoms induced by dopamine antagonists elsewhere in the brain. Hence, abnormalities of thought and mood (largely mammalian capacities of positive and negative symptoms) can be ameliorated without significant effect on lower reptilian circuits evident in involuntary motor symptoms. Thus, novel antipsychotics improve psychosis and mood with few motor effects (5-HT_2 antagonism in tandem with D_4; Janssen et al., 1988). There is, likewise, a significant calculus of social rank hierarchy and particulars of serotonin-dopamine neurotransmission further exemplified by animal escalation and de-escalation behavior (Gawin and Ellenwood, 1988; Wyatt et al., 1988; Kosten, 1993). For example, cocaine is mimetic of manic and depressive symptoms. Acute administration increases synaptic dopamine—via the inhibition of presynaptic dopamine reuptake—which escalates mood and activity. Yet chronic overstimulation of D_2 eventually induces down-regulated physical dependence. Abrupt cessation of cocaine depletes dopamine and induces acute agitated depression, but a chronic syndrome of anhedonia, dysphoria, lethargy, somnolence, and apathy can extend for up to a year. All bioamine receptor subtypes are expressed in the CNS, typically within discrete circuits. Thus, bioamine receptor diversification was a key genetic mechanism fostering encephalization of the vertebrate CNS, particularly as such diversification would enable novel functions. Duplicate receptors are templates for exaptational changes in function arising in response to environmental challenge. These changes may, in part, be mediated by tissue-specific regulatory transacting factors (Stoka, 1999).

That morphological evolution progresses via gene duplication and subsequent alteration in molecular regulation—rather than only via gene mutation—is an appealing if elusive concept. It is appealing as the best plausible explanation for the robust and extravagant course of neuromental evolution among the eusocial mammals (E.O. Wilson, 1975), but it is elusive, as proof of direct evolutionary consequences for gene regulation will require years of detailed laboratory study. Still, confirmation of molecular mechanisms for abrupt emergence of novel yet salubrious adaption casts new light toward long-dark alleys of evolutionary science reminiscent but not repetitive of Haeckel's (1866) "hopeful monsters."

INTEGRATING NEUROTRANSMITTER BIOLOGY AND HAWK-DOVE GAME MATHEMATICS

In the emerging field of evolutionary psychiatry developments, progress converges in genetics and neuroscience, notably specification of how "social competition" affected the evolved basis of social behavior in humans (Price et al., 1994; D.R. Wilson and Price, 2006). Moreover, social competition has strong correlations with *(1)* tripartite hierarchy of assemblages of brain and mind (MacLean, 1990), *(2)* game-theoretical mathematical analyses (Price et al., 1994), and *(3)* evolutionary epidemiological-population genetic assessments (D.R. Wilson, 1998).

At this juncture, it is useful to summarize essential elements of the social competition model before relating it to kinship genetics or neuroscience. There is general agreement among evolutionary psychiatrists that mood disorders constitute some contemporary phenotypic expression of a phylogenetically healthy behavioral repertory (Lewis, 1934; Hill, 1968; Gilbert, 1992; D.R. Wilson, 1993b; D.R. Wilson and Price, 2006). That is, some variant phenotypes of current mood disorders performed adaptive functions among ancestral hominids. Phylogenetic precursors of what are now diagnosed "disorders" can be better appreciated to have assisted function in social competition (Price, 1967; Sloman, 1976; Gardner, 1982; Gilbert, 1992; D.R. Wilson, 1993b). The essential result of social competition in any taxon is that winners behave differently than losers (Price et al., 1994). Yet phylogeny appears to have modulated competitive drives as a key step in the emergence of sociality (Hamilton, 1963). Indeed, recent trends in studies of behavioral ecology posit that most social mammals cooperate or compete in one of two basic social modes (Chance, 1988). In clinical terms, these two modes, the agonic or hedonic, respectively, relate closely to syndromes of depression or mania and, in extreme elaborations, to psychosis. Clinical depression is readily identified in evolutionary psychological terms as a strategy of de-escalation or loss, while mania is a strategy of winning via engagement and assertion (Price et al., 1994). A further definition of the hypothesis is that humans retain, among other possibilities, a phylogenetically structured capacity to yield (become depressed) or assert (become expansive) in the face of socially competitive situations. Such social competition can be specified at several levels, and the hypothesis linking mood disorders to social competition may be expressed in hierarchical fashion. The hierarchy subsumes sexual selection, social stratification, ritualized antagonistic behavior, resource-holding potential, and social attention-holding potential, among other domains. These are skillfully detailed elsewhere (Gilbert, 1992; Price et al., 1994).

In the most fundamental sense, mood disorders appear to have emerged *(1)* in taxonomic terms at the reptilian-mammalian interface and *(2)* in neurobiological terms at the subcortical-limbic interface. Yet such interfaces are not, in themselves, defining aspects of mammalo-primatoid psychology. In the hominoid line, attainment of social dominance via appeal and prestige rather than hierarchical threat has come to characterize social behavior (Barkow, 1989; Gilbert, 1992). Put differently, influence rather than intimidation is the avenue to social dominance among primates. In humans, social competition induces yielding or assertion that may cause dysregulation, especially when there is a crescendo of interpersonal affects. More modulated escalations or de-escalations may have been adaptive in the environment of evolutionary adaptation. However in the context of contemporary culture, further dysregulation may constitute a syndrome of clinical depression or mania. Consequently, neurotransmitter genomics of mood disorders are relevant in that these molecules subserve crucial variations in the phenotypic expression of behavior. In most mammals, reproductive success depends on success in various social roles. One key role is in besting others who are pursing the same resources (Barash, 1977; Gilbert, 1989; Trivers, 1971). As noted earlier, primate social hierarchy is a key factor in reproductive and social success. Those higher up have more breeding opportunities and often make the more attractive allies than those lower down. Navigation of hierarchical relationships wherein some are more powerful than others has been a selective pressure for millions of years. Social neuromentalities evolved in the context of either competition or cooperation. Further, these evolved neuromentalities propitiate adoption of predictable, context-dependent roles and behaviors that modulate competition and cooperation (Nesse, 1990). In some respects, social neuromentalities are synonymous with the everyday term *state of mind* to the extent that each embodies algorithms of social roles. Gradations in states of mind are to be expected between individuals across the social hierarchy—the state of mind of a dominant surely differs from that of subordinates. The consequences can be profound. Most remarkably, in some fish, inhibition can cause change of sex (significantly, a subordinate's genes can be maintained by mating with dominants; Keenleyside, 1979). Likewise, dominant naked mole rats and New World monkeys have been observed to directly suppress sexual reproductive physiology in subordinates (Abbott et al., 1989). Studies have also documented major biological distinctions between dominant and subordinate baboons, notably stress hormones that have been linked to the pathophysiology of affective and anxiety disorders (Sapolsky, 1989, 1990a, 1990b; Ray and Sapolsky, 1992). Biological profiles of subordinates differ from those of more dominant animals in other species (Henry and Stephens, 1977; Henry, 1982). Pharmacological probes are also revealing. Drug effects vary between dominant and subordinate animals, sometimes quite markedly. For example, the social rank of rhesus monkeys given amphetamine determines key aspects of response. Dominants showed increased threat, chase, and attack behaviors, whereas subordinates showed increased submissive behavior—for example, fear grimaces and turning away (Harbor et al., 1981). Likewise, amphetamine was given to a female rhesus monkey that moved between two groups. In the first group, she was highly subordinate, isolative, and fearful, with quite limited affiliation. Amphetamine accentuated all of these submissive behavioral patterns quite dramatically. However, when moved to a new group, she was conspicuously favored by the alpha male. Her behavior changed her markedly with this increased rank. When administered amphetamine, in this novel social milieu her threats as the dominant female increased dramatically, and she did not submit as before but instead increased her social assertion. Other empirical studies confirm that social competition psychobiologically modulates mood states and cognition in primates. A recent review of neuroendocrine correlates of social rank confirms that endocrine states are highly sensitive to social feedback (Sapolsky, 1993). Hormone levels in dominant and subordinate animals vary as a function of group stability. However, instability of the social rank hierarchy affects individuals differently with respect to directional trends in rank (going up vs. down) as well as basic temperament (Sapolsky, 1994). In this sense, dominance-subordination is controlled by sociophysiological feedback in the environment. Perhaps the most significant evidence to date is the correlation of the primate social rank spectrum with serotonin parameters that mirror human mood swings. Physiological changes can be the cause and consequence of rank changes (Raleigh et al., 1984; Hartmann, 1992). Blood levels of serotonin are significantly higher in dominant male vervet monkeys as compared to their subordinates (Raleigh et al., 1984). Sham deposition of the alpha male was followed by a sharp fall in his serotonin blood level but a sharp rise in that of the subordinate male who was raised to dominant status. Restoration some weeks later of the formerly dominant male was marked by a reversal of these serotonin findings as well as his renewed tenure as the group alpha. Significantly, restoration led to a fall in social rank and serotonin level of the "new" dominant below that of his original beta baseline. Social ascendance with subsequent fall in rank leaves subordinates in a lower biosocial status than if no change had occurred. Sex hormones similarly reflect such social contexts. Androgen levels in humans, male and female, vary at baseline, both depending on the degree of social competition or cooperation, and also vary directly with success in competitive games (Kemper, 1984). These rises can include even nonphysical contests such as chess (Mazure et al., 1992). Thus, neurotransmitter and endocrine parameters not only reflect general features of social status, affect, and mood but also directly link to reproductive biology itself. With this, it is useful to begin to integrate the social competition with general patterns of neurotransmitter genomics and game mathematics within a tripartite hierarchy (Table 87.2).

Although this chapter is of necessity only a preliminary cross-correlation of data and models, clearly major subtypes of neurotransmitter receptors have unique anatomical distributions and functional consequences, as seems particularly true of serotonin and dopamine. Such consequences are quite germane to, among other concerns, the resolution of phenotypic challenges engendered by competition within an increasingly complex social milieu as well as diverse nosological conundra (Wilson, 1993b; Miller et al., 2006). This resolution is most often accomplished via innovative capacities for cognitive-affective assessment and behavior. These capacities increasingly typified the brains and psychology of first reptiles, then social mammals, and most distinctively, the primates (Dunbar, 1988; Mithen, 1996) in a manner almost wholly compatible with and anticipated by MacLean (1990). The evolutionary epidemiology and functional anatomy of neurotransmitters sketched here contextualize the neurobiology of psychopathology, particularly as arises when the phylogenetically hierarchical triune brain meets novel ontogenic demands. Thus, some psychopathology is phenotypic reactivity of enduring population polymorphisms—polygenic or Mendelian—of a human genome increasingly mismatched in the contemporary environs. Major subtypes of neurotransmitter receptors have anatomical distributions and behavioral consequences greatly affecting resolution of social competition via innovative affective talents that increasingly characterize the neuromentality of social mammals.

It has long been assumed that the brain evolved gradually with later accretions controlling earlier parts, generally by inhibition. MacLean (1990) noted that the forebrain had three distinct and relatively independent "central processing assemblies" to address subsequent environmental challenges. Ever-more-subtle neuromentalities successively overlay assemblages of basic vertebrates, classic reptiles, and then early mammals. Classic reptilian forebrain, as noted above, evolved 250 mya from fish, amphibian, and even earlier eumetazoan neural systems. Insofar as reptiles socially relate, it is for mating with the opposite sex or agonistic competition with the same sex. In humans, a reptilian brain remains in the basal ganglia. Thereafter, a paleomammalian brain, or limbic system, evolved to facilitate mammalian social life, parent/offspring bonds, play, and other social activity not seen in reptiles. But this assemblage also had to address issues faced by reptiles, that is, mate courtship and rival competition. Soon a neomammalian brain, or cortex, evolved in eusocial animals to subserve rational thought and decision making. These capacities are essential to problems in the modern world—technology, litigation, or politics. But they, too, affect problems as addressed by reptilian and paleomammalian brains, if in a (generally) more sophisticated and rational manner. At least 120 million years of mammalian evolution has brought about extraordinary innovations such as thermoregulation, complex hormones for birth, lactation, and the thalamocingulate gyrus that together cement mother–child bonds—all as the basis for greater eusociality mediated via paleolimbic and neuroendocrine structures. Thereafter, from some 50 mya, primate evolution optimized the social brain (Gardner and Wilson, 2004), with skills deriving from life in small, rather egalitarian, kinship bands of foragers. The evolving limbic system and cortex enabled the emergence of complex, abstract intellect, language, and other domain-specific talents such as artistic, mathematical, and musical abilities as well as religiosity and tale-telling. In this environment of evolutionary adaptation, the limbic system and neocortex expanded with

TABLE 87.2 *Neuroethological Evolutionary Epidemiology: Dual Strategies at Three Brain Levels*

	TWO SOCIAL STRATEGIES	
	Escalate	*De-escalate*
THREE BRAIN LEVELS		
Primatomammalian Cortex		
Game: Social Attention-Holding Potential	Attractive display	Social avoidance
Cognition > affect > instinct	Manic/sociopathic	Depressed/obsessed
Rational, sociotropic, and cognitive	Optimistic, charming	Pessimistic, ashamed
Prestige > agonistic competition		
Prestige – actions	Adopt new goals	Give up goals
	Self-assert	Self-efface
Agonistic – feelings	Stubborn	Submissive
	Courageous	Escapist
Mediators: Advanced hormones and peptides		
$S_2 > S_1$, D_3, $D_4 > D_1$	S_2, D_3, D_4, & NE High	S_2 Low, D_3, D_4, & NE?
Paleomammalian Limbic		
Game: Resource-Holding Potential	Dominant	Submissive
Affect > cognition	Aggressive/sadistic	Morbid/masochistic
Emotionally acquisitive	Confident, likely to win	Unsure, likely to lose
Agonistic > prestige competition		
Prestige – actions	Exhilarated	Shamed and guilty
	Enthusiastic	Sense of failure
Agonistism – feelings	Angry or hostile	Inferiority or anxiety
	Emotions aroused	Emotions depressed
Mediators: Primitive hormones and peptides		
$S_1 > S_2$, D_2, D_3, $D_4 > D_1$, + EPS	S_1, D_3, D_4, & NE High	S_1, D_3, D_4, & NE Low
Reptilian Midbrain		
Game: Ritualized Agonistic Behavior	Fighting	Fleeing
Instinctive territorial	Strident, strong	Cowering, weak
Instinct > affect > cognition	Violent, solipsistic	Frightful, abulic
Agonistic competition	Autonomic dominance	Autonomic meekness
	Mood elevated	Mood depressed
Mediators: Few neurohormones and peptides		
$S_1 >> S_2 << D_1 >> D_2$, D_3, D_4	D_1 and NE High, S?	D_1 and NE Low, S?

S: serotonin, with subtypes; D: dopamine, with subtypes; NE: norepinephrine; EPS: extrapyramidal symptoms.

new variations of neurotransmitters, neurohormones, and other modulators of kin and quasi-kin relationships that endured across the life cycle as personal traits allowed fellow travelers to confer or withhold social esteem. A complex balance between competition and cooperation built on older modules of reptilian and early mammalian neuromentalities "emancipated" brain evolution from a preoccupation with threat assessment and harm avoidance, to turn to play and discovery. Quite amazingly, this proto-hominoid pattern was established by the Miocene Epoch—before India hit Asia and orogenated the Himalayas.

Neurobiology thus must strive to understand three brains dealing with similar problems in somewhat different ways. To some extent, the three cooperate, but there is much autonomy as they attend to different sources of information, make different levels of decisions, and have different cognitive representations. This surprising triune situation is not one that an engineer would design as the most sophisticated thinking machine ever evolved. Perhaps most surprising is that the rational brain has little control over the two lower brains and, quite as Plato noted millennia ago, the driver is in control of neither the horse nor the cart and further affirms Darwin's view that in expression of emotion, the differences "between man and higher animals, great as it is, is one of degree and not of kind" (Darwin, 1872, p. 390).

REFERENCES

Abbott, D.H., Barrette, J., Faulkes, C.G., and George, A. (1989) Social contraception in naked mole rats and marmoset monkeys. *J. Zoology London* 219:703–710.

Adoutte, A., Balavoine, G., Lartillot, N., Lespinet, O., Prud'homme, B., and de Rosa, R. (2000) Special feature: perspective: the new animal phylogeny: reliability and implications *Proc. Natl. Acad. Sci. USA* 97(9):4453–4456.

Aguinaldo, A.M.A., Turbeville, J.M., Linford, L.S., Rivera, M.C., Garey, J.R., Raff, R.A., and Lake, J. A. (1997) Evidence for a clade of nematodes, arthropods and other moulting animals. *Nature* 387:489–493.

Anderson, P.A., and Greenberg, R.M. (2001) Phylogeny of ion channels: clues to structure and function. *Comp. Biochem. Physiol. B Biochem. Mol. Biol.* 129(1):17–28.

Andersson, S.G., Zomorodipour, A., Andersson, J.O., Sicheritz-Ponten, T., Alsmark, U.C., Podowski, R.M., Naslund, A.K., Eriksson, A.S., Winkler, H.H., and Kurland. C.G. (1998) The genome sequence of Rickettsia prowazekii and the origin of mitochondria. *Nature* 396:133–140.

Androutsellis-Theotokis, A., Goldberg, N.R., Ueda, K., Beppu, T., Beckman, M.L., Das, S., Javitch, J.A., and Rudnick, R. (2003) Characterization of a functional bacterial homologue of sodium-dependent neurotransmitter transporters *J. Biol. Chem.* 278(15):12703–12709.

Aravind, L., Anantharaman, V., and Iyer, L.M. (2003) Evolutionary connections between bacterial and eukaryotic signaling systems: a genomic perspective. *Curr. Opin. Microbiol.* 6(5):490–497.

Barash, D.P. (1977) *Sociobiology and behavior*. London: Heineman.

Barkow, J. (1989) *Darwin, sex and status: biological approaches to mind and culture.* Toronto, Canada: University of Toronto Press.

Baker, C.V.H., and Bronner-Fraser, M. (2001) Vertebrate cranial placodes. I. Embryonic induction. *Dev. Biol.* 232:1–6.

Begbie, J., and Graham, A. (2001) Integration between the epibranchial placodes and the hindbrain. *Science* 294:595–598.

Bernal, J.D. (1960) The problem of stages in biopoesis. In: Florkin, M., ed. *Aspects of the Origin of Life.* London: Pergamon Press, pp. 30–45.

Bishop, K.M., Goudreau, G., and O'Leary, D.D. (2000) Regulation of area identity in mammalian neocortex by Emx2 and Pax6. *Science* 288:344–349.

Blair, J.E., and Hedges, S.B. (2005) Molecular phylogeny and divergence times of deuterostome animals. *Mol. Biol. Evol.* 22(11): 2275–2284.

Broca, P. (1878) Anatomie comparée des circonvolutions cérébrales: le grand lobe limbique [Comparative anatomy of cerebral circumvolutions: the great limbic lobe] *Rev. Anthropol.* 1:385–498.

Brocks, J.J, Logan, G.A., Buick, R., and Summons, R.E. (1999) Archean molecular fossils and the early rise of eukaryotes. *Science* 285:1033–1036.

Bruce, E.J., and Ayala, F.J. (1978) Humans and apes are genetically very similar. *Nature* 276(5685):264–265.

Brugmann, S.A., and Moody, S.A. (2005) Induction and specification of the vertebrate ectodermal placodes: precursors of the cranial sensory organs. *Biol. Cell.* 97(5):303–319.

Burnstock, G. (1969) Evolution of the autonomic innervation of visceral and cardiovascular systems in vertebrates. *Pharmacol. Rev.* 21:247–324.

Butterfield, N.J. (2000) *Bangiomorpha pubescens* n. gen., n. sp.: implications for the evolution of sex, multicellularity, and the Mesoproterozoic/Neoproterozoic radiation of eukaryotes. *Paleobiology* 26(3):386–404.

Cardinaud, B., Gibert, J.M., Sugamori, K.S., Vincent, J.D., Niznik, H.B., and Vernier P. (1998) Review. Comparative aspects of dopaminergic neurotransmission in vertebrates. *Ann. N. Y. Acad. Sci.* 839:47–52.

Cardinaud, B., Sugamori, K.S., Coudouel, S., Vincent, J.D., Niznik, H.B., and Vernier, P. (1997) Early emergence of three dopamine D1 receptor subtypes in vertebrates. Molecular phylogenetic, pharmacological, and functional criteria defining D1A, D1B, and D1C receptors in European eel Anguilla anguilla. *J. Biol. Chem.* 272(5):2778–2787.

Carpenter, M.B., Carleton, S.C., Keller, J.T., and Conte, P. (1981) Connections of the subthalamic nucleus in the monkey. *Brain Res.* 224:1–29.

Caveney, S., Cladman, W., Verellen, L., and Donly, C. (2006) Ancestry of neuronal monoamine transporters in the Metazoa. *J. Exp. Biol.* 209:4858–4868.

Cavalier-Smith, T., Allsopp, M.T.E.P., Chao, E.E., Boury, E.N., and Vacelet, J. (1996) Sponge phylogeny, animal monophyly, and the origin of the nervous system: 18S rRNA evidence. *Can. J. Zool.* 74:2031–2045.

Chance, M. (1988) *Social fabrics of the mind.* Hove, UK: Lawrence Erlbaum.

Chang, F.M., Kidd, J.R., Livak, K.J., Pakstis, A.J., and Kidd, K.K. (1996) The world-wide distribution of allele frequencies at the human dopamine D4 receptor locus. *Hum. Genet.* 98(1):91–101.

Chio, C.L., Hess, G.F., Graham, R.S., and Huff, R.M. (1990) A second molecular form of D2 dopamine receptor in rat and bovine caudate nucleus. *Nature* 343(6255):266–269.

Damasio, A.R. (1998) *The feeling of what happens. Body and emotion in the making of consciousness.* New York: Harcourt Brace.

Darwin, C. (1859) *On the origin of species by means of natural selection.* London: John Murray.

Darwin, C. (1871) *The descent of man, and selection in relation to sex.* London: John Murray.

Darwin, C. (1872) *The expression of the emotions in man and animals.* London: John Murray.

Davis, K.L., Kahn, R.S., Ko, G., and Davidson, M. (1991) Dopamine in schizophrenia: a review and reconceptualization. *Am. J. Psych.* 148:1474–1486.

Dawkins, R. (1989) *The extended phenotype.* Oxford, UK: Oxford University Press.

Deamer, D.W., and Pashley, R.M. (1989) Amphiphilic components of carbonaceous meteorites. *Orig. Life Evol. Biosph.* 19:21–33.

Denes, A.S., Jékely, G., Steinmetz, P.R., Raible, F., Snyman, H., Prud'homme, B., Ferrier, D.E., Balavoine, G., and Arendt, D. (2007) Molecular architecture of annelid nerve cord supports common origin of nervous system centralization in bilateria. *Cell* 129(2): 277–288.

Dickinson, W.J. (1988) On the architecture of regulatory systems: evolutionary insights and implications. *Bio. Essays* 8:204–208.

Dobzhansky, T. (1964) Biology, molecular and organismic. *Amer. Zool.* 4:443–452.

Dohrn, A.F. (1875) *Der Ursprung der Wirbelthiere und das Princip des Functionswechsels: Genealogische Skizzen* [The origin of

Vertebrate Animals and the principal of functional change: Genealogical sketches]. Leipzig, Germany: Engelmann.

Dunbar, R.I.M. (1988) *Primate social systems*. London: Croom Helm.

Dworkin, J.P., Deamer, D.W., Sandford, S.A., and Allamandola, L.A. (2001) Self-assembling amphiphilic molecules: Synthesis in simulated interstellar/precometary ices. *Proc. Natl. Acad. Sci. USA* 98(3):815–819.

Edelman, G.M. (1988) *Neural Darwinism: The theory of neuronal group selection*. New York: Basic Books.

Eigen, M. (1972) Molekulare selbstorganisation und evolution [Molecular self-organization and evolution]. *Naturwissenschaften* 58(10):465–523.

Eigen, M., and Schuster, P. (1971) *The hypercycle: A principle of natural self-organization*. Berlin, Germany: Springer.

Engelmann, T.W. (1882) Über Sauerstoffausscheidung von Pflanzenzellen im Mikrospectrum [About oxygen excretion of microplant cells]. *Bot. Zeit.* 40:419–426.

Erwin, D.H. (1993) *The great Paleozoic crisis: Life and death in the Permian*. New York: Columbia University Press.

Fryxell, K.J. (1995) The evolutionary divergence of neurotransmitter receptors and second messenger pathways. *J. Mol. Evol.* 41(1): 85–97.

Garber, R.L., Kuroiwa, A., and Gehring, W.J. (1983) Genomic and cDNA clones of the homeotic locus Antennapedia in *Drosophila. EMBO J* (11):2027–2036. PMID 6416827.

Gardner, R.J. (1982) Mechanisms in major depressive disorder: an evolutionary model. *Arch. Gen. Psychiatry* 39:1436–1441.

Gardner, R.J., and Wilson, D.R. (2004) Sociophysiology and evolutionary aspects of psychiatry. In: Panksepp, J., ed. *Textbook of biological psychiatry*. New York: John Wiley, pp. 597–625.

Garrison, F.H. (1917) *An introduction to the history of medicine: with medical chronology, suggestions for study and bibliographic data*. Philadelphia: W.B. Saunders.

Gawin, F.A., and Ellenwood, E.H. (1988) Cocaine and other stimulants. *N. Eng. J. Med.* 318:1173–1182.

Gazzaniga, M. (1992) *Nature's mind*. New York: Basic Books.

Gehring, W.J. (1998) *Master control genes in development and evolution: the homeobox story*. New Haven, CT: Yale University Press.

Gilbert, P. (1989) *Human nature and suffering*. London: Lawrence Erlbaum.

Gilbert, P. (1992) *Depression: the evolution of powerlessness*. New York: Guilford.

Golden, A.L. (2002) Evolution of voltage-gated Na(+) channels. *J. Exp. Biol.* 205(Pt 5):575–584.

Goodrich, E. (1930) *Studies on the structure and development of vertebrates*. London: Macmillan.

Graham, A., Begbie, J., and McGonnell, I. (2004) Significance of the cranial neural crest. *Dev. Dyn.* 229(1):5–13.

Haeckel, E.H.P.A. (1866) *Generelle morphologie der organismen*. Berlin, Germany: G. Reimer.

Hamilton, W.D. (1963) The evolution of altruistic behavior. *Am. Nat.* 97:354–356.

Hanczyc, M.M., and Szostak, J.W. (2004) Replicating vesicles as models of primitive cell growth and division. *Curr. Opin. Chem. Biol.* 8:660–664.

Harbor, S.N., Barchas, P.R., and Barchas, J. (1981) The regulatory effects of social rank on behavior after amphetamine administration. In: Barchas, P., ed. *Social hierarchies: essays toward a sociophysiological perspective*. Westport, CT: Greenwood Press.

Hartmann, L. (1992) Reflections on humane values and biopsychosocial integration. *Am. J. Psychiatry* 149:1135–1147.

Heckman, D.S., Geiser, D.M., Eidell, B.R., Stauffer, R.L., Kardos, N.L., and Hedges, S.B. (2001) Molecular evidence for the early colonization of land by fungi and plants. *Science* 293:1129–1133.

Hegemann, P. (1997) Vision in microalgae. *Planta* 203(3):265–274.

Hen, R. (1993) Structural and functional conservation of serotonin receptors throughout evolution. *EXS* 63:266–278.

Henry, J.P. (1982) The relation of social to biological processes in disease. *Soc. Sci. Med.* 16:369–380.

Henry, J.P., and Stephens, P.M. (1977) *Stress, health and the social environment*. New York: Springer-Verlag.

Hill, D. (1968) Depression: disease, reaction or posture? *Am. J. Psychiatry* 125:445–456.

Hille, B. (2001) *Ion channels of excitable membranes* (3rd ed.). Sunderland, MA: Sinauer.

Hirabayashi, J., and Kasai, K. (1993) The family of metazoan metal-independent b-galactoside-binding lectins: structure, function and molecular evolution. *Glycobiology* 3:297–304.

Holzschuh, J., Wada, N., Wada, C., Schaffer, A., Javidan, Y., Tallafuss, A., Bally-Cuif, L., and Schilling, T.F. (2005) Requirements for endoderm and BMP signaling in sensory neurogenesis in zebrafish. *Development* 132:3731–3742.

Huxley, L. (1918). *The life and letters of Sir Joseph Dalton Hooker*, Volumes 1 & 2. London: John Murray, Volume 1, p. 526.

Huxley, J., Mayr, E., Osmond, H., and Hoffer, A. (1964) Schizophrenia as a genetic morphism. *Nature* 204:220–221.

Hyman, S. and Nestler, E. (1993) *Foundations of molecular psychiatry*. Washington, DC: American Psychiatric Association.

Jacob, F. (1977) Evolution and tinkering. *Science* 196:1161–1166.

Jan, L.Y., and Jan, Y.N. (1992) Tracing the roots of ion channels. *Cell* 69:715–718.

Janssen, P.A.J., Niemegeers, C.J.E., and Awouters, F. (1988) Pharmacology of risperidone (R64 766), a new antipsychotic with serotonin-S2 and dopamine-D2 antagonist properties. *J. Pharm. Exper. Therap.* 244:685–693.

Jaspers, K. (1963) *General psychopathology* (Hoenig, J., and Hamilton, M.W., trans. of *Allgemeine Psychopathologie*, Berlin, 1913). Manchester, UK: University of Manchester Press.

John Paul II. (1996, October 30) Message on evolution: Address to the Pontifical Academy of Sciences. *L'Osservatore Romano Weekly Edition in English*.

Kalyani, A.J., and Rao, M.S. (1998) Review. Cell lineage in the developing neural tube. *Biochem. Cell Biol.* 76(6):1051–1068.

Kalyani, A.J., Piper, D., Mujtaba, T., Lucero, M.T., and Rao, M.S. (1998) Spinal cord neuronal precursors generate multiple neuronal phenotypes in culture. *J. Neurosci.* 18(19):7856–7868.

Karol, K.G., McCourt, R.M., Cimino, M.T., and Delwiche, C.F. (2001) The closest living relatives of land plants. *Science* 294:2351–2353.

Keenleyside, M.H.A. (1979) *Diversity and adaptation in fish behavior*. Berlin, Germany: Springer.

Kemper, T.D. (1984) Power, status and emotions: A sociobiological contribution to a psychological domain. In: Scherer, K., and Ekman, P., eds. *Approaches to emotion*. Hillsdale, NJ: Lawrence Erlbaum, pp. 369–384.

King, M.C., and Wilson, A.C. (1975) Evolution at two levels in humans and chimpanzees. *Science* 88(4184):107–116.

Kinnier Wilson, S.A. (1914) An experimental research into the anatomy and physiology of the corpus striatum. *Brain* 36:427–492.

Kirk, D.L. (2005) A twelve-step program for evolving multicellularity and a division of labor. *Bioessays* 27(3):299–310.

Kirschvink, J.L. (1992) Late Proterozoic low-latitude global glaciation: The snowball Earth. In: Schopf, J.W., and Klein, C., eds. *The Proterozoic biosphere: A multidisciplinary study*. Cambridge, UK: Cambridge University Press, pp. 51–52.

Knoll, A.H. (1992) The early evolution of eukaryotes: A geological perspective. *Science* 256(5057):622–627.

Knoll, A.H., and Carroll, S.B. (1999) Early animal evolution: emerging views from comparative biology and geology. *Science* 284(5423): 2129–2137.

Knoll, A.H., Walter, M.R., Narbonne, G.M., and Christie-Blick, N. (2004) A new period for the geologic time scale. *Science* 305(5684):621–622.

Koshland, D.E. (1988) Chemotaxis as a model second-messenger system. *Biochem.* 27:5829–5834.

Kosten, T.R. (1993) Pharmacotherapies for cocaine abuse: neurobiological abnormalities reversed with drug intervention. *Psychia. Times* 10:25.

Kumar, S., and Rzhetsky, A. (1996) Evolutionary relationships of eukaryotic kingdoms. *J. Mol. Evol.* 42:183–193.

LeDouarin, N.M. (1982) *The neural crest.* Cambridge, UK: Cambridge University Press.

Lewis, A. (1934) Melancholia: a historical review. *J. Mental Science*, 80:1–42.

Lewis, L.A., and McCourt, R.M. (2004) Green alga and the origin of land plants. *Am. J. Bot.* 91(10):1535–1556.

Liu, Y., Engelman, D.M., and Gerstein, M. (2002) Genomic analysis of membrane protein families: abundance and conserved motifs. *Genome Biol.* Epub: research0054.1–research0054.12.

Livak, K.J., Rogers, J., and Lichter, J.B. (1995) Variability of dopamine D4 receptor (DRD4) gene sequence within and among nonhuman primate species. *Proc. Natl. Acad. Sci. USA* 92(2):427–431.

Lo, L., Morin, X., Brunet, J.F., and Anderson, D.J. (1999) Specification of neurotransmitter identity by Phox2 proteins in neural crest stem cells. *Neuron* 22(4):693–705.

Loewi, O. (1921) Uber humorale Ubertragbarkeit der Herznervenwirkung [Nervous humoral effects on the heart]. I *Pflugers Archiv.* 189:239–242.

MacLean, P.D. (1952) Some psychiatric implications of physiological studies on frontotemporal portion of limbic system (visceral brain). *Electroencephalogr. Clin. Neurophysiol. Suppl.* 4(4):407–418.

MacLean, P.D. (1990). *The triune brain in evolution: role in paleocerebral functions.* New York: Plenum Press.

Marchese, A., George, S., Kolakowski, L.F., Lynch, K.R., and O'Dowd, B.F (1999). Novel GPCRs and their endogenous ligands: expanding the boundaries of physiology and pharmacology. *Trends in Pharmacological Sciences* 20(9)370–375.

Maynard Smith, J. (1974) The theory of games and the evolution of animal conflict. *J. Theor. Biol.* 47:209–221.

Maynard Smith, J. (1976) Evolution and the theory of games. *Am. Scientist* 64:41–45.

Maynard Smith, J. (1982) *Evolution and the theory of games.* Cambridge, UK: Cambridge University Press.

Maynard Smith, J., and Parker, G.A. (1976) The logic of assymetric contests. *Nature* 246:15–18.

Maynard Smith, J., and Price, G.R. (1973) The logic of animal conflict. *Nature* 246:15–18.

Mayr, E. (1963) The new versus the classical in science. *Science* 141(3583):765.

Mazet, F. (2006) The evolution of sensory placodes. *Scientific World Journal* 4(6):1841–1850.

Mazure, A., Booth, A., and Dabbs, J.M. (1992) Testosterone and chess competition. *Soc. Psychol. Quar.* 55:70–77.

McGinnis, W., Levine, M.S., Hafen, E., Kuroiwa, A., and Gehring, W.J. (1984) A conserved DNA sequence in homeotic genes of the Drosophila Antennapedia and bithorax complex. *Nature* 308: 428–433.

Meinhardt, H. (2002) The radial-symmetric hydra and the evolution of the bilateral body plan: an old body became a young brain. *Bioessays* 2:185–191.

Meltzer, H. (1992) The importance of serotonin-dopamine interactions in the action of clozapine. *Br. J. Psychiatry* 160(Suppl 170): 22–29.

Miljkovic-Licina, M., Gauchat, D., and Galliot, B. (2004) Neuronal evolution: analysis of regulatory genes in a first-evolved nervous system, the hydra nervous system. *Biosystems* 76(1/3):75–87.

Miller, F.A., Begbie, M.E., Giacomini, M., Ahern, C., and Harvey, E.A. (2006) Redefining disease? The nosologic implications of molecular genetic knowledge. *Perspect. Biol. Med.* 49(1):99–114.

Miller S.L. (1953) Production of amino acids under possible primitive earth conditions. *Science* 117:528.

Miller S.L., and Urey, H.C (1959) Organic compound synthesis on the primitive earth. *Science* 130:245.

Mithen, S. (1996) *Prehistory of the mind.* London: Thames and Hudson.

Müller, W.E., and Müller, I.M. (2003) Analysis of the sponge [Porifera] gene repertoire: implications for the evolution of the metazoan body plan. *Prog. Mol. Subcell. Biol.* 37:1–33.

National Research Council Committee on Planetary Biology and Chemical Evolution. (1990) *The search for life's origins: progress and future directions in planetary biology and chemical evolution.* Retrieved July 25, 2007, from http://nationalacademies.org/evolution/.

Nelson, R.D., Kuan, G., Saier, M.H., and Montal, M. (1999) Modular assembly of voltage-gated channel proteins: a sequence analysis and phylogenetic study. *J. Mol. Microbiol. Biotechnol.* 1(2):281–287.

Nesse, R.M. (1990) Evolutionary explanations of emotions. *Human Nature* 1:261–289.

Nielsen, K. (2001) *Animal evolution: Interrelationships of the living phyla* (2nd ed.). Oxford, UK: Oxford University Press.

Ohta, T. (1989) Role of gene duplication in evolution. *Genome* 31(1):304-310.

Oparin, A.I. (1952) *The origin of life.* New York: Dover.

Owens, M.J., and Risch, S.C. (1995) Atypical antipsychotics. In: Schatzberg, A.F., and Nemeroff, C., eds. *Psychopharmacology.* Washington, DC: American Psychological Association, pp. 263–280.

Papez, J.W. (1937) A proposed mechanism of emotions. *Arch. Neurol. Psychiatry* 79:217–224.

Patten, C., Clayton, C.L., Blakemore, S.J., Trower, M.K., Wallace, D.M., and Hagan, R.M. (1999) Identification of two novel diurnal genes by screening of a rat brain cDNA library. *Neuroreport* 10(5):1155–1161.

Parent, A. (1986) *Comparative neurobiology of the basal ganglia.* New York: Wiley.

Peroutka, S.J., and Howell, T.A. (1994) The molecular evolution of G protein-coupled receptors: focus on 5-hydroxytryptamine receptors. *Neuropharmacol.* 33(3/4):319–324.

Piggott, M.A., Marshall, E.F., Thomas, N., Lloyd, S., Court, J.A., Jaros, E., Costa, D., Perry, R.H., and Perry, E.K. (1999) Dopaminergic activities in the human striatum: rostrocaudal gradients of uptake sites and of D1 and D2 but not of D3 receptor binding or dopamine. *Neurosci.* 90(2):433–445.

Pohorille, A. (2007) Protocells as universal ancestors of living systems. In: Rasmussen, S., Bedau, M., Chen, L., Deamer, D., Krakauer, D., Packard, N., and Shuster, P., eds. *Protocells: Bridging nonliving and living matter.* Cambridge, MA: MIT Press, pp. 301–316.

Pohorille, A., Wilson, M.A., and Chipot, C. (2003) Membrane peptides and their role in protobiological evolution. *Orig. Life Evol. Biosph.* 33:173–197.

Pratt, L.R., and Pohorille, A. (2002) Hydrophobic effects and modeling of biophysical aqueous solution interfaces. *Chem. Rev.* 102: 2671–2692.

Previc, F.H. (1999) Dopamine and the origins of human intelligence. *Brain Cogn.* 41(3):299–350.

Price, J. (1967) Hypothesis: the dominance hierarchy and the evolution of mental illness. *Lancet* 2:243–246.

Price, J., Sloman, L., Gardner, R., Gilbert, P., and Rhode, P. (1994) The social competition hypothesis of depression. *Br. J. Psychiatry* 164:309–315.

Raleigh, M., McGuire, M., Brammer, G., and Yuwiler, A. (1984) Social status and whole blood serotonin in vervets. *Arch. Gen. Psych.* 41:405–410.

Ramón y Cajal, S. (1911) *Histologie du systeme nerveux de l'homme et des vertebretes* [Histology of the nervous system of humans and vertebretes], Vols. 1 & 2. Paris: A. Maloine.

Rasmussen, S., Chen, L., Nilsson, M., and Abe, S. (2003) Bridging nonliving and living matter. *J. Artif. Life* 9(3):269-316.

Rasmussen, S.L., Holland, L.Z., Schubert, M., Beaster-Jones, L., and Holland, N.D. (2007) Amphioxus AmphiDelta: evolution of Delta protein structure, segmentation, and neurogenesis. *Genesis* 45(3): 113–122.

Ray, J.C., and Sapolsky, R.M. (1992) Styles of social behavior and endocrine correlates among high-ranking wild baboons. *Am. J. Prim.* 28:231–250.

Reiner, A., Medina, L., and Veenman, C.L. (1998) Structural and functional evolution of the basal ganglia in vertebrates. *Brain Res. Brain Res. Rev.* 28(3):235–285.

Rodin, S.N., and Riggs, A.D. (2003) Epigenetic silencing may aid evolution by gene duplication. *J. Mol. Evol.* 6(6):718–729.

Rutherford, E. (1939) *Rutherford: Being the life and letters of the Rt. Hon. Lord Rutherford, O.M.* Cambridge, UK: Cambridge University Press.

Saier, M.H. (1999) A functional-phylogenetic system for the classification of transport proteins. *J. Cell. Biochem.* 75(32):84–94.

Saier, M.H. (2003) Tracing pathways of transport protein evolution. *Mol. Microbiol.* 48:1145–1156.

Saier, M.H., Tran, C.V., and Barabote, R.D. (2006) TCDB: The transporter classification database for membrane transport protein analyses and information. *Nucleic Acids Res.* 34:D181–D186.

Sakarya, O., Armstrong, K.A., Adamska, M., Adamski, M., Wang, I.F., Tidor, B., Degnan, B.M., Oakley, T.H., and Kosik, K.S. (2007) A post-synaptic scaffold at the origin of the animal kingdom. *PLoS ONE* 6(2):e506.

Sanderson, M.J. (2003) Molecular data from 27 proteins do not support a Precambrian origin of land plants. *Am. J. Bot.* 90: 954–956.

Sapolsky, R.M. (1989) Hypercortisolism among socially subordinate wild baboons originates at the CNS level. *Arch. Gen. Psych.* 46: 1047–1051.

Sapolsky, R.M. (1990a) Adrenocortial function, social rank and personality among wild baboons. *Biol. Psychiatry* 28:862–878.

Sapolsky, R.M. (1990b) Stress in the wild. *Sci. Am.* 1:106–113.

Sapolsky, R.M. (1993) Endocrine alfresco: Psychoendocrine studies of wild baboons. *Recent Progress in Hormone Research* 48: 437–468.

Sapolsky, R.M. (1994) Individual differences in the stress response. *Sem. Neurosci.* 6:261–269.

Schlosser, G. (2005) Evolutionary origins of vertebrate placodes: insights from developmental studies and from comparisons with other deuterostomes. *J. Exp. Zoolog. B Mol. Dev. Evol.* 304(4): 347–399.

Seaman, M.I., Fisher, J.B., Chang, F., and Kidd, K.K. (1999) Tandem duplication polymorphism upstream of the dopamine D4 receptor gene (DRD4). *Am. J. Med. Genet.* 88(6):705–709.

Seilacher, A., Bose, P.K., and Pflüger, F. (1998) Triploblastic animals more than 1 billion years ago: trace fossil evidence from India. *Science* 282(5386):80–83.

Sloman, L. (1976) The role of neurosis in phylogenetic adaptation with particular reference to early man. *Am. J. Psychiatry* 133: 543–547.

Smeets, W.J., and González, A. (1992) Comparative aspects of basal forebrain organization in vertebrates. *Eur. J. Morphol.* 30(1): 23–36.

Smeets, W.J., and González, A. (2000) Catecholamine systems in the brain of vertebrates: new perspectives through a comparative approach. *Brain Res. Rev.* 33(2/3):308–379.

Sperry, R.W. (1964) *Problems outstanding in the evolution of brain function. James Arthur Lecture.* New York: American Museum of Natural History.

Spudich, J.L., and Jung, K.-H. (2005) A functional-phylogenetic system for the classification of transport proteins. In: W. Briggs and J.L. Spudich, eds., *Handbook of photosensory receptors.* Weinheim, Germany: Wiley-VCH Verlag, pp. 1–21.

Stoka, A.M. (1999) Phylogeny and evolution of chemical communication. *J. Mol. End.* 22:207–225.

Szostak, J.W., Bartel, D.P., and Luisi, P.L. (2001) Synthesizing life. *Nature* 409:387–390.

Tam, R., and Saier, M.H. (1993) Structural, functional, and evolutionary relationships among extracellular solute-binding receptors of bacteria. *Microbiol. Rev.* 57:320–346.

Tasmees, A., Iyer, L.M., Jakobsson, E., and Aravind, L. (2005) Identification of the prokaryotic ligand-gated ion channels and their implications for the mechanisms and origins of animal Cys-loop ion channels. *Genome Biol.* 6(1):R4.

Trivers, R.L. (1971) The evolution of reciprocal altruism. *Q. Rev. Bio.* 46:35–57.

Tsankova, N., Renthal, W., Kumar, A., and Nestler, E.J. (2007) Epigenetic regulation in psychiatric disorders. *Nat. Rev. Neurosci.* 8(5):355–367

Vaglia, J.L., and Hall, B.K. (1999) Regulation of neural crest cell populations: occurrence, distribution and underlying mechanisms. *Int. J. Dev. Biol.* 43(2):95–110.

Valentine, J.W. (1994) The Cambrian explosion. In: Bengtson, S., ed. *Early life on earth.* New York: Columbia University Press, pp. 401–412.

Valentine, J.W., and Campbell, C.A. (1975) Genetic regulation and the fossil record. *Am. Sci.* 63(6):673–680.

Valentine, J.W., Erwin, D.H., and Jablonski, D. (1996) Developmental evolution of metazoan body plan: the fossil evidence. *Dev. Biol.* 173:373–381.

Vernier, P., Cardinaud, B., Valdenaire, O., Philippe, H., and Vincent, J.D. (1995) Review. An evolutionary view of drug-receptor interaction: the bioamine receptor family. *Trends Pharmacol. Sci.* 16(11):375–381.

Vincent, J.D., Cardinaud, B., and Vernier P. (1998) Evolution of monoamine receptors and the origin of motivational and emotional systems in vertebrates. *Bull. Natl. Acad. Med.* 182(7): 1505–1514; discussion 1515–1516.

Vogt, C. (1911) Quelques considérations générales à propos du syndrôme du corps strié [Some general considerations about the striatal syndrome]. *Journal für Psychologie und Neurologie* 18:479–488.

Wada, H., Saiga, H., Satoh, N., and Holland, P.W. (1998) Tripartite organization of the ancestral chordate brain and the antiquity of placodes: insights from ascidian Pax-2/5/8, Hox and Otx genes. *Development* 125(6):1113–1122.

Walde, P., Goto, A., Monnard, P.A., Wessicken, M., and Luisi, P.L. (1994) Oparin's reactions revisited—enzymatic synthesis of poly (adenylic acid) in micelles and self-reproducing vesicles. *J. Am. Chem. Soc.* 116:7541–7547.

Walde, P., Wick, R., Fresta, A., Mangone, A., and Luisi, P.L. (1994) Autopoietic self reproduction of fatty acid vesicles. *J. Am. Chem. Soc.* 116:11649–11654.

Wallin, E., and von Heijne, G. (1998) Genome-wide analysis of integral membrane proteins from eubacterial, archaean, and eukaryotic organisms. *Protein Sci.* 7:1029–1038.

Wilson, E.O. (1975) *Sociobiology.* Cambridge, MA: Harvard/Belknap Press.

Wilson, D.R. (1993a) Autologous clones: The evolutionary exaptation of endocrine and immune systems from neural ectoderm homeobox genes. *Acta Biotheoretica* 41:267–269.

Wilson, D.R. (1993b) Evolutionary epidemiology: Darwinian theory in the service of medicine and psychiatry. *Acta Biotheoretica* 41:205–218.

Wilson, D.R. (1994) The Darwinian roots of human neurosis. *Acta Biotheoretica* 42:49–62.

Wilson, D.R. (1998) Evolutionary epidemiology and manic-depression. *B. J. Med. Psychol.* 71:375–396.

Wilson, D.R. (2006) The evolution of evolutionary epidemiology: A defense of pluralistic epigenetic modes of transmission. *Behav. Brain Sci.* 29(4):427–429

Wilson, D.R., and Cory, G.A. (2007) *Evolutionary epidemiology of mania, depression and normality*. New York: Mellen.

Wilson, D.R., and Price, J. (2006) Evolutionary epidemiology of endophenotypes in the bipolar spectrum: Evolved neuropsychological mechanisms of social rank. *Current Psychosis and Therapeutics Reports* 4(4):176–180.

Wilson, D.R., Stanton, S., and Wilson S.L. (1999) Phylogeny of neurotransmission: Serotonin, dopamine and the evolution of sociophyiological neurotransmission. In: van der Dennen, J., Smillie, D., and Wilson, D.R., eds. *Sociobiology and the Darwinian heritage*. Westport, CT: Greenwood Press, pp. 309–318.

Wray, G.A., Jeffrey S., and Levinton, L.H. (1996) Shapiro molecular evidence for deep precambrian divergences among metazoan phyla. *Science* 274(5287):568–573.

Wyatt, R.J., Karoum, F., Suddath, R., and Hitri, A. (1988) The role of cocaine in dopamine use and abuse. *Psychiatr. Ann.* 18:531–534.

Yoon, H.S., Hackett, C., Ciniglia, G., and Pinto, D. (2004) A molecular timeline for the origin of photosynthetic eukaryotes. *Mol. Biol. Evol.* 21:809–818.

Zuckerkandl, E., and Pauling, L. (1965) Molecules as documents of evolutionary history. *J. Theor. Biol.* 8(2):357–366.

Index

Note: Page numbers followed by *f* indicate figures; page numbers followed by *t* indicate tables.